PROFESSIONAL EDITION

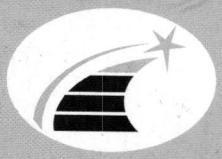

2017 ICD-10-CM FOR HOSPITALS

INCLUDES NETTER'S ANATOMY ART

Carol J. Buck
MS, CPC, CCS-P

Former Program Director
Medical Secretary Programs
Northwest Technical College
East Grand Forks, Minnesota

ELSEVIER

ELSEVIER

3251 Riverport Lane
St. Louis, Missouri 63043

2017 ICD-10-CM HOSPITAL EDITION

ISBN: 978-0-323-43121-7

Copyright © 2017, Elsevier Inc.
All Rights Reserved.
Previous editions copyrighted 2016, 2015, 2014, 2013, 2010

Some material was previously published.

All rights reserved. No part of this publication may be reproduced or transmitted in any form or by any means, electronic or mechanical, including photocopying, recording, or any information storage and retrieval system, without permission in writing from the publisher. Details on how to seek permission, further information about the Publisher's permissions policies and our arrangements with organizations such as the Copyright Clearance Center and the Copyright Licensing Agency can be found at our website: www.elsevier.com/permissions.

This book and the individual contributions contained in it are protected under copyright by the Publisher (other than as may be noted herein).

Notice

Knowledge and best practice in this field are constantly changing. As new research and experience broaden our understanding, changes in research methods, professional practices, or medical treatment may become necessary.

Practitioners and researchers must always rely on their own experience and knowledge in evaluating and using any information, methods, compounds, or experiments described herein. In using such information or methods they should be mindful of their own safety and the safety of others, including parties for whom they have a professional responsibility.

With respect to any drug or pharmaceutical products identified, readers are advised to check the most current information provided (i) on procedures featured or (ii) by the manufacturer of each product to be administered, to verify the recommended dose or formula, the method and duration of administration, and contraindications. It is the responsibility of practitioners, relying on their own experience and knowledge of their patients, to make diagnoses, to determine dosages and the best treatment for each individual patient, and to take all appropriate safety precautions.

To the fullest extent of the law, neither the Publisher nor the authors, contributors, or editors, assume any liability for any injury and/or damage to persons or property as a matter of products liability, negligence or otherwise, or from any use or operation of any methods, products, instructions, or ideas contained in the material herein.

Library of Congress Cataloging-in-Publication Data
Names: Buck, Carol J., author.
Title: 2017 ICD-10-CM for hospitals / Carol J. Buck.
Other titles: ICD-10-CM for hospitals
Description: Professional edition. | St. Louis, Missouri : Elsevier, [2017]
|
Includes index. | Preceded by 2016 ICD-10-CM for hospitals / Carol J. Buck. Professional edition. [2015].
Identifiers: LCCN 2016016060 | ISBN 9780323431217 (pbk.)
Subjects: | MESH: International statistical classification of diseases and related health problems. 10th revision. Clinical modification. | Disease--classification | International Classification of Diseases | Medical Records | Forms and Records Control--methods
Classification: LCC RB115 | NLM WB 15 | DDC 616.001/2--dc23 LC record available at https://lccn.loc.gov/2016016060

Director, Private Sector Education & Professional/References: Jeanne R. Olson
Content Development Manager: Luke Held
Associate Content Development Specialist: Anna Miller
Publishing Services Manager: Jeffrey Patterson
Project Manager: Lisa A. P. Bushey
Design Manager: Julia Dummitt

Printed in the United States of America

Last digit is the print number: 9 8 7 6 5 4 3 2 1

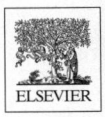

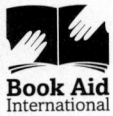

Working together to grow libraries in developing countries

www.elsevier.com • www.bookaid.org

DEDICATION

To all the brave medical coders who transitioned the nation into a new coding system.
Decades of waiting finally concluded with the implementation of I-10,
and you have been the pioneers leading the way.

With greatest appreciations for your efforts!

Carol J. Buck, MS, CPC, CCS-P

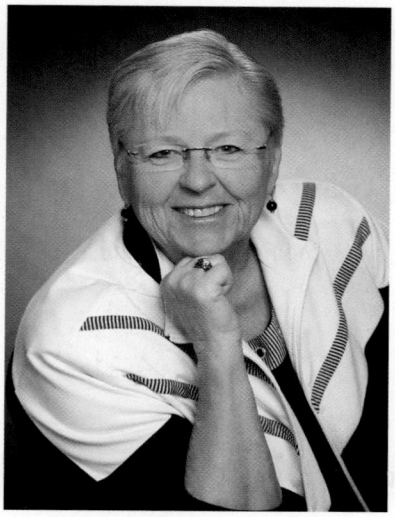

DEVELOPMENT OF THIS EDITION

Query Team

Patricia Cordy Henricksen, MS, CHCA, CPC-I, CPC, CCP-P, ASC-PM
Auditing and Coding Educator
Soterion Medical Services
Lexington, Kentucky

Jackie L. Grass, CPC
Coding and Reimbursement Specialist
Grand Forks, North Dakota

Kathleen Buchda, CPC, CPMA
Revenue Recognition
New Richmond, Wisconsin

Editorial Consultant

Jenna Price, CPC-A
President
Price Editorial Services, LLC
St. Louis, Missouri

Elsevier/MC Strategies Revenue Cycle, Coding and Compliance Staff

"Experts in providing e-learning on revenue cycle, coding and compliance."

Deborah Neville, RHIA, CCS-P
Director

Lynn-Marie D. Wozniak, MS, RHIT
Content Manager

Sandra L. Macica, MS, RHIA, CCS, ROCC
Content Manager

CONTENTS

ICD-10-CM

Guide to Using the 2017 ICD-10-CM for Hospitals vi
Symbols and Conventions viii
Guide to the 2017 Updates xiii

Part I Introduction 1

ICD-10-CM Official Guidelines for Coding and Reporting 1
Netter's Anatomy Illustrations 49

Part II Alphabetic Index 81

Index to Diseases and Injuries 81
Table of Neoplasms 465
Table of Drugs and Chemicals 493
External Cause of Injuries Index 589

Part III Tabular List of Diseases and Injuries 633

Chapter 1 Certain Infectious and Parasitic Diseases (A00-B99) 634
Chapter 2 Neoplasms (C00-D49) 669
Chapter 3 Diseases of the Blood and Blood-Forming Organs and Certain Disorders Involving the Immune Mechanism (D50-D89) 720
Chapter 4 Endocrine, Nutritional and Metabolic Diseases (E00-E89) 731
Chapter 5 Mental, Behavioral and Neurodevelopmental Disorders (F01-F99) 757
Chapter 6 Diseases of the Nervous System (G00-G99) 784
Chapter 7 Diseases of the Eye and Adnexa (H00-H59) 809
Chapter 8 Diseases of the Ear and Mastoid Process (H60-H95) 854
Chapter 9 Diseases of the Circulatory System (I00-I99) 867
Chapter 10 Diseases of the Respiratory System (J00-J99) 917
Chapter 11 Diseases of the Digestive System (K00-K95) 935
Chapter 12 Diseases of the Skin and Subcutaneous Tissue (L00-L99) 962
Chapter 13 Diseases of the Musculoskeletal System and Connective Tissue (M00-M99) 986
Chapter 14 Diseases of the Genitourinary System (N00-N99) 1091
Chapter 15 Pregnancy, Childbirth and the Puerperium (O00-O9A) 1113
Chapter 16 Certain Conditions Originating in the Perinatal Period (P00-P96) 1159
Chapter 17 Congenital Malformations, Deformations and Chromosomal Abnormalities (Q00-Q99) 1173
Chapter 18 Symptoms, Signs and Abnormal Clinical and Laboratory Findings, Not Elsewhere Classified (R00-R99) 1194
Chapter 19 Injury, Poisoning and Certain Other Consequences of External Causes (S00-T88) 1217
Chapter 20 External Causes of Morbidity (V00-Y99) 1516
Chapter 21 Factors Influencing Health Status and Contact with Health Services (Z00-Z99) 1602

GUIDE TO USING THE 2017 ICD-10-CM FOR HOSPITALS

Medical coding has long been a part of the health care profession. Through the years medical coding systems have become more complex and extensive. Today, medical coding is an intricate and immense process that is present in every health care setting. The increased use of electronic submissions for health care services only increases the need for coders who understand the coding process.

2017 ICD-10-CM for Hospitals, Professional Edition was developed to help meet the needs of coding professionals at all levels by offering a comprehensive coding text at a reasonable price.

All material strictly adheres to the latest government versions available at the time of printing. Updates from the *Definitions of Medicare Code Edits* (MCE) will be posted to the companion website (www. codingupdates.com) when available.

Illustrations and Items

The ICD-10-CM Tabular List contains illustrations, pictures, and items to assist you in understanding difficult terminology, diseases/conditions, or coding in a specific category. Items are always printed in [redacted] ink so that the added material is not mistaken for official notations or instructions. [redacted] ink is used for other annotations in the text. Your ideas on what other descriptions or illustrations should be in future editions of this text are always appreciated.

Instructional Notations

Includes Notes

Includes

The word 'Includes' appears immediately under certain categories to further define, or give examples of, the content of the category.

Excludes Notes

The ICD-10-CM has two types of excludes notes. Each note has a different definition for use, but they are both similar in that they indicate that codes excluded from each other are independent of each other.

Excludes1

A type 1 Excludes note is a pure excludes. It means "NOT CODED HERE!" An Excludes1 note indicates that the code excluded should never be used at the same time as the code above the Excludes1 note. An Excludes1 is for use when two conditions cannot occur together, such as a congenital form versus an acquired form of the same condition.

Excludes2

A type 2 Excludes note represents "NOT INCLUDED HERE." An Excludes2 note indicates that the condition excluded is not part of the condition it is excluded from but a patient may have both conditions at the same time. When an Excludes2 note appears under a code, it is acceptable to use both the code and the excluded code together.

Code First/Use Additional Code notes (etiology/manifestation paired codes)

Certain conditions have both an underlying etiology and multiple body system manifestations due to the underlying etiology. For such conditions the ICD-10-CM has a coding convention that requires the underlying condition be sequenced first, followed by the manifestation. Wherever such a combination exists, there is a "use additional code" note at the etiology code, and a "code first" note at the manifestation code. These instructional notes indicate the proper sequencing order of the codes, etiology followed by manifestation.

In most cases the manifestation codes will have in the code title, "in diseases classified elsewhere." Codes with this title are a component of the etiology/manifestation convention. The code title indicates that it is a manifestation code. "In diseases classified elsewhere" codes are never permitted to be used as first-listed or principal diagnosis codes. They must be used in conjunction with an underlying condition code, and they must be listed following the underlying condition.

Use additional

The words indicate an instructional note that another code may be needed.

Code first

The words indicate an instructional note that directs the coder to sequence the underlying condition before the manifestation.

Code also

A "code also" note instructs that two codes may be required to fully describe a condition, but the sequencing of the two codes is discretionary, depending on the severity of the conditions and the reason for the encounter.

Unspecified

The highlight indicates that although the code is valid as a principal (first-listed) diagnosis, it is not as specific as other codes without the highlight.

7th characters and placeholder X

For codes less than 6 characters that require a 7th character a placeholder X should be assigned for all characters less than 6. The 7th character must always be the 7th character of a code.

Annotated

Throughout the manual, revisions, additions, and deleted codes or words are indicated by the following symbols:

Revised: Revisions within the line or code from the previous edition are indicated by the arrow.

◀ **New:** Additions to the previous edition are indicated by the triangle.

~~deleted~~ **Deleted:** Deletions from the previous edition are struck through.

ICD-10-CM Tabular List Symbols

● **Use Additional Character(s):** The red stop sign cautions that the code requires additional character(s) to ensure the greatest specificity.

X For codes less than 6 characters that require a 7th character, a placeholder X should be assigned for all characters less than 6. The 7th character must always be the 7th character of a code.

● **Unacceptable Principal Diagnosis:** These codes have a blue dot before them and give additional information or describe the circumstances affecting the health care encounter but are unacceptable as principal diagnosis in the *Definitions of Medicare Code Edits* (MCE) for inpatient admission.

OGCR The ***Official Guidelines for Coding and Reporting*** symbol includes the placement of a portion of a guideline as that guideline pertains to the code by which it is located. The complete OGCR are located in Part I.

Indicates **complications and comorbidities and major complications and comorbidities** according to the *Medicare Severity Diagnosis Related Groups (MS-DRGs), Definitions Manual.*

Ex Indicates exclusions to complications and comorbidities (CC) and major complications and comorbidities (MCC) for both primary and secondary diagnoses, according to the *Medicare Severity Diagnosis Related Groups (MS-DRGs), Definitions Manual.*

PDX as its own CC/MCC Indicates a combination code that when assigned as the Principal Diagnosis, it includes a condition that also qualifies as a CC/MCC according to the *Medicare Severity Diagnosis Related Groups (MS-DRGs), Definitions Manual.*

HAC is a **Hospital-Acquired Condition** that, when present as a secondary diagnosis in an inpatient setting, is a higher cost, higher volume, or both and results in a higher MS-DRG assignment according to the *Medicare Severity Diagnosis Related Groups (MS-DRGs), Definitions Manual.*

Manifestation Code: Describes the manifestation of an underlying disease, not the disease itself, and therefore should not be assigned as a principal diagnosis, according to the *Definitions of Medicare Code Edits* (MCE).

Age conflict: The *Definitions of Medicare Code Edits* (MCE) detects inconsistencies between a patient's age and diagnosis. For example, a 5-year-old patient with benign prostatic hypertrophy or a 78-year-old pregnant female.

The diagnosis is clinically and virtually impossible in a patient of the stated age. Therefore, either the diagnosis or the age is presumed to be incorrect. There are four age categories for diagnoses in the *Definitions of Medicare Code Edits* (MCE):

N • Newborn. Age of Ø years; a subset of diagnoses intended only for newborns and neonates (e.g., fetal distress, perinatal jaundice).

P • Pediatric. Age range is Ø-17 years inclusive (e.g., Reye's syndrome, routine child health exam).

M • Maternity. Age range is 12-55 years inclusive (e.g., diabetes in pregnancy, antepartum pulmonary complication).

A • Adult. Age range is 15-124 years inclusive (e.g., senile delirium, mature cataract).

♀♂ **Sex conflict:** *Definitions of Medicare Code Edits* (MCE) detects inconsistencies between a patient's sex and any diagnosis or procedure on the patient's record. For example, a male patient with cervical cancer (diagnosis) or a female patient with a prostatectomy (procedure). In both instances, the indicated diagnosis or the procedure conflicts with the stated sex of the patient. Therefore, either the patient's diagnosis, procedure, or sex is presumed to be incorrect.

Coding Clinic Identifies the year, quarter, and page number that presents information about an ICD-10-CM code in the American Hospital Association's *Coding Clinic®* for ICD-10-CM.

Visit codingupdates.com for the full list of 2017 Present on Admission codes.

SYMBOLS AND CONVENTIONS

ICD-10-CM Tabular

Use Additional Character(s): The red stop sign cautions you that the code requires additional character(s) to ensure greatest specificity.

Volume 1, Tabular List

● **K22 Other diseases of esophagus**

Excludes2 esophageal varices (I85.-)

Placeholder X: The red X reminds you that for codes less than 6 characters that require a 7th character, a placeholder X should be assigned to all characters less than 6.

X● **V00.01 Pedestrian on foot injured in collision with roller-skater**

A02.20 Localized salmonella infection, unspecified

Unspecified: These codes are for use when the information in the medical record is insufficient to assign a more specific code. For those categories for which an unspecified code is not provided, the "other specified" code may represent both other and unspecified.

Unacceptable Principal Diagnosis: These codes have a blue dot before them and are not permitted as a first-listed or principal diagnosis. They must be assigned in conjunction with an underlying condition code, and they must be listed following the underlying condition.

● **B95.0 Streptococcus, group A, as the cause of diseases classified elsewhere**

A48.3 Toxic shock syndrome

Use additional code to identify the organism (B95, B96)

Use additional code: Located at the etiology code and directs you to assign a manifestation code.

Code first indicates the etiology code is to be first-listed before the manifestation code.

B39 Histoplasmosis

Code first associated AIDS (B20)

Notes define terms or give coding instructions.

E34.0 Carcinoid syndrome

Note: May be used as an additional code to identify functional activity associated with a carcinoid tumor.

Codes or index entries are for purposes of illustration only and may not be current.

OGCR Section I.C.6.B.5.

Neoplasm Related Pain Code G89.3 is assigned to pain documented as being related, associated or due to cancer, primary or secondary malignancy, or tumor. This code is assigned regardless of whether the pain is acute or chronic.

OGCR: The *Official Guidelines for Coding and Reporting* are placed near the codes to which they refer and are highlighted.

I70.2 Atherosclerosis of native arteries of the extremities
Mönckeberg's (medial) sclerosis

Use additional code, if applicable, to identify chronic total occlusion of artery of extremity (I70.92)

code, if applicable, directs the coder to other conditions that may be appropriate to report.

The word "and" should be interpreted to mean either "and" or "or" when it appears in a statement.

I74 Arterial embolism and thrombosis

Includes embolic infarction
embolic occlusion
thrombotic infarction
thrombotic occlusion

Bold typeface is used on all codes and titles.

I83.001 Varicose veins of unspecified lower extremity with ulcer of thigh

"with" should be interpreted to mean "associated with" or "due to."

K73.2 Chronic active hepatitis, not elsewhere classified

"not elsewhere classified" or **NEC** identifies a code that is assigned only when the information at hand specifies a condition for which no more specific code is available.

"not otherwise specified" or **NOS** is equivalent to unspecified.

W13.9 Fall from, out of or through building, not otherwise specified

Codes or index entries are for purposes of illustration only and may not be current.

Excludes1 means "NOT CODED HERE!" An Excludes1 note indicates that the code excluded should never be assigned at the same time as the code above the Excludes1 note.

M19 Other and unspecified osteoarthritis

Excludes1 polyarthritis (M15.-)

Excludes2 arthrosis of spine (M47.-)
hallux rigidus (M20.2)
osteoarthritis of spine (M47.-)

Excludes2 represents "NOT INCLUDED HERE." An Excludes2 note indicates that the condition excluded is not part of the condition represented by the code, but a patient may have both conditions at the same time and it is acceptable to use both the code and the excluded code together, when appropriate.

Includes: This note appears immediately under a three-character code title to further define, or give examples of, the content.

A06 Amebiasis

Includes infection due to Entamoeba histolytica

E26.01 Conn's syndrome

Code also adrenal adenoma (D35.0)

Code also instructs that two codes may be required to fully describe a condition, but this note does not provide sequencing direction.

Codes titled "other" or "other specified" are for use when the information in the medical record provides detail for which a specific code does not exist.

E25.8 Other adrenogenital disorders

O00.2 Ovarian pregnancy M

Maternity DX (Diagnosis) for ages 12-55 according to the *Definitions of Medicare Code Edits* (MCE).

P02.20 Newborn (suspected to be) affected by unspecified morphological and functional abnormalities of placenta N

Newborn, Age 0, according to the *Definitions of Medicare Code Edits* (MCE).

L21.0 Seborrhea capitis P
Cradle cap

Pediatric Age, 0-17, according to the *Definitions of Medicare Code Edits* (MCE).

G30.1 Alzheimer's disease with late onset A

Adult Age, 15-124, according to the *Definitions of Medicare Code Edits* (MCE).

Females Only according to the *Definitions of Medicare Code Edits* (MCE).

B37.3 Candidiasis of vulva and vagina ♀

C60.1 Malignant neoplasm of glans penis ♂

Males Only according to the *Definitions of Medicare Code Edits* (MCE).

Codes or index entries are for purposes of illustration only and may not be current.

Manifestation according to the *Definitions of Medicare Code Edits* (MCE).

H22 Disorders of iris and ciliary body in diseases classified elsewhere

Code first underlying disease, such as:
gout (M1A-, M1Ø.-)

G14 Postpolio syndrome

Includes Postpolio myelitic syndrome

Excludes1 sequelae of poliomyelitis (B91)

T81.512 Adhesions due to foreign body accidentally left in body following kidney dialysis

Hospital-Acquired Condition according to the *Medicare Severity Diagnosis Related Groups (MS-DRGs).*

Major Complication/ Comorbidity (MCC) according to the *Medicare Severity Diagnosis Related Groups (MS-DRGs).*

R57.1 Hypovolemic shock

Complication/ Comorbidity (CC) according to the *Medicare Severity Diagnosis Related Groups (MS-DRGs).*

B25.1 Cytomegaloviral hepatitis

B96.5 Pseudomonas (aeruginosa) (mallei) (pseudomallei) as the cause of diseases classified elsewhere

Coding Clinic: 2015, Q1, P18

Coding Clinic identifies the year, quarter, and page number that presents information about an ICD-10-PCS code in the American Hospital Association's *Coding Clinic®*.

Codes or index entries are for purposes of illustration only and may not be current.

Alphabetic Index

Main terms are in **bold** typeface.

Aberrant (congenital) —*see also* Malposition, congenital
adrenal gland Q89.1

Etiology code first followed by the manifestation code in **brackets**. The code in brackets is always to be sequenced second.

Amyloid heart (disease) E85.4 *[I43]*

Amylophagia —*see* Pica

"see" indicates another term should be referenced.

Angiofibroma —*see also* Neoplasm, benign, by site

"see also" follows a main term and instructs that there is another main term that may also be referenced.

Appendicitis (pneumococcal) (retrocecal) K37
with
perforation or rupture K35.2
peritoneal abscess K35.3

A default code is listed next to the main term and represents that condition most commonly associated with the main term. If a condition is documented in a medical record without any additional information, such as acute or chronic, the default code should be assigned.

Codes or index entries are for purposes of illustration only and may not be current.

GUIDE TO THE 2017 ICD-10-CM UPDATES

CHAPTER 1

CERTAIN INFECTIOUS AND PARASITIC DISEASES (A00-B99)

A40 Streptococcal sepsis
Code first
Revised postprocedural streptococcal sepsis (T81.4-)

A41 Other sepsis
Code first
Revised postprocedural sepsis (T81.4-)
Deleted **Excludes1** sepsis NOS (A41.9)

New **A92.5 Zika virus disease**
New Zika virus fever
New Zika virus infection
New Zika NOS

B17.9 Acute viral hepatitis, unspecified
New Acute infectious hepatitis NOS

B18 Chronic viral hepatitis
New **Includes** Carrier of viral hepatitis

B18.1 Chronic viral hepatitis B without delta-agent
New Carrier of viral hepatitis B

B18.2 Chronic viral hepatitis C
New Carrier of viral hepatitis C

B18.8 Other chronic viral hepatitis
New Carrier of other viral hepatitis

B18.9 Chronic viral hepatitis, unspecified
New Carrier of unspecified viral hepatitis

CHAPTER 2

NEOPLASMS (C00-D49)

C00 Malignant neoplasm of lip
C01 Malignant neoplasm of base of tongue
C02 Malignant neoplasm of other and unspecified parts of tongue
C03 Malignant neoplasm of gum
C04 Malignant neoplasm of floor of mouth
C05 Malignant neoplasm of palate
C06 Malignant neoplasm of other and unspecified parts of mouth
C07 Malignant neoplasm of parotid gland
C08 Malignant neoplasm of other and unspecified major salivary glands
C09 Malignant neoplasm of tonsil
C10 Malignant neoplasm of oropharynx
C11 Malignant neoplasm of nasopharynx
C12 Malignant neoplasm of pyriform sinus
C13 Malignant neoplasm of hypopharynx
C14 Malignant neoplasm of other and ill-defined sites in the lip, oral cavity and pharynx
Use additional code to identify:
Revised history of tobacco dependence (Z87.891)

MALIGNANT NEOPLASM OF DIGESTIVE ORGANS (C15-C26)

New **Excludes2** gastrointestinal stromal tumors (C49.A-)

C25 Malignant neoplasm of pancreas
New Code also exocrine pancreatic insufficiency (K86.81)

C32 Malignant neoplasm of larynx
C33 Malignant neoplasm of trachea
C34 Malignant neoplasm of bronchus and lung
C39 Malignant neoplasm of other and ill-defined sites in the respiratory system and intrathoracic organs
Use additional code to identify:
Revised history of tobacco dependence (Z87.891)

New **C49.A Gastrointestinal stromal tumor**
New **C49.A0 Gastrointestinal stromal tumor, unspecified site**
New **C49.A1 Gastrointestinal stromal tumor of esophagus**
New **C49.A2 Gastrointestinal stromal tumor of stomach**
New **C49.A3 Gastrointestinal stromal tumor of small intestine**
New **C49.A4 Gastrointestinal stromal tumor of large intestine**
New **C49.A5 Gastrointestinal stromal tumor of rectum**
New **C49.A9 Gastrointestinal stromal tumor of other sites**

C61 Malignant neoplasm of prostate
New Use additional code to identify:
New hormone sensitivity status (Z19.1-Z19.2)
New rising PSA following treatment for malignant neoplasm of prostate (R97.21)

Revised **C7A.094 Malignant carcinoid tumor of the foregut unspecified**
Revised **C7A.095 Malignant carcinoid tumor of the midgut unspecified**
Revised **C7A.096 Malignant carcinoid tumor of the hindgut unspecified**

C78 Secondary malignant neoplasm of respiratory and digestive organs
Deleted **Excludes1** lymph node metastases (C77.0)
New **Excludes2** lymph node metastases (C77.0)

C78.89 Secondary malignant neoplasm of other digestive organs
New Code also exocrine pancreatic insufficiency (K86.81)

C79 Secondary malignant neoplasm of other and unspecified sites
Deleted **Excludes1** lymph node metastases (C77.0)
New **Excludes2** lymph node metastases (C77.0)

Revised **C81.1 Nodular sclerosis Hodgkin lymphoma**
New Nodular sclerosis classical Hodgkin lymphoma
Revised **C81.10 Nodular sclerosis Hodgkin lymphoma, unspecified site**
Revised **C81.11 Nodular sclerosis Hodgkin lymphoma, lymph nodes of head, face, and neck**
Revised **C81.12 Nodular sclerosis Hodgkin lymphoma, intrathoracic lymph nodes**
Revised **C81.13 Nodular sclerosis Hodgkin lymphoma, intra-abdominal lymph nodes**
Revised **C81.14 Nodular sclerosis Hodgkin lymphoma, lymph nodes of axilla and upper limb**
Revised **C81.15 Nodular sclerosis Hodgkin lymphoma, lymph nodes of inguinal region and lower limb**
Revised **C81.16 Nodular sclerosis Hodgkin lymphoma, intrapelvic lymph nodes**
Revised **C81.17 Nodular sclerosis Hodgkin lymphoma, spleen**
Revised **C81.18 Nodular sclerosis Hodgkin lymphoma, lymph nodes of multiple sites**
Revised **C81.19 Nodular sclerosis Hodgkin lymphoma, extranodal and solid organ sites**

Revised **C81.2 Mixed cellularity Hodgkin lymphoma**
New Mixed cellularity classical Hodgkin lymphoma
Revised **C81.20 Mixed cellularity Hodgkin lymphoma, unspecified site**
Revised **C81.21 Mixed cellularity Hodgkin lymphoma, lymph nodes of head, face, and neck**
Revised **C81.22 Mixed cellularity Hodgkin lymphoma, intrathoracic lymph nodes**
Revised **C81.23 Mixed cellularity Hodgkin lymphoma, intra-abdominal lymph nodes**
Revised **C81.24 Mixed cellularity Hodgkin lymphoma, lymph nodes of axilla and upper limb**
Revised **C81.25 Mixed cellularity Hodgkin lymphoma, lymph nodes of inguinal region and lower limb**
Revised **C81.26 Mixed cellularity Hodgkin lymphoma, intrapelvic lymph nodes**
Revised **C81.27 Mixed cellularity Hodgkin lymphoma, spleen**
Revised **C81.28 Mixed cellularity Hodgkin lymphoma, lymph nodes of multiple sites**
Revised **C81.29 Mixed cellularity Hodgkin lymphoma, extranodal and solid organ sites**

Revised **C81.3 Lymphocyte depleted Hodgkin lymphoma**
New Lymphocyte depleted classical Hodgkin lymphoma
Revised **C81.30 Lymphocyte depleted Hodgkin lymphoma, unspecified site**
Revised **C81.31 Lymphocyte depleted Hodgkin lymphoma, lymph nodes of head, face, and neck**
Revised **C81.32 Lymphocyte depleted Hodgkin lymphoma, intrathoracic lymph nodes**
Revised **C81.33 Lymphocyte depleted Hodgkin lymphoma, intra-abdominal lymph nodes**
Revised **C81.34 Lymphocyte depleted Hodgkin lymphoma, lymph nodes of axilla and upper limb**
Revised **C81.35 Lymphocyte depleted Hodgkin lymphoma, lymph nodes of inguinal region and lower limb**
Revised **C81.36 Lymphocyte depleted Hodgkin lymphoma, intrapelvic lymph nodes**
Revised **C81.37 Lymphocyte depleted Hodgkin lymphoma, spleen**
Revised **C81.38 Lymphocyte depleted Hodgkin lymphoma, lymph nodes of multiple sites**
Revised **C81.39 Lymphocyte depleted Hodgkin lymphoma, extranodal and solid organ sites**

Revised **C81.4 Lymphocyte-rich Hodgkin lymphoma**
New Lymphocyte-rich classical Hodgkin lymphoma
Revised **C81.40 Lymphocyte-rich Hodgkin lymphoma, unspecified site**
Revised **C81.41 Lymphocyte-rich Hodgkin lymphoma, lymph nodes of head, face, and neck**
Revised **C81.42 Lymphocyte-rich Hodgkin lymphoma, intrathoracic lymph nodes**
Revised **C81.43 Lymphocyte-rich Hodgkin lymphoma, intra-abdominal lymph nodes**
Revised **C81.44 Lymphocyte-rich Hodgkin lymphoma, lymph nodes of axilla and upper limb**
Revised **C81.45 Lymphocyte-rich Hodgkin lymphoma, lymph nodes of inguinal region and lower limb**
Revised **C81.46 Lymphocyte-rich Hodgkin lymphoma, intrapelvic lymph nodes**
Revised **C81.47 Lymphocyte-rich Hodgkin lymphoma, spleen**
Revised **C81.48 Lymphocyte-rich Hodgkin lymphoma, lymph nodes of multiple sites**
Revised **C81.49 Lymphocyte-rich Hodgkin lymphoma, extranodal and solid organ sites**

Revised **C81.7 Other Hodgkin lymphoma**
New Other classical Hodgkin lymphoma
Revised **C81.70 Other Hodgkin lymphoma, unspecified site**
Revised **C81.71 Other Hodgkin lymphoma, lymph nodes of head, face, and neck**
Revised **C81.72 Other Hodgkin lymphoma, intrathoracic lymph nodes**
Revised **C81.73 Other Hodgkin lymphoma, intra-abdominal lymph nodes**
Revised **C81.74 Other Hodgkin lymphoma, lymph nodes of axilla and upper limb**
Revised **C81.75 Other Hodgkin lymphoma, lymph nodes of inguinal region and lower limb**
Revised **C81.76 Other Hodgkin lymphoma, intrapelvic lymph nodes**
Revised **C81.77 Other Hodgkin lymphoma, spleen**
Revised **C81.78 Other Hodgkin lymphoma, lymph nodes of multiple sites**
Revised **C81.79 Other Hodgkin lymphoma, extranodal and solid organ sites**

Revised **C94.20 Acute megakaryoblastic leukemia not having achieved remission**
Acute megakaryoblastic leukemia with failed remission

Revised **D00.0 Carcinoma in situ of lip, oral cavity and pharynx**
Use additional code to identify:
history of tobacco dependence (Z87.891)

New **D01.3 Carcinoma in situ of anus and anal canal**
New Anal intraepithelial neoplasia III [AIN III]
New Severe dysplasia of anus
Excludes1 anal intraepithelial neoplasia I and II [AIN I and AIN II] (K62.82)

Revised **D02 Carcinoma in situ of middle ear and respiratory system**
Use additional code to identify:
history of tobacco dependence (Z87.891)

D07.5 Carcinoma in situ of prostate

Revised **Excludes1** dysplasia (mild) (moderate) of prostate (N42.3-)

New prostatic intraepithelial neoplasia II [PIN II] (N42.3-)

Revised **D10.3 Benign neoplasm of other and unspecified parts of mouth**

D16.4 Benign neoplasm of bones of skull and face

Deleted **Excludes1** benign neoplasm of lower jaw bone (D16.5)

New **Excludes2** benign neoplasm of lower jaw bone (D16.5)

D27 Benign neoplasm of ovary

Revised **Excludes2** corpus albicans cyst (N83.2-)

Revised corpus luteum cyst (N83.1-)

Revised follicular (atretic) cyst (N83.0-)

Revised graafian follicle cyst (N83.0-)

Revised ovarian cyst NEC (N83.2-)

Revised ovarian retention cyst (N83.2-)

Revised **D3A.094 Benign carcinoid tumor of the foregut, unspecified**

Revised **D3A.095 Benign carcinoid tumor of the midgut, unspecified**

Revised **D3A.096 Benign carcinoid tumor of the hindgut, unspecified**

Revised **D46.2 Refractory anemia with excess of blasts [RAEB]**

New **D47.Z2 Castleman disease**

New Code also if applicable human herpesvirus 8 infection (B10.89)

New **Excludes2** Kaposi's sarcoma (C46-)

D49.2 Neoplasm of unspecified behavior of bone, soft tissue, and skin

Revised **Excludes1** neoplasm of unspecified behavior of skin of genital organs (D49.59)

New **D49.51 Neoplasm of unspecified behavior of kidney**

New **D49.511 Neoplasm of unspecified behavior of right kidney**

New **D49.512 Neoplasm of unspecified behavior of left kidney**

New **D49.519 Neoplasm of unspecified behavior of unspecified kidney**

New **D49.59 Neoplasm of unspecified behavior of other genitourinary organ**

CHAPTER 3

DISEASES OF THE BLOOD AND BLOOD-FORMING ORGANS AND CERTAIN DISORDERS INVOLVING THE IMMUNE MECHANISM (D50-D89)

D61.81 Pancytopenia

Deleted **Excludes1** pancytopenia (due to) (with) myelodysplastic syndromes (D46.-)

New **Excludes2** pancytopenia (due to) (with) myelodysplastic syndromes (D46.-)

D64.81 Anemia due to antineoplastic chemotherapy

Deleted **Excludes1** anemia in neoplastic disease (D63.0)

New **Excludes2** anemia in neoplastic disease (D63.0)

D68.62 Lupus anticoagulant syndrome

Revised **Excludes1** lupus anticoagulant (LAC) finding without diagnosis (R76.0)

D76 Other specified diseases with participation of lymphoreticular and reticulohistiocytic tissue

New **Excludes1** histiocytic medullary reticulosis (C96.9)

New leukemic reticuloendotheliosis (C91.4-)

New lipomelanotic reticulosis (I89.8)

Deleted leukemic reticuloendotheliosis or reticulosis (C91.4-)

Deleted lipomelanotic reticuloendotheliosis or reticulosis (I89.8)

New malignant reticulosis (C86.0)

New nonlipid reticuloendotheliosis (C96.0)

Revised **D78.2 Postprocedural hemorrhage of the spleen following a procedure**

Revised **D78.21 Postprocedural hemorrhage of the spleen following a procedure on the spleen**

Revised **D78.22 Postprocedural hemorrhage of the spleen following other procedure**

New **D78.3 Postprocedural hematoma and seroma of the spleen following a procedure**

New **D78.31 Postprocedural hematoma of the spleen following a procedure on the spleen**

New **D78.32 Postprocedural hematoma of the spleen following other procedure**

New **D78.33 Postprocedural seroma of the spleen following a procedure on the spleen**

New **D78.34 Postprocedural seroma of the spleen following other procedure**

New **D89.4 Mast cell activation syndrome and related disorders**

New **Excludes1** aggressive systemic mastocytosis (C96.2)

New cutaneous mastocytosis (Q82.2)

New indolent systemic mastocytosis (D47.0)

New malignant mastocytoma (C96.2)

New mast cell leukemia (C94.3-)

New mastocytoma (D47.0)

New systemic mastocytosis associated with a clonal hematologic non-mast cell lineage disease (SM-AHNMD) (D47.0)

New **D89.40 Mast cell activation, unspecified**

New Mast cell activation disorder, unspecified

New Mast cell activation syndrome, NOS

New **D89.41 Monoclonal mast cell activation syndrome**

New **D89.42 Idiopathic mast cell activation syndrome**

New **D89.43 Secondary mast cell activation**

New Secondary mast cell activation syndrome

New Code also underlying etiology, if known

New **D89.49 Other mast cell activation disorder**

New Other mast cell activation syndrome

CHAPTER 4

ENDOCRINE, NUTRITIONAL AND METABOLIC DISEASES (E00-E89)

E08 Diabetes mellitus due to underlying condition

Revised Use additional code to identify control using:
New insulin (Z79.4)
New oral antidiabetic drugs (Z79.84)
New oral hypoglycemic drugs (Z79.84)

E08.32 Diabetes mellitus due to underlying condition with mild nonproliferative diabetic retinopathy

New One of the following 7th characters is to be assigned to codes in subcategory E08.32 to designate laterality of the disease:

New 1 right eye
New 2 left eye
New 3 bilateral
New 9 unspecified eye

E08.33 Diabetes mellitus due to underlying condition with moderate nonproliferative diabetic retinopathy

New One of the following 7th characters is to be assigned to codes in subcategory E08.33 to designate laterality of the disease:

New 1 right eye
New 2 left eye
New 3 bilateral
New 9 unspecified eye

E08.34 Diabetes mellitus due to underlying condition with severe nonproliferative diabetic retinopathy

New One of the following 7th characters is to be assigned to codes in subcategory E08.34 to designate laterality of the disease:

New 1 right eye
New 2 left eye
New 3 bilateral
New 9 unspecified eye

E08.35 Diabetes mellitus due to underlying condition with proliferative diabetic retinopathy

New One of the following 7th characters is to be assigned to codes in subcategory E08.35 to designate laterality of the disease:

New 1 right eye
New 2 left eye
New 3 bilateral
New 9 unspecified eye

New **E08.352 Diabetes mellitus due to underlying condition with proliferative diabetic retinopathy with traction retinal detachment involving the macula**

New **E08.353 Diabetes mellitus due to underlying condition with proliferative diabetic retinopathy with traction retinal detachment not involving the macula**

New **E08.354 Diabetes mellitus due to underlying condition with proliferative diabetic retinopathy with combined traction retinal detachment and rhegmatogenous retinal detachment**

New **E08.355 Diabetes mellitus due to underlying condition with stable proliferative diabetic retinopathy**

New **E08.37 Diabetes mellitus due to underlying condition with diabetic macular edema, resolved following treatment**

New One of the following 7th characters is to be assigned to code E08.37 to designate laterality of the disease:

New 1 right eye
New 2 left eye
New 3 bilateral
New 9 unspecified eye

E09 Drug or chemical induced diabetes mellitus

Revised Use additional code to identify control using:
New insulin (Z79.4)
New oral antidiabetic drugs (Z79.84)
New oral hypoglycemic drugs (Z79.84)

E09.32 Drug or chemical induced diabetes mellitus with mild nonproliferative diabetic retinopathy

New One of the following 7th characters is to be assigned to codes in subcategory E09.32 to designate laterality of the disease:

New 1 right eye
New 2 left eye
New 3 bilateral
New 9 unspecified eye

E09.33 Drug or chemical induced diabetes mellitus with moderate nonproliferative diabetic retinopathy

New One of the following 7th characters is to be assigned to codes in subcategory E09.33 to designate laterality of the disease:

New 1 right eye
New 2 left eye
New 3 bilateral
New 9 unspecified eye

E09.34 Drug or chemical induced diabetes mellitus with severe nonproliferative diabetic retinopathy

New One of the following 7th characters is to be assigned to codes in subcategory E09.34 to designate laterality of the disease:

New 1 right eye
New 2 left eye
New 3 bilateral
New 9 unspecified eye

E09.35 Drug or chemical induced diabetes mellitus with proliferative diabetic retinopathy

New One of the following 7th characters is to be assigned to codes in subcategory E09.35 to designate laterality of the disease:

New 1	right eye
New 2	left eye
New 3	bilateral
New 9	unspecified eye

New **E09.352 Drug or chemical induced diabetes mellitus with proliferative diabetic retinopathy with traction retinal detachment involving the macula**

New **E09.353 Drug or chemical induced diabetes mellitus with proliferative diabetic retinopathy with traction retinal detachment not involving the macula**

New **E09.354 Drug or chemical induced diabetes mellitus with proliferative diabetic retinopathy with combined traction retinal detachment and rhegmatogenous retinal detachment**

New **E09.355 Drug or chemical induced diabetes mellitus with stable proliferative diabetic retinopathy**

New **E09.37 Drug or chemical induced diabetes mellitus with diabetic macular edema, resolved following treatment**

New One of the following 7th characters is to be assigned to code E09.37 to designate laterality of the disease:

New 1	right eye
New 2	left eye
New 3	bilateral
New 9	unspecified eye

E10.32 Type 1 diabetes mellitus with mild nonproliferative diabetic retinopathy

New One of the following 7th characters is to be assigned to codes in subcategory E10.32 to designate laterality of the disease:

New 1	right eye
New 2	left eye
New 3	bilateral
New 9	unspecified eye

E10.33 Type 1 diabetes mellitus with moderate nonproliferative diabetic retinopathy

New One of the following 7th characters is to be assigned to codes in subcategory E10.33 to designate laterality of the disease:

New 1	right eye
New 2	left eye
New 3	bilateral
New 9	unspecified eye

E10.34 Type 1 diabetes mellitus with severe nonproliferative diabetic retinopathy

New One of the following 7th characters is to be assigned to codes in subcategory E10.34 to designate laterality of the disease:

New 1	right eye
New 2	left eye
New 3	bilateral
New 9	unspecified eye

E10.35 Type 1 diabetes mellitus with proliferative diabetic retinopathy

New One of the following 7th characters is to be assigned to codes in subcategory E10.35 to designate laterality of the disease:

New 1	right eye
New 2	left eye
New 3	bilateral
New 9	unspecified eye

New **E10.352 Type 1 diabetes mellitus with proliferative diabetic retinopathy with traction retinal detachment involving the macula**

New **E10.353 Type 1 diabetes mellitus with proliferative diabetic retinopathy with traction retinal detachment not involving the macula**

New **E10.354 Type 1 diabetes mellitus with proliferative diabetic retinopathy with combined traction retinal detachment and rhegmatogenous retinal detachment**

New **E10.355 Type 1 diabetes mellitus with stable proliferative diabetic retinopathy**

New **E10.37 Type 1 diabetes mellitus with diabetic macular edema, resolved following treatment**

One of the following 7th characters is to be assigned to code E10.37 to designate laterality of the disease:

New 1	right eye
New 2	left eye
New 3	bilateral
New 9	unspecified eye

E11 Type 2 diabetes mellitus

Revised Use additional code to identify control using:
New insulin (Z79.4)
New oral antidiabetic drugs (Z79.84)
New oral hypoglycemic drugs (Z79.84)

E11.32 Type 2 diabetes mellitus with mild nonproliferative diabetic retinopathy

New One of the following 7th characters is to be assigned to codes in subcategory E11.32 to designate laterality of the disease:

New 1	right eye
New 2	left eye
New 3	bilateral
New 9	unspecified eye

New **E11.33 Type 2 diabetes mellitus with moderate nonproliferative diabetic retinopathy**

New One of the following 7th characters is to be assigned to codes in subcategory E11.33 to designate laterality of the disease:

New 1 right eye
New 2 left eye
New 3 bilateral
New 9 unspecified eye

New **E11.34 Type 2 diabetes mellitus with severe nonproliferative diabetic retinopathy**

New One of the following 7th characters is to be assigned to codes in subcategory E11.34 to designate laterality of the disease:

New 1 right eye
New 2 left eye
New 3 bilateral
New 9 unspecified eye

New **E11.35 Type 2 diabetes mellitus with proliferative diabetic retinopathy**

New One of the following 7th characters is to be assigned to codes in subcategory E11.35 to designate laterality of the disease:

New 1 right eye
New 2 left eye
New 3 bilateral
New 9 unspecified eye

New **E11.352 Type 2 diabetes mellitus with proliferative diabetic retinopathy with traction retinal detachment involving the macula**

New **E11.353 Type 2 diabetes mellitus with proliferative diabetic retinopathy with traction retinal detachment not involving the macula**

New **E11.354 Type 2 diabetes mellitus with proliferative diabetic retinopathy with combined traction retinal detachment and rhegmatogenous retinal detachment**

New **E11.355 Type 2 diabetes mellitus with stable proliferative diabetic retinopathy**

New **E11.37 Type 2 diabetes mellitus with diabetic macular edema, resolved following treatment**

New One of the following 7th characters is to be assigned to code E11.37 to designate laterality of the disease:

New 1 right eye
New 2 left eye
New 3 bilateral
New 9 unspecified eye

Revised **E13 Other specified diabetes mellitus**

New Use additional code to identify control using:
New insulin (Z79.4)
New oral antidiabetic drugs (Z79.84)
New oral hypoglycemic drugs (Z79.84)

New **Excludes1** type 1 diabetes mellitus (E10.-)

New **E13.32 Other specified diabetes mellitus with mild nonproliferative diabetic retinopathy**

New One of the following 7th characters is to be assigned to codes in subcategory E13.32 to designate laterality of the disease:

New 1 right eye
New 2 left eye
New 3 bilateral
New 9 unspecified eye

New **E13.33 Other specified diabetes mellitus with moderate nonproliferative diabetic retinopathy**

New One of the following 7th characters is to be assigned to codes in subcategory E13.33 to designate laterality of the disease:

New 1 right eye
New 2 left eye
New 3 bilateral
New 9 unspecified eye

New **E13.34 Other specified diabetes mellitus with severe nonproliferative diabetic retinopathy**

New One of the following 7th characters is to be assigned to codes in subcategory E13.34 to designate laterality of the disease:

New 1 right eye
New 2 left eye
New 3 bilateral
New 9 unspecified eye

New **E13.35 Other specified diabetes mellitus with proliferative diabetic retinopathy**

New One of the following 7th characters is to be assigned to codes in subcategory E13.35 to designate laterality of the disease:

New 1 right eye
New 2 left eye
New 3 bilateral
New 9 unspecified eye

New **E13.352 Other specified diabetes mellitus with proliferative diabetic retinopathy with traction retinal detachment involving the macula**

New **E13.353 Other specified diabetes mellitus with proliferative diabetic retinopathy with traction retinal detachment not involving the macula**

New **E13.354 Other specified diabetes mellitus with proliferative diabetic retinopathy with combined traction retinal detachment and rhegmatogenous retinal detachment**

New **E13.355 Other specified diabetes mellitus with stable proliferative diabetic retinopathy**

New **E13.37 Other specified diabetes mellitus with diabetic macular edema, resolved following treatment**

New One of the following 7th characters is to be assigned to code E13.37 to designate laterality of the disease:

New	1	right eye
New	2	left eye
New	3	bilateral
New	9	unspecified eye

E16.0 Drug-induced hypoglycemia without coma

New **Excludes1** diabetes with hypoglycemia without coma (E09.692)

E16.1 Other hypoglycemia

New **Excludes1** diabetes with hypoglycemia (E08.649, E10.649, E11.649, E13.649)

E16.2 Hypoglycemia, unspecified

New **Excludes1** diabetes with hypoglycemia (E08.649, E10.649, E11.649, E13.649)

E29 Testicular dysfunction

Revised **Excludes1** Klinefelter's syndrome (Q98.0-Q98.1, Q98.4)

E66.2 Morbid (severe) obesity with alveolar hypoventilation

New Obesity hypoventilation syndrome (OHS)

E78.0 Pure hypercholesterolemia

Deleted Familial hypercholesterolemia
Deleted Fredrickson's hyperlipoproteinemia, type IIa
Deleted Hyperbetalipoproteinemia
Deleted Hyperlipidemia, Group A
Deleted Low-density-lipoprotein-type [LDL] hyperlipoproteinemia

New **E78.00 Pure hypercholesterolemia, unspecified**

New Fredrickson's hyperlipoproteinemia, type IIa
New Hyperbetalipoproteinemia
New Low-density-lipoprotein-type [LDL] hyperlipoproteinemia

New **E78.01 Familial hypercholesterolemia**

E84 Cystic fibrosis

New Code also exocrine pancreatic insufficiency (K86.81)

E85.0 Non-neuropathic heredofamilial amyloidosis

Deleted Familial Mediterranean fever

E86 Volume depletion

New Use additional code(s) for any associated disorders of electrolyte and acid-base balance (E87.-)

E88.42 MERRF syndrome

Revised Code also progressive myoclonic epilepsy (G40.3-)

Revised **E89.81 Postprocedural hemorrhage of an endocrine system organ or structure following a procedure**

Revised **E89.810 Postprocedural hemorrhage of an endocrine system organ or structure following an endocrine system procedure**

Revised **E89.811 Postprocedural hemorrhage of an endocrine system organ or structure following other procedure**

New **E89.82 Postprocedural hematoma and seroma of an endocrine system organ or structure**

New **E89.820 Postprocedural hematoma of an endocrine system organ or structure following an endocrine system procedure**

New **E89.821 Postprocedural hematoma of an endocrine system organ or structure following other procedure**

New **E89.822 Postprocedural seroma of an endocrine system organ or structure following an endocrine system procedure**

New **E89.823 Postprocedural seroma of an endocrine system organ or structure following other procedure**

CHAPTER 5

MENTAL, BEHAVIORAL AND NEURODEVELOPMENTAL DISORDERS (F01-F99)

F01.50 Vascular dementia without behavioral disturbance

New Major neurocognitive disorder without behavioral disturbance

F01.51 Vascular dementia with behavioral disturbance

New Major neurocognitive disorder due to vascular disease, with behavioral disturbance
New Major neurocognitive disorder with aggressive behavior
New Major neurocognitive disorder with combative behavior
New Major neurocognitive disorder with violent behavior

F02 Dementia in other diseases classified elsewhere

Code first the underlying physiological condition, such as:
New dementia with Parkinsonism (G31.83)
New Huntington's disease (G10)
New prion disease (A81.9)
New traumatic brain injury (S06.-)

New **Includes** Major neurocognitive disorder in other diseases classified elsewhere

Deleted **Excludes1** dementia with Parkinsonism (G31.83)

F02.80 Dementia in other diseases classified elsewhere without behavioral disturbance *New*
Major neurocognitive disorder in other diseases classified elsewhere *New*

F02.81 Dementia in other diseases classified elsewhere with behavioral disturbance *New*
Major neurocognitive disorder in other diseases classified elsewhere with aggressive behavior *New*
Major neurocognitive disorder in other diseases classified elsewhere with combative behavior *New*
Major neurocognitive disorder in other diseases classified elsewhere with violent behavior *New*

F06.1 Catatonic disorder due to known physiological condition *New*
Catatonia associated with another mental disorder *New*
Catatonia NOS *New*

F10.10 Alcohol abuse, uncomplicated *New*
Alcohol use disorder, mild *New*

F10.14 Alcohol abuse with alcohol-induced mood disorder *New*
Alcohol use disorder, mild, with alcohol-induced bipolar or related disorder *New*
Alcohol use disorder, mild, with alcohol-induced depressive disorder *New*

F10.20 Alcohol dependence, uncomplicated *New*
Alcohol use disorder, moderate *New*
Alcohol use disorder, severe *New*

F10.22 Alcohol dependence with intoxication *New*
Acute drunkenness (in alcoholism) *Deleted*
Excludes1 alcohol dependence with withdrawal (F10.23-) *New*
Excludes2 alcohol dependence with withdrawal (F10.23-) *New*

F10.23 Alcohol dependence with withdrawal *Deleted*
Excludes1 alcohol dependence with intoxication (F10.22-) *New*
Excludes2 alcohol dependence with intoxication (F10.22-) *New*

F10.24 Alcohol dependence with alcohol-induced mood disorder *New*
Alcohol use disorder, moderate, with alcohol-induced bipolar or related disorder *New*
Alcohol use disorder, moderate, with alcohol-induced depressive disorder *New*
Alcohol use disorder, severe, with alcohol-induced bipolar or related disorder *New*
Alcohol use disorder, severe, with alcohol-induced depressive disorder *New*

F10.26 Alcohol dependence with alcohol-induced persisting amnestic disorder *New*
Alcohol use disorder, moderate, with alcohol-induced major neurocognitive disorder, amnestic-confabulatory type *New*
Alcohol use disorder, severe, with alcohol-induced major neurocognitive disorder, amnestic-confabulatory type *New*

F10.27 Alcohol dependence with alcohol-induced persisting dementia *New*
Alcohol use disorder, moderate, with alcohol-induced major neurocognitive disorder, nonamnestic-confabulatory type *New*
Alcohol use disorder, severe, with alcohol-induced major neurocognitive disorder, nonamnestic-confabulatory type *New*

F10.288 Alcohol dependence with other alcohol-induced disorder *New*
Alcohol use disorder, moderate, with alcohol-induced mild neurocognitive disorder *New*
Alcohol use disorder, severe, with alcohol-induced mild neurocognitive disorder *New*

F10.94 Alcohol use, unspecified with alcohol-induced mood disorder *New*
Alcohol-induced bipolar or related disorder, without use disorder *New*
Alcohol-induced depressive disorder, without use disorder *New*

F10.959 Alcohol use, unspecified with alcohol-induced psychotic disorder, unspecified *New*
Alcohol-induced psychotic disorder without use disorder *New*

F10.96 Alcohol use, unspecified with alcohol-induced persisting amnestic disorder *New*
Alcohol-induced major neurocognitive disorder, amnestic-confabulatory type, without use disorder *New*

F10.97 Alcohol use, unspecified with alcohol-induced persisting dementia *New*
Alcohol-induced major neurocognitive disorder, nonamnestic-confabulatory type, without use disorder *New*

F10.980 Alcohol use, unspecified with alcohol-induced anxiety disorder *New*
Alcohol-induced anxiety disorder, without use disorder *New*

F10.981 Alcohol use, unspecified with alcohol-induced sexual dysfunction *New*
Alcohol-induced sexual dysfunction, without use disorder *New*

F10.982 Alcohol use, unspecified with alcohol-induced sleep disorder *New*
Alcohol-induced sleep disorder, without use disorder *New*

F10.988 Alcohol use, unspecified with other alcohol-induced disorder *New*
Alcohol-induced mild neurocognitive disorder, without use disorder *New*

F11.10 Opioid abuse, uncomplicated *New*
Opioid use disorder, mild *New*

F11.14 Opioid abuse with opioid-induced mood disorder *New*
Opioid use disorder, mild, with opioid-induced depressive disorder *New*

F11.20 Opioid dependence, uncomplicated
New Opioid use disorder, moderate
New Opioid use disorder, severe

F11.24 Opioid dependence with opioid-induced mood disorder
New Opioid use disorder, moderate, with opioid-induced depressive disorder

F11.921 Opioid use, unspecified with intoxication delirium
New Opioid-induced delirium

F11.94 Opioid use, unspecified with opioid-induced mood disorder
New Opioid-induced depressive disorder, without use disorder

F11.981 Opioid use, unspecified with opioid-induced sexual dysfunction
New Opioid-induced sexual dysfunction, without use disorder

F11.982 Opioid use, unspecified with opioid-induced sleep disorder
New Opioid-induced sleep disorder, without use disorder

F11.988 Opioid use, unspecified with other opioid-induced disorder
New Opioid-induced anxiety disorder, without use disorder

F12.10 Cannabis abuse, uncomplicated
New Cannabis use disorder, mild

F12.188 Cannabis abuse with other cannabis-induced disorder
New Cannabis use disorder, mild, with cannabis-induced sleep disorder

F12.2 Cannabis dependence

F12.20 Cannabis dependence, uncomplicated
New Cannabis use disorder, moderate
New Cannabis use disorder, severe

F12.288 Cannabis dependence with other cannabis-induced disorder
New Cannabis use disorder, moderate, with cannabis-induced sleep disorder
New Cannabis use disorder, severe, with cannabis-induced sleep disorder
New Cannabis withdrawal

F12.959 Cannabis use, unspecified with psychotic disorder, unspecified
New Cannabis-induced psychotic disorder, without use disorder

F12.980 Cannabis use, unspecified with anxiety disorder
New Cannabis-induced anxiety disorder, without use disorder

F12.988 Cannabis use, unspecified with other cannabis-induced disorder
New Cannabis-induced sleep disorder, without use disorder

F13.10 Sedative, hypnotic or anxiolytic abuse, uncomplicated
New Sedative, hypnotic, or anxiolytic use disorder, mild

F13.14 Sedative, hypnotic or anxiolytic abuse with sedative, hypnotic or anxiolytic-induced mood disorder
New Sedative, hypnotic, or anxiolytic use disorder, mild, with sedative, hypnotic, or anxiolytic-induced bipolar or related disorder
New Sedative, hypnotic, or anxiolytic use disorder, mild, with sedative, hypnotic, or anxiolytic-induced depressive disorder

F13.23 Sedative, hypnotic or anxiolytic dependence with withdrawal
New Sedative, hypnotic, or anxiolytic use disorder, moderate
New Sedative, hypnotic, or anxiolytic use disorder, severe

F13.232 Sedative, hypnotic or anxiolytic dependence with withdrawal with perceptual disturbance
New Sedative, hypnotic, or anxiolytic withdrawal with perceptual disturbances

F13.239 Sedative, hypnotic or anxiolytic dependence with withdrawal, unspecified
New Sedative, hypnotic, or anxiolytic withdrawal without perceptual disturbances

F13.24 Sedative, hypnotic or anxiolytic dependence with sedative, hypnotic or anxiolytic-induced mood disorder
New Sedative, hypnotic, or anxiolytic use disorder, moderate, with sedative, hypnotic, or anxiolytic-induced bipolar or related disorder
New Sedative, hypnotic, or anxiolytic use disorder, moderate, with sedative, hypnotic, or anxiolytic-induced depressive disorder
New Sedative, hypnotic, or anxiolytic use disorder, severe, with sedative, hypnotic, or anxiolytic-induced bipolar or related disorder
New Sedative, hypnotic, or anxiolytic use disorder, severe, with sedative, hypnotic, or anxiolytic-induced depressive disorder

F13.27 Sedative, hypnotic or anxiolytic dependence with sedative, hypnotic or anxiolytic-induced persisting dementia
New Sedative, hypnotic, or anxiolytic use disorder, moderate, with sedative, hypnotic, or anxiolytic-induced major neurocognitive disorder
New Sedative, hypnotic, or anxiolytic use disorder, severe, with sedative, hypnotic, or anxiolytic-induced major neurocognitive disorder

F13.288 Sedative, hypnotic or anxiolytic dependence with other sedative, hypnotic or anxiolytic-induced disorder

New Sedative, hypnotic, or anxiolytic use disorder, moderate, with sedative, hypnotic, or anxiolytic-induced mild neurocognitive disorder

New Sedative, hypnotic, or anxiolytic use disorder, severe, with sedative, hypnotic, or anxiolytic-induced mild neurocognitive disorder

F13.921 Sedative, hypnotic or anxiolytic use, unspecified with intoxication delirium

New Sedative, hypnotic, or anxiolytic-induced delirium

F13.94 Sedative, hypnotic or anxiolytic use, unspecified with sedative, hypnotic or anxiolytic-induced mood disorder

New Sedative, hypnotic, or anxiolytic-induced bipolar or related disorder, without use disorder

New Sedative, hypnotic, or anxiolytic-induced depressive disorder, without use disorder

F13.959 Sedative, hypnotic or anxiolytic use, unspecified with sedative, hypnotic or anxiolytic-induced psychotic disorder, unspecified

New Sedative, hypnotic, or anxiolytic-induced psychotic disorder, without use disorder

F13.97 Sedative, hypnotic or anxiolytic use, unspecified with sedative, hypnotic or anxiolytic-induced persisting dementia

New Sedative, hypnotic, or anxiolytic-induced major neurocognitive disorder, without use disorder

F13.980 Sedative, hypnotic or anxiolytic use, unspecified with sedative, hypnotic or anxiolytic-induced anxiety disorder

New Sedative, hypnotic, or anxiolytic-induced anxiety disorder, without use disorder

F13.981 Sedative, hypnotic or anxiolytic use, unspecified with sedative, hypnotic or anxiolytic-induced sexual dysfunction

New Sedative, hypnotic, or anxiolytic-induced sexual dysfunction disorder, without use disorder

F13.982 Sedative, hypnotic or anxiolytic use, unspecified with sedative, hypnotic or anxiolytic-induced sleep disorder

New Sedative, hypnotic, or anxiolytic-induced sleep disorder, without use disorder

F13.988 Sedative, hypnotic or anxiolytic use, unspecified with other sedative, hypnotic or anxiolytic-induced disorder

New Sedative, hypnotic, or anxiolytic-induced mild neurocognitive disorder

F14.10 Cocaine abuse, uncomplicated

New Cocaine use disorder, mild

F14.14 Cocaine abuse with cocaine-induced mood disorder

New Cocaine use disorder, mild, with cocaine-induced bipolar or related disorder

New Cocaine use disorder, mild, with cocaine-induced depressive disorder

F14.188 Cocaine abuse with other cocaine-induced disorder

New Cocaine use disorder, mild, with cocaine-induced obsessive-compulsive or related disorder

F14.20 Cocaine dependence, uncomplicated

New Cocaine use disorder, moderate

New Cocaine use disorder, severe

F14.24 Cocaine dependence with cocaine-induced mood disorder

New Cocaine use disorder, moderate, with cocaine-induced bipolar or related disorder

New Cocaine use disorder, moderate, with cocaine-induced depressive disorder

New Cocaine use disorder, severe, with cocaine-induced bipolar or related disorder

New Cocaine use disorder, severe, with cocaine-induced depressive disorder

F14.288 Cocaine dependence with other cocaine-induced disorder

New Cocaine use disorder, moderate, with cocaine-induced obsessive-compulsive or related disorder

New Cocaine use disorder, severe, with cocaine-induced obsessive-compulsive or related disorder

F14.94 Cocaine use, unspecified with cocaine-induced mood disorder

New Cocaine-induced bipolar or related disorder, without use disorder

New Cocaine-induced depressive disorder, without use disorder

New **F14.959 Cocaine use, unspecified with cocaine-induced psychotic disorder, unspecified**
Cocaine-induced psychotic disorder, without use disorder

New **F14.980 Cocaine use, unspecified with cocaine-induced anxiety disorder**
Cocaine-induced anxiety disorder, without use disorder

New **F14.981 Cocaine use, unspecified with cocaine-induced sexual dysfunction**
Cocaine-induced sexual dysfunction, without use disorder

New **F14.982 Cocaine use, unspecified with cocaine-induced sleep disorder**
Cocaine-induced sleep disorder, without use disorder

New **F14.988 Cocaine use, unspecified with other cocaine-induced disorder**
Cocaine-induced obsessive-compulsive or related disorder

F15.10 Other stimulant abuse, uncomplicated
New Amphetamine type substance use disorder, mild
New Other or unspecified stimulant use disorder, mild

New **F15.122 Other stimulant abuse with intoxication with perceptual disturbance**
Amphetamine or other stimulant use disorder, mild, with amphetamine or other stimulant intoxication, with perceptual disturbances

New **F15.129 Other stimulant abuse with intoxication, unspecified**
Amphetamine or other stimulant use disorder, mild, with amphetamine or other stimulant intoxication, without perceptual disturbances

F15.14 Other stimulant abuse with stimulant-induced mood disorder
New Amphetamine or other stimulant use disorder, mild, with amphetamine or other stimulant-induced bipolar or related disorder
New Amphetamine or other stimulant use disorder, mild, with amphetamine or other stimulant-induced depressive disorder

New **F15.188 Other stimulant abuse with other stimulant-induced disorder**
Amphetamine or other stimulant use disorder, mild, with amphetamine or other stimulant-induced obsessive-compulsive or related disorder

F15.20 Other stimulant dependence, uncomplicated
New Amphetamine type substance use disorder, moderate
New Amphetamine type substance use disorder, severe
New Other or unspecified stimulant use disorder, moderate
New Other or unspecified stimulant use disorder, severe

New **F15.222 Other stimulant dependence with intoxication with perceptual disturbance**
Amphetamine or other stimulant use disorder, moderate, with amphetamine or other stimulant intoxication, with perceptual disturbances
Amphetamine or other stimulant use disorder, severe, with amphetamine or other stimulant intoxication, with perceptual disturbances

New **F15.229 Other stimulant dependence with intoxication, unspecified**
Amphetamine or other stimulant use disorder, moderate, with amphetamine or other stimulant intoxication, without perceptual disturbances
Amphetamine or other stimulant use disorder, severe, with amphetamine or other stimulant intoxication, without perceptual disturbances

F15.23 Other stimulant dependence with withdrawal
Amphetamine or other stimulant withdrawal

F15.24 Other stimulant dependence with stimulant-induced mood disorder
New Amphetamine or other stimulant use disorder, moderate, with amphetamine or other stimulant-induced bipolar or related disorder
New Amphetamine or other stimulant use disorder, moderate, with amphetamine or other stimulant-induced depressive disorder
New Amphetamine or other stimulant use disorder, severe, with amphetamine or other stimulant-induced bipolar or related disorder
New Amphetamine or other stimulant use disorder, severe, with amphetamine or other stimulant-induced depressive disorder

F15.288 Other stimulant dependence with other stimulant-induced disorder

New Amphetamine or other stimulant use disorder, moderate, with amphetamine or other stimulant-induced obsessive-compulsive or related disorder

New Amphetamine or other stimulant use disorder, severe, with amphetamine or other stimulant-induced obsessive-compulsive or related disorder

F15.921 Other stimulant use, unspecified with intoxication delirium

New Amphetamine or other stimulant-induced delirium

F15.929 Other stimulant use, unspecified with intoxication, unspecified

New Caffeine intoxication

F15.93 Other stimulant use, unspecified with withdrawal

New Caffeine withdrawal

F15.94 Other stimulant use, unspecified with stimulant-induced mood disorder

New Amphetamine or other stimulant-induced bipolar or related disorder, without use disorder

New Amphetamine or other stimulant-induced depressive disorder, without use disorder

F15.959 Other stimulant use, unspecified with stimulant-induced psychotic disorder, unspecified

New Amphetamine or other stimulant-induced psychotic disorder, without use disorder

F15.980 Other stimulant use, unspecified with stimulant-induced anxiety disorder

New Amphetamine or other stimulant-induced anxiety disorder, without use disorder

New Caffeine-induced anxiety disorder, without use disorder

F15.981 Other stimulant use, unspecified with stimulant-induced sexual dysfunction

New Amphetamine or other stimulant-induced sexual dysfunction, without use disorder

F15.982 Other stimulant use, unspecified with stimulant-induced sleep disorder

New Amphetamine or other stimulant-induced sleep disorder, without use disorder

New Caffeine-induced sleep disorder, without use disorder

F15.988 Other stimulant use, unspecified with other stimulant-induced disorder

New Amphetamine or other stimulant-induced obsessive-compulsive or related disorder, without use disorder

F16.10 Hallucinogen abuse, uncomplicated

New Other hallucinogen use disorder, mild

New Phencyclidine use disorder, mild

F16.14 Hallucinogen abuse with hallucinogen-induced mood disorder

New Other hallucinogen use disorder, mild, with other hallucinogen-induced bipolar or related disorder

New Other hallucinogen use disorder, mild, with other hallucinogen-induced depressive disorder

New Phencyclidine use disorder, mild, with phencyclidine-induced bipolar or related disorder

New Phencyclidine use disorder, mild, with phencyclidine-induced depressive disorder

F16.20 Hallucinogen dependence, uncomplicated

New Other hallucinogen use disorder, moderate

New Other hallucinogen use disorder, severe

New Phencyclidine use disorder, moderate

New Phencyclidine use disorder, severe

F16.24 Hallucinogen dependence with hallucinogen-induced mood disorder

New Other hallucinogen use disorder, moderate, with other hallucinogen-induced bipolar or related disorder

New Other hallucinogen use disorder, moderate, with other hallucinogen-induced depressive disorder

New Other hallucinogen use disorder, severe, with other hallucinogen-induced bipolar or related disorder

New Other hallucinogen use disorder, severe, with other hallucinogen-induced depressive disorder

New Phencyclidine use disorder, moderate, with phencyclidine-induced bipolar or related disorder

New Phencyclidine use disorder, moderate, with phencyclidine-induced depressive disorder

New Phencyclidine use disorder, severe, with phencyclidine-induced bipolar or related disorder

New Phencyclidine use disorder, severe, with phencyclidine-induced depressive disorder

F16.921 Hallucinogen use, unspecified with intoxication with delirium
New Other hallucinogen intoxication delirium

F16.94 Hallucinogen use, unspecified with hallucinogen-induced mood disorder
New Other hallucinogen-induced bipolar or related disorder, without use disorder
New Other hallucinogen-induced depressive disorder, without use disorder
New Phencyclidine-induced bipolar or related disorder, without use disorder
New Phencyclidine-induced depressive disorder, without use disorder

F16.959 Hallucinogen use, unspecified with hallucinogen-induced psychotic disorder, unspecified
New Other hallucinogen-induced psychotic disorder, without use disorder
New Phencyclidine-induced psychotic disorder, without use disorder

F16.980 Hallucinogen use, unspecified with hallucinogen-induced anxiety disorder
New Other hallucinogen-induced anxiety disorder, without use disorder
New Phencyclidine-induced anxiety disorder, without use disorder

F17.200 Nicotine dependence, unspecified, uncomplicated
New Tobacco use disorder, mild
New Tobacco use disorder, moderate
New Tobacco use disorder, severe

F17.203 Nicotine dependence unspecified, with withdrawal
New Tobacco withdrawal

F18.10 Inhalant abuse, uncomplicated
New Inhalant use disorder, mild

F18.14 Inhalant abuse with inhalant-induced mood disorder
New Inhalant use disorder, mild, with inhalant-induced depressive disorder

F18.17 Inhalant abuse with inhalant-induced dementia
New Inhalant use disorder, mild, with inhalant-induced major neurocognitive disorder

F18.188 Inhalant abuse with other inhalant-induced disorder
New Inhalant use disorder, mild, with inhalant-induced mild neurocognitive disorder

F18.20 Inhalant dependence, uncomplicated
New Inhalant use disorder, moderate
New Inhalant use disorder, severe

F18.24 Inhalant dependence with inhalant-induced mood disorder
New Inhalant use disorder, moderate, with inhalant-induced depressive disorder
New Inhalant use disorder, severe, with inhalant-induced depressive disorder

F18.27 Inhalant dependence with inhalant-induced dementia
New Inhalant use disorder, moderate, with inhalant-induced major neurocognitive disorder
New Inhalant use disorder, severe, with inhalant-induced major neurocognitive disorder

F18.288 Inhalant dependence with other inhalant-induced disorder
New Inhalant use disorder, moderate, with inhalant-induced mild neurocognitive disorder
New Inhalant use disorder, severe, with inhalant-induced mild neurocognitive disorder

F18.94 Inhalant use, unspecified with inhalant-induced mood disorder
New Inhalant-induced depressive disorder

F18.97 Inhalant use, unspecified with inhalant-induced persisting dementia
New Inhalant-induced major neurocognitive disorder

F18.988 Inhalant use, unspecified with other inhalant-induced disorder
New Inhalant-induced mild neurocognitive disorder

F19.10 Other psychoactive substance abuse, uncomplicated
New Other (or unknown) substance use disorder, mild

F19.14 Other psychoactive substance abuse with psychoactive substance-induced mood disorder
New Other (or unknown) substance use disorder, mild, with other (or unknown) substance-induced bipolar or related disorder
New Other (or unknown) substance use disorder, mild, with other (or unknown) substance-induced depressive disorder

F19.17 Other psychoactive substance abuse with psychoactive substance-induced persisting dementia
New Other (or unknown) substance use disorder, mild, with other (or unknown) substance-induced major neurocognitive disorder

F19.188 Other psychoactive substance abuse with other psychoactive substance-induced disorder

New Other (or unknown) substance use disorder, mild, with other (or unknown) substance-induced mild neurocognitive disorder

New Other (or unknown) substance use disorder, mild, with other (or unknown) substance-induced obsessive-compulsive or related disorder

F19.20 Other psychoactive substance dependence, uncomplicated

New Other (or unknown) substance use disorder, moderate

New Other (or unknown) substance use disorder, severe

F19.24 Other psychoactive substance dependence with psychoactive substance-induced mood disorder

New Other (or unknown) substance use disorder, moderate, with other (or unknown) substance-induced bipolar or related disorder

New Other (or unknown) substance use disorder, moderate, with other (or unknown) substance-induced depressive disorder

New Other (or unknown) substance use disorder, severe, with other (or unknown) substance-induced bipolar or related disorder

New Other (or unknown) substance use disorder, severe, with other (or unknown) substance-induced depressive disorder

F19.27 Other psychoactive substance dependence with psychoactive substance-induced persisting dementia

New Other (or unknown) substance use disorder, moderate, with other (or unknown) substance-induced major neurocognitive disorder

New Other (or unknown) substance use disorder, severe, with other (or unknown) substance-induced major neurocognitive disorder

F19.288 Other psychoactive substance dependence with other psychoactive substance-induced disorder

New Other (or unknown) substance use disorder, moderate, with other (or unknown) substance-induced mild neurocognitive disorder

New Other (or unknown) substance use disorder, severe, with other (or unknown) substance-induced mild neurocognitive disorder

New Other (or unknown) substance use disorder, moderate, with other (or unknown) substance-induced obsessive-compulsive or related disorder

New Other (or unknown) substance use disorder, severe, with other (or unknown) substance-induced obsessive-compulsive or related disorder

F19.921 Other psychoactive substance use, unspecified with intoxication with delirium

New Other (or unknown) substance-induced delirium

F19.94 Other psychoactive substance use, unspecified with psychoactive substance-induced mood disorder

New Other (or unknown) substance-induced bipolar or related disorder, without use disorder

New Other (or unknown) substance-induced depressive disorder, without use disorder

F19.959 Other psychoactive substance use, unspecified with psychoactive substance-induced psychotic disorder, unspecified

New Other or unknown substance-induced psychotic disorder, without use disorder

F19.97 Other psychoactive substance use, unspecified with psychoactive substance-induced persisting dementia

New Other (or unknown) substance-induced major neurocognitive disorder, without use disorder

F19.980 Other psychoactive substance use, unspecified with psychoactive substance-induced anxiety disorder

New Other (or unknown) substance-induced anxiety disorder, without use disorder

F19.981 Other psychoactive substance use, unspecified with psychoactive substance-induced sexual dysfunction

New Other (or unknown) substance-induced sexual dysfunction, without use disorder

F19.982 Other psychoactive substance use, unspecified with psychoactive substance-induced sleep disorder

New Other (or unknown) substance-induced sleep disorder, without use disorder

F19.988 Other psychoactive substance use, unspecified with other psychoactive substance-induced disorder

New Other (or unknown) substance-induced mild neurocognitive disorder, without use disorder

New Other (or unknown) substance-induced obsessive-compulsive or related disorder, without use disorder

F20.3 Undifferentiated schizophrenia

Revised **Excludes2** post-schizophrenic depression (F32.89)

F32.8 Other depressive episodes
Deleted Atypical depression
Deleted Post-schizophrenic depression
Deleted Single episode of 'masked' depression NOS
New **F32.81 Premenstrual dysphoric disorder**
New **Excludes1** premenstrual tension syndrome (N94.3)
New **F32.89 Other specified depressive episodes**
New Atypical depression
New Post-schizophrenic depression
New Single episode of 'masked' depression NOS

F34.1 Dysthymic disorder
New Persistent depressive disorder

F34.8 Other persistent mood [affective] disorders
New **F34.81 Disruptive mood dysregulation disorder**
New **F34.89 Other specified persistent mood disorders**

F42 Obsessive-compulsive disorder
Deleted Anancastic neurosis
Deleted Obsessive-compulsive neurosis

New **F42.2 Mixed obsessional thoughts and acts**
New **F42.3 Hoarding disorder**
New **F42.4 Excoriation (skin-picking) disorder**
New **Excludes1** factitial dermatitis (L98.1)
New other specified behavioral and emotional disorders with onset usually occurring in early childhood and adolescence (F98.8)

New **F42.8 Other obsessive-compulsive disorder**
New Anancastic neurosis
New Obsessive-compulsive neurosis

New **F42.9 Obsessive-compulsive disorder, unspecified**

F43.8 Other reactions to severe stress
New Other specified trauma and stressor-related disorder

F43.9 Reaction to severe stress, unspecified
New Trauma and stressor-related disorder, NOS

F44.0 Dissociative amnesia
New **Excludes1** dissociative amnesia with dissociative fugue (F44.1)

F44.1 Dissociative fugue
Dissociative amnesia with dissociative fugue

F45.1 Undifferentiated somatoform disorder
New Somatic symptom disorder
F45.21 Hypochondriasis
New Illness anxiety disorder

F50.0 Anorexia nervosa
Revised **Excludes1** psychogenic loss of appetite (F50.89)

F50.8 Other eating disorders
Deleted Pica in adults
Deleted Psychogenic loss of appetite

New **F50.81 Binge eating disorder**
New **F50.89 Other specified eating disorder**
New Pica in adults
New Psychogenic loss of appetite

F52.0 Hypoactive sexual desire disorder
Deleted Anhedonia (sexual)
New Sexual anhedonia
F52.22 Female sexual arousal disorder
Deleted Frigidity
F52.32 Male orgasmic disorder
New Delayed ejaculation

F52.6 Dyspareunia not due to a substance or known physiological condition
New Genito-pelvic pain penetration disorder
Revised **Excludes2** dyspareunia (due to a known physiological condition) (N94.1-)

F60.5 Obsessive-compulsive personality disorder
Revised **Excludes2** obsessive-compulsive disorder (F42-)

New **F64.0 Transsexualism**
New Gender identity disorder in adolescence and adulthood
New Gender dysphoria in adolescents and adults
Revised **F64.1 Dual role transvestism**
Deleted Dual role transvestism
Deleted Transvestism
F64.2 Gender identity disorder of childhood
New Gender dysphoria in children
Revised **Excludes1** gender identity disorder in adolescence and adulthood (F64.0)

F80.0 Phonological disorder
New Speech-sound disorder
F80.8 Other developmental disorders of speech or language
New **F80.82 Social pragmatic communication disorder**
New **Excludes1** Asperger's syndrome (F84.5)
New autistic disorder (F84.0)

F84.0 Autistic disorder
New Autism spectrum disorder

F88 Other disorders of psychological development
New Global developmental delay
New Other specified neurodevelopmental disorder

F89 Unspecified disorder of psychological development
New Neurodevelopmental disorder NOS

F91.8 Other conduct disorders
New Other specified conduct disorder
New Other specified disruptive disorder
F91.9 Conduct disorder, unspecified
New Disruptive disorder NOS

F95.0 Transient tic disorder
New Provisional tic disorder

F98 Other behavioral and emotional disorders with onset usually occurring in childhood and adolescence
Revised **Excludes2** obsessive-compulsive disorder (F42-)
F98.4 Stereotyped movement disorders
Revised **Excludes2** compulsions in obsessive-compulsive disorder (F42-)

CHAPTER 6

DISEASES OF THE NERVOUS SYSTEM (G00-G99)

G00.1 Pneumococcal meningitis
New Meningitis due to Streptococcal pneumoniae

G31.84 Mild cognitive impairment, so stated
Revised **Excludes1** cognitive deficits following (sequelae of) cerebral hemorrhage or infarction (I69.01-, I69.11-, I69.21-, I69.31-, I69.81-, I69.91-)

G40 Epilepsy and recurrent seizures

Deleted **Excludes1** hippocampal sclerosis (G93.81)
Deleted mesial temporal sclerosis (G93.81)
Deleted temporal sclerosis (G93.81)
Deleted Todd's paralysis (G83.8)

New **Excludes2** hippocampal sclerosis (G93.81)
New mesial temporal sclerosis (G93.81)
New temporal sclerosis (G93.81)
New Todd's paralysis (G83.84)

G56.0 Carpal tunnel syndrome

New **G56.03 Carpal tunnel syndrome, bilateral upper limbs**

G56.1 Other lesions of median nerve

New **G56.13 Other lesions of median nerve, bilateral upper limbs**

G56.2 Lesion of ulnar nerve

New **G56.23 Lesion of ulnar nerve, bilateral upper limbs**

G56.3 Lesion of radial nerve

New **G56.33 Lesion of radial nerve, bilateral upper limbs**

G56.4 Causalgia of upper limb

New **G56.43 Causalgia of bilateral upper limbs**

G56.8 Other specified mononeuropathies of upper limb

New **G56.83 Other specified mononeuropathies of bilateral upper limbs**

G56.9 Unspecified mononeuropathy of upper limb

New **G56.93 Unspecified mononeuropathy of bilateral upper limbs**

G57.0 Lesion of sciatic nerve

New **G57.03 Lesion of sciatic nerve, bilateral lower limbs**

G57.1 Meralgia paresthetica

New **G57.13 Meralgia paresthetica, bilateral lower limbs**

G57.2 Lesion of femoral nerve

New **G57.23 Lesion of femoral nerve, bilateral lower limbs**

G57.3 Lesion of lateral popliteal nerve

New **G57.33 Lesion of lateral popliteal nerve, bilateral lower limbs**

G57.4 Lesion of medial popliteal nerve

New **G57.43 Lesion of medial popliteal nerve, bilateral lower limbs**

G57.5 Tarsal tunnel syndrome

New **G57.53 Tarsal tunnel syndrome, bilateral lower limbs**

G57.6 Lesion of plantar nerve

New **G57.63 Lesion of plantar nerve, bilateral lower limbs**

G57.7 Causalgia of lower limb

New **G57.73 Causalgia of bilateral lower limbs**

G57.8 Other specified mononeuropathies of lower limb

New **G57.83 Other specified mononeuropathies of bilateral lower limbs**

G57.9 Unspecified mononeuropathy of lower limb

New **G57.93 Unspecified mononeuropathy of bilateral lower limbs**

G61.8 Other inflammatory polyneuropathies

New **G61.82 Multifocal motor neuropathy**
New MMN

G89 Pain, not elsewhere classified

Revised **Excludes2** pain from prosthetic devices, implants, and grafts (T82.84, T83.84, T84.84, T85.84-)

G97 Intraoperative and postprocedural complications and disorders of nervous system, not elsewhere classified

Revised **G97.5 Postprocedural hemorrhage of a nervous system organ or structure following a procedure**

Revised **G97.51 Postprocedural hemorrhage of a nervous system organ or structure following a nervous system procedure**

Revised **G97.52 Postprocedural hemorrhage of a nervous system organ or structure following other procedure**

New **G97.6 Postprocedural hematoma and seroma of a nervous system organ or structure following a procedure**

New **G97.61 Postprocedural hematoma of a nervous system organ or structure following a nervous system procedure**

New **G97.62 Postprocedural hematoma of a nervous system organ or structure following other procedure**

New **G97.63 Postprocedural seroma of a nervous system organ or structure following a nervous system procedure**

New **G97.64 Postprocedural seroma of a nervous system organ or structure following other procedure**

CHAPTER 7

DISEASES OF THE EYE AND ADNEXA (H00-H59)

H34.81 Central retinal vein occlusion

New One of the following 7th characters is to be assigned to codes in subcategory H34.81 to designate the severity of the occlusion:

New 0 with macular edema
New 1 with retinal neovascularization
New 2 stable
New Old central retinal vein occlusion

H34.83 Tributary (branch) retinal vein occlusion

New One of the following 7th characters is to be assigned to codes in subcategory H34.83 to designate the severity of the occlusion:

New 0 with macular edema
New 1 with retinal neovascularization
New 2 stable
New Old tributary (branch) retinal vein occlusion

H35.31 Nonexudative age-related macular degeneration

New Dry age-related macular degeneration

New One of the following 7th characters is to be assigned to codes in subcategory H35.31 to designate the stage of the disease:

New	0	stage unspecified
New	1	early dry stage
New	2	intermediate dry stage
New	3	advanced atrophic without subfoveal involvement
New		advanced dry stage
New	4	advanced atrophic with subfoveal involvement

New **H35.311 Nonexudative age-related macular degeneration, right eye**

New **H35.312 Nonexudative age-related macular degeneration, left eye**

New **H35.313 Nonexudative age-related macular degeneration, bilateral**

New **H35.319 Nonexudative age-related macular degeneration, unspecified eye**

H35.32 Exudative age-related macular degeneration

New Wet age-related macular degeneration

New One of the following 7th characters is to be assigned to codes in subcategory H35.32 to designate the stage of the disease:

New	0	stage unspecified
New	1	with active choroidal neovascularization
New	2	with inactive choroidal neovascularization
New		with involuted or regressed neovascularization
New	3	with inactive scar

New **H35.321 Exudative age-related macular degeneration, right eye**

New **H35.322 Exudative age-related macular degeneration, left eye**

New **H35.323 Exudative age-related macular degeneration, bilateral**

New **H35.329 Exudative age-related macular degeneration, unspecified eye**

H40.11 Primary open-angle glaucoma

New **H40.111 Primary open-angle glaucoma, right eye**

New **H40.112 Primary open-angle glaucoma, left eye**

New **H40.113 Primary open-angle glaucoma, bilateral**

New **H40.119 Primary open-angle glaucoma, unspecified eye**

H42 Glaucoma in diseases classified elsewhere

Revised **Excludes1** glaucoma (in) onchocerciasis (B73.02)

Deleted diabetes mellitus (E08.39, E09.39, E10.39, E11.39, E13.39)

Deleted onchocerciasis (B73.02)

Revised glaucoma (in) syphilis (A52.71)

Revised glaucoma (in) tuberculous (A18.59)

New **Excludes2** glaucoma (in) diabetes mellitus (E08.39, E09.39, E10.39, E11.39, E13.39)

H53.0 Amblyopia ex anopsia

New **H53.04 Amblyopia suspect**

New **H53.041 Amblyopia suspect, right eye**

New **H53.042 Amblyopia suspect, left eye**

New **H53.043 Amblyopia suspect, bilateral**

H53.049 Amblyopia suspect, unspecified eye

H59 Intraoperative and postprocedural complications and disorders of eye and adnexa, not elsewhere classified

Revised **H59.3 Postprocedural hemorrhage, hematoma, and seroma of eye and adnexa following other procedure**

Revised **H59.31 Postprocedural hemorrhage of eye and adnexa following an ophthalmic procedure**

Revised **H59.311 Postprocedural hemorrhage of right eye and avdnexa following an ophthalmic procedure**

Revised **H59.312 Postprocedural hemorrhage of left eye and adnexa following an ophthalmic procedure**

Revised **H59.313 Postprocedural hemorrhage of eye and adnexa following an ophthalmic procedure, bilateral**

Revised **H59.319 Postprocedural hemorrhage of unspecified eye and adnexa following an ophthalmic procedure**

Revised **H59.32 Postprocedural hemorrhage of eye and adnexa following other procedure**

Revised **H59.321 Postprocedural hemorrhage of right eye and adnexa following other procedure**

Revised **H59.322 Postprocedural hemorrhage of left eye and adnexa following other procedure**

Revised **H59.323 Postprocedural hemorrhage of eye and adnexa following other procedure, bilateral**

Revised **H59.329 Postprocedural hemorrhage of unspecified eye and adnexa following other procedure**

New **H59.33 Postprocedural hematoma of eye and adnexa following an ophthalmic procedure**

New **H59.331 Postprocedural hematoma of right eye and adnexa following an ophthalmic procedure**

New **H59.332 Postprocedural hematoma of left eye and adnexa following an ophthalmic procedure**

New **H59.333 Postprocedural hematoma of eye and adnexa following an ophthalmic procedure, bilateral**

New **H59.339 Postprocedural hematoma of unspecified eye and adnexa following an ophthalmic procedure**

New **H59.34 Postprocedural hematoma of eye and adnexa following other procedure**

New **H59.341 Postprocedural hematoma of right eye and adnexa following other procedure**

New **H59.342 Postprocedural hematoma of left eye and adnexa following other procedure**

New **H59.343 Postprocedural hematoma of eye and adnexa following other procedure, bilateral**

New **H59.349 Postprocedural hematoma of unspecified eye and adnexa following other procedure**

New H59.35 Postprocedural seroma of eye and adnexa following an ophthalmic procedure

New H59.351 Postprocedural seroma of right eye and adnexa following an ophthalmic procedure

New H59.352 Postprocedural seroma of left eye and adnexa following an ophthalmic procedure

New H59.353 Postprocedural seroma of eye and adnexa following an ophthalmic procedure, bilateral

New H59.359 Postprocedural seroma of unspecified eye and adnexa following an ophthalmic procedure

New H59.36 Postprocedural seroma of eye and adnexa following other procedure

New H59.361 Postprocedural seroma of right eye and adnexa following other procedure

New H59.362 Postprocedural seroma of left eye and adnexa following other procedure

New H59.363 Postprocedural seroma of eye and adnexa following other procedure, bilateral

New H59.369 Postprocedural seroma of unspecified eye and adnexa following other procedure

CHAPTER 8

DISEASES OF THE EAR AND MASTOID PROCESS (H60-H95)

H65 Nonsuppurative otitis media

H66 Suppurative and unspecified otitis media

Use additional code to identify:

New history of tobacco dependence (Z87.891)

H90 Conductive and sensorineural hearing loss

New H90.A Conductive and sensorineural hearing loss with restricted hearing on the contralateral side

New H90.A1 Conductive hearing loss, unilateral, with restricted hearing on the contralateral side

New H90.A11 Conductive hearing loss, unilateral, right ear with restricted hearing on the contralateral side

New H90.A12 Conductive hearing loss, unilateral, left ear with restricted hearing on the contralateral side

New H90.A2 Sensorineural hearing loss, unilateral, with restricted hearing on the contralateral side

New H90.A21 Sensorineural hearing loss, unilateral, right ear, with restricted hearing on the contralateral side

New H90.A22 Sensorineural hearing loss, unilateral, left ear, with restricted hearing on the contralateral side

New H90.A3 Mixed conductive and sensorineural hearing loss, unilateral with restricted hearing on the contralateral side

New H90.A31 Mixed conductive and sensorineural hearing loss, unilateral, right ear with restricted hearing on the contralateral side

New H90.A32 Mixed conductive and sensorineural hearing loss, unilateral, left ear with restricted hearing on the contralateral side

H93 Other disorders of ear, not elsewhere classified

New H93.A Pulsatile tinnitus

New H93.A1 Pulsatile tinnitus, right ear

New H93.A2 Pulsatile tinnitus, left ear

New H93.A3 Pulsatile tinnitus, bilateral

New H93.A9 Pulsatile tinnitus, unspecified ear

H95 Intraoperative and postprocedural complications and disorders of ear and mastoid process, not elsewhere classified

Revised H95.4 Postprocedural hemorrhage of ear and mastoid process following a procedure

Revised H95.41 Postprocedural hemorrhage of ear and mastoid process following a procedure on the ear and mastoid process

Revised H95.42 Postprocedural hemorrhage of ear and mastoid process following other procedure

New H95.5 Postprocedural hematoma and seroma of ear and mastoid process following a procedure

New H95.51 Postprocedural hematoma of ear and mastoid process following a procedure on the ear and mastoid process

New H95.52 Postprocedural hematoma of ear and mastoid process following other procedure

New H95.53 Postprocedural seroma of ear and mastoid process following a procedure on the ear and mastoid process

New H95.54 Postprocedural seroma of ear and mastoid process following other procedure

CHAPTER 9 DISEASES OF THE CIRCULATORY SYSTEM (I00-I99)

This chapter contains the following blocks:

Revised I10-I16 Hypertensive diseases

HYPERTENSIVE DISEASES (I10-I16)

Use additional code to identify:

Revised history of tobacco dependence (Z87.891)

New **Excludes2** hypertensive disease complicating pregnancy, childbirth and the puerperium (O10-O11, O13-O16)

New I16 Hypertensive crisis

New Code also any identified hypertensive disease (I10-I15)

New I16.0 Hypertensive urgency

New I16.1 Hypertensive emergency

New I16.9 Hypertensive crisis, unspecified

ISCHEMIC HEART DISEASES (I20-I25)

Revised Use additional code to identify presence of hypertension (I10-I16)

I20 Angina pectoris

Use additional code to identify:
Revised history of tobacco dependence (Z87.891)

I20.8 Other forms of angina pectoris
New Stable angina

I21 ST elevation (STEMI) and non-ST elevation (NSTEMI) myocardial infarction

I22 Subsequent ST elevation (STEMI) and non-ST elevation (NSTEMI) myocardial infarction

I25 Chronic ischemic heart disease

Use additional code to identify:
Revised history of tobacco dependence (Z87.891)

I42 Cardiomyopathy

Deleted **Excludes1** ischemic cardiomyopathy (I25.5)
Deleted peripartum cardiomyopathy (O90.3)
New **Excludes2** ischemic cardiomyopathy (I25.5)
New peripartum cardiomyopathy (O90.3)

I50 Heart failure

Deleted **Excludes1** cardiac arrest (I46.-)
New **Excludes2** cardiac arrest (I46.-)

I50.9 Heart failure, unspecified

Deleted **Excludes1** fluid overload (E87.70)
New **Excludes2** fluid overload (E87.70)

CEREBROVASCULAR DISEASES (I60-I69)

Use additional code to identify presence of:
Revised history of tobacco dependence (Z87.891)

I60 Nontraumatic subarachnoid hemorrhage

Deleted **Excludes1** sequelae of subarachnoid hemorrhage (I69.0-)
New **Excludes2** sequelae of subarachnoid hemorrhage (I69.0-)

I60.2 Nontraumatic subarachnoid hemorrhage from anterior communicating artery

Deleted ~~I60.20 Nontraumatic subarachnoid hemorrhage from unspecified anterior communicating artery~~
Deleted ~~I60.21 Nontraumatic subarachnoid hemorrhage from right anterior communicating artery~~
Deleted ~~I60.22 Nontraumatic subarachnoid hemorrhage from left anterior communicating artery~~

I61 Nontraumatic intracerebral hemorrhage

Deleted **Excludes1** sequelae of intracerebral hemorrhage (I69.1-)
New **Excludes2** sequelae of intracerebral hemorrhage (I69.1-)

I62 Other and unspecified nontraumatic intracranial hemorrhage

Deleted **Excludes1** sequelae of intracerebral hemorrhage (I69.2)
New **Excludes2** sequelae of intracranial hemorrhage (I69.2)

I63 Cerebral infarction

New Use additional code, if known, to indicate National Institutes of Health Stroke Scale (NIHSS) score (R29.7-)

Deleted **Excludes1** sequelae of cerebral infarction (I69.3-)
New **Excludes2** sequelae of cerebral infarction (I69.3-)

New **I63.013 Cerebral infarction due to thrombosis of bilateral vertebral arteries**

I63.03 Cerebral infarction due to thrombosis of carotid artery

New **I63.033 Cerebral infarction due to thrombosis of bilateral carotid arteries**

New **I63.113 Cerebral infarction due to embolism of bilateral vertebral arteries**

New **I63.133 Cerebral infarction due to embolism of bilateral carotid arteries**

New **I63.213 Cerebral infarction due to unspecified occlusion or stenosis of bilateral vertebral arteries**

New **I63.233 Cerebral infarction due to unspecified occlusion or stenosis of bilateral carotid arteries**

New **I63.313 Cerebral infarction due to thrombosis of bilateral middle cerebral arteries**

New **I63.323 Cerebral infarction due to thrombosis of bilateral anterior arteries**

New **I63.333 Cerebral infarction to thrombosis of bilateral posterior arteries**

New **I63.343 Cerebral infarction to thrombosis of bilateral cerebellar arteries**

New **I63.413 Cerebral infarction due to embolism of bilateral middle cerebral arteries**

New **I63.423 Cerebral infarction due to embolism of bilateral anterior cerebral arteries**

New **I63.433 Cerebral infarction due to embolism of bilateral posterior cerebral arteries**

New **I63.443 Cerebral infarction due to embolism of bilateral cerebellar arteries**

New **I63.513 Cerebral infarction due to unspecified occlusion or stenosis of bilateral middle arteries**

New **I63.523** **Cerebral infarction due to unspecified occlusion or stenosis of bilateral anterior arteries**

New **I63.533** **Cerebral infarction due to unspecified occlusion or stenosis of bilateral posterior arteries**

New **I63.543** **Cerebral infarction due to unspecified occlusion or stenosis of bilateral cerebellar arteries**

I67 Other cerebrovascular diseases

Deleted **Excludes1** sequelae of the listed conditions (I69.8)

New **Excludes2** sequelae of the listed conditions (I69.8)

New **I69.010** **Attention and concentration deficit following nontraumatic subarachnoid hemorrhage**

New **I69.011** **Memory deficit following nontraumatic subarachnoid hemorrhage**

New **I69.012** **Visuospatial deficit and spatial neglect following nontraumatic subarachnoid hemorrhage**

New **I69.013** **Psychomotor deficit following nontraumatic subarachnoid hemorrhage**

New **I69.014** **Frontal lobe and executive function deficit following nontraumatic subarachnoid hemorrhage**

New **I69.015** **Cognitive social or emotional deficit following nontraumatic subarachnoid hemorrhage**

New **I69.018** **Other symptoms and signs involving cognitive functions following nontraumatic subarachnoid hemorrhage**

New **I69.019** **Unspecified symptoms and signs involving cognitive functions following nontraumatic subarachnoid hemorrhage**

New **I69.110** **Attention and concentration deficit following nontraumatic intracerebral hemorrhage**

New **I69.111** **Memory deficit following nontraumatic intracerebral hemorrhage**

New **I69.112** **Visuospatial deficit and spatial neglect following nontraumatic intracerebral hemorrhage**

New **I69.113** **Psychomotor deficit following nontraumatic intracerebral hemorrhage**

New **I69.114** **Frontal lobe and executive function deficit following nontraumatic intracerebral hemorrhage**

New **I69.115** **Cognitive social or emotional deficit following nontraumatic intracerebral hemorrhage**

New **I69.118** **Other symptoms and signs involving cognitive functions following nontraumatic intracerebral hemorrhage**

New **I69.119** **Unspecified symptoms and signs involving cognitive functions following nontraumatic intracerebral hemorrhage**

I69.123 **Fluency disorder following nontraumatic intracerebral hemorrhage**

Revised Stuttering following nontraumatic intracerebral hemorrhage

I69.21 **Cognitive deficits following other nontraumatic intracranial hemorrhage**

New **I69.210** **Attention and concentration deficit following other nontraumatic intracranial hemorrhage**

New **I69.211** **Memory deficit following other nontraumatic intracranial hemorrhage**

New **I69.212** **Visuospatial deficit and spatial neglect following other nontraumatic intracranial hemorrhage**

New **I69.213** **Psychomotor deficit following other nontraumatic intracranial hemorrhage**

New **I69.214** **Frontal lobe and executive function deficit following other nontraumatic intracranial hemorrhage**

New **I69.215** **Cognitive social or emotional deficit following other nontraumatic intracranial hemorrhage**

New **I69.218** **Other symptoms and signs involving cognitive functions following other nontraumatic intracranial hemorrhage**

New **I69.219** **Unspecified symptoms and signs involving cognitive functions following other nontraumatic intracranial hemorrhage**

I69.223 **Fluency disorder following other nontraumatic intracranial hemorrhage**

Revised Stuttering following other nontraumatic intracranial hemorrhage

New **I69.310** **Attention and concentration deficit following cerebral infarction**

New **I69.311** **Memory deficit following cerebral infarction**

New **I69.312** **Visuospatial deficit and spatial neglect following cerebral infarction**

New **I69.313** **Psychomotor deficit following cerebral infarction**

New **I69.314** **Frontal lobe and executive function deficit following cerebral infarction**

New **I69.315** **Cognitive social or emotional deficit following cerebral infarction**

New **I69.318** **Other symptoms and signs involving cognitive functions following cerebral infarction**

New **I69.319** **Unspecified symptoms and signs involving cognitive functions following cerebral infarction**

Revised **I69.323 Fluency disorder following cerebral infarction**
Stuttering following cerebral infarction

New **I69.810 Attention and concentration deficit following other cerebrovascular disease**

New **I69.811 Memory deficit following other cerebrovascular disease**

New **I69.812 Visuospatial deficit and spatial neglect following other cerebrovascular disease**

New **I69.813 Psychomotor deficit following other cerebrovascular disease**

New **I69.814 Frontal lobe and executive function deficit following other cerebrovascular disease**

New **I69.815 Cognitive social or emotional deficit following other cerebrovascular disease**

New **I69.818 Other symptoms and signs involving cognitive functions following other cerebrovascular disease**

New **I69.819 Unspecified symptoms and signs involving cognitive functions following other cerebrovascular disease**

I69.823 Fluency disorder following other cerebrovascular disease
Revised Stuttering following other cerebrovascular disease

New **I69.910 Attention and concentration deficit following unspecified cerebrovascular disease**

New **I69.911 Memory deficit following unspecified cerebrovascular disease**

New **I69.912 Visuospatial deficit and spatial neglect following unspecified cerebrovascular disease**

New **I69.913 Psychomotor deficit following unspecified cerebrovascular disease**

New **I69.914 Frontal lobe and executive function deficit following unspecified cerebrovascular disease**

New **I69.915 Cognitive social or emotional deficit following unspecified cerebrovascular disease**

New **I69.918 Other symptoms and signs involving cognitive functions following unspecified cerebrovascular disease**

New **I69.919 Unspecified symptoms and signs involving cognitive functions following unspecified cerebrovascular disease**

I69.923 Fluency disorder following unspecified cerebrovascular disease
Revised Stuttering following unspecified cerebrovascular disease

I70 Atherosclerosis
Use additional code to identify:
Revised history of tobacco dependence (Z87.891)

I72 Other aneurysm
New **Excludes2** dissection of precerebral artery, congenital (nonruptured) (Q28.1)

New **I72.5 Aneurysm of other precerebral arteries**
New Aneurysm of basilar artery (trunk)
New **Excludes2** aneurysm of carotid artery (I72.0)
New aneurysm of vertebral artery (I72.6)
New dissection of carotid artery (I77.71)
New dissection of other precerebral arteries (I77.75)
New dissection of vertebral artery (I77.74)

New **I72.6 Aneurysm of vertebral artery**
New **Excludes2** dissection of vertebral artery (I77.74)

I74 Arterial embolism and thrombosis
Revised **Excludes2** mesenteric embolism and thrombosis (K55.0-)

New **I77.70 Dissection of unspecified artery**

I77.74 Dissection of vertebral artery
New **Excludes2** aneurysm of vertebral artery (I72.6)

New **I77.75 Dissection of other precerebral arteries**
New Dissection of basilar artery (trunk)
New **Excludes2** aneurysm of carotid artery (I72.0)
New aneurysm of other precerebral arteries (I72.5)
New aneurysm of vertebral artery (I72.6)
New dissection of carotid artery (I77.71)
New dissection of vertebral artery (I77.74)

New **I77.76 Dissection of artery of upper extremity**

New **I77.77 Dissection of artery of lower extremity**

Revised **I77.79 Dissection of other specified artery**

I82 Other venous embolism and thrombosis
Revised **Excludes2** mesenteric (K55.0-)

Deleted **I83.1 Varicose veins of lower extremities with inflammation**
Stasis dermatitis

New **I87.2 Venous insufficiency (chronic) (peripheral)**
Stasis dermatitis
New **Excludes1** stasis dermatitis with varicose veins of lower extremities (I83.1-, I83.2-)

I89 Other noninfective disorders of lymphatic vessels and lymph nodes
Revised **Excludes1** chylocele, tunica vaginalis (nonfilarial) NOS (N50.89)

I96 Gangrene, not elsewhere classified
Revised **Excludes1** gangrene in diabetes mellitus (E08-E13 with .52)

Revised **I97.6 Postprocedural hemorrhage, hematoma and seroma of a circulatory system organ or structure following a procedure**

Revised **I97.61 Postprocedural hemorrhage of a circulatory system organ or structure following a circulatory system procedure**

Revised **I97.610 Postprocedural hemorrhage of a circulatory system organ or structure following a cardiac catheterization**

Revised **I97.611 Postprocedural hemorrhage of a circulatory system organ or structure following cardiac bypass**

Revised **I97.618 Postprocedural hemorrhage of a circulatory system organ or structure following other circulatory system procedure**

Revised **I97.62 Postprocedural hemorrhage, hematoma and seroma of a circulatory system organ or structure following other procedure**

New **I97.620 Postprocedural hemorrhage of a circulatory system organ or structure following other procedure**

New **I97.621 Postprocedural hematoma of a circulatory system organ or structure following other procedure**

New **I97.622 Postprocedural seroma of a circulatory system organ or structure following other procedure**

New **I97.63 Postprocedural hematoma of a circulatory system organ or structure following a circulatory system procedure**

New **I97.630 Postprocedural hematoma of a circulatory system organ or structure following a cardiac catheterization**

New **I97.631 Postprocedural hematoma of a circulatory system organ or structure following cardiac bypass**

New **I97.638 Postprocedural hematoma of a circulatory system organ or structure following other circulatory system procedure**

New **I97.64 Postprocedural seroma of a circulatory system organ or structure following a circulatory system procedure**

New **I97.640 Postprocedural seroma of a circulatory system organ or structure following a cardiac catheterization**

New **I97.641 Postprocedural seroma of a circulatory system organ or structure following cardiac bypass**

New **I97.648 Postprocedural seroma of a circulatory system organ or structure following other circulatory system procedure**

Revised **I97.820 Postprocedural cerebrovascular infarction following cardiac surgery**

Revised **I97.821 Postprocedural cerebrovascular infarction following other surgery**

CHAPTER 10

DISEASES OF THE RESPIRATORY SYSTEM (J00-J99)

J31 Chronic rhinitis, nasopharyngitis and pharyngitis

J32 Chronic sinusitis

J33 Nasal polyp

J35 Chronic diseases of tonsils and adenoids

J37 Chronic laryngitis and laryngotracheitis

J38 Diseases of vocal cords and larynx, not elsewhere classified

J40 Bronchitis, not specified as acute or chronic

J41 Simple and mucopurulent chronic bronchitis

J42 Unspecified chronic bronchitis

J43 Emphysema

J44 Other chronic obstructive pulmonary disease

Revised Use additional code to identify: history of tobacco dependence (Z87.891)

Deleted **Excludes1** lung diseases due to external agents (J60-J70)

New **Excludes2** lung diseases due to external agents (J60-J70)

J45 Asthma

J47 Bronchiectasis

Revised Use additional code to identify: history of tobacco dependence (Z87.891)

J47.0 Bronchiectasis with acute lower respiratory infection

New Use additional code to identify the infection

J81 Pulmonary edema

Revised Use additional code to identify: history of tobacco dependence (Z87.891)

J84.89 Other specified interstitial pulmonary diseases

Deleted Organizing pneumonia due to known underlying cause

Revised **J95.83 Postprocedural hemorrhage of a respiratory system organ or structure following a procedure**

Revised **J95.830 Postprocedural hemorrhage of a respiratory system organ or structure following a respiratory system procedure**

Revised **J95.831 Postprocedural hemorrhage of a respiratory system organ or structure following other procedure**

New **J95.86 Postprocedural hematoma and seroma of a respiratory system organ or structure following a procedure**

New **J95.860 Postprocedural hematoma of a respiratory system organ or structure following a respiratory system procedure**

New **J95.861 Postprocedural hematoma of a respiratory system organ or structure following other procedure**

New **J95.862 Postprocedural seroma of a respiratory system organ or structure following a respiratory system procedure**

New **J95.863 Postprocedural seroma of a respiratory system organ or structure following other procedure**

J98 Other respiratory disorders
Use additional code to identify:
Revised history of tobacco dependence (Z87.891)

J98.5 Diseases of mediastinum, not elsewhere classified
Deleted Fibrosis of mediastinum
Deleted Hernia of mediastinum
Deleted Retraction of mediastinum
Deleted Mediastinitis

New **J98.51 Mediastinitis**
New *Code first underlying condition, if applicable, such as postoperative mediastinitis (T81.-)*

New **J98.59 Other diseases of mediastinum, not elsewhere classified**
New Fibrosis of mediastinum
New Hernia of mediastinum
New Retraction of mediastinum

CHAPTER 11

DISEASES OF THE DIGESTIVE SYSTEM (K00-K95)

K02 Dental caries
New **Includes** caries of dentine
New dental cavities
New early childhood caries
New pre-eruptive caries
New recurrent caries (dentino enamel junction) (enamel) (to the pulp)

K02.52 Dental caries on pit and fissure surface penetrating into dentin
New Primary dental caries, cervical origin

K04.0 Pulpitis
Deleted Reversible pulpitis
Deleted Irreversible pulpitis
New **K04.01 Reversible pulpitis**
New **K04.02 Irreversible pulpitis**

K05 Gingivitis and periodontal diseases
Use additional code to identify:
Revised history of tobacco dependence (Z87.891)

K05.00 Acute gingivitis, plaque induced
New Plaque induced gingival disease

K05.1 Chronic gingivitis
New Pregnancy associated gingivitis
New *Code first, if applicable, diseases of the digestive system complicating pregnancy (O99.61-)*

New **K05.211 Aggressive periodontitis, localized, slight**
New **K05.212 Aggressive periodontitis, localized, moderate**
New **K05.213 Aggressive periodontitis, localized, severe**
New **K05.219 Aggressive periodontitis, localized, unspecified severity**

New **K05.221 Aggressive periodontitis, generalized, slight**
New **K05.222 Aggressive periodontitis, generalized, moderate**
New **K05.223 Aggressive periodontitis, generalized, severe**
New **K05.229 Aggressive periodontitis, generalized, unspecified severity**

New **K05.311 Chronic periodontitis, localized, slight**
New **K05.312 Chronic periodontitis, localized, moderate**
New **K05.313 Chronic periodontitis, localized, severe**
New **K05.319 Chronic periodontitis, localized, unspecified severity**

New **K05.321 Chronic periodontitis, generalized, slight**
New **K05.322 Chronic periodontitis, generalized, moderate**
New **K05.323 Chronic periodontitis, generalized, severe**
New **K05.329 Chronic periodontitis, generalized, unspecified severity**

K05.5 Other periodontal diseases
New Combined periodontic-endodontic lesion
New Narrow gingival width (of periodontal soft tissue)

New **K06.3 Horizontal alveolar bone loss**

K06.8 Other specified disorders of gingiva and edentulous alveolar ridge
New Vertical ridge deficiency

K08.8 Other specified disorders of teeth and supporting structures
Deleted Enlargement of alveolar ridge NOS
Deleted Irregular alveolar process
Deleted Toothache NOS
New **K08.81 Primary occlusal trauma**
New **K08.82 Secondary occlusal trauma**
New **K08.89 Other specified disorders of teeth and supporting structures**
New Enlargement of alveolar ridge NOS
New Insufficient anatomic crown height
New Insufficient clinical crown length
New Irregular alveolar process
New Toothache NOS

K11 Diseases of salivary glands
K12 Stomatitis and related lesions
K13 Other diseases of lip and oral mucosa
K14 Diseases of tongue
Use additional code to identify:
Revised history of tobacco dependence (Z87.891)

K35.3 Acute appendicitis with localized peritonitis
Revised Acute appendicitis with or without perforation or rupture with peritonitis NOS

NONINFECTIVE ENTERITIS AND COLITIS (K50-K52)

Revised **Excludes1** megacolon (K59.3-)

K52.2 Allergic and dietetic gastroenteritis and colitis
New **Excludes2** allergic eosinophilic colitis (K52.82)
New allergic eosinophilic esophagitis (K20.0)
New allergic eosinophilic gastritis (K52.81)
New allergic eosinophilic gastroenteritis (K52.81)
New food protein-induced proctocolitis (K52.82)

New **K52.21 Food protein-induced enterocolitis syndrome**
New Use additional code for hypovolemic shock, if present (R57.1)

New **K52.22 Food protein-induced enteropathy**

K52.29 Other allergic and dietetic gastroenteritis and colitis
New Food hypersensitivity gastroenteritis or colitis
New Immediate gastrointestinal hypersensitivity

New **K52.3 Indeterminate colitis**
New Colonic inflammatory bowel disease unclassified (IBDU)
New **Excludes1** unspecified colitis (K52.9)

K52.81 Eosinophilic gastritis or gastroenteritis
Eosinophilic enteritis
Deleted **Excludes1** eosinophilic esophagitis (K20.0)
New **Excludes2** eosinophilic esophagitis (K20.0)

K52.82 Eosinophilic colitis
New Allergic proctocolitis
New Food-induced eosinophilic proctocolitis
New Food protein-induced proctocolitis
New Milk protein-induced proctocolitis

New **K52.83 Microscopic colitis**
New **K52.831 Collagenous colitis**
New **K52.832 Lymphocytic colitis**
New **K52.838 Other microscopic colitis**
New **K52.839 Microscopic colitis, unspecified**

K52.89 Other specified noninfective gastroenteritis and colitis
Deleted Collagenous colitis
Deleted Lymphocytic colitis
Deleted Microscopic colitis (collagenous or lymphocytic)

K55.0 Acute vascular disorders of intestine
Deleted Acute fulminant ischemic colitis
Deleted Acute intestinal infarction
Deleted Acute small intestine ischemia
Deleted Necrosis of intestine
Deleted Subacute ischemic colitis

New **K55.01 Acute (reversible) ischemia of small intestine**
New **K55.011 Focal (segmental) acute (reversible) ischemia of small intestine**
New **K55.012 Diffuse acute (reversible) ischemia of small intestine**
New **K55.019 Acute (reversible) ischemia of small intestine, extent unspecified**

New **K55.02 Acute infarction of small intestine**
New Gangrene of small intestine
New Necrosis of small intestine
New **K55.021 Focal (segmental) acute infarction of small intestine**
New **K55.022 Diffuse acute infarction of small intestine**
New **K55.029 Acute infarction of small intestine, extent unspecified**

New **K55.03 Acute (reversible) ischemia of large intestine**
New Acute fulminant ischemic colitis
New Subacute ischemic colitis
New **K55.031 Focal (segmental) acute (reversible) ischemia of large intestine**
New **K55.032 Diffuse acute (reversible) ischemia of large intestine**
New **K55.039 Acute (reversible) ischemia of large intestine, extent unspecified**

New **K55.04 Acute infarction of large intestine**
New Gangrene of large intestine
New Necrosis of large intestine
New **K55.041 Focal (segmental) acute infarction of large intestine**
New **K55.042 Diffuse acute infarction of large intestine**
New **K55.049 Acute infarction of large intestine, extent unspecified**

New **K55.05 Acute (reversible) ischemia of intestine, part unspecified**
New **K55.051 Focal (segmental) acute (reversible) ischemia of intestine, part unspecified**
New **K55.052 Diffuse acute (reversible) ischemia of intestine, part unspecified**
New **K55.059 Acute (reversible) ischemia of intestine, part and extent unspecified**

New **K55.06 Acute infarction of intestine, part unspecified**
New Acute intestinal infarction
New Gangrene of intestine
New Necrosis of intestine
New **K55.061 Focal (segmental) acute infarction of intestine, part unspecified**
New **K55.062 Diffuse acute infarction of intestine, part unspecified**
New **K55.069 Acute infarction of intestine, part and extent unspecified**

New **K55.3 Necrotizing enterocolitis**
New **Excludes1** necrotizing enterocolitis of newborn (P77.-)
New **Excludes2** necrotizing enterocolitis due to Clostridium difficile (A04.7)

New **K55.30 Necrotizing enterocolitis, unspecified**
New Necrotizing enterocolitis, NOS
New **K55.31 Stage 1 necrotizing enterocolitis**
New Necrotizing enterocolitis without pneumatosis, without perforation
New **K55.32 Stage 2 necrotizing enterocolitis**
New Necrotizing enterocolitis with pneumatosis, without perforation
New **K55.33 Stage 3 necrotizing enterocolitis**
New Necrotizing enterocolitis with perforation
New Necrotizing enterocolitis with pneumatosis and perforation

New **K58.1 Irritable bowel syndrome with constipation**
New **K58.2 Mixed irritable bowel syndrome**
New **K58.8 Other irritable bowel syndrome**

K59.0 Constipation
New Use additional code for adverse effect, if applicable, to identify drug (T36-T50 with fifth or sixth character 5)

New **K59.03 Drug induced constipation**
New Use additional code for adverse effect, if applicable, to identify drug (T36-T50 with fifth or sixth character 5)
New **K59.04 Chronic idiopathic constipation**
New Functional constipation
New **K59.09 Other constipation**
New Chronic constipation

K59.3 Megacolon, not elsewhere classified
Deleted Toxic colon

New **K59.31 Toxic megacolon**
New **K59.39 Other megacolon**
New Megacolon NOS

K72 Hepatic failure, not elsewhere classified

Deleted **Includes** acute hepatitis NEC, with hepatic failure

Deleted **Excludes1** viral hepatitis with hepatic coma (B15-B19)

New **Excludes2** viral hepatitis with hepatic coma (B15-B19)

K72.0 Acute and subacute hepatic failure

New Acute non-viral hepatitis NOS

K75.0 Abscess of liver

New **Excludes2** acute or subacute hepatitis NOS (B17.9)

New acute or subacute non-viral hepatitis (K72.0)

New chronic hepatitis NEC (K73.8)

K76.7 Hepatorenal syndrome

Revised **Excludes1** postprocedural hepatorenal syndrome (K91.83)

K85 Acute pancreatitis

Deleted **Includes** abscess of pancreas

Deleted acute necrosis of pancreas

Deleted gangrene of (gangrenous) pancreas

Deleted hemorrhagic pancreatitis

Deleted infective necrosis of pancreas

Deleted suppurative pancreatitis

New **K85.00 Idiopathic acute pancreatitis without necrosis or infection**

New **K85.01 Idiopathic acute pancreatitis with uninfected necrosis**

New **K85.02 Idiopathic acute pancreatitis with infected necrosis**

New **K85.10 Biliary acute pancreatitis without necrosis or infection**

New **K85.11 Biliary acute pancreatitis with uninfected necrosis**

New **K85.12 Biliary acute pancreatitis with infected necrosis**

New **K85.20 Alcohol induced acute pancreatitis without necrosis or infection**

New **K85.21 Alcohol induced acute pancreatitis with uninfected necrosis**

New **K85.22 Alcohol induced acute pancreatitis with infected necrosis**

New **K85.30 Drug induced acute pancreatitis without necrosis or infection**

New **K85.31 Drug induced acute pancreatitis with uninfected necrosis**

New **K85.32 Drug induced acute pancreatitis with infected necrosis**

New **K85.80 Other acute pancreatitis without necrosis or infection**

New **K85.81 Other acute pancreatitis with uninfected necrosis**

New **K85.82 Other acute pancreatitis with infected necrosis**

New **K85.90 Acute pancreatitis without necrosis or infection, unspecified**

New **K85.91 Acute pancreatitis with uninfected necrosis, unspecified**

New **K85.92 Acute pancreatitis with infected necrosis, unspecified**

K86.0 Alcohol-induced chronic pancreatitis

New Code also exocrine pancreatic insufficiency (K86.81)

Revised **Excludes2** alcohol induced acute pancreatitis (K85.2-)

K86.1 Other chronic pancreatitis

New Code also exocrine pancreatic insufficiency (K86.81)

K86.8 Other specified diseases of pancreas

Deleted Aseptic pancreatic necrosis

Deleted Atrophy of pancreas

Deleted Calculus of pancreas

Deleted Cirrhosis of pancreas

Deleted Fibrosis of pancreas

Deleted Pancreatic fat necrosis

Deleted Pancreatic infantilism

Deleted Pancreatic necrosis NOS

New **K86.81 Exocrine pancreatic insufficiency**

New **K86.89 Other specified diseases of pancreas**

New Aseptic pancreatic necrosis, unrelated to acute pancreatitis

New Atrophy of pancreas

New Calculus of pancreas

New Cirrhosis of pancreas

New Fibrosis of pancreas

New Pancreatic fat necrosis, unrelated to acute pancreatitis

New Pancreatic infantilism

New Pancreatic necrosis NOS, unrelated to acute pancreatitis

K90.0 Celiac disease

New Celiac disease with steatorrhea

Deleted Idiopathic steatorrhea

New Code also exocrine pancreatic insufficiency (K86.81)

K90.4 Other malabsorption due to intolerance

Deleted Malabsorption due to intolerance to carbohydrate

Deleted Malabsorption due to intolerance to fat

Deleted Malabsorption due to intolerance to protein

Deleted Malabsorption due to intolerance to starch

New **K90.41 Non-celiac gluten sensitivity**

New Gluten sensitivity NOS

New Non-celiac gluten sensitive enteropathy

New **K90.49 Malabsorption due to intolerance, not elsewhere classified**

New Malabsorption due to intolerance to carbohydrate

New Malabsorption due to intolerance to fat

New Malabsorption due to intolerance to protein

New Malabsorption due to intolerance to starch

Revised **K91.61 Intraoperative hemorrhage and hematoma of a digestive system organ or structure complicating a digestive system procedure**

Revised **K91.84 Postprocedural hemorrhage of a digestive system organ or structure following a procedure**

Revised **K91.840 Postprocedural hemorrhage of a digestive system organ or structure following a digestive system procedure**

Revised **K91.841 Postprocedural hemorrhage of a digestive system organ or structure following other procedure**

New **K91.87 Postprocedural hematoma and seroma of a digestive system organ or structure following a procedure**

New **K91.870 Postprocedural hematoma of a digestive system organ or structure following a digestive system procedure**

New **K91.871 Postprocedural hematoma of a digestive system organ or structure following other procedure**

New **K91.872 Postprocedural seroma of a digestive system organ or structure following a digestive system procedure**

New **K91.873 Postprocedural seroma of a digestive system organ or structure following other procedure**

CHAPTER 12

DISEASES OF THE SKIN AND SUBCUTANEOUS TISSUE (L00-L99)

L02.2 Cutaneous abscess, furuncle and carbuncle of trunk

Revised **Excludes2** abscess of breast (N61.1)

L03.211 Cellulitis of face

New **Excludes2** abscess of orbit (H05.01-)

Revised cellulitis of orbit (H05.01-)

New **L03.213 Periorbital cellulitis**

New Preseptal cellulitis

L03.31 Cellulitis of trunk

Revised **Excludes2** cellulitis of breast NOS (N61.0)

L05.01 Pilonidal cyst with abscess

Deleted Parasacral dimple with abscess

New **Excludes2** congenital sacral dimple (Q82.6)

New parasacral dimple (Q82.6)

L05.91 Pilonidal cyst without abscess

Deleted Parasacral dimple

New **Excludes2** congenital sacral dimple (Q82.6)

New parasacral dimple (Q82.6)

DERMATITIS AND ECZEMA (L20-L30)

Revised **Excludes2** stasis dermatitis (I87.2)

L30 Other and unspecified dermatitis

Revised **Excludes2** stasis dermatitis (I87.2)

L50.2 Urticaria due to cold and heat

New **Excludes2** familial cold urticaria (M04.2)

L70 Acne

Revised **L70.5 Acné excoriée**

New Acné excoriée des jeunes filles

Revised **L76.2 Postprocedural hemorrhage of skin and subcutaneous tissue following a procedure**

Revised **L76.21 Postprocedural hemorrhage of skin and subcutaneous tissue following a dermatologic procedure**

Revised **L76.22 Postprocedural hemorrhage of skin and subcutaneous tissue following other procedure**

New **L76.3 Postprocedural hematoma and seroma of skin and subcutaneous tissue following a procedure**

New **L76.31 Postprocedural hematoma of skin and subcutaneous tissue following a dermatologic procedure**

New **L76.32 Postprocedural hematoma of skin and subcutaneous tissue following other procedure**

New **L76.33 Postprocedural seroma of skin and subcutaneous tissue following a dermatologic procedure**

New **L76.34 Postprocedural seroma of skin and subcutaneous tissue following other procedure**

L82 Seborrheic keratosis

New **Includes** basal cell papilloma

L89.521 Pressure ulcer of left ankle, stage 1

Revised Pressure pre-ulcer skin changes limited to persistent focal edema, left ankle

L98.1 Factitial dermatitis

New **Excludes1** Excoriation (skin-picking) disorder (F42.4)

New **L98.7 Excessive and redundant skin and subcutaneous tissue**

New Loose or sagging skin following bariatric surgery weight loss

New Loose or sagging skin following dietary weight loss

New Loose or sagging skin, NOS

New **Excludes2** acquired excess or redundant skin of eyelid (H02.3-)

New congenital excess or redundant skin of eyelid (Q10.3)

New skin changes due to chronic exposure to nonionizing radiation (L57.-)

CHAPTER 13

DISEASES OF THE MUSCULOSKELETAL SYSTEM AND CONNECTIVE TISSUE (M00-M99)

This chapter contains the following blocks:

New	M04	Autoinflammatory syndromes
New	M97	Periprosthetic fracture around internal prosthetic joint

New ### AUTOINFLAMMATORY SYNDROMES (M04)

New **M04 Autoinflammatory syndromes**

New **Excludes2** Crohn's disease (K50.-)

New **M04.1 Periodic fever syndromes**

New Familial Mediterranean fever

New Hyperimmunoglobin D syndrome

New Mevalonate kinase deficiency

New Tumor necrosis factor receptor associated periodic syndrome [TRAPS]

New **M04.2 Cryopyrin-associated periodic syndromes**

New Chronic infantile neurological, cutaneous and articular syndrome [CINCA]

New Familial cold autoinflammatory syndrome

New Familial cold urticaria

New Muckle-Wells syndrome

New Neonatal onset multisystemic inflammatory disorder [NOMID]

New **M04.8 Other autoinflammatory syndromes**
New Blau syndrome
New Deficiency of interleukin 1 receptor antagonist [DIRA]
New Majeed syndrome
New Periodic fever, aphthous stomatitis, pharyngitis, and adenopathy syndrome [PFAPA]
New Pyogenic arthritis, pyoderma gangrenosum, and acne syndrome [PAPA]
New **M04.9 Autoinflammatory syndrome, unspecified**

M1A Chronic gout
Deleted **Excludes1** acute gout (M10.-)
New **Excludes2** acute gout (M10.-)

M10 Gout
Deleted Gout NOS
Deleted **Excludes1** chronic gout (M1A.-)
New **Excludes2** chronic gout (M1A.-)

M20.1 Hallux valgus (acquired)
Deleted Bunion
New **Excludes2** bunion (M21.6-)

M21.1 Varus deformity, not elsewhere classified
Revised **Excludes1** metatarsus varus (Q66.22)
M21.6 Other acquired deformities of foot
Revised **Excludes2** deformities of toe (acquired) (M20.1-M20.6-)
New **M21.61 Bunion**
New **M21.611 Bunion of right foot**
New **M21.612 Bunion of left foot**
New **M21.619 Bunion of unspecified foot**
New **M21.62 Bunionette**
New **M21.621 Bunionette of right foot**
New **M21.622 Bunionette of left foot**
New **M21.629 Bunionette of unspecified foot**

New **M25.5 Pain in joint**
New **M25.54 Pain in joints of hand**
New **M25.541 Pain in joints of right hand**
New **M25.542 Pain in joints of left hand**
New **M25.549 Pain in joints of unspecified hand**
New Pain in joints of hand NOS

New **M26.601 Right temporomandibular joint disorder, unspecified**
New **M26.602 Left temporomandibular joint disorder, unspecified**
New **M26.603 Bilateral temporomandibular joint disorder, unspecified**
New **M26.609 Unspecified temporomandibular joint disorder, unspecified side**
New Temporomandibular joint disorder NOS

New **M26.611 Adhesions and ankylosis of right temporomandibular joint**
New **M26.612 Adhesions and ankylosis of left temporomandibular joint**
New **M26.613 Adhesions and ankylosis of bilateral temporomandibular joint**
New **M26.619 Adhesions and ankylosis of temporomandibular joint, unspecified side**

New **M26.621 Arthralgia of right temporomandibular joint**
New **M26.622 Arthralgia of left temporomandibular joint**
New **M26.623 Arthralgia of bilateral temporomandibular joint**
New **M26.629 Arthralgia of temporomandibular joint, unspecified side**

New **M26.631 Articular disc disorder of right temporomandibular joint**
New **M26.632 Articular disc disorder of left temporomandibular joint**
New **M26.633 Articular disc disorder of bilateral temporomandibular joint**
New **M26.639 Articular disc disorder of temporomandibular joint, unspecified side**

M48.5 Collapsed vertebra, not elsewhere classified
New Compression fracture of vertebra NOS

M50.02 Cervical disc disorder with myelopathy, mid-cervical region
Deleted C4-C5 disc disorder with myelopathy
Deleted C5-C6 disc disorder with myelopathy
Deleted C6-C7 disc disorder with myelopathy
M50.020 Cervical disc disorder with myelopathy, mid-cervical region, unspecified level
M50.021 Cervical disc disorder at C4-C5 level with myelopathy
C4-C5 disc disorder with myelopathy
M50.022 Cervical disc disorder at C5-C6 level with myelopathy
C5-C6 disc disorder with myelopathy
M50.023 Cervical disc disorder at C6-C7 level with myelopathy
C6-C7 disc disorder with myelopathy

M50.12 Cervical disc disorder with radiculopathy, mid-cervical region
Deleted C4-C5 disc disorder with radiculopathy
Deleted C5 radiculopathy due to disc disorder
Deleted C5-C6 disc disorder with radiculopathy
Deleted C6 radiculopathy due to disc disorder
Deleted C6-C7 disc disorder with radiculopathy
Deleted C7 radiculopathy due to disc disorder
New **M50.120 Mid-cervical disc disorder, unspecified**
New **M50.121 Cervical disc disorder at C4-C5 level with radiculopathy**
New C4-C5 disc disorder with radiculopathy
New C5 radiculopathy due to disc disorder
New **M50.122 Cervical disc disorder at C5-C6 level with radiculopathy**
New C5-C6 disc disorder with radiculopathy
New C6 radiculopathy due to disc disorder
New **M50.123 Cervical disc disorder at C6-C7 level with radiculopathy**
New C6-C7 disc disorder with radiculopathy
New C7 radiculopathy due to disc disorder

M50.22 Other cervical disc displacement, mid-cervical region
Deleted Other C4-C5 cervical disc displacement
Deleted Other C5-C6 cervical disc displacement
Deleted Other C6-C7 cervical disc displacement
New **M50.220 Other cervical disc displacement, mid-cervical region, unspecified level**
New **M50.221 Other cervical disc displacement at C4-C5 level**
New Other C4-C5 cervical disc displacement
New **M50.222 Other cervical disc displacement at C5-C6 level**
New Other C5-C6 cervical disc displacement
New **M50.223 Other cervical disc displacement at C6-C7 level**
New Other C6-C7 cervical disc displacement

M50.32 Other cervical disc degeneration, mid-cervical region
Deleted Other C4-C5 cervical disc displacement
Deleted Other C5-C6 cervical disc displacement
Deleted Other C6-C7 cervical disc displacement
New **M50.320 Other cervical disc degeneration, mid-cervical region, unspecified level**
New **M50.321 Other cervical disc degeneration at C4-C5 level**
New Other C4-C5 cervical disc degeneration
New **M50.322 Other cervical disc degeneration at C5-C6 level**
New Other C5-C6 cervical disc degeneration
New **M50.323 Other cervical disc degeneration at C6-C7 level**
New Other C6-C7 cervical disc degeneration

M50.82 Other cervical disc disorders, mid-cervical region
Deleted Other C4-C5 cervical disc disorders
Deleted Other C5-C6 cervical disc disorders
Deleted Other C6-C7 cervical disc disorders
New **M50.820 Other cervical disc disorders, mid-cervical region, unspecified level**
New **M50.821 Other cervical disc disorders at C4-C5 level**
New Other C4-C5 cervical disc disorders
New **M50.822 Other cervical disc disorders at C5-C6 level**
New Other C5-C6 cervical disc disorders
New **M50.823 Other cervical disc disorders at C6-C7 level**
New Other C6-C7 cervical disc disorders

M50.92 Cervical disc disorder, unspecified, mid-cervical region
Deleted C4-C5 cervical disc disorder, unspecified
Deleted C5-C6 cervical disc disorder, unspecified
Deleted C6-C7 cervical disc disorder, unspecified
New **M50.920 Unspecified cervical disc disorder, mid-cervical region, unspecified level**
New **M50.921 Unspecified cervical disc disorder at C4-C5 level**
New Unspecified C4-C5 cervical disc disorder
New **M50.922 Unspecified cervical disc disorder at C5-C6 level**
New Unspecified C5-C6 cervical disc disorder
New **M50.923 Unspecified cervical disc disorder at C6-C7 level**
New Unspecified C6-C7 cervical disc disorder

M62.5 Muscle wasting and atrophy, not elsewhere classified
New **Excludes1** sarcopenia (M62.84)

M62.81 Muscle weakness (generalized)
New **Excludes1** muscle weakness in sarcopenia (M62.84)

New **M62.84 Sarcopenia**
New Age-related sarcopenia
New *Code first underlying disease, if applicable, such as:*
New disorders of myoneural junction and muscle disease in diseases classified elsewhere (G73.-)
New other and unspecified myopathies (G72.-)
New primary disorders of muscles (G71.-)

M71.5 Other bursitis, not elsewhere classified
Revised **Excludes2** bursitis of shoulder (M75.5)
bursitis of tibial collateral [Pellegrini-Stieda] (M76.4-)

New **M84.7 Nontraumatic fracture, not elsewhere classified**
New **M84.75 Atypical femoral fracture**
New The appropriate 7th character is to be added to each code from M84.75:

A	initial encounter for fracture
D	subsequent encounter for fracture with routine healing
G	subsequent encounter for fracture with delayed healing
K	subsequent encounter for fracture with nonunion
P	subsequent encounter for fracture with malunion
S	sequela

New **M84.750 Atypical femoral fracture, unspecified**
New **M84.751 Incomplete atypical femoral fracture, right leg**
New **M84.752 Incomplete atypical femoral fracture, left leg**
New **M84.753 Incomplete atypical femoral fracture, unspecified leg**
New **M84.754 Complete transverse atypical femoral fracture, right leg**
New **M84.755 Complete transverse atypical femoral fracture, left leg**
New **M84.756 Complete transverse atypical femoral fracture, unspecified leg**
New **M84.757 Complete oblique atypical femoral fracture, right leg**
New **M84.758 Complete oblique atypical femoral fracture, left leg**
New **M84.759 Complete oblique atypical femoral fracture, unspecified leg**

M90 Osteopathies in diseases classified elsewhere
Revised **Excludes1** diabetes mellitus (E08-E13 with .69-)

M96 Intraoperative and postprocedural complications and disorders of musculoskeletal system, not elsewhere classified

New **Excludes2** periprosthetic fracture around internal prosthetic joint (M97.-)

Revised **M96.83 Postprocedural hemorrhage of a musculoskeletal structure following a procedure**

Revised **M96.830 Postprocedural hemorrhage of a musculoskeletal structure following a musculoskeletal system procedure**

Revised **M96.831 Postprocedural hemorrhage of a musculoskeletal structure following other procedure**

New **M96.84 Postprocedural hematoma and seroma of a musculoskeletal structure following a procedure**

New **M96.840 Postprocedural hematoma of a musculoskeletal structure following a musculoskeletal system procedure**

New **M96.841 Postprocedural hematoma of a musculoskeletal structure following other procedure**

New **M96.842 Postprocedural seroma of a musculoskeletal structure following a musculoskeletal system procedure**

New **M96.843 Postprocedural seroma of a musculoskeletal structure following other procedure**

New **PERIPROSTHETIC FRACTURE AROUND INTERNAL PROSTHETIC JOINT (M97)**

New **M97 Periprosthetic fracture around internal prosthetic joint**

New **Excludes2** fracture of bone following insertion of orthopedic implant, joint prosthesis or bone plate (M96.6-)

New breakage (fracture) of prosthetic joint (T84.01-)

New The appropriate 7th character is to be added to each code from category M97:

New A	initial encounter
New D	subsequent encounter
New S	sequela

New **M97.0 Periprosthetic fracture around internal prosthetic hip joint**

New **M97.01 Periprosthetic fracture around internal prosthetic right hip joint**

New **M97.02 Periprosthetic fracture around internal prosthetic left hip joint**

New **M97.1 Periprosthetic fracture around internal prosthetic knee joint**

New **M97.11 Periprosthetic fracture around internal prosthetic right knee joint**

New **M97.12 Periprosthetic fracture around internal prosthetic left knee joint**

New **M97.2 Periprosthetic fracture around internal prosthetic ankle joint**

New **M97.21 Periprosthetic fracture around internal prosthetic right ankle joint**

New **M97.22 Periprosthetic fracture around internal prosthetic left ankle joint**

New **M97.3 Periprosthetic fracture around internal prosthetic shoulder joint**

New **M97.31 Periprosthetic fracture around internal prosthetic right shoulder joint**

New **M97.32 Periprosthetic fracture around internal prosthetic left shoulder joint**

New **M97.4 Periprosthetic fracture around internal prosthetic elbow joint**

New **M97.41 Periprosthetic fracture around internal prosthetic right elbow joint**

New **M97.42 Periprosthetic fracture around internal prosthetic left elbow joint**

New **M97.8 Periprosthetic fracture around other internal prosthetic joint**

New Periprosthetic fracture around internal prosthetic finger joint

New Periprosthetic fracture around internal prosthetic spinal joint

New Periprosthetic fracture around internal prosthetic toe joint

New Periprosthetic fracture around internal prosthetic wrist joint

New Use additional code to identify the joint (Z96.6-)

New **M97.9 Periprosthetic fracture around unspecified internal prosthetic joint**

CHAPTER 14

DISEASES OF THE GENITOURINARY SYSTEM (N00-N99)

Revised **N10 Acute pyelonephritis**

Revised Acute tubulo-interstitial nephritis

New **N13.0 Hydronephrosis with ureteropelvic junction obstruction**

New Hydronephrosis due to acquired occlusion of ureteropelvic junction

New **Excludes2** Hydronephrosis with ureteropelvic junction obstruction due to calculus (N13.2)

Revised **N13.6 Pyonephrosis**

Conditions in N13.0-N13.5 with infection

N36.0 Urethral fistula

New **Excludes1** urethroscrotal fistula (N50.89)

N36.8 Other specified disorders of urethra

New **Excludes1** congenital urethrocele (Q64.7)

New female urethrocele (N81.0)

N39.42 Incontinence without sensory awareness

New Insensible (urinary) incontinence

N39.49 Other specified urinary incontinence

New **N39.491 Coital incontinence**

New **N39.492 Postural (urinary) incontinence**

N40 Benign prostatic hyperplasia

Deleted **Includes** benign prostatic hyperplasia

New enlarged prostate

Revised **N40.0 Benign prostatic hyperplasia without lower urinary tract symptoms**

Revised **N40.1 Benign prostatic hyperplasia with lower urinary tract symptoms**

N42.3 Dysplasia of prostate

Deleted Prostatic intraepithelial neoplasia I (PIN I)

Deleted Prostatic intraepithelial neoplasia II (PIN II)

Deleted **Excludes1** prostatic intraepithelial neoplasia III (PIN III) (D07.5)

New **N42.30 Unspecified dysplasia of prostate**

New **N42.31 Prostatic intraepithelial neoplasia**

New PIN

New Prostatic intraepithelial neoplasia I (PIN I)

New Prostatic intraepithelial neoplasia II (PIN II)

New **Excludes1** prostatic intraepithelial neoplasia III (PIN III) (D07.5)

New **N42.32 Atypical small acinar proliferation of prostate**

New **N42.39 Other dysplasia of prostate**

N50.8 Other specified disorders of male genital organs
Deleted Atrophy of scrotum, seminal vesicle, spermatic cord, tunica vaginalis and vas deferens
Deleted Edema of scrotum, seminal vesicle, spermatic cord, testis, tunica vaginalis and vas deferens
Deleted Hypertrophy of scrotum, seminal vesicle, spermatic cord, testis, tunica vaginalis and vas deferens
Deleted Ulcer of scrotum, seminal vesicle, spermatic cord, testis, tunica vaginalis and vas deferens
Deleted Chylocele, tunica vaginalis (nonfilarial) NOS
Deleted Urethroscrotal fistula
Deleted Stricture of spermatic cord, tunica vaginalis, and vas deferens

New **N50.81 Testicular pain**
New **N50.811 Right testicular pain**
New **N50.812 Left testicular pain**
New **N50.819 Testicular pain, unspecified**
New **N50.82 Scrotal pain**
New **N50.89 Other specified disorders of the male genital organs**
New Atrophy of scrotum, seminal vesicle, spermatic cord, tunica vaginalis and vas deferens
New Chylocele, tunica vaginalis (nonfilarial) NOS
New Edema of scrotum, seminal vesicle, spermatic cord, tunica vaginalis and vas deferens
New Hypertrophy of scrotum, seminal vesicle, spermatic cord, tunica vaginalis and vas deferens
New Stricture of spermatic cord, tunica vaginalis, and vas deferens
New Ulcer of scrotum, seminal vesicle, spermatic cord, testis, tunica vaginalis and vas deferens
New Urethroscrotal fistula

Revised **N52.3 Postprocedural erectile dysfunction**
New **N52.35 Erectile dysfunction following radiation therapy**
New **N52.36 Erectile dysfunction following interstitial seed therapy**
New **N52.37 Erectile dysfunction following prostate ablative therapy**
New Erectile dysfunction following cryotherapy
New Erectile dysfunction following other prostate ablative therapies
New Erectile dysfunction following ultrasound ablative therapies
Revised **N52.39 Other and unspecified postprocedural erectile dysfunction**

N61 Inflammatory disorders of breast
Deleted Abscess (acute) (chronic) (nonpuerperal) of areola
Deleted Abscess (acute) (chronic) (nonpuerperal) of breast
Deleted Carbuncle of breast
Deleted Infective mastitis (acute) (subacute) (nonpuerperal)
Deleted Mastitis (acute) (subacute) (nonpuerperal) NOS
New **N61.0 Mastitis without abscess**
New Infective mastitis (acute) (nonpuerperal) (subacute)
New Mastitis (acute) (nonpuerperal) (subacute) NOS
New Cellulitis (acute) (nonpuerperal) (subacute) of breast NOS
New Cellulitis (acute) (nonpuerperal) (subacute) of nipple NOS

New **N61.1 Abscess of the breast and nipple**
New Abscess (acute) (chronic) (nonpuerperal) of areola
New Abscess (acute) (chronic) (nonpuerperal) of breast
New Carbuncle of breast
New Mastitis with abscess

N64.1 Fat necrosis of breast
Revised *Code first breast necrosis due to breast graft (T85.898)*

N81 Female genital prolapse
Revised **Excludes1** prolapse and hernia of ovary and fallopian tube (N83.4-)

New **N83.00 Follicular cyst of ovary, unspecified side**
New **N83.01 Follicular cyst of right ovary**
New **N83.02 Follicular cyst of left ovary**
New **N83.10 Corpus luteum cyst of ovary, unspecified side**
New **N83.11 Corpus luteum cyst of right ovary**
New **N83.12 Corpus luteum cyst of left ovary**
N83.20 Unspecified ovarian cysts
New **N83.201 Unspecified ovarian cyst, right side**
New **N83.202 Unspecified ovarian cyst, left side**
New **N83.209 Unspecified ovarian cyst, unspecified side**
New Ovarian cyst, NOS
New **N83.291 Other ovarian cyst, right side**
New **N83.292 Other ovarian cyst, left side**
New **N83.299 Other ovarian cyst, unspecified side**
New **N83.311 Acquired atrophy of right ovary**
New **N83.312 Acquired atrophy of left ovary**
New **N83.319 Acquired atrophy of ovary, unspecified side**
New Acquired atrophy of ovary, NOS
New **N83.321 Acquired atrophy of right fallopian tube**
New **N83.322 Acquired atrophy of left fallopian tube**
New **N83.329 Acquired atrophy of fallopian tube, unspecified side**
New Acquired atrophy of fallopian tube, NOS
New **N83.331 Acquired atrophy of right ovary and fallopian tube**
New **N83.332 Acquired atrophy of left ovary and fallopian tube**
New **N83.339 Acquired atrophy of ovary and fallopian tube, unspecified side**
New Acquired atrophy of ovary and fallopian tube, NOS
New **N83.40 Prolapse and hernia of ovary and fallopian tube, unspecified side**
New Prolapse and hernia of ovary and fallopian tube, NOS

New **N83.41 Prolapse and hernia of right ovary and fallopian tube**

New **N83.42 Prolapse and hernia of left ovary and fallopian tube**

New **N83.511 Torsion of right ovary and ovarian pedicle**

New **N83.512 Torsion of left ovary and ovarian pedicle**

New **N83.519 Torsion of ovary and ovarian pedicle, unspecified side**

New Torsion of ovary and ovarian pedicle, NOS

New **N83.521 Torsion of right fallopian tube**

New **N83.522 Torsion of left fallopian tube**

New **N83.529 Torsion of fallopian tube, unspecified side**

New Torsion of fallopian tube, NOS

N83.6 Hematosalpinx

Revised **Excludes1** tubal pregnancy (O00.1-)

N90.6 Hypertrophy of vulva

Deleted Hypertrophy of labia

New **N90.60 Unspecified hypertrophy of vulva**

New Unspecified hypertrophy of labia

New **N90.61 Childhood asymmetric labium majus enlargement**

New CALME

New **N90.69 Other specified hypertrophy of vulva**

New Other specified hypertrophy of labia

New **N93.1 Pre-pubertal vaginal bleeding**

New **N94.10 Unspecified dyspareunia**

New **N94.11 Superficial (introital) dyspareunia**

New **N94.12 Deep dyspareunia**

New **N94.19 Other specified dyspareunia**

N94.3 Premenstrual tension syndrome

New **Excludes1** Premenstrual dysphoric disorder (F32.81)

Revised **N99.113 Postprocedural anterior bulbous urethral stricture**

New **N99.115 Postprocedural fossa navicularis urethral stricture**

N99.5 Complications of stoma of urinary tract

Revised **Excludes2** mechanical complication of urinary catheter (T83.0-)

Revised **N99.52 Complication of incontinent external stoma of urinary tract**

Revised **N99.520 Hemorrhage of incontinent external stoma of urinary tract**

Revised **N99.521 Infection of incontinent external stoma of urinary tract**

Revised **N99.522 Malfunction of incontinent external stoma of urinary tract**

New **N99.523 Herniation of incontinent stoma of urinary tract**

New **N99.524 Stenosis of incontinent stoma of urinary tract**

Revised **N99.528 Other complication of incontinent external stoma of urinary tract**

Revised **N99.53 Complication of continent stoma of urinary tract**

Revised **N99.530 Hemorrhage of continent stoma of urinary tract**

Revised **N99.531 Infection of continent stoma of urinary tract**

Revised **N99.532 Malfunction of continent stoma of urinary tract**

New **N99.533 Herniation of continent stoma of urinary tract**

New **N99.534 Stenosis of continent stoma of urinary tract**

Revised **N99.538 Other complication of continent stoma of urinary tract**

Revised **N99.82 Postprocedural hemorrhage of a genitourinary system organ or structure following a procedure**

Revised **N99.820 Postprocedural hemorrhage of a genitourinary system organ or structure following a genitourinary system procedure**

Revised **N99.821 Postprocedural hemorrhage of a genitourinary system organ or structure following other procedure**

New **N99.84 Postprocedural hematoma and seroma of a genitourinary system organ or structure following a procedure**

New **N99.840 Postprocedural hematoma of a genitourinary system organ or structure following a genitourinary system procedure**

New **N99.841 Postprocedural hematoma of a genitourinary system organ or structure following other procedure**

New **N99.842 Postprocedural seroma of a genitourinary system organ or structure following a genitourinary system procedure**

New **N99.843 Postprocedural seroma of a genitourinary system organ or structure following other procedure**

CHAPTER 15

PREGNANCY, CHILDBIRTH AND THE PUERPERIUM (O00-O9A)

Revised Use additional code from category Z3A, Weeks of gestation, to identify the specific week of the pregnancy, if known.

O00.0 Abdominal pregnancy

New **O00.00 Abdominal pregnancy without intrauterine pregnancy**

New Abdominal pregnancy NOS

New **O00.01 Abdominal pregnancy with intrauterine pregnancy**

O00.1 Tubal pregnancy

New **O00.10 Tubal pregnancy without intrauterine pregnancy**

New Tubal pregnancy NOS

New **O00.11 Tubal pregnancy with intrauterine pregnancy**

O00.2 Ovarian pregnancy

New O00.20 Ovarian pregnancy without intrauterine pregnancy

New Ovarian pregnancy NOS

New O00.21 Ovarian pregnancy with intrauterine pregnancy

New O00.8 Other ectopic pregnancy

New O00.80 Other ectopic pregnancy without intrauterine pregnancy

New Other ectopic pregnancy NOS

New O00.81 Other ectopic pregnancy with intrauterine pregnancy

New O00.9 Ectopic pregnancy, unspecified

New O00.90 Unspecified ectopic pregnancy without intrauterine pregnancy

New Ectopic pregnancy NOS

New O00.91 Unspecified ectopic pregnancy with intrauterine pregnancy

Revised O09.1 Supervision of pregnancy with history of ectopic pregnancy

Revised O09.10 Supervision of pregnancy with history of ectopic pregnancy, unspecified trimester

Revised O09.11 Supervision of pregnancy with history of ectopic pregnancy, first trimester

Revised O09.12 Supervision of pregnancy with history of ectopic pregnancy, second trimester

Revised O09.13 Supervision of pregnancy with history of ectopic pregnancy, third trimester

New O09.A Supervision of pregnancy with history of molar pregnancy

New O09.A0 Supervision of pregnancy with history of molar pregnancy, unspecified trimester

New O09.A1 Supervision of pregnancy with history of molar pregnancy, first trimester

New O09.A2 Supervision of pregnancy with history of molar pregnancy, second trimester

New O09.A3 Supervision of pregnancy with history of molar pregnancy, third trimester

O09.81 Supervision of pregnancy resulting from assisted reproductive technology

New **Excludes2** gestational carrier status (Z33.3)

New O11.4 Pre-existing hypertension with pre-eclampsia, complicating childbirth

New O11.5 Pre-existing hypertension with pre-eclampsia, complicating the puerperium

New O12.04 Gestational edema, complicating childbirth

New O12.05 Gestational edema, complicating the puerperium

New O12.14 Gestational proteinuria, complicating childbirth

New O12.15 Gestational proteinuria, complicating the puerperium

New O12.24 Gestational edema with proteinuria, complicating childbirth

New O12.25 Gestational edema with proteinuria, complicating the puerperium

O13 Gestational [pregnancy-induced] hypertension without significant proteinuria

New **Includes** transient hypertension of pregnancy

New O13.4 Gestational [pregnancy-induced] hypertension without significant proteinuria, complicating childbirth

New O13.5 Gestational [pregnancy-induced] hypertension without significant proteinuria, complicating the puerperium

New O14.04 Mild to moderate pre-eclampsia, complicating childbirth

New O14.05 Mild to moderate pre-eclampsia, complicating the puerperium

New O14.14 Severe pre-eclampsia complicating childbirth

New O14.15 Severe pre-eclampsia, complicating the puerperium

New O14.24 HELLP syndrome, complicating childbirth

New O14.25 HELLP syndrome, complicating the puerperium

New O14.94 Unspecified pre-eclampsia, complicating childbirth

New O14.95 Unspecified pre-eclampsia, complicating the puerperium

Revised O15.0 Eclampsia complicating pregnancy

Revised O15.00 Eclampsia complicating pregnancy, unspecified trimester

Revised O15.02 Eclampsia complicating pregnancy, second trimester

Revised O15.03 Eclampsia complicating pregnancy, third trimester

Revised O15.1 Eclampsia complicating labor

Revised O15.2 Eclampsia complicating the puerperium

New O16.4 Unspecified maternal hypertension, complicating childbirth

New O16.5 Unspecified maternal hypertension, complicating the puerperium

Revised O24.0 Pre-existing type 1 diabetes mellitus, in pregnancy, childbirth and the puerperium

Revised O24.01 Pre-existing type 1 diabetes mellitus, in pregnancy

Revised O24.011 Pre-existing type 1 diabetes mellitus, in pregnancy, first trimester

Revised O24.012 Pre-existing type 1 diabetes mellitus, in pregnancy, second trimester

Revised O24.013 Pre-existing type 1 diabetes mellitus, in pregnancy, third trimester

Revised O24.019 Pre-existing type 1 diabetes mellitus, in pregnancy, unspecified trimester

Revised O24.02 Pre-existing type 1 diabetes mellitus, in childbirth

Revised O24.03 Pre-existing type 1 diabetes mellitus, in the puerperium

Revised O24.1 Pre-existing type 2 diabetes mellitus, in pregnancy, childbirth and the puerperium

Revised **O24.11 Pre-existing type 2 diabetes mellitus, in pregnancy**

Revised **O24.111 Pre-existing type 2 diabetes mellitus, in pregnancy, first trimester**

Revised **O24.112 Pre-existing type 2 diabetes mellitus, in pregnancy, second trimester**

Revised **O24.113 Pre-existing type 2 diabetes mellitus, in pregnancy, third trimester**

Revised **O24.119 Pre-existing type 2 diabetes mellitus, in pregnancy, unspecified trimester**

Revised **O24.12 Pre-existing type 2 diabetes mellitus, in childbirth**

Revised **O24.13 Pre-existing type 2 diabetes mellitus, in the puerperium**

New **O24.415 Gestational diabetes mellitus in pregnancy, controlled by oral hypoglycemic drugs**

New Gestational diabetes mellitus in pregnancy, controlled by oral antidiabetic drugs

New **O24.425 Gestational diabetes mellitus in childbirth, controlled by oral hypoglycemic drugs**

New Gestational diabetes mellitus in childbirth, controlled by oral antidiabetic drugs

New **O24.435 Gestational diabetes mellitus in puerperium, controlled by oral hypoglycemic drugs**

New Gestational diabetes mellitus in puerperium, controlled by oral antidiabetic drugs

O33.7 Maternal care for disproportion due to other fetal deformities

New One of the following 7th characters is to be assigned to code O33.7. 7th character 0 is for single gestations and multiple gestations where the fetus is unspecified. 7th characters 1 through 9 are for cases of multiple gestations to identify the fetus for which the code applies. The appropriate code from category O30, Multiple gestation, must also be assigned when assigning code O33.7 with a 7th character of 1 through 9.

New	0	not applicable or unspecified
New	1	fetus 1
New	2	fetus 2
New	3	fetus 3
New	4	fetus 4
New	5	fetus 5
New	9	other fetus

O34.0 Maternal care for congenital malformation of uterus

New Maternal care for double uterus

New Maternal care for uterus bicornis

New **O34.211 Maternal care for low transverse scar from previous cesarean delivery**

New **O34.212 Maternal care for vertical scar from previous cesarean delivery**

New Maternal care for classical scar from previous cesarean delivery

New **O34.219 Maternal care for unspecified type scar from previous cesarean delivery**

New **O34.29 Maternal care due to uterine scar from other previous surgery**

New Maternal care due to uterine scar from other transmural uterine incision

O42.02 Full-term premature rupture of membranes, onset of labor within 24 hours of rupture

Revised Premature rupture of membranes at or after 37 completed weeks of gestation, onset of labor within 24 hours of rupture

O42.12 Full-term premature rupture of membranes, onset of labor more than 24 hours following rupture

Revised Premature rupture of membranes at or after 37 completed weeks of gestation, onset of labor more than 24 hours following rupture

O42.92 Full-term premature rupture of membranes, unspecified as to length of time between rupture and onset of labor

Revised Premature rupture of membranes at or after 37 completed weeks of gestation, unspecified as to length of time between rupture and onset of labor

Revised **O44.0 Complete placenta previa NOS or without hemorrhage**

Deleted Low implantation of placenta specified as without hemorrhage

New Placenta previa NOS

Revised **O44.00 Complete placenta previa NOS or without hemorrhage, unspecified trimester**

Revised **O44.01 Complete placenta previa NOS or without hemorrhage, first trimester**

Revised **O44.02 Complete placenta previa NOS or without hemorrhage, second trimester**

Revised **O44.03 Complete placenta previa NOS or without hemorrhage, third trimester**

Revised **O44.1 Complete placenta previa with hemorrhage**

Deleted Complete placenta previa with hemorrhage

Deleted Low implantation of placenta, NOS or with hemorrhage

Deleted Marginal placenta previa, NOS or with hemorrhage

Deleted Partial placenta previa, NOS or with hemorrhage

Deleted Total placenta previa, NOS or with hemorrhage

Revised **O44.10 Complete placenta previa with hemorrhage, unspecified trimester**

Revised **O44.11 Complete placenta previa with hemorrhage, first trimester**

Revised **O44.12 Complete placenta previa with hemorrhage, second trimester**

Revised **O44.13 Complete placenta previa with hemorrhage, third trimester**

New **O44.2 Partial placenta previa without hemorrhage**
Marginal placenta previa, NOS or without hemorrhage

New **O44.20 Partial placenta previa NOS or without hemorrhage, unspecified trimester**

New **O44.21 Partial placenta previa NOS or without hemorrhage, first trimester**

New **O44.22 Partial placenta previa NOS or without hemorrhage, second trimester**

New **O44.23 Partial placenta previa NOS or without hemorrhage, third trimester**

New **O44.3 Partial placenta previa with hemorrhage**
New Marginal placenta previa with hemorrhage

New **O44.30 Partial placenta previa with hemorrhage, unspecified trimester**

New **O44.31 Partial placenta previa with hemorrhage, first trimester**

New **O44.32 Partial placenta previa with hemorrhage, second trimester**

New **O44.33 Partial placenta previa with hemorrhage, third trimester**

New **O44.4 Low lying placenta NOS or without hemorrhage**
New Low implantation of placenta NOS or without hemorrhage

New **O44.40 Low lying placenta NOS or without hemorrhage, unspecified trimester**

New **O44.41 Low lying placenta NOS or without hemorrhage, first trimester**

New **O44.42 Low lying placenta NOS or without hemorrhage, second trimester**

New **O44.43 Low lying placenta NOS or without hemorrhage, third trimester**

New **O44.5 Low lying placenta with hemorrhage**
New Low implantation of placenta with hemorrhage

New **O44.50 Low lying placenta with hemorrhage, unspecified trimester**

New **O44.51 Low lying placenta with hemorrhage, first trimester**

New **O44.52 Low lying placenta with hemorrhage, second trimester**

New **O44.53 Low lying placenta with hemorrhage, third trimester**

New **O70.20 Third degree perineal laceration during delivery, unspecified**

New **O70.21 Third degree perineal laceration during delivery, IIIa**
New Third degree perineal laceration during delivery with less than 50% of external anal sphincter (EAS) thickness torn

New **O70.22 Third degree perineal laceration during delivery, IIIb**
New Third degree perineal laceration during delivery with more than 50% external anal sphincter (EAS) thickness torn

New **O70.23 Third degree perineal laceration during delivery, IIIc**
New Third degree perineal laceration during delivery with both external anal sphincter (EAS) and internal anal sphincter (IAS) torn

Revised **O99.33 Tobacco use disorder complicating pregnancy, childbirth, and the puerperium**
New Smoking complicating pregnancy, childbirth, and the puerperium
New Use additional code from category F17 to identify type of tobacco nicotine dependence

O99.6 Diseases of the digestive system complicating pregnancy, childbirth and the puerperium
New **Excludes2** hemorrhoids in pregnancy (O22.4-)

O99.82 Streptococcus B carrier state complicating pregnancy, childbirth and the puerperium
New **Excludes1** Carrier of streptococcus group B (GBS) in a nonpregnant woman (Z22.330)

CHAPTER 16

CERTAIN CONDITIONS ORIGINATING IN THE PERINATAL PERIOD (P00-P96)

NEWBORN AFFECTED BY MATERNAL FACTORS AND BY COMPLICATIONS OF PREGNANCY, LABOR, AND DELIVERY (P00–P04)

Revised **Note:** These codes are for use when the listed maternal conditions are specified as the cause of confirmed morbidity or potential morbidity which have their origin in the perinatal period (before birth through the first 28 days after birth).

Revised **P00 Newborn affected by maternal conditions that may be unrelated to present pregnancy**
New **Excludes2** encounter for observation of newborn for suspected diseases and conditions ruled out (Z05.-)
New newborn affected by maternal complications of pregnancy (P01.-)

Revised **P00.0 Newborn affected by maternal hypertensive disorders**
Revised Newborn affected by maternal conditions classifiable to O10-O11, O13-O16

Revised **P00.1 Newborn affected by maternal renal and urinary tract diseases**
Revised Newborn affected by maternal conditions classifiable to N00-N39

Revised **P00.2 Newborn affected by maternal infectious and parasitic diseases**
Revised Newborn affected by maternal infectious disease classifiable to A00-B99, J09 and J10

Revised **P00.3 Newborn affected by other maternal circulatory and respiratory diseases**
Revised Newborn affected by maternal conditions classifiable to I00-I99, J00-J99, Q20-Q34 and not included in P00.0, P00.2

Revised **P00.4 Newborn affected by maternal nutritional disorders**
Revised Newborn affected by maternal disorders classifiable to E40-E64

Revised **P00.5 Newborn affected by maternal injury**
Revised Newborn affected by maternal conditions classifiable to O9A.2-

Revised **P00.6 Newborn affected by surgical procedure on mother**
Revised Newborn affected by amniocentesis

Revised **P00.7 Newborn affected by other medical procedures on mother, not elsewhere classified**
Revised Newborn affected by radiation to mother

Revised **P00.8 Newborn affected by other maternal conditions**
Revised **P00.81 Newborn affected by periodontal disease in mother**

Revised **P00.89 Newborn affected by other maternal conditions**
Revised Newborn affected by conditions classifiable to T80-T88
Revised Newborn affected by maternal genital tract or other localized infections
Revised Newborn affected by maternal systemic lupus erythematosus

Revised **P00.9 Newborn affected by unspecified maternal condition**

Revised **P01 Newborn affected by maternal complications of pregnancy**

New **Excludes2** encounter for observation of newborn for suspected diseases and conditions ruled out (Z05.-)

Revised **P01.0 Newborn affected by incompetent cervix**

Revised **P01.1 Newborn affected by premature rupture of membranes**

Revised **P01.2 Newborn affected by oligohydramnios**

Revised **P01.3 Newborn affected by polyhydramnios**

Revised Newborn affected by hydramnios

Revised **P01.4 Newborn affected by ectopic pregnancy**

Revised Newborn affected by abdominal pregnancy

Revised **P01.5 Newborn affected by multiple pregnancy**

Revised Newborn affected by triplet (pregnancy)

Revised Newborn affected by twin (pregnancy)

Revised **P01.6 Newborn affected by maternal death**

Revised **P01.7 Newborn affected by malpresentation before labor**

Revised Newborn affected by breech presentation before labor

Revised Newborn affected by external version before labor

Revised Newborn affected by face presentation before labor

Revised Newborn affected by transverse lie before labor

Revised Newborn affected by unstable lie before labor

Revised **P01.8 Newborn affected by other maternal complications of pregnancy**

Revised **P01.9 Newborn affected by maternal complication of pregnancy, unspecified**

Revised **P02 Newborn affected by complications of placenta, cord and membranes**

New **Excludes2** encounter for observation of newborn for suspected diseases and conditions ruled out (Z05.-)

Revised **P02.0 Newborn affected by placenta previa**

Revised **P02.1 Newborn affected by other forms of placental separation and hemorrhage**

Revised Newborn affected by abruptio placenta

Revised Newborn affected by accidental hemorrhage

Revised Newborn affected by antepartum hemorrhage

Revised Newborn affected by damage to placenta from amniocentesis, cesarean delivery or surgical induction

Revised Newborn affected by maternal blood loss

Revised Newborn affected by premature separation of placenta

Revised **P02.2 Newborn affected by other and unspecified morphological and functional abnormalities of placenta**

Revised **P02.20 Newborn affected by unspecified morphological and functional abnormalities of placenta**

Revised **P02.29 Newborn affected by other morphological and functional abnormalities of placenta**

Revised Newborn affected by placental dysfunction

Revised Newborn affected by placental infarction

Revised Newborn affected by placental insufficiency

Revised **P02.3 Newborn affected by placental transfusion syndromes**

Revised Newborn affected by placental and cord abnormalities resulting in twin-to-twin or other transplacental transfusion

Revised **P02.4 Newborn affected by prolapsed cord**

Revised **P02.5 Newborn affected by other compression of umbilical cord**

Revised Newborn affected by umbilical cord (tightly) around neck

Revised Newborn affected by entanglement of umbilical cord

Revised Newborn affected by knot in umbilical cord

Revised **P02.6 Newborn affected by other and unspecified conditions of umbilical cord**

Revised **P02.60 Newborn affected by unspecified conditions of umbilical cord**

Revised **P02.69 Newborn affected by other conditions of umbilical cord**

Revised Newborn affected by short umbilical cord

Revised Newborn affected by vasa previa

Revised **P02.7 Newborn affected by chorioamnionitis**

Revised Newborn affected by amnionitis

Revised Newborn affected by membranitis

Revised Newborn affected by placentitis

Revised **P02.8 Newborn affected by other abnormalities of membranes**

Revised **P02.9 Newborn affected by abnormality of membranes, unspecified**

Revised **P03 Newborn affected by other complications of labor and delivery**

New **Excludes2** encounter for observation of newborn for suspected diseases and conditions ruled out (Z05.-)

Revised **P03.0 Newborn affected by breech delivery and extraction**

Revised **P03.1 Newborn affected by other malpresentation, malposition and disproportion during labor and delivery**

Revised Newborn affected by contracted pelvis

Revised Newborn affected by conditions classifiable to O64-O66

Revised Newborn affected by persistent occipitoposterior

Revised Newborn affected by transverse lie

Revised **P03.2 Newborn affected by forceps delivery**

Revised **P03.3 Newborn affected by delivery by vacuum extractor [ventouse]**

Revised **P03.4 Newborn affected by Cesarean delivery**

Revised **P03.5 Newborn affected by precipitate delivery**

Revised Newborn affected by rapid second stage

Revised **P03.6 Newborn affected by abnormal uterine contractions**

Revised Newborn affected by conditions classifiable to O62.-, except O62.3

Revised Newborn affected by hypertonic labor

Revised Newborn affected by uterine inertia

Revised **P03.8 Newborn affected by other specified complications of labor and delivery**

Revised **P03.81 Newborn affected by abnormality in fetal (intrauterine) heart rate or rhythm**

Revised **P03.810 Newborn affected by abnormality in fetal (intrauterine) heart rate or rhythm before the onset of labor**

Revised **P03.811 Newborn affected by abnormality in fetal (intrauterine) heart rate or rhythm during labor**

Revised **P03.819 Newborn affected by abnormality in fetal (intrauterine) heart rate or rhythm, unspecified as to time of onset**

Revised **P03.89 Newborn affected by other specified complications of labor and delivery**
Revised Newborn affected by abnormality of maternal soft tissues
Revised Newborn affected by conditions classifiable to O60-O75 and by procedures used in labor and delivery not included in P02.- and P03.0-P03.6
Revised Newborn affected by induction of labor
Revised **P03.9 Newborn affected by complication of labor and delivery, unspecified**

Revised **P04 Newborn affected by noxious substances transmitted via placenta or breast milk**
New **Excludes2** congenital malformations (Q00-Q99)
encounter for observation of newborn for suspected diseases and conditions ruled out (Z05.-)

Revised **P04.0 Newborn affected by maternal anesthesia and analgesia in pregnancy, labor and delivery**
Newborn affected by reactions and intoxications from maternal opiates and tranquilizers administered during labor and delivery

Revised **P04.1 Newborn affected by other maternal medication**
Revised Newborn affected by cancer chemotherapy
Revised Newborn affected by cytotoxic drugs

Revised **P04.2 Newborn affected by maternal use of tobacco**
Newborn affected by exposure in utero to tobacco smoke

Revised **P04.3 Newborn affected by maternal use of alcohol**

Revised **P04.4 Newborn affected by maternal use of drugs of addiction**
Revised **P04.41 Newborn affected by maternal use of cocaine**
Revised **P04.49 Newborn affected by maternal use of other drugs of addiction**
Revised **Excludes2** newborn affected by maternal anesthesia and analgesia (P04.0)

Revised **P04.5 Newborn affected by maternal use of nutritional chemical substances**

Revised **P04.6 Newborn affected by maternal exposure to environmental chemical substances**

Revised **P04.8 Newborn affected by other maternal noxious substances**

Revised **P04.9 Newborn affected by maternal noxious substance, unspecified**

P05.0 Newborn light for gestational age
New Weight below but length above 10th percentile for gestational age

New **P05.09 Newborn light for gestational age, 2500 grams and over**
New Newborn light for gestational age, other

P05.1 Newborn small for gestational age
New Weight and length below 10th percentile for gestational age

New **P05.19 Newborn small for gestational age, other**
New Newborn small for gestational age, 2500 grams and over

P07 Disorders of newborn related to short gestation and low birth weight, not elsewhere classified
Deleted **Excludes1** low birth weight due to slow fetal growth and fetal malnutrition (P05.-)

P07.0 Extremely low birth weight newborn
New **Excludes1** low birth weight due to slow fetal growth and fetal malnutrition (P05.-)

P07.1 Other low birth weight newborn
New **Excludes1** low birth weight due to slow fetal growth and fetal malnutrition (P05.-)

P96.5 Complication to newborn due to (fetal) intrauterine procedure
Revised **Excludes2** newborn affected by amniocentesis (P00.6)

CHAPTER 17

CONGENITAL MALFORMATIONS, DEFORMATIONS AND CHROMOSOMAL ABNORMALITIES (Q00-Q99)

Q25.1 Coarctation of aorta
New Stenosis of aorta

Q25.2 Atresia of aorta
New **Q25.21 Interruption of aortic arch**
New Atresia of aortic arch
New **Q25.29 Other atresia of aorta**
New Atresia of aorta

Q25.4 Other congenital malformations of aorta
Deleted Absence of aorta
Deleted Aneurysm of sinus of Valsalva (ruptured)
Deleted Aplasia of aorta
Deleted Congenital aneurysm of aorta
Deleted Congenital malformations of aorta
Deleted Congenital dilatation of aorta
Deleted Double aortic arch [vascular ring of aorta]
Deleted Hypoplasia of aorta
Deleted Persistent convolutions of aortic arch
Deleted Persistent right aortic arch
New **Q25.40 Congenital malformation of aorta unspecified**
New **Q25.41 Absence and aplasia of aorta**
New **Q25.42 Hypoplasia of aorta**
New **Q25.43 Congenital aneurysm of aorta**
Congenital aneurysm of aortic root
Congenital aneurysm of aortic sinus
New **Q25.44 Congenital dilation of aorta**
New **Q25.45 Double aortic arch**
Vascular ring of aorta
New **Q25.46 Tortuous aortic arch**
Persistent convolutions of aortic arch
New **Q25.47 Right aortic arch**
Persistent right aortic arch
New **Q25.48 Anomalous origin of subclavian artery**
New **Q25.49 Other congenital malformations of aorta**

Q52.12 Longitudinal vaginal septum
Deleted Longitudinal vaginal septum with or without obstruction
New **Q52.120 Longitudinal vaginal septum, nonobstructing**
New **Q52.121 Longitudinal vaginal septum, obstructing, right side**

New **Q52.122 Longitudinal vaginal septum, obstructing, left side**

New **Q52.123 Longitudinal vaginal septum, microperforate, right side**

New **Q52.124 Longitudinal vaginal septum, microperforate, left side**

New **Q52.129 Other and unspecified longitudinal vaginal septum**

New **Q66.21 Congenital metatarsus primus varus**

New **Q66.22 Congenital metatarsus adductus**
Congenital metatarsus varus

New **Q82.6 Congenital sacral dimple**
New Parasacral dimple
New **Excludes2** pilonidal cyst with abscess (L05.01)
New pilonidal cyst without abscess (L05.91)

New **Q87.82 Arterial tortuosity syndrome**

CHAPTER 18

SYMPTOMS, SIGNS AND ABNORMAL CLINICAL AND LABORATORY FINDINGS, NOT ELSEWHERE CLASSIFIED (R00-R99)

R00 Abnormalities of heart beat

Deleted **Excludes1** specified arrhythmias (I47-I49)
New **Excludes2** specified arrhythmias (I47-I49)

R01.1 Cardiac murmur, unspecified
New Systolic murmur NOS

SYMPTOMS AND SIGNS INVOLVING THE DIGESTIVE SYSTEM AND ABDOMEN (R10-R19)

Deleted **Excludes1** congenital or infantile pylorospasm (Q40.0)
Deleted gastrointestinal hemorrhage (K92.0-K92.2)
Deleted intestinal obstruction (K56.-)
Deleted newborn gastrointestinal hemorrhage (P54.0-P54.3)
Deleted newborn intestinal obstruction (P76.-)
Deleted pylorospasm (K31.3)
Deleted signs and symptoms involving the urinary system (R30-R39)
Deleted symptoms referable to female genital organs (N94.-)
Deleted symptoms referable to male genital organs (N48-N50)

New **Excludes2** congenital or infantile pylorospasm (Q40.0)
New gastrointestinal hemorrhage (K92.0-K92.2)
New intestinal obstruction (K56.-)
New newborn gastrointestinal hemorrhage (P54.0-P54.3)
New newborn intestinal obstruction (P76.-)
New pylorospasm (K31.3)
New signs and symptoms involving the urinary system (R30-R39)
New symptoms referable to female genital organs (N94.-)
New symptoms referable to male genital organs (N48-N50)

R11 Nausea and vomiting

Revised **Excludes1** psychogenic vomiting (F50.89)

New **R29.7 National Institutes of Health Stroke Scale (NIHSS) score**
New *Code first the type of cerebral infarction (I63-)*
New **R29.70 NIHSS score 0-9**
New **R29.700 NIHSS score 0**
New **R29.701 NIHSS score 1**
New **R29.702 NIHSS score 2**
New **R29.703 NIHSS score 3**
New **R29.704 NIHSS score 4**
New **R29.705 NIHSS score 5**
New **R29.706 NIHSS score 6**
New **R29.707 NIHSS score 7**
New **R29.708 NIHSS score 8**
New **R29.709 NIHSS score 9**
New **R29.71 NIHSS score 10-19**
New **R29.710 NIHSS score 10**
New **R29.711 NIHSS score 11**
New **R29.712 NIHSS score 12**
New **R29.713 NIHSS score 13**
New **R29.714 NIHSS score 14**
New **R29.715 NIHSS score 15**
New **R29.716 NIHSS score 16**
New **R29.717 NIHSS score 17**
New **R29.718 NIHSS score 18**
New **R29.719 NIHSS score 19**
New **R29.72 NIHSS score 20-29**
New **R29.720 NIHSS score 20**
New **R29.721 NIHSS score 21**
New **R29.722 NIHSS score 22**
New **R29.723 NIHSS score 23**
New **R29.724 NIHSS score 24**
New **R29.725 NIHSS score 25**
New **R29.726 NIHSS score 26**
New **R29.727 NIHSS score 27**
New **R29.728 NIHSS score 28**
New **R29.729 NIHSS score 29**
New **R29.73 NIHSS score 30-39**
New **R29.730 NIHSS score 30**
New **R29.731 NIHSS score 31**
New **R29.732 NIHSS score 32**
New **R29.733 NIHSS score 33**
New **R29.734 NIHSS score 34**
New **R29.735 NIHSS score 35**
New **R29.736 NIHSS score 36**
New **R29.737 NIHSS score 37**
New **R29.738 NIHSS score 38**
New **R29.739 NIHSS score 39**
New **R29.74 NIHSS score 40-42**
New **R29.740 NIHSS score 40**
New **R29.741 NIHSS score 41**
New **R29.742 NIHSS score 42**

New **R31.21 Asymptomatic microscopic hematuria**
New AMH
New **R31.29 Other microscopic hematuria**

R39.19 Other difficulties with micturition
New **R39.191 Need to immediately re-void**
New **R39.192 Position dependent micturition**
New **R39.198 Other difficulties with micturition**

New **R39.82 Chronic bladder pain**

SYMPTOMS AND SIGNS INVOLVING COGNITION, PERCEPTION, EMOTIONAL STATE AND BEHAVIOR (R40-R46)

Deleted **Excludes1** symptoms and signs constituting part of a pattern of mental disorder (F01-F99)

New **Excludes2** symptoms and signs constituting part of a pattern of mental disorder (F01-F99)

R40.2 Coma

Revised **Note:** One code from each subcategory R40.21-R40-23 is required to complete the coma scale

R40.24 Glasgow coma scale, total score

Deleted Use codes R40.21- through R40.23- only when the individual score(s) are documented

New Note: Assign a code from subcategory R40.24, when only the total coma score is documented

New The following appropriate 7th character is to be added to subcategory R40.24-:

New 0	unspecified time
New 1	in the field [EMT or ambulance]
New 2	at arrival to emergency department
New 3	at hospital admission
New 4	24 hours or more after hospital admission

R41.84 Other specified cognitive deficit

New **Excludes1** cognitive deficits as sequelae of cerebrovascular disease (I69.01-, I69.11-, I69.21-, I69.31-, I69.81-, I69.91-)

R46.81 Obsessive-compulsive behavior

Revised **Excludes1** obsessive-compulsive disorder (F42-)

R50.82 Postprocedural fever

Revised **Excludes1** postprocedural infection (T81.4-)

R53.1 Weakness

New **Excludes1** sarcopenia (M62.84)

R54 Age-related physical debility

New **Excludes1** sarcopenia (M62.84)

R63.0 Anorexia

Revised **Excludes1** loss of appetite of nonorganic origin (F50.89)

R65.2 Severe sepsis

Revised *Code first underlying infection, such as:* infection following a procedure (T81.4-)

R68.84 Jaw pain

Revised **Excludes1** temporomandibular joint arthralgia (M26.62-)

ABNORMAL FINDINGS ON EXAMINATION OF BLOOD, WITHOUT DIAGNOSIS (R70-R79)

Deleted **Excludes1** abnormalities (of)(on):

Deleted abnormal findings on antenatal screening of mother (O28.-)

Deleted coagulation hemorrhagic disorders (D65-D68)

Deleted lipids (E78.-)

Deleted platelets and thrombocytes (D69.-)

Deleted white blood cells classified elsewhere (D70-D72)

Deleted diagnostic abnormal findings classified elsewhere - see Alphabetical Index

Deleted hemorrhagic and hematological disorders of newborn (P50-P61)

New **Excludes2** abnormal findings on antenatal screening of mother (O28.-)

New abnormalities of lipids (E78.-)

New abnormalities of platelets and thrombocytes (D69.-)

New abnormalities of white blood cells classified elsewhere (D70-D72)

New coagulation hemorrhagic disorders (D65-D68)

New diagnostic abnormal findings classified elsewhere —*see* Alphabetical Index

New hemorrhagic and hematological disorders of newborn (P50-P61)

R73.03 Prediabetes

New Latent diabetes

R73.09 Other abnormal glucose

New Latent diabetes

Deleted Prediabetes

R78.81 Bacteremia

Revised **Excludes1** sepsis-code to specified infection

R82.7 Abnormal findings on microbiological examination of urine

Deleted Positive culture findings of urine

New **R82.71 Bacteriuria**

New **R82.79 Other abnormal findings on microbiological examination of urine**

New Positive culture findings of urine

R93.4 Abnormal findings on diagnostic imaging of urinary organs

Deleted Filling defect of bladder found on diagnostic imaging

Deleted Filling defect of kidney found on diagnostic imaging

Deleted Filling defect of ureter found on diagnostic imaging

Deleted **Excludes1** hypertrophy of kidney (N28.81)

New **Excludes2** hypertrophy of kidney (N28.81)

New **R93.41 Abnormal radiologic findings on diagnostic imaging of renal pelvis, ureter, or bladder**

New Filling defect of bladder found on diagnostic imaging

New Filling defect of renal pelvis found on diagnostic imaging

New Filling defect of ureter found on diagnostic imaging

New R93.42 Abnormal radiologic findings on diagnostic imaging of kidney

New R93.421 Abnormal radiologic findings on diagnostic imaging of right kidney

New R93.422 Abnormal radiologic findings on diagnostic imaging of left kidney

New R93.429 Abnormal radiologic findings on diagnostic imaging of unspecified kidney

New R93.49 Abnormal radiologic findings on diagnostic imaging of other urinary organs

New R97.20 Elevated prostate specific antigen [PSA]

New R97.21 Rising PSA following treatment for malignant neoplasm of prostate

CHAPTER 19

INJURY, POISONING AND CERTAIN OTHER CONSEQUENCES OF EXTERNAL CAUSES (S00-T88)

S00.8 Superficial injury of other parts of head

New Superficial injuries of face [any part]

New S02.101 Fracture of base of skull, right side

New S02.102 Fracture of base of skull, left side

New S02.109 Fracture of base of skull, unspecified side

Revised S02.110 Type I occipital condyle fracture, unspecified side

Revised S02.111 Type II occipital condyle fracture, unspecified side

Revised S02.112 Type III occipital condyle fracture, unspecified side

Revised S02.118 Other fracture of occiput, unspecified side

New S02.11A Type I occipital condyle fracture, right side

New S02.11B Type I occipital condyle fracture, left side

New S02.11C Type II occipital condyle fracture, right side

New S02.11D Type II occipital condyle fracture, left side

New S02.11E Type III occipital condyle fracture, right side

New S02.11F Type III occipital condyle fracture, left side

New S02.11G Other fracture of occiput, right side

New S02.11H Other fracture of occiput, left side

New S02.30 Fracture of orbital floor, unspecified side

New S02.31 Fracture of orbital floor, right side

New S02.32 Fracture of orbital floor, left side

Revised S02.400 Malar fracture, unspecified side

Revised S02.401 Maxillary fracture, unspecified side

Revised S02.402 Zygomatic fracture, unspecified side

New S02.40A Malar fracture, right side

New S02.40B Malar fracture, left side

New S02.40C Maxillary fracture, right side

New S02.40D Maxillary fracture, left side

New S02.40E Zygomatic fracture, right side

New S02.40F Zygomatic fracture, left side

Revised S02.600 Fracture of unspecified part of body of mandible, unspecified side

New S02.601 Fracture of unspecified part of body of right mandible

New S02.602 Fracture of unspecified part of body of left mandible

New S02.610 Fracture of condylar process of mandible, unspecified side

New S02.611 Fracture of condylar process of right mandible

New S02.612 Fracture of condylar process of left mandible

New S02.620 Fracture of subcondylar process of mandible, unspecified side

New S02.621 Fracture of subcondylar process of right mandible

New S02.622 Fracture of subcondylar process of left mandible

New S02.630 Fracture of coronoid process of mandible, unspecified side

New S02.631 Fracture of coronoid process of right mandible

New S02.632 Fracture of coronoid process of left mandible

New S02.640 Fracture of ramus of mandible, unspecified side

New S02.641 Fracture of ramus of right mandible

New S02.642 Fracture of ramus of left mandible

New S02.650 Fracture of angle of mandible, unspecified side

New S02.651 Fracture of angle of right mandible

New S02.652 Fracture of angle of left mandible

New S02.670 Fracture of alveolus of mandible, unspecified side

New S02.671 Fracture of alveolus of right mandible

New S02.672 Fracture of alveolus of left mandible

New S02.80 Fracture of other specified skull and facial bones, unspecified side

New S02.81 Fracture of other specified skull and facial bones, right side

New S02.82 Fracture of other specified skull and facial bones, left side

New S03.00 Dislocation of jaw, unspecified side

New S03.01 Dislocation of jaw, right side

New S03.02 Dislocation of jaw, left side

New S03.03 Dislocation of jaw, bilateral side

New **S03.40 Sprain of jaw, unspecified side**
New **S03.41 Sprain of jaw, right side**
New **S03.42 Sprain of jaw, left side**
New **S03.43 Sprain of jaw, bilateral side**

S06.0 Concussion

Revised **Excludes1** concussion with other intracranial injuries classified in subcategories S06.1- to S06.6- , S06.81- and S06.82- code to specified intracranial injury

Deleted ~~S06.0X2 Concussion with loss of consciousness of 31 minutes to 59 minutes~~

Deleted ~~S06.0X3 Concussion with loss of consciousness of 1 hour to 5 hours 59 minutes~~

Deleted ~~S06.0X4 Concussion with loss of consciousness of 6 hours to 24 hours~~

Deleted ~~S06.0X5 Concussion with loss of consciousness greater than 24 hours with return to pre-existing conscious level~~

Deleted ~~S06.0X6 Concussion with loss of consciousness greater than 24 hours without return to pre-existing conscious level with patient surviving~~

Deleted ~~S06.0X7 Concussion with loss of consciousness of any duration with death due to brain injury prior to regaining consciousness~~

Deleted ~~S06.0X8 Concussion with loss of consciousness of any duration with death due to other cause prior to regaining consciousness~~

S06.89 Other specified intracranial injury

New **Excludes1** concussion (S06.0X-)

S06.9 Unspecified intracranial injury

New Traumatic brain injury NOS

New **Excludes1** conditions classifiable to S06.0- to S06.8-code to specified intracranial injury

S34.101 Unspecified injury to L_1 level of lumbar spinal cord

New Unspecified injury to lumbar spinal cord level 1

S34.102 Unspecified injury to L_2 level of lumbar spinal cord

New Unspecified injury to lumbar spinal cord level 2

S34.103 Unspecified injury to L_3 level of lumbar spinal cord

New Unspecified injury to lumbar spinal cord level 3

S34.104 Unspecified injury to L_4 level of lumbar spinal cord

New Unspecified injury to lumbar spinal cord level 4

S34.105 Unspecified injury to L_5 level of lumbar spinal cord

New Unspecified injury to lumbar spinal cord level 5

S34.111 Complete lesion of L_1 level of lumbar spinal cord

New Complete lesion of lumbar spinal cord level 1

S34.112 Complete lesion of L_2 level of lumbar spinal cord

New Complete lesion of lumbar spinal cord level 2

S34.113 Complete lesion of L_3 level of lumbar spinal cord

New Complete lesion of lumbar spinal cord level 3

S34.114 Complete lesion of L_4 level of lumbar spinal cord

New Complete lesion of lumbar spinal cord level 4

S34.115 Complete lesion of L_5 level of lumbar spinal cord

New Complete lesion of lumbar spinal cord level 5

S34.121 Incomplete lesion of L_1 level of lumbar spinal cord

New Incomplete lesion of lumbar spinal cord level 1

S34.122 Incomplete lesion of L_2 level of lumbar spinal cord

New Incomplete lesion of lumbar spinal cord level 2

S34.123 Incomplete lesion of L_3 level of lumbar spinal cord

New Incomplete lesion of lumbar spinal cord level 3

S34.124 Incomplete lesion of L_4 level of lumbar spinal cord

New Incomplete lesion of lumbar spinal cord level 4

S34.125 Incomplete lesion of L_5 level of lumbar spinal cord

New Incomplete lesion of lumbar spinal cord level 5

Revised **S49.031 Salter-Harris Type III physeal fracture of upper end of humerus, right arm**

Revised **S49.032 Salter-Harris Type III physeal fracture of upper end of humerus, left arm**

Revised **S49.039 Salter-Harris Type III physeal fracture of upper end of humerus, unspecified arm**

Revised **S49.13 Salter-Harris Type III physeal fracture of lower end of humerus**

Revised **S49.131 Salter-Harris Type III physeal fracture of lower end of humerus, right arm**

Revised **S49.132 Salter-Harris Type III physeal fracture of lower end of humerus, left arm**

Revised **S49.139 Salter-Harris Type III physeal fracture of lower end of humerus, unspecified arm**

Revised **S54.8X Injury of other nerves at forearm level**

Revised **S54.8X1 Injury of other nerves at forearm level, right arm**

Revised **S54.8X2 Injury of other nerves at forearm level, left arm**

Revised **S54.8X9 Injury of other nerves at forearm level, unspecified arm**

S92.0 Fracture of calcaneus

New **Excludes2** Physeal fracture of calcaneus (S99.0-)

S92.3 Fracture of metatarsal bone(s)

New **Excludes2** Physeal fracture of metatarsal (S99.1-)

New **S92.4 Fracture of great toe**

Excludes2 Physeal fracture of phalanx of toe (S99.2-)

New **S92.5 Fracture of lesser toe(s)**

Excludes2 Physeal fracture of phalanx of toe (S99.2-)

New **S92.8 Other fracture of foot, except ankle**

New **S92.81 Other fracture of foot**

Sesamoid fracture of foot

New **S92.811 Other fracture of right foot**

New **S92.812 Other fracture of left foot**

New **S92.819 Other fracture of unspecified foot**

S99 Other and unspecified injuries of ankle and foot

Deleted The appropriate 7th character is to be added to each code from subcategories S99

Deleted A initial encounter
Deleted D subsequent encounter
Deleted S sequela

New **S99.0 Physeal fracture of calcaneus**

New The appropriate 7th character is to be added to each code from subcategories S99.0

New A initial encounter for closed fracture
New B initial encounter for open fracture
New D subsequent encounter for fracture with routine healing
New G subsequent encounter for fracture with delayed healing
New K subsequent encounter for fracture with nonunion
New P subsequent encounter for fracture with malunion
New S sequela

New **S99.00 Unspecified physeal fracture of calcaneus**

New **S99.001 Unspecified physeal fracture of right calcaneus**

New **S99.002 Unspecified physeal fracture of left calcaneus**

New **S99.009 Unspecified physeal fracture of unspecified calcaneus**

New **S99.01 Salter-Harris Type I physeal fracture of calcaneus**

New **S99.011 Salter-Harris Type I physeal fracture of right calcaneus**

New **S99.012 Salter-Harris Type I physeal fracture of left calcaneus**

New **S99.019 Salter-Harris Type I physeal fracture of unspecified calcaneus**

New **S99.02 Salter-Harris Type II physeal fracture of calcaneus**

New **S99.021 Salter-Harris Type II physeal fracture of right calcaneus**

New **S99.022 Salter-Harris Type II physeal fracture of left calcaneus**

New **S99.029 Salter-Harris Type II physeal fracture of unspecified calcaneus**

New **S99.03 Salter-Harris Type III physeal fracture of calcaneus**

New **S99.031 Salter-Harris Type III physeal fracture of right calcaneus**

New **S99.032 Salter-Harris Type III physeal fracture of left calcaneus**

New **S99.039 Salter-Harris Type III physeal fracture of unspecified calcaneus**

New **S99.04 Salter-Harris Type IV physeal fracture of calcaneus**

New **S99.041 Salter-Harris Type IV physeal fracture of right calcaneus**

New **S99.042 Salter-Harris Type IV physeal fracture of left calcaneus**

New **S99.049 Salter-Harris Type IV physeal fracture of unspecified calcaneus**

New **S99.09 Other physeal fracture of calcaneus**

New **S99.091 Other physeal fracture of right calcaneus**

New **S99.092 Other physeal fracture of left calcaneus**

New **S99.099 Other physeal fracture of unspecified calcaneus**

New **S99.1 Physeal fracture of metatarsal**

New The appropriate 7th character is to be added to each code from subcategories S99.1

New A initial encounter for closed fracture
New B initial encounter for open fracture
New D subsequent encounter for fracture with routine healing
New G subsequent encounter for fracture with delayed healing
New K subsequent encounter for fracture with nonunion
New P subsequent encounter for fracture with malunion
New S sequela

New **S99.10 Unspecified physeal fracture of metatarsal**

New **S99.101 Unspecified physeal fracture of right metatarsal**

New **S99.102 Unspecified physeal fracture of left metatarsal**

New **S99.109 Unspecified physeal fracture of unspecified metatarsal**

New **S99.11 Salter-Harris Type I physeal fracture of metatarsal**

New **S99.111 Salter-Harris Type I physeal fracture of right metatarsal**

New **S99.112 Salter-Harris Type I physeal fracture of left metatarsal**

New **S99.119 Salter-Harris Type I physeal fracture of unspecified metatarsal**

New **S99.12 Salter-Harris Type II physeal fracture of metatarsal**

New **S99.121 Salter-Harris Type II physeal fracture of right metatarsal**

New **S99.122 Salter-Harris Type II physeal fracture of left metatarsal**

New **S99.129 Salter-Harris Type II physeal fracture of unspecified metatarsal**

New **S99.13 Salter-Harris Type III physeal fracture of metatarsal**

New **S99.131 Salter-Harris Type III physeal fracture of right metatarsal**

New **S99.132 Salter-Harris Type III physeal fracture of left metatarsal**

New **S99.139 Salter-Harris Type III physeal fracture of unspecified metatarsal**

New **S99.14 Salter-Harris Type IV physeal fracture of metatarsal**

New **S99.141 Salter-Harris Type IV physeal fracture of right metatarsal**

New **S99.142 Salter-Harris Type IV physeal fracture of left metatarsal**

New **S99.149 Salter-Harris Type IV physeal fracture of unspecified metatarsal**

New **S99.19 Other physeal fracture of metatarsal**

New **S99.191 Other physeal fracture of right metatarsal**

New **S99.192 Other physeal fracture of left metatarsal**

New **S99.199 Other physeal fracture of unspecified metatarsal**

New **S99.2 Physeal fracture of phalanx of toe**

New The appropriate 7th character is to be added to each code from subcategories S99.2

New	A	initial encounter for closed fracture
New	B	initial encounter for open fracture
New	D	subsequent encounter for fracture with routine healing
New	G	subsequent encounter for fracture with delayed healing
New	K	subsequent encounter for fracture with nonunion
New	P	subsequent encounter for fracture with malunion
New	S	sequela

New **S99.20 Unspecified physeal fracture of phalanx of toe**

New **S99.201 Unspecified physeal fracture of phalanx of right toe**

New **S99.202 Unspecified physeal fracture of phalanx of right toe**

New **S99.209 Unspecified physeal fracture of phalanx of unspecified toe**

New **S99.21 Salter-Harris Type I physeal fracture of phalanx of toe**

New **S99.211 Salter-Harris Type I physeal fracture of phalanx of right toe**

New **S99.212 Salter-Harris Type I physeal fracture of phalanx of left toe**

New **S99.219 Salter-Harris Type I physeal fracture of phalanx of unspecified toe**

New **S99.22 Salter-Harris Type II physeal fracture of phalanx of toe**

New **S99.221 Salter-Harris Type II physeal fracture of phalanx of right toe**

New **S99.222 Salter-Harris Type II physeal fracture of phalanx of left toe**

New **S99.229 Salter-Harris Type II physeal fracture of phalanx of unspecified toe**

New **S99.23 Salter-Harris Type III physeal fracture of phalanx of toe**

New **S99.231 Salter-Harris Type III physeal fracture of phalanx of right toe**

New **S99.232 Salter-Harris Type III physeal fracture of phalanx of left toe**

New **S99.239 Salter-Harris Type III physeal fracture of phalanx of unspecified toe**

New **S99.24 Salter-Harris Type IV physeal fracture of phalanx of toe**

New **S99.241 Salter-Harris Type IV physeal fracture of phalanx of right toe**

New **S99.242 Salter-Harris Type IV physeal fracture of phalanx of left toe**

New **S99.249 Salter-Harris Type IV physeal fracture of phalanx of unspecified toe**

New **S99.29 Other physeal fracture of phalanx of toe**

New **S99.291 Other physeal fracture of phalanx of right toe**

New **S99.292 Other physeal fracture of phalanx of left toe**

New **S99.299 Other physeal fracture of phalanx of unspecified toe**

New **S99.8 Other specified injuries of ankle and foot**

New The appropriate 7th character is to be added to each code from subcategory S99.8

New	A	initial encounter
New	D	subsequent encounter
New	S	sequela

S99.9 Unspecified injury of ankle and foot

New The appropriate 7th character is to be added to each code from subcategory S99.9

New	A	initial encounter
New	D	subsequent encounter
New	S	sequela

T17.32 Food in larynx

Revised Bones in larynx

T61 Toxic effect of noxious substances eaten as seafood

Excludes1 allergic reaction to food, such as:

Deleted gastroenteritis (noninfective) (K52.2)

New food protein-induced enterocolitis syndrome (K52.21)

New food protein-induced enteropathy (K52.22)

New gastroenteritis (noninfective) (K52.29)

T62 Toxic effect of other noxious substances eaten as food

Excludes1 allergic reaction to food, such as:

Deleted gastroenteritis (noninfective) (K52.2)

New food protein-induced enterocolitis syndrome (K52.21)

New food protein-induced enteropathy (K52.22)

New gastroenteritis (noninfective) (K52.29)

T78.05 Anaphylactic reaction due to tree nuts and seeds

Deleted **Excludes1** anaphylactic reaction due to peanuts (T78.01)

New **Excludes2** anaphylactic reaction due to peanuts (T78.01)

T78.1 Other adverse food reactions, not elsewhere classified

Revised Use additional code to identify the type of reaction, if applicable

Revised **Excludes2** allergic and dietetic gastroenteritis and colitis (K52.29)

New food protein-induced enterocolitis syndrome (K52.21)

New food protein-induced enteropathy (K52.22)

T78.4 Other and unspecified allergy

Excludes1 specified types of allergic reaction such as:

Revised allergic diarrhea (K52.29)

Revised allergic gastroenteritis and colitis (K52.29)

New food protein-induced enterocolitis syndrome (K52.21)

New food protein-induced enteropathy (K52.22)

T80.1 Vascular complications following infusion, transfusion and therapeutic injection

Revised **Excludes2** vascular complications specified as due to prosthetic devices, implants and grafts (T82.8-, T83.8-, T84.8-, T85.8-)

T80.2 Infections following infusion, transfusion and therapeutic injection

Revised **Excludes2** postprocedural infections (T81.4-)

T80.21 Infection due to central venous catheter

New Infection due to pulmonary artery catheter (Swan-Ganz catheter)

T80.211 Bloodstream infection due to central venous catheter

New Bloodstream infection due to pulmonary artery catheter

T80.212 Local infection due to central venous catheter

New Local infection due to pulmonary artery catheter

T80.218 Other infection due to central venous catheter

New Other infection due to pulmonary artery catheter

T80.219 Unspecified infection due to central venous catheter

New Unspecified infection due to pulmonary artery catheter

T80.6 Other serum reactions

Revised **Excludes2** serum hepatitis (B16-B19)

T81.12 Postprocedural septic shock

Revised Postprocedural endotoxic shock resulting from a procedure, not elsewhere classified

Revised Postprocedural gram-negative shock resulting from a procedure, not elsewhere classified

T81.7 Vascular complications following a procedure, not elsewhere classified

Revised **Excludes2** embolism due to prosthetic devices, implants and grafts (T82.8-, T83.81, T84.8-, T85.1-)

Revised **T82.81 Embolism due to cardiac and vascular prosthetic devices, implants and grafts**

Revised **T82.817 Embolism due to cardiac prosthetic devices, implants and grafts**

Revised **T82.818 Embolism due to vascular prosthetic devices, implants and grafts**

Revised **T82.82 Fibrosis due to cardiac and vascular prosthetic devices, implants and grafts**

Revised **T82.827 Fibrosis due to cardiac prosthetic devices, implants and grafts**

Revised **T82.828 Fibrosis due to vascular prosthetic devices, implants and grafts**

Revised **T82.83 Hemorrhage due to cardiac and vascular prosthetic devices, implants and grafts**

Revised **T82.837 Hemorrhage due to cardiac prosthetic devices, implants and grafts**

Revised **T82.838 Hemorrhage due to vascular prosthetic devices, implants and grafts**

Revised **T82.84 Pain due to cardiac and vascular prosthetic devices, implants and grafts**

Revised **T82.847 Pain due to cardiac prosthetic devices, implants and grafts**

Revised **T82.848 Pain due to vascular prosthetic devices, implants and grafts**

Revised **T82.85 Stenosis due to cardiac and vascular prosthetic devices, implants and grafts**

New **T82.855 Stenosis of coronary artery stent**

New In-stent stenosis (restenosis) of coronary artery stent

New Restenosis of coronary artery stent

New **T82.856 Stenosis of peripheral vascular stent**

New In-stent stenosis (restenosis) of peripheral vascular stent

New Restenosis of peripheral vascular stent

Revised **T82.857 Stenosis of other cardiac prosthetic devices, implants and grafts**

Revised **T82.858 Stenosis of other vascular prosthetic devices, implants and grafts**

Revised **T82.86 Thrombosis of cardiac and vascular prosthetic devices, implants and grafts**

Revised **T82.867 Thrombosis due to cardiac prosthetic devices, implants and grafts**

Revised **T82.868 Thrombosis due to vascular prosthetic devices, implants and grafts**

Revised **T83.0 Mechanical complication of urinary catheter**

Revised **T83.01 Breakdown (mechanical) of urinary catheter**

New **T83.011 Breakdown (mechanical) of indwelling urethral catheter**

New **T83.012 Breakdown (mechanical) of nephrostomy catheter**

Revised **T83.018 Breakdown (mechanical) of other urinary catheter**

New Breakdown (mechanical) of Hopkins catheter

New Breakdown (mechanical) of ileostomy catheter

New Breakdown (mechanical) urostomy catheter

Revised **T83.02 Displacement of urinary catheter**
Revised Malposition of urinary catheter
New **T83.021 Displacement of indwelling urethral catheter**
New **T83.022 Displacement of nephrostomy catheter**
Revised **T83.028 Displacement of other urinary catheter**
New Displacement of Hopkins catheter
New Displacement of ileostomy catheter
New Displacement of urostomy catheter
Revised **T83.03 Leakage of urinary catheter**
New **T83.031 Leakage of indwelling urethral catheter**
New **T83.032 Leakage of nephrostomy catheter**
Revised **T83.038 Leakage of other urinary catheter**
New Leakage of Hopkins catheter
New Leakage of ileostomy catheter
New Leakage of urostomy catheter
Revised **T83.09 Other mechanical complication of urinary catheter**
Revised Obstruction (mechanical) of urinary catheter
Revised Perforation of urinary catheter
Revised Protrusion of urinary catheter
New **T83.091 Other mechanical complication of indwelling urethral catheter**
New **T83.092 Other mechanical complication of nephrostomy catheter**
Revised **T83.098 Other mechanical complication of other urinary catheter**
New Other mechanical complication of Hopkins catheter
New Other mechanical complication of ileostomy catheter
New Other mechanical complication of urostomy catheter

T83.110 Breakdown (mechanical) of urinary electronic stimulator device
New **Excludes2** Breakdown (mechanical) of electrode (lead) for sacral nerve neuro-stimulator (T85.111)
New Breakdown (mechanical) of implanted electronic sacral neuro-stimulator, pulse generator or receiver (T85.113)
Revised **T83.111 Breakdown (mechanical) of implanted urinary sphincter**
Revised **T83.112 Breakdown (mechanical) of indwelling ureteral stent**
New **T83.113 Breakdown (mechanical) of other urinary stents**
New Breakdown (mechanical) of ileal conduit stent
New Breakdown (mechanical) of nephroureteral stent

T83.120 Displacement of urinary electronic stimulator device
New **Excludes2** Displacement of electrode (lead) for sacral nerve neuro-stimulator (T85.121)
New Displacement of implanted electronic sacral neuro-stimulator, pulse generator or receiver (T85.123)
Revised **T83.121 Displacement of implanted urinary sphincter**
Revised **T83.122 Displacement of indwelling ureteral stent**
New **T83.123 Displacement of other urinary stents**
New Displacement of ileal conduit stent
New Displacement of nephroureteral stent

T83.190 Other mechanical complication of urinary electronic stimulator device
New **Excludes2** Other mechanical complication of electrode (lead) for sacral nerve neuro-stimulator (T85.191)
New Other mechanical complication of implanted electronic sacral neuro-stimulator, pulse generator or receiver (T85.193)
Revised **T83.191 Other mechanical complication of implanted urinary sphincter**
Revised **T83.192 Other mechanical complication of indwelling ureteral stent**
New **T83.193 Other mechanical complication of other urinary stent**
New Other mechanical complication of ileal conduit stent
New Other mechanical complication of nephroureteral stent

New **T83.24 Erosion of graft of urinary organ**

New **T83.25 Exposure of graft of urinary organ**

T83.32 Displacement of intrauterine contraceptive device

New Missing string of intrauterine contraceptive device

Revised **T83.410 Breakdown (mechanical) of implanted penile prosthesis**

New Breakdown (mechanical) of penile prosthesis cylinder

New Breakdown (mechanical) of penile prosthesis pump

New Breakdown (mechanical) of penile prosthesis reservoir

New **T83.411 Breakdown (mechanical) of implanted testicular prosthesis**

Revised **T83.420 Displacement of implanted penile prosthesis**

New Displacement of penile prosthesis cylinder

New Displacement of penile prosthesis pump

New Displacement of penile prosthesis reservoir

New **T83.421 Displacement of implanted testicular prosthesis**

Revised **T83.490 Other mechanical complication of implanted penile prosthesis**

New Other mechanical complication of penile prosthesis cylinder

New Other mechanical complication of penile prosthesis pump

New Other mechanical complication of penile prosthesis reservoir

New **T83.491 Other mechanical complication of implanted testicular prosthesis**

Revised **T83.51 Infection and inflammatory reaction due to urinary catheter**

New **T83.510 Infection and inflammatory reaction due to cystostomy catheter**

New **T83.511 Infection and inflammatory reaction due to indwelling urethral catheter**

New **T83.512 Infection and inflammatory reaction due to nephrostomy catheter**

New **T83.518 Infection and inflammatory reaction due to other urinary catheter**

New Infection and inflammatory reaction due to Hopkins catheter

New Infection and inflammatory reaction due to ileostomy catheter

New Infection and inflammatory reaction due to urostomy catheter

New **T83.590 Infection and inflammatory reaction due to implanted urinary neurostimulation device**

New **Excludes2** Infection and inflammatory reaction due to electrode lead of sacral nerve neurostimulator (T85.732)

New Infection and inflammatory reaction due to pulse generator or receiver of sacral nerve neurostimulator (T85.734)

New **T83.591 Infection and inflammatory reaction due to implanted urinary sphincter**

New **T83.592 Infection and inflammatory reaction due to indwelling ureteral stent**

New **T83.593 Infection and inflammatory reaction due to other urinary stents**

New Infection and inflammatory reaction due to ileal conduit stents

New Infection and inflammatory reaction due to nephroureteral stent

New **T83.598 Infection and inflammatory reaction due to other prosthetic device, implant and graft in urinary system**

New **T83.61 Infection and inflammatory reaction due to implanted penile prosthesis**

New Infection and inflammatory reaction due to penile prosthesis cylinder

New Infection and inflammatory reaction due to penile prosthesis pump

New Infection and inflammatory reaction due to penile prosthesis reservoir

New **T83.62 Infection and inflammatory reaction due to implanted testicular prosthesis**

New **T83.69 Infection and inflammatory reaction due to other prosthetic device, implant and graft in genital tract**

Revised **T83.711 Erosion of implanted vaginal mesh to surrounding organ or tissue**

Revised Erosion of implanted vaginal mesh into pelvic floor muscles

New **T83.712 Erosion of implanted urethral mesh to surrounding organ or tissue**

New Erosion of implanted female urethral sling

New Erosion of implanted male urethral sling

New Erosion of implanted urethral mesh into pelvic floor muscles

New **T83.713 Erosion of implanted urethral bulking agent to surrounding organ or tissue**

New **T83.714 Erosion of implanted ureteral bulking agent to surrounding organ or tissue**

Revised **T83.718 Erosion of other implanted mesh to organ or tissue**

New **T83.719 Erosion of other prosthetic materials to surrounding organ or tissue**

T83.72 Exposure of implanted mesh and other prosthetic materials into surrounding organ or tissue

New Extrusion of implanted mesh

Revised **T83.721 Exposure of implanted vaginal mesh into vagina**

Revised Exposure of implanted vaginal mesh through vaginal wall

New **T83.722 Exposure of implanted urethral mesh into urethra**

New Exposure of implanted female urethral sling

New Exposure of implanted male urethral sling

New Exposure of implanted urethral mesh through urethral wall

New **T83.723 Exposure of implanted urethral bulking agent into urethra**

New **T83.724 Exposure of implanted ureteral bulking agent into ureter**

Revised **T83.728 Exposure of other implanted mesh into organ or tissue**

New **T83.729 Exposure of other prosthetic materials into organ or tissue**

New **T83.79 Other specified complications due to other genitourinary prosthetic materials**

T83.8 Other specified complications of genitourinary prosthetic devices, implants and grafts

Revised **T83.81 Embolism due to genitourinary prosthetic devices, implants and grafts**

Revised **T83.82 Fibrosis due to genitourinary prosthetic devices, implants and grafts**

Revised **T83.83 Hemorrhage due to genitourinary prosthetic devices, implants and grafts**

Revised **T83.84 Pain due to genitourinary prosthetic devices, implants and grafts**

Revised **T83.85 Stenosis due to genitourinary prosthetic devices, implants and grafts**

Revised **T83.86 Thrombosis due to genitourinary prosthetic devices, implants and grafts**

Deleted ~~T84.04 Periprosthetic fracture around internal prosthetic joint~~

Deleted **Excludes2** breakage (fracture) of prosthetic joint (T84.01)

Deleted ~~T84.040 Periprosthetic fracture around internal prosthetic right hip joint~~

Deleted ~~T84.041 Periprosthetic fracture around internal prosthetic left hip joint~~

Deleted ~~T84.042 Periprosthetic fracture around internal prosthetic right knee joint~~

Deleted ~~T84.043 Periprosthetic fracture around internal prosthetic left knee joint~~

Deleted ~~T84.048 Periprosthetic fracture around other internal prosthetic joint~~

Deleted Use additional code to identify the joint (Z96.6-)

Deleted ~~T84.049 Periprosthetic fracture around unspecified internal prosthetic joint~~

Revised **T85.110 Breakdown (mechanical) of implanted electronic neurostimulator of brain electrode (lead)**

Revised **T85.111 Breakdown (mechanical) of implanted electronic neurostimulator of peripheral nerve electrode (lead)**

New Breakdown of electrode (lead) for cranial nerve neurostimulators

New Breakdown of electrode (lead) for gastric neurostimulator

New Breakdown of electrode (lead) for sacral nerve neurostimulator

New Breakdown of electrode (lead) for vagal nerve neurostimulators

Revised **T85.112 Breakdown (mechanical) of implanted electronic neurostimulator of spinal cord electrode (lead)**

New **T85.113 Breakdown (mechanical) of implanted electronic neurostimulator, generator**

New Breakdown (mechanical) of implanted electronic neurostimuator generator, brain, peripheral, gastric, spinal

New Breakdown (mechanical) of implanted electronic sacral neurostimulator, pulse generator or receiver

Revised **T85.120 Displacement of implanted electronic neurostimulator of brain electrode (lead)**

Revised **T85.121 Displacement of implanted electronic neurostimulator of peripheral nerve electrode (lead)**

New Displacement of electrode (lead) for cranial nerve neurostimulators

New Displacement of electrode (lead) for gastric neurostimulator

New Displacement of electrode (lead) for sacral nerve neurostimulator

New Displacement of electrode (lead) for vagal nerve neurostimulators

Revised **T85.122 Displacement of implanted electronic neurostimulator of spinal cord electrode (lead)**

New **T85.123 Displacement of implanted electronic neurostimulator, generator**

New Displacement of implanted electronic neurostimulator generator, brain, peripheral, gastric, spinal

New Displacement of implanted electronic sacral neurostimulator, pulse generator or receiver

Revised **T85.190 Other mechanical complication of implanted electronic neurostimulator of brain electrode (lead)**

Revised **T85.191 Other mechanical complication of implanted electronic neurostimulator of peripheral nerve electrode (lead)**

New Other mechanical complication of electrode (lead) for cranial nerve neurostimulators

New Other mechanical complication of electrode (lead) for gastric neurostimulator

New Other mechanical complication of electrode (lead) for sacral nerve neurostimulator

New Other mechanical complication of electrode (lead) for vagal nerve neurostimulators

Revised **T85.192 Other mechanical complication of implanted electronic neurostimulator of spinal cord electrode (lead)**

New **T85.193 Other mechanical complication of implanted electronic neurostimulator, generator**

New Other mechanical complication of implanted electronic neurostimulator generator, brain, peripheral, gastric, spinal

New Other mechanical complication of implanted electronic sacral neurostimulator, pulse generator or receiver

Revised **T85.610 Breakdown (mechanical) of cranial or spinal infusion catheter**

New Breakdown (mechanical) of epidural infusion catheter

New Breakdown (mechanical) of intrathecal infusion catheter

New Breakdown (mechanical) of subarachnoid infusion catheter

New Breakdown (mechanical) of subdural infusion catheter

New **T85.615 Breakdown (mechanical) of other nervous system device, implant or graft**

New Breakdown (mechanical) of intrathecal infusion pump

Revised **T85.620 Displacement of cranial or spinal infusion catheter**

New Displacement of epidural infusion catheter

New Displacement of intrathecal infusion catheter

New Displacement of subarachnoid infusion catheter

New Displacement of subdural infusion catheter

New **T85.625 Displacement of other nervous system device, implant or graft**

New Displacement of intrathecal infusion pump

Revised **T85.630 Leakage of cranial or spinal infusion catheter**

New Leakage of epidural infusion catheter

New Leakage of intrathecal infusion catheter

New Leakage of subdural infusion catheter

New Leakage of subarachnoid infusion catheter

New **T85.635 Leakage of other nervous system device, implant or graft**

New Leakage of intrathecal infusion pump

Revised **T85.690 Other mechanical complication of cranial or spinal infusion catheter**

New Other mechanical complication of epidural infusion catheter

New Other mechanical complication of intrathecal infusion catheter

New Other mechanical complication of subarachnoid infusion catheter

New Other mechanical complication of subdural infusion catheter

New **T85.695 Other mechanical complication of other nervous system device, implant or graft**

New Other mechanical complication of intrathecal infusion pump

New **T85.73 Infection and inflammatory reaction due to nervous system devices, implants and graft**

New **T85.730 Infection and inflammatory reaction due to ventricular intracranial (communicating) shunt**

New **T85.731 Infection and inflammatory reaction due to implanted electronic neurostimulator of brain, electrode (lead)**

New **T85.732 Infection and inflammatory reaction due to implanted electronic neurostimulator of peripheral nerve, electrode (lead)**

New Infection and inflammatory reaction due to electrode (lead) for cranial nerve neurostimulators

New Infection and inflammatory reaction due to electrode (lead) for gastric neurostimulator

New Infection and inflammatory reaction due to electrode (lead) for sacral nerve neurostimulator

New Infection and inflammatory reaction due to electrode (lead) for vagal nerve neurostimulators

New **T85.733 Infection and inflammatory reaction due to implanted electronic neurostimulator of spinal cord, electrode (lead)**

New **T85.734 Infection and inflammatory reaction due to implanted electronic neurostimulator, generator**

New Generator pocket infection

New **T85.735 Infection and inflammatory reaction due to cranial or spinal infusion catheter**

New Infection and inflammatory reaction due to epidural catheter

New Infection and inflammatory reaction due to intrathecal infusion catheter

New Infection and inflammatory reaction due to subarachnoid catheter

New Infection and inflammatory reaction due to subdural catheter

New **T85.738 Infection and inflammatory reaction due to other nervous system device, implant or graft**

New Infection and inflammatory reaction due to intrathecal infusion pump

New **T85.810 Embolism due to nervous system prosthetic devices, implants and grafts**

New **T85.818 Embolism due to other internal prosthetic devices, implants and grafts**

New **T85.820 Fibrosis due to nervous system prosthetic devices, implants and grafts**

New **T85.828 Fibrosis due to other internal prosthetic devices, implants and grafts**

New **T85.830 Hemorrhage due to nervous system prosthetic devices, implants and grafts**

New **T85.838 Hemorrhage due to other internal prosthetic devices, implants and grafts**

New **T85.840 Pain due to nervous system prosthetic devices, implants and grafts**

New **T85.848 Pain due to other internal prosthetic devices, implants and grafts**

New **T85.850 Stenosis due to nervous system prosthetic devices, implants and grafts**

New **T85.858 Stenosis due to other internal prosthetic devices, implants and grafts**

New **T85.860 Thrombosis due to nervous system prosthetic devices, implants and grafts**

New **T85.868 Thrombosis due to other internal prosthetic devices, implants and grafts**

T85.89 Other specified complication of internal prosthetic devices, implants and grafts, not elsewhere classified

New Erosion or breakdown of subcutaneous device pocket

New **T85.890 Other specified complication of nervous system prosthetic devices, implants and grafts**

New **T85.898 Other specified complication of other internal prosthetic devices, implants and grafts**

New **T88.53 Unintended awareness under general anesthesia during procedure**

New **Excludes2** personal history of unintended awareness under general anesthesia (Z92.84)

CHAPTER 20

EXTERNAL CAUSES OF MORBIDITY (V00-Y99)

This chapter contains the following blocks:

New	X50	Overexertion and strenuous or repetitive movements
Revised	X92-Y09	Assault

TRANSPORT ACCIDENTS (V00-V99)

Deleted **Note:** This section is structured in 12 groups. Those relating to land transport accidents (V01-V89) reflect the victim's mode of transport and are subdivided to identify the victim's 'counterpart' or the type of event. The vehicle of which the injured person is an occupant is identified in the first two characters since it is seen as the most important factor to identify for prevention purposes. A transport accident is one in which the vehicle involved must be moving or running or in use for transport purposes at the time of the accident.

New **Note:** This section is structured in 12 groups. Those relating to land transport accidents (V00-V89) reflect the victim's mode of transport and are subdivided to identify the victim's 'counterpart' or the type of event. The vehicle of which the injured person is an occupant is identified in the first two characters since it is seen as the most important factor to identify for prevention purposes. A transport accident is one in which the vehicle involved must be moving or running or in use for transport purposes at the time of the accident.

Revised **Note:** Definitions related to transport accidents:

Revised (a) A transport accident (V00-V99) is any accident involving a device designed primarily for, or used at the time primarily for, conveying persons or good from one place to another.

Revised (e) A pedestrian is any person involved in an accident who was not at the time of the accident riding in or on a motor vehicle, railway train, streetcar or animal-drawn or other vehicle, or on a pedal cycle or animal. This includes, a person changing a tire, working on a parked car, or a person on foot. It also includes the user of a pedestrian conveyance such as a baby-stroller, ice-skates, skis, sled, roller skates, a skateboard, nonmotorized or motorized wheelchair, motorized mobility scooter, or nonmotorized scooter.

Revised (h) A person on the outside of a vehicle is any person being transported by a vehicle but not occupying the space normally reserved for the driver or passengers, or the space intended for the transport of property. This includes a person travelling on the bodywork, bumper, fender, roof, running board or step of a vehicle, as well as, hanging on the outside of the vehicle.

Revised (k) A motorcycle is a two-wheeled motor vehicle with one or two riding saddles and sometimes with a third wheel for the support of a sidecar. The sidecar is considered part of the motorcycle. This includes a moped, motor scooter, or motorized bicycle.

Revised (n) A car [automobile] is a four-wheeled motor vehicle designed primarily for carrying up to 7 persons. A trailer being towed by the car is considered part of the car. It does not include a van or minivan—see definition (o)

Revised (t) A special vehicle mainly used on industrial premises is a motor vehicle designed primarily for use within the buildings and premises of industrial or commercial establishments. This includes battery-powered airport passenger vehicles or baggage/mail trucks, forklifts, coal-cars in a coal mine, logging cars and trucks used in mines or quarries.

Revised (w) A special all-terrain vehicle is a motor vehicle of special design to enable it to negotiate over rough or soft terrain, snow or sand. Examples of special design are high construction, special wheels and tires, tracks, and support on a cushion of air. This includes snow mobiles, all-terrain vehicles (ATV), and dune buggies. It does not include passenger vehicle designated as sport utility vehicles (SUV).

Deleted ~~V47.01 Driver of sport utility vehicle injured in collision with fixed or stationary object in nontraffic accident~~

Deleted ~~V47.02 Driver of other type car injured in collision with fixed or stationary object in nontraffic accident~~

Deleted ~~V47.11 Passenger of sport utility vehicle injured in collision with fixed or stationary object in nontraffic accident~~

Deleted ~~V47.12 Passenger of other type car injured in collision with fixed or stationary object in nontraffic accident~~

Deleted ~~V47.31 Unspecified occupant of sport utility vehicle injured in collision with fixed or stationary object in nontraffic accident~~

Deleted ~~V47.32 Unspecified occupant of other type car injured in collision with fixed or stationary object in nontraffic accident~~

Deleted ~~V47.51 Driver of sport utility vehicle injured in collision with fixed or stationary object in traffic accident~~

Deleted ~~V47.52 Driver of other type car injured in collision with fixed or stationary object in traffic accident~~

Deleted ~~V47.61 Passenger of sport utility vehicle injured in collision with fixed or stationary object in traffic accident~~

Deleted ~~V47.62 Passenger of other type car injured in collision with fixed or stationary object in traffic accident~~

Deleted ~~V47.91 Unspecified occupant of sport utility vehicle injured in collision with fixed or stationary object in traffic accident~~

Deleted ~~V47.92 Unspecified occupant of other type car injured in collision with fixed or stationary object in traffic accident~~

EXPOSURE TO INANIMATE MECHANICAL FORCES (W20-W49)

Revised **Excludes1** assault (X92-Y09)

W25 Contact with sharp glass

Excludes2 glass embedded in skin (W45)

Revised **W26 Contact with other sharp objects**

New **Excludes2** sharp object(s) embedded in skin (W45)

New **W26.2 Contact with edge of stiff paper**

New Paper cut

New **W26.8 Contact with other sharp object(s), not elsewhere classified**

New Contact with tin can lid

New **W26.9 Contact with unspecified sharp object(s)**

W45 Foreign body or object entering through skin

New **Includes** foreign body or object embedded in skin
nail embedded in skin

Revised **Excludes2** contact with other sharp object(s) (W26.-)

Deleted ~~W45.1 Paper entering through skin~~

Deleted ~~Paper cut~~

Deleted ~~W45.2 Lid of can entering through skin~~

W89 Exposure to man-made visible and ultraviolet light

Deleted **Excludes2** exposure to sunlight (X32)

New **Excludes1** exposure to sunlight (X32)

X32 Exposure to sunlight

Deleted **Excludes1** radiation-related disorders of the skin and subcutaneous tissue (L55-L59)

X39.0 Exposure to natural radiation

Revised **Excludes1** contact with and (suspected) exposure to radon and other naturally occuring radiation (Z77.123)

New **OVEREXERTION AND STRENUOUS OR REPETITIVE MOVEMENTS (X50)**

New **X50 Overexertion and strenuous or repetitive movements**

New The appropriate 7th character is to be added to each code from category X50

New A initial encounter
New D subsequent encounter
New S sequela

New **X50.0 Overexertion from strenuous movement or load**

New Lifting heavy objects

New Lifting weights

New **X50.1 Overexertion from prolonged static or awkward postures**

New Prolonged bending

New Prolonged kneeling

New Prolonged reaching

New Prolonged sitting

New Prolonged standing

New Prolonged twisting

New Static bending

New Static kneeling

New Static reaching

New Static sitting

New Static standing

New Static twisting

New **X50.3 Overexertion from repetitive movements**
New Use of hand as hammer
New **Excludes2** Overuse from prolonged static or awkward postures (X50.1)

New **X50.9 Other and unspecified overexertion or strenuous movements or postures**
New Contact pressure
New Contact stress

Deleted **ASSAULT (X92-Y08)**

New **ASSAULT (X92-Y09)**

MISADVENTURES TO PATIENTS DURING SURGICAL AND MEDICAL CARE (Y62-Y69)

New **Excludes1** surgical and medical procedures as the cause of abnormal reaction of the patient, without mention of misadventure at the time of the procedure (Y83-Y84)

Deleted **Excludes2** surgical and medical procedures as the cause of abnormal reaction of the patient, without mention of misadventure at the time of the procedure (Y83-Y84)

MEDICAL DEVICES ASSOCIATED WITH ADVERSE INCIDENTS IN DIAGNOSTIC AND THERAPEUTIC USE (Y70-Y82)

Deleted **Excludes1** misadventure to patients during surgical and medical care, classifiable to (Y62-Y69)
Deleted later complications following use of medical devices without breakdown or malfunctioning of device (Y83-Y84)

New **Excludes2** breakdown or malfunctioning of medical device (after implantation) (during procedure) (ongoing use) (Y70-Y82)
New later complications following use of medical devices without breakdown or malfunctioning of device (Y83-Y84)
New misadventure to patients during surgical and medical care, classifiable to (Y62-Y69)
New surgical and other medical procedures as the cause of abnormal reaction of the patient, or of later complication, without mention of misadventure at the time of the procedure (Y83-Y84)

SURGICAL AND OTHER MEDICAL PROCEDURES AS THE CAUSE OF ABNORMAL REACTION OF THE PATIENT, OR OF LATER COMPLICATION, WITHOUT MENTION OF MISADVENTURE AT THE TIME OF THE PROCEDURE (Y83-Y84)

New **Excludes2** breakdown or malfunctioning of medical device (after implantation) (during procedure) (ongoing use) (Y70-Y82)

Revised **Y92.4 Street, highway and other paved roadways as the place of occurrence of the external cause**

New **Y93.85 Activity, choking game**
New Activity, blackout game
New Activity, fainting game
New Activity, pass out game

CHAPTER 21

FACTORS INFLUENCING HEALTH STATUS AND CONTACT WITH HEALTH SERVICES (Z00-Z99)

This chapter contains the following blocks:

Deleted	Z20-Z28	Persons with potential health hazards related to communicable diseases
New	Z19	Hormone sensitivity malignancy status
New	Z20-Z29	Persons with potential health hazards related to communicable diseases

Z01.411 Encounter for gynecological examination (general) (routine) with abnormal findings
New Use additional code to identify any abnormal findings

Z01.419 Encounter for gynecological examination (general) (routine) without abnormal findings
Deleted Use additional code to identify any abnormal findings

New **Z05 Encounter for observation and evaluation of newborn for suspected diseases and conditions ruled out**
New This category is to be used for newborns, within the neonatal period (the first 28 days of life), who are suspected of having an abnormal condition unrelated to exposure from the mother or the birth process, but without signs or symptoms, and which, after examination and observation, is ruled out.
New **Excludes2** newborn observation for suspected condition, related to exposure from the mother or birth process (P00-P04)

New **Z05.0 Observation and evaluation of newborn for suspected cardiac condition ruled out**
New **Z05.1 Observation and evaluation of newborn for suspected infectious condition ruled out**
New **Z05.2 Observation and evaluation of newborn for suspected neurological condition ruled out**
New **Z05.3 Observation and evaluation of newborn for suspected respiratory condition ruled out**
New **Z05.4 Observation and evaluation of newborn for suspected genetic, metabolic or immunologic condition ruled out**
New **Z05.41 Observation and evaluation of newborn for suspected genetic condition ruled out**
New **Z05.42 Observation and evaluation of newborn for suspected metabolic condition ruled out**
New **Z05.43 Observation and evaluation of newborn for suspected immunologic condition ruled out**
New **Z05.5 Observation and evaluation of newborn for suspected gastrointestinal condition ruled out**
New **Z05.6 Observation and evaluation of newborn for suspected genitourinary condition ruled out**
New **Z05.7 Observation and evaluation of newborn for suspected skin, subcutaneous, musculoskeletal and connective tissue condition ruled out**
New **Z05.71 Observation and evaluation of newborn for suspected skin and subcutaneous tissue condition ruled out**
New **Z05.72 Observation and evaluation of newborn for suspected musculoskeletal condition ruled out**
New **Z05.73 Observation and evaluation of newborn for suspected connective tissue condition ruled out**
New **Z05.8 Observation and evaluation of newborn for other specified suspected condition ruled out**
New **Z05.9 Observation and evaluation of newborn for unspecified suspected condition ruled out**

Z12.4 Encounter for screening for malignant neoplasm of cervix
Deleted **Excludes1** encounter for screening for human papillomavirus (Z11.51)
New **Excludes2** encounter for screening for human papillomavirus (Z11.51)

New **HORMONE SENSITIVITY MALIGNANCY STATUS (Z19)**

New **Z19 Hormone sensitivity malignancy status**

New *Code first* malignant neoplasm —*see* Table of Neoplasms, by site, malignant

New **Z19.1 Hormone sensitive malignancy status**

New **Z19.2 Hormone resistant malignancy status**

New Castrate resistant prostate malignancy status

Deleted **PERSONS WITH POTENTIAL HEALTH HAZARDS RELATED TO COMMUNICABLE DISEASES (Z20-Z28)**

New **PERSONS WITH POTENTIAL HEALTH HAZARDS RELATED TO COMMUNICABLE DISEASES (Z20-Z29)**

Z22 Carrier of infectious disease

New **Excludes2** carrier of viral hepatitis (B18.-)

Z22.330 Carrier of Group B streptococcus

New **Excludes1** Carrier of streptococcus group B (GBS) complicating pregnancy, childbirth and the puerperium (O99.82-)

Deleted ~~Z22.5 Carrier of viral hepatitis~~

Deleted ~~Z22.50 Carrier of unspecified viral hepatitis~~

Deleted ~~Z22.51 Carrier of viral hepatitis B~~

Deleted ~~Hepatitis B surface antigen [HBsAg] carrier~~

Deleted ~~Z22.52 Carrier of viral hepatitis C~~

Deleted ~~Z22.59 Carrier of other viral hepatitis~~

New **Z29 Encounter for other prophylactic measures**

New **Excludes1** desensitization to allergens (Z51.6)

New prophylactic surgery (Z40.-)

New **Z29.1 Encounter for prophylactic immunotherapy**

New Encounter for administration of immunoglobulin

New **Z29.11 Encounter for prophylactic immunotherapy for respiratory syncytial virus (RSV)**

New **Z29.12 Encounter for prophylactic antivenin**

New **Z29.13 Encounter for prophylactic Rho(D) immune globulin**

New **Z29.14 Encounter for prophylactic rabies immune globin**

New **Z29.3 Encounter for prophylactic fluoride administration**

New **Z29.8 Encounter for other specified prophylactic measures**

New **Z29.9 Encounter for prophylactic measures, unspecified**

New **Z30.015 Encounter for initial prescription of vaginal ring hormonal contraceptive**

New **Z30.016 Encounter for initial prescription of transdermal patch hormonal contraceptive device**

New **Z30.017 Encounter for initial prescription of implantable subdermal contraceptive**

New **Z30.018 Encounter for initial prescription of other contraceptives**

New Encounter for initial prescription of barrier contraception

New Encounter for initial prescription of diaphragm

New **Z30.44 Encounter for surveillance of vaginal ring hormonal contraceptive device**

New **Z30.45 Encounter for surveillance of transdermal patch hormonal contraceptive device**

New **Z30.46 Encounter for surveillance of implantable subdermal contraceptive**

New Encounter for checking, reinsertion or removal of implantable subdermal contraceptive

New **Z30.49 Encounter for surveillance of other contraceptives**

New Encounter for surveillance of barrier contraception

New Encounter for surveillance of diaphragm

New **Z31.7 Encounter for procreative management and counseling for gestational carrier**

New **Excludes1** pregnant state, gestational carrier (Z33.3)

Z33.1 Pregnant state, incidental

New **Excludes1** pregnant state, gestational carrier (Z33.3)

New **Z33.3 Pregnant state, gestational carrier**

New **Excludes1** encounter for procreative management and counseling for gestational carrier (Z31.7)

Z3A Weeks of gestation

Revised **Note:** Codes from category Z3A are for use, only on the maternal record, to indicate the weeks of gestation of the pregnancy, if known.

Z45.01 Encounter for adjustment and management of cardiac pacemaker

New Encounter for adjustment and management of cardiac resynchronization therapy pacemaker (CRT-P)

Z45.02 Encounter for adjustment and management of automatic implantable cardiac defibrillator

New Encounter for adjustment and management of cardiac resynchronization therapy defibrillator (CRT-D)

Revised **Z51 Encounter for other aftercare and medical care**

New **Z51.6 Encounter for desensitization to allergens**

New **Z53.3 Procedure converted to open procedure**

New **Z53.31 Laparoscopic surgical procedure converted to open procedure**

New **Z53.32 Thoracoscopic surgical procedure converted to open procedure**

New **Z53.33 Arthroscopic surgical procedure converted to open procedure**

New **Z53.39 Other specified procedure converted to open procedure**

Z77 Other contact with and (suspected) exposures hazardous to health

Revised **Excludes2** newborn affected by noxious substances transmitted via placenta or breast milk (P04.-)

Z79 Long term (current) drug therapy

New **Excludes2** long term (current) use of oral antidiabetic drugs (Z79.84)

New long term (current) use of oral hypoglycemic drugs (Z79.84)

New **Z79.84 Long term (current) use of oral hypoglycemic drugs**

New Long term (current) use of oral antidiabetic drugs

New **Excludes2** long term (current) use of insulin (Z79.4)

Z79.891 Long term (current) use of opiate analgesic

Revised **Excludes1** methodone use NOS (F11.9-)

New **Z83.42 Family history of familial hypercholesterolemia**

New **Z84.82 Family history of sudden infant death syndrome**

New Family history of SIDS

Z85 Personal history of malignant neoplasm

Use additional code to identify:

Revised history of tobacco dependence (Z87.891)

Z85.8 Personal history of malignant neoplasms of other organs and systems

Revised Conditions classifiable to C00-C14, C40-C49, C69-C75, C7A.098, C76-C79

Z86.00 Personal history of in-situ neoplasm

New Conditions classifiable to D00-D09

Z86.001 Personal history of in-situ neoplasm of cervix uteri

New Personal history of cervical intraepithelial neoplasia III [CIN III]

Z86.008 Personal history of in-situ neoplasm of other site

New Personal history of vaginal intraepithelial neoplasia III [VAIN III]

New Personal history of vulvar intraepithelial neoplasia III [VIN III]

Z87.41 Personal history of dysplasia of the female genital tract

New **Excludes1** personal history of intraepithelial neoplasia III of female genital tract (Z87.001, Z87.008)

Z90.41 Acquired absence of pancreas

New Code also exocrine pancreatic insufficiency (K86.81)

New **Z92.84 Personal history of unintended awareness under general anesthesia**

New **Excludes2** unintended awareness under general anesthesia during procedure (T88.53)

Z95.0 Presence of cardiac pacemaker

New Presence of cardiac resynchronization therapy (CRT-P) pacemaker

New **Excludes1** adjustment or management of cardiac device (Z45.0-)

Z95.1 Presence of aortocoronary bypass graft

New Presence of coronary artery bypass graft

Z95.810 Presence of automatic (implantable) cardiac defibrillator

New Presence of cardiac resynchronization therapy defibrillator (CRT-D)

New Presence of cardioverter-defribillator (ICD)

Z97.5 Presence of (intrauterine) contraceptive device

Revised **Excludes1** checking, reinsertion or removal of implantable subdermal contraceptive (Z30.46)

New checking, reinsertion or removal of intrauterine contraceptive device (Z30.43-)

Z98.89 Other specified postprocedural states

Deleted Personal history of surgery, not elsewhere classified

New **Z98.890 Other specified postprocedural states**

New Personal history of surgery, not elsewhere classified

New **Z98.891 History of uterine scar from previous surgery**

New **Excludes1** Maternal care due to uterine scar from previous surgery (O34.2-)

Z99.2 Dependence on renal dialysis

Deleted **Excludes1** noncompliance with renal dialysis (Z91.15)

New **Excludes2** noncompliance with renal dialysis (Z91.15)

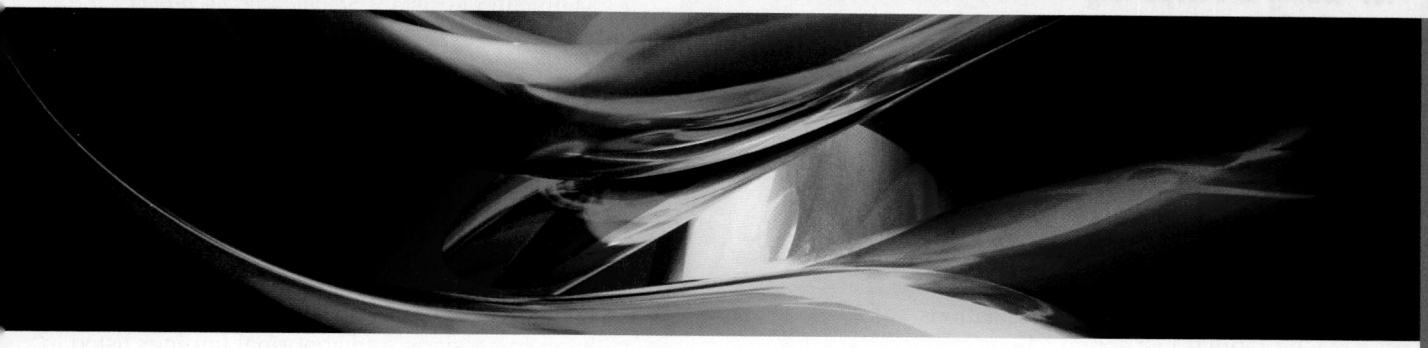

Introduction

ICD-10-CM Official Guidelines for Coding and Reporting 2017

Narrative changes appear in bold text
Items underlined have been moved within the guidelines since the 2016 version
***Italics* are used to indicate revisions to heading changes**

The Centers for Medicare and Medicaid Services (CMS) and the National Center for Health Statistics (NCHS), two departments within the U.S. Federal Government's Department of Health and Human Services (DHHS) provide the following guidelines for coding and reporting using the International Classification of Diseases, 10th Revision, Clinical Modification (ICD-10-CM). These guidelines should be used as a companion document to the official version of the ICD-10-CM as published on the NCHS website. The ICD-10-CM is a morbidity classification published by the United States for classifying diagnoses and reason for visits in all health care settings. The ICD-10-CM is based on the ICD-10, the statistical classification of disease published by the World Health Organization (WHO).

These guidelines have been approved by the four organizations that make up the Cooperating Parties for the ICD-10-CM: the American Hospital Association (AHA), the American Health Information Management Association (AHIMA), CMS, and NCHS.

These guidelines are a set of rules that have been developed to accompany and complement the official conventions and instructions provided within the ICD-10-CM itself. The instructions and conventions of the classification take precedence over guidelines. These guidelines are based on the coding and sequencing instructions in the Tabular List and Alphabetic Index of ICD-10-CM, but provide additional instruction. Adherence to these guidelines when assigning ICD-10-CM diagnosis codes is required under the Health Insurance Portability and Accountability Act (HIPAA). The diagnosis codes (Tabular List and Alphabetic Index) have been adopted under HIPAA for all healthcare settings. A joint effort between the healthcare provider and the coder is essential to achieve complete and accurate documentation, code assignment, and reporting of diagnoses and procedures. These guidelines have been developed to assist both the healthcare provider and the coder in identifying those diagnoses that are to be reported. The importance of consistent, complete documentation in the medical record cannot be overemphasized. Without such documentation accurate coding cannot be achieved. The entire record should be reviewed to determine the specific reason for the encounter and the conditions treated.

The term encounter is used for all settings, including hospital admissions. In the context of these guidelines, the term provider is used throughout the guidelines to mean physician or any qualified health care practitioner who is legally accountable for establishing the patient's diagnosis. Only this set of guidelines, approved by the Cooperating Parties, is official.

The guidelines are organized into sections. Section I includes the structure and conventions of the classification and general guidelines that apply to the entire classification, and chapter-specific guidelines that correspond to the chapters as they are arranged in the classification. Section II includes guidelines for selection of principal diagnosis for non-outpatient settings. Section III includes guidelines for reporting additional diagnoses in non-outpatient settings. Section IV is for outpatient coding and reporting. It is necessary to review all sections of the guidelines to fully understand all of the rules and instructions needed to code properly.

ICD-10-CM Official Guidelines for Coding and Reporting

Section I. Conventions, general coding guidelines and chapter specific guidelines

A. Conventions for the ICD-10-CM
   1. The Alphabetic Index and Tabular List
   2. Format and Structure:
   3. Use of codes for reporting purposes
   4. Placeholder character
   5. 7th Characters
   6. Abbreviations
      a. Alphabetic Index abbreviations
      b. Tabular List abbreviations
   7. Punctuation
   8. Use of "and"
   9. Other and Unspecified codes
      a. "Other" codes
      b. "Unspecified" codes
   10. Includes Notes
   11. Inclusion terms
   12. Excludes Notes
      a. Excludes1
      b. Excludes2
   13. Etiology/manifestation convention ("code first", "use additional code" and "in diseases classified elsewhere" notes)
   14. "And"
   15. "With"
   16. "See" and "See Also"
   17. "Code also note"
   18. Default codes
   19. Code assignment and Clinical Criteria

B. General Coding Guidelines
   1. Locating a code in the ICD-10-CM
   2. Level of Detail in Coding
   3. Code or codes from A00.0 through T88.9, Z00-Z99.8
   4. Signs and symptoms
   5. Conditions that are an integral part of a disease process
   6. Conditions that are not an integral part of a disease process
   7. Multiple coding for a single condition
   8. Acute and Chronic Conditions
   9. Combination Code
   10. Sequela (Late Effects)
   11. Impending or Threatened Condition
   12. Reporting Same Diagnosis Code More than Once
   13. Laterality
   14. Documentation for BMI, *Depth of* Non-pressure ulcers, Pressure Ulcer Stages, Coma Scale, and *NIH Stroke Scale*
   15. Syndromes
   16. Documentation of Complications of Care
   17. Borderline Diagnosis
   18. Use of Sign/Symptom/Unspecified Codes

C. Chapter-Specific Coding Guidelines
   1. Chapter 1: Certain Infectious and Parasitic Diseases (A00-B99)
      a. Human Immunodeficiency Virus (HIV) Infections
      b. Infectious agents as the cause of diseases classified to other chapters
      c. Infections resistant to antibiotics
      d. Sepsis, Severe Sepsis, and Septic Shock
      e. Methicillin Resistant *Staphylococcus aureus* (MRSA) Conditions
      f. Zika virus infection
   2. Chapter 2: Neoplasms (C00-D49)
      a. Treatment directed at the malignancy
      b. Treatment of secondary site
      c. Coding and sequencing of complications
      d. Primary malignancy previously excised
      e. Admissions/Encounters involving chemotherapy, immunotherapy and radiation therapy
      f. Admission/encounter to determine extent of malignancy
      g. Symptoms, signs, and abnormal findings listed in Chapter 18 associated with neoplasms
      h. Admission/encounter for pain control/management
      i. Malignancy in two or more noncontiguous sites
      j. Disseminated malignant neoplasm, unspecified
      k. Malignant neoplasm without specification of site
      l. Sequencing of neoplasm codes
      m. Current malignancy versus personal history of malignancy
      n. Leukemia, Multiple Myeloma, and Malignant Plasma Cell Neoplasms in remission versus personal history
      o. Aftercare following surgery for neoplasm
      p. Follow-up care for completed treatment of a malignancy
      q. Prophylactic organ removal for prevention of malignancy
      r. Malignant neoplasm associated with transplanted organ
   3. Chapter 3: Disease of the blood and blood-forming organs and certain disorders involving the immune mechanism (D50-D89)
   4. Chapter 4: Endocrine, Nutritional, and Metabolic Diseases (E00-E89)
      a. Diabetes mellitus
   5. Chapter 5: Mental, Behavioral and Neurodevelopmental disorders (F01 – F99)
      a. Pain disorders related to psychological factors
      b. Mental and behavioral disorders due to psychoactive substance use
   6. Chapter 6: Diseases of the Nervous System (G00-G99)
      a. Dominant/nondominant side
      b. Pain - Category G89
   7. Chapter 7: Diseases of the Eye and Adnexa (H00-H59)
      a. Glaucoma
   8. Chapter 8: Diseases of the Ear and Mastoid Process (H60-H95)
   9. Chapter 9: Diseases of the Circulatory System (I00-I99)
      a. Hypertension
      b. Atherosclerotic Coronary Artery Disease and Angina
      c. Intraoperative and Postprocedural Cerebrovascular Accident
      d. Sequelae of Cerebrovascular Disease
      e. Acute myocardial infarction (AMI)

10. Chapter 10: Diseases of the Respiratory System (J00-J99)
    a. Chronic Obstructive Pulmonary Disease [COPD] and Asthma
    b. Acute Respiratory Failure
    c. Influenza due to certain identified influenza viruses
    d. Ventilator associated Pneumonia
11. Chapter 11: Diseases of the Digestive System (K00-K95)
12. Chapter 12: Diseases of the Skin and Subcutaneous Tissue (L00-L99)
    a. Pressure ulcer stage codes
13. Chapter 13: Diseases of the Musculoskeletal System and Connective Tissue (M00-M99)
    a. Site and laterality
    b. Acute traumatic versus chronic or recurrent musculoskeletal conditions
    c. Coding of Pathologic Fractures
    d. Osteoporosis
14. Chapter 14: Diseases of Genitourinary System (N00-N99)
    a. Chronic kidney disease
15. Chapter 15: Pregnancy, Childbirth, and the Puerperium (O00-O9A)
    a. General Rules for Obstetric Cases
    b. Selection of OB Principal or First-listed Diagnosis
    c. Pre-existing conditions versus conditions due to the pregnancy
    d. Pre-existing hypertension in pregnancy
    e. Fetal Conditions Affecting the Management of the Mother
    f. HIV Infection in Pregnancy, Childbirth and the Puerperium
    g. Diabetes mellitus in pregnancy
    h. Long term use of insulin and oral hypoglycemics
    i. Gestational (pregnancy induced) diabetes
    j. Sepsis and septic shock complicating abortion, pregnancy, childbirth and the puerperium
    k. Puerperal sepsis
    l. Alcohol and tobacco use during pregnancy, childbirth and the puerperium
    m. Poisoning, toxic effects, adverse effects and underdosing in a pregnant patient
    n. Normal Delivery, Code O80
    o. The Peripartum and Postpartum Periods
    p. Code O94, Sequelae of complication of pregnancy, childbirth, and the puerperium
    q. Termination of Pregnancy and Spontaneous abortions
    r. Abuse in a pregnant patient
16. Chapter 16: Certain Conditions Originating in the Perinatal Period (P00-P96)
    a. General Perinatal Rules
    b. Observation and Evaluation of Newborns for Suspected Conditions not Found
    c. Coding Additional Perinatal Diagnoses
    d. Prematurity and Fetal Growth Retardation
    e. Low birth weight and immaturity status
    f. Bacterial Sepsis of Newborn
    g. Stillbirth
17. Chapter 17: Congenital malformations, deformations, and chromosomal abnormalities (Q00-Q99)
18. Chapter 18: Symptoms, signs, and abnormal clinical and laboratory findings, not elsewhere classified (R00-R99)
    a. Use of symptom codes
    b. Use of a symptom code with a definitive diagnosis code
    c. Combination codes that include symptoms
    d. Repeated falls
    e. Coma scale
    f. Functional quadriplegia
    g. SIRS due to Non-Infectious Process
    h. Death NOS
    i. NIHSS Stroke Scale
19. Chapter 19: Injury, poisoning, and certain other consequences of external causes (S00-T88)
    a. Application of 7th Characters in Chapter 19
    b. Coding of Injuries
    c. Coding of Traumatic Fractures
    d. Coding of Burns and Corrosions
    e. Adverse Effects, Poisoning, Underdosing and Toxic Effects
    f. Adult and child abuse, neglect and other maltreatment
    g. Complications of care
20. Chapter 20: External Causes of Morbidity (V00-Y99)
    a. General External Cause Coding Guidelines
    b. Place of Occurrence Guideline
    c. Activity Code
    d. Place of Occurrence, Activity, and Status Codes Used with other External Cause Code
    e. If the Reporting Format Limits the Number of External Cause Codes
    f. Multiple External Cause Coding Guidelines
    g. Child and Adult Abuse Guideline
    h. Unknown or Undetermined Intent Guideline
    i. Sequelae (Late Effects) of External Cause Guidelines
    j. Terrorism Guidelines
    k. External cause status
21. Chapter 21: Factors influencing health status and contact with health services (Z00-Z99)
    a. Use of Z codes in any healthcare setting
    b. Z Codes indicate a reason for an encounter
    c. Categories of Z Codes

Section II. Selection of Principal Diagnosis

A. Codes for symptoms, signs, and ill-defined conditions
B. Two or more interrelated conditions, each potentially meeting the definition for principal diagnosis
C. Two or more diagnoses that equally meet the definition for principal diagnosis
D. Two or more comparative or contrasting conditions
E. A symptom(s) followed by contrasting/comparative diagnoses
F. Original treatment plan not carried out
G. Complications of surgery and other medical care
H. Uncertain Diagnosis

I. Admission from Observation Unit
   1. Admission Following Medical Observation
   2. Admission Following Post-Operative Observation
J. Admission from Outpatient Surgery
K. Admissions/Encounters for Rehabilitation

Section III. Reporting Additional Diagnoses

A. Previous conditions
B. Abnormal findings
C. Uncertain Diagnosis

Section IV. Diagnostic Coding and Reporting Guidelines for Outpatient Services

A. Selection of first-listed condition
   1. Outpatient Surgery
   2. Observation Stay
B. Codes from A00.0 through T88.9, Z00-Z99
C. Accurate reporting of ICD-10-CM diagnosis codes
D. Codes that describe symptoms and signs
E. Encounters for circumstances other than a disease or injury
F. Level of Detail in Coding
   1. ICD-10-CM codes with 3, 4, 5, 6, or 7 characters
   2. Use of full number of characters required for a code
G. ICD-10-CM code for the diagnosis, condition, problem, or other reason for encounter/visit
H. Uncertain diagnosis
I. Chronic diseases
J. Code all documented conditions that coexist
K. Patients receiving diagnostic services only
L. Patients receiving therapeutic services only
M. Patients receiving preoperative evaluations only
N. Ambulatory surgery
O. Routine outpatient prenatal visits
P. Encounters for general medical examinations with abnormal findings
Q. Encounters for routine health screenings

Appendix I: Present on Admission Reporting Guidelines

Section I. Conventions, general coding guidelines and chapter specific guidelines

The conventions, general guidelines and chapter-specific guidelines are applicable to all health care settings unless otherwise indicated. The conventions and instructions of the classification take precedence over guidelines.

A. Conventions for the ICD-10-CM

The conventions for the ICD-10-CM are the general rules for use of the classification independent of the guidelines. These conventions are incorporated within the Alphabetic Index and Tabular List of the ICD-10-CM as instructional notes.

1. The Alphabetic Index and Tabular List

The ICD-10-CM is divided into the Alphabetic Index, an alphabetical list of terms and their corresponding code, and the Tabular List, a structured list of codes divided into chapters based on body system or condition. The Alphabetic Index consists of the following parts: the Index of Diseases and Injury, the Index of External Causes of Injury, the Table of Neoplasms and the Table of Drugs and Chemicals.

See Section I.C2. General guidelines

See Section I.C.19. Adverse effects, poisoning, underdosing and toxic effects

2. Format and Structure:

The ICD-10-CM Tabular List contains categories, subcategories and codes. Characters for categories, subcategories and codes may be either a letter or a number. All categories are 3 characters. A three-character category that has no further subdivision is equivalent to a code. Subcategories are either 4 or 5 characters. Codes may be 3, 4, 5, 6 or 7 characters. That is, each level of subdivision after a category is a subcategory. The final level of subdivision is a code. Codes that have applicable 7th characters are still referred to as codes, not subcategories. A code that has an applicable 7th character is considered invalid without the 7th character.

The ICD-10-CM uses an indented format for ease in reference

3. Use of codes for reporting purposes

For reporting purposes only codes are permissible, not categories or subcategories, and any applicable 7th character is required.

4. Placeholder character

The ICD-10-CM utilizes a placeholder character "X". The "X" is used as a placeholder at certain codes to allow for future expansion. An example of this is at the poisoning, adverse effect and underdosing codes, categories T36-T50. Where a placeholder exists, the X must be used in order for the code to be considered a valid code.

5. 7th Characters

Certain ICD-10-CM categories have applicable 7th characters. The applicable 7th character is required for all codes within the category, or as the notes in the Tabular List instruct. The 7th character must always be the 7th character in the data field. If a code that requires a 7th character is not 6 characters, a placeholder X must be used to fill in the empty characters.

6. Abbreviations

a. Alphabetic Index abbreviations

NEC "Not elsewhere classifiable"
This abbreviation in the Alphabetic Index represents "other specified". When a specific code is not available for a condition the Alphabetic Index directs the coder to the "other specified" code in the Tabular List.

NOS "Not otherwise specified"
This abbreviation is the equivalent of unspecified.

b. Tabular List abbreviations

NEC "Not elsewhere classifiable"
This abbreviation in the Tabular List represents "other specified". When a specific code is not available for a condition, the Tabular List includes an NEC entry under a code to identify the code as the "other specified" code.

NOS "Not otherwise specified"
This abbreviation is the equivalent of unspecified.

7. Punctuation

[ ] Brackets are used in the Tabular List to enclose synonyms, alternative wording or explanatory phrases. Brackets are used in the Alphabetic Index to identify manifestation codes.

( ) Parentheses are used in both the Alphabetic Index and Tabular List to enclose supplementary words that may be present or absent in the statement of a disease or procedure without affecting the code number to which it is assigned. The terms within the parentheses are referred to as nonessential modifiers.
The nonessential modifiers in the Alphabetic Index to Diseases apply to subterms following a main term except when a nonessential modifier and a subentry are mutually exclusive, the subentry takes precedence. For example, in the ICD-10-CM Alphabetic Index under the main term Enteritis, "acute" is a nonessential modifier and "chronic" is a subentry. In this case, the nonessential modifier "acute" does not apply to the subentry "chronic".

: Colons are used in the Tabular List after an incomplete term which needs one or more of the modifiers following the colon to make it assignable to a given category.

8. Use of "and".

See Section I.A.14. Use of the term "And"

9. Other and Unspecified codes

a. "Other" codes

Codes titled "other" or "other specified" are for use when the information in the medical record provides detail for which a specific code does not exist. Alphabetic Index entries with NEC in the line designate "other" codes in the Tabular List. These Alphabetic Index entries represent specific disease entities for which no specific code exists so the term is included within an "other" code.

b. "Unspecified" codes

Codes titled "unspecified" are for use when the information in the medical record is insufficient to assign a more specific code. For those categories for which an unspecified code is not provided, the "other specified" code may represent both other and unspecified.

See Section I.B.18 Use of Signs/Symptom/Unspecified Codes

10. Includes Notes

This note appears immediately under a three-character code title to further define, or give examples of, the content of the category.

11. Inclusion terms

List of terms is included under some codes. These terms are the conditions for which that code is to be used. The terms may be synonyms of the code title, or, in the case of "other specified" codes, the terms are a list of the various conditions assigned to that code. The inclusion terms are not necessarily exhaustive. Additional terms found only in the Alphabetic Index may also be assigned to a code.

12. Excludes Notes

The ICD-10-CM has two types of excludes notes. Each type of note has a different definition for use but they are all similar in that they indicate that codes excluded from each other are independent of each other.

a. Excludes1

A type 1 Excludes note is a pure excludes note. It means "NOT CODED HERE!" An Excludes1 note indicates that the code excluded should never be used at the same time as the code above the Excludes1 note. An Excludes1 is used when two conditions cannot occur together, such as a congenital form versus an acquired form of the same condition.

An exception to the Excludes1 definition is the circumstance when the two conditions are unrelated to each other. If it is not clear whether the two conditions involving an Excludes1 note are related or not, query the provider. For example, code F45.8, Other somatoform disorders, has an Excludes1 note for "sleep related teeth grinding (G47.63)," because "teeth grinding" is an inclusion term under F45.8. Only one of these two codes should be assigned for teeth grinding. However psychogenic dysmenorrhea is also an inclusion term under F45.8, and a patient could have both this condition and sleep related teeth grinding. In this case, the two conditions are clearly unrelated to each other, and so it would be appropriate to report F45.8 and G47.63 together.

b. Excludes2

A Type 2 Excludes note represents "Not included here." An excludes2 note indicates that the condition excluded is not part of the condition represented by the code, but a patient may have both conditions at the same time. When an Excludes2 note appears under a code, it is acceptable to use both the code and the excluded code together, when appropriate.

13. Etiology/manifestation convention ("code first", "use additional code" and "in diseases classified elsewhere" notes)

Certain conditions have both an underlying etiology and multiple body system manifestations due to the underlying etiology. For such conditions, the ICD-10-CM has a coding convention that requires the underlying condition be sequenced first, **if applicable,** followed by the manifestation. Wherever such a combination exists, there is a "use additional code" note at the etiology code, and a "code first" note at the manifestation code. These instructional notes indicate the proper sequencing order of the codes, etiology followed by manifestation.

In most cases the manifestation codes will have in the code title, "in diseases classified elsewhere." Codes with this title are a component of the etiology/ manifestation convention. The code title indicates that it is a manifestation code. "In diseases classified elsewhere" codes are never permitted to be used as first-listed or principal diagnosis codes. They must be used in conjunction with an underlying condition code and they must be listed following the underlying condition. See category F02, Dementia in other diseases classified elsewhere, for an example of this convention.

There are manifestation codes that do not have "in diseases classified elsewhere" in the title. For such codes, there is a "use additional code" note at the etiology code and a "code first" note at the manifestation code and the rules for sequencing apply.

In addition to the notes in the Tabular List, these conditions also have a specific Alphabetic Index entry structure. In the Alphabetic Index both conditions are listed together with the etiology code first followed by the manifestation codes in brackets. The code in brackets is always to be sequenced second.

An example of the etiology/manifestation convention is dementia in Parkinson's disease. In the Alphabetic Index, code G20 is listed first, followed by code F02.80 or F02.81 in brackets. Code G20 represents the underlying etiology, Parkinson's disease, and must be sequenced first, whereas codes F02.80 and F02.81 represent the manifestation of dementia in diseases classified elsewhere, with or without behavioral disturbance.

"Code first" and "Use additional code" notes are also used as sequencing rules in the classification for certain codes that are not part of an etiology/manifestation combination.

See Section I.B.7. Multiple coding for a single condition.

14. "And"

The word "and" should be interpreted to mean either "and" or "or" when it appears in a title.

For example, cases of "tuberculosis of bones", "tuberculosis of joints" and "tuberculosis of bones and joints" are classified to subcategory A18.0, Tuberculosis of bones and joints.

15. "With"

The word "with" should be interpreted to mean "associated with" or "due to" when it appears in a code title, the Alphabetic Index, or an instructional note in the Tabular List. **The classification presumes a causal relationship between the two conditions linked by these terms in the Alphabetic Index or Tabular List. These conditions should be coded as related even in the absence of provider documentation explicitly linking them, unless the documentation clearly states the conditions are unrelated. For conditions not specifically linked by these relational terms in the classification, provider documentation must link the conditions in order to code them as related.**

The word "with" in the Alphabetic Index is sequenced immediately following the main term, not in alphabetical order.

16. "See" and "See Also"

The "see" instruction following a main term in the Alphabetic Index indicates that another term should be referenced. It is necessary to go to the main term referenced with the "see" note to locate the correct code.

A "see also" instruction following a main term in the Alphabetic Index instructs that there is another main term that may also be referenced that may provide additional Alphabetic Index entries that may be useful. It is not necessary to follow the "see also" note when the original main term provides the necessary code.

17. "Code also" note

A "code also" note instructs that two codes may be required to fully describe a condition, but this note does not provide sequencing direction.

18. Default codes

A code listed next to a main term in the ICD-10-CM Alphabetic Index is referred to as a default code. The default code represents that condition that is most commonly associated with the main term, or is the unspecified code for the condition. If a condition is documented in a medical record (for example, appendicitis) without any additional information, such as acute or chronic, the default code should be assigned.

19. Code assignment and Clinical Criteria

The assignment of a diagnosis code is based on the provider's diagnostic statement that the condition exists. The provider's statement that the patient has a particular condition is sufficient. Code assignment is not based on clinical criteria used by the provider to establish the diagnosis.

B. General Coding Guidelines

1. Locating a code in the ICD-10-CM

To select a code in the classification that corresponds to a diagnosis or reason for visit documented in a medical record, first locate the term in the Alphabetic Index, and then verify the code in the Tabular List. Read and be guided by instructional notations that appear in both the Alphabetic Index and the Tabular List.

It is essential to use both the Alphabetic Index and Tabular List when locating and assigning a code. The Alphabetic Index does not always provide the full code. Selection of the full code, including laterality and any applicable 7th character can only be done in the Tabular List. A dash (-) at the end of an Alphabetic Index entry indicates that additional characters are required. Even if a dash is not included at the Alphabetic Index entry, it is necessary to refer to the Tabular List to verify that no 7th character is required.

2. **Level of Detail in Coding**
Diagnosis codes are to be used and reported at their highest number of characters available.

ICD-10-CM diagnosis codes are composed of codes with 3, 4, 5, 6 or 7 characters. Codes with three characters are included in ICD-10-CM as the heading of a category of codes that may be further subdivided by the use of fourth and/or fifth characters and/or sixth characters, which provide greater detail.

A three-character code is to be used only if it is not further subdivided. A code is invalid if it has not been coded to the full number of characters required for that code, including the 7th character, if applicable.

3. **Code or codes from A00.0 through T88.9, Z00-Z99.8**
The appropriate code or codes from A00.0 through T88.9, Z00-Z99.8 must be used to identify diagnoses, symptoms, conditions, problems, complaints or other reason(s) for the encounter/visit.

4. **Signs and symptoms**
Codes that describe symptoms and signs, as opposed to diagnoses, are acceptable for reporting purposes when a related definitive diagnosis has not been established (confirmed) by the provider. Chapter 18 of ICD-10-CM, Symptoms, Signs, and Abnormal Clinical and Laboratory Findings, Not Elsewhere Classified (codes R00.0 - R99) contains many, but not all codes for symptoms.

See Section I.B.18 Use of Signs/Symptom/ Unspecified Codes

5. **Conditions that are an integral part of a disease process**
Signs and symptoms that are associated routinely with a disease process should not be assigned as additional codes, unless otherwise instructed by the classification.

6. **Conditions that are not an integral part of a disease process**
Additional signs and symptoms that may not be associated routinely with a disease process should be coded when present.

7. **Multiple coding for a single condition**
In addition to the etiology/manifestation convention that requires two codes to fully describe a single condition that affects multiple body systems, there are other single conditions that also require more than one code. "Use additional code" notes are found in the Tabular List at codes that are not part of an etiology/manifestation pair where a secondary code is useful to fully describe a condition. The sequencing rule is the same as the etiology/manifestation pair, "use additional code" indicates that a secondary code should be added.

For example, for bacterial infections that are not included in chapter 1, a secondary code from category B95, Streptococcus, Staphylococcus, and Enterococcus, as the cause of diseases classified elsewhere, or B96, Other bacterial agents as the cause of diseases classified elsewhere, may be required to identify the bacterial organism causing the infection. A "use additional code" note will normally be found at the infectious disease code, indicating a need for the organism code to be added as a secondary code.

"Code first" notes are also under certain codes that are not specifically manifestation codes but may be due to an underlying cause. When there is a "code first" note and an underlying condition is present, the underlying condition should be sequenced first.

"Code, if applicable, any causal condition first," notes indicate that this code may be assigned as a principal diagnosis when the causal condition is unknown or not applicable. If a causal condition is known, then the code for that condition should be sequenced as the principal or first-listed diagnosis.

Multiple codes may be needed for sequela, complication codes and obstetric codes to more fully describe a condition. See the specific guidelines for these conditions for further instruction.

8. **Acute and Chronic Conditions**
If the same condition is described as both acute (subacute) and chronic, and separate subentries exist in the Alphabetic Index at the same indentation level, code both and sequence the acute (subacute) code first.

9. **Combination Code**
A combination code is a single code used to classify:

Two diagnoses, or

A diagnosis with an associated secondary process (manifestation)

A diagnosis with an associated complication

Combination codes are identified by referring to subterm entries in the Alphabetic Index and by reading the inclusion and exclusion notes in the Tabular List.

Assign only the combination code when that code fully identifies the diagnostic conditions involved or when the Alphabetic Index so directs. Multiple coding should not be used when the classification provides a combination code that clearly identifies all of the elements documented in the diagnosis. When the combination code lacks necessary specificity in describing the manifestation or complication, an additional code should be used as a secondary code.

10. **Sequela (Late Effects)**
A sequela is the residual effect (condition produced) after the acute phase of an illness or injury has terminated. There is no time limit on when a sequela code can be used. The residual may

be apparent early, such as in cerebral infarction, or it may occur months or years later, such as that due to a previous injury. Examples of sequela include: scar formation resulting from a burn, deviated septum due to a nasal fracture, and infertility due to tubal occlusion from old tuberculosis. Coding of sequela generally requires two codes sequenced in the following order: the condition or nature of the sequela is sequenced first. The sequela code is sequenced second.

An exception to the above guidelines are those instances where the code for the sequela is followed by a manifestation code identified in the Tabular List and title, or the sequela code has been expanded (at the fourth, fifth or sixth character levels) to include the manifestation(s). The code for the acute phase of an illness or injury that led to the sequela is never used with a code for the late effect.

See Section I.C.9. Sequelae of cerebrovascular disease

See Section I.C.15. Sequelae of complication of pregnancy, childbirth and the puerperium

See Section I.C.19. Application of 7th characters for Chapter 19

11. Impending or Threatened Condition

Code any condition described at the time of discharge as "impending" or "threatened" as follows:

If it did occur, code as confirmed diagnosis.

If it did not occur, reference the Alphabetic Index to determine if the condition has a subentry term for "impending" or "threatened" and also reference main term entries for "Impending" and for "Threatened."

If the subterms are listed, assign the given code.

If the subterms are not listed, code the existing underlying condition(s) and not the condition described as impending or threatened.

12. Reporting Same Diagnosis Code More than Once

Each unique ICD-10-CM diagnosis code may be reported only once for an encounter. This applies to bilateral conditions when there are no distinct codes identifying laterality or two different conditions classified to the same ICD-10-CM diagnosis code.

13. Laterality

Some ICD-10-CM codes indicate laterality, specifying whether the condition occurs on the left, right or is bilateral. If no bilateral code is provided and the condition is bilateral, assign separate codes for both the left and right side. If the side is not identified in the medical record, assign the code for the unspecified side.

When a patient has a bilateral condition and each side is treated during separate encounters, assign the "bilateral" code (as the condition still exists on both sides), including for the encounter to treat the first side. For the second encounter for treatment after one side has previously been treated and the condition no longer exists on that side, assign the appropriate unilateral code for the side where the condition still exists (e.g., cataract surgery performed on each eye in separate encounters). The bilateral code would not be assigned for the subsequent encounter, as the patient no longer has the condition in the previously-treated site. If the treatment on the first side did not completely resolve the condition, then the bilateral code would still be appropriate.

14. Documentation for BMI, *Depth of* Non-pressure ulcers, Pressure Ulcer Stages, Coma Scale, *and NIH Stroke Scale*

For the Body Mass Index (BMI), depth of non-pressure chronic ulcers, pressure ulcer stage, **coma scale, and NIH stroke scale (NIHSS) codes,** code assignment may be based on medical record documentation from clinicians who are not the patient's provider (i.e., physician or other qualified healthcare practitioner legally accountable for establishing the patient's diagnosis), since this information is typically documented by other clinicians involved in the care of the patient (e.g., a dietitian often documents the BMI, a nurse often documents the pressure ulcer stages**, and an emergency medical technician often documents the coma scale**). However, the associated diagnosis (such as overweight, obesity, **acute stroke,** or pressure ulcer) must be documented by the patient's provider. If there is conflicting medical record documentation, either from the same clinician or different clinicians, the patient's attending provider should be queried for clarification.

The BMI**, coma scale, and NIHSS** codes should only be reported as secondary diagnoses.

15. Syndromes

Follow the Alphabetic Index guidance when coding syndromes. In the absence of Alphabetic Index guidance, assign codes for the documented manifestations of the syndrome. Additional codes for manifestations that are not an integral part of the disease process may also be assigned when the condition does not have a unique code.

16. Documentation of Complications of Care

Code assignment is based on the provider's documentation of the relationship between the condition and the care or procedure**, unless otherwise instructed by the classification.** The guideline extends to any complications of care, regardless of the chapter the code is located in. It is important to note that not all conditions that occur during or following medical care or surgery are classified as complications. There must be a cause-and-effect relationship between the care provided and the condition, and an indication in the documentation that it is a complication. Query the provider for clarification, if the complication is not clearly documented.

17. Borderline Diagnosis

If the provider documents a "borderline" diagnosis at the time of discharge, the diagnosis is coded as confirmed, unless the classification provides a specific entry (e.g., borderline diabetes). If a borderline condition has a specific index entry in ICD-10-CM, it should be coded as such. Since borderline conditions are not uncertain diagnoses, no distinction is made between the care setting (inpatient versus outpatient). Whenever the documentation is unclear regarding a borderline condition, coders are encouraged to query for clarification.

18. **Use of Sign/Symptom/Unspecified Codes**
Sign/symptom and "unspecified" codes have acceptable, even necessary, uses. While specific diagnosis codes should be reported when they are supported by the available medical record documentation and clinical knowledge of the patient's health condition, there are instances when signs/symptoms or unspecified codes are the best choices for accurately reflecting the healthcare encounter. Each healthcare encounter should be coded to the level of certainty known for that encounter.

If a definitive diagnosis has not been established by the end of the encounter, it is appropriate to report codes for sign(s) and/or symptom(s) in lieu of a definitive diagnosis. When sufficient clinical information isn't known or available about a particular health condition to assign a more specific code, it is acceptable to report the appropriate "unspecified" code (e.g., a diagnosis of pneumonia has been determined, but not the specific type). Unspecified codes should be reported when they are the codes that most accurately reflect what is known about the patient's condition at the time of that particular encounter. It would be inappropriate to select a specific code that is not supported by the medical record documentation or conduct medically unnecessary diagnostic testing in order to determine a more specific code.

C. **Chapter-Specific Coding Guidelines**
In addition to general coding guidelines, there are guidelines for specific diagnoses and/or conditions in the classification. Unless otherwise indicated, these guidelines apply to all health care settings. Please refer to Section II for guidelines on the selection of principal diagnosis.

1. **Chapter 1: Certain Infectious and Parasitic Diseases (A00-B99)**

a. **Human Immunodeficiency Virus (HIV) Infections**

1) **Code only confirmed cases**
Code only confirmed cases of HIV infection/illness. This is an exception to the hospital inpatient guideline Section II, H.

In this context, "confirmation" does not require documentation of positive serology or culture for HIV; the provider's diagnostic statement that the patient is HIV positive, or has an HIV-related illness is sufficient.

2) **Selection and sequencing of HIV codes**

(a) **Patient admitted for HIV-related condition**
If a patient is admitted for an HIV-related condition, the principal diagnosis should be B20, Human immunodeficiency virus [HIV] disease followed by additional diagnosis codes for all reported HIV-related conditions.

(b) **Patient with HIV disease admitted for unrelated condition**
If a patient with HIV disease is admitted for an unrelated condition (such as a traumatic injury), the code for the unrelated condition (e.g., the nature of injury code) should be the principal diagnosis. Other diagnoses would be B20 followed by additional diagnosis codes for all reported HIV-related conditions.

(c) **Whether the patient is newly diagnosed**
Whether the patient is newly diagnosed or has had previous admissions/encounters for HIV conditions is irrelevant to the sequencing decision.

(d) **Asymptomatic human immunodeficiency virus**
Z21, Asymptomatic human immunodeficiency virus [HIV] infection status, is to be applied when the patient without any documentation of symptoms is listed as being "HIV positive," "known HIV," "HIV test positive," or similar terminology. Do not use this code if the term "AIDS" is used or if the patient is treated for any HIV-related illness or is described as having any condition(s) resulting from his/her HIV positive status; use B20 in these cases.

(e) **Patients with inconclusive HIV serology**
Patients with inconclusive HIV serology, but no definitive diagnosis or manifestations of the illness, may be assigned code R75, Inconclusive laboratory evidence of human immunodeficiency virus [HIV].

(f) **Previously diagnosed HIV-related illness**
Patients with any known prior diagnosis of an HIV-related illness should be coded to B20. Once a patient has developed an HIV-related illness, the patient should always be assigned code B20 on every subsequent admission/encounter. Patients previously diagnosed with any HIV illness (B20) should never be assigned to R75 or Z21, Asymptomatic human immunodeficiency virus [HIV] infection status.

(g) **HIV Infection in Pregnancy, Childbirth and the Puerperium**
During pregnancy, childbirth or the puerperium, a patient admitted (or presenting for a health care encounter) because of an HIV-related illness should receive a principal diagnosis code of O98.7-, Human immunodeficiency [HIV] disease complicating pregnancy, childbirth and the puerperium, followed by B20 and the code(s) for the HIV-related illness(es). Codes from Chapter 15 always take sequencing priority.

Patients with asymptomatic HIV infection status admitted (or presenting for a health care encounter) during pregnancy, childbirth, or the puerperium should receive codes of O98.7- and Z21.

(h) Encounters for testing for HIV

If a patient is being seen to determine his/her HIV status, use code Z11.4, Encounter for screening for human immunodeficiency virus [HIV]. Use additional codes for any associated high risk behavior.

If a patient with signs or symptoms is being seen for HIV testing, code the signs and symptoms. An additional counseling code Z71.7, Human immunodeficiency virus [HIV] counseling, may be used if counseling is provided during the encounter for the test.

When a patient returns to be informed of his/her HIV test results and the test result is negative, use code Z71.7, Human immunodeficiency virus [HIV] counseling.

If the results are positive, see previous guidelines and assign codes as appropriate.

b. Infectious agents as the cause of diseases classified to other chapters

Certain infections are classified in chapters other than Chapter 1 and no organism is identified as part of the infection code. In these instances, it is necessary to use an additional code from Chapter 1 to identify the organism. A code from category B95, Streptococcus, Staphylococcus, and Enterococcus as the cause of diseases classified to other chapters, B96, Other bacterial agents as the cause of diseases classified to other chapters, or B97, Viral agents as the cause of diseases classified to other chapters, is to be used as an additional code to identify the organism. An instructional note will be found at the infection code advising that an additional organism code is required.

c. Infections resistant to antibiotics

Many bacterial infections are resistant to current antibiotics. It is necessary to identify all infections documented as antibiotic resistant. Assign a code from category Z16, Resistance to antimicrobial drugs, following the infection code only if the infection code does not identify drug resistance.

d. Sepsis, Severe Sepsis, and Septic Shock

1) Coding of Sepsis and Severe Sepsis

(a) Sepsis

For a diagnosis of sepsis, assign the appropriate code for the underlying systemic infection. If the type of infection or causal organism is not further specified, assign code A41.9, Sepsis, unspecified organism.

A code from subcategory R65.2, Severe sepsis, should not be assigned unless severe sepsis or an associated acute organ dysfunction is documented.

(i) Negative or inconclusive blood cultures and sepsis
Negative or inconclusive blood cultures do not preclude a diagnosis of sepsis in patients with clinical evidence of the condition, however, the provider should be queried.

(ii) Urosepsis
The term urosepsis is a nonspecific term. It is not to be considered synonymous with sepsis. It has no default code in the Alphabetic Index. Should a provider use this term, he/she must be queried for clarification.

(iii) Sepsis with organ dysfunction
If a patient has sepsis and associated acute organ dysfunction or multiple organ dysfunction (MOD), follow the instructions for coding severe sepsis.

(iv) Acute organ dysfunction that is not clearly associated with the sepsis
If a patient has sepsis and an acute organ dysfunction, but the medical record documentation indicates that the acute organ dysfunction is related to a medical condition other than the sepsis, do not assign a code from subcategory R65.2, Severe sepsis. An acute organ dysfunction must be associated with the sepsis in order to assign the severe sepsis code. If the documentation is not clear as to whether an acute organ dysfunction is related to the sepsis or another medical condition, query the provider.

(b) Severe sepsis

The coding of severe sepsis requires a minimum of 2 codes: first a code for the underlying systemic infection, followed by a code from subcategory R65.2, Severe sepsis. If the causal organism is not documented, assign code A41.9, Sepsis, unspecified organism, for the infection. Additional code(s) for the associated acute organ dysfunction are also required.

Due to the complex nature of severe sepsis, some cases may require querying the provider prior to assignment of the codes.

2) Septic shock

(a) Septic shock generally refers to circulatory failure associated with severe sepsis, and therefore, it represents a type of acute organ dysfunction.

For all cases of septic shock, the code for the systemic infection should be sequenced first, followed by code R65.21, Severe sepsis with septic shock or code T81.12, Postprocedural septic shock. Any additional codes for the other acute organ dysfunctions should also be assigned. As noted in the sequencing instructions in the Tabular List, the code for septic shock cannot be assigned as a principal diagnosis.

3) Sequencing of severe sepsis

If severe sepsis is present on admission, and meets the definition of principal diagnosis, the underlying systemic infection should be assigned as principal diagnosis followed by the appropriate code from subcategory R65.2 as required by the sequencing rules in the Tabular List. A code from subcategory R65.2 can never be assigned as a principal diagnosis.

When severe sepsis develops during an encounter (it was not present on admission) the underlying systemic infection and the appropriate code from subcategory R65.2 should be assigned as secondary diagnoses.

Severe sepsis may be present on admission but the diagnosis may not be confirmed until sometime after admission. If the documentation is not clear whether severe sepsis was present on admission, the provider should be queried.

4) Sepsis and severe sepsis with a localized infection

If the reason for admission is both sepsis or severe sepsis and a localized infection, such as pneumonia or cellulitis, a code(s) for the underlying systemic infection should be assigned first and the code for the localized infection should be assigned as a secondary diagnosis. If the patient has severe sepsis, a code from subcategory R65.2 should also be assigned as a secondary diagnosis. If the patient is admitted with a localized infection, such as pneumonia, and sepsis/severe sepsis doesn't develop until after admission, the localized infection should be assigned first, followed by the appropriate sepsis/severe sepsis codes.

5) Sepsis due to a postprocedural infection

(a) Documentation of causal relationship

As with all postprocedural complications, code assignment is based on the provider's documentation of the relationship between the infection and the procedure.

(b) Sepsis due to a postprocedural infection

For such cases, the postprocedural infection code, such as, T80.2, Infections following infusion, transfusion, and therapeutic injection, T81.4, Infection following a procedure, T88.0, Infection following immunization, or O86.0, Infection of obstetric surgical wound, should be coded first, followed by the code for the specific infection. If the patient has severe sepsis the appropriate code from subcategory R65.2 should also be assigned with the additional code(s) for any acute organ dysfunction.

(c) Postprocedural infection and postprocedural septic shock

In cases where a postprocedural infection has occurred and has resulted in severe sepsis the code for the precipitating complication such as code T81.4, Infection following a procedure, or O86.0, Infection of obstetrical surgical wound should be coded first followed by code R65.20, Severe sepsis without septic shock. A Code for the systemic infection should also be assigned.

If a postprocedural infection has resulted in postprocedural septic shock, the code for the precipitating complication such as code T81.4, Infection following a procedure, or O86.0, Infection of obstetrical surgical wound should be coded first followed by code T81.12-, Postprocedural septic shock. A code for the systemic infection should also be assigned.

6) Sepsis and severe sepsis associated with a noninfectious process (condition)

In some cases a noninfectious process (condition), such as trauma, may lead to an infection which can result in sepsis or severe sepsis. If sepsis or severe sepsis is documented as associated with a noninfectious condition, such as a burn or serious injury, and this condition meets the definition for principal diagnosis, the code for the noninfectious condition should be sequenced first, followed by the code for the resulting infection. If severe sepsis is present, a code from subcategory R65.2 should also be assigned with any associated organ dysfunction(s) codes. It is not necessary to assign a code from subcategory R65.1, Systemic inflammatory response syndrome (SIRS) of non-infectious origin, for these cases.

If the infection meets the definition of principal diagnosis it should be sequenced before the non-infectious condition. When both the associated non-infectious condition and the infection meet the definition of principal diagnosis either may be assigned as principal diagnosis.

Only one code from category R65, Symptoms and signs specifically associated with systemic inflammation and infection, should be assigned. Therefore, when a non-infectious condition leads to an infection resulting in severe sepsis, assign the appropriate code from subcategory R65.2, Severe sepsis. Do not additionally assign a code from subcategory R65.1, Systemic inflammatory response syndrome (SIRS) of non-infectious origin.

See Section I.C.18. SIRS due to non-infectious process

7) Sepsis and septic shock complicating abortion, pregnancy, childbirth, and the puerperium

See Section I.C.15. Sepsis and septic shock complicating abortion, pregnancy, childbirth and the puerperium

8) Newborn sepsis

See Section I.C.16. f. Bacterial sepsis of Newborn

e. Methicillin Resistant Staphylococcus aureus (MRSA) Conditions

1) Selection and sequencing of MRSA codes

(a) Combination codes for MRSA infection

When a patient is diagnosed with an infection that is due to methicillin resistant *Staphylococcus aureus* (MRSA), and that infection has a combination code that includes the causal organism (e.g., sepsis, pneumonia) assign the appropriate combination code for the condition (e.g., code A41.02, Sepsis due to Methicillin resistant Staphylococcus aureus or code J15.212, Pneumonia due to Methicillin resistant Staphylococcus aureus). Do not assign code B95.62, Methicillin resistant Staphylococcus aureus infection as the cause of diseases classified elsewhere, as an additional code because the combination code includes the type of infection and the MRSA organism. Do not assign a code from subcategory Z16.11, Resistance to penicillins, as an additional diagnosis.

See Section C.1. for instructions on coding and sequencing of sepsis and severe sepsis.

(b) Other codes for MRSA infection

When there is documentation of a current infection (e.g., wound infection, stitch abscess, urinary tract infection) due to MRSA, and that infection does not have a combination code that includes the causal organism, assign the appropriate code to identify the condition along with code B95.62, Methicillin resistant Staphylococcus aureus infection as the cause of diseases classified elsewhere for the MRSA infection. Do not assign a code from subcategory Z16.11, Resistance to penicillins.

(c) Methicillin susceptible Staphylococcus aureus (MSSA) and MRSA colonization

The condition or state of being colonized or carrying MSSA or MRSA is called colonization or carriage, while an individual person is described as being colonized or being a carrier. Colonization means that MSSA or MSRA is present on or in the body without necessarily causing illness. A positive MRSA colonization test might be documented by the provider as "MRSA screen positive" or "MRSA nasal swab positive".

Assign code Z22.322, Carrier or suspected carrier of Methicillin resistant Staphylococcus aureus, for patients documented as having MRSA colonization. Assign code Z22.321, Carrier or suspected carrier of Methicillin susceptible Staphylococcus aureus, for patient documented as having MSSA colonization. Colonization is not necessarily indicative of a disease process or as the cause of a specific condition the patient may have unless documented as such by the provider.

(d) MRSA colonization and infection

If a patient is documented as having both MRSA colonization and infection during a hospital admission, code Z22.322, Carrier or suspected carrier of Methicillin resistant Staphylococcus aureus, and a code for the MRSA infection may both be assigned.

f. Zika virus infections

1) Code only confirmed cases

Code only a confirmed diagnosis of Zika virus (A92.5, Zika virus disease) as documented by the provider. This is an exception to the hospital inpatient guideline Section II, H.

In this context, "confirmation" does not require documentation of the type of test performed; the physician's diagnostic statement that the condition is confirmed is sufficient. This code should be assigned regardless of the stated mode of transmission.

If the provider documents "suspected", "possible" or "probable" Zika, do not assign code A92.5. Assign a code(s) explaining the reason for encounter (such as fever, rash, or joint pain) or Z20.828, Contact with and (suspected) exposure to other viral communicable diseases.

2. Chapter 2: Neoplasms (C00-D49)

General guidelines

Chapter 2 of the ICD-10-CM contains the codes for most benign and all malignant neoplasms. Certain benign neoplasms, such as prostatic adenomas, may be found in the specific body system chapters. To properly code a neoplasm it is necessary to determine from the record if the neoplasm is benign, in-situ, malignant, or of uncertain histologic behavior. If malignant, any secondary (metastatic) sites should also be determined.

Primary malignant neoplasms overlapping site boundaries

A primary malignant neoplasm that overlaps two or more contiguous (next to each other) sites should be classified to the subcategory/code .8 ('overlapping lesion'), unless the combination is specifically indexed elsewhere. For multiple neoplasms of the same site that are not contiguous such as tumors in different quadrants of the same breast, codes for each site should be assigned.

Malignant neoplasm of ectopic tissue

Malignant neoplasms of ectopic tissue are to be coded to the site of origin mentioned, e.g., ectopic pancreatic malignant neoplasms involving the stomach are coded to pancreas, unspecified (C25.9).

The neoplasm table in the Alphabetic Index should be referenced first. However, if the histological term is documented, that term should be referenced first, rather than going immediately to the Neoplasm Table, in order to determine which column in the Neoplasm Table is appropriate. For example, if the documentation indicates "adenoma," refer to the term in the Alphabetic Index to review the entries under this term and the instructional note to "see also neoplasm, by site, benign." The table provides the proper code based on the type of neoplasm and the site. It is important to select the proper column in the table that corresponds to the type of neoplasm. The Tabular List should then be referenced to verify that the correct code has been selected from the table and that a more specific site code does not exist.

See Section I.C.21. Factors influencing health status and contact with health services, Status, for information regarding Z15.0, codes for genetic susceptibility to cancer.

a. Treatment directed at the malignancy
If the treatment is directed at the malignancy, designate the malignancy as the principal diagnosis.

The only exception to this guideline is if a patient admission/encounter is solely for the administration of chemotherapy, immunotherapy or radiation therapy, assign the appropriate Z51.— code as the first-listed or principal diagnosis, and the diagnosis or problem for which the service is being performed as a secondary diagnosis.

b. Treatment of secondary site
When a patient is admitted because of a primary neoplasm with metastasis and treatment is directed toward the secondary site only, the secondary neoplasm is designated as the principal diagnosis even though the primary malignancy is still present.

c. Coding and sequencing of complications
Coding and sequencing of complications associated with the malignancies or with the therapy thereof are subject to the following guidelines:

1) Anemia associated with malignancy
When admission/encounter is for management of an anemia associated with the malignancy, and the treatment is only for anemia, the appropriate code for the malignancy is sequenced as the principal or first-listed diagnosis followed by the appropriate code for the anemia (such as code D63.Ø, Anemia in neoplastic disease).

2) Anemia associated with chemotherapy, immunotherapy and radiation therapy
When the admission/encounter is for management of an anemia associated with an adverse effect of the administration of chemotherapy or immunotherapy and the only treatment is for the anemia, the anemia code is sequenced first followed by the appropriate codes for the neoplasm and the adverse effect (T45.1X5, Adverse effect of antineoplastic and immunosuppressive drugs).

When the admission/encounter is for management of an anemia associated with an adverse effect of radiotherapy, the anemia code should be sequenced first, followed by the appropriate neoplasm code and code Y84.2, Radiological procedure and radiotherapy as the cause of abnormal reaction of the patient, or of later complication, without mention of misadventure at the time of the procedure.

3) Management of dehydration due to the malignancy
When the admission/encounter is for management of dehydration due to the malignancy and only the dehydration is being treated (intravenous rehydration), the dehydration is sequenced first, followed by the code(s) for the malignancy.

4) Treatment of a complication resulting from a surgical procedure
When the admission/encounter is for treatment of a complication resulting from a surgical procedure, designate the complication as the principal or first-listed diagnosis if treatment is directed at resolving the complication.

d. Primary malignancy previously excised
When a primary malignancy has been previously excised or eradicated from its site and there is no further treatment directed to that site and there is no evidence of any existing primary malignancy, a code from category Z85, Personal history of malignant neoplasm, should be used to indicate the former site of the malignancy. Any mention of extension, invasion, or metastasis to another site is coded as a secondary malignant neoplasm to that site. The secondary site may be the principal or first-listed with the Z85 code used as a secondary code.

e. Admissions/Encounters involving chemotherapy, immunotherapy and radiation therapy

1) Episode of care involves surgical removal of neoplasm
When an episode of care involves the surgical removal of a neoplasm, primary or secondary site, followed by adjunct chemotherapy or radiation treatment during the same episode of care, the code for the neoplasm should be assigned as principal or first-listed diagnosis.

2) Patient admission/encounter solely for administration of chemotherapy, immunotherapy and radiation therapy
If a patient admission/encounter is solely for the administration of chemotherapy, immunotherapy or radiation therapy assign code Z51.Ø, Encounter for antineoplastic radiation therapy, or Z51.11, Encounter for antineoplastic chemotherapy, or Z51.12, Encounter for antineoplastic immunotherapy as the first-listed or principal diagnosis. If a patient receives more than one of these therapies during the same admission more than one of these codes may be assigned, in any sequence.

The malignancy for which the therapy is being administered should be assigned as a secondary diagnosis.

3) Patient admitted for radiation therapy, chemotherapy or immunotherapy and develops complications
When a patient is admitted for the purpose of radiotherapy, immunotherapy or chemotherapy and develops complications such as uncontrolled nausea and vomiting or dehydration, the principal or first-listed diagnosis is Z51.Ø, Encounter for antineoplastic radiation therapy, or Z51.11, Encounter for antineoplastic chemotherapy, or Z51.12, Encounter for antineoplastic immunotherapy followed by any codes for the complications.

f. Admission/encounter to determine extent of malignancy
When the reason for admission/encounter is to determine the extent of the malignancy, or for a procedure such as paracentesis or thoracentesis, the primary malignancy or appropriate metastatic site is designated as the principal or first-listed diagnosis, even though chemotherapy or radiotherapy is administered.

g. Symptoms, signs, and abnormal findings listed in Chapter 18 associated with neoplasms

Symptoms, signs, and ill-defined conditions listed in Chapter 18 characteristic of, or associated with, an existing primary or secondary site malignancy cannot be used to replace the malignancy as principal or first-listed diagnosis, regardless of the number of admissions or encounters for treatment and care of the neoplasm.

See section I.C.21. Factors influencing health status and contact with health services, Encounter for prophylactic organ removal.

h. Admission/encounter for pain control/management

See Section I.C.6. for information on coding admission/encounter for pain control/management.

i. Malignancy in two or more noncontiguous sites

A patient may have more than one malignant tumor in the same organ. These tumors may represent different primaries or metastatic disease, depending on the site. Should the documentation be unclear, the provider should be queried as to the status of each tumor so that the correct codes can be assigned.

j. Disseminated malignant neoplasm, unspecified

Code C8Ø.Ø, Disseminated malignant neoplasm, unspecified, is for use only in those cases where the patient has advanced metastatic disease and no known primary or secondary sites are specified. It should not be used in place of assigning codes for the primary site and all known secondary sites.

k. Malignant neoplasm without specification of site

Code C8Ø.1, Malignant (primary) neoplasm, unspecified, equates to Cancer, unspecified. This code should only be used when no determination can be made as to the primary site of a malignancy. This code should rarely be used in the inpatient setting.

l. Sequencing of neoplasm codes

1) Encounter for treatment of primary malignancy

If the reason for the encounter is for treatment of a primary malignancy, assign the malignancy as the principal/first-listed diagnosis. The primary site is to be sequenced first, followed by any metastatic sites.

2) Encounter for treatment of secondary malignancy

When an encounter is for a primary malignancy with metastasis and treatment is directed toward the metastatic (secondary) site(s) only, the metastatic site(s) is designated as the principal/first-listed diagnosis. The primary malignancy is coded as an additional code.

3) Malignant neoplasm in a pregnant patient

When a pregnant woman has a malignant neoplasm, a code from subcategory O9A.1-, Malignant neoplasm complicating pregnancy, childbirth, and the puerperium, should be sequenced first, followed by the appropriate code from Chapter 2 to indicate the type of neoplasm.

4) Encounter for complication associated with a neoplasm

When an encounter is for management of a complication associated with a neoplasm, such as dehydration, and the treatment is only for the complication, the complication is coded first, followed by the appropriate code(s) for the neoplasm.

The exception to this guideline is anemia. When the admission/encounter is for management of an anemia associated with the malignancy, and the treatment is only for anemia, the appropriate code for the malignancy is sequenced as the principal or first-listed diagnosis followed by code D63.Ø, Anemia in neoplastic disease.

5) Complication from surgical procedure for treatment of a neoplasm

When an encounter is for treatment of a complication resulting from a surgical procedure performed for the treatment of the neoplasm, designate the complication as the principal/first-listed diagnosis. See guideline regarding the coding of a current malignancy versus personal history to determine if the code for the neoplasm should also be assigned.

6) Pathologic fracture due to a neoplasm

When an encounter is for a pathological fracture due to a neoplasm, and the focus of treatment is the fracture, a code from subcategory M84.5, Pathological fracture in neoplastic disease, should be sequenced first, followed by the code for the neoplasm.

If the focus of treatment is the neoplasm with an associated pathological fracture, the neoplasm code should be sequenced first, followed by a code from M84.5 for the pathological fracture.

m. Current malignancy versus personal history of malignancy

When a primary malignancy has been excised but further treatment, such as an additional surgery for the malignancy, radiation therapy or chemotherapy is directed to that site, the primary malignancy code should be used until treatment is completed.

When a primary malignancy has been previously excised or eradicated from its site, there is no further treatment (of the malignancy) directed to that site, and there is no evidence of any existing primary malignancy, a code from category Z85, Personal history of malignant neoplasm, should be used to indicate the former site of the malignancy.

See Section I.C.21. Factors influencing health status and contact with health services, History (of)

n. Leukemia, Multiple Myeloma, and Malignant Plasma Cell Neoplasms in remission versus personal history

The categories for leukemia, and category C9Ø, Multiple myeloma and malignant plasma cell neoplasms, have codes indicating whether or not the leukemia has achieved remission. There are also codes Z85.6, Personal history of leukemia, and Z85.79, Personal history of other malignant neoplasms of lymphoid, hematopoietic and related tissues. If the documentation is unclear, as to whether the leukemia has achieved remission, the provider should be queried.

See Section I.C.21. Factors influencing health status and contact with health services, History (of)

o. Aftercare following surgery for neoplasm

See Section I.C.21. Factors influencing health status and contact with health services, Aftercare

p. Follow-up care for completed treatment of a malignancy

See Section I.C.21. Factors influencing health status and contact with health services, Follow-up

q. Prophylactic organ removal for prevention of malignancy

See Section I.C. 21, Factors influencing health status and contact with health services, Prophylactic organ removal

r. Malignant neoplasm associated with transplanted organ

A malignant neoplasm of a transplanted organ should be coded as a transplant complication. Assign first the appropriate code from category T86.-, Complications of transplanted organs and tissue, followed by code C80.2, Malignant neoplasm associated with transplanted organ. Use an additional code for the specific malignancy.

3. Chapter 3: Disease of the blood and blood-forming organs and certain disorders involving the immune mechanism (D50-D89)

Reserved for future guideline expansion

4. Chapter 4: Endocrine, Nutritional, and Metabolic Diseases (E00-E89)

a. Diabetes mellitus

The diabetes mellitus codes are combination codes that include the type of diabetes mellitus, the body system affected, and the complications affecting that body system. As many codes within a particular category as are necessary to describe all of the complications of the disease may be used. They should be sequenced based on the reason for a particular encounter. Assign as many codes from categories E08 – E13 as needed to identify all of the associated conditions that the patient has.

1) Type of diabetes

The age of a patient is not the sole determining factor, though most type 1 diabetics develop the condition before reaching puberty. For this reason type 1 diabetes mellitus is also referred to as juvenile diabetes.

2) Type of diabetes mellitus not documented

If the type of diabetes mellitus is not documented in the medical record the default is E11.-, Type 2 diabetes mellitus.

3) Diabetes mellitus and the use of insulin oral hypoglycemics

If the documentation in a medical record does not indicate the type of diabetes but does indicate that the patient uses insulin, code E11, Type 2 diabetes mellitus, should be assigned. Code Z79.4, Long-term (current) use of insulin, **or Z79.84, Long term (current) use of oral hypoglycemic drugs,** should also be assigned to indicate that the patient uses insulin **or hypoglycemic drugs**. Code Z79.4 should not be assigned if insulin is given temporarily to bring a type 2 patient's blood sugar under control during an encounter.

4) Diabetes mellitus in pregnancy and gestational diabetes

See Section I.C.15. Diabetes mellitus in pregnancy.

See Section I.C.15. Gestational (pregnancy induced) diabetes

5) Complications due to insulin pump malfunction

(a) Underdose of insulin due to insulin pump failure

An underdose of insulin due to an insulin pump failure should be assigned to a code from subcategory T85.6, Mechanical complication of other specified internal and external prosthetic devices, implants and grafts, that specifies the type of pump malfunction, as the principal or first-listed code, followed by code T38.3X6-, Underdosing of insulin and oral hypoglycemic [antidiabetic] drugs. Additional codes for the type of diabetes mellitus and any associated complications due to the underdosing should also be assigned.

(b) Overdose of insulin due to insulin pump failure

The principal or first-listed code for an encounter due to an insulin pump malfunction resulting in an overdose of insulin, should also be T85.6-, Mechanical complication of other specified internal and external prosthetic devices, implants and grafts, followed by code T38.3X1-, Poisoning by insulin and oral hypoglycemic [antidiabetic] drugs, accidental (unintentional).

6) Secondary diabetes mellitus

Codes under categories E08, Diabetes mellitus due to underlying condition, E09, Drug or chemical induced diabetes mellitus and E13, Other specified diabetes mellitus, identify complications/manifestations associated with secondary diabetes mellitus. Secondary diabetes is always caused by another condition or event (e.g., cystic fibrosis, malignant neoplasm of pancreas, pancreatectomy, adverse effect of drug, or poisoning).

(a) Secondary diabetes mellitus and the use of insulin or hypoglycemic drugs

For patients who routinely use insulin **or hypoglycemic drugs,** code Z79.4, Long-term (current) use of insulin, **or Z79.84, Long term (current) use of oral hypoglycemic drugs** should also be assigned. Code Z79.4 should not be assigned if insulin is given temporarily to bring a patient's blood sugar under control during an encounter.

(b) Assigning and sequencing secondary diabetes codes and its causes

The sequencing of the secondary diabetes codes in relationship to codes for the cause of the diabetes is based on the Tabular List instructions for categories E08, E09 and E13.

(i) **Secondary diabetes mellitus due to pancreatectomy** For postpancreatectomy diabetes mellitus (lack of insulin due to the surgical removal of all or part of the pancreas), assign code E89.1, Postprocedural hypoinsulinemia. Assign a code from category E13 and a code from subcategory Z90.41-, Acquired absence of pancreas, as additional codes.

(ii) **Secondary diabetes due to drugs** Secondary diabetes may be caused by an adverse effect of correctly administered medications, poisoning or sequela of poisoning.

See section I.C.19.e for coding of adverse effects and poisoning, and section I.C.20 for external cause code reporting.

5. **Chapter 5: Mental, Behavioral and Neurodevelopmental disorders (F01 – F99)**

a. Pain disorders related to psychological factors

Assign code F45.41, for pain that is exclusively related to psychological disorders. As indicated by the Excludes 1 note under category G89, a code from category G89 should not be assigned with code F45.41

Code F45.42, Pain disorders with related psychological factors, should be used with a code from category G89, Pain, not elsewhere classified, if there is documentation of a psychological component for a patient with acute or chronic pain.

See Section I.C.6. Pain

c. Mental and behavioral disorders due to psychoactive substance use

1) In Remission

Selection of codes for "in remission" for categories F10-F19, Mental and behavioral disorders due to psychoactive substance use (categories F10-F19 with -.21) requires the provider's clinical judgment. The appropriate codes for "in remission" are assigned only on the basis of provider documentation (as defined in the Official Guidelines for Coding and Reporting).

2) Psychoactive Substance Use, Abuse And Dependence

When the provider documentation refers to use, abuse and dependence of the same substance (e.g. alcohol, opioid, cannabis, etc.), only one code should be assigned to identify the pattern of use based on the following hierarchy:

- If both use and abuse are documented, assign only the code for abuse
- If both abuse and dependence are documented, assign only the code for dependence
- If use, abuse and dependence are all documented, assign only the code for dependence
- If both use and dependence are documented, assign only the code for dependence.

3) Psychoactive Substance Use

As with all other diagnoses, the codes for psychoactive substance use (F10.9-, F11.9-, F12.9-, F13.9-, F14.9-, F15.9-, F16.9-) should only be assigned based on provider documentation and when they meet the definition of a reportable diagnosis (see Section III, Reporting Additional Diagnoses). The codes are to be used only when the psychoactive substance use is associated with a mental or behavioral disorder, and such a relationship is documented by the provider.

6. **Chapter 6: Diseases of the Nervous System (G00-G99)**

a. Dominant/nondominant side

Codes from category G81, Hemiplegia and hemiparesis, and subcategories, G83.1, Monoplegia of lower limb, G83.2, Monoplegia of upper limb, and G83.3, Monoplegia, unspecified, identify whether the dominant or nondominant side is affected. Should the affected side be documented, but not specified as dominant or nondominant, and the classification system does not indicate a default, code selection is as follows:

- For ambidextrous patients, the default should be dominant.
- If the left side is affected, the default is non-dominant.
- If the right side is affected, the default is dominant.

b. Pain - Category G89

1) General coding information

Codes in category G89, Pain, not elsewhere classified, may be used in conjunction with codes from other categories and chapters to provide more detail about acute or chronic pain and neoplasm-related pain, unless otherwise indicated below.

If the pain is not specified as acute or chronic, post-thoracotomy, postprocedural, or neoplasm-related, do not assign codes from category G89.

A code from category G89 should not be assigned if the underlying (definitive) diagnosis is known, unless the reason for the encounter is pain control/management and not management of the underlying condition.

When an admission or encounter is for a procedure aimed at treating the underlying condition (e.g., spinal fusion, kyphoplasty), a code for the underlying condition (e.g., vertebral fracture, spinal stenosis) should be assigned as the principal diagnosis. No code from category G89 should be assigned.

(a) Category G89 Codes as Principal or First-Listed Diagnosis

Category G89 codes are acceptable as principal diagnosis or the first-listed code:

- When pain control or pain management is the reason for the admission/encounter (e.g., a patient with displaced intervertebral disc, nerve impingement and severe back pain presents for injection of steroid into the spinal canal). The underlying cause of the pain should be reported as an additional diagnosis, if known.

- When a patient is admitted for the insertion of a neurostimulator for pain control, assign the appropriate pain code as the principal or first-listed diagnosis. When an admission or encounter is for a procedure aimed at treating the underlying condition and a neurostimulator is inserted for pain control during the same admission/encounter, a code for the underlying condition should be assigned as the principal diagnosis and the appropriate pain code should be assigned as a secondary diagnosis.

(b) Use of Category G89 Codes in Conjunction with Site Specific Pain Codes

(i) Assigning Category G89 and Site-Specific Pain Codes

Codes from category G89 may be used in conjunction with codes that identify the site of pain (including codes from chapter 18) if the category G89 code provides additional information. For example, if the code describes the site of the pain, but does not fully describe whether the pain is acute or chronic, then both codes should be assigned.

(ii) Sequencing of Category G89 Codes with Site-Specific Pain Codes

The sequencing of category G89 codes with site-specific pain codes (including chapter 18 codes), is dependent on the circumstances of the encounter/admission as follows:

- If the encounter is for pain control or pain management, assign the code from category G89 followed by the code identifying the specific site of pain (e.g., encounter for pain management for acute neck pain from trauma is assigned code G89.11, Acute pain due to trauma, followed by code M54.2, Cervicalgia, to identify the site of pain).
- If the encounter is for any other reason except pain control or pain management, and a related definitive diagnosis has not been established (confirmed) by the provider, assign the code for the specific site of pain first, followed by the appropriate code from category G89.

2) Pain due to devices, implants and grafts

See Section I.C.19. Pain due to medical devices

3) Postoperative Pain

The provider's documentation should be used to guide the coding of postoperative pain, as well as *Section III. Reporting Additional Diagnoses* and *Section IV. Diagnostic Coding and Reporting in the Outpatient Setting.*

The default for post-thoracotomy and other postoperative pain not specified as acute or chronic is the code for the acute form.

Routine or expected postoperative pain immediately after surgery should not be coded.

(a) Postoperative pain not associated with specific postoperative complication

Postoperative pain not associated with a specific postoperative complication is assigned to the appropriate postoperative pain code in category G89.

(b) Postoperative pain associated with specific postoperative complication

Postoperative pain associated with a specific postoperative complication (such as painful wire sutures) is assigned to the appropriate code(s) found in Chapter 19, Injury, poisoning, and certain other consequences of external causes. If appropriate, use additional code(s) from category G89 to identify acute or chronic pain (G89.18 or G89.28).

4) Chronic pain

Chronic pain is classified to subcategory G89.2. There is no time frame defining when pain becomes chronic pain. The provider's documentation should be used to guide use of these codes.

5) Neoplasm Related Pain

Code G89.3 is assigned to pain documented as being related, associated or due to cancer, primary or secondary malignancy, or tumor. This code is assigned regardless of whether the pain is acute or chronic.

This code may be assigned as the principal or first-listed code when the stated reason for the admission/encounter is documented as pain control/pain management. The underlying neoplasm should be reported as an additional diagnosis.

When the reason for the admission/encounter is management of the neoplasm and the pain associated with the neoplasm is also documented, code G89.3 may be assigned as an additional diagnosis. It is not necessary to assign an additional code for the site of the pain.

See Section I.C.2 for instructions on the sequencing of neoplasms for all other stated reasons for the admission/encounter (except for pain control/pain management).

6) Chronic pain syndrome

Central pain syndrome (G89.0) and chronic pain syndrome (G89.4) are different than the term "chronic pain," and therefore codes should only be used when the provider has specifically documented this condition.

See Section I.C.5. Pain disorders related to psychological factors

7. Chapter 7: Diseases of the Eye and Adnexa (H00-H59)

a. Glaucoma

1) Assigning Glaucoma Codes

Assign as many codes from category H40, Glaucoma, as needed to identify the type of glaucoma, the affected eye, and the glaucoma stage.

2) Bilateral glaucoma with same type and stage

When a patient has bilateral glaucoma and both eyes are documented as being the same type and stage, and there is a code for bilateral glaucoma, report only the code for the type of glaucoma, bilateral, with the seventh character for the stage.

When a patient has bilateral glaucoma and both eyes are documented as being the same type and stage, and the classification does not provide a code for bilateral glaucoma (i.e. subcategories H40.10, H40.11 and H40.20) report only one code for the type of glaucoma with the appropriate seventh character for the stage.

3) Bilateral glaucoma stage with different types or stages

When a patient has bilateral glaucoma and each eye is documented as having a different type or stage, and the classification distinguishes laterality, assign the appropriate code for each eye rather than the code for bilateral glaucoma.

When a patient has bilateral glaucoma and each eye is documented as having a different type, and the classification does not distinguish laterality (i.e. subcategories H40.10, H40.11 and H40.20), assign one code for each type of glaucoma with the appropriate seventh character for the stage.

When a patient has bilateral glaucoma and each eye is documented as having the same type, but different stage, and the classification does not distinguish laterality (i.e. subcategories H40.10, H40.11 and H40.20), assign a code for the type of glaucoma for each eye with the seventh character for the specific glaucoma stage documented for each eye.

4) Patient admitted with glaucoma and stage evolves during the admission

If a patient is admitted with glaucoma and the stage progresses during the admission, assign the code for highest stage documented.

5) Indeterminate stage glaucoma

Assignment of the seventh character "4" for "indeterminate stage" should be based on the clinical documentation. The seventh character "4" is used for glaucomas whose stage cannot be clinically determined. This seventh character should not be confused with the seventh character "0", unspecified, which should be assigned when there is no documentation regarding the stage of the glaucoma.

8. **Chapter 8: Diseases of the Ear and Mastoid Process (H60-H95)**

Reserved for future guideline expansion

9. **Chapter 9: Diseases of the Circulatory System (I00-I99)**

a. Hypertension

The classification presumes a causal relationship between hypertension and heart involvement and between hypertension and kidney involvement, as the two conditions are linked by the term "with" in the Alphabetic Index. These conditions should be coded as related even in the absence of provider documentation explicitly linking them, unless the documentation clearly states the conditions are unrelated.

For hypertension and conditions not specifically linked by relational terms such as "with," "associated with" or "due to" in the classification, provider documentation must link the conditions in order to code them as related.

1) Hypertension with Heart Disease

Hypertension with heart conditions classified to I50.- or I51.4-I51.9, are assigned to, a code from category I11, Hypertensive heart disease. Use an additional code from category I50, Heart failure, to identify the type of heart failure in those patients with heart failure.

The same heart conditions (I50.-, I51.4-I51.9) with hypertension are coded separately **if the provider has specifically documented a different cause**. Sequence according to the circumstances of the admission/encounter.

2) Hypertensive Chronic Kidney Disease

Assign codes from category I12, Hypertensive chronic kidney disease, when both hypertension and a condition classifiable to category N18, Chronic kidney disease (CKD), are present. **CKD should not be coded as hypertensive if the physician has specifically documented a different cause.**

The appropriate code from category N18 should be used as a secondary code with a code from category I12 to identify the stage of chronic kidney disease.

See Section I.C.14. Chronic kidney disease.

If a patient has hypertensive chronic kidney disease and acute renal failure, an additional code for the acute renal failure is required.

3) Hypertensive Heart and Chronic Kidney Disease

Assign codes from combination category I13, Hypertensive heart and chronic kidney disease, when **there is hypertension with both heart and kidney involvement.** If heart failure is present, assign an additional code from category I50 to identify the type of heart failure.

The appropriate code from category N18, Chronic kidney disease, should be used as a secondary code with a code from category I13 to identify the stage of chronic kidney disease.

See Section I.C.14. Chronic kidney disease.

The codes in category I13, Hypertensive heart and chronic kidney disease, are combination codes that include hypertension, heart disease and chronic kidney disease. The Includes note at I13 specifies that the conditions included at I11 and I12 are included together in I13. If a patient has hypertension, heart disease and chronic kidney disease then a code from I13 should be used, not individual codes for hypertension, heart disease and chronic kidney disease, or codes from I11 or I12.

For patients with both acute renal failure and chronic kidney disease an additional code for acute renal failure is required.

4) Hypertensive Cerebrovascular Disease
For hypertensive cerebrovascular disease, first assign the appropriate code from categories I60-I69, followed by the appropriate hypertension code.

5) Hypertensive Retinopathy
Subcategory H35.0, Background retinopathy and retinal vascular changes, should be used with a code from category I10 – I15, Hypertensive disease to include the systemic hypertension. The sequencing is based on the reason for the encounter.

6) Hypertension, Secondary
Secondary hypertension is due to an underlying condition. Two codes are required: one to identify the underlying etiology and one from category I15 to identify the hypertension. Sequencing of codes is determined by the reason for admission/encounter.

7) Hypertension, Transient
Assign code R03.0, Elevated blood pressure reading without diagnosis of hypertension, unless patient has an established diagnosis of hypertension. Assign code O13.-, Gestational [pregnancy-induced] hypertension without significant proteinuria, or O14.-, Pre-eclampsia, for transient hypertension of pregnancy.

8) Hypertension, Controlled
This diagnostic statement usually refers to an existing state of hypertension under control by therapy. Assign the appropriate code from categories I10-I15, Hypertensive diseases.

9) Hypertension, Uncontrolled
Uncontrolled hypertension may refer to untreated hypertension or hypertension not responding to current therapeutic regimen. In either case, assign the appropriate code from categories I10-I15, Hypertensive diseases.

10) Hypertensive Crisis
Assign a code from category I16, Hypertensive crisis, for documented hypertensive urgency, hypertensive emergency or unspecified hypertensive crisis. Code also any identified hypertensive disease (I10-I15). The sequencing is based on the reason for the encounter.

b. Atherosclerotic Coronary Artery Disease and Angina
ICD-10-CM has combination codes for atherosclerotic heart disease with angina pectoris. The subcategories for these codes are I25.11, Atherosclerotic heart disease of native coronary artery with angina pectoris and I25.7, Atherosclerosis of coronary artery bypass graft(s) and coronary artery of transplanted heart with angina pectoris.

When using one of these combination codes it is not necessary to use an additional code for angina pectoris. A causal relationship can be assumed in a patient with both atherosclerosis and angina pectoris, unless the documentation indicates the angina is due to something other than the atherosclerosis.

If a patient with coronary artery disease is admitted due to an acute myocardial infarction (AMI), the AMI should be sequenced before the coronary artery disease.

See Section I.C.9. Acute myocardial infarction (AMI)

c. Intraoperative and Postprocedural Cerebrovascular Accident
Medical record documentation should clearly specify the cause-and-effect relationship between the medical intervention and the cerebrovascular accident in order to assign a code for intraoperative or postprocedural cerebrovascular accident.

Proper code assignment depends on whether it was an infarction or hemorrhage and whether it occurred intraoperatively or postoperatively. If it was a cerebral hemorrhage, code assignment depends on the type of procedure performed.

d. Sequelae of Cerebrovascular Disease

1) Category I69, Sequelae of Cerebrovascular disease
Category I69 is used to indicate conditions classifiable to categories I60-I67 as the causes of sequela (neurologic deficits), themselves classified elsewhere. These "late effects" include neurologic deficits that persist after initial onset of conditions classifiable to categories I60-I67. The neurologic deficits caused by cerebrovascular disease may be present from the onset or may arise at any time after the onset of the condition classifiable to categories I60-I67.

Codes from category I69, Sequelae of cerebrovascular disease, that specify hemiplegia, hemiparesis and monoplegia identify whether the dominant or nondominant side is affected. Should the affected side be documented, but not specified as dominant or nondominant, and the classification system does not indicate a default, code selection is as follows:

- For ambidextrous patients, the default should be dominant.
- If the left side is affected, the default is non-dominant.
- If the right side is affected, the default is dominant.

2) Codes from category I69 with codes from I60-I67
Codes from category I69 may be assigned on a health care record with codes from I60-I67, if the patient has a current cerebrovascular disease and deficits from an old cerebrovascular disease.

3) Codes from category I69 and Personal history of transient ischemic attack (TIA) and cerebral infarction (Z86.73)
Codes from category I69 should not be assigned if the patient does not have neurologic deficits.

See Section I.C.21. 4. History (of) for use of personal history codes

e. Acute myocardial infarction (AMI)

1) ST elevation myocardial infarction (STEMI) and non ST elevation myocardial infarction (NSTEMI)

The ICD-10-CM codes for acute myocardial infarction (AMI) identify the site, such as anterolateral wall or true posterior wall. Subcategories I21.Ø-I21.2 and code I21.3 are used for ST elevation myocardial infarction (STEMI). Code I21.4, Non-ST elevation (NSTEMI) myocardial infarction, is used for non ST elevation myocardial infarction (NSTEMI) and nontransmural MIs.

If NSTEMI evolves to STEMI, assign the STEMI code. If STEMI converts to NSTEMI due to thrombolytic therapy, it is still coded as STEMI.

For encounters occurring while the myocardial infarction is equal to, or less than, four weeks old, including transfers to another acute setting or a postacute setting, and the myocardial infarction **meets the definition for "other diagnoses" (see Section III, Reporting Additional Diagnoses)**, codes from category I21 may continue to be reported. For encounters after the 4 week time frame and the patient is still receiving care related to the myocardial infarction, the appropriate aftercare code should be assigned, rather than a code from category I21. For old or healed myocardial infarctions not requiring further care, code I25.2, Old myocardial infarction, may be assigned.

2) Acute myocardial infarction, unspecified

Code I21.3, ST elevation (STEMI) myocardial infarction of unspecified site, is the default for unspecified acute myocardial infarction. If only STEMI or transmural MI without the site is documented, assign code I21.3.

3) AMI documented as nontransmural or subendocardial but site provided

If an AMI is documented as nontransmural or subendocardial, but the site is provided, it is still coded as a subendocardial AMI.

See Section I.C.21.3 for information on coding status post administration of tPA in a different facility within the last 24 hours.

4) Subsequent acute myocardial infarction

A code from category I22, Subsequent ST elevation (STEMI) and non ST elevation (NSTEMI) myocardial infarction, is to be used when a patient who has suffered an AMI has a new AMI within the 4 week time frame of the initial AMI. A code from category I22 must be used in conjunction with a code from category I21. The sequencing of the I22 and I21 codes depends on the circumstances of the encounter.

1Ø. Chapter 1Ø: Diseases of the Respiratory System (JØØ-J99)

a. Chronic Obstructive Pulmonary Disease [COPD] and Asthma

1) Acute exacerbation of chronic obstructive bronchitis and asthma

The codes in categories J44 and J45 distinguish between uncomplicated cases and those in acute exacerbation. An acute exacerbation is a worsening or a decompensation of a chronic condition. An acute exacerbation is not equivalent to an infection superimposed on a chronic condition, though an exacerbation may be triggered by an infection.

b. Acute Respiratory Failure

1) Acute respiratory failure as principal diagnosis

A code from subcategory J96.Ø, Acute respiratory failure, or subcategory J96.2, Acute and chronic respiratory failure, may be assigned as a principal diagnosis when it is the condition established after study to be chiefly responsible for occasioning the admission to the hospital, and the selection is supported by the Alphabetic Index and Tabular List. However, chapter-specific coding guidelines (such as obstetrics, poisoning, HIV, newborn) that provide sequencing direction take precedence.

2) Acute respiratory failure as secondary diagnosis

Respiratory failure may be listed as a secondary diagnosis if it occurs after admission, or if it is present on admission, but does not meet the definition of principal diagnosis.

3) Sequencing of acute respiratory failure and another acute condition

When a patient is admitted with respiratory failure and another acute condition, (e.g., myocardial infarction, cerebrovascular accident, aspiration pneumonia), the principal diagnosis will not be the same in every situation. This applies whether the other acute condition is a respiratory or nonrespiratory condition. Selection of the principal diagnosis will be dependent on the circumstances of admission. If both the respiratory failure and the other acute condition are equally responsible for occasioning the admission to the hospital, and there are no chapter-specific sequencing rules, the guideline regarding two or more diagnoses that equally meet the definition for principal diagnosis *(Section II, C.)* may be applied in these situations.

If the documentation is not clear as to whether acute respiratory failure and another condition are equally responsible for occasioning the admission, query the provider for clarification.

c. Influenza due to certain identified influenza viruses

Code only confirmed cases of influenza due to certain identified influenza viruses (category JØ9), and due to other identified influenza virus (category J1Ø). This is an exception to the hospital inpatient guideline Section II, H. (Uncertain Diagnosis).

In this context, "confirmation" does not require documentation of positive laboratory testing specific for avian or other novel influenza A or other identified influenza virus. However, coding should be based on the provider's diagnostic statement that the patient has avian influenza, or other novel influenza A, for category JØ9, or has another particular identified strain of influenza, such as H1N1 or H3N2, but not identified as novel or variant, for category J10.

If the provider records "suspected" or "possible" or "probable" avian influenza, or novel influenza, or other identified influenza, then the appropriate influenza code from category J11, Influenza due to unidentified influenza virus, should be assigned. A code from category J09, Influenza due to certain identified influenza viruses, should not be assigned nor should a code from category J10, Influenza due to other identified influenza virus.

d. Ventilator associated Pneumonia

1) Documentation of Ventilator associated Pneumonia

As with all procedural or postprocedural complications, code assignment is based on the provider's documentation of the relationship between the condition and the procedure.

Code J95.851, Ventilator associated pneumonia, should be assigned only when the provider has documented ventilator associated pneumonia (VAP). An additional code to identify the organism (e.g., Pseudomonas aeruginosa, code B96.5) should also be assigned. Do not assign an additional code from categories J12-J18 to identify the type of pneumonia.

Code J95.851 should not be assigned for cases where the patient has pneumonia and is on a mechanical ventilator and the provider has not specifically stated that the pneumonia is ventilator-associated pneumonia. If the documentation is unclear as to whether the patient has a pneumonia that is a complication attributable to the mechanical ventilator, query the provider.

2) Ventilator associated Pneumonia Develops after Admission

A patient may be admitted with one type of pneumonia (e.g., code J13, Pneumonia due to Streptococcus pneumonia) and subsequently develop VAP. In this instance, the principal diagnosis would be the appropriate code from categories J12-J18 for the pneumonia diagnosed at the time of admission. Code J95.851, Ventilator associated pneumonia, would be assigned as an additional diagnosis when the provider has also documented the presence of ventilator associated pneumonia.

11. Chapter 11: Diseases of the Digestive System (K00-K95)

Reserved for future guideline expansion

12. Chapter 12: Diseases of the Skin and Subcutaneous Tissue (L00-L99)

a. Pressure ulcer stage codes

1) Pressure ulcer stages

Codes from category L89, Pressure ulcer, identify the site of the pressure ulcer as well as the stage of the ulcer.

The ICD-10-CM classifies pressure ulcer stages based on severity, which is designated by stages 1-4, unspecified stage and unstageable.

Assign as many codes from category L89 as needed to identify all the pressure ulcers the patient has, if applicable.

2) Unstageable pressure ulcers

Assignment of the code for unstageable pressure ulcer (L89.--0) should be based on the clinical documentation. These codes are used for pressure ulcers whose stage cannot be clinically determined (e.g., the ulcer is covered by eschar or has been treated with a skin or muscle graft) and pressure ulcers that are documented as deep tissue injury but not documented as due to trauma. This code should not be confused with the codes for unspecified stage (L89.--9). When there is no documentation regarding the stage of the pressure ulcer, assign the appropriate code for unspecified stage (L89.--9).

3) Documented pressure ulcer stage

Assignment of the pressure ulcer stage code should be guided by clinical documentation of the stage or documentation of the terms found in the Alphabetic Index. For clinical terms describing the stage that are not found in the Alphabetic Index, and there is no documentation of the stage, the provider should be queried.

4) Patients admitted with pressure ulcers documented as healed

No code is assigned if the documentation states that the pressure ulcer is completely healed.

5) Patients admitted with pressure ulcers documented as healing

Pressure ulcers described as healing should be assigned the appropriate pressure ulcer stage code based on the documentation in the medical record. If the documentation does not provide information about the stage of the healing pressure ulcer, assign the appropriate code for unspecified stage.

If the documentation is unclear as to whether the patient has a current (new) pressure ulcer or if the patient is being treated for a healing pressure ulcer, query the provider.

For ulcers that were present on admission but healed at the time of discharge, assign the code for the site and stage of the pressure ulcer at the time of admission.

6) Patient admitted with pressure ulcer evolving into another stage during the admission

If a patient is admitted with a pressure ulcer at one stage and it progresses to a higher stage, **two separate codes should be assigned: one code for the site and stage of the ulcer on admission and a second code for the same ulcer site and the highest stage reported during the stay.**

13. Chapter 13: Diseases of the Musculoskeletal System and Connective Tissue (M00-M99)

a. Site and laterality

Most of the codes within Chapter 13 have site and laterality designations. The site represents the bone, joint or the muscle involved. For some conditions where more than one bone, joint or muscle is usually involved, such as osteoarthritis, there is a "multiple sites" code available. For categories where no multiple site code is provided and more than one bone, joint or muscle is involved, multiple codes should be used to indicate the different sites involved.

1) Bone versus joint

For certain conditions, the bone may be affected at the upper or lower end, (e.g., avascular necrosis of bone, M87, Osteoporosis, M8Ø, M81). Though the portion of the bone affected may be at the joint, the site designation will be the bone, not the joint.

b. Acute traumatic versus chronic or recurrent musculoskeletal conditions

Many musculoskeletal conditions are a result of previous injury or trauma to a site, or are recurrent conditions. Bone, joint or muscle conditions that are the result of a healed injury are usually found in chapter 13. Recurrent bone, joint or muscle conditions are also usually found in chapter 13. Any current, acute injury should be coded to the appropriate injury code from chapter 19. Chronic or recurrent conditions should generally be coded with a code from chapter 13. If it is difficult to determine from the documentation in the record which code is best to describe a condition, query the provider.

c. Coding of Pathologic Fractures

7th character A is for use as long as the patient is receiving active treatment for the fracture. While the patient may be seen by a new or different provider over the course of treatment for a pathological fracture, assignment of the 7th character is based on whether the patient is undergoing active treatment and not whether the provider is seeing the patient for the first time.

7th character, D is to be used for encounters after the patient has completed active treatment. The other 7th characters, listed under each subcategory in the Tabular List, are to be used for subsequent encounters for **routine care of fractures during the healing and recovery phase as well as** treatment of problems associated with the healing, such as malunions, nonunions, and sequelae.

Care for complications of surgical treatment for fracture repairs during the healing or recovery phase should be coded with the appropriate complication codes.

See Section I.C.19. Coding of traumatic fractures.

d. Osteoporosis

Osteoporosis is a systemic condition, meaning that all bones of the musculoskeletal system are affected. Therefore, site is not a component of the codes under category M81, Osteoporosis without current pathological fracture. The site codes under category M8Ø, Osteoporosis with current pathological fracture, identify the site of the fracture, not the osteoporosis.

1) Osteoporosis without pathological fracture

Category M81, Osteoporosis without current pathological fracture, is for use for patients with osteoporosis who do not currently have a pathologic fracture due to the osteoporosis, even if they have had a fracture in the past. For patients with a history of osteoporosis fractures, status code Z87.31Ø, Personal history of (healed) osteoporosis fracture, should follow the code from M81.

2) Osteoporosis with current pathological fracture

Category M8Ø, Osteoporosis with current pathological fracture, is for patients who have a current pathologic fracture at the time of an encounter. The codes under M8Ø identify the site of the fracture. A code from category M8Ø, not a traumatic fracture code, should be used for any patient with known osteoporosis who suffers a fracture, even if the patient had a minor fall or trauma, if that fall or trauma would not usually break a normal, healthy bone.

14. Chapter 14: Diseases of Genitourinary System (NØØ-N99)

a. Chronic kidney disease

1) Stages of chronic kidney disease (CKD)

The ICD-10-CM classifies CKD based on severity. The severity of CKD is designated by stages 1-5. Stage 2, code N18.2, equates to mild CKD; stage 3, code N18.3, equates to moderate CKD; and stage 4, code N18.4, equates to severe CKD. Code N18.6, End stage renal disease (ESRD), is assigned when the provider has documented end-stage-renal disease (ESRD).

If both a stage of CKD and ESRD are documented, assign code N18.6 only.

2) Chronic kidney disease and kidney transplant status

Patients who have undergone kidney transplant may still have some form of chronic kidney disease CKD because the kidney transplant may not fully restore kidney function. Therefore, the presence of CKD alone does not constitute a transplant complication. Assign the appropriate N18 code for the patient's stage of CKD and code Z94.Ø, Kidney transplant status. If a transplant complication such as failure or rejection or other transplant complication is documented, see section I.C.19.g for information on coding complications of a kidney transplant. If the documentation is unclear as to whether the patient has a complication of the transplant, query the provider.

3) Chronic kidney disease with other conditions

Patients with CKD may also suffer from other serious conditions, most commonly diabetes mellitus and hypertension. The sequencing of the CKD code in relationship to codes for other contributing conditions is based on the conventions in the Tabular List.

See I.C.9. Hypertensive chronic kidney disease.

See I.C.19. Chronic kidney disease and kidney transplant complications.

15. Chapter 15: Pregnancy, Childbirth, and the Puerperium (O00-O9A)

a. General Rules for Obstetric Cases

1) Codes from chapter 15 and sequencing priority

Obstetric cases require codes from chapter 15, codes in the range O00-O9A, Pregnancy, Childbirth, and the Puerperium. Chapter 15 codes have sequencing priority over codes from other chapters. Additional codes from other chapters may be used in conjunction with chapter 15 codes to further specify conditions. Should the provider document that the pregnancy is incidental to the encounter, then code Z33.1, Pregnant state, incidental, should be used in place of any chapter 15 codes. It is the provider's responsibility to state that the condition being treated is not affecting the pregnancy.

2) Chapter 15 codes used only on the maternal record

Chapter 15 codes are to be used only on the maternal record, never on the record of the newborn.

3) Final character for trimester

The majority of codes in Chapter 15 have a final character indicating the trimester of pregnancy. The timeframes for the trimesters are indicated at the beginning of the chapter. If trimester is not a component of a code it is because the condition always occurs in a specific trimester, or the concept of trimester of pregnancy is not applicable. Certain codes have characters for only certain trimesters because the condition does not occur in all trimesters, but it may occur in more than just one.

Assignment of the final character for trimester should be based on the provider's documentation of the trimester (or number of weeks) for the current admission/encounter. This applies to the assignment of trimester for pre-existing conditions as well as those that develop during or are due to the pregnancy. The provider's documentation of the number of weeks may be used to assign the appropriate code identifying the trimester.

Whenever delivery occurs during the current admission, and there is an "in childbirth" option for the obstetric complication being coded, the "in childbirth" code should be assigned.

4) Selection of trimester for inpatient admissions that encompass more than one trimester

In instances when a patient is admitted to a hospital for complications of pregnancy during one trimester and remains in the hospital into a subsequent trimester, the trimester character for the antepartum complication code should be assigned on the basis of the trimester when the complication developed, not the trimester of the discharge. If the condition developed prior to the current admission/encounter or represents a pre-existing condition, the trimester character for the trimester at the time of the admission/encounter should be assigned.

5) Unspecified trimester

Each category that includes codes for trimester has a code for "unspecified trimester." The "unspecified trimester" code should rarely be used, such as when the documentation in the record is insufficient to determine the trimester and it is not possible to obtain clarification.

6) 7th character for Fetus Identification

Where applicable, a 7th character is to be assigned for certain categories (O31, O32, O33.3 - O33.6, O35, O36, O40, O41, O60.1, O60.2, O64, and O69) to identify the fetus for which the complication code applies.

Assign 7th character "0":

- For single gestations
- When the documentation in the record is insufficient to determine the fetus affected and it is not possible to obtain clarification.
- When it is not possible to clinically determine which fetus is affected.

b. Selection of OB Principal or First-listed Diagnosis

1) Routine outpatient prenatal visits

For routine outpatient prenatal visits when no complications are present, a code from category Z34, Encounter for supervision of normal pregnancy, should be used as the first-listed diagnosis. These codes should not be used in conjunction with chapter 15 codes.

2) *Supervision of High-Risk Pregnancy*

Codes from category O09, Supervision of high-risk pregnancy, are intended for use only during the prenatal period. For complications during the labor or delivery episode as a result of a high-risk pregnancy, assign the applicable complication codes from Chapter 15. If there are no complications during the labor or delivery episode, assign code O80, Encounter for full-term uncomplicated delivery.

For routine prenatal outpatient visits for patients with high-risk pregnancies, a code from category O09, Supervision of high-risk pregnancy, should be used as the first-listed diagnosis. Secondary chapter 15 codes may be used in conjunction with these codes if appropriate.

3) Episodes when no delivery occurs

In episodes when no delivery occurs, the principal diagnosis should correspond to the principal complication of the pregnancy which necessitated the encounter. Should more than one complication exist, all of which are treated or monitored, any of the complications codes may be sequenced first.

4) When a delivery occurs

When an obstetric patient is admitted and delivers during that admission, the condition that prompted the admission should be sequenced as the principal diagnosis. If multiple conditions prompted the admission, sequence the one most related to the delivery as the principal

diagnosis. A code for any complication of the delivery should be assigned as an additional diagnosis. In cases of cesarean delivery, if the patient was admitted with a condition that resulted in the performance of a cesarean procedure, that condition should be selected as the principal diagnosis. If the reason for the admission was unrelated to the condition resulting in the cesarean delivery, the condition related to the reason for the admission should be selected as the principal diagnosis.

5) Outcome of delivery

A code from category Z37, Outcome of delivery, should be included on every maternal record when a delivery has occurred. These codes are not to be used on subsequent records or on the newborn record.

c. Pre-existing conditions versus conditions due to the pregnancy

Certain categories in Chapter 15 distinguish between conditions of the mother that existed prior to pregnancy (pre-existing) and those that are a direct result of pregnancy. When assigning codes from Chapter 15, it is important to assess if a condition was pre-existing prior to pregnancy or developed during or due to the pregnancy in order to assign the correct code.

Categories that do not distinguish between pre-existing and pregnancy-related conditions may be used for either. It is acceptable to use codes specifically for the puerperium with codes complicating pregnancy and childbirth if a condition arises postpartum during the delivery encounter.

d. Pre-existing hypertension in pregnancy

Category O10, Pre-existing hypertension complicating pregnancy, childbirth and the puerperium, includes codes for hypertensive heart and hypertensive chronic kidney disease. When assigning one of the O10 codes that includes hypertensive heart disease or hypertensive chronic kidney disease, it is necessary to add a secondary code from the appropriate hypertension category to specify the type of heart failure or chronic kidney disease.

See Section I.C.9. Hypertension.

e. Fetal Conditions Affecting the Management of the Mother

1) Codes from categories O35 and O36

Codes from categories O35, Maternal care for known or suspected fetal abnormality and damage, and O36, Maternal care for other fetal problems, are assigned only when the fetal condition is actually responsible for modifying the management of the mother, i.e., by requiring diagnostic studies, additional observation, special care, or termination of pregnancy. The fact that the fetal condition exists does not justify assigning a code from this series to the mother's record.

2) In utero surgery

In cases when surgery is performed on the fetus, a diagnosis code from category O35, Maternal care for known or suspected fetal abnormality and damage, should be assigned identifying the fetal condition. Assign the appropriate procedure code for the procedure performed.

No code from Chapter 16, the perinatal codes, should be used on the mother's record to identify fetal conditions. Surgery performed in utero on a fetus is still to be coded as an obstetric encounter.

f. HIV Infection in Pregnancy, Childbirth and the Puerperium

During pregnancy, childbirth or the puerperium, a patient admitted because of an HIV-related illness should receive a principal diagnosis from subcategory O98.7-, Human immunodeficiency [HIV] disease complicating pregnancy, childbirth and the puerperium, followed by the code(s) for the HIV-related illness(es).

Patients with asymptomatic HIV infection status admitted during pregnancy, childbirth, or the puerperium should receive codes of O98.7- and Z21, Asymptomatic human immunodeficiency virus [HIV] infection status.

g. Diabetes mellitus in pregnancy

Diabetes mellitus is a significant complicating factor in pregnancy. Pregnant women who are diabetic should be assigned a code from category O24, Diabetes mellitus in pregnancy, childbirth, and the puerperium, first, followed by the appropriate diabetes code(s) (E08-E13) from Chapter 4.

h. Long term use of insulin and oral hypoglycemics

Code Z79.4, Long-term (current) use of insulin, or **code Z79.84, Long-term (current) use of oral hypoglycemic drugs,** should also be assigned if the diabetes mellitus is being treated with insulin **or oral medications. If the patient is treated with both oral medications and insulin, only the code for insulin-controlled should be assigned.**

i. Gestational (pregnancy induced) diabetes

Gestational (pregnancy induced) diabetes can occur during the second and third trimester of pregnancy in women who were not diabetic prior to pregnancy. Gestational diabetes can cause complications in the pregnancy similar to those of pre-existing diabetes mellitus. It also puts the woman at greater risk of developing diabetes after the pregnancy. Codes for gestational diabetes are in subcategory O24.4, Gestational diabetes mellitus. No other code from category O24, Diabetes mellitus in pregnancy, childbirth, and the puerperium, should be used with a code from O24.4.

The codes under subcategory O24.4 include diet controlled, insulin controlled**, and controlled by oral hypoglycemic drugs.** If a patient with gestational diabetes is treated with both diet and insulin, only the code for insulin-controlled is required. **If a patient with gestational diabetes is treated with both diet and oral hypoglycemic medications, only the code for "controlled by oral hypoglycemic drugs" is required.** Code Z79.4, Long-term (current) use of insulin **or code Z79.84, Long-term (current) use of oral hypoglycemic drugs,** should not be assigned with codes from subcategory O24.4.

An abnormal glucose tolerance in pregnancy is assigned a code from subcategory O99.81, Abnormal glucose complicating pregnancy, childbirth, and the puerperium.

j. Sepsis and septic shock complicating abortion, pregnancy, childbirth and the puerperium

When assigning a chapter 15 code for sepsis complicating abortion, pregnancy, childbirth, and the puerperium, a code for the specific type of infection should be assigned as an additional diagnosis. If severe sepsis is present, a code from subcategory R65.2, Severe sepsis, and code(s) for associated organ dysfunction(s) should also be assigned as additional diagnoses.

k. Puerperal sepsis

Code O85, Puerperal sepsis, should be assigned with a secondary code to identify the causal organism (e.g., for a bacterial infection, assign a code from category B95-B96, Bacterial infections in conditions classified elsewhere). A code from category A40, Streptococcal sepsis, or A41, Other sepsis, should not be used for puerperal sepsis. If applicable, use additional codes to identify severe sepsis (R65.2-) and any associated acute organ dysfunction.

l. Alcohol and tobacco use during pregnancy, childbirth and the puerperium

1) Alcohol use during pregnancy, childbirth and the puerperium

Codes under subcategory O99.31, Alcohol use complicating pregnancy, childbirth, and the puerperium, should be assigned for any pregnancy case when a mother uses alcohol during the pregnancy or postpartum. A secondary code from category F10, Alcohol related disorders, should also be assigned to identify manifestations of the alcohol use.

2) Tobacco use during pregnancy, childbirth and the puerperium

Codes under subcategory O99.33, Smoking (tobacco) complicating pregnancy, childbirth, and the puerperium, should be assigned for any pregnancy case when a mother uses any type of tobacco product during the pregnancy or postpartum. A secondary code from category F17, Nicotine dependence, should also be assigned to identify the type of nicotine dependence.

m. Poisoning, toxic effects, adverse effects and underdosing in a pregnant patient

A code from subcategory O9A.2, Injury, poisoning and certain other consequences of external causes complicating pregnancy, childbirth, and the puerperium, should be sequenced first, followed by the appropriate injury, poisoning, toxic effect, adverse effect or underdosing code, and then the additional code(s) that specifies the condition caused by the poisoning, toxic effect, adverse effect or underdosing.

See Section I.C.19. Adverse effects, poisoning, underdosing and toxic effects.

n. Normal Delivery, Code O80

1) Encounter for full term uncomplicated delivery

Code O80 should be assigned when a woman is admitted for a full-term normal delivery and delivers a single, healthy infant without any complications antepartum, during the delivery, or postpartum during the delivery episode. Code O80 is always a principal diagnosis. It is not to be used if any other code from chapter 15 is needed to describe a current complication of the antenatal, delivery, or perinatal period. Additional codes from other chapters may be used with code O80 if they are not related to or are in any way complicating the pregnancy.

2) Uncomplicated delivery with resolved antepartum complication

Code O80 may be used if the patient had a complication at some point during the pregnancy, but the complication is not present at the time of the admission for delivery.

3) Outcome of delivery for O80

Z37.0, Single live birth, is the only outcome of delivery code appropriate for use with O80.

o. The Peripartum and Postpartum Periods

1) Peripartum and Postpartum periods

The postpartum period begins immediately after delivery and continues for six weeks following delivery. The peripartum period is defined as the last month of pregnancy to five months postpartum.

2) Peripartum and postpartum complication

A postpartum complication is any complication occurring within the six-week period.

3) Pregnancy-related complications after 6 week period

Chapter 15 codes may also be used to describe pregnancy-related complications after the peripartum or postpartum period if the provider documents that a condition is pregnancy related.

4) Admission for routine postpartum care following delivery outside hospital

When the mother delivers outside the hospital prior to admission and is admitted for routine postpartum care and no complications are noted, code Z39.0, Encounter for care and examination of mother immediately after delivery, should be assigned as the principal diagnosis.

5) Pregnancy associated cardiomyopathy

Pregnancy associated cardiomyopathy, code O9Ø.3, is unique in that it may be diagnosed in the third trimester of pregnancy but may continue to progress months after delivery. For this reason, it is referred to as peripartum cardiomyopathy. Code O9Ø.3 is only for use when the cardiomyopathy develops as a result of pregnancy in a woman who did not have pre-existing heart disease.

p. Code O94, Sequelae of complication of pregnancy, childbirth, and the puerperium

1) Code O94

Code O94, Sequelae of complication of pregnancy, childbirth, and the puerperium, is for use in those cases when an initial complication of a pregnancy develops a sequelae requiring care or treatment at a future date.

2) After the initial postpartum period

This code may be used at any time after the initial postpartum period.

3) Sequencing of Code O94

This code, like all sequela codes, is to be sequenced following the code describing the sequelae of the complication.

q. ***Termination of Pregnancy and Spontaneous abortions***

1) Abortion with Liveborn Fetus

When an attempted termination of pregnancy results in a liveborn fetus assign code Z33.2, Encounter for elective termination of pregnancy and a code from category Z37, Outcome of Delivery.

2) Retained Products of Conception following an abortion

Subsequent encounters for retained products of conception following a spontaneous abortion or elective termination of pregnancy are assigned the appropriate code from category OØ3, Spontaneous abortion, or codes OØ7.4, Failed attempted termination of pregnancy without complication and Z33.2, Encounter for elective termination of pregnancy. This advice is appropriate even when the patient was discharged previously with a discharge diagnosis of complete abortion.

3) Complications leading to abortion

Codes from Chapter 15 may be used as additional codes to identify any documented complications of the pregnancy in conjunction with codes in categories in OØ7 and OØ8.

r. Abuse in a pregnant patient

For suspected or confirmed cases of abuse of a pregnant patient, a code(s) from subcategories O9A.3, Physical abuse complicating pregnancy, childbirth, and the puerperium, O9A.4, Sexual abuse complicating pregnancy, childbirth, and the puerperium, and O9A.5, Psychological abuse complicating pregnancy, childbirth, and the puerperium, should be sequenced first, followed by the appropriate codes (if applicable) to identify any associated current injury due to physical abuse, sexual abuse, and the perpetrator of abuse.

See Section I.C.19. Adult and child abuse, neglect and other maltreatment.

16. Chapter 16: Certain Conditions Originating in the Perinatal Period (PØØ-P96)

For coding and reporting purposes the perinatal period is defined as before birth through the 28th day following birth. The following guidelines are provided for reporting purposes

a. General Perinatal Rules

1) Use of Chapter 16 Codes

Codes in this chapter are never for use on the maternal record. Codes from Chapter 15, the obstetric chapter, are never permitted on the newborn record. Chapter 16 codes may be used throughout the life of the patient if the condition is still present.

2) Principal Diagnosis for Birth Record

When coding the birth episode in a newborn record, assign a code from category Z38, Liveborn infants according to place of birth and type of delivery, as the principal diagnosis. A code from category Z38 is assigned only once, to a newborn at the time of birth. If a newborn is transferred to another institution, a code from category Z38 should not be used at the receiving hospital.

A code from category Z38 is used only on the newborn record, not on the mother's record.

3) Use of Codes from other Chapters with Codes from Chapter 16

Codes from other chapters may be used with codes from chapter 16 if the codes from the other chapters provide more specific detail. Codes for signs and symptoms may be assigned when a definitive diagnosis has not been established. If the reason for the encounter is a perinatal condition, the code from chapter 16 should be sequenced first.

4) Use of Chapter 16 Codes after the Perinatal Period

Should a condition originate in the perinatal period, and continue throughout the life of the patient, the perinatal code should continue to be used regardless of the patient's age.

5) Birth process or community acquired conditions

If a newborn has a condition that may be either due to the birth process or community acquired and the documentation does not indicate which it is, the default is due to the birth process and the code from Chapter 16 should be used. If the condition is community-acquired, a code from Chapter 16 should not be assigned.

6) Code all clinically significant conditions

All clinically significant conditions noted on routine newborn examination should be coded. A condition is clinically significant if it requires:

- clinical evaluation; or
- therapeutic treatment; or
- diagnostic procedures; or

- extended length of hospital stay; or
- increased nursing care and/or monitoring; or
- has implications for future health care needs

Note: The perinatal guidelines listed above are the same as the general coding guidelines for "additional diagnoses", except for the final point regarding implications for future health care needs. Codes should be assigned for conditions that have been specified by the provider as having implications for future health care needs.

b. Observation and Evaluation of Newborns for Suspected Conditions not Found

1) Assign a code from category Z05, Observation and evaluation of newborns and infants for suspected conditions ruled out, to identify those instances when a healthy newborn is evaluated for a suspected condition that is determined after study not to be present. Do not use a code from category Z05 when the patient has identified signs or symptoms of a suspected problem; in such cases code the sign or symptom.

2) A code from category Z05 may also be assigned as a principal or first-listed code for readmissions or encounters when the code from category Z38 code no longer applies. Codes from category Z05 are for use only for healthy newborns and infants for which no condition after study is found to be present.

3) Z05 on a birth record

A code from category Z05 is to be used as a secondary code after the code from category Z38, Liveborn infants according to place of birth and type of delivery.

c. Coding Additional Perinatal Diagnoses

1) Assigning codes for conditions that require treatment

Assign codes for conditions that require treatment or further investigation, prolong the length of stay, or require resource utilization.

2) Codes for conditions specified as having implications for future health care needs

Assign codes for conditions that have been specified by the provider as having implications for future health care needs.

Note: This guideline should not be used for adult patients.

d. Prematurity and Fetal Growth Retardation

Providers utilize different criteria in determining prematurity. A code for prematurity should not be assigned unless it is documented. Assignment of codes in categories P05, Disorders of newborn related to slow fetal growth and fetal malnutrition, and P07, Disorders of newborn related to short gestation and low birth weight, not elsewhere classified, should be based on the recorded birth weight and estimated gestational age. Codes from category P05 should not be assigned with codes from category P07.

When both birth weight and gestational age are available, two codes from category P07 should be assigned, with the code for birth weight sequenced before the code for gestational age.

e. Low birth weight and immaturity status

Codes from category P07, Disorders of newborn related to short gestation and low birth weight, not elsewhere classified, are for use for a child or adult who was premature or had a low birth weight as a newborn and this is affecting the patient's current health status.

See Section I.C.21. Factors influencing health status and contact with health services, Status.

f. Bacterial Sepsis of Newborn

Category P36, Bacterial sepsis of newborn, includes congenital sepsis. If a perinate is documented as having sepsis without documentation of congenital or community acquired, the default is congenital and a code from category P36 should be assigned. If the P36 code includes the causal organism, an additional code from category B95, Streptococcus, Staphylococcus, and Enterococcus as the cause of diseases classified elsewhere, or B96, Other bacterial agents as the cause of diseases classified elsewhere, should not be assigned. If the P36 code does not include the causal organism, assign an additional code from category B96. If applicable, use additional codes to identify severe sepsis (R65.2-) and any associated acute organ dysfunction.

g. Stillbirth

Code P95, Stillbirth, is only for use in institutions that maintain separate records for stillbirths. No other code should be used with P95. Code P95 should not be used on the mother's record.

17. Chapter 17: Congenital malformations, deformations, and chromosomal abnormalities (Q00-Q99)

Assign an appropriate code(s) from categories Q00-Q99, Congenital malformations, deformations, and chromosomal abnormalities when a malformation/deformation or chromosomal abnormality is documented. A malformation/deformation/or chromosomal abnormality may be the principal/first-listed diagnosis on a record or a secondary diagnosis.

When a malformation/deformation/or chromosomal abnormality does not have a unique code assignment, assign additional code(s) for any manifestations that may be present.

When the code assignment specifically identifies the malformation/deformation/or chromosomal abnormality, manifestations that are an inherent component of the anomaly should not be coded separately. Additional codes should be assigned for manifestations that are not an inherent component.

Codes from Chapter 17 may be used throughout the life of the patient. If a congenital malformation or deformity has been corrected, a personal history code should be used to identify the history of the malformation or deformity. Although present at birth, malformation/deformation/or chromosomal abnormality may not be identified until later in life. Whenever the condition is diagnosed by the physician, it is appropriate to assign a code from codes Q00-Q99.

For the birth admission, the appropriate code from category Z38, Liveborn infants, according to place of birth and type of delivery, should be sequenced as the principal diagnosis, followed by any congenital anomaly codes, Q00-Q99.

18. Chapter 18: Symptoms, signs, and abnormal clinical and laboratory findings, not elsewhere classified (R00-R99)

Chapter 18 includes symptoms, signs, abnormal results of clinical or other investigative procedures, and ill-defined conditions regarding which no diagnosis classifiable elsewhere is recorded. Signs and symptoms that point to a specific diagnosis have been assigned to a category in other chapters of the classification.

a. Use of symptom codes

Codes that describe symptoms and signs are acceptable for reporting purposes when a related definitive diagnosis has not been established (confirmed) by the provider.

b. Use of a symptom code with a definitive diagnosis code

Codes for signs and symptoms may be reported in addition to a related definitive diagnosis when the sign or symptom is not routinely associated with that diagnosis, such as the various signs and symptoms associated with complex syndromes. The definitive diagnosis code should be sequenced before the symptom code.

Signs or symptoms that are associated routinely with a disease process should not be assigned as additional codes, unless otherwise instructed by the classification.

c. Combination codes that include symptoms

ICD-10-CM contains a number of combination codes that identify both the definitive diagnosis and common symptoms of that diagnosis. When using one of these combination codes, an additional code should not be assigned for the symptom.

d. Repeated falls

Code R29.6, Repeated falls, is for use for encounters when a patient has recently fallen and the reason for the fall is being investigated.

Code Z91.81, History of falling, is for use when a patient has fallen in the past and is at risk for future falls. When appropriate, both codes R29.6 and Z91.81 may be assigned together.

e. Coma scale

The coma scale codes (R40.2-) can be used in conjunction with traumatic brain injury codes, acute cerebrovascular disease or sequelae of cerebrovascular disease codes. These codes are primarily for use by trauma registries, but they may be used in any setting where this information is collected. **The coma scale may also be used to assess the status of the central nervous system for other non-trauma conditions, such as monitoring patients in the intensive care unit regardless of medical condition.** The coma scale codes should be sequenced after the diagnosis code(s).

These codes, one from each subcategory, are needed to complete the scale. The 7th character indicates when the scale was recorded. The 7th character should match for all three codes.

At a minimum, report the initial score documented on presentation at your facility. This may be a score from the emergency medicine technician (EMT) or in the emergency department. If desired, a facility may choose to capture multiple coma scale scores.

Assign code R40.24, Glasgow coma scale, total score, when only the total score is documented in the medical record and not the individual score(s).

f. Functional quadriplegia

Functional quadriplegia (code R53.2) is the lack of ability to use one's limbs or to ambulate due to extreme debility. It is not associated with neurologic deficit or injury, and code R53.2 should not be used for cases of neurologic quadriplegia. It should only be assigned if functional quadriplegia is specifically documented in the medical record.

g. SIRS due to Non-Infectious Process

The systemic inflammatory response syndrome (SIRS) can develop as a result of certain non-infectious disease processes, such as trauma, malignant neoplasm, or pancreatitis. When SIRS is documented with a noninfectious condition, and no subsequent infection is documented, the code for the underlying condition, such as an injury, should be assigned, followed by code R65.10, Systemic inflammatory response syndrome (SIRS) of non-infectious origin without acute organ dysfunction, or code R65.11, Systemic inflammatory response syndrome (SIRS) of non-infectious origin with acute organ dysfunction. If an associated acute organ dysfunction is documented, the appropriate code(s) for the specific type of organ dysfunction(s) should be assigned in addition to code R65.11. If acute organ dysfunction is documented, but it cannot be determined if the acute organ dysfunction is associated with SIRS or due to another condition (e.g., directly due to the trauma), the provider should be queried.

h. Death NOS

Code R99, Ill-defined and unknown cause of mortality, is only for use in the very limited circumstance when a patient who has already died is brought into an emergency department or other healthcare facility and is pronounced dead upon arrival. It does not represent the discharge disposition of death.

i. NIHSS Stroke Scale

The NIH stroke scale (NIHSS) codes (R29.7- -) can be used in conjunction with acute stroke codes (I63) to identify the patient's neurological status and the severity of the stroke. The stroke scale codes should be sequenced after the acute stroke diagnosis code(s).

At a minimum, report the initial score documented. If desired, a facility may choose to capture multiple stroke scale scores.

See Section I.B.14. for information concerning the medical record documentation that may be used for assignment of the NIHSS codes.

19. Chapter 19: Injury, poisoning, and certain other consequences of external causes (S00-T88)

a. Application of 7th Characters in Chapter 19

Most categories in chapter 19 have a 7th character requirement for each applicable code. Most categories in this chapter have three 7th character values (with the exception of fractures): A, initial encounter, D, subsequent encounter and S, sequela. Categories for traumatic fractures have additional 7th character values. While the patient may be seen by a new or different provider over the course of treatment for an injury, assignment of the 7th character is based on whether the patient is undergoing active treatment and not whether the provider is seeing the patient for the first time.

For complication codes, active treatment refers to treatment for the condition described by the code, even though it may be related to an earlier precipitating problem. For example, code T84.50XA, Infection and inflammatory reaction due to unspecified internal joint prosthesis, initial encounter, is used when active treatment is provided for the infection, even though the condition relates to the prosthetic device, implant or graft that was placed at a previous encounter.

7th character "A", initial encounter is used **for each encounter where** the patient is receiving active treatment for the condition.

7th character "D" subsequent encounter is used for encounters after the patient has **completed** active treatment of the condition and is receiving routine care for the condition during the healing or recovery phase.

The aftercare Z codes should not be used for aftercare for conditions such as injuries or poisonings, where 7th characters are provided to identify subsequent care. For example, for aftercare of an injury, assign the acute injury code with the 7th character "D" (subsequent encounter).

7th character "S", sequela, is for use for complications or conditions that arise as a direct result of a condition, such as scar formation after a burn. The scars are sequelae of the burn. When using 7th character "S", it is necessary to use both the injury code that precipitated the sequela and the code for the sequela itself. The "S" is added only to the injury code, not the sequela code. The 7th character "S" identifies the injury responsible for the sequela. The specific type of sequela (e.g. scar) is sequenced first, followed by the injury code.

See Section I.B.10. Sequelae, (Late Effects)

b. Coding of Injuries

When coding injuries, assign separate codes for each injury unless a combination code is provided, in which case the combination code is assigned. Code T07, Unspecified multiple injuries should not be assigned in the inpatient setting unless information for a more specific code is not available. Traumatic injury codes (S00-T14.9) are not to be used for normal, healing surgical wounds or to identify complications of surgical wounds.

The code for the most serious injury, as determined by the provider and the focus of treatment, is sequenced first.

1) Superficial injuries

Superficial injuries such as abrasions or contusions are not coded when associated with more severe injuries of the same site.

2) Primary injury with damage to nerves/ blood vessels

When a primary injury results in minor damage to peripheral nerves or blood vessels, the primary injury is sequenced first with additional code(s) for injuries to nerves and spinal cord (such as category S04), and/or injury to blood vessels (such as category S15). When the primary injury is to the blood vessels or nerves, that injury should be sequenced first.

c. Coding of Traumatic Fractures

The principles of multiple coding of injuries should be followed in coding fractures. Fractures of specified sites are coded individually by site in accordance with both the provisions within categories S02, S12, S22, S32, S42, S49, S52, S59, S62, S72, S79, S82, S89, S92 and the level of detail furnished by medical record content.

A fracture not indicated as open or closed should be coded to closed. A fracture not indicated whether displaced or not displaced should be coded to displaced.

More specific guidelines are as follows:

1) Initial vs. Subsequent Encounter for Fractures

Traumatic fractures are coded using the appropriate 7th character for initial encounter (A, B, C) **for each encounter where** the patient is receiving active treatment for the fracture. The appropriate 7th character for initial encounter should also be assigned for a patient who delayed seeking treatment for the fracture or nonunion.

Fractures are coded using the appropriate 7th character for subsequent care for encounters after the patient has completed active treatment of the fracture and is receiving routine care for the fracture during the healing or recovery phase.

Care for complications of surgical treatment for fracture repairs during the healing or recovery phase should be coded with the appropriate complication codes.

Care of complications of fractures, such as malunion and nonunion, should be reported with the appropriate 7th character for subsequent care with nonunion (K, M, N,) or subsequent care with malunion (P, Q, R).

Malunion/nonunion: The appropriate 7th character for initial encounter should also be assigned for a patient who delayed seeking treatment for the fracture or nonunion.

The open fracture designations in the assignment of the 7th character for fractures of the forearm, femur and lower leg, including ankle are based on the Gustilo open fracture classification. When the Gustilo classification type is not specified for an open fracture, the 7th character for open fracture type I or II should be assigned (B, E, H, M, Q).

A code from category M8Ø, not a traumatic fracture code, should be used for any patient with known osteoporosis who suffers a fracture, even if the patient had a minor fall or trauma, if that fall or trauma would not usually break a normal, healthy bone.

See Section I.C.13. Osteoporosis.

The aftercare Z codes should not be used for aftercare for traumatic fractures. For aftercare of a traumatic fracture, assign the acute fracture code with the appropriate 7th character.

2) Multiple fractures sequencing

Multiple fractures are sequenced in accordance with the severity of the fracture.

d. Coding of Burns and Corrosions

The ICD-10-CM makes a distinction between burns and corrosions. The burn codes are for thermal burns, except sunburns, that come from a heat source, such as a fire or hot appliance. The burn codes are also for burns resulting from electricity and radiation. Corrosions are burns due to chemicals. The guidelines are the same for burns and corrosions.

Current burns (T2Ø-T25) are classified by depth, extent and by agent (X code). Burns are classified by depth as first degree (erythema), second degree (blistering), and third degree (full-thickness involvement). Burns of the eye and internal organs (T26-T28) are classified by site, but not by degree.

1) Sequencing of burn and related condition codes

Sequence first the code that reflects the highest degree of burn when more than one burn is present.

a. When the reason for the admission or encounter is for treatment of external multiple burns, sequence first the code that reflects the burn of the highest degree.

b. When a patient has both internal and external burns, the circumstances of admission govern the selection of the principal diagnosis or first-listed diagnosis.

c. When a patient is admitted for burn injuries and other related conditions such as smoke inhalation and/or respiratory failure, the circumstances of admission govern the selection of the principal or first-listed diagnosis.

2) Burns of the same local site

Classify burns of the same local site (three-character category level, T2Ø-T28) but of different degrees to the subcategory identifying the highest degree recorded in the diagnosis.

3) Non-healing burns

Non-healing burns are coded as acute burns.

Necrosis of burned skin should be coded as a non-healed burn.

4) Infected Burn

For any documented infected burn site, use an additional code for the infection.

5) Assign separate codes for each burn site

When coding burns, assign separate codes for each burn site. Category T3Ø, Burn and corrosion, body region unspecified is extremely vague and should rarely be used.

6) Burns and Corrosions Classified According to Extent of Body Surface Involved

Assign codes from category T31, Burns classified according to extent of body surface involved, or T32, Corrosions classified according to extent of body surface involved, when the site of the burn is not specified or when there is a need for additional data. It is advisable to use category T31 as additional coding when needed to provide data for evaluating burn mortality, such as that needed by burn units. It is also advisable to use category T31 as an additional code for reporting purposes when there is mention of a third-degree burn involving 2Ø percent or more of the body surface.

Categories T31 and T32 are based on the classic "rule of nines" in estimating body surface involved: head and neck are assigned nine percent, each arm nine percent, each leg 18 percent, the anterior trunk 18 percent, posterior trunk 18 percent, and genitalia one percent. Providers may change these percentage assignments where necessary to accommodate infants and children who have proportionately larger heads than adults, and patients who have large buttocks, thighs, or abdomen that involve burns.

7) Encounters for treatment of sequela of burns

Encounters for the treatment of the late effects of burns or corrosions (i.e., scars or joint contractures) should be coded with a burn or corrosion code with the 7th character "S" for sequela.

8) Sequelae with a late effect code and current burn

When appropriate, both a code for a current burn or corrosion with 7th character "A" or "D" and a burn or corrosion code with 7th character "S" may be assigned on the same record (when both a current burn and sequelae of an old burn exist). Burns and corrosions do not heal at the same rate and a current healing wound may still exist with sequela of a healed burn or corrosion.

See Section I.B.1Ø. Sequela, (Late Effects)

9) Use of an external cause code with burns and corrosions

An external cause code should be used with burns and corrosions to identify the source and intent of the burn, as well as the place where it occurred.

e. Adverse Effects, Poisoning , Underdosing and Toxic Effects

Codes in categories T36-T65 are combination codes that include the substance that was taken as well as the intent. No additional external cause code is required for poisonings, toxic effects, adverse effects and underdosing codes.

1) Do not code directly from the Table of Drugs

Do not code directly from the Table of Drugs and Chemicals. Always refer back to the Tabular List.

2) Use as many codes as necessary to describe

Use as many codes as necessary to describe completely all drugs, medicinal or biological substances.

3) If the same code would describe the causative agent

If the same code would describe the causative agent for more than one adverse reaction, poisoning, toxic effect or underdosing, assign the code only once.

4) If two or more drugs, medicinal or biological substances

If two or more drugs, medicinal or biological substances are reported, code each individually unless a combination code is listed in the Table of Drugs and Chemicals.

5) The occurrence of drug toxicity is classified in ICD-10-CM as follows:

(a) Adverse Effect

When coding an adverse effect of a drug that has been correctly prescribed and properly administered, assign the appropriate code for the nature of the adverse effect followed by the appropriate code for the adverse effect of the drug (T36-T50). The code for the drug should have a 5th or 6th character "5" (for example T36.0X5-) Examples of the nature of an adverse effect are tachycardia, delirium, gastrointestinal hemorrhaging, vomiting, hypokalemia, hepatitis, renal failure, or respiratory failure.

(b) Poisoning

When coding a poisoning or reaction to the improper use of a medication (e.g., overdose, wrong substance given or taken in error, wrong route of administration), first assign the appropriate code from categories T36-T50. The poisoning codes have an associated intent as their 5th or 6th character (accidental, intentional self-harm, assault and undetermined). **If the intent of the poisoning is unknown or unspecified, code the intent as accidental intent. The undetermined intent is only for use if the documentation in the record specifies that the intent cannot be determined.** Use additional code(s) for all manifestations of poisonings.

If there is also a diagnosis of abuse or dependence of the substance, the abuse or dependence is assigned as an additional code.

Examples of poisoning include:

(i) Error was made in drug prescription Errors made in drug prescription or in the administration of the drug by provider, nurse, patient, or other person.

(ii) Overdose of a drug intentionally taken If an overdose of a drug was intentionally taken or administered and resulted in drug toxicity, it would be coded as a poisoning.

(iii) Nonprescribed drug taken with correctly prescribed and properly administered drug.
If a nonprescribed drug or medicinal agent was taken in combination with a correctly prescribed and properly administered drug, any drug toxicity or other reaction resulting from the interaction of the two drugs would be classified as a poisoning.

(iv) Interaction of drug(s) and alcohol.
When a reaction results from the interaction of a drug(s) and alcohol, this would be classified as poisoning.

See Section I.C.4. if poisoning is the result of insulin pump malfunctions.

(c) Underdosing

Underdosing refers to taking less of a medication than is prescribed by a provider or a manufacturer's instruction. For underdosing, assign the code from categories T36-T50 (fifth or sixth character "6").

Codes for underdosing should never be assigned as principal or first-listed codes. If a patient has a relapse or exacerbation of the medical condition for which the drug is prescribed because of the reduction in dose, then the medical condition itself should be coded.

Noncompliance (Z91.12-, Z91.13-) or complication of care (Y63.6-Y63.9) codes are to be used with an underdosing code to indicate intent, if known.

(d) Toxic Effects

When a harmful substance is ingested or comes in contact with a person, this is classified as a toxic effect. The toxic effect codes are in categories T51-T65.

Toxic effect codes have an associated intent: accidental, intentional self-harm, assault and undetermined.

f. Adult and child abuse, neglect and other maltreatment

Sequence first the appropriate code from categories T74.- (Adult and child abuse, neglect and other maltreatment, confirmed) or T76.- (Adult and child abuse, neglect and other maltreatment, suspected) for abuse, neglect and other maltreatment, followed by any accompanying mental health or injury code(s).

If the documentation in the medical record states abuse or neglect it is coded as confirmed (T74.-). It is coded as suspected if it is documented as suspected (T76.-).

For cases of confirmed abuse or neglect an external cause code from the assault section (X92-**Y09**) should be added to identify the cause of any physical injuries. A perpetrator code (Y07) should be added when the perpetrator of the abuse is known. For suspected cases of abuse or neglect, do not report external cause or perpetrator code.

If a suspected case of abuse, neglect or mistreatment is ruled out during an encounter code Z04.71, Encounter for examination and observation following alleged physical adult abuse, ruled out, or code Z04.72, Encounter for examination and observation following alleged child physical abuse, ruled out, should be used, not a code from T76.

If a suspected case of alleged rape or sexual abuse is ruled out during an encounter code Z04.41, Encounter for examination and observation following alleged **adult rape** or code Z04.42, Encounter for examination and observation following alleged **child** rape, should be used, not a code from T76.

See Section I.C.15. Abuse in a pregnant patient.

g. Complications of care

1) General guidelines for complications of care

(a) Documentation of complications of care

See Section I.B.16. for information on documentation of complications of care.

2) Pain due to medical devices

Pain associated with devices, implants or grafts left in a surgical site (for example painful hip prosthesis) is assigned to the appropriate code(s) found in Chapter 19, Injury, poisoning, and certain other consequences of external causes. Specific codes for pain due to medical devices are found in the T code section of the ICD-10-CM. Use additional code(s) from category G89 to identify acute or chronic pain due to presence of the device, implant or graft (G89.18 or G89.28).

3) Transplant complications

(a) Transplant complications other than kidney

Codes under category T86, Complications of transplanted organs and tissues, are for use for both complications and rejection of transplanted organs. A transplant complication code is only assigned if the complication affects the function of the transplanted organ. Two codes are required to fully describe a transplant complication: the appropriate code from category T86 and a secondary code that identifies the complication.

Pre-existing conditions or conditions that develop after the transplant are not coded as complications unless they affect the function of the transplanted organs.

See I.C.21. for transplant organ removal status

See I.C.2. for malignant neoplasm associated with transplanted organ.

(b) Kidney transplant complications

Patients who have undergone kidney transplant may still have some form of chronic kidney disease (CKD) because the kidney transplant may not fully restore kidney function. Code T86.1- should be assigned for documented complications of a kidney transplant, such as transplant failure or rejection or other transplant complication. Code T86.1- should not be assigned for post kidney transplant patients who have chronic kidney (CKD) unless a transplant complication such as transplant failure or rejection is documented. If the documentation is unclear as to whether the patient has a complication of the transplant, query the provider.

Conditions that affect the function of the transplanted kidney, other than CKD, should be assigned a code from subcategory T86.1, Complications of transplanted organ, Kidney, and a secondary code that identifies the complication.

For patients with CKD following a kidney transplant, but who do not have a complication such as failure or rejection, *see section I.C.14. Chronic kidney disease and kidney transplant status.*

4) Complication codes that include the external cause

As with certain other T codes, some of the complications of care codes have the external cause included in the code. The code includes the nature of the complication as well as the type of procedure that caused the complication. No external cause code indicating the type of procedure is necessary for these codes.

5) Complications of care codes within the body system chapters

Intraoperative and postprocedural complication codes are found within the body system chapters with codes specific to the organs and structures of that body system. These codes should be sequenced first, followed by a code(s) for the specific complication, if applicable.

20. Chapter 20: External Causes of Morbidity (V00-Y99)

The external causes of morbidity codes should never be sequenced as the first-listed or principal diagnosis.

External cause codes are intended to provide data for injury research and evaluation of injury prevention strategies. These codes capture how the injury or health condition happened (cause), the intent (unintentional or accidental; or intentional, such as suicide or assault), the place where the event occurred the activity of the patient at the time of the event, and the person's status (e.g., civilian, military).

There is no national requirement for mandatory ICD-10-CM external cause code reporting. Unless a provider is subject to a state-based external cause code reporting mandate or these codes are required by a particular payer, reporting of ICD-10-CM codes in Chapter 20, External Causes of Morbidity, is not required. In the absence of a mandatory reporting requirement, providers are encouraged to voluntarily report external cause codes, as they provide valuable data for injury research and evaluation of injury prevention strategies.

a. General External Cause Coding Guidelines

1) Used with any code in the range of A00.0-T88.9, Z00-Z99

An external cause code may be used with any code in the range of A00.0-T88.9, Z00-Z99, classification that is a health condition due to an external cause. Though they are most applicable to injuries, they are also valid for use with such things as infections or diseases due to an external source, and other health conditions, such as a heart attack that occurs during strenuous physical activity.

2) External cause code used for length of treatment

Assign the external cause code, with the appropriate 7th character (initial encounter, subsequent encounter or sequela) for each encounter for which the injury or condition is being treated.

Most categories in chapter 20 have a 7th character requirement for each applicable code. Most categories in this chapter have three 7th character values: A, initial encounter, D, subsequent encounter and S, sequela. While the patient may be seen by a new or different provider over the course of treatment for an injury or condition, assignment of the 7th character for external cause should match the 7th character of the code assigned for the associated injury or condition for the encounter.

3) Use the full range of external cause codes

Use the full range of external cause codes to completely describe the cause, the intent, the place of occurrence and if applicable, the activity of the patient at the time of the event, and the patient's status, for all injuries, and other health conditions due to an external cause.

4) Assign as many external cause codes as necessary

Assign as many external cause codes as necessary to fully explain each cause. If only one external code can be recorded, assign the code most related to the principal diagnosis.

5) The selection of the appropriate external cause code

The selection of the appropriate external cause code is guided by the Alphabetic Index of External Causes and by Inclusion and Exclusion notes in the Tabular List.

6) External cause code can never be a principal diagnosis

An external cause code can never be a principal (first-listed) diagnosis.

7) Combination external cause codes

Certain of the external cause codes are combination codes that identify sequential events that result in an injury, such as a fall which results in striking against an object. The injury may be due to either event or both. The combination external cause code used should correspond to the sequence of events regardless of which caused the most serious injury.

8) No external cause code needed in certain circumstances

No external cause code from Chapter 20 is needed if the external cause and intent are included in a code from another chapter (e.g. T36.0X1- Poisoning by penicillins, accidental (unintentional)).

b. Place of Occurrence Guideline

Codes from category Y92, Place of occurrence of the external cause, are secondary codes for use after other external cause codes to identify the location of the patient at the time of injury or other condition.

Generally, a place of occurrence code is assigned only once, at the initial encounter for treatment. However, in the rare instance that a new injury occurs during hospitalization, an additional place of occurrence code may be assigned. No 7th characters are used for Y92. Only one code from Y92 should be recorded on a medical record.

Do not use place of occurrence code Y92.9 if the place is not stated or is not applicable.

c. Activity Code

Assign a code from category Y93, Activity code, to describe the activity of the patient at the time the injury or other health condition occurred.

An activity code is used only once, at the initial encounter for treatment. Only one code from Y93 should be recorded on a medical record.

The activity codes are not applicable to poisonings, adverse effects, misadventures or sequela.

Do not assign Y93.9, Unspecified activity, if the activity is not stated.

A code from category Y93 is appropriate for use with external cause and intent codes if identifying the activity provides additional information about the event.

d. Place of Occurrence, Activity, and Status Codes Used with other External Cause Code

When applicable, place of occurrence, activity, and external cause status codes are sequenced after the main external cause code(s). Regardless of the number of external cause codes assigned, there should be only one place of occurrence code, one activity code, and one external cause status code assigned to an encounter.

e. If the Reporting Format Limits the Number of External Cause Codes

If the reporting format limits the number of external cause codes that can be used in reporting clinical data, report the code for the cause/intent most related to the principal diagnosis. If the format permits capture of additional external cause codes, the cause/intent, including medical misadventures, of the additional events should be reported rather than the codes for place, activity, or external status.

f. Multiple External Cause Coding Guidelines

More than one external cause code is required to fully describe the external cause of an illness or injury. The assignment of external cause codes should be sequenced in the following priority:

If two or more events cause separate injuries, an external cause code should be assigned for each cause. The first-listed external cause code will be selected in the following order:

External codes for child and adult abuse take priority over all other external cause codes.

See Section I.C.19., Child and Adult abuse guidelines.

External codes for terrorism events take priority over all other external cause codes except child and adult abuse.

External cause codes for cataclysmic events take priority over all other external cause codes except child and adult abuse and terrorism.

External cause codes for transport accidents take priority over all other external cause codes except cataclysmic events, child and adult abuse and terrorism.

Activity and external cause status codes are assigned following all causal (intent) external cause codes.

The first-listed external cause code should correspond to the cause of the most serious diagnosis due to an assault, accident, or self-harm, following the order of hierarchy listed above.

g. Child and Adult Abuse Guideline

Adult and child abuse, neglect and maltreatment are classified as assault. Any of the assault codes may be used to indicate the external cause of any injury resulting from the confirmed abuse.

For confirmed cases of abuse, neglect and maltreatment, when the perpetrator is known, a code from Y07, Perpetrator of maltreatment and neglect, should accompany any other assault codes.

See Section I.C.19. Adult and child abuse, neglect and other maltreatment

h. Unknown or Undetermined Intent Guideline

If the intent (accident, self-harm, assault) of the cause of an injury or other condition is unknown or unspecified, code the intent as accidental intent. All transport accident categories assume accidental intent.

1) Use of undetermined intent

External cause codes for events of undetermined intent are only for use if the documentation in the record specifies that the intent cannot be determined.

i. Sequelae (Late Effects) of External Cause Guidelines

1) Sequelae external cause codes

Sequela are reported using the external cause code with the 7th character "S" for sequela. These codes should be used with any report of a late effect or sequela resulting from a previous injury.

See Section I.B.10. Sequela, (Late Effects)

2) Sequela external cause code with a related current injury

A sequela external cause code should never be used with a related current nature of injury code.

3) Use of sequela external cause codes for subsequent visits

Use a late effect external cause code for subsequent visits when a late effect of the initial injury is being treated. Do not use a late effect external cause code for subsequent visits for follow-up care (e.g., to assess healing, to receive rehabilitative therapy) of the injury when no late effect of the injury has been documented.

j. Terrorism Guidelines

1) Cause of injury identified by the Federal Government (FBI) as terrorism

When the cause of an injury is identified by the Federal Government (FBI) as terrorism, the first-listed external cause code should be a code from category Y38, Terrorism. The definition of terrorism employed by the FBI is found at the inclusion note at the beginning of category Y38. Use additional code for place of occurrence (Y92.-). More than one Y38 code may be assigned if the injury is the result of more than one mechanism of terrorism.

2) Cause of an injury is suspected to be the result of terrorism

When the cause of an injury is suspected to be the result of terrorism a code from category Y38 should not be assigned. Suspected cases should be classified as assault.

3) Code Y38.9, Terrorism, secondary effects

Assign code Y38.9, Terrorism, secondary effects, for conditions occurring subsequent to the terrorist event. This code should not be assigned for conditions that are due to the initial terrorist act.

It is acceptable to assign code Y38.9 with another code from Y38 if there is an injury due to the initial terrorist event and an injury that is a subsequent result of the terrorist event.

k. External cause status

A code from category Y99, External cause status, should be assigned whenever any other external cause code is assigned for an encounter, including an Activity code, except for the events noted below. Assign a code from category Y99, External cause status, to indicate the work status of the person at the time the event occurred. The status code indicates whether the event occurred during military activity, whether a non-military person was at work, whether an individual including a student or volunteer was involved in a non-work activity at the time of the causal event.

A code from Y99, External cause status, should be assigned, when applicable, with other external cause codes, such as transport accidents and falls. The external cause status codes are not applicable to poisonings, adverse effects, misadventures or late effects.

Do not assign a code from category Y99 if no other external cause codes (cause, activity) are applicable for the encounter.

An external cause status code is used only once, at the initial encounter for treatment. Only one code from Y99 should be recorded on a medical record.

Do not assign code Y99.9, Unspecified external cause status, if the status is not stated.

21. Chapter 21: Factors influencing health status and contact with health services (Z00-Z99)

Note: The chapter specific guidelines provide additional information about the use of Z codes for specified encounters.

a. Use of Z codes in any healthcare setting

Z codes are for use in any healthcare setting. Z codes may be used as either a first-listed (principal diagnosis code in the inpatient setting) or secondary code, depending on the circumstances of the encounter. Certain Z codes may only be used as first-listed or principal diagnosis.

b. Z Codes indicate a reason for an encounter

Z codes are not procedure codes. A corresponding procedure code must accompany a Z code to describe any procedure performed.

c. Categories of Z Codes

1) Contact/Exposure

Category Z20 indicates contact with, and suspected exposure to, communicable diseases. These codes are for patients who do not show any sign or symptom of a disease but are suspected to have been exposed to it by close personal contact with an infected individual or are in an area where a disease is epidemic.

Category Z77, Other contact with and (suspected) exposures hazardous to health, indicates contact with and suspected exposures hazardous to health.

Contact/exposure codes may be used as a first-listed code to explain an encounter for testing, or, more commonly, as a secondary code to identify a potential risk.

2) Inoculations and vaccinations

Code Z23 is for encounters for inoculations and vaccinations. It indicates that a patient is being seen to receive a prophylactic inoculation against a disease. Procedure codes are required to identify the actual administration of the injection and the type(s) of immunizations given. Code Z23 may be used as a secondary code if the inoculation is given as a routine part of preventive health care, such as a well-baby visit.

3) Status

Status codes indicate that a patient is either a carrier of a disease or has the sequelae or residual of a past disease or condition. This includes such things as the presence of prosthetic or mechanical devices resulting from past treatment. A status code is informative, because the status may affect the course of treatment and its outcome. A status code is distinct from a history code. The history code indicates that the patient no longer has the condition.

A status code should not be used with a diagnosis code from one of the body system chapters, if the diagnosis code includes the information provided by the status code. For example, code Z94.1, Heart transplant status, should not be used with a code from subcategory T86.2, Complications of heart transplant. The status code does not provide additional information. The complication code indicates that the patient is a heart transplant patient.

For encounters for weaning from a mechanical ventilator, assign a code from subcategory J96.1, Chronic respiratory failure, followed by code Z99.11, Dependence on respirator [ventilator] status.

The status Z codes/categories are:

Z14 Genetic carrier
Genetic carrier status indicates that a person carries a gene, associated with a particular disease, which may be passed to offspring who may develop that disease. The person does not have the disease and is not at risk of developing the disease.

Z15 Genetic susceptibility to disease Genetic susceptibility indicates that a person has a gene that increases the risk of that person developing the disease.

Codes from category Z15 should not be used as principal or first-listed codes. If the patient has the condition to which he/she is susceptible, and that condition is the reason for the encounter, the code for the current condition should be sequenced first. If the patient is being seen for follow-up after completed treatment for this condition, and the condition no longer exists, a follow-up code should be sequenced first, followed by the appropriate personal history and genetic susceptibility codes. If the purpose of the encounter is genetic counseling associated with procreative management, code Z31.5, Encounter for genetic counseling, should be assigned as the first-listed code, followed by a code from category Z15. Additional codes should be assigned for any applicable family or personal history.

Z16 Resistance to antimicrobial drugs
This code indicates that a patient has a condition that is resistant to antimicrobial drug treatment. Sequence the infection code first.

Z17 Estrogen receptor status
Z18 Retained foreign body fragments
Z19 Hormone sensitivity malignancy status
Z21 Asymptomatic HIV infection status This code indicates that a patient has tested positive for HIV but has manifested no signs or symptoms of the disease.
Z22 Carrier of infectious disease Carrier status indicates that a person harbors the specific organisms of a disease without manifest symptoms and is capable of transmitting the infection.
Z28.3 Underimmunization status
Z33.1 Pregnant state, incidental This code is a secondary code only for use when the pregnancy is in no way complicating the reason for visit. Otherwise, a code from the obstetric chapter is required.
Z66 Do not resuscitate

This code may be used when it is documented by the provider that a patient is on do not resuscitate status at any time during the stay.

Z67 Blood type
Z68 Body mass index (BMI)
As with all other secondary diagnosis codes, the BMI codes should only be assigned when they meet the definition of a reportable diagnosis (see Section III, Reporting Additional Diagnoses).
Z74.01 Bed confinement status
Z76.82 Awaiting organ transplant status
Z78 Other specified health status

Code Z78.1, Physical restraint status, may be used when it is documented by the provider that a patient has been put in restraints during the current encounter. Please note that this code should not be reported when it is documented by the provider that a patient is temporarily restrained during a procedure.

Z79 Long-term (current) drug therapy

Codes from this category indicate a patient's continuous use of a prescribed drug (including such things as aspirin therapy) for the long-term treatment of a condition or for prophylactic use. It is not for use for patients who have addictions to drugs. This subcategory is not for use of medications for detoxification or maintenance programs to prevent withdrawal symptoms in patients with drug dependence (e.g., methadone maintenance for opiate dependence). Assign the appropriate code for the drug dependence instead.

Assign a code from Z79 if the patient is receiving a medication for an extended period as a prophylactic measure (such as for the prevention of deep vein thrombosis) or as treatment of a chronic condition (such as arthritis) or a disease requiring a lengthy course of treatment (such as cancer). Do not assign a code from category Z79 for medication being administered for a brief period of time to treat an acute illness or injury (such as a course of antibiotics to treat acute bronchitis).

Z88 Allergy status to drugs, medicaments and biological substances Except: Z88.9, Allergy status to unspecified drugs, medicaments and biological substances status
Z89 Acquired absence of limb
Z90 Acquired absence of organs, not elsewhere classified
Z91.0- Allergy status, other than to drugs and biological substances
Z92.82 Status post administration of tPA (rtPA) in a different facility within the last 24 hours prior to admission to a current facility Assign code Z92.82, Status post administration of tPA (rtPA) in a different facility within the last 24 hours prior to admission to current facility, as a secondary diagnosis when a patient is received by transfer into a facility and documentation indicates they were administered tissue plasminogen activator (tPA) within the last 24 hours prior to admission to the current facility. This guideline applies even if the patient is still receiving the tPA at the time they are received into the current facility. The appropriate code for the condition for which the tPA was administered (such as cerebrovascular disease or myocardial infarction) should be assigned first. Code Z92.82 is only applicable to the receiving facility record and not to the transferring facility record.
Z93 Artificial opening status
Z94 Transplanted organ and tissue status
Z95 Presence of cardiac and vascular implants and grafts
Z96 Presence of other functional implants
Z97 Presence of other devices
Z98 Other postprocedural states

Assign code Z98.85, Transplanted organ removal status, to indicate that a transplanted organ has been previously removed. This code should not be assigned for the encounter in which the transplanted organ is removed. The complication necessitating removal of the transplant organ should be assigned for that encounter.

See section I.C.19. for information on the coding of organ transplant complications.

Z99 Dependence on enabling machines and devices, not elsewhere classified

Note: Categories Z89-Z90 and Z93-Z99 are for use only if there are no complications or malfunctions of the organ or tissue replaced, the amputation site or the equipment on which the patient is dependent.

4) History (of)

There are two types of history Z codes, personal and family. Personal history codes explain a patient's past medical condition that no longer exists and is not receiving any treatment, but that has the potential for recurrence, and therefore may require continued monitoring.

Family history codes are for use when a patient has a family member(s) who has had a particular disease that causes the patient to be at higher risk of also contracting the disease.

Personal history codes may be used in conjunction with follow-up codes and family history codes may be used in conjunction with screening codes to explain the need for a test or procedure. History codes are also acceptable on any medical record regardless of the reason for visit. A history of an illness, even if no longer present, is important information that may alter the type of treatment ordered.

The history Z code categories are:

- Z8Ø Family history of primary malignant neoplasm
- Z81 Family history of mental and behavioral disorders
- Z82 Family history of certain disabilities and chronic diseases (leading to disablement)
- Z83 Family history of other specific disorders
- Z84 Family history of other conditions
- Z85 Personal history of malignant neoplasm
- Z86 Personal history of certain other diseases
- Z87 Personal history of other diseases and conditions
- Z91.4- Personal history of psychological trauma, not elsewhere classified
- Z91.5 Personal history of self-harm
- Z91.8- Other specified personal risk factors, not elsewhere classified
  Exception:
  Z91.83, Wandering in diseases classified elsewhere
- Z92 Personal history of medical treatment Except: Z92.Ø, Personal history of contraception Except: Z92.82, Status post administration of tPA (rtPA) in a different facility within the last 24 hours prior to admission to a current facility

5) Screening

Screening is the testing for disease or disease precursors in seemingly well individuals so that early detection and treatment can be provided for those who test positive for the disease (e.g., screening mammogram).

The testing of a person to rule out or confirm a suspected diagnosis because the patient has some sign or symptom is a diagnostic examination, not a screening. In these cases, the sign or symptom is used to explain the reason for the test.

A screening code may be a first-listed code if the reason for the visit is specifically the screening exam. It may also be used as an additional code if the screening is done during an office visit for other health problems. A screening code is not necessary if the screening is inherent to a routine examination, such as a pap smear done during a routine pelvic examination.

Should a condition be discovered during the screening then the code for the condition may be assigned as an additional diagnosis.

The Z code indicates that a screening exam is planned. A procedure code is required to confirm that the screening was performed.

The screening Z codes/categories:

- Z11 Encounter for screening for infectious and parasitic diseases
- Z12 Encounter for screening for malignant neoplasms
- Z13 Encounter for screening for other diseases and disorders Except: Z13.9, Encounter for screening, unspecified
- Z36 Encounter for antenatal screening for mother

6) Observation

There are **three** observation Z code categories. They are for use in very limited circumstances when a person is being observed for a suspected condition that is ruled out. The observation codes are not for use if an injury or illness or any signs or symptoms related to the suspected condition are present. In such cases the diagnosis/symptom code is used with the corresponding external cause code.

The observation codes are to be used as principal diagnosis only. **The only exception to this is when the principal diagnosis is required to be a code from category Z38, Liveborn infants according to place of birth and type of delivery. Then a code from category ZØ5, Encounter for observation and evaluation of newborn for suspected diseases and conditions ruled out, is sequenced after the Z38 code.** Additional codes may be used in addition to the observation code, but only if they are unrelated to the suspected condition being observed.

Codes from subcategory ZØ3.7 Encounter for suspected maternal and fetal conditions ruled out, may either be used as a first-listed or as an additional code assignment depending on the case. They are for use in very limited circumstances on a maternal record when an encounter is for a suspected maternal or fetal condition that is ruled out during that encounter (for example, a maternal or fetal condition may be suspected due to an abnormal test result). These codes should not be used when the condition is confirmed. In those cases, the confirmed condition should be coded. In addition, these codes are not for use if an illness or any signs or symptoms related to the suspected condition or problem are present. In such cases the diagnosis/symptom code is used.

Additional codes may be used in addition to the code from subcategory Z03.7, but only if they are unrelated to the suspected condition being evaluated.

Codes from subcategory Z03.7 may not be used for encounters for antenatal screening of mother. *See Section I.C.21. Screening.*

For encounters for suspected fetal condition that are inconclusive following testing and evaluation, assign the appropriate code from category O35, O36, O40 or O41.

The observation Z code categories:

Z03 Encounter for medical observation for suspected diseases and conditions ruled out

Z04 Encounter for examination and observation for other reasons Except: Z04.9, Encounter for examination and observation for unspecified reason

Z05 Encounter for observation and evaluation of newborn for suspected diseases and conditions ruled out

7) Aftercare

Aftercare visit codes cover situations when the initial treatment of a disease has been performed and the patient requires continued care during the healing or recovery phase, or for the long-term consequences of the disease. The aftercare Z code should not be used if treatment is directed at a current, acute disease. The diagnosis code is to be used in these cases.

Exceptions to this rule are codes Z51.0, Encounter for antineoplastic radiation therapy, and codes from subcategory Z51.1, Encounter for antineoplastic chemotherapy and immunotherapy. These codes are to be first-listed, followed by the diagnosis code when a patient's encounter is solely to receive radiation therapy, chemotherapy, or immunotherapy for the treatment of a neoplasm. If the reason for the encounter is more than one type of antineoplastic therapy, code Z51.0 and a code from subcategory Z51.1 may be assigned together, in which case one of these codes would be reported as a secondary diagnosis.

The aftercare Z codes should also not be used for aftercare for injuries. For aftercare of an injury, assign the acute injury code with the appropriate 7th character (for subsequent encounter).

The aftercare codes are generally first-listed to explain the specific reason for the encounter. An aftercare code may be used as an additional code when some type of aftercare is provided in addition to the reason for admission and no diagnosis code is applicable. An example of this would be the closure of a colostomy during an encounter for treatment of another condition.

Aftercare codes should be used in conjunction with other aftercare codes or diagnosis codes to provide better detail on the specifics of an aftercare encounter visit, unless otherwise directed by the classification. Should a patient receive multiple types of antineoplastic therapy during the same encounter, code Z51.0, Encounter for antineoplastic radiation therapy, and codes from subcategory Z51.1, Encounter for antineoplastic chemotherapy and immunotherapy, may be used together on a record. The sequencing of multiple aftercare codes depends on the circumstances of the encounter.

Certain aftercare Z code categories need a secondary diagnosis code to describe the resolving condition or sequelae. For others, the condition is included in the code title.

Additional Z code aftercare category terms include fitting and adjustment, and attention to artificial openings.

Status Z codes may be used with aftercare Z codes to indicate the nature of the aftercare. For example code Z95.1, Presence of aortocoronary bypass graft, may be used with code Z48.812, Encounter for surgical aftercare following surgery on the circulatory system, to indicate the surgery for which the aftercare is being performed. A status code should not be used when the aftercare code indicates the type of status, such as using Z43.0, Encounter for attention to tracheostomy, with Z93.0, Tracheostomy status.

The aftercare Z category/codes:

Z42 Encounter for plastic and reconstructive surgery following medical procedure or healed injury

Z43 Encounter for attention to artificial openings

Z44 Encounter for fitting and adjustment of external prosthetic device

Z45 Encounter for adjustment and management of implanted device

Z46 Encounter for fitting and adjustment of other devices

Z47 Orthopedic aftercare

Z48 Encounter for other postprocedural aftercare

Z49 Encounter for care involving renal dialysis

Z51 Encounter for other aftercare **and medical care**

8) Follow-up

The follow-up codes are used to explain continuing surveillance following completed treatment of a disease, condition, or injury. They imply that the condition has been fully treated and no longer exists. They should not be confused with aftercare codes, or injury codes with a 7th character for subsequent encounter, that explain ongoing care of a healing condition or its sequelae. Follow-up codes may be used in conjunction with history codes to provide the full picture of the healed condition and its treatment. The follow-up code is sequenced first, followed by the history code.

A follow-up code may be used to explain multiple visits. Should a condition be found to have recurred on the follow-up visit, then the diagnosis code for the condition should be assigned in place of the follow-up code.

The follow-up Z code categories:

Z08 Encounter for follow-up examination after completed treatment for malignant neoplasm

Z09 Encounter for follow-up examination after completed treatment for conditions other than malignant neoplasm

Z39 Encounter for maternal postpartum care and examination

9) Donor

Codes in category Z52, Donors of organs and tissues, are used for living individuals who are donating blood or other body tissue. These codes are only for individuals donating for others, not for self-donations. They are not used to identify cadaveric donations.

10) Counseling

Counseling Z codes are used when a patient or family member receives assistance in the aftermath of an illness or injury, or when support is required in coping with family or social problems. They are not used in conjunction with a diagnosis code when the counseling component of care is considered integral to standard treatment.

The counseling Z codes/categories:

Z30.0- Encounter for general counseling and advice on contraception

Z31.5 Encounter for genetic counseling

Z31.6- Encounter for general counseling and advice on procreation

Z32.2 Encounter for childbirth instruction

Z32.3 Encounter for childcare instruction

Z69 Encounter for mental health services for victim and perpetrator of abuse

Z70 Counseling related to sexual attitude, behavior and orientation

Z71 Persons encountering health services for other counseling and medical advice, not elsewhere classified

Z76.81 Expectant mother prebirth pediatrician visit

11) Encounters for Obstetrical and Reproductive Services

See Section I.C.15. Pregnancy, Childbirth, and the Puerperium, for further instruction on the use of these codes.

Z codes for pregnancy are for use in those circumstances when none of the problems or complications included in the codes from the Obstetrics chapter exist (a routine prenatal visit or postpartum care). Codes in category Z34, Encounter for supervision of normal pregnancy, are always first listed and are not to be used with any other code from the OB chapter.

Codes in category Z3A, Weeks of gestation, may be assigned to provide additional information about the pregnancy. **Category Z3A codes should not be assigned for pregnancies with abortive outcomes (categories O00-O08), elective termination of pregnancy (code Z33.32), nor for postpartum conditions, as category Z3A is not applicable to these conditions.** The date of the admission should be used to determine weeks of gestation for inpatient admissions that encompass more than one gestational week.

The outcome of delivery, category Z37, should be included on all maternal delivery records. It is always a secondary code. Codes in category Z37 should not be used on the newborn record.

Z codes for family planning (contraceptive) or procreative management and counseling should be included on an obstetric record either during the pregnancy or the postpartum stage, if applicable.

Z codes/categories for obstetrical and reproductive services:

Z30 Encounter for contraceptive management

Z31 Encounter for procreative management

Z32.2 Encounter for childbirth instruction

Z32.3 Encounter for childcare instruction

Z33 Pregnant state

Z34 Encounter for supervision of normal pregnancy

Z36 Encounter for antenatal screening of mother

Z3A Weeks of gestation

Z37 Outcome of delivery

Z39 Encounter for maternal postpartum care and examination

Z76.81 Expectant mother prebirth pediatrician visit

12) Newborns and Infants

See Section I.C.16. Newborn (Perinatal) Guidelines, for further instruction on the use of these codes.

Newborn Z codes/categories:

Z76.1 Encounter for health supervision and care of foundling

Z00.1- Encounter for routine child health examination

Z38 Liveborn infants according to place of birth and type of delivery

13) Routine and administrative examinations

The Z codes allow for the description of encounters for routine examinations, such as, a general check-up, or, examinations for administrative purposes, such as, a pre-employment physical. The codes are not to be used if the examination is for diagnosis of a suspected condition or for treatment purposes. In such cases the diagnosis code is used. During a routine exam, should a diagnosis or condition be discovered, it should be coded as an additional code. Pre-existing and chronic conditions and history codes may also be included as additional codes as long as the examination is for administrative purposes and not focused on any particular condition.

Some of the codes for routine health examinations distinguish between "with" and "without" abnormal findings. Code assignment depends on the information that is known at the time the encounter is being coded. For example, if no abnormal findings were found during the examination, but the encounter is being coded before test results are back, it is acceptable to assign the code for "without abnormal findings." When assigning a code for "with abnormal findings," additional code(s) should be assigned to identify the specific abnormal finding(s).

Pre-operative examination and pre-procedural laboratory examination Z codes are for use only in those situations when a patient is being cleared for a procedure or surgery and no treatment is given.

The Z codes/categories for routine and administrative examinations:

- Z00 Encounter for general examination without complaint, suspected or reported diagnosis
- Z01 Encounter for other special examination without complaint, suspected or reported diagnosis
- Z02 Encounter for administrative examination
  Except: Z02.9, Encounter for administrative examinations, unspecified
- Z32.0- Encounter for pregnancy test

14) Miscellaneous Z codes

The miscellaneous Z codes capture a number of other health care encounters that do not fall into one of the other categories. Certain of these codes identify the reason for the encounter; others are for use as additional codes that provide useful information on circumstances that may affect a patient's care and treatment.

Prophylactic Organ Removal

For encounters specifically for prophylactic removal of an organ (such as prophylactic removal of breasts due to a genetic susceptibility to cancer or a family history of cancer), the principal or first-listed code should be a code from category Z40, Encounter for prophylactic surgery, followed by the appropriate codes to identify the associated risk factor (such as genetic susceptibility or family history).

If the patient has a malignancy of one site and is having prophylactic removal at another site to prevent either a new primary malignancy or metastatic disease, a code for the malignancy should also be assigned in addition to a code from subcategory Z40.0, Encounter for prophylactic surgery for risk factors related to malignant neoplasms. A Z40.0 code should not be assigned if the patient is having organ removal for treatment of a malignancy, such as the removal of the testes for the treatment of prostate cancer.

Miscellaneous Z codes/categories:

- Z28 Immunization not carried out
  Except: Z28.3, Underimmunization status
- **Z29 Encounter for other prophylactic measures**
- Z40 Encounter for prophylactic surgery
- Z41 Encounter for procedures for purposes other than remedying health state
  Except: Z41.9, Encounter for procedure for purposes other than remedying health state, unspecified
- Z53 Persons encountering health services for specific procedures and treatment, not carried out
- Z55 Problems related to education and literacy
- Z56 Problems related to employment and unemployment
- Z57 Occupational exposure to risk factors
- Z58 Problems related to physical environment
- Z59 Problems related to housing and economic circumstances
- Z60 Problems related to social environment
- Z62 Problems related to upbringing
- Z63 Other problems related to primary support group, including family circumstances
- Z64 Problems related to certain psychosocial circumstances
- Z65 Problems related to other psychosocial circumstances
- Z72 Problems related to lifestyle
  Note: These codes should be assigned only when the documentation specifies that the patient has an associated problem
- Z73 Problems related to life management difficulty
- Z74 Problems related to care provider dependency Except: Z74.01, Bed confinement status
- Z75 Problems related to medical facilities and other health care
- Z76.0 Encounter for issue of repeat prescription
- Z76.3 Healthy person accompanying sick person
- Z76.4 Other boarder to healthcare facility
- Z76.5 Malingerer [conscious simulation]
- Z91.1- Patient's noncompliance with medical treatment and regimen
- Z91.83 Wandering in diseases classified elsewhere
- Z91.89 Other specified personal risk factors, not elsewhere classified

15) Nonspecific Z codes

Certain Z codes are so non-specific, or potentially redundant with other codes in the classification, that there can be little justification for their use in the inpatient setting. Their use in the outpatient setting should be limited to those instances when there is no further documentation to permit more precise coding. Otherwise, any sign or symptom or any other reason for visit that is captured in another code should be used.

Nonspecific Z codes/categories:

- Z02.9 Encounter for administrative examinations, unspecified
- Z04.9 Encounter for examination and observation for unspecified reason
- Z13.9 Encounter for screening, unspecified

Z41.9 Encounter for procedure for purposes other than remedying health state, unspecified
Z52.9 Donor of unspecified organ or tissue
Z86.59 Personal history of other mental and behavioral disorders
Z88.9 Allergy status to unspecified drugs, medicaments and biological substances status
Z92.0 Personal history of contraception

16) Z Codes That May Only be Principal/First-Listed Diagnosis

The following Z codes/categories may only be reported as the principal/first-listed diagnosis, except when there are multiple encounters on the same day and the medical records for the encounters are combined:

Z00 Encounter for general examination without complaint, suspected or reported diagnosis
Except: Z00.6
Z01 Encounter for other special examination without complaint, suspected or reported diagnosis
Z02 Encounter for administrative examination
Z03 Encounter for medical observation for suspected diseases and conditions ruled out
Z04 Encounter for examination and observation for other reasons
Z33.2 Encounter for elective termination of pregnancy
Z31.81 Encounter for male factor infertility in female patient
Z31.83 Encounter for assisted reproductive fertility procedure cycle
Z31.84 Encounter for fertility preservation procedure
Z34 Encounter for supervision of normal pregnancy
Z39 Encounter for maternal postpartum care and examination
Z38 Liveborn infants according to place of birth and type of delivery
Z42 Encounter for plastic and reconstructive surgery following medical procedure or healed injury
Z51.0 Encounter for antineoplastic radiation therapy
Z51.1- Encounter for antineoplastic chemotherapy and immunotherapy
Z52 Donors of organs and tissues Except: Z52.9, Donor of unspecified organ or tissue
Z76.1 Encounter for health supervision and care of foundling
Z76.2 Encounter for health supervision and care of other healthy infant and child
Z99.12 Encounter for respirator [ventilator] dependence during power failure

Section II. Selection of Principal Diagnosis

The circumstances of inpatient admission always govern the selection of principal diagnosis. The principal diagnosis is defined in the Uniform Hospital Discharge Data Set (UHDDS) as "that condition established after study to be chiefly responsible for occasioning the admission of the patient to the hospital for care."

The UHDDS definitions are used by hospitals to report inpatient data elements in a standardized manner. These data elements and their definitions can be found in the July 31, 1985, Federal Register (Vol. 50, No, 147), pp. 31038-40.

Since that time the application of the UHDDS definitions has been expanded to include all nonoutpatient settings (acute care, short term, long term care and psychiatric hospitals; home health agencies; rehab facilities; nursing homes, etc). **The UHDDS definitions also apply to hospice services (all levels of care).**

In determining principal diagnosis, coding conventions in the ICD-10-CM, the Tabular List and Alphabetic Index take precedence over these official coding guidelines.

(See Section I.A., Conventions for the ICD-10-CM)

The importance of consistent, complete documentation in the medical record cannot be overemphasized. Without such documentation the application of all coding guidelines is a difficult, if not impossible, task.

A. Codes for symptoms, signs, and ill-defined conditions

Codes for symptoms, signs, and ill-defined conditions from Chapter 18 are not to be used as principal diagnosis when a related definitive diagnosis has been established.

B. Two or more interrelated conditions, each potentially meeting the definition for principal diagnosis.

When there are two or more interrelated conditions (such as diseases in the same ICD-10-CM chapter or manifestations characteristically associated with a certain disease) potentially meeting the definition of principal diagnosis, either condition may be sequenced first, unless the circumstances of the admission, the therapy provided, the Tabular List, or the Alphabetic Index indicate otherwise.

C. Two or more diagnoses that equally meet the definition for principal diagnosis

In the unusual instance when two or more diagnoses equally meet the criteria for principal diagnosis as determined by the circumstances of admission, diagnostic workup and/or therapy provided, and the Alphabetic Index, Tabular List, or another coding guidelines does not provide sequencing direction, any one of the diagnoses may be sequenced first.

D. Two or more comparative or contrasting conditions.

In those rare instances when two or more contrasting or comparative diagnoses are documented as "either/or" (or similar terminology), they are coded as if the diagnoses were confirmed and the diagnoses are sequenced according to the circumstances of the admission. If no further determination can be made as to which diagnosis should be principal, either diagnosis may be sequenced first.

E. A symptom(s) followed by contrasting/ comparative diagnoses
GUIDELINE HAS BEEN DELETED EFFECTIVE OCTOBER 1, 2014

F. Original treatment plan not carried out
Sequence as the principal diagnosis the condition, which after study occasioned the admission to the hospital, even though treatment may not have been carried out due to unforeseen circumstances.

G. Complications of surgery and other medical care
When the admission is for treatment of a complication resulting from surgery or other medical care, the complication code is sequenced as the principal diagnosis. If the complication is classified to the T80-T88 series and the code lacks the necessary specificity in describing the complication, an additional code for the specific complication should be assigned.

H. Uncertain Diagnosis
If the diagnosis documented at the time of discharge is qualified as "probable", "suspected", "likely", "questionable", "possible", or "still to be ruled out", or other similar terms indicating uncertainty, code the condition as if it existed or was established. The bases for these guidelines are the diagnostic workup, arrangements for further workup or observation, and initial therapeutic approach that correspond most closely with the established diagnosis.

Note: This guideline is applicable only to inpatient admissions to short-term, acute, long-term care and psychiatric hospitals.

I. Admission from Observation Unit

1. Admission Following Medical Observation
When a patient is admitted to an observation unit for a medical condition, which either worsens or does not improve, and is subsequently admitted as an inpatient of the same hospital for this same medical condition, the principal diagnosis would be the medical condition which led to the hospital admission.

2. Admission Following Post-Operative Observation
When a patient is admitted to an observation unit to monitor a condition (or complication) that develops following outpatient surgery, and then is subsequently admitted as an inpatient of the same hospital, hospitals should apply the Uniform Hospital Discharge Data Set (UHDDS) definition of principal diagnosis as "that condition established after study to be chiefly responsible for occasioning the admission of the patient to the hospital for care."

J. Admission from Outpatient Surgery
When a patient receives surgery in the hospital's outpatient surgery department and is subsequently admitted for continuing inpatient care at the same hospital, the following guidelines should be followed in selecting the principal diagnosis for the inpatient admission:

- If the reason for the inpatient admission is a complication, assign the complication as the principal diagnosis.
- If no complication, or other condition, is documented as the reason for the inpatient admission, assign the reason for the outpatient surgery as the principal diagnosis.
- If the reason for the inpatient admission is another condition unrelated to the surgery, assign the unrelated condition as the principal diagnosis.

K. Admissions/Encounters for Rehabilitation
When the purpose for the admission/encounter is rehabilitation, sequence first the code for the condition for which the service is being performed. For example, for an admission/encounter for rehabilitation for right-sided dominant hemiplegia following a cerebrovascular infarction, report code I69.351, Hemiplegia and hemiparesis following cerebral infarction affecting right dominant side, as the first-listed or principal diagnosis.

If the condition for which the rehabilitation service is no longer present, report the appropriate aftercare code as the first-listed or principal diagnosis. For example, if a patient with severe degenerative osteoarthritis of the hip, underwent hip replacement and the current encounter/ admission is for rehabilitation, report code Z47.1, Aftercare following joint replacement surgery, as the first-listed or principal diagnosis.

See Section I.C.21.c.7, Factors influencing health states and contact with health services, Aftercare.

Section III. Reporting Additional Diagnoses

GENERAL RULES FOR OTHER (ADDITIONAL) DIAGNOSES

For reporting purposes the definition for "other diagnoses" is interpreted as additional conditions that affect patient care in terms of requiring:

clinical evaluation; or
therapeutic treatment; or
diagnostic procedures; or
extended length of hospital stay; or
increased nursing care and/or monitoring.

The UHDDS item #11-b defines Other Diagnoses as "all conditions that coexist at the time of admission, that develop subsequently, or that affect the treatment received and/or the length of stay. Diagnoses that relate to an earlier episode which have no bearing on the current hospital stay are to be excluded." UHDDS definitions apply to inpatients in acute care, short-term, long term care and psychiatric hospital setting. The UHDDS definitions are used by acute care short-term hospitals to report inpatient data elements in a standardized manner. These data elements and their definitions can be found in the July 31, 1985, Federal Register (Vol. 50, No, 147), pp. 31038-40.

Since that time the application of the UHDDS definitions has been expanded to include all nonoutpatient settings (acute care, short term, long term care and psychiatric hospitals; home health agencies; rehab facilities; nursing homes, etc). **The UHDDS definitions also apply to hospice services (all levels of care).**

The following guidelines are to be applied in designating "other diagnoses" when neither the Alphabetic Index nor the Tabular List in ICD-10-CM provide direction. The listing of the diagnoses in the patient record is the responsibility of the attending provider.

A. Previous conditions

If the provider has included a diagnosis in the final diagnostic statement, such as the discharge summary or the face sheet, it should ordinarily be coded. Some providers include in the diagnostic statement resolved conditions or diagnoses and status-post procedures from previous admission that have no bearing on the current stay. Such conditions are not to be reported and are coded only if required by hospital policy.

However, history codes (categories Z80-Z87) may be used as secondary codes if the historical condition or family history has an impact on current care or influences treatment.

B. Abnormal findings

Abnormal findings (laboratory, x-ray, pathologic, and other diagnostic results) are not coded and reported unless the provider indicates their clinical significance. If the findings are outside the normal range and the attending provider has ordered other tests to evaluate the condition or prescribed treatment, it is appropriate to ask the provider whether the abnormal finding should be added.

Please note: This differs from the coding practices in the outpatient setting for coding encounters for diagnostic tests that have been interpreted by a provider.

C. Uncertain Diagnosis

If the diagnosis documented at the time of discharge is qualified as "probable", "suspected", "likely", "questionable", "possible", or "still to be ruled out" or other similar terms indicating uncertainty, code the condition as if it existed or was established. The bases for these guidelines are the diagnostic workup, arrangements for further workup or observation, and initial therapeutic approach that correspond most closely with the established diagnosis.

Note: This guideline is applicable only to inpatient admissions to short-term, acute, long-term care and psychiatric hospitals.

Section IV. Diagnostic Coding and Reporting Guidelines for Outpatient Services

These coding guidelines for outpatient diagnoses have been approved for use by hospitals/ providers in coding and reporting hospital-based outpatient services and provider-based office visits. **Guidelines in Section I, Conventions, general coding guidelines and chapter-specific guidelines, should also be applied for outpatient services and office visits.**

Information about the use of certain abbreviations, punctuation, symbols, and other conventions used in the ICD-10-CM Tabular List (code numbers and titles), can be found in Section IA of these guidelines, under "Conventions Used in the Tabular List." Section I.B. contains general guidelines that apply to the entire classification. Section I.C. contains chapter-specific guidelines that correspond to the chapters as they are arranged in the classification. Information about the correct sequence to use in finding a code is also described in Section I.

The terms encounter and visit are often used interchangeably in describing outpatient service contacts and, therefore, appear together in these guidelines without distinguishing one from the other.

Though the conventions and general guidelines apply to all settings, coding guidelines for outpatient and provider reporting of diagnoses will vary in a number of instances from those for inpatient diagnoses, recognizing that:

The Uniform Hospital Discharge Data Set (UHDDS) definition of principal diagnosis **does not apply to hospital-based outpatient services and provider-based office visits.**

Coding guidelines for inconclusive diagnoses (probable, suspected, rule out, etc.) were developed for inpatient reporting and do not apply to outpatients.

A. Selection of first-listed condition

In the outpatient setting, the term first-listed diagnosis is used in lieu of principal diagnosis.

In determining the first-listed diagnosis the coding conventions of ICD-10-CM, as well as the general and disease specific guidelines take precedence over the outpatient guidelines.

Diagnoses often are not established at the time of the initial encounter/visit. It may take two or more visits before the diagnosis is confirmed.

The most critical rule involves beginning the search for the correct code assignment through the Alphabetic Index. Never begin searching initially in the Tabular List as this will lead to coding errors.

1. Outpatient Surgery

When a patient presents for outpatient surgery (same day surgery), code the reason for the surgery as the first-listed diagnosis (reason for the encounter), even if the surgery is not performed due to a contraindication.

2. Observation Stay

When a patient is admitted for observation for a medical condition, assign a code for the medical condition as the first-listed diagnosis.

When a patient presents for outpatient surgery and develops complications requiring admission to observation, code the reason for the surgery as the first reported diagnosis (reason for the encounter), followed by codes for the complications as secondary diagnoses.

B. Codes from A00.0 through T88.9, Z00-Z99
The appropriate code(s) from A00.0 through T88.9, Z00-Z99 must be used to identify diagnoses, symptoms, conditions, problems, complaints, or other reason(s) for the encounter/visit.

C. Accurate reporting of ICD-10-CM diagnosis codes
For accurate reporting of ICD-10-CM diagnosis codes, the documentation should describe the patient's condition, using terminology which includes specific diagnoses as well as symptoms, problems, or reasons for the encounter. There are ICD-10-CM codes to describe all of these.

D. Codes that describe symptoms and signs
Codes that describe symptoms and signs, as opposed to diagnoses, are acceptable for reporting purposes when a diagnosis has not been established (confirmed) by the provider. Chapter 18 of ICD-10-CM, Symptoms, Signs, and Abnormal Clinical and Laboratory Findings Not Elsewhere Classified (codes R00-R99) contain many, but not all codes for symptoms.

E. Encounters for circumstances other than a disease or injury
ICD-10-CM provides codes to deal with encounters for circumstances other than a disease or injury. The Factors Influencing Health Status and Contact with Health Services codes (Z00-Z99) are provided to deal with occasions when circumstances other than a disease or injury are recorded as diagnosis or problems.

See Section I.C.21. Factors influencing health status and contact with health services.

F. Level of Detail in Coding

1. ICD-10-CM codes with 3, 4, 5, 6 or 7 characters
ICD-10-CM is composed of codes with 3, 4, 5, 6 or 7 characters. Codes with three characters are included in ICD-10-CM as the heading of a category of codes that may be further subdivided by the use of fourth, fifth, sixth or seventh characters to provide greater specificity.

2. Use of full number of characters required for a code
A three-character code is to be used only if it is not further subdivided. A code is invalid if it has not been coded to the full number of characters required for that code, including the 7th character, if applicable.

G. ICD-10-CM code for the diagnosis, condition, problem, or other reason for encounter/visit
List first the ICD-10-CM code for the diagnosis, condition, problem, or other reason for encounter/visit shown in the medical record to be chiefly responsible for the services provided. List additional codes that describe any coexisting conditions. In some cases the first-listed diagnosis may be a symptom when a diagnosis has not been established (confirmed) by the physician.

H. Uncertain diagnosis
Do not code diagnoses documented as "probable", "suspected," "questionable," "rule out," or "working diagnosis" or other similar terms indicating uncertainty. Rather, code the condition(s) to the highest degree of certainty for that encounter/visit, such as symptoms, signs, abnormal test results, or other reason for the visit.

Please note: This differs from the coding practices used by short-term, acute care, long-term care and psychiatric hospitals.

I. Chronic diseases
Chronic diseases treated on an ongoing basis may be coded and reported as many times as the patient receives treatment and care for the condition(s)

J. Code all documented conditions that coexist
Code all documented conditions that coexist at the time of the encounter/visit, and require or affect patient care treatment or management. Do not code conditions that were previously treated and no longer exist. However, history codes (categories Z80-Z87) may be used as secondary codes if the historical condition or family history has an impact on current care or influences treatment.

K. Patients receiving diagnostic services only
For patients receiving diagnostic services only during an encounter/visit, sequence first the diagnosis, condition, problem, or other reason for encounter/visit shown in the medical record to be chiefly responsible for the outpatient services provided during the encounter/visit. Codes for other diagnoses (e.g., chronic conditions) may be sequenced as additional diagnoses.

For encounters for routine laboratory/radiology testing in the absence of any signs, symptoms, or associated diagnosis, assign Z01.89, Encounter for other specified special examinations. If routine testing is performed during the same encounter as a test to evaluate a sign, symptom, or diagnosis, it is appropriate to assign both the Z code and the code describing the reason for the non-routine test.

For outpatient encounters for diagnostic tests that have been interpreted by a physician, and the final report is available at the time of coding, code any confirmed or definitive diagnosis(es) documented in the interpretation. Do not code related signs and symptoms as additional diagnoses.

Please note: This differs from the coding practice in the hospital inpatient setting regarding abnormal findings on test results.

L. Patients receiving therapeutic services only
For patients receiving therapeutic services only during an encounter/visit, sequence first the diagnosis, condition, problem, or other reason for encounter/visit shown in the medical record to be chiefly responsible for the outpatient services provided during the encounter/visit. Codes for other diagnoses (e.g., chronic conditions) may be sequenced as additional diagnoses.

The only exception to this rule is that when the primary reason for the admission/encounter is chemotherapy or radiation therapy, the appropriate Z code for the service is listed first, and the diagnosis or problem for which the service is being performed listed second.

M. Patients receiving preoperative evaluations only
For patients receiving preoperative evaluations only, sequence first a code from subcategory Z01.81, Encounter for pre-procedural examinations, to describe the pre-op consultations. Assign a code for the condition to describe the reason for the surgery as an additional diagnosis. Code also any findings related to the pre-op evaluation.

N. Ambulatory surgery
For ambulatory surgery, code the diagnosis for which the surgery was performed. If the postoperative diagnosis is known to be different from the preoperative diagnosis at the time the diagnosis is confirmed, select the postoperative diagnosis for coding, since it is the most definitive.

O. Routine outpatient prenatal visits
See Section I.C.15. Routine outpatient prenatal visits.

P. Encounters for general medical examinations with abnormal findings
The subcategories for encounters for general medical examinations, Z00.0-, provide codes for with and without abnormal findings. Should a general medical examination result in an abnormal finding, the code for general medical examination with abnormal finding should be assigned as the first-listed diagnosis. **An examination with abnormal findings refers to a condition/diagnosis that is newly identified or a change in severity of a chronic condition (such as uncontrolled hypertension, or an acute exacerbation of chronic obstructive pulmonary disease) during a routine physical examination.** A secondary code for the abnormal finding should also be coded.

Q. Encounters for routine health screenings
See Section I.C.21. Factors influencing health status and contact with health services, Screening

Appendix I
Present on Admission Reporting Guidelines

Introduction

These guidelines are to be used as a supplement to the *ICD-10-CM Official Guidelines for Coding and Reporting* to facilitate the assignment of the Present on Admission (POA) indicator for each diagnosis and external cause of injury code reported on claim forms (UB-04 and 837 Institutional).

These guidelines are not intended to replace any guidelines in the main body of the *ICD-10-CM Official Guidelines for Coding and Reporting*. The POA guidelines are not intended to provide guidance on when a condition should be coded, but rather, how to apply the POA indicator to the final set of diagnosis codes that have been assigned in accordance with Sections I, II, and III of the official coding guidelines. Subsequent to the assignment of the ICD-10-CM codes, the POA indicator should then be assigned to those conditions that have been coded.

As stated in the Introduction to the ICD-10-CM Official Guidelines for Coding and Reporting, a joint effort between the healthcare provider and the coder is essential to achieve complete and accurate documentation, code assignment, and reporting of diagnoses and procedures. The importance of consistent, complete documentation in the medical record cannot be overemphasized. Medical record documentation from any provider involved in the care and treatment of the patient may be used to support the determination of whether a condition was present on admission or not. In the context of the official coding guidelines, the term "provider" means a physician or any qualified healthcare practitioner who is legally accountable for establishing the patient's diagnosis.

These guidelines are not a substitute for the provider's clinical judgment as to the determination of whether a condition was/was not present on admission. The provider should be queried regarding issues related to the linking of signs/symptoms, timing of test results, and the timing of findings.

Please see the CDC website for the detailed list of ICD-10-CM codes that do not require the use of a POA indicator (ftp://ftp.cdc.gov/pub/Health_Statistics/NCHS/Publications/ICD10CM/2017/). The conditions on this exempt list represent categories and/or codes for circumstances regarding the healthcare encounter or factors influencing health status that do not represent a current disease or injury or are always present on admission.

General Reporting Requirements

All claims involving inpatient admissions to general acute care hospitals or other facilities that are subject to a law or regulation mandating collection of present on admission information.

Present on admission is defined as present at the time the order for inpatient admission occurs—conditions that develop during an outpatient encounter, including emergency department, observation, or outpatient surgery, are considered as present on admission.

POA indicator is assigned to principal and secondary diagnoses (as defined in Section II of the Official Guidelines for Coding and Reporting) and the external cause of injury codes.

Issues related to inconsistent, missing, conflicting or unclear documentation must still be resolved by the provider.

If a condition would not be coded and reported based on UHDDS definitions and current official coding guidelines, then the POA indicator would not be reported.

Reporting Options

Y - Yes

N - No

U - Unknown

W - Clinically undetermined

Unreported/Not used - (Exempt from POA reporting)

Reporting Definitions

Y = present at the time of inpatient admission

N = not present at the time of inpatient admission

U = documentation is insufficient to determine if condition is present on admission

W = provider is unable to clinically determine whether condition was present on admission or not

Timeframe for POA Identification and Documentation

There is no required timeframe as to when a provider (per the definition of "provider" used in these guidelines) must identify or document a condition to be present on admission. In some clinical situations, it may not be possible for a provider to make a definitive diagnosis (or a condition may not be recognized or reported by the patient) for a period of time after admission. In some cases it may be several days before the provider arrives at a definitive diagnosis. This does not mean that the condition was not present on admission. Determination of whether the condition was present on admission or not will be based on the applicable POA guideline as identified in this document, or on the provider's best clinical judgment.

If at the time of code assignment the documentation is unclear as to whether a condition was present on admission or not, it is appropriate to query the provider for clarification.

Assigning the POA Indicator

Condition is on the "Exempt from Reporting" list

Leave the "present on admission" field blank if the condition is on the list of ICD-10-CM codes for which this field is not applicable. This is the only circumstance in which the field may be left blank.

POA Explicitly Documented

Assign Y for any condition the provider explicitly documents as being present on admission.

Assign N for any condition the provider explicitly documents as not present at the time of admission.

Conditions diagnosed prior to inpatient admission

Assign "Y" for conditions that were diagnosed prior to admission (example: hypertension, diabetes mellitus, asthma)

Conditions diagnosed during the admission but clearly present before admission

Assign "Y" for conditions diagnosed during the admission that were clearly present but not diagnosed until after admission occurred.

Diagnoses subsequently confirmed after admission are considered present on admission if at the time of admission they are documented as suspected, possible, rule out, differential diagnosis, or constitute an underlying cause of a symptom that is present at the time of admission.

Condition develops during outpatient encounter prior to inpatient admission

Assign Y for any condition that develops during an outpatient encounter prior to a written order for inpatient admission.

Documentation does not indicate whether condition was present on admission

Assign "U" when the medical record documentation is unclear as to whether the condition was present on admission. "U" should not be routinely assigned and used only in very limited circumstances. Coders are encouraged to query the providers when the documentation is unclear.

Documentation states that it cannot be determined whether the condition was or was not present on admission

Assign "W" when the medical record documentation indicates that it cannot be clinically determined whether or not the condition was present on admission.

Chronic condition with acute exacerbation during the admission

If a single code identifies both the chronic condition and the acute exacerbation, see POA guidelines pertaining to **codes that contain multiple clinical concepts**.

If a single code only identifies the chronic condition and not the acute exacerbation (e.g., acute exacerbation of chronic leukemia), assign "Y."

Conditions documented as possible, probable, suspected, or rule out at the time of discharge

If the final diagnosis contains a possible, probable, suspected, or rule out diagnosis, and this diagnosis was based on signs, symptoms or clinical findings suspected at the time of inpatient admission, assign "Y."

If the final diagnosis contains a possible, probable, suspected, or rule out diagnosis, and this diagnosis was based on signs, symptoms or clinical findings that were not present on admission, assign "N".

Conditions documented as impending or threatened at the time of discharge

If the final diagnosis contains an impending or threatened diagnosis, and this diagnosis is based on symptoms or clinical findings that were present on admission, assign "Y".

If the final diagnosis contains an impending or threatened diagnosis, and this diagnosis is based on symptoms or clinical findings that were not present on admission, assign "N".

Acute and Chronic Conditions

Assign "Y" for acute conditions that are present at time of admission and N for acute conditions that are not present at time of admission.

Assign "Y" for chronic conditions, even though the condition may not be diagnosed until after admission.

If a single code identifies both an acute and chronic condition, see the POA guidelines for codes **that contain multiple clinical concepts.**

Codes **That Contain Multiple Clinical Concepts**

Assign "N" if at least one of the clinical concepts included in the code was not present on admission (e.g., COPD with acute exacerbation and the exacerbation was not present on admission; gastric ulcer that does not start bleeding until after admission; asthma patient develops status asthmaticus after admission).

Assign "Y" if all of the **clinical concepts included in the code** were present on admission (e.g., **duodenal ulcer that perforates prior to admission**).

For infection codes that include the causal organism, assign "Y" if the infection (or signs of the infection) **were** present on admission, even though the culture results may not be known until after admission (e.g., patient is admitted with pneumonia and the provider documents Pseudomonas as the causal organism a few days later).

Same Diagnosis Code for Two or More Conditions

When the same ICD-10-CM diagnosis code applies to two or more conditions during the same encounter (e.g. two separate conditions classified to the same ICD-10-CM diagnosis code):

Assign "Y" if all conditions represented by the single ICD-10-CM code were present on admission (e.g. bilateral unspecified age-related cataracts).

Assign "N" if any of the conditions represented by the single ICD-10-CM code was not present on admission (e.g. traumatic secondary and recurrent hemorrhage and seroma is assigned to a single code T79.2, but only one of the conditions was present on admission).

Obstetrical conditions

Whether or not the patient delivers during the current hospitalization does not affect assignment of the POA indicator. The determining factor for POA assignment is whether the pregnancy complication or obstetrical condition described by the code was present at the time of admission or not.

If the pregnancy complication or obstetrical condition was present on admission (e.g., patient admitted in preterm labor), assign "Y".

If the pregnancy complication or obstetrical condition was not present on admission (e.g., 2nd degree laceration during delivery, postpartum hemorrhage that occurred during current hospitalization, fetal distress develops after admission), assign "N".

If the obstetrical code includes more than one diagnosis and any of the diagnoses identified by the code were not present on admission assign "N".

(e.g., Category O11, Pre-existing hypertension with pre-eclampsia)

Perinatal conditions

Newborns are not considered to be admitted until after birth. Therefore, any condition present at birth or that developed in utero is considered present at admission and should be assigned "Y". This includes conditions that occur during delivery (e.g., injury during delivery, meconium aspiration, exposure to streptococcus B in the vaginal canal).

Congenital conditions and anomalies

Assign "Y" for congenital conditions and anomalies except for categories Q00-Q99, Congenital anomalies, which are on the exempt list. Congenital conditions are always considered present on admission.

External cause of injury codes

Assign "Y" for any external cause code representing an external cause of morbidity that occurred prior to inpatient admission (e.g., patient fell out of bed at home, patient fell out of bed in emergency room prior to admission).

Assign "N" for any external cause code representing an external cause of morbidity that occurred during inpatient hospitalization (e.g., patient fell out of hospital bed during hospital stay, patient experienced an adverse reaction to a medication administered after inpatient admission).

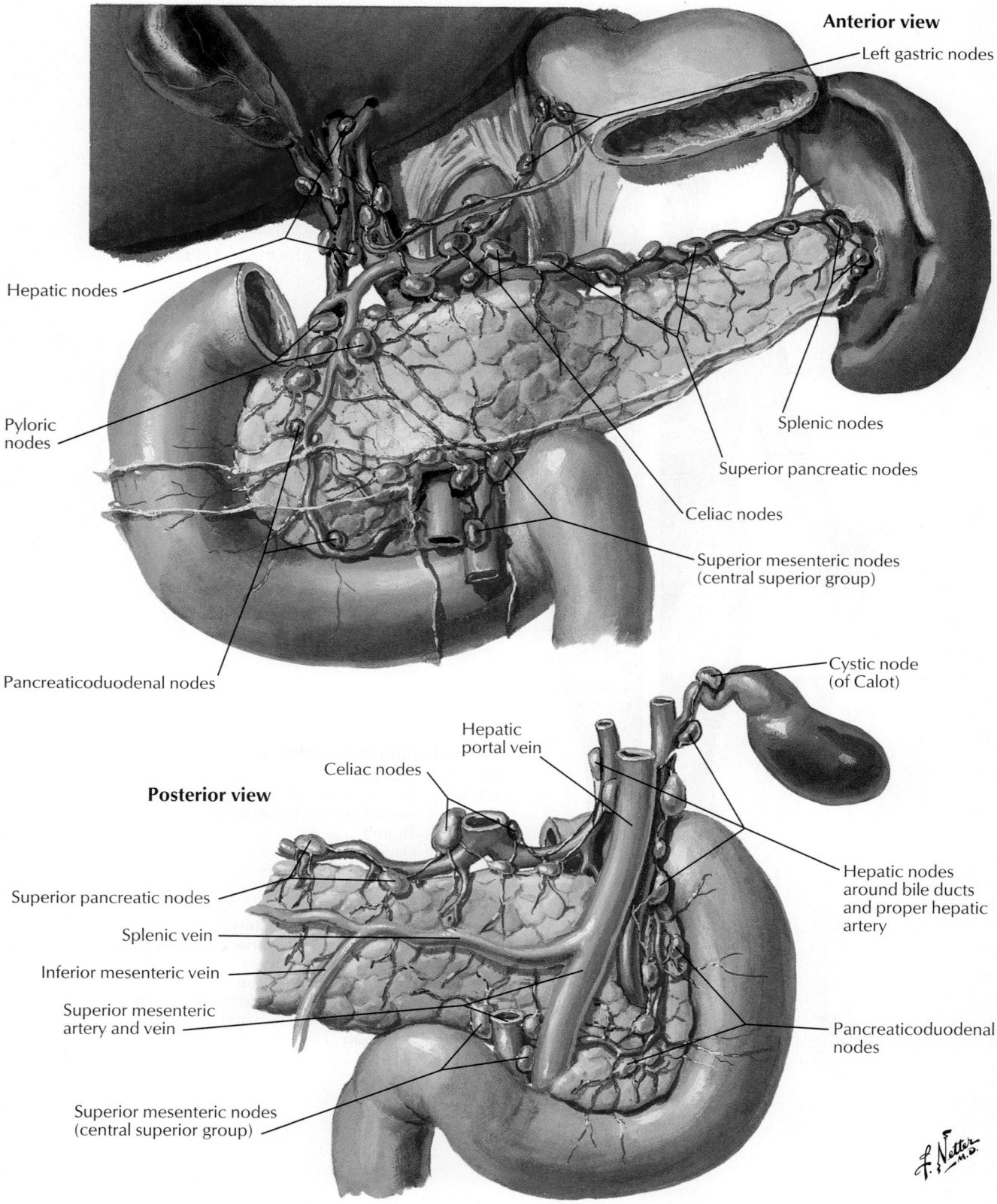

Plate 315 Lymph Vessels and Nodes of Pancreas. (Netter: Atlas of Human Anatomy, 4 ed, 2006, Saunders.)

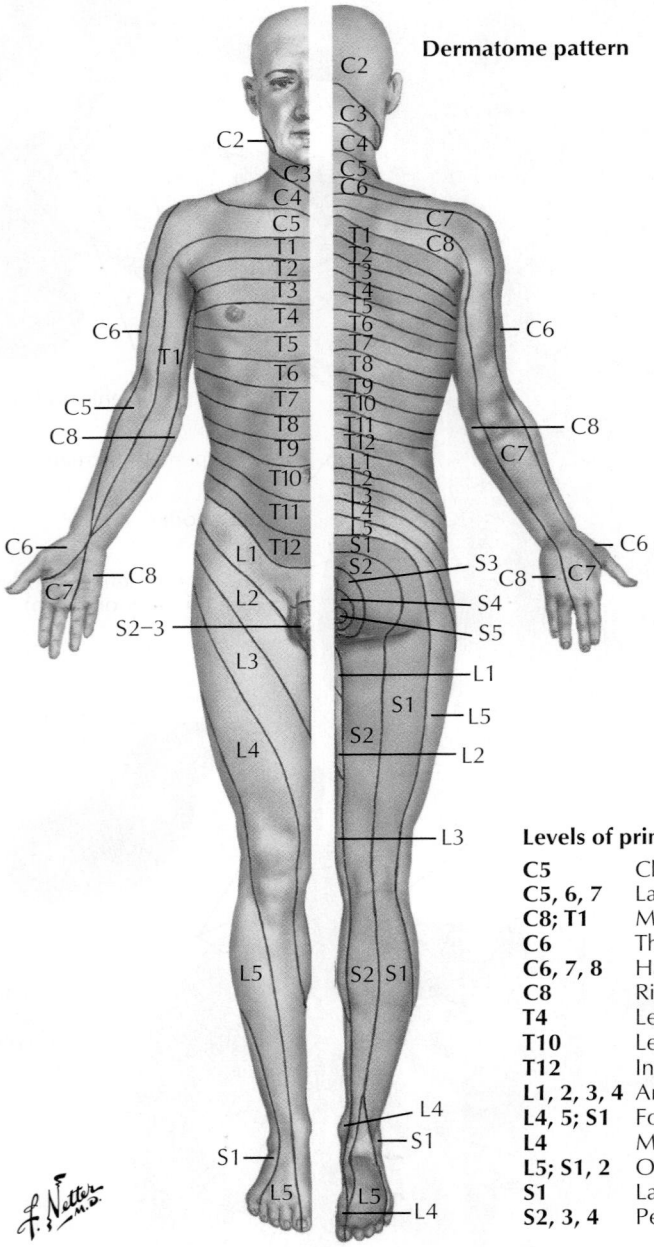

Levels of principal dermatomes

C5	Clavicles
C5, 6, 7	Lateral parts of upper limbs
C8; T1	Medial sides of upper limbs
C6	Thumb
C6, 7, 8	Hand
C8	Ring and little fingers
T4	Level of nipples
T10	Level of umbilicus
T12	Inguinal or groin regions
L1, 2, 3, 4	Anterior and inner surfaces of lower limbs
L4, 5; S1	Foot
L4	Medial side of great toe
L5; S1, 2	Outer and posterior sides of lower limbs
S1	Lateral margin of foot and little toe
S2, 3, 4	Perineum

Plate 164 Dermatomes. (Netter: Atlas of Human Anatomy, 4 ed, 2006, Saunders.)

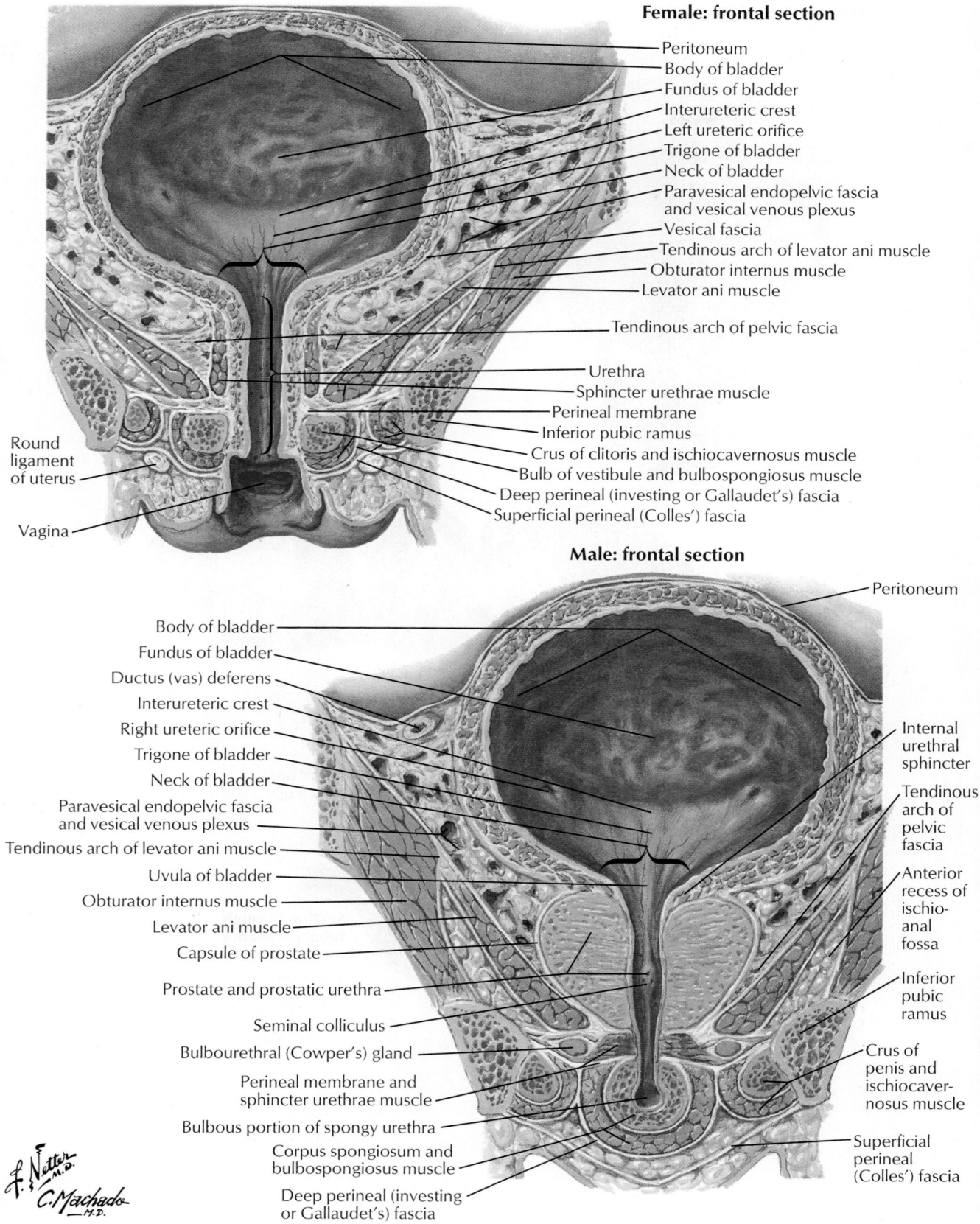

Plate 366 Urinary Bladder: Female and Male. (Netter: Atlas of Human Anatomy, 4 ed, 2006, Saunders.)

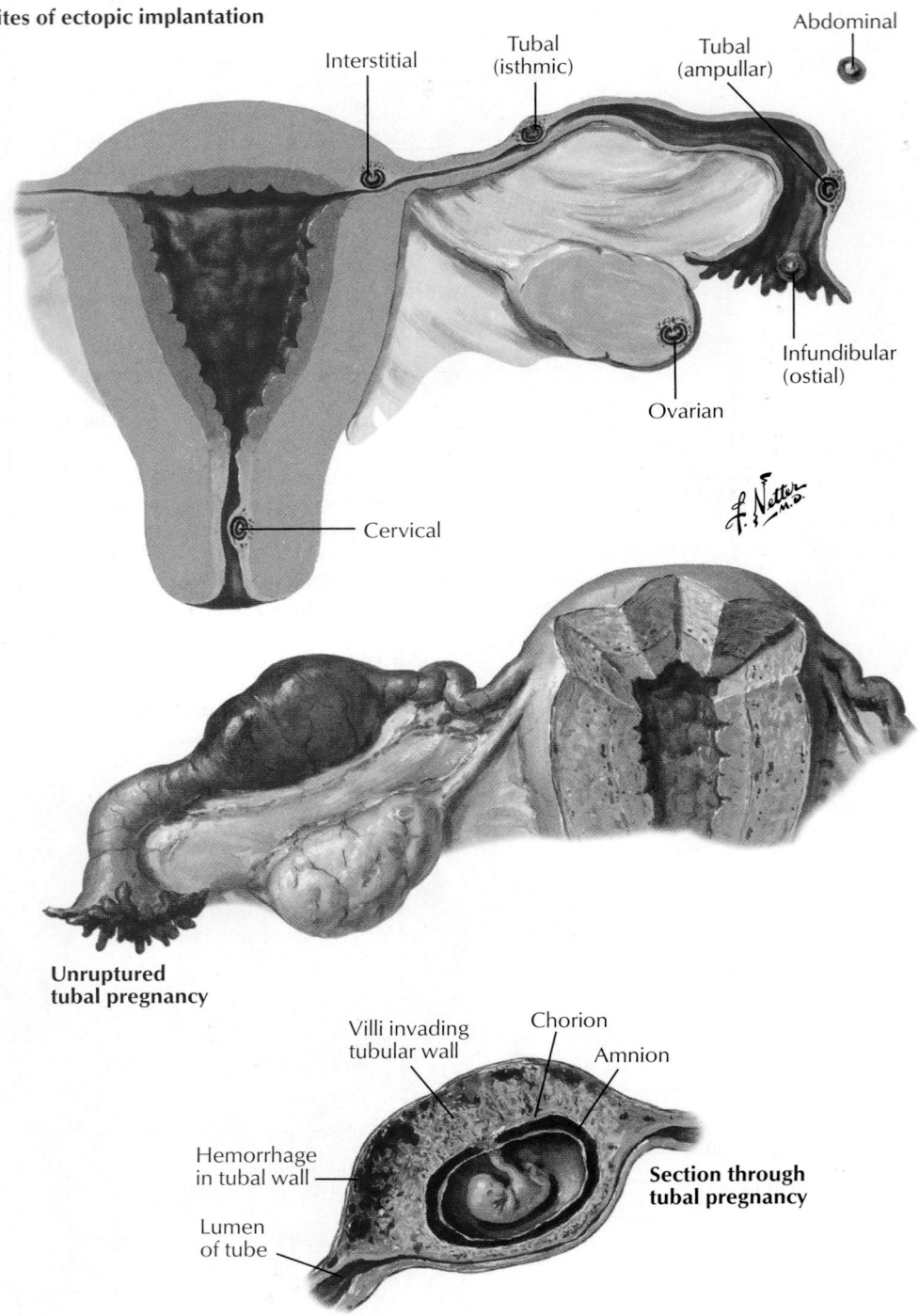

Plate 375 Ectopic Pregnancy. (Netter: Atlas of Human Anatomy, 4 ed, 2006, Saunders.)

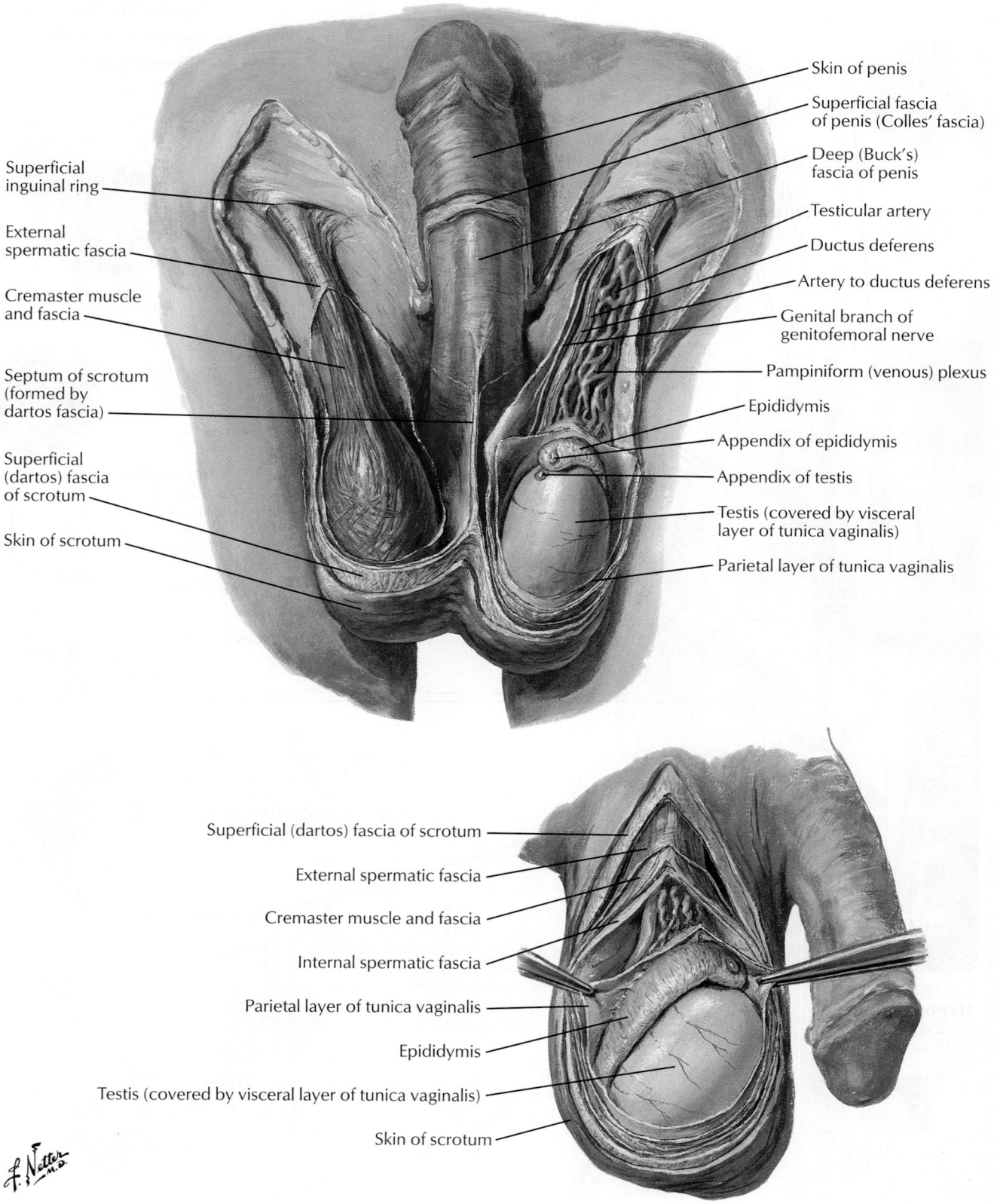

Plate 387 Scrotum and Contents. (Netter: Atlas of Human Anatomy, 4 ed, 2006, Saunders.)

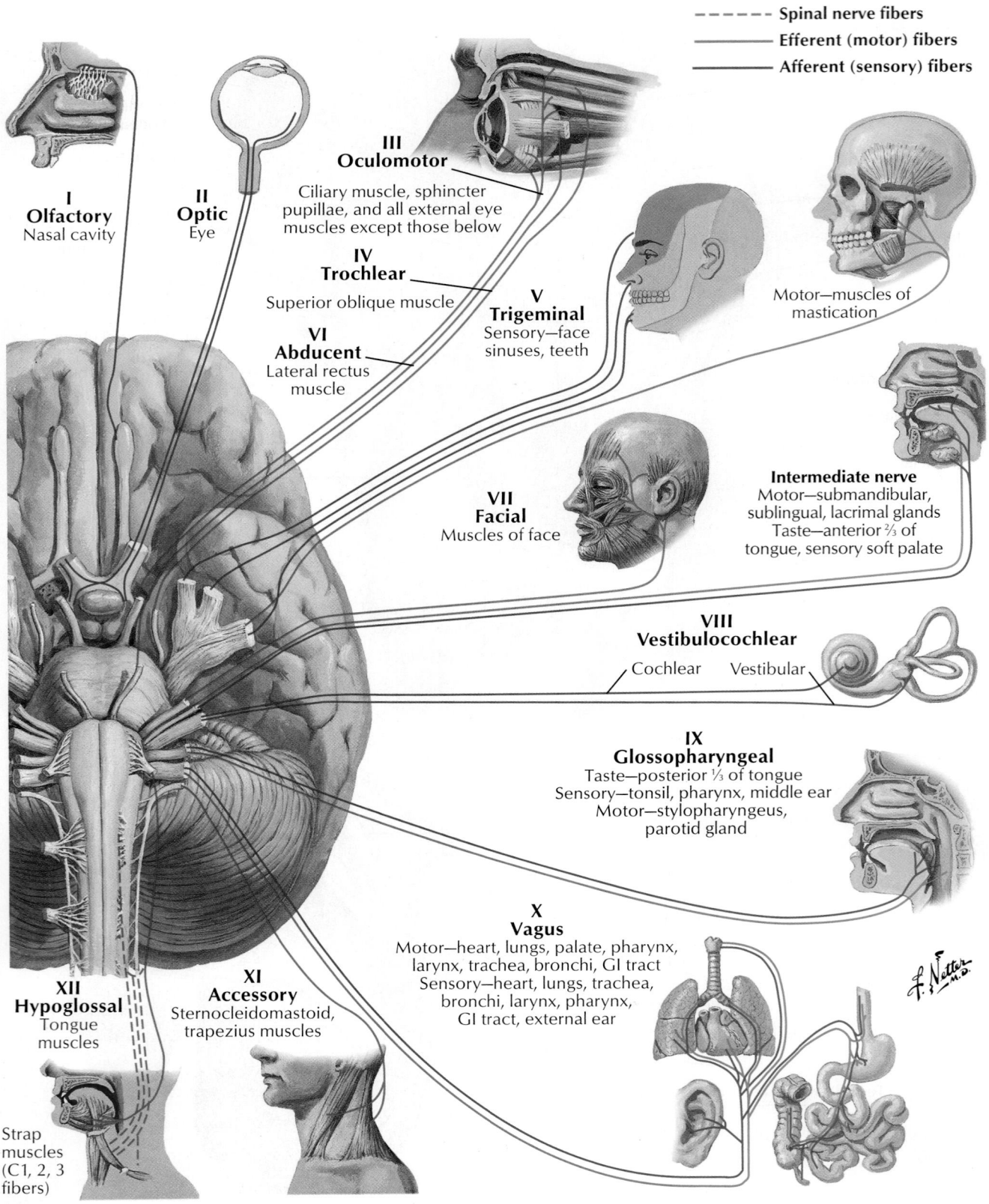

Plate 118 Cranial Nerves (Motor and Sensory Distribution): Schema. (Netter: Atlas of Human Anatomy, 4 ed, 2006, Saunders.)

Superior view

Supratrochlear nerve
Medial rectus muscle
Superior oblique muscle
Infratrochlear nerve
Nasociliary nerve
Trochlear nerve (IV)
Common tendinous ring
Ophthalmic nerve (V_1)
Optic nerve (II)
Internal carotid artery and nerve plexus
Oculomotor nerve (III)
Trochlear nerve (IV)
Abducent nerve (VI)
Tentorium cerebelli

Medial branch
Lateral branch
} Supraorbital nerve
Levator palpebrae superioris muscle
Superior rectus muscle
Lacrimal gland
Lacrimal nerve
Lateral rectus muscle
Frontal nerve
Maxillary nerve (V_2)
Meningeal branch of maxillary nerve
Mandibular nerve (V_3)
Lesser petrosal nerve
Meningeal branch of mandibular nerve
Greater petrosal nerve
Trigeminal (semilunar) ganglion
Tentorial (meningeal) branch of ophthalmic nerve

Superior view:
levator palpebrae superioris, superior rectus, and superior oblique muscles partially cut away

Supratrochlear nerve *(cut)*
Supraorbital nerve branches *(cut)*
Infratrochlear nerve
Anterior ethmoidal nerve
Optic nerve (II)
Posterior ethmoidal nerve
Superior branch of oculomotor nerve (III) *(cut)*
Nasociliary nerve
Internal carotid plexus
Trochlear nerve (IV) *(cut)*
Oculomotor nerve (III)
Abducent nerve (VI)

Long ciliary nerves
Short ciliary nerves
Lacrimal nerve
Ciliary ganglion
Parasympathetic root of ciliary ganglion (from inferior branch of oculomotor nerve)
Sympathetic root of ciliary ganglion (from internal carotid plexus)
Sensory root of ciliary ganglion (from nasociliary nerve)
Branches to inferior and medial rectus muscles
Abducent nerve (VI)
Inferior branch of oculomotor nerve (III)
Lacrimal nerve
Frontal nerve *(cut)*
Ophthalmic nerve (V_1)

F. Netter M.D.

Plate 86 Nerves of Orbit. (Netter: Atlas of Human Anatomy, 4 ed, 2006, Saunders.)

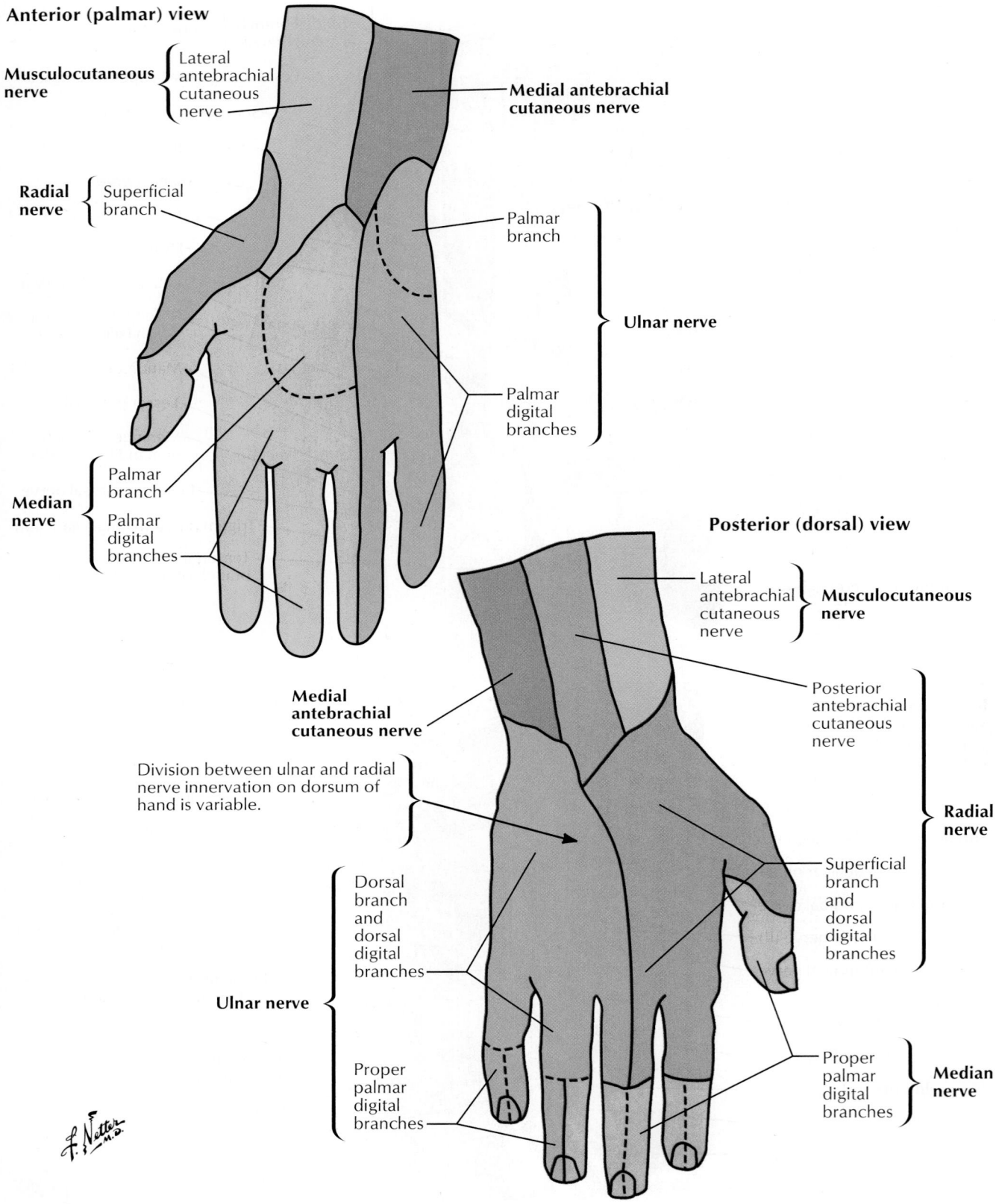

Plate 472 Cutaneous Innervation of Wrist and Hand. (Netter: Atlas of Human Anatomy, 4 ed, 2006, Saunders.)

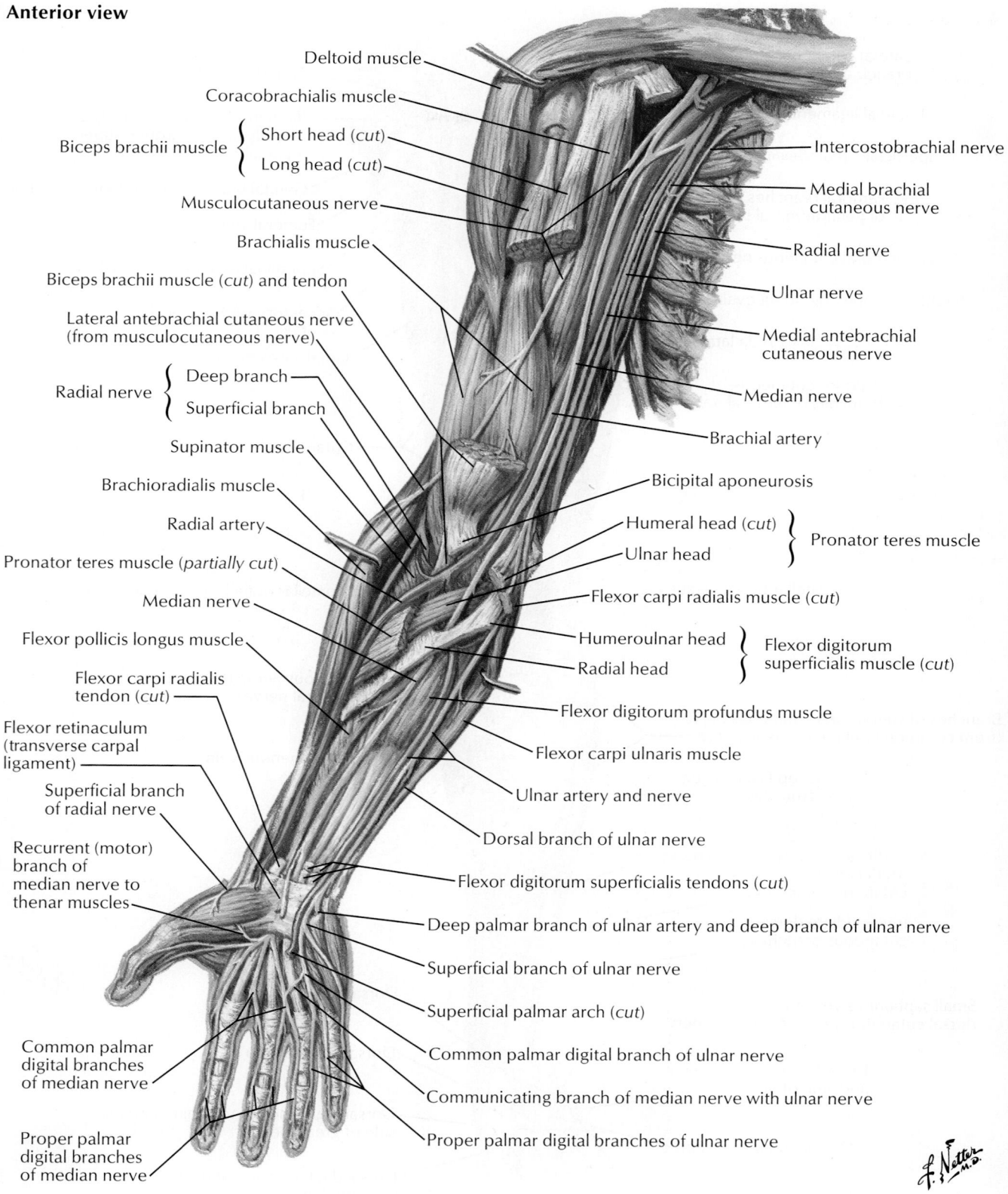

Plate 473 Arteries and Nerves of Upper Limb. (Netter: Atlas of Human Anatomy, 4 ed, 2006, Saunders.)

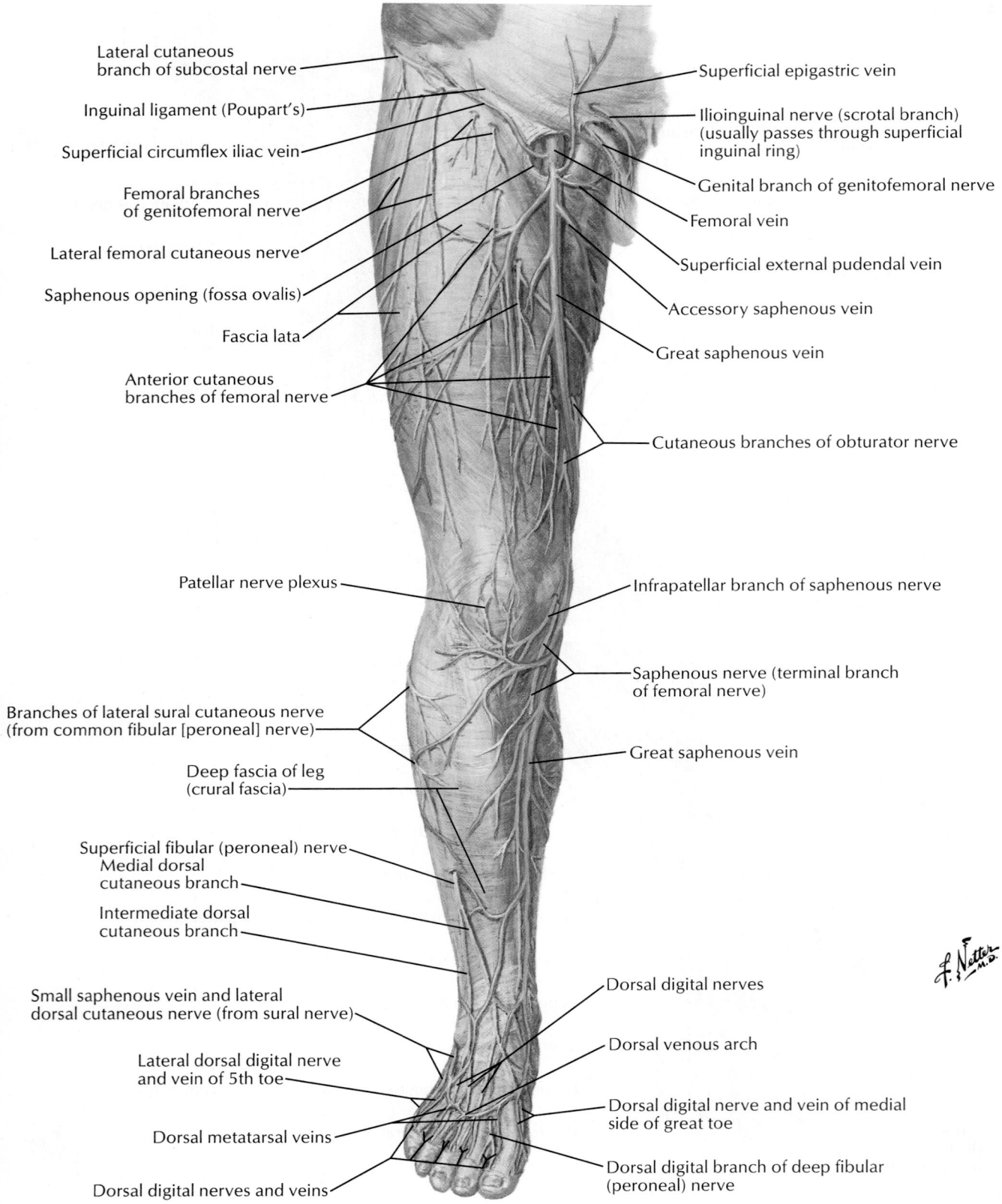

Plate 544 Superficial Nerves and Veins of Lower Limb: Anterior View. (Netter: Atlas of Human Anatomy, 4 ed, 2006, Saunders.)

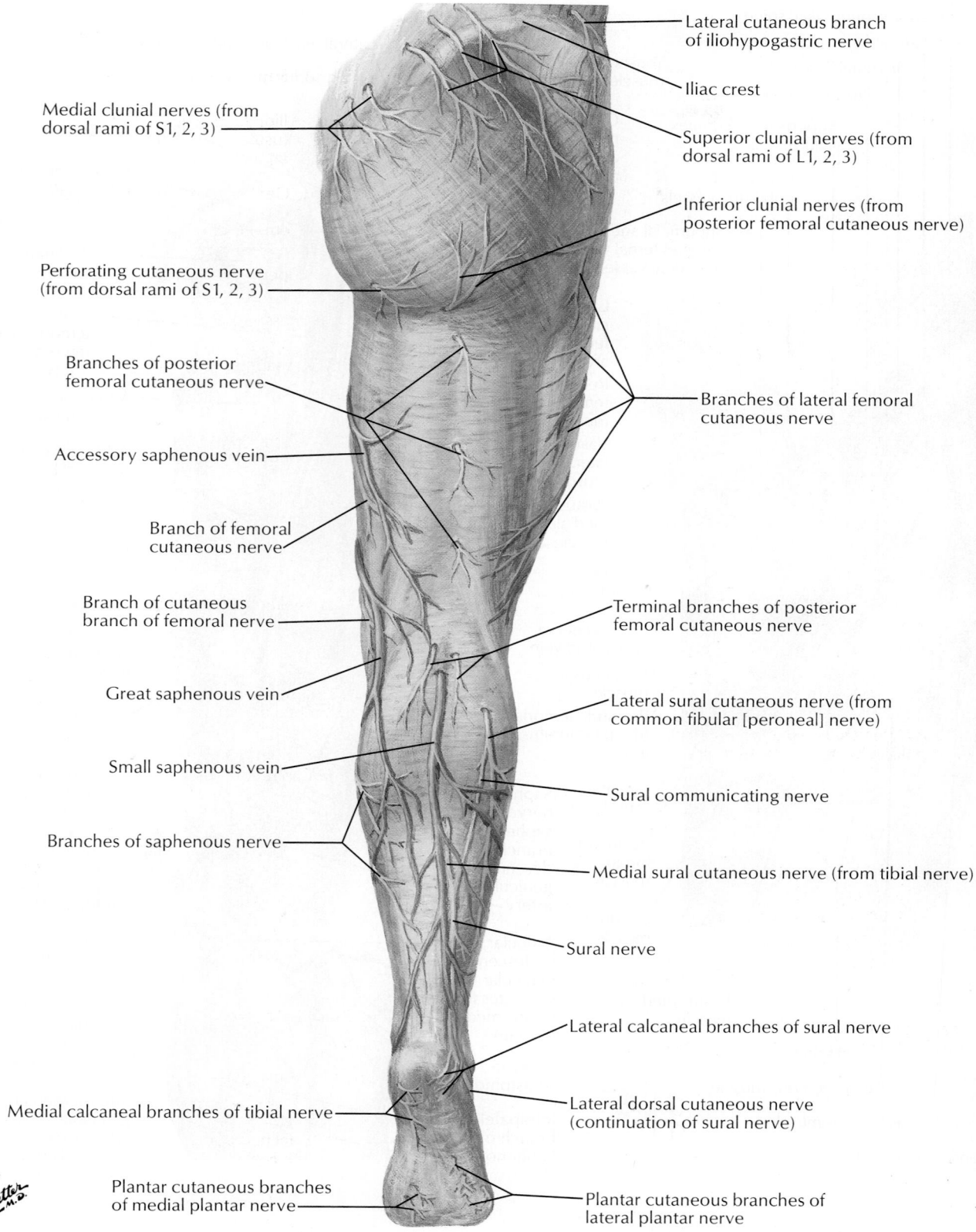

Plate 545 Superficial Nerves and Veins of Lower Limb: Posterior View. (Netter: Atlas of Human Anatomy, 4 ed, 2006, Saunders.)

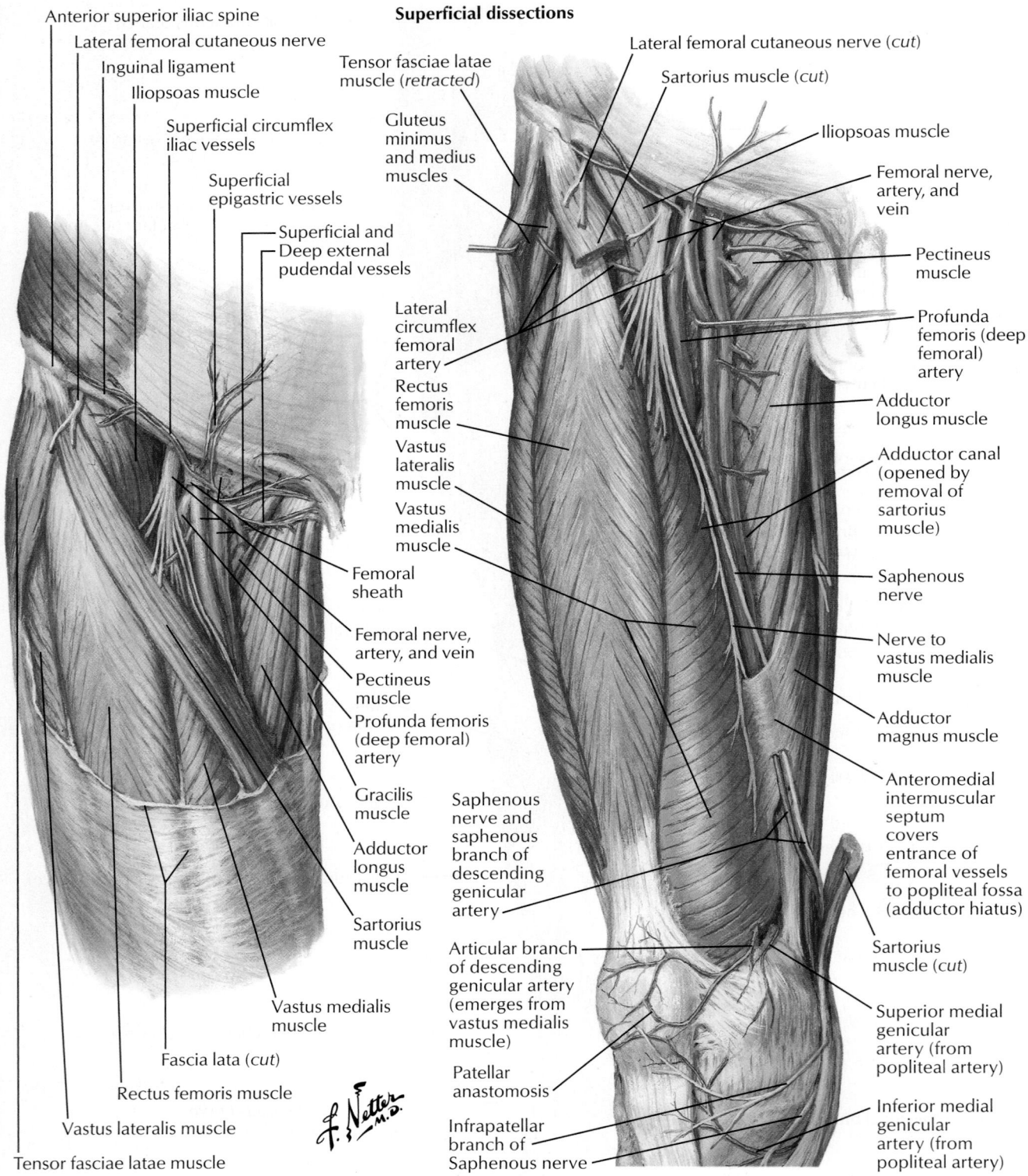

Plate 500 Arteries and Nerves of Thigh: Anterior Views. (Netter: Atlas of Human Anatomy, 4 ed, 2006, Saunders.)

Deep dissection

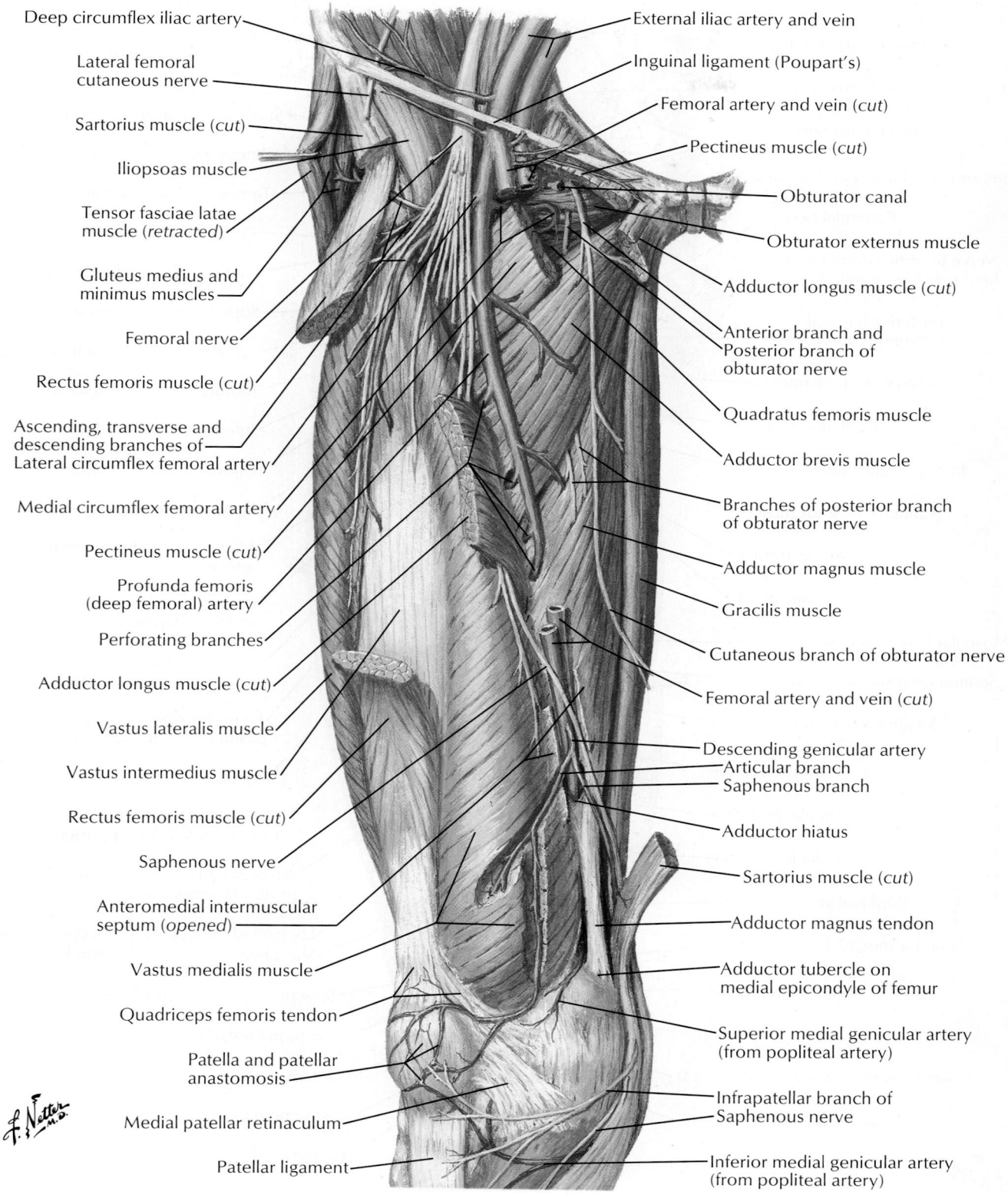

Plate 501 Arteries and Nerves of Thigh: Posterior View. (Netter: Atlas of Human Anatomy, 4 ed, 2006, Saunders.)

Deep dissection

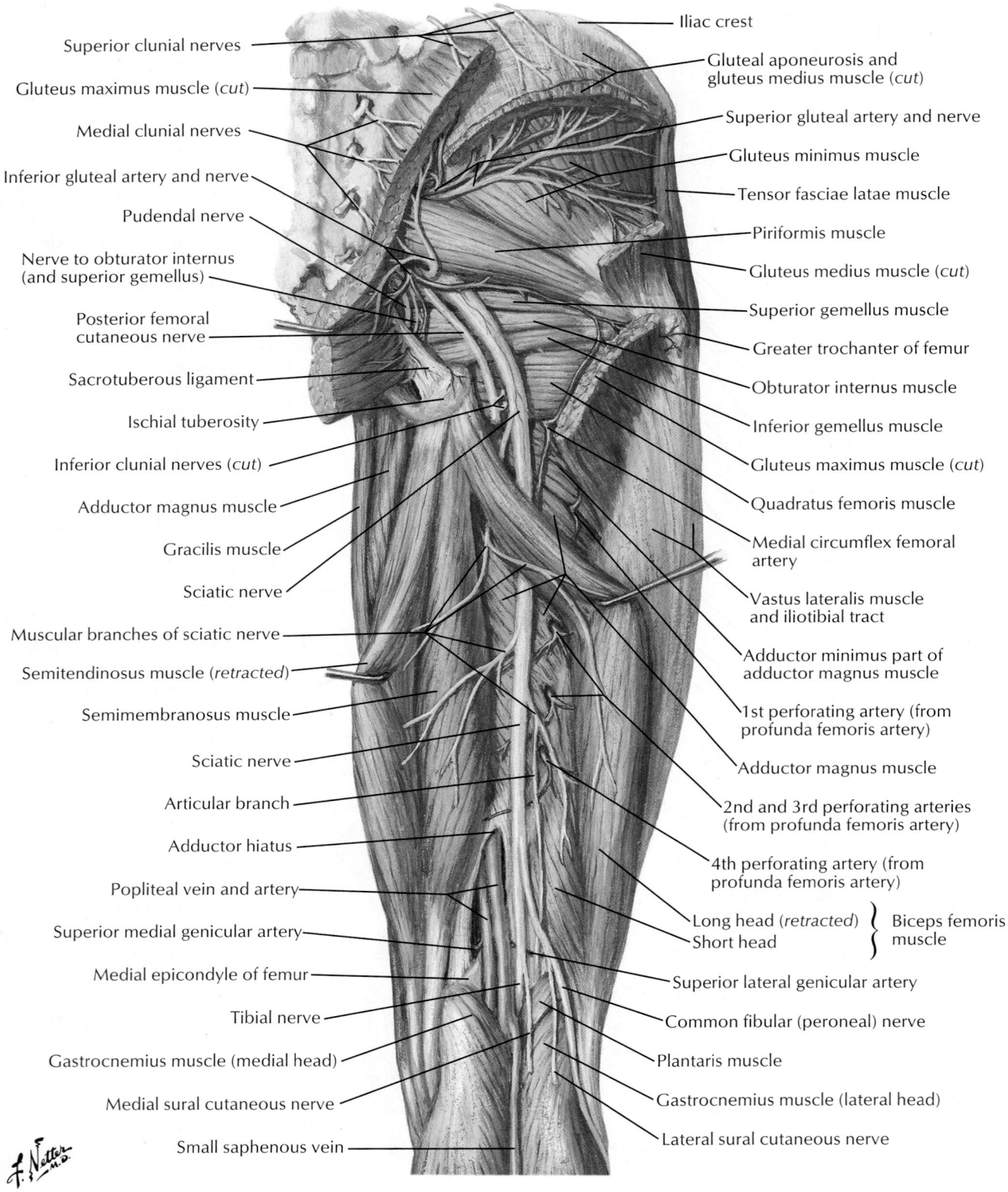

Plate 502 Arteries and Nerves of Thigh: Posterior View. (Netter: Atlas of Human Anatomy, 4 ed, 2006, Saunders.)

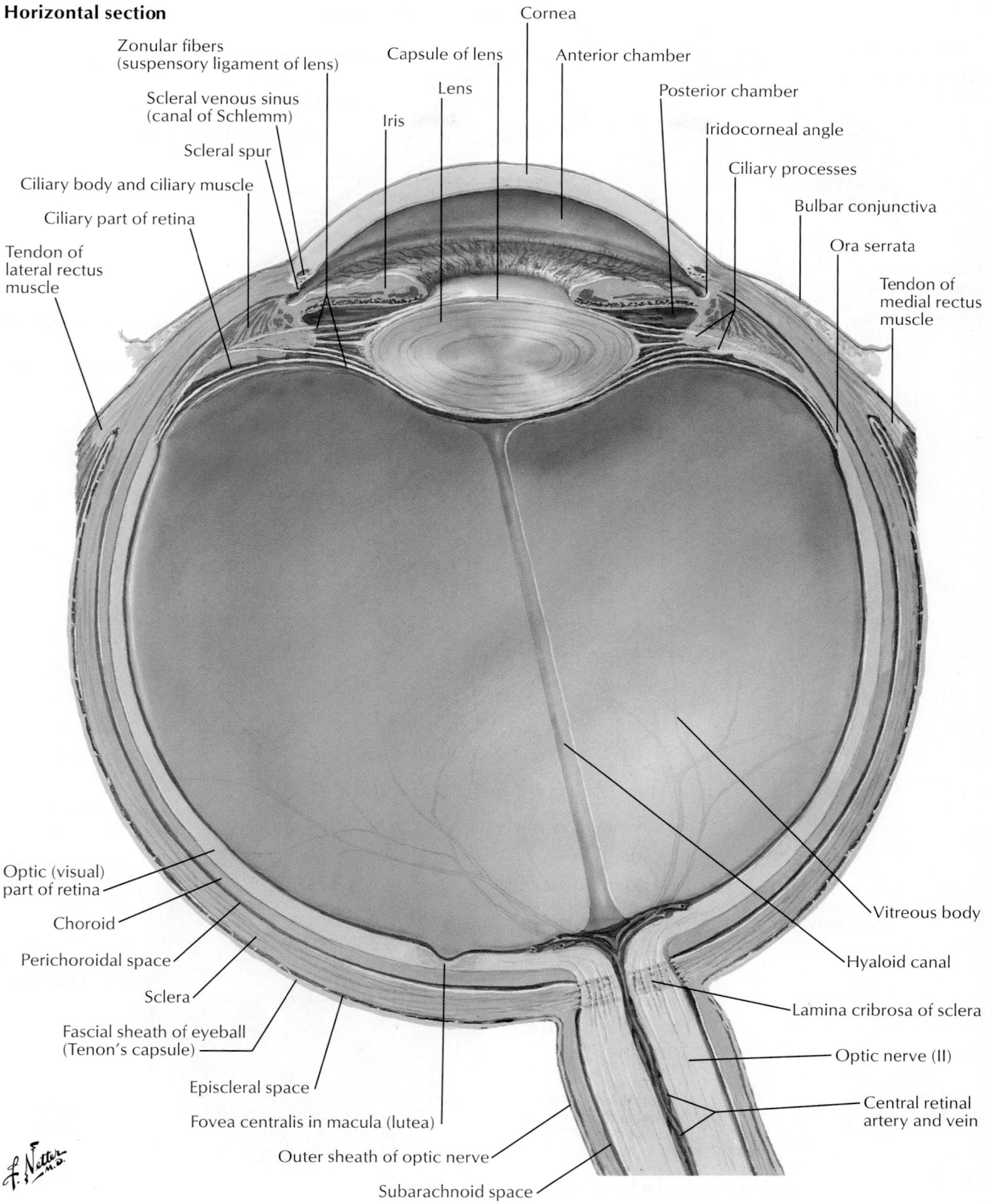

Plate 87 Eyeball. (Netter: Atlas of Human Anatomy, 4 ed, 2006, Saunders.)

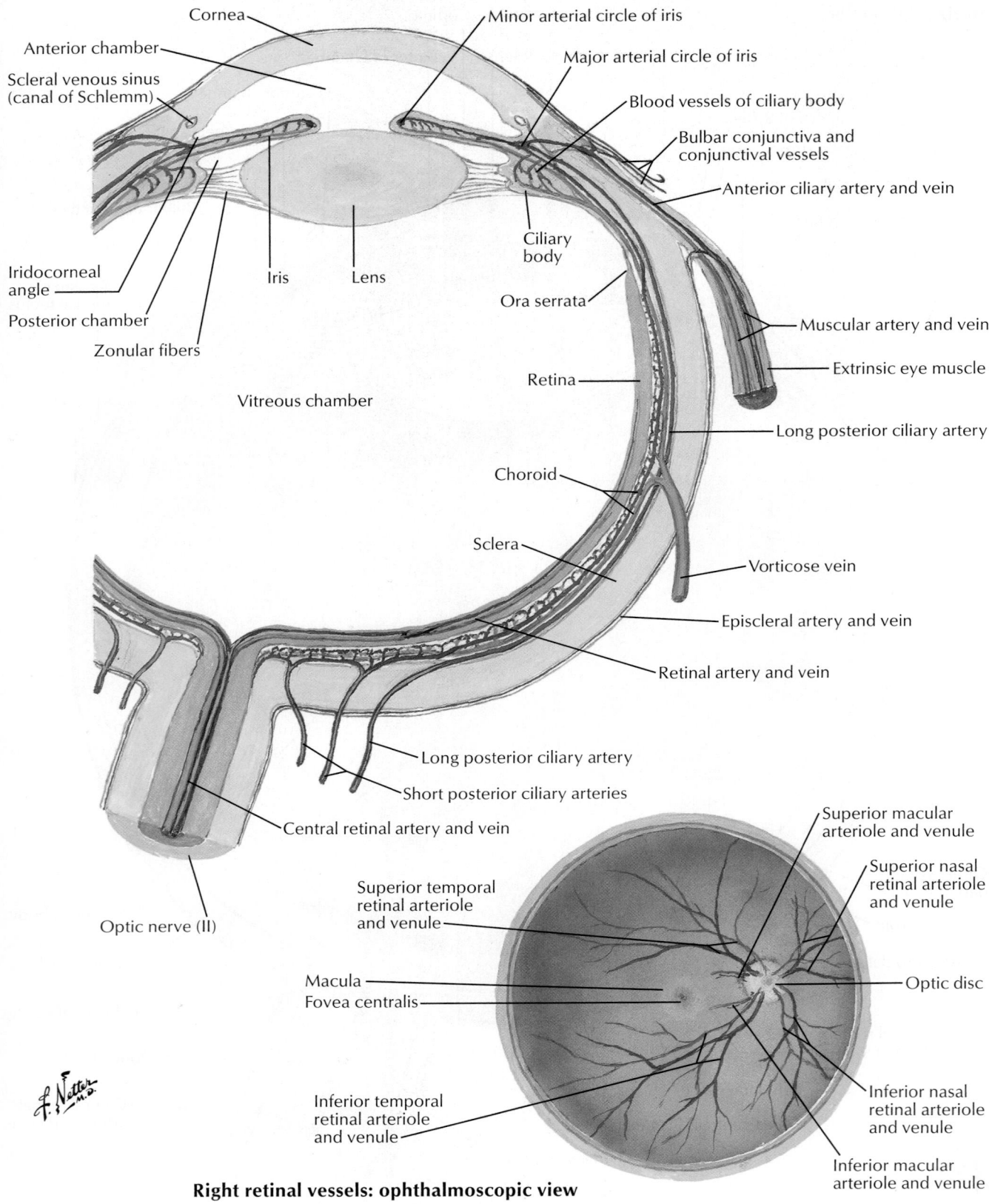

Right retinal vessels: ophthalmoscopic view

Plate 90 Intrinsic Arteries and Veins of Eye. (Netter: Atlas of Human Anatomy, 4 ed, 2006, Saunders.)

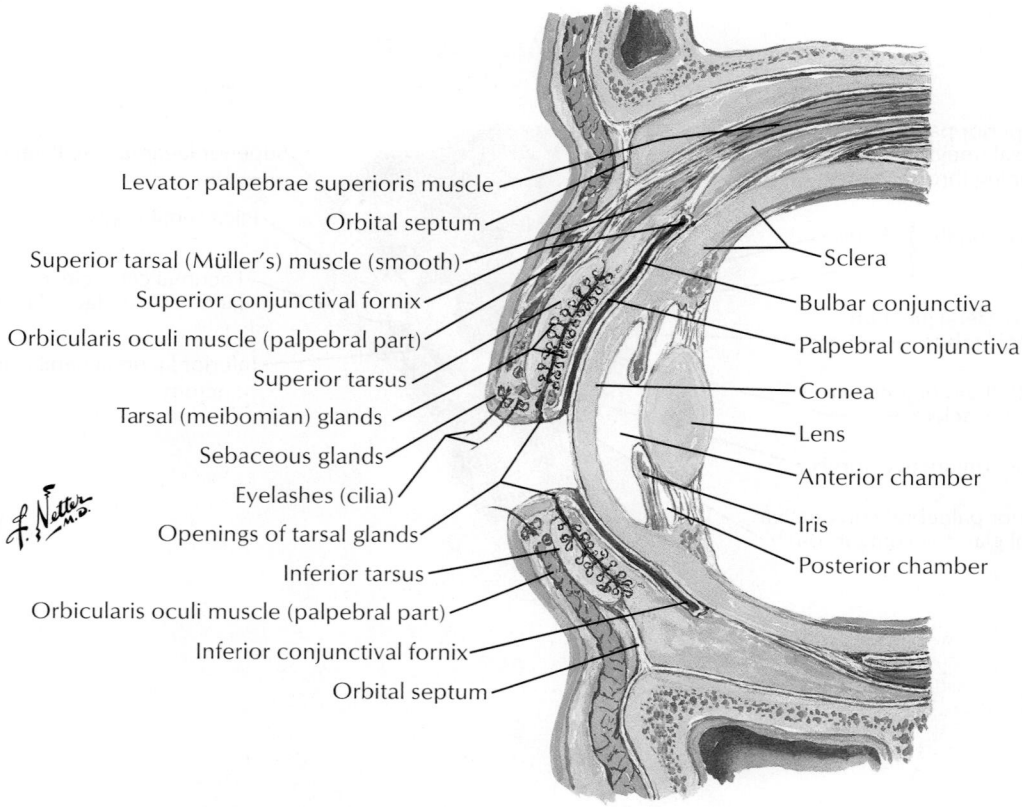

Plate 81, Middle Eyelids. (Netter: Atlas of Human Anatomy, 4 ed, 2006, Saunders.)

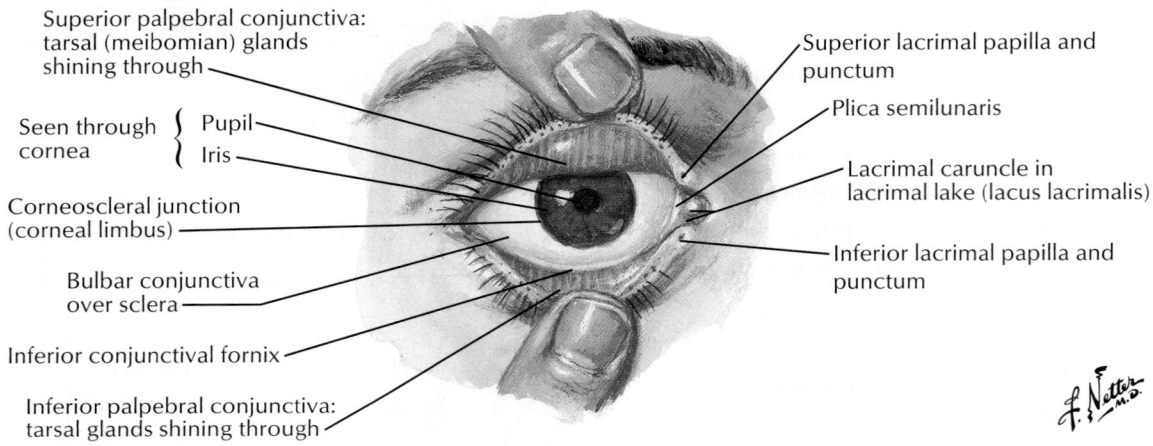

Plate 81, Upper Eyelid. (Netter: Atlas of Human Anatomy, 4 ed, 2006, Saunders.)

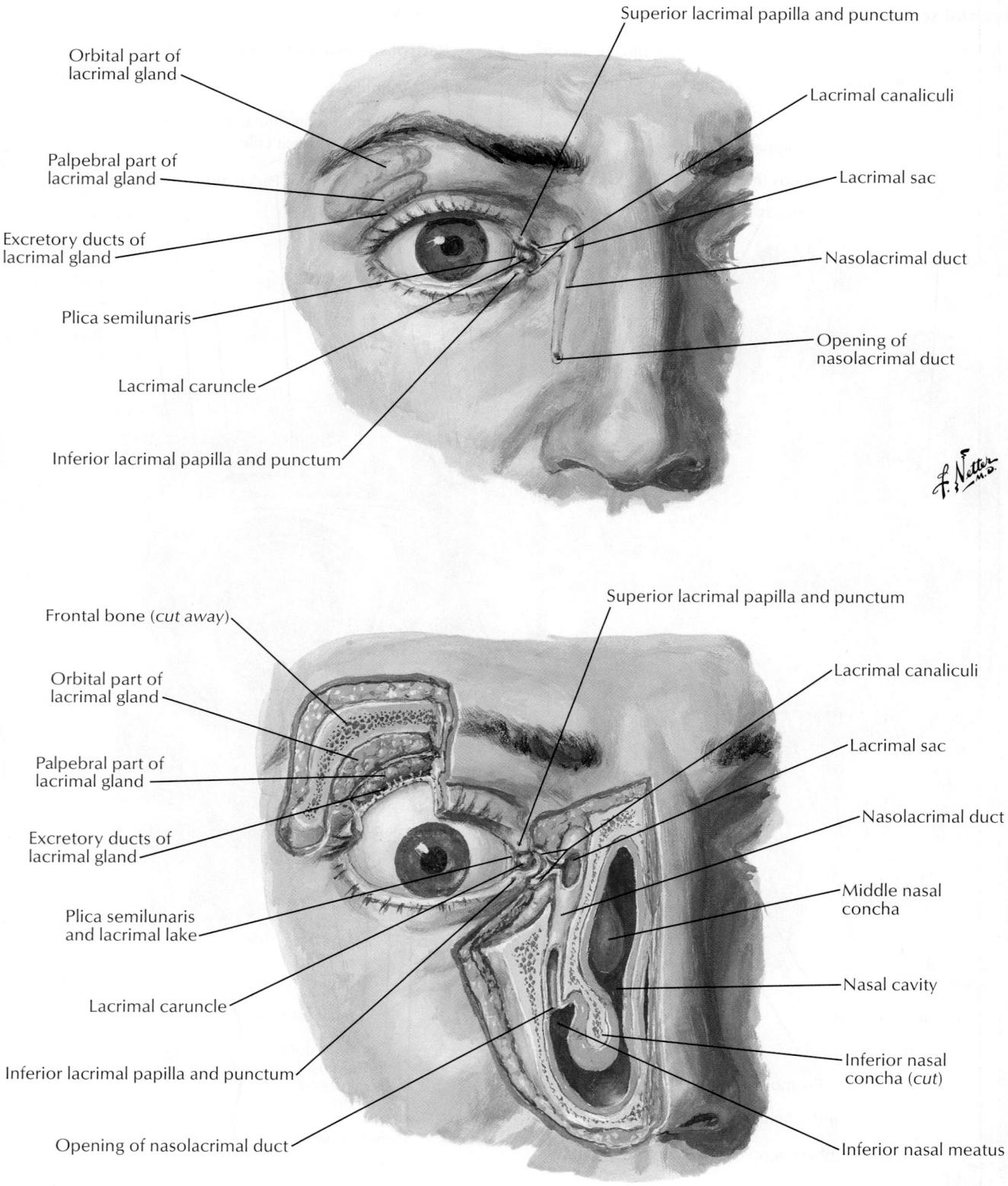

Plate 82 Lacrimal Apparatus. (Netter: Atlas of Human Anatomy, 4 ed, 2006, Saunders.)

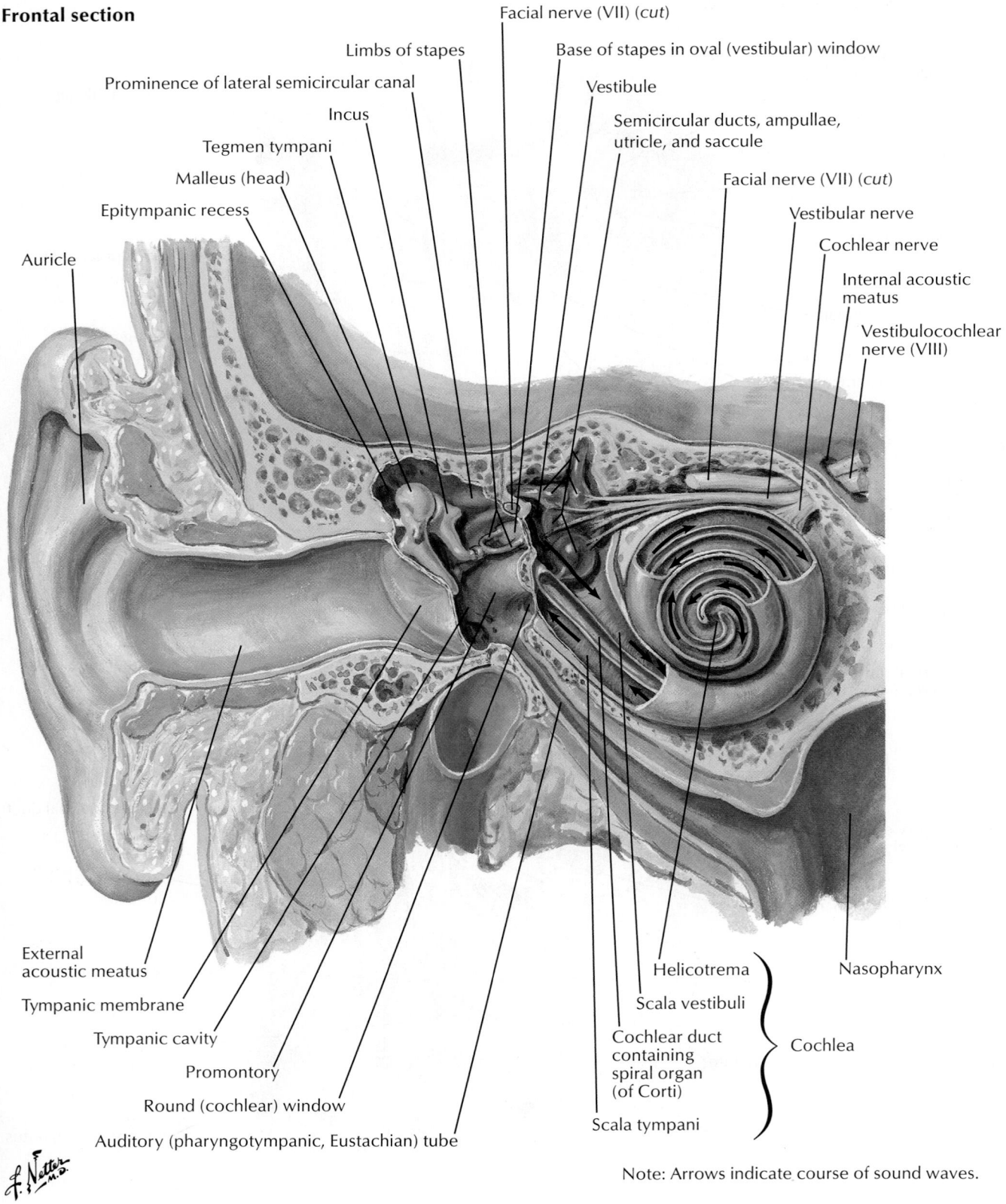

Plate 92 Pathway of Sound Reception. (Netter: Atlas of Human Anatomy, 4 ed, 2006, Saunders.)

Medial wall of tympanic cavity: lateral view

Prominence of lateral semicircular canal
Prominence of facial canal
Mastoid antrum
Geniculum (geniculate ganglion) of facial nerve
Base of stapes in fossa of oval (vestibular) window
Greater petrosal nerve
Tensor tympani muscle (*tendon cut*)
Limbs of stapes
Pyramidal eminence
Auditory (pharyngotympanic, Eustachian) tube
Chorda tympani nerve (*cut*)
Levator veli palatini muscle
Mastoid cells
Tendon of stapedius muscle
Promontory with tympanic nerve (of Jacobson) and plexus under mucosa
Fossa of round (cochlear) window
Jugular fossa
Internal carotid artery
Facial nerve (VII) in stylomastoid foramen
Tympanic cells

Plate 94 Tympanic Cavity. (Netter: Atlas of Human Anatomy, 4 ed, 2006, Saunders.)

Otoscopic view of right tympanic membrane

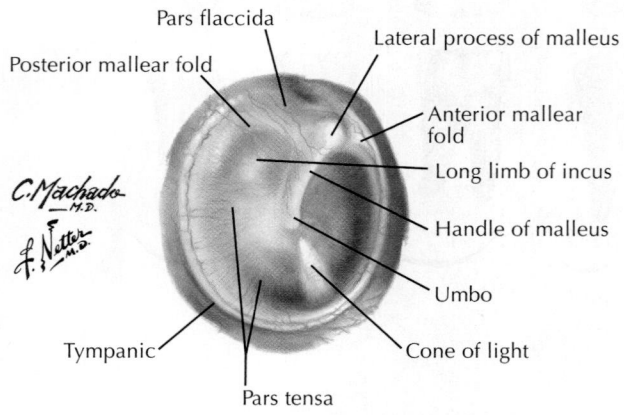

Plate 93 Tympanic Cavity. (Netter: Atlas of Human Anatomy, 4 ed, 2006, Saunders.)

Dissected right bony labyrinth (otic capsule): membranous labyrinth removed

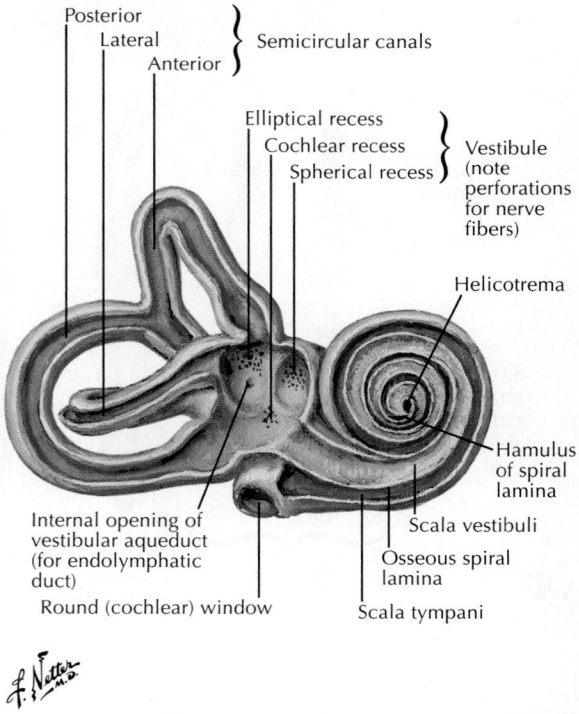

Plate 95 Bony Membranous Labyrinth. (Netter: Atlas of Human Anatomy, 4 ed, 2006, Saunders.)

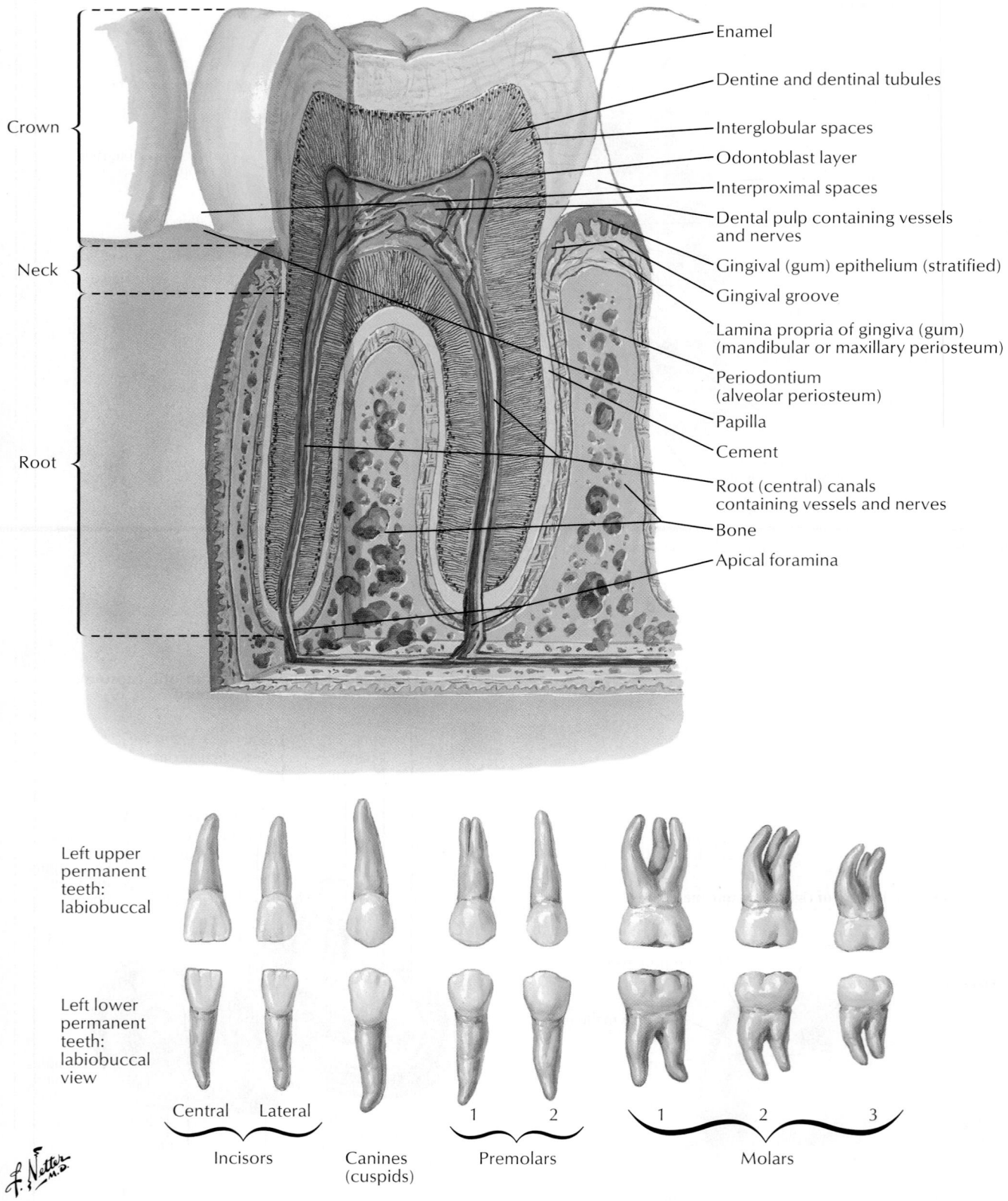

Plate 57 Teeth. (Netter: Atlas of Human Anatomy, 4 ed, 2006, Saunders.)

Tongue

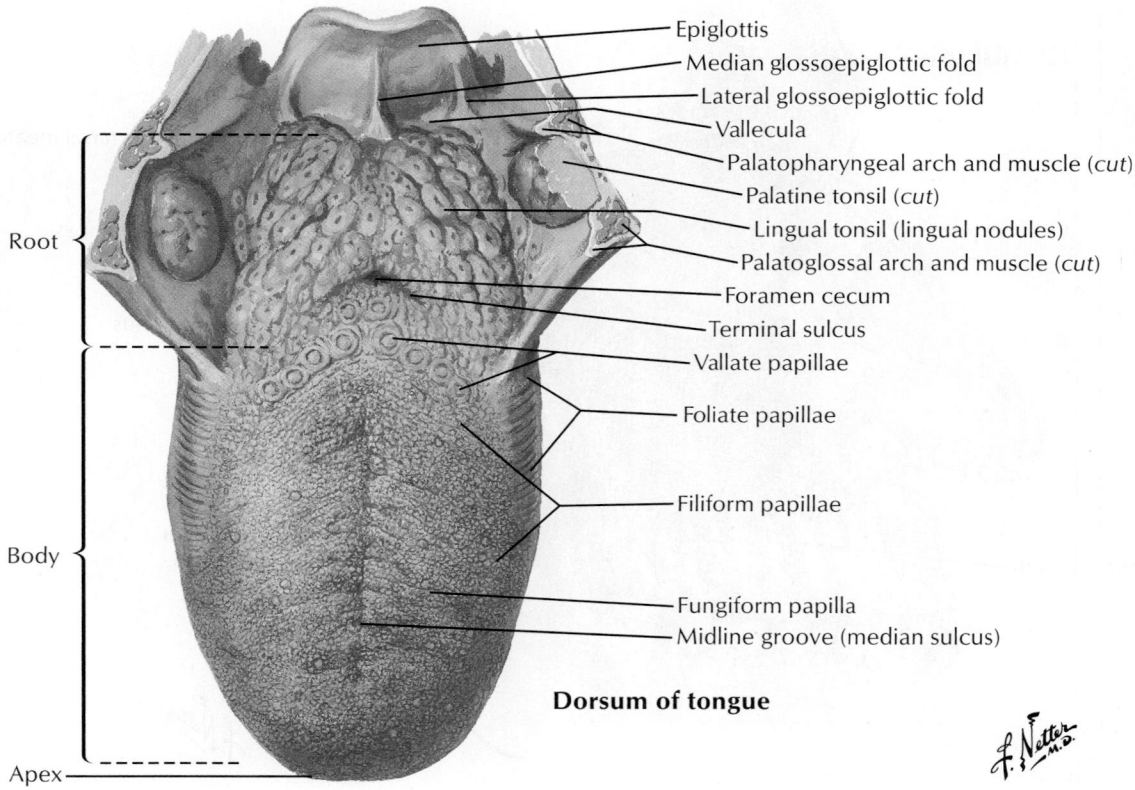

Plate 58 Tongue. (Netter: Atlas of Human Anatomy, 4 ed, 2006, Saunders.)

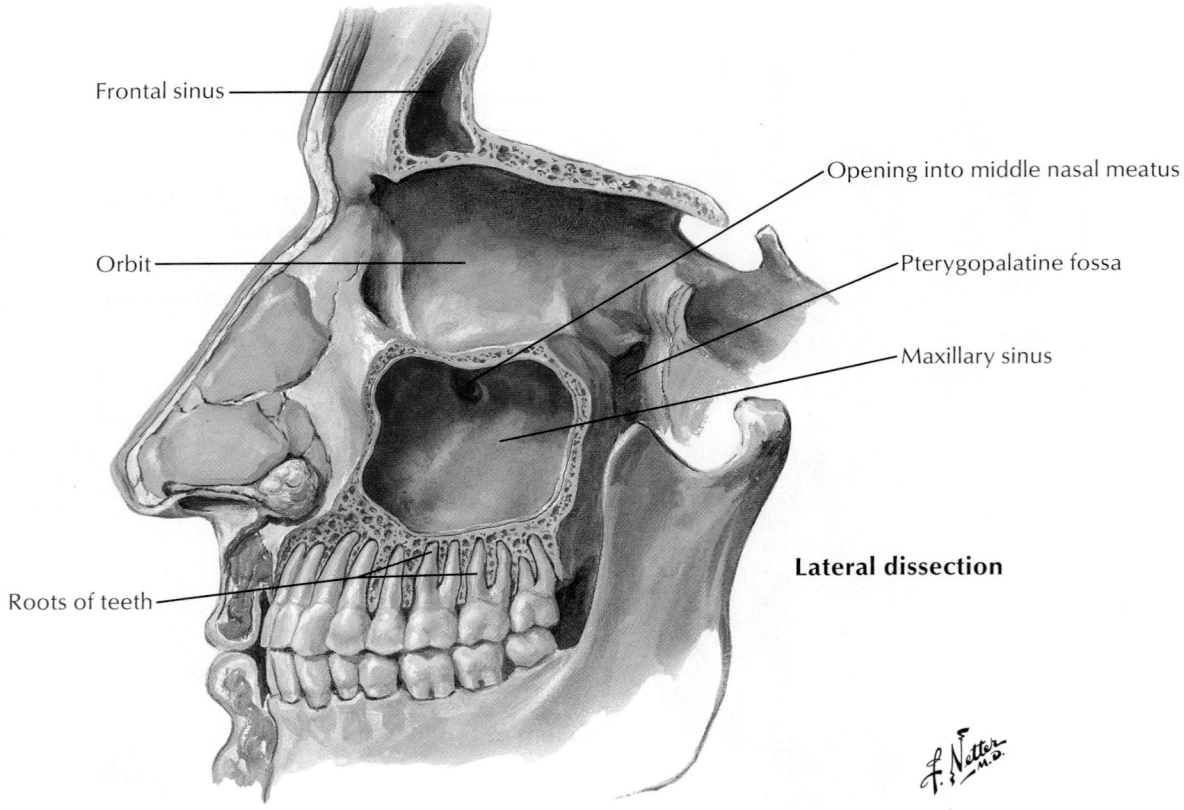

Plate 49 Paranasal Sinuses. (Netter: Atlas of Human Anatomy, 4 ed, 2006, Saunders.)

Superficial temporal artery and vein and auriculotemporal nerve
Branches of facial nerve
Transverse facial artery
Accessory parotid gland
Parotid duct
Buccinator muscle (*cut*)
Masseter muscle
Lingual nerve
Submandibular ganglion
Tongue
Frenulum of tongue
Sublingual fold with openings of sublingual ducts
Sublingual caruncle with opening of submandibular duct
Sublingual gland
Submandibular duct
Sublingual artery and vein
Mylohyoid muscle (*cut*)
Digastric muscle (anterior belly)
Submandibular gland
Facial artery and vein
Hyoid bone
Parotid gland
Retromandibular vein (anterior and posterior branches)
Digastric muscle (posterior belly)
Stylohyoid muscle
External jugular vein
Sternocleidomastoid muscle
Common trunk receiving facial, anterior branch of retromandibular, and lingual veins (common facial vein)
Internal jugular vein
External carotid artery

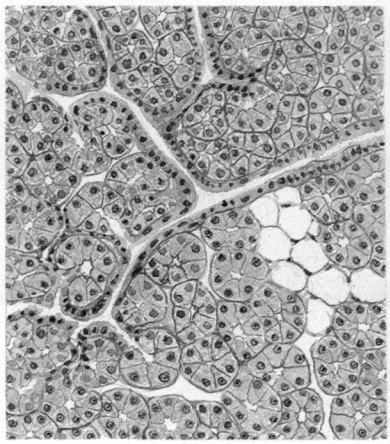

Parotid gland: totally serous

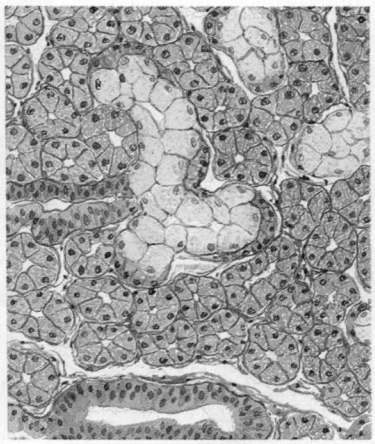

Submandibular gland: mostly serous, partially mucous

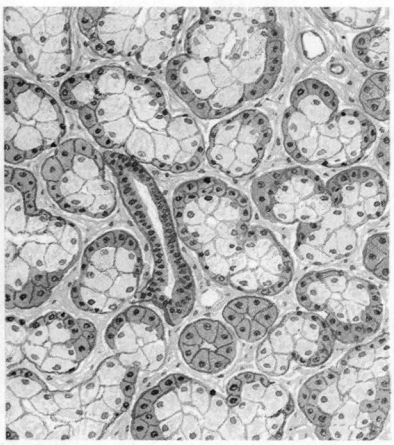

Sublingual gland: almost completely mucous

Plate 61 Salivary Glands. (Netter: Atlas of Human Anatomy, 4 ed, 2006, Saunders.)

Coronary Arteries: Arteriographic Views

Right coronary artery: left anterior oblique view

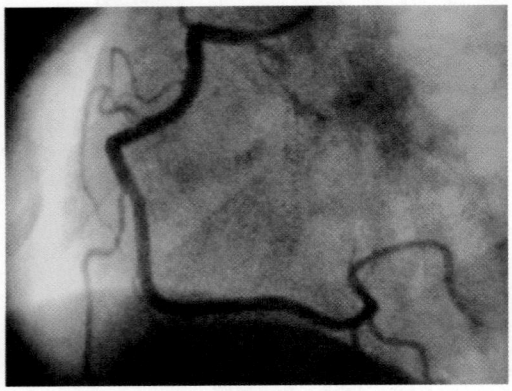

Arteriogram

Sinuatrial (SA) nodal branch

Right coronary artery

Atrioventricular (AV) nodal branch

Branches to back of left ventricle

Right marginal branch

Posterior interventricular branch (posterior descending artery)

Right coronary artery: right anterior oblique view

Sinuatrial (SA) nodal branch

Conus (arteriosus) branch

Right coronary artery

Right marginal branch

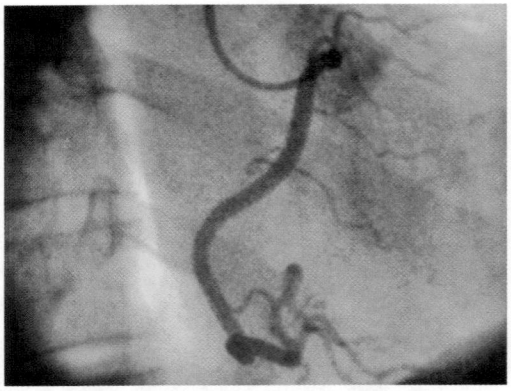

Arteriogram

Atrioventricular (AV) nodal branch

Right posterolateral branches (to back of left ventricle)

Posterior interventricular branch (posterior descending artery)

F. Netter M.D. © ICON LEARNING SYSTEMS

Plate 218 Coronary Arteries: Arteriographic Views. (Netter: Atlas of Human Anatomy, 4 ed, 2006, Saunders.)

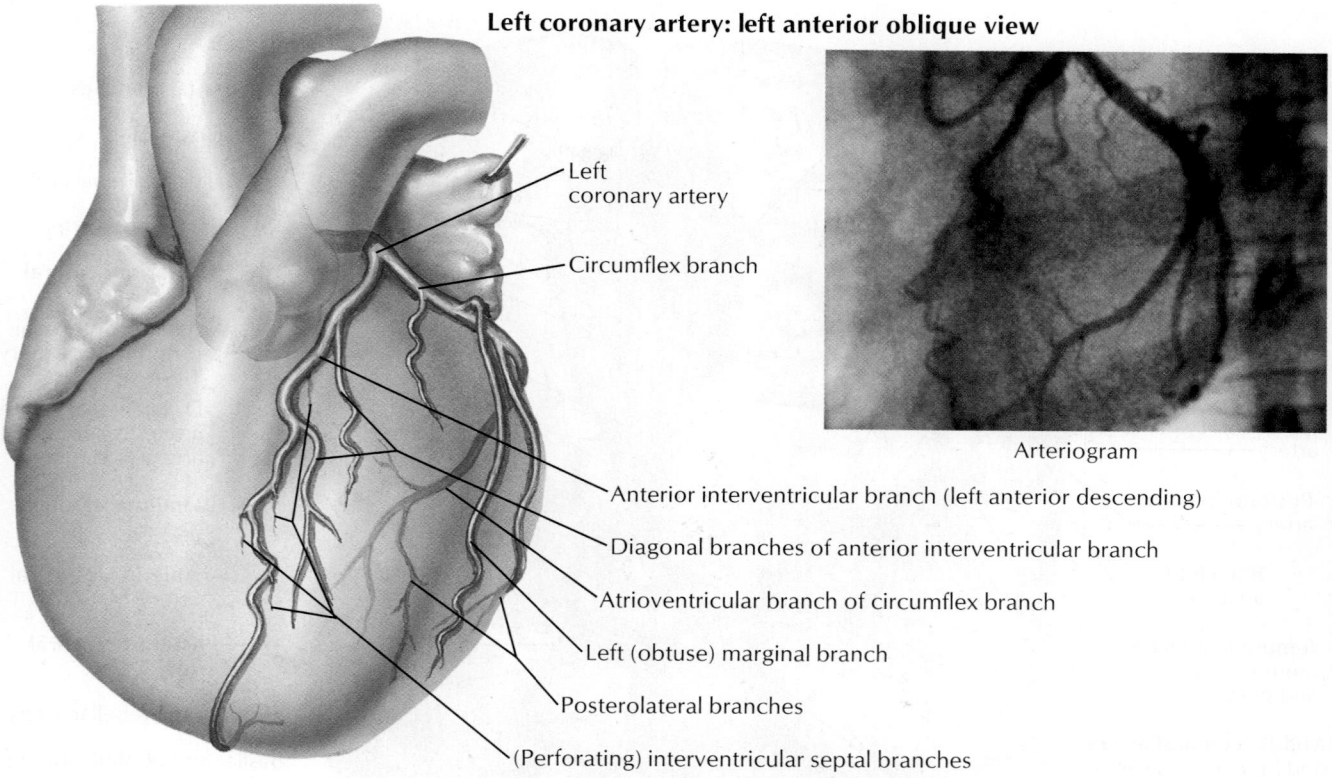

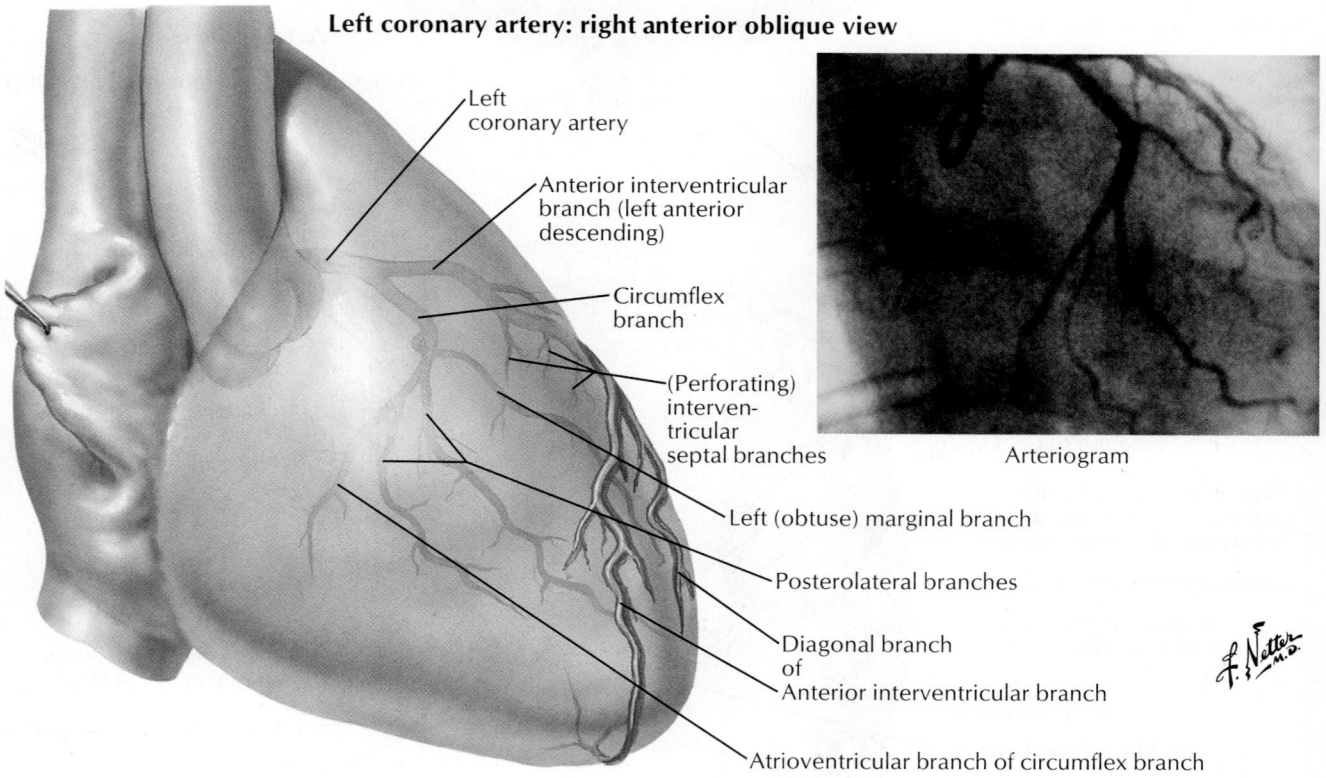

Plate 219 Coronary Arteries: Arteriographic Views. (Netter: Atlas of Human Anatomy, 4 ed, 2006, Saunders.)

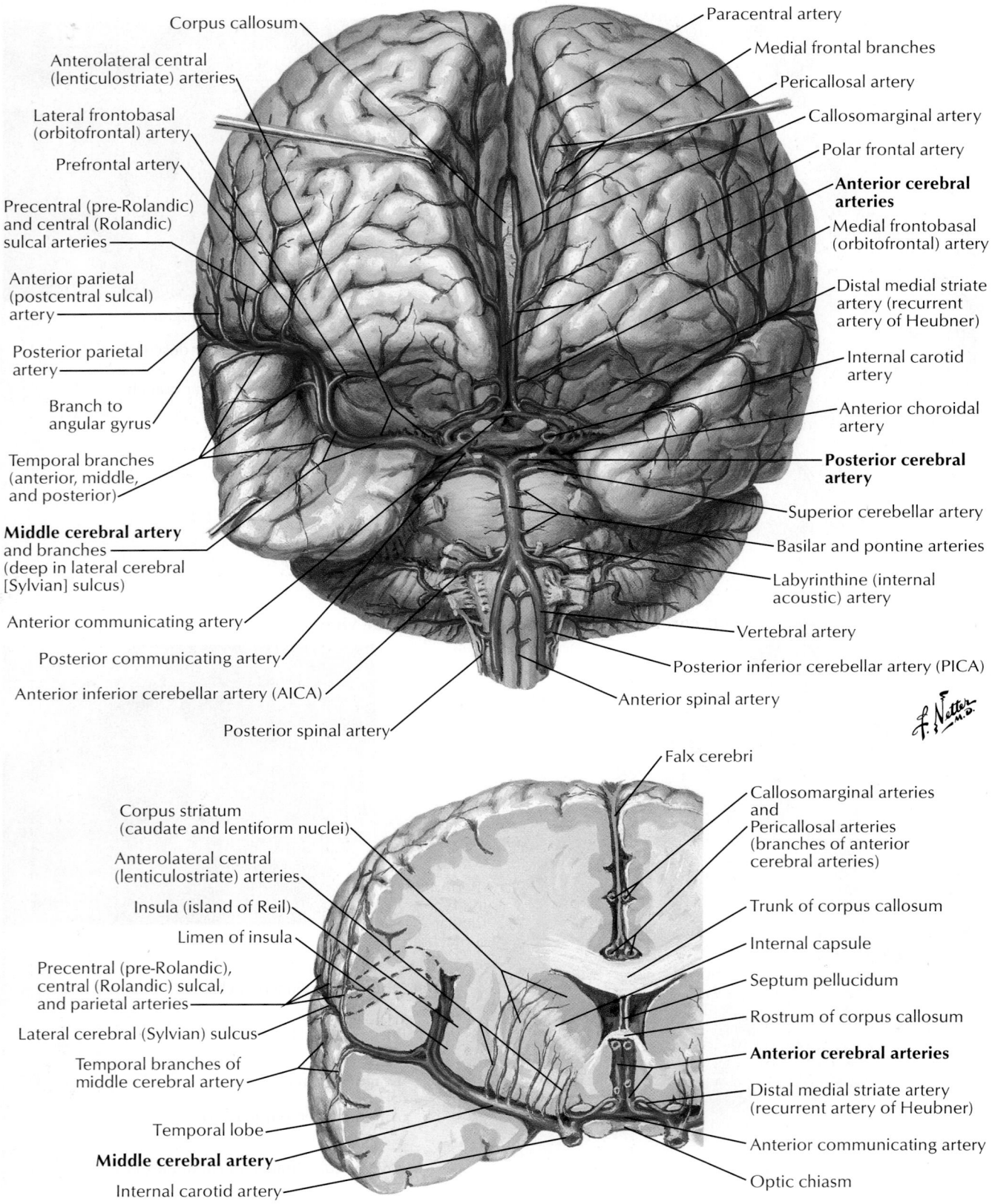

Plate 141 Arteries of Brain: Frontal View and Section. (Netter: Atlas of Human Anatomy, 4 ed, 2006, Saunders.)

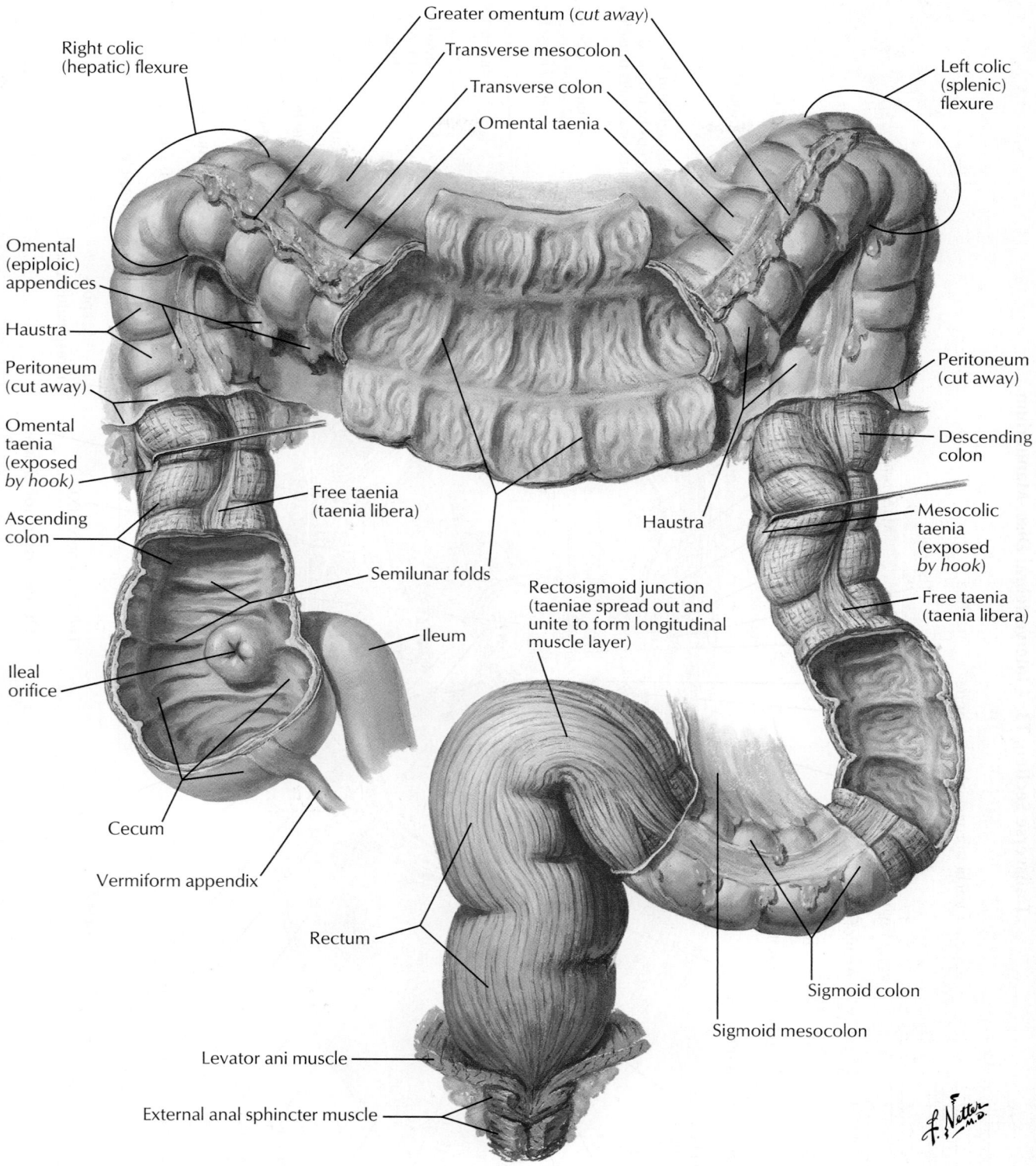

Plate 284 Mucosa and Musculature of Large Intestine. (Netter: Atlas of Human Anatomy, 4 ed, 2006, Saunders.)

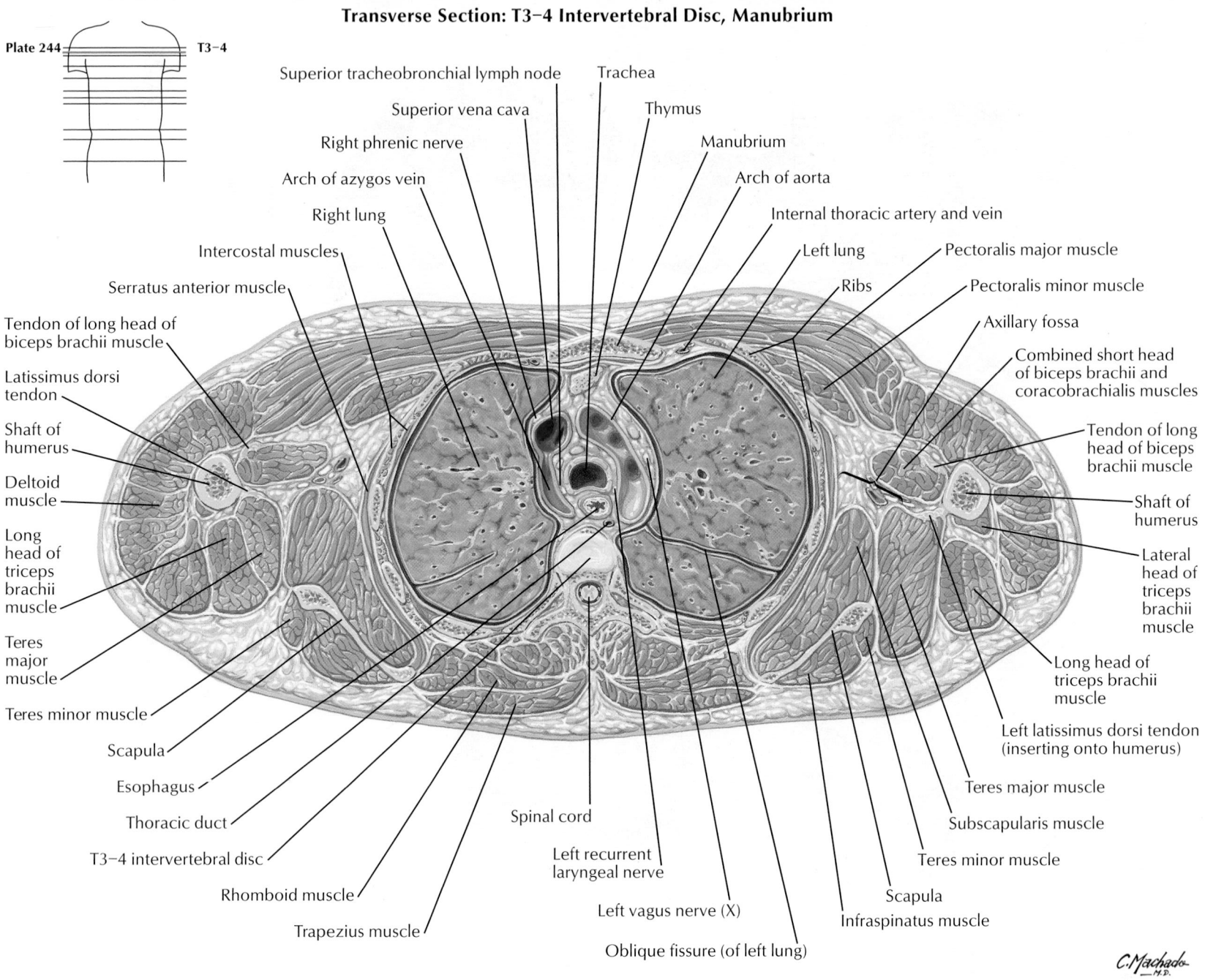

Plate 244 Cross Section of Thorax at T3-4 Disc Level. (Netter: Atlas of Human Anatomy, 4 ed, 2006, Saunders.)

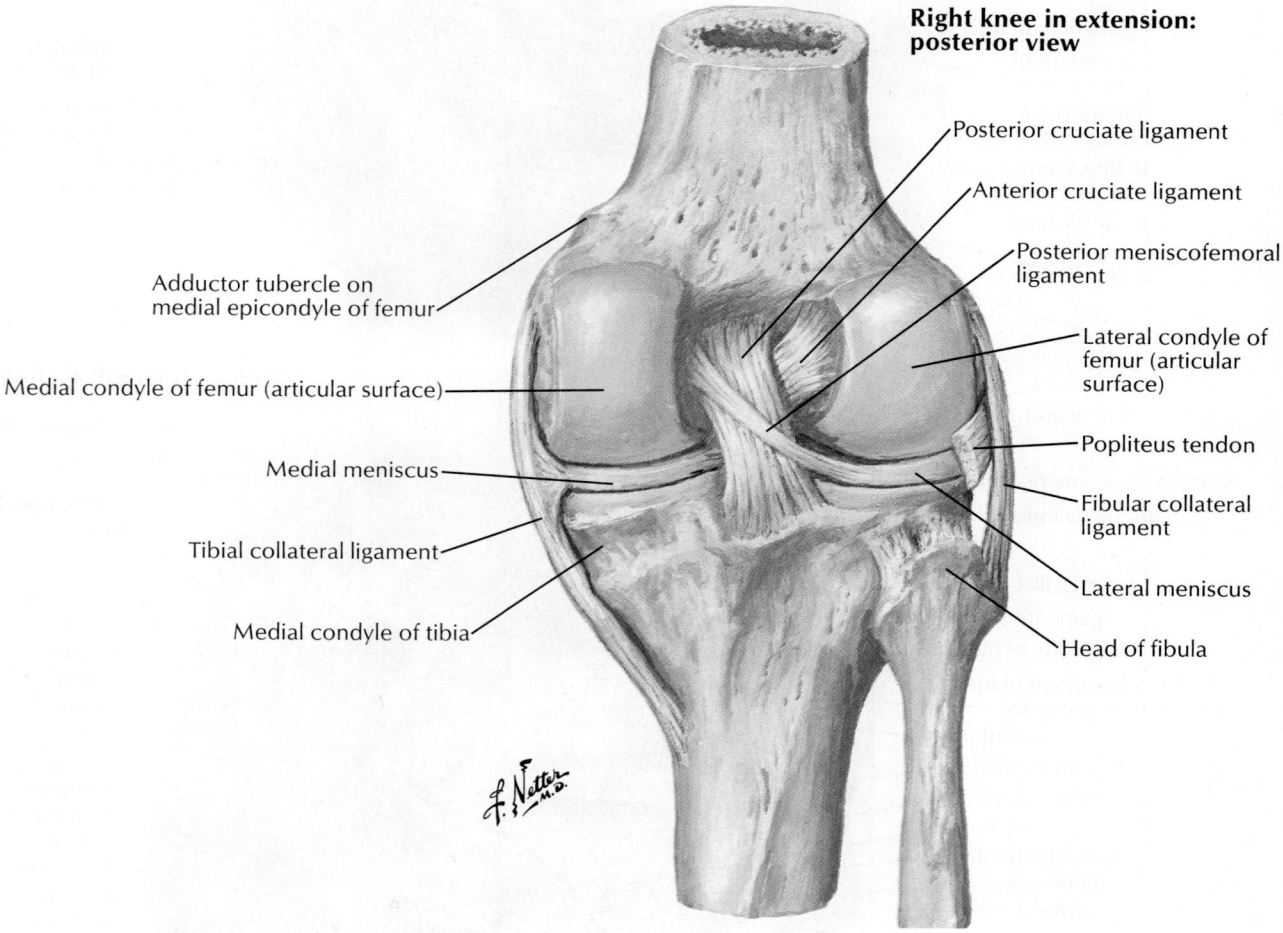

Plate 509 Knee: Cruciate and Collateral Ligaments. (Netter: Atlas of Human Anatomy, 4 ed, 2006, Saunders.)

Paramedian (sagittal) dissection

Ureter
Uterine (fallopian) tube
Ovary
Ligament of ovary
Round ligament of uterus
Broad ligament (*cut*)
Superior pubic ramus (*cut*)
Inferior pubic ramus (*cut*)
Ischiocavernosus muscle
Body of clitoris
Labia minora
Labium majus

Rectouterine pouch (of Douglas)
Peritoneum (*cut edge*)
Vesicouterine pouch
Rectum
Ureter
Urinary bladder
Vagina
Pelvic diaphragm (levator ani muscle)
Deep transverse perineal muscle (*cut*)
External anal sphincter muscle

Median (sagittal) section

Sacral promontory
Ureter
Suspensory ligament of ovary
Uterine (fallopian) tube
Ovary
External iliac vessels
Ligament of ovary
Body of uterus
Round ligament of uterus (ligamentum teres)
Fundus of uterus
Urinary bladder
Pubic symphysis
Urethra
Sphincter urethrae
Deep transverse perineal muscle
Deep dorsal vein of clitoris
Crus of clitoris
External urethral orifice
Superficial transverse perineal muscle
Labium minus
Labium majus

Uterosacral ligament
Vesicouterine pouch
Rectouterine pouch (of Douglas)
Cervix of uterus
Posterior part of vaginal fornix
Anterior part of vaginal fornix
Rectum
Vagina
Perineal membrane
Levator ani muscle
Anal canal
External anal sphincter muscle
Anus
Vaginal orifice

F. Netter M.D.
C. Machado M.D.

Plate 360 Pelvic Viscera and Perineum: Female. (Netter: Atlas of Human Anatomy, 4 ed, 2006, Saunders.)

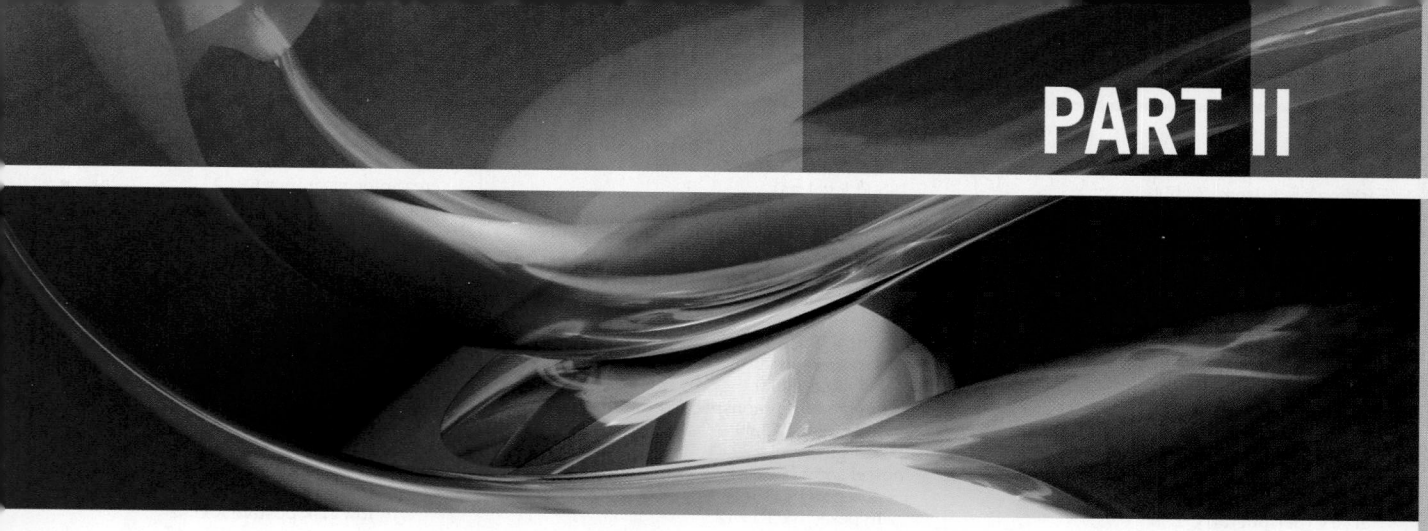

PART II

Alphabetic Index -volume 2

A

Aarskog's syndrome Q87.1
Abandonment —*see* Maltreatment
Abasia (-astasia) (hysterical) F44.4
Abderhalden-Kaufmann-Lignac syndrome (cystinosis) E72.04
Abdomen, abdominal —*see also* condition
  acute R10.0
  angina K55.1
  muscle deficiency syndrome Q79.4
Abdominalgia —*see* Pain, abdominal
Abduction contracture, hip or other joint —*see* Contraction, joint
Aberrant (congenital) —*see also* Malposition, congenital
  adrenal gland Q89.1
  artery (peripheral) Q27.8
    basilar NEC Q28.1
    cerebral Q28.3
    coronary Q24.5
    digestive system Q27.8
    eye Q15.8
    lower limb Q27.8
    precerebral Q28.1
    pulmonary Q25.79
    renal Q27.2
    retina Q14.1
    specified site NEC Q27.8
    subclavian Q27.8
    upper limb Q27.8
    vertebral Q28.1
  breast Q83.8
  endocrine gland NEC Q89.2
  hepatic duct Q44.5
  pancreas Q45.3
  parathyroid gland Q89.2
  pituitary gland Q89.2
  sebaceous glands, mucous membrane, mouth, congenital Q38.6
  spleen Q89.09
  subclavian artery Q27.8
  thymus (gland) Q89.2
  thyroid gland Q89.2
  vein (peripheral) NEC Q27.8
    cerebral Q28.3
    digestive system Q27.8
    lower limb Q27.8
    precerebral Q28.1
    specified site NEC Q27.8
    upper limb Q27.8
Aberration
  distantial —*see* Disturbance, visual
  mental F99
Abetalipoproteinemia E78.6
Abiotrophy R68.89
Ablatio, ablation
  retinae —*see* Detachment, retina
Ablepharia, ablepharon Q10.3
Abnormal, abnormality, abnormalities —*see also* Anomaly
  acid-base balance (mixed) E87.4
  albumin R77.0
  alphafetoprotein R77.2
  alveolar ridge K08.9
  anatomical relationship Q89.9
  apertures, congenital, diaphragm Q79.1
  auditory perception H93.29-
    diplacusis —*see* Diplacusis
    hyperacusis —*see* Hyperacusis
    recruitment —*see* Recruitment, auditory
    threshold shift —*see* Shift, auditory threshold
  autosomes Q99.9
    fragile site Q95.5
  basal metabolic rate R94.8
  biosynthesis, testicular androgen E29.1
  bleeding time R79.1

Abnormal, abnormality, abnormalities — *(Continued)*
  blood level (of)
    cobalt R79.0
    copper R79.0
    iron R79.0
    lithium R78.89
    magnesium R79.0
    mineral NEC R79.0
    zinc R79.0
  blood pressure
    elevated R03.0
    low reading (nonspecific) R03.1
  blood sugar R73.09
  blood-gas level R79.81
  bowel sounds R19.15
    absent R19.11
    hyperactive R19.12
  brain scan R94.02
  breathing R06.9
  caloric test R94.138
  cerebrospinal fluid R83.9
    cytology R83.6
    drug level R83.2
    enzyme level R83.0
    hormones R83.1
    immunology R83.4
    microbiology R83.5
    nonmedicinal level R83.3
    specified type NEC R83.8
  chemistry, blood R79.9
    C-reactive protein R79.82
    drugs —*see* Findings, abnormal, in blood
    gas level R79.81
    minerals R79.0
    pancytopenia D61.818
    PTT R79.1
    specified NEC R79.89
    toxins —*see* Findings, abnormal, in blood
  chest sounds (friction) (rales) R09.89
  chromosome, chromosomal Q99.9
    with more than three X chromosomes, female Q97.1
    analysis result R89.8
      bronchial washings R84.8
      cerebrospinal fluid R83.8
      cervix uteri NEC R87.89
      nasal secretions R84.8
      nipple discharge R89.8
      peritoneal fluid R85.89
      pleural fluid R84.8
      prostatic secretions R86.8
      saliva R85.89
      seminal fluid R86.8
      sputum R84.8
      synovial fluid R89.8
      throat scrapings R84.8
      vagina R87.89
      vulva R87.89
      wound secretions R89.8
    dicentric replacement Q93.2
    ring replacement Q93.2
    sex Q99.8
      female phenotype Q97.9
        specified NEC Q97.8
      male phenotype Q98.9
        specified NEC Q98.8
      structural male Q98.6
    specified NEC Q99.8
  clinical findings NEC R68.89
  coagulation D68.9
    newborn, transient P61.6
    profile R79.1
    time R79.1
  communication —*see* Fistula
  conjunctiva, vascular H11.41-
  coronary artery Q24.5
  cortisol-binding globulin E27.8
  course, eustachian tube Q17.8

Abnormal, abnormality, abnormalities — *(Continued)*
  creatinine clearance R94.4
  cytology
    anus R85.619
      atypical squamous cells cannot exclude high grade squamous intraepithelial lesion (ASC-H) R85.611
      atypical squamous cells of undetermined significance (ASC-US) R85.610
      cytologic evidence of malignancy R85.614
      high grade squamous intraepithelial lesion (HGSIL) R85.613
      human papillomavirus (HPV) DNA test
        high risk positive R85.81
        low risk postive R85.82
      inadequate smear R85.615
      low grade squamous intraepithelial lesion (LGSIL) R85.612
      satisfactory anal smear but lacking transformation zone R85.616
      specified NEC R85.618
      unsatisfactory smear R85.615
    female genital organs —*see* Abnormal, Papanicolaou (smear)
  dark adaptation curve H53.61
  dentofacial NEC —*see* Anomaly, dentofacial
  development, developmental Q89.9
    central nervous system Q07.9
  diagnostic imaging
    abdomen, abdominal region NEC R93.5
    biliary tract R93.2
    bladder R93.41 ◀
    breast R92.8
    central nervous system NEC R90.89
    cerebrovascular NEC R90.89
    coronary circulation R93.1
    digestive tract NEC R93.3
    gastrointestinal (tract) R93.3
    genitourinary organs R93.8
    head R93.0
    heart R93.1
    intrathoracic organ NEC R93.8
    kidney R93.42- ◀
    limbs R93.6
    liver R93.2
    lung (field) R91.8
    musculoskeletal system NEC R93.7
    renal pelvis R93.41 ◀
    retroperitoneum R93.5
    site specified NEC R93.8
    skin and subcutaneous tissue R93.8
    skull R93.0
    ~~urinary organs R93.4~~
    urinary organs specified NEC R93.49 ◀
    ureter R93.41 ◀
  direction, teeth, fully erupted M26.30
  ear ossicles, acquired NEC H74.39-
    ankylosis —*see* Ankylosis, ear ossicles
    discontinuity —*see* Discontinuity, ossicles, ear
    partial loss —*see* Loss, ossicles, ear (partial)
  Ebstein Q22.5
  echocardiogram R93.1
  echoencephalogram R90.81
  echogram —*see* Abnormal, diagnostic imaging
  electrocardiogram [ECG] [EKG] R94.31
  electroencephalogram [EEG] R94.01
  electrolyte —*see* Imbalance, electrolyte
  electromyogram [EMG] R94.131
  electro-oculogram [EOG] R94.110
  electrophysiological intracardiac studies R94.39
  electroretinogram [ERG] R94.111
  erythrocytes
    congenital, with perinatal jaundice D58.9
  feces (color) (contents) (mucus) R19.5

◀ New ⇐ Revised ~~deleted~~ Deleted

Abnormal, abnormality, abnormalities — *(Continued)*
finding —*see* Findings, abnormal, without diagnosis
fluid
amniotic —*see* Abnormal, specimen, specified
cerebrospinal —*see* Abnormal, cerebrospinal fluid
peritoneal —*see* Abnormal, specimen, digestive organs
pleural —*see* Abnormal, specimen, respiratory organs
synovial —*see* Abnormal, specimen, specified
thorax (bronchial washings) (pleural fluid) —*see* Abnormal, specimen, respiratory organs
vaginal —*see* Abnormal, specimen, female genital organs
form
teeth K00.2
uterus —*see* Anomaly, uterus
function studies
auditory R94.120
bladder R94.8
brain R94.09
cardiovascular R94.30
ear R94.128
endocrine NEC R94.7
eye NEC R94.118
kidney R94.4
liver R94.5
nervous system
central NEC R94.09
peripheral NEC R94.138
pancreas R94.8
placenta R94.8
pulmonary R94.2
special senses NEC R94.128
spleen R94.8
thyroid R94.6
vestibular R94.121
gait —*see* Gait
hysterical F44.4
gastrin secretion E16.4
globulin R77.1
cortisol-binding E27.8
thyroid-binding E07.89
glomerular, minor —*see also* N00-N07 with fourth character .0 N05.0
glucagon secretion E16.3
glucose tolerance (test) (non-fasting) R73.09
gravitational (G) forces or states (effect of) T75.81
hair (color) (shaft) L67.9
specified NEC L67.8
hard tissue formation in pulp (dental) K04.3
head movement R25.0
heart
rate R00.9
specified NEC R00.8
shadow R93.1
sounds NEC R01.2
hemoglobin (disease) —*see also* Disease, hemoglobin D58.2
trait —*see* Trait, hemoglobin, abnormal
histology NEC R89.7
immunological findings R89.4
in serum R76.9
specified NEC R76.8
increase in appetite R63.2
involuntary movement —*see* Abnormal, movement, involuntary
jaw closure M26.51
karyotype R89.8
kidney function test R94.4
knee jerk R29.2
leukocyte (cell) (differential) NEC D72.9

Abnormal, abnormality, abnormalities — *(Continued)*
liver
loss of
height R29.890
weight R63.4
mammogram NEC R92.8
calcification (calculus) R92.1
microcalcification R92.0
Mantoux test R76.11
movement (disorder) —*see also* Disorder, movement
head R25.0
involuntary R25.9
fasciculation R25.3
of head R25.0
spasm R25.2
specified type NEC R25.8
tremor R25.1
myoglobin (Aberdeen) (Annapolis) R89.7
neonatal screening P09
oculomotor study R94.113
palmar creases Q82.8
Papanicolaou (smear)
anus R85.619
atypical squamous cells cannot exclude high grade squamous intraepithelial lesion (ASC-H) R85.611
atypical squamous cells of undetermined significance (ASC-US) R85.610
cytologic evidence of malignancy R85.614
high grade squamous intraepithelial lesion (HGSIL) R85.613
human papillomavirus (HPV) DNA test
high risk positive R85.81
low risk postive R85.82
inadequate smear R85.615
low grade squamous intraepithelial lesion (LGSIL) R85.612
satisfactory anal smear but lacking transformation zone R85.616
specified NEC R85.618
unsatisfactory smear R85.615
bronchial washings R84.6
cerebrospinal fluid R83.6
cervix R87.619
atypical squamous cells cannot exclude high grade squamous intraepithelial lesion (ASC-H) R87.611
atypical squamous cells of undetermined significance (ASC-US) R87.610
cytologic evidence of malignancy R87.614
high grade squamous intraepithelial lesion (HGSIL) R87.613
inadequate smear R87.615
low grade squamous intraepithelial lesion (LGSIL) R87.612
non-atypical endometrial cells R87.618
satisfactory cervical smear but lacking transformation zone R87.616
specified NEC R87.618
thin preparaton R87.619
unsatisfactory smear R87.615
nasal secretions R84.6
nipple discharge R89.6
peritoneal fluid R85.69
pleural fluid R84.6
prostatic secretions R86.6
saliva R85.69
seminal fluid R86.6
sites NEC R89.6
sputum R84.6
synovial fluid R89.6
throat scrapings R84.6

Abnormal, abnormality, abnormalities — *(Continued)*
Papanicolaou (smear) *(Continued)*
vagina R87.629
atypical squamous cells cannot exclude high grade squamous intraepithelial lesion (ASC-H) R87.621
atypical squamous cells of undetermined significance (ASC-US) R87.620
cytologic evidence of malignancy R87.624
high grade squamous intraepithelial lesion (HGSIL) R87.623
inadequate smear R87.625
low grade squamous intraepithelial lesion (LGSIL) R87.622
specified NEC R87.628
thin preparation R87.629
unsatisfactory smear R87.625
vulva R87.69
wound secretions R89.6
partial thromboplastin time (PTT) R79.1
pelvis (bony) —*see* Deformity, pelvis
percussion, chest (tympany) R09.89
periods (grossly) —*see* Menstruation
phonocardiogram R94.39
plantar reflex R29.2
plasma
protein R77.9
specified NEC R77.8
viscosity R70.1
pleural (folds) Q34.0
posture R29.3
product of conception O02.9
specified type NEC O02.89
prothrombin time (PT) R79.1
pulmonary
artery, congenital Q25.79
function, newborn P28.89
test results R94.2
pulsations in neck R00.2
pupillary H21.56-
function (reaction) (reflex) —*see* Anomaly, pupil, function
radiological examination —*see* Abnormal, diagnostic imaging
red blood cell (s) (morphology) (volume) R71.8
reflex —*see* Reflex
renal function test R94.4
response to nerve stimulation R94.130
retinal correspondence H53.31
retinal function study R94.111
rhythm, heart —*see also* Arrhythmia
saliva —*see* Abnormal, specimen, digestive organs
scan
kidney R94.4
liver R93.2
thyroid R94.6
secretion
gastrin E16.4
glucagon E16.3
semen, seminal fluid —*see* Abnormal, specimen, male genital organs
serum level (of)
acid phosphatase R74.8
alkaline phosphatase R74.8
amylase R74.8
enzymes R74.9
specified NEC R74.8
lipase R74.8
triacylglycerol lipase R74.8
shape
gravid uterus —*see* Anomaly, uterus
sinus venosus Q21.1
size, tooth, teeth K00.2
spacing, tooth, teeth, fully erupted M26.30

Abnormal, abnormality, abnormalities — *(Continued)*
specimen
digestive organs (peritoneal fluid) (saliva) R85.9
cytology R85.69
drug level R85.2
enzyme level R85.0
histology R85.7
hormones R85.1
immunology R85.4
microbiology R85.5
nonmedicinal level R85.3
specified type NEC R85.89
female genital organs (secretions) (smears) R87.9
cytology R87.69
cervix R87.619
human papillomavirus (HPV) DNA test
high risk positive R87.810
low risk positive R87.820
inadequate (unsatisfactory) smear R87.615
non-atypical endometrial cells R87.618
specified NEC R87.618
vagina R87.629
human papillomavirus (HPV) DNA test
high risk positive R87.811
low risk positive R87.821
inadequate (unsatisfactory) smear R87.625
vulva R87.69
drug level R87.2
enzyme level R87.0
histological R87.7
hormones R87.1
immunology R87.4
microbiology R87.5
nonmedicinal level R87.3
specified type NEC R87.89
male genital organs (prostatic secretions) (semen) R86.9
cytology R86.6
drug level R86.2
enzyme level R86.0
histological R86.7
hormones R86.1
immunology R86.4
microbiology R86.5
nonmedicinal level R86.3
specified type NEC R86.8
nipple discharge —*see* Abnormal, specimen, specified
respiratory organs (bronchial washings) (nasal secretions) (pleural fluid) (sputum) R84.9
cytology R84.6
drug level R84.2
enzyme level R84.0
histology R84.7
hormones R84.1
immunology R84.4
microbiology R84.5
nonmedicinal level R84.3
specified type NEC R84.8
specified organ, system and tissue NOS R89.9
cytology R89.6
drug level R89.2
enzyme level R89.0
histology R89.7
hormones R89.1
immunology R89.4
microbiology R89.5
nonmedicinal level R89.3
specified type NEC R89.8
synovial fluid —*see* Abnormal, specimen, specified

Abnormal, abnormality, abnormalities — *(Continued)*
specimen *(Continued)*
thorax (bronchial washings) (pleural fluids) —*see* Abnormal, specimen, respiratory organs
vagina (secretion) (smear) R87.629
vulva (secretion) (smear) R87.69
wound secretion —*see* Abnormal, specimen, specified
spermatozoa —*see* Abnormal, specimen, male genital organs
sputum (amount) (color) (odor) R09.3
stool (color) (contents) (mucus) R19.5
bloody K92.1
guaiac positive R19.5
synchondrosis Q78.8
thermography —*see also* Abnormal, diagnostic imaging R93.8
thyroid-binding globulin E07.89
tooth, teeth (form) (size) K00.2
toxicology (findings) R78.9
transport protein E88.09
tumor marker NEC R97.8
ultrasound results —*see* Abnormal, diagnostic imaging
umbilical cord complicating delivery O69.9
urination NEC R39.198 ◀
urine (constituents) R82.90
bile R82.2
cytological examination R82.8
drugs R82.5
fat R82.0
glucose R81
heavy metals R82.6
hemoglobin R82.3
histological examination R82.8
ketones R82.4
microbiological examination (culture) R82.79 ◀
myoglobin R82.1
positive culture R82.79 ◀
protein —*see* Proteinuria
specified substance NEC R82.99
chromoabnormality NEC R82.91
substances nonmedical R82.6
uterine hemorrhage —*see* Hemorrhage, uterus
vectorcardiogram R94.39
visually evoked potential (VEP) R94.112
white blood cells D72.9
specified NEC D72.89
X-ray examination —*see* Abnormal, diagnostic imaging
Abnormity (any organ or part) —*see* Anomaly
Abocclusion M26.29
hemolytic disease (newborn) P55.1
incompatibility reaction ABO —*see* Complication (s), transfusion, incompatibility reaction, ABO
Abolition, language R48.8
Aborter, habitual or recurrent —*see* Loss (of), pregnancy, recurrent
Abortion (complete) (spontaneous) O03.9
with
retained products of conception - see Abortion, incomplete
attempted (elective) (failed) O07.4
complicated by O07.30
afibrinogenemia O07.1
cardiac arrest O07.36
chemical damage of pelvic organ (s) O07.34
circulatory collapse O07.31
cystitis O07.38
defibrination syndrome O07.1
electrolyte imbalance O07.33
embolism (air) (amniotic fluid) (blood clot) (fat) (pulmonary) (septic) (soap) O07.2
endometritis O07.0

Abortion *(Continued)*
attempted *(Continued)*
complicated by *(Continued)*
genital tract and pelvic infection O07.0
hemolysis O07.1
hemorrhage (delayed) (excessive) O07.1
infection
genital tract or pelvic O07.0
urinary tract tract O07.38
intravascular coagulation O07.1
laceration of pelvic organ(s) O07.34
metabolic disorder O07.33
oliguria O07.32
oophoritis O07.0
parametritis O07.0
pelvic peritonitis O07.0
perforation of pelvic organ(s) O07.34
renal failure or shutdown O07.32
salpingitis or salpingo-oophoritis O07.0
sepsis O07.37
shock O07.31
specified condition NEC O07.39
tubular necrosis (renal) O07.32
uremia O07.32
urinary tract infection O07.38
venous complication NEC O07.35
embolism (air) (amniotic fluid) (blood clot) (fat) (pulmonary) (septic) (soap) O07.2
complicated (by) (following) O03.80
afibrinogenemia O03.6
cardiac arrest O03.86
chemical damage of pelvic organ (s) O03.84
circulatory collapse O03.81
cystitis O03.88
defibrination syndrome O03.6
electrolyte imbalance O03.83
embolism (air) (amniotic fluid) (blood clot) (fat) (pulmonary) (septic) (soap) O03.7
endometritis O03.5
genital tract and pelvic infection O03.5
hemolysis O03.6
hemorrhage (delayed) (excessive) O03.6
infection
genital tract or pelvic O03.5
urinary tract O03.88
intravascular coagulation O03.6
laceration of pelvic organ (s) O03.84
metabolic disorder O03.83
oliguria O03.82
oophoritis O03.5
parametritis O03.5
pelvic peritonitis O03.5
perforation of pelvic organ (s) O03.84
renal failure or shutdown O03.82
salpingitis or salpingo-oophoritis O03.5
sepsis O03.87
shock O03.81
specified condition NEC O03.89
tubular necrosis (renal) O03.82
uremia O03.82
urinary tract infection O03.88
venous complication NEC O03.85
embolism (air) (amniotic fluid) (blood clot) (fat) (pulmonary) (septic) (soap) O03.7
failed —*see* Abortion, attempted
habitual or recurrent N96
with current abortion —*see* categories O03-O06
without current pregnancy N96
care in current pregnancy O26.2-
incomplete (spontaneous) O03.4
complicated (by) (following) O03.30
afibrinogenemia O03.1
cardiac arrest O03.36
chemical damage of pelvic organ (s) O03.34
circulatory collapse O03.31
cystitis O03.38

◀ New ◀ Revised ~~deleted~~ Deleted

Abortion *(Continued)*
incomplete *(Continued)*
complicated *(Continued)*
defibrination syndrome O03.1
electrolyte imbalance O03.33
embolism (air) (amniotic fluid) (blood clot) (fat) (pulmonary) (septic) (soap) O03.2
endometritis O03.0
genital tract and pelvic infection O03.0
hemolysis O03.1
hemorrhage (delayed) (excessive) O03.1
infection
genital tract or pelvic O03.0
urinary tract O03.38
intravascular coagulation O03.1
laceration of pelvic organ (s) O03.34
metabolic disorder O03.33
oliguria O03.32
oophoritis O03.0
parametritis O03.0
pelvic peritonitis O03.0
perforation of pelvic organ (s) O03.34
renal failure or shutdown O03.32
salpingitis or salpingo-oophoritis O03.0
sepsis O03.37
shock O03.31
specified condition NEC O03.39
tubular necrosis (renal) O03.32
uremia O03.32
urinary infection O03.38
venous complication NEC O03.35
embolism (air) (amniotic fluid) (blood clot) (fat) (pulmonary) (septic) (soap) O03.2
induced (encounter for) Z33.2
complicated by O04.80
afibrinogenemia O04.6
cardiac arrest O04.86
chemical damage of pelvic organ (s) O04.84
circulatory collapse O04.81
cystitis O04.88
defibrination syndrome O04.6
electrolyte imbalance O04.83
embolism (air) (amniotic fluid) (blood clot) (fat) (pulmonary) (septic) (soap) O04.7
endometritis O04.5
genital tract and pelvic infection O04.5
hemolysis O04.6
hemorrhage (delayed) (excessive) O04.6
infection
genital tract or pelvic O04.5
urinary tract O04.88
intravascular coagulation O04.6
laceration of pelvic organ (s) O04.84
metabolic disorder O04.83
oliguria O04.82
oophoritis O04.5
parametritis O04.5
pelvic peritonitis O04.5
perforation of pelvic organ (s) O04.84
renal failure or shutdown O04.82
salpingitis or salpingo-oophoritis O04.5
sepsis O04.87
shock O04.81
specified condition NEC O04.89
tubular necrosis (renal) O04.82
uremia O04.82
urinary tract infection O04.88
venous complication NEC O04.85
embolism (air) (amniotic fluid) (blood clot) (fat) (pulmonary) (septic) (soap) O04.7
missed O02.1
spontaneous —*see* Abortion (complete) (spontaneous)
threatened O20.0
threatened (spontaneous) O20.0

Abortion *(Continued)*
tubal O00.10
with intrauterine pregnancy O00.11
Abortus fever A23.1
Aboulomania F60.7
Abrami's disease D59.8
Abramov-Fiedler myocarditis (acute isolated myocarditis) I40.1
Abrasion T14.8
abdomen, abdominal (wall) S30.811
alveolar process S00.512
ankle S90.51-
antecubital space —*see* Abrasion, elbow
anus S30.817
arm (upper) S40.81-
auditory canal —*see* Abrasion, ear
auricle —*see* Abrasion, ear
axilla —*see* Abrasion, arm
back, lower S30.810
breast S20.11-
brow S00.81
buttock S30.810
calf —*see* Abrasion, leg
canthus —*see* Abrasion, eyelid
cheek S00.81
internal S00.512
chest wall —*see* Abrasion, thorax
chin S00.81
clitoris S30.814
cornea S05.0-
costal region —*see* Abrasion, thorax
dental K03.1
digit (s)
foot —*see* Abrasion, toe
hand —*see* Abrasion, finger
ear S00.41-
elbow S50.31-
epididymis S30.813
epigastric region S30.811
epiglottis S10.11
esophagus (thoracic) S27.818
cervical S10.11
eyebrow —*see* Abrasion, eyelid
eyelid S00.21-
face S00.81
finger (s) S60.41-
index S60.41-
little S60.41-
middle S60.41-
ring S60.41-
flank S30.811
foot (except toe (s) alone) S90.81-
toe —*see* Abrasion, toe
forearm S50.81-
elbow only —*see* Abrasion, elbow
forehead S00.81
genital organs, external
female S30.816
male S30.815
groin S30.811
gum S00.512
hand S60.51-
head S00.91
ear —*see* Abrasion, ear
eyelid —*see* Abrasion, eyelid
lip S00.511
nose S00.31
oral cavity S00.512
scalp S00.01
specified site NEC S00.81
heel —*see* Abrasion, foot
hip S70.21-
inguinal region S30.811
interscapular region S20.419
jaw S00.81
knee S80.21-
labium (majus) (minus) S30.814
larynx S10.11
leg (lower) S80.81-
knee —*see* Abrasion, knee
upper —*see* Abrasion, thigh

Abrasion *(Continued)*
lip S00.511
lower back S30.810
lumbar region S30.810
malar region S00.81
mammary —*see* Abrasion, breast
mastoid region S00.81
mouth S00.512
nail
finger —*see* Abrasion, finger
toe —*see* Abrasion, toe
nape S10.81
nasal S00.31
neck S10.91
specified site NEC S10.81
throat S10.11
nose S00.31
occipital region S00.01
oral cavity S00.512
orbital region —*see* Abrasion, eyelid
palate S00.512
palm —*see* Abrasion, hand
parietal region S00.01
pelvis S30.810
penis S30.812
perineum
female S30.814
male S30.810
periocular area —*see* Abrasion, eyelid
phalanges
finger —*see* Abrasion, finger
toe —*see* Abrasion, toe
pharynx S10.11
pinna —*see* Abrasion, ear
popliteal space —*see* Abrasion, knee
prepuce S30.812
pubic region S30.810
pudendum
female S30.816
male S30.815
sacral region S30.810
scalp S00.01
scapular region —*see* Abrasion, shoulder
scrotum S30.813
shin —*see* Abrasion, leg
shoulder S40.21-
skin NEC T14.8
sternal region S20.319
submaxillary region S00.81
submental region S00.81
subungual
finger (s) —*see* Abrasion, finger
toe (s) —*see* Abrasion, toe
supraclavicular fossa S10.81
supraorbital S00.81
temple S00.81
temporal region S00.81
testis S30.813
thigh S70.31-
thorax, thoracic (wall) S20.91
back S20.41-
front S20.31-
throat S10.11
thumb S60.31-
toe (s) (lesser) S90.416
great S90.41-
tongue S00.512
tooth, teeth (dentifrice) (habitual) (hard tissues) (occupational) (ritual) (traditional) K03.1
trachea S10.11
tunica vaginalis S30.813
tympanum, tympanic membrane —*see* Abrasion, ear
uvula S00.512
vagina S30.814
vocal cords S10.11
vulva S30.814
wrist S60.81-
Abrism —*see* Poisoning, food, noxious, plant

Abruptio placentae O45.9-
with
afibrinogenemia O45.01-
coagulation defect O45.00-
specified NEC O45.09-
disseminated intravascular coagulation O45.02-
hypofibrinogenemia O45.01-
specified NEC O45.8-
Abruption, placenta —*see* Abruptio placentae
Abscess (connective tissue) (embolic) (fistulous) (infective) (metastatic) (multiple) (pernicious) (pyogenic) (septic) L02.91
with
diverticular disease (intestine) K57.80
with bleeding K57.81
large intestine K57.20
with
bleeding K57.21
small intestine K57.40
with bleeding K57.41
small intestine K57.00
with
bleeding K57.01
large intestine K57.40
with bleeding K57.41
lymphangitis - code by site under Abscess
abdomen, abdominal
cavity K65.1
wall L02.211
abdominopelvic K65.1
accessory sinus —*see* Sinusitis
adrenal (capsule) (gland) E27.8
alveolar K04.7
with sinus K04.6
amebic A06.4
brain (and liver or lung abscess) A06.6
genitourinary tract A06.82
liver (without mention of brain or lung abscess) A06.4
lung (and liver) (without mention of brain abscess) A06.5
specified site NEC A06.89
spleen A06.89
anerobic A48.0
ankle —*see* Abscess, lower limb
anorectal K61.2
antecubital space —*see* Abscess, upper limb
antrum (chronic) (Highmore) —*see* Sinusitis, maxillary
anus K61.0
apical (tooth) K04.7
with sinus (alveolar) K04.6
appendix K35.3
areola (acute) (chronic) (nonpuerperal) N61.1 ◀
puerperal, postpartum or gestational —*see* Infection, nipple
arm (any part) —*see* Abscess, upper limb
artery (wall) I77.89
atheromatous I77.2
auricle, ear —*see* Abscess, ear, external
axilla (region) L02.41-
lymph gland or node L04.2
back (any part, except buttock) L02.212
Bartholin's gland N75.1
with
abortion —*see* Abortion, by type complicated by, sepsis
ectopic or molar pregnancy O08.0
following ectopic or molar pregnancy O08.0
Bezold's —*see* Mastoiditis, acute
bilharziasis B65.1
bladder (wall) —*see* Cystitis, specified type NEC
bone (subperiosteal) —*see also* Osteomyelitis, specified type NEC
accessory sinus (chronic) —*see* Sinusitis
chronic or old —*see* Osteomyelitis, chronic
jaw (lower) (upper) M27.2

Abscess *(Continued)*
bone *(Continued)*
mastoid —*see* Mastoiditis, acute, subperiosteal
petrous —*see* Petrositis
spinal (tuberculous) A18.01
nontuberculous —*see* Osteomyelitis, vertebra
bowel K63.0
brain (any part) (cystic) (otogenic) G06.0
amebic (with abscess of any other site) A06.6
gonococcal A54.82
pheomycotic (chromomycotic) B43.1
tuberculous A17.81
breast (acute) (chronic) (nonpuerperal) N61.1 ◀
newborn P39.0
puerperal, postpartum, gestational —*see* Mastitis, obstetric, purulent
broad ligament N73.2
acute N73.0
chronic N73.1
Brodie's (localized) (chronic) M86.8X-
bronchi J98.09
buccal cavity K12.2
bulbourethral gland N34.0
bursa M71.00
ankle M71.07-
elbow M71.02-
foot M71.07-
hand M71.04-
hip M71.05-
knee M71.06-
multiple sites M71.09
pharyngeal J39.1
shoulder M71.01-
specified site NEC M71.08
wrist M71.03-
buttock L02.31
canthus —*see* Blepharoconjunctivitis
cartilage —*see* Disorder, cartilage, specified type NEC
cecum K35.3
cerebellum, cerebellar G06.0
sequelae G09
cerebral (embolic) G06.0
sequelae G09
cervical (meaning neck) L02.11
lymph gland or node L04.0
cervix (stump) (uteri) —*see* Cervicitis
cheek (external) L02.01
inner K12.2
chest J86.9
with fistula J86.0
wall L02.213
chin L02.01
choroid —*see* Inflammation, chorioretinal
circumtonsillar J36
cold (lung) (tuberculous) —*see also* Tuberculosis, abscess, lung
articular —*see* Tuberculosis, joint
colon (wall) K63.0
colostomy K94.02
conjunctiva —*see* Conjunctivitis, acute
cornea H16.31-
corpus
cavernosum N48.21
luteum —*see* Oophoritis
Cowper's gland N34.0
cranium G06.0
cul-de-sac (Douglas') (posterior) —*see* Peritonitis, pelvic, female
cutaneous —*see* Abscess, by site
dental K04.7
with sinus (alveolar) K04.6
dentoalveolar K04.7
with sinus K04.6
diaphragm, diaphragmatic K65.1
Douglas' cul-de-sac or pouch —*see* Peritonitis, pelvic, female
Dubois A50.59

Abscess *(Continued)*
ear (middle) —*see also* Otitis, media, suppurative
acute —*see* Otitis, media, suppurative, acute
external H60.0-
entamebic —*see* Abscess, amebic
enterostomy K94.12
epididymis N45.4
epidural G06.2
brain G06.0
spinal cord G06.1
epiglottis J38.7
epiploon, epiploic K65.1
erysipelatous —*see* Erysipelas
esophagus K20.8
ethmoid (bone) (chronic) (sinus) J32.2
external auditory canal —*see* Abscess, ear, external
extradural G06.2
brain G06.0
sequelae G09
spinal cord G06.1
extraperitoneal K68.19
eye —*see* Endophthalmitis, purulent
eyelid H00.03-
face (any part, except ear, eye and nose) L02.01
fallopian tube —*see* Salpingitis
fascia M72.8
fauces J39.1
fecal K63.0
femoral (region) —*see* Abscess, lower limb
filaria, filarial —*see* Infestation, filarial
finger (any) —*see also* Abscess, hand
nail —*see* Cellulitis, finger
foot L02.61-
forehead L02.01
frontal sinus (chronic) J32.1
gallbladder K81.0
genital organ or tract
female (external) N76.4
male N49.9
multiple sites N49.8
specified NEC N49.8
gestational mammary O91.11-
gestational subareolar O91.11-
gingival —*see* Peridontitis, aggressive, localized ◀
gland, glandular (lymph) (acute) —*see* Lymphadenitis, acute
gluteal (region) L02.31
gonorrheal —*see* Gonococcus
groin L02.214
gum —*see* Peridontitis, aggressive, localized ◀
hand L02.51-
head NEC L02.811
face (any part, except ear, eye and nose) L02.01
heart —*see* Carditis
heel —*see* Abscess, foot
helminthic —*see* Infestation, helminth
hepatic (cholangitic) (hematogenic) (lymphogenic) (pylephlebitic) K75.0
amebic A06.4
hip (region) —*see* Abscess, lower limb
ileocecal K35.3
ileostomy (bud) K94.12
iliac (region) L02.214
fossa K35.3
infraclavicular (fossa) —*see* Abscess, upper limb
inguinal (region) L02.214
lymph gland or node L04.1
intestine, intestinal NEC K63.0
rectal K61.1
intra-abdominal —*see also* Abscess, peritoneum K65.1
~~postoperative T81.4~~
~~retroperitoneal K68.11~~
postprocedural T81.43 ◀
retroperitoneal K68.11 ◀
intra-muscular, postprocedural T81.42 ◀

◀ New ◀ Revised ~~deleted~~ Deleted

Abscess *(Continued)*
intracranial G06.0
intramammary —*see* Abscess, breast
intraorbital —*see* Abscess, orbit
intraperitoneal K65.1
intrasphincteric (anus) K61.4
intraspinal G06.1
intratonsillar J36
ischiorectal (fossa) K61.3
jaw (bone) (lower) (upper) M27.2
joint —*see* Arthritis, pyogenic or pyemic
spine (tuberculous) A18.01
nontuberculous —*see* Spondylopathy, infective
kidney N15.1
with calculus N20.0
with hydronephrosis N13.6
puerperal (postpartum) O86.21
knee —*see also* Abscess, lower limb
joint M00.9
labium (majus) (minus) N76.4
lacrimal
caruncle —*see* Inflammation, lacrimal, passages, acute
gland —*see* Dacryoadenitis
passages (duct) (sac) —*see* Inflammation, lacrimal, passages, acute
lacunar N34.0
larynx J38.7
lateral (alveolar) K04.7
with sinus K04.6
leg (any part) —*see* Abscess, lower limb
lens H27.8
lingual K14.0
tonsil J36
lip K13.0
Littre's gland N34.0
liver (cholangitic) (hematogenic) (lymphogenic) (pylephlebitic) (pyogenic) K75.0
amebic (due to Entamoeba histolytica) (dysenteric) (tropical) A06.4
with
brain abscess (and liver or lung abscess) A06.6
lung abscess A06.5
loin (region) L02.211
lower limb L02.41-
lumbar (tuberculous) A18.01
nontuberculous L02.212
lung (miliary) (putrid) J85.2
with pneumonia J85.1
due to specified organism (*see* Pneumonia, in (due to))
amebic (with liver abscess) A06.5
with
brain abscess A06.6
pneumonia A06.5
lymph, lymphatic, gland or node (acute) —*see also* Lymphadenitis, acute
mesentery I88.0
malar M27.2
mammary gland —*see* Abscess, breast
marginal, anus K61.0
mastoid —*see* Mastoiditis, acute
maxilla, maxillary M27.2
molar (tooth) K04.7
with sinus K04.6
premolar K04.7
sinus (chronic) J32.0
mediastinum J85.3
meibomian gland —*see* Hordeolum
meninges G06.2
mesentery, mesenteric K65.1
mesosalpinx —*see* Salpingitis
mons pubis L02.215
mouth (floor) K12.2
muscle —*see* Myositis, infective
myocardium I40.0
nabothian (follicle) —*see* Cervicitis
nasal J32.9
nasopharyngeal J39.1

Abscess *(Continued)*
navel L02.216
newborn P38.9
with mild hemorrhage P38.1
without hemorrhage P38.9
neck (region) L02.11
lymph gland or node L04.0
nephritic —*see* Abscess, kidney
nipple N61.1 ⇐
associated with
lactation —*see* Pregnancy, complicated by ⇐
pregnancy —*see* Pregnancy, complicated by
nose (external) (fossa) (septum) J34.0
sinus (chronic) —*see* Sinusitis
omentum K65.1
operative wound T81.40 ⇐
orbit, orbital —*see* Cellulitis, orbit
otogenic G06.0
ovary, ovarian (corpus luteum) —*see* Oophoritis
oviduct —*see* Oophoritis
palate (soft) K12.2
hard M27.2
palmar (space) —*see* Abscess, hand
pancreas (duct) —*see* Pancreatitis, acute
parafrenal N48.21
parametric, parametrium N73.2
acute N73.0
chronic N73.1
paranephric N15.1
parapancreatic —*see* Pancreatitis, acute
parapharyngeal J39.0
pararectal K61.1
parasinus —*see* Sinusitis
parauterine (*see also* Disease, pelvis, inflammatory) N73.2
paravaginal —*see* Vaginitis
parietal region (scalp) L02.811
parodontal —*see* Peridontitis, aggressive, localized ⇐
parotid (duct) (gland) K11.3
region K12.2
pectoral (region) L02.213
pelvis, pelvic
female —*see* Disease, pelvis, inflammatory
male, peritoneal K65.1
penis N48.21
gonococcal (accessory gland) (periurethral) A54.1
perianal K61.0
periapical K04.7
with sinus (alveolar) K04.6
periappendicular K35.3
pericardial I30.1
pericecal K35.3
pericemental —*see* Peridontitis, aggressive, localized ⇐
pericholecystic —*see* Cholecystitis, acute
pericoronal —*see* Peridontitis, aggressive, localized ⇐
peridental —*see* Peridontitis, aggressive, localized ⇐
perimetric —*see also* Disease, pelvis, inflammatory N73.2
perinephric, perinephritic —*see* Abscess, kidney
perineum, perineal (superficial) L02.215
urethra N34.0
periodontal (parietal) —*see* Peridontitis, aggressive, localized ⇐
apical K04.7
periosteum, periosteal —*see also* Osteomyelitis, specified type NEC
with osteomyelitis —*see also* Osteomyelitis, specified type NEC
acute —*see* Osteomyelitis, acute
chronic —*see* Osteomyelitis, chronic
peripharyngeal J39.0
peripleuritic J86.9
with fistula J86.0

Abscess *(Continued)*
periprostatic N41.2
perirectal K61.1
perirenal (tissue) —*see* Abscess, kidney
perisinuous (nose) —*see* Sinusitis
peritoneum, peritoneal (perforated) (ruptured) K65.1
with appendicitis K35.3
pelvic
female —*see* Peritonitis, pelvic, female
male K65.1
postoperative T81.43 ⇐
puerperal, postpartum, childbirth O85
tuberculous A18.31
peritonsillar J36
perityphlic K35.3
periureteral N28.89
periurethral N34.0
gonococcal (accessory gland) (periurethral) A54.1
periuterine —*see also* Disease, pelvis, inflammatory N73.2
perivesical —*see* Cystitis, specified type NEC
petrous bone —*see* Petrositis
phagedenic NOS L02.91
chancroid A57
pharynx, pharyngeal (lateral) J39.1
pilonidal L05.01
pituitary (gland) E23.6
pleura J86.9
with fistula J86.0
popliteal —*see* Abscess, lower limb
postcecal K35.3
postlaryngeal J38.7
postnasal J34.0
postoperative (any site) T81.40 ⇐
retroperitoneal K68.11
postpharyngeal J39.0
posttonsillar J36
post-typhoid A01.09
pouch of Douglas —*see* Peritonitis, pelvic, female
premammary —*see* Abscess, breast
prepatellar —*see* Abscess, lower limb
prostate N41.2
gonococcal (acute) (chronic) A54.22
psoas muscle K68.12
puerperal - code by site under Puerperal, abscess
pulmonary —*see* Abscess, lung
pulp, pulpal (dental) K04.01 ⇐
irreversible K04.02 ◀
reversible K04.01 ◀
rectovaginal septum K63.0
rectovesical —*see* Cystitis, specified type NEC
rectum K61.1
renal —*see* Abscess, kidney
retina —*see* Inflammation, chorioretinal
retrobulbar —*see* Abscess, orbit
retrocecal K65.1
retrolaryngeal J38.7
retromammary —*see* Abscess, breast
retroperitoneal NEC K68.19
postprocedural K68.11
retropharyngeal J39.0
retrouterine —*see* Peritonitis, pelvic, female
retrovesical —*see* Cystitis, specified type NEC
root, tooth K04.7
with sinus (alveolar) K04.6
round ligament —*see also* Disease, pelvis, inflammatory N73.2
rupture (spontaneous) NOS L02.91
sacrum (tuberculous) A18.01
nontuberculous M46.28
salivary (duct) (gland) K11.3
scalp (any part) L02.811
scapular —*see* Osteomyelitis, specified type NEC
sclera —*see* Scleritis
scrofulous (tuberculous) A18.2
scrotum N49.2

Abscess *(Continued)*
seminal vesicle N49.0
septal, dental K04.7
with sinus (alveolar) K04.6
serous —*see* Periostitis
shoulder (region) —*see* Abscess, upper limb
sigmoid K63.0
sinus (accessory) (chronic) (nasal) —*see also* Sinusitis
intracranial venous (any) G06.0
Skene's duct or gland N34.0
skin —*see* Abscess, by site
specified site NEC L02.818
spermatic cord N49.1
sphenoidal (sinus) (chronic) J32.3
spinal cord (any part) (staphylococcal) G06.1
tuberculous A17.81
spine (column) (tuberculous) A18.01
epidural G06.1
nontuberculous —*see* Osteomyelitis, vertebra
spleen D73.3
amebic A06.89
stitch T81.48 ◀
subarachnoid G06.2
brain G06.0
spinal cord G06.1
subareolar —*see* Abscess, breast
subcecal K35.3
subcutaneous —*see also* Abscess, by site
pheomycotic (chromomycotic) B43.2
postprocedural T81.41 ◀
subdiaphragmatic K65.1
subdural G06.2
brain G06.0
sequelae G09
spinal cord G06.1
subgaleal L02.811
subhepatic K65.1
sublingual K12.2
gland K11.3
submammary —*see* Abscess, breast
submandibular (region) (space) (triangle) K12.2
gland K11.3
submaxillary (region) L02.01
gland K11.3
submental L02.01
gland K11.3
subperiosteal —*see* Osteomyelitis, specified type NEC
subphrenic K65.1
postoperative T81.43 ◀
suburethral N34.0
sudoriparous L75.8
supraclavicular (fossa) —*see* Abscess, upper limb
suprapelvic, acute N73.0
suprarenal (capsule) (gland) E27.8
sweat gland L74.8
tear duct —*see* Inflammation, lacrimal, passages, acute
temple L02.01
temporal region L02.01
temporosphenoidal G06.0
tendon (sheath) M65.00
ankle M65.07-
foot M65.07-
forearm M65.03-
hand M65.04-
lower leg M65.06-
pelvic region M65.05-
shoulder region M65.01-
specified site NEC M65.08
thigh M65.05-
upper arm M65.02-
testis N45.4
thigh —*see* Abscess, lower limb
thorax J86.9
with fistula J86.0
throat J39.1
thumb —*see also* Abscess, hand
nail —*see* Cellulitis, finger

Abscess *(Continued)*
thymus (gland) E32.1
thyroid (gland) E06.0
toe (any) —*see also* Abscess, foot
nail —*see* Cellulitis, toe
tongue (staphylococcal) K14.0
tonsil (s) (lingual) J36
tonsillopharyngeal J36
tooth, teeth (root) K04.7
with sinus (alveolar) K04.6
supporting structures NEC —*see* Peridontitis, aggressive, localized ◀
trachea J39.8
trunk L02.219
abdominal wall L02.211
back L02.212
chest wall L02.213
groin L02.214
perineum L02.215
umbilicus L02.216
tubal —*see* Salpingitis
tuberculous —*see* Tuberculosis, abscess
tubo-ovarian —*see* Salpingo-oophoritis
tunica vaginalis N49.1
umbilicus L02.216
upper
limb L02.41-
respiratory J39.8
urethral (gland) N34.0
urinary N34.0
uterus, uterine (wall) —*see also* Endometritis
ligament —*see also* Disease, pelvis, inflammatory N73.2
neck —*see* Cervicitis
uvula K12.2
vagina (wall) —*see* Vaginitis
vaginorectal —*see* Vaginitis
vas deferens N49.1
vermiform appendix K35.3
vertebra (column) (tuberculous) A18.01
nontuberculous —*see* Osteomyelitis, vertebra
vesical —*see* Cystitis, specified type NEC
vesico-uterine pouch —*see* Peritonitis, pelvic, female
vitreous (humor) —*see* Endophthalmitis, purulent
vocal cord J38.3
von Bezold's —*see* Mastoiditis, acute
vulva N76.4
vulvovaginal gland N75.1
web space —*see* Abscess, hand
wound T81.40 ◀
wrist —*see* Abscess, upper limb

Absence (of) (organ or part) (complete or partial)
adrenal (gland) (congenital) Q89.1
acquired E89.6
albumin in blood E88.09
alimentary tract (congenital) Q45.8
upper Q40.8
alveolar process (acquired) —*see* Anomaly, alveolar
ankle (acquired) Z89.44-
anus (congenital) Q42.3
with fistula Q42.2
aorta (congenital) Q25.41 ◀
appendix, congenital Q42.8
arm (acquired) Z89.20-
above elbow Z89.22-
congenital (with hand present) —*see* Agenesis, arm, with hand present
and hand —*see* Agenesis, forearm, and hand
below elbow Z89.21-
congenital (with hand present) —*see* Agenesis, arm, with hand present
and hand —*see* Agenesis, forearm, and hand
congenital —*see* Defect, reduction, upper limb

Absence *(Continued)*
arm *(Continued)*
shoulder (following explantation of shoulder joint prosthesis) (joint) (with or without presence of antibiotic-impregnated cement spacer) Z89.23-
congenital (with hand present) —*see* Agenesis, arm, with hand present
artery (congenital) (peripheral) Q27.8
brain Q28.3
coronary Q24.5
pulmonary Q25.79
specified NEC Q27.8
umbilical Q27.0
atrial septum (congenital) Q21.1
auditory canal (congenital) (external) Q16.1
auricle (ear), congenital Q16.0
bile, biliary duct, congenital Q44.5
bladder (acquired) Z90.6
congenital Q64.5
bowel sounds R19.11
brain Q00.0
part of Q04.3
breast (s) (and nipple (s)) (acquired) Z90.1-
congenital Q83.8
broad ligament Q50.6
bronchus (congenital) Q32.4
canaliculus lacrimalis, congenital Q10.4
cerebellum (vermis) Q04.3
cervix (acquired) (with uterus) Z90.710
with remaining uterus Z90.712
congenital Q51.5
chin, congenital Q18.8
cilia (congenital) Q10.3
acquired —*see* Madarosis
clitoris (congenital) Q52.6
coccyx, congenital Q76.49
cold sense R20.8
congenital
lumen —*see* Atresia
organ or site NEC —*see* Agenesis
septum —*see* Imperfect, closure
corpus callosum Q04.0
cricoid cartilage, congenital Q31.8
diaphragm (with hernia), congenital Q79.1
digestive organ (s) or tract, congenital Q45.8
acquired NEC Z90.49
upper Q40.8
ductus arteriosus Q28.8
duodenum (acquired) Z90.49
congenital Q41.0
ear, congenital Q16.9
acquired H93.8-
auricle Q16.0
external Q16.0
inner Q16.5
lobe, lobule Q17.8
middle, except ossicles Q16.4
ossicles Q16.3
ossicles Q16.3
ejaculatory duct (congenital) Q55.4
endocrine gland (congenital) NEC Q89.2
acquired E89.89
epididymis (congenital) Q55.4
acquired Z90.79
epiglottis, congenital Q31.8
esophagus (congenital) Q39.8
acquired (partial) Z90.49
eustachian tube (congenital) Q16.2
extremity (acquired) Z89.9
congenital Q73.0
knee (following explantation of knee joint prosthesis) (joint) (with or without presence of antibiotic-impregnated cement spacer) Z89.52-
lower (above knee) Z89.619
below knee Z89.51-
upper —*see* Absence, arm
eye (acquired) Z90.01
congenital Q11.1
muscle (congenital) Q10.3

◀ New ◀ Revised ~~deleted~~ Deleted

Absence *(Continued)*
eyeball (acquired) Z90.01
eyelid (fold) (congenital) Q10.3
acquired Z90.01
face, specified part NEC Q18.8
fallopian tube (s) (acquired) Z90.79
congenital Q50.6
family member (causing problem in home) NEC —*see also* Disruption, family Z63.32
femur, congenital —*see* Defect, reduction, lower limb, longitudinal, femur
fibrinogen (congenital) D68.2
acquired D65
finger (s) (acquired) Z89.02-
congenital —*see* Agenesis, hand
foot (acquired) Z89.43-
congenital —*see* Agenesis, foot
forearm (acquired) —*see* Absence, arm, below elbow
gallbladder (acquired) Z90.49
congenital Q44.0
gamma globulin in blood D80.1
hereditary D80.0
genital organs
acquired (female) (male) Z90.79
female, congenital Q52.8
external Q52.71
internal NEC Q52.8
male, congenital Q55.8
genitourinary organs, congenital NEC
female Q52.8
male Q55.8
globe (acquired) Z90.01
congenital Q11.1
glottis, congenital Q31.8
hand and wrist (acquired) Z89.11-
congenital —*see* Agenesis, hand
head, part (acquired) NEC Z90.09
heat sense R20.8
hip (following explantation of hip joint prosthesis) (joint) (with or without presence of antibiotic-impregnated cement spacer) Z89.62-
hymen (congenital) Q52.4
ileum (acquired) Z90.49
congenital Q41.2
immunoglobulin, isolated NEC D80.3
IgA D80.2
IgG D80.3
IgM D80.4
incus (acquired) —*see* Loss, ossicles, ear
congenital Q16.3
inner ear, congenital Q16.5
intestine (acquired) (small) Z90.49
congenital Q41.9
specified NEC Q41.8
large Z90.49
congenital Q42.9
specified NEC Q42.8
iris, congenital Q13.1
jejunum (acquired) Z90.49
congenital Q41.1
joint
acquired
hip (following explantation of hip joint prosthesis) (with or without presence of antibiotic-impregnated cement spacer) Z89.62-
knee (following explantation of knee joint prosthesis) (with or without presence of antibiotic-impregnated cement spacer) Z89.52-
shoulder (following explantation of shoulder joint prosthesis) (with or without presence of antibiotic-impregnated cement spacer) Z89.23-
congenital NEC Q74.8
kidney (s) (acquired) Z90.5
congenital Q60.2
bilateral Q60.1
unilateral Q60.0

Absence *(Continued)*
knee (following explantation of knee joint prosthesis) (joint) (with or without presence of antibiotic-impregnated cement spacer) Z89.52-
labyrinth, membranous Q16.5
larynx (congenital) Q31.8
acquired Z90.02
leg (acquired) (above knee) Z89.61-
below knee (acquired) Z89.51-
congenital —*see* Defect, reduction, lower limb
lens (acquired) —*see also* Aphakia
congenital Q12.3
post cataract extraction Z98.4-
limb (acquired) —*see* Absence, extremity
lip Q38.6
liver (congenital) Q44.7
lung (fissure) (lobe) (bilateral) (unilateral) (congenital) Q33.3
acquired (any part) Z90.2
menstruation —*see* Amenorrhea
muscle (congenital) (pectoral) Q79.8
ocular Q10.3
neck, part Q18.8
neutrophil —*see* Agranulocytosis
nipple (s) (with breast (s)) (acquired) Z90.1-
congenital Q83.2
nose (congenital) Q30.1
acquired Z90.09
organ
of Corti, congenital Q16.5
or site, congenital NEC Q89.8
acquired NEC Z90.89
osseous meatus (ear) Q16.4
ovary (acquired)
bilateral Z90.722
congenital
bilateral Q50.02
unilateral Q50.01
unilateral Z90.721
oviduct (acquired)
bilateral Z90.722
congenital Q50.6
unilateral Z90.721
pancreas (congenital) Q45.0
acquired Z90.410
complete Z90.410
partial Z90.411
total Z90.410
parathyroid gland (acquired) E89.2
congenital Q89.2
patella, congenital Q74.1
penis (congenital) Q55.5
acquired Z90.79
pericardium (congenital) Q24.8
pituitary gland (congenital) Q89.2
acquired E89.3
prostate (acquired) Z90.79
congenital Q55.4
pulmonary valve Q22.0
punctum lacrimale (congenital) Q10.4
radius, congenital —*see* Defect, reduction, upper limb, longitudinal, radius
rectum (congenital) Q42.1
with fistula Q42.0
acquired Z90.49
respiratory organ NOS Q34.9
rib (acquired) Z90.89
congenital Q76.6
sacrum, congenital Q76.49
salivary gland (s), congenital Q38.4
scrotum, congenital Q55.29
seminal vesicles (congenital) Q55.4
acquired Z90.79
septum
atrial (congenital) Q21.1
between aorta and pulmonary artery Q21.4
ventricular (congenital) Q20.4
sex chromosome
female phenotype Q97.8
male phenotype Q98.8

Absence *(Continued)*
skull bone (congenital) Q75.8
with
anencephaly Q00.0
encephalocele —*see* Encephalocele
hydrocephalus Q03.9
with spina bifida —*see* Spina bifida, by site, with hydrocephalus
microcephaly Q02
spermatic cord, congenital Q55.4
spine, congenital Q76.49
spleen (congenital) Q89.01
acquired Z90.81
sternum, congenital Q76.7
stomach (acquired) (partial) Z90.3
congenital Q40.2
superior vena cava, congenital Q26.8
teeth, tooth (congenital) K00.0
acquired (complete) K08.109
class I K08.101
class II K08.102
class III K08.103
class IV K08.104
due to
caries K08.139
class I K08.131
class II K08.132
class III K08.133
class IV K08.134
periodontal disease K08.129
class I K08.121
class II K08.122
class III K08.123
class IV K08.124
specified NEC K08.199
class I K08.191
class II K08.192
class III K08.193
class IV K08.194
trauma K08.119
class I K08.111
class II K08.112
class III K08.113
class IV K08.114
partial K08.409
class I K08.401
class II K08.402
class III K08.403
class IV K08.404
due to
caries K08.439
class I K08.431
class II K08.432
class III K08.433
class IV K08.434
periodontal disease K08.429
class I K08.421
class II K08.422
class III K08.423
class IV K08.424
specified NEC K08.499
class I K08.491
class II K08.492
class III K08.493
class IV K08.494
trauma K08.419
class I K08.411
class II K08.412
class III K08.413
class IV K08.414
tendon (congenital) Q79.8
testis (congenital) Q55.0
acquired Z90.79
thumb (acquired) Z89.01-
congenital —*see* Agenesis, hand
thymus gland Q89.2
thyroid (gland) (acquired) E89.0
cartilage, congenital Q31.8
congenital E03.1

Absence *(Continued)*
toe (s) (acquired) Z89.42-
with foot —*see* Absence, foot and ankle
congenital —*see* Agenesis, foot
great Z89.41-
tongue, congenital Q38.3
trachea (cartilage), congenital Q32.1
transverse aortic arch, congenital Q25.49 ◄
tricuspid valve Q22.4
umbilical artery, congenital Q27.0
upper arm and forearm with hand present, congenital —*see* Agenesis, arm, with hand present
ureter (congenital) Q62.4
acquired Z90.6
urethra, congenital Q64.5
uterus (acquired) Z90.710
with cervix Z90.710
with remaining cervical stump Z90.711
congenital Q51.0
uvula, congenital Q38.5
vagina, congenital Q52.0
vas deferens (congenital) Q55.4
acquired Z90.79
vein (peripheral) congenital NEC Q27.8
cerebral Q28.3
digestive system Q27.8
great Q26.8
lower limb Q27.8
portal Q26.5
precerebral Q28.1
specified site NEC Q27.8
upper limb Q27.8
vena cava (inferior) (superior), congenital Q26.8
ventricular septum Q20.4
vertebra, congenital Q76.49
vulva, congenital Q52.71
wrist (acquired) Z89.12-
Absorbent system disease I87.8
Absorption
carbohydrate, disturbance K90.49 ◄
chemical —*see* Table of Drugs and Chemicals
through placenta (newborn) P04.9
environmental substance P04.6
nutritional substance P04.5
obstetric anesthetic or analgesic drug P04.0
drug NEC —*see* Table of Drugs and Chemicals
addictive
through placenta (newborn) P04.49
cocaine P04.41
medicinal
through placenta (newborn) P04.1
through placenta (newborn) P04.1
obstetric anesthetic or analgesic drug P04.0
fat, disturbance K90.49 ◄
pancreatic K90.3
noxious substance —*see* Table of Drugs and Chemicals
protein, disturbance K90.49 ◄
starch, disturbance K90.49 ◄
toxic substance —*see* Table of Drugs and Chemicals
uremic —*see* Uremia
Abstinence symptoms, syndrome
alcohol F10.239
with delirium F10.231
cocaine F14.23
neonatal P96.1
nicotine —*see* Dependence, drug, nicotine, with, withdrawal
opioid F11.93
with dependence F11.23
Abstinence symptoms, syndrome *(Continued)*
psychoactive NEC F19.939
with
delirium F19.931
dependence F19.239
with
delirium F19.231
perceptual disturbance F19.232
uncomplicated F19.230
perceptual disturbance F19.932
uncomplicated F19.930
sedative F13.939
with
delirium F13.931
dependence F13.239
with
delirium F13.231
perceptual disturbance F13.232
uncomplicated F13.230
perceptual disturbance F13.932
uncomplicated F13.930
stimulant NEC F15.93
with dependence F15.23
Abulia R68.89
Abulomania F60.7
Abuse
adult —*see* Maltreatment, adult
as reason for
couple seeking advice (including offender) Z63.0
alcohol (non-dependent) F10.10
with
anxiety disorder F10.180
intoxication F10.129
with delirium F10.121
uncomplicated F10.120
mood disorder F10.14
other specified disorder F10.188
psychosis F10.159
delusions F10.150
hallucinations F10.151
sexual dysfunction F10.181
sleep disorder F10.182
unspecified disorder F10.19
counseling and surveillance Z71.41
amphetamine (or related substance) —*see* Abuse, drug, stimulant NEC
analgesics (non-prescribed) (over the counter) F55.8
antacids F55.0
antidepressants —*see* Abuse, drug, psychoactive NEC
anxiolytic —*see* Abuse, drug, sedative
barbiturates —*see* Abuse, drug, sedative
caffeine —*see* Abuse, drug, stimulant NEC
cannabis, cannabinoids —*see* Abuse, drug, cannabis
child —*see* Maltreatment, child
cocaine —*see* Abuse, drug, cocaine
drug NEC (non-dependent) F19.10
with sleep disorder F19.182
amphetamine type —*see* Abuse, drug, stimulant NEC
analgesics (non-prescribed) (over the counter) F55.8
antacids F55.0
antidepressants —*see* Abuse, drug, psychoactive NEC
anxiolytics —*see* Abuse, drug, sedative
barbiturates —*see* Abuse, drug, sedative
caffeine —*see* Abuse, drug, stimulant NEC
cannabis F12.10
with
anxiety disorder F12.180
intoxication F12.129
with
delirium F12.121
perceptual disturbance F12.122
uncomplicated F12.120
other specified disorder F12.188
Abuse *(Continued)*
drug NEC *(Continued)*
cannabis *(Continued)*
with *(Continued)*
psychosis F12.159
delusions F12.150
hallucinations F12.151
unspecified disorder F12.19
cocaine F14.10
with
anxiety disorder F14.180
intoxication F14.129
with
delirium F14.121
perceptual disturbance F14.122
uncomplicated F14.120
mood disorder F14.14
other specified disorder F14.188
psychosis F14.159
delusions F14.150
hallucinations F14.151
sexual dysfunction F14.181
sleep disorder F14.182
unspecified disorder F14.19
counseling and surveillance Z71.51
hallucinogen F16.10
with
anxiety disorder F16.180
flashbacks F16.183
intoxication F16.129
with
delirium F16.121
perceptual disturbance F16.122
uncomplicated F16.120
mood disorder F16.14
other specified disorder F16.188
perception disorder, persisting F16.183
psychosis F16.159
delusions F16.150
hallucinations F16.151
unspecified disorder F16.19
hashish —*see* Abuse, drug, cannabis
herbal or folk remedies F55.1
hormones F55.3
hypnotics —*see* Abuse, drug, sedative
inhalant F18.10
with
anxiety disorder F18.180
dementia, persisting F18.17
intoxication F18.129
with delirium F18.121
uncomplicated F18.120
mood disorder F18.14
other specified disorder F18.188
psychosis F18.159
delusions F18.150
hallucinations F18.151
unspecified disorder F18.19
laxatives F55.2
LSD —*see* Abuse, drug, hallucinogen
marihuana —*see* Abuse, drug, cannabis
morphine type (opioids) —*see* Abuse, drug, opioid
opioid F11.10
with
intoxication F11.129
with
delirium F11.121
perceptual disturbance F11.122
uncomplicated F11.120
mood disorder F11.14
other specified disorder F11.188
psychosis F11.159
delusions F11.150
hallucinations F11.151
sexual dysfunction F11.181
sleep disorder F11.182
unspecified disorder F11.19
PCP (phencyclidine) (or related substance) —*see* Abuse, drug, hallucinogen

◄ New ◄ Revised ~~deleted~~ Deleted

Abuse *(Continued)*
drug NEC *(Continued)*
psychoactive NEC F19.10
with
amnestic disorder F19.16
anxiety disorder F19.180
dementia F19.17
intoxication F19.129
with
delirium F19.121
perceptual disturbance F19.122
uncomplicated F19.120
mood disorder F19.14
other specified disorder F19.188
psychosis F19.159
delusions F19.150
hallucinations F19.151
sexual dysfunction F19.181
sleep disorder F19.182
unspecified disorder F19.19
sedative, hypnotic or anxiolytic F13.10
with
anxiety disorder F13.180
intoxication F13.129
with delirium F13.121
uncomplicated F13.120
mood disorder F13.14
other specified disorder F13.188
psychosis F13.159
delusions F13.150
hallucinations F13.151
sexual dysfunction F13.181
sleep disorder F13.182
unspecified disorder F13.19
solvent —*see* Abuse, drug, inhalant
steroids F55.3
stimulant NEC F15.10
with
anxiety disorder F15.180
intoxication F15.129
with
delirium F15.121
perceptual disturbance F15.122
uncomplicated F15.120
mood disorder F15.14
other specified disorder F15.188
psychosis F15.159
delusions F15.150
hallucinations F15.151
sexual dysfunction F15.181
sleep disorder F15.182
unspecified disorder F15.19
tranquilizers —*see* Abuse, drug, sedative
vitamins F55.4
hallucinogens —*see* Abuse, drug, hallucinogen
hashish —*see* Abuse, drug, cannabis
herbal or folk remedies F55.1
hormones F55.3
hypnotic —*see* Abuse, drug, sedative
inhalant —*see* Abuse, drug, inhalant
laxatives F55.2
LSD —*see* Abuse, drug, hallucinogen
marihuana —*see* Abuse, drug, cannabis
morphine type (opioids) —*see* Abuse, drug, opioid
non-psychoactive substance NEC F55.8
antacids F55.0
folk remedies F55.1
herbal remedies F55.1
hormones F55.3
laxatives F55.2
steroids F55.3
vitamins F55.4
opioids —*see* Abuse, drug, opioid
PCP (phencyclidine) (or related substance) —*see* Abuse, drug, hallucinogen
physical (adult) (child) —*see* Maltreatment
psychoactive substance —*see* Abuse, drug, psychoactive NEC

Abuse *(Continued)*
psychological (adult) (child) —*see* Maltreatment
sedative —*see* Abuse, drug, sedative
sexual —*see* Maltreatment
solvent —*see* Abuse, drug, inhalant
steroids F55.3
vitamins F55.4
Acalculia R48.8
developmental F81.2
Acanthamebiasis (with) B60.10
conjunctiva B60.12
keratoconjunctivitis B60.13
meningoencephalitis B60.11
other specified B60.19
Acanthocephaliasis B83.8
Acanthocheilonemiasis B74.4
Acanthocytosis E78.6
Acantholysis L11.9
Acanthosis (acquired) (nigricans) L83
benign Q82.8
congenital Q82.8
seborrheic L82.1
inflamed L82.0
tongue K14.3
Acapnia E87.3
Acarbia E87.2
Acardia, acardius Q89.8
Acardiacus amorphus Q89.8
Acardiotrophia I51.4
Acariasis B88.0
scabies B86
Acarodermatitis (urticarioides) B88.0
Acarophobia F40.218
Acatalasemia, acatalasia E80.3
Acathisia (drug induced) G25.71
Accelerated atrioventricular conduction I45.6
Accentuation of personality traits (type A) Z73.1
Accessory (congenital)
adrenal gland Q89.1
anus Q43.4
appendix Q43.4
atrioventricular conduction I45.6
auditory ossicles Q16.3
auricle (ear) Q17.0
biliary duct or passage Q44.5
bladder Q64.79
blood vessels NEC Q27.9
coronary Q24.5
bone NEC Q79.8
breast tissue, axilla Q83.1
carpal bones Q74.0
cecum Q43.4
chromosome (s) NEC (nonsex) Q92.9
with complex rearrangements NEC Q92.5
seen only at prometaphase Q92.8
13 —*see* Trisomy, 13
18 —*see* Trisomy, 18
21 —*see* Trisomy, 21
partial Q92.9
sex
female phenotype Q97.8
coronary artery Q24.5
cusp (s), heart valve NEC Q24.8
pulmonary Q22.3
cystic duct Q44.5
digit (s) Q69.9
ear (auricle) (lobe) Q17.0
endocrine gland NEC Q89.2
eye muscle Q10.3
eyelid Q10.3
face bone (s) Q75.8
fallopian tube (fimbria) (ostium) Q50.6
finger (s) Q69.0
foreskin N47.8
frontonasal process Q75.8

Accessory *(Continued)*
gallbladder Q44.1
genital organ (s)
female Q52.8
external Q52.79
internal NEC Q52.8
male Q55.8
genitourinary organs NEC Q89.8
female Q52.8
male Q55.8
hallux Q69.2
heart Q24.8
valve NEC Q24.8
pulmonary Q22.3
hepatic ducts Q44.5
hymen Q52.4
intestine (large) (small) Q43.4
kidney Q63.0
lacrimal canal Q10.6
leaflet, heart valve NEC Q24.8
ligament, broad Q50.6
liver Q44.7
duct Q44.5
lobule (ear) Q17.0
lung (lobe) Q33.1
muscle Q79.8
navicular of carpus Q74.0
nervous system, part NEC Q07.8
nipple Q83.3
nose Q30.8
organ or site not listed —*see* Anomaly, by site
ovary Q50.31
oviduct Q50.6
pancreas Q45.3
parathyroid gland Q89.2
parotid gland (and duct) Q38.4
pituitary gland Q89.2
preauricular appendage Q17.0
prepuce N47.8
renal arteries (multiple) Q27.2
rib Q76.6
cervical Q76.5
roots (teeth) K00.2
salivary gland Q38.4
sesamoid bones Q74.8
foot Q74.2
hand Q74.0
skin tags Q82.8
spleen Q89.09
sternum Q76.7
submaxillary gland Q38.4
tarsal bones Q74.2
teeth, tooth K00.1
tendon Q79.8
thumb Q69.1
thymus gland Q89.2
thyroid gland Q89.2
toes Q69.2
tongue Q38.3
tooth, teeth K00.1
tragus Q17.0
ureter Q62.5
urethra Q64.79
urinary organ or tract NEC Q64.8
uterus Q51.2
vagina Q52.10
valve, heart NEC Q24.8
pulmonary Q22.3
vertebra Q76.49
vocal cords Q31.8
vulva Q52.79
Accident
birth —*see* Birth, injury
cardiac —*see* Infarct, myocardium
cerebral I63.9
cerebrovascular (embolic) (ischemic) (thrombotic) I63.9
aborted I63.9
hemorrhagic —*see* Hemorrhage, intracranial, intracerebral

A

Accident *(Continued)*
cerebrovascular *(Continued)*
old (without sequelae) Z86.73
with sequelae (of) —*see* Sequelae, infarction, cerebral
coronary —*see* Infarct, myocardium
craniovascular I63.9
vascular, brain I63.9
Accidental —*see* condition
Accommodation (disorder) —*see also* condition
hysterical paralysis of F44.89
insufficiency of H52.4
paresis —*see* Paresis, of accommodation
spasm —*see* Spasm, of accommodation
Accouchement —*see* Delivery
Accreta placenta O43.21-
Accretio cordis (nonrheumatic) I31.0
Accretions, tooth, teeth K03.6
Acculturation difficulty Z60.3
Accumulation secretion, prostate N42.89
Acephalia, acephalism, acephalus, acephaly Q00.0
Acephalobrachia monster Q89.8
Acephalochirus monster Q89.8
Acephalogaster Q89.8
Acephalostomus monster Q89.8
Acephalothorax Q89.8
Acerophobia F40.298
Acetonemia R79.89
in Type 1 diabetes E10.10
with coma E10.11
Acetonuria R82.4
Achalasia (cardia) (esophagus) K22.0
congenital Q39.5
pylorus Q40.0
sphincteral NEC K59.8
Ache (s) —*see* Pain
Acheilia Q38.6
Achillobursitis —*see* Tendinitis, Achilles
Achillodynia —*see* Tendinitis, Achilles
Achlorhydria, achlorhydric (neurogenic) K31.83
anemia D50.8
diarrhea K31.83
psychogenic F45.8
secondary to vagotomy K91.1
Achluophobia F40.228
Acholia K82.8
Acholuric jaundice (familial) (splenomegalic) —*see also* Spherocytosis
acquired D59.8
Achondrogenesis Q77.0
Achondroplasia (osteosclerosis congenita) Q77.4
Achroma, cutis L80
Achromat (ism), achromatopsia (acquired) (congenital) H53.51
Achromia, congenital —*see* Albinism
Achromia parasitica B36.0
Achylia gastrica K31.89
psychogenic F45.8
Acid
burn —*see* Corrosion
deficiency
amide nicotinic E52
ascorbic E54
folic E53.8
nicotinic E52
pantothenic E53.8
intoxication E87.2
peptic disease K30
phosphatase deficiency E83.39
stomach K30
psychogenic F45.8
Acidemia E87.2
argininosuccinic E72.22
isovaleric E71.110
metabolic (newborn) P19.9
first noted before onset of labor P19.0
first noted during labor P19.1
noted at birth P19.2
Acidemia *(Continued)*
methylmalonic E71.120
pipecolic E72.3
propionic E71.121
Acidity, gastric (high) K30
psychogenic F45.8
Acidocytopenia —*see* Agranulocytosis
Acidocytosis D72.1
Acidopenia —*see* Agranulocytosis
Acidosis (lactic) (respiratory) E87.2
in Type 1 diabetes E10.10
with coma E10.11
kidney, tubular N25.89
lactic E87.2
metabolic NEC E87.2
with respiratory acidosis E87.4
late, of newborn P74.0
mixed metabolic and respiratory, newborn P84
newborn P84
renal (hyperchloremic) (tubular) N25.89
respiratory E87.2
complicated by
metabolic
acidosis E87.4
alkalosis E87.4
Aciduria
argininosuccinic E72.22
glutaric (type I) E72.3
type II E71.313
type III E71.5-
orotic (congenital) (hereditary) (pyrimidine deficiency) E79.8
anemia D53.0
Acladiosis (skin) B36.0
Aclasis, diaphyseal Q78.6
Acleistocardia Q21.1
Aclusion —*see* Anomaly, dentofacial, malocclusion
Acne L70.9
artificialis L70.8
atrophica L70.2
cachecticorum (Hebra) L70.8
conglobata L70.1
cystic L70.0
decalvans L66.2
~~excoriée des jeunes filles L70.5~~
excoriée (des jeunes filles) L70.5 ◀
frontalis L70.2
indurata L70.0
infantile L70.4
keloid L73.0
lupoid L70.2
necrotic, necrotica (miliaris) L70.2
neonatal L70.4
nodular L70.0
occupational L70.8
picker's L70.5
pustular L70.0
rodens L70.2
rosacea L71.9
specified NEC L70.8
tropica L70.3
varioliformis L70.2
vulgaris L70.0
Acnitis (primary) A18.4
Acosta's disease T70.29
Acoustic —*see* condition
Acousticophobia F40.298
Acquired —*see also* condition
immunodeficiency syndrome (AIDS) B20
Acrania Q00.0
Acroangiodermatitis I78.9
Acroasphyxia, chronic I73.89
Acrobystitis N47.7
Acrocephalopolysyndactyly Q87.0
Acrocephalosyndactyly Q87.0
Acrocephaly Q75.0
Acrochondrohyperplasia —*see* Syndrome, Marfan's
Acrocyanosis I73.8
newborn P28.2
meaning transient blue hands and feet - omit code
Acrodermatitis L30.8
atrophicans (chronica) L90.4
continua (Hallopeau) L40.2
enteropathica (hereditary) E83.2
Hallopeau's L40.2
infantile papular L44.4
perstans L40.2
pustulosa continua L40.2
recalcitrant pustular L40.2
Acrodynia —*see* Poisoning, mercury
Acromegaly, acromegalia E22.0
Acromelalgia I73.81
Acromicria, acromikria Q79.8
Acronyx L60.0
Acropachy, thyroid —*see* Thyrotoxicosis
Acroparesthesia (simple) (vasomotor) I73.89
Acropathy, thyroid —*see* Thyrotoxicosis
Acrophobia F40.241
Acroposthitis N47.7
Acroscleriasis, acroscleroderma, acrosclerosis —*see* Sclerosis, systemic
Acrosphacelus I96
Acrospiroma, eccrine —*see* Neoplasm, skin, benign
Acrostealgia —*see* Osteochondropathy
Acrotrophodynia —*see* Immersion
ACTH ectopic syndrome E24.3
Actinic —*see* condition
Actinobacillosis, actinobacillus A28.8
mallei A24.0
muris A25.1
Actinomyces israelii (infection) —*see* Actinomycosis
Actinomycetoma (foot) B47.1
Actinomycosis, actinomycotic A42.9
with pneumonia A42.0
abdominal A42.1
cervicofacial A42.2
cutaneous A42.89
gastrointestinal A42.1
pulmonary A42.0
sepsis A42.7
specified site NEC A42.89
Actinoneuritis G62.82
Action, heart
disorder I49.9
irregular I49.9
psychogenic F45.8
Activated protein C resistance D68.51
Activation ◀
mast cell (disorder) (syndrome) D89.40 ◀
idiopathic D89.42 ◀
monoclonal D89.41 ◀
secondary D89.43 ◀
specified type NEC D89.49 ◀
Active —*see* condition
Acute —*see also* condition
abdomen R10.0
gallbladder —*see* Cholecystitis, acute
Acyanotic heart disease (congenital) Q24.9
Acystia Q64.5
Adair-Dighton syndrome (brittle bones and blue sclera, deafness) Q78.0
Adamantinoblastoma —*see* Ameloblastoma
Adamantinoma —*see also* Cyst, calcifying odontogenic
long bones C40.90
lower limb C40.2-
upper limb C40.0-
malignant C41.1
jaw (bone) (lower) C41.1
upper C41.0
tibial C40.2-
Adamantoblastoma —*see* Ameloblastoma
Adams-Stokes (-Morgagni) disease or syndrome I45.9
Adaption reaction —*see* Disorder, adjustment

Addiction —*see also* Dependence F19.20
alcohol, alcoholic (ethyl) (methyl) (wood) (without remission) F10.20
with remission F10.21
drug —*see* Dependence, drug
ethyl alcohol (without remission) F10.20
with remission F10.21
heroin —*see* Dependence, drug, opioid
methyl alcohol (without remission) F10.20
with remission F10.21
methylated spirit (without remission) F10.20
with remission F10.21
morphine(-like substances) —*see* Dependence, drug, opioid
nicotine —*see* Dependence, drug, nicotine
opium and opioids —*see* Dependence, drug, opioid
tobacco —*see* Dependence, drug, nicotine
Addisonian crisis E27.2
Addison's
anemia (pernicious) D51.0
disease (bronze) or syndrome E27.1
tuberculous A18.7
keloid L94.0
Addison-Biermer anemia (pernicious) D51.0
Addison-Schilder complex E71.528
Additional —*see also* Accessory
chromosome (s) Q99.8
21 —*see* Trisomy, 21
sex —*see* Abnormal, chromosome, sex
Adduction contracture, hip or other joint —*see* Contraction, joint
Adenitis —*see also* Lymphadenitis
acute, unspecified site L04.9
axillary I88.9
acute L04.2
chronic or subacute I88.1
Bartholin's gland N75.8
bulbourethral gland —*see* Urethritis
cervical I88.9
acute L04.0
chronic or subacute I88.1
chancroid (Hemophilus ducreyi) A57
chronic, unspecified site I88.1
Cowper's gland —*see* Urethritis
due to Pasteurella multocida (p. septica) A28.0
epidemic, acute B27.09
gangrenous L04.9
gonorrheal NEC A54.89
groin I88.9
acute L04.1
chronic or subacute I88.1
infectious (acute) (epidemic) B27.09
inguinal I88.9
acute L04.1
chronic or subacute I88.1
lymph gland or node, except mesenteric I88.9
acute —*see* Lymphadenitis, acute
chronic or subacute I88.1
mesenteric (acute) (chronic) (nonspecific) (subacute) I88.0
parotid gland (suppurative) —*see* Sialoadenitis
salivary gland (any) (suppurative) —*see* Sialoadenitis
scrofulous (tuberculous) A18.2
Skene's duct or gland —*see* Urethritis
strumous, tuberculous A18.2
subacute, unspecified site I88.1
sublingual gland (suppurative) —*see* Sialoadenitis
submandibular gland (suppurative) —*see* Sialoadenitis
submaxillary gland (suppurative) —*see* Sialoadenitis
tuberculous —*see* Tuberculosis, lymph gland
urethral gland —*see* Urethritis
Wharton's duct (suppurative) —*see* Sialoadenitis
Adenoacanthoma —*see* Neoplasm, malignant, by site
Adenoameloblastoma —*see* Cyst, calcifying odontogenic
Adenocarcinoid (tumor) —*see* Neoplasm, malignant, by site
Adenocarcinoma —*see also* Neoplasm, malignant, by site
acidophil
specified site —*see* Neoplasm, malignant, by site
unspecified site C75.1
adrenal cortical C74.0-
alveolar —*see* Neoplasm, lung, malignant
apocrine
breast —*see* Neoplasm, breast, malignant
in situ
breast D05.8-
specified site NEC —*see* Neoplasm, skin, in situ
unspecified site D04.9
specified site NEC —*see* Neoplasm, skin, malignant
unspecified site C44.99
basal cell
specified site —*see* Neoplasm, skin, malignant
unspecified site C08.9
basophil
specified site —*see* Neoplasm, malignant, by site
unspecified site C75.1
bile duct type C22.1
liver C22.1
specified site NEC —*see* Neoplasm, malignant, by site
unspecified site C22.1
bronchiolar —*see* Neoplasm, lung, malignant
bronchioloalveolar —*see* Neoplasm, lung, malignant
ceruminous C44.29-
cervix, in situ (*see also* Carcinoma, cervix uteri, in situ) D06.9
chromophobe
specified site —*see* Neoplasm, malignant, by site
unspecified site C75.1
diffuse type
specified site —*see* Neoplasm, malignant, by site
unspecified site C16.9
duct
infiltrating
with Paget's disease —*see* Neoplasm, breast, malignant
specified site —*see* Neoplasm, malignant, by site
unspecified site (female) C50.91-
male C50.92-
specified site —*see* Neoplasm, malignant, by site
unspecified site
female C56.9
male C61
eosinophil
specified site —*see* Neoplasm, malignant, by site
unspecified site C75.1
follicular
with papillary C73
moderately differentiated C73
specified site —*see* Neoplasm, malignant, by site
trabecular C73
unspecified site C73
well differentiated C73
Hurthle cell C73
in
adenomatous
polyposis coli C18.9
infiltrating duct
with Paget's disease —*see* Neoplasm, breast, malignant
Adenocarcinoma *(Continued)*
infiltrating duct *(Continued)*
specified site —*see* Neoplasm, malignant, by site
unspecified site (female) C50.91-
male C50.92-
inflammatory
specified site —*see* Neoplasm, malignant, by site
unspecified site (female) C50.91-
male C50.92-
intestinal type
specified site —*see* Neoplasm, malignant, by site
unspecified site C16.9
intracystic papillary
intraductal
breast D05.1-
noninfiltrating
breast D05.1-
papillary
with invasion
specified site —*see* Neoplasm, malignant, by site
unspecified site (female) C50.91-
male C50.92-
breast D05.1-
specified site NEC —*see* Neoplasm, in situ, by site
unspecified site D05.1-
specified site NEC —*see* Neoplasm, in situ, by site
unspecified site D05.1-
papillary
with invasion
specified site —*see* Neoplasm, malignant, by site
unspecified site (female) C50.91-
male C50.92-
breast D05.1-
specified site —*see* Neoplasm, in situ, by site
unspecified site D05.1-
specified site NEC —*see* Neoplasm, in situ, by site
unspecified site D05.1-
islet cell
with exocrine, mixed
specified site —*see* Neoplasm, malignant, by site
unspecified site C25.9
pancreas C25.4
specified site NEC —*see* Neoplasm, malignant, by site
unspecified site C25.4
lobular
in situ
breast D05.0-
specified site NEC —*see* Neoplasm, in situ, by site
unspecified site D05.0-
specified site —*see* Neoplasm, malignant, by site
unspecified site (female) C50.91-
male C50.92-
mucoid —*see also* Neoplasm, malignant, by site
cell
specified site —*see* Neoplasm, malignant, by site
unspecified site C75.1
nonencapsulated sclerosing C73
papillary
with follicular C73
follicular variant C73
intraductal (noninfiltrating)
with invasion
specified site —*see* Neoplasm, malignant, by site
unspecified site (female) C50.91-
male C50.92-
breast D05.1-

Adenocarcinoma *(Continued)*
papillary *(Continued)*
intraductal *(Continued)*
specified site NEC —*see* Neoplasm, in situ, by site
unspecified site D05.1-
serous
specified site —*see* Neoplasm, malignant, by site
unspecified site C56.9
papillocystic
specified site —*see* Neoplasm, malignant, by site
unspecified site C56.9
pseudomucinous
specified site —*see* Neoplasm, malignant, by site
unspecified site C56.9
renal cell C64-
sebaceous —*see* Neoplasm, skin, malignant, by site
serous —*see also* Neoplasm, malignant, by site
papillary
specified site —*see* Neoplasm, malignant, by site
unspecified site C56.9
sweat gland —*see* Neoplasm, skin, malignant
water-clear cell C75.0
Adenocarcinoma-in-situ —*see also* Neoplasm, in situ, by site
breast D05.9-
Adenofibroma
clear cell —*see* Neoplasm, benign, by site
endometrioid D27.9
borderline malignancy D39.10
malignant C56-
mucinous
specified site —*see* Neoplasm, benign, by site
unspecified site D27.9
papillary
specified site —*see* Neoplasm, benign, by site
unspecified site D27.9
prostate —*see* Enlargement, enlarged, prostate
serous
specified site —*see* Neoplasm, benign, by site
unspecified site D27.9
specified site —*see* Neoplasm, benign, by site
unspecified site D27.9
Adenofibrosis
breast —*see* Fibroadenosis, breast
endometrioid N80.0
Adenoiditis (chronic) J35.02
with tonsillitis J35.03
acute J03.90
recurrent J03.91
specified organism NEC J03.80
recurrent J03.81
staphylococcal J03.80
recurrent J03.81
streptococcal J03.00
recurrent J03.01
Adenoids —*see* condition
Adenolipoma —*see* Neoplasm, benign, by site
Adenolipomatosis, Launois-Bensaude E88.89
Adenolymphoma
specified site —*see* Neoplasm, benign, by site
unspecified site D11.9
Adenoma —*see also* Neoplasm, benign, by site
acidophil
specified site —*see* Neoplasm, benign, by site
unspecified site D35.2
acidophil-basophil, mixed
specified site —*see* Neoplasm, benign, by site
unspecified site D35.2

Adenoma *(Continued)*
adrenal (cortical) D35.00
clear cell D35.00
compact cell D35.00
glomerulosa cell D35.00
heavily pigmented variant D35.00
mixed cell D35.00
alpha-cell
pancreas D13.7
specified site NEC —*see* Neoplasm, benign, by site
unspecified site D13.7
alveolar D14.30
apocrine
breast D24-
specified site NEC —*see* Neoplasm, skin, benign, by site
unspecified site D23.9
basal cell D11.9
basophil
specified site —*see* Neoplasm, benign, by site
unspecified site D35.2
basophil-acidophil, mixed
specified site —*see* Neoplasm, benign, by site
unspecified site D35.2
beta-cell
pancreas D13.7
specified site NEC —*see* Neoplasm, benign, by site
unspecified site D13.7
bile duct D13.4
common D13.5
extrahepatic D13.5
intrahepatic D13.4
specified site NEC —*see* Neoplasm, benign, by site
unspecified site D13.4
black D35.00
bronchial D38.1
cylindroid type —*see* Neoplasm, lung, malignant
ceruminous D23.2-
chief cell D35.1
chromophobe
specified site —*see* Neoplasm, benign, by site
unspecified site D35.2
colloid
specified site —*see* Neoplasm, benign, by site
unspecified site D34
duct
eccrine, papillary —*see* Neoplasm, skin, benign
endocrine, multiple
single specified site —*see* Neoplasm, uncertain behavior, by site
two or more specified sites D44-
unspecified site D44.9
endometrioid —*see also* Neoplasm, benign
borderline malignancy —*see* Neoplasm, uncertain behavior, by site
eosinophil
specified site —*see* Neoplasm, malignant, by site
unspecified site D35.2
fetal
specified site —*see* Neoplasm, benign, by site
unspecified site D34
follicular
specified site —*see* Neoplasm, benign, by site
unspecified site D34
hepatocellular D13.4
Hurthle cell D34
islet cell
pancreas D13.7
specified site NEC —*see* Neoplasm, benign, by site
unspecified site D13.7

Adenoma *(Continued)*
liver cell D13.4
macrofollicular
specified site —*see* Neoplasm, benign, by site
unspecified site D34
malignant, malignum —*see* Neoplasm, malignant, by site
microcystic
pancreas D13.6 ⇐
specified site NEC —*see* Neoplasm, benign, by site
unspecified site D13.6 ⇐
microfollicular
specified site —*see* Neoplasm, benign, by site
unspecified site D34
mucoid cell
specified site —*see* Neoplasm, benign, by site
unspecified site D35.2
multiple endocrine
single specified site —*see* Neoplasm, uncertain behavior, by site
two or more specified sites D44-
unspecified site D44.9
nipple D24-
papillary —*see also* Neoplasm, benign, by site
eccrine —*see* Neoplasm, skin, benign, by site
Pick's tubular
specified site —*see* Neoplasm, benign, by site
unspecified site
female D27.9
male D29.20
pleomorphic
carcinoma in —*see* Neoplasm, salivary gland, malignant
specified site —*see* Neoplasm, malignant, by site
unspecified site C08.9
polypoid —*see also* Neoplasm, benign
adenocarcinoma in —*see* Neoplasm, malignant, by site
adenocarcinoma in situ —*see* Neoplasm, in situ, by site
prostate —*see* Neoplasm, benign, prostate
rete cell D29.20
sebaceous —*see* Neoplasm, skin, benign
Sertoli cell
specified site —*see* Neoplasm, benign, by site
unspecified site
female D27.9
male D29.20
skin appendage —*see* Neoplasm, skin, benign
sudoriferous gland —*see* Neoplasm, skin, benign
sweat gland —*see* Neoplasm, skin, benign
testicular
specified site —*see* Neoplasm, benign, by site
unspecified site
female D27.9
male D29.20
tubular —*see also* Neoplasm, benign, by site
adenocarcinoma in —*see* Neoplasm, malignant, by site
adenocarcinoma in situ —*see* Neoplasm, in situ, by site
Pick's
specified site —*see* Neoplasm, benign
unspecified site
female D27.9
male D29.20
tubulovillous —*see also* Neoplasm, benign, by site
adenocarcinoma in —*see* Neoplasm, malignant, by site
adenocarcinoma in situ —*see* Neoplasm, in situ, by site

◀ New ⇐ Revised ~~deleted~~ Deleted

Adenoma *(Continued)*
villous —*see* Neoplasm, uncertain behavior, by site
adenocarcinoma in —*see* Neoplasm, malignant, by site
adenocarcinoma in situ —*see* Neoplasm, in situ, by site
water-clear cell D35.1
Adenomatosis
endocrine (multiple) E31.20
single specified site —*see* Neoplasm, uncertain behavior, by site
erosive of nipple D24-
pluriendocrine —*see* Adenomatosis, endocrine
pulmonary D38.1
malignant —*see* Neoplasm, lung, malignant
specified site —*see* Neoplasm, benign, by site
unspecified site D12.6
Adenomatous
goiter (nontoxic) E04.9
with hyperthyroidism —*see* Hyperthyroidism, with, goiter, nodular
toxic —*see* Hyperthyroidism, with, goiter, nodular
Adenomyoma —*see also* Neoplasm, benign, by site
prostate —*see* Enlarged, prostate
Adenomyometritis N80.0
Adenomyosis N80.0
Adenopathy (lymph gland) R59.9
generalized R59.1
inguinal R59.0
localized R59.0
mediastinal R59.0
mesentery R59.0
syphilitic (secondary) A51.49
tracheobronchial R59.0
tuberculous A15.4
primary (progressive) A15.7
tuberculous —*see also* Tuberculosis, lymph gland
tracheobronchial A15.4
primary (progressive) A15.7
Adenosalpingitis —*see* Salpingitis
Adenosarcoma —*see* Neoplasm, malignant, by site
Adenosclerosis I88.8
Adenosis (sclerosing) **breast** —*see* Fibroadenosis, breast
Adenovirus, as cause of disease classified elsewhere B97.0
Adentia (complete) (partial) —*see* Absence, teeth
Adherent —*see also* Adhesions
labia (minora) N90.89
pericardium (nonrheumatic) I31.0
rheumatic I09.2
placenta (with hemorrhage) O72.0
without hemorrhage O73.0
prepuce, newborn N47.0
scar (skin) L90.5
tendon in scar L90.5
Adhesions, adhesive (postinfective) K66.0
with intestinal obstruction K56.5
abdominal (wall) —*see* Adhesions, peritoneum
appendix K38.8
bile duct (common) (hepatic) K83.8
bladder (sphincter) N32.89
bowel —*see* Adhesions, peritoneum
cardiac I31.0
rheumatic I09.2
cecum —*see* Adhesions, peritoneum
cervicovaginal N88.1
congenital Q52.8
postpartal O90.89
old N88.1
cervix N88.1
ciliary body NEC —*see* Adhesions, iris
Adhesions, adhesive *(Continued)*
clitoris N90.89
colon —*see* Adhesions, peritoneum
common duct K83.8
congenital —*see also* Anomaly, by site
fingers —*see* Syndactylism, complex, fingers
omental, anomalous Q43.3
peritoneal Q43.3
tongue (to gum or roof of mouth) Q38.3
conjunctiva (acquired) H11.21-
congenital Q15.8
cystic duct K82.8
diaphragm —*see* Adhesions, peritoneum
due to foreign body —*see* Foreign body
duodenum —*see* Adhesions, peritoneum
ear
middle H74.1-
epididymis N50.89 ◄
epidural —*see* Adhesions, meninges
epiglottis J38.7
eyelid H02.59
female pelvis N73.6
gallbladder K82.8
globe H44.89
heart I31.0
rheumatic I09.2
ileocecal (coil) —*see* Adhesions, peritoneum
ileum —*see* Adhesions, peritoneum
intestine —*see also* Adhesions, peritoneum
with obstruction K56.5
intra-abdominal —*see* Adhesions, peritoneum
iris H21.50-
anterior H21.51-
goniosynechiae H21.52-
posterior H21.54-
to corneal graft T85.898 ◄
joint —*see* Ankylosis
knee M23.8X
temporomandibular M26.61- ◄
labium (majus) (minus), congenital Q52.5
liver —*see* Adhesions, peritoneum
lung J98.4
mediastinum J98.59 ◄
meninges (cerebral) (spinal) G96.12
congenital Q07.8
tuberculous (cerebral) (spinal) A17.0
mesenteric —*see* Adhesions, peritoneum
nasal (septum) (to turbinates) J34.89
ocular muscle —*see* Strabismus, mechanical
omentum —*see* Adhesions, peritoneum
ovary N73.6
congenital (to cecum, kidney or omentum) Q50.39
paraovarian N73.6
pelvic (peritoneal)
female N73.6
postprocedural N99.4
male —*see* Adhesions, peritoneum
postpartal (old) N73.6
tuberculous A18.17
penis to scrotum (congenital) Q55.8
periappendiceal —*see also* Adhesions, peritoneum
pericardium (nonrheumatic) I31.0
focal I31.8
rheumatic I09.2
tuberculous A18.84
pericholecystic K82.8
perigastric —*see* Adhesions, peritoneum
periovarian N73.6
periprostatic N42.89
perirectal —*see* Adhesions, peritoneum
perirenal N28.89
peritoneum, peritoneal (postinfective) (postprocedural) K66.0
with obstruction (intestinal) K56.5
congenital Q43.3
pelvic, female N73.6
postprocedural N99.4
Adhesions, adhesive *(Continued)*
peritoneum, peritoneal *(Continued)*
postpartal, pelvic N73.6
to uterus N73.6
peritubal N73.6
periureteral N28.89
periuterine N73.6
perivesical N32.89
perivesicular (seminal vesicle) N50.89 ◄
pleura, pleuritic J94.8
tuberculous NEC A15.6
pleuropericardial J94.8
postoperative (gastrointestinal tract) K66.0
with obstruction K91.3
due to foreign body accidentally left in wound —*see* Foreign body, accidentally left during a procedure
pelvic peritoneal N99.4
urethra —*see* Stricture, urethra, postprocedural
vagina N99.2
postpartal, old (vulva or perineum) N90.89
preputial, prepuce N47.5
pulmonary J98.4
pylorus —*see* Adhesions, peritoneum
sciatic nerve —*see* Lesion, nerve, sciatic
seminal vesicle N50.89 ◄
shoulder (joint) —*see* Capsulitis, adhesive
sigmoid flexure —*see* Adhesions, peritoneum
spermatic cord (acquired) N50.89 ◄
congenital Q55.4
spinal canal G96.12
stomach —*see* Adhesions, peritoneum
subscapular —*see* Capsulitis, adhesive
temporomandibular M26.61- ◄
tendinitis —*see also* Tenosynovitis, specified type NEC
shoulder —*see* Capsulitis, adhesive
testis N44.8
tongue, congenital (to gum or roof of mouth) Q38.3
acquired K14.8
trachea J39.8
tubo-ovarian N73.6
tunica vaginalis N44.8
uterus N73.6
internal N85.6
to abdominal wall N73.6
vagina (chronic) N89.5
postoperative N99.2
vitreomacular H43.82-
vitreous H43.89
vulva N90.89
Adiaspiromycosis B48.8
Adie (-Holmes) **pupil or syndrome** —*see* Anomaly, pupil, function, tonic pupil
Adiponecrosis neonatorum P83.8
Adiposis —*see also* Obesity
cerebralis E23.6
dolorosa E88.2
Adiposity —*see also* Obesity
heart —*see* Degeneration, myocardial
localized E65
Adiposogenital dystrophy E23.6
Adjustment
disorder —*see* Disorder, adjustment
implanted device —*see* Encounter (for), adjustment (of)
prosthesis, external —*see* Fitting
reaction —*see* Disorder, adjustment
Administration of tPA (rtPA) in a different facility within the last 24 hours prior to admission to current facility Z92.82
Admission (for) —*see also* Encounter (for)
adjustment (of)
artificial
arm Z44.00-
complete Z44.01-
partial Z44.02-
eye Z44.2

A

Admission *(Continued)*
adjustment *(Continued)*
artificial *(Continued)*
leg Z44.10-
complete Z44.11-
partial Z44.12-
brain neuropacemaker Z46.2
implanted Z45.42
breast
implant Z45.81
prosthesis (external) Z44.3
colostomy belt Z46.89
contact lenses Z46.0
cystostomy device Z46.6
dental prosthesis Z46.3
device NEC
abdominal Z46.89
implanted Z45.89
cardiac Z45.09
defibrillator (with synchronous cardiace pacemaker) Z45.02
pacemaker (cardiac resynchronization therapy (CRT-P)) Z45.018
pulse generator Z45.010
resynchronization therapy defibrillator (CRT-D) Z45.02 ◀
hearing device Z45.328
bone conduction Z45.320
cochlear Z45.321
infusion pump Z45.1
nervous system Z45.49
CSF drainage Z45.41
hearing device —*see* Admission, adjustment, device, implanted, hearing device
neuropacemaker Z45.42
visual substitution Z45.31
specified NEC Z45.89
vascular access Z45.2
visual substitution Z45.31
nervous system Z46.2
implanted —*see* Admission, adjustment, device, implanted, nervous system
orthodontic Z46.4
prosthetic Z44.9
arm —*see* Admission, adjustment, artificial, arm
breast Z44.3
dental Z46.3
eye Z44.2
leg —*see* Admission, adjustment, artificial, leg
specified type NEC Z44.8
substitution
auditory Z46.2
implanted —*see* Admission, adjustment, device, implanted, hearing device
nervous system Z46.2
implanted —*see* Admission, adjustment, device, implanted, nervous system
visual Z46.2
implanted Z45.31
urinary Z46.6
hearing aid Z46.1
implanted —*see* Admission, adjustment, device, implanted, hearing device
ileostomy device Z46.89
intestinal appliance or device NEC Z46.89
neuropacemaker (brain) (peripheral nerve) (spinal cord) Z46.2
implanted Z45.42
orthodontic device Z46.4
orthopedic (brace) (cast) (device) (shoes) Z46.89
pacemaker (cardiac resynchronization therapy (CRT-P))
cardiac Z45.018
pulse generator Z45.010

Admission *(Continued)*
adjustment *(Continued)*
pacemaker *(Continued)*
nervous system Z46.2
implanted Z45.42
portacath (port-a-cath) Z45.2
prosthesis Z44.9
arm —*see* Admission, adjustment, artificial, arm
breast Z44.3
dental Z46.3
eye Z44.2
leg —*see* Admission, adjustment, artificial, leg
specified NEC Z44.8
spectacles Z46.0
aftercare (*see also* Aftercare) Z51.89
postpartum
immediately after delivery Z39.0
routine follow-up Z39.2
radiation therapy (antineoplastic) Z51.0
attention to artificial opening (of) Z43.9
artificial vagina Z43.7
colostomy Z43.3
cystostomy Z43.5
enterostomy Z43.4
gastrostomy Z43.1
ileostomy Z43.2
jejunostomy Z43.4
nephrostomy Z43.6
specified site NEC Z43.8
intestinal tract Z43.4
urinary tract Z43.6
tracheostomy Z43.0
ureterostomy Z43.6
urethrostomy Z43.6
breast augmentation or reduction Z41.1
breast reconstruction following mastectomy Z42.1
change of
dressing (nonsurgical) Z48.00
neuropacemaker device (brain) (peripheral nerve) (spinal cord) Z46.2
implanted Z45.42
surgical dressing Z48.01
circumcision, ritual or routine (in absence of diagnosis) Z41.2
clinical research investigation (control) (normal comparison) (participant) Z00.6
contraceptive management Z30.9
cosmetic surgery NEC Z41.1
counseling (*see also* Counseling)
dietary Z71.3
gestational carrier Z31.7 ◀
HIV Z71.7
human immunodeficiency virus Z71.7
nonattending third party Z71.0
procreative management NEC Z31.69
delivery, full-term, uncomplicated O80
cesarean, without indication O82
desensitization to allergens Z51.6 ◀
dietary surveillance and counseling Z71.3
ear piercing Z41.3
examination at health care facility (adult) —*see also* Examination Z00.00
with abnormal findings Z00.01
clinical research investigation (control) (normal comparison) (participant) Z00.6
dental Z01.20
with abnormal findings Z01.21
donor (potential) Z00.5
ear Z01.10
with abnormal findings NEC Z01.118
eye Z01.00
with abnormal findings Z01.01
general, specified reason NEC Z00.8
hearing Z01.10
with abnormal findings NEC Z01.118
postpartum checkup Z39.2
psychiatric (general) Z00.8
requested by authority Z04.6

Admission *(Continued)*
examination at health care facility *(Continued)*
vision Z01.00
with abnormal findings Z01.01
fitting (of)
artificial
arm —*see* Admission, adjustment, artificial, arm
eye Z44.2
leg —*see* Admission, adjustment, artificial, leg
brain neuropacemaker Z46.2
implanted Z45.42
breast prosthesis (external) Z44.3
colostomy belt Z46.89
contact lenses Z46.0
cystostomy device Z46.6
dental prosthesis Z46.3
dentures Z46.3
device NEC
abdominal Z46.89
nervous system Z46.2
implanted —*see* Admission, adjustment, device, implanted, nervous system
orthodontic Z46.4
prosthetic Z44.9
breast Z44.3
dental Z46.3
eye Z44.2
substitution
auditory Z46.2
implanted —*see* Admission, adjustment, device, implanted, hearing device
nervous system Z46.2
implanted —*see* Admission, adjustment, device, implanted, nervous system
visual Z46.2
implanted Z45.31
hearing aid Z46.1
ileostomy device Z46.89
intestinal appliance or device NEC Z46.89
neuropacemaker (brain) (peripheral nerve) (spinal cord) Z46.2
implanted Z45.42
orthodontic device Z46.4
orthopedic device (brace) (cast) (shoes) Z46.89
prosthesis Z44.9
arm —*see* Admission, adjustment, artificial, arm
breast Z44.3
dental Z46.3
eye Z44.2
leg —*see* Admission, adjustment, artificial, leg
specified type NEC Z44.8
spectacles Z46.0
follow-up examination Z09
intrauterine device management Z30.431
initial prescription Z30.014
mental health evaluation Z00.8
requested by authority Z04.6
observation —*see* Observation
Papanicolaou smear, cervix Z12.4
for suspected malignant neoplasm Z12.4
plastic and reconstructive surgery following medical procedure or healed injury NEC Z42.8
plastic surgery, cosmetic NEC Z41.1
postpartum observation
immediately after delivery Z39.0
routine follow-up Z39.2
poststerilization (for restoration) Z31.0
aftercare Z31.42
procreative management Z31.9
prophylactic (measure) —*see also* Encounter, prophylactic measures
organ removal Z40.00
breast Z40.01
ovary Z40.02

A

◀ New ◀ Revised ~~deleted~~ Deleted

Admission *(Continued)*
prophylactic *(Continued)*
organ removal *(Continued)*
specified organ NEC Z40.09
testes Z40.09
vaccination Z23
psychiatric examination (general) Z00.8
requested by authority Z04.6
radiation therapy (antineoplastic) Z51.0
reconstructive surgery following medical procedure or healed injury NEC Z42.8
removal of
cystostomy catheter Z43.5
drains Z48.03
dressing (nonsurgical) Z48.00
implantable subdermal contraceptive Z30.46 ◀
intrauterine contraceptive device Z30.432
neuropacemaker (brain) (peripheral nerve) (spinal cord) Z46.2
implanted Z45.42
staples Z48.02
surgical dressing Z48.01
sutures Z48.02
ureteral stent Z46.6
respirator [ventilator] use during power failure Z99.12
restoration of organ continuity (poststerilization) Z31.0
aftercare Z31.42
sensitivity test —*see also* Test, skin
allergy NEC Z01.82
Mantoux Z11.1
tuboplasty following previous sterilization Z31.0
aftercare Z31.42
vasoplasty following previous sterilization Z31.0
aftercare Z31.42
vision examination Z01.00
with abnormal findings Z01.01
waiting period for admission to other facility Z75.1
Adnexitis (suppurative) —*see* Salpingo-oophoritis
Adolescent X-linked adrenoleukodystrophy E71.521
Adrenal (gland) —*see* condition
Adrenalism, tuberculous A18.7
Adrenalitis, adrenitis E27.8
autoimmune E27.1
meningococcal, hemorrhagic A39.1
Adrenarche, premature E27.0
Adrenocortical syndrome —*see* Cushing's, syndrome
Adrenogenital syndrome E25.9
acquired E25.8
congenital E25.0
salt loss E25.0
Adrenogenitalism, congenital E25.0
Adrenoleukodystrophy E71.529
neonatal E71.511
X-linked E71.529
Addison only phenotype E71.528
Addison-Schilder E71.528
adolescent E71.521
adrenomyeloneuropathy E71.522
childhood cerebral E71.520
other specified E71.528
Adrenomyeloneuropathy E71.522
Adventitious bursa —*see* Bursopathy, specified type NEC
Adverse effect —*see* Table of Drugs and Chemicals, categories T36-T50, with 6th character 5
Advice —*see* Counseling
Adynamia (episodica) (hereditary) (periodic) G72.3
Aeration lung imperfect, newborn —*see* Atelectasis
Aerobullosis T70.3
Aerocele —*see* Embolism, air
Aerodermectasia
subcutaneous (traumatic) T79.7
Aerodontalgia T70.29
Aeroembolism T70.3
Aerogenes capsulatus infection A48.0
Aero-otitis media T70.0
Aerophagy, aerophagia (psychogenic) F45.8
Aerophobia F40.228
Aerosinusitis T70.1
Aerotitis T70.0
Affection —*see* Disease
Afibrinogenemia —*see also* Defect, coagulation D68.8
acquired D65
congenital D68.2
following ectopic or molar pregnancy O08.1
in abortion —*see* Abortion, by type, complicated by, afibrinogenemia
puerperal O72.3
African
sleeping sickness B56.9
tick fever A68.1
trypanosomiasis B56.9
gambian B56.0
rhodesian B56.1
Aftercare —*see also* Care Z51.89
following surgery (for) (on)
amputation Z47.81
attention to
drains Z48.03
dressings (nonsurgical) Z48.00
surgical Z48.01
sutures Z48.02
circulatory system Z48.812
delayed (planned) wound closure Z48.1
digestive system Z48.815
explantation of joint prosthesis (staged procedure)
hip Z47.32
knee Z47.33
shoulder Z47.31
genitourinary system Z48.816
joint replacement Z47.1
neoplasm Z48.3
nervous system Z48.811
oral cavity Z48.814
organ transplant
bone marrow Z48.290
heart Z48.21
heart-lung Z48.280
kidney Z48.22
liver Z48.23
lung Z48.24
multiple organs NEC Z48.288
specified NEC Z48.298
orthopedic NEC Z47.89
planned wound closure Z48.1
removal of internal fixation device Z47.2
respiratory system Z48.813
scoliosis Z47.82
sense organs Z48.810
skin and subcutaneous tissue Z48.817
specified body system
circulatory Z48.812
digestive Z48.815
genitourinary Z48.816
nervous Z48.811
oral cavity Z48.814
respiratory Z48.813
sense organs Z48.810
skin and subcutaneous tissue Z48.817
teeth Z48.814
specified NEC Z48.89
spinal Z48.89
teeth Z48.814
fracture — code to fracture with seventh character D
involving
removal of
drains Z48.03
dressings (nonsurgical) Z48.00
Aftercare *(Continued)*
involving *(Continued)*
removal of *(Continued)*
staples Z48.02
surgical dressings Z48.01
sutures Z48.02
neuropacemaker (brain) (peripheral nerve) (spinal cord) Z46.2
implanted Z45.42
orthopedic NEC Z47.89
postprocedural —*see* Aftercare, following surgery
After-cataract —*see* Cataract, secondary
Agalactia (primary) O92.3
elective, secondary or therapeutic O92.5
Agammaglobulinemia (acquired (secondary)) (nonfamilial) D80.1
with
immunoglobulin-bearing B-lymphocytes D80.1
lymphopenia D81.9
autosomal recessive (Swiss type) D80.0
Bruton's X-linked D80.0
common variable (CVAgamma) D80.1
congenital sex-linked D80.0
hereditary D80.0
lymphopenic D81.9
Swiss type (autosomal recessive) D80.0
X-linked (with growth hormone deficiency) (Bruton) D80.0 ⟸
Aganglionosis (bowel) (colon) Q43.1
Age (old) —*see* Senility
Agenesis
adrenal (gland) Q89.1
alimentary tract (complete) (partial) NEC Q45.8
upper Q40.8
anus, anal (canal) Q42.3
with fistula Q42.2
aorta Q25.41 ⟸
appendix Q42.8
arm (complete) Q71.0-
with hand present Q71.1-
artery (peripheral) Q27.9
brain Q28.3
coronary Q24.5
pulmonary Q25.79
specified NEC Q27.8
umbilical Q27.0
auditory (canal) (external) Q16.1
auricle (ear) Q16.0
bile duct or passage Q44.5
bladder Q64.5
bone Q79.9
brain Q00.0
part of Q04.3
breast (with nipple present) Q83.8
with absent nipple Q83.0
bronchus Q32.4
canaliculus lacrimalis Q10.4
carpus —*see* Agenesis, hand
cartilage Q79.9
cecum Q42.8
cerebellum Q04.3
cervix Q51.5
chin Q18.8
cilia Q10.3
circulatory system, part NOS Q28.9
clavicle Q74.0
clitoris Q52.6
coccyx Q76.49
colon Q42.9
specified NEC Q42.8
corpus callosum Q04.0
cricoid cartilage Q31.8
diaphragm (with hernia) Q79.1
digestive organ (s) or tract (complete) (partial) NEC Q45.8
upper Q40.8
ductus arteriosus Q28.8
duodenum Q41.0

A

Agenesis *(Continued)*
ear Q16.9
auricle Q16.0
lobe Q17.8
ejaculatory duct Q55.4
endocrine (gland) NEC Q89.2
epiglottis Q31.8
esophagus Q39.8
eustachian tube Q16.2
eye Q11.1
adnexa Q15.8
eyelid (fold) Q10.3
face
bones NEC Q75.8
specified part NEC Q18.8
fallopian tube Q50.6
femur —*see* Defect, reduction, lower limb, longitudinal, femur
fibula —*see* Defect, reduction, lower limb, longitudinal, fibula
finger (complete) (partial) —*see* Agenesis, hand
foot (and toes) (complete) (partial) Q72.3-
forearm (with hand present) —*see* Agenesis, arm, with hand present
and hand Q71.2-
gallbladder Q44.0
gastric Q40.2
genitalia, genital (organ (s))
female Q52.8
external Q52.71
internal NEC Q52.8
male Q55.8
glottis Q31.8
hair Q84.0
hand (and fingers) (complete) (partial) Q71.3-
heart Q24.8
valve NEC Q24.8
pulmonary Q22.0
hepatic Q44.7
humerus —*see* Defect, reduction, upper limb
hymen Q52.4
ileum Q41.2
incus Q16.3
intestine (small) Q41.9
large Q42.9
specified NEC Q42.8
iris (dilator fibers) Q13.1
jaw M26.09
jejunum Q41.1
kidney (s) (partial) Q60.2
bilateral Q60.1
unilateral Q60.0
labium (majus) (minus) Q52.71
labyrinth, membranous Q16.5
lacrimal apparatus Q10.4
larynx Q31.8
leg (complete) Q72.0-
with foot present Q72.1-
lower leg (with foot present) —*see* Agenesis, leg, with foot present
and foot Q72.2-
lens Q12.3
limb (complete) Q73.0
lower —*see* Agenesis, leg
upper —*see* Agenesis, arm
lip Q38.0
liver Q44.7
lung (fissure) (lobe) (bilateral) (unilateral) Q33.3
mandible, maxilla M26.09
metacarpus —*see* Agenesis, hand
metatarsus —*see* Agenesis, foot
muscle Q79.8
eyelid Q10.3
ocular Q15.8
musculoskeletal system NEC Q79.8
nail (s) Q84.3
neck, part Q18.8
nerve Q07.8
nervous system, part NEC Q07.8

Agenesis *(Continued)*
nipple Q83.2
nose Q30.1
nuclear Q07.8
organ
of Corti Q16.5
or site not listed —*see* Anomaly, by site
osseous meatus (ear) Q16.1
ovary
bilateral Q50.02
unilateral Q50.01
oviduct Q50.6
pancreas Q45.0
parathyroid (gland) Q89.2
parotid gland (s) Q38.4
patella Q74.1
pelvic girdle (complete) (partial) Q74.2
penis Q55.5
pericardium Q24.8
pituitary (gland) Q89.2
prostate Q55.4
punctum lacrimale Q10.4
radioulnar —*see* Defect, reduction, upper limb
radius —*see* Defect, reduction, upper limb, longitudinal, radius
rectum Q42.1
with fistula Q42.0
renal Q60.2
bilateral Q60.1
unilateral Q60.0
respiratory organ NEC Q34.8
rib Q76.6
roof of orbit Q75.8
round ligament Q52.8
sacrum Q76.49
salivary gland Q38.4
scapula Q74.0
scrotum Q55.29
seminal vesicles Q55.4
septum
atrial Q21.1
between aorta and pulmonary artery Q21.4
ventricular Q20.4
shoulder girdle (complete) (partial) Q74.0
skull (bone) Q75.8
with
anencephaly Q00.0
encephalocele —*see* Encephalocele
hydrocephalus Q03.9
with spina bifida —*see* Spina bifida, by site, with hydrocephalus
microcephaly Q02
spermatic cord Q55.4
spinal cord Q06.0
spine Q76.49
spleen Q89.01
sternum Q76.7
stomach Q40.2
submaxillary gland (s) (congenital) Q38.4
tarsus —*see* Agenesis, foot
tendon Q79.8
testicle Q55.0
thymus (gland) Q89.2
thyroid (gland) E03.1
cartilage Q31.8
tibia —*see* Defect, reduction, lower limb, longitudinal, tibia
tibiofibular —*see* Defect, reduction, lower limb, specified type NEC
toe (and foot) (complete) (partial) —*see* Agenesis, foot
tongue Q38.3
trachea (cartilage) Q32.1
ulna —*see* Defect, reduction, upper limb, longitudinal, ulna
upper limb —*see* Agenesis, arm
ureter Q62.4
urethra Q64.5
urinary tract NEC Q64.8

Agenesis *(Continued)*
uterus Q51.0
uvula Q38.5
vagina Q52.0
vas deferens Q55.4
vein (s) (peripheral) Q27.9
brain Q28.3
great NEC Q26.8
portal Q26.5
vena cava (inferior) (superior) Q26.8
vermis of cerebellum Q04.3
vertebra Q76.49
vulva Q52.71
Ageusia R43.2
Agitated —*see* condition
Agitation R45.1
Aglossia (congenital) Q38.3
Aglossia-adactylia syndrome Q87.0
Aglycogenosis E74.00
Agnosia (body image) (other senses) (tactile) R48.1
developmental F88
verbal R48.1
auditory R48.1
developmental F80.2
developmental F80.2
visual (object) R48.3
Agoraphobia F40.00
with panic disorder F40.01
without panic disorder F40.02
Agrammatism R48.8
Agranulocytopenia —*see* Agranulocytosis
Agranulocytosis (chronic) (cyclical) (genetic) (infantile) (periodic) (pernicious) (*see also* Neutropenia) D70.9
congenital D70.0
cytoreductive cancer chemotherapy sequela D70.1
drug-induced D70.2
due to cytoreductive cancer chemotherapy D70.1
due to infection D70.3
secondary D70.4
drug-induced D70.2
due to cytoreductive cancer chemotherapy D70.1
Agraphia (absolute) R48.8
with alexia R48.0
developmental F81.81
Ague (dumb) —*see* Malaria
Agyria Q04.3
Ahumada-del Castillo syndrome E23.0
Aichomophobia F40.298
AIDS (related complex) B20
Ailment heart —*see* Disease, heart
Ailurophobia F40.218
Ainhum (disease) L94.6
AIN —*see* Neoplasia, intraepithelial, anal ◀
AIPHI (acute idiopathic pulmonary hemorrhage in infants (over 28 days old)) R04.81
Air
anterior mediastinum J98.2
compressed, disease T70.3
conditioner lung or pneumonitis J67.7
embolism (artery) (cerebral) (any site) T79.0
with ectopic or molar pregnancy O08.2
due to implanted device NEC —*see* Complications, by site and type, specified NEC
following
abortion —*see* Abortion by type, complicated by, embolism
ectopic or molar pregnancy O08.2
infusion, therapeutic injection or transfusion T80.0
in pregnancy, childbirth or puerperium —*see* Embolism, obstetric
traumatic T79.0
hunger, psychogenic F45.8
rarefied, effects of —*see* Effect, adverse, high altitude
sickness T75.3

A

◀ New ◀ Revised ~~deleted~~ Deleted

Airplane sickness T75.3
Akathisia (drug-induced) (treatment- induced) G25.71
neuroleptic induced (acute) G25.71
Akinesia R29.898
Akinetic mutism R41.89
Akureyri's disease G93.3
Alactasia, congenital E73.0
Alagille's syndrome Q44.7
Alastrim B03
Albers-Schönberg syndrome Q78.2
Albert's syndrome —*see* Tendinitis, Achilles
Albinism, albino E70.30
with hematologic abnormality E70.339
Chédiak-Higashi syndrome E70.330
Hermansky-Pudlak syndrome E70.331
other specified E70.338
I E70.320
II E70.321
ocular E70.319
autosomal recessive E70.311
other specified E70.318
X-linked E70.310
oculocutaneous E70.329
other specified E70.328
tyrosinase (ty) negative E70.320
tyrosinase (ty) positive E70.321
other specified E70.39
Albinismus E70.30
Albright (-McCune)(-Sternberg) syndrome Q78.1
Albuminous —*see* condition
Albuminuria, albuminuric (acute) (chronic) (subacute) —*see also* Proteinuria R80.9
complicating pregnancy —*see* Proteinuria, gestational
with
gestational hypertension —*see* Pre-eclampsia
pre-existing hypertension —*see* Hypertension, complicating pregnancy, pre-existing, with, pre-eclampsia
gestational —*see* Proteinuria, gestational
with
gestational hypertension —*see* Pre-eclampsia
pre-existing hypertension —*see* Hypertension, complicating pregnancy, pre-existing, with, pre-eclampsia
orthostatic R80.2
postural R80.2
pre-eclamptic —*see* Pre-eclampsia
scarlatinal A38.8
Albuminurophobia F40.298
Alcaptonuria E70.29
Alcohol, alcoholic, alcohol-induced
addiction (without remission) F10.20
with remission F10.21
amnestic disorder, persisting F10.96
with dependence F10.26
anxiety disorder F10.980 ◀
bipolar and related disorder F10.94 ◀
brain syndrome, chronic F10.97
with dependence F10.27
cardiopathy I42.6
counseling and surveillance Z71.41
family member Z71.42
delirium (acute) (tremens) (withdrawal) F10.231
with intoxication F10.921
in
abuse F10.121
dependence F10.221
dementia F10.97
with dependence F10.27
depressive disorder F10.94 ◀
deterioration F10.97
with dependence F10.27
Alcohol, alcoholic, alcohol-induced *(Continued)*
hallucinosis (acute) F10.951
in
abuse F10.151
dependence F10.251
insanity F10.959
intoxication (acute) (without dependence) F10.129
with
delirium F10.121
dependence F10.229
with delirium F10.221
uncomplicated F10.220
uncomplicated F10.120
jealousy F10.988
Korsakoff's, Korsakov's, Korsakow's F10.26
liver K70.9
acute —*see* Disease, liver, alcoholic, hepatitis
major neurocognitive disorder, amnestic-confabulatory type F10.96 ◀
major neurocognitive disorder, nonamnestic-confabulatory type F10.97 ◀
mania (acute) (chronic) F10.959
mild neurocognitive disorder F10.988 ◀
paranoia, paranoid (type) psychosis F10.950
pellagra E52
poisoning, accidental (acute) NEC —*see* Table of Drugs and Chemicals, alcohol, poisoning
psychosis —*see* Psychosis, alcoholic
psychotic disorder F10.959 ◀
sexual dysfunction F10.981 ◀
sleep disorder F10.982 ◀
withdrawal (without convulsions) F10.239
with delirium F10.231
Alcoholism (chronic) (without remission) F10.20
with
psychosis —*see* Psychosis, alcoholic
remission F10.21
Korsakov's F10.96
with dependence F10.26
Alder (-Reilly) anomaly or syndrome (leukocyte granulation) D72.0
Aldosteronism E26.9
familial (type I) E26.02
glucocorticoid-remediable E26.02
primary (due to (bilateral) adrenal hyperplasia) E26.09
primary NEC E26.09
secondary E26.1
specified NEC E26.89
Aldosteronoma D44.10
Aldrich(-Wiskott) syndrome (eczema-thrombocytopenia) D82.0
Alektorophobia F40.218
Aleppo boil B55.1
Aleukemic —*see* condition Aleukia
congenital D70.0
hemorrhagica D61.9
congenital D61.09
splenica D73.1
Alexia R48.0
developmental F81.0
secondary to organic lesion R48.0
Algoneurodystrophy M89.00
ankle M89.07-
foot M89.07-
forearm M89.03-
hand M89.04-
lower leg M89.06-
multiple sites M89.0-
shoulder M89.01-
specified site NEC M89.08
thigh M89.05-
upper arm M89.02-
Algophobia F40.298
Alienation, mental —*see* Psychosis
Alkalemia E87.3
Alkalosis E87.3
metabolic E87.3
with respiratory acidosis E87.4
respiratory E87.3
Alkaptonuria E70.29
Allen-Masters syndrome N83.8
Allergy, allergic (reaction) (to) T78.40
air-borne substance NEC (rhinitis) J30.89
alveolitis (extrinsic) J67.9
due to
Aspergillus clavatus J67.4
Cryptostroma corticale J67.6
organisms (fungal, thermophilic actinomycete) growing in ventilation (air conditioning) systems J67.7
specified type NEC J67.8
anaphylactic reaction or shock T78.2
angioneurotic edema T78.3
animal (dander) (epidermal) (hair) (rhinitis) J30.81
bee sting (anaphylactic shock) —*see* Toxicity, venom, arthropod, bee
biological —*see* Allergy, drug
colitis —*see also* Colitis, allergic K52.29 ⬅
dander (animal) (rhinitis) J30.81
dandruff (rhinitis) J30.81
dental restorative material (existing) K08.55
dermatitis —*see* Dermatitis, contact, allergic
diathesis —*see* History, allergy
drug, medicament & biological (any) (external) (internal) T78.40
correct substance properly administered —*see* Table of Drugs and Chemicals, by drug, adverse effect
wrong substance given or taken NEC (by accident) —*see* Table of Drugs and Chemicals, by drug, poisoning
due to pollen J30.1
dust (house) (stock) (rhinitis) J30.89
with asthma —*see* Asthma, allergic extrinsic
eczema —*see* Dermatitis, contact, allergic
epidermal (animal) (rhinitis) J30.81
feathers (rhinitis) J30.89
food (any) (ingested) NEC T78.1
anaphylactic shock —*see* Shock, anaphylactic, due to food
dermatitis —*see* Dermatitis, due to, food
dietary counseling and surveillance Z71.3
in contact with skin L23.6
rhinitis J30.5
status (without reaction) Z91.018
eggs Z91.012
milk products Z91.011
peanuts Z91.010
seafood Z91.013
specified NEC Z91.018
gastrointestinal —*see also* specific type of allergic reaction ⬅
meaning colitis —*see also* Colitis, allergic) K52.29 ◀
meaning gastroenteritis —*see also* Gastroenteritis, allergic) K52.29 ◀
meaning other adverse food reaction not elsewhere classified T78.1 ◀
grain J30.1
grass (hay fever) (pollen) J30.1
asthma —*see* Asthma, allergic extrinsic
hair (animal) (rhinitis) J30.81
history (of) —*see* History, allergy
horse serum —*see* Allergy, serum
inhalant (rhinitis) J30.89
pollen J30.1
kapok (rhinitis) J30.89
medicine —*see* Allergy, drug
milk protein —*see also* Allergy, food Z91.011 ⬅
anaphylactic reaction T78.07 ◀
dermatitis L27.2 ◀
enterocolitis syndrome K52.21 ◀
enteropathy K52.22 ◀
gastroenteritis K52.29 ◀

A

Allergy, allergic *(Continued)*
milk protein *(Continued)*
gastroesophageal reflux —*see also* Reaction, adverse, food) K21.9 ◀
with esophagitis K21.0 ◀
proctocolitis K52.82 ◀]
nasal, seasonal due to pollen J30.1
pneumonia J82
pollen (any) (hay fever) J30.1
asthma —*see* Asthma, allergic extrinsic
primrose J30.1
primula J30.1
proctocolitis K52.82 ◀
purpura D69.0
ragweed (hay fever) (pollen) J30.1
asthma —*see* Asthma, allergic extrinsic
rose (pollen) J30.1
seasonal NEC J30.2
Senecio jacobae (pollen) J30.1
serum —*see also* Reaction, serum T80.69
anaphylactic shock T80.59
shock (anaphylactic) T78.2
due to
administration of blood and blood products T80.51
adverse effect of correct medicinal substance properly administered T88.6
immunization T80.52
serum NEC T80.59
vaccination T80.52
specific NEC T78.49
tree (any) (hay fever) (pollen) J30.1
asthma —*see* Asthma, allergic extrinsic
upper respiratory J30.9
urticaria L50.0
vaccine —*see* Allergy, serum
wheat —*see* Allergy, food
Allescheriasis B48.2
Alligator skin disease Q80.9
Allocheiria, allochiria R20.8
Almeida's disease —*see* Paracoccidioidomycosis
Alopecia (hereditaria) (seborrheica) L65.9
androgenic L64.9
drug-induced L64.0
specified NEC L64.8
areata L63.9
ophiasis L63.2
specified NEC L63.8
totalis L63.0
universalis L63.1
cicatricial L66.9
specified NEC L66.8
circumscripta L63.9
congenital, congenitalis Q84.0
due to cytotoxic drugs NEC L65.8
mucinosa L65.2
postinfective NEC L65.8
postpartum L65.0
premature L64.8
specific (syphilitic) A51.32
specified NEC L65.8
syphilitic (secondary) A51.32
totalis (capitis) L63.0
universalis (entire body) L63.1
X-ray L58.1
Alpers' disease G31.81
Alpine sickness T70.29
Alport syndrome Q87.81
ALTE (apparent life threatening event) in newborn and infant R68.13
Alteration (of), **Altered**
~~awareness, transient R40.4~~
awareness ◀
transient R40.4 ◀
unintended under general anesthesia, during procedure T88.53 ◀
mental status R41.82
pattern of family relationships affecting child Z62.898
Alteration (of), **Altered** *(Continued)*
sensation
following
cerebrovascular disease I69.998
cerebral infarction I69.398
intracerebral hemorrhage I69.198
nontraumatic intracranial hemorrhage NEC I69.298
specified disease NEC I69.898
subarachnoid hemorrhage I69.098
Alternating —*see* condition
Altitude, high (effects) —*see* Effect, adverse, high altitude
Aluminosis (of lung) J63.0
Alveolitis
allergic (extrinsic) —*see* Pneumonitis, hypersensitivity
due to
Aspergillus clavatus J67.4
Cryptostroma corticale J67.6
fibrosing (cryptogenic) (idiopathic) J84.112
jaw M27.3
sicca dolorosa M27.3
Alveolus, alveolar —*see* condition
Alymphocytosis D72.810
thymic (with immunodeficiency) D82.1
Alymphoplasia, thymic D82.1
Alzheimer's disease or sclerosis —*see* Disease, Alzheimer's
Amastia (with nipple present) Q83.8
with absent nipple Q83.0
Amathophobia F40.228
Amaurosis (acquired) (congenital) —*see also* Blindness
fugax G45.3
hysterical F44.6
Leber's congenital H35.50
uremic —*see* Uremia
Amaurotic idiocy (infantile) (juvenile) (late) E75.4
Amaxophobia F40.248
Ambiguous genitalia Q56.4
Amblyopia (congenital) (ex anopsia) (partial) (suppression) H53.00-
anisometropic —*see* Amblyopia, refractive
deprivation H53.01-
hysterical F44.6
nocturnal —*see also* Blindness, night
vitamin A deficiency E50.5
refractive H53.02-
strabismic H53.03-
suspect H53.04- ◀
tobacco H53.8
toxic NEC H53.8
uremic —*see* Uremia
Ameba, amebic (histolytica) —*see also* Amebiasis
abscess (liver) A06.4
Amebiasis A06.9
with abscess —*see* Abscess, amebic
acute A06.0
chronic (intestine) A06.1
with abscess —*see* Abscess, amebic
cutaneous A06.7
cutis A06.7
cystitis A06.81
genitourinary tract NEC A06.82
hepatic —*see* Abscess, liver, amebic
intestine A06.0
nondysenteric colitis A06.2
skin A06.7
specified site NEC A06.89
Ameboma (of intestine) A06.3
Amelia Q73.0
lower limb —*see* Agenesis, leg
upper limb —*see* Agenesis, arm
Ameloblastoma —*see also* Cyst, calcifying odontogenic
long bones C40.9-
lower limb C40.2-
upper limb C40.0-
malignant C41.1
jaw (bone) (lower) C41.1
upper C41.0
tibial C40.2-
Amelogenesis imperfecta K00.5
nonhereditaria (segmentalis) K00.4
Amenorrhea N91.2
hyperhormonal E28.8
primary N91.0
secondary N91.1
Amentia —*see* Disability, intellectual
Meynert's (nonalcoholic) F04
American
leishmaniasis B55.2
mountain tick fever A93.2
Ametropia —*see* Disorder, refraction
AMH (asymptomatic microscopic hematuria) R31.21 ◀
Amianthosis J61
Amimia R48.8
Amino-acid disorder E72.9
anemia D53.0
Aminoacidopathy E72.9
Aminoaciduria E72.9
Amnes (t)ic syndrome (post-traumatic) F04
induced by
alcohol F10.96
with dependence F10.26
psychoactive NEC F19.96
with
abuse F19.16
dependence F19.26
sedative F13.96
with dependence F13.26
Amnesia R41.3
anterograde R41.1
auditory R48.8
dissociative F44.0
with dissociative fugue F44.1 ◀
hysterical F44.0
postictal in epilepsy —*see* Epilepsy
psychogenic F44.0
retrograde R41.2
transient global G45.4
Amnion, amniotic —*see* condition
Amnionitis —*see* Pregnancy, complicated by
Amok F68.8
Amoral traits F60.89
Amphetamine (or other stimulant) — induced ◀
anxiety disorder F15.980 ◀
bipolar and related disorder F15.94 ◀
delirium F15.921 ◀
depressive disorder F15.94 ◀
obsessive-compulsive and related disorder F15.988 ◀
psychotic disorder F15.959 ◀
sexual dysfunction F15.981 ◀
sleep disorder F15.982 ◀
stimulant withdrawal F15.23 ◀
Ampulla
lower esophagus K22.8
phrenic K22.8
Amputation —*see also* Absence, by site, acquired
neuroma (postoperative) (traumatic) —*see* Complications, amputation stump, neuroma
stump (surgical)
abnormal, painful, or with complication (late) —*see* Complications, amputation stump
healed or old NOS Z89.9
traumatic (complete) (partial)
arm (upper) (complete) S48.91-
at
elbow S58.01-
partial S58.02-
shoulder joint (complete) S48.01-
partial S48.02-
between
elbow and wrist (complete) S58.11-
partial S58.12-
shoulder and elbow (complete) S48.11-
partial S48.12-
partial S48.92-

◀ New ⇐ Revised ~~deleted~~ Deleted

Amputation *(Continued)*
traumatic *(Continued)*
breast (complete) S28.21-
partial S28.22-
clitoris (complete) S38.211
partial S38.212
ear (complete) S08.11-
partial S08.12-
finger (complete) (metacarpophalangeal) S68.11-
index S68.11-
little S68.11-
middle S68.11-
partial S68.12-
index S68.12-
little S68.12-
middle S68.12-
ring S68.12-
ring S68.11-
thumb —*see* Amputation, traumatic, thumb
transphalangeal (complete) S68.61-
index S68.61-
little S68.61-
middle S68.61-
partial S68.62-
index S68.62-
little S68.62-
middle S68.62-
ring S68.62-
ring S68.61-
foot (complete) S98.91-
at ankle level S98.01-
partial S98.02-
midfoot S98.31-
partial S98.32-
partial S98.92-
forearm (complete) S58.91-
at elbow level (complete) S58.01-
partial S58.02-
between elbow and wrist (complete) S58.11-
partial S58.12-
partial S58.92-
genital organ (s) (external)
female (complete) S38.211
partial S38.212
male
penis (complete) S38.221
partial S38.222
scrotum (complete) S38.231
partial S38.232
testes (complete) S38.231
partial S38.232
hand (complete) (wrist level) S68.41-
finger (s) alone —*see* Amputation, traumatic, finger
partial S68.42-
thumb alone —*see* Amputation, traumatic, thumb
transmetacarpal (complete) S68.71-
partial S68.72-
head
ear —*see* Amputation, traumatic, ear
nose (partial) S08.812
complete S08.811
part S08.89
scalp S08.0
hip (and thigh) (complete) S78.91-
at hip joint (complete) S78.01-
partial S78.02-
between hip and knee (complete) S78.11-
partial S78.12-
partial S78.92-
labium (majus) (minus) (complete) S38.21-
partial S38.21-
leg (lower) S88.91-
at knee level S88.01-
partial S88.02-
between knee and ankle S88.11-
partial S88.12-
partial S88.92-

Amputation *(Continued)*
traumatic *(Continued)*
nose (partial) S08.812
complete S08.811
penis (complete) S38.221
partial S38.222
scrotum (complete) S38.231
partial S38.232
shoulder —*see* Amputation, traumatic, arm
at shoulder joint —*see* Amputation, traumatic, arm, at shoulder joint
testes (complete) S38.231
partial S38.232
thigh —*see* Amputation, traumatic, hip
thorax, part of S28.1
breast —*see* Amputation, traumatic, breast
thumb (complete) (metacarpophalangeal) S68.01-
partial S68.02-
transphalangeal (complete) S68.51-
partial S68.52-
toe (lesser) S98.13-
great S98.11-
partial S98.12-
more than one S98.21-
partial S98.22-
partial S98.14-
vulva (complete) S38.211
partial S38.212
Amputee (bilateral) (old) Z89.9
Amsterdam dwarfism Q87.1
Amusia R48.8
developmental F80.89
Amyelencephalus, amyelencephaly Q00.0
Amyelia Q06.0
Amygdalitis —*see* Tonsillitis
Amygdalolith J35.8
Amyloid heart (disease) E85.4 *[I43]*
Amyloidosis (generalized) (primary) E85.9
with lung involvement E85.4 *[J99]*
familial E85.2
genetic E85.2
heart E85.4 *[I43]*
hemodialysis-associated E85.3
liver E85.4 *[K77]*
localized E85.4
neuropathic heredofamilial E85.1
non-neuropathic heredofamilial E85.0
organ limited E85.4
Portuguese E85.1
pulmonary E85.4 *[J99]*
secondary systemic E85.3
skin (lichen) (macular) E85.4 *[L99]*
specified NEC E85.8
subglottic E85.4 *[J99]*
Amylopectinosis (brancher enzyme deficiency) E74.03
Amylophagia —*see* Pica
Amyoplasia congenita Q79.8
Amyotonia M62.89
congenita G70.2
Amyotrophia, amyotrophy, amyotrophic G71.8
congenita Q79.8
diabetic —*see* Diabetes, amyotrophy
lateral sclerosis G12.21
neuralgic G54.5
spinal progressive G12.21
Anacidity, gastric K31.83
psychogenic F45.8
Anaerosis of newborn P28.89
Analbuminemia E88.09
Analgesia —*see* Anesthesia
Analphalipoproteinemia E78.6
Anaphylactic
purpura D69.0
shock or reaction —*see* Shock, anaphylactic
Anaphylactoid shock or reaction —*see* Shock, anaphylactic
Anaphylactoid syndrome of pregnancy O88.01-

Anaphylaxis —*see* Shock, anaphylactic
Anaplasia cervix —*see also* Dysplasia, cervix N87.9
Anaplasmosis, human A77.49
Anarthria R47.1
Anasarca R60.1
cardiac —*see* Failure, heart, congestive
lung J18.2
newborn P83.2
nutritional E43
pulmonary J18.2
renal N04.9
Anastomosis
aneurysmal —*see* Aneurysm
arteriovenous ruptured brain I60.8
intestinal K63.89
complicated NEC K91.89
involving urinary tract N99.89
retinal and choroidal vessels (congenital) Q14.8
Anatomical narrow angle H40.03-
Ancylostoma, ancylostomiasis (braziliense) (caninum) (ceylanicum) (duodenale) B76.0
Necator americanus B76.1
Andersen's disease (glycogen storage) E74.09
Anderson-Fabry disease E75.21
Andes disease T70.29
Andrews' disease (bacterid) L08.89
Androblastoma
benign
specified site —*see* Neoplasm, benign, by site
unspecified site
female D27.9
male D29.20
malignant
specified site —*see* Neoplasm, malignant, by site
unspecified site
female C56.9
male C62.90
specified site —*see* Neoplasm, uncertain behavior, by site
tubular
with lipid storage
specified site —*see* Neoplasm, benign, by site
unspecified site
female D27.9
male D29.20
specified site —*see* Neoplasm, benign, by site
unspecified site
female D27.9
male D29.20
unspecified site
female D39.10
male D40.10
Androgen insensitivity syndrome —*see also* Syndrome, androgen insensitivity E34.50
Androgen resistance syndrome —*see also* Syndrome, androgen insensitivity E34.50
Android pelvis Q74.2
with disproportion (fetopelvic) O33.3
causing obstructed labor O65.3
Androphobia F40.290
Anectasis, pulmonary (newborn) —*see* Atelectasis
Anemia (essential) (general) (hemoglobin deficiency) (infantile) (primary) (profound) D64.9
with (due to) (in)
disorder of
anaerobic glycolysis D55.2
pentose phosphate pathway D55.1
koilonychia D50.9
achlorhydric D50.8
achrestic D53.1
Addison (-Biermer) (pernicious) D51.0
agranulocytic —*see* Agranulocytosis
amino-acid-deficiency D53.0

Anemia *(Continued)*
aplastic D61.9
congenital D61.09
drug-induced D61.1
due to
drugs D61.1
external agents NEC D61.2
infection D61.2
radiation D61.2
idiopathic D61.3
red cell (pure) D60.9
chronic D60.0
congenital D61.01
specified type NEC D60.8
transient D60.1
specified type NEC D61.89
toxic D61.2
aregenerative
congenital D61.09
asiderotic D50.9
atypical (primary) D64.9
Baghdad spring D55.0
Balantidium coli A07.0
Biermer's (pernicious) D51.0
blood loss (chronic) D50.0
acute D62
bothriocephalus B70.0 *[D63.8]*
brickmaker's B76.9 *[D63.8]*
cerebral I67.89
childhood D58.9
chlorotic D50.8
chronic
blood loss D50.0
hemolytic D58.9
idiopathic D59.9
simple D53.9
chronica congenita aregenerativa D61.09
combined system disease NEC D51.0 *[G32.0]*
due to dietary vitamin B12 deficiency D51.3 *[G32.0]*
complicating pregnancy, childbirth or puerperium —*see* Pregnancy, complicated by (management affected by), anemia
congenital P61.4
aplastic D61.09
due to isoimmunization NOS P55.9
dyserythropoietic, dyshematopoietic D64.4
following fetal blood loss P61.3
Heinz body D58.2
hereditary hemolytic NOS D58.9
pernicious D51.0
spherocytic D58.0
Cooley's (erythroblastic) D56.1
cytogenic D51.0
deficiency D53.9
2, 3 diphosphoglycurate mutase D55.2
2, 3 PG D55.2
6 phosphogluconate dehydrogenase D55.1
6-PGD D55.1
amino-acid D53.0
combined B12 and folate D53.1
enzyme D55.9
drug-induced (hemolytic) D59.2
glucose-6-phosphate dehydrogenase (G6PD) D55.0
glycolytic D55.2
nucleotide metabolism D55.3
related to hexose monophosphate (HMP) shunt pathway NEC D55.1
specified type NEC D55.8
erythrocytic glutathione D55.1
folate D52.9
dietary D52.0
drug-induced D52.1
folic acid D52.9
dietary D52.0
drug-induced D52.1
G SH D55.1
G6PD D55.0
GGS-R D55.1

Anemia *(Continued)*
deficiency *(Continued)*
glucose-6-phosphate dehydrogenase D55.0
glutathione reductase D55.1
glyceraldehyde phosphate dehydrogenase D55.2
hexokinase D55.2
iron D50.9
secondary to blood loss (chronic) D50.0
nutritional D53.9
with
poor iron absorption D50.8
specified deficiency NEC D53.8
phosphofructo-aldolase D55.2
phosphoglycerate kinase D55.2
PK D55.2
protein D53.0
pyruvate kinase D55.2
transcobalamin II D51.2
triose-phosphate isomerase D55.2
vitamin B12 NOS D51.9
dietary D51.3
due to
intrinsic factor deficiency D51.0
selective vitamin B12 malabsorption with proteinuria D51.1
pernicious D51.0
specified type NEC D51.8
Diamond-Blackfan (congenital hypoplastic) D61.01
dibothriocephalus B70.0 *[D63.8]*
dimorphic D53.1
diphasic D53.1
Diphyllobothrium (Dibothriocephalus) B70.0 *[D63.8]*
due to (in) (with)
antineoplastic chemotherapy D64.81
blood loss (chronic) D50.0
acute D62
chemotherapy, antineoplastic D64.81
chronic disease classified elsewhere NEC D63.8
chronic kidney disease D63.1
deficiency
amino-acid D53.0
copper D53.8
folate (folic acid) D52.9
dietary D52.0
drug-induced D52.1
molybdenum D53.8
protein D53.0
zinc D53.8
dietary vitamin B12 deficiency D51.3
disorder of
glutathione metabolism D55.1
nucleotide metabolism D55.3
drug —*see* Anemia, by type —*see also* Table of Drugs and Chemicals
end stage renal disease D63.1
enzyme disorder D55.9
fetal blood loss P61.3
fish tapeworm (D latum) infestation B70.0 *[D63.8]*
hemorrhage (chronic) D50.0
acute D62
impaired absorption D50.9
loss of blood (chronic) D50.0
acute D62
myxedema E03.9 *[D63.8]*
Necator americanus B76.1 *[D63.8]*
prematurity P61.2
selective vitamin B12 malabsorption with proteinuria D51.1
transcobalamin II deficiency D51.2
Dyke-Young type (secondary) (symptomatic) D59.1
dyserythropoietic (congenital) D64.4
dyshematopoietic (congenital) D64.4
Egyptian B76.9 *[D63.8]*
elliptocytosis —*see* Elliptocytosis
enzyme-deficiency, drug-induced D59.2

Anemia *(Continued)*
epidemic —*see also* Ancylostomiasis B76.9 *[D63.8]*
erythroblastic
familial D56.1
newborn —*see also* Disease, hemolytic P55.9
of childhood D56.1
erythrocytic glutathione deficiency D55.1
erythropoietin-resistant anemia (EPO resistant anemia) D63.1
Faber's (achlorhydric anemia) D50.9
factitious (self-induced blood letting) D50.0
familial erythroblastic D56.1
Fanconi's (congenital pancytopenia) D61.09
favism D55.0
fish tapeworm (D. latum) infestation B70.0 *[D63.8]*
folate (folic acid) deficiency D52.9
glucose-6-phosphate dehydrogenase (G6PD) deficiency D55.0
glutathione-reductase deficiency D55.1
goat's milk D52.0
granulocytic —*see* Agranulocytosis
Heinz body, congenital D58.2
hemolytic D58.9
acquired D59.9
with hemoglobinuria NEC D59.6
autoimmune NEC D59.1
infectious D59.4
specified type NEC D59.8
toxic D59.4
acute D59.9
due to enzyme deficiency specified type NEC D55.8
Lederer's D59.1
autoimmune D59.1
drug-induced D59.0
chronic D58.9
idiopathic D59.9
cold type (secondary) (symptomatic) D59.1
congenital (spherocytic) —*see* Spherocytosis
due to
cardiac conditions D59.4
drugs (nonautoimmune) D59.2
autoimmune D59.0
enzyme disorder D55.9
drug-induced D59.2
presence of shunt or other internal prosthetic device D59.4
familial D58.9
hereditary D58.9
due to enzyme disorder D55.9
specified type NEC D55.8
specified type NEC D58.8
idiopathic (chronic) D59.9
mechanical D59.4
microangiopathic D59.4
nonautoimmune D59.4
drug-induced D59.2
nonspherocytic
congenital or hereditary NEC D55.8
glucose-6-phosphate dehydrogenase deficiency D55.0
pyruvate kinase deficiency D55.2
type
I D55.1
II D55.2
type
I D55.1
II D55.2
secondary D59.4
autoimmune D59.1
specified (hereditary) type NEC D58.8
Stransky-Regala type —*see also* Hemoglobinopathy D58.8
symptomatic D59.4
autoimmune D59.1
toxic D59.4
warm type (secondary) (symptomatic) D59.1

Anemia *(Continued)*
hemorrhagic (chronic) D50.0
acute D62
Herrick's D57.1
hexokinase deficiency D55.2
hookworm B76.9 *[D63.8]*
hypochromic (idiopathic) (microcytic) (normoblastic) D50.9
due to blood loss (chronic) D50.0
acute D62
familial sex-linked D64.0
pyridoxine-responsive D64.3
sideroblastic, sex-linked D64.0
hypoplasia, red blood cells D61.9
congenital or familial D61.01
hypoplastic (idiopathic) D61.9
congenital or familial (of childhood) D61.01
hypoproliferative (refractive) D61.9
idiopathic D64.9
aplastic D61.3
hemolytic, chronic D59.9
in (due to) (with)
chronic kidney disease D63.1
end stage renal disease D63.1
failure, kidney (renal) D63.1
neoplastic disease —*see also* Neoplasm D63.0
intertropical —*see also* Ancylostomiasis D63.8
iron deficiency D50.9
secondary to blood loss (chronic) D50.0
acute D62
specified type NEC D50.8
Joseph-Diamond-Blackfan (congenital hypoplastic) D61.01
Lederer's (hemolytic) D59.1
leukoerythroblastic D61.82
macrocytic D53.9
nutritional D52.0
tropical D52.8
malarial (*see also* Malaria) B54 *[D63.8]*
malignant (progressive) D51.0
malnutrition D53.9
marsh (*see also* Malaria) B54 *[D63.8]*
Mediterranean (with other hemoglobinopathy) D56.9
megaloblastic D53.1
combined B12 and folate deficiency D53.1
hereditary D51.1
nutritional D52.0
orotic aciduria D53.0
refractory D53.1
specified type NEC D53.1
megalocytic D53.1
microcytic (hypochromic) D50.9
due to blood loss (chronic) D50.0
acute D62
familial D56.8
microdrepanocytosis D57.40
microelliptopoikilocytic (Rietti-Greppi-Micheli) D56.9
miner's B76.9 *[D63.8]*
myelodysplastic D46.9
myelofibrosis D75.81
myelogenous D64.89
myelopathic D64.89
myelophthisic D61.82
myeloproliferative D47.Z9
newborn P61.4
due to
ABO (antibodies, isoimmunization, maternal/fetal incompatibility) P55.1
Rh (antibodies, isoimmunization, maternal/fetal incompatibility) P55.0
following fetal blood loss P61.3
posthemorrhagic (fetal) P61.3
nonspherocytic hemolytic —*see* Anemia, hemolytic, nonspherocytic

Anemia *(Continued)*
normocytic (infectional) D64.9
due to blood loss (chronic) D50.0
acute D62
myelophthisic D61.82
nutritional (deficiency) D53.9
with
poor iron absorption D50.8
specified deficiency NEC D53.8
megaloblastic D52.0
of prematurity P61.2
orotaciduric (congenital) (hereditary) D53.0
osteosclerotic D64.89
ovalocytosis (hereditary) —*see* Elliptocytosis
paludal —*see also* Malaria B54 *[D63.8]*
pernicious (congenital) (malignant) (progressive) D51.0
pleochromic D64.89
of sprue D52.8
posthemorrhagic (chronic) D50.0
acute D62
newborn P61.3
postoperative (postprocedural)
due to (acute) blood loss D62
chronic blood loss D50.0
specified NEC D64.9
postpartum O90.81
pressure D64.89
progressive D64.9
malignant D51.0
pernicious D51.0
protein-deficiency D53.0
pseudoleukemica infantum D64.89
pure red cell D60.9
congenital D61.01
pyridoxine-responsive D64.3
pyruvate kinase deficiency D55.2
refractory D46.4
with
excess of blasts D46.20
1 (RAEB 1) D46.21
2 (RAEB 2) D46.22
in transformation (RAEB T) —*see* Leukemia, acute myeloblastic
hemochromatosis D46.1
sideroblasts (ring) (RARS) D46.1
without ring sideroblasts, so stated D46.0
without sideroblasts without excess of blasts D46.0
megaloblastic D53.1
sideroblastic D46.1
sideropenic D50.9
Rietti-Greppi-Micheli D56.9
scorbutic D53.2
secondary to
blood loss (chronic) D50.0
acute D62
hemorrhage (chronic) D50.0
acute D62
semiplastic D61.89
sickle-cell —*see* Disease, sickle-cell
sideroblastic D64.3
hereditary D64.0
hypochromic, sex-linked D64.0
pyridoxine-responsive NEC D64.3
refractory D46.1
secondary (due to)
disease D64.1
drugs and toxins D64.2
specified type NEC D64.3
sideropenic (refractory) D50.9
due to blood loss (chronic) D50.0
acute D62
simple chronic D53.9
specified type NEC D64.89
spherocytic (hereditary) —*see* Spherocytosis
splenic D64.89
splenomegalic D64.89
stomatocytosis D58.8
syphilitic (acquired) (late) A52.79 *[D63.8]*
target cell D64.89

Anemia *(Continued)*
thalassemia D56.9
thrombocytopenic —*see* Thrombocytopenia
toxic D61.2
tropical B76.9 *[D63.8]*
macrocytic D52.8
tuberculous A18.89 *[D63.8]*
vegan D51.3
vitamin
B6-responsive D64.3
B12 deficiency (dietary) pernicious D51.0
von Jaksch's D64.89
Witts' (achlorhydric anemia) D50.8
Anemophobia F40.228
Anencephalus, anencephaly Q00.0
Anergasia —*see* Psychosis, organic
Anesthesia, anesthetic R20.0
complication or reaction NEC —*see also* Complications, anesthesia T88.59
due to
correct substance properly administered —*see* Table of Drugs and Chemicals, by drug, adverse effect
overdose or wrong substance given —*see* Table of Drugs and Chemicals, by drug, poisoning
unintended awareness under general anesthesia during procedure T88.53 ◀
personal history of Z92.84 ◀
cornea H18.81-
dissociative F44.6
functional (hysterical) F44.6
hyperesthetic, thalamic G89.0
hysterical F44.6
local skin lesion R20.0
sexual (psychogenic) F52.1
shock (due to) T88.2
skin R20.0
testicular N50.9
Anetoderma (maculosum) (of) L90.8
Jadassohn-Pellizzari L90.2
Schweniger-Buzzi L90.1
Aneurin deficiency E51.9
Aneurysm (anastomotic) (artery) (cirsoid) (diffuse) (false) (fusiform) (multiple) (saccular) I72.9
abdominal (aorta) I71.4
ruptured I71.3
syphilitic A52.01
aorta, aortic (nonsyphilitic) I71.9
abdominal I71.4
ruptured I71.3
arch I71.2
ruptured I71.1
arteriosclerotic I71.9
ruptured I71.8
ascending I71.2
ruptured I71.1
congenital Q25.43 ⇐
descending I71.9
abdominal I71.4
ruptured I71.3
ruptured I71.8
thoracic I71.2
ruptured I71.1
root Q25.43 ◀
ruptured I71.8
sinus, congenital Q25.43 ⇐
syphilitic A52.01
thoracic I71.2
ruptured I71.1
thoracoabdominal I71.6
ruptured I71.5
thorax, thoracic (arch) I71.2
ruptured I71.1
transverse I71.2
ruptured I71.1
valve (heart) —*see also* Endocarditis, aortic I35.8

Aneurysm *(Continued)*
arteriosclerotic I72.9
cerebral I67.1
ruptured —*see* Hemorrhage, intracranial, subarachnoid
arteriovenous (congenital) —*see also* Malformation, arteriovenous
acquired I77.0
brain I67.1
coronary I25.41
pulmonary I28.0
brain Q28.2
ruptured I60.8
peripheral —*see* Malformation, arteriovenous, peripheral
precerebral vessels Q28.0
specified site NEC —*see also* Malformation, arteriovenous
acquired I77.0
basal —*see* Aneurysm, brain
basilar (trunk) I72.5 ◀
berry (congenital) (nonruptured) I67.1
ruptured I60.7
brain I67.1
arteriosclerotic I67.1
ruptured —*see* Hemorrhage, intracranial, subarachnoid
arteriovenous (congenital) (nonruptured) Q28.2
acquired I67.1
ruptured I60.8
ruptured I60.8
berry (congenital) (nonruptured) I67.1
ruptured —*see also* Hemorrhage, intracranial, subarachnoid I60.7
congenital Q28.3
aorta (root) (sinus) Q25.43 ◀
ruptured I60.7
meninges I67.1
ruptured I60.8
miliary (congenital) (nonruptured) I67.1
ruptured —*see also* Hemorrhage, intracranial, subarachnoid I60.7
mycotic I33.0
ruptured —*see* Hemorrhage, intracranial, subarachnoid
syphilitic (hemorrhage) A52.05
cardiac (false) —*see also* Aneurysm, heart I25.3
carotid artery (common) (external) I72.0
internal (intracranial) I67.1
extracranial portion I72.0
ruptured into brain I60.0-
syphilitic A52.09
intracranial A52.05
cavernous sinus I67.1
arteriovenous (congenital) (nonruptured) Q28.3
ruptured I60.8
celiac I72.8
central nervous system, syphilitic A52.05
cerebral —*see* Aneurysm, brain
chest —*see* Aneurysm, thorax
circle of Willis I67.1
congenital Q28.3
ruptured I60.6
ruptured I60.6
common iliac artery I72.3
congenital (peripheral) Q27.8
aorta (root) (sinus) Q25.43 ◀
brain Q28.3
ruptured I60.7
coronary Q24.5
digestive system Q27.8
lower limb Q27.8
pulmonary Q25.79
retina Q14.1
specified site NEC Q27.8
upper limb Q27.8
conjunctiva —*see* Abnormality, conjunctiva, vascular
conus arteriosus —*see* Aneurysm, heart

Aneurysm *(Continued)*
coronary (arteriosclerotic) (artery) I25.41
arteriovenous, congenital Q24.5
congenital Q24.5
ruptured —*see* Infarct, myocardium
syphilitic A52.06
vein I25.89
cylindroid (aorta) I71.9
ruptured I71.8
syphilitic A52.01
ductus arteriosus Q25.0
endocardial, infective (any valve) I33.0
femoral (artery) (ruptured) I72.4
gastroduodenal I72.8
gastroepiploic I72.8
heart (wall) (chronic or with a stated duration of over 4 weeks) I25.3
valve —*see* Endocarditis
hepatic I72.8
iliac (common) (artery) (ruptured) I72.3
infective I72.9
endocardial (any valve) I33.0
innominate (nonsyphilitic) I72.8
syphilitic A52.09
interauricular septum —*see* Aneurysm, heart
interventricular septum —*see* Aneurysm, heart
intrathoracic (nonsyphilitic) I71.2
ruptured I71.1
syphilitic A52.01
lower limb I72.4
lung (pulmonary artery) I28.1
mediastinal (nonsyphilitic) I72.8
syphilitic A52.09
miliary (congenital) I67.1
ruptured —*see* Hemorrhage, intracerebral, subarachnoid, intracranial
mitral (heart) (valve) I34.8
mural —*see* Aneurysm, heart
mycotic I72.9
endocardial (any valve) I33.0
ruptured, brain —*see* Hemorrhage, intracerebral, subarachnoid
myocardium —*see* Aneurysm, heart
neck I72.0
pancreaticoduodenal I72.8
patent ductus arteriosus Q25.0
peripheral NEC I72.8
congenital Q27.8
digestive system Q27.8
lower limb Q27.8
specified site NEC Q27.8
upper limb Q27.8
popliteal (artery) (ruptured) I72.4
~~precerebral, congenital (nonruptured) Q28.1~~
precerebral ◀
congenital (nonruptured) Q28.1 ◀
specified site, NEC I72.5 ◀
pulmonary I28.1
arteriovenous Q25.72
acquired I28.0
syphilitic A52.09
valve (heart) —*see* Endocarditis, pulmonary
racemose (peripheral) I72.9
congenital —*see* Aneurysm, congenital
radial I72.1
Rasmussen NEC A15.0
renal (artery) I72.2
retina —*see also* Disorder, retina, microaneurysms
congenital Q14.1
diabetic —*see* Diabetes, microaneurysms, retinal
sinus of Valsalva Q25.49 ⟸
specified NEC I72.8
spinal (cord) I72.8
syphilitic (hemorrhage) A52.09
splenic I72.8

Aneurysm *(Continued)*
subclavian (artery) (ruptured) I72.8
syphilitic A52.09
superior mesenteric I72.8
syphilitic (aorta) A52.01
central nervous system A52.05
congenital (late) A50.54 *[I79.0]*
spine, spinal A52.09
thoracoabdominal (aorta) I71.6
ruptured I71.5
syphilitic A52.01
thorax, thoracic (aorta) (arch) (nonsyphilitic) I71.2
ruptured I71.1
syphilitic A52.01
traumatic (complication) (early), specified site —*see* Injury, blood vessel
tricuspid (heart) (valve) I07.8
ulnar I72.1
upper limb (ruptured) I72.1
valve, valvular —*see* Endocarditis
visceral NEC I72.8
venous —*see also* Varix I86.8
congenital Q27.8
digestive system Q27.8
lower limb Q27.8
specified site NEC Q27.8
upper limb Q27.8
ventricle —*see* Aneurysm, heart
vertebral artery I72.6 ◀
visceral NEC I72.8
Angelman syndrome Q93.5
Anger R45.4
Angiectasis, angiectopia I99.8
Angiitis I77.6
allergic granulomatous M30.1
hypersensitivity M31.0
necrotizing M31.9
specified NEC M31.8
nervous system, granulomatous I67.7
Angina (attack) (cardiac) (chest) (heart) (pectoris) (syndrome) (vasomotor) I20.9
with
atherosclerotic heart disease —*see* Arteriosclerosis, coronary (artery)
documented spasm I20.1
abdominal K55.1
accelerated —*see* Angina, unstable
agranulocytic —*see* Agranulocytosis
angiospastic —*see* Angina, with documented spasm
aphthous B08.5
crescendo —*see* Angina, unstable
croupous J05.0
cruris I73.9
de novo effort —*see* Angina, unstable
diphtheritic, membranous A36.0
equivalent I20.8
exudative, chronic J37.0
following acute myocardial infarction I23.7
gangrenous diphtheritic A36.0
intestinal K55.1
Ludovici K12.2
Ludwig's K12.2
malignant diphtheritic A36.0
membranous J05.0
diphtheritic A36.0
Vincent's A69.1
mesenteric K55.1
monocytic —*see* Mononucleosis, infectious
of effort —*see* Angina, specified NEC
phlegmonous J36
diphtheritic A36.0
post-infarctional I23.7
pre-infarctional —*see* Angina, unstable
Prinzmetal —*see* Angina, with documented spasm
progressive —*see* Angina, unstable
pseudomembranous A69.1
pultaceous, diphtheritic A36.0

◀ New ⟸ Revised ~~deleted~~ Deleted

Angina *(Continued)*
spasm-induced —*see* Angina, with documented spasm
specified NEC I20.8
stable I20.8 ⬅
stenocardia —*see* Angina, specified NEC
stridulous, diphtheritic A36.2
tonsil J36
trachealis J05.0
unstable I20.0
variant —*see* Angina, with documented spasm
Vincent's A69.1
worsening effort —*see* Angina, unstable
Angioblastoma —*see* Neoplasm, connective tissue, uncertain behavior
Angiocholecystitis —*see* Cholecystitis, acute
Angiocholitis —*see also* Cholecystitis, acute K83.0
Angiodysgenesis spinalis G95.19
Angiodysplasia (cecum) (colon) K55.20
with bleeding K55.21
duodenum (and stomach) K31.819
with bleeding K31.811
stomach (and duodenum) K31.819
with bleeding K31.811
Angioedema (allergic) (any site) (with urticaria) T78.3
hereditary D84.1
Angioendothelioma —*see* Neoplasm, uncertain behavior, by site
benign D18.00
intra-abdominal D18.03
intracranial D18.02
skin D18.01
specified site NEC D18.09
bone —*see* Neoplasm, bone, malignant
Ewing's —*see* Neoplasm, bone, malignant
Angioendotheliomatosis C85.8-
Angiofibroma —*see also* Neoplasm, benign, by site
juvenile
specified site —*see* Neoplasm, benign, by site
unspecified site D10.6
Angiohemophilia (A) (B) D68.0
Angioid streaks (choroid) (macula) (retina) H35.33
Angiokeratoma —*see* Neoplasm, skin, benign
corporis diffusum E75.21
Angioleiomyoma —*see* Neoplasm, connective tissue, benign
Angiolipoma —*see also* Lipoma
infiltrating —*see* Lipoma
Angioma —*see also* Hemangioma, by site
capillary I78.1
hemorrhagicum hereditaria I78.0
intra-abdominal D18.03
intracranial D18.02
malignant —*see* Neoplasm, connective tissue, malignant
plexiform D18.00
intra-abdominal D18.03
intracranial D18.02
skin D18.01
specified site NEC D18.09
senile I78.1
serpiginosum L81.7
skin D18.01
specified site NEC D18.09
spider I78.1
stellate I78.1
venous Q28.3
Angiomatosis Q82.8
bacillary A79.89
encephalotrigeminal Q85.8
hemorrhagic familial I78.0
hereditary familial I78.0
liver K76.4
Angiomyolipoma —*see* Lipoma
Angiomyoliposarcoma —*see* Neoplasm, connective tissue, malignant
Angiomyoma —*see* Neoplasm, connective tissue, benign
Angiomyosarcoma —*see* Neoplasm, connective tissue, malignant
Angiomyxoma —*see* Neoplasm, connective tissue, uncertain behavior
Angioneurosis F45.8
Angioneurotic edema (allergic) (any site) (with urticaria) T78.3
hereditary D84.1
Angiopathia, angiopathy I99.9
cerebral I67.9
amyloid E85.4 *[I68.0]*
diabetic (peripheral) —*see* Diabetes, angiopathy
peripheral I73.9
diabetic —*see* Diabetes, angiopathy
specified type NEC I73.89
retinae syphilitica A52.05
retinalis (juvenilis)
diabetic —*see* Diabetes, retinopathy
proliferative —*see* Retinopathy, proliferative
Angiosarcoma —*see also* Neoplasm, connective tissue, malignant
liver C22.3
Angiosclerosis —*see* Arteriosclerosis
Angiospasm (peripheral) (traumatic) (vessel) I73.9
brachial plexus G54.0
cerebral G45.9
cervical plexus G54.2
nerve
arm —*see* Mononeuropathy, upper limb
axillary G54.0
median —*see* Lesion, nerve, median
ulnar —*see* Lesion, nerve, ulnar
axillary G54.0
leg —*see* Mononeuropathy, lower limb
median —*see* Lesion, nerve, median
plantar —*see* Lesion, nerve, plantar
ulnar —*see* Lesion, nerve, ulnar
Angiospastic disease or edema I73.9
Angiostrongyliasis
due to
Parastrongylus
cantonensis B83.2
costaricensis B81.3
intestinal B81.3
Anguillulosis —*see* Strongyloidiasis
Angulation
cecum —*see* Obstruction, intestine
coccyx (acquired) —*see also* subcategory M43.8
congenital NEC Q76.49
femur (acquired) —*see also* Deformity, limb, specified type NEC, thigh
congenital Q74.2
intestine (large) (small) —*see* Obstruction, intestine
sacrum (acquired) —*see also* subcategory M43.8
congenital NEC Q76.49
sigmoid (flexure) —*see* Obstruction, intestine
spine —*see* Dorsopathy, deforming, specified NEC
tibia (acquired) —*see also* Deformity, limb, specified type NEC, lower leg
congenital Q74.2
ureter N13.5
with infection N13.6
wrist (acquired) —*see also* Deformity, limb, specified type NEC, forearm
congenital Q74.0
Angulus infectiosus (lips) K13.0
Anhedonia R45.84
sexual F52.0 ◀
Anhidrosis L74.4
~~Anhydration, anhydremia E86.0~~
~~with~~
~~hypernatremia E87.0~~
~~hyponatremia E87.1~~
Anhydration E86.0 ◀
Anhydremia E86.0
~~with~~
~~hypernatremia E87.0~~
~~hyponatremia E87.1~~
Anidrosis L74.4
Aniridia (congenital) Q13.1
Anisakiasis (infection) (infestation) B81.0
Anisakis larvae infestation B81.0
Aniseikonia H52.32
Anisocoria (pupil) H57.02
congenital Q13.2
Anisocytosis R71.8
Anisometropia (congenital) H52.31
Ankle —*see* condition
Ankyloblepharon (eyelid) (acquired) —*see also* Blepharophimosis
filiforme (adnatum) (congenital) Q10.3
total Q10.3
Ankyloglossia Q38.1
Ankylosis (fibrous) (osseous) (joint) M24.60
ankle M24.67-
arthrodesis status Z98.1
cricoarytenoid (cartilage) (joint) (larynx) J38.7
dental K03.5
ear ossicles H74.31-
elbow M24.62-
foot M24.67-
hand M24.64-
hip M24.65-
incostapedial joint (infectional) —*see* Ankylosis, ear ossicles
jaw (temporomandibular) M26.61- ⬅
knee M24.66-
lumbosacral (joint) M43.27
postoperative (status) Z98.1
produced by surgical fusion, status Z98.1
sacro-iliac (joint) M43.28
shoulder M24.61-
spine (joint) —*see also* Fusion, spine
spondylitic —*see* Spondylitis, ankylosing
surgical Z98.1
temporomandibular M26.61- ⬅
tooth, teeth (hard tissues) K03.5
wrist M24.63-
Ankylostoma —*see* Ancylostoma
Ankylostomiasis —*see* Ancylostomiasis
Ankylurethria —*see* Stricture, urethra
Annular —*see also* condition
detachment, cervix N88.8
organ or site, congenital NEC —*see* Distortion
pancreas (congenital) Q45.1
Anodontia (complete) (partial) (vera) K00.0
acquired K08.10
Anomaly, anomalous (congenital) (unspecified type) Q89.9
abdominal wall NEC Q79.59
acoustic nerve Q07.8
adrenal (gland) Q89.1
Alder (-Reilly) (leukocyte granulation) D72.0
alimentary tract Q45.9
upper Q40.9
alveolar M26.70
hyperplasia M26.79
mandibular M26.72
maxillary M26.71
hypoplasia M26.79
mandibular M26.74
maxillary M26.73
ridge (process) M26.79
specified NEC M26.79
ankle (joint) Q74.2
anus Q43.9
aorta (arch) NEC Q25.40 ⬅
coarctation (preductal) (postductal) Q25.1
aortic cusp or valve Q23.9
appendix Q43.8
apple peel syndrome Q41.1
aqueduct of Sylvius Q03.0
with spina bifida —*see* Spina bifida, with hydrocephalus

Anomaly, anomalous *(Continued)*
arm Q74.0
arteriovenous NEC
coronary Q24.5
gastrointestinal Q27.33
acquired —*see* Angiodysplasia
artery (peripheral) Q27.9
basilar NEC Q28.1
cerebral Q28.3
coronary Q24.5
digestive system Q27.8
eye Q15.8
great Q25.9
specified NEC Q25.8
lower limb Q27.8
peripheral Q27.9
specified NEC Q27.8
pulmonary NEC Q25.79
renal Q27.2
retina Q14.1
specified site NEC Q27.8
subclavian Q27.8
origin Q25.48 ◀
umbilical Q27.0
upper limb Q27.8
vertebral NEC Q28.1
aryteno-epiglottic folds Q31.8
atrial
bands or folds Q20.8
septa Q21.1
atrioventricular
excitation I45.6
septum Q21.0
auditory canal Q17.8
auricle
ear Q17.8
causing impairment of hearing Q16.9
heart Q20.8
Axenfeld's Q15.0
back Q89.9
band
atrial Q20.8
heart Q24.8
ventricular Q24.8
Bartholin's duct Q38.4
biliary duct or passage Q44.5
bladder Q64.70
absence Q64.5
diverticulum Q64.6
exstrophy Q64.10
cloacal Q64.12
extroversion Q64.19
specified type NEC Q64.19
supravesical fissure Q64.11
neck obstruction Q64.31
specified type NEC Q64.79
bone Q79.9
arm Q74.0
face Q75.9
leg Q74.2
pelvic girdle Q74.2
shoulder girdle Q74.0
skull Q75.9
with
anencephaly Q00.0
encephalocele —*see* Encephalocele
hydrocephalus Q03.9
with spina bifida —*see* Spina bifida, by site, with hydrocephalus
microcephaly Q02
brain (multiple) Q04.9
vessel Q28.3
breast Q83.9
broad ligament Q50.6
bronchus Q32.4
bulbus cordis Q21.9
bursa Q79.9
canal of Nuck Q52.4
canthus Q10.3
capillary Q27.9

Anomaly, anomalous *(Continued)*
cardiac Q24.9
chambers Q20.9
specified NEC Q20.8
septal closure Q21.9
specified NEC Q21.8
valve NEC Q24.8
pulmonary Q22.3
cardiovascular system Q28.8
carpus Q74.0
caruncle, lacrimal Q10.6
cascade stomach Q40.2
cauda equina Q06.3
cecum Q43.9
cerebral Q04.9
vessels Q28.3
cervix Q51.9
Chédiak-Higashi(-Steinbrinck) (congenital gigantism of peroxidase granules) E70.330
cheek Q18.9
chest wall Q67.8
bones Q76.9
chin Q18.9
chordae tendineae Q24.8
choroid Q14.3
plexus Q07.8
chromosomes, chromosomal Q99.9
D (1) —*see* condition, chromosome 13
E (3) —*see* condition, chromosome 18
G —*see* condition, chromosome 21
sex
female phenotype Q97.8
gonadal dysgenesis (pure) Q99.1
Klinefelter's Q98.4
male phenotype Q98.9
Turner's Q96.9
specified NEC Q99.8
cilia Q10.3
circulatory system Q28.9
clavicle Q74.0
clitoris Q52.6
coccyx Q76.49
colon Q43.9
common duct Q44.5
communication
coronary artery Q24.5
left ventricle with right atrium Q21.0
concha (ear) Q17.3
connection
portal vein Q26.5
pulmonary venous Q26.4
partial Q26.3
total Q26.2
renal artery with kidney Q27.2
cornea (shape) Q13.4
coronary artery or vein Q24.5
cranium —*see* Anomaly, skull
cricoid cartilage Q31.8
cystic duct Q44.5
dental
alveolar —*see* Anomaly, alveolar
arch relationship M26.20
specified NEC M26.29
dentofacial M26.9
alveolar —*see* Anomaly, alveolar
dental arch relationship M26.20
specified NEC M26.29
functional M26.50
specified NEC M26.59
jaw-cranial base relationship M26.10
asymmetry M26.12
maxillary M26.11
specified type NEC M26.19
jaw size M26.00
macrogenia M26.05
mandibular
hyperplasia M26.03
hypoplasia M26.04
maxillary
hyperplasia M26.01
hypoplasia M26.02

Anomaly, anomalous *(Continued)*
dentofacial *(Continued)*
jaw size *(Continued)*
microgenia M26.06
specified type NEC M26.09
malocclusion M26.4
dental arch relationship NEC M26.29
jaw-cranial base relationship —*see* Anomaly, dentofacial, jaw-cranial base relationship
jaw size —*see* Anomaly, dentofacial, jaw size
specified type NEC M26.89
temporomandibular joint M26.60- ⟸
adhesions M26.61- ⟸
ankylosis M26.61- ⟸
arthralgia M26.62- ⟸
articular disc M26.63- ⟸
specified type NEC M26.69
tooth position, fully erupted M26.30
specified NEC M26.39
dermatoglyphic Q82.8
diaphragm (apertures) NEC Q79.1
digestive organ (s) or tract Q45.9
lower Q43.9
upper Q40.9
distance, interarch (excessive) (inadequate) M26.25
distribution, coronary artery Q24.5
ductus
arteriosus Q25.0
botalli Q25.0
duodenum Q43.9
dura (brain) Q04.9
spinal cord Q06.9
ear (external) Q17.9
causing impairment of hearing Q16.9
inner Q16.5
middle (causing impairment of hearing) Q16.4
ossicles Q16.3
Ebstein's (heart) (tricuspid valve) Q22.5
ectodermal Q82.9
Eisenmenger's (ventricular septal defect) Q21.8
ejaculatory duct Q55.4
elbow Q74.0
endocrine gland NEC Q89.2
epididymis Q55.4
epiglottis Q31.8
esophagus Q39.9
eustachian tube Q17.8
eye Q15.9
anterior segment Q13.9
specified NEC Q13.89
posterior segment Q14.9
specified NEC Q14.8
ptosis (eyelid) Q10.0
specified NEC Q15.8
eyebrow Q18.8
eyelid Q10.3
ptosis Q10.0
face Q18.9
bone(s) Q75.9
fallopian tube Q50.6
fascia Q79.9
femur NEC Q74.2
fibula NEC Q74.2
finger Q74.0
fixation, intestine Q43.3
flexion (joint) NOS Q74.9
hip or thigh Q65.89
foot NEC Q74.2
varus (congenital) Q66.3
foramen
Botalli Q21.1
ovale Q21.1
forearm Q74.0
forehead Q75.8
form, teeth K00.2
fovea centralis Q14.1

◀ New ⟸ Revised ~~deleted~~ Deleted

Anomaly, anomalous *(Continued)*
frontal bone —*see* Anomaly, skull
gallbladder (position) (shape) (size) Q44.1
Gartner's duct Q52.4
gastrointestinal tract Q45.9
genitalia, genital organ (s) or system
female Q52.9
external Q52.70
internal NOS Q52.9
male Q55.9
hydrocele P83.5
specified NEC Q55.8
genitourinary NEC
female Q52.9
male Q55.9
Gerbode Q21.0
glottis Q31.8
granulation or granulocyte, genetic (constitutional) (leukocyte) D72.0
gum Q38.6
gyri Q07.9
hair Q84.2
hand Q74.0
hard tissue formation in pulp K04.3
head —*see* Anomaly, skull
heart Q24.9
auricle Q20.8
bands or folds Q24.8
fibroelastosis cordis I42.4
obstructive NEC Q22.6
patent ductus arteriosus (Botalli) Q25.0
septum Q21.9
auricular Q21.1
interatrial Q21.1
interventricular Q21.0
with pulmonary stenosis or atresia, dextraposition of aorta and hypertrophy of right ventricle Q21.3
specified NEC Q21.8
ventricular Q21.0
with pulmonary stenosis or atresia, dextraposition of aorta and hypertrophy of right ventricle Q21.3
tetralogy of Fallot Q21.3
valve NEC Q24.8
aortic
bicuspid valve Q23.1
insufficiency Q23.1
stenosis Q23.0
subaortic Q24.4
mitral
insufficiency Q23.3
stenosis Q23.2
pulmonary Q22.3
atresia Q22.0
insufficiency Q22.2
stenosis Q22.1
infundibular Q24.3
subvalvular Q24.3
tricuspid
atresia Q22.4
stenosis Q22.4
ventricle Q20.8
heel NEC Q74.2
Hegglin's D72.0
hemianencephaly Q00.0
hemicephaly Q00.0
hemicrania Q00.0
hepatic duct Q44.5
hip NEC Q74.2
hourglass stomach Q40.2
humerus Q74.0
hydatid of Morgagni
female Q50.5
male (epididymal) Q55.4
testicular Q55.29
hymen Q52.4
hypersegmentation of neutrophils, hereditary D72.0

Anomaly, anomalous *(Continued)*
hypophyseal Q89.2
ileocecal (coil) (valve) Q43.9
ileum Q43.9
ilium NEC Q74.2
integument Q84.9
specified NEC Q84.8
interarch distance (excessive) (inadequate) M26.25
intervertebral cartilage or disc Q76.49
intestine (large) (small) Q43.9
with anomalous adhesions, fixation or malrotation Q43.3
iris Q13.2
ischium NEC Q74.2
jaw —*see* Anomaly, dentofacial
alveolar —*see* Anomaly, alveolar
jaw-cranial base relationship —*see* Anomaly, dentofacial, jaw-cranial base relationship
jejunum Q43.8
joint Q74.9
specified NEC Q74.8
Jordan's D72.0
kidney(s) (calyx) (pelvis) Q63.9
artery Q27.2
specified NEC Q63.8
Klippel-Feil (brevicollis) Q76.1
knee Q74.1
labium (majus) (minus) Q52.70
labyrinth, membranous Q16.5
lacrimal apparatus or duct Q10.6
larynx, laryngeal (muscle) Q31.9
web (bed) Q31.0
lens Q12.9
leukocytes, genetic D72.0
granulation (constitutional) D72.0
lid (fold) Q10.3
ligament Q79.9
broad Q50.6
round Q52.8
limb Q74.9
lower NEC Q74.2
reduction deformity —*see* Defect, reduction, lower limb
upper Q74.0
lip Q38.0
liver Q44.7
duct Q44.5
lower limb NEC Q74.2
lumbosacral (joint) (region) Q76.49
kyphosis —*see* Kyphosis, congenital
lordosis —*see* Lordosis, congenital
lung (fissure) (lobe) Q33.9
mandible —*see* Anomaly, dentofacial
maxilla —*see* Anomaly, dentofacial
May (-Hegglin) D72.0
meatus urinarius NEC Q64.79
meningeal bands or folds Q07.9
constriction of Q07.8
spinal Q06.9
meninges Q07.9
cerebral Q04.8
spinal Q06.9
meningocele Q05.9
mesentery Q45.9
metacarpus Q74.0
metatarsus NEC Q74.2
middle ear Q16.4
ossicles Q16.3
mitral (leaflets) (valve) Q23.9
insufficiency Q23.3
specified NEC Q23.8
stenosis Q23.2
mouth Q38.6
Müllerian —*see also* Anomaly, by site
uterus NEC Q51.818
multiple NEC Q89.7
muscle Q79.9
eyelid Q10.3
musculoskeletal system, except limbs Q79.9

Anomaly, anomalous *(Continued)*
myocardium Q24.8
nail Q84.6
narrowness, eyelid Q10.3
nasal sinus (wall) Q30.8
neck (any part) Q18.9
nerve Q07.9
acoustic Q07.8
optic Q07.8
nervous system (central) Q07.9
nipple Q83.9
nose, nasal (bones) (cartilage) (septum) (sinus) Q30.9
specified NEC Q30.8
ocular muscle Q15.8
omphalomesenteric duct Q43.0
opening, pulmonary veins Q26.4
optic
disc Q14.2
nerve Q07.8
opticociliary vessels Q13.2
orbit (eye) Q10.7
organ Q89.9
of Corti Q16.5
origin
artery
innominate Q25.8
pulmonary Q25.79
renal Q27.2
subclavian Q25.48 ◄
osseous meatus (ear) Q16.1
ovary Q50.39
oviduct Q50.6
palate (hard) (soft) NEC Q38.5
pancreas or pancreatic duct Q45.3
papillary muscles Q24.8
parathyroid gland Q89.2
paraurethral ducts Q64.79
parotid (gland) Q38.4
patella Q74.1
Pelger-Huët (hereditary hyposegmentation) D72.0
pelvic girdle NEC Q74.2
pelvis (bony) NEC Q74.2
rachitic E64.3
penis (glans) Q55.69
pericardium Q24.8
peripheral vascular system Q27.9
Peter's Q13.4
pharynx Q38.8
pigmentation L81.9
congenital Q82.8
pituitary (gland) Q89.2
pleural (folds) Q34.0
portal vein Q26.5
connection Q26.5
position, tooth, teeth, fully erupted M26.30
specified NEC M26.39
precerebral vessel Q28.1
prepuce Q55.69
prostate Q55.4
pulmonary Q33.9
artery NEC Q25.79
valve Q22.3
atresia Q22.0
insufficiency Q22.2
specified type NEC Q22.3
stenosis Q22.1
infundibular Q24.3
subvalvular Q24.3
venous connection Q26.4
partial Q26.3
total Q26.2
pupil Q13.2
function H57.00
anisocoria H57.02
Argyll Robertson pupil H57.01
miosis H57.03
mydriasis H57.04
specified type NEC H57.09
tonic pupil H57.05-

A

◄ New ◄ Revised ~~deleted~~ Deleted

Anomaly, anomalous *(Continued)*
pylorus Q40.3
radius Q74.0
rectum Q43.9
reduction (extremity) (limb)
femur (longitudinal) —*see* Defect, reduction, lower limb, longitudinal, femur
fibula (longitudinal) —*see* Defect, reduction, lower limb, longitudinal, fibula
lower limb —*see* Defect, reduction, lower limb
radius (longitudinal) —*see* Defect, reduction, upper limb, longitudinal, radius
tibia (longitudinal) —*see* Defect, reduction, lower limb, longitudinal, tibia
ulna (longitudinal) —*see* Defect, reduction, upper limb, longitudinal, ulna
upper limb —*see* Defect, reduction, upper limb
refraction —*see* Disorder, refraction
renal Q63.9
artery Q27.2
pelvis Q63.9
specified NEC Q63.8
respiratory system Q34.9
specified NEC Q34.8
retina Q14.1
rib Q76.6
cervical Q76.5
Rieger's Q13.81
rotation —*see* Malrotation
hip or thigh Q65.89
round ligament Q52.8
sacroiliac (joint) NEC Q74.2
sacrum NEC Q76.49
kyphosis —*see* Kyphosis, congenital
lordosis —*see* Lordosis, congenital
saddle nose, syphilitic A50.57
salivary duct or gland Q38.4
scapula Q74.0
scrotum —*see* Malformation, testis and scrotum
sebaceous gland Q82.9
seminal vesicles Q55.4
sense organs NEC Q07.8
sex chromosomes NEC —*see also* Anomaly, chromosomes
female phenotype Q97.8
male phenotype Q98.9
shoulder (girdle) (joint) Q74.0
sigmoid (flexure) Q43.9
simian crease Q82.8
sinus of Valsalva Q25.49 ◀
skeleton generalized Q78.9
skin (appendage) Q82.9
skull Q75.9
with
anencephaly Q00.0
encephalocele —*see* Encephalocele
hydrocephalus Q03.9
with spina bifida —*see* Spina bifida, by site, with hydrocephalus
microcephaly Q02
specified organ or site NEC Q89.8
spermatic cord Q55.4
spine, spinal NEC Q76.49
column NEC Q76.49
kyphosis —*see* Kyphosis, congenital
lordosis —*see* Lordosis, congenital
cord Q06.9
nerve root Q07.8
spleen Q89.09
agenesis Q89.01
stenonian duct Q38.4
sternum NEC Q76.7
stomach Q40.3
submaxillary gland Q38.4
tarsus NEC Q74.2

Anomaly, anomalous *(Continued)*
tendon Q79.9
testis —*see* Malformation, testis and scrotum
thigh NEC Q74.2
thorax (wall) Q67.8
bony Q76.9
throat Q38.8
thumb Q74.0
thymus gland Q89.2
thyroid (gland) Q89.2
cartilage Q31.8
tibia NEC Q74.2
saber A50.56
toe Q74.2
tongue Q38.3
tooth, teeth K00.9
eruption K00.6
position, fully erupted M26.30
spacing, fully erupted M26.30
trachea (cartilage) Q32.1
tragus Q17.9
tricuspid (leaflet) (valve) Q22.9
atresia or stenosis Q22.4
Ebstein's Q22.5
Uhl's (hypoplasia of myocardium, right ventricle) Q24.8
ulna Q74.0
umbilical artery Q27.0
union
cricoid cartilage and thyroid cartilage Q31.8
thyroid cartilage and hyoid bone Q31.8
trachea with larynx Q31.8
upper limb Q74.0
urachus Q64.4
ureter Q62.8
obstructive NEC Q62.39
cecoureterocele Q62.32
orthotopic ureterocele Q62.31
urethra Q64.70
absence Q64.5
double Q64.74
fistula to rectum Q64.73
obstructive Q64.39
stricture Q64.32
prolapse Q64.71
specified type NEC Q64.79
urinary tract Q64.9
uterus Q51.9
with only one functioning horn Q51.4
uvula Q38.5
vagina Q52.4
valleculae Q31.8
valve (heart) NEC Q24.8
coronary sinus Q24.5
inferior vena cava Q24.8
pulmonary Q22.3
sinus coronario Q24.5
venae cavae inferioris Q24.8
vas deferens Q55.4
vascular Q27.9
brain Q28.3
ring Q25.45 ◀
vein (s) (peripheral) Q27.9
brain Q28.3
cerebral Q28.3
coronary Q24.5
developmental Q28.3
great Q26.9
specified NEC Q26.8
vena cava (inferior) (superior) Q26.9
venous —*see* Anomaly, vein (s)
venous return Q26.8
ventricular
bands or folds Q24.8
septa Q21.0
vertebra Q76.49
kyphosis —*see* Kyphosis, congenital
lordosis —*see* Lordosis, congenital

Anomaly, anomalous *(Continued)*
vesicourethral orifice Q64.79
vessel (s) Q27.9
optic papilla Q14.2
precerebral Q28.1
vitelline duct Q43.0
vitreous body or humor Q14.0
vulva Q52.70
wrist (joint) Q74.0
Anomia R48.8
Anonychia (congenital) Q84.3
acquired L60.8
Anophthalmos, anophthalmus (congenital) (globe) Q11.1
acquired Z90.01
Anopia, anopsia H53.46-
quadrant H53.46-
Anorchia, anorchism, anorchidism Q55.0
Anorexia R63.0
hysterical F44.89
nervosa F50.00
atypical F50.9
binge-eating type F50.2
with purging F50.02
restricting type F50.01
Anorgasmy, psychogenic (female) F52.31
male F52.32
Anosmia R43.0
hysterical F44.6
postinfectional J39.8
Anosognosia R41.89
Anosteoplasia Q78.9
Anovulatory cycle N97.0
Anoxemia R09.02
newborn P84
Anoxia (pathological) R09.02
altitude T70.29
cerebral G93.1
complicating
anesthesia (general) (local) or other sedation T88.59
in labor and delivery O74.3
in pregnancy O29.21-
postpartum, puerperal O89.2
delivery (cesarean) (instrumental) O75.4
during a procedure G97.81
newborn P84
resulting from a procedure G97.82
due to
drowning T75.1
high altitude T70.29
heart —*see* Insufficiency, coronary
intrauterine P84
myocardial —*see* Insufficiency, coronary
newborn P84
spinal cord G95.11
systemic (by suffocation) (low content in atmosphere) —*see* Asphyxia, traumatic
Anteflexion —*see* Anteversion
Antenatal
care (normal pregnancy) Z34.90
screening (encounter for) of mother Z36
Antepartum —*see* condition
Anterior —*see* condition
Antero-occlusion M26.220
Anteversion
cervix —*see* Anteversion, uterus
femur (neck), congenital Q65.89
uterus, uterine (cervix) (postinfectional) (postpartal, old) N85.4
congenital Q51.818
in pregnancy or childbirth —*see* Pregnancy, complicated by
Anthophobia F40.228
Anthracosilicosis J60
Anthracosis (lung) (occupational) J60
lingua K14.3

A

◀ New ◀ Revised ~~deleted~~ Deleted

Anthrax A22.9
with pneumonia A22.1
cerebral A22.8
colitis A22.2
cutaneous A22.0
gastrointestinal A22.2
inhalation A22.1
intestinal A22.2
meningitis A22.8
pulmonary A22.1
respiratory A22.1
sepsis A22.7
specified manifestation NEC A22.8
Anthropoid pelvis Q74.2
with disproportion (fetopelvic) O33.0
Anthropophobia F40.10
generalized F40.11
Antibodies, maternal (blood group) —*see* Isoimmunization, affecting management of pregnancy
anti-D —*see* Isoimmunization, affecting management of pregnancy, Rh
newborn P55.0
Antibody
anticardiolipin R76.0
with
hemorrhagic disorder D68.312
hypercoagulable state D68.61
antiphosphatidylglycerol R76.0
with
hemorrhagic disorder D68.312
hypercoagulable state D68.61
antiphosphatidylinositol R76.0
with
hemorrhagic disorder D68.312
hypercoagulable state D68.61
antiphosphatidylserine R76.0
with
hemorrhagic disorder D68.312
hypercoagulable state D68.61
antiphospholipid R76.0
with
hemorrhagic disorder D68.312
hypercoagulable state D68.61
Anticardiolipin syndrome D68.61
Anticoagulant, circulating (intrinsic) —*see also* - Disorder, hemorrhagic D68.318
drug-induced (extrinsic) —*see also* - Disorder, hemorrhagic D68.32
iatrogenic D68.32 ◀
Antidiuretic hormone syndrome E22.2
Antimonial cholera —*see* Poisoning, antimony
Antiphospholipid
antibody
with hemorrhagic disorder D68.312
syndrome D68.61
Antisocial personality F60.2
Antithrombinemia —*see* Circulating anticoagulants
Antithromboplastinemia D68.318
Antithromboplastinogenemia D68.318
Antitoxin complication or reaction —*see* Complications, vaccination
Antlophobia F40.228
Antritis J32.0
maxilla J32.0
acute J01.00
recurrent J01.01
stomach K29.60
with bleeding K29.61
Antrum, antral —*see* condition
Anuria R34
calculous (impacted) (recurrent) —*see also* Calculus, urinary N20.9
following
abortion —*see* Abortion by type complicated by, renal failure
ectopic or molar pregnancy O08.4
newborn P96.0
postprocedural N99.0

Anuria *(Continued)*
postrenal N13.8
traumatic (following crushing) T79.5
Anus, anal —*see* condition
Anusitis K62.89
Anxiety F41.9
depression F41.8
episodic paroxysmal F41.0
generalized F41.1
hysteria F41.8
neurosis F41.1
panic type F41.0
reaction F41.1
separation, abnormal (of childhood) F93.0
specified NEC F41.8
state F41.1
Aorta, aortic —*see* condition
Aortectasia —*see* Ectasia, aorta
with aneurysm —*see* Aneurysm, aorta
Aortitis (nonsyphilitic) (calcific) I77.6
arteriosclerotic I70.0
Doehle-Heller A52.02
luetic A52.02
rheumatic —*see* Endocarditis, acute, rheumatic
specific (syphilitic) A52.02
syphilitic A52.02
congenital A50.54 *[I79.1]*
Apathetic thyroid storm —*see* Thyrotoxicosis
Apathy R45.3
Apeirophobia F40.228
Apepsia K30
psychogenic F45.8
Aperistalsis, esophagus K22.0
Apertognathia M26.29
Apert's syndrome Q87.0
Aphagia R13.0
psychogenic F50.9
Aphakia (acquired) (postoperative) H27.0-
congenital Q12.3
Aphasia (amnestic) (global) (nominal) (semantic) (syntactic) R47.01
acquired, with epilepsy (Landau-Kleffner syndrome) —*see* Epilepsy, specified NEC
auditory (developmental) F80.2
developmental (receptive type) F80.2
expressive type F80.1
Wernicke's F80.2
following
cerebrovascular disease I69.920
cerebral infarction I69.320
intracerebral hemorrhage I69.120
nontraumatic intracranial hemorrhage NEC I69.220
specified disease NEC I69.820
subarachnoid hemorrhage I69.020
primary progressive G31.01 *[F02.80]*
with behavioral disturbance G31.01 *[F02.81]*
progressive isolated G31.01 *[F02.80]*
with behavioral disturbance G31.01 *[F02.81]*
sensory F80.2
syphilis, tertiary A52.19
Wernicke's (developmental) F80.2
Aphonia (organic) R49.1
hysterical F44.4
psychogenic F44.4
Aphthae, aphthous —*see also* condition
Bednar's K12.0
cachectic K14.0
epizootic B08.8
fever B08.8
oral (recurrent) K12.0
stomatitis (major) (minor) K12.0
thrush B37.0
ulcer (oral) (recurrent) K12.0
genital organ (s) NEC
female N76.6
male N50.89 ⇐
larynx J38.7

Apical —*see* condition
Apiphobia F40.218
Aplasia —*see also* Agenesis
abdominal muscle syndrome Q79.4
alveolar process (acquired) —*see* Anomaly, alveolar
congenital Q38.6
aorta (congenital) Q25.41 ⇐
axialis extracorticalis (congenita) E75.29
bone marrow (myeloid) D61.9
congenital D61.01
brain Q00.0
part of Q04.3
bronchus Q32.4
cementum K00.4
cerebellum Q04.3
cervix (congenital) Q51.5
congenital pure red cell D61.01
corpus callosum Q04.0
cutis congenita Q84.8
erythrocyte congenital D61.01
extracortical axial E75.29
eye Q11.1
fovea centralis (congenital) Q14.1
gallbladder, congenital Q44.0
iris Q13.1
labyrinth, membranous Q16.5
limb (congenital) Q73.8
lower —*see* Defect, reduction, lower limb
upper —*see* Agenesis, arm
lung, congenital (bilateral) (unilateral) Q33.3
pancreas Q45.0
parathyroid-thymic D82.1
Pelizaeus-Merzbacher E75.29
penis Q55.5
prostate Q55.4
red cell (with thymoma) D60.9
acquired D60.9
due to drugs D60.9
adult D60.9
chronic D60.0
congenital D61.01
constitutional D61.01
due to drugs D60.9
hereditary D61.01
of infants D61.01
primary D61.01
pure D61.01
due to drugs D60.9
specified type NEC D60.8
transient D60.1
round ligament Q52.8
skin Q84.8
spermatic cord Q55.4
spleen Q89.01
testicle Q55.0
thymic, with immunodeficiency D82.1
thyroid (congenital) (with myxedema) E03.1
uterus Q51.0
ventral horn cell Q06.1
Apnea, apneic (of) (spells) R06.81
newborn NEC P28.4
obstructive P28.4
sleep (central) (obstructive) (primary) P28.3
prematurity P28.4
sleep G47.30
central (primary) G47.31
in conditions classified elsewhere G47.37
obstructive (adult) (pediatric) G47.33
primary central G47.31
specified NEC G47.39
Apneumatosis, newborn P28.0
Apocrine metaplasia (breast) —*see* Dysplasia, mammary, specified type NEC
Apophysitis (bone) —*see also* Osteochondropathy
calcaneus M92.8
juvenile M92.9

A

Apoplectiform convulsions (cerebral ischemia) I67.82
Apoplexia, apoplexy, apoplectic
adrenal A39.1
heart (auricle) (ventricle) —*see* Infarct, myocardium
heat T67.0
hemorrhagic (stroke) —*see* Hemorrhage, intracranial
meninges, hemorrhagic —*see* Hemorrhage, intracranial, subarachnoid
uremic N18.9 *[I68.8]*
Appearance
bizarre R46.1
specified NEC R46.89
very low level of personal hygiene R46.0
Appendage
epididymal (organ of Morgagni) Q55.4
intestine (epiploic) Q43.8
preauricular Q17.0
testicular (organ of Morgagni) Q55.29
Appendicitis (pneumococcal) (retrocecal) K37
with
perforation or rupture K35.2
peritoneal abscess K35.3
peritonitis NEC K35.3
generalized (with perforation or rupture) K35.2
localized (with perforation or rupture) K35.3
acute (catarrhal) (fulminating) (gangrenous) (obstructive) (retrocecal) (suppurative) K35.80
with
peritoneal abscess K35.3
peritonitis NEC K35.3
generalized (with perforation or rupture) K35.2
localized (with perforation or rupture) K35.3
specified NEC K35.89
amebic A06.89
chronic (recurrent) K36
exacerbation —*see* Appendicitis, acute
gangrenous —*see* Appendicitis, acute
healed (obliterative) K36
interval K36
neurogenic K36
obstructive K36
recurrent K36
relapsing K36
subacute (adhesive) K36
subsiding K36
suppurative —*see* Appendicitis, acute
tuberculous A18.32
Appendicopathia oxyurica B80
Appendix, appendicular —*see also* condition
epididymis Q55.4
Morgagni
female Q50.5
male (epididymal) Q55.4
testicular Q55.29
testis Q55.29
Appetite
depraved —*see* Pica
excessive R63.2
lack or loss —*see also* Anorexia R63.0
nonorganic origin F50.89 ◄
psychogenic F50.89 ◄
perverted (hysterical) —*see* Pica
Apple peel syndrome Q41.1
Apprehension state F41.1
Apprehensiveness, abnormal F41.9
Approximal wear K03.0
Apraxia (classic) (ideational) (ideokinetic) (ideomotor) (motor) (verbal) R48.2
following
cerebrovascular disease I69.990
cerebral infarction I69.390
intracerebral hemorrhage I69.190
Apraxia *(Continued)*
following *(Continued)*
cerebrovascular disease *(Continued)*
nontraumatic intracranial hemorrhage NEC I69.290
specified disease NEC I69.890
subarachnoid hemorrhage I69.090
oculomotor, congenital H51.8
Aptyalism K11.7
Apudoma —*see* Neoplasm, uncertain behavior, by site
Aqueous misdirection H40.83-
Arabicum elephantiasis —*see* Infestation, filarial
Arachnitis —*see* Meningitis
Arachnodactyly —*see* Syndrome, Marfan's
Arachnoiditis (acute) (adhesive) (basal) (brain) (cerebrospinal) —*see* Meningitis
Arachnophobia F40.210
Arboencephalitis, Australian A83.4
Arborization block (heart) I45.5
ARC (AIDS-related complex) B20
Arches —*see* condition
Arcuate uterus Q51.810
Arcuatus uterus Q51.810
Arcus (cornea) senilis —*see* Degeneration, cornea, senile
Arc-welder's lung J63.4
Areflexia R29.2
Areola —*see* condition
Argentaffinoma —*see also* Neoplasm, uncertain behavior, by site
malignant —*see* Neoplasm, malignant, by site
syndrome E34.0
Argininemia E72.21
Arginosuccinic aciduria E72.22
Argyll Robertson phenomenon, pupil or syndrome (syphilitic) A52.19
atypical H57.09
nonsyphilitic H57.09
Argyria, argyriasis
conjunctival H11.13-
from drug or medicament —*see* Table of Drugs and Chemicals, by substance
Argyrosis, conjunctival H11.13-
Arhinencephaly Q04.1
Ariboflavinosis E53.0
Arm —*see* condition
Arnold-Chiari disease, obstruction or syndrome (type II) Q07.00
with
hydrocephalus Q07.02
with spina bifida Q07.03
spina bifida Q07.01
with hydrocephalus Q07.03
type III —*see* Encephalocele
type IV Q04.8
Aromatic amino-acid metabolism disorder E70.9
specified NEC E70.8
Arousals, confusional G47.51
Arrest, arrested
cardiac I46.9
complicating
abortion —*see* Abortion, by type, complicated by, cardiac arrest
anesthesia (general) (local) or other sedation —*see* Table of Drugs and Chemicals, by drug
in labor and delivery O74.2
in pregnancy O29.11-
postpartum, puerperal O89.1
delivery (cesarean) (instrumental) O75.4
due to
cardiac condition I46.2
specified condition NEC I46.8
intraoperative I97.71-
newborn P29.81
postprocedural I97.12-
obstetric procedure O75.4
Arrest, arrested *(Continued)*
cardiorespiratory —*see* Arrest, cardiac
circulatory —*see* Arrest, cardiac
deep transverse O64.0
development or growth
bone —*see* Disorder, bone, development or growth
child R62.50
tracheal rings Q32.1
epiphyseal
complete
femur M89.15-
humerus M89.12-
tibia M89.16-
ulna M89.13-
forearm M89.13-
specified NEC M89.13-
ulna —*see* Arrest, epiphyseal, by type, ulna
lower leg M89.16-
specified NEC M89.168
tibia —*see* Arrest, epiphyseal, by type, tibia
partial
femur M89.15-
humerus M89.12-
tibia M89.16-
ulna M89.13-
specified NEC M89.18
granulopoiesis —*see* Agranulocytosis
growth plate —*see* Arrest, epiphyseal
heart —*see* Arrest, cardiac
legal, anxiety concerning Z65.3
physeal —*see* Arrest, epiphyseal
respiratory R09.2
newborn P28.81
sinus I45.5
spermatogenesis (complete) —*see* Azoospermia
incomplete —*see* Oligospermia
transverse (deep) O64.0
Arrhenoblastoma
benign
specified site —*see* Neoplasm, benign, by site
unspecified site
female D27.9
male D29.20
malignant
specified site —*see* Neoplasm, malignant, by site
unspecified site
female C56.9
male C62.90
specified site —*see* Neoplasm, uncertain behavior, by site
unspecified site
female D39.10
male D40.10
Arrhythmia (auricle)(cardiac) (juvenile) (nodal) (reflex)(sinus)(supraventricular) (transitory)(ventricle) I49.9
block I45.9
extrasystolic I49.49
newborn
bradycardia P29.12
occurring before birth P03.819
before onset of labor P03.810
during labor P03.811
tachycardia P29.11
psychogenic F45.8
specified NEC I49.8
vagal R55
ventricular re-entry I47.0
Arrillaga-Ayerza syndrome (pulmonary sclerosis with pulmonary hypertension) I27.0
Arsenical pigmentation L81.8
from drug or medicament —*see* Table of Drugs and Chemicals
Arsenism —*see* Poisoning, arsenic

A

◄ New ◄ Revised ~~deleted~~ Deleted

Arterial —*see* condition
Arteriofibrosis —*see* Arteriosclerosis
Arteriolar sclerosis —*see* Arteriosclerosis
Arteriolith —*see* Arteriosclerosis
Arteriolitis I77.6
  necrotizing, kidney I77.5
  renal —*see* Hypertension, kidney
Arteriolosclerosis —*see* Arteriosclerosis
Arterionephrosclerosis —*see* Hypertension, kidney
Arteriopathy I77.9
Arteriosclerosis, arteriosclerotic (diffuse) (obliterans) (of) (senile) (with calcification) I70.90
  aorta I70.0
  arteries of extremities —*see* Arteriosclerosis, extremities
  brain I67.2
  bypass graft
    coronary —*see* Arteriosclerosis, coronary, bypass graft
    extremities —*see* Arteriosclerosis, extremities, bypass graft
  cardiac —*see* Disease, heart, ischemic, atherosclerotic
  cardiopathy —*see* Disease, heart, ischemic, atherosclerotic
  cardiorenal —*see* Hypertension, cardiorenal
  cardiovascular —*see* Disease, heart, ischemic, atherosclerotic
  carotid —*see also* Occlusion, artery, carotid I65.2-
  central nervous system I67.2
  cerebral I67.2
  cerebrovascular I67.2
  coronary (artery) I25.10
    bypass graft I25.810
      with
        angina pectoris I25.709
          with documented spasm I25.701
          specified type NEC I25.708
          unstable I25.700
        ischemic chest pain I25.709
      autologous artery I25.810
        with
          angina pectoris I25.729
            with documented spasm I25.721
            specified type I25.728
            unstable I25.720
          ischemic chest pain I25.729
      autologous vein I25.810
        with
          angina pectoris I25.719
            with documented spasm I25.711
            specified type I25.718
            unstable I25.710
          ischemic chest pain I25.719
      nonautologous biological I25.810
        with
          angina pectoris I25.739
            with documented spasm I25.731
            specified type I25.738
            unstable I25.730
          ischemic chest pain I25.739
      specified type NEC I25.810
        with
          angina pectoris I25.799
            with documented spasm I25.791
            specified type I25.798
            unstable I25.790
          ischemic chest pain I25.799
    due to
      calcified coronary lesion (severely) I25.84
      lipid rich plaque I25.83
    native vessel
      with
        angina pectoris I25.119
          with documented spasm I25.111
          specified type NEC I25.118
          unstable I25.110
        ischemic chest pain I25.119

Arteriosclerosis, arteriosclerotic *(Continued)*
  coronary *(Continued)*
    transplanted heart I25.811
      bypass graft I25.812
        with
          angina pectoris I25.769
            with documented spasm I25.761
            specified type I25.768
            unstable I25.760
          ischemic chest pain I25.769
      native coronary artery I25.811
        with
          angina pectoris I25.759
            with documented spasm I25.751
            specified type I25.758
            unstable I25.750
          ischemic chest pain I25.759
  extremities (native arteries) I70.209
    bypass graft I70.309
      autologous vein graft I70.409
        leg I70.409
          with
            gangrene (and intermittent claudication, rest pain and ulcer) I70.469
            intermittent claudication I70.419
            rest pain (and intermittent claudication) I70.429
          bilateral I70.403
            with
              gangrene (and intermittent claudication, rest pain and ulcer) I70.463
              intermittent claudication I70.413
              rest pain (and intermittent claudication) I70.423
            specified type NEC I70.493
          left I70.402
            with
              gangrene (and intermittent claudication, rest pain and ulcer) I70.462
              intermittent claudication I70.412
              rest pain (and intermittent claudication) I70.422
              ulceration (and intermittent claudication and rest pain) I70.449
                ankle I70.443
                calf I70.442
                foot site NEC I70.445
                heel I70.444
                lower leg NEC I70.448
                midfoot I70.444
                thigh I70.441
            specified type NEC I70.492
          right I70.401
            with
              gangrene (and intermittent claudication, rest pain and ulcer) I70.461
              intermittent claudication I70.411
              rest pain (and intermittent claudication) I70.421
              ulceration (and intermittent claudication and rest pain) I70.439
                ankle I70.433
                calf I70.432
                foot site NEC I70.435
                heel I70.434
                lower leg NEC I70.438
                midfoot I70.434
                thigh I70.431
            specified type NEC I70.491
          specified type NEC I70.499

Arteriosclerosis, arteriosclerotic *(Continued)*
  extremities *(Continued)*
    bypass graft *(Continued)*
      autologous vein graft *(Continued)*
        specified NEC I70.408
          with
            gangrene (and intermittent claudication, rest pain and ulcer) I70.468
            intermittent claudication I70.418
            rest pain (and intermittent claudication) I70.428
            ulceration (and intermittent claudication and rest pain) I70.45
          specified type NEC I70.498
        leg I70.309
          with
            gangrene (and intermittent claudication, rest pain and ulcer) I70.369
            intermittent claudication I70.319
            rest pain (and intermittent claudication) I70.329
          bilateral I70.303
            with
              gangrene (and intermittent claudication, rest pain and ulcer) I70.363
              intermittent claudication I70.313
              rest pain (and intermittent claudication) I70.323
            specified type NEC I70.393
          left I70.302
            with
              gangrene (and intermittent claudication, rest pain and ulcer) I70.362
              intermittent claudication I70.312
              rest pain (and intermittent claudication) I70.322
              ulceration (and intermittent claudication and rest pain) I70.349
                ankle I70.343
                calf I70.342
                foot site NEC I70.345
                heel I70.344
                lower leg NEC I70.348
                midfoot I70.344
                thigh I70.341
            specified type NEC I70.392
          right I70.301
            with
              gangrene (and intermittent claudication, rest pain and ulcer) I70.361
              intermittent claudication I70.311
              rest pain (and intermittent claudication) I70.321
              ulceration (and intermittent claudication and rest pain) I70.339
                ankle I70.333
                calf I70.332
                foot site NEC I70.335
                heel I70.334
                lower leg NEC I70.338
                midfoot I70.334
                thigh I70.331
            specified type NEC I70.391
          specified type NEC I70.399
        nonautologous biological graft I70.509
          leg I70.509
            with
              gangrene (and intermittent claudication, rest pain and ulcer) I70.569
              intermittent claudication I70.519
              rest pain (and intermittent claudication) I70.529

Arteriosclerosis, arteriosclerotic *(Continued)*
extremities *(Continued)*
bypass graft *(Continued)*
nonautologous biological graft *(Continued)*
leg *(Continued)*
bilateral I70.503
with
gangrene (and intermittent claudication, rest pain and ulcer) I70.563
intermittent claudication I70.513
rest pain (and intermittent claudication) I70.523
specified type NEC I70.593
left I70.502
with
gangrene (and intermittent claudication, rest pain and ulcer) I70.562
intermittent claudication I70.512
rest pain (and intermittent claudication) I70.522
ulceration (and intermittent claudication and rest pain) I70.549
ankle I70.543
calf I70.542
foot site NEC I70.545
heel I70.544
lower leg NEC I70.548
midfoot I70.544
thigh I70.541
specified type NEC I70.592
right I70.501
with
gangrene (and intermittent claudication, rest pain and ulcer) I70.561
intermittent claudication I70.511
rest pain (and intermittent claudication) I70.521
ulceration (and intermittent claudication and rest pain) I70.539
ankle I70.533
calf I70.532
foot site NEC I70.535
heel I70.534
lower leg NEC I70.538
midfoot I70.534
thigh I70.531
specified type NEC I70.591
specified type NEC I70.599
specified NEC I70.508
with
gangrene (and intermittent claudication, rest pain and ulcer) I70.568
intermittent claudication I70.518
rest pain (and intermittent claudication) I70.528
ulceration (and intermittent claudication and rest pain) I70.55
specified type NEC I70.598
nonbiological graft I70.609
leg I70.609
with
gangrene (and intermittent claudication, rest pain and ulcer) I70.669
intermittent claudication I70.619
rest pain (and intermittent claudication) I70.629

Arteriosclerosis, arteriosclerotic *(Continued)*
extremities *(Continued)*
bypass graft *(Continued)*
nonbiological graft *(Continued)*
leg *(Continued)*
bilateral I70.603
with
gangrene (and intermittent claudication, rest pain and ulcer) I70.663
intermittent claudication I70.613
rest pain (and intermittent claudication) I70.623
specified type NEC I70.693
left I70.602
with
gangrene (and intermittent claudication, rest pain and ulcer) I70.662
intermittent claudication I70.612
rest pain (and intermittent claudication) I70.622
ulceration (and intermittent claudication and rest pain) I70.649
ankle I70.643
calf I70.642
foot site NEC I70.645
heel I70.644
lower leg NEC I70.648
midfoot I70.644
thigh I70.641
specified type NEC I70.692
right I70.601
with
gangrene (and intermittent claudication, rest pain and ulcer) I70.661
intermittent claudication I70.611
rest pain (and intermittent claudication) I70.621
ulceration (and intermittent claudication and rest pain) I70.639
ankle I70.633
calf I70.632
foot site NEC I70.635
heel I70.634
lower leg NEC I70.638
midfoot I70.634
thigh I70.631
specified type NEC I70.691
specified type NEC I70.699
specified NEC I70.608
with
gangrene (and intermittent claudication, rest pain and ulcer) I70.668
intermittent claudication I70.618
rest pain (and intermittent claudication) I70.628
ulceration (and intermittent claudication and rest pain) I70.65
specified type NEC I70.698
specified graft NEC I70.709
leg I70.709
with
gangrene (and intermittent claudication, rest pain and ulcer) I70.769
intermittent claudication I70.719
rest pain (and intermittent claudication) I70.729

Arteriosclerosis, arteriosclerotic *(Continued)*
extremities *(Continued)*
bypass graft *(Continued)*
specified graft NEC *(Continued)*
leg *(Continued)*
bilateral I70.703
with
gangrene (and intermittent claudication, rest pain and ulcer) I70.763
intermittent claudication I70.713
rest pain (and intermittent claudication) I70.723
specified type NEC I70.793
left I70.702
with
gangrene (and intermittent claudication, rest pain and ulcer) I70.762
intermittent claudication I70.712
rest pain (and intermittent claudication) I70.722
ulceration (and intermittent claudication and rest pain) I70.749
ankle I70.743
calf I70.742
foot site NEC I70.745
heel I70.744
lower leg NEC I70.748
midfoot I70.744
thigh I70.741
specified type NEC I70.792
right I70.701
with
gangrene (and intermittent claudication, rest pain and ulcer) I70.761
intermittent claudication I70.711
rest pain (and intermittent claudication) I70.721
ulceration (and intermittent claudication and rest pain) I70.739
ankle I70.733
calf I70.732
foot site NEC I70.735
heel I70.734
lower leg NEC I70.738
midfoot I70.734
thigh I70.731
specified type NEC I70.791
specified type NEC I70.799
specified NEC I70.708
with
gangrene (and intermittent claudication, rest pain and ulcer) I70.768
intermittent claudication I70.718
rest pain (and intermittent claudication) I70.728
ulceration (and intermittent claudication and rest pain) I70.75
specified type NEC I70.798
specified NEC I70.308
with
gangrene (and intermittent claudication, rest pain and ulcer) I70.368
intermittent claudication I70.318
rest pain (and intermittent claudication) I70.328
ulceration (and intermittent claudication and rest pain) I70.35
specified type NEC I70.398

Arteriosclerosis, arteriosclerotic *(Continued)*
extremities *(Continued)*
leg I70.209
with
gangrene (and intermittent claudication, rest pain and ulcer) I70.269
intermittent claudication I70.219
rest pain (and intermittent claudication) I70.229
bilateral I70.203
with
gangrene (and intermittent claudication, rest pain and ulcer) I70.263
intermittent claudication I70.213
rest pain (and intermittent claudication) I70.223
specified type NEC I70.293
left I70.202
with
gangrene (and intermittent claudication, rest pain and ulcer) I70.262
intermittent claudication I70.212
rest pain (and intermittent claudication) I70.222
ulceration (and intermittent claudication and rest pain) I70.249
ankle I70.243
calf I70.242
foot site NEC I70.245
heel I70.244
lower leg NEC I70.248
midfoot I70.244
thigh I70.241
specified type NEC I70.292
right I70.201
with
gangrene (and intermittent claudication, rest pain and ulcer) I70.261
intermittent claudication I70.211
rest pain (and intermittent claudication) I70.221
ulceration (and intermittent claudication and rest pain) I70.239
ankle I70.233
calf I70.232
foot site NEC I70.235
heel I70.234
lower leg NEC I70.238
midfoot I70.234
thigh I70.231
specified type NEC I70.291
specified type NEC I70.299
specified site NEC I70.208
with
gangrene (and intermittent claudication, rest pain and ulcer) I70.268
intermittent claudication I70.218
rest pain (and intermittent claudication) I70.228
ulceration (and intermittent claudication and rest pain) I70.25
specified type NEC I70.298
generalized I70.91
heart (disease) —*see* Arteriosclerosis, coronary (artery)
kidney —*see* Hypertension, kidney
medial —*see* Arteriosclerosis, extremities
mesenteric (artery) K55.1
Mönckeberg's —*see* Arteriosclerosis, extremities
myocarditis I51.4
peripheral (of extremities) —*see* Arteriosclerosis, extremities
pulmonary (idiopathic) I27.0

Arteriosclerosis, arteriosclerotic *(Continued)*
renal (arterioles) —*see also* Hypertension, kidney
artery I70.1
retina (vascular) I70.8 *[H35.0-]*
specified artery NEC I70.8
spinal (cord) G95.19
vertebral (artery) I67.2
Arteriospasm I73.9
Arteriovenous —*see* condition
Arteritis I77.6
allergic M31.0
aorta (nonsyphilitic) I77.6
syphilitic A52.02
aortic arch M31.4
brachiocephalic M31.4
brain I67.7
syphilitic A52.04
cerebral I67.7
in
diseases classified elsewhere I68.2
systemic lupus erythematosus M32.19
listerial A32.89
syphilitic A52.04
tuberculous A18.89
coronary (artery) I25.89
rheumatic I01.8
chronic I09.89
syphilitic A52.06
cranial (left) (right), giant cell M31.6
deformans —*see* Arteriosclerosis
giant cell NEC M31.6
with polymyalgia rheumatica M31.5
necrosing or necrotizing M31.9
specified NEC M31.8
nodosa M30.0
obliterans —*see* Arteriosclerosis
pulmonary I28.8
rheumatic —*see* Fever, rheumatic
senile —*see* Arteriosclerosis
suppurative I77.2
syphilitic (general) A52.09
brain A52.04
coronary A52.06
spinal A52.09
temporal, giant cell M31.6
young female aortic arch syndrome M31.4
Artery, arterial —*see also* condition
abscess I77.89
single umbilical Q27.0
Arthralgia (allergic) —*see also* Pain, joint
in caisson disease T70.3
temporomandibular M26.62
Arthritis, arthritic (acute) (chronic) (nonpyogenic) (subacute) M19.90
allergic —*see* Arthritis, specified form NEC
ankylosing (crippling) (spine) —*see also* Spondylitis, ankylosing
sites other than spine —*see* Arthritis, specified form NEC
atrophic —*see* Osteoarthritis
spine —*see* Spondylitis, ankylosing
back —*see* Spondylopathy, inflammatory
blennorrhagic (gonococcal) A54.42
Charcot's —*see* Arthropathy, neuropathic
diabetic —*see* Diabetes, arthropathy, neuropathic
syringomyelic G95.0
chylous (filarial) —*see also* category M01 B74.9
climacteric (any site) NEC —*see* Arthritis, specified form NEC
crystal (-induced) —*see* Arthritis, in, crystals
deformans —*see* Osteoarthritis
degenerative —*see* Osteoarthritis
due to or associated with
acromegaly E22.0
brucellosis —*see* Brucellosis
caisson disease T70.3
diabetes —*see* Diabetes, arthropathy
dracontiasis —*see also* category M01 B72

Arthritis, arthritic *(Continued)*
due to or associated with *(Continued)*
enteritis NEC
regional —*see* Enteritis, regional
erysipelas —*see also* category M01 A46
erythema
epidemic A25.1
nodosum L52
filariasis NOS B74.9
glanders A24.0
helminthiasis —*see also* category M01 B83.9
hemophilia D66 *[M36.2]*
Henoch-(Schönlein) purpura D69.0 *[M36.4]*
human parvovirus —*see also* category M01 B97.6
infectious disease NEC —*see* category M01
leprosy (*see also* category M01) —*see also* Leprosy A30.9
Lyme disease A69.23
mycobacteria —*see also* category M01 A31.8
parasitic disease NEC —*see also* category M01 B89
paratyphoid fever (*see also* category M01) —*see also* Fever, paratyphoid A01.4
rat bite fever —*see also* category M01 A25.1
regional enteritis —*see* Enteritis, regional
respiratory disorder NOS J98.9
serum sickness —*see also* Reaction, serum T80.69
syringomyelia G95.0
typhoid fever A01.04
epidemic erythema A25.1
febrile —*see* Fever, rheumatic
gonococcal A54.42
gouty (acute) —*see* Gout ◄
in (due to)
acromegaly —*see also* subcategory M14.8- E22.0
amyloidosis —*see also* subcategory M14.8- E85.4
bacterial disease —*see also* subcategory M01 A49.9
Behçet's syndrome M35.2
caisson disease —*see also* subcategory M14.8- T70.3
coliform bacilli (Escherichia coli) —*see* Arthritis, in, pyogenic organism NEC
crystals M11.9
dicalcium phosphate —*see* Arthritis, in, crystals, specified type NEC
hydroxyapatite M11.0-
pyrophosphate —*see* Arthritis, in, crystals, specified type NEC
specified type NEC M11.80
ankle M11.87-
elbow M11.82-
foot joint M11.87-
hand joint M11.84-
hip M11.85-
knee M11.86-
multiple sites M11.8-
shoulder M11.81-
vertebrae M11.88
wrist M11.83-
dermatoarthritis, lipoid E78.81
dracontiasis (dracunculiasis) —*see also* category M01 B72
endocrine disorder NEC —*see also* subcategory M14.8- E34.9
enteritis, infectious NEC —*see also* category M01 A09
specified organism NEC —*see also* category M01 A08.8
erythema
multiforme —*see also* subcategory M14.8- L51.9
nodosum —*see also* subcategory M14.8- L52
gout —*see* Gout ◄

A

Arthritis, arthritic *(Continued)*
in *(Continued)*
helminthiasis NEC —*see also* category M01 B83.9
hemochromatosis —*see also* subcategory M14.8- E83.118
hemoglobinopathy NEC D58.2 *[M36.3]*
hemophilia NEC D66 *[M36.2]*
Hemophilus influenzae M00.8- *[B96.3]*
Henoch(-Schönlein) purpura D69.0 *[M36.4]*
hyperparathyroidism NEC —*see also* subcategory M14.8- E21.3
hypersensitivity reaction NEC T78.49 *[M36.4]*
hypogammaglobulinemia —*see also* subcategory M14.8- D80.1
hypothyroidism NEC —*see also* subcategory M14.8- E03.9
infection —*see* Arthritis, pyogenic or pyemic
spine —*see* Spondylopathy, infective
infectious disease NEC —*see* category M01
leprosy —*see also* category M01 A30.9
leukemia NEC C95.9- *[M36.1]*
lipoid dermatoarthritis E78.81
Lyme disease A69.23
Mediterranean fever, familial —*see also* subcategory M14.8- M04.1 ◀
Meningococcus A39.83
metabolic disorder NEC —*see also* subcategory M14.8- E88.9
multiple myelomatosis C90.0- *[M36.1]*
mumps B26.85
mycosis NEC —*see also* category M01 B49
myelomatosis (multiple) C90.0- *[M36.1]*
neurological disorder NEC G98.0
ochronosis —*see also* subcategory M14.8- E70.29
O'nyong-nyong —*see also* category M01 A92.1
parasitic disease NEC —*see also* category M01 B89
paratyphoid fever —*see also* category M01 A01.4
Pseudomonas —*see* Arthritis, pyogenic, bacterial NEC
psoriasis L40.50
pyogenic organism NEC —*see* Arthritis, pyogenic, bacterial NEC
Reiter's disease —*see* Reiter's disease
respiratory disorder NEC —*see also* subcategory M14.8- J98.9
reticulosis, malignant —*see also* subcategory M14.8- C86.0
rubella B06.82
Salmonella (arizonae) (cholerae-suis) (enteritidis) (typhimurium) A02.23
sarcoidosis D86.86
specified bacteria NEC —*see* Arthritis, pyogenic, bacterial NEC
sporotrichosis B42.82
syringomyelia G95.0
thalassemia NEC D56.9 *[M36.3]*
tuberculosis —*see* Tuberculosis, arthritis
typhoid fever A01.04
urethritis, Reiter's —*see* Reiter's disease
viral disease NEC —*see also* category M01 B34.9
infectious or infective —*see also* Arthritis, pyogenic or pyemic
spine —*see* Spondylopathy, infective
juvenile M08.90
with systemic onset —*see* Still's disease
ankle M08.97-
elbow M08.92-
foot joint M08.97-
hand joint M08.94-
hip M08.95-
knee M08.96-
multiple site M08.99

Arthritis, arthritic *(Continued)*
juvenile *(Continued)*
pauciarticular M08.40
ankle M08.47-
elbow M08.42-
foot joint M08.47-
hand joint M08.44-
hip M08.45-
knee M08.46-
shoulder M08.41-
vertebrae M08.48
wrist M08.43-
psoriatic L40.54
rheumatoid —*see* Arthritis, rheumatoid, juvenile
shoulder M08.91-
specified type NEC M08.80
ankle M08.87-
elbow M08.82-
foot joint M08.87-
hand joint M08.84-
hip M08.85-
knee M08.86-
multiple site M08.89
shoulder M08.81-
specified joint NEC M08.88
vertebrae M08.88
wrist M08.83-
vertebra M08.98
wrist M08.93-
meaning osteoarthritis —*see* Osteoarthritis
meningococcal A39.83
menopausal (any site) NEC —*see* Arthritis, specified form NEC
mutilans (psoriatic) L40.52
mycotic NEC —*see also* category M01 B49
neuropathic (Charcot) —*see* Arthropathy, neuropathic
diabetic —*see* Diabetes, arthropathy, neuropathic
nonsyphilitic NEC G98.0
syringomyelic G95.0
ochronotic —*see also* subcategory M14.8- E70.29
palindromic (any site) —*see* Rheumatism, palindromic
pneumococcal M00.10
ankle M00.17-
elbow M00.12-
foot joint —*see* Arthritis, pneumococcal, ankle
hand joint M00.14-
hip M00.15-
knee M00.16-
multiple site M00.19
shoulder M00.11-
vertebra M00.18
wrist M00.13-
postdysenteric —*see* Arthropathy, postdysenteric
postmeningococcal A39.84
postrheumatic, chronic —*see* Arthropathy, postrheumatic, chronic
primary progressive —*see also* Arthritis, specified form NEC
spine —*see* Spondylitis, ankylosing
psoriatic L40.50
purulent (any site except spine) —*see* Arthritis, pyogenic or pyemic
spine —*see* Spondylopathy, infective
pyogenic or pyemic (any site except spine) M00.9
bacterial NEC M00.80
ankle M00.87-
elbow M00.82-
foot joint —*see* Arthritis, pyogenic, bacterial NEC, ankle
hand joint M00.84-
hip M00.85-
knee M00.86-
multiple site M00.89

Arthritis, arthritic *(Continued)*
pyogenic or pyemic *(Continued)*
bacterial NEC *(Continued)*
shoulder M00.81-
vertebra M00.88
wrist M00.83-
pneumococcal —*see* Arthritis, pneumococcal
spine —*see* Spondylopathy, infective
staphylococcal —*see* Arthritis, staphylococcal
streptococcal —*see* Arthritis, streptococcal NEC
pneumococcal —*see* Arthritis, pneumococcal
reactive —*see* Reiter's disease
rheumatic —*see also* Arthritis, rheumatoid
acute or subacute —*see* Fever, rheumatic
rheumatoid M06.9
with
carditis —*see* Rheumatoid, carditis
endocarditis —*see* Rheumatoid, carditis
heart involvement NEC —*see* Rheumatoid, carditis
lung involvement —*see* Rheumatoid, lung
myocarditis —*see* Rheumatoid, carditis
myopathy —*see* Rheumatoid, myopathy
pericarditis —*see* Rheumatoid, carditis
polyneuropathy —*see* Rheumatoid, polyneuropathy
rheumatoid factor —*see* Arthritis, rheumatoid, seropositive
splenoadenomegaly and leukopenia —*see* Felty's syndrome
vasculitis —*see* Rheumatoid, vasculitis
visceral involvement NEC —*see* Rheumatoid, arthritis, with involvement of organs NEC
juvenile (with or without rheumatoid factor) M08.00
ankle M08.07-
elbow M08.02-
foot joint M08.07-
hand joint M08.04-
hip M08.05-
knee M08.06-
multiple site M08.09
shoulder M08.01-
vertebra M08.08
wrist M08.03-
seronegative M06.00
ankle M06.07-
elbow M06.02-
foot joint M06.07-
hand joint M06.04-
hip M06.05-
knee M06.06-
multiple sites M06.09
shoulder M06.01-
vertebra M06.08
wrist M06.03-
seropositive M05.9
without organ involvement M05.70
ankle M05.77-
elbow M05.72-
foot joint M05.77-
hand joint M05.74-
hip M05.75-
knee M05.76-
multiple sites M05.79
shoulder M05.71-
vertebra —*see* Spondylitis, ankylosing
wrist M05.73-
specified NEC M05.80
ankle M05.87-
elbow M05.82-
foot joint M05.87-
hand joint M05.84-
hip M05.85-
knee M05.86-

Arthritis, arthritic *(Continued)*
rheumatoid *(Continued)*
specified NEC *(Continued)*
multiple sites M05.89
shoulder M05.81-
vertebra —*see* Spondylitis, ankylosing
wrist M05.83-
specified type NEC M06.80
ankle M06.87-
elbow M06.82-
foot joint M06.87-
hand joint M06.84-
hip M06.85-
knee M06.86-
multiple site M06.89
shoulder M06.81-
vertebra M06.88
wrist M06.83-
spine —*see* Spondylitis, ankylosing
rubella B06.82
scorbutic —*see also* subcategory M14.8- E54
senile or senescent —*see* Osteoarthritis
septic (any site except spine) —*see* Arthritis, pyogenic or pyemic
spine —*see* Spondylopathy, infective
serum (nontherapeutic) (therapeutic) —*see* Arthropathy, postimmunization
specified form NEC M13.80
ankle M13.87-
elbow M13.82-
foot joint M13.87-
hand joint M13.84-
hip M13.85-
knee M13.86-
multiple site M13.89
shoulder M13.81-
specified joint NEC M13.88
wrist M13.83-
spine —*see also* Spondylopathy, inflammatory
infectious or infective NEC —*see* Spondylopathy, infective
Marie-Strümpell —*see* Spondylitis, ankylosing
pyogenic —*see* Spondylopathy, infective
rheumatoid —*see* Spondylitis, ankylosing
traumatic (old) —*see* Spondylopathy, traumatic
tuberculous A18.01
staphylococcal M00.00
ankle M00.07-
elbow M00.02-
foot joint —*see* Arthritis, staphylococcal, ankle
hand joint M00.04-
hip M00.05-
knee M00.06-
multiple site M00.09
shoulder M00.01-
vertebra M00.08
wrist M00.03-
streptococcal NEC M00.20
ankle M00.27-
elbow M00.22-
foot joint —*see* Arthritis, streptococcal, ankle
hand joint M00.24-
hip M00.25-
knee M00.26-
multiple site M00.29
shoulder M00.21-
vertebra M00.28
wrist M00.23-
suppurative —*see* Arthritis, pyogenic or pyemic
syphilitic (late) A52.16
congenital A50.55 *[M12.80]*
syphilitica deformans (Charcot) A52.16
temporomandibular M26.69
toxic of menopause (any site) —*see* Arthritis, specified form NEC

Arthritis, arthritic *(Continued)*
transient —*see* Arthropathy, specified form NEC
traumatic (chronic) —*see* Arthropathy, traumatic
tuberculous A18.02
spine A18.01
uratic —*see* Gout ◄
urethritica (Reiter's) —*see* Reiter's disease
vertebral —*see* Spondylopathy, inflammatory
villous (any site) —*see* Arthropathy, specified form NEC
Arthrocele —*see* Effusion, joint
Arthrodesis status Z98.1
Arthrodynia —*see also* Pain, joint
Arthrodysplasia Q74.9
Arthrofibrosis, joint —*see* Ankylosis
Arthrogryposis (congenital) Q68.8
multiplex congenita Q74.3
Arthrokatadysis M24.7
Arthropathy (*see also* Arthritis) M12.9
Charcot's —*see* Arthropathy, neuropathic
diabetic —*see* Diabetes, arthropathy, neuropathic
syringomyelic G95.0
cricoarytenoid J38.7
crystal(-induced) —*see* Arthritis, in, crystals
diabetic NEC —*see* Diabetes, arthropathy
distal interphalangeal, psoriatic L40.51
enteropathic M07.60
ankle M07.67-
elbow M07.62-
foot joint M07.67-
hand joint M07.64-
hip M07.65-
knee M07.66-
multiple site M07.69
shoulder M07.61-
vertebra M07.68
wrist M07.63-
following intestinal bypass M02.00
ankle M02.07-
elbow M02.02-
foot joint M02.07-
hand joint M02.04-
hip M02.05-
knee M02.06-
multiple site M02.09
shoulder M02.01-
vertebra M02.08
wrist M02.03-
gouty —*see also* Gout ◄
in (due to)
Lesch-Nyhan syndrome E79.1 *[M14.8-]*
sickle-cell disorders D57- *[M14.8-]*
hemophilic NEC D66 *[M36.2]*
in (due to)
hyperparathyroidism NEC E21.3 *[M14.8-]*
metabolic disease NOS E88.9 *[M14.8-]*
in (due to)
acromegaly E22.0 *[M14.8-]*
amyloidosis E85.4 *[M14.8-]*
blood disorder NOS D75.9 *[M36.3]*
diabetes —*see* Diabetes, arthropathy
endocrine disease NOS E34.9 *[M14.8-]*
erythema
multiforme L51.9 *[M14.8-]*
nodosum L52 *[M14.8-]*
hemochromatosis E83.118 *[M14.8-]*
hemoglobinopathy NEC D58.2 *[M36.3]*
hemophilia NEC D66 *[M36.2]*
Henoch-Schönlein purpura D69.0 *[M36.4]*
hyperthyroidism E05.90 *[M14.8-]*
hypothyroidism E03.9 *[M14.8-]*
infective endocarditis I33.0 *[M12.80]*
leukemia NEC C95.9- *[M36.1]*
malignant histiocytosis C96.A *[M36.1]*
metabolic disease NOS E88.9 *[M14.8-]*
multiple myeloma C90.0- *[M36.1]*
neoplastic disease NOS (*see also* Neoplasm) D49.9 *[M36.1]*

Arthropathy *(Continued)*
hemochromatosis *(Continued)*
nutritional deficiency —*see also* subcategory M14.8- E63.9
psoriasis NOS L40.50
sarcoidosis D86.86
syphilis (late) A52.77
congenital A50.55 *[M12.80]*
thyrotoxicosis —*see also* subcategory M14.8- E05.90
ulcerative colitis K51.90 *[M07.60]*
viral hepatitis (postinfectious) NEC B19.9 *[M12.80]*
Whipple's disease —*see also* subcategory M14.8- K90.81
Jaccoud —*see* Arthropathy, postrheumatic, chronic
juvenile —*see* Arthritis, juvenile
psoriatic L40.54
mutilans (psoriatic) L40.52
neuropathic (Charcot) M14.60
ankle M14.67-
diabetic —*see* Diabetes, arthropathy, neuropathic
elbow M14.62-
foot joint M14.67-
hand joint M14.64-
hip M14.65-
knee M14.66-
multiple site M14.69
nonsyphilitic NEC G98.0
shoulder M14.61-
syringomyelic G95.0
vertebra M14.68
wrist M14.63-
osteopulmonary —*see* Osteoarthropathy, hypertrophic, specified NEC
postdysenteric M02.10
ankle M02.17-
elbow M02.12-
foot joint M02.17-
hand joint M02.14-
hip M02.15-
knee M02.16-
multiple site M02.19
shoulder M02.11-
vertebra M02.18
wrist M02.13-
postimmunization M02.20
ankle M02.27-
elbow M02.22-
foot joint M02.27-
hand joint M02.24-
hip M02.25-
knee M02.26-
multiple site M02.29
shoulder M02.21-
vertebra M02.28
wrist M02.23-
postinfectious NEC B99 *[M12.80]*
in (due to)
enteritis due to Yersinia enterocolitica A04.6 *[M12.80]*
syphilis A52.77
viral hepatitis NEC B19.9 *[M12.80]*
postrheumatic, chronic (Jaccoud) M12.00
ankle M12.07-
elbow M12.02-
foot joint M12.07-
hand joint M12.04-
hip M12.05-
knee M12.06-
multiple site M12.09
shoulder M12.01-
specified joint NEC M12.08
vertebrae M12.08
wrist M12.03-
psoriatic NEC L40.59
interphalangeal, distal L40.51

A

Arthropathy *(Continued)*
reactive M02.9
in (due to)
infective endocarditis I33.0 *[M02.9]*
specified type NEC M02.80
ankle M02.87-
elbow M02.82-
foot joint M02.87-
hand joint M02.84-
hip M02.85-
knee M02.86-
multiple site M02.89
shoulder M02.81-
vertebra M02.88
wrist M02.83-
specified form NEC M12.80
ankle M12.87-
elbow M12.82-
foot joint M12.87-
hand joint M12.84-
hip M12.85-
knee M12.86-
multiple site M12.89
shoulder M12.81-
specified joint NEC M12.88
vertebrae M12.88
wrist M12.83-
syringomyelic G95.0
tabes dorsalis A52.16
tabetic A52.16
transient —*see* Arthropathy, specified form NEC
traumatic M12.50
ankle M12.57-
elbow M12.52-
foot joint M12.57-
hand joint M12.54-
hip M12.55-
knee M12.56-
multiple site M12.59
shoulder M12.51-
specified joint NEC M12.58
vertebrae M12.58
wrist M12.53-
Arthropyosis —*see* Arthritis, pyogenic or pyemic
Arthrosis (deformans) (degenerative) (localized) —*see also* Osteoarthritis M19.90
spine —*see* Spondylosis
Arthus' phenomenon or reaction T78.41
due to
drug —*see* Table of Drugs and Chemicals, by drug
Articular —*see* condition
Articulation, reverse (teeth) M26.24
Artificial
insemination complication —*see* Complications, artificial, fertilization
opening status (functioning) (without complication) Z93.9
anus (colostomy) Z93.3
colostomy Z93.3
cystostomy Z93.50
appendico-vesicostomy Z93.52
cutaneous Z93.51
specified NEC Z93.59
enterostomy Z93.4
gastrostomy Z93.1
ileostomy Z93.2
intestinal tract NEC Z93.4
jejunostomy Z93.4
nephrostomy Z93.6
specified site NEC Z93.8
tracheostomy Z93.0
ureterostomy Z93.6
urethrostomy Z93.6
urinary tract NEC Z93.6
vagina Z93.8
vagina status Z93.8
Arytenoid —*see* condition
Asbestosis (occupational) J61
ASC-H (atypical squamous cells cannot exclude high grade squamous intraepithelial lesion on cytologic smear)
anus R85.611
cervix R87.611
vagina R87.621
ASC-US (atypical squamous cells of undetermined significance on cytologic smear)
anus R85.610
cervix R87.610
vagina R87.620
Ascariasis B77.9
with
complications NEC B77.89
intestinal complications B77.0
pneumonia, pneumonitis B77.81
Ascaridosis, ascaridiasis —*see* Ascariasis
Ascaris (infection) (infestation) (lumbricoides) —*see* Ascariasis
Ascending —*see* condition
Aschoff's bodies —*see* Myocarditis, rheumatic
Ascites (abdominal) R18.8
cardiac I50.9
chylous (nonfilarial) I89.8
filarial —*see* Infestation, filarial
due to
cirrhosis, alcoholic K70.31
hepatitis
alcoholic K70.11
chronic active K71.51
S. japonicum B65.2
heart I50.9
malignant R18.0
pseudochylous R18.8
syphilitic A52.74
tuberculous A18.31
Aseptic —*see* condition
Asherman's syndrome N85.6
Asialia K11.7
Asiatic cholera —*see* Cholera
Asimultagnosia (simultanagnosia) R48.3
Askin's tumor —*see* Neoplasm, connective tissue, malignant
Asocial personality F60.2
Asomatognosia R41.4
Aspartylglucosaminuria E77.1
Asperger's disease or syndrome F84.5
Aspergilloma —*see* Aspergillosis
Aspergillosis (with pneumonia) B44.9
bronchopulmonary, allergic B44.81
disseminated B44.7
generalized B44.7
pulmonary NEC B44.1
allergic B44.81
invasive B44.0
specified NEC B44.89
tonsillar B44.2
Aspergillus (flavus) (fumigatus) (infection) (terreus) —*see* Aspergillosis
Aspermatogenesis —*see* Azoospermia
Aspermia (testis) —*see* Azoospermia
Asphyxia, asphyxiation (by) R09.01
antenatal P84
birth P84
bunny bag —*see* Asphyxia, due to, mechanical threat to breathing, trapped in bed clothes
crushing S28.0
drowning T75.1
gas, fumes, or vapor —*see* Table of Drugs and Chemicals
inhalation —*see* Inhalation
intrauterine P84
local I73.00
with gangrene I73.01
mucus —*see also* Foreign body, respiratory tract, causing asphyxia
newborn P84
Asphyxia, asphyxiation *(Continued)*
pathological R09.01
postnatal P84
mechanical —*see* Asphyxia, due to, mechanical threat to breathing
prenatal P84
reticularis R23.1
strangulation —*see* Asphyxia, due to, mechanical threat to breathing
submersion T75.1
traumatic T71.9
due to
crushed chest S28.0
foreign body (in) —*see* Foreign body, respiratory tract, causing asphyxia
low oxygen content of ambient air T71.20
due to
being trapped in
low oxygen environment T71.29
in car trunk T71.221
circumstances undetermined T71.224
done with intent to harm by another person T71.223
self T71.222
in refrigerator T71.231
circumstances undetermined T71.234
done with intent to harm by another person T71.233
self T71.232
cave-in T71.21
mechanical threat to breathing (accidental) T71.191
circumstances undetermined T71.194
done with intent to harm by
another person T71.193
self T71.192
hanging T71.161
circumstances undetermined T71.164
done with intent to harm by
another person T71.163
self T71.162
plastic bag T71.121
circumstances undetermined T71.124
done with intent to harm by
another person T71.123
self T71.122
smothering
in furniture T71.151
circumstances undetermined T71.154
done with intent to harm by
another person T71.153
self T71.152
under
another person's body T71.141
circumstances undetermined T71.144
done with intent to harm T71.143
pillow T71.111
circumstances undetermined T71.114
done with intent to harm by another person T71.113
self T71.112
trapped in bed clothes T71.131
circumstances undetermined T71.134
done with intent to harm by
another person T71.133
self T71.132
vomiting, vomitus —*see* Foreign body, respiratory tract, causing asphyxia
Aspiration
amniotic (clear) fluid (newborn) P24.10
with
pneumonia (pneumonitis) P24.11
respiratory symptoms P24.11

Aspiration *(Continued)*
blood
newborn (without respiratory symptoms) P24.20
with
pneumonia (pneumonitis) P24.21
respiratory symptoms P24.21
specified age NEC —*see* Foreign body, respiratory tract
bronchitis J69.0
food or foreign body (with asphyxiation) —*see* Asphyxia, food
liquor (amnii) (newborn) P24.10
with
pneumonia (pneumonitis) P24.11
respiratory symptoms P24.11
meconium (newborn) (without respiratory symptoms) P24.00
with
pneumonitis (pneumonitis) P24.01
respiratory symptoms P24.01
milk (newborn) (without respiratory symptoms) P24.30
with
pneumonia (pneumonitis) P24.31
respiratory symptoms P24.31
specified age NEC —*see* Foreign body, respiratory tract
mucus —*see also* Foreign body, by site, causing asphyxia
newborn P24.10
with
pneumonia (pneumonitis) P24.11
respiratory symptoms P24.11
neonatal P24.9
specific NEC (without respiratory symptoms) P24.80
with
pneumonia (pneumonitis) P24.81
respiratory symptoms P24.81
newborn P24.9
specific NEC (without respiratory symptoms) P24.80
with
pneumonia (pneumonitis) P24.81
respiratory symptoms P24.81
pneumonia J69.0
pneumonitis J69.0
syndrome of newborn —*see* Aspiration, by substance, with pneumonia
vernix caseosa (newborn) P24.80
with
pneumonia (pneumonitis) P24.81
respiratory symptoms P24.81
vomitus —*see also* Foreign body, respiratory tract
newborn (without respiratory symptoms) P24.30
with
pneumonia (pneumonitis) P24.31
respiratory symptoms P24.31
Asplenia (congenital) Q89.01
postsurgical Z90.81
Assam fever B55.0
Assault, sexual —*see* Maltreatment
Assmann's focus NEC A15.0
Astasia (-abasia) (hysterical) F44.4
Asteatosis cutis L85.3
Astereognosia, astereognosis R48.1
Asterixis R27.8
in liver disease K71.3
Asteroid hyalitis —*see* Deposit, crystalline
Asthenia, asthenic R53.1
cardiac —*see also* Failure, heart I50.9
psychogenic F45.8
cardiovascular —*see also* Failure, heart I50.9
psychogenic F45.8
heart —*see also* Failure, heart I50.9
psychogenic F45.8

Asthenia, asthenic *(Continued)*
hysterical F44.4
myocardial —*see also* Failure, heart I50.9
psychogenic F45.8
nervous F48.8
neurocirculatory F45.8
neurotic F48.8
psychogenic F48.8
psychoneurotic F48.8
psychophysiologic F48.8
reaction (psychophysiologic) F48.8
senile R54
Asthenopia —*see also* Discomfort, visual
hysterical F44.6
psychogenic F44.6
Asthenospermia —*see* Abnormal, specimen, male genital organs
Asthma, asthmatic (bronchial) (catarrh) (spasmodic) J45.909
with
chronic obstructive bronchitis J44.9
with
acute lower respiratory infection J44.0
exacerbation (acute) J44.1
chronic obstructive pulmonary disease J44.9
with
acute lower respiratory infection J44.0
exacerbation (acute) J44.1
exacerbation (acute) J45.901
hay fever —*see* Asthma, allergic extrinsic
rhinitis, allergic —*see* Asthma, allergic extrinsic
status asthmaticus J45.902
allergic extrinsic J45.909
with
exacerbation (acute) J45.901
status asthmaticus J45.902
atopic —*see* Asthma, allergic extrinsic
cardiac —*see* Failure, ventricular, left
cardiobronchial I50.1
childhood J45.909
with
exacerbation (acute) J45.901
status asthmaticus J45.902
chronic obstructive J44.9
with
acute lower respiratory infection J44.0
exacerbation (acute) J44.1
collier's J60
cough variant J45.991
detergent J69.8
due to
detergent J69.8
inhalation of fumes J68.3
eosinophilic J82
extrinsic, allergic —*see* Asthma, allergic extrinsic
grinder's J62.8
hay —*see* Asthma, allergic extrinsic
heart I50.1
idiosyncratic —*see* Asthma, nonallergic
intermittent (mild) J45.20
with
exacerbation (acute) J45.21
status asthmaticus J45.22
intrinsic, nonallergic —*see* Asthma, nonallergic
Kopp's E32.8
late-onset J45.909
with
exacerbation (acute) J45.901
status asthmaticus J45.902
mild intermittent J45.20
with
exacerbation (acute) J45.21
status asthmaticus J45.22

Asthma, asthmatic *(Continued)*
mild persistent J45.30
with
exacerbation (acute) J45.31
status asthmaticus J45.32
Millar's (laryngismus stridulus) J38.5
miner's J60
mixed J45.909
with
exacerbation (acute) J45.901
status asthmaticus J45.902
moderate persistent J45.40
with
exacerbation (acute) J45.41
status asthmaticus J45.42
nervous —*see* Asthma, nonallergic
nonallergic (intrinsic) J45.909
with
exacerbation (acute) J45.901
status asthmaticus J45.902
persistent
mild J45.30
with
exacerbation (acute) J45.31
status asthmaticus J45.32
moderate J45.40
with
exacerbation (acute) J45.41
status asthmaticus J45.42
severe J45.50
with
exacerbation (acute) J45.51
status asthmaticus J45.52
platinum J45.998
pneumoconiotic NEC J64
potter's J62.8
predominantly allergic J45.909
psychogenic F54
pulmonary eosinophilic J82
red cedar J67.8
Rostan's I50.1
sandblaster's J62.8
sequoiosis J67.8
severe persistent J45.50
with
exacerbation (acute) J45.51
status asthmaticus J45.52
specified NEC J45.998
stonemason's J62.8
thymic E32.8
tuberculous —*see* Tuberculosis, pulmonary
Wichmann's (laryngismus stridulus) J38.5
wood J67.8
Astigmatism (compound) (congenital) H52.20-
irregular H52.21-
regular H52.22-
Astraphobia F40.220
Astroblastoma
specified site —*see* Neoplasm, malignant, by site
unspecified site C71.9
Astrocytoma (cystic)
anaplastic
specified site —*see* Neoplasm, malignant, by site
unspecified site C71.9
fibrillary
specified site —*see* Neoplasm, malignant, by site
unspecified site C71.9
fibrous
specified site —*see* Neoplasm, malignant, by site
unspecified site C71.9
gemistocytic
specified site —*see* Neoplasm, malignant, by site
unspecified site C71.9
juvenile
specified site —*see* Neoplasm, malignant, by site
unspecified site C71.9

A

Astrocytoma *(Continued)*
pilocytic
specified site —*see* Neoplasm, malignant, by site
unspecified site C71.9
piloid
specified site —*see* Neoplasm, malignant, by site
unspecified site C71.9
protoplasmic
specified site —*see* Neoplasm, malignant, by site
unspecified site C71.9
specified site NEC —*see* Neoplasm, malignant, by site
subependymal D43.2
giant cell
specified site —*see* Neoplasm, uncertain behavior, by site
unspecified site D43.2
specified site —*see* Neoplasm, uncertain behavior, by site
unspecified site D43.2
unspecified site C71.9
Astroglioma
specified site —*see* Neoplasm, malignant, by site
unspecified site C71.9
Asymbolia R48.8
Asymmetry —*see also* Distortion
between native and reconstructed breast N65.1
face Q67.0
jaw (lower) —*see* Anomaly, dentofacial, jaw-cranial base relationship, asymmetry
Asynergia, asynergy R27.8
ventricular I51.89
Asystole (heart) —*see* Arrest, cardiac
At risk
for falling Z91.81
Ataxia, ataxy, ataxic R27.0
acute R27.8
brain (hereditary) G11.9
cerebellar (hereditary) G11.9
with defective DNA repair G11.3
alcoholic G31.2
early-onset G11.1
in
alcoholism G31.2
myxedema E03.9 *[G13.2]*
neoplastic disease —*see also* Neoplasm D49.9 *[G32.81]* ◄
specified disease NEC G32.81
late-onset (Marie's) G11.2
cerebral (hereditary) G11.9
congenital nonprogressive G11.0
family, familial —*see* Ataxia, hereditary
following
cerebrovascular disease I69.993
cerebral infarction I69.393
intracerebral hemorrhage I69.193
nontraumatic intracranial hemorrhage NEC I69.293
specified disease NEC I69.893
subarachnoid hemorrhage I69.093
Friedreich's (heredofamilial) (cerebellar) (spinal) G11.1
gait R26.0
hysterical F44.4
general R27.8
gluten M35.9 *[G32.81]*
with celiac disease K90.0 *[G32.81]*
hereditary G11.9
with neuropathy G60.2
cerebellar —*see* Ataxia, cerebellar
spastic G11.4
specified NEC G11.8
spinal (Friedreich's) G11.1
heredofamilial —*see* Ataxia, hereditary
Hunt's G11.1
hysterical F44.4
Ataxia, ataxy, ataxic *(Continued)*
locomotor (progressive) (syphilitic) (partial) (spastic) A52.11
diabetic —*see* Diabetes, ataxia
Marie's (cerebellar) (heredofamilial) (late-onset) G11.2
nonorganic origin F44.4
nonprogressive, congenital G11.0
psychogenic F44.4
Roussy-Lévy G60.0
Sanger-Brown's (hereditary) G11.2
spastic hereditary G11.4
spinal
hereditary (Friedreich's) G11.1
progressive (syphilitic) A52.11
spinocerebellar, X-linked recessive G11.1
telangiectasia (Louis-Bar) G11.3
Ataxia-telangiectasia (Louis-Bar) G11.3
Atelectasis (massive) (partial) (pressure) (pulmonary) J98.11
newborn P28.10
due to resorption P28.11
partial P28.19
primary P28.0
secondary P28.19
primary (newborn) P28.0
tuberculous —*see* Tuberculosis, pulmonary
Atelocardia Q24.9
Atelomyelia Q06.1
Atheroembolism
of
extremities
lower I75.02-
upper I75.01-
kidney I75.81
specified NEC I75.89
Atheroma, atheromatous —*see also* Arteriosclerosis I70.90
aorta, aortic I70.0
valve —*see also* Endocarditis, aortic I35.8
aorto-iliac I70.0
artery —*see* Arteriosclerosis
basilar (artery) I67.2
carotid (artery) (common) (internal) I67.2
cerebral (arteries) I67.2
coronary (artery) I25.10
with angina pectoris —*see* Arteriosclerosis, coronary (artery)
degeneration —*see* Arteriosclerosis
heart, cardiac —*see* Disease, heart, ischemic, atherosclerotic
mitral (valve) I34.8
myocardium, myocardial —*see* Disease, heart, ischemic, atherosclerotic
pulmonary valve (heart) —*see also* Endocarditis, pulmonary I37.8
tricuspid (heart) (valve) I36.8
valve, valvular —*see* Endocarditis
vertebral (artery) I67.2
Atheromatosis —*see* Arteriosclerosis
Atherosclerosis —*see also* Arteriosclerosis
coronary
artery I25.10
with angina pectoris —*see* Arteriosclerosis, coronary (artery), due to
calcified coronary lesion (severely) I25.84
lipid rich plaque I25.83
transplanted heart I25.811
bypass graft I25.812
with angina pectoris —*see* Arteriosclerosis, coronary (artery)
native coronary artery I25.811
with angina pectoris —*see* Arteriosclerosis, coronary (artery)
Athetosis (acquired) R25.8
bilateral (congenital) G80.3
congenital (bilateral) (double) G80.3
double (congenital) G80.3
unilateral R25.8
Athlete's
foot B35.3
heart I51.7
Athrepsia E41
Athyrea (acquired) —*see also* Hypothyroidism
congenital E03.1
Atonia, atony, atonic
bladder (sphincter) (neurogenic) N31.2
capillary I78.8
cecum K59.8
psychogenic F45.8
colon —*see* Atony, intestine
congenital P94.2
esophagus K22.8
intestine K59.8
psychogenic F45.8
stomach K31.89
neurotic or psychogenic F45.8
uterus (during labor) O62.2
with hemorrhage (postpartum) O72.1
postpartum (with hemorrhage) O72.1
without hemorrhage O75.89
Atopy —*see* History, allergy
Atransferrinemia, congenital E88.09
Atresia, atretic
alimentary organ or tract NEC Q45.8
upper Q40.8
ani, anus, anal (canal) Q42.3
with fistula Q42.2
aorta (ring) Q25.29 ◄
aortic (orifice) (valve) Q23.0
arch Q25.21 ◄
congenital with hypoplasia of ascending aorta and defective development of left ventricle (with mitral stenosis) Q23.4
in hypoplastic left heart syndrome Q23.4
aqueduct of Sylvius Q03.0
with spina bifida —*see* Spina bifida, with hydrocephalus
artery NEC Q27.8
cerebral Q28.3
coronary Q24.5
digestive system Q27.8
eye Q15.8
lower limb Q27.8
pulmonary Q25.5
specified site NEC Q27.8
umbilical Q27.0
upper limb Q27.8
auditory canal (external) Q16.1
bile duct (common) (congenital) (hepatic) Q44.2
acquired —*see* Obstruction, bile duct
bladder (neck) Q64.39
obstruction Q64.31
bronchus Q32.4
cecum Q42.8
cervix (acquired) N88.2
congenital Q51.828
in pregnancy or childbirth —*see* Anomaly, cervix, in pregnancy or childbirth
causing obstructed labor O65.5
choana Q30.0
colon Q42.9
specified NEC Q42.8
common duct Q44.2
cricoid cartilage Q31.8
cystic duct Q44.2
acquired K82.8
with obstruction K82.0
digestive organs NEC Q45.8
duodenum Q41.0
ear canal Q16.1
ejaculatory duct Q55.4
epiglottis Q31.8
esophagus Q39.0
with tracheoesophageal fistula Q39.1
eustachian tube Q17.8
fallopian tube (congenital) Q50.6
acquired N97.1

◄ New ◄ Revised ~~deleted~~ Deleted

Atresia, atretic *(Continued)*
follicular cyst N83.0- ◄
foramen of
Luschka Q03.1
with spina bifida —*see* Spina bifida, with hydrocephalus
Magendie Q03.1
with spina bifida —*see* Spina bifida, with hydrocephalus
gallbladder Q44.1
genital organ
external
female Q52.79
male Q55.8
internal
female Q52.8
male Q55.8
glottis Q31.8
gullet Q39.0
with tracheoesophageal fistula Q39.1
heart valve NEC Q24.8
pulmonary Q22.0
tricuspid Q22.4
hymen Q52.3
acquired (postinfective) N89.6
ileum Q41.2
intestine (small) Q41.9
large Q42.9
specified NEC Q42.8
iris, filtration angle Q15.0
jejunum Q41.1
lacrimal apparatus Q10.4
larynx Q31.8
meatus urinarius Q64.33
mitral valve Q23.2
in hypoplastic left heart syndrome Q23.4
nares (anterior) (posterior) Q30.0
nasopharynx Q34.8
nose, nostril Q30.0
acquired J34.89
organ or site NEC Q89.8
osseous meatus (ear) Q16.1
oviduct (congenital) Q50.6
acquired N97.1
parotid duct Q38.4
acquired K11.8
pulmonary (artery) Q25.5
valve Q22.0
pulmonic Q22.0
pupil Q13.2
rectum Q42.1
with fistula Q42.0
salivary duct Q38.4
acquired K11.8
sublingual duct Q38.4
acquired K11.8
submandibular duct Q38.4
acquired K11.8
submaxillary duct Q38.4
acquired K11.8
thyroid cartilage Q31.8
trachea Q32.1
tricuspid valve Q22.4
ureter Q62.10
pelvic junction Q62.11
vesical orifice Q62.12
ureteropelvic junction Q62.11
ureterovesical orifice Q62.12
urethra (valvular) Q64.39
stricture Q64.32
urinary tract NEC Q64.8
uterus Q51.818
acquired N85.8
vagina (congenital) Q52.4
acquired (postinfectional) (senile) N89.5
vas deferens Q55.3
vascular NEC Q27.8
cerebral Q28.3
digestive system Q27.8

Atresia, atretic *(Continued)*
vascular NEC *(Continued)*
lower limb Q27.8
specified site NEC Q27.8
upper limb Q27.8
vein NEC Q27.8
digestive system Q27.8
great Q26.8
lower limb Q27.8
portal Q26.5
pulmonary Q26.3
specified site NEC Q27.8
upper limb Q27.8
vena cava (inferior) (superior) Q26.8
vesicourethral orifice Q64.31
vulva Q52.79
acquired N90.5
Atrichia, atrichosis —*see* Alopecia
Atrophia —*see also* Atrophy
cutis senilis L90.8
due to radiation L57.8
gyrata of choroid and retina H31.23
senilis R54
dermatological L90.8
due to radiation (nonionizing) (solar) L57.8
unguium L60.3
congenita Q84.6
Atrophie blanche (en plaque) (de Milian) L95.0
Atrophoderma, atrophodermia (of) L90.9
diffusum (idiopathic) L90.4
maculatum L90.8
et striatum L90.8
due to syphilis A52.79
syphilitic A51.39
neuriticum L90.8
Pasini and Pierini L90.3
pigmentosum Q82.1
reticulatum symmetricum faciei L66.4
senile L90.8
due to radiation (nonionizing) (solar) L57.8
vermiculata (cheeks) L66.4
Atrophy, atrophic (of)
adrenal (capsule) (gland) E27.49
primary (autoimmune) E27.1
alveolar process or ridge (edentulous) K08.20
anal sphincter (disuse) N81.84
appendix K38.8
arteriosclerotic —*see* Arteriosclerosis
bile duct (common) (hepatic) K83.8
bladder N32.89
neurogenic N31.8
blanche (en plaque) (of Milian) L95.0
bone (senile) NEC —*see also* Disorder, bone, specified type NEC
due to
tabes dorsalis (neurogenic) A52.11
brain (cortex) (progressive) G31.9
frontotemporal circumscribed G31.01 *[F02.80]*
with behavioral disturbance G31.01 *[F02.81]*
senile NEC G31.1
breast N64.2
obstetric —*see* Disorder, breast, specified type NEC
buccal cavity K13.79
cardiac —*see* Degeneration, myocardial
cartilage (infectional) (joint) —*see* Disorder, cartilage, specified NEC
cerebellar —*see* Atrophy, brain
cerebral —*see* Atrophy, brain
cervix (mucosa) (senile) (uteri) N88.8
menopausal N95.8
Charcot-Marie-Tooth G60.0
choroid (central) (macular) (myopic) (retina) H31.10-
diffuse secondary H31.12-
gyrate H31.23
senile H31.11-
ciliary body —*see* Atrophy, iris

Atrophy, atrophic *(Continued)*
conjunctiva (senile) H11.89
corpus cavernosum N48.89
cortical —*see* Atrophy, brain
cystic duct K82.8
Déjérine-Thomas G23.8
disuse NEC —*see* Atrophy, muscle
Duchenne-Aran G12.21
ear H93.8-
edentulous alveolar ridge K08.20
endometrium (senile) N85.8
cervix N88.8
enteric K63.89
epididymis N50.89 ◄
eyeball —*see* Disorder, globe, degenerated condition, atrophy
eyelid (senile) —*see* Disorder, eyelid, degenerative
facial (skin) L90.9
fallopian tube (senile) N83.32- ◄
with ovary N83.33- ◄
fascioscapulohumeral (Landouzy- Déjérine) G71.0
fatty, thymus (gland) E32.8
gallbladder K82.8
gastric K29.40
with bleeding K29.41
gastrointestinal K63.89
glandular I89.8
globe H44.52-
gum —*see also* Recession, gingival K06.0 ◄
hair L67.8
heart (brown) —*see* Degeneration, myocardial
hemifacial Q67.4
Romberg G51.8
infantile E41
paralysis, acute —*see* Poliomyelitis, paralytic
intestine K63.89
iris (essential) (progressive) H21.26-
specified NEC H21.29
kidney (senile) (terminal) —*see also* Sclerosis, renal N26.1
congenital or infantile Q60.5
bilateral Q60.4
unilateral Q60.3
hydronephrotic —*see* Hydronephrosis
lacrimal gland (primary) H04.14-
secondary H04.15-
Landouzy-Déjérine G71.0
laryngitis, infective J37.0
larynx J38.7
Leber's optic (hereditary) H47.22
lip K13.0
liver (yellow) K72.90
with coma K72.91
acute, subacute K72.00
with coma K72.01
chronic K72.10
with coma K72.11
lung (senile) J98.4
macular (dermatological) L90.8
syphilitic, skin A51.39
striated A52.79
mandible (edentulous) K08.20
minimal K08.21
moderate K08.22
severe K08.23
maxilla K08.20
minimal K08.24
moderate K08.25
severe K08.26
muscle, muscular (diffuse) (general) (idiopathic) (primary) M62.50
ankle M62.57-
Duchenne-Aran G12.21
foot M62.57-
forearm M62.53-
hand M62.54-
infantile spinal G12.0
lower leg M62.56-

Atrophy, atrophic *(Continued)*
muscle, muscular *(Continued)*
multiple sites M62.59
myelopathic —*see* Atrophy, muscle, spinal
myotonic G71.11
neuritic G58.9
neuropathic (peroneal) (progressive) G60.0
pelvic (disuse) N81.84
peroneal G60.0
progressive (bulbar) G12.21
adult G12.1
infantile (spinal) G12.0
spinal G12.9
adult G12.1
infantile G12.0
pseudohypertrophic G71.0
shoulder region M62.51-
specified site NEC M62.58
spinal G12.9
adult form G12.1
Aran-Duchenne G12.21
childhood form, type II G12.1
distal G12.1
hereditary NEC G12.1
infantile, type I (Werdnig- Hoffmann) G12.0
juvenile form, type III (Kugelberg-Welander) G12.1
progressive G12.21
scapuloperoneal form G12.1
specified NEC G12.8
syphilitic A52.78
thigh M62.55-
upper arm M62.52-
myocardium —*see* Degeneration, myocardial
myometrium (senile) N85.8
cervix N88.8
myopathic NEC —*see* Atrophy, muscle
myotonia G71.11
nail L60.3
nasopharynx J31.1
nerve —*see also* Disorder, nerve
abducens —*see* Strabismus, paralytic, sixth nerve
accessory G52.8
acoustic or auditory —*see* subcategory H93.3
cranial G52.9
eighth (auditory) —*see* subcategory H93.3
eleventh (accessory) G52.8
fifth (trigeminal) G50.8
first (olfactory) G52.0
fourth (trochlear) —*see* Strabismus, paralytic, fourth nerve
second (optic) H47.20
sixth (abducens) —*see* Strabismus, paralytic, sixth nerve
tenth (pneumogastric) (vagus) G52.2
third (oculomotor) —*see* Strabismus, paralytic, third nerve
twelfth (hypoglossal) G52.3
hypoglossal G52.3
oculomotor —*see* Strabismus, paralytic, third nerve
olfactory G52.0
optic (papillomacular bundle)
syphilitic (late) A52.15
congenital A50.44
pneumogastric G52.2
trigeminal G50.8
trochlear —*see* Strabismus, paralytic, fourth nerve
vagus (pneumogastric) G52.2
neurogenic, bone, tabetic A52.11
nutritional E41
old age R54
olivopontocerebellar G23.8

Atrophy, atrophic *(Continued)*
optic (nerve) H47.20
glaucomatous H47.23-
hereditary H47.22
primary H47.21-
specified type NEC H47.29-
syphilitic (late) A52.15
congenital A50.44
orbit H05.31-
ovary (senile) N83.31- ◄
with fallopian tube N83.33- ◄
oviduct (senile) —*see* Atrophy, fallopian tube
palsy, diffuse (progressive) G12.22
pancreas (duct) (senile) K86.89 ◄
parotid gland K11.0
pelvic muscle N81.84
penis N48.89
pharynx J39.2
pluriglandular E31.8
autoimmune E31.0
polyarthritis M15.9
prostate N42.89
pseudohypertrophic (muscle) G71.0
renal —*see also* Sclerosis, renal N26.1
retina, retinal (postinfectional) H35.89
rhinitis J31.0
salivary gland K11.0
scar L90.5
sclerosis, lobar (of brain) G31.09 *[F02.80]*
with behavioral disturbance G31.09 *[F02.81]*
scrotum N50.89 ◄
seminal vesicle N50.89 ◄
senile R54
due to radiation (nonionizing) (solar) L57.8
skin (patches) (spots) L90.9
degenerative (senile) L90.8
due to radiation (nonionizing) (solar) L57.8
senile L90.8
spermatic cord N50.89 ◄
spinal (acute) (cord) G95.89
muscular —*see* Atrophy, muscle, spinal
paralysis G12.20
acute —*see* Poliomyelitis, paralytic
meaning progressive muscular atrophy G12.21
spine (column) —*see* Spondylopathy, specified NEC
spleen (senile) D73.0
stomach K29.40
with bleeding K29.41
striate (skin) L90.6
syphilitic A52.79
subcutaneous L90.9
sublingual gland K11.0
submandibular gland K11.0
submaxillary gland K11.0
Sudeck's —*see* Algoneurodystrophy
suprarenal (capsule) (gland) E27.49
primary E27.1
systemic affecting central nervous system in
myxedema E03.9 *[G13.2]*
neoplastic disease —*see also* Neoplasm D49.9 *[G13.1]*
specified disease NEC G13.8
tarso-orbital fascia, congenital Q10.3
testis N50.0
thenar, partial —*see* Syndrome, carpal tunnel
thymus (fatty) E32.8
thyroid (gland) (acquired) E03.4
with cretinism E03.1
congenital (with myxedema) E03.1
tongue (senile) K14.8
papillae K14.4
trachea J39.8
tunica vaginalis N50.89 ◄
turbinate J34.89
tympanic membrane (nonflaccid) H73.82-
flaccid H73.81-
upper respiratory tract J39.8

Atrophy, atrophic *(Continued)*
uterus, uterine (senile) N85.8
cervix N88.8
due to radiation (intended effect) N85.8
adverse effect or misadventure N99.89
vagina (senile) N95.2
vas deferens N50.89 ◄
vascular I99.8
vertebra (senile) —*see* Spondylopathy, specified NEC
vulva (senile) N90.5
Werdnig-Hoffmann G12.0
yellow —*see* Failure, hepatic
Attack, attacks
with alteration of consciousness (with automatisms) —*see* Epilepsy, localization-related, symptomatic, with complex partial seizures
without alteration of consciousness —*see* Epilepsy, localization-related, symptomatic, with simple partial seizures
Adams-Stokes I45.9
akinetic —*see* Epilepsy, generalized, specified NEC
angina —*see* Angina
atonic —*see* Epilepsy, generalized, specified NEC
benign shuddering G25.83
cataleptic —*see* Catalepsy
coronary —*see* Infarct, myocardium
cyanotic, newborn P28.2
drop NEC R55
epileptic —*see* Epilepsy
heart —*see* infarct, myocardium
hysterical F44.9
jacksonian —*see* Epilepsy, localization-related, symptomatic, with simple partial seizures
myocardium, myocardial —*see* Infarct, myocardium
myoclonic —*see* Epilepsy, generalized, specified NEC
panic F41.0
psychomotor —*see* Epilepsy, localization-related, symptomatic, with complex partial seizures
salaam —*see* Epilepsy, spasms
schizophreniform, brief F23
shuddering, benign G25.83
Stokes-Adams I45.9
syncope R55
transient ischemic (TIA) G45.9
specified NEC G45.8
unconsciousness R55
hysterical F44.89
vasomotor R55
vasovagal (paroxysmal) (idiopathic) R55
Attention (to)
artificial
opening (of) Z43.9
digestive tract NEC Z43.4
colon Z43.3
ilium Z43.2
stomach Z43.1
specified NEC Z43.8
trachea Z43.0
urinary tract NEC Z43.6
cystostomy Z43.5
nephrostomy Z43.6
ureterostomy Z43.6
urethrostomy Z43.6
vagina Z43.7
colostomy Z43.3
cystostomy Z43.5
deficit disorder or syndrome F98.8
with hyperactivity —*see* Disorder, attention-deficit hyperactivity
gastrostomy Z43.1
ileostomy Z43.2

A

◄ New ◄ Revised ~~deleted~~ Deleted

Attention *(Continued)*
jejunostomy Z43.4
nephrostomy Z43.6
surgical dressings Z48.01
sutures Z48.02
tracheostomy Z43.0
ureterostomy Z43.6
urethrostomy Z43.6
Attrition
gum —*see also* Recession, gingival K06.0 ⬅
tooth, teeth (excessive) (hard tissues) K03.0
Atypical, atypism —*see also* condition
cells (on cytolgocial smear) (endocervical) (endometrial) (glandular)
cervix R87.619
vagina R87.629
cervical N87.9
endometrium N85.9
hyperplasia N85.00
parenting situation Z62.9
Auditory —*see* condition
Aujeszky's disease B33.8
Aurantiasis, cutis E67.1
Auricle, auricular —*see also* condition
cervical Q18.2
Auriculotemporal syndrome G50.8
Austin Flint murmur (aortic insufficiency) I35.1
Australian
Q fever A78
X disease A83.4
Autism, autistic (childhood) (infantile) F84.0
atypical F84.9
spectrum disorder F84.0 ◀
Autodigestion R68.89
Autoerythrocyte sensitization (syndrome) D69.2
Autographism L50.3
Autoimmune
disease (systemic) M35.9
inhibitors to clotting factors D68.311
lymphoproliferative syndrome [ALPS] D89.82
thyroiditis E06.3
Autointoxication R68.89
Automatism G93.89
with temporal sclerosis G93.81
epileptic —*see* Epilepsy, localization- related, symptomatic, with complex partial seizures

Automatism *(Continued)*
paroxysmal, idiopathic —*see* Epilepsy, localization-related, symptomatic, with complex partial seizures
Autonomic, autonomous
bladder (neurogenic) N31.2
hysteria seizure F44.5
Autosensitivity, erythrocyte D69.2
Autosensitization, cutaneous L30.2
Autosome —*see* condition by chromosome involved
Autotopagnosia R48.1
Autotoxemia R68.89
Autumn —*see* condition
Avellis' syndrome G46.8
Aversion
oral R63.3
newborn P92.-
nonorganic origin F98.2
sexual F52.1
Aviator's
disease or sickness —*see* Effect, adverse, high altitude
ear T70.0
Avitaminosis (multiple) —*see also* Deficiency, vitamin E56.9
B E53.9
with
beriberi E51.11
pellagra E52
B2 E53.0
B6 E53.1
B12 E53.8
D E55.9
with rickets E55.0
G E53.0
K E56.1
nicotinic acid E52
AVNRT (atrioventricular nodal re-entrant tachycardia) I47.1
AVRT (atrioventricular nodal re-entrant tachycardia) I47.1
Avulsion (traumatic)
blood vessel —*see* Injury, blood vessel
bone —*see* Fracture, by site
cartilage —*see also* Dislocation, by site
symphyseal (inner), complicating delivery O71.6
external site other than limb —*see* Wound, open, by site

Avulsion *(Continued)*
eye S05.7-
head (intracranial)
external site NEC S08.89
scalp S08.0
internal organ or site —*see* Injury, by site
joint —*see also* Dislocation, by site
capsule —*see* Sprain, by site
kidney S37.06-
ligament —*see* Sprain, by site
limb —*see also* Amputation, traumatic, by site
skin and subcutaneous tissue —*see* Wound, open, by site
muscle —*see* Injury, muscle
nerve (root) —*see* Injury, nerve
scalp S08.0
skin and subcutaneous tissue —*see* Wound, open, by site
spleen S36.032
symphyseal cartilage (inner), complicating delivery O71.6
tendon —*see* Injury, muscle
tooth S03.2
Awareness of heart beat R00.2
Axenfeld's
anomaly or syndrome Q15.0
degeneration (calcareous) Q13.4
Axilla, axillary —*see also* condition
breast Q83.1
Axonotmesis —*see* Injury, nerve
Ayerza's disease or syndrome (pulmonary artery sclerosis with pulmonary hypertension) I27.0
Azoospermia (organic) N46.01
due to
drug therapy N46.021
efferent duct obstruction N46.023
infection N46.022
radiation N46.024
specified cause NEC N46.029
systemic disease N46.025
Azotemia R79.89
meaning uremia N19
Aztec ear Q17.3
Azygos
continuation inferior vena cava Q26.8
lobe (lung) Q33.1

A

B

Baastrup's disease —*see* Kissing spine
Babesiosis B60.0
Babington's disease (familial hemorrhagic telangiectasia) I78.0
Babinski's syndrome A52.79
Baby
crying constantly R68.11
floppy (syndrome) P94.2
Bacillary —*see* condition
Bacilluria R82.71 ◄
Bacillus —*see also* Infection, bacillus
abortus infection A23.1
anthracis infection A22.9
coli infection —*see also* Escherichia coli B96.20
Flexner's A03.1
mallei infection A24.0
Shiga's A03.0
suipestifer infection —*see* Infection, salmonella
Back —*see* condition
Backache (postural) M54.9
sacroiliac M53.3
specified NEC M54.89
Backflow —*see* Reflux
Backward reading (dyslexia) F81.0
Bacteremia R78.81
with sepsis —*see* Sepsis
Bactericholia —*see* Cholecystitis, acute
Bacterid, bacteride (pustular) L40.3
Bacterium, bacteria, bacterial
agent NEC, as cause of disease classified elsewhere B96.89
in blood —*see* Bacteremia
in urine —*see* Bacteriuria
Bacteriuria, bacteruria R82.71 ◄
asymptomatic R82.71 ◄
Bacteroides
fragilis, as cause of disease classified elsewhere B96.6
Bad
heart —*see* Disease, heart
trip
due to drug abuse —*see* Abuse, drug, hallucinogen
due to drug dependence —*see* Dependence, drug, hallucinogen
Baelz's disease (cheilitis glandularis apostematosa) K13.0
Baerensprung's disease (eczema marginatum) B35.6
Bagasse disease or pneumonitis J67.1
Bagassosis J67.1
Baker's cyst —*see* Cyst, Baker's
Bakwin-Krida syndrome (metaphyseal dysplasia) Q78.5 ◄
Balancing side interference M26.56
Balanitis (circinata) (erosiva) (gangrenosa) (phagedenic) (vulgaris) N48.1
amebic A06.82
candidal B37.42
due to Haemophilus ducreyi A57
gonococcal (acute) (chronic) A54.09
xerotica obliterans N48.0
Balanoposthitis N47.6
gonococcal (acute) (chronic) A54.09
ulcerative (specific) A63.8
Balanorrhagia —*see* Balanitis
Balantidiasis, balantidiosis A07.0
Bald tongue K14.4
Baldness —*see also* Alopecia
male-pattern —*see* Alopecia, androgenic
Balkan grippe A78
Balloon disease —*see* Effect, adverse, high altitude
Balo's disease (concentric sclerosis) G37.5
Bamberger-Marie disease —*see* Osteoarthropathy, hypertrophic, specified type NEC
Bancroft's filariasis B74.0
Band (s)
adhesive —*see* Adhesions, peritoneum
anomalous or congenital —*see also* Anomaly, by site
heart (atrial) (ventricular) Q24.8
intestine Q43.3
omentum Q43.3
cervix N88.1
constricting, congenital Q79.8
gallbladder (congenital) Q44.1
intestinal (adhesive) —*see* Adhesions, peritoneum
obstructive
intestine K56.5
peritoneum K56.5
periappendiceal, congenital Q43.3
peritoneal (adhesive) —*see* Adhesions, peritoneum
uterus N73.6
internal N85.6
vagina N89.5
Bandemia D72.825
Bandl's ring (contraction), **complicating delivery** O62.4
Bangkok hemorrhagic fever A91
Bang's disease (brucella abortus) A23.1
Bankruptcy, anxiety concerning Z59.8
Bannister's disease T78.3
hereditary D84.1
Banti's disease or syndrome (with cirrhosis) (with portal hypertension) K76.6
Bar, median, prostate —*see* Enlargement, enlarged, prostate
Barcoo disease or rot —*see* Ulcer, skin
Barlow's disease E54
Barodontalgia T70.29
Baron Münchausen syndrome —*see* Disorder, factitious
Barosinusitis T70.1
Barotitis T70.0
Barotrauma T70.29
odontalgia T70.29
otitic T70.0
sinus T70.1
Barraquer (-Simons) **disease or syndrome** (progressive lipodystrophy) E88.1
Barré-Guillain disease or syndrome G61.0
Barré-Liéou syndrome (posterior cervical sympathetic) M53.0
Barrel chest M95.4
Barrett's
disease —*see* Barrett's, esophagus
esophagus K22.70
with dysplasia K22.719
high grade K22.711
low grade K22.710
without dysplasia K22.70
syndrome —*see* Barrett's, esophagus
ulcer K22.10
with bleeding K22.11
without bleeding K22.10
Barth syndrome E78.71
Bársony (-Polgár) (-Teschendorf) **syndrome** (corkscrew esophagus) K22.4
Bartholinitis (suppurating) N75.8
gonococcal (acute) (chronic) (with abscess) A54.1
Bartonellosis A44.9
cutaneous A44.1
mucocutaneous A44.1
specified NEC A44.8
systemic A44.0
Barton's fracture S52.56-
Bartter's syndrome E26.81
Basal —*see* condition
Basan's (hidrotic) **ectodermal dysplasia** Q82.4
Baseball finger —*see* Dislocation, finger
Basedow's disease (exophthalmic goiter) —*see* Hyperthyroidism, with, goiter
Basic —*see* condition
Basilar —*see* condition
Bason's (hidrotic) **ectodermal dysplasia** Q82.4
Basopenia —*see* Agranulocytosis
Basophilia D72.824
Basophilism (cortico-adrenal) (Cushing's) (pituitary) E24.0
Bassen-Kornzweig disease or syndrome E78.6
Bat ear Q17.5
Bateman's
disease B08.1
purpura (senile) D69.2
Bathing cramp T75.1
Bathophobia F40.248
Batten (-Mayou) **disease** E75.4
retina E75.4 *[H36]*
Batten-Steinert syndrome G71.11
Battered —*see* Maltreatment
Battey Mycobacterium infection A31.0
Battle exhaustion F43.0
Battledore placenta O43.19-
Baumgarten-Cruveilhier cirrhosis, disease or syndrome K74.69
Bauxite fibrosis (of lung) J63.1
Bayle's disease (general paresis) A52.17
Bazin's disease (primary) (tuberculous) A18.4
Beach ear —*see* Swimmer's, ear
Beaded hair (congenital) Q84.1
Béal conjunctivitis or syndrome B30.2
Beard's disease (neurasthenia) F48.8
Beat (s)
atrial, premature I49.1
ectopic I49.49
elbow —*see* Bursitis, elbow
escaped, heart I49.49
hand —*see* Bursitis, hand
knee —*see* Bursitis, knee
premature I49.40
atrial I49.1
auricular I49.1
supraventricular I49.1
Beau's
disease or syndrome —*see* Degeneration, myocardial
lines (transverse furrows on fingernails) L60.4
Bechterev's syndrome —*see* Spondylitis, ankylosing
Beck's syndrome (anterior spinal artery occlusion) I65.8
Becker's
cardiomyopathy I42.8
disease
idiopathic mural endomyocardial disease I42.3
myotonia congenita, recessive form G71.12
dystrophy G71.0
pigmented hairy nevus D22.5
Beckwith-Wiedemann syndrome Q87.3
Bed confinement status Z74.01
Bed sore —*see* Ulcer, pressure, by site
Bedbug bite (s) —*see* Bite (s), by site, superficial, insect
Bedclothes, asphyxiation or suffocation by —*see* Asphyxia, traumatic, due to, mechanical, trapped
Bednar's
aphthae K12.0
tumor —*see* Neoplasm, malignant, by site
Bedridden Z74.01
Bedsore —*see* Ulcer, pressure, by site
Bedwetting —*see* Enuresis
Bee sting (with allergic or anaphylactic shock) —*see* Toxicity, venom, arthropod, bee
Beer drinker's heart (disease) I42.6
Begbie's disease (exophthalmic goiter) —*see* Hyperthyroidism, with, goiter
Behavior
antisocial
adult Z72.811
child or adolescent Z72.810
disorder, disturbance —*see* Disorder, conduct
disruptive —*see* Disorder, conduct

◄ New ◄ Revised ~~deleted~~ Deleted

Behavior *(Continued)*
drug seeking Z76.5 ◀
inexplicable R46.2
marked evasiveness R46.5
obsessive-compulsive R46.81
overactivity R46.3
poor responsiveness R46.4
self-damaging (life-style) Z72.89
sleep-incompatible Z72.821
slowness R46.4
specified NEC R46.89
strange (and inexplicable) R46.2
suspiciousness R46.5
type A pattern Z73.1
undue concern or preoccupation with stressful events R46.6
verbosity and circumstantial detail obscuring reason for contact R46.7
Behcet's disease or syndrome M35.2
Behr's disease —*see* Degeneration, macula
Beigel's disease or morbus (white piedra) B36.2
Bejel A65
Bekhterev's syndrome —*see* Spondylitis, ankylosing
Belching —*see* Eructation
Bell's
mania F30.8
palsy, paralysis G51.0
infant or newborn P11.3
spasm G51.3
Bence Jones albuminuria or proteinuria NEC R80.3
Bends T70.3
Benedikt's paralysis or syndrome G46.3
Benign (*see also* condition)
prostatic hyperplasia —*see* Hyperplasia, prostate
Bennett's fracture (displaced) S62.21-
Benson's disease —*see* Deposit, crystalline
Bent
back (hysterical) F44.4
nose M95.0
congenital Q67.4
Bereavement (uncomplicated) Z63.4
Bergeron's disease (hysterical chorea) F44.4
Berger's disease —*see* Nephropathy, IgA
Beriberi (dry) E51.11
heart (disease) E51.12
polyneuropathy E51.11
wet E51.12
involving circulatory system E51.11
Berlin's disease or edema (traumatic) S05.8X-
Berlock (berloque) dermatitis L56.2
Bernard-Horner syndrome G90.2
Bernard-Soulier disease or thrombopathia D69.1
Bernhardt (-Roth) disease —*see* Mononeuropathy, lower limb, meralgia paresthetica
Bernheim's syndrome —*see* Failure, heart, congestive
Bertielliasis B71.8
Berylliosis (lung) J63.2
Besnier-Boeck (-Schaumann) disease —*see* Sarcoidosis
Besnier's
lupus pernio D86.3
prurigo L20.0
Bestiality F65.89
Best's disease H35.50
Beta-mercaptolactate-cysteine disulfiduria E72.09
Betalipoproteinemia, broad or floating E78.2
Betting and gambling Z72.6
pathological (compulsive) F63.0
Bezoar T18.9
intestine T18.3
stomach T18.2
Bezold's abscess —*see* Mastoiditis, acute
Bianchi's syndrome R48.8
Bicornate or bicornis uterus Q51.3
in pregnancy or childbirth O34.0- ◀
causing obstructed labor O65.5
Bicuspid aortic valve Q23.1
Biedl-Bardet syndrome Q87.89
Bielschowsky (-Jansky) disease E75.4
Biermer's (pernicious) anemia or disease D51.0
Biett's disease L93.0
Bifid (congenital)
apex, heart Q24.8
clitoris Q52.6
kidney Q63.8
nose Q30.2
patella Q74.1
scrotum Q55.29
toe NEC Q74.2
tongue Q38.3
ureter Q62.8
uterus Q51.3
uvula Q35.7
Biforis uterus (suprasimplex) Q51.3
Bifurcation (congenital)
gallbladder Q44.1
kidney pelvis Q63.8
renal pelvis Q63.8
rib Q76.6
tongue, congenital Q38.3
trachea Q32.1
ureter Q62.8
urethra Q64.74
vertebra Q76.49
Big spleen syndrome D73.1
Bigeminal pulse R00.8
Bilateral —*see* condition
Bile
duct —*see* condition
pigments in urine R82.2
Bilharziasis —*see also* Schistosomiasis
chyluria B65.0
cutaneous B65.3
galacturia B65.0
hematochyluria B65.0
intestinal B65.1
lipemia B65.9
lipuria B65.0
oriental B65.2
piarhemia B65.9
pulmonary NOS B65.9 *[J99]*
pneumonia B65.9 *[J17]*
tropical hematuria B65.0
vesical B65.0
Biliary —*see* condition
Bilirubin metabolism disorder E80.7
specified NEC E80.6
Bilirubinemia, familial nonhemolytic E80.4
Bilirubinuria R82.2
Biliuria R82.2
Bilocular stomach K31.2
Binswanger's disease I67.3
Biparta, bipartite
carpal scaphoid Q74.0
patella Q74.1
vagina Q52.10
Bird
face Q75.8
fancier's disease or lung J67.2
Birt-Hogg-Dube syndrome Q87.89
Birth
complications in mother —*see* Delivery, complicated
compression during NOS P15.9
defect —*see* Anomaly
immature (less than 37 completed weeks) —*see* Preterm, newborn
extremely (less than 28 completed weeks) —*see* Immaturity, extreme
inattention, at or after —*see* Maltreatment, child, neglect
injury NOS P15.9
basal ganglia P11.1
brachial plexus NEC P14.3
Birth *(Continued)*
injury NOS *(Continued)*
brain (compression) (pressure) P11.2
central nervous system NOS P11.9
cerebellum P11.1
cerebral hemorrhage P10.1
external genitalia P15.5
eye P15.3
face P15.4
fracture
bone P13.9
specified NEC P13.8
clavicle P13.4
femur P13.2
humerus P13.3
long bone, except femur P13.3
radius and ulna P13.3
skull P13.0
spine P11.5
tibia and fibula P13.3
intracranial P11.2
laceration or hemorrhage P10.9
specified NEC P10.8
intraventricular hemorrhage P10.2
laceration
brain P10.1
by scalpel P15.8
peripheral nerve P14.9
liver P15.0
meninges
brain P11.1
spinal cord P11.5
nerve
brachial plexus P14.3
cranial NEC (except facial) P11.4
facial P11.3
peripheral P14.9
phrenic (paralysis) P14.2
paralysis
facial nerve P11.3
spinal P11.5
penis P15.5
rupture
spinal cord P11.5
scalp P12.9
scalpel wound P15.8
scrotum P15.5
skull NEC P13.1
fracture P13.0
specified type NEC P15.8
spinal cord P11.5
spine P11.5
spleen P15.1
sternomastoid (hematoma) P15.2
subarachnoid hemorrhage P10.3
subcutaneous fat necrosis P15.6
subdural hemorrhage P10.0
tentorial tear P10.4
testes P15.5
vulva P15.5
lack of care, at or after —*see* Maltreatment, child, neglect
neglect, at or after —*see* Maltreatment, child, neglect
palsy or paralysis, newborn, NOS (birth injury) P14.9
premature (infant) —*see* Preterm, newborn
shock, newborn P96.89
trauma —*see* Birth, injury
weight
4000 grams to 4499 grams P08.1
4500 grams or more P08.0
low (2499 grams or less) —*see* Low, birthweight
extremely (999 grams or less) —*see* Low, birthweight, extreme
Birthmark Q82.5
Bisalbuminemia E88.09
Biskra's button B55.1

B

Bite (s) (animal) (human)
abdomen, abdominal
wall S31.159
with penetration into peritoneal cavity S31.659
epigastric region S31.152
with penetration into peritoneal cavity S31.652
left
lower quadrant S31.154
with penetration into peritoneal cavity S31.654
upper quadrant S31.151
with penetration into peritoneal cavity S31.651
periumbilic region S31.155
with penetration into peritoneal cavity S31.655
right
lower quadrant S31.153
with penetration into peritoneal cavity S31.653
upper quadrant S31.150
with penetration into peritoneal cavity S31.650
superficial NEC S30.871
insect S30.861
alveolar (process) —*see* Bite, oral cavity
amphibian (venomous) —*see* Venom, bite, amphibian
animal —*see also* Bite, by site
venomous —*see* Venom
ankle S91.05-
superficial NEC S90.57-
insect S90.56-
antecubital space —*see* Bite, elbow
anus S31.835
superficial NEC S30.877
insect S30.867
arm (upper) S41.15-
lower —*see* Bite, forearm
superficial NEC S40.87-
insect S40.86-
arthropod NEC —*see* Venom, bite, arthropod
auditory canal (external) (meatus) —*see* Bite, ear
auricle, ear —*see* Bite, ear
axilla —*see* Bite, arm
back —*see also* Bite, thorax, back
lower S31.050
with penetration into retroperitoneal space S31.051
superficial NEC S30.870
insect S30.860
bedbug —*see* Bite (s), by site, superficial, insect
breast S21.05-
superficial NEC S20.17-
insect S20.16-
brow —*see* Bite, head, specified site NEC
buttock S31.805
left S31.825
right S31.815
superficial NEC S30.870
insect S30.860
calf —*see* Bite, leg
canaliculus lacrimalis —*see* Bite, eyelid
canthus, eye —*see* Bite, eyelid
centipede —*see* Toxicity, venom, arthropod, centipede
cheek (external) S01.45-
internal —*see* Bite, oral cavity
superficial NEC S00.87
insect S00.86
chest wall —*see* Bite, thorax
chigger B88.0
chin —*see* Bite, head, specified site NEC
clitoris —*see* Bite, vulva
costal region —*see* Bite, thorax

Bite *(Continued)*
digit (s)
hand —*see* Bite, finger
toe —*see* Bite, toe
ear (canal) (external) S01.35-
superficial NEC S00.47-
insect S00.46-
elbow S51.05-
superficial NEC S50.37-
insect S50.36-
epididymis —*see* Bite, testis
epigastric region —*see* Bite, abdomen
epiglottis —*see* Bite, neck, specified site NEC
esophagus, cervical S11.25
superficial NEC S10.17
insect S10.16
eyebrow —*see* Bite, eyelid
eyelid S01.15-
superficial NEC S00.27-
insect S00.26-
face NEC —*see* Bite, head, specified site NEC
finger (s) S61.259
with
damage to nail S61.359
index S61.258
with
damage to nail S61.358
left S61.251
with
damage to nail S61.351
right S61.250
with
damage to nail S61.350
superficial NEC S60.478
insect S60.46-
little S61.25-
with
damage to nail S61.35-
superficial NEC S60.47-
insect S60.46-
middle S61.25-
with
damage to nail S61.35-
superficial NEC S60.47-
insect S60.46-
ring S61.25-
with
damage to nail S61.35-
superficial NEC S60.47-
insect S60.46-
superficial NEC S60.479
insect S60.469
thumb —*see* Bite, thumb
flank —*see* Bite, abdomen, wall
flea —*see* Bite, by site, superficial, insect
foot (except toe (s) alone) S91.35-
superficial NEC S90.87-
insect S90.86-
toe —*see* Bite, toe
forearm S51.85-
elbow only —*see* Bite, elbow
superficial NEC S50.87-
insect S50.86-
forehead —*see* Bite, head, specified site NEC
genital organs, external
female S31.552
superficial NEC S30.876
insect S30.866
vagina and vulva —*see* Bite, vulva
male S31.551
penis —*see* Bite, penis
scrotum —*see* Bite, scrotum
superficial NEC S30.875
insect S30.865
testes —*see* Bite, testis
groin —*see* Bite, abdomen, wall
gum —*see* Bite, oral cavity

Bite *(Continued)*
hand S61.45-
finger —*see* Bite, finger
superficial NEC S60.57-
insect S60.56-
thumb —*see* Bite, thumb
head S01.95
cheek —*see* Bite, cheek
ear —*see* Bite, ear
eyelid —*see* Bite, eyelid
lip —*see* Bite, lip
nose —*see* Bite, nose
oral cavity —*see* Bite, oral cavity
scalp —*see* Bite, scalp
specified site NEC S01.85
superficial NEC S00.87
insect S00.86
superficial NEC S00.97
insect S00.96
temporomandibular area —*see* Bite, cheek
heel —*see* Bite, foot
hip S71.05-
superficial NEC S70.27-
insect S70.26-
hymen S31.45
hypochondrium —*see* Bite, abdomen, wall
hypogastric region —*see* Bite, abdomen, wall
inguinal region —*see* Bite, abdomen, wall
insect —*see* Bite, by site, superficial, insect
instep —*see* Bite, foot
interscapular region —*see* Bite, thorax, back
jaw —*see* Bite, head, specified site NEC
knee S81.05-
superficial NEC S80.27-
insect S80.26-
labium (majus) (minus) —*see* Bite, vulva
lacrimal duct —*see* Bite, eyelid
larynx S11.015
superficial NEC S10.17
insect S10.16
leg (lower) S81.85-
ankle —*see* Bite, ankle
foot —*see* Bite, foot
knee —*see* Bite, knee
superficial NEC S80.87-
insect S80.86-
toe —*see* Bite, toe
upper —*see* Bite, thigh
lip S01.551
superficial NEC S00.571
insect S00.561
lizard (venomous) —*see* Venom, bite, reptile
loin —*see* Bite, abdomen, wall
lower back —*see* Bite, back, lower
lumbar region —*see* Bite, back, lower
malar region —*see* Bite, head, specified site NEC
mammary —*see* Bite, breast
marine animals (venomous) —*see* Toxicity, venom, marine animal
mastoid region —*see* Bite, head, specified site NEC
mouth —*see* Bite, oral cavity
nail
finger —*see* Bite, finger
toe —*see* Bite, toe
nape —*see* Bite, neck, specified site NEC
nasal (septum) (sinus) —*see* Bite, nose
nasopharynx —*see* Bite, head, specified site NEC
neck S11.95
involving
cervical esophagus —*see* Bite, esophagus, cervical
larynx —*see* Bite, larynx
pharynx —*see* Bite, pharynx
thyroid gland S11.15
trachea —*see* Bite, trachea
specified site NEC S11.85
superficial NEC S10.87
insect S10.86

Bite *(Continued)*
neck *(Continued)*
superficial NEC S10.97
insect S10.96
throat S11.85
superficial NEC S10.17
insect S10.16
nose (septum) (sinus) S01.25
superficial NEC S00.37
insect S00.36
occipital region —*see* Bite, scalp
oral cavity S01.552
superficial NEC S00.572
insect S00.562
orbital region —*see* Bite, eyelid
palate —*see* Bite, oral cavity
palm —*see* Bite, hand
parietal region —*see* Bite, scalp
pelvis S31.050
with penetration into retroperitoneal space S31.051
superficial NEC S30.870
insect S30.860
penis S31.25
superficial NEC S30.872
insect S30.862
perineum
female —*see* Bite, vulva
male —*see* Bite, pelvis
periocular area (with or without lacrimal passages) —*see* Bite, eyelid
phalanges
finger —*see* Bite, finger
toe —*see* Bite, toe
pharynx S11.25
superficial NEC S10.17
insect S10.16
pinna —*see* Bite, ear
poisonous —*see* Venom
popliteal space —*see* Bite, knee
prepuce —*see* Bite, penis
pubic region —*see* Bite, abdomen, wall
rectovaginal septum —*see* Bite, vulva
red bug B88.0
reptile NEC —*see also* Venom, bite, reptile
nonvenomous —*see* Bite, by site
snake —*see* Venom, bite, snake
sacral region —*see* Bite, back, lower
sacroiliac region —*see* Bite, back, lower
salivary gland —*see* Bite, oral cavity
scalp S01.05
superficial NEC S00.07
insect S00.06
scapular region —*see* Bite, shoulder
scrotum S31.35
superficial NEC S30.873
insect S30.863
sea-snake (venomous) —*see* Toxicity, venom, snake, sea snake
shin —*see* Bite, leg
shoulder S41.05-
superficial NEC S40.27-
insect S40.26-
snake —*see also* Venom, bite, snake
nonvenomous —*see* Bite, by site
spermatic cord —*see* Bite, testis
spider (venomous) —*see* Toxicity, venom, spider
nonvenomous —*see* Bite, by site, superficial, insect
sternal region —*see* Bite, thorax, front
submaxillary region —*see* Bite, head, specified site NEC
submental region —*see* Bite, head, specified site NEC
subungual
finger (s) —*see* Bite, finger
toe —*see* Bite, toe
superficial —*see* Bite, by site, superficial
supraclavicular fossa S11.85

Bite *(Continued)*
supraorbital —*see* Bite, head, specified site NEC
temple, temporal region —*see* Bite, head, specified site NEC
temporomandibular area —*see* Bite, cheek
testis S31.35
superficial NEC S30.873
insect S30.863
thigh S71.15-
superficial NEC S70.37-
insect S70.36-
thorax, thoracic (wall) S21.95
back S21.25-
with penetration into thoracic cavity S21.45-
breast —*see* Bite, breast
front S21.15-
with penetration into thoracic cavity S21.35-
superficial NEC S20.97
back S20.47-
front S20.37-
insect S20.96
back S20.46-
front S20.36-
throat —*see* Bite, neck, throat
thumb S61.05-
with
damage to nail S61.15-
superficial NEC S60.37-
insect S60.36-
thyroid S11.15
superficial NEC S10.87
insect S10.86
toe (s) S91.15-
with
damage to nail S91.25-
great S91.15-
with
damage to nail S91.25-
lesser S91.15-
with
damage to nail S91.25-
superficial NEC S90.47-
great S90.47-
insect S90.46-
great S90.46-
tongue S01.552
trachea S11.025
superficial NEC S10.17
insect S10.16
tunica vaginalis —*see* Bite, testis
tympanum, tympanic membrane —*see* Bite, ear
umbilical region S31.155
uvula —*see* Bite, oral cavity
vagina —*see* Bite, vulva
venomous —*see* Venom
vocal cords S11.035
superficial NEC S10.17
insect S10.16
vulva S31.45
superficial NEC S30.874
insect S30.864
wrist S61.55-
superficial NEC S60.87-
insect S60.86-
Biting, cheek or lip K13.1
Biventricular failure (heart) I50.9
Björck (-Thorson) **syndrome** (malignant carcinoid) E34.0
Black
death A20.9
eye S00.1-
hairy tongue K14.3
heel (foot) S90.3-
lung (disease) J60
palm (hand) S60.22-
Blackfan-Diamond anemia or syndrome (congenital hypoplastic anemia) D61.01

Blackhead L70.0
Blackout R55
Bladder —*see* condition
Blast (air) (hydraulic) (immersion) (underwater)
blindness S05.8X-
injury
abdomen or thorax —*see* Injury, by site
ear (acoustic nerve trauma) —*see* Injury, nerve, acoustic, specified type NEC
syndrome NEC T70.8
Blastoma —*see* Neoplasm, malignant, by site
pulmonary —*see* Neoplasm, lung, malignant
Blastomycosis, blastomycotic B40.9
Brazilian —*see* Paracoccidioidomycosis
cutaneous B40.3
disseminated B40.7
European —*see* Cryptococcosis
generalized B40.7
keloidal B48.0
North American B40.9
primary pulmonary B40.0
pulmonary B40.2
acute B40.0
chronic B40.1
skin B40.3
South American —*see* Paracoccidioidomycosis
specified NEC B40.89
Bleb (s) R23.8
emphysematous (lung) (solitary) J43.9
endophthalmitis H59.43
filtering (vitreous), after glaucoma surgery Z98.83
inflammed (infected), postprocedural H59.40
stage 1 H59.41
stage 2 H59.42
stage 3 H59.43
lung (ruptured) J43.9
congenital —*see* Atelectasis
newborn P25.8
subpleural (emphysematous) J43.9
Blebitis, postprocedural H59.40
stage 1 H59.41
stage 2 H59.42
stage 3 H59.43
Bleeder (familial) (hereditary) —*see* Hemophilia
Bleeding —*see also* Hemorrhage
anal K62.5
anovulatory N97.0
atonic, following delivery O72.1
capillary I78.8
puerperal O72.2
contact (postcoital) N93.0
due to uterine subinvolution N85.3
ear —*see* Otorrhagia
excessive, associated with menopausal onset N92.4
familial —*see* Defect, coagulation
following intercourse N93.0
gastrointestinal K92.2
hemorrhoids —*see* Hemorrhoids
intermenstrual (regular) N92.3
irregular N92.1
intraoperative —*see* Complication, intraoperative, hemorrhage
irregular N92.6
menopausal N92.4
newborn, intraventricular —*see* Newborn, affected by, hemorrhage, intraventricular
nipple N64.59
nose R04.0
ovulation N92.3
postclimacteric N95.0
postcoital N93.0
postmenopausal N95.0
postoperative —*see* Complication, postprocedural, hemorrhage
preclimacteric N92.4
pre-pubertal vaginal N93.1 ◀
puberty (excessive, with onset of menstrual periods) N92.2

B

Bleeding *(Continued)*
rectum, rectal K62.5
newborn P54.2
tendencies —*see* Defect, coagulation
throat R04.1
tooth socket (post-extraction) K91.840
umbilical stump P51.9
uterus, uterine NEC N93.9
climacteric N92.4
dysfunctional of functional N93.8
menopausal N92.4
preclimacteric or premenopausal N92.4
unrelated to menstrual cycle N93.9
vagina, vaginal (abnormal) N93.9
dysfunctional or functional N93.8
newborn P54.6
pre-pubertal N93.1 ◀
vicarious N94.89
Blennorrhagia, blennorrhagic —*see* Gonorrhea
Blennorrhea (acute) (chronic) —*see also* Gonorrhea
inclusion (neonatal) (newborn) P39.1
lower genitourinary tract (gonococcal) A54.00
neonatorum (gonococcal ophthalmia) A54.31
Blepharelosis —*see* Entropion
Blepharitis (angularis) (ciliaris) (eyelid) (marginal) (nonulcerative) H01.009
herpes zoster B02.39
left H01.006
lower H01.005
upper H01.004
right H01.003
lower H01.002
upper H01.001
squamous H01.029
left H01.026
lower H01.025
upper H01.024
right H01.023
lower H01.022
upper H01.021
ulcerative H01.019
left H01.016
lower H01.015
upper H01.014
right H01.013
lower H01.012
upper H01.011
Blepharochalasis H02.30
congenital Q10.0
left H02.36
lower H02.35
upper H02.34
right H02.33
lower H02.32
upper H02.31
Blepharoclonus H02.59
Blepharoconjunctivitis H10.50-
angular H10.52-
contact H10.53-
ligneous H10.51-
Blepharophimosis (eyelid) H02.529
congenital Q10.3
left H02.526
lower H02.525
upper H02.524
right H02.523
lower H02.522
upper H02.521
Blepharoptosis H02.40-
congenital Q10.0
mechanical H02.41-
myogenic H02.42-
neurogenic H02.43-
paralytic H02.43-
Blepharopyorrhea, gonococcal A54.39
Blepharospasm G24.5
drug induced G24.01
Blighted ovum O02.0
Blind —*see also* Blindness
bronchus (congenital) Q32.4
loop syndrome K90.2
congenital Q43.8
sac, fallopian tube (congenital) Q50.6
spot, enlarged —*see* Defect, visual field, localized, scotoma, blind spot area
tract or tube, congenital NEC —*see* Atresia, by site
Blindness (acquired) (congenital) (both eyes) H54.0
blast S05.8X-
color —*see* Deficiency, color vision
concussion S05.8X-
cortical H47.619
left brain H47.612
right brain H47.611
day H53.11
due to injury (current episode) S05.9-
sequelae — code to injury with seventh character S
eclipse (total) —*see* Retinopathy, solar
emotional (hysterical) F44.6
face H53.16
hysterical F44.6
legal (both eyes) (USA definition) H54.8
mind R48.8
night H53.60
abnormal dark adaptation curve H53.61
acquired H53.62
congenital H53.63
specified type NEC H53.69
vitamin A deficiency E50.5
one eye (other eye normal) H54.40
left (normal vision on right) H54.42
low vision on right H54.12
low vision, other eye H54.10
right (normal vision on left) H54.41
low vision on left H54.11
psychic R48.8
river B73.01
snow —*see* Photokeratitis
sun, solar —*see* Retinopathy, solar
transient —*see* Disturbance, vision, subjective, loss, transient
traumatic (current episode) S05.9-
word (developmental) F81.0
acquired R48.0
secondary to organic lesion R48.0
Blister (nonthermal)
abdominal wall S30.821
alveolar process S00.522
ankle S90.52-
antecubital space —*see* Blister, elbow
anus S30.827
arm (upper) S40.82-
auditory canal —*see* Blister, ear
auricle —*see* Blister, ear
axilla —*see* Blister, arm
back, lower S30.820
beetle dermatitis L24.89
breast S20.12-
brow S00.82
calf —*see* Blister, leg
canthus —*see* Blister, eyelid
cheek S00.82
internal S00.522
chest wall —*see* Blister, thorax
chin S00.82
costal region —*see* Blister, thorax
digit (s)
foot —*see* Blister, toe
hand —*see* Blister, finger
due to burn —*see* Burn, by site, second degree
ear S00.42-
elbow S50.32-
epiglottis S10.12
esophagus, cervical S10.12
eyebrow —*see* Blister, eyelid
eyelid S00.22-
face S00.82
Blister *(Continued)*
fever B00.1
finger (s) S60.429
index S60.42-
little S60.42-
middle S60.42-
ring S60.42-
foot (except toe (s) alone) S90.82-
toe —*see* Blister, toe
forearm S50.82-
elbow only —*see* Blister, elbow
forehead S00.82
fracture - omit code
genital organ
female S30.826
male S30.825
gum S00.522
hand S60.52-
head S00.92
ear —*see* Blister, ear
eyelid —*see* Blister, eyelid
lip S00.521
nose S00.32
oral cavity S00.522
scalp S00.02
specified site NEC S00.82
heel —*see* Blister, foot
hip S70.22-
interscapular region S20.429
jaw S00.82
knee S80.22-
larynx S10.12
leg (lower) S80.82-
knee —*see* Blister, knee
upper —*see* Blister, thigh
lip S00.521
malar region S00.82
mammary —*see* Blister, breast
mastoid region S00.82
mouth S00.522
multiple, skin, nontraumatic R23.8
nail
finger —*see* Blister, finger
toe —*see* Blister, toe
nasal S00.32
neck S10.92
specified site NEC S10.82
throat S10.12
nose S00.32
occipital region S00.02
oral cavity S00.522
orbital region —*see* Blister, eyelid
palate S00.522
palm —*see* Blister, hand
parietal region S00.02
pelvis S30.820
penis S30.822
periocular area —*see* Blister, eyelid
phalanges
finger —*see* Blister, finger
toe —*see* Blister, toe
pharynx S10.12
pinna —*see* Blister, ear
popliteal space —*see* Blister, knee
scalp S00.02
scapular region —*see* Blister, shoulder
scrotum S30.823
shin —*see* Blister, leg
shoulder S40.22-
sternal region S20.329
submaxillary region S00.82
submental region S00.82
subungual
finger (s) —*see* Blister, finger
toe (s) —*see* Blister, toe
supraclavicular fossa S10.82
supraorbital S00.82
temple S00.82
temporal region S00.82
testis S30.823
thermal —*see* Burn, second degree, by site

◀ New ⇐ Revised ~~deleted~~ Deleted

Blister *(Continued)*
thigh S70.32-
thorax, thoracic (wall) S20.92
back S20.42-
front S20.32-
throat S10.12
thumb S60.32-
toe (s) S90.42-
great S90.42-
tongue S00.522
trachea S10.12
tympanum, tympanic membrane —*see* Blister, ear
upper arm —*see* Blister, arm (upper)
uvula S00.522
vagina S30.824
vocal cords S10.12
vulva S30.824
wrist S60.82-
Bloating R14.0
Bloch-Sulzberger disease or syndrome Q82.3
Block, blocked
alveolocapillary J84.10
arborization (heart) I45.5
arrhythmic I45.9
atrioventricular (incomplete) (partial) I44.30
with atrioventricular dissociation I44.2
complete I44.2
congenital Q24.6
congenital Q24.6
first degree I44.0
second degree (types I and II) I44.1
specified NEC I44.39
third degree I44.2
types I and II I44.1
auriculoventricular —*see* Block, atrioventricular
bifascicular (cardiac) I45.2
bundle-branch (complete) (false) (incomplete) I45.4
bilateral I45.2
left I44.7
with right bundle branch block I45.2
hemiblock I44.60
anterior I44.4
posterior I44.5
incomplete I44.7
with right bundle branch block I45.2
right I45.10
with
left bundle branch block I45.2
left fascicular block I45.2
specified NEC I45.19
Wilson's type I45.19
cardiac I45.9
conduction I45.9
complete I44.2
fascicular (left) I44.60
anterior I44.4
posterior I44.5
right I45.0
specified NEC I44.69
foramen Magendie (acquired) G91.1
congenital Q03.1
with spina bifida —*see* Spina bifida, by site, with hydrocephalus
heart I45.9
bundle branch I45.4
bilateral I45.2
complete (atrioventricular) I44.2
congenital Q24.6
first degree (atrioventricular) I44.0
second degree (atrioventricular) I44.1
specified type NEC I45.5
third degree (atrioventricular) I44.2
hepatic vein I82.0
intraventricular (nonspecific) I45.4
bundle branch
bilateral I45.2
kidney N28.9
postcystoscopic or postprocedural N99.0

Block, blocked *(Continued)*
Mobitz (types I and II) I44.1
myocardial —*see* Block, heart
nodal I45.5
organ or site, congenital NEC —*see* Atresia, by site
portal (vein) I81
second degree (types I and II) I44.1
sinoatrial I45.5
sinoauricular I45.5
third degree I44.2
trifascicular I45.3
tubal N97.1
vein NOS I82.90
Wenckebach (types I and II) I44.1
Blockage —*see* Obstruction
Blocq's disease F44.4
Blood
constituents, abnormal R78.9
disease D75.9
donor —*see* Donor, blood
dyscrasia D75.9
with
abortion —*see* Abortion, by type, complicated by, hemorrhage
ectopic pregnancy O08.1
molar pregnancy O08.1
following ectopic or molar pregnancy O08.1
newborn P61.9
puerperal, postpartum O72.3
flukes NEC —*see* Schistosomiasis
in
feces K92.1
occult R19.5
urine —*see* Hematuria
mole O02.0
occult in feces R19.5
pressure
decreased, due to shock following injury T79.4
examination only Z01.30
fluctuating I99.8
high —*see* Hypertension
borderline R03.0
incidental reading, without diagnosis of hypertension R03.0
low —*see also* Hypotension
incidental reading, without diagnosis of hypotension R03.1
spitting —*see* Hemoptysis
staining cornea —*see* Pigmentation, cornea, stromal
transfusion
reaction or complication —*see* Complications, transfusion
type
A (Rh positive) Z67.10
Rh negative Z67.11
AB (Rh positive) Z67.30
Rh negative Z67.31
B (Rh positive) Z67.20
Rh negative Z67.21
O (Rh positive) Z67.40
Rh negative Z67.41
Rh (positive) Z67.90
negative Z67.91
vessel rupture —*see* Hemorrhage
vomiting —*see* Hematemesis
Blood-forming organs, disease D75.9
Bloodgood's disease —*see* Mastopathy, cystic
Bloom (-Machacek)(-Torre) **syndrome** Q82.8
Blount's disease or osteochondrosis —*see* Osteochondrosis, juvenile, tibia
Blue
baby Q24.9
diaper syndrome E72.09
dome cyst (breast) —*see* Cyst, breast
dot cataract Q12.0

Blue *(Continued)*
nevus D22.9
sclera Q13.5
with fragility of bone and deafness Q78.0
toe syndrome I75.02-
Blueness —*see* Cyanosis
Blues, postpartal O90.6
baby O90.6
Blurring, visual H53.8
Blushing (abnormal) (excessive) R23.2
BMI —*see* Body, mass index
Boarder, hospital NEC Z76.4
accompanying sick person Z76.3
healthy infant or child Z76.2
foundling Z76.1
Bockhart's impetigo L01.02
Bodechtel-Guttman disease (subacute sclerosing panencephalitis) A81.1
Boder-Sedgwick syndrome (ataxia-telangiectasia) G11.3
Body, bodies
Aschoff's —*see* Myocarditis, rheumatic
asteroid, vitreous —*see* Deposit, crystalline
cytoid (retina) —*see* Occlusion, artery, retina
drusen (degenerative) (macula) (retinal) —*see also* Degeneration, macula, drusen
optic disc —*see* Drusen, optic disc
foreign —*see* Foreign body
loose
joint, except knee —*see* Loose, body, joint knee M23.4-
sheath, tendon —*see* Disorder, tendon, specified type NEC
mass index (BMI)
adult
19 or less Z68.1
20.0-20.9 Z68.20
21.0-21.9 Z68.21
22.0-22.9 Z68.22
23.0-23.9 Z68.23
24.0-24.9 Z68.24
25.0-25.9 Z68.25
26.0-26.9 Z68.26
27.0-27.9 Z68.27
28.0-28.9 Z68.28
29.0-29.9 Z68.29
30.0-30.9 Z68.30
31.0-31.9 Z68.31
32.0-32.9 Z68.32
33.0-33.9 Z68.33
34.0-34.9 Z68.34
35.0-35.9 Z68.35
36.0-36.9 Z68.36
37.0-37.9 Z68.37
38.0-38.9 Z68.38
39.0-39.9 Z68.39
40.0-44.9 Z68.41
45.0-49.9 Z68.42
50.0-59.9 Z68.43
60.0-69.9 Z68.44
70 and over Z68.45
pediatric
5th percentile to less than 85th percentile for age Z68.52
85th percentile to less than 95th percentile for age Z68.53
greater than or equal to ninety-fifth percentile for age Z68.54
less than fifth percentile for age Z68.51
Mooser's A75.2
rice —*see also* Loose, body, joint knee M23.4-
rocking F98.4
Boeck's
disease or sarcoid —*see* Sarcoidosis
lupoid (miliary) D86.3
Boerhaave's syndrome (spontaneous esophageal rupture) K22.3
Boggy
cervix N88.8
uterus N85.8

Boil —*see also* Furuncle, by site
  Aleppo B55.1
  Baghdad B55.1
  Delhi B55.1
  lacrimal
    gland —*see* Dacryoadenitis
    passages (duct) (sac) —*see* Inflammation, lacrimal, passages, acute
  Natal B55.1
  orbit, orbital —*see* Abscess, orbit
  tropical B55.1
Bold hives —*see* Urticaria
Bombé, iris —*see* Membrane, pupillary
Bone —*see* condition
Bonnevie-Ullrich syndrome —*see also* Turner's syndrome Q87.1 ⟸
Bonnier's syndrome —*see* subcategory H81.8
Bonvale dam fever T73.3
Bony block of joint —*see* Ankylosis
BOOP (bronchiolitis obliterans organized pneumonia) J84.89
Borderline
  diabetes mellitus R73.03 ⟸
  hypertension R03.0
  osteopenia M85.8-
  pelvis, with obstruction during labor O65.1
  personality F60.3
Borna disease A83.9
Bornholm disease B33.0
Boston exanthem A88.0
Botalli, ductus (patent) (persistent) Q25.0
Bothriocephalus latus infestation B70.0
Botulism (foodborne intoxication) A05.1
  infant A48.51
  non-foodborne A48.52
  wound A48.52
Bouba —*see* Yaws
Bouchard's nodes (with arthropathy) M15.2
Bouffée délirante F23
Bouillaud's disease or syndrome (rheumatic heart disease) I01.9
Bourneville's disease Q85.1
Boutonniere deformity (finger) —*see* Deformity, finger, boutonniere
Bouveret (-Hoffmann) **syndrome** (paroxysmal tachycardia) I47.9
Bovine heart —*see* Hypertrophy, cardiac
Bowel —*see* condition
Bowen's
  dermatosis (precancerous) —*see* Neoplasm, skin, in situ
  disease —*see* Neoplasm, skin, in situ
  epithelioma —*see* Neoplasm, skin, in situ
  type
    epidermoid carcinoma-in-situ —*see* Neoplasm, skin, in situ
    intraepidermal squamous cell carcinoma —*see* Neoplasm, skin, in situ
Bowing
  femur —*see also* Deformity, limb, specified type NEC, thigh
    congenital Q68.3
  fibula —*see also* Deformity, limb, specified type NEC, lower leg
    congenital Q68.4
  forearm —*see* Deformity, limb, specified type NEC, forearm
  leg (s), long bones, congenital Q68.5
  radius —*see* Deformity, limb, specified type NEC, forearm
  tibia —*see also* Deformity, limb, specified type NEC, lower leg
    congenital Q68.4
Bowleg (s) (acquired) M21.16-
  congenital Q68.5
  rachitic E64.3
Boyd's dysentery A03.2
Brachial —*see* condition
Brachycardia R00.1
Brachycephaly Q75.0
Bradley's disease A08.19
Bradyarrhythmia, cardiac I49.8
Bradycardia (sinoatrial) (sinus) (vagal) R00.1
  neonatal P29.12
  reflex G90.09
  tachycardia syndrome I49.5
Bradykinesia R25.8
Bradypnea R06.89
Bradytachycardia I49.5
Brailsford's disease or osteochondrosis —*see* Osteochondrosis, juvenile, radius
Brain —*see also* condition
  death G93.82
  syndrome —*see* Syndrome, brain
Branched-chain amino-acid disorder E71.2
Branchial —*see* condition
  cartilage, congenital Q18.2
Branchiogenic remnant (in neck) Q18.0
Brandt's syndrome (acrodermatitis enteropathica) E83.2
Brash (water) R12
Bravais-jacksonian epilepsy —*see* Epilepsy, localization-related, symptomatic, with simple partial seizures
Braxton Hicks contractions —*see* False, labor
Brazilian leishmaniasis B55.2
BRBPR K62.5
Break, retina (without detachment) H33.30-
  with retinal detachment —*see* Detachment, retina
  horseshoe tear H33.31-
  multiple H33.33-
  round hole H33.32-
Breakdown
  device, graft or implant —*see also* Complications, by site and type, mechanical T85.618
    arterial graft NEC —*see* Complication, cardiovascular device, mechanical, vascular
    breast (implant) T85.41
    catheter NEC T85.618
      cystostomy T83.010
      dialysis (renal) T82.41
        intraperitoneal T85.611
      Hopkins T83.018 ◀
      ileostomy T83.018 ◀
      infusion NEC T82.514
        cranial T85.610 ◀
        epidural T85.610 ◀
        intrathecal T85.610 ◀
        spinal T85.610 ⟸
        subarachnoid T85.610 ◀
        subdural T85.610 ◀
      ~~urinary (indwelling) T83.018~~
      nephrostomy T83.012 ◀
      urethral indwelling T83.011 ◀
      urinary NEC T83.018 ◀
      urostomy T83.018 ◀
    electronic (electrode) (pulse generator) (stimulator)
      bone T84.310
      cardiac T82.119
        electrode T82.110
        pulse generator T82.111
        specified type NEC T82.118
      nervous system —*see* Complication, prosthetic device, mechanical, electronic nervous system stimulator
      urinary —*see* Complication, genitourinary, device, urinary, mechanical
    fixation, internal (orthopedic) NEC —*see* Complication, fixation device, mechanical
    gastrointestinal —*see* Complications, prosthetic device, mechanical, gastrointestinal device
    genital NEC T83.418
      intrauterine contraceptive device T83.31
      penile prosthesis (cylinder) (implanted) (pump) (resevoir) T83.410 ⟸
      testicular prosthesis T83.411 ◀
Breakdown *(Continued)*
  device, graft or implant *(Continued)*
    heart NEC —*see* Complication, cardiovascular device, mechanical
    intrathecal infusion pump T85.615 ◀
    joint prosthesis —*see* Complications..., joint prosthesis,internal, mechanical, by site
    nervous system, specified device NEC T85.615 ◀
    ocular NEC —*see* Complications, prosthetic device, mechanical, ocular device
    orthopedic NEC —*see* Complication, orthopedic, device, mechanical
    specified NEC T85.618
    subcutaneous device pocket ◀
      nervous system prosthetic device, implant, or graft T85.890 ◀
      other internal prosthetic device, implant, or graft T85.898 ◀
    sutures, permanent T85.612
      used in bone repair —*see* Complications, fixation device, internal (orthopedic), mechanical
    urinary NEC T83.118 ⟸
      graft T83.21
      sphincter, implanted T83.111 ◀
      stent (ileal conduit) (nephroureteral) T83.113 ◀
        ureteral indwelling T83.112 ◀
    vascular NEC —*see* Complication, cardiovascular device, mechanical
    ventricular intracranial shunt T85.01
  nervous F48.8
  perineum O90.1
  respirator J95.850
    specified NEC J95.859
  ventilator J95.850
    specified NEC J95.859
Breast —*see also* condition
  buds E30.1
    in newborn P96.89
  dense R92.2
  nodule N63
Breath
  foul R19.6
  holder, child R06.89
  holding spell R06.89
  shortness R06.02
Breathing
  labored —*see* Hyperventilation
  mouth R06.5
    causing malocclusion M26.5
  periodic R06.3
    high altitude G47.32
Breathlessness R06.81
Breda's disease —*see* Yaws
Breech presentation (mother) O32.1
  causing obstructed labor O64.1
  footling O32.8
    causing obstructed labor O64.8
  incomplete O32.8
    causing obstructed labor O64.8
Breisky's disease N90.4
Brennemann's syndrome I88.0
Brenner
  tumor (benign) D27.9
    borderline malignancy D39.1-
    malignant C56
    proliferating D39.1
Bretonneau's disease or angina A36.0
Breus' mole O02.0
Brevicollis Q76.49
Brickmakers' anemia B76.9 *[D63.8]*
Bridge, myocardial Q24.5
Bright red blood per rectum (BRBPR) K62.5
Bright's disease —*see also* Nephritis
  arteriosclerotic —*see* Hypertension, kidney
Brill (-Zinsser) **disease** (recrudescent typhus) A75.1
  flea-borne A75.2
  louse-borne A75.1

◀ New ⟸ Revised ~~deleted~~ Deleted

Brill-Symmers' disease C82.90
Brion-Kayser disease —*see* Fever, parathyroid
Briquet's disorder or syndrome F45.0
Brissaud's
  infantilism or dwarfism E23.0
  motor-verbal tic F95.2
Brittle
  bones disease Q78.0
  nails L60.3
    congenital Q84.6
Broad —*see also* condition
  beta disease E78.2
  ligament laceration syndrome N83.8
Broad- or floating-betalipoproteinemia E78.2
Brock's syndrome (atelectasis due to enlarged lymph nodes) J98.19
Brocq-Duhring disease (dermatitis herpetiformis) L13.0
Brodie's abscess or disease M86.8X-
Broken
  arches —*see also* Deformity, limb, flat foot
  arm (meaning upper limb) —*see* Fracture, arm
  back —*see* Fracture, vertebra
  bone —*see* Fracture
  implant or internal device —*see* Complications, by site and type, mechanical
  leg (meaning lower limb) —*see* Fracture, leg
  nose S02.2
  tooth, teeth —*see* Fracture, tooth
Bromhidrosis, bromidrosis L75.0
Bromidism, bromism G92
  chronic (dependence) F13.20
  due to
    correct substance properly administered —*see* Table of Drugs and Chemicals, by drug, adverse effect
    overdose or wrong substance given or taken —*see* Table of Drugs and Chemicals, by drug, poisoning
Bromidrosiphobia F40.298
Bronchi, bronchial —*see* condition
Bronchiectasis (cylindrical) (diffuse) (fusiform) (localized) (saccular) J47.9
  with
    acute
      bronchitis J47.0
      lower respiratory infection J47.0
    exacerbation (acute) J47.1
  congenital Q33.4
  tuberculous NEC —*see* Tuberculosis, pulmonary
Bronchiolectasis —*see* Bronchiectasis
Bronchiolitis (acute) (infective) (subacute) J21.9
  with
    bronchospasm or obstruction J21.9
    influenza, flu or grippe —*see* Influenza, with, respiratory manifestations NEC
  chemical (chronic) J68.4
    acute J68.0
  chronic (fibrosing) (obliterative) J44.9
  due to
    external agent —*see* Bronchitis, acute, due to
    human metapneumovirus J21.1
    respiratory syncytial virus J21.0
    specified organism NEC J21.8
  fibrosa obliterans J44.9
  influenzal —*see* Influenza, with, respiratory manifestations NEC
  obliterans J42
    with organizing pneumonia (BOOP) J84.89
  obliterative (chronic) (subacute) J44.9
    due to chemicals, gases, fumes or vapors (inhalation) J68.4
    due to fumes or vapors J68.4
  respiratory, interstitial lung disease J84.115
Bronchitis (diffuse) (fibrinous) (hypostatic) (infective) (membranous) J40
  with
    influenza, flu or grippe —*see* Influenza, with, respiratory manifestations NEC
Bronchitis *(Continued)*
  with *(Continued)*
    obstruction (airway) (lung) J44.9
    tracheitis (15 years of age and above) J40
      acute or subacute J20.9
      chronic J42
      under 15 years of age J20.9
  acute or subacute (with bronchospasm or obstruction) J20.9
    with
      bronchiectasis J47.0
      chronic obstructive pulmonary disease J44.0
    chemical (due to gases, fumes or vapors) J68.0
    due to
      fumes or vapors J68.0
      Haemophilus influenzae J20.1
      Mycoplasma pneumoniae J20.0
      radiation J70.0
      specified organism NEC J20.8
      Streptococcus J20.2
      virus
        coxsackie J20.3
        echovirus J20.7
        parainfluenzae J20.4
        respiratory syncytial J20.5
        rhinovirus J20.6
    viral NEC J20.8
  allergic (acute) J45.909
    with
      exacerbation (acute) J45.901
      status asthmaticus J45.902
  arachidic T17.528
  aspiration (due to fumes or vapors) J68.0
  asthmatic J45.9
    chronic J44.9
      with
        acute lower respiratory infection J44.0
        exacerbation (acute) J44.1
  capillary —*see* Pneumonia, broncho
  caseous (tuberculous) A15.5
  Castellani's A69.8
  catarrhal (15 years of age and above) J40
    acute —*see* Bronchitis, acute
    chronic J41.0
    under 15 years of age J20.9
  chemical (acute) (subacute) J68.0
    chronic J68.4
    due to fumes or vapors J68.0
      chronic J68.4
  chronic J42
    with
      airways obstruction J44.9
      tracheitis (chronic) J42
    asthmatic (obstructive) J44.9
    catarrhal J41.0
    chemical (due to fumes or vapors) J68.4
    due to
      chemicals, gases, fumes or vapors (inhalation) J68.4
      radiation J70.1
      tobacco smoking J41.0
    emphysematous J44.9
    mucopurulent J41.1
    non-obstructive J41.0
    obliterans J44.9
    obstructive J44.9
    purulent J41.1
    simple J41.0
  croupous —*see* Bronchitis, acute
  due to gases, fumes or vapors (chemical) J68.0
  emphysematous (obstructive) J44.9
  exudative —*see* Bronchitis, acute
  fetid J41.1
  grippal —*see* Influenza, with, respiratory manifestations NEC
  in those under 15 years age —*see* Bronchitis, acute
    chronic —*see* Bronchitis, chronic
Bronchitis *(Continued)*
  influenzal —*see* Influenza, with, respiratory manifestations NEC
  mixed simple and mucopurulent J41.8
  moulder's J62.8
  mucopurulent (chronic) (recurrent) J41.1
    acute or subacute J20.9
    simple (mixed) J41.8
  obliterans (chronic) J44.9
  obstructive (chronic) (diffuse) J44.9
  pituitous J41.1
  pneumococcal, acute or subacute J20.2
  pseudomembranous, acute or subacute —*see* Bronchitis, acute
  purulent (chronic) (recurrent) J41.1
    acute or subacute —*see* Bronchitis, acute
  putrid J41.1
  senile (chronic) J42
  simple and mucopurulent (mixed) J41.8
  smokers' J41.0
  spirochetal NEC A69.8
  subacute —*see* Bronchitis, acute
  suppurative (chronic) J41.1
    acute or subacute —*see* Bronchitis, acute
  tuberculous A15.5
  under 15 years of age —*see* Bronchitis, acute
    chronic —*see* Bronchitis, chronic
  viral NEC, acute or subacute —*see also* Bronchitis, acute J20.8
Bronchoalveolitis J18.0
Bronchoaspergillosis B44.1
Bronchocele meaning goiter E04.0
Broncholithiasis J98.09
  tuberculous NEC A15.5
Bronchomalacia J98.09
  congenital Q32.2
Bronchomycosis NOS B49 *[J99]*
  candidal B37.1
Bronchopleuropneumonia —*see* Pneumonia, broncho
Bronchopneumonia —*see* Pneumonia, broncho
Bronchopneumonitis —*see* Pneumonia, broncho
Bronchopulmonary —*see* condition
Bronchopulmonitis —*see* Pneumonia, broncho
Bronchorrhagia (*see* Hemoptysis)
Bronchorrhea J98.09
  acute J20.9
  chronic (infective) (purulent) J42
Bronchospasm (acute) J98.01
  with
    bronchiolitis, acute J21.9
    bronchitis, acute (conditions in J20) —*see* Bronchitis, acute
  due to external agent —*see* condition, respiratory, acute, due to
  exercise induced J45.990
Bronchospirochetosis A69.8
  Castellani A69.8
Bronchostenosis J98.09
Bronchus —*see* condition
Brontophobia F40.220
Bronze baby syndrome P83.8
Brooke's tumor —*see* Neoplasm, skin, benign
Brown enamel of teeth (hereditary) K00.5
Brown's sheath syndrome H50.61-
Brown-Séquard disease, paralysis or syndrome G83.81
Bruce sepsis A23.0
Brucellosis (infection) A23.9
  abortus A23.1
  canis A23.3
  dermatitis A23.9
  melitensis A23.0
  mixed A23.8
  sepsis A23.9
    melitensis A23.0
    specified NEC A23.8
  suis A23.2
Bruck-de Lange disease Q87.1
Bruck's disease —*see* Deformity, limb

B

Brugsch's syndrome Q82.8
Bruise (skin surface intact) —*see also* Contusion
  with
    open wound —*see* Wound, open
  internal organ —*see* Injury, by site
  newborn P54.5
  scalp, due to birth injury, newborn P12.3
  umbilical cord O69.5
Bruit (arterial) R09.89
  cardiac R01.1
Brush burn —*see* Abrasion, by site
Bruton's X-linked agammaglobulinemia D80.0
Bruxism
  psychogenic F45.8
  sleep related G47.63
Bubbly lung syndrome P27.0
Bubo I88.8
  blennorrhagic (gonococcal) A54.89
  chancroidal A57
  climatic A55
  due to Haemophilus ducreyi A57
  gonococcal A54.89
  indolent (nonspecific) I88.8
  inguinal (nonspecific) I88.8
    chancroidal A57
    climatic A55
    due to H. ducreyi A57
    infective I88.8
  scrofulous (tuberculous) A18.2
  soft chancre A57
  suppurating —*see* Lymphadenitis, acute
  syphilitic (primary) A51.0
    congenital A50.07
  tropical A55
  virulent (chancroidal) A57
Bubonic plague A20.0
Bubonocele —*see* Hernia, inguinal
Buccal —*see* condition
Buchanan's disease or osteochondrosis M91.0
Buchem's syndrome (hyperostosis corticalis) M85.2
Bucket-handle fracture or tear (semilunar cartilage) —*see* Tear, meniscus
Budd-Chiari syndrome (hepatic vein thrombosis) I82.0
Budgerigar fancier's disease or lung J67.2
Buds
  breast E30.1
    in newborn P96.89
Buerger's disease (thromboangiitis obliterans) I73.1
Bulbar —*see* condition
Bulbus cordis (left ventricle) (persistent) Q21.8
Bulimia (nervosa) F50.2
  atypical F50.9
  normal weight F50.9
Bulky
  stools R19.5
  uterus N85.2
Bulla (e) R23.8
  lung (emphysematous) (solitary) J43.9
    newborn P25.8
Bullet wound —*see also* Wound, open
  fracture - code as Fracture, by site
  internal organ —*see* Injury, by site
Bundle
  branch block (complete) (false) (incomplete) —*see* Block, bundle-branch
  of His —*see* condition
Bunion M21.61- ⇐
  tailor's M21.62- ◀
Bunionette M21.62- ◀
Buphthalmia, buphthalmos (congenital) Q15.0
Burdwan fever B55.0
Bürger-Grütz disease or syndrome E78.3
Buried
  penis (congenital) Q55.64
    acquired N48.83
  roots K08.3
Burke's syndrome K86.89 ⇐
Burkitt
  cell leukemia C91.0-
  lymphoma (malignant) C83.7-
    small noncleaved, diffuse C83.7-
    spleen C83.77
    undifferentiated C83.7-
  tumor C83.7-
  type
    acute lymphoblastic leukemia C91.0-
    undifferentiated C83.7-
Burn (electricity) (flame) (hot gas, liquid or hot object) (radiation) (steam) (thermal) T30.0
  abdomen, abdominal (muscle) (wall) T21.02
    first degree T21.12
    second degree T21.22
    third degree T21.32
  above elbow T22.039
    first degree T22.139
    left T22.032
      first degree T22.132
      second degree T22.232
      third degree T22.332
    right T22.031
      first degree T22.131
      second degree T22.231
      third degree T22.331
    second degree T22.239
    third degree T22.339
  acid (caustic) (external) (internal) —*see* Corrosion, by site
  alimentary tract NEC T28.2
    esophagus T28.1
    mouth T28.0
    pharynx T28.0
  alkaline (caustic) (external) (internal) —*see* Corrosion, by site
  ankle T25.019
    first degree T25.119
    left T25.012
      first degree T25.112
      second degree T25.212
      third degree T25.312
    multiple with foot —*see* Burn, lower, limb, multiple, ankle and foot
    right T25.011
      first degree T25.111
      second degree T25.211
      third degree T25.311
    second degree T25.219
    third degree T25.319
  anus —*see* Burn, buttock
  arm (lower) (upper) —*see* Burn, upper, limb
  axilla T22.049
    first degree T22.149
    left T22.042
      first degree T22.142
      second degree T22.242
      third degree T22.342
    right T22.041
      first degree T22.141
      second degree T22.241
      third degree T22.341
    second degree T22.249
    third degree T22.349
  back (lower) T21.04
    first degree T21.14
    second degree T21.24
    third degree T21.34
    upper T21.03
      first degree T21.13
      second degree T21.23
      third degree T21.33
  blisters - code as Burn, second degree, by site
  breast (s) —*see* Burn, chest wall
  buttock (s) T21.05
    first degree T21.15
    second degree T21.25
    third degree T21.35
Burn *(Continued)*
  calf T24.039
    first degree T24.139
    left T24.032
      first degree T24.132
      second degree T24.232
      third degree T24.332
    right T24.031
      first degree T24.131
      second degree T24.231
      third degree T24.331
    second degree T24.239
    third degree T24.339
  canthus (eye) —*see* Burn, eyelid
  caustic acid or alkaline —*see* Corrosion, by site
  cervix T28.3
  cheek T20.06
    first degree T20.16
    second degree T20.26
    third degree T20.36
  chemical (acids) (alkalines) (caustics) (external) (internal) —*see* Corrosion, by site
  chest wall T21.01
    first degree T21.11
    second degree T21.21
    third degree T21.31
  chin T20.03
    first degree T20.13
    second degree T20.23
    third degree T20.33
  colon T28.2
  conjunctiva (and cornea) —*see* Burn, cornea
  cornea (and conjunctiva) T26.1-
    chemical —*see* Corrosion, cornea
  corrosion (external) (internal) —*see* Corrosion, by site
  deep necrosis of underlying tissue - code as Burn, third degree, by site
  dorsum of hand T23.069
    first degree T23.169
    left T23.062
      first degree T23.162
      second degree T23.262
      third degree T23.362
    right T23.061
      first degree T23.161
      second degree T23.261
      third degree T23.361
    second degree T23.269
    third degree T23.369
  due to ingested chemical agent —*see* Corrosion, by site
  ear (auricle) (external) (canal) T20.01
    first degree T20.11
    second degree T20.21
    third degree T20.31
  elbow T22.029
    first degree T22.129
    left T22.022
      first degree T22.122
      second degree T22.222
      third degree T22.322
    right T22.021
      first degree T22.121
      second degree T22.221
      third degree T22.321
    second degree T22.229
    third degree T22.329
  epidermal loss - code as Burn, second degree, by site
  erythema, erythematous - code as Burn, first degree, by site
  esophagus T28.1
  extent (percentage of body surface)
    less than 10 percent T31.0
    10-19 percent T31.10
      with 0-9 percent third degree burns T31.10
      with 10-19 percent third degree burns T31.11

◀ New ⇐ Revised ~~deleted~~ Deleted

Burn *(Continued)*
extent *(Continued)*
20-29 percent T31.20
with 0-9 percent third degree burns T31.20
with 10-19 percent third degree burns T31.21
with 20-29 percent third degree burns T31.22
30-39 percent T31.30
with 0-9 percent third degree burns T31.30
with 10-19 percent third degree burns T31.31
with 20-29 percent third degree burns T31.32
with 30-39 percent third degree burns T31.33
40-49 percent T31.40
with 0-9 percent third degree burns T31.40
with 10-19 percent third degree burns T31.41
with 20-29 percent third degree burns T31.42
with 30-39 percent third degree burns T31.43
with 40-49 percent third degree burns T31.44
50-59 percent T31.50
with 0-9 percent third degree burns T31.50
with 10-19 percent third degree burns T31.51
with 20-29 percent third degree burns T31.52
with 30-39 percent third degree burns T31.53
with 40-49 percent third degree burns T31.54
with 50-59 percent third degree burns T31.55
60-69 percent T31.60
with 0-9 percent third degree burns T31.60
with 10-19 percent third degree burns T31.61
with 20-29 percent third degree burns T31.62
with 30-39 percent third degree burns T31.63
with 40-49 percent third degree burns T31.64
with 50-59 percent third degree burns T31.65
with 60-69 percent third degree burns T31.66
70-79 percent T31.70
with 0-9 percent third degree burns T31.70
with 10-19 percent third degree burns T31.71
with 20-29 percent third degree burns T31.72
with 30-39 percent third degree burns T31.73
with 40-49 percent third degree burns T31.74
with 50-59 percent third degree burns T31.75
with 60-69 percent third degree burns T31.76
with 70-79 percent third degree burns T31.77
80-89 percent T31.80
with 0-9 percent third degree burns T31.80
with 10-19 percent third degree burns T31.81
with 20-29 percent third degree burns T31.82
with 30-39 percent third degree burns T31.83
with 40-49 percent third degree burns T31.84

Burn *(Continued)*
extent *(Continued)*
80-89 percent T31.80 *(Continued)*
with 50-59 percent third degree burns T31.85
with 60-69 percent third degree burns T31.86
with 70-79 percent third degree burns T31.87
with 80-89 percent third degree burns T31.88
90 percent or more T31.90
with 0-9 percent third degree burns T31.90
with 10-19 percent third degree burns T31.91
with 20-29 percent third degree burns T31.92
with 30-39 percent third degree burns T31.93
with 40-49 percent third degree burns T31.94
with 50-59 percent third degree burns T31.95
with 60-69 percent third degree burns T31.96
with 70-79 percent third degree burns T31.97
with 80-89 percent third degree burns T31.98
with 90 percent or more third degree burns T31.99
extremity —*see* Burn, limb
eye (s) and adnexa T26.4-
with resulting rupture and destruction of eyeball T26.2-
conjunctival sac —*see* Burn, cornea
cornea —*see* Burn, cornea
lid —*see* Burn, eyelid
periocular area —*see* Burn, eyelid
specified site NEC T26.3-
eyeball —*see* Burn, eye
eyelid (s) T26.0-
chemical —*see* Corrosion, eyelid
face —*see* Burn, head
finger T23.029
first degree T23.129
left T23.022
first degree T23.122
second degree T23.222
third degree T23.322
multiple sites (without thumb) T23.039
with thumb T23.049
first degree T23.149
left T23.042
first degree T23.142
second degree T23.242
third degree T23.342
right T23.041
first degree T23.141
second degree T23.241
third degree T23.341
second degree T23.249
third degree T23.349
first degree T23.139
left T23.032
first degree T23.132
second degree T23.232
third degree T23.332
right T23.031
first degree T23.131
second degree T23.231
third degree T23.331
second degree T23.239
third degree T23.339
right T23.021
first degree T23.121
second degree T23.221
third degree T23.321
second degree T23.229
third degree T23.329
flank —*see* Burn, abdominal wall

Burn *(Continued)*
foot T25.029
first degree T25.129
left T25.022
first degree T25.122
second degree T25.222
third degree T25.322
multiple with ankle —*see* Burn, lower, limb, multiple, ankle and foot
right T25.021
first degree T25.121
second degree T25.221
third degree T25.321
second degree T25.229
third degree T25.329
forearm T22.019
first degree T22.119
left T22.012
first degree T22.112
second degree T22.212
third degree T22.312
right T22.011
first degree T22.111
second degree T22.211
third degree T22.311
second degree T22.219
third degree T22.319
forehead T20.06
first degree T20.16
second degree T20.26
third degree T20.36
fourth degree - code as Burn, third degree, by site
friction —*see* Burn, by site
from swallowing caustic or corrosive substance NEC —*see* Corrosion, by site
full thickness skin loss - code as Burn, third degree, by site
gastrointestinal tract NEC T28.2
from swallowing caustic or corrosive substance T28.7
genital organs
external
female T21.07
first degree T21.17
second degree T21.27
third degree T21.37
male T21.06
first degree T21.16
second degree T21.26
third degree T21.36
internal T28.3
from caustic or corrosive substance T28.8
groin —*see* Burn, abdominal wall
hand (s) T23.009
back —*see* Burn, dorsum of hand
finger —*see* Burn, finger
first degree T23.109
left T23.002
first degree T23.102
second degree T23.202
third degree T23.302
multiple sites with wrist T23.099
first degree T23.199
left T23.092
first degree T23.192
second degree T23.292
third degree T23.392
right T23.091
first degree T23.191
second degree T23.291
third degree T23.391
second degree T23.299
third degree T23.399
palm —*see* Burn, palm
right T23.001
first degree T23.101
second degree T23.201
third degree T23.301

Burn *(Continued)*
hand *(Continued)*
second degree T23.209
third degree T23.309
thumb —*see* Burn, thumb
head (and face) (and neck) T20.00
cheek —*see* Burn, cheek
chin —*see* Burn, chin
ear —*see* Burn, ear
eye (s) only —*see* Burn, eye
first degree T20.10
forehead —*see* Burn, forehead
lip —*see* Burn, lip
multiple sites T20.09
first degree T20.19
second degree T20.29
third degree T20.39
neck —*see* Burn, neck
nose —*see* Burn, nose
scalp —*see* Burn, scalp
second degree T20.20
third degree T20.30
hip (s) —*see* Burn, thigh
inhalation —*see* Burn, respiratory tract
caustic or corrosive substance (fumes) —*see* Corrosion, respiratory tract
internal organ (s) T28.40
alimentary tract T28.2
esophagus T28.1
eardrum T28.41
esophagus T28.1
from caustic or corrosive substance (swallowing) NEC —*see* Corrosion, by site
genitourinary T28.3
mouth T28.0
pharynx T28.0
respiratory tract —*see* Burn, respiratory tract
specified organ NEC T28.49
interscapular region —*see* Burn, back, upper
intestine (large) (small) T28.2
knee T24.029
first degree T24.129
left T24.022
first degree T24.122
second degree T24.222
third degree T24.322
right T24.021
first degree T24.121
second degree T24.221
third degree T24.321
second degree T24.229
third degree T24.329
labium (majus) (minus) —*see* Burn, genital organs, external, female
lacrimal apparatus, duct, gland or sac —*see* Burn, eye, specified site NEC
larynx T27.0
with lung T27.1
leg (s) (lower) (upper) —*see* Burn, lower, limb
lightning —*see* Burn, by site
limb (s)
lower (except ankle or foot alone) —*see* Burn, lower, limb
upper —*see* Burn, upper limb
lip (s) T20.02
first degree T20.12
second degree T20.22
third degree T20.32
lower
back —*see* Burn, back
limb T24.009
ankle —*see* Burn, ankle
calf —*see* Burn, calf
first degree T24.109
foot —*see* Burn, foot
hip —*see* Burn, thigh
knee —*see* Burn, knee

Burn *(Continued)*
lower *(Continued)*
limb *(Continued)*
left T24.002
first degree T24.102
second degree T24.202
third degree T24.302
multiple sites, except ankle and foot T24.099
ankle and foot T25.099
first degree T25.199
left T25.092
first degree T25.192
second degree T25.292
third degree T25.392
right T25.091
first degree T25.191
second degree T25.291
third degree T25.391
second degree T25.299
third degree T25.399
first degree T24.199
left T24.092
first degree T24.192
second degree T24.292
third degree T24.392
right T24.091
first degree T24.191
second degree T24.291
third degree T24.391
second degree T24.299
third degree T24.399
right T24.001
first degree T24.101
second degree T24.201
third degree T24.301
second degree T24.209
thigh —*see* Burn, thigh
third degree T24.309
toe —*see* Burn, toe
lung (with larynx and trachea) T27.1
mouth T28.0
neck T20.07
first degree T20.17
second degree T20.27
third degree T20.37
nose (septum) T20.04
first degree T20.14
second degree T20.24
third degree T20.34
ocular adnexa —*see* Burn, eye
orbit region —*see* Burn, eyelid
palm T23.059
first degree T23.159
left T23.052
first degree T23.152
second degree T23.252
third degree T23.352
right T23.051
first degree T23.151
second degree T23.251
third degree T23.351
second degree T23.259
third degree T23.359
partial thickness - code as Burn, unspecified degree, by site
pelvis —*see* Burn, trunk
penis —*see* Burn, genital organs, external, male
perineum
female —*see* Burn, genital organs, external, female
male —*see* Burn, genital organs, external, male
periocular area —*see* Burn, eyelid
pharynx T28.0
rectum T28.2
respiratory tract T27.3
larynx —*see* Burn, larynx
specified part NEC T27.2
trachea —*see* Burn, trachea

Burn *(Continued)*
sac, lacrimal —*see* Burn, eye, specified site NEC
scalp T20.05
first degree T20.15
second degree T20.25
third degree T20.35
scapular region T22.069
first degree T22.169
left T22.062
first degree T22.162
second degree T22.262
third degree T22.362
right T22.061
first degree T22.161
second degree T22.261
third degree T22.361
second degree T22.269
third degree T22.369
sclera —*see* Burn, eye, specified site NEC
scrotum —*see* Burn, genital organs, external, male
shoulder T22.059
first degree T22.159
left T22.052
first degree T22.152
second degree T22.252
third degree T22.352
right T22.051
first degree T22.151
second degree T22.251
third degree T22.351
second degree T22.259
third degree T22.359
stomach T28.2
temple —*see* Burn, head
testis —*see* Burn, genital organs, external, male
thigh T24.019
first degree T24.119
left T24.012
first degree T24.112
second degree T24.212
third degree T24.312
right T24.011
first degree T24.111
second degree T24.211
third degree T24.311
second degree T24.219
third degree T24.319
thorax (external) —*see* Burn, trunk
throat (meaning pharynx) T28.0
thumb (s) T23.019
first degree T23.119
left T23.012
first degree T23.112
second degree T23.212
third degree T23.312
multiple sites with fingers T23.049
first degree T23.149
left T23.042
first degree T23.142
second degree T23.242
third degree T23.342
right T23.041
first degree T23.141
second degree T23.241
third degree T23.341
second degree T23.249
third degree T23.349
right T23.011
first degree T23.111
second degree T23.211
third degree T23.311
second degree T23.219
third degree T23.319
toe T25.039
first degree T25.139
left T25.032
first degree T25.132
second degree T25.232
third degree T25.332

Burn *(Continued)*
toe *(Continued)*
right T25.031
first degree T25.131
second degree T25.231
third degree T25.331
second degree T25.239
third degree T25.339
tongue T28.0
tonsil (s) T28.0
trachea T27.0
with lung T27.1
trunk T21.00
abdominal wall —*see* Burn, abdominal wall
anus —*see* Burn, buttock
axilla —*see* Burn, upper limb
back —*see* Burn, back
breast —*see* Burn, chest wall
buttock —*see* Burn, buttock
chest wall —*see* Burn, chest wall
first degree T21.10
flank —*see* Burn, abdominal wall
genital
female —*see* Burn, genital organs, external, female
male —*see* Burn, genital organs, external, male
groin —*see* Burn, abdominal wall
interscapular region —*see* Burn, back, upper
labia —*see* Burn, genital organs, external, female
lower back —*see* Burn, back
penis —*see* Burn, genital organs, external, male
perineum
female —*see* Burn, genital organs, external, female
male —*see* Burn, genital organs, external, male
scapula region —*see* Burn, scapular region
scrotum —*see* Burn, genital organs, external, male
second degree T21.20
specified site NEC T21.09
first degree T21.19
second degree T21.29
third degree T21.39
testes —*see* Burn, genital organs, external, male
third degree T21.30
upper back —*see* Burn, back, upper
vulva —*see* Burn, genital organs, external, female
unspecified site with extent of body surface involved specified
less than 10 percent T31.0
10-19 percent (0-9 percent third degree) T31.10
with 10-19 percent third degree T31.11
20-29 percent (0-9 percent third degree) T31.20
with
10-19 percent third degree T31.21
20-29 percent third degree T31.22
30-39 percent (0-9 percent third degree) T31.30
with
10-19 percent third degree T31.31
20-29 percent third degree T31.32
30-39 percent third degree T31.33
40-49 percent (0-9 percent third degree) T31.40
with
10-19 percent third degree T31.41
20-29 percent third degree T31.42
30-39 percent third degree T31.43
40-49 percent third degree T31.44

Burn *(Continued)*
unspecified site with extent of body surface involved specified *(Continued)*
50-59 percent (0-9 percent third degree) T31.50
with
10-19 percent third degree T31.51
20-29 percent third degree T31.52
30-39 percent third degree T31.53
40-49 percent third degree T31.54
50-59 percent third degree T31.55
60-69 percent (0-9 percent third degree) T31.60
with
10-19 percent third degree T31.61
20-29 percent third degree T31.62
30-39 percent third degree T31.63
40-49 percent third degree T31.64
50-59 percent third degree T31.65
60-69 percent third degree T31.66
70-79 percent (0-9 percent third degree) T31.70
with
10-19 percent third degree T31.71
20-29 percent third degree T31.72
30-39 percent third degree T31.73
40-49 percent third degree T31.74
50-59 percent third degree T31.75
60-69 percent third degree T31.76
70-79 percent third degree T31.77
80-89 percent (0-9 percent third degree) T31.80
with
10-19 percent third degree T31.81
20-29 percent third degree T31.82
30-39 percent third degree T31.83
40-49 percent third degree T31.84
50-59 percent third degree T31.85
60-69 percent third degree T31.86
70-79 percent third degree T31.87
80-89 percent third degree T31.88
90 percent or more (0-9 percent third degree) T31.90
with
10-19 percent third degree T31.91
20-29 percent third degree T31.92
30-39 percent third degree T31.93
40-49 percent third degree T31.94
50-59 percent third degree T31.95
60-69 percent third degree T31.96
70-79 percent third degree T31.97
80-89 percent third degree T31.98
90-99 percent third degree T31.99
upper limb T22.00
above elbow —*see* Burn, above elbow
axilla —*see* Burn, axilla
elbow —*see* Burn, elbow
first degree T22.10
forearm —*see* Burn, forearm
hand —*see* Burn, hand
interscapular region —*see* Burn, back, upper
multiple sites T22.099
first degree T22.199
left T22.092
first degree T22.192
second degree T22.292
third degree T22.392
right T22.091
first degree T22.191
second degree T22.291
third degree T22.391
second degree T22.299
third degree T22.399
scapular region —*see* Burn, scapular region
second degree T22.20
shoulder —*see* Burn, shoulder
third degree T22.30
wrist —*see* Burn, wrist
uterus T28.3
vagina T28.3

Burn *(Continued)*
vulva —*see* Burn, genital organs, external, female
wrist T23.079
first degree T23.179
left T23.072
first degree T23.172
second degree T23.272
third degree T23.372
multiple sites with hand T23.099
first degree T23.199
left T23.092
first degree T23.192
second degree T23.292
third degree T23.392
right T23.091
first degree T23.191
second degree T23.291
third degree T23.391
second degree T23.299
third degree T23.399
right T23.071
first degree T23.171
second degree T23.271
third degree T23.371
second degree T23.279
third degree T23.379
Burnett's syndrome E83.52
Burning
feet syndrome E53.9
sensation R20.8
tongue K14.6
Burn-out (state) Z73.0
Burns' disease or osteochondrosis —*see* Osteochondrosis, juvenile, ulna
Bursa —*see* condition
Bursitis M71.9
Achilles —*see* Tendinitis, Achilles
adhesive —*see* Bursitis, specified NEC
ankle —*see* Enthesopathy, lower limb, ankle, specified type NEC
calcaneal —*see* Enthesopathy, foot, specified type NEC
collateral ligament, tibial —*see* Bursitis, tibial collateral
due to use, overuse, pressure —*see also* Disorder, soft tissue, due to use, specified type NEC
specified NEC —*see* Disorder, soft tissue, due to use, specified NEC
Duplay's M75.0
elbow NEC M70.3-
olecranon M70.2-
finger —*see* Disorder, soft tissue, due to use, specified type NEC, hand
foot —*see* Enthesopathy, foot, specified type NEC
gonococcal A54.49
gouty —*see* Gout ◄
hand M70.1-
hip NEC M70.7-
trochanteric M70.6-
infective NEC M71.10
abscess —*see* Abscess, bursa
ankle M71.17-
elbow M71.12-
foot M71.17-
hand M71.14-
hip M71.15-
knee M71.16-
multiple sites M71.19
shoulder M71.11-
specified site NEC M71.18
wrist M71.13-
ischial —*see* Bursitis, hip
knee NEC M70.5-
prepatellar M70.4-
occupational NEC —*see also* Disorder, soft tissue, due to, use
olecranon —*see* Bursitis, elbow, olecranon
pharyngeal J39.1

Bursitis *(Continued)*
popliteal —*see* Bursitis, knee
prepatellar M70.4-
radiohumeral M77.8
rheumatoid M06.20
ankle M06.27-
elbow M06.22-
foot joint M06.27-
hand joint M06.24-
hip M06.25-
knee M06.26-
multiple site M06.29
shoulder M06.21-
vertebra M06.28
wrist M06.23-
scapulohumeral —*see* Bursitis, shoulder
semimembranous muscle (knee) —*see* Bursitis, knee
shoulder M75.5-
adhesive —*see* Capsulitis, adhesive
specified NEC M71.50
ankle M71.57-
due to use, overuse or pressure —*see* Disorder, soft tissue, due to, use
elbow M71.52-
foot M71.57-
hand M71.54-

Bursitis *(Continued)*
specified NEC *(Continued)*
hip M71.55-
knee M71.56-
shoulder —*see* Bursitis, shoulder
specified site NEC M71.58
tibial collateral M76.4-
wrist M71.53-
subacromial —*see* Bursitis, shoulder
subcoracoid —*see* Bursitis, shoulder
subdeltoid —*see* Bursitis, shoulder
syphilitic A52.78
Thornwaldt, Tornwaldt J39.2
tibial collateral M76.4- ⬅
toe —*see* Enthesopathy, foot, specified type NEC
trochanteric (area) —*see* Bursitis, hip, trochanteric
wrist —*see* Bursitis, hand
Bursopathy M71.9
specified type NEC M71.80
ankle M71.87-
elbow M71.82-
foot M71.87-
hand M71.84-
hip M71.85-
knee M71.86-

Bursopathy *(Continued)*
specified type NEC *(Continued)*
multiple sites M71.89
shoulder M71.81-
specified site NEC M71.88
wrist M71.83-
Burst stitches or sutures (complication of surgery) T81.31
external operation wound T81.31
internal operation wound T81.32
Buruli ulcer A31.1
Bury's disease L95.1
Buschke's
disease B45.3
scleredema —*see* Sclerosis, systemic
Busse-Buschke disease B45.3
Buttock —*see* condition
Button
Biskra B55.1
Delhi B55.1
oriental B55.1
Buttonhole deformity (finger) —*see* Deformity, finger, boutonniere
Bwamba fever A92.8
Byssinosis J66.0
Bywaters' syndrome T79.5

C

Cachexia R64
cancerous R64
cardiac —*see* Disease, heart
dehydration E86.0
with
~~hypernatremia E87.0~~
~~hyponatremia E87.1~~
due to malnutrition R64
exophthalmic —*see* Hyperthyroidism
heart —*see* Disease, heart
hypophyseal E23.0
hypopituitary E23.0
lead —*see* Poisoning, lead
malignant R64
marsh —*see* Malaria
nervous F48.8
old age R54
paludal —*see* Malaria
pituitary E23.0
renal N28.9
saturnine —*see* Poisoning, lead
senile R54
Simmonds' E23.0
splenica D73.0
strumipriva E03.4
tuberculous NEC —*see* Tuberculosis
Café au lait spots L81.3
Caffeine-induced ◀
anxiety disorder F15.980 ◀
sleep disorder F15.982 ◀
Caffey's syndrome Q78.8
Caisson disease T70.3
Cake kidney Q63.1
Caked breast (puerperal, postpartum) O92.79
Calabar swelling B74.3
Calcaneal spur —*see* Spur, bone, calcaneal
Calcaneo-apophysitis M92.8
Calcareous —*see* condition
Calcicosis J62.8
Calciferol (vitamin D) deficiency E55.9
with rickets E55.0
Calcification
adrenal (capsule) (gland) E27.49
tuberculous E35 *[B90.8]*
aorta I70.0
artery (annular) —*see* Arteriosclerosis
auricle (ear) —*see* Disorder, pinna, specified type NEC
basal ganglia G23.8
bladder N32.89
due to Schistosoma hematobium B65.0
brain (cortex) —*see* Calcification, cerebral
bronchus J98.09
bursa M71.40
ankle M71.47-
elbow M71.42-
foot M71.47-
hand M71.44-
hip M71.45-
knee M71.46-
multiple sites M71.49
shoulder M75.3-
specified site NEC M71.48
wrist M71.43-
cardiac —*see* Degeneration, myocardial
cerebral (cortex) G93.89
artery I67.2
cervix (uteri) N88.8
choroid plexus G93.89
conjunctiva —*see* Concretion, conjunctiva
corpora cavernosa (penis) N48.89
cortex (brain) —*see* Calcification, cerebral
dental pulp (nodular) K04.2
dentinal papilla K00.4
fallopian tube N83.8
falx cerebri G96.19
gallbladder K82.8
general E83.59
Calcification *(Continued)*
heart —*see also* Degeneration, myocardial
valve —*see* Endocarditis
idiopathic infantile arterial (IIAC) Q28.8
intervertebral cartilage or disc (postinfective) —*see* Disorder, disc, specified NEC
intracranial —*see* Calcification, cerebral
joint —*see* Disorder, joint, specified type NEC
kidney N28.89
tuberculous N29 *[B90.1]*
larynx (senile) J38.7
lens —*see* Cataract, specified NEC
lung (active) (postinfectional) J98.4
tuberculous B90.9
lymph gland or node (postinfectional) I89.8
tuberculous —*see also* Tuberculosis, lymph gland B90.8
mammographic R92.1
massive (paraplegic) —*see* Myositis, ossificans, in, quadriplegia
medial —*see* Arteriosclerosis, extremities
meninges (cerebral) (spinal) G96.19
metastatic E83.59
Mönckeberg's —*see* Arteriosclerosis, extremities
muscle M61.9
due to burns —*see* Myositis, ossificans, in, burns
paralytic —*see* Myositis, ossificans, in, quadriplegia
specified type NEC M61.40
ankle M61.47-
foot M61.47-
forearm M61.43-
hand M61.44-
lower leg M61.46-
multiple sites M61.49
pelvic region M61.45-
shoulder region M61.41-
specified site NEC M61.48
thigh M61.45-
upper arm M61.42-
myocardium, myocardial —*see* Degeneration, myocardial
ovary N83.8
pancreas K86.89 ⟸
penis N48.89
periarticular —*see* Disorder, joint, specified type NEC
pericardium —*see also* Pericarditis I31.1
pineal gland E34.8
pleura J94.8
postinfectional J94.8
tuberculous NEC B90.9
pulpal (dental) (nodular) K04.2
sclera H15.89
spleen D73.89
subcutaneous L94.2
suprarenal (capsule) (gland) E27.49
tendon (sheath) —*see also* Tenosynovitis, specified type NEC
with bursitis, synovitis or tenosynovitis —*see* Tendinitis, calcific
trachea J39.8
ureter N28.89
vitreous —*see* Deposit, crystalline
Calcified —*see* Calcification
Calcinosis (interstitial) (tumoral) (universalis) E83.59
with Raynaud's phenomenon, esophageal dysfunction, sclerodactyly, telangiectasia (CREST syndrome) M34.1
circumscripta (skin) L94.2
cutis L94.2
Calciphylaxis —*see also* Calcification, by site E83.59
Calcium
deposits —*see* Calcification, by site
metabolism disorder E83.50
salts or soaps in vitreous —*see* Deposit, crystalline
Calciuria R82.99
Calculi —*see* Calculus
Calculosis, intrahepatic —*see* Calculus, bile duct
Calculus, calculi, calculous
ampulla of Vater —*see* Calculus, bile duct
anuria (impacted) (recurrent) —*see also* Calculus, urinary N20.9
appendix K38.1
bile duct (common) (hepatic) K80.50
with
calculus of gallbladder —*see* Calculus, gallbladder and bile duct
cholangitis K80.30
with
cholecystitis —*see* Calculus, bile duct, with cholecystitis
obstruction K80.31
acute K80.32
with
chronic cholangitis K80.36
with obstruction K80.37
obstruction K80.33
chronic K80.34
with
acute cholangitis K80.36
with obstruction K80.37
obstruction K80.35
cholecystitis (with cholangitis) K80.40
with obstruction K80.41
acute K80.42
with
chronic cholecystitis K80.46
with obstruction K80.47
obstruction K80.43
chronic K80.44
with
acute cholecystitis K80.46
with obstruction K80.47
obstruction K80.45
obstruction K80.51
biliary —*see also* Calculus, gallbladder
specified NEC K80.80
with obstruction K80.81
bilirubin, multiple —*see* Calculus, gallbladder
bladder (encysted) (impacted) (urinary) (diverticulum) N21.0
bronchus J98.09
calyx (kidney) (renal) —*see* Calculus, kidney
cholesterol (pure) (solitary) —*see* Calculus, gallbladder
common duct (bile) —*see* Calculus, bile duct
conjunctiva —*see* Concretion, conjunctiva
cystic N21.0
duct —*see* Calculus, gallbladder
dental (subgingival) (supragingival) K03.6
diverticulum
bladder N21.0
kidney N20.0
epididymis N50.89 ⟸
gallbladder K80.20
with
bile duct calculus —*see* Calculus, gallbladder and bile duct
cholecystitis K80.10
with obstruction K80.11
acute K80.00
with
chronic cholecystitis K80.12
with obstruction K80.13
obstruction K80.01
chronic K80.10
with
acute cholecystitis K80.12
with obstruction K80.13
obstruction K80.11
specified NEC K80.18
with obstruction K80.19
obstruction K80.21

Calculus, calculi, calculous *(Continued)*
gallbladder and bile duct K80.70
with
cholecystitis K80.60
with obstruction K80.61
acute K80.62
with
chronic cholecystitis K80.66
with obstruction K80.67
obstruction K80.63
chronic K80.64
with
acute cholecystitis K80.66
with obstruction K80.67
obstruction K80.65
obstruction K80.71
hepatic (duct) —*see* Calculus, bile duct
hepatobiliary K80.80
with obstruction K80.81
ileal conduit N21.8
intestinal (impaction) (obstruction) K56.49
kidney (impacted) (multiple) (pelvis) (recurrent) (staghorn) N20.0
with calculus, ureter N20.2
congenital Q63.8
lacrimal passages —*see* Dacryolith
liver (impacted) —*see* Calculus, bile duct
lung J98.4
mammographic R92.1
nephritic (impacted) (recurrent) —*see* Calculus, kidney
nose J34.89
pancreas (duct) K86.89 ◀
parotid duct or gland K11.5
pelvis, encysted —*see* Calculus, kidney
prostate N42.0
pulmonary J98.4
pyelitis (impacted) (recurrent) N20.0
with hydronephrosis N13.2
pyelonephritis (impacted) (recurrent) —*see* category N20
with hydronephrosis N13.2
renal (impacted) (recurrent) —*see* Calculus, kidney
salivary (duct) (gland) K11.5
seminal vesicle N50.89 ◀
staghorn —*see* Calculus, kidney
Stensen's duct K11.5
stomach K31.89
sublingual duct or gland K11.5
congenital Q38.4
submandibular duct, gland or region K11.5
submaxillary duct, gland or region K11.5
suburethral N21.8
tonsil J35.8
tooth, teeth (subgingival) (supragingival) K03.6
tunica vaginalis N50.89 ◀
ureter (impacted) (recurrent) N20.1
with calculus, kidney N20.2
with hydronephrosis N13.2
with infection N13.6
urethra (impacted) N21.1
urinary (duct) (impacted) (passage) (tract) N20.9
with hydronephrosis N13.2
with infection N13.6
in (due to)
lower N21.9
specified NEC N21.8
vagina N89.8
vesical (impacted) N21.0
Wharton's duct K11.5
xanthine E79.8 *[N22]*
Calicectasis N28.89
Caliectasis N28.89
California
disease B38.9
encephalitis A83.5
Caligo cornea —*see* Opacity, cornea, central
Callositas, callosity (infected) L84
Callus (infected) L84
bone —*see* Osteophyte
excessive, following fracture - code as Sequelae of fracture
CALME (childhood asymmetric labium majus enlargement) N90.61 ◀
Calorie deficiency or malnutrition —*see also* Malnutrition E46
Calvé-Perthes disease —*see* Legg-Calve-Perthes disease
Calvé's disease —*see* Osteochondrosis, juvenile, spine
Calvities —*see* Alopecia, androgenic
Cameroon fever —*see* Malaria
Camptocormia (hysterical) F44.4
Camurati-Engelmann syndrome Q78.3
Canal —*see also* condition
atrioventricular common Q21.2
Canaliculitis (lacrimal) (acute) (subacute) H04.33-
Actinomyces A42.89
chronic H04.42-
Canavan's disease E75.29
Canceled procedure (surgical) Z53.9
because of
contraindication Z53.09
smoking Z53.01
left against medical advice (AMA) Z53.21
patient's decision Z53.20
for reasons of belief or group pressure Z53.1
specified reason NEC Z53.29
specified reason NEC Z53.8
Cancer —*see also* Neoplasm, by site, malignant
bile duct type, liver C22.1
blood —*see* Leukemia
breast —*see also* Neoplasm, breast, malignant C50.91-
hepatocellular C22.0
lung —*see also* Neoplasm, lung, malignant C34.90-
ovarian —*see also* Neoplasm, ovary, malignant C56.9-
unspecified site (primary) C80.1
Cancer (o)phobia F45.29
Cancerous —*see* Neoplasm, malignant, by site
Cancrum oris A69.0
Candidiasis, candidal B37.9
balanitis B37.42
bronchitis B37.1
cheilitis B37.83
congenital P37.5
cystitis B37.41
disseminated B37.7
endocarditis B37.6
enteritis B37.82
esophagitis B37.81
intertrigo B37.2
lung B37.1
meningitis B37.5
mouth B37.0
nails B37.2
neonatal P37.5
onychia B37.2
oral B37.0
osteomyelitis B37.89
otitis externa B37.84
paronychia B37.2
perionyxis B37.2
pneumonia B37.1
proctitis B37.82
pulmonary B37.1
pyelonephritis B37.49
sepsis B37.7
skin B37.2
specified site NEC B37.89
stomatitis B37.0
systemic B37.7
urethritis B37.41
urogenital site NEC B37.49
vagina B37.3
vulva B37.3
vulvovaginitis B37.3
Candidid L30.2
Candidosis —*see* Candidiasis
Candiru infection or infestation B88.8
Canities (premature) L67.1
congenital Q84.2
Canker (mouth) (sore) K12.0
rash A38.9
Cannabinosis J66.2
Cannabis induced ◀
anxiety disorder F12.980 ◀
psychotic disorder F12.959 ◀
sleep disorder F12.988 ◀
Canton fever A75.9
Cantrell's syndrome Q87.89
Capillariasis (intestinal) B81.1
hepatic B83.8
Capillary —*see* condition
Caplan's syndrome —*see* Rheumatoid, lung
Capsule —*see* condition
Capsulitis (joint) —*see also* Enthesopathy
adhesive (shoulder) M75.0-
hepatic K65.8
labyrinthine —*see* Otosclerosis, specified NEC
thyroid E06.9
Caput
crepitus Q75.8
medusae I86.8
succedaneum P12.81
Car sickness T75.3
Carapata (disease) A68.0
Carate —*see* Pinta
Carbon lung J60
Carbuncle L02.93
abdominal wall L02.231
anus K61.0
auditory canal, external —*see* Abscess, ear, external
auricle ear —*see* Abscess, ear, external
axilla L02.43-
back (any part) L02.232
breast N61.1 ◀
buttock L02.33
cheek (external) L02.03
chest wall L02.233
chin L02.03
corpus cavernosum N48.21
ear (any part) (external) (middle) —*see* Abscess, ear, external
external auditory canal —*see* Abscess, ear, external
eyelid —*see* Abscess, eyelid
face NEC L02.03
femoral (region) —*see* Carbuncle, lower limb
finger —*see* Carbuncle, hand
flank L02.231
foot L02.63-
forehead L02.03
genital —*see* Abscess, genital
gluteal (region) L02.33
groin L02.234
hand L02.53-
head NEC L02.831
heel —*see* Carbuncle, foot
hip —*see* Carbuncle, lower limb
kidney —*see* Abscess, kidney
knee —*see* Carbuncle, lower limb
labium (majus) (minus) N76.4
lacrimal
gland —*see* Dacryoadenitis
passages (duct) (sac) —*see* Inflammation, lacrimal, passages, acute
leg —*see* Carbuncle, lower limb
lower limb L02.43-
malignant A22.0
navel L02.236
neck L02.13
nose (external) (septum) J34.0
orbit, orbital —*see* Abscess, orbit
palmar (space) —*see* Carbuncle, hand
partes posteriores L02.33
pectoral region L02.233
penis N48.21

◀ New ◀ Revised ~~deleted~~ Deleted

Carbuncle *(Continued)*
perineum L02.235
pinna —*see* Abscess, ear, external
popliteal —*see* Carbuncle, lower limb
scalp L02.831
seminal vesicle N49.0
shoulder —*see* Carbuncle, upper limb
specified site NEC L02.838
temple (region) L02.03
thumb —*see* Carbuncle, hand
toe —*see* Carbuncle, foot
trunk L02.239
abdominal wall L02.231
back L02.232
chest wall L02.233
groin L02.234
perineum L02.235
umbilicus L02.236
umbilicus L02.236
upper limb L02.43-
urethra N34.0
vulva N76.4
Carbunculus —*see* Carbuncle
Carcinoid (tumor) —*see* Tumor, carcinoid
Carcinoidosis E34.0
Carcinoma (malignant) —*see also* Neoplasm, by site, malignant
acidophil
specified site —*see* Neoplasm, malignant, by site
unspecified site C75.1
acidophil-basophil, mixed
specified site —*see* Neoplasm, malignant, by site
unspecified site C75.1
adnexal (skin) —*see* Neoplasm, skin, malignant
adrenal cortical C74.0-
alveolar —*see* Neoplasm, lung, malignant
cell —*see* Neoplasm, lung, malignant
ameloblastic C41.1
upper jaw (bone) C41.0
apocrine
breast —*see* Neoplasm, breast, malignant
specified site NEC —*see* Neoplasm, skin, malignant
unspecified site C44.99
basal cell (pigmented) (*see also* Neoplasm, skin, malignant) C44.91
fibro-epithelial —*see* Neoplasm, skin, malignant
morphea —*see* Neoplasm, skin, malignant
multicentric —*see* Neoplasm, skin, malignant
basaloid
basal-squamous cell, mixed —*see* Neoplasm, skin, malignant
basophil
specified site —*see* Neoplasm, malignant, by site
unspecified site C75.1
basophil-acidophil, mixed
specified site —*see* Neoplasm, malignant, by site
unspecified site C75.1
basosquamous —*see* Neoplasm, skin, malignant
bile duct
with hepatocellular, mixed C22.0
liver C22.1
specified site NEC —*see* Neoplasm, malignant, by site
unspecified site C22.1
branchial or branchiogenic C10.4
bronchial or bronchogenic —*see* Neoplasm, lung, malignant
bronchiolar —*see* Neoplasm, lung, malignant
bronchioloalveolar —*see* Neoplasm, lung, malignant
C cell
specified site —*see* Neoplasm, malignant, by site
unspecified site C73
ceruminous C44.29-

Carcinoma *(Continued)*
cervix uteri
in situ D06.9
endocervix D06.0
exocervix D06.1
specified site NEC D06.7
chorionic
specified site —*see* Neoplasm, malignant, by site
unspecified site
female C58
male C62.90
chromophobe
specified site —*see* Neoplasm, malignant, by site
unspecified site C75.1
cloacogenic
specified site —*see* Neoplasm, malignant, by site
unspecified site C21.2
diffuse type
specified site —*see* Neoplasm, malignant, by site
unspecified site C16.9
duct (cell)
with Paget's disease —*see* Neoplasm, breast, malignant
infiltrating
with lobular carcinoma (in situ)
specified site —*see* Neoplasm, malignant, by site
unspecified site (female) C50.91-
male C50.92-
specified site —*see* Neoplasm, malignant, by site
unspecified site (female) C50.91-
male C50.92-
ductal
with lobular
specified site —*see* Neoplasm, malignant, by site
unspecified site (female) C50.91-
male C50.92-
ductular, infiltrating
specified site —*see* Neoplasm, malignant, by site
unspecified site (female) C50.91-
male C50.92-
embryonal
liver C22.7
endometrioid
specified site —*see* Neoplasm, malignant, by site
unspecified site
female C56.9
male C61
eosinophil
specified site —*see* Neoplasm, malignant, by site
unspecified site C75.1
epidermoid —*see also* Neoplasm, skin malignant
in situ, Bowen's type —*see* Neoplasm, skin, in situ
fibroepithelial, basal cell —*see* Neoplasm, skin, malignant
follicular
with papillary (mixed) C73
moderately differentiated C73
pure follicle C73
specified site —*see* Neoplasm, malignant, by site
trabecular C73
unspecified site C73
well differentiated C73
generalized, with unspecified primary site C80.0
glycogen-rich —*see* Neoplasm, breast, malignant
granulosa cell C56-
hepatic cell C22.0

Carcinoma *(Continued)*
hepatocellular C22.0
with bile duct, mixed C22.0
fibrolamellar C22.0
hepatocholangiolitic C22.0
Hurthle cell C73
in
adenomatous
polyposis coli C18.9
pleomorphic adenoma —*see* Neoplasm, salivary glands, malignant
situ —*see* Carcinoma-in-situ
infiltrating
duct
with lobular
specified site —*see* Neoplasm, malignant, by site
unspecified site (female) C50.91-
male C50.92-
with Paget's disease —*see* Neoplasm, breast, malignant
specified site —*see* Neoplasm, malignant
unspecified site (female) C50.91-
male C50.92-
ductular
specified site —*see* Neoplasm, malignant
unspecified site (female) C50.91-
male C50.92-
lobular
specified site —*see* Neoplasm, malignant
unspecified site (female) C50.91-
male C50.92-
inflammatory
specified site —*see* Neoplasm, malignant
unspecified site (female) C50.91-
male C50.92-
intestinal type
specified site —*see* Neoplasm, malignant, by site
unspecified site C16.9
intracystic
noninfiltrating —*see* Neoplasm, in situ, by site
intraductal (noninfiltrating)
with Paget's disease —*see* Neoplasm, breast, malignant
breast D05.1-
papillary
with invasion
specified site —*see* Neoplasm, malignant, by site
unspecified site (female) C50.91-
male C50.92-
breast D05.1-
specified site NEC —*see* Neoplasm, in situ, by site
unspecified site (female) D05.1-
specified site NEC —*see* Neoplasm, in situ, by site
unspecified site (female) D05.1-
intraepidermal —*see* Neoplasm, in situ
squamous cell, Bowen's type —*see* Neoplasm, skin, in situ
intraepithelial —*see* Neoplasm, in situ, by site
squamous cell —*see* Neoplasm, in situ, by site
intraosseous C41.1
upper jaw (bone) C41.0
islet cell
with exocrine, mixed
specified site —*see* Neoplasm, malignant, by site
unspecified site C25.9
pancreas C25.4
specified site NEC —*see* Neoplasm, malignant, by site
unspecified site C25.4

Carcinoma *(Continued)*
juvenile, breast —*see* Neoplasm, breast, malignant
large cell
small cell
specified site —*see* Neoplasm, malignant, by site
unspecified site C34.90
Leydig cell (testis)
specified site —*see* Neoplasm, malignant, by site
unspecified site
female C56.9
male C62.90
lipid-rich (female) C50.91-
male C50.92-
liver cell C22.0
liver NEC C22.7
lobular (infiltrating)
with intraductal
specified site —*see* Neoplasm, malignant, by site
unspecified site (female) C50.91-
male C50.92-
noninfiltrating
breast D05.0-
specified site NEC —*see* Neoplasm, in situ, by site
unspecified site D05.0-
specified site —*see* Neoplasm, malignant, by site
unspecified site (female) C50.91-
male C50.92-
medullary
with
amyloid stroma
specified site —*see* Neoplasm, malignant, by site
unspecified site C73
lymphoid stroma
specified site —*see* Neoplasm, malignant, by site
unspecified site (female) C50.91-
male C50.92-
Merkel cell C4A.9
anal margin C4A.51
anal skin C4A.51
canthus C4A.1-
ear and external auricular canal C4A.2-
external auricular canal C4A.2-
eyelid, including canthus C4A.1-
face C4A.30
specified NEC C4A.39
hip C4A.7-
lip C4A.0
lower limb, including hip C4A.7-
neck C4A.4
nodal presentation C7B.1
nose C4A.31
overlapping sites C4A.8
perianal skin C4A.51
scalp C4A.4
secondary C7B.1
shoulder C4A.6-
skin of breast C4A.52
trunk NEC C4A.59
upper limb, including shoulder C4A.6-
visceral metastatic C7B.1
metastatic —*see* Neoplasm, secondary
metatypical —*see* Neoplasm, skin, malignant
morphea, basal cell —*see* Neoplasm, skin, malignant
mucoid
cell
specified site —*see* Neoplasm, malignant, by site
unspecified site C75.1
neuroendocrine —*see also* Tumor, neuroendocrine
high grade, any site C7A.1
poorly differentiated, any site C7A.1

Carcinoma *(Continued)*
nonencapsulated sclerosing C73
noninfiltrating
intracystic —*see* Neoplasm, in situ, by site
intraductal
breast D05.1-
papillary
breast D05.1-
specified site NEC —*see* Neoplasm, in situ, by site
unspecified site D05.1-
specified site —*see* Neoplasm, in situ, by site
unspecified site D05.1-
lobular
breast D05.0-
specified site NEC —*see* Neoplasm, in situ, by site
unspecified site (female) D05.0-
oat cell
specified site —*see* Neoplasm, malignant, by site
unspecified site C34.90
odontogenic C41.1
upper jaw (bone) C41.0
papillary
with follicular (mixed) C73
follicular variant C73
intraductal (noninfiltrating)
with invasion
specified site —*see* Neoplasm, malignant, by site
unspecified site (female) C50.91-
male C50.92-
breast D05.1-
specified site NEC —*see* Neoplasm, in situ, by site
unspecified site D05.1-
serous
specified site —*see* Neoplasm, malignant, by site
surface
specified site —*see* Neoplasm, malignant, by site
unspecified site C56.9
unspecified site C56.9
papillocystic
specified site —*see* Neoplasm, malignant, by site
unspecified site C56.9
parafollicular cell
specified site —*see* Neoplasm, malignant, by site
unspecified site C73
pilomatrix —*see* Neoplasm, skin, malignant
pseudomucinous
specified site —*see* Neoplasm, malignant, by site
unspecified site C56.9
renal cell C64-
Schmincke —*see* Neoplasm, nasopharynx, malignant
Schneiderian
specified site —*see* Neoplasm, malignant, by site
unspecified site C30.0
sebaceous —*see* Neoplasm, skin, malignant
secondary —*see also* Neoplasm, secondary, by site
Merkel cell C7B.1
secretory, breast —*see* Neoplasm, breast, malignant
serous
papillary
specified site —*see* Neoplasm, malignant, by site
unspecified site C56.9
surface, papillary
specified site —*see* Neoplasm, malignant, by site
unspecified site C56.9

Carcinoma *(Continued)*
Sertoli cell
specified site —*see* Neoplasm, malignant, by site
unspecified site C62.90
female C56.9
male C62.90
skin appendage —*see* Neoplasm, skin, malignant
small cell
fusiform cell
specified site —*see* Neoplasm, malignant, by site
unspecified site C34.90
intermediate cell
specified site —*see* Neoplasm, malignant, by site
unspecified site C34.90
large cell
specified site —*see* Neoplasm, malignant, by site
unspecified site C34.90
solid
with amyloid stroma
specified site —*see* Neoplasm, malignant, by site
unspecified site C73
microinvasive
specified site —*see* Neoplasm, malignant, by site
unspecified site C53.9
sweat gland —*see* Neoplasm, skin, malignant
theca cell C56.-
thymic C37
unspecified site (primary) C80.1
water-clear cell C75.0
Carcinoma-in-situ —*see also* Neoplasm, in situ, by site
breast NOS D05.9-
specified type NEC D05.8-
epidermoid —*see also* Neoplasm, in situ, by site
with questionable stromal invasion
cervix D06.9
specified site NEC —*see* Neoplasm, in situ, by site
unspecified site D06.9
Bowen's type —*see* Neoplasm, skin, in situ
intraductal
breast D05.1-
specified site NEC —*see* Neoplasm, in situ, by site
unspecified site D05.1-
lobular
with
infiltrating duct
breast (female) C50.91-
male C50.92-
specified site NEC —*see* Neoplasm, malignant
unspecified site (female) C50.91-
male C50.92-
intraductal
breast D05.8-
specified site NEC —*see* Neoplasm, in situ, by site
unspecified site (female) D05.8-
breast D05.0-
specified site NEC —*see* Neoplasm, in situ, by site
unspecified site D05.0-
squamous cell —*see also* Neoplasm, in situ, by site
with questionable stromal invasion
cervix D06.9
specified site NEC —*see* Neoplasm, in situ, by site
unspecified site D06.9
Carcinomaphobia F45.29

Carcinomatosis C80.0
peritonei C78.6
unspecified site (primary) (secondary) C80.0
Carcinosarcoma —*see* Neoplasm, malignant, by site
embryonal —*see* Neoplasm, malignant, by site
Cardia, cardial —*see* condition
Cardiac —*see also* condition
death, sudden —*see* Arrest, cardiac
pacemaker
in situ Z95.0
management or adjustment Z45.018
tamponade I31.4
Cardialgia —*see* Pain, precordial
Cardiectasis —*see* Hypertrophy, cardiac
Cardiochalasia K21.9
Cardiomalacia I51.5
Cardiomegalia glycogenica diffusa E74.02 *[I43]*
Cardiomegaly —*see also* Hypertrophy, cardiac
congenital Q24.8
glycogen E74.02 *[I43]*
idiopathic I51.7
Cardiomyoliposis I51.5
Cardiomyopathy (familial) (idiopathic) I42.9
alcoholic I42.6
amyloid E85.4 *[I43]*
arteriosclerotic —*see* Disease, heart, ischemic, atherosclerotic
beriberi E51.12
cobalt-beer I42.6
congenital I42.4
congestive I42.0
constrictive NOS I42.5
dilated I42.0
due to
alcohol I42.6
beriberi E51.12
cardiac glycogenosis E74.02 *[I43]*
drugs I42.7
external agents NEC I42.7
Friedreich's ataxia G11.1
myotonia atrophica G71.11 *[I43]*
progressive muscular dystrophy G71.0
glycogen storage E74.02 *[I43]*
hypertensive —*see* Hypertension, heart
hypertrophic (nonobstructive) I42.2
obstructive I42.1
congenital Q24.8
in
Chagas' disease (chronic) B57.2
acute B57.0
sarcoidosis D86.85
ischemic I25.5
metabolic E88.9 *[I43]*
thyrotoxic E05.90 *[I43]*
with thyroid storm E05.91 *[I43]*
newborn I42.8
congenital I42.4
nutritional E63.9 *[I43]*
beriberi E51.12
obscure of Africa I42.8
peripartum O90.3
postpartum O90.3
restrictive NEC I42.5
rheumatic I09.0
secondary I42.9
stress induced I51.81
takotsubo I51.81
thyrotoxic E05.90 *[I43]*
with thyroid storm E05.91 *[I43]*
toxic NEC I42.7
tuberculous A18.84
viral B33.24
Cardionephritis —*see* Hypertension, cardiorenal
Cardionephropathy —*see* Hypertension, cardiorenal
Cardionephrosis —*see* Hypertension, cardiorenal
Cardiopathia nigra I27.0
Cardiopathy —*see also* Disease, heart I51.9
idiopathic I42.9
mucopolysaccharidosis E76.3 *[I52]*
Cardiopericarditis —*see* Pericarditis
Cardiophobia F45.29
Cardiorenal —*see* condition
Cardiorrhexis —*see* Infarct, myocardium
Cardiosclerosis —*see* Disease, heart, ischemic, atherosclerotic
Cardiosis —*see* Disease, heart
Cardiospasm (esophagus) (reflex) (stomach) K22.0
congenital Q39.5
with megaesophagus Q39.5
Cardiostenosis —*see* Disease, heart
Cardiosymphysis I31.0
Cardiovascular —*see* condition
Carditis (acute) (bacterial) (chronic) (subacute) I51.89
meningococcal A39.50
rheumatic —*see* Disease, heart, rheumatic
rheumatoid —*see* Rheumatoid, carditis
viral B33.20
Care (of) (for) (following)
child (routine) Z76.2
family member (handicapped) (sick)
creating problem for family Z63.6
provided away from home for holiday relief Z75.5
unavailable, due to
absence (person rendering care) (sufferer) Z74.2
inability (any reason) of person rendering care Z74.2
foundling Z76.1
holiday relief Z75.5
improper —*see* Maltreatment
lack of (at or after birth) (infant) —*see* Maltreatment, child, neglect
lactating mother Z39.1
palliative Z51.5
postpartum
immediately after delivery Z39.0
routine follow-up Z39.2
respite Z75.5
unavailable, due to
absence of person rendering care Z74.2
inability (any reason) of person rendering care Z74.2
well-baby Z76.2
Caries
bone NEC A18.03
dental (dentino enamel junction) (early childhood) (of dentine) (pre-eruptive) (recurrent) (to the pulp) K02.9 ⇐
arrested (coronal) (root) K02.3
chewing surface
limited to enamel K02.51
penetrating into dentin K02.52
penetrating into pulp K02.53
coronal surface
chewing surface
limited to enamel K02.51
penetrating into dentin K02.52
penetrating into pulp K02.53
pit and fissure surface
limited to enamel K02.51
penetrating into dentin K02.52
penetrating into pulp K02.53
smooth surface
limited to enamel K02.61
penetrating into dentin K02.62
penetrating into pulp K02.63
pit and fissure surface
limited to enamel K02.51
penetrating into dentin K02.52
penetrating into pulp K02.53
primary, cervical origin K02.52 ◀
root K02.7
Caries *(Continued)*
dental *(Continued)*
smooth surface
limited to enamel K02.61
penetrating into dentin K02.62
penetrating into pulp K02.63
external meatus —*see* Disorder, ear, external, specified type NEC
hip (tuberculous) A18.02
initial (tooth)
chewing surface K02.51
pit and fissure surface K02.51
smooth surface K02.61
knee (tuberculous) A18.02
labyrinth —*see* subcategory H83.8
limb NEC (tuberculous) A18.03
mastoid process (chronic) —*see* Mastoiditis, chronic
tuberculous A18.03
middle ear —*see* subcategory H74.8
nose (tuberculous) A18.03
orbit (tuberculous) A18.03
ossicles, ear —*see* Abnormal, ear ossicles
petrous bone —*see* Petrositis
root (dental) (tooth) K02.7
sacrum (tuberculous) A18.01
spine, spinal (column) (tuberculous) A18.01
syphilitic A52.77
congenital (early) A50.02 *[M90.80]*
tooth, teeth —*see* Caries, dental
tuberculous A18.03
vertebra (column) (tuberculous) A18.01
Carious teeth —*see* Caries, dental
Carneous mole O02.0
Carnitine insufficiency E71.40
Carotid body or sinus syndrome G90.01
Carotidynia G90.01
Carotinemia (dietary) E67.1
Carotinosis (cutis) (skin) E67.1
Carpal tunnel syndrome —*see* Syndrome, carpal tunnel
Carpenter's syndrome Q87.0
Carpopedal spasm —*see* Tetany
Carr-Barr-Plunkett syndrome Q97.1
Carrier (suspected) of
amebiasis Z22.1
bacterial disease NEC Z22.39
diphtheria Z22.2
intestinal infectious NEC Z22.1
typhoid Z22.0
meningococcal Z22.31
sexually transmitted Z22.4
specified NEC Z22.39
staphylococcal (Methicillin susceptible) Z22.321
Methicillin resistant Z22.322
streptococcal Z22.338
group B Z22.330
complicating pregnancy or delivery O99.82- ◀
typhoid Z22.0
cholera Z22.1
diphtheria Z22.2
gastrointestinal pathogens NEC Z22.1
genetic Z14.8
cystic fibrosis Z14.1
hemophilia A (asymptomatic) Z14.01
symptomatic Z14.02
gestational, pregnant Z33.1 ◀
gonorrhea Z22.4
HAA (hepatitis Australian-antigen) B18.8 ⇐
HB (c)(s)-AG B18.1 ⇐
hepatitis (viral) B18.9 ⇐
Australia-antigen (HAA) B18.8 ⇐
B surface antigen (HBsAg) B18.1 ⇐
with acute delta- (super)infection B17.0
C B18.2 ⇐
specified NEC B18.8 ⇐
human T-cell lymphotropic virus type-1 (HTLV-1) infection Z22.6

Carrier of *(Continued)*
infectious organism Z22.9
specified NEC Z22.8
meningococci Z22.31
Salmonella typhosa Z22.0
serum hepatitis —*see* Carrier, hepatitis
staphylococci (Methicillin susceptible) Z22.321
Methicillin resistant Z22.322
streptococci Z22.338
group B Z22.330
complicating pregnancy or delivery O99.82- ◀
syphilis Z22.4
typhoid Z22.0
venereal disease NEC Z22.4
Carrion's disease A44.0
Carter's relapsing fever (Asiatic) A68.1
Cartilage —*see* condition
Caruncle (inflamed)
conjunctiva (acute) —*see* Conjunctivitis, acute
labium (majus) (minus) N90.89
lacrimal —*see* Inflammation, lacrimal, passages
myrtiform N89.8
urethral (benign) N36.2
Cascade stomach K31.2
Caseation lymphatic gland (tuberculous) A18.2
Cassidy (-Scholte) **syndrome** (malignant carcinoid) E34.0
Castellani's disease A69.8
Castration, traumatic, male S38.231
Casts in urine R82.99
Cat
cry syndrome Q93.4
ear Q17.3
eye syndrome Q92.8
Catabolism, senile R54
Catalepsy (hysterical) F44.2
schizophrenic F20.2
Cataplexy (idiopathic) —*see* - Narcolepsy
Cataract (cortical) (immature) (incipient) H26.9
with
neovascularization —*see* Cataract, complicated
age-related —*see* Cataract, senile
anterior
and posterior axial embryonal Q12.0
pyramidal Q12.0
associated with
galactosemia E74.21 *[H28]*
myotonic disorders G71.19 *[H28]*
blue Q12.0
central Q12.0
cerulean Q12.0
complicated H26.20
with
neovascularization H26.21-
ocular disorder H26.22-
glaucomatous flecks H26.23-
congenital Q12.0
coraliform Q12.0
coronary Q12.0
crystalline Q12.0
diabetic —*see* Diabetes, cataract
drug-induced H26.3-
due to
ocular disorder —*see* Cataract, complicated
radiation H26.8
electric H26.8
extraction status Z98.4-
glass-blower's H26.8
heat ray H26.8
heterochromic —*see* Cataract, complicated
hypermature —*see* Cataract, senile, morgagnian type
in (due to)
chronic iridocyclitis —*see* Cataract, complicated
diabetes —*see* Diabetes, cataract
endocrine disease E34.9 *[H28]*
eye disease —*see* Cataract, complicated
Cataract *(Continued)*
in (due to) *(Continued)*
hypoparathyroidism E20.9 *[H28]*
malnutrition-dehydration E46 *[H28]*
metabolic disease E88.9 *[H28]*
myotonic disorders G71.19 *[H28]*
nutritional disease E63.9 *[H28]*
infantile —*see* Cataract, presenile
irradiational —*see* Cataract, specified NEC
juvenile —*see* Cataract, presenile
malnutrition-dehydration E46 *[H28]*
morgagnian —*see* Cataract, senile, morgagnian type
myotonic G71.19 *[H28]*
myxedema E03.9 *[H28]*
nuclear
embryonal Q12.0
sclerosis —*see* Cataract, senile, nuclear
presenile H26.00-
combined forms H26.06-
cortical H26.01-
lamellar —*see* Cataract, presenile, cortical
nuclear H26.03-
specified NEC H26.09
subcapsular polar (anterior) H26.04-
posterior H26.05-
zonular —*see* Cataract, presenile, cortical
secondary H26.40
Soemmering's ring H26.41-
specified NEC H26.49-
to eye disease —*see* Cataract, complicated
senile H25.9
brunescens —*see* Cataract, senile, nuclear
combined forms H25.81-
coronary —*see* Cataract, senile, incipient
cortical H25.01-
hypermature —*see* Cataract, senile, morgagnian type
incipient (mature) (total) H25.09-
cortical —*see* Cataract, senile, cortical
subcapsular —*see* Cataract, senile, subcapsular
morgagnian type (hypermature) H25.2-
nuclear (sclerosis) H25.1-
polar subcapsular (anterior) (posterior) —*see* Cataract, senile, incipient
punctate —*see* Cataract, senile, incipient
specified NEC H25.89
subcapsular polar (anterior) H25.03-
posterior H25.04-
snowflake —*see* Diabetes, cataract
specified NEC H26.8
toxic —*see* Cataract, drug-induced
traumatic H26.10-
localized H26.11-
partially resolved H26.12-
total H26.13-
zonular (perinuclear) Q12.0
Cataracta —*see also* Cataract
brunescens —*see* Cataract, senile, nuclear
centralis pulverulenta Q12.0
cerulea Q12.0
complicata —*see* Cataract, complicated
congenita Q12.0
coralliformis Q12.0
coronaria Q12.0
diabetic —*see* Diabetes, cataract
membranacea
accreta —*see* Cataract, secondary
congenita Q12.0
nigra —*see* Cataract, senile, nuclear
sunflower —*see* Cataract, complicated
Catarrh, catarrhal (acute) (febrile) (infectious) (inflammation) (*see also* condition) J00
bronchial —*see* Bronchitis
chest —*see* Bronchitis
chronic J31.0
due to congenital syphilis A50.03
enteric —*see* Enteritis
eustachian H68.009
fauces —*see* Pharyngitis
Catarrh, catarrhal *(Continued)*
gastrointestinal —*see* Enteritis
gingivitis K05.00
nonplaque induced K05.01
plaque induced K05.00
hay —*see* Fever, hay
intestinal —*see* Enteritis
larynx, chronic J37.0
liver B15.9
with hepatic coma B15.0
lung —*see* Bronchitis
middle ear, chronic —*see* Otitis, media, nonsuppurative, chronic, serous
mouth K12.1
nasal (chronic) —*see* Rhinitis
nasobronchial J31.1
nasopharyngeal (chronic) J31.1
acute J00
pulmonary —*see* Bronchitis
spring (eye) (vernal) —*see* Conjunctivitis, acute, atopic
summer (hay) —*see* Fever, hay
throat J31.2
tubotympanal —*see also* Otitis, media, nonsuppurative
chronic —*see* Otitis, media, nonsuppurative, chronic, serous
Catatonia (schizophrenic) F20.2
Catatonic
disorder due to known physiologic condition F06.1
schizophrenia F20.2
stupor R40.1
Cat-scratch —*see also* Abrasion
disease or fever A28.1
Cauda equina —*see* condition
Cauliflower ear M95.1-
Causalgia (upper limb) G56.4-
lower limb G57.7-
Cause
external, general effects T75.89
Caustic burn —*see* Corrosion, by site
Cavare's disease (familial periodic paralysis) G72.3
Cave-in, injury
crushing (severe) —*see* Crush
suffocation —*see* Asphyxia, traumatic, due to low oxygen, due to cave-in
Cavernitis (penis) N48.29
Cavernositis N48.29
Cavernous —*see* condition
Cavitation of lung —*see also* Tuberculosis, pulmonary
nontuberculous J98.4
Cavities, dental —*see* Caries, dental
Cavity
lung —*see* Cavitation of lung
optic papilla Q14.2
pulmonary —*see* Cavitation of lung
Cavovarus foot, congenital Q66.7
Cavus foot (congenital) Q66.7
acquired —*see* Deformity, limb, foot, specified NEC
Cazenave's disease L10.2
Cecitis K52.9
with perforation, peritonitis, or rupture K65.8
Cecum —*see* condition
Celiac
artery compression syndrome I77.4
disease (with steatorrhea) K90.0 ◀
infantilism K90.0
Cell (s), **cellular** —*see also* condition
in urine R82.99
Cellulitis (diffuse) (phlegmonous) (septic) (suppurative) L03.90
abdominal wall L03.311
anaerobic A48.0
ankle —*see* Cellulitis, lower limb
anus K61.0
arm —*see* Cellulitis, upper limb
auricle (ear) —*see* Cellulitis, ear

◀ New ◀ Revised ~~deleted~~ Deleted

Cellulitis *(Continued)*
axilla L03.11-
back (any part) L03.312
breast (acute) (nonpuerperal) (subacute) N61.0 ◀
nipple N61.0 ◀
broad ligament
acute N73.0
buttock L03.317
cervical (meaning neck) L03.221
cervix (uteri) —*see* Cervicitis
cheek (external) L03.211
internal K12.2
chest wall L03.313
chronic L03.90
clostridial A48.0
corpus cavernosum N48.22
digit
finger —*see* Cellulitis, finger
toe —*see* Cellulitis, toe
Douglas' cul-de-sac or pouch
acute N73.0
drainage site (following operation) T81.48 ◀
ear (external) H60.1-
eosinophilic (granulomatous) L98.3
erysipelatous —*see* Erysipelas
external auditory canal —*see* Cellulitis, ear
eyelid —*see* Abscess, eyelid
face NEC L03.211
finger (intrathecal) (periosteal) (subcutaneous) (subcuticular) L03.01-
foot —*see* Cellulitis, lower limb
gangrenous —*see* Gangrene
genital organ NEC
female (external) N76.4
male N49.9
multiple sites N49.8
specified NEC N49.8
gluteal (region) L03.317
gonococcal A54.89
groin L03.314
hand —*see* Cellulitis, upper limb
head NEC L03.811
face (any part, except ear, eye and nose) L03.211
heel —*see* Cellulitis, lower limb
hip —*see* Cellulitis, lower limb
jaw (region) L03.211
knee —*see* Cellulitis, lower limb
labium (majus) (minus) —*see* Vulvitis
lacrimal passages —*see* Inflammation, lacrimal, passages
larynx J38.7
leg —*see* Cellulitis, lower limb
lip K13.0
lower limb L03.11-
toe —*see* Cellulitis, toe
mouth (floor) K12.2
multiple sites, so stated L03.90
nasopharynx J39.1
navel L03.316
newborn P38.9
with mild hemorrhage P38.1
without hemorrhage P38.9
neck (region) L03.221
nipple (acute) (nonpuerperal) (subacute) N61.0 ◀
nose (septum) (external) J34.0
orbit, orbital H05.01-
palate (soft) K12.2
pectoral (region) L03.313
pelvis, pelvic (chronic)
female —*see also* Disease, pelvis, inflammatory N73.2
acute N73.0
following ectopic or molar pregnancy O08.0
male K65.0
penis N48.22
perineal, perineum L03.315
periorbital L03.213 ◀

Cellulitis *(Continued)*
perirectal K61.1
peritonsillar J36
periurethral N34.0
periuterine —*see also* Disease, pelvis, inflammatory N73.2
acute N73.0
pharynx J39.1
preseptal L03.213 ◀
rectum K61.1
retroperitoneal K68.9
round ligament
acute N73.0
scalp (any part) L03.811
scrotum N49.2
seminal vesicle N49.0
shoulder —*see* Cellulitis, upper limb
specified site NEC L03.818
submandibular (region) (space) (triangle) K12.2
gland K11.3
submaxillary (region) K12.2
gland K11.3
thigh —*see* Cellulitis, lower limb
thumb (intrathecal) (periosteal) (subcutaneous) (subcuticular) —*see* Cellulitis, finger
toe (intrathecal) (periosteal) (subcutaneous) (subcuticular) L03.03-
tonsil J36
trunk L03.319
abdominal wall L03.311
back (any part) L03.312
buttock L03.317
chest wall L03.313
groin L03.314
perineal, perineum L03.315
umbilicus L03.316
tuberculous (primary) A18.4
umbilicus L03.316
upper limb L03.11-
axilla —*see* Cellulitis, axilla
finger —*see* Cellulitis, finger
thumb —*see* Cellulitis, finger
vaccinal T88.0
vocal cord J38.3
vulva —*see* Vulvitis
wrist —*see* Cellulitis, upper limb
Cementoblastoma, benign —*see* Cyst, calcifying odontogenic
Cementoma —*see* Cyst, calcifying odontogenic
Cementoperiostitis —*see* Periodontitis
Cementosis K03.4
Central auditory processing disorder H93.25
Central pain syndrome G89.0
Cephalematocele, cephal(o)hematocele
newborn P52.8
birth injury P10.8
traumatic —*see* Hematoma, brain
Cephalematoma, cephalhematoma (calcified)
newborn (birth injury) P12.0
traumatic —*see* Hematoma, brain
Cephalgia, cephalalgia —*see also* Headache
histamine G44.009
intractable G44.001
not intractable G44.009
trigeminal autonomic (TAC) NEC G44.099
intractable G44.091
not intractable G44.099
Cephalic —*see* condition
Cephalitis —*see* Encephalitis
Cephalocele —*see* Encephalocele
Cephalomenia N94.89
Cephalopelvic —*see* condition
Cerclage (with cervical incompetence) in pregnancy —*see* Incompetence, cervix, in pregnancy
Cerebellitis —*see* Encephalitis
Cerebellum, cerebellar —*see* condition
Cerebral —*see* condition
Cerebritis —*see* Encephalitis

Cerebro-hepato-renal syndrome Q87.89
Cerebromalacia —*see* Softening, brain
sequelae of cerebrovascular disease I69.398
Cerebroside lipidosis E75.22
Cerebrospasticity (congenital) G80.1
Cerebrospinal —*see* condition
Cerebrum —*see* condition
Ceroid-lipofuscinosis, neuronal E75.4
Cerumen (accumulation) (impacted) H61.2-
Cervical —*see also* condition
auricle Q18.2
dysplasia in pregnancy —*see* Abnormal, cervix, in pregnancy or childbirth
erosion in pregnancy —*see* Abnormal, cervix, in pregnancy or childbirth
fibrosis in pregnancy —*see* Abnormal, cervix, in pregnancy or childbirth
fusion syndrome Q76.1
rib Q76.5
shortening (complicating pregnancy) O26.87-
Cervicalgia M54.2
Cervicitis (acute) (chronic) (nonvenereal) (senile (atrophic)) (subacute) (with ulceration) N72
with
abortion —*see* Abortion, by type complicated by genital tract and pelvic infection
ectopic pregnancy O08.0
molar pregnancy O08.0
chlamydial A56.09
gonococcal A54.03
herpesviral A60.03
puerperal (postpartum) O86.11
syphilitic A52.76
trichomonal A59.09
tuberculous A18.16
Cervicocolpitis (emphysematosa) (*see also* Cervicitis) N72
Cervix —*see* condition
Cesarean delivery, previous, affecting management of pregnancy O34.219 ◀
classical (vertical) scar O34.212 ◀
low transverse scar O34.211 ◀
Céstan (-Chenais) paralysis or syndrome G46.3
Céstan-Raymond syndrome I65.8
Cestode infestation B71.9
specified type NEC B71.8
Cestodiasis B71.9
Chabert's disease A22.9
Chacaleh E53.8
Chafing L30.4
Chagas' (-Mazza) disease (chronic) B57.2
with
cardiovascular involvement NEC B57.2
digestive system involvement B57.30
megacolon B57.32
megaesophagus B57.31
other specified B57.39
megacolon B57.32
megaesophagus B57.31
myocarditis B57.2
nervous system involvement B57.40
meningitis B57.41
meningoencephalitis B57.42
other specified B57.49
specified organ involvement NEC B57.5
acute (with) B57.1
cardiovascular NEC B57.0
myocarditis B57.0
Chagres fever B50.9
Chairridden Z74.09
Chalasia (cardiac sphincter) K21.9
Chalazion H00.19
left H00.16
lower H00.15
upper H00.14
right H00.13
lower H00.12
upper H00.11

Chalcosis —*see also* Disorder, globe, degenerative, chalcosis
cornea —*see* Deposit, cornea
crystalline lens —*see* Cataract, complicated
retina H35.89
Chalicosis (pulmonum) J62.8
Chancre (any genital site) (hard) (hunterian) (mixed) (primary) (seronegative) (seropositive) (syphilitic) A51.0
congenital A50.07
conjunctiva NEC A51.2
Ducrey's A57
extragenital A51.2
eyelid A51.2
lip A51.2
nipple A51.2
Nisbet's A57
of
carate A67.0
pinta A67.0
yaws A66.0
palate, soft A51.2
phagedenic A57
simple A57
soft A57
bubo A57
palate A51.2
urethra A51.0
yaws A66.0
Chancroid (anus) (genital) (penis) (perineum) (rectum) (urethra) (vulva) A57
Chandler's disease (osteochondritis dissecans, hip) —*see* Osteochondritis, dissecans, hip
Change (s) (in) (of) —*see also* Removal
arteriosclerotic —*see* Arteriosclerosis
bone —*see also* Disorder, bone
diabetic —*see* Diabetes, bone change
bowel habit R19.4
cardiorenal (vascular) —*see* Hypertension, cardiorenal
cardiovascular —*see* Disease, cardiovascular
circulatory I99.9
cognitive (mild) (organic) R41.89
color, tooth, teeth
during formation K00.8
posteruptive K03.7
contraceptive device Z30.433
corneal membrane H18.30
Bowman's membrane fold or rupture H18.31-
Descemet's membrane
fold H18.32-
rupture H18.33-
coronary —*see* Disease, heart, ischemic
degenerative, spine or vertebra —*see* Spondylosis
dental pulp, regressive K04.2
dressing (nonsurgical) Z48.00
surgical Z48.01
heart —*see* Disease, heart
hip joint —*see* Derangement, joint, hip
hyperplastic larynx J38.7
hypertrophic
nasal sinus J34.89
turbinate, nasal J34.3
upper respiratory tract J39.8
indwelling catheter Z46.6
inflammatory —*see also* Inflammation
sacroiliac M46.1
job, anxiety concerning Z56.1
joint —*see* Derangement, joint
life —*see* Menopause
mental status R41.82
minimal (glomerular) —*see also* N00-N07
with fourth character .0 N05.0
myocardium, myocardial —*see* Degeneration, myocardial - of life —*see* Menopause
pacemaker Z45.018
pulse generator Z45.010
Change *(Continued)*
personality (enduring) F68.8
due to (secondary to)
general medical condition F07.0
secondary (nonspecific) F60.89
regressive, dental pulp K04.2
renal —*see* Disease, renal
retina H35.9
myopic H44.2-
sacroiliac joint M53.3
senile —*see also* condition R54
sensory R20.8
skin R23.9
acute, due to ultraviolet radiation L56.9
specified NEC L56.8
chronic, due to nonionizing radiation L57.9
specified NEC L57.8
cyanosis R23.0
flushing R23.2
pallor R23.1
petechiae R23.3
specified change NEC R23.8
swelling —*see* Mass, localized
texture R23.4
trophic
arm —*see* Mononeuropathy, upper limb
leg —*see* Mononeuropathy, lower limb
vascular I99.9
vasomotor I73.9
voice R49.9
psychogenic F44.4
specified NEC R49.8
Changing sleep-work schedule, affecting sleep G47.26
Changuinola fever A93.1
Chapping skin T69.8
Charcot-Marie-Tooth disease, paralysis or syndrome G60.0
Charcot's
arthropathy —*see* Arthropathy, neuropathic
cirrhosis K74.3
disease (tabetic arthropathy) A52.16
joint (disease) (tabetic) A52.16
diabetic —*see* Diabetes, with, arthropathy
syringomyelic G95.0
syndrome (intermittent claudication) I73.9
CHARGE association Q89.8
Charley-horse (quadriceps) M62.831
traumatic (quadriceps) S76.11-
Charlouis' disease —*see* Yaws
Cheadle's disease E54
Checking (of)
cardiac pacemaker (battery) (electrode (s)) Z45.018
pulse generator Z45.010
implantable subdermal contraceptive Z30.46 ◀
intrauterine contraceptive device Z30.431
Check-up —*see* Examination
Chédiak-Higashi (-Steinbrinck) syndrome (congenital gigantism of peroxidase granules) E70.330
Cheek —*see* condition
Cheese itch B88.0
Cheese-washer's lung J67.8
Cheese-worker's lung J67.8
Cheilitis (acute) (angular) (catarrhal) (chronic) (exfoliative) (gangrenous) (glandular) (infectional) (suppurative) (ulcerative) (vesicular) K13.0
actinic (due to sun) L56.8
other than from sun L59.8
candidal B37.83
Cheilodynia K13.0
Cheiloschisis —*see* Cleft, lip
Cheilosis (angular) K13.0
with pellagra E52
due to
vitamin B2 (riboflavin) deficiency E53.0
Cheiromegaly M79.89
Cheiropompholyx L30.1
Cheloid —*see* Keloid
Chemical burn —*see* Corrosion, by site
Chemodectoma —*see* Paraganglioma, nonchromaffin
Chemosis, conjunctiva —*see* Edema, conjunctiva
Chemotherapy (session) (for)
cancer Z51.11
neoplasm Z51.11
Cherubism M27.8
Chest —*see* condition
Cheyne-Stokes breathing (respiration) R06.3
Chiari's
disease or syndrome (hepatic vein thrombosis) I82.0
malformation
type I G93.5
type II —*see* Spina bifida
net Q24.8
Chicago disease B40.9
Chickenpox —*see* Varicella
Chiclero ulcer or sore B55.1
Chigger (infestation) B88.0
Chignon (disease) B36.8
newborn (from vacuum extraction) (birth injury) P12.1
Chilaiditi's syndrome (subphrenic displacement, colon) Q43.3
Chilblain (s) (lupus) T69.1
Child
custody dispute Z65.3
Childbirth —*see* Delivery
Childhood
cerebral X-linked adrenoleukodystrophy E71.520
period of rapid growth Z00.2
Chill (s) R68.83
with fever R50.9
without fever R68.83
congestive in malarial regions B54
Chilomastigiasis A07.8
Chimera 46,XX/46,XY Q99.0
Chin —*see* condition
Chinese dysentery A03.9
Chionophobia F40.228
Chitral fever A93.1
Chlamydia, chlamydial A74.9
cervicitis A56.09
conjunctivitis A74.0
cystitis A56.01
endometritis A56.11
epididymitis A56.19
female
pelvic inflammatory disease A56.11
pelviperitonitis A56.11
orchitis A56.19
peritonitis A74.81
pharyngitis A56.4
proctitis A56.3
psittaci (infection) A70
salpingitis A56.11
sexually-transmitted infection NEC A56.8
specified NEC A74.89
urethritis A56.01
vulvovaginitis A56.02
Chlamydiosis —*see* Chlamydia
Chloasma (skin) (idiopathic) (symptomatic) L81.1
eyelid H02.719
hyperthyroid E05.90 *[H02.719]*
with thyroid storm E05.91 *[H02.719]*
left H02.716
lower H02.715
upper H02.714
right H02.713
lower H02.712
upper H02.711
Chloroma C92.3-
Chlorosis D50.9
Egyptian B76.9 *[D63.8]*
miner's B76.9 *[D63.8]*
Chlorotic anemia D50.8

◀ New ⇐ Revised ~~deleted~~ Deleted

Chocolate cyst (ovary) N80.1
Choked
disc or disk —*see* Papilledema
on food, phlegm, or vomitus NOS —*see* Foreign body, by site
while vomiting NOS —*see* Foreign body, by site
Chokes (resulting from bends) T70.3
Choking sensation R09.89
Cholangiectasis K83.8
Cholangiocarcinoma
with hepatocellular carcinoma, combined C22.0
liver C22.1
specified site NEC —*see* Neoplasm, malignant, by site
unspecified site C22.1
Cholangiohepatitis K83.8
due to fluke infestation B66.1
Cholangiohepatoma C22.0
Cholangiolitis (acute) (chronic) (extrahepatic) (gangrenous) (intrahepatic) K83.0
paratyphoidal —*see* Fever, paratyphoid
typhoidal A01.09
Cholangioma D13.4
malignant —*see* Cholangiocarcinoma
Cholangitis (ascending) (primary) (recurrent) (sclerosing) (secondary) (stenosing) (suppurative) K83.0
with calculus, bile duct —*see* Calculus, bile duct, with cholangitis
chronic nonsuppurative destructive K74.3
Cholecystectasia K82.8
Cholecystitis K81.9
with
calculus, stones in
bile duct (common) (hepatic) —*see* Calculus, bile duct, with cholecystitis
cystic duct —*see* Calculus, gallbladder, with cholecystitis
gallbladder —*see* Calculus, gallbladder, with cholecystitis
choledocholithiasis —*see* Calculus, bile duct, with cholecystitis
cholelithiasis —*see* Calculus, gallbladder, with cholecystitis
acute (emphysematous) (gangrenous) (suppurative) K81.0
with
calculus, stones in
cystic duct —*see* Calculus, gallbladder, with cholecystitis, acute
gallbladder —*see* Calculus, gallbladder, with cholecystitis, acute
choledocholithiasis —*see* Calculus, bile duct, with cholecystitis, acute
cholelithiasis —*see* Calculus, gallbladder, with cholecystitis, acute
chronic cholecystitis K81.2
with gallbladder calculus K80.12
with obstruction K80.13
chronic K81.1
with acute cholecystitis K81.2
with gallbladder calculus K80.12
with obstruction K80.13
emphysematous (acute) —*see* Cholecystitis, acute
gangrenous —*see* Cholecystitis, acute
paratyphoidal, current A01.4
suppurative —*see* Cholecystitis, acute
typhoidal A01.09
Cholecystolithiasis —*see* Calculus, gallbladder
Choledochitis (suppurative) K83.0
Choledocholith —*see* Calculus, bile duct
Choledocholithiasis (common duct) (hepatic duct) —*see* Calculus, bile duct
cystic —*see* Calculus, gallbladder
typhoidal A01.09
Cholelithiasis (cystic duct) (gallbladder) (impacted) (multiple) —*see* Calculus, gallbladder
bile duct (common) (hepatic) —*see* Calculus, bile duct
hepatic duct —*see* Calculus, bile duct
specified NEC K80.80
with obstruction K80.81
Cholemia —*see also* Jaundice
familial (simple) (congenital) E80.4
Gilbert's E80.4
Choleperitoneum, choleperitonitis K65.3
Cholera (Asiatic) (epidemic) (malignant) A00.9
antimonial —*see* Poisoning, antimony
classical A00.0
due to Vibrio cholerae 01 A00.9
biovar cholerae A00.0
biovar eltor A00.1
el tor A00.1
el tor A00.1
Cholerine —*see* Cholera
Cholestasis NEC K83.1
with hepatocyte injury K71.0
due to total parenteral nutrition (TPN) K76.89
pure K71.0
Cholesteatoma (ear) (middle) (with reaction) H71.9-
attic H71.0-
external ear (canal) H60.4-
mastoid H71.2-
postmastoidectomy cavity (recurrent) —*see* Complications, postmastoidectomy, recurrent cholesteatoma
recurrent (postmastoidectomy) —*see* Complications, postmastoidectomy, recurrent cholesteatoma
tympanum H71.1-
Cholesteatosis, diffuse H71.3-
Cholesteremia E78.00 ⇐
Cholesterin in vitreous —*see* Deposit, crystalline
Cholesterol
deposit
retina H35.89
vitreous —*see* Deposit, crystalline
elevated (high) E78.00 ⇐
with elevated (high) triglycerides E78.2
screening for Z13.220
imbibition of gallbladder K82.4
Cholesterolemia (essential) (pure) E78.00 ⇐
familial E78.01 ◀
hereditary E78.01 ◀
Cholesterolosis, cholesterosis (gallbladder) K82.4
cerebrotendinous E75.5
Cholocolic fistula K82.3
Choluria R82.2
Chondritis M94.8X9
aurical H61.03-
costal (Tietze's) M94.0
external ear H61.03-
patella, posttraumatic —*see* Chondromalacia, patella
pinna H61.03-
purulent M94.8X-
tuberculous NEC A18.02
intervertebral A18.01
Chondroblastoma —*see also* Neoplasm, bone, benign
malignant —*see* Neoplasm, bone, malignant
Chondrocalcinosis M11.20
ankle M11.27-
elbow M11.22-
familial M11.10
ankle M11.17-
elbow M11.12-
foot joint M11.17-
hand joint M11.14-
hip M11.15-
knee M11.16-
multiple site M11.19
shoulder M11.11-
Chondrocalcinosis *(Continued)*
familial *(Continued)*
vertebrae M11.18
wrist M11.13-
foot joint M11.27-
hand joint M11.24-
hip M11.25-
knee M11.26-
multiple site M11.29
shoulder M11.21-
specified type NEC M11.20
ankle M11.27-
elbow M11.22-
foot joint M11.27-
hand joint M11.24-
hip M11.25-
knee M11.26-
multiple site M11.29
shoulder M11.21-
vertebrae M11.28
wrist M11.23-
vertebrae M11.28
wrist M11.23-
Chondrodermatitis nodularis helicis or anthelicis —*see* Perichondritis, ear
Chondrodysplasia Q78.9
with hemangioma Q78.4
calcificans congenita Q77.3
fetalis Q77.4
metaphyseal (Jansen's) (McKusick's) (Schmid's) Q78.8 ⇐
punctata Q77.3
Chondrodystrophy, chondrodystrophia (familial) (fetalis) (hypoplastic) Q78.9
calcificans congenita Q77.3
myotonic (congenital) G71.13
punctata Q77.3
Chondroectodermal dysplasia Q77.6
Chondrogenesis imperfecta Q77.4
Chondrolysis M94.35-
Chondroma —*see also* Neoplasm, cartilage, benign
juxtacortical —*see* Neoplasm, bone, benign
periosteal —*see* Neoplasm, bone, benign
Chondromalacia (systemic) M94.20
acromioclavicular joint M94.21-
ankle M94.27-
elbow M94.22-
foot joint M94.27-
glenohumeral joint M94.21-
hand joint M94.24-
hip M94.25-
knee M94.26-
patella M22.4-
multiple sites M94.29
patella M22.4-
rib M94.28
sacroiliac joint M94.259
shoulder M94.21-
sternoclavicular joint M94.21-
vertebral joint M94.28
wrist M94.23-
Chondromatosis —*see also* Neoplasm, cartilage, uncertain behavior
internal Q78.4
Chondromyxosarcoma —*see* Neoplasm, cartilage, malignant
Chondro-osteodysplasia (Morquio-Brailsford type) E76.219
Chondro-osteodystrophy E76.29
Chondro-osteoma —*see* Neoplasm, bone, benign
Chondropathia tuberosa M94.0
Chondrosarcoma —*see* Neoplasm, cartilage, malignant
juxtacortical —*see* Neoplasm, bone, malignant
mesenchymal —*see* Neoplasm, connective tissue, malignant
myxoid —*see* Neoplasm, cartilage, malignant
Chordee (nonvenereal) N48.89
congenital Q54.4
gonococcal A54.09

Chorditis (fibrinous) (nodosa) (tuberosa) J38.2
Chordoma —*see* Neoplasm, vertebral (column), malignant
Chorea (chronic) (gravis) (posthemiplegic) (senile) (spasmodic) G25.5
with
heart involvement I02.0
active or acute (conditions in I01-) I02.0
rheumatic I02.9
with valvular disorder I02.0
rheumatic heart disease (chronic) (inactive) (quiescent) — code to rheumatic heart condition involved
drug-induced G25.4
habit F95.8
hereditary G10
Huntington's G10
hysterical F44.4
minor I02.9
with heart involvement I02.0
progressive G25.5
hereditary G10
rheumatic (chronic) I02.9
with heart involvement I02.0
Sydenham's I02.9
with heart involvement —*see* Chorea, with rheumatic heart disease
nonrheumatic G25.5
Choreoathetosis (paroxysmal) G25.5
Chorioadenoma (destruens) D39.2
Chorioamnionitis O41.12-
Chorioangioma D26.7
Choriocarcinoma —*see* Neoplasm, malignant, by site
combined with
embryonal carcinoma —*see* Neoplasm, malignant, by site
other germ cell elements —*see* Neoplasm, malignant, by site
teratoma —*see* Neoplasm, malignant, by site
specified site —*see* Neoplasm, malignant, by site
unspecified site
female C58
male C62.90
Chorioencephalitis (acute) (lymphocytic) (serous) A87.2
Chorioepithelioma —*see* Choriocarcinoma
Choriomeningitis (acute) (lymphocytic) (serous) A87.2
Chorionepithelioma —*see* Choriocarcinoma
Chorioretinitis —*see also* Inflammation, chorioretinal
disseminated —*see also* Inflammation, chorioretinal, disseminated
in neurosyphilis A52.19
Egyptian B76.9 *[D63.8]*
focal —*see also* Inflammation, chorioretinal, focal
histoplasmic B39.9 *[H32]*
in (due to)
histoplasmosis B39.9 *[H32]*
syphilis (secondary) A51.43
late A52.71
toxoplasmosis (acquired) B58.01
congenital (active) P37.1 *[H32]*
tuberculosis A18.53
juxtapapillary, juxtapapillaris —*see* Inflammation, chorioretinal, focal, juxtapapillary
leprous A30.9 *[H32]*
miner's B76.9 *[D63.8]*
progressive myopia (degeneration) H44.2-
syphilitic (secondary) A51.43
congenital (early) A50.01 *[H32]*
late A50.32
late A52.71
tuberculous A18.53
Chorioretinopathy, central serous H35.71-
Choroid —*see* condition
Choroideremia H31.21
Choroiditis —*see* Chorioretinitis
Choroidopathy —*see* Disorder, choroid
Choroidoretinitis —*see* Chorioretinitis
Choroidoretinopathy, central serous —*see* Chorioretinopathy, central serous
Christian-Weber disease M35.6
Christmas disease D67
Chromaffinoma —*see also* Neoplasm, benign, by site
malignant —*see* Neoplasm, malignant, by site
Chromatopsia —*see* Deficiency, color vision
Chromhidrosis, chromidrosis L75.1
Chromoblastomycosis —*see* Chromomycosis
Chromoconversion R82.91
Chromomycosis B43.9
brain abscess B43.1
cerebral B43.1
cutaneous B43.0
skin B43.0
specified NEC B43.8
subcutaneous abscess or cyst B43.2
Chromophytosis B36.0
Chromosome —*see* condition by chromosome involved
D (1) —*see* condition, chromosome 13
E (3) —*see* condition, chromosome 18
G —*see* condition, chromosome 21
Chromotrichomycosis B36.8
Chronic —*see* condition
fracture —*see* Fracture, pathological
Churg-Strauss syndrome M30.1
Chyle cyst, mesentery I89.8
Chylocele (nonfilarial) I89.8
filarial —*see also* Infestation, filarial B74.9 *[N51]*
tunica vaginalis N50.89 ⇐
filarial —*see also* Infestation, filarial B74.9 *[N51]*
Chylomicronemia (fasting) (with hyperprebetalipoproteinemia) E78.3
Chylopericardium I31.3
acute I30.9
Chylothorax (nonfilarial) I89.8
filarial —*see also* Infestation, filarial B74.9 *[J91.8]*
Chylous —*see* condition
Chyluria (nonfilarial) R82.0
due to
bilharziasis B65.0
Brugia (malayi) B74.1
timori B74.2
schistosomiasis (bilharziasis) B65.0
Wuchereria (bancrofti) B74.0
filarial —*see* Infestation, filarial
Cicatricial (deformity) —*see* Cicatrix
Cicatrix (adherent) (contracted) (painful) (vicious) —*see also* Scar L90.5
adenoid (and tonsil) J35.8
alveolar process M26.79
anus K62.89
auricle —*see* Disorder, pinna, specified type NEC
bile duct (common) (hepatic) K83.8
bladder N32.89
bone —*see* Disorder, bone, specified type NEC
brain G93.89
cervix (postoperative) (postpartal) N88.1
common duct K83.8
cornea H17.9
tuberculous A18.59
duodenum (bulb), obstructive K31.5
esophagus K22.2
eyelid —*see* Disorder, eyelid function
hypopharynx J39.2
lacrimal passages —*see* Obstruction, lacrimal
larynx J38.7
lung J98.4
middle ear —*see* subcategory H74.8
mouth K13.79
Cicatrix *(Continued)*
muscle M62.89
with contracture —*see* Contraction, muscle NEC
nasopharynx J39.2
palate (soft) K13.79
penis N48.89
pharynx J39.2
prostate N42.89
rectum K62.89
retina —*see* Scar, chorioretinal
semilunar cartilage —*see* Derangement, meniscus
seminal vesicle N50.89 ⇐
skin L90.5
infected L08.89
postinfective L90.5
tuberculous B90.8
specified site NEC L90.5
throat J39.2
tongue K14.8
tonsil (and adenoid) J35.8
trachea J39.8
tuberculous NEC B90.9
urethra N36.8
uterus N85.8
vagina N89.8
postoperative N99.2
vocal cord J38.3
wrist, constricting (annular) L90.5
CIDP (chronic inflammatory demyelinating polyneuropathy) G61.81
CIN —*see* Neoplasia, intraepithelial, cervix
CINCA (chronic infantile neurological, cutaneous and articular syndrome) M04.2 ◀
Cinchonism —*see* Deafness, ototoxic
correct substance properly administered —*see* Table of Drugs and Chemicals, by drug, adverse effect
overdose or wrong substance given or taken —*see* Table of Drugs and Chemicals, by drug, poisoning
Circle of Willis —*see* condition
Circular —*see* condition
Circulating anticoagulants —*see also* - Disorder, hemorrhagic D68.318
due to drugs —*see also* - Disorder, hemorrhagic D68.32
following childbirth O72.3
Circulation
collateral, any site I99.8
defective (lower extremity) I99.8
congenital Q28.9
embryonic Q28.9
failure (peripheral) R57.9
newborn P29.89
fetal, persistent P29.3
heart, incomplete Q28.9
Circulatory system —*see* condition
Circulus senilis (cornea) —*see* Degeneration, cornea, senile
Circumcision (in absence of medical indication) (ritual) (routine) Z41.2
Circumscribed —*see* condition
Circumvallate placenta O43.11-
Cirrhosis, cirrhotic (hepatic) (liver) K74.60
alcoholic K70.30
with ascites K70.31
atrophic —*see* Cirrhosis, liver
Baumgarten-Cruveilhier K74.69
biliary (cholangiolitic) (cholangitic) (hypertrophic) (obstructive) (pericholangiolitic) K74.5
due to
Clonorchiasis B66.1
flukes B66.3
primary K74.3
secondary K74.4
cardiac (of liver) K76.1
Charcot's K74.3

◀ New ⇐ Revised ~~deleted~~ Deleted

Cirrhosis, cirrhotic *(Continued)*
cholangiolitic, cholangitic, cholostatic (primary) K74.3
congestive K76.1
Cruveilhier-Baumgarten K74.69
cryptogenic (liver) K74.69
due to
hepatolenticular degeneration E83.01
Wilson's disease E83.01
xanthomatosis E78.2
fatty K76.0
alcoholic K70.0
Hanot's (hypertrophic) K74.3
hepatic —*see* Cirrhosis, liver
hypertrophic K74.3
Indian childhood K74.69
kidney —*see* Sclerosis, renal
Laennec's K70.30
with ascites K70.31
alcoholic K70.30
with ascites K70.31
nonalcoholic K74.69
liver K74.60
alcoholic K70.30
with ascites K70.31
fatty K70.0
congenital P78.81
syphilitic A52.74
lung (chronic) J84.10
macronodular K74.69
alcoholic K70.30
with ascites K70.31
micronodular K74.69
alcoholic K70.30
with ascites K70.31
mixed type K74.69
monolobular K74.3
nephritis —*see* Sclerosis, renal
nutritional K74.69
alcoholic K70.30
with ascites K70.31
obstructive —*see* Cirrhosis, biliary
ovarian N83.8
pancreas (duct) K86.89 ⇐
pigmentary E83.110
portal K74.69
alcoholic K70.30
with ascites K70.31
postnecrotic K74.69
alcoholic K70.30
with ascites K70.31
pulmonary J84.10
renal —*see* Sclerosis, renal
spleen D73.2
stasis K76.1
Todd's K74.3
unilobar K74.3
xanthomatous (biliary) K74.5
due to xanthomatosis (familial) (metabolic) (primary) E78.2
Cistern, subarachnoid R93.0
Citrullinemia E72.23
Citrullinuria E72.23
Civatte's disease or poikiloderma L57.3
Clam digger's itch B65.3
Clammy skin R23.1
Clap —*see* Gonorrhea
Clarke-Hadfield syndrome (pancreatic infantilism) K86.89 ⇐
Clark's paralysis G80.9
Clastothrix L67.8
Claude Bernard-Horner syndrome G90.2
traumatic —*see* Injury, nerve, cervical sympathetic
Claude's disease or syndrome G46.3
Claudicatio venosa intermittens I87.8
~~Claudication, intermittent I73.9~~
~~cerebral (artery) G45.9~~
~~spinal cord (arteriosclerotic) G95.19~~
~~syphilitic A52.09~~
~~venous (axillary) I87.8~~
Claudication (intermittent) I73.9 ◀
cerebral (artery) G45.9 ◀
spinal cord (arteriosclerotic) G95.19 ◀
syphilitic A52.09 ◀
venous (axillary) I87.8 ◀
Claustrophobia F40.240
Clavus (infected) L84
Clawfoot (congenital) Q66.89
acquired —*see* Deformity, limb, clawfoot
Clawhand (acquired) —*see also* Deformity, limb, clawhand
congenital Q68.1
Clawtoe (congenital) Q66.89
acquired —*see* Deformity, toe, specified NEC
Clay eating —*see* Pica
Cleansing of artificial opening —*see* Attention to, artificial, opening
Cleft (congenital) —*see also* Imperfect, closure
alveolar process M26.79
branchial (cyst) (persistent) Q18.2
cricoid cartilage, posterior Q31.8
foot Q72.7 ◀
hand Q71.6 ◀
lip (unilateral) Q36.9
with cleft palate Q37.9
hard Q37.1
with soft Q37.5
soft Q37.3
with hard Q37.5
bilateral Q36.0
with cleft palate Q37.8
hard Q37.0
with soft Q37.4
soft Q37.2
with hard Q37.4
median Q36.1
nose Q30.2
palate Q35.9
with cleft lip (unilateral) Q37.9
bilateral Q37.8
hard Q35.1
with
cleft lip (unilateral) Q37.1
bilateral Q37.0
soft Q35.5
with cleft lip (unilateral) Q37.5
bilateral Q37.4
medial Q35.5
soft Q35.3
with
cleft lip (unilateral) Q37.3
bilateral Q37.2
hard Q35.5
with cleft lip (unilateral) Q37.5
bilateral Q37.4
penis Q55.69
scrotum Q55.29
thyroid cartilage Q31.8
uvula Q35.7
Cleidocranial dysostosis Q74.0
Cleptomania F63.2
Clicking hip (newborn) R29.4
Climacteric (female) —*see also* Menopause
arthritis (any site) NEC —*see* Arthritis, specified form NEC
depression (single episode) F32.89 ⇐
recurrent episode F33.8 ◀
male (symptoms) (syndrome) NEC N50.89 ⇐
melancholia (single episode) F32.89 ◀
recurrent episode F33.8 ◀
paranoid state F22
polyarthritis NEC —*see* Arthritis, specified form NEC
symptoms (female) N95.1
Clinical research investigation (clinical trial) (control subject) (normal comparison) (participant) Z00.6
Clitoris —*see* condition **Cloaca** (persistent) Q43.7
Clonorchiasis, clonorchis infection (liver) B66.1
Clonus R25.8
Closed bite M26.29
Clostridium (C.) **perfringens, as cause of disease classified elsewhere** B96.7
Closure
congenital, nose Q30.0
cranial sutures, premature Q75.0
defective or imperfect NEC —*see* Imperfect, closure
fistula, delayed —*see* Fistula
foramen ovale, imperfect Q21.1
hymen N89.6
interauricular septum, defective Q21.1
interventricular septum, defective Q21.0
lacrimal duct —*see also* Stenosis, lacrimal, duct
congenital Q10.5
nose (congenital) Q30.0
acquired M95.0
of artificial opening —*see* Attention to, artificial, opening
primary angle, without glaucoma damage H40.06-
vagina N89.5
valve —*see* Endocarditis
vulva N90.5
Clot (blood) —*see also* Embolism
artery (obstruction) (occlusion) —*see* Embolism
bladder N32.89
brain (intradural or extradural) —*see* Occlusion, artery, cerebral
circulation I74.9
heart —*see also* Infarct, myocardium
not resulting in infarction I51.3 ⇐
vein —*see* Thrombosis
Clouded state R40.1
epileptic —*see* Epilepsy, specified NEC
paroxysmal —*see* Epilepsy, specified NEC
Cloudy antrum, antra J32.0
Clouston's (hidrotic) **ectodermal dysplasia** Q82.4
Clubbed nail pachydermoperiostosis M89.40 *[L62]*
Clubbing of finger (s) (nails) R68.3
Clubfinger R68.3
congenital Q68.1
Clubfoot (congenital) Q66.89
acquired —*see* Deformity, limb, clubfoot
equinovarus Q66.0
paralytic —*see* Deformity, limb, clubfoot
Clubhand (congenital) (radial) Q71.4-
acquired —*see* Deformity, limb, clubhand
Clubnail R68.3
congenital Q84.6
Clump, kidney Q63.1
Clumsiness, clumsy child syndrome F82
Cluttering F98.81
Clutton's joints A50.51 *[M12.80]*
Coagulation, intravascular (diffuse) (disseminated) —*see also* Defibrination syndrome
complicating abortion —*see* Abortion, by type, complicated by, intravascular coagulation
following ectopic or molar pregnancy O08.1
Coagulopathy —*see also* Defect, coagulation
consumption D65
intravascular D65
newborn P60
Coalition
calcaneo-scaphoid Q66.89
tarsal Q66.89
Coalminer's
elbow —*see* Bursitis, elbow, olecranon
lung or pneumoconiosis J60
Coalworker's lung or pneumoconiosis J60
Coarctation
aorta (preductal) (postductal) Q25.1
pulmonary artery Q25.71
Coated tongue K14.3

Coats' disease (exudative retinopathy) —*see* Retinopathy, exudative
Cocaine-induced ◀
anxiety disorder F14.980 ◀
bipolar and related disorder F14.94 ◀
depressive disorder F14.94 ◀
obsessive-compulsive and related disorder F14.988 ◀
psychotic disorder F14.959 ◀
sleep disorder F14.982 ◀
sexual dysfunction F14.981 ◀
Cocainism —*see* Disorder, cocaine use ⟸
Coccidioidomycosis B38.9
cutaneous B38.3
disseminated B38.7
generalized B38.7
meninges B38.4
prostate B38.81
pulmonary B38.2
acute B38.0
chronic B38.1
skin B38.3
specified NEC B38.89
Coccidioidosis —*see* Coccidioidomycosis
Coccidiosis (intestinal) A07.3
Coccydynia, coccygodynia M53.3
Coccyx —*see* condition
Cochin-China diarrhea K90.1
Cockayne's syndrome Q87.1
Cocked up toe —*see* Deformity, toe, specified NEC
Cock's peculiar tumor L72.3
Codman's tumor —*see* Neoplasm, bone, benign
Coenurosis B71.8
Coffee-worker's lung J67.8
Cogan's syndrome H16.32-
oculomotor apraxia H51.8
Coitus, painful (female) N94.10 ⟸
male N53.12
psychogenic F52.6
Cold J00
with influenza, flu, or grippe —*see* Influenza, with, respiratory manifestations NEC
agglutinin disease or hemoglobinuria (chronic) D59.1
bronchial —*see* Bronchitis
chest —*see* Bronchitis
common (head) J00
effects of T69.9
specified effect NEC T69.8
excessive, effects of T69.9
specified effect NEC T69.8
exhaustion from T69.8
exposure to T69.9
specified effect NEC T69.8
head J00
injury syndrome (newborn) P80.0
on lung —*see* Bronchitis
rose J30.1
sensitivity, auto-immune D59.1
virus J00
Coldsore B00.1
Colibacillosis A49.8
as the cause of other disease (*see also* Escherichia coli) B96.20
generalized A41.50
Colic (bilious) (infantile) (intestinal) (recurrent) (spasmodic) R10.83
abdomen R10.83
psychogenic F45.8
appendix, appendicular K38.8
bile duct —*see* Calculus, bile duct
biliary —*see* Calculus, bile duct
common duct —*see* Calculus, bile duct
cystic duct —*see* Calculus, gallbladder
Devonshire NEC —*see* Poisoning, lead
gallbladder —*see* Calculus, gallbladder
gallstone —*see* Calculus, gallbladder
gallbladder or cystic duct —*see* Calculus, gallbladder
Colic *(Continued)*
hepatic (duct) —*see* Calculus, bile duct
hysterical F45.8
kidney N23
lead NEC —*see* Poisoning, lead
mucous K58.9
with diarrhea K58.0
psychogenic F54
nephritic N23
painter's NEC —*see* Poisoning, lead
pancreas K86.89 ⟸
psychogenic F45.8
renal N23
saturnine NEC —*see* Poisoning, lead
ureter N23
urethral N36.8
due to calculus N21.1
uterus NEC N94.89
menstrual —*see* Dysmenorrhea
worm NOS B83.9
Colicystitis —*see* Cystitis
Colitis (acute) (catarrhal) (chronic) (noninfective) (hemorrhagic) (*see also* Enteritis) K52.9
allergic K52.29 ⟸
with ◀
food protein-induced enterocolitis syndrome K52.21 ◀
proctocolitis K52.82 ◀
amebic (acute) —*see also* Amebiasis A06.0
nondysenteric A06.2
anthrax A22.2
bacillary —*see* Infection, Shigella
balantidial A07.0
Clostridium difficile A04.7
coccidial A07.3
collagenous K52.831 ⟸
cystica superficialis K52.89
dietary counseling and surveillance (for) Z71.3
dietetic —*see also* Colitis, allergic K52.29 ⟸
drug-induced K52.1
due to radiation K52.0
eosinophilic K52.82
food hypersensitivity —*see also* Colitis, allergic K52.29 ⟸
giardial A07.1
granulomatous —*see* Enteritis, regional, large intestine
infectious —*see* Enteritis, infectious
indeterminate, so stated K52.3 ◀
ischemic K55.9
acute (subacute) —*see also* Ischemia, intestine, acute K55.039 ⟸
chronic K55.1
due to mesenteric artery insufficiency K55.1
fulminant (acute) —*see also* Ischemia, intestine, acute K55.039 ⟸
left sided K51.50
with
abscess K51.514
complication K51.519
specified NEC K51.518
fistula K51.513
obstruction K51.512
rectal bleeding K51.511
lymphocytic K52.832 ⟸
membranous
psychogenic F54
microscopic K52.839 ⟸
specified NEC K52.838 ◀
mucous —*see* Syndrome, irritable, bowel
psychogenic F54
noninfective K52.9
specified NEC K52.89
polyposa —*see* Polyp, colon, inflammatory
protozoal A07.9
pseudomembranous A04.7
pseudomucinous —*see* Syndrome, irritable, bowel
Colitis *(Continued)*
regional —*see* Enteritis, regional, large intestine
segmental —*see* Enteritis, regional, large intestine
septic —*see* Enteritis, infectious
spastic K58.9
with diarrhea K58.0
psychogenic F54
staphylococcal A04.8
foodborne A05.0
subacute ischemic —*see also* Ischemia, intestine, acute K55.039 ⟸
thromboulcerative —*see also* Ischemia, intestine, acute K55.039 ⟸
toxic NEC K52.1
due to Clostridium difficile A04.7
transmural —*see* Enteritis, regional, large intestine
trichomonal A07.8
tuberculous (ulcerative) A18.32
ulcerative (chronic) K51.90
with
complication K51.919
abscess K51.914
fistula K51.913
obstruction K51.912
rectal bleeding K51.911
specified complication NEC K51.918
enterocolitis —*see* Enterocolitis, ulcerative
ileocolitis —*see* Ileocolitis, ulcerative
mucosal proctocolitis —*see* Proctocolitis, mucosal
proctitis —*see* Proctitis, ulcerative
pseudopolyposis —*see* Polyp, colon, inflammatory
psychogenic F54
rectosigmoiditis —*see* Rectosigmoiditis, ulcerative
specified type NEC K51.80
with
complication K51.819
abscess K51.814
fistula K51.813
obstruction K51.812
rectal bleeding K51.811
specified complication NEC K51.818
Collagenosis, collagen disease (nonvascular) (vascular) M35.9
cardiovascular I42.8
reactive perforating L87.1
specified NEC M35.8
Collapse R55
adrenal E27.2
cardiorespiratory R57.0
cardiovascular R57.0
newborn P29.89
circulatory (peripheral) R57.9
during or after labor and delivery O75.1
following ectopic or molar pregnancy O08.3
newborn P29.89
during or
after labor and delivery O75.1
resulting from a procedure, not elsewhere classified T81.10
external ear canal —*see* Stenosis, external ear canal
general R55
heart —*see* Disease, heart
heat T67.1
hysterical F44.89
labyrinth, membranous (congenital) Q16.5
lung (massive) —*see also* Atelectasis J98.19
pressure due to anesthesia (general) (local) or other sedation T88.2
during labor and delivery O74.1
in pregnancy O29.02-
postpartum, puerperal O89.09
myocardial —*see* Disease, heart

◀ New ⟸ Revised ~~deleted~~ Deleted

Collapse *(Continued)*
nervous F48.8
neurocirculatory F45.8
nose M95.0
postoperative T81.10
pulmonary —*see also* Atelectasis J98.19
newborn —*see* Atelectasis
trachea J39.8
tracheobronchial J98.09
valvular —*see* Endocarditis
vascular (peripheral) R57.9
during or after labor and delivery O75.1
following ectopic or molar pregnancy O08.3
newborn P29.89
vertebra M48.50-
cervical region M48.52-
cervicothoracic region M48.53-
in (due to)
metastasis —*see* Collapse, vertebra, in, specified disease NEC
osteoporosis —*see also* Osteoporosis M80.88
cervical region M80.88
cervicothoracic region M80.88
lumbar region M80.88
lumbosacral region M80.88
multiple sites M80.88
occipito-atlanto-axial region M80.88
sacrococcygeal region M80.88
thoracic region M80.88
thoracolumbar region M80.88
specified disease NEC M48.50-
cervical region M48.52-
cervicothoracic region M48.53-
lumbar region M48.56-
lumbosacral region M48.57-
occipito-atlanto-axial region M48.51-
sacrococcygeal region M48.58-
thoracic region M48.54-
thoracolumbar region M48.55-
lumbar region M48.56-
lumbosacral region M48.57-
occipito-atlanto-axial region M48.51-
sacrococcygeal region M48.58-
thoracic region M48.54-
thoracolumbar region M48.55-
Collateral —*see also* condition
circulation (venous) I87.8
dilation, veins I87.8
Colles' fracture S52.53-
Collet (-Sicard) syndrome G52.7
Collier's asthma or lung J60
Collodion baby Q80.2
Colloid nodule (of thyroid) (cystic) E04.1
Coloboma (iris) Q13.0
eyelid Q10.3
fundus Q14.8
lens Q12.2
optic disc (congenital) Q14.2
acquired H47.31-
Coloenteritis —*see* Enteritis
Colon —*see* condition
Colonization
MRSA (Methicillin resistant Staphylococcus aureus) Z22.322
MSSA (Methicillin susceptible Staphylococcus aureus) Z22.321
status —*see* Carrier (suspected) of
Coloptosis K63.4
Color blindness —*see* Deficiency, color vision
Colostomy
attention to Z43.3
fitting or adjustment Z46.89
malfunctioning K94.03
status Z93.3
Colpitis (acute) —*see* Vaginitis
Colpocele N81.5
Colpocystitis —*see* Vaginitis
Colpospasm N94.2
Column, spinal, vertebral —*see* condition
Coma R40.20
with
motor response (none) R40.231
abnormal R40.233
extension R40.232
flexion withdrawal R40.234
motor response (none) *(Continued)*
localizes pain R40.235
obeys commands R40.236
opening of eyes (never) R40.211
in response to
pain R40.212
sound R40.213
spontaneous R40.214
verbal response (none) R40.221
confused conversation R40.224
inappropriate words R40.223
incomprehensible words R40.222
oriented R40.225
eclamptic —*see* Eclampsia
epileptic —*see* Epilepsy
Glasgow, scale score —*see* Glasgow coma scale
hepatic —*see* Failure, hepatic, by type, with coma
hyperglycemic (diabetic) —*see* Diabetes, by type, with hyperosmolarity, with coma ◄
hyperosmolar (diabetic) —*see* Diabetes, by type, with hyperosmolarity, with coma ◄
hypoglycemic (diabetic) —*see* Diabetes, by type, with hypoglycemia, with coma ◄
nondiabetic E15
in diabetes —*see* Diabetes, coma
insulin-induced —*see* Coma, hypoglycemic
myxedematous E03.5
newborn P91.5
persistent vegetative state R40.3
specified NEC, without documented Glasgow coma scale score, or with partial Glasgow coma scale score reported R40.244
Comatose —*see* Coma
Combat fatigue F43.0
Combined —*see* condition
Comedo, comedones (giant) L70.0
Comedocarcinoma —*see also* Neoplasm, breast, malignant
noninfiltrating
breast D05.8-
specified site —*see* Neoplasm, in situ, by site
unspecified site D05.8-
Comedomastitis —*see* Ectasia, mammary duct
Comminuted fracture - code as Fracture, closed
Common
arterial trunk Q20.0
atrioventricular canal Q21.2
atrium Q21.1
cold (head) J00
truncus (arteriosus) Q20.0
variable immunodeficiency —*see* Immunodeficiency, common variable
ventricle Q20.4
Commotio, commotion (current)
brain —*see* Injury, intracranial, concussion
cerebri —*see* Injury, intracranial, concussion
retinae S05.8X-
spinal cord —*see* Injury, spinal cord, by region
spinalis —*see* Injury, spinal cord, by region
Communication
between
base of aorta and pulmonary artery Q21.4
left ventricle and right atrium Q20.5
pericardial sac and pleural sac Q34.8
pulmonary artery and pulmonary vein, congenital Q25.72
congenital between uterus and digestive or urinary tract Q51.7
Compartment syndrome (deep) (posterior) (traumatic) T79.A0
abdomen T79.A3
lower extremity (hip, buttock, thigh, leg, foot, toes) T79.A2
nontraumatic
abdomen M79.A3
lower extremity (hip, buttock, thigh, leg, foot, toes) M79.A2-
specified site NEC M79.A9
upper extremity (shoulder, arm, forearm, wrist, hand, fingers) M79.A1-
specified site NEC T79.A9
upper extremity (shoulder, arm, forearm, wrist, hand, fingers) T79.A1
Compensation
failure —*see* Disease, heart
neurosis, psychoneurosis —*see* Disorder, factitious
Complaint —*see also* Disease
bowel, functional K59.9
psychogenic F45.8
intestine, functional K59.9
psychogenic F45.8
kidney —*see* Disease, renal
miners' J60
Complete —*see* condition
Complex
Addison-Schilder E71.528
cardiorenal —*see* Hypertension, cardiorenal
Costen's M26.69
disseminated mycobacterium avium-intracellulare (DMAC) A31.2
Eisenmenger's (ventricular septal defect) I27.89
hypersexual F52.8
jumped process, spine —*see* Dislocation, vertebra
primary, tuberculous A15.7
Schilder-Addison E71.528
subluxation (vertebral) M99.19
abdomen M99.19
acromioclavicular M99.17
cervical region M99.11
cervicothoracic M99.11
costochondral M99.18
costovertebral M99.18
head region M99.10
hip M99.15
lower extremity M99.16
lumbar region M99.13
lumbosacral M99.13
occipitocervical M99.10
pelvic region M99.15
pubic M99.15
rib cage M99.18
sacral region M99.14
sacrococcygeal M99.14
sacroiliac M99.14
specified NEC M99.19
sternochondral M99.18
sternoclavicular M99.17
thoracic region M99.12
thoracolumbar M99.12
upper extremity M99.17
Taussig-Bing (transposition, aorta and overriding pulmonary artery) Q20.1
Complication (s) (from) (of)
accidental puncture or laceration during a procedure (of) —*see* Complications, intraoperative (intraprocedural), puncture or laceration
amputation stump (surgical) (late) NEC T87.9
dehiscence T87.81
infection or inflammation T87.40
lower limb T87.4-
upper limb T87.4-
necrosis T87.50
lower limb T87.5-
upper limb T87.5-

Complication *(Continued)*
amputation stump (surgical) (late) (NEC) *(Continued)*
neuroma T87.30
lower limb T87.3-
upper limb T87.3-
specified type NEC T87.89
anastomosis (and bypass) —*see also* Complications, prosthetic device or implant
intestinal (internal) NEC K91.89
involving urinary tract N99.89
urinary tract (involving intestinal tract) N99.89
vascular —*see* Complications, cardiovascular device or implant
anesthesia, anesthetic —*see also* Anesthesia, complication T88.59
brain, postpartum, puerperal O89.2
cardiac
in
labor and delivery O74.2
pregnancy O29.19-
postpartum, puerperal O89.1
central nervous system
in
labor and delivery O74.3
pregnancy O29.29-
postpartum, puerperal O89.2
difficult or failed intubation T88.4
in pregnancy O29.6-
failed sedation (conscious) (moderate) during procedure T88.52
general, unintended awareness during procedure T88.53 ◀
hyperthermia, malignant T88.3
hypothermia T88.51
intubation failure T88.4
malignant hyperthermia T88.3
pulmonary
in
labor and delivery O74.1
pregnancy NEC O29.09-
postpartum, puerperal O89.09
shock T88.2
spinal and epidural
in
labor and delivery NEC O74.6
headache O74.5
pregnancy NEC O29.5X-
postpartum, puerperal NEC O89.5
headache O89.4
unintended awareness under general anesthesia during procedure T88.53 ◀
anti-reflux device —*see* Complications, esophageal anti-reflux device
aortic (bifurcation) graft —*see* Complications, graft, vascular
aortocoronary (bypass) graft —*see* Complications, coronary artery (bypass) graft
aortofemoral (bypass) graft —*see* Complications, extremity artery (bypass) graft
arteriovenous
fistula, surgically created T82.9
embolism T82.818
fibrosis T82.828
hemorrhage T82.838
infection or inflammation T82.7
mechanical
breakdown T82.510
displacement T82.520
leakage T82.530
malposition T82.520
obstruction T82.590
perforation T82.590
protrusion T82.590
pain T82.848
specified type NEC T82.898
stenosis T82.858
thrombosis T82.868

Complication *(Continued)*
arteriovenous *(Continued)*
shunt, surgically created T82.9
embolism T82.818
fibrosis T82.828
hemorrhage T82.838
infection or inflammation T82.7
mechanical
breakdown T82.511
displacement T82.521
leakage T82.531
malposition T82.521
obstruction T82.591
perforation T82.591
protrusion T82.591
pain T82.848
specified type NEC T82.898
stenosis T82.858
thrombosis T82.868
arthroplasty —*see* Complications, joint prosthesis
artificial
fertilization or insemination N98.9
attempted introduction (of)
embryo in embryo transfer N98.3
ovum following in vitro fertilization N98.2
hyperstimulation of ovaries N98.1
infection N98.0
specified NEC N98.8
heart T82.9
embolism T82.817
fibrosis T82.827
hemorrhage T82.837
infection or inflammation T82.7
mechanical
breakdown T82.512
displacement T82.522
leakage T82.532
malposition T82.522
obstruction T82.592
perforation T82.592
protrusion T82.592
pain T82.847
specified type NEC T82.897
stenosis T82.857
thrombosis T82.867
opening
cecostomy —*see* Complications, colostomy
colostomy —*see* Complications, colostomy
cystostomy —*see* Complications, cystostomy
enterostomy —*see* Complications, enterostomy
gastrostomy —*see* Complications, gastrostomy
ileostomy —*see* Complications, enterostomy
jejunostomy —*see* Complications, enterostomy
nephrostomy —*see* Complications, stoma, urinary tract
tracheostomy —*see* Complications, tracheostomy
ureterostomy —*see* Complications, stoma, urinary tract
urethrostomy —*see* Complications, stoma, urinary tract
balloon implant or device
gastrointestinal T85.9
embolism T85.818 ⇐
fibrosis T85.828 ⇐
hemorrhage T85.838 ⇐
infection and inflammation T85.79
pain T85.848 ⇐
specified type NEC T85.898 ⇐
stenosis T85.858 ⇐
thrombosis T85.868 ⇐

Complication *(Continued)*
balloon implant or device *(Continued)*
vascular (counterpulsation) T82.9
embolism T82.818
fibrosis T82.828
hemorrhage T82.838
infection or inflammation T82.7
mechanical
breakdown T82.513
displacement T82.523
leakage T82.533
malposition T82.523
obstruction T82.593
perforation T82.593
protrusion T82.593
pain T82.848
specified type NEC T82.898
stenosis T82.858
thrombosis T82.868
bariatric procedure
gastric band procedure K95.09
infection K95.01
specified procedure NEC K95.89
infection K95.81
bile duct implant (prosthetic) T85.9
embolism T85.818 ⇐
fibrosis T85.828 ⇐
hemorrhage T85.838 ⇐
infection and inflammation T85.79
mechanical
breakdown T85.510
displacement T85.520
malfunction T85.510
malposition T85.520
obstruction T85.590
perforation T85.590
protrusion T85.590
specified NEC T85.590
pain T85.848 ⇐
specified type NEC T85.898 ⇐
stenosis T85.858 ⇐
thrombosis T85.868 ⇐
bladder device (auxiliary) —*see* Complications, genitourinary, device or implant, urinary system
bleeding (postoperative) —*see* Complication, postoperative, hemorrhage
intraoperative —*see* Complication, intraoperative, hemorrhage
blood vessel graft —*see* Complications, graft, vascular
bone
device NEC T84.9
embolism T84.81
fibrosis T84.82
hemorrhage T84.83
infection or inflammation T84.7
mechanical
breakdown T84.318
displacement T84.328
malposition T84.328
obstruction T84.398
perforation T84.398
protrusion T84.398
pain T84.84
specified type NEC T84.89
stenosis T84.85
thrombosis T84.86
graft —*see* Complications, graft, bone
growth stimulator (electrode) —*see* Complications, electronic stimulator device, bone
marrow transplant —*see* Complications, transplant, bone, marrow
brain neurostimulator (electrode) —*see* Complications, electronic stimulator device, brain
breast implant (prosthetic) T85.9
capsular contracture T85.44
embolism T85.818 ⇐
fibrosis T85.828 ⇐

◀ New ⇐ Revised ~~deleted~~ Deleted

Complication *(Continued)*
breast implant (prosthetic) *(Continued)*
hemorrhage T85.838 ⇐
infection and inflammation T85.79
mechanical
breakdown T85.41
displacement T85.42
leakage T85.43
malposition T85.42
obstruction T85.49
perforation T85.49
protrusion T85.49
specified NEC T85.49
pain T85.848 ⇐
specified type NEC T85.898 ⇐
stenosis T85.858 ⇐
thrombosis T85.868 ⇐
bypass —*see also* Complications, prosthetic device or implant
aortocoronary —*see* Complications, coronary artery (bypass) graft
arterial —*see also* Complications, graft, vascular
extremity —*see* Complications, extremity artery (bypass) graft
cardiac —*see also* Disease, heart
device, implant or graft T82.9
embolism T82.817
fibrosis T82.827
hemorrhage T82.837
infection or inflammation T82.7
valve prosthesis T82.6
mechanical
breakdown T82.519
specified device NEC T82.518
displacement T82.529
specified device NEC T82.528
leakage T82.539
specified device NEC T82.538
malposition T82.529
specified device NEC T82.528
obstruction T82.599
specified device NEC T82.598
perforation T82.599
specified device NEC T82.598
protrusion T82.599
specified device NEC T82.598
pain T82.847
specified type NEC T82.897
stenosis T82.857
thrombosis T82.867
cardiovascular device, graft or implant T82.9
aortic graft —*see* Complications, graft, vascular
arteriovenous
fistula, artificial —*see* Complication, arteriovenous, fistula, surgically created
shunt —*see* Complication, arteriovenous, shunt, surgically created
artificial heart —*see* Complication, artificial, heart
balloon (counterpulsation) device —*see* Complication, balloon implant, vascular
carotid artery graft —*see* Complications, graft, vascular
coronary bypass graft —*see* Complication, coronary artery (bypass) graft
dialysis catheter (vascular) —*see* Complication, catheter, dialysis
electronic T82.9
electrode T82.9
embolism T82.817
fibrosis T82.827
hemorrhage T82.837
infection T82.7
mechanical
breakdown T82.110
displacement T82.120

Complication *(Continued)*
cardiovascular device, graft or implant *(Continued)*
electronic *(Continued)*
electrode *(Continued)*
mechanical *(Continued)*
leakage T82.190
obstruction T82.190
perforation T82.190
protrusion T82.190
specified type NEC T82.190
pain T82.847
specified NEC T82.897
stenosis T82.857
thrombosis T82.867
embolism T82.817
fibrosis T82.827
hemorrhage T82.837
infection T82.7
mechanical
breakdown T82.119
displacement T82.129
leakage T82.199
obstruction T82.199
perforation T82.199
protrusion T82.199
specified type NEC T82.199
pain T82.847
pulse generator T82.9
embolism T82.817
fibrosis T82.827
hemorrhage T82.837
infection T82.7
mechanical
breakdown T82.111
displacement T82.121
leakage T82.191
obstruction T82.191
perforation T82.191
protrusion T82.191
specified type NEC T82.191
pain T82.847
specified NEC T82.897
stenosis T82.857
thrombosis T82.867
specified condition NEC T82.897
specified device NEC T82.9
embolism T82.817
fibrosis T82.827
hemorrhage T82.837
infection T82.7
mechanical
breakdown T82.118
displacement T82.128
leakage T82.198
obstruction T82.198
perforation T82.198
protrusion T82.198
specified type NEC T82.198
pain T82.847
specified NEC T82.897
stenosis T82.857
thrombosis T82.867
stenosis T82.857
thrombosis T82.867
extremity artery graft —*see* Complication, extremity artery (bypass) graft
femoral artery graft —*see* Complication, extremity artery (bypass) graft
heart
transplant —*see* Complication, transplant, heart
valve —*see* Complication, prosthetic device, heart valve
graft —*see* Complication, heart, valve, graft
heart-lung transplant —*see* Complication, transplant, heart, with lung
infection or inflammation T82.7
umbrella device —*see* Complication, umbrella device, vascular

Complication *(Continued)*
cardiovascular device, graft or implant *(Continued)*
vascular graft (or anastomosis) —*see* Complication, graft, vascular
carotid artery (bypass) graft —*see* Complications, graft, vascular
catheter (device) NEC —*see also* Complications, prosthetic device or implant
cranial infusion ◀
infection and inflammation T85.735 ◀
mechanical ◀
breakdown T85.610 ◀
displacement T85.620 ◀
leakage T85.630 ◀
malfunction T85.690 ◀
malposition T85.620 ◀
obstruction T85.690 ◀
perforation T85.690 ◀
protrusion T85.690 ◀
specified NEC T85.690 ◀
cystostomy T83.9
embolism T83.81
fibrosis T83.82
hemorrhage T83.83
infection and inflammation T83.510 ⇐
mechanical
breakdown T83.010
displacement T83.020
leakage T83.030
malposition T83.020
obstruction T83.090
perforation T83.090
protrusion T83.090
specified NEC T83.090
pain T83.84
specified type NEC T83.89
stenosis T83.85
thrombosis T83.86
dialysis (vascular) T82.9
embolism T82.818
fibrosis T82.828
hemorrhage T82.838
infection and inflammation T82.7
intraperitoneal —*see* Complications, catheter, intraperitoneal
mechanical
breakdown T82.41
displacement T82.42
leakage T82.43
malposition T82.42
obstruction T82.49
perforation T82.49
protrusion T82.49
pain T82.848
specified type NEC T82.898
stenosis T82.858
thrombosis T82.868
epidural infusion T85.9
embolism T85.810 ⇐
fibrosis T85.820 ⇐
hemorrhage T85.830 ⇐
infection and inflammation T85.735 ⇐
mechanical
breakdown T85.610
displacement T85.620
leakage T85.630
malfunction T85.610
malposition T85.620
obstruction T85.690
perforation T85.690
protrusion T85.690
specified NEC T85.690
pain T85.840 ⇐
specified type NEC T85.890 ⇐
stenosis T85.850 ⇐
thrombosis T85.860 ⇐
intraperitoneal dialysis T85.9
embolism T85.818 ⇐
fibrosis T85.828 ⇐

C

Complication *(Continued)*
catheter NEC *(Continued)*
intraperitoneal dialysis *(Continued)*
hemorrhage T85.838 ⇐
infection and inflammation T85.71
mechanical
breakdown T85.611
displacement T85.621
leakage T85.631
malfunction T85.611
malposition T85.621
obstruction T85.691
perforation T85.691
protrusion T85.691
specified NEC T85.691
pain T85.848 ⇐
specified type NEC T85.898 ⇐
stenosis T85.858 ⇐
thrombosis T85.868 ⇐
intrathecal infusion ◀
infection and inflammation T85.735 ◀
mechanical ◀
breakdown T85.610 ◀
displacement T85.620 ◀
leakage T85.630 ◀
malfunction T85.690 ◀
malposition T85.620 ◀
obstruction T85.690 ◀
perforation T85.690 ◀
protrusion T85.690 ◀
specified NEC T85.690 ◀
intravenous infusion T82.9
embolism T82.818
fibrosis T82.828
hemorrhage T82.838
infection or inflammation T82.7
mechanical
breakdown T82.514
displacement T82.524
leakage T82.534
malposition T82.524
obstruction T82.594
perforation T82.594
protrusion T82.594
pain T82.848
specified type NEC T82.898
stenosis T82.858
thrombosis T82.868
spinal infusion ◀
infection and inflammation T85.735 ◀
mechanical ◀
breakdown T85.610 ◀
displacement T85.620 ◀
leakage T85.630 ◀
malfunction T85.690 ◀
malposition T85.620 ◀
obstruction T85.690 ◀
perforation T85.690 ◀
protrusion T85.690 ◀
specified NEC T85.690 ◀
subarachnoid infusion ◀
infection and inflammation T85.735 ◀
mechanical ◀
breakdown T85.610 ◀
displacement T85.620 ◀
leakage T85.630 ◀
malfunction T85.690 ◀
malposition T85.620 ◀
obstruction T85.690 ◀
perforation T85.690 ◀
protrusion T85.690 ◀
specified NEC T85.690 ◀
subdural infusion T85.9
embolism T85.810 ⇐
fibrosis T85.820 ⇐
hemorrhage T85.830 ⇐
infection and inflammation T85.735 ⇐
mechanical
breakdown T85.610
displacement T85.620
leakage T85.630

Complication *(Continued)*
catheter NEC *(Continued)*
subdural infusion *(Continued)*
mechanical *(Continued)*
malfunction T85.610
malposition T85.620
obstruction T85.690
perforation T85.690
protrusion T85.690
specified NEC T85.690
pain T85.840 ⇐
specified type NEC T85.890 ⇐
stenosis T85.850 ⇐
thrombosis T85.860 ⇐
~~urethral, indwelling T83.9~~
~~displacement T83.028~~
~~embolism T83.81~~
~~fibrosis T83.82~~
~~hemorrhage T83.83~~
~~infection and inflammation T83.51~~
~~leakage T83.038~~
~~malposition T83.028~~
~~mechanical~~
~~breakdown T83.018~~
~~obstruction (mechanical) T83.098~~
~~pain T83.84~~
~~perforation T83.098~~
~~protrusion T83.098~~
~~specified type NEC T83.098~~
~~stenosis T83.85~~
~~thrombosis T83.86~~
~~urinary (indwelling) —see Complications, catheter, urethral, indwelling~~
urethral T83.9 ◀
displacement T83.028 ◀
embolism T83.81 ◀
fibrosis T83.82 ◀
hemorrhage T83.83 ◀
indwelling ◀
breakdown T83.011 ◀
displacement T83.021 ◀
infection and inflammation T83.511 ◀
leakage T83.031 ◀
specified complication NEC T83.091 ◀
infection and inflammation T83.511 ◀
leakage T83.038 ◀
malposition T83.028 ◀
mechanical ◀
breakdown T83.011 ◀
obstruction (mechanical) T83.091 ◀
pain T83.84 ◀
perforation T83.091 ◀
protrusion T83.091 ◀
specified type NEC T83.091 ◀
stenosis T83.85 ◀
thrombosis T83.86 ◀
urinary NEC ◀
breakdown T83.018 ◀
displacement T83.028 ◀
infection and inflammation T83.518 ◀
leakage T83.038 ◀
specified complication NEC T83.098 ◀
cecostomy (stoma) —*see* Complications, colostomy
cesarean delivery wound NEC O90.89
disruption O90.0
hematoma O90.2
infection (following delivery) O86.0
chemotherapy (antineoplastic) NEC T88.7
chin implant (prosthetic) —*see* Complication, prosthetic device or implant, specified NEC
circulatory system I99.8
intraoperative I97.88
postprocedural I97.89
following cardiac surgery I97.19-
postcardiotomy syndrome I97.0
hypertension I97.3
lymphedema after mastectomy I97.2
postcardiotomy syndrome I97.0
specified NEC I97.89

Complication *(Continued)*
colostomy (stoma) K94.00
hemorrhage K94.01
infection K94.02
malfunction K94.03
mechanical K94.03
specified complication NEC K94.09
contraceptive device, intrauterine —*see* Complications, intrauterine, contraceptive device
cord (umbilical) —*see* Complications, umbilical cord
corneal graft —*see* Complications, graft, cornea
coronary artery (bypass) graft T82.9
atherosclerosis —*see* Arteriosclerosis, coronary (artery)
embolism T82.818
fibrosis T82.828
hemorrhage T82.838
infection and inflammation T82.7
mechanical
breakdown T82.211
displacement T82.212
leakage T82.213
malposition T82.212
obstruction T82.218
perforation T82.218
protrusion T82.218
specified NEC T82.218
pain T82.848
specified type NEC T82.898 ⇐
stenosis T82.858
thrombosis T82.868
counterpulsation device (balloon), intra-aortic —*see* Complications, balloon implant, vascular
cystostomy (stoma) N99.518
catheter —*see* Complications, catheter, cystostomy
hemorrhage N99.510
infection N99.511
malfunction N99.512
specified type NEC N99.518
delivery —*see also* Complications, obstetric O75.9
procedure (instrumental) (manual) (surgical) O75.4
specified NEC O75.89
dialysis (peritoneal) (renal) —*see also* Complications, infusion
catheter (vascular) —*see* Complication, catheter, dialysis
peritoneal, intraperitoneal —*see* Complications, catheter, intraperitoneal
dorsal column (spinal) neurostimulator —*see* Complications, electronic stimulator device, spinal cord
drug NEC T88.7
ear procedure —*see also* Disorder, ear
intraoperative H95.88-
hematoma —*see* Complications, intraoperative, hematoma (of), ear ⇐
hemorrhage —*see* Complications, intraoperative, hemorrhage (of), ear ⇐
laceration —*see* Complications, intraoperative, puncture or laceration..., ear
seroma —*see* Complications, postprocedural, seroma (of), mastoid process ◀
specified NEC H95.88-
postoperative H95.89-
external ear canal stenosis H95.81-
hematoma —*see* Complications, postprocedural, hemorrhage (hematoma) (of), ear

◀ New ⇐ Revised ~~deleted~~ Deleted

Complication *(Continued)*
ear procedure *(Continued)*
postoperative *(Continued)*
hemorrhage —*see* Complications, postprocedural, hemorrhage (hematoma) (of), ear
postmastoidectomy —*see* Complications, postmastoidectomy
specified NEC H95.89-
ectopic pregnancy O08.9
damage to pelvic organs O08.6
embolism O08.2
genital infection O08.0
hemorrhage (delayed) (excessive) O08.1
metabolic disorder O08.5
renal failure O08.4
shock O08.3
specified type NEC O08.0
venous complication NEC O08.7
electronic stimulator device
bladder (urinary) —*see* Complications, electronic stimulator device, urinary
bone T84.9
breakdown T84.310
displacement T84.320
embolism T84.81
fibrosis T84.82
hemorrhage T84.83
infection or inflammation T84.7
malfunction T84.310
malposition T84.320
mechanical NEC T84.390
obstruction T84.390
pain T84.84
perforation T84.390
protrusion T84.390
specified type NEC T84.89
stenosis T84.85
thrombosis T84.86
brain T85.9
embolism T85.810 ⟸
fibrosis T85.820 ⟸
hemorrhage T85.830 ⟸
infection and inflammation T85.731 ⟸
mechanical
breakdown T85.110
displacement T85.120
leakage T85.190
malposition T85.120
obstruction T85.190
perforation T85.190
protrusion T85.190
specified NEC T85.190
pain T85.840 ⟸
specified type NEC T85.890 ⟸
stenosis T85.850 ⟸
thrombosis T85.860 ⟸
cardiac (defibrillator) (pacemaker) —*see* Complications, cardiovascular device or implant, electronic
generator (brain) (gastric) (peripheral) (sacral) (spinal) ◀
breakdown T85.113 ◀
displacement T85.123 ◀
leakage T85.193 ◀
malposition T85.123 ◀
obstruction T85.193 ◀
perforation T85.193 ◀
protrusion T85.193 ◀
specified type NEC T85.193 ◀
muscle T84.9
breakdown T84.418
displacement T84.428
embolism T84.81
fibrosis T84.82
hemorrhage T84.83
infection or inflammation T84.7
mechanical NEC T84.498
pain T84.84
specified type NEC T84.89
stenosis T84.85
thrombosis T84.86

Complication *(Continued)*
electronic stimulator device *(Continued)*
nervous system T85.9
brain —*see* Complications, electronic stimulator device, brain
cranial nerve —*see* Complications, electronic stimulator device, peripheral nerve ◀
embolism T85.810 ⟸
fibrosis T85.820 ⟸
gastric nerve —*see* Complications, electronic stimulator device, peripheral nerve ◀
hemorrhage T85.830 ⟸
infection and inflammation T85.738 ⟸
mechanical
breakdown T85.118
displacement T85.128
leakage T85.199
malposition T85.128
obstruction T85.199
perforation T85.199
protrusion T85.199
specified NEC T85.199
pain T85.840 ⟸
peripheral nerve —*see* Complications, electronic stimulator device, peripheral nerve
sacral nerve —*see* Complications, electronic stimulator device, peripheral nerve ◀
specified type NEC T85.890 ⟸
spinal cord —*see* Complications, electronic stimulator device, spinal cord
stenosis T85.850 ⟸
thrombosis T85.860 ⟸
vagal nerve —*see* Complications, electronic stimulator device, peripheral nerve ◀
peripheral nerve T85.9
embolism T85.810 ⟸
fibrosis T85.820 ⟸
hemorrhage T85.830 ⟸
infection and inflammation T85.732 ⟸
mechanical
breakdown T85.111
displacement T85.121
leakage T85.191
malposition T85.121
obstruction T85.191
perforation T85.191
protrusion T85.191
specified NEC T85.191
pain T85.840 ⟸
specified type NEC T85.890 ⟸
stenosis T85.850 ⟸
thrombosis T85.860 ⟸
spinal cord T85.9
embolism T85.810 ⟸
fibrosis T85.820 ⟸
hemorrhage T85.830 ⟸
infection and inflammation T85.733 ⟸
mechanical
breakdown T85.112
displacement T85.122
leakage T85.192
malposition T85.122
obstruction T85.192
perforation T85.192
protrusion T85.192
specified NEC T85.192
pain T85.840 ⟸
specified type NEC T85.890 ⟸
stenosis T85.850 ⟸
thrombosis T85.860 ⟸
urinary T83.9
embolism T83.81
fibrosis T83.82
hemorrhage T83.83
infection and inflammation T83.598 ⟸

Complication *(Continued)*
electronic stimulator device *(Continued)*
urinary *(Continued)*
mechanical
breakdown T83.110
displacement T83.120
malposition T83.120
perforation T83.190
protrusion T83.190
specified NEC T83.190
pain T83.84
specified type NEC T83.89
stenosis T83.85
thrombosis T83.86
electroshock therapy T88.9
specified NEC T88.8
endocrine E34.9
postprocedural
adrenal hypofunction E89.6
hypoinsulinemia E89.1
hypoparathyroidism E89.2
hypopituitarism E89.3
hypothyroidism E89.0
ovarian failure E89.40
asymptomatic E89.40
symptomatic E89.41
specified NEC E89.89
testicular hypofunction E89.5
endodontic treatment NEC M27.59
enterostomy (stoma) K94.10
hemorrhage K94.11
infection K94.12
malfunction K94.13
mechanical K94.13
specified complication NEC K94.19
episiotomy, disruption O90.1
esophageal anti-reflux device T85.9
embolism T85.818 ⟸
fibrosis T85.828 ⟸
hemorrhage T85.838 ⟸
infection and inflammation T85.79
mechanical
breakdown T85.511
displacement T85.521
malfunction T85.511
malposition T85.521
obstruction T85.591
perforation T85.591
protrusion T85.591
specified NEC T85.591
pain T85.848 ⟸
specified type NEC T85.898 ⟸
stenosis T85.858 ⟸
thrombosis T85.868 ⟸
esophagostomy K94.30
hemorrhage K94.31
infection K94.32
malfunction K94.33
mechanical K94.33
specified complication NEC K94.39
extracorporeal circulation T80.90
extremity artery (bypass) graft T82.9
arteriosclerosis —*see* Arteriosclerosis, extremities, bypass graft
embolism T82.818
fibrosis T82.828
hemorrhage T82.838
infection and inflammation T82.7
mechanical
breakdown T82.318
femoral artery T82.312
displacement T82.328
femoral artery T82.322
leakage T82.338
femoral artery T82.332
malposition T82.328
femoral artery T82.322
obstruction T82.398
femoral artery T82.392
perforation T82.398
femoral artery T82.392

◀ New ⟸ Revised ~~deleted~~ Deleted

Complication *(Continued)*
extremity artery (bypass) graft *(Continued)*
mechanical *(Continued)*
protrusion T82.398
femoral artery T82.392
pain T82.848
specified type NEC T82.898
stenosis T82.858
thrombosis T82.868
eye H57.9
corneal graft —*see* Complications, graft, cornea
implant (prosthetic) T85.9
embolism T85.818 ◀
fibrosis T85.828 ◀
hemorrhage T85.838 ◀
infection and inflammation T85.79
mechanical
breakdown T85.318
displacement T85.328
leakage T85.398
malposition T85.328
obstruction T85.398
perforation T85.398
protrusion T85.398
specified NEC T85.398
pain T85.848 ◀
specified type NEC T85.898 ◀
stenosis T85.858 ◀
thrombosis T85.868 ◀
intraocular lens —*see* Complications, intraocular lens
orbital prosthesis —*see* Complications, orbital prosthesis
female genital N94.9
device, implant or graft NEC —*see* Complications, genitourinary, device or implant, genital tract
femoral artery (bypass) graft —*see* Complication, extremity artery (bypass) graft
fixation device, internal (orthopedic) T84.9
infection and inflammation T84.60
arm T84.61-
humerus T84.61-
radius T84.61-
ulna T84.61-
leg T84.629
femur T84.62-
fibula T84.62-
tibia T84.62-
specified site NEC T84.69
spine T84.63
mechanical
breakdown
limb T84.119
carpal T84.210
femur T84.11-
fibula T84.11-
humerus T84.11-
metacarpal T84.210
metatarsal T84.213
phalanx
foot T84.213
hand T84.210
radius T84.11-
tarsal T84.213
tibia T84.11-
ulna T84.11-
specified bone NEC T84.218
spine T84.216
displacement
limb T84.129
carpal T84.220
femur T84.12-
fibula T84.12-
humerus T84.12-
metacarpal T84.220
metatarsal T84.223
phalanx
foot T84.223
hand T84.220

Complication *(Continued)*
fixation device, internal *(Continued)*
mechanical *(Continued)*
displacement *(Continued)*
limb *(Continued)*
radius T84.12-
tarsal T84.223
tibia T84.12-
ulna T84.12-
specified bone NEC T84.228
spine T84.226
malposition —*see* Complications, fixation device, internal, mechanical, displacement
obstruction —*see* Complications, fixation device, internal, mechanical, specified type NEC
perforation —*see* Complications, fixation device, internal, mechanical, specified type NEC
protrusion —*see* Complications, fixation device, internal, mechanical, specified type NEC
specified type NEC
limb T84.199
carpal T84.290
femur T84.19-
fibula T84.19-
humerus T84.19-
metacarpal T84.290
metatarsal T84.293
phalanx
foot T84.293
hand T84.290
radius T84.19-
tarsal T84.293
tibia T84.19-
ulna T84.19-
specified bone NEC T84.298
vertebra T84.296
specified type NEC T84.89
embolism T84.81
fibrosis T84.82
hemorrhage T84.83
pain T84.84
specified complication NEC T84.89
stenosis T84.85
thrombosis T84.86
following
acute myocardial infarction NEC I23.8
aneurysm (false) (of cardiac wall) (of heart wall) (ruptured) I23.3
angina I23.7
atrial
septal defect I23.1
thrombosis I23.6
cardiac wall rupture I23.3
chordae tendinae rupture I23.4
defect
septal
atrial (heart) I23.1
ventricular (heart) I23.2
hemopericardium I23.0
papillary muscle rupture I23.5
rupture
cardiac wall I23.3
with hemopericardium I23.0
chordae tendineae I23.4
papillary muscle I23.5
specified NEC I23.8
thrombosis
atrium I23.6
auricular appendage I23.6
ventricle (heart) I23.6
ventricular
septal defect I23.2
thrombosis I23.6
ectopic or molar pregnancy O08.9
cardiac arrest O08.81
sepsis O08.82

Complication *(Continued)*
following *(Continued)*
ectopic or molar pregnancy *(Continued)*
specified type NEC O08.89
urinary tract infection O08.83
termination of pregnancy —*see* Abortion
gastrointestinal K92.9
bile duct prosthesis —*see* Complications, bile duct implant
esophageal anti-reflux device —*see* Complications, esophageal anti-reflux device
postoperative
colostomy —*see* Complications, colostomy
dumping syndrome K91.1
enterostomy —*see* Complications, enterostomy
gastrostomy —*see* Complications, gastrostomy
malabsorption NEC K91.2
obstruction K91.3
postcholecystectomy syndrome K91.5
specified NEC K91.89
vomiting after GI surgery K91.0
prosthetic device or implant
bile duct prosthesis —*see* Complications, bile duct implant
esophageal anti-reflux device —*see* Complications, esophageal anti-reflux device
specified type NEC
embolism T85.818 ◀
fibrosis T85.828 ◀
hemorrhage T85.838 ◀
mechanical
breakdown T85.518
displacement T85.528
malfunction T85.518
malposition T85.528
obstruction T85.598
perforation T85.598
protrusion T85.598
specified NEC T85.598
pain T85.848 ◀
specified complication NEC T85.898 ◀
stenosis T85.858 ◀
thrombosis T85.868 ◀
gastrostomy (stoma) K94.20
hemorrhage K94.21
infection K94.22
malfunction K94.23
mechanical K94.23
specified complication NEC K94.29
genitourinary
device or implant T83.9
genital tract T83.9
infection or inflammation T83.69 ◀
intrauterine contraceptive device —*see* Complications, intrauterine, contraceptive device
mechanical —*see* Complications, by device, mechanical
mesh —*see* Complications, mesh
penile prosthesis —*see* Complications, prosthetic device, penile
specified type NEC T83.89
embolism T83.81
fibrosis T83.82
hemorrhage T83.83
pain T83.84
specified complication NEC T83.89
stenosis T83.85
thrombosis T83.86
vaginal mesh —*see* Complications, mesh
urinary system T83.9
cystostomy catheter —*see* Complication, catheter, cystostomy

C

◀ New ◀ Revised ~~deleted~~ Deleted

Complication *(Continued)*
genitourinary *(Continued)*
device or implant *(Continued)*
urinary system *(Continued)*
electronic stimulator —*see* Complications, electronic stimulator device, urinary
indwelling urethral catheter —*see* Complications, catheter, urethral, indwelling
infection or inflammation T83.598 ⇐
~~indwelling urinary catheter T83.51~~
indwelling urethral catheter T83.511 ◀
kidney transplant —*see* Complication, transplant, kidney
organ graft —*see* Complication, graft, urinary organ
specified type NEC T83.89
embolism T83.81
fibrosis T83.82
hemorrhage T83.83
mechanical T83.198
breakdown T83.118
displacement T83.128
malfunction T83.118
malposition T83.128
obstruction T83.198
perforation T83.198
protrusion T83.198
specified NEC T83.198
sphincter, implanted T83.191 ◀
stent (ileal conduit) (nephroureteral) T83.193 ◀
ureteral indwelling T83.192 ◀
pain T83.84
specified complication NEC T83.89
stenosis T83.85
thrombosis T83.86
sphincter implant —*see* Complications, implant, urinary sphincter
postprocedural
pelvic peritoneal adhesions N99.4
renal failure N99.0
specified NEC N99.89
stoma —*see* Complications, stoma, urinary tract
urethral stricture —*see* Stricture, urethra, postprocedural
vaginal
adhesions N99.2
vault prolapse N99.3
graft (bypass) (patch) —*see also* Complications, prosthetic device or implant
aorta —*see* Complications, graft, vascular
arterial —*see* Complication, graft, vascular
bone T86.839
failure T86.831
infection T86.832
mechanical T84.318
breakdown T84.318
displacement T84.328
protrusion T84.398
specified type NEC T84.398
rejection T86.830
specified type NEC T86.838
carotid artery —*see* Complications, graft, vascular
cornea T86.849
failure T86.841
infection T86.842
mechanical T85.398
breakdown T85.318
displacement T85.328
protrusion T85.398
specified type NEC T85.398
rejection T86.840
retroprosthetic membrane T85.398
specified type NEC T86.848

Complication *(Continued)*
graft *(Continued)*
femoral artery (bypass) —*see* Complication, extremity artery (bypass) graft
genital organ or tract —*see* Complications, genitourinary, device or implant, genital tract
muscle T84.9
breakdown T84.410
displacement T84.420
embolism T84.81
fibrosis T84.82
hemorrhage T84.83
infection and inflammation T84.7
mechanical NEC T84.490
pain T84.84
specified type NEC T84.89
stenosis T84.85
thrombosis T84.86
nerve —*see* Complication, prosthetic device or implant, specified NEC
skin —*see* Complications, prosthetic device or implant, skin graft
tendon T84.9
breakdown T84.410
displacement T84.420
embolism T84.81
fibrosis T84.82
hemorrhage T84.83
infection and inflammation T84.7
mechanical NEC T84.490
pain T84.84
specified type NEC T84.89
stenosis T84.85
thrombosis T84.86
urinary organ T83.9
embolism T83.81
fibrosis T83.82
hemorrhage T83.83
infection and inflammation T83.598 ⇐
indwelling urethral catheter T83.511 ⇐
mechanical
breakdown T83.21
displacement T83.22
erosion T83.24 ◀
exposure T83.25 ◀
leakage T83.23
malposition T83.22
obstruction T83.29
perforation T83.29
protrusion T83.29
specified NEC T83.29
pain T83.84
specified type NEC T83.89
stenosis T83.85
thrombosis T83.86
vascular T82.9
embolism T82.818
femoral artery —*see* Complication, extremity artery (bypass) graft
fibrosis T82.828
hemorrhage T82.838
mechanical
breakdown T82.319
aorta (bifurcation) T82.310
carotid artery T82.311
specified vessel NEC T82.318
displacement T82.329
aorta (bifurcation) T82.320
carotid artery T82.321
specified vessel NEC T82.328
leakage T82.339
aorta (bifurcation) T82.330
carotid artery T82.331
specified vessel NEC T82.338
malposition T82.329
aorta (bifurcation) T82.320
carotid artery T82.321
specified vessel NEC T82.328

Complication *(Continued)*
graft *(Continued)*
vascular *(Continued)*
mechanical *(Continued)*
obstruction T82.399
aorta (bifurcation) T82.390
carotid artery T82.391
specified vessel NEC T82.398
perforation T82.399
aorta (bifurcation) T82.390
carotid artery T82.391
specified vessel NEC T82.398
protrusion T82.399
aorta (bifurcation) T82.390
carotid artery T82.391
specified vessel NEC T82.398
pain T82.848
specified complication NEC T82.898
stenosis T82.858
thrombosis T82.868
heart I51.9
assist device
infection and inflammation T82.7
following acute myocardial infarction —*see* Complications, following, acute myocardial infarction
postoperative —*see* Complications, circulatory system
transplant —*see* Complication, transplant, heart
and lung (s) —*see* Complications, transplant, heart, with lung
valve
graft (biological) T82.9
embolism T82.817
fibrosis T82.827
hemorrhage T82.837
infection and inflammation T82.7
mechanical T82.228
breakdown T82.221
displacement T82.222
leakage T82.223
malposition T82.222
obstruction T82.228
perforation T82.228
protrusion T82.228
pain T82.847
specified type NEC T82.897
stenosis T82.857
thrombosis T82.867
prosthesis T82.9
embolism T82.817
fibrosis T82.827
hemorrhage T82.837
infection or inflammation T82.6
mechanical T82.09
breakdown T82.01
displacement T82.02
leakage T82.03
malposition T82.02
obstruction T82.09
perforation T82.09
protrusion T82.09
pain T82.847
specified type NEC T82.897
mechanical T82.09
stenosis T82.857
thrombosis T82.867
hematoma
intraoperative —*see* Complication, intraoperative, hemorrhage
postprocedural —*see* Complication, postprocedural, hematoma ⇐
hemodialysis —*see* Complications, dialysis
hemorrhage
intraoperative —*see* Complication, intraoperative, hemorrhage
postprocedural —*see* Complication, postprocedural, hemorrhage

Complication *(Continued)*
ileostomy (stoma) —*see* Complications, enterostomy
immunization (procedure) —*see* Complications, vaccination
implant —*see also* Complications, by site and type
urinary sphincter T83.9
embolism T83.81
fibrosis T83.82
hemorrhage T83.83
infection and inflammation T83.591 ◀
mechanical
breakdown T83.111
displacement T83.121
leakage T83.191
malposition T83.121
obstruction T83.191
perforation T83.191
protrusion T83.191
specified NEC T83.191
pain T83.84
specified type NEC T83.89
stenosis T83.85
thrombosis T83.86
infusion (procedure) T80.90
air embolism T80.0
blood —*see* Complications, transfusion
catheter —*see* Complications, catheter
infection T80.29
pump —*see* Complications, cardiovascular, device or implant
sepsis T80.29
serum reaction —*see also* Reaction, serum T80.69
anaphylactic shock —*see also* Shock, anaphylactic T80.59
specified type NEC T80.89
inhalation therapy NEC T81.81
injection (procedure) T80.90
drug reaction —*see* Reaction, drug
infection T80.29
sepsis T80.29
serum (prophylactic) (therapeutic) —*see* Complications, vaccination
specified type NEC T80.89
vaccine (any) —*see* Complications, vaccination
inoculation (any) —*see* Complications, vaccination
insulin pump
infection and inflammation T85.72
mechanical
breakdown T85.614
displacement T85.624
leakage T85.633
malposition T85.624
obstruction T85.694
perforation T85.694
protrusion T85.694
specified NEC T85.694
intestinal pouch NEC K91.858
intraocular lens (prosthetic) T85.9
embolism T85.818 ◀
fibrosis T85.828 ◀
hemorrhage T85.838 ◀
infection and inflammation T85.79
mechanical
breakdown T85.21
displacement T85.22
malposition T85.22
obstruction T85.29
perforation T85.29
protrusion T85.29
specified NEC T85.29
pain T85.848 ◀
specified type NEC T85.898 ◀
stenosis T85.858 ◀
thrombosis T85.868 ◀

Complication *(Continued)*
intraoperative (intraprocedural)
cardiac arrest
during cardiac surgery I97.710
during other surgery I97.711
cardiac functional disturbance NEC
during cardiac surgery I97.790
during other surgery I97.791
hemorrhage (hematoma) (of)
circulatory system organ or structure
during cardiac bypass I97.411
during cardiac catheterization I97.410
during other circulatory system procedure I97.418
during other procedure I97.42
digestive system organ
during procedure on digestive system K91.61
during procedure on other organ K91.62
ear
during procedure on ear and mastoid process H95.21
during procedure on other organ H95.22
endocrine system organ or structure
during procedure on endocrine system organ or structure E36.01
during procedure on other organ E36.02
eye and adnexa
during ophthalmic procedure H59.11-
during other procedure H59.12-
genitourinary organ or structure
during procedure on genitourinary organ or structure N99.61
during procedure on other organ N99.62
mastoid process
during procedure on ear and mastoid process H95.21
during procedure on other organ H95.22
musculoskeletal structure
during musculoskeletal surgery M96.810
during non-orthopedic surgery M96.811
during orthopedic surgery M96.810
nervous system
during a nervous system procedure G97.31
during other procedure G97.32
respiratory system
during other procedure J95.62
during procedure on respiratory system organ or structure J95.61
skin and subcutaneous tissue
during a dermatologic procedure L76.01
during a procedure on other organ L76.02
spleen
during a procedure on other organ D78.02
during a procedure on the spleen D78.01
puncture or laceration (accidental) (unintentional) (of)
brain
during a nervous system procedure G97.48
during other procedure G97.49
circulatory system organ or structure
during circulatory system procedure I97.51
during other procedure I97.52
digestive system
during procedure on digestive system K91.71
during procedure on other organ K91.72

Complication *(Continued)*
intraoperative *(Continued)*
puncture or laceration *(Continued)*
ear
during procedure on ear and mastoid process H95.31
during procedure on other organ H95.32
endocrine system organ or structure
during procedure on endocrine system organ or structure E36.11
during procedure on other organ E36.12
eye and adnexa
during ophthalmic procedure H59.21-
during other procedure H59.22-
genitourinary organ or structure
during procedure on genitourinary organ or structure N99.71
during procedure on other organ N99.72
mastoid process
during procedure on ear and mastoid process H95.31
during procedure on other organ H95.32
musculoskeletal structure
during musculoskeletal surgery M96.820
during non-orthopedic surgery M96.821
during orthopedic surgery M96.820
nervous system
during a nervous system procedure G97.48
during other procedure G97.49
respiratory system
during other procedure J95.72
during procedure on respiratory system organ or structure J95.71
skin and subcutaneous tissue
during a dermatologic procedure L76.11
during a procedure on other organ L76.12
spleen
during a procedure on other organ D78.12
during a procedure on the spleen D78.11
specified NEC
circulatory system I97.88
digestive system K91.81
ear H95.88
endocrine system E36.8
eye and adnexa H59.88
genitourinary system N99.81
mastoid process H95.88
musculoskeletal structure M96.89
nervous system G97.81
respiratory system J95.88
skin and subcutaneous tissue L76.81
spleen D78.81
intraperitoneal catheter (dialysis) (infusion) —*see* Complications, catheter, intraperitoneal
intrathecal infusion pump ◀
infection and inflammation T85.738 ◀
mechanical ◀
breakdown T85.615 ◀
displacement T85.625 ◀
leakage T85.635 ◀
malfunction T85.695 ◀
malposition T85.625 ◀
obstruction T85.695 ◀
perforation T85.695 ◀
protrusion T85.695 ◀
specified NEC T85.695 ◀
intrauterine
contraceptive device
embolism T83.81
fibrosis T83.82

◀ New ◀ Revised ~~deleted~~ Deleted

Complication *(Continued)*
intrauterine *(Continued)*
contraceptive device *(Continued)*
hemorrhage T83.83
infection and inflammation T83.69
mechanical
breakdown T83.31
displacement T83.32
malposition T83.32
obstruction T83.39
perforation T83.39
protrusion T83.39
specified NEC T83.39
pain T83.84
specified type NEC T83.89
stenosis T83.85
thrombosis T83.86
procedure (fetal), to newborn P96.5
jejunostomy (stoma) —*see* Complications, enterostomy
joint prosthesis, internal T84.9
breakage (fracture) T84.01-
dislocation T84.02-
fracture T84.01-
infection or inflammation T84.50
hip T84.5-
knee T84.5-
specified joint NEC T84.59
instability T84.02-
malposition —*see* Complications, joint prosthesis, mechanical, displacement
mechanical
breakage, broken T84.01-
dislocation T84.02-
fracture T84.01-
instability T84.02-
leakage —*see* Complications, joint prosthesis, mechanical, specified NEC
loosening T84.039
hip T84.03-
knee T84.03-
specified joint NEC T84.038
obstruction —*see* Complications, joint prosthesis, mechanical, specified NEC
perforation —*see* Complications, joint prosthesis, mechanical, specified NEC
~~periprosthetic~~
~~fracture T84.049~~
~~hip T84.04-~~
~~knee T84.04-~~
~~other specified joint T84.048~~
osteolysis T84.059 ◀
hip T84.05- ◀
knee T84.05- ◀
other specified joint T84.058 ◀
protrusion —*see* Complications, joint prosthesis, mechanical, specified NEC
specified complication NEC T84.099
hip T84.09-
knee T84.09-
other specified joint T84.098
subluxation T84.02-
wear of articular bearing surface T84.069
hip T84.06-
knee T84.06-
other specified joint T84.068
specified joint NEC T84.89
embolism T84.81
fibrosis T84.82
hemorrhage T84.83
pain T84.84
specified complication NEC T84.89
stenosis T84.85
thrombosis T84.86
subluxation T84.02-
kidney transplant —*see* Complications, transplant, kidney

Complication *(Continued)*
labor O75.9
specified NEC O75.89
liver transplant (immune or nonimmune) —*see* Complications, transplant, liver
lumbar puncture G97.1
cerebrospinal fluid leak G97.0
headache or reaction G97.1
lung transplant —*see* Complications, transplant, lung
and heart —*see* Complications, transplant, lung, with heart
male genital N50.9
device, implant or graft —*see* Complications, genitourinary, device or implant, genital tract
postprocedural or postoperative —*see* Complications, genitourinary, postprocedural
specified NEC N99.89
mastoid (process) procedure
intraoperative H95.88-
hematoma —*see* Complications, intraoperative, hemorrhage (hematoma) (of), mastoid process
hemorrhage —*see* Complications, intraoperative, hemorrhage (hematoma) (of), mastoid process
laceration —*see* Complications, intraoperative, puncture or laceration..., mastoid process
specified NEC H95.88-
postmastoidectomy —*see* Complications, postmastoidectomy
postoperative H95.89-
external ear canal stenosis H95.81-
hematoma —*see* Complications..., postprocedural, hematoma (of), mastoid process
hemorrhage —*see* Complications..., postprocedural, hemorrhage (of), mastoid process
postmastoidectomy —*see* Complications, postmastoidectomy
seroma —*see* Complications, postprocedural, seroma (of), mastoid process ◀
specified NEC H95.89-
mastoidectomy cavity —*see* Complications, postmastoidectomy
mechanical —*see* Complications, by site and type, mechanical
medical procedures (*see also* Complication(s), intraoperative) T88.9
metabolic E88.9
postoperative E89.89
specified NEC E89.89
molar pregnancy NOS O08.9
damage to pelvic organs O08.6
embolism O08.2
genital infection O08.0
hemorrhage (delayed) (excessive) O08.1
metabolic disorder O08.5
renal failure O08.4
shock O08.3
specified type NEC O08.0
venous complication NEC O08.7
musculoskeletal system —*see also* Complication, intraoperative (intraprocedural), by site
device, implant or graft NEC —*see* Complications, orthopedic, device or implant
internal fixation (nail) (plate) (rod) —*see* Complications, fixation device, internal
joint prosthesis —*see* Complications, joint prosthesis

Complication *(Continued)*
musculoskeletal system *(Continued)*
postoperative (postprocedural) M96.89
with osteoporosis —*see* Osteoporosis
fracture following insertion of device —*see* Fracture, following insertion of orthopedic implant, joint prosthesis or bone plate
joint instability after prosthesis removal M96.89
lordosis M96.4
postlaminectomy syndrome NEC M96.1
kyphosis M96.2
pseudarthrosis M96.0
specified complication NEC M96.89
post radiation M96.89
kyphosis M96.3
scoliosis M96.5
specified complication NEC M96.89
nephrostomy (stoma) —*see* Complications, stoma, urinary tract, external NEC
nervous system G98.8
central G96.9
device, implant or graft —*see also* Complication, prosthetic device or implant, specified NEC
electronic stimulator (electrode (s)) —*see* Complications, electronic stimulator device
specified NEC ◀
infection and inflammation T85.738 ◀
mechanical T85.695 ◀
breakdown T85.615 ◀
displacement T85.625 ◀
leakage T85.635 ◀
malfunction T85.695 ◀
malposition T85.625 ◀
obstruction T85.695 ◀
perforation T85.695 ◀
protrusion T85.695 ◀
specified NEC T85.695 ◀
ventricular shunt —*see* Complications, ventricular shunt
electronic stimulator (electrode (s)) —*see* Complications, electronic stimulator device
postprocedural G97.82
intracranial hypotension G97.2
specified NEC G97.82
spinal fluid leak G97.0
newborn, due to intrauterine (fetal) procedure P96.5
nonabsorbable (permanent) sutures —*see* Complication, sutures, permanent
obstetric O75.9
procedure (instrumental) (manual) (surgical) specified NEC O75.4
specified NEC O75.89
surgical wound NEC O90.89
hematoma O90.2
infection O86.0
ocular lens implant —*see* Complications, intraocular lens
ophthalmologic
postprocedural bleb —*see* Blebitis
orbital prosthesis T85.9
embolism T85.818
fibrosis T85.828
hemorrhage T85.838
infection and inflammation T85.79
mechanical
breakdown T85.31-
displacement T85.32-
malposition T85.32-
obstruction T85.39-
perforation T85.39-
protrusion T85.39-
specified NEC T85.39-
pain T85.848
specified type NEC T85.898
stenosis T85.858
thrombosis T85.868

◀ New Revised ~~deleted~~ Deleted

Complication *(Continued)*
organ or tissue transplant (partial) (total) —*see* Complications, transplant
orthopedic —*see also* Disorder, soft tissue
device or implant T84.9
bone
device or implant —*see* Complication, bone, device NEC
graft —*see* Complication, graft, bone
breakdown T84.418
displacement T84.428
electronic bone stimulator —*see* Complications, electronic stimulator device, bone
embolism T84.81
fibrosis T84.82
fixation device —*see* Complication, fixation device, internal
hemorrhage T84.83
infection or inflammation T84.7
joint prosthesis —*see* Complication, joint prosthesis, internal
malfunction T84.418
malposition T84.428
mechanical NEC T84.498
muscle graft —*see* Complications, graft, muscle
obstruction T84.498
pain T84.84
perforation T84.498
protrusion T84.498
specified complication NEC T84.89
stenosis T84.85
tendon graft —*see* Complications, graft, tendon
thrombosis T84.86
fracture (following insertion of device) —*see* Fracture, following insertion of orthopedic implant, joint prosthesis or bone plate
postprocedural M96.89
fracture —*see* Fracture, following insertion of orthopedic implant, joint prosthesis or bone plate
postlaminectomy syndrome NEC M96.1
kyphosis M96.3
lordosis M96.4
postradiation
kyphosis M96.2
scoliosis M96.5
pseudarthrosis post-fusion M96.0
specified type NEC M96.89
pacemaker (cardiac) —*see* Complications, cardiovascular device or implant, electronic
pancreas transplant —*see* Complications, transplant, pancreas
penile prosthesis (implant) —*see* Complications, prosthetic device, penile
perfusion NEC T80.90
perineal repair (obstetrical) NEC O90.89
disruption O90.1
hematoma O90.2
infection (following delivery) O86.0
phototherapy T88.9
specified NEC T88.8
postmastoidectomy NEC H95.19-
cyst, mucosal H95.13-
granulation H95.12-
inflammation, chronic H95.11-
recurrent cholesteatoma H95.0-
postoperative —*see* Complications, postprocedural
circulatory —*see* Complications, circulatory system
ear —*see* Complications, ear
endocrine —*see* Complications, endocrine
eye —*see* Complications, eye
lumbar puncture G97.1
cerebrospinal fluid leak G97.0

Complication *(Continued)*
postoperative *(Continued)*
nervous system (central) (peripheral) —*see* Complications, nervous system
respiratory system —*see* Complications, respiratory system
postprocedural —*see also* Complications, surgical procedure
cardiac arrest
following cardiac surgery I97.120
following other surgery I97.121
cardiac functional disturbance NEC
following cardiac surgery I97.190
following other surgery I97.191
cardiac insufficiency
following cardiac surgery I97.110
following other surgery I97.111
chorioretinal scars following retinal surgery H59.81-
following cataract surgery
cataract (lens) fragments H59.02-
cystoid macular edema H59.03-
specified NEC H59.09-
vitreous (touch) syndrome H59.01-
heart failure
following cardiac surgery I97.130
following other surgery I97.131
hematoma (of) ◀
circulatory system organ or structure ◀
following cardiac bypass I97.631 ◀
following cardiac catheterization I97.630 ◀
following other circulatory system procedure I97.638 ◀
following other procedure I97.621 ◀
digestive system ◀
following procedure on digestive system K91.870 ◀
following procedure on other organ K91.871 ◀
ear ◀
following other procedure H95.52 ◀
following procedure on ear and mastoid process H95.51 ◀
endocrine system ◀
following endocrine system procedure E89.820 ◀
following other procedure E89.821 ◀
eye and adnexa ◀
following ophthalmic procedure H59.33- ◀
following other procedure H59.34- ◀
genitourinary organ or structure ◀
following procedure on genitourinary organ or structure N99.840 ◀
following procedure on other organ N99.841 ◀
mastoid process ◀
following other procedure H95.52 ◀
following procedure on ear and mastoid process H95.51 ◀
musculoskeletal structure ◀
following musculoskeletal surgery M96.840 ◀
following non-orthopedic surgery M96.841 ◀
following orthopedic surgery M96.840 ◀
nervous system ◀
following nervous system procedure G97.61 ◀
following other procedure G97.62 ◀
respiratory system ◀
following other procedure J95.861 ◀
following procedure on respiratory system organ or structure J95.860 ◀
skin and subcutaneous tissue ◀
following dermatologic procedure L76.31 ◀
following procedure on other organ L76.32 ◀

Complication *(Continued)*
postprocedural *(Continued)*
hematoma *(Continued)*
spleen ◀
following procedure on other organ D78.32 ◀
following procedure on the spleen D78.31 ◀
hemorrhage (of) ◀
circulatory system organ or structure
~~following a cardiac bypass I97.611~~
~~following a cardiac catheterization I97.610~~
following cardiac bypass I97.611 ◀
following cardiac catheterization I97.610 ◀
following other circulatory system procedure I97.618
following other procedure I97.620 ◀
digestive system
following procedure on digestive system K91.840
following procedure on other organ K91.841
ear
following other procedure H95.42
following procedure on ear and mastoid process H95.41
endocrine system
following endocrine system procedure E89.810
following other procedure E89.811
eye and adnexa
following ophthalmic procedure H59.31-
following other procedure H59.32-
genitourinary organ or structure
following procedure on genitourinary organ or structure N99.820
following procedure on other organ N99.821
mastoid process
following other procedure H95.42
following procedure on ear and mastoid process H95.41
musculoskeletal structure
following musculoskeletal surgery M96.830
following non-orthopedic surgery M96.831
following orthopedic surgery M96.830
nervous system
~~following a nervous system procedure G97.51~~
following nervous system procedure G97.51 ◀
following other procedure G97.52
respiratory system
following other procedure J95.831
following procedure on respiratory system organ or structure J95.830
skin and subcutaneous tissue
~~following a dermatologic procedure L76.21~~
following dermatologic procedure L76.21 ◀
following a procedure on other organ L76.22
spleen
following procedure on other organ D78.22
following procedure on the spleen D78.21
seroma (of) ◀
circulatory system organ or structure ◀
following cardiac bypass I97.641 ◀
following cardiac catheterization I97.640 ◀
following other circulatory system procedure I97.648 ◀
following other procedure I97.622 ◀

◀ New ◀ Revised ~~deleted~~ Deleted

Complication *(Continued)*
postprocedural *(Continued)*
seroma *(Continued)*
digestive system ◀
following procedure on digestive system K91.872 ◀
following procedure on other organ K91.873 ◀
ear ◀
following other procedure H95.54 ◀
following procedure on ear and mastoid process H95.53 ◀
endocrine system ◀
following endocrine system procedure E89.822 ◀
following other procedure E89.823 ◀
eye and adnexa ◀
following ophthalmic procedure H59.35- ◀
following other procedure H59.36- ◀
genitourinary organ or structure ◀
following procedure on genitourinary organ or structure N99.842 ◀
following procedure on other organ N99.843 ◀
mastoid process ◀
following other procedure H95.54 ◀
following procedure on ear and mastoid process H95.53 ◀
musculoskeletal structure ◀
following musculoskeletal surgery M96.842 ◀
following non-orthopedic surgery M96.843 ◀
following orthopedic surgery M96.842 ◀
nervous system ◀
following nervous system procedure G97.63 ◀
following other procedure G97.64 ◀
respiratory system ◀
following other procedure J95.863 ◀
following procedure on respiratory system organ or structure J95.862 ◀
skin and subcutaneous tissue ◀
following dermatologic procedure L76.33 ◀
following procedure on other organ L76.34 ◀
spleen ◀
following procedure on other organ D78.34 ◀
following procedure on the spleen D78.33 ◀
specified NEC
circulatory system I97.89
digestive K91.89
ear H95.89
endocrine E89.89
eye and adnexa H59.89
genitourinary N99.89
mastoid process H95.89
metabolic E89.89
musculoskeletal structure M96.89
nervous system G97.82
respiratory system J95.89
skin and subcutaneous tissue L76.82
spleen D78.89
pregnancy NEC —*see* Pregnancy, complicated by
prosthetic device or implant T85.9
bile duct —*see* Complications, bile duct implant
breast —*see* Complications, breast implant
bulking agent ◀
ureteral ◀
erosion T83.714 ◀
exposure T83.724 ◀
urethral ◀
erosion T83.713 ◀
exposure T83.723 ◀

Complication *(Continued)*
prosthetic device or implant *(Continued)*
cardiac and vascular NEC —*see* Complications, cardiovascular device or implant
corneal transplant —*see* Complications, graft, cornea
electronic nervous system stimulator —*see* Complications, electronic stimulator device
epidural infusion catheter —*see* Complications, catheter, epidural
esophageal anti-reflux device —*see* Complications, esophageal anti-reflux device
genital organ or tract —*see* Complications, genitourinary, device or implant, genital tract
specified NEC T83.79 ◀
heart valve —*see* Complications, heart, valve, prosthesis
infection or inflammation T85.79
intestine transplant T86.892
liver transplant T86.43
lung transplant T86.812
pancreas transplant T86.892
skin graft T86.822
intraocular lens —*see* Complications, intraocular lens
intraperitoneal (dialysis) catheter —*see* Complications, catheter, intraperitoneal
joint —*see* Complications, joint prosthesis, internal
mechanical NEC T85.698
dialysis catheter (vascular) —*see also* Complication, catheter, dialysis, mechanical
peritoneal —*see* Complication, catheter, intraperitoneal, mechanical
gastrointestinal device T85.598
ocular device T85.398
subdural (infusion) catheter T85.690
suture, permanent T85.692
that for bone repair —*see* Complications, fixation device, internal (orthopedic), mechanical
ventricular shunt
breakdown T85.01
displacement T85.02
leakage T85.03
malposition T85.02
obstruction T85.09
perforation T85.09
protrusion T85.09
specified NEC T85.09
mesh
erosion (to surrounding organ or tissue) T83.717 ⟸
urethral (into pelvic floor muscles) T83.712 ◀
vaginal (into pelvic floor muscles) T83.711
exposure (into surrounding organ or tissue) T83.727 ⟸
urethral (through urethral wall) T83.722 ◀
vaginal (into vagina) (through vaginal wall) T83.721
orbital —*see* Complications, orbital prosthesis
penile T83.9
embolism T83.81
fibrosis T83.82
hemorrhage T83.83
infection and inflammation T83.61 ⟸
mechanical
breakdown T83.410
displacement T83.420
leakage T83.490
malposition T83.420

Complication *(Continued)*
prosthetic device or implant *(Continued)*
penile *(Continued)*
mechanical *(Continued)*
obstruction T83.490
perforation T83.490
protrusion T83.490
specified NEC T83.490
pain T83.84
specified type NEC T83.89
stenosis T83.85
thrombosis T83.86
prosthetic materials NEC
erosion (to surrounding organ or tissue) T83.718
~~vaginal (into pelvic floor muscles) T83.711~~
exposure (into surrounding organ or tissue) T83.728
~~vaginal (into vagina) (through vaginal wall) T83.721~~
skin graft T86.829
artificial skin or decellularized allodermis
embolism T85.818 ⟸
fibrosis T85.828 ⟸
hemorrhage T85.838 ⟸
infection and inflammation T85.79
mechanical
breakdown T85.613
displacement T85.623
malfunction T85.613
malposition T85.623
obstruction T85.693
perforation T85.693
protrusion T85.693
specified NEC T85.693
pain T85.848 ⟸
specified type NEC T85.898 ⟸
stenosis T85.858 ⟸
thrombosis T85.868 ⟸
failure T86.821
infection T86.822
rejection T86.820
specified NEC T86.828
sling ◀
urethral (female) (male) ◀
erosion T83.712 ◀
exposure T83.722 ◀
specified NEC T85.9
embolism T85.818 ⟸
fibrosis T85.828 ⟸
hemorrhage T85.838 ⟸
infection and inflammation T85.79
mechanical
breakdown T85.618
displacement T85.628
leakage T85.638
malfunction T85.618
malposition T85.628
obstruction T85.698
perforation T85.698
protrusion T85.698
specified NEC T85.698
pain T85.848 ⟸
specified type NEC T85.898 ⟸
stenosis T85.858 ⟸
thrombosis T85.868 ⟸
subdural infusion catheter —*see* Complications, catheter, subdural
sutures —*see* Complications, sutures
urinary organ or tract NEC —*see* Complications, genitourinary, device or implant, urinary system
vascular —*see* Complications, cardiovascular device or implant
ventricular shunt —*see* Complications, ventricular shunt (device)
puerperium —*see* Puerperal
puncture, spinal G97.1
cerebrospinal fluid leak G97.0
headache or reaction G97.1

Complication *(Continued)*
pyelogram N99.89
radiation
kyphosis M96.2
scoliosis M96.5
reattached
extremity (infection) (rejection)
lower T87.1X-
upper T87.0X-
specified body part NEC T87.2
reconstructed breast
asymmetry between native and reconstructed breast N65.1
deformity N65.0
disproportion between native and reconstructed breast N65.1
excess tissue N65.0
misshappen N65.0
reimplant NEC —*see also* Complications, prosthetic device or implant
limb (infection) (rejection) —*see* Complications, reattached, extremity
organ (partial) (total) —*see* Complications, transplant
prosthetic device NEC —*see* Complications, prosthetic device
renal N28.9
allograft —*see* Complications, transplant, kidney
dialysis —*see* Complications, dialysis
respirator
mechancial J95.850
specified NEC J95.859
respiratory system J98.9
device, implant or graft —*see* Complication, prosthetic device or implant, specified NEC
lung transplant —*see* Complications, prosthetic device or implant, lung transplant
postoperative J95.89
air leak J95.812
Mendelson's syndrome (chemical pneumonitis) J95.4
pneumothorax J95.811
pulmonary insufficiency (acute) (after nonthoracic surgery) J95.2
chronic J95.3
following thoracic surgery J95.1
respiratory failure (acute) J95.821
acute and chronic J95.822
specified NEC J95.89
subglottic stenosis J95.5
tracheostomy complication —*see* Complications, tracheostomy
therapy T81.89
sedation during labor and delivery O74.9
cardiac O74.2
central nervous system O74.3
pulmonary NEC O74.1
shunt —*see also* Complications, prosthetic device or implant
arteriovenous —*see* Complications, arteriovenous, shunt
ventricular (communicating) —*see* Complications, ventricular shunt
skin
graft T86.829
failure T86.821
infection T86.822
rejection T86.820
specified type NEC T86.828
spinal
anesthesia —*see* Complications, anesthesia, spinal
catheter (epidural) (subdural) —*see* Complications, catheter
puncture or tap G97.1
cerebrospinal fluid leak G97.0
headache or reaction G97.1

Complication *(Continued)*
stent
bile duct —*see* Complications, bile duct prosthesis
ureteral indwelling ◀
breakdown T83.112 ◀
displacement T83.122 ◀
leakage T83.192 ◀
malposition T83.122 ◀
obstruction T83.192 ◀
perforation T83.192 ◀
protrusion T83.192 ◀
specified NEC T83.192 ◀
urinary (ileal conduit) (nephroureteral) T83.193 ◀
embolism T83.81 ◀
fibrosis T83.82 ◀
hemorrhage T83.83 ◀
infection and inflammation T83.593 ◀
mechanical ◀
breakdown T83.113 ◀
displacement T83.123 ◀
leakage T83.193 ◀
malposition T83.123 ◀
obstruction T83.193 ◀
perforation T83.193 ◀
protrusion T83.193 ◀
specified NEC T83.193 ◀
pain T83.84 ◀
specified type NEC T83.89 ◀
stenosis T83.85 ◀
thrombosis T83.86 ◀
vascular ◀
end stent stenosis —*see* Restenosis, stent ◀
in stent stenosis —*see* Restenosis, stent ◀
stoma
digestive tract
colostomy —*see* Complications, colostomy
enterostomy —*see* Complications, enterostomy
esophagostomy —*see* Complications, esophagostomy
gastrostomy —*see* Complications, gastrostomy
urinary tract N99.528 ⟸
continent N99.538 ◀
hemorrhage N99.530 ◀
herniation N99.533 ◀
infection N99.531 ◀
malfunction N99.532 ◀
specified type NEC N99.538 ◀
stenosis N99.534 ◀
cystostomy —*see* Complications, cystostomy
external NOS N99.528
~~hemorrhage N99.520~~
~~infection N99.521~~
~~malfunction N99.522~~
~~specified type NEC N99.528~~
hemorrhage N99.520 ⟸
herniation N99.523 ◀
incontinent N99.528 ◀
hemorrhage N99.520 ◀
herniation N99.523 ◀
infection N99.521 ◀
malfunction N99.522 ◀
specified type NEC N99.528 ◀
stenosis N99.524 ◀
infection N99.521 ⟸
malfunction N99.522 ⟸
specified type NEC N99.528 ⟸
stenosis N99.524 ◀
stomach banding —*see* Complication (s), bariatric procedure
stomach stapling —*see* Complication (s), bariatric procedure
surgical material, nonabsorbable —*see* Complication, suture, permanent

Complication *(Continued)*
surgical procedure (on) T81.9
amputation stump (late) —*see* Complications, amputation stump
cardiac —*see* Complications, circulatory system
cholesteatoma, recurrent —*see* Complications, postmastoidectomy, recurrent cholesteatoma
circulatory (early) —*see* Complications, circulatory system
digestive system —*see* Complications, gastrointestinal
dumping syndrome (postgastrectomy) K91.1
ear —*see* Complications, ear
elephantiasis or lymphedema I97.89
postmastectomy I97.2
emphysema (surgical) T81.82
endocrine —*see* Complications, endocrine
eye —*see* Complications, eye
fistula (persistent postoperative) T81.83
foreign body inadvertently left in wound (sponge) (suture) (swab) —*see* Foreign body, accidentally left during a procedure
gastrointestinal —*see* Complications, gastrointestinal
genitourinary NEC N99.89
hematoma
intraoperative —*see* Complication, intraoperative, hemorrhage
postprocedural —*see* Complication, postprocedural, hematoma ⟸
hemorrhage
intraoperative —*see* Complication, intraoperative, hemorrhage
postprocedural —*see* Complication, postprocedural, hemorrhage
hepatic failure K91.82
hyperglycemia (postpancreatectomy) E89.1
hypoinsulinemia (postpancreatectomy) E89.1
hypoparathyroidism (postparathyroidectomy) E89.2
hypopituitarism (posthypophysectomy) E89.3
hypothyroidism (post-thyroidectomy) E89.0
intestinal obstruction K91.3
intracranial hypotension following ventricular shunting (ventriculostomy) G97.2
lymphedema I97.89
postmastectomy I97.2
malabsorption (postsurgical) NEC K91.2
osteoporosis —*see* Osteoporosis, postsurgical malabsorption
mastoidectomy cavity NEC —*see* Complications, postmastoidectomy
metabolic E89.89
specified NEC E89.89
musculoskeletal —*see* Complications, musculoskeletal system
nervous system (central) (peripheral) —*see* Complications, nervous system
ovarian failure E89.40
asymptomatic E89.40
symptomatic E89.41
peripheral vascular —*see* Complications, surgical procedure, vascular
postcardiotomy syndrome I97.0
postcholecystectomy syndrome K91.5
postcommissurotomy syndrome I97.0
postgastrectomy dumping syndrome K91.1
postlaminectomy syndrome NEC M96.1
kyphosis M96.3
postmastectomy lymphedema syndrome I97.2
postmastoidectomy cholesteatoma —*see* Complications, postmastoidectomy, recurrent cholesteatoma

◀ New ⟸ Revised ~~deleted~~ Deleted

Complication *(Continued)*
surgical procedure *(Continued)*
postvagotomy syndrome K91.1
postvalvulotomy syndrome I97.0
pulmonary insufficiency (acute) J95.2
chronic J95.3
following thoracic surgery J95.1
reattached body part —*see* Complications, reattached
respiratory —*see* Complications, respiratory system
shock (hypovolemic) T81.19
spleen (postoperative) D78.89
intraoperative D78.81
stitch abscess T81.48 ◄
subglottic stenosis (postsurgical) J95.5
testicular hypofunction E89.5
transplant —*see* Complications, organ or tissue transplant
urinary NEC N99.89
vaginal vault prolapse (posthysterectomy) N99.3
vascular (peripheral)
artery T81.719
mesenteric T81.710
renal T81.711
specified NEC T81.718
vein T81.72
wound infection T81.40 ◄
suture, permanent (wire) NEC T85.9
with repair of bone —*see* Complications, fixation device, internal
embolism T85.818 ◄
fibrosis T85.828 ◄
hemorrhage T85.838 ◄
infection and inflammation T85.79
mechanical
breakdown T85.612
displacement T85.622
malfunction T85.612
malposition T85.622
obstruction T85.692
perforation T85.692
protrusion T85.692
specified NEC T85.692
pain T85.848 ◄
specified type NEC T85.898 ◄
stenosis T85.858 ◄
thrombosis T85.868 ◄
tracheostomy J95.00
granuloma J95.09
hemorrhage J95.01
infection J95.02
malfunction J95.03
mechanical J95.03
obstruction J95.03
specified type NEC J95.09
tracheo-esophageal fistula J95.04
transfusion (blood) (lymphocytes) (plasma) T80.92
air embolism T80.0
circulatory overload E87.71
febrile nonhemolytic transfusion reaction R50.84
hemochromatosis E83.111
hemolysis T80.89
hemolytic reaction (antigen unspecified) T80.919
incompatibility reaction (antigen unspecified) T80.919
ABO T80.30
delayed serologic (DSTR) T80.39
hemolytic transfusion reaction (HTR) (unspecified time after transfusion) T80.319
acute (AHTR) (less than 24 hours after transfusion) T80.310
delayed (DHTR) (24 hours or more after transfusion) T80.311
specified NEC T80.39

Complication *(Continued)*
transfusion *(Continued)*
incompatibility reaction *(Continued)*
acute (antigen unspecified) T80.910
delayed (antigen unspecified) T80.911
delayed serologic (DSTR) T80.89
Non-ABO (minor antigens (Duffy) (Kell) (Kidd) (Lewis) (M) (N) (P) (S)) T80.A0
delayed serologic (DSTR) T80.A9
hemolytic transfusion reaction (HTR) (unspecified time after transfusion) T80.A19
acute (AHTR) (less than 24 hours after transfusion) T80.A10
delayed (DHTR) (24 hours or more after transfusion) T80.A11
specified NEC T80.A9
Rh (antigens (C) (c) (D) (E) (e)) (factor) T80.40
delayed serologic (DSTR) T80.49
hemolytic transfusion reaction (HTR) (unspecified time after transfusion) T80.419
acute (AHTR) (less than 24 hours after transfusion) T80.410
delayed (DHTR) (24 hours or more after transfusion) T80.411
specified NEC T80.49
infection T80.29
acute T80.22
reaction NEC T80.89
sepsis T80.29
shock T80.89
transplant T86.90
bone T86.839
failure T86.831
infection T86.832
rejection T86.830
specified type NEC T86.838
bone marrow T86.00
failure T86.02
infection T86.03
rejection T86.01
specified type NEC T86.09
cornea T86.849
failure T86.841
infection T86.842
rejection T86.840
specified type NEC T86.848
failure T86.92
heart T86.20
with lung T86.30
cardiac allograft vasculopathy T86.290
failure T86.32
infection T86.33
rejection T86.31
specified type NEC T86.39
failure T86.22
infection T86.23
rejection T86.21
specified type NEC T86.298
infection T86.93
intestine T86.859
failure T86.851
infection T86.852
rejection T86.850
specified type NEC T86.858
kidney T86.10
failure T86.12
infection T86.13
rejection T86.11
specified type NEC T86.19
liver T86.40
failure T86.42
infection T86.43
rejection T86.41
specified type NEC T86.49
lung T86.819
with heart T86.30
failure T86.32
infection T86.33

Complication *(Continued)*
transplant *(Continued)*
lung *(Continued)*
with heart *(Continued)*
rejection T86.31
specified type NEC T86.39
failure T86.811
infection T86.812
rejection T86.810
specified type NEC T86.818
malignant neoplasm C80.2
pancreas T86.899
failure T86.891
infection T86.892
rejection T86.890
specified type NEC T86.898
peripheral blood stem cells T86.5
post-transplant lymphoproliferative disorder (PTLD) D47.Z1
rejection T86.91
skin T86.829
failure T86.821
infection T86.822
rejection T86.820
specified type NEC T86.828
specified
tissue T86.899
failure T86.891
infection T86.892
rejection T86.890
specified type NEC T86.898
type NEC T86.99
stem cell (from peripheral blood) (from umbilical cord) T86.5
umbilical cord stem cells T86.5
trauma (early) T79.9
specified NEC T79.8
ultrasound therapy NEC T88.9
umbilical cord NEC
complicating delivery O69.9
specified NEC O69.89
umbrella device, vascular T82.9
embolism T82.818
fibrosis T82.828
hemorrhage T82.838
infection or inflammation T82.7
mechanical
breakdown T82.515
displacement T82.525
leakage T82.535
malposition T82.525
obstruction T82.595
perforation T82.595
protrusion T82.595
pain T82.848
specified type NEC T82.898
stenosis T82.858
thrombosis T82.868
urethral catheter —*see* Complications, catheter, urethral, indwelling
vaccination T88.1
anaphylaxis NEC T80.52
arthropathy —*see* Arthropathy, postimmunization
cellulitis T88.0
encephalitis or encephalomyelitis G04.02
infection (general) (local) NEC T88.0
meningitis G03.8
myelitis G04.02 ◄
protein sickness T80.62
rash T88.1
reaction (allergic) T88.1
serum T80.62
sepsis T88.0
serum intoxication, sickness, rash, or other serum reaction NEC T80.62
anaphylactic shock T80.52
shock (allergic) (anaphylactic) T80.52
vaccinia (generalized) (localized) T88.1
vas deferens device or implant —*see* Complications, genitourinary, device or implant, genital tract

C

Complication *(Continued)*
vascular I99.9
device or implant T82.9
embolism T82.818
fibrosis T82.828
hemorrhage T82.838
infection or inflammation T82.7
mechanical
breakdown T82.519
specified device NEC T82.518
displacement T82.529
specified device NEC T82.528
leakage T82.539
specified device NEC T82.538
malposition T82.529
specified device NEC T82.528
obstruction T82.599
specified device NEC T82.598
perforation T82.599
specified device NEC T82.598
protrusion T82.599
specified device NEC T82.598
pain T82.848
specified type NEC T82.898
stenosis T82.858
thrombosis T82.868
dialysis catheter —*see* Complication, catheter, dialysis
following infusion, therapeutic injection or transfusion T80.1
graft T82.9
embolism T82.818
fibrosis T82.828
hemorrhage T82.838
mechanical
breakdown T82.319
aorta (bifurcation) T82.310
carotid artery T82.311
specified vessel NEC T82.318
displacement T82.329
aorta (bifurcation) T82.320
carotid artery T82.321
specified vessel NEC T82.328
leakage T82.339
aorta (bifurcation) T82.330
carotid artery T82.331
specified vessel NEC T82.338
malposition T82.329
aorta (bifurcation) T82.320
carotid artery T82.321
specified vessel NEC T82.328
obstruction T82.399
aorta (bifurcation) T82.390
carotid artery T82.391
specified vessel NEC T82.398
perforation T82.399
aorta (bifurcation) T82.390
carotid artery T82.391
specified vessel NEC T82.398
protrusion T82.399
aorta (bifurcation) T82.390
carotid artery T82.391
specified vessel NEC T82.398
pain T82.848
specified complication NEC T82.898
stenosis T82.858
thrombosis T82.868
postoperative —*see* Complications, postoperative, circulatory
vena cava device (filter) (sieve) (umbrella) —*see* Complications, umbrella device, vascular
ventilation therapy NEC T81.81
ventilator
mechanical J95.850
specified NEC J95.859
ventricular (communicating) shunt (device) T85.9
embolism T85.810 ⇐
fibrosis T85.820 ⇐
hemorrhage T85.830 ⇐

Complication *(Continued)*
ventricular shunt *(Continued)*
infection and inflammation T85.730 ⇐
mechanical
breakdown T85.01
displacement T85.02
leakage T85.03
malposition T85.02
obstruction T85.09
perforation T85.09
protrusion T85.09
specified NEC T85.09
pain T85.840 ⇐
specified type NEC T85.890 ⇐
stenosis T85.850 ⇐
thrombosis T85.860 ⇐
wire suture, permanent (implanted) —*see* Complications, suture, permanent
Compressed air disease T70.3
Compression
with injury - code by Nature of injury
artery I77.1
celiac, syndrome I77.4
brachial plexus G54.0
brain (stem) G93.5
due to
contusion (diffuse) —*see* Injury, intracranial, diffuse
focal —*see* Injury, intracranial, focal
injury NEC —*see* Injury, intracranial, diffuse
traumatic —*see* Injury, intracranial, diffuse
bronchus J98.09
cauda equina G83.4
celiac (artery) (axis) I77.4
cerebral —*see* Compression, brain
cervical plexus G54.2
cord
spinal —*see* Compression, spinal
umbilical —*see* Compression, umbilical cord
cranial nerve G52.9
eighth —*see* subcategory H93.3
eleventh G52.8
fifth G50.8
first G52.0
fourth —*see* Strabismus, paralytic, fourth nerve
ninth G52.1
second —*see* Disorder, nerve, optic
seventh G52.8
sixth —*see* Strabismus, paralytic, sixth nerve
tenth G52.2
third —*see* Strabismus, paralytic, third nerve
twelfth G52.3
diver's squeeze T70.3
during birth (newborn) P15.9
esophagus K22.2
eustachian tube —*see* Obstruction, eustachian tube, cartilaginous
facies Q67.1
fracture
nontraumatic NOS —*see* Collapse, vertebra ◀
pathological —*see* Fracture, pathological ◀
traumatic —*see* Fracture, traumatic ◀
heart —*see* Disease, heart
intestine —*see* Obstruction, intestine
laryngeal nerve, recurrent G52.2
with paralysis of vocal cords and larynx J38.00
bilateral J38.02
unilateral J38.01
lumbosacral plexus G54.1
lung J98.4
lymphatic vessel I89.0
medulla —*see* Compression, brain
nerve —*see also* Disorder, nerve G58.9
arm NEC —*see* Mononeuropathy, upper limb

Compression *(Continued)*
nerve *(Continued)*
axillary G54.0
cranial —*see* Compression, cranial nerve
leg NEC —*see* Mononeuropathy, lower limb
median (in carpal tunnel) —*see* Syndrome, carpal tunnel
optic —*see* Disorder, nerve, optic
plantar —*see* Lesion, nerve, plantar
posterior tibial (in tarsal tunnel) —*see* Syndrome, tarsal tunnel
root or plexus NOS (in) G54.9
intervertebral disc disorder NEC —*see* Disorder, disc, with, radiculopathy
with myelopathy —*see* Disorder, disc, with, myelopathy
neoplastic disease —*see also* Neoplasm D49.9 *[G55]*
spondylosis —*see* Spondylosis, with radiculopathy
sciatic (acute) —*see* Lesion, nerve, sciatic
sympathetic G90.8
traumatic —*see* Injury, nerve
ulnar —*see* Lesion, nerve, ulnar
upper extremity NEC —*see* Mononeuropathy, upper limb
spinal (cord) G95.20
by displacement of intervertebral disc NEC —*see also* Disorder, disc, with, myelopathy
nerve root NOS G54.9
due to displacement of intervertebral disc NEC —*see* Disorder, disc, with, radiculopathy
with myelopathy —*see* Disorder, disc, with, myelopathy
specified NEC G95.29
spondylogenic (cervical) (lumbar, lumbosacral) (thoracic) —*see* Spondylosis, with myelopathy NEC
anterior —*see* Syndrome, anterior, spinal artery, compression
traumatic —*see* Injury, spinal cord, by region
subcostal nerve (syndrome) —*see* Mononeuropathy, upper limb, specified NEC
sympathetic nerve NEC G90.8
syndrome T79.5
trachea J39.8
ulnar nerve (by scar tissue) —*see* Lesion, nerve, ulnar
umbilical cord
complicating delivery O69.2
cord around neck O69.1
prolapse O69.0
specified NEC O69.2
ureter N13.5
vein I87.1
vena cava (inferior) (superior) I87.1
Compulsion, compulsive
gambling F63.0
neurosis F42.8 ⇐
personality F60.5
states F42.8 ⇐
swearing F42.8 ⇐
in Gilles de la Tourette's syndrome F95.2
tics and spasms F95.9
Concato's disease (pericardial polyserositis) A19.9
nontubercular I31.1
pleural —*see* Pleurisy, with effusion
Concavity chest wall M95.4
Concealed penis Q55.69
Concern (normal) **about sick person in family** Z63.6
Concrescence (teeth) K00.2
Concretio cordis I31.1
rheumatic I09.2

◀ New ⇐ Revised ~~deleted~~ Deleted

Concretion —*see also* Calculus
appendicular K38.1
canaliculus —*see* Dacryolith
clitoris N90.89
conjunctiva H11.12-
eyelid —*see* Disorder, eyelid, specified type NEC
lacrimal passages —*see* Dacryolith
prepuce (male) N47.8
salivary gland (any) K11.5
seminal vesicle N50.89 ⬅
tonsil J35.8
Concussion (brain) (cerebral) (current) S06.0X9 ⬅
with ◀
loss of consciousness of 30 minutes or less S06.0X1 ◀
loss of consciousness of unspecified duration S06.0X9 ◀
blast (air) (hydraulic) (immersion) (underwater)
abdomen or thorax —*see* Injury, blast, by site
ear with acoustic nerve injury —*see* Injury, nerve, acoustic, specified type NEC
cauda equina S34.3
conus medullaris S34.02
ocular S05.8X-
spinal (cord)
cervical S14.0
lumbar S34.01
sacral S34.02
thoracic S24.0
syndrome F07.81
Without loss of consciousness S06.0X0 ◀
Condition —*see* Disease
Conditions arising in the perinatal period —*see* Newborn, affected by
Conduct disorder —*see* Disorder, conduct
Condyloma A63.0
acuminatum A63.0
gonorrheal A54.09
latum A51.31
syphilitic A51.31
congenital A50.07
venereal, syphilitic A51.31
Conflagration —*see also* Burn
asphyxia (by inhalation of gases, fumes or vapors) —*see also* Table of Drugs and Chemicals T59.9-
Conflict (with) —*see also* Discord
family Z73.9
marital Z63.0
involving divorce or estrangement Z63.5
parent-child Z62.820
parent-adopted child Z62.821
parent-biological child Z62.820
parent-foster child Z62.822
social role NEC Z73.5
Confluent —*see* condition
Confusion, confused R41.0
epileptic F05
mental state (psychogenic) F44.89
psychogenic F44.89
reactive (from emotional stress, psychological trauma) F44.89
Confusional arousals G47.51
Congelation T69.9
Congenital —*see also* condition
aortic septum Q25.49 ⬅
intrinsic factor deficiency D51.0
malformation —*see* Anomaly
Congestion, congestive
bladder N32.89
bowel K63.89
brain G93.89
breast N64.59
bronchial J98.09
catarrhal J31.0
chest R09.89
chill, malarial —*see* Malaria

Congestion, congestive *(Continued)*
circulatory NEC I99.8
duodenum K31.89
eye —*see* Hyperemia, conjunctiva
facial, due to birth injury P15.4
general R68.89
glottis J37.0
heart —*see* Failure, heart, congestive
hepatic K76.1
hypostatic (lung) —*see* Edema, lung
intestine K63.89
kidney N28.89
labyrinth —*see* subcategory H83.8
larynx J37.0
liver K76.1
lung R09.89
active or acute —*see* Pneumonia
malaria, malarial —*see* Malaria
nasal R09.81
nose R09.81
orbit, orbital —*see also* Exophthalmos
inflammatory (chronic) —*see* Inflammation, orbit
ovary N83.8
pancreas K86.89 ⬅
pelvic, female N94.89
pleural J94.8
prostate (active) N42.1
pulmonary —*see* Congestion, lung
renal N28.89
retina H35.81
seminal vesicle N50.1
spinal cord G95.19
spleen (chronic) D73.2
stomach K31.89
trachea —*see* Tracheitis
urethra N36.8
uterus N85.8
with subinvolution N85.3
venous (passive) I87.8
viscera R68.89
Congestive —*see* Congestion
Conical
cervix (hypertrophic elongation) N88.4
cornea —*see* Keratoconus
teeth K00.2
Conjoined twins Q89.4
Conjugal maladjustment Z63.0
involving divorce or estrangement Z63.5
Conjunctiva —*see* condition
Conjunctivitis (staphylococcal) (streptococcal) NOS H10.9
Acanthamoeba B60.12
acute H10.3-
atopic H10.1-
chemical —*see also* Corrosion, cornea H10.21-
mucopurulent H10.02-
follicular H10.01-
pseudomembranous H10.22-
serous except viral H10.23-
viral —*see* Conjunctivitis, viral
toxic H10.21-
adenoviral (acute) (follicular) B30.1
allergic (acute) —*see* Conjunctivitis, acute, atopic
chronic H10.45
vernal H10.44
anaphylactic —*see* Conjunctivitis, acute, atopic
Apollo B30.3
atopic (acute) —*see* Conjunctivitis, acute, atopic
Béal's B30.2
blennorrhagic (gonococcal) (neonatorum) A54.31
chemical (acute) —*see also* Corrosion, cornea H10.21-
chlamydial A74.0
due to trachoma A71.1
neonatal P39.1

Conjunctivitis *(Continued)*
chronic (nodosa) (petrificans) (phlyctenular) H10.40-
allergic H10.45
vernal H10.44
follicular H10.43-
giant papillary H10.41-
simple H10.42-
vernal H10.44
coxsackievirus 24 B30.3
diphtheritic A36.86
due to
dust —*see* Conjunctivitis, acute, atopic
filariasis B74.9
mucocutaneous leishmaniasis B55.2
enterovirus type 70 (hemorrhagic) B30.3
epidemic (viral) B30.9
hemorrhagic B30.3
gonococcal (neonatorum) A54.31
granular (trachomatous) A71.1
sequelae (late effect) B94.0
hemorrhagic (acute) (epidemic) B30.3
herpes zoster B02.31
in (due to)
Acanthamoeba B60.12
adenovirus (acute) (follicular) B30.1
Chlamydia A74.0
coxsackievirus 24 B30.3
diphtheria A36.86
enterovirus type 70 (hemorrhagic) B30.3
filariasis B74.9
gonococci A54.31
herpes (simplex) virus B00.53
zoster B02.31
infectious disease NEC B99
meningococci A39.89
mucocutaneous leishmaniasis B55.2
rosacea L71.9
syphilis (late) A52.71
zoster B02.31
inclusion A74.0
infantile P39.1
gonococcal A54.31
Koch-Weeks' —*see* Conjunctivitis, acute, mucopurulent
light —*see* Conjunctivitis, acute, atopic
ligneous —*see* Blepharoconjunctivitis, ligneous
meningococcal A39.89
mucopurulent —*see* Conjunctivitis, acute, mucopurulent
neonatal P39.1
gonococcal A54.31
Newcastle B30.8
of Béal B30.2
parasitic
filariasis B74.9
mucocutaneous leishmaniasis B55.2
Parinaud's H10.89
petrificans H10.89
rosacea L71.9
specified NEC H10.89
swimming-pool B30.1
trachomatous A71.1
acute A71.0
sequelae (late effect) B94.0
traumatic NEC H10.89
tuberculous A18.59
tularemic A21.1
tularensis A21.1
viral B30.9
due to
adenovirus B30.1
enterovirus B30.3
specified NEC B30.8
Conjunctivochalasis H11.82-
Connective tissue —*see* condition
Conn's syndrome E26.01
Conradi (-Hunermann) **disease** Q77.3
Consanguinity Z84.3
counseling Z71.89

Conscious simulation (of illness) Z76.5
Consecutive —*see* condition
Consolidation lung (base) —*see* Pneumonia, lobar
Constipation (atonic) (neurogenic) (simple) (spastic) K59.00
  chronic K59.09 ◀
    idiopathic K59.04 ◀
  drug-induced K59.03 ◀
  functional K59.04 ◀
  outlet dysfunction K59.02
  psychogenic F45.8
  slow transit K59.01
  specified NEC K59.09
Constitutional —*see also* condition
  substandard F60.7
Constitutionally substandard F60.7
Constriction —*see also* Stricture
  auditory canal —*see* Stenosis, external ear canal
  bronchial J98.09
  duodenum K31.5
  esophagus K22.2
  external
    abdomen, abdominal (wall) S30.841
    alveolar process S00.542
    ankle S90.54-
    antecubital space —*see* Constriction, external, forearm
    arm (upper) S40.84-
    auricle —*see* Constriction, external, ear
    axilla —*see* Constriction, external, arm
    back, lower S30.840
    breast S20.14-
    brow S00.84
    buttock S30.840
    calf —*see* Constriction, external, leg
    canthus —*see* Constriction, external, eyelid
    cheek S00.84
      internal S00.542
    chest wall —*see* Constriction, external, thorax
    chin S00.84
    clitoris S30.844
    costal region —*see* Constriction, external, thorax
    digit (s)
      foot —*see* Constriction, external, toe
      hand —*see* Constriction, external, finger
    ear S00.44-
    elbow S50.34-
    epididymis S30.843
    epigastric region S30.841
    esophagus, cervical S10.14
    eyebrow —*see* Constriction, external, eyelid
    eyelid S00.24-
    face S00.84
    finger (s) S60.44-
      index S60.44-
      little S60.44-
      middle S60.44-
      ring S60.44-
    flank S30.841
    foot (except toe (s) alone) S90.84-
      toe —*see* Constriction, external, toe
    forearm S50.84-
      elbow only —*see* Constriction, external, elbow
    forehead S00.84
    genital organs, external
      female S30.846
      male S30.845
    groin S30.841
    gum S00.542
    hand S60.54-
    head S00.94
      ear —*see* Constriction, external, ear
      eyelid —*see* Constriction, external, eyelid
      lip S00.541
      nose S00.34
      oral cavity S00.542
Constriction *(Continued)*
  external *(Continued)*
    head *(Continued)*
      scalp S00.04
      specified site NEC S00.84
    heel —*see* Constriction, external, foot
    hip S70.24-
    inguinal region S30.841
    interscapular region S20.449
    jaw S00.84
    knee S80.24-
    labium (majus) (minus) S30.844
    larynx S10.14
    leg (lower) S80.84-
      knee —*see* Constriction, external, knee
      upper —*see* Constriction, external, thigh
    lip S00.541
    lower back S30.840
    lumbar region S30.840
    malar region S00.84
    mammary —*see* Constriction, external, breast
    mastoid region S00.84
    mouth S00.542
    nail
      finger —*see* Constriction, external, finger
      toe —*see* Constriction, external, toe
    nasal S00.34
    neck S10.94
      specified site NEC S10.84
      throat S10.14
    nose S00.34
    occipital region S00.04
    oral cavity S00.542
    orbital region —*see* Constriction, external, eyelid
    palate S00.542
    palm —*see* Constriction, external, hand
    parietal region S00.04
    pelvis S30.840
    penis S30.842
    perineum
      female S30.844
      male S30.840
    periocular area —*see* Constriction, external, eyelid
    phalanges
      finger —*see* Constriction, external, finger
      toe —*see* Constriction, external, toe
    pharynx S10.14
    pinna —*see* Constriction, external, ear
    popliteal space —*see* Constriction, external, knee
    prepuce S30.842
    pubic region S30.840
    pudendum
      female S30.846
      male S30.845
    sacral region S30.840
    scalp S00.04
    scapular region —*see* Constriction, external, shoulder
    scrotum S30.843
    shin —*see* Constriction, external, leg
    shoulder S40.24-
    sternal region S20.349
    submaxillary region S00.84
    submental region S00.84
    subungual
      finger (s) —*see* Constriction, external, finger
      toe (s) —*see* Constriction, external, toe
    supraclavicular fossa S10.84
    supraorbital S00.84
    temple S00.84
    temporal region S00.84
    testis S30.843
    thigh S70.34-
    thorax, thoracic (wall) S20.94
      back S20.44-
      front S20.34-
Constriction *(Continued)*
  external *(Continued)*
    throat S10.14
    thumb S60.34-
    toe (s) (lesser) S90.44-
      great S90.44-
    tongue S00.542
    trachea S10.14
    tunica vaginalis S30.843
    uvula S00.542
    vagina S30.844
    vulva S30.844
    wrist S60.84-
  gallbladder —*see* Obstruction, gallbladder
  intestine —*see* Obstruction, intestine
  larynx J38.6
    congenital Q31.8
      specified NEC Q31.8
      subglottic Q31.1
  organ or site, congenital NEC —*see* Atresia, by site
  prepuce (acquired) (congenital) N47.1
  pylorus (adult hypertrophic) K31.1
    congenital or infantile Q40.0
    newborn Q40.0
  ring dystocia (uterus) O62.4
  spastic —*see also* Spasm
    ureter N13.5
  ureter N13.5
    with infection N13.6
  urethra —*see* Stricture, urethra
  visual field (peripheral) (functional) —*see* Defect, visual field
Constrictive —*see* condition
Consultation
  without complaint or sickness Z71.9
    feared complaint unfounded Z71.1
    specified reason NEC Z71.89
  medical —*see* Counseling, medical
  religious Z71.81
  specified reason NEC Z71.89
  spiritual Z71.81
Consumption —*see* Tuberculosis
Contact (with) —*see also* Exposure (to)
  acariasis Z20.7
  AIDS virus Z20.6
  air pollution Z77.110
  algae and algae toxins Z77.121
  algae bloom Z77.121
  anthrax Z20.810
  aromatic (hazardous) compounds NEC Z77.028
  aromatic amines Z77.020
  aromatic dyes NOS Z77.028
  arsenic Z77.010
  asbestos Z77.090
  bacterial disease NEC Z20.818
  benzene Z77.021
  blue-green algae bloom Z77.121
  body fluids (potentially hazardous) Z77.21
  brown tide Z77.121
  chemicals (chiefly nonmedicinal) (hazardous) NEC Z77.098
  cholera Z20.09
  chromium compounds Z77.018
  communicable disease Z20.9
    bacterial NEC Z20.818
    specified NEC Z20.89
    viral NEC Z20.828
  cyanobacteria bloom Z77.121
  dyes Z77.098
  Escherichia coli (E. coli) Z20.01
  fiberglass —*see* Table of Drugs and Chemicals, fiberglass
  German measles Z20.4
  gonorrhea Z20.2
  hazardous metals NEC Z77.018
  hazardous substances NEC Z77.29
  hazards in the physical environment NEC Z77.128
  hazards to health NEC Z77.9

◀ New ◀ Revised ~~deleted~~ Deleted

Contact *(Continued)*
HIV Z20.6
HTLV-III/LAV Z20.6
human immunodeficiency virus (HIV) Z20.6
infection Z20.9
specified NEC Z20.89
infestation (parasitic) NEC Z20.7
intestinal infectious disease NEC Z20.09
Escherichia coli (E. coli) Z20.01
lead Z77.011
meningococcus Z20.811
mold (toxic) Z77.120
nickel dust Z77.018
noise Z77.122
parasitic disease Z20.7
pediculosis Z20.7
pfiesteria piscicida Z77.121
poliomyelitis Z20.89
pollution
air Z77.110
environmental NEC Z77.118
soil Z77.112
water Z77.111
polycyclic aromatic hydrocarbons Z77.028
rabies Z20.3
radiation, naturally occurring NEC Z77.123
radon Z77.123
red tide (Florida) Z77.121
rubella Z20.4
sexually-transmitted disease Z20.2
smallpox (laboratory) Z20.89
syphilis Z20.2
tuberculosis Z20.1
uranium Z77.012
varicella Z20.820
venereal disease Z20.2
viral disease NEC Z20.828
viral hepatitis Z20.5
water pollution Z77.111
Contamination, food —*see* Intoxication, foodborne
Contraception, contraceptive
advice Z30.09
counseling Z30.09
device (intrauterine) (in situ) Z97.5
causing menorrhagia T83.83
checking Z30.431
complications —*see* Complications, intrauterine, contraceptive device
in place Z97.5
initial prescription Z30.014
reinsertion Z30.433
removal Z30.432
replacement Z30.433
emergency (postcoital) Z30.012
initial prescription Z30.019
barrier Z30.018 ◀
diaphragm Z30.018 ◀
injectable Z30.013
intrauterine device Z30.014
pills Z30.011
postcoital (emergency) Z30.012
specified type NEC Z30.018
subdermal implantable Z30.017 ⟸
transdermal patch hormonal Z30.016 ◀
vaginal ring hormonal Z30.015 ◀
maintenance Z30.40
barrier Z30.49 ◀
diaphragm Z30.49 ◀
examination Z30.8
injectable Z30.42
intrauterine device Z30.431
pills Z30.41
specified type NEC Z30.49
subdermal implantable Z30.46 ⟸
transdermal patch hormonal Z30.45 ◀
vaginal ring hormonal Z30.44 ◀
management Z30.9
specified NEC Z30.8
postcoital (emergency) Z30.012
prescription Z30.019
repeat Z30.40
Contraception, contraceptive *(Continued)*
sterilization Z30.2
surveillance (drug) —*see* Contraception, maintenance
Contraction (s), contracture, contracted
Achilles tendon —*see also* Short, tendon, Achilles
congenital Q66.89
amputation stump (surgical) (flexion) (late) next proximal joint T87.89
anus K59.8
bile duct (common) (hepatic) K83.8
bladder N32.89
neck or sphincter N32.0
bowel, cecum, colon or intestine, any part —*see* Obstruction, intestine
Braxton Hicks —*see* False, labor
breast implant, capsular T85.44
bronchial J98.09
burn (old) —*see* Cicatrix
cervix —*see* Stricture, cervix
cicatricial —*see* Cicatrix
conjunctiva, trachomatous, active A71.1
sequelae (late effect) B94.0
Dupuytren's M72.0
eyelid —*see* Disorder, eyelid function
fascia (lata) (postural) M72.8
Dupuytren's M72.0
palmar M72.0
plantar M72.2
finger NEC —*see also* Deformity, finger
congenital Q68.1
joint —*see* Contraction, joint, hand
flaccid —*see* Contraction, paralytic
gallbladder K82.0
heart valve —*see* Endocarditis
hip —*see* Contraction, joint, hip
hourglass
bladder N32.89
congenital Q64.79
gallbladder K82.0
congenital Q44.1
stomach K31.89
congenital Q40.2
psychogenic F45.8
uterus (complicating delivery) O62.4
hysterical F44.4
internal os —*see* Stricture, cervix
joint (abduction) (acquired) (adduction) (flexion) (rotation) M24.50
ankle M24.57-
congenital NEC Q68.8
hip Q65.89
elbow M24.52-
foot joint M24.57-
hand joint M24.54-
hip M24.55-
congenital Q65.89
hysterical F44.4
knee M24.56-
shoulder M24.51-
wrist M24.53-
kidney (granular) (secondary) N26.9
congenital Q63.8
hydronephritic —*see* Hydronephrosis
Page N26.2
pyelonephritic —*see* Pyelitis, chronic
tuberculous A18.11
ligament —*see also* Disorder, ligament
congenital Q79.8
muscle (postinfective) (postural) NEC M62.40
with contracture of joint —*see* Contraction, joint
ankle M62.47-
congenital Q79.8
sternocleidomastoid Q68.0
extraocular —*see* Strabismus
eye (extrinsic) —*see* Strabismus
foot M62.47-
forearm M62.43-
hand M62.44-
Contraction, contracture, contracted *(Continued)*
muscle *(Continued)*
hysterical F44.4
ischemic (Volkmann's) T79.6
lower leg M62.46-
multiple sites M62.49
pelvic region M62.45-
posttraumatic —*see* Strabismus, paralytic
psychogenic F45.8
conversion reaction F44.4
shoulder region M62.41-
specified site NEC M62.48
thigh M62.45-
upper arm M62.42-
neck —*see* Torticollis
ocular muscle —*see* Strabismus
organ or site, congenital NEC —*see* Atresia, by site
outlet (pelvis) —*see* Contraction, pelvis
palmar fascia M72.0
paralytic
joint —*see* Contraction, joint
muscle —*see also* Contraction, muscle NEC
ocular —*see* Strabismus, paralytic
pelvis (acquired) (general) M95.5
with disproportion (fetopelvic) O33.1
causing obstructed labor O65.1
inlet O33.2
mid-cavity O33.3
outlet O33.3
plantar fascia M72.2
premature
atrium I49.1
auriculoventricular I49.49
heart I49.49
junctional I49.2
supraventricular I49.1
ventricular I49.3
prostate N42.89
pylorus NEC —*see also* Pylorospasm
psychogenic F45.8
rectum, rectal (sphincter) K59.8
ring (Bandl's) (complicating delivery) O62.4
scar —*see* Cicatrix
spine —*see* Dorsopathy, deforming
sternocleidomastoid (muscle), congenital Q68.0
stomach K31.89
hourglass K31.89
congenital Q40.2
psychogenic F45.8
psychogenic F45.8
tendon (sheath) M62.40
with contracture of joint —*see* Contraction, joint
Achilles —*see* Short, tendon, Achilles
ankle M62.47-
Achilles —*see* Short, tendon, Achilles
foot M62.47-
forearm M62.43-
hand M62.44-
lower leg M62.46-
multiple sites M62.49
neck M62.48
pelvic region M62.45-
shoulder region M62.41-
specified site NEC M62.48
thigh M62.45-
thorax M62.48
trunk M62.48
upper arm M62.42-
toe —*see* Deformity, toe, specified NEC
ureterovesical orifice (postinfectional) N13.5
with infection N13.6
urethra —*see also* Stricture, urethra
orifice N32.0
uterus N85.8
abnormal NEC O62.9
clonic (complicating delivery) O62.4
dyscoordinate (complicating delivery) O62.4

Contraction, contracture, contracted *(Continued)*
uterus *(Continued)*
hourglass (complicating delivery) O62.4
hypertonic O62.4
hypotonic NEC O62.2
inadequate
primary O62.0
secondary O62.1
incoordinate (complicating delivery) O62.4
poor O62.2
tetanic (complicating delivery) O62.4
vagina (outlet) N89.5
vesical N32.89
neck or urethral orifice N32.0
visual field —*see* Defect, visual field, generalized
Volkmann's (ischemic) T79.6
Contusion (skin surface intact) T14.8
abdomen, abdominal (muscle) (wall) S30.1
adnexa, eye NEC S05.8X-
adrenal gland S37.812
alveolar process S00.532
ankle S90.0-
antecubital space —*see* Contusion, forearm
anus S30.3
arm (upper) S40.02-
lower (with elbow) —*see* Contusion, forearm
auditory canal —*see* Contusion, ear
auricle —*see* Contusion, ear
axilla —*see* Contusion, arm, upper
back —*see also* Contusion, thorax, back
lower S30.0
bile duct S36.13
bladder S37.22
bone NEC T14.8
brain (diffuse) —*see* Injury, intracranial, diffuse
focal —*see* Injury, intracranial, focal
brainstem S06.38-
breast S20.0-
broad ligament S37.892
brow S00.83
buttock S30.0
canthus, eye S00.1-
cauda equina S34.3
cerebellar, traumatic S06.37-
cerebral S06.33-
left side S06.32-
right side S06.31-
cheek S00.83
internal S00.532
chest (wall) —*see* Contusion, thorax
chin S00.83
clitoris S30.23
colon —*see* Injury, intestine, large, contusion
common bile duct S36.13
conjunctiva S05.1-
with foreign body (in conjunctival sac) —*see* Foreign body, conjunctival sac
conus medullaris (spine) S34.139
cornea —*see* Contusion, eyeball
with foreign body —*see* Foreign body, cornea
corpus cavernosum S30.21
cortex (brain) (cerebral) —*see* Injury, intracranial, diffuse
focal —*see* Injury, intracranial, focal
costal region —*see* Contusion, thorax
cystic duct S36.13
diaphragm S27.802
duodenum S36.420
ear S00.43-
elbow S50.0-
with forearm —*see* Contusion, forearm
epididymis S30.22
epigastric region S30.1
epiglottis S10.0
esophagus (thoracic) S27.812
cervical S10.0
eyeball S05.1-
Contusion *(Continued)*
eyebrow S00.1-
eyelid (and periocular area) S00.1-
face NEC S00.83
fallopian tube S37.529
bilateral S37.522
unilateral S37.521
femoral triangle S30.1
finger (s) S60.00
with damage to nail (matrix) S60.10
index S60.02-
with damage to nail S60.12-
little S60.05-
with damage to nail S60.15-
middle S60.03-
with damage to nail S60.13-
ring S60.04-
with damage to nail S60.14-
thumb —*see* Contusion, thumb
flank S30.1
foot (except toe (s) alone) S90.3-
toe —*see* Contusion, toe
forearm S50.1-
elbow only —*see* Contusion, elbow
forehead S00.83
gallbladder S36.122
genital organs, external
female S30.202
male S30.201
globe (eye) —*see* Contusion, eyeball
groin S30.1
gum S00.532
hand S60.22-
finger (s) —*see* Contusion, finger
wrist —*see* Contusion, wrist
head S00.93
ear —*see* Contusion, ear
eyelid —*see* Contusion, eyelid
lip S00.531
nose S00.33
oral cavity S00.532
scalp S00.03
specified part NEC S00.83
heart —*see also* Injury, heart S26.91 ◀
heel —*see* Contusion, foot
hepatic duct S36.13
hip S70.0-
ileum S36.428
iliac region S30.1
inguinal region S30.1
interscapular region S20.229
intra-abdominal organ S36.92
colon —*see* Injury, intestine, large, contusion
liver S36.112
pancreas —*see* Contusion, pancreas
rectum S36.62
small intestine —*see* Injury, intestine, small, contusion
specified organ NEC S36.892
spleen —*see* Contusion, spleen
stomach S36.32
iris (eye) —*see* Contusion, eyeball
jaw S00.83
jejunum S36.428
kidney S37.01-
major (greater than 2 cm) S37.02-
minor (less than 2 cm) S37.01-
knee S80.0-
labium (majus) (minus) S30.23
lacrimal apparatus, gland or sac S05.8X-
larynx S10.0
leg (lower) S80.1-
knee —*see* Contusion, knee
lens —*see* Contusion, eyeball
lip S00.531
liver S36.112
lower back S30.0
lumbar region S30.0
lung S27.329
bilateral S27.322
unilateral S27.321
Contusion *(Continued)*
malar region S00.83
mastoid region S00.83
membrane, brain —*see* Injury, intracranial, diffuse
focal —*see* Injury, intracranial, focal
mesentery S36.892
mesosalpinx S37.892
mouth S00.532
muscle —*see* Contusion, by site
nail
finger —*see* Contusion, finger, with damage to nail
toe —*see* Contusion, toe, with damage to nail
nasal S00.33
neck S10.93
specified site NEC S10.83
throat S10.0
nerve —*see* Injury, nerve
newborn P54.5
nose S00.33
occipital
lobe (brain) —*see* Injury, intracranial, diffuse
focal —*see* Injury, intracranial, focal
region (scalp) S00.03
orbit (region) (tissues) S05.1-
ovary S37.429
bilateral S37.422
unilateral S37.421
palate S00.532
pancreas S36.229
body S36.221
head S36.220
tail S36.222
parietal
lobe (brain) —*see* Injury, intracranial, diffuse
focal —*see* Injury, intracranial, focal
region (scalp) S00.03
pelvic organ S37.92
adrenal gland S37.812
bladder S37.22
fallopian tube —*see* Contusion, fallopian tube
kidney —*see* Contusion, kidney
ovary —*see* Contusion, ovary
prostate S37.822
specified organ NEC S37.892
ureter S37.12
urethra S37.32
uterus S37.62
pelvis S30.0
penis S30.21
perineum
female S30.23
male S30.0
periocular area S00.1-
peritoneum S36.81
periurethral tissue —*see* Contusion, urethra
pharynx S10.0
pinna —*see* Contusion, ear
popliteal space —*see* Contusion, knee
prepuce S30.21
prostate S37.822
pubic region S30.1
pudendum
female S30.202
male S30.201
quadriceps femoris —*see* Contusion, thigh
rectum S36.62
retroperitoneum S36.892
round ligament S37.892
sacral region S30.0
scalp S00.03
due to birth injury P12.3
scapular region —*see* Contusion, shoulder
sclera —*see* Contusion, eyeball

Contusion *(Continued)*
scrotum S30.22
seminal vesicle S37.892
shoulder S40.01-
skin NEC T14.8
small intestine —*see* Injury, intestine, small, contusion
spermatic cord S30.22
spinal cord —*see* Injury, spinal cord, by region
cauda equina S34.3
conus medullaris S34.139
spleen S36.029
major S36.021
minor S36.020
sternal region S20.219
stomach S36.32
subconjunctival S05.1-
subcutaneous NEC T14.8
submaxillary region S00.83
submental region S00.83
subperiosteal NEC T14.8
subungual
finger —*see* Contusion, finger, with damage to nail
toe —*see* Contusion, toe, with damage to nail
supraclavicular fossa S10.83
supraorbital S00.83
suprarenal gland S37.812
temple (region) S00.83
temporal
lobe (brain) —*see* Injury, intracranial, diffuse
focal —*see* Injury, intracranial, focal
region S00.83
testis S30.22
thigh S70.1-
thorax (wall) S20.20
back S20.22-
front S20.21-
throat S10.0
thumb S60.01-
with damage to nail S60.11-
toe (s) (lesser) S90.12-
with damage to nail S90.22-
great S90.11-
with damage to nail S90.21-
specified type NEC S90.221
tongue S00.532
trachea (cervical) S10.0
thoracic S27.52
tunica vaginalis S30.22
tympanum, tympanic membrane —*see* Contusion, ear
ureter S37.12
urethra S37.32
urinary organ NEC S37.892
uterus S37.62
uvula S00.532
vagina S30.23
vas deferens S37.892
vesical S37.22
vocal cord (s) S10.0
vulva S30.23
wrist S60.21-
Conus (congenital) (any type) Q14.8
cornea —*see* Keratoconus
medullaris syndrome G95.81
Conversion hysteria, neurosis or reaction F44.9
Converter, tuberculosis (test reaction) R76.11
Conviction (legal), anxiety concerning Z65.0
with imprisonment Z65.1
Convulsions (idiopathic) —*see also* Seizure(s) R56.9
apoplectiform (cerebral ischemia) I67.82
~~benign neonatal (familial) —see Epilepsy, generalized, idiopathic~~
dissociative F44.5
epileptic —*see* Epilepsy
epileptiform, epileptoid —*see* Seizure, epileptiform

Convulsions *(Continued)*
ether (anesthetic) —*see* Table of Drugs and Chemicals, by drug
febrile R56.00
with status epilepticus G40.901
complex R56.01
with status epilepticus G40.901
simple R56.00
hysterical F44.5
infantile P90
epilepsy —*see* Epilepsy
jacksonian —*see* Epilepsy, localization-related, symptomatic, with simple partial seizures
myoclonic G25.3
~~neonatal, benign (familial) —see Epilepsy, generalized, idiopathic~~
newborn P90
obstetrical (nephritic) (uremic) —*see* Eclampsia
paretic A52.17
post traumatic R56.1
psychomotor —*see* Epilepsy, localization-related, symptomatic, with complex partial seizures
recurrent R56.9
reflex R25.8
scarlatinal A38.8
tetanus, tetanic —*see* Tetanus
thymic E32.8
Convulsive —*see also* Convulsions
Cooley's anemia D56.1
Coolie itch B76.9
Cooper's
disease —*see* Mastopathy, cystic
hernia —*see* Hernia, abdomen, specified site NEC
Copra itch B88.0
Coprophagy F50.89 ⬅
Coprophobia F40.298
Coproporphyria, hereditary E80.29
Cor
biloculare Q20.8
bovis, bovinum —*see* Hypertrophy, cardiac
pulmonale (chronic) I27.81
acute I26.09
triatriatum, triatrium Q24.2
triloculare Q20.8
biatrium Q20.4
biventriculare Q21.1
Corbus' disease (gangrenous balanitis) N48.1
Cord —*see also* condition
around neck (tightly) (with compression) complicating delivery O69.1
bladder G95.89
tabetic A52.19
Cordis ectopia Q24.8
Corditis (spermatic) N49.1
Corectopia Q13.2
Cori's disease (glycogen storage) E74.03
Corkhandler's disease or lung J67.3
Corkscrew esophagus K22.4
Corkworker's disease or lung J67.3
Corn (infected) L84
Cornea —*see also* condition
donor Z52.5
plana Q13.4
Cornelia de Lange syndrome Q87.1
Cornu cutaneum L85.8
Cornual gestation or pregnancy O00.80 ⬅
with intrauterine pregnancy O00.81 ◀
Coronary (artery) —*see* condition
Coronavirus, as cause of disease classified elsewhere B97.29
SARS-associated B97.21
Corpora —*see also* condition
amylacea, prostate N42.89
cavernosa —*see* condition
Corpulence —*see* Obesity
Corpus —*see* condition
Corrected transposition Q20.5

Corrosion (injury) (acid) (caustic) (chemical) (lime) (external) (internal) T30.4
abdomen, abdominal (muscle) (wall) T21.42
first degree T21.52
second degree T21.62
third degree T21.72
above elbow T22.439
first degree T22.539
left T22.432
first degree T22.532
second degree T22.632
third degree T22.732
right T22.431
first degree T22.531
second degree T22.631
third degree T22.731
second degree T22.639
third degree T22.739
alimentary tract NEC T28.7
ankle T25.419
first degree T25.519
left T25.412
first degree T25.512
second degree T25.612
third degree T25.712
multiple with foot —*see* Corrosion, lower, limb, multiple, ankle and foot
right T25.411
first degree T25.511
second degree T25.611
third degree T25.711
second degree T25.619
third degree T25.719
anus —*see* Corrosion, buttock
arm (s) (meaning upper limb (s)) —*see* Corrosion, upper limb
axilla T22.449
first degree T22.549
left T22.442
first degree T22.542
second degree T22.642
third degree T22.742
right T22.441
first degree T22.541
second degree T22.641
third degree T22.741
second degree T22.649
third degree T22.749
back (lower) T21.44
first degree T21.54
second degree T21.64
third degree T21.74
upper T21.43
first degree T21.53
second degree T21.63
third degree T21.73
blisters - code as Corrosion, second degree, by site
breast (s) —*see* Corrosion, chest wall
buttock (s) T21.45
first degree T21.55
second degree T21.65
third degree T21.75
calf T24.439
first degree T24.539
left T24.432
first degree T24.532
second degree T24.632
third degree T24.732
right T24.431
first degree T24.531
second degree T24.631
third degree T24.731
second degree T24.639
third degree T24.739
canthus (eye) —*see* Corrosion, eyelid
cervix T28.8
cheek T20.46
first degree T20.56
second degree T20.66
third degree T20.76

C

◀ New ⬅ Revised ~~deleted~~ Deleted

Corrosion *(Continued)*
chest wall T21.41
first degree T21.51
second degree T21.61
third degree T21.71
chin T20.43
first degree T20.53
second degree T20.63
third degree T20.73
colon T28.7
conjunctiva (and cornea) —*see* Corrosion, cornea
cornea (and conjunctiva) T26.6-
deep necrosis of underlying tissue - code as Corrosion, third degree, by site
dorsum of hand T23.469
first degree T23.569
left T23.462
first degree T23.562
second degree T23.662
third degree T23.762
right T23.461
first degree T23.561
second degree T23.661
third degree T23.761
second degree T23.669
third degree T23.769
ear (auricle) (external) (canal) T20.41
drum T28.91
first degree T20.51
second degree T20.61
third degree T20.71
elbow T22.429
first degree T22.529
left T22.422
first degree T22.522
second degree T22.622
third degree T22.722
right T22.421
first degree T22.521
second degree T22.621
third degree T22.721
second degree T22.629
third degree T22.729
entire body —*see* Corrosion, multiple body regions
epidermal loss - code as Corrosion, second degree, by site
epiglottis T27.4
erythema, erythematous - code as Corrosion, first degree, by site
esophagus T28.6
extent (percentage of body surface)
less than 10 percent T32.0
10-19 percent (0-9 percent third degree) T32.10
with 10-19 percent third degree T32.11
20-29 percent (0-9 percent third degree) T32.20
with
10-19 percent third degree T32.21
20-29 percent third degree T32.22
30-39 percent (0-9 percent third degree) T32.30
with
10-19 percent third degree T32.31
20-29 percent third degree T32.32
30-39 percent third degree T32.33
40-49 percent (0-9 percent third degree) T32.40
with
10-19 percent third degree T32.41
20-29 percent third degree T32.42
30-39 percent third degree T32.43
40-49 percent third degree T32.44
50-59 percent (0-9 percent third degree) T32.50
with
10-19 percent third degree T32.51
20-29 percent third degree T32.52

Corrosion *(Continued)*
extent *(Continued)*
50-59 percent *(Continued)*
with *(Continued)*
30-39 percent third degree T32.53
40-49 percent third degree T32.54
50-59 percent third degree T32.55
60-69 percent (0-9 percent third degree) T32.60
with
10-19 percent third degree T32.61
20-29 percent third degree T32.62
30-39 percent third degree T32.63
40-49 percent third degree T32.64
50-59 percent third degree T32.65
60-69 percent third degree T32.66
70-79 percent (0-9 percent third degree) T32.70
with
10-19 percent third degree T32.71
20-29 percent third degree T32.72
30-39 percent third degree T32.73
40-49 percent third degree T32.74
50-59 percent third degree T32.75
60-69 percent third degree T32.76
70-79 percent third degree T32.77
80-89 percent (0-9 percent third degree) T32.80
with
10-19 percent third degree T32.81
20-29 percent third degree T32.82
30-39 percent third degree T32.83
40-49 percent third degree T32.84
50-59 percent third degree T32.85
60-69 percent third degree T32.86
70-79 percent third degree T32.87
80-89 percent third degree T32.88
90 percent or more (0-9 percent third degree) T32.90
with
10-19 percent third degree T32.91
20-29 percent third degree T32.92
30-39 percent third degree T32.93
40-49 percent third degree T32.94
50-59 percent third degree T32.95
60-69 percent third degree T32.96
70-79 percent third degree T32.97
80-89 percent third degree T32.98
90-99 percent third degree T32.99
extremity —*see* Corrosion, limb
eye (s) and adnexa T26.9-
with resulting rupture and destruction of eyeball T26.7-
conjunctival sac —*see* Corrosion, cornea
cornea —*see* Corrosion, cornea
lid —*see* Corrosion, eyelid
periocular area —*see* Corrosion eyelid
specified site NEC T26.8-
eyeball —*see* Corrosion, eye
eyelid (s) T26.5-
face —*see* Corrosion, head
finger T23.429
first degree T23.529
left T23.422
first degree T23.522
second degree T23.622
third degree T23.722
multiple sites (without thumb) T23.439
with thumb T23.449
first degree T23.549
left T23.442
first degree T23.542
second degree T23.642
third degree T23.742
right T23.441
first degree T23.541
second degree T23.641
third degree T23.741
second degree T23.649
third degree T23.749

Corrosion *(Continued)*
finger *(Continued)*
multiple sites *(Continued)*
first degree T23.539
left T23.432
first degree T23.532
second degree T23.632
third degree T23.732
right T23.431
first degree T23.531
second degree T23.631
third degree T23.731
second degree T23.639
third degree T23.739
right T23.421
first degree T23.521
second degree T23.621
third degree T23.721
second degree T23.629
third degree T23.729
flank —*see* Corrosion, abdomen
foot T25.429
first degree T25.529
left T25.422
first degree T25.522
second degree T25.622
third degree T25.722
multiple with ankle —*see* Corrosion, lower, limb, multiple, ankle and foot
right T25.421
first degree T25.521
second degree T25.621
third degree T25.721
second degree T25.629
third degree T25.729
forearm T22.419
first degree T22.519
left T22.412
first degree T22.512
second degree T22.612
third degree T22.712
right T22.411
first degree T22.511
second degree T22.611
third degree T22.711
second degree T22.619
third degree T22.719
forehead T20.46
first degree T20.56
second degree T20.66
third degree T20.76
fourth degree - code as Corrosion, third degree, by site
full thickness skin loss - code as Corrosion, third degree, by site
gastrointestinal tract NEC T28.7
genital organs
external
female T21.47
first degree T21.57
second degree T21.67
third degree T21.77
male T21.46
first degree T21.56
second degree T21.66
third degree T21.76
internal T28.8
groin —*see* Corrosion, abdominal wall
hand (s) T23.409
back —*see* Corrosion, dorsum of hand
finger —*see* Corrosion, finger
first degree T23.509
left T23.402
first degree T23.502
second degree T23.602
third degree T23.702
multiple sites with wrist T23.499
first degree T23.599
left T23.492
first degree T23.592
second degree T23.692
third degree T23.792

Corrosion *(Continued)*
hand (s) *(Continued)*
multiple sites *(Continued)*
right T23.491
first degree T23.591
second degree T23.691
third degree T23.791
second degree T23.699
third degree T23.799
palm —*see* Corrosion, palm
right T23.401
first degree T23.501
second degree T23.601
third degree T23.701
second degree T23.609
third degree T23.709
thumb —*see* Corrosion, thumb
head (and face) (and neck) T20.40
cheek —*see* Corrosion, cheek
chin —*see* Corrosion, chin
ear —*see* Corrosion, ear
eye (s) only —*see* Corrosion, eye
first degree T20.50
forehead —*see* Corrosion, forehead
lip —*see* Corrosion, lip
multiple sites T20.49
first degree T20.59
second degree T20.69
third degree T20.79
neck —*see* Corrosion, neck
nose —*see* Corrosion, nose
scalp —*see* Corrosion, scalp
second degree T20.60
third degree T20.70
hip (s) —*see* Corrosion, lower, limb
inhalation —*see* Corrosion, respiratory tract
internal organ (s) (*see also* Corrosion, by site) T28.90
alimentary tract T28.7
esophagus T28.6
esophagus T28.6
genitourinary T28.8
mouth T28.5
pharynx T28.5
specified organ NEC T28.99
interscapular region —*see* Corrosion, back, upper
intestine (large) (small) T28.7
knee T24.429
first degree T24.529
left T24.422
first degree T24.522
second degree T24.622
third degree T24.722
right T24.421
first degree T24.521
second degree T24.621
third degree T24.721
second degree T24.629
third degree T24.729
labium (majus) (minus) —*see* Corrosion, genital organs, external, female
lacrimal apparatus, duct, gland or sac —*see* Corrosion, eye, specified site NEC
larynx T27.4
with lung T27.5
leg (s) (meaning lower limb (s)) —*see* Corrosion, lower limb
limb (s)
lower —*see* Corrosion, lower, limb
upper —*see* Corrosion, upper limb
lip (s) T20.42
first degree T20.52
second degree T20.62
third degree T20.72
lower
back —*see* Corrosion, back
limb T24.409
ankle —*see* Corrosion, ankle
calf —*see* Corrosion, calf

Corrosion *(Continued)*
lower *(Continued)*
limb *(Continued)*
first degree T24.509
foot —*see* Corrosion, foot
hip —*see* Corrosion, thigh
knee —*see* Corrosion, knee
left T24.402
first degree T24.502
second degree T24.602
third degree T24.702
multiple sites, except ankle and foot T24.499
ankle and foot T25.499
first degree T25.599
left T25.492
first degree T25.592
second degree T25.692
third degree T25.792
right T25.491
first degree T25.591
second degree T25.691
third degree T25.791
second degree T25.699
third degree T25.799
first degree T24.599
left T24.492
first degree T24.592
second degree T24.692
third degree T24.792
right T24.491
first degree T24.591
second degree T24.691
third degree T24.791
second degree T24.699
third degree T24.799
right T24.401
first degree T24.501
second degree T24.601
third degree T24.701
second degree T24.609
thigh —*see* Corrosion, thigh
third degree T24.709
lung (with larynx and trachea) T27.5
mouth T28.5
neck T20.47
first degree T20.57
second degree T20.67
third degree T20.77
nose (septum) T20.44
first degree T20.54
second degree T20.64
third degree T20.74
ocular adnexa —*see* Corrosion, eye
orbit region —*see* Corrosion, eyelid
palm T23.459
first degree T23.559
left T23.452
first degree T23.552
second degree T23.652
third degree T23.752
right T23.451
first degree T23.551
second degree T23.651
third degree T23.751
second degree T23.659
third degree T23.759
partial thickness - code as Corrosion, unspecified degree, by site
pelvis —*see* Corrosion, trunk
penis —*see* Corrosion, genital organs, external, male
perineum
female —*see* Corrosion, genital organs, external, female
male —*see* Corrosion, genital organs, external, male
periocular area —*see* Corrosion, eyelid
pharynx T28.5
rectum T28.7

Corrosion *(Continued)*
respiratory tract T27.7
larynx —*see* Corrosion, larynx
specified part NEC T27.6
trachea —*see* Corrosion, larynx
sac, lacrimal —*see* Corrosion, eye, specified site NEC
scalp T20.45
first degree T20.55
second degree T20.65
third degree T20.75
scapular region T22.469
first degree T22.569
left T22.462
first degree T22.562
second degree T22.662
third degree T22.762
right T22.461
first degree T22.561
second degree T22.661
third degree T22.761
second degree T22.669
third degree T22.769
sclera —*see* Corrosion, eye, specified site NEC
scrotum —*see* Corrosion, genital organs, external, male
shoulder T22.459
first degree T22.559
left T22.452
first degree T22.552
second degree T22.652
third degree T22.752
right T22.451
first degree T22.551
second degree T22.651
third degree T22.751
second degree T22.659
third degree T22.759
stomach T28.7
temple —*see* Corrosion, head
testis —*see* Corrosion, genital organs, external, male
thigh T24.419
first degree T24.519
left T24.412
first degree T24.512
second degree T24.612
third degree T24.712
right T24.411
first degree T24.511
second degree T24.611
third degree T24.711
second degree T24.619
third degree T24.719
thorax (external) —*see* Corrosion, trunk
throat (meaning pharynx) T28.5
thumb (s) T23.419
first degree T23.519
left T23.412
first degree T23.512
second degree T23.612
third degree T23.712
multiple sites with fingers T23.449
first degree T23.549
left T23.442
first degree T23.542
second degree T23.642
third degree T23.742
right T23.441
first degree T23.541
second degree T23.641
third degree T23.741
second degree T23.649
third degree T23.749
right T23.411
first degree T23.511
second degree T23.611
third degree T23.711
second degree T23.619
third degree T23.719

Corrosion *(Continued)*
toe T25.439
first degree T25.539
left T25.432
first degree T25.532
second degree T25.632
third degree T25.732
right T25.431
first degree T25.531
second degree T25.631
third degree T25.731
second degree T25.639
third degree T25.739
tongue T28.5
tonsil (s) T28.5
total body —*see* Corrosion, multiple body regions
trachea T27.4
with lung T27.5
trunk T21.40
abdominal wall —*see* Corrosion, abdominal wall
anus —*see* Corrosion, buttock
axilla —*see* Corrosion, upper limb
back —*see* Corrosion, back
breast —*see* Corrosion, chest wall
buttock —*see* Corrosion, buttock
chest wall —*see* Corrosion, chest wall
first degree T21.50
flank —*see* Corrosion, abdominal wall
genital
female —*see* Corrosion, genital organs, external, female
male —*see* Corrosion, genital organs, external, male
groin —*see* Corrosion, abdominal wall
interscapular region —*see* Corrosion, back, upper
labia —*see* Corrosion, genital organs, external, female
lower back —*see* Corrosion, back
penis —*see* Corrosion, genital organs, external, male
perineum
female —*see* Corrosion, genital organs, external, female
male —*see* Corrosion, genital organs, external, male
scapular region —*see* Corrosion, upper limb
scrotum —*see* Corrosion, genital organs, external, male
second degree T21.60
shoulder —*see* Corrosion, upper limb
specified site NEC T21.49
first degree T21.59
second degree T21.69
third degree T21.79
testes —*see* Corrosion, genital organs, external, male
third degree T21.70
upper back —*see* Corrosion, back, upper
vagina T28.8
vulva —*see* Corrosion, genital organs, external, female
unspecified site with extent of body surface involved specified
less than 10 percent T32.0
10-19 percent (0-9 percent third degree) T32.10
with 10-19 percent third degree T32.11
20-29 percent (0-9 percent third degree) T32.20
with
10-19 percent third degree T32.21
20-29 percent third degree T32.22
30-39 percent (0-9 percent third degree) T32.30
with
10-19 percent third degree T32.31
20-29 percent third degree T32.32
30-39 percent third degree T32.33

Corrosion *(Continued)*
unspecified site with extent of body surface involved specified *(Continued)*
40-49 percent (0-9 percent third degree) T32.40
with
10-19 percent third degree T32.41
20-29 percent third degree T32.42
30-39 percent third degree T32.43
40-49 percent third degree T32.44
50-59 percent (0-9 percent third degree) T32.50
with
10-19 percent third degree T32.51
20-29 percent third degree T32.52
30-39 percent third degree T32.53
40-49 percent third degree T32.54
50-59 percent third degree T32.55
60-69 percent (0-9 percent third degree) T32.60
with
10-19 percent third degree T32.61
20-29 percent third degree T32.62
30-39 percent third degree T32.63
40-49 percent third degree T32.64
50-59 percent third degree T32.65
60-69 percent third degree T32.66
70-79 percent (0-9 percent third degree) T32.70
with
10-19 percent third degree T32.71
20-29 percent third degree T32.72
30-39 percent third degree T32.73
40-49 percent third degree T32.74
50-59 percent third degree T32.75
60-69 percent third degree T32.76
70-79 percent third degree T32.77
80-89 percent (0-9 percent third degree) T32.80
with
10-19 percent third degree T32.81
20-29 percent third degree T32.82
30-39 percent third degree T32.83
40-49 percent third degree T32.84
50-59 percent third degree T32.85
60-69 percent third degree T32.86
70-79 percent third degree T32.87
80-89 percent third degree T32.88
90 percent or more (0-9 percent third degree) T32.90
with
10-19 percent third degree T32.91
20-29 percent third degree T32.92
30-39 percent third degree T32.93
40-49 percent third degree T32.94
50-59 percent third degree T32.95
60-69 percent third degree T32.96
70-79 percent third degree T32.97
80-89 percent third degree T32.98
90-99 percent third degree T32.99
upper limb (axilla) (scapular region) T22.40
above elbow —*see* Corrosion, above elbow
axilla —*see* Corrosion, axilla
elbow —*see* Corrosion, elbow
first degree T22.50
forearm —*see* Corrosion, forearm
hand —*see* Corrosion, hand
interscapular region —*see* Corrosion, back, upper
multiple sites T22.499
first degree T22.599
left T22.492
first degree T22.592
second degree T22.692
third degree T22.792
right T22.491
first degree T22.591
second degree T22.691
third degree T22.791
second degree T22.699
third degree T22.799

Corrosion *(Continued)*
upper limb (axilla) (scapular region) *(Continued)*
scapular region —*see* Corrosion, scapular region
second degree T22.60
shoulder —*see* Corrosion, shoulder
third degree T22.70
wrist —*see* Corrosion, hand
uterus T28.8
vagina T28.8
vulva —*see* Corrosion, genital organs, external, female
wrist T23.479
first degree T23.579
left T23.472
first degree T23.572
second degree T23.672
third degree T23.772
multiple sites with hand T23.499
first degree T23.599
left T23.492
first degree T23.592
second degree T23.692
third degree T23.792
right T23.491
first degree T23.591
second degree T23.691
third degree T23.791
second degree T23.699
third degree T23.799
right T23.471
first degree T23.571
second degree T23.671
third degree T23.771
second degree T23.679
third degree T23.779
Corrosive burn —*see* Corrosion
Corsican fever —*see* Malaria
Cortical —*see* condition
Cortico-adrenal —*see* condition
Coryza (acute) J00
with grippe or influenza —*see* Influenza, with, respiratory manifestations NEC
syphilitic
congenital (chronic) A50.05
Costen's syndrome or complex M26.69
Costiveness —*see* Constipation
Costochondritis M94.0
Cot death R99
Cotard's syndrome F22
Cotia virus B08.8
Cotton wool spots (retinal) H35.81
Cotungo's disease —*see* Sciatica
Cough (affected) (chronic) (epidemic) (nervous) R05
with hemorrhage —*see* Hemoptysis
bronchial R05
with grippe or influenza —*see* Influenza, with, respiratory manifestations NEC
functional F45.8
hysterical F45.8
laryngeal, spasmodic R05
psychogenic F45.8
smokers' J41.0
tea taster's B49
Counseling (for) Z71.9
abuse NEC
perpetrator Z69.82
victim Z69.81
alcohol abuser Z71.41
family Z71.42
child abuse
nonparental
perpetrator Z69.021
victim Z69.020
parental
perpetrator Z69.011
victim Z69.010

Counseling *(Continued)*
consanguinity Z71.89
contraceptive Z30.09
dietary Z71.3
drug abuser Z71.51
family member Z71.52
family Z71.89
fertility preservation (prior to cancer therapy) (prior to removal of gonads) Z31.62
for non-attending third party Z71.0
related to sexual behavior or orientation Z70.2
genetic NEC Z31.5
gestational carrier Z31.7 ◀
health (advice) (education) (instruction) —*see* Counseling, medical
human immunodeficiency virus (HIV) Z71.7
impotence Z70.1
insulin pump use Z46.81
medical (for) Z71.9
boarding school resident Z59.3
consanguinity Z71.89
feared complaint and no disease found Z71.1
human immunodeficiency virus (HIV) Z71.7
institutional resident Z59.3
on behalf of another Z71.0
related to sexual behavior or orientation Z70.2
person living alone Z60.2
specified reason NEC Z71.89
natural family planning
procreative Z31.61
to avoid pregnancy Z30.02
perpetrator (of)
abuse NEC Z69.82
child abuse
non-parental Z69.021
parental Z69.011
rape NEC Z69.82
spousal abuse Z69.12
procreative NEC Z31.69
fertility preservation (prior to cancer therapy) (prior to removal of gonads) Z31.62
using natural family planning Z31.61
promiscuity Z70.1
rape victim Z69.81
religious Z71.81
sex, sexual (related to) Z70.9
attitude (s) Z70.0
behavior or orientation Z70.1
combined concerns Z70.3
non-responsiveness Z70.1
on behalf of third party Z70.2
specified reason NEC Z70.8
specified reason NEC Z71.89
spiritual Z71.81
spousal abuse (perpetrator) Z69.12
victim Z69.11
substance abuse Z71.89
alcohol Z71.41
drug Z71.51
tobacco Z71.6
tobacco use Z71.6
use (of)
insulin pump Z46.81
victim (of)
abuse Z69.81
child abuse
by parent Z69.010
non-parental Z69.020
rape NEC Z69.81
Coupled rhythm R00.8
Couvelaire syndrome or uterus (complicating delivery) O45.8X-
Cowperitis —*see* Urethritis
Cowper's gland —*see* condition
Cowpox B08.010
due to vaccination T88.1
Coxa
magna M91.4-
plana M91.2-
valga (acquired) —*see also* Deformity, limb, specified type NEC, thigh
congenital Q65.81
sequelae (late effect) of rickets E64.3
vara (acquired) —*see also* Deformity, limb, specified type NEC, thigh
congenital Q65.82
sequelae (late effect) of rickets E64.3
Coxalgia, coxalgic (nontuberculous) —*see also* Pain, joint, hip
tuberculous A18.02
Coxitis —*see* Monoarthritis, hip
Coxsackie (virus) (infection) B34.1
as cause of disease classified elsewhere B97.11
carditis B33.20
central nervous system NEC A88.8
endocarditis B33.21
enteritis A08.39
meningitis (aseptic) A87.0
myocarditis B33.22
pericarditis B33.23
pharyngitis B08.5
pleurodynia B33.0
specific disease NEC B33.8
Crabs, meaning pubic lice B85.3
Crack baby P04.41
Cracked nipple N64.0
associated with
lactation O92.13
pregnancy O92.11-
puerperium O92.12
Cracked tooth K03.81
Cradle cap L21.0
Craft neurosis F48.8
Cramp (s) R25.2
abdominal —*see* Pain, abdominal
bathing T75.1
colic R10.83
psychogenic F45.8
due to immersion T75.1
fireman T67.2
heat T67.2
immersion T75.1
intestinal —*see* Pain, abdominal
psychogenic F45.8
leg, sleep related G47.62
limb (lower) (upper) NEC R25.2
sleep related G47.62
linotypist's F48.8
organic G25.89
muscle (limb) (general) R25.2
due to immersion T75.1
psychogenic F45.8
occupational (hand) F48.8
organic G25.89
salt-depletion E87.1
sleep related, leg G47.62
stoker's T67.2
swimmer's T75.1
telegrapher's F48.8
organic G25.89
typist's F48.8
organic G25.89
uterus N94.89
menstrual —*see* Dysmenorrhea
writer's F48.8
organic G25.89
Cranial —*see* condition
Craniocleidodysostosis Q74.0
Craniofenestria (skull) Q75.8
Craniolacunia (skull) Q75.8
Craniopagus Q89.4
Craniopathy, metabolic M85.2
Craniopharyngeal —*see* condition
Craniopharyngioma D44.4
Craniorachischisis (totalis) Q00.1
Cranioschisis Q75.8
Craniostenosis Q75.0
Craniosynostosis Q75.0
Craniotabes (cause unknown) M83.8
neonatal P96.3
rachitic E64.3
syphilitic A50.56
Cranium —*see* condition
Craw-craw —*see* Onchocerciasis
Creaking joint —*see* Derangement, joint, specified type NEC
Creeping
eruption B76.9
palsy or paralysis G12.22
Crenated tongue K14.8
Creotoxism A05.9
Crepitus
caput Q75.8
joint —*see* Derangement, joint, specified type NEC
Crescent or conus choroid, congenital Q14.3
CREST syndrome M34.1
Cretin, cretinism (congenital) (endemic) (nongoitrous) (sporadic) E00.9
pelvis
with disproportion (fetopelvic) O33.0
causing obstructed labor O65.0
type
hypothyroid E00.1
mixed E00.2
myxedematous E00.1
neurological E00.0
Creutzfeldt-Jakob disease or syndrome (with dementia) A81.00
familial A81.09
iatrogenic A81.09
specified NEC A81.09
sporadic A81.09
variant (vCJD) A81.01
Crib death R99
Cribriform hymen Q52.3
Cri-du-chat syndrome Q93.4
Crigler-Najjar disease or syndrome E80.5
Crime, victim of Z65.4
Crimean hemorrhagic fever A98.0
Criminalism F60.2
Crisis
abdomen R10.0
acute reaction F43.0
addisonian E27.2
adrenal (cortical) E27.2
celiac K90.0
Dietl's N13.8
emotional —*see also* Disorder, adjustment
acute reaction to stress F43.0
specific to childhood and adolescence F93.8
glaucomatocyclitic —*see* Glaucoma, secondary, inflammation
heart —*see* Failure, heart
nitritoid I95.2
correct substance properly administered —*see* Table of Drugs and Chemicals, by drug, adverse effect
overdose or wrong substance given or taken —*see* Table of Drugs and Chemicals, by drug, poisoning
oculogyric H51.8
psychogenic F45.8
Pel's (tabetic) A52.11
psychosexual identity F64.2
renal N28.0
sickle-cell D57.00
with
acute chest syndrome D57.01
splenic sequestration D57.02
state (acute reaction) F43.0
tabetic A52.11
thyroid —*see* Thyrotoxicosis with thyroid storm
thyrotoxic —*see* Thyrotoxicosis with thyroid storm

C

Crocq's disease (acrocyanosis) I73.89
Crohn's disease —*see* Enteritis, regional
Crooked septum, nasal J34.2
Cross syndrome E70.328
Crossbite (anterior) (posterior) M26.24
Cross-eye —*see* Strabismus, convergent concomitant
Croup, croupous (catarrhal) (infectious) (inflammatory) (nondiphtheritic) J05.0
  bronchial J20.9
  diphtheritic A36.2
  false J38.5
  spasmodic J38.5
    diphtheritic A36.2
  stridulous J38.5
    diphtheritic A36.2
Crouzon's disease Q75.1
Crowding, tooth, teeth, fully erupted M26.31
CRST syndrome M34.1
Cruchet's disease A85.8
Cruelty in children —*see also* Disorder, conduct
Crural ulcer —*see* Ulcer, lower limb
Crush, crushed, crushing T14.8
  abdomen S38.1
  ankle S97.0-
  arm (upper) (and shoulder) S47.-
  axilla —*see* Crush, arm
  back, lower S38.1
  buttock S38.1
  cheek S07.0
  chest S28.0
  cranium S07.1
  ear S07.0
  elbow S57.0-
  extremity
    lower
      ankle —*see* Crush, ankle
      below knee —*see* Crush, leg
      foot —*see* Crush, foot
      hip —*see* Crush, hip
      knee —*see* Crush, knee
      thigh —*see* Crush, thigh
      toe —*see* Crush, toe
    upper
      below elbow S67.9-
      elbow —*see* Crush, elbow
      finger —*see* Crush, finger
      forearm —*see* Crush, forearm
      hand —*see* Crush, hand
      thumb —*see* Crush, thumb
      upper arm —*see* Crush, arm
      wrist —*see* Crush, wrist
  face S07.0
  finger (s) S67.1-
    with hand (and wrist) —*see* Crush, hand, specified site NEC
    index S67.19-
    little S67.19-
    middle S67.19-
    ring S67.19-
    thumb —*see* Crush, thumb
  foot S97.8-
    toe —*see* Crush, toe
  forearm S57.8-
  genitalia, external
    female S38.002
      vagina S38.03
      vulva S38.03
    male S38.001
      penis S38.01
      scrotum S38.02
      testis S38.02
  hand (except fingers alone) S67.2-
    with wrist S67.4-
  head S07.9
    specified NEC S07.8
  heel —*see* Crush, foot
  hip S77.0-
    with thigh S77.2-
  internal organ (abdomen, chest, or pelvis) NEC T14.8
Crush, crushed, crushing *(Continued)*
  knee S87.0-
  labium (majus) (minus) S38.03
  larynx S17.0
  leg (lower) S87.8-
    knee —*see* Crush, knee
  lip S07.0
  lower
    back S38.1
    leg —*see* Crush, leg
  neck S17.9
  nerve —*see* Injury, nerve
  nose S07.0
  pelvis S38.1
  penis S38.01
  scalp S07.8
  scapular region —*see* Crush, arm
  scrotum S38.02
  severe, unspecified site T14.8
  shoulder (and upper arm) —*see* Crush, arm
  skull S07.1
  syndrome (complication of trauma) T79.5
  testis S38.02
  thigh S77.1-
    with hip S77.2-
  throat S17.8
  thumb S67.0-
    with hand (and wrist) —*see* Crush, hand, specified site NEC
  toe (s) S97.10-
    great S97.11-
    lesser S97.12-
  trachea S17.0
  vagina S38.03
  vulva S38.03
  wrist S67.3-
    with hand S67.4-
Crusta lactea L21.0
Crusts R23.4
Crutch paralysis —*see* Injury, brachial plexus
Cruveilhier-Baumgarten cirrhosis, disease or syndrome K74.69
Cruveilhier's atrophy or disease G12.8
Crying (constant) (continuous) (excessive)
  child, adolescent, or adult R45.83
  infant (baby) (newborn) R68.11
Cryofibrinogenemia D89.2
Cryoglobulinemia (essential) (idiopathic) (mixed) (primary) (purpura) (secondary) (vasculitis) D89.1
  with lung involvement D89.1 *[J99]*
Cryptitis (anal) (rectal) K62.89
Cryptococcosis, cryptococcus (infection) (neoformans) B45.9
  bone B45.3
  cerebral B45.1
  cutaneous B45.2
  disseminated B45.7
  generalized B45.7
  meningitis B45.1
  meningocerebralis B45.1
  osseous B45.3
  pulmonary B45.0
  skin B45.2
  specified NEC B45.8
Cryptopapillitis (anus) K62.89
Cryptophthalmos Q11.2
  syndrome Q87.0
Cryptorchid, cryptorchism, cryptorchidism Q53.9
  bilateral Q53.20
    abdominal Q53.21
    perineal Q53.22
  unilateral Q53.10
    abdominal Q53.11
    perineal Q53.12
Cryptosporidiosis A07.2
  hepatobiliary B88.8
  respiratory B88.8
Cryptostromosis J67.6
Crystalluria R82.99
Cubitus
  congenital Q68.8
  valgus (acquired) M21.0-
    congenital Q68.8
    sequelae (late effect) of rickets E64.3
  varus (acquired) M21.1-
    congenital Q68.8
    sequelae (late effect) of rickets E64.3
Cultural deprivation or shock Z60.3
Curling esophagus K22.4
Curling's ulcer —*see* Ulcer, peptic, acute
Curschmann (-Batten) (-Steinert) **disease or syndrome** G71.11
Curse, Ondine's —*see* Apnea, sleep
Curvature
  organ or site, congenital NEC —*see* Distortion
  penis (lateral) Q55.61
  Pott's (spinal) A18.01
  radius, idiopathic, progressive (congenital) Q74.0
  spine (acquired) (angular) (idiopathic) (incorrect) (postural) —*see* Dorsopathy, deforming
    congenital Q67.5
    due to or associated with
      Charcot-Marie-Tooth disease —*see also* subcategory M49.8 G60.0
      osteitis
        deformans M88.88
        fibrosa cystica —*see also* subcategory M49.8 E21.0
      tuberculosis (Pott's curvature) A18.01
    sequelae (late effect) of rickets E64.3
    tuberculous A18.01
Cushingoid due to steroid therapy E24.2
  correct substance properly administered —*see* Table of Drugs and Chemicals, by drug, adverse effect
  overdose or wrong substance given or taken —*see* Table of Drugs and Chemicals, by drug, poisoning
Cushing's
  syndrome or disease E24.9
    drug-induced E24.2
    iatrogenic E24.2
    pituitary-dependent E24.0
    specified NEC E24.8
  ulcer —*see* Ulcer, peptic, acute
Cusp, Carabelli - omit code
Cut (external) —*see also* Laceration
  muscle —*see* Injury, muscle
Cutaneous —*see also* condition
  hemorrhage R23.3
  larva migrans B76.9
Cutis —*see also* condition
  hyperelastica Q82.8
    acquired L57.4
  laxa (hyperelastica) —*see* Dermatolysis
  marmorata R23.8
  osteosis L94.2
  pendula —*see* Dermatolysis
  rhomboidalis nuchae L57.2
  verticis gyrata Q82.8
    acquired L91.8
Cyanosis R23.0
  due to
    patent foramen botalli Q21.1
    persistent foramen ovale Q21.1
  enterogenous D74.8
  paroxysmal digital —*see* Raynaud's disease
    with gangrene I73.01
  retina, retinal H35.89
Cyanotic heart disease I24.9
  congenital Q24.9
Cycle
  anovulatory N97.0
  menstrual, irregular N92.6
Cyclencephaly Q04.9
Cyclical vomiting (*see also* Vomiting, cyclical) G43.A0
  psychogenic F50.89 ◄

◄ New ◄ Revised ~~deleted~~ Deleted

Cyclitis —*see also* Iridocyclitis H20.9
chronic —*see* Iridocyclitis, chronic
Fuchs' heterochromic H20.81-
granulomatous —*see* Iridocyclitis, chronic
lens-induced —*see* Iridocyclitis, lens-induced
posterior H30.2-
Cycloid personality F34.0
Cyclophoria H50.54
Cyclopia, cyclops Q87.0
Cyclopism Q87.0
Cyclosporiasis A07.4
Cyclothymia F34.0
Cyclothymic personality F34.0
Cyclotropia H50.41-
Cylindroma —*see also* Neoplasm, malignant, by site
eccrine dermal —*see* Neoplasm, skin, benign
skin —*see* Neoplasm, skin, benign
Cylindruria R82.99
Cynanche
diphtheritic A36.2
tonsillaris J36
Cynophobia F40.218
Cynorexia R63.2
Cyphosis —*see* Kyphosis
Cyprus fever —*see* Brucellosis
Cyst (colloid) (mucous) (simple) (retention)
adenoid (infected) J35.8
adrenal gland E27.8
congenital Q89.1
air, lung J98.4
allantoic Q64.4
alveolar process (jaw bone) M27.40
amnion, amniotic O41.8X-
aneurysmal M27.49 ◀
anterior
chamber (eye) —*see* Cyst, iris
nasopalatine K09.1
antrum J34.1
anus K62.89
apical (tooth) (periodontal) K04.8
appendix K38.8
arachnoid, brain (acquired) G93.0
congenital Q04.6
arytenoid J38.7
Baker's M71.2-
ruptured M66.0
tuberculous A18.02
Bartholin's gland N75.0
bile duct (common) (hepatic) K83.5
bladder (multiple) (trigone) N32.89
blue dome (breast) —*see* Cyst, breast
bone (local) NEC M85.60
aneurysmal M85.50
ankle M85.57-
foot M85.57-
forearm M85.53-
hand M85.54-
jaw M27.49
lower leg M85.56-
multiple site M85.59
neck M85.58
rib M85.58
shoulder M85.51-
skull M85.58
specified site NEC M85.58
thigh M85.55-
toe M85.57-
upper arm M85.52-
vertebra M85.58
solitary M85.40
ankle M85.47-
fibula M85.46-
foot M85.47-
hand M85.44-
humerus M85.42-
jaw M27.49
neck M85.48
pelvis M85.45-

Cyst *(Continued)*
bone NEC *(Continued)*
solitary *(Continued)*
radius M85.43-
rib M85.48
shoulder M85.41-
skull M85.48
specified site NEC M85.48
tibia M85.46-
toe M85.47-
ulna M85.43-
vertebra M85.48
specified type NEC M85.60
ankle M85.67-
foot M85.67-
forearm M85.63-
hand M85.64-
jaw M27.40
developmental (nonodontogenic) K09.1
odontogenic K09.0
latent M27.0
lower leg M85.66-
multiple site M85.69
neck M85.68
rib M85.68
shoulder M85.61-
skull M85.68
specified site NEC M85.68
thigh M85.65-
toe M85.67-
upper arm M85.62-
vertebra M85.68
brain (acquired) G93.0
congenital Q04.6
hydatid B67.99 *[G94]*
third ventricle (colloid), congenital Q04.6
branchial (cleft) Q18.0
branchiogenic Q18.0
breast (benign) (blue dome) (pedunculated) (solitary) N60.0-
involution —*see* Dysplasia, mammary, specified type NEC
sebaceous —*see* Dysplasia, mammary, specified type NEC
broad ligament (benign) N83.8
bronchogenic (mediastinal) (sequestration) J98.4
congenital Q33.0
buccal K09.8
bulbourethral gland N36.8
bursa, bursal NEC M71.30
with rupture —*see* Rupture, synovium
ankle M71.37-
elbow M71.32-
foot M71.37-
hand M71.34-
hip M71.35-
multiple sites M71.39
pharyngeal J39.2
popliteal space —*see* Cyst, Baker's
shoulder M71.31-
specified site NEC M71.38
wrist M71.33-
calcifying odontogenic D16.5
upper jaw (bone) (maxilla) D16.4
canal of Nuck (female) N94.89
congenital Q52.4
canthus —*see* Cyst, conjunctiva
carcinomatous —*see* Neoplasm, malignant, by site
cauda equina G95.89
cavum septi pellucidi —*see* Cyst, brain
celomic (pericardium) Q24.8
cerebellopontine (angle) —*see* Cyst, brain
cerebellum —*see* Cyst, brain
cerebral —*see* Cyst, brain
cervical lateral Q18.0 ⟸
cervix NEC N88.8
embryonic Q51.6
nabothian N88.8

Cyst *(Continued)*
chiasmal optic NEC —*see* Disorder, optic, chiasm
chocolate (ovary) N80.1
choledochus, congenital Q44.4
chorion O41.8X-
choroid plexus G93.0
ciliary body —*see* Cyst, iris
clitoris N90.7
colon K63.89
common (bile) duct K83.5
congenital NEC Q89.8
adrenal gland Q89.1
epiglottis Q31.8
esophagus Q39.8
fallopian tube Q50.4
kidney Q61.00
more than one (multiple) Q61.02
specified as polycystic Q61.3
adult type Q61.2
infantile type NEC Q61.19
collecting duct dilation Q61.11
solitary Q61.01
larynx Q31.8
liver Q44.6
lung Q33.0
mediastinum Q34.1
ovary Q50.1
oviduct Q50.4
periurethral (tissue) Q64.79
prepuce Q55.69
salivary gland (any) Q38.4
sublingual Q38.6
submaxillary gland Q38.6
thymus (gland) Q89.2
tongue Q38.3
ureterovesical orifice Q62.8
vulva Q52.79
conjunctiva H11.44-
cornea H18.89-
corpora quadrigemina G93.0
corpus
albicans N83.29- ⟸
luteum (hemorrhagic) (ruptured) N83.1- ⟸
Cowper's gland (benign) (infected) N36.8
cranial meninges G93.0
craniobuccal pouch E23.6
craniopharyngeal pouch E23.6
cystic duct K82.8
Cysticercus —*see* Cysticercosis
Dandy-Walker Q03.1
with spina bifida —*see* Spina bifida
dental (root) K04.8
developmental K09.0
eruption K09.0
primordial K09.0
dentigerous (mandible) (maxilla) K09.0
dermoid —*see* Neoplasm, benign, by site
with malignant transformation C56.-
implantation
external area or site (skin) NEC L72.0
iris —*see* Cyst, iris, implantation
vagina N89.8
vulva N90.7
mouth K09.8
oral soft tissue K09.8
sacrococcygeal —*see* Cyst, pilonidal
developmental K09.1
odontogenic K09.0
oral region (nonodontogenic) K09.1
ovary, ovarian Q50.1
dura (cerebral) G93.0
spinal G96.19
ear (external) Q18.1
echinococcal —*see* Echinococcus
embryonic
cervix uteri Q51.6
fallopian tube Q50.4
vagina Q51.6

◀ New ⟸ Revised ~~deleted~~ Deleted

Cyst *(Continued)*
endometrium, endometrial (uterus) N85.8
ectopic —*see* Endometriosis
enterogenous Q43.8
epidermal, epidermoid (inclusion) (*see also* Cyst, skin) L72.0
mouth K09.8
oral soft tissue K09.8
epididymis N50.3
epiglottis J38.7
epiphysis cerebri E34.8
epithelial (inclusion) L72.0
epoophoron Q50.5
eruption K09.0
esophagus K22.8
ethmoid sinus J34.1
external female genital organs NEC N90.7
eye NEC H57.8
congenital Q15.8
eyelid (sebaceous) H02.829
infected —*see* Hordeolum
left H02.826
lower H02.825
upper H02.824
right H02.823
lower H02.822
upper H02.821
fallopian tube N83.8
congenital Q50.4
fimbrial (twisted) Q50.4
fissural (oral region) K09.1
follicle (graafian) (hemorrhagic) N83.0- ⇐
nabothian N88.8
follicular (atretic) (hemorrhagic) (ovarian) N83.0- ⇐
dentigerous K09.0
odontogenic K09.0
skin L72.9
specified NEC L72.8
frontal sinus J34.1
gallbladder K82.8
ganglion —*see* Ganglion
Gartner's duct Q52.4
gingiva K09.0
gland of Moll —*see* Cyst, eyelid
globulomaxillary K09.1
graafian follicle (hemorrhagic) N83.0- ⇐
granulosal lutein (hemorrhagic) N83.1- ⇐
hemangiomatous D18.00
intra-abdominal D18.03
intracranial D18.02
skin D18.01
specified site NEC D18.09
hemorrhagic M27.49 ◀
hydatid —*see also* Echinococcus B67.90
brain B67.99 *[G94]*
liver —*see also* Cyst, liver, hydatid B67.8
lung NEC B67.99 *[J99]*
Morgagni
female Q50.5
male (epididymal) Q55.4
testicular Q55.29
specified site NEC B67.99
hymen N89.8
embryonic Q52.4
hypopharynx J39.2
hypophysis, hypophyseal (duct) (recurrent) E23.6
cerebri E23.6
implantation (dermoid)
external area or site (skin) NEC L72.0
iris —*see* Cyst, iris, implantation
vagina N89.8
vulva N90.7
incisive canal K09.1
inclusion (epidermal) (epithelial) (epidermoid) (squamous) L72.0
not of skin - code under Cyst, by site
intestine (large) (small) K63.89
intracranial —*see* Cyst, brain
intraligamentous —*see also* Disorder, ligament
knee —*see* Derangement, knee

Cyst *(Continued)*
intrasellar E23.6
iris H21.309
exudative H21.31-
idiopathic H21.30-
implantation H21.32-
parasitic H21.33-
pars plana (primary) H21.34-
exudative H21.35-
jaw (bone) M27.40
aneurysmal M27.49
developmental (odontogenic) K09.0
fissural K09.1
hemorrhagic M27.49
traumatic M27.49
joint NEC —*see* Disorder, joint, specified type NEC
kidney (acquired) N28.1
calyceal —*see* Hydronephrosis
congenital Q61.00
more than one (multiple) Q61.02
specified as polycystic Q61.3
adult type (autosomal dominant) Q61.2
infantile type (autosomal recessive) NEC Q61.19
collecting duct dilation Q61.11
pyelogenic —*see* Hydronephrosis
simple N28.1
solitary (single) Q61.01
acquired N28.1
labium (majus) (minus) N90.7
sebaceous N90.7
lacrimal —*see also* Disorder, lacrimal system, specified NEC
gland H04.13-
passages or sac —*see* Disorder, lacrimal system, specified NEC
larynx J38.7
lateral periodontal K09.0
lens H27.8
congenital Q12.8
lip (gland) K13.0
liver (idiopathic) (simple) K76.89
congenital Q44.6
hydatid B67.8
granulosus B67.0
multilocularis B67.5
lung J98.4
congenital Q33.0
giant bullous J43.9
lutein N83.1- ⇐
lymphangiomatous D18.1
lymphoepithelial, oral soft tissue K09.8
macula —*see* Degeneration, macula, hole
malignant —*see* Neoplasm, malignant, by site
mammary gland —*see* Cyst, breast
mandible M27.40
dentigerous K09.0
radicular K04.8
maxilla M27.40
dentigerous K09.0
radicular K04.8
medial, face and neck Q18.8
median
anterior maxillary K09.1
palatal K09.1
mediastinum, congenital Q34.1
meibomian (gland) —*see* Chalazion
infected —*see* Hordeolum
membrane, brain G93.0
meninges (cerebral) G93.0
spinal G96.19
meniscus, knee —*see* Derangement, knee, meniscus, cystic
mesentery, mesenteric K66.8
chyle I89.8
mesonephric duct
female Q50.5
male Q55.4
milk N64.89

Cyst *(Continued)*
Morgagni (hydatid)
female Q50.5
male (epididymal) Q55.4
testicular Q55.29
mouth K09.8
Müllerian duct Q50.4
appendix testis Q55.29
cervix Q51.6
fallopian tube Q50.4
female Q50.4
male Q55.29
prostatic utricle Q55.4
vagina (embryonal) Q52.4
multilocular (ovary) D39.10
benign —*see* Neoplasm, benign, by site
myometrium N85.8
nabothian (follicle) (ruptured) N88.8
nasoalveolar K09.1
nasolabial K09.1
nasopalatine (anterior) (duct) K09.1
nasopharynx J39.2
neoplastic —*see* Neoplasm, uncertain behavior, by site
benign —*see* Neoplasm, benign, by site
nervous system NEC G96.8
neuroenteric (congenital) Q06.8
nipple —*see* Cyst, breast
nose (turbinates) J34.1
sinus J34.1
odontogenic, developmental K09.0
omentum (lesser) K66.8
congenital Q45.8
ora serrata —*see* Cyst, retina, ora serrata
oral
region K09.9
developmental (nonodontogenic) K09.1
specified NEC K09.8
soft tissue K09.9
specified NEC K09.8
orbit H05.81-
ovary, ovarian (twisted) N83.20- ⇐
adherent N83.20- ⇐
chocolate N80.1
corpus
albicans N83.29- ⇐
luteum (hemorrhagic) N83.1- ⇐
dermoid D27.9
developmental Q50.1
due to failure of involution NEC N83.20- ⇐
endometrial N80.1
follicular (graafian) (hemorrhagic) N83.0- ⇐
hemorrhagic N83.20- ⇐
in pregnancy or childbirth O34.8-
with obstructed labor O65.5
multilocular D39.10
pseudomucinous D27.9
retention N83.29- ⇐
serous N83.20- ⇐
specified NEC N83.29- ⇐
theca lutein (hemorrhagic) N83.1- ⇐
tuberculous A18.18
oviduct N83.8
palate (median) (fissural) K09.1
palatine papilla (jaw) K09.1
pancreas, pancreatic (hemorrhagic) (true) K86.2
congenital Q45.2
false K86.3
paralabral
hip M24.85-
shoulder S43.43-
paramesonephric duct Q50.4
female Q50.4
male Q55.29
paranephric N28.1
paraphysis, cerebri, congenital Q04.6
parasitic B89
parathyroid (gland) E21.4
paratubal N83.8
paraurethral duct N36.8
paroophoron Q50.5

◀ New ⇐ Revised ~~deleted~~ Deleted

Cyst *(Continued)*
parotid gland K11.6
parovarian Q50.5
pelvis, female N94.89
in pregnancy or childbirth O34.8-
causing obstructed labor O65.5
penis (sebaceous) N48.89
periapical K04.8
pericardial (congenital) Q24.8
acquired (secondary) I31.8
pericoronal K09.0
periodontal K04.8
lateral K09.0
peripelvic (lymphatic) N28.1
peritoneum K66.8
chylous I89.8
periventricular, acquired, newborn P91.1
pharynx (wall) J39.2
pilar L72.11
pilonidal (infected) (rectum) L05.91
with abscess L05.01
malignant C44.59-
pituitary (duct) (gland) E23.6
placenta O43.19-
pleura J94.8
popliteal —*see* Cyst, Baker's
porencephalic Q04.6
acquired G93.0
postanal (infected) —*see* Cyst, pilonidal
postmastoidectomy cavity (mucosal) —*see* Complications, postmastoidectomy, cyst
preauricular Q18.1
prepuce N47.4
congenital Q55.69
primordial (jaw) K09.0
prostate N42.83
pseudomucinous (ovary) D27.9
pupillary, miotic H21.27-
radicular (residual) K04.8
radiculodental K04.8
ranular K11.8
Rathke's pouch E23.6
rectum (epithelium) (mucous) K62.89
renal —*see* Cyst, kidney
residual (radicular) K04.8
retention (ovary) N83.29- ◄
salivary gland K11.6
retina H33.19-
ora serrata H33.11-
parasitic H33.12-
retroperitoneal K68.9
sacrococcygeal (dermoid) —*see* Cyst, pilonidal
salivary gland or duct (mucous extravasation or retention) K11.6
Sampson's N80.1
sclera H15.89
scrotum L72.9
sebaceous L72.3
sebaceous (duct) (gland) L72.3
breast —*see* Dysplasia, mammary, specified type NEC
eyelid —*see* Cyst, eyelid
genital organ NEC
female N94.89
male N50.89 ◄
scrotum L72.3
semilunar cartilage (knee) (multiple) —*see* Derangement, knee, meniscus, cystic
seminal vesicle N50.89 ◄
serous (ovary) N83.20- ◄
sinus (accessory) (nasal) J34.1
Skene's gland N36.8
skin L72.9
breast —*see* Dysplasia, mammary, specified type NEC
epidermal, epidermoid L72.0
epithelial L72.0
eyelid —*see* Cyst, eyelid
genital organ NEC
female N90.7
male N50.89 ◄

Cyst *(Continued)*
skin *(Continued)*
inclusion L72.0
scrotum L72.9
sebaceous L72.3
sweat gland or duct L74.8
solitary
bone —*see* Cyst, bone, solitary
jaw M27.40
kidney N28.1
spermatic cord N50.89 ◄
sphenoid sinus J34.1
spinal meninges G96.19
spleen NEC D73.4
congenital Q89.09
hydatid —*see also* Echinococcus B67.99 *[D77]*
Stafne's M27.0
subarachnoid intrasellar R93.0
subcutaneous, pheomycotic (chromomycotic) B43.2
subdural (cerebral) G93.0
spinal cord G96.19
sublingual gland K11.6
submandibular gland K11.6
submaxillary gland K11.6
suburethral N36.8
suprarenal gland E27.8
suprasellar —*see* Cyst, brain
sweat gland or duct L74.8
synovial —*see also* Cyst, bursa
ruptured —*see* Rupture, synovium
tarsal —*see* Chalazion
tendon (sheath) —*see* Disorder, tendon, specified type NEC
testis N44.2
tunica albuginea N44.1
theca lutein (ovary) N83.1- ◄
Thornwaldt's J39.2
thymus (gland) E32.8
thyroglossal duct (infected) (persistent) Q89.2
thyroid (gland) E04.1
thyrolingual duct (infected) (persistent) Q89.2
tongue K14.8
tonsil J35.8
tooth —*see* Cyst, dental
Tornwaldt's J39.2
trichilemmal (proliferating) L72.12
trichodermal L72.12
tubal (fallopian) N83.8
inflammatory —*see* Salpingitis, chronic
tubo-ovarian N83.8
inflammatory N70.13
tunica
albuginea testis N44.1
vaginalis N50.89 ◄
turbinate (nose) J34.1
Tyson's gland N48.89
urachus, congenital Q64.4
ureter N28.89
ureterovesical orifice N28.89
urethra, urethral (gland) N36.8
uterine ligament N83.8
uterus (body) (corpus) (recurrent) N85.8
embryonic Q51.818
cervix Q51.6
vagina, vaginal (implantation) (inclusion) (squamous cell) (wall) N89.8
embryonic Q52.4
vallecula, vallecular (epiglottis) J38.7
vesical (orifice) N32.89
vitreous body H43.89
vulva (implantation) (inclusion) N90.7
congenital Q52.79
sebaceous gland N90.7
vulvovaginal gland N90.7
wolffian
female Q50.5
male Q55.4

Cystadenocarcinoma —*see* Neoplasm, malignant, by site
bile duct C22.1
endometrioid —*see* Neoplasm, malignant, by site
specified site —*see* Neoplasm, malignant, by site
unspecified site
female C56.9
male C61
mucinous
papillary
specified site —*see* Neoplasm, malignant, by site
unspecified site C56.9
specified site —*see* Neoplasm, malignant, by site
unspecified site C56.9
papillary
mucinous
specified site —*see* Neoplasm, malignant, by site
unspecified site C56.9
pseudomucinous
specified site —*see* Neoplasm, malignant, by site
unspecified site C56.9
serous
specified site —*see* Neoplasm, malignant, by site
unspecified site C56.9
specified site —*see* Neoplasm, malignant, by site
unspecified site C56.9
pseudomucinous
papillary
specified site —*see* Neoplasm, malignant, by site
unspecified site C56.9
specified site —*see* Neoplasm, malignant, by site
unspecified site C56.9
serous
papillary
specified site —*see* Neoplasm, malignant, by site
unspecified site C56.9
specified site —*see* Neoplasm, malignant, by site
unspecified site C56.9
Cystadenofibroma
clear cell —*see* Neoplasm, benign, by site
endometrioid D27.9
borderline malignancy D39.1-
malignant C56.-
mucinous
specified site —*see* Neoplasm, benign, by site
unspecified site D27.9
serous
specified site —*see* Neoplasm, benign, by site
unspecified site D27.9
specified site —*see* Neoplasm, benign, by site
unspecified site D27.9
Cystadenoma —*see also* Neoplasm, benign, by site
bile duct D13.4
endometrioid —*see* Neoplasm, benign, by site
borderline malignancy —*see* Neoplasm, uncertain behavior, by site
malignant —*see* Neoplasm, malignant, by site
mucinous
borderline malignancy
ovary C56.-
specified site NEC —*see* Neoplasm, uncertain behavior, by site
unspecified site C56.9
papillary
borderline malignancy
ovary C56.-
specified site NEC —*see* Neoplasm, uncertain behavior, by site
unspecified site C56.9

Cystadenoma *(Continued)*
mucinous *(Continued)*
papillary *(Continued)*
specified site —*see* Neoplasm, benign, by site
unspecified site D27.9
specified site —*see* Neoplasm, benign, by site
unspecified site D27.9
papillary
borderline malignancy
ovary C56-
specified site NEC —*see* Neoplasm, uncertain behavior, by site
unspecified site C56.9
lymphomatosum
specified site —*see* Neoplasm, benign, by site
unspecified site D11.9
mucinous
borderline malignancy
ovary C56.-
specified site NEC —*see* Neoplasm, uncertain behavior, by site
unspecified site C56.9
specified site —*see* Neoplasm, benign, by site
unspecified site D27.9
pseudomucinous
borderline malignancy
ovary C56.-
specified site NEC —*see* Neoplasm, uncertain behavior, by site
unspecified site C56.9
specified site —*see* Neoplasm, benign, by site
unspecified site D27.9
serous
borderline malignancy
ovary C56.-
specified site NEC —*see* Neoplasm, uncertain behavior, by site
unspecified site C56.9
specified site —*see* Neoplasm, benign, by site
unspecified site D27.9
specified site —*see* Neoplasm, benign, by site
unspecified site D27.9
pseudomucinous
borderline malignancy
ovary C56.-
specified site NEC —*see* Neoplasm, uncertain behavior, by site
unspecified site C56.9
papillary
borderline malignancy
ovary C56.-
specified site NEC —*see* Neoplasm, uncertain behavior, by site
unspecified site C56.9
specified site —*see* Neoplasm, benign, by site
unspecified site D27.9
specified site —*see* Neoplasm, benign, by site
unspecified site D27.9
serous
borderline malignancy
ovary C56.-
specified site NEC —*see* Neoplasm, uncertain behavior, by site
unspecified site C56.9
papillary
borderline malignancy
ovary C56.-
specified site NEC —*see* Neoplasm, uncertain behavior, by site
unspecified site C56.9
specified site —*see* Neoplasm, benign, by site
unspecified site D27.9
specified site —*see* Neoplasm, benign, by site
unspecified site D27.9
Cystathionine synthase deficiency E72.11
Cystathioninemia E72.19
Cystathioninuria E72.19
Cystic —*see also* condition
breast (chronic) —*see* Mastopathy, cystic
corpora lutea (hemorrhagic) N83.1- ◄
duct —*see* condition
eyeball (congenital) Q11.0
fibrosis —*see* Fibrosis, cystic
kidney (congenital) Q61.9
adult type Q61.2
infantile type NEC Q61.19
collecting duct dilatation Q61.11
medullary Q61.5
liver, congenital Q44.6
lung disease J98.4
congenital Q33.0
mastitis, chronic —*see* Mastopathy, cystic
medullary, kidney Q61.5
meniscus —*see* Derangement, knee, meniscus, cystic
ovary N83.20- ◄
Cysticercosis, cysticerciasis B69.9
with
epileptiform fits B69.0
myositis B69.81
brain B69.0
central nervous system B69.0
cerebral B69.0
ocular B69.1
specified NEC B69.89
Cysticercus cellulose infestation —*see* Cysticercosis
Cystinosis (malignant) E72.04
Cystinuria E72.01
Cystitis (exudative) (hemorrhagic) (septic) (suppurative) N30.90
with
fibrosis —*see* Cystitis, chronic, interstitial
hematuria N30.91
leukoplakia —*see* Cystitis, chronic, interstitial
malakoplakia —*see* Cystitis, chronic, interstitial
metaplasia —*see* Cystitis, chronic, interstitial
prostatitis N41.3
acute N30.00
with hematuria N30.01
of trigone N30.30
with hematuria N30.31
allergic —*see* Cystitis, specified type NEC
amebic A06.81
bilharzial B65.9 *[N33]*
blennorrhagic (gonococcal) A54.01
bullous —*see* Cystitis, specified type NEC
calculous N21.0
chlamydial A56.01
chronic N30.20
with hematuria N30.21
interstitial N30.10
with hematuria N30.11
of trigone N30.30
with hematuria N30.31
specified NEC N30.20
with hematuria N30.21
cystic (a) —*see* Cystitis, specified type NEC
diphtheritic A36.85
echinococcal
granulosus B67.39
multilocularis B67.69
emphysematous —*see* Cystitis, specified type NEC
encysted —*see* Cystitis, specified type NEC
eosinophilic —*see* Cystitis, specified type NEC
follicular —*see* Cystitis, of trigone
gangrenous —*see* Cystitis, specified type NEC
glandularis —*see* Cystitis, specified type NEC
Cystitis *(Continued)*
gonococcal A54.01
incrusted —*see* Cystitis, specified type NEC
interstitial (chronic) —*see* Cystitis, chronic, interstitial
irradiation N30.40
with hematuria N30.41
irritation —*see* Cystitis, specified type NEC
malignant —*see* Cystitis, specified type NEC
of trigone N30.30
with hematuria N30.31
panmural —*see* Cystitis, chronic, interstitial
polyposa —*see* Cystitis, specified type NEC
prostatic N41.3
puerperal (postpartum) O86.22
radiation —*see* Cystitis, irradiation
specified type NEC N30.80
with hematuria N30.81
subacute —*see* Cystitis, chronic
submucous —*see* Cystitis, chronic, interstitial
syphilitic (late) A52.76
trichomonal A59.03
tuberculous A18.12
ulcerative —*see* Cystitis, chronic, interstitial
Cystocele (-urethrocele)
female N81.10
with prolapse of uterus —*see* Prolapse, uterus
lateral N81.12
midline N81.11
paravaginal N81.12
in pregnancy or childbirth O34.8-
causing obstructed labor O65.5
male N32.89
Cystolithiasis N21.0
Cystoma —*see also* Neoplasm, benign, by site
endometrial, ovary N80.1
mucinous
specified site —*see* Neoplasm, benign, by site
unspecified site D27.9
serous
specified site —*see* Neoplasm, benign, by site
unspecified site D27.9
simple (ovary) N83.29- ◄
Cystoplegia N31.2
Cystoptosis N32.89
Cystopyelitis —*see* Pyelonephritis
Cystorrhagia N32.89
Cystosarcoma phyllodes D48.6-
benign D24-
malignant —*see* Neoplasm, breast, malignant
Cystostomy
attention to Z43.5
complication —*see* Complications, cystostomy
status Z93.50
appendico-vesicostomy Z93.52
cutaneous Z93.51
specified NEC Z93.59
Cystourethritis —*see* Urethritis
Cystourethrocele —*see also* Cystocele
female N81.10
with uterine prolapse —*see* Prolapse, uterus
lateral N81.12
midline N81.11
paravaginal N81.12
male N32.89
Cytomegalic inclusion disease
congenital P35.1
Cytomegalovirus infection B25.9
Cytomycosis (reticuloendothelial) B39.4
Cytopenia D75.9
refractory
with multilineage dysplasia D46.A
and ring sideroblasts (RCMD RS) D46.B
Czerny's disease (periodic hydrarthrosis of the knee) —*see* Effusion, joint, knee

◄ New ◄ Revised ~~deleted~~ Deleted

D

Daae (-Finsen) **disease** (epidemic pleurodynia) B33.0
Dabney's grip B33.0
Da Costa's syndrome F45.8
Dacryoadenitis, dacryadenitis H04.00-
acute H04.01-
chronic H04.02-
Dacryocystitis H04.30-
acute H04.32-
chronic H04.41-
neonatal P39.1
phlegmonous H04.31-
syphilitic A52.71
congenital (early) A50.01
trachomatous, active A71.1
sequelae (late effect) B94.0
Dacryocystoblenorrhea —*see* Inflammation, lacrimal, passages, chronic
Dacryocystocele —*see* Disorder, lacrimal system, changes
Dacryolith, dacryolithiasis H04.51-
Dacryoma —*see* Disorder, lacrimal system, changes
Dacryopericystitis —*see* Dacryocystitis
Dacryops H04.11-
Dacryostenosis —*see also* Stenosis, lacrimal
congenital Q10.5
Dactylitis
bone —*see* Osteomyelitis
sickle-cell D57.00
Hb C D57.219
Hb SS D57.00
specified NEC D57.819
skin L08.9
syphilitic A52.77
tuberculous A18.03
Dactylolysis spontanea (ainhum) L94.6
Dactylosymphysis Q70.9
fingers —*see* Syndactylism, complex, fingers
toes —*see* Syndactylism, complex, toes
Damage
arteriosclerotic —*see* Arteriosclerosis
brain (nontraumatic) G93.9
anoxic, hypoxic G93.1
resulting from a procedure G97.82
child NEC G80.9
due to birth injury P11.2
cardiorenal (vascular) —*see* Hypertension, cardiorenal
cerebral NEC —*see* Damage, brain
coccyx, complicating delivery O71.6
coronary —*see* Disease, heart, ischemic
eye, birth injury P15.3
liver (nontraumatic) K76.9
alcoholic K70.9
due to drugs —*see* Disease, liver, toxic
toxic —*see* Disease, liver, toxic
medication T88.7
pelvic
joint or ligament, during delivery O71.6
organ NEC
during delivery O71.5
following ectopic or molar pregnancy O08.6
renal —*see* Disease, renal
subendocardium, subendocardial —*see* Degeneration, myocardial
vascular I99.9
Dana-Putnam syndrome (subacute combined sclerosis with pernicious anemia) —*see* Degeneration, combined
Danbolt (-Cross) **syndrome** (acrodermatitis enteropathica) E83.2
Dandruff L21.0
Dandy-Walker syndrome Q03.1
with spina bifida —*see* Spina bifida
Danlos' syndrome Q79.6
Darier (-White) **disease** (congenital) Q82.8
meaning erythema annulare centrifugum L53.1
Darier-Roussy sarcoid D86.3
Darling's disease or histoplasmosis B39.4
Darwin's tubercle Q17.8
Dawson's (inclusion body) **encephalitis** A81.1
De Beurmann (-Gougerot) **disease** B42.1
De la Tourette's syndrome F95.2
De Lange's syndrome Q87.1
De Morgan's spots (senile angiomas) I78.1
De Quervain's
disease (tendon sheath) M65.4
syndrome E34.51
thyroiditis (subacute granulomatous thyroiditis) E06.1
De Toni-Fanconi (-Debré) **syndrome** E72.09
with cystinosis E72.04
Dead
fetus, retained (mother) O36.4
early pregnancy O02.1
labyrinth —*see* subcategory H83.2
ovum, retained O02.0
Deaf nonspeaking NEC H91.3
Deafmutism (acquired) (congenital) NEC H91.3
hysterical F44.6
syphilitic, congenital —*see also* subcategory H94.8 A50.09
Deafness (acquired) (complete) (hereditary) (partial) H91.9-
with blue sclera and fragility of bone Q78.0
auditory fatigue —*see* Deafness, specified type NEC
aviation T70.0
nerve injury —*see* Injury, nerve, acoustic, specified type NEC
boilermaker's —*see* subcategory H83.3
central —*see* Deafness, sensorineural
conductive H90.2
~~and sensorineural, mixed H90.8~~
~~bilateral H90.6~~
and sensorineural ◀
mixed H90.8 ◀
bilateral H90.6 ◀
bilateral H90.0
unilateral H90.1-
with restricted hearing on the contralateral side H90.A- ◀
congenital H90.5
with blue sclera and fragility of bone Q78.0
due to toxic agents —*see* Deafness, ototoxic
emotional (hysterical) F44.6
functional (hysterical) F44.6
high frequency H91.9-
hysterical F44.6
low frequency H91.9-
mental R48.8
mixed conductive and sensorineural H90.8
bilateral H90.6
unilateral H90.7-
nerve —*see* Deafness, sensorineural
neural —*see* Deafness, sensorineural
noise-induced —*see also* subcategory H83.3
nerve injury —*see* Injury, nerve, acoustic, specified type NEC
nonspeaking H91.3
ototoxic —*see* subcategory H91.0
perceptive —*see* Deafness, sensorineural
psychogenic (hysterical) F44.6
sensorineural H90.5
~~and conductive, mixed H90.8~~
~~bilateral H90.6~~
and conductive ◀
mixed H90.8 ◀
bilateral H90.6 ◀
bilateral H90.3
unilateral H90.4-
with restricted hearing on the contralateral side H90.A- ◀
sensory —*see* Deafness, sensorineural
specified type NEC —*see* subcategory H91.8
sudden (idiopathic) H91.2-
Deafness *(Continued)*
syphilitic A52.15
transient ischemic H93.01-
traumatic —*see* Injury, nerve, acoustic, specified type NEC
word (developmental) H93.25
Death (cause unknown) (of) (unexplained) (unspecified cause) R99
brain G93.82
cardiac (sudden) (with successful resuscitation) — code to underlying disease
family history of Z82.41
personal history of Z86.74
family member (assumed) Z63.4
Debility (chronic) (general) (nervous) R53.81
congenital or neonatal NOS P96.9
nervous R53.81
old age R54
senile R54
Débove's disease (splenomegaly) R16.1
Decalcification
bone —*see* Osteoporosis
teeth K03.89
Decapsulation, kidney N28.89
Decay
dental —*see* Caries, dental
senile R54
tooth, teeth —*see* Caries, dental
Deciduitis (acute)
following ectopic or molar pregnancy O08.0
Decline (general) —*see* Debility
cognitive, age-associated R41.81
Decompensation
cardiac (acute) (chronic) —*see* Disease, heart
cardiovascular —*see* Disease, cardiovascular
heart —*see* Disease, heart
hepatic —*see* Failure, hepatic
myocardial (acute) (chronic) —*see* Disease, heart
respiratory J98.8
Decompression sickness T70.3
Decrease (d)
absolute neutrophile count —*see* Neutropenia
blood
platelets —*see* Thrombocytopenia
pressure R03.1
due to shock following
injury T79.4
operation T81.19
estrogen E28.39
postablative E89.40
asymptomatic E89.40
symptomatic E89.41
fragility of erythrocytes D58.8
function
lipase (pancreatic) K90.3
ovary in hypopituitarism E23.0
parenchyma of pancreas K86.89 ⇐
pituitary (gland) (anterior) (lobe) E23.0
posterior (lobe) E23.0
functional activity R68.89
glucose R73.09
hematocrit R71.0
hemoglobin R71.0
leukocytes D72.819
specified NEC D72.818
libido R68.82
lymphocytes D72.810
platelets D69.6
respiration, due to shock following injury T79.4
sexual desire R68.82
tear secretion NEC —*see* Syndrome, dry eye
tolerance
fat K90.49 ⇐
glucose R73.09
pancreatic K90.3
salt and water E87.8
vision NEC H54.7
white blood cell count D72.819
specified NEC D72.818

Decubitus (ulcer) —*see* Ulcer, pressure, by site
cervix N86
Deepening acetabulum —*see* Derangement, joint, specified type NEC, hip
Defect, defective Q89.9
3-beta-hydroxysteroid dehydrogenase E25.0
11-hydroxylase E25.0
21-hydroxylase E25.0
abdominal wall, congenital Q79.59
antibody immunodeficiency D80.9
aorticopulmonary septum Q21.4
atrial septal (ostium secundum type) Q21.1
following acute myocardial infarction (current complication) I23.1
ostium primum type Q21.2
atrioventricular
canal Q21.2
septum Q21.2
auricular septal Q21.1
bilirubin excretion NEC E80.6
biosynthesis, androgen (testicular) E29.1
bulbar septum Q21.0
catalase E80.3
cell membrane receptor complex (CR3) D71
circulation I99.9
congenital Q28.9
newborn Q28.9
coagulation (factor) —*see also* Deficiency, factor D68.9
with
ectopic pregnancy O08.1
molar pregnancy O08.1
acquired D68.4
antepartum with hemorrhage —*see* Hemorrhage, antepartum, with coagulation defect
due to
liver disease D68.4
vitamin K deficiency D68.4
hereditary NEC D68.2
intrapartum O67.0
newborn, transient P61.6
postpartum O72.3
specified type NEC D68.8
complement system D84.1
conduction (heart) I45.9
bone —*see* Deafness, conductive
congenital, organ or site not listed —*see* Anomaly, by site
coronary sinus Q21.1
cushion, endocardial Q21.2
degradation, glycoprotein E77.1
dental bridge, crown, fillings —*see* Defect, dental restoration
dental restoration K08.50
specified NEC K08.59
dentin (hereditary) K00.5
Descemet's membrane, congenital Q13.89
developmental —*see also* Anomaly
cauda equina Q06.3
diaphragm
with elevation, eventration or hernia —*see* Hernia, diaphragm
congenital Q79.1
with hernia Q79.0
gross (with hernia) Q79.0
ectodermal, congenital Q82.9
Eisenmenger's Q21.8
enzyme
catalase E80.3
peroxidase E80.3
esophagus, congenital Q39.9
extensor retinaculum M62.89
fibrin polymerization D68.2
filling
bladder R93.41 ⇐
kidney R93.42- ⇐
renal pelvis R93.41 ◀
stomach R93.3
ureter R93.41 ⇐
urinary organs, specified NEC R93.49 ◀

Defect, defective *(Continued)*
Gerbode Q21.0
glycoprotein degradation E77.1
Hageman (factor) D68.2
hearing —*see* Deafness
high grade F70
interatrial septal Q21.1
interauricular septal Q21.1
interventricular septal Q21.0
with dextroposition of aorta, pulmonary stenosis and hypertrophy of right ventricle Q21.3
in tetralogy of Fallot Q21.3
learning (specific) —*see* Disorder, learning
lymphocyte function antigen-1 (LFA-1) D84.0
lysosomal enzyme, post-translational modification E77.0
major osseous M89.70
ankle M89.77-
carpus M89.74-
clavicle M89.71-
femur M89.75-
fibula M89.76-
fingers M89.74-
foot M89.77-
forearm M89.73-
hand M89.74-
humerus M89.72-
lower leg M89.76-
metacarpus M89.74-
metatarsus M89.77-
multiple sites M89.79
pelvic region M89.75-
pelvis M89.75-
radius M89.73-
scapula M89.71-
shoulder region M89.71-
specified NEC M89.78
tarsus M89.77-
thigh M89.75-
tibia M89.76-
toes M89.77-
ulna M89.73-
mental —*see* Disability, intellectual
modification, lysosomal enzymes, post-translational E77.0
obstructive, congenital
renal pelvis Q62.39
ureter Q62.39
atresia —*see* Atresia, ureter
cecoureterocele Q62.32
megaureter Q62.2
orthotopic ureterocele Q62.31
osseous, major M89.70
ankle M89.77-
carpus M89.74-
clavicle M89.71-
femur M89.75-
fibula M89.76-
fingers M89.74-
foot M89.77-
forearm M89.73-
hand M89.74-
humerus M89.72-
lower leg M89.76-
metacarpus M89.74-
metatarsus M89.77-
multiple sites M89.9
pelvic region M89.75-
pelvis M89.75-
radius M89.73-
scapula M89.71-
shoulder region M89.71-
specified NEC M89.78
tarsus M89.77-
thigh M89.75-
tibia M89.76-
toes M89.77-
ulna M89.73-
osteochondral NEC —*see also* Deformity M95.8-

Defect, defective *(Continued)*
ostium
primum Q21.2
secundum Q21.1
peroxidase E80.3
placental blood supply —*see* Insufficiency, placental
platelets, qualitative D69.1
constitutional D68.0
postural NEC, spine —*see* Dorsopathy, deforming
reduction
limb Q73.8
lower Q72.9-
absence —*see* Agenesis, leg
foot —*see* Agenesis, foot
longitudinal
femur Q72.4-
fibula Q72.6-
tibia Q72.5-
specified type NEC Q72.89-
split foot Q72.7-
specified type NEC Q73.8
upper Q71.9-
absence —*see* Agenesis, arm
forearm —*see* Agenesis, forearm
hand —*see* Agenesis, hand
lobster-claw hand Q71.6-
longitudinal
radius Q71.4-
ulna Q71.5-
specified type NEC Q71.89-
renal pelvis Q63.8
obstructive Q62.39
respiratory system, congenital Q34.9
restoration, dental K08.50
specified NEC K08.59
retinal nerve bundle fibers H35.89
septal (heart) NOS Q21.9
acquired (atrial) (auricular) (ventricular) (old) I51.0
atrial Q21.1
concurrent with acute myocardial infarction —*see* Infarct, myocardium
following acute myocardial infarction (current complication) I23.1
ventricular —*see also* Defect, ventricular septal Q21.0
sinus venosus Q21.1
speech R47.9
developmental F80.9
specified NEC R47.89
Taussig-Bing (aortic transposition and overriding pulmonary artery) Q20.1
teeth, wedge K03.1
vascular (local) I99.9
congenital Q27.9
ventricular septal Q21.0
concurrent with acute myocardial infarction —*see* Infarct, myocardium
following acute myocardial infarction (current complication) I23.2
in tetralogy of Fallot Q21.3
vision NEC H54.7
visual field H53.40
bilateral
heteronymous H53.47
homonymous H53.46-
generalized contraction H53.48-
localized
arcuate H53.43-
scotoma (central area) H53.41-
blind spot area H53.42-
sector H53.43-
specified type NEC H53.45-
voice R49.9
specified NEC R49.8
wedge, tooth, teeth (abrasion) K03.1
Deferentitis N49.1
gonorrheal (acute) (chronic) A54.23

◀ New ⇐ Revised ~~deleted~~ Deleted

Defibrination (syndrome) D65
antepartum —*see* Hemorrhage, antepartum, with coagulation defect, disseminated intravascular coagulation
following ectopic or molar pregnancy O08.1
intrapartum O67.0
newborn P60
postpartum O72.3
Deficiency, deficient
3-beta hydroxysteroid dehydrogenase E25.0
11-hydroxylase E25.0
21-hydroxylase E25.0
5-alpha reductase (with male pseudohermaphroditism) E29.1
abdominal muscle syndrome Q79.4
AC globulin (congenital) (hereditary) D68.2
acquired D68.4
accelerator globulin (Ac G) (blood) D68.2
acid phosphatase E83.39
activating factor (blood) D68.2
adenosine deaminase (ADA) D81.3
aldolase (hereditary) E74.19
alpha-1-antitrypsin E88.01
amino-acids E72.9
anemia —*see* Anemia
aneurin E51.9
antibody with
hyperimmunoglobulinemia D80.6
near-normal immunoglobins D80.6
antidiuretic hormone E23.2
anti-hemophilic
factor (A) D66
B D67
C D68.1
globulin (AHG) NEC D66
antithrombin (antithrombin III) D68.59
ascorbic acid E54
attention (disorder) (syndrome) F98.8
with hyperactivity —*see* Disorder, attention-deficit hyperactivity
autoprothrombin
I D68.2
II D67
C D68.2
beta-glucuronidase E76.29
biotin E53.8
biotin-dependent carboxylase D81.819
biotinidase D81.810
brancher enzyme (amylopectinosis) E74.03
C1 esterase inhibitor (C1-INH) D84.1
calciferol E55.9
with
adult osteomalacia M83.8
rickets —*see* Rickets
calcium (dietary) E58
calorie, severe E43
with marasmus E41
and kwashiorkor E42
cardiac —*see* Insufficiency, myocardial
carnitine E71.40
due to
hemodialysis E71.43
inborn errors of metabolism E71.42
Valproic acid therapy E71.43
iatrogenic E71.43
muscle palmityltransferase E71.314
primary E71.41
secondary E71.448
carotene E50.9
central nervous system G96.8
ceruloplasmin (Wilson) E83.01
choline E53.8
Christmas factor D67
chromium E61.4
clotting (blood) —*see also* Deficiency, coagulation factor D68.9
clotting factor NEC (hereditary) —*see also* Deficiency, factor D68.2
coagulation NOS D68.9
with
ectopic pregnancy O08.1
molar pregnancy O08.1
Deficiency, deficient *(Continued)*
coagulation NOS *(Continued)*
acquired (any) D68.4
antepartum hemorrhage —*see* Hemorrhage, antepartum, with coagulation defect
clotting factor NEC —*see also* Deficiency, factor D68.2
due to
hyperprothrombinemia D68.4
liver disease D68.4
vitamin K deficiency D68.4
newborn, transient P61.6
postpartum O72.3
specified NEC D68.8
cognitive F09
color vision H53.50
achromatopsia H53.51
acquired H53.52
deuteranomaly H53.53
protanomaly H53.54
specified type NEC H53.59
tritanomaly H53.55
combined glucocorticoid and mineralocorticoid E27.49
contact factor D68.2
copper (nutritional) E61.0
corticoadrenal E27.40
primary E27.1
craniofacial axis Q75.0
cyanocobalamin E53.8
debrancher enzyme (limit dextrinosis) E74.03
dehydrogenase
long chain/very long chain acyl CoA E71.310
medium chain acyl CoA E71.311
short chain acyl CoA E71.312
diet E63.9
dihydropyrimidine dehydrogenase (DPD) E88.89
disaccharidase E73.9
edema —*see* Malnutrition, severe
endocrine E34.9
energy-supply —*see* Malnutrition
enzymes, circulating NEC E88.09
ergosterol E55.9
with
adult osteomalacia M83.8
rickets —*see* Rickets
essential fatty acid (EFA) E63.0
factor —*see also* Deficiency, coagulation
Hageman D68.2
I (congenital) (hereditary) D68.2
II (congenital) (hereditary) D68.2
IX (congenital) (functional) (hereditary) (with functional defect) D67
multiple (congenital) D68.8
acquired D68.4
V (congenital) (hereditary) D68.2
VII (congenital) (hereditary) D68.2
VIII (congenital) (functional) (hereditary) (with functional defect) D66
with vascular defect D68.0
X (congenital) (hereditary) D68.2
XI (congenital) (hereditary) D68.1
XII (congenital) (hereditary) D68.2
XIII (congenital) (hereditary) D68.2
femoral, proximal focal (congenital) —*see* Defect, reduction, lower limb, longitudinal, femur
fibrin-stabilizing factor (congenital) (hereditary) D68.2
acquired D68.4
fibrinase D68.2
fibrinogen (congenital) (hereditary) D68.2
acquired D65
folate E53.8
folic acid E53.8
foreskin N47.3
fructokinase E74.11
fructose 1,6-diphosphatase E74.19
Deficiency, deficient *(Continued)*
fructose-1-phosphate aldolase E74.19
galactokinase E74.29
galactose-1-phosphate uridyl transferase E74.29
gammaglobulin in blood D80.1
hereditary D80.0
glass factor D68.2
glucocorticoid E27.49
mineralocorticoid E27.49
glucose-6-phosphatase E74.01
glucose-6-phosphate dehydrogenase anemia D55.0
glucuronyl transferase E80.5
glycogen synthetase E74.09
gonadotropin (isolated) E23.0
growth hormone (idiopathic) (isolated) E23.0
Hageman factor D68.2
hemoglobin D64.9
hepatophosphorylase E74.09
homogentisate 1,2-dioxygenase E70.29
hormone
anterior pituitary (partial) NEC E23.0
growth E23.0
growth (isolated) E23.0
pituitary E23.0
testicular E29.1
hypoxanthine-(guanine)-phosphoribosyltransferase (HG-PRT) (total HG-PRT) E79.1
immunity D84.9
cell-mediated D84.8
with thrombocytopenia and eczema D82.0
combined D81.9
humoral D80.9
IgA (secretory) D80.2
IgG D80.3
IgM D80.4
immuno —*see* Immunodeficiency
immunoglobulin, selective
A (IgA) D80.2
G (IgG) (subclasses) D80.3
M (IgM) D80.4
inositol (B complex) E53.8
intrinsic
factor (congenital) D51.0
sphincter N36.42
with urethral hypermobility N36.43
iodine E61.8
congenital syndrome —*see* Syndrome, iodine-deficiency, congenital
iron E61.1
anemia D50.9
kalium E87.6
kappa-light chain D80.8
labile factor (congenital) (hereditary) D68.2
acquired D68.4
lacrimal fluid (acquired) —*see also* Syndrome, dry eye
congenital Q10.6
lactase
congenital E73.0
secondary E73.1
Laki-Lorand factor D68.2
lecithin cholesterol acyltransferase E78.6
lipocaic K86.89 ⇐
lipoprotein (familial) (high density) E78.6
liver phosphorylase E74.09
lysosomal alpha-1, 4 glucosidase E74.02
magnesium E61.2
major histocompatibility complex
class I D81.6
class II D81.7
manganese E61.3
menadione (vitamin K) E56.1
newborn P53
mental (familial) (hereditary) —*see* Disability, intellectual
methylenetetrahydrofolate reductase (MTHFR) E72.12

Deficiency, deficient *(Continued)*
mevalonate kinase M04.1 ◀
mineral NEC E61.8
mineralocorticoid E27.49
with glucocorticoid E27.49
molybdenum (nutritional) E61.5
moral F60.2
multiple nutrient elements E61.7
muscle
carnitine (palmityltransferase) E71.314
phosphofructokinase E74.09
myoadenylate deaminase E79.2
myocardial —*see* Insufficiency, myocardial
myophosphorylase E74.04
NADH diaphorase or reductase (congenital) D74.0
NADH-methemoglobin reductase (congenital) D74.0
natrium E87.1
niacin (amide) (-tryptophan) E52
nicotinamide E52
nicotinic acid E52
number of teeth —*see* Anodontia
nutrient element E61.9
multiple E61.7
specified NEC E61.8
nutrition, nutritional E63.9
sequelae —*see* Sequelae, nutritional deficiency
specified NEC E63.8
of interleukin 1 receptor antagonist [DIRA] M04.8 ◀
ornithine transcarbamylase E72.4
ovarian E28.39
oxygen —*see* Anoxia
pantothenic acid E53.8
parathyroid (gland) E20.9
perineum (female) N81.89
phenylalanine hydroxylase E70.1
phosphoenolpyruvate carboxykinase E74.4
phosphofructokinase E74.19
phosphomannomutuse E74.8
phosphomannose isomerase E74.8
phosphomannosyl mutase E74.8
phosphorylase kinase, liver E74.09
pituitary hormone (isolated) E23.0
plasma thromboplastin
antecedent (PTA) D68.1
component (PTC) D67
platelet NEC D69.1
constitutional D68.0
polyglandular E31.8
autoimmune E31.0
potassium (K) E87.6
prepuce N47.3
proaccelerin (congenital) (hereditary) D68.2
acquired D68.4
proconvertin factor (congenital) (hereditary) D68.2
acquired D68.4
protein —*see also* Malnutrition E46
anemia D53.0
C D68.59
S D68.59
prothrombin (congenital) (heredItary) D68.2
acquired D68.4
Prower factor D68.2
pseudocholinesterase E88.09
PTA (plasma thromboplastin antecedent) D68.1
PTC (plasma thromboplastin component) D67
purine nucleoside phosphorylase (PNP) D81.5
pyracin (alpha) (beta) E53.1
pyridoxal E53.1
pyridoxamine E53.1
pyridoxine (derivatives) E53.1
pyruvate
carboxylase E74.4
dehydrogenase E74.4
riboflavin (vitamin B2) E53.0

Deficiency, deficient *(Continued)*
salt E87.1
secretion
ovary E28.39
salivary gland (any) K11.7
urine R34
selenium (dietary) E59
serum antitrypsin, familial E88.01
short stature homeobox gene (SHOX)
with
dyschondrosteosis Q78.8
short stature (idiopathic) E34.3
Turner's syndrome Q96.9
sodium (Na) E87.1
SPCA (factor VII) D68.2
sphincter, intrinsic N36.42
with urethral hypermobility N36.43
stable factor (congenital) (hereditary) D68.2
acquired D68.4
Stuart-Prower (factor X) D68.2
sucrase E74.39
sulfatase E75.29
sulfite oxidase E72.19
thiamin, thiaminic (chloride) E51.9
beriberi (dry) E51.11
wet E51.12
thrombokinase D68.2
newborn P53
thyroid (gland) —*see* Hypothyroidism
tocopherol E56.0
tooth bud K00.0
transcobalamine II (anemia) D51.2
vanadium E61.6
vascular I99.9
vasopressin E23.2
vertical ridge K06.8 ◀
viosterol —*see* Deficiency, calciferol
vitamin (multiple) NOS E56.9
A E50.9
with
Bitot's spot (corneal) E50.1
follicular keratosis E50.8
keratomalacia E50.4
manifestations NEC E50.8
night blindness E50.5
scar of cornea, xerophthalmic E50.6
xeroderma E50.8
xerophthalmia E50.7
xerosis
conjunctival E50.0
and Bitot's spot E50.1
cornea E50.2
and ulceration E50.3
sequelae E64.1
B (complex) NOS E53.9
with
beriberi (dry) E51.11
wet E51.12
pellagra E52
B1 NOS E51.9
beriberi (dry) E51.11
with circulatory system manifestations E51.11
wet E51.12
B12 E53.8
B2 (riboflavin) E53.0
B6 E53.1
C E54
sequelae E64.2
D E55.9
with
adult osteomalacia M83.8
rickets —*see* Rickets
25-hydroxylase E83.32
E E56.0
folic acid E53.8
G E53.0
group B E53.9
specified NEC E53.8

Deficiency, deficient *(Continued)*
vitamin *(Continued)*
H (biotin) E53.8
K E56.1
of newborn P53
nicotinic E52
P E56.8
PP (pellagra-preventing) E52
specified NEC E56.8
thiamin E51.9
beriberi —*see* Beriberi
zinc, dietary E60
Deficit —*see also* Deficiency
attention and concentration R41.840
following ◀
cerebral infarction I69.310 ◀
cerebrovascular disease I69.910 ◀
specified disease NEC I69.810 ◀
nontraumatic ◀
intracerebral hemorrhage I69.110 ◀
specified intracranial hemorrhage NEC I69.210 ◀
subarachnoid hemorrhage I69.010 ◀
disorder —*see* Attention, deficit
~~cognitive communication R41.841~~
cognitive ◀
communication R41.841 ◀
emotional ◀
following ◀
cerebral infarction I69.315 ◀
cerebrovascular disease I69.915 ◀
specified disease NEC I69.815 ◀
nontraumatic ◀
intracerebral hemorrhage I69.115 ◀
specified intracranial hemorrhage NEC I69.215 ◀
subarachnoid hemorrhage I69.015 ◀
following ◀
cerebral infarction I69.319 ◀
cerebrovascular disease I69.919 ◀
specified disease NEC I69.819 ◀
nontraumatic ◀
intracerebral hemorrhage I69.119 ◀
specified intracranial hemorrhage NEC I69.219 ◀
subarachnoid hemorrhage I69.019 ◀
social ◀
following ◀
cerebral infarction I69.315 ◀
cerebrovascular disease I69.915 ◀
specified disease NEC I69.815 ◀
nontraumatic ◀
intracerebral hemorrhage I69.115 ◀
specified intracranial hemorrhage NEC I69.215 ◀
subarachnoid hemorrhage I69.015 ◀
cognitive NEC R41.89
following
cerebral infarction I69.318 ◀
cerebrovascular disease I69.918 ◀
specified disease NEC I69.818 ◀
~~intracerebral hemorrhage I69.11~~
~~nontraumatic intracranial hemorrhage NEC I69.21~~
nontraumatic ◀
intracerebral hemorrhage I69.118 ◀
specified intracranial hemorrhage NEC I69.218 ◀
subarachnoid hemorrhage I69.018 ◀
~~subarachnoid hemorrhage I69.01~~
concentration R41.840
executive function R41.844
following ◀
cerebral infarction I69.314 ◀
cerebrovascular disease I69.914 ◀
specified disease NEC I69.814 ◀
nontraumatic ◀
intracerebral hemorrhage I69.114 ◀
specified intracranial hemorrhage NEC I69.214 ◀
subarachnoid hemorrhage I69.014 ◀

◀ New ◀ Revised ~~deleted~~ Deleted

Deficit *(Continued)*
frontal lobe R41.844
following ◀
cerebral infarction I69.314 ◀
cerebrovascular disease I69.914 ◀
specified disease NEC I69.814 ◀
nontraumatic ◀
intracerebral hemorrhage I69.114 ◀
specified intracranial hemorrhage NEC I69.214 ◀
subarachnoid hemorrhage I69.014 ◀
memory ◀
following ◀
cerebral infarction I69.311 ◀
cerebrovascular disease I69.911 ◀
specified disease NEC I69.811 ◀
nontraumatic ◀
intracerebral hemorrhage I69.111 ◀
specified intracranial hemorrhage NEC I69.211 ◀
subarachnoid hemorrhage I69.011 ◀
neurologic NEC R29.818
ischemic
reversible (RIND) I63.9
prolonged (PRIND) I63.9
oxygen R09.02
prolonged reversible ischemic neurologic (PRIND) I63.9
psychomotor R41.843
following ◀
cerebral infarction I69.313 ◀
cerebrovascular disease I69.913 ◀
specified disease NEC I69.813 ◀
nontraumatic ◀
intracerebral hemorrhage I69.113 ◀
specified intracranial hemorrhage NEC I69.213 ◀
subarachnoid hemorrhage I69.013 ◀
visuospatial R41.842
following ◀
cerebral infarction I69.312 ◀
cerebrovascular disease I69.912 ◀
specified disease NEC I69.812 ◀
nontraumatic ◀
intracerebral hemorrhage I69.112 ◀
specified intracranial hemorrhage NEC I69.212 ◀
subarachnoid hemorrhage I69.012 ◀
Deflection
radius —*see* Deformity, limb, specified type NEC, forearm
septum (acquired) (nasal) (nose) J34.2
spine —*see* Curvature, spine
turbinate (nose) J34.2
Defluvium
capillorum —*see* Alopecia
ciliorum —*see* Madarosis
unguium L60.8
Deformity Q89.9
abdomen, congenital Q89.9
abdominal wall
acquired M95.8
congenital Q79.59
acquired (unspecified site) M95.9
adrenal gland Q89.1
alimentary tract, congenital Q45.9
upper Q40.9
ankle (joint) (acquired) —*see also* Deformity, limb, lower leg
abduction —*see* Contraction, joint, ankle
congenital Q68.8
contraction —*see* Contraction, joint, ankle
specified type NEC —*see* Deformity, limb, foot, specified NEC
anus (acquired) K62.89
congenital Q43.9
aorta (arch) (congenital) Q25.40 ⇐
acquired I77.89

Deformity *(Continued)*
aortic
arch, acquired I77.89
cusp or valve (congenital) Q23.8
acquired —*see also* Endocarditis, aortic I35.8
arm (acquired) (upper) —*see also* Deformity, limb, upper arm
congenital Q68.8
forearm —*see* Deformity, limb, forearm
artery (congenital) (peripheral) NOS Q27.9
acquired I77.89
coronary (acquired) I25.9
congenital Q24.5
umbilical Q27.0
atrial septal Q21.1
auditory canal (external) (congenital) —*see also* Malformation, ear, external
acquired —*see* Disorder, ear, external, specified type NEC
auricle
ear (congenital) —*see also* Malformation, ear, external
acquired —*see* Disorder, pinna, deformity
back —*see* Dorsopathy, deforming
bile duct (common) (congenital) (hepatic) Q44.5
acquired K83.8
biliary duct or passage (congenital) Q44.5
acquired K83.8
bladder (neck) (trigone) (sphincter) (acquired) N32.89
congenital Q64.79
bone (acquired) NOS M95.9
congenital Q79.9
turbinate M95.0
brain (congenital) Q04.9
acquired G93.89
reduction Q04.3
breast (acquired) N64.89
congenital Q83.9
reconstructed N65.0
bronchus (congenital) Q32.4
acquired NEC J98.09
bursa, congenital Q79.9
canaliculi (lacrimalis) (acquired) —*see also* Disorder, lacrimal system, changes
congenital Q10.6
canthus, acquired —*see* Disorder, eyelid, specified type NEC
capillary (acquired) I78.8
cardiovascular system, congenital Q28.9
caruncle, lacrimal (acquired) —*see also* Disorder, lacrimal system, changes
congenital Q10.6
cascade, stomach K31.2
cecum (congenital) Q43.9
acquired K63.89
cerebral, acquired G93.89
congenital Q04.9
cervix (uterus) (acquired) NEC N88.8
congenital Q51.9
cheek (acquired) M95.2
congenital Q18.9
chest (acquired) (wall) M95.4
congenital Q67.8
sequelae (late effect) of rickets E64.3
chin (acquired) M95.2
congenital Q18.9
choroid (congenital) Q14.3
acquired H31.8
plexus Q07.8
acquired G96.19
cicatricial —*see* Cicatrix
cilia, acquired —*see* Disorder, eyelid, specified type NEC
clavicle (acquired) M95.8
congenital Q68.8
clitoris (congenital) Q52.6
acquired N90.89
clubfoot —*see* Clubfoot

Deformity *(Continued)*
coccyx (acquired) —*see* subcategory M43.8
colon (congenital) Q43.9
acquired K63.89
concha (ear), congenital —*see also* Malformation, ear, external
acquired —*see* Disorder, pinna, deformity
cornea (acquired) H18.70
congenital Q13.4
descemetocele —*see* Descemetocele
ectasia —*see* Ectasia, cornea
specified NEC H18.79-
staphyloma —*see* Staphyloma, cornea
coronary artery (acquired) I25.9
congenital Q24.5
cranium (acquired) —*see* Deformity, skull
cricoid cartilage (congenital) Q31.8
acquired J38.7
cystic duct (congenital) Q44.5
acquired K82.8
Dandy-Walker Q03.1
with spina bifida —*see* Spina bifida
diaphragm (congenital) Q79.1
acquired J98.6
digestive organ NOS Q45.9
ductus arteriosus Q25.0
duodenal bulb K31.89
duodenum (congenital) Q43.9
acquired K31.89
dura —*see* Deformity, meninges
ear (acquired) —*see also* Disorder, pinna, deformity
congenital (external) Q17.9
internal Q16.5
middle Q16.4
ossicles Q16.3
ossicles Q16.3
ectodermal (congenital) NEC Q84.9
ejaculatory duct (congenital) Q55.4
acquired N50.89 ⇐
elbow (joint) (acquired) —*see also* Deformity, limb, upper arm
congenital Q68.8
contraction —*see* Contraction, joint, elbow
endocrine gland NEC Q89.2
epididymis (congenital) Q55.4
acquired N50.89 ⇐
epiglottis (congenital) Q31.8
acquired J38.7
esophagus (congenital) Q39.9
acquired K22.8
eustachian tube (congenital) NEC Q17.8
eye, congenital Q15.9
eyebrow (congenital) Q18.8
eyelid (acquired) —*see also* Disorder, eyelid, specified type NEC
congenital Q10.3
face (acquired) M95.2
congenital Q18.9
fallopian tube, acquired N83.8
femur (acquired) —*see* Deformity, limb, specified type NEC, thigh
fetal
with fetopelvic disproportion O33.7
causing obstructed labor O66.3
finger (acquired) M20.00-
boutonniere M20.02-
congenital Q68.1
flexion contracture —*see* Contraction, joint, hand
mallet finger M20.01-
specified NEC M20.09-
swan-neck M20.03-
flexion (joint) (acquired) —*see also* Deformity, limb, flexion M21.20
congenital NOS Q74.9
hip Q65.89
foot (acquired) —*see also* Deformity, limb, lower leg
cavovarus (congenital) Q66.1
congenital NOS Q66.9
specified type NEC Q66.89

◀ New ⇐ Revised ~~deleted~~ Deleted

Deformity *(Continued)*
foot *(Continued)*
specified type NEC —*see* Deformity, limb, foot, specified NEC
valgus (congenital) Q66.6
acquired —*see* Deformity, valgus, ankle
varus (congenital) NEC Q66.3
acquired —*see* Deformity, varus, ankle
forearm (acquired) —*see also* Deformity, limb, forearm
congenital Q68.8
forehead (acquired) M95.2
congenital Q75.8
frontal bone (acquired) M95.2
congenital Q75.8
gallbladder (congenital) Q44.1
acquired K82.8
gastrointestinal tract (congenital) NOS Q45.9
acquired K63.89
genitalia, genital organ (s) or system NEC
female (congenital) Q52.9
acquired N94.89
external Q52.70
male (congenital) Q55.9
acquired N50.89 ◀
globe (eye) (congenital) Q15.8
acquired H44.89
gum, acquired NEC K06.8
hand (acquired) —*see* Deformity, limb, hand
congenital Q68.1
head (acquired) M95.2
congenital Q75.8
heart (congenital) Q24.9
septum Q21.9
auricular Q21.1
ventricular Q21.0
valve (congenital) NEC Q24.8
acquired —*see* Endocarditis
heel (acquired) —*see* Deformity, foot
hepatic duct (congenital) Q44.5
acquired K83.8
hip (joint) (acquired) —*see also* Deformity, limb, thigh
congenital Q65.9
due to (previous) juvenile osteochondrosis —*see* Coxa, plana
flexion —*see* Contraction, joint, hip
hourglass —*see* Contraction, hourglass
humerus (acquired) M21.82-
congenital Q74.0
hypophyseal (congenital) Q89.2
ileocecal (coil) (valve) (acquired) K63.89
congenital Q43.9
ileum (congenital) Q43.9
acquired K63.89
ilium (acquired) M95.5
congenital Q74.2
integument (congenital) Q84.9
intervertebral cartilage or disc (acquired) —*see* Disorder, disc, specified NEC
intestine (large) (small) (congenital) NOS Q43.9
acquired K63.89
intrinsic minus or plus (hand) —*see* Deformity, limb, specified type NEC, forearm
iris (acquired) H21.89
congenital Q13.2
ischium (acquired) M95.5
congenital Q74.2
jaw (acquired) (congenital) M26.9
joint (acquired) NEC M21.90
congenital Q68.8
elbow M21.92-
hand M21.94-
hip M21.95-
knee M21.96-
shoulder M21.92-
wrist M21.93-

Deformity *(Continued)*
kidney (s) (calyx) (pelvis) (congenital) Q63.9
acquired N28.89
artery (congenital) Q27.2
acquired I77.89
Klippel-Feil (brevicollis) Q76.1
knee (acquired) NEC —*see also* Deformity, limb, lower leg
congenital Q68.2
labium (majus) (minus) (congenital) Q52.79
acquired N90.89
lacrimal passages or duct (congenital) NEC Q10.6
acquired —*see* Disorder, lacrimal system, changes
larynx (muscle) (congenital) Q31.8
acquired J38.7
web (glottic) Q31.0
leg (upper) (acquired) NEC —*see also* Deformity, limb, thigh
congenital Q68.8
lower leg —*see* Deformity, limb, lower leg
lens (acquired) H27.8
congenital Q12.9
lid (fold) (acquired) —*see also* Disorder, eyelid, specified type NEC
congenital Q10.3
ligament (acquired) —*see* Disorder, ligament
congenital Q79.9
limb (acquired) M21.90
clawfoot M21.53-
clawhand M21.51-
clubfoot M21.54-
clubhand M21.52-
congenital, except reduction deformity Q74.9
flat foot M21.4-
flexion M21.20
ankle M21.27-
elbow M21.22-
finger M21.24-
hip M21.25-
knee M21.26-
shoulder M21.21-
toe M21.27-
wrist M21.23-
foot
claw —*see* Deformity, limb, clawfoot
club —*see* Deformity, limb, clubfoot
drop M21.37-
flat —*see* Deformity, limb, flat foot
specified NEC M21.6X-
forearm M21.93-
hand M21.94-
lower leg M21.96-
specified type NEC M21.80
forearm M21.83-
lower leg M21.86-
thigh M21.85-
upper arm M21.82-
thigh M21.95-
unequal length M21.70
short site is
femur M21.75-
fibula M21.76-
humerus M21.72-
radius M21.73-
tibia M21.76-
ulna M21.73-
upper arm M21.92-
valgus —*see* Deformity, valgus
varus —*see* Deformity, varus
wrist drop M21.33-
lip (acquired) NEC K13.0
congenital Q38.0
liver (congenital) Q44.7
acquired K76.89
lumbosacral (congenital) (joint) (region) Q76.49
acquired —*see* subcategory M43.8
kyphosis —*see* Kyphosis, congenital
lordosis —*see* Lordosis, congenital

Deformity *(Continued)*
lung (congenital) Q33.9
acquired J98.4
lymphatic system, congenital Q89.9
Madelung's (radius) Q74.0
mandible (acquired) (congenital) M26.9
maxilla (acquired) (congenital) M26.9
meninges or membrane (congenital) Q07.9
cerebral Q04.8
acquired G96.19
spinal cord (congenital) G96.19
acquired G96.19
metacarpus (acquired) —*see* Deformity, limb, forearm
congenital Q74.0
metatarsus (acquired) —*see* Deformity, foot
congenital Q66.9
middle ear (congenital) Q16.4
ossicles Q16.3
mitral (leaflets) (valve) I05.8
parachute Q23.2
stenosis, congenital Q23.2
mouth (acquired) K13.79
congenital Q38.6
multiple, congenital NEC Q89.7
muscle (acquired) M62.89
congenital Q79.9
sternocleidomastoid Q68.0
musculoskeletal system (acquired) M95.9
congenital Q79.9
specified NEC M95.8
nail (acquired) L60.8
congenital Q84.6
nasal —*see* Deformity, nose
neck (acquired) M95.3
congenital Q18.9
sternocleidomastoid Q68.0
nervous system (congenital) Q07.9
nipple (congenital) Q83.9
acquired N64.89
nose (acquired) (cartilage) M95.0
bone (turbinate) M95.0
congenital Q30.9
bent or squashed Q67.4
saddle M95.0
syphilitic A50.57
septum (acquired) J34.2
congenital Q30.8
sinus (wall) (congenital) Q30.8
acquired M95.0
syphilitic (congenital) A50.57
late A52.73
ocular muscle (congenital) Q10.3
acquired —*see* Strabismus, mechanical
opticociliary vessels (congenital) Q13.2
orbit (eye) (acquired) H05.30
atrophy —*see* Atrophy, orbit
congenital Q10.7
due to
bone disease NEC H05.32-
trauma or surgery H05.33-
enlargement —*see* Enlargement, orbit
exostosis —*see* Exostosis, orbit
organ of Corti (congenital) Q16.5
ovary (congenital) Q50.39
acquired N83.8
oviduct, acquired N83.8
palate (congenital) Q38.5
acquired M27.8
cleft (congenital) —*see* Cleft, palate
pancreas (congenital) Q45.3
acquired K86.89 ◀
parathyroid (gland) Q89.2
parotid (gland) (congenital) Q38.4
acquired K11.8
patella (acquired) —*see* Disorder, patella, specified NEC
pelvis, pelvic (acquired) (bony) M95.5
with disproportion (fetopelvic) O33.0
causing obstructed labor O65.0

◀ New ◀ Revised ~~deleted~~ Deleted

Deformity *(Continued)*
pelvis, pelvic *(Continued)*
congenital Q74.2
rachitic sequelae (late effect) E64.3
penis (glans) (congenital) Q55.69
acquired N48.89
pericardium (congenital) Q24.8
acquired —*see* Pericarditis
pharynx (congenital) Q38.8
acquired J39.2
pinna, acquired —*see also* Disorder, pinna, deformity
congenital Q17.9
pituitary (congenital) Q89.2
posture —*see* Dorsopathy, deforming
prepuce (congenital) Q55.69
acquired N47.8
prostate (congenital) Q55.4
acquired N42.89
pupil (congenital) Q13.2
acquired —*see* Abnormality, pupillary
pylorus (congenital) Q40.3
acquired K31.89
rachitic (acquired), old or healed E64.3
radius (acquired) —*see also* Deformity, limb, forearm
congenital Q68.8
rectum (congenital) Q43.9
acquired K62.89
reduction (extremity) (limb), congenital (*see also* condition and site) Q73.8
brain Q04.3
lower —*see* Defect, reduction, lower limb
upper —*see* Defect, reduction, upper limb
renal —*see* Deformity, kidney
respiratory system (congenital) Q34.9
rib (acquired) M95.4
congenital Q76.6
cervical Q76.5
rotation (joint) (acquired) —*see* Deformity, limb, specified site NEC
congenital Q74.9
hip —*see* Deformity, limb, specified type NEC, thigh
congenital Q65.89
sacroiliac joint (congenital) Q74.2
acquired —*see* subcategory M43.8
sacrum (acquired) —*see* subcategory M43.8
saddle
back —*see* Lordosis
nose M95.0
syphilitic A50.57
salivary gland or duct (congenital) Q38.4
acquired K11.8
scapula (acquired) M95.8
congenital Q68.8
scrotum (congenital) —*see also* Malformation, testis and scrotum
acquired N50.89 ◄
seminal vesicles (congenital) Q55.4
acquired N50.89 ◄
septum, nasal (acquired) J34.2
shoulder (joint) (acquired) —*see* Deformity, limb, upper arm
congenital Q74.0
contraction —*see* Contraction, joint, shoulder
sigmoid (flexure) (congenital) Q43.9
acquired K63.89
skin (congenital) Q82.9
skull (acquired) M95.2
congenital Q75.8
with
anencephaly Q00.0
encephalocele —*see* Encephalocele
hydrocephalus Q03.9
with spina bifida —*see* Spina bifida, by site, with hydrocephalus
microcephaly Q02

Deformity *(Continued)*
soft parts, organs or tissues (of pelvis)
in pregnancy or childbirth NEC O34.8-
causing obstructed labor O65.5
spermatic cord (congenital) Q55.4
acquired N50.89 ◄
torsion —*see* Torsion, spermatic cord
spinal —*see* Dorsopathy, deforming
column (acquired) —*see* Dorsopathy, deforming
congenital Q67.5
cord (congenital) Q06.9
acquired G95.89
nerve root (congenital) Q07.9
spine (acquired) —*see also* Dorsopathy, deforming
congenital Q67.5
rachitic E64.3
specified NEC —*see* Dorsopathy, deforming, specified NEC
spleen
acquired D73.89
congenital Q89.09
Sprengel's (congenital) Q74.0
sternocleidomastoid (muscle), congenital Q68.0
sternum (acquired) M95.4
congenital NEC Q76.7
stomach (congenital) Q40.3
acquired K31.89
submandibular gland (congenital) Q38.4
submaxillary gland (congenital) Q38.4
acquired K11.8
talipes —*see* Talipes
testis (congenital) —*see also* Malformation, testis and scrotum
acquired N44.8
torsion —*see* Torsion, testis
thigh (acquired) —*see also* Deformity, limb, thigh
congenital NEC Q68.8
thorax (acquired) (wall) M95.4
congenital Q67.8
sequelae of rickets E64.3
thumb (acquired) —*see also* Deformity, finger
congenital NEC Q68.1
thymus (tissue) (congenital) Q89.2
thyroid (gland) (congenital) Q89.2
cartilage Q31.8
acquired J38.7
tibia (acquired) —*see also* Deformity, limb, specified type NEC, lower leg
congenital NEC Q68.8
saber (syphilitic) A50.56
toe (acquired) M20.6-
congenital Q66.9
hallux rigidus M20.2-
hallux valgus M20.1-
hallux varus M20.3-
hammer toe M20.4-
specified NEC M20.5X-
tongue (congenital) Q38.3
acquired K14.8
tooth, teeth K00.2
trachea (rings) (congenital) Q32.1
acquired J39.8
transverse aortic arch (congenital) Q25.49 ◄
tricuspid (leaflets) (valve) I07.8
atresia or stenosis Q22.4
Ebstein's Q22.5
trunk (acquired) M95.8
congenital Q89.9
ulna (acquired) —*see also* Deformity, limb, forearm
congenital NEC Q68.8
urachus, congenital Q64.4
ureter (opening) (congenital) Q62.8
acquired N28.89
urethra (congenital) Q64.79
acquired N36.8

Deformity *(Continued)*
urinary tract (congenital) Q64.9
urachus Q64.4
uterus (congenital) Q51.9
acquired N85.8
uvula (congenital) Q38.5
vagina (acquired) N89.8
congenital Q52.4
valgus NEC M21.00
ankle M21.07-
elbow M21.02-
hip M21.05-
knee M21.06-
valve, valvular (congenital) (heart) Q24.8
acquired —*see* Endocarditis
varus NEC M21.10
ankle M21.17-
elbow M21.12-
hip M21.15
knee M21.16-
tibia —*see* Osteochondrosis, juvenile, tibia
vas deferens (congenital) Q55.4
acquired N50.89 ◄
vein (congenital) Q27.9
great Q26.9
vertebra —*see* Dorsopathy, deforming
vertical talus (congenital) Q66.80
left foot Q66.82
right foot Q66.81
vesicourethral orifice (acquired) N32.89
congenital NEC Q64.79
vessels of optic papilla (congenital) Q14.2
visual field (contraction) —*see* Defect, visual field
vitreous body, acquired H43.89
vulva (congenital) Q52.79
acquired N90.89
wrist (joint) (acquired) —*see also* Deformity, limb, forearm
congenital Q68.8
contraction —*see* Contraction, joint, wrist

Degeneration, degenerative
adrenal (capsule) (fatty) (gland) (hyaline) (infectional) E27.8
amyloid —*see also* Amyloidosis E85.9
anterior cornua, spinal cord G12.29
anterior labral S43.49-
aorta, aortic I70.0
fatty I77.89
aortic valve (heart) —*see* Endocarditis, aortic
arteriovascular —*see* Arteriosclerosis
artery, arterial (atheromatous) (calcareous) —*see also* Arteriosclerosis
cerebral, amyloid E85.4 *[I68.0]*
medial —*see* Arteriosclerosis, extremities
articular cartilage NEC —*see* Derangement, joint, articular cartilage, by site
atheromatous —*see* Arteriosclerosis
basal nuclei or ganglia G23.9
specified NEC G23.8
bone NEC —*see* Disorder, bone, specified type NEC
brachial plexus G54.0
brain (cortical) (progressive) G31.9
alcoholic G31.2
arteriosclerotic I67.2
childhood G31.9
specified NEC G31.89
cystic G31.89
congenital Q04.6
in
alcoholism G31.2
beriberi E51.2
cerebrovascular disease I67.9
congenital hydrocephalus Q03.9
with spina bifida —*see also* Spina bifida
Fabry-Anderson disease E75.21
Gaucher's disease E75.22
Hunter's syndrome E76.1

Degeneration, degenerative *(Continued)*
brain *(Continued)*
in *(Continued)*
lipidosis
cerebral E75.4
generalized E75.6
mucopolysaccharidosis —*see* Mucopolysaccharidosis
myxedema E03.9 *[G32.89]*
neoplastic disease —*see also* Neoplasm D49.6 *[G32.89]*
Niemann-Pick disease E75.249 *[G32.89]*
sphingolipidosis E75.3 *[G32.89]*
vitamin B12 deficiency E53.8 *[G32.89]*
senile NEC G31.1
breast N64.89
Bruch's membrane —*see* Degeneration, choroid
capillaries (fatty) I78.8
amyloid E85.8 *[I79.8]*
cardiac —*see also* Degeneration, myocardial
valve, valvular —*see* Endocarditis
cardiorenal —*see* Hypertension, cardiorenal
cardiovascular —*see also* Disease, cardiovascular
renal —*see* Hypertension, cardiorenal
cerebellar NOS G31.9
alcoholic G31.2
primary (hereditary) (sporadic) G11.9
cerebral —*see* Degeneration, brain
cerebrovascular I67.9
due to hypertension I67.4
cervical plexus G54.2
cervix N88.8
due to radiation (intended effect) N88.8
adverse effect or misadventure N99.89
chamber angle H21.21-
changes, spine or vertebra —*see* Spondylosis
chorioretinal —*see also* Degeneration, choroid
hereditary H31.20
choroid (colloid) (drusen) H31.10-
atrophy —*see* Atrophy, choroidal
hereditary —*see* Dystrophy, choroidal, hereditary
ciliary body H21.22-
cochlear —*see* subcategory H83.8
combined (spinal cord) (subacute) E53.8 *[G32.0]*
with anemia (pernicious) D51.0 *[G32.0]*
due to dietary vitamin B12 deficiency D51.3 *[G32.0]*
in (due to)
vitamin B12 deficiency E53.8 *[G32.0]*
anemia D51.9 *[G32.0]*
conjunctiva H11.10
concretions —*see* Concretion, conjunctiva
deposits —*see* Deposit, conjunctiva
pigmentations —*see* Pigmentation, conjunctiva
pinguecula —*see* Pinguecula
xerosis —*see* Xerosis, conjunctiva
cornea H18.40
calcerous H18.43
band keratopathy H18.42-
familial, hereditary —*see* Dystrophy, cornea
hyaline (of old scars) H18.49
keratomalacia —*see* Keratomalacia
nodular H18.45-
peripheral H18.46-
senile H18.41-
specified type NEC H18.49
cortical (cerebellar) (parenchymatous) G31.89
alcoholic G31.2
diffuse, due to arteriopathy I67.2
corticobasal G31.85
cutis L98.8
amyloid E85.4 *[L99]*
dental pulp K04.2
disc disease —*see* Degeneration, intervertebral disc NEC

Degeneration, degenerative *(Continued)*
dorsolateral (spinal cord) —*see* Degeneration, combined
extrapyramidal G25.9
eye, macular —*see also* Degeneration, macula
congenital or hereditary —*see* Dystrophy, retina
facet joints —*see* Spondylosis
fatty
liver NEC K76.0
alcoholic K70.0
grey matter (brain) (Alpers') G31.81
heart —*see also* Degeneration, myocardial
amyloid E85.4 *[I43]*
atheromatous —*see* Disease, heart, ischemic, atherosclerotic
ischemic —*see* Disease, heart, ischemic
hepatolenticular (Wilson's) E83.01
hepatorenal K76.7
hyaline (diffuse) (generalized)
localized —*see* Degeneration, by site
infrapatellar fat pad M79.4
intervertebral disc NOS
with
myelopathy —*see* Disorder, disc, with, myelopathy
radiculitis or radiculopathy —*see* Disorder, disc, with, radiculopathy
cervical, cervicothoracic —*see* Disorder, disc, cervical, degeneration
with
myelopathy —*see* Disorder, disc, cervical, with myelopathy
neuritis, radiculitis or radiculopathy —*see* Disorder, disc, cervical, with neuritis
lumbar region M51.36
with
myelopathy M51.06
neuritis, radiculitis, radiculopathy or sciatica M51.16
lumbosacral region M51.37
with
neuritis, radiculitis, radiculopathy or sciatica M51.17
sacrococcygeal region M53.3
thoracic region M51.34
with
myelopathy M51.04
neuritis, radiculitis, radiculopathy M51.14
thoracolumbar region M51.35
with
myelopathy M51.05
neuritis, radiculitis, radiculopathy M51.15
intestine, amyloid E85.4
iris (pigmentary) H21.23-
ischemic —*see* Ischemia
joint disease —*see* Osteoarthritis
kidney N28.89
amyloid E85.4 *[N29]*
cystic, congenital Q61.9
fatty N28.89
polycystic Q61.3
adult type (autosomal dominant) Q61.2
infantile type (autosomal recessive) NEC Q61.19
collecting duct dilatation Q61.11
Kuhnt-Junius —*see also* Degeneration, macula H35.32- ⬅
lens —*see* Cataract
lenticular (familial) (progressive) (Wilson's) (with cirrhosis of liver) E83.01
liver (diffuse) NEC K76.89
amyloid E85.4 *[K77]*
cystic K76.89
congenital Q44.6
fatty NEC K76.0
alcoholic K70.0

Degeneration, degenerative *(Continued)*
liver *(Continued)*
hypertrophic K76.89
parenchymatous, acute or subacute K72.00
with coma K72.01
pigmentary K76.89
toxic (acute) K71.9
lung J98.4
lymph gland I89.8
hyaline I89.8
macula, macular (acquired) (age-related) (senile) H35.30
angioid streaks H35.33
atrophic age-related H35.31- ⬅
congenital or hereditary —*see* Dystrophy, retina
cystoid H35.35-
drusen H35.36-
dry age-related H35.31- ◀
exudative H35.32- ⬅
hole H35.34-
nonexudative H35.31- ⬅
puckering H35.37-
toxic H35.38-
wet age-related H35.32- ◀
membranous labyrinth, congenital (causing impairment of hearing) Q16.5
meniscus —*see* Derangement, meniscus
mitral —*see* Insufficiency, mitral
Mönckeberg's —*see* Arteriosclerosis, extremities
motor centers, senile G31.1
multi-system G90.3
mural —*see* Degeneration, myocardial
muscle (fatty) (fibrous) (hyaline) (progressive) M62.89
heart —*see* Degeneration, myocardial
myelin, central nervous system G37.9
myocardial, myocardium (fatty) (hyaline) (senile) I51.5
with rheumatic fever (conditions in I00) I09.0
active, acute or subacute I01.2
with chorea I02.0
inactive or quiescent (with chorea) I09.0
hypertensive —*see* Hypertension, heart
rheumatic —*see* Degeneration, myocardial, with rheumatic fever
syphilitic A52.06
nasal sinus (mucosa) J32.9
frontal J32.1
maxillary J32.0
nerve —*see* Disorder, nerve
nervous system G31.9
alcoholic G31.2
amyloid E85.4 *[G99.8]*
autonomic G90.9
fatty G31.89
specified NEC G31.89
nipple N64.89
olivopontocerebellar (hereditary) (familial) G23.8
osseous labyrinth —*see* subcategory H83.8
ovary N83.8
cystic N83.20- ⬅
microcystic N83.20- ⬅
pallidal pigmentary (progressive) G23.0
pancreas K86.89 ⬅
tuberculous A18.83
penis N48.89
pigmentary (diffuse) (general)
localized —*see* Degeneration, by site
pallidal (progressive) G23.0
pineal gland E34.8
pituitary (gland) E23.6
popliteal fat pad M79.4
posterolateral (spinal cord) —*see* Degeneration, combined
pulmonary valve (heart) I37.8
pulp (tooth) K04.2

◀ New ⬅ Revised ~~deleted~~ Deleted

Degeneration, degenerative *(Continued)*
pupillary margin H21.24-
renal —*see* Degeneration, kidney
retina H35.9
hereditary (cerebroretinal) (congenital) (juvenile) (macula) (peripheral) (pigmentary) —*see* Dystrophy, retina
Kuhnt-Junius —*see also* Degeneration, macula H35.32- ◀
macula (cystic) (exudative) (hole) (nonexudative) (pseudohole) (senile) (toxic) —*see* Degeneration, macula
peripheral H35.40
lattice H35.41-
microcystoid H35.42-
paving stone H35.43-
secondary
pigmentary H35.45-
vitreoretinal H35.46-
senile reticular H35.44-
pigmentary (primary) —*see also* Dystrophy, retina
secondary —*see* Degeneration, retina, peripheral, secondary
posterior pole —*see* Degeneration, macula
saccule, congenital (causing impairment of hearing) Q16.5
senile R54
brain G31.1
cardiac, heart or myocardium —*see* Degeneration, myocardial
motor centers G31.1
vascular —*see* Arteriosclerosis
sinus (cystic) —*see also* Sinusitis
polypoid J33.1
skin L98.8
amyloid E85.4 *[L99]*
colloid L98.8
spinal (cord) G31.89
amyloid E85.4 *[G32.89]*
combined (subacute) —*see* Degeneration, combined
dorsolateral —*see* Degeneration, combined
familial NEC G31.89
fatty G31.89
funicular —*see* Degeneration, combined
posterolateral —*see* Degeneration, combined
subacute combined —*see* Degeneration, combined
tuberculous A17.81
spleen D73.0
amyloid E85.4 *[D77]*
stomach K31.89
striatonigral G23.2
suprarenal (capsule) (gland) E27.8
synovial membrane (pulpy) —*see* Disorder, synovium, specified type NEC
tapetoretinal —*see* Dystrophy, retina
thymus (gland) E32.8
fatty E32.8
thyroid (gland) E07.89
tricuspid (heart) (valve) I07.9
tuberculous NEC —*see* Tuberculosis
turbinate J34.89
uterus (cystic) N85.8
vascular (senile) —*see* Arteriosclerosis
hypertensive —*see* Hypertension
vitreoretinal, secondary —*see* Degeneration, retina, peripheral, secondary, vitreoretinal
vitreous (body) H43.81-
Wallerian —*see* Disorder, nerve
Wilson's hepatolenticular E83.01
Deglutition
paralysis R13.0
hysterical F44.4
pneumonia J69.0
Degos' disease I77.89
Dehiscence (of)
amputation stump T87.81
cesarean wound O90.0

Dehiscence *(Continued)*
closure of
cornea T81.31
craniotomy T81.32
fascia (muscular) (superficial) T81.32
internal organ or tissue T81.32
laceration (external) (internal) T81.33
ligament T81.32
mucosa T81.31
muscle or muscle flap T81.32
ribs or rib cage T81.32
skin and subcutaneous tissue (full-thickness) (superficial) T81.31
skull T81.32
sternum (sternotomy) T81.32
tendon T81.32
traumatic laceration (external) (internal) T81.33
episiotomy O90.1
operation wound NEC T81.31
external operation wound (superficial) T81.31
internal operation wound (deep) T81.32
perineal wound (postpartum) O90.1
traumatic injury wound repair T81.33
wound T81.30
traumatic repair T81.33
Dehydration E86.0
~~hypertonic E87.0~~
~~hypotonic E87.1~~
newborn P74.1
Déjérine-Roussy syndrome G93.89
Déjérine-Sottas disease or neuropathy (hypertrophic) G60.0
Déjérine-Thomas atrophy G23.8
Delay, delayed
any plane in pelvis
complicating delivery O66.9
birth or delivery NOS O63.9
closure, ductus arteriosus (Botalli) P29.3
coagulation —*see* Defect, coagulation
conduction (cardiac) (ventricular) I45.9
delivery, second twin, triplet, etc O63.2
development R62.50
global F88
intellectual (specific) F81.9
language F80.9
due to hearing loss F80.4
learning F81.9
pervasive F84.9
physiological R62.50
specified stage NEC R62.0
reading F81.0
sexual E30.0
speech F80.9
due to hearing loss F80.4
spelling F81.81
ejaculation F52.32 ◀
gastric emptying K30
menarche E30.0
menstruation (cause unknown) N91.0
milestone R62.0
passage of meconium (newborn) P76.0
primary respiration P28.9
puberty (constitutional) E30.0
separation of umbilical cord P96.82
sexual maturation, female E30.0
sleep phase syndrome G47.21
union, fracture —*see* Fracture, by site
vaccination Z28.9
Deletion (s)
autosome Q93.9
identified by fluorescence in situ hybridization (FISH) Q93.89
identified by in situ hybridization (ISH) Q93.89
chromosome
with complex rearrangements NEC Q93.7
part of NEC Q93.5
seen only at prometaphase Q93.89

Deletion *(Continued)*
chromosome *(Continued)*
short arm
4 Q93.3
5p Q93.4
22q11.2 Q93.81
specified NEC Q93.89
long arm chromosome 18 or 21 Q93.89
with complex rearrangements NEC Q93.7
microdeletions NEC Q93.88
Delhi boil or button B55.1
Delinquency (juvenile) (neurotic) F91.8
group Z72.810
Delinquent immunization status Z28.3
Delirium, delirious (acute or subacute) (not alcohol or drug-induced) (with dementia) R41.0
alcoholic (acute) (tremens) (withdrawal) F10.921
with intoxication F10.921
in
abuse F10.121
dependence F10.221
due to (secondary to)
alcohol
intoxication F10.921
in
abuse F10.121
dependence F10.221
withdrawal F10.231
amphetamine intoxication F15.921
in
abuse F15.121
dependence F15.221
anxiolytic
intoxication F13.921
in
abuse F13.121
dependence F13.221
withdrawal F13.231
cannabis intoxication (acute) F12.921
in
abuse F12.121
dependence F12.221
cocaine intoxication (acute) F14.921
in
abuse F14.121
dependence F14.221
general medical condition F05
hallucinogen intoxication F16.921
in
abuse F16.121
dependence F16.221
hypnotic
intoxication F13.921
in
abuse F13.121
dependence F13.221
withdrawal F13.231
inhalant intoxication (acute) F18.921
in
abuse F18.121
dependence F18.221
multiple etiologies F05
opioid intoxication (acute) F11.921
in
abuse F11.121
dependence F11.221
other (or unknown) substance F19.921 ◀
phencyclidine intoxication (acute) F16.921
in
abuse F16.121
dependence F16.221
psychoactive substance NEC intoxication (acute) F19.921
in
abuse F19.121
dependence F19.221

Delirium, delirious *(Continued)*
due to *(Continued)*
sedative
intoxication F13.921
in
abuse F13.121
dependence F13.221
withdrawal F13.231
unknown etiology F05
exhaustion F43.0
hysterical F44.89
postprocedural (postoperative) F05
puerperal F05
thyroid —*see* Thyrotoxicosis with thyroid storm
traumatic —*see* Injury, intracranial
tremens (alcohol-induced) F10.231
sedative-induced F13.231
Delivery (childbirth) (labor)
arrested active phase O62.1
cesarean (for)
without indication O82
abnormal
pelvis (bony) (deformity) (major) NEC
with disproportion (fetopelvic) O33.0
with obstructed labor O65.0
presentation or position O32.9
abruptio placentae —*see also* Abruptio placentae 045.9-
acromion presentation O32.2
atony, uterus O62.2
breech presentation O32.1
incomplete O32.8
brow presentation O32.3
cephalopelvic disproportion O33.9
cerclage O34.3-
chin presentation O32.3
cicatrix of cervix O34.4-
contracted pelvis (general)
inlet O33.2
outlet O33.3
cord presentation or prolapse O69.0
cystocele O34.8-
deformity (acquired) (congenital)
pelvic organs or tissues NEC O34.8-
pelvis (bony) NEC O33.0
disproportion NOS O33.9
eclampsia —*see* Eclampsia
face presentation O32.3
failed
forceps O66.5
induction of labor O61.9
instrumental O61.1
mechanical O61.1
medical O61.0
specified NEC O61.8
surgical O61.1
trial of labor NOS O66.40
following previous cesarean delivery O66.41
vacuum extraction O66.5
ventouse O66.5
fetal-maternal hemorrhage O43.01-
hemorrhage (intrapartum) O67.9
with coagulation defect O67.0
specified cause NEC O67.8
high head at term O32.4
hydrocephalic fetus O33.6
incarceration of uterus O34.51-
incoordinate uterine action O62.4
increased size, fetus O33.5
inertia, uterus O62.2
primary O62.0
secondary O62.1
lateroversion, uterus O34.59-
mal lie O32.9
malposition
fetus O32.9
pelvic organs or tissues NEC O34.8-
uterus NEC O34.59-
Delivery *(Continued)*
cesarean *(Continued)*
malpresentation NOS O32.9
oblique presentation O32.2
occurring after 37 completed weeks of gestation but before 39 completed weeks gestation due to (spontaneous) onset of labor O75.82
oversize fetus O33.5
pelvic tumor NEC O34.8-
placenta previa O44.0- ⇐
complete O44.0- ◀
with hemorrhage O44.1- ◀
~~without hemorrhage O44.0-~~
placental insufficiency O36.51-
planned, occurring after 37 completed weeks of gestation but before 39 completed weeks gestation due to (spontaneous) onset of labor O75.82
polyp, cervix O34.4-
causing obstructed labor O65.5
poor dilatation, cervix O62.0
pre-eclampsia O14.94 ⇐
mild O14.04 ⇐
moderate O14.04 ⇐
severe O14.14 ⇐
with hemolysis, elevated liver enzymes and low platelet count (HELLP) O14.24 ⇐
previous
cesarean delivery O34.219 ⇐
classical (vertical) scar O34.212 ◀
low transverse scar O34.211 ◀
surgery (to)
cervix O34.4-
gynecological NEC O34.8-
rectum O34.7-
uterus O34.29
vagina O34.6-
prolapse
arm or hand O32.2
uterus O34.52-
prolonged labor NOS O63.9
rectocele O34.8-
retroversion
uterus O34.53-
rigid
cervix O34.4-
pelvic floor O34.8-
perineum O34.7-
vagina O34.6-
vulva O34.7-
sacculation, pregnant uterus O34.59-
scar (s)
cervix O34.4-
cesarean delivery O34.219 ⇐
classical (vertical) O34.212 ◀
low transverse O34.211 ◀
transmural uterine O34.29 ◀
uterus O34.29
Shirodkar suture in situ O34.3-
shoulder presentation O32.2
stenosis or stricture, cervix O34.4-
~~streptococcus B carrier state O99.824~~
streptococcus group B (GBS) carrier state O99.824 ◀
transmural uterine scar O34.29 ◀
transverse presentation or lie O32.2
tumor, pelvic organs or tissues NEC O34.8-
cervix O34.4-
umbilical cord presentation or prolapse O69.0
completely normal case O80
complicated O75.9
by
abnormal, abnormality (of)
forces of labor O62.9
specified type NEC O62.8
glucose O99.814
uterine contractions NOS O62.9
abruptio placentae —*see also* Abruptio placentae O45.9-
Delivery *(Continued)*
complicated *(Continued)*
by *(Continued)*
abuse
physical O9A.32
psychological O9A.52
sexual O9A.42
adherent placenta O72.0
without hemorrhage O73.0
alcohol use O99.314
anemia (pre-existing) O99.02
anesthetic death O74.8
annular detachment of cervix O71.3
atony, uterus O62.2
attempted vacuum extraction and forceps O66.5
Bandl's ring O62.4
bariatric surgery status O99.844
biliary tract disorder O26.62
bleeding —*see* Delivery, complicated by, hemorrhage
blood disorder NEC O99.12
cervical dystocia (hypotonic) O62.2
primary O62.0
secondary O62.1
circulatory system disorder O99.42
compression of cord (umbilical) NEC O69.2
condition NEC O99.89
contraction, contracted ring O62.4
cord (umbilical)
around neck
with compression O69.1
without compression O69.81
bruising O69.5
complication O69.9
specified NEC O69.89
compression NEC O69.2
entanglement O69.2
without compression O69.82
hematoma O69.5
presentation O69.0
prolapse O69.0
short O69.3
thrombosis (vessels) O69.5
vascular lesion O69.5
Couvelaire uterus O45.8X-
damage to (injury to) NEC
perineum O71.82
periurethral tissue O71.82
vulva O71.82
delay following rupture of membranes (spontaneous) —*see* Pregnancy, complicated by, premature rupture of membranes
depressed fetal heart tones O76
diabetes O24.92
gestational O24.429
diet controlled O24.420
insulin controlled O24.424
oral drug controlled (antidiabetic) (hypoglycemic) O24.425 ◀
pre-existing O24.32
specified NEC O24.82
type 1 O24.02
type 2 O24.12
diastasis recti (abdominis) O71.89
dilatation
bladder O66.8
cervix incomplete, poor or slow O62.0
disease NEC O99.89
disruptio uteri —*see* Delivery, complicated by, rupture, uterus
drug use O99.324
dysfunction, uterus NOS O62.9
hypertonic O62.4
hypotonic O62.2
primary O62.0
secondary O62.1
incoordinate O62.4
eclampsia O15.1
embolism (pulmonary) —*see* Embolism, obstetric

◀ New ⇐ Revised ~~deleted~~ Deleted

Delivery *(Continued)*
complicated *(Continued)*
by *(Continued)*
endocrine, nutritional or metabolic disease NEC O99.284
failed
attempted vaginal birth after previous cesarean delivery O66.41
induction of labor O61.9
instrumental O61.1
mechanical O61.1
medical O61.0
specified NEC O61.8
surgical O61.1
trial of labor O66.40
female genital mutilation O65.5
fetal
abnormal acid-base balance O68
acidemia O68
acidosis O68
alkalosis O68
death, early O02.1
deformity O66.3
heart rate or rhythm (abnormal) (non-reassuring) O76
hypoxia O77.8
stress O77.9
due to drug administration O77.1
electrocardiographic evidence of O77.8
specified NEC O77.8
ultrasound evidence of O77.8
fever during labor O75.2
gastric banding status O99.844
gastric bypass status O99.844
gastrointestinal disease NEC O99.62
~~gestational diabetes O24.429~~
~~diet controlled O24.420~~
~~insulin (and diet) controlled O24.424~~
gestational ◀
diabetes O24.429 ◀
diet controlled O24.420 ◀
insulin (and diet) controlled O24.424 ◀
oral drug controlled (antidiabetic) (hypoglycemic) O24.425 ◀
edema O12.04 ◀
with proteinuria O12.24 ◀
proteinuria O12.14 ◀
gonorrhea O98.22
hematoma O71.7
ischial spine O71.7
pelvic O71.7
vagina O71.7
vulva or perineum O71.7
hemorrhage (uterine) O67.9
associated with
afibrinogenemia O67.0
coagulation defect O67.0
hyperfibrinolysis O67.0
hypofibrinogenemia O67.0
due to
low implantation of placenta O44.5- ◀
low-lying placenta O44.5- ⇐
placenta previa O44.1-
marginal O44.3- ◀
partial O44.3- ◀
premature separation of placenta (normally implanted) (*see also* Abruptio placentae) O45.9-
retained placenta O72.0
uterine leiomyoma O67.8
placenta NEC O67.8
postpartum NEC (atonic) (immediate) O72.1
with retained or trapped placenta O72.0
delayed O72.2
secondary O72.2
third stage O72.0

Delivery *(Continued)*
complicated *(Continued)*
by *(Continued)*
hourglass contraction, uterus O62.4
hypertension, hypertensive (pre-existing) —*see* Hypertension, complicated by, childbirth (labor)
hypotension O26.5-
incomplete dilatation (cervix) O62.0
incoordinate uterus contractions O62.4
inertia, uterus O62.2
during latent phase of labor O62.0
primary O62.0
secondary O62.1
infection (maternal) O98.92
carrier state NEC O99.834
gonorrhea O98.22
human immunodeficiency virus (HIV) O98.72
sexually transmitted NEC O98.32
specified NEC O98.82
syphilis O98.12
tuberculosis O98.02
viral hepatitis O98.42
viral NEC O98.52
injury (to mother) (*see also* Delivery, complicated, by, damage to) O71.9
nonobstetric O9A.22
caused by abuse —*see* Delivery, complicated by, abuse
intrauterine fetal death, early O02.1
inversion, uterus O71.2
laceration (perineal) O70.9
anus (sphincter) O70.4
with third degree laceration —*see also* Delivery, complicated, by, laceration, perineum, third degree O70.20 ⇐
with mucosa O70.3
without third degree laceration O70.4
bladder (urinary) O71.5
bowel O71.5
cervix (uteri) O71.3
fourchette O70.0
hymen O70.0
labia O70.0
pelvic
floor O70.1
organ NEC O71.5
perineum, perineal O70.9
first degree O70.0
fourth degree O70.3
muscles O70.1
second degree O70.1
skin O70.0
slight O70.0
third degree O70.20 ⇐
with ◀
both external anal sphincter (EAS) and internal anal sphincter (IAS) torn (IIIc) O70.23 ◀
less than 50% of external anal sphincter (EAS) thickness torn (IIIa) O70.21 ◀
more than 50% external anal sphincter (EAS) thickness torn (IIIb) O70.22 ◀
IIIa O70.21 ◀
IIIb O70.22 ◀
IIIc O70.23 ◀
peritoneum (pelvic) O71.5
rectovaginal (septum) (without perineal laceration) O71.4
with perineum —*see also* Delivery, complicated, by, laceration, perineum, third degree O70.20 ⇐
with anal or rectal mucosa O70.3

Delivery *(Continued)*
complicated *(Continued)*
by *(Continued)*
laceration *(Continued)*
specified NEC O71.89
sphincter ani —*see* Delivery, complicated, by, laceration, anus (sphincter)
urethra O71.5
uterus O71.81
before labor O71.81
vagina, vaginal (deep) (high) (without perineal laceration) O71.4
with perineum O70.0
muscles, with perineum O70.1
vulva O70.0
liver disorder O26.62
malignancy O9A.12
malnutrition O25.2
malposition, malpresentation
without obstruction O32.9 —*see also* Delivery, complicated by, obstruction
breech O32.1
compound O32.6
face (brow) (chin) O32.3
footling O38.8
high head O32.4
oblique O32.2
specified NEC O32.8
transverse O32.2
unstable lie O32.0
placenta O44.0- ⇐
~~without hemorrhage O44.0-~~
with hemorrhage O44.1- ◀
uterus or cervix O65.5
meconium in amniotic fluid O77.0
mental disorder NEC O99.344
metrorrhexis —*see* Delivery, complicated by, rupture, uterus
nervous system disorder O99.354
obesity (pre-existing) O99.214
obesity surgery status O99.844
obstetric trauma O71.9
specified NEC O71.89
obstructed labor
due to
breech (complete) (frank) presentation O64.1
incomplete O64.8
brow presenation O64.3
buttock presentation O64.1
chin presentation O64.2
compound presentation O64.5
contracted pelvis O65.1
deep transverse arrest O64.0
deformed pelvis O65.0
dystocia (fetal) O66.9
due to
conjoined twins O66.3
fetal
abnormality NEC O66.3
ascites O66.3
hydrops O66.3
meningomyelocele O66.3
sacral teratoma O66.3
tumor O66.3
hydrocephalic fetus O66.3
shoulder O66.0
face presentation O64.2
fetopelvic disproportion O65.4
footling presentation O64.8
impacted shoulders O66.0
incomplete rotation of fetal head O64.0
large fetus O66.2
locked twins O66.1
malposition O64.9
specified NEC O64.8
malpresentation O64.9
specified NEC O64.8

Delivery *(Continued)*
complicated *(Continued)*
by *(Continued)*
obstructed labor *(Continued)*
due to *(Continued)*
multiple fetuses NEC O66.6
pelvic
abnormality (maternal) O65.9
organ O65.5
specified NEC O65.8
contraction
inlet O65.2
mid-cavity O65.3
outlet O65.3
persistent (position)
occipitoiliac O64.0
occipitoposterior O64.0
occipitosacral O64.0
occipitotransverse O64.0
prolapsed arm O64.4
shoulder presentation O64.4
specified NEC O66.8
pathological retraction ring, uterus O62.4
penetration, pregnant uterus by instrument O71.1
perforation —*see* Delivery, complicated by, laceration
placenta, placental
ablatio —*see also* Abruptio placentae O45.9-
abnormality O43.9-
specified NEC O43.89-
abruptio —*see also* Abruptio placentae O45.9-
accreta O43.21-
adherent (with hemorrhage) O72.0
without hemorrhage O73.0
detachment (premature) —*see also* Abruptio placentae O45.9-
disorder O43.9-
specified NEC O43.89-
hemorrhage NEC O67.8
increta O43.22-
low (implantation) (lying) O44.4- ⟸
~~without hemorrhage O44.0-~~
with hemorrhage O44.5- ◀
malformation O43.10-
malposition O44.0- ⟸
without hemorrhage O44.1- ⟸
percreta O43.23-
previa (central) (complete) (lateral) (total) O44.0- ⟸
~~without hemorrhage O44.0-~~
with hemorrhage O44.1- ◀
marginal O44.2- ◀
with hemorrhage O44.3- ◀
partial O44.2- ◀
with hemorrhage O44.3- ◀
retained (with hemorrhage) O72.0
without hemorrhage O73.0
separation (premature) O45.9-
specified NEC O45.8X-
vicious insertion O44.1-
precipitate labor O62.3
premature rupture, membranes (*see also* Pregnancy, complicated by, premature rupture of membranes) O42.90
prolapse
arm or hand O32.2
cord (umbilical) O69.0
foot or leg O32.8
uterus O34.52-
prolonged labor O63.9
first stage O63.0
second stage O63.1
protozoal disease (maternal) O98.62
respiratory disease NEC O99.52
retained membranes or portions of placenta O72.2
without hemorrhage O73.1
retarded birth O63.9

Delivery *(Continued)*
complicated *(Continued)*
by *(Continued)*
retention of secundines (with hemorrhage) O72.0
without hemorrhage O73.0
partial O72.2
without hemorrhage O73.1
rupture
bladder (urinary) O71.5
cervix O71.3
pelvic organ NEC O71.5
urethra O71.5
uterus (during or after labor) O71.1
before labor O71.0-
separation, pubic bone (symphysis pubis) O71.6
shock O75.1
shoulder presentation O64.4
skin disorder NEC O99.72
spasm, cervix O62.4
stenosis or stricture, cervix O65.5
~~streptococcus B carrier state O99.824~~
streptococcus group B (GBS) carrier state O99.824 ◀
subluxation of symphysis (pubis) O26.72
syphilis (maternal) O98.12
tear —*see* Delivery, complicated by, laceration
tetanic uterus O62.4
trauma (obstetrical) —*see also* Delivery, complicated, by, damage to O71.9
non-obstetric O9A.22
periurethral O71.82
specified NEC O71.89
tuberculosis (maternal) O98.02
tumor, pelvic organs or tissues NEC O65.5
umbilical cord around neck
with compression O69.1
without compression O69.81
uterine inertia O62.2
during latent phase of labor O62.0
primary O62.0
secondary O62.1
vasa previa O69.4
velamentous insertion of cord O43.12-
specified complication NEC O75.89
delayed NOS O63.9
following rupture of membranes
artificial O75.5
second twin, triplet, etc. O63.2
forceps, low following failed vacuum extraction O66.5
missed (at or near term) O36.4
normal O80
obstructed —*see* Delivery, complicated by, obstruction
precipitate O62.3
preterm —*see also* Pregnancy, complicated by, preterm labor O60.10
spontaneous O80
term pregnancy NOS O80
uncomplicated O80
vaginal, following previous cesarean delivery O34.219 ⟸
classical (vertical) scar O34.212 ◀
low transverse scar O34.211 ◀
Delusions (paranoid) —*see* Disorder, delusional
Dementia (degenerative (primary)) (old age) (persisting) F03.90
with
aggressive behavior F03.91
behavioral disturbance F03.91
combative behavior F03.91
Lewy bodies G31.83 *[F02.80]*
with behavioral disturbance G31.83 *[F02.81]*
Parkinson's disease G20 *[F02.80]*
with behavioral disturbance G20 *[F02.81]*

Dementia *(Continued)*
with *(Continued)*
Parkinsonism G31.83 *[F02.80]*
with behavioral disturbance G31.83 *[F02.81]*
violent behavior F03.91
alcoholic F10.97
with dependence F10.27
Alzheimer's type —*see* Disease, Alzheimer's
arteriosclerotic —*see* Dementia, vascular
atypical, Alzheimer's type —*see* Disease, Alzheimer's, specified NEC
congenital —*see* Disability, intellectual
frontal (lobe) G31.09 *[F02.80]*
with behavioral disturbance G31.09 *[F02.81]*
frontotemporal G31.09 *[F02.80]*
with behavioral disturbance G31.09 *[F02.81]*
specified NEC G31.09 *[F02.80]*
with behavioral disturbance G31.09 *[F02.81]*
in (due to)
alcohol F10.97
with dependence F10.27
Alzheimer's disease —*see* Disease, Alzheimer's
arteriosclerotic brain disease —*see* Dementia, vascular
cerebral lipidoses E75.- *[F02.80]*
with behavioral disturbance E75.- *[F02.81]*
Creutzfeldt-Jakob disease —*see also* Creutzfeldt-Jakob disease or syndrome (with dementia) A81.00
epilepsy G40.- *[F02.80]*
with behavioral disturbance G40.- *[F02.81]*
hepatolenticular degeneration E83.01 *[F02.80]*
with behavioral disturbance E83.01 *[F02.81]*
human immunodeficiency virus (HIV) disease B20 *[F02.80]*
with behavioral disturbance B20 *[F02.81]*
Huntington's disease or chorea G10
hypercalcemia E83.52 *[F02.80]*
with behavioral disturbance E83.52 *[F02.81]*
hypothyroidism, acquired E03.9 *[F02.80]*
with behavioral disturbance E03.9 *[F02.81]*
due to iodine deficiency E01.8 *[F02.80]*
with behavioral disturbance E01.8 *[F02.81]*
inhalants F18.97
with dependence F18.27
multiple
etiologies F03
sclerosis G35 *[F02.80]*
with behavioral disturbance G35 *[F02.81]*
neurosyphilis A52.17 *[F02.80]*
with behavioral disturbance A52.17 *[F02.81]*
juvenile A50.49 *[F02.80]*
with behavioral disturbance A50.49 *[F02.81]*
niacin deficiency E52 *[F02.80]*
with behavioral disturbance E52 *[F02.81]*
paralysis agitans G20 *[F02.80]*
with behavioral disturbance G20 *[F02.81]*
Parkinson's disease G20 *[F02.80]*
pellagra E52 *[F02.80]*
with behavioral disturbance E52 *[F02.81]*
Pick's G31.01 *[F02.80]*
with behavioral disturbance G31.01 *[F02.81]*
polyarteritis nodosa M30.0 *[F02.80]*
with behavioral disturbance M30.0 *[F02.81]*

◀ New ⟸ Revised ~~deleted~~ Deleted

Dementia *(Continued)*
in *(Continued)*
psychoactive drug F19.97
with dependence F19.27
inhalants F18.97
with dependence F18.27
sedatives, hypnotics or anxiolytics F13.97
with dependence F13.27
sedatives, hypnotics or anxiolytics F13.97
with dependence F13.27
systemic lupus erythematosus M32.- *[F02.80]*
with behavioral disturbance M32.- *[F02.81]*
trypanosomiasis
African B56.9 *[F02.80]*
with behavioral disturbance B56.9 *[F02.81]*
unknown etiology F03
vitamin B12 deficiency E53.8 *[F02.80]*
with behavioral disturbance E53.8 *[F02.81]*
volatile solvents F18.97
with dependence F18.27
infantile, infantilis F84.3
Lewy body G31.83 *[F02.80]*
with behavioral disturbance G31.83 *[F02.81]*
multi-infarct —*see* Dementia, vascular
paralytica, paralytic (syphilitic) A52.17 *[F02.80]*
with behavioral disturbance A52.17 *[F02.81]*
juvenilis A50.45
paretic A52.17
praecox —*see* Schizophrenia
presenile F03
Alzheimer's type —*see* Disease, Alzheimer's, early onset
primary degenerative F03
progressive, syphilitic A52.17
senile F03
with acute confusional state F05
Alzheimer's type —*see* Disease, Alzheimer's, late onset
depressed or paranoid type F03
vascular (acute onset) (mixed) (multi-infarct) (subcortical) F01.50
with behavioral disturbance F01.51
Demineralization, bone —*see* Osteoporosis
Demodex folliculorum (infestation) B88.0
Demophobia F40.248
Demoralization R45.3
Demyelination, demyelinization
central nervous system G37.9
specified NEC G37.8
corpus callosum (central) G37.1
disseminated, acute G36.9
specified NEC G36.8
global G35
in optic neuritis G36.0
Dengue (classical) (fever) A90
hemorrhagic A91
sandfly A93.1
Dennie-Marfan syphilitic syndrome A50.45
Dens evaginatus, in dente or invaginatus K00.2
Dense breasts R92.2
Density
increased, bone (disseminated) (generalized) (spotted) —*see* Disorder, bone, density and structure, specified type NEC
lung (nodular) J98.4
Dental —*see also* condition
examination Z01.20
with abnormal findings Z01.21
restoration
aesthetically inadequate or displeasing K08.56

Dental *(Continued)*
restoration *(Continued)*
defective K08.50
specified NEC K08.59
failure of marginal integrity K08.51
failure of periodontal anatomical integrity K08.54
Dentia praecox K00.6
Denticles (pulp) K04.2
Dentigerous cyst K09.0
Dentin
irregular (in pulp) K04.3
opalescent K00.5
secondary (in pulp) K04.3
sensitive K03.89
Dentinogenesis imperfecta K00.5
Dentinoma —*see* Cyst, calcifying odontogenic
Dentition (syndrome) K00.7
delayed K00.6
difficult K00.7
precocious K00.6
premature K00.6
retarded K00.6
Dependence (on) (syndrome) F19.20
with remission F19.21
alcohol (ethyl) (methyl) (without remission) F10.20
with
amnestic disorder, persisting F10.26
anxiety disorder F10.280
dementia, persisting F10.27
intoxication F10.229
with delirium F10.221
uncomplicated F10.220
mood disorder F10.24
psychotic disorder F10.259
with
delusions F10.250
hallucinations F10.251
remission F10.21
sexual dysfunction F10.281
sleep disorder F10.282
specified disorder NEC F10.288
withdrawal F10.239
with
delirium F10.231
perceptual disturbance F10.232
uncomplicated F10.230
counseling and surveillance Z71.41
amobarbital —*see* Dependence, drug, sedative
amphetamine (s) (type) —*see* Dependence, drug, stimulant NEC
amytal (sodium) —*see* Dependence, drug, sedative
analgesic NEC F55.8
anesthetic (agent) (gas) (general) (local) NEC —*see* Dependence, drug, psychoactive NEC
anxiolytic NEC —*see* Dependence, drug, sedative
barbital (s) —*see* Dependence, drug, sedative
barbiturate (s) (compounds) (drugs classifiable to T42) —*see* Dependence, drug, sedative
benzedrine —*see* Dependence, drug, stimulant NEC
bhang —*see* Dependence, drug, cannabis
bromide (s) NEC —*see* Dependence, drug, sedative
caffeine —*see* Dependence, drug, stimulant NEC
cannabis (sativa) (indica) (resin) (derivatives) (type) —*see* Dependence, drug, cannabis
chloral (betaine) (hydrate) —*see* Dependence, drug, sedative
chlordiazepoxide —*see* Dependence, drug, sedative
coca (leaf) (derivatives) —*see* Dependence, drug, cocaine
cocaine —*see* Dependence, drug, cocaine

Dependence *(Continued)*
codeine —*see* Dependence, drug, opioid
combinations of drugs F19.20
dagga —*see* Dependence, drug, cannabis
demerol —*see* Dependence, drug, opioid
dexamphetamine —*see* Dependence, drug, stimulant NEC
dexedrine —*see* Dependence, drug, stimulant NEC
dextromethorphan —*see* Dependence, drug, opioid
dextromoramide —*see* Dependence, drug, opioid
dextro-nor-pseudo-ephedrine —*see* Dependence, drug, stimulant NEC
dextrorphan —*see* Dependence, drug, opioid
diazepam —*see* Dependence, drug, sedative
dilaudid —*see* Dependence, drug, opioid
D-lysergic acid diethylamide —*see* Dependence, drug, hallucinogen
drug NEC F19.20
with sleep disorder F19.282
cannabis F12.20
with
anxiety disorder F12.280
intoxication F12.229
with
delirium F12.221
perceptual disturbance F12.222
uncomplicated F12.220
other specified disorder F12.288
psychosis F12.259
delusions F12.250
hallucinations F12.251
unspecified disorder F12.29
in remission F12.21
cocaine F14.20
with
anxiety disorder F14.280
intoxication F14.229
with
delirium F14.221
perceptual disturbance F14.222
uncomplicated F14.220
mood disorder F14.24
other specified disorder F14.288
psychosis F14.259
delusions F14.250
hallucinations F14.251
sexual dysfunction F14.281
sleep disorder F14.282
unspecified disorder F14.29
withdrawal F14.23
in remission F14.21
withdrawal symptoms in newborn P96.1
counseling and surveillance Z71.51
hallucinogen F16.20
with
anxiety disorder F16.280
flashbacks F16.283
intoxication F16.229
with delirium F16.221
uncomplicated F16.220
mood disorder F16.24
other specified disorder F16.288
perception disorder, persisting F16.283
psychosis F16.259
delusions F16.250
hallucinations F16.251
unspecified disorder F16.29
in remission F16.21
in remission F19.21
inhalant F18.20
with
anxiety disorder F18.280
dementia, persisting F18.27
intoxication F18.229
with delirium F18.221
uncomplicated F18.220
mood disorder F18.24
other specified disorder F18.288

Dependence *(Continued)*
drug NEC *(Continued)*
inhalant *(Continued)*
with *(Continued)*
psychosis F18.259
delusions F18.250
hallucinations F18.251
unspecified disorder F18.29
in remission F18.21
nicotine F17.200
with disorder F17.209
remission F17.201
specified disorder NEC F17.208
withdrawal F17.203
chewing tobacco F17.220
with disorder F17.229
remission F17.221
specified disorder NEC F17.228
withdrawal F17.223
cigarettes F17.210
with disorder F17.219
remission F17.211
specified disorder NEC F17.218
withdrawal F17.213
specified product NEC F17.290
with disorder F17.299
remission F17.291
specified disorder NEC F17.298
withdrawal F17.293
opioid F11.20
with
intoxication F11.229
with
delirium F11.221
perceptual disturbance F11.222
uncomplicated F11.220
mood disorder F11.24
other specified disorder F11.288
psychosis F11.259
delusions F11.250
hallucinations F11.251
sexual dysfunction F11.281
sleep disorder F11.282
unspecified disorder F11.29
withdrawal F11.23
in remission F11.21
psychoactive NEC F19.20
with
amnestic disorder F19.26
anxiety disorder F19.280
dementia F19.27
intoxication F19.229
with
delirium F19.221
perceptual disturbance F19.222
uncomplicated F19.220
mood disorder F19.24
other specified disorder F19.288
psychosis F19.259
delusions F19.250
hallucinations F19.251
sexual dysfunction F19.281
sleep disorder F19.282
unspecified disorder F19.29
withdrawal F19.239
with
delirium F19.231
perceptual disturbance F19.232
uncomplicated F19.230
sedative, hypnotic or anxiolytic F13.20
with
amnestic disorder F13.26
anxiety disorder F13.280
dementia, persisting F13.27
intoxication F13.229
with delirium F13.221
uncomplicated F13.220
mood disorder F13.24
other specified disorder F13.288

Dependence *(Continued)*
drug NEC *(Continued)*
sedative, hypnotic or anxiolytic *(Continued)*
with *(Continued)*
psychosis F13.259
delusions F13.250
hallucinations F13.251
sexual dysfunction F13.281
sleep disorder F13.282
unspecified disorder F13.29
withdrawal F13.239
with
delirium F13.231
perceptual disturbance F13.232
uncomplicated F13.230
in remission F13.21
stimulant NEC F15.20
with
anxiety disorder F15.280
intoxication F15.229
with
delirium F15.221
perceptual disturbance F15.222
uncomplicated F15.220
mood disorder F15.24
other specified disorder F15.288
psychosis F15.259
delusions F15.250
hallucinations F15.251
sexual dysfunction F15.281
sleep disorder F15.282
unspecified disorder F15.29
withdrawal F15.23
in remission F15.21
ethyl
alcohol (without remission) F10.20
with remission F10.21
bromide —*see* Dependence, drug, sedative
carbamate F19.20
chloride F19.20
morphine —*see* Dependence, drug, opioid
ganja —*see* Dependence, drug, cannabis
glue (airplane) (sniffing) —*see* Dependence, drug, inhalant
glutethimide —*see* Dependence, drug, sedative
hallucinogenics —*see* Dependence, drug, hallucinogen
hashish —*see* Dependence, drug, cannabis
hemp —*see* Dependence, drug, cannabis
heroin (salt) (any) —*see* Dependence, drug, opioid
hypnotic NEC —*see* Dependence, drug, sedative
Indian hemp —*see* Dependence, drug, cannabis
inhalants —*see* Dependence, drug, inhalant
khat —*see* Dependence, drug, stimulant NEC
laudanum —*see* Dependence, drug, opioid
LSD (-25) (derivatives) —*see* Dependence, drug, hallucinogen
luminal —*see* Dependence, drug, sedative
lysergic acid —*see* Dependence, drug, hallucinogen
maconha —*see* Dependence, drug, cannabis
marihuana —*see* Dependence, drug, cannabis
meprobamate —*see* Dependence, drug, sedative
mescaline —*see* Dependence, drug, hallucinogen
methadone —*see* Dependence, drug, opioid
methamphetamine (s) —*see* Dependence, drug, stimulant NEC
methaqualone —*see* Dependence, drug, sedative
methyl
alcohol (without remission) F10.20
with remission F10.21
bromide —*see* Dependence, drug, sedative
morphine —*see* Dependence, drug, opioid

Dependence *(Continued)*
methyl *(Continued)*
phenidate —*see* Dependence, drug, stimulant NEC
sulfonal —*see* Dependence, drug, sedative
morphine (sulfate) (sulfite) (type) —*see* Dependence, drug, opioid
narcotic (drug) NEC —*see* Dependence, drug, opioid
nembutal —*see* Dependence, drug, sedative
neraval —*see* Dependence, drug, sedative
neravan —*see* Dependence, drug, sedative
neurobarb —*see* Dependence, drug, sedative
nicotine —*see* Dependence, drug, nicotine
nitrous oxide F19.20
nonbarbiturate sedatives and tranquilizers with similar effect —*see* Dependence, drug, sedative
on
artificial heart (fully implantable) (mechanical) Z95.812
aspirator Z99.0
care provider (because of) Z74.9
impaired mobility Z74.09
need for
assistance with personal care Z74.1
continuous supervision Z74.3
no other household member able to render care Z74.2
specified reason NEC Z74.8
machine Z99.89
enabling NEC Z99.89
specified type NEC Z99.89
renal dialysis (hemodialysis) (peritoneal) Z99.2
respirator Z99.11
ventilator Z99.11
wheelchair Z99.3
opiate —*see* Dependence, drug, opioid
opioids —*see* Dependence, drug, opioid
opium (alkaloids) (derivatives) (tincture) —*see* Dependence, drug, opioid
oxygen (long-term) (supplemental) Z99.81
paraldehyde —*see* Dependence, drug, sedative
paregoric —*see* Dependence, drug, opioid
PCP (phencyclidine) (or related substance) —*see* Dependence, drug, hallucinogen ◄
pentobarbital —*see* Dependence, drug, sedative
pentobarbitone (sodium) —*see* Dependence, drug, sedative
pentothal —*see* Dependence, drug, sedative
peyote —*see* Dependence, drug, hallucinogen
phencyclidine (PCP) (or related substance) —*see* Dependence, drug, hallucinogen ◄
phenmetrazine —*see* Dependence, drug, stimulant NEC
phenobarbital —*see* Dependence, drug, sedative
polysubstance F19.20
psilocibin, psilocin, psilocyn, psilocyline —*see* Dependence, drug, hallucinogen
psychostimulant NEC —*see* Dependence, drug, stimulant NEC
secobarbital —*see* Dependence, drug, sedative
seconal —*see* Dependence, drug, sedative
sedative NEC —*see* Dependence, drug, sedative
specified drug NEC —*see* Dependence, drug
stimulant NEC —*see* Dependence, drug, stimulant NEC
substance NEC —*see* Dependence, drug
supplemental oxygen Z99.81
tobacco —*see* Dependence, drug, nicotine
counseling and surveillance Z71.6
tranquilizer NEC —*see* Dependence, drug, sedative
vitamin B6 E53.1
volatile solvents —*see* Dependence, drug, inhalant

◄ New ◄ Revised ~~deleted~~ Deleted

Dependency
care-provider Z74.9
passive F60.7
reactions (persistent) F60.7
Depersonalization (in neurotic state) (neurotic) (syndrome) F48.1
Depletion
extracellular fluid E86.9
plasma E86.1
potassium E87.6
nephropathy N25.89
salt or sodium E87.1
causing heat exhaustion or prostration T67.4
nephropathy N28.9
volume NOS E86.9
Deployment (current) (military) status Z56.82
in theater or in support of military war, peacekeeping and humanitarian operations Z56.82
personal history of Z91.82
military war, peacekeeping and humanitarian deployment (current or past conflict) Z91.82
returned from Z91.82
Depolarization, premature I49.40
atrial I49.1
junctional I49.2
specified NEC I49.49
ventricular I49.3
Deposit
bone in Boeck's sarcoid D86.89
calcareous, calcium —*see* Calcification
cholesterol
retina H35.89
vitreous (body) (humor) —*see* Deposit, crystalline
conjunctiva H11.11-
cornea H18.00-
argentous H18.02-
due to metabolic disorder H18.03-
Kayser-Fleischer ring H18.04-
pigmentation —*see* Pigmentation, cornea
crystalline, vitreous (body) (humor) H43.2-
hemosiderin in old scars of cornea —*see* Pigmentation, cornea, stromal
metallic in lens —*see* Cataract, specified NEC
skin R23.8
tooth, teeth (betel) (black) (green) (materia alba) (orange) (tobacco) K03.6
urate, kidney —*see* Calculus, kidney
Depraved appetite —*see* Pica
Depressed
HDL cholesterol E78.6
Depression (acute) (mental) F32.9
agitated (single episode) F32.2
anaclitic —*see* Disorder, adjustment
anxiety F41.8
persistent F34.1
arches —*see also* Deformity, limb, flat foot
atypical (single episode) F32.89 ⇐
recurrent episode F33.8 ◀
basal metabolic rate R94.8
bone marrow D75.89
central nervous system R09.2
cerebral R29.818
newborn P91.4
cerebrovascular I67.9
chest wall M95.4
climacteric (single episode) F32.89 ⇐
recurrent episode F33.8 ◀
endogenous (without psychotic symptoms) F33.2
with psychotic symptoms F33.3
functional activity R68.89
hysterical F44.89
involutional (single episode) F32.89 ⇐
recurrent episode F33.8 ◀
major F32.9
with psychotic symptoms F32.3
recurrent —*see* Disorder, depressive, recurrent
Depression *(Continued)*
manic-depressive —*see* Disorder, depressive, recurrent
masked (single episode) F32.89 ⇐
medullary G93.89
menopausal (single episode) F32.89 ⇐
recurrent episode F33.8 ◀
metatarsus —*see* Depression, arches
monopolar F33.9
nervous F34.1
neurotic F34.1
nose M95.0
postnatal F53
postpartum F53
post-psychotic of schizophrenia F32.89 ⇐
post-schizophrenic F32.89 ⇐
psychogenic (reactive) (single episode) F32.9
psychoneurotic F34.1
psychotic (single episode) F32.3
recurrent F33.3
reactive (psychogenic) (single episode) F32.9
psychotic (single episode) F32.3
recurrent —*see* Disorder, depressive, recurrent
respiratory center G93.89
seasonal —*see* Disorder, depressive, recurrent
senile F03
severe, single episode F32.2
situational F43.21
skull Q67.4
specified NEC (single episode) F32.89 ⇐
sternum M95.4
visual field —*see* Defect, visual field
vital (recurrent) (without psychotic symptoms) F33.2
with psychotic symptoms F33.3
single episode F32.2
Deprivation
cultural Z60.3
effects NOS T73.9
specified NEC T73.8
emotional NEC Z65.8
affecting infant or child —*see* Maltreatment, child, psychological
food T73.0
protein —*see* Malnutrition
sleep Z72.820
social Z60.4
affecting infant or child —*see* Maltreatment, child, psychological
specified NEC T73.8
vitamins —*see* Deficiency, vitamin
water T73.1
Derangement
ankle (internal) —*see* Derangement, joint, ankle
cartilage (articular) NEC —*see* Derangement, joint, articular cartilage, by site
recurrent —*see* Dislocation, recurrent
cruciate ligament, anterior, current injury —*see* Sprain, knee, cruciate, anterior
elbow (internal) —*see* Derangement, joint, elbow
hip (joint) (internal) (old) —*see* Derangement, joint, hip
joint (internal) M24.9
ankylosis —*see* Ankylosis
articular cartilage M24.10
ankle M24.17-
elbow M24.12-
foot M24.17-
hand M24.14-
hip M24.15-
knee NEC M23.9-
loose body —*see* Loose, body
shoulder M24.11-
wrist M24.13-
contracture —*see* Contraction, joint
current injury —*see also* Dislocation
knee, meniscus or cartilage —*see* Tear, meniscus
Derangement *(Continued)*
joint *(Continued)*
dislocation
pathological —*see* Dislocation, pathological
recurrent —*see* Dislocation, recurrent
knee —*see* Derangement, knee
ligament —*see* Disorder, ligament
loose body —*see* Loose, body
recurrent —*see* Dislocation, recurrent
specified type NEC M24.80
ankle M24.87-
elbow M24.82-
foot joint M24.87-
hand joint M24.84-
hip M24.85-
shoulder M24.81-
wrist M24.83-
temporomandibular M26.69
knee (recurrent) M23.9-
ligament disruption, spontaneous M23.60-
anterior cruciate M23.61-
capsular M23.67-
instability, chronic M23.5-
lateral collateral M23.64-
medial collateral M23.63-
posterior cruciate M23.62-
loose body M23.4-
meniscus M23.30-
cystic M23.00-
lateral M23.002
anterior horn M23.04-
posterior horn M23.05-
specified NEC M23.06-
medial M23.005
anterior horn M23.01-
posterior horn M23.02-
specified NEC M23.03-
degenerate —*see* Derangement, knee, meniscus, specified NEC
detached —*see* Derangement, knee, meniscus, specified NEC
due to old tear or injury M23.20-
lateral M23.20-
anterior horn M23.24-
posterior horn M23.25-
specified NEC M23.26-
medial M23.20-
anterior horn M23.21-
posterior horn M23.22-
specified NEC M23.23-
retained —*see* Derangement, knee, meniscus, specified NEC
specified NEC M23.30-
lateral M23.30-
anterior horn M23.34-
posterior horn M23.35-
specified NEC M23.36-
medial M23.30-
anterior horn M23.31-
posterior horn M23.32-
specified NEC M23.33-
old M23.8X-
specified NEC —*see* subcategory M23.8
low back NEC —*see* Dorsopathy, specified NEC
meniscus —*see* Derangement, knee, meniscus
mental —*see* Psychosis
patella, specified NEC —*see* Disorder, patella, derangement NEC
semilunar cartilage (knee) —*see* Derangement, knee, meniscus, specified NEC
shoulder (internal) —*see* Derangement, joint, shoulder
Dercum's disease E88.2
Derealization (neurotic) F48.1
Dermal —*see* condition
Dermaphytid —*see* Dermatophytosis

Dermatitis (eczematous) L30.9
ab igne L59.0
acarine B88.0
actinic (due to sun) L57.8
other than from sun L59.8
allergic —*see* Dermatitis, contact, allergic
ambustionis, due to burn or scald —*see* Burn
amebic A06.7
ammonia L22
arsenical (ingested) L27.8
artefacta L98.1
psychogenic F54
atopic L20.9
psychogenic F54
specified NEC L20.89
autoimmune progesterone L30.8
berlock, berloque L56.2
blastomycotic B40.3
blister beetle L24.89
bullous, bullosa L13.9
mucosynechial, atrophic L12.1
seasonal L30.8
specified NEC L13.8
calorica L59.0
due to burn or scald —*see* Burn
caterpillar L24.89
cercarial B65.3
combustionis L59.0
due to burn or scald —*see* Burn
congelationis T69.1
contact (occupational) L25.9
allergic L23.9
due to
adhesives L23.1
cement L23.5
chemical products NEC L23.5
chromium L23.0
cosmetics L23.2
dander (cat) (dog) L23.81
drugs in contact with skin L23.3
dyes L23.4
food in contact with skin L23.6
hair (cat) (dog) L23.81
insecticide L23.5
metals L23.0
nickel L23.0
plants, non-food L23.7
plastic L23.5
rubber L23.5
specified agent NEC L23.89
due to
cement L25.3
chemical products NEC L25.3
cosmetics L25.0
dander (cat) (dog) L23.81
drugs in contact with skin L25.1
dyes L25.2
food in contact with skin L25.4
hair (cat) (dog) L23.81
plants, non-food L25.5
specified agent NEC L25.8
irritant L24.9
due to
cement L24.5 ◀
chemical products NEC L24.5
cosmetics L24.3
detergents L24.0
drugs in contact with skin L24.4
food in contact with skin L24.6
oils and greases L24.1
plants, non-food L24.7
solvents L24.2
specified agent NEC L24.89
contusiformis L52
diabetic —*see* E08-E13 with .620
diaper L22
diphtheritica A36.3
dry skin L85.3
due to
acetone (contact) (irritant) L24.2
acids (contact) (irritant) L24.5

Dermatitis *(Continued)*
due to *(Continued)*
adhesive (s) (allergic) (contact) (plaster) L23.1
irritant L24.5
alcohol (irritant) (skin contact) (substances in category T51) L24.2
taken internally L27.8
alkalis (contact) (irritant) L24.5
arsenic (ingested) L27.8
carbon disulfide (contact) (irritant) L24.2
caustics (contact) (irritant) L24.5
cement (contact) L25.3
cereal (ingested) L27.2
chemical (s) NEC L25.3
taken internally L27.8
chlorocompounds L24.2
chromium (contact) (irritant) L24.81
coffee (ingested) L27.2
cold weather L30.8
cosmetics (contact) L25.0
allergic L23.2
irritant L24.3
cyclohexanes L24.2
dander (cat) (dog) L23.81
Demodex species B88.0
Dermanyssus gallinae B88.0
detergents (contact) (irritant) L24.0
dichromate L24.81
drugs and medicaments (generalized) (internal use) L27.0
external —*see* Dermatitis, due to, drugs, in contact with skin
in contact with skin L25.1
allergic L23.3
irritant L24.4
localized skin eruption L27.1
specified substance —*see* Table of Drugs and Chemicals
dyes (contact) L25.2
allergic L23.4
irritant L24.89
epidermophytosis —*see* Dermatophytosis
esters L24.2
external irritant NEC L24.9
fish (ingested) L27.2
flour (ingested) L27.2
food (ingested) L27.2
in contact with skin L25.4
fruit (ingested) L27.2
furs (allergic) (contact) L23.81
glues —*see* Dermatitis, due to, adhesives
glycols L24.2
greases NEC (contact) (irritant) L24.1
hair (cat) (dog) L23.81
hot
objects and materials —*see* Burn
weather or places L59.0
hydrocarbons L24.2
infrared rays L59.8
ingestion, ingested substance L27.9
chemical NEC L27.8
drugs and medicaments —*see* Dermatitis, due to, drugs
food L27.2
specified NEC L27.8
insecticide in contact with skin L24.5
internal agent L27.9
drugs and medicaments (generalized) —*see* Dermatitis, due to, drugs
food L27.2
irradiation —*see* Dermatitis, due to, radioactive substance
ketones L24.2
lacquer tree (allergic) (contact) L23.7
light (sun) NEC L57.8
acute L56.8
other L59.8
Liponyssoides sanguineus B88.0
low temperature L30.8
meat (ingested) L27.2

Dermatitis *(Continued)*
due to *(Continued)*
metals, metal salts (contact) (irritant) L24.81
milk (ingested) L27.2
nickel (contact) (irritant) L24.81
nylon (contact) (irritant) L24.5
oils NEC (contact) (irritant) L24.1
paint solvent (contact) (irritant) L24.2
petroleum products (contact) (irritant) (substances in T52) L24.2
plants NEC (contact) L25.5
allergic L23.7
irritant L24.7
plasters (adhesive) (any) (allergic) (contact) L23.1
irritant L24.5
plastic (contact) L25.3
preservatives (contact) —*see* Dermatitis, due to, chemical, in contact with skin
primrose (allergic) (contact) L23.7
primula (allergic) (contact) L23.7
radiation L59.8
nonionizing (chronic exposure) L57.8
sun NEC L57.8
acute L56.8
radioactive substance L58.9
acute L58.0
chronic L58.1
radium L58.9
acute L58.0
chronic L58.1
ragweed (allergic) (contact) L23.7
Rhus (allergic) (contact) (diversiloba) (radicans) (toxicodendron) (venenata) (verniciflua) L23.7
rubber (contact) L24.5
Senecio jacobaea (allergic) (contact) L23.7
solvents (contact) (irritant) (substances in categories T52) L24.2
specified agent NEC (contact) L25.8
allergic L23.89
irritant L24.89
sunshine NEC L57.8
acute L56.8
tetrachlorethylene (contact) (irritant) L24.2
toluene (contact) (irritant) L24.2
turpentine (contact) L24.2
ultraviolet rays (sun NEC) (chronic exposure) L57.8
acute L56.8
vaccine or vaccination L27.0
specified substance —*see* Table of Drugs and Chemicals
varicose veins —*see* Varix, leg, with, inflammation
X-rays L58.9
acute L58.0
chronic L58.1
dyshydrotic L30.1
dysmenorrheica N94.6
escharotica —*see* Burn
exfoliative, exfoliativa (generalized) L26
neonatorum L00
eyelid —*see also* Dermatosis, eyelid
allergic H01.119
left H01.116
lower H01.115
upper H01.114
right H01.113
lower H01.112
upper H01.111
contact —*see* Dermatitis, eyelid, allergic
due to
Demodex species B88.0
herpes (zoster) B02.39
simplex B00.59

◀ New ⇐ Revised ~~deleted~~ Deleted

Dermatitis *(Continued)*
eyelid *(Continued)*
eczematous H01.139
left H01.136
lower H01.135
upper H01.134
right H01.133
lower H01.132
upper H01.131
facta, factitia, factitial L98.1
psychogenic F54
flexural NEC L20.82
friction L30.4
fungus B36.9
specified type NEC B36.8
gangrenosa, gangrenous infantum L08.0
harvest mite B88.0
heat L59.0
herpesviral, vesicular (ear) (lip) B00.1
herpetiformis (bullous) (erythematous) (pustular) (vesicular) L13.0
juvenile L12.2
senile L12.0
hiemalis L30.8
hypostatic, hypostatica —*see* Varix, leg, with, inflammation
infectious eczematoid L30.3
infective L30.3
irritant —*see* Dermatitis, contact, irritant
Jacquet's (diaper dermatitis) L22
Leptus B88.0
lichenified NEC L28.0
medicamentosa (generalized) (internal use) —*see* Dermatitis, due to drugs
mite B88.0
multiformis L13.0
juvenile L12.2
napkin L22
neurotica L13.0
nummular L30.0
papillaris capillitii L73.0
pellagrous E52
perioral L71.0
photocontact L56.2
polymorpha dolorosa L13.0
pruriginosa L13.0
pruritic NEC L30.8
psychogenic F54
purulent L08.0
pustular
contagious B08.02
subcorneal L13.1
pyococcal L08.0
pyogenica L08.0
repens L40.2
Ritter's (exfoliativa) L00
Schamberg's L81.7
schistosome B65.3
seasonal bullous L30.8
seborrheic L21.9
infantile L21.1
specified NEC L21.8
sensitization NOS L23.9
septic L08.0
solare L57.8
specified NEC L30.8
stasis I87.2
~~with varicose ulcer —see Varix, leg, with ulcer, with inflammation~~
with ◀
varicose ulcer —*see* Varix, leg, with ulcer, with inflammation ◀
varicose veins —*see* Varix, leg, with, inflammation ◀
due to postthrombotic syndrome —*see* Syndrome, postthrombotic
suppurative L08.0
traumatic NEC L30.4
trophoneurotica L13.0
ultraviolet (sun) (chronic exposure) L57.8
acute L56.8

Dermatitis *(Continued)*
varicose —*see* Varix, leg, with, inflammation
vegetans L10.1
verrucosa B43.0
vesicular, herpesviral B00.1
Dermatoarthritis, lipoid E78.81
Dermatochalasis, eyelid H02.839
left H02.836
lower H02.835
upper H02.834
right H02.833
lower H02.832
upper H02.831
Dermatofibroma (lenticulare) —*see* Neoplasm, skin, benign
protuberans —*see* Neoplasm, skin, uncertain behavior
Dermatofibrosarcoma (pigmented) (protuberans) —*see* Neoplasm, skin, malignant
Dermatographia L50.3
Dermatolysis (exfoliativa) (congenital) Q82.8
acquired L57.4
eyelids —*see* Blepharochalasis
palpebrarum —*see* Blepharochalasis
senile L57.4
Dermatomegaly NEC Q82.8
Dermatomucosomyositis M33.10
with
myopathy M33.12
respiratory involvement M33.11
specified organ involvement NEC M33.19
Dermatomycosis B36.9
furfuracea B36.0
specified type NEC B36.8
Dermatomyositis (acute) (chronic) —*see also* Dermatopolymyositis
in (due to) neoplastic disease —*see also* Neoplasm D49.9 *[M36.0]*
Dermatoneuritis of children —*see* Poisoning, mercury
Dermatophilosis A48.8
Dermatophytid L30.2
Dermatophytide —*see* Dermatophytosis
Dermatophytosis (epidermophyton) (infection) (Microsporum) (tinea) (Trichophyton) B35.9
beard B35.0
body B35.4
capitis B35.0
corporis B35.4
deep-seated B35.8
disseminated B35.8
foot B35.3
granulomatous B35.8
groin B35.6
hand B35.2
nail B35.1
perianal (area) B35.6
scalp B35.0
specified NEC B35.8
Dermatopolymyositis M33.90
with
myopathy M33.92
respiratory involvement M33.91
specified organ involvement NEC M33.99
in neoplastic disease (*see also* Neoplasm) D49.9 *[M36.0]*
juvenile M33.00
with
myopathy M33.02
respiratory involvement M33.01
specified organ involvement NEC M33.09
specified NEC M33.10
myopathy M33.12
respiratory involvement M33.11
specified organ involvement NEC M33.19

Dermatopolyneuritis —*see* Poisoning, mercury
Dermatorrhexis Q79.6
acquired L57.4
Dermatosclerosis —*see also* Scleroderma
localized L94.0
Dermatosis L98.9
Andrews' L08.89
Bowen's —*see* Neoplasm, skin, in situ
bullous L13.9
specified NEC L13.8
exfoliativa L26
eyelid (noninfectious)
dermatitis —*see* Dermatitis, eyelid
discoid lupus erythematosus —*see* Lupus, erythematosus, eyelid
xeroderma —*see* Xeroderma, acquired, eyelid
factitial L98.1
febrile neutrophilic L98.2
gonococcal A54.89
herpetiformis L13.0
juvenile L12.2
linear IgA L13.8
menstrual NEC L98.8
neutrophilic, febrile L98.2
occupational —*see* Dermatitis, contact
papulosa nigra L82.1
pigmentary L81.9
progressive L81.7
Schamberg's L81.7
psychogenic F54
purpuric, pigmented L81.7
pustular, subcorneal L13.1
transient acantholytic L11.1
Dermographia, dermographism L50.3
Dermoid (cyst) —*see also* Neoplasm, benign, by site
with malignant transformation C56-
due to radiation (nonionizing) L57.8
Dermopathy
infiltrative with thyrotoxicosis —*see* Thyrotoxicosis
nephrogenic fibrosing L90.8
Dermophytosis —*see* Dermatophytosis
Descemetocele H18.73-
Descemet's membrane —*see* condition
Descending —*see* condition
Descensus uteri —*see* Prolapse, uterus
Desert
rheumatism B38.0
sore —*see* Ulcer, skin
Desertion (newborn) —*see* Maltreatment
Desmoid (extra-abdominal) (tumor) —*see* Neoplasm, connective tissue, uncertain behavior
abdominal D48.1
Despondency F32.9
Desquamation, skin R23.4
Destruction, destructive —*see also* Damage
articular facet —*see also* Derangement, joint, specified type NEC
knee M23.8X-
vertebra —*see* Spondylosis
bone —*see also* Disorder, bone, specified type NEC
syphilitic A52.77
joint —*see also* Derangement, joint, specified type NEC
sacroiliac M53.3
rectal sphincter K62.89
septum (nasal) J34.89
tuberculous NEC —*see* Tuberculosis
tympanum, tympanic membrane (nontraumatic) —*see* Disorder, tympanic membrane, specified NEC
vertebral disc —*see* Degeneration, intervertebral disc
Destructiveness —*see also* Disorder, conduct
adjustment reaction —*see* Disorder, adjustment

Desultory labor O62.2
Detachment
cartilage —*see* Sprain
cervix, annular N88.8
complicating delivery O71.3
choroid (old) (postinfectional) (simple) (spontaneous) H31.40-
hemorrhagic H31.41-
serous H31.42-
ligament —*see* Sprain
meniscus (knee) —*see also* Derangement, knee, meniscus, specified NEC
current injury —*see* Tear, meniscus
due to old tear or injury —*see* Derangement, knee, meniscus, due to old tear
retina (without retinal break) (serous) H33.2-
with retinal:
break H33.00-
giant H33.03-
multiple H33.02-
single H33.01-
dialysis H33.04-
pigment epithelium —*see* Degeneration, retina, separation of layers, pigment epithelium detachment
rhegmatogenous —*see* Detachment, retina, with retinal, break
specified NEC H33.8
total H33.05-
traction H33.4-
vitreous (body) H43.81
Detergent asthma J69.8
Deterioration
epileptic F06.8
general physical R53.81
heart, cardiac —*see* Degeneration, myocardial
mental —*see* Psychosis
myocardial, myocardium —*see* Degeneration, myocardial
senile (simple) R54
Deuteranomaly (anomalous trichromat) H53.53
Deuteranopia (complete) (incomplete) H53.53
Development
abnormal, bone Q79.9
arrested R62.50
bone —*see* Arrest, development or growth, bone
child R62.50
due to malnutrition E45
defective, congenital —*see also* Anomaly, by site
cauda equina Q06.3
left ventricle Q24.8
in hypoplastic left heart syndrome Q23.4
valve Q24.8
pulmonary Q22.3
delayed (*see also* Delay, development) R62.50
arithmetical skills F81.2
language (skills) (expressive) F80.1
learning skill F81.9
mixed skills F88
motor coordination F82
reading F81.0
specified learning skill NEC F81.89
speech F80.9
spelling F81.81
written expression F81.81
imperfect, congenital —*see also* Anomaly, by site
heart Q24.9
lungs Q33.6
incomplete
bronchial tree Q32.4
organ or site not listed —*see* Hypoplasia, by site
respiratory system Q34.9
sexual, precocious NEC E30.1
tardy, mental (*see also* Disability, intellectual) F79
Developmental —*see* condition
~~testing, child —see Examination, child~~
testing, infant or child —*see* Examination, child ◀
Devergie's disease (pityriasis rubra pilaris) L44.0
Deviation (in)
conjugate palsy (eye) (spastic) H51.0
esophagus (acquired) K22.8
eye, skew H51.8
midline (jaw) (teeth) (dental arch) M26.29
specified site NEC —*see* Malposition
nasal septum J34.2
congenital Q67.4
opening and closing of the mandible M26.53
organ or site, congenital NEC —*see* Malposition, congenital
septum (nasal) (acquired) J34.2
congenital Q67.4
sexual F65.9
bestiality F65.89
erotomania F52.8
exhibitionism F65.2
fetishism, fetishistic F65.0
transvestism F65.1
frotteurism F65.81
masochism F65.51
multiple F65.89
necrophilia F65.89
nymphomania F52.8
pederosis F65.4
pedophilia F65.4
sadism, sadomasochism F65.52
satyriasis F52.8
specified type NEC F65.89
transvestism F64.1
voyeurism F65.3
teeth, midline M26.29
trachea J39.8
ureter, congenital Q62.61
Device
cerebral ventricle (communicating) in situ Z98.2
contraceptive —*see* Contraceptive, device
drainage, cerebrospinal fluid, in situ Z98.2
Devic's disease G36.0
Devil's
grip B33.0
pinches (purpura simplex) D69.2
Devitalized tooth K04.99
Devonshire colic —*see* Poisoning, lead
Dextraposition, aorta Q20.3
in tetralogy of Fallot Q21.3
Dextrinosis, limit (debrancher enzyme deficiency) E74.03
Dextrocardia (true) Q24.0
with
complete transposition of viscera Q89.3
situs inversus Q89.3
Dextrotransposition, aorta Q20.3
d-glycericacidemia E72.59
Dhat syndrome F48.8
Dhobi itch B35.6
Di George's syndrome D82.1
Di Guglielmo's disease C94.0-
Diabetes, diabetic (mellitus) (sugar) E11.9
with
amyotrophy E11.44
arthropathy NEC E11.618
autonomic (poly)neuropathy E11.43
cataract E11.36
Charcot's joints E11.610
chronic kidney disease E11.22
circulatory complication NEC E11.59
complication E11.8
specified NEC E11.69
dermatitis E11.620
foot ulcer E11.621
gangrene E11.52
gastroparalysis E11.43 ◀
gastroparesis E11.43
Diabetes, diabetic *(Continued)*
with *(Continued)*
glomerulonephrosis, intracapillary E11.21
glomerulosclerosis, intercapillary E11.21
hyperglycemia E11.65
hyperosmolarity E11.00
with coma E11.01
hypoglycemia E11.649
with coma E11.641
kidney complications NEC E11.29
Kimmelsteil-Wilson disease E11.21
loss of protective sensation (LOPS) —*see* Diabetes, by type, with neuropathy
mononeuropathy E11.41
myasthenia E11.44
necrobiosis lipoidica E11.620
nephropathy E11.21
neuralgia E11.42
neurologic complication NEC E11.49
neuropathic arthropathy E11.610
neuropathy E11.40
ophthalmic complication NEC E11.39
oral complication NEC E11.638
osteomyelitis E11.69 ◀
periodontal disease E11.630
peripheral angiopathy E11.51
with gangrene E11.52
polyneuropathy E11.42
renal complication NEC E11.29
renal tubular degeneration E11.29
retinopathy E11.319
with macular edema E11.311
resolved following treatment E11.37 ◀
nonproliferative E11.329
with macular edema E11.321
mild E11.329
with macular edema E11.321
moderate E11.339
with macular edema E11.331
severe E11.349
with macular edema E11.341
proliferative E11.359
~~with macular edema E11.351~~
with ◀
combined traction retinal detachment and rhegmatogenous retinal detachment E11.354 ◀
macular edema E11.351 ◀
stable proliferative diabetic retinopathy E11.355 ◀
traction retinal detachment involving the macula E11.352 ◀
traction retinal detachment not involving the macula E11.353 ◀
skin complication NEC E11.628
skin ulcer NEC E11.622
brittle —*see* Diabetes, type 1 ◀
bronzed E83.110
complicating pregnancy —*see* Pregnancy, complicated by, diabetes
dietary counseling and surveillance Z71.3
due to ◀
autoimmune process —*see* Diabetes, type 1 ◀
immune mediated pancreatic islet beta-cell destruction —*see* Diabetes, type 1 ◀
due to drug or chemical E09.9
with
amyotrophy E09.44
arthropathy NEC E09.618
autonomic (poly)neuropathy E09.43
cataract E09.36
Charcot's joints E09.610
chronic kidney disease E09.22
circulatory complication NEC E09.59
complication E09.8
specified NEC E09.69

Diabetes, diabetic *(Continued)*
due to drug or chemical *(Continued)*
with *(Continued)*
dermatitis E09.620
foot ulcer E09.621
gangrene E09.52
gastroparalysis E09.43 ◀
gastroparesis E09.43
glomerulonephrosis, intracapillary E09.21
glomerulosclerosis, intercapillary E09.21
hyperglycemia E09.65
hyperosmolarity E09.00
with coma E09.01
hypoglycemia E09.649
with coma E09.641
ketoacidosis E09.10
with coma E09.11
kidney complications NEC E09.29
Kimmelsteil-Wilson disease E09.21
mononeuropathy E09.41
myasthenia E09.44
necrobiosis lipoidica E09.620
nephropathy E09.21
neuralgia E09.42
neurologic complication NEC E09.49
neuropathic arthropathy E09.610
neuropathy E09.40
ophthalmic complication NEC E09.39
oral complication NEC E09.638
periodontal disease E09.630
peripheral angiopathy E09.51
with gangrene E09.52
polyneuropathy E09.42
renal complication NEC E09.29
renal tubular degeneration E09.29
retinopathy E09.319
with macular edema E09.311
resolved following treatment E09.37 ◀
nonproliferative E09.329
with macular edema E09.321
mild E09.329
with macular edema E09.321
moderate E09.339
with macular edema E09.331
severe E09.349
with macular edema E09.341
proliferative E09.359
~~with macular edema E09.351~~
with ◀
combined traction retinal detachment and rhegmatogenous retinal detachment E09.354 ◀
macular edema E09.351 ◀
stable proliferative diabetic retinopathy E09.355 ◀
traction retinal detachment involving the macula E09.352 ◀
traction retinal detachment not involving the macula E09.353 ◀
skin complication NEC E09.628
skin ulcer NEC E09.622
due to underlying condition E08.9
with
amyotrophy E08.44
arthropathy NEC E08.618
autonomic (poly)neuropathy E08.43
cataract E08.36
Charcot's joints E08.610
chronic kidney disease E08.22
circulatory complication NEC E08.59
complication E08.8
specified NEC E08.69
dermatitis E08.620
foot ulcer E08.621
gangrene E08.52
gastroparalysis E08.43 ◀

Diabetes, diabetic *(Continued)*
due to underlying condition *(Continued)*
with *(Continued)*
gastroparesis E08.43
glomerulonephrosis, intracapillary E08.21
glomerulosclerosis, intercapillary E08.21
hyperglycemia E08.69
hyperosmolarity E08.00
with coma E08.01
hypoglycemia E08.649
with coma E08.641
ketoacidosis E08.10
with coma E08.11
kidney complications NEC E08.29
Kimmelsteil-WIlson disease E08.21
mononeuropathy E08.41
myasthenia E08.44
necrobiosis lipoidica E08.620
nephropathy E08.21
neuralgia E08.42
neurologic complication NEC E08.49
neuropathic arthropathy E08.610
neuropathy E08.40
ophthalmic complication NEC E08.39
oral complication NEC E08.638
periodontal disease E08.630
peripheral angiopathy E08.51
with gangrene E08.52
polyneuropathy E08.42
renal complication NEC E08.29
renal tubular degeneration E08.29
retinopathy E08.319
with macular edema E08.311
resolved following treatment E08.37 ◀
nonproliferative E08.329
with macular edema E08.321
mild E08.329
with macular edema E08.321
moderate E08.339
with macular edema E08.331
severe E08.349
with macular edema E08.341
proliferative E08.359
~~with macular edema E08.351~~
with ◀
combined traction retinal detachment and rhegmatogenous retinal detachment E08.354 ◀
macular edema E08.351 ◀
stable proliferative diabetic retinopathy E08.355 ◀
traction retinal detachment involving the macula E08.352 ◀
traction retinal detachment not involving the macula E08.353 ◀
skin complication NEC E08.628
skin ulcer NEC E08.622
gestational (in pregnancy) O24.419
affecting newborn P70.0
diet-controlled O24.410
in childbirth O24.429
diet-controlled O24.420
insulin (and diet) controlled O24.424
oral drug controlled (antidiabetic) (hypoglycemic) O24.425 ◀
insulin (and diet) controlled O24.414
oral drug controlled (antidiabetic) (hypoglycemic) O24.415 ◀
puerperal O24.439
diet-controlled O24.430
insulin (and diet) controlled O24.434
oral drug controlled (antidiabetic) (hypoglycemic) O24.435 ◀
hepatogenous E13.9
idiopathic —*see* Diabetes, type 1 ◀

Diabetes, diabetic *(Continued)*
inadequately controlled — code to Diabetes, by type, with hyperglycemia
insipidus E23.2
nephrogenic N25.1
pituitary E23.2
vasopressin resistant N25.1
insulin dependent — code to type of diabetes
juvenile-onset —*see* Diabetes, type 1
ketosis-prone —*see* Diabetes, type 1
latent R73.03 ⬅
neonatal (transient) P70.2
non-insulin dependent — code to type of diabetes
out of control — code to Diabetes, by type, with hyperglycemia
phosphate E83.39
poorly controlled — code to Diabetes, by type, with hyperglycemia
postpancreatectomy —*see* Diabetes, specified type NEC
postprocedural —*see* Diabetes, specified type NEC
secondary diabetes mellitus NEC —*see* Diabetes, specified type NEC
specified type NEC E13.9
with
amyotrophy E13.44
arthropathy NEC E13.618
autonomic (poly)neuropathy E13.43
cataract E13.36
Charcot's joints E13.610
chronic kidney disease E13.22
circulatory complication NEC E13.59
complication E13.8
specified NEC E13.69
dermatitis E13.620
foot ulcer E13.621
gangrene E13.52
gastroparalysis E13.43 ◀
gastroparesis E13.43
glomerulonephrosis, intracapillary E13.21
glomerulosclerosis, intercapillary E13.21
hyperglycemia E13.65
hyperosmolarity E13.00
with coma E13.01
hypoglycemia E13.649
with coma E13.641
ketoacidosis E13.10
with coma E13.11
kidney complications NEC E13.29
Kimmelsteil-Wilson disease E13.21
mononeuropathy E13.41
myasthenia E13.44
necrobiosis lipoidica E13.620
nephropathy E13.21
neuralgia E13.42
neurologic complication NEC E13.49
neuropathic arthropathy E13.610
neuropathy E13.40
ophthalmic complication NEC E13.39
oral complication NEC E13.638
periodontal disease E13.630
peripheral angiopathy E13.51
with gangrene E13.52
polyneuropathy E13.42
renal complication NEC E13.29
renal tubular degeneration E13.29
retinopathy E13.319
with macular edema E13.311
resolved following treatment E13.37 ◀
nonproliferative E13.329
with macular edema E13.321
mild E13.329
with macular edema E13.321
moderate E13.339
with macular edema E13.331
severe E13.349
with macular edema E13.341

Diabetes, diabetic *(Continued)*
specified type NEC *(Continued)*
with *(Continued)*
retinopathy *(Continued)*
proliferative E13.359
~~with macular edema E13.351~~
with ◀
combined traction retinal detachment and rhegmatogenous retinal detachment E13.354 ◀
macular edema E13.351 ◀
stable proliferative diabetic retinopathy E13.355 ◀
traction retinal detachment involving the macula E13.352 ◀
traction retinal detachment not involving the macula E13.353 ◀
skin complication NEC E13.628
skin ulcer NEC E13.622
steroid-induced —*see* Diabetes, due to, drug or chemical
type 1 E10.9
with
amyotrophy E10.44
arthropathy NEC E10.618
autonomic (poly)neuropathy E10.43
cataract E10.36
Charcot's joints E10.610
chronic kidney disease E10.22
circulatory complication NEC E10.59
complication E10.8
specified NEC E10.69
dermatitis E10.620
foot ulcer E10.621
gangrene E10.52
gastroparalysis E10.43 ◀
gastroparesis E10.43
glomerulonephrosis, intracapillary E10.21
glomerulosclerosis, intercapillary E10.21
hyperglycemia E10.65
hypoglycemia E10.649
with coma E10.641
ketoacidosis E10.10
with coma E10.11
kidney complications NEC E10.29
Kimmelsteil-Wilson disease E10.21
mononeuropathy E10.41
myasthenia E10.44
necrobiosis lipoidica E10.620
nephropathy E10.21
neuralgia E10.42
neurologic complication NEC E10.49
neuropathic arthropathy E10.610
neuropathy E10.40
ophthalmic complication NEC E10.39
oral complication NEC E10.638
periodontal disease E10.630
peripheral angiopathy E10.51
with gangrene E10.52
polyneuropathy E10.42
renal complication NEC E10.29
renal tubular degeneration E10.29
retinopathy E10.319
with macular edema E10.311
resolved following treatment E10.37 ◀
nonproliferative E10.329
with macular edema E10.321
mild E10.329
with macular edema E10.321
moderate E10.339
with macular edema E10.331
severe E10.349
with macular edema E10.341

Diabetes, diabetic *(Continued)*
type 1 *(Continued)*
with *(Continued)*
retinopathy *(Continued)*
proliferative E10.359
~~with macular edema E10.351~~
with ◀
combined traction retinal detachment and rhegmatogenous retinal detachment E13.354 ◀
macular edema E13.351 ◀
stable proliferative diabetic retinopathy E13.355 ◀
traction retinal detachment involving the macula E13.352 ◀
traction retinal detachment not involving the macula E13.353 ◀
skin complication NEC E10.628
skin ulcer NEC E10.622
type 2 E11.9
with
amyotrophy E11.44
arthropathy NEC E11.618
autonomic (poly)neuropathy E11.43
cataract E11.36
Charcot's joints E11.610
chronic kidney disease E11.22
circulatory complication NEC E11.59
complication E11.8
specified NEC E11.69
dermatitis E11.620
foot ulcer E11.621
gangrene E11.52
gastroparalysis E11.43 ◀
gastroparesis E11.43
glomerulonephrosis, intracapillary E11.21
glomerulosclerosis, intercapillary E11.21
hyperglycemia E11.65
hyperosmolarity E11.00
with coma E11.01
hypoglycemia E11.649
with coma E11.641
kidney complications NEC E11.29
Kimmelsteil-Wilson disease E11.21
mononeuropathy E11.41
myasthenia E11.44
necrobiosis lipoidica E11.620
nephropathy E11.21
neuralgia E11.42
neurologic complication NEC E11.49
neuropathic arthropathy E11.610
neuropathy E11.40
ophthalmic complication NEC E11.39
oral complication NEC E11.638
periodontal disease E11.630
peripheral angiopathy E11.51
with gangrene E11.52
polyneuropathy E11.42
renal complication NEC E11.29
renal tubular degeneration E11.29
retinopathy E11.319
with macular edema E11.311
resolved following treatment E11.37 ◀
nonproliferative E11.329
with macular edema E11.321
mild E11.329
with macular edema E11.321
moderate E11.339
with macular edema E11.331
severe E11.349
with macular edema E11.341
proliferative E11.359
~~with macular edema E11.351~~
with ◀
combined traction retinal detachment and rhegmatogenous retinal detachment E11.354 ◀

Diabetes, diabetic *(Continued)*
type 2 *(Continued)*
with *(Continued)*
retinopathy *(Continued)*
proliferative *(Continued)*
with *(Continued)*
macular edema E11.351 ◀
stable proliferative diabetic retinopathy E11.355 ◀
traction retinal detachment involving the macula E11.352 ◀
traction retinal detachment not involving the macula E11.353 ◀
skin complication NEC E11.628
skin ulcer NEC E11.622
uncontrolled ◀
meaning ◀
hyperglycemia —*see* Diabetes, by type, with, hyperglycemia ◀
hypoglycemia —*see* Diabetes, by type, with, hypoglycemia ◀
Diacyclothrombopathia D69.1
Diagnosis deferred R69
Dialysis (intermittent) (treatment)
noncompliance (with) Z91.15
renal (hemodialysis) (peritoneal), status Z99.2
retina, retinal —*see* Detachment, retina, with retinal, dialysis
Diamond-Blackfan anemia (congenital hypoplastic) D61.01
Diamond-Gardener syndrome (autoerythrocyte sensitization) D69.2
Diaper rash L22
Diaphoresis (excessive) R61
Diaphragm —*see* condition
Diaphragmalgia R07.1
Diaphragmatitis, diaphragmitis J98.6
Diaphysial aclasis Q78.6
Diaphysitis —*see* Osteomyelitis, specified type NEC
Diarrhea, diarrheal (disease) (infantile) (inflammatory) R19.7
achlorhydric K31.83
allergic K52.29 ⬅
due to ◀
colitis —*see* Colitis, allergic ◀
enteritis —*see* Enteritis, allergic ◀
amebic —*see also* Amebiasis A06.0
with abscess —*see* Abscess, amebic
acute A06.0
chronic A06.1
nondysenteric A06.2
bacillary —*see* Dysentery, bacillary
balantidial A07.0
cachectic NEC K52.89
Chilomastix A07.8
choleriformis A00.1
chronic (noninfectious) K52.9
coccidial A07.3
Cochin-China K90.1
strongyloidiasis B78.0
Dientamoeba A07.8
dietetic —*see also* Diarrhea, allergic K52.29 ⬅
drug-induced K52.1
due to
bacteria A04.9
specified NEC A04.8
Campylobacter A04.5
Capillaria philippinensis B81.1
Clostridium difficile A04.7
Clostridium perfringens (C) (F) A04.8
Cryptosporidium A07.2
drugs K52.1
Escherichia coli A04.4
enteroaggregative A04.4
enterohemorrhagic A04.3
enteroinvasive A04.2
enteropathogenic A04.0

◀ New ⬅ Revised ~~deleted~~ Deleted

Diarrhea, diarrheal *(Continued)*
due to *(Continued)*
Escherichia coli *(Continued)*
enterotoxigenic A04.1
specified NEC A04.4
food hypersensitivity —*see also* Diarrhea, allergic K52.29 ◀
Necator americanus B76.1
S. japonicum B65.2
specified organism NEC A08.8
bacterial A04.8
viral A08.39
Staphylococcus A04.8
Trichuris trichiuria B79
virus —*see* Enteritis, viral
Yersinia enterocolitica A04.6
dysenteric A09
endemic A09
epidemic A09
flagellate A07.9
Flexner's (ulcerative) A03.1
functional K59.1
following gastrointestinal surgery K91.89
psychogenic F45.8
Giardia lamblia A07.1
giardial A07.1
hill K90.1
infectious A09
malarial —*see* Malaria
mite B88.0
mycotic NEC B49
neonatal (noninfectious) P78.3
nervous F45.8
neurogenic K59.1
noninfectious K52.9
postgastrectomy K91.1
postvagotomy K91.1
protozoal A07.9
specified NEC A07.8
psychogenic F45.8
specified
bacterium NEC A04.8
virus NEC A08.39
strongyloidiasis B78.0
toxic K52.1
trichomonal A07.8
tropical K90.1
tuberculous A18.32
viral —*see* Enteritis, viral
Diastasis
cranial bones M84.88
congenital NEC Q75.8
joint (traumatic) —*see* Dislocation
muscle M62.00
ankle M62.07-
congenital Q79.8
foot M62.07-
forearm M62.03-
hand M62.04-
lower leg M62.06-
pelvic region M62.05-
shoulder region M62.01-
specified site NEC M62.08
thigh M62.05-
upper arm M62.02-
recti (abdomen)
complicating delivery O71.89
congenital Q79.59
Diastema, tooth, teeth, fully erupted M26.32
Diastematomyelia Q06.2
Diataxia, cerebral G80.4
Diathesis
allergic —*see* History, allergy
bleeding (familial) D69.9
cystine (familial) E72.00
gouty —*see* Gout
hemorrhagic (familial) D69.9
newborn NEC P53
spasmophilic R29.0
Diaz's disease or osteochondrosis (juvenile) (talus) —*see* Osteochondrosis, juvenile, tarsus
Dibothriocephalus, dibothriocephaliasis (latus) (infection) (infestation) B70.0
larval B70.1
Dicephalus, dicephaly Q89.4
Dichotomy, teeth K00.2
Dichromat, dichromatopsia (congenital) —*see* Deficiency, color vision
Dichuchwa A65
Dicroceliasis B66.2
Didelphia, didelphys —*see* Double uterus
Didymytis N45.1
with orchitis N45.3
Dietary
inadequacy or deficiency E63.9
surveillance and counseling Z71.3
Dietl's crisis N13.8
Dieulafoy lesion (hemorrhagic)
duodenum K31.82
esophagus K22.8
intestine (colon) K63.81
stomach K31.82
Difficult, difficulty (in)
acculturation Z60.3
feeding R63.3
newborn P92.9
breast P92.5
specified NEC P92.8
nonorganic (infant or child) F98.29
intubation, in anesthesia T88.4
mechanical, gastroduodenal stoma K91.89
causing obstruction K91.3
micturition ◀
need to immediately re-void R39.191 ◀
position dependent R39.192 ◀
specified NEC R39.198 ◀
reading (developmental) F81.0
secondary to emotional disorders F93.9
spelling (specific) F81.81
with reading disorder F81.89
due to inadequate teaching Z55.8
swallowing —*see* Dysphagia
walking R26.2
work
conditions NEC Z56.5
schedule Z56.3
Diffuse —*see* condition
DiGeorge's syndrome (thymic hypoplasia) D82.1
Digestive —*see* condition
Dihydropyrimidine dehydrogenase disease (DPD) E88.89
Diktyoma —*see* Neoplasm, malignant, by site
Dilaceration, tooth K00.4
Dilatation
anus K59.8
venule —*see* Hemorrhoids
aorta (focal) (general) —*see* Ectasia, aorta
with aneurysm —*see* Aneurysm, aorta
congenital Q25.44 ◀
artery —*see* Aneurysm
bladder (sphincter) N32.89
congenital Q64.79
blood vessel I99.8
bronchial J47.9
with
exacerbation (acute) J47.1
lower respiratory infection J47.0
calyx (due to obstruction) —*see* Hydronephrosis
capillaries I78.8
cardiac (acute) (chronic) —*see also* Hypertrophy, cardiac
congenital Q24.8
valve NEC Q24.8
pulmonary Q22.3
valve —*see* Endocarditis
cavum septi pellucidi Q06.8
cervix (uteri) —*see also* Incompetency, cervix
incomplete, poor, slow complicating delivery O62.0
Dilatation *(Continued)*
colon K59.39 ◀
congenital Q43.1
psychogenic F45.8
toxic K59.31 ◀
common duct (acquired) K83.8
congenital Q44.5
cystic duct (acquired) K82.8
congenital Q44.5
duct, mammary —*see* Ectasia, mammary duct
duodenum K59.8
esophagus K22.8
congenital Q39.5
due to achalasia K22.0
eustachian tube, congenital Q17.8
gallbladder K82.8
gastric —*see* Dilatation, stomach
heart (acute) (chronic) —*see also* Hypertrophy, cardiac
congenital Q24.8
valve —*see* Endocarditis
ileum K59.8
psychogenic F45.8
jejunum K59.8
psychogenic F45.8
kidney (calyx) (collecting structures) (cystic) (parenchyma) (pelvis) (idiopathic) N28.89
lacrimal passages or duct —*see* Disorder, lacrimal system, changes
lymphatic vessel I89.0
mammary duct —*see* Ectasia, mammary duct
Meckel's diverticulum (congenital) Q43.0
malignant —*see* Table of Neoplasms, small intestine, malignant
myocardium (acute) (chronic) —*see* Hypertrophy, cardiac organ or site, congenital NEC —*see* Distortion
pancreatic duct K86.89 ◀
pericardium —*see* Pericarditis
pharynx J39.2
prostate N42.89
pulmonary
artery (idiopathic) I28.8
valve, congenital Q22.3
pupil H57.04
rectum K59.39 ◀
saccule, congenital Q16.5
salivary gland (duct) K11.8
sphincter ani K62.89
stomach K31.89
acute K31.0
psychogenic F45.8
submaxillary duct K11.8
trachea, congenital Q32.1
ureter (idiopathic) N28.82
congenital Q62.2
due to obstruction N13.4
urethra (acquired) N36.8
vasomotor I73.9
vein I86.8
ventricular, ventricle (acute) (chronic) —*see also* Hypertrophy, cardiac
cerebral, congenital Q04.8
venule NEC I86.8
vesical orifice N32.89
Dilated, dilation —*see* Dilatation
Diminished, diminution
hearing (acuity) —*see* Deafness
sense or sensation (cold) (heat) (tactile) (vibratory) R20.8
vision NEC H54.7
vital capacity R94.2
Diminuta taenia B71.0
Dimitri-Sturge-Weber disease Q85.8
Dimple
~~parasacral, pilonidal or postanal —see Cyst, pilonidal~~
congenital sacral Q82.6 ◀
parasacral Q82.6 ◀
pilonidal or postanal —*see* Cyst, pilonidal ◀

Dioctophyme renalis (infection) (infestation) B83.8
Dipetalonemiasis B74.4
Diphallus Q55.69
Diphtheria, diphtheritic (gangrenous) (hemorrhagic) A36.9
carrier (suspected) Z22.2
cutaneous A36.3
faucial A36.0
infection of wound A36.3
laryngeal A36.2
myocarditis A36.81
nasal, anterior A36.89
nasopharyngeal A36.1
neurological complication A36.89
pharyngeal A36.0
specified site NEC A36.89
tonsillar A36.0
Diphyllobothriasis (intestine) B70.0
larval B70.1
Diplacusis H93.22-
Diplegia (upper limbs) G83.0
congenital (cerebral) G80.8
facial G51.0
lower limbs G82.20
spastic G80.1
Diplococcus, diplococcal —*see* condition
Diplopia H53.2
Dipsomania F10.20
with
psychosis —*see* Psychosis, alcoholic
remission F10.21
Dipylidiasis B71.1
DIRA (deficiency of interleukin 1 receptor antagonist) M04.8 ◀
Direction, teeth, abnormal, fully erupted M26.30
Dirofilariasis B74.8
Dirt-eating child F98.3
Disability, disabilities
heart —*see* Disease, heart
intellectual F79
with
autistic features F84.9
mild (I.Q. 50-69) F70
moderate (I.Q. 35-49) F71
profound (I.Q. under 20) F73
severe (I.Q. 20-34) F72
specified level NEC F78
knowledge acquisition F81.9
learning F81.9
limiting activities Z73.6
spelling, specific F81.81
Disappearance of family member Z63.4
Disarticulation —*see* Amputation
meaning traumatic amputation —*see* Amputation, traumatic
Discharge (from)
abnormal finding in —*see* Abnormal, specimen
breast (female) (male) N64.52
diencephalic autonomic idiopathic —*see* Epilepsy, specified NEC
ear —*see also* Otorrhea
blood —*see* Otorrhagia
excessive urine R35.8
nipple N64.52
penile R36.9
postnasal R09.82
prison, anxiety concerning Z65.2
urethral R36.9
without blood R36.0
hematospermia R36.1
vaginal N89.8
Discitis, diskitis M46.40
cervical region M46.42
cervicothoracic region M46.43
lumbar region M46.46
lumbosacral region M46.47
multiple sites M46.49
occipito-atlanto-axial region M46.41
Discitis, diskitis *(Continued)*
pyogenic —*see* Infection, intervertebral disc, pyogenic
sacrococcygeal region M46.48
thoracic region M46.44
thoracolumbar region M46.45
Discoid
meniscus (congenital) Q68.6
semilunar cartilage (congenital) —*see* Derangement, knee, meniscus, specified NEC
Discoloration
nails L60.8
teeth (posteruptive) K03.7
during formation K00.8
Discomfort
chest R07.89
visual H53.14-
Discontinuity, ossicles, ear H74.2-
Discord (with)
boss Z56.4
classmates Z55.4
counselor Z64.4
employer Z56.4
family Z63.8
fellow employees Z56.4
in-laws Z63.1
landlord Z59.2
lodgers Z59.2
neighbors Z59.2
probation officer Z64.4
social worker Z64.4
teachers Z55.4
workmates Z56.4
Discordant connection
atrioventricular (congenital) Q20.5
ventriculoarterial Q20.3
Discrepancy
centric occlusion maximum intercuspation M26.55
leg length (acquired) —*see* Deformity, limb, unequal length
congenital —*see* Defect, reduction, lower limb
uterine size date O26.84-
Discrimination
ethnic Z60.5
political Z60.5
racial Z60.5
religious Z60.5
sex Z60.5
Disease, diseased —*see also* Syndrome
absorbent system I87.8
acid-peptic K30
Acosta's T70.29
Adams-Stokes (-Morgagni) (syncope with heart block) I45.9
Addison's anemia (pernicious) D51.0
adenoids (and tonsils) J35.9
adrenal (capsule) (cortex) (gland) (medullary) E27.9
hyperfunction E27.0
specified NEC E27.8
ainhum L94.6
airway
obstructive, chronic J44.9
due to
cotton dust J66.0
specific organic dusts NEC J66.8
reactive —*see* Asthma
akamushi (scrub typhus) A75.3
Albers-Schönberg (marble bones) Q78.2
Albert's —*see* Tendinitis, Achilles
alimentary canal K63.9
alligator-skin Q80.9
acquired L85.0
alpha heavy chain C88.3
alpine T70.29
altitude T70.20
Disease, diseased *(Continued)*
alveolar ridge
edentulous K06.9
specified NEC K06.8
alveoli, teeth K08.9
Alzheimer's G30.9 *[F02.80]*
with behavioral disturbance G30.9 *[F02.81]*
early onset G30.0 *[F02.80]*
with behavioral disturbance G30.0 *[F02.81]*
late onset G30.1 *[F02.80]*
with behavioral disturbance G30.1 *[F02.81]*
specified NEC G30.8 *[F02.80]*
with behavioral disturbance G30.8 *[F02.81]*
amyloid —*see* Amyloidosis
Andersen's (glycogenosis IV) E74.09
Andes T70.29
Andrews' (bacterid) L08.89
angiospastic I73.9
cerebral G45.9
vein I87.8
anterior
chamber H21.9
horn cell G12.29
antiglomerular basement membrane (anti-GBM) antibody M31.0
tubulo-interstitial nephritis N12
antral —*see* Sinusitis, maxillary
anus K62.9
specified NEC K62.89
aorta (nonsyphilitic) I77.9
syphilitic NEC A52.02
aortic (heart) (valve) I35.9
rheumatic I06.9
Apollo B30.3
aponeuroses —*see* Enthesopathy
appendix K38.9
specified NEC K38.8
aqueous (chamber) H21.9
Arnold-Chiari —*see* Arnold-Chiari disease
arterial I77.9
occlusive —*see* Occlusion, by site due to stricture or stenosis I77.1
arteriocardiorenal —*see* Hypertension, cardiorenal
arteriolar (generalized) (obliterative) I77.9
arteriorenal —*see* Hypertension, kidney
arteriosclerotic —*see also* Arteriosclerosis
cardiovascular —*see* Disease, heart, ischemic, atherosclerotic
coronary (artery) —*see* Disease, heart, ischemic, atherosclerotic
heart —*see* Disease, heart, ischemic, atherosclerotic
artery I77.9
cerebral I67.9
coronary I25.10
with angina pectoris —*see* Arteriosclerosis, coronary (artery),
arthropod-borne NOS (viral) A94
specified type NEC A93.8
atticoantral, chronic H66.20
left H66.22
with right H66.23
right H66.21
with left H66.23
auditory canal —*see* Disorder, ear, external
auricle, ear NEC —*see* Disorder, pinna
Australian X A83.4
autoimmune (systemic) NOS M35.9
hemolytic (cold type) (warm type) D59.1
drug-induced D59.0
thyroid E06.3
aviator's —*see* Effect, adverse, high altitude
~~Ayala's Q78.5~~
Ayerza's (pulmonary artery sclerosis with pulmonary hypertension) I27.0

◀ New ◀ Revised ~~deleted~~ Deleted

Disease, diseased *(Continued)*
Babington's (familial hemorrhagic telangiectasia) I78.0
bacterial A49.9
specified NEC A48.8
zoonotic A28.9
specified type NEC A28.8
Baelz's (cheilitis glandularis apostematosa) K13.0
bagasse J67.1
balloon —*see* Effect, adverse, high altitude
Bang's (brucella abortus) A23.1
Bannister's T78.3
barometer makers' —*see* Poisoning, mercury
Barraquer (-Simons') (progressive lipodystrophy) E88.1
Barrett's —*see* Barrett's, esophagus
Bartholin's gland N75.9
basal ganglia G25.9
degenerative G23.9
specified NEC G23.8
specified NEC G25.89
Basedow's (exophthalmic goiter) —*see* Hyperthyroidism, with, goiter (diffuse)
Bateman's B08.1
Batten-Steinert G71.11
Battey A31.0
Beard's (neurasthenia) F48.8
Becker
idiopathic mural endomyocardial I42.3
myotonia congenita G71.12
Begbie's (exophthalmic goiter) —*see* Hyperthyroidism, with, goiter (diffuse)
behavioral, organic F07.9
Beigel's (white piedra) B36.2
Benson's —*see* Deposit, crystalline
Bernard-Soulier (thrombopathy) D69.1
Bernhardt (-Roth) —*see* Mononeuropathy, lower limb, meralgia paresthetica
Biermer's (pernicious anemia) D51.0
bile duct (common) (hepatic) K83.9
with calculus, stones —*see* Calculus, bile duct
specified NEC K83.8
biliary (tract) K83.9
specified NEC K83.8
Billroth's —*see* Spina bifida
bird fancier's J67.2
black lung J60
bladder N32.9
in (due to)
schistosomiasis (bilharziasis) B65.0 *[N33]*
specified NEC N32.89
bleeder's D66
blood D75.9
forming organs D75.9
vessel I99.9
Bloodgood's —*see* Mastopathy, cystic
Bodechtel-Guttmann (subacute sclerosing panencephalitis) A81.1
bone —*see also* Disorder, bone
aluminum M83.4
fibrocystic NEC
jaw M27.49
bone-marrow D75.9
Borna A83.9
Bornholm (epidemic pleurodynia) B33.0
Bouchard's (myopathic dilatation of the stomach) K31.0
Bouillaud's (rheumatic heart disease) I01.9
Bourneville (-Brissaud) (tuberous sclerosis) Q85.1
Bouveret (-Hoffmann) (paroxysmal tachycardia) I47.9
bowel K63.9
functional K59.9
psychogenic F45.8
brain G93.9
arterial, artery I67.9
arteriosclerotic I67.2
congenital Q04.9

Disease, diseased *(Continued)*
brain *(Continued)*
degenerative —*see* Degeneration, brain
inflammatory —*see* Encephalitis
organic G93.9
arteriosclerotic I67.2
parasitic NEC B71.9 *[G94]*
senile NEC G31.1
specified NEC G93.89
breast (*see also* Disorder, breast) N64.9
cystic (chronic) —*see* Mastopathy, cystic
fibrocystic —*see* Mastopathy, cystic
Paget's
female, unspecified side C50.91-
male, unspecified side C50.92-
specified NEC N64.89
Breda's —*see* Yaws
Bretonneau's (diphtheritic malignant angina) A36.0
Bright's —*see* Nephritis
arteriosclerotic —*see* Hypertension, kidney
Brill's (recrudescent typhus) A75.1
Brill-Zinsser (recrudescent typhus) A75.1
Brion-Kayser —*see* Fever, paratyphoid
broad
beta E78.2
ligament (noninflammatory) N83.9
inflammatory —*see* Disease, pelvis, inflammatory
specified NEC N83.8
Brocq-Duhring (dermatitis herpetiformis) L13.0
Brocq's
meaning
dermatitis herpetiformis L13.0
prurigo L28.2
bronchopulmonary J98.4
bronchus NEC J98.09
bronze Addison's E27.1
tuberculous A18.7
budgerigar fancier's J67.2
Buerger's (thromboangiitis obliterans) I73.1
bullous L13.9
chronic of childhood L12.2
specified NEC L13.8
Bürger-Grütz (essential familial hyperlipemia) E78.3
bursa —*see* Bursopathy
caisson T70.3
California —*see* Coccidioidomycosis
capillaries I78.9
specified NEC I78.8
Carapata A68.0
cardiac —*see* Disease, heart
cardiopulmonary, chronic I27.9
cardiorenal (hepatic) (hypertensive) (vascular) —*see* Hypertension, cardiorenal
cardiovascular (atherosclerotic) I25.10
with angina pectoris —*see* Arteriosclerosis, coronary (artery),
congenital Q28.9
hypertensive —*see* Hypertension, heart
newborn P29.9
specified NEC P29.89
renal (hypertensive) —*see* Hypertension, cardiorenal
syphilitic (asymptomatic) A52.00
cartilage —*see* Disorder, cartilage
Castellani's A69.8
Castleman (unicentric) (multicentric) D47.Z2 ◀
HHV-8-associated —*see also* Herpesvirus, human, 8 D47.Z2 ◀
cat-scratch A28.1
Cavare's (familial periodic paralysis) G72.3
cecum K63.9
celiac (adult) (infantile) (with steatorrhea) K90.0 ⇐
cellular tissue L98.9

Disease, diseased *(Continued)*
central core G71.2
cerebellar, cerebellum —*see* Disease, brain
cerebral —*see also* Disease, brain
degenerative —*see* Degeneration, brain
cerebrospinal G96.9
cerebrovascular I67.9
acute I67.89
embolic I63.4-
thrombotic I63.3-
arteriosclerotic I67.2
specified NEC I67.89
cervix (uteri) (noninflammatory) N88.9
inflammatory —*see* Cervicitis
specified NEC N88.8
Chabert's A22.9
Chandler's (osteochondritis dissecans, hip) —*see* Osteochondritis, dissecans, hip
Charlouis —*see* Yaws
Chédiak-Steinbrinck (-Higashi) (congenital gigantism of peroxidase granules) E70.330
chest J98.9
Chiari's (hepatic vein thrombosis) I82.0
Chicago B40.9
Chignon B36.8
chigo, chigoe B88.1
childhood granulomatous D71
Chinese liver fluke B66.1
chlamydial A74.9
specified NEC A74.89
cholecystic K82.9
choroid H31.9
specified NEC H31.8
Christmas D67
chronic bullous of childhood L12.2
chylomicron retention E78.3
ciliary body H21.9
specified NEC H21.89
circulatory (system) NEC I99.8
newborn P29.9
syphilitic A52.00
congenital A50.54
coagulation factor deficiency (congenital) —*see* Defect, coagulation
coccidioidal —*see* Coccidioidomycosis
cold
agglutinin or hemoglobinuria D59.1
paroxysmal D59.6
hemagglutinin (chronic) D59.1
collagen NOS (nonvascular) (vascular) M35.9
specified NEC M35.8
colon K63.9
functional K59.9
congenital Q43.2
ischemic —*see also* Ischemia, intestine, acute K55.039 ⇐
colonic inflammatory bowel, unclassified (IBDU) K52.3 ◀
combined system —*see* Degeneration, combined
compressed air T70.3
Concato's (pericardial polyserositis) A19.9
nontubercular I31.1
pleural —*see* Pleurisy, with effusion
conjunctiva H11.9
chlamydial A74.0
specified NEC H11.89
viral B30.9
specified NEC B30.8
connective tissue, systemic (diffuse) M35.9
in (due to)
hypogammaglobulinemia D80.1 *[M36.8]*
ochronosis E70.29 *[M36.8]*
specified NEC M35.8
Conor and Bruch's (boutonneuse fever) A77.1
Cooper's —*see* Mastopathy, cystic
Cori's (glycogenosis III) E74.03
corkhandler's or corkworker's J67.3
cornea H18.9
specified NEC H18.89-

Disease, diseased *(Continued)*
coronary (artery) —*see* Disease, heart, ischemic, atherosclerotic
congenital Q24.5
ostial, syphilitic (aortic) (mitral) (pulmonary) A52.03
corpus cavernosum N48.9
specified NEC N48.89
Cotugno's —*see* Sciatica
coxsackie (virus) NEC B34.1
cranial nerve NOS G52.9
Creutzfeldt-Jakob —*see* Creutzfeldt- Jakob disease or syndrome
Crocq's (acrocyanosis) I73.89
Crohn's —*see* Enteritis, regional
Curschmann G71.11
cystic
breast (chronic) —*see* Mastopathy, cystic
kidney, congenital Q61.9
liver, congenital Q44.6
lung J98.4
congenital Q33.0
cytomegalic inclusion (generalized) B25.9
with pneumonia B25.0
congenital P35.1
cytomegaloviral B25.9
specified NEC B25.8
Czerny's (periodic hydrarthrosis of the knee) —*see* Effusion, joint, knee
Daae (-Finsen) (epidemic pleurodynia) B33.0
Darling's —*see* Histoplasmosis capsulati
Débove's (splenomegaly) R16.1
deer fly —*see* Tularemia
Degos' I77.8
demyelinating, demyelinizating (nervous system) G37.9
multiple sclerosis G35
specified NEC G37.8
dense deposit —*see also* N00-N07 with fourth character .6 N05.6
deposition, hydroxyapatite —*see* Disease, hydroxyapatite deposition
de Quervain's (tendon sheath) M65.4
thyroid (subacute granulomatous thyroiditis) E06.1
Devergie's (pityriasis rubra pilaris) L44.0
Devic's G36.0
diaphorase deficiency D74.0
diaphragm J98.6
diarrheal, infectious NEC A09
digestive system K92.9
specified NEC K92.89
disc, degenerative —*see* Degeneration, intervertebral disc
discogenic —*see also* Displacement, intervertebral disc NEC
with myelopathy —*see* Disorder, disc, with, myelopathy
diverticular —*see* Diverticula
Dubois (thymus) A50.59 *[E35]*
Duchenne-Griesinger G71.0
Duchenne's
muscular dystrophy G71.0
pseudohypertrophy, muscles G71.0
ductless glands E34.9
Duhring's (dermatitis herpetiformis) L13.0
duodenum K31.9
specified NEC K31.89
Dupré's (meningism) R29.1
Dupuytren's (muscle contracture) M72.0
Durand-Nicholas-Favre (climatic bubo) A55
Duroziez's (congenital mitral stenosis) Q23.2
ear —*see* Disorder, ear
Eberth's —*see* Fever, typhoid
Ebola (virus) A98.4
Ebstein's heart Q22.5
Echinococcus —*see* Echinococcus
echovirus NEC B34.1
Eddowes' (brittle bones and blue sclera) Q78.0
edentulous (alveolar) ridge K06.9
specified NEC K06.8

Disease, diseased *(Continued)*
Edsall's T67.2
Eichstedt's (pityriasis versicolor) B36.0
Ellis-van Creveld (chondroectodermal dysplasia) Q77.6
end stage renal (ESRD) N18.6
due to hypertension I12.0
endocrine glands or system NEC E34.9
endomyocardial (eosinophilic) I42.3
English (rickets) E55.0
enteroviral, enterovirus NEC B34.1
central nervous system NEC A88.8
epidemic B99.9
specified NEC B99.8
epididymis N50.9
Erb (-Landouzy) G71.0
Erdheim-Chester (ECD) E88.89
esophagus K22.9
functional K22.4
psychogenic F45.8
specified NEC K22.8
Eulenburg's (congenital paramyotonia) G71.19
eustachian tube —*see* Disorder, eustachian tube
external
auditory canal —*see* Disorder, ear, external
ear —*see* Disorder, ear, external
extrapyramidal G25.9
specified NEC G25.89
eye H57.9
anterior chamber H21.9
inflammatory NEC H57.8
muscle (external) —*see* Strabismus
specified NEC H57.8
syphilitic —*see* Oculopathy, syphilitic
eyeball H44.9
specified NEC H44.89
eyelid —*see* Disorder, eyelid
specified NEC —*see* Disorder, eyelid, specified type NEC
eyeworm of Africa B74.3
facial nerve (seventh) G51.9
newborn (birth injury) P11.3
Fahr (of brain) G23.8
Fahr Volhard (of kidney) I12.-
fallopian tube (noninflammatory) N83.9
inflammatory —*see* Salpingo-oophoritis
specified NEC N83.8
familial periodic paralysis G72.3
Fanconi's (congenital pancytopenia) D61.09
fascia NEC —*see also* Disorder, muscle
inflammatory —*see* Myositis
specified NEC M62.89
Fauchard's (periodontitis) —*see* Periodontitis
Favre-Durand-Nicolas (climatic bubo) A55
Fede's K14.0
Feer's —*see* Poisoning, mercury
female pelvic inflammatory —*see also* Disease, pelvis, inflammatory N73.9
syphilitic (secondary) A51.42
tuberculous A18.17
Fernels' (aortic aneurysm) I71.9
fibrocaseous of lung —*see* Tuberculosis, pulmonary
fibrocystic —*see* Fibrocystic disease
Fiedler's (leptospiral jaundice) A27.0
fifth B08.3
file-cutter's —*see* Poisoning, lead
fish-skin Q80.9
acquired L85.0
Flajani (-Basedow) (exophthalmic goiter) —*see* Hyperthyroidism, with, goiter (diffuse)
flax-dresser's J66.1
fluke —*see* Infestation, fluke
foot and mouth B08.8
foot process N04.9
Forbes' (glycogenosis III) E74.03
Fordyce-Fox (apocrine miliaria) L75.2
Fordyce's (ectopic sebaceous glands) (mouth) Q38.6

Disease, diseased *(Continued)*
Forestier's (rhizomelic pseudopolyarthritis) M35.3
meaning ankylosing hyperostosis —*see* Hyperostosis, ankylosing
Fothergill's
neuralgia —*see* Neuralgia, trigeminal
scarlatina anginosa A38.9
Fournier (gangrene) N49.3
female N76.89
fourth B08.8
Fox (-Fordyce) (apocrine miliaria) L75.2
Francis' —*see* Tularemia
Franklin C88.2
Frei's (climatic bubo) A55
Friedreich's
combined systemic or ataxia G11.1
myoclonia G25.3
frontal sinus —*see* Sinusitis, frontal
fungus NEC B49
Gaisböck's (polycythemia hypertonica) D75.1
gallbladder K82.9
calculus —*see* Calculus, gallbladder
cholecystitis —*see* Cholecystitis
cholesterolosis K82.4
fistula —*see* Fistula, gallbladder
hydrops K82.1
obstruction —*see* Obstruction, gallbladder
perforation K82.2
specified NEC K82.8
gamma heavy chain C88.2
Gamna's (siderotic splenomegaly) D73.2
Gamstorp's (adynamia episodica hereditaria) G72.3
Gandy-Nanta (siderotic splenomegaly) D73.2
ganister J62.8
gastric —*see* Disease, stomach
gastroesophageal reflux (GERD) K21.9
with esophagitis K21.0
gastrointestinal (tract) K92.9
amyloid E85.4
functional K59.9
psychogenic F45.8
specified NEC K92.89
Gee (-Herter) (-Heubner) (-Thaysen) (nontropical sprue) K90.0
genital organs
female N94.9
male N50.9
Gerhardt's (erythromelalgia) I73.81
Gibert's (pityriasis rosea) L42
Gierke's (glycogenosis I) E74.01
Gilles de la Tourette's (motor-verbal tic) F95.2
gingiva K06.9
plaque induced K05.00 ◀
specified NEC K06.8
gland (lymph) I89.9
Glanzmann's (hereditary hemorrhagic thrombasthenia) D69.1
glass-blower's (cataract) —*see* Cataract, specified NEC
salivary gland hypertrophy K11.1
Glisson's —*see* Rickets
globe H44.9
specified NEC H44.89
glomerular —*see also* Glomerulonephritis
with edema —*see* Nephrosis
acute —*see* Nephritis, acute
chronic —*see* Nephritis, chronic
minimal change N05.0
rapidly progressive N01.9
glycogen storage E74.00
Andersen's E74.09
Cori's E74.03
Forbes' E74.03
generalized E74.00
glucose-6-phosphatase deficiency E74.01
heart E74.02 *[I43]*
hepatorenal E74.09
Hers' E74.09
liver and kidney E74.09

◀ New ◀ Revised ~~deleted~~ Deleted

Disease, diseased *(Continued)*
glycogen storage *(Continued)*
McArdle's E74.04
muscle phosphofructokinase E74.09
myocardium E74.02 *[143]*
Pompe's E74.02
Tauri's E74.09
type 0 E74.09
type I E74.01
type II E74.02
type III E74.03
type IV E74.09
type V E74.04
type VI-XI E74.09
Von Gierke's E74.01
Goldstein's (familial hemorrhagic telangiectasia) I78.0
gonococcal NOS A54.9
graft-versus-host (GVH) D89.813
acute D89.810
acute on chronic D89.812
chronic D89.811
grainhandler's J67.8
granulomatous (childhood) (chronic) D71
Graves' (exophthalmic goiter) —*see* Hyperthyroidism, with, goiter (diffuse)
Griesinger's —*see* Ancylostomiasis
Grisel's M43.6
Gruby's (tinea tonsurans) B35.0
Guillain-Barré G61.0
Guinon's (motor-verbal tic) F95.2
gum K06.9
gynecological N94.9
H (Hartnup's) E72.02
Haff —*see* Poisoning, mercury
Hageman (congenital factor XII deficiency) D68.2
hair (color) (shaft) L67.9
follicles L73.9
specified NEC L73.8
Hamman's (spontaneous mediastinal emphysema) J98.2
hand, foot and mouth B08.4
Hansen's —*see* Leprosy
Hantavirus, with pulmonary manifestations B33.4
with renal manifestations A98.5
Harada's H30.81-
Hartnup (pellagra-cerebellar ataxia-renal aminoaciduria) E72.02
Hart's (pellagra-cerebellar ataxia-renal aminoaciduria) E72.02
Hashimoto's (struma lymphomatosa) E06.3
Hb —*see* Disease, hemoglobin
heart (organic) I51.9
with
pulmonary edema (acute) —*see also* Failure, ventricular, left I50.1
rheumatic fever (conditions in I00)
active I01.9
with chorea I02.0
specified NEC I01.8
inactive or quiescent (with chorea) I09.9
specified NEC I09.89
amyloid E85.4 *[143]*
aortic (valve) I35.9
arteriosclerotic or sclerotic (senile) —*see* Disease, heart, ischemic, atherosclerotic
artery, arterial —*see* Disease, heart, ischemic, atherosclerotic
beer drinkers' I42.6
beriberi (wet) E51.12
black I27.0
congenital Q24.9
cyanotic Q24.9
specified NEC Q24.8
coronary —*see* Disease, heart, ischemic
cryptogenic I51.9

Disease, diseased *(Continued)*
heart *(Continued)*
fibroid —*see* Myocarditis
functional I51.89
psychogenic F45.8
glycogen storage E74.02 *[143]*
gonococcal A54.83
hypertensive —*see* Hypertension, heart
hyperthyroid —*see also* Hyperthyroidism E05.90 *[143]*
with thyroid storm E05.91 *[143]*
ischemic (chronic or with a stated duration of over 4 weeks) I25.9
atherosclerotic (of) I25.10
with angina pectoris —*see* Arteriosclerosis, coronary (artery)
coronary artery bypass graft —*see* Arteriosclerosis, coronary (artery),
cardiomyopathy I25.5
diagnosed on ECG or other special investigation, but currently presenting no symptoms I25.6
silent I25.6
specified form NEC I25.89
kyphoscoliotic I27.1
meningococcal A39.50
endocarditis A39.51
myocarditis A39.52
pericarditis A39.53
mitral I05.9
specified NEC I05.8
muscular —*see* Degeneration, myocardial
psychogenic (functional) F45.8
pulmonary (chronic) I27.9
in schistosomiasis B65.9 *[I52]*
specified NEC I27.89
rheumatic (chronic) (inactive) (old) (quiescent) (with chorea) I09.9
active or acute I01.9
with chorea (acute) (rheumatic) (Sydenham's) I02.0
specified NEC I09.89
senile —*see* Myocarditis
syphilitic A52.06
aortic A52.03
aneurysm A52.01
congenital A50.54 *[I52]*
thyrotoxic —*see also* Thyrotoxicosis E05.90 *[143]*
with thyroid storm E05.91 *[143]*
valve, valvular (obstructive) (regurgitant) —*see also* Endocarditis
congenital NEC Q24.8
pulmonary Q22.3
vascular —*see* Disease, cardiovascular
heavy chain NEC C88.2
alpha C88.3
gamma C88.2
mu C88.2
Hebra's
pityriasis
maculata et circinata L42
rubra pilaris L44.0
prurigo L28.2
hematopoietic organs D75.9
hemoglobin or Hb
abnormal (mixed) NEC D58.2
with thalassemia D56.9
AS genotype D57.3
Bart's D56.0
C (Hb-C) D58.2
with other abnormal hemoglobin NEC D58.2
elliptocytosis D58.1
Hb-S D57.2-
sickle-cell D57.2-
thalassemia D56.8
Constant Spring D58.2
D (Hb-D) D58.2

Disease, diseased *(Continued)*
hemoglobin or Hb *(Continued)*
E (Hb-E) D58.2
E-beta thalassemia D56.5
elliptocytosis D58.1
H (Hb-H) (thalassemia) D56.0
with other abnormal hemoglobin NEC D56.9
Constant Spring D56.0
I thalassemia D56.9
M D74.0
S or SS D57.1
SC D57.2-
SD D57.8-
SE D57.8-
spherocytosis D58.0
unstable, hemolytic D58.2
hemolytic (newborn) P55.9
autoimmune (cold type) (warm type) D59.1
drug-induced D59.0
due to or with
incompatibility
ABO (blood group) P55.1
blood (group) (Duffy) (K(ell)) (Kidd) (Lewis) (M) (S) NEC P55.8
Rh (blood group) (factor) P55.0
Rh negative mother P55.0
specified type NEC P55.8
unstable hemoglobin D58.2
hemorrhagic D69.9
newborn P53
Henoch (-Schönlein) (purpura nervosa) D69.0
hepatic —*see* Disease, liver
hepatobiliary K83.9
toxic K71.9
hepatolenticular E83.01
heredodegenerative NEC
spinal cord G95.89
herpesviral, disseminated B00.7
Hers' (glycogenosis VI) E74.09
Herter (-Gee) (-Heubner) (nontropical sprue) K90.0
Heubner-Herter (nontropical sprue) K90.0
high fetal gene or hemoglobin thalassemia D56.9
Hildenbrand's —*see* Typhus
hip (joint) M25.9
congenital Q65.89
suppurative M00.9
tuberculous A18.02
His (-Werner) (trench fever) A79.0
Hodgson's I71.2
ruptured I71.1
Holla —*see* Spherocytosis
hookworm B76.9
specified NEC B76.8
host-versus-graft D89.813
acute D89.810
acute on chronic D89.812
chronic D89.811
human immunodeficiency virus (HIV) B20
Huntington's G10
Hutchinson's (cheiropompholyx) —*see* Hutchinson's disease
hyaline (diffuse) (generalized)
membrane (lung) (newborn) P22.0
adult J80
hydatid —*see* Echinococcus
hydroxyapatite deposition M11.00
ankle M11.07-
elbow M11.02-
foot joint M11.07-
hand joint M11.04-
hip M11.05-
knee M11.06-
multiple site M11.09
shoulder M11.01-
vertebra M11.08
wrist M11.03-
hyperkinetic —*see* Hyperkinesia
hypertensive —*see* Hypertension

Disease, diseased *(Continued)*
hypophysis E23.7
Iceland G93.3
I-cell E77.0
immune D89.9
immunoproliferative (malignant) C88.9
small intestinal C88.3
specified NEC C88.8
inclusion B25.9
salivary gland B25.9
infectious, infective B99.9
congenital P37.9
specified NEC P37.8
viral P35.9
specified type NEC P35.8
specified NEC B99.8
inflammatory
penis N48.29
abscess N48.21
cellulitis N48.22
prepuce N47.7
balanoposthitis N47.6
tubo-ovarian —*see* Salpingo-oophoritis
intervertebral disc —*see also* Disorder, disc
with myelopathy —*see* Disorder, disc, with, myelopathy
cervical, cervicothoracic —*see* Disorder, disc, cervical
with
myelopathy —*see* Disorder, disc, cervical, with myelopathy
neuritis, radiculitis or radiculopathy —*see* Disorder, disc, cervical, with neuritis
specified NEC —*see* Disorder, disc, cervical, specified type NEC
lumbar (with)
myelopathy M51.06
neuritis, radiculitis, radiculopathy or sciatica M51.16
specified NEC M51.86
lumbosacral (with)
neuritis, radiculitis, radiculopathy or sciatica M51.17
specified NEC M51.87
specified NEC —*see* Disorder, disc, specified NEC
thoracic (with)
myelopathy M51.04
neuritis, radiculitis or radiculopathy M51.14
specified NEC M51.84
thoracolumbar (with)
myelopathy M51.05
neuritis, radiculitis or radiculopathy M51.15
specified NEC M51.85
intestine K63.9
functional K59.9
psychogenic F45.8
specified NEC K59.8
organic K63.9
protozoal A07.9
specified NEC K63.89
iris H21.9
specified NEC H21.89
iron metabolism or storage E83.10
island (scrub typhus) A75.3
itai-itai —*see* Poisoning, cadmium
Jakob-Creutzfeldt —*see* Creutzfeldt- Jakob disease or syndrome
jaw M27.9
fibrocystic M27.49
specified NEC M27.8
jigger B88.1
joint —*see also* Disorder, joint
Charcot's —*see* Arthropathy, neuropathic (Charcot)
degenerative —*see* Osteoarthritis
multiple M15.9
spine —*see* Spondylosis

Disease, diseased *(Continued)*
joint *(Continued)*
hypertrophic —*see* Osteoarthritis
sacroiliac M53.3
specified NEC —*see* Disorder, joint, specified type NEC
spine NEC —*see* Dorsopathy
suppurative —*see* Arthritis, pyogenic or pyemic
Jourdain's (acute gingivitis) K05.00
nonplaque induced K05.01
plaque induced K05.00
Kaschin-Beck (endemic polyarthritis) M12.10
ankle M12.17-
elbow M12.12-
foot joint M12.17-
hand joint M12.14-
hip M12.15-
knee M12.16-
multiple site M12.19
shoulder M12.11-
vertebra M12.18
wrist M12.13-
Katayama B65.2
Kedani (scrub typhus) A75.3
Keshan E59
kidney (functional) (pelvis) N28.9
chronic N18.9
hypertensive —*see* Hypertension, kidney
stage 1 N18.1
stage 2 (mild) N18.2
stage 3 (moderate) N18.3
stage 4 (severe) N18.4
stage 5 N18.5
complicating pregnancy —*see* Pregnancy, complicated by, renal disease
cystic (congenital) Q61.9
diabetic - see E08-E13 with .22
fibrocystic (congenital) Q61.8
hypertensive —*see* Hypertension, kidney
in (due to)
schistosomiasis (bilharziasis) B65.9 *[N29]*
multicystic Q61.4
polycystic Q61.3
adult type Q61.2
childhood type NEC Q61.19
collecting duct dilatation Q61.11
Kimmelstiel (-Wilson) (intercapillary polycystic (congenital) glomerulosclerosis) —*see* E08-E13 with .21
Kimura D21.9
specified site (see Neoplasm, connective tissue benign)
Kinnier Wilson's (hepatolenticular degeneration) E83.01
kissing —*see* Mononucleosis, infectious
Klebs' —*see also* Glomerulonephritis N05.-
Klippel-Feil (brevicollis) Q76.1
Köhler-Pellegrini-Stieda (calcification, knee joint) —*see* Bursitis, tibial collateral
Kok Q89.8
König's (osteochondritis dissecans) —*see* Osteochondritis, dissecans
Korsakoff's (nonalcoholic) F04
alcoholic F10.96
with dependence F10.26
Kostmann's (infantile genetic agranulocytosis) D70.0
kuru A81.81
Kyasanur Forest A98.2
labyrinth, ear —*see* Disorder, ear, inner
lacrimal system —*see* Disorder, lacrimal system
Lafora's —*see* Epilepsy, generalized, idiopathic
Lancereaux-Mathieu (leptospiral jaundice) A27.0
Landry's G61.0
Larrey-Weil (leptospiral jaundice) A27.0
larynx J38.7

Disease, diseased *(Continued)*
legionnaires' A48.1
nonpneumonic A48.2
Lenegre's I44.2
lens H27.9
specified NEC H27.8
Lev's (acquired complete heart block) I44.2
Lewy body (dementia) G31.83 *[F02.80]*
with behavioral disturbance G31.83 *[F02.81]*
Lichtheim's (subacute combined sclerosis with pernicious anemia) D51.0
Lightwood's (renal tubular acidosis) N25.89
Lignac's (cystinosis) E72.04
lip K13.0
lipid-storage E75.6
specified NEC E75.5
Lipschütz's N76.6
liver (chronic) (organic) K76.9
alcoholic (chronic) K70.9
acute —*see* Disease, liver, alcoholic, hepatitis
cirrhosis K70.30
with ascites K70.31
failure K70.40
with coma K70.41
fatty liver K70.0
fibrosis K70.2
hepatitis K70.10
with ascites K70.11
sclerosis K70.2
cystic, congenital Q44.6
drug-induced (idiosyncratic) (toxic) (predictable) (unpredictable) —*see* Disease, liver, toxic
end stage K72.90
due to hepatitis —*see* Hepatitis
fatty, nonalcoholic (NAFLD) K76.0
alcoholic K70.0
fibrocystic (congenital) Q44.6
fluke
Chinese B66.1
oriental B66.1
sheep B66.3
glycogen storage E74.09 *[K77]*
in (due to)
schistosomiasis (bilharziasis) B65.9 *[K77]*
inflammatory K75.9
alcoholic K70.1
specified NEC K75.89
polycystic (congenital) Q44.6
toxic K71.9
with
cholestasis K71.0
cirrhosis (liver) K71.7
fibrosis (liver) K71.7
focal nodular hyperplasia K71.8
hepatic granuloma K71.8
hepatic necrosis K71.10
with coma K71.11
hepatitis NEC K71.6
acute K71.2
chronic
active K71.50
with ascites K71.51
lobular K71.4
persistent K71.3
lupoid K71.50
with ascites K71.51
peliosis hepatis K71.8
veno-occlusive disease (VOD) of liver K71.8
veno-occlusive K76.5
Lobo's (keloid blastomycosis) B48.0
Lobstein's (brittle bones and blue sclera) Q78.0
Ludwig's (submaxillary cellulitis) K12.2
lumbosacral region M53.87
lung J98.4
black J60
congenital Q33.9
cystic J98.4
congenital Q33.0

Disease, diseased *(Continued)*
lung *(Continued)*
fibroid (chronic) —*see* Fibrosis, lung
fluke B66.4
oriental B66.4
in
amyloidosis E85.4 *[J99]*
sarcoidosis D86.0
Sjögren's syndrome M35.02
systemic
lupus erythematosus M32.13
sclerosis M34.81
interstitial J84.9
of childhood, specified NEC J84.848
respiratory bronchiolitis J84.115
specified NEC J84.89
obstructive (chronic) J44.9
with
acute
bronchitis J44.0
exacerbation NEC J44.1
lower respiratory infection J44.0
alveolitis, allergic J67.9
asthma J44.9
bronchiectasis J47.9
with
exacerbation (acute) J47.1
lower respiratory infection J47.0
bronchitis J44.9
with
exacerbation (acute) J44.1
lower respiratory infection J44.0
emphysema J44.9
hypersensitivity pneumonitis J67.9
decompensated J44.1
with
exacerbation (acute) J44.1
polycystic J98.4
congenital Q33.0
rheumatoid (diffuse) (interstitial) —*see* Rheumatoid, lung
Lutembacher's (atrial septal defect with mitral stenosis) Q21.1
Lyme A69.20
lymphatic (gland) (system) (channel) (vessel) I89.9
lymphoproliferative D47.9
specified NEC D47.Z9
T-gamma D47.Z9
X-linked D82.3
Magitot's M27.2
malarial —*see* Malaria
malignant —*see also* Neoplasm, malignant, by site
Manson's B65.1
maple bark J67.6
maple-syrup-urine E71.0
Marburg (virus) A98.3
Marion's (bladder neck obstruction) N32.0
Marsh's (exophthalmic goiter) —*see* Hyperthyroidism, with, goiter (diffuse)
mastoid (process) —*see* Disorder, ear, middle
Mathieu's (leptospiral jaundice) A27.0
Maxcy's A75.2
McArdle (-Schmid-Pearson) (glycogenosis V) E74.04
mediastinum J98.59 ⇐
medullary center (idiopathic) (respiratory) G93.89
Meige's (chronic hereditary edema) Q82.0
meningococcal —*see* Infection, meningococcal
mental F99
organic F09
mesenchymal M35.9
mesenteric embolic —*see also* Ischemia, intestine, acute K55.039 ⇐
metabolic, metabolism E88.9
bilirubin E80.7
metal-polisher's J62.8
metastatic —*see also* Neoplasm, secondary, by site C79.9

Disease, diseased *(Continued)*
microvascular — code to condition
microvillus
atrophy Q43.8
inclusion (MVD) Q43.8
middle ear —*see* Disorder, ear, middle
Mikulicz' (dryness of mouth, absent or decreased lacrimation) K11.8
Milroy's (chronic hereditary edema) Q82.0
Minamata —*see* Poisoning, mercury
minicore G71.2
Minor's G95.19
Minot's (hemorrhagic disease, newborn) P53
Minot-von Willebrand-Jürgens (angiohemophilia) D68.0
Mitchell's (erythromelalgia) I73.81
mitral (valve) I05.9
nonrheumatic I34.9
mixed connective tissue M35.1
moldy hay J67.0
Monge's T70.29
Morgagni-Adams-Stokes (syncope with heart block) I45.9
Morgagni's (syndrome) (hyperostosis frontalis interna) M85.2
Morton's (with metatarsalgia) —*see* Lesion, nerve, plantar
Morvan's G60.8
motor neuron (bulbar) (familial) (mixed type) (spinal) G12.20
amyotrophic lateral sclerosis G12.21
progressive bulbar palsy G12.22
specified NEC G12.29
moyamoya I67.5
mu heavy chain disease C88.2
multicore G71.2
muscle —*see also* Disorder, muscle
inflammatory —*see* Myositis
ocular (external) —*see* Strabismus
musculoskeletal system, soft tissue —*see also* Disorder, soft tissue
specified NEC —*see* Disorder, soft tissue, specified type NEC
mushroom workers' J67.5
mycotic B49
myelodysplastic, not classified C94.6
myeloproliferative, not classified C94.6
chronic D47.1
myocardium, myocardial —*see also* Degeneration, myocardial I51.5
primary (idiopathic) I42.9
myoneural G70.9
Naegeli's D69.1
nails L60.9
specified NEC L60.8
Nairobi (sheep virus) A93.8
nasal J34.9
nemaline body G71.2
nerve —*see* Disorder, nerve
nervous system G98.8
autonomic G90.9
central G96.9
specified NEC G96.8
congenital Q07.9
parasympathetic G90.9
specified NEC G98.8
sympathetic G90.9
vegetative G90.9
neuromuscular system G70.9
Newcastle B30.8
Nicolas (-Durand)-Favre (climatic bubo) A55
nipple N64.9
Paget's C50.01-
female C50.01-
male C50.02-
Nishimoto (-Takeuchi) I67.5
nonarthropod-borne NOS (viral) B34.9
enterovirus NEC B34.1
nonautoimmune hemolytic D59.4
drug-induced D59.2

Disease, diseased *(Continued)*
Nonne-Milroy-Meige (chronic hereditary edema) Q82.0
nose J34.9
nucleus pulposus —*see* Disorder, disc
nutritional E63.9
oast-house-urine E72.19
ocular
herpesviral B00.50
zoster B02.30
obliterative vascular I77.1
Ohara's —*see* Tularemia
Opitz's (congestive splenomegaly) D73.2
Oppenheim-Urbach (necrobiosis lipoidica diabeticorum) —*see* E08-E13 with .620
optic nerve NEC —*see* Disorder, nerve, optic
orbit —*see* Disorder, orbit
Oriental liver fluke B66.1
Oriental lung fluke B66.4
Ormond's N13.5
Oropouche virus A93.0
Osler-Rendu (familial hemorrhagic telangiectasia) I78.0
osteofibrocystic E21.0
Otto's M24.7
outer ear —*see* Disorder, ear, external
ovary (noninflammatory) N83.9
cystic N83.20- ⇐
inflammatory —*see* Salpingo-oophoritis
polycystic E28.2
specified NEC N83.8
Owren's (congenital) —*see* Defect, coagulation
pancreas K86.9
cystic K86.2
fibrocystic E84.9
specified NEC K86.89 ⇐
panvalvular I08.9
specified NEC I08.8
parametrium (noninflammatory) N83.9
parasitic B89
cerebral NEC B71.9 *[G94]*
intestinal NOS B82.9
mouth B37.0
skin NOS B88.9
specified type —*see* Infestation
tongue B37.0
parathyroid (gland) E21.5
specified NEC E21.4
Parkinson's G20
parodontal K05.6
Parrot's (syphilitic osteochondritis) A50.02
Parry's (exophthalmic goiter) —*see* Hyperthyroidism, with, goiter (diffuse)
Parson's (exophthalmic goiter) —*see* Hyperthyroidism, with, goiter (diffuse)
Paxton's (white piedra) B36.2
pearl-worker's —*see* Osteomyelitis, specified type NEC
Pellegrini-Stieda (calcification, knee joint) —*see* Bursitis, tibial collateral
pelvis, pelvic
female NOS N94.9
specified NEC N94.89
gonococcal (acute) (chronic) A54.24
inflammatory (female) N73.9
acute N73.0
chlamydial A56.11 ◀
chronic N73.1
specified NEC N73.8
syphilitic (secondary) A51.42
late A52.76
tuberculous A18.17
organ, female N94.9
peritoneum, female NEC N94.89
penis N48.9
inflammatory N48.29
abscess N48.21
cellulitis N48.22
specified NEC N48.89

◀ New ⇐ Revised ~~deleted~~ Deleted

Disease, diseased *(Continued)*
periapical tissues NOS K04.90
periodontal K05.6
specified NEC K05.5
periosteum —*see* Disorder, bone, specified type NEC
peripheral
arterial I73.9
autonomic nervous system G90.9
nerves —*see* Polyneuropathy
vascular NOS I73.9
peritoneum K66.9
pelvic, female NEC N94.89
specified NEC K66.8
persistent mucosal (middle ear) H66.20
left H66.22
with right H66.23
right H66.21
with left H66.23
Petit's —*see* Hernia, abdomen, specified site NEC
pharynx J39.2
specified NEC J39.2
Phocas' —*see* Mastopathy, cystic
photochromogenic (acid-fast bacilli) (pulmonary) A31.0
nonpulmonary A31.9
Pick's G31.01 *[F02.80]*
with behavioral disturbance G31.01 *[F02.81]*
brain G31.01 *[F02.80]* ◀
with behavioral disturbance G31.01 *[F02.81]* ◀
of pericardium (pericardial pseudocirrhosis of liver) I31.1 ◀
pigeon fancier's J67.2
pineal gland E34.8
pink —*see* Poisoning, mercury
Pinkus' (lichen nitidus) L44.1
pinworm B80
Piry virus A93.8
pituitary (gland) E23.7
pituitary-snuff-taker's J67.8
pleura (cavity) J94.9
specified NEC J94.8
pneumatic drill (hammer) T75.21
Pollitzer's (hidradenitis suppurativa) L73.2
polycystic
kidney or renal Q61.3
adult type Q61.2
childhood type NEC Q61.19
collecting duct dilatation Q61.11
liver or hepatic Q44.6
lung or pulmonary J98.4
congenital Q33.0
ovary, ovaries E28.2
spleen Q89.09
polyethylene T84.05-
Pompe's (glycogenosis II) E74.02
Posadas-Wernicke B38.9
Potain's (pulmonary edema) —*see* Edema, lung
prepuce N47.8
inflammatory N47.7
balanoposthitis N47.6
Pringle's (tuberous sclerosis) Q85.1
prion, central nervous system A81.9
specified NEC A81.89
prostate N42.9
specified NEC N42.89
protozoal B64
acanthamebiasis —*see* Acanthamebiasis
African trypanosomiasis —*see* African trypanosomiasis
babesiosis B60.0
Chagas disease —*see* Chagas disease
intestine, intestinal A07.9
leishmaniasis —*see* Leishmaniasis
malaria —*see* Malaria
naegleriasis B60.2

Disease, diseased *(Continued)*
protozoal *(Continued)*
pneumocystosis B59
specified organism NEC B60.8
toxoplasmosis —*see* Toxoplasmosis
pseudo-Hurler's E77.0
psychiatric F99
psychotic —*see* Psychosis
Puente's (simple glandular cheilitis) K13.0
puerperal —*see also* Puerperal O90.89
pulmonary —*see also* Disease, lung
artery I28.9
chronic obstructive J44.9
with
acute bronchitis J44.0
exacerbation (acute) J44.1
lower respiratory infection (acute) J44.0
decompensated J44.1
with
exacerbation (acute) J44.1
heart I27.9
specified NEC I27.89
hypertensive (vascular) I27.0
valve I37.9
rheumatic I09.89
pulp (dental) NOS K04.90
pulseless M31.4
Putnam's (subacute combined sclerosis with pernicious anemia) D51.0
Pyle (-Cohn) (metaphyseal dysplasia) Q78.5 ⇐
ragpicker's or ragsorter's A22.1
Raynaud's —*see* Raynaud's disease
reactive airway —*see* Asthma
Reclus' (cystic) —*see* Mastopathy, cystic
rectum K62.9
specified NEC K62.89
Refsum's (heredopathia atactica polyneuritiformis) G60.1
renal (functional) (pelvis) —*see also* Disease, kidney N28.9
with
edema —*see* Nephrosis
glomerular lesion —*see* Glomerulonephritis
with edema —*see* Nephrosis
interstitial nephritis N12
acute N28.9
chronic —*see also* Disease, kidney, chronic N18.9
cystic, congenital Q61.9
diabetic —*see* E08-E13 with .22
end-stage (failure) N18.6
due to hypertension I12.0
fibrocystic (congenital) Q61.8
hypertensive —*see* Hypertension, kidney
lupus M32.14
phosphate-losing (tubular) N25.0
polycystic (congenital) Q61.3
adult type Q61.2
childhood type NEC Q61.19
collecting duct dilatation Q61.11
rapidly progressive N01.9
subacute N01.9
Rendu-Osler-Weber (familial hemorrhagic telangiectasia) I78.0
renovascular (arteriosclerotic) —*see* Hypertension, kidney
respiratory (tract) J98.9
acute or subacute NOS J06.9
due to
chemicals, gases, fumes or vapors (inhalation) J68.3
external agent J70.9
specified NEC J70.8
radiation J70.0
smoke inhalation J70.5
noninfectious J39.8

Disease, diseased *(Continued)*
respiratory *(Continued)*
chronic NOS J98.9
due to
chemicals, gases, fumes or vapors J68.4
external agent J70.9
specified NEC J70.8
radiation J70.1
newborn P27.9
specified NEC P27.8
due to
chemicals, gases, fumes or vapors J68.9
acute or subacute NEC J68.3
chronic J68.4
external agent J70.9
specified NEC J70.8
newborn P28.9
specified type NEC P28.89
upper J39.9
acute or subacute J06.9
noninfectious NEC J39.8
specified NEC J39.8
streptococcal J06.9
retina, retinal H35.9
Batten's or Batten-Mayou E75.4 *[H36]*
specified NEC H35.89
rheumatoid —*see* Arthritis, rheumatoid
rickettsial NOS A79.9
specified type NEC A79.89
Riga (-Fede) (cachectic aphthae) K14.0
Riggs' (compound periodontitis) —*see* Periodontitis
Ritter's L00
Rivalta's (cervicofacial actinomycosis) A42.2
Robles' (onchocerciasis) B73.01
Roger's (congenital interventricular septal defect) Q21.0
Rosenthal's (factor XI deficiency) D68.1
Ross River B33.1
Rossbach's (hyperchlorhydria) K30
Rotes Quérol —*see* Hyperostosis, ankylosing
Roth (-Bernhardt) —*see* Mononeuropathy, lower limb, meralgia paresthetica
Runeberg's (progressive pernicious anemia) D51.0
sacroiliac NEC M53.3
salivary gland or duct K11.9
inclusion B25.9
specified NEC K11.8
virus B25.9
sandworm B76.9
Schimmelbusch's —*see* Mastopathy, cystic
Schmorl's —*see* Schmorl's disease or nodes
Schönlein (-Henoch) (purpura rheumatica) D69.0
Schottmüller's —*see* Fever, paratyphoid
Schultz's (agranulocytosis) —*see* Agranulocytosis
Schwalbe-Ziehen-Oppenheim G24.1
Schwartz-Jampel G71.13
sclera H15.9
specified NEC H15.89
scrofulous (tuberculous) A18.2
scrotum N50.9
sebaceous glands L73.9
semilunar cartilage, cystic —*see also* Derangement, knee, meniscus, cystic
seminal vesicle N50.9
serum NEC —*see also* Reaction, serum T80.69
sexually transmitted A64
anogenital
herpesviral infection —*see* Herpes, anogenital
warts A63.0
chancroid A57
chlamydial infection —*see* Chlamydia
gonorrhea —*see* Gonorrhea
granuloma inguinale A58
specified organism NEC A63.8

◀ New ⇐ Revised ~~deleted~~ Deleted

Disease, diseased *(Continued)*
sexually transmitted *(Continued)*
syphilis —*see* Syphilis
trichomoniasis —*see* Trichomoniasis
Sézary C84.1-
shimamushi (scrub typhus) A75.3
shipyard B30.0
sickle-cell D57.1
with crisis (vasoocclusive pain) D57.00
with
acute chest syndrome D57.01
splenic sequestration D57.02
elliptocytosis D57.8-
Hb-C D57.20
with crisis (vasoocclusive pain) D57.219
with
acute chest syndrome D57.211
splenic sequestration D57.212
without crisis D57.20
Hb-SD D57.80
with crisis D57.819
with
acute chest syndrome D57.811
splenic sequestration D57.812
Hb-SE D57.80
with crisis D57.819
with
acute chest syndrome D57.811
splenic sequestration D57.812
specified NEC D57.80
with crisis D57.819
with
acute chest syndrome D57.811
splenic sequestration D57.812
spherocytosis D57.80
with crisis D57.819
with
acute chest syndrome D57.811
splenic sequestration D57.812
thalassemia D57.40
with crisis (vasoocclusive pain) D57.419
with
acute chest syndrome D57.411
splenic sequestration D57.412
without crisis D57.40
silo-filler's J68.8
bronchitis J68.0
pneumonitis J68.0
pulmonary edema J68.1
simian B B00.4
Simons' (progressive lipodystrophy) E88.1
sin nombre virus B33.4
sinus —*see* Sinusitis
Sirkari's B55.0
sixth B08.20
due to human herpesvirus 6 B08.21
due to human herpesvirus 7 B08.22
skin L98.9
due to metabolic disorder NEC E88.9 *[L99]*
specified NEC L98.8
slim (HIV) B20
small vessel I73.9
Sneddon-Wilkinson (subcorneal pustular dermatosis) L13.1
South African creeping B88.0
spinal (cord) G95.9
congenital Q06.9
specified NEC G95.89
spine —*see also* Spondylopathy
joint —*see* Dorsopathy
tuberculous A18.01
spinocerebellar (hereditary) G11.9
specified NEC G11.8
spleen D73.9
amyloid E85.4 *[D77]*
organic D73.9
polycystic Q89.09
postinfectional D73.89
sponge-diver's —*see* Toxicity, venom, marine animal, sea anemone

Disease, diseased *(Continued)*
Startle Q89.8
Steinert's G71.11
Sticker's (erythema infectiosum) B08.3
Stieda's (calcification, knee joint) —*see* Bursitis, tibial collateral
Stokes' (exophthalmic goiter) —*see* Hyperthyroidism, with, goiter (diffuse)
Stokes-Adams (syncope with heart block) I45.9
stomach K31.9
functional, psychogenic F45.8
specified NEC K31.89
stonemason's J62.8
storage
glycogen —*see* Disease, glycogen storage
mucopolysaccharide —*see* Mucopolysaccharidosis
striatopallidal system NEC G25.89
Stuart-Prower (congenital factor X deficiency) D68.2
Stuart's (congenital factor X deficiency) D68.2
subcutaneous tissue —*see* Disease, skin
supporting structures of teeth K08.9
specified NEC K08.89 ◀
suprarenal (capsule) (gland) E27.9
hyperfunction E27.0
specified NEC E27.8
sweat glands L74.9
specified NEC L74.8
Sweeley-Klionsky E75.21
Swift (-Feer) —*see* Poisoning, mercury
swimming-pool granuloma A31.1
Sylvest's (epidemic pleurodynia) B33.0
sympathetic nervous system G90.9
synovium —*see* Disorder, synovium
syphilitic —*see* Syphilis
systemic tissue mast cell C96.2
tanapox (virus) B08.71
Tangier E78.6
Tarral-Besnier (pityriasis rubra pilaris) L44.0
Tauri's E74.09
tear duct —*see* Disorder, lacrimal system
tendon, tendinous —*see also* Disorder, tendon
nodular —*see* Trigger finger
terminal vessel I73.9
testis N50.9
thalassemia Hb-S —*see* Disease, sickle-cell, thalassemia
Thaysen-Gee (nontropical sprue) K90.0
Thomsen G71.12
throat J39.2
septic J02.0
thromboembolic —*see* Embolism
thymus (gland) E32.9
specified NEC E32.8
thyroid (gland) E07.9
heart —*see also* Hyperthyroidism E05.90 *[I43]*
with thyroid storm E05.91 *[I43]*
specified NEC E07.8
Tietze's M94.0
tongue K14.9
specified NEC K14.89
tonsils, tonsillar (and adenoids) J35.9
tooth, teeth K08.9
hard tissues K03.9
specified NEC K03.89
pulp NEC K04.99
specified NEC K08.89 ◀
Tourette's F95.2
trachea NEC J39.8
tricuspid I07.9
nonrheumatic I36.9
triglyceride-storage E75.5
trophoblastic —*see* Mole, hydatidiform
tsutsugamushi A75.3
tube (fallopian) (noninflammatory) N83.9
inflammatory —*see* Salpingitis
specified NEC N83.8
tuberculous NEC —*see* Tuberculosis

Disease, diseased *(Continued)*
tubo-ovarian (noninflammatory) N83.9
inflammatory —*see* Salpingo-oophoritis
specified NEC N83.8
tubotympanic, chronic —*see* Otitis, media, suppurative, chronic, tubotympanic
tubulo-interstitial N15.9
specified NEC N15.8
tympanum —*see* Disorder, tympanic membrane
Uhl's Q24.8
Underwood's (sclerema neonatorum) P83.0
Unverricht (-Lundborg) —*see* Epilepsy, generalized, idiopathic
Urbach-Oppenheim (necrobiosis lipoidica diabeticorum) —*see* E08-E13 with .620
ureter N28.9
in (due to)
schistosomiasis (bilharziasis) B65.0 *[N29]*
urethra N36.9
specified NEC N36.8
urinary (tract) N39.9
bladder N32.9
specified NEC N32.89
specified NEC N39.8
uterus (noninflammatory) N85.9
infective —*see* Endometritis
inflammatory —*see* Endometritis
specified NEC N85.8
uveal tract (anterior) H21.9
posterior H31.9
vagabond's B85.1
vagina, vaginal (noninflammatory) N89.9
inflammatory NEC N76.89
specified NEC N89.8
valve, valvular I38
multiple I08.9
specified NEC I08.8
van Creveld-von Gierke (glycogenosis I) E74.01
vas deferens N50.9
vascular I99.9
arteriosclerotic —*see* Arteriosclerosis
ciliary body NEC —*see* Disorder, iris, vascular
hypertensive —*see* Hypertension
iris NEC —*see* Disorder, iris, vascular
obliterative I77.1
peripheral I73.9
occlusive I99.8
peripheral (occlusive) I73.9
in diabetes mellitus —*see* E08-E13 with .51
vasomotor I73.9
vasospastic I73.9
vein I87.9
venereal —*see also* Disease, sexually transmitted A64
chlamydial NEC A56.8
anus A56.3
genitourinary NOS A56.2
pharynx A56.4
rectum A56.3
fifth A55
sixth A55
specified nature or type NEC A63.8
vertebra, vertebral —*see also* Spondylopathy
disc —*see* Disorder, disc
vibration —*see* Vibration, adverse effects
viral, virus —*see also* Disease, by type of virus B34.9
arbovirus NOS A94
arthropod-borne NOS A94
congenital P35.9
specified NEC P35.8
Hanta (with renal manifestations) (Dobrava) (Puumala) (Seoul) A98.5
with pulmonary manifestations (Andes) (Bayou) (Bermejo) (Black Creek Canal) (Choclo) (Juquitiba) (Laguna negra) (Lechiguanas) (New York) (Oran) (Sin nombre) B33.4

Disease, diseased *(Continued)*
viral, virus *(Continued)*
Hantaan (Korean hemorrhagic fever) A98.5
human immunodeficiency (HIV) B20
Kunjin A83.4
nonarthropod-borne NOS B34.9
Powassan A84.8
Rocio (encephalitis) A83.6
Sin nombre (Hantavirus) (cardio)-pulmonary syndrome B33.4
Tahyna B33.8
vesicular stomatitis A93.8
vitreous H43.9
specified NEC H43.89
vocal cord J38.3
Volkmann's, acquired T79.6
von Eulenburg's (congenital paramyotonia) G71.19
von Gierke's (glycogenosis I) E74.01
von Graefe's —*see* Strabismus, paralytic, ophthalmoplegia, progressive
von Willebrand (-Jürgens) (angiohemophilia) D68.0
Vrolik's (osteogenesis imperfecta) Q78.0
vulva (noninflammatory) N90.9
inflammatory NEC N76.89
specified NEC N90.89
Wallgren's (obstruction of splenic vein with collateral circulation) I87.8
Wassilieff's (leptospiral jaundice) A27.0
wasting NEC R64
due to malnutrition E41
Waterhouse-Friderichsen A39.1
Wegner's (syphilitic osteochondritis) A50.02
Weil's (leptospiral jaundice of lung) A27.0
Weir Mitchell's (erythromelalgia) I73.81
Werdnig-Hoffmann G12.0
Wermer's E31.21
Werner-His (trench fever) A79.0
Werner-Schultz (neutropenic splenomegaly) D73.81
Wernicke-Posadas B38.9
whipworm B79
white blood cells D72.9
specified NEC D72.89
white matter R90.82
white-spot, meaning lichen sclerosus et atrophicus L90.0
penis N48.0
vulva N90.4
Wilkie's K55.1
Wilkinson-Sneddon (subcorneal pustular dermatosis) L13.1
Willis' —*see* Diabetes
Wilson's (hepatolenticular degeneration) E83.01
woolsorter's A22.1
yaba monkey tumor B08.72
yaba pox (virus) B08.72
Zika virus A92.5 ◀
zoonotic, bacterial A28.9
specified type NEC A28.8
Disfigurement (due to scar) L90.5
Disgerminoma —*see* Dysgerminoma
DISH (diffuse idiopathic skeletal hyperostosis) —*see* Hyperostosis, ankylosing
Disinsertion, retina —*see* Detachment, retina
Dislocatable hip, congenital Q65.6
Dislocation (articular)
with fracture —*see* Fracture
acromioclavicular (joint) S43.10-
with displacement
100%-200% S43.12-
more than 200% S43.13-
inferior S43.14-
posterior S43.15-
ankle S93.0-
astragalus —*see* Dislocation, ankle
atlantoaxial S13.121
atlantooccipital S13.111

Dislocation *(Continued)*
atloidooccipital S13.111
breast bone S23.29
capsule, joint code by site under Dislocation
carpal (bone) —*see* Dislocation, wrist
carpometacarpal (joint) NEC S63.05-
thumb S63.04-
cartilage (joint) - code by site under Dislocation
cervical spine (vertebra) —*see* Dislocation, vertebra, cervical
chronic —*see* Dislocation, recurrent
clavicle —*see* Dislocation, acromioclavicular joint
coccyx S33.2
congenital NEC Q68.8
coracoid —*see* Dislocation, shoulder
costal cartilage S23.29
costochondral S23.29
cricoarytenoid articulation S13.29
cricothyroid articulation S13.29
dorsal vertebra —*see* Dislocation, vertebra, thoracic
ear ossicle —*see* Discontinuity, ossicles, ear
elbow S53.10-
congenital Q68.8
pathological —*see* Dislocation, pathological NEC, elbow
radial head alone —*see* Dislocation, radial head
recurrent —*see* Dislocation, recurrent, elbow
traumatic S53.10-
anterior S53.11-
lateral S53.14-
medial S53.13-
posterior S53.12-
specified type NEC S53.19-
eye, nontraumatic —*see* Luxation, globe
eyeball, nontraumatic —*see* Luxation, globe
femur
distal end —*see* Dislocation, knee
proximal end —*see* Dislocation, hip
fibula
distal end —*see* Dislocation, ankle
proximal end —*see* Dislocation, knee
finger S63.25-
index S63.25-
interphalangeal S63.27-
distal S63.29-
index S63.29-
little S63.29-
middle S63.29-
ring S63.29-
index S63.27-
little S63.27-
middle S63.27-
proximal S63.28-
index S63.28-
little S63.28-
middle S63.28-
ring S63.28-
ring S63.27-
little S63.25-
metacarpophalangeal S63.26-
index S63.26-
little S63.26-
middle S63.26-
ring S63.26-
middle S63.25-
recurrent —*see* Dislocation, recurrent, finger
ring S63.25-
thumb —*see* Dislocation, thumb
foot S93.30-
recurrent —*see* Dislocation, recurrent, foot
specified site NEC S93.33-
tarsal joint S93.31-
tarsometatarsal joint S93.32-
toe —*see* Dislocation, toe

Dislocation *(Continued)*
fracture —*see* Fracture
glenohumeral (joint) —*see* Dislocation, shoulder
glenoid —*see* Dislocation, shoulder
habitual —*see* Dislocation, recurrent
hip S73.00-
anterior S73.03-
obturator S73.02-
central S73.04-
congenital (total) Q65.2
bilateral Q65.1
partial Q65.5
bilateral Q65.4
unilateral Q65.3-
unilateral Q65.0-
developmental M24.85-
pathological —*see* Dislocation, pathological NEC, hip
posterior S73.01-
recurrent —*see* Dislocation, recurrent, hip
humerus, proximal end —*see* Dislocation, shoulder
incomplete —*see* Subluxation, by site
incus —*see* Discontinuity, ossicles, ear
infracoracoid —*see* Dislocation, shoulder
innominate (pubic junction) (sacral junction) S33.39
acetabulum —*see* Dislocation, hip
interphalangeal (joint (s))
finger S63.279
distal S63.29-
index S63.29-
little S63.29-
middle S63.29-
ring S63.29-
index S63.27-
little S63.27-
middle S63.27-
proximal S63.28-
index S63.28-
little S63.28-
middle S63.28-
ring S63.28-
ring S63.27-
foot or toe —*see* Dislocation, toe
thumb S63.12-
distal joint S63.14-
proximal joint S63.13-
jaw (cartilage) (meniscus) S03.0- ⇐
joint prosthesis —*see* Complications, joint prosthesis, mechanical, displacement, by site
knee S83.106
cap —*see* Dislocation, patella
congenital Q68.2
old M23.8X-
patella —*see* Dislocation, patella
pathological —*see* Dislocation, pathological NEC, knee
proximal tibia
anteriorly S83.11-
laterally S83.14-
medially S83.13-
posteriorly S83.12-
recurrent —*see also* Derangement, knee, specified NEC
specified type NEC S83.19-
lacrimal gland H04.16-
lens (complete) H27.10-
anterior H27.12-
congenital Q12.1
ocular implant —*see* Complications, intraocular lens
partial H27.11-
posterior H27.13-
traumatic S05.8X-
ligament code by site under Dislocation
lumbar (vertebra) —*see* Dislocation, vertebra, lumbar

◀ New ⇐ Revised ~~deleted~~ Deleted

Dislocation *(Continued)*
lumbosacral (vertebra) —*see also* Dislocation, vertebra, lumbar
congenital Q76.49
mandible S03.0- ◄
meniscus (knee) —*see* Tear, meniscus
other sites code by site under Dislocation
metacarpal (bone)
distal end —*see* Dislocation, finger
proximal end S63.06-
metacarpophalangeal (joint)
finger S63.26-
index S63.26-
little S63.26-
middle S63.26-
ring S63.26-
thumb S63.11-
metatarsal (bone) —*see* Dislocation, foot
metatarsophalangeal (joint (s)) —*see* Dislocation, toe
midcarpal (joint) S63.03-
midtarsal (joint) —*see* Dislocation, foot
neck S13.20
specified site NEC S13.29
vertebra —*see* Dislocation, vertebra, cervical
nose (septal cartilage) S03.1
occipitoatloid S13.111
old —*see* Derangement, joint, specified type NEC
ossicles, ear —*see* Discontinuity, ossicles, ear
partial —*see* Subluxation, by site
patella S83.006
congenital Q74.1
lateral S83.01-
recurrent (nontraumatic) M22.0-
incomplete M22.1-
specified type NEC S83.09-
pathological NEC M24.30
ankle M24.37-
elbow M24.32-
foot joint M24.37-
hand joint M24.34-
hip M24.35-
knee M24.36-
lumbosacral joint —*see* subcategory M53.2
pelvic region —*see* Dislocation, pathological, hip
sacroiliac —*see* subcategory M53.2
shoulder M24.31-
wrist M24.33-
pelvis NEC S33.30
specified NEC S33.39
phalanx
finger or hand —*see* Dislocation, finger
foot or toe —*see* Dislocation, toe
prosthesis, internal —*see* Complications, prosthetic device, by site, mechanical
radial head S53.006
anterior S53.01-
posterior S53.02-
specified type NEC S53.09-
radiocarpal (joint) S63.02-
radiohumeral (joint) —*see* Dislocation, radial head
radioulnar (joint)
distal S63.01-
proximal —*see* Dislocation, elbow
radius
distal end —*see* Dislocation, wrist
proximal end —*see* Dislocation, radial head
recurrent M24.40
ankle M24.47-
elbow M24.42-
finger M24.44-
foot joint M24.47-
hand joint M24.44-
hip M24.45-
knee M24.46-
patella —*see* Dislocation, patella, recurrent

Dislocation *(Continued)*
recurrent *(Continued)*
patella —*see* Dislocation, patella, recurrent
sacroiliac —*see* subcategory M53.2
shoulder M24.41-
toe M24.47-
vertebra —*see also* subcategory M43.5
atlantoaxial M43.4
with myelopathy M43.3
wrist M24.43-
rib (cartilage) S23.29
sacrococcygeal S33.2
sacroiliac (joint) (ligament) S33.2
congenital Q74.2
recurrent —*see* subcategory M53.2
sacrum S33.2
scaphoid (bone) (hand) (wrist) —*see* Dislocation, wrist
foot —*see* Dislocation, foot
scapula —*see* Dislocation, shoulder, girdle, scapula
semilunar cartilage, knee —*see* Tear, meniscus
septal cartilage (nose) S03.1
septum (nasal) (old) J34.2
sesamoid bone code by site under Dislocation
shoulder (blade) (ligament) (joint) (traumatic) S43.006
acromioclavicular —*see* Dislocation, acromioclavicular
chronic —*see* Dislocation, recurrent, shoulder
congenital Q68.8
girdle S43.30-
scapula S43.31-
specified site NEC S43.39-
humerus S43.00-
anterior S43.01-
inferior S43.03-
posterior S43.02-
pathological —*see* Dislocation, pathological NEC, shoulder
recurrent —*see* Dislocation, recurrent, shoulder
specified type NEC S43.08-
spine
cervical —*see* Dislocation, vertebra, cervical
congenital Q76.49
due to birth trauma P11.5
lumbar —*see* Dislocation, vertebra, lumbar
thoracic —*see* Dislocation, vertebra, thoracic
spontaneous —*see* Dislocation, pathological
sternoclavicular (joint) S43.206
anterior S43.21-
posterior S43.22-
sternum S23.29
subglenoid —*see* Dislocation, shoulder
symphysis pubis S33.4
talus —*see* Dislocation, ankle
tarsal (bone (s)) (joint (s)) —*see* Dislocation, foot
tarsometatarsal (joint (s)) —*see* Dislocation, foot
temporomandibular (joint) S03.0- ◄
thigh, proximal end —*see* Dislocation, hip
thorax S23.20
specified site NEC S23.29
vertebra —*see* Dislocation, vertebra
thumb S63.10-
interphalangeal joint —*see* Dislocation, interphalangeal (joint), thumb
metacarpophalangeal joint —*see* Dislocation, metacarpophalangeal (joint), thumb
thyroid cartilage S13.29
tibia
distal end —*see* Dislocation, ankle
proximal end —*see* Dislocation, knee
tibiofibular (joint)
distal —*see* Dislocation, ankle
superior —*see* Dislocation, knee

Dislocation *(Continued)*
toe (s) S93.106
great S93.10-
interphalangeal joint S93.11-
metatarsophalangeal joint S93.12-
interphalangeal joint S93.119
lesser S93.106
interphalangeal joint S93.11-
metatarsophalangeal joint S93.12-
metatarsophalangeal joint S93.12-
tooth S03.2
trachea S23.29
ulna
distal end S63.07-
proximal end —*see* Dislocation, elbow
ulnohumeral (joint) —*see* Dislocation, elbow
vertebra (articular process) (body) (traumatic)
cervical S13.101
atlantoaxial joint S13.121
atlantooccipital joint S13.111
atloidooccipital joint S13.111
joint between
C0 and C1 S13.111
C1 and C2 S13.121
C2 and C3 S13.131
C3 and C4 S13.141
C4 and C5 S13.151
C5 and C6 S13.161
C6 and C7 S13.171
C7 and T1 S13.181
occipitoatloid joint S13.111
congenital Q76.49
lumbar S33.101
joint between
L1 and L2 S33.111
L2 and L3 S33.121
L3 and L4 S33.131
L4 and L5 S33.141
nontraumatic —*see* Displacement, intervertebral disc
partial —*see* Subluxation, by site
recurrent NEC —*see* subcategory M43.5
thoracic S23.101
joint between
T1 and T2 S23.111
T2 and T3 S23.121
T3 and T4 S23.123
T4 and T5 S23.131
T5 and T6 S23.133
T6 and T7 S23.141
T7 and T8 S23.143
T8 and T9 S23.151
T9 and T10 S23.153
T10 and T11 S23.161
T11 and T12 S23.163
T12 and L1 S23.171
wrist (carpal bone) S63.006
carpometacarpal joint —*see* Dislocation, carpometacarpal (joint)
distal radioulnar joint —*see* Dislocation, radioulnar (joint), distal
metacarpal bone, proximal —*see* Dislocation, metacarpal (bone), proximal end
midcarpal —*see* Dislocation, midcarpal (joint)
radiocarpal joint —*see* Dislocation, radiocarpal (joint)
recurrent —*see* Dislocation, recurrent, wrist
specified site NEC S63.09-
ulna —*see* Dislocation, ulna, distal end
xiphoid cartilage S23.29
Disorder (of) —*see also* Disease
acantholytic L11.9
specified NEC L11.8
acute
psychotic —*see* Psychosis, acute
stress F43.0

Disorder *(Continued)*
adjustment (grief) F43.20
with
anxiety F43.22
with depressed mood F43.23
conduct disturbance F43.24
with emotional disturbance F43.25
depressed mood F43.21
with anxiety F43.23
other specified symptom F43.29
adrenal (capsule) (gland) (medullary) E27.9
specified NEC E27.8
adrenogenital E25.9
drug-induced E25.8
iatrogenic E25.8
idiopathic E25.8
adult personality (and behavior) F69
specified NEC F68.8
affective (mood) —*see* Disorder, mood
aggressive, unsocialized F91.1
alcohol-related F10.99
with
amnestic disorder, persisting F10.96
anxiety disorder F10.980
dementia, persisting F10.97
intoxication F10.929
with delirium F10.921
uncomplicated F10.920
mood disorder F10.94
other specified F10.988
psychotic disorder F10.959
with
delusions F10.950
hallucinations F10.951
sexual dysfunction F10.981
sleep disorder F10.982
alcohol use ◀
mild F10.10 ◀
with ◀
alcohol-induced ◀
anxiety disorder F10.180 ◀
bipolar and related disorder F10.14 ◀
depressive disorder F10.14 ◀
psychotic disorder F10.159 ◀
sexual dysfunction F10.181 ◀
sleep disorder F10.182 ◀
alcohol intoxication F10.129 ◀
delirium F10.121 ◀
moderate or severe F10.20 ◀
with ◀
alcohol-induced ◀
anxiety disorder F10.280 ◀
bipolar and related disorder F10.24 ◀
depressive disorder F10.24 ◀
major neurocognitive disorder, amnestic-confabulatory type F10.26 ◀
major neurocognitive disorder, nonamnestic-confabulatory type F10.27 ◀
mild neurocognitive disorder F10.288 ◀
psychotic disorder F10.259 ◀
sexual dysfunction F10.281 ◀
sleep disorder F10.282 ◀
alcohol intoxication F10.229 ◀
delirium F10.221 ◀
allergic —*see* Allergy
alveolar NEC J84.09
amino-acid
cystathioninuria E72.19
cystinosis E72.04
cystinuria E72.01
glycinuria E72.09
homocystinuria E72.11
metabolism —*see* Disturbance, metabolism, amino-acid
specified NEC E72.8
neonatal, transitory P74.8

Disorder *(Continued)*
amino-acid *(Continued)*
renal transport NEC E72.09
transport NEC E72.09
amnesic, amnestic
alcohol-induced F10.96
with dependence F10.26
due to (secondary to) general medical condition F04
psychoactive NEC-induced F19.96
with
abuse F19.16
dependence F19.26
sedative, hypnotic or anxiolytic-induced F13.96
with dependence F13.26
amphetamine-type substance use ◀
mild F15.10 ◀
moderate F15.20 ◀
severe F15.20 ◀
amphetamine (or other stimulant) use ◀
mild ◀
with ◀
amphetamine (or other stimulant) -induced ◀
anxiety disorder F15.180 ◀
bipolar and related disorder F15.14 ◀
depressive disorder F15.14 ◀
obsessive-compulsive and related disorder F15.188 ◀
psychotic disorder F15.159 ◀
sexual dysfunction F15.181 ◀
amphetamine, cocaine, or other stimulant intoxication ◀
with perceptual disturbances F15.122 ◀
without perceptual disturbances F15.129 ◀
intoxication delirium F15.121 ◀
moderate or severe ◀
with ◀
amphetamine (or other stimulant) -induced ◀
anxiety disorder F15.280 ◀
obsessive-compulsive and related disorder F15.288 ◀
sexual dysfunction F15.281 ◀
bipolar and related disorder F15.24 ◀
depressive disorder F15.24 ◀
psychotic disorder F15.259 ◀
amphetamine, cocaine, or other stimulant intoxication ◀
with perceptual disturbances F15.222 ◀
without perceptual disturbances F15.229 ◀
intoxication delirium F15.221 ◀
anaerobic glycolysis with anemia D55.2
anxiety F41.9
due to (secondary to)
alcohol F10.980
amphetamine F15.980
in
abuse F15.180
dependence F15.280
anxiolytic F13.980
in
abuse F13.180
dependence F13.280
caffeine F15.980
in
abuse F15.180
dependence F15.280
cannabis F12.980
in
abuse F12.180
dependence F12.280

Disorder *(Continued)*
anxiety *(Continued)*
due to *(Continued)*
cocaine F14.980
in
abuse F14.180
dependence F14.180
general medical condition F06.4
hallucinogen F16.980
in
abuse F16.180
dependence F16.280
hypnotic F13.980
in
abuse F13.180
dependence F13.280
inhalant F18.980
in
abuse F18.180
dependence F18.280
phencyclidine F16.980
in
abuse F16.180
dependence F16.280
psychoactive substance NEC F19.980
in
abuse F19.180
dependence F19.280
sedative F13.980
in
abuse F13.180
dependence F13.280
volatile solvents F18.980
in
abuse F18.180
dependence F18.280
generalized F41.1
illness F45.21 ◀
mixed
with depression (mild) F41.8
specified NEC F41.3
organic F06.4
phobic F40.9
of childhood F40.8
specified NEC F41.8
aortic valve —*see* Endocarditis, aortic
aromatic amino-acid metabolism E70.9
specified NEC E70.8
arteriole NEC I77.89
artery NEC I77.89
articulation —*see* Disorder, joint
attachment (childhood)
disinhibited F94.2
reactive F94.1
attention-deficit hyperactivity (adolescent) (adult) (child) F98.8 ◀
combined type F90.2
hyperactive type F90.1
inattentive type F90.0
specified type NEC F90.8
attention-deficit without hyperactivity (adolescent) (adult) (child) F90.0
auditory processing (central) H93.25
autism spectrum F84.0 ◀
autistic F84.0
autonomic nervous system G90.9
specified NEC G90.8
~~avoidant, child or adolescent F40.10~~
avoidant ◀
child or adolescent F40.10 ◀
restrictive food intake F50.89 ◀
balance
acid-base E87.8
mixed E87.4
electrolyte E87.8
fluid NEC E87.8
behavioral (disruptive) —*see* Disorder, conduct
beta-amino-acid metabolism E72.8
bile acid and cholesterol metabolism E78.70
Barth syndrome E78.71
other specified E78.79
Smith-Lemli-Opitz syndrome E78.72

◀ New ◀ Revised ~~deleted~~ Deleted

Disorder *(Continued)*
bilirubin excretion E80.6
binge eating F50.81 ◀
binocular
movement H51.9
convergence
excess H51.12
insufficiency H51.11
internuclear ophthalmoplegia —*see* Ophthalmoplegia, internuclear
palsy of conjugate gaze H51.0
specified type NEC H51.8
vision NEC —*see* Disorder, vision, binocular
bipolar (I) F31.9
current episode
depressed F31.9
with psychotic features F31.5
without psychotic features F31.30
mild F31.31
moderate F31.32
severe (without psychotic features) F31.4
with psychotic features F31.5
hypomanic F31.0
manic F31.9
with psychotic features F31.2
without psychotic features F31.10
mild F31.11
moderate F31.12
severe (without psychotic features) F31.13
with psychotic features F31.2
mixed F31.60
mild F31.61
moderate F31.62
severe (without psychotic features) F31.63
with psychotic features F31.64
severe depression (without psychotic features) F31.4
with psychotic features F31.5
II F31.81
in remission (currently) F31.70
in full remission
most recent episode
depressed F31.76
hypomanic F31.72
manic F31.74
mixed F31.78
in partial remission
most recent episode
depressed F31.75
hypomanic F31.71
manic F31.73
mixed F31.77
organic F06.30
single manic episode F30.9
mild F30.11
moderate F30.12
hhsevere (without psychotic symptoms) F30.13
with psychotic symptoms F30.2
specified NEC F31.89
bladder N32.9
functional NEC N31.9
in schistosomiasis B65.0 *[N33]*
specified NEC N32.89
bleeding D68.9
blood D75.9
in congenital early syphilis A50.09 *[D77]*
body dysmorphic F45.22
bone M89.9
continuity M84.9
specified type NEC M84.80
ankle M84.87-
fibula M84.86-
foot M84.87-
hand M84.84-

Disorder *(Continued)*
bone *(Continued)*
continuity *(Continued)*
specified type *(Continued)*
humerus M84.82-
neck M84.88
pelvis M84.859
radius M84.83-
rib M84.88
shoulder M84.81-
skull M84.88
thigh M84.85-
tibia M84.86-
ulna M84.83-
vertebra M84.88
density and structure M85.9
cyst —*see also* Cyst, bone, specified type NEC
aneurysmal —*see* Cyst, bone, aneurysmal
solitary —*see* Cyst, bone, solitary
diffuse idiopathic skeletal hyperostosis —*see* Hyperostosis, ankylosing
fibrous dysplasia (monostotic) —*see* Dysplasia, fibrous, bone
fluorosis —*see* Fluorosis, skeletal
hyperostosis of skull M85.2
osteitis condensans —*see* Osteitis, condensans
specified type NEC M85.8-
ankle M85.87-
foot M85.87-
forearm M85.83-
hand M85.84-
lower leg M85.86-
multiple sites M85.89
neck M85.88
rib M85.88
shoulder M85.81-
skull M85.88
thigh M85.85-
upper arm M85.82-
vertebra M85.88
development and growth NEC M89.20
carpus M89.24-
clavicle M89.21-
femur M89.25-
fibula M89.26-
finger M89.24-
humerus M89.22-
ilium M89.259
ischium M89.259
metacarpus M89.24-
metatarsus M89.27-
multiple sites M89.29
neck M89.28
radius M89.23-
rib M89.28
scapula M89.21-
skull M89.28
tarsus M89.27-
tibia M89.26-
toe M89.27-
ulna M89.23-
vertebra M89.28
specified type NEC M89.8X-
brachial plexus G54.0
branched-chain amino-acid metabolism E71.2
specified NEC E71.19
breast N64.9
agalactia —*see* Agalactia
associated with
lactation O92.70
specified NEC O92.79
pregnancy O92.20
specified NEC O92.29
puerperium O92.20
specified NEC O92.29

Disorder *(Continued)*
breast *(Continued)*
cracked nipple —*see* Cracked nipple
galactorrhea —*see* Galactorrhea
hypogalactia O92.4
lactation disorder NEC O92.79
mastitis —*see* Mastitis
nipple infection —*see* Infection, nipple
retracted nipple —*see* Retraction, nipple
specified type NEC N64.89
Briquet's F45.0
bullous, in diseases classified elsewhere L14
caffeine use ◀
mild ◀
with ◀
caffeine-induced ◀
anxiety disorder F15.180 ◀
sleep disorder F15.182 ◀
moderate or severe ◀
with ◀
caffeine-induced ◀
anxiety disorder F15.280 ◀
sleep disorder F15.282 ◀
cannabis use
~~due to drug abuse — see Abuse, drug, cannabis~~
~~due to drug dependence — see Dependence, drug, cannabis~~
mild F12.10 ◀
with ◀
cannabis-induced ◀
anxiety disorder F12.180 ◀
psychotic disorder F12.159 ◀
sleep disorder F12.188 ◀
cannabis intoxication delirium F12.121 ◀
with perceptual disturbances F12.122 ◀
without perceptual disturbances F12.129 ◀
moderate or severe F12.20 ◀
with ◀
cannabis-induced ◀
anxiety disorder F12.280 ◀
psychotic disorder F12.259 ◀
sleep disorder F12.288 ◀
cannabis intoxication ◀
with perceptual disturbances F12.222 ◀
without perceptual disturbances F12.229 ◀
delirium F12.221 ◀
carbohydrate
absorption, intestinal NEC E74.39
metabolism (congenital) E74.9
specified NEC E74.8
cardiac, functional I51.89
carnitine metabolism E71.40
cartilage M94.9
articular NEC —*see* Derangement, joint, articular cartilage
chondrocalcinosis —*see* Chondrocalcinosis
specified type NEC M94.8X-
articular —*see* Derangement, joint, articular cartilage
multiple sites M94.8X0
catatonia (due to known physiological condition) (with another mental disorder) F06.1 ◀
catatonic
due to (secondary to) known physiological condition F06.1
organic F06.1
central auditory processing H93.25
cervical
region NEC M53.82
root (nerve) NEC G54.2
character NOS F60.9
childhood disintegrative NEC F84.3

Disorder *(Continued)*
cholesterol and bile acid metabolism E78.70
Barth syndrome E78.71
other specified E78.79
Smith-Lemli-Opitz syndrome E78.72
choroid H31.9
atrophy —*see* Atrophy, choroid
degeneration —*see* Degeneration, choroid
detachment —*see* Detachment, choroid
dystrophy —*see* Dystrophy, choroid
hemorrhage —*see* Hemorrhage, choroid
rupture —*see* Rupture, choroid
scar —*see* Scar, chorioretinal
solar retinopathy —*see* Retinopathy, solar
specified type NEC H31.8
ciliary body —*see* Disorder, iris
degeneration —*see* Degeneration, ciliary body
coagulation (factor) (*see also* Defect, coagulation) D68.9
newborn, transient P61.6
cocaine use ◀
mild F14.10 ◀
with ◀
amphetamine, cocaine, or other stimulant intoxication ◀
with perceptual disturbances F14.122 ◀
without perceptual disturbances F14.129 ◀
cocaine-induced ◀
anxiety disorder F14.180 ◀
bipolar and related disorder F14.14 ◀
depressive disorder F14.14 ◀
obsessive-compulsive and related disorder F14.188 ◀
psychotic disorder F14.159 ◀
sexual dysfunction F14.181 ◀
sleep disorder F14.182 ◀
cocaine intoxication delirium F14.121 ◀
moderate or severe F14.20 ◀
with ◀
amphetamine, cocaine, or other stimulant intoxication ◀
with perceptual disturbances F14.222 ◀
without perceptual disturbances F14.229 ◀
cocaine-induced ◀
anxiety disorder F14.280 ◀
bipolar and related disorder F14.24 ◀
depressive disorder F14.24 ◀
obsessive-compulsive and related disorder F14.288 ◀
psychotic disorder F14.259 ◀
sexual dysfunction F14.281 ◀
sleep disorder F14.282 ◀
cocaine intoxication delirium F14.221 ◀
coccyx NEC M53.3
cognitive F09
due to (secondary to) general medical condition F09
persisting R41.89
due to
alcohol F10.97
with dependence F10.27
anxiolytics F13.97
with dependence F13.27
hypnotics F13.97
with dependence F13.27
sedatives F13.97
with dependence F13.27
specified substance NEC F19.97
with
abuse F19.17
dependence F19.27

Disorder *(Continued)*
communication F80.9
social pragmatic F80.82 ◀
conduct (childhood) F91.9
adjustment reaction —*see* Disorder, adjustment
adolescent onset type F91.2
childhood onset type F91.1
compulsive F63.9
confined to family context F91.0
depressive F91.8
group type F91.2
hyperkinetic —*see* Disorder, attention-deficit hyperactivity
oppositional defiance F91.3
socialized F91.2
solitary aggressive type F91.1
specified NEC F91.8
unsocialized (aggressive) F91.1
conduction, heart I45.9
congenital glycosylation (CDG) E74.8
conjunctiva H11.9
infection —*see* Conjunctivitis
connective tissue, localized L94.9
specified NEC L94.8
conversion (functional neurological symptom disorder) ⬅
with ◀
abnormal movement F44.4 ◀
anesthesia or sensory loss F44.6 ◀
attacks or seizures F44.5 ◀
mixed symptoms F44.7 ◀
special sensory symptoms F44.6 ◀
speech symptoms F44.4 ◀
swallowing symptoms F44.4 ◀
weakness or paralysis F44.4 ◀
convulsive (secondary) —*see* Convulsions
cornea H18.9
deformity —*see* Deformity, cornea
degeneration —*see* Degeneration, cornea
deposits —*see* Deposit, cornea
due to contact lens H18.82-
specified as edema —*see* Edema, cornea
edema —*see* Edema, cornea
keratitis —*see* Keratitis
keratoconjunctivitis —*see* Keratoconjunctivitis
membrane change —*see* Change, corneal membrane
neovascularization —*see* Neovascularization, cornea
scar —*see* Opacity, cornea
specified type NEC H18.89-
ulcer —*see* Ulcer, cornea
corpus cavernosum N48.9
cranial nerve —*see* Disorder, nerve, cranial
cyclothymic F34.0
defiant oppositional F91.3
delusional (persistent) (systematized) F22
induced F24
depersonalization F48.1
depressive F32.9
major F32.9
with psychotic symptoms F32.3
in remission (full) F32.5
partial F32.4
recurrent F33.9
single episode F32.9
mild F32.0
moderate F32.1
severe (without psychotic symptoms) F32.2
with psychotic symptoms F32.3
organic F06.31
persistent F34.1 ◀
recurrent F33.9
current episode
mild F33.0
moderate F33.1

Disorder *(Continued)*
depressive *(Continued)*
recurrent *(Continued)*
current episode *(Continued)*
severe (without psychotic symptoms) F33.2
with psychotic symptoms F33.3
in remission F33.40
full F33.42
partial F33.41
specified NEC F33.8
single episode —*see* Episode, depressive
specified NEC F32.89 ◀
developmental F89
arithmetical skills F81.2
coordination (motor) F82
expressive writing F81.81
language F80.9
expressive F80.1
mixed receptive and expressive F80.2
receptive type F80.2
specified NEC F80.89
learning F81.9
arithmetical F81.2
reading F81.0
mixed F88
motor coordination or function F82
pervasive F84.9
specified NEC F84.8
phonological F80.0
reading F81.0
scholastic skills —*see also* Disorder, learning
mixed F81.89
specified NEC F88
speech F80.9
articulation F80.0
specified NEC F80.89
written expression F81.81
diaphragm J98.6
digestive (system) K92.9
newborn P78.9
specified NEC P78.89
postprocedural —*see* Complication, gastrointestinal
psychogenic F45.8
disc (intervertebral) M51.9
with
myelopathy
cervical region M50.00
cervicothoracic region M50.03
high cervical region M50.01
lumbar region M51.06
mid-cervical region M50.020 ⬅
sacrococcygeal region M53.3
thoracic region M51.04
thoracolumbar region M51.05
radiculopathy
cervical region M50.10
cervicothoracic region M50.13
high cervical region M50.11
lumbar region M51.16
lumbosacral region M51.17
mid-cervical region M50.120 ⬅
sacrococcygeal region M53.3
thoracic region M51.14
thoracolumbar region M51.15
cervical M50.90
with
myelopathy M50.00
C2-C3 M50.01
C3-C4 M50.01
C4-C5 M50.021 ⬅
C5-C6 M50.022 ⬅
C6-C7 M50.023 ⬅
C7-T1 M50.03
cervicothoracic region M50.03
high cervical region M50.01
mid-cervical region M50.020 ⬅

◀ New ⬅ Revised ~~deleted~~ Deleted

Disorder *(Continued)*
disc *(Continued)*
cervical *(Continued)*
with *(Continued)*
neuritis, radiculitis or radiculopathy M50.10
C2-C3 M50.11
C3-C4 M50.11
C4-C5 M50.121 ⟸
C5-C6 M50.122 ⟸
C6-C7 M50.123 ⟸
C7-T1 M50.13
cervicothoracic region M50.13
high cervical region M50.11
mid-cervical region M50.120 ⟸
C2-C3 M50.91
C3-C4 M50.91
C4-C5 M50.921 ⟸
C5-C6 M50.922 ⟸
C6-C7 M50.923 ⟸
C7-T1 M50.93
cervicothoracic region M50.93
degeneration M50.30
C2-C3 M50.31
C3-C4 M50.31
C4-C5 M50.321 ⟸
C5-C6 M50.322 ⟸
C6-C7 M50.323 ⟸
C7-T1 M50.33
cervicothoracic region M50.33
high cervical region M50.31
mid-cervical region M50.320 ⟸
displacement M50.20
C2-C3 M50.21
C3-C4 M50.21
C4-C5 M50.221 ⟸
C5-C6 M50.222 ⟸
C6-C7 M50.223 ⟸
C7-T1 M50.23
cervicothoracic region M50.23
high cervical region M50.21
mid-cervical region M50.220 ⟸
high cervical region M50.91
mid-cervical region M50.920 ⟸
specified type NEC M50.80
C2-C3 M50.81
C3-C4 M50.81
C4-C5 M50.821 ⟸
C5-C6 M50.822 ⟸
C6-C7 M50.823 ⟸
C7-T1 M50.83
cervicothoracic region M50.83
high cervical region M50.81
mid-cervical region M50.820 ⟸
specified NEC
lumbar region M51.86
lumbosacral region M51.87
sacrococcygeal region M53.3
thoracic region M51.84
thoracolumbar region M51.85
disinhibited attachment (childhood) F94.2
disintegrative, childhood NEC F84.3
disruptive F91.9 ◀
mood dysregulation F34.81 ◀
specified NEC F91.8 ◀
disruptive behavior F91.9 ⟸
dissocial personality F60.2
dissociative F44.9
affecting
motor function F44.4
and sensation F44.7
sensation F44.6
and motor function F44.7
brief reactive F43.0
due to (secondary to) general medical condition F06.8
mixed F44.7
organic F06.8
other specified NEC F44.89
double heterozygous sickling —*see* Disease, sickle-cell

Disorder *(Continued)*
dream anxiety F51.5
drug induced hemorrhagic D68.32
drug related F19.99
abuse —*see* Abuse, drug
dependence —*see* Dependence, drug
dysmorphic body F45.22 ⟸
dysthymic F34.1
ear H93.9-
bleeding —*see* Otorrhagia
deafness —*see* Deafness
degenerative H93.09-
discharge —*see* Otorrhea
external H61.9-
auditory canal stenosis —*see* Stenosis, external ear canal
exostosis —*see* Exostosis, external ear canal
impacted cerumen —*see* Impaction, cerumen
otitis —*see* Otitis, externa
perichondritis —*see* Perichondritis, ear
pinna —*see* Disorder, pinna
specified type NEC H61.89-
in diseases classified elsewhere H62.8X-
inner H83.9-
vestibular dysfunction —*see* Disorder, vestibular function
middle H74.9-
adhesive H74.1-
ossicle —*see* Abnormal, ear ossicles
polyp —*see* Polyp, ear (middle)
specified NEC, in diseases classified elsewhere H75.8-
postprocedural —*see* Complications, ear, procedure
specified NEC, in diseases classified elsewhere H94.8-
eating (adult) (psychogenic) F50.9
anorexia —*see* Anorexia
binge F50.81 ◀
bulimia F50.2
child F98.29
pica F98.3
rumination disorder F98.21
pica F50.89 ⟸
childhood F98.3
electrolyte (balance) NEC E87.8
with
abortion —*see* Abortion by type complicated by specified condition NEC
ectopic pregnancy O08.5
molar pregnancy O08.5
acidosis (metabolic) (respiratory) E87.2
alkalosis (metabolic) (respiratory) E87.3
elimination, transepidermal L87.9
specified NEC L87.8
emotional (persistent) F34.9
of childhood F93.9
specified NEC F93.8
endocrine E34.9
postprocedural E89.89
specified NEC E89.89
erectile (male) (organic) —*see also* Dysfunction, sexual, male, erectile N52.9
nonorganic F52.21
erythematous —*see* Erythema
esophagus K22.9
functional K22.4
psychogenic F45.8
eustachian tube H69.9-
infection —*see* Salpingitis, eustachian
obstruction —*see* Obstruction, eustachian tube
patulous —*see* Patulous, eustachian tube
specified NEC H69.8-

Disorder *(Continued)*
extrapyramidal G25.9
in diseases classified elsewhere —*see* category G26
specified type NEC G25.89
eye H57.9
postprocedural —*see* Complication, postprocedural, eye
eyelid H02.9
cyst —*see* Cyst, eyelid
degenerative H02.70
chloasma —*see* Chloasma, eyelid
madarosis —*see* Madarosis
specified type NEC H02.79
vitiligo —*see* Vitiligo, eyelid
xanthelasma —*see* Xanthelasma
dermatochalasis —*see* Dermato-chalasis
edema —*see* Edema, eyelid
elephantiasis —*see* Elephantiasis, eyelid
foreign body, retained —*see* Foreign body, retained, eyelid
function H02.59
abnormal innervation syndrome —*see* Syndrome, abnormal innervation
blepharochalasis —*see* Blepharochalasis
blepharoclonus —*see* Blepharoclonus
blepharophimosis —*see* Blepharophimosis
blepharoptosis —*see* Blepharoptosis
lagophthalmos —*see* Lagophthalmos
lid retraction —*see* Retraction, lid
hypertrichosis —*see* Hypertrichosis, eyelid
specified type NEC H02.89
vascular H02.879
left H02.876
lower H02.875
upper H02.874
right H02.873
lower H02.872
upper H02.871
factitious F68.10
with predominantly
physical symptoms F68.12
with psychological symptoms F68.13
psychological symptoms F68.11
with physical symptoms F68.13
factor, coagulation —*see* Defect, coagulation
fatty acid
metabolism E71.30
specified NEC E71.39
oxidation
LCAD E71.310
MCAD E71.311
SCAD E71.312
specified deficiency NEC E71.318
feeding (infant or child) —*see also* Disorder, eating R63.3-
feigned (with obvious motivation) Z76.5
without obvious motivation —*see* Disorder, factitious
female
hypoactive sexual desire F52.0
orgasmic F52.31
sexual arousal F52.22
fibroblastic M72.9
specified NEC M72.8
fluency
adult onset F98.5
childhood onset F80.81
following
cerebral infarction I69.323
cerebrovascular disease I69.923
specified disease NEC I69.823
intracerebral hemorrhage I69.123
nontraumatic intracranial hemorrhage NEC I69.223
subarachnoid hemorrhage I69.023
in conditions classified elsewhere R47.82
fluid balance E87.8
follicular (skin) L73.9
specified NEC L73.8

Disorder *(Continued)*
fructose metabolism E74.10
essential fructosuria E74.11
fructokinase deficiency E74.11
fructose-1, 6-diphosphatase deficiency E74.19
hereditary fructose intolerance E74.12
other specified E74.19
functional polymorphonuclear neutrophils D71
gallbladder, biliary tract and pancreas in diseases classified elsewhere K87
gamma-glutamyl cycle E72.8
gastric (functional) K31.9
motility K30
psychogenic F45.8
secretion K30
gastrointestinal (functional) NOS K92.9
newborn P78.9
psychogenic F45.8
gender-identity or -role F64.9
childhood F64.2
effect on relationship F66
of adolescence or adulthood F64.0 ⟸
nontranssexual F64.8 ◀
specified NEC F64.8
uncertainty F66
genito-pelvic pain penetration F52.6 ◀
genitourinary system
female N94.9
male N50.9
psychogenic F45.8
globe H44.9
degenerated condition H44.50
absolute glaucoma H44.51-
atrophy H44.52-
leucocoria H44.53-
degenerative H44.30
chalcosis H44.31-
myopia H44.2-
siderosis H44.32-
specified type NEC H44.39-
endophthalmitis —*see* Endophthalmitis
foreign body, retained —*see* Foreign body, intraocular, old, retained
hemophthalmos —*see* Hemophthalmos
hypotony H44.40
due to
ocular fistula H44.42-
specified disorder NEC H44.43-
flat anterior chamber H44.41-
primary H44.44-
luxation —*see* Luxation, globe
specified type NEC H44.89
glomerular (in) N05.9
amyloidosis E85.4 *[N08]*
cryoglobulinemia D89.1 *[N08]*
disseminated intravascular coagulation D65 *[N08]*
Fabry's disease E75.21 *[N08]*
familial lecithin cholesterol acyltransferase deficiency E78.6 *[N08]*
Goodpasture's syndrome M31.0
hemolytic-uremic syndrome D59.3
Henoch (-Schönlein) purpura D69.0 *[N08]*
malariae malaria B52.0
microscopic polyangiitis M31.7 *[N08]*
multiple myeloma C90.0- *[N08]*
mumps B26.83
schistosomiasis B65.9 *[N08]*
sepsis NEC A41.- *[N08]*
streptococcal A40.- *[N08]*
sickle-cell disorders D57.- *[N08]*
strongyloidiasis B78.9 *[N08]*
subacute bacterial endocarditis I33.0 *[N08]*
syphilis A52.75
systemic lupus erythematosus M32.14
thrombotic thrombocytopenic purpura M31.1 *[N08]*
Waldenström macroglobulinemia C88.0 *[N08]*
Wegener's granulomatosis M31.31

Disorder *(Continued)*
gluconeogenesis E74.4
glucosaminoglycan metabolism — *see* Disorder, metabolism, glucosaminoglycan
glycine metabolism E72.50
d-glycericacidemia E72.59
hyperhydroxyprolinemia E72.59
hyperoxaluria E72.53
hyperprolinemia E72.59
non-ketotic hyperglycinemia E72.51
oxalosis E72.53
oxaluria E72.53
sarcosinemia E72.59
trimethylaminuria E72.52
glycoprotein metabolism E77.9
specified NEC E77.8
habit (and impulse) F63.9
involving sexual behavior NEC F65.9
specified NEC F63.89
hallucinogen use ◀
mild F16.10 ◀
with ◀
hallucinogen-induced ◀
anxiety disorder F16.180 ◀
bipolar and related disorder F16.14 ◀
depressive disorder F16.14 ◀
psychotic disorder F16.159 ◀
hallucinogen intoxication delirium F16.121 ◀
other hallucinogen intoxication F16.129 ◀
moderate or severe F16.20 ◀
with ◀
hallucinogen-induced ◀
anxiety disorder F16.280 ◀
bipolar and related disorder F16.24 ◀
depressive disorder F16.24 ◀
psychotic disorder F16.259 ◀
hallucinogen intoxication delirium F16.221 ◀
other hallucinogen intoxication F16.229 ◀
heart action I49.9
hematological D75.9
newborn (transient) P61.9
specified NEC P61.8
hematopoietic organs D75.9
hemorrhagic NEC D69.9
drug-induced D68.32
due to
extrinsic circulating anticoagulants D68.32
increase in
anti-IIa D68.32
anti-Xa D68.32
intrinsic
circulating anticoagulants D68.318
increase in
antithrombin D68.318
anti-VIIIa D68.318
anti-IXa D68.318
anti-XIa D68.318
following childbirth O72.3
hemostasis —*see* Defect, coagulation
histidine metabolism E70.40
histidinemia E70.41
other specified E70.49
hoarding F42.3 ◀
hyperkinetic —*see* Disorder, attention-deficit hyperactivity
hyperleucine-isoleucinemia E71.19
hypervalinemia E71.19
hypoactive sexual desire F52.0
hypochondriacal F45.20
body dysmorphic F45.22
neurosis F45.21
other specified F45.29

Disorder *(Continued)*
identity
dissociative F44.81
illness anxiety F45.21 ◀
of childhood F93.8
immune mechanism (immunity) D89.9
specified type NEC D89.89
impaired renal tubular function N25.9
specified NEC N25.89
impulse (control) F63.9
inflammatory
pelvic, in diseases classified elsewhere — *see* category N74
penis N48.29
abscess N48.21
cellulitis N48.22
inhalant use ◀
mild F18.10 ◀
with ◀
inhalant-induced ◀
anxiety disorder F18.180 ◀
depressive disorder F18.14 ◀
major neurocognitive disorder F18.17 ◀
mild neurocognitive disorder F18.188 ◀
psychotic disorder F18.159 ◀
inhalant intoxication F18.129 ◀
inhalant intoxication delirium F18.121 ◀
moderate or severe F18.20 ◀
with ◀
inhalant-induced ◀
anxiety disorder F18.280 ◀
depressive disorder F18.24 ◀
major neurocognitive disorder F18.27 ◀
mild neurocognitive disorder F18.288 ◀
psychotic disorder F18.259 ◀
inhalant intoxication F18.229 ◀
inhalant intoxication delirium F18.221 ◀
integument, newborn P83.9
specified NEC P83.8
intermittent explosive F63.81
internal secretion pancreas —*see* Increased, secretion, pancreas, endocrine
intestine, intestinal
carbohydrate absorption NEC E74.39
postoperative K91.2
functional NEC K59.9
postoperative K91.89
psychogenic F45.8
vascular K55.9
chronic K55.1
specified NEC K55.8
intraoperative (intraprocedural) —*see* Complications, intraoperative
involuntary emotional expression (IEED) F48.2
iris H21.9
adhesions —*see* Adhesions, iris
atrophy —*see* Atrophy, iris
chamber angle recession —*see* Recession, chamber angle
cyst —*see* Cyst, iris
degeneration —*see* Degeneration, iris
in diseases classified elsewhere H22
iridodialysis —*see* Iridodialysis
iridoschisis —*see* Iridoschisis
miotic pupillary cyst —*see* Cyst, pupillary
pupillary
abnormality —*see* Abnormality, pupillary
membrane —*see* Membrane, pupillary
specified type NEC H21.89
vascular NEC H21.1X-
iron metabolism E83.10
specified NEC E83.19

◀ New ⟸ Revised ~~deleted~~ Deleted

Disorder *(Continued)*
isovaleric acidemia E71.110
jaw, developmental M27.0
temporomandibular —*see also* Anomaly, dentofacial, temporomandibular joint M26.60- ◀
joint M25.9
derangement —*see* Derangement, joint
effusion —*see* Effusion, joint
fistula —*see* Fistula, joint
hemarthrosis —*see* Hemarthrosis
instability —*see* Instability, joint
osteophyte —*see* Osteophyte
pain —*see* Pain, joint
psychogenic F45.8
specified type NEC M25.80
ankle M25.87-
elbow M25.82-
foot joint M25.87-
hand joint M25.84-
hip M25.85-
knee M25.86-
shoulder M25.81-
wrist M25.83-
stiffness —*see* Stiffness, joint
ketone metabolism E71.32
kidney N28.9
functional (tubular) N25.9
in
schistosomiasis B65.9 *[N29]*
tubular function N25.9
specified NEC N25.89
lacrimal system H04.9
changes H04.69
fistula —*see* Fistula, lacrimal
gland H04.19
atrophy —*see* Atrophy, lacrimal gland
cyst —*see* Cyst, lacrimal, gland
dacryops —*see* Dacryops
dislocation —*see* Dislocation, lacrimal gland
dry eye syndrome —*see* Syndrome, dry eye
infection —*see* Dacryoadenitis
granuloma —*see* Granuloma, lacrimal
inflammation —*see* Inflammation, lacrimal
obstruction —*see* Obstruction, lacrimal
specified NEC H04.89
lactation NEC O92.79
language (developmental) F80.9
expressive F80.1
mixed receptive and expressive F80.2
receptive F80.2
late luteal phase dysphoric N94.89
learning (specific) F81.9
acalculia R48.8
alexia R48.0
mathematics F81.2
reading F81.0
specified NEC F81.89
spelling F81.81
written expression F81.81
lens H27.9
aphakia —*see* Aphakia
cataract —*see* Cataract
dislocation —*see* Dislocation, lens
specified type NEC H27.8
ligament M24.20
ankle M24.27-
attachment, spine —*see* Enthesopathy, spinal
elbow M24.22-
foot joint M24.27-
hand joint M24.24-
hip M24.25-
knee —*see* Derangement, knee, specified NEC
shoulder M24.21-
vertebra M24.28
wrist M24.23-

Disorder *(Continued)*
ligamentous attachments —*see also* Enthesopathy
spine —*see* Enthesopathy, spinal
lipid
metabolism, congenital E78.9
storage E75.6
specified NEC E75.5
lipoprotein
deficiency (familial) E78.6
metabolism E78.9
specified NEC E78.89
liver K76.9
malarial B54 *[K77]*
low back —*see also* Dorsopathy, specified NEC
lumbosacral
plexus G54.1
root (nerve) NEC G54.4
lung, interstitial, drug-induced J70.4
acute J70.2
chronic J70.3
lymphoproliferative, post-transplant (PTLD) D47.Z1
lysine and hydroxylysine metabolism E72.3
major neurocognitive —*see* Dementia, in (due to) ◀
male
erectile (organic) —*see also* Dysfunction, sexual, male, erectile N52.9
nonorganic F52.21
hypoactive sexual desire F52.0
orgasmic F52.32
manic F30.9
organic F06.33
mast cell activation —*see* Activation, mast cell ◀
mastoid —*see also* Disorder, ear, middle
postprocedural —*see* Complications, ear, procedure
meniscus —*see* Derangement, knee, meniscus
menopausal N95.9
specified NEC N95.8
menstrual N92.6
psychogenic F45.8
specified NEC N92.5
mental (or behavioral) (nonpsychotic) F99
due to (secondary to)
amphetamine
due to drug abuse —*see* Abuse, drug, stimulant
due to drug dependence —*see* Dependence, drug, stimulant
brain disease, damage and dysfunction F09
caffeine use
due to drug abuse —*see* Abuse, drug, stimulant
due to drug dependence —*see* Dependence, drug, stimulant
cannabis use
due to drug abuse —*see* Abuse, drug, cannabis
due to drug dependence —*see* Dependence, drug, cannabis
general medical condition F09
sedative or hypnotic use
due to drug abuse —*see* Abuse, drug, sedative
due to drug dependence —*see* Dependence, drug, sedative
tobacco (nicotine) use —*see* Dependence, drug, nicotine
following organic brain damage F07.9
frontal lobe syndrome F07.0
personality change F07.0
postconcussional syndrome F07.81
specified NEC F07.89
infancy, childhood or adolescence F98.9
neurotic —*see* Neurosis
organic or symptomatic F09

Disorder *(Continued)*
mental *(Continued)*
presenile, psychotic F03
problem NEC
psychoneurotic —*see* Neurosis
psychotic —*see* Psychosis
puerperal F53
senile, psychotic NEC F03
metabolic, amino acid, transitory, newborn P74.8
metabolism NOS E88.9
amino-acid E72.9
aromatic E70.9
albinism —*see* Albinism
histidine E70.40
histidinemia E70.41
other specified E70.49
hyperphenylalaninemia E70.1
classical phenylketonuria E70.0
other specified E70.8
tryptophan E70.5
tyrosine E70.20
hypertyrosinemia E70.21
other specified E70.29
branched chain E71.2
3-methylglutaconic aciduria E71.111
hyperleucine-isoleucinemia E71.19
hypervalinemia E71.19
isovaleric acidemia E71.110
maple syrup urine disease E71.0
methylmalonic acidemia E71.120
organic aciduria NEC E71.118
other specified E71.19
proprionate NEC E71.128
proprionic acidemia E71.121
glycine E72.50
d-glycericacidemia E72.59
hyperhydroxyprolinemia E72.59
hyperoxaluria E72.53
hyperprolinemia E72.59
non-ketotic hyperglycinemia E72.51
other specified E72.59
sarcosinemia E72.59
trimethylaminuria E72.52
hydroxylysine E72.3
lysine E72.3
ornithine E72.4
other specified E72.8
beta-amino acid E72.8
gamma-glutamyl cycle E72.8
straight-chain E72.8
sulfur-bearing E72.10
homocystinuria E72.11
methylenetetrahydrofolate reductase deficiency E72.12
other specified E72.19
bile acid and cholesterol metabolism E78.70
bilirubin E80.7
specified NEC E80.6
calcium E83.50
hypercalcemia E83.52
hypocalcemia E83.51
other specified E83.59
carbohydrate E74.9
specified NEC E74.8
cholesterol and bile acid metabolism E78.70
congenital E88.9
copper E83.00
specified type NEC E83.09
Wilson's disease E83.01
cystinuria E72.01
fructose E74.10
galactose E74.20
glucosaminoglycan E76.9
mucopolysaccharidosis —*see* Mucopolysaccharidosis
specified NEC E76.8
glutamine E72.8
glycine E72.50

Disorder *(Continued)*
metabolism *(Continued)*
glycogen storage (hepatorenal) E74.09
glycoprotein E77.9
specified NEC E77.8
glycosaminoglycan E76.9
specified NEC E76.8
in labor and delivery O75.89
iron E83.10
isoleucine E71.19
leucine E71.19
lipoid E78.9
lipoprotein E78.9
specified NEC E78.89
magnesium E83.40
hypermagnesemia E83.41
hypomagnesemia E83.42
other specified E83.49
mineral E83.9
specified NEC E83.89
mitochondrial E88.40
MELAS syndrome E88.41
MERRF syndrome (myoclonic epilepsy associated with ragged-red fibers) E88.42
other specified E88.49
ornithine E72.4
phosphatases E83.30
phosphorus E83.30
acid phosphatase deficiency E83.39
hypophosphatasia E83.39
hypophosphatemia E83.39
familial E83.31
other specified E83.39
pseudovitamin D deficiency E83.32
plasma protein NEC E88.09
porphyrin —*see* Porphyria
postprocedural E89.89
specified NEC E89.89
purine E79.9
specified NEC E79.8
pyrimidine E79.9
specified NEC E79.8
pyruvate E74.4
serine E72.8
sodium E87.8
specified NEC E88.89
threonine E72.8
valine E71.19
zinc E83.2
methylmalonic acidemia E71.120
micturition NEC —*see also* Difficulty, micturition R39.198 ⇐
feeling of incomplete emptying R39.14
hesitancy R39.11
poor stream R39.12
psychogenic F45.8
split stream R39.13
straining R39.16
urgency R39.15
mild neurocognitive G31.84 ◀
mitochondrial metabolism E88.40
mitral (valve) —*see* Endocarditis, mitral
mixed
anxiety and depressive F41.8
of scholastic skills (developmental) F81.89
receptive expressive language F80.2
mood F39
bipolar —*see* Disorder, bipolar
depressive —*see* Disorder, depressive
due to (secondary to)
alcohol F10.94
amphetamine F15.94
in
abuse F15.14
dependence F15.24
anxiolytic F13.94
in
abuse F13.14
dependence F13.24

Disorder *(Continued)*
mood *(Continued)*
due to *(Continued)*
cocaine F14.94
in
abuse F14.14
dependence F14.24
general medical condition F06.30
hallucinogen F16.94
in
abuse F16.14
dependence F16.24
hypnotic F13.94
in
abuse F13.14
dependence F13.24
inhalant F18.94
in
abuse F18.14
dependence F18.24
opioid F11.94
in
abuse F11.14
dependence F11.24
phencyclidine (PCP) F16.94
in
abuse F16.14
dependence F16.24
physiological condition F06.30
with
depressive features F06.31
major depressive-like episode F06.32
manic features F06.33
mixed features F06.34
psychoactive substance NEC F19.94
in
abuse F19.14
dependence F19.24
sedative F13.94
in
abuse F13.14
dependence F13.24
volatile solvents F18.94
in
abuse F18.14
dependence F18.24
manic episode F30.9
with psychotic symptoms F30.2
without psychotic symptoms F30.10
mild F30.11
moderate F30.12
severe F30.13
in remission (full) F30.4
partial F30.3
specified type NEC F30.8
organic F06.30
right hemisphere F07.89
persistent F34.9
cyclothymia F34.0
dysthymia F34.1
specified type NEC F34.89 ⇐
recurrent F39
right hemisphere organic F07.89
movement G25.9
drug-induced G25.70
akathisia G25.71
specified NEC G25.79
hysterical F44.4
in diseases classified elsewhere —*see* category G26
periodic limb G47.61
sleep related G47.61
sleep related NEC G47.69
specified NEC G25.89
stereotyped F98.4
treatment-induced G25.9
multiple personality F44.81
muscle M62.9
attachment, spine —*see* Enthesopathy, spinal

Disorder *(Continued)*
muscle *(Continued)*
in trichinellosis —*see* Trichinellosis, with muscle disorder
psychogenic F45.8
specified type NEC M62.89
tone, newborn P94.9
specified NEC P94.8
muscular
attachments —*see also* Enthesopathy
spine —*see* Enthesopathy, spinal
urethra N36.44
musculoskeletal system, soft tissue —*see* Disorder, soft tissue
postprocedural M96.89
psychogenic F45.8
myoneural G70.9
due to lead G70.1
specified NEC G70.89
toxic G70.1
myotonic NEC G71.19
nail, in diseases classified elsewhere L62
neck region NEC —*see* Dorsopathy, specified NEC
neonatal onset multisystemic inflammatory (NOMID) M04.2 ◀
nerve G58.9
abducent NEC —*see* Strabismus, paralytic, sixth nerve
accessory G52.8
acoustic —*see* subcategory H93.3
auditory —*see* subcategory H93.3
auriculotemporal G50.8
axillary G54.0
cerebral —*see* Disorder, nerve, cranial
cranial G52.9
eighth —*see* subcategory H93.3
eleventh G52.8
fifth G50.9
first G52.0
fourth NEC —*see* Strabismus, paralytic, fourth nerve
multiple G52.7
ninth G52.1
second NEC —*see* Disorder, nerve, optic
seventh NEC G51.8
sixth NEC —*see* Strabismus, paralytic, sixth nerve
specified NEC G52.8
tenth G52.2
third NEC —*see* Strabismus, paralytic, third nerve
twelfth G52.3
entrapment —*see* Neuropathy, entrapment
facial G51.9
specified NEC G51.8
femoral —*see* Lesion, nerve, femoral
glossopharyngeal NEC G52.1
hypoglossal G52.3
intercostal G58.0
lateral
cutaneous of thigh —*see* Mononeuropathy, lower limb, meralgia paresthetica
popliteal —*see* Lesion, nerve, popliteal
lower limb —*see* Mononeuropathy, lower limb
medial popliteal —*see* Lesion, nerve, popliteal, medial
median NEC —*see* Lesion, nerve, median
multiple G58.7
oculomotor NEC —*see* Strabismus, paralytic, third nerve
olfactory G52.0
optic NEC H47.09-
hemorrhage into sheath —*see* Hemorrhage, optic nerve
ischemic H47.01-
peroneal —*see* Lesion, nerve, popliteal
phrenic G58.8
plantar —*see* Lesion, nerve, plantar

◀ New ⇐ Revised ~~deleted~~ Deleted

Disorder *(Continued)*
nerve *(Continued)*
pneumogastric G52.2
posterior tibial —*see* Syndrome, tarsal tunnel
radial —*see* Lesion, nerve, radial
recurrent laryngeal G52.2
root G54.9
cervical G54.2
lumbosacral G54.1
specified NEC G54.8
thoracic G54.3
sciatic NEC —*see* Lesion, nerve, sciatic
specified NEC G58.8
lower limb —*see* Mononeuropathy, lower limb, specified NEC
upper limb —*see* Mononeuropathy, upper limb, specified NEC
sympathetic G90.9
tibial —*see* Lesion, nerve, popliteal, medial
trigeminal G50.9
specified NEC G50.8
trochlear NEC —*see* Strabismus, paralytic, fourth nerve
ulnar —*see* Lesion, nerve, ulnar
upper limb —*see* Mononeuropathy, upper limb
vagus G52.2
nervous system G98.8
autonomic (peripheral) G90.9
specified NEC G90.8
central G96.9
specified NEC G96.8
parasympathetic G90.9
specified NEC G98.8
sympathetic G90.9
vegetative G90.9
neurocognitive ◀
major ◀
with ◀
aggressive behavior F01.51 ◀
combative behavior F01.51 ◀
violent behavior F01.51 ◀
due to vascular disease, with behavioral disturbance F01.51 ◀
in (due to) (other diseases classified elsewhere) —*see also* Dementia, in (due to) F02.80 ◀
with ◀
aggressive behavior F02.81 ◀
combative behavior F02.81 ◀
violent behavior F02.81 ◀
without behavioral disturbance F01.50 ◀
mild G31.84 ◀
neurodevelopmental F89 ◀
specified NEC F88 ◀
neurohypophysis NEC E23.3
neurological NEC R29.818
neuromuscular G70.9
hereditary NEC G71.9
specified NEC G70.89
toxic G70.1
neurotic F48.9
specified NEC F48.8
neutrophil, polymorphonuclear D71
nicotine use —*see* Dependence, drug, nicotine
nightmare F51.5
nose J34.9
specified NEC J34.89
obsessive-compulsive F42.9 ◀
odontogenesis NOS K00.9
opioid use
with
opioid-induced psychotic disorder F11.959
with
delusions F11.950
hallucinations F11.951

Disorder *(Continued)*
opioid use *(Continued)*
due to drug abuse —*see* Abuse, drug, opioid
due to drug dependence —*see* Dependence, drug, opioid
mild F11.10 ◀
with ◀
opioid-induced ◀
anxiety disorder F11.188 ◀
depressive disorder F11.14 ◀
sexual dysfunction F11.181 ◀
opioid intoxication ◀
with perceptual disturbances F11.122 ◀
delirium F11.121 ◀
without perceptual disturbances F11.129 ◀
moderate or severe F11.20 ◀
with ◀
opioid-induced ◀
anxiety disorder F11.288 ◀
anxiety disorder F11.988 ◀
depressive disorder F11.24 ◀
depressive disorder F11.94 ◀
sexual dysfunction F11.281 ◀
sexual dysfunction F11.981 ◀
opioid intoxication ◀
with perceptual disturbances F11.222 ◀
delirium F11.221 ◀
without perceptual disturbances F11.229 ◀
oppositional defiant F91.3
optic
chiasm H47.49
due to
inflammatory disorder H47.41
neoplasm H47.42
vascular disorder H47.43
disc H47.39-
coloboma —*see* Coloboma, optic disc
drusen —*see* Drusen, optic disc
pseudopapilledema —*see* Pseudopapilledema
radiations —*see* Disorder, visual, pathway
tracts —*see* Disorder, visual, pathway
orbit H05.9
cyst —*see* Cyst, orbit
deformity —*see* Deformity, orbit
edema —*see* Edema, orbit
enophthalmos —*see* Enophthalmos
exophthalmos —*see* Exophthalmos
hemorrhage —*see* Hemorrhage, orbit
inflammation —*see* Inflammation, orbit
myopathy —*see* Myopathy, extraocular muscles
retained foreign body —*see* Foreign body, orbit, old
specified type NEC H05.89
organic
anxiety F06.4
catatonic F06.1
delusional F06.2
dissociative F06.8
emotionally labile (asthenic) F06.8
mood (affective) F06.30
schizophrenia-like F06.2
orgasmic (female) F52.31
male F52.32
ornithine metabolism E72.4
overanxious F41.1
of childhood F93.8
pain
with related psychological factors F45.42
exclusively related to psychological factors F45.41
genito-pelvic penetration disorder F52.6 ◀
pancreatic internal secretion E16.9
specified NEC E16.8

Disorder *(Continued)*
panic F41.0
with agoraphobia F40.01
papulosquamous L44.9
in diseases classified elsewhere L45
specified NEC L44.8
paranoid F22
induced F24
shared F24
parathyroid (gland) E21.5
specified NEC E21.4
parietoalveolar NEC J84.09
paroxysmal, mixed R56.9
patella M22.9-
chondromalacia —*see* Chondromalacia, patella
derangement NEC M22.3X-
recurrent
dislocation —*see* Dislocation, patella, recurrent
subluxation —*see* Dislocation, patella, recurrent, incomplete
specified NEC M22.8X-
patellofemoral M22.2X-
pentose phosphate pathway with anemia D55.1
perception, due to hallucinogens F16.983
in
abuse F16.183
dependence F16.283
peripheral nervous system NEC G64
peroxisomal E71.50
biogenesis
neonatal adrenoleukodystrophy E71.511
specified disorder NEC E71.518
Zellweger syndrome E71.510
rhizomelic chondrodysplasia punctata E71.540
specified form NEC E71.548
group 1 E71.518
group 2 E71.53
group 3 E71.542
X-linked adrenoleukodystrophy E71.529
adolescent E71.521
adrenomyeloneuropathy E71.522
childhood E71.520
specified form NEC E71.528
Zellweger-like syndrome E71.541
persistent
(somatoform) pain F45.41
affective (mood) F34.9
personality —*see also* Personality F60.9
affective F34.0
aggressive F60.3
amoral F60.2
anankastic F60.5
antisocial F60.2
anxious F60.6
asocial F60.2
asthenic F60.7
avoidant F60.6
borderline F60.3
change (secondary) due to general medical condition F07.0
compulsive F60.5
cyclothymic F34.0
dependent (passive) F60.7
depressive F34.1
dissocial F60.2
emotional instability F60.3
expansive paranoid F60.0
explosive F60.3
following organic brain damage F07.9
histrionic F60.4
hyperthymic F34.0
hypothymic F34.1
hysterical F60.4
immature F60.89
inadequate F60.7

Disorder *(Continued)*
personality *(Continued)*
labile F60.3
mixed (nonspecific) F60.89
moral deficiency F60.2
narcissistic F60.81
negativistic F60.89
obsessional F60.5
obsessive (-compulsive) F60.5
organic F07.9
overconscientious F60.5
paranoid F60.0
passive (-dependent) F60.7
passive-aggressive F60.89
pathological NEC F60.9
pseudosocial F60.2
psychopathic F60.2
schizoid F60.1
schizotypal F21
self-defeating F60.7
specified NEC F60.89
type A F60.5
unstable (emotional) F60.3
pervasive, developmental F84.9
phencyclidine use ◀
mild F16.10 ◀
with ◀
phencyclidine-induced ◀
anxiety disorder F16.180 ◀
bipolar and related disorder F16.14 ◀
depressive disorder F16.14 ◀
psychotic disorder F16.159 ◀
phencyclidine intoxication F16.129 ◀
phencyclidine intoxication delirium F16.121 ◀
moderate or severe F16.20 ◀
with ◀
phencyclidine-induced ◀
anxiety disorder F16.280 ◀
bipolar and related disorder F16.24 ◀
depressive disorder F16.24 ◀
psychotic disorder F16.259 ◀
phencyclidine intoxication F16.229 ◀
phencyclidine intoxication delirium F16.221 ◀
phobic anxiety, childhood F40.8
phosphate-losing tubular N25.0
pigmentation L81.9
choroid, congenital Q14.3
diminished melanin formation L81.6
iron L81.8
specified NEC L81.8
pinna (noninfective) H61.10-
deformity, acquired H61.11-
hematoma H61.12-
perichondritis —*see* Perichondritis, ear
specified type NEC H61.19-
pituitary gland E23.7
iatrogenic (postprocedural) E89.3
specified NEC E23.6
platelets D69.1
plexus G54.9
specified NEC G54.8
polymorphonuclear neutrophils D71
porphyrin metabolism —*see* Porphyria
postconcussional F07.81
posthallucinogen perception F16.983
in
abuse F16.183
dependence F16.283
postmenopausal N95.9
specified NEC N95.8
postprocedural (postoperative) —*see* Complications, postprocedural
post-transplant lymphoproliferative D47.z1
post-traumatic stress (PTSD) F43.10
acute F43.11
chronic F43.12

Disorder *(Continued)*
premenstrual dysphoric (PMDD) F32.81 ⇐
prepuce N47.8
propionic acidemia E71.121
prostate N42.9
specified NEC N42.89
psychogenic NOS —*see also* condition F45.9
anxiety F41.8
appetite F50.9
asthenic F48.8
cardiovascular (system) F45.8
compulsive F42.8 ⇐
cutaneous F54
depressive F32.9
digestive (system) F45.8
dysmenorrheic F45.8
dyspneic F45.8
endocrine (system) F54
eye NEC F45.8
feeding —*see* Disorder, eating
functional NEC F45.8
gastric F45.8
gastrointestinal (system) F45.8
genitourinary (system) F45.8
heart (function) (rhythm) F45.8
hyperventilatory F45.8
hypochondriacal —*see* Disorder, hypochondriacal
intestinal F45.8
joint F45.8
learning F81.9
limb F45.8
lymphatic (system) F45.8
menstrual F45.8
micturition F45.8
monoplegic NEC F44.4
motor F44.4
muscle F45.8
musculoskeletal F45.8
neurocirculatory F45.8
obsessive F42.8 ⇐
occupational F48.8
organ or part of body NEC F45.8
paralytic NEC F44.4
phobic F40.9
physical NEC F45.8
rectal F45.8
respiratory (system) F45.8
rheumatic F45.8
sexual (function) F52.9
skin (allergic) (eczematous) F54
sleep F51.9
specified part of body NEC F45.8
stomach F45.8
psychological F99
associated with
disease classified elsewhere F54
sexual
development F66
relationship F66
uncertainty about gender identity F64.9 ⇐
psychomotor NEC F44.4
hysterical F44.4
psychoneurotic —*see also* Neurosis
mixed NEC F48.8
psychophysiologic —*see* Disorder, somatoform
psychosexual F65.9
development F66
identity of childhood F64.2
psychosomatic NOS —*see* Disorder, somatoform
multiple F45.0
undifferentiated F45.1
psychotic —*see* Psychosis
transient (acute) F23
puberty E30.9
specified NEC E30.8
pulmonary (valve) —*see* Endocarditis, pulmonary

Disorder *(Continued)*
purine metabolism E79.9
pyrimidine metabolism E79.9
pyruvate metabolism E74.4
reactive attachment (childhood) F94.1
reading R48.0
developmental (specific) F81.0
receptive language F80.2
receptor, hormonal, peripheral —*see also* Syndrome, androgen insensitivity E34.50
recurrent brief depressive F33.8
reflex R29.2
refraction H52.7
aniseikonia H52.32
anisometropia H52.31
astigmatism —*see* Astigmatism
hypermetropia —*see* Hypermetropia
myopia —*see* Myopia
presbyopia H52.4
specified NEC H52.6
relationship F68.8
due to sexual orientation F66
REM sleep behavior G47.52
renal function, impaired (tubular) N25.9
resonance R49.9
specified NEC R49.8
respiratory function, impaired —*see also* Failure, respiration
postprocedural —*see* Complication, postoperative, respiratory system
psychogenic F45.8
retina H35.9
angioid streaks H35.33
changes in vascular appearance H35.01-
degeneration —*see* Degeneration, retina
dystrophy (hereditary) —*see* Dystrophy, retina
edema H35.81
hemorrhage —*see* Hemorrhage, retina
ischemia H35.82
macular degeneration —*see* Degeneration, macula
microaneurysms H35.04-
microvascular abnormality NEC H35.09
neovascularization —*see* Neovascularization, retina
retinopathy —*see* Retinopathy
separation of layers H35.70
central serous chorioretinopathy H35.71-
pigment epithelium detachment (serous) H35.72-
hemorrhagic H35.73-
specified type NEC H35.89
telangiectasis —*see* Telangiectasis, retina
vasculitis —*see* Vasculitis, retina
retroperitoneal K68.9
right hemisphere organic affective F07.89
rumination (infant or child) F98.21
sacrum, sacrococcygeal NEC M53.3
schizoaffective F25.9
bipolar type F25.0
depressive type F25.1
manic type F25.0
mixed type F25.0
specified NEC F25.8
schizoid of childhood F84.5
schizophreniform F20.81
brief F23
schizotypal (personality) F21
secretion, thyrocalcitonin E07.0
sedative, hypnotic, or anxiolytic use ◀
mild F13.10 ◀
with ◀
sedative, hypnotic, or anxiolytic-induced ◀
anxiety disorder F13.180 ◀
bipolar and related disorder F13.14 ◀

◀ New ⇐ Revised ~~deleted~~ Deleted

Disorder *(Continued)*
sedative, hypnotic, or anxiolytic use *(Continued)*
mild *(Continued)*
with *(Continued)*
sedative, hypnotic, or anxiolytic-induced *(Continued)*
depressive disorder F13.14 ◀
psychotic disorder F13.159 ◀
sexual dysfunction F13.181 ◀
sedative, hypnotic, or anxiolytic intoxication F13.129 ◀
sedative, hypnotic, or anxiolytic intoxication delirium F13.121 ◀
moderate or severe F13.20 ◀
with ◀
sedative, hypnotic, or anxiolytic-induced ◀
anxiety disorder F13.280 ◀
bipolar and related disorder F13.24 ◀
depressive disorder F13.24 ◀
major neurocognitive disorder F13.27 ◀
mild neurocognitive disorder F13.288 ◀
psychotic disorder F13.259 ◀
sexual dysfunction F13.281 ◀
sedative, hypnotic, or anxiolytic intoxication F13.229 ◀
sedative, hypnotic, or anxiolytic intoxication delirium F13.221 ◀
seizure —*see also* Epilepsy G40.909
intractable G40.919
with status epilepticus G40.911
semantic pragmatic F80.89
with autism F84.0
sense of smell R43.1
psychogenic F45.8
separation anxiety, of childhood F93.0
sexual
arousal, female F52.22
aversion F52.1
function, psychogenic F52.9
maturation F66
nonorganic F52.9
preference —*see also* Deviation, sexual F65.9
fetishistic transvestism F65.1
relationship F66
shyness, of childhood and adolescence F40.10
sibling rivalry F93.8
sickle-cell (sickling) (homozygous) —*see* Disease, sickle-cell
heterozygous D57.3
specified type NEC D57.8-
trait D57.3
sinus (nasal) J34.9
specified NEC J34.89
skin L98.9
atrophic L90.9
specified NEC L90.8
granulomatous L92.9
specified NEC L92.8
hypertrophic L91.9
specified NEC L91.8
infiltrative NEC L98.6
newborn P83.9
specified NEC P83.8
picking F42.4 ◀
psychogenic (allergic) (eczematous) F54
sleep G47.9
breathing-related —*see* Apnea, sleep
circadian rhythm G47.20
advance sleep phase type G47.22
delayed sleep phase type G47.21
due to
alcohol
abuse F10.182
dependence F10.282
use F10.982

Disorder *(Continued)*
sleep *(Continued)*
circadian rhythm *(Continued)*
due to *(Continued)*
amphetamines
abuse F15.182
dependence F15.282
use F15.982
caffeine
abuse F15.182
dependence F15.282
use F15.982
cocaine
abuse F14.182
dependence F14.282
use F14.982
drug NEC
abuse F19.182
dependence F19.282
use F19.982
opioid
abuse F11.182
dependence F11.282
use F11.982
psychoactive substance NEC
abuse F19.182
dependence F19.282
use F19.982
sedative, hypnotic, or anxiolytic
abuse F13.182
dependence F13.282
use F13.982
stimulant NEC
abuse F15.182
dependence F15.282
use F15.982
free running type G47.24
in conditions classified elsewhere G47.27
irregular sleep wake type G47.23
jet lag type G47.25
shift work type G47.26
specified NEC G47.29
due to
alcohol
abuse F10.182
dependence F10.282
use F10.982
amphetamine
abuse F15.182
dependence F15.282
use F15.982
anxiolytic
abuse F13.182
dependence F13.282
use F13.982
caffeine
abuse F15.182
dependence F15.282
use F15.982
cocaine
abuse F14.182
dependence F14.282
use F14.982
drug NEC
abuse F19.182
dependence F19.282
use F19.982
hypnotic
abuse F13.182
dependence F13.282
use F13.982
opioid
abuse F11.182
dependence F11.282
use F11.982
psychoactive substance NEC
abuse F19.182
dependence F19.282
use F19.982

Disorder *(Continued)*
sleep *(Continued)*
due to *(Continued)*
sedative
abuse F13.182
dependence F13.282
use F13.982
stimulant NEC
abuse F15.182
dependence F15.282
use F15.982
emotional F51.9
excessive somnolence —*see* Hypersomnia
hypersomnia type —*see* Hypersomnia
initiating or maintaining —*see* Insomnia
nightmares F51.5
nonorganic F51.9
specified NEC F51.8
parasomnia type G47.50
specified NEC G47.8
terrors F51.4
walking F51.3
sleep-wake pattern or schedule —*see* Disorder, sleep, circadian rhythm
social
anxiety of childhood F40.10
functioning in childhood F94.9
specified NEC F94.8
pragmatic F80.82 ◀
soft tissue M79.9
ankle M79.9
due to use, overuse and pressure M70.90
ankle M70.97-
bursitis —*see* Bursitis
foot M70.97-
forearm M70.93-
hand M70.94-
lower leg M70.96-
multiple sites M70.99
pelvic region M70.95-
shoulder region M70.91-
specified site NEC M70.98
specified type NEC M70.80
ankle M70.87-
foot M70.87-
forearm M70.83-
hand M70.84-
lower leg M70.86-
multiple sites M70.89
pelvic region M70.85-
shoulder region M70.81-
specified site NEC M70.88
thigh M70.85-
upper arm M70.82-
thigh M70.95-
upper arm M70.92-
foot M79.9
forearm M79.9
hand M79.9
lower leg M79.9
multiple sites M79.9
occupational —*see* Disorder, soft tissue, due to use, overuse and pressure
pelvic region M79.9
shoulder region M79.9
specified type NEC M79.89
thigh M79.9
upper arm M79.9
somatic symptom F45.1 ◀
somatization F45.0
somatoform F45.9
pain (persistent) F45.41
somatization (multiple) (long-lasting) F45.0
specified NEC F45.8
undifferentiated F45.1
somnolence, excessive —*see* Hypersomnia
specific
arithmetical F81.2
developmental, of motor F82
reading F81.0

Disorder *(Continued)*
specific *(Continued)*
speech and language F80.9
spelling F81.81
written expression F81.81
speech R47.9
articulation (functional) (specific) F80.0
developmental F80.9
specified NEC R47.89
speech-sound F80.0 ◀
spelling (specific) F81.81
spine —*see also* Dorsopathy
ligamentous or muscular attachments, peripheral —*see* Enthesopathy, spinal
specified NEC —*see* Dorsopathy, specified NEC
stereotyped, habit or movement F98.4
stimulant use (other) (unspecified) ◀
mild F15.10 ◀
moderate or severe F15.20 ◀
stomach (functional) —*see* Disorder, gastric
stress F43.9
acute F43.0 ◀
post-traumatic F43.10
acute F43.11
chronic F43.12
substance use (other) (unknown) ◀
mild F19.10 ◀
with substance-induced ◀
anxiety disorder F19.180 ◀
bipolar and related disorder F19.14 ◀
depressive disorder F19.14 ◀
major neurocognitive disorder F19.17 ◀
mild neurocognitive disorder F19.188 ◀
obsessive-compulsive and related disorder F19.188 ◀
sexual dysfunction F19.181 ◀
substance intoxication F19.129 ◀
substance intoxication delirium F19.121 ◀
moderate or severe F19.20 ◀
with substance-induced ◀
anxiety disorder F19.280 ◀
bipolar and related disorder F19.24 ◀
depressive disorder F19.24 ◀
major neurocognitive disorder F19.27 ◀
mild neurocognitive disorder F19.288 ◀
obsessive-compulsive and related disorder F19.288 ◀
sexual dysfunction F19.281 ◀
substance intoxication F19.229 ◀
substance intoxication delirium F19.221 ◀
sulfur-bearing amino-acid metabolism E72.10
sweat gland (eccrine) L74.9
apocrine L75.9
specified NEC L75.8
specified NEC L74.8
synovium M67.90
acromioclavicular M67.91-
ankle M67.97-
elbow M67.92-
foot M67.97-
forearm M67.93-
hand M67.94-
hip M67.95-
knee M67.96-
multiple sites M67.99
rupture —*see* Rupture, synovium
shoulder M67.91-
specified type NEC M67.80
acromioclavicular M67.81-
ankle M67.87-
elbow M67.82-
foot M67.87-
hand M67.84-
hip M67.85-

Disorder *(Continued)*
synovium *(Continued)*
specified type *(Continued)*
knee M67.86-
multiple sites M67.89
wrist M67.83-
synovitis —*see* Synovitis
upper arm M67.92-
wrist M67.93-
temperature regulation, newborn P81.9
specified NEC P81.8
temporomandibular joint M26.60- ◀
tendon M67.90
acromioclavicular M67.91-
ankle M67.97-
contracture —*see* Contracture, tendon
elbow M67.92-
foot M67.97-
forearm M67.93-
hand M67.94-
hip M67.95-
knee M67.96-
multiple sites M67.99
rupture —*see* Rupture, tendon
shoulder M67.91-
specified type NEC M67.80
acromioclavicular M67.81-
ankle M67.87-
elbow M67.82-
foot M67.87-
hand M67.84-
hip M67.85-
knee M67.86-
multiple sites M67.89
trunk M67.88
wrist M67.83-
synovitis —*see* Synovitis
tendinitis —*see* Tendinitis
tenosynovitis —*see* Tenosynovitis
trunk M67.98
upper arm M67.92-
wrist M67.93-
thoracic root (nerve) NEC G54.3
thyrocalcitonin hypersecretion E07.0
thyroid (gland) E07.9
function NEC, neonatal, transitory P72.2
iodine-deficiency related E01.8
specified NEC E07.89
tic —*see* Tic
tobacco use ◀
mild Z72.0 ◀
moderate F17.200 ◀
severe F17.200 ◀
tooth K08.9
development K00.9
specified NEC K00.8
eruption K00.6
Tourette's F95.2
trance and possession F44.89
trauma and stressor-related F43.9 ◀
other specified F43.8 ◀
tricuspid (valve) —*see* Endocarditis, tricuspid
tryptophan metabolism E70.5
tubular, phosphate-losing N25.0
tubulo-interstitial (in)
brucellosis A23.9 *[N16]*
cystinosis E72.04
diphtheria A36.84
glycogen storage disease E74.00 *[N16]*
leukemia NEC C95.9- *[N16]*
lymphoma NEC C85.9- *[N16]*
mixed cryoglobulinemia D89.1 *[N16]*
multiple myeloma C90.0- *[N16]*
Salmonella infection A02.25
sarcoidosis D86.84
sepsis A41.9 *[N16]*
streptococcal A40.9 *[N16]*
systemic lupus erythematosus M32.15
toxoplasmosis B58.83
transplant rejection T86.91 *[N16]*
Wilson's disease E83.01 *[N16]*

Disorder *(Continued)*
tubulo-renal function, impaired N25.9
specified NEC N25.89
tympanic membrane H73.9-
atrophy —*see* Atrophy, tympanic membrane
infection —*see* Myringitis
perforation —*see* Perforation, tympanum
specified NEC H73.89-
unsocialized aggressive F91.1
urea cycle metabolism E72.20
argininemia E72.21
arginosuccinic aciduria E72.22
citrullinemia E72.23
ornithine transcarbamylase deficiency E72.4
other specified E72.29
ureter (in) N28.9
schistosomiasis B65.0 *[N29]*
tuberculosis A18.11
urethra N36.9
specified NEC N36.8
urinary system N39.9
specified NEC N39.8
valve, heart
aortic —*see* Endocarditis, aortic
mitral —*see* Endocarditis, mitral
pulmonary —*see* Endocarditis, pulmonary
rheumatic
aortic —*see* Endocarditis, aortic, rheumatic
mitral —*see* Endocarditis, mitral
pulmonary —*see* Endocarditis, pulmonary, rheumatic
tricuspid —*see* Endocarditis, tricuspid
tricuspid —*see* Endocarditis, tricuspid
vestibular function H81.9-
specified NEC —*see* subcategory H81.8
in diseases classified elsewhere H82.-
vertigo —*see* Vertigo
vision, binocular H53.30
abnormal retinal correspondence H53.31
diplopia H53.2
fusion with defective stereopsis H53.32
simultaneous perception H53.33
suppression H53.34
visual
cortex
blindness H47.619
left brain H47.612
right brain H47.611
due to
inflammatory disorder H47.629
left brain H47.622
right brain H47.621
neoplasm H47.639
left brain H47.632
right brain H47.631
vascular disorder H47.649
left brain H47.642
right brain H47.641
pathway H47.9
due to
inflammatory disorder H47.51-
neoplasm H47.52-
vascular disorder H47.53-
optic chiasm —*see* Disorder, optic, chiasm
vitreous body H43.9
crystalline deposits —*see* Deposit, crystalline
degeneration —*see* Degeneration, vitreous
hemorrhage —*see* Hemorrhage, vitreous
opacities —*see* Opacity, vitreous
prolapse —*see* Prolapse, vitreous
specified type NEC H43.89
voice R49.9
specified type NEC R49.8
volatile solvent use
due to drug abuse —*see* Abuse, drug, inhalant
due to drug dependence —*see* Dependence, drug, inhalant

◀ New ◀ Revised ~~deleted~~ Deleted

Disorder *(Continued)*
white blood cells D72.9
specified NEC D72.89
withdrawing, child or adolescent F40.10
Disorientation R41.0
Displacement, displaced
acquired traumatic of bone, cartilage, joint, tendon NEC —*see* Dislocation
adrenal gland (congenital) Q89.1
appendix, retrocecal (congenital) Q43.8
auricle (congenital) Q17.4
bladder (acquired) N32.89
congenital Q64.19
brachial plexus (congenital) Q07.8
brain stem, caudal (congenital) Q04.8
canaliculus (lacrimalis), congenital Q10.6
cardia through esophageal hiatus (congenital) Q40.1
cerebellum, caudal (congenital) Q04.8
cervix —*see* Malposition, uterus
colon (congenital) Q43.3
device, implant or graft —*see also* Complications, by site and type, mechanical T85.628
arterial graft NEC —*see* Complication, cardiovascular device, mechanical, vascular
breast (implant) T85.42
catheter NEC T85.628
dialysis (renal) T82.42
intraperitoneal T85.621
infusion NEC T82.524
spinal (epidural) (subdural) T85.620
urinary ◀
cystostomy T83.020
Hopkins T83.028 ◀
ileostomy T83.028 ◀
indwelling T83.021 ◀
nephrostomy T83.022 ◀
specified NEC T83.028 ◀
urostomy T83.028 ◀
electronic (electrode) (pulse generator) (stimulator) —*see* Complication, electronic stimulator
fixation, internal (orthopedic) NEC —*see* Complication, fixation device, mechanical
gastrointestinal —*see* Complications, prosthetic device, mechanical, gastrointestinal device
genital NEC T83.428
intrauterine contraceptive device (string) T83.32 ◀
penile prosthesis (cylinder) (implanted) (pump) (resevoir) T83.420 ◀
testicular prosthesis T83.421 ◀
heart NEC —*see* Complication, cardiovascular device, mechanical
joint prosthesis —*see* Complications, joint prosthesis, mechanical
ocular —*see* Complications, prosthetic device, mechanical, ocular device
orthopedic NEC —*see* Complication, orthopedic, device or graft, mechanical
specified NEC T85.628
urinary NEC T83.128 ◀
graft T83.22
sphincter, implanted T83.121 ◀
stent (ileal conduit) (nephroureteral) T83.123 ◀
ureteral indwelling T83.122 ◀
vascular NEC —*see* Complication, cardiovascular device, mechanical
ventricular intracranial shunt T85.02
electronic stimulator
bone T84.320
cardiac —*see* Complications, cardiac device, electronic

Displacement, displaced *(Continued)*
electronic stimulator *(Continued)*
nervous system —*see* Complication, prosthetic device, mechanical, electronic nervous system stimulator
urinary —*see* Complications, electronic stimulator, urinary
esophageal mucosa into cardia of stomach, congenital Q39.8
esophagus (acquired) K22.8
congenital Q39.8
eyeball (acquired) (lateral) (old) —*see* Displacement, globe
congenital Q15.8
current —*see* Avulsion, eye
fallopian tube (acquired) N83.4- ◀
congenital Q50.6
opening (congenital) Q50.6
gallbladder (congenital) Q44.1
gastric mucosa (congenital) Q40.2
globe (acquired) (old) (lateral) H05.21-
current —*see* Avulsion, eye
heart (congenital) Q24.8
acquired I51.89
hymen (upward) (congenital) Q52.4
intervertebral disc NEC
with myelopathy —*see* Disorder, disc, with, myelopathy
cervical, cervicothoracic (with) M50.20
myelopathy —*see* Disorder, disc, cervical, with myelopathy
neuritis, radiculitis or radiculopathy —*see* Disorder, disc, cervical, with neuritis
due to trauma —*see* Dislocation, vertebra
lumbar region M51.26
with
neuritis, radiculitis, radiculopathy or sciatica M51.16
lumbosacral region M51.27
with
myelopathy M51.07
neuritis, radiculitis, radiculopathy or sciatica M51.17
sacrococcygeal region M53.3
thoracic region M51.24
with
myelopathy M51.04
neuritis, radiculitis, radiculopathy M51.14
thoracolumbar region M51.25
with
myelopathy M51.05
neuritis, radiculitis, radiculopathy M51.15
intrauterine device (string) T83.32 ◀
kidney (acquired) N28.83
congenital Q63.2
lachrymal, lacrimal apparatus or duct (congenital) Q10.6
lens, congenital Q12.1
macula (congenital) Q14.1
Meckel's diverticulum Q43.0
malignant —*see* Table of Neoplasms, small intestine, malignant
nail (congenital) Q84.6
acquired L60.8
opening of Wharton's duct in mouth Q38.4
organ or site, congenital NEC —*see* Malposition, congenital
ovary (acquired) N83.4- ◀
congenital Q50.39
free in peritoneal cavity (congenital) Q50.39
into hernial sac N83.4- ◀
oviduct (acquired) N83.4- ◀
congenital Q50.6
parathyroid (gland) E21.4
parotid gland (congenital) Q38.4

Displacement, displaced *(Continued)*
punctum lacrimale (congenital) Q10.6
sacro-iliac (joint) (congenital) Q74.2
current injury S33.2
old —*see* subcategory M53.2
salivary gland (any) (congenital) Q38.4
spleen (congenital) Q89.09
stomach, congenital Q40.2
sublingual duct Q38.4
tongue (downward) (congenital) Q38.3
tooth, teeth, fully erupted M26.30
horizontal M26.33
vertical M26.34
trachea (congenital) Q32.1
ureter or ureteric opening or orifice (congenital) Q62.62
uterine opening of oviducts or fallopian tubes Q50.6
uterus, uterine —*see* Malposition, uterus
ventricular septum Q21.0
with rudimentary ventricle Q20.4
Disproportion
between native and reconstructed breast N65.1
fiber-type G71.2
Disruptio uteri —*see* Rupture, uterus
Disruption (of)
ciliary body NEC H21.89
closure of
cornea T81.31
craniotomy T81.32
fascia (muscular) (superficial) T81.32
internal organ or tissue T81.32
laceration (external) (internal) T81.33
ligament T81.32
mucosa T81.31
muscle or muscle flap T81.32
ribs or rib cage T81.32
skin and subcutaneous tissue (full-thickness) (superficial) T81.31
skull T81.32
sternum (sternotomy) T81.32
tendon T81.32
traumatic laceration (external) (internal) T81.33
family Z63.8
due to
absence of family member due to military deployment Z63.31
absence of family member NEC Z63.32
alcoholism and drug addiction in family Z63.72
bereavement Z63.4
death (assumed) or disappearance of family member Z63.4
divorce or separation Z63.5
drug addiction in family Z63.72
return of family member from military deployment (current or past conflict) Z63.71
stressful life events NEC Z63.79
iris NEC H21.89
ligament (s) —*see also* Sprain
knee
current injury —*see* Dislocation, knee
old (chronic) —*see* Derangement, knee, ligament, instability, chronic
spontaneous NEC —*see* Derangement, knee, disruption ligament
ossicular chain —*see* Discontinuity, ossicles, ear
pelvic ring (stable) S32.810
unstable S32.811
traumatic injury wound repair T81.33
wound T81.30
episiotomy O90.1
operation T81.31
cesarean O90.0
external operation wound (superficial) T81.31
internal operation wound (deep) T81.32
perineal (obstetric) O90.1
traumatic injury repair T81.33

Dissatisfaction with
  employment Z56.9
  school environment Z55.4
Dissecting —*see* condition
Dissection
  aorta I71.00
    abdominal I71.02
    thoracic I71.01
    thoracoabdominal I71.03
  artery I77.70 ⬅
    basilar (trunk) I77.75 ◀
    carotid I77.71
    cerebral (nonruptured) I67.0
      ruptured —*see* Hemorrhage, intracranial, subarachnoid
    coronary I25.42
    extremity ◀
      lower I77.77 ◀
      upper I77.76 ◀
    iliac I77.72
    precerebral ◀
      congenital (nonruptured) Q28.1 ◀
      specified site NEC I77.75 ◀
    renal I77.73
    specified NEC I77.79
    vertebral I77.74
  traumatic —*see* Wound, open, by site
  vascular I99.8
  wound —*see* Wound, open
Disseminated —*see* condition
Dissociation
  auriculoventricular or atrioventricular (AV) (any degree) (isorhythmic) I45.89
    with heart block I44.2
  interference I45.89
Dissociative reaction, state F44.9
Dissolution, vertebra —*see* Osteoporosis
Distension, distention
  abdomen R14.0
  bladder N32.89
  cecum K63.89
  colon K63.89
  gallbladder K82.8
  intestine K63.89
  kidney N28.89
  liver K76.89
  seminal vesicle N50.89 ⬅
  stomach K31.89
    acute K31.0
    psychogenic F45.8
  ureter —*see* Dilatation, ureter
  uterus N85.8
Distoma hepaticum infestation B66.3
Distomiasis B66.9
  bile passages B66.3
  hemic B65.9
  hepatic B66.3
    due to Clonorchis sinensis B66.1
  intestinal B66.5
  liver B66.3
    due to Clonorchis sinensis B66.1
  lung B66.4
  pulmonary B66.4
Distomolar (fourth molar) K00.1
Disto-occlusion (Division I) (Division II) M26.212
Distortion (s) (congenital)
  adrenal (gland) Q89.1
  arm NEC Q68.8
  bile duct or passage Q44.5
  bladder Q64.79
  brain Q04.9
  cervix (uteri) Q51.9
  chest (wall) Q67.8
    bones Q76.8
  clavicle Q74.0
  clitoris Q52.6
  coccyx Q76.49
  common duct Q44.5
  coronary Q24.5
  cystic duct Q44.5

Distortion *(Continued)*
  ear (auricle) (external) Q17.3
    inner Q16.5
    middle Q16.4
      ossicles Q16.3
  endocrine NEC Q89.2
  eustachian tube Q17.8
  eye (adnexa) Q15.8
  face bone (s) NEC Q75.8
  fallopian tube Q50.6
  femur NEC Q68.8
  fibula NEC Q68.8
  finger (s) Q68.1
  foot Q66.9
  genitalia, genital organ (s)
    female Q52.8
      external Q52.79
      internal NEC Q52.8
  gyri Q04.8
  hand bone (s) Q68.1
  heart (auricle) (ventricle) Q24.8
    valve (cusp) Q24.8
  hepatic duct Q44.5
  humerus NEC Q68.8
  hymen Q52.4
  intrafamilial communications Z63.8
  jaw NEC M26.89
  labium (majus) (minus) Q52.79
  leg NEC Q68.8
  lens Q12.8
  liver Q44.7
  lumbar spine Q76.49
    with disproportion O33.8
      causing obstructed labor O65.0
  lumbosacral (joint) (region) Q76.49
    kyphosis —*see* Kyphosis, congenital
    lordosis —*see* Lordosis, congenital
  nerve Q07.8
  nose Q30.8
  organ
    of Corti Q16.5
    or site not listed —*see* Anomaly, by site
      ossicles, ear Q16.3
  oviduct Q50.6
  pancreas Q45.3
  parathyroid (gland) Q89.2
  pituitary (gland) Q89.2
  radius NEC Q68.8
  sacroiliac joint Q74.2
  sacrum Q76.49
  scapula Q74.0
  shoulder girdle Q74.0
  skull bone (s) NEC Q75.8
    with
      anencephalus Q00.0
      encephalocele —*see* Encephalocele
      hydrocephalus Q03.9
        with spina bifida —*see* Spina bifida, with hydrocephalus
      microcephaly Q02
  spinal cord Q06.8
  spine Q76.49
    kyphosis —*see* Kyphosis, congenital
    lordosis —*see* Lordosis, congenital
  spleen Q89.09
  sternum NEC Q76.7
  thorax (wall) Q67.8
    bony Q76.8
  thymus (gland) Q89.2
  thyroid (gland) Q89.2
  tibia NEC Q68.8
  toe (s) Q66.9
  tongue Q38.3
  trachea (cartilage) Q32.1
  ulna NEC Q68.8
  ureter Q62.8
  urethra Q64.79
    causing obstruction Q64.39
  uterus Q51.9
  vagina Q52.4

Distortion *(Continued)*
  vertebra Q76.49
    kyphosis —*see* Kyphosis, congenital
    lordosis —*see* Lordosis, congenital
  visual —*see also* Disturbance, vision
    shape and size H53.15
  vulva Q52.79
  wrist (bones) (joint) Q68.8
Distress
  abdomen —*see* Pain, abdominal
  acute respiratory R06.00 ⬅
    syndrome (adult) (child) J80 ◀
  epigastric R10.13
  fetal P84
    complicating pregnancy —*see* Stress, fetal
  gastrointestinal (functional) K30
    psychogenic F45.8
  intestinal (functional) NOS K59.9
    psychogenic F45.8
  maternal, during labor and delivery O75.0
  respiratory (adult) (child) R06.00 ⬅
    ~~adult J80~~
    ~~child J80~~
    newborn P22.9
      specified NEC P22.8
    orthopnea R06.01
    psychogenic F45.8
    shortness of breath R06.02
    specified type NEC R06.09
Distribution vessel, atypical Q27.9
  coronary artery Q24.5
  precerebral Q28.1
Districhiasis L68.8
Disturbance (s) —*see also* Disease
  absorption K90.9
    calcium E58
    carbohydrate K90.49 ⬅
    fat K90.49 ⬅
      pancreatic K90.3
    protein K90.49 ⬅
    starch K90.49 ⬅
    vitamin —*see* Deficiency, vitamin
  acid-base equilibrium E87.8
    mixed E87.4
  activity and attention (with hyperkinesis) —*see* Disorder, attention-deficit hyperactivity
  amino acid transport E72.00
  assimilation, food K90.9
  auditory nerve, except deafness —*see* subcategory H93.3
  behavior —*see* Disorder, conduct
  blood clotting (mechanism) —*see also* Defect, coagulation D68.9
  cerebral
    nerve —*see* Disorder, nerve, cranial
    status, newborn P91.9
      specified NEC P91.8
  circulatory I99.9
  conduct —*see also* Disorder, conduct F91.9
    adjustment reaction —*see* Disorder, adjustment
    compulsive F63.9
    disruptive F91.9
    hyperkinetic —*see* Disorder, attention-deficit hyperactivity
    socialized F91.2
    specified NEC F91.8
    unsocialized F91.1
  coordination R27.8
  cranial nerve —*see* Disorder, nerve, cranial
  deep sensibility —*see* Disturbance, sensation
  digestive K30
    psychogenic F45.8
  electrolyte —*see also* Imbalance, electrolyte
    newborn, transitory P74.4
      hyperammonemia P74.6
      potassium balance P74.3
      sodium balance P74.2
      specified type NEC P74.4

◀ New ⬅ Revised ~~deleted~~ Deleted

Disturbance *(Continued)*
emotions specific to childhood and adolescence F93.9
with
anxiety and fearfulness NEC F93.8
elective mutism F94.0
oppositional disorder F91.3
sensitivity (withdrawal) F40.10
shyness F40.10
social withdrawal F40.10
involving relationship problems F93.8
mixed F93.8
specified NEC F93.8
endocrine (gland) E34.9
neonatal, transitory P72.9
specified NEC P72.8
equilibrium R42
fructose metabolism E74.10
gait —*see* Gait
hysterical F44.4
psychogenic F44.4
gastrointestinal (functional) K30
psychogenic F45.8
habit, child F98.9
hearing, except deafness and tinnitus —*see* Abnormal, auditory perception
heart, functional (conditions in I44-I50)
due to presence of (cardiac) prosthesis I97.19-
postoperative I97.89
cardiac surgery I97.19-
hormones E34.9
innervation uterus (parasympathetic) (sympathetic) N85.8
keratinization NEC
gingiva K05.10
nonplaque induced K05.11
plaque induced K05.10
lip K13.0
oral (mucosa) (soft tissue) K13.29
tongue K13.29
learning (specific) —*see* Disorder, learning
memory —*see* Amnesia
mild, following organic brain damage F06.8
mental F99
associated with diseases classified elsewhere F54
metabolism E88.9
with
abortion —*see* Abortion, by type with other specified complication
ectopic pregnancy O08.5
molar pregnancy O08.5
amino-acid E72.9
aromatic E70.9
branched-chain E71.2
straight-chain E72.8
sulfur-bearing E72.10
ammonia E72.20
arginine E72.21
arginosuccinic acid E72.22
carbohydrate E74.9
cholesterol E78.9
citrulline E72.23
cystathionine E72.19
general E88.9
glutamine E72.8
histidine E70.40
homocystine E72.19
hydroxylysine E72.3
in labor or delivery O75.89
iron E83.10
lipoid E78.9
lysine E72.3
methionine E72.19
neonatal, transitory P74.9
calcium and magnesium P71.9
specified type NEC P71.8

Disturbance *(Continued)*
metabolism *(Continued)*
neonatal, transitory *(Continued)*
carbohydrate metabolism P70.9
specified type NEC P70.8
specified NEC P74.8
ornithine E72.4
phosphate E83.39
sodium NEC E87.8
threonine E72.8
tryptophan E70.5
tyrosine E70.20
urea cycle E72.20
motor R29.2
nervous, functional R45.0
neuromuscular mechanism (eye), due to syphilis A52.15
nutritional E63.9
nail L60.3
ocular motion H51.9
psychogenic F45.8
oculogyric H51.8
psychogenic F45.8
oculomotor H51.9
psychogenic F45.8
olfactory nerve R43.1
optic nerve NEC —*see* Disorder, nerve, optic
oral epithelium, including tongue NEC K13.29
perceptual due to
alcohol withdrawal F10.232
amphetamine intoxication F15.922
in
abuse F15.122
dependence F15.222
anxiolytic withdrawal F13.232
cannabis intoxication (acute) F12.922
in
abuse F12.122
dependence F12.222
cocaine intoxication (acute) F14.922
in
abuse F14.122
dependence F14.222
hypnotic withdrawal F13.232
opioid intoxication (acute) F11.922
in
abuse F11.122
dependence F11.222
phencyclidine intoxication (acute) F16.122 ◀
~~in~~
~~abuse F19.122~~
~~dependence F19.222~~
sedative withdrawal F13.232
personality (pattern) (trait) —*see also* Disorder, personality F60.9
following organic brain damage F07.9
polyglandular E31.9
specified NEC E31.8
potassium balance, newborn P74.3
psychogenic F45.9
psychomotor F44.4
psychophysical visual H53.16
pupillary —*see* Anomaly, pupil, function
reflex R29.2
rhythm, heart I49.9
salivary secretion K11.7
sensation (cold) (heat) (localization) (tactile discrimination) (texture) (vibratory) NEC R20.9
hysterical F44.6
skin R20.9
anesthesia R20.0
hyperesthesia R20.3
hypoesthesia R20.1
paresthesia R20.2
specified type NEC R20.8
smell R43.9
and taste (mixed) R43.8
anosmia R43.0

Disturbance *(Continued)*
sensation *(Continued)*
smell *(Continued)*
parosmia R43.1
specified NEC R43.8
taste R43.9
and smell (mixed) R43.8
parageusia R43.2
specified NEC R43.8
sensory —*see* Disturbance, sensation
situational (transient) —*see also* Disorder, adjustment
acute F43.0
sleep G47.9
nonorganic origin F51.9
smell —*see* Disturbance, sensation, smell
sociopathic F60.2
sodium balance, newborn P74.2
speech R47.9
developmental F80.9
specified NEC R47.89
stomach (functional) K31.9
sympathetic (nerve) G90.9
taste —*see* Disturbance, sensation, taste
temperature
regulation, newborn P81.9
specified NEC P81.8
sense R20.8
hysterical F44.6
tooth
eruption K00.6
formation K00.4
structure, hereditary NEC K00.5
touch —*see* Disturbance, sensation
vascular I99.9
arteriosclerotic —*see* Arteriosclerosis
vasomotor I73.9
vasospastic I73.9
vision, visual H53.9
following
cerebral infarction I69.398
cerebrovascular disease I69.998
specified NEC I69.898
intracerebral hemorrhage I69.198
nontraumatic intracranial hemorrhage NEC I69.298
specified disease NEC I69.898
subarachnoid hemorrhage I69.098
psychophysical H53.16
specified NEC H53.8
subjective H53.10
day blindness H53.11
discomfort H53.14-
distortions of shape and size H53.15
loss
sudden H53.13-
transient H53.12-
specified type NEC H53.19
voice R49.9
psychogenic F44.4
specified NEC R49.8
Diuresis R35.8
Diver's palsy, paralysis or squeeze T70.3
Diverticulitis (acute) K57.92
bladder —*see* Cystitis
ileum —*see* Diverticulitis, intestine, small
intestine K57.92
with
abscess, perforation or peritonitis K57.80
with bleeding K57.81
bleeding K57.93
congenital Q43.8
large K57.32
with
abscess, perforation or peritonitis K57.20
with bleeding K57.21

Diverticulitis *(Continued)*
intestine *(Continued)*
large *(Continued)*
with *(Continued)*
bleeding K57.33
small intestine K57.52
with
abscess, perforation or peritonitis K57.40
with bleeding K57.41
bleeding K57.53
small K57.12
with
abscess, perforation or peritonitis K57.00
with bleeding K57.01
bleeding K57.13
large intestine K57.52
with
abscess, perforation or peritonitis K57.40
with bleeding K57.41
bleeding K57.53
Diverticulosis K57.90
with bleeding K57.91
large intestine K57.30
with
bleeding K57.31
small intestine K57.50
with bleeding K57.51
small intestine K57.10
with
bleeding K57.11
large intestine K57.50
with bleeding K57.51
Diverticulum, diverticula (multiple) K57.90
appendix (noninflammatory) K38.2
bladder (sphincter) N32.3
congenital Q64.6
bronchus (congenital) Q32.4
acquired J98.09
calyx, calyceal (kidney) N28.89
cardia (stomach) K31.4
cecum —*see* Diverticulosis, intestine, large
congenital Q43.8
colon —*see* Diverticulosis, intestine, large
congenital Q43.8
duodenum —*see* Diverticulosis, intestine, small
congenital Q43.8
epiphrenic (esophagus) K22.5
esophagus (congenital) Q39.6
acquired (epiphrenic) (pulsion) (traction) K22.5
eustachian tube —*see* Disorder, eustachian tube, specified NEC
fallopian tube N83.8
gastric K31.4
heart (congenital) Q24.8
ileum —*see* Diverticulosis, intestine, small
jejunum —*see* Diverticulosis, intestine, small
kidney (pelvis) (calyces) N28.89
with calculus —*see* Calculus, kidney
Meckel's (displaced) (hypertrophic) Q43.0
malignant —*see* Table of Neoplasms, small intestine, malignant
midthoracic K22.5
organ or site, congenital NEC —*see* Distortion
pericardium (congenital) (cyst) Q24.8
acquired I31.8
pharyngoesophageal (congenital) Q39.6
acquired K22.5
pharynx (congenital) Q38.7
rectosigmoid —*see* Diverticulosis, intestine, large
congenital Q43.8
rectum —*see* Diverticulosis, intestine, large
Rokitansky's K22.5
seminal vesicle N50.89
sigmoid —*see* Diverticulosis, intestine, large
congenital Q43.8
Diverticulum, diverticula *(Continued)*
stomach (acquired) K31.4
congenital Q40.2
trachea (acquired) J39.8
ureter (acquired) N28.89
congenital Q62.8
ureterovesical orifice N28.89
urethra (acquired) N36.1
congenital Q64.79
ventricle, left (congenital) Q24.8
vesical N32.3
congenital Q64.6
Zenker's (esophagus) K22.5
Division
cervix uteri (acquired) N88.8
glans penis Q55.69
labia minora (congenital) Q52.79
ligament (partial or complete) (current) —*see also* Sprain
with open wound —*see* Wound, open
muscle (partial or complete) (current) —*see also* Injury, muscle
with open wound —*see* Wound, open
nerve (traumatic) —*see* Injury, nerve
spinal cord —*see* Injury, spinal cord, by region
vein I87.8
Divorce, causing family disruption Z63.5
Dix-Hallpike neurolabyrinthitis —*see* Neuronitis, vestibular
Dizziness R42
hysterical F44.89
psychogenic F45.8
DMAC (disseminated mycobacterium avium-intracellulare complex) A31.2
DNR (do not resuscitate) Z66
Doan-Wiseman syndrome (primary splenic neutropenia) —*see* Agranulocytosis
Doehle-Heller aortitis A52.02
Dog bite —*see* Bite
Dohle body panmyelopathic syndrome D72.0
Dolichocephaly Q67.2
Dolichocolon Q43.8
Dolichostenomelia —*see* Syndrome, Marfan's
Donohue's syndrome E34.8
Donor (organ or tissue) Z52.9
blood (whole) Z52.000
autologous Z52.010
specified component (lymphocytes) (platelets) NEC Z52.008
autologous Z52.018
specified donor NEC Z52.098
specified donor NEC Z52.090
stem cells Z52.001
autologous Z52.011
specified donor NEC Z52.091
bone Z52.20
autologous Z52.21
marrow Z52.3
specified type NEC Z52.29
cornea Z52.5
egg (Oocyte) Z52.819
age 35 and over Z52.812
anonymous recipient Z52.812
designated recipient Z52.813
under age 35 Z52.810
anonymous recipient Z52.810
designated recipient Z52.811
kidney Z52.4
liver Z52.6
lung Z52.89
lymphocyte —*see* Donor, blood, specified components NEC
Oocyte —*see* Donor, egg
platelets Z52.008
potential, examination of Z00.5
semen Z52.89
skin Z52.10
autologous Z52.11
specified type NEC Z52.19
Donor *(Continued)*
specified organ or tissue NEC Z52.89
sperm Z52.89
Donovanosis A58
Dorsalgia M54.9
psychogenic F45.41
specified NEC M54.89
Dorsopathy M53.9
deforming M43.9
specified NEC —*see* subcategory M43.8
specified NEC M53.80
cervical region M53.82
cervicothoracic region M53.83
lumbar region M53.86
lumbosacral region M53.87
occipito-atlanto-axial region M53.81
sacrococcygeal region M53.88
thoracic region M53.84
thoracolumbar region M53.85
Double
albumin E88.09
aortic arch Q25.45
auditory canal Q17.8
auricle (heart) Q20.8
bladder Q64.79
cervix Q51.820
with doubling of uterus (and vagina) Q51.10
with obstruction Q51.11
inlet ventricle Q20.4
kidney with double pelvis (renal) Q63.0
meatus urinarius Q64.75
monster Q89.4
outlet
left ventricle Q20.2
right ventricle Q20.1
pelvis (renal) with double ureter Q62.5
tongue Q38.3
ureter (one or both sides) Q62.5
with double pelvis (renal) Q62.5
urethra Q64.74
urinary meatus Q64.75
uterus Q51.2
with
doubling of cervix (and vagina) Q51.10
with obstruction Q51.11
in pregnancy or childbirth O34.59-causing obstructed labor O65.5
vagina Q52.10
with doubling of uterus (and cervix) Q51.10
with obstruction Q51.11
vision H53.2
vulva Q52.79
Douglas' pouch, cul-de-sac —*see* condition
Down syndrome Q90.9
meiotic nondisjunction Q90.0
mitotic nondisjunction Q90.1
mosaicism Q90.1
translocation Q90.2
DPD (dihydropyrimidine dehydrogenase deficiency) E88.89
Dracontiasis B72
Dracunculiasis, dracunculosis B72
Dream state, hysterical F44.89
Drepanocytic anemia —*see* Disease, sickle-cell
Dresbach's syndrome (elliptocytosis) D58.1
Dreschlera (hawaiiensis) (infection) B43.8
Dressler's syndrome I24.1
Drift, ulnar —*see* Deformity, limb, specified type NEC, forearm
Drinking (alcohol)
excessive, to excess NEC (without dependence) F10.10
habitual (continual) (without remission) F10.20
with remission F10.21
Drip, postnasal (chronic) R09.82
due to
allergic rhinitis —*see* Rhinitis, allergic
common cold J00

Drip, postnasal *(Continued)*
due to *(Continued)*
gastroesophageal reflux —*see* Reflux, gastroesophageal
nasopharyngitis —*see* Nasopharyngitis
other known condition — code to condition
sinusitis —*see* Sinusitis
Droop
facial R29.81Ø
cerebrovascular disease I69.992
cerebral infarction I69.392
intracerebral hemorrhage I69.192
nontraumatic intracranial hemorrhage NEC I69.292
specified disease NEC I69.892
subarachnoid hemorrhage I69.Ø92
Drop (in)
attack NEC R55
finger —*see* Deformity, finger
foot —*see* Deformity, limb, foot, drop
hematocrit (precipitous) R71.Ø
hemoglobin R71.Ø
toe —*see* Deformity, toe, specified NEC
wrist —*see* Deformity, limb, wrist drop
Dropped heart beats I45.9
Dropsy, dropsical —*see also* Hydrops
abdomen R18.8
brain —*see* Hydrocephalus
cardiac, heart —*see* Failure, heart, congestive
gangrenous —*see* Gangrene
heart —*see* Failure, heart, congestive
kidney —*see* Nephrosis
lung —*see* Edema, lung
newborn due to isoimmunization P56.Ø
pericardium —*see* Pericarditis
Drowned, drowning (near) T75.1
Drowsiness R4Ø.Ø
Drug
abuse counseling and surveillance Z71.51
addiction —*see* Dependence
dependence —*see* Dependence
habit —*see* Dependence
harmful use —*see* Abuse, drug
induced fever R5Ø.2
overdose —*see* Table of Drugs and Chemicals, by drug, poisoning
poisoning —*see* Table of Drugs and Chemicals, by drug, poisoning
resistant organism infection —*see also* Resistant, organism, to, drug Z16.3Ø
therapy
long term (current) (prophylactic) —*see* Therapy, drug long-term (current) (prophylactic)
short term - omit code
wrong substance given or taken in error —*see* Table of Drugs and Chemicals, by drug, poisoning
Drunkenness (without dependence) F1Ø.129
acute in alcoholism F1Ø.229
chronic (without remission) F1Ø.2Ø
with remission F1Ø.21
pathological (without dependence) F1Ø.129
with dependence F1Ø.229
sleep F51.9
Drusen
macula (degenerative) (retina) —*see* Degeneration, macula, drusen
optic disc H47.32-
Dry, dryness —*see also* condition
larynx J38.7
mouth R68.2
due to dehydration E86.Ø
nose J34.89
socket (teeth) M27.3
throat J39.2
DSAP L56.5
Duane's syndrome H5Ø.81-
Dubin-Johnson disease or syndrome E8Ø.6
Dubois' disease (thymus gland) A5Ø.59 *[E35]*
Dubowitz' syndrome Q87.1
Duchenne-Aran muscular atrophy G12.21
Duchenne-Griesinger disease G71.Ø
Duchenne's
disease or syndrome
motor neuron disease G12.22
muscular dystrophy G71.Ø
locomotor ataxia (syphilitic) A52.11
paralysis
birth injury P14.Ø
due to or associated with
motor neuron disease G12.22
muscular dystrophy G71.Ø
Ducrey's chancre A57
Duct, ductus —*see* condition
Duhring's disease (dermatitis herpetiformis) L13.Ø
Dullness, cardiac (decreased) (increased) RØ1.2
Dumb ague —*see* Malaria
Dumbness —*see* Aphasia
Dumdum fever B55.Ø
Dumping syndrome (postgastrectomy) K91.1
Duodenitis (nonspecific) (peptic) K29.8Ø
with bleeding K29.81
Duodenocholangitis —*see* Cholangitis
Duodenum, duodenal —*see* condition
Duplay's bursitis or periarthritis —*see* Tendinitis, calcific, shoulder
Duplication, duplex —*see also* Accessory
alimentary tract Q45.8
anus Q43.4
appendix (and cecum) Q43.4
biliary duct (any) Q44.5
bladder Q64.79
cecum (and appendix) Q43.4
cervix Q51.82Ø
chromosome NEC
with complex rearrangements NEC Q92.5
seen only at prometaphase Q92.8
cystic duct Q44.5
digestive organs Q45.8
esophagus Q39.8
frontonasal process Q75.8
intestine (large) (small) Q43.4
kidney Q63.Ø
liver Q44.7
pancreas Q45.3
penis Q55.69
respiratory organs NEC Q34.8
salivary duct Q38.4
spinal cord (incomplete) Q06.2
stomach Q4Ø.2
Dupré's disease (meningism) R29.1
Dupuytren's contraction or disease M72.Ø
Durand-Nicolas-Favre disease A55
Durotomy (inadvertent) (incidental) G97.41
Duroziez's disease (congenital mitral stenosis) Q23.2
Dutton's relapsing fever (West African) A68.1
Dwarfism E34.3
achondroplastic Q77.4
congenital E34.3
constitutional E34.3
hypochondroplastic Q77.4
hypophyseal E23.Ø
infantile E34.3
Laron-type E34.3
Lorain (-Levi) type E23.Ø
metatropic Q77.8
nephrotic-glycosuric (with hypophosphatemic rickets) E72.Ø9
nutritional E45
pancreatic K86.89 ⇐
pituitary E23.Ø
renal N25.Ø
thanatophoric Q77.1
Dyke-Young anemia (secondary) (symptomatic) D59.1
Dysacusis —*see* Abnormal, auditory perception
Dysadrenocortism E27.9
hyperfunction E27.Ø
Dysarthria R47.1
following
cerebral infarction I69.322
cerebrovascular disease I69.922
specified disease NEC I69.822
intracerebral hemorrhage I69.122
nontraumatic intracranial hemorrhage NEC I69.222
subarachnoid hemorrhage I69.Ø22
Dysautonomia (familial) G9Ø.1
Dysbarism T7Ø.3
Dysbasia R26.2
angiosclerotica intermittens I73.9
hysterical F44.4
lordotica (progressiva) G24.1
nonorganic origin F44.4
psychogenic F44.4
Dysbetalipoproteinemia (familial) E78.2
Dyscalculia R48.8
developmental F81.2
Dyschezia K59.ØØ
Dyschondroplasia (with hemangiomata) Q78.4
Dyschromia (skin) L81.9
Dyscollagenosis M35.9
Dyscranio-pygo-phalangy Q87.Ø
Dyscrasia
blood (with) D75.9
antepartum hemorrhage —*see* Hemorrhage, antepartum, with coagulation defect
intrapartum hemorrhage O67.Ø
newborn P61.9
specified type NEC P61.8
puerperal, postpartum O72.3
polyglandular, pluriglandular E31.9
Dysendocrinism E34.9
Dysentery, dysenteric (catarrhal) (diarrhea) (epidemic) (hemorrhagic) (infectious) (sporadic) (tropical) AØ9
abscess, liver AØ6.4
amebic —*see also* Amebiasis AØ6.Ø
with abscess —*see* Abscess, amebic
acute AØ6.Ø
chronic AØ6.1
arthritis —*see also* category MØ1 AØ9
bacillary —*see also* category MØ1 AØ3.9
bacillary AØ3.9
arthritis —*see also* category MØ1 AØ3.9
Boyd AØ3.2
Flexner AØ3.1
Schmitz (-Stutzer) AØ3.Ø
Shiga (-Kruse) AØ3.Ø
Shigella AØ3.9
boydii AØ3.2
dysenteriae AØ3.Ø
flexneri AØ3.1
group A AØ3.Ø
group B AØ3.1
group C AØ3.2
group D AØ3.3
sonnei AØ3.3
specified type NEC AØ3.8
Sonne AØ3.3
specified type NEC AØ3.8
balantidial AØ7.Ø
Balantidium coli AØ7.Ø
Boyd's AØ3.2
candidal B37.82
Chilomastix AØ7.8
Chinese AØ3.9
coccidial AØ7.3
Dientamoeba (fragilis) AØ7.8
Embadomonas AØ7.8
Entamoeba, entamebic —*see* Dysentery, amebic
Flexner-Boyd AØ3.2
Flexner's AØ3.1

Dysentery, dysenteric *(Continued)*
Giardia lamblia A07.1
Hiss-Russell A03.1
Lamblia A07.1
leishmanial B55.0
malarial —*see* Malaria
metazoal B82.0
monilial B37.82
protozoal A07.9
Salmonella A02.0
schistosomal B65.1
Schmitz (-Stutzer) A03.0
Shiga (-Kruse) A03.0
Shigella NOS —*see* Dysentery, bacillary
Sonne A03.3
strongyloidiasis B78.0
trichomonal A07.8
viral —*see also* Enteritis, viral A08.4
Dysequilibrium R42
Dysesthesia R20.8
hysterical F44.6
Dysfibrinogenemia (congenital) D68.2
Dysfunction
adrenal E27.9
hyperfunction E27.0
autonomic
due to alcohol G31.2
somatoform F45.8
bladder N31.9
neurogenic NOS —*see* Dysfunction, bladder, neuromuscular
neuromuscular NOS N31.9
atonic (motor) (sensory) N31.2
autonomous N31.2
flaccid N31.2
nonreflex N31.2
reflex N31.1
specified NEC N31.8
uninhibited N31.0
bleeding, uterus N93.8
cerebral G93.89
colon K59.9
psychogenic F45.8
colostomy K94.03
cystic duct K82.8
cystostomy (stoma) —*see* Complications, cystostomy
ejaculatory N53.19
anejaculatory orgasm N53.13
painful N53.12
premature F52.4
retarded N53.11
endocrine NOS E34.9
endometrium N85.8
enterostomy K94.13
erectile —*see* Dysfunction, sexual, male, erectile ◀
gallbladder K82.8
gastrostomy (stoma) K94.23
gland, glandular NOS E34.9
heart I51.89
hemoglobin D75.89
hepatic K76.89
hypophysis E23.7
hypothalamic NEC E23.3
ileostomy (stoma) K94.13
jejunostomy (stoma) K94.13
kidney —*see* Disease, renal
labyrinthine —*see* subcategory H83.2
left ventricular, following sudden emotional stress I51.81
liver K76.89
male —*see* Dysfunction, sexual, male
orgasmic (female) F52.31
male F52.32
ovary E28.9
specified NEC E28.8
papillary muscle I51.89
parathyroid E21.4
physiological NEC R68.89
psychogenic F59

Dysfunction *(Continued)*
pineal gland E34.8
pituitary (gland) E23.3
platelets D69.1
polyglandular E31.9
specified NEC E31.8
psychophysiologic F59
psychosexual F52.9
with
dyspareunia F52.6
premature ejaculation F52.4
vaginismus F52.5
pylorus K31.9
rectum K59.9
psychogenic F45.8
reflex (sympathetic) —*see* Syndrome, pain, complex regional I
segmental —*see* Dysfunction, somatic
senile R54
sexual (due to) R37
alcohol F10.981
amphetamine F15.981
in
abuse F15.181
dependence F15.281
anxiolytic F13.981
in
abuse F13.181
dependence F13.281
cocaine F14.981
in
abuse F14.181
dependence F14.281
excessive sexual drive F52.8
failure of genital response (male) F52.21
female F52.22
female N94.9
aversion F52.1
dyspareunia N94.10 ◀
psychogenic F52.6
frigidity F52.22
nymphomania F52.8
orgasmic F52.31
psychogenic F52.9
aversion F52.1
dyspareunia F52.6
frigidity F52.22
nymphomania F52.8
orgasmic F52.31
vaginismus F52.5
vaginismus N94.2
psychogenic F52.5
hypnotic F13.981
in
abuse F13.181
dependence F13.281
inhibited orgasm (female) F52.31
male F52.32
lack
of sexual enjoyment F52.1
or loss of sexual desire F52.0
male N53.9
anejaculatory orgasm N53.13
ejaculatory N53.19
painful N53.12
premature F52.4
retarded N53.11
erectile N52.9
drug induced N52.2
due to
disease classified elsewhere N52.1
drug N52.2
postoperative (postprocedural) N52.39
following
cryotherapy N52.37 ◀
interstitial seed therapy N52.36 ◀
prostate ablative therapy N52.37 ◀
prostatectomy N52.34
radical N52.31

Dysfunction *(Continued)*
sexual *(Continued)*
male *(Continued)*
erectile *(Continued)*
postoperative *(Continued)*
following *(Continued)*
radiation therapy N52.35 ◀
radical cystectomy N52.32
ultrasound ablative therapy N52.37 ◀
urethral surgery N52.33
psychogenic F52.21
specified cause NEC N52.8
vasculogenic
arterial insufficiency N52.01
with corporo-venous occlusive N52.03
corporo-venous occlusive N52.02
with arterial insufficiency N52.03
impotence —*see* Dysfunction, sexual, male, erectile
psychogenic F52.9
aversion F52.1
erectile F52.21
orgasmic F52.32
premature ejaculation F52.4
satyriasis F52.8
specified type NEC F52.8
specified type NEC N53.8
nonorganic F52.9
specified NEC F52.8
opioid F11.981
in
abuse F11.181
dependence F11.281
orgasmic dysfunction (female) F52.31
male F52.32
premature ejaculation F52.4
psychoactive substances NEC F19.981
in
abuse F19.181
dependence F19.281
psychogenic F52.9
sedative F13.981
in
abuse F13.181
dependence F13.281
sexual aversion F52.1
vaginismus (nonorganic) (psychogenic) F52.5
sinoatrial node I49.5
somatic M99.09
abdomen M99.09
acromioclavicular M99.07
cervical region M99.01
cervicothoracic M99.01
costochondral M99.08
costovertebral M99.08
head region M99.00
hip M99.05
lower extremity M99.06
lumbar region M99.03
lumbosacral M99.03
occipitocervical M99.00
pelvic region M99.05
pubic M99.05
rib cage M99.08
sacral region M99.04
sacrococcygeal M99.04
sacroiliac M99.04
specified NEC M99.09
sternochondral M99.08
sternoclavicular M99.07
thoracic region M99.02
thoracolumbar M99.02
upper extremity M99.07
somatoform autonomic F45.8
stomach K31.89
psychogenic F45.8
suprarenal E27.9
hyperfunction E27.0

◀ New ◀ Revised ~~deleted~~ Deleted

Dysfunction *(Continued)*
symbolic R48.9
specified type NEC R48.8
temporomandibular (joint) M26.69
joint-pain syndrome M26.62-
testicular (endocrine) E29.9
specified NEC E29.8
thymus E32.9
thyroid E07.9
ureterostomy (stoma) —*see* Complications, stoma, urinary tract
urethrostomy (stoma) —*see* Complications, stoma, urinary tract
uterus, complicating delivery O62.9
hypertonic O62.4
hypotonic O62.2
primary O62.0
secondary O62.1
ventricular I51.9
with congestive heart failure I50.9-
left, reversible, following sudden emotional stress I51.81
Dysgenesis
gonadal (due to chromosomal anomaly) Q96.9
pure Q99.1
renal Q60.5
bilateral Q60.4
unilateral Q60.3
reticular D72.0
tidal platelet D69.3
Dysgerminoma
specified site —*see* Neoplasm, malignant, by site
unspecified site
female C56.9
male C62.90
Dysgeusia R43.2
Dysgraphia R27.8
Dyshidrosis, dysidrosis L30.1
Dyskaryotic cervical smear R87.619
Dyskeratosis L85.8
cervix —*see* Dysplasia, cervix
congenital Q82.8
uterus NEC N85.8
Dyskinesia G24.9
biliary (cystic duct or gallbladder) K82.8
drug induced
orofacial G24.01
esophagus K22.4
hysterical F44.4
intestinal K59.8
nonorganic origin F44.4
orofacial (idiopathic) G24.4
drug induced G24.01
psychogenic F44.4
subacute, drug induced G24.01
tardive G24.01
neuroleptic induced G24.01
trachea J39.8
tracheobronchial J98.09
Dyslalia (developmental) F80.0
Dyslexia R48.0
developmental F81.0
Dyslipidemia E78.5
depressed HDL cholesterol E78.6
elevated fasting triglycerides E78.1
Dysmaturity —*see also* Light for dates
pulmonary (newborn) (Wilson-Mikity) P27.0
Dysmenorrhea (essential) (exfoliative) N94.6
congestive (syndrome) N94.6
primary N94.4
psychogenic F45.8
secondary N94.5
Dysmetabolic syndrome X E88.81
Dysmetria R27.8
Dysmorphism (due to)
alcohol Q86.0
exogenous cause NEC Q86.8
hydantoin Q86.1
warfarin Q86.2
Dysmorphophobia (nondelusional) F45.22
delusional F22
Dysnomia R47.01
Dysorexia R63.0
psychogenic F50.89
Dysostosis
cleidocranial, cleidocranialis Q74.0
craniofacial Q75.1
Fairbank's (idiopathic familial generalized osteophytosis) Q78.9
mandibulofacial (incomplete) Q75.4
multiplex E76.01
oculomandibular Q75.5
Dyspareunia (female) N94.10
deep N94.12
male N53.12
nonorganic F52.6
psychogenic F52.6
secondary N94.19
specified NEC N94.19
superficial (introital) N94.11
Dyspepsia R10.13
atonic K30
functional (allergic) (congenital) (gastrointestinal) (occupational) (reflex) K30
intestinal K59.8
nervous F45.8
neurotic F45.8
psychogenic F45.8
Dysphagia R13.10
cervical R13.19
following
cerebral infarction I69.391
cerebrovascular disease I69.991
specified NEC I69.891
intracerebral hemorrhage I69.191
nontraumatic intracranial hemorrhage NEC I69.291
specified disease NEC I69.891
subarachnoid hemorrhage I69.091
functional (hysterical) F45.8
hysterical F45.8
nervous (hysterical) F45.8
neurogenic R13.19
oral phase R13.11
oropharyngeal phase R13.12
pharyneal phase R13.13
pharyngoesophageal phase R13.14
psychogenic F45.8
sideropenic D50.1
spastica K22.4
specified NEC R13.19
Dysphagocytosis, congenital D71
Dysphasia R47.02
developmental
expressive type F80.1
receptive type F80.2
following
cerebrovascular disease I69.921
cerebral infarction I69.321
intracerebral hemorrhage I69.121
nontraumatic intracranial hemorrhage NEC I69.221
specified disease NEC I69.821
subarachnoid hemorrhage I69.021
Dysphonia R49.0
functional F44.4
hysterical F44.4
psychogenic F44.4
spastica J38.3
~~Dysphoria, postpartal O90.6~~
Dysphoria
gender
in
adolescence and adulthood F64.0
children F64.2
postpartal O90.6
Dyspituitarism E23.3
Dysplasia —*see also* Anomaly
acetabular, congenital Q65.89
alveolar capillary, with vein misalignment J84.843
anus (histologically confirmed) (mild) (moderate) K62.82
severe D01.3
arrhythmogenic right ventricular I42.8
arterial, fibromuscular I77.3
asphyxiating thoracic (congenital) Q77.2
brain Q07.9
bronchopulmonary, perinatal P27.1
cervix (uteri) N87.9
mild N87.0
moderate N87.1
severe D06.9
chondroectodermal Q77.6
colon D12.6
craniometaphyseal Q78.58
dentinal K00.5
diaphyseal, progressive Q78.3
dystrophic Q77.5
ectodermal (anhidrotic) (congenital) (hereditary) Q82.4
hydrotic Q82.8
epithelial, uterine cervix —*see* Dysplasia, cervix
eye (congenital) Q11.2
fibrous
bone NEC (monostotic) M85.00
ankle M85.07-
foot M85.07-
forearm M85.03-
hand M85.04-
lower leg M85.06-
multiple site M85.09
neck M85.08
rib M85.08
shoulder M85.01-
skull M85.08
specified site NEC M85.08
thigh M85.05-
toe M85.07-
upper arm M85.02-
vertebra M85.08
diaphyseal, progressive Q78.3
jaw M27.8
polyostotic Q78.1
florid osseous —*see also* Cyst, calcifying odontogenic
high grade, focal D12.6
hip, congenital Q65.89
joint, congenital Q74.8
kidney Q61.4
multicystic Q61.4
leg Q74.2
lung, congenital (not associated with short gestation) Q33.6
mammary (gland) (benign) N60.9-
cyst (solitary) —*see* Cyst, breast
cystic —*see* Mastopathy, cystic
duct ectasia —*see* Ectasia, mammary duct
fibroadenosis —*see* Fibroadenosis, breast
fibrosclerosis —*see* Fibrosclerosis, breast
specified type NEC N60.8-
metaphyseal Q78.5
muscle Q79.8
oculodentodigital Q87.0
periapical (cemental) (cemento-osseous) —*see* Cyst, calcifying odontogenic
periosteum —*see* Disorder, bone, specified type NEC
polyostotic fibrous Q78.1
prostate —*see also* Neoplasia, intraepithelial, prostate N42.30
severe D07.5
specified NEC N42.39
renal Q61.4
multicystic Q61.4
retinal, congenital Q14.1

Dysplasia *(Continued)*
right ventricular, arrhythmogenic I42.8
septo-optic Q04.4
skin L98.8
spinal cord Q06.1
spondyloepiphyseal Q77.7
thymic, with immunodeficiency D82.1
vagina N89.3
mild N89.0
moderate N89.1
severe NEC D07.2
vulva N90.3
mild N90.0
moderate N90.1
severe NEC D07.1
Dyspnea (nocturnal) (paroxysmal) R06.00
asthmatic (bronchial) J45.909
with
bronchitis J45.909
with
exacerbation (acute) J45.901
status asthmaticus J45.902
chronic J44.9
exacerbation (acute) J45.901
status asthmaticus J45.902
cardiac —*see* Failure, ventricular, left
cardiac —*see* Failure, ventricular, left
functional F45.8
hyperventilation R06.4
hysterical F45.8
newborn P28.89
psychogenic F45.8
shortness of breath R06.02
specified type NEC R06.09
Dyspraxia R27.8
developmental (syndrome) F82
Dysproteinemia E88.09
Dysreflexia, autonomic G90.4
Dysrhythmia
cardiac I49.9
newborn
bradycardia P29.12
occurring before birth P03.819
before onset of labor P03.810
during labor P03.811
tachycardia P29.11
postoperative I97.89
cerebral or cortical —*see* Epilepsy
Dyssomnia —*see* Disorder, sleep
Dyssynergia
biliary K83.8
bladder sphincter N36.44
cerebellaris myoclonica (Hunt's ataxia) G11.1
Dysthymia F34.1
Dysthyroidism E07.9
Dystocia O66.9
affecting newborn P03.1
cervical (hypotonic) O62.2
affecting newborn P03.6
primary O62.0
secondary O62.1
contraction ring O62.4
Dystocia *(Continued)*
fetal O66.9
abnormality NEC O66.3
conjoined twins O66.3
oversize O66.2
maternal O66.9
positional O64.9
shoulder (girdle) O66.0
causing obstructed labor O66.0
uterine NEC O62.4
Dystonia G24.9
deformans progressiva G24.1
drug induced NEC G24.09
acute G24.02
specified NEC G24.09
familial G24.1
idiopathic G24.1
familial G24.1
nonfamilial G24.2
orofacial G24.4
lenticularis G24.8
musculorum deformans G24.1
neuroleptic induced (acute) G24.02
orofacial (idiopathic) G24.4
oromandibular G24.4
due to drug G24.01
specified NEC G24.8
torsion (familial) (idiopathic) G24.1
acquired G24.8
genetic G24.1
symptomatic (nonfamilial) G24.2
Dystonic movements R25.8
Dystrophy, dystrophia
adiposogenital E23.6
Becker's type G71.0
cervical sympathetic G90.2
choroid (hereditary) H31.20
central areolar H31.22
choroideremia H31.21
gyrate atrophy H31.23
specified type NEC H31.29
cornea (hereditary) H18.50
endothelial H18.51
epithelial H18.52
granular H18.53
lattice H18.54
macular H18.55
specified type NEC H18.59
Duchenne's type G71.0
due to malnutrition E45
Erb's G71.0
Fuchs' H18.51
Gower's muscular G71.0
hair L67.8
infantile neuraxonal G31.89
Landouzy-Déjérine G71.0
Leyden-Möbius G71.0
muscular G71.0
benign (Becker type) G71.0
congenital (hereditary) (progressive) (with specific morphological abnormalities of the muscle fiber) G71.0
myotonic G71.11
Dystrophy, dystrophia *(Continued)*
muscular *(Continued)*
distal G71.0
Duchenne type G71.0
Emery-Dreifuss G71.0
Erb type G71.0
facioscapulohumeral G71.0
Gower's G71.0
hereditary (progressive) G71.0
Landouzy-Déjérine type G71.0
limb-girdle G71.0
myotonic G71.11
progressive (hereditary) G71.0
Charcot-Marie (-Tooth) type G60.0
pseudohypertrophic (infantile) G71.0
severe (Duchenne type) G71.0
myocardium, myocardial —*see* Degeneration, myocardial
nail L60.3
congenital Q84.6
nutritional E45
ocular G71.0
oculocerebrorenal E72.03
oculopharyngeal G71.0
ovarian N83.8
polyglandular E31.8
reflex (neuromuscular) (sympathetic) —*see* Syndrome, pain, complex regional I
retinal (hereditary) H35.50
in
lipid storage disorders E75.6 *[H36]*
systemic lipidoses E75.6 *[H36]*
involving
pigment epithelium H35.54
sensory area H35.53
pigmentary H35.52
vitreoretinal H35.51
Salzmann's nodular —*see* Degeneration, cornea, nodular
scapuloperoneal G71.0
skin NEC L98.8
sympathetic (reflex) —*see* Syndrome, pain, complex regional I
cervical G90.2
tapetoretinal H35.54
thoracic, asphyxiating Q77.2
unguium L60.3
congenital Q84.6
vitreoretinal H35.51
vulva N90.4
yellow (liver) —*see* Failure, hepatic
Dysuria R30.0
psychogenic F45.8

E

Eales' disease H35.06-
Ear —*see also* condition
piercing Z41.3
~~tropical B36.8~~
tropical NEC B36.9 *[H62.40]* ◀
in ◀
aspergillosis B44.89 ◀
candidiasis B37.84 ◀
moniliasis B37.84 ◀
wax (impacted) H61.20
left H61.22
with right H61.23
right H61.21
with left H61.23
Earache —*see* subcategory H92.0
Early satiety R68.81
Eaton-Lambert syndrome—*see* Syndrome, Lambert-Eaton
Eberth's disease (typhoid fever) A01.00
Ebola virus disease A98.4
Ebstein's anomaly or syndrome (heart) Q22.5
Eccentro-osteochondrodysplasia E76.29
Ecchondroma —*see* Neoplasm, bone, benign
Ecchondrosis D48.0
Ecchymosis R58
conjunctiva —*see* Hemorrhage, conjunctiva
eye (traumatic) —*see* Contusion, eyeball
eyelid (traumatic) —*see* Contusion, eyelid
newborn P54.5
spontaneous R23.3
traumatic —*see* Contusion
Echinococciasis —*see* Echinococcus
Echinococcosis —*see* Echinococcus
Echinococcus (infection) B67.90
granulosus B67.4
bone B67.2
liver B67.0
lung B67.1
multiple sites B67.32
specified site NEC B67.39
thyroid B67.31 ⬅
liver NOS B67.8
granulosus B67.0
multilocularis B67.5
lung NEC B67.99
granulosus B67.1
multilocularis B67.69
multilocularis B67.7
liver B67.5
multiple sites B67.61
specified site NEC B67.69
specified site NEC B67.99
granulosus B67.39
multilocularis B67.69
thyroid NEC B67.99
granulosus B67.31 ⬅
multilocularis B67.69 *[E35]*
Echinorhynchiasis B83.8
Echinostomiasis B66.8
Echolalia R48.8
Echovirus, as cause of disease classified elsewhere B97.12
Eclampsia, eclamptic (coma) (convulsions) (delirium) (with hypertension) NEC O15.9
complicating ◀
labor and delivery O15.1 ◀
postpartum O15.2 ◀
pregnancy O15.0- ◀
puerperium O15.2 ◀
~~during labor and delivery O15.1~~
~~postpartum O15.2~~
~~pregnancy O15.0-~~
~~puerperal O15.2~~
Economic circumstances affecting care Z59.9
Economo's disease A85.8
Ectasia, ectasis
annuloaortic I35.8
aorta I77.819
with aneurysm —*see* Aneurysm, aorta
abdominal I77.811
Ectasia, ectasis *(Continued)*
aorta *(Continued)*
thoracic I77.810
thoracoabdominal I77.812
breast —*see* Ectasia, mammary duct
capillary I78.8
cornea H18.71-
gastric antral vascular (GAVE) K31.819
with hemorrhage K31.811
without hemorrhage K31.819
mammary duct N60.4-
salivary gland (duct) K11.8
sclera —*see* Sclerectasia
Ecthyma L08.0
contagiosum B08.02
gangrenosum L08.0
infectiosum B08.02
Ectocardia Q24.8
Ectodermal dysplasia (anhidrotic) Q82.4
Ectodermosis erosiva pluriorificialis L51.1
Ectopic, ectopia (congenital)
abdominal viscera Q45.8
due to defect in anterior abdominal wall Q79.59
ACTH syndrome E24.3
adrenal gland Q89.1
anus Q43.5
atrial beats I49.1
beats I49.49
atrial I49.1
ventricular I49.3
bladder Q64.10
bone and cartilage in lung Q33.5
brain Q04.8
breast tissue Q83.8
cardiac Q24.8
cerebral Q04.8
cordis Q24.8
endometrium —*see* Endometriosis
gastric mucosa Q40.2
gestation —*see* Pregnancy, by site
heart Q24.8
hormone secretion NEC E34.2
kidney (crossed) (pelvis) Q63.2
lens, lentis Q12.1
mole —*see* Pregnancy, by site
organ or site NEC —*see* Malposition, congenital
pancreas Q45.3
pregnancy —*see* Pregnancy, ectopic
pupil —*see* Abnormality, pupillary
renal Q63.2
sebaceous glands of mouth Q38.6
spleen Q89.09
testis Q53.00
bilateral Q53.02
unilateral Q53.01
thyroid Q89.2
tissue in lung Q33.5
ureter Q62.63
ventricular beats I49.3
vesicae Q64.10
Ectromelia Q73.8
lower limb —*see* Defect, reduction, limb, lower, specified type NEC
upper limb —*see* Defect, reduction, limb, upper, specified type NEC
Ectropion H02.109
cervix N86
with cervicitis N72
congenital Q10.1
eyelid (paralytic) H02.109
cicatricial H02.119
left H02.116
lower H02.115
upper H02.114
right H02.113
lower H02.112
upper H02.111
congenital Q10.1
Ectropion *(Continued)*
eyelid *(Continued)*
left H02.106
lower H02.105
upper H02.104
mechanical H02.129
left H02.126
lower H02.125
upper H02.124
right H02.123
lower H02.122
upper H02.121
right H02.103
lower H02.102
upper H02.101
senile H02.139
left H02.136
lower H02.135
upper H02.134
right H02.133
lower H02.132
upper H02.131
spastic H02.149
left H02.146
lower H02.145
upper H02.144
right H02.143
lower H02.142
upper H02.141
iris H21.89
lip (acquired) K13.0
congenital Q38.0
urethra N36.8
uvea H21.89
Eczema (acute) (chronic) (erythematous) (fissum) (rubrum) (squamous) (*see also* Dermatitis) L30.9
contact —*see* Dermatitis, contact
dyshydrotic L30.1
external ear —*see* Otitis, externa, acute, eczematoid
flexural L20.82
herpeticum B00.0
hypertrophicum L28.0
hypostatic —*see* Varix, leg, with, inflammation
impetiginous L01.1
infantile (due to any substance) L20.83
intertriginous L21.1
seborrheic L21.1
intertriginous NEC L30.4
infantile L21.1
intrinsic (allergic) L20.84
lichenified NEC L28.0
marginatum (hebrae) B35.6
pustular L30.3
stasis I87.2 ⬅
with varicose veins —*see* Varix, leg, with, inflammation ◀
vaccination, vaccinatum T88.1
varicose —*see* Varix, leg, with, inflammation
Eczematid L30.2
Eddowes (-Spurway) syndrome Q78.0
Edema, edematous (infectious) (pitting) (toxic) R60.9
with nephritis —*see* Nephrosis
allergic T78.3
amputation stump (surgical) (sequelae (late effect)) T87.89
angioneurotic (allergic) (any site) (with urticaria) T78.3
hereditary D84.1
angiospastic I73.9
Berlin's (traumatic) S05.8X-
brain (cytotoxic) (vasogenic) G93.6
due to birth injury P11.0
newborn (anoxia or hypoxia) P52.4
birth injury P11.0
traumatic —*see* Injury, intracranial, cerebral edema
cardiac —*see* Failure, heart, congestive

Edema, edematous *(Continued)*
cardiovascular —*see* Failure, heart, congestive
cerebral —*see* Edema, brain
cerebrospinal —*see* Edema, brain
cervix (uteri) (acute) N88.8
puerperal, postpartum O90.89
chronic hereditary Q82.0
circumscribed, acute T78.3
hereditary D84.1
conjunctiva H11.42-
cornea H18.2-
idiopathic H18.22-
secondary H18.23-
due to contact lens H18.21-
due to
lymphatic obstruction I89.0
salt retention E87.0
epiglottis —*see* Edema, glottis
essential, acute T78.3
hereditary D84.1
extremities, lower —*see* Edema, legs
eyelid NEC H02.849
left H02.846
lower H02.845
upper H02.844
right H02.843
lower H02.842
upper H02.841
familial, hereditary Q82.0
famine —*see* Malnutrition, severe
generalized R60.1
glottis, glottic, glottidis (obstructive) (passive) J38.4
allergic T78.3
hereditary D84.1
heart —*see* Failure, heart, congestive
heat T67.7
hereditary Q82.0
inanition —*see* Malnutrition, severe
intracranial G93.6
iris H21.89
joint —*see* Effusion, joint
larynx —*see* Edema, glottis
legs R60.0
due to venous obstruction I87.1
hereditary Q82.0
localized R60.0
due to venous obstruction I87.1
lower limbs —*see* Edema, legs
lung J81.1
with heart condition or failure —*see* Failure, ventricular, left
acute J81.0
chemical (acute) J68.1
chronic J68.1
chronic J81.1
due to
chemicals, gases, fumes or vapors (inhalation) J68.1
external agent J70.9
specified NEC J70.8
radiation J70.1
due to
chemicals, fumes or vapors (inhalation) J68.1
external agent J70.9
specified NEC J70.8
high altitude T70.29
near drowning T75.1
radiation J70.0
meaning failure, left ventricle I50.1
lymphatic I89.0
due to mastectomy I97.2
macula H35.81
cystoid, following cataract surgery —*see* Complications, postprocedural, following cataract surgery
diabetic —*see* Diabetes, by type, with, retinopathy, with macular edema
malignant —*see* Gangrene, gas
Milroy's Q82.0

Edema, edematous *(Continued)*
nasopharynx J39.2
newborn P83.30
hydrops fetalis —*see* Hydrops, fetalis
specified NEC P83.39
nutritional —*see also* Malnutrition, severe with dyspigmentation, skin and hair E40
optic disc or nerve —*see* Papilledema
orbit H05.22-
pancreas K86.89 ⇐
papilla, optic —*see* Papilledema
penis N48.89
periodic T78.3
hereditary D84.1
pharynx J39.2
pulmonary —*see* Edema, lung
Quincke's T78.3
hereditary D84.1
renal —*see* Nephrosis
retina H35.81
diabetic —*see* Diabetes, by type, with, retinopathy, with macular edema
salt E87.0
scrotum N50.89 ⇐
seminal vesicle N50.89 ⇐
spermatic cord N50.89 ⇐
spinal (cord) (vascular) (nontraumatic) G95.19
starvation —*see* Malnutrition, severe
stasis —*see* Hypertension, venous, (chronic)
subglottic —*see* Edema, glottis
supraglottic —*see* Edema, glottis
testis N44.8
tunica vaginalis N50.89 ⇐
vas deferens N50.89 ⇐
vulva (acute) N90.89
Edentulism —*see* Absence, teeth, acquired
Edsall's disease T67.2
Educational handicap Z55.9
specified NEC Z55.8
Edward's syndrome —*see* Trisomy, 18
Effect, adverse
abnormal gravitational (G) forces or states T75.81
abuse —*see* Maltreatment
air pressure T70.9
specified NEC T70.8
altitude (high) —*see* Effect, adverse, high altitude
anesthesia —*see also* Anesthesia T88.59
in labor and delivery O74.9
~~in pregnancy NEC O29.3-~~
local, toxic
in labor and delivery O74.4-
in pregnancy NEC O29.3- ◀
postpartum, puerperal O89.3
postpartum, puerperal O89.9
specified NEC T88.59
in labor and delivery O74.8
postpartum, puerperal O89.8
spinal and epidural T88.59
headache T88.59
in labor and delivery O74.5
postpartum, puerperal O89.4
specified NEC
in labor and delivery O74.6
postpartum, puerperal O89.5
antitoxin —*see* Complications, vaccination
atmospheric pressure T70.9
due to explosion T70.8
high T70.3
low —*see* Effect, adverse, high altitude
specified effect NEC T70.8
biological, correct substance properly administered —*see* Effect, adverse, drug
blood (derivatives) (serum) (transfusion) —*see* Complications, transfusion
chemical substance —*see* Table of Drugs and Chemicals
cold (temperature) (weather) T69.9
chilblains T69.1
frostbite —*see* Frostbite
specified effect NEC T69.8

Effect, adverse *(Continued)*
drugs and medicaments T88.7
specified drug —*see* Table of Drugs and Chemicals, by drug, adverse effect
specified effect — code to condition
electric current, electricity (shock) T75.4
burn —*see* Burn
exertion (excessive) T73.3
exposure —*see* Exposure
external cause NEC T75.89
foodstuffs T78.1
allergic reaction —*see* Allergy, food
causing anaphylaxis —*see* Shock, anaphylactic, due to food
noxious —*see* Poisoning, food, noxious
gases, fumes, or vapors T59.9-
specified agent —*see* Table of Drugs and Chemicals
glue (airplane) sniffing
due to drug abuse —*see* Abuse, drug, inhalant
due to drug dependence —*see* Dependence, drug, inhalant
heat —*see* Heat
high altitude NEC T70.29
anoxia T70.29
on
ears T70.0
sinuses T70.1
polycythemia D75.1
high pressure fluids T70.4
hot weather —*see* Heat
hunger T73.0
immersion, foot —*see* Immersion
immunization —*see* Complications, vaccination
immunological agents —*see* Complications, vaccination
infrared (radiation) (rays) NOS T66
dermatitis or eczema L59.8
infusion —*see* Complications, infusion
lack of care of infants —*see* Maltreatment, child
lightning —*see* Lightning
medical care T88.9
specified NEC T88.8
medicinal substance, correct, properly administered —*see* Effect, adverse, drug
motion T75.3
noise, on inner ear —*see* subcategory H83.3
overheated places —*see* Heat
psychosocial, of work environment Z56.5
radiation (diagnostic) (infrared) (natural source) (therapeutic) (ultraviolet) (X-ray) NOS T66
dermatitis or eczema —*see* Dermatitis, due to, radiation
fibrosis of lung J70.1
pneumonitis J70.0
pulmonary manifestations
acute J70.0
chronic J70.1
skin L59.9
radioactive substance NOS
dermatitis or eczema —*see* Radiodermatitis
reduced temperature T69.9
immersion foot or hand —*see* Immersion
specified effect NEC T69.8
serum NEC (*see also* Reaction, serum) T80.69
specified NEC T78.8
external cause NEC T75.89
strangulation —*see* Asphyxia, traumatic
submersion T75.1
thirst T73.1
toxic —*see* Toxicity
transfusion —*see* Complications, transfusion
ultraviolet (radiation) (rays) NOS T66
burn —*see* Burn
dermatitis or eczema —*see* Dermatitis, due to, ultraviolet rays
acute L56.8

E

◀ New ⇐ Revised ~~deleted~~ Deleted

Effect, adverse *(Continued)*
vaccine (any) —*see* Complications, vaccination
vibration —*see* Vibration, adverse effects
water pressure NEC T70.9
specified NEC T70.8
weightlessness T75.82
whole blood —*see* Complications, transfusion
work environment Z56.5
Effect (s) (of) (from) —*see* Effect, adverse NEC
Effects, late —*see* Sequelae
Effluvium
anagen L65.1
telogen L65.0
Effort syndrome (psychogenic) F45.8
Effusion
amniotic fluid —*see* Pregnancy, complicated by, prematue rupture of membranes
brain (serous) G93.6
bronchial —*see* Bronchitis
cerebral G93.6
cerebrospinal —*see also* Meningitis
vessel G93.6
chest —*see* Effusion, pleura
chylous, chyliform (pleura) J94.0
intracranial G93.6
joint M25.40
ankle M25.47-
elbow M25.42-
foot joint M25.47-
hand joint M25.44-
hip M25.45-
knee M25.46-
shoulder M25.41-
specified joint NEC M25.48
wrist M25.43-
malignant pleural J91.0
meninges —*see* Meningitis
pericardium, pericardial (noninflammatory) I31.3
acute —*see* Pericarditis, acute
peritoneal (chronic) R18.8
pleura, pleurisy, pleuritic, pleuropericardial J90
chylous, chyliform J94.0
due to systemic lupus erythematosis M32.13
influenzal —*see* Influenza, with, respiratory manifestations NEC
malignant J91.0
newborn P28.89
tuberculous NEC A15.6
primary (progressive) A15.7
spinal —*see* Meningitis
thorax, thoracic —*see* Effusion, pleura
Egg shell nails L60.3
congenital Q84.6
Egyptian splenomegaly B65.1
Ehlers-Danlos syndrome Q79.6
Ehrlichiosis A77.40
due to
E. chafeensis A77.41
E. sennetsu A79.81
specified organism NEC A77.49
Eichstedt's disease B36.0
Eisenmenger's
complex or syndrome I27.89
defect Q21.8
Ejaculation
delayed F52.32 ◀
painful N53.12
premature F52.4
retarded N53.11
retrograde N53.14
semen, painful N53.12
psychogenic F52.6
Ekbom's syndrome (restless legs) G25.81
Ekman's syndrome (brittle bones and blue sclera) Q78.0
Elastic skin Q82.8
acquired L57.4
Elastofibroma —*see* Neoplasm, connective tissue, benign
Elastoma (juvenile) Q82.8
Miescher's L87.2
Elastomyofibrosis I42.4
Elastosis
actinic, solar L57.8
atrophicans (senile) L57.4
perforans serpiginosa L87.2
senilis L57.4
Elbow —*see* condition
Electric current, electricity, effects (concussion) (fatal) (nonfatal) (shock) T75.4
burn —*see* Burn
Electric feet syndrome E53.8
Electrocution T75.4
from electroshock gun (taser) T75.4
Electrolyte imbalance E87.8
with
abortion —*see* Abortion by type, complicated by, electrolyte imbalance
ectopic pregnancy O08.5
molar pregnancy O08.5
Elephantiasis (nonfilarial) I89.0
arabicum —*see* Infestation, filarial
bancroftian B74.0
congenital (any site) (hereditary) Q82.0
due to
Brugia (malayi) B74.1
timori B74.2
mastectomy I97.2
Wuchereria (bancrofti) B74.0
eyelid H02.859
left H02.856
lower H02.855
upper H02.854
right H02.853
lower H02.852
upper H02.851
filarial, filariensis —*see* Infestation, filarial
glandular I89.0
graecorum A30.9
lymphangiectatic I89.0
lymphatic vessel I89.0
due to mastectomy I97.2
scrotum (nonfilarial) I89.0
streptococcal I89.0
surgical I97.89
postmastectomy I97.2
telangiectodes I89.0
vulva (nonfilarial) N90.89
Elevated, elevation
antibody titer R76.0
basal metabolic rate R94.8
blood pressure —*see also* Hypertension
reading (incidental) (isolated) (nonspecific), no diagnosis of hypertension R03.0
blood sugar R73.9
body temperature (of unknown origin) R50.9
C-reactive protein (CRP) R79.82
cancer antigen 125 [CA 125] R97.1
carcinoembryonic antigen [CEA] R97.0
cholesterol E78.00 ⟸
with high triglycerides E78.2
conjugate, eye H51.0
diaphragm, congenital Q79.1
erythrocyte sedimentation rate R70.0
fasting glucose R73.01
fasting triglycerides E78.1
finding on laboratory examination —*see* Findings, abnormal, inconclusive, without diagnosis, by type of exam
GFR (glomerular filtration rate) —*see* Findings, abnormal, inconclusive, without diagnosis, by type of exam
glucose tolerance (oral) R73.02
immunoglobulin level R76.8
indoleacetic acid R82.5
lactic acid dehydrogenase (LDH) level R74.0
leukocytes D72.829
lipoprotein a level E78.8
Elevated, elevation *(Continued)*
liver function
study R94.5
test R79.89
alkaline phosphatase R74.8
aminotransferase R74.0
bilirubin R17
hepatic enzyme R74.8
lactate dehydrogenase R74.0
lymphocytes D72.820
prostate specific antigen [PSA] R97.20 ⟸
Rh titer —*see* Complication (s), transfusion, incompatibility reaction, Rh (factor)
scapula, congenital Q74.0
sedimentation rate R70.0
SGOT R74.0
SGPT R74.0
transaminase level R74.0
triglycerides E78.1
with high cholesterol E78.2
tumor associated antigens [TAA] NEC R97.8
tumor specific antigens [TSA] NEC R97.8
urine level of
17-ketosteroids R82.5
catecholamine R82.5
indoleacetic acid R82.5
steroids R82.5
vanillylmandelic acid (VMA) R82.5
venous pressure I87.8
white blood cell count D72.829
specified NEC D72.828
Elliptocytosis (congenital) (hereditary) D58.1
Hb C (disease) D58.1
hemoglobin disease D58.1
sickle-cell (disease) D57.8-
trait D57.3
Ellison-Zollinger syndrome E16.4
Ellis-van Creveld syndrome (chondroectodermal dysplasia) Q77.6
Elongated, elongation (congenital) —*see also* Distortion
bone Q79.9
cervix (uteri) Q51.828
acquired N88.4
hypertrophic N88.4
colon Q43.8
common bile duct Q44.5
cystic duct Q44.5
frenulum, penis Q55.69
labia minora (acquired) N90.69 ⟸
ligamentum patellae Q74.1
petiolus (epiglottidis) Q31.8
tooth, teeth K00.2
uvula Q38.6
Eltor cholera A00.1
Emaciation (due to malnutrition) E41
Embadomoniasis A07.8
Embedded tooth, teeth K01.0
root only K08.3
Embolic —*see* condition
Embolism (multiple) (paradoxical) I74.9
air (any site) (traumatic) T79.0
following
abortion —*see* Abortion by type complicated by embolism
ectopic pregnancy O08.2
infusion, therapeutic injection or transfusion T80.0
molar pregnancy O08.2
procedure NEC
artery T81.719
mesenteric T81.710
renal T81.711
specified NEC T81.718
vein T81.72
in pregnancy, childbirth or puerperium —*see* Embolism, obstetric
amniotic fluid (pulmonary) —*see also* Embolism, obstetric
following
abortion —*see* Abortion by type complicated by embolism

E

◀ New ⟸ Revised ~~deleted~~ Deleted

Embolism *(Continued)*
amniotic fluid *(Continued)*
following *(Continued)*
ectopic pregnancy O08.2
molar pregnancy O08.2
aorta, aortic I74.10
abdominal I74.09
saddle I74.01
bifurcation I74.09
saddle I74.01
thoracic I74.11
artery I74.9
auditory, internal I65.8
basilar —*see* Occlusion, artery, basilar
carotid (common) (internal) —*see* Occlusion, artery, carotid
cerebellar (anterior inferior) (posterior inferior) (superior) I66.3
cerebral —*see* Occlusion, artery, cerebral
choroidal (anterior) I66.8
communicating posterior I66.8
coronary —*see also* Infarct, myocardium
not resulting in infarction I24.0
extremity I74.4
lower I74.3
upper I74.2
hypophyseal I66.8
iliac I74.5
limb I74.4
lower I74.3
upper I74.2
mesenteric (with gangrene) —*see also* Ischemia, intestine, acute K55.09 ◄
ophthalmic —*see* Occlusion, artery, retina
peripheral I74.4
pontine I66.8
precerebral —*see* Occlusion, artery, precerebral
pulmonary —*see* Embolism, pulmonary
renal N28.0
retinal —*see* Occlusion, artery, retina
septic I76
specified NEC I74.8
vertebral —*see* Occlusion, artery, vertebral
basilar (artery) I65.1
blood clot
following
abortion —*see* Abortion by type complicated by embolism
ectopic or molar pregnancy O08.2
in pregnancy, childbirth or puerperium —*see* Embolism, obstetric
brain —*see also* Occlusion, artery, cerebral
following
abortion —*see* Abortion by type complicated by embolism
ectopic or molar pregnancy O08.2
puerperal, postpartum, childbirth —*see* Embolism, obstetric
capillary I78.8
cardiac —*see also* Infarct, myocardium
not resulting in infarction I51.3 ◄
carotid (artery) (common) (internal) —*see* Occlusion, artery, carotid
cavernous sinus (venous) —*see* Embolism, intracranial venous sinus
cerebral —*see* Occlusion, artery, cerebral
cholesterol —*see* Atheroembolism
coronary (artery or vein) (systemic) —*see* Occlusion, coronary
due to device, implant or graft —*see also* Complications, by site and type, specified NEC
arterial graft NEC T82.818
breast (implant) T85.818 ◄
catheter NEC T85.818 ◄
dialysis (renal) T82.818
intraperitoneal T85.818 ◄
infusion NEC T82.818
spinal (epidural) (subdural) T85.810 ◄
urinary (indwelling) T83.81

Embolism *(Continued)*
due to device, implant or graft *(Continued)*
electronic (electrode) (pulse generator) (stimulator)
bone T84.81
cardiac T82.817
nervous system (brain) (peripheral nerve) (spinal) T85.810 ◄
urinary T83.81
fixation, internal (orthopedic) NEC T84.81
gastrointestinal (bile duct) (esophagus) T85.818 ◄
genital NEC T83.81
heart (graft) (valve) T82.817
joint prosthesis T84.81
ocular (corneal graft) (orbital implant) T85.818 ◄
orthopedic (bone graft) NEC T86.838
specified NEC T85.818 ◄
urinary (graft) NEC T83.81
vascular NEC T82.818
ventricular intracranial shunt T85.810 ◄
extremities
lower —*see* Embolism, vein, lower extremity
arterial I74.3
upper I74.2
eye H34.9
fat (cerebral) (pulmonary) (systemic) T79.1
complicating delivery —*see* Embolism, obstetric
following
abortion —*see* Abortion by type complicated by embolism
ectopic or molar pregnancy O08.2
following
abortion —*see* Abortion by type complicated by embolism
ectopic or molar pregnancy O08.2
infusion, therapeutic injection or transfusion
air T80.0
heart (fatty) —*see also* Infarct, myocardium
not resulting in infarction I51.3 ◄
hepatic (vein) I82.0
in pregnancy, childbirth or puerperium —*see* Embolism, obstetric
intestine (artery) (vein) (with gangrene) —*see also* Ischemia, intestine, acute K55.039 ◄
intracranial —*see also* Occlusion, artery, cerebral
venous sinus (any) G08
nonpyogenic I67.6
intraspinal venous sinuses or veins G08
nonpyogenic G95.19
kidney (artery) N28.0
lateral sinus (venous) —*see* Embolism, intracranial, venous sinus
leg —*see* Embolism, vein, lower extremity
arterial I74.3
longitudinal sinus (venous) —*see* Embolism, intracranial, venous sinus
lung (massive) —*see* Embolism, pulmonary
meninges I66.8
mesenteric (artery) (vein) (with gangrene) —*see also* Ischemia, intestine, acute K55.059 ◄
obstetric (in) (pulmonary)
childbirth O88.22 ◄
air O88.02
amniotic fluid O88.12
blood clot O88.22
fat O88.82
pyemic O88.32
septic O88.32
specified type NEC O88.82
pregnancy O88.21- ◄
air O88.01-
amniotic fluid O88.11-
blood clot O88.21-
fat O88.81-

Embolism *(Continued)*
obstetric *(Continued)*
pregnancy *(Continued)*
pyemic O88.31-
septic O88.31-
specified type NEC O88.81-
puerperal O88.23 ◄
air O88.03
amniotic fluid O88.13
blood clot O88.23
fat O88.83
pyemic O88.33
septic O88.33
specified type NEC O88.83
ophthalmic —*see* Occlusion, artery, retina
penis N48.81
peripheral artery NOS I74.4
pituitary E23.6
popliteal (artery) I74.3
portal (vein) I81
postoperative, postprocedural
artery T81.719
mesenteric T81.710
renal T81.711
specified NEC T81.718
vein T81.72
precerebral artery —*see* Occlusion, artery, precerebral
puerperal —*see* Embolism, obstetric
pulmonary (acute) (artery) (vein) I26.99
with acute cor pulmonale I26.09
chronic I27.82
following
abortion —*see* Abortion by type complicated by embolism
ectopic or molar pregnancy O08.2
healed or old Z86.711
in pregnancy, childbirth or puerperium —*see* Embolism, obstetric
personal history of Z86.711
saddle I26.92
with acute cor pulmonale I26.02
septic I26.90
with acute cor pulmonale I26.01
pyemic (multiple) I76
following
abortion —*see* Abortion by type complicated by embolism
ectopic or molar pregnancy O08.2
Hemophilus influenzae A41.3
pneumococcal A40.3
with pneumonia J13
puerperal, postpartum, childbirth (any organism) —*see* Embolism, obstetric
specified organism NEC A41.89
staphylococcal A41.2
streptococcal A40.9
renal (artery) N28.0
vein I82.3
retina, retinal —*see* Occlusion, artery, retina
saddle
abdominal aorta I74.01
pulmonary artery I26.92
with acute cor pulmonale I26.02
septic (arterial) I76
complicating abortion —*see* Abortion, by type, complicated by, embolism
sinus —*see* Embolism, intracranial, venous sinus
soap complicating abortion —*see* Abortion, by type, complicated by, embolism
spinal cord G95.19
pyogenic origin G06.1
spleen, splenic (artery) I74.8
upper extremity I74.2
vein (acute) I82.90
antecubital I82.61-
chronic I82.71-
axillary I82.A1-
chronic I82.A2-

E

◄ New ◄ Revised ~~deleted~~ Deleted

Embolism *(Continued)*
vein *(Continued)*
basilic I82.61-
chronic I82.71-
brachial I82.62-
chronic I82.72-
brachiocephalic (innominate) I82.290
chronic I82.291
cephalic I82.61-
chronic I82.71-
chronic I82.91
deep (DVT) I82.40-
calf I82.4Z-
chronic I82.5Z-
lower leg I82.4Z-
chronic I82.5Z-
thigh I82.4Y-
chronic I82.5Y-
upper leg I82.4Y
chronic I82.5y--
femoral I82.41-
chronic I82.51-
iliac (iliofemoral) I82.42-
chronic I82.52-
innominate I82.290
chronic I82.291
internal jugular I82.C1-
chronic I82.C2-
lower extremity
deep I82.40-
chronic I82.50-
specified NEC I82.49-
chronic NEC I82.59-
distal
deep I82.4Z-
proximal
deep I82.4Y-
chronic I82.5Y-
superficial I82.81-
popliteal I82.43-
chronic I82.53-
radial I82.62-
chronic I82.72-
renal I82.3
saphenous (greater) (lesser) I82.81-
specified NEC I82.890
chronic NEC I82.891
subclavian I82.B1-
chronic I82.B2-
thoracic NEC I82.290
chronic I82.291
tibial I82.44-
chronic I82.54-
ulnar I82.62-
chronic I82.72-
upper extremity I82.60-
chronic I82.70-
deep I82.62-
chronic I82.72-
superficial I82.61-
chronic I82.71-
vena cava
inferior (acute) I82.220
chronic I82.221
superior (acute) I82.210
chronic I82.211
venous sinus G08
vessels of brain —*see* Occlusion, artery, cerebral
Embolus —*see* Embolism
Embryoma —*see also* Neoplasm, uncertain behavior, by site
benign —*see* Neoplasm, benign, by site
kidney C64.-
liver C22.0
malignant —*see also* Neoplasm, malignant, by site
kidney C64.-
liver C22.0
testis C62.9-
descended (scrotal) C62.1-
undescended C62.0-

Embryoma *(Continued)*
testis C62.9-
descended (scrotal) C62.1-
undescended C62.0-
Embryonic
circulation Q28.9
heart Q28.9
vas deferens Q55.4
Embryopathia NOS Q89.9
Embryotoxon Q13.4
Emesis —*see* Vomiting
Emotional lability R45.86
Emotionality, pathological F60.3
Emotogenic disease —*see* Disorder, psychogenic
Emphysema (atrophic) (bullous) (chronic) (interlobular) (lung) (obstructive) (pulmonary) (senile) (vesicular) J43.9
cellular tissue (traumatic) T79.7
surgical T81.82
centrilobular J43.2
compensatory J98.3
congenital (interstitial) P25.0
conjunctiva H11.89
connective tissue (traumatic) T79.7
surgical T81.82
due to chemicals, gases, fumes or vapors J68.4
eyelid (s) —*see* Disorder, eyelid, specified type NEC
surgical T81.82
traumatic T79.7
interstitial J98.2
congenital P25.0
perinatal period P25.0
laminated tissue T79.7
surgical T81.82
mediastinal J98.2
newborn P25.2
orbit, orbital —*see* Disorder, orbit, specified type NEC
panacinar J43.1
panlobular J43.1
specified NEC J43.8
subcutaneous (traumatic) T79.7
nontraumatic J98.2
postprocedural T81.82
surgical T81.82
surgical T81.82
thymus (gland) (congenital) E32.8
traumatic (subcutaneous) T79.7
unilateral J43.0
Empty nest syndrome Z60.0
Empyema (acute) (chest) (double) (pleura) (supradiaphragmatic) (thorax) J86.9
with fistula J86.0
accessory sinus (chronic) —*see* Sinusitis
antrum (chronic) —*see* Sinusitis, maxillary
brain (any part) —*see* Abscess, brain
ethmoidal (chronic) (sinus) —*see* Sinusitis, ethmoidal
extradural —*see* Abscess, extradural
frontal (chronic) (sinus) —*see* Sinusitis, frontal
gallbladder K81.0
mastoid (process) (acute) —*see* Mastoiditis, acute
maxilla, maxillary M27.2
sinus (chronic) —*see* Sinusitis, maxillary
nasal sinus (chronic) —*see* Sinusitis
sinus (accessory) (chronic) (nasal) —*see* Sinusitis
sphenoidal (sinus) (chronic) —*see* Sinusitis, sphenoidal
subarachnoid —*see* Abscess, extradural
subdural —*see* Abscess, subdural
tuberculous A15.6
ureter —*see* Ureteritis
ventricular —*see* Abscess, brain

En coup de sabre lesion L94.1
Enamel pearls K00.2
Enameloma K00.2
Enanthema, viral B09
Encephalitis (chronic) (hemorrhagic) (idiopathic) (nonepidemic) (spurious) (subacute) G04.90
acute —*see also* Encephalitis, viral A86
disseminated G04.00
infectious G04.01
noninfectious G04.81
postimmunization (postvaccination) G04.02
postinfectious G04.01
inclusion body A85.8
necrotizing hemorrhagic G04.30
postimmunization G04.32
postinfectious G04.31
specified NEC G04.39
arboviral, arbovirus NEC A85.2
arthropod-borne NEC (viral) A85.2
Australian A83.4
California (virus) A83.5
Central European (tick-borne) A84.1
Czechoslovakian A84.1
Dawson's (inclusion body) A81.1
diffuse sclerosing A81.1
disseminated, acute G04.00
due to
cat scratch disease A28.1
human immunodeficiency virus (HIV) disease B20 *[G05.3]*
malaria —*see* Malaria
rickettsiosis —*see* Rickettsiosis
smallpox inoculation G04.02
typhus —*see* Typhus
Eastern equine A83.2
endemic (viral) A86
epidemic NEC (viral) A86
equine (acute) (infectious) (viral) A83.9
Eastern A83.2
Venezuelan A92.2
Western A83.1
Far Eastern (tick-borne) A84.0
following vaccination or other immunization procedure G04.02
herpes zoster B02.0
herpesviral B00.4
due to herpesvirus 6 B10.01
due to herpesvirus 7 B10.09
specified NEC B10.09
Ilheus (virus) A83.8
in (due to)
actinomycosis A42.82
adenovirus A85.1
African trypanosomiasis B56.9 *[G05.3]*
Chagas' disease (chronic) B57.42
cytomegalovirus B25.8
enterovirus A85.0
herpes (simplex) virus B00.4
due to herpesvirus 6 B10.01
due to herpesvirus 7 B10.09
specified NEC B10.09
infectious disease NEC B99 *[G05.3]*
influenza —*see* Influenza, with, encephalopathy
listeriosis A32.12
measles B05.0
mumps B26.2
naegleriasis B60.2
parasitic disease NEC B89 *[G05.3]*
poliovirus A80.9 *[G05.3]*
rubella B06.01
syphilis
congenital A50.42
late A52.14
systemic lupus erythematosus M32.19
toxoplasmosis (acquired) B58.2
congenital P37.1
tuberculosis A17.82
zoster B02.0

Encephalitis *(Continued)*
inclusion body A81.1
infectious (acute) (virus) NEC A86
Japanese (B type) A83.0
La Crosse A83.5
lead —*see* Poisoning, lead
lethargica (acute) (infectious) A85.8
louping ill A84.8
lupus erythematosus, systemic M32.19
lymphatica A87.2
Mengo A85.8
meningococcal A39.81
Murray Valley A83.4
otitic NEC H66.40 *[G05.3]*
parasitic NOS B71.9
periaxial G37.0
periaxialis (concentrica) (diffuse) G37.5
postchickenpox B01.11
postexanthematous NEC B09
postimmunization G04.02
postinfectious NEC G04.01
postmeasles B05.0
postvaccinal G04.02
postvaricella B01.11
postviral NEC A86
Powassan A84.8
Rasmussen G04.81
Rio Bravo A85.8
Russian
autumnal A83.0
spring-summer (taiga) A84.0
saturnine —*see* Poisoning, lead
specified NEC G04.81
St. Louis A83.3
subacute sclerosing A81.1
summer A83.0
suppurative G04.81
tick-borne A84.9
Torula, torular (cryptococcal) B45.1
toxic NEC G92
trichinosis B75 *[G05.3]*
type
B A83.0
C A83.3
van Bogaert's A81.1
Venezuelan equine A92.2
Vienna A85.8
viral, virus A86
arthropod-borne NEC A85.2
mosquito-borne A83.9
Australian X disease A83.4
California virus A83.5
Eastern equine A83.2
Japanese (B type) A83.0
Murray Valley A83.4
specified NEC A83.8
St. Louis A83.3
type B A83.0
type C A83.3
Western equine A83.1
tick-borne A84.9
biundulant A84.1
central European A84.1
Czechoslovakian A84.1
diphasic meningoencephalitis A84.1
Far Eastern A84.0
Russian spring-summer (taiga) A84.0
specified NEC A84.8
specified type NEC A85.8
Western equine A83.1
Encephalocele Q01.9
frontal Q01.0
nasofrontal Q01.1
occipital Q01.2
specified NEC Q01.8
Encephalocystocele —*see* Encephalocele
Encephaloduroarteriomyosynangiosis (EDAMS) I67.5
Encephalomalacia (brain) (cerebellar) (cerebral) —*see* Softening, brain
Encephalomeningitis —*see* Meningoencephalitis
Encephalomeningocele —*see* Encephalocele
Encephalomeningomyelitis —*see* Meningoencephalitis
Encephalomyelitis —*see also* Encephalitis G04.90
acute disseminated G04.00
infectious G04.01
noninfectious G04.81
postimmunization G04.02
postinfectious G04.01
acute necrotizing hemorrhagic G04.30
postimmunization G04.32
postinfectious G04.31
specified NEC G04.39
benign myalgic G93.3
equine A83.9
Eastern A83.2
Venezuelan A92.2
Western A83.1
in diseases classified elsewhere G05.3
myalgic, benign G93.3
postchickenpox B01.11
postinfectious NEC G04.01
postmeasles B05.0
postvaccinal G04.02
postvaricella B01.11
rubella B06.01
specified NEC G04.81
Venezuelan equine A92.2
Encephalomyelocele —*see* Encephalocele
Encephalomyelomeningitis —*see* Meningoencephalitis
Encephalomyelopathy G96.9
Encephalomyeloradiculitis (acute) G61.0
Encephalomyeloradiculoneuritis (acute) (Guillain-Barré) G61.0
Encephalomyeloradiculopathy G96.9
Encephalopathia hyperbilirubinemica, newborn P57.9
due to isoimmunization (conditions in P55) P57.0
Encephalopathy (acute) G93.40
acute necrotizing hemorrhagic G04.30
postimmunization G04.32
postinfectious G04.31
specified NEC G04.39
alcoholic G31.2
anoxic —*see* Damage, brain, anoxic
arteriosclerotic I67.2
centrolobar progressive (Schilder) G37.0
congenital Q07.9
degenerative, in specified disease NEC G32.89
due to
drugs (*see also* Table of Drugs and Chemicals) G92
demyelinating callosal G37.1
hepatic —*see* Failure, hepatic
hyperbilirubinemic, newborn P57.9
due to isoimmunization (conditions in P55) P57.0
hypertensive I67.4
hypoglycemic E16.2
hypoxic —*see* Damage, brain, anoxic
hypoxic ischemic P91.60
mild P91.61
moderate P91.62
severe P91.63
in (due to) (with)
birth injury P11.1
hyperinsulinism E16.1 *[G94]*
influenza —*see* Influenza, with, encephalopathy
lack of vitamin (*see also* Deficiency, vitamin) E56.9 *[G32.89]*
neoplastic disease (*see also* Neoplasm) D49.9 *[G13.1]*
serum (*see also* Reaction, serum) T80.69
syphilis A52.17
Encephalopathy *(Continued)*
in *(Continued)*
trauma (postconcussional) F07.81
current injury —*see* Injury, intracranial
vaccination G04.02
lead —*see* Poisoning, lead
metabolic G93.41
drug induced G92
toxic G92
myoclonic, early, symptomatic —*see* Epilepsy, generalized, specified NEC
necrotizing, subacute (Leigh) G31.82
pellagrous E52 *[G32.89]*
portosystemic —*see* Failure, hepatic
postcontusional F07.81
current injury —*see* Injury, intracranial, diffuse
posthypoglycemic (coma) E16.1 *[G94]*
postradiation G93.89
saturnine —*see* Poisoning, lead
septic G93.41
specified NEC G93.49
spongioform, subacute (viral) A81.09
toxic G92
metabolic G92
traumatic (postconcussional) F07.81
current injury —*see* Injury, intracranial
vitamin B deficiency NEC E53.9 *[G32.89]*
vitamin B1 E51.2
Wernicke's E51.2
Encephalorrhagia —*see* Hemorrhage, intracranial, intracerebral
Encephalosis, posttraumatic F07.81
Enchondroma —*see also* Neoplasm, bone, benign
Enchondromatosis (cartilaginous) (multiple) Q78.4
Encopresis R15.9
functional F98.1
nonorganic origin F98.1
psychogenic F98.1
Encounter (with health service) (for) Z76.89
adjustment and management (of)
breast implant Z45.81
implanted device NEC Z45.89
myringotomy device (stent) (tube) Z45.82
administrative purpose only Z02.9
examination for
adoption Z02.82
armed forces Z02.3
disability determination Z02.71
driving license Z02.4
employment Z02.1
insurance Z02.6
medical certificate NEC Z02.79
paternity testing Z02.81
residential institution admission Z02.2
school admission Z02.0
sports Z02.5
specified reason NEC Z02.89
aftercare —*see* Aftercare
antenatal screening Z36
assisted reproductive fertility procedure cycle Z31.83
blood typing Z01.83
Rh typing Z01.83
breast augmentation or reduction Z41.1
breast implant exchange (different material) (different size) Z45.81
breast reconstruction following mastectomy Z42.1
check-up —*see* Examination
chemotherapy for neoplasm Z51.11
colonoscopy, screening Z12.11
counseling —*see* Counseling
delivery, full-term, uncomplicated O80
cesarean, without indication O82
desensitization to allergens Z51.6 ◀
ear piercing Z41.3
examination —*see* Examination

E

◀ New ◀ Revised ~~deleted~~ Deleted

Encounter *(Continued)*
expectant parent (s) (adoptive) pre-birth pediatrician visit Z76.81
fertility preservation procedure (prior to cancer therapy) (prior to removal of gonads) Z31.84
fitting (of) —*see* Fitting (and adjustment) (of)
genetic
counseling Z31.5
testing —*see* Test, genetic
hearing conservation and treatment Z01.12
immunotherapy for neoplasm Z51.12
in vitro fertilization cycle Z31.83
instruction (in)
child care (postpartal) (prenatal) Z32.3
childbirth Z32.2
natural family planning
procreative Z31.61
to avoid pregnancy Z30.02
insulin pump titration Z46.81
joint prosthesis insertion following prior explantation of joint prosthesis (staged procedure)
hip Z47.32
knee Z47.33
shoulder Z47.31
laboratory (as part of a general medical examination) Z00.00
with abnormal findings Z00.01
mental health services (for)
abuse NEC
perpetrator Z69.82
victim Z69.81
child abuse
nonparental
perpetrator Z69.021
victim Z69.020
parental
perpetrator Z69.011
victim Z69.010
spousal or partner abuse
perpetrator Z69.12
victim Z69.11
observation (for) (ruled out)
exposure to (suspected)
anthrax Z03.810
biological agent NEC Z03.818
pediatrician visit, by expectant parent (s) (adoptive) Z76.81
plastic and reconstructive surgery following medical procedure or healed injury NEC Z42.8
pregnancy
supervision of —*see* Pregnancy, supervision of
test Z32.00
result negative Z32.02
result positive Z32.01
procreative management and counseling for gestational carrier Z31.7 ◀
prophylactic measures Z29.9 ◀
antivenin Z29.12 ◀
fluoride administration Z29.3 ◀
immunotherapy for respiratory syncytial virus (RSV) Z29.11 ◀
rabies immune globin Z29.14 ◀
Rho (D) immune globulin Z29.13 ◀
specified NEC Z29.8 ◀
radiation therapy (antineoplastic) Z51.0
radiological (as part of a general medical examination) Z00.00
with abnormal findings Z00.01
reconstructive surgery following medical procedure or healed injury NEC Z42.8
removal (of) —*see also* Removal
artificial
arm Z44.00-
complete Z44.01-
partial Z44.02-

Encounter *(Continued)*
removal *(Continued)*
artificial *(Continued)*
eye Z44.2-
leg Z44.10-
complete Z44.11-
partial Z44.12-
breast implant Z45.81
tissue expander (without synchronous insertion of permanent implant) Z45.81
device Z46.9
specified NEC Z46.89
external
fixation device — code to fracture with seventh character D
prosthesis, prosthetic device Z44.9
breast Z44.3-
specified NEC Z44.8
implanted device NEC Z45.89
insulin pump Z46.81
internal fixation device Z47.2
myringotomy device (stent) (tube) Z45.82
nervous system device NEC Z46.2
brain neuropacemaker Z46.2
visual substitution device Z46.2
implanted Z45.31
non-vascular catheter Z46.82
orthodontic device Z46.4
stent
ureteral Z46.6
urinary device Z46.6
repeat cervical smear to confirm findings of recent normal smear following initial abnormal smear Z01.42
respirator [ventilator] use during power failure (Z99.12)
Rh typing Z01.83
screening —*see* Screening
specified NEC Z76.89
sterilization Z30.2
suspected condition, ruled out
amniotic cavity and membrane Z03.71
cervical shortening Z03.75
fetal anomaly Z03.73
fetal growth Z03.74
maternal and fetal conditions NEC Z03.79
oligohydramnios Z03.71
placental problem Z03.72
polyhydramnios Z03.71
suspected exposure (to), ruled out
anthrax Z03.810
biological agents NEC Z03.818
termination of pregnancy, elective Z33.2
testing —*see* Test
therapeutic drug level monitoring Z51.81
titration, insulin pump Z46.81
to determine fetal viability of pregnancy O36.80
training
insulin pump Z46.81
X-ray of chest (as part of a general medical examination Z00.00)
with abnormal findings Z00.01
Encystment —*see* Cyst
Endarteritis (bacterial, subacute) (infective) I77.6
brain I67.7
cerebral or cerebrospinal I67.7
deformans —*see* Arteriosclerosis
embolic —*see* Embolism
obliterans —*see also* Arteriosclerosis
pulmonary I28.8
pulmonary I28.8
retina —*see* Vasculitis, retina
senile —*see* Arteriosclerosis
syphilitic A52.09
brain or cerebral A52.04
congenital A50.54 *[I79.8]*
tuberculous A18.89
Endemic —*see* condition

Endocarditis (chronic) (marantic) (nonbacterial) (thrombotic) (valvular) I38
with rheumatic fever (conditions in I00)
active —*see* Endocarditis, acute, rheumatic
inactive or quiescent (with chorea) I09.1
acute or subacute I33.9
infective I33.0
rheumatic (aortic) (mitral) (pulmonary) (tricuspid) I01.1
with chorea (acute) (rheumatic) (Sydenham's) I02.0
aortic (heart) (nonrheumatic) (valve) I35.8
with
mitral disease I08.0
with tricuspid (valve) disease I08.3
active or acute I01.1
with chorea (acute) (rheumatic) (Sydenham's) I02.0
rheumatic fever (conditions in I00)
active —*see* Endocarditis, acute, rheumatic
inactive or quiescent (with chorea) I06.9
tricuspid (valve) disease I08.2
with mitral (valve) disease I08.3
acute or subacute I33.9
arteriosclerotic I35.8
rheumatic I06.9
with mitral disease I08.0
with tricuspid (valve) disease I08.3
active or acute I01.1
with chorea (acute) (rheumatic) (Sydenham's) I02.0
active or acute I01.1
with chorea (acute) (rheumatic) (Sydenham's) I02.0
specified NEC I06.8
specified cause NEC I35.8
syphilitic A52.03
arteriosclerotic I38
atypical verrucous (Libman-Sacks) M32.11
bacterial (acute) (any valve) (subacute) I33.0
candidal B37.6
congenital Q24.8
constrictive I33.0
Coxiella burnetii A78 *[I39]*
Coxsackie B33.21
due to
prosthetic cardiac valve T82.6
Q fever A78 *[I39]*
Serratia marcescens I33.0
typhoid (fever) A01.02
gonococcal A54.83
infectious or infective (acute) (any valve) (subacute) I33.0
lenta (acute) (any valve) (subacute) I33.0
Libman-Sacks M32.11
listerial A32.82
Löffler's I42.3
malignant (acute) (any valve) (subacute) I33.0
meningococcal A39.51
mitral (chronic) (double) (fibroid) (heart) (inactive) (valve) (with chorea) I05.9
with
aortic (valve) disease I08.0
with tricuspid (valve) disease I08.3
active or acute I01.1
with chorea (acute) (rheumatic) (Sydenham's) I02.0
rheumatic fever (conditions in I00)
active —*see* Endocarditis, acute, rheumatic
inactive or quiescent (with chorea) I05.9
tricuspid (valve) disease I08.1
with aortic (valve) disease I08.3
active or acute I01.1
with chorea (acute) (rheumatic) (Sydenham's) I02.0
bacterial I33.0

E

Endocarditis *(Continued)*
mitral *(Continued)*
arteriosclerotic I34.8
nonrheumatic I34.8
acute or subacute I33.9
specified NEC I05.8
monilial B37.6
multiple valves I08.9
specified disorders I08.8
mycotic (acute) (any valve) (subacute) I33.0
pneumococcal (acute) (any valve) (subacute) I33.0
pulmonary (chronic) (heart) (valve) I37.8
with rheumatic fever (conditions in I00)
active —*see* Endocarditis, acute, rheumatic
inactive or quiescent (with chorea) I09.89
with aortic, mitral or tricuspid disease I08.8
acute or subacute I33.9
rheumatic I01.1
with chorea (acute) (rheumatic) (Sydenham's) I02.0
arteriosclerotic I37.8
congenital Q22.2
rheumatic (chronic) (inactive) (with chorea) I09.89
active or acute I01.1
with chorea (acute) (rheumatic) (Sydenham's) I02.0
syphilitic A52.03
purulent (acute) (any valve) (subacute) I33.0
Q fever A78 *[I39]*
rheumatic (chronic) (inactive) (with chorea) I09.1
active or acute (aortic) (mitral) (pulmonary) (tricuspid) I01.1
with chorea (acute) (rheumatic) (Sydenham's) I02.0
rheumatoid —*see* Rheumatoid, carditis
septic (acute) (any valve) (subacute) I33.0
streptococcal (acute) (any valve) (subacute) I33.0
subacute —*see* Endocarditis, acute
suppurative (acute) (any valve) (subacute) I33.0
syphilitic A52.03
toxic I33.9
tricuspid (chronic) (heart) (inactive) (rheumatic) (valve) (with chorea) I07.9
with
aortic (valve) disease I08.2
mitral (valve) disease I08.3
mitral (valve) disease I08.1
aortic (valve) disease I08.3
rheumatic fever (conditions in I00)
active —*see* Endocarditis, acute, rheumatic
inactive or quiescent (with chorea) I07.8
active or acute I01.1
with chorea (acute) (rheumatic) (Sydenham's) I02.0
arteriosclerotic I36.8
nonrheumatic I36.8
acute or subacute I33.9
specified cause, except rheumatic I36.8
tuberculous —*see* Tuberculosis, endocarditis
typhoid A01.02
ulcerative (acute) (any valve) (subacute) I33.0
vegetative (acute) (any valve) (subacute) I33.0
verrucous (atypical) (nonbacterial) (nonrheumatic) M32.11
Endocardium, endocardial —*see also* condition
cushion defect Q21.2
Endocervicitis —*see also* Cervicitis
due to intrauterine (contraceptive) device T83.69 ◀
hyperplastic N72
Endocrine —*see* condition
Endocrinopathy, pluriglandular E31.9
Endodontic
overfill M27.52
underfill M27.53
Endodontitis K04.01 ◀
irreversible K04.02 ◀
reversible K04.01 ◀
Endomastoiditis —*see* Mastoiditis
Endometrioma N80.9
Endometriosis N80.9
appendix N80.5
bladder N80.8
bowel N80.5
broad ligament N80.3
cervix N80.0
colon N80.5
cul-de-sac (Douglas') N80.3
exocervix N80.0
fallopian tube N80.2
female genital organ NEC N80.8
gallbladder N80.8
in scar of skin N80.6
internal N80.0
intestine N80.5
lung N80.8
myometrium N80.0
ovary N80.1
parametrium N80.3
pelvic peritoneum N80.3
peritoneal (pelvic) N80.3
rectovaginal septum N80.4
rectum N80.5
round ligament N80.3
skin (scar) N80.6
specified site NEC N80.8
stromal D39.0
umbilicus N80.8
uterus (internal) N80.0
vagina N80.4
vulva N80.8
Endometritis (decidual) (nonspecific) (purulent) (senile (atrophic) (suppurative) N71.9
with ectopic pregnancy O08.0
acute N71.0
blenorrhagic (gonococcal) (acute) (chronic) A54.24
cervix, cervical (with erosion or ectropion) —*see also* Cervicitis
hyperplastic N72
chlamydial A56.11
chronic N71.1
following
abortion —*see* Abortion by type complicated by genital infection
ectopic or molar pregnancy O08.0
gonococcal, gonorrheal (acute) (chronic) A54.24
hyperplastic —*see also* Hyperplasia, endometrial N85.00-
cervix N72
puerperal, postpartum, childbirth O86.12
subacute N71.0
tuberculous A18.17
Endometrium —*see* condition
Endomyocardiopathy, South African I42.3
Endomyocarditis —*see* Endocarditis
Endomyofibrosis I42.3
Endomyometritis —*see* Endometritis
Endopericarditis —*see* Endocarditis
Endoperineuritis —*see* Disorder, nerve
Endophlebitis —*see* Phlebitis
Endophthalmia —*see* Endophthalmitis, purulent
Endophthalmitis (acute) (infective) (metastatic) (subacute) H44.009
bleb associated H59.4 —*see also* Bleb, inflammed (infected), postprocedural
gonorrheal A54.39
in (due to)
cysticercosis B69.1
onchocerciasis B73.01
toxocariasis B83.0
Endophthalmitis *(Continued)*
panuveitis —*see* Panuveitis
parasitic H44.12-
purulent H44.00-
panophthalmitis —*see* Panophthalmitis
vitreous abscess H44.02-
specified NEC H44.19
sympathetic —*see* Uveitis, sympathetic
Endosalpingioma D28.2
Endosalpingiosis N94.89
Endosteitis —*see* Osteomyelitis
Endothelioma, bone —*see* Neoplasm, bone, malignant
Endotheliosis (hemorrhagic infectional) D69.8
Endotoxemia — code to condition
Endotrachelitis —*see* Cervicitis
Engelmann (-Camurati) syndrome Q78.3
English disease —*see* Rickets
Engman's disease L30.3
Engorgement
breast N64.59
newborn P83.4
puerperal, postpartum O92.79
lung (passive) —*see* Edema, lung
pulmonary (passive) —*see* Edema, lung
stomach K31.89
venous, retina —*see* Occlusion, retina, vein, engorgement
Enlargement, enlarged —*see also* Hypertrophy
adenoids J35.2
with tonsils J35.3
alveolar ridge K08.89 ◀
congenital —*see* Anomaly, alveolar
apertures of diaphragm (congenital) Q79.1
gingival K06.1
heart, cardiac —*see* Hypertrophy, cardiac
labium majus, childhood asymmetric (CALME) N90.61 ◀
lacrimal gland, chronic H04.03-
liver —*see* Hypertrophy, liver
lymph gland or node R59.9
generalized R59.1
localized R59.0
orbit H05.34-
organ or site, congenital NEC —*see* Anomaly, by site
parathyroid (gland) E21.0
pituitary fossa R93.0
prostate N40.0
with lower urinary tract symptoms (LUTS) N40.1
without lower urinary tract symptoms (LUTS) N40.0
sella turcica R93.0
spleen —*see* Splenomegaly
thymus (gland) (congenital) E32.0
thyroid (gland) —*see* Goiter
tongue K14.8
tonsils J35.1
with adenoids J35.3
uterus N85.2
Enophthalmos H05.40-
due to
orbital tissue atrophy H05.41-
trauma or surgery H05.42-
Enostosis M27.8
Entamebic, entamebiasis —*see* Amebiasis
Entanglement
umbilical cord (s) O69.2
with compression O69.2
without compression O69.82
around neck (with compression) O69.1
without compression O69.81
of twins in monoamniotic sac O69.2
Enteralgia —*see* Pain, abdominal
Enteric —*see* condition
Enteritis (acute) (diarrheal) (hemorrhagic) (noninfective) K52.9 ◀
adenovirus A08.2
aertrycke infection A02.0

E

◀ New ◀ Revised ~~deleted~~ Deleted

Enteritis *(Continued)*
allergic K52.29
with
eosinophilic gastritis or gastroenteritis K52.81
food protein-induced enterocolitis syndrome K52.21
food protein-induced enteropathy K52.22
amebic (acute) A06.0
with abscess —*see* Abscess, amebic
chronic A06.1
with abscess —*see* Abscess, amebic
nondysenteric A06.2
nondysenteric A06.2
astrovirus A08.32
bacillary NOS A03.9
bacterial A04.9
specified NEC A04.8
calicivirus A08.31
candidal B37.82
Chilomastix A07.8
choleriformis A00.1
chronic (noninfectious) K52.9
ulcerative —*see* Colitis, ulcerative
cicatrizing (chronic) —*see* Enteritis, regional, small intestine
Clostridium
botulinum (food poisoning) A05.1
difficile A04.7
coccidial A07.3
coxsackie virus A08.39
dietetic —*see also* Enteritis, allergic K52.29
drug-induced K52.1
due to
astrovirus A08.32
calicivirus A08.31
coxsackie virus A08.39
drugs K52.1
echovirus A08.39
enterovirus NEC A08.39
food hypersensitivity —*see also* Enteritis, allergic K52.29
infectious organism (bacterial) (viral) —*see* Enteritis, infectious
torovirus A08.39
Yersinia enterocolitica A04.6
echovirus A08.39
eltor A00.1
enterovirus NEC A08.39
eosinophilic K52.81
epidemic (infectious) A09
fulminant —*see also* Ischemia, intestine, acute K55.019
gangrenous —*see* Enteritis, infectious
giardial A07.1
infectious NOS A09
due to
adenovirus A08.2
Aerobacter aerogenes A04.8
Arizona (bacillus) A02.0
bacteria NOS A04.9
specified NEC A04.8
Campylobacter A04.5
Clostridium difficile A04.7
Clostridium perfringens A04.8
Enterobacter aerogenes A04.8
enterovirus A08.39
Escherichia coli A04.4
enteroaggregative A04.4
enterohemorrhagic A04.3
enteroinvasive A04.2
enteropathogenic A04.0
enterotoxigenic A04.1
specified NEC A04.4
specified
bacteria NEC A04.8
virus NEC A08.39
Staphylococcus A04.8

Enteritis *(Continued)*
infectious NOS *(Continued)*
due to *(Continued)*
virus NEC A08.4
specified type NEC A08.39
Yersinia enterocolitica A04.6
specified organism NEC A08.8
influenzal —*see* Influenza, with, digestive manifestations
ischemic K55.9
acute —*see also* Ischemia, intestine, acute K55.019
chronic K55.1
microsporidial A07.8
mucomembranous, myxomembranous —*see* Syndrome, irritable bowel
mucous —*see* Syndrome, irritable bowel
necroticans A05.2
necrotizing of newborn —*see* Enterocolitis, necrotizing, in newborn
neurogenic —*see* Syndrome, irritable bowel
newborn necrotizing —*see* Enterocolitis, necrotizing, in newborn
noninfectious K52.9
norovirus A08.11
parasitic NEC B82.9
paratyphoid (fever) —*see* Fever, paratyphoid
protozoal A07.9
specified NEC A07.8
radiation K52.0
regional (of) K50.90
with
complication K50.919
abscess K50.914
fistula K50.913
intestinal obstruction K50.912
rectal bleeding K50.911
specified complication NEC K50.918
colon —*see* Enteritis, regional, large intestine
duodenum —*see* Enteritis, regional, small intestine
ileum —*see* Enteritis, regional, small intestine
jejunum —*see* Enteritis, regional, small intestine
large bowel —*see* Enteritis, regional, large intestine
large intestine (colon) (rectum) K50.10
with
complication K50.119
abscess K50.114
fistula K50.113
intestinal obstruction K50.112
rectal bleeding K50.111
small intestine (duodenum) (ileum) (jejunum) involvement K50.80
with
complication K50.819
abscess K50.814
fistula K50.813
intestinal obstruction K50.812
rectal bleeding K50.811
specified complication NEC K50.818
specified complication NEC K50.118
rectum —*see* Enteritis, regional, large intestine
small intestine (duodenum) (ileum) (jejunum) K50.00
with
complication K50.019
abscess K50.014
fistula K50.013
intestinal obstruction K50.012

Enteritis *(Continued)*
regional *(Continued)*
small intestine *(Continued)*
with *(Continued)*
complication *(Continued)*
large intestine (colon) (rectum) involvement K50.80
with
complication K50.819
abscess K50.814
fistula K50.813
intestinal obstruction K50.812
rectal bleeding K50.811
specified complication NEC K50.818
rectal bleeding K50.011
specified complication NEC K50.018
rotaviral A08.0
Salmonella, salmonellosis (arizonae) (cholerae-suis) (enteritidis) (typhimurium) A02.0
segmental —*see* Enteritis, regional
septic A09
Shigella —*see* Infection, Shigella
small round structured NEC A08.19
spasmodic, spastic —*see* Syndrome, irritable bowel
staphylococcal A04.8
due to food A05.0
torovirus A08.39
toxic NEC K52.1
due to Clostridium difficile A04.7
trichomonal A07.8
tuberculous A18.32
typhosa A01.00
ulcerative (chronic) —*see* Colitis, ulcerative
viral A08.4
adenovirus A08.2
enterovirus A08.39
Rotavirus A08.0
small round structured NEC A08.19
specified NEC A08.39
virus specified NEC A08.39
Enterobiasis B80
Enterobius vermicularis (infection) (infestation) B80
Enterocele —*see also* Hernia, abdomen
pelvic, pelvis (acquired) (congenital) N81.5
vagina, vaginal (acquired) (congenital) NEC N81.5
Enterocolitis —*see also* Enteritis K52.9
due to Clostridium difficile A04.7
fulminant ischemic —*see also* Ischemia, intestine, acute K55.059
granulomatous —*see* Enteritis, regional
hemorrhagic (acute) —*see also* Ischemia, intestine, acute K55.059
chronic K55.1
infectious NEC A09
ischemic K55.9
necrotizing K55.30
with
perforation K55.33
pneumatosis K55.32
and perforation K55.33
due to Clostridium difficile A04.7
in non-newborn K55.30
stage 1 (without pneumatosis, without perforation) K55.31
stage 2 (with pneumatosis, without perforation) K55.32
stage 3 (with pneumatosis, with perforation) K55.33
in newborn P77.9
stage 1 (without pneumatosis, without perforation) P77.1
stage 2 (with pneumatosis, without perforation) P77.2
stage 3 (with pneumatosis, with perforation) P77.3
without pneumatosis or perforation K55.31

Enterocolitis *(Continued)*
noninfectious K52.9
newborn —*see* Enterocolitis, necrotizing, in newborn
pseudomembranous (newborn) A04.7
radiation K52.0
newborn —*see* Enterocolitis, necrotizing, in newborn
ulcerative (chronic) —*see* Pancolitis, ulcerative (chronic)
Enterogastritis —*see* Enteritis
Enteropathy K63.9
food protein-induced enterocolitis K52.22 ◀
gluten-sensitive K90.0
non-celiac K90.41 ◀
hemorrhagic, terminal —*see also* Ischemia, intestine, acute K55.059 ⟸
protein-losing K90.49 ⟸
Enteroperitonitis —*see* Peritonitis
Enteroptosis K63.4
Enterorrhagia K92.2
Enterospasm —*see also* Syndrome, irritable, bowel
psychogenic F45.8
Enterostenosis —*see also* Obstruction, intestine K56.69
Enterostomy
complication —*see* Complication, enterostomy
status Z93.4
Enterovirus, as cause of disease classified elsewhere B97.10
coxsackievirus B97.11
echovirus B97.12
other specified B97.19
Enthesopathy (peripheral) M77.9
Achilles tendinitis —*see* Tendinitis, Achilles
ankle and tarsus M77.9
specified type NEC —*see* Enthesopathy, foot, specified type NEC
anterior tibial syndrome M76.81-
calcaneal spur —*see* Spur, bone, calcaneal
elbow region M77.8
lateral epicondylitis —*see* Epicondylitis, lateral
medial epicondylitis —*see* Epicondylitis, medial
foot NEC M77.9
metatarsalgia —*see* Metatarsalgia
specified type NEC M77.5-
forearm M77.9
gluteal tendinitis —*see* Tendinitis, gluteal
hand M77.9
hip —*see* Enthesopathy, lower limb, specified type NEC
iliac crest spur —*see* Spur, bone, iliac crest
iliotibial band syndrome —*see* Syndrome, iliotibial band
knee —*see* Enthesopathy, lower limb, lower leg, specified type NEC
lateral epicondylitis —*see* Epicondylitis, lateral
lower limb (excluding foot) M76.9
Achilles tendinitis —*see* Tendinitis, Achilles
anterior tibial syndrome M76.81-
gluteal tendinitis —*see* Tendinitis, gluteal
iliac crest spur —*see* Spur, bone, iliac crest
iliotibial band syndrome —*see* Syndrome, iliotibial band
patellar tendinitis —*see* Tendinitis, patellar
pelvic region —*see* Enthesopathy, lower limb, specified type NEC
peroneal tendinitis —*see* Tendinitis, peroneal
posterior tibial syndrome M76.82-
psoas tendinitis —*see* Tendinitis, psoas
shoulder M77.9
specified type NEC M76.89-
tibial collateral bursitis —*see* Bursitis, tibial collateral
Enthesopathy *(Continued)*
medial epicondylitis —*see* Epicondylitis, medial
multiple sites M77.9
patellar tendinitis —*see* Tendinitis, patellar
pelvis M77.9
periarthritis of wrist —*see* Periarthritis, wrist
peroneal tendinitis —*see* Tendinitis, peroneal
posterior tibial syndrome M76.82-
psoas tendinitis —*see* Tendinitis, psoas
shoulder region —*see* Lesion, shoulder
specified site NEC M77.9
specified type NEC M77.8
spinal M46.00
cervical region M46.02
cervicothoracic region M46.03
lumbar region M46.06
lumbosacral region M46.07
multiple sites M46.09
occipito-atlanto-axial region M46.01
sacrococcygeal region M46.08
thoracic region M46.04
thoracolumbar region M46.05
tibial collateral bursitis —*see* Bursitis, tibial collateral
upper arm M77.9
wrist and carpus NEC M77.8
calcaneal spur —*see* Spur, bone, calcaneal
periarthritis of wrist —*see* Periarthritis, wrist
Entomophobia F40.218
Entomophthoromycosis B46.8
Entrance, air into vein —*see* Embolism, air
Entrapment, nerve —*see* Neuropathy, entrapment
Entropion (eyelid) (paralytic) H02.009
cicatricial H02.019
left H02.016
lower H02.015
upper H02.014
right H02.013
lower H02.012
upper H02.011
congenital Q10.2
left H02.006
lower H02.005
upper H02.004
mechanical H02.029
left H02.026
lower H02.025
upper H02.024
right H02.023
lower H02.022
upper H02.021
right H02.003
lower H02.002
upper H02.001
senile H02.039
left H02.036
lower H02.035
upper H02.034
right H02.033
lower H02.032
upper H02.031
spastic H02.049
left H02.046
lower H02.045
upper H02.044
right H02.043
lower H02.042
upper H02.041
Enucleated eye (traumatic, current) S05.7-
Enuresis R32
functional F98.0
habit disturbance F98.0
nocturnal N39.44
psychogenic F98.0
nonorganic origin F98.0
psychogenic F98.0
Eosinopenia —*see* Agranulocytosis
Eosinophilia (allergic) (hereditary) (idiopathic) (secondary) D72.1
with
angiolymphoid hyperplasia (ALHE) D18.01
infiltrative J82
Löffler's J82
peritoneal —*see* Peritonitis, eosinophilic
pulmonary NEC J82
tropical (pulmonary) J82
Eosinophilia-myalgia syndrome M35.8
Ependymitis (acute) (cerebral) (chronic) (granular) —*see* Encephalomyelitis
Ependymoblastoma
specified site —*see* Neoplasm, malignant, by site
unspecified site C71.9
Ependymoma (epithelial) (malignant)
anaplastic
specified site —*see* Neoplasm, malignant, by site
unspecified site C71.9
benign
specified site —*see* Neoplasm, benign, by site
unspecified site D33.2
myxopapillary D43.2
specified site —*see* Neoplasm, uncertain behavior, by site
unspecified site D43.2
papillary D43.2
specified site —*see* Neoplasm, uncertain behavior, by site
unspecified site D43.2
specified site —*see* Neoplasm, malignant, by site
unspecified site C71.9
Ependymopathy G93.89
Ephelis, ephelides L81.2
Epiblepharon (congenital) Q10.3
Epicanthus, epicanthic fold (eyelid) (congenital) Q10.3
Epicondylitis (elbow)
lateral M77.1-
medial M77.0-
Epicystitis —*see* Cystitis
Epidemic —*see* condition
Epidermidalization, cervix —*see* Dysplasia, cervix
Epidermis, epidermal —*see* condition
Epidermodysplasia verruciformis B07.8
Epidermolysis
bullosa (congenital) Q81.9
acquired L12.30
drug-induced L12.31
specified cause NEC L12.35
dystrophica Q81.2
letalis Q81.1
simplex Q81.0
specified NEC Q81.8
necroticans combustiformis L51.2
due to drug —*see* Table of Drugs and Chemicals, by drug
Epidermophytid —*see* Dermatophytosis
Epidermophytosis (infected) —*see* Dermatophytosis
Epididymis —*see* condition
Epididymitis (acute) (nonvenereal) (recurrent) (residual) N45.1
with orchitis N45.3
blennorrhagic (gonococcal) A54.23
caseous (tuberculous) A18.15
chlamydial A56.19
filarial —*see also* Infestation, filarial B74.9 *[N51]*
gonococcal A54.23
syphilitic A52.76
tuberculous A18.15
Epididymo-orchitis —*see also* Epididymitis N45.3
Epidural —*see* condition

E

◀ New ⟸ Revised ~~deleted~~ Deleted

Epigastrium, epigastric —*see* condition
Epigastrocele —*see* Hernia, ventral
Epiglottis —*see* condition
Epiglottitis, epiglottiditis (acute) J05.10
with obstruction J05.11
chronic J37.0
Epignathus Q89.4
Epilepsia partialis continua —*see also* Kozhevnikof's epilepsy G40.1-
Epilepsy, epileptic, epilepsia (attack) (cerebral) (convulsion) (fit) (seizure) G40.909

Note: the following terms are to be considered equivalent to intractable: pharmacoresistant (pharmacologically resistant), treatment resistant, refractory (medically) and poorly controlled

with
complex partial seizures —*see* Epilepsy, localization-related, symptomatic, with complex partial seizures
grand mal seizures on awakening —*see* Epilepsy, generalized, specified NEC
myoclonic absences —*see* Epilepsy, generalized, specified NEC
myoclonic-astatic seizures —*see* Epilepsy, generalized, specified NEC
simple partial seizures —*see* Epilepsy, localization-related, symptomatic, with simple partial seizures
akinetic —*see* Epilepsy, generalized, specified NEC
benign childhood with centrotemporal EEG spikes —*see* Epilepsy, localization-related, idiopathic
benign myoclonic in infancy G40.80-
Bravais-jacksonian —*see* Epilepsy, localization-related, symptomatic, with simple partial seizures
childhood
with occipital EEG paroxysms —*see* Epilepsy, localization-related, idiopathic
absence G40.A09
intractable G40.A19
with status epilepticus G40.A11
without status epilepticus G40.A19
not intractable G40.A09
with status epilepticus G40.A01
without status epilepticus G40.A09
climacteric —*see* Epilepsy, specified NEC
cysticercosis B69.0
deterioration (mental) F06.8
due to syphilis A52.19
focal —*see* Epilepsy, localization-related, symptomatic, with simple partial seizures
generalized
idiopathic G40.309
intractable G40.319
with status epilepticus G40.311
without status epilepticus G40.319
not intractable G40.309
with status epilepticus G40.301
without status epilepticus G40.309
specified NEC G40.409
intractable G40.419
with status epilepticus G40.411
without status epilepticus G40.419
not intractable G40.409
with status epilepticus G40.401
without status epilepticus G40.409
impulsive petit mal —*see* Epilepsy, juvenile myoclonic
intractable G40.919
with status epilepticus G40.911
without status epilepticus G40.919

Epilepsy, epileptic, epilepsia *(Continued)*
juvenile absence G40.A09
intractable G40.A19
with status epilepticus G40.A11
without status epilepticus G40.A19
not intractable G40.A09
with status epilepticus G40.A01
without status epilepticus G40.A09
juvenile myoclonic G40.B11
intractable G40.B19
with status epilepticus G40.B11
without status epilepticus G40.B19
not intractable G40.B09
with status epilepticus G40.B01
without status epilepticus G40.B09
localization-related (focal) (partial)
idiopathic G40.009
with seizures of localized onset G40.009
intractable G40.019
with status epilepticus G40.011
without status epilepticus G40.019
not intractable G40.009
with status epilepticus G40.001
without status epilepticus G40.009
symptomatic
with complex partial seizures G40.209
intractable G40.219
with status epilepticus G40.211
without status epilepticus G40.219
not intractable G40.209
with status epilepticus G40.201
without status epilepticus G40.209
with simple partial seizures G40.109
intractable G40.119
with status epilepticus G40.111
without status epilepticus G40.119
not intractable G40.109
with status epilepticus G40.101
without status epilepticus G40.109
myoclonus, myoclonic —*see* Epilepsy, generalized, specified NEC ⇐
progressive —*see* Epilepsy, generalized, idiopathic ◀
not intractable G40.909
with status epilepticus G40.901
without status epilepticus G40.909
on awakening —*see* Epilepsy, generalized, specified NEC
parasitic NOS B71.9 *[G94]*
partialis continua —*see also* Kozhevnikof's epilepsy G40.1-
peripheral —*see* Epilepsy, specified NEC
procursiva —*see* Epilepsy, localization-related, symptomatic, with simple partial seizures
progressive (familial) myoclonic —*see* Epilepsy, generalized, idiopathic
reflex —*see* Epilepsy, specified NEC
related to
alcohol G40.509
not intractable G40.509
with status epilepticus G40.501
without status epilepticus G40.509
drugs G40.509
not intractable G40.509
with status epilepticus G40.501
without status epilepticus G40.509
external causes G40.509
not intractable G40.509
with status epilepticus G40.501
without status epilepticus G40.509
hormonal changes G40.509
not intractable G40.509
with status epilepticus G40.501
without status epilepticus G40.509
sleep deprivation G40.509
not intractable G40.509
with status epilepticus G40.501
without status epilepticus G40.509

Epilepsy, epileptic, epilepsia *(Continued)*
related to *(Continued)*
stress G40.509
not intractable G40.509
with status epilepticus G40.501
without status epilepticus G40.509
somatomotor —*see* Epilepsy, localization-related, symptomatic, with simple partial seizures
somatosensory —*see* Epilepsy, localization-related, symptomatic, with simple partial seizures
spasms G40.822
intractable G40.824
with status epilepticus G40.823
without status epilepticus G40.824
not intractable G40.822
with status epilepticus G40.821
without status epilepticus G40.822
specified NEC G40.802
intractable G40.804
with status epilepticus G40.803
without status epilepticus G40.804
not intractable G40.802
with status epilepticus G40.801
without status epilepticus G40.802
syndromes
generalized
idiopathic G40.309
intractable G40.319
with status epilepticus G40.311
without status epilepticus G40.319
not intractable G40.309
with status epilepticus G40.301
without status epilepticus G40.309
specified NEC G40.409
intractable G40.419
with status epilepticus G40.411
without status epilepticus G40.419
not intractable G40.409
with status epilepticus G40.401
without status epilepticus G40.409
localization-related (focal) (partial)
idiopathic G40.009
with seizures of localized onset G40.009
intractable G40.019
with status epilepticus G40.011
without status epilepticus G40.019
not intractable G40.009
with status epilepticus G40.001
without status epilepticus G40.009
symptomatic
with complex partial seizures G40.209
intractable G40.219
with status epilepticus G40.211
without status epilepticus G40.219
not intractable G40.209
with status epilepticus G40.201
without status epilepticus G40.209
with simple partial seizures G40.109
intractable G40.119
with status epilepticus G40.111
without status epilepticus G40.119
not intractable G40.109
with status epilepticus G40.101
without status epilepticus G40.109
specified NEC G40.802
intractable G40.804
with status epilepticus G40.803
without status epilepticus G40.804
not intractable G40.802
with status epilepticus G40.801
without status epilepticus G40.802
tonic (-clonic) —*see* Epilepsy, generalized, specified NEC
twilight F05

Epilepsy, epileptic, epilepsia *(Continued)*
uncinate (gyrus) —*see* Epilepsy, localization-related, symptomatic, with complex partial seizures
Unverricht (-Lundborg) (familial myoclonic) —*see* Epilepsy, generalized, idiopathic
visceral —*see* Epilepsy, specified NEC
visual —*see* Epilepsy, specified NEC
Epiloia Q85.1
Epimenorrhea N92.0
Epipharyngitis —*see* Nasopharyngitis
Epiphora H04.20-
due to
excess lacrimation H04.21-
insufficient drainage H04.22-
Epiphyseal arrest —*see* Arrest, epiphyseal
Epiphyseolysis, epiphysiolysis —*see* Osteochondropathy
Epiphysitis —*see also* Osteochondropathy
juvenile M92.9
syphilitic (congenital) A50.02
Epiplocele —*see* Hernia, abdomen
Epiploitis —*see* Peritonitis
Epiplosarcomphalocele —*see* Hernia, umbilicus
Episcleritis (suppurative) H15.10-
in (due to)
syphilis A52.71
tuberculosis A18.51
nodular H15.12-
periodica fugax H15.11-
angioneurotic —*see* Edema, angioneurotic
syphilitic (late) A52.71
tuberculous A18.51
Episode
affective, mixed F39
depersonalization (in neurotic state) F48.1
depressive F32.9
major F32.9
mild F32.0
moderate F32.1
severe (without psychotic symptoms) F32.2
with psychotic symptoms F32.3
recurrent F33.9
brief F33.8
specified NEC F32.89 ◀
hypomanic F30.8
manic F30.9
with
psychotic symptoms F30.2
remission (full) F30.4
partial F30.3
without psychotic symptoms F30.10
mild F30.11
moderate F30.12
severe (without psychotic symptoms) F30.13
with psychotic symptoms F30.2
other specified F30.8
recurrent F31.89
psychotic F23
organic F06.8
schizophrenic (acute) NEC, brief F23
Epispadias (female) (male) Q64.0
Episplenitis D73.89
Epistaxis (multiple) R04.0
hereditary I78.0
vicarious menstruation N94.89
Epithelioma (malignant) —*see also* Neoplasm, malignant, by site
adenoides cysticum —*see* Neoplasm, skin, benign
basal cell —*see* Neoplasm, skin, malignant
benign —*see* Neoplasm, benign, by site
Bowen's —*see* Neoplasm, skin, in situ
calcifying, of Malherbe —*see* Neoplasm, skin, benign
external site —*see* Neoplasm, skin, malignant
intraepidermal, Jadassohn —*see* Neoplasm, skin, benign
squamous cell —*see* Neoplasm, malignant, by site
Epitheliomatosis pigmented Q82.1
Epitheliopathy, multifocal placoid pigment H30.14-
Epithelium, epithelial —*see* condition
Epituberculosis (with atelectasis) (allergic) A15.7
Eponychia Q84.6
Epstein's
nephrosis or syndrome —*see* Nephrosis
pearl K09.8
Epulis (gingiva) (fibrous) (giant cell) K06.8
Equinia A24.0
Equinovarus (congenital) (talipes) Q66.0
acquired —*see* Deformity, limb, clubfoot
Equivalent
convulsive (abdominal) —*see* Epilepsy, specified NEC
epileptic (psychic) —*see* Epilepsy, localization-related, symptomatic, with complex partial seizures
Erb (-Duchenne) paralysis (birth injury) (newborn) P14.0
Erb's
disease G71.0
palsy, paralysis (brachial) (birth) (newborn) P14.0
spinal (spastic) syphilitic A52.17
pseudohypertrophic muscular dystrophy G71.0
Erb-Goldflam disease or syndrome G70.00
with exacerbation (acute) G70.01
in crisis G70.01
Erdheim's syndrome (acromegalic macrospondylitis) E22.0
Erection, painful (persistent) —*see* Priapism
Ergosterol deficiency (vitamin D) E55.9
with
adult osteomalacia M83.8
rickets —*see* Rickets
Ergotism —*see also* Poisoning, food, noxious, plant
from ergot used as drug (migraine therapy) —*see* Table of Drugs and Chemicals
Erosio interdigitalis blastomycetica B37.2
Erosion
artery I77.2
without rupture I77.89
bone —*see* Disorder, bone, density and structure, specified NEC
bronchus J98.09
cartilage (joint) —*see* Disorder, cartilage, specified type NEC
cervix (uteri) (acquired) (chronic) (congenital) N86
with cervicitis N72
cornea (nontraumatic) —*see* Ulcer, cornea
recurrent H18.83-
traumatic —*see* Abrasion, cornea
dental (idiopathic) (occupational) (due to diet, drugs or vomiting) K03.2
duodenum, postpyloric —*see* Ulcer, duodenum
esophagus K22.10
with bleeding K22.11
gastric —*see* Ulcer, stomach
gastrojejunal —*see* Ulcer, gastrojejunal
implanted mesh —*see* Complications, mesh
intestine K63.3
lymphatic vessel I89.8
pylorus, pyloric (ulcer) —*see* Ulcer, stomach
spine, aneurysmal A52.09
stomach —*see* Ulcer, stomach
subcutaneous device pocket ◀
nervous system prosthetic device, implant, or graft T85.890 ◀
other internal prosthetic device, implant, or graft T85.898 ◀
teeth (idiopathic) (occupational) (due to diet, drugs or vomiting) K03.2
urethra N36.8
uterus N85.8
Erotomania F52.8
Error
metabolism, inborn —*see* Disorder, metabolism
refractive —*see* Disorder, refraction
Eructation R14.2
nervous or psychogenic F45.8
Eruption
creeping B76.9
drug (generalized) (taken internally) L27.0
fixed L27.1
in contact with skin —*see* Dermatitis, due to drugs
localized L27.1
Hutchinson, summer L56.4
Kaposi's varicelliform B00.0
napkin L22
polymorphous light (sun) L56.4
recalcitrant pustular L13.8
ringed R23.8
skin (nonspecific) R21
creeping (meaning hookworm) B76.9
due to inoculation/vaccination (generalized) —*see also* Dermatitis, due to, vaccine L27.0
localized L27.1
erysipeloid A26.0
feigned L98.1
Kaposi's varicelliform B00.0
lichenoid L28.0
meaning dermatitis —*see* Dermatitis
toxic NEC L53.0
tooth, teeth, abnormal (incomplete) (late) (premature) (sequence) K00.6
vesicular R23.8
Erysipelas (gangrenous) (infantile) (newborn) (phlegmonous) (suppurative) A46
external ear A46 *[H62.40]*
puerperal, postpartum O86.89
Erysipeloid A26.9
cutaneous (Rosenbach's) A26.0
disseminated A26.8
sepsis A26.7
specified NEC A26.8
Erythema, erythematous (infectional) (inflammation) L53.9
ab igne L59.0
annulare (centrifugum) (rheumaticum) L53.1
arthriticum epidemicum A25.1
brucellum —*see* Brucellosis
chronic figurate NEC L53.3
chronicum migrans (Borrelia burgdorferi) A69.20
diaper L22
due to
chemical NEC L53.0
in contact with skin L24.5
drug (internal use) —*see* Dermatitis, due to, drugs
elevatum diutinum L95.1
endemic E52
epidemic, arthritic A25.1
figuratum perstans L53.3
gluteal L22
heat - code by site under Burn, first degree
ichthyosiforme congenitum bullous Q80.3
in diseases classified elsewhere L54
induratum (nontuberculous) L52
tuberculous A18.4
infectiosum B08.3
intertrigo L30.4
iris L51.9
marginatum L53.2
in (due to) acute rheumatic fever I00
medicamentosum —*see* Dermatitis, due to, drugs
migrans A26.0
chronicum A69.20
tongue K14.1

E

◀ New ◀ Revised ~~deleted~~ Deleted

Erythema, erythematous *(Continued)*
multiforme (major) (minor) L51.9
bullous, bullosum L51.1
conjunctiva L51.1
nonbullous L51.0
pemphigoides L12.0
specified NEC L51.8
napkin L22
neonatorum P83.8
toxic P83.1
nodosum L52
tuberculous A18.4
palmar L53.8
pernio T69.1
rash, newborn P83.8
scarlatiniform (recurrent) (exfoliative) L53.8
solare L55.0
specified NEC L53.8
toxic, toxicum NEC L53.0
newborn P83.1
tuberculous (primary) A18.4
Erythematous, erythematosus —*see* condition
Erythermalgia (primary) I73.81
Erythralgia I73.81
Erythrasma L08.1
Erythredema (polyneuropathy) —*see* Poisoning, mercury
Erythremia (acute) C94.0-
chronic D45
secondary D75.1
Erythroblastopenia —*see also* Aplasia, red cell D60.9
congenital D61.01
Erythroblastophthisis D61.09
Erythroblastosis (fetalis) (newborn) P55.9
due to
ABO (antibodies) (incompatibility) (isoimmunization) P55.1
Rh (antibodies) (incompatibility) (isoimmunization) P55.0
Erythrocyanosis (crurum) I73.89
Erythrocythemia —*see* Erythremia
Erythrocytosis (megalosplenic) (secondary) D75.1
familial D75.0
oval, hereditary —*see* Elliptocytosis
secondary D75.1
stress D75.1
Erythroderma (secondary) —*see also* Erythema L53.9
bullous ichthyosiform, congenital Q80.3
desquamativum L21.1
ichthyosiform, congenital (bullous) Q80.3
neonatorum P83.8
psoriaticum L40.8
Erythrodysesthesia, palmar plantar (PPE) L27.1
Erythrogenesis imperfecta D61.09
Erythroleukemia C94.0-
Erythromelalgia I73.81
Erythrophagocytosis D75.89
Erythrophobia F40.298
Erythroplakia, oral epithelium, and tongue K13.29
Erythroplasia (Queyrat) D07.4
specified site —*see* Neoplasm, skin, in situ
unspecified site D07.4
Escherichia coli (E. coli), as cause of disease classified elsewhere B96.20
non-O157 Shiga toxin-producing (with known O group) B96.22
non-Shiga toxin-producing B96.29
O157 with confirmation of Shiga toxin when H antigen is unknown, or is not H7 B96.21
O157:H- (nonmotile) with confirmation of Shiga toxin B96.21
O157:H7 with or without confirmation of Shiga toxin-production B96.21
Shiga toxin-producing (with unspecified O group) (STEC) B96.23
Escherichia coli *(Continued)*
O157 B96.21
O157:H7 with or without confirmation of Shiga toxin-production B96.21
specified NEC B96.22
specified NEC B96.29
Esophagismus K22.4
Esophagitis (acute) (alkaline) (chemical) (chronic) (infectional) (necrotic) (peptic) (postoperative) K20.9
candidal B37.81
due to gastrointestinal reflux disease K21.0
eosinophilic K20.0
reflux K21.0
specified NEC K20.8
tuberculous A18.83
ulcerative K22.10
with bleeding K22.11
Esophagocele K22.5
Esophagomalacia K22.8
Esophagospasm K22.4
Esophagostenosis K22.2
Esophagostomiasis B81.8
Esophagotracheal —*see* condition
Esophagus —*see* condition
Esophoria H50.51
convergence, excess H51.12
divergence, insufficiency H51.8
Esotropia —*see* Strabismus, convergent concomitant
Espundia B55.2
Essential —*see* condition
Esthesioneuroblastoma C30.0
Esthesioneurocytoma C30.0
Esthesioneuroepithelioma C30.0
Esthiomene A55
Estivo-autumnal malaria (fever) B50.9
Estrangement (marital) Z63.5
parent-child NEC Z62.890
Estriasis —*see* Myiasis
Ethanolism —*see* Alcoholism
Etherism —*see* Dependence, drug, inhalant
Ethmoid, ethmoidal —*see* condition
Ethmoiditis (chronic) (nonpurulent) (purulent) —*see also* Sinusitis, ethmoidal
influenzal —*see* Influenza, with, respiratory manifestations NEC
Woakes' J33.1
Ethylism —*see* Alcoholism
Eulenburg's disease (congenital paramyotonia) G71.19
Eumycetoma B47.0
Eunuchoidism E29.1
hypogonadotropic E23.0
European blastomycosis —*see* Cryptococcosis
Eustachian —*see* condition
Evaluation (for) (of)
development state
adolescent Z00.3
period of
delayed growth in childhood Z00.70
with abnormal findings Z00.71
rapid growth in childhood Z00.2
puberty Z00.3
growth and developmental state (period of rapid growth) Z00.2
delayed growth Z00.70
with abnormal findings Z00.71
mental health (status) Z00.8
requested by authority Z04.6
period of
delayed growth in childhood Z00.70
with abnormal findings Z00.71
rapid growth in childhood Z00.2
suspected condition —*see* Observation
Evans syndrome D69.41
Event, apparent life threatening in newborn and infant (ALTE) R68.13
Eventration —*see also* Hernia, ventral
colon into chest —*see* Hernia, diaphragm
diaphragm (congenital) Q79.1
Eversion
bladder N32.89
cervix (uteri) N86
with cervicitis N72
foot NEC —*see also* Deformity, valgus, ankle congenital Q66.6
punctum lacrimale (postinfectional) (senile) H04.52-
ureter (meatus) N28.89
urethra (meatus) N36.8
uterus N81.4
Evidence
cytologic
of malignancy on anal smear R85.614
of malignancy on cervical smear R87.614
of malignancy on vaginal smear R87.624
Evisceration
birth injury P15.8
traumatic NEC
eye —*see* Enucleated eye
Evulsion —*see* Avulsion
Ewing's sarcoma or tumor —*see* Neoplasm, bone, malignant
Examination (for) (following) (general) (of) (routine) Z00.00
with abnormal findings Z00.01
abuse, physical (alleged), ruled out
adult Z04.71
child Z04.72
adolescent (development state) Z00.3
alleged rape or sexual assault (victim), ruled out
adult Z04.41
child Z04.42
allergy Z01.82
annual (adult) (periodic) (physical) Z00.00
with abnormal findings Z00.01
gynecological Z01.419
with abnormal findings Z01.411
antibody response Z01.84
blood —*see* Examination, laboratory
blood pressure Z01.30
with abnormal findings Z01.31
cancer staging —*see* Neoplasm, malignant, by site
cervical Papanicolaou smear Z12.4
as part of routine gynecological examination Z01.419
with abnormal findings Z01.411
child (over 28 days old) Z00.129
with abnormal findings Z00.121
under 28 days old —*see* Newborn, examination
clinical research control or normal comparison (control) (participant) Z00.6
contraceptive (drug) maintenance (routine) Z30.8
device (intrauterine) Z30.431
dental Z01.20
with abnormal findings Z01.21
developmental —*see* Examination, child
donor (potential) Z00.5
ear Z01.10
with abnormal findings NEC Z01.118
eye Z01.00
with abnormal findings Z01.01
following
accident NEC Z04.3
transport Z04.1
work Z04.2
assault, alleged, ruled out
adult Z04.71
child Z04.72
motor vehicle accident Z04.1
treatment (for) Z09
combined NEC Z09
fracture Z09
malignant neoplasm Z08
malignant neoplasm Z08
mental disorder Z09
specified condition NEC Z09

Examination *(Continued)*
follow-up (routine) (following) Z09
chemotherapy NEC Z09
malignant neoplasm Z08
fracture Z09
malignant neoplasm Z08
postpartum Z39.2
psychotherapy Z09
radiotherapy NEC Z09
malignant neoplasm Z08
surgery NEC Z09
malignant neoplasm Z08
gynecological Z01.419
with abnormal findings Z01.411
for contraceptive maintenance Z30.8
health —*see* Examination, medical
hearing Z01.10
with abnormal findings NEC Z01.118
following failed hearing screening Z01.110
immunity status testing Z01.84
laboratory (as part of a general medical examination) Z00.00
with abnormal findings Z00.01
preprocedural Z01.812
lactating mother Z39.1
medical (adult) (for) (of) Z00.00
with abnormal findings Z00.01
administrative purpose only Z02.9
specified NEC Z02.89
admission to
armed forces Z02.3
old age home Z02.2
prison Z02.89
residential institution Z02.2
school Z02.0
following illness or medical treatment Z02.0
summer camp Z02.89
adoption Z02.82
blood alcohol or drug level Z02.83
camp (summer) Z02.89
clinical research, normal subject (control) (participant) Z00.6
control subject in clinical research (normal comparison) (participant) Z00.6
donor (potential) Z00.5
driving license Z02.4
general (adult) Z00.00
with abnormal findings Z00.01
immigration Z02.89
insurance purposes Z02.6
marriage Z02.89
medicolegal reasons NEC Z04.8
naturalization Z02.89
participation in sport Z02.5
paternity testing Z02.81
population survey Z00.8
pre-employment Z02.1
pre-operative —*see* Examination, pre-procedural
pre-procedural
cardiovascular Z01.810
respiratory Z01.811
specified NEC Z01.818
preschool children
for admission to school Z02.0
prisoners
for entrance into prison Z02.89
recruitment for armed forces Z02.3
specified NEC Z00.8
sport competition Z02.5
medicolegal reason NEC Z04.8
newborn —*see* Newborn, examination
pelvic (annual) (periodic) Z01.419
with abnormal findings Z01.411
period of rapid growth in childhood Z00.2
periodic (adult) (annual) (routine) Z00.00
with abnormal findings Z00.01
physical (adult) —*see also* Examination, medical Z00.00
sports Z02.5

Examination *(Continued)*
postpartum
immediately after delivery Z39.0
routine follow-up Z39.2
pre-chemotherapy (antineoplastic) Z01.818
prenatal (normal pregnancy) —*see also* Pregnancy, normal Z34.9-
pre-procedural (pre-operative)
cardiovascular Z01.810
laboratory Z01.812
respiratory Z01.811
specified NEC Z01.818
prior to chemotherapy (antineoplastic) Z01.818
psychiatric NEC Z00.8
follow-up not needing further care Z09
requested by authority Z04.6
radiological (as part of a general medical examination) Z00.00
with abnormal findings Z00.01
repeat cervical smear to confirm findings of recent normal smear following initial abnormal smear Z01.42
skin (hypersensitivity) Z01.82
special —*see also* Examination, by type Z01.89
specified type NEC Z01.89
specified type or reason NEC Z04.8
teeth Z01.20
with abnormal findings Z01.21
urine —*see* Examination, laboratory
vision Z01.00
with abnormal findings Z01.01
Exanthem, exanthema —*see also* Rash
with enteroviral vesicular stomatitis B08.4
Boston A88.0
epidemic with meningitis A88.0 *[G02]*
subitum B08.20
due to human herpesvirus 6 B08.21
due to human herpesvirus 7 B08.22
viral, virus B09
specified type NEC B08.8
Excess, excessive, excessively
alcohol level in blood R78.0
androgen (ovarian) E28.1
attrition, tooth, teeth K03.0
carotene, carotin (dietary) E67.1
cold, effects of T69.9
specified effect NEC T69.8
convergence H51.12
crying
in child, adolescent, or adult R45.83
in infant R68.11
development, breast N62
divergence H51.8
drinking (alcohol) NEC (without dependence) F10.10
habitual (continual) (without remission) F10.20
eating R63.2
estrogen E28.0
fat —*see also* Obesity
in heart —*see* Degeneration, myocardial
localized E65
foreskin N47.8
gas R14.0
glucagon E16.3
heat —*see* Heat
intermaxillary vertical dimension of fully erupted teeth M26.37
interocclusal distance of fully erupted teeth M26.37
kalium E87.5
large
colon K59.39 ◀
congenital Q43.8
infant P08.0
organ or site, congenital NEC —*see* Anomaly, by site
long
organ or site, congenital NEC —*see* Anomaly, by site

Excess, excessive, excessively *(Continued)*
menstruation (with regular cycle) N92.0
with irregular cycle N92.1
napping Z72.821
natrium E87.0
number of teeth K00.1
nutrient (dietary) NEC R63.2
potassium (K) E87.5
salivation K11.7
secretion —*see also* Hypersecretion
milk O92.6
sputum R09.3
sweat R61
sexual drive F52.8
short
organ or site, congenital NEC —*see* Anomaly, by site
umbilical cord in labor or delivery O69.3
~~skin, eyelid (acquired) —see Blepharochalasis congenital Q10.3~~
skin L98.7 ◀
and subcutaneous tissue L98.7 ◀
eyelid (acquired) —*see* Blepharochalasis ◀
congenital Q10.3 ◀
sodium (Na) E87.0
spacing of fully erupted teeth M26.32
sputum R09.3
sweating R61
thirst R63.1
due to deprivation of water T73.1
tuberosity of jaw M26.07
vitamin
A (dietary) E67.0
administered as drug (prolonged intake) —*see* Table of Drugs and Chemicals, vitamins, adverse effect
overdose or wrong substance given or taken —*see* Table of Drugs and Chemicals, vitamins, poisoning
D (dietary) E67.3
administered as drug (prolonged intake) —*see* Table of Drugs and Chemicals, vitamins, adverse effect
overdose or wrong substance given or taken —*see* Table of Drugs and Chemicals, vitamins, poisoning
weight
gain R63.5
loss R63.4
Excitability, abnormal, under minor stress (personality disorder) F60.3
Excitation
anomalous atrioventricular I45.6
psychogenic F30.8
reactive (from emotional stress, psychological trauma) F30.8
Excitement
hypomanic F30.8
manic F30.9
mental, reactive (from emotional stress, psychological trauma) F30.8
state, reactive (from emotional stress, psychological trauma) F30.8
Excoriation (traumatic) —*see also* Abrasion
neurotic L98.1
skin picking disorder F42.4 ◀
Exfoliation
due to erythematous conditions according to extent of body surface involved L49.0
10-19 percent of body surface L49.1
20-29 percent of body surface L49.2
30-39 percent of body surface L49.3
40-49 percent of body surface L49.4
50-59 percent of body surface L49.5
60-69 percent of body surface L49.6
70-79 percent of body surface L49.7
80-89 percent of body surface L49.8
90-99 percent of body surface L49.9
less than 10 percent of body surface L49.0
teeth, due to systemic causes K08.0

◀ New ⇐ Revised ~~deleted~~ Deleted

Exfoliative —*see* condition
Exhaustion, exhaustive (physical NEC) R53.83
battle F43.0
cardiac —*see* Failure, heart
delirium F43.0
due to
cold T69.8
excessive exertion T73.3
exposure T73.2
neurasthenia F48.8
heart —*see* Failure, heart
heat —*see also* Heat, exhaustion T67.5
due to
salt depletion T67.4
water depletion T67.3
maternal, complicating delivery O75.81
mental F48.8
myocardium, myocardial —*see* Failure, heart
nervous F48.8
old age R54
psychogenic F48.8
psychosis F43.0
senile R54
vital NEC Z73.0
Exhibitionism F65.2
Exocervicitis —*see* Cervicitis
Exomphalos Q79.2
meaning hernia —*see* Hernia, umbilicus
Exophoria H50.52
convergence, insufficiency H51.11
divergence, excess H51.8
Exophthalmos H05.2-
congenital Q15.8
constant NEC H05.24-
displacement, globe —*see* Displacement, globe
due to thyrotoxicosis (hyperthyroidism) —*see* Hyperthyroidism, with, goiter (diffuse)
dysthyroid —*see* Hyperthyroidism, with, goiter (diffuse)
goiter —*see* Hyperthyroidism, with, goiter (diffuse)
intermittent NEC H05.25-
malignant —*see* Hyperthyroidism, with, goiter (diffuse)
orbital
edema —*see* Edema, orbit
hemorrhage —*see* Hemorrhage, orbit
pulsating NEC H05.26-
thyrotoxic, thyrotropic —*see* Hyperthyroidism, with, goiter (diffuse)
Exostosis —*see also* Disorder, bone
cartilaginous —*see* Neoplasm, bone, benign
congenital (multiple) Q78.6
external ear canal H61.81-
gonococcal A54.49
jaw (bone) M27.8
multiple, congenital Q78.6
orbit H05.35-
osteocartilaginous —*see* Neoplasm, bone, benign
syphilitic A52.77
Exotropia —*see* Strabismus, divergent concomitant
Explanation of
investigation finding Z71.2
medication Z71.89
Exposure (to) —*see also* Contact, with T75.89
acariasis Z20.7
AIDS virus Z20.6
air pollution Z77.110
algae and algae toxins Z77.121
algae bloom Z77.121
anthrax Z20.810
aromatic amines Z77.020
aromatic (hazardous) compounds NEC Z77.028
aromatic dyes NOS Z77.028
Exposure *(Continued)*
arsenic Z77.010
asbestos Z77.090
bacterial disease NEC Z20.818
benzene Z77.021
blue-green algae bloom Z77.121
body fluids (potentially hazardous) Z77.21
brown tide Z77.121
chemicals (chiefly nonmedicinal) (hazardous) NEC Z77.098
cholera Z20.09
chromium compounds Z77.018
cold, effects of T69.9
specified effect NEC T69.8
communicable disease Z20.9
bacterial NEC Z20.818
specified NEC Z20.89
viral NEC Z20.828
cyanobacteria bloom Z77.121
disaster Z65.5
discrimination Z60.5
dyes Z77.098
effects of T73.9
environmental tobacco smoke (acute) (chronic) Z77.22
Escherichia coli (E. coli) Z20.01
exhaustion due to T73.2
fiberglass —*see* Table of Drugs and Chemicals, fiberglass
German measles Z20.4
gonorrhea Z20.2
hazardous metals NEC Z77.018
hazardous substances NEC Z77.29
hazards in the physical environment NEC Z77.128
hazards to health NEC Z77.9
human immunodeficiency virus (HIV) Z20.6
human T-lymphotropic virus type-1 (HTLV-1) Z20.89
implanted
mesh —*see* Complications, mesh
prosthetic materials NEC —*see* Complications, prosthetic materials NEC
infestation (parasitic) NEC Z20.7
intestinal infectious disease NEC Z20.09
Escherichia coli (E. coli) Z20.01
lead Z77.011
meningococcus Z20.811
mold (toxic) Z77.120
nickel dust Z77.018
noise Z77.122
occupational
air contaminants NEC Z57.39
dust Z57.2
environmental tobacco smoke Z57.31
extreme temperature Z57.6
noise Z57.0
radiation Z57.1
risk factors Z57.9
specified NEC Z57.8
toxic agents (gases) (liquids) (solids) (vapors) in agriculture Z57.4
toxic agents (gases) (liquids) (solids) (vapors) in industry NEC Z57.5
vibration Z57.7
parasitic disease NEC Z20.7
pediculosis Z20.7
persecution Z60.5
pfiesteria piscicida Z77.121
poliomyelitis Z20.89
pollution
air Z77.110
environmental NEC Z77.118
soil Z77.112
water Z77.111
polycyclic aromatic hydrocarbons Z77.028
Exposure *(Continued)*
prenatal (drugs) (toxic chemicals) —*see* Newborn, affected by, noxious substances transmitted via placenta or breast milk ◄
rabies Z20.3
radiation, naturally occurring NEC Z77.123
radon Z77.123
red tide (Florida) Z77.121
rubella Z20.4
second hand tobacco smoke (acute) (chronic) Z77.22
in the perinatal period P96.81
sexually-transmitted disease Z20.2
smallpox (laboratory) Z20.89
syphilis Z20.2
terrorism Z65.4
torture Z65.4
tuberculosis Z20.1
uranium Z77.012
varicella Z20.820
venereal disease Z20.2
viral disease NEC Z20.828
war Z65.5
water pollution Z77.111
Exsanguination —*see* Hemorrhage
Exstrophy
abdominal contents Q45.8
bladder Q64.10
cloacal Q64.12
specified type NEC Q64.19
supravesical fissure Q64.11
Extensive —*see* condition
Extra —*see also* Accessory
marker chromosomes (normal individual) Q92.61
in abnormal individual Q92.62
rib Q76.6
cervical Q76.5
Extrasystoles (supraventricular) I49.49
atrial I49.1
auricular I49.1
junctional I49.2
ventricular I49.3
Extrauterine gestation or pregnancy —*see* Pregnancy, by site
Extravasation
blood R58
chyle into mesentery I89.8
pelvicalyceal N13.8
pyelosinus N13.8
urine (from ureter) R39.0
vesicant agent
antineoplastic chemotherapy T80.810
other agent NEC T80.818
Extremity —*see* condition, limb
Extrophy —*see* Exstrophy
Extroversion
bladder Q64.19
uterus N81.4
complicating delivery O71.2
postpartal (old) N81.4
Extruded tooth (teeth) M26.34
Extrusion
breast implant (prosthetic) T85.42
eye implant (globe) (ball) T85.328
intervertebral disc —*see* Displacement, intervertebral disc
ocular lens implant (prosthetic) —*see* Complications, intraocular lens
vitreous —*see* Prolapse, vitreous
Exudate
pleural —*see* Effusion, pleura
retina H35.89
Exudative —*see* condition
Eye, eyeball, eyelid —*see* condition
Eyestrain —*see* Disturbance, vision, subjective
Eyeworm disease of Africa B74.3

F

Faber's syndrome (achlorhydric anemia) D50.9
Fabry (-Anderson) disease E75.21
Faciocephalalgia, autonomic —*see also* Neuropathy, peripheral, autonomic G90.09
Factor (s)
psychic, associated with diseases classified elsewhere F54
psychological
affecting physical conditions F54
or behavioral
affecting general medical condition F54
associated with disorders or diseases classified elsewhere F54
Fahr disease (of brain) G23.8
Fahr Volhard disease (of kidney) I12.-
Failure, failed
abortion —*see* Abortion, attempted
aortic (valve) I35.8
rheumatic I06.8
attempted abortion —*see* Abortion, attempted
biventricular I50.9
bone marrow —*see* Anemia, aplastic
cardiac —*see* Failure, heart
cardiorenal (chronic) I50.9
hypertensive I13.2
cardiorespiratory (*see also* Failure, heart) R09.2
cardiovascular (chronic) —*see* Failure, heart
cerebrovascular I67.9
cervical dilatation in labor O62.0
circulation, circulatory (peripheral) R57.9
newborn P29.89
compensation —*see* Disease, heart
compliance with medical treatment or regimen —*see* Noncompliance
congestive —*see* Failure, heart, congestive
dental implant (endosseous) M27.69
due to
failure of dental prosthesis M27.63
lack of attached gingiva M27.62
occlusal trauma (poor prosthetic design) M27.62
parafunctional habits M27.62
periodontal infection (peri-implantitis) M27.62
poor oral hygiene M27.62
osseointegration M27.61
due to
complications of systemic disease M27.61
poor bone quality M27.61
iatrogenic M27.61
post-osseointegration
biological M27.62
due to complications of systemic disease M27.62
iatrogenic M27.62
mechanical M27.63
pre-integration M27.61
pre-osseointegration M27.61
specified NEC M27.69
descent of head (at term) of pregnancy (mother) O32.4
endosseous dental implant —*see* Failure, dental implant
engagement of head (term of pregnancy) (mother) O32.4
erection (penile) —*see also* Dysfunction, sexual, male, erectile N52.9
~~nonorganic F52.21~~
nonorganic F52.21 ◀
examination (s), anxiety concerning Z55.2
expansion terminal respiratory units (newborn) (primary) P28.0
forceps NOS (with subsequent cesarean delivery) O66.5
gain weight (child over 28 days old) R62.51
adult R62.7
newborn P92.6

Failure, failed *(Continued)*
genital response (male) F52.21
female F52.22
heart (acute) (senile) (sudden) I50.9
with
acute pulmonary edema —*see* Failure, ventricular, left
decompensation —*see* Failure, heart, congestive
dilatation —*see* Disease, heart
arteriosclerotic I70.90
biventricular I50.9
combined left-right sided I50.9
compensated I50.9
complicating
anesthesia (general) (local) or other sedation
in labor and delivery O74.2
in pregnancy O29.12-
postpartum, puerperal O89.1
delivery (cesarean) (instrumental) O75.4
congestive (compensated) (decompensated) I50.9
with rheumatic fever (conditions in I00)
active I01.8
inactive or quiescent (with chorea) I09.81
newborn P29.0
rheumatic (chronic) (inactive) (with chorea) I09.81
active or acute I01.8
with chorea I02.0
decompensated I50.9
degenerative —*see* Degeneration, myocardial
diastolic (congestive) I50.30
acute (congestive) I50.31
and (on) chronic (congestive) I50.33
chronic (congestive) I50.32
and (on) acute (congestive) I50.33
combined with systolic (congestive) I50.40
acute (congestive) I50.41
and (on) chronic (congestive) I50.43
chronic (congestive) I50.42
and (on) acute (congestive) I50.43
due to presence of cardiac prosthesis I97.13-
following cardiac surgery I97.13-
high output NOS I50.9
hypertensive —*see* Hypertension, heart
left (ventricular) —*see* Failure, ventricular, left
low output (syndrome) NOS I50.9
newborn P29.0
organic —*see* Disease, heart
peripartum O90.3
postprocedural I97.13-
rheumatic (chronic) (inactive) I09.9
right (ventricular) (secondary to left heart failure) —*see* Failure, heart, congestive
systolic (congestive) I50.20
acute (congestive) I50.21
and (on) chronic (congestive) I50.23
chronic (congestive) I50.22
and (on) acute (congestive) I50.23
combined with diastolic (congestive) I50.40
acute (congestive) I50.41
and (on) chronic (congestive) I50.43
chronic (congestive) I50.42
and (on) acute (congestive) I50.43
thyrotoxic —*see also* Thyrotoxicosis E05.90 *[I43]*
with thyroid storm E05.91 *[I43]*
valvular —*see* Endocarditis

Failure, failed *(Continued)*
hepatic K72.90
with coma K72.91
acute or subacute K72.00
with coma K72.01
due to drugs K71.10
with coma K71.11
alcoholic (acute) (chronic) (subacute) K70.40
with coma K70.41
chronic K72.10
with coma K72.11
due to drugs (acute) (subacute) (chronic) K71.10
with coma K71.11
due to drugs (acute) (subacute) (chronic) K71.10
with coma K71.11
postprocedural K91.82
hepatorenal K76.7
induction (of labor) O61.9
abortion —*see* Abortion, attempted
by
oxytocic drugs O61.0
prostaglandins O61.0
instrumental O61.1
mechanical O61.1
medical O61.0
specified NEC O61.8
surgical O61.1
intubation during anesthesia T88.4
in pregnancy O29.6-
labor and delivery O74.7
postpartum, puerperal O89.6
involution, thymus (gland) E32.0
kidney —*see also* Disease, kidney, chronic N19
acute —*see also* Failure, renal, acute N17.9-
diabetic —*see* E08-E13 with .22
lactation (complete) O92.3
partial O92.4
Leydig's cell, adult E29.1
liver —*see* Failure, hepatic
menstruation at puberty N91.0
mitral I05.8
myocardial, myocardium —*see also* Failure, heart I50.9
chronic —*see also* Failure, heart, congestive I50.9
congestive —*see also* Failure, heart, congestive I50.9
orgasm (female) (psychogenic) F52.31
male F52.32
ovarian (primary) E28.39
iatrogenic E89.40
asymptomatic E89.40
symptomatic E89.41
postprocedural (postablative) (postirradiation) (postsurgical) E89.40
asymptomatic E89.40
symptomatic E89.41
ovulation causing infertility N97.0
polyglandular, autoimmune E31.0
prosthetic joint implant —*see* Complications, joint prosthesis, mechanical, breakdown, by site
renal N19
with
tubular necrosis (acute) N17.0
acute N17.9
with
cortical necrosis N17.1
medullary necrosis N17.2
tubular necrosis N17.0
specified NEC N17.8
chronic N18.9
hypertensive —*see* Hypertension, kidney
congenital P96.0
end stage (chronic) N18.6
due to hypertension I12.0

◀ New ◀ Revised ~~deleted~~ Deleted

Failure, failed *(Continued)*
renal *(Continued)*
following
abortion —*see* Abortion by type complicated by specified condition NEC
crushing T79.5
ectopic or molar pregnancy O08.4
labor and delivery (acute) O90.4
hypertensive —*see* Hypertension, kidney
postprocedural N99.0
respiration, respiratory J96.9
with
hypercapnia J96.92
hypoxia J96.91
acute J96.00
with
hypercapnia J96.02
hypoxia J96.01
acute and (on) chronic J96.20
with
hypercapnia J96.22
hypoxia J96.21
center G93.89
chronic J96.10
with
hypercapnia J96.12
hypoxia J96.11
newborn P28.5
postprocedural (acute) J95.821
acute and chronic J95.822
rotation
cecum Q43.3
colon Q43.3
intestine Q43.3
kidney Q63.2
sedation (conscious) (moderate) during procedure T88.52
history of Z92.83
segmentation —*see also* Fusion
fingers —*see* Syndactylism, complex, fingers
vertebra Q76.49
with scoliosis Q76.3
seminiferous tubule, adult E29.1
senile (general) R54
sexual arousal (male) F52.21
female F52.22
testicular endocrine function E29.1
to thrive (child over 28 days old) R62.51
adult R62.7
newborn P92.6
transplant T86.92
bone T86.831
marrow T86.02
cornea T86.841
heart T86.22
with lung (s) T86.32
intestine T86.851
kidney T86.12
liver T86.42
lung (s) T86.811
with heart T86.32
pancreas T86.891
skin (allograft) (autograft) T86.821
specified organ or tissue NEC T86.891
stem cell (peripheral blood) (umbilical cord) T86.5
trial of labor (with subsequent cesarean delivery) O66.40
following previous cesarean delivery O66.41
tubal ligation N99.89
urinary —*see* Disease, kidney, chronic
vacuum extraction NOS (with subsequent cesarean delivery) O66.5
vasectomy N99.89
ventouse NOS (with subsequent cesarean delivery) O66.5

Failure, failed *(Continued)*
ventricular —*see also* Failure, heart I50.9
left I50.1
with rheumatic fever (conditions in I00)
active I01.8
with chorea I02.0
inactive or quiescent (with chorea) I09.81
rheumatic (chronic) (inactive) (with chorea) I09.81
active or acute I01.8
with chorea I02.0
right —*see also* Failure, heart, congestive I50.9
vital centers, newborn P91.8
Fainting (fit) R55
Fallen arches —*see* Deformity, limb, flat foot
Falling, falls (repeated) R29.6
any organ or part —*see* Prolapse
Fallopian
insufflation Z31.41
tube —*see* condition
Fallot's
pentalogy Q21.8
tetrad or tetralogy Q21.3
triad or trilogy Q22.3
False —*see also* condition
croup J38.5
joint —*see* Nonunion, fracture
labor (pains) O47.9
at or after 37 completed weeks of gestation O47.1
before 37 completed weeks of gestation O47.0-
passage, urethra (prostatic) N36.5
pregnancy F45.8
Family, familial —*see also* condition
disruption Z63.8
involving divorce or separation Z63.5
Li-Fraumeni (syndrome) Z15.01
planning advice Z30.09
problem Z63.9
specified NEC Z63.8
retinoblastoma C69.2-
Famine (effects of) T73.0
edema —*see* Malnutrition, severe
Fanconi (-de Toni)(-Debré) syndrome E72.09
with cystinosis E72.04
Fanconi's anemia (congenital pancytopenia) D61.09
Farber's disease or syndrome E75.29
Farcy A24.0
Farmer's
lung J67.0
skin L57.8
Farsightedness —*see* Hypermetropia
Fascia —*see* condition
Fasciculation R25.3
Fasciitis M72.9
diffuse (eosinophilic) M35.4
infective M72.8
necrotizing M72.6
necrotizing M72.6
nodular M72.4
perirenal (with ureteral obstruction) N13.5
with infection N13.6
plantar M72.2
specified NEC M72.8
traumatic (old) M72.8
current - code by site under Sprain
Fascioliasis B66.3
Fasciolopsis, fasciolopsiasis (intestinal) B66.5
Fascioscapulohumeral myopathy G71.0
Fast pulse R00.0
Fat
embolism —*see* Embolism, fat
excessive —*see also* Obesity
in heart —*see* Degeneration, myocardial
in stool R19.5

Fat *(Continued)*
localized (pad) E65
heart —*see* Degeneration, myocardial
knee M79.4
retropatellar M79.4
necrosis
breast N64.1
mesentery K65.4
omentum K65.4
pad E65
knee M79.4
Fatigue R53.83
auditory deafness —*see* Deafness
chronic R53.82
combat F43.0
general R53.83
psychogenic F48.8
heat (transient) T67.6
muscle M62.89
myocardium —*see* Failure, heart
neoplasm-related R53.0
nervous, neurosis F48.8
operational F48.8
psychogenic (general) F48.8
senile R54
voice R49.8
Fatness —*see* Obesity
Fatty —*see also* condition
apron E65
degeneration —*see* Degeneration, fatty
heart (enlarged) —*see* Degeneration, myocardial
liver NEC K76.0
alcoholic K70.0
nonalcoholic K76.0
necrosis —*see* Degeneration, fatty
Fauces —*see* condition
Fauchard's disease (periodontitis) —*see* Periodontitis
Faucitis J02.9
Favism (anemia) D55.0
Favus —*see* Dermatophytosis
Fazio-Londe disease or syndrome G12.1
Fear complex or reaction F40.9
Fear of —*see* Phobia
Feared complaint unfounded Z71.1
Febris, febrile —*see also* Fever
flava —*see also* Fever, yellow A95.9
melitensis A23.0
pestis —*see* Plague
recurrens —*see* Fever, relapsing
rubra A38.9
Fecal
incontinence R15.9
smearing R15.1
soiling R15.1
urgency R15.2
Fecalith (impaction) K56.41
appendix K38.1
congenital P76.8
Fede's disease K14.0
Feeble rapid pulse due to shock following injury T79.4
Feeble-minded F70
Feeding
difficulties R63.3
problem R63.3
newborn P92.9
specified NEC P92.8
nonorganic (adult) —*see* Disorder, eating
Feeling (of)
foreign body in throat R09.89
Feer's disease —*see* Poisoning, mercury
Feet —*see* condition
Feigned illness Z76.5
Feil-Klippel syndrome (brevicollis) Q76.1
Feinmesser's (hidrotic) ectodermal dysplasia Q82.4
Felinophobia F40.218

F

Felon —*see also* Cellulitis, digit
with lymphangitis —*see* Lymphangitis, acute, digit
Felty's syndrome M05.00
ankle M05.07-
elbow M05.02-
foot joint M05.07-
hand joint M05.04-
hip M05.05-
knee M05.06-
multiple site M05.09
shoulder M05.01-
vertebra —*see* Spondylitis, ankylosing
wrist M05.03-
Female genital cutting status —*see* Female genital mutilation status (FGM)
Female genital mutilation status (FGM) N90.810
specified NEC N90.818
type I (clitorectomy status) N90.811
type II (clitorectomy with excision of labia minora status) N90.812
type III (infibulation status) N90.813
type IV N90.818
Femur, femoral —*see* condition
Fenestration, fenestrated —*see also* Imperfect, closure
aortico-pulmonary Q21.4
cusps, heart valve NEC Q24.8
pulmonary Q22.3
pulmonic cusps Q22.3
Fernell's disease (aortic aneurysm) I71.9
Fertile eunuch syndrome E23.0
Fetid
breath R19.6
sweat L75.0
Fetishism F65.0
transvestic F65.1
Fetus, fetal —*see also* condition
alcohol syndrome (dysmorphic) Q86.0
compressus O31.0-
hydantoin syndrome Q86.1
lung tissue P28.0
papyraceous O31.0-
Fever (inanition) (of unknown origin) (persistent) (with chills) (with rigor) R50.9
abortus A23.1
Aden (dengue) A90
African tick-borne A68.1
American
mountain (tick) A93.2
spotted A77.0
aphthous B08.8
arbovirus, arboviral A94
hemorrhagic A94
specified NEC A93.8
Argentinian hemorrhagic A96.0
Assam B55.0
Australian Q A78
Bangkok hemorrhagic A91
Barmah forest A92.8
Bartonella A44.0
bilious, hemoglobinuric B50.8
blackwater B50.8
blister B00.1
Bolivian hemorrhagic A96.1
Bonvale dam T73.3
boutonneuse A77.1
brain —*see* Encephalitis
Brazilian purpuric A48.4
breakbone A90
Bullis A77.0
Bunyamwera A92.8
Burdwan B55.0
Bwamba A92.8
Cameroon —*see* Malaria
Canton A75.9
catarrhal (acute) J00
chronic J31.0
cat-scratch A28.1
Central Asian hemorrhagic A98.0
cerebral —*see* Encephalitis

Fever *(Continued)*
cerebrospinal meningococcal A39.0
Chagres B50.9
Chandipura A92.8
Changuinola A93.1
Charcot's (biliary) (hepatic) (intermittent) —*see* Calculus, bile duct
Chikungunya (viral) (hemorrhagic) A92.0
Chitral A93.1
Colombo —*see* Fever, paratyphoid
Colorado tick (virus) A93.2
congestive (remittent) —*see* Malaria
Congo virus A98.0
continued malarial B50.9
Corsican —*see* Malaria
Crimean-Congo hemorrhagic A98.0
Cyprus —*see* Brucellosis
dandy A90
deer fly —*see* Tularemia
dengue (virus) A90
hemorrhagic A91
sandfly A93.1
desert B38.0
drug induced R50.2
due to
conditions classified elsewhere R50.81
heat T67.0
enteric A01.00
enteroviral exanthematous (Boston exanthem) A88.0
ephemeral (of unknown origin) R50.9
epidemic hemorrhagic A98.5
erysipelatous —*see* Erysipelas
estivo-autumnal (malarial) B50.9
famine A75.0
five day A79.0
following delivery O86.4
Fort Bragg A27.89
gastroenteric A01.00
gastromalarial —*see* Malaria
Gibraltar —*see* Brucellosis
glandular —*see* Mononucleosis, infectious
Guama (viral) A92.8
Haverhill A25.1
hay (allergic) J30.1
with asthma (bronchial) J45.909
with
exacerbation (acute) J45.901
status asthmaticus J45.902
due to
allergen other than pollen J30.89
pollen, any plant or tree J30.1
heat (effects) T67.0
hematuric, bilious B50.8
hemoglobinuric (malarial) (bilious) B50.8
hemorrhagic (arthropod-borne) NOS A94
with renal syndrome A98.5
arenaviral A96.9
specified NEC A96.8
Argentinian A96.0
Bangkok A91
Bolivian A96.1
Central Asian A98.0
Chikungunya A92.0
Crimean-Congo A98.0
dengue (virus) A91
epidemic A98.5
Junin (virus) A96.0
Korean A98.5
Kyasanur forest A98.2
Machupo (virus) A96.1
mite-borne A93.8
mosquito-borne A92.8
Omsk A98.1
Philippine A91
Russian A98.5
Singapore A91
Southeast Asia A91
Thailand A91

Fever *(Continued)*
hemorrhagic NOS *(Continued)*
tick-borne NEC A93.8
viral A99
specified NEC A98.8
hepatic —*see* Cholecystitis
herpetic —*see* Herpes
icterohemorrhagic A27.0
Indiana A93.8
infective B99.9
specified NEC B99.8
intermittent (bilious) —*see also* Malaria
of unknown origin R50.9
pernicious B50.9
iodide R50.2
Japanese river A75.3
jungle —*see also* Malaria
yellow A95.0
Junin (virus) hemorrhagic A96.0
Katayama B65.2
kedani A75.3
Kenya (tick) A77.1
Kew Garden A79.1
Korean hemorrhagic A98.5
Lassa A96.2
Lone Star A77.0
Machupo (virus) hemorrhagic A96.1
malaria, malarial —*see* Malaria
Malta A23.9
Marseilles A77.1
marsh —*see* Malaria
Mayaro (viral) A92.8
Mediterranean —*see also* Brucellosis A23.9
familial M04.1 ⇐
tick A77.1
meningeal —*see* Meningitis
Meuse A79.0
Mexican A75.2
mianeh A68.1
miasmatic —*see* Malaria
mosquito-borne (viral) A92.9
hemorrhagic A92.8
mountain —*see also* Brucellosis
meaning Rocky Mountain spotted fever A77.0
tick (American) (Colorado) (viral) A93.2
Mucambo (viral) A92.8
mud A27.9
Neapolitan —*see* Brucellosis
neutropenic D70.9
newborn P81.9
environmental P81.0
Nine-Mile A78
non-exanthematous tick A93.2
North Asian tick-borne A77.2
Omsk hemorrhagic A98.1
O'nyong-nyong (viral) A92.1
Oropouche (viral) A93.0
Oroya A44.0
paludal —*see* Malaria
Panama (malarial) B50.9
Pappataci A93.1
paratyphoid A01.4
A A01.1
B A01.2
C A01.3
parrot A70
periodic (Mediterranean) M04.1 ⇐
persistent (of unknown origin) R50.9
petechial A39.0
pharyngoconjunctival B30.2
Philippine hemorrhagic A91
phlebotomus A93.1
Piry (virus) A93.8
Pixuna (viral) A92.8
Plasmodium ovale B53.0
polioviral (nonparalytic) A80.4
Pontiac A48.2
postimmunization R50.83
postoperative R50.82
due to infection T81.40 ⇐

◀ New ⇐ Revised ~~deleted~~ Deleted

Fever *(Continued)*
posttransfusion R50.84
postvaccination R50.83
presenting with conditions classified elsewhere R50.81
pretibial A27.89
puerperal O86.4
Q A78
quadrilateral A78
quartan (malaria) B52.9
Queensland (coastal) (tick) A77.3
quintan A79.0
rabbit —*see* Tularemia
rat-bite A25.9
due to
Spirillum A25.0
Streptobacillus moniliformis A25.1
recurrent —*see* Fever, relapsing
relapsing (Borrelia) A68.9
Carter's (Asiatic) A68.1
Dutton's (West African) A68.1
Koch's A68.9
louse-borne A68.0
Novy's
louse-borne A68.0
tick-borne A68.1
Obermeyer's (European) A68.0
tick-borne A68.1
remittent (bilious) (congestive) (gastric) —*see* Malaria
rheumatic (active) (acute) (chronic) (subacute) I00
with central nervous system involvement I02.9
active with heart involvement —*see* category I01
inactive or quiescent with
cardiac hypertrophy I09.89
carditis I09.9
endocarditis I09.1
aortic (valve) I06.9
with mitral (valve) disease I08.0
mitral (valve) I05.9
with aortic (valve) disease I08.0
pulmonary (valve) I09.89
tricuspid (valve) I07.8
heart disease NEC I09.89
heart failure (congestive) (conditions in I50.9) I09.81
left ventricular failure (conditions in I50.1) I09.81
myocarditis, myocardial degeneration (conditions in I51.4) I09.0
pancarditis I09.9
pericarditis I09.2
Rift Valley (viral) A92.4
Rocky Mountain spotted A77.0
rose J30.1
Ross River B33.1
Russian hemorrhagic A98.5
San Joaquin (Valley) B38.0
sandfly A93.1
Sao Paulo A77.0
scarlet A38.9
seven day (leptospirosis) (autumnal) (Japanese) A27.89
dengue A90
shin-bone A79.0
Singapore hemorrhagic A91
solar A90
Songo A98.5
sore B00.1
South African tick-bite A68.1
Southeast Asia hemorrhagic A91
spinal —*see* Meningitis
spirillary A25.0
splenic —*see* Anthrax
spotted A77.9
American A77.0
Brazilian A77.0
cerebrospinal meningitis A39.0

Fever *(Continued)*
spotted *(Continued)*
Colombian A77.0
due to Rickettsia
australis A77.3
conorii A77.1
rickettsii A77.0
sibirica A77.2
specified type NEC A77.8
Ehrlichiosis A77.40
due to
E. chafeensis A77.41
specified organism NEC A77.49
Rocky Mountain A77.0
steroid R50.2
streptobacillary A25.1
subtertian B50.9
Sumatran mite A75.3
sun A90
swamp A27.9
swine A02.8
sylvatic, yellow A95.0
Tahyna B33.8
tertian —*see* Malaria, tertian
Thailand hemorrhagic A91
thermic T67.0
three-day A93.1
tick
American mountain A93.2
Colorado A93.2
Kemerovo A93.8
Mediterranean A77.1
mountain A93.2
nonexanthematous A93.2
Quaranfil A93.8
tick-bite NEC A93.8
tick-borne (hemorrhagic) NEC A93.8
trench A79.0
tsutsugamushi A75.3
typhogastric A01.00
typhoid (abortive) (hemorrhagic) (intermittent) (malignant) A01.00
complicated by
arthritis A01.04
heart involvement A01.02
meningitis A01.01
osteomyelitis A01.05
pneumonia A01.03
specified NEC A01.09
typhomalarial —*see* Malaria
typhus —*see* Typhus (fever)
undulant —*see* Brucellosis
unknown origin R50.9
uveoparotid D86.89
valley B38.0
Venezuelan equine A92.2
vesicular stomatitis A93.8
viral hemorrhagic —*see* Fever, hemorrhagic, by type of virus
Volhynian A79.0
Wesselsbron (viral) A92.8
West
African B50.8
Nile (viral) A92.30
with
complications NEC A92.39
cranial nerve disorders A92.32
encephalitis A92.31
encephalomyelitis A92.31
neurologic manifestation NEC A92.32
optic neuritis A92.32
polyradiculitis A92.32
Whitmore's —*see* Melioidosis
Wolhynian A79.0
worm B83.9
yellow A95.9
jungle A95.0
sylvatic A95.0
urban A95.1
Zika virus A92.5 ◀

Fibrillation
atrial or auricular (established) I48.91
chronic I48.2
paroxysmal I48.0
permanent I48.2
persistent I48.1
cardiac I49.8
heart I49.8
muscular M62.89
ventricular I49.01
Fibrin
ball or bodies, pleural (sac) J94.1
chamber, anterior (eye) (gelatinous exudate) —*see* Iridocyclitis, acute
Fibrinogenolysis —*see* Fibrinolysis
Fibrinogenopenia D68.8
acquired D65
congenital D68.2
Fibrinolysis (hemorrhagic) (acquired) D65
antepartum hemorrhage —*see* Hemorrhage, antepartum, with coagulation defect
following
abortion —*see* Abortion by type complicated by hemorrhage
ectopic or molar pregnancy O08.1
intrapartum O67.0
newborn, transient P60
postpartum O72.3
Fibrinopenia (hereditary) D68.2
acquired D68.4
Fibrinopurulent —*see* condition
Fibrinous —*see* condition
Fibroadenoma
cellular intracanalicular D24-
giant D24-
intracanalicular
cellular D24-
giant D24-
specified site —*see* Neoplasm, benign, by site
unspecified site D24-
juvenile D24-
pericanalicular
specified site —*see* Neoplasm, benign, by site
unspecified site D24-
phyllodes D24-
prostate D29.1
specified site NEC —*see* Neoplasm, benign, by site
unspecified site D24-
Fibroadenosis, breast (chronic) (cystic) (diffuse) (periodic) (segmental) N60.2-
Fibroangioma —*see also* Neoplasm, benign, by site
juvenile
specified site —*see* Neoplasm, benign, by site
unspecified site D10.6
Fibrochondrosarcoma —*see* Neoplasm, cartilage, malignant
Fibrocystic
disease —*see also* Fibrosis, cystic
breast —*see* Mastopathy, cystic
jaw M27.49
kidney (congenital) Q61.8
liver Q44.6
pancreas E84.9
kidney (congenital) Q61.8
Fibrodysplasia ossificans progressiva —*see* Myositis, ossificans, progressiva
Fibroelastosis (cordis) (endocardial) (endomyocardial) I42.4
Fibroid (tumor) —*see also* Neoplasm, connective tissue, benign
disease, lung (chronic) —*see* Fibrosis, lung
heart (disease) —*see* Myocarditis
in pregnancy or childbirth O34.1-
causing obstructed labor O65.5
induration, lung (chronic) —*see* Fibrosis, lung
lung —*see* Fibrosis, lung

Fibroid *(Continued)*
pneumonia (chronic) —*see* Fibrosis, lung
uterus D25.9
Fibrolipoma —*see* Lipoma
Fibroliposarcoma —*see* Neoplasm, connective tissue, malignant
Fibroma —*see also* Neoplasm, connective tissue, benign
ameloblastic —*see* Cyst, calcifying odontogenic
bone (nonossifying) —*see* Disorder, bone, specified type NEC
ossifying —*see* Neoplasm, bone, benign
cementifying —*see* Neoplasm, bone, benign
chondromyxoid —*see* Neoplasm, bone, benign
desmoplastic —*see* Neoplasm, connective tissue, uncertain behavior
durum —*see* Neoplasm, connective tissue, benign
fascial —*see* Neoplasm, connective tissue, benign
invasive —*see* Neoplasm, connective tissue, uncertain behavior
molle —*see* Lipoma
myxoid —*see* Neoplasm, connective tissue, benign
nasopharynx, nasopharyngeal (juvenile) D10.6
nonosteogenic (nonossifying) —*see* Dysplasia, fibrous
odontogenic (central) —*see* Cyst, calcifying odontogenic
ossifying —*see* Neoplasm, bone, benign
periosteal —*see* Neoplasm, bone, benign
soft —*see* Lipoma
Fibromatosis M72.9
abdominal —*see* Neoplasm, connective tissue, uncertain behavior
aggressive —*see* Neoplasm, connective tissue, uncertain behavior
congenital generalized —*see* Neoplasm, connective tissue, uncertain behavior
Dupuytren's M72.0
gingival K06.1
palmar (fascial) M72.0
plantar (fascial) M72.2
pseudosarcomatous (proliferative) (subcutaneous) M72.4
retroperitoneal D48.3
specified NEC M72.8
Fibromyalgia M79.7
Fibromyoma —*see also* Neoplasm, connective tissue, benign
uterus (corpus) —*see also* Leiomyoma, uterus
in pregnancy or childbirth —*see* Fibroid, in pregnancy or childbirth
causing obstructed labor O65.5
Fibromyositis M79.7
Fibromyxolipoma D17.9
Fibromyxoma —*see* Neoplasm, connective tissue, benign
Fibromyxosarcoma —*see* Neoplasm, connective tissue, malignant
Fibro-odontoma, ameloblastic —*see* Cyst, calcifying odontogenic
Fibro-osteoma —*see* Neoplasm, bone, benign
Fibroplasia, retrolental H35.17
Fibropurulent —*see* condition
Fibrosarcoma —*see also* Neoplasm, connective tissue, malignant
ameloblastic C41.1
upper jaw (bone) C41.0
congenital —*see* Neoplasm, connective tissue, malignant
fascial —*see* Neoplasm, connective tissue, malignant
infantile —*see* Neoplasm, connective tissue, malignant
Fibrosarcoma *(Continued)*
odontogenic C41.1
upper jaw (bone) C41.0
periosteal —*see* Neoplasm, bone, malignant
Fibrosclerosis
breast N60.3-
multifocal M35.5
penis (corpora cavernosa) N48.6
Fibrosis, fibrotic
adrenal (gland) E27.8
amnion O41.8X-
anal papillae K62.89
arteriocapillary —*see* Arteriosclerosis
bladder N32.89
interstitial —*see* Cystitis, chronic, interstitial
localized submucosal —*see* Cystitis, chronic, interstitial
panmural —*see* Cystitis, chronic, interstitial
breast —*see* Fibrosclerosis, breast
capillary —*see also* Arteriosclerosis I70.90
lung (chronic) —*see* Fibrosis, lung
cardiac —*see* Myocarditis
cervix N88.8
chorion O41.8X-
corpus cavernosum (sclerosing) N48.6
cystic (of pancreas) E84.9
with
distal intestinal obstruction syndrome E84.19
fecal impaction E84.19
intestinal manifestations NEC E84.19
pulmonary manifestations E84.0
specified manifestations NEC E84.8
due to device, implant or graft —*see also* Complications, by site and type, specified NEC T85.828 ◄
arterial graft NEC T82.828
breast (implant) T85.828 ◄
catheter NEC T85.828 ◄
dialysis (renal) T82.828
intraperitoneal T85.828 ◄
infusion NEC T82.828
spinal (epidural) (subdural) T85.820 ◄
urinary (indwelling) T83.82
electronic (electrode) (pulse generator) (stimulator)
bone T84.82
cardiac T82.827
nervous system (brain) (peripheral nerve) (spinal) T85.820 ◄
urinary T83.82
fixation, internal (orthopedic) NEC T84.82
gastrointestinal (bile duct) (esophagus) T85.828 ◄
genital NEC T83.82
heart NEC T82.827
joint prosthesis T84.82
ocular (corneal graft) (orbital implant) NEC T85.828 ◄
orthopedic NEC T84.82
specified NEC T85.828 ◄
urinary NEC T83.82
vascular NEC T82.828
ventricular intracranial shunt T85.820 ◄
ejaculatory duct N50.89 ◄
endocardium —*see* Endocarditis
endomyocardial (tropical) I42.3
epididymis N50.89 ◄
eye muscle —*see* Strabismus, mechanical
heart —*see* Myocarditis
hepatic —*see* Fibrosis, liver
hepatolienal (portal hypertension) K76.6
hepatosplenic (portal hypertension) K76.6
infrapatellar fat pad M79.4
intrascrotal N50.89 ◄
kidney N26.9
liver K74.0
with sclerosis K74.2
alcoholic K70.2
Fibrosis, fibrotic *(Continued)*
lung (atrophic) (chronic) (confluent) (massive) (perialveolar) (peribronchial) J84.10
with
anthracosilicosis J60
anthracosis J60
asbestosis J61
bagassosis J67.1
bauxite J63.1
berylliosis J63.2
byssinosis J66.0
calcicosis J62.8
chalicosis J62.8
dust reticulation J64
farmer's lung J67.0
ganister disease J62.8
graphite J63.3
pneumoconiosis NOS J64
siderosis J63.4
silicosis J62.8
capillary J84.10
congenital P27.8
diffuse (idiopathic) J84.10
chemicals, gases, fumes or vapors (inhalation) J68.4
interstitial J84.10
acute J84.114
talc J62.0
following radiation J70.1
idiopathic J84.112
postinflammatory J84.10
silicotic J62.8
tuberculous —*see* Tuberculosis, pulmonary
lymphatic gland I89.8
median bar —*see* Hyperplasia, prostate
mediastinum (idiopathic) J98.59 ◄
meninges G96.19
myocardium, myocardial —*see* Myocarditis
ovary N83.8
oviduct N83.8
pancreas K86.89 ◄
penis NEC N48.6
pericardium I31.0
perineum, in pregnancy or childbirth O34.7- causing obstructed labor O65.5
pleura J94.1
popliteal fat pad M79.4
prostate (chronic) —*see* Hyperplasia, prostate
pulmonary —*see also* Fibrosis, lung J84.10
congenital P27.8
idiopathic J84.112
rectal sphincter K62.89
retroperitoneal, idiopathic (with ureteral obstruction) N13.5
with infection N13.6
sclerosing mesenteric (idiopathic) K65.4
scrotum N50.89 ◄
seminal vesicle N50.89 ◄
senile R54
skin L90.5
spermatic cord N50.89 ◄
spleen D73.89
in schistosomiasis (bilharziasis) B65.9 *[D77]*
subepidermal nodular —*see* Neoplasm, skin, benign
submucous (oral) (tongue) K13.5
testis N44.8
chronic, due to syphilis A52.76
thymus (gland) E32.8
tongue, submucous K13.5
tunica vaginalis N50.89 ◄
uterus (non-neoplastic) N85.8
vagina N89.8
valve, heart —*see* Endocarditis
vas deferens N50.89 ◄
vein I87.8
Fibrositis (periarticular) M79.7
nodular, chronic (Jaccoud's) (rheumatoid) —*see* Arthropathy, postrheumatic, chronic

◄ New ◄ Revised ~~deleted~~ Deleted

Fibrothorax J94.1
Fibrotic —*see* Fibrosis
Fibrous —*see* condition
Fibroxanthoma —*see also* Neoplasm, connective tissue, benign
  atypical —*see* Neoplasm, connective tissue, uncertain behavior
  malignant —*see* Neoplasm, connective tissue, malignant
Fibroxanthosarcoma —*see* Neoplasm, connective tissue, malignant
Fiedler's
  disease (icterohemorrhagic leptospirosis) A27.0
  myocarditis (acute) I40.1
Fifth disease B08.3
  venereal A55
Filaria, filarial, filariasis —*see* Infestation, filarial
Filatov's disease —*see* Mononucleosis, infectious
File-cutter's disease —*see* Poisoning, lead
Filling defect
  biliary tract R93.2
  bladder R93.41 ◀
  duodenum R93.3
  gallbladder R93.2
  gastrointestinal tract R93.3
  intestine R93.3
  kidney R93.42- ◀
  stomach R93.3
  ureter R93.41 ◀
  urinary organs, specified NEC R93.49 ◀
Fimbrial cyst Q50.4
Financial problem affecting care NOS Z59.9
  bankruptcy Z59.8
  foreclosure on loan Z59.8
Findings, abnormal, inconclusive, without diagnosis —*see also* Abnormal
  17-ketosteroids, elevated R82.5
  acetonuria R82.4
  alcohol in blood R78.0
  anisocytosis R71.8
  antenatal screening of mother O28.9
    biochemical O28.1
    chromosomal O28.5
    cytological O28.2
    genetic O28.5
    hematological O28.0
    radiological O28.4
    specified NEC O28.8
    ultrasonic O28.3
  antibody titer, elevated R76.0
  anticardiolipin antibody R76.0
  antiphosphatidylglycerol antibody R76.0
  antiphosphatidylinositol antibody R76.0
  antiphosphatidylserine antibody R76.0
  antiphospholipid antibody R76.0
  bacteriuria R82.71 ◀
  bicarbonate E87.8
  bile in urine R82.2
  blood sugar R73.09
    high R73.9
    low (transient) E16.2
  body fluid or substance, specified NEC R88.8
  casts, urine R82.99
  catecholamines R82.5
  cells, urine R82.99
  chloride E87.8
  cholesterol E78.9
    high E78.00 ◀
      with high triglycerides E78.2
  chyluria R82.0
  cloudy
    dialysis effluent R88.0
    urine R82.90
  creatinine clearance R94.4
  crystals, urine R82.99
  culture
    blood R78.81
    positive —*see* Positive, culture
  echocardiogram R93.1
Findings, abnormal, inconclusive, without diagnosis *(Continued)*
  electrolyte level, urinary R82.99
  function study NEC R94.8
    bladder R94.8
    endocrine NEC R94.7
      thyroid R94.6
    kidney R94.4
    liver R94.5
    pancreas R94.8
    placenta R94.8
    pulmonary R94.2
    spleen R94.8
  gallbladder, nonvisualization R93.2
  glucose (tolerance test) (non-fasting) R73.09
  glycosuria R81
  heart
    shadow R93.1
    sounds R01.2
  hematinuria R82.3
  hematocrit drop (precipitous) R71.0
  hemoglobinuria R82.3
  human papillomavirus (HPV) DNA test positive
    cervix
      high risk R87.810
      low risk R87.820
    vagina
      high risk R87.811
      low risk R87.821
  in blood (of substance not normally found in blood) R78.9
    addictive drug NEC R78.4
    alcohol (excessive level) R78.0
    cocaine R78.2
    hallucinogen R78.3
    heavy metals (abnormal level) R78.79
    lead R78.71
    lithium (abnormal level) R78.89
    opiate drug R78.1
    psychotropic drug R78.5
    specified substance NEC R78.89
    steroid agent R78.6
  indoleacetic acid, elevated R82.5
  ketonuria R82.4
  lactic acid dehydrogenase (LDH) R74.0
  liver function test R79.89
  mammogram NEC R92.8
    calcification (calculus) R92.1
    inconclusive result (due to dense breasts) R92.2
    microcalcification R92.0
  mediastinal shift R93.8
  melanin, urine R82.99
  myoglobinuria R82.1
  neonatal screening P09
  nonvisualization of gallbladder R93.2
  odor of urine NOS R82.90
  Papanicolaou cervix R87.619
    non-atypical endometrial cells R87.618
  pneumoencephalogram R93.0
  poikilocytosis R71.8
  potassium (deficiency) E87.6
    excess E87.5
  PPD R76.11
  radiologic (X-ray) R93.8
    abdomen R93.5
    biliary tract R93.2
    breast R92.8
    gastrointestinal tract R93.3
    genitourinary organs R93.8
    head R93.0
    inconclusive due to excess body fat of patient R93.9
    intrathoracic organs NEC R93.1
    placenta R93.8
    retroperitoneum R93.5
    skin R93.8
    skull R93.0
    subcutaneous tissue R93.8
Findings, abnormal, inconclusive, without diagnosis *(Continued)*
  red blood cell (count) (morphology) (sickling) (volume) R71.8
  scan NEC R94.8
    bladder R94.8
    bone R94.8
    kidney R94.4
    liver R93.2
    lung R94.2
    pancreas R94.8
    placental R94.8
    spleen R94.8
    thyroid R94.6
  sedimentation rate, elevated R70.0
  SGOT R74.0
  SGPT R74.0
  sodium (deficiency) E87.1
    excess E87.0
  specified body fluid NEC R88.8
  stress test R94.39
  thyroid (function) (metabolic rate) (scan) (uptake) R94.6
  transaminase (level) R74.0
  triglycerides E78.9
    high E78.1
      with high cholesterol E78.2
  tuberculin skin test (without active tuberculosis) R76.11
  urine R82.90
    acetone R82.4
    bacteria R82.71 ◀
    bile R82.2
    casts or cells R82.99
    chyle R82.0
    culture positive R82.79 ◀
    glucose R81
    hemoglobin R82.3
    ketone R82.4
    sugar R81
  vanillylmandelic acid (VMA), elevated R82.5
  vectorcardiogram (VCG) R94.39
  ventriculogram R93.0
  white blood cell (count) (differential) (morphology) D72.9
  xerography R92.8
Finger —*see* condition
Fire, Saint Anthony's —*see* Erysipelas
Fire-setting
  pathological (compulsive) F63.1
Fish hook stomach K31.89
Fishmeal-worker's lung J67.8
Fissure, fissured
  anus, anal K60.2
    acute K60.0
    chronic K60.1
    congenital Q43.8
  ear, lobule, congenital Q17.8
  epiglottis (congenital) Q31.8
  larynx J38.7
    congenital Q31.8
  lip K13.0
    congenital —*see* Cleft, lip
  nipple N64.0
    associated with
      lactation O92.13
      pregnancy O92.11-
      puerperium O92.12
  nose Q30.2
  palate (congenital) —*see* Cleft, palate
  skin R23.4
  spine (congenital) —*see also* Spina bifida
    with hydrocephalus —*see* Spina bifida, by site, with hydrocephalus
  tongue (acquired) K14.5
    congenital Q38.3
Fistula (cutaneous) L98.8
  abdomen (wall) K63.2
    bladder N32.2
    intestine NEC K63.2

F

Fistula *(Continued)*
abdomen *(Continued)*
ureter N28.89
uterus N82.5
abdominorectal K63.2
abdominosigmoidal K63.2
abdominothoracic J86.0
abdominouterine N82.5
congenital Q51.7
abdominovesical N32.2
accessory sinuses —*see* Sinusitis
actinomycotic —*see* Actinomycosis
alveolar antrum —*see* Sinusitis, maxillary
alveolar process K04.6
anorectal K60.5
antrobuccal —*see* Sinusitis, maxillary
antrum —*see* Sinusitis, maxillary
anus, anal (recurrent) (infectional) K60.3
congenital Q43.6
with absence, atresia and stenosis Q42.2
tuberculous A18.32
aorta-duodenal I77.2
appendix, appendicular K38.3
arteriovenous (acquired) (nonruptured) I77.0
brain I67.1
congenital Q28.2
ruptured I60.8
ruptured I60.8
cerebral —*see* Fistula, arteriovenous, brain
congenital (peripheral) —*see also* Malformation, arteriovenous
brain Q28.2
ruptured I60.8
coronary Q24.5
pulmonary Q25.72
coronary I25.41
congenital Q24.5
pulmonary I28.0
congenital Q25.72
surgically created (for dialysis) Z99.2
complication —*see* Complication, arteriovenous, fistula, surgically created
traumatic —*see* Injury, blood vessel
artery I77.2
aural (mastoid) —*see* Mastoiditis, chronic
auricle —*see also* Disorder, pinna, specified type NEC
congenital Q18.1
Bartholin's gland N82.8
bile duct (common) (hepatic) K83.3
with calculus, stones —*see* Calculus, bile duct
biliary (tract) —*see* Fistula, bile duct
bladder (sphincter) NEC —*see also* Fistula, vesico- N32.2
into seminal vesicle N32.2
bone —*see also* Disorder, bone, specified type NEC
with osteomyelitis, chronic —*see* Osteomyelitis, chronic, with draining sinus
brain G93.89
arteriovenous (acquired) I67.1
congenital Q28.2
branchial (cleft) Q18.0
branchiogenous Q18.0
breast N61.0 ◄
puerperal, postpartum or gestational, due to mastitis (purulent) —*see* Mastitis, obstetric, purulent
bronchial J86.0
bronchocutaneous, bronchomediastinal, bronchopleural, bronchopleuromediastinal (infective) J86.0
tuberculous NEC A15.5
bronchoesophageal J86.0
congenital Q39.2
with atresia of esophagus Q39.1
bronchovisceral J86.0

Fistula *(Continued)*
buccal cavity (infective) K12.2
cecosigmoidal K63.2
cecum K63.2
cerebrospinal (fluid) G96.0
cervical, lateral Q18.1
cervicoaural Q18.1
cervicosigmoidal N82.4
cervicovesical N82.1
cervix N82.8
chest (wall) J86.0
cholecystenteric —*see* Fistula, gallbladder
cholecystocolic —*see* Fistula, gallbladder
cholecystocolonic —*see* Fistula, gallbladder
cholecystoduodenal —*see* Fistula, gallbladder
cholecystogastric —*see* Fistula, gallbladder
cholecystointestinal —*see* Fistula, gallbladder
choledochoduodenal —*see* Fistula, bile duct
cholocolic K82.3
coccyx —*see* Sinus, pilonidal
colon K63.2
colostomy K94.09
common duct —*see* Fistula, bile duct
congenital, site not listed —*see* Anomaly, by site
coronary, arteriovenous I25.41
congenital Q24.5
costal region J86.0
cul-de-sac, Douglas' N82.8
cystic duct —*see also* Fistula, gallbladder
congenital Q44.5
dental K04.6
diaphragm J86.0
duodenum K31.6
ear (external) (canal) —*see* Disorder, ear, external, specified type NEC
enterocolic K63.2
enterocutaneous K63.2
enterouterine N82.4
congenital Q51.7
enterovaginal N82.4
congenital Q52.2
large intestine N82.3
small intestine N82.2
enterovesical N32.1
epididymis N50.89 ◄
tuberculous A18.15
esophagobronchial J86.0
congenital Q39.2
with atresia of esophagus Q39.1
esophagocutaneous K22.8
esophagopleural-cutaneous J86.0
esophagotracheal J86.0
congenital Q39.2
with atresia of esophagus Q39.1
esophagus K22.8
congenital Q39.2
with atresia of esophagus Q39.1
ethmoid —*see* Sinusitis, ethmoidal
eyeball (cornea) (sclera) —*see* Disorder, globe, hypotony
eyelid H01.8
fallopian tube, external N82.5
fecal K63.2
congenital Q43.6
from periapical abscess K04.6
frontal sinus —*see* Sinusitis, frontal
gallbladder K82.3
with calculus, cholelithiasis, stones —*see* Calculus, gallbladder
gastric K31.6
gastrocolic K31.6
congenital Q40.2
tuberculous A18.32
gastroenterocolic K31.6
gastroesophageal K31.6
gastrojejunal K31.6
gastrojejunocolic K31.6

Fistula *(Continued)*
genital tract (female) N82.9
specified NEC N82.8
to intestine NEC N82.4
to skin N82.5
hepatic artery-portal vein, congenital Q26.6
hepatopleural J86.0
hepatopulmonary J86.0
ileorectal or ileosigmoidal K63.2
ileovaginal N82.2
ileovesical N32.1
ileum K63.2
in ano K60.3
tuberculous A18.32
inner ear (labyrinth) —*see* subcategory H83.1
intestine NEC K63.2
intestinocolonic (abdominal) K63.2
intestinoureteral N28.89
intestinouterine N82.4
intestinovaginal N82.4
large intestine N82.3
small intestine N82.2
intestinovesical N32.1
ischiorectal (fossa) K61.3
jejunum K63.2
joint M25.10
ankle M25.17-
elbow M25.12-
foot joint M25.17-
hand joint M25.14-
hip M25.15-
knee M25.16-
shoulder M25.11-
specified joint NEC M25.18
tuberculous —*see* Tuberculosis, joint
vertebrae M25.18
wrist M25.13-
kidney N28.89
labium (majus) (minus) N82.8
labyrinth —*see* subcategory H83.1
lacrimal (gland) (sac) H04.61-
lacrimonasal duct —*see* Fistula, lacrimal
laryngotracheal, congenital Q34.8
larynx J38.7
lip K13.0
congenital Q38.0
lumbar, tuberculous A18.01
lung J86.0
lymphatic I89.8
mammary (gland) N61.0 ◄
mastoid (process) (region) —*see* Mastoiditis, chronic
maxillary J32.0
medial, face and neck Q18.8
mediastinal J86.0
mediastinobronchial J86.0
mediastinocutaneous J86.0
middle ear —*see* subcategory H74.8
mouth K12.2
nasal J34.89
sinus —*see* Sinusitis
nasopharynx J39.2
nipple N64.0
nose J34.89
oral (cutaneous) K12.2
maxillary J32.0
nasal (with cleft palate) —*see* Cleft, palate
orbit, orbital —*see* Disorder, orbit, specified type NEC
oroantral J32.0
oviduct, external N82.5
palate (hard) M27.8
pancreatic K86.89 ◄
pancreaticoduodenal K86.89 ◄
parotid (gland) K11.4
region K12.2
penis N48.89
perianal K60.3
pericardium (pleura) (sac) —*see* Pericarditis
pericecal K63.2
perineorectal K60.4
perineosigmoidal K63.2

◄ New ◄ Revised ~~deleted~~ Deleted

Fistula *(Continued)*
perineum, perineal (with urethral involvement) NEC N36.0
tuberculous A18.13
ureter N28.89
perirectal K60.4
tuberculous A18.32
peritoneum K65.9
pharyngoesophageal J39.2
pharynx J39.2
branchial cleft (congenital) Q18.0
pilonidal (infected) (rectum) —*see* Sinus, pilonidal
pleura, pleural, pleurocutaneous, pleuroperitoneal J86.0
tuberculous NEC A15.6
pleuropericardial I31.8
portal vein-hepatic artery, congenital Q26.6
postauricular H70.81-
postoperative, persistent T81.83
specified site —*see* Fistula, by site
preauricular (congenital) Q18.1
prostate N42.89
pulmonary J86.0
arteriovenous I28.0
congenital Q25.72
tuberculous —*see* Tuberculosis, pulmonary
pulmonoperitoneal J86.0
rectolabial N82.4
rectosigmoid (intercommunicating) K63.2
rectoureteral N28.89
rectourethral N36.0
congenital Q64.73
rectouterine N82.4
congenital Q51.7
rectovaginal N82.3
congenital Q52.2
tuberculous A18.18
rectovesical N32.1
congenital Q64.79
rectovesicovaginal N82.3
rectovulval N82.4
congenital Q52.79
rectum (to skin) K60.4
congenital Q43.6
with absence, atresia and stenosis Q42.0
tuberculous A18.32
renal N28.89
retroauricular —*see* Fistula, postauricular
salivary duct or gland (any) K11.4
congenital Q38.4
scrotum (urinary) N50.89 ⇐
tuberculous A18.15
semicircular canals —*see* subcategory H83.1
sigmoid K63.2
to bladder N32.1
sinus —*see* Sinusitis
skin L98.8
to genital tract (female) N82.5
splenocolic D73.89
stercoral K63.2
stomach K31.6
sublingual gland K11.4
submandibular gland K11.4
submaxillary (gland) K11.4
region K12.2
thoracic J86.0
duct I89.8
thoracoabdominal J86.0
thoracogastric J86.0
thoracointestinal J86.0
thorax J86.0
thyroglossal duct Q89.2
thyroid E07.89
trachea, congenital (external) (internal) Q32.1
tracheoesophageal J86.0
congenital Q39.2
with atresia of esophagus Q39.1
following tracheostomy J95.04
traumatic arteriovenous —*see* Injury, blood vessel, by site

Fistula *(Continued)*
tuberculous - code by site under Tuberculosis
typhoid A01.09
umbilicourinary Q64.8
urachus, congenital Q64.4
ureter (persistent) N28.89
ureteroabdominal N28.89
ureterorectal N28.89
ureterosigmoido-abdominal N28.89
ureterovaginal N82.1
ureterovesical N32.2
urethra N36.0
congenital Q64.79
tuberculous A18.13
urethroperineal N36.0
urethroperineovesical N32.2
urethrorectal N36.0
congenital Q64.73
urethroscrotal N50.89 ⇐
urethrovaginal N82.1
urethrovesical N32.2
urinary (tract) (persistent) (recurrent) N36.0
uteroabdominal N82.5
congenital Q51.7
uteroenteric, uterointestinal N82.4
congenital Q51.7
uterorectal N82.4
congenital Q51.7
uteroureteric N82.1
uterourethral Q51.7
uterovaginal N82.8
uterovesical N82.1
congenital Q51.7
uterus N82.8
vagina (postpartal) (wall) N82.8
vaginocutaneous (postpartal) N82.5
vaginointestinal NEC N82.4
large intestine N82.3
small intestine N82.2
vaginoperineal N82.5
vasocutaneous, congenital Q55.7
vesical NEC N32.2
vesicoabdominal N32.2
vesicocervicovaginal N82.1
vesicocolic N32.1
vesicocutaneous N32.2
vesicoenteric N32.1
vesicointestinal N32.1
vesicometrorectal N82.4
vesicoperineal N32.2
vesicorectal N32.1
congenital Q64.79
vesicosigmoidal N32.1
vesicosigmoidovaginal N82.3
vesicoureteral N32.2
vesicoureterovaginal N82.1
vesicourethral N32.2
vesicourethrorectal N32.1
vesicouterine N82.1
congenital Q51.7
vesicovaginal N82.0
vulvorectal N82.4
congenital Q52.79
Fit R56.9
epileptic —*see* Epilepsy
fainting R55
hysterical F44.5
newborn P90
Fitting (and adjustment) (of)
artificial
arm —*see* Admission, adjustment, artificial, arm
breast Z44.3
eye Z44.2
leg —*see* Admission, adjustment, artificial, leg
automatic implantable cardiac defibrillator (with synchronous cardiac pacemaker) Z45.02

Fitting *(Continued)*
brain neuropacemaker Z46.2
implanted Z45.42
cardiac defibrillator —*see* Fitting (and adjustment) (of), automatic implantable cardiac defibrillator
catheter, non-vascular Z46.82
colostomy belt Z46.89
contact lenses Z46.0
CRT-D (resynchronization therapy defibrillator) Z45.02 ◀
CRT-P (cardiac resynchronization therapy pacemaker) Z45.018 ◀
pulse generator Z45.010 ◀
cystostomy device Z46.6
defibrillator, cardiac —*see* Fitting (and adjustment) (of), automatic implantable cardiac defibrillator
dentures Z46.3
device NOS Z46.9
abdominal Z46.89
gastrointestinal NEC Z46.59
implanted NEC Z45.89
nervous system Z46.2
implanted —*see* Admission, adjustment, device, implanted, nervous system
orthodontic Z46.4
orthoptic Z46.0
orthotic Z46.89
prosthetic (external) Z44.9
breast Z44.3
dental Z46.3
eye Z44.2
specified NEC Z44.8
specified NEC Z46.89
substitution
auditory Z46.2
implanted —*see* Admission, adjustment, device, implanted, hearing device
nervous system Z46.2
implanted —*see* Admission, adjustment, device, implanted, nervous system
visual Z46.2
implanted Z45.31
urinary Z46.6
gastric lap band Z46.51
gastrointestinal appliance NEC Z46.59
glasses (reading) Z46.0
hearing aid Z46.1
ileostomy device Z46.89
insulin pump Z46.81
intestinal appliance NEC Z46.89
myringotomy device (stent) (tube) Z45.82
neuropacemaker Z46.2
implanted Z45.42
non-vascular catheter Z46.82
orthodontic device Z46.4
orthopedic device (brace) (cast) (corset) (shoes) Z46.89
pacemaker (cardiac) (cardiac resynchronization therapy (CRT-P)) Z45.018 ⇐
nervous system (brain) (peripheral nerve) (spinal cord) Z46.2
implanted Z45.42
pulse generator Z45.010
portacath (port-a-cath) Z45.2
prosthesis (external) Z44.9
arm —*see* Admission, adjustment, artificial, arm
breast Z44.3
dental Z46.3
eye Z44.2
leg —*see* Admission, adjustment, artificial, leg
specified NEC Z44.8
spectacles Z46.0
wheelchair Z46.89

F

Fitzhugh-Curtis syndrome
due to
Chlamydia trachomatis A74.81
Neisseria gonorrhorea (gonococcal peritonitis) A54.85
Fitz's syndrome (acute hemorrhagic pancreatitis) —*see also* Pancreatitis, acute K85.80 ◀
Fixation
joint —*see* Ankylosis
larynx J38.7
stapes —*see* Ankylosis, ear ossicles
deafness —*see* Deafness, conductive
uterus (acquired) —*see* Malposition, uterus
vocal cord J38.3
Flabby ridge K06.8
Flaccid —*see also* condition
palate, congenital Q38.5
Flail
chest S22.5-
newborn (birth injury) P13.8
joint (paralytic) M25.20
ankle M25.27-
elbow M25.22-
foot joint M25.27-
hand joint M25.24-
hip M25.25-
knee M25.26-
shoulder M25.21-
specified joint NEC M25.28
wrist M25.23-
Flajani's disease —*see* Hyperthyroidism, with, goiter (diffuse)
Flap, liver K71.3
Flashbacks (residual to hallucinogen use) F16.283
Flat
chamber (eye) —*see* Disorder, globe, hypotony, flat anterior chamber
chest, congenital Q67.8
foot (acquired) (fixed type) (painful) (postural) —*see also* Deformity, limb, flat foot
congenital (rigid) (spastic (everted)) Q66.5-
rachitic sequelae (late effect) E64.3
organ or site, congenital NEC —*see* Anomaly, by site
pelvis M95.5
with disproportion (fetopelvic) O33.0
causing obstructed labor O65.0
congenital Q74.2
Flatau-Schilder disease G37.0
Flatback syndrome M40.30
lumbar region M40.36
lumbosacral region M40.37
thoracolumbar region M40.35
Flattening
head, femur M89.8X5
hip —*see* Coxa, plana
lip (congenital) Q18.8
nose (congenital) Q67.4
acquired M95.0
Flatulence R14.3
psychogenic F45.8
Flatus R14.3
vaginalis N89.8
Flax-dresser's disease J66.1
Flea bite —*see* Injury, bite, by site, superficial, insect
Flecks, glaucomatous (subcapsular) —*see* Cataract, complicated
Fleischer (-Kayser) ring (cornea) H18.04-
Fleshy mole O02.0
Flexibilitas cerea —*see* Catalepsy
Flexion
amputation stump (surgical) T87.89
cervix —*see* Malposition, uterus
contracture, joint —*see* Contraction, joint
deformity, joint —*see also* Deformity, limb, flexion M21.20
hip, congenital Q65.89
uterus —*see also* Malposition, uterus
lateral —*see* Lateroversion, uterus
Flexner-Boyd dysentery A03.2
Flexner's dysentery A03.1
Flexure —*see* Flexion
Flint murmur (aortic insufficiency) I35.1
Floater, vitreous —*see* Opacity, vitreous
Floating
cartilage (joint) —*see also* Loose, body, joint
knee —*see* Derangement, knee, loose body
gallbladder, congenital Q44.1
kidney N28.89
congenital Q63.8
spleen D73.89
Flooding N92.0
Floor —*see* condition
Floppy
baby syndrome (nonspecific) P94.2
iris syndrome (intraoperative) (IFIS) H21.81
nonrheumatic mitral valve syndrome I34.1
Flu —*see also* Influenza
avian —*see also* Influenza, due to, identified novel influenza A virus J09.X2
bird —*see also* Influenza, due to, identified novel influenza A virus J09.X2
intestinal NEC A08.4
swine (viruses that normally cause infections in pigs) —*see also* Influenza, due to, identified novel influenza A virus J09.X2
Fluctuating blood pressure I99.8
Fluid
abdomen R18.8
chest J94.8
heart —*see* Failure, heart, congestive
joint —*see* Effusion, joint
loss (acute) E86.9
~~with~~
~~hypernatremia E87.0~~
~~hyponatremia E87.1~~
lung —*see* Edema, lung
overload E87.70
specified NEC E87.79
peritoneal cavity R18.8
pleural cavity J94.8
retention R60.9
Flukes NEC —*see also* Infestation, fluke
blood NEC —*see* Schistosomiasis
liver B66.3
Fluor (vaginalis) N89.8
trichomonal or due to Trichomonas (vaginalis) A59.00
Fluorosis
dental K00.3
skeletal M85.10
ankle M85.17-
foot M85.17-
forearm M85.13-
hand M85.14-
lower leg M85.16-
multiple site M85.19
neck M85.18
rib M85.18
shoulder M85.11-
skull M85.18
specified site NEC M85.18
thigh M85.15-
toe M85.17-
upper arm M85.12-
vertebra M85.18
Flush syndrome E34.0
Flushing R23.2
menopausal N95.1
Flutter
atrial or auricular I48.92
atypical I48.4
type I I48.3
type II I48.4
typical I48.3
heart I49.8
atrial or auricular I48.92
atypical I48.4
type I I48.3
Fistula *(Continued)*
heart *(Continued)*
atrial or auricular *(Continued)*
type II I48.4
typical I48.3
ventricular I49.02
ventricular I49.02
FNHTR (febrile nonhemolytic transfusion reaction) R50.84
Fochier's abscess - code by site under Abscess
Focus, Assmann's —*see* Tuberculosis, pulmonary
Fogo selvagem L10.3
Foix-Alajouanine syndrome G95.19
Fold, folds (anomalous) —*see also* Anomaly, by site
Descemet's membrane —*see* Change, corneal membrane, Descemet's, fold
epicanthic Q10.3
heart Q24.8
Folie à deux F24
Follicle
cervix (nabothian) (ruptured) N88.8
graafian, ruptured, with hemorrhage N83.0- ◀
nabothian N88.8
Follicular —*see* condition
Folliculitis (superficial) L73.9
abscedens et suffodiens L66.3
cyst N83.0- ◀
decalvans L66.2
deep —*see* Furuncle, by site
gonococcal (acute) (chronic) A54.01
keloid, keloidalis L73.0
pustular L01.02
ulerythematosa reticulata L66.4
Folliculome lipidique
specified site —*see* Neoplasm, benign, by site
unspecified site
female D27.9
male D29.20
Følling's disease E70.0
Follow-up —*see* Examination, follow-up
Fong's syndrome (hereditary osteo-onychodysplasia) Q87.2 ◀
Food
allergy L27.2
asphyxia (from aspiration or inhalation) —*see* Foreign body, by site
choked on —*see* Foreign body, by site
deprivation T73.0
specified kind of food NEC E63.8
intoxication —*see* Poisoning, food
lack of T73.0
poisoning —*see* Poisoning, food
rejection NEC —*see* Disorder, eating
strangulation or suffocation —*see* Foreign body, by site
toxemia —*see* Poisoning, food
Foot —*see* condition
Foramen ovale (nonclosure) (patent) (persistent) Q21.1
Forbes' glycogen storage disease E74.03
Fordyce-Fox disease L75.2
Fordyce's disease (mouth) Q38.6
Forearm —*see* condition
Foreign body
with
laceration —*see* Laceration, by site, with foreign body
puncture wound —*see* Puncture, by site, with foreign body
accidentally left following a procedure T81.509
aspiration T81.506
resulting in
adhesions T81.516
obstruction T81.526
perforation T81.536
specified complication NEC T81.596

◀ New ◀ Revised ~~deleted~~ Deleted

Foreign body *(Continued)*
accidentally left following a procedure *(Continued)*
cardiac catheterization T81.505
resulting in
acute reaction T81.60
aseptic peritonitis T81.61
specified NEC T81.69
adhesions T81.515
obstruction T81.525
perforation T81.535
specified complication NEC T81.595
causing
acute reaction T81.60
aseptic peritonitis T81.61
specified complication NEC T81.69
adhesions T81.519
aseptic peritonitis T81.61
obstruction T81.529
perforation T81.539
specified complication NEC T81.599
endoscopy T81.504
resulting in
adhesions T81.514
obstruction T81.524
perforation T81.534
specified complication NEC T81.594
immunization T81.503
resulting in
adhesions T81.513
obstruction T81.523
perforation T81.533
specified complication NEC T81.593
infusion T81.501
resulting in
adhesions T81.511
obstruction T81.521
perforation T81.531
specified complication NEC T81.591
injection T81.503
resulting in
adhesions T81.513
obstruction T81.523
perforation T81.533
specified complication NEC T81.593
kidney dialysis T81.502
resulting in
adhesions T81.512
obstruction T81.522
perforation T81.532
specified complication NEC T81.592
packing removal T81.507
resulting in
acute reaction T81.60
aseptic peritonitis T81.61
specified NEC T81.69
adhesions T81.517
obstruction T81.527
perforation T81.537
specified complication NEC T81.597
puncture T81.506
resulting in
adhesions T81.516
obstruction T81.526
perforation T81.536
specified complication NEC T81.596
specified procedure NEC T81.508
resulting in
acute reaction T81.60
aseptic peritonitis T81.61
specified NEC T81.69
adhesions T81.518
obstruction T81.528
perforation T81.538
specified complication NEC T81.598
surgical operation T81.500
resulting in
acute reaction T81.60
aseptic peritonitis T81.61
specified NEC T81.69

Foreign body *(Continued)*
accidentally left following a procedure *(Continued)*
surgical operation *(Continued)*
resulting in *(Continued)*
adhesions T81.510
obstruction T81.520
perforation T81.530
specified complication NEC T81.590
transfusion T81.501
resulting in
adhesions T81.511
obstruction T81.521
perforation T81.531
specified complication NEC T81.591
alimentary tract T18.9
anus T18.5
colon T18.4
esophagus —*see* Foreign body, esophagus
mouth T18.0
multiple sites T18.8
rectosigmoid (junction) T18.5
rectum T18.5
small intestine T18.3
specified site NEC T18.8
stomach T18.2
anterior chamber (eye) S05.5-
auditory canal —*see* Foreign body, entering through orifice, ear
bronchus T17.508
causing
asphyxiation T17.500
food (bone) (seed) T17.520
gastric contents (vomitus) T17.510
specified type NEC T17.590
injury NEC T17.508
food (bone) (seed) T17.528
gastric contents (vomitus) T17.518
specified type NEC T17.598
canthus —*see* Foreign body, conjunctival sac
ciliary body (eye) S05.5-
conjunctival sac T15.1-
cornea T15.0-
entering through orifice
accessory sinus T17.0
alimentary canal T18.9
multiple parts T18.8
specified part NEC T18.8
alveolar process T18.0
antrum (Highmore's) T17.0
anus T18.5
appendix T18.4
auditory canal —*see* Foreign body, entering through orifice, ear
auricle —*see* Foreign body, entering through orifice, ear
bladder T19.1
bronchioles —*see* Foreign body, respiratory tract, specified site NEC
bronchus (main) —*see* Foreign body, bronchus
buccal cavity T18.0
canthus (inner) —*see* Foreign body, conjunctival sac
cecum T18.4
cervix (canal) (uteri) T19.3
colon T18.4
conjunctival sac —*see* Foreign body, conjunctival sac
cornea —*see* Foreign body, cornea
digestive organ or tract NOS T18.9
multiple parts T18.8
specified part NEC T18.8
duodenum T18.3
ear (external) T16.-
esophagus —*see* Foreign body, esophagus
eye (external) NOS T15.9-
conjunctival sac —*see* Foreign body, conjunctival sac
cornea —*see* Foreign body, cornea
specified part NEC T15.8-

Foreign body *(Continued)*
entering through orifice *(Continued)*
eyeball —*see also* Foreign body, entering through orifice, eye, specified part NEC
with penetrating wound —*see* Puncture, eyeball
eyelid —*see also* Foreign body, conjunctival sac
with
laceration —*see* Laceration, eyelid, with foreign body
puncture —*see* Puncture, eyelid, with foreign body
superficial injury —*see* Foreign body, superficial, eyelid
gastrointestinal tract T18.9
multiple parts T18.8
specified part NEC T18.8
genitourinary tract T19.9
multiple parts T19.8
specified part NEC T19.8
globe —*see* Foreign body, entering through orifice, eyeball
gum T18.0
Highmore's antrum T17.0
hypopharynx —*see* Foreign body, pharynx
ileum T18.3
intestine (small) T18.3
large T18.4
lacrimal apparatus (punctum) —*see* Foreign body, entering through orifice, eye, specified part NEC
large intestine T18.4
larynx —*see* Foreign body, larynx
lung —*see* Foreign body, respiratory tract, specified site NEC
maxillary sinus T17.0
mouth T18.0
nasal sinus T17.0
nasopharynx —*see* Foreign body, pharynx
nose (passage) T17.1
nostril T17.1
oral cavity T18.0
palate T18.0
penis T19.4
pharynx —*see* Foreign body, pharynx
piriform sinus —*see* Foreign body, pharynx
rectosigmoid (junction) T18.5
rectum T18.5
respiratory tract —*see* Foreign body, respiratory tract
sinus (accessory) (frontal) (maxillary) (nasal) T17.0
piriform —*see* Foreign body, pharynx
small intestine T18.3
stomach T18.2
suffocation by —*see* Foreign body, by site
tear ducts or glands —*see* Foreign body, entering through orifice, eye, specified part NEC
throat —*see* Foreign body, pharynx
tongue T18.0
tonsil, tonsillar (fossa) —*see* Foreign body, pharynx
trachea —*see* Foreign body, trachea
ureter T19.8
urethra T19.0
uterus (any part) T19.3
vagina T19.2
vulva T19.2
esophagus T18.108
causing
injury NEC T18.108
food (bone) (seed) T18.128
gastric contents (vomitus) T18.118
specified type NEC T18.198
tracheal compression T18.100
food (bone) (seed) T18.120
gastric contents (vomitus) T18.110
specified type NEC T18.190

F

Foreign body *(Continued)*
felling of, in throat R09.89
fragment —*see* Retained, foreign body fragments (type of)
genitourinary tract T19.9
bladder T19.1
multiple parts T19.8
penis T19.4
specified site NEC T19.8
urethra T19.0
uterus T19.3
IUD Z97.5
vagina T19.2
contraceptive device Z97.5
vulva T19.2
granuloma (old) (soft tissue) —*see also* Granuloma, foreign body
skin L92.3
in
laceration —*see* Laceration, by site, with foreign body
puncture wound —*see* Puncture, by site, with foreign body
soft tissue (residual) M79.5
inadvertently left in operation wound —*see* Foreign body, accidentally left during a procedure
ingestion, ingested NOS T18.9
inhalation or inspiration —*see* Foreign body, by site
internal organ, not entering through a natural orifice - code as specific injury with foreign body
intraocular S05.5-
old, retained (nonmagnetic) H44.70-
anterior chamber H44.71-
ciliary body H44.72-
iris H44.72-
lens H44.73-
magnetic H44.60-
anterior chamber H44.61-
ciliary body H44.62-
iris H44.62-
lens H44.63-
posterior wall H44.64-
specified site NEC H44.69-
vitreous body H44.65-
posterior wall H44.74-
specified site NEC H44.79-
vitreous body H44.75-
iris —*see* Foreign body, intraocular
lacrimal punctum —*see* Foreign body, entering through orifice, eye, specified part NEC
larynx T17.308
causing
asphyxiation T17.300
food (bone) (seed) T17.320
gastric contents (vomitus) T17.310
specified type NEC T17.390
injury NEC T17.308
food (bone) (seed) T17.328
gastric contents (vomitus) T17.318
specified type NEC T17.398
lens —*see* Foreign body, intraocular
ocular muscle S05.4-
old, retained —*see* Foreign body, orbit, old
old or residual
soft tissue (residual) M79.5
operation wound, left accidentally —*see* Foreign body, accidentally left during a procedure
orbit S05.4-
old, retained H05.5-
pharynx T17.208
causing
asphyxiation T17.200
food (bone) (seed) T17.220
gastric contents (vomitus) T17.210
specified type NEC T17.290

Foreign body *(Continued)*
pharynx *(Continued)*
causing *(Continued)*
injury NEC T17.208
food (bone) (seed) T17.228
gastric contents (vomitus) T17.218
specified type NEC T17.298
respiratory tract T17.908
bronchioles —*see* Foreign body, respiratory tract, specified site NEC
bronchus —*see* Foreign body, bronchus
causing
asphyxiation T17.900
food (bone) (seed) T17.920
gastric contents (vomitus) T17.910
specified type NEC T17.990
injury NEC T17.908
food (bone) (seed) T17.928
gastric contents (vomitus) T17.918
specified type NEC T17.998
larynx —*see* Foreign body, larynx
lung —*see* Foreign body, respiratory tract, specified site NEC
multiple parts —*see* Foreign body, respiratory tract, specified site NEC
nasal sinus T17.0
nasopharynx —*see* Foreign body, pharynx
nose T17.1
nostril T17.1
pharynx —*see* Foreign body, pharynx
specified site NEC T17.808
causing
asphyxiation T17.800
food (bone) (seed) T17.820
gastric contents (vomitus) T17.810
specified type NEC T17.890
injury NEC T17.808
food (bone) (seed) T17.828
gastric contents (vomitus) T17.818
specified type NEC T17.898
throat —*see* Foreign body, pharynx
trachea —*see* Foreign body, trachea
retained (old) (nonmagnetic) (in)
anterior chamber (eye) —*see* Foreign body, intraocular, old, retained, anterior chamber
magnetic —*see* Foreign body, intraocular, old, retained, magnetic, anterior chamber
ciliary body —*see* Foreign body, intraocular, old, retained, ciliary body
magnetic —*see* Foreign body, intraocular, old, retained, magnetic, ciliary body
eyelid H02.819
left H02.816
lower H02.815
upper H02.814
right H02.813
lower H02.812
upper H02.811
fragments —*see* Retained, foreign body fragments (type of)
globe —*see* Foreign body, intraocular, old, retained
magnetic —*see* Foreign body, intraocular, old, retained, magnetic
intraocular —*see* Foreign body, intraocular, old, retained
magnetic —*see* Foreign body, intraocular, old, retained, magnetic
iris —*see* Foreign body, intraocular, old, retained, iris
magnetic —*see* Foreign body, intraocular, old, retained, magnetic, iris
lens —*see* Foreign body, intraocular, old, retained, lens
magnetic —*see* Foreign body, intraocular, old, retained, magnetic, lens
muscle —*see* Foreign body, retained, soft tissue

Foreign body *(Continued)*
retained *(Continued)*
orbit —*see* Foreign body, orbit, old
posterior wall of globe —*see* Foreign body, intraocular, old, retained, posterior wall
magnetic —*see* Foreign body, intraocular, old, retained, magnetic, posterior wall
retrobulbar —*see* Foreign body, orbit, old, retrobulbar
soft tissue M79.5
vitreous —*see* Foreign body, intraocular, old, retained, vitreous body
magnetic —*see* Foreign body, intraocular, old, retained, magnetic, vitreous body
retina S05.5-
superficial, without open wound
abdomen, abdominal (wall) S30.851
alveolar process S00.552
ankle S90.55-
antecubital space —*see* Foreign body, superficial, forearm
anus S30.857
arm (upper) S40.85-
auditory canal —*see* Foreign body, superficial, ear
auricle —*see* Foreign body, superficial, ear
axilla —*see* Foreign body, superficial, arm
back, lower S30.850
breast S20.15-
brow S00.85
buttock S30.850
calf —*see* Foreign body, superficial, leg
canthus —*see* Foreign body, superficial, eyelid
cheek S00.85
internal S00.552
chest wall —*see* Foreign body, superficial, thorax
chin S00.85
clitoris S30.854
costal region —*see* Foreign body, superficial, thorax
digit (s)
foot —*see* Foreign body, superficial, toe
hand —*see* Foreign body, superficial, finger
ear S00.45-
elbow S50.35-
epididymis S30.853
epigastric region S30.851
epiglottis S10.15
esophagus, cervical S10.15
eyebrow —*see* Foreign body, superficial, eyelid
eyelid S00.25-
face S00.85
finger (s) S60.459
index S60.45-
little S60.45-
middle S60.45-
ring S60.45-
flank S30.851
foot (except toe (s) alone) S90.85-
toe —*see* Foreign body, superficial, toe
forearm S50.85-
elbow only —*see* Foreign body, superficial, elbow
forehead S00.85
genital organs, external
female S30.856
male S30.855
groin S30.851
gum S00.552
hand S60.55-
head S00.95
ear —*see* Foreign body, superficial, ear
eyelid —*see* Foreign body, superficial, eyelid

F

Foreign body *(Continued)*
superficial, without open wound *(Continued)*
head *(Continued)*
lip S00.551
nose S00.35
oral cavity S00.552
scalp S00.05
specified site NEC S00.85
heel —*see* Foreign body, superficial, foot
hip S70.25-
inguinal region S30.851
interscapular region S20.459
jaw S00.85
knee S80.25-
labium (majus) (minus) S30.854
larynx S10.15
leg (lower) S80.85-
knee —*see* Foreign body, superficial, knee
upper —*see* Foreign body, superficial, thigh
lip S00.551
lower back S30.850
lumbar region S30.850
malar region S00.85
mammary —*see* Foreign body, superficial, breast
mastoid region S00.85
mouth S00.552
nail
finger —*see* Foreign body, superficial, finger
toe —*see* Foreign body, superficial, toe
nape S10.85
nasal S00.35
neck S10.95
specified site NEC S10.85
throat S10.15
nose S00.35
occipital region S00.05
oral cavity S00.552
orbital region —*see* Foreign body, superficial, eyelid
palate S00.552
palm —*see* Foreign body, superficial, hand
parietal region S00.05
pelvis S30.850
penis S30.852
perineum
female S30.854
male S30.850
periocular area —*see* Foreign body, superficial, eyelid
phalanges
finger —*see* Foreign body, superficial, finger
toe —*see* Foreign body, superficial, toe
pharynx S10.15
pinna —*see* Foreign body, superficial, ear
popliteal space —*see* Foreign body, superficial, knee
prepuce S30.852
pubic region S30.850
pudendum
female S30.856
male S30.855
sacral region S30.850
scalp S00.05
scapular region —*see* Foreign body, superficial, shoulder
scrotum S30.853
shin —*see* Foreign body, superficial, leg
shoulder S40.25-
sternal region S20.359
submaxillary region S00.85
submental region S00.85
subungual
finger (s) —*see* Foreign body, superficial, finger
toe (s) —*see* Foreign body, superficial, toe

Foreign body *(Continued)*
superficial, without open wound *(Continued)*
supraclavicular fossa S10.85
supraorbital S00.85
temple S00.85
temporal region S00.85
testis S30.853
thigh S70.35-
thorax, thoracic (wall) S20.95
back S20.45-
front S20.35-
throat S10.15
thumb S60.35-
toe (s) (lesser) S90.456
great S90.45-
tongue S00.552
trachea S10.15
tunica vaginalis S30.853
tympanum, tympanic membrane —*see* Foreign body, superficial, ear
uvula S00.552
vagina S30.854
vocal cords S10.15
vulva S30.854
wrist S60.85-
swallowed T18.9
trachea T17.408
causing
asphyxiation T17.400
food (bone) (seed) T17.420
gastric contents (vomitus) T17.410
specified type NEC T17.490
injury NEC T17.408
food (bone) (seed) T17.428
gastric contents (vomitus) T17.418
specified type NEC T17.498
type of fragment —*see* Retained, foreign body fragments (type of)
vitreous (humor) S05.5-
Forestier's disease (rhizomelic pseudopolyarthritis) M35.3-
meaning ankylosing hyperostosis —*see* Hyperostosis, ankylosing
Formation
hyalin in cornea —*see* Degeneration, cornea
sequestrum in bone (due to infection) —*see* Osteomyelitis, chronic
valve
colon, congenital Q43.8
ureter (congenital) Q62.39
Formication R20.2
Fort Bragg fever A27.89
Fossa —*see also* condition
pyriform —*see* condition
Foster-Kennedy syndrome H47.14-
Fothergill's
disease (trigeminal neuralgia) —*see also* Neuralgia, trigeminal
scarlatina anginosa A38.9
Foul breath R19.6
Foundling Z76.1
Fournier disease or gangrene N49.3
female N76.89
Fourth
cranial nerve —*see* condition
molar K00.1
Foville's (peduncular) disease or syndrome G46.3
Fox (-Fordyce) disease (apocrine miliaria) L75.2
Fracture, burst —*see* Fracture, traumatic, by site
Fracture, chronic —*see* Fracture, pathological
Fracture, insufficiency —*see* Fracture, pathologic, by site
Fracture, nontraumatic, NEC ◀
atypical ◀
femur M84.750- ◀
complete ◀
oblique M84.759 ◀
left side M84.758 ◀
right side M84.757 ◀

Fracture, nontraumatic *(Continued)*
atypical *(Continued)*
femur *(Continued)*
complete *(Continued)*
transverse M84.756 ◀
left side M84.755 ◀
right side M84.754 ◀
incomplete M84.753 ◀
left side M84.752 ◀
right side M84.751 ◀
Fracture, pathological (pathologic) —*see also* Fracture, traumatic M84.40
ankle M84.47-
carpus M84.44-
clavicle M84.41-
compression (not due to trauma) —*see also* Collapse, vertebra M48.50- ◀
dental implant M27.63
dental restorative material K08.539
with loss of material K08.531
without loss of material K08.530
due to
neoplastic disease NEC —*see also* Neoplasm M84.50
ankle M84.57-
carpus M84.54-
clavicle M84.51-
femur M84.55-
fibula M84.56-
finger M84.54-
hip M84.559
humerus M84.52-
ilium M84.550
ischium M84.550
metacarpus M84.54-
metatarsus M84.57-
neck M84.58
pelvis M84.550
radius M84.53-
rib M84.58
scapula M84.51-
skull M84.58
specified site NEC M84.58
tarsus M84.57-
tibia M84.56-
toe M84.57-
ulna M84.53-
vertebra M84.58
osteoporosis M80.00 ◀
disuse —*see* Osteoporosis, specified type NEC, with pathological fracture
drug-induced —*see* Osteoporosis, drug induced, with pathological fracture
idiopathic —*see* Osteoporosis, specified type NEC, with pathological fracture
postmenopausal —*see* Osteoporosis, postmenopausal, with pathological fracture
postoophorectomy —*see* Osteoporosis, postoophorectomy, with pathological fracture
postsurgical malabsorption —*see* Osteoporosis, specified type NEC, with pathological fracture
specified cause NEC —*see* Osteoporosis, specified type NEC, with pathological fracture
specified disease NEC M84.60
ankle M84.67-
carpus M84.64-
clavicle M84.61-
femur M84.65-
fibula M84.66-
finger M84.64-
hip M84.65-
humerus M84.62-
ilium M84.650
ischium M84.650
metacarpus M84.64-
metatarsus M84.67-

F

Fracture, pathological *(Continued)*
due to *(Continued)*
specified disease NEC *(Continued)*
neck M84.68
radius M84.63-
rib M84.68
scapula M84.61-
skull M84.68
tarsus M84.67-
tibia M84.66-
toe M84.67-
ulna M84.63-
vertebra M84.68
femur M84.45-
fibula M84.46-
finger M84.44-
hip M84.459
humerus M84.42-
ilium M84.454
ischium M84.454
joint prosthesis —*see* Complications, joint prosthesis, mechanical, breakdown, by site
periprosthetic —*see* Fracture, pathological, periprosthetic
metacarpus M84.44-
metatarsus M84.47-
neck M84.48
pelvis M84.454
periprosthetic M97.9 ◀
ankle M97.2- ◀
elbow M97.4- ◀
finger M97.8 ◀
hip M97.0- ◀
knee M97.1- ◀
other specified joint M97.8 ◀
shoulder M97.3- ◀
spinal joint M97.8 ◀
toe joint M97.8 ◀
wrist joint M97.8 ◀
radius M84.43-
restorative material (dental) K08.539
with loss of material K08.531
without loss of material K08.530
rib M84.48
scapula M84.41-
skull M84.48
tarsus M84.47-
tibia M84.46-
toe M84.47-
ulna M84.43-
vertebra M84.48
Fracture, traumatic (abduction) (adduction) (separation) —*see also* Fracture, pathological T14.8
acetabulum S32.40-
column
anterior (displaced) (iliopubic) S32.43-
nondisplaced S32.436
posterior (displaced) (ilioischial) S32.443
nondisplaced S32.44-
dome (displaced) S32.48-
nondisplaced S32.48
specified NEC S32.49-
transverse (displaced) S32.45-
with associated posterior wall fracture (displaced) S32.46-
nondisplaced S32.46-
nondisplaced S32.45-
wall
anterior (displaced) S32.41-
nondisplaced S32.41-
medial (displaced) S32.47-
nondisplaced S32.47-
posterior (displaced) S32.42-
with associated transverse fracture (displaced) S32.46-
nondisplaced S32.46-
nondisplaced S32.42-

Fracture, traumatic *(Continued)*
acromion —*see* Fracture, scapula, acromial process
ankle S82.899
bimalleolar (displaced) S82.84-
nondisplaced S82.84-
lateral malleolus only (displaced) S82.6-
nondisplaced S82.6-
medial malleolus (displaced) S82.5-
associated with Maisonneuve's fracture —*see* Fracture, Maisonneuve's
nondisplaced S82.5-
talus —*see* Fracture, tarsal, talus
trimalleolar (displaced) S82.85-
nondisplaced S82.85-
arm (upper) —*see also* Fracture, humerus, shaft
humerus —*see* Fracture, humerus
radius —*see* Fracture, radius
ulna —*see* Fracture, ulna
astragalus —*see* Fracture, tarsal, talus
atlas —*see* Fracture, neck, cervical vertebra, first
axis —*see* Fracture, neck, cervical vertebra, second
back —*see* Fracture, vertebra
Barton's —*see* Barton's fracture
base of skull —*see* Fracture, skull, base
basicervical (basal) (femoral) S72.0
Bennett's —*see* Bennett's fracture
bimalleolar —*see* Fracture, ankle, bimalleolar
blow-out S02.3-
bone NEC T14.8
birth injury P13.9
following insertion of orthopedic implant, joint prosthesis or bone plate —*see* Fracture, following insertion of orthopedic implant, joint prosthesis or bone plate
in (due to) neoplastic disease NEC —*see* Fracture, pathological, due to, neoplastic disease
pathological (cause unknown) —*see* Fracture, pathological
breast bone —*see* Fracture, sternum
bucket handle (semilunar cartilage) —*see* Tear, meniscus
burst —*see* Fracture, traumatic, by site
calcaneus —*see* Fracture, tarsal, calcaneus
carpal bone (s) S62.10-
capitate (displaced) S62.13-
nondisplaced S62.13-
cuneiform —*see* Fracture, carpal bone, triquetrum
hamate (body) (displaced) S62.143
hook process (displaced) S62.15-
nondisplaced S62.15-
nondisplaced S62.14-
larger multangular —*see* Fracture, carpal bones, trapezium
lunate (displaced) S62.12-
nondisplaced S62.12-
navicular S62.00-
distal pole (displaced) S62.01-
nondisplaced S62.01-
middle third (displaced) S62.02-
nondisplaced S62.02-
proximal third (displaced) S62.03-
nondisplaced S62.03-
volar tuberosity —*see* Fracture, carpal bones, navicular, distal pole
os magnum —*see* Fracture, carpal bones, capitate
pisiform (displaced) S62.16-
nondisplaced S62.16-
semilunar —*see* Fracture, carpal bones, lunate
smaller multangular —*see* Fracture, carpal bones, trapezoid

Fracture, traumatic *(Continued)*
carpal bone (s) *(Continued)*
trapezium (displaced) S62.17-
nondisplaced S62.17-
trapezoid (displaced) S62.18-
nondisplaced S62.18-
triquetrum (displaced) S62.11-
nondisplaced S62.11-
unciform —*see* Fracture, carpal bones, hamate
cervical —*see* Fracture, vertebra, cervical
clavicle S42.00-
acromial end (displaced) S42.03-
nondisplaced S42.03-
birth injury P13.4
lateral end —*see* Fracture, clavicle, acromial end
shaft (displaced) S42.02-
nondisplaced S42.02-
sternal end (anterior) (displaced) S42.01-
nondisplaced S42.01-
posterior S42.01-
coccyx S32.2
collapsed —*see* Collapse, vertebra
collar bone —*see* Fracture, clavicle
Colles' —*see* Colles' fracture
~~compression, not due to trauma —see Collapse, vertebra~~
coronoid process —*see* Fracture, ulna, upper end, coronoid process
corpus cavernosum penis S39.840
costochondral cartilage S23.41
costochondral, costosternal junction —*see* Fracture, rib
cranium —*see* Fracture, skull
cricoid cartilage S12.8
cuboid (ankle) —*see* Fracture, tarsal, cuboid
cuneiform
foot —*see* Fracture, tarsal, cuneiform
wrist —*see* Fracture, carpal, triquetrum
delayed union —*see* Delay, union, fracture
dental restorative material K08.539
with loss of material K08.531
without loss of material K08.530
due to
birth injury —*see* Birth, injury, fracture
osteoporosis —*see* Osteoporosis, with fracture
Dupuytren's —*see* Fracture, ankle, lateral malleolus
elbow S42.40-
ethmoid (bone) (sinus) —*see* Fracture, skull, base
face bone S02.92
fatigue —*see also* Fracture, stress
vertebra M48.40
cervical region M48.42
cervicothoracic region M48.43
lumbar region M48.46
lumbosacral region M48.47
occipito-atlanto-axial region M48.41
sacrococcygeal region M48.48
thoracic region M48.44
thoracolumbar region M48.45
femur, femoral S72.9-
basicervical (basal) S72.0
birth injury P13.2
capital epiphyseal S79.01-
condyles, epicondyles —*see* Fracture, femur, lower end
distal end —*see* Fracture, femur, lower end
epiphysis
head —*see* Fracture, femur, upper end, epiphysis
lower —*see* Fracture, femur, lower end, epiphysis
upper —*see* Fracture, femur, upper end, epiphysis
following insertion of implant, prosthesis or plate M96.66-

◀ New ◀ Revised ~~deleted~~ Deleted

Fracture, traumatic *(Continued)*
femur, femoral *(Continued)*
head —*see* Fracture, femur, upper end, head
intertrochanteric —*see* Fracture, femur, trochanteric
intratrochanteric —*see* Fracture, femur, trochanteric
lower end S72.40-
condyle (displaced) S72.41-
lateral (displaced) S72.42-
nondisplaced S72.42-
medial (displaced) S72.43-
nondisplaced S72.43-
nondisplaced S72.41-
epiphysis (displaced) S72.44-
nondisplaced S72.44-
physeal S79.10-
Salter-Harris
Type I S79.11-
Type II S79.12-
Type III S79.13-
Type IV S79.14-
specified NEC S79.19-
specified NEC S72.49-
supracondylar (displaced) S72.45-
with intracondylar extension (displaced) S72.46-
nondisplaced S72.46-
nondisplaced S72.45-
torus S72.47-
neck —*see* Fracture, femur, upper end, neck
pertrochanteric —*see* Fracture, femur, trochanteric
shaft (lower third) (middle third) (upper third) S72.30-
comminuted (displaced) S72.35-
nondisplaced S72.35-
oblique (displaced) S72.33-
nondisplaced S72.33-
segmental (displaced) S72.36-
nondisplaced S72.36-
specified NEC S72.39-
spiral (displaced) S72.34-
nondisplaced S72.34-
transverse (displaced) S72.32-
nondisplaced S72.32-
specified site NEC —*see* subcategory S72.8
subcapital (displaced) S72.01-
subtrochanteric (region) (section) (displaced) S72.2-
nondisplaced S72.2-
transcervical —*see* Fracture, femur, upper end, neck
transtrochanteric —*see* Fracture, femur, trochanteric
trochanteric S72.10-
apophyseal (displaced) S72.13-
nondisplaced S72.13-
greater trochanter (displaced) S72.11-
nondisplaced S72.11-
intertrochanteric (displaced) S72.14-
nondisplaced S72.14-
lesser trochanter (displaced) S72.12-
nondisplaced S72.12-
upper end S72.00-
apophyseal (displaced) S72.13-
nondisplaced S72.13-
cervicotrochanteric —*see* Fracture, femur, upper end, neck, base
epiphysis (displaced) S72.02-
nondisplaced S72.02-
head S72.05-
articular (displaced) S72.06-
nondisplaced S72.06-
specified NEC S72.09-
intertrochanteric (displaced) S72.14-
nondisplaced S72.14-
intracapsular S72.01-
midcervical (displaced) S72.03-
nondisplaced S72.03-

Fracture, traumatic *(Continued)*
femur, femoral *(Continued)*
upper end *(Continued)*
neck S72.00-
base (displaced) S72.04-
nondisplaced S72.04-
specified NEC S72.09-
pertrochanteric —*see* Fracture, femur, upper end, trochanteric
physeal S79.00-
Salter-Harris type I S79.01-
specified NEC S79.09-
subcapital (displaced) S72.01-
subtrochanteric (displaced) S72.2-
nondisplaced S72.2-
transcervical —*see* Fracture, femur, upper end, midcervical
trochanteric S72.10-
greater (displaced) S72.11-
nondisplaced S72.11-
lesser (displaced) S72.12-
nondisplaced S72.12-
fibula (shaft) (styloid) S82.40-
comminuted (displaced) S82.45-
nondisplaced S82.45-
following insertion of implant, prosthesis or plate M96.67-
involving ankle or malleolus —*see* Fracture, fibula, lateral malleolus
lateral malleolus (displaced) S82.6-
nondisplaced S82.6-
lower end
physeal S89.30-
Salter-Harris
Type I S89.31-
Type II S89.32-
specified NEC S89.39-
specified NEC S82.83-
torus S82.82-
oblique (displaced) S82.43-
nondisplaced S82.43-
segmental (displaced) S82.46-
nondisplaced S82.46-
specified NEC S82.49-
spiral (displaced) S82.44-
nondisplaced S82.44-
transverse (displaced) S82.42-
nondisplaced S82.42-
upper end
physeal S89.20-
Salter-Harris
Type I S89.21-
Type II S89.22-
specified NEC S89.29-
specified NEC S82.83-
torus S82.81-
finger (except thumb) S62.60-
distal phalanx (displaced) S62.63-
nondisplaced S62.66-
index S62.60-
distal phalanx (displaced) S62.63-
nondisplaced S62.66-
medial phalanx (displaced) S62.62-
nondisplaced S62.65-
proximal phalanx (displaced) S62.61-
nondisplaced S62.64-
little S62.60-
distal phalanx (displaced) S62.63-
nondisplaced S62.66-
medial phalanx (displaced) S62.62-
nondisplaced S62.65-
proximal phalanx (displaced) S62.61-
nondisplaced S62.64-
medial phalanx (displaced) S62.62-
nondisplaced S62.65-
middle S62.60-
distal phalanx (displaced) S62.63-
nondisplaced S62.66-
medial phalanx (displaced) S62.62-
nondisplaced S62.65-

Fracture, traumatic *(Continued)*
finger *(Continued)*
middle *(Continued)*
proximal phalanx (displaced) S62.61-
nondisplaced S62.64-
proximal phalanx (displaced) S62.61-
nondisplaced S62.64-
ring S62.60-
distal phalanx (displaced) S62.63-
nondisplaced S62.66-
medial phalanx (displaced) S62.62-
nondisplaced S62.65-
proximal phalanx (displaced) S62.61-
nondisplaced S62.64-
thumb —*see* Fracture, thumb
following insertion (intraoperative) (postoperative) of orthopedic implant, joint prosthesis or bone plate M96.69
femur M96.66-
fibula M96.67-
humerus M96.62-
pelvis M96.65
radius M96.63-
specified bone NEC M96.69
tibia M96.67-
ulna M96.63-
foot S92.90-
astragalus —*see* Fracture, tarsal, talus
calcaneus —*see* Fracture, tarsal, calcaneus
cuboid —*see* Fracture, tarsal, cuboid
cuneiform —*see* Fracture, tarsal, cuneiform
metatarsal —*see* Fracture, metatarsal
navicular —*see* Fracture, tarsal, navicular
sesamoid S92.81- ◀
specified NEC S92.81- ◀
talus —*see* Fracture, tarsal, talus
tarsal —*see* Fracture, tarsal
toe —*see* Fracture, toe
forearm S52.9-
radius —*see* Fracture, radius
ulna —*see* Fracture, ulna
fossa (anterior) (middle) (posterior) S02.19
frontal (bone) (skull) S02.0
sinus S02.19
glenoid (cavity) (scapula) —*see* Fracture, scapula, glenoid cavity
greenstick —*see* Fracture, by site
hallux —*see* Fracture, toe, great
hand S62.9-
carpal —*see* Fracture, carpal bone
finger (except thumb) —*see* Fracture, finger
metacarpal —*see* Fracture, metacarpal
navicular (scaphoid) (hand) —*see* Fracture, carpal bone, navicular
thumb —*see* Fracture, thumb
healed or old
with complications - code by Nature of the complication
heel bone —*see* Fracture, tarsal, calcaneus
Hill-Sachs S42.29-
hip —*see* Fracture, femur, neck
humerus S42.30-
anatomical neck —*see* Fracture, humerus, upper end
articular process —*see* Fracture, humerus, lower end
capitellum —*see* Fracture, humerus, lower end, condyle, lateral
distal end —*see* Fracture, humerus, lower end
epiphysis
lower —*see* Fracture, humerus, lower end, physeal
upper —*see* Fracture, humerus, upper end, physeal
external condyle —*see* Fracture, humerus, lower end, condyle, lateral
following insertion of implant, prosthesis or plate M96.62-
great tuberosity —*see* Fracture, humerus, upper end, greater tuberosity

Fracture, traumatic *(Continued)*
humerus *(Continued)*
intercondylar —*see* Fracture, humerus, lower end
internal epicondyle —*see* Fracture, humerus, lower end, epicondyle, medial
lesser tuberosity —*see* Fracture, humerus, upper end, lesser tuberosity
lower end S42.40-
condyle
lateral (displaced) S42.45-
nondisplaced S42.45-
medial (displaced) S42.46-
nondisplaced S42.46-
epicondyle
lateral (displaced) S42.43-
nondisplaced S42.43-
medial (displaced) S42.44-
incarcerated S42.44-
nondisplaced S42.44-
physeal S49.10-
Salter-Harris
Type I S49.11-
Type II S49.12-
Type III S49.13-
Type IV S49.14-
specified NEC S49.19-
specified NEC (displaced) S42.49-
nondisplaced S42.49-
supracondylar (simple) (displaced) S42.41-
with intercondylar fracture —*see* Fracture, humerus, lower end ◀
comminuted (displaced) S42.42-
nondisplaced S42.42-
nondisplaced S42.41-
torus S42.48-
transcondylar (displaced) S42.47-
nondisplaced S42.47-
proximal end —*see* Fracture, humerus, upper end
shaft S42.30-
comminuted (displaced) S42.35-
nondisplaced S42.35-
greenstick S42.31-
oblique (displaced) S42.33-
nondisplaced S42.33-
segmental (displaced) S42.36-
nondisplaced S42.36-
specified NEC S42.39-
spiral (displaced) S42.34-
nondisplaced S42.34-
transverse (displaced) S42.32-
nondisplaced S42.32-
supracondylar —*see* Fracture, humerus, lower end
surgical neck —*see* Fracture, humerus, upper end, surgical neck
trochlea —*see* Fracture, humerus, lower end, condyle, medial
tuberosity —*see* Fracture, humerus, upper end
upper end S42.20-
anatomical neck —*see* Fracture, humerus, upper end, specified NEC
articular head —*see* Fracture, humerus, upper end, specified NEC
epiphysis —*see* Fracture, humerus, upper end, physeal
greater tuberosity (displaced) S42.25-
nondisplaced S42.25-
lesser tuberosity (displaced) S42.26-
nondisplaced S42.26-
physeal S49.00-
Salter-Harris
Type I S49.01-
Type II S49.02-
Type III S49.03-
Type IV S49.04-
specified NEC S49.09-

Fracture, traumatic *(Continued)*
humerus *(Continued)*
upper end *(Continued)*
specified NEC (displaced) S42.29-
nondisplaced S42.29-
surgical neck (displaced) S42.21-
four-part S42.24-
nondisplaced S42.21-
three-part S42.23-
two-part (displaced) S42.22-
nondisplaced S42.22-
torus S42.27-
transepiphyseal —*see* Fracture, humerus, upper end, physeal
hyoid bone S12.8
ilium S32.30-
with disruption of pelvic ring —*see* Disruption, pelvic ring
avulsion (displaced) S32.31-
nondisplaced S32.31-
specified NEC S32.39-
impaction, impacted - code as Fracture, by site
innominate bone —*see* Fracture, ilium
instep —*see* Fracture, foot
ischium S32.60-
with disruption of pelvic ring —*see* Disruption, pelvic ring
avulsion (displaced) S32.61-
nondisplaced S32.61-
specified NEC S32.69-
jaw (bone) (lower) —*see* Fracture, mandible
upper —*see* Fracture, maxilla
joint prosthesis —*see* Complications, joint prosthesis, mechanical, breakdown, by site
periprosthetic —*see* Fracture, traumatic, periprosthetic ⬅
knee cap —*see* Fracture, patella
larynx S12.8
late effects —*see* Sequelae, fracture
leg (lower) S82.9-
ankle —*see* Fracture, ankle
femur —*see* Fracture, femur
fibula —*see* Fracture, fibula
malleolus —*see* Fracture, ankle
patella —*see* Fracture, patella
specified site NEC S82.89-
tibia —*see* Fracture, tibia
lumbar spine —*see* Fracture, vertebra, lumbar
lumbosacral spine S32.9
Maisonneuve's (displaced) S82.86-
nondisplaced S82.86-
malar bone —*see also* Fracture, maxilla S02.400
left side S02.40B ◀
right side S02.40A ◀
malleolus —*see* Fracture, ankle
malunion —*see* Fracture, by site
mandible (lower jawbone) S02.609
alveolus S02.67- ⬅
angle (of jaw) S02.65- ⬅
body, unspecified S02.600-
left side S02.602 ◀
right side S02.601 ◀
condylar process S02.61- ⬅
coronoid process S02.63- ⬅
ramus, unspecified S02.64- ⬅
specified site NEC S02.69
subcondylar process S02.62- ⬅
symphysis S02.66
manubrium (sterni) S22.21
dissociation from sternum S22.23
march —*see* Fracture, traumatic, stress, by site
maxilla, maxillary (bone) (sinus) (superior) (upper jaw) S02.401
alveolus S02.42
inferior —*see* Fracture, mandible
LeFort I S02.411
LeFort II S02.412
LeFort III S02.413

Fracture, traumatic *(Continued)*
maxilla, maxillary *(Continued)*
left side S02.40D ◀
right side S02.40C ◀
metacarpal S62.309
base (displaced) S62.319
nondisplaced S62.349
fifth S62.30-
base (displaced) S62.31-
nondisplaced S62.34-
neck (displaced) S62.33-
nondisplaced S62.36-
shaft (displaced) S62.32-
nondisplaced S62.35-
specified NEC S62.398
first S62.20-
base NEC (displaced) S62.23-
nondisplaced S62.23-
Bennett's —*see* Bennett's fracture
neck (displaced) S62.25-
nondisplaced S62.25-
shaft (displaced) S62.24-
nondisplaced S62.24-
specified NEC S62.29-
fourth S62.30-
base (displaced) S62.31-
nondisplaced S62.34-
neck (displaced) S62.33-
nondisplaced S62.36-
shaft (displaced) S62.32-
nondisplaced S62.35-
specified NEC S62.39-
neck (displaced) S62.33-
nondisplaced S62.36-
Rolando's —*see* Rolando's fracture
second S62.30-
base (displaced) S62.31-
nondisplaced S62.34-
neck (displaced) S62.33-
nondisplaced S62.36-
shaft (displaced) S62.32-
nondisplaced S62.35-
specified NEC S62.39-
shaft (displaced) S62.32-
nondisplaced S62.35-
specified NEC S62.399
third S62.30-
base (displaced) S62.31-
nondisplaced S62.34-
neck (displaced) S62.33-
nondisplaced S62.36-
shaft (displaced) S62.32-
nondisplaced S62.35-
specified NEC S62.39-
metastatic —*see* Fracture, pathological, due to, neoplastic disease —*see also* Neoplasm
metatarsal bone S92.30-
fifth (displaced) S92.35-
nondisplaced S92.35-
first (displaced) S92.31-
nondisplaced S92.31-
fourth (displaced) S92.34-
nondisplaced S92.34-
physeal S99.10- ◀
Salter-Harris ◀
Type I S99.11- ◀
Type II S99.12- ◀
Type III S99.13- ◀
Type IV S99.14- ◀
specified NEC S99.19- ◀
second (displaced) S92.32-
nondisplaced S92.32-
third (displaced) S92.33-
nondisplaced S92.33-
Monteggia's —*see* Monteggia's fracture
multiple
hand (and wrist) NEC —*see* Fracture, by site
ribs —*see* Fracture, rib, multiple

◀ New ⬅ Revised ~~deleted~~ Deleted

Fracture, traumatic *(Continued)*
nasal (bone (s)) S02.2
navicular (scaphoid) (foot) —*see also* Fracture, tarsal, navicular
hand —*see* Fracture, carpal, navicular
neck S12.9
cervical vertebra S12.9
fifth (displaced) S12.400
nondisplaced S12.401
specified type NEC (displaced) S12.490
nondisplaced S12.491
first (displaced) S12.000
burst (stable) S12.01
unstable S12.02
lateral mass (displaced) S12.040
nondisplaced S12.041
nondisplaced S12.001
posterior arch (displaced) S12.030
nondisplaced S12.031
specified type NEC (displaced) S12.090
nondisplaced S12.091
fourth (displaced) S12.300
nondisplaced S12.301
specified type NEC (displaced) S12.390
nondisplaced S12.391
second (displaced) S12.100
dens (anterior) (displaced) (type II) S12.110
nondisplaced S12.112
posterior S12.111
specified type NEC (displaced) S12.120
nondisplaced S12.121
nondisplaced S12.101
specified type NEC (displaced) S12.190
nondisplaced S12.191
seventh (displaced) S12.600
nondisplaced S12.601
specified type NEC (displaced) S12.690
~~displaced S12.691~~
nondisplaced S12.691 ◀
sixth (displaced) S12.500
nondisplaced S12.501
specified type NEC (displaced) S12.590
~~displaced S12.591~~
nondisplaced S12.591 ◀
third (displaced) S12.200
nondisplaced S12.201
specified type NEC (displaced) S12.290
~~displaced S12.291~~
nondisplaced S12.291 ◀
hyoid bone S12.8
larynx S12.8
specified site NEC S12.8
thyroid cartilage S12.8
trachea S12.8
neoplastic NEC —*see* Fracture, pathological, due to, neoplastic disease
neural arch —*see* Fracture, vertebra
newborn —*see* Birth, injury, fracture
nontraumatic —*see* Fracture, pathological
nonunion —*see* Nonunion, fracture
nose, nasal (bone) (septum) S02.2
occiput —*see* Fracture, skull, base, occiput
odontoid process —*see* Fracture, neck, cervical vertebra, second
olecranon (process) (ulna) —*see* Fracture, ulna, upper end, olecranon process
orbit, orbital (bone) (region) S02.8- ⟸
floor (blow-out) S02.3- ⟸
roof S02.19
os
calcis —*see* Fracture, tarsal, calcaneus
magnum —*see* Fracture, carpal, capitate
pubis —*see* Fracture, pubis
palate S02.8- ⟸
parietal bone (skull) S02.0

Fracture, traumatic *(Continued)*
patella S82.00-
comminuted (displaced) S82.04-
nondisplaced S82.04-
longitudinal (displaced) S82.02-
nondisplaced S82.02-
osteochondral (displaced) S82.01-
nondisplaced S82.01-
specified NEC S82.09-
transverse (displaced) S82.03-
nondisplaced S82.03-
pedicle (of vertebral arch) —*see* Fracture, vertebra
pelvis, pelvic (bone) S32.9
acetabulum —*see* Fracture, acetabulum
circle —*see* Disruption, pelvic ring
following insertion of implant, prosthesis or plate M96.65
ilium —*see* Fracture, ilium
ischium —*see* Fracture, ischium
multiple
with disruption of pelvic ring (circle) —*see* Disruption, pelvic ring
without disruption of pelvic ring (circle) S32.82
pubis —*see* Fracture, pubis
sacrum —*see* Fracture, sacrum
specified site NEC S32.89
periprosthetic, around internal prosthetic joint M97.9 ◀
ankle M97.2- ◀
elbow M97.4- ◀
finger M97.8 ◀
hip M97.0- ◀
knee M97.1-- ◀
shoulder M97.3- ◀
specified joint NEC M97.8 ◀
spine M97.8 ◀
toe M97.8 ◀
wrist M97.8 ◀
phalanx
foot —*see* Fracture, toe
hand —*see* Fracture, finger
pisiform —*see* Fracture, carpal, pisiform
pond —*see* Fracture, skull
prosthetic device, internal —*see* Complications, prosthetic device, by site, mechanical
pubis S32.50-
with disruption of pelvic ring —*see* Disruption, pelvic ring
specified site NEC S32.59-
superior rim S32.59-
radius S52.9-
distal end —*see* Fracture, radius, lower end
following insertion of implant, prosthesis or plate M96.63-
head —*see* Fracture, radius, upper end, head
lower end S52.50-
Barton's —*see* Barton's fracture
Colles' —*see* Colles' fracture
extraarticular NEC S52.55-
intraarticular NEC S52.57-
physeal S59.20-
Salter-Harris
Type I S59.21-
Type II S59.22-
Type III S59.23-
Type IV S59.24-
specified NEC S59.29-
Smith's —*see* Smith's fracture
specified NEC S52.59-
styloid process (displaced) S52.51-
nondisplaced S52.51-
torus S52.52-
neck —*see* Fracture, radius, upper end
proximal end —*see* Fracture, radius, upper end

Fracture, traumatic *(Continued)*
radius *(Continued)*
shaft S52.30-
bent bone S52.38-
comminuted (displaced) S52.35-
nondisplaced S52.35-
Galeazzi's —*see* Galeazzi's fracture
greenstick S52.31-
oblique (displaced) S52.33-
nondisplaced S52.33-
segmental (displaced) S52.36-
nondisplaced S52.36-
specified NEC S52.39-
spiral (displaced) S52.34-
nondisplaced S52.34-
transverse (displaced) S52.32-
nondisplaced S52.32-
upper end S52.10-
head (displaced) S52.12-
nondisplaced S52.12-
neck (displaced) S52.13-
nondisplaced S52.13-
physeal S59.10-
Salter-Harris
Type I S59.11-
Type II S59.12-
Type III S59.13-
Type IV S59.14-
specified NEC S59.19-
specified NEC S52.18-
torus S52.11-
ramus
inferior or superior, pubis —*see* Fracture, pubis
mandible —*see* Fracture, mandible
restorative material (dental) K08.539
with loss of material K08.531
without loss of material K08.530
rib S22.3-
with flail chest —*see* Flail, chest
multiple S22.4-
with flail chest —*see* Flail, chest
root, tooth —*see* Fracture, tooth
sacrum S32.10
specified NEC S32.19
Type
1 S32.14
2 S32.15
3 S32.16
4 S32.17
Zone
I S32.119
displaced (minimally) S32.111
severely S32.112
nondisplaced S32.110
II S32.129
displaced (minimally) S32.121
severely S32.122
nondisplaced S32.120
III S32.139
displaced (minimally) S32.131
severely S32.132
nondisplaced S32.130
scaphoid (hand) —*see also* Fracture, carpal, navicular
foot —*see* Fracture, tarsal, navicular
scapula S42.10-
acromial process (displaced) S42.12-
nondisplaced S42.12-
body (displaced) S42.11-
nondisplaced S42.11-
coracoid process (displaced) S42.13-
nondisplaced S42.13-
glenoid cavity (displaced) S42.14-
nondisplaced S42.14-
neck (displaced) S42.15-
nondisplaced S42.15-
specified NEC S42.19-
semilunar bone, wrist —*see* Fracture, carpal, lunate
sequelae —*see* Sequelae, fracture

Fracture, traumatic *(Continued)*
sesamoid bone
foot S92.81- ◀
hand —*see* Fracture, carpal
other —*see* Fracture, traumatic, by site ◀
~~other - code by site under Fracture~~
shepherd's —*see* Fracture, tarsal, talus
shoulder (girdle) S42.9-
blade —*see* Fracture, scapula
sinus (ethmoid) (frontal) S02.19
skull S02.91
base S02.10- ⇐
occiput S02.119
condyle S02.113
type I S02.110
left side S02.11B ◀
right side S02.11A ◀
type II S02.111
left side S02.11D ◀
right side S02.11C ◀
type III S02.112
left side S02.11F ◀
right side S02.11E ◀
specified NEC S02.118 ◀
left side S02.11H ◀
right side S02.11G ◀
~~specified NEC S02.118~~
specified NEC S02.19- ⇐
birth injury P13.0
frontal bone S02.0
parietal bone S02.0
specified site NEC S02.8
temporal bone S02.19
vault S02.0
Smith's —*see* Smith's fracture
sphenoid (bone) (sinus) S02.19
spine —*see* Fracture, vertebra
spinous process —*see* Fracture, vertebra
spontaneous (cause unknown) —*see* Fracture, pathological
stave (of thumb) —*see* Fracture, metacarpal, first
sternum S22.20
with flail chest —*see* Flail, chest
body S22.22
manubrium S22.21
xiphoid (process) S22.24
stress M84.30
ankle M84.37-
carpus M84.34-
clavicle M84.31-
femoral neck M84.359
femur M84.35-
fibula M84.36-
finger M84.34-
hip M84.359
humerus M84.32-
ilium M84.350
ischium M84.350
metacarpus M84.34-
metatarsus M84.37-
neck —*see* Fracture, fatigue, vertebra
pelvis M84.350
radius M84.33-
rib M84.38
scapula M84.31-
skull M84.38
tarsus M84.37-
tibia M84.36-
toe M84.37-
ulna M84.33-
vertebra —*see* Fracture, fatigue, vertebra
supracondylar, elbow —*see* Fracture, humerus, lower end, supracondylar
symphysis pubis —*see* Fracture, pubis
talus (ankle bone) —*see* Fracture, tarsal, talus
tarsal bone (s) S92.20-
astragalus —*see* Fracture, tarsal, talus
calcaneus S92.00-
anterior process (displaced) S92.02-
nondisplaced S92.02-

Fracture, traumatic *(Continued)*
tarsal bone *(Continued)*
calcaneus *(Continued)*
body (displaced) S92.01-
nondisplaced S92.01-
extraarticular NEC (displaced) S92.05-
nondisplaced S92.05-
intraarticular (displaced) S92.06-
nondisplaced S92.06-
physeal S99.00- ◀
Salter-Harris ◀
Type I S99.01- ◀
Type II S99.02- ◀
Type III S99.03- ◀
Type IV S99.04- ◀
specified NEC S99.09- ◀
tuberosity (displaced) S92.04-
avulsion (displaced) S92.03-
nondisplaced S92.03-
nondisplaced S92.04-
cuboid (displaced) S92.21-
nondisplaced S92.21-
cuneiform
intermediate (displaced) S92.23-
nondisplaced S92.23-
lateral (displaced) S92.22-
nondisplaced S92.22-
medial (displaced) S92.24-
nondisplaced S92.24-
navicular (displaced) S92.25-
nondisplaced S92.25-
scaphoid —*see* Fracture, tarsal, navicular
talus S92.10-
avulsion (displaced) S92.15-
nondisplaced S92.15-
body (displaced) S92.12-
nondisplaced S92.12-
dome (displaced) S92.14-
nondisplaced S92.14-
head (displaced) S92.12-
nondisplaced S92.12-
lateral process (displaced) S92.14-
nondisplaced S92.14-
neck (displaced) S92.11-
nondisplaced S92.11-
posterior process (displaced) S92.13-
nondisplaced S92.13-
specified NEC S92.19-
temporal bone (styloid) S02.19
thorax (bony) S22.9
with flail chest —*see* Flail, chest
rib S22.3-
multiple S22.4-
with flail chest —*see* Flail, chest
sternum S22.20
body S22.22
manubrium S22.21
xiphoid process S22.24
vertebra (displaced) S22.009
burst (stable) S22.001
unstable S22.002
eighth S22.069
burst (stable) S22.061
unstable S22.062
specified type NEC S22.068
wedge compression S22.060
eleventh S22.089
burst (stable) S22.081
unstable S22.082
specified type NEC S22.088
wedge compression S22.080
fifth S22.059
burst (stable) S22.051
unstable S22.052
specified type NEC S22.058
wedge compression S22.050
first S22.019
burst (stable) S22.011
unstable S22.012
specified type NEC S22.018
wedge compression S22.010

Fracture, traumatic *(Continued)*
thorax *(Continued)*
vertebra *(Continued)*
fourth S22.049
burst (stable) S22.041
unstable S22.042
specified type NEC S22.048
wedge compression S22.040
ninth S22.079
burst (stable) S22.071
unstable S22.072
specified type NEC S22.078
wedge compression S22.070
nondisplaced S22.001
second S22.029
burst (stable) S22.021
unstable S22.022
specified type NEC S22.028
wedge compression S22.020
seventh S22.069
burst (stable) S22.061
unstable S22.062
specified type NEC S22.068
wedge compression S22.060
sixth S22.059
burst (stable) S22.051
unstable S22.052
specified type NEC S22.058
wedge compression S22.050
specified type NEC S22.008
tenth S22.079
burst (stable) S22.071
unstable S22.072
specified type NEC S22.078
wedge compression S22.070
third S22.039
burst (stable) S22.031
unstable S22.032
specified type NEC S22.038
wedge compression S22.030
twelfth S22.089
burst (stable) S22.081
unstable S22.082
specified type NEC S22.088
wedge compression S22.080
wedge compression S22.000
thumb S62.50-
distal phalanx (displaced) S62.52-
nondisplaced S62.52-
proximal phalanx (displaced) S62.51-
nondisplaced S62.51-
thyroid cartilage S12.8
tibia (shaft) S82.20-
comminuted (displaced) S82.25-
nondisplaced S82.25-
condyles —*see* Fracture, tibia, upper end
distal end —*see* Fracture, tibia, lower end
epiphysis
lower —*see* Fracture, tibia, lower end
upper —*see* Fracture, tibia, upper end
following insertion of implant, prosthesis or plate M96.67-
head (involving knee joint) —*see* Fracture, tibia, upper end
intercondyloid eminence —*see* Fracture, tibia, upper end
involving ankle or malleolus —*see* Fracture, ankle, medial malleolus
lower end S82.30-
physeal S89.10-
Salter-Harris
Type I S89.11-
Type II S89.12-
Type III S89.13-
Type IV S89.14-
specified NEC S89.19-
pilon (displaced) S82.87-
nondisplaced S82.87-
specified NEC S82.39-
torus S82.31-

Fracture, traumatic *(Continued)*
tibia *(Continued)*
malleolus —*see* Fracture, ankle, medial malleolus
oblique (displaced) S82.23-
nondisplaced S82.23-
pilon —*see* Fracture, tibia, lower end, pilon
proximal end —*see* Fracture, tibia, upper end
segmental (displaced) S82.26-
nondisplaced S82.26-
specified NEC S82.29-
spine —*see* Fracture, upper end, spine
spiral (displaced) S82.24-
nondisplaced S82.24-
transverse (displaced) S82.22-
nondisplaced S82.22-
tuberosity —*see* Fracture, tibia, upper end, tuberosity
upper end S82.10-
bicondylar (displaced) S82.14-
nondisplaced S82.14-
lateral condyle (displaced) S82.12-
nondisplaced S82.12-
medial condyle (displaced) S82.13-
nondisplaced S82.13-
physeal S89.00-
Salter-Harris
Type I S89.01-
Type II S89.02-
Type III S89.03-
Type IV S89.04-
specified NEC S89.09-
plateau —*see* Fracture, tibia, upper end, bicondylar
specified NEC S82.19-
spine (displaced) S82.11-
nondisplaced S82.11-
torus S82.16-
tuberosity (displaced) S82.15-
nondisplaced S82.15-
toe S92.91-
great (displaced) S92.40-
distal phalanx (displaced) S92.42-
nondisplaced S92.42-
nondisplaced S92.40-
proximal phalanx (displaced) S92.41-
nondisplaced S92.41-
specified NEC S92.49-
lesser (displaced) S92.50-
distal phalanx (displaced) S92.53-
nondisplaced S92.53-
medial phalanx (displaced) S92.52-
nondisplaced S92.52-
nondisplaced S92.50-
proximal phalanx (displaced) S92.51-
nondisplaced S92.51-
specified NEC S92.59-
physeal ◀
phalanx S99.20- ◀
Salter-Harris ◀
Type I S99.21- ◀
Type II S99.22- ◀
Type III S99.23- ◀
Type IV S99.24- ◀
specified NEC S99.29- ◀
tooth (root) S02.5
trachea (cartilage) S12.8
transverse process —*see* Fracture, vertebra
trapezium or trapezoid bone —*see* Fracture, carpal
trimalleolar —*see* Fracture, ankle, trimalleolar
triquetrum (cuneiform of carpus) —*see* Fracture, carpal, triquetrum
trochanter —*see* Fracture, femur, trochanteric
tuberosity (external) —*see* Fracture, traumatic, by site ⬅

Fracture, traumatic *(Continued)*
ulna (shaft) S52.20-
bent bone S52.28-
coronoid process —*see* Fracture, ulna, upper end, coronoid process
distal end —*see* Fracture, ulna, lower end
following insertion of implant, prosthesis or plate M96.63-
head S52.00-
lower end S52.60-
physeal S59.00-
Salter-Harris
Type I S59.01-
Type II S59.02-
Type III S59.03-
Type IV S59.04-
specified NEC S59.09-
specified NEC S52.69-
styloid process (displaced) S52.61-
nondisplaced S52.61-
torus S52.62-
proximal end —*see* Fracture, ulna, upper end
shaft S52.20-
comminuted (displaced) S52.25-
nondisplaced S52.25-
greenstick S52.21-
Monteggia's —*see* Monteggia's fracture
oblique (displaced) S52.23-
nondisplaced S52.23-
segmental (displaced) S52.26-
nondisplaced S52.26-
specified NEC S52.29-
spiral (displaced) S52.24-
nondisplaced S52.24-
transverse (displaced) S52.22-
nondisplaced S52.22-
upper end S52.00-
coronoid process (displaced) S52.04-
nondisplaced S52.04-
olecranon process (displaced) S52.02-
with intraarticular extension S52.03-
nondisplaced S52.02-
with intraarticular extension S52.03-
specified NEC S52.09-
torus S52.01-
unciform —*see* Fracture, carpal, hamate
vault of skull S02.0
vertebra, vertebral (arch) (body) (column) (neural arch) (pedicle) (spinous process) (transverse process)
atlas —*see* Fracture, neck, cervical vertebra, first
axis —*see* Fracture, neck, cervical vertebra, second
cervical (teardrop) S12.9
axis —*see* Fracture, neck, cervical vertebra, second
first (atlas) —*see* Fracture, neck, cervical vertebra, first
second (axis) —*see* Fracture, neck, cervical vertebra, second
chronic M84.48
coccyx S32.2
dorsal —*see* Fracture, thorax, vertebra
lumbar S32.009
burst (stable) S32.001
unstable S32.002
fifth S32.059
burst (stable) S32.051
unstable S32.052
specified type NEC S32.058
wedge compression S32.050
first S32.019
burst (stable) S32.011
unstable S32.012
specified type NEC S32.018
wedge compression S32.010

Fracture, traumatic *(Continued)*
vertebra, vertebral *(Continued)*
lumbar *(Continued)*
fourth S32.049
burst (stable) S32.041
unstable S32.042
specified type NEC S32.048
wedge compression S32.040
second S32.029
burst (stable) S32.021
unstable S32.022
specified type NEC S32.028
wedge compression S32.020
specified type NEC S32.008
third S32.039
burst (stable) S32.031
unstable S32.032
specified type NEC S32.038
wedge compression S32.030
wedge compression S32.000
metastatic —*see* Collapse, vertebra, in, specified disease NEC —*see also* Neoplasm
newborn (birth injury) P11.5
sacrum S32.10
specified NEC S32.19
Type
1 S32.14
2 S32.15
3 S32.16
4 S32.17
Zone
I S32.119
displaced (minimally) S32.111
severely S32.112
nondisplaced S32.110
II S32.129
displaced (minimally) S32.121
severely S32.122
nondisplaced S32.120
III S32.139
displaced (minimally) S32.131
severely S32.132
nondisplaced S32.130
thoracic —*see* Fracture, thorax, vertebra
vertex S02.0
vomer (bone) S02.2
wrist S62.10-
carpal —*see* Fracture, carpal bone
navicular (scaphoid) (hand) —*see* Fracture, carpal, navicular
xiphisternum, xiphoid (process) S22.24
zygoma S02.442
left side S02.40F ◀
right side S02.40E ◀
Fragile, fragility
autosomal site Q95.5
bone, congenital (with blue sclera) Q78.0
capillary (hereditary) D69.8
hair L67.8
nails L60.3
non-sex chromosome site Q95.5
X chromosome Q99.2
Fragilitas
crinium L67.8
ossium (with blue sclerae) (hereditary) Q78.0
unguium L60.3
congenital Q84.6
Fragments, cataract (lens), following cataract surgery H59.02-
retained foreign body —*see* Retained, foreign body fragments (type of)
Frailty (frail) R54
mental R41.81
Frambesia, frambesial (tropica) —*see also* Yaws
initial lesion or ulcer A66.0
primary A66.0
Frambeside
gummatous A66.4
of early yaws A66.2

F

Frambesioma A66.1
Franceschetti-Klein (-Wildervanck) disease or syndrome Q75.4
Francis' disease —*see* Tularemia
Franklin disease C88.2
Frank's essential thrombocytopenia D69.3
Fraser's syndrome Q87.0
Freckle (s) L81.2
  malignant melanoma in —*see* Melanoma
  melanotic (Hutchinson's) —*see* Melanoma, in situ
  retinal D49.81
Frederickson's hyperlipoproteinemia, type
  I and V E78.3
  IIA E78.00 ◄
  IIB and III E78.2
  IV E78.1
Freeman Sheldon syndrome Q87.0
Freezing —*see also* Effect, adverse, cold T69.9
Freiberg's disease (infraction of metatarsal head or osteochondrosis) —*see* Osteochondrosis, juvenile, metatarsus
Frei's disease A55
Fremitus, friction, cardiac R01.2
Frenum, frenulum
  external os Q51.828
  tongue (shortening) (congenital) Q38.1
Frequency micturition (nocturnal) R35.0
  psychogenic F45.8
Frey's syndrome
  auriculotemporal G50.8
  hyperhidrosis L74.52
Friction
  burn —*see* Burn, by site
  fremitus, cardiac R01.2
  precordial R01.2
  sounds, chest R09.89
Friderichsen-Waterhouse syndrome or disease A39.1
Friedländer's B (bacillus) NEC —*see also* condition A49.8
Friedreich's
  ataxia G11.1
  combined systemic disease G11.1
  facial hemihypertrophy Q67.4
  sclerosis (cerebellum) (spinal cord) G11.1
Frigidity F52.22
Fröhlich's syndrome E23.6
Frontal —*see also* condition
  lobe syndrome F07.0
Frostbite (superficial) T33.90
  with
    partial thickness skin loss —*see* Frostbite (superficial), by site
    tissue necrosis T34.90
  abdominal wall T33.3
    with tissue necrosis T34.3
  ankle T33.81-
    with tissue necrosis T34.81-
  arm T33.4-
  with tissue necrosis T34.4-
    finger (s) —*see* Frostbite, finger
    hand —*see* Frostbite, hand
    wrist —*see* Frostbite, wrist
  ear T33.01-
    with tissue necrosis T34.01-
  face T33.09
    with tissue necrosis T34.09
  finger T33.53-
    with tissue necrosis T34.53-
  foot T33.82-
    with tissue necrosis T34.82-
  hand T33.52-
    with tissue necrosis T34.52-
  head T33.09
    with tissue necrosis T34.09
    ear —*see* Frostbite, ear
    nose —*see* Frostbite, nose
  hip (and thigh) T33.6-
    with tissue necrosis T34.6-
Frostbite *(Continued)*
  knee T33.7-
    with tissue necrosis T34.7-
  leg T33.9-
    with tissue necrosis T34.9-
    ankle —*see* Frostbite, ankle
    foot —*see* Frostbite, foot
    knee —*see* Frostbite, knee
    lower T33.7-
      with tissue necrosis T34.7-
    thigh —*see* Frostbite, hip
    toe —*see* Frostbite, toe
  limb
    lower T33.99
      with tissue necrosis T34.99
    upper —*see* Frostbite, arm
  neck T33.1
    with tissue necrosis T34.1
  nose T33.02
    with tissue necrosis T34.02
  pelvis T33.3
    with tissue necrosis T34.3
  specified site NEC T33.99
    with tissue necrosis T34.99
  thigh —*see* Frostbite, hip
  thorax T33.2
    with tissue necrosis T34.2
  toes T33.83-
    with tissue necrosis T34.83-
  trunk T33.99
    with tissue necrosis T34.99
  wrist T33.51-
    with tissue necrosis T34.51-
Frotteurism F65.81
Frozen —*see also* Effect, adverse, cold T69.9
  pelvis (female) N94.89
    male K66.8
  shoulder —*see* Capsulitis, adhesive
Fructokinase deficiency E74.11
Fructose 1,6 diphosphatase deficiency E74.19
Fructosemia (benign) (essential) E74.12
Fructosuria (benign) (essential) E74.11
Fuchs'
  black spot (myopic) H44.2-
  dystrophy (corneal endothelium) H18.51
  heterochromic cyclitis —*see* Cyclitis, Fuchs' heterochromic
Fucosidosis E77.1
Fugue R68.89
  dissociative F44.1
  hysterical (dissociative) F44.1
  postictal in epilepsy —*see* Epilepsy
  reaction to exceptional stress (transient) F43.0
Fulminant, fulminating —*see* condition
Functional —*see also* condition
  bleeding (uterus) N93.8
Functioning, intellectual, borderline R41.83
Fundus —*see* condition
Fungemia NOS B49
Fungus, fungous
  cerebral G93.89
  disease NOS B49
  infection —*see* Infection, fungus
Funiculitis (acute) (chronic) (endemic) N49.1
  gonococcal (acute) (chronic) A54.23
  tuberculous A18.15
Funnel
  breast (acquired) M95.4
    congenital Q67.6
    sequelae (late effect) of rickets E64.3
  chest (acquired) M95.4
    congenital Q67.6
    sequelae (late effect) of rickets E64.3
  pelvis (acquired) M95.5
    with disproportion (fetopelvic) O33.3
      causing obstructed labor O65.3
    congenital Q74.2
FUO (fever of unknown origin) R50.9
Furfur L21.0
  microsporon B36.0
Furrier's lung J67.8
Furrowed K14.5
  nail (s) (transverse) L60.4
    congenital Q84.6
  tongue K14.5
    congenital Q38.3
Furuncle L02.92
  abdominal wall L02.221
  ankle —*see* Furuncle, lower limb
  antecubital space —*see* Furuncle, upper limb
  anus K61.0
  arm —*see* Furuncle, upper limb
  auditory canal, external —*see* Abscess, ear, external
  auricle (ear) —*see* Abscess, ear, external
  axilla (region) L02.42-
  back (any part) L02.222
  breast N61.1 ◄
  buttock L02.32
  cheek (external) L02.02
  chest wall L02.223
  chin L02.02
  corpus cavernosum N48.21
  ear, external —*see* Abscess, ear, external
  external auditory canal —*see* Abscess, ear, external
  eyelid —*see* Abscess, eyelid
  face L02.02
  femoral (region) —*see* Furuncle, lower limb
  finger —*see* Furuncle, hand
  flank L02.221
  foot L02.62-
  forehead L02.02
  gluteal (region) L02.32
  groin L02.224
  hand L02.52-
  head L02.821
    face L02.02
  hip —*see* Furuncle, lower limb
  kidney —*see* Abscess, kidney
  knee —*see* Furuncle, lower limb
  labium (majus) (minus) N76.4
  lacrimal
    gland —*see* Dacryoadenitis
    passages (duct) (sac) —*see* Inflammation, lacrimal, passages, acute
  leg (any part) —*see* Furuncle, lower limb
  lower limb L02.42-
  malignant A22.0
  mouth K12.2
  navel L02.226
  neck L02.12
  nose J34.0
  orbit, orbital —*see* Abscess, orbit
  palmar (space) —*see* Furuncle, hand
  partes posteriores L02.32
  pectoral region L02.223
  penis N48.21
  perineum L02.225
  pinna —*see* Abscess, ear, external
  popliteal —*see* Furuncle, lower limb
  prepatellar —*see* Furuncle, lower limb
  scalp L02.821
  seminal vesicle N49.0
  shoulder —*see* Furuncle, upper limb
  specified site NEC L02.828
  submandibular K12.2
  temple (region) L02.02
  thumb —*see* Furuncle, hand
  toe —*see* Furuncle, foot
  trunk L02.229
    abdominal wall L02.221
    back L02.222
    chest wall L02.223
    groin L02.224
    perineum L02.225
    umbilicus L02.226
  umbilicus L02.226
  upper limb L02.42-
  vulva N76.4

◄ New ◄ Revised ~~deleted~~ Deleted

Furunculosis —*see* Furuncle
Fused —*see* Fusion, fused
Fusion, fused (congenital)
astragaloscaphoid Q74.2
atria Q21.1
auditory canal Q16.1
auricles, heart Q21.1
binocular with defective stereopsis H53.32
bone Q79.8
cervical spine M43.22
choanal Q30.0
commissure, mitral valve Q23.2
cusps, heart valve NEC Q24.8
mitral Q23.2
pulmonary Q22.1
tricuspid Q22.4
ear ossicles Q16.3
fingers Q70.0-
hymen Q52.3
joint (acquired) —*see also* Ankylosis
congenital Q74.8
kidneys (incomplete) Q63.1
labium (majus) (minus) Q52.5
larynx and trachea Q34.8

Fusion, fused *(Continued)*
limb, congenital Q74.8
lower Q74.2
upper Q74.0
lobes, lung Q33.8
lumbosacral (acquired) M43.27
arthrodesis status Z98.1
congenital Q76.49
postprocedural status Z98.1
nares, nose, nasal, nostril (s) Q30.0
organ or site not listed —*see* Anomaly, by site
ossicles Q79.9
auditory Q16.3
pulmonic cusps Q22.1
ribs Q76.6
sacroiliac (joint) (acquired) M43.28
arthrodesis status Z98.1
congenital Q74.2
postprocedural status Z98.1
spine (acquired) NEC M43.20
arthrodesis status Z98.1
cervical region M43.22
cervicothoracic region M43.23
congenital Q76.49

Fusion, fused *(Continued)*
spine *(Continued)*
lumbar M43.26
lumbosacral region M43.27
occipito-atlanto-axial region M43.21
postoperative status Z98.1
sacrococcygeal region M43.28
thoracic region M43.24
thoracolumbar region M43.25
sublingual duct with submaxillary duct at opening in mouth Q38.4
testes Q55.1
toes Q70.2
tooth, teeth K00.2
trachea and esophagus Q39.8
twins Q89.4
vagina Q52.4
ventricles, heart Q21.0
vertebra (arch) —*see* Fusion, spine
vulva Q52.5
Fusospirillosis (mouth) (tongue) (tonsil) A69.1
Fussy baby R68.12

F

G

Gain in weight (abnormal) (excessive) —*see also* Weight, gain
Gaisböck's disease (polycythemia hypertonica) D75.1
Gait abnormality R26.9
  ataxic R26.0
  falling R29.6
  hysterical (ataxic) (staggering) F44.4
  paralytic R26.1
  spastic R26.1
  specified type NEC R26.89
  staggering R26.0
  unsteadiness R26.81
  walking difficulty NEC R26.2
Galactocele (breast) N64.89
  puerperal, postpartum O92.79
Galactokinase deficiency E74.29
Galactophoritis N61.0 ⇐
  gestational, puerperal, postpartum O91.2-
Galactorrhea O92.6
  not associated with childbirth N64.3
Galactosemia (classic) (congenital) E74.21
Galactosuria E74.29
Galacturia R82.0
  schistosomiasis (bilharziasis) B65.0
Galeazzi's fracture S52.37-
Galen's vein —*see* condition
Galeophobia F40.218
Gall duct —*see* condition
Gallbladder —*see also* condition
  acute K81.0
Gallop rhythm R00.8
Gallstone (colic) (cystic duct) (gallbladder) (impacted) (multiple) —*see also* Calculus, gallbladder
  with
    cholecystitis —*see* Calculus, gallbladder, with cholecystitis
  bile duct (common) (hepatic) —*see* Calculus, bile duct
  causing intestinal obstruction K56.3
  specified NEC K80.80
    with obstruction K80.81
Gambling Z72.6
  pathological (compulsive) F63.0
Gammopathy (of undetermined significance [MGUS]) D47.2
  associated with lymphoplasmacytic dyscrasia D47.2
  monoclonal D47.2
  polyclonal D89.0
Gamna's disease (siderotic splenomegaly) D73.1
Gamophobia F40.298
Gampsodactylia (congenital) Q66.7
Gamstorp's disease (adynamia episodica hereditaria) G72.3
Gandy-Nanta disease (siderotic splenomegaly) D73.1
Gang
  membership offenses Z72.810
Gangliocytoma D36.10
Ganglioglioma —*see* Neoplasm, uncertain behavior, by site
Ganglion (compound) (diffuse) (joint) (tendon (sheath)) M67.40
  ankle M67.47-
  foot M67.47-
  forearm M67.43-
  hand M67.44-
  lower leg M67.46-
  multiple sites M67.49
  of yaws (early) (late) A66.6
  pelvic region M67.45-
  periosteal —*see* Periostitis
  shoulder region M67.41-
  specified site NEC M67.48
  thigh region M67.45-
  tuberculous A18.09
  upper arm M67.42-
  wrist M67.43-
Ganglioneuroblastoma —*see* Neoplasm, nerve, malignant
Ganglioneuroma D36.10
  malignant —*see* Neoplasm, nerve, malignant
Ganglioneuromatosis D36.10
Ganglionitis
  fifth nerve —*see* Neuralgia, trigeminal
  gasserian (postherpetic) (postzoster) B02.21
  geniculate G51.1
    newborn (birth injury) P11.3
    postherpetic, postzoster B02.21
  herpes zoster B02.21
  postherpetic geniculate B02.21
Gangliosidosis E75.10
  GM1 E75.19
  GM2 E75.00
    other specified E75.09
    Sandhoff disease E75.01
    Tay-Sachs disease E75.02
  GM3 E75.19
  mucolipidosis IV E75.11
Gangosa A66.5
Gangrene, gangrenous (connective tissue) (dropsical) (dry) (moist) (skin) (ulcer) —*see also* Necrosis I96
  with diabetes (mellitus) —*see* Diabetes, gangrene
  abdomen (wall) I96
  alveolar M27.3
  appendix K35.80
    with
      perforation or rupture K35.2
      peritoneal abscess K35.3
      peritonitis NEC K35.3
        generalized (with perforation or rupture) K35.2
        localized (with perforation or rupture) K35.3
  arteriosclerotic (general) (senile) —*see* Arteriosclerosis, extremities, with, gangrene
  auricle I96
  Bacillus welchii A48.0
  bladder (infectious) —*see* Cystitis, specified type NEC
  bowel, cecum, or colon —*see* Gangrene, intestine
  Clostridium perfringens or welchii A48.0
  cornea H18.89-
  corpora cavernosa N48.29
    noninfective N48.89
  cutaneous, spreading I96
  decubital —*see* Ulcer, pressure, by site
  diabetic (any site) —*see* Diabetes, gangrene
  emphysematous —*see* Gangrene, gas
  epidemic —*see* Poisoning, food, noxious, plant
  epididymis (infectional) N45.1
  erysipelas —*see* Erysipelas
  extremity (lower) (upper) I96
  Fournier N49.3
    female N76.89
  fusospirochetal A69.0
  gallbladder —*see* Cholecystitis, acute
  gas (bacillus) A48.0
    following
      abortion —*see* Abortion by type complicated by infection
      ectopic or molar pregnancy O08.0
  glossitis K14.0
  hernia —*see* Hernia, by site, with gangrene
  intestine, intestinal (hemorrhagic) (massive) —*see also* Infarct, intestine K55.069 ⇐
    with
      mesenteric embolism —*see also* Infarct, intestine K55.069 ⇐
      obstruction —*see* Obstruction, intestine
  laryngitis J04.0
  limb (lower) (upper) I96
Gangrene, gangrenous *(Continued)*
  lung J85.0
    spirochetal A69.8
  lymphangitis I89.1
  Meleney's (synergistic) —*see* Ulcer, skin
  mesentery —*see also* Infarct, intestine K55.069 ⇐
    with
      embolism —*see also* Infarct, intestine K55.069 ⇐
      intestinal obstruction —*see* Obstruction, intestine
  mouth A69.0
  ovary —*see* Oophoritis
  pancreas —*see* Pancreatitis, acute ⇐
  penis N48.29
    noninfective N48.89
  perineum I96
  pharynx —*see also* Pharyngitis
    Vincent's A69.1
  presenile I73.1
  progressive synergistic —*see* Ulcer, skin
  pulmonary J85.0
  pulpal (dental) K04.1
  quinsy J36
  Raynaud's (symmetric gangrene) I73.01
  retropharyngeal J39.2
  scrotum N49.3
    noninfective N50.89 ⇐
  senile (atherosclerotic) —*see* Arteriosclerosis, extremities, with, gangrene
  spermatic cord N49.1
    noninfective N50.89 ⇐
  spine I96
  spirochetal NEC A69.8
  spreading cutaneous I96
  stomatitis A69.0
  symmetrical I73.01
  testis (infectional) N45.2
    noninfective N44.8
  throat —*see also* Pharyngitis
    diphtheritic A36.0
    Vincent's A69.1
  thyroid (gland) E07.89
  tooth (pulp) K04.1
  tuberculous NEC —*see* Tuberculosis
  tunica vaginalis N49.1
    noninfective N50.89 ⇐
  umbilicus I96
  uterus —*see* Endometritis
  uvulitis K12.2
  vas deferens N49.1
    noninfective N50.89 ⇐
  vulva N76.89
Ganister disease J62.8
Ganser's syndrome (hysterical) F44.89
Gardner-Diamond syndrome (autoerythrocyte sensitization) D69.2
Gargoylism E76.01
Garré's disease, osteitis (sclerosing), osteomyelitis —*see* Osteomyelitis, specified type NEC
Garrod's pad, knuckle M72.1
Gartner's duct
  cyst Q52.4
  persistent Q50.6
Gas R14.3
  asphyxiation, inhalation, poisoning, suffocation NEC —*see* Table of Drugs and Chemicals
  excessive R14.0
  gangrene A48.0
    following
      abortion —*see* Abortion by type complicated by infection
      ectopic or molar pregnancy O08.0
  on stomach R14.0
  pains R14.1
Gastralgia —*see also* Pain, abdominal
Gastrectasis K31.0
  psychogenic F45.8
Gastric —*see* condition

◀ New ⇐ Revised ~~deleted~~ Deleted

Gastrinoma
malignant
pancreas C25.4
specified site NEC —*see* Neoplasm, malignant, by site
unspecified site C25.4
specified site —*see* Neoplasm, uncertain behavior
unspecified site D37.9
Gastritis (simple) K29.70
with bleeding K29.71
acute (erosive) K29.00
with bleeding K29.01
alcoholic K29.20
with bleeding K29.21
allergic K29.60
with bleeding K29.61
atrophic (chronic) K29.40
with bleeding K29.41
chronic (antral) (fundal) K29.50
with bleeding K29.51
atrophic K29.40
with bleeding K29.41
superficial K29.30
with bleeding K29.31
dietary counseling and surveillance Z71.3
due to diet deficiency E63.9
eosinophilic K52.81
giant hypertrophic K29.60
with bleeding K29.61
granulomatous K29.60
with bleeding K29.61
hypertrophic (mucosa) K29.60
with bleeding K29.61
nervous F54
spastic K29.60
with bleeding K29.61
specified NEC K29.60
with bleeding K29.61
superficial chronic K29.30
with bleeding K29.31
tuberculous A18.83
viral NEC A08.4
Gastrocarcinoma —*see* Neoplasm, malignant, stomach
Gastrocolic —*see* condition
Gastrodisciasis, gastrodiscoidiasis B66.8
Gastroduodenitis K29.90
with bleeding K29.91
virus, viral A08.4
specified type NEC A08.39
Gastrodynia —*see* Pain, abdominal
Gastroenteritis (acute) (chronic) (noninfectious) (*see also* Enteritis) K52.9
allergic K52.29 ⇐
with ◀
eosinophilic gastritis or gastroenteritis K52.81 ◀
food protein-induced enterocolitis syndrome K52.21 ◀
food protein-induced enteropathy K52.22 ◀
dietetic —*see also* Gastroenteritis, allergic K52.29 ⇐
drug-induced K52.1
due to
Cryptosporidium A07.2
drugs K52.1
food poisoning —*see* Intoxication, foodborne
radiation K52.0
eosinophilic K52.81
epidemic (infectious) A09
food hypersensitivity —*see also* Gastroenteritis, allergic K52.29 ⇐
infectious —*see* Enteritis, infectious
influenzal —*see* Influenza, with gastroenteritis
noninfectious K52.9
specified NEC K52.89
rotaviral A08.0
Gastroenteritis *(Continued)*
Salmonella A02.0
toxic K52.1
viral NEC A08.4
acute infectious A08.39
type Norwalk A08.11
infantile (acute) A08.39
Norwalk agent A08.11
rotaviral A08.0
severe of infants A08.39
specified type NEC A08.39
Gastroenteropathy —*see also* Gastroenteritis K52.9
acute, due to Norovirus A08.11
acute, due to Norwalk agent A08.11
infectious A09
Gastroenteroptosis K63.4
Gastroesophageal laceration-hemorrhage syndrome K22.6
Gastrointestinal —*see* condition
Gastrojejunal —*see* condition
Gastrojejunitis —*see also* Enteritis K52.9
Gastrojejunocolic —*see* condition
Gastroliths K31.89
Gastromalacia K31.89
Gastroparalysis K31.84
diabetic —*see* Diabetes, gastroparalysis
Gastroparesis K31.84
diabetic —*see* Diabetes, by type, with gastroparesis
Gastropathy K31.9
congestive portal K31.89
erythematous K29.70
exudative K90.89
portal hypertensive K31.89
Gastroptosis K31.89
Gastrorrhagia K92.2
psychogenic F45.8
Gastroschisis (congenital) Q79.3
Gastrospasm (neurogenic) (reflex) K31.89
neurotic F45.8
psychogenic F45.8
Gastrostaxis —*see* Gastritis, with bleeding
Gastrostenosis K31.89
Gastrostomy
attention to Z43.1
status Z93.1
Gastrosuccorrhea (continuous) (intermittent) K31.89
neurotic F45.8
psychogenic F45.8
Gatophobia F40.218
Gaucher's disease or splenomegaly (adult) (infantile) E75.22
Gee (-Herter)(-Thaysen) disease (nontropical sprue) K90.0
Gélineau's syndrome G47.419
with cataplexy G47.411
Gemination, tooth, teeth K00.2
Gemistocytoma
specified site —*see* Neoplasm, malignant, by site
unspecified site C71.9
General, generalized —*see* condition
Genetic
carrier (status)
cystic fibrosis Z14.1
hemophilia A (asymptomatic) Z14.01
symptomatic Z14.02
specified NEC Z14.8
susceptibility to disease NEC Z15.89
malignant neoplasm Z15.09
breast Z15.01
endometrium Z15.04
ovary Z15.02
prostate Z15.03
specified NEC Z15.09
multiple endocrine neoplasia Z15.81
Genital —*see* condition
Genito-anorectal syndrome A55
Genitourinary system —*see* condition
Genu
congenital Q74.1
extrorsum (acquired) —*see also* Deformity, varus, knee
congenital Q74.1
sequelae (late effect) of rickets E64.3
introrsum (acquired) —*see also* Deformity, valgus, knee
congenital Q74.1
sequelae (late effect) of rickets E64.3
rachitic (old) E64.3
recurvatum (acquired) —*see also* Deformity, limb, specified type NEC, lower leg
congenital Q68.2
sequelae (late effect) of rickets E64.3
valgum (acquired) (knock-knee) M21.06-
congenital Q74.1
sequelae (late effect) of rickets E64.3
varum (acquired) (bowleg) M21.16-
congenital Q74.1
sequelae (late effect) of rickets E64.3
Geographic tongue K14.1
Geophagia —*see* Pica
Geotrichosis B48.3
stomatitis B48.3
Gephyrophobia F40.242
Gerbode defect Q21.0
GERD (gastroesophageal reflux disease) K21.9
Gerhardt's
disease (erythromelalgia) I73.81
syndrome (vocal cord paralysis) J38.00
bilateral J38.02
unilateral J38.01
German measles —*see also* Rubella
exposure to Z20.4
Germinoblastoma (diffuse) C85.9-
follicular C82.9-
Germinoma —*see* Neoplasm, malignant, by site
Gerontoxon —*see* Degeneration, cornea, senile
Gerstmann-Sträussler-Scheinker syndrome (GSS) A81.82
Gerstmann's syndrome R48.8
developmental F81.2
Gestation (period) —*see also* Pregnancy
ectopic —*see* Pregnancy, by site
multiple O30.9-
greater than quadruplets —*see* Pregnancy, multiple (gestation), specified NEC
specified NEC —*see* Pregnancy, multiple (gestation), specified NEC
Gestational
mammary abscess O91.11-
purulent mastitis O91.11-
subareolar abscess O91.11-
Ghon tubercle, primary infection A15.7
Ghost
teeth K00.4
vessels (cornea) H16.41-
Ghoul hand A66.3
Gianotti-Crosti disease L44.4
Giant
cell
epulis K06.8
peripheral granuloma K06.8
esophagus, congenital Q39.5
kidney, congenital Q63.3
urticaria T78.3
hereditary D84.1
Giardiasis A07.1
Gibert's disease or pityriasis L42
Giddiness R42
hysterical F44.89
psychogenic F45.8
Gierke's disease (glycogenosis I) E74.01
Gigantism (cerebral) (hypophyseal) (pituitary) E22.0
constitutional E34.4
Gilbert's disease or syndrome E80.4
Gilchrist's disease B40.9
Gilford-Hutchinson disease E34.8

G

Gilles de la Tourette's disease or syndrome (motor-verbal tic) F95.2
Gingivitis K05.10
acute (catarrhal) K05.00
necrotizing A69.1
nonplaque induced K05.01
plaque induced K05.00
chronic (desquamative) (hyperplastic) (simple marginal) (pregnancy associated) (ulcerative) K05.10 ◄
nonplaque induced K05.11
plaque induced K05.10
expulsiva —*see* Periodontitis
necrotizing ulcerative (acute) A69.1
pellagrous E52
acute necrotizing A69.1
Vincent's A69.1
Gingivoglossitis K14.0
Gingivopericementitis —*see* Periodontitis
Gingivosis —*see* Gingivitis, chronic
Gingivostomatitis K05.10
herpesviral B00.2
necrotizing ulcerative (acute) A69.1
Gland, glandular —*see* condition
Glanders A24.0
Glanzmann (-Naegeli) disease or thrombasthenia D69.1
Glasgow coma scale
total score
3-8 R40.243
9-12 R40.242
13-15 R40.241
Glass-blower's disease (cataract) —*see* Cataract, specified NEC
Glaucoma H40.9
with
increased episcleral venous pressure H40.81-
pseudoexfoliation of lens —*see* Glaucoma, open angle, primary, capsular
absolute H44.51-
angle-closure (primary) H40.20-
acute (attack) (crisis) H40.21-
chronic H40.22-
intermittent H40.23-
residual stage H40.24-
borderline H40.00-
capsular (with pseudoexfoliation of lens) —*see* Glaucoma, open angle, primary, capsular
childhood Q15.0
closed angle —*see* Glaucoma, angle-closure
congenital Q15.0
corticosteroid-induced —*see* Glaucoma, secondary, drugs
hypersecretion H40.82-
in (due to)
amyloidosis E85.4 *[H42]*
aniridia Q13.1 *[H42]*
concussion of globe —*see* Glaucoma, secondary, trauma
dislocation of lens —*see* Glaucoma, secondary
disorder of lens NEC —*see* Glaucoma, secondary
drugs —*see* Glaucoma, secondary, drugs
endocrine disease NOS E34.9 *[H42]*
eye
inflammation —*see* Glaucoma, secondary, inflammation
trauma —*see* Glaucoma, secondary, trauma
hypermature cataract —*see* Glaucoma, secondary
iridocyclitis —*see* Glaucoma, secondary, inflammation
lens disorder —*see* Glaucoma, secondary, Lowe's syndrome E72.03 *[H42]*
metabolic disease NOS E88.9 *[H42]*
ocular disorders NEC —*see* Glaucoma, secondary
Glaucoma *(Continued)*
in (due to) *(Continued)*
onchocerciasis B73.02
pupillary block —*see* Glaucoma, secondary
retinal vein occlusion —*see* Glaucoma, secondary
Rieger's anomaly Q13.81 *[H42]*
rubeosis of iris —*see* Glaucoma, secondary
tumor of globe —*see* Glaucoma, secondary
infantile Q15.0
low tension —*see* Glaucoma, open angle, primary, low-tension
malignant H40.83-
narrow angle —*see* Glaucoma, angle-closure
newborn Q15.0
noncongestive (chronic) —*see* Glaucoma, open angle
nonobstructive —*see* Glaucoma, open angle
obstructive —*see also* Glaucoma, angle-closure
due to lens changes —*see* Glaucoma, secondary
open angle H40.10-
primary H40.11-
capsular (with pseudoexfoliation of lens) H40.14-
low-tension H40.12-
pigmentary H40.13-
residual stage H40.15-
phacolytic —*see* Glaucoma, secondary
pigmentary —*see* Glaucoma, open angle, primary, pigmentary
postinfectious —*see* Glaucoma, secondary, inflammation
secondary (to) H40.5-
drugs H40.6-
inflammation H40.4-
trauma H40.3-
simple (chronic) H40.11- ◄
simplex H40.11- ◄
specified type NEC H40.89
suspect H40.00-
syphilitic A52.71
traumatic —*see also* Glaucoma, secondary, trauma
newborn (birth injury) P15.3
tuberculous A18.59
Glaucomatous flecks (subcapsular) —*see* Cataract, complicated
Glazed tongue K14.4
Gleet (gonococcal) A54.01
Glénard's disease K63.4
Glioblastoma (multiforme)
with sarcomatous component
specified site —*see* Neoplasm, malignant, by site
unspecified site C71.9
giant cell
specified site —*see* Neoplasm, malignant, by site
unspecified site C71.9
specified site —*see* Neoplasm, malignant, by site
unspecified site C71.9
Glioma (malignant)
astrocytic
specified site —*see* Neoplasm, malignant, by site
unspecified site C71.9
mixed
specified site —*see* Neoplasm, malignant, by site
unspecified site C71.9
nose Q30.8
specified site NEC —*see* Neoplasm, malignant, by site
subependymal D43.2
specified site —*see* Neoplasm, uncertain behavior, by site
unspecified site D43.2
unspecified site C71.9
Gliomatosis cerebri C71.0
Glioneuroma —*see* Neoplasm, uncertain behavior, by site
Gliosarcoma
specified site —*see* Neoplasm, malignant, by site
unspecified site C71.9
Gliosis (cerebral) G93.89
spinal G95.89
Glisson's disease —*see* Rickets
Globinuria R82.3
Globus (hystericus) F45.8
Glomangioma D18.00
intra-abdominal D18.03
intracranial D18.02
skin D18.01
specified site NEC D18.09
Glomangiomyoma D18.00
intra-abdominal D18.03
intracranial D18.02
skin D18.01
specified site NEC D18.09
Glomangiosarcoma —*see* Neoplasm, connective tissue, malignant
Glomerular
disease in syphilis A52.75
nephritis —*see* Glomerulonephritis
Glomerulitis —*see* Glomerulonephritis
Glomerulonephritis —*see also* Nephritis N05.9
with
edema —*see* Nephrosis
minimal change N05.0
minor glomerular abnormality N05.0
acute N00.9
chronic N03.9
crescentic (diffuse) NEC —*see also* N00-N07 with fourth character .7 N05.7
dense deposit —*see also* N00-N07 with fourth character .6 N05.6
diffuse
crescentic —*see also* N00-N07 with fourth character .7 N05.7
endocapillary proliferative —*see also* N00N07 with fourth character .4 N05.4
membranous —*see also* N00-N07 with fourth character .2 N05.2
mesangial proliferative —*see also* N00-N07 with fourth character .3 N05.3
mesangiocapillary —*see also* N00-N07 with fourth character .5 N05.5
sclerosing N05.8
endocapillary proliferative (diffuse) NEC —*see also* N00-N07 with fourth character .4 N05.4
extracapillary NEC —*see also* N00-N07 with fourth character .7 N05.7
focal (and segmental) —*see also* N00-N07 with fourth character .1 N05.1
hypocomplementemic —*see* Glomerulonephritis, membranoproliferative
IgA —*see* Nephropathy, IgA
immune complex (circulating) NEC N05.8
in (due to)
amyloidosis E85.4 *[N08]*
bilharziasis B65.9 *[N08]*
cryoglobulinemia D89.1 *[N08]*
defibrination syndrome D65 *[N08]*
diabetes mellitus —*see* Diabetes, glomerulosclerosis
disseminated intravascular coagulation D65 *[N08]*
Fabry (-Anderson) disease E75.21 *[N08]*
Goodpasture's syndrome M31.0
hemolytic-uremic syndrome D59.3
Henoch (-Schönlein) purpura D69.0 *[N08]*
lecithin cholesterol acyltransferase deficiency E78.6 *[N08]*

◄ New ◄ Revised ~~deleted~~ Deleted

Glomerulonephritis *(Continued)*
in *(Continued)*
microscopic polyangiitis M31.7 *[N08]*
multiple myeloma C90.0- *[N08]*
Plasmodium malariae B52.0
schistosomiasis B65.9 *[N08]*
sepsis A41.9- *[N08]*
streptococcal A40- *[N08]*
sickle-cell disorders D57.- *[N08]*
strongyloidiasis B78.9 *[N08]*
subacute bacterial endocarditis I33.0 *[N08]*
syphilis (late) congenital A50.59 *[N08]*
systemic lupus erythematosus M32.14
thrombotic thrombocytopenic purpura M31.1 *[N08]*
typhoid fever A01.09
Waldenström macroglobulinemia C88.0 *[N08]*
Wegener's granulomatosis M31.31
latent or quiescent N03.9
lobular, lobulonodular —*see* Glomerulonephritis, membranoproliferative
membranoproliferative (diffuse) (type 1 or 3) —*see also* N00-N07 with fourth character .5 N05.5
dense deposit (type 2) NEC —*see also* N00-N07 with fourth character .6 N05.6
membranous (diffuse) NEC —*see also* N00-N07 with fourth character .2 N05.2
mesangial
IgA/IgG —*see* Nephropathy, IgA
proliferative (diffuse) NEC —*see also* N00-N07 with fourth character .3 N05.3
mesangiocapillary (diffuse) NEC —*see also* N00-N07 with fourth character .5 N05.5
necrotic, necrotizing NEC —*see also* N00-N07 with fourth character .8 N05.8
nodular —*see* Glomerulonephritis, membranoproliferative
poststreptococcal NEC N05.9
acute N00.9
chronic N03.9
rapidly progressive N01.9
proliferative NEC —*see also* N00-N07 with fourth character .8 N05.8
diffuse (lupus) M32.14
rapidly progressive N01.9
sclerosing, diffuse N05.8
specified pathology NEC —*see also* N00-N07 with fourth character .8 N05.8
subacute N01.9
Glomerulopathy —*see* Glomerulonephritis
Glomerulosclerosis —*see also* Sclerosis, renal
intercapillary (nodular) (with diabetes) —*see* Diabetes, glomerulosclerosis
intracapillary —*see* Diabetes, glomerulosclerosis
Glossagra K14.6
Glossalgia K14.6
Glossitis (chronic superficial) (gangrenous) (Moeller's) K14.0
areata exfoliativa K14.1
atrophic K14.4
benign migratory K14.1
cortical superficial, sclerotic K14.0
Hunter's D51.0
interstitial, sclerous K14.0
median rhomboid K14.2
pellagrous E52
superficial, chronic K14.0
Glossocele K14.8
Glossodynia K14.6
exfoliativa K14.4
Glossoncus K14.8
Glossopathy K14.9
Glossophytia K14.3
Glossoplegia K14.8
Glossoptosis K14.8
Glossopyrosis K14.6
Glossotrichia K14.3
Glossy skin L90.8
Glottis —*see* condition
Glottitis —*see also* Laryngitis J04.0
Glucagonoma
pancreas
benign D13.7
malignant C25.4
uncertain behavior D37.8
specified site NEC
benign —*see* Neoplasm, benign, by site
malignant —*see* Neoplasm, malignant, by site
uncertain behavior —*see* Neoplasm, uncertain behavior, by site
unspecified site
benign D13.7
malignant C25.4
uncertain behavior D37.8
Glucoglycinuria E72.51
Glucose-galactose malabsorption E74.39
Glue
ear —*see* Otitis, media, nonsuppurative, chronic, mucoid
sniffing (airplane) —*see* Abuse, drug, inhalant
dependence —*see* Dependence, drug, inhalant
Glutaric aciduria E72.3
Glycinemia E72.51
Glycinuria (renal) (with ketosis) E72.09
Glycogen
infiltration —*see* Disease, glycogen storage
storage disease —*see* Disease, glycogen storage
Glycogenosis (diffuse) (generalized) —*see also* Disease, glycogen storage
cardiac E74.02 *[I43]*
diabetic, secondary —*see* Diabetes, glycogenosis, secondary
pulmonary interstitial J84.842
Glycopenia E16.2
Glycosuria R81
renal E74.8
Gnathostoma spinigerum (infection) (infestation), gnathostomiasis (wandering swelling) B83.1
Goiter (plunging) (substernal) E04.9
with
hyperthyroidism (recurrent) —*see* Hyperthyroidism, with, goiter
thyrotoxicosis —*see* Hyperthyroidism, with, goiter
adenomatous —*see* Goiter, nodular
cancerous C73
congenital (nontoxic) E03.0
diffuse E03.0
parenchymatous E03.0
transitory, with normal functioning P72.0
cystic E04.2
due to iodine-deficiency E01.1
due to
enzyme defect in synthesis of thyroid hormone E07.1
iodine-deficiency (endemic) E01.2
dyshormonogenetic (familial) E07.1
endemic (iodine-deficiency) E01.2
diffuse E01.0
multinodular E01.1
exophthalmic —*see* Hyperthyroidism, with, goiter
iodine-deficiency (endemic) E01.2
diffuse E01.0
multinodular E01.1
nodular E01.1
lingual Q89.2
lymphadenoid E06.3
malignant C73
Goiter *(Continued)*
multinodular (cystic) (nontoxic) E04.2
toxic or with hyperthyroidism E05.20
with thyroid storm E05.21
neonatal NEC P72.0
nodular (nontoxic) (due to) E04.9
with
hyperthyroidism E05.20
with thyroid storm E05.21
thyrotoxicosis E05.20
with thyroid storm E05.21
endemic E01.1
iodine-deficiency E01.1
sporadic E04.9
toxic E05.20
with thyroid storm E05.21
nontoxic E04.9
diffuse (colloid) E04.0
multinodular E04.2
simple E04.0
specified NEC E04.8
uninodular E04.1
simple E04.0
toxic —*see* Hyperthyroidism, with, goiter
uninodular (nontoxic) E04.1
toxic or with hyperthyroidism E05.10
with thyroid storm E05.11
Goiter-deafness syndrome E07.1
Goldberg syndrome Q89.8
Goldberg-Maxwell syndrome E34.51
Goldblatt's hypertension or kidney I70.1
Goldenhar (-Gorlin) syndrome Q87.0
Goldflam-Erb disease or syndrome G70.00
with exacerbation (acute) G70.01
in crisis G70.01
Goldscheider's disease Q81.8
Goldstein's disease (familial hemorrhagic telangiectasia) I78.0
Golfer's elbow —*see* Epicondylitis, medial
Gonadoblastoma
specified site —*see* Neoplasm, uncertain behavior, by site
unspecified site
female D39.10
male D40.10
Gonecystitis —*see* Vesiculitis
Gongylonemiasis B83.8
Goniosynechiae —*see* Adhesions, iris, goniosynechiae
Gonococcemia A54.86
Gonococcus, gonococcal (disease) (infection) —*see also* condition A54.9
anus A54.6
bursa, bursitis A54.49
conjunctiva, conjunctivitis (neonatorum) A54.31
endocardium A54.83
eye A54.30
conjunctivitis A54.31
iridocyclitis A54.32
keratitis A54.33
newborn A54.31
other specified A54.39
fallopian tubes (acute) (chronic) A54.24
genitourinary (organ) (system) (tract) (acute)
lower A54.00
with abscess (accessory gland) (periurethral) A54.1
upper —*see also* condition A54.29
heart A54.83
iridocyclitis A54.32
joint A54.42
lymphatic (gland) (node) A54.89
meninges, meningitis A54.81
musculoskeletal A54.40
arthritis A54.42
osteomyelitis A54.43
other specified A54.49
spondylopathy A54.41
pelviperitonitis A54.24
pelvis (acute) (chronic) A54.24

G

Gonococcus, gonococcal *(Continued)*
pharynx A54.5
proctitis A54.6
pyosalpinx (acute) (chronic) A54.24
rectum A54.6
skin A54.89
specified site NEC A54.89
tendon sheath A54.49
throat A54.5
urethra (acute) (chronic) A54.01
with abscess (accessory gland) (periurethral) A54.1
vulva (acute) (chronic) A54.02
Gonocytoma
specified site —*see* Neoplasm, uncertain behavior, by site
unspecified site
female D39.10
male D40.10
Gonorrhea (acute) (chronic) A54.9
Bartholin's gland (acute) (chronic) (purulent) A54.02
with abscess (accessory gland) (periurethral) A54.1
bladder A54.01
cervix A54.03
conjunctiva, conjunctivitis (neonatorum) A54.31
contact Z20.2
Cowper's gland (with abscess) A54.1
exposure to Z20.2
fallopian tube (acute) (chronic) A54.24
kidney (acute) (chronic) A54.21
lower genitourinary tract A54.00
with abscess (accessory gland) (periurethral) A54.1
ovary (acute) (chronic) A54.24
pelvis (acute) (chronic) A54.24
female pelvic inflammatory disease A54.24
penis A54.09
prostate (acute) (chronic) A54.22
seminal vesicle (acute) (chronic) A54.23
specified site not listed —*see also* Gonococcus A54.89
spermatic cord (acute) (chronic) A54.23
urethra A54.01
with abscess (accessory gland) (periurethral) A54.1
vagina A54.02
vas deferens (acute) (chronic) A54.23
vulva A54.02
Goodall's disease A08.19
Goodpasture's syndrome M31.0
Gopalan's syndrome (burning feet) E53.0
Gorlin-Chaudry-Moss syndrome Q87.0
Gottron's papules L94.4
Gougerot's syndrome (trisymptomatic) L81.7
Gougerot-Blum syndrome (pigmented purpuric lichenoid dermatitis) L81.7
Gougerot-Carteaud disease or syndrome (confluent reticulate papillomatosis) L83
Gouley's syndrome (constrictive pericarditis) I31.1
Goundou A66.6
Gout, chronic (*see also* Gout, gouty) M1A.9-
drug-induced M1A.20
ankle M1A.27-
elbow M1A.22-
foot joint M1A.27-
hand joint M1A.24-
hip M1A.25-
knee M1A.26-
multiple site M1A.29-
shoulder M1A.21-
vertebrae M1A.28
wrist M1A.23-
idiopathic M1A.00
ankle M1A.07-
elbow M1A.02-
foot joint M1A.07-
hand joint M1A.04-
Gout, chronic *(Continued)*
idiopathic *(Continued)*
hip M1A.05-
knee M1A.06-
multiple site M1A.09
shoulder M1A.01-
vertebrae M1A.08
wrist M1A.03-
in (due to) renal impairment M1A.30
ankle M1A.37-
elbow M1A.32-
foot joint M1A.37-
hand joint M1A.34-
hip M1A.35-
knee M1A.36-
multiple site M1A.39
shoulder M1A.31-
vertebrae M1A.38
wrist M1A.33-
lead-induced M1A.10
ankle M1A.17-
elbow M1A.12-
foot joint M1A.17-
hand joint M1A.14-
hip M1A.15-
knee M1A.16-
multiple site M1A.19
shoulder M1A.11-
vertebrae M1A.18
wrist M1A.13-
primary —*see* Gout, chronic, idiopathic
saturnine —*see* Gout, chronic, lead-induced
secondary NEC M1A.40
ankle M1A.47-
elbow M1A.42-
foot joint M1A.47-
hand joint M1A.44-
hip M1A.45-
knee M1A.46-
multiple site M1A.49
shoulder M1A.41-
vertebrae M1A.48
wrist M1A.43-
syphilitic —*see also* subcategory M14.8- A52.77
tophi M1A.9
Gout, gouty (acute) (attack) (flare) —*see also* Gout, chronic M10.9-
drug-induced M10.20
ankle M10.27-
elbow M10.22-
foot joint M10.27-
hand joint M10.24-
hip M10.25-
knee M10.26-
multiple site M10.29
shoulder M10.21-
vertebrae M10.28
wrist M10.23-
idiopathic M10.00
ankle M10.07-
elbow M10.02-
foot joint M10.07-
hand joint M10.04-
hip M10.05-
knee M10.06-
multiple site M10.09
shoulder M10.01-
vertebrae M10.08
wrist M10.03-
in (due to) renal impairment M10.30
ankle M10.37-
elbow M10.32-
foot joint M10.37-
hand joint M10.34-
hip M10.35-
knee M10.36-
multiple site M10.39
shoulder M10.31-
vertebrae M10.38
wrist M10.33-
Gout, gouty *(Continued)*
lead-induced M10.10
ankle M10.17-
elbow M10.12-
foot joint M10.17-
hand joint M10.14-
hip M10.15-
knee M10.16-
multiple site M10.19
shoulder M10.11-
vertebrae M10.18
wrist M10.13-
primary —*see* Gout, idiopathic
saturnine —*see* Gout, lead-induced
secondary NEC M10.40
ankle M10.47-
elbow M10.42-
foot joint M10.47-
hand joint M10.44-
hip M10.45-
knee M10.46-
multiple site M10.49
shoulder M10.41-
vertebrae M10.48
wrist M10.43-
syphilitic —*see also* subcategory M14.8- A52.77
tophi NEC —*see* Gout, chronic
Gower's
muscular dystrophy G71.0
syndrome (vasovagal attack) R55
Gradenigo's syndrome —*see* Otitis, media, suppurative, acute
Graefe's disease —*see* Strabismus, paralytic, ophthalmoplegia, progressive
Graft-versus-host disease D89.813
acute D89.810
acute on chronic D89.812
chronic D89.811
Grain mite (itch) B88.0
Grainhandler's disease or lung J67.8
Grand mal —*see* Epilepsy, generalized, specified NEC
Grand multipara status only (not pregnant) Z64.1
pregnant —*see* Pregnancy, complicated by, grand multiparity
Granite worker's lung J62.8
Granular —*see also* condition
inflammation, pharynx J31.2
kidney (contracting) —*see* Sclerosis, renal
liver K74.69
Granulation tissue (abnormal) (excessive) L92.9
postmastoidectomy cavity —*see* Complications, postmastoidectomy, granulation
Granulocytopenia (primary) (malignant) —*see* Agranulocytosis
Granuloma L92.9
abdomen K66.8
from residual foreign body L92.3
pyogenicum L98.0
actinic L57.5
annulare (perforating) L92.0
apical K04.5
aural —*see* Otitis, externa, specified NEC
beryllium (skin) L92.3
bone
eosinophilic C96.6
from residual foreign body —*see* Osteomyelitis, specified type NEC
lung C96.6
brain (any site) G06.0
schistosomiasis B65.9 *[G07]*
canaliculus lacrimalis —*see* Granuloma, lacrimal
candidal (cutaneous) B37.2
cerebral (any site) G06.0
coccidioidal (primary) (progressive) B38.7
lung B38.1
meninges B38.4

Granuloma *(Continued)*
colon K63.89
conjunctiva H11.22-
dental K04.5
ear, middle —*see* Cholesteatoma
eosinophilic C96.6
bone C96.6
lung C96.6
oral mucosa K13.4
skin L92.2
eyelid H01.8
facial (e) L92.2
foreign body (in soft tissue) NEC M60.20
ankle M60.27-
foot M60.27-
forearm M60.23-
hand M60.24-
in operation wound —*see* Foreign body, accidentally left during a procedure
lower leg M60.26-
pelvic region M60.25-
shoulder region M60.21-
skin L92.3
specified site NEC M60.28
subcutaneous tissue L92.3
thigh M60.25-
upper arm M60.22-
gangraenescens M31.2
genito-inguinale A58
giant cell (central) (reparative) (jaw) M27.1
gingiva (peripheral) K06.8
gland (lymph) I88.8
hepatic NEC K75.3
in (due to)
berylliosis J63.2 *[K77]*
sarcoidosis D86.89
Hodgkin C81.9
ileum K63.89
infectious B99.9
specified NEC B99.8
inguinale (Donovan) (venereal) A58
intestine NEC K63.89
intracranial (any site) G06.0
intraspinal (any part) G06.1
iridocyclitis —*see* Iridocyclitis, chronic
jaw (bone) (central) M27.1
reparative giant cell M27.1
kidney —*see also* Infection, kidney N15.8
lacrimal H04.81-
larynx J38.7
lethal midline (faciale (e)) M31.2
liver NEC —*see* Granuloma, hepatic
lung (infectious) —*see also* Fibrosis, lung
coccidioidal B38.1
eosinophilic C96.6
Majocchi's B35.8
malignant (facial (e)) M31.2
mandible (central) M27.1
midline (lethal) M31.2
monilial (cutaneous) B37.2
nasal sinus —*see* Sinusitis
operation wound T81.89
foreign body —*see* Foreign body, accidentally left during a procedure
stitch T81.89
talc —*see* Foreign body, accidentally left during a procedure
oral mucosa K13.4
orbit, orbital H05.11-
paracoccidioidal B41.8
penis, venereal A58
periapical K04.5
peritoneum K66.8
due to ova of helminths NOS —*see also* Helminthiasis B83.9 *[K67]*
postmastoidectomy cavity —*see* Complications, postmastoidectomy, recurrent cholesteatoma
prostate N42.89
pudendi (ulcerating) A58
pulp, internal (tooth) K03.3

Granuloma *(Continued)*
pyogenic, pyogenicum (of) (skin) L98.0
gingiva K06.8
maxillary alveolar ridge K04.5
oral mucosa K13.4
rectum K62.89
reticulohistiocytic D76.3
rubrum nasi L74.8
Schistosoma —*see* Schistosomiasis
septic (skin) L98.0
silica (skin) L92.3
sinus (accessory) (infective) (nasal) —*see* Sinusitis
skin L92.9
from residual foreign body L92.3
pyogenicum L98.0
spine
syphilitic (epidural) A52.19
tuberculous A18.01
stitch (postoperative) T81.89
suppurative (skin) L98.0
swimming pool A31.1
talc —*see also* Granuloma, foreign body
in operation wound —*see* Foreign body, accidentally left during a procedure
telangiectaticum (skin) L98.0
tracheostomy J95.09
trichophyticum B35.8
tropicum A66.4
umbilicus L92.9
urethra N36.8
uveitis —*see* Iridocyclitis, chronic
vagina A58
venereum A58
vocal cord J38.3
Granulomatosis L92.9
lymphoid C83.8-
miliary (listerial) A32.89
necrotizing, respiratory M31.30
progressive septic D71
specified NEC L92.8
Wegener's M31.30
with renal involvement M31.31
Granulomatous tissue (abnormal) (excessive) L92.9
Granulosis rubra nasi L74.8
Graphite fibrosis (of lung) J63.3
Graphospasm F48.8
organic G25.89
Grating scapula M89.8X1
Gravel (urinary) —*see* Calculus, urinary
Graves' disease —*see* Hyperthyroidism, with, goiter
Gravis —*see* condition
Grawitz tumor C64.-
Gray syndrome (newborn) P93.0
Grayness, hair (premature) L67.1
congenital Q84.2
Green sickness D50.8
Greenfield's disease
meaning
concentric sclerosis (encephalitis periaxialis concentrica) G37.5
metachromatic leukodystrophy E75.25
Greenstick fracture - code as Fracture, by site
Grey syndrome (newborn) P93.0
Grief F43.21
prolonged F43.29
reaction —*see also* Disorder, adjustment F43.20
Griesinger's disease B76.9
Grinder's lung or pneumoconiosis J62.8
Grinding, teeth
psychogenic F45.8
sleep related G47.63
Grip
Dabney's B33.0
devil's B33.0
Grippe, grippal —*see also* Influenza
Balkan A78
summer, of Italy A93.1
Grisel's disease M43.6
Groin —*see* condition

Grooved tongue K14.5
Ground itch B76.9
Grover's disease or syndrome L11.1
Growing pains, children R29.898
Growth (fungoid) (neoplastic) (new) —*see also* Neoplasm
adenoid (vegetative) J35.8
benign —*see* Neoplasm, benign, by site
malignant —*see* Neoplasm, malignant, by site
rapid, childhood Z00.2
secondary —*see* Neoplasm, secondary, by site
Gruby's disease B35.0
Gubler-Millard paralysis or syndrome G46.3
Guerin-Stern syndrome Q74.3
Guidance, insufficient anterior (occlusal) M26.54
Guillain-Barré disease or syndrome G61.0
sequelae G65.0
Guinea worms (infection) (infestation) B72
Guinon's disease (motor-verbal tic) F95.2
Gull's disease E03.4
Gum —*see* condition
Gumboil K04.7
with sinus K04.6
Gumma (syphilitic) A52.79
artery A52.09
cerebral A52.04
bone A52.77
of yaws (late) A66.6
brain A52.19
cauda equina A52.19
central nervous system A52.3
ciliary body A52.71
congenital A50.59
eyelid A52.71
heart A52.06
intracranial A52.19
iris A52.71
kidney A52.75
larynx A52.73
leptomeninges A52.19
liver A52.74
meninges A52.19
myocardium A52.06
nasopharynx A52.73
neurosyphilitic A52.3
nose A52.73
orbit A52.71
palate (soft) A52.79
penis A52.76
pericardium A52.06
pharynx A52.73
pituitary A52.79
scrofulous (tuberculous) A18.4
skin A52.79
specified site NEC A52.79
spinal cord A52.19
tongue A52.79
tonsil A52.73
trachea A52.73
tuberculous A18.4
ulcerative due to yaws A66.4
ureter A52.75
yaws A66.4
bone A66.6
Gunn's syndrome Q07.8
Gunshot wound —*see also* Wound, open
fracture - code as Fracture, by site
internal organs —*see* Injury, by site
Gynandrism Q56.0
Gynandroblastoma
specified site —*see* Neoplasm, uncertain behavior, by site
unspecified site
female D39.10
male D40.10
Gynecological examination (periodic) (routine) Z01.419
with abnormal findings Z01.411
Gynecomastia N62
Gynephobia F40.291
Gyrate scalp Q82.8

H

H (Hartnup's) **disease** E72.02
Haas' disease or osteochondrosis (juvenile) (head of humerus) —*see* Osteochondrosis, juvenile, humerus
Habit, habituation
bad sleep Z72.821
chorea F95.8
disturbance, child F98.9
drug —*see* Dependence, drug
irregular sleep Z72.821
laxative F55.2
spasm —*see* Tic
tic —*see* Tic
Haemophilus (H.) **influenzae, as cause of disease classified elsewhere** B96.3
Haff disease —*see* Poisoning, mercury
Hageman's factor defect, deficiency or disease D68.2
Haglund's disease or osteochondrosis (juvenile) (os tibiale externum) —*see* Osteochondrosis, juvenile, tarsus
Hailey-Hailey disease Q82.8
Hair —*see also* condition
plucking F63.3
in stereotyped movement disorder F98.4
tourniquet syndrome —*see also* Constriction, external, by site
finger S60.44-
penis S30.842
thumb S60.34-
toe S90.44-
Hairball in stomach T18.2
Hair-pulling, pathological (compulsive) F63.3
Hairy black tongue K14.3
Half vertebra Q76.49
Halitosis R19.6
Hallerman-Streiff syndrome Q87.0
Hallervorden-Spatz disease G23.0
Hallopeau's acrodermatitis or disease L40.2
Hallucination R44.3
auditory R44.0
gustatory R44.2
olfactory R44.2
specified NEC R44.2
tactile R44.2
visual R44.1
Hallucinosis (chronic) F28
alcoholic (acute) F10.951
in
abuse F10.151
dependence F10.251
drug-induced F19.951
cannabis F12.951
cocaine F14.951
hallucinogen F16.151
in
abuse F19.151
cannabis F12.151
cocaine F14.151
hallucinogen F16.151
inhalant F18.151
opioid F11.151
sedative, anxiolytic or hypnotic F13.151
stimulant NEC F15.151
dependence F19.251
cannabis F12.251
cocaine F14.251
hallucinogen F16.251
inhalant F18.251
opioid F11.251
sedative, anxiolytic or hypnotic F13.251
stimulant NEC F15.251
inhalant F18.951
opioid F11.951
sedative, anxiolytic or hypnotic F13.951
stimulant NEC F15.951
organic F06.0
Hallux
deformity (acquired) NEC M20.5X-
limitus M20.5X-
malleus (acquired) NEC M20.3-
rigidus (acquired) M20.2-
congenital Q74.2
sequelae (late effect) of rickets E64.3
valgus (acquired) M20.1-
congenital Q66.6
varus (acquired) M20.3-
congenital Q66.3
Halo, visual H53.19
Hamartoma, hamartoblastoma Q85.9
epithelial (gingival), odontogenic, central or peripheral —*see* Cyst, calcifying odontogenic
Hamartosis Q85.9
Hamman-Rich syndrome J84.114
Hammer toe (acquired) **NEC** —*see also* Deformity, toe, hammer toe
congenital Q66.89
sequelae (late effect) of rickets E64.3
Hand —*see* condition
Hand-foot syndrome L27.1
Handicap, handicapped
educational Z55.9
specified NEC Z55.8
Hand-Schüller-Christian disease or syndrome C96.5
Hanging (asphyxia) (strangulation) (suffocation) —*see* Asphyxia, traumatic, due to mechanical threat
Hangnail —*see also* Cellulitis, digit
with lymphangitis —*see* Lymphangitis, acute, digit
Hangover (alcohol) F10.129
Hanhart's syndrome Q87.0
Hanot-Chauffard (-Troisier) **syndrome** E83.19
Hanot's cirrhosis or disease K74.3
Hansen's disease —*see* Leprosy
Hantaan virus disease (Korean hemorrhagic fever) A98.5
Hantavirus disease (with renal manifestations) (Dobrava) (Puumala) (Seoul) A98.5
with pulmonary manifestations (Andes) (Bayou) (Bermejo) (Black Creek Canal) (Choclo) (Juquitiba) (Laguna negra) (Lechiguanas) (New York) (Oran) (Sin nombre) B33.4
Happy puppet syndrome Q93.5
Harada's disease or syndrome H30.81-
Hardening
artery —*see* Arteriosclerosis
brain G93.89
Harelip (complete) (incomplete) —*see* Cleft, lip
Harlequin (newborn) Q80.4
Harley's disease D59.6
Harmful use (of)
alcohol F10.10
anxiolytics —*see* Abuse, drug, sedative
cannabinoids —*see* Abuse, drug, cannabis
cocaine —*see* Abuse, drug, cocaine
drug —*see* Abuse, drug
hallucinogens —*see* Abuse, drug, hallucinogen
hypnotics —*see* Abuse, drug, sedative - opioids —*see* Abuse, drug, opioid
PCP (phencyclidine) —*see* Abuse, drug, hallucinogen
sedatives —*see* Abuse, drug, sedative
stimulants NEC —*see* Abuse, drug, stimulant
Harris' lines —*see* Arrest, epiphyseal
Hartnup's disease E72.02
Harvester's lung J67.0
Harvesting ovum for in vitro fertilization Z31.83
Hashimoto's disease or thyroiditis E06.3
Hashitoxicosis (transient) E06.3
Hassal-Henle bodies or warts (cornea) H18.49
Haut mal —*see* Epilepsy, generalized, specified NEC
Haverhill fever A25.1
Hay fever —*see also* Fever, hay J30.1
Hayem-Widal syndrome D59.8
Haygarth's nodes M15.8
Haymaker's lung J67.0
Hb (abnormal)
Bart's disease D56.0
disease —*see* Disease, hemoglobin
trait —*see* Trait
Head —*see* condition
Headache R51
allergic NEC G44.89
associated with sexual activity G44.82
chronic daily R51
cluster G44.009
chronic G44.029
intractable G44.021
not intractable G44.029
episodic G44.019
intractable G44.011
not intractable G44.019
intractable G44.001
not intractable G44.009
cough (primary) G44.83
daily chronic R51
drug-induced NEC G44.40
intractable G44.41
not intractable G44.40
exertional (primary) G44.84
histamine G44.009
intractable G44.001
not intractable G44.009
hypnic G44.81
lumbar puncture G97.1
medication overuse G44.40
intractable G44.41
not intractable G44.40
menstrual —*see* Migraine, menstrual
migraine (type) —*see also* Migraine G43.909
nasal septum R51
neuralgiform, short lasting unilateral, with conjunctival injection and tearing (SUNCT) G44.059
intractable G44.051
not intractable G44.059
new daily persistent (NDPH) G44.52
orgasmic G44.82
periodic syndromes in adults and children G43.C0
with refractory migraine G43.C1
intractable G43.C1
not intractable G43.C0
without refractory migraine G43.C0
postspinal puncture G97.1
post-traumatic G44.309
acute G44.319
intractable G44.311
not intractable G44.319
chronic G44.329
intractable G44.321
not intractable G44.329
intractable G44.301
not intractable G44.309
pre-menstrual —*see* Migraine, menstrual
preorgasmic G44.82
primary
cough G44.83
exertional G44.84
stabbing G44.85
thunderclap G44.53
rebound G44.40
intractable G44.41
not intractable G44.40
short lasting unilateral neuralgiform, with conjunctival injection and tearing (SUNCT) G44.059
intractable G44.051
not intractable G44.059
specified syndrome NEC G44.89

Headache *(Continued)*
spinal and epidural anesthesia - induced T88.59
in labor and delivery O74.5
in pregnancy O29.4-
postpartum, puerperal O89.4
spinal fluid loss (from puncture) G97.1
stabbing (primary) G44.85
tension (-type) G44.2Ø9
chronic G44.229
intractable G44.221
not intractable G44.229
episodic G44.219
intractable G44.211
not intractable G44.219
intractable G44.2Ø1
not intractable G44.2Ø9
thunderclap (primary) G44.53
vascular NEC G44.1
Healthy
infant
accompanying sick mother Z76.3
receiving care Z76.2
person accompanying sick person Z76.3
Hearing examination ZØ1.1Ø
with abnormal findings NEC ZØ1.118
following failed hearing screening ZØ1.11Ø
for hearing conservation and treatment ZØ1.12
Heart —*see* condition
Heart beat
abnormality RØØ.9
specified NEC RØØ.8
awareness RØØ.2
rapid RØØ.Ø
slow RØØ.1
Heartburn R12
psychogenic F45.8
Heat (effects) T67.9
apoplexy T67.Ø
burn —*see also* Burn L55.9
collapse T67.1
cramps T67.2
dermatitis or eczema L59.Ø
edema T67.7
erythema - code by site under Burn, first degree
excessive T67.9
specified effect NEC T67.8
exhaustion T67.5
anhydrotic T67.3
due to
salt (and water) depletion T67.4
water depletion T67.3
with salt depletion T67.4
fatigue (transient) T67.6
fever T67.Ø
hyperpyrexia T67.Ø
prickly L74.Ø
prostration —*see* Heat, exhaustion
pyrexia T67.Ø
rash L74.Ø
specified effect NEC T67.8
stroke T67.Ø
sunburn —*see* Sunburn
syncope T67.1
Heavy-for-dates NEC (infant) (4ØØØg to 4499g) PØ8.1
exceptionally (45ØØg or more) PØ8.Ø
Hebephrenia, hebephrenic (schizophrenia) F2Ø.1
Heberden's disease or nodes (with arthropathy) M15.1
Hebra's
pityriasis L26
prurigo L28.2
Heel —*see* condition
Heerfordt's disease D86.89
Hegglin's anomaly or syndrome D72.Ø
Heilmeyer-Schoner disease D45
Heine-Medin disease AØØ.9
Heinz body anemia, congenital D58.2
Heliophobia F4Ø.228
Heller's disease or syndrome F84.3
HELLP syndrome (hemolysis, elevated liver enzymes and low platelet count) O14.2-
complicating ◀
childbirth O14.24 ◀
puerperium O14.25 ◀
Helminthiasis —*see also* Infestation, helminth
Ancylostoma B76.Ø
intestinal B82.Ø
mixed types (types classifiable to more than one of the titles B65.Ø-B81.3 and B81.8) B81.4
specified type NEC B81.8
mixed types (intestinal) (types classifiable to more than one of the titles B65.Ø-B81.3 and B81.8) B81.4
Necator (americanus) B76.1
specified type NEC B83.8
Heloma L84
Hemangioblastoma —*see* Neoplasm, connective tissue, uncertain behavior
malignant —*see* Neoplasm, connective tissue, malignant
Hemangioendothelioma —*see also* Neoplasm, uncertain behavior, by site
benign D18.ØØ
intra-abdominal D18.Ø3
intracranial D18.Ø2
skin D18.Ø1
specified site NEC D18.Ø9
bone (diffuse) —*see* Neoplasm, bone, malignant
epithelioid —*see also* Neoplasm, uncertain behavior, by site
malignant —*see* Neoplasm, malignant, by site
malignant —*see* Neoplasm, connective tissue, malignant
Hemangiofibroma —*see* Neoplasm, benign, by site
Hemangiolipoma —*see* Lipoma
Hemangioma D18.ØØ
arteriovenous D18.ØØ
intra-abdominal D18.Ø3
intracranial D18.Ø2
skin D18.Ø1
specified site NEC D18.Ø9
capillary D18.ØØ
intra-abdominal D18.Ø3
intracranial D18.Ø2
skin D18.Ø1
specified site NEC D18.Ø9
cavernous D18.ØØ
intra-abdominal D18.Ø3
intracranial D18.Ø2
skin D18.Ø1
specified site NEC D18.Ø9
epithelioid D18.ØØ
intra-abdominal D18.Ø3
intracranial D18.Ø2
skin D18.Ø1
specified site NEC D18.Ø9
histiocytoid D18.ØØ
intra-abdominal D18.Ø3
intracranial D18.Ø2
skin D18.Ø1
specified site NEC D18.Ø9
infantile D18.ØØ
intra-abdominal D18.Ø3
intracranial D18.Ø2
skin D18.Ø1
specified site NEC D18.Ø9
intra-abdominal D18.Ø3
intracranial D18.Ø2
intramuscular D18.ØØ
intra-abdominal D18.Ø3
intracranial D18.Ø2
skin D18.Ø1
specified site NEC D18.Ø9
Hemangioma *(Continued)*
intrathoracic structures D18.Ø9 ◀
juvenile D18.ØØ
malignant —*see* Neoplasm, connective tissue, malignant
plexiform D18.ØØ
intra-abdominal D18.Ø3
intracranial D18.Ø2
skin D18.Ø1
specified site NEC D18.Ø9
racemose D18.ØØ
intra-abdominal D18.Ø3
intracranial D18.Ø2
skin D18.Ø1
specified site NEC D18.Ø9
sclerosing —*see* Neoplasm, skin, benign
simplex D18.ØØ
intra-abdominal D18.Ø3
intracranial D18.Ø2
skin D18.Ø1
specified site NEC D18.Ø9
skin D18.Ø1
specified site NEC D18.Ø9
venous D18.ØØ
intra-abdominal D18.Ø3
intracranial D18.Ø2
skin D18.Ø1
specified site NEC D18.Ø9
verrucous keratotic D18.ØØ
intra-abdominal D18.Ø3
intracranial D18.Ø2
skin D18.Ø1
specified site NEC D18.Ø9
Hemangiomatosis (systemic) I78.8
involving single site —*see* Hemangioma
Hemangiopericytoma —*see also* Neoplasm, connective tissue, uncertain behavior
benign —*see* Neoplasm, connective tissue, benign
malignant —*see* Neoplasm, connective tissue, malignant
Hemangiosarcoma —*see* Neoplasm, connective tissue, malignant
Hemarthrosis (nontraumatic) M25.ØØ
ankle M25.Ø7-
elbow M25.Ø2-
foot joint M25.Ø7-
hand joint M25.Ø4-
hip M25.Ø5-
in hemophilic arthropathy —*see* Arthropathy, hemophilic
knee M25.Ø6-
shoulder M25.Ø1-
specified joint NEC M25.Ø8
traumatic —*see* Sprain, by site
vertebrae M25.Ø8
wrist M25.Ø3-
Hematemesis K92.Ø
with ulcer - code by site under Ulcer, with hemorrhage K27.4
newborn, neonatal P54.Ø
due to swallowed maternal blood P78.2
Hematidrosis L74.8
Hematinuria —*see also* Hemoglobinuria
malarial B5Ø.8
Hematobilia K83.8
Hematocele
female NEC N94.89
with ectopic pregnancy OØØ.9Ø ◀
with intrauterine pregnancy OØØ.91 ◀
ovary N83.8
male N5Ø.1
Hematochezia —*see also* Melena K92.1
Hematochyluria —*see also* Infestation, filarial
schistosomiasis (bilharziasis) B65.Ø
Hematocolpos (with hematometra or hematosalpinx) N89.7
Hematocornea —*see* Pigmentation, cornea, stromal
Hematogenous —*see* condition

H

Hematoma (traumatic) (skin surface intact) —*see also* Contusion
with
injury of internal organs —*see* Injury, by site
open wound —*see* Wound, open
amputation stump (surgical) (late) T87.89
aorta, dissecting I71.00
abdominal I71.02
thoracic I71.01
thoracoabdominal I71.03
aortic intramural —*see* Dissection, aorta
arterial (complicating trauma) —*see* Injury, blood vessel, by site
auricle —*see* Contusion, ear
nontraumatic —*see* Disorder, pinna, hematoma
birth injury NEC P15.8
brain (traumatic)
with
cerebral laceration or contusion (diffuse) —*see* Injury, intracranial, diffuse
focal —*see* Injury, intracranial, focal
cerebellar, traumatic S06.37-
intracerebral, traumatic —*see* Injury, intracranial, intracerebral hemorrhage
newborn NEC P52.4
birth injury P10.1
nontraumatic —*see* Hemorrhage, intracranial
subarachnoid, arachnoid, traumatic —*see* Injury, intracranial, subarachnoid hemorrhage
subdural, traumatic —*see* Injury, intracranial, subdural hemorrhage
breast (nontraumatic) N64.89
broad ligament (nontraumatic) N83.7
traumatic S37.892
cerebellar, traumatic S06.37-
cerebral —*see* Hematoma, brain
cerebrum S06.36-
left S06.35-
right S06.34-
cesarean delivery wound O90.2
complicating delivery (perineal) (pelvic) (vagina) (vulva) O71.7
corpus cavernosum (nontraumatic) N48.89
epididymis (nontraumatic) N50.1
epidural (traumatic) —*see* Injury, intracranial, epidural hemorrhage
spinal —*see* Injury, spinal cord, by region
episiotomy O90.2
face, birth injury P15.4
genital organ NEC (nontraumatic)
female (nonobstetric) N94.89
traumatic S30.202
male N50.1
traumatic S30.201
internal organs —*see* Injury, by site
intracerebral, traumatic —*see* Injury, intracranial, intracerebral hemorrhage
intraoperative —*see* Complications, intraoperative, hemorrhage
labia (nontraumatic) (nonobstetric) N90.8
liver (subcapsular) (nontraumatic) K76.89
birth injury P15.0
mediastinum —*see* Injury, intrathoracic
mesosalpinx (nontraumatic) N83.7
traumatic S37.898
muscle - code by site under Contusion
nontraumatic
muscle M79.81
soft tissue M79.81
obstetrical surgical wound O90.2
orbit, orbital (nontraumatic) —*see also* Hemorrhage, orbit
traumatic —*see* Contusion, orbit
pelvis (female) (nontraumatic) (nonobstetric) N94.89
obstetric O71.7
traumatic —*see* Injury, by site

Hematoma *(Continued)*
penis (nontraumatic) N48.89
birth injury P15.5
perianal (nontraumatic) K64.5
perineal S30.23
complicating delivery O71.7
perirenal —*see* Injury, kidney
pinna —*see* Contusion, ear
nontraumatic —*see* Disorder, pinna, hematoma
placenta O43.89-
postoperative (postprocedural) —*see* Complication, postprocedural, hematoma ◀
retroperitoneal (nontraumatic) K66.1
traumatic S36.892
scrotum, superficial S30.22
birth injury P15.5
seminal vesicle (nontraumatic) N50.1
traumatic S37.892
spermatic cord (traumatic) S37.892
nontraumatic N50.1
spinal (cord) (meninges) —*see also* Injury, spinal cord, by region
newborn (birth injury) P11.5
spleen D73.5
intraoperative —*see* Complications, intraoperative, hemorrhage, spleen
postprocedural (postoperative) —*see* Complications, postprocedural, hemorrhage, spleen
sternocleidomastoid, birth injury P15.2
sternomastoid, birth injury P15.2
subarachnoid (traumatic) —*see* Injury, intracranial, subarachnoid hemorrhage
newborn (nontraumatic) P52.5
due to birth injury P10.3
nontraumatic —*see* Hemorrhage, intracranial, subarachnoid
subdural (traumatic) —*see* Injury, intracranial, subdural hemorrhage
newborn (localized) P52.8
birth injury P10.0
nontraumatic —*see* Hemorrhage, intracranial, subdural
superficial, newborn P54.5
testis (nontraumatic) N50.1
birth injury P15.5
tunica vaginalis (nontraumatic) N50.1
umbilical cord, complicating delivery O69.5
uterine ligament (broad) (nontraumatic) N83.7
traumatic S37.892
vagina (ruptured) (nontraumatic) N89.8
complicating delivery O71.7
vas deferens (nontraumatic) N50.1
traumatic S37.892
vitreous —*see* Hemorrhage, vitreous
vulva (nontraumatic) (nonobstetric) N90.89
complicating delivery O71.7
newborn (birth injury) P15.5
Hematometra N85.7
with hematocolpos N89.7
Hematomyelia (central) G95.19
newborn (birth injury) P11.5
traumatic T14.8
Hematomyelitis G04.90
Hematoperitoneum —*see* Hemoperitoneum
Hematophobia F40.230
Hematopneumothorax (*see* Hemothorax)
Hematopoiesis, cyclic D70.4
Hematoporphyria —*see* Porphyria
Hematorachis, hematorrhachis G95.19
newborn (birth injury) P11.5
Hematosalpinx N83.6
with
hematocolpos N89.7
hematometra N85.7
with hematocolpos N89.7
infectional —*see* Salpingitis

Hematospermia R36.1
Hematothorax (*see* Hemothorax)
Hematuria R31.9
benign (familial) (of childhood) —*see also* Hematuria, idiopathic
essential microscopic R31.1
due to sulphonamide, sulfonamide —*see* Table of Drugs and Chemicals, by drug
endemic —*see also* Schistosomiasis B65.0
gross R31.0
idiopathic N02.9
with glomerular lesion
crescentic (diffuse) glomerulonephritis N02.7
dense deposit disease N02.6
endocapillary proliferative glomerulonephritis N02.4
focal and segmental hyalinosis or sclerosis N02.1
membranoproliferative (diffuse) N02.5
membranous (diffuse) N02.2
mesangial proliferative (diffuse) N02.3
mesangiocapillary (diffuse) N02.5
minor abnormality N02.0
proliferative NEC N02.8
specified pathology NEC N02.8
intermittent —*see* Hematuria, idiopathic
malarial B50.8
microscopic NEC (with symptoms) R31.29 ◀
asymptomatic R31.21 ◀
benign essential R31.1
paroxysmal —*see also* Hematuria, idiopathic
nocturnal D59.5
persistent —*see* Hematuria, idiopathic
recurrent —*see* Hematuria, idiopathic
tropical —*see also* Schistosomiasis B65.0
tuberculous A18.13
Hemeralopia (day blindness) H53.11
vitamin A deficiency E50.5
Hemi-akinesia R41.4
Hemianalgesia R20.0
Hemianencephaly Q00.0
Hemianesthesia R20.0
Hemianopia, hemianopsia (heteronymous) H53.47
homonymous H53.46-
syphilitic A52.71
Hemiathetosis R25.8
Hemiatrophy R68.89
cerebellar G31.9
face, facial, progressive (Romberg) G51.8
tongue K14.8
Hemiballism (us) G25.5
Hemicardia Q24.8
Hemicephalus, hemicephaly Q00.0
Hemichorea G25.5
Hemicolitis, left —*see* Colitis, left sided
Hemicrania
congenital malformation Q00.0
continua G44.51
meaning migraine —*see also* Migraine G43.909
paroxysmal G44.039
chronic G44.049
intractable G44.041
not intractable G44.049
episodic G44.039
intractable G44.031
not intractable G44.039
intractable G44.031
not intractable G44.039
Hemidystrophy —*see* Hemiatrophy
Hemiectromelia Q73.8
Hemihypalgesia R20.8
Hemihypesthesia R20.1
Hemi-inattention R41.4
Hemimelia Q73.8
lower limb —*see* Defect, reduction, lower limb, specified type NEC
upper limb —*see* Defect, reduction, upper limb, specified type NEC
Hemiparalysis —*see* Hemiplegia
Hemiparesis —*see* Hemiplegia

◀ New ◀ Revised ~~deleted~~ Deleted

Hemiparesthesia R20.2
Hemiparkinsonism G20
Hemiplegia G81.9-
alternans facialis G83.89
ascending NEC G81.90
spinal G95.89
congenital (cerebral) G80.8
spastic G80.2
embolic (current episode) I63.4-
flaccid G81.0-
following
cerebrovascular disease I69.959
cerebral infarction I69.35-
intracerebral hemorrhage I69.15-
nontraumatic intracranial hemorrhage NEC I69.25-
specified disease NEC I69.85-
stroke NOS I69.35-
subarachnoid hemorrhage I69.05-
hysterical F44.4
newborn NEC P91.8
birth injury P11.9
spastic G81.1-
congenital G80.2
thrombotic (current episode) I63.3- ◄
Hemisection, spinal cord —*see* Injury, spinal cord, by region
Hemispasm (facial) R25.2
Hemisporosis B48.8
Hemitremor R25.1
Hemivertebra Q76.49
failure of segmentation with scoliosis Q76.3
fusion with scoliosis Q76.3
Hemochromatosis E83.119
with refractory anemia D46.1
due to repeated red blood cell transfusion E83.111
hereditary (primary) E83.110
primary E83.110
specified NEC E83.118
Hemoglobin —*see also* condition
abnormal (disease) —*see* Disease, hemoglobin
AS genotype D57.3
Constant Spring D58.2
E-beta thalassemia D56.5
fetal, hereditary persistence (HPFH) D56.4
H Constant Spring D56.0
low NOS D64.9
S (Hb S), heterozygous D57.3
Hemoglobinemia D59.9
due to blood transfusion T80.89
paroxysmal D59.6
nocturnal D59.5
Hemoglobinopathy (mixed) D58.2
with thalassemia D56.8
sickle-cell D57.1
with thalassemia D57.40
with crisis (vasoocclusive pain) D57.419
with
acute chest syndrome D57.411
splenic sequestration D57.412
without crisis D57.40
Hemoglobinuria R82.3
with anemia, hemolytic, acquired (chronic) NEC D59.6
cold (agglutinin) (paroxysmal) (with Raynaud's syndrome) D59.6
due to exertion or hemolysis NEC D59.6
intermittent D59.6
malarial B50.8
march D59.6
nocturnal (paroxysmal) D59.5
paroxysmal (cold) D59.6
nocturnal D59.5
Hemolymphangioma D18.1
Hemolysis
intravascular
with
abortion —*see* Abortion, by type, complicated by, hemorrhage
ectopic or molar pregnancy O08.1

Hemolysis *(Continued)*
intravascular *(Continued)*
with *(Continued)*
hemorrhage
antepartum —*see* Hemorrhage, antepartum, with coagulation defect
intrapartum —*see also* Hemorrhage, complicating, delivery O67.0
postpartum O72.3
neonatal (excessive) P58.9
specified NEC P58.8
Hemolytic —*see* condition
Hemopericardium I31.2
following acute myocardial infarction (current complication) I23.0
newborn P54.8
traumatic —*see* Injury, heart, with hemopericardium
Hemoperitoneum K66.1
infectional K65.9
traumatic S36.899
with open wound —*see* Wound, open, with penetration into peritoneal cavity
Hemophilia (classical) (familial) (hereditary) D66
A D66
B D67
C D68.1
acquired D68.311
autoimmune D68.311
calcipriva —*see also* Defect, coagulation D68.4
nonfamilial —*see also* Defect, coagulation D68.4
secondary D68.311
vascular D68.0
Hemophthalmos H44.81-
Hemopneumothorax —*see also* Hemothorax
traumatic S27.2
Hemoptysis R04.2
newborn P26.9
tuberculous —*see* Tuberculosis, pulmonary
Hemorrhage, hemorrhagic (concealed) R58
abdomen R58
accidental antepartum —*see* Hemorrhage, antepartum
acute idiopathic pulmonary, in infants R04.81
adenoid J35.8
adrenal (capsule) (gland) E27.49
medulla E27.8
newborn P54.4
after delivery —*see* Hemorrhage, postpartum
alveolar
lung, newborn P26.8
process K08.89 ◄
alveolus K08.89 ◄
amputation stump (surgical) T87.89
anemia (chronic) D50.0
acute D62
antepartum (with) O46.90
with coagulation defect O46.00-
afibrinogenemia O46.01-
disseminated intravascular coagulation O46.02-
hypofibrinogenemia O46.01-
specified defect NEC O46.09-
before 20 weeks gestation O20.9
specified type NEC O20.8
threatened abortion O20.0
due to
abruptio placenta —*see also* Abruptio placentae O45.9-
leiomyoma, uterus —*see* Hemorrhage, antepartum, specified cause NEC
placenta previa O44.1-
specified cause NEC —*see* subcategory O46.8X-
anus (sphincter) K62.5
apoplexy (stroke) —*see* Hemorrhage, intracranial, intracerebral

Hemorrhage, hemorrhagic *(Continued)*
arachnoid —*see* Hemorrhage, intracranial, subarachnoid
artery R58
brain —*see* Hemorrhage, intracranial, intracerebral
basilar (ganglion) I61.0
bladder N32.89
bowel K92.2
newborn P54.3
brain (miliary) (nontraumatic) —*see* Hemorrhage, intracranial, intracerebral
due to
birth injury P10.1
syphilis A52.05
epidural or extradural (traumatic) —*see* Injury, intracranial, epidural hemorrhage
newborn P52.4
birth injury P10.1
subarachnoid —*see* Hemorrhage, intracranial, subarachnoid
subdural —*see* Hemorrhage, intracranial, subdural
brainstem (nontraumatic) I61.3
traumatic S06.38-
breast N64.59
bronchial tube —*see* Hemorrhage, lung
bronchopulmonary —*see* Hemorrhage, lung
bronchus —*see* Hemorrhage, lung
bulbar I61.5
capillary I78.8
primary D69.8
cecum K92.2
cerebellar, cerebellum (nontraumatic) I61.4
newborn P52.6
traumatic S06.37-
cerebral, cerebrum —*see also* Hemorrhage, intracranial, intracerebral
lobe I61.1
newborn (anoxic) P52.4
birth injury P10.1
cerebromeningeal I61.8
cerebrospinal —*see* Hemorrhage, intracranial, intracerebral
cervix (uteri) (stump) NEC N88.8
chamber, anterior (eye) —*see* Hyphema
childbirth —*see* Hemorrhage, complicating, delivery
choroid H31.30-
expulsive H31.31-
ciliary body —*see* Hyphema
cochlea —*see* subcategory H83.8
colon K92.2
complicating
abortion —*see* Abortion, by type, complicated by, hemorrhage
delivery O67.9
associated with coagulation defect (afibrinogenemia) (DIC) (hyperfibrinolysis) O67.0
specified cause NEC O67.8
surgical procedure —*see* Hemorrhage, intraoperative
conjunctiva H11.3-
newborn P54.8
cord, newborn (stump) P51.9
corpus luteum (ruptured) cyst N83.1- ◄
cortical (brain) I61.1
cranial —*see* Hemorrhage, intracranial
cutaneous R23.3
due to autosensitivity, erythrocyte D69.2
newborn P54.5
delayed
following ectopic or molar pregnancy O08.1
postpartum O72.2
diathesis (familial) D69.9
disease D69.9
newborn P53
specified type NEC D69.8

H

Hemorrhage, hemorrhagic *(Continued)*
due to or associated with
afibrinogenemia or other coagulation defect (conditions in categories D65-D69)
antepartum —*see* Hemorrhage, antepartum, with coagulation defect
intrapartum O67.0
dental implant M27.61
device, implant or graft —*see also* Complications, by site and type, specified NEC T85.838 ◄
arterial graft NEC T82.838
breast T85.838 ◄
catheter NEC T85.838 ◄
dialysis (renal) T82.838
intraperitoneal T85.838 ◄
infusion NEC T82.838
spinal (epidural) (subdural) T85.830 ◄
urinary (indwelling) T83.83
electronic (electrode) (pulse generator) (stimulator)
bone T84.83
cardiac T82.837
nervous system (brain) (peripheral nerve) (spinal) T85.830 ◄
urinary T83.83
fixation, internal (orthopedic) NEC T84.83
gastrointestinal (bile duct) (esophagus) T85.838 ◄
genital NEC T83.83
heart NEC T82.837
joint prosthesis T84.83
ocular (corneal graft) (orbital implant) NEC T85.838 ◄
orthopedic NEC T84.83
bone graft T86.838
specified NEC T85.838 ◄
urinary NEC T83.83
vascular NEC T82.838
ventricular intracranial shunt T85.838 ◄
duodenum, duodenal K92.2
ulcer —*see* Ulcer, duodenum, with hemorrhage
dura mater —*see* Hemorrhage, intracranial, subdural
endotracheal —*see* Hemorrhage, lung
epicranial subaponeurotic (massive), birth injury P12.2
epidural (traumatic) —*see also* Injury, intracranial, epidural hemorrhage
nontraumatic I62.1
esophagus K22.8
varix I85.01
secondary I85.11
excessive, following ectopic gestation (subsequent episode) O08.1
extradural (traumatic) —*see* Injury, intracranial, epidural hemorrhage
birth injury P10.8
newborn (anoxic) (nontraumatic) P52.8
nontraumatic I62.1
eye NEC H57.8
fundus —*see* Hemorrhage, retina
lid —*see* Disorder, eyelid, specified type NEC
fallopian tube N83.6
fibrinogenolysis —*see* Fibrinolysis
fibrinolytic (acquired) —*see* Fibrinolysis
from
ear (nontraumatic) —*see* Otorrhagia
tracheostoma stoma J95.01
fundus, eye —*see* Hemorrhage, retina
funis —*see* Hemorrhage, umbilicus, cord
gastric —*see* Hemorrhage, stomach
gastroenteric K92.2
newborn P54.3
gastrointestinal (tract) K92.2
newborn P54.3
genital organ, male N50.1

Hemorrhage, hemorrhagic *(Continued)*
genitourinary (tract) NOS R31.9
gingiva K06.8
globe (eye) —*see* Hemophthalmos
graafian follicle cyst (ruptured) N83.0- ◄
gum K06.8
heart I51.89
hypopharyngeal (throat) R04.1
intermenstrual (regular) N92.3
irregular N92.1
internal (organs) NEC R58
capsule I61.0
ear —*see* subcategory H83.8
newborn P54.8
intestine K92.2
newborn P54.3
intra-abdominal R58
intra-alveolar (lung), newborn P26.8
intracerebral (nontraumatic) —*see* Hemorrhage, intracranial, intracerebral
intracranial (nontraumatic) I62.9
birth injury P10.9
epidural, nontraumatic I62.1
extradural, nontraumatic I62.1
intracerebral (nontraumatic) (in) I61.9
brain stem I61.3
cerebellum I61.4
hemisphere I61.2
cortical (superficial) I61.1
subcortical (deep) I61.0
intraoperative
during a nervous system procedure G97.31
during other procedure G97.32
intraventricular I61.5
multiple localized I61.6
newborn P52.4
birth injury P10.1
postprocedural
following a nervous system procedure G97.51
following other procedure G97.52
specified NEC I61.8
superficial I61.1
traumatic (diffuse) —*see* Injury, intracranial, diffuse
focal —*see* Injury, intracranial, focal
newborn P52.9
specified NEC P52.8
subarachnoid (nontraumatic) (from) I60.9
intracranial (cerebral) artery I60.7
anterior communicating I60.2 ◄
basilar I60.4
carotid siphon and bifurcation I60.0-
communicating I60.7
anterior I60.2 ◄
posterior I60.3-
middle cerebral I60.1-
posterior communicating I60.3-
specified artery NEC I60.6
vertebral I60.5-
newborn P52.5
birth injury P10.3
specified NEC I60.8
traumatic S06.6X-
subdural (nontraumatic) I62.00
acute I62.01
birth injury P10.0
chronic I62.03
newborn (anoxic) (hypoxic) P52.8
birth injury P10.0
spinal G95.19
subacute I62.02
traumatic —*see* Injury, intracranial, subdural hemorrhage
traumatic —*see* Injury, intracranial, focal brain injury

Hemorrhage, hemorrhagic *(Continued)*
intramedullary NEC G95.19
intraocular —*see* Hemophthalmos
intraoperative, intraprocedural —*see* Complication, hemorrhage (hematoma), intraoperative (intraprocedural), by site
intrapartum —*see* Hemorrhage, complicating, delivery
intrapelvic
female N94.89
male K66.1
intraperitoneal K66.1
intrapontine I61.3
intraprocedural —*see* Complication, hemorrhage (hematoma), intraoperative (intraprocedural), by site
intrauterine N85.7
complicating delivery —*see also* Hemorrhage, complicating, delivery O67.9
postpartum —*see* Hemorrhage, postpartum
intraventricular I61.5
newborn (nontraumatic) —*see also* Newborn, affected by, hemorrhage P52.3
due to birth injury P10.2
grade
1 P52.0
2 P52.1
3 P52.21
4 P52.22
intravesical N32.89
iris (postinfectional) (postinflammatory) (toxic) —*see* Hyphema
joint (nontraumatic) —*see* Hemarthrosis
kidney N28.89
knee (joint) (nontraumatic) —*see* Hemarthrosis, knee
labyrinth —*see* subcategory H83.8
lenticular striate artery I61.0
ligature, vessel —*see* Hemorrhage, postoperative
liver K76.89
lung R04.89
newborn P26.9
massive P26.1
specified NEC P26.8
tuberculous —*see* Tuberculosis, pulmonary
massive umbilical, newborn P51.0
mediastinum —*see* Hemorrhage, lung
medulla I61.3
membrane (brain) I60.8
spinal cord —*see* Hemorrhage, spinal cord
meninges, meningeal (brain) (middle) I60.8
spinal cord —*see* Hemorrhage, spinal cord
mesentery K66.1
metritis —*see* Endometritis
mouth K13.79
mucous membrane NEC R58
newborn P54.8
muscle M62.89
nail (subungual) L60.8
nasal turbinate R04.0
newborn P54.8
navel, newborn P51.9
newborn P54.9
specified NEC P54.8
nipple N64.59
nose R04.0
newborn P54.8
omentum K66.1
optic nerve (sheath) H47.02-
orbit, orbital H05.23-
ovary NEC N83.8
oviduct N83.6
pancreas K86.89 ◄
parathyroid (gland) (spontaneous) E21.4
parturition —*see* Hemorrhage, complicating, delivery
penis N48.89
pericardium, pericarditis I31.2
peritoneum, peritoneal K66.1
peritonsillar tissue J35.8
due to infection J36

◄ New ◄ Revised ~~deleted~~ Deleted

Hemorrhage, hemorrhagic *(Continued)*
petechial R23.3
due to autosensitivity, erythrocyte D69.2
pituitary (gland) E23.6
pleura —*see* Hemorrhage, lung
polioencephalitis, superior E51.2
polymyositis —*see* Polymyositis
pons, pontine I61.3
posterior fossa (nontraumatic) I61.8
newborn P52.6
postmenopausal N95.0
postnasal R04.0
postoperative —*see* Complications, postprocedural, hemorrhage, by site
postpartum NEC (following delivery of placenta) O72.1
delayed or secondary O72.2
retained placenta O72.0
third stage O72.0
pregnancy —*see* Hemorrhage, antepartum
preretinal —*see* Hemorrhage, retina
prostate N42.1
puerperal —*see* Hemorrhage, postpartum
delayed or secondary O72.2
pulmonary R04.89
newborn P26.9
massive P26.1
specified NEC P26.8
tuberculous —*see* Tuberculosis, pulmonary
purpura (primary) D69.3
rectum (sphincter) K62.5
newborn P54.2
recurring, following initial hemorrhage at time of injury T79.2
renal N28.89
respiratory passage or tract R04.9
specified NEC R04.89
retina, retinal (vessels) H35.6-
diabetic —*see* Diabetes, retinal, hemorrhage
retroperitoneal R58
scalp R58
scrotum N50.1
secondary (nontraumatic) R58
following initial hemorrhage at time of injury T79.2
seminal vesicle N50.1
skin R23.3
newborn P54.5
slipped umbilical ligature P51.8
spermatic cord N50.1
spinal (cord) G95.19
newborn (birth injury) P11.5
spleen D73.5
intraoperative —*see* Complications, intraoperative, hemorrhage, spleen
postprocedural —*see* Complications, postprocedural, hemorrhage, spleen
stomach K92.2
newborn P54.3
ulcer —*see* Ulcer, stomach, with hemorrhage
subarachnoid (nontraumatic) —*see* Hemorrhage, intracranial, subarachnoid
subconjunctival —*see also* Hemorrhage, conjunctiva
birth injury P15.3
subcortical (brain) I61.0
subcutaneous R23.3
subdiaphragmatic R58
subdural (acute) (nontraumatic) —*see* Hemorrhage, intracranial, subdural
subependymal
newborn P52.0
with intraventricular extension P52.1
and intracerebral extension P52.22
subgaleal P12.2 ◀
subhyaloid —*see* Hemorrhage, retina
subperiosteal —*see* Disorder, bone, specified type NEC
subretinal —*see* Hemorrhage, retina
subtentorial —*see* Hemorrhage, intracranial, subdural

Hemorrhage, hemorrhagic *(Continued)*
subungual L60.8
suprarenal (capsule) (gland) E27.49
newborn P54.4
tentorium (traumatic) NEC —*see* Hemorrhage, brain
newborn (birth injury) P10.4
testis N50.1
third stage (postpartum) O72.0
thorax —*see* Hemorrhage, lung
throat R04.1
thymus (gland) E32.8
thyroid (cyst) (gland) E07.89
tongue K14.8
tonsil J35.8
trachea —*see* Hemorrhage, lung
tracheobronchial R04.89
newborn P26.0
traumatic — code to specific injury
cerebellar —*see* Hemorrhage, brain
intracranial —*see* Hemorrhage, brain
recurring or secondary (following initial hemorrhage at time of injury) T79.2
tuberculous NEC —*see also* Tuberculosis, pulmonary A15.0
tunica vaginalis N50.1
ulcer - code by site under Ulcer, with hemorrhage K27.4
umbilicus, umbilical
cord
after birth, newborn P51.9
complicating delivery O69.5
newborn P51.9
massive P51.0
slipped ligature P51.8
stump P51.9
urethra (idiopathic) N36.8
uterus, uterine (abnormal) N93.9
climacteric N92.4
complicating delivery —*see* Hemorrhage, complicating, delivery
dysfunctional or functional N93.8
intermenstrual (regular) N92.3
irregular N92.1
postmenopausal N95.0
postpartum —*see* Hemorrhage, postpartum
preclimacteric or premenopausal N92.4
prepubertal N93.8
pubertal N92.2
vagina (abnormal) N93.9
newborn P54.6
vas deferens N50.1
vasa previa O69.4
ventricular I61.5
vesical N32.89
viscera NEC R58
newborn P54.8
vitreous (humor) (intraocular) H43.1-
vulva N90.89
Hemorrhoids (bleeding) (without mention of degree) K64.9
1st degree (grade/stage I) (without prolapse outside of anal canal) K64.0
2nd degree (grade/stage II) (that prolapse with straining but retract spontaneously) K64.1
3rd degree (grade/stage III) (that prolapse with straining and require manual replacement back inside anal canal) K64.2
4th degree (grade/stage IV) (with prolapsed tissue that cannot be manually replaced) K64.3
complicating
pregnancy O22.4
puerperium O87.2
external K64.4
with
thrombosis K64.5

Hemorrhoids *(Continued)*
internal (without mention of degree) K64.8
prolapsed K64.8
skin tags
anus K64.4
residual K64.4
specified NEC K64.8
strangulated —*see also* Hemorrhoids, by degree K64.8
thrombosed —*see also* Hemorrhoids, by degree K64.5
ulcerated —*see also* Hemorrhoids, by degree K64.8
Hemosalpinx N83.6
with
hematocolpos N89.7
hematometra N85.7
with hematocolpos N89.7
Hemosiderosis (dietary) E83.19
pulmonary, idiopathic E83.1 *[J84.03]*
transfusion T80.89
Hemothorax (bacterial) (nontuberculous) J94.2
newborn P54.8
traumatic S27.1
with pneumothorax S27.2
tuberculous NEC A15.6
Henoch (-Schönlein) disease or syndrome (purpura) D69.0
Henpue, henpuye A66.6
Hepar lobatum (syphilitic) A52.74
Hepatalgia K76.89
Hepatitis K75.9
acute B17.9
with coma K72.01
with hepatic failure —*see* Failure, hepatic
alcoholic —*see* Hepatitis, alcoholic
infectious B15.9 ◀
~~with hepatic coma B15.0~~
non-viral K72.0 ◀
viral B17.9
alcoholic (acute) (chronic) K70.10
with ascites K70.11
amebic —*see* Abscess, liver, amebic
anicteric (viral) —*see* Hepatitis, viral
antigen-associated (HAA) —*see* Hepatitis, B
Australia-antigen (positive) —*see* Hepatitis, B
autoimmune K75.4
B B19.10
with hepatic coma B19.11
acute B16.9
with
delta-agent (coinfection) (without hepatic coma) B16.1
with hepatic coma B16.0
hepatic coma (without delta-agent coinfection) B16.2
chronic B18.1
with delta-agent B18.0
bacterial NEC K75.89
C (viral) B19.20
with hepatic coma B19.21
acute B17.10
with hepatic coma B17.11
chronic B18.2
catarrhal (acute) B15.9
with hepatic coma B15.0
cholangiolitic K75.89
cholestatic K75.89
chronic K73.9
active NEC K73.2
lobular NEC K73.1
persistent NEC K73.0
specified NEC K73.8
cytomegaloviral B25.1
due to ethanol (acute) (chronic) —*see* Hepatitis, alcoholic
epidemic B15.9
with hepatic coma B15.0
fulminant NEC (viral) —*see* Hepatitis, viral
granulomatous NEC K75.3
herpesviral B00.81

H

Hepatitis *(Continued)*
history of
B Z86.19
C Z86.19
homologous serum —*see* Hepatitis, viral, type B
in (due to)
mumps B26.81
toxoplasmosis (acquired) B58.1
congenital (active) P37.1 *[K77]*
infectious, infective B15.9 ⬅
~~with hepatic coma B15.0~~
acute (subacute) B17.9 ◀
chronic B18.9 ◀
inoculation —*see* Hepatitis, viral, type B
interstitial (chronic) K74.69
lupoid NEC K75.2
malignant NEC (with hepatic failure) K72.90
with coma K72.91
neonatal giant cell P59.29
neonatal (idiopathic) (toxic) P59.29
newborn P59.29
postimmunization —*see* Hepatitis, viral, type B
post-transfusion —*see* Hepatitis, viral, type B
reactive, nonspecific K75.2
serum —*see* Hepatitis, viral, type B
specified type NEC
with hepatic failure —*see* Failure, hepatic
syphilitic (late) A52.74
congenital (early) A50.08 *[K77]*
late A50.59 *[K77]*
secondary A51.45
toxic —*see also* Disease, liver, toxic K71.6
tuberculous A18.83
viral, virus B19.9
with hepatic coma B19.0
acute B17.9
chronic B18.9
specified NEC B18.8
type
B B18.1
with delta-agent B18.0
C B18.2
congenital P35.3
coxsackie B33.8 *[K77]*
cytomegalic inclusion B25.1
in remission, any type — code to Hepatitis, chronic, by type
non-A, non-B B17.8
specified type NEC (with or without coma) B17.8
type
A B15.9
with hepatic coma B15.0
B B19.10
with hepatic coma B19.11
acute B16.9
with
delta-agent (coinfection) (without hepatic coma) B16.1
with hepatic coma B16.0
hepatic coma (without delta-agent coinfection) B16.2
chronic B18.1
with delta-agent B18.0
C B19.20
with hepatic coma B19.21
acute B17.10
with hepatic coma B17.11
chronic B18.2
E B17.2
non-A, non-B B17.8
Hepatization lung (acute) —*see* Pneumonia, lobar
Hepatoblastoma C22.2
Hepatocarcinoma C22.0
Hepatocholangiocarcinoma C22.0
Hepatocholangioma, benign D13.4
Hepatocholangitis K75.89
Hepatolenticular degeneration E83.01
Hepatoma (malignant) C22.0
benign D13.4
embryonal C22.0
Hepatomegaly —*see also* Hypertrophy, liver
with splenomegaly R16.2
congenital Q44.7
in mononucleosis
gammaherpesviral B27.09
infectious specified NEC B27.89
Hepatoptosis K76.89
Hepatorenal syndrome following labor and delivery O90.4
Hepatosis K76.89
Hepatosplenomegaly R16.2
hyperlipemic (Bürger-Grütz type) E78.3 *[K77]*
Hereditary —*see* condition
Heredodegeneration, macular —*see* Dystrophy, retina
Heredopathia atactica polyneuritiformis G60.1
Heredosyphilis —*see* Syphilis, congenital
Herlitz' syndrome Q81.1
Hermansky-Pudlak syndrome E70.331
Hermaphrodite, hermaphroditism (true) Q56.0
46,XX with streak gonads Q99.1
46,XX/46,XY Q99.0
46,XY with streak gonads Q99.1
chimera 46,XX/46,XY Q99.0
Hernia, hernial (acquired) (recurrent) K46.9
with
gangrene —*see* Hernia, by site, with, gangrene
incarceration —*see* Hernia, by site, with, obstruction
irreducible —*see* Hernia, by site, with, obstruction
obstruction —*see* Hernia, by site, with, obstruction
strangulation —*see* Hernia, by site, with, obstruction
abdomen, abdominal K46.9
with
gangrene (and obstruction) K46.1
obstruction K46.0
femoral —*see* Hernia, femoral
incisional —*see* Hernia, incisional
inguinal —*see* Hernia, inguinal
specified site NEC K45.8
with
gangrene (and obstruction) K45.1
obstruction K45.0
umbilical —*see* Hernia, umbilical
wall —*see* Hernia, ventral
appendix —*see* Hernia, abdomen
bladder (mucosa) (sphincter)
congenital (female) (male) Q79.51
female —*see* Cystocele
male N32.89
brain, congenital —*see* Encephalocele
cartilage, vertebra —*see* Displacement, intervertebral disc
cerebral, congenital —*see also* Encephalocele
endaural Q01.8
ciliary body (traumatic) S05.2-
colon —*see* Hernia, abdomen
Cooper's —*see* Hernia, abdomen, specified site NEC
crural —*see* Hernia, femoral
diaphragm, diaphragmatic K44.9
with
gangrene (and obstruction) K44.1
obstruction K44.0
congenital Q79.0
direct (inguinal) —*see* Hernia, inguinal
diverticulum, intestine —*see* Hernia, abdomen
double (inguinal) —*see* Hernia, inguinal, bilateral
due to adhesions (with obstruction) K56.5
epigastric —*see also* Hernia, ventral K43.9
esophageal hiatus —*see* Hernia, hiatal
Hernia, hernial *(Continued)*
external (inguinal) —*see* Hernia, inguinal
fallopian tube N83.4- ⬅
fascia M62.89
femoral K41.90
with
gangrene (and obstruction) K41.40
not specified as recurrent K41.40
recurrent K41.41
obstruction K41.30
not specified as recurrent K41.30
recurrent K41.31
bilateral K41.20
with
gangrene (and obstruction) K41.10
not specified as recurrent K41.10
recurrent K41.11
obstruction K41.00
not specified as recurrent K41.00
recurrent K41.01
not specified as recurrent K41.20
recurrent K41.21
not specified as recurrent K41.90
recurrent K41.91
unilateral K41.90
with
gangrene (and obstruction) K41.40
not specified as recurrent K41.40
recurrent K41.41
obstruction K41.30
not specified as recurrent K41.30
recurrent K41.31
not specified as recurrent K41.90
recurrent K41.91
foramen magnum G93.5
congenital Q01.8
funicular (umbilical) —*see also* Hernia, umbilicus
spermatic (cord) —*see* Hernia, inguinal
gastrointestinal tract —*see* Hernia, abdomen
Hesselbach's —*see* Hernia, femoral, specified site NEC
hiatal (esophageal) (sliding) K44.9
with
gangrene (and obstruction) K44.1
obstruction K44.0
congenital Q40.1
hypogastric —*see* Hernia, ventral
incarcerated —*see also* Hernia, by site, with obstruction
with gangrene —*see* Hernia, by site, with gangrene
incisional K43.92
with
gangrene (and obstruction) K43.1
obstruction K43.0
indirect (inguinal) —*see* Hernia, inguinal
inguinal (direct) (external) (funicular) (indirect) (internal) (oblique) (scrotal) (sliding) K40.90
with
gangrene (and obstruction) K40.40
not specified as recurrent K40.40
recurrent K40.41
obstruction K40.30
not specified as recurrent K40.30
recurrent K40.31
bilateral K40.20
with
gangrene (and obstruction) K40.10
not specified as recurrent K40.10
recurrent K40.11
obstruction K40.00
not specified as recurrent K40.00
recurrent K40.01
not specified as recurrent K40.20
recurrent K40.21
not specified as recurrent K40.90
recurrent K40.91

◀ New ⬅ Revised ~~deleted~~ Deleted

Hernia, hernial *(Continued)*
inguinal *(Continued)*
unilateral K40.90
with
gangrene (and obstruction) K40.40
not specified as recurrent K40.40
recurrent K40.41
obstruction K40.30
not specified as recurrent K40.30
recurrent K40.31
not specified as recurrent K40.90
recurrent K40.91
internal —*see also* Hernia, abdomen
inguinal —*see* Hernia, inguinal
interstitial —*see* Hernia, abdomen
intervertebral cartilage or disc —*see* Displacement, intervertebral disc
intestine, intestinal —*see* Hernia, by site
intra-abdominal —*see* Hernia, abdomen
iris (traumatic) S05.2-
irreducible —*see also* Hernia, by site, with obstruction
with gangrene —*see* Hernia, by site, with gangrene
ischiatic —*see* Hernia, abdomen, specified site NEC
ischiorectal —*see* Hernia, abdomen, specified site NEC
lens (traumatic) S05.2-
linea (alba) (semilunaris) —*see* Hernia, ventral
Littre's —*see* Hernia, abdomen
lumbar —*see* Hernia, abdomen, specified site NEC
lung (subcutaneous) J98.4
mediastinum J98.59 ◄
mesenteric (internal) —*see* Hernia, abdomen
midline —*see* Hernia, ventral
muscle (sheath) M62.89
nucleus pulposus —*see* Displacement, intervertebral disc
oblique (inguinal) —*see* Hernia, inguinal
obstructive —*see also* Hernia, by site, with obstruction
with gangrene —*see* Hernia, by site, with gangrene
obturator —*see* Hernia, abdomen, specified site NEC
omental —*see* Hernia, abdomen
ovary N83.4- ◄
oviduct N83.4- ◄
paraesophageal —*see also* Hernia, diaphragm
congenital Q40.1
parastomal K43.5
with
gangrene (and obstruction) K43.4
obstruction K43.3
paraumbilical —*see* Hernia, umbilicus
perineal —*see* Hernia, abdomen, specified site NEC
Petit's —*see* Hernia, abdomen, specified site NEC
postoperative —*see* Hernia, incisional
pregnant uterus —*see* Abnormal, uterus in pregnancy or childbirth
prevesical N32.89
properitoneal —*see* Hernia, abdomen, specified site NEC
pudendal —*see* Hernia, abdomen, specified site NEC
rectovaginal N81.6
retroperitoneal —*see* Hernia, abdomen, specified site NEC
Richter's —*see* Hernia, abdomen, with obstruction
Rieux's, Riex's —*see* Hernia, abdomen, specified site NEC
sac condition (adhesion) (dropsy) (inflammation) (laceration) (suppuration) - code by site under Hernia

Hernia, hernial *(Continued)*
sciatic —*see* Hernia, abdomen, specified site NEC
scrotum, scrotal —*see* Hernia, inguinal
sliding (inguinal) —*see also* Hernia, inguinal
hiatus —*see* Hernia, hiatal
spigelian —*see* Hernia, ventral
spinal —*see* Spina bifida
strangulated —*see also* Hernia, by site, with obstruction
with gangrene —*see* Hernia, by site, with gangrene
subxiphoid —*see* Hernia, ventral
supra-umbilicus —*see* Hernia, ventral
tendon —*see* Disorder, tendon, specified type NEC
Treitz's (fossa) —*see* Hernia, abdomen, specified site NEC
tunica vaginalis Q55.29
umbilicus, umbilical K42.9
with
gangrene (and obstruction) K42.1
obstruction K42.0
ureter N28.89
urethra, congenital Q64.79
urinary meatus, congenital Q64.79
uterus N81.4
pregnant —*see* Abnormal, uterus in pregnancy or childbirth
vaginal (anterior) (wall) —*see* Cystocele
Velpeau's —*see* Hernia, femoral
ventral K43.9
with
gangrene (and obstruction) K43.7
obstruction K43.6
incisional K43.2
with
gangrene (and obstruction) K43.1
obstruction K43.0
recurrent —*see* Hernia, incisional
specified NEC K43.9
with
gangrene (and obstruction) K43.7
obstruction K43.6
vesical
congenital (female) (male) Q79.51
female —*see* Cystocele
male N32.89
vitreous (into wound) S05.2-
into anterior chamber —*see* Prolapse, vitreous
Herniation —*see also* Hernia
brain (stem) G93.5
cerebral G93.5
mediastinum J98.59 ◄
nucleus pulposus —*see* Displacement, intervertebral disc
Herpangina B08.5
Herpes, herpesvirus, herpetic B00.9
anogenital A60.9
perianal skin A60.1
rectum A60.1
urogenital tract A60.00
cervix A60.03
male genital organ NEC A60.02
penis A60.01
specified site NEC A60.09
vagina A60.04
vulva A60.04
blepharitis (zoster) B02.39
simplex B00.59
circinatus B35.4
bullosus L12.0
conjunctivitis (simplex) B00.53
zoster B02.31
cornea B02.33
encephalitis B00.4
due to herpesvirus 6 B10.01
due to herpesvirus 7 B10.09
specified NEC B10.09

Herpes, herpesvirus, herpetic *(Continued)*
eye (zoster) B02.30
simplex B00.50
eyelid (zoster) B02.39
simplex B00.59
facialis B00.1
febrilis B00.1
geniculate ganglionitis B02.21
genital, genitalis A60.00
female A60.09
male A60.02
gestational, gestationis O26.4-
gingivostomatitis B00.2
human B00.9
1 —*see* Herpes, simplex
2 —*see* Herpes, simplex
3 —*see* Varicella
4 —*see* Mononucleosis, Epstein-Barr (virus)
5 —*see* Disease, cytomegalic inclusion (generalized)
6
encephalitis B10.01
specified NEC B10.81
7
encephalitis B10.09
specified NEC B10.82
8 B10.89
infection NEC B10.89
Kaposi's sarcoma associated B10.89
iridocyclitis (simplex) B00.51
zoster B02.32
iris (vesicular erythema multiforme) L51.9
iritis (simplex) B00.51
Kaposi's sarcoma associated B10.89
keratitis (simplex) (dendritic) (disciform) (interstitial) B00.52
zoster (interstitial) B02.33
keratoconjunctivitis (simplex) B00.52
zoster B02.33
labialis B00.1
lip B00.1
meningitis (simplex) B00.3
zoster B02.1
ophthalmicus (zoster) NEC B02.30
simplex B00.50
penis A60.01
perianal skin A60.1
pharyngitis, pharyngotonsillitis B00.2
rectum A60.1
scrotum A60.02
sepsis B00.7
simplex B00.9
complicated NEC B00.89
congenital P35.2
conjunctivitis B00.53
external ear B00.1
eyelid B00.59
hepatitis B00.81
keratitis (interstitial) B00.52
myleitis B00.82
specified complication NEC B00.89
visceral B00.89
stomatitis B00.2
tonsurans B35.0
visceral B00.89
vulva A60.04
whitlow B00.89
zoster —*see also* condition B02.9
auricularis B02.21
complicated NEC B02.8
conjunctivitis B02.31
disseminated B02.7
encephalitis B02.0
eye(lid) B02.39
geniculate ganglionitis B02.21
keratitis (interstitial) B02.33
meningitis B02.1
myelitis B02.24
neuritis, neuralgia B02.29
ophthalmicus NEC B02.30
oticus B02.21

H

Herpes, herpesvirus, herpetic *(Continued)*
zoster *(Continued)*
polyneuropathy B02.23
specified complication NEC B02.8
trigeminal neuralgia B02.22
Herpesvirus (human) —*see* Herpes
Herpetophobia F40.218
Herrick's anemia —*see* Disease, sickle-cell
Hers' disease E74.09
Herter-Gee syndrome K90.0
Herxheimer's reaction R68.89
Hesitancy
of micturition R39.11
urinary R39.11
Hesselbach's hernia —*see* Hernia, femoral, specified site NEC
Heterochromia (congenital) Q13.2
cataract —*see* Cataract, complicated
cyclitis (Fuchs) —*see* Cyclitis, Fuchs' heterochromic
hair L67.1
iritis —*see* Cyclitis, Fuchs' heterochromic
retained metallic foreign body (nonmagnetic) —*see* Foreign body, intraocular, old, retained
magnetic —*see* Foreign body, intraocular, old, retained, magnetic
uveitis —*see* Cyclitis, Fuchs' heterochromic
Heterophoria —*see* Strabismus, heterophoria
Heterophyes, heterophyiasis (small intestine) B66.8
Heterotopia, heterotopic —*see also* Malposition, congenital
cerebralis Q04.8
Heterotropia —*see* Strabismus
Heubner-Herter disease K90.0
Hexadactylism Q69.9
HGSIL (cytology finding) (high grade squamous intraepithelial lesion on cytologic smear) (Pap smear finding)
anus R85.613
cervix R87.613
biopsy (histology) finding — *see* Neoplasia, intraepithelial, cervix, grade II or grade III ⇐
vagina R87.623
biopsy (histology) finding — *see* Neoplasia, intraepithelial, vagina, grade II or grade III ⇐
Hibernoma —*see* Lipoma
Hiccup, hiccough R06.6
epidemic B33.0
psychogenic F45.8
Hidden penis (congenital) Q55.64
acquired N48.83
Hidradenitis (axillaris) (suppurative) L73.2
Hidradenoma (nodular) —*see also* Neoplasm, skin, benign
clear cell —*see* Neoplasm, skin, benign
papillary —*see* Neoplasm, skin, benign
Hidrocystoma —*see* Neoplasm, skin, benign
High
altitude effects T70.20
anoxia T70.29
on
ears T70.0
sinuses T70.1
polycythemia D75.1
arch
foot Q66.7
palate, congenital Q38.5
arterial tension —*see* Hypertension
basal metabolic rate R94.8
blood pressure —*see also* Hypertension
borderline R03.0
reading (incidental) (isolated) (nonspecific), without diagnosis of hypertension R03.0
cholesterol E78.00 ⇐
with high triglycerides E78.2
diaphragm (congenital) Q79.1
High *(Continued)*
expressed emotional level within family Z63.8
head at term O32.4
palate, congenital Q38.5
risk
infant NEC Z76.2
sexual behavior (heterosexual) Z72.51
bisexual Z72.53
homosexual Z72.52
temperature (of unknown origin) R50.9
thoracic rib Q76.6
triglycerides E78.1
with high cholesterol E78.2
Hildenbrand's disease A75.0
Hilum —*see* condition
Hip —*see* condition
Hippel's disease Q85.8
Hippophobia F40.218
Hippus H57.09
Hirschsprung's disease or megacolon Q43.1
Hirsutism, hirsuties L68.0
Hirudiniasis
external B88.3
internal B83.4
Hiss-Russell dysentery A03.1
Histidinemia, histidinuria E70.41
Histiocytoma —*see also* Neoplasm, skin, benign
fibrous —*see also* Neoplasm, skin, benign
atypical —*see* Neoplasm, connective tissue, uncertain behavior
malignant —*see* Neoplasm, connective tissue, malignant
Histiocytosis D76.3
acute differentiated progressive C96.0
Langerhans' cell NEC C96.6
multifocal X
multisystemic (disseminated) C96.0
unisystemic C96.5
pulmonary, adult (adult PLCH) J84.82
unifocal (X) C96.6
lipid, lipoid D76.3
essential E75.29
malignant C96.A
mononuclear phagocytes NEC D76.1
Langerhans' cells C96.6
non-Langerhans cell D76.3
polyostotic sclerosing D76.3
sinus, with massive lymphadenopathy D76.3
syndrome NEC D76.3
X NEC C96.6
acute (progressive) C96.0
chronic C96.6
multifocal C96.5
multisystemic C96.0
unifocal C96.6
Histoplasmosis B39.9
with pneumonia NEC B39.2
African B39.5
American —*see* Histoplasmosis, capsulati
capsulati B39.4
disseminated B39.3
generalized B39.3
pulmonary B39.2
acute B39.0
chronic B39.1
Darling's B39.4
duboisii B39.5
lung NEC B39.2
History
family (of) —*see also* History, personal (of)
alcohol abuse Z81.1
allergy NEC Z84.89
anemia Z83.2
arthritis Z82.61
asthma Z82.5
blindness Z82.1
cardiac death (sudden) Z82.41
carrier of genetic disease Z84.81
chromosomal anomaly Z82.79
History *(Continued)*
family *(Continued)*
chronic
disabling disease NEC Z82.8
lower respiratory disease Z82.5
colonic polyps Z83.71
congenital malformations and deformations Z82.79
polycystic kidney Z82.71
consanguinity Z84.3
deafness Z82.2
diabetes mellitus Z83.3
disability NEC Z82.8
disease or disorder (of)
allergic NEC Z84.89
behavioral NEC Z81.8
blood and blood-forming organs Z83.2
cardiovascular NEC Z82.49
chronic disabling NEC Z82.8
digestive Z83.79
ear NEC Z83.52
endocrine NEC Z83.49
eye NEC Z83.518
glaucoma Z83.511
familial hypercholesterolemia Z83.42 ◀
genitourinary NEC Z84.2
glaucoma Z83.511
hematological Z83.2
immune mechanism Z83.2
infectious NEC Z83.1
ischemic heart Z82.49
kidney Z84.1
mental NEC Z81.8
metabolic Z83.49
musculoskeletal NEC Z82.69
neurological NEC Z82.0
nutritional Z83.49
parasitic NEC Z83.1
psychiatric NEC Z81.8
respiratory NEC Z83.6
skin and subcutaneous tissue NEC Z84.0
specified NEC Z84.89
drug abuse NEC Z81.3
epilepsy Z82.0
familial hypercholesterolemia Z83.42 ◀
genetic disease carrier Z84.81
glaucoma Z83.511
hearing loss Z82.2
human immunodeficiency virus (HIV) infection Z83.0
Huntington's chorea Z82.0
intellectual disability Z81.0
leukemia Z80.6
malignant neoplasm (of) NOS Z80.9
bladder Z80.52
breast Z80.3
bronchus Z80.1
digestive organ Z80.0
gastrointestinal tract Z80.0
genital organ Z80.49
ovary Z80.41
prostate Z80.42
specified organ NEC Z80.49
testis Z80.43
hematopoietic NEC Z80.7
intrathoracic organ NEC Z80.2
kidney Z80.51
lung Z80.1
lymphatic NEC Z80.7
ovary Z80.41
prostate Z80.42
respiratory organ NEC Z80.2
specified site NEC Z80.8
testis Z80.43
trachea Z80.1
urinary organ or tract Z80.59
bladder Z80.52
kidney Z80.51
mental
disorder NEC Z81.8
multiple endocrine neoplasia (MEN) syndrome Z83.41

◀ New ⇐ Revised ~~deleted~~ Deleted

History *(Continued)*
family *(Continued)*
osteoporosis Z82.62
polycystic kidney Z82.71
polyps (colon) Z83.71
psychiatric disorder Z81.8
psychoactive substance abuse NEC Z81.3
respiratory condition NEC Z83.6
asthma and other lower respiratory conditions Z82.5
self-harmful behavior Z81.8
SIDS (sudden infant death syndrome) Z84.82 ◀
skin condition Z84.0
specified condition NEC Z84.89
stroke (cerebrovascular) Z82.3
substance abuse NEC Z81.4
alcohol Z81.1
drug NEC Z81.3
psychoactive NEC Z81.3
tobacco Z81.2
~~sudden cardiac death Z82.41~~
sudden ◀
cardiac death Z82.41 ◀
infant death syndrome (SIDS) Z84.82 ◀
tobacco abuse Z81.2
violence, violent behavior Z81.8
visual loss Z82.1
personal (of) —*see also* History, family (of)
abuse
adult Z91.419
physical and sexual Z91.410
psychological Z91.411
childhood Z62.819
physical Z62.810
psychological Z62.811
sexual Z62.810
alcohol dependence F10.21
allergy (to) Z88.9
analgesic agent NEC Z88.6
anesthetic Z88.4
antibiotic agent NEC Z88.1
anti-infective agent NEC Z88.3
contrast media Z91.041
drugs, medicaments and biological substances Z88.9
specified NEC Z88.8
food Z91.018
additives Z91.02
eggs Z91.012
milk products Z91.011
peanuts Z91.010
seafood Z91.013
specified food NEC Z91.018
insect Z91.038
bee Z91.030
latex Z91.040
medicinal agents Z88.9
specified NEC Z88.8
narcotic agent NEC Z88.5
nonmedicinal agents Z91.048
penicillin Z88.0
serum Z88.7
specified NEC Z91.09
sulfonamides Z88.2
vaccine Z88.7
anaphylactic shock Z87.892
anaphylaxis Z87.892
behavioral disorders Z86.59
benign carcinoid tumor Z86.012
benign neoplasm Z86.018
brain Z86.011
carcinoid Z86.012
colonic polyps Z86.010
brain injury (traumatic) Z87.820
breast implant removal Z98.86
calculi, renal Z87.442
cancer —*see* History, personal (of), malignant neoplasm (of)
cardiac arrest (death), successfully resuscitated Z86.74

History *(Continued)*
personal *(Continued)*
cerebral infarction without residual deficit Z86.73
cervical dysplasia Z87.410
chemotherapy for neoplastic condition Z92.21
childhood abuse —*see* History, personal (of), abuse
cleft lip (corrected) Z87.730
cleft palate (corrected) Z87.730
collapsed vertebra (healed) Z87.311
due to osteoporosis Z87.310
combat and operational stress reaction Z86.51
congenital malformation (corrected) Z87.798
circulatory system (corrected) Z87.74
digestive system (corrected) NEC Z87.738
ear (corrected) Z87.720
eye (corrected) Z87.721
face and neck (corrected) Z87.790
genitourinary system (corrected) NEC Z87.718
heart (corrected) Z87.74
integument (corrected) Z87.76
limb (s) (corrected) Z87.76
musculoskeletal system (corrected) Z87.76
neck (corrected) Z87.790
nervous system (corrected) NEC Z87.728
respiratory system (corrected) Z87.75
sense organs (corrected) NEC Z87.728
specified NEC Z87.798
contraception Z92.0
deployment (military) Z91.82
diabetic foot ulcer Z86.31
disease or disorder (of) Z87.898
blood and blood-forming organs Z86.2
circulatory system Z86.79
specified condition NEC Z86.79
connective tissue NEC Z87.39
digestive system Z87.19
colonic polyp Z86.010
peptic ulcer disease Z87.11
specified condition NEC Z87.19
ear Z86.69
endocrine Z86.39
diabetic foot ulcer Z86.31
gestational diabetes Z86.32
specified type NEC Z86.39
eye Z86.69
genital (track) system NEC
female Z87.42
male Z87.438
hematological Z86.2
Hodgkin Z85.71
immune mechanism Z86.2
infectious Z86.19
malaria Z86.13
Methicillin resistant Staphylococcus aureus (MRSA) Z86.14
poliomyelitis Z86.12
specified NEC Z86.19
tuberculosis Z86.11
mental NEC Z86.59
metabolic Z86.39
diabetic foot ulcer Z86.31
gestational diabetes Z86.32
specified type NEC Z86.39
musculoskeletal NEC Z87.39
nervous system Z86.69
nutritional Z86.39
parasitic Z86.19
respiratory system NEC Z87.09
sense organs Z86.69
skin Z87.2
specified site or type NEC Z87.898
subcutaneous tissue Z87.2

History *(Continued)*
personal *(Continued)*
disease or disorder (of) *(Continued)*
trophoblastic Z87.59
urinary system NEC Z87.448
drug dependence —*see* Dependence, drug, by type, in remission
drug therapy
antineoplastic chemotherapy Z92.21
estrogen Z92.23
immunosupression Z92.25
inhaled steroids Z92.240
monoclonal drug Z92.22
specified NEC Z92.29
steroid Z92.241
systemic steroids Z92.241
dysplasia
cervical (mild) (moderate) Z87.410 ⟸
severe (grade III) Z86.001 ◀
prostatic Z87.430
vaginal Z87.411
vulvar (mild) (moderate) Z87.412 ⟸
severe (grade III) Z86.008 ◀
embolism (venous) Z86.718
pulmonary Z86.711
encephalitis Z86.61
estrogen therapy Z92.23
extracorporeal membrane oxygenation (ECMO) Z92.81
failed conscious sedation Z92.83
failed moderate sedation Z92.83
fall, falling Z91.81
fracture (healed)
fatigue Z87.312
fragility Z87.310
osteoporosis Z87.310
pathological NEC Z87.311
stress Z87.312
traumatic Z87.81
gestational diabetes Z86.32
hepatitis
B Z86.19
C Z86.19
Hodgkin disease Z85.71
hyperthermia, malignant Z88.4
hypospadias (corrected) Z87.710
hysterectomy Z90.710
immunosupression therapy Z92.25
in situ neoplasm
breast Z86.000
cervix uteri Z86.001
specified NEC Z86.008
infection NEC Z86.19
central nervous system Z86.61
Methicillin resistant Staphylococcus aureus (MRSA) Z86.14
urinary (tract) Z87.41
injury NEC Z87.828
in utero procedure during pregnancy Z98.870
in utero procedure while a fetus Z98.871
irradiation Z92.3
kidney stones Z87.442
leukemia Z85.6
lymphoma (non-Hodgkin) Z85.72
malignant melanoma (skin) Z85.820
malignant neoplasm (of) Z85.9
accessory sinuses Z85.22
anus NEC Z85.048
carcinoid Z85.040
bladder Z85.51
bone Z85.830
brain Z85.841
breast Z85.3
bronchus NEC Z85.118
carcinoid Z85.110
carcinoid —*see* History, personal (of), malignant neoplasm, by site, carcinioid
cervix Z85.41
colon NEC Z85.038
carcinoid Z85.030

H

History *(Continued)*
personal *(Continued)*
malignant neoplasm *(Continued)*
digestive organ Z85.00
specified NEC Z85.09
endocrine gland NEC Z85.858
epididymis Z85.48
esophagus Z85.01
eye Z85.840
gastrointestinal tract —*see* History, malignant neoplasm, digestive organ
genital organ
female Z85.40
specified NEC Z85.44
male Z85.45
specified NEC Z85.49
hematopoietic NEC Z85.79
intrathoracic organ Z85.20-
kidney NEC Z85.528
carcinoid Z85.520
large intestine NEC Z85.038
carcinoid Z85.030
larynx Z85.21
liver Z85.05
lung NEC Z85.118
carcinoid Z85.110
mediastinum Z85.29
Merkel cell Z85.821
middle ear Z85.22
nasal cavities Z85.22
nervous system NEC Z85.848
oral cavity Z85.819
specified site NEC Z85.818
ovary Z85.43
pancreas Z85.07
pelvis Z85.53
pharynx Z85.819
specified site NEC Z85.818
pleura Z85.29
prostate Z85.46
rectosigmoid junction NEC Z85.048
carcinoid Z85.040
rectum NEC Z85.048
carcinoid Z85.040
respiratory organ Z85.20
sinuses, accessory Z85.22
skin NEC Z85.828
melanoma Z85.820
Merkel cell Z85.821
small intestine NEC Z85.068
carcinoid Z85.060
soft tissue Z85.831
specified site NEC Z85.89
stomach NEC Z85.028
carcinoid Z85.020
testis Z85.47
thymus NEC Z85.238
carcinoid Z85.230
thyroid Z85.850
tongue Z85.810
trachea Z85.12
ureter Z85.54
urinary organ or tract Z85.50
specified NEC Z85.59
uterus Z85.42
maltreatment Z91.89
medical treatment NEC Z92.89
melanoma (malignant) (skin) Z85.820
meningitis Z86.61
mental disorder Z86.59
Merkel cell carcinoma (skin) Z85.821
Methicillin resistant Staphylococcus aureus (MRSA) Z86.14
military deployment Z91.82
military war, peacekeeping and humanitarian deployment (current or past conflict) Z91.82
myocardial infarction (old) I25.2
neglect (in)
adult Z91.412
childhood Z62.812

History *(Continued)*
personal *(Continued)*
neoplasm
benign Z86.018
brain Z86.011
colon polyp Z86.010
in situ
breast Z86.000
cervix uteri Z86.001
specified NEC Z86.008
malignant —*see* History of, malignant neoplasm
uncertain behavior Z86.03
nephrotic syndrome Z87.441
nicotine dependence Z87.891
noncompliance with medical treatment or regimen —*see* Noncompliance
nutritional deficiency Z86.39
obstetric complications Z87.59
childbirth Z87.59
pregnancy Z87.59
pre-term labor Z87.51
puerperium Z87.59
osteoporosis fractures Z87.31
parasuicide (attempt) Z91.5
physical trauma NEC Z87.828
self-harm or suicide attempt Z91.5
pneumonia (recurrent) Z87.01
poisoning NEC Z91.89
self-harm or suicide attempt Z91.5
poor personal hygiene Z91.89
preterm labor Z87.51
procedure during pregnancy Z98.870
procedure while a fetus Z98.871
prolonged reversible ischemic neurologic deficit (PRINO) Z86.73
prostatic dysplasia Z87.430
psychiatric disorder NEC Z87.89
psychological
abuse
adult Z91.411
child Z62.811
trauma, specified NEC Z91.49
radiation therapy Z92.3
removal
implant
breast Z98.86
renal calculi Z87.442
respiratory condition NEC Z87.09
retained foreign body fully removed Z87.821
risk factors NEC Z91.89
self-harm Z91.5
self-poisoning attempt Z91.5
sex reassignment Z87.890
sleep-wake cycle problem Z72.821
specified NEC Z87.898
steroid therapy (systemic) Z92.241
inhaled Z92.240
stroke without residual deficits Z86.73
substance abuse NEC F10-F19 with fifth character 1
sudden cardiac arrest Z86.74
sudden cardiac death successfully resuscitated Z86.74
suicide attempt Z91.5
surgery NEC Z98.890 ⇐
with uterine scar Z98.891 ◀
sex reassignment Z87.890
transplant —*see* Transplant
thrombophlebitis Z86.72
thrombosis (venous) Z86.718
pulmonary Z86.711
tobacco dependence Z87.891
transient ischemic attack (TIA) without residual deficits Z86.73
trauma (physical) NEC Z87.828
psychological NEC Z91.49
self-harm Z91.5
traumatic brain injury Z87.820
unhealthy sleep-wake cycle Z72.821

History *(Continued)*
personal *(Continued)*
unintended awareness under general anesthesia Z92.84 ◀
urinary (recurrent) (tract) infection (s) Z87.440
urinary calculi Z87.42
uterine scar from previous surgery Z98.891 ◀
vaginal dysplasia Z87.411
venous thrombosis or embolism Z86.718
pulmonary Z86.711
vulvar dysplasia Z87.412
His-Werner disease A79.0
HIV —*see also* Human, immunodeficiency virus B20
laboratory evidence (nonconclusive) R75
nonconclusive test (in infants) R75
positive, seropositive Z21
Hives (bold) —*see* Urticaria
Hoarseness R49.0
Hobo Z59.0
Hodgkin disease —*see* Lymphoma, Hodgkin
Hodgson's disease I71.2
ruptured I71.1
Hoffa-Kastert disease E88.89
Hoffa's disease E88.89
Hoffmann-Bouveret syndrome I47.9
Hoffmann's syndrome E03.9 *[G73.7]*
Hole (round)
macula H35.34-
retina (without detachment) —*see* Break, retina, round hole
with detachment —*see* Detachment, retina, with retinal, break
Holiday relief care Z75.5
Hollenhorst's plaque —*see* Occlusion, artery, retina
Hollow foot (congenital) Q66.7
acquired —*see* Deformity, limb, foot, specified NEC
Holoprosencephaly Q04.2
Holt-Oram syndrome Q87.2
Homelessness Z59.0
Homesickness —*see* Disorder, adjustment
Homocystinemia, homocystinuria E72.11
Homogentisate 1,2-dioxygenase deficiency E70.29
Homologous serum hepatitis (prophylactic) (therapeutic) —*see* Hepatitis, viral, type B
Honeycomb lung J98.4
congenital Q33.0
Hooded
clitoris Q52.6
penis Q55.69
Hookworm (anemia) (disease) (infection) (infestation) B76.9
specified NEC B76.8
Hordeolum (eyelid) (externum) (recurrent) H00.019
internum H00.029
left H00.026
lower H00.025
upper H00.024
right H00.023
lower H00.022
upper H00.021
left H00.016
lower H00.015
upper H00.014
right H00.013
lower H00.012
upper H00.011
Horn
cutaneous L85.8
nail L60.2
congenital Q84.6
Horner (-Claude Bernard) syndrome G90.2
traumatic —*see* Injury, nerve, cervical sympathetic

Horseshoe kidney (congenital) Q63.1
Horton's headache or neuralgia G44.099
intractable G44.091
not intractable G44.099
Hospital hopper syndrome —*see* Disorder, factitious
Hospitalism in children —*see* Disorder, adjustment
Hostility R45.5
towards child Z62.3
Hot flashes
menopausal N95.1
Hourglass (contracture) —*see also* Contraction, hourglass
stomach K31.89
congenital Q40.2
stricture K31.2
Household, housing circumstance affecting care Z59.9
specified NEC Z59.8
Housemaid's knee —*see* Bursitis, prepatellar
Hudson (-Stähli) **line** (cornea) —*see* Pigmentation, cornea, anterior
Human
bite (open wound) —*see also* Bite
intact skin surface —*see* Bite, superficial
herpesvirus —*see* Herpes
immunodeficiency virus (HIV) disease (infection) B20
asymptomatic status Z21
contact Z20.6
counseling Z71.7
dementia B20 *[F02.80]*
with behavioral disturbance B20 *[F02.81]*
exposure to Z20.6
laboratory evidence R75
type-2 (HIV 2) as cause of disease classified elsewhere B97.35
papillomavirus (HPV)
DNA test positive
high risk
cervix R87.810
vagina R87.811
low risk
cervix R87.820
vagina R87.821
screening for Z11.51
T-cell lymphotropic virus
type-1 (HTLV-I) infection B33.3
as cause of disease classified elsewhere B97.33
carrier Z22.6
type-2 (HTLV-II) as cause of disease classified elsewhere B97.34
Humidifier lung or pneumonitis J67.7
Humiliation (experience) **in childhood** Z62.898
Humpback (acquired) —*see* Kyphosis
Hunchback (acquired) —*see* Kyphosis
Hunger T73.0
air, psychogenic F45.8
Hungry bone syndrome E83.81
Hunner's ulcer —*see* Cystitis, chronic, interstitial
Hunter's
glossitis D51.0
syndrome E76.1
Huntington's disease or chorea G10
with dementia G10 *[F02.80]*
with behavioral disturbance G10 *[F02.81]*
Hunt's
disease or syndrome (herpetic geniculate ganglionitis) B02.21
dyssynergia cerebellaris myoclonica G11.1
neuralgia B02.21
Hurler (-Scheie) **disease or syndrome** E76.02
Hurst's disease G36.1
Hurthle cell
adenocarcinoma C73
adenoma D34
carcinoma C73
tumor D34
Hutchinson-Boeck disease or syndrome —*see* Sarcoidosis
Hutchinson-Gilford disease or syndrome E34.8
Hutchinson's
disease, meaning
angioma serpiginosum L81.7
pompholyx (cheiropompholyx) L30.1
prurigo estivalis L56.4
summer eruption or summer prurigo L56.4
melanotic freckle —*see* Melanoma, in situ
malignant melanoma in —*see* Melanoma
teeth or incisors (congenital syphilis) A50.52
triad (congenital syphilis) A50.53
Hyalin plaque, sclera, senile H15.89
Hyaline membrane (disease) (lung) (pulmonary) (newborn) P22.0
Hyalinosis
cutis (et mucosae) E78.89
focal and segmental (glomerular) —*see also* N00-N07 with fourth character .1 N05.1
Hyalitis, hyalosis, asteroid —*see also* Deposit, crystalline
syphilitic (late) A52.71
Hydatid
cyst or tumor —*see* Echinococcus
mole —*see* Hydatidiform mole
Morgagni
female Q50.5
male (epididymal) Q55.4
testicular Q55.29
Hydatidiform mole (benign) (complicating pregnancy) (delivered) (undelivered) O01.9
classical O01.0
complete O01.0
incomplete O01.1
invasive D39.2
malignant D39.2
partial O01.1
Hydatidosis —*see* Echinococcus
Hydradenitis (axillaris) (suppurative) L73.2
Hydradenoma —*see* Hidradenoma
Hydramnios O40.-
Hydrancephaly, hydranencephaly Q04.3
with spina bifida —*see* Spina bifida, with hydrocephalus
Hydrargyrism NEC —*see* Poisoning, mercury
Hydrarthrosis —*see also* Effusion, joint
gonococcal A54.42
intermittent M12.40
ankle M12.47-
elbow M12.42-
foot joint M12.47-
hand joint M12.44-
hip M12.45-
knee M12.46-
multiple site M12.49
shoulder M12.41-
specified joint NEC M12.48
wrist M12.43-
of yaws (early) (late) —*see also* subcategory M14.8- A66.6
syphilitic (late) A52.77
congenital A50.55 *[M12.80]*
Hydremia D64.89
Hydrencephalocele (congenital) —*see* Encephalocele
Hydrencephalomeningocele (congenital) —*see* Encephalocele
Hydroa R23.8
aestivale L56.4
vacciniforme L56.4
Hydroadenitis (axillaris) (suppurative) L73.2
Hydrocalycosis —*see* Hydronephrosis
Hydrocele (spermatic cord) (testis) (tunica vaginalis) N43.3
canal of Nuck N94.89
communicating N43.2
congenital P83.5
congenital P83.5
encysted N43.0
Hydrocele *(Continued)*
female NEC N94.89
infected N43.1
newborn P83.5
round ligament N94.89
specified NEC N43.2
spinalis —*see* Spina bifida
vulva N90.89
Hydrocephalus (acquired) (external) (internal) (malignant) (recurrent) G91.9
aqueduct Sylvius stricture Q03.0
causing disproportion O33.6
with obstructed labor O66.3
communicating G91.0
congenital (external) (internal) Q03.9
with spina bifida Q05.4
cervical Q05.0
dorsal Q05.1
lumbar Q05.2
lumbosacral Q05.2
sacral Q05.3
thoracic Q05.1
thoracolumbar Q05.1
specified NEC Q03.8
due to toxoplasmosis (congenital) P37.1
foramen Magendie block (acquired) G91.1
congenital —*see also* Hydrocephalus, congenital Q03.1
in (due to)
infectious disease NEC B89 *[G91.4]*
neoplastic disease NEC (*see also* Neoplasm) G91.4
parasitic disease B89 *[G91.4]*
newborn Q03.9
with spina bifida —*see* Spina bifida, with hydrocephalus
noncommunicating G91.1
normal pressure G91.2
secondary G91.0
obstructive G91.1
otitic G93.2
post-traumatic NEC G91.3
secondary G91.4
post-traumatic G91.3
specified NEC G91.8
syphilitic, congenital A50.49
Hydrocolpos (congenital) N89.8
Hydrocystoma —*see* Neoplasm, skin, benign
Hydroencephalocele (congenital) —*see* Encephalocele
Hydroencephalomeningocele (congenital) —*see* Encephalocele
Hydrohematopneumothorax —*see* Hemothorax
Hydromeningitis —*see* Meningitis
Hydromeningocele (spinal) —*see also* Spina bifida
cranial —*see* Encephalocele
Hydrometra N85.8
Hydrometrocolpos N89.8
Hydromicrocephaly Q02
Hydromphalos (since birth) Q45.8
Hydromyelia Q06.4
Hydromyelocele —*see* Spina bifida
Hydronephrosis (atrophic) (early) (functionless) (intermittent) (primary) (secondary) NEC N13.30
with
infection N13.6
obstruction (by) (of)
renal calculus N13.2
with infection N13.6
ureteral NEC N13.1
with infection N13.6
calculus N13.2
with infection N13.6
ureteropelvic junction (congenital) Q62.0
~~with infection N13.6~~
acquired N13.0 ◀
with infection N13.6 ◀
ureteral stricture NEC N13.1
with infection N13.6

Hydronephrosis NEC *(Continued)*
congenital Q62.0
due to acquired occlusion of ureteropelvic junction N13.0 ◀
specified type NEC N13.39
tuberculous A18.11
Hydropericarditis —*see* Pericarditis
Hydropericardium —*see* Pericarditis
Hydroperitoneum R18.8
Hydrophobia —*see* Rabies
Hydrophthalmos Q15.0
Hydropneumohemothorax —*see* Hemothorax
Hydropneumopericarditis —*see* Pericarditis
Hydropneumopericardium —*see* Pericarditis
Hydropneumothorax J94.8
traumatic —*see* Injury, intrathoracic, lung
tuberculous NEC A15.6
Hydrops R60.9
abdominis R18.8
articulorum intermittens —*see* Hydrarthrosis, intermittent
cardiac —*see* Failure, heart, congestive
causing obstructed labor (mother) O66.3
endolymphatic H81.0-
fetal —*see* Pregnancy, complicated by, hydrops, fetalis
fetalis P83.2
due to
ABO isoimmunization P56.0
alpha thalassemia D56.0
hemolytic disease P56.90
specified NEC P56.99
isoimmunization (ABO) (Rh) P56.0
other specified nonhemolytic disease NEC P83.2
Rh incompatibility P56.0
during pregnancy —*see* Pregnancy, complicated by, hydrops, fetalis
gallbladder K82.1
joint —*see* Effusion, joint
labyrinth H81.0
newborn (idiopathic) P83.2
due to
ABO isoimmunization P56.0
alpha thalassemia D56.0
hemolytic disease P56.90
specified NEC P56.99
isoimmunization (ABO) (Rh) P56.0
Rh incompatibility P56.0
nutritional —*see* Malnutrition, severe
pericardium —*see* Pericarditis
pleura —*see* Hydrothorax
spermatic cord —*see* Hydrocele
Hydropyonephrosis N13.6
Hydrorachis Q06.4
Hydrorrhea (nasal) J34.89
pregnancy —*see* Rupture, membranes, premature
Hydrosadenitis (axillaris) (suppurative) L73.2
Hydrosalpinx (fallopian tube) (follicularis) N70.11
Hydrothorax (double) (pleura) J94.8
chylous (nonfilarial) I89.8
filarial —*see also* Infestation, filarial B74.9 *[J91.8]*
traumatic —*see* Injury, intrathoracic
tuberculous NEC (non primary) A15.6
Hydroureter —*see also* Hydronephrosis N13.4
with infection N13.6
congenital Q62.39
Hydroureteronephrosis —*see* Hydronephrosis
Hydrourethra N36.8
Hydroxykynureninuria E70.8
Hydroxylysinemia E72.3
Hydroxyprolinemia E72.59
Hygiene, sleep
abuse Z72.821
inadequate Z72.821
poor Z72.821
Hygroma (congenital) (cystic) D18.1
praepatellare, prepatellar —*see* Bursitis, prepatellar
Hymen —*see* condition
Hymenolepis, hymenolepiasis (diminuta) (infection) (infestation) (nana) B71.0
Hypalgesia R20.8
Hyperacidity (gastric) K31.89
psychogenic F45.8
Hyperactive, hyperactivity F90.9
basal cell, uterine cervix —*see* Dysplasia, cervix
bowel sounds R19.12
cervix epithelial (basal) —*see* Dysplasia, cervix
child F90.9
attention deficit —*see* Disorder, attention-deficit hyperactivity
detrusor muscle N32.81
gastrointestinal K31.89
psychogenic F45.8
nasal mucous membrane J34.3
stomach K31.89
thyroid (gland) —*see* Hyperthyroidism
Hyperacusis H93.23-
Hyperadrenalism E27.5
Hyperadrenocorticism E24.9
congenital E25.0
iatrogenic E24.2
correct substance properly administered —*see* Table of Drugs and Chemicals, by drug, adverse effect
overdose or wrong substance given or taken —*see* Table of Drugs and Chemicals, by drug, poisoning
not associated with Cushing's syndrome E27.0
pituitary-dependent E24.0
Hyperaldosteronism E26.9
familial (type I) E26.02
glucocorticoid-remediable E26.02
primary (due to (bilateral) adrenal hyperplasia) E26.09
primary NEC E26.09
secondary E26.1
specified NEC E26.89
Hyperalgesia R20.8
Hyperalimentation R63.2
carotene, carotin E67.1
specified NEC E67.8
vitamin
A E67.0
D E67.3
Hyperaminoaciduria
arginine E72.21
cystine E72.01
lysine E72.3
ornithine E72.4
Hyperammonemia (congenital) E72.20
Hyperazotemia —*see* Uremia
Hyperbetalipoproteinemia (familial) E78.00 ⟸
with prebetalipoproteinemia E78.2
Hyperbilirubinemia
constitutional E80.6
familial conjugated E80.6
neonatal (transient) —*see* Jaundice, newborn
Hypercalcemia, hypocalciuric, familial E83.52
Hypercalciuria, idiopathic E83.52
Hypercapnia R06.89
newborn P84
Hypercarotenemia, hypercarotinemia (dietary) E67.1
Hypercementosis K03.4
Hyperchloremia E87.8
Hyperchlorhydria K31.89
neurotic F45.8
psychogenic F45.8
Hypercholesterinemia —*see* Hypercholesterolemia
Hypercholesterolemia (essential) (primary) (pure) E78.00 ⟸
with hyperglyceridemia, endogenous E78.2
dietary counseling and surveillance Z71.3
familial E78.01 ◀
hereditary E78.01 ◀
Hyperchylia gastrica, psychogenic F45.8
Hyperchylomicronemia (familial) (primary) E78.3
with hyperbetalipoproteinemia E78.3
Hypercoagulable (state) D68.59
activated protein C resistance D68.51
antithrombin (III) deficiency D68.59
factor V Leiden mutation D68.51
primary NEC D68.59
protein C deficiency D68.59
protein S deficiency D68.59
prothrombin gene mutation D68.52
secondary D68.69
specified NEC D68.69
Hypercoagulation (state) D68.59
Hypercorticalism, pituitary-dependent E24.0
Hypercorticosolism —*see* Cushing's, syndrome
Hypercorticosteronism E24.2
correct substance properly administered —*see* Table of Drugs and Chemicals, by drug, adverse effect
overdose or wrong substance given or taken —*see* Table of Drugs and Chemicals, by drug, poisoning
Hypercortisonism E24.2
correct substance properly administered —*see* Table of Drugs and Chemicals, by drug, adverse effect
overdose or wrong substance given or taken —*see* Table of Drugs and Chemicals, by drug, poisoning
Hyperekplexia Q89.8
Hyperelectrolytemia E87.8
Hyperemesis R11.10
with nausea R11.2
gravidarum (mild) O21.0
with
carbohydrate depletion O21.1
dehydration O21.1
electrolyte imbalance O21.1
metabolic disturbance O21.1
severe (with metabolic disturbance) O21.1
projectile R11.12
psychogenic F45.8
Hyperemia (acute) (passive) R68.89
anal mucosa K62.89
bladder N32.89
cerebral I67.89
conjunctiva H11.43-
ear internal, acute —*see* subcategory H83.0
enteric K59.8
eye —*see* Hyperemia, conjunctiva
eyelid (active) (passive) —*see* Disorder, eyelid, specified type NEC
intestine K59.8
iris —*see* Disorder, iris, vascular
kidney N28.89
labyrinth —*see* subcategory H83.0
liver (active) K76.89
lung (passive) —*see* Edema, lung
pulmonary (passive) —*see* Edema, lung
renal N28.89
retina H35.89
stomach K31.89
Hyperesthesia (body surface) R20.3
larynx (reflex) J38.7
hysterical F44.89
pharynx (reflex) J39.2
hysterical F44.89
Hyperestrogenism (drug-induced) (iatrogenic) E28.0
Hyperexplexia Q89.8
Hyperfibrinolysis —*see* Fibrinolysis
Hyperfructosemia E74.19
Hyperfunction
adrenal cortex, not associated with Cushing's syndrome E27.0
medulla E27.5
adrenomedullary E27.5
virilism E25.9
congenital E25.0

◀ New ⟸ Revised ~~deleted~~ Deleted

Hyperfunction *(Continued)*
ovarian E28.8
pancreas K86.89 ◄
parathyroid (gland) E21.3
pituitary (gland) (anterior) E22.9
specified NEC E22.8
polyglandular E31.1
testicular E29.0
Hypergammaglobulinemia D89.2
polyclonal D89.0
Waldenström D89.0
Hypergastrinemia E16.4
Hyperglobulinemia R77.1
Hyperglycemia, hyperglycemic (transient) R73.9
coma —*see* Diabetes, by type, with coma
postpancreatectomy E89.1
Hyperglyceridemia (endogenous) (essential) (familial) (hereditary) (pure) E78.1
mixed E78.3
Hyperglycinemia (non-ketotic) E72.51
Hypergonadism
ovarian E28.8
testicular (primary) (infantile) E29.0
Hyperheparinemia D68.32
Hyperhidrosis, hyperidrosis R61
focal
primary L74.519
axilla L74.510
face L74.511
palms L74.512
soles L74.513
secondary L74.52
generalized R61
localized
primary L74.519
axilla L74.510
face L74.511
palms L74.512
soles L74.513
secondary L74.52
psychogenic F45.8
secondary R61
focal L74.52
Hyperhistidinemia E70.41
Hyperhomocysteinemia E72.11
Hyperhydroxyprolinemia E72.59
Hyperinsulinism (functional) E16.1
with
coma (hypoglycemic) E15
encephalopathy E16.1 *[G94]*
ectopic E16.1
therapeutic misadventure (from administration of insulin) —*see* subcategory T38.3
Hyperkalemia E87.5
Hyperkeratosis —*see also* Keratosis L85.9
cervix N88.0
due to yaws (early) (late) (palmar or plantar) A66.3
follicularis Q82.8
penetrans (in cutem) L87.0
palmoplantaris climacterica L85.1
pinta A67.1
senile (with pruritus) L57.0
universalis congenita Q80.8
vocal cord J38.3
vulva N90.4
Hyperkinesia, hyperkinetic (disease) (reaction) (syndrome) (childhood) (adolescence) —*see also* Disorder, attention-deficit hyperactivity
heart I51.89
Hyperleucine-isoleucinemia E71.19
Hyperlipemia, hyperlipidemia E78.5
combined E78.2
familial E78.4
group
A E78.00 ◄
B E78.1
C E78.2
D E78.3
mixed E78.2
specified NEC E78.4
Hyperlipidosis E75.6
hereditary NEC E75.5
Hyperlipoproteinemia E78.5
Fredrickson's type
I E78.3
IIa E78.00 ◄
IIb E78.2
III E78.2
IV E78.1
V E78.3
low-density-lipoprotein-type (LDL) E78.00 ◄
very-low-density-lipoprotein-type (VLDL) E78.1
Hyperlucent lung, unilateral J43.0
Hyperlysinemia E72.3
Hypermagnesemia E83.41
neonatal P71.8
Hypermenorrhea N92.0
Hypermethioninemia E72.19
Hypermetropia (congenital) H52.0-
Hypermobility, hypermotility
cecum —*see* Syndrome, irritable bowel
coccyx —*see* subcategory M53.2
colon —*see* Syndrome, irritable bowel
psychogenic F45.8
ileum K58.9
intestine —*see also* Syndrome, irritable bowel K58.9
psychogenic F45.8
meniscus (knee) —*see* Derangement, knee, meniscus
scapula —*see* Instability, joint, shoulder
stomach K31.89
psychogenic F45.8
syndrome M35.7
urethra N36.41
with intrinsic sphincter deficiency N36.43
Hypernasality R49.21
Hypernatremia E87.0
Hypernephroma C64.-
Hyperopia —*see* Hypermetropia
Hyperorexia nervosa F50.2
Hyperornithinemia E72.4
Hyperosmia R43.1
Hyperosmolality E87.0
Hyperostosis (monomelic) —*see also* Disorder, bone, density and structure, specified NEC
ankylosing (spine) M48.10
cervical region M48.12
cervicothoracic region M48.13
lumbar region M48.16
lumbosacral region M48.17
multiple sites M48.19
occipito-atlanto-axial region M48.11
sacrococcygeal region M48.18
thoracic region M48.14
thoracolumbar region M48.15
cortical (skull) M85.2
infantile M89.8X-
frontal, internal of skull M85.2
interna frontalis M85.2
skeletal, diffuse idiopathic —*see* Hyperostosis, ankylosing
skull M85.2
congenital Q75.8
vertebral, ankylosing —*see* Hyperostosis, ankylosing
Hyperovarism E28.8
Hyperoxaluria (primary) E72.53
Hyperparathyroidism E21.3
primary E21.0
secondary (renal) N25.81
non-renal E21.1
specified NEC E21.2
tertiary E21.2
Hyperpathia R20.8
Hyperperistalsis R19.2
psychogenic F45.8
Hyperpermeability, capillary I78.8
Hyperphagia R63.2
Hyperphenylalaninemia NEC E70.1
Hyperphoria (alternating) H50.53
Hyperphosphatemia E83.39
Hyperpiesis, hyperpiesia —*see* Hypertension
Hyperpigmentation —*see also* Pigmentation
melanin NEC L81.4
postinflammatory L81.0
Hyperpinealism E34.8
Hyperpituitarism E22.9
Hyperplasia, hyperplastic
adenoids J35.2
adrenal (capsule) (cortex) (gland) E27.8
with
sexual precocity (male) E25.9
congenital E25.0
virilism, adrenal E25.9
congenital E25.0
virilization (female) E25.9
congenital E25.0
congenital E25.0
salt-losing E25.0
adrenomedullary E27.5
angiolymphoid, eosinophilia (ALHE) D18.01
appendix (lymphoid) K38.0
artery, fibromuscular I77.3
bone —*see also* Hypertrophy, bone
marrow D75.89
breast —*see also* Hypertrophy, breast
ductal (atypical) N60.9-
C-cell, thyroid E07.0
cementation (tooth) (teeth) K03.4
cervical gland R59.0
cervix (uteri) (basal cell) (endometrium) (polypoid) —*see also* Dysplasia, cervix
congenital Q51.828
clitoris, congenital Q52.6
denture K06.2
endocervicitis N72
endometrium, endometrial (adenomatous) (benign) (cystic) (glandular) (glandular-cystic) (polypoid) N85.00
with atypia N85.02
cervix —*see* Dysplasia, cervix
complex (without atypia) N85.01
simple (without atypia) N85.01
epithelial L85.9
focal, oral, including tongue K13.29
nipple N62
skin L85.9
tongue K13.29
vaginal wall N89.3
erythroid D75.89
fibromuscular of artery (carotid) (renal) I77.3
genital
female NEC N94.89
male N50.89 ◄
gingiva K06.1
glandularis cystica uteri (interstitialis) —*see also* Hyperplasia, endometrial N85.00-
gum K06.1
hymen, congenital Q52.4
irritative, edentulous (alveolar) K06.2
jaw M26.09
alveolar M26.79
lower M26.03
alveolar M26.72
upper M26.01
alveolar M26.71
kidney (congenital) Q63.3
labia N90.69 ◄
epithelial N90.3
liver (congenital) Q44.7
nodular, focal K76.89
lymph gland or node R59.9
mandible, mandibular M26.03
alveolar M26.72
unilateral condylar M27.8
maxilla, maxillary M26.01
alveolar M26.71
myometrium, myometrial N85.2
neuroendocrine cell, of infancy J84.841

H

Hyperplasia, hyperplastic *(Continued)*
nose
lymphoid J34.89
polypoid J33.9
oral mucosa (irritative) K13.6
organ or site, congenital NEC —*see* Anomaly, by site
ovary N83.8
palate, papillary (irritative) K13.6
pancreatic islet cells E16.9
alpha E16.8
with excess
gastrin E16.4
glucagon E16.3
beta E16.1
parathyroid (gland) E21.0
pharynx (lymphoid) J39.2
prostate (adenofibromatous) (nodular) N40.0
with lower urinary tract symptoms (LUTS) N40.1
without lower urinary tract symptoms (LUTS) N40.0
renal artery I77.89
reticulo-endothelial (cell) D75.89
salivary gland (any) K11.1
Schimmelbusch's —*see* Mastopathy, cystic
suprarenal capsule (gland) E27.8
thymus (gland) (persistent) E32.0
thyroid (gland) —*see* Goiter
tonsils (faucial) (infective) (lingual) (lymphoid) J35.1
with adenoids J35.3
unilateral condylar M27.8
uterus, uterine N85.2
endometrium (glandular) —*see also* Hyperplasia, endometrial N85.00-
vulva N90.69 ⇐
epithelial N90.3
Hyperpnea —*see* Hyperventilation
Hyperpotassemia E87.5
Hyperprebetalipoproteinemia (familial) E78.1
Hyperprolactinemia E22.1
Hyperprolinemia (type I) (type II) E72.59
Hyperproteinemia E88.09
Hyperprothrombinemia, causing coagulation factor deficiency D68.4
Hyperpyrexia R50.9
heat (effects) T67.0
malignant, due to anesthetic T88.3
rheumatic —*see* Fever, rheumatic
unknown origin R50.9
Hyper-reflexia R29.2
Hypersalivation K11.7
Hypersecretion
ACTH (not associated with Cushing's syndrome) E27.0
pituitary E24.0
adrenaline E27.5
adrenomedullary E27.5
androgen (testicular) E29.0
ovarian (drug-induced) (iatrogenic) E28.1
calcitonin E07.0
catecholamine E27.5
corticoadrenal E24.9
cortisol E24.9
epinephrine E27.5
estrogen E28.0
gastric K31.89
psychogenic F45.8
gastrin E16.4
glucagon E16.3
hormone (s)
ACTH (not associated with Cushing's syndrome) E27.0
pituitary E24.0
antidiuretic E22.2
growth E22.0

Hypersecretion *(Continued)*
hormone *(Continued)*
intestinal NEC E34.1
ovarian androgen E28.1
pituitary E22.9
testicular E29.0
thyroid stimulating E05.80
with thyroid storm E05.81
insulin —*see* Hyperinsulinism
lacrimal glands —*see* Epiphora
medulloadrenal E27.5
milk O92.6
ovarian androgens E28.1
salivary gland (any) K11.7
thyrocalcitonin E07.0
upper respiratory J39.8
Hypersegmentation, leukocytic, hereditary D72.0
Hypersensitive, hypersensitiveness, hypersensitivity —*see also* Allergy
carotid sinus G90.01
colon —*see* Irritable, colon
drug T88.7
gastrointestinal K52.29 ⇐
immediate K52.29 ◀
psychogenic F45.8
labyrinth —*see* subcategory H83.2
pain R20.8
pneumonitis —*see* Pneumonitis, allergic
reaction T78.40
upper respiratory tract NEC J39.3
Hypersomnia (organic) G47.10
due to
alcohol
abuse F10.182
dependence F10.282
use F10.982
amphetamines
abuse F15.182
dependence F15.282
use F15.982
caffeine
abuse F15.182
dependence F15.282
use F15.982
cocaine
abuse F14.182
dependence F14.282
use F14.982
drug NEC
abuse F19.182
dependence F19.282
use F19.982
medical condition G47.14
mental disorder F51.13
opioid
abuse F11.182
dependence F11.282
use F11.982
psychoactive substance NEC
abuse F19.182
dependence F19.282
use F19.982
sedative, hypnotic, or anxiolytic
abuse F13.182
dependence F13.282
use F13.982
stimulant NEC
abuse F15.182
dependence F15.282
use F15.982
idiopathic G47.11
with long sleep time G47.11
without long sleep time G47.12
menstrual related G47.13
nonorganic origin F51.11
specified NEC F51.19
not due to a substance or known physiological condition F51.11
specified NEC F51.19

Hypersomnia *(Continued)*
primary F51.11
recurrent G47.13
specified NEC G47.19
Hypersplenia, hypersplenism D73.1
Hyperstimulation, ovaries (associated with induced ovulation) N98.1
Hypersusceptibility —*see* Allergy
Hypertelorism (ocular) (orbital) Q75.2
Hypertension, hypertensive (accelerated) (benign) (essential) (idiopathic) (malignant) (systemic) I10
with
heart involvement (conditions in I51.4-I51.9 due to hypertension) —*see* Hypertension, heart
kidney involvement —*see* Hypertension, kidney
benign, intracranial G93.2
borderline R03.0
cardiorenal (disease) I13.10
with heart failure I13.0
with stage 1 through stage 4 chronic kidney disease I13.0
with stage 5 or end stage renal disease I13.2
without heart failure I13.10
with stage 1 through stage 4 chronic kidney disease I13.10
with stage 5 or end stage renal disease I13.11
cardiovascular
disease (arteriosclerotic) (sclerotic) —*see* Hypertension, heart
renal (disease) —*see* Hypertension, cardiorenal
chronic venous —*see* Hypertension, venous (chronic)
complicating
childbirth (labor) O16.4 ⇐
~~with~~
~~heart disease O10.12~~
~~with renal disease O10.32~~
~~renal disease O10.22~~
~~with heart disease O10.32~~
~~essential O10.02~~
pre-existing O10.92 ◀
with ◀
heart disease O10.12 ◀
with renal disease O10.32 ◀
pre-eclampsia O11.4 ◀
renal disease O10.22 ◀
with heart disease O10.32 ◀
essential O10.02 ◀
secondary O10.42
pregnancy O16.-
with edema —*see also* Pre-eclampsia O14.9-
gestational (pregnancy induced) (without proteinuria) O13.- ⇐
with proteinuria O14.9-
mild pre-eclampsia O14.0-
moderate pre-eclampsia O14.0-
severe pre-eclampsia O14.1-
with hemolysis, elevated liver enzymes and low platelet count (HELLP) O14.2-
pre-existing O10.91-
with
heart disease O10.11-
with renal disease O10.31-
pre-eclampsia —*see* category O11 ⇐
renal disease O10.21-
with heart disease O10.31-
essential O10.01-
secondary O10.41-
transient O13.- ◀

◀ New ⇐ Revised ~~deleted~~ Deleted

Hypertension, hypertensive *(Continued)*
complicating *(Continued)*
puerperium pre-existing O16.5 ◀
~~with~~
~~heart disease O10.13~~
~~with renal disease O10.33~~
~~renal disease O10.23~~
~~with heart disease O10.33~~
~~essential O10.03~~
pre-existing ◀
with ◀
heart disease O10.13 ◀
with renal disease O10.33 ◀
pre-eclampsia O11.5 ◀
renal disease O10.23 ◀
with heart disease O10.33 ◀
essential O10.03 ◀
pregnancy-induced O13.9
secondary O10.43
crisis I16.9 ◀
due to
endocrine disorders I15.2
pheochromocytoma I15.2
renal disorders NEC I15.1
arterial I15.0
renovascular disorders I15.0
specified disease NEC I15.8
emergency I16.2 ◀
encephalopathy I67.4
gestational (without significant proteinuria) (pregnancy-induced) (transient) O13.-
with significant proteinuria —*see* Pre-eclampsia
complicating ◀
delivery O13.4 ◀
puerperium O13.5 ◀
Goldblatt's I70.1
heart (disease) (conditions in I51.4-I51.9 due to hypertension) I11.9
with
heart failure (congestive) I11.0
kidney disease (chronic) —*see* Hypertension, cardiorenal
intracranial (benign) G93.2
kidney I12.9
with
heart disease —*see* Hypertension, cardiorenal
stage 1 through stage 4 chronic kidney disease I12.9
stage 5 chronic kidney disease (CKD) or end stage renal disease (ESRD) I12.0
lesser circulation I27.0
maternal O16.- ◀
newborn P29.2
pulmonary (persistent) P29.3
ocular H40.05-
pancreatic duct — code to underlying condition
with chronic pancreatitis K86.1
portal (due to chronic liver disease) (idiopathic) K76.6
gastropathy K31.89
in (due to) schistosomiasis (bilharziasis) B65.9 *[K77]*
postoperative I97.3
psychogenic F45.8
pulmonary (artery) (secondary) NEC I27.2
with
cor pulmonale (chronic) I27.2
acute I26.09
right heart ventricular strain/failure I27.2
acute I26.09
of newborn (persistent) P29.3
primary (idiopathic) I27.0
renal —*see* Hypertension, kidney
renovascular I15.0

Hypertension, hypertensive *(Continued)*
secondary NEC I15.9
due to
endocrine disorders I15.2
pheochromocytoma I15.2
renal disorders NEC I15.1
arterial I15.0
renovascular disorders I15.0
specified NEC I15.8
transient, of pregnancy O13.- ◀
urgency I16.0 ◀
venous (chronic)
due to
deep vein thrombosis —*see* Syndrome, postthrombotic
idiopathic I87.309
with
inflammation I87.32-
with ulcer I87.33-
specified complication NEC I87.39-
ulcer I87.31-
with inflammation I87.33-
asymptomatic I87.30-
Hypertensive urgency —*see* Hypertension
Hyperthecosis ovary E28.8
Hyperthermia (of unknown origin) —*see also* Hyperpyrexia
malignant, due to anesthesia T88.3
newborn P81.9
environmental P81.0
Hyperthyroid (recurrent) —*see* Hyperthyroidism
Hyperthyroidism (latent) (pre-adult) (recurrent) E05.90
with
goiter (diffuse) E05.00
with thyroid storm E05.01
nodular (multinodular) E05.20
with thyroid storm E05.21
uninodular E05.10
with thyroid storm E05.11
storm E05.91
due to ectopic thyroid tissue E05.30
with thyroid storm E05.31
neonatal, transitory P72.1
specified NEC E05.80
with thyroid storm E05.81
Hypertony, hypertonia, hypertonicity
bladder N31.8
congenital P94.1
stomach K31.89
psychogenic F45.8
uterus, uterine (contractions) (complicating delivery) O62.4
Hypertrichosis L68.9
congenital Q84.2
eyelid H02.869
left H02.866
lower H02.865
upper H02.864
right H02.863
lower H02.862
upper H02.861
lanuginosa Q84.2
acquired L68.1
localized L68.2
specified NEC L68.8
Hypertriglyceridemia, essential E78.1
Hypertrophy, hypertrophic
adenofibromatous, prostate —*see* Enlargement, enlarged, prostate
adenoids (infective) J35.2
with tonsils J35.3
adrenal cortex E27.8
alveolar process or ridge —*see* Anomaly, alveolar
anal papillae K62.89
artery I77.89
congenital NEC Q27.8
digestive system Q27.8
lower limb Q27.8

Hypertrophy, hypertrophic *(Continued)*
artery *(Continued)*
congenital NEC *(Continued)*
specified site NEC Q27.8
upper limb Q27.8
auricular —*see* Hypertrophy, cardiac
Bartholin's gland N75.8
bile duct (common) (hepatic) K83.8
bladder (sphincter) (trigone) N32.89
bone M89.30
carpus M89.34-
clavicle M89.31-
femur M89.35-
fibula M89.36-
finger M89.34-
humerus M89.32-
ilium M89.359
ischium M89.359
metacarpus M89.34-
metatarsus M89.37-
multiple sites M89.39
neck M89.38
radius M89.33-
rib M89.38
scapula M89.31-
skull M89.38
tarsus M89.37-
tibia M89.36-
toe M89.37-
ulna M89.33-
vertebra M89.38
brain G93.89
breast N62
cystic —*see* Mastopathy, cystic
newborn P83.4
pubertal, massive N62
puerperal, postpartum —*see* Disorder, breast, specified type NEC
senile (parenchymatous) N62
cardiac (chronic) (idiopathic) I51.7
with rheumatic fever (conditions in I00)
active I01.8
inactive or quiescent (with chorea) I09.89
congenital NEC Q24.8
fatty —*see* Degeneration, myocardial
hypertensive —*see* Hypertension, heart
rheumatic (with chorea) I09.89
active or acute I01.8
with chorea I02.0
valve —*see* Endocarditis
cartilage —*see* Disorder, cartilage, specified type NEC
cecum —*see* Megacolon
cervix (uteri) N88.8
congenital Q51.828
elongation N88.4
clitoris (cirrhotic) N90.89
congenital Q52.6
colon —*see also* Megacolon
congenital Q43.2
conjunctiva, lymphoid H11.89
corpora cavernosa N48.89
cystic duct K82.8
duodenum K31.89
endometrium (glandular) —*see also* Hyperplasia, endometrial N85.00-
cervix N88.8
epididymis N50.89 ◀
esophageal hiatus (congenital) Q79.1
with hernia —*see* Hernia, hiatal
eyelid —*see* Disorder, eyelid, specified type NEC
fat pad E65
knee (infrapatellar) (popliteal) (prepatellar) (retropatellar) M79.4
foot (congenital) Q74.2
frenulum, frenum (tongue) K14.8
lip K13.0
gallbladder K82.8
gastric mucosa K29.60
with bleeding K29.61

H

Hypertrophy, hypertrophic *(Continued)*
gland, glandular R59.9
generalized R59.1
localized R59.0
gum (mucous membrane) K06.1
heart (idiopathic) —*see also* Hypertrophy, cardiac
valve —*see also* Endocarditis I38
hemifacial Q67.4
hepatic —*see* Hypertrophy, liver
hiatus (esophageal) Q79.1
hilus gland R59.0
hymen, congenital Q52.4
ileum K63.89
intestine NEC K63.89
jejunum K63.89
kidney (compensatory) N28.81
congenital Q63.3
labium (majus) (minus) N90.60 ◄
ligament —*see* Disorder, ligament
lingual tonsil (infective) J35.1
with adenoids J35.3
lip K13.0
congenital Q18.6
liver R16.0
acute K76.89
cirrhotic —*see* Cirrhosis, liver
congenital Q44.7
fatty —*see* Fatty, liver
lymph, lymphatic gland R59.9
generalized R59.1
localized R59.0
tuberculous —*see* Tuberculosis, lymph gland
mammary gland —*see* Hypertrophy, breast
Meckel's diverticulum (congenital) Q43.0
malignant —*see* Table of Neoplasms, small intestine, malignant
median bar —*see* Hyperplasia, prostate
meibomian gland —*see* Chalazion
meniscus, knee, congenital Q74.1
metatarsal head —*see* Hypertrophy, bone, metatarsus
metatarsus —*see* Hypertrophy, bone, metatarsus
mucous membrane
alveolar ridge K06.2
gum K06.1
nose (turbinate) J34.3
muscle M62.89
muscular coat, artery I77.89
myocardium —*see also* Hypertrophy, cardiac
idiopathic I42.2
myometrium N85.2
nail L60.2
congenital Q84.5
nasal J34.89
alae J34.89
bone J34.89
cartilage J34.89
mucous membrane (septum) J34.3
sinus J34.89
turbinate J34.3
nasopharynx, lymphoid (infectional) (tissue) (wall) J35.2
nipple N62
organ or site, congenital NEC —*see* Anomaly, by site - ovary N83.8
palate (hard) M27.8
soft K13.79
pancreas, congenital Q45.3
parathyroid (gland) E21.0
parotid gland K11.1
penis N48.89
pharyngeal tonsil J35.2
pharynx J39.2
lymphoid (infectional) (tissue) (wall) J35.2
pituitary (anterior) (fossa) (gland) E23.6
prepuce (congenital) N47.8
female N90.89

Hypertrophy, hypertrophic *(Continued)*
prostate —*see* Enlargement, enlarged, prostate
congenital Q55.4
pseudomuscular G71.0
pylorus (adult) (muscle) (sphincter) K31.1
congenital or infantile Q40.0
rectal, rectum (sphincter) K62.89
rhinitis (turbinate) J31.0
salivary gland (any) K11.1
congenital Q38.4
scaphoid (tarsal) —*see* Hypertrophy, bone, tarsus
scar L91.0
scrotum N50.89 ◄
seminal vesicle N50.89 ◄
sigmoid —*see* Megacolon
skin L91.9
specified NEC L91.8
spermatic cord N50.89 ◄
spleen —*see* Splenomegaly
spondylitis —*see* Spondylosis
stomach K31.89
sublingual gland K11.1
submandibular gland K11.1
suprarenal cortex (gland) E27.8
synovial NEC M67.20
acromioclavicular M67.21-
ankle M67.27-
elbow M67.22-
foot M67.27-
hand M67.24-
hip M67.25-
knee M67.26-
multiple sites M67.29
specified site NEC M67.28
wrist M67.23-
tendon —*see* Disorder, tendon, specified type NEC
testis N44.8
congenital Q55.29
thymic, thymus (gland) (congenital) E32.0
thyroid (gland) —*see* Goiter
toe (congenital) Q74.2
acquired —*see also* Deformity, toe, specified NEC
tongue K14.8
congenital Q38.2
papillae (foliate) K14.3
tonsils (faucial) (infective) (lingual) (lymphoid) J35.1
with adenoids J35.3
tunica vaginalis N50.89 ◄
ureter N28.89
urethra N36.8
uterus N85.2
neck (with elongation) N88.4
puerperal O90.89
uvula K13.79
vagina N89.8
vas deferens N50.89 ◄
vein I87.8
ventricle, ventricular (heart) —*see also* Hypertrophy, cardiac
congenital Q24.8
in tetralogy of Fallot Q21.3
verumontanum N36.8
vocal cord J38.3
vulva N90.60 ◄
stasis (nonfilarial) N90.69 ◄
Hypertropia H50.2-
Hypertyrosinemia E70.21
Hyperuricemia (asymptomatic) E79.0
Hypervalinemia E71.19
Hyperventilation (tetany) R06.4
hysterical F45.8
psychogenic F45.8
syndrome F45.8

Hypervitaminosis (dietary) NEC E67.8
A E67.0
administered as drug (prolonged intake) —*see* Table of Drugs and Chemicals, vitamins, adverse effect
overdose or wrong substance given or taken —*see* Table of Drugs and Chemicals, vitamins, poisoning
B6 E67.2
D E67.3
administered as drug (prolonged intake) —*see* Table of Drugs and Chemicals, vitamins, adverse effect
overdose or wrong substance given or taken —*see* Table of Drugs and Chemicals, vitamins, poisoning
K E67.8
administered as drug (prolonged intake) —*see* Table of Drugs and Chemicals, vitamins, adverse effect
overdose or wrong substance given or taken —*see* Table of Drugs and Chemicals, vitamins, poisoning
Hypervolemia E87.70
specified NEC E87.79
Hypesthesia R20.1
cornea —*see* Anesthesia, cornea
Hyphema H21.0-
traumatic S05.1-
Hypoacidity, gastric K31.89
psychogenic F45.8
Hypoadrenalism, hypoadrenia E27.40
primary E27.1
tuberculous A18.7
Hypoadrenocorticism E27.40
pituitary E23.0
primary E27.1
Hypoalbuminemia E88.09
Hypoaldosteronism E27.40
Hypoalphalipoproteinemia E78.6
Hypobarism T70.29
Hypobaropathy T70.29
Hypobetalipoproteinemia (familial) E78.6
Hypocalcemia E83.51
dietary E58
neonatal P71.1
due to cow's milk P71.0
phosphate-loading (newborn) P71.1
Hypochloremia E87.8
Hypochlorhydria K31.89
neurotic F45.8
psychogenic F45.8
Hypochondria, hypochondriac, hypochondriasis (reaction) F45.21
sleep F51.03
Hypochondrogenesis Q77.0
Hypochondroplasia Q77.4
Hypochromasia, blood cells D50.8
Hypodontia —*see* Anodontia
Hypoeosinophilia D72.89
Hypoesthesia R20.1
Hypofibrinogenemia D68.8
acquired D65
congenital (hereditary) D68.2
Hypofunction
adrenocortical E27.40
drug-induced E27.3
postprocedural E89.6
primary E27.1
adrenomedullary, postprocedural E89.6
cerebral R29.818
corticoadrenal NEC E27.40
intestinal K59.8
labyrinth —*see* subcategory H83.2
ovary E28.39
pituitary (gland) (anterior) E23.0
testicular E29.1
postprocedural (postsurgical) (postirradiation) (iatrogenic) E89.5
Hypogalactia O92.4

◄ New ◄ Revised ~~deleted~~ Deleted

Hypogammaglobulinemia —*see also* Agammaglobulinemia D80.1
hereditary D80.0
nonfamilial D80.1
transient, of infancy D80.7
Hypogenitalism (congenital) —*see* Hypogonadism
Hypoglossia Q38.3
Hypoglycemia (spontaneous) E16.2
coma E15
diabetic —*see* Diabetes, coma
diabetic —*see* Diabetes, hypoglycemia
dietary counseling and surveillance Z71.3
drug-induced E16.0
with coma (nondiabetic) E15
due to insulin E16.0
with coma (nondiabetic) E15
therapeutic misadventure —*see* subcategory T38.3
functional, nonhyperinsulinemic E16.1
iatrogenic E16.0
with coma (nondiabetic) E15
in infant of diabetic mother P70.1
gestational diabetes P70.0
infantile E16.1
leucine-induced E71.19
neonatal (transitory) P70.4
iatrogenic P70.3
reactive (not drug-induced) E16.1
transitory neonatal P70.4
Hypogonadism
female E28.39
hypogonadotropic E23.0
male E29.1
ovarian (primary) E28.39
pituitary E23.0
testicular (primary) E29.1
Hypohidrosis, hypoidrosis L74.4
Hypoinsulinemia, postprocedural E89.1
Hypokalemia E87.6
Hypoleukocytosis —*see* Agranulocytosis
Hypolipoproteinemia (alpha) (beta) E78.6
Hypomagnesemia E83.42
neonatal P71.2
Hypomania, hypomanic reaction F30.8
Hypomenorrhea —*see* Oligomenorrhea
Hypometabolism R63.8
Hypomotility
gastrointestinal (tract) K31.89
psychogenic F45.8
intestine K59.8
psychogenic F45.8
stomach K31.89
psychogenic F45.8
Hyponasality R49.22
Hyponatremia E87.1
Hypo-osmolality E87.1
Hypo-ovarianism, hypo-ovarism E28.39
Hypoparathyroidism E20.9
familial E20.8
idiopathic E20.0
neonatal, transitory P71.4
postprocedural E89.2
specified NEC E20.8
Hypoperfusion (in)
newborn P96.89
Hypopharyngitis —*see* Laryngopharyngitis
Hypophoria H50.53
Hypophosphatemia, hypophosphatasia (acquired) (congenital) (renal) E83.39
familial E83.31
Hypophyseal, hypophysis —*see also* condition
dwarfism E23.0
gigantism E22.0
Hypopiesis —*see* Hypotension
Hypopinealism E34.8
Hypopituitarism (juvenile) E23.0
drug-induced E23.1
due to
hypophysectomy E89.3
radiotherapy E89.3
Hypopituitarism *(Continued)*
iatrogenic NEC E23.1
postirradiation E89.3
postpartum O99.285 ◄
postprocedural E89.3
Hypoplasia, hypoplastic
adrenal (gland), congenital Q89.1
alimentary tract, congenital Q45.8
upper Q40.8
anus, anal (canal) Q42.3
with fistula Q42.2
aorta, aortic Q25.42 ◄
ascending, in hypoplastic left heart syndrome Q23.4
valve Q23.1
in hypoplastic left heart syndrome Q23.4
areola, congenital Q83.8
arm (congenital) —*see* Defect, reduction, upper limb
artery (peripheral) Q27.8
brain (congenital) Q28.3
coronary Q24.5
digestive system Q27.8
lower limb Q27.8
pulmonary Q25.79
functional, unilateral J43.0
retinal (congenital) Q14.1
specified site NEC Q27.8
umbilical Q27.0
upper limb Q27.8
auditory canal Q17.8
causing impairment of hearing Q16.9
biliary duct or passage Q44.5
bone NOS Q79.9
face Q75.8
marrow D61.9
megakaryocytic D69.49
skull —*see* Hypoplasia, skull
brain Q02
gyri Q04.3
part of Q04.3
breast (areola) N64.82
bronchus Q32.4
cardiac Q24.8
carpus —*see* Defect, reduction, upper limb, specified type NEC
cartilage hair Q78.8 ◄
cecum Q42.8
cementum K00.4
cephalic Q02
cerebellum Q04.3
cervix (uteri), congenital Q51.821
clavicle (congenital) Q74.0
coccyx Q76.49
colon Q42.9
specified NEC Q42.8
corpus callosum Q04.0
cricoid cartilage Q31.2
digestive organ (s) or tract NEC Q45.8
upper (congenital) Q40.8
ear (auricle) (lobe) Q17.2
middle Q16.4
enamel of teeth (neonatal) (postnatal) (prenatal) K00.4
endocrine (gland) NEC Q89.2
endometrium N85.8
epididymis (congenital) Q55.4
epiglottis Q31.2
erythroid, congenital D61.01
esophagus (congenital) Q39.8
eustachian tube Q17.8
eye Q11.2
eyelid (congenital) Q10.3
face Q18.8
bone (s) Q75.8
femur (congenital) —*see* Defect, reduction, lower limb, specified type NEC
fibula (congenital) —*see* Defect, reduction, lower limb, specified type NEC
Hypoplasia, hypoplastic *(Continued)*
finger (congenital) —*see* Defect, reduction, upper limb, specified type NEC
focal dermal Q82.8
foot —*see* Defect, reduction, lower limb, specified type NEC
gallbladder Q44.0
genitalia, genital organ (s)
female, congenital Q52.8
external Q52.79
internal NEC Q52.8
in adiposogenital dystrophy E23.6
glottis Q31.2
hair Q84.2
hand (congenital) —*see* Defect, reduction, upper limb, specified type NEC
heart Q24.8
humerus (congenital) —*see* Defect, reduction, upper limb, specified type NEC
intestine (small) Q41.9
large Q42.9
specified NEC Q42.8
jaw M26.09
alveolar M26.79
lower M26.04
alveolar M26.74
upper M26.02
alveolar M26.73
kidney (s) Q60.5
bilateral Q60.4
unilateral Q60.3
labium (majus) (minus), congenital Q52.79
larynx Q31.2
left heart syndrome Q23.4
leg (congenital) —*see* Defect, reduction, lower limb
limb Q73.8
lower (congenital) —*see* Defect, reduction, lower limb
upper (congenital) —*see* Defect, reduction, upper limb
liver Q44.7
lung (lobe) (not associated with short gestation) Q33.6
associated with immaturity, low birth weight, prematurity, or short gestation P28.0
mammary (areola), congenital Q83.8
mandible, mandibular M26.04
alveolar M26.74
unilateral condylar M27.8
maxillary M26.02
alveolar M26.73
medullary D61.9
megakaryocytic D69.49
metacarpus —*see* Defect, reduction, upper limb, specified type NEC
metatarsus —*see* Defect, reduction, lower limb, specified type NEC
muscle Q79.8
nail (s) Q84.6
nose, nasal Q30.1
optic nerve H47.03-
osseous meatus (ear) Q17.8
ovary, congenital Q50.39
pancreas Q45.0
parathyroid (gland) Q89.2
parotid gland Q38.4
patella Q74.1
pelvis, pelvic girdle Q74.2
penis (congenital) Q55.62
peripheral vascular system Q27.8
digestive system Q27.8
lower limb Q27.8
specified site NEC Q27.8
upper limb Q27.8
pituitary (gland) (congenital) Q89.2
pulmonary (not associated with short gestation) Q33.6
artery, functional J43.0
associated with short gestation P28.0

H

Hypoplasia, hypoplastic *(Continued)*
radioulnar —*see* Defect, reduction, upper limb, specified type NEC
radius —*see* Defect, reduction, upper limb
rectum Q42.1
with fistula Q42.0
respiratory system NEC Q34.8
rib Q76.6
right heart syndrome Q22.6
sacrum Q76.49
scapula Q74.0
scrotum Q55.1
shoulder girdle Q74.0
skin Q82.8
skull (bone) Q75.8
with
anencephaly Q00.0
encephalocele —*see* Encephalocele
hydrocephalus Q03.9
with spina bifida —*see* Spina bifida, by site, with hydrocephalus
microcephaly Q02
spinal (cord) (ventral horn cell) Q06.1
spine Q76.49
sternum Q76.7
tarsus —*see* Defect, reduction, lower limb, specified type NEC
testis Q55.1
thymic, with immunodeficiency D82.1
thymus (gland) Q89.2
with immunodeficiency D82.1
thyroid (gland) E03.1
cartilage Q31.2
tibiofibular (congenital) —*see* Defect, reduction, lower limb, specified type NEC
toe —*see* Defect, reduction, lower limb, specified type NEC
tongue Q38.3
Turner's K00.4
ulna (congenital) —*see* Defect, reduction, upper limb
umbilical artery Q27.0
unilateral condylar M27.8
ureter Q62.8
uterus, congenital Q51.811
vagina Q52.4
vascular NEC peripheral Q27.8
brain Q28.3
digestive system Q27.8
lower limb Q27.8
specified site NEC Q27.8
upper limb Q27.8
vein (s) (peripheral) Q27.8
brain Q28.3
digestive system Q27.8
great Q26.8
lower limb Q27.8
specified site NEC Q27.8
upper limb Q27.8
vena cava (inferior) (superior) Q26.8
vertebra Q76.49
vulva, congenital Q52.79
zonule (ciliary) Q12.8

Hypopotassemia E87.6
Hypoproconvertinemia, congenital (hereditary) D68.2
Hypoproteinemia E77.8
Hypoprothrombinemia (congenital) (hereditary) (idiopathic) D68.2
acquired D68.4
newborn, transient P61.6
Hypoptyalism K11.7
Hypopyon (eye) (anterior chamber) —*see* Iridocyclitis, acute, hypopyon
Hypopyrexia R68.0
Hyporeflexia R29.2
Hyposecretion
ACTH E23.0
antidiuretic hormone E23.2
ovary E28.39
salivary gland (any) K11.7
vasopressin E23.2
Hyposegmentation, leukocytic, hereditary D72.0
Hyposiderinemia D50.9
Hypospadias Q54.9
balanic Q54.0
coronal Q54.0
glandular Q54.0
penile Q54.1
penoscrotal Q54.2
perineal Q54.3
specified NEC Q54.8
Hypospermatogenesis —*see* Oligospermia
Hyposplenism D73.0
Hypostasis pulmonary, passive —*see* Edema, lung
Hypostatic —*see* condition
Hyposthenuria N28.89
Hypotension (arterial) (constitutional) I95.9
chronic I95.89
drug-induced I95.2
due to (of) hemodialysis I95.3
iatrogenic I95.89
idiopathic (permanent) I95.0
intracranial, following ventricular shunting (ventriculostomy) G97.2
intra-dialytic I95.3
maternal, syndrome (following labor and delivery) O26.5-
neurogenic, orthostatic G90.3
orthostatic (chronic) I95.1
due to drugs I95.2
neurogenic G90.3
postoperative I95.81
postural I95.1
specified NEC I95.89
Hypothermia (accidental) T68
due to anesthesia, anesthetic T88.51
low environmental temperature T68
neonatal P80.9
environmental (mild) NEC P80.8
mild P80.8
severe (chronic) (cold injury syndrome) P80.0
specified NEC P80.8
not associated with low environmental temperature R68.0

Hypothyroidism (acquired) E03.9
congenital (without goiter) E03.1
with goiter (diffuse) E03.0
due to
exogenous substance NEC E03.2
iodine-deficiency, acquired E01.8
subclinical E02
irradiation therapy E89.0
medicament NEC E03.2
P-aminosalicylic acid (PAS) E03.2
phenylbutazone E03.2
resorcinol E03.2
sulfonamide E03.2
surgery E89.0
thiourea group drugs E03.2
iatrogenic NEC E03.2
iodine-deficiency (acquired) E01.8
congenital —*see* Syndrome, iodine-deficiency, congenital
subclinical E02
neonatal, transitory P72.2
postinfectious E03.3
postirradiation E89.0
postprocedural E89.0
postsurgical E89.0
specified NEC E03.8
subclinical, iodine-deficiency related E02
Hypotonia, hypotonicity, hypotony
bladder N31.2
congenital (benign) P94.2
eye —*see* Disorder, globe, hypotony
Hypotrichosis —*see* Alopecia
Hypotropia H50.2-
Hypoventilation R06.89
congenital central alveolar G47.35
sleep related
idiopathic nonobstructive alveolar G47.34
in conditions classified elsewhere G47.36
Hypovitaminosis —*see* Deficiency, vitamin
Hypovolemia E86.1
surgical shock T81.19
traumatic (shock) T79.4
Hypoxemia R09.02
newborn P84
sleep related, in conditions classified elsewhere G47.36
Hypoxia —*see also* Anoxia R09.02
cerebral, during a procedure NEC G97.81
postprocedural NEC G97.82
intrauterine P84
myocardial —*see* Insufficiency, coronary
newborn P84
sleep-related G47.34
Hypsarhythmia —*see* Epilepsy, generalized, specified NEC
Hysteralgia, pregnant uterus O26.89-
Hysteria, hysterical (conversion) (dissociative state) F44.9
anxiety F41.8
convulsions F44.5
psychosis, acute F44.9
Hysteroepilepsy F44.5

H

I

IBDU (colonic inflammatory bowel dissease unclassified) K52.3 ◀
Ichthyoparasitism due to Vandellia cirrhosa B88.8
Ichthyosis (congenital) Q80.9
acquired L85.0
fetalis Q80.4
hystrix Q80.8
lamellar Q80.2
lingual K13.29
palmaris and plantaris Q82.8
simplex Q80.0
vera Q80.8
vulgaris Q80.0
X-linked Q80.1
Ichthyotoxism —*see* Poisoning, fish
bacterial —*see* Intoxication, foodborne
Icteroanemia, hemolytic (acquired) D59.9
congenital —*see* Spherocytosis
Icterus —*see also* Jaundice
conjunctiva R17
gravis, newborn P55.0
hematogenous (acquired) D59.9
hemolytic (acquired) D59.9
congenital —*see* Spherocytosis
hemorrhagic (acute) (leptospiral) (spirochetal) A27.0
newborn P53
infectious B15.9
with hepatic coma B15.0
leptospiral A27.0
spirochetal A27.0
neonatorum —*see* Jaundice, newborn
newborn P59.9
spirochetal A27.0
Ictus solaris, solis T67.0
Ideation
homicidal R45.850
suicidal R45.851
Identity disorder (child) F64.9
gender role F64.2
psychosexual F64.2
Idioglossia F80.0
Idiopathic —*see* condition
Idiot, idiocy (congenital) F73
amaurotic (Bielschowsky(-Jansky)) (family) (infantile (late)) (juvenile (late)) (Vogt-Spielmeyer) E75.4
microcephalic Q02
Id reaction (due to bacteria) L30.2
IgE asthma J45.909
IIAC (idiopathic infantile arterial calcification) Q28.8
Ileitis (chronic) (noninfectious) —*see also* Enteritis K52.9
backwash —*see* Pancolitis, ulcerative (chronic)
infectious A09
regional (ulcerative) —*see* Enteritis, regional, small intestine
segmental —*see* Enteritis, regional
terminal (ulcerative) —*see* Enteritis, regional, small intestine
Ileocolitis —*see also* Enteritis K52.9
infectious A09
regional —*see* Enteritis, regional
Ileostomy
attention to Z43.2
malfunctioning K94.13
status Z93.2
with complication —*see* Complications, enterostomy
Ileotyphus —*see* Typhoid
Ileum —*see* condition
Ileus (bowel) (colon) (inhibitory) (intestine) K56.7
adynamic K56.0
due to gallstone (in intestine) K56.3
duodenal (chronic) K31.5
Ileus *(Continued)*
gallstone K56.3
mechanical NEC K56.69
meconium P76.0
in cystic fibrosis E84.11
meaning meconium plug (without cystic fibrosis) P76.0
myxedema K59.8
neurogenic K56.0
Hirschsprung's disease or megacolon Q43.1
newborn
due to meconium P76.0
in cystic fibrosis E84.11
meaning meconium plug (without cystic fibrosis) P76.0
transitory P76.1
obstructive K56.69
paralytic K56.0
Iliac —*see* condition
Iliotibial band syndrome M76.3-
Illiteracy Z55.0
Illness—*see also* Disease R69
manic-depressive —*see* Disorder, bipolar
Imbalance R26.89
autonomic G90.8
constituents of food intake E63.1
electrolyte E87.8
with
abortion —*see* Abortion by type, complicated by, electrolyte imbalance
molar pregnancy O08.5
due to hyperemesis gravidarum O21.1
following ectopic or molar pregnancy O08.5
neonatal, transitory NEC P74.4
potassium P74.3
sodium P74.2
endocrine E34.9
eye muscle NOS H50.9
hormone E34.9
hysterical F44.4
labyrinth —*see* subcategory H83.2
posture R29.3
protein-energy —*see* Malnutrition
sympathetic G90.8
Imbecile, imbecility (I.Q. 35-49) F71
Imbedding, intrauterine device T83.39
Imbibition, cholesterol (gallbladder) K82.4
Imbrication, teeth, fully erupted M26.30
Imerslund (-Gräsbeck) syndrome D51.1
Immature —*see also* Immaturity
birth (less than 37 completed weeks) —*see* Preterm, newborn
extremely (less than 28 completed weeks) —*see* Immaturity, extreme
personality F60.89
Immaturity (less than 37 completed weeks) —*see also* Preterm, newborn
extreme of newborn (less than 28 completed weeks of gestation) (less than 196 completed days of gestation) (unspecified weeks of gestation) P07.20
gestational age
23 completed weeks (23 weeks, 0 days through 23 weeks, 6 days) P07.22
24 completed weeks (24 weeks, 0 days through 24 weeks, 6 days) P07.23
25 completed weeks (25 weeks, 0 days through 25 weeks, 6 days) P07.24
26 completed weeks (26 weeks, 0 days through 26 weeks, 6 days) P07.25
27 completed weeks (27 weeks, 0 days through 27 weeks, 6 days) P07.26
less than 23 completed weeks P07.21
fetus or infant light-for-dates —*see* Light-for-dates
lung, newborn P28.0
organ or site NEC —*see* Hypoplasia
pulmonary, newborn P28.0
reaction F60.89
sexual (female) (male), after puberty E30.0
Immersion T75.1
foot T69.02-
hand T69.01-
Immobile, immobility
complete, due to severe physical disability or frailty R53.2
intestine K59.8
syndrome (paraplegic) M62.3
Immune reconstitution (inflammatory) syndrome [IRIS] D89.3
Immunization —*see also* Vaccination
ABO —*see* Incompatibility, ABO
in newborn P55.1
complication —*see* Complications, vaccination
encounter for Z23
not done (not carried out) Z28.9
because (of)
acute illness of patient Z28.01
allergy to vaccine (or component) Z28.04
caregiver refusal Z28.82
chronic illness of patient Z28.02
contraindication NEC Z28.09
group pressure Z28.1
guardian refusal Z28.82
immune compromised state of patient Z28.03
parent refusal Z28.82
patient's belief Z28.1
patient had disease being vaccinated against Z28.81
patient refusal Z28.21
religious beliefs of patient Z28.1
specified reason NEC Z28.89
of patient Z28.29
unspecified patient reason Z28.20
Rh factor
affecting management of pregnancy NEC O36.09-
anti-D antibody O36.01-
from transfusion —*see* Complication (s), transfusion, incompatibility reaction, Rh (factor)
Immunocytoma C83.0-
Immunodeficiency D84.9
with
adenosine-deaminase deficiency D81.3
antibody defects D80.9
specified type NEC D80.8
hyperimmunoglobulinemia D80.6
increased immunoglobulin M (IgM) D80.5
major defect D82.9
specified type NEC D82.8
partial albinism D82.8
short-limbed stature D82.2
thrombocytopenia and eczema D82.0
antibody with
hyperimmunoglobulinemia D80.6
near-normal immunoglobulins D80.6
autosomal recessive, Swiss type D80.0
combined D81.9
biotin-dependent carboxylase D81.819
biotinidase D81.810
holocarboxylase synthetase D81.818
specified type NEC D81.818
severe (SCID) D81.9
with
low or normal B-cell numbers D81.2
low T- and B-cell numbers D81.1
reticular dysgenesis D81.0
specified type NEC D81.89
common variable D83.9
with
abnormalities of B-cell numbers and function D83.0
autoantibodies to B- or T-cells D83.2
immunoregulatory T-cell disorders D83.1
specified type NEC D83.8
following hereditary defective response to Epstein-Barr virus (EBV) D82.3

Immunodeficiency *(Continued)*
selective, immunoglobulin
A (IgA) D80.2
G (IgG) (subclasses) D80.3
M (IgM) D80.4
severe combined (SCID) D81.9
specified type NEC D84.8
X-linked, with increased IgM D80.5
Immunotherapy (encounter for)
antineoplastic Z51.12
Impaction, impacted
bowel, colon, rectum —*see also* Impaction, fecal K56.49
by gallstone K56.3
calculus —*see* Calculus
cerumen (ear) (external) H61.2-
cuspid —*see* Impaction, tooth
dental (same or adjacent tooth) K01.1
fecal, feces K56.41
fracture —*see* Fracture, by site
gallbladder —*see* Calculus, gallbladder
gallstone (s) —*see* Calculus, gallbladder
bile duct (common) (hepatic) —*see* Calculus, bile duct
cystic duct —*see* Calculus, gallbladder
in intestine, with obstruction (any part) K56.3
intestine (calculous) NEC —*see also* Impaction, fecal K56.49
gallstone, with ileus K56.3
intrauterine device (IUD) T83.39
molar —*see* Impaction, tooth
shoulder, causing obstructed labor O66.0
tooth, teeth K01.1
turbinate J34.89
Impaired, impairment (function)
auditory discrimination —*see* Abnormal, auditory perception
cognitive, mild, so stated G31.84
dual sensory Z73.82
fasting glucose R73.01
glucose tolerance (oral) R73.02
hearing —*see* Deafness
heart —*see* Disease, heart
kidney N28.9
disorder resulting from N25.9
specified NEC N25.89
liver K72.90
with coma K72.91
mastication K08.89 ◄
mild cognitive, so stated G31.84
mobility
ear ossicles —*see* Ankylosis, ear ossicles
requiring care provider Z74.09
myocardium, myocardial —*see* Insufficiency, myocardial
rectal sphincter R19.8
renal (acute) (chronic) N28.9
disorder resulting from N25.9
specified NEC N25.89
vision NEC H54.7
both eyes H54.3
Impediment, speech R47.9
psychogenic (childhood) F98.8
slurring R47.81
specified NEC R47.89
Impending
coronary syndrome I20.0
delirium tremens F10.239
myocardial infarction I20.0
Imperception auditory (acquired) —*see also* Deafness
congenital H93.25
Imperfect
aeration, lung (newborn) NEC —*see* Atelectasis
closure (congenital)
alimentary tract NEC Q45.8
lower Q43.8
upper Q40.8
atrioventricular ostium Q21.2

Imperfect *(Continued)*
closure *(Continued)*
atrium (secundum) Q21.1
branchial cleft or sinus Q18.0
choroid Q14.3
cricoid cartilage Q31.8
cusps, heart valve NEC Q24.8
pulmonary Q22.3
ductus
arteriosus Q25.0
Botalli Q25.0
ear drum (causing impairment of hearing) Q16.4
esophagus with communication to bronchus or trachea Q39.1
eyelid Q10.3
foramen
botalli Q21.1
ovale Q21.1
genitalia, genital organ (s) or system
female Q52.8
external Q52.79
internal NEC Q52.8
male Q55.8
glottis Q31.8
interatrial ostium or septum Q21.1
interauricular ostium or septum Q21.1
interventricular ostium or septum Q21.0
larynx Q31.8
lip —*see* Cleft, lip
nasal septum Q30.3
nose Q30.2
omphalomesenteric duct Q43.0
optic nerve entry Q14.2
organ or site not listed —*see* Anomaly, by site
ostium
interatrial Q21.1
interauricular Q21.1
interventricular Q21.0
palate —*see* Cleft, palate
preauricular sinus Q18.1
retina Q14.1
roof of orbit Q75.8
sclera Q13.5
septum
aorticopulmonary Q21.4
atrial (secundum) Q21.1
between aorta and pulmonary artery Q21.4
heart Q21.9
interatrial (secundum) Q21.1
interauricular (secundum) Q21.1
interventricular Q21.0
in tetralogy of Fallot Q21.3
nasal Q30.3
ventricular Q21.0
with pulmonary stenosis or atresia, dextraposition of aorta, and hypertrophy of right ventricle Q21.3
in tetralogy of Fallot Q21.3
skull Q75.0
with
anencephaly Q00.0
encephalocele —*see* Encephalocele
hydrocephalus Q03.9
with spina bifida —*see* Spina bifida, by site, with hydrocephalus
microcephaly Q02
spine (with meningocele) —*see* Spina bifida
trachea Q32.1
tympanic membrane (causing impairment of hearing) Q16.4
uterus Q51.818
vitelline duct Q43.0
erection —*see* Dysfunction, sexual, male, erectile
fusion —*see* Imperfect, closure
inflation, lung (newborn) —*see* Atelectasis

Imperfect *(Continued)*
posture R29.3
rotation, intestine Q43.3
septum, ventricular Q21.0
Imperfectly descended testis —*see* Cryptorchid
Imperforate (congenital) —*see also* Atresia
anus Q42.3
with fistula Q42.2
cervix (uteri) Q51.828
esophagus Q39.0
with tracheoesophageal fistula Q39.1
hymen Q52.3
jejunum Q41.1
pharynx Q38.8
rectum Q42.1
with fistula Q42.0
urethra Q64.39
vagina Q52.4
Impervious (congenital) —*see also* Atresia
anus Q42.3
with fistula Q42.2
bile duct Q44.2
esophagus Q39.0
with tracheoesophageal fistula Q39.1
intestine (small) Q41.9
large Q42.9
specified NEC Q42.8
rectum Q42.1
with fistula Q42.0
ureter —*see* Atresia, ureter
urethra Q64.39
Impetiginization of dermatoses L01.1
Impetigo (any organism) (any site) (circinate) (contagiosa) (simplex) (vulgaris) L01.00
Bockhart's L01.02
bullous, bullosa L01.03
external ear L01.00 *[H62.40]*
follicularis L01.02
furfuracea L30.5
herpetiformis L40.1
nonobstetrical L40.1
neonatorum L01.03
nonbullous L01.01
specified type NEC L01.09
ulcerative L01.09
Impingement (on teeth)
soft tissue
anterior M26.81
posterior M26.82
Implant, endometrial N80.9
Implantation
anomalous —*see* Anomaly, by site
ureter Q62.63
cyst
external area or site (skin) NEC L72.0
iris —*see* Cyst, iris, implantation
vagina N89.8
vulva N90.7
dermoid (cyst) —*see* Implantation, cyst
Impotence (sexual) N52.9
counseling Z70.1
organic origin —*see also* Dysfunction, sexual, male, erectile N52.9
psychogenic F52.21
Impression, basilar Q75.8
Imprisonment, anxiety concerning Z65.1
Improper care (child) (newborn) —*see* Maltreatment
Improperly tied umbilical cord (causing hemorrhage) P51.8
Impulsiveness (impulsive) R45.87
Inability to swallow —*see* Aphagia
Inaccessible, inaccessibility
health care NEC Z75.3
due to
waiting period Z75.2
for admission to facility elsewhere Z75.1
other helping agencies Z75.4
Inactive —*see* condition

◄ New ◄ Revised ~~deleted~~ Deleted

Inadequate, inadequacy
aesthetics of dental restoration K08.56
biologic, constitutional, functional, or social F60.7
development
child R62.50
genitalia
after puberty NEC E30.0
congenital
female Q52.8
external Q52.79
internal Q52.8
male Q55.8
lungs Q33.6
associated with short gestation P28.0
organ or site not listed —*see* Anomaly, by site
diet (causing nutritional deficiency) E63.9
eating habits Z72.4
environment, household Z59.1
family support Z63.8
food (supply) NEC Z59.4
hunger effects T73.0
functional F60.7
household care, due to
family member
handicapped or ill Z74.2
on vacation Z75.5
temporarily away from home Z74.2
technical defects in home Z59.1
temporary absence from home of person rendering care Z74.2
housing (heating) (space) Z59.1
income (financial) Z59.6
intrafamilial communication Z63.8
material resources Z59.9
mental —*see* Disability, intellectual
parental supervision or control of child Z62.0
personality F60.7
pulmonary
function R06.89
newborn P28.5
ventilation, newborn P28.5
sample of cytologic smear
anus R85.615
cervix R87.615
vagina R87.625
social F60.7
insurance Z59.7
skills NEC Z73.4
supervision of child by parent Z62.0
teaching affecting education Z55.8
welfare support Z59.7
Inanition R64
with edema —*see* Malnutrition, severe
due to
deprivation of food T73.0
malnutrition —*see* Malnutrition
fever R50.9
Inappropriate
change in quantitative human chorionic gonadotropin (hCG) in early pregnancy O02.81
diet or eating habits Z72.4
level of quantitative human chorionic gonadotropin (hCG) for gestational age in early pregnancy O02.81
secretion
antidiuretic hormone (ADH) (excessive) E22.2
deficiency E23.2
pituitary (posterior) E22.2
Inattention at or after birth —*see* Neglect
Incarceration, incarcerated
enterocele K46.0
gangrenous K46.1
epiplocele K46.0
gangrenous K46.1
exomphalos K42.0 ◀
gangrenous K42.1 ◀
~~exophthalmos K42.0~~
~~gangrenous K42.1~~

Incarceration, incarcerated *(Continued)*
hernia —*see also* Hernia, by site, with obstruction
with gangrene —*see* Hernia, by site, with gangrene
iris, in wound —*see* Injury, eye, laceration, with prolapse
lens, in wound —*see* Injury, eye, laceration, with prolapse
omphalocele K42.0
prison, anxiety concerning Z65.1
rupture —*see* Hernia, by site
sarcoepiplocele K46.0
gangrenous K46.1
sarcoepiplomphalocele K42.0
with gangrene K42.1
uterus N85.8
gravid O34.51-
causing obstructed labor O65.5
Incised wound
external —*see* Laceration
internal organs —*see* Injury, by site
Incision, incisional
hernia K43.2
with
gangrene (and obstruction) K43.1
obstruction K43.0
surgical, complication —*see* Complications, surgical procedure
traumatic
external —*see* Laceration
internal organs —*see* Injury, by site
Inclusion
azurophilic leukocytic D72.0
blennorrhea (neonatal) (newborn) P39.1
gallbladder in liver (congenital) Q44.1
Incompatibility
ABO
affecting management of pregnancy O36.11-
anti-A sensitization O36.11-
anti-B sensitization O36.19-
specified NEC O36.19-
infusion or transfusion reaction —*see* Complication (s), transfusion, incompatibility reaction, ABO
newborn P55.1
blood (group) (Duffy) (K(ell)) (Kidd) (Lewis) (M) (S) NEC
affecting management of pregnancy O36.11-
anti-A sensitization O36.11-
anti-B sensitization O36.19-
infusion or transfusion reaction T80.89
newborn P55.8
divorce or estrangement Z63.5
Rh (blood group) (factor) Z31.82
affecting management of pregnancy NEC O36.09-
anti-D antibody O36.01-
infusion or transfusion reaction —*see* Complication (s), transfusion, incompatibility reaction, Rh (factor)
newborn P55.0
rhesus —*see* Incompatibility, Rh
Incompetency, incompetent, incompetence
annular
aortic (valve) —*see* Insufficiency, aortic
mitral (valve) I34.0
pulmonary valve (heart) I37.1
aortic (valve) —*see* Insufficiency, aortic
cardiac valve —*see* Endocarditis
cervix, cervical (os) N88.3
in pregnancy O34.3-
chronotropic I45.89
with
autonomic dysfunction G90.8
ischemic heart disease I25.89
left ventricular dysfunction I51.89
sinus node dysfunction I49.8
esophagogastric (junction) (sphincter) K22.0

Incompetency, incompetent, incompetence *(Continued)*
mitral (valve) —*see* Insufficiency, mitral
pelvic fundus N81.89
pubocervical tissue N81.82
pulmonary valve (heart) I37.1
congenital Q22.3
rectovaginal tissue N81.83
tricuspid (annular) (valve) —*see* Insufficiency, tricuspid
valvular —*see* Endocarditis
congenital Q24.8
vein, venous (saphenous) (varicose) —*see* Varix, leg
Incomplete —*see also* condition
bladder, emptying R33.9
defecation R15.0
expansion lungs (newborn) NEC —*see* Atelectasis
rotation, intestine Q43.3
Inconclusive
diagnostic imaging due to excess body fat of patient R93.9
findings on diagnostic imaging of breast NEC R92.8
mammogram (due to dense breasts) R92.2
Incontinence R32
anal sphincter R15.9
coital N39.491 ◀
feces R15.9
nonorganic origin F98.1
insensible (urinary) N39.42 ◀
overflow N39.490
postural (urinary) N39.492 ◀
psychogenic F45.8
rectal R15.9
reflex N39.498
stress (female) (male) N39.3
and urge N39.46
urethral sphincter R32
urge N39.41
and stress (female) (male) N39.46
urine (urinary) R32
continuous N39.45
due to cognitive impairment, or severe physical disability or immobility R39.81
functional R39.81
insensible N39.42 ◀
mixed (stress and urge) N39.46
nocturnal N39.44
nonorganic origin F98.0
overflow N39.490
post dribbling N39.43
postural N39.492 ◀
reflex N39.498
specified NEC N39.498
stress (female) (male) N39.3
and urge N39.46
total N39.498
unaware N39.42
urge N39.41
and stress (female) (male) N39.46
Incontinentia pigmenti Q82.3
Incoordinate, incoordination
esophageal-pharyngeal (newborn) —*see* Dysphagia
muscular R27.8
uterus (action) (contractions) (complicating delivery) O62.4
Increase, increased
abnormal, in development R63.8
androgens (ovarian) E28.1
anticoagulants (antithrombin) (anti-VIIIa) (anti-IXa) (anti-Xa) (anti-XIa) —*see* Circulating anticoagulants
cold sense R20.8
estrogen E28.0
function
adrenal
cortex —*see* Cushing's, syndrome
medulla E27.5

Increase, increased *(Continued)*
function *(Continued)*
pituitary (gland) (anterior) (lobe) E22.9
posterior E22.2
heat sense R20.8
intracranial pressure (benign) G93.2
permeability, capillaries I78.8
pressure, intracranial G93.2
secretion
gastrin E16.4
glucagon E16.3
pancreas, endocrine E16.9
growth hormone-releasing hormone E16.8
pancreatic polypeptide E16.8
somatostatin E16.8
vasoactive-intestinal polypeptide E16.8
sphericity, lens Q12.4
splenic activity D73.1
venous pressure I87.8
portal K76.6
Increta placenta O43.22-
Incrustation, cornea, foreign body (lead) (zinc) —*see* Foreign body, cornea
Incyclophoria H50.54
Incyclotropia —*see* Cyclotropia
Indeterminate sex Q56.4
India rubber skin Q82.8
Indigestion (acid) (bilious) (functional) K30
catarrhal K31.89
due to decomposed food NOS A05.9
nervous F45.8
psychogenic F45.8
Indirect —*see* condition
Induratio penis plastica N48.6
Induration, indurated
brain G93.89
breast (fibrous) N64.51
puerperal, postpartum O92.29
broad ligament N83.8
chancre
anus A51.1
congenital A50.07
extragenital NEC A51.2
corpora cavernosa (penis) (plastic) N48.6
liver (chronic) K76.89
lung (black) (chronic) (fibroid) —*see also* Fibrosis, lung J84.10
essential brown J84.03
penile (plastic) N48.6
phlebitic —*see* Phlebitis
skin R23.4
Inebriety (without dependence) —*see* Alcohol, intoxication
Inefficiency, kidney N28.9
Inelasticity, skin R23.4
Inequality, leg (length) (acquired) —*see also* Deformity, limb, unequal length
congenital —*see* Defect, reduction, lower limb
lower leg —*see* Deformity, limb, unequal length
Inertia
bladder (neurogenic) N31.2
stomach K31.89
psychogenic F45.8
uterus, uterine during labor O62.2
during latent phase of labor O62.0
primary O62.0
secondary O62.1
vesical (neurogenic) N31.2
Infancy, infantile, infantilism —*see also* condition
celiac K90.0
genitalia, genitals (after puberty) E30.0
Herter's (nontropical sprue) K90.0
intestinal K90.0
Lorain E23.0
pancreatic K86.89 ⇐
pelvis M95.5
with disproportion (fetopelvic) O33.1
causing obstructed labor O65.1
Infancy, infantile, infantilism *(Continued)*
pituitary E23.0
renal N25.0
uterus —*see* Infantile, genitalia
Infant (s) —*see also* Infancy
excessive crying R68.11
irritable child R68.12
lack of care —*see* Neglect
liveborn (singleton) Z38.2
born in hospital Z38.00
by cesarean Z38.01
born outside hospital Z38.1
multiple NEC Z38.8
born in hospital Z38.68
by cesarean Z38.69
born outside hospital Z38.7
quadruplet Z38.8
born in hospital Z38.63
by cesarean Z38.64
born outside hospital Z38.7
quintuplet Z38.8
born in hospital Z38.65
by cesarean Z38.66
born outside hospital Z38.7
triplet Z38.8
born in hospital Z38.61
by cesarean Z38.62
born outside hospital Z38.7
twin Z38.5
born in hospital Z38.30
by cesarean Z38.31
born outside hospital Z38.4
of diabetic mother (syndrome of) P70.1
gestational diabetes P70.0
Infantile —*see also* condition
genitalia, genitals E30.0
os, uterine E30.0
penis E30.0
testis E29.1
uterus E30.0
Infantilism —*see* Infancy
Infarct, infarction
adrenal (capsule) (gland) E27.49
appendices epiploicae —*see also* Infarct, intestine K55.069 ⇐
bowel —*see also* Infarct, intestine K55.069 ⇐
brain (stem) —*see* Infarct, cerebral
breast N64.89
brewer's (kidney) N28.0
cardiac —*see* Infarct, myocardium
cerebellar —*see* Infarct, cerebral
cerebral —*see also* Occlusion, artery cerebral or precerebral, with infarction I63.9-
aborted I63.9
cortical I63.9
due to
cerebral venous thrombosis, nonpyogenic I63.6
embolism
cerebral arteries I63.4-
precerebral arteries I63.1-
occlusion NEC
cerebral arteries I63.5-
precerebral arteries I63.2-
stenosis NEC
cerebral arteries I63.5-
precerebral arteries I63.2-
thrombosis
cerebral artery I63.3-
precerebral artery I63.0-
intraoperative
during cardiac surgery I97.810
during other surgery I97.811
postprocedural
following cardiac surgery I97.820
following other surgery I97.821
specified NEC I63.8
colon (acute) (agnogenic) (embolic) (hemorrhagic) (nonocclusive) (nonthrombotic) (occlusive) (segmental) (thrombotic) (with gangrene) —*see also* Infarct, intestine K55.049 ⇐
Infarct, infarction *(Continued)*
coronary artery —*see* Infarct, myocardium
embolic —*see* Embolism
fallopian tube N83.8
gallbladder K82.8
heart —*see* Infarct, myocardium
hepatic K76.3
hypophysis (anterior lobe) E23.6
impending (myocardium) I20.0
intestine (acute) (agnogenic) (embolic) (hemorrhagic) (nonocclusive) (nonthrombotic) (occlusive) (thrombotic) (with gangrene) K55.069 ⇐
diffuse K55.062 ◀
focal K55.061 ◀
large K55.049 ◀
diffuse K55.042 ◀
focal K55.041 ◀
small K55.029 ◀
diffuse K55.022 ◀
focal K55.021 ◀
kidney N28.0
liver K76.3
lung (embolic) (thrombotic) —*see* Embolism, pulmonary
lymph node I89.8
mesentery, mesenteric (embolic) (thrombotic) (with gangrene) —*see also* Infarct, intestine K55.069 ⇐
muscle (ischemic) M62.20
ankle M62.27-
foot M62.27-
forearm M62.23-
hand M62.24-
lower leg M62.26-
pelvic region M62.25-
shoulder region M62.21-
specified site NEC M62.28
thigh M62.25-
upper arm M62.22-
myocardium, myocardial (acute) (with stated duration of 4 weeks or less) I21.3
diagnosed on ECG, but presenting no symptoms I25.2
healed or old I25.2
intraoperative
during cardiac surgery I97.790
during other surgery I97.791
non-Q wave I21.4
non-ST elevation (NSTEMI) I21.4
subsequent I22.2
nontransmural I21.4
past (diagnosed on ECG or other investigation, but currently presenting no symptoms) I25.2
postprocedural
following cardiac surgery I97.190
following other surgery I97.191
Q wave (*see also*, Infarct, myocardium, by site) I21.3
ST elevation (STEMI) I21.3
anterior (anteroapical) (anterolateral) (anteroseptal) (Q wave) (wall) I21.09
subsequent I22.0
inferior (diaphragmatic) (inferolateral) (inferoposterior) (wall) NEC I21.19
subsequent I22.1
inferoposterior transmural (Q wave) I21.11
involving
coronary artery of anterior wall NEC I21.09
coronary artery of inferior wall NEC I21.19
diagonal coronary artery I21.02
left anterior descending coronary artery I21.02
left circumflex coronary artery I21.21
left main coronary artery I21.01

◀ New ⇐ Revised ~~deleted~~ Deleted

Infarct, infarction *(Continued)*
myocardium, myocardial *(Continued)*
ST elevation (STEMI) *(Continued)*
involving *(Continued)*
oblique marginal coronary artery I21.21
right coronary artery I21.11
lateral (apical-lateral) (basal-lateral) (high) I21.29
subsequent I22.8
posterior (posterobasal) (posterolateral) (posteroseptal) (true) I21.29
subsequent I22.8
septal I21.29
subsequent I22.8
specified NEC I21.29
subsequent I22.8
subsequent I22.9
subsequent (recurrent) (reinfarction) I22.9
anterior (anteroapical) (anterolateral) (anteroseptal) (wall) I22.0
diaphragmatic (wall) I22.1
inferior (diaphragmatic) (inferolateral) (inferoposterior) (wall) I22.1
lateral (apical-lateral) (basal-lateral) (high) I22.8
non-ST elevation (NSTEMI) I22.2
posterior (posterobasal) (posterolateral) (posteroseptal) (true) I22.8
septal I22.8
specified NEC I22.8
ST elevation I22.9
anterior (anteroapical) (anterolateral) (anteroseptal) (wall) I22.0
inferior (diaphragmatic) (inferolateral) (inferoposterior) (wall) I22.1
specified NEC I22.8
subendocardial I22.2
transmural I22.9
anterior (anteroapical) (anterolateral) (anteroseptal) (wall) I22.0
diaphragmatic (wall) I22.1
inferior (diaphragmatic) (inferolateral) (inferoposterior) (wall) I22.1
lateral (apical-lateral) (basal-lateral) (high) I22.8
posterior (posterobasal) (posterolateral) (posteroseptal) (true) I22.8
specified NEC I22.8
syphilitic A52.06
transmural I21.3
anterior (anteroapical) (anterolateral) (anteroseptal) (Q wave) (wall) NEC I21.09
inferior (diaphragmatic) (inferolateral) (inferoposterior) (Q wave) (wall) NEC I21.19
inferoposterior (Q wave) I21.11
lateral (apical-lateral) (basal-lateral) (high) NEC I21.29
posterior (posterobasal) (posterolateral) (posteroseptal) (true) NEC I21.29
septal NEC I21.29
specified NEC I21.29
nontransmural I21.4
omentum —*see also* Infarct, intestine K55.069 ◀
ovary N83.8
pancreas K86.89 ◀
papillary muscle —*see* Infarct, myocardium
parathyroid gland E21.4
pituitary (gland) E23.6
placenta O43.81-
prostate N42.89
pulmonary (artery) (vein) (hemorrhagic) —*see* Embolism, pulmonary
renal (embolic) (thrombotic) N28.0
retina, retinal (artery) —*see* Occlusion, artery, retina
spinal (cord) (acute) (embolic) (nonembolic) G95.11

Infarct, infarction *(Continued)*
spleen D73.5
embolic or thrombotic I74.8
subendocardial (acute) (nontransmural) I21.4
suprarenal (capsule) (gland) E27.49
testis N50.1
thrombotic —*see also* Thrombosis
artery, arterial —*see* Embolism
thyroid (gland) E07.89
ventricle (heart) —*see* Infarct, myocardium
Infecting —*see* condition
Infection, infected, infective (opportunistic) B99.9
with
drug resistant organism —*see* Resistance (to), drug —*see also* specific organism
lymphangitis —*see* Lymphangitis
organ dysfunction (acute) R65.20
with septic shock R65.21
abscess (skin) - code by site under Abscess
Absidia —*see* Mucormycosis
Acanthamoeba —*see* Acanthamebiasis
Acanthocheilonema (perstans) (streptocerca) B74.4
accessory sinus (chronic) —*see* Sinusitis
achorion —*see* Dermatophytosis
Acremonium falciforme B47.0
acromioclavicular M00.9
Actinobacillus (actinomycetem-comitans) A28.8
mallei A24.0
muris A25.1
Actinomadura B47.1
Actinomyces (israelii) —*see also* Actinomycosis A42.9
Actinomycetales —*see* Actinomycosis
actinomycotic NOS —*see* Actinomycosis
adenoid (and tonsil) J03.90
chronic J35.02
adenovirus NEC
as cause of disease classified elsewhere B97.0
unspecified nature or site B34.0
aerogenes capsulatus A48.0
aertrycke —*see* Infection, salmonella
alimentary canal NOS —*see* Enteritis, infectious
Allescheria boydii B48.2
Alternaria B48.8
alveolus, alveolar (process) K04.7
Ameba, amebic (histolytica) —*see* Amebiasis
amniotic fluid, sac or cavity O41.10-
chorioamnionitis O41.12-
placentitis O41.14-
amputation stump (surgical) —*see* Complication, amputation stump, infection
Ancylostoma (duodenalis) B76.0
Anisakiasis, Anisakis larvae B81.0
anthrax —*see* Anthrax
antrum (chronic) —*see* Sinusitis, maxillary
anus, anal (papillae) (sphincter) K62.89
arbovirus (arbor virus) A94
specified type NEC A93.8
artificial insemination N98.0
Ascaris lumbricoides —*see* Ascariasis
Ascomycetes B47.0
Aspergillus (flavus) (fumigatus) (terreus) —*see* Aspergillosis
atypical
acid-fast (bacilli) —*see* Mycobacterium, atypical
mycobacteria —*see* Mycobacterium, atypical
virus A81.9
specified type NEC A81.89
auditory meatus (external) —*see* Otitis, externa, infective
auricle (ear) —*see* Otitis, externa, infective
axillary gland (lymph) L04.2

Infection, infected, infective *(Continued)*
Bacillus A49.9
abortus A23.1
anthracis —*see* Anthrax
Ducrey's (any location) A57
Flexner's A03.1
Friedländer's NEC A49.8
gas (gangrene) A48.0
mallei A24.0
melitensis A23.0
paratyphoid, paratyphosus A01.4
A A01.1
B A01.2
C A01.3
Shiga (-Kruse) A03.0
suipestifer —*see* Infection, salmonella
swimming pool A31.1
typhosa A01.00
welchii —*see* Gangrene, gas
bacterial NOS A49.9
as cause of disease classified elsewhere B96.89
Bacteroides fragilis [B. fragilis] B96.6
Clostridium perfringens [C. perfringens] B96.7
Enterobacter sakazakii B96.89
Enterococcus B95.2
Escherichia coli [E. coli] (*see also* Escherichia coli) B96.20
Helicobacter pylori [H.pylori] B96.81
Hemophilus influenzae [H. influenzae] B96.3
Klebsiella pneumoniae [K. pneumoniae] B96.1
Mycoplasma pneumoniae [M. pneumoniae] B96.0
Proteus (mirabilis) (morganii) B96.4
Pseudomonas (aeruginosa) (mallei) (pseudomallei) B96.5
Staphylococcus B95.8
aureus (methicillin susceptible) (MSSA) B95.61
methicillin resistant (MRSA) B95.62
specified NEC B95.7
Streptococcus B95.5
group A B95.0
group B B95.1
pneumoniae B95.3
specified NEC B95.4
Vibrio vulnificus B96.82
specified NEC A48.8
Bacterium
paratyphosum A01.4
A A01.1
B A01.2
C A01.3
typhosum A01.00
Bacteroides NEC A49.8
fragilis, as cause of disease classified elsewhere B96.6
Balantidium coli A07.0
Bartholin's gland N75.8
Basidiobolus B46.8
bile duct (common) (hepatic) —*see* Cholangitis
bladder —*see* Cystitis
Blastomyces, blastomycotic —*see also* Blastomycosis
brasiliensis —*see* Paracoccidioidomycosis
dermatitidis —*see* Blastomycosis
European —*see* Cryptococcosis
Loboi B48.0
North American B40.9
South American —*see* Paracoccidioidomycosis
bleb, postprocedure —*see* Blebitis
bone —*see* Osteomyelitis
Bordetella —*see* Whooping cough
Borrelia bergdorfi A69.20

Infection, infected, infective *(Continued)*
brain —*see also* Encephalitis G04.90
membranes —*see* Meningitis
septic G06.0
meninges —*see* Meningitis, bacterial
branchial cyst Q18.0
breast —*see* Mastitis
bronchus —*see* Bronchitis
Brucella A23.9
abortus A23.1
canis A23.3
melitensis A23.0
mixed A23.8
specified NEC A23.8
suis A23.2
Brugia (malayi) B74.1
timori B74.2
bursa —*see* Bursitis, infective
buttocks (skin) L08.9
Campylobacter, intestinal A04.5
as cause of disease classified elsewhere B96.81
Candida (albicans) (tropicalis) —*see* Candidiasis
candiru B88.8
Capillaria (intestinal) B81.1
hepatica B83.8
philippinensis B81.1
cartilage —*see* Disorder, cartilage, specified type NEC
catheter-related bloodstream (CRBSI) T80.211
cat liver fluke B66.0
cellulitis - code by site under Cellulitis
central line-associated T80.219
bloodstream (CLABSI) T80.211
specified NEC T80.218
Cephalosporium falciforme B47.0
cerebrospinal —*see* Meningitis
cervical gland (lymph) L04.0
cervix —*see* Cervicitis
cesarean delivery wound (puerperal) O86.0
cestodes —*see* Infestation, cestodes
chest J22
Chilomastix (intestinal) A07.8
Chlamydia, chlamydial A74.9
anus A56.3
genitourinary tract A56.2
lower A56.00
specified NEC A56.19
lymphogranuloma A55
pharynx A56.4
psittaci A70
rectum A56.3
sexually transmitted NEC A56.8
cholera —*see* Cholera
Cladosporium
bantianum (brain abscess) B43.1
carrionii B43.0
castellanii B36.1
trichoides (brain abscess) B43.1
werneckii B36.1
Clonorchis (sinensis) (liver) B66.1
Clostridium NEC
bifermentans A48.0
botulinum (food poisoning) A05.1
infant A48.51
wound A48.52
difficile
as cause of disease classified elsewhere B96.89
foodborne (disease) A04.7
gas gangrene A48.0
necrotizing enterocolitis A04.7
sepsis A41.4
gas-forming NEC A48.0
histolyticum A48.0
novyi, causing gas gangrene A48.0
oedematiens A48.0
perfringens
as cause of disease classified elsewhere B96.7
due to food A05.2

Infection, infected, infective *(Continued)*
Clostridium *(Continued)*
perfringens *(Continued)*
foodborne (disease) A05.2
gas gangrene A48.0
sepsis A41.4
septicum, causing gas gangrene A48.0
sordellii, causing gas gangrene A48.0
welchii
as cause of disease classified elsewhere B96.7
foodborne (disease) A05.2
gas gangrene A48.0
necrotizing enteritis A05.2
sepsis A41.4
Coccidioides (immitis) —*see* Coccidioidomycosis
colon —*see* Enteritis, infectious
colostomy K94.02
common duct —*see* Cholangitis
congenital P39.9
Candida (albicans) P37.5
cytomegalovirus P35.1
hepatitis, viral P35.3
herpes simplex P35.2
infectious or parasitic disease P37.9
specified NEC P37.8
listeriosis (disseminated) P37.2
malaria NEC P37.4
falciparum P37.3
Plasmodium falciparum P37.3
poliomyelitis P35.8
rubella P35.0
skin P39.4
toxoplasmosis (acute) (subacute) (chronic) P37.1
tuberculosis P37.0
urinary (tract) P39.3
vaccinia P35.8
virus P35.9
specified type NEC P35.8
Conidiobolus B46.8
coronavirus NEC B34.2
as cause of disease classified elsewhere B97.29
severe acute respiratory syndrome (SARS associated) B97.21
corpus luteum —*see* Salpingo-oophoritis
Corynebacterium diphtheriae —*see* Diphtheria
cotia virus B08.8
Coxiella burnetii A78
coxsackie —*see* Coxsackie
Cryptococcus neoformans —*see* Cryptococcosis
Cryptosporidium A07.2
Cunninghamella —*see* Mucormycosis
cyst —*see* Cyst
cystic duct —*see also* Cholecystitis K81.9
Cysticercus cellulosae —*see* Cysticercosis
cytomegalovirus, cytomegaloviral B25.9
congenital P35.1
maternal, maternal care for (suspected) damage to fetus O35.3
mononucleosis B27.10
with
complication NEC B27.19
meningitis B27.12
polyneuropathy B27.11
delta-agent (acute), in hepatitis B carrier B17.0
dental (pulpal origin) K04.7
Deuteromycetes B47.0
Dicrocoelium dendriticum B66.2
Dipetalonema (perstans) (streptocerca) B74.4
diphtherial —*see* Diphtheria
Diphyllobothrium (adult) (latum) (pacificum) B70.0
larval B70.1
Diplogonoporus (grandis) B71.8
Dipylidium caninum B67.4

Infection, infected, infective *(Continued)*
Dirofilaria B74.8
Dracunculus medinensis B72
Drechslera (hawaiiensis) B43.8
Ducrey Haemophilus (any location) A57
due to or resulting from
artificial insemination N98.0
central venous catheter T80.219
bloodstream T80.211
exit or insertion site T80.212
localized T80.212
port or reservoir T80.212
specified NEC T80.218
tunnel T80.212
device, implant or graft —*see also* Complications, by site and type, infection or inflammation T85.79
arterial graft NEC T82.7
breast (implant) T85.79
catheter NEC T85.79
dialysis (renal) T82.7
intraperitoneal T85.71
infusion NEC T82.7
cranial T85.735 ◀
intrathecal T85.735 ◀
spinal (epidural) (subdural) T85.735 ⇐
subarachnoid T85.735 ◀
urinary T83.518 ⇐
cystostomy T83.510 ◀
Hopkins T83.518 ◀
ileostomy T83.518 ◀
nephrostomy T83.512 ◀
specified NEC T83.518 ◀
urethral indwelling T83.511 ◀
urostomy T83.518 ◀
electronic (electrode) (pulse generator) (stimulator)
bone T84.7
cardiac T82.7
nervous system T85.738 ⇐
brain T85.731 ◀
cranial nerve T85.732 ◀
gastric nerve T85.732 ◀
generator pocket T85.734 ◀
neurostimulator generator T85.734 ◀
peripheral nerve T85.732 ◀
sacral nerve T85.732 ◀
spinal cord T85.733 ◀
vagal nerve T85.732 ◀
urinary T83.590 ⇐
fixation, internal (orthopedic) NEC —*see* Complication, fixation device, infection
gastrointestinal (bile duct) (esophagus) T85.79
neurostimulator electrode (lead) T85.732 ◀
genital NEC T83.69 ⇐
heart NEC T82.7
valve (prosthesis) T82.6
graft T82.7
joint prosthesis —*see* Complication, joint prosthesis, infection
ocular (corneal graft) (orbital implant) NEC T85.79
orthopedic NEC T84.7
penile (cylinder) (pump) (resevoir) T83.61 ◀
specified NEC T85.79
testicular T83.62 ◀
urinary NEC T83.598 ⇐
ileal conduit stent T83.593 ◀
implanted neurostimulation T83.590 ◀
implanted sphincter T83.591 ◀
indwelling ureteral stent T83.592 ◀
nephroureteral stent T83.593 ◀
specified stent NEC T83.593 ◀

◀ New ⇐ Revised ~~deleted~~ Deleted

Infection, infected, infective *(Continued)*
due to or resulting from *(Continued)*
device, implant or graft *(Continued)*
vascular NEC T82.7
~~ventricular intracranial shunt T85.79~~
ventricular intracranial (communicating) shunt T85.730 ◀
Hickman catheter T80.219
bloodstream T80.211
localized T80.212
specified NEC T80.218
immunization or vaccination T88.0
infusion, injection or transfusion NEC T80.29
acute T80.22
injury NEC - code by site under Wound, open
peripherally inserted central catheter (PICC) T80.219
bloodstream T80.211
localized T80.212
specified NEC T80.218
portacath (port-a-cath) T80.219
bloodstream T80.211
localized T80.212
specified NEC T80.218
pulmonary artery catheter —*see* Infection, due to or resulting from, central venous catheter ◀
surgery T81.40 ⟸
Swan Ganz catheter —*see* Infection, due to or resulting from, central venous catheter ◀
triple lumen catheter T80.219
bloodstream T80.211
localized T80.212
specified NEC T80.218
umbilical venous catheter T80.219
bloodstream T80.211
localized T80.212
specified NEC T80.218
during labor NEC O75.3
ear (middle) —*see also* Otitis media
external —*see* Otitis, externa, infective
inner —*see* subcategory H83.0
Eberthella typhosa A01.00
Echinococcus —*see* Echinococcus
echovirus
as cause of disease classified elsewhere B97.12
unspecified nature or site B34.1
endocardium I33.0
endocervix —*see* Cervicitis
Entamoeba —*see* Amebiasis
enteric —*see* Enteritis, infectious
Enterobacter sakazakii B96.89
Enterobius vermicularis B80
enterostomy K94.12
enterovirus B34.1
as cause of disease classified elsewhere B97.10
coxsackievirus B97.11
echovirus B97.12
specified NEC B97.19
Entomophthora B46.8
Epidermophyton —*see* Dermatophytosis
epididymis —*see* Epididymitis
episiotomy (puerperal) O86.0
Erysipelothrix (insidiosa) (rhusiopathiae) —*see* Erysipeloid
erythema infectiosum B08.3
Escherichia (E.) coli NEC A49.8
as cause of disease classified elsewhere —*see also* Escherichia coli B96.20
congenital P39.8
sepsis P36.4
generalized A41.51
intestinal —*see* Enteritis, infectious, due to, Escherichia coli
ethmoidal (chronic) (sinus) —*see* Sinusitis, ethmoidal

Infection, infected, infective *(Continued)*
eustachian tube (ear) —*see* Salpingitis, eustachian
external auditory canal (meatus) NEC —*see* Otitis, externa, infective
eye (purulent) —*see* Endophthalmitis, purulent
eyelid —*see* Inflammation, eyelid
fallopian tube —*see* Salpingo-oophoritis
Fasciola (gigantica) (hepatica) (indica) B66.3
Fasciolopsis (buski) B66.5
filarial —*see* Infestation, filarial
finger (skin) L08.9
nail L03.01-
fungus B35.1
fish tapeworm B70.0
larval B70.1
flagellate, intestinal A07.9
fluke —*see* Infestation, fluke
focal
teeth (pulpal origin) K04.7
tonsils J35.01
Fonsecaea (compactum) (pedrosoi) B43.0
food —*see* Intoxication, foodborne
foot (skin) L08.9
dermatophytic fungus B35.3
Francisella tularensis —*see* Tularemia
frontal (sinus) (chronic) —*see* Sinusitis, frontal
fungus NOS B49
beard B35.0
dermatophytic —*see* Dermatophytosis
foot B35.3
groin B35.6
hand B35.2
nail B35.1
pathogenic to compromised host only B48.8
perianal (area) B35.6
scalp B35.0
skin B36.9
foot B35.3
hand B35.2
toenails B35.1
Fusarium B48.8
gallbladder —*see* Cholecystitis
gas bacillus —*see* Gangrene, gas
gastrointestinal —*see* Enteritis, infectious
generalized NEC —*see* Sepsis
generator pocket, implanted electronic neurostimulator T85.734 ◀
genital organ or tract
female —*see* Disease, pelvis, inflammatory
male N49.9
multiple sites N49.8
specified NEC N49.8
Ghon tubercle, primary A15.7
Giardia lamblia A07.1
gingiva (chronic) K05.10
acute K05.00
nonplaque induced K05.01
plaque induced K05.00
nonplaque induced K05.11
plaque induced K05.10
glanders A24.0
glenosporopsis B48.0
Gnathostoma (spinigerum) B83.1
Gongylonema B83.8
gonococcal —*see* Gonococcus
gram-negative bacilli NOS A49.9
guinea worm B72
gum (chronic) K05.10
acute K05.00
nonplaque induced K05.01
plaque induced K05.00
nonplaque induced K05.11
plaque induced K05.10
Haemophilus —*see* Infection, Hemophilus
heart —*see* Carditis

Infection, infected, infective *(Continued)*
Helicobacter pylori A04.8
as cause of disease classified elsewhere B96.81
helminths B83.9
intestinal B82.0
mixed (types classifiable to more than one of the titles B65.0-B81.3 and B81.8) B81.4
specified type NEC B81.8
specified type NEC B83.8
Hemophilus
aegyptius, systemic A48.4
ducrey (any location) A57
generalized A41.3
influenzae NEC A49.2
as cause of disease classified elsewhere B96.3
herpes (simplex) —*see also* Herpes
congenital P35.2
disseminated B00.7
zoster B02.9
herpesvirus, herpesviral —*see* Herpes
Heterophyes (heterophyes) B66.8
hip (joint) NEC M00.9
due to internal joint prosthesis
left T84.52
right T84.51
skin NEC L08.9
Histoplasma —*see* Histoplasmosis
American B39.4
capsulatum B39.4
hookworm B76.9
human
papilloma virus A63.0
T-cell lymphotropic virus type-1 (HTLV-1) B33.3
hydrocele N43.0
Hymenolepis B71.0
hypopharynx —*see* Pharyngitis
inguinal (lymph) glands L04.1
due to soft chancre A57
intervertebral disc, pyogenic M46.30
cervical region M46.32
cervicothoracic region M46.33
lumbar region M46.36
lumbosacral region M46.37
multiple sites M46.39
occipito-atlanto-axial region M46.31
sacrococcygeal region M46.38
thoracic region M46.34
thoracolumbar region M46.35
intestine, intestinal —*see* Enteritis, infectious
specified NEC A08.8
intra-amniotic affecting newborn NEC P39.2
Isospora belli or hominis A07.3
Japanese B encephalitis A83.0
jaw (bone) (lower) (upper) M27.2
joint NEC M00.9
due to internal joint prosthesis T84.50
kidney (cortex) (hematogenous) N15.9
with calculus N20.0
with hydronephrosis N13.6
following ectopic gestation O08.83
pelvis and ureter (cystic) N28.85
puerperal (postpartum) O86.21
specified NEC N15.8
Klebsiella (K.) pneumoniae NEC A49.8
as cause of disease classified elsewhere B96.1
knee (joint) NEC M00.9
due to internal joint prosthesis
left T84.54
right T84.53
joint M00.9
skin L08.9
Koch's —*see* Tuberculosis
labia (majora) (minora) (acute) —*see* Vulvitis
lacrimal
gland —*see* Dacryoadenitis
passages (duct) (sac) —*see* Inflammation, lacrimal, passages

Infection, infected, infective *(Continued)*
lancet fluke B66.2
larynx NEC J38.7
leg (skin) NOS L08.9
Legionella pneumophila A48.1
nonpneumonic A48.2
Leishmania —*see also* Leishmaniasis
aethiopica B55.1
braziliensis B55.2
chagasi B55.0
donovani B55.0
infantum B55.0
major B55.1
mexicana B55.1
tropica B55.1
lentivirus, as cause of disease classified elsewhere B97.31
Leptosphaeria senegalensis B47.0
Leptospira interrogans A27.9
autumnalis A27.89
canicola A27.89
hebdomadis A27.89
icterohaemorrhagiae A27.0
pomona A27.89
specified type NEC A27.89
leptospirochetal NEC —*see* Leptospirosis
Listeria monocytogenes —*see also* Listeriosis
congenital P37.2
Loa loa B74.3
with conjunctival infestation B74.3
eyelid B74.3
Loboa loboi B48.0
local, skin (staphylococcal) (streptococcal) L08.9
abscess - code by site under Abscess
cellulitis - code by site under Cellulitis
specified NEC L08.89
ulcer —*see* Ulcer, skin
Loefflerella mallei A24.0
lung —*see also* Pneumonia J18.9
atypical Mycobacterium A31.0
spirochetal A69.8
tuberculous —*see* Tuberculosis, pulmonary
virus —*see* Pneumonia, viral
lymph gland —*see also* Lymphadenitis, acute
mesenteric I88.0
lymphoid tissue, base of tongue or posterior pharynx, NEC (chronic) J35.03
Madurella (grisea) (mycetomii) B47.0
major
following ectopic or molar pregnancy O08.0
puerperal, postpartum, childbirth O85
Malassezia furfur B36.0
Malleomyces
mallei A24.0
pseudomallei (whitmori) —*see* Melioidosis
mammary gland N61.0 ⇐
Mansonella (ozzardi) (perstans) (streptocerca) B74.4
mastoid —*see* Mastoiditis
maxilla, maxillary M27.2
sinus (chronic) —*see* Sinusitis, maxillary
mediastinum J98.51 ⇐
Medina (worm) B72
meibomian cyst or gland —*see* Hordeolum
meninges —*see* Meningitis, bacterial
meningococcal —*see also* condition A39.9
adrenals A39.1
brain A39.81
cerebrospinal A39.0
conjunctiva A39.89
endocardium A39.51
heart A39.50
endocardium A39.51
myocardium A39.52
pericardium A39.53

Infection, infected, infective *(Continued)*
meningococcal *(Continued)*
joint A39.83
meninges A39.0
meningococcemia A39.4
acute A39.2
chronic A39.3
myocardium A39.52
pericardium A39.53
retrobulbar neuritis A39.82
specified site NEC A39.89
mesenteric lymph nodes or glands NEC I88.0
Metagonimus B66.8
metatarsophalangeal M00.9
methicillin
resistant Staphylococcus aureus (MRSA) A49.02
susceptible Staphylococcus aureus (MSSA) A49.01
Microsporum, microsporic —*see* Dermatophytosis
mixed flora (bacterial) NEC A49.8
Monilia —*see* Candidiasis
Monosporium apiospermum B48.2
mouth, parasitic B37.0
Mucor —*see* Mucormycosis
muscle NEC —*see* Myositis, infective
mycelium NOS B49
mycetoma B47.9
actinomycotic NEC B47.1
mycotic NEC B47.0
Mycobacterium, mycobacterial —*see* Mycobacterium
Mycoplasma NEC A49.3
pneumoniae, as cause of disease classified elsewhere B96.0
mycotic NOS B49
pathogenic to compromised host only B48.8
skin NOS B36.9
myocardium NEC I40.0
nail (chronic)
with lymphangitis —*see* Lymphangitis, acute, digit
finger L03.01-
fungus B35.1
ingrowing L60.0
toe L03.03-
fungus B35.1
nasal sinus (chronic) —*see* Sinusitis
nasopharynx —*see* Nasopharyngitis
navel L08.82
Necator americanus B76.1
Neisseria —*see* Gonococcus
Neotestudina rosatii B47.0
newborn P39.9
intra-amniotic NEC P39.2
skin P39.4
specified type NEC P39.8
nipple N61.0 ⇐
associated with
lactation O91.03
pregnancy O91.01-
puerperium O91.02
Nocardia —*see* Nocardiosis
obstetrical surgical wound (puerperal) O86.0
Oesophagostomum (apiostomum) B81.8
Oestrus ovis —*see* Myiasis
Oidium albicans B37.9
Onchocerca (volvulus) —*see* Onchocerciasis - oncovirus, as cause of disease classified elsewhere B97.32
operation wound T81.40 ⇐
Opisthorchis (felineus) (viverrini) B66.0
orbit, orbital —*see* Inflammation, orbit
orthopoxvirus NEC B08.09
ovary —*see* Salpingo-oophoritis
Oxyuris vermicularis B80

Infection, infected, infective *(Continued)*
pancreas (acute) —see Pancreatitis, acute ⇐
abscess —*see* Pancreatitis, acute
specified NEC —*see also* Pancreatitis, acute K85.80 ⇐
papillomavirus, as cause of disease classified elsewhere B97.7
papovavirus NEC B34.4
Paracoccidioides brasiliensis —*see* Paracoccidioidomycosis
Paragonimus (westermani) B66.4
parainfluenza virus B34.8
parameningococcus NOS A39.9
parapoxvirus B08.60
specified NEC B08.69
parasitic B89
Parastrongylus
cantonensis B83.2
costaricensis B81.3
paratyphoid A01.4
Type A A01.1
Type B A01.2
Type C A01.3
paraurethral ducts N34.2
parotid gland —*see* Sialoadenitis
parvovirus NEC B34.3
as cause of disease classified elsewhere B97.6
Pasteurella NEC A28.0
multocida A28.0
pestis —*see* Plague
pseudotuberculosis A28.0
septica (cat bite) (dog bite) A28.0
tularensis —*see* Tularemia
pelvic, female —*see* Disease, pelvis, inflammatory
Penicillium (marneffei) B48.4
penis (glans) (retention) NEC N48.29
periapical K04.5
peridental, periodontal K05.20
generalized —*see* Peridontitis, aggressive, generalized ⇐
localized —*see* Peridontitis, aggressive, localized ⇐
perinatal period P39.9
specified type NEC P39.8
perineal repair (puerperal) O86.0
periorbital —*see* Inflammation, orbit
perirectal K62.89
perirenal —*see* Infection, kidney
peritoneal —*see* Peritonitis
periureteral N28.89
Petriellidium boydii B48.2
pharynx —*see also* Pharyngitis
coxsackievirus B08.5
posterior, lymphoid (chronic) J35.03
Phialophora
gougerotii (subcutaneous abscess or cyst) B43.2
jeanselmei (subcutaneous abscess or cyst) B43.2
verrucosa (skin) B43.0
Piedraia hortae B36.3
pinta A67.9
intermediate A67.1
late A67.2
mixed A67.3
primary A67.0
pinworm B80
pityrosporum furfur B36.0
pleuro-pneumonia-like organism (PPLO) NEC A49.3
as cause of disease classified elsewhere B96.0
pneumococcus, pneumococcal NEC A49.1
as cause of disease classified elsewhere B95.3
generalized (purulent) A40.3
with pneumonia J13
Pneumocystis carinii (pneumonia) B59
Pneumocystis jiroveci (pneumonia) B59

◀ New ⇐ Revised ~~deleted~~ Deleted

Infection, infected, infective *(Continued)*
port or reservoir T80.212
postoperative T81.40 ⬅
postoperative wound T81.40 ⬅
postprocedural T81.40 ⬅
deep incisional surgical site T81.42 ◀
organ and space surgical site T81.43 ◀
sepsis T81.49 ◀
specified surgical site NEC T81.48 ◀
superficial incisional surgical site T81.41 ◀
postvaccinal T88.0
prepuce NEC N47.7
with penile inflammation N47.6
prion —*see* Disease, prion, central nervous system
prostate (capsule) —*see* Prostatitis
Proteus (mirabilis) (morganii) (vulgaris) NEC A49.8
as cause of disease classified elsewhere B96.4
protozoal NEC B64
intestinal A07.9
specified NEC A07.8
specified NEC B60.8
Pseudoallescheria boydii B48.2
Pseudomonas NEC A49.8
as cause of disease classified elsewhere B96.5
mallei A24.0
pneumonia J15.1
pseudomallei —*see* Melioidosis
puerperal O86.4
genitourinary tract NEC O86.89
major or generalized O85
minor O86.4
specified NEC O86.89
pulmonary —*see* Infection, lung
purulent —*see* Abscess
Pyrenochaeta romeroi B47.0
Q fever A78
rectum (sphincter) K62.89
renal —*see also* Infection, kidney
pelvis and ureter (cystic) N28.85
reovirus, as cause of disease classified elsewhere B97.5
respiratory (tract) NEC J98.8
acute J22
chronic J98.8
influenzal (upper) (acute) —*see* Influenza, with, respiratory manifestations NEC
lower (acute) J22
chronic —*see* Bronchitis, chronic
rhinovirus J00
syncytial virus, as cause of disease classified elsewhere B97.4
upper (acute) NOS J06.9
chronic J39.8
streptococcal J06.9
viral NOS J06.9
resulting from
presence of internal prosthesis, implant, graft —*see* Complications, by site and type, infection
retortamoniasis A07.8
retroperitoneal NEC K68.9
retrovirus B33.3
as cause of disease classified elsewhere B97.30
human
immunodeficiency, type 2 (HIV 2) B97.35
T-cell lymphotropic
type I (HTLV-I) B97.33
type II (HTLV-II) B97.34
lentivirus B97.31
oncovirus B97.32
specified NEC B97.39
Rhinosporidium (seeberi) B48.1
rhinovirus
as cause of disease classified elsewhere B97.89
unspecified nature or site B34.8

Infection, infected, infective *(Continued)*
Rhizopus —*see* Mucormycosis
rickettsial NOS A79.9
roundworm (large) NEC B82.0
Ascariasis —*see also* Ascariasis B77.9
rubella —*see* Rubella
Saccharomyces —*see* Candidiasis
salivary duct or gland (any) —*see* Sialoadenitis
Salmonella (aertrycke) (arizonae) (callinarum) (cholerae-suis) (enteritidis) (suipestifer) (typhimurium) A02.9
with
(gastro) enteritis A02.0
sepsis A02.1
specified manifestation NEC A02.8
due to food (poisoning) A02.9
hirschfeldii A01.3
localized A02.20
arthritis A02.23
meningitis A02.21
osteomyelitis A02.24
pneumonia A02.22
pyelonephritis A02.25
specified NEC A02.29
paratyphi A01.4
A A01.1
B A01.2
C A01.3
schottmuelleri A01.2
typhi, typhosa —*see* Typhoid
Sarcocystis A07.8
scabies B86
Schistosoma —*see* Infestation, Schistosoma
scrotum (acute) NEC N49.2
seminal vesicle —*see* Vesiculitis
septic
localized, skin —*see* Abscess
sheep liver fluke B66.3
Shigella A03.9
boydii A03.2
dysenteriae A03.0
flexneri A03.1
group
A A03.0
B A03.1
C A03.2
D A03.3
Schmitz (-Stutzer) A03.0
schmitzii A03.0
shigae A03.0
sonnei A03.3
specified NEC A03.8
shoulder (joint) NEC M00.9
due to internal joint prosthesis T84.59
skin NEC L08.9
sinus (accessory) (chronic) (nasal) —*see also* Sinusitis
pilonidal —*see* Sinus, pilonidal
skin NEC L08.89
Skene's duct or gland —*see* Urethritis
skin (local) (staphylococcal) (streptococcal) L08.9
abscess - code by site under Abscess
cellulitis - code by site under Cellulitis
due to fungus B36.9
specified type NEC B36.8
mycotic B36.9
specified type NEC B36.8
newborn P39.4
ulcer —*see* Ulcer, skin
slow virus A81.9
specified NEC A81.89
Sparganum (mansoni) (proliferum) (baxteri) B70.1
specific —*see also* Syphilis
to perinatal period —*see* Infection, congenital
specified NEC B99.8
spermatic cord NEC N49.1

Infection, infected, infective *(Continued)*
sphenoidal (sinus) —*see* Sinusitis, sphenoidal
spinal cord NOS —*see also* Myelitis G04.91
abscess G06.1
meninges —*see* Meningitis
streptococcal G04.89
Spirillum A25.0
spirochetal NOS A69.9
lung A69.8
specified NEC A69.8
Spirometra larvae B70.1
spleen D73.89
Sporotrichum, Sporothrix (schenckii) —*see* Sporotrichosis
staphylococcal, unspecified site
aureus (methicillin susceptible) (MSSA) A49.01
methicillin resistant (MRSA) A49.02
as cause of disease classified elsewhere B95.8
aureus (methicillin susceptible) (MSSA) B95.61
methicillin resistant (MRSA) B95.62
specified NEC B95.7
food poisoning A05.0
generalized (purulent) A41.2
pneumonia —*see* Pneumonia, staphylococcal
Stellantchasmus falcatus B66.8
streptobacillus moniliformis A25.1
streptococcal NEC A49.1
as cause of disease classified elsewhere B95.5
B genitourinary complicating
childbirth O98.82
pregnancy O98.81-
puerperium O98.83
congenital
sepsis P36.10
group B P36.0
specified NEC P36.19
generalized (purulent) A40.9
Streptomyces B47.1
Strongyloides (stercoralis) —*see* Strongyloidiasis
stump (amputation) (surgical) —*see* Complication, amputation stump, infection
subcutaneous tissue, local L08.9
suipestifer —*see* Infection, salmonella
swimming pool bacillus A31.1
Taenia —*see* Infestation, Taenia
Taeniarhynchus saginatus B68.1
tapeworm —*see* Infestation, tapeworm
tendon (sheath) —*see* Tenosynovitis, infective NEC
Ternidens diminutus B81.8
testis —*see* Orchitis
threadworm B80
throat —*see* Pharyngitis
thyroglossal duct K14.8
toe (skin) L08.9
cellulitis L03.03-
fungus B35.1
nail L03.03-
fungus B35.1
tongue NEC K14.0
parasitic B37.0
tonsil (and adenoid) (faucial) (lingual) (pharyngeal) —*see* Tonsillitis
tooth, teeth K04.7
irreversible K04.02 ◀
periapical K04.7
peridental, periodontal K05.20
generalized —*see* Peridontitis, aggressive, generalized ⬅
localized —*see* Peridontitis, aggressive, localized ⬅

Infection, infected, infective *(Continued)*
tooth, teeth *(Continued)*
pulp K04.01 ⬅
reversible K04.01 ◀
socket M27.3
TORCH —*see* Infection, congenital
without active infection P00.2
Torula histolytica —*see* Cryptococcosis
Toxocara (canis) (cati) (felis) B83.0
Toxoplasma gondii —*see* Toxoplasma
trachea, chronic J42
trematode NEC —*see* Infestation, fluke
trench fever A79.0
Treponema pallidum —*see* Syphilis
Trichinella (spiralis) B75
Trichomonas A59.9
cervix A59.09
intestine A07.8
prostate A59.02
specified site NEC A59.8
urethra A59.03
urogenitalis A59.00
vagina A59.01
vulva A59.01
Trichophyton, trichophytic —*see* Dermatophytosis
Trichosporon (beigelii) cutaneum B36.2
Trichostrongylus B81.2
Trichuris (trichiura) B79
Trombicula (irritans) B88.0
Trypanosoma
brucei
gambiense B56.0
rhodesiense B56.1
cruzi —*see* Chagas' disease
tubal —*see* Salpingo-oophoritis
tuberculous NEC —*see* Tuberculosis
tubo-ovarian —*see* Salpingo-oophoritis
tunica vaginalis N49.1
tunnel T80.212
tympanic membrane NEC —*see* Myringitis
typhoid (abortive) (ambulant) (bacillus) —*see* Typhoid
typhus A75.9
flea-borne A75.2
mite-borne A75.3
recrudescent A75.1
tick-borne A77.9
African A77.1
North Asian A77.2
umbilicus L08.82
ureter N28.86
urethra —*see* Urethritis
urinary (tract) N39.0
bladder —*see* Cystitis
complicating
pregnancy O23.4-
specified type NEC O23.3-
kidney —*see* Infection, kidney
newborn P39.3
puerperal (postpartum) O86.20
tuberculous A18.13
urethra —*see* Urethritis
uterus, uterine —*see* Endometritis
vaccination T88.0
vaccinia not from vaccination B08.011
vagina (acute) —*see* Vaginitis
varicella B01.9
varicose veins —*see* Varix
vas deferens NEC N49.1
vesical —*see* Cystitis
Vibrio
cholerae A00.0
El Tor A00.1
parahaemolyticus (food poisoning) A05.3
vulnificus
as cause of disease classified elsewhere B96.82
foodborne intoxication A05.5
Vincent's (gum) (mouth) (tonsil) A69.1

Infection, infected, infective *(Continued)*
virus, viral NOS B34.9
adenovirus
as cause of disease classified elsewhere B97.0
unspecified nature or site B34.0
arborvirus, arbovirus arthropod-borne A94
as cause of disease classified elsewhere B97.89
adenovirus B97.0
coronavirus B97.29
SARS-associated B97.21
coxsackievirus B97.11
echovirus B97.12
enterovirus B97.10
coxsackievirus B97.11
echovirus B97.12
specified NEC B97.19
human
immunodeficiency, type 2 (HIV 2) B97.35
metapneumovirus B97.81
T-cell lymphotropic,
type I (HTLV-I) B97.33
type II (HTLV-II) B97.34
papillomavirus B97.7
parvovirus B97.6
reovirus B97.5
respiratory syncytial B97.4
retrovirus B97.30
human
immunodeficiency, type 2 (HIV 2) B97.35
T-cell lymphotropic,
type I (HTLV-I) B97.33
type II (HTLV-II) B97.34
lentivirus B97.31
oncovirus B97.32
specified NEC B97.39
specified NEC B97.89
central nervous system A89
atypical A81.9
specified NEC A81.89
enterovirus NEC A88.8
meningitis A87.0
slow virus A81.9
specified NEC A81.89
specified NEC A88.8
chest J98.8
cotia B08.8
coxsackie —*see also* Infection, coxsackie B34.1
as cause of disease classified elsewhere B97.11
ECHO
as cause of disease classified elsewhere B97.12
unspecified nature or site B34.1
encephalitis, tick-borne A84.9
enterovirus, as cause of disease classified elsewhere B97.10
coxsackievirus B97.11
echovirus B97.12
specified NEC B97.19
exanthem NOS B09
human metapneumovirus as cause of disease classified elsewhere B97.81
human papilloma as cause of disease classified elsewhere B97.7
intestine —*see* Enteritis, viral
respiratory syncytial
as cause of disease classified elsewhere B97.4
bronchopneumonia J12.1
common cold syndrome J00
nasopharyngitis (acute) J00
rhinovirus
as cause of disease classified elsewhere B97.89
unspecified nature or site B34.8
slow A81.9
specified NEC A81.89

Infection, infected, infective *(Continued)*
virus, viral NOS *(Continued)*
specified type NEC B33.8
as cause of disease classified elsewhere B97.89
unspecified nature or site B34.8
unspecified nature or site B34.9
West Nile —*see* Virus, West Nile
vulva (acute) —*see* Vulvitis
West Nile —*see* Virus, West Nile
whipworm B79
worms B83.9
specified type NEC B83.8
Wuchereria (bancrofti) B74.0
malayi B74.1
yatapoxvirus B08.70
specified NEC B08.79
yeast (*see also* Candidiasis) B37.9
yellow fever —*see* Fever, yellow
Yersinia
enterocolitica (intestinal) A04.6
pestis —*see* Plague
pseudotuberculosis A28.2
Zeis' gland —*see* Hordeolum
Zika virus A92.5 ◀
zoonotic bacterial NOS A28.9
Zopfia senegalensis B47.0
Infective, infectious —*see* condition
Infertility
female N97.9
age-related N97.8
associated with
anovulation N97.0
cervical (mucus) disease or anomaly N88.3
congenital anomaly
cervix N88.3
fallopian tube N97.1
uterus N97.2
vagina N97.8
dysmucorrhea N88.3
fallopian tube disease or anomaly N97.1
pituitary-hypothalamic origin E23.0
specified origin NEC N97.8
Stein-Leventhal syndrome E28.2
uterine disease or anomaly N97.2
vaginal disease or anomaly N97.8
due to
cervical anomaly N88.3
fallopian tube anomaly N97.1
ovarian failure E28.39
Stein-Leventhal syndrome E28.2
uterine anomaly N97.2
vaginal anomaly N97.8
nonimplantation N97.2
origin
cervical N88.3
tubal (block) (occlusion) (stenosis) N97.1
uterine N97.2
vaginal N97.8
male N46.9
azoospermia N46.01
extratesticular cause N46.029
drug therapy N46.021
efferent duct obstruction N46.023
infection N46.022
radiation N46.024
specified cause NEC N46.029
systemic disease N46.025
oligospermia N46.11
extratesticular cause N46.129
drug therapy N46.121
efferent duct obstruction N46.123
infection N46.122
radiation N46.124
specified cause NEC N46.129
systemic disease N46.125
specified type NEC N46.8
Infestation B88.9
Acanthocheilonema (perstans) (streptocerca) B74.4

◀ New ⬅ Revised ~~deleted~~ Deleted

Infestation *(Continued)*
Acariasis B88.0
demodex folliculorum B88.0
sarcoptes scabiei B86
trombiculae B88.0
Agamofilaria streptocerca B74.4
Ancylostoma, ankylostoma (braziliense) (caninum) (ceylanicum) (duodenale) B76.0
americanum B76.1
new world B76.1
Anisakis larvae, anisakiasis B81.0
arthropod NEC B88.2
Ascaris lumbricoides —*see* Ascariasis
Balantidium coli A07.0
beef tapeworm B68.1
Bothriocephalus (latus) B70.0
larval B70.1
broad tapeworm B70.0
larval B70.1
Brugia (malayi) B74.1
timori B74.2
candiru B88.8
Capillaria
hepatica B83.8
philippinensis B81.1
cat liver fluke B66.0
cestodes B71.9
diphyllobothrium —*see* Infestation, diphyllobothrium
dipylidiasis B71.1
hymenolepiasis B71.0
specified type NEC B71.8
chigger B88.0
chigo, chigoe B88.1
Clonorchis (sinensis) (liver) B66.1
coccidial A07.3
crab-lice B85.3
Cysticercus cellulosae —*see* Cysticercosis
Demodex (folliculorum) B88.0
Dermanyssus gallinae B88.0
Dermatobia (hominis) —*see* Myiasis
Dibothriocephalus (latus) B70.0
larval B70.1
Dicrocoelium dendriticum B66.2
Diphyllobothrium (adult) (latum) (intestinal) (pacificum) B70.0
larval B70.1
Diplogonoporus (grandis) B71.8
Dipylidium caninum B67.4
Distoma hepaticum B66.3
dog tapeworm B67.4
Dracunculus medinensis B72
dragon worm B72
dwarf tapeworm B71.0
Echinococcus —*see* Echinococcus
Echinostomum ilocanum B66.8
Entamoeba (histolytica) —*see* Infection, Ameba
Enterobius vermicularis B80
eyelid
in (due to)
leishmaniasis B55.1
loiasis B74.3
onchocerciasis B73.09
phthiriasis B85.3
parasitic NOS B89
eyeworm B74.3
Fasciola (gigantica) (hepatica) (indica) B66.3
Fasciolopsis (buski) (intestine) B66.5
filarial B74.9
bancroftian B74.0
conjunctiva B74.9
due to
Acanthocheilonema (perstans) (streptocerca) B74.4
Brugia (malayi) B74.1
timori B74.2
Dracunculus medinensis B72
guinea worm B72
loa loa B74.3

Infestation *(Continued)*
filarial *(Continued)*
due to *(Continued)*
Mansonella (ozzardi) (perstans) (streptocerca) B74.4
Onchocerca volvulus B73.00
eye B73.00
eyelid B73.09
Wuchereria (bancrofti) B74.0
Malayan B74.1
ozzardi B74.4
specified type NEC B74.8
fish tapeworm B70.0
larval B70.1
fluke B66.9
blood NOS —*see* Schistosomiasis
cat liver B66.0
intestinal B66.5
lancet B66.2
liver (sheep) B66.3
cat B66.0
Chinese B66.1
due to clonorchiasis B66.1
oriental B66.1
lung (oriental) B66.4
sheep liver B66.3
specified type NEC B66.8
fly larvae —*see* Myiasis
Gasterophilus (intestinalis) —*see* Myiasis
Gastrodiscoides hominis B66.8
Giardia lamblia A07.1
Gnathostoma (spinigerum) B83.1
Gongylonema B83.8
guinea worm B72
helminth B83.9
angiostrongyliasis B83.2
intestinal B81.3
gnathostomiasis B83.1
hirudiniasis, internal B83.4
intestinal B82.0
angiostrongyliasis B81.3
anisakiasis B81.0
ascariasis —*see* Ascariasis
capillariasis B81.1
cysticercosis —*see* Cysticercosis
diphyllobothriasis —*see* Infestation, diphyllobothriasis
dracunculiasis B72
echinococcus —*see* Echinococcosis
enterobiasis B80
filariasis —*see* Infestation, filarial
fluke —*see* Infestation, fluke
hookworm —*see* Infestation, hookworm
mixed (types classifiable to more than one of the titles B65.0-B81.3 and B81.8) B81.4
onchocerciasis —*see* Onchocerciasis
schistosomiasis —*see* Infestation, schistosoma
specified
cestode NEC —*see* Infestation, cestode type NEC B81.8
strongyloidiasis —*see* Strongyloidiasis
taenia —*see* Infestation, taenia
trichinellosis B75
trichostrongyliasis B81.2
trichuriasis B79
specified type NEC B83.8
syngamiasis B83.3
visceral larva migrans B83.0
Heterophyes (heterophyes) B66.8
hookworm B76.9
ancylostomiasis B76.0
necatoriasis B76.1
specified type NEC B76.8
Hymenolepis (diminuta) (nana) B71.0
intestinal NEC B82.9
leeches (aquatic) (land) —*see* Hirudiniasis
Leishmania —*see* Leishmaniasis
lice, louse —*see* Infestation, Pediculus
Linguatula B88.8

Infestation *(Continued)*
Liponyssoides sanguineus B88.0
Loa loa B74.3
conjunctival B74.3
eyelid B74.3
louse —*see* Infestation, Pediculus
maggots —*see* Myiasis
Mansonella (ozzardi) (perstans) (streptocerca) B74.4
Medina (worm) B72
Metagonimus (yokogawai) B66.8
microfilaria streptocerca —*see* Onchocerciasis
eye B73.00
eyelid B73.09
mites B88.9
scabic B86
Monilia (albicans) —*see* Candidiasis
mouth B37.0
Necator americanus B76.1
nematode NEC (intestinal) B82.0
Ancylostoma B76.0
conjunctiva NEC B83.9
Enterobius vermicularis B80
Gnathostoma spinigerum B83.1
physaloptera B80
specified NEC B81.8
trichostrongylus B81.2
trichuris (trichuria) B79
Oesophagostomum (apiostomum) B81.8
Oestrus ovis —*see also* Myiasis B87.9
Onchocerca (volvulus) —*see* Onchocerciasis
Opisthorchis (felineus) (viverrini) B66.0
orbit, parasitic NOS B89
Oxyuris vermicularis B80
Paragonimus (westermani) B66.4
parasite, parasitic B89
eyelid B89
intestinal NOS B82.9
mouth B37.0
skin B88.9
tongue B37.0
Parastrongylus
cantonensis B83.2
costaricensis B81.3
Pediculus B85.2
body B85.1
capitis (humanus) (any site) B85.0
corporis (humanus) (any site) B85.1
head B85.0
mixed (classifiable to more than one of the titles B85.0-B85.3) B85.4
pubis (any site) B85.3
Pentastoma B88.8
Phthirus (pubis) (any site) B85.3
with any infestation classifiable to B85.0-B85.2 B85.4
pinworm B80
pork tapeworm (adult) B68.0
protozoal NEC B64
intestinal A07.9
specified NEC A07.8
specified NEC B60.8
pubic, louse B85.3
rat tapeworm B71.0
red bug B88.0
roundworm (large) NEC B82.0
Ascariasis —*see also* Ascariasis B77.9
sandflea B88.1
Sarcoptes scabiei B86
scabies B86
Schistosoma B65.9
bovis B65.8
cercariae B65.3
haematobium B65.0
intercalatum B65.8
japonicum B65.2
mansoni B65.1
mattheei B65.8
mekongi B65.8
specified type NEC B65.8
spindale B65.8

Infestation *(Continued)*
screw worms —*see* Myiasis
skin NOS B88.9
Sparganum (mansoni) (proliferum) (baxteri) B70.1
larval B70.1
specified type NEC B88.8
Spirometra larvae B70.1
Stellantchasmus falcatus B66.8
Strongyloides stercoralis —*see* Strongyloidiasis
Taenia B68.9
diminuta B71.0
echinococcus —*see* Echinococcus
mediocanellata B68.1
nana B71.0
saginata B68.1
solium (intestinal form) B68.0
larval form —*see* Cysticercosis
Taeniarhynchus saginatus B68.1
tapeworm B71.9
beef B68.1
broad B70.0
larval B70.1
dog B67.4
dwarf B71.0
fish B70.0
larval B70.1
pork B68.0
rat B71.0
Ternidens diminutus B81.8
Tetranychus molestissimus B88.0
threadworm B80
tongue B37.0
Toxocara (canis) (cati) (felis) B83.0
trematode (s) NEC —*see* Infestation, fluke
Trichinella (spiralis) B75
Trichocephalus B79
Trichomonas —*see* Trichomoniasis
Trichostrongylus B81.2
Trichuris (trichiura) B79
Trombicula (irritans) B88.0
Tunga penetrans B88.1
Uncinaria americana B76.1
Vandellia cirrhosa B88.8
whipworm B79
worms B83.9
intestinal B82.0
Wuchereria (bancrofti) B74.0
Infiltrate, infiltration
amyloid (generalized) (localized) —*see* Amyloidosis
calcareous NEC R89.7
localized —*see* Degeneration, by site
calcium salt R89.7
cardiac
fatty —*see* Degeneration, myocardial
glycogenic E74.02 *[I43]*
corneal —*see* Edema, cornea
eyelid —*see* Inflammation, eyelid
glycogen, glycogenic —*see* Disease, glycogen storage
heart, cardiac
fatty —*see* Degeneration, myocardial
glycogenic E74.02 *[I43]*
inflammatory in vitreous H43.89
kidney N28.89
leukemic —*see* Leukemia
liver K76.89
fatty —*see* Fatty, liver NEC
glycogen —*see also* Disease, glycogen storage E74.03 *[K77]*
lung R91.8
eosinophilic J82
lymphatic —*see also* Leukemia, lymphatic C91.9-
gland I88.9
muscle, fatty M62.89
myocardium, myocardial
fatty —*see* Degeneration, myocardial
glycogenic E74.02 *[I43]*
Infiltrate, infiltration *(Continued)*
on chest x-ray R91.8
pulmonary R91.8
with eosinophilia J82
skin (lymphocytic) L98.6
thymus (gland) (fatty) E32.8
urine R39.0
vesicant agent
antineoplastic chemotherapy T80.810
other agent NEC T80.818
vitreous body H43.89
Infirmity R68.89
senile R54
Inflammation, inflamed, inflammatory (with exudation)
abducent (nerve) —*see* Strabismus, paralytic, sixth nerve
accessory sinus (chronic) —*see* Sinusitis
adrenal (gland) E27.8
alveoli, teeth M27.3
scorbutic E54
anal canal, anus K62.89
antrum (chronic) —*see* Sinusitis, maxillary
appendix —*see* Appendicitis
arachnoid —*see* Meningitis
areola N61.0 ⇐
puerperal, postpartum or gestational —*see* Infection, nipple
areolar tissue NOS L08.9
artery —*see* Arteritis
auditory meatus (external) —*see* Otitis, externa
Bartholin's gland N75.8
bile duct (common) (hepatic) or passage —*see* Cholangitis
bladder —*see* Cystitis
bone —*see* Osteomyelitis
brain —*see also* Encephalitis
membrane —*see* Meningitis
breast N61.0 ⇐
puerperal, postpartum, gestational —*see* Mastitis, obstetric
broad ligament —*see* Disease, pelvis, inflammatory
bronchi —*see* Bronchitis
catarrhal J00
cecum —*see* Appendicitis
cerebral —*see also* Encephalitis
membrane —*see* Meningitis
cerebrospinal
meningococcal A39.0
cervix (uteri) —*see* Cervicitis
chest J98.8
chorioretinal H30.9-
cyclitis —*see* Cyclitis
disseminated H30.10-
generalized H30.13-
peripheral H30.12-
posterior pole H30.11-
epitheliopathy —*see* Epitheliopathy
focal H30.00-
juxtapapillary H30.01-
macular H30.04-
paramacular —*see* Inflammation, chorioretinal, focal, macular
peripheral H30.03-
posterior pole H30.02-
specified type NEC H30.89-
choroid —*see* Inflammation, chorioretinal
chronic, postmastoidectomy cavity —*see* Complications, postmastoidectomy, inflammation
colon —*see* Enteritis
connective tissue (diffuse) NEC —*see* Disorder, soft tissue, specified type NEC
cornea —*see* Keratitis
corpora cavernosa N48.29
cranial nerve —*see* Disorder, nerve, cranial
Douglas' cul-de-sac or pouch (chronic) N73.0
Inflammation, inflamed, inflammatory *(Continued)*
due to device, implant or graft —*see also* Complications, by site and type, infection or inflammation
arterial graft T82.7
breast (implant) T85.79
catheter T85.79
dialysis (renal) T82.7
intraperitoneal T85.71
infusion T82.7
cranial T85.735 ◀
intrathecal T85.735 ◀
spinal (epidural) (subdural) T85.735 ⇐
subarachnoid T85.735 ◀
urinary T83.518 ⇐
cystostomy T83.510 ◀
Hopkins T83.518 ◀
ileostomy T83.518 ◀
nephrostomy T83.512 ◀
specified NEC T83.518 ◀
urethral indwelling T83.511 ◀
urostomy T83.518 ◀
electronic (electrode) (pulse generator) (stimulator)
bone T84.7
cardiac T82.7
nervous system T85.738 ⇐
brain T85.731 ◀
cranial nerve T85.732 ◀
gastric nerve T85.732 ◀
neurostimulator generator T85.734 ◀
peripheral nerve T85.732 ◀
sacral nerve T85.732 ◀
spinal cord T85.733 ◀
vagal nerve T85.732 ◀
urinary T83.590 ⇐
fixation, internal (orthopedic) NEC —*see* Complication, fixation device, infection
gastrointestinal (bile duct) (esophagus) T85.79
neurostimulator electrode (lead) T85.732 ◀
genital NEC T83.69 ⇐
heart NEC T82.7
valve (prosthesis) T82.6
graft T82.7
joint prosthesis —*see* Complication, joint prosthesis, infection
ocular (corneal graft) (orbital implant) NEC T85.79
orthopedic NEC T84.7
penile (cylinder) (pump) (reservoir) T83.61 ◀
specified NEC T85.79
testicular T83.62 ◀
urinary NEC T83.598 ⇐
ileal conduit stent T83.593 ◀
implanted neurostimulation T83.590 ◀
implanted sphincter T83.591 ◀
indwelling ureteral stent T83.592 ◀
nephroureteral stent T83.593 ◀
specified stent NEC T83.593 ◀
vascular NEC T82.7
~~ventricular intracranial shunt T85.79~~
ventricular intracranial (communicating) shunt T85.730 ◀
duodenum K29.80
with bleeding K29.81
dura mater —*see* Meningitis
ear (middle) —*see also* Otitis, media
external —*see* Otitis, externa
inner —*see* subcategory H83.0
epididymis —*see* Epididymitis
esophagus K20.9
ethmoidal (sinus) (chronic) —*see* Sinusitis, ethmoidal
eustachian tube (catarrhal) —*see* Salpingitis, eustachian

◀ New ⇐ Revised ~~deleted~~ Deleted

Inflammation, inflamed, inflammatory *(Continued)*
eyelid H01.9
abscess —*see* Abscess, eyelid
blepharitis —*see* Blepharitis
chalazion —*see* Chalazion
dermatosis (noninfectious) —*see* Dermatosis, eyelid
hordeolum —*see* Hordeolum
specified NEC H01.8
fallopian tube —*see* Salpingo-oophoritis
fascia —*see* Myositis
follicular, pharynx J31.2
frontal (sinus) (chronic) —*see* Sinusitis, frontal
gallbladder —*see* Cholecystitis
gastric —*see* Gastritis
gastrointestinal —*see* Enteritis
genital organ (internal) (diffuse)
female —*see* Disease, pelvis, inflammatory
male N49.9
multiple sites N49.8
specified NEC N49.8
gland (lymph) —*see* Lymphadenitis
glottis —*see* Laryngitis
granular, pharynx J31.2
gum K05.10
nonplaque induced K05.11
plaque induced K05.10
heart —*see* Carditis
hepatic duct —*see* Cholangitis
ileoanal (internal) pouch K91.850
ileum —*see also* Enteritis
regional or terminal —*see* Enteritis, regional
intestinal pouch K91.850
intestine (any part) —*see* Enteritis
jaw (acute) (bone) (chronic) (lower) (suppurative) (upper) M27.2
joint NEC —*see* Arthritis
sacroiliac M46.1
kidney —*see* Nephritis
knee (joint) M13.169
tuberculous A18.02
labium (majus) (minus) —*see* Vulvitis
lacrimal
gland —*see* Dacryoadenitis
passages (duct) (sac) —*see also* Dacryocystitis
canaliculitis —*see* Canaliculitis, lacrimal
larynx —*see* Laryngitis
leg NOS L08.9
lip K13.0
liver (capsule) —*see also* Hepatitis
chronic K73.9
suppurative K75.0
lung (acute) —*see also* Pneumonia
chronic J98.4
lymphatic vessel —*see* Lymphangitis
lymph gland or node —*see* Lymphadenitis
maxilla, maxillary M27.2
sinus (chronic) —*see* Sinusitis, maxillary
membranes of brain or spinal cord —*see* Meningitis
meninges —*see* Meningitis
mouth K12.1
muscle —*see* Myositis
myocardium —*see* Myocarditis
nasal sinus (chronic) —*see* Sinusitis
nasopharynx —*see* Nasopharyngitis
navel L08.82
nerve NEC —*see* Neuralgia
nipple N61.0 ⇐
puerperal, postpartum or gestational —*see* Infection, nipple
nose —*see* Rhinitis
oculomotor (nerve) —*see* Strabismus, paralytic, third nerve
optic nerve —*see* Neuritis, optic
orbit (chronic) H05.10
acute H05.00
abscess —*see* Abscess, orbit
cellulitis —*see* Cellulitis, orbit

Inflammation, inflamed, inflammatory *(Continued)*
orbit (chronic) *(Continued)*
acute *(Continued)*
osteomyelitis —*see* Osteomyelitis, orbit
periostitis —*see* Periostitis, orbital
tenonitis —*see* Tenonitis, eye
granuloma —*see* Granuloma, orbit
myositis —*see* Myositis, orbital
ovary —*see* Salpingo-oophoritis
oviduct —*see* Salpingo-oophoritis
pancreas (acute) —*see* Pancreatitis
parametrium N73.0
parotid region L08.9
pelvis, female —*see* Disease, pelvis, inflammatory
penis (corpora cavernosa) N48.29
perianal K62.89
pericardium —*see* Pericarditis
perineum (female) (male) L08.9
perirectal K62.89
peritoneum —*see* Peritonitis
periuterine —*see* Disease, pelvis, inflammatory
perivesical —*see* Cystitis
petrous bone (acute) (chronic) —*see* Petrositis
pharynx (acute) —*see* Pharyngitis
pia mater —*see* Meningitis
pleura —*see* Pleurisy
polyp, colon —*see also* Polyp, colon, inflammatory K51.40
prostate —*see also* Prostatitis
specified type NEC N41.8
rectosigmoid —*see* Rectosigmoiditis
rectum —*see also* Proctitis K62.89
respiratory, upper —*see also* Infection, respiratory, upper J06.9
acute, due to radiation J70.0
chronic, due to external agent —*see* condition, respiratory, chronic, due to
due to
chemicals, gases, fumes or vapors (inhalation) J68.2
radiation J70.1
retina —*see* Chorioretinitis
retrocecal —*see* Appendicitis
retroperitoneal —*see* Peritonitis
salivary duct or gland (any) (suppurative) —*see* Sialoadenitis
scorbutic, alveoli, teeth E54
scrotum N49.2
seminal vesicle —*see* Vesiculitis
sigmoid —*see* Enteritis
sinus —*see* Sinusitis
Skene's duct or gland —*see* Urethritis
skin L08.9
spermatic cord N49.1
sphenoidal (sinus) —*see* Sinusitis, sphenoidal
spinal
cord —*see* Encephalitis
membrane —*see* Meningitis
nerve —*see* Disorder, nerve
spine —*see* Spondylopathy, inflammatory
spleen (capsule) D73.89
stomach —*see* Gastritis
subcutaneous tissue L08.9
suprarenal (gland) E27.8
synovial —*see* Tenosynovitis
tendon (sheath) NEC —*see* Tenosynovitis
testis —*see* Orchitis
throat (acute) —*see* Pharyngitis
thymus (gland) E32.8
thyroid (gland) —*see* Thyroiditis
tongue K14.0
tonsil —*see* Tonsillitis
trachea —*see* Tracheitis
trochlear (nerve) —*see* Strabismus, paralytic, fourth nerve
tubal —*see* Salpingo-oophoritis
tuberculous NEC —*see* Tuberculosis

Inflammation, inflamed, inflammatory *(Continued)*
tubo-ovarian —*see* Salpingo-oophoritis
tunica vaginalis N49.1
tympanic membrane —*see* Tympanitis
umbilicus, umbilical L08.82
uterine ligament —*see* Disease, pelvis, inflammatory
uterus (catarrhal) —*see* Endometritis
uveal tract (anterior) NOS —*see also* Iridocyclitis
posterior —*see* Chorioretinitis
vagina —*see* Vaginitis
vas deferens N49.1
vein —*see also* Phlebitis
intracranial or intraspinal (septic) G08
thrombotic I80.9
leg —*see* Phlebitis, leg
lower extremity —*see* Phlebitis, leg
vocal cord J38.3
vulva —*see* Vulvitis
Wharton's duct (suppurative) —*see* Sialoadenitis
Inflation, lung, imperfect (newborn) —*see* Atelectasis
Influenza (bronchial) (epidemic) (respiratory (upper)) (unidentified influenza virus) J11.1
with
digestive manifestations J11.2
encephalopathy J11.81
enteritis J11.2
gastroenteritis J11.2
gastrointestinal manifestations J11.2
laryngitis J11.1
myocarditis J11.82
otitis media J11.83
pharyngitis J11.1
pneumonia J11.00
specified type J11.08
respiratory manifestations NEC J11.1
specified manifestation NEC J11.89
A/H5N1 —*see also* Influenza, due to, identified novel influenza A virus J09.X2
avian —*see also* Influenza, due to, identified novel influenza A virus J09.X2
bird —*see also* Influenza, due to, identified novel influenza A virus J09.X2
novel (2009) H1N1 influenza —*see also* Influenza, due to, identified influenza virus NEC J10.1
novel influenza A/H1N1 —*see also* Influenza, due to, identified influenza virus NEC J10.1
due to
avian (*see also* Influenza, due to, identified novel influenza A virus) J09.X2
identified influenza virus NEC J10.1
with
digestive manifestations J10.2
encephalopathy J10.81
enteritis J10.2
gastroenteritis J10.2
gastrointestinal manifestations J10.2
laryngitis J10.1
myocarditis J10.82
otitis media J10.83
pharyngitis J10.1
pneumonia (unspecified type) J10.00
with same identified influenza virus J10.01
specified type NEC J10.08
respiratory manifestations NEC J10.1
specified manifestation NEC J10.89
identified novel influenza A virus J09.X2
with
digestive manifestations J09.X3
encephalopathy J09.X9
enteritis J09.X3
gastroenteritis J09.X3
gastrointestinal manifestations J09.X3

Influenza *(Continued)*
due to *(Continued)*
identified novel influenza A virus *(Continued)*
with *(Continued)*
laryngitis J09.X2
myocarditis J09.X9
otitis media J09.X9
pharyngitis J09.X2
pneumonia J09.X1
respiratory manifestations NEC J09.X2
specified manifestation NEC J09.X9
upper respiratory symptoms J09.X2
of other animal origin, not bird or swine (*see also* Influenza, due to, identified novel influenza A virus) J09.X2
swine (viruses that normally cause infections in pigs) —*see also* Influenza, due to, identified novel influenza A virus J09.X2
Influenza-like disease —*see* Influenza
Influenzal —*see* Influenza
Infraction, Freiberg's (metatarsal head) —*see* Osteochondrosis, juvenile, metatarsus
Infraeruption of tooth (teeth) M26.34
Infusion complication, misadventure, or reaction —*see* Complications, infusion
Ingestion
chemical —*see* Table of Drugs and Chemicals, by substance, poisoning
drug or medicament
correct substance properly administered —*see* Table of Drugs and Chemicals, by drug, adverse effect
overdose or wrong substance given or taken —*see* Table of Drugs and Chemicals, by drug, poisoning
foreign body —*see* Foreign body, alimentary tract
tularemia A21.3
Ingrowing
hair (beard) L73.1
nail (finger) (toe) L60.0
Inguinal —*see also* condition
testicle Q53.9
bilateral Q53.21
unilateral Q53.11
Inhalant-induced ◀
anxiety disorder F18.980 ◀
depressive disorder F18.94 ◀
major neurocognitive disorder F18.97 ◀
mild neurocognitive disorder F18.988 ◀
psychotic disorder F18.959 ◀
Inhalation
anthrax A22.1
flame T27.3
food or foreign body —*see* Foreign body, by site
gases, fumes, or vapors NEC T59.9-
specified agent —*see* Table of Drugs and Chemicals, by substance
liquid or vomitus —*see* Asphyxia
meconium (newborn) P24.00
with
with respiratory symptoms P24.01
pneumonia (pneumonitis) P24.01
mucus —*see* Asphyxia, mucus
oil or gasoline (causing suffocation) —*see* Foreign body, by site
smoke J70.5
due to chemicals, gases, fumes and vapors J68.9
steam —*see* Toxicity, vapors
stomach contents or secretions —*see* Foreign body, by site
due to anesthesia (general) (local) or other sedation T88.59
in labor and delivery O74.0
in pregnancy O29.01-
postpartum, puerperal O89.01
Inhibition, orgasm
female F52.31
male F52.32
Inhibitor, systemic lupus erythematosus (presence of) D68.62
Iniencephalus, iniencephaly Q00.2
Injection, traumatic jet (air) (industrial) (water) (paint or dye) T70.4
Injury —*see also* specified injury type T14.90
abdomen, abdominal S39.91
blood vessel —*see* Injury, blood vessel, abdomen
cavity —*see* Injury, intra-abdominal
contusion S30.1
internal —*see* Injury, intra-abdominal
intra-abdominal organ —*see* Injury, intra-abdominal
nerve —*see* Injury, nerve, abdomen
open —*see* Wound, open, abdomen
specified NEC S39.81
superficial —*see* Injury, superficial, abdomen
Achilles tendon S86.00-
laceration S86.02-
specified type NEC S86.09-
strain S86.01-
acoustic, resulting in deafness —*see* Injury, nerve, acoustic
adrenal (gland) S37.819
contusion S37.812
laceration S37.813
specified type NEC S37.818
alveolar (process) S09.93
ankle S99.91-
contusion —*see* Contusion, ankle
dislocation —*see* Dislocation, ankle
fracture —*see* Fracture, ankle
nerve —*see* Injury, nerve, ankle
open —*see* Wound, open, ankle
specified type NEC S99.81-
sprain —*see* Sprain, ankle
superficial —*see* Injury, superficial, ankle
anterior chamber, eye —*see* Injury, eye, specified site NEC
anus —*see* Injury, abdomen
aorta (thoracic) S25.00
abdominal S35.00
laceration (minor) (superficial) S35.01
major S35.02
specified type NEC S35.09
laceration (minor) (superficial) S25.01
major S25.02
specified type NEC S25.09
arm (upper) S49.9-
blood vessel —*see* Injury, blood vessel, arm
contusion —*see* Contusion, arm, upper
fracture —*see* Fracture, humerus
lower —*see* Injury, forearm
muscle —*see* Injury, muscle, shoulder
nerve —*see* Injury, nerve, arm
open —*see* Wound, open, arm
specified type NEC S49.8-
superficial —*see* Injury, superficial, arm
artery (complicating trauma) —*see also* Injury, blood vessel, by site
cerebral or meningeal —*see* Injury, intracranial
auditory canal (external) (meatus) S09.91
auricle, auris, ear S09.91
axilla —*see* Injury, shoulder
back —*see* Injury, back, lower
bile duct S36.13
birth —*see also* Birth, injury P15.9
bladder (sphincter) S37.20
at delivery O71.5
contusion S37.22
laceration S37.23
obstetrical trauma O71.5
specified type NEC S37.29
Injury *(Continued)*
blast (air) (hydraulic) (immersion) (underwater) NEC T14.8
acoustic nerve trauma —*see* Injury, nerve, acoustic
bladder —*see* Injury, bladder
brain —*see* Concussion
colon —*see* Injury, intestine, large, blast injury
ear (primary) S09.31-
secondary S09.39-
generalized T70.8
lung —*see* Injury, intrathoracic, lung, blast injury
multiple body organs T70.8
peritoneum S36.81
rectum S36.61
retroperitoneum S36.898
small intestine S36.419
duodenum S36.410
specified site NEC S36.418
specified
intra-abdominal organ NEC S36.898
pelvic organ NEC S37.899
blood vessel NEC T14.8
abdomen S35.9-
aorta —*see* Injury, aorta, abdominal
celiac artery —*see* Injury, blood vessel, celiac artery
iliac vessel —*see* Injury, blood vessel, iliac
laceration S35.91
mesenteric vessel —*see* Injury, mesenteric
portal vein —*see* Injury, blood vessel, portal vein
renal vessel —*see* Injury, blood vessel, renal
specified vessel NEC S35.8X-
splenic vessel —*see* Injury, blood vessel, splenic
vena cava —*see* Injury, vena cava, inferior
ankle —*see* Injury, blood vessel, foot
aorta (abdominal) (thoracic) —*see* Injury, aorta
arm (upper) NEC S45.90-
forearm —*see* Injury, blood vessel, forearm
laceration S45.91-
specified
site NEC S45.80-
laceration S45.81-
specified type NEC S45.89-
type NEC S45.99-
superficial vein S45.30-
laceration S45.31-
specified type NEC S45.39-
axillary
artery S45.00-
laceration S45.01-
specified type NEC S45.09-
vein S45.20-
laceration S45.21-
specified type NEC S45.29-
azygos vein —*see* Injury, blood vessel, thoracic, specified site NEC
brachial
artery S45.10-
laceration S45.11-
specified type NEC S45.19-
vein S45.20-
laceration S45.219
specified type NEC S45.29-
carotid artery (common) (external) (internal, extracranial) S15.00-
internal, intracranial S06.8-
laceration (minor) (superficial) S15.01-
major S15.02-
specified type NEC S15.09-

Injury *(Continued)*
blood vessel NEC *(Continued)*
celiac artery S35.219
branch S35.299
laceration (minor) (superficial) S35.291
major S35.292
specified NEC S35.298
laceration (minor) (superficial) S35.211
major S35.212
specified type NEC S35.218
cerebral —*see* Injury, intracranial
deep plantar —*see* Injury, blood vessel, plantar artery
digital (hand) —*see* Injury, blood vessel, finger
dorsal
artery (foot) S95.00-
laceration S95.01-
specified type NEC S95.09-
vein (foot) S95.20-
laceration S95.21-
specified type NEC S95.29-
due to accidental laceration during procedure —*see* Laceration, accidental complicating surgery
extremity —*see* Injury, blood vessel, limb
femoral
artery (common) (superficial) S75.00-
laceration (minor) (superficial) S75.01-
major S75.02-
specified type NEC S75.09-
vein (hip level) (thigh level) S75.10-
laceration (minor) (superficial) S75.11-
major S75.12-
specified type NEC S75.19-
finger S65.50-
index S65.50-
laceration S65.51-
specified type NEC S65.59-
laceration S65.51-
little S65.50-
laceration S65.51-
specified type NEC S65.59-
middle S65.50-
laceration S65.51-
specified type NEC S65.59-
specified type NEC S65.59-
thumb —*see* Injury, blood vessel, thumb
foot S95.90-
dorsal
artery —*see* Injury, blood vessel, dorsal, artery
vein —*see* Injury, blood vessel, dorsal, vein
laceration S95.91-
plantar artery —*see* Injury, blood vessel, plantar artery
specified
site NEC S95.80-
laceration S95.81-
specified type NEC S95.89-
specified type NEC S95.99-
forearm S55.90-
laceration S55.91-
radial artery —*see* Injury, blood vessel, radial artery
specified
site NEC S55.80-
laceration S55.81-
specified type NEC S55.89-
type NEC S55.99-
ulnar artery —*see* Injury, blood vessel, ulnar artery
vein S55.20-
laceration S55.21-
specified type NEC S55.29-
gastric
artery —*see* Injury, mesenteric, artery, branch
vein —*see* Injury, blood vessel, abdomen

Injury *(Continued)*
blood vessel NEC *(Continued)*
gastroduodenal artery —*see* Injury, mesenteric, artery, branch
greater saphenous vein (lower leg level) S85.30-
hip (and thigh) level S75.20-
laceration (minor) (superficial) S75.21-
major S75.22-
specified type NEC S75.29-
laceration S85.31-
specified type NEC S85.39-
hand (level) S65.90-
finger —*see* Injury, blood vessel, finger
laceration S65.91-
palmar arch —*see* Injury, blood vessel, palmar arch
radial artery —*see* Injury, blood vessel, radial artery, hand
specified
site NEC S65.80-
laceration S65.81-
specified type NEC S65.89-
type NEC S65.99-
thumb —*see* Injury, blood vessel, thumb
ulnar artery —*see* Injury, blood vessel, ulnar artery, hand
head S09.0
intracranial —*see* Injury, intracranial
multiple S09.0
hepatic
artery —*see* Injury, mesenteric, artery
vein —*see* Injury, vena cava, inferior
hip S75.90-
femoral artery —*see* Injury, blood vessel, femoral, artery
femoral vein —*see* Injury, blood vessel, femoral, vein
greater saphenous vein —*see* Injury, blood vessel, greater saphenous, hip level
laceration S75.91-
specified
site NEC S75.80-
laceration S75.81-
specified type NEC S75.89-
type NEC S75.99-
hypogastric (artery) (vein) —*see* Injury, blood vessel, iliac
iliac S35.5-
artery S35.51-
specified vessel NEC S35.5-
uterine vessel —*see* Injury, blood vessel, uterine
vein S35.51-
innominate —*see* Injury, blood vessel, thoracic, innominate
intercostal (artery) (vein) —*see* Injury, blood vessel, thoracic, intercostal
jugular vein (external) S15.20-
internal S15.30-
laceration (minor) (superficial) S15.31-
major S15.32-
specified type NEC S15.39-
laceration (minor) (superficial) S15.21-
major S15.22-
specified type NEC S15.29-
leg (level) (lower) S85.90-
greater saphenous —*see* Injury, blood vessel, greater saphenous
laceration S85.91-
lesser saphenous —*see* Injury, blood vessel, lesser saphenous
peroneal artery —*see* Injury, blood vessel, peroneal artery
popliteal
artery —*see* Injury, blood vessel, popliteal, artery
vein —*see* Injury, blood vessel, popliteal, vein

Injury *(Continued)*
blood vessel NEC *(Continued)*
leg (level) (lower) *(Continued)*
specified
site NEC S85.80-
laceration S85.81-
specified type NEC S85.89-
type NEC S85.99-
thigh —*see* Injury, blood vessel, hip
tibial artery —*see* Injury, blood vessel, tibial artery
lesser saphenous vein (lower leg level) S85.40-
laceration S85.41-
specified type NEC S85.49-
limb
lower —*see* Injury, blood vessel, leg
upper —*see* Injury, blood vessel, arm
lower back —*see* Injury, blood vessel, abdomen
specified NEC —*see* Injury, blood vessel, abdomen, specified, site NEC
mammary (artery) (vein) —*see* Injury, blood vessel, thoracic, specified site NEC
mesenteric (inferior) (superior)
artery —*see* Injury, mesenteric, artery
vein —*see* Injury, mesenteric, vein
neck S15.9
specified site NEC S15.8
ovarian (artery) (vein) —*see* subcategory S35.8
palmar arch (superficial) S65.20-
deep S65.30-
laceration S65.31-
specified type NEC S65.39-
laceration S65.21-
specified type NEC S65.29-
pelvis —*see* Injury, blood vessel, abdomen
specified NEC —*see* Injury, blood vessel, abdomen, specified, site NEC
peroneal artery S85.20-
laceration S85.21-
specified type NEC S85.29-
plantar artery (deep) (foot) S95.10-
laceration S95.11-
specified type NEC S95.19-
popliteal
artery S85.00-
laceration S85.01-
specified type NEC S85.09-
vein S85.50-
laceration S85.51-
specified type NEC S85.59-
portal vein S35.319
laceration S35.311
specified type NEC S35.318
precerebral —*see* Injury, blood vessel, neck
pulmonary (artery) (vein) —*see* Injury, blood vessel, thoracic, pulmonary
radial artery (forearm level) S55.10-
hand and wrist (level) S65.10-
laceration S65.11-
specified type NEC S65.19-
laceration S55.11-
specified type NEC S55.19-
renal
artery S35.40-
laceration S35.41-
specified NEC S35.49-
vein S35.40-
laceration S35.41-
specified NEC S35.49-
saphenous vein (greater) (lower leg level) —*see* Injury, blood vessel, greater saphenous
hip and thigh level —*see* Injury, blood vessel, greater saphenous, hip level
lesser —*see* Injury, blood vessel, lesser saphenous

Injury *(Continued)*
blood vessel NEC *(Continued)*
shoulder
specified NEC —*see* Injury, blood vessel, arm, specified site NEC
superficial vein —*see* Injury, blood vessel, arm, superficial vein
specified NEC T14.8
splenic
artery —*see* Injury, blood vessel, celiac artery, branch
vein S35.329
laceration S35.321
specified NEC S35.328
subclavian —*see* Injury, blood vessel, thoracic, innominate
thigh —*see* Injury, blood vessel, hip
thoracic S25.90
aorta S25.00
laceration (minor) (superficial) S25.01
major S25.02
specified type NEC S25.09
azygos vein —*see* Injury, blood vessel, thoracic, specified, site NEC
innominate
artery S25.10-
laceration (minor) (superficial) S25.11-
major S25.12-
specified type NEC S25.19-
vein S25.30-
laceration (minor) (superficial) S25.31-
major S25.32-
specified type NEC S25.39-
intercostal S25.50-
laceration S25.51-
specified type NEC S25.59-
laceration S25.91
mammary vessel —*see* Injury, blood vessel, thoracic, specified, site NEC
pulmonary S25.40-
laceration (minor) (superficial) S25.41-
major S25.42-
specified type NEC S25.49-
specified
site NEC S25.80-
laceration S25.81-
specified type NEC S25.89-
type NEC S25.99
subclavian —*see* Injury, blood vessel, thoracic, innominate
vena cava (superior) S25.20
laceration (minor) (superficial) S25.21
major S25.22
specified type NEC S25.29
thumb S65.40-
laceration S65.41-
specified type NEC S65.49-
tibial artery S85.10-
anterior S85.13-
laceration S85.14-
specified injury NEC S85.15-
laceration S85.11-
posterior S85.16-
laceration S85.17-
specified injury NEC S85.18-
specified injury NEC S85.12-
ulnar artery (forearm level) S55.00-
hand and wrist (level) S65.00-
laceration S65.01-
specified type NEC S65.09-
laceration S55.01-
specified type NEC S55.09-
upper arm (level) —*see* Injury, blood vessel, arm
superficial vein —*see* Injury, blood vessel, arm, superficial vein
uterine S35.5-
artery S35.53-
vein S35.53-

Injury *(Continued)*
blood vessel NEC *(Continued)*
vena cava —*see* Injury, vena cava
vertebral artery S15.10-
laceration (minor) (superficial) S15.11-
major S15.12-
specified type NEC S15.19-
wrist (level) —*see* Injury, blood vessel, hand
brachial plexus S14.3
newborn P14.3
brain (traumatic) S06.9-
diffuse (axonal) S06.2X-
focal S06.30-
~~traumatic —see category S06~~
brainstem S06.38-
breast NOS S29.9
broad ligament —*see* Injury, pelvic organ, specified site NEC
bronchus, bronchi —*see* Injury, intrathoracic, bronchus
brow S09.90
buttock S39.92
canthus, eye S05.90
cardiac plexus —*see* Injury, nerve, thorax, sympathetic
cauda equina S34.3
cavernous sinus —*see* Injury, intracranial
cecum —*see* Injury, colon
celiac ganglion or plexus —*see* Injury, nerve, lumbosacral, sympathetic
cerebellum —*see* Injury, intracranial
cerebral —*see* Injury, intracranial
cervix (uteri) —*see* Injury, uterus
cheek (wall) S09.93
chest —*see* Injury, thorax
childbirth (newborn) —*see also* Birth, injury
maternal NEC O71.9
chin S09.93
choroid (eye) —*see* Injury, eye, specified site NEC
clitoris S39.94
coccyx —*see also* Injury, back, lower
complicating delivery O71.6
colon —*see* Injury, intestine, large
common bile duct —*see* Injury, liver
conjunctiva (superficial) —*see* Injury, eye, conjunctiva
conus medullaris —*see* Injury, spinal, sacral
cord
spermatic (pelvic region) S37.898
scrotal region S39.848
spinal —*see* Injury, spinal cord, by region
cornea —*see* Injury, eye, specified site NEC
abrasion —*see* Injury, eye, cornea, abrasion
cortex (cerebral) —*see also* Injury, intracranial
visual —*see* Injury, nerve, optic
costal region NEC S29.9
costochondral NEC S29.9
cranial
cavity —*see* Injury, intracranial
nerve —*see* Injury, nerve, cranial
crushing —*see* Crush
cutaneous sensory nerve
cystic duct —*see* Injury, liver
deep tissue —*see* Contusion, by site
meaning pressure ulcer —*see* Ulcer, pressure, unstageable, by site
delivery (newborn) P15.9
maternal NEC O71.9
Descemet's membrane —*see* Injury, eyeball, penetrating
diaphragm —*see* Injury, intrathoracic, diaphragm
duodenum —*see* Injury, intestine, small, duodenum
ear (auricle) (external) (canal) S09.91
abrasion —*see* Abrasion, ear
bite —*see* Bite, ear
blister —*see* Blister, ear
bruise —*see* Contusion, ear

Injury *(Continued)*
ear *(Continued)*
contusion —*see* Contusion, ear
external constriction —*see* Constriction, external, ear
hematoma —*see* Hematoma, ear
inner —*see* Injury, ear, middle
laceration —*see* Laceration, ear
middle S09.30-
blast —*see* Injury, blast, ear
specified NEC S09.39-
puncture —*see* Puncture, ear
superficial —*see* Injury, superficial, ear
eighth cranial nerve (acoustic or auditory) —*see* Injury, nerve, acoustic
elbow S59.90-
contusion —*see* Contusion, elbow
dislocation —*see* Dislocation, elbow
fracture —*see* Fracture, ulna, upper end
open —*see* Wound, open, elbow
specified NEC S59.80-
sprain —*see* Sprain, elbow
superficial —*see* Injury, superficial, elbow
eleventh cranial nerve (accessory) —*see* Injury, nerve, accessory
epididymis S39.94
epigastric region S39.91
epiglottis NEC S19.89
esophageal plexus —*see* Injury, nerve, thorax, sympathetic
esophagus (thoracic part) —*see also* Injury, intrathoracic, esophagus
cervical NEC S19.85
eustachian tube S09.30-
eye S05.9-
avulsion S05.7-
ball —*see* Injury, eyeball
conjunctiva S05.0-
cornea
abrasion S05.0-
laceration S05.3-
with prolapse S05.2-
lacrimal apparatus S05.8X-
orbit penetration S05.4-
specified site NEC S05.8X-
eyeball S05.8X-
contusion S05.1-
penetrating S05.6-
with
foreign body S05.5-
prolapse or loss of intraocular tissue S05.2-
without prolapse or loss of intraocular tissue S05.3-
specified type NEC S05.8-
eyebrow S09.93
eyelid S09.93
abrasion —*see* Abrasion, eyelid
contusion —*see* Contusion, eyelid
open —*see* Wound, open, eyelid
face S09.93
fallopian tube S37.509
bilateral S37.502
blast injury S37.512
contusion S37.522
laceration S37.532
specified type NEC S37.592
blast injury (primary) S37.519
bilateral S37.512
secondary —*see* Injury, fallopian tube, specified type NEC
unilateral S37.511
contusion S37.529
bilateral S37.522
unilateral S37.521
laceration S37.539
bilateral S37.532
unilateral S37.531
specified type NEC S37.599
bilateral S37.592
unilateral S37.591

Injury *(Continued)*
fallopian tube *(Continued)*
unilateral S37.501
blast injury S37.511
contusion S37.521
laceration S37.531
specified type NEC S37.591
fascia —*see* Injury, muscle
fifth cranial nerve (trigeminal) —*see* Injury, nerve, trigeminal
finger (nail) S69.9-
blood vessel —*see* Injury, blood vessel, finger
contusion —*see* Contusion, finger
dislocation —*see* Dislocation, finger
fracture —*see* Fracture, finger
muscle —*see* Injury, muscle, finger
nerve —*see* Injury, nerve, digital, finger
open —*see* Wound, open, finger
specified NEC S69.8-
sprain —*see* Sprain, finger
superficial —*see* Injury, superficial, finger
first cranial nerve (olfactory) —*see* Injury, nerve, olfactory
flank —*see* Injury, abdomen
foot S99.92-
blood vessel —*see* Injury, blood vessel, foot
contusion —*see* Contusion, foot
dislocation —*see* Dislocation, foot
fracture —*see* Fracture, foot
muscle —*see* Injury, muscle, foot
open —*see* Wound, open, foot
specified type NEC S99.82-
sprain —*see* Sprain, foot
superficial —*see* Injury, superficial, foot
forceps NOS P15.9
forearm S59.91-
blood vessel —*see* Injury, blood vessel, forearm
contusion —*see* Contusion, forearm
fracture —*see* Fracture, forearm
muscle —*see* Injury, muscle, forearm
nerve —*see* Injury, nerve, forearm
open —*see* Wound, open, forearm
specified NEC S59.81-
superficial —*see* Injury, superficial, forearm
forehead S09.90
fourth cranial nerve (trochlear) —*see* Injury, nerve, trochlear
gallbladder S36.129
contusion S36.122
laceration S36.123
specified NEC S36.128
ganglion
celiac, coeliac —*see* Injury, nerve, lumbosacral, sympathetic
gasserian —*see* Injury, nerve, trigeminal
stellate —*see* Injury, nerve, thorax, sympathetic
thoracic sympathetic —*see* Injury, nerve, thorax, sympathetic
gasserian ganglion —*see* Injury, nerve, trigeminal
gastric artery —*see* Injury, blood vessel, celiac artery, branch
gastroduodenal artery —*see* Injury, blood vessel, celiac artery, branch
gastrointestinal tract —*see* Injury, intra-abdominal
with open wound into abdominal cavity —*see* Wound, open, with penetration into peritoneal cavity
colon —*see* Injury, intestine, large
rectum —*see* Injury, intestine, large, rectum
with open wound into abdominal cavity S36.61
small intestine —*see* Injury, intestine, small
specified site NEC —*see* Injury, intra-abdominal, specified, site NEC
stomach —*see* Injury, stomach

Injury *(Continued)*
genital organ (s)
external S39.94
specified NEC S39.848
internal S37.90
fallopian tube —*see* Injury, fallopian tube
ovary —*see* Injury, ovary
prostate —*see* Injury, prostate
seminal vesicle —*see* Injury, pelvis, organ, specified site NEC
uterus —*see* Injury, uterus
vas deferens —*see* Injury, pelvis, organ, specified site NEC
obstetrical trauma O71.9
gland
lacrimal laceration —*see* Injury, eye, specified site NEC
salivary S09.93 ◀
thyroid NEC S19.84
globe (eye) S05.90
specified NEC S05.8X-
groin —*see* Injury, abdomen
gum S09.90
hand S69.9-
blood vessel —*see* Injury, blood vessel, hand
contusion —*see* Contusion, hand
fracture —*see* Fracture, hand
muscle —*see* Injury, muscle, hand
nerve —*see* Injury, nerve, hand
open —*see* Wound, open, hand
specified NEC S69.8-
sprain —*see* Sprain, hand
superficial —*see* Injury, superficial, hand
head S09.90
with loss of consciousness S06.9-
specified NEC S09.8-
heart S26.90
with hemopericardium S26.00
contusion S26.01
laceration (mild) S26.020
major S26.022
moderate S26.021
specified type NEC S26.09
without hemopericardium S26.10
contusion S26.11
laceration S26.12
specified type NEC S26.19
contusion S26.91
laceration S26.92
specified type NEC S26.99
heel —*see* Injury, foot
hepatic
artery —*see* Injury, blood vessel, celiac artery, branch
duct —*see* Injury, liver
vein —*see* Injury, vena cava, inferior
hip S79.91-
blood vessel —*see* Injury, blood vessel, hip
contusion —*see* Contusion, hip
dislocation —*see* Dislocation, hip
fracture —*see* Fracture, femur, neck
muscle —*see* Injury, muscle, hip
nerve —*see* Injury, nerve, hip
open —*see* Wound, open, hip
specified NEC S79.81-
sprain —*see* Sprain, hip
superficial —*see* Injury, superficial, hip
hymen S39.94
hypogastric
blood vessel —*see* Injury, blood vessel, iliac
plexus —*see* Injury, nerve, lumbosacral, sympathetic
ileum —*see* Injury, intestine, small
iliac region S39.91
instrumental (during surgery) —*see* Laceration, accidental complicating surgery
birth injury —*see* Birth, injury
nonsurgical —*see* Injury, by site

Injury *(Continued)*
instrumental *(Continued)*
obstetrical O71.9
bladder O71.5
cervix O71.3
high vaginal O71.4
perineal NOS O70.9
urethra O71.5
uterus O71.5
with rupture or perforation O71.1
internal T14.8
aorta —*see* Injury, aorta
bladder (sphincter) —*see* Injury, bladder
with ectopic or molar pregnancy O08.6
following ectopic or molar pregnancy O08.6
obstetrical trauma O71.5
bronchus, bronchi —*see* Injury, intrathoracic, bronchus
cecum —*see* Injury, intestine, large
cervix (uteri) —*see also* Injury, uterus
with ectopic or molar pregnancy O08.6
following ectopic or molar pregnancy O08.6
obstetrical trauma O71.3
chest —*see* Injury, intrathoracic
gastrointestinal tract —*see* Injury, intra-abdominal
heart —*see* Injury, heart
intestine NEC —*see* Injury, intestine
intrauterine —*see* Injury, uterus
mesentery —*see* Injury, intra-abdominal, specified, site NEC
pelvis, pelvic (organ) S37.90
following ectopic or molar pregnancy (subsequent episode) O08.6
obstetrical trauma NEC O71.5
rupture or perforation O71.1
specified NEC S39.83
rectum —*see* Injury, intestine, large, rectum
stomach —*see* Injury, stomach
ureter —*see* Injury, ureter
urethra (sphincter) following ectopic or molar pregnancy O08.6
uterus —*see* Injury, uterus
interscapular area —*see* Injury, thorax
intestine
large S36.509
ascending (right) S36.500
blast injury (primary) S36.510
secondary S36.590
contusion S36.520
laceration S36.530
specified type NEC S36.590
blast injury (primary) S36.519
ascending (right) S36.510
descending (left) S36.512
rectum S36.61
sigmoid S36.513
specified site NEC S36.518
transverse S36.511
contusion S36.529
ascending (right) S36.520
descending (left) S36.522
rectum S36.62
sigmoid S36.523
specified site NEC S36.528
transverse S36.521
descending (left) S36.502
blast injury (primary) S36.512
secondary S36.592
contusion S36.522
laceration S36.532
specified type NEC S36.592
laceration S36.539
ascending (right) S36.530
descending (left) S36.532
rectum S36.63
sigmoid S36.533

Injury *(Continued)*
intestine *(Continued)*
large *(Continued)*
laceration *(Continued)*
specified site NEC S36.538
transverse S36.531
rectum S36.60
blast injury (primary) S36.61
secondary S36.69
contusion S36.62
laceration S36.63
specified type NEC S36.69
sigmoid S36.503
blast injury (primary) S36.513
secondary S36.593
contusion S36.523
laceration S36.533
specified type NEC S36.593
specified
site NEC S36.508
blast injury (primary) S36.518
secondary S36.598
contusion S36.528
laceration S36.538
specified type NEC S36.598
type NEC S36.599
ascending (right) S36.590
descending (left) S36.592
rectum S36.69
sigmoid S36.593
specified site NEC S36.598
transverse S36.591
transverse S36.501
blast injury (primary) S36.511
secondary S36.591
contusion S36.521
laceration S36.531
specified type NEC S36.591
small S36.409
blast injury (primary) S36.419
duodenum S36.410
secondary S36.499
duodenum S36.490
specified site NEC S36.498
specified site NEC S36.418
contusion S36.429
duodenum S36.420
specified site NEC S36.428
duodenum S36.400
blast injury (primary) S36.410
secondary S36.490
contusion S36.420
laceration S36.430
specified NEC S36.490
laceration S36.439
duodenum S36.430
specified site NEC S36.438
specified
site NEC S36.408
type NEC S36.499
duodenum S36.490
specified site NEC S36.498
intra-abdominal S36.90
adrenal gland —*see* Injury, adrenal gland
bladder —*see* Injury, bladder
colon —*see* Injury, intestine, large
contusion S36.92
fallopian tube —*see* Injury, fallopian tube
gallbladder —*see* Injury, gallbladder
intestine —*see* Injury, intestine
kidney —*see* Injury, kidney
laceration S36.93
liver —*see* Injury, liver
ovary —*see* Injury, ovary
pancreas —*see* Injury, pancreas
pelvic NOS S37.90
peritoneum —*see* Injury, intra-abdominal, specified, site NEC
prostate —*see* Injury, prostate
rectum —*see* Injury, intestine, large, rectum

Injury *(Continued)*
intra-abdominal *(Continued)*
retroperitoneum —*see* Injury, intra-abdominal, specified, site NEC
seminal vesicle —*see* Injury, pelvis, organ, specified site NEC
small intestine —*see* Injury, intestine, small
specified
pelvic S37.90
specified
site NEC S37.899
specified type NEC S37.898
type NEC S37.99
site NEC S36.899
contusion S36.892
laceration S36.893
specified type NEC S36.898
type NEC S36.99
spleen —*see* Injury, spleen
stomach —*see* Injury, stomach
ureter —*see* Injury, ureter
urethra —*see* Injury, urethra
uterus —*see* Injury, uterus
vas deferens —*see* Injury, pelvis, organ, specified site NEC
intracranial (traumatic) S06.9-
cerebellar hemorrhage, traumatic —*see* Injury, intracranial, focal
cerebral edema, traumatic S06.1X-
diffuse S06.1X-
focal S06.1X-
diffuse (axonal) S06.2X-
epidural hemorrhage (traumatic) S06.4X-
focal brain injury S06.30-
contusion —*see* Contusion, cerebral
laceration —*see* Laceration, cerebral
intracerebral hemorrhage, traumatic S06.36-
left side S06.35-
right side S06.34-
subarachnoid hemorrhage, traumatic S06.6X-
subdural hemorrhage, traumatic S06.5X-
intraocular —*see* Injury, eyeball, penetrating
intrathoracic S27.9
bronchus S27.409
bilateral S27.402
blast injury (primary) S27.419
bilateral S27.412
secondary —*see* Injury, intrathoracic, bronchus, specified type NEC
unilateral S27.411
contusion S27.429
bilateral S27.422
unilateral S27.421
laceration S27.439
bilateral S27.432
unilateral S27.431
specified type NEC S27.499
bilateral S27.492
unilateral S27.491
unilateral S27.401
diaphragm S27.809
contusion S27.802
laceration S27.803
specified type NEC S27.808
esophagus (thoracic) S27.819
contusion S27.812
laceration S27.813
specified type NEC S27.818
heart —*see* Injury, heart
hemopneumothorax S27.2
hemothorax S27.1
lung S27.309
aspiration J69.0
bilateral S27.302
blast injury (primary) S27.319
bilateral S27.312
secondary —*see* Injury, intrathoracic, lung, specified type NEC
unilateral S27.311

Injury *(Continued)*
intrathoracic *(Continued)*
bronchus *(Continued)*
contusion S27.329
bilateral S27.322
unilateral S27.321
laceration S27.339
bilateral S27.332
unilateral S27.331
specified type NEC S27.399
bilateral S27.392
unilateral S27.391
unilateral S27.301
pleura S27.60
laceration S27.63
specified type NEC S27.69
pneumothorax S27.0
specified organ NEC S27.899
contusion S27.892
laceration S27.893
specified type NEC S27.898
thoracic duct —*see* Injury, intrathoracic, specified organ NEC
thymus gland —*see* Injury, intrathoracic, specified organ NEC
trachea, thoracic S27.50
blast (primary) S27.51
contusion S27.52
laceration S27.53
specified type NEC S27.59
iris —*see* Injury, eye, specified site NEC
penetrating —*see* Injury, eyeball, penetrating
jaw S09.93
jejunum —*see* Injury, intestine, small
joint NOS T14.8
old or residual —*see* Disorder, joint, specified type NEC
kidney S37.00-
acute (nontraumatic) N17.9
contusion —*see* Contusion, kidney
laceration —*see* Laceration, kidney
specified NEC S37.09-
knee S89.9-
contusion —*see* Contusion, knee
dislocation —*see* Dislocation, knee
meniscus (lateral) (medial) —*see* Sprain, knee, specified site NEC
old injury or tear —*see* Derangement, knee, meniscus, due to old injury
open —*see* Wound, open, knee
specified NEC S89.8-
sprain —*see* Sprain, knee
superficial —*see* Injury, superficial, knee
labium (majus) (minus) S39.94
labyrinth, ear S09.30-
lacrimal apparatus, duct, gland, or sac —*see* Injury, eye, specified site NEC
larynx NEC S19.81
leg (lower) S89.9-
blood vessel —*see* Injury, blood vessel, leg
contusion —*see* Contusion, leg
fracture —*see* Fracture, leg
muscle —*see* Injury, muscle, leg
nerve —*see* Injury, nerve, leg
open —*see* Wound, open, leg
specified NEC S89.8-
superficial —*see* Injury, superficial, leg
lens, eye —*see* Injury, eye, specified site NEC
penetrating —*see* Injury, eyeball, penetrating
limb NEC T14.8
lip S09.93
liver S36.119
contusion S36.112
laceration S36.113
major (stellate) S36.116
minor S36.114
moderate S36.115
specified NEC S36.118
lower back S39.92
specified NEC S39.82

◀ New ⬅ Revised ~~deleted~~ Deleted

Injury *(Continued)*
lumbar, lumbosacral (region) S39.92
plexus —*see* Injury, lumbosacral plexus
lumbosacral plexus S34.4
lung —*see also* Injury, intrathoracic, lung
aspiration J69.0
transfusion-related (TRALI) J95.84
lymphatic thoracic duct —*see* Injury, intrathoracic, specified organ NEC
malar region S09.93
mastoid region S09.90
maxilla S09.93
mediastinum —*see* Injury, intrathoracic, specified organ NEC
membrane, brain —*see* Injury, intracranial
meningeal artery —*see* Injury, intracranial, subdural hemorrhage
meninges (cerebral) —*see* Injury, intracranial
mesenteric
artery
branch S35.299
laceration (minor) (superficial) S35.291
major S35.292
specified NEC S35.298
inferior S35.239
laceration (minor) (superficial) S35.231
major S35.232
specified NEC S35.238
superior S35.229
laceration (minor) (superficial) S35.221
major S35.222
specified NEC S35.228
plexus (inferior) (superior) —*see* Injury, nerve, lumbosacral, sympathetic
vein
inferior S35.349
laceration S35.341
specified NEC S35.348
superior S35.339
laceration S35.331
specified NEC S35.338
mesentery —*see* Injury, intra-abdominal, specified site NEC
mesosalpinx —*see* Injury, pelvic organ, specified site NEC
middle ear S09.30-
midthoracic region NOS S29.9
mouth S09.93
multiple NOS T07
muscle (and fascia) (and tendon)
abdomen S39.001
laceration S39.021
specified type NEC S39.091
strain S39.011
abductor
thumb, forearm level —*see* Injury, muscle, thumb, abductor
adductor
thigh S76.20-
laceration S76.22-
specified type NEC S76.29-
strain S76.21-
ankle —*see* Injury, muscle, foot
anterior muscle group, at leg level (lower) S86.20-
laceration S86.22-
specified type NEC S86.29-
strain S86.21-
arm (upper) —*see* Injury, muscle, shoulder
biceps (parts NEC) S46.20-
laceration S46.22-
long head S46.10-
laceration S46.12-
specified type NEC S46.19-
strain S46.11-
specified type NEC S46.29-
strain S46.21-
extensor
finger (s) (other than thumb) —*see* Injury, muscle, finger by site, extensor

Injury *(Continued)*
muscle *(Continued)*
extensor *(Continued)*
forearm level, specified NEC —*see* Injury, muscle, forearm, extensor
thumb —*see* Injury, muscle, thumb, extensor
toe (large) (ankle level) (foot level) —*see* Injury, muscle, toe, extensor
finger
extensor (forearm level) S56.40-
hand level S66.309
laceration S66.329
specified type NEC S66.399
strain S66.319
laceration S56.429
specified type NEC S56.499
strain S56.419
flexor (forearm level) S56.10-
hand level S66.109
laceration S66.129
specified type NEC S66.199
strain S66.119
laceration S56.129
specified type NEC S56.199
strain S56.119
index
extensor (forearm level)
hand level S66.308
laceration S66.32-
specified type NEC S66.39-
strain S66.31-
specified type NEC S56.492-
flexor (forearm level)
hand level S66.108
laceration S66.12-
specified type NEC S66.19-
strain S66.11-
specified type NEC S56.19-
strain S56.11-
intrinsic S66.50-
laceration S66.52-
specified type NEC S66.59-
strain S66.51-
intrinsic S66.509
laceration S66.529
specified type NEC S66.599
strain S66.519
little
extensor (forearm level)
hand level S66.30-
laceration S66.32-
specified type NEC S66.39-
strain S66.31-
laceration S56.42-
specified type NEC S56.49-
strain S56.41-
flexor (forearm level)
hand level S66.10-
laceration S66.12-
specified type NEC S66.19-
strain S66.11-
laceration S56.12-
specified type NEC S56.19-
strain S56.11-
intrinsic S66.50-
laceration S66.52-
specified type NEC S66.59-
strain S66.51-
middle
extensor (forearm level)
hand level S66.30-
laceration S66.32-
specified type NEC S66.39-
strain S66.31-
laceration S56.42-
specified type NEC S56.49-
strain S56.41-

Injury *(Continued)*
muscle *(Continued)*
finger *(Continued)*
middle *(Continued)*
flexor (forearm level)
hand level S66.10-
laceration S66.12-
specified type NEC S66.19-
strain S66.11-
laceration S56.12-
specified type NEC S56.19-
strain S56.11-
intrinsic S66.50-
laceration S66.52-
specified type NEC S66.59-
strain S66.51-
ring
extensor (forearm level)
hand level S66.30-
laceration S66.32-
specified type NEC S66.39-
strain S66.31-
laceration S56.42-
specified type NEC S56.49-
strain S56.41-
flexor (forearm level)
hand level S66.10-
laceration S66.12-
specified type NEC S66.19-
strain S66.11-
laceration S56.12-
specified type NEC S56.19-
strain S56.11-
intrinsic S66.50-
laceration S66.52-
specified type NEC S66.59-
strain S66.51-
flexor
finger(s) (other than thumb) — *see* Injury, muscle, finger
forearm level, specified NEC — *see* Injury, muscle, forearm, flexor
thumb —*see* Injury, muscle, thumb, flexor
toe (long) (ankle level) (foot level) —*see* Injury, muscle, toe, flexor
foot S96.90-
intrinsic S96.20-
laceration S96.22-
specified type NEC S96.29-
strain S96.21-
laceration S96.92-
long extensor, toe —*see* Injury, muscle, toe, extensor
long flexor, toe —*see* Injury, muscle, toe, flexor
specified
site NEC S96.80-
laceration S96.82-
specified type NEC S96.89-
strain S96.81-
type NEC S96.99-
strain S96.91-
forearm (level) S56.90-
extensor S56.50-
laceration S56.52-
specified type NEC S56.59-
strain S56.51-
flexor S56.20-
laceration S56.22-
specified type NEC S56.29-
strain S56.21-
laceration S56.92-
specified S56.99-
site NEC S56.80-
laceration S56.82-
strain S56.81-
type NEC S56.89-
strain S56.91-

Injury *(Continued)*
muscle *(Continued)*
hand (level) S66.90-
laceration S66.92-
specified
site NEC S66.80-
laceration S66.82-
specified type NEC S66.89-
strain S66.81-
type NEC S66.99-
strain S66.91-
head S09.10
laceration S09.12
specified type NEC S09.19
strain S09.11
hip NEC S76.00-
laceration S76.02-
specified type NEC S76.09-
strain S76.01-
intrinsic
ankle and foot level —*see* Injury, muscle, foot, intrinsic
finger (other than thumb) —*see* Injury, muscle, finger by site, intrinsic
foot (level) —*see* Injury, muscle, foot, intrinsic
thumb —*see* Injury, muscle, thumb, intrinsic
leg (level) (lower) S86.90-
Achilles tendon —*see* Injury, Achilles tendon
anterior muscle group —*see* Injury, muscle, anterior muscle group
laceration S86.92-
peroneal muscle group —*see* Injury, muscle, peroneal muscle group
posterior muscle group —*see* Injury, muscle, posterior muscle group, leg level
specified
site NEC S86.80-
laceration S86.82-
specified type NEC S86.89-
strain S86.81-
type NEC S86.99-
strain S86.91-
long
extensor toe, at ankle and foot level —*see* Injury, muscle, toe, extensor
flexor, toe, at ankle and foot level —*see* Injury, muscle, toe, flexor
head, biceps —*see* Injury, muscle, biceps, long head
lower back S39.002
laceration S39.022
specified type NEC S39.092
strain S39.012
neck (level) S16.9
laceration S16.2
specified type NEC S16.8
strain S16.1
pelvis S39.003
laceration S39.023
specified type NEC S39.093
strain S39.013
peroneal muscle group, at leg level (lower) S86.30-
laceration S86.32-
specified type NEC S86.39-
strain S86.31-
posterior muscle (group)
leg level (lower) S86.10-
laceration S86.12-
specified type NEC S86.19-
strain S86.11-
thigh level S76.30-
laceration S76.32-
specified type NEC S76.39-
strain S76.31-

Injury *(Continued)*
muscle *(Continued)*
quadriceps (thigh) S76.10-
laceration S76.12-
specified type NEC S76.19-
strain S76.11-
shoulder S46.90-
laceration S46.92-
rotator cuff —*see* Injury, rotator cuff
specified site NEC S46.80-
laceration S46.82-
specified type NEC S46.89-
strain S46.81-
specified type NEC S46.99-
strain S46.91-
thigh NEC (level) S76.90-
adductor —*see* Injury, muscle, adductor, thigh
laceration S76.92-
posterior muscle (group) —*see* Injury, muscle, posterior muscle, thigh level
quadriceps —*see* Injury, muscle, quadriceps
specified
site NEC S76.80-
laceration S76.82-
specified type NEC S76.89-
strain S76.81-
type NEC S76.99-
strain S76.91-
thorax (level) S29.009
back wall S29.002
front wall S29.001
laceration S29.029
back wall S29.022
front wall S29.021
specified type NEC S29.099
back wall S29.092
front wall S29.091
strain S29.019
back wall S29.012
front wall S29.011
thumb
abductor (forearm level) S56.30-
laceration S56.32-
specified type NEC S56.39-
strain S56.31-
extensor (forearm level) S56.30-
hand level S66.20-
laceration S66.22-
specified type NEC S66.29-
strain S66.21-
laceration S56.32-
specified type NEC S56.39-
strain S56.31-
flexor (forearm level) S56.00-
hand level S66.00-
laceration S66.02-
specified type NEC S66.09-
strain S66.01-
laceration S56.02-
specified type NEC S56.09-
strain S56.01-
wrist level —*see* Injury, muscle, thumb, flexor, hand level
intrinsic S66.40-
laceration S66.42-
specified type NEC S66.49-
strain S66.41-
toe —*see also* Injury, muscle, foot
extensor, long S96.10-
laceration S96.12-
specified type NEC S96.19-
strain S96.11-
flexor, long S96.00-
laceration S96.02-
specified type NEC S96.09-
strain S96.01-

Injury *(Continued)*
muscle *(Continued)*
triceps S46.30-
laceration S46.32-
specified type NEC S46.39-
strain S46.31-
wrist (and hand) level —*see* Injury, muscle, hand
musculocutaneous nerve —*see* Injury, nerve, musculocutaneous
myocardium —*see* Injury, heart
nape —*see* Injury, neck
nasal (septum) (sinus) S09.92
nasopharynx S09.92
neck S19.9
specified NEC S19.80
specified site NEC S19.89
nerve NEC T14.8
abdomen S34.9
peripheral S34.6
specified site NEC S34.8
abducens S04.4-
contusion S04.4-
laceration S04.4-
specified type NEC S04.4-
abducent —*see* Injury, nerve, abducens
accessory S04.7-
contusion S04.7-
laceration S04.7-
specified type NEC S04.7-
acoustic S04.6-
contusion S04.6-
laceration S04.6-
specified type NEC S04.6-
ankle S94.9-
cutaneous sensory S94.3-
specified site NEC —*see* subcategory S94.8
anterior crural, femoral —*see* Injury, nerve, femoral
arm (upper) S44.9-
axillary —*see* Injury, nerve, axillary
cutaneous —*see* Injury, nerve, cutaneous, arm
median —*see* Injury, nerve, median, upper arm
musculocutaneous —*see* Injury, nerve, musculocutaneous
radial —*see* Injury, nerve, radial, upper arm
specified site NEC —*see* subcategory S44.8
ulnar —*see* Injury, nerve, ulnar, arm
auditory —*see* Injury, nerve, acoustic
axillary S44.3-
brachial plexus —*see* Injury, brachial plexus
cervical sympathetic S14.5
cranial S04.9
contusion S04.9
eighth (acoustic or auditory) —*see* Injury, nerve, acoustic
eleventh (accessory) —*see* Injury, nerve, accessory
fifth (trigeminal) —*see* Injury, nerve, trigeminal
first (olfactory) —*see* Injury, nerve, olfactory
fourth (trochlear) —*see* Injury, nerve, trochlear
laceration S04.9
ninth (glossopharyngeal) —*see* Injury, nerve, glossopharyngeal
second (optic) —*see* Injury, nerve, optic
seventh (facial) —*see* Injury, nerve, facial
sixth (abducent) —*see* Injury, nerve, abducens
specified
nerve NEC S04.89-
contusion S04.89-
laceration S04.89-
specified type NEC S04.89-
type NEC S04.9

Injury *(Continued)*
nerve NEC *(Continued)*
cranial *(Continued)*
tenth (pneumogastric or vagus) —*see* Injury, nerve, vagus
third (oculomotor) —*see* Injury, nerve, oculomotor
twelfth (hypoglossal) —*see* Injury, nerve, hypoglossal
cutaneous sensory
ankle (level) S94.3-
arm (upper) (level) S44.5-
foot (level) —*see* Injury, nerve, cutaneous sensory, ankle
forearm (level) S54.3-
hip (level) S74.2-
leg (lower level) S84.2-
shoulder (level) —*see* Injury, nerve, cutaneous sensory, arm
thigh (level) —*see* Injury, nerve, cutaneous sensory, hip
deep peroneal —*see* Injury, nerve, peroneal, foot
digital
finger S64.4-
index S64.49-
little S64.49-
middle S64.49-
ring S64.49-
thumb S64.3-
toe —*see* Injury, nerve, ankle, specified site NEC
eighth cranial (acoustic or auditory) —*see* Injury, nerve, acoustic
eleventh cranial (accessory) —*see* Injury, nerve, accessory
facial S04.5-
contusion S04.5-
laceration S04.5-
newborn P11.3
specified type NEC S04.5-
femoral (hip level) (thigh level) S74.1-
fifth cranial (trigeminal) —*see* Injury, nerve, trigeminal
finger (digital) —*see* Injury, nerve, digital, finger
first cranial (olfactory) —*see* Injury, nerve, olfactory
foot S94.9-
cutaneous sensory S94.3-
deep peroneal S94.2-
lateral plantar S94.0-
medial plantar S94.1-
specified site NEC —*see* subcategory S94.8
forearm (level) S54.9-
cutaneous sensory —*see* Injury, nerve, cutaneous sensory, forearm
median —*see* Injury, nerve, median
radial —*see* Injury, nerve, radial
specified site NEC —*see* subcategory S54.8
ulnar —*see* Injury, nerve, ulnar
fourth cranial (trochlear) —*see* Injury, nerve, trochlear
glossopharyngeal S04.89-
specified type NEC S04.89-
hand S64.9-
median —*see* Injury, nerve, median, hand
radial —*see* Injury, nerve, radial, hand
specified NEC —*see* subcategory S64.8
ulnar —*see* Injury, nerve, ulnar, hand
hip (level) S74.9-
cutaneous sensory —*see* Injury, nerve, cutaneous sensory, hip
femoral —*see* Injury, nerve, femoral
sciatic —*see* Injury, nerve, sciatic
specified site NEC —*see* subcategory S74.8

Injury *(Continued)*
nerve NEC *(Continued)*
hypoglossal S04.89-
specified type NEC S04.89-
lateral plantar S94.0-
leg (lower) S84.9-
cutaneous sensory —*see* Injury, nerve, cutaneous sensory, leg
peroneal —*see* Injury, nerve, peroneal
specified site NEC —*see* subcategory S84.8
tibial —*see* Injury, nerve, tibial
upper —*see* Injury, nerve, thigh
lower
back —*see* Injury, nerve, abdomen, specified site NEC
peripheral —*see* Injury, nerve, abdomen, peripheral
limb —*see* Injury, nerve, leg
lumbar plexus —*see* Injury, nerve, lumbosacral, sympathetic
lumbar spinal —*see* Injury, nerve, spinal, lumbar
lumbosacral
plexus —*see* Injury, nerve, lumbosacral, sympathetic
sympathetic S34.5
medial plantar S94.1-
median (forearm level) S54.1-
hand (level) S64.1-
upper arm (level) S44.1-
wrist (level) —*see* Injury, nerve, median, hand
musculocutaneous S44.4-
musculospiral (upper arm level) —*see* Injury, nerve, radial, upper arm
neck S14.9
peripheral S14.4
specified site NEC S14.8
sympathetic S14.5
ninth cranial (glossopharyngeal) —*see* Injury, nerve, glossopharyngeal
oculomotor S04.1-
contusion S04.1-
laceration S04.1-
specified type NEC S04.1-
olfactory S04.81-
specified type NEC S04.81-
optic S04.01-
contusion S04.01-
laceration S04.01-
specified type NEC S04.01-
pelvic girdle —*see* Injury, nerve, hip
pelvis —*see* Injury, nerve, abdomen, specified site NEC
peripheral —*see* Injury, nerve, abdomen, peripheral
peripheral NEC T14.8
abdomen —*see* Injury, nerve, abdomen, peripheral
lower back —*see* Injury, nerve, abdomen, peripheral
neck —*see* Injury, nerve, neck, peripheral
pelvis —*see* Injury, nerve, abdomen, peripheral
specified NEC T14.8
peroneal (lower leg level) S84.1-
foot S94.2-
plexus
brachial —*see* Injury, brachial plexus
celiac, coeliac —*see* Injury, nerve, lumbosacral, sympathetic
mesenteric, inferior —*see* Injury, nerve, lumbosacral, sympathetic
sacral —*see* Injury, lumbosacral plexus
spinal
brachial —*see* Injury, brachial plexus
lumbosacral —*see* Injury, lumbosacral plexus

Injury *(Continued)*
nerve NEC *(Continued)*
pneumogastric —*see* Injury, nerve, vagus
radial (forearm level) S54.2-
hand (level) S64.2-
upper arm (level) S44.2-
wrist (level) —*see* Injury, nerve, radial, hand
root —*see* Injury, nerve, spinal, root
sacral plexus —*see* Injury, lumbosacral plexus
sacral spinal —*see* Injury, nerve, spinal, sacral
sciatic (hip level) (thigh level) S74.0-
second cranial (optic) —*see* Injury, nerve, optic
seventh cranial (facial) —*see* Injury, nerve, facial
shoulder —*see* Injury, nerve, arm
sixth cranial (abducent) —*see* Injury, nerve, abducens
spinal
plexus —*see* Injury, nerve, plexus, spinal
root
cervical S14.2
dorsal S24.2
lumbar S34.21
sacral S34.22
thoracic —*see* Injury, nerve, spinal, root, dorsal
splanchnic —*see* Injury, nerve, lumbosacral, sympathetic
sympathetic NEC —*see* Injury, nerve, lumbosacral, sympathetic
cervical —*see* Injury, nerve, cervical sympathetic
tenth cranial (pneumogastric or vagus) —*see* Injury, nerve, vagus
thigh (level) —*see* Injury, nerve, hip
cutaneous sensory —*see* Injury, nerve, cutaneous sensory, hip
femoral —*see* Injury, nerve, femoral
sciatic —*see* Injury, nerve, sciatic
specified NEC —*see* Injury, nerve, hip
third cranial (oculomotor) —*see* Injury, nerve, oculomotor
thorax S24.9
peripheral S24.3
specified site NEC S24.8
sympathetic S24.4
thumb, digital —*see* Injury, nerve, digital, thumb
tibial (lower leg level) (posterior) S84.0-
toe —*see* Injury, nerve, ankle
trigeminal S04.3-
contusion S04.3-
laceration S04.3-
specified type NEC S04.3-
trochlear S04.2-
contusion S04.2-
laceration S04.2-
specified type NEC S04.2-
twelfth cranial (hypoglossal) —*see* Injury, nerve, hypoglossal
ulnar (forearm level) S54.0-
arm (upper) (level) S44.0-
hand (level) S64.0-
wrist (level) —*see* Injury, nerve, ulnar, hand
vagus S04.89-
specified type NEC S04.89-
wrist (level) —*see* Injury, nerve, hand
ninth cranial nerve (glossopharyngeal) —*see* Injury, nerve, glossopharyngeal
nose (septum) S09.92
obstetrical O71.9
specified NEC O71.89
occipital (region) (scalp) S09.90
lobe —*see* Injury, intracranial
optic chiasm S04.02
optic radiation S04.03-

Injury *(Continued)*
optic tract and pathways S04.03-
orbit, orbital (region) —*see* Injury, eye
penetrating (with foreign body) —*see* Injury, eye, orbit, penetrating
specified NEC —*see* Injury, eye, specified site NEC
ovary, ovarian S37.409
bilateral S37.402
contusion S37.422
laceration S37.432
specified type NEC S37.492
blood vessel —*see* Injury, blood vessel, ovarian
contusion S37.429
bilateral S37.422
unilateral S37.421
laceration S37.439
bilateral S37.432
unilateral S37.431
specified type NEC S37.499
bilateral S37.492
unilateral S37.491
unilateral S37.401
contusion S37.421
laceration S37.431
specified type NEC S37.491
palate (hard) (soft) S09.93
pancreas S36.209
body S36.201
contusion S36.221
laceration S36.231
major S36.261
minor S36.241
moderate S36.251
specified type NEC S36.291
contusion S36.229
head S36.200
contusion S36.220
laceration S36.230
major S36.260
minor S36.240
moderate S36.250
specified type NEC S36.290
laceration S36.239
major S36.269
minor S36.249
moderate S36.259
specified type NEC S36.299
tail S36.202
contusion S36.222
laceration S36.232
major S36.262
minor S36.242
moderate S36.252
specified type NEC S36.292
parietal (region) (scalp) S09.90
lobe —*see* Injury, intracranial
patellar ligament (tendon) S76.10-
laceration S76.12-
specified NEC S76.19-
strain S76.11-
pelvis, pelvic (floor) S39.93
complicating delivery O70.1
joint or ligament, complicating delivery O71.6
organ S37.90
with ectopic or molar pregnancy O08.6
complication of abortion —*see* Abortion
contusion S37.92
following ectopic or molar pregnancy O08.6
laceration S37.93
obstetrical trauma NEC O71.5
specified
site NEC S37.899
contusion S37.892
laceration S37.893
specified type NEC S37.898
type NEC S37.99
specified NEC S39.83

Injury *(Continued)*
penis S39.94
perineum S39.94
peritoneum S36.81
laceration S36.893
periurethral tissue —*see* Injury, urethra
complicating delivery O71.82
phalanges
foot —*see* Injury, foot
hand —*see* Injury, hand
pharynx NEC S19.85
pleura —*see* Injury, intrathoracic, pleura
plexus
brachial —*see* Injury, brachial plexus
cardiac —*see* Injury, nerve, thorax, sympathetic
celiac, coeliac —*see* Injury, nerve, lumbosacral, sympathetic
esophageal —*see* Injury, nerve, thorax, sympathetic
hypogastric —*see* Injury, nerve, lumbosacral, sympathetic
lumbar, lumbosacral —*see* Injury, lumbosacral plexus
mesenteric —*see* Injury, nerve, lumbosacral, sympathetic
pulmonary —*see* Injury, nerve, thorax, sympathetic
postcardiac surgery (syndrome) I97.0
prepuce S39.94
prostate S37.829
contusion S37.822
laceration S37.823
specified type NEC S37.828
pubic region S39.94
pudendum S39.94
pulmonary plexus —*see* Injury, nerve, thorax, sympathetic
rectovaginal septum NEC S39.83
rectum —*see* Injury, intestine, large, rectum
retina —*see* Injury, eye, specified site NEC
penetrating —*see* Injury, eyeball, penetrating
retroperitoneal —*see* Injury, intra-abdominal, specified site NEC
rotator cuff (muscle (s)) (tendon (s)) S46.00-
laceration S46.02-
specified type NEC S46.09-
strain S46.01-
round ligament —*see* Injury, pelvic organ, specified site NEC
sacral plexus —*see* Injury, lumbosacral plexus
salivary duct or gland S09.93
scalp S09.90
newborn (birth injury) P12.9
due to monitoring (electrode) (sampling incision) P12.4
specified NEC P12.89
caput succedaneum P12.81
scapular region —*see* Injury, shoulder
sclera —*see* Injury, eye, specified site NEC
penetrating —*see* Injury, eyeball, penetrating
scrotum S39.94
second cranial nerve (optic) —*see* Injury, nerve, optic
seminal vesicle —*see* Injury, pelvic organ, specified site NEC
seventh cranial nerve (facial) —*see* Injury, nerve, facial
shoulder S49.9-
blood vessel —*see* Injury, blood vessel, arm
contusion —*see* Contusion, shoulder
dislocation —*see* Dislocation, shoulder
fracture —*see* Fracture, shoulder
muscle —*see* Injury, muscle, shoulder
nerve —*see* Injury, nerve, shoulder
open —*see* Wound, open, shoulder
specified type NEC S49.8-

Injury *(Continued)*
shoulder *(Continued)*
sprain —*see* Sprain, shoulder girdle
superficial —*see* Injury, superficial, shoulder
sinus
cavernous —*see* Injury, intracranial
nasal S09.92
sixth cranial nerve (abducent) —*see* Injury, nerve, abducens
skeleton, birth injury P13.9
specified part NEC P13.8
skin NEC T14.8
surface intact —*see* Injury, superficial
skull NEC S09.90
specified NEC T14.8
spermatic cord (pelvic region) S37.898
scrotal region S39.848
spinal (cord)
cervical (neck) S14.109
anterior cord syndrome S14.139
C1 level S14.131
C2 level S14.132
C3 level S14.133
C4 level S14.134
C5 level S14.135
C6 level S14.136
C7 level S14.137
C8 level S14.138
Brown-Séquard syndrome S14.149
C1 level S14.141
C2 level S14.142
C3 level S14.143
C4 level S14.144
C5 level S14.145
C6 level S14.146
C7 level S14.147
C8 level S14.148
C1 level S14.101
C2 level S14.102
C3 level S14.103
C4 level S14.104
C5 level S14.105
C6 level S14.106
C7 level S14.107
C8 level S14.108
central cord syndrome S14.129
C1 level S14.121
C2 level S14.122
C3 level S14.123
C4 level S14.124
C5 level S14.125
C6 level S14.126
C7 level S14.127
C8 level S14.128
complete lesion S14.119
C1 level S14.111
C2 level S14.112
C3 level S14.113
C4 level S14.114
C5 level S14.115
C6 level S14.116
C7 level S14.117
C8 level S14.118
concussion S14.0
edema S14.0
incomplete lesion specified NEC S14.159
C1 level S14.151
C2 level S14.152
C3 level S14.153
C4 level S14.154
C5 level S14.155
C6 level S14.156
C7 level S14.157
C8 level S14.158
posterior cord syndrome S14.159
C1 level S14.151
C2 level S14.152
C3 level S14.153
C4 level S14.154
C5 level S14.155

Injury *(Continued)*
spinal *(Continued)*
cervical *(Continued)*
posterior cord syndrome *(Continued)*
C6 level S14.156
C7 level S14.157
C8 level S14.158
dorsal —*see* Injury, spinal, thoracic
lumbar S34.109
complete lesion S34.119
L1 level S34.111
L2 level S34.112
L3 level S34.113
L4 level S34.114
L5 level S34.115
concussion S34.01
edema S34.01
incomplete lesion S34.129
L1 level S34.121
L2 level S34.122
L3 level S34.123
L4 level S34.124
L5 level S34.125
L1 level S34.101
L2 level S34.102
L3 level S34.103
L4 level S34.104
L5 level S34.105
nerve root NEC
cervical —*see* Injury, nerve, spinal, root, cervical
dorsal —*see* Injury, nerve, spinal, root, dorsal
lumbar S34.21
sacral S34.22
thoracic —*see* Injury, nerve, spinal, root, dorsal
plexus
brachial —*see* Injury, brachial plexus
lumbosacral —*see* Injury, lumbosacral plexus
sacral S34.139
complete lesion S34.131
incomplete lesion S34.132
thoracic S24.109
anterior cord syndrome S24.139
T1 level S24.131
T2-T6 level S24.132
T7-T10 level S24.133
T11-T12 level S24.134
Brown-Séquard syndrome S24.149
T1 level S24.141
T2-T6 level S24.142
T7-T10 level S24.143
T11-T12 level S24.144
complete lesion S24.119
T1 level S24.111
T2-T6 level S24.112
T7-T10 level S24.113
T11-T12 level S24.114
concussion S24.0
edema S24.0
incomplete lesion specified NEC S24.159
T1 level S24.151
T2-T6 level S24.152
T7-T10 level S24.153
T11-T12 level S24.154
posterior cord syndrome S24.159
T1 level S24.151
T2-T6 level S24.152
T7-T10 level S24.153
T11-T12 level S24.154
T1 level S24.101
T2-T6 level S24.102
T7-T10 level S24.103
T11-T12 level S24.104
splanchnic nerve —*see* Injury, nerve, lumbosacral, sympathetic

Injury *(Continued)*
spleen S36.00
contusion S36.029
major S36.021
minor S36.020
laceration S36.039
major (massive) (stellate) S36.032
moderate S36.031
superficial (capsular) (minor) S36.030
specified type NEC S36.09
splenic artery —*see* Injury, blood vessel, celiac artery, branch
stellate ganglion —*see* Injury, nerve, thorax, sympathetic
sternal region S29.9
stomach S36.30
contusion S36.32
laceration S36.33
specified type NEC S36.39
subconjunctival —*see* Injury, eye, conjunctiva
subcutaneous NEC T14.8
submaxillary region S09.93
submental region S09.93
subungual
fingers —*see* Injury, hand
toes —*see* Injury, foot
superficial NEC T14.8
abdomen, abdominal (wall) S30.92
abrasion S30.811
bite S30.871
insect S30.861
contusion S30.1
external constriction S30.841
foreign body S30.851
abrasion —*see* Abrasion, by site
adnexa, eye NEC —*see* Injury, eye, specified site NEC
alveolar process —*see* Injury, superficial, oral cavity
ankle S90.91-
abrasion —*see* Abrasion, ankle
bite —*see* Bite, ankle
blister —*see* Blister, ankle
contusion —*see* Contusion, ankle
external constriction —*see* Constriction, external, ankle
foreign body —*see* Foreign body, superficial, ankle
anus S30.98
arm (upper) S40.92-
abrasion —*see* Abrasion, arm
bite —*see* Bite, superficial, arm
blister —*see* Blister, arm (upper)
contusion —*see* Contusion, arm
external constriction —*see* Constriction, external, arm
foreign body —*see* Foreign body, superficial, arm
auditory canal (external) (meatus) —*see* Injury, superficial, ear
auricle —*see* Injury, superficial, ear
axilla —*see* Injury, superficial, arm
back —*see also* Injury, superficial, thorax, back
lower S30.91
abrasion S30.810
contusion S30.0
external constriction S30.840
superficial
bite NEC S30.870
insect S30.860
foreign body S30.850
bite NEC —*see* Bite, superficial NEC, by site
blister —*see* Blister, by site
breast S20.10-
abrasion —*see* Abrasion, breast
bite —*see* Bite, superficial, breast
contusion —*see* Contusion, breast
external constriction —*see* Constriction, external, breast
foreign body —*see* Foreign body, superficial, breast

Injury *(Continued)*
superficial NEC *(Continued)*
brow —*see* Injury, superficial, head, specified NEC
buttock S30.91
calf —*see* Injury, superficial, leg
canthus, eye —*see* Injury, superficial, periocular area
cheek (external) —*see* Injury, superficial, head, specified NEC
internal —*see* Injury, superficial, oral cavity
chest wall —*see* Injury, superficial, thorax
chin —*see* Injury, superficial, head NEC
clitoris S30.95
conjunctiva —*see* Injury, eye, conjunctiva
with foreign body (in conjunctival sac) —*see* Foreign body, conjunctival sac
contusion —*see* Contusion, by site
costal region —*see* Injury, superficial, thorax
digit (s)
hand —*see* Injury, superficial, finger
ear (auricle) (canal) (external) S00.40-
abrasion —*see* Abrasion, ear
bite —*see* Bite, superficial, ear
contusion —*see* Contusion, ear
external constriction —*see* Constriction, external, ear
foreign body —*see* Foreign body, superficial, ear
elbow S50.90-
abrasion —*see* Abrasion, elbow
bite —*see* Bite, superficial, elbow
blister —*see* Blister, elbow
contusion —*see* Contusion, elbow
external constriction —*see* Constriction, external, elbow
foreign body —*see* Foreign body, superficial, elbow
epididymis S30.94
epigastric region S30.92
epiglottis —*see* Injury, superficial, throat
esophagus
cervical —*see* Injury, superficial, throat
external constriction —*see* Constriction, external, by site
extremity NEC T14.8
eyeball NEC —*see* Injury, eye, specified site NEC
eyebrow —*see* Injury, superficial, periocular area
eyelid S00.20-
abrasion —*see* Abrasion, eyelid
bite —*see* Bite, superficial, eyelid
contusion —*see* Contusion, eyelid
external constriction —*see* Constriction, external, eyelid
foreign body —*see* Foreign body, superficial, eyelid
face NEC —*see* Injury, superficial, head, specified NEC
finger (s) S60.949
abrasion —*see* Abrasion, finger
bite —*see* Bite, superficial, finger
blister —*see* Blister, finger
contusion —*see* Contusion, finger
external constriction —*see* Constriction, external, finger
foreign body —*see* Foreign body, superficial, finger
index S60.94-
insect bite —*see* Bite, by site, superficial, insect
little S60.94-
middle S60.94-
ring S60.94-
flank S30.92
foot S90.92-
abrasion —*see* Abrasion, foot
bite —*see* Bite, foot

Injury *(Continued)*
superficial NEC *(Continued)*
foot *(Continued)*
blister —*see* Blister, foot
contusion —*see* Contusion, foot
external constriction —*see* Constriction, external, foot
foreign body —*see* Foreign body, superficial, foot
forearm S50.91-
abrasion —*see* Abrasion, forearm
bite —*see* Bite, forearm, superficial
blister —*see* Blister, forearm
contusion —*see* Contusion, forearm
elbow only —*see* Injury, superficial, elbow
external constriction —*see* Constriction, external, forearm
foreign body —*see* Foreign body, superficial, forearm
forehead —*see* Injury, superficial, head NEC
foreign body —*see* Foreign body, superficial
genital organs, external
female S30.97
male S30.96
globe (eye) —*see* Injury, eye, specified site NEC
groin S30.92
gum —*see* Injury, superficial, oral cavity
hand S60.92-
abrasion —*see* Abrasion, hand
bite —*see* Bite, superficial, hand
contusion —*see* Contusion, hand
external constriction —*see* Constriction, external, hand
foreign body —*see* Foreign body, superficial, hand
head S00.90
ear —*see* Injury, superficial, ear
eyelid —*see* Injury, superficial, eyelid
nose S00.30
oral cavity S00.502
scalp S00.00
specified site NEC S00.80
heel —*see* Injury, superficial, foot
hip S70.91-
abrasion —*see* Abrasion, hip
bite —*see* Bite, superficial, hip
blister —*see* Blister, hip
contusion —*see* Contusion, hip
external constriction —*see* Constriction, external, hip
foreign body —*see* Foreign body, superficial, hip
iliac region —*see* Injury, superficial, abdomen
inguinal region —*see* Injury, superficial, abdomen
insect bite —*see* Bite, by site, superficial, insect
interscapular region —*see* Injury, superficial, thorax, back
jaw —*see* Injury, superficial, head, specified NEC
knee S80.91-
abrasion —*see* Abrasion, knee
bite —*see* Bite, superficial, knee
blister —*see* Blister, knee
contusion —*see* Contusion, knee
external constriction —*see* Constriction, external, knee
foreign body —*see* Foreign body, superficial, knee
labium (majus) (minus) S30.95
lacrimal (apparatus) (gland) (sac) —*see* Injury, eye, specified site NEC
larynx —*see* Injury, superficial, throat
leg (lower) S80.92-
abrasion —*see* Abrasion, leg
bite —*see* Bite, superficial, leg

Injury *(Continued)*
superficial NEC *(Continued)*
leg *(Continued)*
contusion —*see* Contusion, leg
external constriction —*see* Constriction, external, leg
foreign body —*see* Foreign body, superficial, leg
knee —*see* Injury, superficial, knee
limb NEC T14.8
lip S00.501
lower back S30.91
lumbar region S30.91
malar region —*see* Injury, superficial, head, specified NEC
mammary —*see* Injury, superficial, breast
mastoid region —*see* Injury, superficial, head, specified NEC
mouth —*see* Injury, superficial, oral cavity
muscle NEC T14.8
nail NEC T14.8
finger —*see* Injury, superficial, finger
toe —*see* Injury, superficial, toe
nasal (septum) —*see* Injury, superficial, nose
neck S10.90
specified site NEC S10.80
nose (septum) S00.30
occipital region —*see* Injury, superficial, scalp
oral cavity S00.502
orbital region —*see* Injury, superficial, periocular area
palate —*see* Injury, superficial, oral cavity
palm —*see* Injury, superficial, hand
parietal region —*see* Injury, superficial, scalp
pelvis S30.91
girdle —*see* Injury, superficial, hip
penis S30.93
perineum
female S30.95
male S30.91
periocular area S00.20-
abrasion —*see* Abrasion, eyelid
bite —*see* Bite, superficial, eyelid
contusion —*see* Contusion, eyelid
external constriction —*see* Constriction, external, eyelid
foreign body —*see* Foreign body, superficial, eyelid
phalanges
finger —*see* Injury, superficial, finger
toe —*see* Injury, superficial, toe
pharynx —*see* Injury, superficial, throat
pinna —*see* Injury, superficial, ear
popliteal space —*see* Injury, superficial, knee
prepuce S30.93
pubic region S30.91
pudendum
female S30.97
male S30.96
sacral region S30.91
scalp S00.00
scapular region —*see* Injury, superficial, shoulder
sclera —*see* Injury, eye, specified site NEC
scrotum S30.94
shin —*see* Injury, superficial, leg
shoulder S40.91-
abrasion —*see* Abrasion, shoulder
bite —*see* Bite, superficial, shoulder
blister —*see* Blister, shoulder
contusion —*see* Contusion, shoulder
external constriction —*see* Constriction, external, shoulder
foreign body —*see* Foreign body, superficial, shoulder

Injury *(Continued)*
superficial NEC *(Continued)*
skin NEC T14.8
sternal region —*see* Injury, superficial, thorax, front
subconjunctival —*see* Injury, eye, specified site NEC
subcutaneous NEC T14.8
submaxillary region —*see* Injury, superficial, head, specified NEC
submental region —*see* Injury, superficial, head, specified NEC
subungual
finger (s) —*see* Injury, superficial, finger
toe (s) —*see* Injury, superficial, toe
supraclavicular fossa —*see* Injury, superficial, neck
supraorbital —*see* Injury, superficial, head, specified NEC
temple —*see* Injury, superficial, head, specified NEC
temporal region —*see* Injury, superficial, head, specified NEC
testis S30.94
thigh S70.92-
abrasion —*see* Abrasion, thigh
bite —*see* Bite, superficial, thigh
blister —*see* Blister, thigh
contusion —*see* Contusion, thigh
external constriction —*see* Constriction, external, thigh
foreign body —*see* Foreign body, superficial, thigh
thorax, thoracic (wall) S20.90
abrasion —*see* Abrasion, thorax
back S20.40-
bite —*see* Bite, thorax, superficial
blister —*see* Blister, thorax
contusion —*see* Contusion, thorax
external constriction —*see* Constriction, external, thorax
foreign body —*see* Foreign body, superficial, thorax
front S20.30-
throat S10.10
abrasion S10.11
bite S10.17
insect S10.16
blister S10.12
contusion S10.0
external constriction S10.14
foreign body S10.15
thumb S60.93-
abrasion —*see* Abrasion, thumb
bite —*see* Bite, superficial, thumb
blister —*see* Blister, thumb
contusion —*see* Contusion, thumb
external constriction —*see* Constriction, external, thumb
foreign body —*see* Foreign body, superficial, thumb
insect bite —*see* Bite, by site, superficial, insect
specified type NEC S60.39-
toe (s) S90.93-
abrasion —*see* Abrasion, toe
bite —*see* Bite, toe
blister —*see* Blister, toe
contusion —*see* Contusion, toe
external constriction —*see* Constriction, external, toe
foreign body —*see* Foreign body, superficial, toe
great S90.93-
tongue —*see* Injury, superficial, oral cavity
tooth, teeth —*see* Injury, superficial, oral cavity
trachea S10.10
tunica vaginalis S30.94
tympanum, tympanic membrane —*see* Injury, superficial, ear

◀ New ◀ Revised ~~deleted~~ Deleted

Injury *(Continued)*
superficial NEC *(Continued)*
uvula —*see* Injury, superficial, oral cavity
vagina S30.95
vocal cords —*see* Injury, superficial, throat
vulva S30.95
wrist S60.91-
supraclavicular region —*see* Injury, neck
supraorbital S09.93
suprarenal gland (multiple) —*see* Injury, adrenal
surgical complication (external or internal site) —*see* Laceration, accidental complicating surgery
temple S09.90
temporal region S09.90
tendon —*see also* Injury, muscle, by site
abdomen —*see* Injury, muscle, abdomen
Achilles —*see* Injury, Achilles tendon
lower back —*see* Injury, muscle, lower back
pelvic organs —*see* Injury, muscle, pelvis
tenth cranial nerve (pneumogastric or vagus) —*see* Injury, nerve, vagus
testis S39.94
thigh S79.92-
blood vessel —*see* Injury, blood vessel, hip
contusion —*see* Contusion, thigh
fracture —*see* Fracture, femur
muscle —*see* Injury, muscle, thigh
nerve —*see* Injury, nerve, thigh
open —*see* Wound, open, thigh
specified NEC S79.82-
superficial —*see* Injury, superficial, thigh
third cranial nerve (oculomotor) —*see* Injury, nerve, oculomotor
thorax, thoracic S29.9
blood vessel —*see* Injury, blood vessel, thorax
cavity —*see* Injury, intrathoracic
dislocation —*see* Dislocation, thorax
external (wall) S29.9
contusion —*see* Contusion, thorax
nerve —*see* Injury, nerve, thorax
open —*see* Wound, open, thorax
specified NEC S29.8
sprain —*see* Sprain, thorax
superficial —*see* Injury, superficial, thorax
fracture —*see* Fracture, thorax
internal —*see* Injury, intrathoracic
intrathoracic organ —*see* Injury, intrathoracic
sympathetic ganglion —*see* Injury, nerve, thorax, sympathetic
throat —*see also* Injury, neck S19.9
thumb S69.9-
blood vessel —*see* Injury, blood vessel, thumb
contusion —*see* Contusion, thumb
dislocation —*see* Dislocation, thumb
fracture —*see* Fracture, thumb
muscle —*see* Injury, muscle, thumb
nerve —*see* Injury, nerve, digital, thumb
open —*see* Wound, open, thumb
specified NEC S69.8-
sprain —*see* Sprain, thumb
superficial —*see* Injury, superficial, thumb
thymus (gland) —*see* Injury, intrathoracic, specified organ NEC
thyroid (gland) NEC S19.84
toe S99.92-
contusion —*see* Contusion, toe
dislocation —*see* Dislocation, toe
fracture —*see* Fracture, toe
muscle —*see* Injury, muscle, toe
open —*see* Wound, open, toe
specified type NEC S99.82-
sprain —*see* Sprain, toe
superficial —*see* Injury, superficial, toe
tongue S09.93
tonsil S09.93

Injury *(Continued)*
tooth S09.93
trachea (cervical) NEC S19.82
thoracic —*see* Injury, intrathoracic, trachea, thoracic
transfusion-related acute lung (TRALI) J95.84
tunica vaginalis S39.94
twelfth cranial nerve (hypoglossal) —*see* Injury, nerve, hypoglossal
ureter S37.10
contusion S37.12
laceration S37.13
specified type NEC S37.19
urethra (sphincter) S37.30
at delivery O71.5
contusion S37.32
laceration S37.33
specified type NEC S37.38
urinary organ S37.899
contusion S37.92
laceration S37.93
specified
site NEC S37.899
contusion S37.892
laceration S37.893
specified type NEC S37.898
type NEC S37.99
uterus, uterine S37.60
with ectopic or molar pregnancy O08.6
blood vessel —*see* Injury, blood vessel, iliac
contusion S37.62
laceration S37.63
cervix at delivery O71.3
rupture associated with obstetrics —*see* Rupture, uterus
specified type NEC S37.69
uvula S09.93
vagina S39.93
abrasion S30.814
bite S31.45
insect S30.864
superficial NEC S30.874
contusion S30.23
crush S38.03
during delivery —*see* Laceration, vagina, during delivery
external constriction S30.844
insect bite S30.864
laceration S31.41
with foreign body S31.42
open wound S31.40
puncture S31.43
with foreign body S31.44
superficial S30.95
foreign body S30.854
vas deferens —*see* Injury, pelvic organ, specified site NEC
vascular NEC T14.8
vein —*see* Injury, blood vessel
vena cava (superior) S25.20
inferior S35.10
laceration (minor) (superficial) S35.11
major S35.12
specified type NEC S35.19
laceration (minor) (superficial) S25.21
major S25.22
specified type NEC S25.29
vesical (sphincter) —*see* Injury, bladder
visual cortex S04.04-
vitreous (humor) S05.90
specified NEC S05.8X-
vocal cord NEC S19.83
vulva S39.94
abrasion S30.814
bite S31.45
insect S30.864
superficial NEC S30.874
contusion S30.23
crush S38.03
during delivery —*see* Laceration, perineum, female, during delivery

Injury *(Continued)*
vulva *(Continued)*
external constriction S30.844
insect bite S30.864
laceration S31.41
with foreign body S31.42
open wound S31.40
puncture S31.43
with foreign body S31.44
superficial S30.95
foreign body S30.854
whiplash (cervical spine) S13.4
wrist S69.9-
blood vessel —*see* Injury, blood vessel, hand
contusion —*see* Contusion, wrist
dislocation —*see* Dislocation, wrist
fracture —*see* Fracture, wrist
muscle —*see* Injury, muscle, hand
nerve —*see* Injury, nerve, hand
open —*see* Wound, open, wrist
specified NEC S69.8-
sprain —*see* Sprain, wrist
superficial —*see* Injury, superficial, wrist
Inoculation —*see also* Vaccination
complication or reaction —*see* Complications, vaccination
Insanity, insane —*see also* Psychosis
adolescent —*see* Schizophrenia
confusional F28
acute or subacute F05
delusional F22
senile F03
Insect
bite —*see* Bite, by site, superficial, insect
venomous, poisoning NEC (by) —*see* Venom, arthropod
Insensitivity
adrenocorticotropin hormone (ACTH) E27.49
androgen E34.50
complete E34.51
partial E34.52
Insertion
cord (umbilical) lateral or velamentous O43.12-
intrauterine contraceptive device (encounter for) —*see* Intrauterine contraceptive device
Insolation (sunstroke) T67.0
Insomnia (organic) G47.00
without objective findings F51.02
adjustment F51.02
adjustment disorder F51.02
behavioral, of childhood Z73.819
combined type Z73.812
limit setting type Z73.811
sleep-onset association type Z73.810
childhood Z73.819
chronic F51.04
somatized tension F51.04
conditioned F51.04
due to
alcohol
abuse F10.182
dependence F10.282
use F10.982
amphetamines
abuse F15.182
dependence F15.282
use F15.982
anxiety disorder F51.05
caffeine
abuse F15.182
dependence F15.282
use F15.982
cocaine
abuse F14.182
dependence F14.282
use F14.982
depression F51.05

Insomnia *(Continued)*
due to *(Continued)*
drug NEC
abuse F19.182
dependence F19.282
use F19.982
medical condition G47.01
mental disorder NEC F51.05
opioid
abuse F11.182
dependence F11.282
use F11.982
psychoactive substance NEC
abuse F19.182
dependence F19.282
use F19.982
sedative, hypnotic, or anxiolytic
abuse F13.182
dependence F13.282
use F13.982
stimulant NEC
abuse F15.182
dependence F15.282
use F15.982
fatal familial (FFI) A81.83
idiopathic F51.01
learned F51.3
nonorganic origin F51.01
not due to a substance or known physiological condition F51.01
specified NEC F51.09
paradoxical F51.03
primary F51.01
psychiatric F51.05
psychophysiologic F51.04
related to psychopathology F51.05
short-term F51.02
specified NEC G47.09
stress-related F51.02
transient F51.02
Inspiration
food or foreign body —*see* Foreign body, by site
mucus —*see* Asphyxia, mucus
Inspissated bile syndrome (newborn) P59.1
Instability
emotional (excessive) F60.3
joint (post-traumatic) M25.30
ankle M25.37-
due to old ligament injury —*see* Disorder, ligament
elbow M25.32-
flail —*see* Flail, joint
foot M25.37-
hand M25.34-
hip M25.35-
knee M25.36-
lumbosacral —*see* subcategory M53.2
prosthesis —*see* Complications, joint prosthesis, mechanical, displacement, by site
sacroiliac —*see* subcategory M53.2
secondary to
old ligament injury —*see* Disorder, ligament
removal of joint prosthesis M96.89
shoulder (region) M25.31-
spine —*see* subcategory M53.2
wrist M25.33-
knee (chronic) M23.5-
lumbosacral —*see* subcategory M53.2
nervous F48.8
personality (emotional) F60.3
spine —*see* Instability, joint, spine
vasomotor R55
Institutional syndrome (childhood) F94.2
Institutionalization, affecting child Z62.22
disinhibited attachment F94.2

Insufficiency, insufficient
accommodation, old age H52.4
adrenal (gland) E27.40
primary E27.1
adrenocortical E27.40
drug-induced E27.3
iatrogenic E27.3
primary E27.1
anatomic crown height K08.89 ◀
anterior (occlusal) guidance M26.54
anus K62.89
aortic (valve) I35.1
with
mitral (valve) disease I08.0
with tricuspid (valve) disease I08.3
stenosis I35.2
tricuspid (valve) disease I08.2
with mitral (valve) disease I08.3
congenital Q23.1
rheumatic I06.1
with
mitral (valve) disease I08.0
with tricuspid (valve) disease I08.3
stenosis I06.2
with mitral (valve) disease I08.0
with tricuspid (valve) disease I08.3
tricuspid (valve) disease I08.2
with mitral (valve) disease I08.3
specified cause NEC I35.1
syphilitic A52.03
arterial I77.1
basilar G45.0
carotid (hemispheric) G45.1
cerebral I67.81
coronary (acute or subacute) I24.8
mesenteric K55.1
peripheral I73.9
precerebral (multiple) (bilateral) G45.2
vertebral G45.0
arteriovenous I99.8
biliary K83.8
cardiac —*see also* Insufficiency, myocardial
due to presence of (cardiac) prosthesis I97.11-
postprocedural I97.11-
cardiorenal, hypertensive I13.2
cardiovascular —*see* Disease, cardiovascular
cerebrovascular (acute) I67.81
with transient focal neurological signs and symptoms G45.8
circulatory NEC I99.8
newborn P29.89
clinical crown length K08.89 ◀
convergence H51.11
coronary (acute or subacute) I24.8
chronic or with a stated duration of over 4 weeks I25.89
corticoadrenal E27.40
primary E27.1
dietary E63.9
divergence H51.8
food T73.0
gastroesophageal K22.8
gonadal
ovary E28.39
testis E29.1
heart —*see also* Insufficiency, myocardial
newborn P29.0
valve —*see* Endocarditis
hepatic —*see* Failure, hepatic
idiopathic autonomic G90.09
interocclusal distance of fully erupted teeth (ridge) M26.36
kidney N28.9
acute N28.9
chronic N18.9
lacrimal (secretion) H04.12-
passages —*see* Stenosis, lacrimal
liver —*see* Failure, hepatic

Insufficiency, insufficient *(Continued)*
lung —*see* Insufficiency, pulmonary
mental (congenital) —*see* Disability, intellectual
mesenteric K55.1
mitral (valve) I34.0
with
aortic valve disease I08.0
with tricuspid (valve) disease I08.3
obstruction or stenosis I05.2
with aortic valve disease I08.0
tricuspid (valve) disease I08.1
with aortic (valve) disease I08.3
congenital Q23.3
rheumatic I05.1
with
aortic valve disease I08.0
with tricuspid (valve) disease I08.3
obstruction or stenosis I05.2
with aortic valve disease I08.0
with tricuspid (valve) disease I08.3
tricuspid (valve) disease I08.1
with aortic (valve) disease I08.3
active or acute I01.1
with chorea, rheumatic (Sydenham's) I02.0
specified cause, except rheumatic I34.0
muscle —*see also* Disease, muscle
heart —*see* Insufficiency, myocardial
ocular NEC H50.9
myocardial, myocardium (with arteriosclerosis) I50.9
with
rheumatic fever (conditions in I00) I09.0
active, acute or subacute I01.2
with chorea I02.0
inactive or quiescent (with chorea) I09.0
congenital Q24.8
hypertensive —*see* Hypertension, heart
newborn P29.0
rheumatic I09.0
active, acute, or subacute I01.2
syphilitic A52.06
nourishment T73.0
pancreatic K86.89 ⇐
exocrine K86.81 ◀
parathyroid (gland) E20.9
peripheral vascular (arterial) I73.9
pituitary E23.0
placental (mother) O36.51-
platelets D69.6
prenatal care affecting management of pregnancy O09.3-
progressive pluriglandular E31.0
pulmonary J98.4
acute, following surgery (nonthoracic) J95.2
thoracic J95.1
chronic, following surgery J95.3
following
shock J98.4
trauma J98.4
newborn P28.5
valve I37.1
with stenosis I37.2
congenital Q22.2
rheumatic I09.89
with aortic, mitral or tricuspid (valve) disease I08.8
pyloric K31.89
renal (acute) N28.9
chronic N18.9
respiratory R06.89
newborn P28.5
rotation —*see* Malrotation
sleep syndrome F51.12

◀ New ⇐ Revised ~~deleted~~ Deleted

Insufficiency, insufficient *(Continued)*
social insurance Z59.7
suprarenal E27.40
primary E27.1
tarso-orbital fascia, congenital Q10.3
testis E29.1
thyroid (gland) (acquired) E03.9
congenital E03.1
tricuspid (valve) (rheumatic) I07.1
with
aortic (valve) disease I08.2
with mitral (valve) disease I08.3
mitral (valve) disease I08.1
with aortic (valve) disease I08.3
obstruction or stenosis I07.2
with aortic (valve) disease I08.2
with mitral (valve) disease I08.3
congenital Q22.8
nonrheumatic I36.1
with stenosis I36.2
urethral sphincter R32
valve, valvular (heart) —*see* Endocarditis
congenital Q24.8
vascular I99.8
intestine K55.9
acute —*see also* Ischemia, intestine, acute K55.059 ⇐
mesenteric K55.1
peripheral I73.9
renal —*see* Hypertension, kidney
velopharyngeal
acquired K13.79
congenital Q38.8
venous (chronic) (peripheral) I87.2
ventricular —*see* Insufficiency, myocardial
welfare support Z59.7
Insufflation, fallopian Z31.41
Insular —*see* condition
Insulinoma
pancreas
benign D13.7
malignant C25.4
uncertain behavior D37.8
specified site
benign —*see* Neoplasm, by site, benign
malignant —*see* Neoplasm, by site, malignant
uncertain behavior —*see* Neoplasm, by site, uncertain behavior
unspecified site
benign D13.7
malignant C25.4
uncertain behavior D37.8
Insuloma —*see* Insulinoma
Interference
balancing side M26.56
non-working side M26.56
Intermenstrual —*see* condition
Intermittent —*see* condition
Internal —*see* condition
Interrogation
cardiac defibrillator (automatic) (implantable) Z45.02
cardiac pacemaker Z45.018
cardiac (event) (loop) recorder Z45.09
infusion pump (implanted) (intrathecal) Z45.1
neurostimulator Z46.2
Interruption
aortic arch Q25.21 ◀
phase-shift, sleep cycle —*see* Disorder, sleep, circadian rhythm
sleep phase-shift, or 24 hour sleep-wake cycle —*see* Disorder, sleep, circadian rhythm
Interstitial —*see* condition
Intertrigo L30.4
labialis K13.0
Intervertebral disc —*see* condition
Intestine, intestinal —*see* condition
Intolerance
carbohydrate K90.49 ⇐
disaccharide, hereditary E73.0
fat NEC K90.49 ⇐
pancreatic K90.3
food K90.49 ⇐
dietary counseling and surveillance Z71.3
fructose E74.10
hereditary E74.12
glucose(-galactose) E74.39
gluten K90.01 ⇐
lactose E73.9
specified NEC E73.8
lysine E72.3
milk NEC K90.49 ⇐
lactose E73.9
protein K90.49 ⇐
starch NEC K90.49 ⇐
sucrose (-isomaltose) E74.31
Intoxicated NEC (without dependence) —*see* Alcohol, intoxication
Intoxication
acid E87.2
alcoholic (acute) (without dependence) —*see* Alcohol, intoxication
alimentary canal K52.1
amphetamine (without dependence) —*see* Abuse, drug, stimulant, with intoxication
with dependence —*see* Dependence, drug, stimulant, with intoxication
anxiolytic (acute) (without dependence) —*see* Abuse, drug, sedative, with intoxication
with dependence —*see* Dependence, drug, sedative, with intoxication
caffeine F15.929 ⇐
with dependence —*see* Dependence, drug, stimulant, with intoxication
cannabinoids (acute) (without dependence) —*see* Use, cannabis, with intoxication ⇐
~~with dependence — see Dependence, drug, cannabis, with intoxication~~
with ◀
abuse —*see* Abuse, drug, cannabis, with intoxication ◀
dependence —*see* Dependence, drug, cannabis, with intoxication ◀
chemical —*see* Table of Drugs and Chemicals
via placenta or breast milk —*see* - Absorption, chemical, through placenta
cocaine (acute) (without dependence) —*see* Abuse, drug, cocaine, with intoxication
with dependence —*see* Dependence, drug, cocaine, with intoxication
drug
acute (without dependence) —*see* Abuse, drug, by type with intoxication
with dependence —*see* Dependence, drug, by type with intoxication
addictive
via placenta or breast milk —*see* Absorption, drug, addictive, through placenta
newborn P93.8
gray baby syndrome P93.0
overdose or wrong substance given or taken —*see* Table of Drugs and Chemicals, by drug, poisoning
enteric K52.1
foodborne A05.9
bacterial A05.9
classical (Clostridium botulinum) A05.1
due to
Bacillus cereus A05.4
bacterium A05.9
specified NEC A05.8
Clostridium
botulinum A05.1
perfringens A05.2
welchii A05.2
Intoxication *(Continued)*
foodborne *(Continued)*
due to *(Continued)*
Salmonella A02.9
with
(gastro) enteritis A02.0
localized infection (s) A02.20
arthritis A02.23
meningitis A02.21
osteomyelitis A02.24
pneumonia A02.22
pyelonephritis A02.25
specified NEC A02.29
sepsis A02.1
specified manifestation NEC A02.8
Staphylococcus A05.0
Vibrio
parahaemolyticus A05.3
vulnificus A05.5
enterotoxin, staphylococcal A05.0
noxious —*see* Poisoning, food, noxious
gastrointestinal K52.1
hallucinogenic (without dependence) —*see* Abuse, drug, hallucinogen, with intoxication
with dependence —*see* Dependence, drug, hallucinogen, with intoxication
hypnotic (acute) (without dependence) —*see* Abuse, drug, sedative, with intoxication
with dependence —*see* Dependence, drug, sedative, with intoxication
inhalant (acute) (without dependence) —*see* Abuse, drug, inhalant, with intoxication
with dependence —*see* Dependence, drug, inhalant, with intoxication
meaning
inebriation —*see* category F10
poisoning —*see* Table of Drugs and Chemicals
methyl alcohol (acute) (without dependence) —*see* Alcohol, intoxication
opioid (acute) (without dependence) —*see* Abuse, drug, opioid, with intoxication
with dependence —*see* Dependence, drug, opioid, with intoxication
pathologic NEC (without dependence) —*see* Alcohol, intoxication
phencyclidine (without dependence) —*see* Abuse, drug, hallucinogen, with intoxication ⇐
with dependence —*see* Dependence, drug, hallucinogen, with intoxication ⇐
potassium (K) E87.5
psychoactive substance NEC (without dependence) —*see* Abuse, drug, psychoactive NEC, with intoxication
with dependence —*see* Dependence, drug, psychoactive NEC, with intoxication
sedative (acute) (without dependence) —*see* Abuse, drug, sedative, with intoxication
with dependence —*see* Dependence, drug, sedative, with intoxication
serum —*see also* Reaction, serum T80.69
uremic —*see* Uremia
volatile solvents (acute) (without dependence) —*see* Abuse, drug, inhalant, with intoxication
with dependence —*see* Dependence, drug, inhalant, with intoxication
water E87.79
Intracranial —*see* condition
Intrahepatic gallbladder Q44.1
Intraligamentous —*see* condition
Intrathoracic —*see also* condition
kidney Q63.2
Intrauterine contraceptive device
checking Z30.431
in situ Z97.5
insertion Z30.430
immediately following removal Z30.433

Intrauterine contraceptive device *(Continued)*
management Z30.431
reinsertion Z30.433
removal Z30.432
replacement Z30.433
retention in pregnancy O26.3-
Intraventricular —*see* condition
Intrinsic deformity —*see* Deformity
Intubation, difficult or failed T88.4
Intumescence, lens (eye) (cataract) —*see* Cataract
Intussusception (bowel) (colon) (enteric) (ileocecal) (ileocolic) (intestine) (rectum) K56.1
appendix K38.8
congenital Q43.8
ureter (with obstruction) N13.5
Invagination (bowel, colon, intestine or rectum) K56.1
Inversion
albumin-globulin (A-G) ratio E88.09
bladder N32.89
cecum —*see* Intussusception
cervix N88.8
chromosome in normal individual Q95.1
circadian rhythm —*see* Disorder, sleep, circadian rhythm
nipple N64.59
congenital Q83.8
gestational —*see* Retraction, nipple
puerperal, postpartum —*see* Retraction, nipple
nyctohemeral rhythm —*see* Disorder, sleep, circadian rhythm
optic papilla Q14.2
organ or site, congenital NEC —*see* Anomaly, by site
sleep rhythm —*see* Disorder, sleep, circadian rhythm
testis (congenital) Q55.29
uterus (chronic) (postinfectional) (postpartal, old) N85.5
postpartum O71.2
vagina (posthysterectomy) N99.3
ventricular Q20.5
Investigation —*see also* Examination Z04.9
clinical research subject (control) (normal comparison) (participant) Z00.6
Involuntary movement, abnormal R25.9
Involution, involutional —*see also* condition
breast, cystic —*see* Dysplasia, mammary, specified type NEC
depression (single episode) F32.89 ⇐
recurrent episode F33.9
melancholia (single episode) F32.89 ⇐
recurrent episode F33.8 ◀
ovary, senile —*see* Atrophy, ovary
thymus failure E32.8
I.Q.
under 20 F73
20-34 F72
35-49 F71
50-69 F70
IRDS (type I) P22.0
type II P22.1
Irideremia Q13.1
Iridis rubeosis —*see* Disorder, iris, vascular
Iridochoroiditis (panuveitis) —*see* Panuveitis
Iridocyclitis H20.9-
acute H20.0-
hypopyon H20.05-
primary H20.01-
recurrent H20.02-
secondary (noninfectious) H20.04-
infectious H20.03-
chronic H20.1-
due to allergy —*see* Iridocyclitis, acute, secondary
endogenous —*see* Iridocyclitis, acute, primary
Fuchs' —*see* Cyclitis, Fuchs' heterochromic
gonococcal A54.32
granulomatous —*see* Iridocyclitis, chronic
herpes, herpetic (simplex) B00.51
zoster B02.32
Iridocyclitis *(Continued)*
hypopyon —*see* Iridocyclitis, acute, hypopyon
in (due to)
ankylosing spondylitis M45.9
gonococcal infection A54.32
herpes (simplex) virus B00.51
zoster B02.32
infectious disease NOS B99
parasitic disease NOS B89 *[H22]*
sarcoidosis D86.83
syphilis A51.43
tuberculosis A18.54
zoster B02.32
lens-induced H20.2-
nongranulomatous —*see* Iridocyclitis, acute
recurrent —*see* Iridocyclitis, acute, recurrent
rheumatic —*see* Iridocyclitis, chronic
subacute —*see* Iridocyclitis, acute
sympathetic —*see* Uveitis, sympathetic
syphilitic (secondary) A51.43
tuberculous (chronic) A18.54
Vogt-Koyanagi H20.82-
Iridocyclochoroiditis (panuveitis) —*see* Panuveitis
Iridodialysis H21.53-
Iridodonesis H21.89
Iridoplegia (complete) (partial) (reflex) H57.09
Iridoschisis H21.25-
Iris —*see also* condition
bombé —*see* Membrane, pupillary
Iritis —*see also* Iridocyclitis
chronic —*see* Iridocyclitis, chronic
diabetic —*see* E08-E13 with .39
due to
herpes simplex B00.51
leprosy A30.9 *[H22]*
gonococcal A54.32
gouty —*see also* Gout, by type M10.9 *[H22]* ⇐
granulomatous —*see* Iridocyclitis, chronic
lens induced —*see* Iridocyclitis, lens-induced
papulosa (syphilitic) A52.71
rheumatic —*see* Iridocyclitis, chronic
syphilitic (secondary) A51.43
congenital (early) A50.01
late A52.71
tuberculous A18.54
Iron —*see* condition
Iron-miner's lung J63.4
Irradiated enamel (tooth, teeth) K03.89
Irradiation effects, adverse T66
Irreducible, irreducibility —*see* condition
Irregular, irregularity
action, heart I49.9
alveolar process K08.89 ⇐
bleeding N92.6
breathing R06.89
contour of cornea (acquired) —*see* Deformity, cornea
congenital Q13.4
contour, reconstructed breast N65.0
dentin (in pulp) K04.3
eye movements H55.89
nystagmus —*see* Nystagmus
saccadic H55.81
labor O62.2
menstruation (cause unknown) N92.6
periods N92.6
prostate N42.9
pupil —*see* Abnormality, pupillary
reconstructed breast N65.0
respiratory R06.89
septum (nasal) J34.2
shape, organ or site, congenital NEC —*see* Distortion
sleep-wake pattern (rhythm) G47.23
Irritable, irritability R45.4
bladder N32.89
bowel (syndrome) K58.9
~~with diarrhea K58.0~~
with ◀
constipation K58.1 ◀
diarrhea K58.0 ◀
Irritable, irritability *(Continued)*
bowel (syndrome) *(Continued)*
mixed K58.2 ◀
psychogenic F45.8
specified NEC K58.8 ◀
bronchial —*see* Bronchitis
cerebral, in newborn P91.3
colon —*see also* Irritable, bowel K58.9 ⇐
with diarrhea K58.0
psychogenic F45.8
duodenum K59.8
heart (psychogenic) F45.8
hip —*see* Derangement, joint, specified type NEC, hip
ileum K59.8
infant R68.12
jejunum K59.8
rectum K59.8
stomach K31.89
psychogenic F45.8
sympathetic G90.8
urethra N36.8
Irritation
anus K62.89
axillary nerve G54.0
bladder N32.89
brachial plexus G54.0
bronchial —*see* Bronchitis
cervical plexus G54.2
cervix —*see* Cervicitis
choroid, sympathetic —*see* Endophthalmitis
cranial nerve —*see* Disorder, nerve, cranial
gastric K31.89
psychogenic F45.8
globe, sympathetic —*see* Uveitis, sympathetic
labyrinth —*see* subcategory H83.2
lumbosacral plexus G54.1
meninges (traumatic) —*see* Injury, intracranial
nontraumatic —*see* Meningismus
nerve —*see* Disorder, nerve
nervous R45.0
penis N48.89
perineum NEC L29.3
peripheral autonomic nervous system G90.8
peritoneum —*see* Peritonitis
pharynx J39.2
plantar nerve —*see* Lesion, nerve, plantar
spinal (cord) (traumatic) —*see also* Injury, spinal cord, by region
nerve G58.9
root NEC —*see* Radiculopathy
nontraumatic —*see* Myelopathy
stomach K31.89
psychogenic F45.8
sympathetic nerve NEC G90.8
ulnar nerve —*see* Lesion, nerve, ulnar
vagina N89.8
Ischemia, ischemic I99.8
bowel (transient)
acute —*see also* Ischemia, intestine, acute K55.059 ⇐
chronic K55.1
due to mesenteric artery insufficiency K55.1
brain —*see* Ischemia, cerebral
cardiac (*see* Disease, heart, ischemic)
cardiomyopathy I25.5
cerebral (chronic) (generalized) I67.82
arteriosclerotic I67.2
intermittent G45.9
newborn P91.0
recurrent focal G45.8
transient G45.9
colon chronic (due to mesenteric artery insufficiency) K55.1
coronary —*see* Disease, heart, ischemic
demand (coronary) —*see also* Angina I24.8
heart (chronic or with a stated duration of over 4 weeks) I25.9
acute or with a stated duration of 4 weeks or less I24.9
subacute I24.9

◀ New ⇐ Revised ~~deleted~~ Deleted

Ischemia, ischemic *(Continued)*
infarction, muscle —*see* Infarct, muscle
intestine (large) (small) (transient) K55.9
acute K55.Ø59 ⟸
diffuse K55.Ø52 ◀
focal K55.Ø51 ◀
large K55.Ø39 ◀
diffuse K55.Ø32 ◀
focal K55.Ø31 ◀
small K55.Ø19 ◀
diffuse K55.Ø12 ◀
focal K55.Ø11 ◀
chronic K55.1
due to mesenteric artery insufficiency K55.1
kidney N28.Ø
mesenteric, acute —*see also* Ischemia, intestine, acute K55.Ø59 ⟸
muscle, traumatic T79.6
myocardium, myocardial (chronic or with a stated duration of over 4 weeks) I25.9
acute, without myocardial infarction I51.3 ⟸
silent (asymptomatic) I25.6
transient of newborn P29.4
renal N28.Ø
retina, retinal —*see* Occlusion, artery, retina
small bowel
acute K55.Ø19 ⟸
diffuse K55.Ø12 ◀
focal K55.Ø11 ◀
chronic K55.1
due to mesenteric artery insufficiency K55.1
spinal cord G95.11
subendocardial —*see* Insufficiency, coronary
supply (coronary) —*see also* Angina I25.9
due to vasospasm I2Ø.1
Ischial spine —*see* condition
Ischialgia —*see* Sciatica
Ischiopagus Q89.4
Ischium, ischial —*see* condition
Ischuria R34
Iselin's disease or osteochondrosis —*see* Osteochondrosis, juvenile, metatarsus
Islands of
parotid tissue in
lymph nodes Q38.6
neck structures Q38.6
submaxillary glands in
fascia Q38.6
lymph nodes Q38.6
neck muscles Q38.6
Islet cell tumor, pancreas D13.7
Isoimmunization NEC —*see also* Incompatibility
affecting management of pregnancy (ABO) (with hydrops fetalis) O36.11-
anti-A sensitization O36.11-
anti-B sensitization O36.19-
anti-c sensitization O36.Ø9-
anti-C sensitization O36.Ø9-
anti-e sensitization O36.Ø9-
anti-E sensitization O36.Ø9-
Rh NEC O36.Ø9-
anti-D antibody O36.Ø1-
specified NEC O36.19-
newborn P55.9
with
hydrops fetalis P56.Ø
kernicterus P57.Ø
ABO (blood groups) P55.1
Rhesus (Rh) factor P55.Ø
specified type NEC P55.8
Isolation, isolated
dwelling Z59.8
family Z63.79
social Z6Ø.4
Isoleucinosis E71.19
Isomerism atrial appendages (with asplenia or polysplenia) Q2Ø.6
Isosporiasis, isosporosis AØ7.3
Isovaleric acidemia E71.11Ø
Issue of
medical certificate ZØ2.79
for disability determination ZØ2.71
Issue of *(Continued)*
repeat prescription (appliance) (glasses) (medicinal substance, medicament, medicine) Z76.Ø
contraception —*see* Contraception
Itch, itching —*see also* Pruritus
baker's L23.6
barber's B35.Ø
bricklayer's L24.5
cheese B88.Ø
clam digger's B65.3
coolie B76.9
copra B88.Ø
dew B76.9
dhobi B35.6
filarial —*see* Infestation, filarial
grain B88.Ø
grocer's B88.Ø
ground B76.9
harvest B88.Ø
jock B35.6
Malabar B35.5
beard B35.Ø
foot B35.3
scalp B35.Ø
meaning scabies B86
Norwegian B86
perianal L29.Ø
poultrymen's B88.Ø
sarcoptic B86
scabies B86
scrub B88.Ø
straw B88.Ø
swimmer's B65.3
water B76.9
winter L29.8
Ivemark's syndrome (asplenia with congenital heart disease) Q89.Ø1
Ivory bones Q78.2
Ixodiasis NEC B88.8

◀ New ⟸ Revised ~~deleted~~ Deleted

J

Jaccoud's syndrome —*see* Arthropathy, postrheumatic, chronic
Jackson's
membrane Q43.3
paralysis or syndrome G83.89
veil Q43.3
Jacquet's dermatitis (diaper dermatitis) L22
Jadassohn-Pellizari's disease or anetoderma L90.2
Jadassohn's
blue nevus —*see* Nevus
intraepidermal epithelioma —*see* Neoplasm, skin, benign
Jaffe-Lichtenstein (-Uehlinger) **syndrome** —*see* Dysplasia, fibrous, bone NEC
Jakob-Creutzfeldt disease or syndrome —*see* Creutzfeldt-Jakob disease or syndrome
Jaksch-Luzet disease D64.89
Jamaican
neuropathy G92
paraplegic tropical ataxic-spastic syndrome G92
Janet's disease F48.8
Janiceps Q89.4
Jansky-Bielschowsky amaurotic idiocy E75.4
Japanese
B-type encephalitis A83.0
river fever A75.3
Jaundice (yellow) R17
acholuric (familial) (splenomegalic) —*see also* Spherocytosis
acquired D59.8
breast-milk (inhibitor) P59.3
catarrhal (acute) B15.9
with hepatic coma B15.0
cholestatic (benign) R17
due to or associated with
delayed conjugation P59.8
associated with (due to) preterm delivery P59.0
preterm delivery P59.0
epidemic (catarrhal) B15.9
with hepatic coma B15.0
leptospiral A27.0
spirochetal A27.0
familial nonhemolytic (congenital) (Gilbert) E80.4
Crigler-Najjar E80.5
febrile (acute) B15.9
with hepatic coma B15.0
leptospiral A27.0
spirochetal A27.0
hematogenous D59.9
hemolytic (acquired) D59.9
congenital —*see* Spherocytosis

Jaundice *(Continued)*
hemorrhagic (acute) (leptospiral) (spirochetal) A27.0
infectious (acute) (subacute) B15.9
with hepatic coma B15.0
leptospiral A27.0
spirochetal A27.0
leptospiral (hemorrhagic) A27.0
malignant (without coma) K72.90
with coma K72.91
neonatal —*see* Jaundice, newborn
newborn P59.9
due to or associated with
ABO
antibodies P55.1
incompatibility, maternal/fetal P55.1
isoimmunization P55.1
absence or deficiency of enzyme system for bilirubin conjugation (congenital) P59.8
bleeding P58.1
breast milk inhibitors to conjugation P59.3
associated with preterm delivery P59.0
bruising P58.0
Crigler-Najjar syndrome E80.5
delayed conjugation P59.8
associated with preterm delivery P59.0
drugs or toxins
given to newborn P58.42
transmitted from mother P58.41
excessive hemolysis P58.9
due to
bleeding P58.1
bruising P58.0
drugs or toxins
given to newborn P58.42
transmitted from mother P58.41
infection P58.2
polycythemia P58.3
swallowed maternal blood P58.5
specified type NEC P58.8
galactosemia E74.21
Gilbert syndrome E80.4
hemolytic disease P55.9
ABO isoimmunization P55.1
Rh isoimmunization P55.0
specified NEC P55.8
hepatocellular damage P59.20
specified NEC P59.29
hereditary hemolytic anemia P58.8
hypothyroidism, congenital E03.1
incompatibility, maternal/fetal NOS P55.9
infection P58.2

Jaundice *(Continued)*
newborn *(Continued)*
due to or associated with *(Continued)*
inspissated bile syndrome P59.1
isoimmunization NOS P55.9
mucoviscidosis E84.9
polycythemia P58.3
preterm delivery P59.0
Rh
antibodies P55.0
incompatibility, maternal/fetal P55.0
isoimmunization P55.0
specified cause NEC P59.8
swallowed maternal blood P58.5
spherocytosis (congenital) D58.0
nonhemolytic congenital familial (Gilbert) E80.4
nuclear, newborn —*see also* Kernicterus of newborn P57.9
obstructive —*see also* Obstruction, bile duct K83.1
post-immunization —*see* Hepatitis, viral, type, B
post-transfusion —*see* Hepatitis, viral, type, B
regurgitation —*see also* Obstruction, bile duct K83.1
serum (homologous) (prophylactic) (therapeutic) —*see* Hepatitis, viral, type, B
spirochetal (hemorrhagic) A27.0
symptomatic R17
newborn P59.9
Jaw —*see* condition
Jaw-winking phenomenon or syndrome Q07.8
Jealousy
alcoholic F10.988
childhood F93.8
sibling F93.8
Jejunitis —*see* Enteritis
Jejunostomy status Z93.4
Jejunum, jejunal —*see* condition
Jensen's disease —*see* Inflammation, chorioretinal, focal, juxtapapillary
Jerks, myoclonic G25.3
Jervell-Lange-Nielsen syndrome I45.81
Jeune's disease Q77.2
Jigger disease B88.1
Job's syndrome (chronic granulomatous disease) D71
Joint —*see also* condition
mice —*see* Loose, body, joint
knee M23.4-
Jordan's anomaly or syndrome D72.0
Joseph-Diamond-Blackfan anemia (congenital hypoplastic) D61.01
Jungle yellow fever A95.0
Jüngling's disease —*see* Sarcoidosis
Juvenile —*see* condition

K

Kahler's disease C90.0-
Kakke E51.11
Kala-azar B55.0
Kallmann's syndrome E23.0
Kanner's syndrome (autism) —*see* Psychosis, childhood
Kaposi's
dermatosis (xeroderma pigmentosum) Q82.1
lichen ruber L44.0
acuminatus L44.0
sarcoma
colon C46.4
connective tissue C46.1
gastrointestinal organ C46.4
lung C46.5-
lymph node (multiple) C46.3
palate (hard) (soft) C46.2
rectum C46.4
skin (multiple sites) C46.0
specified site NEC C46.7
stomach C46.4
unspecified site C46.9
varicelliform eruption B00.0
vaccinia T88.1
Kartagener's syndrome or triad (sinusitis, bronchiectasis, situs inversus) Q89.3
Karyotype
with abnormality except iso (Xq) Q96.2
45,X Q96.0
46,X
iso (Xq) Q96.1
46,XX Q98.3
with streak gonads Q50.32
hermaphrodite (true) Q99.1
male Q98.3
46,XY
with streak gonads Q56.1
female Q97.3
hermaphrodite (true) Q99.1
47,XXX Q97.0
47,XXY Q98.0
47,XYY Q98.5
Kaschin-Beck disease —*see* Disease, Kaschin-Beck
Katayama's disease or fever B65.2
Kawasaki's syndrome M30.3
Kayser-Fleischer ring (cornea) (pseudosclerosis) H18.04-
Kaznelson's syndrome (congenital hypoplastic anemia) D61.01
Kearns-Sayre syndrome H49.81-
Kedani fever A75.3
Kelis L91.0
Kelly (-Patterson) **syndrome** (sideropenic dysphagia) D50.1
Keloid, cheloid L91.0
acne L73.0
Addison's L94.0
cornea —*see* Opacity, cornea
Hawkin's L91.0
scar L91.0
Keloma L91.0
Kenya fever A77.1
Keratectasia —*see also* Ectasia, cornea
congenital Q13.4
Keratinization of alveolar ridge mucosa
excessive K13.23
minimal K13.22
Keratinized residual ridge mucosa
excessive K13.23
minimal K13.22
Keratitis (nodular) (nonulcerative) (simple) (zonular) H16.9
with ulceration (central) (marginal) (perforated) (ring) —*see* Ulcer, cornea
actinic —*see* Photokeratitis
arborescens (herpes simplex) B00.52
areolar H16.11-
bullosa H16.8
Keratitis *(Continued)*
deep H16.309
specified type NEC H16.399
dendritic (a) (herpes simplex) B00.52
disciform (is) (herpes simplex) B00.52
varicella B01.81
filamentary H16.12-
gonococcal (congenital or prenatal) A54.33
herpes, herpetic (simplex) B00.52
zoster B02.33
in (due to)
acanthamebiasis B60.13
adenovirus B30.0
exanthema —*see also* Exanthem B09
herpes (simplex) virus B00.52
measles B05.81
syphilis A50.31
tuberculosis A18.52
zoster B02.33
interstitial (nonsyphilitic) H16.30-
diffuse H16.32-
herpes, herpetic (simplex) B00.52
zoster B02.33
sclerosing H16.33-
specified type NEC H16.39-
syphilitic (congenital) (late) A50.31
tuberculous A18.52
macular H16.11-
nummular H16.11-
oyster shuckers' H16.8
parenchymatous —*see* Keratitis, interstitial
petrificans H16.8
postmeasles B05.81
punctata
leprosa A30.9 *[H16.14-]*
syphilitic (profunda) A50.31
punctate H16.14-
purulent H16.8
rosacea L71.8
sclerosing H16.33-
specified type NEC H16.8
stellate H16.11-
striate H16.11-
superficial H16.10-
with conjunctivitis —*see* Keratoconjunctivitis
due to light —*see* Photokeratitis
suppurative H16.8
syphilitic (congenital) (prenatal) A50.31
trachomatous A71.1
sequelae B94.0
tuberculous A18.52
vesicular H16.8
xerotic —*see also* Keratomalacia H16.8
vitamin A deficiency E50.4
Keratoacanthoma L85.8
Keratocele —*see* Descemetocele
Keratoconjunctivitis H16.20-
Acanthamoeba B60.13
adenoviral B30.0
epidemic B30.0
exposure H16.21-
herpes, herpetic (simplex) B00.52
zoster B02.33
in exanthema —*see also* Exanthem B09
infectious B30.0
lagophthalmic —*see* Keratoconjunctivitis, specified type NEC
neurotrophic H16.23-
phlyctenular H16.25-
postmeasles B05.81
shipyard B30.0
sicca (Sjogren's) M35.0-
not Sjogren's H16.22-
specified type NEC H16.29-
tuberculous (phlyctenular) A18.52
vernal H16.26-
Keratoconus H18.60-
congenital Q13.4
stable H18.61-
unstable H18.62-
Keratocyst (dental) (odontogenic) —*see* Cyst, calcifying odontogenic
Keratoderma, keratodermia (congenital) (palmaris et plantaris) (symmetrical) Q82.8
acquired L85.1
in diseases classified elsewhere L86
climactericum L85.1
gonococcal A54.89
gonorrheal A54.89
punctata L85.2
Reiter's —*see* Reiter's disease
Keratodermatocele —*see* Descemetocele
Keratoglobus H18.79
congenital Q15.8
with glaucoma Q15.0
Keratohemia —*see* Pigmentation, cornea, stromal
Keratoiritis —*see also* Iridocyclitis
syphilitic A50.39
tuberculous A18.54
Keratoma L57.0
palmaris and plantaris hereditarium Q82.8
senile L57.0
Keratomalacia H18.44-
vitamin A deficiency E50.4
Keratomegaly Q13.4
Keratomycosis B49
nigrans, nigricans (palmaris) B36.1
Keratopathy H18.9
band H18.42-
bullous H18.1-
bullous (aphakic), following cataract surgery H59.01-
Keratoscleritis, tuberculous A18.52
Keratosis L57.0
actinic L57.0
arsenical L85.8
congenital, specified NEC Q80.8
female genital NEC N94.89
follicularis Q82.8
acquired L11.0
congenita Q82.8
et parafollicularis in cutem penetrans L87.0
spinulosa (decalvans) Q82.8
vitamin A deficiency E50.8
gonococcal A54.89
male genital (external) N50.89 ◄
nigricans L83
obturans, external ear (canal) —*see* Cholesteatoma, external ear
palmaris et plantaris (inherited) (symmetrical) Q82.8
acquired L85.1
penile N48.89
pharynx J39.2
pilaris, acquired L85.8
punctata (palmaris et plantaris) L85.2
scrotal N50.89 ◄
seborrheic L82.1
inflamed L82.0
senile L57.0
solar L57.0
tonsillaris J35.8
vagina N89.4
vegetans Q82.8
vitamin A deficiency E50.8
vocal cord J38.3
Kerato-uveitis —*see* Iridocyclitis
Kerion (celsi) B35.0
Kernicterus of newborn (not due to isoimmunization) P57.9
due to isoimmunization (conditions in P55.0-P55.9) P57.0
specified type NEC P57.8
Kerunoparalysis T75.09
Keshan disease E59
Ketoacidosis E87.2
diabetic —*see* Diabetes, by type, with ketoacidosis
Ketonuria R82.4

Ketosis NEC E88.89
diabetic —*see* Diabetes, by type, with ketoacidosis
Kew Garden fever A79.1
Kidney —*see* condition
Kienböck's disease —*see also* Osteochondrosis, juvenile, hand, carpal lunate
adult M93.1
Kimmelstiel (-Wilson) disease —*see* Diabetes, Kimmelstiel (-Wilson) disease
Kimura disease D21.9
specified site (see Neoplasm, connective tissue benign)
Kink, kinking
artery I77.1
hair (acquired) L67.8
ileum or intestine —*see* Obstruction, intestine
Lane's —*see* Obstruction, intestine
organ or site, congenital NEC —*see* Anomaly, by site
ureter (pelvic junction) N13.5
with
hydronephrosis N13.1
with infection N13.6
pyelonephritis (chronic) N11.1
congenital Q62.39
vein (s) I87.8
caval I87.1
peripheral I87.1
Kinnier Wilson's disease (hepatolenticular degeneration) E83.01
Kissing spine M48.20
cervical region M48.22
cervicothoracic region M48.23
lumbar region M48.26
lumbosacral region M48.27
occipito-atlanto-axial region M48.21
thoracic region M48.24
thoracolumbar region M48.25
Klatskin's tumor C24.0
Klauder's disease A26.8
Klebs' disease —*see also* Glomerulonephritis N05.-
Klebsiella (K.) pneumoniae, as cause of disease classified elsewhere B96.1
Klein (e)-Levin syndrome G47.13
Kleptomania F63.2
Klinefelter's syndrome Q98.4
karyotype 47,XXY Q98.0
male with more than two X chromosomes Q98.1
Klippel-Feil deficiency, disease, or syndrome (brevicollis) Q76.1
Klippel's disease I67.2
Klippel-Trenaunay (-Weber) syndrome Q87.2
Klumpke (-Déjerine) palsy, paralysis (birth) (newborn) P14.1
Knee —*see* condition
Knock knee (acquired) M21.06-
congenital Q74.1
Knot (s)
intestinal, syndrome (volvulus) K56.2
surfer S89.8-
umbilical cord (true) O69.2
Knotting (of)
hair L67.8
intestine K56.2
Knuckle pad (Garrod's) M72.1
Koch's
infection —*see* Tuberculosis
relapsing fever A68.9
Koch-Weeks' conjunctivitis —*see* Conjunctivitis, acute, mucopurulent
Köebner's syndrome Q81.8
Köenig's disease (osteochondritis dissecans) —*see* Osteochondritis, dissecans
Köhler-Pellegrini-Steida disease or syndrome (calcification, knee joint) —*see* Bursitis, tibial collateral
Köhler's disease
patellar —*see* Osteochondrosis, juvenile, patella
tarsal navicular —*see* Osteochondrosis, juvenile, tarsus
Koilonychia L60.3
congenital Q84.6
Kojevnikov's, epilepsy —*see* Kozhevnikof's epilepsy
Koplik's spots B05.9
Kopp's asthma E32.8
Korsakoff's (Wernicke) disease, psychosis or syndrome (alcoholic) F10.96
with dependence F10.26
drug-induced
due to drug abuse —*see* Abuse, drug, by type, with amnestic disorder
due to drug dependence —*see* Dependence, drug, by type, with amnestic disorder
nonalcoholic F04
Korsakov's disease, psychosis or syndrome —*see* Korsakoff's disease
Korsakow's disease, psychosis or syndrome —*see* Korsakoff's disease
Kostmann's disease or syndrome (infantile genetic agranulocytosis) —*see* Agranulocytosis
Kozhevnikof's epilepsy G40.109
intractable G40.119
with status epilepticus G40.111
without status epilepticus G40.119
not intractable G40.109
with status epilepticus G40.101
without status epilepticus G40.109
Krabbe's
disease E75.23
syndrome, congenital muscle hypoplasia Q79.8
Kraepelin-Morel disease —*see* Schizophrenia
Kraft-Weber-Dimitri disease Q85.8
Kraurosis
ani K62.89
penis N48.0
Kraurosis *(Continued)*
vagina N89.8
vulva N90.4
Kreotoxism A05.9
Krukenberg's
spindle —*see* Pigmentation, cornea, posterior
tumor C79.6-
Kufs' disease E75.4
Kugelberg-Welander disease G12.1
Kuhnt-Junius degeneration —*see also* Degeneration, macula H35.32- ⬅
Kümmell's disease or spondylitis —*see* Spondylopathy, traumatic
Kupffer cell sarcoma C22.3
Kuru A81.81
Kussmaul's
disease M30.0
respiration E87.2
in diabetic acidosis —*see* Diabetes, by type, with ketoacidosis
Kwashiorkor E40
marasmic, marasmus type E42
Kyasanur Forest disease A98.2
Kyphoscoliosis, kyphoscoliotic (acquired) —*see also* Scoliosis M41.9
congenital Q67.5
heart (disease) I27.1
sequelae of rickets E64.3
tuberculous A18.01
Kyphosis, kyphotic (acquired) M40.209
cervical region M40.202
cervicothoracic region M40.203
congenital Q76.419
cervical region Q76.412
cervicothoracic region Q76.413
occipito-atlanto-axial region Q76.411
thoracic region Q76.414
thoracolumbar region Q76.415
Morquio-Brailsford type (spinal) —*see also* subcategory M49.8 E76.219
postlaminectomy M96.3
postradiation therapy M96.2
postural (adolescent) M40.00
cervicothoracic region M40.03
thoracic region M40.04
thoracolumbar region M40.05
secondary NEC M40.10
cervical region M40.12
cervicothoracic region M40.13
thoracic region M40.14
thoracolumbar region M40.15
sequelae of rickets E64.3
specified type NEC M40.299
cervical region M40.292
cervicothoracic region M40.293
thoracic region M40.294
thoracolumbar region M40.295
syphilitic, congenital A50.56
thoracic region M40.204
thoracolumbar region M40.205
tuberculous A18.01
Kyrle disease L87.0

◀ New ⬅ Revised ~~deleted~~ Deleted

L

Labia, labium —*see* condition
Labile
blood pressure R09.89
vasomotor system I73.9
Labioglossal paralysis G12.29
Labium leporinum —*see* Cleft, lip
Labor —*see* Delivery
Labored breathing —*see* Hyperventilation
Labyrinthitis (circumscribed) (destructive) (diffuse) (inner ear) (latent) (purulent) (suppurative) (*see also* subcategory) H83.0
syphilitic A52.79
Laceration
with abortion —*see* Abortion, by type, complicated by laceration of pelvic organs
abdomen, abdominal
wall S31.119
with
foreign body S31.129
penetration into peritoneal cavity S31.619
with foreign body S31.629
epigastric region S31.112
with
foreign body S31.122
penetration into peritoneal cavity S31.612
with foreign body S31.622
left
lower quadrant S31.114
with
foreign body S31.124
penetration into peritoneal cavity S31.614
with foreign body S31.624
upper quadrant S31.111
with
foreign body S31.121
penetration into peritoneal cavity S31.611
with foreign body S31.621
periumbilic region S31.115
with
foreign body S31.125
penetration into peritoneal cavity S31.615
with foreign body S31.625
right
lower quadrant S31.113
with
foreign body S31.123
penetration into peritoneal cavity S31.613
with foreign body S31.623
upper quadrant S31.110
with
foreign body S31.120
penetration into peritoneal cavity S31.610
with foreign body S31.620
accidental, complicating surgery —*see* Complications, surgical, accidental puncture or laceration
Achilles tendon S86.02-
adrenal gland S37.813
alveolar (process) —*see* Laceration, oral cavity
ankle S91.01-
with
foreign body S91.02-
antecubital space —*see* Laceration, elbow
anus (sphincter) S31.831
with
ectopic or molar pregnancy O08.6
foreign body S31.832
complicating delivery —*see* Delivery, complicated, by, laceration, anus (sphincter)

Laceration *(Continued)*
anus *(Continued)*
following ectopic or molar pregnancy O08.6
nontraumatic, nonpuerperal —*see* Fissure, anus
arm (upper) S41.11-
with foreign body S41.12-
lower —*see* Laceration, forearm
auditory canal (external) (meatus) —*see* Laceration, ear
auricle, ear —*see* Laceration, ear
axilla —*see* Laceration, arm
back —*see also* Laceration, thorax, back
lower S31.010
with
foreign body S31.020
with penetration into retroperitoneal space S31.021
penetration into retroperitoneal space S31.011
bile duct S36.13
bladder S37.23
with ectopic or molar pregnancy O08.6
following ectopic or molar pregnancy O08.6
obstetrical trauma O71.5
blood vessel —*see* Injury, blood vessel
bowel —*see also* Laceration, intestine
with ectopic or molar pregnancy O08.6
complicating abortion —*see* Abortion, by type, complicated by, specified condition NEC
following ectopic or molar pregnancy O08.6
obstetrical trauma O71.5
brain (any part) (cortex) (diffuse) (membrane) —*see also* Injury, intracranial, diffuse
during birth P10.8
with hemorrhage P10.1
focal —*see* Injury, intracranial, focal brain injury
brainstem S06.38-
breast S21.01-
with foreign body S21.02-
broad ligament S37.893
with ectopic or molar pregnancy O08.6
following ectopic or molar pregnancy O08.6
laceration syndrome N83.8
obstetrical trauma O71.6
syndrome (laceration) N83.8
buttock S31.801
with foreign body S31.802
left S31.821
with foreign body S31.822
right S31.811
with foreign body S31.812
calf —*see* Laceration, leg
canaliculus lacrimalis —*see* Laceration, eyelid
canthus, eye —*see* Laceration, eyelid
capsule, joint —*see* Sprain
causing eversion of cervix uteri (old) N86
central (perineal), complicating delivery O70.9
cerebellum, traumatic S06.37-
cerebral S06.33-
during birth P10.8
with hemorrhage P10.1
left side S06.32-
right side S06.31-
cervix (uteri)
with ectopic or molar pregnancy O08.6
following ectopic or molar pregnancy O08.6
nonpuerperal, nontraumatic N88.1
obstetrical trauma (current) O71.3
old (postpartal) N88.1
traumatic S37.63

Laceration *(Continued)*
cheek (external) S01.41-
with foreign body S01.42-
internal —*see* Laceration, oral cavity
chest wall —*see* Laceration, thorax
chin —*see* Laceration, head, specified site NEC
chordae tendinae NEC I51.1
concurrent with acute myocardial infarction —*see* Infarct, myocardium
following acute myocardial infarction (current complication) I23.4
clitoris —*see* Laceration, vulva
colon —*see* Laceration, intestine, large, colon
common bile duct S36.13
cortex (cerebral) —*see* Injury, intracranial, diffuse
costal region —*see* Laceration, thorax
cystic duct S36.13
diaphragm S27.803
digit (s)
foot —*see* Laceration, toe
hand —*see* Laceration, finger
duodenum S36.430
ear (canal) (external) S01.31-
with foreign body S01.32-
drum S09.2-
elbow S51.01-
with
foreign body S51.02-
epididymis —*see* Laceration, testis
epigastric region —*see* Laceration, abdomen, wall, epigastric region
esophagus K22.8
traumatic
cervical S11.21
with foreign body S11.22
thoracic S27.813
eye (ball) S05.3-
with prolapse or loss of intraocular tissue S05.2-
penetrating S05.6-
eyebrow —*see* Laceration, eyelid
eyelid S01.11-
with foreign body S01.12-
face NEC —*see* Laceration, head, specified site NEC
fallopian tube S37.539
bilateral S37.532
unilateral S37.531
finger (s) S61.219
with
damage to nail S61.319
with
foreign body S61.329
foreign body S61.229
index S61.218
with
damage to nail S61.318
with
foreign body S61.328
foreign body S61.228
left S61.211
with
damage to nail S61.311
with
foreign body S61.321
foreign body S61.221
right S61.210
with
damage to nail S61.310
with
foreign body S61.320
foreign body S61.220
little S61.218
with
damage to nail S61.318
with
foreign body S61.328
foreign body S61.228

Laceration *(Continued)*
finger *(Continued)*
little *(Continued)*
left S61.217
with
damage to nail S61.317
with
foreign body S61.327
foreign body S61.227
right S61.216
with
damage to nail S61.316
with
foreign body S61.326
foreign body S61.226
middle S61.218
with
damage to nail S61.318
with
foreign body S61.328
foreign body S61.228
left S61.213
with
damage to nail S61.313
with
foreign body S61.323
foreign body S61.223
right S61.212
with
damage to nail S61.312
with
foreign body S61.322
foreign body S61.222
ring S61.218
with
damage to nail S61.318
with
foreign body S61.328
foreign body S61.228
left S61.215
with
damage to nail S61.315
with
foreign body S61.325
foreign body S61.225
right S61.214
with
damage to nail S61.314
with
foreign body S61.324
foreign body S61.224
flank S31.119
with foreign body S31.129
foot (except toe (s) alone) S91.319
with foreign body S91.329
left S91.312
with foreign body S91.322
right S91.311
with foreign body S91.321
toe —*see* Laceration, toe
forearm S51.819
with
foreign body S51.829
elbow only —*see* Laceration, elbow
left S51.812
with
foreign body S51.822
right S51.811
with
foreign body S51.821
forehead S01.81
with foreign body S01.82
fourchette O70.0
with ectopic or molar pregnancy O08.6
complicating delivery O70.0
following ectopic or molar pregnancy O08.6
gallbladder S36.123

Laceration *(Continued)*
genital organs, external
female S31.512
with foreign body S31.522
vagina —*see* Laceration, vagina
vulva —*see* Laceration, vulva
male S31.511
with foreign body S31.521
penis —*see* Laceration, penis
scrotum —*see* Laceration, scrotum
testis —*see* Laceration, testis
groin —*see* Laceration, abdomen, wall
gum —*see* Laceration, oral cavity
hand S61.419
with
foreign body S61.429
finger —*see* Laceration, finger
left S61.412
with
foreign body S61.422
right S61.411
with
foreign body S61.421
thumb —*see* Laceration, thumb
head S01.91
with foreign body S01.92
cheek —*see* Laceration, cheek
ear —*see* Laceration, ear
eyelid —*see* Laceration, eyelid
lip —*see* Laceration, lip
nose —*see* Laceration, nose
oral cavity —*see* Laceration, oral cavity
scalp S01.01
with foreign body S01.02
specified site NEC S01.81
with foreign body S01.82
temporomandibular area —*see* Laceration, cheek
heart —*see* Injury, heart, laceration
heel —*see* Laceration, foot
hepatic duct S36.13
hip S71.019
with foreign body S71.029
left S71.012
with foreign body S71.022
right S71.011
with foreign body S71.021
hymen —*see* Laceration, vagina
hypochondrium —*see* Laceration, abdomen, wall
hypogastric region —*see* Laceration, abdomen, wall
ileum S36.438
inguinal region —*see* Laceration, abdomen, wall
instep —*see* Laceration, foot
internal organ —*see* Injury, by site
interscapular region —*see* Laceration, thorax, back
intestine
large
colon S36.539
ascending S36.530
descending S36.532
sigmoid S36.533
specified site NEC S36.538
rectum S36.63
transverse S36.531
small S36.439
duodenum S36.430
specified site NEC S36.438
intra-abdominal organ S36.93
intestine —*see* Laceration, intestine
liver —*see* Laceration, liver
pancreas —*see* Laceration, pancreas
peritoneum S36.81
specified site NEC S36.893
spleen —*see* Laceration, spleen
stomach —*see* Laceration, stomach

Laceration *(Continued)*
intracranial NEC —*see also* Injury, intracranial, diffuse
birth injury P10.9
jaw —*see* Laceration, head, specified site NEC
jejunum S36.438
joint capsule —*see* Sprain, by site
kidney S37.03-
major (greater than 3 cm) (massive) (stellate) S37.06-
minor (less than 1 cm) S37.04-
moderate (1 to 3 cm) S37.05-
multiple S37.06-
knee S81.01-
with foreign body S81.02-
labium (majus) (minus) —*see* Laceration, vulva
lacrimal duct —*see* Laceration, eyelid
large intestine —*see* Laceration, intestine, large
larynx S11.011
with foreign body S11.012
leg (lower) S81.819
with foreign body S81.829
foot —*see* Laceration, foot
knee —*see* Laceration, knee
left S81.812
with foreign body S81.822
right S81.811
with foreign body S81.821
upper —*see* Laceration, thigh
ligament —*see* Sprain
lip S01.511
with foreign body S01.521
liver S36.113
major (stellate) S36.116
minor S36.114
moderate S36.115
loin —*see* Laceration, abdomen, wall
lower back —*see* Laceration, back, lower
lumbar region —*see* Laceration, back, lower
lung S27.339
bilateral S27.332
unilateral S27.331
malar region —*see* Laceration, head, specified site NEC
mammary —*see* Laceration, breast
mastoid region —*see* Laceration, head, specified site NEC
meninges —*see* Injury, intracranial, diffuse
meniscus —*see* Tear, meniscus
mesentery S36.893
mesosalpinx S37.893
mouth —*see* Laceration, oral cavity
muscle —*see* Injury, muscle, by site, laceration
nail
finger —*see* Laceration, finger, with damage to nail
toe —*see* Laceration, toe, with damage to nail
nasal (septum) (sinus) —*see* Laceration, nose
nasopharynx —*see* Laceration, head, specified site NEC
neck S11.91
with foreign body S11.92
involving
cervical esophagus S11.21
with foreign body S11.22
larynx —*see* Laceration, larynx
pharynx —*see* Laceration, pharynx
thyroid gland —*see* Laceration, thyroid gland
trachea —*see* Laceration, trachea
specified site NEC S11.81
with foreign body S11.82
nerve —*see* Injury, nerve
nose (septum) (sinus) S01.21
with foreign body S01.22
ocular NOS S05.3-
adnexa NOS S01.11-

Laceration *(Continued)*
oral cavity S01.512
with foreign body S01.522
orbit (eye) —*see* Wound, open, ocular, orbit
ovary S37.439
bilateral S37.432
unilateral S37.431
palate —*see* Laceration, oral cavity
palm —*see* Laceration, hand
pancreas S36.239
body S36.231
major S36.261
minor S36.241
moderate S36.251
head S36.230
major S36.260
minor S36.240
moderate S36.250
major S36.269
minor S36.249
moderate S36.259
tail S36.232
major S36.262
minor S36.242
moderate S36.252
pelvic S31.010
with
foreign body S31.020
penetration into retroperitoneal cavity S31.021
penetration into retroperitoneal cavity S31.011
floor —*see also* Laceration, back, lower
with ectopic or molar pregnancy O08.6
complicating delivery O70.1
following ectopic or molar pregnancy O08.6
old (postpartal) N81.89
organ S37.93
with ectopic or molar pregnancy O08.6
adrenal gland S37.813
bladder S37.23
fallopian tube —*see* Laceration, fallopian tube
following ectopic or molar pregnancy O08.6
kidney —*see* Laceration, kidney
obstetrical trauma O71.5
ovary —*see* Laceration, ovary
prostate S37.823
specified site NEC S37.893
ureter S37.13
urethra S37.33
uterus S37.63
penis S31.21
with foreign body S31.22
perineum
female S31.41
with
ectopic or molar pregnancy O08.6
foreign body S31.42
during delivery O70.9
first degree O70.0
fourth degree O70.3
second degree O70.1
third degree —*see also* Delivery, complicated, by, laceration, perineum, third degree O70.20 ◀
old (postpartal) N81.89
postpartal N81.89
secondary (postpartal) O90.1
male S31.119
with foreign body S31.129
periocular area (with or without lacrimal passages) —*see* Laceration, eyelid
peritoneum S36.893
periumbilic region —*see* Laceration, abdomen, wall, periumbilic

Laceration *(Continued)*
periurethral tissue —*see* Laceration, urethra
phalanges
finger —*see* Laceration, finger
toe —*see* Laceration, toe
pharynx S11.21
with foreign body S11.22
pinna —*see* Laceration, ear
popliteal space —*see* Laceration, knee
prepuce —*see* Laceration, penis
prostate S37.823
pubic region S31.119
with foreign body S31.129
pudendum —*see* Laceration, genital organs, external
rectovaginal septum —*see* Laceration, vagina
rectum S36.63
retroperitoneum S36.893
round ligament S37.893
sacral region —*see* Laceration, back, lower
sacroiliac region —*see* Laceration, back, lower
salivary gland —*see* Laceration, oral cavity
scalp S01.01
with foreign body S01.02
scapular region —*see* Laceration, shoulder
scrotum S31.31
with foreign body S31.32
seminal vesicle S37.893
shin —*see* Laceration, leg
shoulder S41.019
with foreign body S41.029
left S41.012
with foreign body S41.022
right S41.011
with foreign body S41.021
small intestine —*see* Laceration, intestine, small
spermatic cord —*see* Laceration, testis
spinal cord (meninges) —*see also* Injury, spinal cord, by region
due to injury at birth P11.5
newborn (birth injury) P11.5
spleen S36.039
major (massive) (stellate) S36.032
moderate S36.031
superficial (minor) S36.030
sternal region —*see* Laceration, thorax, front
stomach S36.33
submaxillary region —*see* Laceration, head, specified site NEC
submental region —*see* Laceration, head, specified site NEC
subungual
finger (s) —*see* Laceration, finger, with damage to nail
toe (s) —*see* Laceration, toe, with damage to nail
suprarenal gland —*see* Laceration, adrenal gland
temple, temporal region —*see* Laceration, head, specified site NEC
temporomandibular area —*see* Laceration, cheek
tendon —*see* Injury, muscle, by site, laceration
Achilles S86.02-
tentorium cerebelli —*see* Injury, intracranial, diffuse
testis S31.31
with foreign body S31.32
thigh S71.11-
with foreign body S71.12-
thorax, thoracic (wall) S21.91
with foreign body S21.92
back S21.22-
with penetration into thoracic cavity S21.42-
front S21.12-
with penetration into thoracic cavity S21.32-

Laceration *(Continued)*
thorax, thoracic *(Continued)*
back S21.21-
with
foreign body S21.22-
with penetration into thoracic cavity S21.42-
penetration into thoracic cavity S21.41-
breast —*see* Laceration, breast
front S21.11-
with
foreign body S21.12-
with penetration into thoracic cavity S21.32-
penetration into thoracic cavity S21.31-
thumb S61.019
with
damage to nail S61.119
with
foreign body S61.129
foreign body S61.029
left S61.012
with
damage to nail S61.112
with
foreign body S61.122
foreign body S61.022
right S61.011
with
damage to nail S61.111
with
foreign body S61.121
foreign body S61.021
thyroid gland S11.11
with foreign body S11.12
toe (s) S91.119
with
damage to nail S91.219
with
foreign body S91.229
foreign body S91.129
great S91.113
with
damage to nail S91.213
with
foreign body S91.223
foreign body S91.123
left S91.112
with
damage to nail S91.212
with
foreign body S91.222
foreign body S91.122
right S91.111
with
damage to nail S91.211
with
foreign body S91.221
foreign body S91.121
lesser S91.116
with
damage to nail S91.216
with
foreign body S91.226
foreign body S91.126
left S91.115
with
damage to nail S91.215
with
foreign body S91.225
foreign body S91.125
right S91.114
with
damage to nail S91.214
with
foreign body S91.224
foreign body S91.124
tongue —*see* Laceration, oral cavity

Laceration *(Continued)*
trachea S11.021
with foreign body S11.022
tunica vaginalis —*see* Laceration, testis
tympanum, tympanic membrane —*see* Laceration, ear, drum
umbilical region S31.115
with foreign body S31.125
ureter S37.13
urethra S37.33
with or following ectopic or molar pregnancy O08.6
obstetrical trauma O71.5
urinary organ NEC S37.893
uterus S37.63
with ectopic or molar pregnancy O08.6
following ectopic or molar pregnancy O08.6
nonpuerperal, nontraumatic N85.8
obstetrical trauma NEC O71.81
old (postpartal) N85.8
uvula —*see* Laceration, oral cavity
vagina S31.41
with
ectopic or molar pregnancy O08.6
foreign body S31.42
during delivery O71.4
with perineal laceration —*see* Laceration, perineum, female, during delivery
following ectopic or molar pregnancy O08.6
nonpuerperal, nontraumatic N89.8
old (postpartal) N89.8
vas deferens S37.893
vesical —*see* Laceration, bladder
vocal cords S11.031
with foreign body S11.032
vulva S31.41
with
ectopic or molar pregnancy O08.6
foreign body S31.42
complicating delivery O70.0
following ectopic or molar pregnancy O08.6
nonpuerperal, nontraumatic N90.89
old (postpartal) N90.89
wrist S61.519
with
foreign body S61.529
left S61.512
with
foreign body S61.522
right S61.511
with
foreign body S61.521
Lack of
achievement in school Z55.3
adequate
food Z59.4
intermaxillary vertical dimension of fully erupted teeth M26.36
sleep Z72.820
appetite (*see* Anorexia) R63.0
awareness R41.9
care
in home Z74.2
of infant (at or after birth) T76.02
confirmed T74.02
cognitive functions R41.9
coordination R27.9
ataxia R27.0
specified type NEC R27.8
development (physiological) R62.50
failure to thrive (child over 28 days old) R62.51
adult R62.7
newborn P92.6
short stature R62.52
specified type NEC R62.59
energy R53.83
financial resources Z59.6
Lack of *(Continued)*
food T73.0
growth R62.52
heating Z59.1
housing (permanent) (temporary) Z59.0
adequate Z59.1
learning experiences in childhood Z62.898
leisure time (affecting life-style) Z73.2
material resources Z59.9
memory —*see also* Amnesia
mild, following organic brain damage F06.8
ovulation N97.0
parental supervision or control of child Z62.0
person able to render necessary care Z74.2
physical exercise Z72.3
play experience in childhood Z62.898
posterior occlusal support M26.57
relaxation (affecting life-style) Z73.2
sexual
desire F52.0
enjoyment F52.1
shelter Z59.0
sleep (adequate) Z72.820
supervision of child by parent Z62.0
support, posterior occlusal M26.57
water T73.1
Lacrimal —*see* condition
Lacrimation, abnormal —*see* Epiphora
Lacrimonasal duct —*see* condition
Lactation, lactating (breast) (puerperal, postpartum)
associated
cracked nipple O92.13
retracted nipple O92.03
defective O92.4
disorder NEC O92.79
excessive O92.6
failed (complete) O92.3
partial O92.4
mastitis NEC —*see* Mastitis, obstetric
mother (care and/or examination) Z39.1
nonpuerperal N64.3
Lacticemia, excessive E87.2
Lacunar skull Q75.8
Laennec's cirrhosis K70.30 ⬅
~~alcoholic K70.30~~
~~with ascites K70.31~~
with ascites K70.31 ◀
nonalcoholic K74.69 ◀
Lafora's disease —*see* Epilepsy, generalized, idiopathic
Lag, lid (nervous) —*see* Retraction, lid
Lagophthalmos (eyelid) (nervous) H02.209
cicatricial H02.219
left H02.216
lower H02.215
upper H02.214
right H02.213
lower H02.212
upper H02.211
keratoconjunctivitis —*see* Keratoconjunctivitis
left H02.206
lower H02.205
upper H02.204
mechanical H02.229
left H02.226
lower H02.225
upper H02.224
right H02.223
lower H02.222
upper H02.221
paralytic H02.239
left H02.236
lower H02.235
upper H02.234
right H02.233
lower H02.232
upper H02.231
right H02.203
lower H02.202
upper H02.201
Laki-Lorand factor deficiency —*see* Defect, coagulation, specified type NEC
Lalling F80.0
Lambert-Eaton syndrome —*see* Syndrome, Lambert-Eaton
Lambliasis, lambliosis A07.1
Landau-Kleffner syndrome —*see* Epilepsy, specified NEC
Landouzy-Déjérine dystrophy or facioscapulohumeral atrophy G71.0
Landouzy's disease (icterohemorrhagic leptospirosis) A27.0
Landry-Guillain-Barré, syndrome or paralysis G61.0
Landry's disease or paralysis G61.0
Lane's
band Q43.3
kink —*see* Obstruction, intestine
syndrome K90.2
Langdon Down's syndrome —*see* Trisomy, 21
Lapsed immunization schedule status Z28.3
Large
baby (regardless of gestational age) (4000g to 4499g) P08.1
ear, congenital Q17.1
physiological cup Q14.2
stature R68.89
Large-for-dates NEC (infant) (4000g to 4499g) P08.1
affecting management of pregnancy O36.6-
exceptionally (4500g or more) P08.0
Larsen-Johansson disease
orosteochondrosis —*see* Osteochondrosis, juvenile, patella
Larsen's syndrome (flattened facies and multiple congenital dislocations) Q74.8
Larva migrans
cutaneous B76.9
Ancylostoma B76.0
visceral B83.0
Laryngeal —*see* condition
Laryngismus (stridulus) J38.5
congenital P28.89
diphtheritic A36.2
Laryngitis (acute) (edematous) (fibrinous) (infective) (infiltrative) (malignant) (membranous) (phlegmonous) (pneumococcal) (pseudomembranous) (septic) (subglottic) (suppurative) (ulcerative) J04.0
with
influenza, flu, or grippe —*see* Influenza, with, laryngitis
tracheitis (acute) —*see* Laryngotracheitis
atrophic J37.0
catarrhal J37.0
chronic J37.0
with tracheitis (chronic) J37.1
diphtheritic A36.2
due to external agent —*see* Inflammation, respiratory, upper, due to
Hemophilus influenzae J04.0
H. influenzae J04.0
hypertrophic J37.0
influenzal —*see* Influenza, with, respiratory manifestations NEC
obstructive J05.0
sicca J37.0
spasmodic J05.0
acute J04.0
streptococcal J04.0
stridulous J05.0
syphilitic (late) A52.73
congenital A50.59 *[J99]*
early A50.03 *[J99]*
tuberculous A15.5
Vincent's A69.1
Laryngocele (congenital) (ventricular) Q31.3
Laryngofissure J38.7
congenital Q31.8
Laryngomalacia (congenital) Q31.5

◀ New ⬅ Revised ~~deleted~~ Deleted

Laryngopharyngitis (acute) J06.0
chronic J37.0
due to external agent —*see* Inflammation, respiratory, upper, due to
Laryngoplegia J38.00
bilateral J38.02
unilateral J38.01
Laryngoptosis J38.7
Laryngospasm J38.5
Laryngostenosis J38.6
Laryngotracheitis (acute) (Infectional) (infective) (viral) J04.2
atrophic J37.1
catarrhal J37.1
chronic J37.1
diphtheritic A36.2
due to external agent —*see* Inflammation, respiratory, upper, due to
Hemophilus influenzae J04.2
hypertrophic J37.1
influenzal —*see* Influenza, with, respiratory manifestations NEC
pachydermic J38.7
sicca J37.1
spasmodic J38.5
acute J05.0
streptococcal J04.2
stridulous J38.5
syphilitic (late) A52.73
congenital A50.59 *[J99]*
early A50.03 *[J99]*
tuberculous A15.5
Vincent's A69.1
Laryngotracheobronchitis —*see* Bronchitis
Larynx, laryngeal —*see* condition
Lassa fever A96.2
Lassitude —*see* Weakness
Late
talker R62.0
walker R62.0
Late effect (s) —*see* Sequelae
Latent —*see* condition
Laterocession —*see* Lateroversion
Lateroflexion —*see* Lateroversion
Lateroversion
cervix —*see* Lateroversion, uterus
uterus, uterine (cervix) (postinfectional) (postpartal, old) N85.4
congenital Q51.818
in pregnancy or childbirth O34.59-
Lathyrism —*see* Poisoning, food, noxious, plant
Launois' syndrome (pituitary gigantism) E22.0
Launois-Bensaude adenolipomatosis E88.89
Laurence-Moon (-Bardet)-Biedl syndrome Q87.89
Lax, laxity —*see also* Relaxation
ligament (ous) —*see also* Disorder, ligament
familial M35.7
knee —*see* Derangement, knee
skin (acquired) L57.4
congenital Q82.8
Laxative habit F55.2
Lazy leukocyte syndrome D70.8
Lead miner's lung J63.6
Leak, leakage
air NEC J93.82
postprocedural J95.812
amniotic fluid —*see* Rupture, membranes, premature
blood (microscopic), fetal, into maternal circulation affecting management of pregnancy —*see* Pregnancy, complicated by
cerebrospinal fluid G96.0
from spinal (lumbar) puncture G97.0
device, implant or graft —*see also* Complications, by site and type, mechanical
arterial graft NEC —*see* Complication, cardiovascular device, mechanical, vascular

Leak, leakage *(Continued)*
device, implant or graft *(Continued)*
breast (implant) T85.43
catheter NEC T85.638
dialysis (renal) T82.43
intraperitoneal T85.631
infusion NEC T82.534
spinal (epidural) (subdural) T85.630
~~urinary, indwelling T83.038~~
~~cystostomy T83.030~~
urinary T83.038 ◀
cystostomy T83.030 ◀
Hopkins T83.038 ◀
ileostomy T83.038 ◀
indwelling T83.031 ◀
nephrostomy T83.032 ◀
specified NEC T83.038 ◀
urostomy T83.038 ◀
gastrointestinal —*see* Complications, prosthetic device, mechanical, gastrointestinal device
genital NEC T83.498
penile prosthesis (cylinder) (implanted) (pump) (resevoir) T83.490 ⟸
testicular prosthesis T83.491 ◀
heart NEC —*see* Complication, cardiovascular device, mechanical
joint prosthesis —*see* Complications, joint prosthesis, mechanical, specified NEC, by site
ocular NEC —*see* Complications, prosthetic device, mechanical, ocular device
orthopedic NEC —*see* Complication, orthopedic, device, mechanical
persistent air J93.82
specified NEC T85.638
urinary NEC —*see also* Complication, genitourinary, device, urinary, mechanical
graft T83.23
vascular NEC —*see* Complication, cardiovascular device, mechanical
ventricular intracranial shunt T85.03
urine —*see* Incontinence
Leaky heart —*see* Endocarditis
Learning defect (specific) F81.9
Leather bottle stomach C16.9
Leber's
congenital amaurosis H35.50
optic atrophy (hereditary) H47.22
Lederer's anemia D59.1
Leeches (external) —*see* Hirudiniasis
Leg —*see* condition
Legg (-Calvé)-Perthes disease, syndrome or osteochondrosis M91.1-
Legionellosis A48.1
nonpneumonic A48.2
Legionnaires'
disease A48.1
nonpneumonic A48.2
pneumonia A48.1
Leigh's disease G31.82
Leiner's disease L21.1
Leiofibromyoma —*see* Leiomyoma
Leiomyoblastoma —*see* Neoplasm, connective tissue, benign
Leiomyofibroma —*see also* Neoplasm, connective tissue, benign
uterus (cervix) (corpus) D25.9
Leiomyoma —*see also* Neoplasm, connective tissue, benign
bizarre —*see* Neoplasm, connective tissue, benign
cellular —*see* Neoplasm, connective tissue, benign
epithelioid —*see* Neoplasm, connective tissue, benign
uterus (cervix) (corpus) D25.9
intramural D25.1
submucous D25.0
subserosal D25.2

Leiomyoma *(Continued)*
vascular —*see* Neoplasm, connective tissue, benign
Leiomyoma, leiomyomatosis (intravascular) —*see* Neoplasm, connective tissue, uncertain behavior
Leiomyosarcoma —*see also* Neoplasm, connective tissue, malignant
epithelioid —*see* Neoplasm, connective tissue, malignant
myxoid —*see* Neoplasm, connective tissue, malignant
Leishmaniasis B55.9
American (mucocutaneous) B55.2
cutaneous B55.1
Asian Desert B55.1
Brazilian B55.2
cutaneous (any type) B55.1
dermal —*see also* Leishmaniasis, cutaneous
post-kala-azar B55.0
eyelid B55.1
infantile B55.0
Mediterranean B55.0
mucocutaneous (American) (New World) B55.2
naso-oral B55.2
nasopharyngeal B55.2
old world B55.1
tegumentaria diffusa B55.1
visceral B55.0
Leishmanoid, dermal —*see also* Leishmaniasis, cutaneous
post-kala-azar B55.0
Lenegre's disease I44.2
Lengthening, leg —*see* Deformity, limb, unequal length
Lennert's lymphoma —*see* Lymphoma, Lennert's
Lennox-Gastaut syndrome G40.812
intractable G40.814
with status epilepticus G40.813
without status epilepticus G40.814
not intractable G40.812
with status epilepticus G40.811
without status epilepticus G40.812
Lens —*see* condition
Lenticonus (anterior) (posterior) (congenital) Q12.8
Lenticular degeneration, progressive E83.01
Lentiglobus (posterior) (congenital) Q12.8
Lentigo (congenital) L81.4
maligna —*see also* Melanoma, in situ
melanoma —*see* Melanoma
Lentivirus, as cause of disease classified elsewhere B97.31
Leontiasis
ossium M85.2
syphilitic (late) A52.78
congenital A50.59
Lepothrix A48.8
Lepra —*see* Leprosy
Leprechaunism E34.8
Leprosy A30.-
with muscle disorder A30.9 *[M63.80]*
ankle A30.9 *[M63.87-]*
foot A30.9 *[M63.87-]*
forearm A30.9 *[M63.83-]*
hand A30.9 *[M63.84-]*
lower leg A30.9 *[M63.86-]*
multiple sites A30.9 *[M63.89]*
pelvic region A30.9 *[M63.85-]*
shoulder region A30.9 *[M63.81-]*
specified site NEC A30.9 *[M63.88]*
thigh A30.9 *[M63.85-]*
upper arm A30.9 *[M63.82-]*
anesthetic A30.9
BB A30.3
BL A30.4
borderline (infiltrated) (neuritic) A30.3
lepromatous A30.4
tuberculoid A30.2

Leprosy *(Continued)*
BT A30.2
dimorphous (infiltrated) (neuritic) A30.3
I A30.0
indeterminate (macular) (neuritic) A30.0
lepromatous (diffuse) (infiltrated) (macular) (neuritic) (nodular) A30.5
LL A30.5
macular (early) (neuritic) (simple) A30.9
maculoanesthetic A30.9
mixed A30.3
neural A30.9
nodular A30.5
primary neuritic A30.3
specified type NEC A30.8
TT A30.1
tuberculoid (major) (minor) A30.1
Leptocytosis, hereditary D56.9
Leptomeningitis (chronic) (circumscribed) (hemorrhagic) (nonsuppurative) —*see* Meningitis
Leptomeningopathy G96.19
Leptospiral —*see* condition
Leptospirochetal —*see* condition
Leptospirosis A27.9
canicola A27.89
due to Leptospira interrogans serovar icterohaemorrhagiae A27.0
icterohemorrhagica A27.0
pomona A27.89
Weil's disease A27.0
Leptus dermatitis B88.0
Leriche's syndrome (aortic bifurcation occlusion) I74.09
Leri's pleonosteosis Q78.8
Leri-Weill syndrome Q77.8
Lermoyez' syndrome —*see* Vertigo, peripheral NEC
Lesch-Nyhan syndrome E79.1
Leser-Trélat disease L82.1
inflamed L82.0
Lesion (s) (nontraumatic)
abducens nerve —*see* Strabismus, paralytic, sixth nerve
alveolar process K08.9
angiocentric immunoproliferative D47.Z9
anorectal K62.9
aortic (valve) I35.9
auditory nerve —*see* subcategory H93.3
basal ganglion G25.9
bile duct —*see* Disease, bile duct
biomechanical M99.9
specified type NEC M99.89
abdomen M99.89
acromioclavicular M99.87
cervical region M99.81
cervicothoracic M99.81
costochondral M99.88
costovertebral M99.88
head region M99.80
hip M99.85
lower extremity M99.86
lumbar region M99.83
lumbosacral M99.83
occipitocervical M99.80
pelvic region M99.85
pubic M99.85
rib cage M99.88
sacral region M99.84
sacrococcygeal M99.84
sacroiliac M99.84
specified NEC M99.89
sternochondral M99.88
sternoclavicular M99.87
thoracic region M99.82
thoracolumbar M99.82
upper extremity M99.87
bladder N32.9
bone —*see* Disorder, bone
brachial plexus G54.0

Lesion *(Continued)*
brain G93.9
congenital Q04.9
vascular I67.9
degenerative I67.9
hypertensive I67.4
buccal cavity K13.79
calcified —*see* Calcification
canthus —*see* Disorder, eyelid
carate —*see* Pinta, lesions
cardia K31.9 ◀
cardiac —*see also* Disease, heart I51.9
congenital Q24.9
valvular —*see* Endocarditis
cauda equina G83.4
cecum K63.9
cerebral —*see* Lesion, brain
cerebrovascular I67.9
degenerative I67.9
hypertensive I67.4
cervical (nerve) root NEC G54.2
chiasmal —*see* Disorder, optic, chiasm
chorda tympani G51.8
coin, lung R91.1
colon K63.9
combined periodontic - endodontic K05.5 ◀
congenital —*see* Anomaly, by site
conjunctiva H11.9
conus medullaris —*see* Injury, conus medullaris
coronary artery —*see* Ischemia, heart
cranial nerve G52.9
eighth —*see* Disorder, ear
eleventh G52.9
fifth G50.9
first G52.0
fourth —*see* Strabismus, paralytic, fourth nerve
seventh G51.9
sixth —*see* Strabismus, paralytic, sixth nerve
tenth G52.2
twelfth G52.3
cystic —*see* Cyst
degenerative —*see* Degeneration
duodenum K31.9
edentulous (alveolar) ridge, associated with trauma, due to traumatic occlusion K06.2
en coup de sabre L94.1
eyelid —*see* Disorder, eyelid
gasserian ganglion G50.8
gastric K31.9
gastroduodenal K31.9
gastrointestinal K63.9
gingiva, associated with trauma K06.2
glomerular
focal and segmental —*see also* N00-N07 with fourth character .1 N05.1
minimal change —*see also* N00-N07 with fourth character .0 N05.0
heart (organic) —*see* Disease, heart
hyperchromic, due to pinta (carate) A67.1
hyperkeratotic —*see* Hyperkeratosis
hypothalamic E23.7
ileocecal K63.9
ileum K63.9
iliohypogastric nerve G57.8-
inflammatory —*see* Inflammation
intestine K63.9
intracerebral —*see* Lesion, brain
intrachiasmal (optic) —*see* Disorder, optic, chiasm
intracranial, space-occupying R90.0
joint —*see* Disorder, joint
sacroiliac (old) M53.3
keratotic —*see* Keratosis
kidney —*see* Disease, renal
laryngeal nerve (recurrent) G52.2
lip K13.0

Lesion *(Continued)*
liver K76.9
lumbosacral
plexus G54.1
root (nerve) NEC G54.4
lung (coin) R91.1
maxillary sinus J32.0
mitral I05.9
Morel-Lavallée —*see* Hematoma, by site
motor cortex NEC G93.89
mouth K13.79
nerve G58.9
femoral G57.2-
median G56.1-
carpal tunnel syndrome —*see* Syndrome, carpal tunnel
plantar G57.6-
popliteal (lateral) G57.3-
medial G57.4-
radial G56.3-
sciatic G57.0-
spinal —*see* Injury, nerve, spinal
ulnar G56.2-
nervous system, congenital Q07.9
nonallopathic —*see* Lesion, biomechanical
nose (internal) J34.89
obstructive —*see* Obstruction
obturator nerve G57.8-
oral mucosa K13.70
organ or site NEC —*see* Disease, by site
osteolytic —*see* Osteolysis
peptic K27.9
periodontal, due to traumatic occlusion K05.5
pharynx J39.2
pigment, pigmented (skin) L81.9
pinta —*see* Pinta, lesions
polypoid —*see* Polyp
prechiasmal (optic) —*see* Disorder, optic, chiasm
primary —*see also* Syphilis, primary A51.0
carate A67.0
pinta A67.0
yaws A66.0
pulmonary J98.4
valve I37.9
pylorus K31.9
rectosigmoid K63.9
retina, retinal H35.9
sacroiliac (joint) (old) M53.3
salivary gland K11.9
benign lymphoepithelial K11.8
saphenous nerve G57.8-
sciatic nerve G57.0-
secondary —*see* Syphilis, secondary
shoulder (region) M75.9-
specified NEC M75.8-
sigmoid K63.9
sinus (accessory) (nasal) J34.89
skin L98.9
suppurative L08.0
SLAP S43.43-
spinal cord G95.9
congenital Q06.9
spleen D73.89
stomach K31.9
superior glenoid labrum S43.43-
syphilitic —*see* Syphilis
tertiary —*see* Syphilis, tertiary
thoracic root (nerve) NEC G54.3
tonsillar fossa J35.9
tooth, teeth K08.9
white spot
chewing surface K02.51
pit and fissure surface K02.51
smooth surface K02.61
traumatic —*see* specific type of injury by site
tricuspid (valve) I07.9
nonrheumatic I36.9
trigeminal nerve G50.9

◀ New ◀ Revised ~~deleted~~ Deleted

Lesion *(Continued)*
ulcerated or ulcerative —*see* Ulcer, skin
uterus N85.9
vagus nerve G52.2
valvular —*see* Endocarditis
vascular I99.9
affecting central nervous system I67.9
following trauma NEC T14.8
umbilical cord, complicating delivery O69.5
warty —*see* Verruca
white spot (tooth)
chewing surface K02.51
pit and fissure surface K02.51
smooth surface K02.61
Lethargic —*see* condition
Lethargy R53.83
Letterer-Siwe's disease C96.0
Leukemia, leukemic C95.9-
acute basophilic C94.8-
acute bilineal C95.0-
acute erythroid C94.0-
acute lymphoblastic C91.0-
acute megakaryoblastic C94.2-
acute megakaryocytic C94.2-
acute mixed lineage C95.0-
acute monoblastic (monoblastic/monocytic) C93.0-
acute monocytic (monoblastic/monocytic) C93.0-
acute myeloblastic (minimal differentiation) (with maturation) C92.0-
acute myeloid
with
11q23-abnormality C92.6-
dysplasia of remaining hematopoesis and/or myelodysplastic disease in its history C92.A-
multilineage dysplasia C92.A-
variation of MLL-gene C92.6-
M6 (a)(b) C94.0-
M7 C94.2-
acute myelomonocytic C92.5-
acute promyelocytic C92.4-
adult T-cell (HTLV-1-associated) (acute variant) (chronic variant) (lymphomatoid variant) (smouldering variant) C91.5-
aggressive NK-cell C94.8-
AML (1/ETO) (M0) (M1) (M2) (without a FAB classification) C92.0-
AML M3 C92.4-
AML M4 (Eo with inv(16) or t(16;16)) C92.5-
AML M5 C93.0-
AML M5a C93.0-
AML M5b C93.0-
AML Me with t (15;17) and variants C92.4-
atypical chronic myeloid, BCR/ABL-negative C92.2-
biphenotypic acute C95.0-
blast cell C95.0-
Burkitt-type, mature B-cell C91.A-
chronic lymphocytic, of B-cell type C91.1-
chronic monocytic C93.1-
chronic myelogenous (Philadelphia chromosome (Ph1) positive) (t(9;22)) (q34;q11) (with crisis of blast cells) C92.1-
chronic myeloid, BCR/ABL-positive C92.1-
atypical, BCR/ABL-negative C92.2-
chronic myelomonocytic C93.1-
chronic neutrophilic D47.1
CMML (-1) (-2) (with eosinophilia) C93.1-
granulocytic —*see also* Category C92 C92.9-
hairy-cell C91.4-
juvenile myelomonocytic C93.3-
lymphoid C91.9-
specified NEC C91.Z-
mast cell C94.3-
mature B-cell, Burkitt-type C91.A-
Leukemia, leukemic *(Continued)*
monocytic (subacute) C93.9-
specified NEC C93.Z-
myelogenous —*see also* Category C92 C92.9-
myeloid C92.9-
specified NEC C92.Z-
plasma cell C90.1-
plasmacytic C90.1-
prolymphocytic
of B-cell type C91.3-
of T-cell type C91.6-
specified NEC C94.8-
stem cell, of unclear lineage C95.0-
subacute lymphocytic C91.9-
T-cell large granular lymphocytic C91.Z-
unspecified cell type C95.9-
acute C95.0-
chronic C95.1-
Leukemoid reaction —*see also* Reaction, leukemoid D72.823-
Leukoaraiosis (hypertensive) I67.81
Leukoariosis —*see* Leukoaraiosis
Leukocoria —*see* Disorder, globe, degenerated condition, leucocoria
Leukocytopenia D72.819
Leukocytosis D72.829
eosinophilic D72.1
Leukoderma, leukodermia NEC L81.5
syphilitic A51.39
late A52.79
Leukodystrophy E75.29
Leukoedema, oral epithelium K13.29
Leukoencephalitis G04.81
acute (subacute) hemorrhagic G36.1
postimmunization or postvaccinal G04.02
postinfectious G04.01
subacute sclerosing A81.1
van Bogaert's (sclerosing) A81.1
Leukoencephalopathy —*see also* Encephalopathy G93.49
Binswanger's I67.3
heroin vapor G92
metachromatic E75.25
multifocal (progressive) A81.2
postimmunization and postvaccinal G04.02
progressive multifocal A81.2
reversible, posterior G93.6
van Bogaert's (sclerosing) A81.1
vascular, progressive I67.3
Leukoerythroblastosis D75.9
Leukokeratosis —*see also* Leukoplakia
mouth K13.21
nicotina palati K13.24
oral mucosa K13.21
tongue K13.21
vocal cord J38.3
Leukokraurosis vulva (e) N90.4
Leukoma (cornea) —*see also* Opacity, cornea
adherent H17.0-
interfering with central vision —*see* Opacity, cornea, central
Leukomalacia, cerebral, newborn P91.2
periventricular P91.2
Leukomelanopathy, hereditary D72.0
Leukonychia (punctata) (striata) L60.8
congenital Q84.4
Leukopathia unguium L60.8
congenital Q84.4
Leukopenia D72.819
basophilic D72.818
chemotherapy (cancer) induced D70.1
congenital D70.0
cyclic D70.0
drug induced NEC D70.2
due to cytoreductive cancer chemotherapy D70.1
eosinophilic D72.818
familial D70.0
infantile genetic D70.0
malignant D70.9
periodic D70.0
transitory neonatal P61.5
Leukopenic —*see* condition
Leukoplakia
anus K62.89
bladder (postinfectional) N32.89
buccal K13.21
cervix (uteri) N88.0
esophagus K22.8
gingiva K13.21
hairy (oral mucosa) (tongue) K13.3
kidney (pelvis) N28.89
larynx J38.7
lip K13.21
mouth K13.21
oral epithelium, including tongue (mucosa) K13.21
palate K13.21
pelvis (kidney) N28.89
penis (infectional) N48.0
rectum K62.89
syphilitic (late) A52.79
tongue K13.21
ureter (postinfectional) N28.89
urethra (postinfectional) N36.8
uterus N85.8
vagina N89.4
vocal cord J38.3
vulva N90.4
Leukorrhea N89.8
due to Trichomonas (vaginalis) A59.00
trichomonal A59.00
Leukosarcoma C85.9
Levocardia (isolated) Q24.1
with situs inversus Q89.3
Levotransposition Q20.5
Lev's disease or syndrome (acquired complete heart block) I44.2
Levulosuria —*see* Fructosuria
Levurid L30.2
Lewy body (ies) (dementia) (disease) G31.83
Leyden-Moebius dystrophy G71.0
Leydig cell
carcinoma
specified site —*see* Neoplasm, malignant, by site
unspecified site
female C56.9-
male C62.9-
tumor
benign
specified site —*see* Neoplasm, benign, by site
unspecified site
female D27.-
male D29.2-
malignant
specified site —*see* Neoplasm, malignant, by site
unspecified site
female C56.-
male C62.9-
specified site —*see* Neoplasm, uncertain behavior, by site
unspecified site
female D39.1-
male D40.1-
Leydig-Sertoli cell tumor
specified site —*see* Neoplasm, benign, by site
unspecified site
female D27.-
male D29.2-
LGSIL (Low grade squamous intraepithelial lesion on cytologic smear of)
anus R85.612
cervix R87.612
vagina R87.622
Liar, pathologic F60.2
Libido
decreased R68.82

Libman-Sacks disease M32.11
Lice (infestation) B85.2
  body (Pediculus corporis) B85.1
  crab B85.3
  head (Pediculus capitis) B85.0
  mixed (classifiable to more than one of the titles B85.0-B85.3) B85.4
  pubic (Phthirus pubis) B85.3
Lichen L28.0
  albus L90.0
    penis N48.0
    vulva N90.4
  amyloidosis E85.4 *[L99]*
  atrophicus L90.0
    penis N48.0
    vulva N90.4
  congenital Q82.8
  myxedematosus L98.5
  nitidus L44.1
  pilaris Q82.8
    acquired L85.8
  planopilaris L66.1
  planus (chronicus) L43.9
    annularis L43.8
    bullous L43.1
    follicular L66.1
    hypertrophic L43.0
    moniliformis L44.3
    of Wilson L43.9
    specified NEC L43.8
    subacute (active) L43.3
    tropicus L43.3
  ruber
    acuminatus L44.0
    moniliformis L44.3
    planus L43.9
  sclerosus (et atrophicus) L90.0
    penis N48.0
    vulva N90.4
  scrofulosus (primary) (tuberculous) A18.4
  simplex (chronicus) (circumscriptus) L28.0
  striatus L44.2
  urticatus L28.2
Lichenification L28.0
Lichenoides tuberculosis (primary) A18.4
Lichtheim's disease or syndrome —*see* Degeneration, combined
Lien migrans D73.89
Ligament —*see* condition
Light
  for gestational age —*see* Light for dates
  headedness R42
Light-for-dates (infant) P05.00
  with weight of
    499 grams or less P05.01
    500-749 grams P05.02
    750-999 grams P05.03
    1000-1249 grams P05.04
    1250-1499 grams P05.05
    1500-1749 grams P05.06
    1750-1999 grams P05.07
    2000-2499 grams P05.08
    2500 grams and over P05.09 ◀
  affecting management of pregnancy O36.59-
  and small-for-dates —*see* Small for dates
  specified NEC P05.09 ◀
Lightning (effects) (stroke) (struck by) T75.00
  burn —*see* Burn
  foot E53.8
  shock T75.01
  specified effect NEC T75.09
Lightwood-Albright syndrome N25.89
Lightwood's disease or syndrome (renal tubular acidosis) N25.89
Lignac (-de Toni) (-Fanconi) (-Debré) disease or syndrome E72.09
  with cystinosis E72.04
Ligneous thyroiditis E06.5
Likoff's syndrome I20.8
Limb —*see* condition
Limbic epilepsy personality syndrome F07.0
Limitation, limited
  activities due to disability Z73.6
  cardiac reserve —*see* Disease, heart
  eye muscle duction, traumatic —*see* Strabismus, mechanical
  mandibular range of motion M26.52
Lindau (-von Hippel) disease Q85.8
Line (s)
  Beau's L60.4
  Harris' —*see* Arrest, epiphyseal
  Hudson's (cornea) —*see* Pigmentation, cornea, anterior
  Stähli's (cornea) —*see* Pigmentation, cornea, anterior
Linea corneae senilis —*see* Change, cornea, senile
Lingua
  geographica K14.1
  nigra (villosa) K14.3
  plicata K14.5
  tylosis K13.29
Lingual —*see* condition
Linguatulosis B88.8
Linitis (gastric) plastica C16.9
Lip —*see* condition
Lipedema —*see* Edema
Lipemia —*see also* Hyperlipidemia
  retina, retinalis E78.3
Lipidosis E75.6
  cerebral (infantile) (juvenile) (late) E75.4
  cerebroretinal E75.4
  cerebroside E75.22
  cholesterol (cerebral) E75.5
  glycolipid E75.21
  hepatosplenomegalic E78.3
  sphingomyelin —*see* Niemann-Pick disease or syndrome
  sulfatide E75.29
Lipoadenoma —*see* Neoplasm, benign, by site
Lipoblastoma —*see* Lipoma
Lipoblastomatosis —*see* Lipoma
Lipochondrodystrophy E76.01
Lipochrome histiocytosis (familial) D71
Lipodermatosclerosis —*see* Varix, leg, with, inflammation
  ulcerated —*see* Varix, leg, with, ulcer, with inflammation by site
Lipodystrophia progressiva E88.1
Lipodystrophy (progressive) E88.1
  insulin E88.1
  intestinal K90.81
  mesenteric K65.4
Lipofibroma —*see* Lipoma
Lipofuscinosis, neuronal (with ceroidosis) E75.4
Lipogranuloma, sclerosing L92.8
Lipogranulomatosis E78.89
Lipoid —*see also* condition
  histiocytosis D76.3
    essential E75.29
  nephrosis N04.9
  proteinosis of Urbach E78.89
Lipoidemia —*see* Hyperlipidemia
Lipoidosis —*see* Lipidosis
Lipoma D17.9
  fetal D17.9
    fat cell D17.9
  infiltrating D17.9
  intramuscular D17.9
  pleomorphic D17.9
  site classification
    arms (skin) (subcutaneous) D17.2-
    connective tissue D17.30
      intra-abdominal D17.5
      intrathoracic D17.4
      peritoneum D17.79
      retroperitoneum D17.79
      specified site NEC D17.39
      spermatic cord D17.6
    face (skin) (subcutaneous) D17.0
    genitourinary organ NEC D17.72
Lipoma *(Continued)*
  site classification *(Continued)*
    head (skin) (subcutaneous) D17.0
    intra-abdominal D17.5
    intrathoracic D17.4
    kidney D17.71
    legs (skin) (subcutaneous) D17.2-
    neck (skin) (subcutaneous) D17.0
    peritoneum D17.79
    retroperitoneum D17.79
    skin D17.30
      specified site NEC D17.39
    specified site NEC D17.79
    spermatic cord D17.6
    subcutaneous D17.30
      specified site NEC D17.39
    trunk (skin) (subcutaneous) D17.1
    unspecified D17.9
  spindle cell D17.9
Lipomatosis E88.2
  dolorosa (Dercum) E88.2
  fetal —*see* Lipoma
  Launois-Bensaude E88.89
Lipomyoma —*see* Lipoma
Lipomyxoma —*see* Lipoma
Lipomyxosarcoma —*see* Neoplasm, connective tissue, malignant
Lipoprotein metabolism disorder E78.9
Lipoproteinemia E78.5
  broad-beta E78.2
  floating-beta E78.2
  hyper-pre-beta E78.1
Liposarcoma —*see also* Neoplasm, connective tissue, malignant
  dedifferentiated —*see* Neoplasm, connective tissue, malignant
  differentiated type —*see* Neoplasm, connective tissue, malignant
  embryonal —*see* Neoplasm, connective tissue, malignant
  mixed type —*see* Neoplasm, connective tissue, malignant
  myxoid —*see* Neoplasm, connective tissue, malignant
  pleomorphic —*see* Neoplasm, connective tissue, malignant
  round cell —*see* Neoplasm, connective tissue, malignant
  well differentiated type —*see* Neoplasm, connective tissue, malignant
Liposynovitis prepatellaris E88.89
Lipping, cervix N86
Lipschütz disease or ulcer N76.6
Lipuria R82.0
  schistosomiasis (bilharziasis) B65.0
Lisping F80.0
Lissauer's paralysis A52.17
Lissencephalia, lissencephaly Q04.3
Listeriosis, listerellosis A32.9
  congenital (disseminated) P37.2
  cutaneous A32.0
  neonatal, newborn (disseminated) P37.2
  oculoglandular A32.81
  specified NEC A32.89
Lithemia E79.0
Lithiasis —*see* Calculus
Lithosis J62.8
Lithuria R82.99
Litigation, anxiety concerning Z65.3
Little leaguer's elbow —*see* Epicondylitis, medial
Little's disease G80.9
Littre's
  gland —*see* condition
  hernia —*see* Hernia, abdomen
Littritis —*see* Urethritis
Livedo (annularis) (racemosa) (reticularis) R23.1
Liver —*see* condition
Living alone (problems with) Z60.2
  with handicapped person Z74.2

◀ New ◀ Revised ~~deleted~~ Deleted

Lloyd's syndrome —*see* Adenomatosis, endocrine
Loa loa, loaiasis, loasis B74.3
Lobar —*see* condition
Lobomycosis B48.0
Lobo's disease B48.0
Lobotomy syndrome F07.0
Lobstein (-Ekman) **disease or syndrome** Q78.0
Lobster-claw hand Q71.6-
Lobulation (congenital) —*see also* Anomaly, by site
kidney, Q63.1
liver, abnormal Q44.7
spleen Q89.09
Lobule, lobular —*see* condition
Local, localized —*see* condition
Locked twins causing obstructed labor O66.1
Locked-in state G83.5
Locking
joint —*see* Derangement, joint, specified type NEC
knee —*see* Derangement, knee
Lockjaw —*see* Tetanus
Löffler's
endocarditis I42.3
eosinophilia J82
pneumonia J82
syndrome (eosinophilic pneumonitis) J82
Loiasis (with conjunctival infestation) (eyelid) B74.3
Lone Star fever A77.0
Long
labor O63.9
first stage O63.0
second stage O63.1
QT syndrome I45.81
Long-term (current) (prophylactic) drug therapy (use of)
agents affecting estrogen receptors and estrogen levels NEC Z79.818
anastrozole (Arimidex) Z79.811
antibiotics Z79.2
short-term use - omit code
anticoagulants Z79.01
anti-inflammatory, non-steroidal (NSAID) Z79.1
antiplatelet Z79.02
antithrombotics Z79.02
aromatase inhibitors Z79.811
aspirin Z79.82
birth control pill or patch Z79.3
bisphosphonates Z79.83
contraceptive, oral Z79.3
drug, specified NEC Z79.899
estrogen receptor downregulators Z79.818
Evista Z79.810
exemestane (Aromasin) Z79.811
Fareston Z79.810
fulvestrant (Faslodex) Z79.818
gonadotropin-releasing hormone (GnRH) agonist Z79.818
goserelin acetate (Zoladex) Z79.818
hormone replacement (postmenopausal) Z79.890
insulin Z79.4
letrozole (Femara) Z79.811
leuprolide acetate (leuprorelin) (Lupron) Z79.818
megestrol acetate (Megace) Z79.818
methadone for pain management Z79.891
Nolvadex Z79.810
non-steroidal anti-inflammatories (NSAID) Z79.1
opiate analgesic Z79.891
~~oral contraceptive Z79.3~~
oral ◀
antidiabetic Z79.84 ◀
contraceptive Z79.3 ◀
hypoglycemic Z79.84 ◀
raloxifene (Evista) Z79.810

Long-term *(Continued)*
selective estrogen receptor modulators (SERMs) Z79.810
steroids
inhaled Z79.51
systemic Z79.52
tamoxifen (Nolvadex) Z79.810
toremifene (Fareston) Z79.810
Longitudinal stripes or grooves, nails L60.8
congenital Q84.6
Loop
intestine —*see* Volvulus
vascular on papilla (optic) Q14.2
Loose —*see also* condition
body
joint M24.00
ankle M24.07-
elbow M24.02-
hand M24.04-
hip M24.05-
knee M23.4-
shoulder (region) M24.01-
specified site NEC M24.08
toe M24.07-
vertebra M24.08
wrist M24.03-
knee M23.4-
sheath, tendon —*see* Disorder, tendon, specified type NEC
cartilage —*see* Loose, body, joint
skin and subcutaneous tissue (following bariatric surgery weight loss) (following dietary weight loss) L98.7 ◀
tooth, teeth K08.89 ◀
Loosening
aseptic
joint prosthesis —*see* Complications, joint prosthesis, mechanical, loosening, by site
epiphysis —*see* Osteochondropathy
mechanical
joint prosthesis —*see* Complications, joint prosthesis, mechanical, loosening, by site
Looser-Milkman (-Debray) **syndrome** M83.8
Lop ear (deformity) Q17.3
Lorain (-Levi) **short stature syndrome** E23.0
Lordosis M40.50
acquired —*see* Lordosis, specified type NEC
congenital Q76.429
lumbar region Q76.426
lumbosacral region Q76.427
sacral region Q76.428
sacrococcygeal region Q76.428
thoracolumbar region Q76.425
lumbar region M40.56
lumbosacral region M40.57
postsurgical M96.4
postural —*see* Lordosis, specified type NEC
rachitic (late effect) (sequelae) E64.3
sequelae of rickets E64.3
specified type NEC M40.40
lumbar region M40.46
lumbosacral region M40.47
thoracolumbar region M40.45
thoracolumbar region M40.55
tuberculous A18.01
Loss (of)
appetite (*see* Anorexia) R63.0
hysterical F50.89 ◀
nonorganic origin F50.89 ◀
psychogenic F50.89 ◀
blood —*see* Hemorrhage
bone —*see* Loss, substance of, bone ◀
consciousness, transient R55
traumatic —*see* Injury, intracranial
control, sphincter, rectum R15.9
nonorganic origin F98.1
elasticity, skin R23.4

Loss *(Continued)*
family (member) in childhood Z62.898
fluid (acute) E86.9
~~with~~
~~hypernatremia E87.0~~
~~hyponatremia E87.1~~
function of labyrinth —*see* subcategory H83.2
hair, nonscarring —*see* Alopecia
hearing —*see also* Deafness
central NOS H90.5
conductive H90.2 ◀
bilateral H90.0 ◀
unilateral ◀
with ◀
restricted hearing on the contralateral side H90.A1- ◀
unrestricted hearing on the contralateral side H90.1- ◀
mixed conductive and sensorineural hearing loss H90.8 ◀
bilateral H90.6 ◀
unilateral ◀
with ◀
restricted hearing on the contralateral side H90.A3- ◀
unrestricted hearing on the contralateral side H90.7- ◀
neural NOS H90.5
perceptive NOS H90.5
sensorineural NOS H90.5
bilateral H90.3 ◀
unilateral ◀
with ◀
restricted hearing on the contralateral side H90.A2- ◀
unrestricted hearing on the contralateral side H90.4- ◀
sensory NOS H90.5
height R29.890
limb or member, traumatic, current —*see* Amputation, traumatic
love relationship in childhood Z62.898
memory —*see also* Amnesia
mild, following organic brain damage F06.8
mind —*see* Psychosis
occlusal vertical dimension of fully erupted teeth M26.37
organ or part —*see* Absence, by site, acquired
ossicles, ear (partial) H74.32-
parent in childhood Z63.4
pregnancy, recurrent N96
without current pregnancy N96
care in current pregnancy O26.2-
recurrent pregnancy —*see* Loss, pregnancy, recurrent
self-esteem, in childhood Z62.898
sense of
smell —*see* Disturbance, sensation, smell
taste —*see* Disturbance, sensation, taste
touch R20.8
sensory R44.9
dissociative F44.6
sexual desire F52.0
sight (acquired) (complete) (congenital) —*see* Blindness
substance of
bone —*see* Disorder, bone, density and structure, specified NEC
horizontal alveolar K06.3 ◀
cartilage —*see* Disorder, cartilage, specified type NEC
auricle (ear) —*see* Disorder, pinna, specified type NEC
vitreous (humor) H15.89
tooth, teeth —*see* Absence, teeth, acquired
vision, visual H54.7
both eyes H54.3
one eye H54.60
left (normal vision on right) H54.62
right (normal vision on left) H54.61

Loss *(Continued)*
vision, visual *(Continued)*
specified as blindness —*see* Blindness
subjective
sudden H53.13-
transient H53.12-
vitreous —*see* Prolapse, vitreous
voice —*see* Aphonia
weight (abnormal) (cause unknown) R63.4
Louis-Bar syndrome (ataxia-telangiectasia) G11.3
Louping ill (encephalitis) A84.8
Louse, lousiness —*see* Lice
Low
achiever, school Z55.3
back syndrome M54.5
basal metabolic rate R94.8
birthweight (2499 grams or less) P07.10
with weight of
1000-1249 grams P07.14
1250-1499 grams P07.15
1500-1749 grams P07.16
1750-1999 grams P07.17
2000-2499 grams P07.18
extreme (999 grams or less) P07.00
with weight of
499 grams or less P07.01
500-749 grams P07.02
750-999 grams P07.03
for gestational age —*see* Light for dates
blood pressure —*see also* Hypotension
reading (incidental) (isolated) (nonspecific) R03.1
cardiac reserve —*see* Disease, heart
function —*see also* Hypofunction
kidney N28.9
hematocrit D64.9
hemoglobin D64.9
income Z59.6
level of literacy Z55.0
lying
kidney N28.89
organ or site, congenital —*see* Malposition, congenital
output syndrome (cardiac) —*see* Failure, heart
platelets (blood) —*see* Thrombocytopenia
reserve, kidney N28.89
salt syndrome E87.1
self esteem R45.81
set ears Q17.4
vision H54.2
one eye (other eye normal) H54.50
left (normal vision on right) H54.52
other eye blind —*see* Blindness
right (normal vision on left) H54.51
Low-density-lipoprotein-type (LDL) **hyperlipoproteinemia** E78.00 ⟸
Lowe's syndrome E72.03
Lown-Ganong-Levine syndrome I45.6
LSD reaction (acute) (without dependence) F16.90
with dependence F16.20
L-shaped kidney Q63.8
Ludwig's angina or disease K12.2
Lues (venerea), **luetic** —*see* Syphilis
Luetscher's syndrome (dehydration) E86.0
Lumbago, lumbalgia M54.5
with sciatica M54.4-
due to intervertebral disc disorder M51.17
due to displacement, intervertebral disc M51.27
with sciatica M51.17
Lumbar —*see* condition
Lumbarization, vertebra, congenital Q76.49
Lumbermen's itch B88.0
Lump —*see* Mass
Lunacy —*see* Psychosis
Lung —*see* condition
Lupoid (miliary) **of Boeck** D86.3
Lupus
anticoagulant D68.62
with
hemorrhagic disorder D68.312
hypercoagulable state D68.62
finding without diagnosis R76.0
discoid (local) L93.0
erythematosus (discoid) (local) L93.0
disseminated —*see* Lupus, erythematosus, systemic
eyelid H01.129
left H01.126
lower H01.125
upper H01.124
right H01.123
lower H01.122
upper H01.121
profundus L93.2
specified NEC L93.2
subacute cutaneous L93.1
systemic M32.9
with organ or system involvement M32.10
endocarditis M32.11
lung M32.13
pericarditis M32.12
renal (glomerular) M32.14
tubulo-interstitial M32.15
specified organ or system NEC M32.19
drug-induced M32.0
inhibitor (presence of) D68.62
with
hemorrhagic disorder D68.312
hypercoagulable state D68.62
finding without diagnosis R76.0
specified NEC M32.8
exedens A18.4
hydralazine M32.0
correct substance properly administered —*see* Table of Drugs and Chemicals, by drug, adverse effect
overdose or wrong substance given or taken —*see* Table of Drugs and Chemicals, by drug, poisoning
nephritis (chronic) M32.14
nontuberculous, not disseminated L93.0
panniculitis L93.2
pernio (Besnier) D86.3
systemic —*see* Lupus, erythematosus, systemic
tuberculous A18.4
eyelid A18.4
vulgaris A18.4
eyelid A18.4
Luteinoma D27.-
Lutembacher's disease or syndrome (atrial septal defect with mitral stenosis) Q21.1
Luteoma D27.-
Lutz (-Splendore-de Almeida) **disease** —*see* Paracoccidioidomycosis
Luxation —*see also* Dislocation
eyeball (nontraumatic) —*see* Luxation, globe
birth injury P15.3
globe, nontraumatic H44.82-
lacrimal gland —*see* Dislocation, lacrimal gland
lens (old) (partial) (spontaneous)
congenital Q12.1
syphilitic A50.39
Lycanthropy F22
Lyell's syndrome L51.2
due to drug L51.2
correct substance properly administered —*see* Table of Drugs and Chemicals, by drug, adverse effect
overdose or wrong substance given or taken —*see* Table of Drugs and Chemicals, by drug, poisoning
Lyme disease A69.20
Lymph
gland or node —*see* condition
scrotum —*see* Infestation, filarial
Lymphadenitis I88.9
with ectopic or molar pregnancy O08.0
acute L04.9
axilla L04.2
face L04.0
head L04.0
hip L04.3
limb
lower L04.3
upper L04.2
neck L04.0
shoulder L04.2
specified site NEC L04.8
trunk L04.1
anthracosis (occupational) J60
any site, except mesenteric I88.9
chronic I88.1
subacute I88.1
breast
gestational —*see* Mastitis, obstetric
puerperal, postpartum (nonpurulent) O91.22
chancroidal (congenital) A57
chronic I88.1
mesenteric I88.0
due to
Brugia (malayi) B74.1
timori B74.2
chlamydial lymphogranuloma A55
diphtheria (toxin) A36.89
lymphogranuloma venereum A55
Wuchereria bancrofti B74.0
following ectopic or molar pregnancy O08.0
gonorrheal A54.89
infective —*see* Lymphadenitis, acute
mesenteric (acute) (chronic) (nonspecific) (subacute) I88.0
due to Salmonella typhi A01.09
tuberculous A18.39
mycobacterial A31.8
purulent —*see* Lymphadenitis, acute
pyogenic —*see* Lymphadenitis, acute
regional, nonbacterial I88.8
septic —*see* Lymphadenitis, acute
subacute, unspecified site I88.1
suppurative —*see* Lymphadenitis, acute
syphilitic (early) (secondary) A51.49
late A52.79
tuberculous —*see* Tuberculosis, lymph gland
venereal (chlamydial) A55
Lymphadenoid goiter E06.3
Lymphadenopathy (generalized) R59.1
angioimmunoblastic, with dysproteinemia (AILD) C86.5
due to toxoplasmosis (acquired) B58.89
congenital (acute) (subacute) (chronic) P37.1
localized R59.0
syphilitic (early) (secondary) A51.49
Lymphadenosis R59.1
Lymphangiectasis I89.0
conjunctiva H11.89
postinfectional I89.0
scrotum I89.0
Lymphangiectatic elephantiasis, nonfilarial I89.0
Lymphangioendothelioma D18.1
malignant —*see* Neoplasm, connective tissue, malignant
Lymphangioleiomyomatosis J84.81
Lymphangioma D18.1
capillary D18.1
cavernous D18.1
cystic D18.1
malignant —*see* Neoplasm, connective tissue, malignant
Lymphangiomyoma D18.1
Lymphangiomyomatosis J84.81

◀ New ⟸ Revised ~~deleted~~ Deleted

Lymphangiosarcoma —*see* Neoplasm, connective tissue, malignant
Lymphangitis I89.1
with
abscess - code by site under Abscess
cellulitis - code by site under Cellulitis
ectopic or molar pregnancy O08.0
acute L03.91
abdominal wall L03.321
ankle —*see* Lymphangitis, acute, lower limb
arm —*see* Lymphangitis, acute, upper limb
auricle (ear) —*see* Lymphangitis, acute, ear
axilla L03.12-
back (any part) L03.322
buttock L03.327
cervical (meaning neck) L03.222
cheek (external) L03.212
chest wall L03.323
digit
finger —*see* Lymphangitis, acute, finger
toe —*see* Lymphangitis, acute, toe
ear (external) H60.1-
external auditory canal —*see* Lymphangitis, acute, ear
eyelid —*see* Abscess, eyelid
face NEC L03.212
finger (intrathecal) (periosteal) (subcutaneous) (subcuticular) L03.02-
foot —*see* Lymphangitis, acute, lower limb
gluteal (region) L03.327
groin L03.324
hand —*see* Lymphangitis, acute, upper limb
head NEC L03.891
face (any part, except ear, eye and nose) L03.212
heel —*see* Lymphangitis, acute, lower limb
hip —*see* Lymphangitis, acute, lower limb
jaw (region) L03.212
knee —*see* Lymphangitis, acute, lower limb
leg —*see* Lymphangitis, acute, lower limb
lower limb L03.12-
toe —*see* Lymphangitis, acute, toe
navel L03.326
neck (region) L03.222
orbit, orbital —*see* Cellulitis, orbit
pectoral (region) L03.323
perineal, perineum L03.325
scalp (any part) L03.891
shoulder —*see* Lymphangitis, acute, upper limb
specified site NEC L03.898
thigh —*see* Lymphangitis, acute, lower limb
thumb (intrathecal) (periosteal) (subcutaneous) (subcuticular) —*see* Lymphangitis, acute, finger
toe (intrathecal) (periosteal) (subcutaneous) (subcuticular) L03.04-
trunk L03.329
abdominal wall L03.321
back (any part) L03.322
buttock L03.327
chest wall L03.323
groin L03.324
perineal, perineum L03.325
umbilicus L03.326
umbilicus L03.326
upper limb L03.12-
axilla —*see* Lymphangitis, acute, axilla
finger —*see* Lymphangitis, acute, finger
thumb —*see* Lymphangitis, acute, finger
wrist —*see* Lymphangitis, acute, upper limb
breast
gestational —*see* Mastitis, obstetric
chancroidal A57
chronic (any site) I89.1

Lymphangitis *(Continued)*
due to
Brugia (malayi) B74.1
timori B74.2
Wuchereria bancrofti B74.0
following ectopic or molar pregnancy O08.89
penis
acute N48.29
gonococcal (acute) (chronic) A54.09
puerperal, postpartum, childbirth O86.89
strumous, tuberculous A18.2
subacute (any site) I89.1
tuberculous —*see* Tuberculosis, lymph gland
Lymphatic (vessel) —*see* condition
Lymphatism E32.8
Lymphectasia I89.0
Lymphedema (acquired) —*see also* Elephantiasis
congenital Q82.0
hereditary (chronic) (idiopathic) Q82.0
postmastectomy I97.2
praecox I89.0
secondary I89.0
surgical NEC I97.89
postmastectomy (syndrome) I97.2
Lymphoblastic —*see* condition
Lymphoblastoma (diffuse) —*see* Lymphoma, lymphoblastic (diffuse)
giant follicular —*see* Lymphoma, lymphoblastic (diffuse)
macrofollicular —*see* Lymphoma, lymphoblastic (diffuse)
Lymphocele I89.8
Lymphocytic
chorioencephalitis (acute) (serous) A87.2
choriomeningitis (acute) (serous) A87.2
meningoencephalitis A87.2
Lymphocytoma, benign cutis L98.8
Lymphocytopenia D72.810
Lymphocytosis (symptomatic) D72.820
infectious (acute) B33.8
Lymphoepithelioma —*see* Neoplasm, malignant, by site
Lymphogranuloma (malignant) —*see also* Lymphoma, Hodgkin
chlamydial A55
inguinale A55
venereum (any site) (chlamydial) (with stricture of rectum) A55
Lymphogranulomatosis (malignant) —*see also* Lymphoma, Hodgkin
benign (Boeck's sarcoid) (Schaumann's) D86.1
Lymphohistiocytosis, hemophagocytic (familial) D76.1
Lymphoid —*see* condition
Lymphoma (of) (malignant) C85.90
adult T-cell (HTLV-1-associated) (acute variant) (chronic variant) (lymphomatoid variant) (smouldering variant) C91.5-
anaplastic large cell
ALK-negative C84.7-
ALK-positive C84.6-
CD30-positive C84.6-
primary cutaneous C86.6
angioimmunoblastic T-cell C86.5
BALT C88.4
B-cell C85.1-
B-precursor C83.5-
blastic NK-cell C86.4
bronchial-associated lymphoid tissue [BALT-lymphoma] C88.4
Burkitt (atypical) C83.7-
Burkitt-like C83.7-
centrocytic C83.1-
cutaneous follicle center C82.6-
cutaneous T-cell C84.A-
diffuse follicle center C82.5-
diffuse large cell C83.3-
anaplastic C83.3-
B-cell C83.3-

Lymphoma *(Continued)*
diffuse large cell *(Continued)*
CD30-positive C83.3-
centroblastic C83.3-
immunoblastic C83.3-
plasmablastic C83.3-
subtype not specified C83.3-
T-cell rich C83.3-
enteropathy-type (associated) (intestinal) T-cell C86.2
extranodal marginal zone B-cell lymphoma of mucosa-associated lymphoid tissue [MALT-lymphoma] C88.4
extranodal NK/T-cell, nasal type C86.0
follicular C82.9-
grade
I C82.0-
II C82.1-
III C82.2-
IIIa C82.3-
IIIb C82.4-
specified NEC C82.8-
hepatosplenic T-cell (alpha-beta) (gamma-delta) C86.1
histiocytic C85.9-
true C96.A
Hodgkin C81.9
~~classical C81.7-~~
~~lymphocyte-rich C81.4-~~
~~lymphocytic depletion C81.3-~~
~~mixed cellularity C81.2-~~
~~nodular sclerosis C81.1-~~
~~specified NEC C81.7-~~
lymphocyte-rich (classical) C81.4- ◀
lymphocyte depleted (classical) C81.3- ◀
mixed cellularity (classical) C81.2- ◀
nodular sclerosis (classical) C81.1- ◀
specified NEC (classical) C81.7- ◀
lymphocyte-rich classical C81.4-
lymphocyte depleted classical C81.3-
mixed cellularity classical C81.2-
nodular
lymphocyte predominant C81.0-
~~sclerosis classical C81.1-~~
sclerosis (classical) C81.1- ◀
intravascular large B-cell C83.8-
Lennert's C84.4-
lymphoblastic (diffuse) C83.5-
lymphoblastic B-cell C83.5-
lymphoblastic T-cell C83.5-
lymphoepithelioid C84.4-
lymphoplasmacytic C83.0-
with IgM-production C88.0
MALT C88.4
mantle cell C83.1-
mature T-cell NEC C84.4-
mature T/NK-cell C84.9-
specified NEC C84.Z-
mediastinal (thymic) large B-cell C85.2-
Mediterranean C88.3
mucosa-associated lymphoid tissue [MALT-lymphoma] C88.4
NK/T cell C84.9-
nodal marginal zone C83.0-
non-follicular (diffuse) C83.9-
specified NEC C83.8-
non-Hodgkin —*see also* Lymphoma, by type C85.9-
specified NEC C85.8-
non-leukemic variant of B-CLL C83.0-
peripheral T-cell, not classified C84.4-
primary cutaneous
anaplastic large cell C86.6
CD30-positive large T-cell C86.6
primary effusion B-cell C83.8-
SALT C88.4
skin-associated lymphoid tissue [SALT-lymphoma] C88.4

Lymphoma *(Continued)*
small cell B-cell C83.0-
splenic marginal zone C83.0-
subcutaneous panniculitis-like T-cell C86.3
T-precursor C83.5-
true histiocytic C96.A
Lymphomatosis —*see* Lymphoma
Lymphopathia venereum, veneris A55
Lymphopenia D72.810
Lymphoplasmacytic leukemia —*see* Leukemia, chronic lymphocytic, B-cell type
Lymphoproliferation, X-linked disease D82.3
Lymphoreticulosis, benign (of inoculation) A28.1
Lymphorrhea I89.8
Lymphosarcoma (diffuse) —*see also* Lymphoma C85.9-
Lymphostasis I89.8
Lypemania —*see* Melancholia
Lysine and hydroxylysine metabolism disorder E72.3
Lyssa —*see* Rabies

◀ New ⬅ Revised ~~deleted~~ Deleted

M

Macacus ear Q17.3
Maceration, wet feet, tropical (syndrome) T69.02-
MacLeod's syndrome J43.0
Macrocephalia, macrocephaly Q75.3
Macrocheilia, macrochilia (congenital)Q18.6
Macrocolon —*see also* Megacolon Q43.1
Macrocornea Q15.8
with glaucoma Q15.0
Macrocytic —*see* condition
Macrocytosis D75.89
Macrodactylia, macrodactylism (fingers) (thumbs) Q74.0
toes Q74.2
Macrodontia K00.2
Macrogenia M26.05
Macrogenitosomia (adrenal) (male) (praecox) E25.9
congenital E25.0
Macroglobulinemia (idiopathic) (primary) C88.0
monoclonal (essential) D47.2
Waldenström C88.0
Macroglossia (congenital) Q38.2
acquired K14.8
Macrognathia, macrognathism (congenital) (mandibular) (maxillary) M26.09
Macrogyria (congenital) Q04.8
Macrohydrocephalus —*see* Hydrocephalus
Macromastia —*see* Hypertrophy, breast
Macrophthalmos Q11.3
in congenital glaucoma Q15.0
Macropsia H53.15
Macrosigmoid K59.39 ◄
congenital Q43.2
Macrospondylitis, acromegalic E22.0
Macrostomia (congenital) Q18.4
Macrotia (external ear) (congenital) Q17.1
Macula
cornea, corneal —*see* Opacity, cornea
degeneration (atrophic) (exudative) (senile) —*see also* Degeneration, macula
hereditary —*see* Dystrophy, retina
Maculae ceruleae — B85.1
Maculopathy, toxic —*see* Degeneration, macula, toxic
Madarosis (eyelid) H02.729
left H02.726
lower H02.725
upper H02.724
right H02.723
lower H02.722
upper H02.721
Madelung's
deformity (radius) Q74.0
disease
radial deformity Q74.0
symmetrical lipomas, neck E88.89
Madness —*see* Psychosis
Madura
foot B47.9
actinomycotic B47.1
mycotic B47.0
Maduromycosis B47.0
Maffucci's syndrome Q78.4
Magnesium metabolism disorder —*see* Disorder, metabolism, magnesium
Main en griffe (acquired) —*see also* Deformity, limb, clawhand
congenital Q74.0
Maintenance (encounter for)
antineoplastic chemotherapy Z51.11
antineoplastic radiation therapy Z51.0
methadone F11.20
Majocchi's
disease L81.7
granuloma B35.8
Major —*see* condition
Malabar itch (any site) B35.5
Malabsorption K90.9
calcium K90.89
carbohydrate K90.49 ◄
disaccharide E73.9
fat K90.49 ◄
galactose E74.20
glucose(-galactose) E74.39
intestinal K90.9
specified NEC K90.89
isomaltose E74.31
lactose E73.9
methionine E72.19
monosaccharide E74.39
postgastrectomy K91.2
postsurgical K91.2
protein K90.49 ◄
starch K90.49 ◄
sucrose E74.39
syndrome K90.9
postsurgical K91.2
Malacia, bone (adult) M83.9
juvenile —*see* Rickets
Malacoplakia
bladder N32.89
pelvis (kidney) N28.89
ureter N28.89
urethra N36.8
Malacosteon, juvenile —*see* Rickets
Maladaptation —*see* Maladjustment
Maladie de Roger Q21.0
Maladjustment
conjugal Z63.0
involving divorce or estrangement Z63.5
educational Z55.4
family Z63.9
marital Z63.0
involving divorce or estrangement Z63.5
occupational NEC Z56.89
simple, adult —*see* Disorder, adjustment
situational —*see* Disorder, adjustment
social Z60.9
due to
acculturation difficulty Z60.3
discrimination and persecution (perceived) Z60.5
exclusion and isolation Z60.4
life-cycle (phase of life) transition Z60.0
rejection Z60.4
specified reason NEC Z60.8
Malaise R53.81
Malakoplakia —*see* Malacoplakia
Malaria, malarial (fever) B54
with
blackwater fever B50.8
hemoglobinuric (bilious) B50.8
hemoglobinuria B50.8
accidentally induced (therapeutically) - code by type under Malaria
algid B50.9
cerebral B50.0 *[G94]*
clinically diagnosed (without parasitological confirmation) B54
congenital NEC P37.4
falciparum P37.3
congestion, congestive B54
continued (fever) B50.9
estivo-autumnal B50.9
falciparum B50.9
with complications NEC B50.8
cerebral B50.0 *[G94]*
severe B50.8
hemorrhagic B54
malariae B52.9
with
complications NEC B52.8
glomerular disorder B52.0
malignant (tertian) —*see* Malaria, falciparum
mixed infections — code to first listed type in B50-B53
ovale B53.0
parasitologically confirmed NEC B53.8
Malaria, malarial *(Continued)*
pernicious, acute —*see* Malaria, falciparum
Plasmodium (P.)
falciparum NEC —*see* Malaria, falciparum
malariae NEC B52.9
with Plasmodium
falciparum (and or vivax) —*see* Malaria, falciparum
vivax —*see also* Malaria, vivax
and falciparum —*see* Malaria, falciparum
ovale B53.0
with Plasmodium malariae —*see also* Malaria, malariae
and vivax —*see also* Malaria, vivax
and falciparum —*see* Malaria, falciparum
simian B53.1
with Plasmodium malariae —*see also* Malaria, malariae
and vivax —*see also* Malaria, vivax
and falciparum —*see* Malaria, falciparum
vivax NEC B51.9
with Plasmodium falciparum —*see* Malaria, falciparum
quartan —*see* Malaria, malariae
quotidian —*see* Malaria, falciparum
recurrent B54
remittent B54
specified type NEC (parasitologically confirmed) B53.8
spleen B54
subtertian (fever) —*see* Malaria, falciparum
tertian (benign) —*see also* Malaria, vivax
malignant B50.9
tropical B50.9
typhoid B54
vivax B51.9
with
complications NEC B51.8
ruptured spleen B51.0
Malassez's disease (cystic) N50.89 ◄
Malassimilation K90.9
Mal de los pintos —*see* Pinta
Mal de mer T75.3
Maldescent, testis Q53.9
bilateral Q53.20
abdominal Q53.21
perineal Q53.22
unilateral Q53.10
abdominal Q53.11
perineal Q53.12
Maldevelopment —*see also* Anomaly
brain Q07.9
colon Q43.9
hip Q74.2
congenital dislocation Q65.2
bilateral Q65.1
unilateral Q65.0-
mastoid process Q75.8
middle ear Q16.4
except ossicles Q16.4
ossicles Q16.3
ossicles Q16.3
spine Q76.49
toe Q74.2
Male type pelvis Q74.2
with disproportion (fetopelvic) O33.3
causing obstructed labor O65.3
Malformation (congenital) —*see also* Anomaly
adrenal gland Q89.1
affecting multiple systems with skeletal changes NEC Q87.5
alimentary tract Q45.9
specified type NEC Q45.8
upper Q40.9
specified type NEC Q40.8
aorta Q25.40 ◄
absence Q25.41 ◄
aneurysm, congenital Q25.43 ◄

M

Malformation *(Continued)*
aorta *(Continued)*
aplasia Q25.41 ◀
atresia Q25.29 ⇐
aortic arch Q25.21 ◀
coarctation (preductal) (postductal) Q25.1
dilatation, congenital Q25.44 ◀
hypoplasia Q25.42 ◀
patent ductus arteriosus Q25.0
specified type NEC Q25.49 ⇐
stenosis Q25.1 ⇐
supravalvular Q25.3 ◀
aortic valve Q23.9
specified NEC Q23.8
arteriovenous, aneurysmatic (congenital) Q27.30
brain Q28.2
cerebral Q28.2
peripheral Q27.30
digestive system Q27.33
lower limb Q27.32
other specified site Q27.39
renal vessel Q27.34
upper limb Q27.31
precerebral vessels (nonruptured) Q28.0
auricle
ear (congenital) Q17.3
acquired H61.119
left H61.112
with right H61.113
right H61.111
with left H61.113
bile duct Q44.5
bladder Q64.79
aplasia Q64.5
diverticulum Q64.6
exstrophy —*see* Exstrophy, bladder
neck obstruction Q64.31
bone Q79.9
face Q75.9
specified type NEC Q75.8
skull Q75.9
specified type NEC Q75.8
brain (multiple) Q04.9
arteriovenous Q28.2
specified type NEC Q04.8
branchial cleft Q18.2
breast Q83.9
specified type NEC Q83.8
broad ligament Q50.6
bronchus Q32.4
bursa Q79.9
cardiac
chambers Q20.9
specified type NEC Q20.8
septum Q21.9
specified type NEC Q21.8
cerebral Q04.9
vessels Q28.3
cervix uteri Q51.9
specified type NEC Q51.828
Chiari
Type I G93.5
Type II Q07.01
choroid (congenital) Q14.3
plexus Q07.8
circulatory system Q28.9
cochlea Q16.5
cornea Q13.4
coronary vessels Q24.5
corpus callosum (congenital) Q04.0
diaphragm Q79.1
digestive system NEC, specified type NEC Q45.8
dura Q07.9
brain Q04.9
spinal Q06.9
ear Q17.9
causing impairment of hearing Q16.9

Malformation *(Continued)*
ear *(Continued)*
external Q17.9
accessory auricle Q17.0
causing impairment of hearing Q16.9
absence of
auditory canal Q16.1
auricle Q16.0
macrotia Q17.1
microtia Q17.2
misplacement Q17.4
misshapen NEC Q17.3
prominence Q17.5
specified type NEC Q17.8
inner Q16.5
middle Q16.4
absence of eustachian tube Q16.2
ossicles (fusion) Q16.3
ossicles Q16.3
specified type NEC Q17.8
epididymis Q55.4
esophagus Q39.9
specified type NEC Q39.8
eye Q15.9
lid Q10.3
specified NEC Q15.8
fallopian tube Q50.6
genital organ —*see* Anomaly, genitalia
great
artery Q25.9
aorta —*see* Malformation, aorta
pulmonary artery —*see* Malformation, pulmonary, artery
specified type NEC Q25.8
vein Q26.9
anomalous
portal venous connection Q26.5
pulmonary venous connection Q26.4
partial Q26.3
total Q26.2
persistent left superior vena cava Q26.1
portal vein-hepatic artery fistula Q26.6
specified type NEC Q26.8
vena cava stenosis, congenital Q26.0
gum Q38.6
hair Q84.2
heart Q24.9
specified type NEC Q24.8
integument Q84.9
specified type NEC Q84.8
internal ear Q16.5
intestine Q43.9
specified type NEC Q43.8
iris Q13.2
joint Q74.9
ankle Q74.2
lumbosacral Q76.49
sacroiliac Q74.2
specified type NEC Q74.8
kidney Q63.9
accessory Q63.0
giant Q63.3
horseshoe Q63.1
hydronephrosis Q62.0
malposition Q63.2
specified type NEC Q63.8
lacrimal apparatus Q10.6
lingual Q38.3
lip Q38.0
liver Q44.7
lung Q33.9
meninges or membrane (congenital) Q07.9
cerebral Q04.8
spinal (cord) Q06.9
middle ear Q16.4
ossicles Q16.3
mitral valve Q23.9
specified NEC Q23.8
Mondini's (congenital) (malformation, cochlea) Q16.5

Malformation *(Continued)*
mouth (congenital) Q38.6
multiple types NEC Q89.7
musculoskeletal system Q79.9
myocardium Q24.8
nail Q84.6
nervous system (central) Q07.9
nose Q30.9
specified type NEC Q30.8
optic disc Q14.2
orbit Q10.7
ovary Q50.39
palate Q38.5
parathyroid gland Q89.2
pelvic organs or tissues NEC
in pregnancy or childbirth O34.8-
causing obstructed labor O65.5
penis Q55.69
aplasia Q55.5
curvature (lateral) Q55.61
hypoplasia Q55.62
pericardium Q24.8
peripheral vascular system Q27.9
specified type NEC Q27.8
pharynx Q38.8
precerebral vessels Q28.1
prostate Q55.4
pulmonary
arteriovenous Q25.72
artery Q25.9
atresia Q25.5
specified type NEC Q25.79
stenosis Q25.6
valve Q22.3
renal artery Q27.2
respiratory system Q34.9
retina Q14.1
scrotum —*see* Malformation, testis and scrotum
seminal vesicles Q55.4
sense organs NEC Q07.9
skin Q82.9
specified NEC Q89.8
spinal
cord Q06.9
nerve root Q07.8
spine Q76.49
kyphosis —*see* Kyphosis, congenital
lordosis —*see* Lordosis, congenital
spleen Q89.09
stomach Q40.3
specified type NEC Q40.2
teeth, tooth K00.9
tendon Q79.9
testis and scrotum Q55.20
aplasia Q55.0
hypoplasia Q55.1
polyorchism Q55.21
retractile testis Q55.22
scrotal transposition Q55.23
specified NEC Q55.29
thorax, bony Q76.9
throat Q38.8
thyroid gland Q89.2
tongue (congenital) Q38.3
hypertrophy Q38.2
tie Q38.1
trachea Q32.1
tricuspid valve Q22.9
specified type NEC Q22.8
umbilical cord NEC (complicating delivery) O69.89
umbilicus Q89.9
ureter Q62.8
agenesis Q62.4
duplication Q62.5
malposition —*see* Malposition, congenital, ureter
obstructive defect —*see* Defect, obstructive, ureter
vesico-uretero-renal reflux Q62.7

◀ New ⇐ Revised ~~deleted~~ Deleted

Malformation *(Continued)*
urethra Q64.79
aplasia Q64.5
duplication Q64.74
posterior valves Q64.2
prolapse Q64.71
stricture Q64.32
urinary system Q64.9
uterus Q51.9
specified type NEC Q51.818
vagina Q52.4
vascular system, peripheral Q27.9
vas deferens Q55.4
atresia Q55.3
venous —*see* Anomaly, vein (s)
vulva Q52.70
Malfunction —*see also* Dysfunction
cardiac electronic device T82.119
electrode T82.110
pulse generator T82.111
specified type NEC T82.118
catheter device NEC T85.618
cystostomy T83.010
dialysis (renal) (vascular) T82.41
intraperitoneal T85.611
infusion NEC T82.514
cranial T85.610 ◀
epidural T85.610 ◀
intrathecal T85.610 ◀
spinal T85.610 ⟸
subarachnoid T85.610 ◀
subdural T85.610 ◀
~~urinary, indwelling T83.018~~
urinary —*see also* Breakdown, device, catheter T83.018 ◀
colostomy K94.03
valve K94.03
cystostomy (stoma) N99.512
catheter T83.010
enteric stoma K94.13
enterostomy K94.13
esophagostomy K94.33
gastroenteric K31.89
gastrostomy K94.23
ileostomy K94.13
valve K94.13
intrathecal infusion pump T85.615 ◀
jejunostomy K94.13
nervous system device, implant or graft, specified NEC T85.615 ◀
pacemaker —*see* Malfunction, cardiac electronic device
prosthetic device, internal —*see* Complications, prosthetic device, by site, mechanical
tracheostomy J95.03
urinary device NEC —*see* Complication, genitourinary, device, urinary, mechanical
valve
colostomy K94.03
heart T82.09
ileostomy K94.13
vascular graft or shunt NEC —*see* Complication, cardiovascular device, mechanical, vascular
ventricular (communicating shunt) T85.01
Malherbe's tumor —*see* Neoplasm, skin, benign
Malibu disease L98.8-
Malignancy —*see also* Neoplasm, malignant, by site
unspecified site (primary) C80.1
Malignant —*see* condition
Malingerer, malingering Z76.5
Mallet finger (acquired) —*see* Deformity, finger, mallet finger
congenital Q74.0
sequelae of rickets E64.3
Malleus A24.0
Mallory's bodies R89.7
Mallory-Weiss syndrome K22.6

Malnutrition E46
degree
first E44.1
mild (protein) E44.1
moderate (protein) E44.0
second E44.0
severe (protein-energy) E43
intermediate form E42
with
kwashiorkor (and marasmus) E42
marasmus E41
third E43
following gastrointestinal surgery K91.2
intrauterine
light-for-dates —*see* Light for dates
small-for-dates —*see* Small for dates
lack of care, or neglect (child) (infant) T76.02
confirmed T74.02
malignant E40
protein E46
calorie E46
mild E44.1
moderate E44.0
severe E43
intermediate form E42
with
kwashiorkor (and marasmus) E42
marasmus E41
energy E46
mild E44.1
moderate E44.0
severe E43
intermediate form E42
with
kwashiorkor (and marasmus) E42
marasmus E41
severe (protein-energy) E43
with
kwashiorkor (and marasmus) E42
marasmus E41
Malocclusion (teeth) M26.4
Angle's M26.219
class I M26.211
class II M26.212
class III M26.213
due to
abnormal swallowing M26.59
mouth breathing M26.59
tongue, lip or finger habits M26.59
temporomandibular (joint) M26.69
Malposition
cervix —*see* Malposition, uterus
congenital
adrenal (gland) Q89.1
alimentary tract Q45.8
lower Q43.8
upper Q40.8
aorta Q25.49 ⟸
appendix Q43.8
arterial trunk Q20.0
artery (peripheral) Q27.8
coronary Q24.5
digestive system Q27.8
lower limb Q27.8
pulmonary Q25.79
specified site NEC Q27.8
upper limb Q27.8
auditory canal Q17.8
causing impairment of hearing Q16.9
auricle (ear) Q17.4
causing impairment of hearing Q16.9
cervical Q18.2
biliary duct or passage Q44.5
bladder (mucosa) —*see* Exstrophy, bladder
brachial plexus Q07.8
brain tissue Q04.8
breast Q83.8
bronchus Q32.4

Malposition *(Continued)*
congenital *(Continued)*
cecum Q43.8
clavicle Q74.0
colon Q43.8
digestive organ or tract NEC Q45.8
lower Q43.8
upper Q40.8
ear (auricle) (external) Q17.4
ossicles Q16.3
endocrine (gland) NEC Q89.2
epiglottis Q31.8
eustachian tube Q17.8
eye Q15.8
facial features Q18.8
fallopian tube Q50.6
finger (s) Q68.1
supernumerary Q69.0
foot Q66.9
gallbladder Q44.1
gastrointestinal tract Q45.8
genitalia, genital organ (s) or tract
female Q52.8
external Q52.79
internal NEC Q52.8
male Q55.8
glottis Q31.8
hand Q68.1
heart Q24.8
dextrocardia Q24.0
with complete transposition of viscera Q89.3
hepatic duct Q44.5
hip (joint) Q65.89
intestine (large) (small) Q43.8
with anomalous adhesions, fixation or malrotation Q43.3
joint NEC Q68.8
kidney Q63.2
larynx Q31.8
limb Q68.8
lower Q68.8
upper Q68.8
liver Q44.7
lung (lobe) Q33.8
nail (s) Q84.6
nerve Q07.8
nervous system NEC Q07.8
nose, nasal (septum) Q30.8
organ or site not listed —*see* Anomaly, by site
ovary Q50.39
pancreas Q45.3
parathyroid (gland) Q89.2
patella Q74.1
peripheral vascular system Q27.8
pituitary (gland) Q89.2
respiratory organ or system NEC Q34.8
rib (cage) Q76.6
supernumerary in cervical region Q76.5
scapula Q74.0
shoulder Q74.0
spinal cord Q06.8
spleen Q89.09
sternum NEC Q76.7
stomach Q40.2
symphysis pubis Q74.2
thymus (gland) Q89.2
thyroid (gland) (tissue) Q89.2
cartilage Q31.8
toe (s) Q66.9
supernumerary Q69.2
tongue Q38.3
trachea Q32.1
ureter Q62.60
deviation Q62.61
displacement Q62.62
ectopia Q62.63
specified type NEC Q62.69

Malposition *(Continued)*
congenital *(Continued)*
uterus Q51.818
vein (s) (peripheral) Q27.8
great Q26.8
vena cava (inferior) (superior) Q26.8
device, implant or graft —*see also* Complications, by site and type, mechanical T85.628
arterial graft NEC —*see* Complication, cardiovascular device, mechanical, vascular
breast (implant) T85.42
catheter NEC T85.628
cystostomy T83.020
dialysis (renal) T82.42
intraperitoneal T85.621
infusion NEC T82.524
spinal (epidural) (subdural) T85.620
~~urinary, indwelling T83.028~~
urinary —*see also* Displacement, device, catheter, urinary T83.028 ◀
electronic (electrode) (pulse generator) (stimulator)
bone T84.320
cardiac T82.129
electrode T82.120
pulse generator T82.121
specified type NEC T82.128
nervous system —*see* Complication, prosthetic device, mechanical, electronic nervous system stimulator
urinary —*see* Complication, genitourinary, device, urinary, mechanical
fixation, internal (orthopedic) NEC —*see* Complication, fixation device, mechanical
gastrointestinal —*see* Complications, prosthetic device, mechanical, gastrointestinal device
genital NEC T83.428
intrauterine contraceptive device (string) T83.32 ⇐
penile prosthesis (cylinder) (implanted) (pump) (resevoir) T83.420 ⇐
testicular prosthesis T83.421 ◀
heart NEC —*see* Complication, cardiovascular device, mechanical
joint prosthesis —*see* Complication, joint prosthesis, mechanical
ocular NEC —*see* Complications, prosthetic device, mechanical, ocular device
orthopedic NEC —*see* Complication, orthopedic, device, mechanical
specified NEC T85.628
urinary NEC —*see also* Complication, genitourinary, device, urinary, mechanical
graft T83.22
vascular NEC —*see* Complication, cardiovascular device, mechanical
ventricular intracranial shunt T85.02
fetus —*see* Pregnancy, complicated by (management affected by), presentation, fetal
gallbladder K82.8
gastrointestinal tract, congenital Q45.8
heart, congenital NEC Q24.8
joint prosthesis —*see* Complications, joint prosthesis, mechanical, displacement, by site
stomach K31.89
congenital Q40.2
tooth, teeth, fully erupted M26.30
uterus (acute) (acquired) (adherent) (asymptomatic) (postinfectional) (postpartal, old) N85.4
anteflexion or anteversion N85.4
congenital Q51.818

Malposition *(Continued)*
uterus *(Continued)*
flexion N85.4
lateral —*see* Lateroversion, uterus
inversion N85.5
lateral (flexion) (version) —*see* Lateroversion, uterus
in pregnancy or childbirth —*see* subcategory O34.5
retroflexion or retroversion —*see* Retroversion, uterus
Malposture R29.3
Malrotation
cecum Q43.3
colon Q43.3
intestine Q43.3
kidney Q63.2
Malta fever —*see* Brucellosis
Maltreatment
adult
abandonment
confirmed T74.01
suspected T76.01
confirmed T74.91
history of Z91.419
neglect
confirmed T74.01
suspected T76.01
physical abuse
confirmed T74.11
suspected T76.11
psychological abuse
confirmed T74.31
history of Z91.411
suspected T76.31
sexual abuse
confirmed T74.21
suspected T76.21
suspected T76.91
child
abandonment
confirmed T74.02
suspected T76.02
confirmed T74.92
history of —*see* History, personal (of), abuse
neglect
confirmed T74.02
history of —*see* History, personal (of), abuse
suspected T76.02
physical abuse
confirmed T74.12
history of —*see* History, personal (of), abuse
suspected T76.12
psychological abuse
confirmed T74.32
history of —*see* History, personal (of), abuse
suspected T76.32
sexual abuse
confirmed T74.22
history of —*see* History, personal (of), abuse
suspected T76.22
suspected T76.92
personal history of Z91.89
Maltworker's lung J67.4
Malunion, fracture —*see* Fracture, by site
Mammillitis N61.0 ⇐
puerperal, postpartum O91.02
Mammitis —*see* Mastitis
Mammogram (examination) Z12.39
routine Z12.31
Mammoplasia N62
Management (of)
bone conduction hearing device (implanted) Z45.320
cardiac pacemaker NEC Z45.018
cerebrospinal fluid drainage device Z45.41

Management *(Continued)*
cochlear device (implanted) Z45.321
contraceptive Z30.9
specified NEC Z30.8
implanted device Z45.9
specified NEC Z45.89
infusion pump Z45.1
procreative Z31.9
male factor infertility in female Z31.81
specified NEC Z31.89
prosthesis (external) —*see also* Fitting Z44.9
implanted Z45.9
specified NEC Z45.89
renal dialysis catheter Z49.01
vascular access device Z45.2
Mangled —*see* specified injury by site
Mania (monopolar) —*see also* Disorder, mood, manic episode
with psychotic symptoms F30.2
without psychotic symptoms F30.10
mild F30.11
moderate F30.12
severe F30.13
Bell's F30.8
chronic (recurrent) F31.89
hysterical F44.89
puerperal F30.8
recurrent F31.89
Manic-depressive insanity, psychosis, or syndrome —*see* Disorder, bipolar
Mannosidosis E77.1
Mansonelliasis, mansonellosis B74.4
Manson's
disease B65.1
schistosomiasis B65.1
Manual —*see* condition
Maple-bark-stripper's lung (disease) J67.6
Maple-syrup-urine disease E71.0
Marable's syndrome (celiac artery compression) I77.4
Marasmus E41
due to malnutrition E41
intestinal E41
nutritional E41
senile R54
tuberculous NEC —*see* Tuberculosis
Marble
bones Q78.2
skin R23.8
Marburg virus disease A98.3
March
fracture —*see* Fracture, traumatic, stress, by site
hemoglobinuria D59.6
Marchesani (-Weill) syndrome Q87.0
Marchiafava (-Bignami) syndrome or disease G37.1
Marchiafava-Micheli syndrome D59.5
Marcus Gunn's syndrome Q07.8
Marfan's syndrome —*see* Syndrome, Marfan's
Marie-Bamberger disease —*see* Osteoarthropathy, hypertrophic, specified NEC
Marie-Charcot-Tooth neuropathic muscular atrophy G60.0
Marie's
cerebellar ataxia (late-onset) G11.2
disease or syndrome (acromegaly) E22.0
Marie-Strümpell arthritis, disease or spondylitis —*see* Spondylitis, ankylosing
Marion's disease (bladder neck obstruction) N32.0
Marital conflict Z63.0
Mark
port wine Q82.5
raspberry Q82.5
strawberry Q82.5
stretch L90.6
tattoo L81.8
Marker heterochromatin —*see* Extra, marker chromosomes

◀ New ⇐ Revised ~~deleted~~ Deleted

Maroteaux-Lamy syndrome (mild) (severe) E76.29
Marrow (bone)
arrest D61.9
poor function D75.89
Marseilles fever A77.1
Marsh fever —*see* Malaria
Marshall's (hidrotic) ectodermal dysplasia Q82.4
Marsh's disease (exophthalmic goiter) E05.00
with storm E05.01
Masculinization (female) with adrenal hyperplasia E25.9
congenital E25.0
Masculinovoblastoma D27.-
Masochism (sexual) F65.51
Mason's lung J62.8
Mass
abdominal R19.00
epigastric R19.06
generalized R19.07
left lower quadrant R19.04
left upper quadrant R19.02
periumbilic R19.05
right lower quadrant R19.03
right upper quadrant R19.01
specified site NEC R19.09
breast N63
chest R22.2
cystic —*see* Cyst
ear H93.8-
head R22.0
intra-abdominal (diffuse) (generalized) —*see* Mass, abdominal
kidney N28.89
liver R16.0
localized (skin) R22.9
chest R22.2
head R22.0
limb
lower R22.4-
upper R22.3-
neck R22.1
trunk R22.2
lung R91.8
malignant —*see* Neoplasm, malignant, by site
neck R22.1
pelvic (diffuse) (generalized) —*see* Mass, abdominal
specified organ NEC —*see* Disease, by site
splenic R16.1
substernal thyroid —*see* Goiter
superficial (localized) R22.9
umbilical (diffuse) (generalized) R19.09
Massive —*see* condition
Mast cell
disease, systemic tissue D47.0
leukemia C94.3-
sarcoma C96.2
tumor D47.0
malignant C96.2
Mastalgia N64.4
Masters-Allen syndrome N83.8
Mastitis (acute) (diffuse) (nonpuerperal) (subacute) N61.0 ⇐
with abscess N61.1 ◀
chronic (cystic) —*see* Mastopathy, cystic
cystic (Schimmelbusch's type) —*see* Mastopathy, cystic
fibrocystic —*see* Mastopathy, cystic
infective N61.0 ⇐
newborn P39.0
interstitial, gestational or puerperal —*see* Mastitis, obstetric
neonatal (noninfective) P83.4
infective P39.0
obstetric (interstitial) (nonpurulent)
associated with
lactation O91.23
pregnancy O91.21-
puerperium O91.22
Mastitis *(Continued)*
obstetric *(Continued)*
purulent
associated with
lactation O91.13
pregnancy O91.11-
puerperium O91.12
periductal —*see* Ectasia, mammary duct
phlegmonous —*see* Mastopathy, cystic
plasma cell —*see* Ectasia, mammary duct
without abscess N61.0 ◀
Mastocytoma D47.0
malignant C96.2
Mastocytosis Q82.2
aggressive systemic C96.2
indolent systemic D47.0
malignant C96.2
systemic, associated with clonal hematopoetic non-mast-cell disease (SM-AHNMD) D47.0
Mastodynia N64.4
Mastoid —*see* condition
Mastoidalgia —*see* subcategory H92.0
Mastoiditis (coalescent) (hemorrhagic) (suppurative) H70.9-
acute, subacute H70.00-
complicated NEC H70.09-
subperiosteal H70.01-
chronic (necrotic) (recurrent) H70.1-
in (due to)
infectious disease NEC B99 *[H75.0-]*
parasitic disease NEC B89 *[H75.0-]*
tuberculosis A18.03
petrositis —*see* Petrositis
postauricular fistula —*see* Fistula, postauricular
specified NEC H70.89-
tuberculous A18.03
Mastopathy, mastopathia N64.9
chronica cystica —*see* Mastopathy, cystic
cystic (chronic) (diffuse) N60.1
with epithelial proliferation N60.3-
diffuse cystic —*see* Mastopathy, cystic
estrogenic, oestrogenica N64.89
ovarian origin N64.89
Mastoplasia, mastoplastia N62
Masturbation (excessive) F98.8
Maternal care (for) —*see* Pregnancy (complicated by) (management affected by)
Matheiu's disease (leptospiral jaundice) A27.0
Mauclaire's disease or osteochondrosis —*see* Osteochondrosis, juvenile, hand, metacarpal
Maxcy's disease A75.2
Maxilla, maxillary —*see* condition
May (-Hegglin) anomaly or syndrome D72.0
McArdle (-Schmid)(-Pearson) disease (glycogen storage) E74.04
McCune-Albright syndrome Q78.1
McQuarrie's syndrome (idiopathic familial hypoglycemia) E16.2
Meadow's syndrome Q86.1
Measles (black) (hemorrhagic) (suppressed) B05.9
with
complications NEC B05.89
encephalitis B05.0
intestinal complications B05.4
keratitis (keratoconjunctivitis) B05.81
meningitis B05.1
otitis media B05.3
pneumonia B05.2
French —*see* Rubella
German —*see* Rubella
Liberty —*see* Rubella
Meatitis, urethral —*see* Urethritis
Meatus, meatal —*see* condition
Meat-wrappers' asthma J68.9
Meckel-Gruber syndrome Q61.9
Meckel's diverticulitis, diverticulum (displaced) (hypertrophic) Q43.0
Meconium
ileus, newborn P76.0
in cystic fibrosis E84.11
meaning meconium plug (without cystic fibrosis) P76.0
obstruction, newborn P76.0
due to fecaliths P76.0
in mucoviscidosis E84.11
peritonitis P78.0
plug syndrome (newborn) NEC P76.0
Median —*see also* condition
arcuate ligament syndrome I77.4
bar (prostate) (vesical orifice) —*see* Hyperplasia, prostate
rhomboid glossitis K14.2
Mediastinal shift R93.8
Mediastinitis (acute) (chronic) J98.51 ⇐
syphilitic A52.73
tuberculous A15.8
Mediastinopericarditis —*see also* Pericarditis
acute I30.9
adhesive I31.0
chronic I31.8
rheumatic I09.2
Mediastinum, mediastinal —*see* condition
Medicine poisoning —*see* Table of Drugs and Chemicals, by drug, poisoning
Mediterranean
fever —*see* Brucellosis
familial M04.1 ⇐
tick A77.1
kala-azar B55.0
leishmaniasis B55.0
tick fever A77.1
Medulla —*see* condition
Medullary cystic kidney Q61.5
Medullated fibers
optic (nerve) Q14.8
retina Q14.1
Medulloblastoma
desmoplastic C71.6
specified site —*see* Neoplasm, malignant, by site
unspecified site C71.6
Medulloepithelioma —*see also* Neoplasm, malignant, by site
teratoid —*see* Neoplasm, malignant, by site
Medullomyoblastoma
specified site —*see* Neoplasm, malignant, by site
unspecified site C71.6
Meekeren-Ehlers-Danlos syndrome Q79.6
Megacolon (acquired) (functional) (not Hirschsprung's disease) (in) K59.39 ⇐
Chagas' disease B57.32
congenital, congenitum (aganglionic) Q43.1
Hirschsprung's (disease) Q43.1
toxic NEC K59.31 ⇐
due to Clostridium difficile A04.7
Megaesophagus (functional) K22.0
congenital Q39.5
in (due to) Chagas' disease B57.31
Megalencephaly Q04.5
Megalerythema (epidemic) B08.3
Megaloappendix Q43.8
Megalocephalus, megalocephaly NEC Q75.3
Megalocornea Q15.8
with glaucoma Q15.0
Megalocytic anemia D53.1
Megalodactylia (fingers) (thumbs) (congenital) Q74.0
toes Q74.2
Megaloduodenum Q43.8
Megaloesophagus (functional) K22.0
congenital Q39.5

M

Megalogastria (acquired) K31.89
congenital Q40.2
Megalophthalmos Q11.3
Megalopsia H53.15
Megalosplenia —*see* Splenomegaly
Megaloureter N28.82
congenital Q62.2
Megarectum K62.89
Megasigmoid K59.39 ◄
congenital Q43.2
Megaureter N28.82
congenital Q62.2
Megavitamin-B6 syndrome E67.2
Megrim —*see* Migraine
Meibomian
cyst, infected —*see* Hordeolum
gland —*see* condition
sty, stye —*see* Hordeolum
Meibomitis —*see* Hordeolum
Meige-Milroy disease (chronic hereditary edema) Q82.0
Meige's syndrome Q82.0
Melalgia, nutritional E53.8
Melancholia F32.9
climacteric (single episode) F32.89 ◄
recurrent episode F33.8 ◄
hypochondriac F45.29
intermittent (single episode) F32.89 ◄
recurrent episode F33.8 ◄
involutional (single episode) F32.89 ◄
recurrent episode F33.8 ◄
menopausal (single episode) F32.89 ◄
recurrent episode F33.8 ◄
puerperal F32.89 ◄
reactive (emotional stress or trauma) F32.3
recurrent F33.9
senile F03
stuporous (single episode) F32.89 ◄
recurrent episode F33.8 ◄
Melanemia R79.89
Melanoameloblastoma —*see* Neoplasm, bone, benign
Melanoblastoma —*see* Melanoma
Melanocarcinoma —*see* Melanoma
Melanocytoma, eyeball D31.9- ◄
Melanocytosis, neurocutaneous Q82.8
Melanoderma, melanodermia L81.4
Melanodontia, infantile K03.89
Melanodontoclasia K03.89
Melanoepithelioma —*see* Melanoma
Melanoma (malignant) C43.9
acral lentiginous, malignant —*see* Melanoma, skin, by site
amelanotic —*see* Melanoma, skin, by site
balloon cell —*see* Melanoma, skin, by site
benign —*see* Nevus
desmoplastic, malignant —*see* Melanoma, skin, by site
epithelioid cell —*see* Melanoma, skin, by site
with spindle cell, mixed —*see* Melanoma, skin, by site
in
giant pigmented nevus —*see* Melanoma, skin, by site
Hutchinson's melanotic freckle —*see* Melanoma, skin, by site
junctional nevus —*see* Melanoma, skin, by site
precancerous melanosis —*see* Melanoma, skin, by site
in situ D03.9
abdominal wall D03.59
ala nasi D03.39
ankle D03.7-
anus, anal (margin) (skin) D03.51
arm D03.6-
auditory canal D03.2-
auricle (ear) D03.2-
auricular canal (external) D03.2-
axilla, axillary fold D03.59
back D03.59

Melanoma *(Continued)*
in situ *(Continued)*
breast D03.52
brow D03.39
buttock D03.59
canthus (eye) D03.1-
cheek (external) D03.39
chest wall D03.59
chin D03.39
choroid D03.8
conjunctiva D03.8
ear (external) D03.2-
external meatus (ear) D03.2-
eye D03.8
eyebrow D03.39
eyelid (lower) (upper) D03.1-
face D03.30
specified NEC D03.39
female genital organ (external) NEC D03.8
finger D03.6-
flank D03.59
foot D03.7-
forearm D03.6-
forehead D03.39
foreskin D03.8
gluteal region D03.59
groin D03.59
hand D03.6-
heel D03.7-
helix D03.2-
hip D03.7-
interscapular region D03.59
iris D03.8
jaw D03.39
knee D03.7-
labium (majus) (minus) D03.8
lacrimal gland D03.8
leg D03.7-
lip (lower) (upper) D03.0
lower limb NEC D03.7-
male genital organ (external) NEC D03.8
nail D03.9
finger D03.6-
toe D03.7-
neck D03.4
nose (external) D03.39
orbit D03.8
penis D03.8
perianal skin D03.51
perineum D03.51
pinna D03.2-
popliteal fossa or space D03.7-
prepuce D03.8
pudendum D03.8
retina D03.8
retrobulbar D03.8
scalp D03.4
scrotum D03.8
shoulder D03.6-
specified site NEC D03.8
submammary fold D03.52
temple D03.39
thigh D03.7-
toe D03.7-
trunk NEC D03.59
umbilicus D03.59
upper limb NEC D03.6-
vulva D03.8
juvenile —*see* Nevus
malignant, of soft parts except skin —*see* Neoplasm, connective tissue, malignant
metastatic
breast C79.81
genital organ C79.82
specified site NEC C79.89
neurotropic, malignant —*see* Melanoma, skin, by site
nodular —*see* Melanoma, skin, by site
regressing, malignant —*see* Melanoma, skin, by site

Melanoma *(Continued)*
skin C43.9
abdominal wall C43.59
ala nasi C43.31
ankle C43.7-
anus, anal (skin) C43.51
arm C43.6-
auditory canal (external) C43.2-
auricle (ear) C43.2-
auricular canal (external) C43.2-
axilla, axillary fold C43.59
back C43.59
breast (female) (male) C43.52
brow C43.39
buttock C43.59
canthus (eye) C43.1-
cheek (external) C43.39
chest wall C43.59
chin C43.39
ear (external) C43.2-
elbow C43.6-
external meatus (ear) C43.2-
eyebrow C43.39
eyelid (lower) (upper) C43.1-
face C43.30
specified NEC C43.39
female genital organ (external) NEC C51.9
finger C43.6-
flank C43.59
foot C43.7-
forearm C43.6-
forehead C43.39
foreskin C60.0
glabella C43.39
gluteal region C43.59
groin C43.59
hand C43.6-
heel C43.7-
helix C43.2-
hip C43.7-
interscapular region C43.59
jaw (external) C43.39
knee C43.7-
labium C51.9
majus C51.0
minus C51.1
leg C43.7-
lip (lower) (upper) C43.0
lower limb NEC C43.7-
male genital organ (external) NEC C63.9
nail
finger C43.6-
toe C43.7-
nasolabial groove C43.39
nates C43.59
neck C43.4
nose (external) C43.31
overlapping site C43.8
palpebra C43.1-
penis C60.9
perianal skin C43.51
perineum C43.51
pinna C43.2-
popliteal fossa or space C43.7-
prepuce C60.0
pudendum C51.9
scalp C43.4
scrotum C63.2
shoulder C43.6-
skin NEC C43.9
submammary fold C43.52
temple C43.39
thigh C43.7-
toe C43.7-
trunk NEC C43.59
umbilicus C43.59
upper limb NEC C43.6-
vulva C51.9
overlapping sites C51.8

◄ New ◄ Revised ~~deleted~~ Deleted

Melanoma *(Continued)*
spindle cell
with epithelioid, mixed —*see* Melanoma, skin, by site
type A C69.4-
type B C69.4-
superficial spreading —*see* Melanoma, skin, by site
Melanosarcoma —*see also* Melanoma
epithelioid cell —*see* Melanoma
Melanosis L81.4
addisonian E27.1
tuberculous A18.7
adrenal E27.1
colon K63.89
conjunctiva —*see* Pigmentation, conjunctiva
congenital Q13.89
cornea (presenile) (senile) —*see also* Pigmentation, cornea
congenital Q13.4
eye NEC H57.8
congenital Q15.8
lenticularis progressiva Q82.1
liver K76.89
precancerous —*see also* Melanoma, in situ
malignant melanoma in —*see* Melanoma
Riehl's L81.4
sclera H15.89
congenital Q13.89
suprarenal E27.1
tar L81.4
toxic L81.4
Melanuria R82.99
MELAS syndrome E88.41
Melasma L81.1
adrenal (gland) E27.1
suprarenal (gland) E27.1
Melena K92.1
with ulcer - code by site under Ulcer, with hemorrhage K27.4
due to swallowed maternal blood P78.2
newborn, neonatal P54.1
due to swallowed maternal blood P78.2
Meleney's
gangrene (cutaneous) —*see* Ulcer, skin
ulcer (chronic undermining) —*see* Ulcer, skin
Melioidosis A24.9
acute A24.1
chronic A24.2
fulminating A24.1
pneumonia A24.1
pulmonary (chronic) A24.2
acute A24.1
subacute A24.2
sepsis A24.1
specified NEC A24.3
subacute A24.2
Melitensis, febris A23.0
Melkersson (-Rosenthal) **syndrome** G51.2
Mellitus, diabetes —*see* Diabetes
Melorheostosis (bone) —*see* Disorder, bone, density and structure, specified NEC
Meloschisis Q18.4
Melotia Q17.4
Membrana
capsularis lentis posterior Q13.89
epipapillaris Q14.2
Membranacea placenta O43.19-
Membranaceous uterus N85.8
Membrane (s), **membranous** —*see also* condition
cyclitic —*see* Membrane, pupillary
folds, congenital —*see* Web
Jackson's Q43.3
over face of newborn P28.9
premature rupture —*see* Rupture, membranes, premature
pupillary H21.4-
persistent Q13.89
retained (with hemorrhage) (complicating delivery) O72.2
without hemorrhage O73.1
Membrane (s), **membranous** *(Continued)*
secondary cataract —*see* Cataract, secondary
unruptured (causing asphyxia) —*see* Asphyxia, newborn
vitreous —*see* Opacity, vitreous, membranes and strands
Membranitis —*see* Chorioamnionitis
Memory disturbance, lack or loss —*see also* Amnesia
mild, following organic brain damage F06.8
Menadione deficiency E56.1
Menarche
delayed E30.0
precocious E30.1
Mendacity, pathologic F60.2
Mendelson's syndrome (due to anesthesia) J95.4
in labor and delivery O74.0
in pregnancy O29.01-
obstetric O74.0
postpartum, puerperal O89.01
Ménétrier's disease or syndrome K29.60
with bleeding K29.61
Ménière's disease, syndrome or vertigo H81.0-
Meninges, meningeal —*see* condition
Meningioma —*see also* Neoplasm, meninges, benign
angioblastic —*see* Neoplasm, meninges, benign
angiomatous —*see* Neoplasm, meninges, benign
endotheliomatous —*see* Neoplasm, meninges, benign
fibroblastic —*see* Neoplasm, meninges, benign
fibrous —*see* Neoplasm, meninges, benign
hemangioblastic —*see* Neoplasm, meninges, benign
hemangiopericytic —*see* Neoplasm, meninges, benign
malignant —*see* Neoplasm, meninges, malignant
meningiothelial —*see* Neoplasm, meninges, benign
meningotheliomatous —*see* Neoplasm, meninges, benign
mixed —*see* Neoplasm, meninges, benign
multiple —*see* Neoplasm, meninges, uncertain behavior
papillary —*see* Neoplasm, meninges, uncertain behavior
psammomatous —*see* Neoplasm, meninges, benign
syncytial —*see* Neoplasm, meninges, benign
transitional —*see* Neoplasm, meninges, benign
Meningiomatosis (diffuse) —*see* Neoplasm, meninges, uncertain behavior
Meningism —*see* Meningismus
Meningismus (infectional) (pneumococcal) R29.1
due to serum or vaccine R29.1
influenzal —*see* Influenza, with, manifestations NEC
Meningitis (basal) (basic) (brain) (cerebral) (cervical) (congestive) (diffuse) (hemorrhagic) infantile) (membranous) (metastatic) (nonspecific) (pontine) (progressive) (simple) (spinal) (subacute) (sympathetic) (toxic) G03.9
abacterial G03.0
actinomycotic A42.81
adenoviral A87.1
arbovirus A87.8
aseptic (acute) G03.0
bacterial G00.9
Escherichia coli (E. coli) G00.8
Friedländer (bacillus) G00.8
gram-negative G00.9
H. influenzae G00.0
Klebsiella G00.8
Meningitis *(Continued)*
bacterial *(Continued)*
pneumococcal G00.1
specified organism NEC G00.8
staphylococcal G00.3
streptococcal (acute) G00.2
benign recurrent (Mollaret) G03.2
candidal B37.5
caseous (tuberculous) A17.0
cerebrospinal A39.0
chronic NEC G03.1
clear cerebrospinal fluid NEC G03.0
coxsackievirus A87.0
cryptococcal B45.1
diplococcal (gram positive) A39.0
echovirus A87.0
enteroviral A87.0
eosinophilic B83.2
epidemic NEC A39.0
Escherichia coli (E. coli) G00.8
fibrinopurulent G00.9
specified organism NEC G00.8
Friedländer (bacillus) G00.8
gonococcal A54.81
gram-negative cocci G00.9
gram-positive cocci G00.9
Haemophilus (influenzae) G00.0
H. influenzae G00.0
in (due to)
adenovirus A87.1
African trypanosomiasis B56.9 *[G02]*
anthrax A22.8
bacterial disease NEC A48.8 *[G01]*
Chagas' disease (chronic) B57.41
chickenpox B01.0
coccidioidomycosis B38.4
Diplococcus pneumoniae G00.1
enterovirus A87.0
herpes (simplex) virus B00.3
zoster B02.1
infectious mononucleosis B27.92
leptospirosis A27.81
Listeria monocytogenes A32.11
Lyme disease A69.21
measles B05.1
mumps (virus) B26.1
neurosyphilis (late) A52.13
parasitic disease NEC B89 *[G02]*
poliovirus A80.9 *[G02]*
preventive immunization, inoculation or vaccination G03.8
rubella B06.02
Salmonella infection A02.21
specified cause NEC G03.8
Streptococcal pneumoniae G00.1 ◀
typhoid fever A01.01
varicella B01.0
viral disease NEC A87.8
whooping cough A37.90
zoster B02.1
infectious G00.9
influenzal (H. influenzae) G00.0
Klebsiella G00.8
leptospiral (aseptic) A27.81
lymphocytic (acute) (benign) (serous) A87.2
meningococcal A39.0
Mima polymorpha G00.8
Mollaret (benign recurrent) G03.2
monilial B37.5
mycotic NEC B49 *[G02]*
Neisseria A39.0
nonbacterial G03.0
nonpyogenic NEC G03.0
ossificans G96.19
~~pneumococcal G00.1~~
pneumococcal streptococcus pneumoniae G00.1 ◀
poliovirus A80.9 *[G02]*
postmeasles B05.1
purulent G00.9
specified organism NEC G00.8

M

Meningitis *(Continued)*
pyogenic G00.9
specified organism NEC G00.8
Salmonella (arizonae) (Cholerae-Suis) (enteritidis) (typhimurium) A02.21
septic G00.9
specified organism NEC G00.8
serosa circumscripta NEC G03.0
serous NEC G93.2
specified organism NEC G00.8
sporotrichosis B42.81
staphylococcal G00.3
sterile G03.0
Streptococcal (acute) G00.2 ⇐
pneumoniae G00.1 ◀
suppurative G00.9
specified organism NEC G00.8
syphilitic (late) (tertiary) A52.13
acute A51.41
congenital A50.41
secondary A51.41
Torula histolytica (cryptococcal) B45.1
traumatic (complication of injury) T79.8
tuberculous A17.0
typhoid A01.01
viral NEC A87.9
Yersinia pestis A20.3
Meningocele (spinal) —*see also* Spina bifida
with hydrocephalus —*see* Spina bifida, by site, with hydrocephalus
acquired (traumatic) G96.19
cerebral —*see* Encephalocele
Meningocerebritis —*see* Meningoencephalitis
Meningococcemia A39.4
acute A39.2
chronic A39.3
Meningococcus, meningococcal —*see also* condition A39.9
adrenalitis, hemorrhagic A39.1
carrier (suspected) of Z22.31
meningitis (cerebrospinal) A39.0
Meningoencephalitis —*see also* Encephalitis G04.90
acute NEC —*see also* Encephalitis, viral A86
bacterial NEC G04.2
California A83.5
diphasic A84.1
eosinophilic B83.2
epidemic A39.81
herpesviral, herpetic B00.4
due to herpesvirus 6 B10.01
due to herpesvirus 7 B10.09
specified NEC B10.09
in (due to)
blastomycosis NEC B40.81
diseases classified elsewhere G05.3
free-living amebae B60.2
Hemophilus influenzae (H. influenzae) G00.0 ⇐
herpes B00.4
due to herpesvirus 6 B10.01
due to herpesvirus 7 B10.09
specified NEC B10.09
H. influenzae G00.0
Lyme disease A69.22
mercury —*see* subcategory T56.1
mumps B26.2
Naegleria (amebae) (organisms) (fowleri) B60.2
Parastrongylus cantonensis B83.2
toxoplasmosis (acquired) B58.2
congenital P37.1
infectious (acute) (viral) A86
influenzal (H. influenzae) G00.0 ⇐
Listeria monocytogenes A32.12
lymphocytic (serous) A87.2
mumps B26.2
parasitic NEC B89 *[G05.3]*
pneumococcal G04.2 ⇐
primary amebic B60.2

Meningoencephalitis *(Continued)*
specific (syphilitic) A52.14
specified organism NEC G04.81
staphylococcal G04.2
streptococcal G04.2
syphilitic A52.14
toxic NEC G92
due to mercury —*see* subcategory T56.1
tuberculous A17.82
virus NEC A86
Meningoencephalocele —*see also* Encephalocele
syphilitic A52.19
congenital A50.49
Meningoencephalomyelitis —*see also* Meningoencephalitis
acute NEC (viral) A86
disseminated G04.00
postimmunization or postvaccination G04.02
postinfectious G04.01
due to
actinomycosis A42.82
Torula B45.1
Toxoplasma or toxoplasmosis (acquired) B58.2
congenital P37.1
postimmunization or postvaccination G04.02
Meningoencephalomyelopathy G96.9
Meningoencephalopathy G96.9
Meningomyelitis —*see also* Meningoencephalitis
bacterial NEC G04.2
blastomycotic NEC B40.81
cryptococcal B45.1
in diseases classified elsewhere G05.4
meningococcal A39.81
syphilitic A52.14
tuberculous A17.82
Meningomyelocele —*see also* Spina bifida
syphilitic A52.19
Meningomyeloneuritis —*see* Meningoencephalitis
Meningoradiculitis —*see* Meningitis
Meningovascular —*see* condition
Menkes' disease or syndrome E83.09
meaning maple-syrup-urine disease E71.0
Menometrorrhagia N92.1
Menopause, menopausal (asymptomatic) (state) Z78.0
arthritis (any site) NEC —*see* Arthritis, specified form NEC
bleeding N92.4
depression (single episode) F32.89 ⇐
agitated (single episode) F32.2
recurrent episode F33.9
psychotic (single episode) F32.89 ⇐
recurrent episode F33.8 ⇐
recurrent episode F33.9
melancholia (single episode) F32.89 ⇐
recurrent episode F33.8 ⇐
paranoid state F22
premature E28.319
asymptomatic E28.319
postirradiation E89.40
postsurgical E89.40
symptomatic E28.310
postirradiation E89.41
postsurgical E89.41
psychosis NEC F28
symptomatic N95.1
toxic polyarthritis NEC —*see* Arthritis, specified form NEC
Menorrhagia (primary) N92.0
climacteric N92.4
menopausal N92.4
menopausal N92.4
postclimacteric N95.0
postmenopausal N95.0
preclimacteric or premenopausal N92.4
pubertal (menses retained) N92.2

Menostaxis N92.0
Menses, retention N94.89
Menstrual —*see* Menstruation
Menstruation
absent —*see* Amenorrhea
anovulatory N97.0
cycle, irregular N92.6
delayed N91.0
disorder N93.9
psychogenic F45.8
during pregnancy O20.8
excessive (with regular cycle) N92.0
with irregular cycle N92.1
at puberty N92.2
frequent N92.0
infrequent —*see* Oligomenorrhea
irregular N92.6
specified NEC N92.5
latent N92.5
membranous N92.5
painful —*see also* Dysmenorrhea N94.6
primary N94.4
psychogenic F45.8
secondary N94.5
passage of clots N92.0
precocious E30.1
protracted N92.5
rare —*see* Oligomenorrhea
retained N94.89
retrograde N92.5
scanty —*see* Oligomenorrhea
suppression N94.89
vicarious (nasal) N94.89
Mental —*see also* condition
deficiency —*see* Disability, intellectual
deterioration —*see* Psychosis
disorder —*see* Disorder, mental
exhaustion F48.8
insufficiency (congenital) —*see* Disability, intellectual
observation without need for further medical care Z03.89
retardation —*see* Disability, intellectual
subnormality —*see* Disability, intellectual
upset —*see* Disorder, mental
Meralgia paresthetica G57.1-
Mercurial —*see* condition
Mercurialism —*see* subcategory T56.1
MERRF syndrome (myoclonic epilepsy associated with ragged-red fiber) E88.42
Merkel cell tumor —*see* Carcinoma, Merkel cell
Merocele —*see* Hernia, femoral
Meromelia
lower limb —*see* Defect, reduction, lower limb
intercalary
femur —*see* Defect, reduction, lower limb, specified type NEC
tibiofibular (complete) (incomplete) —*see* Defect, reduction, lower limb
upper limb —*see* Defect, reduction, upper limb
intercalary, humeral, radioulnar —*see* Agenesis, arm, with hand present
Merzbacher-Pelizaeus disease E75.29
Mesaortitis —*see* Aortitis
Mesarteritis —*see* Arteritis
Mesencephalitis —*see* Encephalitis
Mesenchymoma —*see also* Neoplasm, connective tissue, uncertain behavior
benign —*see* Neoplasm, connective tissue, benign
malignant —*see* Neoplasm, connective tissue, malignant
Mesenteritis
retractile K65.4
sclerosing K65.4
Mesentery, mesenteric —*see* condition

◀ New ⇐ Revised ~~deleted~~ Deleted

Mesiodens, mesiodentes K00.1
Mesio-occlusion M26.213
Mesocolon —*see* condition
Mesonephroma (malignant) —*see* Neoplasm, malignant, by site
benign —*see* Neoplasm, benign, by site
Mesophlebitis —*see* Phlebitis
Mesostromal dysgenesia Q13.89
Mesothelioma (malignant) C45.9
benign
mesentery D19.1
mesocolon D19.1
omentum D19.1
peritoneum D19.1
pleura D19.0
specified site NEC D19.7
unspecified site D19.9
biphasic C45.9
benign
mesentery D19.1
mesocolon D19.1
omentum D19.1
peritoneum D19.1
pleura D19.0
specified site NEC D19.7
unspecified site D19.9
cystic D48.4
epithelioid C45.9
benign
mesentery D19.1
mesocolon D19.1
omentum D19.1
peritoneum D19.1
pleura D19.0
specified site NEC D19.7
unspecified site D19.9
fibrous C45.9
benign
mesentery D19.1
mesocolon D19.1
omentum D19.1
peritoneum D19.1
pleura D19.0
specified site NEC D19.7
unspecified site D19.9
site classification
liver C45.7
lung C45.7
mediastinum C45.7
mesentery C45.1
mesocolon C45.1
omentum C45.1
pericardium C45.2
peritoneum C45.1
pleura C45.0
parietal C45.0
retroperitoneum C45.7
specified site NEC C45.7
unspecified C45.9
Metabolic syndrome E88.81
Metagonimiasis B66.8
Metagonimus infestation (intestine) B66.8
Metal
pigmentation L81.8
polisher's disease J62.8
Metamorphopsia H53.15
Metaplasia
apocrine (breast) —*see* Dysplasia, mammary, specified type NEC
cervix (squamous) —*see* Dysplasia, cervix
endometrium (squamous) (uterus) N85.8
esophagus K22.7-
kidney (pelvis) (squamous) N28.89
myelogenous D73.1
myeloid (agnogenic) (megakaryocytic) D73.1
spleen D73.1
squamous cell, bladder N32.89
Metastasis, metastatic
abscess —*see* Abscess
calcification E83.59
Metastasis, metastatic *(Continued)*
cancer
from specified site —*see* Neoplasm, malignant, by site
to specified site —*see* Neoplasm, secondary, by site
deposits (in) —*see* Neoplasm, secondary, by site
disease (*see also* Neoplasm, secondary, by site) C79.9
spread (to) —*see* Neoplasm, secondary, by site
Metastrongyliasis B83.8
Metatarsalgia M77.4-
anterior G57.6-
Morton's G57.6-
Metatarsus, metatarsal —*see also* condition
adductus, congenital Q66.22 ◀
valgus (abductus), congenital Q66.6
varus (congenital) Q66.22
primus Q66.21 ◀
Methadone use —*see* Use, opioid
Methemoglobinemia D74.9
acquired (with sulfhemoglobinemia) D74.8
congenital D74.0
enzymatic (congenital) D74.0
Hb M disease D74.0
hereditary D74.0
toxic D74.8
Methemoglobinuria —*see* Hemoglobinuria
Methioninemia E72.19
Methylmalonic acidemia E71.120
Metritis (catarrhal) (hemorrhagic) (septic) (suppurative) —*see also* Endometritis
cervical —*see* Cervicitis
Metropathia hemorrhagica N93.8
Metroperitonitis —*see* Peritonitis, pelvic, female
Metrorrhagia N92.1
climacteric N92.4
menopausal N92.4
postpartum NEC (atonic) (following delivery of placenta) O72.1
delayed or secondary O72.2
preclimacteric or premenopausal N92.4
psychogenic F45.8
Metrorrhexis —*see* Rupture, uterus
Metrosalpingitis N70.91
Metrostaxis N93.8
Metrovaginitis —*see* Endometritis
Meyer-Schwickerath and Weyers syndrome Q87.0
Meynert's amentia (nonalcoholic) F04
alcoholic F10.96
with dependence F10.26
Mibelli's disease (porokeratosis) Q82.8
Mice, joint —*see* Loose, body, joint
knee M23.4
Micrencephalon, micrencephaly Q02
Microalbuminuria R80.9
Microaneurysm, retinal —*see also* Disorder, retina, microaneurysms
diabetic —*see* E08-E13 with .31
Microangiopathy (peripheral) I73.9
thrombotic M31.1
Microcalcifications, breast R92.0
Microcephalus, microcephalic, microcephaly Q02
due to toxoplasmosis (congenital) P37.1
Microcheilia Q18.7
Microcolon (congenital) Q43.8
Microcornea (congenital) Q13.4
Microcytic —*see* condition D57.40
Microdeletions NEC Q93.88
Microdontia K00.2
Microdrepanocytosis D57.40
with crisis (vasoocclusive pain) D57.419
with
acute chest syndrome D57.411
splenic sequestration D57.412
Microembolism
atherothrombotic —*see* Atheroembolism
retinal —*see* Occlusion, artery, retina
Microencephalon Q02
Microfilaria streptocerca infestation —*see* Onchocerciasis
Microgastria (congenital) Q40.2
Microgenia M26.06
Microgenitalia, congenital
female Q52.8
male Q55.8
Microglioma —*see* Lymphoma, non-Hodgkin, specified NEC
Microglossia (congenital) Q38.3
Micrognathia, micrognathism (congenital) (mandibular) (maxillary) M26.09
Microgyria (congenital) Q04.3
Microinfarct of heart —*see* Insufficiency, coronary
Microlentia (congenital) Q12.8
Microlithiasis, alveolar, pulmonary J84.02
Micromastia N64.82
Micromyelia (congenital) Q06.8
Micropenis Q55.62
Microphakia (congenital) Q12.8
Microphthalmos, microphthalmia (congenital) Q11.2
due to toxoplasmosis P37.1
Micropsia H53.15
Microscopic polyangiitis (polyarteritis) M31.7
Microsporidiosis B60.8
intestinal A07.8
Microsporon furfur infestation B36.0
Microsporosis —*see also* Dermatophytosis
nigra B36.1
Microstomia (congenital) Q18.5
Microtia (congenital) (external ear) Q17.2
Microtropia H50.40
Microvillus inclusion disease (MVD) (MVID) Q43.8
Micturition
disorder NEC —*see also* Difficulty, micturition R39.198
psychogenic F45.8
frequency R35.0
psychogenic F45.8
hesitancy R39.11
incomplete emptying R39.14
nocturnal R35.1
painful R30.9
dysuria R30.0
psychogenic F45.8
tenesmus R30.1
poor stream R39.12
position dependent R39.192 ◀
split stream R39.13
straining R39.16
urgency R39.15
Mid plane —*see* condition
Middle
ear —*see* condition
lobe (right) syndrome J98.19
Miescher's elastoma L87.2
Mietens' syndrome Q87.2
Migraine (idiopathic) G43.909
with refractory migraine G43.919
with status migrainosus G43.911
without status migrainosus G43.919
with aura (acute-onset) (prolonged) (typical) (without headache) G43.109
with refractory migraine G43.119
with status migrainosus G43.111
without status migrainosus G43.119
intractable G43.119
with status migrainosus G43.111
without status migrainosus G43.119
not intractable G43.109
with status migrainosus G43.101
without status migrainosus G43.109
persistent G43.509
with cerebral infarction G43.609
with refractory migraine G43.619
with status migrainosus G43.611
without status migrainosus G43.619

Migraine *(Continued)*
with aura *(Continued)*
persistent *(Continued)*
with cerebral infarction *(Continued)*
intractable G43.619
with status migrainosus G43.611
without status migrainosus G43.619
not intractable G43.609
with status migrainosus G43.601
without status migrainosus G43.609
without refractory migraine G43.609
with status migrainosus G43.601
without status migrainosus G43.609
without cerebral infarction G43.509
with refractory migraine G43.519
with status migrainosus G43.511
without status migrainosus G43.519
intractable G43.519
with status migrainosus G43.511
without status migrainosus G43.519
not intractable G43.509
with status migrainosus G43.501
without status migrainosus G43.509
without refractory migraine G43.509
with status migrainosus G43.501
without status migrainosus G43.509
without mention of refractory migraine G43.109
with status migrainosus G43.101
without status migrainosus G43.109
abdominal G43.D0
with refractory migraine G43.D1
intractable G43.D1
not intractable G43.D0
without refractory migraine G43.D0
basilar —*see* Migraine, with aura
classical —*see* Migraine, with aura
common —*see* Migraine, without aura
complicated G43.109
equivalents —*see* Migraine, with aura
familiar —*see* Migraine, hemiplegic
hemiplegic G43.409
with refractory migraine G43.419
with status migrainosus G43.411
without status migrainosus G43.419
intractable G43.419
with status migrainosus G43.411
without status migrainosus G43.419
not intractable G43.409
with status migrainosus G43.401
without status migrainosus G43.409
without refractory migraine G43.409
with status migrainosus G43.401
without status migrainosus G43.409
intractable G43.919
with status migrainosus G43.911
without status migrainosus G43.919
menstrual G43.829
with refractory migraine G43.839
with status migrainosus G43.831
without status migrainosus G43.839
intractable G43.839
with status migrainosus G43.831
without status migrainosus G43.839
not intractable G43.829
with status migrainosus G43.821
without status migrainosus G43.829
without refractory migraine G43.829
with status migrainosus G43.821
without status migrainosus G43.829
menstrually related —*see* Migraine, menstrual
not intractable G43.909
with status migrainosus G43.901
without status migrainosus G43.919
ophthalmoplegic G43.B0
with refractory migraine G43.B1
intractable G43.B1
not intractable G43.B0
without refractory migraine G43.B0

Migraine *(Continued)*
persistent aura (with, without) cerebral infarction —*see* Migraine, with aura, persistent
preceded or accompanied by transient focal neurological phenomena —*see* Migraine, with aura
pre-menstrual —*see* Migraine, menstrual
pure menstrual —*see* Migraine, menstrual
retinal —*see* Migraine, with aura
specified NEC G43.809
intractable G43.819
with status migrainosus G43.811
without status migrainosus G43.819
not intractable G43.809
with status migrainosus G43.801
without status migrainosus G43.809
sporadic —*see* Migraine, hemiplegic
transformed —*see* Migraine, without aura, chronic
triggered seizures —*see* Migraine, with aura
without aura G43.009
with refractory migraine G43.019
with status migrainosus G43.011
without status migrainosus G43.019
chronic G43.709
with refractory migraine G43.719
with status migrainosus G43.711
without status migrainosus G43.719
intractable
with status migrainosus G43.711
without status migrainosus G43.719
not intractable
with status migrainosus G43.701
without status migrainosus G43.709
without refractory migraine G43.709
with status migrainosus G43.701
without status migrainosus G43.709
intractable
with status migrainosus G43.011
without status migrainosus G43.019
not intractable
with status migrainosus G43.001
without status migrainosus G43.009
without mention of refractory migraine G43.009
with status migrainosus G43.001
without status migrainosus G43.009
without refractory migraine G43.909
with status migrainosus G43.901
without status migrainosus G43.919
Migrant, social Z59.0
Migration, anxiety concerning Z60.3
Migratory, migrating —*see also* condition
person Z59.0
testis Q55.29
Mikity-Wilson disease or syndrome P27.0
Mikulicz' disease or syndrome K11.8
Miliaria L74.3
alba L74.1
apocrine L75.2
crystallina L74.1
profunda L74.2
rubra L74.0
tropicalis L74.2
Miliary —*see* condition
Milium L72.0
colloid L57.8
Milk
crust L21.0
excessive secretion O92.6
poisoning —*see* Poisoning, food, noxious
retention O92.79
sickness —*see* Poisoning, food, noxious
spots I31.0
Milk-alkali disease or syndrome E83.52
Milk-leg (deep vessels) (nonpuerperal) —*see* Embolism, vein, lower extremity
complicating pregnancy O22.3-
puerperal, postpartum, childbirth O87.1

Milkman's disease or syndrome M83.8
Milky urine —*see* Chyluria
Millard-Gubler (-Foville) paralysis or syndrome G46.3
Millar's asthma J38.5
Miller-Fisher syndrome G61.0
Mills' disease —*see* Hemiplegia
Millstone maker's pneumoconiosis J62.8
Milroy's disease (chronic hereditary edema) Q82.0
Minamata disease T56.1- ⬅
Miners' asthma or lung J60
Minkowski-Chauffard syndrome —*see* Spherocytosis
Minor —*see* condition
Minor's disease (hematomyelia) G95.19
Minot's disease (hemorrhagic disease), newborn P53
Minot-von Willebrand-Jurgens disease or syndrome (angiohemophilia) D68.0
Minus (and plus) hand (intrinsic) —*see* Deformity, limb, specified type NEC, forearm
Miosis (pupil) H57.03
Mirizzi's syndrome (hepatic duct stenosis) K83.1
Mirror writing F81.0
Misadventure (of) (prophylactic) (therapeutic) —*see also* Complications T88.9
administration of insulin (by accident) —*see* subcategory T38.3
infusion —*see* Complications, infusion
local applications (of fomentations, plasters, etc.) T88.9
burn or scald —*see* Burn
specified NEC T88.8
medical care (early) (late) T88.9
adverse effect of drugs or chemicals —*see* Table of Drugs and Chemicals
medical care (early) (late)
burn or scald —*see* Burn
specified NEC T88.8
specified NEC T88.8
surgical procedure (early) (late) —*see* Complications, surgical procedure
transfusion —*see* Complications, transfusion
vaccination or other immunological procedure —*see* Complications, vaccination
Miscarriage O03.9
Misdirection, aqueous H40.83-
Misperception, sleep state F51.02
Misplaced, misplacement
ear Q17.4
kidney (acquired) N28.89
congenital Q63.2
organ or site, congenital NEC —*see* Malposition, congenital
Missed
abortion O02.1
delivery O36.4
Missing —*see also* Absence ⬅
string of intrauterine contraceptive device T83.32 ◀
Misuse of drugs F19.99
Mitchell's disease (erythromelalgia) I73.81
Mite (s) (infestation) B88.9
diarrhea B88.0
grain (itch) B88.0
hair follicle (itch) B88.0
in sputum B88.0
Mitral —*see* condition
Mittelschmerz N94.0
Mixed —*see* condition
MMN (multifocal motor neuropathy) G61.82 ◀
MNGIE (Mitochondrial Neurogastrointestinal Encephalopathy) syndrome E88.49
Mobile, mobility
cecum Q43.3
excessive —*see* Hypermobility
gallbladder, congenital Q44.1

◀ New ⬅ Revised ~~deleted~~ Deleted

Mobile, mobility *(Continued)*
kidney N28.89
organ or site, congenital NEC —*see* Malposition, congenital
Mobitz heart block (atrioventricular) I44.1
Moebius, Möbius
disease (ophthalmoplegic migraine) —*see* Migraine, ophthalmoplegic
syndrome Q87.0
congenital oculofacial paralysis (with other anomalies) Q87.0
ophthalmoplegic migraine —*see* Migraine, ophthalmoplegic
Moeller's glossitis K14.0
Mohr's syndrome (Types I and II) Q87.0
Mola destruens D39.2
Molar pregnancy O02.0
Molarization of premolars K00.2
Molding, head (during birth) - omit code
Mole (pigmented) —*see also* Nevus
blood O02.0
Breus' O02.0
cancerous —*see* Melanoma
carneous O02.0
destructive D39.2
fleshy O02.0
hydatid, hydatidiform (benign) (complicating pregnancy) (delivered) (undelivered) O01.9
classical O01.0
complete O01.0
incomplete O01.1
invasive D39.2
malignant D39.2
partial O01.1
intrauterine O02.0
invasive (hydatidiform) D39.2
malignant
meaning
malignant hydatidiform mole D39.2
melanoma —*see* Melanoma
nonhydatidiform O02.0
nonpigmented —*see* Nevus
pregnancy NEC O02.0
skin —*see* Nevus
tubal O00.10 ⇐
with intrauterine pregnancy O00.11 ◀
vesicular —*see* Mole, hydatidiform
Molimen, molimina (menstrual) N94.3
Molluscum contagiosum (epitheliale) B08.1
Mönckeberg's arteriosclerosis, disease, or sclerosis —*see* Arteriosclerosis, extremities
Mondini's malformation (cochlea) Q16.5
Mondor's disease I80.8
Monge's disease T70.29
Monilethrix (congenital) Q84.1
Moniliasis —*see also* Candidiasis B37.9
neonatal P37.5
Monitoring (encounter for)
therapeutic drug level Z51.81
Monkey malaria B53.1
Monkeypox B04
Monoarthritis M13.10
ankle M13.17-
elbow M13.12-
foot joint M13.17-
hand joint M13.14-
hip M13.15-
knee M13.16-
shoulder M13.11-
wrist M13.13-
Monoblastic —*see* condition
Monochromat (ism), **monochromatopsia** (acquired) (congenital) H53.51
Monocytic —*see* condition
Monocytopenia D72.818
Monocytosis (symptomatic) D72.821
Monomania —*see* Psychosis
Mononeuritis G58.9
cranial nerve —*see* Disorder, nerve, cranial
Mononeuritis *(Continued)*
femoral nerve G57.2-
lateral
cutaneous nerve of thigh G57.1-
popliteal nerve G57.3-
lower limb G57.9-
specified nerve NEC G57.8-
medial popliteal nerve G57.4-
median nerve G56.1-
multiplex G58.7
plantar nerve G57.6-
posterior tibial nerve G57.5-
radial nerve G56.3-
sciatic nerve G57.0-
specified NEC G58.8
tibial nerve G57.4-
ulnar nerve G56.2-
upper limb G56.9-
specified nerve NEC G56.8-
vestibular —*see* subcategory H93.3
Mononeuropathy G58.9
carpal tunnel syndrome —*see* Syndrome, carpal tunnel
diabetic NEC —*see* E08-E13 with .41
femoral nerve —*see* Lesion, nerve, femoral
ilioinguinal nerve G57.8-
in diseases classified elsewhere —*see* category G59
intercostal G58.0
lower limb G57.9-
causalgia —*see* Causalgia, lower limb
femoral nerve —*see* Lesion, nerve, femoral
meralgia paresthetica G57.1-
plantar nerve —*see* Lesion, nerve, plantar
popliteal nerve —*see* Lesion, nerve, popliteal
sciatic nerve —*see* Lesion, nerve, sciatic
specified NEC G57.8-
tarsal tunnel syndrome —*see* Syndrome, tarsal tunnel
median nerve —*see* Lesion, nerve, median
multiplex G58.7
obturator nerve G57.8-
popliteal nerve —*see* Lesion, nerve, popliteal
radial nerve —*see* Lesion, nerve, radial
saphenous nerve G57.8-
specified NEC G58.8
tarsal tunnel syndrome —*see* Syndrome, tarsal tunnel
tuberculous A17.83
ulnar nerve —*see* Lesion, nerve, ulnar
upper limb G56.9-
carpal tunnel syndrome —*see* Syndrome, carpal tunnel
causalgia —*see* Causalgia
median nerve —*see* Lesion, nerve, median
radial nerve —*see* Lesion, nerve, radial
specified site NEC G56.8-
ulnar nerve —*see* Lesion, nerve, ulnar
Mononucleosis, infectious B27.90
with
complication NEC B27.99
meningitis B27.92
polyneuropathy B27.91
cytomegaloviral B27.10
with
complication NEC B27.19
meningitis B27.12
polyneuropathy B27.11
Epstein-Barr (virus) B27.00
with
complication NEC B27.09
meningitis B27.02
polyneuropathy B27.01
gammaherpesviral B27.00
with
complication NEC B27.09
meningitis B27.02
polyneuropathy B27.01
Mononucleosis, infectious *(Continued)*
specified NEC B27.80
with
complication NEC B27.89
meningitis B27.82
polyneuropathy B27.81
Monoplegia G83.3-
congenital (cerebral) G80.8
spastic G80.1
embolic (current episode) I63.4- ⇐
following
cerebrovascular disease
cerebral infarction
lower limb I69.34-
upper limb I69.33-
intracerebral hemorrhage
lower limb I69.14-
upper limb I69.13-
lower limb I69.94-
nontraumatic intracranial hemorrhage NEC
lower limb I69.24-
upper limb I69.23-
specified disease NEC
lower limb I69.84-
upper limb I69.83-
stroke NOS
lower limb I69.34-
upper limb I69.33-
subarachnoid hemorrhage
lower limb I69.04-
upper limb I69.03-
upper limb I69.93-
hysterical (transient) F44.4
lower limb G83.1-
psychogenic (conversion reaction) F44.4
thrombotic (current episode) I63.3- ⇐
transient R29.818
upper limb G83.2-
Monorchism, monorchidism Q55.0
Monosomy —*see also* Deletion, chromosome Q93.9
specified NEC Q93.89
whole chromosome
meiotic nondisjunction Q93.0
mitotic nondisjunction Q93.1
mosaicism Q93.1
X Q96.9
Monster, monstrosity (single) Q89.7
acephalic Q00.0
twin Q89.4
Monteggia's fracture (-dislocation) S52.27-
Mooren's ulcer (cornea) —*see* Ulcer, cornea, Mooren's
Moore's syndrome —*see* Epilepsy, specified NEC
Mooser-Neill reaction A75.2
Mooser's bodies A75.2
Morbidity not stated or unknown R69
Morbilli —*see* Measles
Morbus —*see also* Disease
angelicus, anglorum E55.0
Beigel B36.2
caducus —*see* Epilepsy
celiacus K90.0
comitialis —*see* Epilepsy
cordis —*see also* Disease, heart I51.9
valvulorum —*see* Endocarditis
coxae senilis M16.9
tuberculous A18.02
hemorrhagicus neonatorum P53
maculosus neonatorum P54.5
Morel (-Stewart)(-Morgagni) **syndrome** M85.2
Morel-Kraepelin disease —*see* Schizophrenia
Morel-Moore syndrome M85.2
Morgagni's
cyst, organ, hydatid, or appendage
female Q50.5
male (epididymal) Q55.4
testicular Q55.29
syndrome M85.2

M

Morgagni-Stewart-Morel syndrome M85.2
Morgagni-Stokes-Adams syndrome I45.9
Morgagni-Turner (-Albright) **syndrome** Q96.9
Moria F07.0
Moron (I.Q. 50-69) F70
Morphea L94.0
Morphinism (without remission) F11.20
  with remission F11.21
Morphinomania (without remission) F11.20
  with remission F11.21
Morquio (-Ullrich)(-Brailsford) **disease or syndrome** —*see* Mucopolysaccharidosis
Mortification (dry) (moist) —*see* Gangrene
Morton's metatarsalgia (neuralgia)(neuroma) (syndrome) G57.6
Morvan's disease or syndrome G60.8
Mosaicism, mosaic (autosomal) (chromosomal)
  45,X/46,XX Q96.3
  45,X/other cell lines NEC with abnormal sex chromosome Q96.4
  sex chromosome
    female Q97.8
    lines with various numbers of X chromosomes Q97.2
    male Q98.7
  XY Q96.3
Moschowitz' disease M31.1
Mother yaw A66.0
Motion sickness (from travel, any vehicle) (from roundabouts or swings) T75.3
Mottled, mottling, teeth (enamel) (endemic) (nonendemic) K00.3
Mounier-Kuhn syndrome Q32.4
  with bronchiectasis J47.9
    exacerbation (acute) J47.1
    lower respiratory infection J47.0
  acquired J98.09
    with bronchiectasis J47.9
      with
        exacerbation (acute) J47.1
        lower respiratory infection J47.0
Mountain
  sickness T70.29
    with polycythemia , acquired (acute) D75.1
  tick fever A93.2
Mouse, joint —*see* Loose, body, joint
  knee M23.4-
Mouth —*see* condition
Movable
  coccyx —*see* subcategory M53.2
  kidney N28.89
    congenital Q63.8
  spleen D73.89
Movements, dystonic R25.8
Moyamoya disease I67.5
MRSA (Methicillin resistant Staphylococcus aureus)
  infection A49.02
    as the cause of diseases classified elsewhere B95.62
  sepsis A41.02
MSSA (Methicillin susceptible Staphylococcus aureus)
  infection A49.01
    as the cause of diseases classified elsewhere B95.61
  sepsis A41.01
Mucha-Habermann disease L41.0
Mucinosis (cutaneous) (focal) (papular) (reticular erythematous) (skin) L98.5
  oral K13.79
Mucocele
  appendix K38.8
  buccal cavity K13.79
  gallbladder K82.1
  lacrimal sac, chronic H04.43-
  nasal sinus J34.1
  nose J34.1
  salivary gland (any) K11.6
  sinus (accessory) (nasal) J34.1
  turbinate (bone) (middle) (nasal) J34.1
  uterus N85.8
Mucolipidosis
  I E77.1
  II, III E77.0
  IV E75.11
Mucopolysaccharidosis E76.3
  beta-gluduronidase deficiency E76.29
  cardiopathy E76.3 *[I52]*
  Hunter's syndrome E76.1
  Hurler's syndrome E76.01
  Hurler-Scheie syndrome E76.02
  Maroteaux-Lamy syndrome E76.29
  Morquio syndrome E76.219
    A E76.210
    B E76.211
    classic E76.210
  Sanfilippo syndrome E76.22
  Scheie's syndrome E76.03
  specified NEC E76.29
  type
    I
      Hurler's syndrome E76.01
      Hurler-Scheie syndrome E76.02
      Scheie's syndrome E76.03
    II E76.1
    III E76.22
    IV E76.219
    IVA E76.210
    IVB E76.211
    VI E76.29
    VII E76.29
Mucormycosis B46.5
  cutaneous B46.3
  disseminated B46.4
  gastrointestinal B46.2
  generalized B46.4
  pulmonary B46.0
  rhinocerebral B46.1
  skin B46.3
  subcutaneous B46.3
Mucositis (ulcerative) K12.30
  due to drugs NEC K12.32
  gastrointestinal K92.81
  mouth (oral) (oropharyngeal) K12.30
    due to antineoplastic therapy K12.31
    due to drugs NEC K12.32
    due to radiation K12.33
    specified NEC K12.39
    viral K12.39
  nasal J34.81
  oral cavity —*see* Mucositis, mouth
  oral soft tissues —*see* Mucositis, mouth
  vagina and vulva N76.81
Mucositis necroticans agranulocytica —*see* Agranulocytosis
Mucous —*see also* condition
  patches (syphilitic) A51.39
    congenital A50.07
Mucoviscidosis E84.9
  with meconium obstruction E84.11
Mucus
  asphyxia or suffocation —*see* Asphyxia, mucus
  in stool R19.5
  plug —*see* Asphyxia, mucus
Muguet B37.0
Mulberry molars (congenital syphilis) A50.52
Müllerian mixed tumor
  specified site —*see* Neoplasm, malignant, by site
  unspecified site C54.9
Multicystic kidney (development) Q61.4
Multiparity (grand) Z64.1
  affecting management of pregnancy, labor and delivery (supervision only) O09.4-
  requiring contraceptive management —*see* Contraception
Multipartita placenta O43.19-
Multiple, multiplex —*see also* condition
  digits (congenital) Q69.9
Multiple, multiplex *(Continued)*
  endocrine neoplasia —*see* Neoplasia, endocrine, multiple [MEN]
  personality F44.81
Mumps B26.9
  arthritis B26.85
  complication NEC B26.89
  encephalitis B26.2
  hepatitis B26.81
  meningitis (aseptic) B26.1
  meningoencephalitis B26.2
  myocarditis B26.82
  oophoritis B26.89
  orchitis B26.0
  pancreatitis B26.3
  polyneuropathy B26.84
Mumu —*see also* Infestation, filarial B74.9 *[N51]*
Münchhausen's syndrome —*see* Disorder, factitious
Münchmeyer's syndrome —*see* Myositis, ossificans, progressiva
Mural —*see* condition
Murmur (cardiac) (heart) (organic) R01.1
  abdominal R19.15
  aortic (valve) —*see* Endocarditis, aortic
  benign R01.0
  diastolic —*see* Endocarditis
  Flint I35.1
  functional R01.0
  Graham Steell I37.1
  innocent R01.0
  mitral (valve) —*see* Insufficiency, mitral
  nonorganic R01.0
  presystolic, mitral —*see* Insufficiency, mitral
  pulmonic (valve) I37.8
  systolic R01.1 ⬅
  tricuspid (valve) I07.9
  valvular —*see* Endocarditis
Murri's disease (intermittent hemoglobinuria) D59.6
Muscle, muscular —*see also* condition
  carnitine (palmityltransferase) deficiency E71.314
Musculoneuralgia —*see* Neuralgia
Mushroom-workers' (pickers') **disease or lung** J67.5
Mushrooming hip —*see* Derangement, joint, specified NEC, hip
Mutation (s)
  factor V Leiden D68.51
  surfactant, of lung J84.83
  prothrombin gene D68.52
Mutism —*see also* Aphasia
  deaf (acquired) (congenital) NEC H91.3
  elective (adjustment reaction) (childhood) F94.0
  hysterical F44.4
  selective (childhood) F94.0
MVD (microvillus inclusion disease) Q43.8
MVID (microvillus inclusion disease) Q43.8
Myalgia M79.1
  epidemic (cervical) B33.0
  traumatic NEC T14.8
Myasthenia G70.9
  congenital G70.2
  cordis —*see* Failure, heart
  developmental G70.2
  gravis G70.00
    with exacerbation (acute) G70.01
    in crisis G70.01
    neonatal, transient P94.0
    pseudoparalytica G70.00
      with exacerbation (acute) G70.01
      in crisis G70.01
  stomach, psychogenic F45.8
  syndrome
    in
      diabetes mellitus —*see* E08-E13 with .44
      neoplastic disease —*see also* Neoplasm D49.9 *[G73.3]*

◀ New ⬅ Revised ~~deleted~~ Deleted

Myasthenia *(Continued)*
syndrome *(Continued)*
in *(Continued)*
pernicious anemia D51.0 *[G73.3]*
thyrotoxicosis E05.90 *[G73.3]*
with thyroid storm E05.91 *[G73.3]*
Myasthenic M62.81
Mycelium infection B49
Mycetismus —*see* Poisoning, food, noxious, mushroom
Mycetoma B47.9
actinomycotic B47.1
bone (mycotic) B47.9 *[M90.80]*
eumycotic B47.0
foot B47.9
actinomycotic B47.1
mycotic B47.0
madurae NEC B47.9
mycotic B47.0
maduromycotic B47.0
mycotic B47.0
nocardial B47.1
Mycobacteriosis —*see* Mycobacterium
Mycobacterium, mycobacterial (infection) A31.9
anonymous A31.9
atypical A31.9
cutaneous A31.1
pulmonary A31.0
tuberculous —*see* Tuberculosis, pulmonary
specified site NEC A31.8
avium (intracellulare complex) A31.0
balnei A31.1
Battey A31.0
chelonei A31.8
cutaneous A31.1
extrapulmonary systemic A31.8
fortuitum A31.8
intracellulare (Battey bacillus) A31.0
kakaferifu A31.8
kansasii (yellow bacillus) A31.0
kasongo A31.8
leprae —*see also* Leprosy A30.9
luciflavum A31.1
marinum (M. balnei) A31.1
nonspecific —*see* Mycobacterium, atypical
pulmonary (atypical) A31.0
tuberculous —*see* Tuberculosis, pulmonary
scrofulaceum A31.8
simiae A31.8
systemic, extrapulmonary A31.8
szulgai A31.8
terrae A31.8
triviale A31.8
tuberculosis (human, bovine) —*see* Tuberculosis
ulcerans A31.1
xenopi A31.8
Mycoplasma (M.) pneumoniae, as cause of disease classified elsewhere B96.0
Mycosis, mycotic B49
cutaneous NEC B36.9
ear B36.9 ⇐
in ◀
aspergillosis B44.89 ◀
candidiasis B37.84 ◀
moniliasis B37.84 ◀
fungoides (extranodal) (solid organ) C84.0-
mouth B37.0
nails B35.1
opportunistic B48.8
skin NEC B36.9
specified NEC B48.8
stomatitis B37.0
vagina, vaginitis (candidal) B37.3
Mydriasis (pupil) H57.04
Myelatelia Q06.1
Myelinolysis, pontine, central G37.2
Myelitis (acute) (ascending) (childhood) (chronic) (descending) (diffuse) (disseminated) (idiopathic) (pressure) (progressive) (spinal cord) (subacute) —*see also* Encephalitis G04.91
herpes simplex B00.82
herpes zoster B02.24
in diseases classified elsewhere G05.4
necrotizing, subacute G37.4
optic neuritis in G36.0
postchickenpox B01.12
postherpetic B02.24
postimmunization G04.02
postinfectious NEC G04.89
postvaccinal G04.02
specified NEC G04.89
syphilitic (transverse) A52.14
toxic G92
transverse (in demyelinating diseases of central nervous system) G37.3
tuberculous A17.82
varicella B01.12
Myeloblastic —*see* condition
Myeloblastoma
granular cell —*see also* Neoplasm, connective tissue
malignant —*see* Neoplasm, connective tissue, malignant
tongue D10.1
Myelocele —*see* Spina bifida
Myelocystocele —*see* Spina bifida
Myelocytic —*see* condition
Myelodysplasia D46.9
specified NEC D46.Z
spinal cord (congenital) Q06.1
Myelodysplastic syndrome D46.9
with
5q deletion D46.C
isolated del (5q) chromosomal abnormality C46.C
specified NEC D46.Z
Myeloencephalitis —*see* Encephalitis
Myelofibrosis D75.81
with myeloid metaplasia D47.4
acute C94.4-
idiopathic (chronic) D47.4
primary D47.1
secondary D75.81
in myeloproliferative disease D47.4
Myelogenous —*see* condition
Myeloid —*see* condition
Myelokathexis D70.9
Myeloleukodystrophy E75.29
Myelolipoma —*see* Lipoma
Myeloma (multiple) C90.0-
monostotic C90.3
plasma cell C90.0-
plasma cell C90.0-
solitary —*see also* Plasmacytoma, solitary C90.3-
Myelomalacia G95.89
Myelomatosis C90.0-
Myelomeningitis —*see* Meningoencephalitis
Myelomeningocele (spinal cord) —*see* Spina bifida
Myelo-osteo-musculodysplasia hereditaria Q79.8
Myelopathic
anemia D64.89
muscle atrophy —*see* Atrophy, muscle, spinal
pain syndrome G89.0
Myelopathy (spinal cord) G95.9
drug-induced G95.89
in (due to)
degeneration or displacement, intervertebral disc NEC —*see* Disorder, disc, with, myelopathy
infection —*see* Encephalitis
intervertebral disc disorder —*see also* Disorder, disc, with, myelopathy
mercury —*see* subcategory T56.1
Myelopathy *(Continued)*
in (due to) *(Continued)*
neoplastic disease —*see also* Neoplasm D49.9 *[G99.2]*
pernicious anemia D51.0 *[G99.2]*
spondylosis —*see* Spondylosis, with myelopathy NEC
necrotic (subacute) (vascular) G95.19
radiation-induced G95.89
spondylogenic NEC —*see* Spondylosis, with myelopathy NEC
toxic G95.89
transverse, acute G37.3
vascular G95.19
vitamin B12 E53.8 *[G32.0]*
Myelophthisis D61.82
Myeloradiculitis G04.91
Myeloradiculodysplasia (spinal) Q06.1
Myelosarcoma C92.3-
Myelosclerosis D75.89
with myeloid metaplasia D47.4
disseminated, of nervous system G35
megakaryocytic D47.4
with myeloid metaplasia D47.4
Myelosis
acute C92.0-
aleukemic C92.9-
chronic D47.1
erythremic (acute) C94.0-
megakaryocytic C94.2-
nonleukemic D72.828
subacute C92.9-
Myiasis (cavernous) B87.9
aural B87.4
creeping B87.0
cutaneous B87.0
dermal B87.0
ear (external) (middle) B87.4
eye B87.2
genitourinary B87.81
intestinal B87.82
laryngeal B87.3
nasopharyngeal B87.3
ocular B87.2
orbit B87.2
skin B87.0
specified site NEC B87.89
traumatic B87.1
wound B87.1
Myoadenoma, prostate —*see* Hyperplasia, prostate
Myoblastoma
granular cell —*see also* Neoplasm, connective tissue, benign
malignant —*see* Neoplasm, connective tissue, malignant
tongue D10.1
Myocardial —*see* condition
Myocardiopathy (congestive) (constrictive) (familial) (hypertrophic nonobstructive) (idiopathic) (infiltrative) (obstructive) (primary) (restrictive) (sporadic) —*see also* Cardiomyopathy I42.9
alcoholic I42.6
cobalt-beer I42.6
glycogen storage E74.02 *[I43]*
hypertrophic obstructive I42.1
in (due to)
beriberi E51.12
cardiac glycogenosis E74.02 *[I43]*
Friedreich's ataxia G11.1 *[I43]*
myotonia atrophica G71.11 *[I43]*
progressive muscular dystrophy G71.0 *[I43]*
obscure (African) I42.8
secondary I42.9
thyrotoxic E05.90 *[I43]*
with storm E05.91 *[I43]*
toxic NEC I42.7

M

Myocarditis (with arteriosclerosis) (chronic) (fibroid) (interstitial) (old) (progressive) (senile) I51.4
with
rheumatic fever (conditions in I00) I09.0
active —*see* Myocarditis, acute, rheumatic
inactive or quiescent (with chorea) I09.0
active I40.9
rheumatic I01.2
with chorea (acute) (rheumatic) (Sydenham's) I02.0
acute or subacute (interstitial) I40.9
due to
streptococcus (beta-hemolytic) I01.2
idiopathic I40.1
rheumatic I01.2
with chorea (acute) (rheumatic) (Sydenham's) I02.0
specified NEC I40.8
aseptic of newborn B33.22
bacterial (acute) I40.0
Coxsackie (virus) B33.22
diphtheritic A36.81
eosinophilic I40.1
epidemic of newborn (Coxsackie) B33.22
Fiedler's (acute) (isolated) I40.1
giant cell (acute) (subacute) I40.1
gonococcal A54.83
granulomatous (idiopathic) (isolated) (nonspecific) I40.1
hypertensive —*see* Hypertension, heart
idiopathic (granulomatous) I40.1
in (due to)
diphtheria A36.81
epidemic louse-borne typhus A75.0 *[I41]*
Lyme disease A69.29
sarcoidosis D86.85
scarlet fever A38.1
toxoplasmosis (acquired) B58.81
typhoid A01.02
typhus NEC A75.9 *[I41]*
infective I40.0
influenzal —*see* Influenza, with, myocarditis
isolated (acute) I40.1
meningococcal A39.52
mumps B26.82
nonrheumatic, active I40.9
parenchymatous I40.9
pneumococcal I40.0
rheumatic (chronic) (inactive) (with chorea) I09.0
active or acute I01.2
with chorea (acute) (rheumatic) (Sydenham's) I02.0
rheumatoid —*see* Rheumatoid, carditis
septic I40.0
staphylococcal I40.0
suppurative I40.0
syphilitic (chronic) A52.06
toxic I40.8
rheumatic —*see* Myocarditis, acute, rheumatic
tuberculous A18.84
typhoid A01.02
valvular —*see* Endocarditis
virus, viral I40.0
of newborn (Coxsackie) B33.22
Myocardium, myocardial —*see* condition
Myocardosis —*see* Cardiomyopathy
Myoclonus, myoclonic, myoclonia (familial) (essential) (multifocal) (simplex) G25.3
drug-induced G25.3
epilepsy —*see also* Epilepsy, generalized, specified NEC G40.4-
familial (progressive) G25.3
epileptica G40.409
with status epilepticus G40.401
facial G51.3
familial progressive G25.3
Friedreich's G25.3
Myoclonus, myoclonic, myoclonia *(Continued)*
jerks G25.3
massive G25.3
palatal G25.3
pharyngeal G25.3
Myocytolysis I51.5
Myodiastasis —*see* Diastasis, muscle
Myoendocarditis —*see* Endocarditis
Myoepithelioma —*see* Neoplasm, benign, by site
Myofasciitis (acute) —*see* Myositis
Myofibroma —*see also* Neoplasm, connective tissue, benign
uterus (cervix) (corpus) —*see* Leiomyoma
Myofibromatosis D48.1
infantile Q89.8
Myofibrosis M62.89
heart —*see* Myocarditis
scapulohumeral —*see* Lesion, shoulder, specified NEC
Myofibrositis M79.7
scapulohumeral —*see* Lesion, shoulder, specified NEC
Myoglobulinuria, myoglobinuria (primary) R82.1
Myokymia, facial G51.4
Myolipoma —*see* Lipoma
Myoma —*see also* Neoplasm, connective tissue, benign
malignant —*see* Neoplasm, connective tissue, malignant
prostate D29.1
uterus (cervix) (corpus) —*see* Leiomyoma
Myomalacia M62.89
Myometritis —*see* Endometritis
Myometrium —*see* condition
Myonecrosis, clostridial A48.0
Myopathy G72.9
acute
necrotizing G72.81
quadriplegic G72.81
alcoholic G72.1
benign congenital G71.2
central core G71.2
centronuclear G71.2
congenital (benign) G71.2
critical illness G72.81
distal G71.0
drug-induced G72.0
endocrine NEC E34.9 *[G73.7]*
extraocular muscles H05.82-
facioscapulohumeral G71.0
hereditary G71.9
specified NEC G71.8
immune NEC G72.49
in (due to)
Addison's disease E27.1 *[G73.7]*
alcohol G72.1
amyloidosis E85.0 *[G73.7]*
cretinism E00.9 *[G73.7]*
Cushing's syndrome E24.9 *[G73.7]*
drugs G72.0
endocrine disease NEC E34.9 *[G73.7]*
giant cell arteritis M31.6 *[G73.7]*
glycogen storage disease E74.00 *[G73.7]*
hyperadrenocorticism E24.9 *[G73.7]*
hyperparathyroidism NEC E21.3 *[G73.7]*
hypoparathyroidism E20.9 *[G73.7]*
hypopituitarism E23.0 *[G73.7]*
hypothyroidism E03.9 *[G73.7]*
infectious disease NEC B99 *[G73.7]*
lipid storage disease E75.6 *[G73.7]*
metabolic disease NEC E88.9 *[G73.7]*
myxedema E03.9 *[G73.7]*
parasitic disease NEC B89 *[G73.7]*
polyarteritis nodosa M30.0 *[G73.7]*
rheumatoid arthritis —*see* Rheumatoid, myopathy
sarcoidosis D86.87
scleroderma M34.82
sicca syndrome M35.03
Myopathy *(Continued)*
in (due to) *(Continued)*
Sjögren's syndrome M35.03
systemic lupus erythematosus M32.19
thyrotoxicosis (hyperthyroidism) E05.90 *[G73.7]*
with thyroid storm E05.91 *[G73.7]*
toxic agent NEC G72.2
inflammatory NEC G72.49
intensive care (ICU) G72.81
limb-girdle G71.0
mitochondrial NEC G71.3
myotubular G71.2
mytonic, proximal (PROMM) G71.11
nemaline G71.2
ocular G71.0
oculopharyngeal G71.0
of critical illness G72.81
primary G71.9
specified NEC G71.8
progressive NEC G72.89
proximal myotonic (PROMM) G71.11
rod G71.2
scapulohumeral G71.0
specified NEC G72.89
toxic G72.2
Myopericarditis —*see also* Pericarditis
chronic rheumatic I09.2
Myopia (axial) (congenital) H52.1-
degenerative (malignant) H44.2-
malignant H44.2-
pernicious H44.2-
progressive high (degenerative) H44.2-
Myosarcoma —*see* Neoplasm, connective tissue, malignant
Myosis (pupil) H57.03
stromal (endolymphatic) D39.0
Myositis M60.9
clostridial A48.0
due to posture —*see* Myositis, specified type NEC
epidemic B33.0
fibrosa or fibrous (chronic), Volkmann's T79.6
foreign body granuloma —*see* Granuloma, foreign body
in (due to)
bilharziasis B65.9 *[M63.8-]*
cysticercosis B69.81
leprosy A30.9 *[M63.8-]*
mycosis B49 *[M63.8-]*
sarcoidosis D86.87
schistosomiasis B65.9 *[M63.8-]*
syphilis
late A52.78
secondary A51.49
toxoplasmosis (acquired) B58.82
trichinellosis B75 *[M63.8-]*
tuberculosis A18.09
inclusion body [IBM] G72.41
infective M60.009
arm M60.002
left M60.001
right M60.000
leg M60.005
left M60.004
right M60.003
lower limb M60.005
ankle M60.07-
foot M60.07-
lower leg M60.06-
thigh M60.05-
toe M60.07-
multiple sites M60.09
specified site NEC M60.08
upper limb M60.002
finger M60.04-
forearm M60.03-
hand M60.04-
shoulder region M60.01-
upper arm M60.02-

Myositis *(Continued)*
interstitial M60.10
ankle M60.17-
foot M60.17-
forearm M60.13-
hand M60.14-
lower leg M60.16-
multiple sites M60.19
shoulder region M60.11-
specified site NEC M60.18
thigh M60.15-
upper arm M60.12-
mycotic B49 *[M63.8-]*
ossificans or ossifying (circumscripta) —*see also* Ossification, muscle, specified NEC
in (due to)
burns M61.30
ankle M61.37-
foot M61.37-
forearm M61.33-
hand M61.34-
lower leg M61.36-
multiple sites M61.39
pelvic region M61.35-
shoulder region M61.31-
specified site NEC M61.38
thigh M61.35-
upper arm M61.32-
quadriplegia or paraplegia M61.20
ankle M61.27-
foot M61.27-
forearm M61.23-
hand M61.24-
lower leg M61.26-
multiple sites M61.29
pelvic region M61.25-
shoulder region M61.21-
specified site NEC M61.28
thigh M61.25-
upper arm M61.22-
progressiva M61.10
ankle M61.17-
finger M61.14-
foot M61.17-
forearm M61.13-
hand M61.14-
lower leg M61.16-

Myositis *(Continued)*
ossificans or ossifying *(Continued)*
progressiva *(Continued)*
multiple sites M61.19
pelvic region M61.15-
shoulder region M61.11-
specified site NEC M61.18
thigh M61.15-
toe M61.17-
upper arm M61.12-
traumatica M61.00
ankle M61.07-
foot M61.07-
forearm M61.03-
hand M61.04-
lower leg M61.06-
multiple sites M61.09
pelvic region M61.05-
shoulder region M61.01-
specified site NEC M61.08
thigh M61.05-
upper arm M61.02-
purulent —*see* Myositis, infective
specified type NEC M60.80
ankle M60.87-
foot M60.87-
forearm M60.83-
hand M60.84-
lower leg M60.86-
multiple sites M60.89
pelvic region M60.85-
shoulder region M60.81-
specified site NEC M60.88
thigh M60.85-
upper arm M60.82-
suppurative —*see* Myositis, infective
traumatic (old) —*see* Myositis, specified type NEC
Myospasia impulsiva F95.2
Myotonia (acquisita) (intermittens) M62.89
atrophica G71.11
chondrodystrophic G71.13
congenita (acetazolamide responsive) (dominant) (recessive) G71.12
drug-induced G71.14
dystrophica G71.11
fluctuans G71.19

Myotonia *(Continued)*
levior G71.12
permanens G71.19
symptomatic G71.19
Myotonic pupil —*see* Anomaly, pupil, function, tonic pupil
Myriapodiasis B88.2
Myringitis H73.2-
with otitis media —*see* Otitis, media
acute H73.00-
bullous H73.01-
specified NEC H73.09-
bullous —*see* Myringitis, acute, bullous
chronic H73.1-
Mysophobia F40.228
Mytilotoxism —*see* Poisoning, fish
Myxadenitis labialis K13.0
Myxedema (adult) (idiocy) (infantile) (juvenile) —*see also* Hypothyroidism E03.9
circumscribed E05.90
with storm E05.91
coma E03.5
congenital E00.1
cutis L98.5
localized (pretibial) E05.90
with storm E05.91
papular L98.5
Myxochondrosarcoma —*see* Neoplasm, cartilage, malignant
Myxofibroma —*see* Neoplasm, connective tissue, benign
odontogenic —*see* Cyst, calcifying odontogenic
Myxofibrosarcoma —*see* Neoplasm, connective tissue, malignant
Myxolipoma D17.9
Myxoliposarcoma —*see* Neoplasm, connective tissue, malignant
Myxoma —*see also* Neoplasm, connective tissue, benign
nerve sheath —*see* Neoplasm, nerve, benign
odontogenic —*see* Cyst, calcifying odontogenic
Myxosarcoma —*see* Neoplasm, connective tissue, malignant

N

Naegeli's
disease Q82.8
leukemia, monocytic C93.1-
Naegleriasis (with meningoencephalitis) B60.2
Naffziger's syndrome G54.0
Naga sore —*see* Ulcer, skin
Nägele's pelvis M95.5
with disproportion (fetopelvic) O33.0
causing obstructed labor O65.0
Nail —*see also* condition
biting F98.8
patella syndrome Q87.2
Nanism, nanosomia —*see* Dwarfism
Nanophyetiasis B66.8
Nanukayami A27.89
Napkin rash L22
Narcolepsy G47.419
with cataplexy G47.411
in conditions classified elsewhere G47.429
with cataplexy G47.421
Narcosis R06.89
Narcotism —*see* Dependence
NARP (Neuropathy, Ataxia and Retinitis pigmentosa) syndrome E88.49
Narrow
anterior chamber angle H40.03-
gingival width (of periodontal soft tissue) K05.5 ◀
pelvis —*see* Contraction, pelvis
Narrowing —*see also* Stenosis
artery I77.1
auditory, internal I65.8
basilar —*see* Occlusion, artery, basilar
carotid —*see* Occlusion, artery, carotid
cerebellar —*see* Occlusion, artery, cerebellar
cerebral —*see* Occlusion artery, cerebral
choroidal —*see* Occlusion, artery, cerebral, specified NEC
communicating posterior —*see* Occlusion, artery, cerebral, specified NEC
coronary —*see also* Disease, heart, ischemic, atherosclerotic
congenital Q24.5
syphilitic A50.54 *[I52]*
due to syphilis NEC A52.06
hypophyseal —*see* Occlusion, artery, cerebral, specified NEC
pontine —*see* Occlusion, artery, cerebral, specified NEC
precerebral —*see* Occlusion, artery, precerebral
vertebral —*see* Occlusion, artery, vertebral
auditory canal (external) —*see* Stenosis, external ear canal
eustachian tube —*see* Obstruction, eustachian tube
eyelid —*see* Disorder, eyelid function
larynx J38.6
mesenteric artery —*see also* Ischemia, intestine, acute K55.059 ⇐
palate M26.89
palpebral fissure —*see* Disorder, eyelid function
ureter N13.5
with infection N13.6
urethra —*see* Stricture, urethra
Narrowness, abnormal, eyelid Q10.3
Nasal —*see* condition
Nasolachrymal, nasolacrimal —*see* condition
Nasopharyngeal —*see also* condition
pituitary gland Q89.2
torticollis M43.6
Nasopharyngitis (acute) (infective) (streptococcal) (subacute) J00
chronic (suppurative) (ulcerative) J31.1
Nasopharynx, nasopharyngeal —*see* condition
Natal tooth, teeth K00.6
Nausea (without vomiting) R11.0
with vomiting R11.2
gravidarum —*see* Hyperemesis, gravidarum
marina T75.3
navalis T75.3
Navel —*see* condition
Neapolitan fever —*see* Brucellosis
Near drowning T75.1
Nearsightedness —*see* Myopia
Near-syncope R55
Nebula, cornea —*see* Opacity, cornea
Necator americanus infestation B76.1
Necatoriasis B76.1
Neck —*see* condition
Necrobiosis R68.89
lipoidica NEC L92.1
with diabetes —*see* E08-E13 with .620
Necrolysis, toxic epidermal L51.2
due to drug
correct substance properly administered —*see* Table of Drugs and Chemicals, by drug, adverse effect
overdose or wrong substance given or taken —*see* Table of Drugs and Chemicals, by drug, poisoning
Necrophilia F65.89
Necrosis, necrotic (ischemic) —*see also* Gangrene
adrenal (capsule) (gland) E27.49
amputation stump (surgical) (late) T87.50
arm T87.5-
leg T87.5-
antrum J32.0
aorta (hyaline) —*see also* Aneurysm, aorta
cystic medial —*see* Dissection, aorta
artery I77.5
bladder (aseptic) (sphincter) N32.89
bone —*see also* Osteonecrosis M87.9
aseptic or avascular —*see* Osteonecrosis
idiopathic M87.00
ethmoid J32.2
jaw M27.2
tuberculous —*see* Tuberculosis, bone
brain I67.89
breast (aseptic) (fat) (segmental) N64.1
bronchus J98.09
central nervous system NEC I67.89
cerebellar I67.89
cerebral I67.89
colon —*see also* Infarct, intestine K55.049 ⇐
cornea H18.89- ⇐
cortical (acute) (renal) N17.1
cystic medial (aorta) —*see* Dissection, aorta
dental pulp K04.1
esophagus K22.8
ethmoid (bone) J32.2
eyelid —*see* Disorder, eyelid, degenerative
fat, fatty (generalized) —*see also* Disorder, soft tissue, specified type NEC
abdominal wall K65.4
breast (aseptic) (segmental) N64.1
localized —*see* Degeneration, by site, fatty
mesentery K65.4
omentum K65.4
pancreas K86.89 ⇐
peritoneum K65.4
skin (subcutaneous), newborn P83.0
subcutaneous, due to birth injury P15.6
gallbladder —*see* Cholecystitis, acute
heart —*see* Infarct, myocardium
hip, aseptic or avascular —*see* Osteonecrosis, by type, femur
intestine (acute) (hemorrhagic) (massive) —*see also* Infarct, intestine K55.069 ⇐
jaw M27.2
kidney (bilateral) N28.0
acute N17.9
cortical (acute) (bilateral) N17.1
with ectopic or molar pregnancy O08.4
medullary (bilateral) (in acute renal failure) (papillary) N17.2
Necrosis, necrotic *(Continued)*
kidney *(Continued)*
papillary (bilateral) (in acute renal failure) N17.2
tubular N17.0
with ectopic or molar pregnancy O08.4
complicating
abortion —*see* Abortion, by type, complicated by, tubular necrosis
ectopic or molar pregnancy O08.4
pregnancy —*see* Pregnancy, complicated by, diseases of, specified type or system NEC
following ectopic or molar pregnancy O08.4
traumatic T79.5
larynx J38.7
liver (with hepatic failure) (cell) —*see* Failure, hepatic
hemorrhagic, central K76.2
lung J85.0
lymphatic gland —*see* Lymphadenitis, acute
mammary gland (fat) (segmental) N64.1
mastoid (chronic) —*see* Mastoiditis, chronic
medullary (acute) (renal) N17.2
mesentery —*see also* Infarct, intestine K55.069 ⇐
fat K65.4
mitral valve —*see* Insufficiency, mitral
myocardium, myocardial —*see* Infarct, myocardium
nose J34.0
omentum (with mesenteric infarction) —*see also* Infarct, intestine K55.069 ⇐
fat K65.4
orbit, orbital —*see* Osteomyelitis, orbit
ossicles, ear —*see* Abnormal, ear ossicles
ovary N70.92
pancreas (aseptic) (duct) (fat) K86.89 ⇐
acute (infective) —*see* Pancreatitis, acute
infective —*see* Pancreatitis, acute
papillary (acute) (renal) N17.2
perineum N90.89
peritoneum (with mesenteric infarction) —*see also* Infarct, intestine K55.069 ⇐
fat K65.4
pharynx J02.9
in granulocytopenia —*see* Neutropenia
Vincent's A69.1
phosphorus —*see* subcategory T54.2
pituitary (gland) E23.0 ⇐
postpartum O99.285 ◀
Sheehan O99.285 ◀
pressure —*see* Ulcer, pressure, by site
pulmonary J85.0
pulp (dental) K04.1
radiation —*see* Necrosis, by site
radium —*see* Necrosis, by site
renal —*see* Necrosis, kidney
sclera H15.89
scrotum N50.89 ⇐
skin or subcutaneous tissue NEC I96
spine, spinal (column) —*see also* Osteonecrosis, by type, vertebra
cord G95.19
spleen D73.5
stomach K31.89
stomatitis (ulcerative) A69.0
subcutaneous fat, newborn P83.8
subendocardial (acute) I21.4
chronic I25.89
suprarenal (capsule) (gland) E27.49
testis N50.89 ⇐
thymus (gland) E32.8
tonsil J35.8
trachea J39.8
tuberculous NEC —*see* Tuberculosis
tubular (acute) (anoxic) (renal) (toxic) N17.0
postprocedural N99.0
vagina N89.8

◀ New ⇐ Revised ~~deleted~~ Deleted

Necrosis, necrotic *(Continued)*
vertebra —*see also* Osteonecrosis, by type, vertebra
tuberculous A18.01
vulva N90.89
X-ray —*see* Necrosis, by site
Necrospermia —*see* Infertility, male
Need (for)
care provider because (of)
assistance with personal care Z74.1
continuous supervision required Z74.3
impaired mobility Z74.09
no other household member able to render care Z74.2
specified reason NEC Z74.8
immunization —*see* Vaccination
vaccination —*see* Vaccination
Neglect
adult
confirmed T74.01
history of Z91.412
suspected T76.01
child (childhood)
confirmed T74.02
history of Z62.812
suspected T76.02
emotional, in childhood Z62.898
hemispatial R41.4
left-sided R41.4
sensory R41.4
visuospatial R41.4
Neisserian infection NEC —*see* Gonococcus
Nelaton's syndrome G60.8
Nelson's syndrome E24.1
Nematodiasis (intestinal) B82.0
Ancylostoma B76.0
Neonatal —*see also* Newborn
acne L70.4
bradycardia P29.12
screening, abnormal findings on P09
tachycardia P29.11
tooth, teeth K00.6
Neonatorum —*see* condition
Neoplasia
endocrine, multiple (MEN) E31.20
type I E31.21
type IIA E31.22
type IIB E31.23
intraepithelial (histologically confirmed)
anal (AIN) (histologically confirmed) K62.82
grade I K62.82
grade II K62.82
severe D01.3
cervical glandular (histologically confirmed) D06.9
cervix (uteri) (CIN) (histologically confirmed) N87.9
glandular D06.9
grade I N87.0
grade II N87.1
grade III (severe dysplasia) —*see also* Carcinoma, cervix uteri, in situ D06.9
prostate (histologically confirmed) (PIN) N42.31 ⟸
grade I N42.31 ⟸
grade II N42.31 ⟸
grade III (severe dysplasia) D07.5 ◀
~~severe D07.5~~
vagina (histologically confirmed) (VAIN) N89.3
grade I N89.0
grade II N89.1
grade III (severe dysplasia) D07.2
vulva (histologically confirmed) (VIN) N90.3
grade I N90.0
grade II N90.1
grade III (severe dysplasia) D07.1
Neoplasm, neoplastic —*see also* Table of Neoplasms
lipomatous, benign —*see* Lipoma
Neovascularization
ciliary body —*see* Disorder, iris, vascular
cornea H16.40-
deep H16.44-
ghost vessels —*see* Ghost, vessels
localized H16.43-
pannus —*see* Pannus
iris —*see* Disorder, iris, vascular
retina H35.05-
Nephralgia N23
Nephritis, nephritic (albuminuric) (azotemic) (congenital) (disseminated) (epithelial) (familial) (focal) (granulomatous) (hemorrhagic) (infantile) (nonsuppurative, excretory) (uremic) N05.9
with
dense deposit disease N05.6
diffuse
crescentic glomerulonephritis N05.7
endocapillary proliferative glomerulonephritis N05.4
membranous glomerulonephritis N05.2
mesangial proliferative glomerulonephritis N05.3
mesangiocapillary glomerulonephritis N05.5
edema —*see* Nephrosis
focal and segmental glomerular lesions N05.1
foot process disease N04.9
glomerular lesion
diffuse sclerosing N05.8
hypocomplementemic —*see* Nephritis, membranoproliferative
IgA —*see* Nephropathy, IgA
lobular, lobulonodular —*see* Nephritis, membranoproliferative
nodular —*see* Nephritis, membranoproliferative
lesion of
glomerulonephritis, proliferative N05.8
renal necrosis N05.9
minor glomerular abnormality N05.0
specified morphological changes NEC N05.8
acute N00.9
with
dense deposit disease N00.6
diffuse
crescentic glomerulonephritis N00.7
endocapillary proliferative glomerulonephritis N00.4
membranous glomerulonephritis N00.2
mesangial proliferative glomerulonephritis N00.3
mesangiocapillary glomerulonephritis N00.5
focal and segmental glomerular lesions N00.1
minor glomerular abnormality N00.0
specified morphological changes NEC N00.8
amyloid E85.4 *[N08]*
antiglomerular basement membrane (anti-GBM) antibody NEC
in Goodpasture's syndrome M31.0
antitubular basement membrane (tubulo-interstitial) NEC N12
toxic —*see* Nephropathy, toxic
arteriolar —*see* Hypertension, kidney
arteriosclerotic —*see* Hypertension, kidney
ascending —*see* Nephritis, tubulo-interstitial
atrophic N03.9
Nephritis, nephritic *(Continued)*
Balkan (endemic) N15.0
calculous, calculus —*see* Calculus, kidney
cardiac —*see* Hypertension, kidney
cardiovascular —*see* Hypertension, kidney
chronic N03.9
with
dense deposit disease N03.6
diffuse
crescentic glomerulonephritis N03.7
endocapillary proliferative glomerulonephritis N03.4
membranous glomerulonephritis N03.2
mesangial proliferative glomerulonephritis N03.3
mesangiocapillary glomerulonephritis N03.5
focal and segmental glomerular lesions N03.1
minor glomerular abnormality N03.0
specified morphological changes NEC N03.8
arteriosclerotic —*see* Hypertension, kidney
cirrhotic N26.9
complicating pregnancy O26.83-
croupous N00.9
degenerative —*see* Nephrosis
diffuse sclerosing N05.8
due to
diabetes mellitus —*see* E08-E13 with .21
subacute bacterial endocarditis I33.0
systemic lupus erythematosus (chronic) M32.14
typhoid fever A01.09
gonococcal (acute) (chronic) A54.21
hypocomplementemic —*see* Nephritis, membranoproliferative
IgA —*see* Nephropathy, IgA
immune complex (circulating) NEC N05.8
infective —*see* Nephritis, tubulo-interstitial
interstitial —*see* Nephritis, tubulo-interstitial
lead N14.3
membranoproliferative (diffuse) (type 1 or 3) —*see also* N00-N07 with fourth character .5 N05.5
type 2 —*see also* N00-N07 with fourth character .6 N05.6
minimal change N05.0
necrotic, necrotizing NEC —*see also* N00-N07 with fourth character .8 N05.8
nephrotic —*see* Nephrosis
nodular —*see* Nephritis, membranoproliferative
polycystic Q61.3
adult type Q61.2
autosomal
dominant Q61.2
recessive NEC Q61.19
childhood type NEC Q61.19
infantile type NEC Q61.19
poststreptococcal N05.9
acute N00.9
chronic N03.9
rapidly progressive N01.9
proliferative NEC —*see also* N00-N07 with fourth character .8 N05.8
purulent —*see* Nephritis, tubulo-interstitial
rapidly progressive N01.9
with
dense deposit disease N01.6
diffuse
crescentic glomerulonephritis N01.7
endocapillary proliferative glomerulonephritis N01.4

◀ New ⟸ Revised ~~deleted~~ Deleted

Nephritis, nephritic *(Continued)*
rapidly progressive *(Continued)*
with *(Continued)*
diffuse *(Continued)*
membranous glomerulonephritis N01.2
mesangial proliferative glomerulonephritis N01.3
mesangiocapillary glomerulonephritis N01.5
focal and segmental glomerular lesions N01.1
minor glomerular abnormality N01.0
specified morphological changes NEC N01.8
salt losing or wasting NEC N28.89
saturnine N14.3
sclerosing, diffuse N05.8
septic —*see* Nephritis, tubulo-interstitial
specified pathology NEC —*see also* N00-N07 with fourth character .8 N05.8
subacute N01.9
suppurative —*see* Nephritis, tubulo-interstitial
syphilitic (late) A52.75
congenital A50.59 *[N08]*
early (secondary) A51.44
toxic —*see* Nephropathy, toxic
tubal, tubular —*see* Nephritis, tubulo-interstitial
tuberculous A18.11
tubulo-interstitial (in) N12
acute (infectious) N10
chronic (infectious) N11.9
nonobstructive N11.8
reflux-associated N11.0
obstructive N11.1
specified NEC N11.8
due to
brucellosis A23.9 *[N16]*
cryoglobulinemia D89.1 *[N16]*
glycogen storage disease E74.00 *[N16]*
Sjögren's syndrome M35.04
vascular —*see* Hypertension, kidney
war N00.9
Nephroblastoma (epithelial) (mesenchymal) C64-
Nephrocalcinosis E83.59 *[N29]*
Nephrocystitis, pustular —*see* Nephritis, tubulo-interstitial
Nephrolithiasis (congenital) (pelvis) (recurrent) —*see also* Calculus, kidney
Nephroma C64-
mesoblastic D41.0-
Nephronephritis —*see* Nephrosis
Nephronophthisis Q61.5
Nephropathia epidemica A98.5
Nephropathy —*see also* Nephritis N28.9
with
edema —*see* Nephrosis
glomerular lesion —*see* Glomerulonephritis
amyloid, hereditary E85.0
analgesic N14.0
with medullary necrosis, acute N17.2
Balkan (endemic) N15.0
chemical —*see* Nephropathy, toxic
diabetic —*see* E08-E13 with .21
drug-induced N14.2
specified NEC N14.1
focal and segmental hyalinosis or sclerosis N02.1
heavy metal-induced N14.3
hereditary NEC N07.9
with
dense deposit disease N07.6
diffuse
crescentic glomerulonephritis N07.7
endocapillary proliferative glomerulonephritis N07.4
Nephropathy *(Continued)*
hereditary NEC *(Continued)*
with *(Continued)*
diffuse *(Continued)*
membranous glomerulonephritis N07.2
mesangial proliferative glomerulonephritis N07.3
mesangiocapillary glomerulonephritis N07.5
focal and segmental glomerular lesions N07.1
minor glomerular abnormality N07.0
specified morphological changes NEC N07.8
hypercalcemic N25.89
hypertensive —*see* Hypertension, kidney
hypokalemic (vacuolar) N25.89
IgA N02.8
with glomerular lesion N02.9
focal and segmental hyalinosis or sclerosis N02.1
membranoproliferative (diffuse) N02.5
membranous (diffuse) N02.2
mesangial proliferative (diffuse) N02.3
mesangiocapillary (diffuse) N02.5
proliferative NEC N02.8
specified pathology NEC N02.8
lead N14.3
membranoproliferative (diffuse) N02.5
membranous (diffuse) N02.2
mesangial (IgA/IgG) —*see* Nephropathy, IgA
proliferative (diffuse) N02.3
mesangiocapillary (diffuse) N02.5
obstructive N13.8
phenacetin N17.2
phosphate-losing N25.0
potassium depletion N25.89
pregnancy-related O26.83-
proliferative NEC (*see also* N00-N07 with fourth character .8) N05.8
protein-losing N25.89
saturnine N14.3
sickle-cell D57.- *[N08]*
toxic NEC N14.4
due to
drugs N14.2
analgesic N14.0
specified NEC N14.1
heavy metals N14.3
vasomotor N17.0
water-losing N25.89
Nephroptosis N28.83
Nephropyosis —*see* Abscess, kidney
Nephrorrhagia N28.89
Nephrosclerosis (arteriolar) (arteriosclerotic) (chronic) (hyaline) —*see also* Hypertension, kidney
hyperplastic —*see* Hypertension, kidney
senile N26.9
Nephrosis, nephrotic (Epstein's) (syndrome) (congenital) N04.9
with
foot process disease N04.9
glomerular lesion N04.1
hypocomplementemic N04.5
acute N04.9
anoxic —*see* Nephrosis, tubular
chemical —*see* Nephrosis, tubular
cholemic K76.7
diabetic —*see* E08-E13 with .21
Finnish type (congenital) Q89.8
hemoglobin N10
hemoglobinuric —*see* Nephrosis, tubular
in
amyloidosis E85.4 *[N08]*
diabetes mellitus —*see* E08-E13 with .21
epidemic hemorrhagic fever A98.5
malaria (malariae) B52.0
ischemic —*see* Nephrosis, tubular
lipoid N04.9
Nephrosis, nephrotic *(Continued)*
lower nephron —*see* Nephrosis, tubular
malarial (malariae) B52.0
minimal change N04.0
myoglobin N10
necrotizing —*see* Nephrosis, tubular
osmotic (sucrose) N25.89
radiation N04.9
syphilitic (late) A52.75
toxic —*see* Nephrosis, tubular
tubular (acute) N17.0
postprocedural N99.0
radiation N04.9
Nephrosonephritis, hemorrhagic (endemic) A98.5
Nephrostomy
attention to Z43.6
status Z93.6
Nerve —*see also* condition
injury —*see* Injury, nerve, by body site
Nerves R45.0
Nervous —*see also* condition R45.0
heart F45.8
stomach F45.8
tension R45.0
Nervousness R45.0
Nesidioblastoma
pancreas D13.7
specified site NEC —*see* Neoplasm, benign, by site
unspecified site D13.7
Nettleship's syndrome Q82.2
Neumann's disease or syndrome L10.1
Neuralgia, neuralgic (acute) M79.2
accessory (nerve) G52.8
acoustic (nerve) —*see* subcategory H93.3
auditory (nerve) —*see* subcategory H93.3
ciliary G44.009
intractable G44.001
not intractable G44.009
cranial
nerve —*see also* Disorder, nerve, cranial
fifth or trigeminal —*see* Neuralgia, trigeminal
postherpetic, postzoster B02.29
ear —*see* subcategory H92.0
facialis vera G51.1
Fothergill's —*see* Neuralgia, trigeminal
glossopharyngeal (nerve) G52.1
Horton's G44.099
intractable G44.091
not intractable G44.099
Hunt's B02.21
hypoglossal (nerve) G52.3
infraorbital —*see* Neuralgia, trigeminal
malarial —*see* Malaria
migrainous G44.009
intractable G44.001
not intractable G44.009
Morton's G57.6-
nerve, cranial —*see* Disorder, nerve, cranial
nose G52.0
occipital M54.81
olfactory G52.0
penis N48.9
perineum R10.2
postherpetic NEC B02.29
trigeminal B02.22
pubic region R10.2
scrotum R10.2
Sluder's G44.89
specified nerve NEC G58.8
spermatic cord R10.2
sphenopalatine (ganglion) G90.09
trifacial —*see* Neuralgia, trigeminal
trigeminal G50.0
postherpetic, postzoster B02.22
vagus (nerve) G52.2
writer's F48.8
organic G25.89

Neurapraxia —*see* Injury, nerve
Neurasthenia F48.8
cardiac F45.8
gastric F45.8
heart F45.8
Neurilemmoma —*see also* Neoplasm, nerve, benign
acoustic (nerve) D33.3
malignant —*see also* Neoplasm, nerve, malignant
acoustic (nerve) C72.4
Neurilemmosarcoma —*see* Neoplasm, nerve, malignant
Neurinoma —*see* Neoplasm, nerve, benign
Neurinomatosis —*see* Neoplasm, nerve, uncertain behavior
Neuritis (rheumatoid) M79.2
abducens (nerve) —*see* Strabismus, paralytic, sixth nerve
accessory (nerve) G52.8
acoustic (nerve) —*see also* subcategory H93.3
in (due to)
infectious disease NEC B99 *[H94.0-]*
parasitic disease NEC B89 *[H94.0-]*
syphilitic A52.15
alcoholic G62.1
with psychosis —*see* Psychosis, alcoholic
amyloid, any site E85.4 *[G63]*
auditory (nerve) —*see* subcategory H93.3
brachial —*see* Radiculopathy
due to displacement, intervertebral disc —*see* Disorder, disc, cervical, with neuritis
cranial nerve
due to Lyme disease A69.22
eighth or acoustic or auditory —*see* subcategory H93.3
eleventh or accessory G52.8
fifth or trigeminal G51.0
first or olfactory G52.0
fourth or trochlear —*see* Strabismus, paralytic, fourth nerve
second or optic —*see* Neuritis, optic
seventh or facial G51.8
newborn (birth injury) P11.3
sixth or abducent —*see* Strabismus, paralytic, sixth nerve
tenth or vagus G52.2
third or oculomotor —*see* Strabismus, paralytic, third nerve
twelfth or hypoglossal G52.3
Déjérine-Sottas G60.0
diabetic (mononeuropathy) —*see* E08-E13 with .41
polyneuropathy —*see* E08-E13 with .42
due to
beriberi E51.11
displacement, prolapse or rupture, intervertebral disc —*see* Disorder, disc, with, radiculopathy
herniation, nucleus pulposus M51.9 *[G55]*
endemic E51.11
facial G51.8
newborn (birth injury) P11.3
general —*see* Polyneuropathy
geniculate ganglion G51.1
due to herpes (zoster) B02.21
gouty —*see also* Gout, by type M10.9 *[G63]* ◄
hypoglossal (nerve) G52.3
ilioinguinal (nerve) G57.9-
infectious (multiple) NEC G61.0
interstitial hypertrophic progressive G60.0
lumbar M54.16
lumbosacral M54.17
multiple —*see also* Polyneuropathy
endemic E51.11
infective, acute G61.0
multiplex endemica E51.11
nerve root —*see* Radiculopathy
oculomotor (nerve) —*see* Strabismus, paralytic, third nerve
Neuritis *(Continued)*
olfactory nerve G52.0
optic (nerve) (hereditary) (sympathetic) H46.9
with demyelination G36.0
in myelitis G36.0
nutritional H46.2
papillitis —*see* Papillitis, optic
retrobulbar H46.1-
specified type NEC H46.8
toxic H46.3
peripheral (nerve) G62.9
multiple —*see* Polyneuropathy
single —*see* Mononeuritis
pneumogastric (nerve) G52.2
postherpetic, postzoster B02.29
progressive hypertrophic interstitial G60.0
retrobulbar —*see also* Neuritis, optic, retrobulbar
in (due to)
late syphilis A52.15
meningococcal infection A39.82
meningococcal A39.82
syphilitic A52.15
sciatic (nerve) —*see also* Sciatica
due to displacement of intervertebral disc —*see* Disorder, disc, with, radiculopathy
serum —*see also* Reaction, serum T80.69
shoulder-girdle G54.5
specified nerve NEC G58.8
spinal (nerve) root —*see* Radiculopathy
syphilitic A52.15
thenar (median) G56.1-
thoracic M54.14
toxic NEC G62.2
trochlear (nerve) —*see* Strabismus, paralytic, fourth nerve
vagus (nerve) G52.2
Neuroastrocytoma —*see* Neoplasm, uncertain behavior, by site
Neuroavitaminosis E56.9 *[G99.8]*
Neuroblastoma
olfactory C30.0
specified site —*see* Neoplasm, malignant, by site
unspecified site C74.90
Neurochorioretinitis —*see* Chorioretinitis
Neurocirculatory asthenia F45.8
Neurocysticercosis B69.0
Neurocytoma —*see* Neoplasm, benign, by site
Neurodermatitis (circumscribed) (circumscripta) (local) L28.0
atopic L20.81
diffuse (Brocq) L20.81
disseminated L20.81
Neuroencephalomyelopathy, optic G36.0
Neuroepithelioma —*see also* Neoplasm, malignant, by site
olfactory C30.0
Neurofibroma —*see also* Neoplasm, nerve, benign
melanotic —*see* Neoplasm, nerve, benign
multiple —*see* Neurofibromatosis
plexiform —*see* Neoplasm, nerve, benign
Neurofibromatosis (multiple) (nonmalignant) Q85.00
acoustic Q85.02
malignant —*see* Neoplasm, nerve, malignant
specified NEC Q85.09
type 1 (von Recklinghausen) Q85.01
type 2 Q85.02
Neurofibrosarcoma —*see* Neoplasm, nerve, malignant
Neurogenic —*see also* condition
bladder (*see also* Dysfunction, bladder, neuromuscular) N31.9
cauda equina syndrome G83.4
bowel NEC K59.2
heart F45.8
Neuroglioma —*see* Neoplasm, uncertain behavior, by site
Neurolabyrinthitis (of Dix and Hallpike) —*see* Neuronitis, vestibular
Neurolathyrism —*see* Poisoning, food, noxious, plant
Neuroleprosy A30.9
Neuroma —*see also* Neoplasm, nerve, benign
acoustic (nerve) D33.3
amputation (stump) (traumatic) (surgical complication) (late) T87.3-
arm T87.3-
leg T87.3-
digital (toe) G57.6-
interdigital G58.8 ◄
lower limb toe G57.8- ◄
upper limb G56.8-
intermetatarsal G57.8-
Morton's G57.6-
nonneoplastic
arm G56.9-
leg G57.9-
lower extremity G57.9-
upper extremity G56.9-
optic (nerve) D33.3
plantar G57.6-
plexiform —*see* Neoplasm, nerve, benign
surgical (nonneoplastic)
arm G56.9-
leg G57.9-
lower extremity G57.9-
upper extremity G56.9-
Neuromyalgia —*see* Neuralgia
Neuromyasthenia (epidemic) (postinfectious) G93.3
Neuromyelitis G36.9
ascending G61.0
optica G36.0
Neuromyopathy G70.9
paraneoplastic D49.9 *[G13.0]*
Neuromyotonia (Isaacs) G71.19
Neuronevus —*see* Nevus
Neuronitis G58.9
ascending (acute) G57.2-
vestibular H81.2-
Neuroparalytic —*see* condition
Neuropathy, neuropathic G62.9
acute motor G62.81
alcoholic G62.1
with psychosis —*see* Psychosis, alcoholic
arm G56.9-
autonomic, peripheral —*see* Neuropathy, peripheral, autonomic
axillary G56.9-
bladder N31.9
atonic (motor) (sensory) N31.2
autonomous N31.2
flaccid N31.2
nonreflex N31.2
reflex N31.1
uninhibited N31.0
brachial plexus G54.0
cervical plexus G54.2
chronic
progressive segmentally demyelinating G62.89
relapsing demyelinating G62.89
Déjérine-Sottas G60.0
diabetic —*see* E08-E13 with .40
mononeuropathy —*see* E08-E13 with .41
polyneuropathy —*see* E08-E13 with .42
entrapment G58.9
iliohypogastric nerve G57.8-
ilioinguinal nerve G57.8-
lateral cutaneous nerve of thigh G57.1-
median nerve G56.0-
obturator nerve G57.8-
peroneal nerve G57.3-
posterior tibial nerve G57.5-
saphenous nerve G57.8-
ulnar nerve G56.2-

Neuropathy, neuropathic *(Continued)*
facial nerve G51.9
hereditary G60.9
motor and sensory (types I-IV) G60.0
sensory G60.8
specified NEC G60.8
hypertrophic G60.0
Charcot-Marie-Tooth G60.0
Déjérine-Sottas G60.0
interstitial progressive G60.0
of infancy G60.0
Refsum G60.1
idiopathic G60.9
progressive G60.3
specified NEC G60.8
in association with hereditary ataxia G60.2
intercostal G58.0
ischemic —*see* Disorder, nerve
Jamaica (ginger) G62.2
leg NEC G57.9-
lower extremity G57.9-
lumbar plexus G54.1
median nerve G56.1-
motor and sensory —*see also* Polyneuropathy
hereditary (types I-IV) G60.0
multifocal motor (MMN) G61.82 ◀
multiple (acute) (chronic) —*see* Polyneuropathy
optic (nerve) —*see also* Neuritis, optic
ischemic H47.01-
paraneoplastic (sensorial) (Denny Brown) D49.9 *[G13.0]*
peripheral (nerve) —*see also* Polyneuropathy G62.9
autonomic G90.9
idiopathic G90.09
in (due to)
amyloidosis E85.4 *[G99.0]*
diabetes mellitus —*see* E08-E13 with .43
endocrine disease NEC E34.9 *[G99.0]*
gout M10.00 *[G99.0]*
hyperthyroidism E05.90 *[G99.0]*
with thyroid storm E05.91 *[G99.0]*
metabolic disease NEC E88.9 *[G99.0]*
idiopathic G60.9
progressive G60.3
in (due to)
antitetanus serum G62.0
arsenic G62.2
drugs NEC G62.0
lead G62.2
organophosphate compounds G62.2
toxic agent NEC G62.2
plantar nerves G57.6-
progressive
hypertrophic interstitial G60.0
inflammatory G62.81
radicular NEC —*see* Radiculopathy
sacral plexus G54.1
sciatic G57.0-
serum G61.1
toxic NEC G62.2
trigeminal sensory G50.8
ulnar nerve G56.2-
uremic N18.9 *[G63]*
vitamin B12 E53.8 *[G63]*
with anemia (pernicious) D51.0 *[G63]*
due to dietary deficiency D51.3 *[G63]*
Neurophthisis —*see also* Disorder, nerve
peripheral, diabetic —*see* E08-E13 with .42
Neuroretinitis —*see* Chorioretinitis
Neuroretinopathy, hereditary optic H47.22
Neurosarcoma —*see* Neoplasm, nerve, malignant
Neurosclerosis —*see* Disorder, nerve
Neurosis, neurotic F48.9
anankastic F42.8 ⇐
anxiety (state) F41.1
panic type F41.0
asthenic F48.8
bladder F45.8

Neurosis, neurotic *(Continued)*
cardiac (reflex) F45.8
cardiovascular F45.8
character F60.9
colon F45.8
compensation F68.1
compulsive, compulsion F42.8 ⇐
conversion F44.9
craft F48.8
cutaneous F45.8
depersonalization F48.1
depressive (reaction) (type) F34.1
environmental F48.8
excoriation L98.1
fatigue F48.8
functional —*see* Disorder, somatoform
gastric F45.8
gastrointestinal F45.8
heart F45.8
hypochondriacal F45.21
hysterical F44.9
incoordination F45.8
larynx F45.8
vocal cord F45.8
intestine F45.8
larynx (sensory) F45.8
hysterical F44.4
mixed NEC F48.8
musculoskeletal F45.8
obsessional F42.8 ⇐
obsessive-compulsive F42.8 ⇐
occupational F48.8
ocular NEC F45.8
organ —*see* Disorder, somatoform
pharynx F45.8
phobic F40.9
posttraumatic (situational) F43.10
acute F43.11
chronic F43.12
psychasthenic (type) F48.8
railroad F48.8
rectum F45.8
respiratory F45.8
rumination F45.8
sexual F65.9
situational F48.8
social F40.10
generalized F40.11
specified type NEC F48.8
state F48.9
with depersonalization episode F48.1
stomach F45.8
traumatic F43.10
acute F43.11
chronic F43.12
vasomotor F45.8
visceral F45.8
war F48.8
Neurospongioblastosis diffusa Q85.1
Neurosyphilis (arrested) (early) (gumma) (late) (latent) (recurrent) (relapse) A52.3
with ataxia (cerebellar) (locomotor) (spastic) (spinal) A52.19
aneurysm (cerebral) A52.05
arachnoid (adhesive) A52.13
arteritis (any artery) (cerebral) A52.04
asymptomatic A52.2
congenital A50.40
dura (mater) A52.13
general paresis A52.17
hemorrhagic A52.05
juvenile (asymptomatic) (meningeal) A50.40
leptomeninges (aseptic) A52.13
meningeal, meninges (adhesive) A52.13
meningitis A52.13
meningovascular (diffuse) A52.13
optic atrophy A52.15
parenchymatous (degenerative) A52.19
paresis, paretic A52.17
juvenile A50.45

Neurosyphilis *(Continued)*
remission in (sustained) A52.3
serological (without symptoms) A52.2
specified nature or site NEC A52.19
tabes, tabetic (dorsalis) A52.11
juvenile A50.45
taboparesis A52.17
juvenile A50.45
thrombosis (cerebral) A52.05
vascular (cerebral) NEC A52.05
Neurothekeoma —*see* Neoplasm, nerve, benign
Neurotic —*see* Neurosis
Neurotoxemia —*see* Toxemia
Neutroclusion M26.211
Neutropenia, neutropenic (chronic) (genetic) (idiopathic) (immune) (infantile) (malignant) (pernicious) (splenic) D70.9
congenital (primary) D70.0
cyclic D70.4
cytoreductive cancer chemotherapy sequela D70.1
drug-induced D70.2
due to cytoreductive cancer chemotherapy D70.1
due to infection D70.3
fever D70.9
neonatal, transitory (isoimmune) (maternal transfer) P61.5
periodic D70.4
secondary (cyclic) (periodic) (splenic) D70.4
drug-induced D70.2
due to cytoreductive cancer chemotherapy D70.1
toxic D70.8
Neutrophilia, hereditary giant D72.0
Nevocarcinoma —*see* Melanoma
Nevus D22.9
achromic —*see* Neoplasm, skin, benign
amelanotic —*see* Neoplasm, skin, benign
angiomatous D18.00
intra-abdominal D18.03
intracranial D18.02
skin D18.01
specified site NEC D18.09
araneus I78.1
balloon cell —*see* Neoplasm, skin, benign
bathing trunk D48.5
blue —*see* Neoplasm, skin, benign
cellular —*see* Neoplasm, skin, benign
giant —*see* Neoplasm, skin, benign
Jadassohn's —*see* Neoplasm, skin, benign
malignant —*see* Melanoma
capillary D18.00
intra-abdominal D18.03
intracranial D18.02
skin D18.01
specified site NEC D18.09
cavernous D18.00
intra-abdominal D18.03
intracranial D18.02
skin D18.01
specified site NEC D18.09
cellular —*see* Neoplasm, skin, benign
blue —*see* Neoplasm, skin, benign
choroid D31.3-
comedonicus Q82.5
conjunctiva D31.0-
dermal —*see* Neoplasm, skin, benign
with epidermal nevus —*see* Neoplasm, skin, benign
dysplastic —*see* Neoplasm, skin, benign
eye D31.9-
flammeus Q82.5
hemangiomatous D18.00
intra-abdominal D18.03
intracranial D18.02
skin D18.01
specified site NEC D18.09
iris D31.4-
lacrimal gland D31.5-
lymphatic D18.1

◀ New ⇐ Revised ~~deleted~~ Deleted

Nevus *(Continued)*
magnocellular
specified site —*see* Neoplasm, benign, by site
unspecified site D31.40
malignant —*see* Melanoma
meaning hemangioma D18.00
intra-abdominal D18.03
intracranial D18.02
skin D18.01
specified site NEC D18.09
mouth (mucosa) D10.30
specified site NEC D10.39
white sponge Q38.6
multiplex Q85.1
non-neoplastic I78.1
oral mucosa D10.30
specified site NEC D10.39
white sponge Q38.6
orbit D31.6-
pigmented
giant —*see also* Neoplasm, skin, uncertain behavior D48.5
malignant melanoma in —*see* Melanoma
portwine Q82.5
retina D31.2-
retrobulbar D31.6-
sanguineous Q82.5
senile I78.1
skin D22.9
abdominal wall D22.5
ala nasi D22.39
ankle D22.7-
anus, anal D22.5
arm D22.6-
auditory canal (external) D22.2-
auricle (ear) D22.2-
auricular canal (external) D22.2-
axilla, axillary fold D22.5
back D22.5
breast D22.5
brow D22.39
buttock D22.5
canthus (eye) D22.1-
cheek (external) D22.39
chest wall D22.5
chin D22.39
ear (external) D22.2-
external meatus (ear) D22.2-
eyebrow D22.39
eyelid (lower) (upper) D22.1-
face D22.30
specified NEC D22.39
female genital organ (external) NEC D28.0
finger D22.6-
flank D22.5
foot D22.7-
forearm D22.6-
forehead D22.39
foreskin D29.0
genital organ (external) NEC
female D28.0
male D29.9
gluteal region D22.5
groin D22.5
hand D22.6-
heel D22.7-
helix D22.2-
hip D22.7-
interscapular region D22.5
jaw D22.39
knee D22.7-
labium (majus) (minus) D28.0
leg D22.7-
lip (lower) (upper) D22.0
lower limb D22.7-
male genital organ (external) D29.9
nail D22.9
finger D22.6-
toe D22.7-
nasolabial groove D22.39
nates D22.5

Nevus *(Continued)*
skin *(Continued)*
neck D22.4
nose (external) D22.39
palpebra D22.1-
penis D29.0
perianal skin D22.5
perineum D22.5
pinna D22.2-
popliteal fossa or space D22.7-
prepuce D29.0
pudendum D28.0
scalp D22.4
scrotum D29.4
shoulder D22.6-
submammary fold D22.5
temple D22.39
thigh D22.7-
toe D22.7-
trunk NEC D22.5
umbilicus D22.5
upper limb D22.6-
vulva D28.0
specified site NEC —*see* Neoplasm, benign, by site
spider I78.1
stellar I78.1
strawberry Q82.5
Sutton's —*see* Neoplasm, skin, benign
unius lateris Q82.5
Unna's Q82.5
vascular Q82.5
verrucous Q82.5
Newborn (infant) (liveborn) (singleton) Z38.2
abstinence syndrome P96.1
acne L70.4
affected by ◄
abnormalities of membranes P02.9
specified NEC P02.8
abruptio placenta P02.1
amino-acid metabolic disorder, transitory P74.8
amniocentesis (while in utero) P00.6
amnionitis P02.7
apparent life threatening event (ALTE) R68.13
bleeding (into)
cerebral cortex P52.22
germinal matrix P52.0
ventricles P52.1
breech delivery P03.0
cardiac arrest P29.81
cardiomyopathy I42.8
congenital I42.4
cerebral ischemia P91.0
Cesarean delivery P03.4
chemotherapy agents P04.1
chorioamnionitis P02.7
cocaine (crack) P04.41
complications of labor and delivery P03.9
specified NEC P03.89
compression of umbilical cord NEC P02.5
contracted pelvis P03.1
delivery P03.9
Cesarean P03.4
forceps P03.2
vacuum extractor P03.3
entanglement (knot) in umbilical cord P02.5
environmental chemicals P04.6
fetal (intrauterine)
growth retardation P05.9
malnutrition not light or small for gestational age P05.2
forceps delivery P03.2
heart rate abnormalities
bradycardia P29.12
intrauterine P03.819
before onset of labor P03.810
during labor P03.811
tachycardia P29.11

Newborn *(Continued)*
affected by *(Continued)*
hemorrhage (antepartum) P02.1
cerebellar (nontraumatic) P52.6
intracerebral (nontraumatic) P52.4
intracranial (nontraumatic) P52.9
specified NEC P52.8
intraventricular (nontraumatic) P52.3
grade 1 P52.0
grade 2 P52.1
grade 3 P52.21
grade 4 P52.22
posterior fossa (nontraumatic) P52.6
subarachnoid (nontraumatic) P52.5
subependymal P52.0
with intracerebral extension P52.22
with intraventricular extension P52.1
with enlargment of ventricles P52.21
without intraventricular extension P52.0
hypoxic ischemic encephalopathy [HIE] P91.60
mild P91.61
moderate P91.62
severe P91.63
induction of labor P03.89
intestinal perforation P78.0
intrauterine (fetal) blood loss P50.9
due to (from)
cut end of co-twin cord P50.5
hemorrhage into
co-twin P50.3
maternal circulation P50.4
placenta P50.2
ruptured cord blood P50.1
vasa previa P50.0
specified NEC P50.8
intrauterine (fetal) hemorrhage P50.9
intrauterine (in utero) procedure P96.5
malpresentation (malposition) NEC P03.1
maternal (complication of) (use of)
alcohol P04.3
analgesia (maternal) P04.0
anesthesia (maternal) P04.0
blood loss P02.1
circulatory disease P00.3
condition P00.9
specified NEC P00.89
delivery P03.9
Cesarean P03.4
forceps P03.2
vacuum extractor P03.3
diabetes mellitus (pre-existing) P70.1
disorder P00.9
specified NEC P00.89
drugs (addictive) (illegal) NEC P04.49
ectopic pregnancy P01.4
gestational diabetes P70.0
hemorrhage P02.1
hypertensive disorder P00.0
incompetent cervix P01.0
infectious disease P00.2
injury P00.5
labor and delivery P03.9
malpresentation before labor P01.7
maternal death P01.6
medical procedure P00.7
medication P04.1
multiple pregnancy P01.5
nutritional disorder P00.4
oligohydramnios P01.2
parasitic disease P00.2
periodontal disease P00.81
placenta previa P02.0
polyhydramnios P01.3
precipitate delivery P03.5
pregnancy P01.9
specified P01.8
premature rupture of membranes P01.1
renal disease P00.1

N

Newborn *(Continued)*
affected by *(Continued)*
maternal *(Continued)*
respiratory disease P00.3
surgical procedure P00.6
urinary tract disease P00.1
uterine contraction (abnormal) P03.6
meconium peritonitis P78.0
medication (legal) (maternal use) (prescribed) P04.1
membrane abnormalities P02.9
specified NEC P02.8
membranitis P02.7
methamphetamine (s) P04.49
mixed metabolic and respiratory acidosis P84
neonatal abstinence syndrome P96.1
noxious substances transmitted via placenta or breast milk P04.9
specified NEC P04.8
nutritional supplements P04.5
placenta previa P02.0
placental
abnormality (functional) (morphological) P02.20
specified NEC P02.29
dysfunction P02.29
infarction P02.29
insufficiency P02.29
separation NEC P02.1
transfusion syndromes P02.3
placentitis P02.7
precipitate delivery P03.5
prolapsed cord P02.4
respiratory arrest P28.81
slow intrauterine growth P05.9
tobacco P04.2
twin to twin transplacental transfusion P02.3
umbilical cord (tightly) around neck P02.5
umbilical cord condition P02.60
short cord P02.69
specified NEC P02.69
uterine contractions (abnormal) P03.6
vasa previa P02.69
from intrauterine blood loss P50.0
apnea P28.4 ⬅
obstructive P28.4
primary P28.3
~~specified P28.4~~
sleep (central) (obstructive) (primary) P28.3 ◀
born in hospital Z38.00
by cesarean Z38.01
born outside hospital Z38.1
breast buds P96.89
breast engorgement P83.4
check-up —*see* Newborn, examination
convulsion P90
dehydration P74.1
examination
8 to 28 days old Z00.111
under 8 days old Z00.110
fever P81.9
environmentally-induced P81.0
hyperbilirubinemia P59.9
of prematurity P59.0
hypernatremia P74.2
hyponatremia P74.2
infection P39.9
candidal P37.5
specified NEC P39.8
urinary tract P39.3
jaundice P59.9 ⬅
due to
breast milk inhibitor P59.3
hepatocellular damage P59.20
specified NEC P59.29
preterm delivery P59.0
of prematurity P59.0
specified NEC P59.8

Newborn *(Continued)*
late metabolic acidosis P74.0
mastitis P39.0
infective P39.0
noninfective P83.4
multiple born NEC Z38.8
born in hospital Z38.68
by cesarean Z38.69
born outside hospital Z38.7
omphalitis P38.9
with mild hemorrhage P38.1
without hemorrhage P38.9
post-term P08.21
prolonged gestation (over 42 completed weeks) P08.22
quadruplet Z38.8
born in hospital Z38.63
by cesarean Z38.64
born outside hospital Z38.7
quintuplet Z38.8
born in hospital Z38.65
by cesarean Z38.66
born outside hospital Z38.7
seizure P90
sepsis (congenital) P36.9
due to
anaerobes NEC P36.5
Escherichia coli P36.4
Staphylococcus P36.30
aureus P36.2
specified NEC P36.39
Streptococcus P36.10
group B P36.0
specified NEC P36.19
specified NEC P36.8
triplet Z38.8
born in hospital Z38.61
by cesarean Z38.62
born outside hospital Z38.7
twin Z38.5
born in hospital Z38.30
by cesarean Z38.31
born outside hospital Z38.4
vomiting P92.09
bilious P92.01
weight check Z00.111
Newcastle conjunctivitis or disease B30.8
Nezelof's syndrome (pure alymphocytosis) D81.4
Niacin (amide) **deficiency** E52
Nicolas (-Durand)-**Favre disease** A55
Nicotine —*see* Tobacco
Nicotinic acid deficiency E52
Niemann-Pick disease or syndrome E75.249
specified NEC E75.248
type
A E75.240
B E75.241
C E75.242
D E75.243
Night
blindness —*see* Blindness, night
sweats R61
terrors (child) F51.4
Nightmares (REM sleep type) F51.5
NIHSS (National Institutes of Health Stroke Scale) **score** R29.7- ◀
Nipple —*see* condition
Nisbet's chancre A57
Nishimoto (-Takeuchi) disease I67.5
Nitritoid crisis or reaction —*see* Crisis, nitritoid
Nitrosohemoglobinemia D74.8
Njovera A65
Nocardiosis, nocardiasis A43.9
cutaneous A43.1
lung A43.0
pneumonia A43.0
pulmonary A43.0
specified site NEC A43.8
Nocturia R35.1
psychogenic F45.8

Nocturnal —*see* condition
Nodal rhythm I49.8
Node (s) —*see also* Nodule
Bouchard's (with arthropathy) M15.2
Haygarth's M15.8
Heberden's (with arthropathy) M15.1
larynx J38.7
lymph —*see* condition
milker's B08.03
Osler's I33.0
Schmorl's —*see* Schmorl's disease
singer's J38.2
teacher's J38.2
tuberculous —*see* Tuberculosis, lymph gland
vocal cord J38.2
Nodule (s), **nodular**
actinomycotic —*see* Actinomycosis
breast NEC N63
colloid (cystic), thyroid E04.1
cutaneous —*see* Swelling, localized
endometrial (stromal) D26.1
Haygarth's M15.8
inflammatory —*see* Inflammation
juxta-articular
syphilitic A52.77
yaws A66.7
larynx J38.7
lung, solitary (subsegmental branch of the bronchial tree) R91.1
multiple R91.8
milker's B08.03
prostate N40.2
with lower urinary tract symptoms (LUTS) N40.3
without lower urinary tract symptoms (LUTS) N40.2
pulmonary, solitary (subsegmental branch of the bronchial tree) R91.1
retrocardiac R09.89
rheumatoid M06.30
ankle M06.37-
elbow M06.32-
foot joint M06.37-
hand joint M06.34-
hip M06.35-
knee M06.36-
multiple site M06.39
shoulder M06.31-
vertebra M06.38
wrist M06.33-
scrotum (inflammatory) N49.2
singer's J38.2
solitary, lung (subsegmental branch of the bronchial tree) R91.1
multiple R91.8
subcutaneous —*see* Swelling, localized
teacher's J38.2
thyroid (cold) (gland) (nontoxic) E04.1
with thyrotoxicosis E05.20
with thyroid storm E05.21
toxic or with hyperthyroidism E05.20
with thyroid storm E05.21
vocal cord J38.2
Noma (gangrenous) (hospital) (infective) A69.0
auricle I96
mouth A69.0
pudendi N76.89
vulvae N76.89
Nomad, nomadism Z59.0
NOMID (neonatal onset multisystemic inflammatory disorder) M04.2 ◀
Nonautoimmune hemolytic anemia D59.4
drug-induced D59.2
Nonclosure —*see also* Imperfect, closure
ductus arteriosus (Botallo's) Q25.0
foramen
botalli Q21.1
ovale Q21.1

◀ New ⬅ Revised ~~deleted~~ Deleted

Noncompliance Z91.19
with
dialysis Z91.15
dietary regimen Z91.11
medical treatment Z91.19
medication regimen NEC Z91.14
underdosing —*see also* Table of Drugs and Chemicals, categories T36-T50, with final character 6 Z91.14
intentional NEC Z91.128
due to financial hardship of patient Z91.120
unintentional NEC Z91.138
due to patient's age related debility Z91.130
renal dialysis Z91.15
Nondescent (congenital) —*see also* Malposition, congenital
cecum Q43.3
colon Q43.3
testicle Q53.9
bilateral Q53.20
abdominal Q53.21
perineal Q53.22
unilateral Q53.10
abdominal Q53.11
perineal Q53.12
Nondevelopment
brain Q02
part of Q04.3
heart Q24.8
organ or site, congenital NEC —*see* Hypoplasia
Nonengagement
head NEC O32.4
in labor, causing obstructed labor O64.8
Nonexanthematous tick fever A93.2
Nonexpansion, lung (newborn) P28.0
Nonfunctioning
cystic duct —*see also* Disease, gallbladder K82.8
gallbladder —*see also* Disease, gallbladder K82.8
kidney N28.9
labyrinth —*see* subcategory H83.2
Non-Hodgkin lymphoma NEC —*see* Lymphoma, non-Hodgkin
Nonimplantation, ovum N97.2
Noninsufflation, fallopian tube N97.1
Non-ketotic hyperglycinemia E72.51
Nonne-Milroy syndrome Q82.0
Nonovulation N97.0
Nonpatent fallopian tube N97.1
Nonpneumatization, lung NEC P28.0
Nonrotation —*see* Malrotation
Nonsecretion, urine —*see* Anuria
Nonunion
fracture —*see* Fracture, by site
joint, following fusion or arthrodesis M96.0 ◀
organ or site, congenital NEC —*see* Imperfect, closure
symphysis pubis, congenital Q74.2
Nonvisualization, gallbladder R93.2
Nonvital, nonvitalized tooth K04.99
Non-working side interference M26.56
Noonan's syndrome Q87.1
Normocytic anemia (infectional) due to blood loss (chronic) D50.0
acute D62
Norrie's disease (congenital) Q15.8
North American blastomycosis B40.9
Norwegian itch B86
Nose, nasal —*see* condition
Nosebleed R04.0
Nose-picking F98.8
Nosomania F45.21
Nosophobia F45.22
Nostalgia F43.20
Notch of iris Q13.2
Notching nose, congenital (tip) Q30.2
Nothnagel's
syndrome —*see* Strabismus, paralytic, third nerve
vasomotor acroparesthesia I73.89
Novy's relapsing fever A68.9
louse-borne A68.0
tick-borne A68.1
Noxious
foodstuffs, poisoning by —*see* Poisoning, food, noxious, plant
substances transmitted through placenta or breast milk P04.9
Nucleus pulposus —*see* condition
Numbness R20.0
Nuns' knee —*see* Bursitis, prepatellar
Nursemaid's elbow S53.03-
Nutcracker esophagus K22.4
Nutmeg liver K76.1
Nutrient element deficiency E61.9
specified NEC E61.8
Nutrition deficient or insufficient —*see also* Malnutrition E46
due to
insufficient food T73.0
lack of
care (child) T76.02
adult T76.01
food T73.0
Nutritional stunting E45
Nyctalopia (night blindness) —*see* Blindness, night
Nycturia R35.1
psychogenic F45.8
Nymphomania F52.8
Nystagmus H55.00
benign paroxysmal —*see* Vertigo, benign paroxysmal
central positional H81.4-
congenital H55.01
dissociated H55.04
latent H55.02
miners' H55.09
positional
benign paroxysmal H81.4-
central H81.4-
specified form NEC H55.09
visual deprivation H55.03

O

Obermeyer's relapsing fever (European) A68.0
Obesity E66.9
~~with alveolar hyperventilation E66.2~~
with alveolar hypoventilation E66.2 ◀
adrenal E27.8
complicating
childbirth O99.214
pregnancy O99.21-
puerperium O99.215
constitutional E66.8
dietary counseling and surveillance Z71.3
drug-induced E66.1
due to
drug E66.1
excess calories E66.09
morbid E66.01
severe E66.01
endocrine E66.8
endogenous E66.8
exogenous E66.09 ◀
familial E66.8
glandular E66.8
hypothyroid —*see* Hypothyroidism
hypoventilation syndrome (OHS) E66.2 ◀
morbid E66.01
~~with alveolar hypoventilation E66.2~~
with ◀
alveolar hypoventilation E66.2 ◀
obesity hypoventilation syndrome (OHS) E66.2 ◀
due to excess calories E66.01
nutritional E66.09
pituitary E23.6
severe E66.01
specified type NEC E66.8
Oblique —*see* condition
Obliteration
appendix (lumen) K38.8
artery I77.1
bile duct (noncalculous) K83.1
common duct (noncalculous) K83.1
cystic duct —*see* Obstruction, gallbladder
disease, arteriolar I77.1
endometrium N85.8
eye, anterior chamber —*see* Disorder, globe, hypotony
fallopian tube N97.1
lymphatic vessel I89.0
due to mastectomy I97.2
organ or site, congenital NEC —*see* Atresia, by site
ureter N13.5
with infection N13.6
urethra —*see* Stricture, urethra
vein I87.8
vestibule (oral) K08.89 ⇐
Observation (following) (for) (without need for further medical care) Z04.9
accident NEC Z04.3
at work Z04.2
transport Z04.1
adverse effect of drug Z03.6
alleged rape or sexual assault (victim), ruled out
adult Z04.41
child Z04.42
criminal assault Z04.8
development state
adolescent Z00.3
period of rapid growth in childhood Z00.2
puberty Z00.3
disease, specified NEC Z03.89
following work accident Z04.2
growth and development state —*see* Observation, development state
injuries (accidental) NEC —*see also* Observation, accident
Observation *(Continued)*
newborn (for) ⇐
suspected condition, related to exposure from the mother or birth process —*see* Newborn, affected by, maternal ◀
ruled out Z05.9 ◀
cardiac Z05.0 ◀
connective tissue Z05.73 ◀
gastrointestinal Z05.5 ◀
genetic Z05.41 ◀
genitourinary Z05.6 ◀
immunologic Z05.43 ◀
infectious Z05.1 ◀
metabolic Z05.42 ◀
musculoskeletal Z05.72 ◀
neurological Z05.2 ◀
respiratory Z05.3 ◀
skin and subcutaneous tissue Z05.71 ◀
specified condition NEC Z05.8 ◀
postpartum
immediately after delivery Z39.0
routine follow-up Z39.2
pregnancy (normal) (without complication) Z34.9-
high risk O09.9-
suicide attempt, alleged NEC Z03.89
self-poisoning Z03.6
suspected, ruled out —*see also* Suspected condition, ruled out
abuse, physical
adult Z04.71
child Z04.72
accident at work Z04.2
adult battering victim Z04.71
child battering victim Z04.72
condition NEC Z03.89
newborn —*see also* Observation, newborn (for), suspected condition, ruled out Z05.9 ⇐
drug poisoning or adverse effect Z03.6
exposure (to)
anthrax Z03.810
biological agent NEC Z03.818
inflicted injury NEC Z04.8
suicide attempt, alleged Z03.89
self-poisoning Z03.6
toxic effects from ingested substance (drug) (poison) Z03.6
toxic effects from ingested substance (drug) (poison) Z03.6
Obsession, obsessional state F42.8 ⇐
mixed thoughts and acts F42.2 ◀
Obsessive-compulsive neurosis or reaction F42.8 ⇐
Obstetric embolism, septic —*see* Embolism, obstetric, septic
Obstetrical trauma (complicating delivery) O71.9
with or following ectopic or molar pregnancy O08.6
specified type NEC O71.89
Obstipation —*see* Constipation
Obstruction, obstructed, obstructive
airway J98.8
with
allergic alveolitis J67.9
asthma J45.909
with
exacerbation (acute) J45.901
status asthmaticus J45.902
bronchiectasis J47.9
with
exacerbation (acute) J47.1
lower respiratory infection J47.0
bronchitis (chronic) J44.9
emphysema J43.9
Obstruction, obstructed, obstructive *(Continued)*
airway *(Continued)*
chronic J44.9
with
allergic alveolitis —*see* Pneumonitis, hypersensitivity
bronchiectasis J47.9
with
exacerbation (acute) J47.1
lower respiratory infection J47.0
due to
foreign body —*see* Foreign body, by site, causing asphyxia
inhalation of fumes or vapors J68.9
laryngospasm J38.5
ampulla of Vater K83.1
aortic (heart) (valve) —*see* Stenosis, aortic
aortoiliac I74.09
aqueduct of Sylvius G91.1
congenital Q03.0
with spina bifida —*see* Spina bifida, by site, with hydrocephalus
Arnold-Chiari —*see* Arnold-Chiari disease
artery (*see also* Embolism, artery) I74.9
basilar (complete) (partial) —*see* Occlusion, artery, basilar
carotid (complete) (partial) —*see* Occlusion, artery, carotid
cerebellar —*see* Occlusion, artery, cerebellar
cerebral (anterior) (middle) (posterior) —*see* Occlusion, artery, cerebral
precerebral —*see* Occlusion, artery, precerebral
renal N28.0
retinal NEC —*see* Occlusion, artery, retina
stent —*see* Restenosis, stent ◀
vertebral (complete) (partial) —*see* Occlusion, artery, vertebral
band (intestinal) K56.69
bile duct or passage (common) (hepatic) (noncalculous) K83.1
with calculus K80.51
congenital (causing jaundice) Q44.3
biliary (duct) (tract) K83.1
gallbladder K82.0
bladder-neck (acquired) N32.0
congenital Q64.31
due to hyperplasia (hypertrophy) of prostate —*see* Hyperplasia, prostate
bowel —*see* Obstruction, intestine
bronchus J98.09
canal, ear —*see* Stenosis, external ear canal
cardia K22.2
caval veins (inferior) (superior) I87.1
cecum —*see* Obstruction, intestine
circulatory I99.8
colon —*see* Obstruction, intestine
common duct (noncalculous) K83.1
coronary (artery) —*see* Occlusion, coronary
cystic duct —*see also* Obstruction, gallbladder
with calculus K80.21
device, implant or graft —*see also* Complications, by site and type, mechanical T85.698
arterial graft NEC —*see* Complication, cardiovascular device, mechanical, vascular
catheter NEC T85.628
cystostomy T83.090
dialysis (renal) T82.49
intraperitoneal T85.691
Hopkins T83.098 ◀
ileostomy T83.098 ◀
infusion NEC T82.594
spinal (epidural) (subdural) T85.690
nephrostomy T83.092 ◀
urethral indwelling T83.091 ◀
urinary T83.098 ◀
~~urinary, indwelling T83.098~~
urostomy T83.098 ◀

◀ New ⇐ Revised ~~deleted~~ Deleted

Obstruction, obstructed, obstructive *(Continued)*
device, implant or graft *(Continued)*
due to infection T85.79
gastrointestinal —*see* Complications, prosthetic device, mechanical, gastrointestinal device
genital NEC T83.498
intrauterine contraceptive device T83.39
penile prosthesis (cylinder) (implanted) (pump) (resevoir) T83.490 ◀
testicular prosthesis T83.491 ◀
heart NEC —*see* Complication, cardiovascular device, mechanical
joint prosthesis —*see* Complications, joint prosthesis, mechanical, specified NEC, by site
orthopedic NEC —*see* Complication, orthopedic, device, mechanical
specified NEC T85.628
urinary NEC —*see also* Complication, genitourinary, device, urinary, mechanical
graft T83.29
vascular NEC —*see* Complication, cardiovascular device, mechanical
ventricular intracranial shunt T85.09
due to foreign body accidentally left in operative wound T81.529
duodenum K31.5
ejaculatory duct N50.89 ◀
esophagus K22.2
eustachian tube (complete) (partial) H68.10-
cartilagenous (extrinsic) H68.13-
intrinsic H68.12-
osseous H68.11-
fallopian tube (bilateral) N97.1
fecal K56.41
with hernia —*see* Hernia, by site, with obstruction
foramen of Monro (congenital) Q03.8
with spina bifida —*see* Spina bifida, by site, with hydrocephalus
foreign body —*see* Foreign body
gallbladder K82.0
with calculus, stones K80.21
congenital Q44.1
gastric outlet K31.1
gastrointestinal —*see* Obstruction, intestine
hepatic K76.89
duct (noncalculous) K83.1
hepatobiliary K83.1
ileum —*see* Obstruction, intestine
iliofemoral (artery) I74.5
intestine K56.60
with
adhesions (intestinal) (peritoneal) K56.5
adynamic K56.0
by gallstone K56.3
congenital (small) Q41.9
large Q42.9
specified part NEC Q42.8
neurogenic K56.0
Hirschsprung's disease or megacolon Q43.1
newborn P76.9
due to
fecaliths P76.8
inspissated milk P76.2
meconium (plug) P76.0
in mucoviscidosis E84.11
specified NEC P76.8
postoperative K91.3
reflex K56.0
specified NEC K56.69
volvulus K56.2
intracardiac ball valve prosthesis T82.09
jejunum —*see* Obstruction, intestine
joint prosthesis —*see* Complications, joint prosthesis, mechanical, specified NEC, by site

Obstruction, obstructed, obstructive *(Continued)*
kidney (calices) N28.89
labor —*see* Delivery
lacrimal (passages) (duct)
by
dacryolith —*see* Dacryolith
stenosis —*see* Stenosis, lacrimal
congenital Q10.5
neonatal H04.53-
lacrimonasal duct —*see* Obstruction, lacrimal
lacteal, with steatorrhea K90.2
laryngitis —*see* Laryngitis
larynx NEC J38.6
congenital Q31.8
lung J98.4
disease, chronic J44.9
lymphatic I89.0
meconium (plug)
newborn P76.0
due to fecaliths P76.0
in mucoviscidosis E84.11
mitral —*see* Stenosis, mitral
nasal J34.89
nasolacrimal duct —*see also* Obstruction, lacrimal
congenital Q10.5
nasopharynx J39.2
nose J34.89
organ or site, congenital NEC —*see* Atresia, by site
pancreatic duct K86.89 ◀
parotid duct or gland K11.8
pelviureteral junction N13.5
with hydronephrosis N13.0 ◀
congenital Q62.39
pharynx J39.2
portal (circulation) (vein) I81
prostate —*see also* Hyperplasia, prostate
valve (urinary) N32.0
pulmonary valve (heart) I37.0
pyelonephritis (chronic) N11.1
pylorus
adult K31.1
congenital or infantile Q40.0
rectosigmoid —*see* Obstruction, intestine
rectum K62.4
renal N28.89
outflow N13.8
pelvis, congenital Q62.39
respiratory J98.8
chronic J44.9
retinal (vessels) H34.9
salivary duct (any) K11.8
with calculus K11.5
sigmoid —*see* Obstruction, intestine
sinus (accessory) (nasal) J34.89
Stensen's duct K11.8
stomach NEC K31.89
acute K31.0
congenital Q40.2
due to pylorospasm K31.3
submandibular duct K11.8
submaxillary gland K11.8
with calculus K11.5
thoracic duct I89.0
thrombotic —*see* Thrombosis
trachea J39.8
tracheostomy airway J95.03
tricuspid (valve) —*see* Stenosis, tricuspid
upper respiratory, congenital Q34.8
ureter (functional) (pelvic junction) NEC N13.5
with
hydronephrosis N13.1
with infection N13.6
pyelonephritis (chronic) N11.1
congenital Q62.39
due to calculus —*see* Calculus, ureter

Obstruction, obstructed, obstructive *(Continued)*
urethra NEC N36.8
congenital Q64.39
urinary (moderate) N13.9
due to hyperplasia (hypertrophy) of prostate —*see* Hyperplasia, prostate
organ or tract (lower) N13.9
prostatic valve N32.0
specified NEC N13.8
uropathy N13.9
uterus N85.8
vagina N89.5
valvular —*see* Endocarditis
vein, venous I87.1
caval (inferior) (superior) I87.1
thrombotic —*see* Thrombosis
vena cava (inferior) (superior) I87.1
vesical NEC N32.0
vesicourethral orifice N32.0
congenital Q64.31
vessel NEC I99.8
stent —*see* Restenosis, stent ◀
Obturator —*see* condition
Occlusal wear, teeth K03.0
Occlusio pupillae —*see* Membrane, pupillary
Occlusion, occluded
anus K62.4
congenital Q42.3
with fistula Q42.2
aortoiliac (chronic) I74.09
aqueduct of Sylvius G91.1
congenital Q03.0
with spina bifida —*see* Spina bifida, by site, with hydrocephalus
artery —*see also* Embolism, artery I74.9
auditory, internal I65.8
basilar I65.1
with
infarction I63.22
due to
embolism I63.12
thrombosis I63.02
brain or cerebral I66.9
with infarction (due to) I63.5- ◀
embolism I63.4- ◀
thrombosis I63.3- ◀
carotid I65.2-
with
infarction I63.23-
due to
embolism I63.13-
thrombosis I63.03-
cerebellar (anterior inferior) (posterior inferior) (superior) I66.3
with infarction I63.54-
due to
embolism I63.44-
thrombosis I63.34-
cerebral I66.9
with infarction I63.50
due to
embolism I63.40
specified NEC I63.49
thrombosis I63.30
specified NEC I63.39
anterior I66.1-
with infarction I63.52-
due to
embolism I63.42-
thrombosis I63.32-
middle I66.0-
with infarction I63.51-
due to
embolism I63.41-
thrombosis I63.31-
posterior I66.2-
with infarction I63.53-
due to
embolism I63.43-
thrombosis I63.33-

Occlusion, occluded *(Continued)*
artery *(Continued)*
cerebral *(Continued)*
specified NEC I66.8
with infarction I63.59
due to
embolism I63.4- ⬅
thrombosis I63.3- ⬅
choroidal (anterior) —*see* Occlusion, artery, cerebral, specified NEC
communicating posterior —*see* Occlusion, artery, precerebral, specified NEC
complete
coronary I25.82
extremities I7Ø.92
coronary (acute) (thrombotic) (without myocardial infarction) I24.Ø
with myocardial infarction —*see* Infarction, myocardium
chronic total I25.82
complete I25.82
healed or old I25.2
total (chronic) I25.82
hypophyseal —*see* Occlusion, artery, precerebral, specified NEC
iliac I74.5
lower extremities due to stenosis or stricture I77.1
mesenteric (embolic) (thrombotic) —*see also* Infarct, intestine K55.Ø69 ⬅
perforating —*see* Occlusion, artery, cerebral, specified NEC
peripheral I77.9
thrombotic or embolic I74.4
pontine —*see* Occlusion, artery, cerebral, specified NEC
precerebral I65.9
with infarction I63.2Ø
due to
embolism I63.1Ø
specified NEC I63.19
thrombosis I63.ØØ
specified NEC I63.Ø9
specified NEC I63.29
basilar —*see* Occlusion, artery, basilar
carotid —*see* Occlusion, artery, carotid
puerperal O88.23
specified NEC I65.8
with infarction I63.29
due to
embolism I63.19
thrombosis I63.ØØ
vertebral —*see* Occlusion, artery, vertebral
renal N28.Ø
retinal
branch H34.23-
central H34.1-
partial H34.21-
transient H34.Ø-
spinal —*see* Occlusion, artery, precerebral, vertebral
total (chronic)
coronary I25.82
extremities I7Ø.92
vertebral I65.Ø-
with
infarction I63.21-
due to
embolism I63.11-
thrombosis I63.Ø1-
basilar artery —*see* Occlusion, artery, basilar
bile duct (common) (hepatic) (noncalculous) K83.1
bowel —*see* Obstruction, intestine
carotid (artery) (common) (internal) —*see* Occlusion, artery, carotid
centric (of teeth) M26.59
maximum intercuspation discrepancy M26.55

Occlusion, occluded *(Continued)*
cerebellar (artery) —*see* Occlusion, artery, cerebellar
cerebral (artery) —*see* Occlusion, artery, cerebral
cerebrovascular —*see also* Occlusion, artery, cerebral
with infarction I63.5- ⬅
cervical canal —*see* Stricture, cervix
cervix (uteri) —*see* Stricture, cervix
choanal Q3Ø.Ø
choroidal (artery) —*see* Occlusion, artery, precerebral, specified NEC
colon —*see* Obstruction, intestine
communicating posterior artery —*see* Occlusion, artery, precerebral, specified NEC
coronary (artery) (vein) (thrombotic) —*see also* Infarct, myocardium
chronic total I25.82
healed or old I25.2
not resulting in infarction I24.Ø
total (chronic) I25.82
cystic duct —*see* Obstruction, gallbladder
embolic —*see* Embolism
fallopian tube N97.1
congenital Q5Ø.6
gallbladder —*see also* Obstruction, gallbladder
congenital (causing jaundice) Q44.1
gingiva, traumatic KØ6.2
hymen N89.6
congenital Q52.3
hypophyseal (artery) —*see* Occlusion, artery, precerebral, specified NEC
iliac artery I74.5
intestine —*see* Obstruction, intestine
lacrimal passages —*see* Obstruction, lacrimal
lung J98.4
lymph or lymphatic channel I89.Ø
mammary duct N64.89
mesenteric artery (embolic) (thrombotic) —*see also* Infarct, intestine K55.Ø69 ⬅
nose J34.89
congenital Q3Ø.Ø
organ or site, congenital NEC —*see* Atresia, by site
oviduct N97.1
congenital Q5Ø.6
peripheral arteries
due to stricture or stenosis I77.1
upper extremity I74.2
pontine (artery) —*see* Occlusion, artery, precerebral, specified NEC
posterior lingual, of mandibular teeth M26.29
precerebral artery —*see* Occlusion, artery, precerebral
punctum lacrimale —*see* Obstruction, lacrimal
pupil —*see* Membrane, pupillary
pylorus, adult —*see also* Stricture, pylorus K31.1
renal artery N28.Ø
retina, retinal
artery —*see* Occlusion, artery, retinal
vein (central) H34.81-
engorgement H34.82-
tributary H34.83-
vessels H34.9
spinal artery —*see* Occlusion, artery, precerebral, vertebral
teeth (mandibular) (posterior lingual) M26.29
thoracic duct I89.Ø
thrombotic —*see* Thrombosis, artery
traumatic
edentulous (alveolar) ridge KØ6.2
gingiva KØ6.2
periodontal KØ5.5
tubal N97.1
ureter (complete) (partial) N13.5
congenital Q62.1Ø

Occlusion, occluded *(Continued)*
ureteropelvic junction N13.5
congenital Q62.11
ureterovesical orifice N13.5
congenital Q62.12
urethra —*see* Stricture, urethra
uterus N85.8
vagina N89.5
vascular NEC I99.8
vein —*see* Thrombosis
retinal —*see* Occlusion, retinal, vein
vena cava (inferior) (superior) —*see* Embolism, vena cava
ventricle (brain) NEC G91.1
vertebral (artery) —*see* Occlusion, artery, vertebral
vessel (blood) I99.8
vulva N9Ø.5
Occult
blood in feces (stools) R19.5
Occupational
problems NEC Z56.89
Ochlophobia —*see* Agoraphobia
Ochronosis (endogenous) E7Ø.29
Ocular muscle —*see* condition
Oculogyric crisis or disturbance H51.8
psychogenic F45.8
Oculomotor syndrome H51.9
Oculopathy
syphilitic NEC A52.71
congenital
early A5Ø.Ø1
late A5Ø.3Ø
early (secondary) A51.43
late A52.71
Oddi's sphincter spasm K83.4
Odontalgia KØ8.89 ⬅
Odontoameloblastoma —*see* Cyst, calcifying odontogenic
Odontoclasia KØ3.89
Odontodysplasia, regional KØØ.4
Odontogenesis imperfecta KØØ.5
Odontoma (ameloblastic) (complex) (compound) (fibroameloblastic) —*see* Cyst, calcifying odontogenic
Odontomyelitis (closed) (open) KØ4.Ø1 ⬅
irreversible KØ4.Ø2 ◀
reversible KØ4.Ø1 ◀
Odontorrhagia KØ8.89 ⬅
Odontosarcoma, ameloblastic C41.1
upper jaw (bone) C41.Ø
Oestriasis —*see* Myiasis
Oguchi's disease H53.63
Ohara's disease —*see* Tularemia
OHS (obesity hypoventilation syndrome) E66.2 ◀
Oidiomycosis —*see* Candidiasis
Oidium albicans infection —*see* Candidiasis
Old (previous) myocardial infarction I25.2
Old age (without mention of debility) R54-
dementia FØ3
Olfactory —*see* condition
Oligemia —*see* Anemia
Oligoastrocytoma
specified site —*see* Neoplasm, malignant, by site
unspecified site C71.9
Oligocythemia D64.9
Oligodendroblastoma
specified site —*see* Neoplasm, malignant
unspecified site C71.9
Oligodendroglioma
anaplastic type
specified site —*see* Neoplasm, malignant, by site
unspecified site C71.9
specified site —*see* Neoplasm, malignant, by site
unspecified site C71.9
Oligodontia —*see* Anodontia

◀ New ⬅ Revised ~~deleted~~ Deleted

Oligoencephalon Q02
Oligohidrosis L74.4
Oligohydramnios O41.0-
Oligohydrosis L74.4
Oligomenorrhea N91.5
primary N91.3
secondary N91.4
Oligophrenia —*see also* Disability, intellectual
phenylpyruvic E70.0
Oligospermia N46.11
due to
drug therapy N46.121
efferent duct obstruction N46.123
infection N46.122
radiation N46.124
specified cause NEC N46.129
systemic disease N46.125
Oligotrichia —*see* Alopecia
Oliguria R34
with, complicating or following ectopic or molar pregnancy O08.4
postprocedural N99.0
Ollier's disease Q78.4
Omenotocele —*see* Hernia, abdomen, specified site NEC
Omentitis —*see* Peritonitis
Omentum, omental —*see* condition
Omphalitis (congenital) (newborn) P38.9
with mild hemorrhage P38.1
without hemorrhage P38.9
not of newborn L08.82
tetanus A33
Omphalocele Q79.2
Omphalomesenteric duct, persistent Q43.0
Omphalorrhagia, newborn P51.9
Omsk hemorrhagic fever A98.1
Onanism (excessive) F98.8
Onchocerciasis, onchocercosis B73.1
with
eye disease B73.00
endophthalmitis B73.01
eyelid B73.09
glaucoma B73.02
specified NEC B73.09
eye NEC B73.00
eyelid B73.09
Oncocytoma —*see* Neoplasm, benign, by site
Oncovirus, as cause of disease classified elsewhere B97.32
Ondine's curse —*see* Apnea, sleep
Oneirophrenia F23
Onychauxis L60.2
congenital Q84.5
Onychia —*see also* Cellulitis, digit
with lymphangitis —*see* Lymphangitis, acute, digit
candidal B37.2
dermatophytic B35.1
Onychitis —*see also* Cellulitis, digit
with lymphangitis —*see* Lymphangitis, acute, digit
Onychocryptosis L60.0
Onychodystrophy L60.3
congenital Q84.6
Onychogryphosis, onychogryposis L60.2
Onycholysis L60.1
Onychomadesis L60.8
Onychomalacia L60.3
Onychomycosis (finger) (toe) B35.1
Onycho-osteodysplasia Q87.2 ◀
Onychophagia F98.8
Onychophosis L60.8
Onychoptosis L60.8
Onychorrhexis L60.3
congenital Q84.6
Onychoschizia L60.3
Onyxis (finger) (toe) L60.0
Onyxitis —*see also* Cellulitis, digit
with lymphangitis —*see* Lymphangitis, acute, digit
Oophoritis (cystic) (infectional) (interstitial) N70.92
with salpingitis N70.93
acute N70.02
with salpingitis N70.03
chronic N70.12
with salpingitis N70.13
complicating abortion —*see* Abortion, by type, complicated by, oophoritis
Oophorocele N83.4- ◀
Opacity, opacities
cornea H17.-
central H17.1-
congenital Q13.3
degenerative —*see* Degeneration, cornea
hereditary —*see* Dystrophy, cornea
inflammatory —*see* Keratitis
minor H17.81-
peripheral H17.82-
sequelae of trachoma (healed) B94.0
specified NEC H17.89
enamel (teeth) (fluoride) (nonfluoride) K00.3
lens —*see* Cataract
snowball —*see* Deposit, crystalline
vitreous (humor) NEC H43.39-
congenital Q14.0
membranes and strands H43.31-
Opalescent dentin (hereditary) K00.5
Open, opening
abnormal, organ or site, congenital —*see* Imperfect, closure
angle with
borderline
findings
high risk H40.02-
low risk H40.01-
intraocular pressure H40.00-
cupping of discs H40.01-
glaucoma (primary) —*see* Glaucoma, open angle
bite
anterior M26.220
posterior M26.221
false —*see* Imperfect, closure
margin on tooth restoration K08.51
restoration margins of tooth K08.51
wound —*see* Wound, open
Operational fatigue F48.8
Operative —*see* condition
Operculitis —*see* Periodontitis
Operculum —*see* Break, retina
Ophiasis L63.2
Ophthalmia —*see also* Conjunctivitis H10.9
actinic rays —*see* Photokeratitis
allergic (acute) —*see* Conjunctivitis, acute, atopic
blennorrhagic (gonococcal) (neonatorum) A54.31
diphtheritic A36.86
Egyptian A71.1
electrica —*see* Photokeratitis
gonococcal (neonatorum) A54.31
metastatic —*see* Endophthalmitis, purulent
migraine —*see* Migraine, ophthalmoplegic
neonatorum, newborn P39.1
gonococcal A54.31
nodosa H16.24-
purulent —*see* Conjunctivitis, acute, mucopurulent
spring —*see* Conjunctivitis, acute, atopic
sympathetic —*see* Uveitis, sympathetic
Ophthalmitis —*see* Ophthalmia
Ophthalmocele (congenital) Q15.8
Ophthalmoneuromyelitis G36.0
Ophthalmoplegia —*see also* Strabismus, paralytic
anterior internuclear —*see* Ophthalmoplegia, internuclear
ataxia-areflexia G61.0
diabetic —*see* E08-E13 with .39
Ophthalmoplegia *(Continued)*
exophthalmic E05.00
with thyroid storm E05.01
external H49.88-
progressive H49.4-
with pigmentary retinopathy —*see* Kearns-Sayre syndrome
total H49.3-
internal (complete) (total) H52.51-
internuclear H51.2-
migraine —*see* Migraine, ophthalmoplegic
Parinaud's H49.88-
progressive external —*see* Ophthalmoplegia, external, progressive
supranuclear, progressive G23.1
total (external) —*see* Ophthalmoplegia, external, total
Opioid (s)
abuse —*see* Abuse, drug, opioids
dependence —*see* Dependence, drug, opioids
induced, without use disorder ◀
anxiety disorder F11.988 ◀
delirium F11.921 ◀
depressive disorder F11.94 ◀
sexual dysfunction F11.981 ◀
sleep disorder F11.982 ◀
Opisthognathism M26.09
Opisthorchiasis (felineus) (viverrini) B66.0
Opitz' disease D73.2
Opiumism —*see* Dependence, drug, opioid
Oppenheim's disease G70.2
Oppenheim-Urbach disease (necrobiosis lipoidica diabeticorum) —*see* E08-E13 with .620
Optic nerve —*see* condition
Orbit —*see* condition
Orchioblastoma C62.9-
Orchitis (gangrenous) (nonspecific) (septic) (suppurative) N45.2
blennorrhagic (gonococcal) (acute) (chronic) A54.23
chlamydial A56.19
filarial —*see also* Infestation, filarial B74.9 *[N51]*
gonococcal (acute) (chronic) A54.23
mumps B26.0
syphilitic A52.76
tuberculous A18.15
Orf (virus disease) B08.02
Organic —*see also* condition
brain syndrome F09
heart —*see* Disease, heart
mental disorder F09
psychosis F09
Orgasm
anejaculatory N53.13
Oriental
bilharziasis B65.2
schistosomiasis B65.2
Orifice —*see* condition
Origin of both great vessels from right ventricle Q20.1
Ormond's disease (with ureteral obstruction) N13.5
with infection N13.6
Ornithine metabolism disorder E72.4
Ornithinemia (Type I) (Type II) E72.4
Ornithosis A70
Orotaciduria, oroticaciduria (congenital) (hereditary) (pyrimidine deficiency) E79.8
anemia D53.0
Orthodontics
adjustment Z46.4
fitting Z46.4
Orthopnea R06.01
Orthopoxvirus B08.09
specified NEC B08.09
Os, uterus —*see* condition
Osgood-Schlatter disease or osteochondrosis —*see* Osteochondrosis, juvenile, tibia

◀ New ◀ Revised ~~deleted~~ Deleted

Osler (-Weber)-Rendu disease I78.0
Osler's nodes I33.0
Osmidrosis L75.0
Osseous —*see* condition
Ossification
artery —*see* Arteriosclerosis
auricle (ear) —*see* Disorder, pinna, specified type NEC
bronchial J98.09
cardiac —*see* Degeneration, myocardial
cartilage (senile) —*see* Disorder, cartilage, specified type NEC
coronary (artery) —*see* Disease, heart, ischemic, atherosclerotic
diaphragm J98.6
ear, middle —*see* Otosclerosis
falx cerebri G96.19
fontanel, premature Q75.0
heart —*see also* Degeneration, myocardial
valve —*see* Endocarditis
larynx J38.7
ligament —*see* Disorder, tendon, specified type NEC
posterior longitudinal —*see* Spondylopathy, specified NEC
meninges (cerebral) (spinal) G96.19
multiple, eccentric centers —*see* Disorder, bone, development or growth
muscle —*see also* Calcification, muscle
due to burns —*see* Myositis, ossificans, in, burns
paralytic —*see* Myositis, ossificans, in, quadriplegia
progressive —*see* Myositis, ossificans, progressiva
specified NEC M61.50
ankle M61.57-
foot M61.57-
forearm M61.53-
hand M61.54-
lower leg M61.56-
multiple sites M61.59
pelvic region M61.55-
shoulder region M61.51-
specified site NEC M61.58
thigh M61.55-
upper arm M61.52-
traumatic —*see* Myositis, ossificans, traumatica
myocardium, myocardial —*see* Degeneration, myocardial
penis N48.89
periarticular —*see* Disorder, joint, specified type NEC
pinna —*see* Disorder, pinna, specified type NEC
rider's bone —*see* Ossification, muscle, specified NEC
sclera H15.89
subperiosteal, post-traumatic M89.8X-
tendon —*see* Disorder, tendon, specified type NEC
trachea J39.8
tympanic membrane —*see* Disorder, tympanic membrane, specified NEC
vitreous (humor) —*see* Deposit, crystalline
Osteitis —*see also* Osteomyelitis
alveolar M27.3
condensans M85.30
ankle M85.37-
foot M85.37-
forearm M85.33-
hand M85.34-
lower leg M85.36-
multiple site M85.39
neck M85.38
rib M85.38
shoulder M85.31-
skull M85.38
Osteitis *(Continued)*
condensans *(Continued)*
specified site NEC M85.38
thigh M85.35-
toe M85.37-
upper arm M85.32-
vertebra M85.38
deformans M88.9
in (due to)
malignant neoplasm of bone C41.9 *[M90.60]*
neoplastic disease —*see also* Neoplasm D49.9 *[M90.60]*
carpus D49.9 *[M90.64-]*
clavicle D49.9 *[M90.61-]*
femur D49.9 *[M90.65-]*
fibula D49.9 *[M90.66-]*
finger D49.9 *[M90.64-]*
humerus D49.9 *[M90.62-]*
ilium D49.9 *[M90.65-]*
ischium D49.9 *[M90.65-]*
metacarpus D49.9 *[M90.64-]*
metatarsus D49.9 *[M90.67-]*
multiple sites D49.9 *[M90.69]*
neck D49.9 *[M90.68]*
radius D49.9 *[M90.63-]*
rib D49.9 *[M90.68]*
scapula D49.9 *[M90.61-]*
skull D49.9 *[M90.68]*
tarsus D49.9 *[M90.67-]*
tibia D49.9 *[M90.66-]*
toe D49.9 *[M90.67-]*
ulna D49.9 *[M90.63-]*
vertebra D49.9 *[M90.68]*
skull M88.0
specified NEC —*see* Paget's disease, bone, by site
vertebra M88.1
due to yaws A66.6
fibrosa NEC —*see* Cyst, bone, by site
circumscripta —*see* Dysplasia, fibrous, bone NEC
cystica (generalisata) E21.0
disseminata Q78.1
osteoplastica E21.0
fragilitans Q78.0
Garr's (sclerosing) —*see* Osteomyelitis, specified type NEC
jaw (acute) (chronic) (lower) (suppurative) (upper) M27.2
parathyroid E21.0
petrous bone (acute) (chronic) —*see* Petrositis
sclerotic, nonsuppurative —*see* Osteomyelitis, specified type NEC
tuberculosa A18.09
cystica D86.89
multiplex cystoides D86.89
Osteoarthritis M19.90
ankle M19.07-
elbow M19.02-
foot joint M19.07-
generalized M15.9
erosive M15.4
primary M15.0
specified NEC M15.8
hand joint M19.04-
first carpometacarpal joint M18.9-
hip M16.1-
bilateral M16.0
due to hip dysplasia (unilateral) M16.3-
bilateral M16.2
interphalangeal
distal (Heberden) M15.1
proximal (Bouchard) M15.2
knee M17.9-
bilateral M17.0
post-traumatic NEC M19.92
ankle M19.17-
elbow M19.12-
foot joint M19.17-
Osteoarthritis *(Continued)*
post-traumatic NEC *(Continued)*
hand joint M19.14-
first carpometacarpal joint M18.3-
bilateral M18.2
hip M16.5-
bilateral M16.4
knee M17.3-
bilateral M17.2
shoulder M19.11-
wrist M19.13-
primary M19.91
ankle M19.07-
elbow M19.02-
foot joint M19.07-
hand joint M19.04-
first carpometacarpal joint M18.1-
bilateral M18.0
hip M16.1-
bilateral M16.0
knee M17.1-
bilateral M17.0
shoulder M19.01-
spine —*see* Spondylosis
wrist M19.03-
secondary M19.93
ankle M19.27-
elbow M19.22-
foot joint M19.27-
hand joint M19.24-
first carpometacarpal joint M18.5-
bilateral M18.4
hip M16.7
bilateral M16.6
knee M17.5
bilateral M17.4
multiple M15.3
shoulder M19.21-
spine —*see* Spondylosis
wrist M19.23-
shoulder M19.01-
spine —*see* Spondylosis
wrist M19.03-
Osteoarthropathy (hypertrophic) M19.90
ankle —*see* Osteoarthritis, primary, ankle
elbow —*see* Osteoarthritis, primary, elbow
foot joint —*see* Osteoarthritis, primary, foot
hand joint —*see* Osteoarthritis, primary, hand joint
knee joint —*see* Osteoarthritis, primary, knee
multiple site —*see* Osteoarthritis, primary, multiple joint
pulmonary —*see also* Osteoarthropathy, specified type NEC
hypertrophic —*see* Osteoarthropathy, hypertrophic, specified type NEC
secondary —*see* Osteoarthropathy, specified type NEC
secondary hypertrophic —*see* Osteoarthropathy, specified type NEC
shoulder —*see* Osteoarthritis, primary, shoulder
specified joint NEC —*see* Osteoarthritis, primary, specified joint NEC
specified type NEC M89.40
carpus M89.44-
clavicle M89.41-
femur M89.45-
fibula M89.46-
finger M89.44-
humerus M89.42-
ilium M89.459
ischium M89.459
metacarpus M89.44-
metatarsus M89.47-
multiple sites M89.49
neck M89.48
radius M89.43-
rib M89.48
scapula M89.41-
skull M89.48

Osteoarthropathy *(Continued)*
specified type NEC *(Continued)*
tarsus M89.47-
tibia M89.46-
toe M89.47-
ulna M89.43-
vertebra M89.48
spine —*see* Spondylosis
wrist —*see* Osteoarthritis, primary, wrist
Osteoarthrosis (degenerative) (hypertrophic) (joint) —*see also* Osteoarthritis
deformans alkaptonurica E70.29 *[M36.8]*
erosive M15.4
generalized M15.9
primary M15.0
polyarticular M15.9
spine —*see* Spondylosis
Osteoblastoma —*see* Neoplasm, bone, benign
aggressive —*see* Neoplasm, bone, uncertain behavior
Osteochondroarthrosis deformans endemica —*see* Disease, Kaschin-Beck
Osteochondritis —*see also* Osteochondropathy, by site
Brailsford's —*see* Osteochondrosis, juvenile, radius
dissecans M93.20
ankle M93.27-
elbow M93.22-
foot M93.27-
hand M93.24-
hip M93.25-
knee M93.26-
multiple sites M93.29
shoulder joint M93.21-
specified site NEC M93.28
wrist M93.23-
juvenile M92.9
patellar —*see* Osteochondrosis, juvenile, patella
syphilitic (congenital) (early) A50.02 *[M90.80]*
ankle A50.02 *[M90.87-]*
elbow A50.02 *[M90.82-]*
foot A50.02 *[M90.87-]*
forearm A50.02 *[M90.83-]*
hand A50.02 *[M90.84-]*
hip A50.02 *[M90.85-]*
knee A50.02 *[M90.86-]*
multiple sites A50.02 *[M90.89]*
shoulder joint A50.02 *[M90.81-]*
specified site NEC A50.02 *[M90.88]*
Osteochondrodysplasia Q78.9
with defects of growth of tubular bones and spine Q77.9
specified NEC Q77.8
specified NEC Q78.8
Osteochondrodystrophy E78.9
Osteochondrolysis —*see* Osteochondritis, dissecans
Osteochondroma —*see* Neoplasm, bone, benign
Osteochondromatosis D48.0
syndrome Q78.4
Osteochondromyxosarcoma —*see* Neoplasm, bone, malignant
Osteochondropathy M93.90
ankle M93.97-
elbow M93.92-
foot M93.97-
hand M93.94-
hip M93.95-
Kienböck's disease of adults M93.1
knee M93.96-
multiple joints M93.99
osteochondritis dissecans —*see* Osteochondritis, dissecans
osteochondrosis —*see* Osteochondrosis
shoulder region M93.91-
slipped upper femoral epiphysis —*see* Slipped, epiphysis, upper femoral
specified joint NEC M93.98

Osteochondropathy *(Continued)*
specified type NEC M93.80
ankle M93.87-
elbow M93.82-
foot M93.87-
hand M93.84-
hip M93.85-
knee M93.86-
multiple joints M93.89
shoulder region M93.81-
specified joint NEC M93.88
wrist M93.83-
syphilitic, congenital
early A50.02 *[M90.80]*
late A50.56 *[M90.80]*
wrist M93.93-
Osteochondrosarcoma —*see* Neoplasm, bone, malignant
Osteochondrosis —*see also* Osteochondropathy, by site
acetabulum (juvenile) M91.0
adult —*see* Osteochondropathy, specified type NEC, by site
astragalus (juvenile) —*see* Osteochondrosis, juvenile, tarsus
Blount's —*see* Osteochondrosis, juvenile, tibia
Buchanan's M91.0
Burns' —*see* Osteochondrosis, juvenile, ulna
calcaneus (juvenile) —*see* Osteochondrosis, juvenile, tarsus
capitular epiphysis (femur) (juvenile) —*see* Legg-Calvé-Perthes disease
carpal (juvenile) (lunate) (scaphoid) —*see* Osteochondrosis, juvenile, hand, carpal lunate
adult M93.1
coxae juvenilis —*see* Legg-Calvé-Perthes disease
deformans juvenilis, coxae —*see* Legg-Calvé-Perthes disease
Diaz's —*see* Osteochondrosis, juvenile, tarsus
dissecans (knee) (shoulder) —*see* Osteochondritis, dissecans
femoral capital epiphysis (juvenile) —*see* Legg-Calvé-Perthes disease
femur (head), juvenile —*see* Legg-Calvé-Perthes disease
fibula (juvenile) —*see* Osteochondrosis, juvenile, fibula
foot NEC (juvenile) M92.8
Freiberg's —*see* Osteochondrosis, juvenile, metatarsus
Haas' (juvenile) —*see* Osteochondrosis, juvenile, humerus
Haglund's —*see* Osteochondrosis, juvenile, tarsus
hip (juvenile) —*see* Legg-Calvé-Perthes disease
humerus (capitulum) (head) (juvenile) —*see* Osteochondrosis, juvenile, humerus
ilium, iliac crest (juvenile) M91.0
ischiopubic synchondrosis M91.0
Iselin's —*see* Osteochondrosis, juvenile, metatarsus
juvenile, juvenilis M92.9
after congenital dislocation of hip reduction —*see* Osteochondrosis, juvenile, hip, specified NEC
arm —*see* Osteochondrosis, juvenile, upper limb NEC
capitular epiphysis (femur) —*see* Legg-Calvé-Perthes disease
clavicle, sternal epiphysis —*see* Osteochondrosis, juvenile, upper limb NEC
coxae —*see* Legg-Calvé-Perthes disease
deformans M92.9
fibula M92.5-
foot NEC M92.8

Osteochondrosis *(Continued)*
juvenile, juvenilis *(Continued)*
hand M92.20-
carpal lunate M92.21-
metacarpal head M92.22-
specified site NEC M92.29-
head of femur —*see* Legg-Calvé-Perthes disease
hip and pelvis M91.9-
coxa plana —*see* Coxa, plana
femoral head —*see* Legg-Calvé-Perthes disease
pelvis M91.0
pseudocoxalgia —*see* Pseudocoxalgia
specified NEC M91.8-
humerus M92.0-
limb
lower NEC M92.8
upper NEC —*see* Osteochondrosis, juvenile, upper limb NEC
medial cuneiform bone —*see* Osteochondrosis, juvenile, tarsus
metatarsus M92.7-
patella M92.4-
radius M92.1-
specified site NEC M92.8
spine M42.00
cervical region M42.02
cervicothoracic region M42.03
lumbar region M42.06
lumbosacral region M42.07
multiple sites M42.09
occipito-atlanto-axial region M42.01
sacrococcygeal region M42.08
thoracic region M42.04
thoracolumbar region M42.05
tarsus M92.6-
tibia M92.5-
ulna M92.1-
upper limb NEC M92.3-
vertebra (body) (epiphyseal plates) (Calvé's) (Scheuermann's) —*see* Osteochondrosis, juvenile, spine
Kienböck's —*see* Osteochondrosis, juvenile, hand, carpal lunate
adult M93.1
Köhler's
patellar —*see* Osteochondrosis, juvenile, patella
tarsal navicular —*see* Osteochondrosis, juvenile, tarsus
Legg-Perthes (-Calvé's) (-Waldenström) —*see* Legg-Calvé-Perthes disease
limb
lower NEC (juvenile) M92.8
upper NEC (juvenile) —*see* Osteochondrosis, juvenile, upper limb NEC
lunate bone (carpal) (juvenile) —*see also* Osteochondrosis, juvenile, hand, carpal lunate
adult M93.1
Mauclaire's —*see* Osteochondrosis, juvenile, hand, metacarpal
metacarpal (head) (juvenile) —*see* Osteochondrosis, juvenile, hand, metacarpal
metatarsus (fifth) (head) (juvenile) (second) —*see* Osteochondrosis, juvenile, metatarsus
navicular (juvenile) —*see* Osteochondrosis, juvenile, tarsus
os
calcis (juvenile) —*see* Osteochondrosis, juvenile, tarsus
tibiale externum (juvenile) —*see* Osteochondrosis, juvenile, tarsus
Osgood-Schlatter —*see* Osteochondrosis, juvenile, tibia
Panner's —*see* Osteochondrosis, juvenile, humerus

Osteochondrosis *(Continued)*
patellar center (juvenile) (primary) (secondary) —*see* Osteochondrosis, juvenile, patella
pelvis (juvenile) M91.0
Pierson's M91.0
radius (head) (juvenile) —*see* Osteochondrosis, juvenile, radius
Scheuermann's —*see* Osteochondrosis, juvenile, spine
Sever's —*see* Osteochondrosis, juvenile, tarsus
Sinding-Larsen —*see* Osteochondrosis, juvenile, patella
spine M42.9
adult M42.10
cervical region M42.12
cervicothoracic region M42.13
lumbar region M42.16
lumbosacral region M42.17
multiple sites M42.19
occipito-atlanto-axial region M42.11
sacrococcygeal region M42.18
thoracic region M42.14
thoracolumbar region M42.15
juvenile —*see* Osteochondrosis, juvenile, spine
symphysis pubis (juvenile) M91.0
syphilitic (congenital) A50.02
talus (juvenile) —*see* Osteochondrosis, juvenile, tarsus
tarsus (navicular) (juvenile) —*see* Osteochondrosis, juvenile, tarsus
tibia (proximal) (tubercle) (juvenile) —*see* Osteochondrosis, juvenile, tibia
tuberculous —*see* Tuberculosis, bone
ulna (lower) (juvenile) —*see* Osteochondrosis, juvenile, ulna
van Neck's M91.0
vertebral —*see* Osteochondrosis, spine
Osteoclastoma D48.0
malignant —*see* Neoplasm, bone, malignant
Osteodynia —*see* Disorder, bone, specified type NEC
Osteodystrophy Q78.9
azotemic N25.0
congenital Q78.9
parathyroid, secondary E21.1
renal N25.0
Osteofibroma —*see* Neoplasm, bone, benign
Osteofibrosarcoma —*see* Neoplasm, bone, malignant
Osteogenesis imperfecta Q78.0
Osteogenic —*see* condition
Osteolysis M89.50
carpus M89.54-
clavicle M89.51-
femur M89.55-
fibula M89.56-
finger M89.54-
humerus M89.52-
ilium M89.559
ischium M89.559
joint prosthesis (periprosthetic) —*see* Complications, joint prosthesis, mechanical, periprosthetic, osteolysis, by site
metacarpus M89.54-
metatarsus M89.57-
multiple sites M89.59
neck M89.58
periprosthetic —*see* Complications, joint prosthesis, mechanical, periprosthetic, osteolysis, by site
radius M89.53-
rib M89.58
scapula M89.51-
skull M89.58
Osteolysis *(Continued)*
tarsus M89.57-
tibia M89.56-
toe M89.57-
ulna M89.53-
vertebra M89.58
Osteoma —*see also* Neoplasm, bone, benign
osteoid —*see also* Neoplasm, bone, benign
giant —*see* Neoplasm, bone, benign
Osteomalacia M83.9
adult M83.9
drug-induced NEC M83.5
due to
malabsorption (postsurgical) M83.2
malnutrition M83.3
specified NEC M83.8
aluminium-induced M83.4
infantile —*see* Rickets
juvenile —*see* Rickets
oncogenic E83.89
pelvis M83.8
puerperal M83.0
senile M83.1
vitamin-D-resistant in adults E83.31 *[M90.8-]*
carpus E83.31 *[M90.84-]*
clavicle E83.31 *[M90.81-]*
femur E83.31 *[M90.85-]*
fibula E83.31 *[M90.86-]*
finger E83.31 *[M90.84-]*
humerus E83.31 *[M90.82-]*
ilium E83.31 *[M90.859]*
ischium E83.31 *[M90.859]*
metacarpus E83.31 *[M90.84-]*
metatarsus E83.31 *[M90.87-]*
multiple sites E83.31 *[M90.89]*
neck E83.31 *[M90.88]*
radius E83.31 *[M90.83-]*
rib E83.31 *[M90.88]*
scapula E83.31 *[M90.819]*
skull E83.31 *[M90.88]*
tarsus E83.31 *[M90.879]*
tibia E83.31 *[M90.869]*
toe E83.31 *[M90.879]*
ulna E83.31 *[M90.839]*
vertebra E83.31 *[M90.88]*
Osteomyelitis (general) (infective) (localized) (neonatal) (purulent) (septic) (staphylococcal) (streptococcal) (suppurative) (with periostitis) M86.9
acute M86.10
carpus M86.14-
clavicle M86.11-
femur M86.15-
fibula M86.16-
finger M86.14-
hematogenous M86.00
carpus M86.04-
clavicle M86.01-
femur M86.05-
fibula M86.06-
finger M86.04-
humerus M86.02-
ilium M86.059
ischium M86.059
mandible M27.2
metacarpus M86.04-
metatarsus M86.07-
multiple sites M86.09
neck M86.08
orbit H05.02-
petrous bone —*see* Petrositis
radius M86.03-
rib M86.08
scapula M86.01-
skull M86.08
tarsus M86.07-
tibia M86.06-
toe M86.07-
ulna M86.03-
vertebra —*see* Osteomyelitis, vertebra
Osteomyelitis *(Continued)*
acute *(Continued)*
humerus M86.12-
ilium M86.159
ischium M86.159
mandible M27.2
metacarpus M86.14-
metatarsus M86.17-
multiple sites M86.19
neck M86.18
orbit H05.02-
petrous bone —*see* Petrositis
radius M86.13-
rib M86.18
scapula M86.11-
skull M86.18
tarsus M86.17-
tibia M86.16-
toe M86.17-
ulna M86.13-
vertebra —*see* Osteomyelitis, vertebra
chronic (or old) M86.60
with draining sinus M86.40
carpus M86.44-
clavicle M86.41-
femur M86.45-
fibula M86.46-
finger M86.44-
humerus M86.42-
ilium M86.459
ischium M86.459
mandible M27.2
metacarpus M86.44-
metatarsus M86.47-
multiple sites M86.49
neck M86.48
orbit H05.02-
petrous bone —*see* Petrositis
radius M86.43-
rib M86.48
scapula M86.41-
skull M86.48
tarsus M86.47-
tibia M86.46-
toe M86.47-
ulna M86.43-
vertebra —*see* Osteomyelitis, vertebra
carpus M86.64-
clavicle M86.61-
femur M86.65-
fibula M86.66-
finger M86.64-
hematogenous NEC M86.50
carpus M86.54-
clavicle M86.51-
femur M86.55-
fibula M86.56-
finger M86.54-
humerus M86.52-
ilium M86.559
ischium M86.559
mandible M27.2
metacarpus M86.54-
metatarsus M86.57-
multifocal M86.30
carpus M86.34-
clavicle M86.31-
femur M86.35-
fibula M86.36-
finger M86.34-
humerus M86.32-
ilium M86.359
ischium M86.359
metacarpus M86.34-
metatarsus M86.37-
multiple sites M86.39
neck M86.38
radius M86.33-
rib M86.38
scapula M86.31-

Osteomyelitis *(Continued)*
chronic *(Continued)*
hematogenous NEC *(Continued)*
multifocal *(Continued)*
skull M86.38
tarsus M86.37-
tibia M86.36-
toe M86.37-
ulna M86.33-
vertebra —*see* Osteomyelitis, vertebra
multiple sites M86.59
neck M86.58
orbit H05.02-
petrous bone —*see* Petrositis
radius M86.53-
rib M86.58
scapula M86.51-
skull M86.58
tarsus M86.57-
tibia M86.56-
toe M86.57-
ulna M86.53-
vertebra —*see* Osteomyelitis, vertebra
humerus M86.62-
ilium M86.659
ischium M86.659
mandible M27.2
metacarpus M86.64-
metatarsus M86.67-
multifocal —*see* Osteomyelitis, chronic, hematogenous, multifocal
multiple sites M86.69
neck M86.68
orbit H05.02-
petrous bone —*see* Petrositis
radius M86.63-
rib M86.68
scapula M86.61-
skull M86.68
tarsus M86.67-
tibia M86.66-
toe M86.67-
ulna M86.63-
vertebra —*see* Osteomyelitis, vertebra
echinococcal B67.2
Garr's —*see* Osteomyelitis, specified type NEC
in diabetes mellitus —*see* E08-E13 with .69 ◀
jaw (acute) (chronic) (lower) (neonatal) (suppurative) (upper) M27.2
nonsuppurating —*see* Osteomyelitis, specified type NEC
orbit H05.02-
petrous bone —*see* Petrositis
Salmonella (arizonae) (cholerae-suis) (enteritidis) (typhimurium) A02.24
sclerosing, nonsuppurative —*see* Osteomyelitis, specified type NEC
specified type NEC —*see also* subcategory M86.8X-
mandible M27.2
orbit H05.02-
petrous bone —*see* Petrositis
vertebra —*see* Osteomyelitis, vertebra
subacute M86.20
carpus M86.24-
clavicle M86.21-
femur M86.25-
fibula M86.26-
finger M86.24-
humerus M86.22-
mandible M27.2
metacarpus M86.24-
metatarsus M86.27-
multiple sites M86.29
neck M86.28
orbit H05.02-
petrous bone —*see* Petrositis
radius M86.23-
rib M86.28
scapula M86.21-

Osteomyelitis *(Continued)*
subacute *(Continued)*
skull M86.28
tarsus M86.27-
tibia M86.26-
toe M86.27-
ulna M86.23-
vertebra —*see* Osteomyelitis, vertebra
syphilitic A52.77
congenital (early) A50.02 *[M90.80]*
tuberculous —*see* Tuberculosis, bone
typhoid A01.05
vertebra M46.20
cervical region M46.22
cervicothoracic region M46.23
lumbar region M46.26
lumbosacral region M46.27
occipito-atlanto-axial region M46.21
sacrococcygeal region M46.28
thoracic region M46.24
thoracolumbar region M46.25
Osteomyelofibrosis D47.4 ⇐
Osteomyelosclerosis D75.89
Osteonecrosis M87.9
due to
drugs —*see* Osteonecrosis, secondary, due to, drugs
trauma —*see* Osteonecrosis, secondary, due to, trauma
idiopathic aseptic M87.00
ankle M87.07-
carpus M87.03-
clavicle M87.01-
femur M87.05-
fibula M87.06-
finger M87.04-
humerus M87.02-
ilium M87.050
ischium M87.050
metacarpus M87.04-
metatarsus M87.07-
multiple sites M87.09
neck M87.08
pelvis M87.050
radius M87.03-
rib M87.08
scapula M87.01-
skull M87.08
tarsus M87.07-
tibia M87.06-
toe M87.07-
ulna M87.03-
vertebra M87.08
secondary NEC M87.30
carpus M87.33-
clavicle M87.31-
due to
drugs M87.10
carpus M87.13-
clavicle M87.11-
femur M87.15-
fibula M87.16-
finger M87.14-
humerus M87.12-
ilium M87.159
ischium M87.159
jaw M87.180
metacarpus M87.14-
metatarsus M87.17-
multiple sites M87.19
neck M87.18
radius M87.13-
rib M87.18
scapula M87.11-
skull M87.18
tarsus M87.17-
tibia M87.16-
toe M87.17-
ulna M87.13-
vertebra M87.18

Osteonecrosis *(Continued)*
secondary NEC *(Continued)*
due to *(Continued)*
hemoglobinopathy NEC D58.2 *[M90.50]*
carpus D58.2 *[M90.54-]*
clavicle D58.2 *[M90.51-]*
femur D58.2 *[M90.55-]*
fibula D58.2 *[M90.56-]*
finger D58.2 *[M90.54-]*
humerus D58.2 *[M90.52-]*
ilium D58.2 *[M90.55-]*
ischium D58.2 *[M90.55-]*
metacarpus D58.2 *[M90.54-]*
metatarsus D58.2 *[M90.57-]*
multiple sites D58.2 *[M90.58]*
neck D58.2 *[M90.58]*
radius D58.2 *[M90.53-]*
rib D58.2 *[M90.58]*
scapula D58.2 *[M90.51-]*
skull D58.2 *[M90.58]*
tarsus D58.2 *[M90.57-]*
tibia D58.2 *[M90.56-]*
toe D58.2 *[M90.57-]*
ulna D58.2 *[M90.53-]*
vertebra D58.2 *[M90.58]*
trauma (previous) M87.20
carpus M87.23-
clavicle M87.21-
femur M87.25-
fibula M87.26-
finger M87.24-
humerus M87.22-
ilium M87.25-
ischium M87.25-
metacarpus M87.24-
metatarsus M87.27-
multiple sites M87.29
neck M87.28
radius M87.23-
rib M87.28
scapula M87.21-
skull M87.28
tarsus M87.27-
tibia M87.26-
toe M87.27-
ulna M87.23-
vertebra M87.28
femur M87.35-
fibula M87.36-
finger M87.34-
humerus M87.32
ilium M87.350
in
caisson disease T70.3 *[M90.50]*
carpus T70.3 *[M90.54-]*
clavicle T70.3 *[M90.51-]*
femur T70.3 *[M90.55-]*
fibula T70.3 *[M90.56-]*
finger T70.3 *[M90.54-]*
humerus T70.3 *[M90.52-]*
ilium T70.3 *[M90.55-]*
ischium T70.3 *[M90.55-]*
metacarpus T70.3 *[M90.54-]*
metatarsus T70.3 *[M90.57-]*
multiple sites T70.3 *[M90.59]*
neck T70.3 *[M90.58]*
radius T70.3 *[M90.53-]*
rib T70.3 *[M90.58]*
scapula T70.3 *[M90.51-]*
skull T70.3 *[M90.58]*
tarsus T70.3 *[M90.57-]*
tibia T70.3 *[M90.56-]*
toe T70.3 *[M90.57-]*
ulna T70.3 *[M90.53-]*
vertebra T70.3 *[M90.58]*
ischium M87.350
metacarpus M87.34-
metatarsus M87.37-
multiple site M87.39
neck M87.38

◀ New ⇐ Revised ~~deleted~~ Deleted

Osteonecrosis *(Continued)*
secondary NEC *(Continued)*
radius M87.33-
rib M87.38
scapula M87.319
skull M87.38
tarsus M87.379
tibia M87.366
toe M87.379
ulna M87.33-
vertebra M87.38
specified type NEC M87.80
carpus M87.83-
clavicle M87.81-
femur M87.85-
fibula M87.86-
finger M87.84-
humerus M87.82-
ilium M87.85-
ischium M87.85-
metacarpus M87.84-
metatarsus M87.87-
multiple sites M87.89
neck M87.88
radius M87.83-
rib M87.88-
scapula M87.81-
skull M87.88
tarsus M87.87-
tibia M87.86-
toe M87.87-
ulna M87.83-
vertebra M87.88
Osteo-onycho-arthro-dysplasia Q87.2 ◀
Osteo-onychodysplasia, hereditary Q87.2 ◀
Osteopathia condensans disseminata Q78.8
Osteopathy —*see also* Osteomyelitis, Osteonecrosis, Osteoporosis
after poliomyelitis M89.60
carpus M89.64-
clavicle M89.61-
femur M89.65-
fibula M89.66-
finger M89.64-
humerus M89.62-
ilium M89.659
ischium M89.659
metacarpus M89.64-
metatarsus M89.67-
multiple sites M89.69
neck M89.68
radius M89.63-
rib M89.68
scapula M89.61-
skull M89.68
tarsus M89.67-
tibia M89.66-
toe M89.67-
ulna M89.63-
vertebra M89.68
in (due to)
renal osteodystrophy N25.0
specified diseases classified elsewhere —*see* subcategory M90.8
Osteopenia M85.8-
borderline M85.8-
Osteoperiostitis —*see* Osteomyelitis, specified type NEC
Osteopetrosis (familial) Q78.2
Osteophyte M25.70
ankle M25.77-
elbow M25.72-
foot joint M25.77-
hand joint M25.74-
hip M25.75-
knee M25.76-
shoulder M25.71-
spine M25.78
vertebrae M25.78
wrist M25.73-
Osteopoikilosis Q78.8
Osteoporosis (female) (male) M81.0
with current pathological fracture M80.00
age-related M81.0
with current pathologic fracture M80.00
carpus M80.04-
clavicle M80.01-
fibula M80.06-
finger M80.04-
humerus M80.02-
ilium M80.05-
ischium M80.05-
metacarpus M80.04-
metatarsus M80.07-
pelvis M80.05-
radius M80.03-
scapula M80.01-
tarsus M80.07-
tibia M80.06-
toe M80.07-
ulna M80.03-
vertebra M80.08
disuse M81.8
with current pathological fracture M80.80
carpus M80.84-
clavicle M80.81-
fibula M80.86-
finger M80.84-
humerus M80.82-
ilium M80.85-
ischium M80.85-
metacarpus M80.84-
metatarsus M80.87-
pelvis M80.85-
radius M80.83-
scapula M80.81-
tarsus M80.87-
tibia M80.86-
toe M80.87-
ulna M80.83-
vertebra M80.88
drug-induced —*see* Osteoporosis, specified type NEC
idiopathic —*see* Osteoporosis, specified type NEC
involutional —*see* Osteoporosis, age-related
Lequesne M81.6
localized M81.6
postmenopausal M81.0
with pathological fracture M80.00
carpus M80.04-
clavicle M80.01-
fibula M80.06-
finger M80.04-
humerus M80.02-
ilium M80.05-
ischium M80.05-
metacarpus M80.04-
metatarsus M80.07-
pelvis M80.05-
radius M80.03-
scapula M80.01-
tarsus M80.07-
tibia M80.06-
toe M80.07-
ulna M80.03-
vertebra M80.08
postoophorectomy —*see* Osteoporosis, specified type NEC
postsurgical malabsorption —*see* Osteoporosis, specified type NEC
post-traumatic —*see* Osteoporosis, specified type NEC
senile —*see* Osteoporosis, age-related
specified type NEC M81.8
with pathological fracture M80.80
carpus M80.84-
clavicle M80.81-
fibula M80.86-
finger M80.84-
humerus M80.82-
ilium M80.85-
Osteoporosis *(Continued)*
specified type NEC *(Continued)*
with pathological fracture *(Continued)*
ischium M80.85-
metacarpus M80.84-
metatarsus M80.87-
pelvis M80.85-
radius M80.83-
scapula M80.81-
tarsus M80.87-
tibia M80.86-
toe M80.87-
ulna M80.83-
vertebra M80.88
Osteopsathyrosis (idiopathica) Q78.0
Osteoradionecrosis, jaw (acute) (chronic) (lower) (suppurative) (upper) M27.2
Osteosarcoma (any form) —*see* Neoplasm, bone, malignant
Osteosclerosis Q78.2
acquired M85.8-
congenita Q77.4
fragilitas (generalisata) Q78.2
myelofibrosis D75.81
Osteosclerotic anemia D64.89
Osteosis
cutis L94.2
renal fibrocystic N25.0
Österreicher-Turner syndrome Q87.2
Ostium
atrioventriculare commune Q21.2
primum (arteriosum) (defect) (persistent) Q21.2
secundum (arteriosum) (defect) (patent) (persistent) Q21.1
Ostrum-Furst syndrome Q75.8
Otalgia —*see* subcategory H92.0
Otitis (acute) H66.90
with effusion —*see also* Otitis, media, nonsuppurative
purulent —*see* Otitis, media, suppurative
adhesive —*see* subcategory H74.1
chronic —*see also* Otitis, media, chronic
with effusion —*see also* Otitis, media, nonsuppurative, chronic
externa H60.9-
abscess —*see* Abscess, ear, external
acute (noninfective) H60.50-
actinic H60.51-
chemical H60.52-
contact H60.53-
eczematoid H60.54-
infective —*see* Otitis, externa, infective
reactive H60.55-
specified NEC H60.59-
cellulitis —*see* Cellulitis, ear
chronic H60.6-
diffuse —*see* Otitis, externa, infective, diffuse
hemorrhagic —*see* Otitis, externa, infective, hemorrhagic
in (due to)
aspergillosis B44.89
candidiasis B37.84
erysipelas A46 *[H62.40]*
herpes (simplex) virus infection B00.1
zoster B02.8
impetigo L01.00 *[H62.40]*
infectious disease NEC B99 *[H62.4-]*
mycosis NEC B36.9 *[H62.40]*
parasitic disease NEC B89 *[H62.40]*
viral disease NEC B34.9 *[H62.40]*
zoster B02.8
infective NEC H60.39-
abscess —*see* Abscess, ear, external
cellulitis —*see* Cellulitis, ear
diffuse H60.31-
hemorrhagic H60.32-
swimmer's ear —*see* Swimmer's, ear
malignant H60.2-
~~mycotic B36.9 [H62.40]~~

◀ New ◀ Revised ~~deleted~~ Deleted

Otitis *(Continued)*
externa *(Continued)*
mycotic NEC B36.9 *[H62.40]* ◀
in ◀
aspergillosis B44.89 ◀
candidiasis B37.84 ◀
moniliasis B37.84 ◀
necrotizing —*see* Otitis, externa, malignant
Pseudomonas aeruginosa —*see* Otitis, externa, malignant
reactive —*see* Otitis, externa, acute, reactive
specified NEC —*see* subcategory H60.8
~~tropical B36.8~~
tropical NEC B36.9 *[H62.40]* ◀
in ◀
aspergillosis B44.89 ◀
candidiasis B37.84 ◀
moniliasis B37.84 ◀
insidiosa —*see* Otosclerosis
interna —*see* subcategory H83.0
media (hemorrhagic) (staphylococcal) (streptococcal) H66.9-
with effusion (nonpurulent) —*see* Otitis, media, nonsuppurative
acute, subacute H66.90
allergic —*see* Otitis, media, nonsuppurative, acute, allergic
exudative —*see* Otitis, media, suppurative, acute ⟸
mucoid —*see* Otitis, media, nonsuppurative, acute
necrotizing —*see also* Otitis, media, suppurative, acute
in
measles B05.3
scarlet fever A38.0
nonsuppurative NEC —*see* Otitis, media, nonsuppurative, acute
purulent —*see* Otitis, media, suppurative, acute
sanguinous —*see* Otitis, media, nonsuppurative, acute
secretory —*see* Otitis, media, nonsuppurative, acute, serous
seromucinous —*see* Otitis, media, nonsuppurative, acute
serous —*see* Otitis, media, nonsuppurative, acute, serous
suppurative —*see* Otitis, media, suppurative, acute
allergic —*see* Otitis, media, nonsuppurative
catarrhal —*see* Otitis, media, nonsuppurative
chronic H66.90
with effusion (nonpurulent) —*see* Otitis, media, nonsuppurative, chronic
allergic —*see* Otitis, media, nonsuppurative, chronic, allergic
benign suppurative —*see* Otitis, media, suppurative, chronic, tubotympanic
catarrhal —*see* Otitis, media, nonsuppurative, chronic, serous
exudative —*see* Otitis, media, suppurative, chronic ⟸
mucinous —*see* Otitis, media, nonsuppurative, chronic, mucoid
mucoid —*see* Otitis, media, nonsuppurative, chronic, mucoid
nonsuppurative NEC —*see* Otitis, media, nonsuppurative, chronic
purulent —*see* Otitis, media, suppurative, chronic
secretory —*see* Otitis, media, nonsuppurative, chronic, mucoid
seromucinous —*see* Otitis, media, nonsuppurative, chronic
serous —*see* Otitis, media, nonsuppurative, chronic, serous
suppurative —*see* Otitis, media, suppurative, chronic

Otitis *(Continued)*
media *(Continued)*
chronic *(Continued)*
transudative —*see* Otitis, media, nonsuppurative, chronic, mucoid
exudative —*see* Otitis, media, nonsuppurative
in (due to) (with)
influenza —*see* Influenza, with, otitis media
measles B05.3
scarlet fever A38.0
tuberculosis A18.6
viral disease NEC B34.- *[H67.-]*
mucoid —*see* Otitis, media, nonsuppurative
nonsuppurative H65.9-
acute or subacute NEC H65.19-
allergic H65.11-
recurrent H65.11-
recurrent H65.19-
secretory —*see* Otitis, media, nonsuppurative, serous
serous H65.0-
recurrent H65.0-
chronic H65.49-
allergic H65.41-
mucoid H65.3-
serous H65.2-
postmeasles B05.3
purulent —*see* Otitis, media, suppurative
secretory —*see* Otitis, media, nonsuppurative
seromucinous —*see* Otitis, media, nonsuppurative
serous —*see* Otitis, media, nonsuppurative
suppurative H66.4-
acute H66.00-
with rupture of ear drum H66.01-
recurrent H66.00-
with rupture of ear drum H66.01-
chronic —*see also* subcategory H66.3
atticoantral H66.2-
benign —*see* Otitis, media, suppurative, chronic, tubotympanic
tubotympanic H66.1-
transudative —*see* Otitis, media, nonsuppurative
tuberculous A18.6
Otocephaly Q18.2
Otolith syndrome —*see* subcategory H81.8
Otomycosis (diffuse) NEC B36.9 *[H62.40]*
in
aspergillosis B44.89
candidiasis B37.84
moniliasis B37.84
Otoporosis —*see* Otosclerosis
Otorrhagia (nontraumatic) H92.2-
traumatic - code by Type of injury
Otorrhea H92.1-
cerebrospinal G96.0
Otosclerosis (general) H80.9-
cochlear (endosteal) H80.2-
involving
otic capsule —*see* Otosclerosis, cochlear
oval window
nonobliterative H80.0-
obliterative H80.1-
round window —*see* Otosclerosis, cochlear
nonobliterative —*see* Otosclerosis, involving, oval window, nonobliterative
obliterative —*see* Otosclerosis, involving, oval window, obliterative
specified NEC H80.8-
Otospongiosis —*see* Otosclerosis
Otto's disease or pelvis M24.7
Outcome of delivery Z37.9
multiple births Z37.9
all liveborn Z37.50
quadruplets Z37.52
quintuplets Z37.53

Outcome of delivery *(Continued)*
multiple births *(Continued)*
all liveborn *(Continued)*
sextuplets Z37.54
specified number NEC Z37.59
triplets Z37.51
all stillborn Z37.7
some liveborn Z37.60
quadruplets Z37.62
quintuplets Z37.63
sextuplets Z37.64
specified number NEC Z37.69
triplets Z37.61
single NEC Z37.9
liveborn Z37.0
stillborn Z37.1
twins NEC Z37.9
both liveborn Z37.2
both stillborn Z37.4
one liveborn, one stillborn Z37.3
Outlet —*see* condition
Ovalocytosis (congenital) (hereditary) —*see* Elliptocytosis
Ovarian —*see* Condition
Ovariocele N83.4- ⟸
Ovaritis (cystic) —*see* Oophoritis
Ovary, ovarian —*see also* condition
resistant syndrome E28.39
vein syndrome N13.8
Overactive —*see also* Hyperfunction
adrenal cortex NEC E27.0
bladder N32.81
hypothalamus E23.3
thyroid —*see* Hyperthyroidism
Overactivity R46.3
child —*see* Disorder, attention-deficit hyperactivity
Overbite (deep) (excessive) (horizontal) (vertical) M26.29
Overbreathing —*see* Hyperventilation
Overconscientious personality F60.5
Overdevelopment —*see* Hypertrophy
Overdistension —*see* Distension
Overdose, overdosage (drug) —*see* Table of Drugs and Chemicals, by drug, poisoning
Overeating R63.2
nonorganic origin F50.89 ⟸
psychogenic F50.89 ⟸
Overexertion (effects) (exhaustion) T73.3
Overexposure (effects) T73.9
exhaustion T73.2
Overfeeding —*see* Overeating
newborn P92.4
Overfill, endodontic M27.52
Overgrowth, bone —*see* Hypertrophy, bone
Overhanging of dental restorative material (unrepairable) K08.52
Overheated (places) (effects) —*see* Heat
Overjet (excessive horizontal) M26.23
Overlaid, overlying (suffocation) —*see* Asphyxia, traumatic, due to mechanical threat
Overlap, excessive horizontal (teeth) M26.23
Overl apping toe (acquired) —*see also* Deformity, toe, specified NEC
congenital (fifth toe) Q66.89
Overload
circulatory, due to transfusion (blood) (blood components) (TACO) E87.71
fluid E87.70
due to transfusion (blood) (blood components) E87.71
specified NEC E87.79
iron, due to repeated red blood cell transfusions E83.111
potassium (K) E87.5
sodium (Na) E87.0
Overnutrition —*see* Hyperalimentation
Overproduction —*see also* Hypersecretion
ACTH E27.0
catecholamine E27.5
growth hormone E22.0

Overprotection, child by parent Z62.1
Overriding
aorta Q25.49 ⬅
finger (acquired) —*see* Deformity, finger
congenital Q68.1
toe (acquired) —*see also* Deformity, toe, specified NEC
congenital Q66.89
Overstrained R53.83
heart —*see* Hypertrophy, cardiac
Overuse, muscle NEC M70.8-
Overweight E66.3
Overworked R53.83
Oviduct —*see* condition
Ovotestis Q56.0
Ovulation (cycle)
failure or lack of N97.0
pain N94.0
Ovum —*see* condition
Owren's disease or syndrome (parahemophilia) D68.2
Ox heart —*see* Hypertrophy, cardiac
Oxalosis E72.53
Oxaluria E72.53
Oxycephaly, oxycephalic Q75.0
syphilitic, congenital A50.02
Oxyuriasis B80
Oxyuris vermicularis (infestation) B80
Ozena J31.0

P

Pachyderma, pachydermia L85.9
larynx (verrucosa) J38.7
Pachydermatocele (congenital) Q82.8
Pachydermoperiostosis —*see also* Osteoarthropathy, hypertrophic, specified type NEC
clubbed nail M89.40 *[L62]*
Pachygyria Q04.3
Pachymeningitis (adhesive) (basal) (brain) (cervical) (chronic) (circumscribed) (external) (fibrous) (hemorrhagic) (hypertrophic) (internal) (purulent) (spinal) (suppurative) —*see* Meningitis
Pachyonychia (congenital) Q84.5
Pacinian tumor —*see* Neoplasm, skin, benign
Pad, knuckle or Garrod's M72.1
Paget-Schroetter syndrome I82.890
Paget's disease
with infiltrating duct carcinoma —*see* Neoplasm, breast, malignant
bone M88.9
carpus M88.84-
clavicle M88.81-
femur M88.85-
fibula M88.86-
finger M88.84-
humerus M88.82-
ilium M88.85-
in neoplastic disease —*see* Osteitis, deformans, in neoplastic disease
ischium M88.85-
metacarpus M88.84-
metatarsus M88.87-
multiple sites M88.89
neck M88.88
radius M88.83-
rib M88.88
scapula M88.81-
skull M88.0
tarsus M88.87-
tibia M88.86-
toe M88.87-
ulna M88.83-
vertebra M88.88
breast (female) C50.01-
male C50.02-
extramammary —*see also* Neoplasm, skin, malignant
anus C21.0
margin C44.590
skin C44.590
intraductal carcinoma —*see* Neoplasm, breast, malignant
malignant —*see* Neoplasm, skin, malignant
breast (female) C50.01-
male C50.02-
unspecified site (female) C50.01-
male C50.02-
mammary —*see* Paget's disease, breast
nipple —*see* Paget's disease, breast
osteitis deformans —*see* Paget's disease, bone
Pain(s) —*see also* Painful R52
abdominal R10.9
colic R10.83
generalized R10.84
with acute abdomen R10.0
lower R10.30
left quadrant R10.32
pelvic or perineal R10.2
periumbilical R10.33
right quadrant R10.31
rebound —*see* Tenderness, abdominal, rebound
severe with abdominal rigidity R10.0
tenderness —*see* Tenderness, abdominal
upper R10.10
epigastric R10.13
left quadrant R10.12
right quadrant R10.11

Pain *(Continued)*
acute R52
due to trauma G89.11
neoplasm related G89.3
postprocedural NEC G89.18
post-thoracotomy G89.12
specified by site — code to Pain, by site
adnexa (uteri) R10.2
anginoid —*see* Pain, precordial
anus K62.89
arm —*see* Pain, limb, upper
axillary (axilla) M79.62-
back (postural) M54.9
bladder R39.89
associated with micturition —*see* Micturition, painful
chronic R39.82 ◀
bone —*see* Disorder, bone, specified type NEC
breast N64.4
broad ligament R10.2
cancer associated (acute) (chronic) G89.3
cecum —*see* Pain, abdominal
cervicobrachial M53.1
chest (central) R07.9
anterior wall R07.89
atypical R07.89
ischemic I20.9
musculoskeletal R07.89
non-cardiac R07.89
on breathing R07.1
pleurodynia R07.81
precordial R07.2
wall (anterior) R07.89
chronic G89.29
associated with significant psychosocial dysfunction G89.4
due to trauma G89.21
neoplasm related G89.3
postoperative NEC G89.28
postprocedural NEC G89.28
post-thoracotomy G89.22
specified NEC G89.29
coccyx M53.3
colon —*see* Pain, abdominal
coronary —*see* Angina
costochondral R07.1
diaphragm R07.1
due to cancer G89.3
due to device, implant or graft —*see also* Complications, by site and type, specified NEC T85.848 ⟸
arterial graft NEC T82.848
breast (implant) T85.848 ⟸
catheter NEC T85.848 ⟸
dialysis (renal) T82.848
intraperitoneal T85.848 ⟸
infusion NEC T82.848
spinal (epidural) (subdural) T85.840 ⟸
urinary (indwelling) T83.84
electronic (electrode) (pulse generator) (stimulator)
bone T84.84
cardiac T82.847
nervous system (brain) (peripheral nerve) (spinal) T85.840 ⟸
urinary T83.84
fixation, internal (orthopedic) NEC T84.84
gastrointestinal (bile duct) (esophagus) T85.848 ⟸
genital NEC T83.84
heart NEC T82.847
infusion NEC T85.848 ⟸
joint prosthesis T84.84
ocular (corneal graft) (orbital implant) NEC T85.848 ⟸
orthopedic NEC T84.84
specified NEC T85.848 ⟸
urinary NEC T83.84
vascular NEC T82.848
ventricular intracranial shunt T85.840 ⟸

Pain *(Continued)*
due to malignancy (primary) (secondary) G89.3
ear —*see* subcategory H92.0
epigastric, epigastrium R10.13
eye —*see* Pain, ocular
face, facial R51
atypical G50.1
female genital organs NEC N94.89
finger —*see* Pain, limb, upper
flank —*see* Pain, abdominal
foot —*see* Pain, limb, lower
gallbladder K82.9
gas (intestinal) R14.1
gastric —*see* Pain, abdominal
generalized NOS R52
genital organ
female N94.89
male N50.89 ⟸
groin —*see* Pain, abdominal, lower
hand —*see* Pain, limb, upper
head —*see* Headache
heart —*see* Pain, precordial
infra-orbital —*see* Neuralgia, trigeminal
intercostal R07.82
intermenstrual N94.0
jaw R68.84
joint M25.50
ankle M25.57-
elbow M25.52-
finger M25.54- ⟸
foot M25.57-
hand M25.54- ⟸
hip M25.55-
knee M25.56-
shoulder M25.51-
toe M25.57-
wrist M25.53-
kidney N23
laryngeal R07.0
leg —*see* Pain, limb, lower
limb M79.609
lower M79.60-
foot M79.67-
lower leg M79.66-
thigh M79.65-
toe M79.67-
upper M79.60-
axilla M79.62-
finger M79.64-
forearm M79.63-
hand M79.64-
upper arm M79.62-
loin M54.5
low back M54.5
lumbar region M54.5
mandibular R68.84
mastoid —*see* subcategory H92.0
maxilla R68.84
menstrual —*see also* Dysmenorrhea N94.6
metacarpophalangeal (joint) —*see* Pain, joint, hand
metatarsophalangeal (joint) —*see* Pain, joint, foot
mouth K13.79
muscle —*see* Myalgia
musculoskeletal —*see also* Pain, by site M79.1
myofascial M79.1
nasal J34.89
nasopharynx J39.2
neck NEC M54.2
nerve NEC —*see* Neuralgia
neuromuscular —*see* Neuralgia
nose J34.89
ocular H57.1-
ophthalmic —*see* Pain, ocular
orbital region —*see* Pain, ocular
ovary N94.89
over heart —*see* Pain, precordial
ovulation N94.0
pelvic (female) R10.2

Pain *(Continued)*
penis N48.89
pericardial —*see* Pain, precordial
perineal, perineum R10.2
pharynx J39.2
pleura, pleural, pleuritic R07.81
postoperative NOS G89.18
postprocedural NOS G89.18
post-thoracotomy G89.12
precordial (region) R07.2
premenstrual N94.3
psychogenic (persistent) (any site) F45.41
radicular (spinal) —*see* Radiculopathy
rectum K62.89
respiration R07.1
retrosternal R07.2
rheumatoid, muscular —*see* Myalgia
rib R07.81
root (spinal) —*see* Radiculopathy
round ligament (stretch) R10.2
sacroiliac M53.3
sciatic —*see* Sciatica
scrotum N50.82 ◀
seminal vesicle N50.89 ◀
shoulder M25.51-
spermatic cord N50.89 ◀
spinal root —*see* Radiculopathy
spine M54.9
cervical M54.2
low back M54.5
with sciatica M54.4-
thoracic M54.6
stomach —*see* Pain, abdominal
substernal R07.2
temporomandibular (joint) M26.62- ◀
testis N50.81- ◀
thoracic spine M54.6
with radicular and visceral pain M54.14
throat R07.0
tibia —*see* Pain, limb, lower
toe —*see* Pain, limb, lower
tongue K14.6
tooth K08.89 ◀
trigeminal —*see* Neuralgia, trigeminal
tumor associated G89.3
ureter N23
urinary (organ) (system) N23
uterus NEC N94.89
vagina R10.2
vertebrogenic (syndrome) M54.89
vesical R39.89
associated with micturition —*see* Micturition, painful
vulva R10.2
Painful —*see also* Pain
coitus
female N94.10 ◀
male N53.12
psychogenic F52.6
ejaculation (semen) N53.12
psychogenic F52.6
erection —*see* Priapism
feet syndrome E53.8
joint replacement (hip) (knee) T84.84
menstruation —*see* Dysmenorrhea
psychogenic F45.8
micturition —*see* Micturition, painful
respiration R07.1
scar NEC L90.5
wire sutures T81.89
Painter's colic —*see* subcategory T56.0
Palate —*see* condition
Palatoplegia K13.79
Palatoschisis —*see* Cleft, palate
Palilalia R48.8
Palliative care Z51.5
Pallor R23.1
optic disc, temporal —*see* Atrophy, optic
Palmar —*see also* condition
fascia —*see* condition
Palpable
cecum K63.89
kidney N28.89
ovary N83.8
prostate N42.9
spleen —*see* Splenomegaly
Palpitations (heart) R00.2
psychogenic F45.8
Palsy —*see also* Paralysis G83.9
atrophic diffuse (progressive) G12.22
Bell's —*see also* Palsy, facial
newborn P11.3
brachial plexus NEC G54.0
newborn (birth injury) P14.3
brain —*see* Palsy, cerebral
bulbar (progressive) (chronic) G12.22
of childhood (Fazio-Londe) G12.1
pseudo NEC G12.29
supranuclear (progressive) G23.1
cerebral (congenital) G80.9
ataxic G80.4
athetoid G80.3
choreathetoid G80.3
diplegic G80.8
spastic G80.1
dyskinetic G80.3
athetoid G80.3
choreathetoid G80.3
distonic G80.3
dystonic G80.3
hemiplegic G80.8
spastic G80.2
mixed G80.8
monoplegic G80.8
spastic G80.1
paraplegic G80.8
spastic G80.1
quadriplegic G80.8
spastic G80.0
spastic G80.1
diplegic G80.1
hemiplegic G80.2
monoplegic G80.1
quadriplegic G80.0
specified NEC G80.1
tetrapelgic G80.0
specified NEC G80.8
syphilitic A52.12
congenital A50.49
tetraplegic G80.8
spastic G80.0
cranial nerve —*see also* Disorder, nerve, cranial
multiple G52.7
in
infectious disease B99 *[G53]*
neoplastic disease —*see also* Neoplasm D49.9 *[G53]*
parasitic disease B89 *[G53]*
sarcoidosis D86.82
creeping G12.22
diver's T70.3
Erb's P14.0
facial G51.0
newborn (birth injury) P11.3
glossopharyngeal G52.1
Klumpke (-Déjérine) P14.1
lead —*see* subcategory T56.0
median nerve (tardy) G56.1-
nerve G58.9
specified NEC G58.8
peroneal nerve (acute) (tardy) G57.3-
progressive supranuclear G23.1
pseudobulbar NEC G12.29
radial nerve (acute) G56.3-
seventh nerve —*see also* Palsy, facial
newborn P11.3
shaking —*see* Parkinsonism
spastic (cerebral) (spinal) G80.1
ulnar nerve (tardy) G56.2-
wasting G12.29
Paludism —*see* Malaria
Panangiitis M30.0
Panaris, panaritium —*see also* Cellulitis, digit
with lymphangitis —*see* Lymphangitis, acute, digit
Panarteritis nodosa M30.0
brain or cerebral I67.7
Pancake heart R93.1
with cor pulmonale (chronic) I27.81
Pancarditis (acute) (chronic) I51.89
rheumatic I09.89
active or acute I01.8
Pancoast's syndrome or tumor C34.1-
Pancolitis, ulcerative (chronic) K51.00
with
abscess K51.014
complication K51.019
fistula K51.013
obstruction K51.012
rectal bleeding K51.011
specified complication NEC K51.018
Pancreas, pancreatic —*see* condition
Pancreatitis (annular) (apoplectic) (calcareous) (edematous) (hemorrhagic) (malignant) (recurrent) (subacute) (suppurative) K85.90 ◀
with necrosis (uninfected) K85.91 ◀
infected K85.92 ◀
acute (without necrosis or infection) K85.90 ◀
with necrosis (uninfected) K85.91 ◀
infected K85.92 ◀
alcohol induced (without necrosis or infection) K85.20 ◀
with necrosis (uninfected) K85.21 ◀
infected K85.22 ◀
biliary (without necrosis or infection) K85.10 ◀
with necrosis (uninfected) K85.11 ◀
infected K85.12 ◀
drug induced (without necrosis or infection) K85.30 ◀
with necrosis (uninfected) K85.31 ◀
infected K85.32 ◀
gallstone (without necrosis or infection) K85.10 ◀
with necrosis (uninfected) K85.11 ◀
infected K85.12 ◀
idiopathic (without necrosis or infection) K85.00 ◀
with necrosis (uninfected) K85.01 ◀
infected K85.02 ◀
specified NEC (without necrosis or infection) K85.80 ◀
with necrosis (uninfected) K85.81 ◀
infected K85.82 ◀
chronic (infectious) K86.1
alcohol-induced K86.0
recurrent K86.1
relapsing K86.1
cystic (chronic) K86.1
cytomegaloviral B25.2
fibrous (chronic) K86.1
gallstone (without necrosis or infection) K85.10 ◀
with necrosis (uninfected) K85.11 ◀
infected K85.12 ◀
gangrenous —*see* Pancreatitis, acute ◀
interstitial (chronic) K86.1
acute —*see also* Pancreatitis, acute K85.80 ◀
mumps B26.3
recurrent (chronic) K86.1
relapsing, chronic K86.1
syphilitic A52.74
Pancreatoblastoma —*see* Neoplasm, pancreas, malignant
Pancreolithiasis K86.89 ◀
Pancytolysis D75.89

◀ New ◀ Revised ~~deleted~~ Deleted

Pancytopenia (acquired) D61.818
with
malformations D61.09
myelodysplastic syndrome —*see* Syndrome, myelodysplastic
antineoplastic chemotherapy induced D61.810
congenital D61.09
drug-induced NEC D61.811
Panencephalitis, subacute, sclerosing A81.1
Panhematopenia D61.9
congenital D61.09
constitutional D61.09
splenic, primary D73.1
Panhemocytopenia D61.9
congenital D61.09
constitutional D61.09
Panhypogonadism E29.1
Panhypopituitarism E23.0
prepubertal E23.0
Panic (attack) (state) F41.0
reaction to exceptional stress (transient) F43.0
Panmyelopathy, familial, constitutional D61.09
Panmyelophthisis D61.82
congenital D61.09
Panmyelosis (acute) (with myelofibrosis) C94.4-
Panner's disease —*see* Osteochondrosis, juvenile, humerus
Panneuritis endemica E51.11
Panniculitis (nodular) (nonsuppurative) M79.3
back M54.00
cervical region M54.02
cervicothoracic region M54.03
lumbar region M54.06
lumbosacral region M54.07
multiple sites M54.09
occipito-atlanto-axial region M54.01
sacrococcygeal region M54.08
thoracic region M54.04
thoracolumbar region M54.05
lupus L93.2
mesenteric K65.4
neck M54.02
cervicothoracic region M54.03
occipito-atlanto-axial region M54.01
relapsing M35.6
Panniculus adiposus (abdominal) E65
Pannus (allergic) (cornea) (degenerativus) (keratic) H16.42-
abdominal (symptomatic) E65
trachomatosus, trachomatous (active) A71.1
Panophthalmitis H44.01-
Pansinusitis (chronic) (hyperplastic) (nonpurulent) (purulent) J32.4
acute J01.40
recurrent J01.41
tuberculous A15.8
Panuveitis (sympathetic) H44.11-
Panvalvular disease I08.9
specified NEC I08.8
PAPA (pyogenic arthritis, pyoderma gangrenosum, and acne syndrome) M04.8 ◀
Papanicolaou smear, cervix Z12.4
as part of routine gynecological examination Z01.419
with abnormal findings Z01.411
for suspected neoplasm Z12.4
nonspecific abnormal finding R87.619
routine Z01.419
with abnormal findings Z01.411
Papilledema (choked disc) H47.10
associated with
decreased ocular pressure H47.12
increased intracranial pressure H47.11
retinal disorder H47.13
Foster-Kennedy syndrome H47.14-
Papillitis H46.00
anus K62.89
chronic lingual K14.4
necrotizing, kidney N17.2
optic H46.0-
rectum K62.89
renal, necrotizing N17.2
tongue K14.0
Papilloma —*see also* Neoplasm, benign, by site
acuminatum (female) (male) (anogenital) A63.0
basal cell L82.1 ◀
inflamed L82.0 ◀
benign pinta (primary) A67.0
bladder (urinary) (transitional cell) D41.4
choroid plexus (lateral ventricle) (third ventricle) D33.0
anaplastic C71.5
fourth ventricle D33.1
malignant C71.5
renal pelvis (transitional cell) D41.1-
benign D30.1-
Schneiderian
specified site —*see* Neoplasm, benign, by site
unspecified site D14.0
serous surface
borderline malignancy
specified site —*see* Neoplasm, uncertain behavior, by site
unspecified site D39.10
specified site —*see* Neoplasm, benign, by site
unspecified site D27.9
transitional (cell)
bladder (urinary) D41.4
inverted type —*see* Neoplasm, uncertain behavior, by site
renal pelvis D41.1-
ureter D41.2-
ureter (transitional cell) D41.2-
benign D30.2-
urothelial —*see* Neoplasm, uncertain behavior, by site
villous —*see* Neoplasm, uncertain behavior, by site
adenocarcinoma in —*see* Neoplasm, malignant, by site
in situ —*see* Neoplasm, in situ
yaws, plantar or palmar A66.1
Papillomata, multiple, of yaws A66.1
Papillomatosis —*see also* Neoplasm, benign, by site
confluent and reticulated L83
cystic, breast —*see* Mastopathy, cystic
ductal, breast —*see* Mastopathy, cystic
intraductal (diffuse) —*see* Neoplasm, benign, by site
subareolar duct D24-
Papillomavirus, as cause of disease classified elsewhere B97.7
Papillon-Léage and Psaume syndrome Q87.0
Papule (s) R23.8
carate (primary) A67.0
fibrous, of nose D22.39
Gottron's L94.4
pinta (primary) A67.0
Papulosis
lymphomatoid C86.6
malignant I77.89
Papyraceous fetus O31.0-
Para-albuminemia E88.09
Paracephalus Q89.7
Parachute mitral valve Q23.2
Paracoccidioidomycosis B41.9
disseminated B41.7
generalized B41.7
mucocutaneous-lymphangitic B41.8
pulmonary B41.0
Paracoccidioidomycosis *(Continued)*
specified NEC B41.8
visceral B41.8
Paradentosis K05.4
Paraffinoma T88.8
Paraganglioma D44.7
adrenal D35.0-
malignant C74.1-
aortic body D44.7
malignant C75.5
carotid body D44.6
malignant C75.4
chromaffin —*see also* Neoplasm, benign, by site
malignant —*see* Neoplasm, malignant, by site
extra-adrenal D44.7
malignant C75.5
specified site —*see* Neoplasm, malignant, by site
unspecified site C75.5
specified site —*see* Neoplasm, uncertain behavior, by site
unspecified site D44.7
gangliocytic D13.2
specified site —*see* Neoplasm, benign, by site
unspecified site D13.2
glomus jugulare D44.7
malignant C75.5
jugular D44.7
malignant C75.5
specified site —*see* Neoplasm, malignant, by site
unspecified site C75.5
nonchromaffin D44.7
malignant C75.5
specified site —*see* Neoplasm, malignant, by site
unspecified site C75.5
specified site —*see* Neoplasm, uncertain behavior, by site
unspecified site D44.7
parasympathetic D44.7
specified site —*see* Neoplasm, uncertain behavior, by site
unspecified site D44.7
specified site —*see* Neoplasm, uncertain behavior, by site
sympathetic D44.7
specified site —*see* Neoplasm, uncertain behavior, by site
unspecified site D44.7
unspecified site D44.7
Parageusia R43.2
psychogenic F45.8
Paragonimiasis B66.4
Paragranuloma, Hodgkin —*see* Lymphoma, Hodgkin, classical, specified NEC
Parahemophilia —*see also* Defect, coagulation D68.2
Parakeratosis R23.4
variegata L41.0
Paralysis, paralytic (complete) (incomplete) G83.9
with
syphilis A52.17
abducens, abducent (nerve) —*see* Strabismus, paralytic, sixth nerve
abductor, lower extremity G57.9-
accessory nerve G52.8
accommodation —*see also* Paresis, of accommodation
hysterical F44.89
acoustic nerve (except Deafness) —*see* subcategory H93.3
agitans —*see also* Parkinsonism G20
arteriosclerotic G21.4
alternating (oculomotor) G83.89
amyotrophic G12.21

Paralysis, paralytic *(Continued)*
ankle G57.9-
anus (sphincter) K62.89
arm —*see* Monoplegia, upper limb
ascending (spinal), acute G61.0
association G12.29
asthenic bulbar G70.00
with exacerbation (acute) G70.01
in crisis G70.01
ataxic (hereditary) G11.9
general (syphilitic) A52.17
atrophic G58.9
infantile, acute —*see* Poliomyelitis, paralytic
progressive G12.22
spinal (acute) —*see* Poliomyelitis, paralytic
axillary G54.0
Babinski-Nageotte's G83.89
Bell's G51.0
newborn P11.3
Benedikt's G46.3
birth injury P14.9
spinal cord P11.5
bladder (neurogenic) (sphincter) N31.2
bowel, colon or intestine K56.0
brachial plexus G54.0
birth injury P14.3
newborn (birth injury) P14.3
brain G83.9
diplegia G83.0
triplegia G83.89
bronchial J98.09
Brown-Séquard G83.81
bulbar (chronic) (progressive) G12.22
infantile —*see* Poliomyelitis, paralytic
poliomyelitic —*see* Poliomyelitis, paralytic
pseudo G12.29
bulbospinal G70.00
with exacerbation (acute) G70.01
in crisis G70.01
cardiac —*see also* Failure, heart I50.9
cerebrocerebellar, diplegic G80.1
cervical
plexus G54.2
sympathetic G90.09
Céstan-Chenais G46.3
Charcot-Marie-Tooth type G60.0
Clark's G80.9
colon K56.0
compressed air T70.3
compression
arm G56.9-
leg G57.9-
lower extremity G57.9-
upper extremity G56.9-
congenital (cerebral) —*see* Palsy, cerebral
conjugate movement (gaze) (of eye) H51.0
cortical (nuclear) (supranuclear) H51.0
cordis —*see* Failure, heart
cranial or cerebral nerve G52.9
creeping G12.22
crossed leg G83.89
crutch —*see* Injury, brachial plexus
deglutition R13.0
hysterical F44.4
dementia A52.17
descending (spinal) NEC G12.29
diaphragm (flaccid) J98.6
due to accidental dissection of phrenic nerve during procedure —*see* Puncture, accidental complicating surgery
digestive organs NEC K59.8
diplegic —*see* Diplegia
divergence (nuclear) H51.8
diver's T70.3
Duchenne's
birth injury P14.0
due to or associated with
motor neuron disease G12.22
muscular dystrophy G71.0

Paralysis, paralytic *(Continued)*
due to intracranial or spinal birth injury —*see* Palsy, cerebral
embolic (current episode) I63.4- ⬅
Erb (-Duchenne) (birth) (newborn) P14.0
Erb's syphilitic spastic spinal A52.17
esophagus K22.8
eye muscle (extrinsic) H49.9
intrinsic —*see also* Paresis, of accommodation
facial (nerve) G51.0
birth injury P11.3
congenital P11.3
following operation NEC —*see* Puncture, accidental complicating surgery
newborn (birth injury) P11.3
familial (recurrent) (periodic) G72.3
spastic G11.4
fauces J39.2
finger G56.9-
gait R26.1
gastric nerve (nondiabetic) G52.2
gaze, conjugate H51.0
general (progressive) (syphilitic) A52.17
juvenile A50.45
glottis J38.00
bilateral J38.02
unilateral J38.01
gluteal G54.1
Gubler (-Millard) G46.3
hand —*see* Monoplegia, upper limb
heart —*see* Arrest, cardiac
hemiplegic —*see* Hemiplegia
hyperkalemic periodic (familial) G72.3
hypoglossal (nerve) G52.3
hypokalemic periodic G72.3
hysterical F44.4
ileus K56.0
infantile —*see also* Poliomyelitis, paralytic A80.30
bulbar —*see* Poliomyelitis, paralytic
cerebral —*see* Palsy, cerebral
spastic —*see* Palsy, cerebral, spastic
infective —*see* Poliomyelitis, paralytic
inferior nuclear G83.9
internuclear —*see* Ophthalmoplegia, internuclear
intestine K56.0
iris H57.09
due to diphtheria (toxin) A36.89
ischemic, Volkmann's (complicating trauma) T79.6
Jackson's G83.89
jake —*see* Poisoning, food, noxious, plant
Jamaica ginger (jake) G62.2
juvenile general A50.45
Klumpke (-Déjérine) (birth) (newborn) P14.1
labioglossal (laryngeal) (pharyngeal) G12.29
Landry's G61.0
laryngeal nerve (recurrent) (superior) (unilateral) J38.00
bilateral J38.02
unilateral J38.01
larynx J38.00
bilateral J38.02
due to diphtheria (toxin) A36.2
unilateral J38.01
lateral G12.21
lead —*see* subcategory T56.0
left side —*see* Hemiplegia
leg G83.1-
both —*see* Paraplegia
crossed G83.89
hysterical F44.4
psychogenic F44.4
transient or transitory R29.818
traumatic NEC —*see* Injury, nerve, leg
levator palpebrae superioris —*see* Blepharoptosis, paralytic
limb —*see* Monoplegia
lip K13.0

Paralysis, paralytic *(Continued)*
Lissauer's A52.17
lower limb —*see* Monoplegia, lower limb
both —*see* Paraplegia
lung J98.4
median nerve G56.1-
medullary (tegmental) G83.89
mesencephalic NEC G83.89
tegmental G83.89
middle alternating G83.89
Millard-Gubler-Foville G46.3
monoplegic —*see* Monoplegia
motor G83.9
muscle, muscular NEC G72.89
due to nerve lesion G58.9
eye (extrinsic) H49.9
intrinsic —*see* Paresis, of accommodation
oblique —*see* Strabismus, paralytic, fourth nerve
iris sphincter H21.9
ischemic (Volkmann's) (complicating trauma) T79.6
progressive G12.21
pseudohypertrophic G71.0
musculocutaneous nerve G56.9-
musculospiral G56.9-
nerve —*see also* Disorder, nerve
abducent —*see* Strabismus, paralytic, sixth nerve
accessory G52.8
auditory (except Deafness) —*see* subcategory H93.3
birth injury P14.9
cranial or cerebral G52.9
facial G51.0
birth injury P11.3
congenital P11.3
newborn (birth injury) P11.3
fourth or trochlear —*see* Strabismus, paralytic, fourth nerve
newborn (birth injury) P14.9
oculomotor —*see* Strabismus, paralytic, third nerve
phrenic (birth injury) P14.2
radial G56.3-
seventh or facial G51.0
newborn (birth injury) P11.3
sixth or abducent —*see* Strabismus, paralytic, sixth nerve
syphilitic A52.15
third or oculomotor —*see* Strabismus, paralytic, third nerve
trigeminal G50.9
trochlear —*see* Strabismus, paralytic, fourth nerve
ulnar G56.2-
normokalemic periodic G72.3
ocular H49.9
alternating G83.89
oculofacial, congenital (Moebius) Q87.0
oculomotor (external bilateral) (nerve) —*see* Strabismus, paralytic, third nerve
palate (soft) K13.79
paratrigeminal G50.9
periodic (familial) (hyperkalemic) (hypokalemic) (myotonic) (normokalemic) (potassium sensitive) (secondary) G72.3
peripheral autonomic nervous system —*see* Neuropathy, peripheral, autonomic
peroneal (nerve) G57.3-
pharynx J39.2
phrenic nerve G56.8-
plantar nerve (s) G57.6-
pneumogastric nerve G52.2
poliomyelitis (current) —*see* Poliomyelitis, paralytic
popliteal nerve G57.3-
postepileptic transitory G83.84

◀ New ⬅ Revised ~~deleted~~ Deleted

Paralysis, paralytic *(Continued)*
progressive (atrophic) (bulbar) (spinal) G12.22
general A52.17
infantile acute —*see* Poliomyelitis, paralytic
supranuclear G23.1
pseudobulbar G12.29
pseudohypertrophic (muscle) G71.0
psychogenic F44.4
quadriceps G57.9-
quadriplegic —*see* Tetraplegia
radial nerve G56.3-
rectus muscle (eye) H49.9
recurrent isolated sleep G47.53
respiratory (muscle) (system) (tract) R06.81
center NEC G93.89
congenital P28.89
newborn P28.89
right side —*see* Hemiplegia
saturnine —*see* subcategory T56.0
sciatic nerve G57.0-
senile G83.9
shaking —*see* Parkinsonism
shoulder G56.9-
sleep, recurrent isolated G47.53
spastic G83.9
cerebral —*see* Palsy, cerebral, spastic
congenital (cerebral) —*see* Palsy, cerebral, spastic
familial G11.4
hereditary G11.4
quadriplegic G80.0
syphilitic (spinal) A52.17
sphincter, bladder —*see* Paralysis, bladder
spinal (cord) G83.9
accessory nerve G52.8
acute —*see* Poliomyelitis, paralytic
ascending acute G61.0
atrophic (acute) —*see also* Poliomyelitis, paralytic
spastic, syphilitic A52.17
congenital NEC —*see* Palsy, cerebral
hereditary G95.89
infantile —*see* Poliomyelitis, paralytic
progressive G12.21
sequelae NEC G83.89
sternomastoid G52.8
stomach K31.84
diabetic —*see* Diabetes, by type, with gastroparesis
nerve G52.2
diabetic —*see* Diabetes, by type, with gastroparesis
stroke —*see* Infarct, brain
subcapsularis G56.8-
supranuclear (progressive) G23.1
sympathetic G90.8
cervical G90.09
nervous system —*see* Neuropathy, peripheral, autonomic
syndrome G83.9
specified NEC G83.89
syphilitic spastic spinal (Erb's) A52.17
thigh G57.9-
throat J39.2
diphtheritic A36.0
muscle J39.2
thrombotic (current episode) I63.3- ⬅
thumb G56.9-
tick —*see* Toxicity, venom, arthropod, specified NEC
Todd's (postepileptic transitory paralysis) G83.84
toe G57.6-
tongue K14.8
transient R29.5
arm or leg NEC R29.818
traumatic NEC —*see* Injury, nerve
trapezius G52.8
traumatic, transient NEC —*see* Injury, nerve

Paralysis, paralytic *(Continued)*
trembling —*see* Parkinsonism
triceps brachii G56.9-
trigeminal nerve G50.9
trochlear (nerve) —*see* Strabismus, paralytic, fourth nerve
ulnar nerve G56.2-
upper limb —*see* Monoplegia, upper limb
uremic N18.9 *[G99.8]*
uveoparotitic D86.89
uvula K13.79
postdiphtheritic A36.0
vagus nerve G52.2
vasomotor NEC G90.8
velum palati K13.79
vesical —*see* Paralysis, bladder
vestibular nerve (except Vertigo) —*see* subcategory H93.3
vocal cords J38.00
bilateral J38.02
unilateral J38.01
Volkmann's (complicating trauma) T79.6
wasting G12.29
Weber's G46.3
wrist G56.9-
Paramedial urethrovesical orifice Q64.79
Paramenia N92.6
Parametritis —*see also* Disease, pelvis, inflammatory N73.2
acute N73.0
complicating abortion —*see* Abortion, by type, complicated by, parametritis
Parametrium, parametric —*see* condition
Paramnesia —*see* Amnesia
Paramolar K00.1
Paramyloidosis E85.8
Paramyoclonus multiplex G25.3
Paramyotonia (congenita) G71.19
Parangi —*see* Yaws
Paranoia (querulans) F22
senile F03
Paranoid
dementia (senile) F03
praecox —*see* Schizophrenia
personality F60.0
psychosis (climacteric) (involutional) (menopausal) F22
psychogenic (acute) F23
senile F03
reaction (acute) F23
chronic F22
schizophrenia F20.0
state (climacteric) (involutional) (menopausal) (simple) F22
senile F03
tendencies F60.0
traits F60.0
trends F60.0
type, psychopathic personality F60.0
Paraparesis —*see* Paraplegia
Paraphasia R47.02
Paraphilia F65.9
Paraphimosis (congenital) N47.2
chancroidal A57
Paraphrenia, paraphrenic (late) F22
schizophrenia F20.0
Paraplegia (lower) G82.20
ataxic —*see* Degeneration, combined, spinal cord
complete G82.21
congenital (cerebral) G80.8
spastic G80.1
familial spastic G11.4
functional (hysterical) F44.4
hereditary, spastic G11.4
hysterical F44.4
incomplete G82.22
Pott's A18.01
psychogenic F44.4

Paraplegia *(Continued)*
spastic
Erb's spinal, syphilitic A52.17
hereditary G11.4
tropical G04.1
syphilitic (spastic) A52.17
tropical spastic G04.1
Parapoxvirus B08.60
specified NEC B08.69
Paraproteinemia D89.2
benign (familial) D89.2
monoclonal D47.2
secondary to malignant disease D47.2
Parapsoriasis L41.9
en plaques L41.4
guttata L41.1
large plaque L41.4
retiform, retiformis L41.5
small plaque L41.3
specified NEC L41.8
varioliformis (acuta) L41.0
Parasitic —*see also* condition
disease NEC B89
stomatitis B37.0
sycosis (beard) (scalp) B35.0
twin Q89.4
Parasitism B89
intestinal B82.9
skin B88.9
specified —*see* Infestation
Parasitophobia F40.218
Parasomnia G47.50
due to
alcohol
abuse F10.182
dependence F10.282
use F10.982
amphetamines
abuse F15.182
dependence F15.282
use F15.982
caffeine
abuse F15.182
dependence F15.282
use F15.982
cocaine
abuse F14.182
dependence F14.282
use F14.982
drug NEC
abuse F19.182
dependence F19.282
use F19.982
opioid
abuse F11.182
dependence F11.282
use F11.982
psychoactive substance NEC
abuse F19.182
dependence F19.282
use F19.982
sedative, hypnotic, or anxiolytic
abuse F13.182
dependence F13.282
use F13.982
stimulant NEC
abuse F15.182
dependence F15.282
use F15.982
in conditions classified elsewhere G47.54
nonorganic origin F51.8
organic G47.50
specified NEC G47.59
Paraspadias Q54.9
Paraspasmus facialis G51.8
Parasuicide (attempt)
history of (personal) Z91.5
in family Z81.8
Parathyroid gland —*see* condition
Parathyroid tetany E20.9
Paratrachoma A74.0

Paratyphilitis —*see* Appendicitis
Paratyphoid (fever) —*see* Fever, paratyphoid
Paratyphus —*see* Fever, paratyphoid
Paraurethral duct Q64.79
  nonorganic origin F51.5
Paraurethritis —*see also* Urethritis
  gonococcal (acute) (chronic) (with abscess) A54.1
Paravaccinia NEC B08.04
Paravaginitis —*see* Vaginitis
Parencephalitis —*see also* Encephalitis
  sequelae G09
Parent-child conflict —*see* Conflict, parent-child
  estrangement NEC Z62.890
Paresis —*see also* Paralysis
  accommodation —*see* Paresis, of accommodation
  Bernhardt's G57.1-
  bladder (sphincter) —*see also* Paralysis, bladder
    tabetic A52.17
  bowel, colon or intestine K56.0
  extrinsic muscle, eye H49.9
  general (progressive) (syphilitic) A52.17
    juvenile A50.45
  heart —*see* Failure, heart
  insane (syphilitic) A52.17
  juvenile (general) A50.45
  of accommodation H52.52-
  peripheral progressive (idiopathic) G60.3
  pseudohypertrophic G71.0
  senile G83.9
  syphilitic (general) A52.17
    congenital A50.45
  vesical NEC N31.2
Paresthesia —*see also* Disturbance, sensation
  Bernhardt G57.1-
Paretic —*see* condition
Parinaud's
  conjunctivitis H10.89
  oculoglandular syndrome H10.89
  ophthalmoplegia H49.88
Parkinsonism (idiopathic) (primary) G20
  with neurogenic orthostatic hypotension (symptomatic) G90.3
  arteriosclerotic G21.4
  dementia G31.83 *[F02.80]*
    with behavioral disturbance G31.83 *[F02.81]*
  due to
    drugs NEC G21.19
      neuroleptic G21.11
  neuroleptic induced G21.11
  postencephalitic G21.3
  secondary G21.9
    due to
      arteriosclerosis G21.4
      drugs NEC G21.19
        neuroleptic G21.11
      encephalitis G21.3
      external agents NEC G21.2
      syphilis A52.19
    specified NEC G21.8
  syphilitic A52.19
  treatment-induced NEC G21.19
  vascular G21.4
Parkinson's disease, syndrome or tremor —*see* Parkinsonism
Parodontitis —*see* Periodontitis
Parodontosis K05.4
Paronychia —*see also* Cellulitis, digit
  with lymphangitis —*see* Lymphangitis, acute, digit
  candidal (chronic) B37.2
  tuberculous (primary) A18.4
Parorexia (psychogenic) F50.89 ◄
Parosmia R43.1
  psychogenic F45.8
Parotid gland —*see* condition
Parotitis, parotiditis (allergic) (nonspecific toxic) (purulent) (septic) (suppurative) —*see also* Sialoadenitis
Parotitis, parotiditis *(Continued)*
  epidemic —*see* Mumps
  infectious —*see* Mumps
  postoperative K91.89
  surgical K91.89
Parrot fever A70
Parrot's disease (early congenital syphilitic pseudoparalysis) A50.02
Parry-Romberg syndrome G51.8
Parry's disease or syndrome E05.00
  with thyroid storm E05.01
Pars planitis —*see* Cyclitis
Parsonage (-Aldren)-Turner syndrome G54.5
Parson's disease (exophthalmic goiter) E05.00
  with thyroid storm E05.01
Particolored infant Q82.8
Parturition —*see* Delivery
Parulis K04.7
  with sinus K04.6
Parvovirus, as cause of disease classified elsewhere B97.6
Pasini and Pierini's atrophoderma L90.3
Passage
  false, urethra N36.5
  meconium (newborn) during delivery P03.82
  of sounds or bougies —*see* Attention to, artificial, opening
Passive —*see* condition
  smoking Z77.22
Pasteurella septica A28.0
Pasteurellosis —*see* Infection, Pasteurella
PAT (paroxysmal atrial tachycardia) I47.1
Patau's syndrome —*see* Trisomy, 13
Patches
  mucous (syphilitic) A51.39
    congenital A50.07
  smokers' (mouth) K13.24
Patellar —*see* condition
Patent —*see also* Imperfect, closure
  canal of Nuck Q52.4
  cervix N88.3
  ductus arteriosus or Botallo's Q25.0
  foramen
    botalli Q21.1
    ovale Q21.1
  interauricular septum Q21.1
  interventricular septum Q21.0
  omphalomesenteric duct Q43.0
  os (uteri) —*see* Patent, cervix
  ostium secundum Q21.1
  urachus Q64.4
  vitelline duct Q43.0
Paterson (-Brown)(-Kelly) syndrome or web D50.1
Pathologic, pathological —*see also* condition
  asphyxia R09.01
  fire-setting F63.1
  gambling F63.0
  ovum O02.0
  resorption, tooth K03.3
  stealing F63.2
Pathology (of) —*see* Disease
  periradicular, associated with previous endodontic treatment NEC M27.59
Pattern, sleep-wake, irregular G47.23
Patulous —*see also* Imperfect, closure (congenital)
  alimentary tract Q45.8
    lower Q43.8
    upper Q40.8
  eustachian tube H69.0-
Pause, sinoatrial I49.5
Paxton's disease B36.2
Pearl (s)
  enamel K00.2
  Epstein's K09.8
Pearl-worker's disease —*see* Osteomyelitis, specified type NEC
Pectenosis K62.4
Pectoral —*see* condition
Pectus
  carinatum (congenital) Q67.7
    acquired M95.4
    rachitic sequelae (late effect) E64.3
  excavatum (congenital) Q67.6
    acquired M95.4
    rachitic sequelae (late effect) E64.3
  recurvatum (congenital) Q67.6
Pedatrophia E41
Pederosis F65.4
Pediculosis (infestation) B85.2
  capitis (head-louse) (any site) B85.0
  corporis (body-louse) (any site) B85.1
  eyelid B85.0
  mixed (classifiable to more than one of the titles B85.0-B85.3) B85.4
  pubis (pubic louse) (any site) B85.3
  vestimenti B85.1
  vulvae B85.3
Pediculus (infestation) —*see* Pediculosis
Pedophilia F65.4
Peg-shaped teeth K00.2
Pelade —*see* Alopecia, areata
Pelger-Huët anomaly or syndrome D72.0
Peliosis (rheumatica) D69.0
  hepatis K76.4
    with toxic liver disease K71.8
Pelizaeus-Merzbacher disease E75.29
Pellagra (alcoholic) (with polyneuropathy) E52
Pellagra-cerebellar-ataxia-renal aminoaciduria syndrome E72.02
Pellegrini (-Stieda) disease or syndrome —*see* Bursitis, tibial collateral
Pellizzi's syndrome E34.8
Pel's crisis A52.11
Pelvic —*see also* condition
  examination (periodic) (routine) Z01.419
    with abnormal findings Z01.411
  kidney, congenital Q63.2
Pelviolithiasis —*see* Calculus, kidney
Pelviperitonitis —*see also* Peritonitis, pelvic
  gonococcal A54.24
  puerperal O85
Pelvis —*see* condition or type
Pemphigoid L12.9
  benign, mucous membrane L12.1
  bullous L12.0
  cicatricial L12.1
  juvenile L12.2
  ocular L12.1
  specified NEC L12.8
Pemphigus L10.9
  benign familial (chronic) Q82.8
  Brazilian L10.3
  circinatus L13.0
  conjunctiva L12.1
  drug-induced L10.5
  erythematosus L10.4
  foliaceous L10.2
  gangrenous —*see* Gangrene
  neonatorum L01.03
  ocular L12.1
  paraneoplastic L10.81
  specified NEC L10.89
  syphilitic (congenital) A50.06
  vegetans L10.1
  vulgaris L10.0
  wildfire L10.3
Pendred's syndrome E07.1
Pendulous
  abdomen, in pregnancy —*see* Pregnancy, complicated by, abnormal, pelvic organs or tissues NEC
  breast N64.89
Penetrating wound —*see also* Puncture
  with internal injury —*see* Injury, by site
  eyeball —*see* Puncture, eyeball
  orbit (with or without foreign body) —*see* Puncture, orbit
  uterus by instrument with or following ectopic or molar pregnancy O08.6

◄ New ◄ Revised ~~deleted~~ Deleted

Penicillosis B48.4
Penis —*see* condition
Penitis N48.29
Pentalogy of Fallot Q21.8
Pentasomy X syndrome Q97.1
Pentosuria (essential) E74.8
Percreta placenta O43.23-
Peregrinating patient —*see* Disorder, factitious
Perforation, perforated (nontraumatic) (of)
accidental during procedure (blood vessel) (nerve) (organ) —*see* Complication, accidental puncture or laceration
antrum —*see* Sinusitis, maxillary
appendix K35.2
with localized peritonitis K35.3 ◀
atrial septum, multiple Q21.1
attic, ear —*see* Perforation, tympanum, attic
bile duct (common) (hepatic) K83.2
cystic K82.2
bladder (urinary)
with or following ectopic or molar pregnancy O08.6
obstetrical trauma O71.5
traumatic S37.29
at delivery O71.5
bowel K63.1
with or following ectopic or molar pregnancy O08.6
newborn P78.0
obstetrical trauma O71.5
traumatic —*see* Laceration, intestine
broad ligament N83.8
with or following ectopic or molar pregnancy O08.6
obstetrical trauma O71.6
by
device, implant or graft —*see also* Complications, by site and type, mechanical T85.628
arterial graft NEC —*see* Complication, cardiovascular device, mechanical, vascular
breast (implant) T85.49
catheter NEC T85.698
cystostomy T83.090
dialysis (renal) T82.49
intraperitoneal T85.691
infusion NEC T82.594
spinal (epidural) (subdural) T85.690
urinary —*see also* Complications, catheter, urinary T83.098 ◀
electronic (electrode) (pulse generator) (stimulator)
bone T84.390
cardiac T82.199
electrode T82.190
pulse generator T82.191
specified type NEC T82.198
nervous system —*see* Complication, prosthetic device, mechanical, electronic nervous system stimulator
urinary —*see* Complication, genitourinary, device, urinary, mechanical
fixation, internal (orthopedic) NEC —*see* Complication, fixation device, mechanical
gastrointestinal —*see* Complications, prosthetic device, mechanical, gastrointestinal device
genital NEC T83.498
intrauterine contraceptive device T83.39
penile prosthesis T83.490
heart NEC —*see* Complication, cardiovascular device, mechanical
joint prosthesis —*see* Complications, joint prosthesis, mechanical, specified NEC, by site

Perforation, perforated *(Continued)*
by *(Continued)*
urinary *(Continued)*
ocular NEC —*see* Complications, prosthetic device, mechanical, ocular device
orthopedic NEC —*see* Complication, orthopedic, device, mechanical
specified NEC T85.628
urinary NEC —*see also* Complication, genitourinary, device, urinary, mechanical
graft T83.29
~~urinary, indwelling T83.098~~
vascular NEC —*see* Complication, cardiovascular device, mechanical
ventricular intracranial shunt T85.09
foreign body left accidentally in operative wound T81.539
instrument (any) during a procedure, accidental —*see* Puncture, accidental complicating surgery
cecum K35.2
with localized peritonitis K35.3 ◀
cervix (uteri) N88.8
with or following ectopic or molar pregnancy O08.6
obstetrical trauma O71.3
colon K63.1
newborn P78.0
obstetrical trauma O71.5
traumatic —*see* Laceration, intestine, large
common duct (bile) K83.2
cornea (due to ulceration) —*see* Ulcer, cornea, perforated
cystic duct K82.2
diverticulum (intestine) K57.80
with bleeding K57.81
large intestine K57.20
with
bleeding K57.21
small intestine K57.40
with bleeding K57.41
small intestine K57.00
with
bleeding K57.01
large intestine K57.40
with bleeding K57.41
ear drum —*see* Perforation, tympanum
esophagus K22.3
ethmoidal sinus —*see* Sinusitis, ethmoidal
frontal sinus —*see* Sinusitis, frontal
gallbladder K82.2
heart valve —*see* Endocarditis
ileum K63.1
newborn P78.0
obstetrical trauma O71.5
traumatic —*see* Laceration, intestine, small
instrumental, surgical (accidental) (blood vessel) (nerve) (organ) —*see* Puncture, accidental complicating surgery
intestine NEC K63.1
with ectopic or molar pregnancy O08.6
newborn P78.0
obstetrical trauma O71.5
traumatic —*see* Laceration, intestine
ulcerative NEC K63.1
newborn P78.0
jejunum, jejunal K63.1
obstetrical trauma O71.5
traumatic —*see* Laceration, intestine, small
ulcer —*see* Ulcer, gastrojejunal, with perforation
joint prosthesis —*see* Complications, joint prosthesis, mechanical, specified NEC, by site
mastoid (antrum) (cell) —*see* Disorder, mastoid, specified NEC
maxillary sinus —*see* Sinusitis, maxillary
membrana tympani —*see* Perforation, tympanum

Perforation, perforated *(Continued)*
nasal
septum J34.89
congenital Q30.3
syphilitic A52.73
sinus J34.89
congenital Q30.8
due to sinusitis —*see* Sinusitis
palate —*see also* Cleft, palate Q35.9
syphilitic A52.79
palatine vault —*see also* Cleft, palate, hard Q35.1
syphilitic A52.79
congenital A50.59
pars flaccida (ear drum) —*see* Perforation, tympanum, attic
pelvic
floor S31.030
with
ectopic or molar pregnancy O08.6
penetration into retroperitoneal space S31.031
retained foreign body S31.040
with penetration into retroperitoneal space S31.041
following ectopic or molar pregnancy O08.6
obstetrical trauma O70.1
organ S37.99
adrenal gland S37.818
bladder —*see* Perforation, bladder
fallopian tube S37.599
bilateral S37.592
unilateral S37.591
kidney S37.09-
obstetrical trauma O71.5
ovary S37.499
bilateral S37.492
unilateral S37.491
prostate S37.828
specified organ NEC S37.898
ureter —*see* Perforation, ureter
urethra —*see* Perforation, urethra
uterus —*see* Perforation, uterus
perineum —*see* Laceration, perineum
pharynx J39.2
rectum K63.1
newborn P78.0
obstetrical trauma O71.5
traumatic S36.63
root canal space due to endodontic treatment M27.51
sigmoid K63.1
newborn P78.0
obstetrical trauma O71.5
traumatic S36.533
sinus (accessory) (chronic) (nasal) J34.89
sphenoidal sinus —*see* Sinusitis, sphenoidal
surgical (accidental) (by instrument) (blood vessel) (nerve) (organ) —*see* Puncture, accidental complicating surgery
traumatic
external —*see* Puncture
eye —*see* Puncture, eyeball
internal organ —*see* Injury, by site
tympanum, tympanic (membrane) (persistent post-traumatic) (postinflammatory) H72.9-
attic H72.1-
multiple —*see* Perforation, tympanum, multiple
total —*see* Perforation, tympanum, total
central H72.0-
multiple —*see* Perforation, tympanum, multiple
total —*see* Perforation, tympanum, total
marginal NEC —*see* subcategory H72.2
multiple H72.81-
pars flaccida —*see* Perforation, tympanum, attic
total H72.82-
traumatic, current episode S09.2-

Perforation, perforated *(Continued)*
typhoid, gastrointestinal —*see* Typhoid
ulcer —*see* Ulcer, by site, with perforation
ureter N28.89
traumatic S37.19
urethra N36.8
with ectopic or molar pregnancy O08.6
following ectopic or molar pregnancy O08.6
obstetrical trauma O71.5
traumatic S37.39
at delivery O71.5
uterus
with ectopic or molar pregnancy O08.6
by intrauterine contraceptive device T83.39
following ectopic or molar pregnancy O08.6
obstetrical trauma O71.1
traumatic S37.69
obstetric O71.1
uvula K13.79
syphilitic A52.79
vagina
obstetrical trauma O71.4
other trauma - see Puncture, vagina
Periadenitis mucosa necrotica recurrens K12.0
Periappendicitis (acute) —*see* Appendicitis
Periarteritis nodosa (disseminated) (infectious) (necrotizing) M30.0
Periarthritis (joint) —*see also* Enthesopathy
Duplay's M75.0-
gonococcal A54.42
humeroscapularis —*see* Capsulitis, adhesive
scapulohumeral —*see* Capsulitis, adhesive
shoulder —*see* Capsulitis, adhesive
wrist M77.2-
Periarthrosis (angioneural) —*see* Enthesopathy
Pericapsulitis, adhesive (shoulder) —*see* Capsulitis, adhesive
Pericarditis (with decompensation) (with effusion) I31.9
with rheumatic fever (conditions in I00)
active —*see* Pericarditis, rheumatic
inactive or quiescent I09.2
acute (hemorrhagic) (nonrheumatic) (Sicca) I30.9
with chorea (acute) (rheumatic) (Sydenham's) I02.0
benign I30.8
nonspecific I30.0
rheumatic I01.0
with chorea (acute) (Sydenham's) I02.0
adhesive or adherent (chronic) (external) (internal) I31.0
acute —*see* Pericarditis, acute
rheumatic I09.2
bacterial (acute) (subacute) (with serous or seropurulent effusion) I30.1
calcareous I31.1
cholesterol (chronic) I31.8
acute I30.9
chronic (nonrheumatic) I31.9
rheumatic I09.2
constrictive (chronic) I31.1
coxsackie B33.23
fibrinocaseous (tuberculous) A18.84
fibrinopurulent I30.1
fibrinous I30.8
fibrous I31.0
gonococcal A54.83
idiopathic I30.0
in systemic lupus erythematosus M32.12
infective I30.1
meningococcal A39.53
neoplastic (chronic) I31.8
acute I30.9
obliterans, obliterating I31.0
plastic I31.0
pneumococcal I30.1

Pericarditis *(Continued)*
postinfarction I24.1
purulent I30.1
rheumatic (active) (acute) (with effusion) (with pneumonia) I01.0
with chorea (acute) (rheumatic) (Sydenham's) I02.0
chronic or inactive (with chorea) I09.2
rheumatoid —*see* Rheumatoid, carditis
septic I30.1
serofibrinous I30.8
staphylococcal I30.1
streptococcal I30.1
suppurative I30.1
syphilitic A52.06
tuberculous A18.84
uremic N18.9 *[I32]*
viral I30.1
Pericardium, pericardial —*see* condition
Pericellulitis —*see* Cellulitis
Pericementitis (chronic) (suppurative) —*see also* Periodontitis
acute K05.20
generalized —*see* Peridontitis, aggressive, generalized ⇐
localized —*see* Peridontitis, aggressive, localized ⇐
Perichondritis
auricle —*see* Perichondritis, ear
bronchus J98.09
ear (external) H61.00-
acute H61.01-
chronic H61.02-
external auditory canal —*see* Perichondritis, ear
larynx J38.7
syphilitic A52.73
typhoid A01.09
nose J34.89
pinna —*see* Perichondritis, ear
trachea J39.8
Periclasia K05.4
Pericoronitis —*see* Periodontitis
Pericystitis N30.90
with hematuria N30.91
Peridiverticulitis (intestine) K57.92
cecum —*see* Diverticulitis, intestine, large
colon —*see* Diverticulitis, intestine, large
duodenum —*see* Diverticulitis, intestine, small
intestine —*see* Diverticulitis, intestine
jejunum —*see* Diverticulitis, intestine, small
rectosigmoid —*see* Diverticulitis, intestine, large
rectum —*see* Diverticulitis, intestine, large
sigmoid —*see* Diverticulitis, intestine, large
Periendocarditis —*see* Endocarditis
Periepididymitis N45.1
Perifolliculitis L01.02
abscedens, caput, scalp L66.3
capitis, abscedens (et suffodiens) L66.3
superficial pustular L01.02
Perihepatitis K65.8
Perilabyrinthitis (acute) —*see* subcategory H83.0
Perimeningitis —*see* Meningitis
Perimetritis —*see* Endometritis
Perimetrosalpingitis —*see* Salpingo-oophoritis
Perineocele N81.81
Perinephric, perinephritic —*see* condition
Perinephritis —*see also* Infection, kidney
purulent —*see* Abscess, kidney
Perineum, perineal —*see* condition
Perineuritis NEC —*see* Neuralgia
Periodic —*see* condition
Periodontitis (chronic) (complex) (compound) (local) (simplex) K05.30
acute K05.20
generalized K05.229 ⇐
moderate K05.222 ◀
severe K05.223 ◀
slight K05.221 ◀

Periodontitis *(Continued)*
acute *(Continued)*
localized K05.219 ⇐
moderate K05.212 ◀
severe K05.213 ◀
slight K05.211 ◀
apical K04.5
acute (pulpal origin) K04.4
generalized K05.329 ⇐
moderate K05.322 ◀
severe K05.323 ◀
slight K05.321 ◀
localized K05.319 ⇐
moderate K05.312 ◀
severe K05.313 ◀
slight K05.311 ◀
Periodontoclasia K05.4
Periodontosis (juvenile) K05.4
Periods —*see also* Menstruation
heavy N92.0
irregular N92.6
shortened intervals (irregular) N92.1
Perionychia —*see also* Cellulitis, digit
with lymphangitis —*see* Lymphangitis, acute, digit
Perioophoritis —*see* Salpingo-oophoritis
Periorchitis N45.2
Periosteum, periosteal —*see* condition
Periostitis (albuminosa) (circumscribed) (diffuse) (infective) (monomelic) —*see also* Osteomyelitis
alveolar M27.3
alveolodental M27.3
dental M27.3
gonorrheal A54.43
jaw (lower) (upper) M27.2
orbit H05.03-
syphilitic A52.77
congenital (early) A50.02 *[M90.80]*
secondary A51.46
tuberculous —*see* Tuberculosis, bone
yaws (hypertrophic) (early) (late) A66.6 *[M90.80]*
Periostosis (hyperplastic) —*see also* Disorder, bone, specified type NEC
with osteomyelitis —*see* Osteomyelitis, specified type NEC
Peripartum
cardiomyopathy O90.3
Periphlebitis —*see* Phlebitis
Periproctitis K62.89
Periprostatitis —*see* Prostatitis
Perirectal —*see* condition
Perirenal —*see* condition
Perisalpingitis —*see* Salpingo-oophoritis
Perisplenitis (infectional) D73.89
Peristalsis, visible or reversed R19.2
Peritendinitis —*see* Enthesopathy
Peritoneum, peritoneal —*see* condition
Peritonitis (adhesive) (bacterial) (fibrinous) (hemorrhagic) (idiopathic) (localized) (perforative) (primary) (with adhesions) (with effusion) K65.9
with or following
abscess K65.1
appendicitis K35.3 ⇐
with perforation or rupture K35.2
generalized K35.2
localized K35.3
diverticular disease (intestine) K57.80
with bleeding K57.81
ectopic or molar pregnancy O08.0
large intestine K57.20
with
bleeding K57.21
small intestine K57.40
with bleeding K57.41
small intestine K57.00
with
bleeding K57.01
large intestine K57.40
with bleeding K57.41

◀ New ⇐ Revised ~~deleted~~ Deleted

Peritonitis *(Continued)*
acute (generalized) K65.0
aseptic T81.61
bile, biliary K65.3
chemical T81.61
chlamydial A74.81
chronic proliferative K65.8
complicating abortion —*see* Abortion, by type, complicated by, pelvic peritonitis
congenital P78.1
diaphragmatic K65.0
diffuse K65.0
diphtheritic A36.89
disseminated K65.0
due to
bile K65.3
foreign
body or object accidentally left during a procedure (instrument) (sponge) (swab) T81.599
substance accidentally left during a procedure (chemical) (powder) (talc) T81.61
talc T81.61
urine K65.8
eosinophilic K65.8
acute K65.0
fibrocaseous (tuberculous) A18.31
fibropurulent K65.0
following ectopic or molar pregnancy O08.0
general (ized) K65.0
gonococcal A54.85
meconium (newborn) P78.0
neonatal P78.1
meconium P78.0
pancreatic K65.0
paroxysmal, familial E85.0
benign E85.0
pelvic
female N73.5
acute N73.3
chronic N73.4
with adhesions N73.6
male K65.0
periodic, familial E85.0
proliferative, chronic K65.8
puerperal, postpartum, childbirth O85
purulent K65.0
septic K65.0
specified NEC K65.8
spontaneous bacterial K65.2
subdiaphragmatic K65.0
subphrenic K65.0
suppurative K65.0
syphilitic A52.74
congenital (early) A50.08 *[K67]*
talc T81.61
tuberculous A18.31
urine K65.8
Peritonsillar —*see* condition
Peritonsillitis J36
Perityphlitis K37
Periureteritis N28.89
Periurethral —*see* condition
Periurethritis (gangrenous) —*see* Urethritis
Periuterine —*see* condition
Perivaginitis —*see* Vaginitis
Perivasculitis, retinal H35.06-
Perivasitis (chronic) N49.1
Perivesiculitis (seminal) —*see* Vesiculitis
Perlèche NEC K13.0
due to
candidiasis B37.83
moniliasis B37.83
riboflavin deficiency E53.0
vitamin B2 (riboflavin) deficiency E53.0
Pernicious —*see* condition
Pernio, perniosis T69.1
Perpetrator (of abuse) —*see* Index to External Causes of Injury, Perpetrator
Persecution
delusion F22
social Z60.5
Perseveration (tonic) R48.8
Persistence, persistent (congenital)
anal membrane Q42.3
with fistula Q42.2
arteria stapedia Q16.3
atrioventricular canal Q21.2
branchial cleft Q18.0
bulbus cordis in left ventricle Q21.8
canal of Cloquet Q14.0
capsule (opaque) Q12.8
cilioretinal artery or vein Q14.8
cloaca Q43.7
communication —*see* Fistula, congenital
convolutions
aortic arch Q25.46 ◄
fallopian tube Q50.6
oviduct Q50.6
uterine tube Q50.6
double aortic arch Q25.45 ◄
ductus arteriosus (Botalli) Q25.0
fetal
circulation P29.3
form of cervix (uteri) Q51.828
hemoglobin, hereditary (HPFH) D56.4
foramen
Botalli Q21.1
ovale Q21.1
Gartner's duct Q52.4
hemoglobin, fetal (hereditary) (HPFH) D56.4
hyaloid
artery (generally incomplete) Q14.0
system Q14.8
hymen, in pregnancy or childbirth —*see* Pregnancy, complicated by, abnormal, vulva
lanugo Q84.2
left
posterior cardinal vein Q26.8
root with right arch of aorta Q25.49 ◄
superior vena cava Q26.1
Meckel's diverticulum Q43.0
malignant —*see* Table of Neoplasms, small intestine, malignant
mucosal disease (middle ear) —*see* Otitis, media, suppurative, chronic, tubotympanic
nail (s), anomalous Q84.6
omphalomesenteric duct Q43.0
organ or site not listed —*see* Anomaly, by site
ostium
atrioventriculare commune Q21.2
primum Q21.2
secundum Q21.1
ovarian rests in fallopian tube Q50.6
pancreatic tissue in intestinal tract Q43.8
primary (deciduous)
teeth K00.6
vitreous hyperplasia Q14.0
pupillary membrane Q13.89
rhesus (Rh)titer —*see* Complication (s), transfusion, incompatibility reaction, Rh (factor)
right aortic arch Q25.47 ◄
sinus
urogenitalis
female Q52.8
male Q55.8
venosus with imperfect incorporation in right auricle Q26.8
thymus (gland) (hyperplasia) E32.0
thyroglossal duct Q89.2
thyrolingual duct Q89.2
truncus arteriosus or communis Q20.0
tunica vasculosa lentis Q12.2
umbilical sinus Q64.4
urachus Q64.4
vitelline duct Q43.0
Person (with)
admitted for clinical research, as a control subject (normal comparison) (participant) Z00.6
awaiting admission to adequate facility elsewhere Z75.1
concern (normal) about sick person in family Z63.6
consulting on behalf of another Z71.0
feigning illness Z76.5
living (in)
without
adequate housing (heating) (space) Z59.1
housing (permanent) (temporary) Z59.0
person able to render necessary care Z74.2
shelter Z59.0
alone Z60.2
boarding school Z59.3
residential institution Z59.3
on waiting list Z75.1
sick or handicapped in family Z63.6
Personality (disorder) F60.9
accentuation of traits (type A pattern) Z73.1
affective F34.0
aggressive F60.3
amoral F60.2
anacastic, anankastic F60.5
antisocial F60.2
anxious F60.6
asocial F60.2
asthenic F60.7
avoidant F60.6
borderline F60.3
change due to organic condition (enduring) F07.0
compulsive F60.5
cycloid F34.0
cyclothymic F34.0
dependent F60.7
depressive F34.1
dissocial F60.2
dual F44.81
eccentric F60.89
emotionally unstable F60.3
expansive paranoid F60.0
explosive F60.3
fanatic F60.0
haltlose type F60.89
histrionic F60.4
hyperthymic F34.0
hypothymic F34.1
hysterical F60.4
immature F60.89
inadequate F60.7
labile (emotional) F60.3
mixed (nonspecific) F60.89 ◄
morally defective F60.2
multiple F44.81
narcissistic F60.81
obsessional F60.5
obsessive (-compulsive) F60.5
organic F07.0
overconscientious F60.5
paranoid F60.0
passive (-dependent) F60.7
passive-aggressive F60.89
pathologic F60.9
pattern defect or disturbance F60.9
pseudopsychopathic (organic) F07.0
pseudoretarded (organic) F07.0
psychoinfantile F60.4
psychoneurotic NEC F60.89
psychopathic F60.2
querulant F60.0
sadistic F60.89
schizoid F60.1
self-defeating F60.7
sensitive paranoid F60.0

P

◄ New ◄ Revised ~~deleted~~ Deleted

Personality *(Continued)*
sociopathic (amoral) (antisocial) (asocial) (dissocial) F60.2
specified NEC F60.89
type A Z73.1
unstable (emotional) F60.3
Perthes' disease —*see* Legg-Calvé-Perthes disease
Pertussis (*see also* Whooping cough) A37.90
Perversion, perverted
appetite F50.89 ◀
psychogenic F50.89 ◀
function
pituitary gland E23.2
posterior lobe E22.2
sense of smell and taste R43.8
psychogenic F45.8
sexual —*see* Deviation, sexual
Pervious, congenital —*see also* Imperfect, closure
ductus arteriosus Q25.0
Pes (congenital) —*see also* Talipes
acquired —*see also* Deformity, limb, foot, specified NEC
planus —*see* Deformity, limb, flat foot
adductus Q66.89
cavus Q66.7
deformity NEC, acquired —*see* Deformity, limb, foot, specified NEC
planus (acquired) (any degree) —*see also* Deformity, limb, flat foot
rachitic sequelae (late effect) E64.3
valgus Q66.6
Pest, pestis —*see* Plague
Petechia, petechiae R23.3
newborn P54.5
Petechial typhus A75.9
Peter's anomaly Q13.4
Petit mal seizure —*see* Epilepsy, generalized, specified NEC
Petit's hernia —*see* Hernia, abdomen, specified site NEC
Petrellidosis B48.2
Petrositis H70.20-
acute H70.21-
chronic H70.22-
Peutz-Jeghers disease or syndrome Q85.8
Peyronie's disease N48.6
PFAPA (periodic fever, aphthous stomatitis, pharyngitis, and adenopathy syndrome) M04.8 ◀
Pfeiffer's disease —*see* Mononucleosis, infectious
Phagedena (dry) (moist) (sloughing) —*see also* Gangrene
geometric L88
penis N48.29
tropical —*see* Ulcer, skin
vulva N76.6
Phagedenic —*see* condition
Phakoma H35.89
Phakomatosis —*see also* specific eponymous syndromes Q85.9
Bourneville's Q85.1
specified NEC Q85.8
Phantom limb syndrome (without pain) G54.7
with pain G54.6
Pharyngeal pouch syndrome D82.1
Pharyngitis (acute) (catarrhal) (gangrenous) (infective) (malignant) (membranous) (phlegmonous) (pseudomembranous) (simple) (subacute) (suppurative) (ulcerative) (viral) J02.9
with influenza, flu, or grippe —*see* Influenza, with, pharyngitis
aphthous B08.5
atrophic J31.2
chlamydial A56.4
chronic (atrophic) (granular) (hypertrophic) J31.2

Pharyngitis *(Continued)*
coxsackievirus B08.5
diphtheritic A36.0
enteroviral vesicular B08.5
follicular (chronic) J31.2
fusospirochetal A69.1
gonococcal A54.5
granular (chronic) J31.2
herpesviral B00.2
hypertrophic J31.2
infectional, chronic J31.2
influenzal —*see* Influenza, with, respiratory manifestations NEC
lymphonodular, acute (enteroviral) B08.8
pneumococcal J02.8
purulent J02.9
putrid J02.9
septic J02.0
sicca J31.2
specified organism NEC J02.8
staphylococcal J02.8
streptococcal J02.0
syphilitic, congenital (early) A50.03
tuberculous A15.8
vesicular, enteroviral B08.5
viral NEC J02.8
Pharyngoconjunctivitis, viral B30.2
Pharyngolaryngitis (acute) J06.0
chronic J37.0
Pharyngoplegia J39.2
Pharyngotonsillitis, herpesviral B00.2
Pharyngotracheitis, chronic J42
Pharynx, pharyngeal —*see* condition
Phencyclidine-induced ◀
anxiety disorder F16.980 ◀
bipolar and related disorder F16.94 ◀
depressive disorder F16.94 ◀
psychotic disorder F16.959 ◀
Phenomenon
Arthus' —*see* Arthus' phenomenon
jaw-winking Q07.8
lupus erythematosus (LE) cell M32.9
Raynaud's (secondary) I73.00
with gangrene I73.01
vasomotor R55
vasospastic I73.9
vasovagal R55
Wenckebach's I44.1
Phenylketonuria E70.1
classical E70.0
maternal E70.1
Pheochromoblastoma
specified site —*see* Neoplasm, malignant, by site
unspecified site C74.10
Pheochromocytoma
malignant
specified site —*see* Neoplasm, malignant, by site
unspecified site C74.10
specified site —*see* Neoplasm, benign, by site
unspecified site D35.00
Pheohyphomycosis —*see* Chromomycosis
Pheomycosis —*see* Chromomycosis
Phimosis (congenital) (due to infection) N47.1
chancroidal A57
Phlebectasia —*see also* Varix
congenital Q27.4
Phlebitis (infective) (pyemic) (septic) (suppurative) I80.9
antepartum —*see* Thrombophlebitis, antepartum
blue —*see* Phlebitis, leg, deep
breast, superficial I80.8
cavernous (venous) sinus —*see* Phlebitis, intracranial (venous) sinus
cerebral (venous) sinus —*see* Phlebitis, intracranial (venous) sinus
chest wall, superficial I80.8
cranial (venous) sinus —*see* Phlebitis, intracranial (venous) sinus

Phlebitis *(Continued)*
deep (vessels) —*see* Phlebitis, leg, deep
due to implanted device —*see* Complications, by site and type, specified NEC
during or resulting from a procedure T81.72
femoral vein (superficial) I80.1-
femoropopliteal vein I80.0-
gestational —*see* Phlebopathy, gestational
hepatic veins I80.8
iliofemoral —*see* Phlebitis, femoral vein
intracranial (venous) sinus (any) G08
nonpyogenic I67.6
intraspinal venous sinuses and veins G08
nonpyogenic G95.19
lateral (venous) sinus —*see* Phlebitis, intracranial (venous) sinus
leg I80.3
antepartum —*see* Thrombophlebitis, antepartum
deep (vessels) NEC I80.20-
iliac I80.21-
popliteal vein I80.22-
specified vessel NEC I80.29-
tibial vein I80.23-
femoral vein (superficial) I80.1-
superficial (vessels) I80.0-
longitudinal sinus —*see* Phlebitis, intracranial (venous) sinus
lower limb —*see* Phlebitis, leg
migrans, migrating (superficial) I82.1
pelvic
with ectopic or molar pregnancy O08.0
following ectopic or molar pregnancy O08.0
puerperal, postpartum O87.1
popliteal vein —*see* Phlebitis, leg, deep, popliteal
portal (vein) K75.1
postoperative T81.72
pregnancy —*see* Thrombophlebitis, antepartum
puerperal, postpartum, childbirth O87.0
deep O87.1
pelvic O87.1
superficial O87.0
retina —*see* Vasculitis, retina
saphenous (accessory) (great) (long) (small) —*see* Phlebitis, leg, superficial
sinus (meninges) —*see* Phlebitis, intracranial (venous) sinus
specified site NEC I80.8
syphilitic A52.09
tibial vein —*see* Phlebitis, leg, deep, tibial
ulcerative I80.9
leg —*see* Phlebitis, leg
umbilicus I80.8
uterus (septic) —*see* Endometritis
varicose (leg) (lower limb) —*see* Varix, leg, with, inflammation
Phlebofibrosis I87.8
Phleboliths I87.8
Phlebopathy
gestational O22.9-
puerperal O87.9
Phlebosclerosis I87.8
Phlebothrombosis —*see also* Thrombosis
antepartum —*see* Thrombophlebitis, antepartum
pregnancy —*see* Thrombophlebitis, antepartum
puerperal —*see* Thrombophlebitis, puerperal
Phlebotomus fever A93.1
Phlegmasia
alba dolens O87.1
nonpuerperal —*see* Phlebitis, femoral vein
cerulea dolens —*see* Phlebitis, leg, deep
Phlegmon —*see* Abscess
Phlegmonous —*see* condition

◀ New ◀ Revised ~~deleted~~ Deleted

Phlyctenulosis (allergic) (keratoconjunctivitis) (nontuberculous) —*see also* Keratoconjunctivitis
cornea —*see* Keratoconjunctivitis
tuberculous A18.52
Phobia, phobic F40.9
animal F40.218
spiders F40.210
examination F40.298
reaction F40.9
simple F40.298
social F40.10
generalized F40.11
specific (isolated) F40.298
animal F40.218
spiders F40.210
blood F40.230
injection F40.231
injury F40.233
men F40.290
natural environment F40.228
thunderstorms F40.220
situational F40.248
bridges F40.242
closed in spaces F40.240
flying F40.243
heights F40.241
specified focus NEC F40.298
transfusion F40.231
women F40.291
specified NEC F40.8
medical care NEC F40.232
state F40.9
Phocas' disease —*see* Mastopathy, cystic
Phocomelia Q73.1
lower limb —*see* Agenesis, leg, with foot present
upper limb —*see* Agenesis, arm, with hand present
Phoria H50.50
Phosphate-losing tubular disorder N25.0
Phosphatemia E83.39
Phosphaturia E83.39
Photodermatitis (sun) L56.8
chronic L57.8
due to drug L56.8
light other than sun L59.8
Photokeratitis H16.13-
Photophobia H53.14-
Photophthalmia —*see* Photokeratitis
Photopsia H53.19
Photoretinitis —*see* Retinopathy, solar
Photosensitivity, photosensitization (sun) **skin** L56.8
light other than sun L59.8
Phrenitis —*see* Encephalitis
Phrynoderma (vitamin A deficiency) E50.8
Phthiriasis (pubis) B85.3
with any infestation classifiable to B85.0-B85.2 B85.4
Phthirus infestation —*see* Phthiriasis
Phthisis —*see also* Tuberculosis
bulbi (infectional) —*see* Disorder, globe, degenerated condition, atrophy
eyeball (due to infection) —*see* Disorder, globe, degenerated condition, atrophy
Phycomycosis —*see* Zygomycosis
Physalopteriasis B81.8
Physical restraint status Z78.1
Phytobezoar T18.9
intestine T18.3
stomach T18.2
Pian —*see* Yaws
Pianoma A66.1
Pica F50.89 ◀
in adults F50.89 ◀
infant or child F98.3
Picking, nose F98.8
Pick-Niemann disease —*see* Niemann-Pick disease or syndrome
Pick's
cerebral atrophy G31.01 *[F02.80]*
with behavioral disturbance G31.01 *[F02.81]*
disease or syndrome (brain) G31.01 *[F02.80]*
with behavioral disturbance G31.01 *[F02.81]*
brain G31.01 *[F02.80]* ◀
with behavioral disturbance G31.01 *[F02.81]* ◀
pericardium (pericardial pseudocirrhosis of liver) I31.1 ◀
syndrome ◀
brain G31.01 *[F02.80]* ◀
with behavioral disturbance G31.01 *[F02.81]* ◀
of heart (pericardial pseudocirrhosis of liver) I31.1 ◀
Pickwickian syndrome E66.2
Piebaldism E70.39
Piedra (beard) (scalp) B36.8
black B36.3
white B36.2
Pierre Robin deformity or syndrome Q87.0
Pierson's disease or osteochondrosis M91.0
Pig-bel A05.2
Pigeon
breast or chest (acquired) M95.4
congenital Q67.7
rachitic sequelae (late effect) E64.3
breeder's disease or lung J67.2
fancier's disease or lung J67.2
toe —*see* Deformity, toe, specified NEC
Pigmentation (abnormal) (anomaly) L81.9
conjunctiva H11.13-
cornea (anterior) H18.01-
posterior H18.05-
stromal H18.06-
diminished melanin formation NEC L81.6
iron L81.8
lids, congenital Q82.8
limbus corneae —*see* Pigmentation, cornea
metals L81.8
optic papilla, congenital Q14.2
retina, congenital (grouped) (nevoid) Q14.1
scrotum, congenital Q82.8
tattoo L81.8
Piles —*see also* Hemorrhoids K64.9
Pili
annulati or torti (congenital) Q84.1
incarnati L73.1
Pill roller hand (intrinsic) —*see* Parkinsonism
Pilomatrixoma —*see* Neoplasm, skin, benign
malignant —*see* Neoplasm, skin, malignant
Pilonidal —*see* condition
Pimple R23.8
PIN —*see* Neoplasia, intraepithelial, prostate ◀
Pinched nerve —*see* Neuropathy, entrapment
Pindborg tumor —*see* Cyst, calcifying odontogenic
Pineal body or gland —*see* condition
Pinealoblastoma C75.3
Pinealoma D44.5
malignant C75.3
Pineoblastoma C75.3
Pineocytoma D44.5
Pinguecula H11.15-
Pingueculitis H10.81-
Pinhole meatus —*see also* Stricture, urethra N35.9
Pink
disease —*see* subcategory T56.1
eye —*see* Conjunctivitis, acute, mucopurulent
Pinkus' disease (lichen nitidus) L44.1
Pinpoint
meatus —*see* Stricture, urethra
os (uteri) —*see* Stricture, cervix
Pins and needles R20.2
Pinta A67.9
cardiovascular lesions A67.2
chancre (primary) A67.0
Pinta *(Continued)*
erythematous plaques A67.1
hyperchromic lesions A67.1
hyperkeratosis A67.1
lesions A67.9
cardiovascular A67.2
hyperchromic A67.1
intermediate A67.1
late A67.2
mixed A67.3
primary A67.0
skin (achromic) (cicatricial) (dyschromic) A67.2
hyperchromic A67.1
mixed (achromic and hyperchromic) A67.3
papule (primary) A67.0
skin lesions (achromic) (cicatricial) (dyschromic) A67.2
hyperchromic A67.1
mixed (achromic and hyperchromic) A67.3
vitiligo A67.2
Pintids A67.1
Pinworm (disease) (infection) (infestation) B80
Piroplasmosis B60.0
Pistol wound —*see* Gunshot wound
Pitchers' elbow —*see* Derangement, joint, specified type NEC, elbow
Pithecoid pelvis Q74.2
with disproportion (fetopelvic) O33.0
causing obstructed labor O65.0
Pithiatism F48.8
Pitted —*see* Pitting
Pitting —*see also* Edema R60.9
lip R60.0
nail L60.8
teeth K00.4
Pituitary gland —*see* condition
Pituitary-snuff-taker's disease J67.8
Pityriasis (capitis) L21.0
alba L30.5
circinata (et maculata) L42
furfuracea L21.0
Hebra's L26
lichenoides L41.0
chronica L41.1
et varioliformis (acuta) L41.0
maculata (et circinata) L30.5
nigra B36.1
pilaris, Hebra's L44.0
rosea L42
rotunda L44.8
rubra (Hebra) pilaris L44.0
simplex L30.5
specified type NEC L30.5
streptogenes L30.5
versicolor (scrotal) B36.0
Placenta, placental —*see* Pregnancy, complicated by (care of) (management affected by), specified condition
Placentitis O41.14-
Plagiocephaly Q67.3
Plague A20.9
abortive A20.8
ambulatory A20.8
asymptomatic A20.8
bubonic A20.0
cellulocutaneous A20.1
cutaneobubonic A20.1
lymphatic gland A20.0
meningitis A20.3
pharyngeal A20.8
pneumonic (primary) (secondary) A20.2
pulmonary, pulmonic A20.2
septicemic A20.7
tonsillar A20.8
septicemic A20.7
Planning, family
contraception Z30.9
procreation Z31.69

P

Plaque (s)
artery, arterial —*see* Arteriosclerosis
calcareous —*see* Calcification
coronary, lipid rich I25.83
epicardial I31.8
erythematous, of pinta A67.1
Hollenhorst's —*see* Occlusion, artery, retina
lipid rich, coronary I25.83
pleural (without asbestos) J92.9
with asbestos J92.0
tongue K13.29
Plasmacytoma C90.3-
extramedullary C90.2-
medullary C90.0-
solitary C90.3-
Plasmacytopenia D72.818
Plasmacytosis D72.822
Plaster ulcer —*see* Ulcer, pressure, by site
Plateau iris syndrome (post-iridectomy) (postprocedural) (without glaucoma) H21.82
with glaucoma H40.22-
Platybasia Q75.8
Platyonychia (congenital) Q84.6
acquired L60.8
Platypelloid pelvis M95.5
with disproportion (fetopelvic) O33.0
causing obstructed labor O65.0
congenital Q74.2
Platyspondylisis Q76.49
Plaut (-Vincent) **disease** —*see also* Vincent's A69.1
Plethora R23.2
newborn P61.1
Pleura, pleural —*see* condition
Pleuralgia R07.81
Pleurisy (acute) (adhesive) (chronic) (costal) (diaphragmatic) (double) (dry) (fibrinous) (fibrous) (interlobar) (latent) (plastic) (primary) (residual) (sicca) (sterile) (subacute) (unresolved) R09.1
with
adherent pleura J86.0
effusion J90
chylous, chyliform J94.0
tuberculous (non primary) A15.6
primary (progressive) A15.7
tuberculosis —*see* Pleurisy, tuberculous (non primary)
encysted —*see* Pleurisy, with effusion
exudative —*see* Pleurisy, with effusion
fibrinopurulent, fibropurulent —*see* Pyothorax
hemorrhagic —*see* Hemothorax
pneumococcal J90
purulent —*see* Pyothorax
septic —*see* Pyothorax
serofibrinous —*see* Pleurisy, with effusion
seropurulent —*see* Pyothorax
serous —*see* Pleurisy, with effusion
staphylococcal J86.9
streptococcal J90
suppurative —*see* Pyothorax
traumatic (post) (current) —*see* Injury, intrathoracic, pleura
tuberculous (with effusion) (non primary) A15.6
primary (progressive) A15.7
Pleuritis sicca —*see* Pleurisy
Pleurobronchopneumonia —*see* Pneumonia, broncho
Pleurodynia R07.81
epidemic B33.0
viral B33.0
Pleuropericarditis —*see also* Pericarditis
acute I30.9
Pleuropneumonia (acute) (bilateral) (double) (septic) —*see also* Pneumonia J18.8
chronic —*see* Fibrosis, lung
Pleuro-pneumonia-like-organism (PPLO), **as cause of disease classified elsewhere** B96.0
Pleurorrhea —*see* Pleurisy, with effusion
Plexitis, brachial G54.0
Plica
polonica B85.0
syndrome, knee M67.5
tonsil J35.8
Plicated tongue K14.5
Plug
bronchus NEC J98.09
meconium (newborn) NEC syndrome P76.0
mucus —*see* Asphyxia, mucus
Plumbism —*see* subcategory T56.0
Plummer's disease E05.20
with thyroid storm E05.21
Plummer-Vinson syndrome D50.1
Pluricarential syndrome of infancy E40
Plus (and minus) **hand** (intrinsic) —*see* Deformity, limb, specified type NEC, forearm
Pneumathemia —*see* Air, embolism
Pneumatic hammer (drill) **syndrome** T75.21
Pneumatocele (lung) J98.4
intracranial G93.89
tension J44.9
Pneumatosis
cystoides intestinalis K63.89
intestinalis K63.89
peritonei K66.8
Pneumaturia R39.89
Pneumoblastoma —*see* Neoplasm, lung, malignant
Pneumocephalus G93.89
Pneumococcemia A40.3
Pneumococcus, pneumococcal —*see* condition
Pneumoconiosis (due to) (inhalation of) J64
with tuberculosis (any type in A15) J65
aluminum J63.0
asbestos J61
bagasse, bagassosis J67.1
bauxite J63.1
beryllium J63.2
coal miners' (simple) J60
coalworkers' (simple) J60
collier's J60
cotton dust J66.0
diatomite (diatomaceous earth) J62.8
dust
inorganic NEC J63.6
lime J62.8
marble J62.8
organic NEC J66.8
fumes or vapors (from silo) J68.9
graphite J63.3
grinder's J62.8
kaolin J62.8
mica J62.8
millstone maker's J62.8
mineral fibers NEC J61
miner's J60
moldy hay J67.0
potter's J62.8
rheumatoid —*see* Rheumatoid, lung
sandblaster's J62.8
silica, silicate NEC J62.8
with carbon J60
stonemason's J62.8
talc (dust) J62.0
Pneumocystis carinii pneumonia B59
Pneumocystis jiroveci (pneumonia) B59
Pneumocystosis (with pneumonia) B59
Pneumohemopericardium I31.2
Pneumohemothorax J94.2
traumatic S27.2
Pneumohydropericardium —*see* Pericarditis
Pneumohydrothorax —*see* Hydrothorax
Pneumomediastinum J98.2
congenital or perinatal P25.2
Pneumomycosis B49 *[J99]*
Pneumonia (acute) (double) (migratory) (purulent) (septic) (unresolved) J18.9
with
influenza —*see* Influenza, with, pneumonia
lung abscess J85.1
due to specified organism —*see* Pneumonia, in (due to)
adenoviral J12.0
adynamic J18.2
alba A50.04
allergic (eosinophilic) J82
alveolar —*see* Pneumonia, lobar
anaerobes J15.8
anthrax A22.1
apex, apical —*see* Pneumonia, lobar
Ascaris B77.81
aspiration J69.0
due to
aspiration of microorganisms
bacterial J15.9
viral J12.9
food (regurgitated) J69.0
gastric secretions J69.0
milk (regurgitated) J69.0
oils, essences J69.1
solids, liquids NEC J69.8
vomitus J69.0
newborn P24.81
amniotic fluid (clear) P24.11
blood P24.21
food (regurgitated) P24.31
liquor (amnii) P24.11
meconium P24.01
milk P24.31
mucus P24.11
specified NEC P24.81
stomach contents P24.31
postprocedural J95.4
atypical NEC J18.9
bacillus J15.9
specified NEC J15.8
bacterial J15.9
specified NEC J15.8
Bacteroides (fragilis) (oralis) (melaninogenicus) J15.8
basal, basic, basilar —*see* Pneumonia, by type
bronchiolitis obliterans organized (BOOP) J84.89
broncho-, bronchial (confluent) (croupous) (diffuse) (disseminated) (hemorrhagic) (involving lobes) (lobar) (terminal) J18.0
allergic (eosinophilic) J82
aspiration —*see* Pneumonia, aspiration
bacterial J15.9
specified NEC J15.8
chronic —*see* Fibrosis, lung
diplococcal J13
Eaton's agent J15.7
Escherichia coli (E. coli) J15.5
Friedländer's bacillus J15.0
Hemophilus influenzae J14
hypostatic J18.2
inhalation (*see also* Pneumonia, aspiration
due to fumes or vapors (chemical) J68.0
of oils or essences J69.1
Klebsiella (pneumoniae) J15.0
lipid, lipoid J69.1
endogenous J84.89
Mycoplasma (pneumoniae) J15.7
pleuro-pneumonia-like-organisms (PPLO) J15.7
pneumococcal J13
Proteus J15.6
Pseudomonas J15.1
Serratia marcescens J15.6
specified organism NEC J16.8
staphylococcal —*see* Pneumonia, staphylococcal
streptococcal NEC J15.4
group B J15.3
pneumoniae J13
viral, virus —*see* Pneumonia, viral

Pneumonia *(Continued)*
Butyrivibrio (fibriosolvens) J15.8
Candida B37.1
caseous —*see* Tuberculosis, pulmonary
catarrhal —*see* Pneumonia, broncho
chlamydial J16.0
congenital P23.1
cholesterol J84.89
cirrhotic (chronic) —*see* Fibrosis, lung
Clostridium (haemolyticum) (novyi) J15.8
confluent —*see* Pneumonia, broncho
congenital (infective) P23.9
due to
bacterium NEC P23.6
Chlamydia P23.1
Escherichia coli P23.4
Haemophilus influenzae P23.6
infective organism NEC P23.8
Klebsiella pneumoniae P23.6
Mycoplasma P23.6
Pseudomonas P23.5
Staphylococcus P23.2
Streptococcus (except group B) P23.6
group B P23.3
viral agent P23.0
specified NEC P23.8
croupous —*see* Pneumonia, lobar
cryptogenic organizing J84.116
cytomegalic inclusion B25.0
cytomegaloviral B25.0
deglutition —*see* Pneumonia, aspiration
desquamative interstitial J84.117
diffuse —*see* Pneumonia, broncho
diplococcal, diplococcus (broncho-) (lobar) J13
disseminated (focal) —*see* Pneumonia, broncho
Eaton's agent J15.7
embolic, embolism —*see* Embolism, pulmonary
Enterobacter J15.6
eosinophilic J82
Escherichia coli (E. coli) J15.5
Eubacterium J15.8
fibrinous —*see* Pneumonia, lobar
fibroid, fibrous (chronic) —*see* Fibrosis, lung
Friedländer's bacillus J15.0
Fusobacterium (nucleatum) J15.8
gangrenous J85.0
giant cell (measles) B05.2
gonococcal A54.84
gram-negative bacteria NEC J15.6
anaerobic J15.8
Hemophilus influenzae (broncho) (lobar) J14
human metapneumovirus J12.3
hypostatic (broncho) (lobar) J18.2
in (due to)
actinomycosis A42.0
adenovirus J12.0
anthrax A22.1
ascariasis B77.81
aspergillosis B44.9
Bacillus anthracis A22.1
Bacterium anitratum J15.6
candidiasis B37.1
chickenpox B01.2
Chlamydia J16.0
neonatal P23.1
coccidioidomycosis B38.2
acute B38.0
chronic B38.1
cytomegalovirus disease B25.0
Diplococcus (pneumoniae) J13
Eaton's agent J15.7
Enterobacter J15.6
Escherichia coli (E. coli) J15.5
Friedländer's bacillus J15.0
fumes and vapors (chemical) (inhalation) J68.0
gonorrhea A54.84
Hemophilus influenzae (H. influenzae) J14

Pneumonia *(Continued)*
in *(Continued)*
Herellea J15.6
histoplasmosis B39.2
acute B39.0
chronic B39.1
human metapneumovirus J12.3
Klebsiella (pneumoniae) J15.0
measles B05.2
Mycoplasma (pneumoniae) J15.7
nocardiosis, nocardiasis A43.0
ornithosis A70
parainfluenza virus J12.2
pleuro-pneumonia-like-organism (PPLO) J15.7
pneumococcus J13
pneumocystosis (Pneumocystis carinii) (Pneumocystis jiroveci) B59
Proteus J15.6
Pseudomonas NEC J15.1
pseudomallei A24.1
psittacosis A70
Q fever A78
respiratory syncytial virus J12.1
rheumatic fever I00 *[J17]*
rubella B06.81
Salmonella (infection) A02.22
typhi A01.03
schistosomiasis B65.9 *[J17]*
Serratia marcescens J15.6
specified
bacterium NEC J15.8
organism NEC J16.8
spirochetal NEC A69.8
Staphylococcus J15.20
aureus (methicillin susceptible) (MSSA) J15.211
methicillin resistant (MRSA) J15.212
specified NEC J15.29
Streptococcus J15.4
group B J15.3
pneumoniae J13
specified NEC J15.4
toxoplasmosis B58.3
tularemia A21.2
typhoid (fever) A01.03
varicella B01.2
virus —*see* Pneumonia, viral
whooping cough A37.91
due to
Bordetella parapertussis A37.11
Bordetella pertussis A37.01
specified NEC A37.81
Yersinia pestis A20.2
inhalation of food or vomit —*see* Pneumonia, aspiration
interstitial J84.9
chronic J84.111
desquamative J84.117
due to
collagen vascular disease J84.17
known underlying cause J84.17
idiopathic NOS J84.111
in disease classified elsewhere J84.17
lymphocytic (due to collagen vascular disease) (in diseases classified elsewhere) J84.17
lymphoid J84.2
non-specific J84.89
due to
collagen vascular disease J84.17
known underlying cause J84.17
idiopathic J84.113
in diseases classified elsewhere J84.17
plasma cell B59
pseudomonas J15.1
usual J84.112
due to collagen vascular disease J84.17
idiopathic J84.112
in diseases classified elsewhere J84.17

Pneumonia *(Continued)*
Klebsiella (pneumoniae) J15.0
lipid, lipoid (exogenous) J69.1
endogenous J84.89
lobar (disseminated) (double) (interstitial) J18.1
bacterial J15.9
specified NEC J15.8
chronic —*see* Fibrosis, lung
Escherichia coli (E. coli) J15.5
Friedländer's bacillus J15.0
Hemophilus influenzae J14
hypostatic J18.2
Klebsiella (pneumoniae) J15.0
pneumococcal J13
Proteus J15.6
Pseudomonas J15.1
specified organism NEC J16.8
staphylococcal —*see* Pneumonia, staphylococcal
streptococcal NEC J15.4
Streptococcus pneumoniae J13
viral, virus —*see* Pneumonia, viral
lobular —*see* Pneumonia, broncho
Löffler's J82
lymphoid interstitial J84.2
massive —*see* Pneumonia, lobar
meconium P24.01
MRSA (Methicillin resistant Staphylococcus aureus) J15.212 ◀
MSSA (methicillin susceptible Staphylococcus aureus) J15.211
multilobar —*see* Pneumonia, by type
Mycoplasma (pneumoniae) J15.7
necrotic J85.0
neonatal P23.9
aspiration —*see* Aspiration, by substance, with pneumonia
nitrogen dioxide J68.0 ⟸
organizing J84.89
due to
collagen vascular disease J84.17
known underlying cause J84.17
in diseases classified elsewhere J84.17
orthostatic J18.2
parainfluenza virus J12.2
parenchymatous —*see* Fibrosis, lung
passive J18.2
patchy —*see* Pneumonia, broncho
Peptococcus J15.8
Peptostreptococcus J15.8
plasma cell (of infants) B59
pleurolobar —*see* Pneumonia, lobar
pleuro-pneumonia-like organism (PPLO) J15.7
pneumococcal (broncho) (lobar) J13
Pneumocystis (carinii) (jiroveci) B59
postinfectional NEC B99 *[J17]*
postmeasles B05.2
Proteus J15.6
Pseudomonas J15.1
psittacosis A70
radiation J70.0
respiratory syncytial virus J12.1
resulting from a procedure J95.89
rheumatic I00 *[J17]*
Salmonella (arizonae) (cholerae-suis) (enteritidis) (typhimurium) A02.22
typhi A01.03
typhoid fever A01.03
SARS-associated coronavirus J12.81
segmented, segmental —*see* Pneumonia, broncho-
Serratia marcescens J15.6
specified NEC J18.8
bacterium NEC J15.8
organism NEC J16.8
virus NEC J12.89
spirochetal NEC A69.8

Pneumonia *(Continued)*
staphylococcal (broncho) (lobar) J15.20
aureus (methicillin susceptible) (MSSA) J15.211
methicillin resistant (MRSA) J15.212
specified NEC J15.29
static, stasis J18.2
streptococcal NEC (broncho) (lobar) J15.4
group
A J15.4
B J15.3
specified NEC J15.4
Streptococcus pneumoniae J13
syphilitic, congenital (early) A50.04
traumatic (complication) (early) (secondary) T79.8
tuberculous (any) —*see* Tuberculosis, pulmonary
tularemic A21.2
varicella B01.2
Veillonella J15.8
ventilator associated J95.851
viral, virus (broncho) (interstitial) (lobar) J12.9
adenoviral J12.0
congenital P23.0
human metapneumovirus J12.3
parainfluenza J12.2
respiratory syncytial J12.1
SARS-associated coronavirus J12.81
specified NEC J12.89
white (congenital) A50.04
Pneumonic —*see* condition
Pneumonitis (acute) (primary) —*see also* Pneumonia
air-conditioner J67.7
allergic (due to) J67.9
organic dust NEC J67.8
red cedar dust J67.8
sequoiosis J67.8
wood dust J67.8
aspiration J69.0
due to
anesthesia J95.4
during
labor and delivery O74.0
pregnancy O29.01-
puerperium O89.01
fumes or gases J68.0
obstetric O74.0
chemical (due to gases, fumes or vapors) (inhalation) J68.0
due to anesthesia J95.4
cholesterol J84.89
chronic —*see* Fibrosis, lung
congenital rubella P35.0
crack (cocaine) J68.0
due to
beryllium J68.0
cadmium J68.0
crack (cocaine) J68.0
detergent J69.8
fluorocarbon-polymer J68.0
food, vomit (aspiration) J69.0
fumes or vapors J68.0
gases, fumes or vapors (inhalation) J68.0
inhalation
blood J69.8
essences J69.1
food (regurgitated), milk, vomit J69.0
oils, essences J69.1
saliva J69.0
solids, liquids NEC J69.8
manganese J68.0
nitrogen dioxide J68.0
oils, essences J69.1
solids, liquids NEC J69.8
toxoplasmosis (acquired) B58.3
congenital P37.1
vanadium J68.0
ventilator J95.851

Pneumonitis *(Continued)*
eosinophilic J82
hypersensitivity J67.9
air conditioner lung J67.7
bagassosis J67.1
bird fancier's lung J67.2
farmer's lung J67.0
maltworker's lung J67.4
maple bark-stripper's lung J67.6
mushroom worker's lung J67.5
specified organic dust NEC J67.8
suberosis J67.3
interstitial (chronic) J84.89
acute J84.114
lymphoid J84.2
non-specific J84.89
idiopathic J84.113
lymphoid, interstitial J84.2
meconium P24.01
postanesthetic J95.4
correct substance properly administered —*see* Table of Drugs and Chemcials, by drug, adverse effect
in labor and delivery O74.0
in pregnancy O29.01-
obstetric O74.0
overdose or wrong substance given or taken (by accident) —*see* Table of Drugs and Chemicals, by drug, poisoning
postpartum, puerperal O89.01
postoperative J95.4
obstetric O74.0
radiation J70.0
rubella, congenital P35.0
ventilation (air-conditioning) J67.7
ventilator associated J95.851
wood-dust J67.8
Pneumonoconiosis —*see* Pneumoconiosis
Pneumoparotid K11.8
Pneumopathy NEC J98.4
alveolar J84.09
due to organic dust NEC J66.8
parietoalveolar J84.09
Pneumopericarditis —*see also* Pericarditis
acute I30.9
Pneumopericardium —*see also* Pericarditis
congenital P25.3
newborn P25.3
traumatic (post) —*see* Injury, heart
Pneumophagia (psychogenic) F45.8
Pneumopleurisy, pneumopleuritis —*see also* Pneumonia J18.8
Pneumopyopericardium I30.1
Pneumopyothorax —*see* Pyopneumothorax
with fistula J86.0
Pneumorrhagia —*see also* Hemorrhage, lung
tuberculous —*see* Tuberculosis, pulmonary
Pneumothorax NOS J93.9
acute J93.83
chronic J93.81
congenital P25.1
perinatal period P25.1
postprocedural J95.811
specified NEC J93.83
spontaneous NOS J93.83
newborn P25.1
primary J93.11
secondary J93.12
tension J93.0
tense valvular, infectional J93.0
tension (spontaneous) J93.0
traumatic S27.0
with hemothorax S27.2
tuberculous —*see* Tuberculosis, pulmonary
Podagra —*see also* Gout M10.9
Podencephalus Q01.9
Poikilocytosis R71.8
Poikiloderma L81.6
Civatte's L57.3
congenital Q82.8
vasculare atrophicans L94.5

Poikilodermatomyositis M33.10
with
myopathy M33.12
respiratory involvement M33.11
specified organ involvement NEC M33.19
Pointed ear (congenital) Q17.3
Poison ivy, oak, sumac or other plant dermatitis (allergic) (contact) L23.7
Poisoning (acute) —*see also* Table of Drugs and Chemicals
algae and toxins T65.82-
Bacillus B (aertrycke) (cholerae (suis)) (paratyphosus) (suipestifer) A02.9
botulinus A05.1
bacterial toxins A05.9
berries, noxious —*see* Poisoning, food, noxious, berries
botulism A05.1
ciguatera fish T61.0-
Clostridium botulinum A05.1
death-cap (Amanita phalloides) (Amanita verna) —*see* Poisoning, food, noxious, mushrooms
drug —*see* Table of Drugs and Chemicals, by drug, poisoning
epidemic, fish (noxious) —*see* Poisoning, seafood
bacterial A05.9
fava bean D55.0
fish (noxious) T61.9-
bacterial —*see* Intoxication, foodborne, by agent
ciguatera fish —*see* Poisoning, ciguatera fish
scombroid fish —*see* Poisoning, scombroid fish
specified type NEC T61.77-
food (acute) (diseased) (infected) (noxious) NEC T62.9-
bacterial —*see* Intoxication, foodborne, by agent
due to
Bacillus (aertrycke) (choleraesuis) (paratyphosus) (suipestifer) A02.9
botulinus A05.1
Clostridium (perfringens) (Welchii) A05.2
salmonella (aertrycke) (callinarum) (choleraesuis) (enteritidis) (paratyphi) (suipestifer) A02.9
with
gastroenteritis A02.0
sepsis A02.1
staphylococcus A05.0
Vibrio
parahaemolyticus A05.3
vulnificus A05.5
noxious or naturally toxic T62.9-
berries —*see* subcategory T62.1-
fish —*see* Poisoning, seafood
mushrooms —*see* subcategory T62.0X-
plants NEC —*see* subcategory T62.2X-
seafood —*see* Poisoning, seafood
specified NEC —*see* subcategory T62.8X-
ichthyotoxism —*see* Poisoning, seafood
kreotoxism, food A05.9
latex T65.81-
lead T56.0-
mushroom —*see* Poisoning, food, noxious, mushroom
mussels —*see also* Poisoning, shellfish
bacterial —*see* Intoxication, foodborne, by agent
nicotine (tobacco) T65.2-
noxious foodstuffs —*see* Poisoning, food, noxious
plants, noxious —*see* Poisoning, food, noxious, plants NEC
ptomaine —*see* Poisoning, food
radiation J70.0

◀ New ⇐ Revised ~~deleted~~ Deleted

Poisoning *(Continued)*
Salmonella (arizonae) (cholerae-suis) (enteritidis) (typhimurium) A02.9
scombroid fish T61.1-
seafood (noxious) T61.9-
bacterial —*see* Intoxication, foodborne, by agent
fish —*see* Poisoning, fish
shellfish —*see* Poisoning, shellfish
specified NEC —*see* subcategory T61.8X-
shellfish (amnesic) (azaspiracid) (diarrheic) (neurotoxic) (noxious) (paralytic) T61.78-
bacterial —*see* Intoxication, foodborne, by agent
ciguatera mollusk —*see* Poisoning, ciguatera fish
specified substance NEC T65.891
Staphylococcus, food A05.0
tobacco (nicotine) T65.2-
water E87.79
Poker spine —*see* Spondylitis, ankylosing
Poland syndrome Q79.8
Polioencephalitis (acute) (bulbar) A80.9
inferior G12.22
influenzal —*see* Influenza, with, encephalopathy
superior hemorrhagic (acute) (Wernicke's) E51.2
Wernicke's E51.2
Polioencephalomyelitis (acute) (anterior) A80.9
with beriberi E51.2
Polioencephalopathy, superior hemorrhagic E51.2
with
beriberi E51.11
pellagra E52
Poliomeningoencephalitis —*see* Meningoencephalitis
Poliomyelitis (acute) (anterior) (epidemic) A80.9
with paralysis (bulbar) —*see* Poliomyelitis, paralytic
abortive A80.4
ascending (progressive) —*see* Poliomyelitis, paralytic
bulbar (paralytic) —*see* Poliomyelitis, paralytic
congenital P35.8
nonepidemic A80.9
nonparalytic A80.4
paralytic A80.30
specified NEC A80.39
vaccine-associated A80.0
wild virus
imported A80.1
indigenous A80.2
spinal, acute A80.9
Poliosis (eyebrow) (eyelashes) L67.1
circumscripta, acquired L67.1
Pollakiuria R35.0
psychogenic F45.8
Pollinosis J30.1
Pollitzer's disease L73.2
Polyadenitis —*see also* Lymphadenitis
malignant A20.0
Polyalgia M79.89
Polyangiitis M30.0
microscopic M31.7
overlap syndrome M30.8
Polyarteritis
microscopic M31.7
nodosa M30.0
with lung involvement M30.1
juvenile M30.2
related condition NEC M30.8
Polyarthralgia —*see* Pain, joint
Polyarthritis, polyarthropathy —*see also* Arthritis M13.0
due to or associated with other specified conditions —*see* Arthritis

Polyarthritis, polyarthropathy *(Continued)*
epidemic (Australian) (with exanthema) B33.1
infective —*see* Arthritis, pyogenic or pyemic
inflammatory M06.4
juvenile (chronic) (seronegative) M08.3
migratory —*see* Fever, rheumatic
rheumatic, acute —*see* Fever, rheumatic
Polyarthrosis M15.9
post-traumatic M15.3
primary M15.0
specified NEC M15.8
Polycarential syndrome of infancy E40
Polychondritis (atrophic) (chronic) —*see also* Disorder, cartilage, specified type NEC
relapsing M94.1
Polycoria Q13.2
Polycystic (disease)
degeneration, kidney Q61.3
autosomal dominant (adult type) Q61.2
autosomal recessive (infantile type) NEC Q61.19
kidney Q61.3
autosomal
dominant Q61.2
recessive NEC Q61.19
autosomal dominant (adult type) Q61.2
autosomal recessive (childhood type) NEC Q61.19
infantile type NEC Q61.19
liver Q44.6
lung J98.4
congenital Q33.0
ovary, ovaries E28.2
spleen Q89.09
Polycythemia (secondary) D75.1
acquired D75.1
benign (familial) D75.0
due to
donor twin P61.1
erythropoietin D75.1
fall in plasma volume D75.1
high altitude D75.1
maternal-fetal transfusion P61.1
stress D75.1
emotional D75.1
erythropoietin D75.1
familial (benign) D75.0
Gaisböck's (hypertonica) D75.1
high altitude D75.1
hypertonica D75.1
hypoxemic D75.1
neonatorum P61.1
nephrogenous D75.1
relative D75.1
secondary D75.1
spurious D75.1
stress D75.1
vera D45
Polycytosis cryptogenica D75.1
Polydactylism, polydactyly Q69.9
toes Q69.2
Polydipsia R63.1
Polydystrophy, pseudo-Hurler E77.0
Polyembryoma —*see* Neoplasm, malignant, by site
Polyglandular
deficiency E31.0
dyscrasia E31.9
dysfunction E31.9
syndrome E31.8
Polyhydramnios O40.-
Polymastia Q83.1
Polymenorrhea N92.0
Polymyalgia M35.3
arteritica, giant cell M31.5
rheumatica M35.3
with giant cell arteritis M31.5

Polymyositis (acute) (chronic) (hemorrhagic) M33.20
with
myopathy M33.22
respiratory involvement M33.21
skin involvement —*see* Dermatopolymyositis
specified organ involvement NEC M33.29
ossificans (generalisata) (progressiva) —*see* Myositis, ossificans, progressiva
Polyneuritis, polyneuritic —*see also* Polyneuropathy
acute (post-)infective G61.0
alcoholic G62.1
cranialis G52.7
demyelinating, chronic inflammatory (CIDP) G61.81
diabetic —*see* Diabetes, polyneuropathy
diphtheritic A36.83
due to lack of vitamin NEC E56.9 *[G63]*
endemic E51.11
erythredema —*see* subcategory T56.1
febrile, acute G61.0
hereditary ataxic G60.1
idiopathic, acute G61.0
infective (acute) G61.0
inflammatory, chronic demyelinating (CIDP) G61.81
nutritional E63.9 *[G63]*
postinfective (acute) G61.0
specified NEC G62.89
Polyneuropathy (peripheral) G62.9
alcoholic G62.1
amyloid (Portuguese) E85.1 *[G63]*
arsenical G62.2
critical illness G62.81
demyelinating, chronic inflammatory (CIDP) G61.81
diabetic —*see* Diabetes, polyneuropathy
drug-induced G62.0
hereditary G60.9
specified NEC G60.8
idiopathic G60.9
progressive G60.3
in (due to)
alcohol G62.1
sequelae G65.2
amyloidosis, familial (Portuguese) E85.1 *[G63]*
antitetanus serum G61.1
arsenic G62.2
sequelae G65.2
avitaminosis NEC E56.9 *[G63]*
beriberi E51.11
collagen vascular disease NEC M35.9 *[G63]*
deficiency (of)
B (-complex) vitamins E53.9 *[G63]*
vitamin B6 E53.1 *[G63]*
diabetes —*see* Diabetes, polyneuropathy
diphtheria A36.83
drug or medicament G62.0
correct substance properly administered —*see* Table of Drugs and Chemicals, by drug, adverse effect
overdose or wrong substance given or taken —*see* Table of Drugs and Chemicals, by drug, poisoning
endocrine disease NEC E34.9 *[G63]*
herpes zoster B02.23
hypoglycemia E16.2 *[G63]*
infectious
disease NEC B99 *[G63]*
mononucleosis B27.91
lack of vitamin NEC E56.9 *[G63]*
lead G62.2
sequelae G65.2
leprosy A30.9 *[G63]*
Lyme disease A69.22
metabolic disease NEC E88.9 *[G63]*
microscopic polyangiitis M31.7 *[G63]*

Polyneuropathy *(Continued)*
in *(Continued)*
mumps B26.84
neoplastic disease —*see also* Neoplasm D49.9 *[G63]*
nutritional deficiency NEC E63.9 *[G63]*
organophosphate compounds G62.2
sequelae G65.2
parasitic disease NEC B89 *[G63]*
pellagra E52 *[G63]*
polyarteritis nodosa M30.0
porphyria E80.20 *[G63]*
radiation G62.82
rheumatoid arthritis —*see* Rheumatoid, polyneuropathy
sarcoidosis D86.89
serum G61.1
syphilis (late) A52.15
congenital A50.43
systemic
connective tissue disorder M35.9 *[G63]*
lupus erythematosus M32.19
toxic agent NEC G62.2
sequelae G65.2
triorthocresyl phosphate G62.2
sequelae G65.2
tuberculosis A17.89
uremia N18.9 *[G63]*
vitamin B12 deficiency E53.8 *[G63]*
with anemia (pernicious) D51.0 *[G63]*
due to dietary deficiency D51.3 *[G63]*
zoster B02.23
inflammatory G61.9
chronic demyelinating (CIDP) G61.81
sequelae G65.1
specified NEC G61.89
lead G62.2
sequelae G65.2
nutritional NEC E63.9 *[G63]*
postherpetic (zoster) B02.23
progressive G60.3
radiation-induced G62.82
sensory (hereditary) (idiopathic) G60.8
specified NEC G62.89
syphilitic (late) A52.15
congenital A50.43
Polyopia H53.8
Polyorchism, polyorchidism Q55.21
Polyosteoarthritis —*see also* Osteoarthritis, generalized M15.9-
post-traumatic M15.3
specified NEC M15.8
Polyostotic fibrous dysplasia Q78.1
Polyotia Q17.0
Polyp, polypus
accessory sinus J33.8
adenocarcinoma in —*see* Neoplasm, malignant, by site
adenocarcinoma in situ in —*see* Neoplasm, in situ, by site
adenoid tissue J33.0
adenomatous —*see also* Neoplasm, benign, by site
adenocarcinoma in —*see* Neoplasm, malignant, by site
adenocarcinoma in situ in —*see* Neoplasm, in situ, by site
carcinoma in —*see* Neoplasm, malignant, by site
carcinoma in situ in —*see* Neoplasm, in situ, by site
multiple —*see* Neoplasm, benign
adenocarcinoma in —*see* Neoplasm, malignant, by site
adenocarcinoma in situ in —*see* Neoplasm, in situ, by site
antrum J33.8
anus, anal (canal) K62.0

Polyp, polypus *(Continued)*
Bartholin's gland N84.3
bladder D41.4
carcinoma in —*see* Neoplasm, malignant, by site
carcinoma in situ in —*see* Neoplasm, in situ, by site
cecum D12.0
cervix (uteri) N84.1
in pregnancy or childbirth —*see* Pregnancy, complicated by, abnormal, cervix
mucous N84.1
nonneoplastic N84.1
choanal J33.0
cholesterol K82.4
clitoris N84.3
colon K63.5
adenomatous D12.6
ascending D12.2
cecum D12.0
descending D12.4
inflammatory K51.40
with
abscess K51.414
complication K51.419
specified NEC K51.418
fistula K51.413
intestinal obstruction K51.412
rectal bleeding K51.411
sigmoid D12.5
transverse D12.3
corpus uteri N84.0
dental K04.01 ◀
irreversible K04.02 ◀
reversible K04.01 ◀
duodenum K31.7
ear (middle) H74.4-
endometrium N84.0
ethmoidal (sinus) J33.8
fallopian tube N84.8
female genital tract N84.9
specified NEC N84.8
frontal (sinus) J33.8
gallbladder K82.4
gingiva, gum K06.8
labia, labium (majus) (minus) N84.3
larynx (mucous) J38.1
adenomatous D14.1
malignant —*see* Neoplasm, malignant, by site
maxillary (sinus) J33.8
middle ear —*see* Polyp, ear (middle)
myometrium N84.0
nares
anterior J33.9
posterior J33.0
nasal (mucous) J33.9
cavity J33.0
septum J33.0
nasopharyngeal J33.0
nose (mucous) J33.9
oviduct N84.8
pharynx J39.2
placenta O90.89
prostate —*see* Enlargement, enlarged, prostate
pudenda, pudendum N84.3
pulpal (dental) K04.01 ◀
irreversible K04.02 ◀
reversible K04.01 ◀
rectum (nonadenomatous) K62.1
adenomatous —*see* Polyp, adenomatous
septum (nasal) J33.0
sinus (accessory) (ethmoidal) (frontal) (maxillary) (sphenoidal) J33.8
sphenoidal (sinus) J33.8
stomach K31.7
adenomatous D13.1
tube, fallopian N84.8
turbinate, mucous membrane J33.8
umbilical, newborn P83.6
ureter N28.89

Polyp, polypus *(Continued)*
urethra N36.2
uterus (body) (corpus) (mucous) N84.0
cervix N84.1
in pregnancy or childbirth —*see* Pregnancy, complicated by, tumor, uterus
vagina N84.2
vocal cord (mucous) J38.1
vulva N84.3
Polyphagia R63.2
Polyploidy Q92.7
Polypoid —*see* condition
Polyposis —*see also* Polyp
coli (adenomatous) D12.6
adenocarcinoma in C18.9
adenocarcinoma in situ in —*see* Neoplasm, in situ, by site
carcinoma in C18.9
colon (adenomatous) D12.6
familial D12.6
adenocarcinoma in situ in —*see* Neoplasm, in situ, by site
intestinal (adenomatous) D12.6
malignant lymphomatous C83.1
multiple, adenomatous —*see also* Neoplasm, benign D36.9
Polyradiculitis —*see* Polyneuropathy
Polyradiculoneuropathy (acute) (postinfective) (segmentally demyelinating) G61.0
Polyserositis
due to pericarditis I31.1
pericardial I31.1
periodic, familial E85.0
tuberculous A19.9
acute A19.1
chronic A19.8
Polysplenia syndrome Q89.09
Polysyndactyly —*see also* Syndactylism, syndactyly Q70.4
Polytrichia L68.3
Polyunguia Q84.6
Polyuria R35.8
nocturnal R35.1
psychogenic F45.8
Pompe's disease (glycogen storage) E74.02
Pompholyx L30.1
Poncet's disease (tuberculous rheumatism) A18.09
Pond fracture —*see* Fracture, skull
Ponos B55.0
Pons, pontine —*see* condition
Poor
aesthetic of existing restoration of tooth K08.56
contractions, labor O62.2
gingival margin to tooth restoration K08.51
personal hygiene R46.0
prenatal care, affecting management of pregnancy —*see* Pregnancy, complicated by, insufficient, prenatal care
sucking reflex (newborn) R29.2
urinary stream R39.12
vision NEC H54.7
Poradenitis, nostras inguinalis or venerea A55
Porencephaly (congenital) (developmental) (true) Q04.6
acquired G93.0
nondevelopmental G93.0
traumatic (post) F07.89
Porocephaliasis B88.8
Porokeratosis Q82.8
Poroma, eccrine —*see* Neoplasm, skin, benign
Porphyria (South African) E80.20
acquired E80.20
acute intermittent (hepatic) (Swedish) E80.21
cutanea tarda (hereditary) (symptomatic) E80.1
due to drugs E80.20
correct substance properly administered —*see* Table of Drugs and Chemicals, by drug, adverse effect

◀ New ◀ Revised ~~deleted~~ Deleted

Porphyria *(Continued)*
due to drugs *(Continued)*
overdose or wrong substance given or taken —*see* Table of Drugs and Chemicals, by drug, poisoning
erythropoietic (congenital) (hereditary) E80.0
hepatocutaneous type E80.1
secondary E80.20
toxic NEC E80.20
variegata E80.20
Porphyrinuria —*see* Porphyria
Porphyruria —*see* Porphyria
Portal —*see* condition
Port wine nevus, mark, or stain Q82.5
Posadas-Wernicke disease B38.9
Positive
culture (nonspecific)
blood R78.81
bronchial washings R84.5
cerebrospinal fluid R83.5
cervix uteri R87.5
nasal secretions R84.5
nipple discharge R89.5
nose R84.5
staphylococcus (Methicillin susceptible) Z22.321
Methicillin resistant Z22.322
peritoneal fluid R85.5
pleural fluid R84.5
prostatic secretions R86.5
saliva R85.5
seminal fluid R86.5
sputum R84.5
synovial fluid R89.5
throat scrapings R84.5
urine R82.79 ⇐
vagina R87.5
vulva R87.5
wound secretions R89.5
PPD (skin test) R76.11
serology for syphilis A53.0
with signs or symptoms - code as Syphilis, by site and stage
false R76.8
skin test, tuberculin (without active tuberculosis) R76.11
test, human immunodeficiency virus (HIV) R75
VDRL A53.0
with signs or symptoms - code by site and stage under Syphilis A53.9
Wassermann reaction A53.0
Postcardiotomy syndrome I97.0
Postcaval ureter Q62.62
Postcholecystectomy syndrome K91.5
Postclimacteric bleeding N95.0
Postcommissurotomy syndrome I97.0
Postconcussional syndrome F07.81
Postcontusional syndrome F07.81
Postcricoid region —*see* condition
Post-dates (40-42 weeks) (pregnancy) (mother) O48.0
more than 42 weeks gestation O48.1
Postencephalitic syndrome F07.89
Posterior —*see* condition
Posterolateral sclerosis (spinal cord) —*see* Degeneration, combined
Postexanthematous —*see* condition
Postfebrile —*see* condition
Postgastrectomy dumping syndrome K91.1
Posthemiplegic chorea —*see* Monoplegia
Posthemorrhagic anemia (chronic) D50.0
acute D62
newborn P61.3
Postherpetic neuralgia (zoster) B02.29
trigeminal B02.22
Posthitis N47.7
Postimmunization complication or reaction —*see* Complications, vaccination
Postinfectious —*see* condition
Postlaminectomy syndrome NEC M96.1
Postleukotomy syndrome F07.0
Postmastectomy lymphedema (syndrome) I97.2
Postmaturity, postmature (over 42 weeks)
maternal (over 42 weeks gestation) O48.1
newborn P08.22
Postmeasles complication NEC —*see also* condition B05.89
Postmenopausal
endometrium (atrophic) N95.8
suppurative —*see also* Endometritis N71.9
osteoporosis —*see* Osteoporosis, postmenopausal
Postnasal drip R09.82
due to
allergic rhinitis —*see* Rhinitis, allergic
common cold J00
gastroesophageal reflux —*see* Reflux, gastroesophageal
nasopharyngitis —*see* Nasopharyngitis
other know condition — code to condition
sinusitis —*see* Sinusitis
Postnatal —*see* condition
Postoperative (postprocedural) —*see* Complication, postoperative
pneumothorax, therapeutic Z98.3
state NEC Z98.890 ⇐
Postpancreatectomy hyperglycemia E89.1
Postpartum —*see* Puerperal
Postphlebitic syndrome —*see* Syndrome, postthrombotic
Postpolio (myelitic) syndrome G14
Postpoliomyelitic —*see also* condition
osteopathy —*see* Osteopathy, after poliomyelitis
Postprocedural —*see also* Postoperative
hypoinsulinemia E89.1
Postschizophrenic depression F32.89 ⇐
Postsurgery status —*see also* Status (post)
pneumothorax, therapeutic Z98.3
Post-term (40-42 weeks) (pregnancy) (mother) O48.0
infant P08.21
more than 42 weeks gestation (mother) O48.1
Post-traumatic brain syndrome, nonpsychotic F07.81
Post-typhoid abscess A01.09
Postures, hysterical F44.2
Postvaccinal reaction or complication —*see* Complications, vaccination
Postvalvulotomy syndrome I97.0
Potain's
disease (pulmonary edema) —*see* Edema, lung
syndrome (gastrectasis with dyspepsia) K31.0
Potter's
asthma J62.8
facies Q60.6
lung J62.8
syndrome (with renal agenesis) Q60.6
Pott's
curvature (spinal) A18.01
disease or paraplegia A18.01
spinal curvature A18.01
tumor, puffy —*see* Osteomyelitis, specified type NEC
Pouch
bronchus Q32.4
Douglas' —*see* condition
esophagus, esophageal, congenital Q39.6
acquired K22.5
gastric K31.4
Hartmann's K82.8
pharynx, pharyngeal (congenital) Q38.7
Pouchitis K91.850
Poultrymen's itch B88.0
Poverty NEC Z59.6
extreme Z59.5
Poxvirus NEC B08.8
Prader-Willi syndrome Q87.1
Preauricular appendage or tag Q17.0
Prebetalipoproteinemia (acquired) (essential) (familial) (hereditary) (primary) (secondary) E78.1
with chylomicronemia E78.3
Precipitate labor or delivery O62.3
Preclimacteric bleeding (menorrhagia) N92.4
Precocious
adrenarche E30.1
menarche E30.1
menstruation E30.1
pubarche E30.1
puberty E30.1
central E22.8
sexual development NEC E30.1
thelarche E30.8
Precocity, sexual (constitutional) (cryptogenic) (female) (idiopathic) (male) E30.1
with adrenal hyperplasia E25.9
congenital E25.0
Precordial pain R07.2
Predeciduous teeth K00.2
Prediabetes, prediabetic R73.03 ⇐
complicating
pregnancy —*see* Pregnancy, complicated by, diseases of, specified type or system NEC
puerperium O99.89
Predislocation status of hip at birth Q65.6
Pre-eclampsia O14.9-
with pre-existing hypertension —*see* Hypertension, complicating pregnancy, pre-existing, with, pre-eclampsia
complicating ◀
childbirth O14.94 ◀
puerperium O14.95 ◀
mild O14.0-
complicating ◀
childbirth O14.04 ◀
puerperium O14.05 ◀
moderate O14.0-
complicating ◀
childbirth O14.04 ◀
puerperium O14.05 ◀
severe O14.1-
with hemolysis, elevated liver enzymes and low platelet count (HELLP) O14.2-
complicating ◀
childbirth O14.24 ◀
puerperium O14.25 ◀
complicating ◀
childbirth O14.14 ◀
puerperium O14.15 ◀
Pre-eruptive color change, teeth, tooth K00.8
Pre-excitation atrioventricular conduction I45.6
Preglaucoma H40.00-
Pregnancy (single) (uterine) —*see also* Delivery and Puerperal

Note: The Tabular must be reviewed for assignment of the appropriate character indicating the trimester of the pregnancy

Note: The Tabular must be reviewed for assignment of appropriate seventh character for multiple gestation codes in Chapter 15

abdominal (ectopic) O00.00 ⇐
with intrauterine pregnancy O00.01 ◀
with viable fetus O36.7-
ampullar O00.10 ⇐
with intrauterine pregnancy O00.11 ◀
biochemical O02.81
broad ligament O00.80 ⇐
with intrauterine pregnancy O00.81 ◀
cervical O00.80 ⇐
with intrauterine pregnancy O00.81 ◀
chemical O02.81
complicated NOS O26.9-

◀ New ⇐ Revised ~~deleted~~ Deleted

Pregnancy *(Continued)*
complicated by (care of) (management affected by)
abnormal, abnormality
cervix O34.4-
causing obstructed labor O65.5
cord (umbilical) O69.9
findings on antenatal screening of mother O28.9
biochemical O28.1
chromosomal O28.5
cytological O28.2
genetic O28.5
hematological O28.0
radiological O28.4
specified NEC O28.8
ultrasonic O28.3
glucose (tolerance) NEC O99.810
pelvic organs O34.9-
specified NEC O34.8-
causing obstructed labor O65.5
pelvis (bony) (major) NEC O33.0
perineum O34.7-
position
placenta O44.0- ◀
~~without hemorrhage O44.0-~~
with hemorrhage O44.1- ◀
uterus O34.59-
uterus O34.59-
causing obstructed labor O65.5
congenital O34.0-
vagina O34.6-
causing obstructed labor O65.5
vulva O34.7-
causing obstructed labor O65.5
abruptio placentae —*see* Abruptio placentae
abscess or cellulitis
bladder O23.1-
breast O91.11-
genital organ or tract O23.9-
abuse
physical O9A.31-
psychological O9A.51-
sexual O9A.41-
adverse effect anesthesia O29.9-
aspiration pneumonitis O29.01-
cardiac arrest O29.11-
cardiac complication NEC O29.19-
cardiac failure O29.12-
central nervous system complication NEC O29.29-
cerebral anoxia O29.21-
failed or difficult intubation O29.6-
inhalation of stomach contents or secretions NOS O29.01-
local, toxic reaction O29.3X
Mendelson's syndrome O29.01-
pressure collapse of lung O29.02-
pulmonary complications NEC O29.09-
specified NEC O29.8X
spinal and epidural type NEC O29.5X
induced headache O29.4-
albuminuria —*see also* Proteinuria, gestational O12.1- ◀
alcohol use O99.31-
amnionitis O41.12-
anaphylactoid syndrome of pregnancy O88.01-
anemia (conditions in D50-D64) (pre-existing) O99.01-
complicating the puerperium O99.03
antepartum hemorrhage O46.9-
with coagulation defect —*see* Hemorrhage, antepartum, with coagulation defect
specified NEC O46.8X-
appendicitis O99.61-
atrophy (yellow) (acute) liver (subacute) O26.61-
bariatric surgery status O99.84- ◀

Pregnancy *(Continued)*
complicated by *(Continued)*
bicornis or bicornuate uterus O34.0- ◀
biliary tract problems O26.61-
breech presentation O32.1
cardiovascular diseases (conditions in I00-I09, I20-I52, I70-I99) O99.41-
cerebrovascular disorders (conditions in I60-I69) O99.41-
cervical shortening O26.87-
cervicitis O23.51-
chloasma (gravidarum) O26.89-
cholecystitis O99.61-
cholestasis (intrahepatic) O26.61-
chorioamnionitis O41.12-
circulatory system disorder (conditions in I00-I09, I20-I99, O99.41-)
compound presentation O32.6
conjoined twins O30.02-
connective system disorders (conditions in M00-M99) O99.89
contracted pelvis (general) O33.1
inlet O33.2
outlet O33.3
convulsions (eclamptic) (uremic) —*see also* Eclampsia O15.9-
cracked nipple O92.11-
cystitis O23.1-
cystocele O34.8-
death of fetus (near term) O36.4
early pregnancy O02.1
of one fetus or more in multiple gestation O31.2-
deciduitis O41.14-
decreased fetal movement O36.81-
dental problems O99.61-
diabetes (mellitus) O24.91-
gestational (pregnancy induced) —*see* Diabetes, gestational
pre-existing O24.31-
specified NEC O24.81-
type 1 O24.01-
type 2 O24.11-
digestive system disorders (conditions in K00-K93) O99.61-
diseases of —*see* Pregnancy, complicated by, specified body system disease
biliary tract O26.61-
blood NEC (conditions in D65-D77) O99.11-
liver O26.61-
specified NEC O99.89
disorders of —*see* Pregnancy, complicated by, specified body system disorder
amniotic fluid and membranes O41.9-
specified NEC O41.8X-
biliary tract O26.61-
ear and mastoid process (conditions in H60-H95) O99.89
eye and adnexa (conditions in H00-H59) O99.89
liver O26.61-
skin (conditions in L00-L99) O99.71-
specified NEC O99.89
displacement, uterus NEC O34.59-
causing obstructed labor O65.5
disproportion (due to) O33.9
~~fetal deformities NEC O33.7~~
fetal (ascites) (hydrops) (meningomyelocele) (sacral teratoma) (tumor) deformities NEC O33.7 ◀
generally contracted pelvis O33.1
hydrocephalic fetus O33.6
inlet contraction of pelvis O33.2
mixed maternal and fetal origin O33.4
specified NEC O33.8
double uterus O34.0- ◀
causing obstructed labor O65.5
drug use (conditions in F11-F19) O99.32-

Pregnancy *(Continued)*
complicated by *(Continued)*
eclampsia, eclamptic (coma) (convulsions) (delirium) (nephritis) (uremia) (*see also* Eclampsia) O15-
ectopic pregnancy —*see* Pregnancy, ectopic
edema O12.0-
with
gestational hypertension, mild —*see also* Pre-eclampsia O14.0-
proteinuria O12.2-
effusion, amniotic fluid —*see* Pregnancy, complicated by, premature rupture of membranes
elderly
multigravida O09.52-
primigravida O09.51-
embolism —*see also* Embolism, obstetric, pregnancy O88.-
endocrine diseases NEC O99.28-
endometritis O86.12
excessive weight gain O26.0-
exhaustion O26.81-
during labor and delivery O75.81
face presentation O32.3
failed induction of labor O61.9
failed or difficult intubation for anesthesia O29.6-
instrumental O61.1
mechanical O61.1
medical O61.0
specified NEC O61.8
surgical O61.1
false labor (pains) O47.9
at or after 37 completed weeks of pregnancy O47.1
before 37 completed weeks of pregnancy O47.0-
fatigue O26.81-
during labor and delivery O75.81
fatty metamorphosis of liver O26.61-
female genital mutilation O34.8- *[N90.81-]*
fetal (maternal care for)
abnormality or damage O35.9
acid-base balance O68
specified type NEC O35.8
acidemia O68
acidosis O68
alkalosis O68
anemia and thrombocytopenia O36.82-
anencephaly O35.0
chromosomal abnormality (conditions in Q90-Q99) O35.1
conjoined twins O30.02-
damage from
amniocentesis O35.7
biopsy procedures O35.7
drug addiction O35.5
hematological investigation O35.7
intrauterine contraceptive device O35.7
maternal
alcohol addiction O35.4
cytomegalovirus infection O35.3
disease NEC O35.8
drug addiction O35.5
listeriosis O35.8
rubella O35.3
toxoplasmosis O35.8
viral infection O35.3
medical procedure NEC O35.7
radiation O35.6
death (near term) O36.4
early pregnancy O02.1
decreased movement O36.81-
disproportion due to deformity (fetal) O33.7
excessive growth (large for dates) O36.6-
growth retardation O36.59-
light for dates O36.59-
small for dates O36.59-

◀ New ◀ Revised ~~deleted~~ Deleted

Pregnancy *(Continued)*
complicated by *(Continued)*
fetal *(Continued)*
heart rate irregularity (bradycardia) (decelerations) (tachycardia) O76
hereditary disease O35.2
hydrocephalus O35.0
intrauterine death O36.4
poor growth O36.59-
light for dates O36.59-
small for dates O36.59-
problem O36.9-
specified NEC O36.89-
reduction (elective) O31.3-
selective termination O31.3-
spina bifida O35.0
thrombocytopenia O36.82-
fibroid (tumor) (uterus) O34.1-
fissure of nipple O92.11-
gallstones O99.61-
gastric banding status O99.84-
gastric bypass status O99.84-
genital herpes (asymptomatic) (history of) (inactive) O98.51-
genital tract infection O23.9-
glomerular diseases (conditions in N00-N07) O26.83-
with hypertension, pre-existing —*see* Hypertension, complicating, pregnancy, pre-existing, with, renal disease
gonorrhea O98.21-
grand multiparity O09.4
habitual aborter —*see* Pregnancy, complicated by, recurrent pregnancy loss
HELLP syndrome (hemolysis, elevated liver enzymes and low platelet count) O14.2-
hemorrhage
antepartum —*see* Hemorrhage, antepartum
before 20 completed weeks gestation O20.9
specified NEC O20.8
due to premature separation, placenta —*see also* Abruptio placentae O45.9-
early O20.9
specified NEC O20.8
threatened abortion O20.0
hemorrhoids O22.4-
hepatitis (viral) O98.41-
herniation of uterus O34.59-
high
head at term O32.4
risk —*see* Supervision (of) (for), high-risk
history of in utero procedure during previous pregnancy O09.82-
HIV O98.71-
human immunodeficiency virus (HIV) disease O98.71-
hydatidiform mole —*see also* Mole, hydatidiform O01.9-
hydramnios O40.-
hydrocephalic fetus (disproportion) O33.6
hydrops
amnii O40.-
fetalis O36.2-
associated with isoimmunization —*see also* Pregnancy, complicated by, isoimmunization O36.11-
hydrorrhea O42.90
hyperemesis (gravidarum) (mild) —*see also* Hyperemesis, gravidarum O21.0-
hypertension —*see* Hypertension, complicating pregnancy
hypertensive
heart and renal disease, pre-existing —*see* Hypertension, complicating, pregnancy, pre-existing, with, heart disease, with renal disease

Pregnancy *(Continued)*
complicated by *(Continued)*
hypertensive *(Continued)*
heart disease, pre-existing —*see* Hypertension, complicating, pregnancy, pre-existing, with, heart disease
renal disease, pre-existing —*see* Hypertension, complicating, pregnancy, pre-existing, with, renal disease
hypotension O26.5-
immune disorders NEC (conditions in D80-D89) O99.11-
incarceration, uterus O34.51-
incompetent cervix O34.3-
inconclusive fetal viability O36.80
infection (s) O98.91-
amniotic fluid or sac O41.10-
bladder O23.1-
carrier state NEC O99.830
streptococcus B O99.820
genital organ or tract O23.9-
specified NEC O23.59-
genitourinary tract O23.9-
gonorrhea O98.21-
hepatitis (viral) O98.41-
HIV O98.71-
human immunodeficiency virus (HIV) O98.71-
kidney O23.0-
nipple O91.01-
parasitic disease O98.91-
specified NEC O98.81-
protozoal disease O98.61-
sexually transmitted NEC O98.31-
specified type NEC O98.81-
syphilis O98.11-
tuberculosis O98.01-
urethra O23.2-
urinary (tract) O23.4-
specified NEC O23.3-
viral disease O98.51-
injury or poisoning (conditions in S00-T88) O9A.21-
due to abuse
physical O9A.31-
psychological O9A.51-
sexual O9A.41-
insufficient
prenatal care O09.3-
weight gain O26.1-
insulin resistance O26.89
intrauterine fetal death (near term) O36.4
early pregnancy O02.1
multiple gestation (one fetus or more) O31.2-
isoimmunization O36.11-
anti-A sensitization O36.11-
anti-B sensitization O36.19-
Rh O36.09-
anti-D antibody O36.01-
specified NEC O36.19-
laceration of uterus NEC O71.81
malformation
placenta, placental (vessel) O43.10-
specified NEC O43.19-
uterus (congenital) O34.0-
malnutrition (conditions in E40-E46) O25.1-
maternal hypotension syndrome O26.5-
mental disorders (conditions in F01-F09, F20-F99) O99.34-
alcohol use O99.31-
drug use O99.32-
smoking O99.33-
mentum presentation O32.3
metabolic disorders O99.28-
missed
abortion O02.1
delivery O36.4

Pregnancy *(Continued)*
complicated by *(Continued)*
multiple gestations O30.9-
conjoined twins O30.02-
quadruplet —*see* Pregnancy, quadruplet
specified complication NEC O31.8X-
specified number of multiples NEC —*see* Pregnancy, multiple (gestation), specified NEC
triplet —*see* Pregnancy, triplet
twin —*see* Pregnancy, twin
musculoskeletal condition (conditions is M00-M99) O99.89
necrosis, liver (conditions in K72) O26.61-
neoplasm
benign
cervix O34.4-
corpus uteri O34.1-
uterus O34.1-
malignant O9A.11-
nephropathy NEC O26.83-
nervous system condition (conditions in G00-G99) O99.35-
nutritional diseases NEC O99.28-
obesity (pre-existing) O99.21-
obesity surgery status O99.84-
oblique lie or presentation O32.2
older mother —*see* Pregnancy, complicated by, elderly
oligohydramnios O41.0-
with premature rupture of membranes —*see also* Pregnancy, complicated by, premature rupture of membranes O42-
onset (spontaneous) of labor after 37 completed weeks of gestation but before 39 completed weeks gestation, with delivery by (planned) cesarean section O75.82
oophoritis O23.52-
overdose, drug —*see also* Table of Drugs and Chemicals, by drug, poisoning O9A.21-
oversize fetus O33.5
papyraceous fetus O31.0-
pelvic inflammatory disease O99.89
periodontal disease O99.61-
peripheral neuritis O26.82-
peritoneal (pelvic) adhesions O99.89
phlebitis O22.9-
phlebopathy O22.9-
phlebothrombosis (superficial) O22.2-
deep O22.3-
placenta accreta O43.21-
placenta increta O43.22-
placenta percreta O43.23-
placenta previa O44.0- ⬅
complete O44.0- ◀
with hemorrhage O44.1- ◀
marginal O44.2- ◀
with hemorrhage O44.3- ◀
partial O44.2- ◀
with hemorrhage O44.3- ◀
~~without hemorrhage O44.0-~~
placental disorder O43.9-
specified NEC O43.89-
placental dysfunction O43.89-
placental infarction O43.81-
placental insufficiency O36.51-
placental transfusion syndromes
fetomaternal O43.01-
fetus to fetus O43.02-
maternofetal O43.01-
placentitis O41.14-
pneumonia O99.51-
poisoning —*see also* Table of Drugs and Chemicals O9A.21-
polyhydramnios O40-
polymorphic eruption of pregnancy O26.86
poor obstetric history NEC O09.29-

◀ New ⬅ Revised ~~deleted~~ Deleted

Pregnancy *(Continued)*
complicated by *(Continued)*
postmaturity (post-term) (40 to 42 weeks) O48.0
more than 42 completed weeks gestation (prolonged) O48.1
pre-eclampsia O14.9-
mild O14.0-
moderate O14.0-
severe O14.1-
with hemolysis, elevated liver enzymes and low platelet count (HELLP) O14.2-
premature labor —*see* Pregnancy, complicated by, preterm labor
premature rupture of membranes O42.90
full-term, unspecified as to length of time between rupture and onset of labor O42.92 ◀
with onset of labor
within 24 hours O42.00
~~after 37 weeks gestation O42.02~~
at or after 37 weeks gestation, onset of labor within 24 hours of rupture O42.02 ◀
pre-term (before 37 completed weeks of gestation) O42.01-
after 24 hours O42.10
~~after 37 weeks gestation O42.12~~
at or after 37 weeks gestation, onset of labor more than 24 hours following rupture O42.12 ◀
pre-term (before 37 completed weeks of gestation) O42.11-
~~after 37 weeks gestation O42.92~~
at or after 37 weeks gestation, unspecified as to length of time between rupture and onset of labor O42.92 ◀
~~full-term O42.92~~
pre-term (before 37 completed weeks of gestation) O42.91-
premature separation of placenta —*see also* Abruptio placentae O45.9-
presentation, fetal —*see* Delivery, complicated by, malposition
preterm delivery O60.10
preterm labor
with delivery O60.10
preterm O60.10
term O60.20
second trimester
with preterm delivery
second trimester O60.12
third trimester O60.13
with term delivery O60.22
without delivery O60.02
third trimester
with term delivery O60.23
with third trimester preterm delivery O60.14
without delivery O60.03
without delivery O60.00
second trimester O60.02
third trimester O60.03
previous history of —*see* Pregnancy, supervision of, high-risk
prolapse, uterus O34.52-
proteinuria (gestational) —*see also* Proteinuria, gestational O12.1- ⬅
with edema O12.2-
pruritic urticarial papules and plaques of pregnancy (PUPPP) O26.86
pruritus (neurogenic) O26.89-
psychosis or psychoneurosis (puerperal) F53
ptyalism O26.89-
PUPPP (pruritic urticarial papules and plaques of pregnancy) O26.86
pyelitis O23.0-
recurrent pregnancy loss O26.2-

Pregnancy *(Continued)*
complicated by *(Continued)*
renal disease or failure NEC O26.83-
with secondary hypertension, pre-existing —*see* Hypertension, complicating, pregnancy, pre-existing, secondary
hypertensive, pre-existing —*see* Hypertension, complicating, pregnancy, pre-existing, with, renal disease
respiratory condition (conditions in J00-J99) O99.51-
retained, retention
dead ovum O02.0
intrauterine contraceptive device O26.3-
retroversion, uterus O34.53-
Rh immunization, incompatibility or sensitization NEC O36.09-
anti-D antibody O36.01-
rupture
amnion (premature) —*see also* Pregnancy, complicated by, premature rupture of membranes O42-
membranes (premature) —*see also* Pregnancy, complicated by, premature rupture of membranes O42-
uterus (during labor) O71.1
before onset of labor O71.0-
salivation (excessive) O26.89-
salpingitis O23.52-
salpingo-oophoritis O23.52-
sepsis (conditions in A40, A41) O98.81-
size date discrepancy (uterine) O26.84-
skin condition (conditions in L00-L99) O99.71-
smoking (tobacco) O99.33-
social problem O09.7-
specified condition NEC O26.89-
spotting O26.85-
~~streptococcus B carrier state O99.820~~
streptococcus group B (GBS) carrier state O99.820 ◀
subluxation of symphysis (pubis) O26.71-
syphilis (conditions in A50-A53) O98.11-
threatened
abortion O20.0
labor O47.9
at or after 37 completed weeks of gestation O47.1
before 37 completed weeks of gestation O47.0-
thrombophlebitis (superficial) O22.2-
thrombosis O22.9-
cerebral venous O22.5-
cerebrovenous sinus O22.5-
deep O22.3-
tobacco use disorder (smoking) O99.33- ◀
torsion of uterus O34.59-
toxemia O14.9-
transverse lie or presentation O32.2
tuberculosis (conditions in A15-A19) O98.01-
tumor (benign)
cervix O34.4-
malignant O9A.11-
uterus O34.1-
unstable lie O32.0
upper respiratory infection O99.51-
urethritis O23.2-
uterine size date discrepancy O26.84-
vaginitis or vulvitis O23.59-
varicose veins (lower extremities) O22.0-
genitals O22.1-
legs O22.0-
perineal O22.1-
vaginal or vulval O22.1-
venereal disease NEC (conditions in A63.8) O98.31-

Pregnancy *(Continued)*
complicated by *(Continued)*
venous disorders O22.9-
specified NEC O22.8X-
very young mother —*see* Pregnancy, complicated by, young mother
viral diseases (conditions in A80-B09, B25-B34) O98.51-
vomiting O21.9
due to diseases classified elsewhere O21.8
hyperemesis gravidarum (mild) —*see also* Hyperemesis, gravidarum O21.0-
late (occurring after 20 weeks of gestation) O21.2
young mother
multigravida O09.62-
primigravida O09.61-
concealed O09.3-
continuing following
elective fetal reduction of one or more fetus O31.3-
intrauterine death of one or more fetus O31.2-
spontaneous abortion of one or more fetus O31.1-
cornual O00.80 ⬅
with intrauterine pregnancy O00.81 ◀
ectopic (ruptured) O00.90 ⬅
with intrauterine pregnancy O00.91 ◀
abdominal O00.00 ⬅
~~with viable fetus O36.7-~~
with ◀
intrauterine pregnancy O00.01 ◀
viable fetus O36.7- ◀
cervical O00.80 ⬅
with intrauterine pregnancy O00.81 ◀
complicated (by) O08.9
afibrinogenemia O08.1
cardiac arrest O08.81
chemical damage of pelvic organ (s) O08.6
circulatory collapse O08.3
defibrination syndrome O08.1
electrolyte imbalance O08.5
embolism (amniotic fluid) (blood clot) (pulmonary) (septic) O08.2
endometritis O08.0
genital tract and pelvic infection O08.0
hemorrhage (delayed) (excessive) O08.1
infection
genital tract or pelvic O08.0
kidney 008.83
urinary tract O08.83
intravascular coagulation O08.1
laceration of pelvic organ (s) O08.6
metabolic disorder O08.5
oliguria O08.4
oophoritis O08.0
parametritis O08.0
pelvic peritonitis O08.0
perforation of pelvic organ (s) O08.6
renal failure or shutdown O08.4
salpingitis or salpingo-oophoritis O08.0
sepsis O08.82
shock O08.83
septic O08.82
specified condition NEC O08.89
tubular necrosis (renal) O08.4
uremia O08.4
urinary infection O08.83
venous complication NEC O08.7
embolism O08.2
cornual O00.80 ⬅
with intrauterine pregnancy O00.81 ◀
intraligamentous O00.80 ⬅
with intrauterine pregnancy O00.81 ◀

P

◀ New ⬅ Revised ~~deleted~~ Deleted

Pregnancy *(Continued)*
complicated by *(Continued)*
mural O00.80 ◀
with intrauterine pregnancy O00.81 ◀
ovarian O00.20 ◀
with intrauterine pregnancy O00.21 ◀
specified site NEC O00.80 ◀
with intrauterine pregnancy O00.81 ◀
tubal (ruptured) O00.10 ◀
with intrauterine pregnancy O00.11 ◀
examination (normal) Z34.9-
first Z34.0-
high-risk —*see* Pregnancy, supervision of, high-risk
specified Z34.8-
extrauterine —*see* Pregnancy, ectopic
fallopian O00.10 ◀
with intrauterine pregnancy O00.11 ◀
false F45.8
gestational carrier Z33.3 ◀
hidden O09.3-
high-risk —*see* Pregnancy, supervision of, high-risk
incidental finding Z33.1
interstitial O00.80 ◀
with intrauterine pregnancy O00.81 ◀
intraligamentous O00.80 ◀
with intrauterine pregnancy O00.81 ◀
intramural O00.80 ◀
with intrauterine pregnancy O00.81 ◀
intraperitoneal O00.00 ◀
with intrauterine pregnancy O00.01 ◀
isthmian O00.10 ◀
with intrauterine pregnancy O00.11 ◀
mesometric (mural) O00.80 ◀
with intrauterine pregnancy O00.81 ◀
molar NEC O02.0
complicated (by) O08.9
afibrinogenemia O08.1
cardiac arrest O08.81
chemical damage of pelvic organ (s) O08.6
circulatory collapse O08.3
defibrination syndrome O08.1
electrolyte imbalance O08.5
embolism (amniotic fluid) (blood clot) (pulmonary) (septic) O08.2
endometritis O08.0
genital tract and pelvic infection O08.0
hemorrhage (delayed) (excessive) O08.1
infection
genital tract or pelvic O08.0
kidney O08.83
urinary tract O08.83
intravascular coagulation O08.1
laceration of pelvic organ (s) O08.6
metabolic disorder O08.5
oliguria O08.4
oophoritis O08.0
parametritis O08.0
pelvic peritonitis O08.0
perforation of pelvic organ (s) O08.6
renal failure or shutdown O08.4
salpingitis or salpingo-oophoritis O08.0
sepsis O08.82
shock O08.3
septic O08.82
specified condition NEC O08.89
tubular necrosis (renal) O08.4
uremia O08.4
urinary infection O08.83
venous complication NEC O08.7
embolism O08.2
hydatidiform —*see also* Mole, hydatidiform O01.9-
multiple (gestation) O30.9-
greater than quadruplets —*see* Pregnancy, multiple (gestation), specified NEC

Pregnancy *(Continued)*
multiple (gestation) *(Continued)*
specified NEC O30.80-
with
two or more monoamniotic fetuses O30.82-
two or more monochorionic fetuses O30.81-
two or more monoamniotic fetuses O30.82-
two or more monochorionic fetuses O30.81-
unable to determine number of placenta and number of amniotic sacs O30.89-
unspecified number of placenta and unspecified number of amniotic sacs O30.80-
mural O00.80 ◀
with intrauterine pregnancy O00.81 ◀
normal (supervision of) Z34.9-
first Z34.0-
high-risk —*see* Pregnancy, supervision of, high-risk
specified Z34.8-
ovarian O00.20 ◀
with intrauterine pregnancy O00.21 ◀
postmature (40 to 42 weeks) O48.0
more than 42 weeks gestation O48.1
post-term (40 to 42 weeks) O48.0
prenatal care only Z34.9-
first Z34.0-
high-risk —*see* Pregnancy, supervision of, high-risk
specified Z34.8-
prolonged (more than 42 weeks gestation) O48.1
quadruplet O30.20-
with
two or more monoamniotic fetuses O30.22-
two or more monochorionic fetuses O30.21-
two or more monoamniotic fetuses O30.22-
two or more monochorionic fetuses O30.21-
unable to determine number of placenta and number of amniotic sacs O30.29-
unspecified number of placenta and unspecified number of amniotic sacs O30.20-
quintuplet —*see* Pregnancy, multiple (gestation), specified NEC
sextuplet —*see* Pregnancy, multiple (gestation), specified NEC
supervision of
concealed pregnancy O09.3-
elderly mother
multigravida O09.52-
primigravida O09.51-
hidden pregnancy O09.3-
high-risk O09.9-
due to (history of)
ectopic pregnancy O09.1-
elderly —*see* Pregnancy, supervision, elderly mother
grand multiparity O09.4
infertility O09.0-
insufficient prenatal care O09.3-
in utero procedure during previous pregnancy O09.82-
in vitro fertilization O09.81-
molar pregnancy O09.A- ◀
multiple previous pregnancies O09.4-
older mother —*see* Pregnancy, supervision of, elderly mother
poor reproductive or obstetric history NEC O09.29-
pre-term labor O09.21-
previous
neonatal death O09.29-

Pregnancy *(Continued)*
supervision of *(Continued)*
high-risk *(Continued)*
due to *(Continued)*
social problems O09.7-
specified NEC O09.89-
very young mother —*see* Pregnancy, supervision, young mother
resulting from in vitro fertilization O09.81-
normal Z34.9-
first Z34.0-
specified NEC Z34.8-
young mother
multigravida O09.62-
primigravida O09.61-
triplet O30.10-
with
two or more monoamniotic fetuses O30.12-
two or more monochorionic fetuses O30.11-
two or more monoamniotic fetuses O30.12-
two or more monochorionic fetuses O30.11-
unable to determine number of placenta and number of amniotic sacs O30.19-
unspecified number of placenta and unspecified number of amniotic sacs O30.10-
tubal (with abortion) (with rupture) O00.10 ◀
with intrauterine pregnancy O00.11 ◀
twin O30.00-
conjoined O30.02-
dichorionic/diamniotic (two placenta, two amniotic sacs) O30.04-
monochorionic/diamniotic (one placenta, two amniotic sacs) O30.03-
monochorionic/monoamniotic (one placenta, one amniotic sac) O30.01-
unable to determine number of placenta and number of amniotic sacs O30.09-
unspecified number of placenta and unspecified number of amniotic sacs O30.00-
unwanted Z64.0
weeks of gestation
8 weeks Z3A.08
9 weeks Z3A.09
10 weeks Z3A.10
11 weeks Z3A.11
12 weeks Z3A.12
13 weeks Z3A.13
14 weeks Z3A.14
15 weeks Z3A.15
16 weeks Z3A.16
17 weeks Z3A.17
18 weeks Z3A.18
19 weeks Z3A.19
20 weeks Z3A.20
21 weeks Z3A.21
22 weeks Z3A.22
23 weeks Z3A.23
24 weeks Z3A.24
25 weeks Z3A.25
26 weeks Z3A.26
27 weeks Z3A.27
28 weeks Z3A.28
29 weeks Z3A.29
30 weeks Z3A.30
31 weeks Z3A.31
32 weeks Z3A.32
33 weeks Z3A.33
34 weeks Z3A.34
35 weeks Z3A.35
36 weeks Z3A.36
37 weeks Z3A.37
38 weeks Z3A.38
39 weeks Z3A.39
40 weeks Z3A.40
41 weeks Z3A.41
42 weeks Z3A.42

Pregnancy *(Continued)*
weeks of gestation *(Continued)*
greater than 42 weeks Z3A.49
less than 8 weeks Z3A.01
not specified Z3A.00
Preiser's disease —*see* Osteonecrosis, secondary, due to, trauma, metacarpus
Pre-kwashiorkor —*see* Malnutrition, severe
Preleukemia (syndrome) D46.9
Preluxation, hip, congenital Q65.6
Premature —*see also* condition
adrenarche E27.0
aging E34.8
beats I49.40
atrial I49.1
auricular I49.1
supraventricular I49.1
birth NEC —*see* Preterm, newborn
closure, foramen ovale Q21.8
contraction
atrial I49.1
atrioventricular I49.49
auricular I49.1
auriculoventricular I49.2
heart (extrasystole) I49.49
junctional I49.2
ventricular I49.3
delivery —*see also* Pregnancy, complicated by, preterm labor O60.10
ejaculation F52.4
infant NEC —*see* Preterm, newborn
light-for-dates —*see* Light for dates
labor —*see* Pregnancy, complicated by, preterm labor
lungs P28.0
menopause E28.319
asymptomatic E28.319
symptomatic E28.310
newborn
extreme (less than 28 completed weeks) —*see* Immaturity, extreme
less than 37 completed weeks —*see* Preterm, newborn
puberty E30.1
rupture membranes or amnion —*see* Pregnancy, complicated by, premature rupture of membranes
senility E34.8
thelarche E30.8
ventricular systole I49.3
Prematurity NEC (less than 37 completed weeks) —*see* Preterm, newborn
extreme (less than 28 completed weeks) —*see* Immaturity, extreme
Premenstrual
dysphoric disorder (PMDD) F32.81 ⟸
tension (syndrome) N94.3
Premolarization, cuspids K00.2
Prenatal
care, normal pregnancy —*see* Pregnancy, normal
screening of mother Z36
teeth K00.6
Preparatory care for subsequent treatment NEC
for dialysis Z49.01
peritoneal Z49.02
Prepartum —*see* condition
Preponderance, left or right ventricular I51.7
Prepuce —*see* condition
PRES (posterior reversible encephalopathy syndrome) I67.83
Presbycardia R54
Presbycusis, presbyacusia H91.1-
Presbyesophagus K22.8
Presbyophrenia F03
Presbyopia H52.4
Prescription of contraceptives (initial) Z30.019
barrier Z30.018 ◀
diaphragm Z30.018 ◀
emergency (postcoital) Z30.012
Prescription of contraceptives *(Continued)*
implantable subdermal Z30.017 ⟸
injectable Z30.013
intrauterine contraceptive device Z30.014
pills Z30.011
postcoital (emergency) Z30.012
repeat Z30.40
barrier Z30.49 ◀
diaphragm Z30.49 ◀
implantable subdermal Z30.46 ⟸
injectable Z30.42
pills Z30.41
specified type NEC Z30.49
transdermal patch hormonal Z30.45 ◀
vaginal ring hormonal Z30.44 ◀
specified type NEC Z30.018
transdermal patch hormonal Z30.016 ◀
vaginal ring hormonal Z30.015 ◀
Presence (of)
ankle-joint implant (functional) (prosthesis) Z96.66-
aortocoronary (bypass) graft Z95.1
arterial-venous shunt (dialysis) Z99.2
artificial
eye (globe) Z97.0
heart (fully implantable) (mechanical) Z95.812
valve Z95.2
larynx Z96.3
lens (intraocular) Z96.1
limb (complete) (partial) Z97.1-
arm Z97.1-
bilateral Z97.15
leg Z97.1-
bilateral Z97.16
audiological implant (functional) Z96.29
bladder implant (functional) Z96.0
bone
conduction hearing device Z96.29
implant (functional) NEC Z96.7
joint (prosthesis) —*see* Presence, joint implant
cardiac
defibrillator (functional) (with synchronous cardiac pacemaker)Z95.810
implant or graft Z95.9
specified type NEC Z95.818
pacemaker Z95.0
resynchronization therapy ◀
defibrillator Z95.810 ◀
pacemaker Z95.0 ◀
cerebrospinal fluid drainage device Z98.2
cochlear implant (functional) Z96.21
contact lens (es) Z97.3
coronary artery graft or prosthesis Z95.5
CRT-D (cardiac resynchronization therapy defibrillator) Z95.810 ◀
CRT-P (cardiac resynchronization therapy pacemaker) Z95.0 ◀
cardioverter-defribillator (ICD) Z95.810 ◀
CSF shunt Z98.2
dental prosthesis device Z97.2
dentures Z97.2
device (external) NEC Z97.8
cardiac NEC Z95.818
heart assist Z95.811
implanted (functional) Z96.9
specified NEC Z96.89
prosthetic Z97.8
ear implant Z96.20
cochlear implant Z96.21
myringotomy tube Z96.22
specified type NEC Z96.29
elbow-joint implant (functional) (prosthesis) Z96.62-
endocrine implant (functional) NEC Z96.49
eustachian tube stent or device (functional) Z96.29
external hearing-aid or device Z97.4
finger-joint implant (functional) (prosthetic) Z96.69-
Presence *(Continued)*
functional implant Z96.9
specified NEC Z96.89
graft
cardiac NEC Z95.818
vascular NEC Z95.828
hearing-aid or device (external) Z97.4
implant (bone) (cochlear) (functional) Z96.21
heart assist device Z95.811
heart valve implant (functional) Z95.2
prosthetic Z95.2
specified type NEC Z95.4
xenogenic Z95.3
hip-joint implant (functional) (prosthesis) Z96.64-
ICD (cardioverter-defribillator) Z95.810 ◀
implanted device (artificial) (functional) (prosthetic) Z96.9
automatic cardiac defibrillator (with synchronous cardiac pacemaker) Z95.810
cardiac pacemaker Z95.0
cochlear Z96.21
dental Z96.5
heart Z95.812
heart valve Z95.2
prosthetic Z95.2
specified NEC Z95.4
xenogenic Z95.3
insulin pump Z96.41
intraocular lens Z96.1
joint Z96.60
ankle Z96.66-
elbow Z96.62-
finger Z96.69-
hip Z96.64-
knee Z96.65-
shoulder Z96.61-
specified NEC Z96.698
wrist Z96.63-
larynx Z96.3
myringotomy tube Z96.22
otological Z96.20
cochlear Z96.21
eustachian stent Z96.29
myringotomy Z96.22
specified NEC Z96.29
stapes Z96.29
skin Z96.81
skull plate Z96.7
specified NEC Z96.89
urogenital Z96.0
insulin pump (functional) Z96.41
intestinal bypass or anastomosis Z98.0
intraocular lens (functional) Z96.1
intrauterine contraceptive device (IUD) Z97.5
intravascular implant (functional) (prosthetic) NEC Z95.9
coronary artery Z95.5
defibrillator (with synchronous cardiac pacemaker) Z95.810
peripheral vessel (with angioplasty) Z95.820
joint implant (prosthetic) (any) Z96.60
ankle —*see* Presence, ankle joint implant
elbow —*see* Presence, elbow joint implant
finger —*see* Presence, finger joint implant
hip —*see* Presence, hip joint implant
knee —*see* Presence, knee joint implant
shoulder —*see* Presence, shoulder joint implant
specified joint NEC Z96.698
wrist —*see* Presence, wrist joint implant
knee-joint implant (functional) (prosthesis) Z96.65-
laryngeal implant (functional) Z96.3
mandibular implant (dental) Z96.5
myringotomy tube (s) Z96.22
orthopedic-joint implant (prosthetic) (any) —*see* Presence, joint implant

◀ New ⟸ Revised ~~deleted~~ Deleted

Presence *(Continued)*
otological implant (functional) Z96.29
shoulder-joint implant (functional) (prosthesis) Z96.61-
skull-plate implant Z96.7
spectacles Z97.3
stapes implant (functional) Z96.29
systemic lupus erythematosus [SLE] inhibitor D68.62
tendon implant (functional) (graft) Z96.7
tooth root (s) implant Z96.5
ureteral stent Z96.0
urethral stent Z96.0
urogenital implant (functional) Z96.0
vascular implant or device Z95.9
access port device Z95.828
specified type NEC Z95.828
wrist-joint implant (functional) (prosthesis) Z96.63-
Presenile —*see also* condition
dementia F03
premature aging E34.8
Presentation, fetal —*see* Delivery, complicated by, malposition
Prespondylolisthesis (congenital) Q76.2
Pressure
area, skin —*see* Ulcer, pressure, by site
brachial plexus G54.0
brain G93.5
injury at birth NEC P11.1
cerebral —*see* Pressure, brain
chest R07.89
cone, tentorial G93.5
hyposystolic —*see also* Hypotension
incidental reading, without diagnosis of hypotension R03.1
increased
intracranial (benign) G93.2
injury at birth P11.0
intraocular H40.05-
lumbosacral plexus G54.1
mediastinum J98.59 ◀
necrosis (chronic) —*see* Ulcer, pressure, by site
parental, inappropriate (excessive) Z62.6
sore (chronic) —*see* Ulcer, pressure, by site
spinal cord G95.20
ulcer (chronic) —*see* Ulcer, pressure, by site
venous, increased I87.8
Pre-syncope R55
Preterm
delivery (*see also* Pregnancy, complicated by, preterm labor) O60.10
labor —*see* Pregnancy, complicated by, preterm labor
newborn (infant) P07.30
gestational age
28 completed weeks (28 weeks, 0 days through 28 weeks, 6 days) P07.31
29 completed weeks (29 weeks, 0 days through 29 weeks, 6 days) P07.32
30 completed weeks (30 weeks, 0 days through 30 weeks, 6 days) P07.33
31 completed weeks (31 weeks, 0 days through 31 weeks, 6 days) P07.34
32 completed weeks (32 weeks, 0 days through 32 weeks, 6 days) P07.35
33 completed weeks (33 weeks, 0 days through 33 weeks, 6 days) P07.36
34 completed weeks (34 weeks, 0 days through 34 weeks, 6 days) P07.37
35 completed weeks (35 weeks, 0 days through 35 weeks, 6 days) P07.38
36 completed weeks (36 weeks, 0 days through 36 weeks, 6 days) P07.39
Previa
placenta (total) (without hemorrhage) O44.0- ◀
~~without hemorrhage O44.0-~~
Previa *(Continued)*
placenta *(Continued)*
with hemorrhage O44.1- ◀
complete O44.0- ◀
with hemorrhage O44.1- ◀
low —*see also* Delivery, complicated, by, placenta, low O44.4- ◀
with hemorrhage O44.5- ◀
marginal O44.2- ◀
with hemorrhage O44.3- ◀
partial O44.2- ◀
with hemorrhage O44.3- ◀
vasa O69.4
Priapism N48.30
due to
disease classified elsewhere N48.32
drug N48.33
specified cause NEC N48.39
trauma N48.31
Prickling sensation (skin) R20.2
Prickly heat L74.0
Primary —*see* condition
Primigravida
elderly, affecting management of pregnancy, labor and delivery (supervision only) —*see* Pregnancy, complicated by, elderly, primigravida
older, affecting management of pregnancy, labor and delivery (supervision only) —*see* Pregnancy, complicated by, elderly, primigravida
very young, affecting management of pregnancy, labor and delivery (supervision only) —*see* Pregnancy, complicated by, young mother, primigravida
Primipara
elderly, affecting management of pregnancy, labor and delivery (supervision only) —*see* Pregnancy, complicated by, elderly, primigravida
older, affecting management of pregnancy, labor and delivery (supervision only) —*see* Pregnancy, complicated by, elderly, primigravida
very young, affecting management of pregnancy, labor and delivery (supervision only) —*see* Pregnancy, complicated by, young mother, primigravida
Primus varus (bilateral) Q66.2
PRIND (Prolonged reversible ischemic neurologic deficit) I63.9
Pringle's disease (tuberous sclerosis)Q85.1
Prinzmetal angina I20.1
Prizefighter ear —*see* Cauliflower ear
Problem (with) (related to)
academic Z55.8
acculturation Z60.3
adjustment (to)
change of job Z56.1
life-cycle transition Z60.0
pension Z60.0
retirement Z60.0
adopted child Z62.821
alcoholism in family Z63.72
atypical parenting situation Z62.9
bankruptcy Z59.8
behavioral (adult) F69
drug seeking Z76.5 ◀
birth of sibling affecting child Z62.898
care (of)
provider dependency Z74.9
specified NEC Z74.8
sick or handicapped person in family or household Z63.6
child
abuse (affecting the child) —*see* Maltreatment, child
custody or support proceedings Z65.3
in care of non-parental family member Z62.21
Problem *(Continued)*
child *(Continued)*
in foster care Z62.21
in welfare custody Z62.21
living in orphanage or group home Z62.22
child-rearing Z62.9
specified NEC Z62.898
communication (developmental) F80.9
conflict or discord (with)
boss Z56.4
classmates Z55.4
counselor Z64.4
employer Z56.4
family Z63.9
specified NEC Z63.8
probation officer Z64.4
social worker Z64.4
teachers Z55.4
workmates Z56.4
conviction in legal proceedings Z65.0
with imprisonment Z65.1
counselor Z64.4
creditors Z59.8
digestive K92.9
drug addict in family Z63.72
ear —*see* Disorder, ear
economic Z59.9
affecting care Z59.9
specified NEC Z59.8
education Z55.9
specified NEC Z55.8
employment Z56.9
change of job Z56.1
discord Z56.4
environment Z56.5
sexual harassment Z56.81
specified NEC Z56.89
stress NEC Z56.6
stressful schedule Z56.3
threat of job loss Z56.2
unemployment Z56.0
enuresis, child F98.0
eye H57.9
failed examinations (school) Z55.2
falling Z91.81
family —*see also* Disruption, family Z63.9-
specified NEC Z63.8
feeding (elderly) (infant) R63.3
newborn P92.9
breast P92.5
overfeeding P92.4
slow P92.2
specified NEC P92.8
underfeeding P92.3
nonorganic F50.89 ◀
finance Z59.9
specified NEC Z59.8
foreclosure on loan Z59.8
foster child Z62.822
frightening experience (s) in childhood Z62.898
genital NEC
female N94.9
male N50.9
health care Z75.9
specified NEC Z75.8
hearing —*see* Deafness
homelessness Z59.0
housing Z59.9
inadequate Z59.1
isolated Z59.8
specified NEC Z59.8
identity (of childhood) F93.8
illegitimate pregnancy (unwanted) Z64.0
illiteracy Z55.0
impaired mobility Z74.09
imprisonment or incarceration Z65.1
inadequate teaching affecting education Z55.8
inappropriate (excessive) parental pressure Z62.6

◀ New ◀ Revised ~~deleted~~ Deleted

Problem *(Continued)*
influencing health status NEC Z78.9
in-law Z63.1
institutionalization, affecting child Z62.22
intrafamilial communication Z63.8
jealousy, child F93.8
landlord Z59.2
language (developmental) F80.9
learning (developmental) F81.9
legal Z65.3
conviction without imprisonment Z65.0
imprisonment Z65.1
release from prison Z65.2
life-management Z73.9
specified NEC Z73.89
life-style Z72.9
gambling Z72.6
high-risk sexual behavior (heterosexual) Z72.51
bisexual Z72.53
homosexual Z72.52
inappropriate eating habits Z72.4
self-damaging behavior NEC Z72.89
specified NEC Z72.89
tobacco use Z72.0
literacy Z55.9
low level Z55.0
specified NEC Z55.8
living alone Z60.2
lodgers Z59.2
loss of love relationship in childhood Z62.898
marital Z63.0
involving
divorce Z63.5
estrangement Z63.5
gender identity F66
mastication K08.89 ◀
medical
care, within family Z63.6
facilities Z75.9
specified NEC Z75.8
mental F48.9
multiparity Z64.1
negative life events in childhood Z62.9
altered pattern of family relationships Z62.898
frightening experience Z62.898
loss of
love relationship Z62.898
self-esteem Z62.898
physical abuse (alleged) —*see* Maltreatment, child
removal from home Z62.29
specified event NEC Z62.898
neighbor Z59.2
neurological NEC R29.818
new step-parent affecting child Z62.898
none (feared complaint unfounded) Z71.1
occupational NEC Z56.89
parent-child —*see* Conflict, parent-child
personal hygiene Z91.89
personality F69
phase-of-life transition, adjustment Z60.0
presence of sick or disabled person in family or household Z63.79
needing care Z63.6
primary support group (family) Z63.9
specified NEC Z63.8
probation officer Z64.4
psychiatric F99
psychosexual (development) F66
psychosocial Z65.9
specified NEC Z65.8
relationship Z63.9
childhood F93.8
release from prison Z65.2
removal from home affecting child Z62.29

Problem *(Continued)*
seeking and accepting known hazardous and harmful
behavioral or psychological interventions Z65.8
chemical, nutritional or physical interventions Z65.8
sexual function (nonorganic) F52.9
sight H54.7
sleep disorder, child F51.9
smell —*see* Disturbance, sensation, smell
social
environment Z60.9
specified NEC Z60.8
exclusion and rejection Z60.4
worker Z64.4
speech R47.9
developmental F80.9
specified NEC R47.89
swallowing —*see* Dysphagia
taste —*see* Disturbance, sensation, taste
tic, child F95.0
underachievement in school Z55.3
unemployment Z56.0
threatened Z56.2
unwanted pregnancy Z64.0
upbringing Z62.9
specified NEC Z62.898
urinary N39.9
voice production R47.89
work schedule (stressful) Z56.3
Procedure (surgical)
converted ◀
arthroscopic to open Z53.33 ◀
laparoscopic to open Z53.31 ◀
specified procedure NEC to open Z53.39 ◀
thoracoscopic to open Z53.32 ◀
for purpose other than remedying health state Z41.9
specified NEC Z41.8
not done Z53.9
because of
administrative reasons Z53.8
contraindication Z53.09
smoking Z53.01
patient's decision Z53.20
for reasons of belief or group pressure Z53.1
left against medical advice (AMA) Z53.21
specified reason NEC Z53.29
specified reason NEC Z53.8
Procidentia (uteri) N81.3
Proctalgia K62.89
fugax K59.4
spasmodic K59.4
Proctitis K62.89
amebic (acute) A06.0
chlamydial A56.3
gonococcal A54.6
granulomatous —*see* Enteritis, regional, large intestine
herpetic A60.1
radiation K62.7
tuberculous A18.32
ulcerative (chronic) K51.20
with
complication K51.219
abscess K51.214
fistula K51.213
obstruction K51.212
rectal bleeding K51.211
specified NEC K51.218
Proctocele
female (without uterine prolapse) N81.6
with uterine prolapse N81.2
complete N81.3
male K62.3
~~Proctocolitis, mucosal — see Rectosigmoiditis, ulcerative~~

Proctocolitis ◀
food-induced eosinophilic K52.82 ◀
food protein-induced K52.82 ◀
milk protein-induced K52.82 ◀
mucosal —*see* Rectosigmoiditis, ulcerative ◀
Proctoptosis K62.3
Proctorrhagia K62.5
Proctosigmoiditis K63.89
ulcerative (chronic) —*see* Rectosigmoiditis, ulcerative
Proctospasm K59.4
psychogenic F45.8
Profichet's disease —*see* Disorder, soft tissue, specified type NEC
Progeria E34.8
Prognathism (mandibular) (maxillary) M26.19
Progonoma (melanotic) —*see* Neoplasm, benign, by site
Progressive —*see* condition
Prolactinoma
specified site —*see* Neoplasm, benign, by site
unspecified site D35.2
Prolapse, prolapsed
anus, anal (canal) (sphincter) K62.2
arm or hand O32.2
causing obstructed labor O64.4
bladder (mucosa) (sphincter) (acquired)
congenital Q79.4
female —*see* Cystocele
male N32.89
breast implant (prosthetic) T85.49
cecostomy K94.09
cecum K63.4
cervix, cervical (hypertrophied) N81.2
anterior lip, obstructing labor O65.5
congenital Q51.828
postpartal, old N81.2
stump N81.85
ciliary body (traumatic) —*see* Laceration, eye(ball), with prolapse or loss of interocular tissue
colon (pedunculated) K63.4
colostomy K94.09
disc (intervertebral) —*see* Displacement, intervertebral disc
eye implant (orbital) T85.398
lens (ocular) —*see* Complications, intraocular lens
fallopian tube N83.4- ◀
gastric (mucosa) K31.89
genital, female N81.9
specified NEC N81.89
globe, nontraumatic —*see* Luxation, globe
ileostomy bud K94.19
intervertebral disc —*see* Displacement, intervertebral disc
intestine (small) K63.4
iris (traumatic) —*see* Laceration, eye(ball), with prolapse or loss of interocular tissue
nontraumatic H21.89
kidney N28.83
congenital Q63.2
laryngeal muscles or ventricle J38.7
liver K76.89
meatus urinarius N36.8
mitral (valve) I34.1
ocular lens implant —*see* Complications, intraocular lens
organ or site, congenital NEC —*see* Malposition, congenital
ovary N83.4- ◀
pelvic floor, female N81.89
perineum, female N81.89
rectum (mucosa) (sphincter) K62.3
due to trichuris trichuria B79
spleen D73.89
stomach K31.89
umbilical cord
complicating delivery O69.0

◀ New ◀ Revised ~~deleted~~ Deleted

Prolapse, prolapsed *(Continued)*
urachus, congenital Q64.4
ureter N28.89
with obstruction N13.5
with infection N13.6
ureterovesical orifice N28.89
urethra (acquired) (infected) (mucosa) N36.8
congenital Q64.71
urinary meatus N36.8
congenital Q64.72
uterovaginal N81.4
complete N81.3
incomplete N81.2
uterus (with prolapse of vagina) N81.4
complete N81.3
congenital Q51.818
first degree N81.2
in pregnancy or childbirth —*see* Pregnancy, complicated by, abnormal, uterus
incomplete N81.2
postpartal (old) N81.4
second degree N81.2
third degree N81.3
uveal (traumatic) —*see* Laceration, eye(ball), with prolapse or loss of interocular tissue
vagina (anterior) (wall) —*see* Cystocele
with prolapse of uterus N81.4
complete N81.3
incomplete N81.2
posterior wall N81.6
posthysterectomy N99.3
vitreous (humor) H43.0-
in wound —*see* Laceration, eye(ball), with prolapse or loss of interocular tissue
womb —*see* Prolapse, uterus
Prolapsus, female N81.9
specified NEC N81.89
Proliferation (s)
primary cutaneous CD30-positive large T-cell C86.6
prostate, atypical small acinar N42.32 ◀
Proliferative —*see* condition
Prolonged, prolongation (of)
bleeding (time) (idiopathic) R79.1
coagulation (time) R79.1
gestation (over 42 completed weeks)
mother O48.1
newborn P08.22
interval I44.0
labor O63.9
first stage O63.0
second stage O63.1
partial thromboplastin time (PTT) R79.1
pregnancy (more than 42 weeks gestation) O48.1
prothrombin time R79.1
QT interval I45.81
uterine contractions in labor O62.4
Prominence, prominent
with disproportion (fetopelvic) O33.0
causing obstructed labor O65.0
auricle (congenital) (ear) Q17.5
ischial spine or sacral promontory
nose (congenital) acquired M95.0
Promiscuity —*see* High, risk, sexual behavior
Pronation
ankle —*see* Deformity, limb, foot, specified NEC
foot —*see also* Deformity, limb, foot, specified NEC
congenital Q74.2
Prophylactic
administration of
antibiotics, long-term Z79.2
short-term use - omit code
drug —*see also* Long-term (current) drug therapy (use of) Z79.899-
medication Z79.899
Prophylactic *(Continued)*
organ removal (for neoplasia management) Z40.00
breast Z40.01
ovary Z40.02
specified site NEC Z40.09
surgery Z40.9
for risk factors related to malignant neoplasm —*see* Prophylactic, organ removal
specified NEC Z40.8
vaccination Z23
Propionic acidemia E71.121
Proptosis (ocular) —*see also* Exophthalmos
thyroid —*see* Hyperthyroidism, with goiter
Prosecution, anxiety concerning Z65.3
Prosopagnosia R48.3
Prostadynia N42.81
Prostate, prostatic —*see* condition
Prostatism —*see* Hyperplasia, prostate
Prostatitis (congestive) (suppurative) (with cystitis) N41.9
acute N41.0
cavitary N41.8
chronic N41.1
diverticular N41.8
due to Trichomonas (vaginalis) A59.02
fibrous N41.1
gonococcal (acute) (chronic) A54.22
granulomatous N41.4
hypertrophic N41.1
subacute N41.1
trichomonal A59.02
tuberculous A18.14
Prostatocystitis N41.3
Prostatorrhea N42.89
Prostatosis N42.82
Prostration R53.83
heat —*see also* Heat, exhaustion
anhydrotic T67.3
due to
salt (and water) depletion T67.4
water depletion T67.3
nervous F48.8
senile R54
Protanomaly (anomalous trichromat) H53.54
Protanopia (complete) (incomplete) H53.54
Protection (against) (from) —*see* Prophylactic
Protein
deficiency NEC —*see* Malnutrition
malnutrition —*see* Malnutrition
sickness —*see also* Reaction, serum T80.69
Proteinemia R77.9
Proteinosis
alveolar (pulmonary) J84.01
lipid or lipoid (of Urbach) E78.89
Proteinuria R80.9
Bence Jones R80.3
complicating pregnancy —*see* Proteinuria, gestational
gestational ◀
~~with edema O12.2-~~
complicating ◀
childbirth O12.14 ◀
pregnancy O12.1- ◀
with edema O12.2- ◀
puerperium O12.15 ◀
idiopathic R80.0
isolated R80.0
with glomerular lesion N06.9
dense deposit disease N06.6
diffuse
crescentic glomerulonephritis N06.7
endocapillary proliferative glomerulonephritis N06.4
mesangiocapillary glomerulonephritis N06.5
focal and segmental hyalinosis or sclerosis N06.1
membranous (diffuse) N06.2
Proteinuria *(Continued)*
isolated *(Continued)*
with glomerular lesion *(Continued)*
mesangial proliferative (diffuse) N06.3
minimal change N06.0
specified pathology NEC N06.8
orthostatic R80.2
with glomerular lesion —*see* Proteinuria, isolated, with glomerular lesion
persistent R80.1
with glomerular lesion —*see* Proteinuria, isolated, with glomerular lesion
postural R80.2
with glomerular lesion —*see* Proteinuria, isolated, with glomerular lesion
pre-eclamptic —*see* Pre-eclampsia
puerperal O12.15 ◀
specified type NEC R80.8
Proteolysis, pathologic D65
Proteus (mirabilis) (morganii), as cause of disease classified elsewhere B96.4
Prothrombin gene mutation D68.52
Protoporphyria, erythropoietic E80.0
Protozoal —*see also* condition
disease B64
specified NEC B60.8
Protrusion, protrusio
acetabuli M24.7
acetabulum (into pelvis) M24.7
device, implant or graft —*see also* Complications, by site and type, mechanical T85.698
arterial graft NEC —*see* Complication, cardiovascular device, mechanical, vascular
breast (implant) T85.49
catheter NEC T85.698
cystostomy T83.090
dialysis (renal) T82.49
intraperitoneal T85.691
infusion NEC T82.594
spinal (epidural) (subdural) T85.690
~~urinary, indwelling T83.098~~
urinary —*see also* Complications, catheter, urinary T83.098 ◀
electronic (electrode) (pulse generator) (stimulator)
bone T84.390
nervous system —*see* Complication, prosthetic device, mechanical, electronic nervous system stimulator
fixation, internal (orthopedic) NEC —*see* Complication, fixation device, mechanical
gastrointestinal —*see* Complications, prosthetic device, mechanical, gastrointestinal device
genital NEC T83.498
intrauterine contraceptive device T83.39
penile prosthesis (cylinder) (implanted) (pump) (resevoir) T83.490 ◀
testicular prosthesis T83.491 ◀
heart NEC —*see* Complication, cardiovascular device, mechanical
joint prosthesis —*see* Complications, joint prosthesis, mechanical, specified NEC, by site
ocular NEC —*see* Complications, prosthetic device, mechanical, ocular device
orthopedic NEC —*see* Complication, orthopedic, device, mechanical
specified NEC T85.628
urinary NEC —*see also* Complication, genitourinary, device, urinary, mechanical
graft T83.29
vascular NEC —*see* Complication, cardiovascular device, mechanical

Protrusion, protrusio *(Continued)*
device, implant or graft *(Continued)*
ventricular intracranial shunt T85.09
intervertebral disc —*see* Displacement, intervertebral disc
joint prosthesis —*see* Complications, joint prosthesis, mechanical, specified NEC, by site
nucleus pulposus —*see* Displacement, intervertebral disc
Prune belly (syndrome) Q79.4
Prurigo (ferox) (gravis) (Hebrae) (Hebra's) (mitis) (simplex) L28.2
Besnier's L20.0
estivalis L56.4
nodularis L28.1
psychogenic F45.8
Pruritus, pruritic (essential) L29.9
ani, anus L29.0
psychogenic F45.8
anogenital L29.3
psychogenic F45.8
due to onchocerca volvulus B73.1
gravidarum —*see* Pregnancy, complicated by, specified pregnancy-related condition NEC
hiemalis L29.8
neurogenic (any site) F45.8
perianal L29.0
psychogenic (any site) F45.8
scroti, scrotum L29.1
psychogenic F45.8
senile, senilis L29.8
specified NEC L29.8
psychogenic F45.8
Trichomonas A59.9
vulva, vulvae L29.2
psychogenic F45.8
Pseudarthrosis, pseudoarthrosis (bone) —*see* Nonunion, fracture
clavicle, congenital Q74.0
joint, following fusion or arthrodesis M96.0
Pseudoaneurysm —*see* Aneurysm
Pseudoangina (pectoris) —*see* Angina
Pseudoangioma I81
Pseudoarteriosus Q28.8
Pseudoarthrosis —*see* Pseudarthrosis
Pseudobulbar affect (PBA) F48.2
Pseudochromhidrosis L67.8
Pseudocirrhosis, liver, pericardial I31.1
Pseudocowpox B08.03
Pseudocoxalgia M91.3-
Pseudocroup J38.5
Pseudo-Cushing's syndrome, alcohol-induced E24.4
Pseudocyesis F45.8
Pseudocyst
lung J98.4
pancreas K86.3
retina —*see* Cyst, retina
Pseudoelephantiasis neuroarthritica Q82.0
Pseudoexfoliation, capsule (lens) —*see* Cataract, specified NEC
Pseudofolliculitis barbae L73.1
Pseudoglioma H44.89
Pseudohemophilia (Bernuth's) (hereditary) (type B) D68.0
Type A D69.8
vascular D69.8
Pseudohermaphroditism Q56.3
adrenal E25.8
female Q56.2
with adrenocortical disorder E25.8
without adrenocortical disorder Q56.2
~~adrenal, congenital E25.0~~
adrenal (congenital) E25.0 ◀
male Q56.1
with
adrenocortical disorder E25.8
androgen resistance E34.51
Pseudohermaphroditism *(Continued)*
male *(Continued)*
with *(Continued)*
cleft scrotum Q56.1
feminizing testis E34.51
5-alpha-reductase deficiency E29.1
without gonadal disorder Q56.1
adrenal E25.8
Pseudo-Hurler's polydystrophy E77.0
Pseudohydrocephalus G93.2
Pseudohypertrophic muscular dystrophy (Erb's) G71.0
Pseudohypertrophy, muscle G71.0
Pseudohypoparathyroidism E20.1
Pseudoinsomnia F51.03
Pseudoleukemia, infantile D64.89
Pseudomembranous —*see* condition
Pseudomeningocele (cerebral) (infective) (post-traumatic) G96.19
postprocedural (spinal) G97.82
Pseudomenses (newborn) P54.6
Pseudomenstruation (newborn) P54.6
Pseudomonas
aeruginosa, as cause of disease classified elsewhere B96.5
mallei infection A24.0
as cause of disease classified elsewhere B96.5
pseudomallei, as cause of disease classified elsewhere B96.5
Pseudomyotonia G71.19
Pseudomyxoma peritonei C78.6
Pseudoneuritis, optic (nerve) (disc) (papilla), **congenital** Q14.2
Pseudo-obstruction intestine (acute) (chronic) (idiopathic) (intermittent secondary) (primary) K59.8
Pseudopapilledema H47.33-
congenital Q14.2
Pseudoparalysis
arm or leg R29.818
atonic, congenital P94.2
Pseudopelade L66.0
Pseudophakia Z96.1
Pseudopolyarthritis, rhizomelic M35.3
Pseudopolycythemia D75.1
Pseudopseudohypoparathyroidism E20.1
Pseudopterygium H11.81-
Pseudoptosis (eyelid) —*see* Blepharochalasis
Pseudopuberty, precocious
female heterosexual E25.8
male isosexual E25.8
Pseudorickets (renal) N25.0
Pseudorubella B08.20
Pseudosclerema, newborn P83.8
Pseudosclerosis (brain)
Jakob's —*see* Creutzfeldt-Jakob disease or syndrome
of Westphal (Strüümpell) E83.01
spastic —*see* Creutzfeldt-Jakob disease or syndrome
Pseudotetanus —*see* Convulsions
Pseudotetany R29.0
hysterical F44.5
Pseudotruncus arteriosus Q25.49 ⟸
Pseudotuberculosis A28.2
enterocolitis A04.8
pasteurella (infection) A28.0
Pseudotumor
cerebri G93.2
orbital H05.11-
Pseudoxanthoma elasticum Q82.8
Psilosis (sprue) (tropical) K90.1
nontropical K90.0
Psittacosis A70
Psoitis M60.88
Psoriasis L40.9
arthropathic L40.50
arthritis mutilans L40.52
distal interphalangeal L40.51
Psoriasis *(Continued)*
arthropathic *(Continued)*
juvenile L40.54
other specified L40.59
spondylitis L40.53
buccal K13.29
flexural L40.8
guttate L40.4
mouth K13.29
nummular L40.0
plaque L40.0
psychogenic F54
pustular (generalized) L40.1
palmaris et plantaris L40.3
specified NEC L40.8
vulgaris L40.0
Psychasthenia F48.8
Psychiatric disorder or problem F99
Psychogenic —*see also* condition
factors associated with physical conditions F54
Psychological and behavioral factors affecting medical condition F59
Psychoneurosis, psychoneurotic —*see also* Neurosis
anxiety (state) F41.1
depersonalization F48.1
hypochondriacal F45.21
hysteria F44.9
neurasthenic F48.8
personality NEC F60.89
Psychopathy, psychopathic
affectionless F94.2
autistic F84.5
constitution, post-traumatic F07.81
personality —*see* Disorder, personality
sexual —*see* Deviation, sexual
state F60.2
Psychosexual identity disorder of childhood F64.2
Psychosis, psychotic F29
acute (transient) F23
hysterical F44.9
affective —*see* Disorder, mood
alcoholic F10.959
with
abuse F10.159
anxiety disorder F10.980
with
abuse F10.180
dependence F10.280
delirium tremens F10.231
delusions F10.950
with
abuse F10.150
dependence F10.250
dementia F10.97
with dependence F10.27
dependence F10.259
hallucinosis F10.951
with
abuse F10.151
dependence F10.251
mood disorder F10.94
with
abuse F10.14
dependence F10.24
paranoia F10.950
with
abuse F10.150
dependence F10.250
persisting amnesia F10.96
with dependence F10.26
amnestic confabulatory F10.96
with dependence F10.26
delirium tremens F10.231
Korsakoff's, Korsakov's, Korsakow's F10.26
paranoid type F10.950
with
abuse F10.150
dependence F10.250

◀ New ⟸ Revised ~~deleted~~ Deleted

Psychosis, psychotic *(Continued)*
anergastic —*see* Psychosis, organic
arteriosclerotic (simple type) (uncomplicated) F01.50
with behavioral disturbance F01.51
childhood F84.0
atypical F84.8
climacteric —*see* Psychosis, involutional
confusional F29
acute or subacute F05
reactive F23
cycloid F23
depressive —*see* Disorder, depressive
disintegrative (childhood) F84.3
drug-induced —*see* F11-F19 with .x59
paranoid and hallucinatory states —*see* F11-F19 with .x50 or .x51
due to or associated with
addiction, drug —*see* F11-F19 with .X59
dependence
alcohol F10.259
drug —*see* F11-F19 with .x59
epilepsy F06.8
Huntington's chorea F06.8
ischemia, cerebrovascular (generalized) F06.8
multiple sclerosis F06.8
physical disease F06.8
presenile dementia F03
senile dementia F03
vascular disease (arteriosclerotic) (cerebral) F01.50
with behavioral disturbance F01.51
epileptic F06.8
episode F23
due to or associated with physical condition F06.8
exhaustive F43.0
hallucinatory, chronic F28
hypomanic F30.8
hysterical (acute) F44.9
induced F24
infantile F84.0
atypical F84.8
infective (acute) (subacute) F05
involutional F28
depressive —*see* Disorder, depressive
melancholic —*see* Disorder, depressive
paranoid (state) F22
Korsakoff's, Korsakov's, Korsakow's (nonalcoholic) F04
alcoholic F10.96
in dependence F10.26
induced by other psychoactive substance —*see* categories F11-F19 with .x5x
mania, manic (single episode) F30.2
recurrent type F31.89
manic-depressive —*see* Disorder, bipolar ◄
menopausal —*see* Psychosis, involutional
mixed schizophrenic and affective F25.8
multi-infarct (cerebrovascular) F01.50
with behavioral disturbance F01.51
nonorganic F29
specified NEC F28
organic F09
due to or associated with
arteriosclerosis (cerebral) —*see* Psychosis, arteriosclerotic
cerebrovascular disease, arteriosclerotic —*see* Psychosis, arteriosclerotic
childbirth —*see* Psychosis, puerperal
Creutzfeldt-Jakob disease or syndrome —*see* Creutzfeldt-Jakob disease or syndrome
dependence, alcohol F10.259
disease
alcoholic liver F10.259
brain, arteriosclerotic —*see* Psychosis, arteriosclerotic

Psychosis, psychotic *(Continued)*
organic *(Continued)*
due to or associated with *(Continued)*
disease *(Continued)*
cerebrovascular F01.50
with behavioral disturbance F01.51
Creutzfeldt-Jakob —*see* Creutzfeldt-Jakob disease or syndrome
endocrine or metabolic F06.8
acute or subacute F05
liver, alcoholic F10.259
epilepsy transient (acute) F05
infection
brain (intracranial) F06.8
acute or subacute F05
intoxication
alcoholic (acute) F10.259
drug F19 with .X59 F11-
ischemia, cerebrovascular (generalized) —*see* Psychosis, arteriosclerotic
puerperium —*see* Psychosis, puerperal
trauma, brain (birth) (from electric current) (surgical) F06.8
acute or subacute F05
infective F06.8
acute or subacute F05
post-traumatic F06.8
acute or subacute F05
paranoiac F22
paranoid (climacteric) (involutional) (menopausal) F22
psychogenic (acute) F23
schizophrenic F20.0
senile F03
postpartum F53
presbyophrenic (type) F03
presenile F03
psychogenic (paranoid) F23
depressive F32.3
puerperal F53
specified type —*see* Psychosis, by type
reactive (brief) (transient) (emotional stress) (psychological trauma) F23
depressive F32.3
recurrent F33.3
excitative type F30.8
schizoaffective F25.9
depressive type F25.1
manic type F25.0
schizophrenia, schizophrenic —*see* Schizophrenia
schizophrenia-like, in epilepsy F06.2
schizophreniform F20.81
affective type F25.9
brief F23
confusional type F23
depressive type F25.1
manic type F25.0
mixed type F25.0
senile NEC F03
depressed or paranoid type F03
simple deterioration F03
specified type — code to condition
shared F24
situational (reactive) F23
symbiotic (childhood) F84.3
symptomatic F09
Psychosomatic —*see* Disorder, psychosomatic
Psychosyndrome, organic F07.9
Psychotic episode due to or associated with physical condition F06.8
Pterygium (eye) H11.00-
amyloid H11.01-
central H11.02-
colli Q18.3
double H11.03-
peripheral
progressive H11.05-
stationary H11.04-
recurrent H11.06-

Ptilosis (eyelid) —*see* Madarosis
Ptomaine (poisoning) —*see* Poisoning, food
Ptosis —*see also* Blepharoptosis
adiposa (false) —*see* Blepharoptosis
breast N64.81
cecum K63.4
colon K63.4
congenital (eyelid) Q10.0
specified site NEC —*see* Anomaly, by site
eyelid —*see* Blepharoptosis
congenital Q10.0
gastric K31.89
intestine K63.4
kidney N28.83
liver K76.89
renal N28.83
splanchnic K63.4
spleen D73.89
stomach K31.89
viscera K63.4
PTP D69.51
Ptyalism (periodic) K11.7
hysterical F45.8
pregnancy —*see* Pregnancy, complicated by, specified pregnancy-related condition NEC
psychogenic F45.8
Ptyalolithiasis K11.5
Pubarche, precocious E30.1
Pubertas praecox E30.1
Puberty (development state) Z00.3
bleeding (excessive) N92.2
delayed E30.0
precocious (constitutional) (cryptogenic) (idiopathic) E30.1
central E22.8
due to
ovarian hyperfunction E28.1
estrogen E28.0
testicular hyperfunction E29.0
premature E30.1
due to
adrenal cortical hyperfunction E25.8
pineal tumor E34.8
pituitary (anterior) hyperfunction E22.8
Puckering, macula —*see* Degeneration, macula, puckering
Pudenda, pudendum —*see* condition
Puente's disease (simple glandular cheilitis) K13.0
Puerperal, puerperium (complicated by, complications)
abnormal glucose (tolerance test) O99.815
abscess
areola O91.02
associated with lactation O91.03
Bartholin's gland O86.19
breast O91.12
associated with lactation O91.13
cervix (uteri) O86.11
genital organ NEC O86.19
kidney O86.21
mammary O91.12
associated with lactation O91.13
nipple O91.02
associated with lactation O91.03
peritoneum O85
subareolar O91.12
associated with lactation O91.13
urinary tract —*see* Puerperal, infection, urinary
uterus O86.12
vagina (wall) O86.13
vaginorectal O86.13
vulvovaginal gland O86.13
adnexitis O86.19
afibrinogenemia, or other coagulation defect O72.3
albuminuria (acute) (subacute) —*see* Proteinuria, gestational
alcohol use O99.315

Puerperal, puerperium *(Continued)*
anemia O90.81
pre-existing (pre-pregnancy) O99.03
anesthetic death O89.8
apoplexy O99.43
bariatric surgery status O99.845
blood disorder NEC O99.13
blood dyscrasia O72.3
cardiomyopathy O90.3
cerebrovascular disorder (conditions in I60-I69) O99.43
cervicitis O86.11
circulatory system disorder O99.43
coagulopathy (any) O72.3
complications O90.9
specified NEC O90.89
convulsions —*see* Eclampsia
cystitis O86.22
cystopyelitis O86.29
delirium NEC F05
diabetes O24.93
gestational —*see* Puerperal, gestational diabetes
pre-existing O24.33
specified NEC O24.83
type 1 O24.03
type 2 O24.13
digestive system disorder O99.63
disease O90.9
breast NEC O92.29
cerebrovascular (acute) O99.43
nonobstetric NEC O99.89
tubo-ovarian O86.19
Valsuani's O99.03
disorder O90.9
biliary tract O26.63
lactation O92.70
liver O26.63
nonobstetric NEC O99.89
disruption
cesarean wound O90.0
episiotomy wound O90.1
perineal laceration wound O90.1
drug use O99.325
eclampsia (with pre-existing hypertension) O15.2
embolism (pulmonary) (blood clot) —*see* Embolism, obstetric, puerperal
endocrine, nutritional or metabolic disease NEC O99.285
endophlebitis —*see* Puerperal, phlebitis
endotrachelitis O86.11
failure
lactation (complete) O92.3
partial O92.4
renal, acute O90.4
fever (of unknown origin) O86.4
septic O85
fissure, nipple O92.12
associated with lactation O92.13
fistula
breast (due to mastitis) O91.12
associated with lactation O91.13
nipple O91.02
associated with lactation O91.03
galactophoritis O91.22
associated with lactation O91.23
galactorrhea O92.6
gastric banding status O99.845
gastric bypass status O99.845
gastrointestinal disease NEC O99.63
~~gestational diabetes O24.439~~
~~diet controlled O24.430~~
~~insulin (and diet) controlled O24.434~~
gestational ◀
diabetes O24.439 ◀
diet controlled O24.430 ◀
insulin (and diet) controlled O24.434 ◀
oral drug controlled (antidiabetic) (hypoglycemic) O24.435 ◀

Puerperal, puerperium *(Continued)*
gestational *(Continued)*
edema O12.05 ◀
with proteinuria O12.25 ◀
proteinuria O12.15 ◀
gonorrhea O98.23
hematoma, subdural O99.43
hemiplegia, cerebral O99.355-
due to cerebrovascular disorder O99.43
hemorrhage O72.1
brain O99.43
bulbar O99.43
cerebellar O99.43
cerebral O99.43
cortical O99.43
delayed or secondary O72.2
extradural O99.43
internal capsule O99.43
intracranial O99.43
intrapontine O99.43
meningeal O99.43
pontine O99.43
retained placenta O72.0
subarachnoid O99.43
subcortical O99.43
subdural O99.43
third stage O72.0
uterine, delayed O72.2
ventricular O99.43
hemorrhoids O87.2
hepatorenal syndrome O90.4
hypertension —*see* Hypertension, complicating, puerperium
hypertrophy, breast O92.29
induration breast (fibrous) O92.29
infection O86.4
cervix O86.11
generalized O85
genital tract NEC O86.19
obstetric surgical wound O86.0
kidney (bacillus coli) O86.21
maternal O98.93
carrier state NEC O99.835
gonorrhea O98.23
human immunodeficiency virus (HIV) O98.73
protozoal O98.63
sexually transmitted NEC O98.33
specified NEC O98.83
~~streptococcus B carrier state O99.825~~
streptococcus group B (GBS) carrier state O99.825 ◀
syphilis O98.13
tuberculosis O98.03
viral hepatitis O98.43
viral NEC O98.53
nipple O91.02
associated with lactation O91.03
peritoneum O85
renal O86.21
specified NEC O86.89
urinary (asymptomatic) (tract) NEC O86.20
bladder O86.22
kidney O86.21
specified site NEC O86.29
urethra O86.22
vagina O86.13
vein —*see* Puerperal, phlebitis
ischemia, cerebral O99.43
lymphangitis O86.89
breast O91.22
associated with lactation O91.23
malignancy O9A.13
malnutrition O25.3
mammillitis O91.02
associated with lactation O91.03
mammitis O91.22
associated with lactation O91.23
mania F30.8

Puerperal, puerperium *(Continued)*
mastitis O91.22
associated with lactation O91.23
purulent O91.12
associated with lactation O91.13
melancholia —*see* Disorder, depressive
mental disorder NEC O99.345
metroperitonitis O85
metrorrhagia —*see* Hemorrhage, postpartum
metrosalpingitis O86.19
metrovaginitis O86.13
milk leg O87.1
monoplegia, cerebral O99.43
mood disturbance O90.6
necrosis, liver (acute) (subacute) (conditions in subcategory K72.0) O26.63 ◀
with renal failure O90.4
nervous system disorder O99.355
neuritis O90.89
obesity (pre-existing prior to pregnancy) O99.215
obesity surgery status O99.845
occlusion, precerebral artery O99.43
paralysis
bladder (sphincter) O90.89
cerebral O99.43
paralytic stroke O99.43
parametritis O85
paravaginitis O86.13
pelviperitonitis O85
perimetritis O86.12
perimetrosalpingitis O86.19
perinephritis O86.21
periphlebitis —*see* Puerperal phlebitis
peritoneal infection O85
peritonitis (pelvic) O85
perivaginitis O86.13
phlebitis O87.0
deep O87.1
pelvic O87.1
superficial O87.0
phlebothrombosis, deep O87.1
phlegmasia alba dolens O87.1
placental polyp O90.89
pneumonia, embolic —*see* Embolism, obstetric, puerperal
pre-eclampsia —*see* Pre-eclampsia
psychosis F53
pyelitis O86.21
pyelocystitis O86.29
pyelonephritis O86.21
pyelonephrosis O86.21
pyemia O85
pyocystitis O86.29
pyohemia O85
pyometra O86.12
pyonephritis O86.21
pyosalpingitis O86.19
pyrexia (of unknown origin) O86.4
renal
disease NEC O90.89
failure O90.4
respiratory disease NEC O99.53
retention
decidua —*see* Retention, decidua
placenta O72.0
secundines —*see* Retention, secundines
retrated nipple O92.02
salpingo-ovaritis O86.19
salpingoperitonitis O85
secondary perineal tear O90.1
sepsis O85
sepsis (pelvic) O85
septic thrombophlebitis O86.81
skin disorder NEC O99.73
specified condition NEC O99.89
stroke O99.43
subinvolution (uterus) O90.89
subluxation of symphysis (pubis) O26.73

◀ New ◀ Revised ~~deleted~~ Deleted

Puerperal, puerperium *(Continued)*
suppuration —*see* Puerperal, abscess
tetanus A34
thelitis O91.02
associated with lactation O91.03
thrombocytopenia O72.3
thrombophlebitis (superficial) O87.0
deep O87.1
pelvic O87.1
septic O86.81
thrombosis (venous) —*see* Thrombosis, puerperal
thyroiditis O90.5
toxemia (eclamptic) (pre-eclamptic) (with convulsions) O15.2
trauma, non-obstetric O9A.23
caused by abuse (physical) (suspected) O9A.33
confirmed O9A.33
psychological (suspected) O9A.53
confirmed O9A.53
sexual (suspected) O9A.43
confirmed O9A.43
uremia (due to renal failure) O90.4
urethritis O86.22
vaginitis O86.13
varicose veins (legs) O87.4
vulva or perineum O87.8
venous O87.9
vulvitis O86.19
vulvovaginitis O86.13
white leg O87.1
Puerperium —*see* Puerperal
Pulmolithiasis J98.4
Pulmonary —*see* condition
Pulpitis (acute) (anachoretic) (chronic) (hyperplastic) (putrescent) (suppurative) (ulcerative) K04.01 ◄
irreversible K04.02 ◄
reversible K04.01 ◄
Pulpless tooth K04.99
Pulse
alternating R00.8
bigeminal R00.8
fast R00.0
feeble, rapid due to shock following injury T79.4
rapid R00.0
weak R09.89
Pulsus alternans or trigeminus R00.8
Punch drunk F07.81
Punctum lacrimale occlusion —*see* Obstruction, lacrimal
Puncture
abdomen, abdominal
wall S31.139
with
foreign body S31.149
penetration into peritoneal cavity S31.639
with foreign body S31.649
epigastric region S31.132
with
foreign body S31.142
penetration into peritoneal cavity S31.632
with foreign body S31.642
left
lower quadrant S31.134
with
foreign body S31.144
penetration into peritoneal cavity S31.634
with foreign body S31.644
upper quadrant S31.131
with
foreign body S31.141
penetration into peritoneal cavity S31.631
with foreign body S31.641

Puncture *(Continued)*
abdomen, abdominal *(Continued)*
wall *(Continued)*
periumbilic region S31.135
with
foreign body S31.145
penetration into peritoneal cavity S31.635
with foreign body S31.645
right
lower quadrant S31.133
with
foreign body S31.143
penetration into peritoneal cavity S31.633
with foreign body S31.643
upper quadrant S31.130
with
foreign body S31.140
penetration into peritoneal cavity S31.630
with foreign body S31.640
accidental, complicating surgery —*see* Complication, accidental puncture or laceration
alveolar (process) —*see* Puncture, oral cavity
ankle S91.039
with
foreign body S91.049
left S91.032
with
foreign body S91.042
right S91.031
with
foreign body S91.041
anus S31.833
with foreign body S31.834
arm (upper) S41.139
with foreign body S41.149
left S41.132
with foreign body S41.142
lower —*see* Puncture, forearm
right S41.131
with foreign body S41.141
auditory canal (external) (meatus) —*see* Puncture, ear
auricle, ear —*see* Puncture, ear
axilla —*see* Puncture, arm
back —*see also* Puncture, thorax, back
lower S31.030
with
foreign body S31.040
with penetration into retroperitoneal space S31.041
penetration into retroperitoneal space S31.031
bladder (traumatic) S37.29
nontraumatic N32.89
breast S21.039
with foreign body S21.049
left S21.032
with foreign body S21.042
right S21.031
with foreign body S21.041
buttock S31.803
with foreign body S31.804
left S31.823
with foreign body S31.824
right S31.813
with foreign body S31.814
by
device, implant or graft —*see* Complications, by site and type, mechanical
foreign body left accidentally in operative wound T81.539
instrument (any) during a procedure, accidental —*see* Puncture, accidental complicating surgery
calf —*see* Puncture, leg
canaliculus lacrimalis —*see* Puncture, eyelid

Puncture *(Continued)*
canthus, eye —*see* Puncture, eyelid
cervical esophagus S11.23
with foreign body S11.24
cheek (external) S01.439
with foreign body S01.449
internal —*see* Puncture, oral cavity
left S01.432
with foreign body S01.442
right S01.431
with foreign body S01.441
chest wall —*see* Puncture, thorax
chin —*see* Puncture, head, specified site NEC
clitoris —*see* Puncture, vulva
costal region —*see* Puncture, thorax
digit (s)
foot —*see* Puncture, toe
hand —*see* Puncture, finger
ear (canal) (external) S01.339
with foreign body S01.349
drum S09.2-
left S01.332
with foreign body S01.342
right S01.331
with foreign body S01.341
elbow S51.039
with
foreign body S51.049
left S51.032
with
foreign body S51.042
right S51.031
with
foreign body S51.041
epididymis —*see* Puncture, testis
epigastric region —*see* Puncture, abdomen, wall, epigastric
epiglottis S11.83
with foreign body S11.84
esophagus
cervical S11.23
with foreign body S11.24
thoracic S27.818
eyeball S05.6-
with foreign body S05.5-
eyebrow —*see* Puncture, eyelid
eyelid S01.13-
with foreign body S01.14-
left S01.132
with foreign body S01.142
right S01.131
with foreign body S01.141
face NEC —*see* Puncture, head, specified site NEC
finger (s) S61.239
with
damage to nail S61.339
with
foreign body S61.349
foreign body S61.249
index S61.238
with
damage to nail S61.338
with
foreign body S61.348
foreign body S61.248
left S61.231
with
damage to nail S61.331
with
foreign body S61.341
foreign body S61.241
right S61.230
with
damage to nail S61.330
with
foreign body S61.340
foreign body S61.240
little S61.238
with
damage to nail S61.338

◄ New ◄ Revised ~~deleted~~ Deleted

Puncture *(Continued)*
finger *(Continued)*
with *(Continued)*
with *(Continued)*
damage to nail *(Continued)*
with
foreign body S61.348
foreign body S61.248
left S61.237
with
damage to nail S61.337
with
foreign body S61.347
foreign body S61.247
right S61.236
with
damage to nail S61.336
with
foreign body S61.346
foreign body S61.246
middle S61.238
with
damage to nail S61.338
with
foreign body S61.348
foreign body S61.248
left S61.233
with
damage to nail S61.333
with
foreign body S61.343
foreign body S61.243
right S61.232
with
damage to nail S61.332
with
foreign body S61.342
foreign body S61.242
ring S61.238
with
damage to nail S61.338
with
foreign body S61.348
foreign body S61.248
left S61.235
with
damage to nail S61.335
with
foreign body S61.345
foreign body S61.245
right S61.234
with
damage to nail S61.334
with
foreign body S61.344
foreign body S61.244
flank S31.139
with foreign body S31.149
foot (except toe (s) alone) S91.339
with foreign body S91.349
left S91.332
with foreign body S91.342
right S91.331
with foreign body S91.341
toe —*see* Puncture, toe
forearm S51.839
with
foreign body S51.849
elbow only —*see* Puncture, elbow
left S51.832
with
foreign body S51.842
right S51.831
with
foreign body S51.841
forehead —*see* Puncture, head, specified site NEC
genital organs, external
female S31.532
with foreign body S31.542
vagina —*see* Puncture, vagina
vulva —*see* Puncture, vulva

Puncture *(Continued)*
genital organs, external *(Continued)*
male S31.531
with foreign body S31.541
penis —*see* Puncture, penis
scrotum —*see* Puncture, scrotum
testis —*see* Puncture, testis
groin —*see* Puncture, abdomen, wall
gum —*see* Puncture, oral cavity
hand S61.439
with
foreign body S61.449
finger —*see* Puncture, finger
left S61.432
with
foreign body S61.442
right S61.431
with
foreign body S61.441
thumb —*see* Puncture, thumb
head S01.93
with foreign body S01.94
cheek —*see* Puncture, cheek
ear —*see* Puncture, ear
eyelid —*see* Puncture, eyelid
lip —*see* Puncture, oral cavity
nose —*see* Puncture, nose
oral cavity —*see* Puncture, oral cavity
scalp S01.03
with foreign body S01.04
specified site NEC S01.83
with foreign body S01.84
temporomandibular area —*see* Puncture, cheek
heart S26.99
with hemopericardium S26.09
without hemopericardium S26.19
heel —*see* Puncture, foot
hip S71.039
with foreign body S71.049
left S71.032
with foreign body S71.042
right S71.031
with foreign body S71.041
hymen —*see* Puncture, vagina
hypochondrium —*see* Puncture, abdomen, wall
hypogastric region —*see* Puncture, abdomen, wall
inguinal region —*see* Puncture, abdomen, wall
instep —*see* Puncture, foot
internal organs —*see* Injury, by site
interscapular region —*see* Puncture, thorax, back
intestine
large
colon S36.599
ascending S36.590
descending S36.592
sigmoid S36.593
specified site NEC S36.598
transverse S36.591
rectum S36.69
small S36.499
duodenum S36.490
specified site NEC S36.498
intra-abdominal organ S36.99
gallbladder S36.128
intestine —*see* Puncture, intestine
liver S36.118
pancreas —*see* Puncture, pancreas
peritoneum S36.81
specified site NEC S36.898
spleen S36.09
stomach S36.39
jaw —*see* Puncture, head, specified site NEC
knee S81.039
with foreign body S81.049
left S81.032
with foreign body S81.042

Puncture *(Continued)*
knee *(Continued)*
right S81.031
with foreign body S81.041
labium (majus) (minus) —*see* Puncture, vulva
lacrimal duct —*see* Puncture, eyelid
larynx S11.013
with foreign body S11.014
leg (lower) S81.839
with foreign body S81.849
foot —*see* Puncture, foot
knee —*see* Puncture, knee
left S81.832
with foreign body S81.842
right S81.831
with foreign body S81.841
upper —*see* Puncture, thigh
lip S01.531
with foreign body S01.541
loin —*see* Puncture, abdomen, wall
lower back —*see* Puncture, back, lower
lumbar region —*see* Puncture, back, lower
malar region —*see* Puncture, head, specified site NEC
mammary —*see* Puncture, breast
mastoid region —*see* Puncture, head, specified site NEC
mouth —*see* Puncture, oral cavity
nail
finger —*see* Puncture, finger, with damage to nail
toe —*see* Puncture, toe, with damage to nail
nasal (septum) (sinus) —*see* Puncture, nose
nasopharynx —*see* Puncture, head, specified site NEC
neck S11.93
with foreign body S11.94
involving
cervical esophagus —*see* Puncture, cervical esophagus
larynx —*see* Puncture, larynx
pharynx —*see* Puncture, pharynx
thyroid gland —*see* Puncture, thyroid gland
trachea —*see* Puncture, trachea
specified site NEC S11.83
with foreign body S11.84
nose (septum) (sinus) S01.23
with foreign body S01.24
ocular —*see* Puncture, eyeball - oral cavity S01.532
with foreign body S01.542
orbit S05.4-
palate —*see* Puncture, oral cavity
palm —*see* Puncture, hand
pancreas S36.299
body S36.291
head S36.290
tail S36.292
pelvis —*see* Puncture, back, lower
penis S31.23
with foreign body S31.24
perineum
female S31.43
with foreign body S31.44
male S31.139
with foreign body S31.149
periocular area (with or without lacrimal passages) —*see* Puncture, eyelid
phalanges
finger —*see* Puncture, finger
toe —*see* Puncture, toe
pharynx S11.23
with foreign body S11.24
pinna —*see* Puncture, ear
popliteal space —*see* Puncture, knee
prepuce —*see* Puncture, penis
pubic region S31.139
with foreign body S31.149

Puncture *(Continued)*
pudendum —*see* Puncture, genital organs, external
rectovaginal septum —*see* Puncture, vagina
sacral region —*see* Puncture, back, lower
sacroiliac region —*see* Puncture, back, lower
salivary gland —*see* Puncture, oral cavity
scalp S01.03
with foreign body S01.04
scapular region —*see* Puncture, shoulder
scrotum S31.33
with foreign body S31.34
shin —*see* Puncture, leg
shoulder S41.039
with foreign body S41.049
left S41.032
with foreign body S41.042
right S41.031
with foreign body S41.041
spermatic cord —*see* Puncture, testis
sternal region —*see* Puncture, thorax, front
submaxillary region —*see* Puncture, head, specified site NEC
submental region —*see* Puncture, head, specified site NEC
subungual
finger (s) —*see* Puncture, finger, with damage to nail
toe —*see* Puncture, toe, with damage to nail
supraclavicular fossa —*see* Puncture, neck, specified site NEC
temple, temporal region —*see* Puncture, head, specified site NEC
temporomandibular area —*see* Puncture, cheek
testis S31.33
with foreign body S31.34
thigh S71.139
with foreign body S71.149
left S71.132
with foreign body S71.142
right S71.131
with foreign body S71.141
thorax, thoracic (wall) S21.93
with foreign body S21.94
back S21.23-
with
foreign body S21.24-
with penetration S21.44
penetration S21.43
breast —*see* Puncture, breast
front S21.13-
with
foreign body S21.14-
with penetration S21.34
penetration S21.33
throat —*see* Puncture, neck
thumb S61.039
with
damage to nail S61.139
with
foreign body S61.149
foreign body S61.049
left S61.032
with
damage to nail S61.132
with
foreign body S61.142
foreign body S61.042
right S61.031
with
damage to nail S61.131
with
foreign body S61.141
foreign body S61.041

Puncture *(Continued)*
thyroid gland S11.13
with foreign body S11.14
toe (s) S91.139
with
damage to nail S91.239
with
foreign body S91.249
foreign body S91.149
great S91.133
with
damage to nail S91.233
with
foreign body S91.243
foreign body S91.143
left S91.132
with
damage to nail S91.232
with
foreign body S91.242
foreign body S91.142
right S91.131
with
damage to nail S91.231
with
foreign body S91.241
foreign body S91.141
lesser S91.136
with
damage to nail S91.236
with
foreign body S91.246
foreign body S91.146
left S91.135
with
damage to nail S91.235
with
foreign body S91.245
foreign body S91.145
right S91.134
with
damage to nail S91.234
with
foreign body S91.244
foreign body S91.144
tongue —*see* Puncture, oral cavity
trachea S11.023
with foreign body S11.024
tunica vaginalis —*see* Puncture, testis
tympanum, tympanic membrane S09.2-
umbilical region S31.135
with foreign body S31.145
uvula —*see* Puncture, oral cavity
vagina S31.43
with foreign body S31.44
vocal cords S11.033
with foreign body S11.034
vulva S31.43
with foreign body S31.44
wrist S61.539
with
foreign body S61.549
left S61.532
with
foreign body S61.542
right S61.531
with
foreign body S61.541
PUO (pyrexia of unknown origin) R50.9
Pupillary membrane (persistent) Q13.89
Pupillotonia —*see* Anomaly, pupil, function, tonic pupil
Purpura D69.2
abdominal D69.0
allergic D69.0
anaphylactoid D69.0
annularis telangiectodes L81.7
arthritic D69.0
autoerythrocyte sensitization D69.2
autoimmune D69.0

Purpura *(Continued)*
bacterial D69.0
Bateman's (senile) D69.2
capillary fragility (hereditary) (idiopathic) D69.8
cryoglobulinemic D89.1
Devil's pinches D69.2
fibrinolytic —*see* Fibrinolysis
fulminans, fulminous D65
gangrenous D65
hemorrhagic, hemorrhagica D69.3
not due to thrombocytopenia D69.0
Henoch (-Schönlein) (allergic) D69.0
hypergammaglobulinemic (benign) (Waldenström's) D89.0
idiopathic (thrombocytopenic) D69.3
nonthrombocytopenic D69.0
immune thrombocytopenic D69.3
infectious D69.0
malignant D69.0
neonatorum P54.5
nervosa D69.0
newborn P54.5
nonthrombocytopenic D69.2
hemorrhagic D69.0
idiopathic D69.0
nonthrombopenic D69.2
peliosis rheumatica D69.0
posttransfusion (post-transfusion) (from (fresh) whole blood or blood products) D69.51
primary D69.49
red cell membrane sensitivity D69.2
rheumatica D69.0
Schönlein (-Henoch) (allergic) D69.0
scorbutic E54 *[D77]*
senile D69.2
simplex D69.2
symptomatica D69.0
telangiectasia annularis L81.7
thrombocytopenic D69.49
congenital D69.42
hemorrhagic D69.3
hereditary D69.42
idiopathic D69.3
immune D69.3
neonatal, transitory P61.0
thrombotic M31.1
thrombohemolytic —*see* Fibrinolysis
thrombolytic —*see* Fibrinolysis
thrombopenic D69.49
thrombotic, thrombocytopenic M31.1
toxic D69.0
vascular D69.0
visceral symptoms D69.0
Purpuric spots R23.3
Purulent —*see* condition
Pus
in
stool R19.5
urine N39.0
tube (rupture) —*see* Salpingo-oophoritis
Pustular rash L08.0
Pustule (nonmalignant) L08.9
malignant A22.0
Pustulosis palmaris et plantaris L40.3
Putnam (-Dana) disease or syndrome —*see* Degeneration, combined
Putrescent pulp (dental) K04.1
Pyarthritis, pyarthrosis —*see* Arthritis, pyogenic or pyemic
tuberculous —*see* Tuberculosis, joint
Pyelectasis —*see* Hydronephrosis
Pyelitis (congenital) (uremic) —*see also* Pyelonephritis
with
calculus —*see* category N20
with hydronephrosis N13.2
contracted kidney N11.9

P

Pyelitis *(Continued)*
acute N10
chronic N11.9
with calculus —*see* category N20
with hydronephrosis N13.2
cystica N28.84
puerperal (postpartum) O86.21
tuberculous A18.11
Pyelocystitis —*see* Pyelonephritis
Pyelonephritis —*see also* Nephritis, tubulo-interstitial
with
calculus —*see* category N20
with hydronephrosis N13.2
contracted kidney N11.9
acute N10
calculous —*see* category N20
with hydronephrosis N13.2
chronic N11.9
with calculus —*see* category N20
with hydronephrosis N13.2
associated with ureteral obstruction or stricture N11.1
nonobstructive N11.8
with reflux (vesicoureteral) N11.0
obstructive N11.1
specified NEC N11.8
in (due to)
brucellosis A23.9 *[N16]*
cryoglobulinemia (mixed) D89.1 *[N16]*
cystinosis E72.04
diphtheria A36.84
glycogen storage disease E74.09 *[N16]*
leukemia NEC C95.9- *[N16]*
lymphoma NEC C85.90 *[N16]*
multiple myeloma C90.0- *[N16]*
obstruction N11.1
Salmonella infection A02.25
sarcoidosis D86.84
sepsis A41.9 *[N16]*
Sjögren's disease M35.04
toxoplasmosis B58.83
transplant rejection T86.91 *[N16]*
Wilson's disease E83.01 *[N16]*
nonobstructive N12
with reflux (vesicoureteral) N11.0
chronic N11.8
syphilitic A52.75
Pyelonephrosis (obstructive) N11.1
chronic N11.9
Pyelophlebitis I80.8
Pyeloureteritis cystica N28.85
Pyemia, pyemic (fever) (infection) (purulent) —*see also* Sepsis
joint —*see* Arthritis, pyogenic or pyemic
liver K75.1
pneumococcal A40.3
portal K75.1
postvaccinal T88.0
puerperal, postpartum, childbirth O85
specified organism NEC A41.89
tuberculous —*see* Tuberculosis, miliary
Pygopagus Q89.4
Pyknoepilepsy (idiopathic) —*see* Pyknolepsy
Pyknolepsy G40.A09
intractable G40.A19
with status epilepticus G40.A11
without status epilepticus G40.A19
not intractable G40.A09
with status epilepticus G40.A01
without status epilepticus G40.A09
Pylephlebitis K75.1
Pyle's syndrome Q78.5
Pylethrombophlebitis K75.1
Pylethrombosis K75.1
Pyloritis K29.90
with bleeding K29.91
Pylorospasm (reflex) NEC K31.3
congenital or infantile Q40.0
neurotic F45.8
newborn Q40.0
psychogenic F45.8
Pylorus, pyloric —*see* condition
Pyoarthrosis —*see* Arthritis, pyogenic or pyemic
Pyocele
mastoid —*see* Mastoiditis, acute
sinus (accessory) —*see* Sinusitis
turbinate (bone) J32.9
urethra —*see also* Urethritis N34.0
Pyocolpos —*see* Vaginitis
Pyocystitis N30.80
with hematuria N30.81
Pyoderma, pyodermia L08.0
gangrenosum L88
newborn P39.4
Pyoderma, pyodermia *(Continued)*
phagedenic L88
vegetans L08.81
Pyodermatitis L08.0
vegetans L08.81
Pyogenic —*see* condition
Pyohydronephrosis N13.6
Pyometra, pyometrium, pyometritis —*see* Endometritis
Pyomyositis (tropical) —*see* Myositis, infective
Pyonephritis N12
Pyonephrosis N13.6
tuberculous A18.11
Pyo-oophoritis —*see* Salpingo-oophoritis
Pyo-ovarium —*see* Salpingo-oophoritis
Pyopericarditis, pyopericardium I30.1
Pyophlebitis —*see* Phlebitis
Pyopneumopericardium I30.1
Pyopneumothorax (infective) J86.9
with fistula J86.0
tuberculous NEC A15.6
Pyosalpinx, pyosalpingitis —*see also* Salpingo-oophoritis
Pyothorax J86.9
with fistula J86.0
tuberculous NEC A15.6
Pyoureter N28.89
tuberculous A18.11
Pyramidopallidonigral syndrome G20
Pyrexia (of unknown origin) R50.9
atmospheric T67.0
during labor NEC O75.2
heat T67.0
newborn P81.9
environmentally-induced P81.0
persistent R50.9
puerperal O86.4
Pyroglobulinemia NEC E88.09
Pyromania F63.1
Pyrosis R12
Pyuria (bacterial) N39.0

◀ New ⇐ Revised ~~deleted~~ Deleted

Q

Q fever A78
  with pneumonia A78
Quadricuspid aortic valve Q23.8
Quadrilateral fever A78
Quadriparesis —*see* Quadriplegia
  meaning muscle weakness M62.81
Quadriplegia G82.50-
  complete
    C1-C4 level G82.51
    C5-C7 level G82.53
  congenital (cerebral) (spinal) G80.8
    spastic G80.0
Quadriplegia *(Continued)*
  embolic (current episode) I63.4- ⇐
  functional R53.2
  incomplete
    C1-C4 level G82.52
    C5-C7 level G82.54
  thrombotic (current episode) I63.3- ⇐
  traumatic — code to injury with seventh character S
    current episode —*see* Injury, spinal (cord), cervical
Quadruplet, pregnancy —*see* Pregnancy, quadruplet
Quarrelsomeness F60.3
Queensland fever A77.3
Quervain's disease M65.4
  thyroid E06.1
Queyrat's erythroplasia D07.4
  penis D07.4
  specified site —*see* Neoplasm, skin, in situ
  unspecified site D07.4
Quincke's disease or edema T78.3
  hereditary D84.1
Quinsy (gangrenous) J36
Quintan fever A79.0
Quintuplet, pregnancy —*see* Pregnancy, quintuplet

R

Rabbit fever —*see* Tularemia
Rabies A82.9
contact Z20.3
exposure to Z20.3
inoculation reaction —*see* Complications, vaccination
sylvatic A82.0
urban A82.1
Rachischisis —*see* Spina bifida
Rachitic —*see also* condition
deformities of spine (late effect) (sequelae) E64.3
pelvis (late effect) (sequelae) E64.3
with disproportion (fetopelvic) O33.0
causing obstructed labor O65.0
Rachitis, rachitism (acute) (tarda) —*see also* Rickets
renalis N25.0
sequelae E64.3
Radial nerve —*see* condition
Radiation
burn —*see* Burn
effects NOS T66
sickness NOS T66
therapy, encounter for Z51.0
Radiculitis (pressure) (vertebrogenic) —*see* Radiculopathy
Radiculomyelitis —*see also* Encephalitis
toxic, due to
Clostridium tetani A35
Corynebacterium diphtheriae A36.82
Radiculopathy M54.10
cervical region M54.12
cervicothoracic region M54.13
due to
disc disorder
C3 M50.11
C4 M50.11
C5 M50.121 ◀
C6 M50.122 ◀
C7 M50.123 ◀
C8 M50.13
displacement of intervertebral disc —*see* Disorder, disc, with, radiculopathy
leg M54.1-
lumbar region M54.16
lumbosacral region M54.17
occipito-atlanto-axial region M54.11
postherpetic B02.29
sacrococcygeal region M54.18
syphilitic A52.11
thoracic region (with visceral pain) M54.14
thoracolumbar region M54.15
Radiodermal burns (acute, chronic, or occupational) —*see* Burn
Radiodermatitis L58.9
acute L58.0
chronic L58.1
Radiotherapy session Z51.0
RAEB (refractory anemia with excess blasts) D46.2- ◀
Rage, meaning rabies —*see* Rabies
Ragpicker's disease A22.1
Ragsorter's disease A22.1
Raillietiniasis B71.8
Railroad neurosis F48.8
Railway spine F48.8
Raised —*see also* Elevated
antibody titer R76.0
Rake teeth, tooth M26.39
Rales R09.89
Ramifying renal pelvis Q63.8
Ramsay-Hunt disease or syndrome —*see also* Hunt's disease B02.21
meaning dyssynergia cerebellaris myoclonica G11.1
Ranula K11.6
congenital Q38.4
Rape
adult
confirmed T74.21
suspected T76.21
alleged, observation or examination, ruled out
adult Z04.41
child Z04.42
child
confirmed T74.22
suspected T76.22
Rapid
feeble pulse, due to shock, following injury T79.4
heart (beat) R00.0
psychogenic F45.8
second stage (delivery) O62.3
time-zone change syndrome —*see* Disorder, sleep, circadian rhythm, psychogenic
Rarefaction, bone —*see* Disorder, bone, density and structure, specified NEC
Rash (toxic) R21
canker A38.9
diaper L22
drug (internal use) L27.0
contact —*see also* Dermatitis, due to, drugs, external L25.1
following immunization T88.1
food —*see* Dermatitis, due to, food
heat L74.0
napkin (psoriasiform) L22
nettle —*see* Urticaria
pustular L08.0
rose R21
epidemic B06.9
scarlet A38.9
serum —*see also* Reaction, serum T80.69
wandering tongue K14.1
Rasmussen aneurysm —*see* Tuberculosis, pulmonary
Rasmussen encephalitis G04.81
Rat-bite fever A25.9
due to Streptobacillus moniliformis A25.1
spirochetal (morsus muris) A25.0
Rathke's pouch tumor D44.3
Raymond (-Céstan) syndrome I65.8
Raynaud's disease, phenomenon or syndrome (secondary) I73.00
with gangrene (symmetric) I73.01
RDS (newborn) (type I) P22.0
type II P22.1
Reaction —*see also* Disorder
adaptation —*see* Disorder, adjustment
adjustment (anxiety) (conduct disorder) (depressiveness) (distress) —*see* Disorder, adjustment
with
mutism, elective (child) (adolescent) F94.0
adverse
food (any) (ingested) NEC T78.1
anaphylactic —*see* Shock, anaphylactic, due to food
anaphylactoid —*see* Shock, anaphylactic
affective —*see* Disorder, mood
allergic —*see* Allergy
anaphylactic —*see* Shock, anaphylactic
anesthesia —*see* Anesthesia, complication
antitoxin (prophylactic) (therapeutic) —*see* Complications, vaccination
anxiety F41.1
Arthus —*see* Arthus' phenomenon
asthenic F48.8
combat and operational stress F43.0
compulsive F42.8 ◀
conversion F44.9
crisis, acute F43.0
deoxyribonuclease (DNA) (DNase) hypersensitivity D69.2
depressive (single episode) F32.9
affective (single episode) F31.4
recurrent episode F33.9
neurotic F34.1
psychoneurotic F34.1
Reaction *(Continued)*
depressive *(Continued)*
psychotic F32.3
recurrent —*see* Disorder, depressive, recurrent
dissociative F44.9
drug NEC T88.7
addictive —*see* Dependence, drug
transmitted via placenta or breast milk —*see* Absorption, drug, addictive, through placenta
allergic —*see* Allergy, drug
lichenoid L43.2
newborn P93.8
gray baby syndrome P93.0
overdose or poisoning (by accident) —*see* Table of Drugs and Chemicals, by drug, poisoning
photoallergic L56.1
phototoxic L56.0
withdrawal —*see* Dependence, by drug, with, withdrawal
infant of dependent mother P96.1
newborn P96.1
wrong substance given or taken (by accident) —*see* Table of Drugs and Chemicals, by drug, poisoning
fear F40.9
child (abnormal) F93.8
febrile nonhemolytic transfusion (FNHTR) R50.84
fluid loss, cerebrospinal G97.1
foreign
body NEC —*see* Granuloma, foreign body
in operative wound (inadvertently left) —*see* Foreign body, accidentally left during a procedure
substance accidentally left during a procedure (chemical) (powder) (talc) T81.60
aseptic peritonitis T81.61
body or object (instrument) (sponge) (swab) —*see* Foreign body, accidentally left during a procedure
specified reaction NEC T81.69
grief —*see* Disorder, adjustment
Herxheimer's R68.89
hyperkinetic —*see* Hyperkinesia
hypochondriacal F45.20
hypoglycemic, due to insulin E16.0
with coma (diabetic) —*see* Diabetes, coma
nondiabetic E15
therapeutic misadventure —*see* subcategory T38.3
hypomanic F30.8
hysterical F44.9
immunization —*see* Complications, vaccination
incompatibility
ABO blood group (infusion) (transfusion) —*see* Complication (s), transfusion, incompatibility reaction, ABO
delayed serologic T80.39
minor blood group (Duffy) (E) (K(ell)) (Kidd) (Lewis) (M) (N) (P) (S) T80.89
Rh (factor) (infusion) (transfusion) —*see* Complication (s), transfusion, incompatibility reaction, Rh (factor)
inflammatory —*see* Infection
infusion —*see* Complications, infusion
inoculation (immune serum) —*see* Complications, vaccination
insulin T38.3-
involutional psychotic —*see* Disorder, depressive
leukemoid D72.823
basophilic D72.823
lymphocytic D72.823
monocytic D72.823
myelocytic D72.823
neutrophilic D72.823

◀ New ◀ Revised ~~deleted~~ Deleted

Reaction *(Continued)*
LSD (acute)
due to drug abuse —*see* Abuse, drug, hallucinogen
due to drug dependence —*see* Dependence, drug, hallucinogen
lumbar puncture G97.1
manic-depressive —*see* Disorder, bipolar
neurasthenic F48.8
neurogenic —*see* Neurosis
neurotic F48.9
neurotic-depressive F34.1
nitritoid —*see* Crisis, nitritoid - obsessive-compulsive F42
nonspecific
to
cell mediated immunity measurement of gamma interferon antigen response without active tuberculosis R76.12
QuantiFERON-TB test (QFT) without active tuberculosis R76.12
tuberculin test —*see also* Reaction, tuberculin skin test R76.11
obsessive-compulsive F42.8 ⇐
organic, acute or subacute —*see* Delirium
paranoid (acute) F23
chronic F22
senile F03
passive dependency F60.7
phobic F40.9
post-traumatic stress, uncomplicated Z73.3
psychogenic F99
psychoneurotic —*see also* Neurosis
compulsive F42.8 ⇐
depersonalization F48.1
depressive F34.1
hypochondriacal F45.20
neurasthenic F48.8
obsessive F42.8 ⇐
psychophysiologic —*see* Disorder, somatoform
psychosomatic —*see* Disorder, somatoform
psychotic —*see* Psychosis
scarlet fever toxin —*see* Complications, vaccination
schizophrenic F23
acute (brief) (undifferentiated) F23
latent F21
undifferentiated (acute) (brief) F23
serological for syphilis —*see* Serology for syphilis
serum T80.69
anaphylactic (immediate) —*see also* Shock, anaphylactic T80.59
specified reaction NEC
due to
administration of blood and blood products T80.61
immunization T80.62
serum specified NEC T80.69
vaccination T80.62
situational —*see* Disorder, adjustment
somatization —*see* Disorder, somatoform
spinal puncture G97.1
stress (severe) F43.9
acute (agitation) ("daze") (disorientation) (disturbance of consciousness) (flight reaction) (fugue) F43.0
specified NEC F43.8
surgical procedure —*see* Complications, surgical procedure
tetanus antitoxin —*see* Complications, vaccination
toxic, to local anesthesia T81.59 ⇐
in labor and delivery O74.4
in pregnancy O29.3X-
postpartum, puerperal O89.3
toxin-antitoxin —*see* Complications, vaccination

Reaction *(Continued)*
transfusion (blood) (bone marrow) (lymphocytes) (allergic) —*see* Complications, transfusion
tuberculin skin test, abnormal R76.11
vaccination (any) —*see* Complications, vaccination
withdrawing, child or adolescent F93.8
Reactive airway disease —*see* Asthma
Reactive depression —*see* Reaction, depressive
Rearrangement
chromosomal
balanced (in) Q95.9
abnormal individual (autosomal) Q95.2
non-sex (autosomal) chromosomes Q95.2
sex/non-sex chromosomes Q95.3
specified NEC Q95.8
Recalcitrant patient —*see* Noncompliance
Recanalization, thrombus —*see* Thrombosis
Recession, receding
chamber angle (eye) H21.55-
chin M26.09
gingival (generalized) (localized) (postinfective) (postoperative) K06.00 ⇐
Miller Class I K06.01 ◀
Miller Class II K06.02 ◀
Miller Class III K06.03 ◀
Miller Class IV K06.04 ◀
Recklinghausen's disease Q85.01
bones E21.0
Reclus' disease (cystic) —*see* Mastopathy, cystic
Recrudescent typhus (fever) A75.1
Recruitment, auditory H93.21-
Rectalgia K62.89
Rectitis K62.89
Rectocele
female (without uterine prolapse) N81.6
with uterine prolapse N81.4
incomplete N81.2
in pregnancy —*see* Pregnancy, complicated by, abnormal, pelvic organs or tissues NEC
male K62.3
Rectosigmoid junction —*see* condition
Rectosigmoiditis K63.89
ulcerative (chronic) K51.30
with
complication K51.319
abscess K51.314
fistula K51.313
obstruction K51.312
rectal bleeding K51.311
specified NEC K51.318
Rectourethral —*see* condition
Rectovaginal —*see* condition
Rectovesical —*see* condition
Rectum, rectal —*see* condition
Recurrent —*see* condition
pregnancy loss —*see* Loss (of), pregnancy, recurrent
Red bugs B88.0
Red-cedar lung or pneumonitis J67.8
Red tide —*see also* Table of Drugs and Chemicals T65.82-
Reduced
mobility Z74.09
ventilatory or vital capacity R94.2
Redundant, redundancy
anus (congenital) Q43.8
clitoris N90.89
colon (congenital) Q43.8
foreskin (congenital) N47.8
intestine (congenital) Q43.8
labia N90.69 ⇐
organ or site, congenital NEC —*see* Accessory
panniculus (abdominal) E65
prepuce (congenital) N47.8
pylorus K31.89
rectum (congenital) Q43.8
scrotum N50.89 ⇐

Redundant, redundancy *(Continued)*
sigmoid (congenital) Q43.8
skin L98.7 ⇐
~~eyelids — see Blepharochalasis~~
and subcutaneous tissue L98.7 ◀
of face L57.4 ◀
eyelids —*see* Blepharochalasis ◀
stomach K31.89
Reduplication —*see* Duplication
Reflex R29.2
hyperactive gag J39.2
pupillary, abnormal —*see* Anomaly, pupil, function
vasoconstriction I73.9
vasovagal R55
Reflux K21.9
acid K21.9
esophageal K21.9
with esophagitis K21.0
newborn P78.83
gastroesophageal K21.9
with esophagitis K21.0
mitral —*see* Insufficiency, mitral
ureteral —*see* Reflux, vesicoureteral
vesicoureteral (with scarring) N13.70
with
nephropathy N13.729
with hydroureter N13.739
bilateral N13.732
unilateral N13.731
without hydroureter N13.729
bilateral N13.722
unilateral N13.721
bilateral N13.722
unilateral N13.721
pyelonephritis (chronic) N11.0
without nephropathy N13.71
congenital Q62.7
Reforming, artificial openings —*see* Attention to, artificial, opening
Refractive error —*see* Disorder, refraction
Refsum's disease or syndrome G60.1
Refusal of
food, psychogenic F50.89 ⇐
treatment (because of) Z53.20
left against medical advice (AMA) Z53.21
patient's decision NEC Z53.29
reasons of belief or group pressure Z53.1
Regional —*see* condition
Regurgitation R11.10
aortic (valve) —*see* Insufficiency, aortic
food —*see also* Vomiting
with reswallowing —*see* Rumination
newborn P92.1
gastric contents —*see* Vomiting
heart —*see* Endocarditis
mitral (valve) —*see* Insufficiency, mitral
congenital Q23.3
myocardial —*see* Endocarditis
pulmonary (valve) (heart) I37.1
congenital Q22.2
syphilitic A52.03
tricuspid —*see* Insufficiency, tricuspid
valve, valvular —*see* Endocarditis
congenital Q24.8
vesicoureteral —*see* Reflux, vesicoureteral
Reichmann's disease or syndrome K31.89
Reifenstein syndrome E34.52
~~Reinsertion, contraceptive device Z30.433~~
Reinsertion ◀
implantable subdermal contraceptive Z30.46 ◀
intrauterine contraceptive device Z30.433 ◀
Reiter's disease, syndrome, or urethritis M02.30
ankle M02.37-
elbow M02.32-
foot joint M02.37-
hand joint M02.34-
hip M02.35-
knee M02.36-
multiple site M02.39

Reiter's disease, syndrome, or urethritis *(Continued)*
shoulder M02.31-
vertebra M02.38
wrist M02.33-
Rejection
food, psychogenic F50.89 ⬅
transplant T86.91
bone T86.830
marrow T86.01
cornea T86.840
heart T86.21
with lung (s) T86.31
intestine T86.850
kidney T86.11
liver T86.41
lung (s) T86.810
with heart T86.31
organ (immune or nonimmune cause) T86.91
pancreas T86.890
skin (allograft) (autograft) T86.820
specified NEC T86.890
stem cell (peripheral blood) (umbilical cord) T86.5
Relapsing fever A68.9
Carter's (Asiatic) A68.1
Dutton's (West African) A68.1
Koch's A68.9
louse-borne (epidemic) A68.0
Novy's (American) A68.1
Obermeyers's (European) A68.0
Spirillum A68.9
tick-borne (endemic) A68.1
Relationship
occlusal
open anterior M26.220
open posterior M26.221
Relaxation
anus (sphincter) K62.89
psychogenic F45.8
arch (foot) —*see also* Deformity, limb, flat foot
back ligaments —*see* Instability, joint, spine
bladder (sphincter) N31.2
cardioesophageal K21.9
cervix —*see* Incompetency, cervix
diaphragm J98.6
joint (capsule) (ligament) (paralytic) —*see* Flail, joint
congenital NEC Q74.8
lumbosacral (joint) —*see* subcategory M53.2
pelvic floor N81.89
perineum N81.89
posture R29.3
rectum (sphincter) K62.89
sacroiliac (joint) —*see* subcategory M53.2
scrotum N50.89 ⬅
urethra (sphincter) N36.44
vesical N31.2
Release from prison, anxiety concerning Z65.2
Remains
canal of Cloquet Q14.0
capsule (opaque) Q14.8
Remittent fever (malarial) B54
Remnant
canal of Cloquet Q14.0
capsule (opaque) Q14.8
cervix, cervical stump (acquired) (postoperative) N88.8
cystic duct, postcholecystectomy K91.5
fingernail L60.8
congenital Q84.6
meniscus, knee —*see* Derangement, knee, meniscus, specified NEC
thyroglossal duct Q89.2
tonsil J35.8
infected (chronic) J35.01
urachus Q64.4
Removal (from) (of)
artificial
arm Z44.00-
complete Z44.01-
partial Z44.02-
eye Z44.2-
leg Z44.10-
complete Z44.11-
partial Z44.12-
breast implant Z45.81
cardiac pulse generator (battery) (end-of-life) Z45.010
catheter (urinary) (indwelling) Z46.6
from artificial opening —*see* Attention to, artificial, opening
non-vascular Z46.82
vascular NEC Z45.2
device Z46.9
contraceptive Z30.432
implantable subdermal Z30.46 ◀
implanted NEC Z45.89
specified NEC Z46.89
drains Z48.03
dressing (nonsurgical) Z48.00
surgical Z48.01
external
fixation device — code to fracture with seventh character D
prosthesis, prosthetic device Z44.9
breast Z44.3-
specified NEC Z44.8
home in childhood (to foster home or institution) Z62.29
ileostomy Z43.2
insulin pump Z46.81
myringotomy device (stent) (tube) Z45.82
nervous system device NEC Z46.2
brain neuropacemaker Z46.2
visual substitution device Z46.2
implanted Z45.31
non-vascular catheter Z46.82
organ, prophylactic (for neoplasia management) —*see* Prophylactic, organ removal
orthodontic device Z46.4
staples Z48.02
stent
ureteral Z46.6
suture Z48.02
urinary device Z46.6
vascular access device or catheter Z45.2
Ren
arcuatus Q63.1
mobile, mobilis N28.89
congenital Q63.8
unguliformis Q63.1
Renal —*see* condition
Rendu-Osler-Weber disease or syndrome I78.0
Reninoma D41.0-
Renon-Delille syndrome E23.3
Reovirus, as cause of disease classified elsewhere B97.5
Repeated falls NEC R29.6
Replaced chromosome by dicentric ring Q93.2
Replacement by artificial or mechanical device or prosthesis of
bladder Z96.0
blood vessel NEC Z95.828
bone NEC Z96.7
cochlea Z96.21
coronary artery Z95.5
eustachian tube Z96.29
eye globe Z97.0
heart Z95.812
valve Z95.2
prosthetic Z95.2
specified NEC Z95.4
xenogenic Z95.3
intestine Z96.89
Replacement by artificial or mechanical device or prosthesis of *(Continued)*
joint Z96.60
hip —*see* Presence, hip joint implant
knee —*see* Presence, knee joint implant
specified site NEC Z96.698
larynx Z96.3
lens Z96.1
limb (s) —*see* Presence, artificial, limb
mandible NEC (for tooth root implant (s)) Z96.5
organ NEC Z96.89
peripheral vessel NEC Z95.828
stapes Z96.29
teeth Z97.2
tendon Z96.7
tissue NEC Z96.89
tooth root (s) Z96.5
vessel NEC Z95.828
coronary (artery) Z95.5
Request for expert evidence Z04.8
Reserve, decreased or low
cardiac —*see* Disease, heart
kidney N28.89
Residual —*see also* condition
ovary syndrome N99.83
state, schizophrenic F20.5
urine R39.198 ⬅
Resistance, resistant (to)
activated protein C D68.51
complicating pregnancy O26.89
insulin E88.81
organism (s)
to
drug Z16.30 ⬅
aminoglycosides Z16.29
amoxicillin Z16.11
ampicillin Z16.11
antibiotic (s) Z16.20
multiple Z16.24
specified NEC Z16.29
antifungal Z16.32
antimicrobial (single) Z16.30
multiple Z16.35
specified NEC Z16.39
~~antimycobacterial (single) Z16.341~~
~~multiple Z16.342~~
antimycobacterial (single) Z16.341 ◀
multiple Z16.342 ◀
antiparasitic Z16.31
antiviral Z16.33
beta lactam antibiotics Z16.10
specified NEC Z16.19
cephalosporins Z16.19
extended beta lactamase (ESBL) Z16.12
fluoroquinolones Z16.23
macrolides Z16.29
methicillin —*see* MRSA
multiple drugs (MDRO)
antibiotics Z16.24
antimicrobial Z16.35 ◀
antimycobacterials Z16.342 ◀
penicillins Z16.11
quinine (and related compounds) Z16.31
quinolones Z16.23
sulfonamides Z16.29
tetracyclines Z16.29
tuberculostatics (single) Z16.341
multiple Z16.342
vancomycin Z16.21
related antibiotics Z16.22
thyroid hormone E07.89
Resorption
dental (roots) K03.3
alveoli M26.79
teeth (external) (internal) (pathological) (roots) K03.3

◀ New ⬅ Revised ~~deleted~~ Deleted

Respiration
Cheyne-Stokes R06.3
decreased due to shock, following injury T79.4
disorder of, psychogenic F45.8
insufficient, or poor R06.89
newborn P28.5
painful R07.1
sighing, psychogenic F45.8
Respiratory —*see also* condition
distress syndrome (newborn) (type I) P22.0
type II P22.1
syncytial virus, as cause of disease classified elsewhere B97.4
Respite care Z75.5
Response (drug)
photoallergic L56.1
phototoxic L56.0
Restenosis ◀
stent ◀
vascular ◀
end stent ◀
adjacent to stent —*see* Arteriosclerosis ◀
within the stent ◀
coronary T82.855 ◀
peripheral T82.856 ◀
in stent ◀
coronary vessel T82.855 ◀
peripheral vessel T82.856 ◀
Restless legs (syndrome) G25.81
Restlessness R45.1
Restoration (of)
dental
aesthetically inadequate or displeasing K08.56
defective K08.50
specified NEC K08.59
failure of marginal integrity K08.51
failure of periodontal anatomical intergrity K08.54
organ continuity from previous sterilization (tuboplasty) (vasoplasty) Z31.0
aftercare Z31.42
tooth (existing)
contours biologically incompatible with oral health K08.54
open margins K08.51
overhanging K08.52
poor aesthetic K08.56
poor gingival margins K08.51
unsatisfactory, of tooth K08.50
specified NEC K08.59
Restorative material (dental)
allergy to K08.55
fractured K08.539
with loss of material K08.531
without loss of material K08.530
unrepairable overhanging of K08.52
Restriction of housing space Z59.1
Rests, ovarian, in fallopian tube Q50.6
Restzustand (schizophrenic) F20.5
Retained —*see also* Retention
cholelithiasis following cholecystectomy K91.86
foreign body fragments (type of) Z18.9
acrylics Z18.2
animal quill (s) or spines Z18.31
cement Z18.83
concrete Z18.83
crystalline Z18.83
depleted isotope Z18.09
depleted uranium Z18.01
diethylhexylphthalates Z18.2
glass Z18.81
isocyanate Z18.2
magnetic metal Z18.11
metal Z18.10
nonmagnetic metal Z18.12
nontherapeutic radioactive Z18.09
Retained *(Continued)*
foreign body fragments *(Continued)*
organic NEC Z18.39
plastic Z18.2
quill (s) (animal) Z18.31
radioactive (nontherapeutic) NEC Z18.09
specified NEC Z18.89
spine (s) (animal) Z18.31
stone Z18.83
tooth (teeth) Z18.32
wood Z18.33
fragments (type of) Z18.9
acrylics Z18.2
animal quill (s) or spines Z18.31
cement Z18.83
concrete Z18.83
crystalline Z18.83
depleted isotope Z18.09
depleted uranium Z18.01
diethylhexylphthalates Z18.2
glass Z18.81
isocyanate Z18.2
magnetic metal Z18.11
metal Z18.10
nonmagnetic metal Z18.12
nontherapeutic radioactive Z18.09
organic NEC Z18.39
plastic Z18.2
quill (s) (animal) Z18.31
radioactive (nontherapeutic) NEC Z18.09
specified NEC Z18.89
spine (s) (animal) Z18.31
stone Z18.83
tooth (teeth) Z18.32
wood Z18.33
gallstones, following cholecystectomy K91.86
Retardation
development, developmental, specific —*see* Disorder, developmental
endochondral bone growth —*see* Disorder, bone, development or growth
growth R62.50
due to malnutrition E45
mental —*see* Disability, intellectual
motor function, specific F82
physical (child) R62.52
due to malnutrition E45
reading (specific) F81.0
spelling (specific) (without reading disorder) F81.81
Retching —*see* Vomiting
Retention —*see also* Retained
bladder —*see* Retention, urine
carbon dioxide E87.2
cholelithiasis following cholecystectomy K91.86
cyst —*see* Cyst
dead
fetus (at or near term) (mother) O36.4
early fetal death O02.1
ovum O02.0
decidua (fragments) (following delivery) (with hemorrhage) O72.2
without hemorrhage O73.1
deciduous tooth K00.6
dental root K08.3
fecal —*see* Constipation
fetus
dead O36.4
early O02.1
fluid R60.9
foreign body —*see also* Foreign body, retained
current trauma - code as Foreign body, by site or type
gallstones, following cholecystectomy K91.86
gastric K31.89
intrauterine contraceptive device, in pregnancy —*see* Pregnancy, complicated by, retention, intrauterine device
Retention *(Continued)*
membranes (complicating delivery) (with hemorrhage) O72.2
with abortion —*see* Abortion, by type without hemorrhage O73.1
meniscus —*see* Derangement, meniscus
menses N94.89
milk (puerperal, postpartum) O92.79
nitrogen, extrarenal R39.2
ovary syndrome N99.83
placenta (total) (with hemorrhage) O72.0
without hemorrhage O73.0
portions or fragments (with hemorrhage) O72.2
without hemorrhage O73.1
products of conception
early pregnancy (dead fetus) O02.1
following
delivery (with hemorrhage) O72.2
without hemorrhage O73.1
secundines (following delivery) (with hemorrhage) O72.0
without hemorrhage O73.0
complicating puerperium (delayed hemorrhage) O72.2
partial O72.2
without hemorrhage O73.1
smegma, clitoris N90.89
urine R33.9
drug-induced R33.0
due to hyperplasia (hypertrophy) of prostate —*see* Hyperplasia, prostate
organic R33.8
drug-induced R33.0
psychogenic F45.8
specified NEC R33.8
water (in tissues) —*see* Edema
Reticular erythematous mucinosis L98.5
Reticulation, dust —*see* Pneumoconiosis
Reticulocytosis R70.1
Reticuloendotheliosis
acute infantile C96.0
leukemic C91.4-
~~malignant C96.9~~
nonlipid C96.0
Reticulohistiocytoma (giant-cell) D76.3
Reticuloid, actinic L57.1
Reticulosis (skin)
acute of infancy C96.0
hemophagocytic, familial D76.1
histiocytic medullary C96.A ⇐
lipomelanotic I89.8
malignant (midline) C86.0
~~nonlipid C96.0~~
polymorphic C86.0
Sézary —*see* Sézary disease
Retina, retinal —*see also* condition
dark area D49.81
Retinitis —*see also* Inflammation, chorioretinal
albuminurica N18.9 *[H32]*
diabetic —*see* Diabetes, retinitis
disciformis —*see* Degeneration, macula
focal —*see* Inflammation, chorioretinal, focal
gravidarum —*see* Pregnancy, complicated by, specified pregnancy-related condition NEC
juxtapapillaris —*see* Inflammation, chorioretinal, focal, juxtapapillary
luetic —*see* Retinitis, syphilitic
pigmentosa H35.52
proliferans —*see* Disorder, globe, degenerative, specified type NEC
proliferating —*see* Disorder, globe, degenerative, specified type NEC
renal N18.9 *[H32]*
syphilitic (early) (secondary) A51.43
central, recurrent A52.71
congenital (early) A50.01 *[H32]*
late A52.71
tuberculous A18.53

Retinoblastoma C69.2-
differentiated C69.2-
undifferentiated C69.2-
Retinochoroiditis —*see also* Inflammation, chorioretinal
disseminated —*see* Inflammation, chorioretinal, disseminated
syphilitic A52.71
focal —*see* Inflammation, chorioretinal
juxtapapillaris —*see* Inflammation, chorioretinal, focal, juxtapapillary
Retinopathy (background) H35.00
arteriosclerotic I70.8 *[H35.0-]*
atherosclerotic I70.8 *[H35.0-]*
central serous —*see* Chorioretinopathy, central serous
Coats H35.02-
diabetic —*see* Diabetes, retinopathy
exudative H35.02-
hypertensive H35.03-
in (due to)
diabetes —*see* Diabetes, retinopathy
sickle-cell disorders D57.- *[H36]*
of prematurity H35.10-
stage 0 H35.11-
stage 1 H35.12-
stage 2 H35.13-
stage 3 H35.14-
stage 4 H35.15-
stage 5 H35.16-
pigmentary, congenital —*see* Dystrophy, retina
proliferative NEC H35.2-
diabetic —*see* Diabetes, retinopathy, proliferative
sickle-cell D57.- *[H36]*
solar H31.02-
Retinoschisis H33.10-
congenital Q14.1
specified type NEC H33.19-
Retortamoniasis A07.8
Retractile testis Q55.22
Retraction
cervix —*see* Retroversion, uterus
drum (membrane) —*see* Disorder, tympanic membrane, specified NEC
finger —*see* Deformity, finger
lid H02.539
left H02.536
lower H02.535
upper H02.534
right H02.533
lower H02.532
upper H02.531
lung J98.4
mediastinum J98.59 ◄
nipple N64.53
associated with
lactation O92.03
pregnancy O92.01-
puerperium O92.02
congenital Q83.8
palmar fascia M72.0
pleura —*see* Pleurisy
ring, uterus (Bandl's) (pathological) O62.4
sternum (congenital) Q76.7
acquired M95.4
uterus —*see* Retroversion, uterus
valve (heart) —*see* Endocarditis
Retrobulbar —*see* condition
Retrocecal —*see* condition
Retrocession —*see* Retroversion
Retrodisplacement —*see* Retroversion
Retroflection, retroflexion —*see* Retroversion
Retrognathia, retrognathism (mandibular) (maxillary) M26.19
Retrograde menstruation N92.5
Retroperineal —*see* condition
Retroperitoneal —*see* condition
Retroperitonitis K68.9
Retropharyngeal —*see* condition
Retroplacental —*see* condition
Retroposition —*see* Retroversion
Retroprosthetic membrane T85.398
Retrosternal thyroid (congenital) Q89.2
Retroversion, retroverted
cervix —*see* Retroversion, uterus
female NEC —*see* Retroversion, uterus
iris H21.89
testis (congenital) Q55.29
uterus (acquired) (acute) (any degree) (asymptomatic) (cervix) (postinfectional) (postpartal, old) N85.4
congenital Q51.818
in pregnancy O34.53-
Retrovirus, as cause of disease classified elsewhere B97.30
human
immunodeficiency, type 2 (HIV 2) B97.35
T-cell lymphotropic
type I (HTLV-I) B97.33
type II (HTLV-II) B97.34
lentivirus B97.31
oncovirus B97.32
specified NEC B97.39
Retrusion, premaxilla (developmental) M26.09
Rett's disease or syndrome F84.2
Reverse peristalsis R19.2
Reye's syndrome G93.7
Rh (factor)
hemolytic disease (newborn) P55.0
incompatibility, immunization or sensitization
affecting management of pregnancy NEC O36.09-
anti-D antibody O36.01-
newborn P55.0
transfusion reaction —*see* Complication (s), transfusion, incompatibility reaction, Rh (factor)
negative mother affecting newborn P55.0
titer elevated —*see* Complication (s), transfusion, incompatibility reaction, Rh (factor)
transfusion reaction —*see* Complication (s), transfusion, incompatibility reaction, Rh (factor)
Rhabdomyolysis (idiopathic) **NEC** M62.82
traumatic T79.6
Rhabdomyoma —*see also* Neoplasm, connective tissue, benign
adult —*see* Neoplasm, connective tissue, benign
fetal —*see* Neoplasm, connective tissue, benign
glycogenic —*see* Neoplasm, connective tissue, benign
Rhabdomyosarcoma (any type) —*see* Neoplasm, connective tissue, malignant
Rhabdosarcoma —*see* Rhabdomyosarcoma
Rhesus (factor) **incompatibility** —*see* Rh, incompatibility
Rheumatic (acute) (subacute) (chronic)
adherent pericardium I09.2
coronary arteritis I01.9
degeneration, myocardium I09.0
fever (acute) —*see* Fever, rheumatic
heart —*see* Disease, heart, rheumatic
myocardial degeneration —*see* Degeneration, myocardium
myocarditis (chronic) (inactive) (with chorea) I09.0
with chorea (acute) (rheumatic) (Sydenham's) I02.0
active or acute I01.2
pancarditis, acute I01.8
with chorea (acute (rheumatic) Sydenham's) I02.0
pericarditis (active) (acute) (with effusion) (with pneumonia) I01.0
with chorea (acute) (rheumatic) (Sydenham's) I02.0
chronic or inactive I09.2
Rheumatic *(Continued)*
pneumonia I00 *[J17]*
torticollis M43.6
typhoid fever A01.09
Rheumatism (articular) (neuralgic) (nonarticular) M79.0
gout —*see* Arthritis, rheumatoid
intercostal, meaning Tietze's disease M94.0
palindromic (any site) M12.30
ankle M12.37-
elbow M12.32-
foot joint M12.37-
hand joint M12.34-
hip M12.35-
knee M12.36-
multiple site M12.39
shoulder M12.31-
specified joint NEC M12.38
vertebrae M12.38
wrist M12.33-
sciatic M54.4-
Rheumatoid —*see also* condition
arthritis —*see also* Arthritis, rheumatoid
with involvement of organs NEC M05.60
ankle M05.67-
elbow M05.62-
foot joint M05.67-
hand joint M05.64-
hip M05.65-
knee M05.66-
multiple site M05.69
shoulder M05.61-
vertebra —*see* Spondylitis, ankylosing
wrist M05.63-
seronegative —*see* Arthritis, rheumatoid, seronegative
seropositive —*see* Arthritis, rheumatoid, seropositive
carditis M05.30
ankle M05.37-
elbow M05.32-
foot joint M05.37-
hand joint M05.34-
hip M05.35-
knee M05.36-
multiple site M05.39
shoulder M05.31-
vertebra —*see* Spondylitis, ankylosing
wrist M05.33-
endocarditis —*see* Rheumatoid, carditis
lung (disease) M05.10
ankle M05.17-
elbow M05.12-
foot joint M05.17-
hand joint M05.14-
hip M05.15-
knee M05.16-
multiple site M05.19
shoulder M05.11-
vertebra —*see* Spondylitis, ankylosing
wrist M05.13-
myocarditis —*see* Rheumatoid, carditis
myopathy M05.40
ankle M05.47-
elbow M05.42-
foot joint M05.47-
hand joint M05.44-
hip M05.45-
knee M05.46-
multiple site M05.49
shoulder M05.41-
vertebra —*see* Spondylitis, ankylosing
wrist M05.43-
pericarditis —*see* Rheumatoid, carditis
polyarthritis —*see* Arthritis, rheumatoid
polyneuropathy M05.50
ankle M05.57-
elbow M05.52-
foot joint M05.57-
hand joint M05.54-
hip M05.55-

◄ New ◄ Revised ~~deleted~~ Deleted

Rheumatoid *(Continued)*
polyneuropathy *(Continued)*
knee M05.56-
multiple site M05.59
shoulder M05.51-
vertebra —*see* Spondylitis, ankylosing
wrist M05.53-
vasculitis M05.20
ankle M05.27-
elbow M05.22-
foot joint M05.27-
hand joint M05.24-
hip M05.25-
knee M05.26-
multiple site M05.29
shoulder M05.21-
vertebra —*see* Spondylitis, ankylosing
wrist M05.23-
Rhinitis (atrophic) (catarrhal) (chronic) (croupous) (fibrinous) (granulomatous) (hyperplastic) (hypertrophic) (membranous) (obstructive) (purulent) (suppurative) (ulcerative) J31.0
with
sore throat —*see* Nasopharyngitis
acute J00
allergic J30.9
with asthma J45.909
with
exacerbation (acute) J45.901
status asthmaticus J45.902
due to
food J30.5
pollen J30.1
nonseasonal J30.89
perennial J30.89
seasonal NEC J30.2
specified NEC J30.89
infective J00
pneumococcal J00
syphilitic A52.73
congenital A50.05 *[J99]*
tuberculous A15.8
vasomotor J30.0
Rhinoantritis (chronic) —*see* Sinusitis, maxillary
Rhinodacryolith —*see* Dacryolith
Rhinolith (nasal sinus) J34.89
Rhinomegaly J34.89
Rhinopharyngitis (acute) (subacute) —*see also* Nasopharyngitis
chronic J31.1
destructive ulcerating A66.5
mutilans A66.5
Rhinophyma L71.1
Rhinorrhea J34.89
cerebrospinal (fluid) G96.0
paroxysmal —*see* Rhinitis, allergic
spasmodic —*see* Rhinitis, allergic
Rhinosalpingitis —*see* Salpingitis, eustachian
Rhinoscleroma A48.8
Rhinosporidiosis B48.1
Rhinovirus infection NEC B34.8
Rhizomelic chondrodysplasia punctata E71.540
Rhythm
atrioventricular nodal I49.8
disorder I49.9
coronary sinus I49.8
ectopic I49.8
nodal I49.8
escape I49.9
heart, abnormal I49.9
idioventricular I44.2
nodal I49.8
sleep, inversion G47.2-
nonorganic origin —*see* Disorder, sleep, circadian rhythm, psychogenic
Rhytidosis facialis L98.8
Rib —*see also* condition
cervical Q76.5
Riboflavin deficiency E53.0
Rice bodies —*see also* Loose, body, joint
knee M23.4-
Richter syndrome —*see* Leukemia, chronic lymphocytic, B-cell type
Richter's hernia —*see* Hernia, abdomen, with obstruction
Ricinism —*see* Poisoning, food, noxious, plant
Rickets (active) (acute) (adolescent) (chest wall) (congenital) (current) (infantile) (intestinal) E55.0
adult —*see* Osteomalacia
celiac K90.0
hypophosphatemic with nephrotic-glycosuric dwarfism E72.09
inactive E64.3
kidney N25.0
renal N25.0
sequelae, any E64.3
vitamin-D-resistant E83.31 *[M90.80]*
Rickettsial disease A79.9
specified type NEC A79.89
Rickettsialpox (Rickettsia akari) A79.1
Rickettsiosis A79.9
due to
Ehrlichia sennetsu A79.81
Rickettsia akari (rickettsialpox) A79.1
specified type NEC A79.89
tick-borne A77.9
vesicular A79.1
Rider's bone —*see* Ossification, muscle, specified NEC
Ridge, alveolus —*see also* condition
flabby K06.8
Ridged ear, congenital Q17.3
Riedel's
lobe, liver Q44.7
struma, thyroiditis or disease E06.5
Rieger's anomaly or syndrome Q13.81
Riehl's melanosis L81.4
Rietti-Greppi-Micheli anemia D56.9
Rieux's hernia —*see* Hernia, abdomen, specified site NEC
Riga (-Fede) disease K14.0
Riggs' disease —*see* Periodontitis
Right aortic arch Q25.47 ◀
Right middle lobe syndrome J98.11
Rigid, rigidity —*see also* condition
abdominal R19.30
with severe abdominal pain R10.0
epigastric R19.36
generalized R19.37
left lower quadrant R19.34
left upper quadrant R19.32
periumbilic R19.35
right lower quadrant R19.33
right upper quadrant R19.31
articular, multiple, congenital Q68.8
cervix (uteri) in pregnancy —*see* Pregnancy, complicated by, abnormal, cervix
hymen (acquired) (congenital) N89.6
nuchal R29.1
pelvic floor in pregnancy —*see* Pregnancy, complicated by, abnormal, pelvic organs or tissues NEC
perineum or vulva in pregnancy —*see* Pregnancy, complicated by, abnormal, vulva
spine —*see* Dorsopathy, specified NEC
vagina in pregnancy —*see* Pregnancy, complicated by, abnormal, vagina
Rigors R68.89
with fever R50.9
Riley-Day syndrome G90.1
RIND (reversible ischemic neurologic deficit) I63.9
Ring (s)
aorta (vascular) Q25.45 ⇐
Bandl's O62.4
contraction, complicating delivery O62.4
Ring (s) *(Continued)*
esophageal, lower (muscular) K22.2
Fleischer's (cornea) H18.04-
hymenal, tight (acquired) (congenital) N89.6
Kayser-Fleischer (cornea) H18.04-
retraction, uterus, pathological O62.4
Schatzki's (esophagus) (lower) K22.2
congenital Q39.3
Soemmerring's —*see* Cataract, secondary
vascular (congenital) Q25.8
aorta Q25.45 ⇐
Ringed hair (congenital) Q84.1
Ringworm B35.9
beard B35.0
black dot B35.0
body B35.4
Burmese B35.5
corporeal B35.4
foot B35.3
groin B35.6
hand B35.2
honeycomb B35.0
nails B35.1
perianal (area) B35.6
scalp B35.0
specified NEC B35.8
Tokelau B35.5
Rise, venous pressure I87.8
Rising, PSA following treatment for malignant neoplasm of prostate R97.21 ◀
Risk, suicidal
meaning personal history of attempted suicide Z91.5
meaning suicidal ideation —*see* Ideation, suicidal
Ritter's disease L00
Rivalry, sibling Z62.891
Rivalta's disease A42.2
River blindness B73.01
Robert's pelvis Q74.2
with disproportion (fetopelvic) O33.0
causing obstructed labor O65.0
Robin (-Pierre) syndrome Q87.0
Robinow-Silvermann-Smith syndrome Q87.1
Robinson's (hidrotic) **ectodermal dysplasia or syndrome** Q82.4
Robles' disease B73.01
Rocky Mountain (spotted) **fever** A77.0
Roetheln —*see* Rubella
Roger's disease Q21.0
Rokitansky-Aschoff sinuses (gallbladder) K82.8
Rolando's fracture (displaced) S62.22-
nondisplaced S62.22-
Romano-Ward (prolonged QT interval) **syndrome** I45.81
Romberg's disease or syndrome G51.8
Roof, mouth —*see* condition
Rosacea L71.9
acne L71.9
keratitis L71.8
specified NEC L71.8
Rosary, rachitic E55.0
Rose
cold J30.1
fever J30.1
rash R21
epidemic B06.9
Rosenbach's erysipeloid A26.0
Rosenthal's disease or syndrome D68.1
Roseola B09
infantum B08.20
due to human herpesvirus 6 B08.21
due to human herpesvirus 7 B08.22
Ross River disease or fever B33.1
Rossbach's disease K31.89
psychogenic F45.8
Rostan's asthma (cardiac) —*see* Failure, ventricular, left
Rotation
anomalous, incomplete or insufficient, intestine Q43.3

R

Rotation *(Continued)*
cecum (congenital) Q43.3
colon (congenital) Q43.3
spine, incomplete or insufficient —*see* Dorsopathy, deforming, specified NEC
tooth, teeth, fully erupted M26.35
vertebra, incomplete or insufficient —*see* Dorsopathy, deforming, specified NEC
Rotes Quérol disease or syndrome —*see* Hyperostosis, ankylosing
Roth (-Bernhardt) **disease or syndrome** —*see* Meralgia paraesthetica
Rothmund (-Thomson) **syndrome** Q82.8
Rotor's disease or syndrome E80.6
Round
back (with wedging of vertebrae) —*see* Kyphosis
sequelae (late effect) of rickets E64.3
worms (large) (infestation) NEC B82.0
Ascariasis —*see also* Ascariasis B77.9
Roussy-Lévy syndrome G60.0
Rubella (German measles) B06.9
complication NEC B06.09
neurological B06.00
congenital P35.0
contact Z20.4
exposure to Z20.4
maternal
care for (suspected) damage to fetus O35.3
manifest rubella in infant P35.0
suspected damage to fetus affecting management of pregnancy O35.3
specified complications NEC B06.89
Rubeola (meaning measles) —*see* Measles
meaning rubella —*see* Rubella
Rubeosis, iris —*see* Disorder, iris, vascular
Rubinstein-Taybi syndrome Q87.2
Rudimentary (congenital) —*see also* Agenesis
arm —*see* Defect, reduction, upper limb
bone Q79.9
cervix uteri Q51.828
eye Q11.2
lobule of ear Q17.3
patella Q74.1
respiratory organs in thoracopagus Q89.4
tracheal bronchus Q32.4
uterus Q51.818
in male Q56.1
vagina Q52.0
Ruled out condition —*see* Observation, suspected
Rumination R11.10
with nausea R11.2
disorder of infancy F98.21
neurotic F42.8 ⬅
newborn P92.1
obsessional F42.8 ⬅
psychogenic F42.8 ⬅
Runeberg's disease D51.0
Runny nose R09.89
Rupia (syphilitic) A51.39
congenital A50.06
tertiary A52.79
Rupture, ruptured
abscess (spontaneous) - code by site under Abscess
aneurysm —*see* Aneurysm
anus (sphincter) —*see* Laceration, anus
aorta, aortic I71.8
abdominal I71.3
arch I71.1
ascending I71.1
descending I71.8
abdominal I71.3
thoracic I71.1
syphilitic A52.01
thoracoabdominal I71.5
thorax, thoracic I71.1
transverse I71.1
traumatic —*see* Injury, aorta, laceration, major

Rupture, ruptured *(Continued)*
aorta, aortic *(Continued)*
valve or cusp —*see also* Endocarditis, aortic I35.8
appendix (with peritonitis) K35.2
with localized peritonitis K35.3 ◀
arteriovenous fistula, brain I60.8
artery I77.2
brain —*see* Hemorrhage, intracranial, intracerebral
coronary —*see* Infarct, myocardium
heart —*see* Infarct, myocardium
pulmonary I28.8
traumatic (complication) —*see* Injury, blood vessel
bile duct (common) (hepatic) K83.2
cystic K82.2
bladder (sphincter) (nontraumatic) (spontaneous) N32.89
following ectopic or molar pregnancy O08.6
obstetrical trauma O71.5
traumatic S37.29
blood vessel —*see also* Hemorrhage
brain —*see* Hemorrhage, intracranial, intracerebral
heart —*see* Infarct, myocardium
traumatic (complication) —*see* Injury, blood vessel, laceration, major, by site
bone —*see* Fracture
bowel (nontraumatic) K63.1
brain
aneurysm (congenital) —*see also* Hemorrhage, intracranial, subarachnoid
syphilitic A52.05
hemorrhagic —*see* Hemorrhage, intracranial, intracerebral
capillaries I78.8
cardiac (auricle) (ventricle) (wall) I23.3
with hemopericardium I23.0
infectional I40.9
traumatic —*see* Injury, heart
cartilage (articular) (current) —*see also* Sprain
knee S83.3-
semilunar —*see* Tear, meniscus
cecum (with peritonitis) K65.0
with peritoneal abscess K35.3
traumatic S36.598
celiac artery, traumatic —*see* Injury, blood vessel, celiac artery, laceration, major
cerebral aneurysm (congenital) (*see* Hemorrhage, intracranial, subarachnoid)
cervix (uteri)
with ectopic or molar pregnancy O08.6
following ectopic or molar pregnancy O08.6
obstetrical trauma O71.3
traumatic S37.69
chordae tendineae NEC I51.1
concurrent with acute myocardial infarction —*see* Infarct, myocardium
following acute myocardial infarction (current complication) I23.4
choroid (direct) (indirect) (traumatic) H31.32-
circle of Willis I60.6
colon (nontraumatic) K63.1
traumatic —*see* Injury, intestine, large
cornea (traumatic) —*see* Injury, eye, laceration
coronary (artery) (thrombotic) —*see* Infarct, myocardium
corpus luteum (infected) (ovary) N83.1- ⬅
cyst —*see* Cyst
cystic duct K82.2
Descemet's membrane —*see* Change, corneal membrane, Descemet's, rupture
traumatic —*see* Injury, eye, laceration
diaphragm, traumatic —*see* Injury, intrathoracic, diaphragm
disc —*see* Rupture, intervertebral disc

Rupture, ruptured *(Continued)*
diverticulum (intestine) K57.80
with bleeding K57.81
bladder N32.3
large intestine K57.20
with
bleeding K57.21
small intestine K57.40
with bleeding K57.41
small intestine K57.00
with
bleeding K57.01
large intestine K57.40
with bleeding K57.41
duodenal stump K31.89
ear drum (nontraumatic) —*see also* Perforation, tympanum
traumatic S09.2-
due to blast injury —*see* Injury, blast, ear
esophagus K22.3
eye (without prolapse or loss of intraocular tissue) —*see* Injury, eye, laceration
fallopian tube NEC (nonobstetric) (nontraumatic) N83.8
due to pregnancy O00.10 ⬅
with intrauterine pregnancy O00.11 ◀
fontanel P13.1
gallbladder K82.2
traumatic S36.128
gastric —*see also* Rupture, stomach
vessel K92.2
globe (eye) (traumatic) —*see* Injury, eye, laceration
graafian follicle (hematoma) N83.0- ⬅
heart —*see* Rupture, cardiac
hymen (nontraumatic) (nonintentional) N89.8
internal organ, traumatic —*see* Injury, by site
intervertebral disc —*see* Displacement, intervertebral disc
traumatic —*see* Rupture, traumatic, intervertebral disc
intestine NEC (nontraumatic) K63.1
traumatic —*see* Injury, intestine
iris —*see also* Abnormality, pupillary
traumatic —*see* Injury, eye, laceration
joint capsule, traumatic —*see* Sprain
kidney (traumatic) S37.06-
birth injury P15.8
nontraumatic N28.89
lacrimal duct (traumatic) —*see* Injury, eye, specified site NEC
lens (cataract) (traumatic) —*see* Cataract, traumatic
ligament, traumatic —*see* Rupture, traumatic, ligament, by site
liver S36.116
birth injury P15.0
lymphatic vessel I89.8
marginal sinus (placental) (with hemorrhage) —*see* Hemorrhage, antepartum, specified cause NEC
membrana tympani (nontraumatic) —*see* Perforation, tympanum
membranes (spontaneous)
artificial
delayed delivery following O75.5
delayed delivery following —*see* Pregnancy, complicated by, premature rupture of membranes
meningeal artery I60.8
meniscus (knee) —*see also* Tear, meniscus
old —*see* Derangement, meniscus
site other than knee - code as Sprain
mesenteric artery, traumatic —*see* Injury, mesenteric, artery, laceration, major
mesentery (nontraumatic) K66.8
traumatic —*see* Injury, intra-abdominal, specified, site NEC
mitral (valve) I34.8

◀ New ⬅ Revised ~~deleted~~ Deleted

Rupture, ruptured *(Continued)*
muscle (traumatic) —*see also* Strain
diastasis —*see* Diastasis, muscle
nontraumatic M62.10
ankle M62.17-
foot M62.17-
forearm M62.13-
hand M62.14-
lower leg M62.16-
pelvic region M62.15-
shoulder region M62.11-
specified site NEC M62.18
thigh M62.15-
upper arm M62.12-
traumatic —*see* Strain, by site
musculotendinous junction NEC, nontraumatic —*see* Rupture, tendon, spontaneous
mycotic aneurysm causing cerebral hemorrhage —*see* Hemorrhage, intracranial, subarachnoid
myocardium, myocardial —*see* Rupture, cardiac
traumatic —*see* Injury, heart
nontraumatic, meaning hernia —*see* Hernia
obstructed —*see* Hernia, by site, obstructed
operation wound —*see* Disruption, wound, operation
ovary, ovarian N83.8
corpus luteum cyst N83.1- ⇐
follicle (graafian) N83.0- ⇐
oviduct (nonobstetric) (nontraumatic) N83.8
due to pregnancy O00.10 ⇐
with intrauterine pregnancy O00.11 ◀
pancreas (nontraumatic) K86.89 ⇐
traumatic S36.299
papillary muscle NEC I51.2
following acute myocardial infarction (current complication) I23.5
pelvic
floor, complicating delivery O70.1
organ NEC, obstetrical trauma O71.5
perineum (nonobstetric) (nontraumatic) N90.89
complicating delivery —*see* Delivery, complicated, by, laceration, anus (sphincter)
postoperative wound —*see* Disruption, wound, operation
prostate (traumatic) S37.828
pulmonary
artery I28.8
valve (heart) I37.8
vein I28.8
vessel I28.8
pus tube —*see* Salpingitis
pyosalpinx —*see* Salpingitis
rectum (nontraumatic) K63.1
traumatic S36.69
retina, retinal (traumatic) (without detachment) —*see also* Break, retina
with detachment —*see* Detachment, retina, with retinal, break
rotator cuff (nontraumatic) M75.10-
complete M75.12-
incomplete M75.11-
sclera —*see* Injury, eye, laceration
sigmoid (nontraumatic) K63.1
traumatic S36.593
spinal cord —*see also* Injury, spinal cord, by region
due to injury at birth P11.5
newborn (birth injury) P11.5
spleen (traumatic) S36.09
birth injury P15.1
congenital (birth injury) P15.1
due to P. vivax malaria B51.0
nontraumatic D73.5
spontaneous D73.5

Rupture, ruptured *(Continued)*
splenic vein R58
traumatic —*see* Injury, blood vessel, splenic vein
stomach (nontraumatic) (spontaneous) K31.89
traumatic S36.39
supraspinatus (complete) (incomplete) (nontraumatic) —*see* Tear, rotator cuff
symphysis pubis
obstetric O71.6
traumatic S33.4
synovium (cyst) M66.10
ankle M66.17-
elbow M66.12-
finger M66.14-
foot M66.17-
forearm M66.13-
hand M66.14-
pelvic region M66.15-
shoulder region M66.11-
specified site NEC M66.18
thigh M66.15-
toe M66.17-
upper arm M66.12-
wrist M66.13-
tendon (traumatic) —*see* Strain
nontraumatic (spontaneous) M66.9
ankle M66.87-
extensor M66.20
ankle M66.27-
foot M66.27-
forearm M66.23-
hand M66.24-
lower leg M66.26-
multiple sites M66.29
pelvic region M66.25-
shoulder region M66.21-
specified site NEC M66.28
thigh M66.25-
upper arm M66.22-
flexor M66.30
ankle M66.37-
foot M66.37-
forearm M66.33-
hand M66.34-
lower leg M66.36-
multiple sites M66.39
pelvic region M66.35-
shoulder region M66.31-
specified site NEC M66.38
thigh M66.35-
upper arm M66.32-
foot M66.87-
forearm M66.83-
hand M66.84-
lower leg M66.86-
multiple sites M66.89
pelvic region M66.85-
shoulder region M66.81-
specified
site NEC M66.88
tendon M66.80
thigh M66.85-
upper arm M66.82-
thoracic duct I89.8
tonsil J35.8
traumatic
aorta —*see* Injury, aorta, laceration, major
diaphragm —*see* Injury, intrathoracic, diaphragm
external site —*see* Wound, open, by site
eye —*see* Injury, eye, laceration
internal organ —*see* Injury, by site
intervertebral disc
cervical S13.0
lumbar S33.0
thoracic S23.0

Rupture, ruptured *(Continued)*
traumatic *(Continued)*
kidney S37.06-
ligament —*see also* Sprain
ankle —*see* Sprain, ankle
carpus —*see* Rupture, traumatic, ligament, wrist
collateral (hand) —*see* Rupture, traumatic, ligament, finger, collateral
finger (metacarpophalangeal) (interphalangeal) S63.40-
collateral S63.41-
index S63.41-
little S63.41-
middle S63.41-
ring S63.41-
index S63.40-
little S63.40-
middle S63.40-
palmar S63.42-
index S63.42-
little S63.42-
middle S63.42-
ring S63.42-
ring S63.40-
specified site NEC S63.499
index S63.49-
little S63.49-
middle S63.49-
ring S63.49-
volar plate S63.43-
index S63.43-
little S63.43-
middle S63.43-
ring S63.43-
foot —*see* Sprain, foot
radial collateral S53.2-
radiocarpal —*see* Rupture, traumatic, ligament, wrist, radiocarpal
ulnar collateral S53.3-
ulnocarpal —*see* Rupture, traumatic, ligament, wrist, ulnocarpal
wrist S63.30-
collateral S63.31-
radiocarpal S63.32-
specified site NEC S63.39-
ulnocarpal (palmar) S63.33-
liver S36.116
membrana tympani —*see* Rupture, ear drum, traumatic
muscle or tendon —*see* Strain
myocardium —*see* Injury, heart
pancreas S36.299
rectum S36.69
sigmoid S36.593
spleen S36.09
stomach S36.39
symphysis pubis S33.4
tympanum, tympanic (membrane) —*see* Rupture, ear drum, traumatic
ureter S37.19
uterus S37.69
vagina —*see* Injury, vagina
vena cava —*see* Injury, vena cava, laceration, major
tricuspid (heart) (valve) I07.8
tube, tubal (nonobstetric) (nontraumatic) N83.8
abscess —*see* Salpingitis
due to pregnancy O00.10 ⇐
with intrauterine pregnancy O00.11 ◀
tympanum, tympanic (membrane) (nontraumatic) —*see also* Perforation, tympanic membrane H72.9-
traumatic —*see* Rupture, ear drum, traumatic
umbilical cord, complicating delivery O69.89
ureter (traumatic) S37.19
nontraumatic N28.89

R

◀ New ⇐ Revised ~~deleted~~ Deleted

Rupture, ruptured *(Continued)*
urethra (nontraumatic) N36.8
with ectopic or molar pregnancy O08.6
following ectopic or molar pregnancy O08.6
obstetrical trauma O71.5
traumatic S37.39
uterosacral ligament (nonobstetric) (nontraumatic) N83.8
uterus (traumatic) S37.69
before labor O71.0-
during or after labor O71.1

Rupture, ruptured *(Continued)*
uterus *(Continued)*
nonpuerperal, nontraumatic N85.8
pregnant (during labor) O71.1
before labor O71.0-
vagina —*see* Injury, vagina
valve, valvular (heart) —*see* Endocarditis
varicose vein —*see* Varix
varix —*see* Varix
vena cava R58
traumatic —*see* Injury, vena cava, laceration, major
vesical (urinary) N32.89

Rupture, ruptured *(Continued)*
vessel (blood) R58
pulmonary I28.8
traumatic —*see* Injury, blood vessel
viscus R19.8
vulva complicating delivery O70.0
Russell-Silver syndrome Q87.1
Russian spring-summer type encephalitis A84.0
Rust's disease (tuberculous cervical spondylitis) A18.01
Ruvalcaba-Myhre-Smith syndrome E71.440
Rytand-Lipsitch syndrome I44.2

R

S

Saber, sabre shin or tibia (syphilitic) A50.56 *[M90.8-]*
Sac lacrimal —*see* condition
Saccharomyces infection B37.9
Saccharopinuria E72.3
Saccular —*see* condition
Sacculation
aorta (nonsyphilitic) —*see* Aneurysm, aorta
bladder N32.3
intralaryngeal (congenital) (ventricular) Q31.3
larynx (congenital) (ventricular) Q31.3
organ or site, congenital —*see* Distortion
pregnant uterus —*see* Pregnancy, complicated by, abnormal, uterus
ureter N28.89
urethra N36.1
vesical N32.3
Sachs' amaurotic familial idiocy or disease E75.02
Sachs-Tay disease E75.02
Sacks-Libman disease M32.11
Sacralgia M53.3
Sacralization Q76.49
Sacrodynia M53.3
Sacroiliac joint —*see* condition
Sacroiliitis NEC M46.1
Sacrum —*see* condition
Saddle
back —*see* Lordosis
embolus
abdominal aorta I74.01
pulmonary artery I26.92
with acute cor pulmonale I26.02
injury — code to condition
nose M95.0
due to syphilis A50.57
Sadism (sexual) F65.52
Sadness, postpartal O90.6
Sadomasochism F65.50
Saemisch's ulcer (cornea) —*see* Ulcer, cornea, central
Sagging ◀
skin and subcutaneous tissue (following bariatric surgery weight loss) (following dietary weight loss) L98.7 ◀
Sahib disease B55.0
Sailors' skin L57.8
Saint
Anthony's fire —*see* Erysipelas
triad —*see* Hernia, diaphragm
Vitus' dance —*see* Chorea, Sydenham's
Salaam
attack (s) —*see* Epilepsy, spasms
tic R25.8
Salicylism
abuse F55.8
overdose or wrong substance given —*see* Table of Drugs and Chemicals, by drug, poisoning
Salivary duct or gland —*see* condition
Salivation, excessive K11.7
Salmonella —*see* Infection, Salmonella
Salmonellosis A02.0
Salpingitis (catarrhal) (fallopian tube) (nodular) (pseudofollicular) (purulent) (septic) N70.91
with oophoritis N70.93
acute N70.01
with oophoritis N70.03
chlamydial A56.11
chronic N70.11
with oophoritis N70.13
complicating abortion —*see* Abortion, by type, complicated by, salpingitis
ear —*see* Salpingitis, eustachian
eustachian (tube) H68.00-
acute H68.01-
chronic H68.02-
Salpingitis *(Continued)*
follicularis N70.11
with oophoritis N70.13
gonococcal (acute) (chronic) A54.24
interstitial, chronic N70.11
with oophoritis N70.13
isthmica nodosa N70.11
with oophoritis N70.13
specific (gonococcal) (acute) (chronic) A54.24
tuberculous (acute) (chronic) A18.17
venereal (gonococcal) (acute) (chronic) A54.24
Salpingocele N83.4- ◀
Salpingo-oophoritis (catarrhal) (purulent) (ruptured) (septic) (suppurative) N70.93
acute N70.03
with ectopic or molar pregnancy O08.0
following ectopic or molar pregnancy O08.0
gonococcal A54.24
chronic N70.13
following ectopic or molar pregnancy O08.0
gonococcal (acute) (chronic) A54.24
puerperal O86.19
specific (gonococcal) (acute) (chronic) A54.24
subacute N70.03
tuberculous (acute) (chronic) A18.17
venereal (gonococcal) (acute) (chronic) A54.24
Salpingo-ovaritis —*see* Salpingo-oophoritis
Salpingoperitonitis —*see* Salpingo-oophoritis
Salzmann's nodular dystrophy —*see* Degeneration, cornea, nodular
Sampson's cyst or tumor N80.1
San Joaquin (Valley) **fever** B38.0
Sandblaster's asthma, lung or pneumoconiosis J62.8
Sander's disease (paranoia) F22
Sandfly fever A93.1
Sandhoff's disease E75.01
Sanfilippo (Type B) (Type C) (Type D) **syndrome** E76.22
Sanger-Brown ataxia G11.2
Sao Paulo fever or typhus A77.0
Saponification, mesenteric K65.8
Sarcocele (benign)
syphilitic A52.76
congenital A50.59
Sarcocystosis A07.8
Sarcoepiplocele —*see* Hernia
Sarcoepiplomphalocele Q79.2
Sarcoid —*see also* Sarcoidosis
arthropathy D86.86
Boeck's D86.9
Darier-Roussy D86.3
iridocyclitis D86.83
meningitis D86.81
myocarditis D86.85
myositis D86.87
pyelonephritis D86.84
Spiegler-Fendt L08.89
Sarcoidosis D86.9
with
cranial nerve palsies D86.82
hepatic granuloma D86.89
polyarthritis D86.86
tubulo-interstitial nephropathy D86.84
combined sites NEC D86.89
lung D86.0
and lymph nodes D86.2
lymph nodes D86.1
and lung D86.2
meninges D86.81
skin D86.3
specified type NEC D86.89
Sarcoma (of) —*see also* Neoplasm, connective tissue, malignant
alveolar soft part —*see* Neoplasm, connective tissue, malignant
ameloblastic C41.1
upper jaw (bone) C41.0
botryoid —*see* Neoplasm, connective tissue, malignant
Sarcoma *(Continued)*
botryoides —*see* Neoplasm, connective tissue, malignant
cerebellar C71.6
circumscribed (arachnoidal) C71.6
circumscribed (arachnoidal) cerebellar C71.6
clear cell —*see also* Neoplasm, connective tissue, malignant
kidney C64.-
dendritic cells (accessory cells) C96.4
embryonal —*see* Neoplasm, connective tissue, malignant
endometrial (stromal) C54.1
isthmus C54.0
epithelioid (cell) —*see* Neoplasm, connective tissue, malignant
Ewing's —*see* Neoplasm, bone, malignant
follicular dendritic cell C96.4
germinoblastic (diffuse) —*see* Lymphoma, diffuse, large cell
follicular —*see* Lymphoma, follicular, specified NEC
giant cell (except of bone) —*see also* Neoplasm, connective tissue, malignant
bone —*see* Neoplasm, bone, malignant
glomoid —*see* Neoplasm, connective tissue, malignant
granulocytic C92.3-
hemangioendothelial —*see* Neoplasm, connective tissue, malignant
hemorrhagic, multiple —*see* Sarcoma, Kaposi's
histiocytic C96.A
Hodgkin —*see* Lymphoma, Hodgkin
immunoblastic (diffuse) —*see* Lymphoma, diffuse large cell
interdigitating dendritic cell C96.4
Kaposi's
colon C46.4
connective tissue C46.1
gastrointestinal organ C46.4
lung C46.5-
lymph node (s) C46.3
palate (hard) (soft) C46.2
rectum C46.4
skin C46.0
specified site NEC C46.7
stomach C46.4
unspecified site C46.9
Kupffer cell C22.3
Langerhans cell C96.4
leptomeningeal —*see* Neoplasm, meninges, malignant
liver NEC C22.4
lymphangioendothelial —*see* Neoplasm, connective tissue, malignant
lymphoblastic —*see* Lymphoma, lymphoblastic (diffuse)
lymphocytic —*see* Lymphoma, small cell B-cell
mast cell C96.2
melanotic —*see* Melanoma
meningeal —*see* Neoplasm, meninges, malignant
meningothelial —*see* Neoplasm, meninges, malignant
mesenchymal —*see also* Neoplasm, connective tissue, malignant
mixed —*see* Neoplasm, connective tissue, malignant
mesothelial —*see* Mesothelioma
monstrocellular
specified site —*see* Neoplasm, malignant, by site
unspecified site C71.9
myeloid C92.3-
neurogenic —*see* Neoplasm, nerve, malignant
odontogenic C41.1
upper jaw (bone) C41.0

Sarcoma *(Continued)*
osteoblastic —*see* Neoplasm, bone, malignant
osteogenic —*see also* Neoplasm, bone, malignant
juxtacortical —*see* Neoplasm, bone, malignant
periosteal —*see* Neoplasm, bone, malignant
periosteal —*see also* Neoplasm, bone, malignant
osteogenic —*see* Neoplasm, bone, malignant
pleomorphic cell —*see* Neoplasm, connective tissue, malignant
reticulum cell (diffuse) —*see* Lymphoma, diffuse large cell
nodular —*see* Lymphoma, follicular
pleomorphic cell type —*see* Lymphoma, diffuse large cell
rhabdoid —*see* Neoplasm, malignant, by site
round cell —*see* Neoplasm, connective tissue, malignant
small cell —*see* Neoplasm, connective tissue, malignant
soft tissue —*see* Neoplasm, connective tissue, malignant
spindle cell —*see* Neoplasm, connective tissue, malignant
stromal (endometrial) C54.1
isthmus C54.0
synovial —*see also* Neoplasm, connective tissue, malignant
biphasic —*see* Neoplasm, connective tissue, malignant
epithelioid cell —*see* Neoplasm, connective tissue, malignant
spindle cell —*see* Neoplasm, connective tissue, malignant
Sarcomatosis
meningeal —*see* Neoplasm, meninges, malignant
specified site NEC —*see* Neoplasm, connective tissue, malignant
unspecified site C80.1
Sarcopenia (age-related) M62.84 ◀
Sarcosinemia E72.59
Sarcosporidiosis (intestinal) A07.8
Satiety, early R68.81
Saturnine —*see* condition
Saturnism
overdose or wrong substance given or taken —*see* Table of Drugs and Chemicals, by drug, poisoning
Satyriasis F52.8
Sauriasis —*see* Ichthyosis
SBE (subacute bacterial endocarditis) I33.0
Scabies (any site) B86
Scabs R23.4
Scaglietti-Dagnini syndrome E22.0
Scald —*see* Burn
Scalenus anticus (anterior) **syndrome** G54.0
Scales R23.4
Scaling, skin R23.4
Scalp —*see* condition
Scapegoating affecting child Z62.3
Scaphocephaly Q75.0
Scapulalgia M89.8X1
Scapulohumeral myopathy G71.0
Scar, scarring —*see also* Cicatrix L90.5
adherent L90.5
atrophic L90.5
cervix
in pregnancy or childbirth —*see* Pregnancy, complicated by, abnormal cervix
cheloid L91.0
chorioretinal H31.00-
posterior pole macula H31.01-
postsurgical H59.81-
solar retinopathy H31.02-
specified type NEC H31.09-
Scar, scarring *(Continued)*
choroid —*see* Scar, chorioretinal
conjunctiva H11.24-
cornea H17.9
xerophthalmic —*see also* Opacity, cornea vitamin A deficiency E50.6
duodenum, obstructive K31.5
hypertrophic L91.0
keloid L91.0
labia N90.89
lung (base) J98.4
macula —*see* Scar, chorioretinal, posterior pole
muscle M62.89
myocardium, myocardial I25.2
painful L90.5
posterior pole (eye) —*see* Scar, chorioretinal, posterior pole
retina —*see* Scar, chorioretinal
trachea J39.8
transmural uterine, in pregnancy O34.29 ◀
uterus N85.8
in pregnancy O34.29
vagina N89.8
postoperative N99.2
vulva N90.89
Scarabiasis B88.2
Scarlatina (anginosa) (maligna) (ulcerosa) A38.9
myocarditis (acute) A38.1
old —*see* Myocarditis
otitis media A38.0
Scarlet fever (albuminuria) (angina) A38.9
Schamberg's disease (progressive pigmentary dermatosis) L81.7
Schatzki's ring (acquired) (esophagus) (lower) K22.2
congenital Q39.3
Schaufenster krankheit I20.8
Schaumann's
benign lymphogranulomatosis D86.1
disease or syndrome —*see* Sarcoidosis
Scheie's syndrome E76.03
Schenck's disease B42.1
Scheuermann's disease or osteochondrosis —*see* Osteochondrosis, juvenile, spine
Schilder (-Flatau) **disease** G37.0
Schilling-type monocytic leukemia C93.0-
Schimmelbusch's disease, cystic mastitis, or hyperplasia —*see* Mastopathy, cystic
Schistosoma infestation —*see* Infestation, Schistosoma
Schistosomiasis B65.9
with muscle disorder B65.9 *[M63.80]*
ankle B65.9 *[M63.87-]*
foot B65.9 *[M63.87-]*
forearm B65.9 *[M63.83-]*
hand B65.9 *[M63.84-]*
lower leg B65.9 *[M63.86-]*
multiple sites B65.9 *[M63.89]*
pelvic region B65.9 *[M63.85-]*
shoulder region B65.9 *[M63.81-]*
specified site NEC B65.9 *[M63.88]*
thigh B65.9 *[M63.85-]*
upper arm B65.9 *[M63.82-]*
Asiatic B65.2
bladder B65.0
chestermani B65.8
colon B65.1
cutaneous B65.3
due to
S. haematobium B65.0
S. japonicum B65.2
S. mansoni B65.1
S. mattheii B65.8
Eastern B65.2
genitourinary tract B65.0
intestinal B65.1
lung NEC B65.9 *[J99]*
pneumonia B65.9 *[J17]*
Manson's (intestinal) B65.1
Schistosomiasis *(Continued)*
oriental B65.2
pulmonary NEC B65.9 *[J99]*
pneumonia B65.9
Schistosoma
haematobium B65.0
japonicum B65.2
mansoni B65.1
specified type NEC B65.8
urinary B65.0
vesical B65.0
Schizencephaly Q04.6
Schizoaffective psychosis F25.9
Schizodontia K00.2
Schizoid personality F60.1
Schizophrenia, schizophrenic F20.9
acute (brief) (undifferentiated) F23
atypical (form) F20.3
borderline F21
catalepsy F20.2
catatonic (type) (excited) (withdrawn) F20.2
cenesthopathic, cenesthesiopathic F20.89
childhood type F84.5
chronic undifferentiated F20.5
cyclic F25.0
disorganized (type) F20.1
flexibilitas cerea F20.2
hebephrenic (type) F20.1
incipient F21
latent F21
negative type F20.5
paranoid (type) F20.0
paraphrenic F20.0
post-psychotic depression F32.89 ⬅
prepsychotic F21
prodromal F21
pseudoneurotic F21
pseudopsychopathic F21
reaction F23
residual (state) (type) F20.5
restzustand F20.5
schizoaffective (type) —*see* Psychosis, schizoaffective
simple (type) F20.89
simplex F20.89
specified type NEC F20.89
stupor F20.2
syndrome of childhood F84.5
undifferentiated (type) F20.3
chronic F20.5
Schizothymia (persistent) F60.1
Schlatter-Osgood disease or osteochondrosis —*see* Osteochondrosis, juvenile, tibia
Schlatter's tibia —*see* Osteochondrosis, juvenile, tibia
Schmidt's syndrome (polyglandular, autoimmune) E31.0
Schmincke's carcinoma or tumor —*see* Neoplasm, nasopharynx, malignant
Schmitz (-Stutzer) **dysentery** A03.0
Schmorl's disease or nodes
lumbar region M51.46
lumbosacral region M51.47
sacrococcygeal region M53.3
thoracic region M51.44
thoracolumbar region M51.45
Schneiderian
papilloma —*see* Neoplasm, nasopharynx benign
specified site —*see* Neoplasm, benign, by site
unspecified site D14.0
specified site —*see* Neoplasm, malignant, by site
unspecified site C30.0
Scholte's syndrome (malignant carcinoid) E34.0
Scholz (-Bielchowsky-Henneberg) **disease or syndrome** E75.25
Schönlein (-Henoch) **disease or purpura** (primary) (rheumatic) D69.0

◀ New ⬅ Revised ~~deleted~~ Deleted

Schottmuller's disease A01.4
Schroeder's syndrome (endocrine hypertensive) E27.0
Schüller-Christian disease or syndrome C96.5
Schultze's type acroparesthesia, simple I73.89
Schultz's disease or syndrome —*see* Agranulocytosis
Schwalbe-Ziehen-Oppenheim disease G24.1
Schwannoma —*see also* Neoplasm, nerve, benign
  malignant —*see also* Neoplasm, nerve, malignant
    with rhabdomyoblastic differentiation —*see* Neoplasm, nerve, malignant
  melanocytic —*see* Neoplasm, nerve, benign
  pigmented —*see* Neoplasm, nerve, benign
Schwannomatosis Q85.03
Schwartz (-Jampel) syndrome G71.13
Schwartz-Bartter syndrome E22.2
Schweniger-Buzzi anetoderma L90.1
Sciatic —*see* condition
Sciatica (infective)
  with lumbago M54.4-
    due to intervertebral disc disorder —*see* Disorder, disc, with, radiculopathy
  due to displacement of intervertebral disc (with lumbago) —*see* Disorder, disc, with, radiculopathy
  wallet M54.3-
Scimitar syndrome Q26.8
Sclera —*see* condition
Sclerectasia H15.84-
Scleredema
  adultorum —*see* Sclerosis, systemic
  Buschke's —*see* Sclerosis, systemic
  newborn P83.0
Sclerema (adiposum) (edematosum) (neonatorum) (newborn) P83.0
  adultorum —*see* Sclerosis, systemic
Scleriasis —*see* Scleroderma
Scleritis H15.00-
  with corneal involvement H15.04-
  anterior H15.01-
  brawny H15.02-
  in (due to) zoster B02.34
  posterior H15.03-
  specified type NEC H15.09-
  syphilitic A52.71
  tuberculous (nodular) A18.51
Sclerochoroiditis H31.8
Scleroconjunctivitis —*see* Scleritis
Sclerocystic ovary syndrome E28.2
Sclerodactyly, sclerodactylia L94.3
Scleroderma, sclerodermia (acrosclerotic) (diffuse) (generalized) (progressive) (pulmonary) —*see also* Sclerosis, systemic M34.9-
  circumscribed L94.0
  linear L94.1
  localized L94.0
  newborn P83.8
  systemic M34.9
Sclerokeratitis H16.8
  tuberculous A18.52
Scleroma nasi A48.8
Scleromalacia (perforans) H15.05-
Scleromyxedema L98.5
Sclérose en plaques G35
Sclerosis, sclerotic
  adrenal (gland) E27.8
  Alzheimer's —*see* Disease, Alzheimer's
  amyotrophic (lateral) G12.21
  aorta, aortic I70.0
    valve —*see* Endocarditis, aortic
  artery, arterial, arteriolar, arteriovascular —*see* Arteriosclerosis
  ascending multiple G35
  brain (generalized) (lobular) G37.9
    artery, arterial I67.2
    diffuse G37.0
    disseminated G35
Sclerosis, sclerotic *(Continued)*
  brain *(Continued)*
    insular G35
    Krabbe's E75.23
    miliary G35
    multiple G35
    presenile (Alzheimer's) —*see* Disease, Alzheimer's, early onset
    senile (arteriosclerotic) I67.2
    stem, multiple G35
    tuberous Q85.1
  bulbar, multiple G35
  bundle of His I44.39
  cardiac —*see* Disease, heart, ischemic, atherosclerotic
  cardiorenal —*see* Hypertension, cardiorenal
  cardiovascular —*see also* Disease, cardiovascular
    renal —*see* Hypertension, cardiorenal
  cerebellar —*see* Sclerosis, brain
  cerebral —*see* Sclerosis, brain
  cerebrospinal (disseminated) (multiple) G35
  cerebrovascular I67.2
  choroid —*see* Degeneration, choroid
  combined (spinal cord) —*see also* Degeneration, combined
    multiple G35
  concentric (Balo) G37.5
  cornea —*see* Opacity, cornea
  coronary (artery) I25.10
    with angina pectoris —*see* Arteriosclerosis, coronary (artery),
  corpus cavernosum
    female N90.89
    male N48.6
  diffuse (brain) (spinal cord) G37.0
  disseminated G35
  dorsal G35
  dorsolateral (spinal cord) —*see* Degeneration, combined
  endometrium N85.5
  extrapyramidal G25.9
  eye, nuclear (senile) —*see* Cataract, senile, nuclear
  focal and segmental (glomerular) —*see also* N00-N07 with fourth character .1
    N05.1
  Friedreich's (spinal cord) G11.1
  funicular (spermatic cord) N50.89 ◀
  general (vascular) —*see* Arteriosclerosis
  gland (lymphatic) I89.8
  hepatic K74.1
    alcoholic K70.2
  hereditary
    cerebellar G11.9
    spinal (Friedreich's ataxia) G11.1
  hippocampal G93.81
  insular G35
  kidney —*see* Sclerosis, renal
  larynx J38.7
  lateral (amyotrophic) (descending) (primary) (spinal) G12.21
  lens, senile nuclear —*see* Cataract, senile, nuclear
  liver K74.1
    with fibrosis K74.2
      alcoholic K70.2
    alcoholic K70.2
    cardiac K76.1
  lung —*see* Fibrosis, lung
  mastoid —*see* Mastoiditis, chronic
  mesial temporal G93.81
  mitral I05.8
  Mönckeberg's (medial) —*see* Arteriosclerosis, extremities
  multiple (brain stem) (cerebral) (generalized) (spinal cord) G35
  myocardium, myocardial —*see* Disease, heart, ischemic, atherosclerotic
  nuclear (senile), eye —*see* Cataract, senile, nuclear
Sclerosis, sclerotic *(Continued)*
  ovary N83.8
  pancreas K86.89 ◀
  penis N48.6
  peripheral arteries —*see* Arteriosclerosis, extremities
  plaques G35
  pluriglandular E31.8
  polyglandular E31.8
  posterolateral (spinal cord) —*see* Degeneration, combined
  presenile (Alzheimer's) —*see* Disease, Alzheimer's, early onset
  primary, lateral G12.29
  progressive, systemic M34.0
  pulmonary —*see* Fibrosis, lung
    artery I27.0
    valve (heart) —*see* Endocarditis, pulmonary
  renal N26.9
    with
      cystine storage disease E72.09
      hypertensive heart disease (conditions in I11) —*see* Hypertension, cardiorenal
    arteriolar (hyaline) (hyperplastic) —*see* Hypertension, kidney
  retina (senile) (vascular) H35.00
  senile (vascular) —*see* Arteriosclerosis
  spinal (cord) (progressive) G95.89
    ascending G61.0
    combined —*see also* Degeneration, combined
      multiple G35
      syphilitic A52.11
    disseminated G35
    dorsolateral —*see* Degeneration, combined
    hereditary (Friedreich's) (mixed form) G11.1
    lateral (amyotrophic) G12.21
    multiple G35
    posterior (syphilitic) A52.11
  stomach K31.89
  subendocardial, congenital I42.4
  systemic M34.9
    with
      lung involvement M34.81
      myopathy M34.82
      polyneuropathy M34.83
    drug-induced M34.2
    due to chemicals NEC M34.2
    progressive M34.0
    specified NEC M34.89
  temporal (mesial) G93.81
  tricuspid (heart) (valve) I07.8
  tuberous (brain) Q85.1
  tympanic membrane —*see* Disorder, tympanic membrane, specified NEC
  valve, valvular (heart) —*see* Endocarditis
  vascular —*see* Arteriosclerosis
  vein I87.8
Scoliosis (acquired) (postural) M41.9
  adolescent (idiopathic) —*see* Scoliosis, idiopathic, adolescent ◀
  congenital Q67.5
    due to bony malformation Q76.3
    failure of segmentation (hemivertebra) Q76.3
    hemivertebra fusion Q76.3
    postural Q67.5
  idiopathic M41.20
    adolescent M41.129
      cervical region M41.122
      cervicothoracic region M41.123
      lumbar region M41.126
      lumbosacral region M41.127
      thoracic region M41.124
      thoracolumbar region M41.125
    cervical region M41.22
    cervicothoracic region M41.23

Scoliosis *(Continued)*
idiopathic *(Continued)*
infantile M41.00
cervical region M41.02
cervicothoracic region M41.03
lumbar region M41.06
lumbosacral region M41.07
sacrococcygeal region M41.08
thoracic region M41.04
thoracolumbar region M41.05
juvenile M41.119
cervical region M41.112
cervicothoracic region M41.113
lumbar region M41.116
lumbosacral region M41.117
thoracic region M41.114
thoracolumbar region M41.115
lumbar region M41.26
lumbosacral region M41.27
thoracic region M41.24
thoracolumbar region M41.25
infantile —*see* Scoliosis, idiopathic, infantile ◀
neuromuscular M41.40
cervical region M41.42
cervicothoracic region M41.43
lumbar region M41.46
lumbosacral region M41.47
occipito-atlanto-axial region M41.41
thoracic region M41.44
thoracolumbar region M41.45
paralytic —*see* Scoliosis, neuromuscular
postradiation therapy M96.5
rachitic (late effect or sequelae) E64.3 *[M49.80]*
cervical region E64.3 *[M49.82]*
cervicothoracic region E64.3 *[M49.83]*
lumbar region E64.3 *[M49.86]*
lumbosacral region E64.3 *[M49.87]*
multiple sites E64.3 *[M49.89]*
occipito-atlanto-axial region E64.3 *[M49.81]*
sacrococcygeal region E64.3 *[M49.88]*
thoracic region E64.3 *[M49.84]*
thoracolumbar region E64.3 *[M49.85]*
sciatic M54.4-
secondary (to) NEC M41.50
cerebral palsy, Friedreich's ataxia, poliomyelitis, neuromuscular disorders —*see* Scoliosis, neuromuscular
cervical region M41.52
cervicothoracic region M41.53
lumbar region M41.56
lumbosacral region M41.57
thoracic region M41.54
thoracolumbar region M41.55
specified form NEC M41.80
cervical region M41.82
cervicothoracic region M41.83
lumbar region M41.86
lumbosacral region M41.87
thoracic region M41.84
thoracolumbar region M41.85
thoracogenic M41.30
thoracic region M41.34
thoracolumbar region M41.35
tuberculous A18.01
Scoliotic pelvis
with disproportion (fetopelvic) O33.0
causing obstructed labor O65.0
Scorbutus, scorbutic —*see also* Scurvy
anemia D53.2
Score, NIHSS (National Institutes of Health Stroke Scale) R29.7- ◀
Scotoma (arcuate) (Bjerrum) (central) (ring) —*see also* Defect, visual field, localized, scotoma
scintillating H53.19
Scratch —*see* Abrasion
Scratchy throat R09.89

Screening (for) Z13.9
alcoholism Z13.89
anemia Z13.0
anomaly, congenital Z13.89
antenatal, of mother Z36
arterial hypertension Z13.6
arthropod-borne viral disease NEC Z11.59
bacteriuria, asymptomatic Z13.89
behavioral disorder Z13.89
brain injury, traumatic Z13.850
bronchitis, chronic Z13.83
brucellosis Z11.2
cardiovascular disorder Z13.6
cataract Z13.5
chlamydial diseases Z11.8
cholera Z11.0
chromosomal abnormalities (nonprocreative) NEC Z13.79
colonoscopy Z12.11
congenital
dislocation of hip Z13.89
eye disorder Z13.5
malformation or deformation Z13.89
contamination NEC Z13.88
cystic fibrosis Z13.228
dengue fever Z11.59
dental disorder Z13.84
depression Z13.89
developmental handicap Z13.42 ⇐
in early childhood Z13.42 ⇐
infant Z13.41 ◀
diabetes mellitus Z13.1
diphtheria Z11.2
disability, intellectual Z13.42 ⇐
infant Z13.41 ◀
disease or disorder Z13.9
bacterial NEC Z11.2
intestinal infectious Z11.0
respiratory tuberculosis Z11.1
blood or blood-forming organ Z13.0
cardiovascular Z13.6
Chagas' Z11.6
chlamydial Z11.8
dental Z13.89
developmental Z13.42 ⇐
in child Z13.42 ◀
infant Z13.41 ◀
digestive tract NEC Z13.818
lower GI Z13.811
upper GI Z13.810
ear Z13.5
endocrine Z13.29
eye Z13.5
genitourinary Z13.89
heart Z13.6
human immunodeficiency virus (HIV) infection Z11.4
immunity Z13.0
infection
intestinal Z11.0
specified NEC Z11.6
infectious Z11.9
mental Z13.89
metabolic Z13.228
neurological Z13.89
nutritional Z13.21
metabolic Z13.228
lipoid disorders Z13.220
protozoal Z11.6
intestinal Z11.0
respiratory Z13.83
rheumatic Z13.828
rickettsial Z11.8
sexually-transmitted NEC Z11.3
human immunodeficiency virus (HIV) Z11.4
sickle-cell (trait) Z13.0
skin Z13.89
specified NEC Z13.89
spirochetal Z11.8
thyroid Z13.29

Screening *(Continued)*
disease or disorder *(Continued)*
vascular Z13.6
venereal Z11.3
viral NEC Z11.59
human immunodeficiency virus (HIV) Z11.4
intestinal Z11.0
elevated titer Z13.89
emphysema Z13.83
encephalitis, viral (mosquito- or tick-borne) Z11.59
exposure to contaminants (toxic) Z13.88
fever
dengue Z11.59
hemorrhagic Z11.59
yellow Z11.59
filariasis Z11.6
galactosemia Z13.228
gastrointestinal condition Z13.818
genetic (nonprocreative)- for procreative management —*see* Testing, genetic, for procreative management
disease carrier status (nonprocreative) Z13.71
specified NEC (nonprocreative) Z13.79
genitourinary condition Z13.89
glaucoma Z13.5
gonorrhea Z11.3
gout Z13.89
helminthiasis (intestinal) Z11.6
hematopoietic malignancy Z12.89
hemoglobinopathies NEC Z13.0
hemorrhagic fever Z11.59
Hodgkin disease Z12.89
human immunodeficiency virus (HIV) Z11.4
human papillomavirus Z11.51
hypertension Z13.6
immunity disorders Z13.0
infection
mycotic Z11.8
parasitic Z11.8
ingestion of radioactive substance Z13.88
intellectual disability Z13.42 ⇐
infant Z13.41 ◀
intestinal
helminthiasis Z11.6
infectious disease Z11.0
leishmaniasis Z11.6
leprosy Z11.2
leptospirosis Z11.8
leukemia Z12.89
lymphoma Z12.89
malaria Z11.6
malnutrition Z13.29
metabolic Z13.228
nutritional Z13.21
measles Z11.59
mental disorder Z13.89
metabolic errors, inborn Z13.228
multiphasic Z13.89
musculoskeletal disorder Z13.828
osteoporosis Z13.820
mycoses Z11.8
myocardial infarction (acute) Z13.6
neoplasm (malignant) (of) Z12.9
bladder Z12.6
blood Z12.89
breast Z12.39
routine mammogram Z12.31
cervix Z12.4
colon Z12.11
genitourinary organs NEC Z12.79
bladder Z12.6
cervix Z12.4
ovary Z12.73
prostate Z12.5
testis Z12.71
vagina Z12.72
hematopoietic system Z12.89

◀ New ⇐ Revised ~~deleted~~ Deleted

Screening *(Continued)*
neoplasm *(Continued)*
intestinal tract Z12.10
colon Z12.11
rectum Z12.12
small intestine Z12.13
lung Z12.2
lymph (glands) Z12.89
nervous system Z12.82
oral cavity Z12.81
prostate Z12.5
rectum Z12.12
respiratory organs Z12.2
skin Z12.83
small intestine Z12.13
specified site NEC Z12.89
stomach Z12.0
nephropathy Z13.89
nervous system disorders NEC Z13.858
neurological condition Z13.89
osteoporosis Z13.820
parasitic infestation Z11.9
specified NEC Z11.8
phenylketonuria Z13.228
plague Z11.2
poisoning (chemical) (heavy metal) Z13.88
poliomyelitis Z11.59
postnatal, chromosomal abnormalities Z13.89
prenatal, of mother Z36
protozoal disease Z11.6
intestinal Z11.0
pulmonary tuberculosis Z11.1
radiation exposure Z13.88
respiratory condition Z13.83
respiratory tuberculosis Z11.1
rheumatoid arthritis Z13.828
rubella Z11.59
schistosomiasis Z11.6
sexually-transmitted disease NEC Z11.3
human immunodeficiency virus (HIV) Z11.4
sickle-cell disease or trait Z13.0
skin condition Z13.89
sleeping sickness Z11.6
special Z13.9
specified NEC Z13.89
syphilis Z11.3
tetanus Z11.2
trachoma Z11.8
traumatic brain injury Z13.850
trypanosomiasis Z11.6
tuberculosis, respiratory Z11.1
venereal disease Z11.3
viral encephalitis (mosquito- or tick-borne) Z11.59
whooping cough Z11.2
worms, intestinal Z11.6
yaws Z11.8
yellow fever Z11.59
Scrofula, scrofulosis (tuberculosis of cervical lymph glands) A18.2
Scrofulide (primary) (tuberculous) A18.4
Scrofuloderma, scrofulodermia (any site) (primary) A18.4
Scrofulosus lichen (primary) (tuberculous) A18.4
Scrofulous —*see* condition
Scrotal tongue K14.5
Scrotum —*see* condition
Scurvy, scorbutic E54
anemia D53.2
gum E54
infantile E54
rickets E55.0 *[M90.80]*
Sealpox B08.62
Seasickness T75.3
Seatworm (infection) (infestation) B80
Sebaceous —*see also* condition
cyst —*see* Cyst, sebaceous
Seborrhea, seborrheic L21.9
capillitii R23.8
capitis L21.0
dermatitis L21.9
infantile L21.1
eczema L21.9
infantile L21.1
sicca L21.0
Seckel's syndrome Q87.1
Seclusion, pupil —*see* Membrane, pupillary
Second hand tobacco smoke exposure (acute) (chronic) Z77.22
in the perinatal period P96.81
Secondary
dentin (in pulp) K04.3
neoplasm, secondaries —*see* Table of Neoplasms, secondary
Secretion
antidiuretic hormone, inappropriate E22.2
catecholamine, by pheochromocytoma E27.5
hormone
antidiuretic, inappropriate (syndrome) E22.2
by
carcinoid tumor E34.0
pheochromocytoma E27.5
ectopic NEC E34.2
urinary
excessive R35.8
suppression R34
Section
nerve, traumatic —*see* Injury, nerve
Sedative, hypnotic, or anxiolytic-induced ◀
anxiety disorder F13.980 ◀
bipolar and related disorder F13.94 ◀
delirium F13.921 ◀
depressive disorder F13.94 ◀
major neurocognitive disorder F13.97 ◀
mild neurocognitive disorder F13.988 ◀
psychotic disorder F13.959 ◀
sexual dysfunction F13.981 ◀
sleep disorder F13.982 ◀
Segmentation, incomplete (congenital) —*see also* Fusion
bone NEC Q78.8
lumbosacral (joint) (vertebra) Q76.49
Seitelberger's syndrome (infantile neuraxonal dystrophy) G31.89
Seizure(s) —*see also* Convulsions R56.9
akinetic —*see* Epilepsy, generalized, specified NEC
atonic —*see* Epilepsy, generalized, specified NEC
autonomic (hysterical) F44.5
convulsive —*see* Convulsions
cortical (focal) (motor) —*see* Epilepsy, localization-related, symptomatic, with simple partial seizures
disorder —*see also* Epilepsy G40.909
due to stroke —*see* Sequelae (of), disease, cerebrovascular, by type, specified NEC
epileptic —*see* Epilepsy
febrile (simple) R56.00
with status epilepticus G40.901
complex (atypical) (complicated) R56.01
with status epilepticus G40.901
grand mal G40.409
intractable G40.419
with status epilepticus G40.411
without status epilepticus G40.419
not intractable G40.409
with status epilepticus G40.401
without status epilepticus G40.409
heart —*see* Disease, heart
hysterical F44.5
intractable G40.919
with status epilepticus G40.911
Jacksonian (focal) (motor type) (sensory type) —*see* Epilepsy, localization-related, symptomatic, with simple partial seizures
Seizure *(Continued)*
newborn P90
nonspecific epileptic
atonic —*see* Epilepsy, generalized, specified NEC
clonic —*see* Epilepsy, generalized, specified NEC
myoclonic —*see* Epilepsy, generalized, specified NEC
tonic —*see* Epilepsy, generalized, specified NEC
tonic-clonic —*see* Epilepsy, generalized, specified NEC
partial, developing into secondarily generalized seizures
complex —*see* Epilepsy, localization-related, symptomatic, with complex partial seizures
simple —*see* Epilepsy, localization-related, symptomatic, with simple partial seizures
petit mal G40.409
intractable G40.419
with status epilepticus G40.411
without status epilepticus G40.419
not intractable G40.409
with status epilepticus G40.401
without status epilepticus G40.409
post traumatic R56.1
recurrent G40.909
specified NEC G40.89
uncinate —*see* Epilepsy, localization-related, symptomatic, with complex partial seizures
Selenium deficiency, dietary E59
Self-damaging behavior (life-style) Z72.89
Self-harm (attempted)
history (personal) Z91.5
in family Z81.8
Self-mutilation (attempted)
history (personal) Z91.5
in family Z81.8
Self-poisoning
history (personal) Z91.5
in family Z81.8
observation following (alleged) attempt Z03.6
Semicoma R40.1
Seminal vesiculitis N49.0
Seminoma C62.9-
specified site —*see* Neoplasm, malignant, by site
Senear-Usher disease or syndrome L10.4
Senectus R54
Senescence (without mention of psychosis) R54
Senile, senility —*see also* condition R41.81
with
acute confusional state F05
mental changes NOS F03
psychosis NEC —*see* Psychosis, senile
asthenia R54
cervix (atrophic) N88.8
debility R54
endometrium (atrophic) N85.8
fallopian tube (atrophic) —*see* Atrophy, fallopian tube
heart (failure) R54
ovary (atrophic) —*see* Atrophy, ovary
premature E34.8
vagina, vaginitis (atrophic) N95.2
wart L82.1
Sensation
burning (skin) R20.8
tongue K14.6
loss of R20.8
prickling (skin) R20.2
tingling (skin) R20.2
Sense loss
smell —*see* Disturbance, sensation, smell
taste —*see* Disturbance, sensation, taste
touch R20.8

◀ New ⇐ Revised ~~deleted~~ Deleted

Sensibility disturbance (cortical) (deep) (vibratory) R20.9
Sensitive, sensitivity —*see also* Allergy
carotid sinus G90.01
child (excessive) F93.8
cold, autoimmune D59.1
dentin K03.89
gluten (non-celiac) K90.41 ◀
latex Z91.040
methemoglobin D74.8
tuberculin, without clinical or radiological symptoms R76.11
visual
glare H53.71
impaired contrast H53.72
Sensitiver Beziehungswahn F22
Sensitization, auto-erythrocytic D69.2
Separation
anxiety, abnormal (of childhood) F93.0
apophysis, traumatic - code as Fracture, by site
choroid —*see* Detachment, choroid
epiphysis, epiphyseal
nontraumatic —*see also* Osteochondropathy, specified type NEC
upper femoral —*see* Slipped, epiphysis, upper femoral
traumatic - code as Fracture, by site
fracture —*see* Fracture
infundibulum cardiac from right ventricle by a partition Q24.3
joint (traumatic) (current) - code by site under Dislocation
pubic bone, obstetrical trauma O71.6
retina, retinal —*see* Detachment, retina
symphysis pubis, obstetrical trauma O71.6
tracheal ring, incomplete, congenital Q32.1
Sepsis (generalized) (unspecified organism) A41.9
with
organ dysfunction (acute) (multiple) R65.20
with septic shock R65.21
actinomycotic A42.7
adrenal hemorrhage syndrome (meningococcal) A39.1
anaerobic A41.4
Bacillus anthracis A22.7
Brucella —*see also* Brucellosis A23.9
candidal B37.7
cryptogenic A41.9
due to device, implant or graft T85.79
arterial graft NEC T82.7
breast (implant) T85.79
catheter NEC T85.79
dialysis (renal) T82.7
intraperitoneal T85.71
infusion NEC T82.7
spinal (cranial) (epidural) (intrathecal) (spinal) (subarachnoid) (subdural) T85.735 ⇐
urethral indwelling T83.511 ◀
urinary T83.518 ⇐
ectopic or molar pregnancy O08.82
electronic (electrode) (pulse generator) (stimulator)
bone T84.7
cardiac T82.7
nervous system T85.738 ⇐
brain T85.731 ◀
neurostimulator generator T85.734 ◀
peripheral nerve T85.732 ◀
spinal cord T85.733 ◀
urinary T83.590 ⇐
fixation, internal (orthopedic) —*see* Complication, fixation device, infection
gastrointestinal (bile duct) (esophagus) T85.79
neurostimulator electrode (lead) T85.732 ◀

Sepsis *(Continued)*
due to device, implant or graft *(Continued)*
genital T83.69 ⇐
heart NEC T82.7
valve (prosthesis) T82.6
graft T82.7
joint prosthesis —*see* Complication, joint prosthesis, infection
ocular (corneal graft) (orbital implant) T85.79
orthopedic NEC T84.7
fixation device, internal —*see* Complication, fixation device, infection
specified NEC T85.79
vascular T82.7
~~ventricular intracranial shunt T85.79~~
ventricular intracranial (communicating) shunt T85.730 ◀
during labor O75.3
Enterococcus A41.81
Erysipelothrix (rhusiopathiae) (erysipeloid) A26.7
Escherichia coli (E. coli) A41.5
extraintestinal yersiniosis A28.2
following
abortion (subsequent episode) O08.0
current episode —*see* Abortion
ectopic or molar pregnancy O08.82
immunization T88.0
infusion, therapeutic injection or transfusion NEC T80.29
gangrenous A41.9
gonococcal A54.86
Gram-negative (organism) A41.5
anaerobic A41.4
Haemophilus influenzae A41.3
herpesviral B00.7
intra-abdominal K65.1
intraocular —*see* Endophthalmitis, purulent
Listeria monocytogenes A32.7
localized — code to specific localized infection
in operation wound T81.49 ⇐
skin —*see* Abscess
malleus A24.0
melioidosis A24.1
meningeal —*see* Meningitis
meningococcal A39.4
acute A39.2
chronic A39.3
MSSA (Methicillin susceptible Staphylococcus aureus) A41.01
newborn P36.9
due to
anaerobes NEC P36.5
Escherichia coli P36.4
Staphylococcus P36.30
aureus P36.2
specified NEC P36.39
Streptococcus P36.10
group B P36.0
specified NEC P36.19
specified NEC P36.8
Pasteurella multocida A28.0
pelvic, puerperal, postpartum, childbirth O85
pneumococcal A40.3
postprocedural T81.49 ⇐
puerperal, postpartum, childbirth (pelvic) O85
Salmonella (arizonae) (cholerae-suis) (enteritidis) (typhimurium) A02.1
severe R65.20
with septic shock R65.21
Shigella (*see also* Dysentery, bacillary) A03.9
skin, localized —*see* Abscess
specified organism NEC A41.89
Staphylococcus, staphylococcal A41.2
aureus (methicillin susceptible) (MSSA) A41.01
methicillin resistant (MRSA) A41.02

Sepsis *(Continued)*
Staphylococcus, staphylococcal *(Continued)*
coagulase-negative A41.1
specified NEC A41.1
Streptococcus, streptococcal A40.9
agalactiae A40.1
group
A A40.0
B A40.1
D A41.81
neonatal P36.10
group B P36.0
specified NEC P36.19
pneumoniae A40.3
pyogenes A40.0
specified NEC A40.8
tracheostomy stoma J95.02
tularemic A21.7
umbilical, umbilical cord (newborn) —*see* Sepsis, newborn
Yersinia pestis A20.7
Septate —*see* Septum
Septic —*see* condition
arm —*see* Cellulitis, upper limb
with lymphangitis —*see* Lymphangitis, acute, upper limb
embolus —*see* Embolism
finger —*see* Cellulitis, digit
with lymphangitis —*see* Lymphangitis, acute, digit
foot —*see* Cellulitis, lower limb
with lymphangitis —*see* Lymphangitis, acute, lower limb
gallbladder (acute) K81.0
hand —*see* Cellulitis, upper limb
with lymphangitis —*see* Lymphangitis, acute, upper limb
joint —*see* Arthritis, pyogenic or pyemic
leg —*see* Cellulitis, lower limb
with lymphangitis —*see* Lymphangitis, acute, lower limb
nail —*see also* Cellulitis, digit
with lymphangitis —*see* Lymphangitis, acute, digit
sore —*see also* Abscess
throat J02.0
streptococcal J02.0
spleen (acute) D73.89
teeth, tooth (pulpal origin) K04.4
throat —*see* Pharyngitis
thrombus —*see* Thrombosis
toe —*see* Cellulitis, digit
with lymphangitis —*see* Lymphangitis, acute, digit
tonsils, chronic J35.01
with adenoiditis J35.03
uterus —*see* Endometritis
Septicemia A41.9
meaning sepsis —*see* Sepsis
Septum, septate (congenital) —*see also* Anomaly, by site
anal Q42.3
with fistula Q42.2
aqueduct of Sylvius Q03.0
with spina bifida —*see* Spina bifida, by site, with hydrocephalus
uterus (complete) (partial) Q51.2
vagina Q52.10
in pregnancy —*see* Pregnancy, complicated by, abnormal vagina
causing obstructed labor O65.5
longitudinal Q52.129 ⇐
microperforate ◀
left side Q52.124 ◀
right side Q52.123 ◀
nonobstruction Q52.120 ◀
obstructing Q52.129 ◀
left side Q52.122 ◀
right side Q52.121 ◀
transverse Q52.11

◀ New ⇐ Revised ~~deleted~~ Deleted

Sequelae (of) —*see also* condition
abscess, intracranial or intraspinal (conditions in G06) G09
amputation — code to injury with seventh character S
burn and corrosion — code to injury with seventh character S
calcium deficiency E64.8
cerebrovascular disease —*see* Sequelae, disease, cerebrovascular
childbirth O94
contusion — code to injury with seventh character S
corrosion —*see* Sequelae, burn and corrosion
crushing injury — code to injury with seventh character S
disease
cerebrovascular I69.90
alteration of sensation I69.998
aphasia I69.920
apraxia I69.990
ataxia I69.993
cognitive deficits I69.91
disturbance of vision I69.998
dysarthria I69.922
dysphagia I69.991
dysphasia I69.921
facial droop I69.992
facial weakness I69.992
fluency disorder I69.923
hemiplegia I69.95-
hemorrhage
intracerebral —*see* Sequelae, hemorrhage, intracerebral
intracranial, nontraumatic NEC —*see* Sequelae, hemorrhage, intracranial, nontraumatic
subarachnoid —*see* Sequelae, hemorrhage, subarachnoid
language deficit I69.928
monoplegia
lower limb I69.84-
upper limb I69.93-
paralytic syndrome I69.96-
specified effect NEC I69.998
specified type NEC I69.80
alteration of sensation I69.898
aphasia I69.820
apraxia I69.890
ataxia I69.893
cognitive deficits I69.81
disturbance of vision I69.898
dysarthria I69.822
dysphagia I69.891
dysphasia I69.821
facial droop I69.892
facial weakness I69.892
fluency disorder I69.823
hemiplegia I69.85-
language deficit I69.828
monoplegia
lower limb I69.84-
upper limb I69.83-
paralytic syndrome I69.86-
specified effect NEC I69.898
speech deficit I69.928
speech deficit I69.828
stroke NOS —*see* Sequelae, stroke NOS
dislocation — code to injury with seventh character S
encephalitis or encephalomyelitis (conditions in G04) G09
in infectious disease NEC B94.8
viral B94.1
external cause — code to injury with seventh character S
foreign body entering natural orifice — code to injury with seventh character S
fracture — code to injury with seventh character S

Sequelae *(Continued)*
frostbite — code to injury with seventh character S
Hansen's disease B92
hemorrhage
intracerebral I69.10
alteration of sensation I69.198
aphasia I69.120
apraxia I69.190
ataxia I69.193
cognitive deficits I69.11
disturbance of vision I69.198
dysarthria I69.122
dysphagia I69.191
dysphasia I69.121
facial droop I69.192
facial weakness I69.192
fluency disorder I69.123
hemiplegia I69.15-
language deficit NEC I69.128
monoplegia
lower limb I69.14-
upper limb I69.13-
paralytic syndrome I69.16-
specified effect NEC I69.198
speech deficit NEC I69.128
intracranial, nontraumatic NEC I69.20
alteration of sensation I69.298
aphasia I69.220
apraxia I69.290
ataxia I69.293
cognitive deficits I69.21
disturbance of vision I69.298
dysarthria I69.222
dysphagia I69.291
dysphasia I69.221
facial droop I69.292
facial weakness I69.292
fluency disorder I69.223
hemiplegia I69.25-
language deficit NEC I69.228
monoplegia
lower limb I69.24-
upper limb I69.23-
paralytic syndrome I69.26-
specified effect NEC I69.298
speech deficit NEC I69.228
subarachnoid I69.00
alteration of sensation I69.098
aphasia I69.020
apraxia I69.090
ataxia I69.093
cognitive deficits —*see* subcategory I69.01- ◄
disturbance of vision I69.098
dysarthria I69.022
dysphagia I69.091
dysphasia I69.021
facial droop I69.092
facial weakness I69.092
fluency disorder I69.023
hemiplegia I69.05-
language deficit NEC I69.028
monoplegia
lower limb I69.04-
upper limb I69.03-
paralytic syndrome I69.06-
specified effect NEC I69.098
speech deficit NEC I69.028
hepatitis, viral B94.2
hyperalimentation E68
infarction
cerebral I69.30
alteration of sensation I69.398
aphasia I69.320
apraxia I69.390
ataxia I69.393
cognitive deficits I69.31
disturbance of vision I69.398
dysarthria I69.322
dysphagia I69.391

Sequelae *(Continued)*
infarction *(Continued)*
cerebral *(Continued)*
dysphasia I69.321
facial droop I69.392
facial weakness I69.392
fluency disorder I69.323
hemiplegia I69.35-
language deficit NEC I69.328
monoplegia
lower limb I69.34-
upper limb I69.33-
paralytic syndrome I69.36-
specified effect NEC I69.398
speech deficit NEC I69.328
infection, pyogenic, intracranial or intraspinal G09
infectious disease B94.9
specified NEC B94.8
injury — code to injury with seventh character S
leprosy B92
meningitis
bacterial (conditions in G00) G09
other or unspecified cause (conditions in G03) G09
muscle (and tendon) injury — code to injury with seventh character S
myelitis —*see* Sequelae, encephalitis
niacin deficiency E64.8
nutritional deficiency E64.9
specified NEC E64.8
obstetrical condition O94
parasitic disease B94.9
phlebitis or thrombophlebitis of intracranial or intraspinal venous sinuses and veins (conditions in G08) G09
poisoning — code to poisoning with seventh character S
nonmedicinal substance —*see* Sequelae, toxic effect, nonmedicinal substance
poliomyelitis (acute) B91
pregnancy O94
protein-energy malnutrition E64.0
puerperium O94
rickets E64.3
selenium deficiency E64.8
sprain and strain — code to injury with seventh character S
stroke NOS I69.30
alteration in sensation I69.398
aphasia I69.320
apraxia I69.390
ataxia I69.393
cognitive deficits I69.31
disturbance of vision I69.398
dysarthria I69.322
dysphagia I69.391
dysphasia I69.321
facial droop I69.392
facial weakness I69.392
hemiplegia I69.35-
language deficit NEC I69.328
monoplegia
lower limb I69.34-
upper limb I69.33-
paralytic syndrome I69.36-
specified effect NEC I69.398
speech deficit NEC I69.328
tendon and muscle injury — code to injury with seventh character S
thiamine deficiency E64.8
trachoma B94.0
tuberculosis B90.9
bones and joints B90.2
central nervous system B90.0
genitourinary B90.1
pulmonary (respiratory) B90.9
specified organs NEC B90.8

S

◄ New ⇐ Revised ~~deleted~~ Deleted

Sequelae *(Continued)*
viral
encephalitis B94.1
hepatitis B94.2
vitamin deficiency NEC E64.8
A E64.1
B E64.8
C E64.2
wound, open — code to injury with seventh character S
Sequestration —*see also* Sequestrum
disk —*see* Displacement, intervertebral disk ◀
lung, congenital Q33.2
Sequestrum
bone —*see* Osteomyelitis, chronic
dental M27.2
jaw bone M27.2
orbit —*see* Osteomyelitis, orbit
sinus (accessory) (nasal) —*see* Sinusitis
Sequoiosis lung or pneumonitis J67.8
Serology for syphilis
doubtful
with signs or symptoms - code by site and stage under Syphilis
follow-up of latent syphilis —*see* Syphilis, latent
negative, with signs or symptoms — code by site and stage under Syphilis
positive A53.0
with signs or symptoms - code by site and stage under Syphilis
reactivated A53.0
Seroma —*see also* Hematoma
postprocedural —*see* Complication, postprocedural, seroma ◀
traumatic, secondary and recurrent T79.2
Seropurulent —*see* condition
Serositis, multiple K65.8
pericardial I31.1
peritoneal K65.8
Serous —*see* condition
Sertoli cell
adenoma
specified site —*see* Neoplasm, benign, by site
unspecified site
female D27.9
male D29.20
carcinoma
specified site —*see* Neoplasm, malignant, by site
unspecified site (male) C62.9-
female C56.9
tumor
with lipid storage
specified site —*see* Neoplasm, benign, by site
unspecified site
female D27.9
male D29.20
specified site —*see* Neoplasm, benign, by site
unspecified site
female D27.9
male D29.20
Sertoli-Leydig cell tumor —*see* Neoplasm, benign, by site
specified site —*see* Neoplasm, benign, by site
unspecified site
female D27.9
male D29.20
Serum
allergy, allergic reaction —*see also* Reaction, serum T80.69
shock —*see also* Shock, anaphylactic T80.59
arthritis —*see also* Reaction, serum T80.69
complication or reaction NEC —*see also* Reaction, serum T80.69

Serum *(Continued)*
disease NEC —*see also* Reaction, serum T80.69
hepatitis —*see also* Hepatitis, viral, type B
carrier (suspected) of B18.1 ⟸
intoxication —*see also* Reaction, serum T80.69
neuritis —*see also* Reaction, serum T80.69
neuropathy G61.1
poisoning NEC —*see also* Reaction, serum T80.69
rash NEC —*see also* Reaction, serum T80.69
reaction NEC —*see also* Reaction, serum T80.69
sickness NEC —*see also* Reaction, serum T80.69
urticaria —*see also* Reaction, serum T80.69
Sesamoiditis M25.8-
Sever's disease or osteochondrosis —*see* Osteochondrosis, juvenile, tarsus
Severe sepsis R65.20
with septic shock R65.21
Sex
chromosome mosaics Q97.8
lines with various numbers of X chromosomes Q97.2
education Z70.8
reassignment surgery status Z87.890
Sextuplet pregnancy —*see* Pregnancy, sextuplet
Sexual
function, disorder of (psychogenic) F52.9
immaturity (female) (male) E30.0
impotence (psychogenic) organic origin NEC —*see* Dysfunction, sexual, male
precocity (constitutional) (cryptogenic) (female) (idiopathic) (male) E30.1
Sexuality, pathologic —*see* Deviation, sexual
Sézary disease C84.1-
Shadow, lung R91.8
Shaking palsy or paralysis —*see* Parkinsonism
Shallowness, acetabulum —*see* Derangement, joint, specified type NEC, hip
Shaver's disease J63.1
Sheath (tendon) —*see* condition
Sheathing, retinal vessels H35.01-
Shedding
nail L60.8
premature, primary (deciduous) teeth K00.6
Sheehan's disease or syndrome E23.0
Shelf, rectal K62.89
Shell teeth K00.5
Shellshock (current) F43.0
lasting state —*see* Disorder, post-traumatic stress
Shield kidney Q63.1
Shift
auditory threshold (temporary) H93.24-
mediastinal R93.8
Shifting sleep-work schedule (affecting sleep) G47.26
Shiga (-Kruse) dysentery A03.0
Shiga's bacillus A03.0
Shigella (dysentery) —*see* Dysentery, bacillary
Shigellosis A03.9
Group A A03.0
Group B A03.1
Group C A03.2
Group D A03.3
Shin splints S86.89
Shingles —*see* Herpes, zoster
Shipyard disease or eye B30.0
Shirodkar suture, in pregnancy —*see* Pregnancy, complicated by, incompetent cervix
Shock R57.9
with ectopic or molar pregnancy O08.3
adrenal (cortical) (Addisonian) E27.2
adverse food reaction (anaphylactic) —*see* Shock, anaphylactic, due to food
allergic —*see* Shock, anaphylactic

Shock *(Continued)*
anaphylactic T78.2
chemical —*see* Table of Drugs and Chemicals
due to drug or medicinal substance
correct substance properly administered T88.6
overdose or wrong substance given or taken (by accident) —*see* Table of Drugs and Chemicals, by drug, poisoning
due to food (nonpoisonous) T78.00
additives T78.06
dairy products T78.07
eggs T78.08
fish T78.03
shellfish T78.02
fruit T78.04
milk T78.07
nuts T78.05
multiple types T78.05 ◀
peanuts T78.01
peanuts T78.01
seeds T78.05
specified type NEC T78.09
vegetable T78.04
following sting (s) —*see* Venom
immunization T80.52
serum T80.59
blood and blood products T80.51
immunization T80.52
specified NEC T80.59
vaccination T80.52
anaphylactoid —*see* Shock, anaphylactic
anesthetic
correct substance properly administered T88.2
overdose or wrong substance given or taken —*see* Table of Drugs and Chemicals, by drug, poisoning
specified anesthetic —*see* Table of Drugs and Chemicals, by drug, poisoning
cardiogenic R57.0
chemical substance —*see* Table of Drugs and Chemicals
complicating ectopic or molar pregnancy O08.3
culture —*see* Disorder, adjustment
drug
due to correct substance properly administered T88.6
overdose or wrong substance given or taken (by accident) —*see* Table of Drugs and Chemicals, by drug, poisoning
during or after labor and delivery O75.1
electric T75.4
(taser) T75.4
endotoxic R65.21
postprocedural (resulting from a procedure, not elsewhere classified) T81.12 ⟸
following
ectopic or molar pregnancy O08.3
injury (immediate) (delayed) T79.4
labor and delivery O75.1
food (anaphylactic) —*see* Shock, anaphylactic, due to food
from electroshock gun (taser) T75.4
gram-negative R65.21
postprocedural (resulting from a procedure, not elsewhere classified) T81.12 ⟸
hematologic R57.8
hemorrhagic
surgery (intraoperative) (postoperative) T81.19
trauma T79.4
hypovolemic R57.1
surgical T81.19
traumatic T79.4

◀ New ⟸ Revised ~~deleted~~ Deleted

Shock *(Continued)*
insulin E15
therapeutic misadventure —*see* subcategory T38.3
kidney N17.0
traumatic (following crushing) T79.5
lightning T75.01
liver K72.00 ◀
lung J80
obstetric O75.1
with ectopic or molar pregnancy O08.3
following ectopic or molar pregnancy O08.3
pleural (surgical) T81.19
due to trauma T79.4
postprocedural (postoperative) T81.10
with ectopic or molar pregnancy O08.3
cardiogenic T81.11
endotoxic T81.12
following ectopic or molar pregnancy O08.3
gram-negative T81.12
hypovolemic T81.19
septic T81.12
specified type NEC T81.19
psychic F43.0
septic (due to severe sepsis) R65.21
specified NEC R57.8
surgical T81.10
taser gun (taser) T75.4
therapeutic misadventure NEC T81.10
thyroxin
overdose or wrong substance given or taken —*see* Table of Drugs and Chemicals, by drug, poisoning
toxic, syndrome A48.3
transfusion —*see* Complications, transfusion
traumatic (immediate) (delayed) T79.4
Shoemaker's chest M95.4
Short, shortening, shortness
arm (acquired) —*see also* Deformity, limb, unequal length
congenital Q71.81-
forearm —*see* Deformity, limb, unequal length
bowel syndrome K91.2
breath R06.02
cervical (complicating pregnancy) O26.87-
non-gravid uterus N88.3
common bile duct, congenital Q44.5
cord (umbilical), complicating delivery O69.3
cystic duct, congenital Q44.5
esophagus (congenital) Q39.8
femur (acquired) —*see* Deformity, limb, unequal length, femur
congenital —*see* Defect, reduction, lower limb, longitudinal, femur
frenum, frenulum, linguae (congenital) Q38.1
hip (acquired) —*see also* Deformity, limb, unequal length
congenital Q65.89
leg (acquired) —*see also* Deformity, limb, unequal length
congenital Q72.81-
lower leg —*see also* Deformity, limb, unequal length
limbed stature, with immunodeficiency D82.2
lower limb (acquired) —*see also* Deformity, limb, unequal length
congenital Q72.81-
organ or site, congenital NEC —*see* Distortion
palate, congenital Q38.5
radius (acquired) —*see also* Deformity, limb, unequal length
congenital —*see* Defect, reduction, upper limb, longitudinal, radius
rib syndrome Q77.2
stature (child) (hereditary) (idiopathic) NEC R62.52
constitutional E34.3
due to endocrine disorder E34.3
Laron-type E34.3

Short, shortening, shortness *(Continued)*
tendon —*see also* Contraction, tendon
with contracture of joint —*see* Contraction, joint
Achilles (acquired) M67.0-
congenital Q66.89
congenital Q79.8
thigh (acquired) —*see also* Deformity, limb, unequal length, femur
congenital —*see* Defect, reduction, lower limb, longitudinal, femur
tibialis anterior (tendon) —*see* Contraction, tendon
umbilical cord
complicating delivery O69.3
upper limb, congenital —*see* Defect, reduction, upper limb, specified type NEC
urethra N36.8
uvula, congenital Q38.5
vagina (congenital) Q52.4
Shortsightedness —*see* Myopia
Shoshin (acute fulminating beriberi) E51.11
Shoulder —*see* condition
Shovel-shaped incisors K00.2
Shower, thromboembolic —*see* Embolism
Shunt
arterial-venous (dialysis) Z99.2
arteriovenous, pulmonary (acquired) I28.0
congenital Q25.72
cerebral ventricle (communicating) in situ Z98.2
surgical, prosthetic, with complications —*see* Complications, cardiovascular, device or implant Shutdown, renal N28.9
Shutdown, renal N28.9
Shy-Drager syndrome G90.3
Sialadenitis, sialadenosis (any gland) (chronic) (periodic) (suppurative) —*see* Sialoadenitis
Sialectasia K11.8
Sialidosis E77.1
Sialitis, silitis (any gland) (chronic) (suppurative) —*see* Sialoadenitis
Sialoadenitis (any gland) (periodic) (suppurative) K11.20
acute K11.21
recurrent K11.22
chronic K11.23
Sialoadenopathy K11.9
Sialoangitis —*see* Sialoadenitis
Sialodochitis (fibrinosa) —*see* Sialoadenitis
Sialodocholithiasis K11.5
Sialolithiasis K11.5
Sialometaplasia, necrotizing K11.8
Sialorrhea —*see also* Ptyalism
periodic —*see* Sialoadenitis
Sialosis K11.7
Siamese twin Q89.4
Sibling rivalry Z62.891
Sicard's syndrome G52.7
Sicca syndrome M35.00
with
keratoconjunctivitis M35.01
lung involvement M35.02
myopathy M35.03
renal tubulo-interstitial disorders M35.04
specified organ involvement NEC M35.09
Sick R69
or handicapped person in family Z63.79
needing care at home Z63.6
sinus (syndrome) I49.5
Sick-euthyroid syndrome E07.81
Sickle-cell
anemia —*see* Disease, sickle-cell
trait D57.3
Sicklemia —*see also* Disease, sickle-cell
trait D57.3
Sickness
air (travel) T75.3
airplane T75.3
alpine T70.29

Sickness *(Continued)*
altitude T70.20
Andes T70.29
aviator's T70.29
balloon T70.29
car T75.3
compressed air T70.3
decompression T70.3
green D50.8
milk —*see* Poisoning, food, noxious
motion T75.3
mountain T70.29
acute D75.1
protein —*see also* Reaction, serum T80.69
radiation T66
roundabout (motion) T75.3
sea T75.3
serum NEC —*see also* Reaction, serum T80.69
sleeping (African) B56.9
by Trypanosoma B56.9
brucei
gambiense B56.0
rhodesiense B56.1
East African B56.1
Gambian B56.0
Rhodesian B56.1
West African B56.0
swing (motion) T75.3
train (railway) (travel) T75.3
travel (any vehicle) T75.3
Sideropenia —*see* Anemia, iron deficiency
Siderosilicosis J62.8
Siderosis (lung) J63.4
eye (globe) —*see* Disorder, globe, degenerative, siderosis
Siemens' syndrome (ectodermal dysplasia) Q82.8
Sighing R06.89
psychogenic F45.8
Sigmoid —*see also* condition
flexure —*see* condition
kidney Q63.1
Sigmoiditis —*see also* Enteritis K52.9
infectious A09
noninfectious K52.9
Silfversköld's syndrome Q78.9
Silicosiderosis J62.8
Silicosis, silicotic (simple) (complicated) J62.8
with tuberculosis J65
Silicotuberculosis J65
Silo-fillers' disease J68.8
bronchitis J68.0
pneumonitis J68.0
pulmonary edema J68.1
Silver's syndrome Q87.1
Simian malaria B53.1
Simmonds' cachexia or disease E23.0
Simons' disease or syndrome (progressive lipodystrophy) E88.1
Simple, simplex —*see* condition
Simulation, conscious (of illness) Z76.5
Simultanagnosia (asimultagnosia) R48.3
Sin Nombre virus disease (Hantavirus) (cardio)-pulmonary syndrome) B33.4
Sinding-Larsen disease or osteochondrosis —*see* Osteochondrosis, juvenile, patella
Singapore hemorrhagic fever A91
Singer's node or nodule J38.2
Single
atrium Q21.2
coronary artery Q24.5
umbilical artery Q27.0
ventricle Q20.4
Singultus R06.6
epidemicus B33.0
Sinus —*see also* Fistula
abdominal K63.89
arrest I45.5
arrhythmia I49.8
bradycardia R00.1
branchial cleft (internal) (external) Q18.0
coccygeal —*see* Sinus, pilonidal

S

Sinus *(Continued)*
dental K04.6
dermal (congenital) Q06.8
with abscess Q06.8
coccygeal, pilonidal —*see* Sinus, coccygeal
infected, skin NEC L08.89
marginal, ruptured or bleeding —*see* Hemorrhage, antepartum, specified cause NEC
medial, face and neck Q18.8
pause I45.5
pericranii Q01.9
pilonidal (infected) (rectum) L05.92
with abscess L05.02
preauricular Q18.1
rectovaginal N82.3
Rokitansky-Aschoff (gallbladder) K82.8
sacrococcygeal (dermoid) (infected) —*see* Sinus, pilonidal
tachycardia R00.0
paroxysmal I47.1
tarsi syndrome M25.57- ◄
testis N50.89 ◄
tract (postinfective) —*see* Fistula
urachus Q64.4
Sinusitis (accessory) (chronic) (hyperplastic) (nasal) (nonpurulent) (purulent) J32.9
acute J01.90
ethmoidal J01.20
recurrent J01.21
frontal J01.10
recurrent J01.11
involving more than one sinus, other than pansinusitis J01.80
recurrent J01.81
maxillary J01.00
recurrent J01.01
pansinusitis J01.40
recurrent J01.41
recurrent J01.91
specified NEC J01.80
recurrent J01.81
sphenoidal J01.30
recurrent J01.31
allergic —*see* Rhinitis, allergic
due to high altitude T70.1
ethmoidal J32.2
acute J01.20
recurrent J01.21
frontal J32.1
acute J01.10
recurrent J01.11
influenzal —*see* Influenza, with, respiratory manifestations NEC
involving more than one sinus but not pansinusitis J32.8
acute J01.80
recurrent J01.81
maxillary J32.0
acute J01.00
recurrent J01.01
sphenoidal J32.3
acute J01.30
recurrent J01.31
tuberculous, any sinus A15.8
Sinusitis-bronchiectasis-situs inversus (syndrome) (triad) Q89.3
Sipple's syndrome E31.22
Sirenomelia (syndrome) Q87.2
Siriasis T67.0
Sirkari's disease B55.0
Siti A65
Situation, psychiatric F99
Situational
disturbance (transient) —*see* Disorder, adjustment
acute F43.0
maladjustment —*see* Disorder, adjustment
reaction —*see* Disorder, adjustment
acute F43.0
Situs inversus or transversus (abdominalis) (thoracis) Q89.3
Sixth disease B08.20
due to human herpesvirus 6 B08.21
due to human herpesvirus 7 B08.22
Sjögren-Larsson syndrome Q87.1
Sjögren's syndrome or disease —*see* Sicca syndrome
Skeletal —*see* condition
Skene's gland —*see* condition
Skenitis —*see* Urethritis
Skerljevo A65
Skevas-Zerfus disease —*see* Toxicity, venom, marine animal, sea anemone
Skin —*see also* condition
clammy R23.1
donor —*see* Donor, skin
hidebound M35.9
Slate-dressers' or slate-miners' lung J62.8
Sleep
apnea —*see* Apnea, sleep
deprivation Z72.820
disorder or disturbance G47.9
child F51.9
nonorganic origin F51.9
specified NEC G47.8
disturbance G47.9
nonorganic origin F51.9
drunkenness F51.9
rhythm inversion G47.2-
terrors F51.4
walking F51.3
hysterical F44.89
Sleep hygiene
abuse Z72.821
inadequate Z72.821
poor Z72.821
Sleeping sickness —*see* Sickness, sleeping
Sleeplessness —*see* Insomnia
menopausal N95.11
Sleep-wake schedule disorder G47.20
Slim disease (in HIV infection) B20
Slipped, slipping
epiphysis (traumatic) —*see also* Osteochondropathy, specified type NEC
capital femoral (traumatic)
acute (on chronic) S79.01-
current traumatic - code as Fracture, by site
upper femoral (nontraumatic) M93.00-
acute M93.01-
on chronic M93.03-
chronic M93.02-
intervertebral disc —*see* Displacement, intervertebral disc
ligature, umbilical P51.8
patella —*see* Disorder, patella, derangement NEC
rib M89.8X8
sacroiliac joint —*see* subcategory M53.2
tendon —*see* Disorder, tendon
ulnar nerve, nontraumatic —*see* Lesion, nerve, ulnar
vertebra NEC —*see* Spondylolisthesis
Slocumb's syndrome E27.0
Sloughing (multiple) (phagedena) (skin) —*see also* Gangrene
abscess —*see* Abscess
appendix K38.8
fascia —*see* Disorder, soft tissue, specified type NEC
scrotum N50.89 ◄
tendon —*see* Disorder, tendon
transplanted organ —*see* Rejection, transplant
ulcer —*see* Ulcer, skin
Slow
feeding, newborn P92.2
flow syndrome, coronary I20.8
heart(beat) R00.1
Slowing, urinary stream R39.198 ◄
Sluder's neuralgia (syndrome) G44.89
Slurred, slurring speech R47.81
Small (ness)
for gestational age —*see* Small for dates
introitus, vagina N89.6
kidney (unknown cause) N27.9
bilateral N27.1
unilateral N27.0
ovary (congenital) Q50.39
pelvis
with disproportion (fetopelvic) O33.1
causing obstructed labor O65.1
uterus N85.8
white kidney N03.9
Small-and-light-for-dates —*see* Small for dates
Small-for-dates (infant) P05.10
with weight of
499 grams or less P05.11
500-749 grams P05.12
750-999 grams P05.13
1000-1249 grams P05.14
1250-1499 grams P05.15
1500-1749 grams P05.16
1750-1999 grams P05.17
2000-2499 grams P05.18
2500 grams and over P05.19 ◄
specified NEC P05.19 ◄
Smallpox B03
Smearing, fecal R15.1
Smith-Lemli-Opitz syndrome E78.72
Smith's fracture S52.54-
Smoker —*see* Dependence, drug, nicotine
Smoker's
bronchitis J41.0
cough J41.0
palate K13.24
throat J31.2
tongue K13.24
Smoking
passive Z77.22
Smothering spells R06.81
Snaggle teeth, tooth M26.39
Snapping
finger —*see* Trigger finger
hip —*see* Derangement, joint, specified type NEC, hip
involving the iliotiblial band M76.3-
knee —*see* Derangement, knee
involving the iliotiblial band M76.3-
Sneddon-Wilkinson disease or syndrome (subcorneal pustular dermatosis) L13.1
Sneezing (intractable) R06.7
Sniffing
cocaine
abuse —*see* Abuse, drug, cocaine
dependence —*see* Dependence, drug, cocaine
gasoline
abuse —*see* Abuse, drug, inhalant
dependence —*see* Dependence, drug, inhalant
glue (airplane)
abuse —*see* Abuse, drug, inhalant
drug dependence —*see* Dependence, drug, inhalant
Sniffles
newborn P28.89
Snoring R06.83
Snow blindness —*see* Photokeratitis
Snuffles (non-syphilitic) R06.5
newborn P28.89
syphilitic (infant) A50.05 *[J99]*
Social
exclusion Z60.4
due to discrimination or persecution (perceived) Z60.5
migrant Z59.0
acculturation difficulty Z60.3
rejection Z60.4
due to discrimination or persecution Z60.5

S

◄ New ◄ Revised ~~deleted~~ Deleted

Social *(Continued)*
role conflict NEC Z73.5
skills inadequacy NEC Z73.4
transplantation Z60.3
Sodoku A25.0
Soemmerring's ring —*see* Cataract, secondary
Soft —*see also* condition
nails L60.3
Softening
bone —*see* Osteomalacia
brain (necrotic) (progressive) G93.89
congenital Q04.8
embolic I63.4- ◄
hemorrhagic —*see* Hemorrhage, intracranial, intracerebral
occlusive I63.5- ◄
thrombotic I63.3- ◄
cartilage M94.2-
patella M22.4-
cerebellar —*see* Softening, brain
cerebral —*see* Softening, brain
cerebrospinal —*see* Softening, brain
myocardial, heart —*see* Degeneration, myocardial
spinal cord G95.89
stomach K31.89
Soldier's
heart F45.8
patches I31.0
Solitary
cyst, kidney N28.1
kidney, congenital Q60.0
Solvent abuse —*see* Abuse, drug, inhalant
dependence —*see* Dependence, drug, inhalant
Somatization reaction, somatic reaction —*see* Disorder, somatoform
Somnambulism F51.3
hysterical F44.89
Somnolence R40.0
nonorganic origin F51.11
Sonne dysentery A03.3
Soor B37.0
Sore
bed —*see* Ulcer, pressure, by site
chiclero B55.1
Delhi B55.1
desert —*see* Ulcer, skin
eye H57.1-
Lahore B55.1
mouth K13.79
canker K12.0
muscle M79.1
Naga —*see* Ulcer, skin
of skin —*see* Ulcer, skin - oriental B55.1
pressure —*see* Ulcer, pressure, by site
skin L98.9
soft A57
throat (acute) —*see also* Pharyngitis
with influenza, flu, or grippe —*see* Influenza, with, respiratory manifestations NEC
chronic J31.2
coxsackie (virus) B08.5
diphtheritic A36.0
herpesviral B00.2
influenzal —*see* Influenza, with, respiratory manifestations NEC
septic J02.0
streptococcal (ulcerative) J02.0
viral NEC J02.8
coxsackie B08.5
tropical —*see* Ulcer, skin
veldt —*see* Ulcer, skin
Soto's syndrome (cerebral gigantism) Q87.3
South African cardiomyopathy syndrome I42.8
Southeast Asian hemorrhagic fever A91
Spacing
abnormal, tooth, teeth, fully erupted M26.30
excessive, tooth, fully erupted M26.32
Spade-like hand (congenital) Q68.1
Spading nail L60.8
congenital Q84.6
Spanish collar N47.1
Sparganosis B70.1
Spasm (s), **spastic, spasticity** —*see also* condition R25.2
accommodation —*see* Spasm, of accommodation
ampulla of Vater K83.4
anus, ani (sphincter) (reflex) K59.4
psychogenic F45.8
artery I73.9
cerebral G45.9
Bell's G51.3
bladder (sphincter, external or internal) N32.89
psychogenic F45.8
bronchus, bronchiole J98.01
cardia K22.0
cardiac I20.1
carpopedal —*see* Tetany
cerebral (arteries) (vascular) G45.9
cervix, complicating delivery O62.4
ciliary body (of accommodation) —*see* Spasm, of accommodation
colon —*see also* Irritable, bowel K58.9 ◄
with diarrhea K58.0
psychogenic F45.8
common duct K83.8
compulsive —*see* Tic
conjugate H51.8
coronary (artery) I20.1
diaphragm (reflex) R06.6
epidemic B33.0
psychogenic F45.8
duodenum K59.8
epidemic diaphragmatic (transient) B33.0
esophagus (diffuse) K22.4
psychogenic F45.8
facial G51.3
fallopian tube N83.8
gastrointestinal (tract) K31.89
psychogenic F45.8
glottis J38.5
hysterical F44.4
psychogenic F45.8
conversion reaction F44.4
reflex through recurrent laryngeal nerve J38.5
habit —*see* Tic
heart I20.1
hemifacial (clonic) G51.3
hourglass —*see* Contraction, hourglass
hysterical F44.4
infantile —*see* Epilepsy, spasms
inferior oblique, eye H51.8
intestinal —*see also* Syndrome, irritable bowel K58.9
psychogenic F45.8
larynx, laryngeal J38.5
hysterical F44.4
psychogenic F45.8
conversion reaction F44.4
levator palpebrae superioris —*see* Disorder, eyelid function
muscle NEC M62.838
back M62.830
nerve, trigeminal G51.0
nervous F45.8
nodding F98.4
occupational F48.8
oculogyric H51.8
psychogenic F45.8
of accommodation H52.53-
ophthalmic artery —*see* Occlusion, artery, retina
perineal, female N94.89
peroneo-extensor —*see also* Deformity, limb, flat foot
pharynx (reflex) J39.2
hysterical F45.8
psychogenic F45.8
Spasm (s), **spastic, spasticity** *(Continued)*
psychogenic F45.8
pylorus NEC K31.3
adult hypertrophic K31.89
congenital or infantile Q40.0
psychogenic F45.8
rectum (sphincter) K59.4
psychogenic F45.8
retinal (artery) —*see* Occlusion, artery, retina
sigmoid —*see also* Syndrome, irritable bowel K58.9
psychogenic F45.8
sphincter of Oddi K83.4
stomach K31.89
neurotic F45.8
throat J39.2
hysterical F45.8
psychogenic F45.8
tic F95.9
chronic F95.1
transient of childhood F95.0
tongue K14.8
torsion (progressive) G24.1
trigeminal nerve —*see* Neuralgia, trigeminal
ureter N13.5
urethra (sphincter) N35.9
uterus N85.8
complicating labor O62.4
vagina N94.2
psychogenic F52.5
vascular I73.9
vasomotor I73.9
vein NEC I87.8
viscera —*see* Pain, abdominal
Spasmodic —*see* condition
Spasmophilia —*see* Tetany
Spasmus nutans F98.4
Spastic, spasticity —*see also* Spasm
child (cerebral) (congenital) (paralysis) G80.1
Speaker's throat R49.8
Specific, specified —*see* condition
Speech
defect, disorder, disturbance, impediment R47.9
psychogenic, in childhood and adolescence F98.8
slurring R47.81
specified NEC R47.89
Spencer's disease A08.19
Spens' syndrome (syncope with heart block) I45.9
Sperm counts (fertility testing) Z31.41
postvasectomy Z30.8
reversal Z31.42
Spermatic cord —*see* condition
Spermatocele N43.40
congenital Q55.4
multiple N43.42
single N43.41
Spermatocystitis N49.0
Spermatocytoma C62.9-
specified site —*see* Neoplasm, malignant, by site
Spermatorrhea N50.89 ◄
Sphacelus —*see* Gangrene
Sphenoidal —*see* condition
Sphenoiditis (chronic) —*see* Sinusitis, sphenoidal
Sphenopalatine ganglion neuralgia G90.09
Sphericity, increased, lens (congenital) Q12.4
Spherocytosis (congenital) (familial) (hereditary) D58.0
hemoglobin disease D58.0
sickle-cell (disease) D57.8-
Spherophakia Q12.4
Sphincter —*see* condition
Sphincteritis, sphincter of Oddi —*see* Cholangitis
Sphingolipidosis E75.3
specified NEC E75.29

S

◄ New ◄ Revised ~~deleted~~ Deleted

Sphingomyelinosis E75.3
Spicule tooth K00.2
Spider
bite —*see* Toxicity, venom, spider
fingers —*see* Syndrome, Marfan's
nevus I78.1
toes —*see* Syndrome, Marfan's
vascular I78.1
Spiegler-Fendt
benign lymphocytoma L98.8
sarcoid L08.89
Spielmeyer-Vogt disease E75.4
Spina bifida (aperta) Q05.9
with hydrocephalus NEC Q05.4
cervical Q05.5
with hydrocephalus Q05.0
dorsal Q05.6
with hydrocephalus Q05.1
lumbar Q05.7
with hydrocephalus Q05.2
lumbosacral Q05.7
with hydrocephalus Q05.2
occulta Q76.0
sacral Q05.8
with hydrocephalus Q05.3
thoracic Q05.6
with hydrocephalus Q05.1
thoracolumbar Q05.6
with hydrocephalus Q05.1
Spindle, Krukenberg's —*see* Pigmentation, cornea, posterior
Spine, spinal —*see* condition
Spiradenoma (eccrine) —*see* Neoplasm, skin, benign
Spirillosis A25.0
Spirillum
minus A25.0
obermeieri infection A68.0
Spirochetal —*see* condition
Spirochetosis A69.9
arthritic, arthritica A69.9
bronchopulmonary A69.8
icterohemorrhagic A27.0
lung A69.8
Spirometrosis B70.1
Spitting blood —*see* Hemoptysis
Splanchnoptosis K63.4
Spleen, splenic —*see* condition
Splenectasis —*see* Splenomegaly
Splenitis (interstitial) (malignant) (nonspecific) D73.89
malarial —*see also* Malaria B54 *[D77]*
tuberculous A18.85
Splenocele D73.89
Splenomegaly, splenomegalia (Bengal) (cryptogenic) (idiopathic) (tropical) R16.1
with hepatomegaly R16.2
cirrhotic D73.2
congenital Q89.09
congestive, chronic D73.2
Egyptian B65.1
Gaucher's E75.22
malarial —*see also* Malaria B54 *[D77]*
neutropenic D73.81
Niemann-Pick —*see* Niemann-Pick disease or syndrome
siderotic D73.2
syphilitic A52.79
congenital (early) A50.08 *[D77]*
Splenopathy D73.9
Splenoptosis D73.89
Splenosis D73.89
Splinter —*see* Foreign body, superficial, by site
Split, splitting
foot Q72.7-
hand Q71.6 ◀
heart sounds R01.2
lip, congenital —*see* Cleft, lip
nails L60.3
urinary stream R39.13
Spondylarthrosis —*see* Spondylosis
Spondylitis (chronic) —*see also* Spondylopathy, inflammatory
ankylopoietica —*see* Spondylitis, ankylosing
ankylosing (chronic) M45.9
with lung involvement M45.9 *[J99]*
cervical region M45.2
cervicothoracic region M45.3
juvenile M08.1
lumbar region M45.6
lumbosacral region M45.7
multiple sites M45.0
occipito-atlanto-axial region M45.1
sacrococcygeal region M45.8
thoracic region M45.4
thoracolumbar region M45.5
atrophic (ligamentous) —*see* Spondylitis, ankylosing
deformans (chronic) —*see* Spondylosis
gonococcal A54.41
gouty —*see also* Gout, by type, vertebrae M10.08 ⟸
in (due to)
brucellosis A23.9 *[M49.80]*
cervical region A23.9 *[M49.82]*
cervicothoracic region A23.9 *[M49.83]*
lumbar region A23.9 *[M49.86]*
lumbosacral region A23.9 *[M49.87]*
multiple sites A23.9 *[M49.89]*
occipito-atlanto-axial region A23.9 *[M49.81]*
sacrococcygeal region A23.9 *[M49.88]*
thoracic region A23.9 *[M49.84]*
thoracolumbar region A23.9 *[M49.85]*
enterobacteria —*see also* subcategory M49.8 A04.9
tuberculosis A18.01
infectious NEC —*see* Spondylopathy, infective
juvenile ankylosing (chronic) M08.1
Kümmell's —*see* Spondylopathy, traumatic
Marie-Strümpell —*see* Spondylitis, ankylosing
muscularis —*see* Spondylopathy, specified NEC
psoriatic L40.53
rheumatoid —*see* Spondylitis, ankylosing
rhizomelica —*see* Spondylitis, ankylosing
sacroiliac NEC M46.1
senescent, senile —*see* Spondylosis
traumatic (chronic) or post-traumatic —*see* Spondylopathy, traumatic
tuberculous A18.01
typhosa A01.05
Spondylolisthesis (acquired) (degenerative) M43.10
with disproportion (fetopelvic) O33.0
causing obstructed labor O65.0
cervical region M43.12
cervicothoracic region M43.13
congenital Q76.2
lumbar region M43.16
lumbosacral region M43.17
multiple sites M43.19
occipito-atlanto-axial region M43.11
sacrococcygeal region M43.18
thoracic region M43.14
thoracolumbar region M43.15
traumatic (old) M43.10
acute
fifth cervical (displaced) S12.430
nondisplaced S12.431
specified type NEC (displaced) S12.450
nondisplaced S12.451
type III S12.44
fourth cervical (displaced) S12.330
nondisplaced S12.331
specified type NEC (displaced) S12.350
nondisplaced S12.351
type III S12.34
Spondylolisthesis *(Continued)*
traumatic *(Continued)*
acute *(Continued)*
second cervical (displaced) S12.130
nondisplaced S12.131
specified type NEC (displaced) S12.150
nondisplaced S12.151
type III S12.14
seventh cervical (displaced) S12.630
nondisplaced S12.631
specified type NEC (displaced) S12.650
nondisplaced S12.651
type III S12.64
sixth cervical (displaced) S12.530
nondisplaced S12.531
specified type NEC (displaced) S12.550
nondisplaced S12.551
type III S12.54
third cervical (displaced) S12.230
nondisplaced S12.231
specified type NEC (displaced) S12.250
nondisplaced S12.251
type III S12.24
Spondylolysis (acquired) M43.00
cervical region M43.02
cervicothoracic region M43.03
congenital Q76.2
lumbar region M43.06
lumbosacral region M43.07
with disproportion (fetopelvic) O33.0
causing obstructed labor O65.8
multiple sites M43.09
occipito-atlanto-axial region M43.01
sacrococcygeal region M43.08
thoracic region M43.04
thoracolumbar region M43.05
Spondylopathy M48.9
infective NEC M46.50
cervical region M46.52
cervicothoracic region M46.53
lumbar region M46.56
lumbosacral region M46.57
multiple sites M46.59
occipito-atlanto-axial region M46.51
sacrococcygeal region M46.58
thoracic region M46.54
thoracolumbar region M46.55
inflammatory M46.90
cervical region M46.92
cervicothoracic region M46.93
lumbar region M46.96
lumbosacral region M46.97
multiple sites M46.99
occipito-atlanto-axial region M46.91
sacrococcygeal region M46.98
specified type NEC M46.80
cervical region M46.82
cervicothoracic region M46.83
lumbar region M46.86
lumbosacral region M46.87
multiple sites M46.89
occipito-atlanto-axial region M46.81
sacrococcygeal region M46.88
thoracic region M46.84
thoracolumbar region M46.85
thoracic region M46.94
thoracolumbar region M46.95
neuropathic, in
syringomyelia and syringobulbia G95.0
tabes dorsalis A52.11
specified NEC —*see* subcategory M48.8
traumatic M48.30
cervical region M48.32
cervicothoracic region M48.33
lumbar region M48.36
lumbosacral region M48.37
occipito-atlanto-axial region M48.31

S

◀ New ⟸ Revised ~~deleted~~ Deleted

Spondylopathy *(Continued)*
traumatic *(Continued)*
sacrococcygeal region M48.38
thoracic region M48.34
thoracolumbar region M48.35
Spondylosis M47.9
with
disproportion (fetopelvic) O33.0
causing obstructed labor O65.0
myelopathy NEC M47.10
cervical region M47.12
cervicothoracic region M47.13
lumbar region M47.16
occipito-atlanto-axial region M47.11
thoracic region M47.14
thoracolumbar region M47.15
radiculopathy M47.20
cervical region M47.22
cervicothoracic region M47.23
lumbar region M47.26
lumbosacral region M47.27
occipito-atlanto-axial region M47.21
sacrococcygeal region M47.28
thoracic region M47.24
thoracolumbar region M47.25
without myelopathy or radiculopathy M47.819
cervical region M47.812
cervicothoracic region M47.813
lumbar region M47.816
lumbosacral region M47.817
occipito-atlanto-axial region M47.811
sacrococcygeal region M47.818
thoracic region M47.814
thoracolumbar region M47.815
specified NEC M47.899
cervical region M47.892
cervicothoracic region M47.893
lumbar region M47.896
lumbosacral region M47.897
occipito-atlanto-axial region M47.891
sacrococcygeal region M47.898
thoracic region M47.894
thoracolumbar region M47.895
traumatic —*see* Spondylopathy, traumatic
Sponge
inadvertently left in operation wound —*see* Foreign body, accidentally left during a procedure
kidney (medullary) Q61.5
Sponge-diver's disease —*see* Toxicity, venom, marine animal, sea anemone
Spongioblastoma (any type) —*see* Neoplasm, malignant, by site
specified site —*see* Neoplasm, malignant, by site
unspecified site C71.9
Spongioneuroblastoma —*see* Neoplasm, malignant, by site
Spontaneous —*see also* condition
fracture (cause unknown) —*see* Fracture, pathological
Spoon nail L60.3
congenital Q84.6
Sporadic —*see* condition
Sporothrix schenckii infection —*see* Sporotrichosis
Sporotrichosis B42.9
arthritis B42.82
disseminated B42.7
generalized B42.7
lymphocutaneous (fixed) (progressive) B42.1
pulmonary B42.0
specified NEC B42.89
Spots, spotting (in) (of)
Bitot's —*see also* Pigmentation, conjunctiva
in the young child E50.1
vitamin A deficiency E50.1
Spots, spotting *(Continued)*
café, au lait L81.3
Cayenne pepper I78.1
cotton wool, retina —*see* Occlusion, artery, retina
de Morgan's (senile angiomas) I78.1
Fuchs' black (myopic) H44.2-
intermenstrual (regular) N92.0
irregular N92.1
Koplik's B05.9
liver L81.4
pregnancy O26.85-
purpuric R23.3
ruby I78.1
Spotted fever —*see* Fever, spotted N92.3
Sprain (joint) (ligament)
acromioclavicular joint or ligament S43.5-
ankle S93.40-
calcaneofibular ligament S93.41-
deltoid ligament S93.42-
internal collateral ligament —*see* Sprain, ankle, specified ligament NEC
specified ligament NEC S93.49-
talofibular ligament —*see* Sprain, ankle, specified ligament NEC
tibiofibular ligament S93.43-
anterior longitudinal, cervical S13.4
atlas, atlanto-axial, atlanto-occipital S13.4
breast bone —*see* Sprain, sternum
calcaneofibular —*see* Sprain, ankle
carpal —*see* Sprain, wrist
carpometacarpal —*see* Sprain, hand, specified site NEC
cartilage
costal S23.41
semilunar (knee) —*see* Sprain, knee, specified site NEC
with current tear —*see* Tear, meniscus
thyroid region S13.5
xiphoid —*see* Sprain, sternum
cervical, cervicodorsal, cervicothoracic S13.4
chondrosternal S23.421
coracoclavicular S43.8-
coracohumeral S43.41-
coronary, knee —*see* Sprain, knee, specified site NEC
costal cartilage S23.41
cricoarytenoid articulation or ligament S13.5
cricothyroid articulation S13.5
cruciate, knee —*see* Sprain, knee, cruciate
deltoid, ankle —*see* Sprain, ankle
dorsal (spine) S23.3
elbow S53.40-
radial collateral ligament S53.43-
radiohumeral S53.41-
rupture
radial collateral ligament —*see* Rupture, traumatic, ligament, radial collateral
ulnar collateral ligament —*see* Rupture, traumatic, ligament, ulnar collateral
specified type NEC S53.49-
ulnar collateral ligament S53.44-
ulnohumeral S53.42-
femur, head —*see* Sprain, hip
fibular collateral, knee —*see* Sprain, knee, collateral
fibulocalcaneal —*see* Sprain, ankle
finger (s) S63.61-
index S63.61-
interphalangeal (joint) S63.63-
index S63.63-
little S63.63-
middle S63.63-
ring S63.63-
little S63.61-
metacarpophalangeal (joint) S63.65-
middle S63.61-
ring S63.61-
Sprain *(Continued)*
finger (s) *(Continued)*
specified site NEC S63.69-
index S63.69-
little S63.69-
middle S63.69-
ring S63.69-
foot S93.60-
specified ligament NEC S93.69-
tarsal ligament S93.61-
tarsometatarsal ligament S93.62-
toe —*see* Sprain, toe
hand S63.9-
finger —*see* Sprain, finger
specified site NEC —*see* subcategory S63.8
thumb —*see* Sprain, thumb
head S03.9
hip S73.10-
iliofemoral ligament S73.11-
ischiocapsular (ligament) S73.12-
specified NEC S73.19-
iliofemoral —*see* Sprain, hip
innominate
acetabulum —*see* Sprain, hip
sacral junction S33.6
internal
collateral, ankle —*see* Sprain, ankle
semilunar cartilage —*see* Sprain, knee, specified site NEC
interphalangeal
finger —*see* Sprain, finger, interphalangeal (joint)
toe —*see* Sprain, toe, interphalangeal joint
ischiocapsular —*see* Sprain, hip
ischiofemoral —*see* Sprain, hip
jaw (articular disc) (cartilage) (meniscus) S03.4- ◄
old M26.69
knee S83.9-
collateral ligament S83.40-
lateral (fibular) S83.42-
medial (tibial) S83.41-
cruciate ligament S83.50-
anterior S83.51-
posterior S83.52-
lateral (fibular) collateral ligament S83.42-
medial (tibial) collateral ligament S83.41-
patellar ligament S76.11-
specified site NEC S83.8X-
superior tibiofibular joint (ligament) S83.6-
lateral collateral, knee —*see* Sprain, knee, collateral
lumbar (spine) S33.5
lumbosacral S33.9
mandible (articular disc) S03.4- ◄
old M26.69
medial collateral, knee —*see* Sprain, knee, collateral
meniscus
jaw S03.4- ◄
old M26.69
knee —*see* Sprain, knee, specified site NEC
with current tear —*see* Tear, meniscus
old —*see* Derangement, knee, meniscus, due to old tear
mandible S03.4- ◄
old M26.69
metacarpal (distal) (proximal) —*see* Sprain, hand, specified site NEC
metacarpophalangeal —*see* Sprain, finger, metacarpophalangeal (joint)
metatarsophalangeal —*see* Sprain, toe, metatarsophalangeal joint
midcarpal —*see* Sprain, hand, specified site NEC
midtarsal —*see* Sprain, foot, specified site NEC
neck S13.9
anterior longitudinal cervical ligament S13.4
atlanto-axial joint S13.4

S

◄ New ◄ Revised ~~deleted~~ Deleted

Sprain *(Continued)*
neck *(Continued)*
atlanto-occipital joint S13.4
cervical spine S13.4
cricoarytenoid ligament S13.5
cricothyroid ligament S13.5
specified site NEC S13.8
thyroid region (cartilage) S13.5
nose S03.8
orbicular, hip —*see* Sprain, hip
patella —*see* Sprain, knee, specified site NEC
patellar ligament S76.11-
pelvis NEC S33.8
phalanx
finger —*see* Sprain, finger
toe —*see* Sprain, toe
pubofemoral —*see* Sprain, hip
radiocarpal —*see* Sprain, wrist
radiohumeral —*see* Sprain, elbow
radius, collateral —*see* Rupture, traumatic, ligament, radial collateral
rib (cage) S23.41
rotator cuff (capsule) S43.42-
sacroiliac (region)
chronic or old —*see* subcategory M53.2
joint S33.6
scaphoid (hand) —*see* Sprain, hand, specified site NEC
scapula (r) —*see* Sprain, shoulder girdle, specified site NEC
semilunar cartilage (knee) —*see* Sprain, knee, specified site NEC
with current tear —*see* Tear, meniscus
old —*see* Derangement, knee, meniscus, due to old tear
shoulder joint S43.40-
acromioclavicular joint (ligament) —*see* Sprain, acromioclavicular joint
blade —*see* Sprain, shoulder, girdle, specified site NEC
coracoclavicular joint (ligament) —*see* Sprain, coracoclavicular joint
coracohumeral ligament —*see* Sprain, coracohumeral joint
girdle S43.9-
specified site NEC S43.8-
rotator cuff —*see* Sprain, rotator cuff
specified site NEC S43.49-
sternoclavicular joint (ligament) —*see* Sprain, sternoclavicular joint
spine
cervical S13.4
lumbar S33.5
thoracic S23.3
sternoclavicular joint S43.6-
sternum S23.429
chondrosternal joint S23.421
specified site NEC S23.428
sternoclavicular (joint) (ligament) S23.420
symphysis
jaw S03.4- ⇐
old M26.69
mandibular S03.4- ⇐
old M26.69
talofibular —*see* Sprain, ankle
tarsal —*see* Sprain, foot, specified site NEC
tarsometatarsal —*see* Sprain, foot, specified site NEC
temporomandibular S03.4- ⇐
old M26.69
thorax S23.9
ribs S23.41
specified site NEC S23.8
spine S23.3
sternum —*see* Sprain, sternum
thumb S63.60-
interphalangeal (joint) S63.62-
metacarpophalangeal (joint) S63.64-
specified site NEC S63.68-
thyroid cartilage or region S13.5

Sprain *(Continued)*
tibia (proximal end) —*see* Sprain, knee, specified site NEC
tibial collateral, knee —*see* Sprain, knee, collateral
tibiofibular
distal —*see* Sprain, ankle
superior —*see* Sprain, knee, specified site NEC
toe (s) S93.50-
great S93.50-
interphalangeal joint S93.51-
great S93.51-
lesser S93.51-
lesser S93.50-
metatarsophalangeal joint S93.52-
great S93.52-
lesser S93.52-
ulna, collateral —*see* Rupture, traumatic, ligament, ulnar collateral
ulnohumeral —*see* Sprain, elbow
wrist S63.50-
carpal S63.51-
radiocarpal S63.52-
specified site NEC S63.59-
xiphoid cartilage —*see* Sprain, sternum
Sprengel's deformity (congenital) Q74.0
Sprue (tropical) K90.1
celiac K90.0
idiopathic K90.49 ⇐
meaning thrush B37.0
nontropical K90.0
Spur, bone —*see also* Enthesopathy
calcaneal M77.3-
iliac crest M76.2-
nose (septum) J34.89
Spurway's syndrome Q78.0
Sputum
abnormal (amount) (color) (odor) (purulent) R09.3
blood-stained R04.2
excessive (cause unknown) R09.3
Squamous —*see also* condition
epithelium in
cervical canal (congenital) Q51.828
uterine mucosa (congenital) Q51.818
Squashed nose M95.0
congenital Q67.4
Squeeze, diver's T70.3
Squint —*see also* Strabismus
accommodative —*see* Strabismus, convergent concomitant
St. Hubert's disease A82.9
Stab —*see also* Laceration
internal organs —*see* Injury, by site
Stafne's cyst or cavity M27.0
Staggering gait R26.0
hysterical F44.4
Staghorn calculus —*see* Calculus, kidney
Stähli's line (cornea) (pigment) —*see* Pigmentation, cornea, anterior
Stain, staining
meconium (newborn) P96.83
port wine Q82.5
tooth, teeth (hard tissues) (extrinsic) K03.6
due to
accretions K03.6
deposits (betel) (black) (green) (materia alba) (orange) (soft) (tobacco) K03.6
metals (copper) (silver) K03.7
nicotine K03.6
pulpal bleeding K03.7
tobacco K03.6
intrinsic K00.8
Stammering —*see also* Disorder, fluency F80.81
Standstill
auricular I45.5
cardiac —*see* Arrest, cardiac
sinoatrial I45.5
ventricular —*see* Arrest, cardiac
Stannosis J63.5

Stanton's disease —*see* Melioidosis
Staphylitis (acute) (catarrhal) (chronic) (gangrenous) (membranous) (suppurative) (ulcerative) K12.2
Staphylococcal scalded skin syndrome L00
Staphylococcemia A41.2
Staphylococcus, staphylococcal —*see also* condition
as cause of disease classified elsewhere B95.8
aureus (methicillin susceptible) (MSSA) B95.61
methicillin resistant (MRSA) B95.62
specified NEC, as cause of disease classified elsewhere B95.7
Staphyloma (sclera)
cornea H18.72-
equatorial H15.81-
localized (anterior) H15.82-
posticum H15.83-
ring H15.85-
Stargardt's disease —*see* Dystrophy, retina
Starvation (inanition) (due to lack of food) T73.0
edema —*see* Malnutrition, severe
Stasis
bile (noncalculous) K83.1
bronchus J98.09
with infection —*see* Bronchitis
cardiac —*see* Failure, heart, congestive
cecum K59.8
colon K59.8
dermatitis I87.2 ⇐
with ◀
varicose ulcer —*see* Varix, leg, with ulcer, with inflammation ◀
varicose veins —*see* Varix, leg, with, inflammation ◀
due to postthrombotic syndrome —*see* Syndrome, postthrombotic ◀
duodenal K31.5
eczema —*see* Varix, leg, with, inflammation
edema —*see* Hypertension, venous (chronic), idiopathic
foot T69.0-
ileocecal coil K59.8
ileum K59.8
intestinal K59.8
jejunum K59.8
kidney N19
liver (cirrhotic) K76.1
lymphatic I89.8
pneumonia J18.2
pulmonary —*see* Edema, lung
rectal K59.8
renal N19
tubular N17.0
ulcer —*see* Varix, leg, with, ulcer
without varicose veins I87.2
urine —*see* Retention, urine
venous I87.8
State (of)
affective and paranoid, mixed, organic psychotic F06.8
agitated R45.1
acute reaction to stress F43.0
anxiety (neurotic) F41.1
apprehension F41.1
burn-out Z73.0
climacteric, female Z78.0
symptomatic N95.1
compulsive F42.8 ⇐
mixed with obsessional thoughts F42.2 ⇐
confusional (psychogenic) F44.89
acute —*see also* Delirium
with
arteriosclerotic dementia F01.50
with behavioral disturbance F01.51
senility or dementia F05
alcoholic F10.231

◀ New ⇐ Revised ~~deleted~~ Deleted

State *(Continued)*
confusional (psychogenic) *(Continued)*
epileptic F05
reactive (from emotional stress, psychological trauma) F44.89
subacute —*see* Delirium
convulsive —*see* Convulsions
crisis F43.0
depressive F32.9
neurotic F34.1
dissociative F44.9
emotional shock (stress) R45.7
hypercoagulation —*see* Hypercoagulable
locked-in G83.5
menopausal Z78.0
symptomatic N95.1
neurotic F48.9
with depersonalization F48.1
obsessional F42.8 ⇐
oneiroid (schizophrenia-like) F23
organic
hallucinatory (nonalcoholic) F06.0
paranoid (-hallucinatory) F06.2
panic F41.0
paranoid F22
climacteric F22
involutional F22
menopausal F22
organic F06.2
senile F03
simple F22
persistent vegetative R40.3
phobic F40.9
postleukotomy F07.0
~~pregnant, incidental Z33.1~~
pregnant ◀
gestational carrier Z33.3 ◀
incidental Z33.1 ◀
psychogenic, twilight F44.89
psychopathic (constitutional) F60.2
psychotic, organic —*see also* Psychosis, organic
mixed paranoid and affective F06.8
senile or presenile F03
transient NEC F06.8
with
depression F06.31
hallucinations F06.0
residual schizophrenic F20.5
restlessness R45.1
stress (emotional) R45.7
tension (mental) F48.9
specified NEC F48.8
transient organic psychotic NEC F06.8
depressive type F06.31
hallucinatory type F06.0 ⇐
twilight
epileptic F05
psychogenic F44.89
vegetative, persistent R40.3
vital exhaustion Z73.0
withdrawal —*see* Withdrawal, state
Status (post) —*see also* Presence (of)
absence, epileptic —*see* Epilepsy, by type, with status epilepticus
administration of tPA (rtPA) in a different facility within the last 24 hours prior to admission to the current facility Z92.82
adrenalectomy (unilateral) (bilateral) E89.6
anastomosis Z98.0
anginosus I20.9
angioplasty (peripheral) Z98.62
with implant Z95.820
coronary artery Z98.61
with implant Z95.5
aortocoronary bypass Z95.1
arthrodesis Z98.1
artificial opening (of) Z93.9
gastrointestinal tract Z93.4
specified NEC Z93.8

Status *(Continued)*
artificial opening (of) *(Continued)*
urinary tract Z93.6
vagina Z93.8
asthmaticus —*see* Asthma, by type, with status asthmaticus
awaiting organ transplant Z76.82
bariatric surgery Z98.84
bed confinement Z74.01
bleb, filtering (vitreous), after glaucoma surgery Z98.83
breast implant Z98.82
removal Z98.86
cataract extraction Z98.4-
cholecystectomy Z90.49
clitorectomy N90.811
with excision of labia minora N90.812
colectomy (complete) (partial) Z90.49
colonization —*see* Carrier (suspected) of
colostomy Z93.3
convulsivus idiopathicus —*see* Epilepsy, by type, with status epilepticus
coronary artery angioplasty —*see* Status, angioplasty, coronary artery
cystectomy (urinary bladder) Z90.6
cystostomy Z93.50
appendico-vesicostomy Z93.52
cutaneous Z93.51
specified NEC Z93.59
delinquent immunization Z28.3
dental Z98.818
crown Z98.811
fillings Z98.811
restoration Z98.811
sealant Z98.810
specified NEC Z98.818
deployment (current) (military) Z56.82
dialysis (hemodialysis) (peritoneal) Z99.2
do not resuscitate (DNR) Z66
donor —*see* Donor
embedded fragments —*see* Retained, foreign body fragments (type of)
embedded splinter —*see* Retained, foreign body fragments (type of)
enterostomy Z93.4
epileptic, epilepticus —*see also* Epilepsy, by type, with status epilepticus G40.901
estrogen receptor
negative Z17.1
positive Z17.0
female genital cutting —*see* Female genital mutilation status
female genital mutilation —*see* Female genital mutilation status
filtering (vitreous) bleb after glaucoma surgery Z98.83
gastrectomy (complete) (partial) Z90.3
gastric banding Z98.84
gastric bypass for obesity Z98.84
gastrostomy Z93.1
human immunodeficiency virus (HIV) infection, asymptomatic Z21
hysterectomy (complete) (total) Z90.710
partial (with remaining cervial stump) Z90.711
ileostomy Z93.2
implant
breast Z98.82
infibulation N90.813
intestinal bypass Z98.0
jejunostomy Z93.4
lapsed immunization schedule Z28.3
laryngectomy Z90.02
lymphaticus E32.8
malignancy ◀
castrate resistant prostate Z19.2 ◀
hormone resistant Z19.2 ◀
hormone sensitive Z19.1 ◀
marmoratus G80.3
mastectomy (unilateral) (bilateral) Z90.1-

Status *(Continued)*
military deployment status (current) Z56.82
in theater or in support of military war, peacekeeping and humanitarian operations Z56.82
nephrectomy (unilateral) (bilateral) Z90.5
nephrostomy Z93.6
obesity surgery Z98.84
oophorectomy
bilateral Z90.722
unilateral Z90.721
organ replacement
by artificial or mechanical device or prosthesis of
artery Z95.828
bladder Z96.0
blood vessel Z95.828
breast Z97.8
eye globe Z97.0
heart Z95.812
valve Z95.2
intestine Z97.8
joint Z96.60
hip —*see* Presence, hip joint implant
knee —*see* Presence, knee joint implant
specified site NEC Z96.698
kidney Z97.8
larynx Z96.3
lens Z96.1
limbs —*see* Presence, artificial, limb
liver Z97.8
lung Z97.8
pancreas Z97.8
by organ transplant (heterologous) (homologous) —*see* Transplant
pacemaker
brain Z96.89
cardiac Z95.0
specified NEC Z96.89
pancreatectomy Z90.410
complete Z90.410
partial Z90.411
total Z90.410
pneumonectomy (complete) (partial) Z90.2
pneumothorax, therapeutic Z98.3
postcommotio cerebri F07.81
postoperative (postprocedural) NEC Z98.890 ⇐
breast implant Z98.82
dental Z98.818
crown Z98.811
fillings Z98.811
restoration Z98.811
sealant Z98.810
specified NEC Z98.818
pneumothorax, therapeutic Z98.3
uterine scar Z98.891 ◀
postpartum (routine follow-up) Z39.2
care immediately after delivery Z39.0
postsurgical (postprocedural) NEC Z98.890 ⇐
pneumothorax, therapeutic Z98.3
pregnancy, incidental Z33.1
prosthesis coronary angioplasty Z95.5
pseudophakia Z96.1
renal dialysis (hemodialysis) (peritoneal) Z99.2
retained foreign body —*see* Retained, foreign body fragments (type of)
reversed jejunal transposition (for bypass Z98.0
salpingo-oophorectomy
bilateral Z90.722
unilateral Z90.721
sex reassignment surgery status Z87.890
shunt
arteriovenous (for dialysis) Z99.2
cerebrospinal fluid Z98.2
ventricular (communicating) (for drainage) Z98.2

S

Status *(Continued)*
splenectomy Z90.81
thymicolymphaticus E32.8
thymicus E32.8
thymolymphaticus E32.8
thyroidectomy (hypothyroidism) E89.0
tooth (teeth) extraction —*see also* Absence, teeth, acquired K08.409
tPA (rtPA) administration in a different facility within the last 24 hours prior to admission to current facility Z92.82
tracheostomy Z93.0
transplant —*see* Transplant
organ removed Z98.85
tubal ligation Z98.51
underimmunization Z28.3
ureterostomy Z93.6
urethrostomy Z93.6
vagina, artificial Z93.8
vasectomy Z98.52
wheelchair confinement Z99.3
Stealing
child problem F91.8
in company with others Z72.810
pathological (compulsive) F63.2
Steam burn —*see* Burn
Steatocystoma multiplex L72.2
Steatohepatitis (nonalcoholic) (NASH) K75.81
Steatoma L72.3
eyelid (cystic) —*see* Dermatosis, eyelid
infected —*see* Hordeolum
Steatorrhea (chronic) K90.9 ⟸
with lacteal obstruction K90.2
idiopathic (adult) (infantile) K90.9 ⟸
pancreatic K90.3
primary K90.0
tropical K90.1
Steatosis E88.89
heart —*see* Degeneration, myocardial
kidney N28.89
liver NEC K76.0
Steele-Richardson-Olszewski disease or syndrome G23.1
Steinbrocker's syndrome G90.8
Steinert's disease G71.11
Stein-Leventhal syndrome E28.2
Stein's syndrome E28.2
STEMI —*see also* - Infarct, myocardium, ST elevation I21.3
Stenocardia I20.8
Stenocephaly Q75.8
Stenosis, stenotic (cicatricial) —*see also* Stricture
ampulla of Vater K83.1
anus, anal (canal) (sphincter) K62.4
and rectum K62.4
congenital Q42.3
with fistula Q42.2
aorta (ascending) (supraventricular) (congenital) Q25.1 ⟸
arteriosclerotic I70.0
calcified I70.0
supravalvular Q25.3 ◀
aortic (valve) I35.0
with insufficiency I35.2
congenital Q23.0
rheumatic I06.0
with
incompetency, insufficiency or regurgitation I06.2
with mitral (valve) disease I08.0
with tricuspid (valve) disease I08.3
mitral (valve) disease I08.0
with tricuspid (valve) disease I08.3
tricuspid (valve) disease I08.2
with mitral (valve) disease I08.3
specified cause NEC I35.0
syphilitic A52.03
Stenosis, stenotic *(Continued)*
aqueduct of Sylvius (congenital) Q03.0
with spina bifida —*see* Spina bifida, by site, with hydrocephalus
acquired G91.1
artery NEC —*see also* Arteriosclerosis I77.1
celiac I77.4
cerebral —*see* Occlusion, artery, cerebral
extremities —*see* Arteriosclerosis, extremities
precerebral —*see* Occlusion, artery, precerebral
pulmonary (congenital) Q25.6
acquired I28.8
renal I70.1
stent ◀
coronary T82.855 ◀
peripheral T82.856 ◀
bile duct (common) (hepatic) K83.1
congenital Q44.3
bladder-neck (acquired) N32.0
congenital Q64.31
brain G93.89
bronchus J98.09
congenital Q32.3
syphilitic A52.72
cardia (stomach) K22.2
congenital Q39.3
cardiovascular —*see* Disease, cardiovascular
caudal M48.08
cervix, cervical (canal) N88.2
congenital Q51.828
in pregnancy or childbirth —*see* Pregnancy, complicated by, abnormal cervix
colon —*see also* Obstruction, intestine
congenital Q42.9
specified NEC Q42.8
colostomy K94.03
common (bile) duct K83.1
congenital Q44.3
coronary (artery) —*see* Disease, heart, ischemic, atherosclerotic
cystic duct —*see* Obstruction, gallbladder
due to presence of device, implant or graft —*see also* Complications, by site and type, specified NEC T85.858 ⟸
arterial graft NEC T82.858
breast (implant) T85.858 ⟸
catheter T85.858 ⟸
dialysis (renal) T82.858
intraperitoneal T85.858 ⟸
infusion NEC T82.858
spinal (epidural) (subdural) T85.850 ⟸
urinary (indwelling) T83.85
fixation, internal (orthopedic) NEC T84.85
gastrointestinal (bile duct) (esophagus) T85.858 ⟸
genital NEC T83.85
heart NEC T82.857
joint prosthesis T84.85
ocular (corneal graft) (orbital implant) NEC T85.858 ⟸
orthopedic NEC T84.85
specified NEC T85.858 ⟸
urinary NEC T83.85
vascular NEC T82.858
ventricular intracranial shunt T85.850 ⟸
duodenum K31.5
congenital Q41.0
ejaculatory duct NEC N50.89 ⟸
endocervical os —*see* Stenosis, cervix
enterostomy K94.13
esophagus K22.2
congenital Q39.3
syphilitic A52.79
congenital A50.59 *[K23]*
eustachian tube —*see* Obstruction, eustachian tube
Stenosis, stenotic *(Continued)*
external ear canal (acquired) H61.30-
congenital Q16.1
due to
inflammation H61.32-
trauma H61.31-
postprocedural H95.81-
specified cause NEC H61.39-
gallbladder —*see* Obstruction, gallbladder
glottis J38.6
heart valve (congenital) Q24.8
aortic Q23.0
mitral Q23.2
pulmonary Q22.1
tricuspid Q22.4
hepatic duct K83.1
hymen N89.6
hypertrophic subaortic (idiopathic) I42.1
ileum K56.69
congenital Q41.2
infundibulum cardia Q24.3
intervertebral foramina —*see also* Lesion, biomechanical, specified NEC
connective tissue M99.79
abdomen M99.79
cervical region M99.71
cervicothoracic M99.71
head region M99.70
lumbar region M99.73
lumbosacral M99.73
occipitocervical M99.70
sacral region M99.74
sacrococcygeal M99.74
sacroiliac M99.74
specified NEC M99.79
thoracic region M99.72
thoracolumbar M99.72
disc M99.79
abdomen M99.79
cervical region M99.71
cervicothoracic M99.71
head region M99.70
lower extremity M99.76
lumbar region M99.73
lumbosacral M99.73
occipitocervical M99.70
pelvic M99.75
rib cage M99.78
sacral region M99.74
sacrococcygeal M99.74
sacroiliac M99.74
specified NEC M99.79
thoracic region M99.72
thoracolumbar M99.72
upper extremity M99.77
osseous M99.69
abdomen M99.69
cervical region M99.61
cervicothoracic M99.61
head region M99.60
lower extremity M99.66
lumbar region M99.63
lumbosacral M99.63
occipitocervical M99.60
pelvic M99.65
rib cage M99.68
sacral region M99.64
sacrococcygeal M99.64
sacroiliac M99.64
specified NEC M99.69
thoracic region M99.62
thoracolumbar M99.62
upper extremity M99.67
subluxation —*see* Stenosis, intervertebral foramina, osseous
intestine —*see also* Obstruction, intestine
congenital (small) Q41.9
large Q42.9
specified NEC Q42.8
specified NEC Q41.8

S

◀ New ⟸ Revised ~~deleted~~ Deleted

Stenosis, stenotic *(Continued)*
jejunum K56.69
congenital Q41.1
lacrimal (passage)
canaliculi H04.54-
congenital Q10.5
duct H04.55-
punctum H04.56-
sac H04.57-
lacrimonasal duct —*see* Stenosis, lacrimal, duct
congenital Q10.5
larynx J38.6
congenital NEC Q31.8
subglottic Q31.1
syphilitic A52.73
congenital A50.59 *[J99]*
mitral (chronic) (inactive) (valve) I05.0
with
aortic valve disease I08.0
incompetency, insufficiency or regurgitation I05.2
active or acute I01.1
with rheumatic or Sydenham's chorea I02.0
congenital Q23.2
specified cause, except rheumatic I34.2
syphilitic A52.03
myocardium, myocardial —*see also* Degeneration, myocardial
hypertrophic subaortic (idiopathic) I42.1
nares (anterior) (posterior) J34.89
congenital Q30.0
nasal duct —*see also* Stenosis, lacrimal, duct
congenital Q10.5
nasolacrimal duct —*see also* Stenosis, lacrimal, duct
congenital Q10.5
neural canal —*see also* Lesion, biomechanical, specified NEC
connective tissue M99.49
abdomen M99.49
cervical region M99.41
cervicothoracic M99.41
head region M99.40
lower extremity M99.46
lumbar region M99.43
lumbosacral M99.43
occipitocervical M99.40
pelvic M99.45
rib cage M99.48
sacral region M99.44
sacrococcygeal M99.44
sacroiliac M99.44
specified NEC M99.49
thoracic region M99.42
thoracolumbar M99.42
upper extremity M99.47
intervertebral disc M99.59
abdomen M99.59
cervical region M99.51
cervicothoracic M99.51
head region M99.50
lower extremity M99.56
lumbar region M99.53
lumbosacral M99.53
occipitocervical M99.50
pelvic M99.55
rib cage M99.58
sacral region M99.54
sacrococcygeal M99.54
sacroiliac M99.54
specified NEC M99.59
thoracic region M99.52
thoracolumbar M99.52
upper extremity M99.57
osseous M99.39
abdomen M99.39
cervical region M99.31
cervicothoracic M99.31
head region M99.30

Stenosis, stenotic *(Continued)*
neural canal *(Continued)*
osseous *(Continued)*
lower extremity M99.36
lumbar region M99.33
lumbosacral M99.33
occipitocervical M99.30
pelvic M99.35
rib cage M99.38
sacral region M99.34
sacrococcygeal M99.34
sacroiliac M99.34
specified NEC M99.39
thoracic region M99.32
thoracolumbar M99.32
upper extremity M99.37
subluxation M99.29
cervical region M99.21
cervicothoracic M99.21
head region M99.20
lower extremity M99.26
lumbar region M99.23
lumbosacral M99.23
occipitocervical M99.20
pelvic M99.25
rib cage M99.28
sacral region M99.24
sacrococcygeal M99.24
sacroiliac M99.24
specified NEC M99.29
thoracic region M99.22
thoracolumbar M99.22
upper extremity M99.27
organ or site, congenital NEC —*see* Atresia, by site
papilla of Vater K83.1
pulmonary (artery) (congenital) Q25.6
with ventricular septal defect, transposition of aorta, and hypertrophy of right ventricle Q21.3
acquired I28.8
in tetralogy of Fallot Q21.3
infundibular Q24.3
subvalvular Q24.3
supravalvular Q25.6
valve I37.0
with insufficiency I37.2
congenital Q22.1
rheumatic I09.89
with aortic, mitral or tricuspid (valve) disease I08.8
vein, acquired I28.8
vessel NEC I28.8
pulmonic (congenital) Q22.1
infundibular Q24.3
subvalvular Q24.3
pylorus (hypertrophic) (acquired) K31.1
adult K31.1
congenital Q40.0
infantile Q40.0
rectum (sphincter) —*see* Stricture, rectum
renal artery I70.1
congenital Q27.1
salivary duct (any) K11.8
sphincter of Oddi K83.1
spinal M48.00
cervical region M48.02
cervicothoracic region M48.03
lumbar region M48.06
lumbosacral region M48.07
occipito-atlanto-axial region M48.01
sacrococcygeal region M48.08
thoracic region M48.04
thoracolumbar region M48.05
stent ◀
vascular ◀
end stent ◀
adjacent to stent —*see* Arteriosclerosis ◀

Stenosis, stenotic *(Continued)*
stent *(Continued)*
vascular *(Continued)*
end stent *(Continued)*
within the stent ◀
coronary T82.855 ◀
peripheral T82.856 ◀
in stent ◀
coronary vessel T82.855 ◀
peripheral vessel T82.856 ◀
stomach, hourglass K31.2
subaortic (congenital) Q24.4
hypertrophic (idiopathic) I42.1
subglottic J38.6
congenital Q31.1
postprocedural J95.5
trachea J39.8
congenital Q32.1
syphilitic A52.73
tuberculous NEC A15.5
tracheostomy J95.03
tricuspid (valve) I07.0
with
aortic (valve) disease I08.2
incompetency, insufficiency or regurgitation I07.2
with aortic (valve) disease I08.2
with mitral (valve) disease I08.3
mitral (valve) disease I08.1
with aortic (valve) disease I08.3
congenital Q22.4
nonrheumatic I36.0
with insufficiency I36.2
tubal N97.1
ureter —*see* Atresia, ureter
ureteropelvic junction, congenital Q62.11
ureterovesical orifice, congenital Q62.12
urethra (valve) —*see also* Stricture, urethra
congenital Q64.32
urinary meatus, congenital Q64.33
vagina N89.5
congenital Q52.4
in pregnancy —*see* Pregnancy, complicated by, abnormal vagina
causing obstructed labor O65.5
valve (cardiac) (heart) —*see also* Endocarditis I38
congenital Q24.8
aortic Q23.0
mitral Q23.2
pulmonary Q22.1
tricuspid Q22.4
vena cava (inferior) (superior) I87.1
congenital Q26.0
vesicourethral orifice Q64.31
vulva N90.5
Stent jail T82.897
Stercolith (impaction) K56.41
appendix K38.1
Stercoraceous, stercoral ulcer K63.3
anus or rectum K62.6
Stereotypies NEC F98.4
Sterility —*see* Infertility
Sterilization —*see* Encounter (for), sterilization
Sternalgia —*see* Angina
Sternopagus Q89.4
Sternum bifidum Q76.7
Steroid
effects (adverse) (adrenocortical) (iatrogenic)
cushingoid E24.2
correct substance properly administered —*see* Table of Drugs and Chemicals, by drug, adverse effect
overdose or wrong substance given or taken —*see* Table of Drugs and Chemicals, by drug, poisoning

S

Steroid *(Continued)*
effects *(Continued)*
diabetes —*see* category E09
correct substance properly administered —*see* Table of Drugs and Chemicals, by drug, adverse effect
overdose or wrong substance given or taken —*see* Table of Drugs and Chemicals, by drug, poisoning
fever R50.2
insufficiency E27.3
correct substance properly administered —*see* Table of Drugs and Chemicals, by drug, adverse effect
overdose or wrong substance given or taken —*see* Table of Drugs and Chemicals, by drug, poisoning
responder H40.04-
Stevens-Johnson disease or syndrome L51.1
toxic epidermal necrolysis overlap L51.3
Stewart-Morel syndrome M85.2
Sticker's disease B08.3
Sticky eye —*see* Conjunctivitis, acute, mucopurulent
Stieda's disease —*see* Bursitis, tibial collateral
Stiff neck —*see* Torticollis
Stiff-man syndrome G25.82
Stiffness, joint NEC M25.60-
ankle M25.67-
ankylosis —*see* Ankylosis, joint
contracture —*see* Contraction, joint
elbow M25.62-
foot M25.67-
hand M25.64-
hip M25.65-
knee M25.66-
shoulder M25.61-
wrist M25.63-
Stigmata congenital syphilis A50.59
Stillbirth P95
Still-Felty syndrome —*see* Felty's syndrome
Still's disease or syndrome (juvenile) M08.20
adult-onset M06.1
ankle M08.27-
elbow M08.22-
foot joint M08.27-
hand joint M08.24-
hip M08.25-
knee M08.26-
multiple site M08.29
shoulder M08.21-
vertebra M08.28
wrist M08.23-
Stimulation, ovary E28.1
Sting (venomous) (with allergic or anaphylactic shock) —*see* Table of Drugs and Chemicals, by animal or substance, poisoning
Stippled epiphyses Q78.8
Stitch
abscess T81.48 ◄
burst (in operation wound) —*see* Disruption, wound, operation
Stokes-Adams disease or syndrome I45.9
Stokes' disease E05.00
with thyroid storm E05.01
Stokvis (-Talma) **disease** D74.8
Stoma malfunction
colostomy K94.03
enterostomy K94.13
gastrostomy K94.23
ileostomy K94.13
tracheostomy J95.03
Stomach —*see* condition
Stomatitis (denture) (ulcerative) K12.1
angular K13.0
due to dietary or vitamin deficiency E53.0
aphthous K12.0
bovine B08.61

Stomatitis *(Continued)*
candidal B37.0
catarrhal K12.1
diphtheritic A36.89
due to
dietary deficiency E53.0
thrush B37.0
vitamin deficiency
B group NEC E53.9
B2 (riboflavin) E53.0
epidemic B08.8
epizootic B08.8
follicular K12.1
gangrenous A69.0
Geotrichum B48.3
herpesviral, herpetic B00.2
herpetiformis K12.0
malignant K12.1
membranous acute K12.1
monilial B37.0
mycotic B37.0
necrotizing ulcerative A69.0
parasitic B37.0
septic K12.1
spirochetal A69.1
suppurative (acute) K12.2
ulceromembranous A69.1
vesicular K12.1
with exanthem (enteroviral) B08.4
virus disease A93.8
Vincent's A69.1
Stomatocytosis D58.8
Stomatomycosis B37.0
Stomatorrhagia K13.79
Stone (s) —*see also* Calculus
bladder (diverticulum) N21.0
cystine E72.09
heart syndrome I50.1
kidney N20.0
prostate N42.0
pulpal (dental) K04.2
renal N20.0
salivary gland or duct (any) K11.5
urethra (impacted) N21.1
urinary (duct) (impacted) (passage) N20.9
bladder (diverticulum) N21.0
lower tract N21.9
specified NEC N21.8
xanthine E79.8 *[N22]*
Stonecutter's lung J62.8
Stonemason's asthma, disease, lung or pneumoconiosis J62.8
Stoppage
heart —*see* Arrest, cardiac
urine —*see* Retention, urine
Storm, thyroid —*see* Thyrotoxicosis
Strabismus (congenital) (nonparalytic) H50.9
concomitant H50.40
convergent —*see* Strabismus, convergent concomitant
divergent —*see* Strabismus, divergent concomitant
convergent concomitant H50.00
accommodative component H50.43
alternating H50.05
with
A pattern H50.06
specified nonconcomitances NEC H50.08
V pattern H50.07
monocular H50.01-
with
A pattern H50.02-
specified nonconcomitances NEC H50.04-
V pattern H50.03-
intermittent H50.31-
alternating H50.32

Strabismus *(Continued)*
cyclotropia H50.41 ◄
divergent concomitant H50.10
alternating H50.15
with
A pattern H50.16
specified noncomitances NEC H50.18
V pattern H50.17
monocular H50.11-
with
A pattern H50.12-
specified noncomitances NEC H50.14-
V pattern H50.13-
intermittent H50.33-
alternating H50.34
Duane's syndrome H50.81-
due to adhesions, scars H50.69
heterophoria H50.50
alternating H50.55
cyclophoria H50.54
esophoria H50.51
exophoria H50.52
vertical H50.53
heterotropia H50.40
intermittent H50.30
hypertropia H50.2-
hypotropia —*see* Hypertropia
latent H50.50
mechanical H50.60
Brown's sheath syndrome H50.61-
specified type NEC H50.69
monofixation syndrome H50.42
paralytic H49.9
abducens nerve H49.2-
fourth nerve H49.1-
Kearns-Sayre syndrome H49.81-
ophthalmoplegia (external)
progressive H49.4-
with pigmentary retinopathy H49.81-
total H49.3-
sixth nerve H49.2-
specified type NEC H49.88-
third nerve H49.0-
trochlear nerve H49.1-
specified type NEC H50.89
vertical H50.2-
Strain
back S39.012
cervical S16.1
eye NEC —*see* Disturbance, vision, subjective
heart —*see* Disease, heart
low back S39.012
mental NOS Z73.3
work-related Z56.6
muscle (tendon) —*see* Injury, muscle, by site, strain
neck S16.1
physical NOS Z73.3
work-related Z56.6
postural —*see also* Disorder, soft tissue, due to use
psychological NEC Z73.3
tendon —*see* Injury, muscle, by site, strain
Straining, on urination R39.16
Strand, vitreous —*see* Opacity, vitreous, membranes and strands
Strangulation, strangulated —*see also* Asphyxia, traumatic
appendix K38.8
bladder-neck N32.0
bowel or colon K56.2
food or foreign body —*see* Foreign body, by site
hemorrhoids —*see* Hemorrhoids, with complication
hernia —*see also* Hernia, by site, with obstruction
with gangrene —*see* Hernia, by site, with gangrene

◄ New ◄ Revised ~~deleted~~ Deleted

Strangulation, strangulated *(Continued)*
intestine (large) (small) K56.2
with hernia —*see also* Hernia, by site, with obstruction
with gangrene —*see* Hernia, by site, with gangrene
mesentery K56.2
mucus —*see* Asphyxia, mucus
omentum K56.2
organ or site, congenital NEC —*see* Atresia, by site
ovary —*see* Torsion, ovary
penis N48.89
foreign body T19.4
rupture —*see* Hernia, by site, with obstruction
stomach due to hernia —*see also* Hernia, by site, with obstruction
with gangrene —*see* Hernia, by site, with gangrene
vesicourethral orifice N32.0
Strangury R30.0
Straw itch B88.0
Strawberry
gallbladder K82.4
mark Q82.5
tongue (red) (white) K14.3
Streak (s)
macula, angioid H35.33
ovarian Q50.32
Strephosymbolia F81.0
secondary to organic lesion R48.8
Streptobacillary fever A25.1
Streptobacillosis A25.1
Streptobacillus moniliformis A25.1
Streptococcus, streptococcal —*see also* condition
as cause of disease classified elsewhere B95.5
group
A, as cause of disease classified elsewhere B95.0
B, as cause of disease classified elsewhere B95.1
D, as cause of disease classified elsewhere B95.2
pneumoniae, as cause of disease classified elsewhere B95.3
specified NEC, as cause of disease classified elsewhere B95.4
Streptomycosis B47.1
Streptotrichosis A48.8
Stress F43.9
family —*see* Disruption, family
fetal P84
complicating pregnancy O77.9
due to drug administration O77.1
mental NEC Z73.3
work-related Z56.6
physical NEC Z73.3
work-related Z56.6
polycythemia D75.1
reaction —*see also* Reaction, stress F43.9
work schedule Z56.3
Stretching, nerve —*see* Injury, nerve
Striae albicantes, atrophicae or distensae (cutis) L90.6
Stricture —*see also* Stenosis
ampulla of Vater K83.1
anus (sphincter) K62.4
congenital Q42.3
with fistula Q42.2
infantile Q42.3
with fistula Q42.2
aorta (ascending) (congenital) Q25.1 ⇐
arteriosclerotic I70.0
calcified I70.0
supravalvular, congenital Q25.3
aortic (valve) —*see* Stenosis, aortic
aqueduct of Sylvius (congenital) Q03.0
with spina bifida —*see* Spina bifida, by site, with hydrocephalus
acquired G91.1

Stricture *(Continued)*
artery I77.1
basilar —*see* Occlusion, artery, basilar
carotid —*see* Occlusion, artery, carotid
celiac I77.4
congenital (peripheral) Q27.8
cerebral Q28.3
coronary Q24.5
digestive system Q27.8
lower limb Q27.8
retinal Q14.1
specified site NEC Q27.8
umbilical Q27.0
upper limb Q27.8
coronary —*see* Disease, heart, ischemic, atherosclerotic
congenital Q24.5
precerebral —*see* Occlusion, artery, precerebral
pulmonary (congenital) Q25.6
acquired I28.8
renal I70.1
vertebral —*see* Occlusion, artery, vertebral
auditory canal (external) (congenital)
acquired —*see* Stenosis, external ear canal
bile duct (common) (hepatic) K83.1
congenital Q44.3
postoperative K91.89
bladder N32.89
neck N32.0
bowel —*see* Obstruction, intestine
brain G93.89
bronchus J98.09
congenital Q32.3
syphilitic A52.72
cardia (stomach) K22.2
congenital Q39.3
cardiac —*see also* Disease, heart
orifice (stomach) K22.2
cecum —*see* Obstruction, intestine
cervix, cervical (canal) N88.2
congenital Q51.828
in pregnancy —*see* Pregnancy, complicated by, abnormal cervix
causing obstructed labor O65.5
colon —*see also* Obstruction, intestine
congenital Q42.9
specified NEC Q42.8
colostomy K94.03
common (bile) duct K83.1
coronary (artery) —*see* Disease, heart, ischemic, atherosclerotic
cystic duct —*see* Obstruction, gallbladder
digestive organs NEC, congenital Q45.8
duodenum K31.5
congenital Q41.0
ear canal (external) (congenital) Q16.1
acquired —*see* Stricture, auditory canal, acquired
ejaculatory duct N50.89 ⇐
enterostomy K94.13
esophagus K22.2
congenital Q39.3
syphilitic A52.79
congenital A50.59 *[K23]*
eustachian tube —*see also* Obstruction, eustachian tube
congenital Q17.8
fallopian tube N97.1
gonococcal A54.24
tuberculous A18.17
gallbladder —*see* Obstruction, gallbladder
glottis J38.6
heart —*see also* Disease, heart
valve (*see also* Endocarditis) I38
aortic Q23.0
mitral Q23.4
pulmonary Q22.1
tricuspid Q22.4
hepatic duct K83.1
hourglass, of stomach K31.2

Stricture *(Continued)*
hymen N89.6
hypopharynx J39.2
ileum K56.69
congenital Q41.2
intestine —*see also* Obstruction, intestine
congenital (small) Q41.9
large Q42.9
specified NEC Q42.8
specified NEC Q41.8
ischemic K55.1
jejunum K56.69
congenital Q41.1
lacrimal passages —*see also* Stenosis, lacrimal
congenital Q10.5
larynx J38.6
congenital NEC Q31.8
subglottic Q31.1
syphilitic A52.73
congenital A50.59 *[J99]*
meatus
ear (congenital) Q16.1
acquired —*see* Stricture, auditory canal, acquired
osseous (ear) (congenital) Q16.1
acquired —*see* Stricture, auditory canal, acquired
urinarius —*see also* Stricture, urethra
congenital Q64.33
mitral (valve) —*see* Stenosis, mitral
myocardium, myocardial I51.5
hypertrophic subaortic (idiopathic) I42.1
nares (anterior) (posterior) J34.89
congenital Q30.0
nasal duct —*see also* Stenosis, lacrimal, duct
congenital Q10.5
nasolacrimal duct —*see also* Stenosis, lacrimal, duct
congenital Q10.5
nasopharynx J39.2
syphilitic A52.73
nose J34.89
congenital Q30.0
nostril (anterior) (posterior) J34.89
congenital Q30.0
syphilitic A52.73
congenital A50.59 *[J99]*
organ or site, congenital NEC —*see* Atresia, by site
os uteri —*see* Stricture, cervix
osseous meatus (ear) (congenital) Q16.1
acquired —*see* Stricture, auditory canal, acquired
oviduct —*see* Stricture, fallopian tube
pelviureteric junction (congenital) Q62.11
acquired, with hydronephrosis N13.0 ◀
penis, by foreign body T19.4
pharynx J39.2
prostate N42.89
pulmonary, pulmonic
artery (congenital) Q25.6
acquired I28.8
noncongenital I28.8
infundibulum (congenital) Q24.3
valve I37.0
congenital Q22.1
vein, acquired I28.8
vessel NEC I28.8
punctum lacrimale —*see also* Stenosis, lacrimal, punctum
congenital Q10.5
pylorus (hypertrophic) K31.1
adult K31.1
congenital Q40.0
infantile Q40.0
rectosigmoid K56.69
rectum (sphincter) K62.4
congenital Q42.1
with fistula Q42.0

S

Stricture *(Continued)*
rectum (sphincter) *(Continued)*
due to
chlamydial lymphogranuloma A55
irradiation K91.89
lymphogranuloma venereum A55
gonococcal A54.6
inflammatory (chlamydial) A55
syphilitic A52.74
tuberculous A18.32
renal artery I70.1
congenital Q27.1
salivary duct or gland (any) K11.8
sigmoid (flexure) —*see* Obstruction, intestine
spermatic cord N50.89 ⬅
stoma (following) (of)
colostomy K94.03
enterostomy K94.13
gastrostomy K94.23
ileostomy K94.13
tracheostomy J95.03
stomach K31.89
congenital Q40.2
hourglass K31.2
subaortic Q24.4
hypertrophic (acquired) (idiopathic) I42.1
subglottic J38.6
syphilitic NEC A52.79
trachea J39.8
congenital Q32.1
syphilitic A52.73
tuberculous NEC A15.5
tracheostomy J95.03
tricuspid (valve) —*see* Stenosis, tricuspid
tunica vaginalis N50.89 ⬅
ureter (postoperative) N13.5
with
hydronephrosis N13.1
with infection N13.6
pyelonephritis (chronic) N11.1
congenital —*see* Atresia, ureter
tuberculous A18.11
ureteropelvic junction (congenital) Q62.11
acquired, with hydronephrosis N13.0 ◀
ureterovesical orifice N13.5
with infection N13.6
urethra (organic) (spasmodic) N35.9
associated with schistosomiasis B65.0 *[N37]*
congenital Q64.39
valvular (posterior) Q64.2
due to
infection —*see* Stricture, urethra, postinfective
trauma —*see* Stricture, urethra, post-traumatic
gonococcal, gonorrheal A54.01
infective NEC —*see* Stricture, urethra, postinfective
late effect (sequelae) of injury —*see* Stricture, urethra, post-traumatic
postcatheterization —*see* Stricture, urethra, postprocedural
postinfective NEC
female N35.12
male N35.119
anterior urethra N35.114
bulbous urethra N35.112
meatal N35.111
membranous urethra N35.113
postobstetric N35.021
postoperative —*see* Stricture, urethra, postprocedural
postprocedural
female N99.12
male N99.114
~~anterior urethra N99.113~~
anterior bulbous urethra N99.113 ◀
bulbous urethra N99.111
fossa navicularis N99.115 ◀
meatal N99.110
membranous urethra N99.112

Stricture *(Continued)*
urethra (organic) (spasmodic) *(Continued)*
post-traumatic
female N35.028
due to childbirth N35.021
male N35.014
anterior urethra N35.013
bulbous urethra N35.011
meatal N35.010
membranous urethra N35.012
sequela (late effect) of
childbirth N35.021
injury —*see* Stricture, urethra, post-traumatic
specified cause NEC N35.8
syphilitic A52.76
traumatic —*see* Stricture, urethra, post-traumatic
valvular (posterior), congenital Q64.2
urinary meatus —*see* Stricture, urethra
uterus, uterine (synechiae) N85.6
os (external) (internal) —*see* Stricture, cervix
vagina (outlet) —*see* Stenosis, vagina
valve (cardiac) (heart) —*see also* Endocarditis
congenital
aortic Q23.0
mitral Q23.2
pulmonary Q22.1
tricuspid Q22.4
vas deferens N50.89 ⬅
congenital Q55.4
vein I87.1
vena cava (inferior) (superior) NEC I87.1
congenital Q26.0
vesicourethral orifice N32.0
congenital Q64.31
vulva (acquired) N90.5
Stridor R06.1
congenital (larynx) P28.89
Stridulous —*see* condition
Stroke (apoplectic) (brain) (embolic) (ischemic) (paralytic) (thrombotic) I63.9
epileptic —*see* Epilepsy
heat T67.0
in evolution I63.9
intraoperative
during cardiac surgery I97.810
during other surgery I97.811
lightning —*see* Lightning
meaning
cerebral hemorrhage — code to Hemorrhage, intracranial
cerebral infarction — code to Infarction, cerebral
postprocedural
following cardiac surgery I97.820
following other surgery I97.821
unspecified (NOS) I63.9
Stromatosis, endometrial D39.0
Strongyloidiasis, strongyloidosis B78.9
cutaneous B78.1
disseminated B78.7
intestinal B78.0
Strophulus pruriginosus L28.2
Struck by lightning —*see* Lightning
Struma —*see also* Goiter
Hashimoto E06.3
lymphomatosa E06.3
nodosa (simplex) E04.9
endemic E01.2
multinodular E01.1
multinodular E04.2
iodine-deficiency related E01.1
toxic or with hyperthyroidism E05.20
with thyroid storm E05.21
multinodular E05.20
with thyroid storm E05.21
uninodular E05.10
with thyroid storm E05.11

Struma *(Continued)*
nodosa (simplex) *(Continued)*
toxicosa E05.20
with thyroid storm E05.21
multinodular E05.20
with thyroid storm E05.21
uninodular E05.10
with thyroid storm E05.11
uninodular E04.1
ovarii D27.-
Riedel's E06.5
Strumipriva cachexia E03.4
Strümpell-Marie spine —*see* Spondylitis, ankylosing
Strümpell-Westphal pseudosclerosis E83.01
Stuart deficiency disease (factor X) D68.2
Stuart-Prower factor deficiency (factor X) D68.2
Student's elbow —*see* Bursitis, elbow, olecranon
Stump —*see* Amputation
Stunting, nutritional E45
Stupor (catatonic) R40.1
depressive (single episode) F32.89 ⬅
recurrent episode F33.8 ◀
dissociative F44.2
manic F30.2
manic-depressive F31.89
psychogenic (anergic) F44.2
reaction to exceptional stress (transient) F43.0
Sturge (-Weber) (-Dimitri) (-Kalischer) **disease or syndrome** Q85.8
Stuttering F80.81
adult onset F98.5
childhood onset F80.81
following cerebrovascular disease — *see* Disorder, fluency, following cerebrovascular disease
in conditions classified elsewhere R47.82
Sty, stye (external) (internal) (meibomian) (zeisian) —*see* Hordeolum
Subacidity, gastric K31.89
psychogenic F45.8
Subacute —*see* condition
Subarachnoid —*see* condition
Subcortical —*see* condition
Subcostal syndrome, nerve compression —*see* Mononeuropathy, upper limb, specified site NEC
Subcutaneous, subcuticular —*see* condition
Subdural —*see* condition
Subendocardium —*see* condition
Subependymoma
specified site —*see* Neoplasm, uncertain behavior, by site
unspecified site D43.2
Suberosis J67.3
Subglossitis —*see* Glossitis
Subhemophilia D66
Subinvolution
breast (postlactational) (postpuerperal) N64.89
puerperal O90.89
uterus (chronic) (nonpuerperal) N85.3
puerperal O90.89
Sublingual —*see* condition
Sublinguitis —*see* Sialoadenitis
Subluxatable hip Q65.6
Subluxation —*see also* Dislocation
acromioclavicular S43.11-
ankle S93.0-
atlantoaxial, recurrent M43.4
with myelopathy M43.3
carpometacarpal (joint) NEC S63.05-
thumb S63.04-
complex, vertebral —*see* Complex, subluxation
congenital —*see also* Malposition, congenital
hip —*see* Dislocation, hip, congenital, partial

S

◀ New ⬅ Revised ~~deleted~~ Deleted

Subluxation *(Continued)*
congenital *(Continued)*
joint (excluding hip)
lower limb Q68.8
shoulder Q68.8
upper limb Q68.8
elbow (traumatic) S53.10-
anterior S53.11-
lateral S53.14-
medial S53.13-
posterior S53.12-
specified type NEC S53.19-
finger S63.20-
index S63.20-
interphalangeal S63.22-
distal S63.24-
index S63.24-
little S63.24-
middle S63.24-
ring S63.24-
index S63.22-
little S63.22-
middle S63.22-
proximal S63.23-
index S63.23-
little S63.23-
middle S63.23-
ring S63.23-
ring S63.22-
little S63.20-
metacarpophalangeal S63.21-
index S63.21-
little S63.21-
middle S63.21-
ring S63.21-
middle S63.20-
ring S63.20-
foot S93.30-
specified site NEC S93.33-
tarsal joint S93.31-
tarsometatarsal joint S93.32-
toe —*see* Subluxation, toe
hip S73.00-
anterior S73.03-
obturator S73.02-
central S73.04-
posterior S73.01-
interphalangeal (joint)
finger S63.22-
distal joint S63.24-
index S63.24-
little S63.24-
middle S63.24-
ring S63.24-
index S63.22-
little S63.22-
middle S63.22-
proximal joint S63.23-
index S63.23-
little S63.23-
middle S63.23-
ring S63.23-
ring S63.22-
thumb S63.12-
distal joint S63.14-
proximal joint S63.13-
toe S93.13-
great S93.13-
lesser S93.13-
joint prosthesis —*see* Complications, joint prosthesis, mechanical, displacement, by site
knee S83.10-
cap —*see* Subluxation, patella
patella —*see* Subluxation, patella
proximal tibia
anteriorly S83.11-
laterally S83.14-
medially S83.13-
posteriorly S83.12-
specified type NEC S83.19-

Subluxation *(Continued)*
lens —*see* Dislocation, lens, partial
ligament, traumatic —*see* Sprain, by site
metacarpal (bone)
proximal end S63.06-
metacarpophalangeal (joint)
finger S63.21-
index S63.21-
little S63.21-
middle S63.21-
ring S63.21-
thumb S63.11-
metatarsophalangeal joint S93.14-
great toe S93.14-
lesser toe S93.14-
midcarpal (joint) S63.03-
patella S83.00-
lateral S83.01-
recurrent (nontraumatic) —*see* Dislocation, patella, recurrent, incomplete
specified type NEC S83.09-
pathological —*see* Dislocation, pathological
radial head S53.00-
anterior S53.01-
nursemaid's elbow S53.03-
posterior S53.02-
specified type NEC S53.09-
radiocarpal (joint) S63.02-
radioulnar (joint)
distal S63.01-
proximal —*see* Subluxation, elbow
shoulder
congenital Q68.8
girdle S43.30-
scapula S43.31-
specified site NEC S43.39-
traumatic S43.00-
anterior S43.01-
inferior S43.03-
posterior S43.02-
specified type NEC S43.08-
sternoclavicular (joint) S43.20-
anterior S43.21-
posterior S43.22-
symphysis (pubis)
thumb S63.103
interphalangeal joint —*see* Subluxation, interphalangeal (joint), thumb
metacarpophalangeal joint —*see* Subluxation, metacarpophalangeal (joint), thumb
toe (s) S93.10-
great S93.10-
interphalangeal joint S93.13-
metatarsophalangeal joint S93.14-
interphalangeal joint S93.13-
lesser S93.10-
interphalangeal joint S93.13-
metatarsophalangeal joint S93.14-
metatarsophalangeal joint S93.149
ulnohumeral joint —*see* Subluxation, elbow
vertebral
recurrent NEC —*see* subcategory M43.5
traumatic
cervical S13.100
atlantoaxial joint S13.120
atlantooccipital joint S13.110
atloidooccipital joint S13.110
joint between
C0 and C1 S13.110
C1 and C2 S13.120
C2 and C3 S13.130
C3 and C4 S13.140
C4 and C5 S13.150
C5 and C6 S13.160
C6 and C7 S13.170
C7 and T1 S13.180
occipitoatloid joint S13.110

Subluxation *(Continued)*
vertebral *(Continued)*
traumatic *(Continued)*
lumbar S33.100
joint between
L1 and L2 S33.110
L2 and L3 S33.120
L3 and L4 S33.130
L4 and L5 S33.140
thoracic S23.100
joint between
T1 and T2 S23.110
T2 and T3 S23.120
T3 and T4 S23.122
T4 and T5 S23.130
T5 and T6 S23.132
T6 and T7 S23.140
T7 and T8 S23.142
T8 and T9 S23.150
T9 and T10 S23.152
T10 and T11 S23.160
T11 and T12 S23.162
T12 and L1 S23.170
ulna
distal end S63.07-
proximal end —*see* Subluxation, elbow
wrist (carpal bone) S63.00-
carpometacarpal joint —*see* Subluxation, carpometacarpal (joint)
distal radioulnar joint —*see* Subluxation, radioulnar (joint), distal
metacarpal bone, proximal —*see* Subluxation, metacarpal (bone), proximal end
midcarpal —*see* Subluxation, midcarpal (joint)
radiocarpal joint —*see* Subluxation, radiocarpal (joint)
recurrent —*see* Dislocation, recurrent, wrist
specified site NEC S63.09-
ulna —*see* Subluxation, ulna, distal end
Submaxillary —*see* condition
Submersion (fatal) (nonfatal) T75.1
Submucous —*see* condition
Subnormal, subnormality
accommodation (old age) H52.4
mental —*see* Disability, intellectual
temperature (accidental) T68
Subphrenic —*see* condition
Subscapular nerve —*see* condition
Subseptus uterus Q51.2
Subsiding appendicitis K36
Substance (other psychoactive) **-induced** ◀
anxiety disorder F19.980 ◀
bipolar and related disorder F19.94 ◀
delirium F19.921 ◀
depressive disorder F19.94 ◀
major neurocognitive disorder F19.97 ◀
mild neurocognitive disorder F19.988 ◀
obsessive-compulsive and related disorder F19.988 ◀
psychotic disorder F19.959 ◀
sexual dysfunction F19.981 ◀
sleep disorder F19.982 ◀
Substernal thyroid E04.9
congenital Q89.2
Substitution disorder F44.9
Subtentorial —*see* condition
Subthyroidism (acquired) —*see also* Hypothyroidism
congenital E03.1
Succenturiate placenta O43.19-
Sucking thumb, child (excessive) F98.8
Sudamen, sudamina L74.1
Sudanese kala-azar B55.0
Sudden
hearing loss —*see* Deafness, sudden
heart failure —*see* Failure, heart
Sudeck's atrophy, disease, or syndrome —*see* Algoneurodystrophy
Suffocation —*see* Asphyxia, traumatic

S

Sugar
blood
high (transient) R73.9
low (transient) E16.2
in urine R81
Suicide, suicidal (attempted) T14.91
by poisoning —*see* Table of Drugs and Chemicals
history of (personal) Z91.5
in family Z81.8
ideation —*see* Ideation, suicidal
risk
meaning personal history of attempted suicide Z91.5
meaning suicidal ideation —*see* Ideation, suicidal
tendencies
meaning personal history of attempted suicide Z91.5
meaning suicidal ideation —*see* Ideation, suicidal
trauma —*see* nature of injury by site
Suipestifer infection —*see* Infection, salmonella
Sulfhemoglobinemia, sulphemoglobinemia (acquired) (with methemoglobinemia) D74.8
Sumatran mite fever A75.3
Summer —*see* condition
Sunburn L55.9
due to ◀
tanning bed (acute) L56.8 ◀
chronic L57.8 ◀
ultraviolet radiation (acute) L56.8 ◀
chronic L57.8 ◀
first degree L55.0
second degree L55.1
third degree L55.2
SUNCT (short lasting unilateral neuralgiform headache with conjunctival injection and tearing) G44.059
intractable G44.051
not intractable G44.059
Sunken acetabulum —*see* Derangement, joint, specified type NEC, hip
Sunstroke T67.0
Superfecundation —*see* Pregnancy, multiple
Superfetation —*see* Pregnancy, multiple
Superinvolution (uterus) N85.8
Supernumerary (congenital)
aortic cusps Q23.8
auditory ossicles Q16.3
bone Q79.8
breast Q83.1
carpal bones Q74.0
cusps, heart valve NEC Q24.8
aortic Q23.8
mitral Q23.2
pulmonary Q22.3
digit (s) Q69.9
ear (lobule) Q17.0
fallopian tube Q50.6
finger Q69.0
hymen Q52.4
kidney Q63.0
lacrimonasal duct Q10.6
lobule (ear) Q17.0
mitral cusps Q23.2
muscle Q79.8
nipple (s) Q83.3
organ or site not listed —*see* Accessory
ossicles, auditory Q16.3
ovary Q50.31
oviduct Q50.6
pulmonary, pulmonic cusps Q22.3
rib Q76.6
cervical or first (syndrome) Q76.5
roots (of teeth) K00.2
spleen Q89.09
tarsal bones Q74.2
teeth K00.1
Supernumerary *(Continued)*
testis Q55.29
thumb Q69.1
toe Q69.2
uterus Q51.2
vagina Q52.1
vertebra Q76.49
Supervision (of)
contraceptive —*see* Prescription, contraceptives
dietary (for) Z71.3
allergy (food) Z71.3
colitis Z71.3
diabetes mellitus Z71.3
food allergy or intolerance Z71.3
gastritis Z71.3
hypercholesterolemia Z71.3
hypoglycemia Z71.3
intolerance (food) Z71.3
obesity Z71.3
specified NEC Z71.3
healthy infant or child Z76.2
foundling Z76.1
high-risk pregnancy —*see* Pregnancy, complicated by, high, risk
lactation Z39.1
pregnancy —*see* Pregnancy, supervision of
Supplemental teeth K00.1
Suppression
binocular vision H53.34
lactation O92.5
menstruation N94.89
ovarian secretion E28.39
renal N28.9
urine, urinary secretion R34
Suppuration, suppurative —*see also* condition
accessory sinus (chronic) —*see* Sinusitis
adrenal gland
antrum (chronic) —*see* Sinusitis, maxillary
bladder —*see* Cystitis
brain G06.0
sequelae G09
breast N61.1 ⟸
puerperal, postpartum or gestational —*see* Mastitis, obstetric, purulent
dental periosteum M27.3
ear (middle) —*see also* Otitis, media
external NEC —*see* Otitis, externa, infective
internal —*see* subcategory H83.0
ethmoidal (chronic) (sinus) —*see* Sinusitis, ethmoidal
fallopian tube —*see* Salpingo-oophoritis
frontal (chronic) (sinus) —*see* Sinusitis, frontal
gallbladder (acute) K81.0
gum K05.20
generalized —*see* Peridontitis, aggressive, generalized ⟸
localized —*see* Peridontitis, aggressive, localized ⟸
intracranial G06.0
joint —*see* Arthritis, pyogenic or pyemic
labyrinthine —*see* subcategory H83.0
lung —*see* Abscess, lung
mammary gland N61.1 ⟸
puerperal, postpartum O91.12
associated with lactation O91.13
maxilla, maxillary M27.2
sinus (chronic) —*see* Sinusitis, maxillary
muscle —*see* Myositis, infective
nasal sinus (chronic) —*see* Sinusitis
pancreas, acute —*see also* Pancreatitis, acute K85.80 ⟸
parotid gland —*see* Sialoadenitis
pelvis, pelvic
female —*see* Disease, pelvis, inflammatory
male K65.0
pericranial —*see* Osteomyelitis
salivary duct or gland (any) —*see* Sialoadenitis
Suppuration, suppurative *(Continued)*
sinus (accessory) (chronic) (nasal) —*see* Sinusitis
sphenoidal sinus (chronic) —*see* Sinusitis, sphenoidal
thymus (gland) E32.1
thyroid (gland) E06.0
tonsil —*see* Tonsillitis
uterus —*see* Endometritis
Supraeruption of tooth (teeth) M26.34
Supraglottitis J04.30
with obstruction J04.31
Suprarenal (gland) —*see* condition
Suprascapular nerve —*see* condition
Suprasellar —*see* condition
Surfer's knots or nodules S89.8-
Surgical
emphysema T81.82
procedures, complication or misadventure —*see* Complications, surgical procedures
shock T81.10
Surveillance (of) (for) —*see also* Observation
alcohol abuse Z71.41
contraceptive —*see* Prescription, contraceptives
dietary Z71.3
drug abuse Z71.51
Susceptibility to disease, genetic Z15.89
malignant neoplasm Z15.09
breast Z15.01
endometrium Z15.04
ovary Z15.02
prostate Z15.03
specified NEC Z15.09
multiple endocrine neoplasia Z15.81
Suspected condition, ruled out —*see also* Observation, suspected
amniotic cavity and membrane Z03.71
cervical shortening Z03.75
fetal anomaly Z03.73
fetal growth Z03.74
maternal and fetal conditions NEC Z03.79
newborn —*see also* Observation, newborn, suspected condition ruled out Z05.9 ◀
oligohydramnios Z03.71
placental problem Z03.72
polyhydramnios Z03.71
Suspended uterus
in pregnancy or childbirth —*see* Pregnancy, complicated by, abnormal uterus
Sutton's nevus D22.9
Suture
burst (in operation wound) T81.31
external operation wound T81.31
internal operation wound T81.32
inadvertently left in operation wound —*see* Foreign body, accidentally left during a procedure
removal Z48.02
Swab inadvertently left in operation wound —*see* Foreign body, accidentally left during a procedure
Swallowed, swallowing
difficulty —*see* Dysphagia
foreign body —*see* Foreign body, alimentary tract
Swan-neck deformity (finger) —*see* Deformity, finger, swan-neck
Swearing, compulsive F42.8 ⟸
in Gilles de la Tourette's syndrome F95.2
Sweat, sweats
fetid L75.0
night R61
Sweating, excessive R61
Sweeley-Klionsky disease E75.21
Sweet's disease or dermatosis L98.2
Swelling (of) R60.9
abdomen, abdominal (not referable to any particular organ) —*see* Mass, abdominal
ankle —*see* Effusion, joint, ankle

◀ New ⟸ Revised ~~deleted~~ Deleted

Swelling *(Continued)*
arm M79.89
forearm M79.89
breast N63
Calabar B74.3
cervical gland R59.0
chest, localized R22.2
ear H93.8-
extremity (lower) (upper) —*see* Disorder, soft tissue, specified type NEC
finger M79.89
foot M79.89
glands R59.9
generalized R59.1
localized R59.0
hand M79.89
head (localized) R22.0
inflammatory —*see* Inflammation
intra-abdominal —*see* Mass, abdominal
joint —*see* Effusion, joint
leg M79.89
lower M79.89
limb —*see* Disorder, soft tissue, specified type NEC
localized (skin) R22.9
chest R22.2
head R22.0
limb
lower —*see* Mass, localized, limb, lower
upper —*see* Mass, localized, limb, upper
neck R22.1
trunk R22.2
neck (localized) R22.1
pelvic —*see* Mass, abdominal
scrotum N50.89 ⇐
splenic —*see* Splenomegaly
testis N50.89 ⇐
toe M79.89
umbilical R19.09
wandering, due to Gnathostoma (spinigerum) B83.1
white —*see* Tuberculosis, arthritis
Swift (-Feer) disease
overdose or wrong substance given or taken —*see* Table of Drugs and Chemicals, by drug, poisoning
Swimmer's
cramp T75.1
ear H60.33-
itch B65.3
Swimming in the head R42
Swollen —*see* Swelling
Swyer syndrome Q99.1
Sycosis L73.8
barbae (not parasitic) L73.8
contagiosa (mycotic) B35.0
lupoides L73.8
mycotic B35.0
parasitic B35.0
vulgaris L73.8
Sydenham's chorea —*see* Chorea, Sydenham's
Sylvatic yellow fever A95.0
Sylvest's disease B33.0
Symblepharon H11.23-
congenital Q10.3
Symond's syndrome G93.2
Sympathetic —*see* condition
Sympatheticotonia G90.8
Sympathicoblastoma
specified site —*see* Neoplasm, malignant, by site
unspecified site C74.90
Sympathogonioma —*see* Sympathicoblastoma
Symphalangy (fingers) (toes) Q70.9
Symptoms NEC R68.89
breast NEC N64.59
development NEC R63.8
factitious, self-induced —*see* Disorder, factitious

Symptoms NEC *(Continued)*
genital organs, female R10.2
involving
abdomen NEC R19.8
appearance NEC R46.89
awareness R41.9
altered mental status R41.82
amnesia —*see* Amnesia
borderline intellectual functioning R41.83
coma —*see* Coma
disorientation R41.0
neurologic neglect syndrome R41.4
senile cognitive decline R41.81
specified symptom NEC R41.89
behavior NEC R46.89
cardiovascular system NEC R09.89
chest NEC R09.89
circulatory system NEC R09.89
cognitive functions R41.9
altered mental status R41.82
amnesia —*see* Amnesia
borderline intellectual functioning R41.83
coma —*see* Coma
disorientation R41.0
neurologic neglect syndrome R41.4
senile cognitive decline R41.81
specified symptom NEC R41.89
development NEC R62.50
digestive system NEC R19.8
emotional state NEC R45.89
emotional lability R45.86
food and fluid intake R63.8
general perceptions and sensations R44.9
specified NEC R44.8
musculoskeletal system R29.91
specified NEC R29.898
nervous system R29.90
specified NEC R29.818
pelvis NEC R19.8
respiratory system NEC R09.89
skin and integument R23.9
urinary system R39.9
menopausal N95.1
metabolism NEC R63.8
neurotic F48.8
of infancy R68.19
pelvis NEC, female R10.2
skin and integument NEC R23.9
subcutaneous tissue NEC R23.9
Sympus Q74.2
Syncephalus Q89.4
Synchondrosis
abnormal (congenital) Q78.8
ischiopubic M91.0
Synchysis (scintillans) (senile) (vitreous body) H43.89
Syncope (near) (pre-) R55
anginosa I20.8
bradycardia R00.1
cardiac R55
carotid sinus G90.01
due to spinal (lumbar) puncture G97.1
heart R55
heat T67.1
laryngeal R05
psychogenic F48.8
tussive R05
vasoconstriction R55
vasodepressor R55
vasomotor R55
vasovagal R55
Syndactylism, syndactyly Q70.9
complex (with synostosis)
fingers Q70.0-
toes Q70.2-
simple (without synostosis)
fingers Q70.1-
toes Q70.3-

Syndrome —*see also* Disease
5q minus NOS D46.C
48,XXXX Q97.1
49,XXXXX Q97.1
abdominal
acute R10.0
muscle deficiency Q79.4
abnormal innervation H02.519
left H02.516
lower H02.515
upper H02.514
right H02.513
lower H02.512
upper H02.511
abstinence, neonatal P96.1
acid pulmonary aspiration, obstetric O74.0
acquired immunodeficiency —*see* Human, immunodeficiency virus (HIV) disease
acute abdominal R10.0
acute respiratory distress (adult) (child) J80
idiopathic J84.114 ◀
Adair-Dighton Q78.0
Adams-Stokes (-Morgagni) I45.9
adiposogenital E23.6
adrenal
hemorrhage (meningococcal) A39.1
meningococcic A39.1
adrenocortical —*see* Cushing's, syndrome
adrenogenital E25.9
congenital, associated with enzyme deficiency E25.0
afferent loop NEC K91.89
Alagille's Q44.7
alcohol withdrawal (without convulsions) —*see* Dependence, alcohol, with, withdrawal
Alder's D72.0
Aldrich (-Wiskott) D82.0
alien hand R41.4
Alport Q87.81
alveolar hypoventilation E66.2
alveolocapillary block J84.10
amnesic, amnestic (confabulatory) (due to) —*see* Disorder, amnesic
amyostatic (Wilson's disease) E83.01
androgen insensitivity E34.50
complete E34.51
partial E34.52
androgen resistance (*see also* Syndrome, androgen insensitivity) E34.50
Angelman Q93.5
anginal —*see* Angina
ankyloglossia superior Q38.1
anterior
chest wall R07.89
cord G83.82
spinal artery G95.19
compression M47.019
cervical region M47.012
cervicothoracic region M47.013
lumbar region M47.016
occipito-atlanto-axial region M47.011
thoracic region M47.014
thoracolumbar region M47.015
tibial M76.81-
antibody deficiency D80.9
agammaglobulinemic D80.1
hereditary D80.0
congenital D80.0
hypogammaglobulinemic D80.1
hereditary D80.0
anticardiolipin (-antibody) D68.61
antiphospholipid (-antibody) D68.61
aortic
arch M31.4
bifurcation I74.09
aortomesenteric duodenum occlusion K31.5
apical ballooning (transient left ventricular) I51.81
arcuate ligament I77.4

S

Syndrome *(Continued)*
argentaffin, argintaffinoma E34.0
Arnold-Chiari —*see* Arnold-Chiari disease
Arrillaga-Ayerza I27.0
arterial tortuosity Q87.82 ◀
arteriovenous steal T82.898- ◀
Asherman's N85.6
aspiration, of newborn —*see* Aspiration, by substance, with pneumonia
meconium P24.01
ataxia-telangiectasia G11.3
auriculotemporal G50.8
autoerythrocyte sensitization (Gardner-Diamond) D69.2
autoimmune lymphoproliferative [ALPS] D89.82
autoimmune polyglandular E31.0
autoinflammatory M04.9 ◀
specified type NEC M04.8 ◀
autosomal —*see* Abnormal, autosomes
Avellis' G46.8
Ayerza (-Arrillaga) I27.0
Babinski-Nageotte G83.89
Bakwin-Krida Q78.5 ⟸
bare lymphocyte D81.6
Barré-Guillain G61.0
Barré-Liéou M53.0
Barrett's —*see* Barrett's, esophagus
Barsony-Polgar K22.4
Barsony-Teschendorf K22.4
Barth E78.71
Bartter's E26.81
basal cell nevus Q87.89
Basedow's E05.00
with thyroid storm E05.01
basilar artery G45.0
Batten-Steinert G71.11
battered
baby or child —*see* Maltreatment, child, physical abuse
spouse —*see* Maltreatment, adult, physical abuse
Beals Q87.40
Beau's I51.5
Beck's I65.8
Benedikt's G46.3
Béquez César (-Steinbrinck-Chédiak-Higashi) D70.330
Bernhardt-Roth —*see* Meralgia paresthetica
Bernheim's I50.9
big spleen D73.1
bilateral polycystic ovarian E28.2
Bing-Horton's —*see* Horton's headache
Birt-Hogg-Dube syndrome Q87.89
Björck (-Thorsen) E34.0
black
lung J60
widow spider bite —*see* Toxicity, venom, spider, black widow
Blackfan-Diamond D61.01
Blau M04.8 ◀
blind loop K90.2
congenital Q43.8
postsurgical K91.2
blue sclera Q78.0
blue toe I75.02-
Boder-Sedgewick G11.3
Boerhaave's K22.3
Borjeson Forssman Lehmann Q89.8
Bouillaud's I01.9
Bourneville (-Pringle) Q85.1
Bouveret (-Hoffman) I47.9
brachial plexus G54.0
bradycardia-tachycardia I49.5
brain (nonpsychotic) F09
with psychosis, psychotic reaction F09
acute or subacute —*see* Delirium
congenital —*see* Disability, intellectual
organic F09
post-traumatic (nonpsychotic) F07.81
psychotic F09

Syndrome *(Continued)*
brain (nonpsychotic) *(Continued)*
personality change F07.0
postcontusional F07.81
post-traumatic, nonpsychotic F07.81
psycho-organic F09
psychotic F06.8
brain stem stroke G46.3
Brandt's (acrodermatitis enteropathica) E83.2
broad ligament laceration N83.8
Brock's J98.11
bronze baby P83.8
Brown-Sequard G83.81
bubbly lung P27.0
Buchem's M85.2
Budd-Chiari I82.0
bulbar (progressive) G12.22
Bürger-Grütz E78.3
Burke's K86.89 ⟸
Burnett's (milk-alkali) E83.52
burning feet E53.9
Bywaters' T79.5
Call-Fleming I67.841
carbohydrate-deficient glycoprotein (CDGS) E77.8
carcinogenic thrombophlebitis I82.1
carcinoid E34.0
cardiac asthma I50.1
cardiacos negros I27.0
cardiofaciocutaneous Q87.89
cardiopulmonary-obesity E66.2
cardiorenal —*see* Hypertension, cardiorenal
cardiorespiratory distress (idiopathic), newborn P22.0
cardiovascular renal —*see* Hypertension, cardiorenal
carotid
artery (hemispheric) (internal) G45.1
body G90.01
sinus G90.01
carpal tunnel G56.0-
Cassidy (-Scholte) E34.0
cat-cry Q93.4
cat eye Q92.8
cauda equina G83.4
causalgia —*see* Causalgia
celiac K90.0
artery compression I77.4
axis I77.4
central pain G89.0
cerebellar
hereditary G11.9
stroke G46.4
cerebellomedullary malformation —*see* Spina bifida
cerebral
artery
anterior G46.1
middle G46.0
posterior G46.2
gigantism E22.0
cervical (root) M53.1
disc —*see* Disorder, disc, cervical, with neuritis
fusion Q76.1
posterior, sympathicus M53.0
rib Q76.5
sympathetic paralysis G90.2
cervicobrachial (diffuse) M53.1
cervicocranial M53.0
cervicodorsal outlet G54.2
cervicothoracic outlet G54.0
Céstan (-Raymond) I65.8
Charcot's (angina cruris) (intermittent claudication) I73.9
Charcot-Weiss-Baker G90.09
CHARGE Q89.8
Chédiak-Higashi (-Steinbrinck) E70.330
chest wall R07.1
Chiari's (hepatic vein thrombosis) I82.0
Chilaiditi's Q43.3

Syndrome *(Continued)*
child maltreatment —*see* Maltreatment, child
chondrocostal junction M94.0
chondroectodermal dysplasia Q77.6
chromosome 4 short arm deletion Q93.3
chromosome 5 short arm deletion Q93.4
chronic
infantile neurological, cutaneous and articular (CINCA) M04.2 ◀
pain G89.4
personality F68.8
Clarke-Hadfield K86.89 ⟸
Clerambault's automatism G93.89
Clouston's (hidrotic ectodermal dysplasia) Q82.4
clumsiness, clumsy child F82
cluster headache G44.009
intractable G44.001
not intractable G44.009
Coffin-Lowry Q89.8
cold injury (newborn) P80.0
combined immunity deficiency D81.9
compartment (deep) (posterior) (traumatic) T79.A0
abdomen T79.A3
lower extremity (hip, buttock, thigh, leg, foot, toes) T79.A2
nontraumatic
abdomen M79.A3
lower extremity (hip, buttock, thigh, leg, foot, toes) M79.A2-
specified site NEC M79.A9
upper extremity (shoulder, arm, forearm, wrist, hand, fingers) M79.A1-
postprocedural —*see* Syndrome compartment, nontraumatic
specified site NEC T79.A9
upper extremity (shoulder, arm, forearm, wrist, hand, fingers) T79.A1
complex regional pain —*see* Syndrome, pain, complex regional
compression T79.5
anterior spinal —*see* Syndrome, anterior, spinal artery, compression
cauda equina G83.4
celiac artery I77.4
vertebral artery M47.029
cervical region M47.022
occipito-atlanto-axial region M47.021
concussion F07.81
congenital
affecting multiple systems NEC Q87.89
central alveolar hypoventilation G47.35
facial diplegia Q87.0
muscular hypertrophy-cerebral Q87.89
oculo-auriculovertebral Q87.0
oculofacial diplegia (Moebius) Q87.0
rubella (manifest) P35.0
congestion-fibrosis (pelvic), female N94.89
congestive dysmenorrhea N94.6
Conn's E26.01
connective tissue M35.9
overlap NEC M35.1
conus medullaris G95.81
cord
anterior G83.82
posterior G83.83
coronary
acute NEC I24.9
insufficiency or intermediate I20.0
slow flow I20.8
Costen's (complex) M26.69
costochondral junction M94.0
costoclavicular G54.0
costovertebral E22.0
Cowden Q85.8
craniovertebral M53.0
Creutzfeldt-Jakob —*see* Creutzfeldt-Jakob disease or syndrome
cri-du-chat Q93.4

◀ New ⟸ Revised ~~deleted~~ Deleted

Syndrome *(Continued)*
crib death R99
cricopharyngeal —*see* Dysphagia
croup J05.0
CRPS I —*see* Syndrome, pain, complex regional I
crush T79.5
cubital tunnel —*see* Lesion, nerve, ulnar
Curschmann (-Batten) (-Steinert) G71.11
Cushing's E24.9
alcohol-induced E24.4
drug-induced E24.2
due to
alcohol
drugs E24.2
ectopic ACTH E24.3
overproduction of pituitary ACTH E24.0
overdose or wrong substance given or taken —*see* Table of Drugs and Chemicals, by drug, poisoning
pituitary-dependent E24.0
specified type NEC E24.8
cryopyrin-associated periodic M04.2 ◀
cryptophthalmos Q87.0
cystic duct stump K91.5
Dana-Putnam D51.0
Danbolt (-Cross) (acrodermatitis enteropathica) E83.2
Dandy-Walker Q03.1
with spina bifida Q07.01
Danlos' Q79.6 ⇐
defibrination —*see also* Fibrinolysis
with
antepartum hemorrhage —*see* Hemorrhage, antepartum, with coagulation defect
intrapartum hemorrhage —*see* Hemorrhage, complicating, delivery
newborn P60
postpartum O72.3
Degos' I77.8
Déjérine-Roussy G89.0
delayed sleep phase G47.21
demyelinating G37.9
dependence —*see* F10-F19 with fourth character .2
depersonalization (-derealization) F48.1
De Quervain E34.51
de Toni-Fanconi (-Debré) E72.09
with cystinosis E72.04
diabetes mellitus-hypertension-nephrosis —*see* Diabetes, nephrosis
diabetes mellitus in newborn infant P70.2
diabetes-nephrosis —*see* Diabetes, nephrosis
diabetic amyotrophy —*see* Diabetes, amyotrophy
dialysis associated steal T82.898- ◀
Diamond-Blackfan D61.01
Diamond-Gardener D69.2
DIC (diffuse or disseminated intravascular coagulopathy) D65
di George's D82.1
Dighton's Q78.0
disequilibrium E87.8
Döhle body-panmyelopathic D72.0
dorsolateral medullary G46.4
double athetosis G80.3
Down (*see also* Down syndrome) Q90.9
Dresbach's (elliptocytosis) D58.1
Dressler's (postmyocardial infarction) I24.1
postcardiotomy I97.0
drug withdrawal, infant of dependent mother P96.1
dry eye H04.12-
due to abnormality
chromosomal Q99.9
sex
female phenotype Q97.9
male phenotype Q98.9
specified NEC Q99.8

Syndrome *(Continued)*
dumping (postgastrectomy) K91.1
nonsurgical K31.89
Dupré's (meningism) R29.1
dysmetabolic X E88.81
dyspraxia, developmental F82
Eagle-Barrett Q79.4
Eaton-Lambert —*see* Syndrome, Lambert-Eaton
Ebstein's Q22.5
ectopic ACTH E24.3
eczema-thrombocytopenia D82.0
Eddowes' Q78.0
effort (psychogenic) F45.8
Ehlers-Danlos Q79.6
Eisenmenger's I27.89
Ekman's Q78.0
electric feet E53.8
Ellis-van Creveld Q77.6
empty nest Z60.0
endocrine-hypertensive E27.0
entrapment —*see* Neuropathy, entrapment
eosinophilia-myalgia M35.8
epileptic —*see also* Epilepsy, by type
absence G40.A09
intractable G40.A19
with status epilepticus G40.A11
without status epilepticus G40.A19
not intractable G40.A09
with status epilepticus G40.A01
without status epilepticus G40.A09
Erdheim-Chester (ECD) E88.89
Erdheim's E22.0
erythrocyte fragmentation D59.4
Evans D69.41
exhaustion F48.8
extrapyramidal G25.9
specified NEC G25.89
eye retraction —*see* Strabismus
eyelid-malar-mandible Q87.0
Faber's D50.9
facial pain, paroxysmal G50.0
Fallot's Q21.3
familial cold autoinflammatory M04.2 ◀
familial eczema-thrombocytopenia (Wiskott-Aldrich) D82.0
Fanconi (-de Toni) (-Debré) E72.09
with cystinosis E72.04
Fanconi's (anemia) (congenital pancytopenia) D61.09
fatigue
chronic R53.82
psychogenic F48.8
faulty bowel habit K59.39 ⇐
Feil-Klippel (brevicollis) Q76.1
Felty's —*see* Felty's syndrome
fertile eunuch E23.0
fetal
alcohol (dysmorphic) Q86.0
hydantoin Q86.1
Fiedler's I40.1
first arch Q87.0
fish odor E72.8
Fisher's G61.0
Fitzhugh-Curtis
due to
Chlamydia trachomatis A74.81
Neisseria gonorrhorea (gonococcal peritonitis) A54.85
Fitz's —*see also* Pancreatitis, acute K85.80 ⇐
Flajani (-Basedow) E05.00
with thyroid storm E05.01
flatback —*see* Flatback syndrome
floppy
baby P94.2
iris (intraoeprative) (IFIS) H21.81
mitral valve I34.1
flush E34.0
Foix-Alajouanine G95.19
Fong's Q87.2 ⇐

Syndrome *(Continued)*
food protein-induced enterocolitis K52.21 ◀
foramen magnum G93.5
Foster-Kennedy H47.14-
Foville's (peduncular) G46.3
fragile X Q99.2
Franceschetti Q75.4
Frey's
auriculotemporal G50.8
hyperhidrosis L74.52
Friderichsen-Waterhouse A39.1
Froin's G95.89
frontal lobe F07.0
Fukuhara E88.49
functional
bowel K59.9
prepubertal castrate E29.1
Gaisböck's D75.1
ganglion (basal ganglia brain) G25.9
geniculi G51.1
Gardner-Diamond D69.2
gastroesophageal
junction K22.0
laceration-hemorrhage K22.6
gastrojejunal loop obstruction K91.89
Gee-Herter-Heubner K90.0
Gelineau's G47.419
with cataplexy G47.411
genito-anorectal A55
Gerstmann-Sträussler-Scheinker (GSS) A81.82
Gianotti-Crosti L44.4
giant platelet (Bernard-Soulier) D69.1
Gilles de la Tourette's F95.2
goiter-deafness E07.1
Goldberg Q89.8
Goldberg-Maxwell E34.51
Good's D83.8
Gopalan' (burning feet) E53.8
Gorlin's Q87.89
Gougerot-Blum L81.7
Gouley's I31.1
Gower's R55
gray or grey (newborn) P93.0
platelet D69.1
Gubler-Millard G46.3
Guillain-Barré (-Strohl) G61.0
gustatory sweating G50.8
Hadfield-Clarke K86.89 ⇐
hair tourniquet —*see* Constriction, external, by site
Hamman's J98.19
hand-foot L27.1
hand-shoulder G90.8
hantavirus (cardio)-pulmonary (HPS) (HCPS) B33.4
happy puppet Q93.5
Harada's H30.81-
Hayem-Faber D50.9
headache NEC G44.89
complicated NEC G44.59
Heberden's I20.8
Hedinger's E34.0
Hegglin's D72.0
HELLP (hemolysis, elevated liver enzymes and low platelet count) O14.2-
complicating ◀
childbirth O14.24 ◀
puerperium O14.25 ◀
hemolytic-uremic D59.3
hemophagocytic, infection-associated D76.2
Henoch-Schönlein D69.0
hepatic flexure K59.8
hepatopulmonary K76.81
hepatorenal K76.7
following delivery O90.4
postoperative or postprocedural K91.83
postpartum, puerperal O90.4
hepatourologic K76.7
Herter (-Gee) (nontropical sprue) K90.0

S

Syndrome *(Continued)*
Heubner-Herter K90.0
Heyd's K76.7
Hilger's G90.09
histamine-like (fish poisoning) —*see* Poisoning, fish
histiocytic D76.3
histiocytosis NEC D76.3
HIV infection, acute B20
Hoffmann-Werdnig G12.0
Hollander-Simons E88.1
Hoppe-Goldflam G70.00
with exacerbation (acute) G70.01
in crisis G70.01
Horner's G90.2
hungry bone E83.81
hunterian glossitis D51.0
Hutchinson's triad A50.53
hyperabduction G54.0
hyperammonemia-hyperornithinemia-homocitrullinemia E72.4
hypereosinophilic (idiopathic) D72.1
hyperimmunoglobulin D M04.1 ◀
hyperimmunoglobulin E (IgE) D82.4
hyperkalemic E87.5
hyperkinetic —*see* Hyperkinesia
hypermobility M35.7
hypernatremia E87.0
hyperosmolarity E87.0
hyperperfusion G97.82
hypersplenic D73.1
hypertransfusion, newborn P61.1
hyperventilation F45.8
hyperviscosity (of serum)
polycythemic D75.1
sclerothymic D58.8
hypoglycemic (familial) (neonatal) E16.2
hypokalemic E87.6
hyponatremic E87.1
hypopituitarism E23.0
hypoplastic left-heart Q23.4
hypopotassemia E87.6
hyposmolality E87.1
hypotension, maternal O26.5-
hypothenar hammer I73.89
hypoventilation, obesity (OHS) E66.2 ◀
ICF (intravascular coagulation-fibrinolysis) D65
idiopathic
cardiorespiratory distress, newborn P22.0
nephrotic (infantile) N04.9
iliotibial band M76.3-
immobility, immobilization (paraplegic) M62.3
immune reconstitution D89.3
immune reconstitution inflammatory [IRIS] D89.3
immunity deficiency, combined D81.9
immunodeficiency
acquired —*see* Human, immunodeficiency virus (HIV) disease
combined D81.9
impending coronary I20.0
impingement, shoulder M75.4-
inappropriate secretion of antidiuretic hormone E22.2
infant
gestational diabetes P70.0
of diabetic mother P70.1
infantilism (pituitary) E23.0
inferior vena cava I87.1
inspissated bile (newborn) P59.1
institutional (childhood) F94.2
insufficient sleep F51.12
intermediate coronary (artery) I20.0
interspinous ligament —*see* Spondylopathy, specified NEC
intestinal
carcinoid E34.0
knot K56.2
intravascular coagulation-fibrinolysis (ICF) D65

Syndrome *(Continued)*
iodine-deficiency, congenital E00.9
type
mixed E00.2
myxedematous E00.1
neurological E00.0
IRDS (idiopathic respiratory distress, newborn) P22.0
irritable
bowel K58.9
~~with diarrhea K58.0~~
with ◀
constipation K58.1 ◀
diarrhea K58.0 ◀
mixed K58.2 ◀
psychogenic F45.8
specified NEC K58.8 ◀
heart (psychogenic) F45.8
weakness F48.8
~~ischemic bowel (transient) K55.9~~
~~chronic K55.1~~
~~due to mesenteric artery insufficiency K55.1~~
ischemic ◀
bowel (transient) K55.9 ◀
chronic K55.1 ◀
due to mesenteric artery insufficiency K55.1 ◀
steal T82.898 ◀
IVC (intravascular coagulopathy) D65
Ivemark's Q89.01
Jaccoud's —*see* Arthropathy, postrheumatic, chronic
Jackson's G83.89
Jakob-Creutzfeldt —*see* Creutzfeldt-Jakob disease or syndrome
jaw-winking Q07.8
Jervell-Lange-Nielsen I45.81
jet lag G47.25
Job's D71
Joseph-Diamond-Blackfan D61.01
jugular foramen G52.7
Kabuki Q89.8
Kanner's (autism) F84.0
Kartagener's Q89.3
Kelly's D50.1
Kimmelsteil-Wilson —*see* Diabetes, specified type, with Kimmelsteil-Wilson disease
Klein (e)-Levine G47.13
Klippel-Feil (brevicollis) Q76.1
Köhler-Pellegrini-Steida —*see* Bursitis, tibial collateral
König's K59.8
Korsakoff (-Wernicke) (nonalcoholic) F04
alcoholic F10.26
Kostmann's D70.0
Krabbe's congenital muscle hypoplasia Q79.8
labyrinthine —*see* subcategory H83.2
lacunar NEC G46.7
Lambert-Eaton G70.80
in
neoplastic disease G73.1
specified disease NEC G70.81
Landau-Kleffner —*see* Epilepsy, specified NEC
Larsen's Q74.8
lateral
cutaneous nerve of thigh G57.1-
medullary G46.4
Launois' E22.0
lazy
leukocyte D70.8
posture M62.3
Lemiere I80.8
Lennox-Gastaut G40.812
intractable G40.814
with status epilepticus G40.813
without status epilepticus G40.814
not intractable G40.812
with status epilepticus G40.811
without status epilepticus G40.812

Syndrome *(Continued)*
lenticular, progressive E83.01
Leopold-Levi's E05.90
Lev's I44.2
Li-Fraumeni Z15.01
Lichtheim's D51.0
Lightwood's N25.89
Lignac (de Toni) (-Fanconi) (-Debré) E72.09
with cystinosis E72.04
Likoff's I20.8
limbic epilepsy personality F07.0
liver-kidney K76.7
lobotomy F07.0
Loffler's J82
long arm 18 or 21 deletion Q93.89
long QT I45.81
Louis-Barré G11.3
low
atmospheric pressure T70.29
back M54.5
output (cardiac) I50.9
lower radicular, newborn (birth injury) P14.8
Luetscher's (dehydration) E86.0
Lupus anticoagulant D68.62
Lutembacher's Q21.1
macrophage activation D76.1
due to infection D76.2
magnesium-deficiency R29.0
Majeed M04.8 ◀
Mal de Debarquement R42
malabsorption K90.9
postsurgical K91.2
malformation, congenital, due to
alcohol Q86.0
exogenous cause NEC Q86.8
hydantoin Q86.1
warfarin Q86.2
malignant
carcinoid E34.0
neuroleptic G21.0
Mallory-Weiss K22.6
mandibulofacial dysostosis Q75.4
manic-depressive —*see* Disorder, bipolar ◀
maple-syrup-urine E71.0
Marable's I77.4
Marfan's Q87.40
with
cardiovascular manifestations Q87.418
aortic dilation Q87.410
ocular manifestations Q87.42
skeletal manifestations Q87.43
Marie's (acromegaly) E22.0
mast cell activation —*see* Activation, mast cell ◀
maternal hypotension —*see* Syndrome, hypotension, maternal
May (-Hegglin) D72.0
McArdle (-Schmidt) (-Pearson) E74.04
McQuarrie's E16.2
meconium plug (newborn) P76.0
median arcuate ligament I77.4
Meekeren-Ehlers-Danlos Q79.6
megavitamin-B6 E67.2
Meige G24.4
MELAS E88.41
Mendelson's O74.0
MERRF (myoclonic epilepsy associated with ragged-red fibers) E88.42
mesenteric
artery (superior) K55.1
vascular insufficiency K55.1
metabolic E88.81
metastatic carcinoid E34.0
micrognathia-glossoptosis Q87.0
midbrain NEC G93.89
middle lobe (lung) J98.19
middle radicular G54.0
migraine —*see also* Migraine G43.909-
Mikulicz' K11.8
milk-alkali E83.52
Millard-Gubler G46.3

◀ New ◀ Revised ~~deleted~~ Deleted

Syndrome *(Continued)*
Miller-Dieker Q93.88
Miller-Fisher G61.0
Minkowski-Chauffard D58.0
Mirizzi's K83.1
MNGIE (Mitochondrial Neurogastrointestinal Encephalopathy) E88.49
Möbius, ophthalmoplegic migraine —*see* Migraine, ophthalmoplegic
monofixation H50.42
Morel-Moore M85.2
Morel-Morgagni M85.2
Morgagni (-Morel) (-Stewart) M85.2
Morgagni-Adams-Stokes I45.9
Mounier-Kuhn Q32.4
with bronchiectasis J47.9
with
exacerbation (acute) J47.1
lower respiratory infection J47.0
acquired J98.09
with bronchiectasis J47.9
with
exacerbation (acute) J47.1
lower respiratory infection J47.0
Muckle-Wells M04.2 ◀
mucocutaneous lymph node (acute febrile) (MCLS) M30.3
multiple endocrine neoplasia (MEN) —*see* Neoplasia, endocrine, multiple (MEN)
multiple operations —*see* Disorder, factitious
myasthenic G70.9
in
diabetes mellitus —*see* Diabetes, amyotrophy
endocrine disease NEC E34.9 *[G73.3]*
neoplastic disease —*see also* Neoplasm D49.9 *[G73.3]*
thyrotoxicosis (hyperthyroidism) E05.90 *[G73.3]*
with thyroid storm E05.91 *[G73.3]*
myelodysplastic D46.9
with
5q deletion D46.C
isolated del (5q) chromosomal abnormality D46.C
lesions, low grade D46.20
specified NEC D46.Z
myelopathic pain G89.0
myeloproliferative (chronic) D47.1
myofascial pain M79.1
Naffziger's G54.0
nail patella Q87.2
NARP (Neuropathy, Ataxia and Retinitis pigmentosa) E88.49
neonatal abstinence P96.1
nephritic —*see also* Nephritis
with edema —*see* Nephrosis
acute N00.9
chronic N03.9
rapidly progressive N01.9
nephrotic (congenital) —*see also* Nephrosis N04.9
with
dense deposit disease N04.6
diffuse
crescentic glomerulonephritis N04.7
endocapillary proliferative glomerulonephritis N04.4
membranous glomerulonephritis N04.2
mesangial proliferative glomerulonephritis N04.3
mesangiocapillary glomerulonephritis N04.5
focal and segmental glomerular lesions N04.1
minor glomerular abnormality N04.0
specified morphological changes NEC N04.8
diabetic —*see* Diabetes, nephrosis

Syndrome *(Continued)*
neurologic neglect R41.4
Nezelof's D81.4
Nonne-Milroy-Meige Q82.0
Nothnagel's vasomotor acroparesthesia I73.89
obesity hypoventilation (OHS) E66.2 ◀
oculomotor H51.9
ophthalmoplegia-cerebellar ataxia —*see* Strabismus, paralytic, third nerve
oral allergy T78.1 ◀
oral-facial-digital Q87.0
organic
affective F06.30
amnesic (not alcohol- or drug-induced) F04
brain F09
depressive F06.31
hallucinosis F06.0
personality F07.0
Ormond's N13.5
oro-facial-digital Q87.0
os trigonum Q68.8
Osler-Weber-Rendu I78.0
osteoporosis-osteomalacia M83.8
Osterreicher-Turner Q87.2 ◀
otolith —*see* subcategory H81.8
oto-palatal-digital Q87.0
outlet (thoracic) G54.0
ovary
polycystic E28.2
resistant E28.39
sclerocystic E28.2
Owren's D68.2
Paget-Schroetter I82.890
pain —*see also* Pain
complex regional I G90.50
lower limb G90.52-
specified site NEC G90.59
upper limb G90.51-
complex regional II —*see* Causalgia
painful
bruising D69.2
feet E53.8
prostate N42.81
paralysis agitans —*see* Parkinsonism
paralytic G83.9
specified NEC G83.89
Parinaud's H51.0
parkinsonian —*see* Parkinsonism
Parkinson's —*see* Parkinsonism
paroxysmal facial pain G50.0
Parry's E05.00
with thyroid storm E05.01
Parsonage (-Aldren)-Turner G54.5
patella clunk M25.86-
Paterson (-Brown) (-Kelly) D50.1
pectoral girdle I77.89
pectoralis minor I77.89
Pelger-Huet D72.0
pellagra-cerebellar ataxia-renal aminoaciduria E72.02
pellagroid E52
Pellegrini-Stieda —*see* Bursitis, tibial collateral
pelvic congestion-fibrosis, female N94.89
penta X Q97.1
peptic ulcer —*see* Ulcer, peptic
perabduction I77.89
periodic fever M04.1 ◀
periodic fever, aphthous stomatitis, pharyngitis, and adenopathy [PFAPA] M04.8 ◀
periodic headache, in adults and children —*see* Headache, periodic syndromes in adults and children
periurethral fibrosis N13.5
phantom limb (without pain) G54.7
with pain G54.6
pharyngeal pouch D82.1
Pick's —*see* Disease, Pick's ◀
Pickwickian E66.2

Syndrome *(Continued)*
PIE (pulmonary infiltration with eosinophilia) J82
pigmentary pallidal degeneration (progressive) G23.0
pineal E34.8
pituitary E22.0
placental transfusion —*see* Pregnancy, complicated by, placental transfusion syndromes
plantar fascia M72.2
plateau iris (post-iridectomy) (postprocedural) H21.82
Plummer-Vinson D50.1
pluricarential of infancy E40
plurideficiency E40
pluriglandular (compensatory) E31.8
autoimmune E31.0
pneumatic hammer T75.21
polyangiitis overlap M30.8
polycarential of infancy E40
polyglandular E31.8
autoimmune E31.0
polysplenia Q89.09
pontine NEC G93.89
popliteal
artery entrapment I77.89
web Q87.89
postcardiac injury
postcardiotomy I97.0
postmyocardial infarction I24.1
postcardiotomy I97.0
post chemoembolization — code to associated conditions
postcholecystectomy K91.5
postcommissurotomy I97.0
postconcussional F07.81
postcontusional F07.81
postencephalitic F07.89
posterior
cervical sympathetic M53.0
cord G83.83
fossa compression G93.5
reversible encephalopathy (PRES) I67.83
postgastrectomy (dumping) K91.1
postgastric surgery K91.1
postinfarction I24.1
postlaminectomy NEC M96.1
postleukotomy F07.0
postmastectomy lymphedema I97.2
postmyocardial infarction I24.1
postoperative NEC T81.9
blind loop K90.2
postpartum panhypopituitary (Sheehan) E23.0
postpolio (myelitic) G14
postthrombotic I87.009
with
inflammation I87.02-
with ulcer I87.03-
specified complication NEC I87.09-
ulcer I87.01-
with inflammation I87.03-
asymptomatic I87.00-
postvagotomy K91.1
postvalvulotomy I97.0
postviral NEC G93.3
fatigue G93.3
Potain's K31.0
potassium intoxication E87.5
precerebral artery (multiple) (bilateral) G45.2
preinfarction I20.0
preleukemic D46.9
premature senility E34.8
premenstrual dysphoric F32.89 ◀
premenstrual tension N94.3
Prinzmetal-Massumi R07.1
prune belly Q79.4
pseudocarpal tunnel (sublimis) —*see* Syndrome, carpal tunnel

S

◀ New ◀ Revised ~~deleted~~ Deleted

Syndrome *(Continued)*
pseudoparalytica G70.00
with exacerbation (acute) G70.01
in crisis G70.01
pseudo -Turner's Q87.1
psycho-organic (nonpsychotic severity) F07.9
acute or subacute F05
depressive type F06.31
hallucinatory type F06.0
nonpsychotic severity F07.0
specified NEC F07.89
pulmonary
arteriosclerosis I27.0
dysmaturity (Wilson-Mikity) P27.0
hypoperfusion (idiopathic) P22.0
renal (hemorrhagic) (Goodpasture's) M31.0
pure
motor lacunar G46.5
sensory lacunar G46.6
Putnam-Dana D51.0
pyogenic arthritis, pyoderma gangrenosum, and acne [PAPA] M04.8 ◀
pyramidopallidonigral G20
pyriformis —*see* Lesion, nerve, sciatic
QT interval prolongation I45.81
radicular NEC —*see* Radiculopathy
upper limbs, newborn (birth injury) P14.3
rapid time-zone change G47.25
Rasmussen G04.81
Raymond (-Céstan) I65.8
Raynaud's I73.00
with gangrene I73.01
RDS (respiratory distress syndrome, newborn) P22.0
reactive airways dysfunction J68.3
Refsum's G60.1
Reifenstein E34.52
renal glomerulohyalinosis-diabetic —*see* Diabetes, nephrosis
Rendu-Osler-Weber I78.0
residual ovary N99.83
resistant ovary E28.39
respiratory
distress
acute J80
adult J80
child J80
idiopathic J84.114 ◀
newborn (idiopathic) (type I) P22.0
type II P22.1
restless legs G25.81
retinoblastoma (familial) C69.2
retroperitoneal fibrosis N13.5
retroviral seroconversion (acute) Z21
Reye's G93.7
Richter —*see* Leukemia, chronic lymphocytic, B-cell type
Ridley's I50.1
right
heart, hypoplastic Q22.6
ventricular obstruction —*see* Failure, heart, congestive
Romano-Ward (prolonged QT interval) I45.81
rotator cuff, shoulder —*see also* Tear, rotator cuff M75.10-
Rotes Quérol —*see* Hyperostosis, ankylosing
Roth —*see* Meralgia paresthetica
rubella (congenital) P35.0
Ruvalcaba-Myhre-Smith E71.440
Rytand-Lipsitch I44.2
salt
depletion E87.1
due to heat NEC T67.8
causing heat exhaustion or prostration T67.4
low E87.1
salt-losing N28.89
Scaglietti-Dagnini E22.0
scalenus anticus (anterior) G54.0
scapulocostal —*see* Mononeuropathy, upper limb, specified site NEC

Syndrome *(Continued)*
scapuloperoneal G71.0
schizophrenic, of childhood NEC F84.5
Schnitzler D47.2
Scholte's E34.0
Schroeder's E27.0
Schüller-Christian C96.5
Schwachman's —*see* Syndrome, Shwachman's
Schwartz (-Jampel) G71.13
Schwartz-Bartter E22.2
scimitar Q26.8
sclerocystic ovary E28.2
Seitelberger's G31.89
septicemic adrenal hemorrhage A39.1
seroconversion, retroviral (acute) Z21
serous meningitis G93.2
severe acute respiratory (SARS) J12.81
shaken infant T74.4
shock (traumatic) T79.4
kidney N17.0
following crush injury T79.5
toxic A48.3
shock-lung J80
Shone's — code to specific anomalies
short
bowel K91.2
rib Q77.2
shoulder-hand —*see* Algoneurodystrophy
Shwachman's D70.4
sicca —*see* Sicca syndrome
sick
cell E87.1
sinus I49.5
sick-euthyroid E07.81
sideropenic D50.1
Siemens' ectodermal dysplasia Q82.4
Silfverskölds Q78.9
Simons' E88.1
sinus tarsi M25.57- ◀
sinusitis-bronchiectasis-situs inversus Q89.3
Sipple's E31.22
sirenomelia Q87.2
Slocumb's E27.0
slow flow, coronary I20.8
Sluder's G44.89
Smith-Magenis Q93.88
Sneddon-Wilkinson L13.1
Sotos' Q87.3 ◀
South African cardiomyopathy I42.8
spasmodic
upward movement, eyes H51.8
winking F95.8
Spen's I45.9
splenic
agenesis Q89.01
flexure K59.8
neutropenia D73.81
Spurway's Q78.0
staphylococcal scalded skin L00
steal ◀
arteriovenous T82.898- ◀
ischemic T82.898- ◀
subclavian G45.8 ◀
Stein-Leventhal E28.2
Stein's E28.2
Stevens-Johnson syndrome L51.1
toxic epidermal necrolysis overlap L51.3
Stewart-Morel M85.2
Stickler Q89.8
stiff baby Q89.8
stiff man G25.82
Still-Felty —*see* Felty's syndrome
Stokes (-Adams) I45.9
stone heart I50.1
straight back, congenital Q76.49
subclavian steal G45.8
subcoracoid-pectoralis minor G54.0
subcostal nerve compression I77.89
subphrenic interposition Q43.3

Syndrome *(Continued)*
superior
cerebellar artery I63.8
mesenteric artery K55.1
semi-circular canal dehiscence H83.8X-
vena cava I87.1
supine hypotensive (maternal) —*see* Syndrome, hypotension, maternal
suprarenal cortical E27.0
supraspinatus —*see also* Tear, rotator cuff M75.10-
Susac G93.49
swallowed blood P78.2
sweat retention L74.0
Swyer Q99.1
Symond's G93.2
sympathetic
cervical paralysis G90.2
pelvic, female N94.89
systemic inflammatory response (SIRS), of non-infectious origin (without organ dysfunction) R65.10
with acute organ dysfunction R65.11
tachycardia-bradycardia I49.5
takotsubo I51.81
TAR (thrombocytopenia with absent radius) Q87.2
tarsal tunnel G57.5-
teething K00.7
tegmental G93.89
telangiectasic-pigmentation-cataract Q82.8
temporal pyramidal apex —*see* Otitis, media, suppurative, acute
temporomandibular joint-pain-dysfunction M26.62- ◀
Terry's H44.2-
testicular feminization —*see also* Syndrome, androgen insensitivity E34.51
thalamic pain (hyperesthetic) G89.0
thoracic outlet (compression) G54.0
Thorson-Björck E34.0
thrombocytopenia with absent radius (TAR) Q87.2
thyroid-adrenocortical insufficiency E31.0
tibial
anterior M76.81-
posterior M76.82-
Tietze's M94.0
time-zone (rapid) G47.25
Toni-Fanconi E72.09
with cystinosis E72.04
Touraine's Q79.8
tourniquet —*see* Constriction, external, by site
toxic shock A48.3
transient left ventricular apical ballooning I51.81
traumatic vasospastic T75.22
Treacher Collins Q75.4
triple X, female Q97.0
trisomy Q92.9
13 Q91.7
meiotic nondisjunction Q91.4
mitotic nondisjunction Q91.5
mosaicism Q91.5
translocation Q91.6
18 Q91.3
meiotic nondisjunction Q91.0
mitotic nondisjunction Q91.1
mosaicism Q91.1
translocation Q91.2
20 (q)(p) Q92.8
21 Q90.9
meiotic nondisjunction Q90.0
mitotic nondisjunction Q90.1
mosaicism Q90.1
translocation Q90.2
22 Q92.8
tropical wet feet T69.0-
Trousseau's I82.1

◀ New ◀ Revised ~~deleted~~ Deleted

Syndrome *(Continued)*
tumor lysis (following antineoplastic chemotherapy) (spontaneous) NEC E88.3
tumor necrosis factor receptor associated periodic (TRAPS) M04.1 ◀
Twiddler's (due to)
automatic implantable defibrillator T82.198
cardiac pacemaker T82.198
Unverricht (-Lundborg) —*see* Epilepsy, generalized, idiopathic
upward gaze H51.8
uremia, chronic —*see also* Disease, kidney, chronic N18.9
urethral N34.3
urethro-oculo-articular —*see* Reiter's disease
urohepatic K76.7
vago-hypoglossal G52.7
van Buchem's M85.2
van der Hoeve's Q78.0
vascular NEC in cerebrovascular disease G46.8
vasoconstriction, reversible cerebrovascular I67.841
vasomotor I73.9
vasospastic (traumatic) T75.22
vasovagal R55
VATER Q87.2
velo-cardio-facial Q93.81
vena cava (inferior) (superior) (obstruction) I87.1
vertebral
artery G45.0
compression —*see* Syndrome, anterior, spinal artery, compression
steal G45.0
vertebro-basilar artery G45.0
vertebrogenic (pain) M54.89
vertiginous —*see* Disorder, vestibular function
Vinson-Plummer D50.1
virus B34.9
visceral larva migrans B83.0
visual disorientation H53.8
vitamin B6 deficiency E53.1
vitreal corneal H59.01-
vitreous (touch) H59.01-
Vogt-Koyanagi H20.82-
Volkmann's T79.6
von Schroetter's I82.890
von Willebrand (-Jürgen) D68.0
Waldenström-Kjellberg D50.1
Wallenberg's G46.3
water retention E87.79
Waterhouse (-Friderichsen) A39.1
Weber-Gubler G46.3
Weber-Leyden G46.3
Weber's G46.3
Wegener's M31.30
with
kidney involvement M31.31
lung involvement M31.30
with kidney involvement M31.31
Weingarten's (tropical eosinophilia) J82
Weiss-Baker G90.09
Werdnig-Hoffman G12.0
Wermer's E31.21
Werner's E34.8
Wernicke-Korsakoff (nonalcoholic) F04
alcoholic F10.26
West's —*see* Epilepsy, spasms
Westphal-Strümpell E83.01
wet
feet (maceration) (tropical) T69.0-
lung, newborn P22.1
whiplash S13.4
whistling face Q87.0
Wilkie's K55.1
Wilkinson-Sneddon L13.1
Willebrand (-Jürgens) D68.0

Syndrome *(Continued)*
Wilson's (hepatolenticular degeneration) E83.01
Wiskott-Aldrich D82.0
withdrawal —*see* Withdrawal, state
drug
infant of dependent mother P96.1
therapeutic use, newborn P96.2
Woakes' (ethmoiditis) J33.1
Wright's (hyperabduction) I77.89
X I20.9
XXXX Q97.1
XXXXX Q97.1
XXXXY Q98.1
XXY Q98.0
yellow nail L60.5
Zahorsky's B08.5
Zellweger syndrome E71.510
Zellweger-like syndrome E71.541
Synechia (anterior) (iris) (posterior) (pupil) —*see also* Adhesions, iris
intra-uterine (traumatic) N85.6
Synesthesia R20.8
Syngamiasis, syngamosis B83.3
Synodontia K00.2
Synorchidism, synorchism Q55.1
Synostosis (congenital) Q78.8
astragalo-scaphoid Q74.2
radioulnar Q74.0
Synovial sarcoma —*see* Neoplasm, connective tissue, malignant
Synovioma (malignant) —*see also* Neoplasm, connective tissue, malignant
benign —*see* Neoplasm, connective tissue, benign
Synoviosarcoma —*see* Neoplasm, connective tissue, malignant
Synovitis —*see also* Tenosynovitis M65.9 ◀
crepitant
hand M70.0-
wrist M70.03-
gonococcal A54.49
gouty —*see* Gout ◀
in (due to)
crystals M65.8-
gonorrhea A54.49
syphilis (late) A52.78
use, overuse, pressure —*see* Disorder, soft tissue, due to use
infective NEC —*see* Tenosynovitis, infective NEC
specified NEC —*see* Tenosynovitis, specified type NEC
syphilitic A52.78
congenital (early) A50.02
toxic —*see* Synovitis, transient
transient M67.3-
ankle M67.37-
elbow M67.32-
foot joint M67.37-
hand joint M67.34-
hip M67.35-
knee M67.36-
multiple site M67.39
pelvic region M67.35-
shoulder M67.31-
specified joint NEC M67.38
wrist M67.33-
traumatic, current —*see* Sprain
tuberculous —*see* Tuberculosis, synovitis
villonodular (pigmented) M12.2-
ankle M12.27-
elbow M12.22-
foot joint M12.27-
hand joint M12.24-
hip M12.25-
knee M12.26-
multiple site M12.29
pelvic region M12.25-
shoulder M12.21-
specified joint NEC M12.28

Synovitis *(Continued)*
villonodular (pigmented) *(Continued)*
vertebrae M12.28
wrist M12.23-
Syphilid A51.39
congenital A50.06
newborn A50.06
tubercular (late) A52.79
Syphilis, syphilitic (acquired) A53.9
abdomen (late) A52.79
acoustic nerve A52.15
adenopathy (secondary) A51.49
adrenal (gland) (with cortical hypofunction) A52.79
age under 2 years NOS —*see also* Syphilis, congenital, early
acquired A51.9
alopecia (secondary) A51.32
anemia (late) A52.79 *[D63.8]*
aneurysm (aorta) (ruptured) A52.01
central nervous system A52.05
congenital A50.54 *[I79.0]*
anus (late) A52.74
primary A51.1
secondary A51.39
aorta (arch) (abdominal) (thoracic) A52.02
aneurysm A52.01
aortic (insufficiency) (regurgitation) (stenosis)A52.03
aneurysm A52.01
arachnoid (adhesive) (cerebral) (spinal) A52.13
asymptomatic —*see* Syphilis, latent
ataxia (locomotor) A52.11
atrophoderma maculatum A51.39
auricular fibrillation A52.06
bladder (late) A52.76
bone A52.77
secondary A51.46
brain A52.17
breast (late) A52.79
bronchus (late) A52.72
bubo (primary) A51.0
bulbar palsy A52.19
bursa (late) A52.78
cardiac decompensation A52.06
cardiovascular A52.00
central nervous system (late) (recurrent) (relapse) (tertiary) A52.3
with
ataxia A52.11
general paralysis A52.17
juvenile A50.45
paresis (general) A52.17
juvenile A50.45
tabes (dorsalis) A52.11
juvenile A50.45
taboparesis A52.17
juvenile A50.45
aneurysm A52.05
congenital A50.40
juvenile A50.40
remission in (sustained) A52.3
serology doubtful, negative, or positive A52.3
specified nature or site NEC A52.19
vascular A52.05
cerebral A52.17
meningovascular A52.13
nerves (multiple palsies) A52.15
sclerosis A52.17
thrombosis A52.05
cerebrospinal (tabetic type) A52.12
cerebrovascular A52.05
cervix (late) A52.76
chancre (multiple) A51.0
extragenital A51.2
Rollet's A51.0
Charcot's joint A52.16
chorioretinitis A51.43
congenital A50.01
late A52.71
prenatal A50.01

S

Syphilis, syphilitic *(Continued)*
choroiditis —*see* Syphilitic chorioretinitis
choroidoretinitis —*see* Syphilitic chorioretinitis
ciliary body (secondary) A51.43
late A52.71
colon (late) A52.74
combined spinal sclerosis A52.11
condyloma (latum) A51.31
congenital A50.9
with
paresis (general) A50.45
tabes (dorsalis) A50.45
taboparesis A50.45
chorioretinitis, choroiditis A50.01 *[H32]*
early, or less than 2 years after birth NEC A50.2
with manifestations —*see* Syphilis, congenital, early, symptomatic
latent (without manifestations) A50.1
negative spinal fluid test A50.1
serology positive A50.1
symptomatic A50.09
cutaneous A50.06
mucocutaneous A50.07
oculopathy A50.01
osteochondropathy A50.02
pharyngitis A50.03
pneumonia A50.04
rhinitis A50.05
visceral A50.08
interstitial keratitis A50.31
juvenile neurosyphilis A50.45
late, or 2 years or more after birth NEC A50.7
chorioretinitis, choroiditis A50.32
interstitial keratitis A50.31
juvenile neurosyphilis A50.45
latent (without manifestations) A50.6
negative spinal fluid test A50.6
serology positive A50.6
symptomatic or with manifestations NEC A50.59
arthropathy A50.55
cardiovascular A50.54
Clutton's joints A50.51
Hutchinson's teeth A50.52
Hutchinson's triad A50.53
osteochondropathy A50.56
saddle nose A50.57
conjugal A53.9
tabes A52.11
conjunctiva (late) A52.71
contact Z20.2
cord bladder A52.19
cornea, late A52.71
coronary (artery) (sclerosis) A52.06
coryza, congenital A50.05
cranial nerve A52.15
multiple palsies A52.15
cutaneous —*see* Syphilis, skin
dacryocystitis (late) A52.71
degeneration, spinal cord A52.12
dementia paralytica A52.17
juvenilis A50.45
destruction of bone A52.77
dilatation, aorta A52.01
due to blood transfusion A53.9
dura mater A52.13
ear A52.79
inner A52.79
nerve (eighth) A52.15
neurorecurrence A52.15
early A51.9
cardiovascular A52.00
central nervous system A52.3
latent (without manifestations) (less than 2 years after infection) A51.5
negative spinal fluid test A51.5
serological relapse after treatment A51.5
serology positive A51.5

Syphilis, syphilitic *(Continued)*
early *(Continued)*
relapse (treated, untreated) A51.9
skin A51.39
symptomatic A51.9
extragenital chancre A51.2
primary, except extragenital chancre A51.0
secondary —*see also* Syphilis, secondary A51.39
relapse (treated, untreated) A51.49
ulcer A51.39
eighth nerve (neuritis) A52.15
endemic A65
endocarditis A52.03
aortic A52.03
pulmonary A52.03
epididymis (late) A52.76
epiglottis (late) A52.73
epiphysitis (congenital) (early) A50.02
episcleritis (late) A52.71
esophagus A52.79
eustachian tube A52.73
exposure to Z20.2
eye A52.71
eyelid (late) (with gumma) A52.71
fallopian tube (late) A52.76
fracture A52.77
gallbladder (late) A52.74
gastric (polyposis) (late) A52.74
general A53.9
paralysis A52.17
juvenile A50.45
genital (primary) A51.0
glaucoma A52.71
gumma NEC A52.79
cardiovascular system A52.00
central nervous system A52.3
congenital A50.59
heart (block) (decompensation) (disease) (failure) A52.06 *[I52]*
valve NEC A52.03
hemianesthesia A52.19
hemianopsia A52.71
hemiparesis A52.17
hemiplegia A52.17
hepatic artery A52.09
hepatis A52.74
hepatomegaly, congenital A50.08
hereditaria tarda —*see* Syphilis, congenital, late
hereditary —*see* Syphilis, congenital
Hutchinson's teeth A50.52
hyalitis A52.71
inactive —*see* Syphilis, latent
infantum —*see* Syphilis, congenital
inherited —*see* Syphilis, congenital
internal ear A52.79
intestine (late) A52.74
iris, iritis (secondary) A51.43
late A52.71
joint (late) A52.77
keratitis (congenital) (interstitial) (late) A50.31
kidney (late) A52.75
lacrimal passages (late) A52.71
larynx (late) A52.73
late A52.9
cardiovascular A52.00
central nervous system A52.3
kidney A52.75
latent or 2 years or more after infection (without manifestations) A52.8
negative spinal fluid test A52.8
serology positive A52.8
paresis A52.17
specified site NEC A52.79
symptomatic or with manifestations A52.79
tabes A52.11
latent A53.0
with signs or symptoms - code by site and stage under Syphilis

Syphilis, syphilitic *(Continued)*
latent *(Continued)*
central nervous system A52.2
date of infection unspecified A53.0
early, or less than 2 years after infection A51.5
follow-up of latent syphilis A53.0
date of infection unspecified A53.0
late, or 2 years or more after infection A52.8
late, or 2 years or more after infection A52.8
positive serology (only finding) A53.0
date of infection unspecified A53.0
early, or less than 2 years after infection A51.5
late, or 2 years or more after infection A52.8
lens (late) A52.71
leukoderma A51.39
late A52.79
lienitis A52.79
lip A51.39
chancre (primary) A51.2
late A52.79
Lissauer's paralysis A52.17
liver A52.74
locomotor ataxia A52.11
lung A52.72
lymph gland (early) (secondary) A51.49
late A52.79
lymphadenitis (secondary) A51.49
macular atrophy of skin A51.39
striated A52.79
mediastinum (late) A52.73
meninges (adhesive) (brain) (spinal cord) A52.13
meningitis A52.13
acute (secondary) A51.41
congenital A50.41
meningoencephalitis A52.14
meningovascular A52.13
congenital A50.41
mesarteritis A52.09
brain A52.04
middle ear A52.77
mitral stenosis A52.03
monoplegia A52.17
mouth (secondary) A51.39
late A52.79
mucocutaneous (secondary) A51.39
late A52.79
mucous
membrane (secondary) A51.39
late A52.79
patches A51.39
congenital A50.07
mulberry molars A50.52
muscle A52.78
myocardium A52.06
nasal sinus (late) A52.73
neonatorum —*see* Syphilis, congenital
nephrotic syndrome (secondary) A51.44
nerve palsy (any cranial nerve) A52.15
multiple A52.15
nervous system, central A52.3
neuritis A52.15
acoustic A52.15
neurorecidive of retina A52.19
neuroretinitis A52.19
newborn —*see* Syphilis, congenital
nodular superficial (late) A52.79
nonvenereal A65
nose (late) A52.73
saddle back deformity A50.57
occlusive arterial disease A52.09
oculopathy A52.71
ophthalmic (late) A52.71
optic nerve (atrophy) (neuritis) (papilla) A52.15

S

Syphilis, syphilitic *(Continued)*
orbit (late) A52.71
organic A53.9
osseous (late) A52.77
osteochondritis (congenital) (early) A50.02 *[M90.80]*
osteoporosis A52.77
ovary (late) A52.76
oviduct (late) A52.76
palate (late) A52.79
pancreas (late) A52.74
paralysis A52.17
general A52.17
juvenile A50.45
paresis (general) A52.17
juvenile A50.45
paresthesia A52.19
Parkinson's disease or syndrome A52.19
paroxysmal tachycardia A52.06
pemphigus (congenital) A50.06
penis (chancre) A51.0
late A52.76
pericardium A52.06
perichondritis, larynx (late) A52.73
periosteum (late) A52.77
congenital (early) A50.02 *[M90.80]*
early (secondary) A51.46
peripheral nerve A52.79
petrous bone (late) A52.77
pharynx (late) A52.73
secondary A51.39
pituitary (gland) A52.79
pleura (late) A52.73
pneumonia, white A50.04
pontine lesion A52.17
portal vein A52.09
primary A51.0
anal A51.1
and secondary —*see* Syphilis, secondary
central nervous system A52.3
extragenital chancre NEC A51.2
fingers A51.2
genital A51.0
lip A51.2
specified site NEC A51.2
tonsils A51.2
prostate (late) A52.76
ptosis (eyelid) A52.71
pulmonary (late) A52.72
artery A52.09
pyelonephritis (late) A52.75
recently acquired, symptomatic A51.9
rectum (late) A52.74
respiratory tract (late) A52.73
retina, late A52.71
retrobulbar neuritis A52.15
salpingitis A52.76
sclera (late) A52.71
sclerosis
cerebral A52.17
coronary A52.06
multiple A52.11
scotoma (central) A52.71
scrotum (late) A52.76

Syphilis, syphilitic *(Continued)*
secondary (and primary) A51.49
adenopathy A51.49
anus A51.39
bone A51.46
chorioretinitis, choroiditis A51.43
hepatitis A51.45
liver A51.45
lymphadenitis A51.49
meningitis (acute) A51.41
mouth A51.39
mucous membranes A51.39
periosteum, periostitis A51.46
pharynx A51.39
relapse (treated, untreated) A51.49
skin A51.39
specified form NEC A51.49
tonsil A51.39
ulcer A51.39
viscera NEC A51.49
vulva A51.39
seminal vesicle (late) A52.76
seronegative with signs or symptoms - code by site and stage under Syphilis
seropositive
with signs or symptoms - code by site and stage under Syphilis
follow-up of latent syphilis —*see* Syphilis, latent
only finding —*see* Syphilis, latent
seventh nerve (paralysis) A52.15
sinus, sinusitis (late) A52.73
skeletal system A52.77
skin (with ulceration) (early) (secondary) A51.39
late or tertiary A52.79
small intestine A52.74
spastic spinal paralysis A52.17
spermatic cord (late) A52.76
spinal (cord) A52.12
spleen A52.79
splenomegaly A52.79
spondylitis A52.77
staphyloma A52.71
stigmata (congenital) A50.59
stomach A52.74
synovium A52.78
tabes dorsalis (late) A52.11
juvenile A50.45
tabetic type A52.11
juvenile A50.45
taboparesis A52.17
juvenile A50.45
tachycardia A52.06
tendon (late) A52.78
tertiary A52.9
with symptoms NEC A52.79
cardiovascular A52.00
central nervous system A52.3
multiple NEC A52.79
specified site NEC A52.79
testis A52.76
thorax A52.73
throat A52.73

Syphilis, syphilitic *(Continued)*
thymus (gland) (late) A52.79
thyroid (late) A52.79
tongue (late) A52.79
tonsil (lingual) (late) A52.73
primary A51.2
secondary A51.39
trachea (late) A52.73
tunica vaginalis (late) A52.76
ulcer (any site) (early) (secondary) A51.39
late A52.79
perforating A52.79
foot A52.11
urethra (late) A52.76
urogenital (late) A52.76
uterus (late) A52.76
uveal tract (secondary) A51.43
late A52.71
uveitis (secondary) A51.43
late A52.71
uvula (late) (perforated) A52.79
vagina A51.0
late A52.76
valvulitis NEC A52.03
vascular A52.00
brain (cerebral) A52.05
ventriculi A52.74
vesicae urinariae (late) A52.76
viscera (abdominal) (late) A52.74
secondary A51.49
vitreous (opacities) (late) A52.71
hemorrhage A52.71
vulva A51.0
late A52.76
secondary A51.39
Syphiloma A52.79
cardiovascular system A52.00
central nervous system A52.3
circulatory system A52.00
congenital A50.59
Syphilophobia F45.29
Syringadenoma —*see also* Neoplasm, skin, benign
papillary —*see* Neoplasm, skin, benign
Syringobulbia G95.0
Syringocystadenoma —*see* Neoplasm, skin, benign
papillary —*see* Neoplasm, skin, benign
Syringoma —*see also* Neoplasm, skin, benign
chondroid —*see* Neoplasm, skin, benign
Syringomyelia G95.0
Syringomyelitis —*see* Encephalitis
Syringomyelocele —*see* Spina bifida
Syringopontia G95.0
System, systemic —*see also* condition
disease, combined —*see* Degeneration, combined
inflammatory response syndrome (SIRS) of non-infectious origin (without organ dysfunction) R65.10
with acute organ dysfunction R65.11
lupus erythematosus M32.9
inhibitor present D68.62

S

T

Tabacism, tabacosis, tabagism —*see also* Poisoning, tobacco
meaning dependence (without remission) F17.200
with
disorder F17.299
remission F17.211
specified disorder NEC F17.298
withdrawal F17.203
Tabardillo A75.9
flea-borne A75.2
louse-borne A75.0
Tabes, tabetic A52.10
with
central nervous system syphilis A52.10
Charcot's joint A52.16
cord bladder A52.19
crisis, viscera (any) A52.19
paralysis, general A52.17
paresis (general) A52.17
perforating ulcer (foot) A52.19
arthropathy (Charcot) A52.16
bladder A52.19
bone A52.11
cerebrospinal A52.12
congenital A50.45
conjugal A52.10
dorsalis A52.11
juvenile A50.49
juvenile A50.49
latent A52.19
mesenterica A18.39
paralysis, insane, general A52.17
spasmodic A52.17
syphilis (cerebrospinal) A52.12
Taboparalysis A52.17
Taboparesis (remission) A52.17
juvenile A50.45
TAC (trigeminal autonomic cephalgia) NEC G44.099
intractable G44.091
not intractable G44.099
Tache noir S60.22-
Tachyalimentation K91.2
Tachyarrhythmia, tachyrhythmia —*see* Tachycardia
Tachycardia R00.0
atrial (paroxysmal) I47.1
auricular I47.1
AV nodal re-entry (re-entrant) I47.1
junctional (paroxysmal) I47.1
newborn P29.11
nodal (paroxysmal) I47.1
non-paroxysmal AV nodal I45.89
paroxysmal (sustained) (nonsustained) I47.9
with sinus bradycardia I49.5
atrial (PAT) I47.1
atrioventricular (AV) (re-entrant) I47.1
psychogenic F54
junctional I47.1
ectopic I47.1
nodal I47.1
psychogenic (atrial) (supraventricular) (ventricular) F54
supraventricular (sustained) I47.1
psychogenic F54
ventricular I47.2
psychogenic F54
psychogenic F45.8
sick sinus I49.5
sinoauricular NOS R00.0
paroxysmal I47.1
sinus [sinusal] NOS R00.0
paroxysmal I47.1
supraventricular I47.1
ventricular (paroxysmal) (sustained) I47.2
psychogenic F54
Tachygastria K31.89
Tachypnea R06.82
hysterical F45.8
newborn (idiopathic) (transitory) P22.1
psychogenic F45.8
transitory, of newborn P22.1
TACO (transfusion associated circulatory overload) E87.71
Taenia (infection) (infestation) B68.9
diminuta B71.0
echinococcal infestation B67.90
mediocanellata B68.1
nana B71.0
saginata B68.1
solium (intestinal form) B68.0
larval form —*see* Cysticercosis
Taeniasis (intestine) —*see* Taenia
Tag (hypertrophied skin) (infected) L91.8
adenoid J35.8
anus K64.4
hemorrhoidal K64.4
hymen N89.8
perineal N90.89
preauricular Q17.0
sentinel K64.4
skin L91.8
accessory (congenital) Q82.8
anus K64.4
congenital Q82.8
preauricular Q17.0
tonsil J35.8
urethra, urethral N36.8
vulva N90.89
Tahyna fever B33.8
Takahara's disease E80.3
Takayasu's disease or syndrome M31.4
Talcosis (pulmonary) J62.0
Talipes (congenital) Q66.89
acquired, planus —*see* Deformity, limb, flat foot
asymmetric Q66.89
calcaneovalgus Q66.4
calcaneovarus Q66.1
calcaneus Q66.89
cavus Q66.7
equinovalgus Q66.6
equinovarus Q66.0
equinus Q66.89
percavus Q66.7
planovalgus Q66.6
planus (acquired) (any degree) —*see also* Deformity, limb, flat foot
congenital Q66.5-
due to rickets (sequelae) E64.3
valgus Q66.6
varus Q66.3
Tall stature, constitutional E34.4
Talma's disease M62.89
Talon noir S90.3-
hand S60.22-
heel S90.3-
toe S90.1-
Tamponade, heart I31.4
Tanapox (virus disease) B08.71
Tangier disease E78.6
Tantrum, child problem F91.8
Tapeworm (infection) (infestation) —*see* Infestation, tapeworm
Tapia's syndrome G52.7
TAR (thrombocytopenia with absent radius) **syndrome** Q87.2
Tarral-Besnier disease L44.0
Tarsal tunnel syndrome —*see* Syndrome, tarsal tunnel
Tarsalgia —*see* Pain, limb, lower
Tarsitis (eyelid) H01.8
syphilitic A52.71
tuberculous A18.4
Tartar (teeth) (dental calculus) K03.6
Tattoo (mark) L81.8
Tauri's disease E74.09
Taurodontism K00.2
Taussig-Bing syndrome Q20.1
Taybi's syndrome Q87.2
Tay-Sachs amaurotic familial idiocy or disease E75.02
TBI (traumatic brain injury) S06.9 ◀
Teacher's node or nodule J38.2
Tear, torn (traumatic) —*see also* Laceration
with abortion —*see* Abortion
annular fibrosis M51.35
anus, anal (sphincter) S31.831
complicating delivery
with third degree perineal laceration —*see also* Delivery, complicated, by, laceration, perineum, third degree O70.20 ◀
with mucosa O70.3
without third degree perineal laceration O70.4
nontraumatic (healed) (old) K62.81
articular cartilage, old —*see* Derangement, joint, articular cartilage, by site
bladder
with ectopic or molar pregnancy O08.6
following ectopic or molar pregnancy O08.6
obstetrical O71.5
traumatic —*see* Injury, bladder
bowel
with ectopic or molar pregnancy O08.6
following ectopic or molar pregnancy O08.6
obstetrical trauma O71.5
broad ligament
with ectopic or molar pregnancy O08.6
following ectopic or molar pregnancy O08.6
obstetrical trauma O71.6
bucket handle (knee) (meniscus) —*see* Tear, meniscus
capsule, joint —*see* Sprain
cartilage —*see also* Sprain
articular, old —*see* Derangement, joint, articular cartilage, by site
cervix
with ectopic or molar pregnancy O08.6
following ectopic or molar pregnancy O08.6
obstetrical trauma (current) O71.3
old N88.1
traumatic —*see* Injury, uterus
dural G97.41
nontraumatic G96.11
internal organ —*see* Injury, by site
knee cartilage
articular (current) S83.3-
old —*see* Derangement, knee, meniscus, due to old tear
ligament —*see* Sprain
meniscus (knee) (current injury) S83.209
bucket-handle S83.20-
lateral
bucket-handle S83.25-
complex S83.27-
peripheral S83.26-
specified type NEC S83.28-
medial
bucket-handle S83.21-
complex S83.23-
peripheral S83.22-
specified type NEC S83.24-
old —*see* Derangement, knee, meniscus, due to old tear
site other than knee - code as Sprain
specified type NEC S83.20-
muscle —*see* Strain
pelvic
floor, complicating delivery O70.1
organ NEC, obstetrical trauma O71.5
with ectopic or molar pregnancy O08.6
following ectopic or molar pregnancy O08.6
perineal, secondary O90.1

◀ New ◀ Revised ~~deleted~~ Deleted

Tear, torn *(Continued)*
periurethral tissue, obstetrical trauma O71.82
with ectopic or molar pregnancy O08.6
following ectopic or molar pregnancy O08.6
rectovaginal septum —*see* Laceration, vagina
retina, retinal (without detachment) (horseshoe) —*see also* Break, retina, horseshoe
with detachment —*see* Detachment, retina, with retinal, break
rotator cuff (nontraumatic) M75.10-
complete M75.12-
incomplete M75.11-
traumatic S46.01-
capsule S43.42-
semilunar cartilage, knee —*see* Tear, meniscus
supraspinatus (complete) (incomplete) (nontraumatic) —*see also* Tear, rotator cuff M75.10-
tendon —*see* Strain
tentorial, at birth P10.4
umbilical cord
complicating delivery O69.89
urethra
with ectopic or molar pregnancy O08.6
following ectopic or molar pregnancy O08.6
obstetrical trauma O71.5
uterus —*see* Injury, uterus
vagina —*see* Laceration, vagina
vessel, from catheter —*see* Puncture, accidental complicating surgery
vulva, complicating delivery O70.0
Tear-stone —*see* Dacryolith
Teeth —*see also* condition
grinding
psychogenic F45.8
sleep related G47.63
Teething (syndrome) K00.7
Telangiectasia, telangiectasis (verrucous) I78.1
ataxic (cerebellar) (Louis-Bar) G11.3
familial I78.0
hemorrhagic, hereditary (congenital) (senile) I78.0
hereditary, hemorrhagic (congenital) (senile) I78.0
juxtafoveal H35.07-
macular H35.07-
parafoveal H35.07-
retinal (idiopathic) (juxtafoveal) (macular) (parafoveal) H35.07-
spider I78.1
Telephone scatologia F65.89
Telescoped bowel or intestine K56.1
congenital Q43.8
Temperature
body, high (of unknown origin) R50.9
cold, trauma from T69.9
newborn P80.0
specified effect NEC T69.8
Temple —*see* condition
Temporal —*see* condition
Temporomandibular joint pain-dysfunction syndrome M26.62- ◄
Temporosphenoidal —*see* condition
Tendency
bleeding —*see* Defect, coagulation
suicide
meaning personal history of attempted suicide Z91.5
meaning suicidal ideation —*see* Ideation, suicidal
to fall R29.6
Tenderness, abdominal R10.819
epigastric R10.816
generalized R10.817
left lower quadrant R10.814
left upper quadrant R10.812
periumbilic R10.815
Tenderness, abdominal *(Continued)*
rebound R10.829
epigastric R10.826
generalized R10.827
left lower quadrant R10.824
left upper quadrant R10.822
periumbilic R10.825
right lower quadrant R10.823
right upper quadrant R10.821
right lower quadrant R10.813
right upper quadrant R10.811
Tendinitis, tendonitis —*see also* Enthesopathy
Achilles M76.6-
adhesive —*see* Tenosynovitis, specified type NEC
shoulder —*see* Capsulitis, adhesive
bicipital M75.2-
calcific M65.2-
ankle M65.27-
foot M65.27-
forearm M65.23-
hand M65.24-
lower leg M65.26-
multiple sites M65.29
pelvic region M65.25-
shoulder M75.3-
specified site NEC M65.28
thigh M65.25-
upper arm M65.22-
due to use, overuse, pressure —*see also* Disorder, soft tissue, due to use
specified NEC —*see* Disorder, soft tissue, due to use, specified NEC
gluteal M76.0-
patellar M76.5-
peroneal M76.7-
psoas M76.1-
tibial (posterior) M76.82-
anterior M76.81-
trochanteric —*see* Bursitis, hip, trochanteric
Tendon —*see* condition
Tendosynovitis —*see* Tenosynovitis
Tenesmus (rectal) R19.8
vesical R30.1
Tennis elbow —*see* Epicondylitis, lateral
Tenonitis —*see also* Tenosynovitis
eye (capsule) H05.04-
Tenontosynovitis —*see* Tenosynovitis
Tenontothecitis —*see* Tenosynovitis
Tenophyte —*see* Disorder, synovium, specified type NEC
Tenosynovitis —*see also* Synovitis M65.9
adhesive —*see* Tenosynovitis, specified type NEC
shoulder —*see* Capsulitis, adhesive
bicipital (calcifying) —*see* Tendinitis, bicipital
gonococcal A54.49
in (due to)
crystals M65.8-
gonorrhea A54.49
syphilis (late) A52.78
use, overuse, pressure —*see also* Disorder, soft tissue, due to use
specified NEC —*see* Disorder, soft tissue, due to use, specified NEC
infective NEC M65.1-
ankle M65.17-
foot M65.17-
forearm M65.13-
hand M65.14-
lower leg M65.16-
multiple sites M65.19
pelvic region M65.15-
shoulder region M65.11-
specified site NEC M65.18
thigh M65.15-
upper arm M65.12-
radial styloid M65.4
shoulder region M65.81-
adhesive —*see* Capsulitis, adhesive
Tenosynovitis *(Continued)*
specified type NEC M65.88-
ankle M65.87-
foot M65.87-
forearm M65.83-
hand M65.84-
lower leg M65.86-
multiple sites M65.89
pelvic region M65.85-
shoulder region M65.81-
specified site NEC M65.88
thigh M65.85-
upper arm M65.82-
tuberculous —*see* Tuberculosis, tenosynovitis
Tenovaginitis —*see* Tenosynovitis
Tension
arterial, high —*see also* Hypertension
without diagnosis of hypertension R03.0
headache G44.209
intractable G44.201
not intractable G44.209
nervous R45.0
pneumothorax J93.0
premenstrual N94.3
state (mental) F48.9
Tentorium —*see* condition
Teratencephalus Q89.8
Teratism Q89.7
Teratoblastoma (malignant) —*see* Neoplasm, malignant, by site
Teratocarcinoma —*see also* Neoplasm, malignant, by site
liver C22.7
Teratoma (solid) —*see also* Neoplasm, uncertain behavior, by site
with embryonal carcinoma, mixed —*see* Neoplasm, malignant, by site
with malignant transformation —*see* Neoplasm, malignant, by site
adult (cystic) —*see* Neoplasm, benign, by site
benign —*see* Neoplasm, benign, by site
combined with choriocarcinoma —*see* Neoplasm, malignant, by site
cystic (adult) —*see* Neoplasm, benign, by site
differentiated —*see* Neoplasm, benign, by site
embryonal —*see also* Neoplasm, malignant, by site
liver C22.7
immature —*see* Neoplasm, malignant, by site
liver C22.7
adult, benign, cystic, differentiated type or mature D13.4
malignant —*see also* Neoplasm, malignant, by site
anaplastic —*see* Neoplasm, malignant, by site
intermediate —*see* Neoplasm, malignant, by site
specified site —*see* Neoplasm, malignant, by site
unspecified site C62.90
undifferentiated —*see* Neoplasm, malignant, by site
mature —*see* Neoplasm, uncertain behavior, by site
malignant —*see* Neoplasm, by site, malignant, by site
ovary D27.-
embryonal, immature or malignant C56-
solid —*see* Neoplasm, uncertain behavior, by site
testis C62.9-
adult, benign, cystic, differentiated type or mature D29.2-
scrotal C62.1-
undescended C62.0-
Termination
anomalous —*see also* Malposition, congenital
right pulmonary vein Q26.3
pregnancy, elective Z33.2

Ternidens diminutus infestation B81.8
Ternidensiasis B81.8
Terror (s) night (child) F51.4
Terrorism, victim of Z65.4
Terry's syndrome H44.2-
Tertiary —*see* condition
Test, tests, testing (for)
adequacy (for dialysis)
hemodialysis Z49.31
peritoneal Z49.32
blood pressure Z01.30
abnormal reading —*see* Blood, pressure
blood typing Z01.83
Rh typing Z01.83
blood-alcohol Z04.8
positive —*see* Findings, abnormal, in blood
blood-drug Z04.8
positive —*see* Findings, abnormal, in blood
cardiac pulse generator (battery) Z45.010
fertility Z31.41
genetic
disease carrier status for procreative management
female Z31.430
male Z31.440
male partner of patient with recurrent pregnancy loss Z31.441
procreative management NEC
female Z31.438
male Z31.448
hearing Z01.10
with abnormal findings NEC Z01.118
HIV (human immunodeficiency virus)
nonconclusive (in infants) R75
positive Z21
seropositive Z21
immunity status Z01.84
intelligence NEC Z01.89
laboratory (as part of a general medical examination) Z00.00
with abnormal finding Z00.01
for medicolegal reason NEC Z04.8
male partner of patient with recurrent pregnancy loss Z31.441
Mantoux (for tuberculosis) Z11.1
abnormal result R76.11
pregnancy, positive first pregnancy —*see* Pregnancy, normal, first
procreative Z31.49
fertility Z31.41
skin, diagnostic
allergy Z01.82
special screening examination —*see* Screening, by name of disease
Mantoux Z11.1
tuberculin Z11.1
specified NEC Z01.89
tuberculin Z11.1
abnormal result R76.11
vision Z01.00
with abnormal findings Z01.01
Wassermann Z11.3
positive —*see* Serology for syphilis, positive
Testicle, testicular, testis —*see also* condition
feminization syndrome —*see also* Syndrome, androgen insensitivity E34.51
migrans Q55.29
Tetanus, tetanic (cephalic) (convulsions) A35
with
abortion A34
ectopic or molar pregnancy O08.0
following ectopic or molar pregnancy O08.0
inoculation reaction (due to serum) —*see* Complications, vaccination
neonatorum A33
obstetrical A34
puerperal, postpartum, childbirth A34
Tetany (due to) R29.0
alkalosis E87.3
associated with rickets E55.0
convulsions R29.0
hysterical F44.5
functional (hysterical) F44.5
hyperkinetic R29.0
hysterical F44.5
hyperpnea R06.4
hysterical F44.5
psychogenic F45.8
hyperventilation —*see also* Hyperventilation R06.4
hysterical F44.5
neonatal (without calcium or magnesium deficiency) P71.3
parathyroid (gland) E20.9
parathyroprival E89.2
post- (para)thyroidectomy E89.2
postoperative E89.2
pseudotetany R29.0
psychogenic (conversion reaction) F44.5
Tetralogy of Fallot Q21.3
Tetraplegia (chronic) —*see also* Quadriplegia G82.50-
Thailand hemorrhagic fever A91
Thalassanemia —*see* Thalassemia
Thalassemia (anemia) (disease) D56.9
with other hemoglobinopathy D56.8
alpha (major) (severe) (triple gene defect) D56.0
minor D56.3
silent carrier D56.3
trait D56.3
beta (severe) D56.1
homozygous D56.1
major D56.1
minor D56.3
trait D56.3
delta-beta (homozygous) D56.2
minor D56.3
trait D56.3
dominant D56.8
hemoglobin
C D56.8
E-beta D56.5
intermedia D56.1
major D56.1
minor D56.3
mixed D56.8
sickle-cell —*see* Disease, sickle-cell, thalassemia
specified type NEC D56.8
trait D56.3
variants D56.8
Thanatophoric dwarfism or short stature Q77.1
Thaysen-Gee disease (nontropical sprue) K90.0
Thaysen's disease K90.0
Thecoma D27-
luteinized D27-
malignant C56-
Thelarche, premature E30.8
Thelaziasis B83.8
Thelitis N61.0 ⇐
puerperal, postpartum or gestational —*see* Infection, nipple
Therapeutic —*see* condition
Therapy
drug, long-term (current) (prophylactic)
agents affecting estrogen receptors and estrogen levels NEC Z79.818
anastrozole (Arimidex) Z79.811
antibiotics Z79.2
short-term use - omit code
anticoagulants Z79.01
anti-inflammatory Z79.1
antiplatelet Z79.02
antithrombotics Z79.02
aromatase inhibitors Z79.811
aspirin Z79.82
birth control pill or patch Z79.3
Therapy *(Continued)*
drug, long-term *(Continued)*
bisphosphonates Z79.83
contraceptive, oral Z79.3
drug, specified NEC Z79.899
estrogen receptor downregulators Z79.818
Evista Z79.810
exemestane (Aromasin) Z79.811
Fareston Z79.810
fulvestrant (Faslodex) Z79.818
gonadotropin-releasing hormone (GnRH) agonist Z79.818
goserelin acetate (Zoladex) Z79.818
hormone replacement (postmenopausal) Z79.890
insulin Z79.4
letrozole (Femara) Z79.811
leuprolide acetate (leuprorelin) (Lupron) Z79.818
megestrol acetate (Megace) Z79.818
methadone
for pain management Z79.891
maintenance therapy F11.20
Nolvadex Z79.810
opiate analgesic Z79.891
oral contraceptive Z79.3
raloxifene (Evista) Z79.810
selective estrogen receptor modulators (SERMs) Z79.810
short term - omit code
steroids
inhaled Z79.51
systemic Z79.52
tamoxifen (Nolvadex) Z79.810
toremifene (Fareston) Z79.810
Thermic —*see* condition
Thermography (abnormal) —*see also* Abnormal, diagnostic imaging R93.8
breast R92.8
Thermoplegia T67.0
Thesaurismosis, glycogen —*see* Disease, glycogen storage
Thiamin deficiency E51.9
specified NEC E51.8
Thiaminic deficiency with beriberi E51.11
Thibierge-Weissenbach syndrome —*see* Sclerosis, systemic
Thickening
bone —*see* Hypertrophy, bone
breast N64.59
endometrium R93.8
epidermal L85.9
specified NEC L85.8
hymen N89.6
larynx J38.7
nail L60.2
congenital Q84.5
periosteal —*see* Hypertrophy, bone
pleura J92.9
with asbestos J92.0
skin R23.4
subepiglottic J38.7
tongue K14.8
valve, heart —*see* Endocarditis
Thigh —*see* condition
Thinning vertebra —*see* Spondylopathy, specified NEC
Thirst, excessive R63.1
due to deprivation of water T73.1
Thomsen disease G71.12
Thoracic —*see also* condition
kidney Q63.2
outlet syndrome G54.0
Thoracogastroschisis (congenital) Q79.8
Thoracopagus Q89.4
Thorax —*see* condition
Thorn's syndrome N28.89
Thorson-Björck syndrome E34.0
Threadworm (infection) (infestation) B80

◀ New ⇐ Revised ~~deleted~~ Deleted

Threatened
abortion O20.0
with subsequent abortion O03.9
job loss, anxiety concerning Z56.2
labor (without delivery) O47.9
~~after 37 completed weeks of gestation O47.1~~
at or after 37 completed weeks of gestation O47.1 ◀
before 37 completed weeks of gestation O47.0-
loss of job, anxiety concerning Z56.2
miscarriage O20.0
unemployment, anxiety concerning Z56.2
Three-day fever A93.1
Threshers' lung J67.0
Thrix annulata (congenital) Q84.1
Throat —*see* condition
Thrombasthenia (Glanzmann) (hemorrhagic) (hereditary) D69.1
Thromboangiitis I73.1
obliterans (general) I73.1
cerebral I67.89
vessels
brain I67.89
spinal cord I67.89
Thromboarteritis —*see* Arteritis
Thromboasthenia (Glanzmann) (hemorrhagic) (hereditary) D69.1
Thrombocytasthenia (Glanzmann) D69.1
Thrombocythemia (essential) (hemorrhagic) (idiopathic) (primary) D47.3
Thrombocytopathy (dystrophic) (granulopenic) D69.1
Thrombocytopenia, thrombocytopenic D69.6
with absent radius (TAR) Q87.2
congenital D69.42
dilutional D69.59
due to
drugs D69.59
extracorporeal circulation of blood D69.59
(massive)blood transfusion D69.59
platelet alloimmunization D69.59
essential D69.3
heparin induced (HIT) D75.82
hereditary D69.42
idiopathic D69.3
neonatal, transitory P61.0
due to
exchange transfusion P61.0
idiopathic maternal thrombocytopenia P61.0
isoimmunization P61.0
primary NEC D69.49
idiopathic D69.3
puerperal, postpartum O72.3
secondary D69.59
transient neonatal P61.0
Thrombocytosis, essential D47.3
primary D47.3
Thromboembolism —*see* Embolism
Thrombopathy (Bernard-Soulier) D69.1
constitutional D68.0
Willebrand-Jurgens D68.0
Thrombopenia —*see* Thrombocytopenia
Thrombophilia D68.59
primary NEC D68.59
secondary NEC D68.69
specified NEC D68.69
Thrombophlebitis I80.9
antepartum O22.2-
deep O22.3-
superficial O22.2-
cavernous (venous) sinus G08
complicating pregnancy O22.5-
nonpyogenic I67.6
cerebral (sinus) (vein) G08
nonpyogenic I67.6
sequelae G09
due to implanted device —*see* Complications, by site and type, specified NEC

Thrombophlebitis *(Continued)*
during or resulting from a procedure NEC T81.72
femoral vein (superficial) I80.1-
femoropopliteal vein I80.0-
hepatic (vein) I80.8
idiopathic, recurrent I82.1
iliofemoral I80.1-
intracranial venous sinus (any) G08
nonpyogenic I67.6
sequelae G09
intraspinal venous sinuses and veins G08
nonpyogenic G95.19
lateral (venous) sinus G08
nonpyogenic I67.6
leg I80.299
superficial I80.0-
longitudinal (venous) sinus G08
nonpyogenic I67.6
lower extremity I80.299
migrans, migrating I82.1
pelvic
with ectopic or molar pregnancy O08.0
following ectopic or molar pregnancy O08.0
puerperal O87.1
popliteal vein —*see* Phlebitis, leg, deep, popliteal
portal (vein) K75.1
postoperative T81.72
pregnancy —*see* Thrombophlebitis, antepartum
puerperal, postpartum, childbirth O87.0
deep O87.1
pelvic O87.1
septic O86.81
superficial O87.0
saphenous (greater) (lesser) I80.0-
sinus (intracranial) G08
nonpyogenic I67.6
specified site NEC I80.8
tibial vein I80.23-
Thrombosis, thrombotic (bland) (multiple) (progressive) (silent) (vessel) I82.90
anal K64.5
antepartum —*see* Thrombophlebitis, antepartum
aorta, aortic I74.10
abdominal I74.09
saddle I74.01
bifurcation I74.09
saddle I74.01
specified site NEC I74.19
terminal I74.09
thoracic I74.11
valve —*see* Endocarditis, aortic
apoplexy I63.3- ⟸
artery, arteries (postinfectional) I74.9
auditory, internal —*see* Occlusion, artery, precerebral, specified NEC
basilar —*see* Occlusion, artery, basilar
carotid (common) (internal) —*see* Occlusion, artery, carotid
cerebellar (anterior inferior) (posterior inferior) (superior) —*see* Occlusion, artery, cerebellar
cerebral —*see* Occlusion, artery, cerebral
choroidal (anterior) —*see* Occlusion, artery, cerebral, specified NEC
communicating, posterior —*see* Occlusion, artery, cerebral, specified NEC
coronary —*see also* Infarct, myocardium
not resulting in infarction I24.0
hepatic I74.8
hypophyseal —*see* Occlusion, artery, cerebral, specified NEC
iliac I74.5
limb I74.4
lower I74.3
upper I74.2

Thrombosis, thrombotic *(Continued)*
artery, arteries *(Continued)*
meningeal, anterior or posterior —*see* Occlusion, artery, cerebral, specified NEC
mesenteric (with gangrene) —*see also* Infarct, intestine K55.069 ⟸
ophthalmic —*see* Occlusion, artery, retina
pontine —*see* Occlusion, artery, cerebral, specified NEC
precerebral —*see* Occlusion, artery, precerebral
pulmonary (iatrogenic) —*see* Embolism, pulmonary
renal N28.0
retinal —*see* Occlusion, artery, retina
spinal, anterior or posterior G95.11
traumatic NEC T14.8
vertebral —*see* Occlusion, artery, vertebral
atrium, auricular —*see also* Infarct, myocardium
following acute myocardial infarction (current complication) I23.6
not resulting in infarction I51.3 ⟸
basilar (artery) —*see* Occlusion, artery, basilar
brain (artery) (stem) —*see also* Occlusion, artery, cerebral
due to syphilis A52.05
puerperal O99.43
sinus —*see* Thrombosis, intracranial venous sinus
capillary I78.8
cardiac —*see also* Infarct, myocardium
not resulting in infarction I51.3 ⟸
valve —*see* Endocarditis
carotid (artery) (common) (internal) —*see* Occlusion, artery, carotid
cavernous (venous) sinus —*see* Thrombosis, intracranial venous sinus
cerebellar artery (anterior inferior) (posterior inferior) (superior) I66.3
cerebral (artery) —*see* Occlusion, artery, cerebral
cerebrovenous sinus —*see also* Thrombosis, intracranial venous sinus
puerperium O87.3
chronic I82.91
coronary (artery) (vein) —*see also* Infarct, myocardium
not resulting in infarction I24.0
corpus cavernosum N48.89
cortical I66.9
deep —*see* Embolism, vein, lower extremity
due to device, implant or graft —*see also* Complications, by site and type, specified NEC T85.868 ⟸
arterial graft NEC T82.868
breast (implant) T85.868 ⟸
catheter NEC T85.868 ⟸
dialysis (renal) T82.868
intraperitoneal T85.868 ⟸
infusion NEC T82.868
spinal (epidural) (subdural) T85.860 ⟸
urinary (indwelling) T83.86
electronic (electrode) (pulse generator) (stimulator)
bone T84.86
cardiac T82.867
nervous system (brain) (peripheral nerve) (spinal) T85.860 ⟸
urinary T83.86
fixation, internal (orthopedic) NEC T84.86
gastrointestinal (bile duct) (esophagus) T85.868 ⟸
genital NEC T83.86
heart T82.867
joint prosthesis T84.86
ocular (corneal graft) (orbital implant) NEC T85.868 ⟸
orthopedic NEC T84.86

◀ New ⟸ Revised ~~deleted~~ Deleted

Thrombosis, thrombotic *(Continued)*
due to device, implant or graft *(Continued)*
specified NEC T85.868
urinary NEC T83.86
vascular NEC T82.868
ventricular intracranial shunt T85.860
during the puerperium —*see* Thrombosis, puerperal
endocardial —*see also* Infarct, myocardium
not resulting in infarction I51.3
eye —*see* Occlusion, retina
genital organ
female NEC N94.89
pregnancy —*see* Thrombophlebitis, antepartum
male N50.1
gestational —*see* Phlebopathy, gestational
heart (chamber) —*see also* Infarct, myocardium
not resulting in infarction I51.3
hepatic (vein) I82.0
artery I74.8
history (of) Z86.718
intestine (with gangrene) —*see also* Infarct, intestine K55.069
intracardiac NEC (apical) (atrial) (auricular) (ventricular) (old) I51.3
intracranial (arterial) I66.9
venous sinus (any) G08
nonpyogenic origin I67.6
puerperium O87.3
intramural —*see also* Infarct, myocardium
not resulting in infarction I51.3
intraspinal venous sinuses and veins G08
nonpyogenic G95.19
kidney (artery) N28.0
lateral (venous) sinus —*see* Thrombosis, intracranial venous sinus
leg —*see* Thrombosis, vein, lower extremity
arterial I74.3
liver (venous) I82.0
artery I74.8
portal vein I81
longitudinal (venous) sinus —*see* Thrombosis, intracranial venous sinus
lower limb —*see* Thrombosis, vein, lower extremity
lung (iatrogenic) (postoperative) —*see* Embolism, pulmonary
meninges (brain) (arterial) I66.8
mesenteric (artery) (with gangrene) —*see also* Infarct, intestine K55.069
vein (inferior) (superior) I81
mitral I34.8
mural —*see also* Infarct, myocardium
due to syphilis A52.06
not resulting in infarction I51.3
omentum (with gangrene) —*see also* Infarct, intestine K55.069
ophthalmic —*see* Occlusion, retina
pampiniform plexus (male) N50.1
parietal —*see also* Infarct, myocardium
not resulting in infarction I24.0
penis, superficial vein N48.81
perianal venous K64.5
peripheral arteries I74.4
upper I74.2
personal history (of) Z86.718
portal I81
due to syphilis A52.09
precerebral artery —*see* Occlusion, artery, precerebral
puerperal, postpartum O87.0
brain (artery) O99.43
venous (sinus) O87.3
cardiac O99.43
cerebral (artery) O99.43
venous (sinus) O87.3
superficial O87.0

Thrombosis, thrombotic *(Continued)*
pulmonary (artery) (iatrogenic) (postoperative) (vein) —*see* Embolism, pulmonary
renal (artery) N28.0
vein I82.3
resulting from presence of device, implant or graft —*see* Complications, by site and type, specified NEC
retina, retinal —*see* Occlusion, retina
scrotum N50.1
seminal vesicle N50.1
sigmoid (venous) sinus —*see* Thrombosis, intracranial venous sinus
sinus, intracranial (any) —*see* Thrombosis, intracranial venous sinus
specified site NEC I82.890
chronic I82.891
spermatic cord N50.1
spinal cord (arterial) G95.11
due to syphilis A52.09
pyogenic origin G06.1
spleen, splenic D73.5
artery I74.8
testis N50.1
traumatic NEC T14.8
tricuspid I07.8
tumor —*see* Neoplasm, by site
tunica vaginalis N50.1
umbilical cord (vessels), complicating delivery O69.5
vas deferens N50.1
vein (acute) I82.90
antecubital I82.61-
chronic I82.71-
axillary I82.A1-
chronic I82.A2-
basilic I82.61-
chronic I82.71-
brachial I82.62-
chronic I82.72-
brachiocephalic (innominate) I82.290
chronic I82.291
cerebral, nonpyogenic I67.6
cephalic I82.61-
chronic I82.71-
chronic I82.91
deep (DVT) I82.40-
calf I82.4Z-
chronic I82.5Z-
lower leg I82.4Z-
chronic I82.5Z-
thigh I82.4Y-
chronic I82.5Y-
upper leg I82.4Y
chronic I82.5y-
femoral I82.41-
chronic I82.51-
iliac (iliofemoral) I82.42-
chronic I82.52-
innominate I82.290
chronic I82.291
internal jugular I82.C1-
chronic I82.C2-
lower extremity
deep I82.40-
chronic I82.50-
specified NEC I82.49-
chronic NEC I82.59-
distal
deep I82.4Z-
proximal
deep I82.4Y-
chronic I82.5Y-
superficial I82.81-
perianal K64.5
popliteal I82.43-
chronic I82.53-
radial I82.62-
chronic I82.72-
renal I82.3

Thrombosis, thrombotic *(Continued)*
vein *(Continued)*
saphenous (greater) (lesser) I82.81-
specified NEC I82.890
chronic NEC I82.891
subclavian I82.B1-
chronic I82.B2-
thoracic NEC I82.290
chronic I82.291
tibial I82.44-
chronic I82.54-
ulnar I82.62-
chronic I82.72-
upper extremity I82.60-
chronic I82.70-
deep I82.62-
chronic I82.72-
superficial I82.61-
chronic I82.71-
vena cava
inferior I82.220
chronic I82.221
superior I82.210
chronic I82.211
venous, perianal K64.5
ventricle —*see also* Infarct, myocardium
following acute myocardial infarction (current complication) I23.6
not resulting in infarction I24.0
Thrombus —*see* Thrombosis
Thrush —*see also* Candidiasis
newborn P37.5
oral B37.0
vaginal B37.3
Thumb —*see also* condition
sucking (child problem) F98.8
Thymitis E32.8
Thymoma (benign) D15.0
malignant C37
Thymus, thymic (gland) —*see* condition
Thyrocele —*see* Goiter
Thyroglossal —*see also* condition
cyst Q89.2
duct, persistent Q89.2
Thyroid (gland) (body) —*see also* condition
hormone resistance E07.89
lingual Q89.2
nodule (cystic) (nontoxic) (single) E04.1
Thyroiditis E06.9
acute (nonsuppurative) (pyogenic) (suppurative) E06.0
autoimmune E06.3
chronic (nonspecific) (sclerosing) E06.5
with thyrotoxicosis, transient E06.2
fibrous E06.5
lymphadenoid E06.3
lymphocytic E06.3
lymphoid E06.3
de Quervain's E06.1
drug-induced E06.4
fibrous (chronic) E06.5
giant-cell (follicular) E06.1
granulomatous (de Quervain) (subacute) E06.1
Hashimoto's (struma lymphomatosa) E06.3
iatrogenic E06.4
ligneous E06.5
lymphocytic (chronic) E06.3
lymphoid E06.3
lymphomatous E06.3
nonsuppurative E06.1
postpartum, puerperal O90.5
pseudotuberculous E06.1
pyogenic E06.0
radiation E06.4
Riedel's E06.5
subacute (granulomatous) E06.1
suppurative E06.0
tuberculous A18.81
viral E06.1
woody E06.5

◀ New ◀ Revised ~~deleted~~ Deleted

Thyrolingual duct, persistent Q89.2
Thyromegaly E01.0
Thyrotoxic
crisis —*see* Thyrotoxicosis
heart disease or failure —*see also* Thyrotoxicosis E05.90 *[I43]*
with thyroid storm E05.91 *[I43]*
storm —*see* Thyrotoxicosis
Thyrotoxicosis (recurrent) E05.90
with
goiter (diffuse) E05.00
with thyroid storm E05.01
adenomatous uninodular E05.10
with thyroid storm E05.11
multinodular E05.20
with thyroid storm E05.21
nodular E05.20
with thyroid storm E05.21
uninodular E05.10
with thyroid storm E05.11
infiltrative
dermopathy E05.00
with thyroid storm E05.01
ophthalmopathy E05.00
with thyroid storm E05.01
single thyroid nodule E05.10
with thyroid storm E05.11
thyroid storm E05.91
due to
ectopic thyroid nodule or tissue E05.30
with thyroid storm E05.31
ingestion of (excessive) thyroid material E05.40
with thyroid storm E05.41
overproduction of thyroid-stimulating hormone E05.80
with thyroid storm E05.81
specified cause NEC E05.80
with thyroid storm E05.81
factitia E05.40
with thyroid storm E05.41
heart E05.90 *[I43]*
with thyroid storm E05.91 *[I43]*
failure E05.90 *[I43]*
neonatal (transient) P72.1
transient with chronic thyroiditis E06.2
Tibia vara —*see* Osteochondrosis, juvenile, tibia
Tic (disorder) F95.9
breathing F95.8
child problem F95.0
compulsive F95.1
de la Tourette F95.2
degenerative (generalized) (localized) G25.69
facial G25.69
disorder
chronic
motor F95.1
vocal F95.1
combined vocal and multiple motor F95.2
transient F95.0
douloureux G50.0
atypical G50.1
postherpetic, postzoster B02.22
drug-induced G25.61
eyelid F95.8
habit F95.9
chronic F95.1
transient of childhood F95.0
lid, transient of childhood F95.0
motor-verbal F95.2
occupational F48.8
orbicularis F95.8
transient of childhood F95.0
organic origin G25.69
postchoreic G25.69
provisional F95.0 ◀
psychogenic, compulsive F95.1
salaam R25.8
spasm (motor or vocal) F95.9
chronic F95.1
transient of childhood F95.0
specified NEC F95.8
Tick-borne —*see* condition
Tietze's disease or syndrome M94.0
Tight, tightness
anus K62.89
chest R07.89
fascia (lata) M62.89
foreskin (congenital) N47.1
hymen, hymenal ring N89.6
introitus (acquired) (congenital) N89.6
rectal sphincter K62.89
tendon —*see* Short, tendon
urethral sphincter N35.9
Tilting vertebra —*see* Dorsopathy, deforming, specified NEC
Timidity, child F93.8
Tin-miner's lung J63.5
Tinea (intersecta) (tarsi) B35.9
amiantacea L44.8
asbestina B35.0
barbae B35.0
beard B35.0
black dot B35.0
blanca B36.2
capitis B35.0
corporis B35.4
cruris B35.6
flava B36.0
foot B35.3
furfuracea B36.0
imbricata (Tokelau) B35.5
kerion B35.0
manuum B35.2
microsporic —*see* Dermatophytosis
nigra B36.1
nodosa —*see* Piedra
pedis B35.3
scalp B35.0
specified site NEC B35.8
sycosis B35.0
tonsurans B35.0
trichophytic —*see* Dermatophytosis
unguium B35.1
versicolor B36.0
Tingling sensation (skin) R20.2
~~Tinnitus (audible) (aurium) (subjective) —see subcategory H93.1~~
Tinnitus NOS H93.1- ◀
audible H93.1- ◀
aurium H93.1- ◀
pulsatile H93.A- ◀
subjective H93.1- ◀
Tipped tooth (teeth) M26.33
Tipping
pelvis M95.5
with disproportion (fetopelvic) O33.0
causing obstructed labor O65.0
tooth (teeth), fully erupted M26.33
Tiredness R53.83
Tissue —*see* condition
Tobacco (nicotine)
abuse —*see* Tobacco, use ◀
dependence —*see* Dependence, drug, nicotine
harmful use Z72.0
heart —*see* Tobacco, toxic effect
maternal use, affecting newborn P04.2
toxic effect —*see* Table of Drugs and Chemicals, by substance, poisoning
chewing tobacco —*see* Table of Drugs and Chemicals, by substance, poisoning
cigarettes —*see* Table of Drugs and Chemicals, by substance, poisoning
use Z72.0
complicating
childbirth O99.334
pregnancy O99.33-
puerperium O99.335
counseling and surveillance Z71.6
history Z87.891 ◀
withdrawal state —*see also* Dependence, drug, nicotine F17.203 ◀
Tocopherol deficiency E56.0
Todd's
cirrhosis K74.3
paralysis (postepileptic) (transitory) G83.84
Toe —*see* condition
Toilet, artificial opening —*see* Attention to, artificial, opening
Tokelau (ringworm) B35.5
Tollwut —*see* Rabies
Tommaselli's disease R31.9
correct substance properly administered —*see* Table of Drugs and Chemicals, by drug, adverse effect
overdose or wrong substance given or taken —*see* Table of Drugs and Chemicals, by drug, poisoning
Tongue —*see also* condition
tie Q38.1
Tonic pupil —*see* Anomaly, pupil, function, tonic pupil
Toni-Fanconi syndrome (cystinosis) E72.09
with cystinosis E72.04
Tonsil —*see* condition
Tonsillitis (acute) (catarrhal) (croupous) (follicular) (gangrenous) (infective) (lacunar) (lingual) (malignant) (membranous) (parenchymatous) (phlegmonous) (pseudomembranous) (purulent) (septic) (subacute) (suppurative) (toxic) (ulcerative) (vesicular) (viral) J03.90
chronic J35.01
with adenoiditis J35.03
diphtheritic A36.0
hypertrophic J35.01
with adenoiditis J35.03
recurrent J03.91
specified organism NEC J03.80
recurrent J03.81
staphylococcal J03.80
recurrent J03.81
streptococcal J03.00
recurrent J03.01
tuberculous A15.8
Vincent's A69.1
Tooth, teeth —*see* condition
Toothache K08.89 ◀
Topagnosis R20.8
Tophi —*see* Gout, chronic
TORCH infection —*see* Infection, congenital
without active infection P00.2
Torn —*see* Tear
Tornwaldt's cyst or disease J39.2
Torsion
accessory tube —*see* Torsion, fallopian tube
adnexa (female) —*see* Torsion, fallopian tube
aorta, acquired I77.1
appendix epididymis N44.04
appendix testis N44.03
bile duct (common) (hepatic) K83.8
congenital Q44.5
bowel, colon or intestine K56.2
cervix —*see* Malposition, uterus
cystic duct K82.8
dystonia —*see* Dystonia, torsion
epididymis (appendix) N44.04
fallopian tube N83.52- ◀
with ovary N83.53
gallbladder K82.8
congenital Q44.1
hydatid of Morgagni
female N83.52- ◀
male N44.03
kidney (pedicle) (leading to infarction) N28.0
Meckel's diverticulum (congenital) Q43.0
malignant —*see* Table of Neoplasms, small intestine, malignant
mesentery K56.2
omentum K56.2
organ or site, congenital NEC —*see* Anomaly, by site

◀ New ◀ Revised ~~deleted~~ Deleted

Torsion *(Continued)*
ovary (pedicle) N83.51- ◀
with fallopian tube N83.53
congenital Q50.2
oviduct —*see* Torsion, fallopian tube
penis (acquired) N48.82
congenital Q55.63
spasm —*see* Dystonia, torsion
spermatic cord N44.02
extravaginal N44.01
intravaginal N44.02
spleen D73.5
testis, testicle N44.00
appendix N44.03
tibia —*see* Deformity, limb, specified type NEC, lower leg
uterus —*see* Malposition, uterus
Torticollis (intermittent) (spastic) M43.6
congenital (sternomastoid) Q68.0
due to birth injury P15.8
hysterical F44.4
ocular R29.891
psychogenic F45.8
conversion reaction F44.4
rheumatic M43.6
rheumatoid M06.88
spasmodic G24.3
traumatic, current S13.4
Tortipelvis G24.1
Tortuous
aortic arch Q25.46 ◀
artery I77.1
organ or site, congenital NEC —*see* Distortion
retinal vessel, congenital Q14.1
ureter N13.8
urethra N36.8
vein —*see* Varix
Torture, victim of Z65.4
Torula, torular (histolytica) (infection) —*see* Cryptococcosis
Torulosis —*see* Cryptococcosis
Torus (mandibularis) (palatinus) M27.0
fracture —*see* Fracture, by site, torus
Touraine's syndrome Q79.8
Tourette's syndrome F95.2
Tourniquet syndrome —*see* Constriction, external, by site
Tower skull Q75.0
with exophthalmos Q87.0
Toxemia R68.89
bacterial —*see* Sepsis
burn —*see* Burn
eclamptic (with pre-existing hypertension) —*see* Eclampsia
erysipelatous —*see* Erysipelas
fatigue R68.89
food —*see* Poisoning, food
gastrointestinal K52.1
intestinal K52.1
kidney —*see* Uremia
malarial —*see* Malaria
myocardial —*see* Myocarditis, toxic
of pregnancy —*see* Pre-eclampsia
pre-eclamptic —*see* Pre-eclampsia
small intestine K52.1
staphylococcal, due to food A05.0
stasis R68.89
uremic —*see* Uremia
urinary —*see* Uremia
Toxemica cerebropathia psychica (nonalcoholic) F04
alcoholic —*see* Alcohol, amnestic disorder
Toxic (poisoning) —*see also* condition T65.91
effect —*see* Table of Drugs and Chemicals, by substance, poisoning
shock syndrome A48.3
thyroid (gland) —*see* Thyrotoxicosis
Toxicemia —*see* Toxemia
Toxicity —*see* Table of Drugs and Chemicals, by substance, poisoning
fava bean D55.0

Toxic *(Continued)*
food, noxious —*see* Poisoning, food
from drug or nonmedicinal substance —*see* Table of Drugs and Chemicals, by drug
Toxicosis —*see also* Toxemia
capillary, hemorrhagic D69.0
Toxinfection, gastrointestinal K52.1
Toxocariasis B83.0
Toxoplasma, toxoplasmosis (acquired) B58.9
with
hepatitis B58.1
meningoencephalitis B58.2
ocular involvement B58.00
other organ involvement B58.89
pneumonia, pneumonitis B58.3
congenital (acute) (subacute) (chronic) P37.1
maternal, manifest toxoplasmosis in infant (acute) (subacute) (chronic) P37.1
tPA (rtPA) administation in a different facility within the last 24 hours prior to admission to current facility Z92.82
Trabeculation, bladder N32.89
Trachea —*see* condition
Tracheitis (catarrhal) (infantile) (membranous) (plastic) (septal) (suppurative) (viral) J04.10
with
bronchitis (15 years of age and above) J40
acute or subacute —*see* Bronchitis, acute
chronic J42
tuberculous NEC A15.5
under 15 years of age J20.9
laryngitis (acute) J04.2
chronic J37.1
tuberculous NEC A15.5
acute J04.10
with obstruction J04.11
chronic J42
with
bronchitis (chronic) J42
laryngitis (chronic) J37.1
diphtheritic (membranous) A36.89
due to external agent —*see* Inflammation, respiratory, upper, due to
syphilitic A52.73
tuberculous A15.5
Trachelitis (nonvenereal) —*see* Cervicitis
Tracheobronchial —*see* condition
Tracheobronchitis (15 years of age and above) —*see also* Bronchitis
due to
Bordetella bronchiseptica A37.80
with pneumonia A37.81
Francisella tularensis A21.8
Tracheobronchomegaly Q32.4
with bronchiectasis J47.9
with
exacerbation (acute) J47.1
lower respiratory infection J47.0
acquired J98.09
with bronchiectasis J47.9
with
exacerbation (acute) J47.1
lower respiratory infection J47.0
Tracheobronchopneumonitis —*see* Pneumonia, broncho-
Tracheocele (external) (internal) J39.8
congenital Q32.1
Tracheomalacia J39.8
congenital Q32.0
Tracheopharyngitis (acute) J06.9
chronic J42
due to external agent —*see* Inflammation, respiratory, upper, due to
Tracheostenosis J39.8
Tracheostomy
complication —*see* Complication, tracheostomy
status Z93.0
attention to Z43.0
malfunctioning J95.03

Trachoma, trachomatous A71.9
active (stage) A71.1
contraction of conjunctiva A71.1
dubium A71.0
healed or sequelae B94.0
initial (stage) A71.0
pannus A71.1
Türck's J37.0
Traction, vitreomacular H43.82-
Train sickness T75.3
Trait (s)
Hb-S D57.3
hemoglobin
abnormal NEC D58.2
with thalassemia D56.3
C —*see* Disease, hemoglobin C
S (Hb-S) D57.3
Lepore D56.3
personality, accentuated Z73.1
sickle-cell D57.3
with elliptocytosis or spherocytosis D57.3
type A personality Z73.1
Tramp Z59.0
Trance R41.89
hysterical F44.89
Transaminasemia R74.0
Transection
abdomen (partial) S38.3
aorta (incomplete) —*see also* Injury, aorta
complete —*see* Injury, aorta, laceration, major
carotid artery (incomplete) —*see also* Injury, blood vessel, carotid, laceration
complete —*see* Injury, blood vessel, carotid, laceration, major
celiac artery (incomplete) S35.211
branch (incomplete) S35.291
complete S35.292
complete S35.212
innominate
artery (incomplete) —*see also* Injury, blood vessel, thoracic, innominate, artery, laceration
complete —*see* Injury, blood vessel, thoracic, innominate, artery, laceration, major
vein (incomplete) —*see also* Injury, blood vessel, thoracic, innominate, vein, laceration
complete —*see* Injury, blood vessel, thoracic, innominate, vein, laceration, major
jugular vein (external) (incomplete) —*see also* Injury, blood vessel, jugular vein, laceration
complete —*see* Injury, blood vessel, jugular vein, laceration, major
internal (incomplete) —*see also* Injury, blood vessel, jugular vein, internal, laceration
complete —*see* Injury, blood vessel, jugular vein, internal, laceration, major
mesenteric artery (incomplete) —*see also* Injury, mesenteric, artery, laceration
complete —*see* Injury, mesenteric artery, laceration, major
pulmonary vessel (incomplete) —*see also* Injury, blood vessel, thoracic, pulmonary, laceration
complete —*see* Injury, blood vessel, thoracic, pulmonary, laceration, major
subclavian —*see* Transection, innominate
vena cava (incomplete) —*see also* Injury, vena cava
complete —*see* Injury, vena cava, laceration, major
vertebral artery (incomplete) —*see also* Injury, blood vessel, vertebral, laceration
complete —*see* Injury, blood vessel, vertebral, laceration, major

Transfusion
associated (red blood cell) hemochromatosis E83.111
blood
ABO incompatible —*see* Complication (s), transfusion, incompatibility reaction, ABO
minor blood group (Duffy) (E) (K(ell)) (Kidd) (Lewis) (M) (N) (P) (S) T80.89
reaction or complication —*see* Complications, transfusion
fetomaternal (mother) —*see* Pregnancy, complicated by, placenta, transfusion syndrome
maternofetal (mother) —*see* Pregnancy, complicated by, placenta, transfusion syndrome
placental (syndrome) (mother) —*see* Pregnancy, complicated by, placenta, transfusion syndrome
reaction (adverse) —*see* Complications, transfusion
related acute lung injury (TRALI) J95.84
twin-to-twin —*see* Pregnancy, complicated by, placenta, transfusion syndrome, fetus to fetus
Transient (meaning homeless) —*see also* condition Z59.0
Translocation
balanced autosomal Q95.9
in normal individual Q95.0
chromosomes NEC Q99.8
balanced and insertion in normal individual Q95.0
Down's syndrome Q90.2
trisomy
13 Q91.6
18 Q91.2
21 Q90.2
Translucency, iris —*see* Degeneration, iris
Transmission of chemical substances through the placenta —*see* Absorption, chemical, through placenta
Transparency, lung, unilateral J43.0
Transplant (ed) (status) Z94.9
awaiting organ Z76.82
bone Z94.6
marrow Z94.81
candidate Z76.82
complication —*see* Complication, transplant
cornea Z94.7
heart Z94.1
and lung (s) Z94.3
valve Z95.2
prosthetic Z95.2
specified NEC Z95.4
xenogenic Z95.3
intestine Z94.82
kidney Z94.0
liver Z94.4
lung (s) Z94.2
and heart Z94.3
organ (failure) (infection) (rejection)Z94.9
removal status Z98.85
pancreas Z94.83
skin Z94.5
social Z60.3
specified organ or tissue NEC Z94.89
stem cells Z94.84
tissue Z94.9
Transplants, ovarian, endometrial N80.1
Transposed —*see* Transposition
Transposition (congenital) —*see also* Malposition, congenital
abdominal viscera Q89.3
aorta (dextra) Q20.3
appendix Q43.8
colon Q43.8
corrected Q20.5
great vessels (complete) (partial) Q20.3
Transposition *(Continued)*
heart Q24.0
with complete transposition of viscera Q89.3
intestine (large) (small) Q43.8
reversed jejunal (for bypass) (status) Z98.0
scrotum Q55.23
stomach Q40.2
with general transposition of viscera Q89.3
tooth, teeth, fully erupted M26.30
vessels, great (complete) (partial) Q20.3
viscera (abdominal) (thoracic) Q89.3
Transsexualism F64.0 ⇐
Transverse —*see also* condition
arrest (deep), in labor O64.0
lie (mother) O32.2
causing obstructed labor O64.8
Transvestism, transvestitism (dual-role) F64.1
fetishistic F65.1
Trapped placenta (with hemorrhage) O72.0
without hemorrhage O73.0
TRAPS (tumor necrosis factor receptor associated periodic syndrome) M04.1 ◀
Trauma, traumatism —*see also* Injury
acoustic —*see* subcategory H83.3
birth —*see* Birth, injury
complicating ectopic or molar pregnancy O08.6
during delivery O71.9
following ectopic or molar pregnancy O08.6
obstetric O71.9
specified NEC O71.89
occlusal ◀
primary K08.81 ◀
secondary K08.82 ◀
Traumatic —*see also* condition
brain injury S06.9 ⇐
Treacher Collins syndrome Q75.4
Treitz's hernia —*see* Hernia, abdomen, specified site NEC
Trematode infestation —*see* Infestation, fluke
Trematodiasis —*see* Infestation, fluke
Trembling paralysis —*see* Parkinsonism
Tremor (s) R25.1
drug induced G25.1
essential (benign) G25.0
familial G25.0
hereditary G25.0
hysterical F44.4
intention G25.2
medication induced postural G25.1
mercurial —*see* subcategory T56.1
Parkinson's —*see* Parkinsonism
psychogenic (conversion reaction) F44.4
senilis R54
specified type NEC G25.2
Trench
fever A79.0
foot —*see* Immersion, foot
mouth A69.1
Treponema pallidum infection —*see* Syphilis
Treponematosis
due to
T. pallidum —*see* Syphilis
T. pertenue —*see* Yaws
Triad
Hutchinson's (congenital syphilis) A50.53
Kartagener's Q89.3
Saint's —*see* Hernia, diaphragm
Trichiasis (eyelid) H02.059
with entropion —*see* Entropion
left H02.056
lower H02.055
upper H02.054
right H02.053
lower H02.052
upper H02.051
Trichinella spiralis (infection) (infestation) B75
Trichinellosis, trichiniasis, trichinelliasis, trichinosis B75
with muscle disorder B75 *[M63.80]*
ankle B75 *[M63.87-]*
foot B75 *[M63.87-]*
forearm B75 *[M63.83-]*
hand B75 *[M63.84-]*
lower leg B75 *[M63.86-]*
multiple sites B75 *[M63.89]*
pelvic region B75 *[M63.85-]*
shoulder region B75 *[M63.81-]*
specified site NEC B75 *[M63.88]*
thigh B75 *[M63.85-]*
upper arm B75 *[M63.82-]*
Trichobezoar T18.9
intestine T18.3
stomach T18.2
Trichocephaliasis, trichocephalosis B79
Trichocephalus infestation B79
Trichoclasis L67.8
Trichoepithelioma —*see also* Neoplasm, skin, benign
malignant —*see* Neoplasm, skin, malignant
Trichofolliculoma —*see* Neoplasm, skin, benign
Tricholemmoma —*see* Neoplasm, skin, benign
Trichomoniasis A59.9
bladder A59.03
cervix A59.09
intestinal A07.8
prostate A59.02
seminal vesicles A59.09
specified site NEC A59.8
urethra A59.03
urogenitalis A59.00
vagina A59.01
vulva A59.01
Trichomycosis
axillaris A48.8
nodosa, nodularis B36.8
Trichonodosis L67.8
Trichophytid, trichophyton infection —*see* Dermatophytosis
Trichophytobezoar T18.9
intestine T18.3
stomach T18.2
Trichophytosis —*see* Dermatophytosis
Trichoptilosis L67.8
Trichorrhexis (nodosa) (invaginata) L67.0
Trichosis axillaris A48.8
Trichosporosis nodosa B36.2
Trichostasis spinulosa (congenital) Q84.1
Trichostrongyliasis, trichostrongylosis (small intestine) B81.2
Trichostrongylus infection B81.2
Trichotillomania F63.3
Trichromat, trichromatopsia, anomalous (congenital) H53.55
Trichuriasis B79
Trichuris trichiura (infection) (infestation) (any site) B79
Tricuspid (valve) —*see* condition
Trifid —*see also* Accessory
kidney (pelvis) Q63.8
tongue Q38.3
Trigeminal neuralgia —*see* Neuralgia, trigeminal
Trigeminy R00.8
Trigger finger (acquired) M65.30
congenital Q74.0
index finger M65.32-
little finger M65.35-
middle finger M65.33-
ring finger M65.34-
thumb M65.31-
Trigonitis (bladder) (chronic) (pseudomembranous) N30.30
with hematuria N30.31
Trigonocephaly Q75.0
Trilocular heart —*see* Cor triloculare

Trimethylaminuria E72.52
Tripartite placenta O43.19-
Triphalangeal thumb Q74.0
Triple —*see also* Accessory
  kidneys Q63.0
  uteri Q51.818
  X, female Q97.0
Triplegia G83.89
  congenital G80.8
Triplet (newborn) —*see also* Newborn, triplet
  complicating pregnancy —*see* Pregnancy, triplet
Triplication —*see* Accessory
Triploidy Q92.7
Trismus R25.2
  neonatorum A33
  newborn A33
Trisomy (syndrome) Q92.9
  13 (partial) Q91.7
    meiotic nondisjunction Q91.4
    mitotic nondisjunction Q91.5
    mosaicism Q91.5
    translocation Q91.6
  18 (partial) Q91.3
    meiotic nondisjunction Q91.0
    mitotic nondisjunction Q91.1
    mosaicism Q91.1
    translocation Q91.2
  20 Q92.8
  21 (partial) Q90.9
    meiotic nondisjunction Q90.0
    mitotic nondisjunction Q90.1
    mosaicism Q90.1
    translocation Q90.2
  22 Q92.8
  autosomes Q92.9
  chromosome specified NEC Q92.8
    partial Q92.2
      due to unbalanced translocation Q92.5
    specified NEC Q92.8
    whole (nonsex chromosome)
      meiotic nondisjunction Q92.0
      mitotic nondisjunction Q92.1
      mosaicism Q92.1
  due to
    dicentrics —*see* Extra, marker chromosomes
    extra rings —*see* Extra, marker chromosomes
    isochromosomes —*see* Extra, marker chromosomes
  specified NEC Q92.8
  whole chromosome Q92.9
    meiotic nondisjunction Q92.0
    mitotic nondisjunction Q92.1
    mosaicism Q92.1
    partial Q92.9
    specified NEC Q92.8
Tritanomaly, tritanopia H53.55
Trombiculosis, trombiculiasis, trombidiosis B88.0
Trophedema (congenital) (hereditary) Q82.0
Trophoblastic disease —*see also* Mole, hydatidiform O01.9
Tropholymphedema Q82.0
Trophoneurosis NEC G96.8
  disseminated M34.9
Tropical —*see* condition
Trouble —*see also* Disease
  heart —*see* Disease, heart
  kidney —*see* Disease, renal
  nervous R45.0
  sinus —*see* Sinusitis
Trousseau's syndrome (thrombophlebitis migrans) I82.1
Truancy, childhood
  from school Z72.810
Truncus
  arteriosus (persistent) Q20.0
  communis Q20.0
Trunk —*see* condition
Trypanosomiasis
  African B56.9
    by Trypanosoma brucei
      gambiense B56.0
      rhodesiense B56.1
  American —*see* Chagas' disease
  Brazilian —*see* Chagas' disease
  by Trypanosoma
    brucei gambiense B56.0
    brucei rhodesiense B56.1
    cruzi —*see* Chagas' disease
  gambiensis, Gambian B56.0
  rhodesiensis, Rhodesian B56.1
  South American —*see* Chagas' disease
  where
    African trypanosomiasis is prevalent B56.9
    Chagas' disease is prevalent B57.2
T-shaped incisors K00.2
Tsutsugamushi (disease) (fever) A75.3
Tube, tubal, tubular —*see* condition
Tubercle —*see also* Tuberculosis
  brain, solitary A17.81
  Darwin's Q17.8
  Ghon, primary infection A15.7
Tuberculid, tuberculide (indurating, subcutaneous) (lichenoid) (miliary) (papulonecrotic) (primary) (skin) A18.4
Tuberculoma —*see also* Tuberculosis
  brain A17.81
  meninges (cerebral) (spinal) A17.1
  spinal cord A17.81
Tuberculosis, tubercular, tuberculous (calcification) (calcified) (caseous) (chromogenic acid-fast bacilli) (degeneration) (fibrocaseous) (fistula) (interstitial) (isolated circumscribed lesions) (necrosis) (parenchymatous) (ulcerative) A15.9
  with pneumoconiosis (any condition in J60-J64) J65
  abdomen (lymph gland) A18.39
  abscess (respiratory) A15.9
    bone A18.03
      hip A18.02
      knee A18.02
      sacrum A18.01
      specified site NEC A18.03
      spinal A18.01
      vertebra A18.01
    brain A17.81
    breast A18.89
    Cowper's gland A18.15
    dura (mater) (cerebral) (spinal) A17.81
    epidural (cerebral) (spinal) A17.81
    female pelvis A18.17
    frontal sinus A15.8
    genital organs NEC A18.10
    genitourinary A18.10
    gland (lymphatic) —*see* Tuberculosis, lymph gland
    hip A18.02
    intestine A18.32
    ischiorectal A18.32
    joint NEC A18.02
      hip A18.02
      knee A18.02
      specified NEC A18.02
      vertebral A18.01
    kidney A18.11
    knee A18.02
    latent R76.11
    lumbar (spine) A18.01
    lung —*see* Tuberculosis, pulmonary
    meninges (cerebral) (spinal) A17.0
    muscle A18.09
    perianal (fistula) A18.32
    perinephritic A18.11
    perirectal A18.32
    rectum A18.32
    retropharyngeal A15.8
    sacrum A18.01
Tuberculosis, tubercular, tuberculous *(Continued)*
  abscess *(Continued)*
    scrofulous A18.2
    scrotum A18.15
    skin (primary) A18.4
    spinal cord A17.81
    spine or vertebra (column) A18.01
    subdiaphragmatic A18.31
    testis A18.15
    urinary A18.13
    uterus A18.17
  accessory sinus —*see* Tuberculosis, sinus
  Addison's disease A18.7
  adenitis —*see* Tuberculosis, lymph gland
  adenoids A15.8
  adenopathy —*see* Tuberculosis, lymph gland
  adherent pericardium A18.84
  adnexa (uteri) A18.17
  adrenal (capsule) (gland) A18.7
  alimentary canal A18.32
  anemia A18.89
  ankle (joint) (bone) A18.02
  anus A18.32
  apex, apical —*see* Tuberculosis, pulmonary
  appendicitis, appendix A18.32
  arachnoid A17.0
  artery, arteritis A18.89
    cerebral A18.89
  arthritis (chronic) (synovial) A18.02
    spine or vertebra (column) A18.01
  articular —*see* Tuberculosis, joint
  ascites A18.31
  asthma —*see* Tuberculosis, pulmonary
  axilla, axillary (gland) A18.2
  bladder A18.12
  bone A18.03
    hip A18.02
    knee A18.02
    limb NEC A18.03
    sacrum A18.01
    spine or vertebral column A18.01
  bowel (miliary) A18.32
  brain A17.81
  breast A18.89
  broad ligament A18.17
  bronchi, bronchial, bronchus A15.5
    ectasia, ectasis (bronchiectasis) —*see* Tuberculosis, pulmonary
    fistula A15.5
      primary (progressive) A15.7
    gland or node A15.4
      primary (progressive) A15.7
    lymph gland or node A15.4
      primary (progressive) A15.7
  bronchiectasis —*see* Tuberculosis, pulmonary
  bronchitis A15.5
  bronchopleural A15.6
  bronchopneumonia, bronchopneumonic —*see* Tuberculosis, pulmonary
  bronchorrhagia A15.5
  bronchotracheal A15.5
  bronze disease A18.7
  buccal cavity A18.83
  bulbourethral gland A18.15
  bursa A18.09
  cachexia A15.9
  cardiomyopathy A18.84
  caries —*see* Tuberculosis, bone
  cartilage A18.02
    intervertebral A18.01
  catarrhal —*see* Tuberculosis, respiratory
  cecum A18.32
  cellulitis (primary) A18.4
  cerebellum A17.81
  cerebral, cerebrum A17.81
  cerebrospinal A17.81
    meninges A17.0
  cervical (lymph gland or node) A18.2
  cervicitis, cervix (uteri) A18.16
  chest —*see* Tuberculosis, respiratory

Tuberculosis, tubercular, tuberculous *(Continued)*
chorioretinitis A18.53
choroid, choroiditis A18.53
ciliary body A18.54
colitis A18.32
collier's J65
colliquativa (primary) A18.4
colon A18.32
complex, primary A15.7
congenital P37.0
conjunctiva A18.59
connective tissue (systemic) A18.89
contact Z20.1
cornea (ulcer) A18.52
Cowper's gland A18.15
coxae A18.02
coxalgia A18.02
cul-de-sac of Douglas A18.17
curvature, spine A18.01
cutis (colliquativa) (primary) A18.4
cyst, ovary A18.18
cystitis A18.12
dactylitis A18.03
diarrhea A18.32
diffuse —*see* Tuberculosis, miliary
digestive tract A18.32
disseminated —*see* Tuberculosis, miliary
duodenum A18.32
dura (mater) (cerebral) (spinal) A17.0
abscess (cerebral) (spinal) A17.81
dysentery A18.32
ear (inner) (middle) A18.6
bone A18.03
external (primary) A18.4
skin (primary) A18.4
elbow A18.02
emphysema —*see* Tuberculosis, pulmonary
empyema A15.6
encephalitis A17.82
endarteritis A18.89
endocarditis A18.84
aortic A18.84
mitral A18.84
pulmonary A18.84
tricuspid A18.84
endocrine glands NEC A18.82
endometrium A18.17
enteric, enterica, enteritis A18.32
enterocolitis A18.32
epididymis, epididymitis A18.15
epidural abscess (cerebral) (spinal) A17.81
epiglottis A15.5
episcleritis A18.51
erythema (induratum) (nodosum) (primary) A18.4
esophagus A18.83
eustachian tube A18.6
exposure (to) Z20.1
exudative —*see* Tuberculosis, pulmonary
eye A18.50
eyelid (primary) (lupus) A18.4
fallopian tube (acute) (chronic) A18.17
fascia A18.09
fauces A15.8
female pelvic inflammatory disease A18.17
finger A18.03
first infection A15.7
gallbladder A18.83
ganglion A18.09
gastritis A18.83
gastrocolic fistula A18.32
gastroenteritis A18.32
gastrointestinal tract A18.32
general, generalized —*see* Tuberculosis, miliary
genital organs A18.10
genitourinary A18.10
genu A18.02
glandula suprarenalis A18.7
glandular, general A18.2

Tuberculosis, tubercular, tuberculous *(Continued)*
glottis A15.5
grinder's J65
gum A18.83
hand A18.03
heart A18.84
hematogenous —*see* Tuberculosis, miliary
hemoptysis —*see* Tuberculosis, pulmonary
hemorrhage NEC —*see* Tuberculosis, pulmonary
hemothorax A15.6
hepatitis A18.83
hilar lymph nodes A15.4
primary (progressive) A15.7
hip (joint) (disease) (bone) A18.02
hydropneumothorax A15.6
hydrothorax A15.6
hypoadrenalism A18.7
hypopharynx A15.8
ileocecal (hyperplastic) A18.32
ileocolitis A18.32
ileum A18.32
iliac spine (superior) A18.03
immunological findings only A15.7
indurativa (primary) A18.4
infantile A15.7
infection A15.9
without clinical manifestations A15.7
infraclavicular gland A18.2
inguinal gland A18.2
inguinalis A18.2
intestine (any part) A18.32
iridocyclitis A18.54
iris, iritis A18.54
ischiorectal A18.32
jaw A18.03
jejunum A18.32
joint A18.02
vertebral A18.01
keratitis (interstitial) A18.52
keratoconjunctivitis A18.52
kidney A18.11
knee (joint) A18.02
kyphosis, kyphoscoliosis A18.01
laryngitis A15.5
larynx A15.5
latent R76.11
leptomeninges, leptomeningitis (cerebral) (spinal) A17.0
lichenoides (primary) A18.4
linguae A18.83
lip A18.83
liver A18.83
lordosis A18.01
lung —*see* Tuberculosis, pulmonary
lupus vulgaris A18.4
lymph gland or node (peripheral) A18.2
abdomen A18.39
bronchial A15.4
primary (progressive) A15.7
cervical A18.2
hilar A15.4
primary (progressive) A15.7
intrathoracic A15.4
primary (progressive) A15.7
mediastinal A15.4
primary (progressive) A15.7
mesenteric A18.39
retroperitoneal A18.39
tracheobronchial A15.4
primary (progressive) A15.7
lymphadenitis —*see* Tuberculosis, lymph gland
lymphangitis —*see* Tuberculosis, lymph gland
lymphatic (gland) (vessel) —*see* Tuberculosis, lymph gland
mammary gland A18.89
marasmus A15.9
mastoiditis A18.03

Tuberculosis, tubercular, tuberculous *(Continued)*
mediastinal lymph gland or node A15.4
primary (progressive) A15.7
mediastinitis A15.8
primary (progressive) A15.7
mediastinum A15.8
primary (progressive) A15.7
medulla A17.81
melanosis, Addisonian A18.7
meninges, meningitis (basilar) (cerebral) (cerebrospinal) (spinal) A17.0
meningoencephalitis A17.82
mesentery, mesenteric (gland or node) A18.39
miliary A19.9
acute A19.2
multiple sites A19.1
single specified site A19.0
chronic A19.8
specified NEC A19.8
millstone makers' J65
miner's J65
molder's J65
mouth A18.83
multiple A19.9
acute A19.1
chronic A19.8
muscle A18.09
myelitis A17.82
myocardium, myocarditis A18.84
nasal (passage) (sinus) A15.8
nasopharynx A15.8
neck gland A18.2
nephritis A18.11
nerve (mononeuropathy) A17.83
nervous system A17.9
nose (septum) A15.8
ocular A18.50
omentum A18.31
oophoritis (acute) (chronic) A18.17
optic (nerve trunk) (papilla) A18.59
orbit A18.59
orchitis A18.15
organ, specified NEC A18.89
osseous —*see* Tuberculosis, bone
osteitis —*see* Tuberculosis, bone
osteomyelitis —*see* Tuberculosis, bone
otitis media A18.6
ovary, ovaritis (acute) (chronic) A18.17
oviduct (acute) (chronic) A18.17
pachymeningitis A17.0
palate (soft) A18.83
pancreas A18.83
papulonecrotic (a) (primary) A18.4
parathyroid glands A18.82
paronychia (primary) A18.4
parotid gland or region A18.83
pelvis (bony) A18.03
penis A18.15
peribronchitis A15.5
pericardium, pericarditis A18.84
perichondritis, larynx A15.5
periostitis —*see* Tuberculosis, bone
perirectal fistula A18.32
peritoneum NEC A18.31
peritonitis A18.31
pharynx, pharyngitis A15.8
phlyctenulosis (keratoconjunctivitis) A18.52
phthisis NEC —*see* Tuberculosis, pulmonary
pituitary gland A18.82
pleura, pleural, pleurisy, pleuritis (fibrinous) (obliterative) (purulent) (simple plastic) (with effusion) A15.6
primary (progressive) A15.7
pneumonia, pneumonic —*see* Tuberculosis, pulmonary
pneumothorax (spontaneous) (tense valvular) —*see* Tuberculosis, pulmonary
polyneuropathy A17.89

Tuberculosis, tubercular, tuberculous *(Continued)*
polyserositis A19.9
acute A19.1
chronic A19.8
potter's J65
prepuce A18.15
primary (complex) A15.7
proctitis A18.32
prostate, prostatitis A18.14
pulmonalis —*see* Tuberculosis, pulmonary
pulmonary (cavitated) (fibrotic) (infiltrative) (nodular) A15.0
childhood type or first infection A15.7
primary (complex) A15.7
pyelitis A18.11
pyelonephritis A18.11
pyemia —*see* Tuberculosis, miliary
pyonephrosis A18.11
pyopneumothorax A15.6
pyothorax A15.6
rectum (fistula) (with abscess) A18.32
reinfection stage —*see* Tuberculosis, pulmonary
renal A18.11
renis A18.11
respiratory A15.9
primary A15.7
specified site NEC A15.8
retina, retinitis A18.53
retroperitoneal (lymph gland or node) A18.39
rheumatism NEC A18.09
rhinitis A15.8
sacroiliac (joint) A18.01
sacrum A18.01
salivary gland A18.83
salpingitis (acute) (chronic) A18.17
sandblaster's J65
sclera A18.51
scoliosis A18.01
scrofulous A18.2
scrotum A18.15
seminal tract or vesicle A18.15
senile A15.9
septic —*see* Tuberculosis, miliary
shoulder (joint) A18.02
blade A18.03
sigmoid A18.32
sinus (any nasal) A15.8
bone A18.03
epididymis A18.15
skeletal NEC A18.03
skin (any site) (primary) A18.4
small intestine A18.32
soft palate A18.83
spermatic cord A18.15
spine, spinal (column) A18.01
cord A17.81
medulla A17.81
membrane A17.0
meninges A17.0
spleen, splenitis A18.85
spondylitis A18.01
sternoclavicular joint A18.02
stomach A18.83
stonemason's J65
subcutaneous tissue (cellular) (primary) A18.4
subcutis (primary) A18.4
subdeltoid bursa A18.83
submaxillary (region) A18.83
supraclavicular gland A18.2
suprarenal (capsule) (gland) A18.7
swelling, joint —*see also* category M01 (*see also* Tuberculosis, joint) A18.02
symphysis pubis A18.02
synovitis A18.09
articular A18.02
spine or vertebra A18.01
systemic —*see* Tuberculosis, miliary

Tuberculosis, tubercular, tuberculous *(Continued)*
tarsitis A18.4
tendon (sheath) —*see* Tuberculosis, tenosynovitis
tenosynovitis A18.09
spine or vertebra A18.01
testis A18.15
throat A15.8
thymus gland A18.82
thyroid gland A18.81
tongue A18.83
tonsil, tonsillitis A15.8
trachea, tracheal A15.5
lymph gland or node A15.4
primary (progressive) A15.7
tracheobronchial A15.5
lymph gland or node A15.4
primary (progressive) A15.7
tubal (acute) (chronic) A18.17
tunica vaginalis A18.15
ulcer (skin) (primary) A18.4
bowel or intestine A18.32
specified NEC - code under Tuberculosis, by site
unspecified site A15.9
ureter A18.11
urethra, urethral (gland) A18.13
urinary organ or tract A18.13
uterus A18.17
uveal tract A18.54
uvula A18.83
vagina A18.18
vas deferens A18.15
verruca, verrucosa (cutis) (primary) A18.4
vertebra (column) A18.01
vesiculitis A18.15
vulva A18.18
wrist (joint) A18.02

Tuberculum
Carabelli —*see* Note at K00.2
occlusal —*see* Note at K00.2
paramolare K00.2

Tuberosity, enitre maxillary M26.07

Tuberous sclerosis (brain) Q85.1

Tubo-ovarian —*see* condition

Tuboplasty, after previous sterilization Z31.0
aftercare Z31.42

Tubotympanitis, catarrhal (chronic) —*see* Otitis, media, nonsuppurative, chronic, serous

Tularemia A21.9
with
conjunctivitis A21.1
pneumonia A21.2
abdominal A21.3
bronchopneumonic A21.2
conjunctivitis A21.1
cryptogenic A21.3
enteric A21.3
gastrointestinal A21.3
generalized A21.7
ingestion A21.3
intestinal A21.3
oculoglandular A21.1
ophthalmic A21.1
pneumonia (any), pneumonic A21.2
pulmonary A21.2
sepsis A21.7
specified NEC A21.8
typhoidal A21.7
ulceroglandular A21.0

Tularensis conjunctivitis A21.1

Tumefaction —*see also* Swelling
liver —*see* Hypertrophy, liver

Tumor —*see also* Neoplasm, unspecified behavior, by site
acinar cell —*see* Neoplasm, uncertain behavior, by site
acinic cell —*see* Neoplasm, uncertain behavior, by site

Tumor *(Continued)*
adenocarcinoid —*see* Neoplasm, malignant, by site
adenomatoid —*see also* Neoplasm, benign, by site
odontogenic —*see* Cyst, calcifying odontogenic
adnexal (skin) —*see* Neoplasm, skin, benign, by site
adrenal
cortical (benign) D35.0-
malignant C74.0-
rest —*see* Neoplasm, benign, by site
alpha-cell
malignant
pancreas C25.4
specified site NEC —*see* Neoplasm, malignant, by site
unspecified site C25.4
pancreas D13.7
specified site NEC —*see* Neoplasm, benign, by site
unspecified site D13.7
aneurysmal —*see* Aneurysm
aortic body D44.7
malignant C75.5
Askin's —*see* Neoplasm, connective tissue, malignant
basal cell —*see also* Neoplasm, skin, uncertain behavior D48.5
Bednar —*see* Neoplasm, skin, malignant
benign (unclassified) —*see* Neoplasm, benign, by site
beta-cell
malignant
pancreas C25.4
specified site NEC —*see* Neoplasm, malignant, by site
unspecified site C25.4
pancreas D13.7
specified site NEC —*see* Neoplasm, benign, by site
unspecified site D13.7
Brenner D27.9
borderline malignancy D39.1-
malignant C56-
proliferating D39.1
bronchial alveolar, intravascular D38.1
Brooke's —*see* Neoplasm, skin, benign
brown fat —*see* Lipoma
Burkitt —*see* Lymphoma, Burkitt
calcifying epithelial odontogenic —*see* Cyst, calcifying odontogenic
carcinoid
benign D3A.00
appendix D3A.020
ascending colon D3A.022
bronchus (lung) D3A.090
cecum D3A.021
colon D3A.029
descending colon D3A.024
duodenum D3A.010
foregut NOS D3A.094
hindgut NOS D3A.096
ileum D3A.012
jejunum D3A.011
kidney D3A.093
large intestine D3A.029
lung (bronchus) D3A.090
midgut NOS D3A.095
rectum D3A.026
sigmoid colon D3A.025
small intestine D3A.019
specified NEC D3A.098
stomach D3A.092
thymus D3A.091
transverse colon D3A.023
malignant C7A.00
appendix C7A.020
ascending colon C7A.022
bronchus (lung) C7A.090

Tumor *(Continued)*
carcinoid *(Continued)*
malignant *(Continued)*
cecum C7A.021
colon C7A.029
descending colon C7A.024
duodenum C7A.010
foregut NOS C7A.094
hindgut NOS C7A.096
ileum C7A.012
jejunum C7A.011
kidney C7A.093
large intestine C7A.029
lung (bronchus) C7A.090
midgut NOS C7A.095
rectum C7A.026
sigmoid colon C7A.025
small intestine C7A.019
specified NEC C7A.098
stomach C7A.092
thymus C7A.091
transverse colon C7A.023
mesentery metastasis C7B.04
secondary C7B.00
bone C7B.03
distant lymph nodes C7B.01
liver C7B.02
peritoneum C7B.04
specified NEC C7B.09
carotid body D44.6
malignant C75.4
cells —*see also* Neoplasm, unspecified behavior, by site
benign —*see* Neoplasm, benign, by site
malignant —*see* Neoplasm, malignant, by site
uncertain whether benign or malignant —*see* Neoplasm, uncertain behavior, by site
cervix, in pregnancy or childbirth —*see* Pregnancy, complicated by, tumor, cervix
chondromatous giant cell —*see* Neoplasm, bone, benign
chromaffin —*see also* Neoplasm, benign, by site
malignant —*see* Neoplasm, malignant, by site
Cock's peculiar L72.3
Codman's —*see* Neoplasm, bone, benign
dentigerous, mixed —*see* Cyst, calcifying odontogenic
dermoid —*see* Neoplasm, benign, by site
with malignant transformation C56-
desmoid (extra-abdominal) —*see also* Neoplasm, connective tissue, uncertain behavior
abdominal —*see* Neoplasm, connective tissue, uncertain behavior
embolus —*see* Neoplasm, secondary, by site
embryonal (mixed) —*see also* Neoplasm, uncertain behavior, by site
liver C22.7
endodermal sinus
specified site —*see* Neoplasm, malignant, by site
unspecified site
female C56.-
male C62.90
epithelial
benign —*see* Neoplasm, benign, by site
malignant —*see* Neoplasm, malignant, by site
Ewing's —*see* Neoplasm, bone, malignant, by site
fatty —*see* Lipoma
fibroid —*see* Leiomyoma

Tumor *(Continued)*
G cell
malignant
pancreas C25.4
specified site NEC —*see* Neoplasm, malignant, by site
unspecified site C25.4
specified site —*see* Neoplasm, uncertain behavior, by site
unspecified site D37.8
germ cell —*see also* Neoplasm, malignant, by site
mixed —*see* Neoplasm, malignant, by site
ghost cell, odontogenic —*see* Cyst, calcifying odontogenic
giant cell —*see also* Neoplasm, uncertain behavior, by site
bone D48.0
malignant —*see* Neoplasm, bone, malignant
chondromatous —*see* Neoplasm, bone, benign
malignant —*see* Neoplasm, malignant, by site
soft parts —*see* Neoplasm, connective tissue, uncertain behavior
malignant —*see* Neoplasm, connective tissue, malignant
glomus D18.00
intra-abdominal D18.03
intracranial D18.02
jugulare D44.7
malignant C75.5
skin D18.01
specified site NEC D18.09
gonadal stromal —*see* Neoplasm, uncertain behavior, by site
granular cell —*see also* Neoplasm, connective tissue, benign
malignant —*see* Neoplasm, connective tissue, malignant
granulosa cell D39.1-
juvenile D39.1-
malignant C56-
granulosa cell-theca cell D39.1-
malignant C56-
Grawitz's C64-
hemorrhoidal —*see* Hemorrhoids
hilar cell D27-
hilus cell D27-
Hurthle cell (benign) D34
malignant C73
hydatid —*see* Echinococcus
hypernephroid —*see also* Neoplasm, uncertain behavior, by site
interstitial cell —*see also* Neoplasm, uncertain behavior, by site
benign —*see* Neoplasm, benign, by site
malignant —*see* Neoplasm, malignant, by site
intravascular bronchial alveolar D38.1
islet cell —*see* Neoplasm, benign, by site
malignant —*see* Neoplasm, malignant, by site
pancreas C25.4
specified site NEC —*see* Neoplasm, malignant, by site
unspecified site C25.4
pancreas D13.7
specified site NEC —*see* Neoplasm, benign, by site
unspecified site D13.7
juxtaglomerular D41.0-
Klatskin's C24.0
Krukenberg's C79.6-
Leydig cell —*see* Neoplasm, uncertain behavior, by site
benign —*see* Neoplasm, benign, by site
specified site —*see* Neoplasm, benign, by site

Tumor *(Continued)*
Leydig cell *(Continued)*
benign *(Continued)*
unspecified site
female D27.9
male D29.20
malignant —*see* Neoplasm, malignant, by site
specified site —*see* Neoplasm, malignant, by site
unspecified site
female C56.9
male C62.90
specified site —*see* Neoplasm, uncertain behavior, by site
unspecified site
female D39.10
male D40.10
lipid cell, ovary D27-
lipoid cell, ovary D27-
malignant —*see also* Neoplasm, malignant, by site C80.1
fusiform cell (type) C80.1
giant cell (type) C80.1
localized, plasma cell —*see* Plasmacytoma, solitary
mixed NEC C80.1
small cell (type) C80.1
spindle cell (type) C80.1
unclassified C80.1
mast cell D47.0
malignant C96.2
melanotic, neuroectodermal —*see* Neoplasm, benign, by site
Merkel cell —*see* Carcinoma, Merkel cell
mesenchymal
malignant —*see* Neoplasm, connective tissue, malignant
mixed —*see* Neoplasm, connective tissue, uncertain behavior
mesodermal, mixed —*see also* Neoplasm, malignant, by site
liver C22.4
mesonephric —*see also* Neoplasm, uncertain behavior, by site
malignant —*see* Neoplasm, malignant, by site
metastatic
from specified site —*see* Neoplasm, malignant, by site
of specified site —*see* Neoplasm, malignant, by site
to specified site —*see* Neoplasm, secondary, by site
mixed NEC —*see also* Neoplasm, benign, by site
malignant —*see* Neoplasm, malignant, by site
mucinous of low malignant potential
specified site —*see* Neoplasm, malignant, by site
unspecified site C56.9
mucocarcinoid
specified site —*see* Neoplasm, malignant, by site
unspecified site C18.1
mucoepidermoid —*see* Neoplasm, uncertain behavior, by site
Müllerian, mixed
specified site —*see* Neoplasm, malignant, by site
unspecified site C54.9
myoepithelial —*see* Neoplasm, benign, by site
neuroectodermal (peripheral) —*see* Neoplasm, malignant, by site
primitive
specified site —*see* Neoplasm, malignant, by site
unspecified site C71.9

Tumor *(Continued)*
neuroendocrine D3A.8
malignant poorly differentiated C7A.1
secondary NEC C7B.8
specified NEC C7A.8
neurogenic olfactory C30.0
nonencapsulated sclerosing C73
odontogenic (adenomatoid) (benign) (calcifying epithelial) (keratocystic) (squamous) —*see* Cyst, calcifying odontogenic
malignant C41.1
upper jaw (bone) C41.0
ovarian stromal D39.1-
ovary, in pregnancy —*see* Pregnancy, complicated by
pacinian —*see* Neoplasm, skin, benign
Pancoast's —*see* Pancoast's syndrome
papillary —*see also* Papilloma
cystic D37.9
mucinous of low malignant potential C56-
specified site —*see* Neoplasm, malignant, by site
unspecified site C56.9
serous of low malignant potential
specified site —*see* Neoplasm, malignant, by site
unspecified site C56.9
pelvic, in pregnancy or childbirth —*see* Pregnancy, complicated by
phantom F45.8
phyllodes D48.6-
benign D24-
malignant —*see* Neoplasm, breast, malignant
Pindborg —*see* Cyst, calcifying odontogenic
placental site trophoblastic D39.2
plasma cell (malignant) (localized) —*see* Plasmacytoma, solitary
polyvesicular vitelline
specified site —*see* Neoplasm, malignant, by site
unspecified site
female C56.9
male C62.90
Pott's puffy —*see* Osteomyelitis, specified NEC
Rathke's pouch D44.3
retinal anlage —*see* Neoplasm, benign, by site
salivary gland type, mixed —*see* Neoplasm, salivary gland, benign
malignant —*see* Neoplasm, salivary gland, malignant
Sampson's N80.1
Schmincke's —*see* Neoplasm, nasopharynx, malignant
sclerosing stromal D27-
sebaceous —*see* Cyst, sebaceous
secondary —*see* Neoplasm, secondary, by site
carcinoid C7B.00
bone C7B.03
distant lymph nodes C7B.01
liver C7B.02
peritoneum C7B.04
specified NEC C7B.09
neuroendocrine NEC C7B.8
serous of low malignant potential
specified site —*see* Neoplasm, malignant, by site
unspecified site C56.9
Sertoli cell —*see* Neoplasm, benign, by site
with lipid storage
specified site —*see* Neoplasm, benign, by site
unspecified site
female D27.9
male D29.20
specified site —*see* Neoplasm, benign, by site
unspecified site
female D27.9
male D29.20

Tumor *(Continued)*
Sertoli-Leydig cell —*see* Neoplasm, benign, by site
specified site —*see* Neoplasm, benign, by site
unspecified site
female D27.9
male D29.20
sex cord(-stromal) —*see* Neoplasm, uncertain behavior, by site
with annular tubules D39.1-
skin appendage —*see* Neoplasm, skin, benign
smooth muscle —*see* Neoplasm, connective tissue, uncertain behavior
soft tissue
benign —*see* Neoplasm, connective tissue, benign
malignant —*see* Neoplasm, connective tissue, malignant
sternomastoid (congenital) Q68.0
stromal
endometrial D39.0
gastric D48.1
benign D21.4
malignant C16.9
uncertain behavior D48.1
gastrointestinal C49.A- ⟸
benign D21.4
esophagus C49.A1 ◀
large intestine C49.A4 ◀
malignant C49.A0 ⟸
colon C49.A4 ◀
duodenum C49.A3 ◀
esophagus C49.A1 ◀
ileum C49.A3 ◀
jejunum C49.A3 ◀
Meckel diverticulum C49.A3 ◀
large intestine C49.A4 ◀
omentum C49.A9 ◀
peritoneum C49.A9 ◀
rectum C49.A5 ◀
small intestine C49.A3 ◀
specified site NEC C49.A9 ◀
stomach C49.A2 ◀
large intestine C49.A4 ◀
rectum C49.A5 ◀
small intestine C49.A3 ◀
specified site NEC C49.A9 ◀
stomach C49.A2 ◀
uncertain behavior D48.1
intestine
benign D21.4
malignant ⟸
large C49.A4 ◀
small C49.A3 ◀
uncertain behavior D48.1
ovarian D39.1-
stomach C49.A2 ⟸
benign D21.4
malignant C49.A2 ⟸
uncertain behavior D48.1
sweat gland —*see also* Neoplasm, skin, uncertain behavior
benign —*see* Neoplasm, skin, benign
malignant —*see* Neoplasm, skin, malignant
syphilitic, brain A52.17
testicular D40.10
testicular stromal D40.1-
theca cell D27.-
theca cell-granulosa cell D39.1-
Triton, malignant —*see* Neoplasm, nerve, malignant
trophoblastic, placental site D39.2
turban D23.4
uterus (body), in pregnancy or childbirth —*see* Pregnancy, complicated by, tumor, uterus
vagina, in pregnancy or childbirth —*see* Pregnancy, complicated by
varicose —*see* Varix

Tumor *(Continued)*
von Recklinghausen's —*see* Neurofibromatosis
vulva or perineum, in pregnancy or childbirth —*see* Pregnancy, complicated by
causing obstructed labor O65.5
Warthin's —*see* Neoplasm, salivary gland, benign
Wilms' C64-
yolk sac —*see* Neoplasm, malignant, by site
specified site —*see* Neoplasm, malignant, by site
unspecified site
female C56.9
male C62.90
Tumor lysis syndrome (following antineoplastic chemotherapy) (spontaneous) NEC E88.3
Tumorlet —*see* Neoplasm, uncertain behavior, by site
Tungiasis B88.1
Tunica vasculosa lentis Q12.2
Turban tumor D23.4
Türck's trachoma J37.0
Turner-Kieser syndrome Q87.2 ⟸
Turner-like syndrome Q87.1
Turner's
hypoplasia (tooth) K00.4
syndrome Q96.9
specified NEC Q96.8
tooth K00.4
Turner-Ullrich syndrome Q96.9
Tussis convulsiva —*see* Whooping cough
Twiddler's syndrome (due to)
automatic implantable defibrillator T82.198
cardiac pacemaker T82.198
Twilight state
epileptic F05
psychogenic F44.89
Twin (newborn) —*see also* Newborn, twin
conjoined Q89.4
pregnancy —*see* Pregnancy, twin, conjoined
Twinning, teeth K00.2
Twist, twisted
bowel, colon or intestine K56.2
hair (congenital) Q84.1
mesentery K56.2
omentum K56.2
organ or site, congenital NEC —*see* Anomaly, by site
ovarian pedicle —*see* Torsion, ovary
Twitching R25.3
Tylosis (acquired) L84
buccalis K13.29
linguae K13.29
palmaris et plantaris (congenital) (inherited) Q82.8
acquired L85.1
Tympanism R14.0
Tympanites (abdominal) (intestinal) R14.0
Tympanitis —*see* Myringitis
Tympanosclerosis —*see* subcategory H74.0
Tympanum —*see* condition
Tympany
abdomen R14.0
chest R09.89
Type A behavior pattern Z73.1
Typhlitis —*see* Appendicitis
Typhoenteritis —*see* Typhoid
Typhoid (abortive) (ambulant) (any site) (clinical) (fever) (hemorrhagic) (infection) (intermittent) (malignant) (rheumatic) (Widal negative) A01.00
with pneumonia A01.03
abdominal A01.09
arthritis A01.04
carrier (suspected) of Z22.0
cholecystitis (current) A01.09
endocarditis A01.02
heart involvement A01.02

◀ New ⟸ Revised ~~deleted~~ Deleted

Typhoid *(Continued)*
inoculation reaction —*see* Complications, vaccination
meningitis A01.01
mesenteric lymph nodes A01.09
myocarditis A01.02
osteomyelitis A01.05
perichondritis, larynx A01.09
pneumonia A01.03
specified NEC A01.09
spine A01.05
ulcer (perforating) A01.09
Typhomalaria (fever) —*see* Malaria
Typhomania A01.00
Typhoperitonitis A01.09
Typhus (fever) A75.9
abdominal, abdominalis —*see* Typhoid
African tick A77.1
amarillic A95.9
brain A75.9 *[G94]*

Typhus *(Continued)*
cerebral A75.9 *[G94]*
classical A75.0
due to Rickettsia
prowazekii A75.0
recrudescent A75.1
tsutsugamushi A75.3
typhi A75.2
endemic (flea-borne) A75.2
epidemic (louse-borne) A75.0
exanthematic NEC A75.0
exanthematicus SAI A75.0
brillii SAI A75.1
mexicanus SAI A75.2
typhus murinus A75.2
flea-borne A75.2
India tick A77.1
Kenya (tick) A77.1
louse-borne A75.0
Mexican A75.2

Typhus *(Continued)*
mite-borne A75.3
murine A75.2
North Asian tick-borne A77.2
petechial A75.9
Queensland tick A77.3
rat A75.2
recrudescent A75.1
recurrens —*see* Fever, relapsing
Sao Paulo A77.0
scrub (China) (India) (Malaysia) (New Guinea) A75.3
shop (of Malaysia) A75.2
Siberian tick A77.2
tick-borne A77.9
tropical (mite-borne) A75.3
Tyrosinemia E70.21
newborn, transitory P74.5
Tyrosinosis E70.21
Tyrosinuria E70.29

T

U

Uhl's anomaly or disease Q24.8
Ulcer, ulcerated, ulcerating, ulceration, ulcerative
alveolar process M27.3
amebic (intestine) A06.1
skin A06.7
anastomotic —*see* Ulcer, gastrojejunal
anorectal K62.6
antral —*see* Ulcer, stomach
anus (sphincter) (solitary) K62.6
aorta —*see* Aneurysm
aphthous (oral) (recurrent) K12.0
genital organ (s)
female N76.6
male N50.89 ◄
artery I77.2
atrophic —*see* Ulcer, skin
decubitus —*see* Ulcer, pressure, by site
back L98.429
with
bone necrosis L98.424
exposed fat layer L98.422
muscle necrosis L98.423
skin breakdown only L98.421
Barrett's (esophagus) K22.10
with bleeding K22.11
bile duct (common) (hepatic) K83.8
bladder (solitary) (sphincter) NEC N32.89
bilharzial B65.9 *[N33]*
in schistosomiasis (bilharzial) B65.9 *[N33]*
submucosal —*see* Cystitis, interstitial
tuberculous A18.12
bleeding K27.4
bone —*see* Osteomyelitis, specified type NEC
bowel —*see* Ulcer, intestine
breast N61.1 ◄
bronchus J98.09
buccal (cavity) (traumatic) K12.1
Buruli A31.1
buttock L98.419
with
bone necrosis L98.414
exposed fat layer L98.412
muscle necrosis L98.413
skin breakdown only L98.411
cancerous —*see* Neoplasm, malignant, by site
cardia K22.10
with bleeding K22.11
cardioesophageal (peptic) K22.10
with bleeding K22.11
cecum —*see* Ulcer, intestine
cervix (uteri) (decubitus) (trophic) N86
with cervicitis N72
chancroidal A57
chiclero B55.1
chronic (cause unknown) —*see* Ulcer, skin
Cochin-China B55.1
colon —*see* Ulcer, intestine
conjunctiva H10.89
cornea H16.00-
with hypopyon H16.03-
central H16.01-
dendritic (herpes simplex) B00.52
marginal H16.04-
Mooren's H16.05-
mycotic H16.06-
perforated H16.07-
ring H16.02-
tuberculous (phlyctenular) A18.52
corpus cavernosum (chronic) N48.5
crural —*see* Ulcer, lower limb
Curling's —*see* Ulcer, peptic, acute
Cushing's —*see* Ulcer, peptic, acute
cystic duct K82.8
cystitis (interstitial) —*see* Cystitis, interstitial
decubitus —*see* Ulcer, pressure, by site
dendritic, cornea (herpes simplex) B00.52
diabetes, diabetic —*see* Diabetes, ulcer
Dieulafoy's K25.0

Ulcer, ulcerated, ulcerating, ulceration, ulcerative *(Continued)*
due to
infection NEC —*see* Ulcer, skin
radiation NEC L59.8
trophic disturbance (any region) —*see* Ulcer, skin
X-ray L58.1
duodenum, duodenal (eroded) (peptic) K26.9
with
hemorrhage K26.4
and perforation K26.6
perforation K26.5
acute K26.3
with
hemorrhage K26.0
and perforation K26.2
perforation K26.1
chronic K26.7
with
hemorrhage K26.4
and perforation K26.6
perforation K26.5
dysenteric A09
elusive —*see* Cystitis, interstitial
endocarditis (acute) (chronic) (subacute) I28.8
epiglottis J38.7
esophagus (peptic) K22.10
with bleeding K22.11
due to
aspirin K22.10
with bleeding K22.11
gastrointestinal reflux disease K21.0
ingestion of chemical or medicament K22.10
with bleeding K22.11
fungal K22.10
with bleeding K22.11
infective K22.10
with bleeding K22.11
varicose —*see* Varix, esophagus
eyelid (region) H01.8
fauces J39.2
Fenwick (-Hunner) (solitary) —*see* Cystitis, interstitial
fistulous —*see* Ulcer, skin
foot (indolent) (trophic) —*see* Ulcer, lower limb
frambesial, initial A66.0
frenum (tongue) K14.0
gallbladder or duct K82.8
gangrenous —*see* Gangrene
gastric —*see* Ulcer, stomach
gastrocolic —*see* Ulcer, gastrojejunal
gastroduodenal —*see* Ulcer, peptic
gastroesophageal —*see* Ulcer, stomach
gastrointestinal —*see* Ulcer, gastrojejunal
gastrojejunal (peptic) K28.9
with
hemorrhage K28.4
and perforation K28.6
perforation K28.5
acute K28.3
with
hemorrhage K28.0
and perforation K28.2
perforation K28.1
chronic K28.7
with
hemorrhage K28.4
and perforation K28.6
perforation K28.5
gastrojejunocolic —*see* Ulcer, gastrojejunal
gingiva K06.8
gingivitis K05.10
nonplaque induced K05.11
plaque induced K05.10
glottis J38.7
granuloma of pudenda A58
gum K06.8
gumma, due to yaws A66.4

Ulcer, ulcerated, ulcerating, ulceration, ulcerative *(Continued)*
heel —*see* Ulcer, lower limb
hemorrhoid —*see also* Hemorrhoids, by degree K64.8
Hunner's —*see* Cystitis, interstitial
hypopharynx J39.2
hypopyon (chronic) (subacute) —*see* Ulcer, cornea, with hypopyon
hypostaticum —*see* Ulcer, varicose
ileum —*see* Ulcer, intestine
intestine, intestinal K63.3
with perforation K63.1
amebic A06.1
duodenal —*see* Ulcer, duodenum
granulocytopenic (with hemorrhage) —*see* Neutropenia
marginal —*see* Ulcer, gastrojejunal
perforating K63.1
newborn P78.0
primary, small intestine K63.3
rectum K62.6
stercoraceous, stercoral K63.3
tuberculous A18.32
typhoid (fever) —*see* Typhoid
varicose I86.8
jejunum, jejunal —*see* Ulcer, gastrojejunal
keratitis —*see* Ulcer, cornea
knee —*see* Ulcer, lower limb
labium (majus) (minus) N76.6
laryngitis —*see* Laryngitis
larynx (aphthous) (contact) J38.7
diphtheritic A36.2
leg —*see* Ulcer, lower limb
lip K13.0
Lipschütz's N76.6
lower limb (atrophic) (chronic) (neurogenic) (perforating) (pyogenic) (trophic) (tropical) L97.909
with
bone necrosis L97.904
exposed fat layer L97.902
muscle necrosis L97.903
skin breakdown only L97.901
ankle L97.309
with
bone necrosis L97.304
exposed fat layer L97.302
muscle necrosis L97.303
skin breakdown only L97.301
left L97.329
with
bone necrosis L97.324
exposed fat layer L97.322
muscle necrosis L97.323
skin breakdown only L97.321
right L97.319
with
bone necrosis L97.314
exposed fat layer L97.312
muscle necrosis L97.313
skin breakdown only L97.311
calf L97.209
with
bone necrosis L97.204
exposed fat layer L97.202
muscle necrosis L97.203
skin breakdown only L97.201
left L97.229
with
bone necrosis L97.224
exposed fat layer L97.222
muscle necrosis L97.223
skin breakdown only L97.221
right L97.219
with
bone necrosis L97.214
exposed fat layer L97.212
muscle necrosis L97.213
skin breakdown only L97.211
decubitus —*see* Ulcer, pressure, by site

◄ New ◄ Revised ~~deleted~~ Deleted

ed, ulcerating, ulceration,
re *(Continued)*
(Continued)
fied NEC L97.509

necrosis L97.504
sed fat layer L97.502
cle necrosis L97.503
breakdown only L97.501
.529

ne necrosis L97.524
posed fat layer L97.522
uscle necrosis L97.523
n breakdown only L97.521
97.519

ne necrosis L97.514
posed fat layer L97.512
uscle necrosis L97.513
n breakdown only L97.511
09

necrosis L97.404
sed fat layer L97.402
le necrosis L97.403
breakdown only L97.401
429

ne necrosis L97.424
osed fat layer L97.422
scle necrosis L97.423
n breakdown only L97.421
7.419

e necrosis L97.414
osed fat layer L97.412
scle necrosis L97.413
n breakdown only L97.411

necrosis L97.924
ed fat layer L97.922
e necrosis L97.923
reakdown only L97.921
IOS L97.909

ecrosis L97.904
d fat layer L97.902
necrosis L97.903
eakdown only L97.901
29

necrosis L97.924
sed fat layer L97.922
cle necrosis L97.923
breakdown only L97.921
919

necrosis L97.914
sed fat layer L97.912
le necrosis L97.913
breakdown only L97.911
site NEC L97.809

necrosis L97.804
sed fat layer L97.802
le necrosis L97.803
breakdown only L97.801
.829

ne necrosis L97.824
osed fat layer L97.822
uscle necrosis L97.823
n breakdown only L97.821
7.819

ne necrosis L97.814
osed fat layer L97.812
scle necrosis L97.813
n breakdown only L97.811

Ulcer, ulcerated, ulcerating, ulceration, ulcerative *(Continued)*
lower limb *(Continued)*
midfoot L97.409
with
bone necrosis L97.404
exposed fat layer L97.402
muscle necrosis L97.403
skin breakdown only L97.401
left L97.429
with
bone necrosis L97.424
exposed fat layer L97.422
muscle necrosis L97.423
skin breakdown only L97.421
right L97.419
with
bone necrosis L97.414
exposed fat layer L97.412
muscle necrosis L97.413
skin breakdown only L97.411
right L97.919
with
bone necrosis L97.914
exposed fat layer L97.912
muscle necrosis L97.913
skin breakdown only L97.911
thigh L97.109
with
bone necrosis L97.104
exposed fat layer L97.102
muscle necrosis L97.103
skin breakdown only L97.101
left L97.129
with
bone necrosis L97.124
exposed fat layer L97.122
muscle necrosis L97.123
skin breakdown only L97.121
right L97.119
with
bone necrosis L97.114
exposed fat layer L97.112
muscle necrosis L97.113
skin breakdown only L97.111
toe L97.509
with
bone necrosis L97.504
exposed fat layer L97.502
muscle necrosis L97.503
skin breakdown only L97.501
left L97.529
with
bone necrosis L97.524
exposed fat layer L97.522
muscle necrosis L97.523
skin breakdown only L97.521
right L97.519
with
bone necrosis L97.514
exposed fat layer L97.512
muscle necrosis L97.513
skin breakdown only L97.511
leprous A30.1
syphilitic A52.19
varicose —*see* Varix, leg, with, ulcer
luetic —*see* Ulcer, syphilitic
lung J98.4
tuberculous —*see* Tuberculosis, pulmonary
malignant —*see* Neoplasm, malignant, by site
marginal NEC —*see* Ulcer, gastrojejunal
meatus (urinarius) N34.2
Meckel's diverticulum Q43.0
malignant —*see* Table of Neoplasms, small intestine, malignant
Meleney's (chronic undermining) —*see* Ulcer, skin
Mooren's (cornea) —*see* Ulcer, cornea, Mooren's
mycobacterial (skin) A31.1
nasopharynx J39.2

Ulcer, ulcerated, ulcerating, ulceration, ulcerative *(Continued)*
neck, uterus N86
neurogenic NEC —*see* Ulcer, skin
nose, nasal (passage) (infective) (septum) J34.0
skin —*see* Ulcer, skin
spirochetal A69.8
varicose (bleeding) I86.8
oral mucosa (traumatic) K12.1
palate (soft) K12.1
penis (chronic) N48.5
peptic (site unspecified) K27.9
with
hemorrhage K27.4
and perforation K27.6
perforation K27.5
acute K27.3
with
hemorrhage K27.0
and perforation K27.2
perforation K27.1
chronic K27.7
with
hemorrhage K27.4
and perforation K27.6
perforation K27.5
esophagus K22.10
with bleeding K22.11
newborn P78.82
perforating K27.5
skin —*see* Ulcer, skin
peritonsillar J35.8
phagedenic (tropical) —*see* Ulcer, skin
pharynx J39.2
phlebitis —*see* Phlebitis
plaster —*see* Ulcer, pressure, by site
popliteal space —*see* Ulcer, lower limb
postpyloric —*see* Ulcer, duodenum
prepuce N47.7
prepyloric —*see* Ulcer, stomach
pressure (pressure area) L89.9-
ankle L89.5-
back L89.1-
buttock L89.3-
coccyx L89.15-
contiguous site of back, buttock, hip L89.4-
elbow L89.0-
face L89.81-
head L89.81-
heel L89.6-
hip L89.2-
sacral region (tailbone) L89.15-
specified site NEC L89.89-
stage 1 (healing) (pre-ulcer skin changes limited to persistent focal edema)
ankle L89.5-
back L89.1-
buttock L89.3-
coccyx L89.15-
contiguous site of back, buttock, hip L89.4-
elbow L89.0-
face L89.81-
head L89.81-
heel L89.6-
hip L89.2-
sacral region (tailbone) L89.15-
specified site NEC L89.89-
stage 2 (healing) (abrasion, blister, partial thickness skin loss involving epidermis and/or dermis)
ankle L89.5-
back L89.1-
buttock L89.3-
coccyx L89.15-
contiguous site of back, buttock, hip L89.4-
elbow L89.0-
face L89.81-
head L89.81-

U

Ulcer, ulcerated, ulcerating, ulceration, ulcerative *(Continued)*
pressure *(Continued)*
stage 2 *(Continued)*
heel L89.6-
hip L89.2-
sacral region (tailbone) L89.15-
specified site NEC L89.89-
stage 3 (healing) (full thickness skin loss involving damage or necrosis of subcutaneous tissue)
ankle L89.5-
back L89.1-
buttock L89.3-
coccyx L89.15-
contiguous site of back, buttock, hip L89.4-
elbow L89.0-
face L89.81-
head L89.81-
heel L89.6-
hip L89.2-
sacral region (tailbone) L89.15-
specified site NEC L89.89-
stage 4 (healing) (necrosis of soft tissues through to underlying muscle, tendon, or bone)
ankle L89.5-
back L89.1-
buttock L89.3-
coccyx L89.15-
contiguous site of back, buttock, hip L89.4-
elbow L89.0-
face L89.81-
head L89.81-
heel L89.6-
hip L89.2-
sacral region (tailbone) L89.15-
specified site NEC L89.89-
unspecified stage
ankle L89.5-
back L89.1-
buttock L89.3-
coccyx L89.15-
contiguous site of back, buttock, hip L89.4-
elbow L89.0-
face L89.81-
head L89.81-
heel L89.6-
hip L89.2-
sacral region (tailbone) L89.15-
specified site NEC L89.89-
unstageable
ankle L89.5-
back L89.1-
buttock L89.3-
coccyx L89.15-
contiguous site of back, buttock, hip L89.4-
elbow L89.0-
face L89.81-
head L89.81-
heel L89.6-
hip L89.2-
sacral region (tailbone) L89.15-
specified site NEC L89.89-
primary of intestine K63.3
with perforation K63.1
prostate N41.9
pyloric —*see* Ulcer, stomach
rectosigmoid K63.3
with perforation K63.1
rectum (sphincter) (solitary) K62.6
stercoraceous, stercoral K62.6
retina —*see* Inflammation, chorioretinal
rodent —*see also* Neoplasm, skin, malignant
sclera —*see* Scleritis
scrofulous (tuberculous) A18.2

Ulcer, ulcerated, ulcerating, ulceration, ulcerative *(Continued)*
scrotum N50.89 ◀
tuberculous A18.15
varicose I86.1
seminal vesicle N50.89 ◀
sigmoid —*see* Ulcer, intestine
skin (atrophic) (chronic) (neurogenic) (non-healing) (perforating) (pyogenic) (trophic) (tropical) L98.499
with gangrene —*see* Gangrene
amebic A06.7
back —*see* Ulcer, back
buttock —*see* Ulcer, buttock
decubitus —*see* Ulcer, pressure
lower limb —*see* Ulcer, lower limb
mycobacterial A31.1
specified site NEC L98.499
with
bone necrosis L98.494
exposed fat layer L98.492
muscle necrosis L98.493
skin breakdown only L98.491
tuberculous (primary) A18.4
varicose —*see* Ulcer, varicose
sloughing —*see* Ulcer, skin
solitary, anus or rectum (sphincter) K62.6
sore throat J02.9
streptococcal J02.0
spermatic cord N50.89 ◀
spine (tuberculous) A18.01
stasis (venous) —*see* Varix, leg, with, ulcer
without varicose veins I87.2
stercoraceous, stercoral K63.3
with perforation K63.1
anus or rectum K62.6
stoma, stomal —*see* Ulcer, gastrojejunal
stomach (eroded) (peptic) (round) K25.9
with
hemorrhage K25.4
and perforation K25.6
perforation K25.5
acute K25.3
with
hemorrhage K25.0
and perforation K25.2
perforation K25.1
chronic K25.7
with
hemorrhage K25.4
and perforation K25.6
perforation K25.5
stomal —*see* Ulcer, gastrojejunal
stomatitis K12.1
stress —*see* Ulcer, peptic
strumous (tuberculous) A18.2
submucosal, bladder —*see* Cystitis, interstitial
syphilitic (any site) (early) (secondary) A51.39
late A52.79
perforating A52.79
foot A52.11
testis N50.89 ◀
thigh —*see* Ulcer, lower limb
throat J39.2
diphtheritic A36.0
toe —*see* Ulcer, lower limb
tongue (traumatic) K14.0
tonsil J35.8
diphtheritic A36.0
trachea J39.8
trophic —*see* Ulcer, skin
tropical —*see* Ulcer, skin
tuberculous —*see* Tuberculosis, ulcer
tunica vaginalis N50.89 ◀
turbinate J34.89
typhoid (perforating) —*see* Typhoid

Ulcer, ulcerated, ulcerati
ulcerative *(Continu*
unspecified site —*see* U
urethra (meatus) —*see*
uterus N85.8
cervix N86
with cervicitis N7
neck N86
with cervicitis N7
vagina N76.5
in Behçet's disease I
pessary N89.8
valve, heart I33.0
varicose (lower limb, Varix, leg, with,
broad ligament I86.
esophagus —*see* Va
inflamed or infecte with ulcer, with inf
nasal septum I86.8
perineum I86.3
scrotum I86.1
specified site NEC
sublingual I86.0
vulva I86.3
vas deferens N50.89 ◀
vulva (acute) (infecti
in (due to)
Behçet's disease
herpesviral (her ion A60.04
tuberculosis A18
vulvobuccal, recurrin
X-ray L58.1
yaws A66.4
Ulcerosa scarlatina A38
Ulcus —*see also* Ulcer
cutis tuberculosum A
duodeni —*see* Ulcer,
durum (syphilitic) A
extragenital A51.2
gastrojejunale —*see* U
hypostaticum —*see* U
molle (cutis) (skin) A
serpens corneae —*se* tral
ventriculi —*see* Ulce
Ulegyria Q04.8
Ulerythema
ophryogenes, conge
sycosiforme L73.8
Ullrich(-Bonnevie)(-Tu —*see also* Turner's syn
Ullrich-Feichtiger syn
Ulnar —*see* condition
Ulorrhagia, ulorrhea F
Umbilicus, umbilical
Unacceptable
contours of tooth K
morphology of toot
Unavailability (of)
bed at medical facili
health service-relate
medical facilities (a
due to
investigation b ency Z75.2
lack of service
remoteness fro
waiting list Z7
home Z75.0
outpatient clinic
schooling Z55.1
social service agen
Uncinaria americana
Uncinariasis B76.9
Uncongenial work Z
Unconscious (ness) –
Underachievement i
Underdevelopment ped
nose Q30.1
sexual E30.0

◀ New ◀ Revised ~~deleted~~ Deleted

Underdosing —*see also* Table of Drugs and Chemicals, categories T36-T50, with final character 6 Z91.14
intentional NEC Z91.128
due to financial hardship of patient Z91.120
unintentional NEC Z91.138
due to patient's age related debility Z91.130
Underfeeding, newborn P92.3
Underfill, endodontic M27.53
Underimmunization status Z28.3
Undernourishment —*see* Malnutrition
Undernutrition —*see* Malnutrition
Under observation —*see* Observation
Underweight R63.6
for gestational age —*see* Light for dates
Underwood's disease P83.0
Undescended —*see also* Malposition, congenital
cecum Q43.3
colon Q43.3
testicle —*see* Cryptorchid
Undeveloped, undevelopment —*see also* Hypoplasia
brain (congenital) Q02
cerebral (congenital) Q02
heart Q24.8
lung Q33.6
testis E29.1
uterus E30.0
Undiagnosed (disease) R69
Undulant fever —*see* Brucellosis
Unemployment, anxiety concerning Z56.0
threatened Z56.2
Unequal length (acquired) (limb) —*see also* Deformity, limb, unequal length
leg —*see also* Deformity, limb, unequal length
congenital Q72.9-
Unextracted dental root K08.3
Unguis incarnatus L60.0
Unhappiness R45.2
Unicornate uterus Q51.4
Unilateral —*see also* condition
development, breast N64.89
organ or site, congenital NEC —*see* Agenesis, by site
Unilocular heart Q20.8
Union, abnormal —*see also* Fusion
larynx and trachea Q34.8
Universal mesentery Q43.3
Unrepairable overhanging of dental restorative materials K08.52
Unsatisfactory
restoration of tooth K08.50
specified NEC K08.59
sample of cytologic smear
anus R85.615
cervix R87.615
vagina R87.625
surroundings Z59.1
work Z56.5
Unsoundness of mind —*see* Psychosis
Unstable
back NEC —*see* Instability, joint, spine
hip (congenital) Q65.6
acquired —*see* Derangement, joint, specified type NEC, hip
joint —*see* Instability, joint
secondary to removal of joint prosthesis M96.89
lie (mother) O32.0
lumbosacral joint (congenital)
acquired —*see* subcategory M53.2
sacroiliac —*see* subcategory M53.2
spine NEC —*see* Instability, joint, spine
Unsteadiness on feet R26.81
Untruthfulness, child problem F91.8
Unverricht(-Lundborg) **disease or epilepsy** —*see* Epilepsy, generalized, idiopathic
Unwanted pregnancy Z64.0
Upbringing, institutional Z62.22
away from parents NEC Z62.29
in care of non-parental family member Z62.21
in foster care Z62.21
in orphanage or group home Z62.22
in welfare custody Z62.21
Upper respiratory —*see* condition
Upset
gastric K30
gastrointestinal K30
psychogenic F45.8
intestinal (large) (small) K59.9
psychogenic F45.8
menstruation N93.9
mental F48.9
stomach K30
psychogenic F45.8
Urachus —*see also* condition
patent or persistent Q64.4
Urbach-Oppenheim disease (necrobiosis lipoidica diabeticorum) —*see* E08-E13 with .620
Urbach's lipoid proteinosis E78.89
Urbach-Wiethe disease E78.89
Urban yellow fever A95.1
Urea
blood, high —*see* Uremia
cycle metabolism disorder —*see* Disorder, urea cycle metabolism
Uremia, uremic N19
with
ectopic or molar pregnancy O08.4
polyneuropathy N18.9 *[G63]*
chronic —*see also* Disease, kidney, chronic N18.9
due to hypertension —*see* Hypertensive, kidney
complicating
ectopic or molar pregnancy O08.4
congenital P96.0
extrarenal R39.2
following ectopic or molar pregnancy O08.4
newborn P96.0
prerenal R39.2
Ureter, ureteral —*see* condition
Ureteralgia N23
Ureterectasis —*see* Hydroureter
Ureteritis N28.89
cystica N28.86
due to calculus N20.1
with calculus, kidney N20.2
with hydronephrosis N13.2
gonococcal (acute) (chronic) A54.21
nonspecific N28.89
Ureterocele N28.89
congenital (orthotopic) Q62.31
ectopic Q62.32
Ureterolith, ureterolithiasis —*see* Calculus, ureter
Ureterostomy
attention to Z43.6
status Z93.6
Urethra, urethral —*see* condition
Urethralgia R39.89
Urethritis (anterior) (posterior) N34.2
calculous N21.1
candidal B37.41
chlamydial A56.01
diplococcal (gonococcal) A54.01
with abscess (accessory gland) (periurethral) A54.1
gonococcal A54.01
with abscess (accessory gland) (periurethral) A54.1
nongonococcal N34.1
Reiter's —*see* Reiter's disease
nonspecific N34.1
nonvenereal N34.1
postmenopausal N34.2
puerperal O86.22
Reiter's —*see* Reiter's disease
Urethritis *(Continued)*
specified NEC N34.2
trichomonal or due to Trichomonas (vaginalis) A59.03
Urethrocele N81.0
with
cystocele —*see* Cystocele
prolapse of uterus —*see* Prolapse, uterus
Urethrolithiasis (with colic or infection) N21.1
Urethrorectal —*see* condition
Urethrorrhagia N36.8
Urethrorrhea R36.9
Urethrostomy
attention to Z43.6
status Z93.6
Urethrotrigonitis —*see* Trigonitis
Urethrovaginal —*see* condition
Urgency
fecal R15.2
hypertensive —*see* Hypertension
urinary N39.15 ◄
Urhidrosis, uridrosis L74.8
Uric acid in blood (increased) E79.0
Uricacidemia (asymptomatic) E79.0
Uricemia (asymptomatic) E79.0
Uricosuria R82.99
Urinary —*see* condition
Urination
frequent R35.0
painful R30.9
Urine
blood in —*see* Hematuria
discharge, excessive R35.8
enuresis, nonorganic origin F98.0
extravasation R39.0
frequency R35.0
incontinence R32
nonorganic origin F98.0
intermittent stream R39.198 ◄
pus in N39.0
retention or stasis R33.9
organic R33.8
drug-induced R33.0
psychogenic F45.8
secretion
deficient R34
excessive R35.8
frequency R35.0
stream
intermittent R39.198 ◄
slowing R39.198 ◄
splitting R39.13
weak R39.12
Urinemia —*see* Uremia
Urinoma, urethra N36.8
Uroarthritis, infectious (Reiter's) —*see* Reiter's disease
Urodialysis R34
Urolithiasis —*see* Calculus, urinary
Uronephrosis —*see* Hydronephrosis
Uropathy N39.9
obstructive N13.9
specified NEC N13.8
reflux N13.9
specified NEC N13.8
vesicoureteral reflux-associated —*see* Reflux, vesicoureteral
Urosepsis — code to condition
Urticaria L50.9
with angioneurotic edema T78.3
hereditary D84.1
allergic L50.0
cholinergic L50.5
chronic L50.8
cold, familial L50.2
contact L50.6
dermatographic L50.3
due to
cold or heat L50.2
drugs L50.0
food L50.0

◄ New ◄ Revised ~~deleted~~ Deleted

Urticaria *(Continued)*
due to *(Continued)*
inhalants L50.0
plants L50.6
serum —*see also* Reaction, serum T80.69
factitial L50.3
familial cold M04.2 ◀
giant T78.3
hereditary D84.1
gigantea T78.3
idiopathic L50.1
larynx T78.3
hereditary D84.1
neonatorum P83.8
nonallergic L50.1
papulosa (Hebra) L28.2
pigmentosa Q82.2
recurrent periodic L50.8
serum —*see also* Reaction, serum T80.69
solar L56.3
specified type NEC L50.8
thermal (cold) (heat) L50.2
vibratory L50.4
xanthelasmoidea Q82.2
Use (of)
alcohol Z72.89 ⟸
~~with sleep disorder F10.982~~
with ◀
intoxication F10.929 ◀
sleep disorder F10.982 ◀
harmful —*see* Abuse, alcohol
amphetamines —*see* Use, stimulant NEC
caffeine —*see* Use, stimulant NEC
cannabis F12.90
with
anxiety disorder F12.980
intoxication F12.929
with
delirium F12.921
perceptual disturbance F12.922
uncomplicated F12.920
other specified disorder F12.988
psychosis F12.959
delusions F12.950
hallucinations F12.951
unspecified disorder F12.99
cocaine F14.90
with
anxiety disorder F14.980
intoxication F14.929
with
delirium F14.921
perceptual disturbance F14.922
uncomplicated F14.920
other specified disorder F14.988
psychosis F14.959
delusions F14.950
hallucinations F14.951
sexual dysfunction F14.981
sleep disorder F14.982
unspecified disorder F14.99
harmful —*see* Abuse, drug, cocaine
drug (s) NEC F19.90
with sleep disorder F19.982
harmful —*see* Abuse, drug, by type
hallucinogen NEC F16.90
with
anxiety disorder F16.980
intoxication F16.929
with
delirium F16.921
uncomplicated F16.920
mood disorder F16.94
other specified disorder F16.988
Use *(Continued)*
hallucinogen NEC *(Continued)*
with *(Continued)*
perception disorder (flashbacks) F16.983
psychosis F16.959
delusions F16.950
hallucinations F16.951
unspecified disorder F16.99
harmful —*see* Abuse, drug, hallucinogen NEC
inhalants F18.90
with
anxiety disorder F18.980
intoxication F18.929
with delirium F18.921
uncomplicated F18.920
mood disorder F18.94
other specified disorder F18.988
persisting dementia F18.97
psychosis F18.959
delusions F18.950
hallucinations F18.951
unspecified disorder F18.99
harmful —*see* Abuse, drug, inhalant
methadone —*see* Use, opioid ⟸
nonprescribed drugs F19.90
harmful —*see* Abuse, non-psychoactive substance
opioid F11.90
with
disorder F11.99
mood F11.94
sleep F11.982
specified type NEC F11.988
intoxication F11.929
with
delirium F11.921
perceptual disturbance F11.922
uncomplicated F11.920
withdrawal F11.93
harmful —*see* Abuse, drug, opioid
patent medicines F19.90
harmful —*see* Abuse, non-psychoactive substance
psychoactive drug NEC F19.90
with
anxiety disorder F19.980
intoxication F19.929
with
delirium F19.921
perceptual disturbance F19.922
uncomplicated F19.920
mood disorder F19.94
other specified disorder F19.988
persisting
amnestic disorder F19.96
dementia F19.97
psychosis F19.959
delusions F19.950
hallucinations F19.951
sexual dysfunction F19.981
sleep disorder F19.982
unspecified disorder F19.99
withdrawal F19.939
with
delirium F19.931
perceptual disturbance F19.932
uncomplicated F19.930
harmful —*see* Abuse, drug NEC, psychoactive NEC
Use *(Continued)*
sedative, hypnotic, or anxiolytic F13.90
with
anxiety disorder F13.980
intoxication F13.929
with
delirium F13.921
uncomplicated F13.920
other specified disorder F13.988
persisting
amnestic disorder F13.96
dementia F13.97
psychosis F13.959
delusions F13.950
hallucinations F13.951
sexual dysfunction F13.981
sleep disorder F13.982
unspecified disorder F13.99
harmful —*see* Abuse, drug, sedative, hypnotic, or anxiolytic
stimulant NEC F15.90
with
anxiety disorder F15.980
intoxication F15.929
with
delirium F15.921
perceptual disturbance F15.922
uncomplicated F15.920
mood disorder F15.94
other specified disorder F15.988
psychosis F15.959
delusions F15.950
hallucinations F15.951
sexual dysfunction F15.981
sleep disorder F15.982
unspecified disorder F15.99
withdrawal F15.93
harmful —*see* Abuse, drug, stimulant NEC
tobacco Z72.0
with dependence —*see* Dependence, drug, nicotine
volatile solvents —*see also* Use, inhalant F18.90
harmful —*see* Abuse, drug, inhalant
Usher-Senear disease or syndrome L10.4
Uta B55.1
Uteromegaly N85.2
Uterovaginal —*see* condition
Uterovesical —*see* condition
Uveal —*see* condition
Uveitis (anterior) —*see also* Iridocyclitis
acute —*see* Iridocyclitis, acute
chronic —*see* Iridocyclitis, chronic
due to toxoplasmosis (acquired) B58.09
congenital P37.1
granulomatous —*see* Iridocyclitis, chronic
heterochromic —*see* Cyclitis, Fuchs' heterochromic
lens-induced —*see* Iridocyclitis, lens-induced
posterior —*see* Chorioretinitis
sympathetic H44.13-
syphilitic (secondary) A51.43
congenital (early) A50.01
late A52.71
tuberculous A18.54
Uveoencephalitis —*see* Inflammation, chorioretinal
Uveokeratitis —*see* Iridocyclitis
Uveoparotitis D86.89
Uvula —*see* condition
Uvulitis (acute) (catarrhal) (chronic) (membranous) (suppurative) (ulcerative) K12.2

◀ New ⟸ Revised ~~deleted~~ Deleted

V

Vaccination (prophylactic)
complication or reaction —*see* Complications, vaccination
delayed Z28.9
encounter for Z23
not done —*see* Immunization, not done, because (of)
Vaccinia (generalized) (localized) T88.1
without vaccination B08.011
congenital P35.8
Vacuum, in sinus (accessory) (nasal) J34.89
Vagabond, vagabondage Z59.0
Vagabond's disease B85.1
Vagina, vaginal —*see* condition
Vaginalitis (tunica) (testis) N49.1
Vaginismus (reflex) N94.2
functional F52.5
nonorganic F52.5
psychogenic F52.5
secondary N94.2
Vaginitis (acute) (circumscribed) (diffuse) (emphysematous) (nonvenereal) (ulcerative) N76.0
with ectopic or molar pregnancy O08.0
amebic A06.82
atrophic, postmenopausal N95.2
bacterial N76.0
blennorrhagic (gonococcal) A54.02
candidal B37.3
chlamydial A56.02
chronic N76.1
due to Trichomonas (vaginalis) A59.01
following ectopic or molar pregnancy O08.0
gonococcal A54.02
with abscess (accessory gland) (periurethral) A54.1
granuloma A58
in (due to)
candidiasis B37.3
herpesviral (herpes simplex) infection A60.04
pinworm infection B80 *[N77.1]*
monilial B37.3
mycotic (candidal) B37.3
postmenopausal atrophic N95.2
puerperal (postpartum) O86.13
senile (atrophic) N95.2
subacute or chronic N76.1
syphilitic (early) A51.0
late A52.76
trichomonal A59.01
tuberculous A18.18
Vaginosis —*see* Vaginitis
Vagotonia G52.2
Vagrancy Z59.0
VAIN —*see* Neoplasia, intraepithelial, vagina
Vallecula —*see* condition
Valley fever B38.0
Valsuani's disease —*see* Anemia, obstetric
Valve, valvular (formation) —*see also* condition
cerebral ventricle (communicating) in situ Z98.2
cervix, internal os Q51.828
congenital NEC —*see* Atresia, by site
ureter (pelvic junction) (vesical orifice) Q62.39
urethra (congenital) (posterior) Q64.2
Valvulitis (chronic) —*see* Endocarditis
Valvulopathy —*see* Endocarditis
Van Bogaert's leukoencephalopathy (sclerosing) (subacute) A81.1
Van Bogaert-Scherer-Epstein disease or syndrome E75.5
Van Buchem's syndrome M85.2
Van Creveld-von Gierke disease E74.01
Van der Hoeve (-de Kleyn) **syndrome** Q78.0
Van der Woude's syndrome Q38.0
Van Neck's disease or osteochondrosis M91.0
Vanishing lung J44.9
Vapor asphyxia or suffocation T59.9
specified agent —*see* Table of Drugs and Chemicals
Variance, lethal ball, prosthetic heart valve T82.09
Variants, thalassemic D56.8
Variations in hair color L67.1
Varicella B01.9
with
complications NEC B01.89
encephalitis B01.11
encephalomyelitis B01.11
meningitis B01.0
myelitis B01.12
pneumonia B01.2
congenital P35.8
Varices —*see* Varix
Varicocele (scrotum) (thrombosed) I86.1
ovary I86.2
perineum I86.3
spermatic cord (ulcerated) I86.1
Varicose
aneurysm (ruptured) I77.0
dermatitis —*see* Varix, leg, with, inflammation
eczema —*see* Varix, leg, with, inflammation
phlebitis —*see* Varix, with, inflammation
tumor —*see* Varix
ulcer (lower limb, any part) —*see also* Varix, leg, with, ulcer
anus —*see also* Hemorrhoids K64.8
esophagus —*see* Varix, esophagus
inflamed or infected —*see* Varix, leg, with ulcer, with inflammation
nasal septum I86.8
perineum I86.3
scrotum I86.1
specified site NEC I86.8
vein —*see* Varix
vessel —*see* Varix, leg
Varicosis, varicosities, varicosity —*see* Varix
Variola (major) (minor) B03
Varioloid B03
Varix (lower limb) (ruptured) I83.90
with
edema I83.899
inflammation I83.10
with ulcer (venous) I83.209
pain I83.819
specified complication NEC I83.899
stasis dermatitis I83.10
with ulcer (venous) I83.209
swelling I83.899
ulcer I83.009
with inflammation I83.209
aneurysmal I77.0
asymptomatic I83.9-
bladder I86.2
broad ligament I86.2
complicating
childbirth (lower extremity) O87.4
anus or rectum O87.2
genital (vagina, vulva or perineum) O87.8
pregnancy (lower extremity) O22.0-
anus or rectum O22.4-
genital (vagina, vulva or perineum) O22.1-
puerperium (lower extremity) O87.4
anus or rectum O87.2
genital (vagina, vulva, perineum) O87.8
congenital (any site) Q27.8
esophagus (idiopathic) (primary) (ulcerated) I85.00
bleeding I85.01
congenital Q27.8
in (due to)
alcoholic liver disease I85.10
bleeding I85.11
cirrhosis of liver I85.10
bleeding I85.11
Varix *(Continued)*
esophagus *(Continued)*
in *(Continued)*
portal hypertension I85.10
bleeding I85.11
schistosomiasis I85.10
bleeding I85.11
toxic liver disease I85.10
bleeding I85.11
secondary I85.10
bleeding I85.11
gastric I86.4
inflamed or infected I83.10
ulcerated I83.209
labia (majora) I86.3
leg (asymptomatic) I83.90
with
edema I83.899
inflammation I83.10
with ulcer —*see* Varix, leg, with, ulcer, with inflammation by site
pain I83.819
specified complication NEC I83.899
swelling I83.899
ulcer I83.009
with inflammation I83.209
ankle I83.003
with inflammation I83.203
calf I83.002
with inflammation I83.202
foot NEC I83.005
with inflammation I83.205
heel I83.004
with inflammation I83.204
lower leg NEC I83.008
with inflammation I83.208
midfoot I83.004
with inflammation I83.204
thigh I83.001
with inflammation I83.201
bilateral (asymptomatic) I83.93
with
edema I83.893
pain I83.813
specified complication NEC I83.893
swelling I83.893
ulcer I83.009
with inflammation I83.209
left (asymptomatic) I83.92
with
edema I83.892
inflammation I83.12
with ulcer —*see* Varix, leg, with, ulcer, with inflammation by site
pain I83.812
specified complication NEC I83.892
swelling I83.892
ulcer I83.029
with inflammation I83.229
ankle I83.023
with inflammation I83.223
calf I83.022
with inflammation I83.222
foot NEC I83.025
with inflammation I83.225
heel I83.024
with inflammation I83.224
lower leg NEC I83.028
with inflammation I83.228
midfoot I83.024
with inflammation I83.224
thigh I83.021
with inflammation I83.221
right (asymptomatic) I83.91
with
edema I83.891
inflammation I83.11
with ulcer —*see* Varix, leg, with, ulcer, with inflammation by site

Varix *(Continued)*
leg *(Continued)*
right *(Continued)*
with *(Continued)*
pain I83.811
specified complication NEC I83.891
swelling I83.891
ulcer I83.019
with inflammation I83.219
ankle I83.013
with inflammation I83.213
calf I83.012
with inflammation I83.212
foot NEC I83.015
with inflammation I83.215
heel I83.014
with inflammation I83.214
lower leg NEC I83.018
with inflammation I83.218
midfoot I83.014
with inflammation I83.214
thigh I83.011
with inflammation I83.211
nasal septum I86.8
orbit I86.8
congenital Q27.8
ovary I86.2
papillary I78.1
pelvis I86.2
perineum I86.3
pharynx I86.8
placenta O43.89-
renal papilla I86.8
retina H35.09
scrotum (ulcerated) I86.1
sigmoid colon I86.8
specified site NEC I86.8
spinal (cord) (vessels) I86.8
spleen, splenic (vein) (with phlebolith) I86.8
stomach I86.4
sublingual I86.0
ulcerated I83.009
inflamed or infected I83.209
uterine ligament I86.2
vagina I86.8
vocal cord I86.8
vulva I86.3
Vas deferens —*see* condition
Vas deferentitis N49.1
Vasa previa O69.4
hemorrhage from, affecting newborn P50.0
Vascular —*see also* condition
loop on optic papilla Q14.2
spasm I73.9
spider I78.1
Vascularization, cornea —*see* Neovascularization, cornea
Vasculitis I77.6
allergic D69.0
cryoglobulinemic D89.1
disseminated I77.6
hypocomplementemic M31.8
kidney I77.89
livedoid L95.0
nodular L95.8
retina H35.06-
rheumatic —*see* Fever, rheumatic
rheumatoid —*see* Rheumatoid, vasculitis
skin (limited to) L95.9
specified NEC L95.8
Vasculopathy, necrotizing M31.9
cardiac allograft T86.290
specified NEC M31.8
Vasitis (nodosa) N49.1
tuberculous A18.15
Vasodilation I73.9
Vasomotor —*see* condition
Vasoplasty, after previous sterilization Z31.0
aftercare Z31.42
Vasospasm (vasoconstriction) I73.9
cerebral (cerebrovascular) (artery) I67.848
reversible I67.841
coronary I20.1
nerve
arm —*see* Mononeuropathy, upper limb
brachial plexus G54.0
cervical plexus G54.2
leg —*see* Mononeuropathy, lower limb
peripheral NOS I73.9
retina (artery) —*see* Occlusion, artery, retina
Vasospastic —*see* condition
Vasovagal attack (paroxysmal) R55
psychogenic F45.8
VATER syndrome Q87.2
Vater's ampulla —*see* condition
Vegetation, vegetative
adenoid (nasal fossa) J35.8
endocarditis (acute) (any valve) (subacute) I33.0
heart (mycotic) (valve) I33.0
Veil
Jackson's Q43.3
Vein, venous —*see* condition
Veldt sore —*see* Ulcer, skin
Velpeau's hernia —*see* Hernia, femoral
Venereal
bubo A55
disease A64
granuloma inguinale A58
lymphogranuloma (Durand-Nicolas-Favre) A55
Venofibrosis I87.8
Venom, venomous —*see* Table of Drugs and Chemicals, by animal or substance, poisoning
Venous —*see* condition
Ventilator lung, newborn P27.8
Ventral —*see* condition
Ventricle, ventricular —*see also* condition
escape I49.3
inversion Q20.5
Ventriculitis (cerebral) —*see also* Encephalitis G04.90
Ventriculostomy status Z98.2
Vernet's syndrome G52.7
Verneuil's disease (syphilitic bursitis) A52.78
Verruca (due to HPV) (filiformis) (simplex) (viral) (vulgaris) B07.9
acuminata A63.0
necrogenica (primary) (tuberculosa) A18.4
plana B07.8
plantaris B07.0
seborrheica L82.1
inflamed L82.0
senile (seborrheic) L82.1
inflamed L82.0
tuberculosa (primary) A18.4
venereal A63.0
Verrucosities —*see* Verruca
Verruga peruana, peruviana A44.1
Version
with extraction
cervix —*see* Malposition, uterus
uterus (postinfectional) (postpartal, old) —*see* Malposition, uterus
Vertebra, vertebral —*see* condition
Vertical talus (congenital) Q66.80
left foot Q66.82
right foot Q66.81
Vertigo R42
auditory —*see* Vertigo, aural
aural H81.31-
benign paroxysmal (positional) H81.1-
central (origin) H81.4-
cerebral H81.4-
Dix and Hallpike (epidemic) —*see* Neuronitis, vestibular
due to infrasound T75.23
Vertigo *(Continued)*
epidemic A88.1
Dix and Hallpike —*see* Neuronitis, vestibular
Pedersen's —*see* Neuronitis, vestibular
vestibular neuronitis —*see* Neuronitis, vestibular
hysterical F44.89
infrasound T75.23
labyrinthine —*see* subcategory H81.0
laryngeal R05
malignant positional H81.4-
Ménière's —*see* subcategory H81.40
menopausal N95.11
otogenic —*see* Vertigo, aural
paroxysmal positional, benign —*see* Vertigo, benign paroxysmal
Pedersen's (epidemic) —*see* Neuronitis, vestibular
peripheral NEC H81.39-
positional
benign paroxysmal —*see* Vertigo, benign paroxysmal
malignant H81.4-
Very-low-density-lipoprotein-type (VLDL) **hyperlipoproteinemia** E78.1
Vesania —*see* Psychosis
Vesical —*see* condition
Vesicle
cutaneous R23.8
seminal —*see* condition
skin R23.8
Vesicocolic —*see* condition
Vesicoperineal —*see* condition
Vesicorectal —*see* condition
Vesicourethrorectal —*see* condition
Vesicovaginal —*see* condition
Vesicular —*see* condition
Vesiculitis (seminal) N49.0
amebic A06.82
gonorrheal (acute) (chronic) A54.23
trichomonal A59.09
tuberculous A18.15
Vestibulitis (ear) —*see also* subcategory H83.0
nose (external) J34.89
vulvar N94.810
Vestibulopathy, acute peripheral (recurrent) —*see* Neuronitis, vestibular
Vestige, vestigial —*see also* Persistence
branchial Q18.0
structures in vitreous Q14.0
Vibration
adverse effects T75.20
pneumatic hammer syndrome T75.21
specified effect NEC T75.29
vasospastic syndrome T75.22
vertigo from infrasound T75.23
exposure (occupational) Z57.7
vertigo T75.23
Vibriosis A28.9
Victim (of)
crime Z65.4
disaster Z65.5
terrorism Z65.4
torture Z65.4
war Z65.5
Vidal's disease L28.0
Villaret's syndrome G52.7
Villous —*see* condition
VIN —*see* Neoplasia, intraepithelial, vulva
Vincent's infection (angina) (gingivitis) A69.1
stomatitis NEC A69.1
Vinson-Plummer syndrome D50.1
Violence, physical R45.6
Viosterol deficiency —*see* Deficiency, calciferol
Vipoma —*see* Neoplasm, malignant, by site
Viremia B34.9
Virilism (adrenal) E25.9
congenital E25.0
Virilization (female) (suprarenal) E25.9
congenital E25.0
isosexual E28.2

◀ New ⇐ Revised ~~deleted~~ Deleted

Virulent bubo A57
Virus, viral —*see also* condition
as cause of disease classified elsewhere B97.89
cytomegalovirus B25.9
human immunodeficiency (HIV) —*see* Human, immunodeficiency virus (HIV) disease
infection —*see* Infection, virus
specified NEC B34.8
~~swine influenza (viruses that normally cause infections in pigs) (see also Influenza, due to, identified novel influenza A virus) J09.X2~~
swine influenza (viruses that normally cause infections in pigs) —*see also* Influenza, due to, identified novel influenza A virus J09.X2 ◀
West Nile (fever) A92.30
with
complications NEC A92.39
cranial nerve disorders A92.32
encephalitis A92.31
encephalomyelitis A92.31
neurologic manifestation NEC A92.32
optic neuritis A92.32
polyradiculitis A92.32
Viscera, visceral —*see* condition
Visceroptosis K63.4
Visible peristalsis R19.2
Vision, visual
binocular, suppression H53.34
blurred, blurring H53.8
hysterical F44.6
defect, defective NEC H54.7
disorientation (syndrome) H53.8
disturbance H53.9
hysterical F44.6
double H53.2
examination Z01.00
with abnormal findings Z01.01
field, limitation (defect) —*see* Defect, visual field
hallucinations R44.1
halos H53.19
loss —*see* Loss, vision
sudden —*see* Disturbance, vision, subjective, loss, sudden
low (both eyes) —*see* Low, vision
perception, simultaneous without fusion H53.33
Vitality, lack or want of R53.83
newborn P96.89
Vitamin deficiency —*see* Deficiency, vitamin
Vitelline duct, persistent Q43.0
Vitiligo L80
eyelid H02.739
left H02.736
lower H02.735
upper H02.734
Vitiligo *(Continued)*
eyelid *(Continued)*
right H02.733
lower H02.732
upper H02.731
pinta A67.2
vulva N90.89
Vitreal corneal syndrome H59.01-
Vitreoretinopathy, proliferative —*see also* Retinopathy, proliferative
with retinal detachment —*see* Detachment, retina, traction
Vitreous —*see also* condition
touch syndrome —*see* Complication, postprocedural, following cataract surgery
Vocal cord —*see* condition
Vogt-Koyanagi syndrome H20.82-
Vogt's disease or syndrome G80.3
Vogt-Spielmeyer amaurotic idiocy or disease E75.4
Voice
change R49.9
specified NEC R49.8
loss —*see* Aphonia
Volhynian fever A79.0
Volkmann's ischemic contracture or paralysis (complicating trauma) T79.6
Volvulus (bowel) (colon) (intestine) K56.2 ⬅
with perforation K56.2
congenital Q43.8
duodenum K31.5 ◀
fallopian tube —*see* Torsion, fallopian tube
oviduct —*see* Torsion, fallopian tube
stomach (due to absence of gastrocolic ligament) K31.89
Vomiting R11.10
with nausea R11.2
without nausea R11.11
asphyxia —*see* Foreign body, by site, causing asphyxia, gastric contents
bilious (cause unknown) R11.14
following gastro-intestinal surgery K91.0
in newborn P92.01
blood —*see* Hematemesis
causing asphyxia, choking, or suffocation —*see* Foreign body, by site
cyclical G43.A0
with refractory migraine G43.A1
intractable G43.A1
not intractable G43.A0
psychogenic F50.89 ⬅
without refractory migraine G43.A0
fecal mater R11.13
following gastrointestinal surgery K91.0
psychogenic F50.89 ⬅
Vomiting *(Continued)*
functional K31.89
hysterical F50.89 ⬅
nervous F50.89 ⬅
neurotic F50.89 ⬅
newborn NEC P92.09
bilious P92.01
periodic R11.10
psychogenic F50.89 ⬅
projectile R11.12
psychogenic F50.89 ⬅
uremic —*see* Uremia
Vomito negro —*see* Fever, yellow
Von Bezold's abscess —*see* Mastoiditis, acute
Von Economo-Cruchet disease A85.8
Von Eulenburg's disease G71.19
Von Gierke's disease E74.01
Von Hippel (-Lindau) **disease or syndrome** Q85.8
Von Jaksch's anemia or disease D64.89
Von Recklinghausen
disease (neurofibromatosis) Q85.01
bones E21.0
Von Schroetter's syndrome I82.890
Von Willebrand (-Jurgens)(-Minot) **disease or syndrome** D68.0
Von Zumbusch's disease L40.1
Voyeurism F65.3
Vrolik's disease Q78.0
Vulva —*see* condition
Vulvismus N94.2
Vulvitis (acute) (allergic) (atrophic) (hypertrophic) (intertriginous) (senile) N76.2
with ectopic or molar pregnancy O08.0
adhesive, congenital Q52.79
blennorrhagic (gonococcal) A54.02
candidal B37.3
chlamydial A56.02
due to Haemophilus ducreyi A57
following ectopic or molar pregnancy O08.0
gonococcal A54.02
with abscess (accessory gland) (periurethral) A54.1
herpesviral A60.04
leukoplakic N90.4
monilial B37.3
puerperal (postpartum) O86.19
subacute or chronic N76.3
syphilitic (early) A51.0
late A52.76
trichomonal A59.01
tuberculous A18.18
Vulvodynia N94.819
specified NEC N94.818
Vulvorectal —*see* condition
Vulvovaginitis (acute) —*see* Vaginitis

W

Waiting list, person on Z75.1
for organ transplant Z76.82
undergoing social agency investigation Z75.2
Waldenström
hypergammaglobulinemia D89.0
syndrome or macroglobulinemia C88.0
Waldenström-Kjellberg syndrome D50.1
Walking
difficulty R26.2
psychogenic F44.4
sleep F51.3
hysterical F44.89
Wall, abdominal —*see* condition
Wallenberg's disease or syndrome G46.3
Wallgren's disease I87.8
Wandering
gallbladder, congenital Q44.1
in diseases classified elsewhere Z91.83
kidney, congenital Q63.8
organ or site, congenital NEC —*see* Malposition, congenital, by site
pacemaker (heart) I49.8
spleen D73.89
War neurosis F48.8
Wart (due to HPV) (filiform) (infectious) (viral) B07.9
anogenital region (venereal) A63.0
common B07.8
external genital organs (venereal) A63.0
flat B07.8
Hassal-Henle's (of cornea) H18.49
Peruvian A44.1
plantar B07.0
prosector (tuberculous) A18.4
seborrheic L82.1
inflamed L82.0
senile (seborrheic) L82.1
inflamed L82.0
tuberculous A18.4
venereal A63.0
Warthin's tumor —*see* Neoplasm, salivary gland, benign
Wassilieff's disease A27.0
Wasting
disease R64
due to malnutrition E41
extreme (due to malnutrition) E41
muscle NEC —*see* Atrophy, muscle
Water
clefts (senile cataract) —*see* Cataract, senile, incipient
deprivation of T73.1
intoxication E87.79
itch B76.9
lack of T73.1
loading E87.70
on
brain —*see* Hydrocephalus
chest J94.8
poisoning E87.79
Waterbrash R12
Waterhouse(-Friderichsen) syndrome or disease (meningococcal) A39.1
Water-losing nephritis N25.89
Watermelon stomach K31.819
with hemorrhage K31.811
without hemorrhage K31.819
Watsoniasis B66.8
Wax in ear —*see* Impaction, cerumen
Weak, weakening, weakness (generalized) R53.1
arches (acquired) —*see also* Deformity, limb, flat foot
bladder (sphincter) R32
facial R29.810
following
cerebrovascular disease I69.992
cerebral infarction I69.392
intracerebral hemorrhage I69.192
Weak, weakening, weakness *(Continued)*
facial *(Continued)*
following *(Continued)*
cerebrovascular disease *(Continued)*
nontraumatic intracranial hemorrhage NEC I69.292
specified disease NEC I69.892
stroke I69.392
subarachnoid hemorrhage I69.092
foot (double) —*see* Weak, arches
heart, cardiac —*see* Failure, heart
mind F70
muscle M62.81
myocardium —*see* Failure, heart
newborn P96.89
pelvic fundus N81.89
pubocervical tissue N81.82
rectovaginal tissue N81.83
senile R54
urinary stream R39.12
valvular —*see* Endocarditis
Wear, worn (with normal or routine use)
articular bearing surface of internal joint prosthesis —*see* Complications, joint prosthesis, mechanical, wear of articular bearing surfaces, by site
device, implant or graft —*see* Complications, by site, mechanical complication
tooth, teeth (approximal) (hard tissues) (interproximal) (occlusal) K03.0
Weather, weathered
effects of
cold T69.9
specified effect NEC T69.8
hot —*see* Heat
skin L57.8
Weaver's syndrome Q87.3
Web, webbed (congenital)
duodenal Q43.8
esophagus Q39.4
fingers Q70.1
larynx (glottic) (subglottic) Q31.0
neck (pterygium colli) Q18.3
Paterson-Kelly D50.1
popliteal syndrome Q87.89
toes Q70.3
Weber-Christian disease M35.6
Weber-Cockayne syndrome (epidermolysis bullosa) Q81.8
Weber-Gubler syndrome G46.3
Weber-Leyden syndrome G46.3
Weber-Osler syndrome I78.0
Weber's paralysis or syndrome G46.3
Wedge-shaped or wedging vertebra —*see* Collapse, vertebra NEC
Wegener's granulomatosis or syndrome M31.30
with
kidney involvement M31.31
lung involvement M31.30
with kidney involvement M31.31
Wegner's disease A50.02
Weight
1000-2499 grams at birth (low) —*see* Low, birthweight
999 grams or less at birth (extremely low) —*see* Low, birthweight, extreme
and length below 10th percentile for gestational age P05.1- ◀
below but length above 10th percentile for gestational age P05.0- ◀
gain (abnormal) (excessive) R63.5
in pregnancy —*see* Pregnancy, complicated by, excessive weight gain
low —*see* Pregnancy, complicated by, insufficient, weight gain
loss (abnormal) (cause unknown) R63.4
Weightlessness (effect of) T75.82
Weil (l)-Marchesani syndrome Q87.1
Weil's disease A27.0
Weingarten's syndrome J82
Weir Mitchell's disease I73.81
Weiss-Baker syndrome G90.09
Wells' disease L98.3
Wen —*see* Cyst, sebaceous
Wenckebach's block or phenomenon I44.1
Werdnig-Hoffmann syndrome (muscular atrophy) G12.0
Werlhof's disease D69.3
Werner-His disease A79.0
Wermer's disease or syndrome E31.21
Werner's disease or syndrome E34.8
Wernicke-Korsakoff's syndrome or psychosis (alcoholic) F10.96
with dependence F10.26
drug-induced
due to drug abuse —*see* Abuse, drug, by type, with amnestic disorder
due to drug dependence —*see* Dependence, drug, by type, with amnestic disorder
nonalcoholic F04
Wernicke-Posadas disease B38.9
Wernicke's
developmental aphasia F80.2
disease or syndrome E51.2
encephalopathy E51.2
polioencephalitis, superior E51.2
West African fever B50.8
Westphal-Strümpell syndrome E83.01
West's syndrome —*see* Epilepsy, spasms
Wet
feet, tropical (maceration) (syndrome) —*see* Immersion, foot
lung (syndrome), newborn P22.1
Wharton's duct —*see* condition
Wheal —*see* Urticaria
Wheezing R06.2
Whiplash injury S13.4
Whipple's disease —*see also* subcategory M14.8- K90.81
Whipworm (disease) (infection) (infestation) B79
Whistling face Q87.0
White —*see also* condition
kidney, small N03.9
leg, puerperal, postpartum, childbirth O87.1
mouth B37.0
patches of mouth K13.29
spot lesions, teeth
chewing surface K02.51
pit and fissure surface K02.51
smooth surface K02.61
Whitehead L70.0
Whitlow —*see also* Cellulitis, digit
with lymphangitis —*see* Lymphangitis, acute, digit
herpesviral B00.89
Whitmore's disease or fever —*see* Melioidosis
Whooping cough A37.90
with pneumonia A37.91
due to Bordetella
bronchiseptica A37.81
parapertussis A37.11
pertussis A37.01
specified organism NEC A37.81
due to
Bordetella
bronchiseptica A37.80
with pneumonia A37.81
parapertussis A37.10
with pneumonia A37.11
pertussis A37.00
with pneumonia A37.01
specified NEC A37.80
with pneumonia A37.81
Wichman's asthma J38.5
Wide cranial sutures, newborn P96.3
Widening aorta —*see* Ectasia, aorta
with aneurysm —*see* Aneurysm, aorta
Wilkie's disease or syndrome K55.1
Wilkinson-Sneddon disease or syndrome L13.1

Willebrand (-Jürgens) thrombopathy D68.0
Willige-Hunt disease or syndrome G23.1
Wilms' tumor C64-
Wilson-Mikity syndrome P27.0
Wilson's
disease or syndrome E83.01
hepatolenticular degeneration E83.01
lichen ruber L43.9
Window —*see also* Imperfect, closure
aorticopulmonary Q21.4
Winter —*see* condition
Wiskott-Aldrich syndrome D82.0
Withdrawal state —*see also* Dependence, drug by type, with withdrawal
alcohol ◀
with perceptual disturbances F10.232 ◀
without perceptual disturbances F10.239 ◀
caffeine F15.93 ◀
cannabis F12.288 ◀
newborn
correct therapeutic substance properly administered P96.2
infant of dependent mother P96.1
therapeutic substance, neonatal P96.2
Witts' anemia D50.8
Witzelsucht F07.0
Woakes' ethmoiditis or syndrome J33.1
Wolff-Hirschorn syndrome Q93.3
Wolff-Parkinson-White syndrome I45.6
Wolhynian fever A79.0
Wolman's disease E75.5
Wood lung or pneumonitis J67.8
Woolly, wooly hair (congenital) (nevus) Q84.1
Woolsorter's disease A22.1
Word
blindness (congenital) (developmental) F81.0
deafness (congenital) (developmental) H93.25
Worm (s) (infection) (infestation) —*see also* Infestation, helminth
guinea B72
in intestine NEC B82.0
Worm-eaten soles A66.3
Worn out —*see* Exhaustion
cardiac
defibrillator (with synchronous cardiac pacemaker) Z45.02
pacemaker
battery Z45.010
lead Z45.018
device, implant or graft —*see* Complications, by site, mechanical
Worried well Z71.1
Worries R45.82
Wound, open
abdomen, abdominal
wall S31.109
with penetration into peritoneal cavity S31.609
bite —*see* Bite, abdomen, wall
epigastric region S31.102
with penetration into peritoneal cavity S31.602
bite —*see* Bite, abdomen, wall, epigastric region
laceration —*see* Laceration, abdomen, wall, epigastric region
puncture —*see* Puncture, abdomen, wall, epigastric region
laceration —*see* Laceration, abdomen, wall
left
lower quadrant S31.104
with penetration into peritoneal cavity S31.604
bite —*see* Bite, abdomen, wall, left, lower quadrant
laceration —*see* Laceration, abdomen, wall, left, lower quadrant
puncture —*see* Puncture, abdomen, wall, left, lower quadrant

Wound, open *(Continued)*
abdomen, abdominal *(Continued)*
wall *(Continued)*
left *(Continued)*
upper quadrant S31.101
with penetration into peritoneal cavity S31.601
bite —*see* Bite, abdomen, wall, left, upper quadrant
laceration —*see* Laceration, abdomen, wall, left, upper quadrant
puncture —*see* Puncture, abdomen, wall, left, upper quadrant
periumbilic region S31.105
with penetration into peritoneal cavity S31.605
bite —*see* Bite, abdomen, wall, periumbilic region
laceration —*see* Laceration, abdomen, wall, periumbilic region
puncture —*see* Puncture, abdomen, wall, periumbilic region
puncture —*see* Puncture, abdomen, wall
right
lower quadrant S31.103
with penetration into peritoneal cavity S31.603
bite —*see* Bite, abdomen, wall, right, lower quadrant
laceration —*see* Laceration, abdomen, wall, right, lower quadrant
puncture —*see* Puncture, abdomen, wall, right, lower quadrant
upper quadrant S31.100
with penetration into peritoneal cavity S31.600
bite —*see* Bite, abdomen, wall, right, upper quadrant
laceration —*see* Laceration, abdomen, wall, right, upper quadrant
puncture —*see* Puncture, abdomen, wall, right, upper quadrant
alveolar (process) —*see* Wound, open, oral cavity
ankle S91.00-
bite —*see* Bite, ankle
laceration —*see* Laceration, ankle
puncture —*see* Puncture, ankle
antecubital space —*see* Wound, open, elbow
anterior chamber, eye —*see* Wound, open, ocular
anus S31.839
bite S31.835
laceration —*see* Laceration, anus
puncture —*see* Puncture, anus
arm (upper) S41.10-
with amputation —*see* Amputation, traumatic, arm
bite —*see* Bite, arm
forearm —*see* Wound, open, forearm
laceration —*see* Laceration, arm
puncture —*see* Puncture, arm
auditory canal (external) (meatus) —*see* Wound, open, ear
auricle, ear —*see* Wound, open, ear
axilla —*see* Wound, open, arm
back —*see also* Wound, open, thorax, back
lower S31.000
with penetration into retroperitoneal space S31.001
bite —*see* Bite, back, lower
laceration —*see* Laceration, back, lower
puncture —*see* Puncture, back, lower
bite —*see* Bite
blood vessel —*see* Injury, blood vessel
breast S21.00-
with amputation —*see* Amputation, traumatic, breast

Wound, open *(Continued)*
breast *(Continued)*
bite —*see* Bite, breast
laceration —*see* Laceration, breast
puncture —*see* Puncture, breast
buttock S31.809
bite —*see* Bite, buttock
laceration —*see* Laceration, buttock
left S31.829
puncture —*see* Puncture, buttock
right S31.819
calf —*see* Wound, open, leg
canaliculus lacrimalis —*see* Wound, open, eyelid
canthus, eye —*see* Wound, open, eyelid
cervical esophagus S11.20
bite S11.25
laceration —*see* Laceration, esophagus, traumatic, cervical
puncture —*see* Puncture, cervical esophagus
cheek (external) S01.40-
bite —*see* Bite, cheek
internal —*see* Wound, open, oral cavity
laceration —*see* Laceration, cheek
puncture —*see* Puncture, cheek
chest wall —*see* Wound, open, thorax
chin —*see* Wound, open, head, specified site NEC
choroid —*see* Wound, open, ocular
ciliary body (eye) —*see* Wound, open, ocular
clitoris S31.40
with amputation —*see* Amputation, traumatic, clitoris
bite S31.45
laceration —*see* Laceration, vulva
puncture —*see* Puncture, vulva
conjunctiva —*see* Wound, open, ocular
cornea —*see* Wound, open, ocular
costal region —*see* Wound, open, thorax
Descemet's membrane —*see* Wound, open, ocular
digit (s)
foot —*see* Wound, open, toe
hand —*see* Wound, open, finger
ear (canal) (external) S01.30-
with amputation —*see* Amputation, traumatic, ear
bite —*see* Bite, ear
drum S09.2-
laceration —*see* Laceration, ear
puncture —*see* Puncture, ear
elbow S51.00-
bite —*see* Bite, elbow
laceration —*see* Laceration, elbow
puncture —*see* Puncture, elbow
epididymis —*see* Wound, open, testis
epigastric region S31.102
with penetration into peritoneal cavity S31.602
bite —*see* Bite, abdomen, wall, epigastric region
laceration —*see* Laceration, abdomen, wall, epigastric region
puncture —*see* Puncture, abdomen, wall, epigastric region
epiglottis —*see* Wound, open, neck, specified site NEC
esophagus (thoracic) S27.819
cervical —*see* Wound, open, cervical esophagus
laceration S27.813
specified type NEC S27.818
eye —*see* Wound, open, ocular
eyeball —*see* Wound, open, ocular
eyebrow —*see* Wound, open, eyelid
eyelid S01.10-
bite —*see* Bite, eyelid
laceration —*see* Laceration, eyelid
puncture —*see* Puncture, eyelid
face NEC —*see* Wound, open, head, specified site NEC

Wound, open *(Continued)*
finger (s) S61.209
with
amputation —*see* Amputation, traumatic, finger
damage to nail S61.309
bite —*see* Bite, finger
index S61.208
with
damage to nail S61.308
left S61.201
with
damage to nail S61.301
right S61.200
with
damage to nail S61.300
laceration —*see* Laceration, finger
little S61.208
with
damage to nail S61.308
left S61.207
with damage to nail S61.307
right S61.206
with damage to nail S61.306
middle S61.208
with
damage to nail S61.308
left S61.203
with damage to nail S61.303
right S61.202
with damage to nail S61.302
puncture —*see* Puncture, finger
ring S61.208
with
damage to nail S61.308
left S61.205
with damage to nail S61.305
right S61.204
with damage to nail S61.304
flank —*see* Wound, open, abdomen, wall
foot (except toe (s) alone) S91.30-
with amputation —*see* Amputation, traumatic, foot
bite —*see* Bite, foot
laceration —*see* Laceration, foot
puncture —*see* Puncture, foot
toe —*see* Wound, open, toe
forearm S51.80-
with
amputation —*see* Amputation, traumatic, forearm
bite —*see* Bite, forearm
elbow only —*see* Wound, open, elbow
laceration —*see* Laceration, forearm
puncture —*see* Puncture, forearm
forehead —*see* Wound, open, head, specified site NEC
genital organs, external
with amputation —*see* Amputation, traumatic, genital organs
bite —*see* Bite, genital organ
female S31.502
vagina S31.40
vulva S31.40
laceration —*see* Laceration, genital organ
male S31.501
penis S31.20
scrotum S31.30
testes S31.30
puncture —*see* Puncture, genital organ
globe (eye) —*see* Wound, open, ocular
groin —*see* Wound, open, abdomen, wall
gum —*see* Wound, open, oral cavity
hand S61.40-
with
amputation —*see* Amputation, traumatic, hand
bite —*see* Bite, hand
finger (s) —*see* Wound, open, finger
laceration —*see* Laceration, hand

Wound, open *(Continued)*
hand *(Continued)*
puncture —*see* Puncture, hand
thumb —*see* Wound, open, thumb
head S01.90
bite —*see* Bite, head
cheek —*see* Wound, open, cheek
ear —*see* Wound, open, ear
eyelid —*see* Wound, open, eyelid
laceration —*see* Laceration, head
lip —*see* Wound, open, lip
nose S01.20
oral cavity —*see* Wound, open, oral cavity
puncture —*see* Puncture, head
scalp —*see* Wound, open, scalp
specified site NEC S01.80
temporomandibular area —*see* Wound, open, cheek
heel —*see* Wound, open, foot
hip S71.00-
with amputation —*see* Amputation, traumatic, hip
bite —*see* Bite, hip
laceration —*see* Laceration, hip
puncture —*see* Puncture, hip
hymen S31.40
bite —*see* Bite, vulva
laceration —*see* Laceration, vagina
puncture —*see* Puncture, vagina
hypochondrium S31.109
bite —*see* Bite, hypochondrium
laceration —*see* Laceration, hypochondrium
puncture —*see* Puncture, hypochondrium
hypogastric region S31.109
bite —*see* Bite, hypogastric region
laceration —*see* Laceration, hypogastric region
puncture —*see* Puncture, hypogastric region
iliac (region) —*see* Wound, open, inguinal region
inguinal region S31.109
bite —*see* Bite, abdomen, wall, lower quadrant
laceration —*see* Laceration, inguinal region
puncture —*see* Puncture, inguinal region
instep —*see* Wound, open, foot
interscapular region —*see* Wound, open, thorax, back
intraocular —*see* Wound, open, ocular
iris —*see* Wound, open, ocular
jaw —*see* Wound, open, head, specified site NEC
knee S81.00-
bite —*see* Bite, knee
laceration —*see* Laceration, knee
puncture —*see* Puncture, knee
labium (majus) (minus) —*see* Wound, open, vulva
laceration —*see* Laceration, by site
lacrimal duct —*see* Wound, open, eyelid
larynx S11.019
bite —*see* Bite, larynx
laceration —*see* Laceration, larynx
puncture —*see* Puncture, larynx
left
lower quadrant S31.104
with penetration into peritoneal cavity S31.604
bite —*see* Bite, abdomen, wall, left, lower quadrant
laceration —*see* Laceration, abdomen, wall, left, lower quadrant
puncture —*see* Puncture, abdomen, wall, left, lower quadrant
upper quadrant S31.101
with penetration into peritoneal cavity S31.601
bite —*see* Bite, abdomen, wall, left, upper quadrant

Wound, open *(Continued)*
left *(Continued)*
upper quadrant *(Continued)*
laceration —*see* Laceration, abdomen, wall, left, upper quadrant
puncture —*see* Puncture, abdomen, wall, left, upper quadrant
leg (lower) S81.80-
with amputation —*see* Amputation, traumatic, leg
ankle —*see* Wound, open, ankle
bite —*see* Bite, leg
foot —*see* Wound, open, foot
knee —*see* Wound, open, knee
laceration —*see* Laceration, leg
puncture —*see* Puncture, leg
toe —*see* Wound, open, toe
upper —*see* Wound, open, thigh
lip S01.501
bite —*see* Bite, lip
laceration —*see* Laceration, lip
puncture —*see* Puncture, lip
loin S31.109
bite —*see* Bite, abdomen, wall
laceration —*see* Laceration, loin
puncture —*see* Puncture, loin
lower back —*see* Wound, open, back, lower
lumbar region —*see* Wound, open, back, lower
malar region —*see* Wound, open, head, specified site NEC
mammary —*see* Wound, open, breast
mastoid region —*see* Wound, open, head, specified site NEC
mouth —*see* Wound, open, oral cavity
nail
finger —*see* Wound, open, finger, with damage to nail
toe —*see* Wound, open, toe, with damage to nail
nape (neck) —*see* Wound, open, neck
nasal (septum) (sinus) —*see* Wound, open, nose
nasopharynx —*see* Wound, open, head, specified site NEC
neck S11.90
bite —*see* Bite, neck
involving
cervical esophagus S11.20
larynx —*see* Wound, open, larynx
pharynx S11.20
thyroid S11.10
trachea (cervical) S11.029
bite —*see* Bite, trachea
laceration S11.021
with foreign body S11.022
puncture S11.023
with foreign body S11.024
laceration —*see* Laceration, neck
puncture —*see* Puncture, neck
specified site NEC S11.80
specified type NEC S11.89
nose (septum) (sinus) S01.20
with amputation —*see* Amputation, traumatic, nose
bite —*see* Bite, nose
laceration —*see* Laceration, nose
puncture —*see* Puncture, nose
ocular S05.90
avulsion (traumatic enucleation) S05.7-
eyeball S05.6-
with foreign body S05.5-
eyelid —*see* Wound, open, eyelid
laceration and rupture S05.3-
with prolapse or loss of intraocular tissue S05.2-
orbit (penetrating) (with or without foreign body) S05.4-
periocular area —*see* Wound, open, eyelid
specified NEC S05.8X-

Wound, open *(Continued)*
oral cavity S01.502
bite S01.552
laceration —*see* Laceration, oral cavity
puncture —*see* Puncture, oral cavity
orbit —*see* Wound, open, ocular, orbit
palate —*see* Wound, open, oral cavity
palm —*see* Wound, open, hand
pelvis, pelvic —*see also* Wound, open, back, lower
girdle —*see* Wound, open, hip
penetrating —*see* Puncture, by site
penis S31.20
with amputation —*see* Amputation, traumatic, penis
bite S31.25
laceration —*see* Laceration, penis
puncture —*see* Puncture, penis
perineum
bite —*see* Bite, perineum
female S31.502
laceration —*see* Laceration, perineum
male S31.501
puncture —*see* Puncture, perineum
periocular area (with or without lacrimal passages) —*see* Wound, open, eyelid
periumbilic region S31.105
with penetration into peritoneal cavity S31.605
bite —*see* Bite, abdomen, wall, periumbilic region
laceration —*see* Laceration, abdomen, wall, periumbilic region
puncture —*see* Puncture, abdomen, wall, periumbilic region
phalanges
finger —*see* Wound, open, finger
toe —*see* Wound, open, toe
pharynx S11.20
pinna —*see* Wound, open, ear
popliteal space —*see* Wound, open, knee
prepuce —*see* Wound, open, penis
pubic region —*see* Wound, open, back, lower
pudendum —*see* Wound, open, genital organs, external
puncture wound —*see* Puncture
rectovaginal septum —*see* Wound, open, vagina
right
lower quadrant S31.103
with penetration into peritoneal cavity S31.603
bite —*see* Bite, abdomen, wall, right, lower quadrant
laceration —*see* Laceration, abdomen, wall, right, lower quadrant
puncture —*see* Puncture, abdomen, wall, right, lower quadrant
upper quadrant S31.100
with penetration into peritoneal cavity S31.600
bite —*see* Bite, abdomen, wall, right, upper quadrant
laceration —*see* Laceration, abdomen, wall, right, upper quadrant
puncture —*see* Puncture, abdomen, wall, right, upper quadrant
sacral region —*see* Wound, open, back, lower
sacroiliac region —*see* Wound, open, back, lower
salivary gland —*see* Wound, open, oral cavity

Wound, open *(Continued)*
scalp S01.00
bite S01.05
laceration —*see* Laceration, scalp
puncture —*see* Puncture, scalp
scalpel, newborn (birth injury) P15.8
scapular region —*see* Wound, open, shoulder
sclera —*see* Wound, open, ocular
scrotum S31.30
with amputation —*see* Amputation, traumatic, scrotum
bite S31.35
laceration —*see* Laceration, scrotum
puncture —*see* Puncture, scrotum
shin —*see* Wound, open, leg
shoulder S41.00-
with amputation —*see* Amputation, traumatic, arm
bite —*see* Bite, shoulder
laceration —*see* Laceration, shoulder
puncture —*see* Puncture, shoulder
skin NOS T14.8
spermatic cord —*see* Wound, open, testis
sternal region —*see* Wound, open, thorax, front wall
submaxillary region —*see* Wound, open, head, specified site NEC
submental region —*see* Wound, open, head, specified site NEC
subungual
finger (s) —*see* Wound, open, finger
toe (s) —*see* Wound, open, toe
supraclavicular region —*see* Wound, open, neck, specified site NEC
temple, temporal region —*see* Wound, open, head, specified site NEC
temporomandibular area —*see* Wound, open, cheek
testis S31.30
with amputation —*see* Amputation, traumatic, testes
bite S31.35
laceration —*see* Laceration, testis
puncture —*see* Puncture, testis
thigh S71.10-
with amputation —*see* Amputation, traumatic, hip
bite —*see* Bite, thigh
laceration —*see* Laceration, thigh
puncture —*see* Puncture, thigh
thorax, thoracic (wall) S21.90
back S21.20-
with penetration S21.40
bite —*see* Bite, thorax
breast —*see* Wound, open, breast
front S21.10-
with penetration S21.30
laceration —*see* Laceration, thorax
puncture —*see* Puncture, thorax
throat —*see* Wound, open, neck
thumb S61.009
with
amputation —*see* Amputation, traumatic, thumb
damage to nail S61.109
bite —*see* Bite, thumb
laceration —*see* Laceration, thumb
left S61.002
with
damage to nail S61.102
puncture —*see* Puncture, thumb
right S61.001
with
damage to nail S61.101

Wound, open *(Continued)*
thyroid (gland) —*see* Wound, open, neck, thyroid
toe (s) S91.109
with
amputation —*see* Amputation, traumatic, toe
damage to nail S91.209
bite —*see* Bite, toe
great S91.103
with
damage to nail S91.203
left S91.102
with
damage to nail S91.202
right S91.101
with
damage to nail S91.201
laceration —*see* Laceration, toe
lesser S91.106
with
damage to nail S91.206
left S91.105
with
damage to nail S91.205
right S91.104
with
damage to nail S91.204
puncture —*see* Puncture, toe
tongue —*see* Wound, open, oral cavity
trachea (cervical region) —*see* Wound, open, neck, trachea
tunica vaginalis —*see* Wound, open, testis
tympanum, tympanic membrane S09.2-
laceration —*see* Laceration, ear, drum
puncture —*see* Puncture, tympanum
umbilical region —*see* Wound, open, abdomen, wall, periumbilic region
uvula —*see* Wound, open, oral cavity
vagina S31.40
bite S31.45
laceration —*see* Laceration, vagina
puncture —*see* Puncture, vagina
vitreous (humor) —*see* Wound, open, ocular
vocal cord S11.039
bite —*see* Bite, vocal cord
laceration S11.031
with foreign body S11.032
puncture S11.033
with foreign body S11.034
vulva S31.40
with amputation —*see* Amputation, traumatic, vulva
bite S31.45
laceration —*see* Laceration, vulva
puncture —*see* Puncture, vulva
wrist S61.50-
bite —*see* Bite, wrist
laceration —*see* Laceration, wrist
puncture —*see* Puncture, wrist
Wound, superficial —*see* Injury (*see also* specified injury type)
Wright's syndrome G54.0
Wrist —*see* condition
Wrong drug (by accident) (given in error) —*see* Table of Drugs and Chemicals, by drug, poisoning
Wry neck —*see* Torticollis
Wuchereria (bancrofti) infestation B74.0
Wuchereriasis B74.0
Wuchernde Struma Langhans C73

X

Xanthelasma (eyelid) (palpebrarum) H02.60
  left H02.66
    lower H02.65
    upper H02.64
  right H02.63
    lower H02.62
    upper H02.61
Xanthelasmatosis (essential) E78.2
Xanthinuria, hereditary E79.8
Xanthoastrocytoma
  specified site —*see* Neoplasm, malignant, by site
  unspecified site C71.9
Xanthofibroma —*see* Neoplasm, connective tissue, benign
Xanthogranuloma D76.3
Xanthoma (s), xanthomatosis (primary) (familial) (hereditary) E75.5
  with
    hyperlipoproteinemia
      Type I E78.3
      Type III E78.2
      Type IV E78.1
      Type V E78.3
  bone (generalisata) C96.5
  cerebrotendinous E75.5
  cutaneotendinous E75.5
Xanthoma (s), xanthomatosis *(Continued)*
  disseminatum (skin) E78.2
  eruptive E78.2
  hypercholesterinemic E78.00 ⟸
  hypercholesterolemic E78.00 ⟸
  hyperlipidemic E78.5
  joint E75.5
  multiple (skin) E78.2
  tendon (sheath) E75.5
  tuberosum E78.2
  tuberous E78.2
  tubo-eruptive E78.2
  verrucous, oral mucosa K13.4
Xanthosis R23.8
Xenophobia F40.10
Xeroderma —*see also* Ichthyosis
  acquired L85.0
    eyelid H01.149
      left H01.146
        lower H01.145
        upper H01.144
      right H01.143
        lower H01.142
        upper H01.141
  pigmentosum Q82.1
  vitamin A deficiency E50.8
Xerophthalmia (vitamin A deficiency) E50.7
  unrelated to vitamin A deficiency —*see* Keratoconjunctivitis
Xerosis
  conjunctiva H11.14-
    with Bitot's spots —*see also* Pigmentation, conjunctiva
      vitamin A deficiency E50.1
    vitamin A deficiency E50.0
  cornea H18.89-
    with ulceration —*see* Ulcer, cornea
      vitamin A deficiency E50.3
    vitamin A deficiency E50.2
  cutis L85.3
  skin L85.3
Xerostomia K11.7
Xiphopagus Q89.4
XO syndrome Q96.9
X-ray (of)
  abnormal findings —*see* Abnormal, diagnostic imaging
  breast (mammogram) (routine) Z12.31
  chest
    routine (as part of a general medical examination) Z00.00
      with abnormal findings Z00.01
  routine (as part of a general medical examination) Z00.00
    with abnormal findings Z00.01
XXXXY syndrome Q98.1
XXY syndrome Q98.0

◀ New ⟸ Revised ~~deleted~~ Deleted

Y

Yaba pox virus disease B08.72
Yatapoxvirus B08.70
  specified NEC B08.79
Yawning R06.89
  psychogenic F45.8
Yaws A66.9
  bone lesions A66.6
  butter A66.1
  chancre A66.0
  cutaneous, less than five years after infection A66.2
  early (cutaneous) (macular) (maculopapular) (micropapular) (papular) A66.2
    frambeside A66.2
    skin lesions NEC A66.2
  eyelid A66.2
  ganglion A66.6
  gangosis, gangosa A66.5
  gumma, gummata A66.4
    bone A66.6
  gummatous
    frambeside A66.4
    osteitis A66.6
    periostitis A66.6
  hydrarthrosis —*see also* subcategory M14.8- A66.6
  hyperkeratosis (early) (late) A66.3
Yaws *(Continued)*
  initial lesions A66.0
  joint lesions —*see also* subcategory M14.8- A66.6
  juxta-articular nodules A66.7
  late nodular (ulcerated) A66.4
  latent (without clinical manifestations) (with positive serology) A66.8
  mother A66.0
  mucosal A66.7
  multiple papillomata A66.1
  nodular, late (ulcerated) A66.4
  osteitis A66.6
  papilloma, plantar or palmar A66.1
  periostitis (hypertrophic) A66.6
  specified NEC A66.7
  ulcers A66.4
  wet crab A66.1
Yeast infection —*see also* Candidiasis B37.9
Yellow
  atrophy (liver) —*see* Failure, hepatic
  fever —*see* Fever, yellow
  jack —*see* Fever, yellow
  jaundice —*see* Jaundice
  nail syndrome L60.5
Yersiniosis —*see also* Infection, Yersinia
  extraintestinal A28.2
  intestinal A04.6

Z

Zahorsky's syndrome (herpangina) B08.5
Zellweger's syndrome Q87.89
Zenker's diverticulum (esophagus) K22.5
Ziehen-Oppenheim disease G24.1
Zieve's syndrome K70.0
Zika NOS A92.5 ◀
Zinc
  deficiency, dietary E60
  metabolism disorder E83.2
Zollinger-Ellison syndrome E16.4
Zona —*see* Herpes, zoster
Zoophobia F40.218
Zoster (herpes) —*see* Herpes, zoster
Zygomycosis B46.9
  specified NEC B46.8
Zymotic —*see* condition

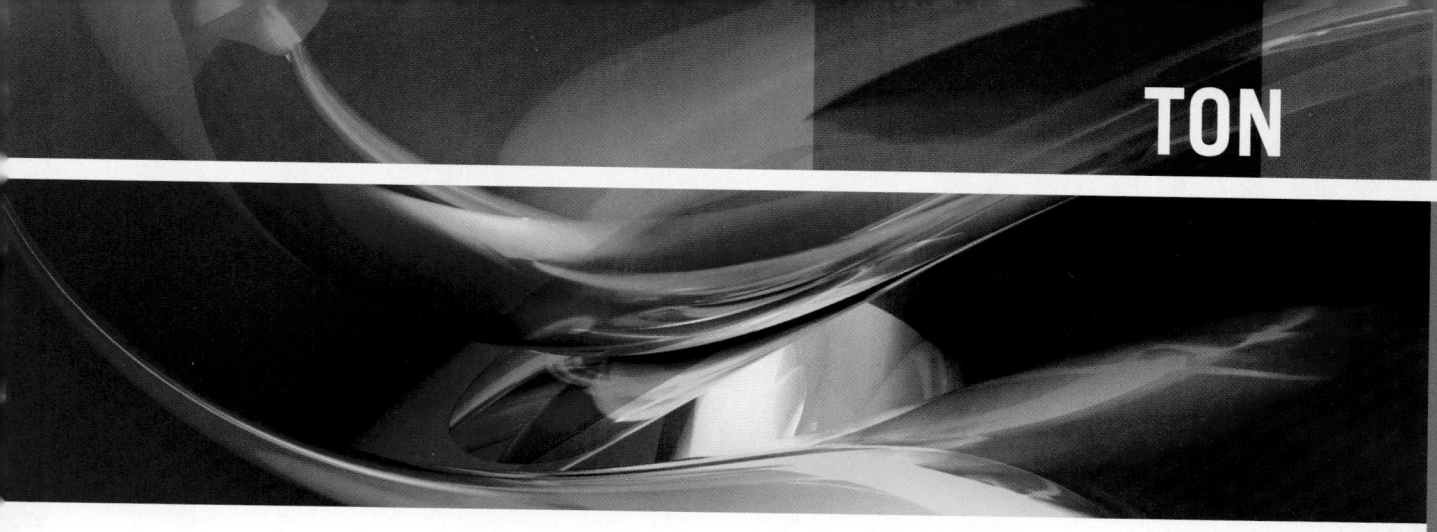

ICD-10-CM Table of Neoplasms

The list below gives the code numbers for neoplasms by anatomical site. For each site there are six possible code numbers according to whether the neoplasm in question is malignant, benign, in situ, of uncertain behavior, or of unspecified nature. The description of the neoplasm will often indicate which of the six columns is appropriate; e.g., malignant melanoma of skin, benign fibroadenoma of breast, carcinoma in situ of cervix uteri.

Where such descriptors are not present, the remainder of the Index should be consulted where guidance is given to the appropriate column for each morphological (histological) variety listed; e.g., Mesonephroma — *see Neoplasm, malignant;* Embryoma — *see also Neoplasm, uncertain behavior;* Disease, Bowen's — *see Neoplasm, skin, in situ.* However, the guidance in the Index can be overridden if one of the descriptors mentioned above is present; e.g., malignant adenoma of colon is coded to C18.9 and not to D12.6 as the adjective "Malignant" overrides the Index entry 'Adenoma — *see also Neoplasm, benign.*'

Codes listed with a dash -, following the code have a required additional character for laterality. The Tablular must be reviewed for the complete code.

	Malignant Primary	Malignant Secondary	Ca in situ	Benign	Uncertain Behavior	Unspecified Behavior
Neoplasm, neoplastic	C80.1	C79.9	D09.9	D36.9	D48.9	D49.9
abdomen, abdominal	C76.2	C79.8-	D09.8	D36.7	D48.7	D49.89
cavity	C76.2	C79.8-	D09.8	D36.7	D48.7	D49.89
organ	C76.2	C79.8-	D09.8	D36.7	D48.7	D49.89
viscera	C76.2	C79.8-	D09.8	D36.7	D48.7	D49.89
wall — *see also Neoplasm, abdomen, wall, skin*	C44.509	C79.2-	D04.5	D23.5	D48.5	D49.2
connective tissue	C49.4	C79.8-	—	D21.4	D48.1	D49.2
skin	C44.509					
basal cell carcinoma	C44.519	—	—	—	—	—
specified type NEC	C44.599	—	—	—	—	—
squamous cell carcinoma	C44.529	—	—	—	—	—
abdominopelvic	C76.8	C79.8-	—	D36.7	D48.7	D49.89
accessory sinus — *see Neoplasm, sinus*						
acoustic nerve	C72.4-	C79.49	—	D33.3	D43.3	D49.7
adenoid (pharynx) (tissue)	C11.1	C79.89	D00.08	D10.6	D37.05	D49.0
adipose tissue — *see also Neoplasm, connective tissue*	C49.4	C79.89	—	D21.9	D48.1	D49.2
adnexa (uterine)	C57.4	C79.89	D07.39	D28.7	D39.8	D49.59
adrenal	C74.9-	C79.7-	D09.3	D35.0-	D44.1-	D49.7
capsule	C74.9-	C79.7-	D09.3	D35.0-	D44.1-	D49.7
cortex	C74.0-	C79.7-	D09.3	D35.0-	D44.1-	D49.7
gland	C74.9-	C79.7-	D09.3	D35.0-	D44.1-	D49.7
medulla	C74.1-	C79.7-	D09.3	D35.0-	D44.1-	D49.7
ala nasi (external) — *see also Neoplasm, skin, nose*	C44.301	C79.2	D04.39	D23.39	D48.5	D49.2
alimentary canal or tract NEC	C26.9	C78.80	D01.9	D13.9	D37.9	D49.0
alveolar	C03.9	C79.89	D00.03	D10.39	D37.09	D49.0
mucosa	C03.9	C79.89	D00.03	D10.39	D37.09	D49.0
lower	C03.1	C79.89	D00.03	D10.39	D37.09	D49.0
upper	C03.0	C79.89	D00.03	D10.39	D37.09	D49.0
ridge or process	C41.1	C79.51	—	D16.5-	D48.0	D49.2
carcinoma	C03.9	C79.8-	—	—	—	—
lower	C03.1	C79.8-	—	—	—	—
upper	C03.0	C79.8-	—	—	—	—
lower	C41.1	C79.51	—	D16.5-	D48.0	D49.2
mucosa	C03.9	C79.89	D00.03	D10.39	D37.09	D49.0
lower	C03.1	C79.89	D00.03	D10.39	D37.09	D49.0
upper	C03.0	C79.89	D00.03	D10.39	D37.09	D49.0
upper	C41.0	C79.51	—	D16.4-	D48.0	D49.2
sulcus	C06.1	C79.89	D00.02	D10.39	D37.09	D49.0
alveolus	C03.9	C79.89	D00.03	D10.39	D37.09	D49.0
lower	C03.1	C79.89	D00.03	D10.39	D37.09	D49.0
upper	C03.0	C79.89	D00.03	D10.39	D37.09	D49.0
ampulla of Vater	C24.1	C78.89	D01.5	D13.5	D37.6	D49.0
ankle NEC	C76.5-	C79.89	D04.7-	D36.7	D48.7	D49.89
anorectum, anorectal (junction)	C21.8	C78.5	D01.3	D12.9	D37.8	D49.0
antecubital fossa or space	C76.4-	C79.89	D04.6-	D36.7	D48.7	D49.89
antrum (Highmore) (maxillary)	C31.0	C78.39	D02.3	D14.0	D38.5	D49.1
pyloric	C16.3	C78.89	D00.2	D13.1	D37.1	D49.0
tympanicum	C30.1	C78.39	D02.3	D14.0	D38.5	D49.1
anus, anal	C21.0	C78.5	D01.3	D12.9	D37.8	D49.0
canal	C21.1	C78.5	D01.3	D12.9	D37.8	D49.0
cloacogenic zone	C21.2	C78.5	D01.3	D12.9	D37.8	D49.0
margin — *see also Neoplasm, anus, skin*	C44.500	C79.2	D04.5	D23.5	D48.5	D49.2
overlapping lesion with rectosigmoid junction or rectum	C21.8	—	—	—	—	—
skin	C44.500	C79.2	D04.5	D23.5	D48.5	D49.2
basal cell carcinoma	C44.510	—	—	—	—	—
specified type NEC	C44.590	—	—	—	—	—
squamous cell carcinoma	C44.520	—	—	—	—	—
sphincter	C21.1	C78.5	D01.3	D12.9	D37.8	D49.0
aorta (thoracic)	C49.3	C79.89	—	D21.3	D48.1	D49.2
abdominal	C49.4	C79.89	—	D21.4	D48.1	D49.2
aortic body	C75.5	C79.89	—	D35.6	D44.7	D49.7
aponeurosis	C49.9	C79.89	—	D21.9	D48.1	D49.2
palmar	C49.1-	C79.89	—	D21.1-	D48.1	D49.2
plantar	C49.2-	C79.89	—	D21.2-	D48.1	D49.2

◀ New ⇐ Revised ~~deleted~~ Deleted

	Malignant Primary	Malignant Secondary	Ca in situ	Benign	Uncertain Behavior	Unspecified Behavior
appendix	C18.1	C78.5	D01.0	D12.1	D37.3	D49.0
arachnoid	C70.9	C79.49	—	D32.9	D42.9	D49.7
cerebral	C70.0	C79.32	—	D32.0	D42.0	D49.7
spinal	C70.1	C79.49	—	D32.1	D42.1	D49.7
areola	C50.0-	C79.81	D05.-	D24.-	D48.6-	D49.3
arm NEC	C76.4-	C79.89	D04.6-	D36.7	D48.7	D49.89
artery — *see Neoplasm, connective tissue*						
aryepiglottic fold	C13.1	C79.89	D00.08	D10.7	D37.05	D49.0
hypopharyngeal aspect	C13.1	C79.89	D00.08	D10.7	D37.05	D49.0
laryngeal aspect	C32.1	C78.39	D02.0	D14.1	D38.0	D49.1
marginal zone	C13.1	C79.89	D00.08	D10.7	D37.05	D49.0
arytenoid (cartilage)	C32.3	C78.39	D02.0	D14.1	D38.0	D49.1
fold — *see Neoplasm, aryepiglottic*						
associated with transplanted organ	C80.2	—	—	—	—	—
atlas	C41.2	C79.51	—	D16.6	D48.0	D49.2
atrium, cardiac	C38.0	C79.89	—	D15.1	D48.7	D49.89
auditory						
canal (external) (skin)	C44.20-	C79.2	D04.2-	D23.2-	D48.5	D49.2
internal	C30.1	C78.39	D02.3	D14.0	D38.5	D49.1
nerve	C72.4-	C79.49	—	D33.3	D43.3	D49.7
tube	C30.1	C78.39	D02.3	D14.0	D38.5	D49.1
opening	C11.2	C79.89	D00.08	D10.6	D37.05	D49.0
auricle, ear — *see also Neoplasm, skin, ear*	C44.20-	C79.2	D04.2-	D23.2-	D48.5	D49.2
auricular canal (external) — *see also Neoplasm, skin, ear*	C44.20-	C79.2	D04.2-	D23.2-	D48.5	D49.2
internal	C30.1	C78.39	D02.3	D14.0	D38.5	D49.2
autonomic nerve or nervous system NEC *(see Neoplasm, nerve, peripheral)*						
axilla, axillary	C76.1	C79.89	D09.8	D36.7	D48.7	D49.89
fold — *see also Neoplasm, skin, trunk*	C44.509	C79.2	D04.5	D23.5	D48.5	D49.2
back NEC	C76.8	C79.89	D04.5	D36.7	D48.7	D49.89
Bartholin's gland	C51.0	C79.82	D07.1	D28.0	D39.8	D49.59
basal ganglia	C71.0	C79.31	—	D33.0	D43.0	D49.6
basis pedunculi	C71.7	C79.31	—	D33.1	D43.1	D49.6
bile or biliary (tract)	C24.9	C78.89	D01.5	D13.5	D37.6	D49.0
canaliculi (biliferi) (intrahepatic)	C22.1	C78.7	D01.5	D13.4	D37.6	D49.0
canals, interlobular	C22.1	C78.89	D01.5	D13.4	D37.6	D49.0

	Malignant Primary	Malignant Secondary	Ca in situ	Benign	Uncertain Behavior	Unspecified Behavior
bile or biliary *(Continued)*						
duct or passage (common) (cystic) (extrahepatic)	C24.0	C78.89	D01.5	D13.5	D37.6	D49.0
interlobular	C22.1	C78.89	D01.5	D13.4	D37.6	D49.0
intrahepatic	C22.1	C78.7	D01.5	D13.4	D37.6	D49.0
and extrahepatic	C24.8	C78.89	D01.5	D13.5	D37.6	D49.0
bladder (urinary)	C67.9	C79.11	D09.0	D30.3	D41.4	D49.4
dome	C67.1	C79.11	D09.0	D30.3	D41.4	D49.4
neck	C67.5	C79.11	D09.0	D30.3	D41.4	D49.4
orifice	C67.9	C79.11	D09.0	D30.3	D41.4	D49.4
ureteric	C67.6	C79.11	D09.0	D30.3	D41.4	D49.4
urethral	C67.5	C79.11	D09.0	D30.3	D41.4	D49.4
overlapping lesion	C67.8	—	—	—	—	—
sphincter	C67.8	C79.11	D09.0	D30.3	D41.4	D49.4
trigone	C67.0	C79.11	D09.0	D30.3	D41.4	D49.4
urachus	C67.7	C79.11	D09.0	D30.3	D41.4	D49.4
wall	C67.9	C79.11	D09.0	D30.3	D41.4	D49.4
anterior	C67.3	C79.11	D09.0	D30.3	D41.4	D49.4
lateral	C67.2	C79.11	D09.0	D30.3	D41.4	D49.4
posterior	C67.4	C79.11	D09.0	D30.3	D41.4	D49.4
blood vessel — *see Neoplasm, connective tissue*						
bone (periosteum)	C41.9	C79.51	—	D16.9-	D48.0	D49.2
acetabulum	C41.4	C79.51	—	D16.8-	D48.0	D49.2
ankle	C40.3-	C79.51	—	D16.3-	—	—
arm NEC	C40.0-	C79.51	—	D16.0-	—	—
astragalus	C40.3-	C79.51	—	D16.3-	—	—
atlas	C41.2	C79.51	—	D16.6-	D48.0	D49.2
axis	C41.2	C79.51	—	D16.6-	D48.0	D49.2
back NEC	C41.2	C79.51	—	D16.6-	D48.0	D49.2
calcaneus	C40.3-	C79.51	—	D16.3-	—	—
calvarium	C41.0	C79.51	—	D16.4-	D48.0	D49.2
carpus (any)	C40.1-	C79.51	—	D16.1-	—	—
cartilage NEC	C41.9	C79.51	—	D16.9-	D48.0	D49.2
clavicle	C41.3	C79.51	—	D16.7-	D48.0	D49.2
clivus	C41.0	C79.51	—	D16.4-	D48.0	D49.2
coccygeal vertebra	C41.4	C79.51	—	D16.8-	D48.0	D49.2
coccyx	C41.4	C79.51	—	D16.8-	D48.0	D49.2
costal cartilage	C41.3	C79.51	—	D16.7-	D48.0	D49.2
costovertebral joint	C41.3	C79.51	—	D16.7-	D48.0	D49.2
cranial	C41.0	C79.51	—	D16.4-	D48.0	D49.2
cuboid	C40.3-	C79.51	—	D16.3-	—	—
cuneiform	C41.9	C79.51	—	D16.9-	D48.0	D49.2
elbow	C40.0-	C79.51	—	D16.0-	—	—

◀ New ⇐ Revised ~~deleted~~ Deleted

	Malignant Primary	Malignant Secondary	Ca in situ	Benign	Uncertain Behavior	Unspecified Behavior
bone *(Continued)*						
ethmoid (labyrinth)	C41.0	C79.51	—	D16.4-	D48.0	D49.2
face	C41.0	C79.51	—	D16.4-	D48.0	D49.2
femur (any part)	C40.2-	C79.51	—	D16.2-	—	—
fibula (any part)	C40.2-	C79.51	—	D16.2-	—	—
finger (any)	C40.1-	C79.51	—	D16.1-	—	—
foot	C40.3-	C79.51	—	D16.3-	—	—
forearm	C40.0-	C79.51	—	D16.0-	—	—
frontal	C41.0	C79.51	—	D16.4-	D48.0	D49.2
hand	C40.1-	C79.51	—	D16.1-	—	—
heel	C40.3-	C79.51	—	D16.3-	—	—
hip	C41.4	C79.51	—	D16.8-	D48.0	D49.2
humerus (any part)	C40.0-	C79.51	—	D16.0-	—	—
hyoid	C41.0	C79.51	—	D16.4-	D48.0	D49.2
ilium	C41.4	C79.51	—	D16.8-	D48.0	D49.2
innominate	C41.4	C79.51	—	D16.8-	D48.0	D49.2
intervertebral cartilage or disc	C41.2	C79.51	—	D16.6-	D48.0	D49.2
ischium	C41.4	C79.51	—	D16.8-	D48.0	D49.2
jaw (lower)	C41.1	C79.51	—	D16.5-	D48.0	D49.2
knee	C40.2-	C79.51	—	D16.2-	—	—
leg NEC	C40.2-	C79.51	—	D16.2-	—	—
limb NEC	C40.9-	C79.51	—	D16.9-	—	—
lower (long bones)	C40.2-	C79.51	—	D16.2-	—	—
short bones	C40.3-	C79.51	—	D16.3-	—	—
upper (long bones)	C40.0-	C79.51	—	D16.0-	—	—
short bones	C40.1-	C79.51	—	D16.1-	—	—
malar	C41.0	C79.51	—	D16.4-	D48.0	D49.2
mandible	C41.1	C79.51	—	D16.5-	D48.0	D49.2
marrow NEC (any bone)	C96.9	C79.52	—	—	D47.9	D49.89
mastoid	C41.0	C79.51	—	D16.4-	D48.0	D49.2
maxilla, maxillary (superior)	C41.0	C79.51	—	D16.4-	D48.0	D49.2
inferior	C41.1	C79.51	—	D16.5-	D48.0	D49.2
metacarpus (any)	C40.1-	C79.51	—	D16.1-	—	—
metatarsus (any)	C40.3-	C79.51	—	D16.3-	—	—
overlapping sites	C40.8-	—	—	—	—	—
navicular						
ankle	C40.3-	C79.51	—	—	—	—
hand	C40.1-	C79.51	—	—	—	—
nose, nasal	C41.0	C79.51	—	D16.4-	D48.0	D49.2
occipital	C41.0	C79.51	—	D16.4-	D48.0	D49.2
orbit	C41.0	C79.51	—	D16.4-	D48.0	D49.2
parietal	C41.0	C79.51	—	D16.4-	D48.0	D49.2
patella	C40.2-	C79.51	—	—	—	—
pelvic	C41.4	C79.51	—	D16.8	D48.0	D49.2

	Malignant Primary	Malignant Secondary	Ca in situ	Benign	Uncertain Behavior	Unspecified Behavior
bone *(Continued)*						
phalanges						
foot	C40.3-	C79.51	—	—	—	—
hand	C40.1-	C79.51	—	—	—	—
pubic	C41.4	C79.51	—	D16.8	D48.0	D49.2
radius (any part)	C40.0-	C79.51	—	D16.0-	—	—
rib	C41.3	C79.51	—	D16.7	D48.0	D49.2
sacral vertebra	C41.4	C79.51	—	D16.8	D48.0	D49.2
sacrum	C41.4	C79.51	—	D16.8	D48.0	D49.2
scaphoid					—	—
of ankle	C40.3-	C79.51	—	—	—	—
of hand	C40.1-	C79.51	—	—	—	—
scapula (any part)	C40.0-	C79.51	—	D16.0-	—	—
sella turcica	C41.0	C79.51	—	D16.4-	D48.0	D49.2
shoulder	C40.0-	C79.51	—	D16.0-	—	—
skull	C41.0	C79.51	—	D16.4-	D48.0	D49.2
sphenoid	C41.0	C79.51	—	D16.4-	D48.0	D49.2
spine, spinal (column)	C41.2	C79.51	—	D16.6	D48.0	D49.2
coccyx	C41.4	C79.51	—	D16.8	D48.0	D49.2
sacrum	C41.4	C79.51	—	D16.8	D48.0	D49.2
sternum	C41.3	C79.51	—	D16.7	D48.0	D49.2
tarsus (any)	C40.3-	C79.51	—	—	—	—
temporal	C41.0	C79.51	—	D16.4-	D48.0	D49.2
thumb	C40.1-	C79.51	—	—	—	—
tibia (any part)	C40.2-	C79.51	—	—	—	—
toe (any)	C40.3-	C79.51	—	—	—	—
trapezium	C40.1-	C79.51	—	—	—	—
trapezoid	C40.1-	C79.51	—	—	—	—
turbinate	C41.0	C79.51	—	D16.4-	D48.0	D49.2
ulna (any part)	C40.0-	C79.51	—	D16.0-	—	—
unciform	C40.1-	C79.51	—	—	—	—
vertebra (column)	C41.2	C79.51	—	D16.6	D48.0	D49.2
coccyx	C41.4	C79.51	—	D16.8	D48.0	D49.2
sacrum	C41.4	C79.51	—	D16.8	D48.0	D49.2
vomer	C41.0	C79.51	—	D16.4-	D48.0	D49.2
wrist	C40.1-	C79.51	—	—	—	—
xiphoid process	C41.3	C79.51	—	D16.7	D48.0	D49.2
zygomatic	C41.0	C79.51	—	D16.4-	D48.0	D49.2
book-leaf (mouth)	C06.89	C79.89	D00.00	D10.39	D37.09	D49.0
bowel — *see Neoplasm, intestine*						
brachial plexus	C47.1-	C79.89	—	D36.12	D48.2	D49.2
brain NEC	C71.9	C79.31	—	D33.2	D43.2	D49.6
basal ganglia	C71.0	C79.31	—	D33.0	D43.0	D49.6
cerebellopontine angle	C71.6	C79.31	—	D33.1	D43.1	D49.6

	Malignant Primary	Malignant Secondary	Ca in situ	Benign	Uncertain Behavior	Unspecified Behavior
brain NEC *(Continued)*						
cerebellum NOS	C71.6	C79.31	—	D33.1	D43.1	D49.6
cerebrum	C71.0	C79.31	—	D33.0	D43.0	D49.6
choroid plexus	C71.7	C79.31	—	D33.1	D43.1	D49.6
corpus callosum	C71.8	C79.31	—	D33.2	D43.2	D49.6
corpus striatum	C71.0	C79.31	—	D33.0	D43.0	D49.6
cortex (cerebral)	C71.0	C79.31	—	D33.0	D43.0	D49.6
frontal lobe	C71.1	C79.31	—	D33.0	D43.0	D49.6
globus pallidus	C71.0	C79.31	—	D33.0	D43.0	D49.6
hippocampus	C71.2	C79.31	—	D33.0	D43.0	D49.6
hypothalamus	C71.0	C79.31	—	D33.0	D43.0	D49.6
internal capsule	C71.0	C79.31	—	D33.0	D43.0	D49.6
medulla oblongata	C71.7	C79.31	—	D33.1	D43.1	D49.6
meninges	C70.0	C79.32	—	D32.0	D42.0	D49.7
midbrain	C71.7	C79.31	—	D33.1	D43.1	D49.6
occipital lobe	C71.4	C79.31	—	D33.0	D43.0	D49.6
overlapping lesion	C71.8	C79.31	—	—	—	—
parietal lobe	C71.3	C79.31	—	D33.0	D43.0	D49.6
peduncle	C71.7	C79.31	—	D33.1	D43.1	D49.6
pons	C71.7	C79.31	—	D33.1	D43.1	D49.6
stem	C71.7	C79.31	—	D33.1	D43.1	D49.6
tapetum	C71.8	C79.31	—	D33.2	D43.2	D49.6
temporal lobe	C71.2	C79.31	—	D33.0	D43.0	D49.6
thalamus	C71.0	C79.31	—	D33.0	D43.0	D49.6
uncus	C71.2	C79.31	—	D33.0	D43.0	D49.6
ventricle (floor)	C71.5	C79.31	—	D33.0	D43.0	D49.6
fourth	C71.7	C79.31	—	D33.1	D43.1	D49.6
branchial (cleft) (cyst) (vestiges)	C10.4	C79.89	D00.08	D10.5	D37.05	D49.0
breast (connective tissue) (glandular tissue) (soft parts)	C50.9-	C79.81	D05.-	D24.-	D48.6-	D49.3
areola	C50.0-	C79.81	D05.-	D24.-	D48.6-	D49.3
axillary tail	C50.6-	C79.81	D05.-	D24.-	D48.6-	D49.3
central portion	C50.1-	C79.81	D05.-	D24.-	D48.6-	D49.3
inner	C50.8-	C79.81	D05.-	D24.-	D48.6-	D49.3
lower	C50.8-	C79.81	D05.-	D24.-	D48.6-	D49.3
lower-inner quadrant	C50.3-	C79.81	D05.-	D24.-	D48.6-	D49.3
lower-outer quadrant	C50.5-	C79.81	D05.-	D24.-	D48.6-	D49.3
mastectomy site (skin) — *see also Neoplasm, breast, skin*	C44.501	C79.2	—	—	—	—
specified as breast tissue	C50.8-	C79.81	—	—	—	—
midline	C50.8-	C79.81	D05.-	D24.-	D48.6-	D49.3
nipple	C50.0-	C79.81	D05.-	D24.-	D48.6-	D49.3
outer	C50.8-	C79.81	D05.-	D24.-	D48.6-	D49.3
overlapping lesion	C50.8-	—	—	—	—	—

	Malignant Primary	Malignant Secondary	Ca in situ	Benign	Uncertain Behavior	Unspecified Behavior
breast *(Continued)*						
skin	C44.501	C79.2	D04.5	D23.5	D48.5	D49.2
basal cell carcinoma	C44.511	—	—	—	—	—
specified type NEC	C44.591	—	—	—	—	—
squamous cell carcinoma	C44.521	—	—	—	—	—
tail (axillary)	C50.6-	C79.81	D05.-	D24.-	D48.6-	D49.3
upper	C50.8-	C79.81	D05.-	D24.-	D48.6-	D49.3
upper-inner quadrant	C50.2-	C79.81	D05.-	D24.-	D48.6-	D49.3
upper-outer quadrant	C50.4-	C79.81	D05.-	D24.-	D48.6-	D49.3
broad ligament	C57.1	C79.82	D07.39	D28.2	D39.8	D49.59 ◄
bronchiogenic, bronchogenic (lung)	C34.9-	C78.0-	D02.2-	D14.3-	D38.1	D49.1
bronchiole	C34.9-	C78.0-	D02.2-	D14.3-	D38.1	D49.1
bronchus	C34.9-	C78.0-	D02.2-	D14.3-	D38.1	D49.1
carina	C34.0-	C78.0-	D02.2-	D14.3-	D38.1	D49.1
lower lobe of lung	C34.3-	C78.0-	D02.2-	D14.3-	D38.1	D49.1
main	C34.0-	C78.0-	D02.2-	D14.3-	D38.1	D49.1
middle lobe of lung	C34.2	C78.0-	D02.21	D14.31	D38.1	D49.1
overlapping lesion	C34.8-	—	—	—	—	—
upper lobe of lung	C34.1-	C78.0-	D02.2-	D14.3-	D38.1	D49.1
brow	C44.309	C79.2	D04.39	D23.39	D48.5	D49.2
basal cell carcinoma	C44.319	—	—	—	—	—
specified type NEC	C44.399	—	—	—	—	—
squamous cell carcinoma	C44.329	—	—	—	—	—
buccal (cavity)	C06.9	C79.89	D00.00	D10.39	D37.09	D49.0
commissure	C06.0	C79.89	D00.02	D10.39	D37.09	D49.0
groove (lower) (upper)	C06.1	C79.89	D00.02	D10.39	D37.09	D49.0
mucosa	C06.0	C79.89	D00.02	D10.39	D37.09	D49.0
sulcus (lower) (upper)	C06.1	C79.89	D00.02	D10.39	D37.09	D49.0
bulbourethral gland	C68.0	C79.19	D09.19	D30.4	D41.3	D49.59 ◄
bursa — *see Neoplasm, connective tissue*						
buttock NEC	C76.3	C79.89	D04.5	D36.7	D48.7	D49.89
calf	C76.5-	C79.89	D04.7-	D36.7	D48.7	D49.89
calvarium	C41.0	C79.51	—	D16.4-	D48.0	D49.2
calyx, renal	C65.-	C79.0-	D09.19	D30.1-	D41.1-	D49.51- ◄
canal						
anal	C21.1	C78.5	D01.3	D12.9	D37.8	D49.0
auditory (external) — *see also Neoplasm, skin, ear*	C44.20-	C79.2	D04.2-	D23.2-	D48.5	D49.2
auricular (external) — *see also Neoplasm, skin, ear*	C44.20-	C79.2	D04.2-	D23.2-	D48.5	D49.2
canaliculi, biliary (biliferi) (intrahepatic)	C22.1	C78.7	D01.5	D13.4	D37.6	D49.0

◄ New ◄ Revised ~~deleted~~ Deleted

	Malignant Primary	Malignant Secondary	Ca in situ	Benign	Uncertain Behavior	Unspecified Behavior
canthus (eye) (inner) (outer)	C44.10-	C79.2	D04.1-	D23.1-	D48.5	D49.2
basal cell carcinoma	C44.11-	—	—	—	—	—
specified type NEC	C44.19-	—	—	—	—	—
squamous cell carcinoma	C44.12-	—	—	—	—	—
capillary — *see Neoplasm, connective tissue*						
caput coli	C18.0	C78.5	D01.0	D12.0	D37.4	D49.0
carcinoid — *see Tumor, carcinoid*						
cardia (gastric)	C16.0	C78.89	D00.2	D13.1	D37.1	D49.0
cardiac orifice (stomach)	C16.0	C78.89	D00.2	D13.1	D37.1	D49.0
cardio-esophageal junction	C16.0	C78.89	D00.2	D13.1	D37.1	D49.0
cardio-esophagus	C16.0	C78.89	D00.2	D13.1	D37.1	D49.0
carina (bronchus)	C34.0-	C78.0-	D02.2-	D14.3-	D38.1	D49.1
carotid (artery)	C49.0	C79.89	—	D21.0	D48.1	D49.2
body	C75.4	C79.89	—	D35.5	D44.6	D49.7
carpus (any bone)	C40.1-	C79.51	—	D16.1-	—	—
cartilage (articular) (joint) NEC — *see also Neoplasm, bone*	C41.9	C79.51	—	D16.9-	D48.0	D49.2
arytenoid	C32.3	C78.39	D02.0	D14.1	D38.0	D49.1
auricular	C49.0	C79.89	—	D21.0	D48.1	D49.2
bronchi	C34.0-	C78.39	—	D14.3-	D38.1	D49.1
costal	C41.3	C79.51	—	D16.7	D48.0	D49.2
cricoid	C32.3	C78.39	D02.0	D14.1	D38.0	D49.1
cuneiform	C32.3	C78.39	D02.0	D14.1	D38.0	D49.1
ear (external)	C49.0	C79.89	—	D21.0	D48.1	D49.2
ensiform	C41.3	C79.51	—	D16.7	D48.0	D49.2
epiglottis	C32.1	C78.39	D02.0	D14.1	D38.0	D49.1
anterior surface	C10.1	C79.89	D00.08	D10.5	D37.05	D49.0
eyelid	C49.0	C79.89	—	D21.0	D48.1	D49.2
intervertebral	C41.2	C79.51	—	D16.6	D48.0	D49.2
larynx, laryngeal	C32.3	C78.39	D02.0	D14.1	D38.0	D49.1
nose, nasal	C30.0	C78.39	D02.3	D14.0	D38.5	D49.1
pinna	C49.0	C79.89	—	D21.0	D48.1	D49.2
rib	C41.3	C79.51	—	D16.7	D48.0	D49.2
semilunar (knee)	C40.2-	C79.51	—	D16.2-	D48.0	D49.2
thyroid	C32.3	C78.39	D02.0	D14.1	D38.0	D49.1
trachea	C33	C78.39	D02.1	D14.2	D38.1	D49.1
cauda equina	C72.1	C79.49	—	D33.4	D43.4	D49.7
cavity						
buccal	C06.9	C79.89	D00.00	D10.30	D37.09	D49.0
nasal	C30.0	C78.39	D02.3	D14.0	D38.5	D49.1
oral	C06.9	C79.89	D00.00	D10.30	D37.09	D49.0
peritoneal	C48.2	C78.6	—	D20.1	D48.4	D49.0
tympanic	C30.1	C78.39	D02.3	D14.0	D38.5	D49.1

	Malignant Primary	Malignant Secondary	Ca in situ	Benign	Uncertain Behavior	Unspecified Behavior
cecum	C18.0	C78.5	D01.0	D12.0	D37.4	D49.0
central nervous system	C72.9	C79.40	—	—	—	—
cerebellopontine (angle)	C71.6	C79.31	—	D33.1	D43.1	D49.6
cerebellum, cerebellar	C71.6	C79.31	—	D33.1	D43.1	D49.6
cerebrum, cerebral (cortex) (hemisphere) (white matter)	C71.0	C79.31	—	D33.0	D43.0	D49.6
meninges	C70.0	C79.32	—	D32.0	D42.0	D49.7
peduncle	C71.7	C79.31	—	D33.1	D43.1	D49.6
ventricle	C71.5	C79.31	—	D33.0	D43.0	D49.6
fourth	C71.7	C79.31	—	D33.1	D43.1	D49.6
cervical region	C76.0	C79.89	D09.8	D36.7	D48.7	D49.89
cervix (cervical) (uteri) (uterus)	C53.9	C79.82	D06.9	D26.0	D39.0	D49.59 ⇐
canal	C53.0	C79.82	D06.0	D26.0	D39.0	D49.59 ⇐
endocervix (canal) (gland)	C53.0	C79.82	D06.0	D26.0	D39.0	D49.59 ⇐
exocervix	C53.1	C79.82	D06.1	D26.0	D39.0	D49.59 ⇐
external os	C53.1	C79.82	D06.1	D26.0	D39.0	D49.59 ⇐
internal os	C53.0	C79.82	D06.0	D26.0	D39.0	D49.59 ⇐
nabothian gland	C53.0	C79.82	D06.0	D26.0	D39.0	D49.59 ⇐
overlapping lesion	C53.8	—	—	—	—	—
squamocolumnar junction	C53.8	C79.82	D06.7	D26.0	D39.0	D49.59 ⇐
stump	C53.8	C79.82	D06.7	D26.0	D39.0	D49.59 ⇐
cheek	C76.0	C79.89	D09.8	D36.7	D48.7	D49.89
external	C44.309	C79.2	D04.39	D23.39	D48.5	D49.2
basal cell carcinoma	C44.319	—	—	—	—	—
specified type NEC	C44.399	—	—	—	—	—
squamous cell carcinoma	C44.329	—	—	—	—	—
inner aspect	C06.0	C79.89	D00.02	D10.39	D37.09	D49.0
internal	C06.0	C79.89	D00.02	D10.39	D37.09	D49.0
mucosa	C06.0	C79.89	D00.02	D10.39	D37.09	D49.0
chest (wall) NEC	C76.1	C79.89	D09.8	D36.7	D48.7	D49.89
chiasma opticum	C72.3-	C79.49	—	D33.3	D43.3	D49.7
chin	C44.309	C79.2	D04.39	D23.39	D48.5	D49.2
basal cell carcinoma	C44.319	—	—	—	—	—
specified type NEC	C44.399	—	—	—	—	—
squamous cell carcinoma	C44.329	—	—	—	—	—
choana	C11.3	C79.89	D00.08	D10.6	D37.05	D49.0
cholangiole	C22.1	C78.89	D01.5	D13.4	D37.6	D49.0
choledochal duct	C24.0	C78.89	D01.5	D13.5	D37.6	D49.0
choroid	C69.3-	C79.49	D09.2-	D31.3-	D48.7	D49.81
plexus	C71.5	C79.31	—	D33.0	D43.0	D49.6
ciliary body	C69.4-	C79.49	D09.2-	D31.4-	D48.7	D49.89
clavicle	C41.3	C79.51	—	D16.7	D48.0	D49.2
clitoris	C51.2	C79.82	D07.1	D28.0	D39.8	D49.59 ⇐
clivus	C41.0	C79.51	—	D16.4-	D48.0	D49.2

◀ New ⇐ Revised ~~deleted~~ Deleted

	Malignant Primary	Malignant Secondary	Ca in situ	Benign	Uncertain Behavior	Unspecified Behavior
cloacogenic zone	C21.2	C78.5	D01.3	D12.9	D37.8	D49.0
coccygeal						
body or glomus	C49.5	C79.89	—	D21.5	D48.1	D49.2
vertebra	C41.4	C79.51	—	D16.8	D48.0	D49.2
coccyx	C41.4	C79.51	—	D16.8	D48.0	D49.2
colon — *see also Neoplasm, intestine, large*	C18.9	C78.5	—	—	—	—
with rectum	C19	C78.5	D01.1	D12.7	D37.5	D49.0
column, spinal — *see Neoplasm, spine*						
columnella — *see also Neoplasm, skin, face*	C44.390	C79.2	D04.39	D23.39	D48.5	D49.2
commissure						
labial, lip	C00.6	C79.89	D00.01	D10.39	D37.01	D49.0
laryngeal	C32.0	C78.39	D02.0	D14.1	D38.0	D49.1
common (bile) duct	C24.0	C78.89	D01.5	D13.5	D37.6	D49.0
concha — *see also Neoplasm, skin, ear*	C44.20-	C79.2	D04.2-	D23.2-	D48.5	D49.2
nose	C30.0	C78.39	D02.3	D14.0	D38.5	D49.1
conjunctiva	C69.0-	C79.49	D09.2-	D31.0-	D48.7	D49.89
connective tissue NEC	C49.9	C79.89	—	D21.9	D48.1	D49.2
Note: For neoplasms of connective tissue (blood vessel, bursa, fascia, ligament, muscle, peripheral nerves, sympathetic and parasympathetic nerves and ganglia, synovia, tendon, etc.) or of morphological types that indicate connective tissue, code according to the list under "Neoplasm, connective tissue". For sites that do not appear in this list, code to neoplasm of that site; e.g., fibrosarcoma, pancreas (C25.9)						
Note: Morphological types that indicate connective tissue appear in their proper place in the alphabetic index with the instruction "*see Neoplasm, connective tissue ....*"						
abdomen	C49.4	C79.89	—	D21.4	D48.1	D49.2
abdominal wall	C49.4	C79.89	—	D21.4	D48.1	D49.2
ankle	C49.2-	C79.89	—	D21.2-	D48.1	D49.2
antecubital fossa or space	C49.1-	C79.89	—	D21.1-	D48.1	D49.2
arm	C49.1-	C79.89	—	D21.1-	D48.1	D49.2
auricle (ear)	C49.0	C79.89	—	D21.0	D48.1	D49.2
axilla	C49.3	C79.89	—	D21.3	D48.1	D49.2
back	C49.6	C79.89	—	D21.6	D48.1	D49.2
breast — *see Neoplasm, breast*						
buttock	C49.5	C79.89	—	D21.5	D48.1	D49.2
calf	C49.2-	C79.89	—	D21.2-	D48.1	D49.2
cervical region	C49.0	C79.89	—	D21.0	D48.1	D49.2
cheek	C49.0	C79.89	—	D21.0	D48.1	D49.2
chest (wall)	C49.3	C79.89	—	D21.3	D48.1	D49.2
chin	C49.0	C79.89	—	D21.0	D48.1	D49.2

	Malignant Primary	Malignant Secondary	Ca in situ	Benign	Uncertain Behavior	Unspecified Behavior
connective tissue NEC *(Continued)*						
diaphragm	C49.3	C79.89	—	D21.3	D48.1	D49.2
ear (external)	C49.0	C79.89	—	D21.0	D48.1	D49.2
elbow	C49.1-	C79.89	—	D21.1-	D48.1	D49.2
extrarectal	C49.5	C79.89	—	D21.5	D48.1	D49.2
extremity	C49.9	C79.89	—	D21.9	D48.1	D49.2
lower	C49.2-	C79.89	—	D21.2-	D48.1	D49.2
upper	C49.1-	C79.89	—	D21.1-	D48.1	D49.2
eyelid	C49.0	C79.89	—	D21.0	D48.1	D49.2
face	C49.0	C79.89	—	D21.0	D48.1	D49.2
finger	C49.1-	C79.89	—	D21.1-	D48.1	D49.2
flank	C49.6	C79.89	—	D21.6	D48.1	D49.2
foot	C49.2-	C79.89	—	D21.2-	D48.1	D49.2
forearm	C49.1-	C79.89	—	D21.1-	D48.1	D49.2
forehead	C49.0	C79.89	—	D21.0	D48.1	D49.2
gastric	C49.4	C79.89	—	D21.4	D48.1	D49.2
gastrointestinal	C49.4	C79.89	—	D21.4	D48.1	D49.2
gluteal region	C49.5	C79.89	—	D21.5	D48.1	D49.2
great vessels NEC	C49.3	C79.89	—	D21.3	D48.1	D49.2
groin	C49.5	C79.89	—	D21.5	D48.1	D49.2
hand	C49.1-	C79.89	—	D21.1-	D48.1	D49.2
head	C49.0	C79.89	—	D21.0	D48.1	D49.2
heel	C49.2-	C79.89	—	D21.2-	D48.1	D49.2
hip	C49.2-	C79.89	—	D21.2-	D48.1	D49.2
hypochondrium	C49.4	C79.89	—	D21.4	D48.1	D49.2
iliopsoas muscle	C49.5	C79.89	—	D21.5	D48.1	D49.2
infraclavicular region	C49.3	C79.89	—	D21.3	D48.1	D49.2
inguinal (canal) (region)	C49.5	C79.89	—	D21.5	D48.1	D49.2
intestinal	C49.4	C79.89	—	D21.4	D48.1	D49.2
intrathoracic	C49.3	C79.89	—	D21.3	D48.1	D49.2
ischiorectal fossa	C49.5	C79.89	—	D21.5	D48.1	D49.2
jaw	C03.9	C79.89	D00.03	D10.39	D48.1	D49.0
knee	C49.2-	C79.89	—	D21.2-	D48.1	D49.2
leg	C49.2-	C79.89	—	D21.2-	D48.1	D49.2
limb NEC	C49.9	C79.89	—	D21.9	D48.1	D49.2
lower	C49.2-	C79.89	—	D21.2-	D48.1	D49.2
upper	C49.1-	C79.89	—	D21.1-	D48.1	D49.2
nates	C49.5	C79.89	—	D21.5	D48.1	D49.2
neck	C49.0	C79.89	—	D21.0	D48.1	D49.2
orbit	C69.6-	C79.49	D09.2-	D31.6-	D48.1	D49.89
overlapping lesion	C49.8	—	—	—	—	—
pararectal	C49.5	C79.89	—	D21.5	D48.1	D49.2
para-urethral	C49.5	C79.89	—	D21.5	D48.1	D49.2
paravaginal	C49.5	C79.89	—	D21.5	D48.1	D49.2

	Malignant Primary	Malignant Secondary	Ca in situ	Benign	Uncertain Behavior	Unspecified Behavior
connective tissue NEC *(Continued)*						
pelvis (floor)	C49.5	C79.89	—	D21.5	D48.1	D49.2
pelvo-abdominal	C49.8	C79.89	—	D21.6	D48.1	D49.2
perineum	C49.5	C79.89	—	D21.5	D48.1	D49.2
perirectal (tissue)	C49.5	C79.89	—	D21.5	D48.1	D49.2
periurethral (tissue)	C49.5	C79.89	—	D21.5	D48.1	D49.2
popliteal fossa or space	C49.2-	C79.89	—	D21.2-	D48.1	D49.2
presacral	C49.5	C79.89	—	D21.5	D48.1	D49.2
psoas muscle	C49.4	C79.89	—	D21.4	D48.1	D49.2
pterygoid fossa	C49.0	C79.89	—	D21.0	D48.1	D49.2
rectovaginal septum or wall	C49.5	C79.89	—	D21.5	D48.1	D49.2
rectovesical	C49.5	C79.89	—	D21.5	D48.1	D49.2
retroperitoneum	C48.0	C78.6	—	D20.0	D48.3	D49.0
sacrococcygeal region	C49.5	C79.89	—	D21.5	D48.1	D49.2
scalp	C49.0	C79.89	—	D21.0	D48.1	D49.2
scapular region	C49.3	C79.89	—	D21.3	D48.1	D49.2
shoulder	C49.1-	C79.89	—	D21.1-	D48.1	D49.2
skin (dermis) NEC — *see also Neoplasm, skin, by site*	C44.90	C79.2	D04.9	D23.9	D48.5	D49.2
stomach	C49.4	C79.89	—	D21.4	D48.1	D49.2
submental	C49.0	C79.89	—	D21.0	D48.1	D49.2
supraclavicular region	C49.0	C79.89	—	D21.0	D48.1	D49.2
temple	C49.0	C79.89	—	D21.0	D48.1	D49.2
temporal region	C49.0	C79.89	—	D21.0	D48.1	D49.2
thigh	C49.2-	C79.89	—	D21.2-	D48.1	D49.2
thoracic (duct) (wall)	C49.3	C79.89	—	D21.3	D48.1	D49.2
thorax	C49.3	C79.89	—	D21.3	D48.1	D49.2
thumb	C49.1-	C79.89	—	D21.1-	D48.1	D49.2
toe	C49.2-	C79.89	—	D21.2-	D48.1	D49.2
trunk	C49.6	C79.89	—	D21.6	D48.1	D49.2
umbilicus	C49.4	C79.89	—	D21.4	D48.1	D49.2
vesicorectal	C49.5	C79.89	—	D21.5	D48.1	D49.2
wrist	C49.1-	C79.89	—	D21.1-	D48.1	D49.2
conus medullaris	C72.0	C79.49	—	D33.4	D43.4	D49.7
cord (true) (vocal)	C32.0	C78.39	D02.0	D14.1	D38.0	D49.1
false	C32.1	C78.39	D02.0	D14.1	D38.0	D49.1
spermatic	C63.1-	C79.82	D07.69	D29.8	D40.8	D49.59
spinal (cervical) (lumbar) (thoracic)	C72.0	C79.49	—	D33.4	D43.4	D49.7
cornea (limbus)	C69.1-	C79.49	D09.2-	D31.1-	D48.7	D49.89
corpus						
albicans	C56.-	C79.6-	D07.39	D27.-	D39.1-	D49.59
callosum, brain	C71.0	C79.31	—	D33.2	D43.2	D49.6
cavernosum	C60.2	C79.82	D07.4	D29.0	D40.8	D49.59

	Malignant Primary	Malignant Secondary	Ca in situ	Benign	Uncertain Behavior	Unspecified Behavior
corpus *(Continued)*						
gastric	C16.2	C78.89	D00.2	D13.1	D37.1	D49.0
overlapping sites	C54.8	—	—	—	—	—
penis	C60.2	C79.82	D07.4	D29.0	D40.8	D49.59
striatum, cerebrum	C71.0	C79.31	—	D33.0	D43.0	D49.6
uteri	C54.9	C79.82	D07.0	D26.1	D39.0	D49.59
isthmus	C54.0	C79.82	D07.0	D26.1	D39.0	D49.59
cortex						
adrenal	C74.0-	C79.7-	D09.3	D35.0-	D44.1-	D49.7
cerebral	C71.0	C79.31	—	D33.0	D43.0	D49.6
costal cartilage	C41.3	C79.51	—	D16.7	D48.0	D49.2
costovertebral joint	C41.3	C79.51	—	D16.7	D48.0	D49.2
Cowper's gland	C68.0	C79.19	D09.19	D30.4	D41.3	D49.59
cranial (fossa, any)	C71.9	C79.31	—	D33.2	D43.2	D49.6
meninges	C70.0	C79.32	—	D32.0	D42.0	D49.7
nerve	C72.50	C79.49	—	D33.3	D43.3	D49.7
specified NEC	C72.59	C79.49	—	D33.3	D43.3	D49.7
craniobuccal pouch	C75.2	C79.89	D09.3	D35.2	D44.3	D49.7
craniopharyngeal (duct) (pouch)	C75.2	C79.89	D09.3	D35.3	D44.4	D49.7
cricoid	C13.0	C79.89	D00.08	D10.7	D37.05	D49.0
cartilage	C32.3	C78.39	D02.0	D14.1	D38.0	D49.1
cricopharynx	C13.0	C79.89	D00.08	D10.7	D37.05	D49.0
crypt of Morgagni	C21.8	C78.5	D01.3	D12.9	D37.8	D49.0
crystalline lens	C69.4-	C79.49	D09.2-	D31.4-	D48.7	D49.89
cul-de-sac (Douglas')	C48.1	C78.6	—	D20.1	D48.4	D49.0
cuneiform cartilage	C32.3	C78.39	D02.0	D14.1	D38.0	D49.1
cutaneous — *see Neoplasm, skin*						
cutis — *see Neoplasm, skin*						
cystic (bile) duct (common)	C24.0	C78.89	D01.5	D13.5	D37.6	D49.0
dermis — *see Neoplasm, skin*						
diaphragm	C49.3	C79.89	—	D21.3	D48.1	D49.2
digestive organs, system, tube, or tract NEC	C26.9	C78.89	D01.9	D13.9	D37.9	D49.0
disc, intervertebral	C41.2	C79.51	—	D16.6	D48.0	D49.2
disease, generalized	C80.0	—	—	—	—	—
disseminated	C80.0	—	—	—	—	—
Douglas' cul-de-sac or pouch	C48.1	C78.6	—	D20.1	D48.4	D49.0
duodenojejunal junction	C17.8	C78.4	D01.49	D13.39	D37.2	D49.0
duodenum	C17.0	C78.4	D01.49	D13.2	D37.2	D49.0
dura (cranial) (mater)	C70.9	C79.49	—	D32.9	D42.9	D49.7
cerebral	C70.0	C79.32	—	D32.0	D42.0	D49.7
spinal	C70.1	C79.49	—	D32.1	D42.1	D49.7

◀ New ⇐ Revised ~~deleted~~ Deleted

	Malignant Primary	Malignant Secondary	Ca in situ	Benign	Uncertain Behavior	Unspecified Behavior
ear (external) — *see also Neoplasm, skin, ear*	C44.20-	C79.2	D04.2-	D23.2-	D48.5	D49.2
auricle or auris — *see also Neoplasm, skin, ear*	C44.20-	C79.2	D04.2-	D23.2-	D48.5	D49.2
canal, external — *see also Neoplasm, skin, ear*	C44.20-	C79.2	D04.2-	D23.2-	D48.5	D49.2
cartilage	C49.0	C79.89	—	D21.0	D48.1	D49.2
external meatus — *see also Neoplasm, skin, ear*	C44.20-	C79.2	D04.2-	D23.2-	D48.5	D49.2
inner	C30.1	C78.39	D02.3	D14.0	D38.5	D49.1
lobule — *see also Neoplasm, skin, ear*	C44.20-	C79.2	D04.2-	D23.2-	D48.5	D49.2
middle	C30.1	C78.39	D02.3	D14.0	D38.5	D49.1
overlapping lesion with accessory sinuses	C31.8	—	—	—	—	—
skin	C44.20-	C79.2	D04.2-	D23.2-	D48.5	D49.2
basal cell carcinoma	C44.21-	—	—	—	—	—
specified type NEC	C44.29-	—	—	—	—	—
squamous cell carcinoma	C44.22-	—	—	—	—	—
earlobe	C44.20-	C79.2	D04.2-	D23.2-	D48.5	D49.2
basal cell carcinoma	C44.21-	—	—	—	—	—
specified type NEC	C44.29-	—	—	—	—	—
squamous cell carcinoma	C44.22-	—	—	—	—	—
ejaculatory duct	C63.7	C79.82	D07.69	D29.8	D40.8	D49.59
elbow NEC	C76.4-	C79.89	D04.6-	D36.7	D48.7	D49.89
endocardium	C38.0	C79.89	—	D15.1	D48.7	D49.89
endocervix (canal) (gland)	C53.0	C79.82	D06.0	D26.0	D39.0	D49.59
endocrine gland NEC	C75.9	C79.89	D09.3	D35.9	D44.9	D49.7
pluriglandular	C75.8	C79.89	D09.3	D35.7	D44.9	D49.7
endometrium (gland) (stroma)	C54.1	C79.82	D07.0	D26.1	D39.0	D49.59
ensiform cartilage	C41.3	C79.51	—	D16.7	D48.0	D49.2
enteric — *see Neoplasm, intestine*						
ependyma (brain)	C71.5	C79.31	—	D33.0	D43.0	D49.6
fourth ventricle	C71.7	C79.31	—	D33.1	D43.1	D49.6
epicardium	C38.0	C79.89	—	D15.1	D48.7	D49.89
epididymis	C63.0-	C79.82	D07.69	D29.3-	D40.8	D49.59
epidural	C72.9	C79.49	—	D33.9	D43.9	D49.7
epiglottis	C32.1	C78.39	D02.0	D14.1	D38.0	D49.1
anterior aspect or surface	C10.1	C79.89	D00.08	D10.5	D37.05	D49.0
cartilage	C32.3	C78.39	D02.0	D14.1	D38.0	D49.1
free border (margin)	C10.1	C79.89	D00.08	D10.5	D37.05	D49.0
junctional region	C10.8	C79.89	D00.08	D10.5	D37.05	D49.0
posterior (laryngeal) surface	C32.1	C78.39	D02.0	D14.1	D38.0	D49.1
suprahyoid portion	C32.1	C78.39	D02.0	D14.1	D38.0	D49.1

	Malignant Primary	Malignant Secondary	Ca in situ	Benign	Uncertain Behavior	Unspecified Behavior
esophagogastric junction	C16.0	C78.89	D00.2	D13.1	D37.1	D49.0
esophagus	C15.9	C78.89	D00.1	D13.0	D37.8	D49.0
abdominal	C15.5	C78.89	D00.1	D13.0	D37.8	D49.0
cervical	C15.3	C78.89	D00.1	D13.0	D37.8	D49.0
distal (third)	C15.5	C78.89	D00.1	D13.0	D37.8	D49.0
lower (third)	C15.5	C78.89	D00.1	D13.0	D37.8	D49.0
middle (third)	C15.4	C78.89	D00.1	D13.0	D37.8	D49.0
overlapping lesion	C15.8	—	—	—	—	—
proximal (third)	C15.3	C78.89	D00.1	D13.0	D37.8	D49.0
thoracic	C15.4	C78.89	D00.1	D13.0	D37.8	D49.0
upper (third)	C15.3	C78.89	D00.1	D13.0	D37.8	D49.0
ethmoid (sinus)	C31.1	C78.39	D02.3	D14.0	D38.5	D49.1
bone or labyrinth	C41.0	C79.51	—	D16.4-	D48.0	D49.2
eustachian tube	C30.1	C78.39	D02.3	D14.0	D38.5	D49.1
exocervix	C53.1	C79.82	D06.1	D26.0	D39.0	D49.59
external						
meatus (ear) — *see also Neoplasm, skin, ear*	C44.20-	C79.2	D04.2-	D23.2-	D48.5	D49.2
os, cervix uteri	C53.1	C79.82	D06.1	D26.0	D39.0	D49.59
extradural	C72.9	C79.49	—	D33.9	D43.9	D49.7
extrahepatic (bile) duct	C24.0	C78.89	D01.5	D13.5	D37.6	D49.0
overlapping lesion with gallbladder	C24.8	—	—	—	—	—
extraocular muscle	C69.6-	C79.49	D09.2-	D31.6-	D48.7	D49.89
extrarectal	C76.3	C79.89	D09.8	D36.7	D48.7	D49.89
extremity	C76.8	C79.89	D04.8	D36.7	D48.7	D49.89
lower	C76.5-	C79.89	D04.7-	D36.7	D48.7	D49.89
upper	C76.4-	C79.89	D04.6-	D36.7	D48.7	D49.89
eye NEC	C69.9-	C79.49	D09.2	D31.9	D48.7	D49.89
overlapping sites	C69.8	—	—	—	—	—
eyeball	C69.9-	C79.49	D09.2-	D31.9-	D48.7	D49.89
eyebrow	C44.309	C79.2	D04.39	D23.39	D48.5	D49.2
basal cell carcinoma	C44.319	—	—	—	—	—
specified type NEC	C44.399	—	—	—	—	—
squamous cell carcinoma	C44.329	—	—	—	—	—
eyelid (lower) (skin) (upper)	C44.10-	—	—	—	—	—
basal cell carcinoma	C44.11-	—	—	—	—	—
cartilage	C49.0	C79.89	—	D21.0	D48.1	D49.2
specified type NEC	C44.19-	—	—	—	—	—
squamous cell carcinoma	C44.12-	—	—	—	—	—
face NEC	C76.0	C79.89	D04.39	D36.7	D48.7	D49.89
fallopian tube (accessory)	C57.0-	C79.82	D07.39	D28.2	D39.8	D49.59
falx (cerebella) (cerebri)	C70.0	C79.32	—	D32.0	D42.0	D49.7

◀ New ⇐ Revised ~~deleted~~ Deleted

	Malignant Primary	Malignant Secondary	Ca in situ	Benign	Uncertain Behavior	Unspecified Behavior
fascia — *see also Neoplasm, connective tissue*						
palmar	C49.1-	C79.89	—	D21.1-	D48.1	D49.2
plantar	C49.2-	C79.89	—	D21.2-	D48.1	D49.2
fatty tissue — *see Neoplasm, connective tissue*						
fauces, faucial NEC	C10.9	C79.89	D00.08	D10.5	D37.05	D49.0
pillars	C09.1	C79.89	D00.08	D10.5	D37.05	D49.0
tonsil	C09.9	C79.89	D00.08	D10.4	D37.05	D49.0
femur (any part)	C40.2-	—	—	D16.2-	—	—
fetal membrane	C58	C79.82	D07.0	D26.7	D39.2	D49.59
fibrous tissue — *see Neoplasm, connective tissue*						
fibula (any part)	C40.2-	C79.51	—	D16.2-	—	—
filum terminale	C72.0	C79.49	—	D33.4	D43.4	D49.7
finger NEC	C76.4-	C79.89	D04.6-	D36.7	D48.7	D49.89
flank NEC	C76.8	C79.89	D04.5	D36.7	D48.7	D49.89
follicle, nabothian	C53.0	C79.82	D06.0	D26.0	D39.0	D49.59
foot NEC	C76.5-	C79.89	D04.7-	D36.7	D48.7	D49.89
forearm NEC	C76.4-	C79.89	D04.6-	D36.7	D48.7	D49.89
forehead (skin)	C44.309	C79.2	D04.39	D23.39	D48.5	D49.2
basal cell carcinoma	C44.319	—	—	—	—	—
specified type NEC	C44.399	—	—	—	—	—
squamous cell carcinoma	C44.329	—	—	—	—	—
foreskin	C60.0	C79.82	D07.4	D29.0	D40.8	D49.59
fornix						
pharyngeal	C11.3	C79.89	D00.08	D10.6	D37.05	D49.0
vagina	C52	C79.82	D07.2	D28.1	D39.8	D49.59
fossa (of)						
anterior (cranial)	C71.9	C79.31	—	D33.2	D43.2	D49.6
cranial	C71.9	C79.31	—	D33.2	D43.2	D49.6
ischiorectal	C76.3	C79.89	D09.8	D36.7	D48.7	D49.89
middle (cranial)	C71.9	C79.31	—	D33.2	D43.2	D49.6
piriform	C12	C79.89	D00.08	D10.7	D37.05	D49.0
pituitary	C75.1	C79.89	D09.3	D35.2	D44.3	D49.7
posterior (cranial)	C71.9	C79.31	—	D33.2	D43.2	D49.6
pterygoid	C49.0	C79.89	—	D21.0	D48.1	D49.2
pyriform	C12	C79.89	D00.08	D10.7	D37.05	D49.0
Rosenmuller	C11.2	C79.89	D00.08	D10.6	D37.05	D49.0
tonsillar	C09.0	C79.89	D00.08	D10.5	D37.05	D49.0
fourchette	C51.9	C79.82	D07.1	D28.0	D39.8	D49.59
frenulum						
labii — *see Neoplasm, lip, internal*						
linguae	C02.2	C79.89	D00.07	D10.1	D37.02	D49.0

	Malignant Primary	Malignant Secondary	Ca in situ	Benign	Uncertain Behavior	Unspecified Behavior
frontal						
bone	C41.0	C79.51	—	D16.4-	D48.0	D49.2
lobe, brain	C71.1	C79.31	—	D33.0	D43.0	D49.6
pole	C71.1	C79.31	—	D33.0	D43.0	D49.6
sinus	C31.2	C78.39	D02.3	D14.0	D38.5	D49.1
fundus						
stomach	C16.1	C78.89	D00.2	D13.1	D37.1	D49.0
uterus	C54.3	C79.82	D07.0	D26.1	D39.0	D49.59
gall duct (extrahepatic)	C24.0	C78.89	D01.5	D13.5	D37.6	D49.0
intrahepatic	C22.1	C78.7	D01.5	D13.4	D37.6	D49.0
gallbladder	C23	C78.89	D01.5	D13.5	D37.6	D49.0
overlapping lesion with extrahepatic bile ducts	C24.8	—	—	—	—	—
ganglia — *see also Neoplasm, nerve, peripheral*	C47.9	C79.89	—	D36.10	D48.2	D49.2
basal	C71.0	C79.31	—	D33.0	D43.0	D49.6
cranial nerve	C72.50	C79.49	—	D33.3	D43.3	D49.7
Gartner's duct	C52	C79.82	D07.2	D28.1	D39.8	D49.59
gastric — *see Neoplasm, stomach*						
gastrocolic	C26.9	C78.89	D01.9	D13.9	D37.9	D49.0
gastroesophageal junction	C16.0	C78.89	D00.2	D13.1	D37.1	D49.0
gastrointestinal (tract) NEC	C26.9	C78.89	D01.9	D13.9	D37.9	D49.0
generalized	C80.0	—	—	—	—	—
genital organ or tract						
female NEC	C57.9	C79.82	D07.30	D28.9	D39.9	D49.59
overlapping lesion	C57.8	—	—	—	—	—
specified site NEC	C57.7	C79.82	D07.39	D28.7	D39.8	D49.59
male NEC	C63.9	C79.82	D07.60	D29.9	D40.9	D49.59
overlapping lesion	C63.8	—	—	—	—	—
specified site NEC	C63.7	C79.82	D07.69	D29.8	D40.8	D49.59
genitourinary tract						
female	C57.9	C79.82	D07.30	D28.9	D39.9	D49.59
male	C63.9	C79.82	D07.60	D29.9	D40.9	D49.59
gingiva (alveolar) (marginal)	C03.9	C79.89	D00.03	D10.39	D37.09	D49.0
lower	C03.1	C79.89	D00.03	D10.39	D37.09	D49.0
mandibular	C03.1	C79.89	D00.03	D10.39	D37.09	D49.0
maxillary	C03.0	C79.89	D00.03	D10.39	D37.09	D49.0
upper	C03.0	C79.89	D00.03	D10.39	D37.09	D49.0
gland, glandular (lymphatic) (system) — *see also Neoplasm, lymph gland*						
endocrine NEC	C75.9	C79.89	D09.3	D35.9	D44.9	D49.7
salivary — *see Neoplasm, salivary gland*						

◀ New ◀ Revised ~~deleted~~ Deleted

	Malignant Primary	Malignant Secondary	Ca in situ	Benign	Uncertain Behavior	Unspecified Behavior
glans penis	C60.1	C79.82	D07.4	D29.0	D40.8	D49.59
globus pallidus	C71.0	C79.31	—	D33.0	D43.0	D49.6
glomus						
coccygeal	C49.5	C79.89	—	D21.5	D48.1	D49.2
jugularis	C75.5	C79.89	—	D35.6	D44.7	D49.7
glosso-epiglottic fold(s)	C10.1	C79.89	D00.08	D10.5	D37.05	D49.0
glossopalatine fold	C09.1	C79.89	D00.08	D10.5	D37.05	D49.0
glossopharyngeal sulcus	C09.0	C79.89	D00.08	D10.5	D37.05	D49.0
glottis	C32.0	C78.39	D02.0	D14.1	D38.0	D49.1
gluteal region	C76.3	C79.89	D04.5	D36.7	D48.7	D49.89
great vessels NEC	C49.3	C79.89	—	D21.3	D48.1	D49.2
groin NEC	C76.3	C79.89	D04.5	D36.7	D48.7	D49.89
gum	C03.9	C79.89	D00.03	D10.39	D37.09	D49.0
lower	C03.1	C79.89	D00.03	D10.39	D37.09	D49.0
upper	C03.0	C79.89	D00.03	D10.39	D37.09	D49.0
hand NEC	C76.4-	C79.89	D04.6-	D36.7	D48.7	D49.89
head NEC	C76.0	C79.89	D04.4	D36.7	D48.7	D49.89
heart	C38.0	C79.89	—	D15.1	D48.7	D49.89
heel NEC	C76.5-	C79.89	D04.7-	D36.7	D48.7	D49.89
helix — *see also Neoplasm, skin, ear*	C44.20-	C79.2	D04.2-	D23.2-	D48.5	D49.2
hematopoietic, hemopoietic tissue NEC	C96.9	—	—	—	—	—
specified NEC	C96.Z	—	—	—	—	—
hemisphere, cerebral	C71.0	C79.31	—	D33.0	D43.0	D49.6
hemorrhoidal zone	C21.1	C78.5	D01.3	D12.9	D37.8	D49.0
hepatic — *see also Index to disease, by histology*	C22.9	C78.7	D01.5	D13.4	D37.6	D49.0
duct (bile)	C24.0	C78.89	D01.5	D13.5	D37.6	D49.0
flexure (colon)	C18.3	C78.5	D01.0	D12.3	D37.4	D49.0
primary	C22.8	C78.7	D01.5	D13.4	D37.6	D49.0
hepatobiliary	C24.9	C79.89	D01.5	D13.5	D37.6	D49.0
hepatoblastoma	C22.2	C78.7	D01.5	D13.4	D37.6	D49.0
hepatoma	C22.0	C78.7	D01.5	D13.4	D37.6	D49.0
hilus of lung	C34.0-	C78.0-	D02.2-	D14.3-	D38.1	D49.1
hip NEC	C76.5-	C79.89	D04.7-	D36.7	D48.7	D49.89
hippocampus, brain	C71.2	C79.31	—	D33.0	D43.0	D49.6
humerus (any part)	C40.0-	C79.51	—	D16.0-	—	—
hymen	C52	C79.82	D07.2	D28.1	D39.8	D49.59
hypopharynx, hypopharyngeal NEC	C13.9	C79.89	D00.08	D10.7	D37.05	D49.0
overlapping lesion	C13.8	—	—	—	—	—
postcricoid region	C13.0	C79.89	D00.08	D10.7	D37.05	D49.0
posterior wall	C13.2	C79.89	D00.08	D10.7	D37.05	D49.0
pyriform fossa (sinus)	C12	C79.89	D00.08	D10.7	D37.05	D49.0
hypophysis	C75.1	C79.89	D09.3	D35.2	D44.3	D49.7

	Malignant Primary	Malignant Secondary	Ca in situ	Benign	Uncertain Behavior	Unspecified Behavior
hypothalamus	C71.0	C79.31	—	D33.0	D43.0	D49.6
ileocecum, ileocecal (coil) (junction) (valve)	C18.0	C78.5	D01.0	D12.0	D37.4	D49.0
ileum	C17.2	C78.4	D01.49	D13.39	D37.2	D49.0
ilium	C41.4	C79.51	—	D16.8	D48.0	D49.2
immunoproliferative NEC	C88.9	—	—	—	—	—
infraclavicular (region)	C76.1	C79.89	D04.5	D36.7	D48.7	D49.89
inguinal (region)	C76.3	C79.89	D04.5	D36.7	D48.7	D49.89
insula	C71.0	C79.31	—	D33.0	D43.0	D49.6
insular tissue (pancreas)	C25.4	C78.89	D01.7	D13.7	D37.8	D49.0
brain	C71.0	C79.31	—	D33.0	D43.0	D49.6
interarytenoid fold	C13.1	C79.89	D00.08	D10.7	D37.05	D49.0
hypopharyngeal aspect	C13.1	C79.89	D00.08	D10.7	D37.05	D49.0
laryngeal aspect	C32.1	C78.39	D02.0	D14.1	D38.0	D49.1
marginal zone	C13.1	C79.89	D00.08	D10.7	D37.05	D49.0
interdental papillae	C03.9	C79.89	D00.03	D10.39	D37.09	D49.0
lower	C03.1	C79.89	D00.03	D10.39	D37.09	D49.0
upper	C03.0	C79.89	D00.03	D10.39	D37.09	D49.0
internal						
capsule	C71.0	C79.31	—	D33.0	D43.0	D49.6
os (cervix)	C53.0	C79.82	D06.0	D26.0	D39.0	D49.59
intervertebral cartilage or disc	C41.2	C79.51	—	D16.6	D48.0	D49.2
intestine, intestinal	C26.0	C78.80	D01.40	D13.9	D37.8	D49.0
large	C18.9	C78.5	D01.0	D12.6	D37.4	D49.0
appendix	C18.1	C78.5	D01.0	D12.1	D37.3	D49.0
caput coli	C18.0	C78.5	D01.0	D12.0	D37.4	D49.0
cecum	C18.0	C78.5	D01.0	D12.0	D37.4	D49.0
colon	C18.9	C78.5	D01.0	D12.6	D37.4	D49.0
and rectum	C19	C78.5	D01.1	D12.7	D37.5	D49.0
ascending	C18.2	C78.5	D01.0	D12.2	D37.4	D49.0
caput	C18.0	C78.5	D01.0	D12.0	D37.4	D49.0
descending	C18.6	C78.5	D01.0	D12.4	D37.4	D49.0
distal	C18.6	C78.5	D01.0	D12.4	D37.4	D49.0
left	C18.6	C78.5	D01.0	D12.4	D37.4	D49.0
overlapping lesion	C18.8	—	—	—	—	—
pelvic	C18.7	C78.5	D01.0	D12.5	D37.4	D49.0
right	C18.2	C78.5	D01.0	D12.2	D37.4	D49.0
sigmoid (flexure)	C18.7	C78.5	D01.0	D12.5	D37.4	D49.0
transverse	C18.4	C78.5	D01.0	D12.3	D37.4	D49.0
hepatic flexure	C18.3	C78.5	D01.0	D12.3	D37.4	D49.0
ileocecum, ileocecal (coil) (valve)	C18.0	C78.5	D01.0	D12.0	D37.4	D49.0
overlapping lesion	C18.8	—	—	—	—	—

◀ New ⇐ Revised ~~deleted~~ Deleted

	Malignant Primary	Malignant Secondary	Ca in situ	Benign	Uncertain Behavior	Unspecified Behavior
intestine, intestinal *(Continued)*						
large *(Continued)*						
sigmoid flexure (lower) (upper)	C18.7	C78.5	D01.0	D12.5	D37.4	D49.0
splenic flexure	C18.5	C78.5	D01.0	D12.3	D37.4	D49.0
small	C17.9	C78.4	D01.40	D13.30	D37.2	D49.0
duodenum	C17.0	C78.4	D01.49	D13.2	D37.2	D49.0
ileum	C17.2	C78.4	D01.49	D13.39	D37.2	D49.0
jejunum	C17.1	C78.4	D01.49	D13.39	D37.2	D49.0
overlapping lesion	C17.8	—	—	—	—	—
tract NEC	C26.0	C78.89	D01.40	D13.9	D37.8	D49.0
intra-abdominal	C76.2	C79.89	D09.8	D36.7	D48.7	D49.89
intracranial NEC	C71.9	C79.31	—	D33.2	D43.2	D49.6
intrahepatic (bile) duct	C22.1	C78.7	D01.5	D13.4	D37.6	D49.0
intraocular	C69.9-	C79.49	D09.2-	D31.9-	D48.7	D49.89
intraorbital	C69.6-	C79.49	D09.2-	D31.6-	D48.7	D49.89
intrasellar	C75.1	C79.89	D09.3	D35.2	D44.3	D49.7
intrathoracic (cavity) (organs)	C76.1	C79.89	D09.8	D15.9	D48.7	D49.89
specified NEC	C76.1	C79.89	D09.8	D15.7	—	—
iris	C69.4-	C79.49	D09.2-	D31.4-	D48.7	D49.89
ischiorectal (fossa)	C76.3	C79.89	D09.8	D36.7	D48.7	D49.89
ischium	C41.4	C79.51	—	D16.8	D48.0	D49.2
island of Reil	C71.0	C79.31	—	D33.0	D43.0	D49.6
islands or islets of Langerhans	C25.4	C78.89	D01.7	D13.7	D37.8	D49.0
isthmus uteri	C54.0	C79.82	D07.0	D26.1	D39.0	D49.59
jaw	C76.0	C79.89	D09.8	D36.7	D48.7	D49.89
bone	C41.1	C79.51	—	D16.5-	D48.0	D49.2
lower	C41.1	C79.51	—	D16.5-	—	—
upper	C41.0	C79.51	—	D16.4-	—	—
carcinoma (any type) (lower) (upper)	C76.0	C79.89	—	—	—	—
skin — *see also Neoplasm, skin, face*	C44.309	C79.2	D04.39	D23.39	D48.5	D49.2
soft tissues	C03.9	C79.89	D00.03	D10.39	D37.09	D49.0
lower	C03.1	C79.89	D00.03	D10.39	D37.09	D49.0
upper	C03.0	C79.89	D00.03	D10.39	D37.09	D49.0
jejunum	C17.1	C78.4	D01.49	D13.39	D37.2	D49.0
joint NEC — *see also Neoplasm, bone*	C41.9	C79.51	—	D16.9-	D48.0	D49.2
acromioclavicular	C40.0-	C79.51	—	D16.0-	—	—
bursa or synovial membrane — *see Neoplasm, connective tissue*						
costovertebral	C41.3	C79.51	—	D16.7	D48.0	D49.2
sternocostal	C41.3	C79.51	—	D16.7	D48.0	D49.2
temporomandibular	C41.1	C79.51	—	D16.5-	D48.0	D49.2

	Malignant Primary	Malignant Secondary	Ca in situ	Benign	Uncertain Behavior	Unspecified Behavior
junction						
anorectal	C21.8	C78.5	D01.3	D12.9	D37.8	D49.0
cardioesophageal	C16.0	C78.89	D00.2	D13.1	D37.1	D49.0
esophagogastric	C16.0	C78.89	D00.2	D13.1	D37.1	D49.0
gastroesophageal	C16.0	C78.89	D00.2	D13.1	D37.1	D49.0
hard and soft palate	C05.9	C79.89	D00.00	D10.39	D37.09	D49.0
ileocecal	C18.0	C78.5	D01.0	D12.0	D37.4	D49.0
pelvirectal	C19	C78.5	D01.1	D12.7	D37.5	D49.0
pelviureteric	C65.-	C79.0-	D09.19	D30.1-	D41.1-	D49.59
rectosigmoid	C19	C78.5	D01.1	D12.7	D37.5	D49.0
squamocolumnar, of cervix	C53.8	C79.82	D06.7	D26.0	D39.0	D49.59
Kaposi's sarcoma — *see Kaposi's, sarcoma*						
kidney (parenchymal)	C64.-	C79.0-	D09.19	D30.0-	D41.0-	D49.51-
calyx	C65.-	C79.0-	D09.19	D30.1-	D41.1-	D49.51-
hilus	C65.-	C79.0-	D09.19	D30.1-	D41.1-	D49.51-
pelvis	C65.-	C79.0-	D09.19	D30.1-	D41.1-	D49.51-
knee NEC	C76.5-	C79.89	D04.7-	D36.7	D48.7	D49.89
labia (skin)	C51.9	C79.82	D07.1	D28.0	D39.8	D49.59
majora	C51.0	C79.82	D07.1	D28.0	D39.8	D49.59
minora	C51.1	C79.82	D07.1	D28.0	D39.8	D49.59
labial — *see also Neoplasm, lip*	C00.9	C79.89	D00.01	D10.0	D37.01	D49.0
sulcus (lower) (upper)	C06.1	C79.89	D00.02	D10.39	D37.09	D49.0
labium (skin)	C51.9	C79.82	D07.1	D28.0	D39.8	D49.59
majus	C51.0	C79.82	D07.1	D28.0	D39.8	D49.59
minus	C51.1	C79.82	D07.1	D28.0	D39.8	D49.59
lacrimal						
canaliculi	C69.5-	C79.49	D09.2-	D31.5-	D48.7	D49.89
duct (nasal)	C69.5-	C79.49	D09.2-	D31.5-	D48.7	D49.89
gland	C69.5-	C79.49	D09.2-	D31.5-	D48.7	D49.89
punctum	C69.5-	C79.49	D09.2-	D31.5-	D48.7	D49.89
sac	C69.5-	C79.49	D09.2-	D31.5-	D48.7	D49.89
Langerhans, islands or islets	C25.4	C78.89	D01.7	D13.7	D37.8	D49.0
laryngopharynx	C13.9	C79.89	D00.08	D10.7	D37.05	D49.0
larynx, laryngeal NEC	C32.9	C78.39	D02.0	D14.1	D38.0	D49.1
aryepiglottic fold	C32.1	C78.39	D02.0	D14.1	D38.0	D49.1
cartilage (arytenoid) (cricoid) (cuneiform) (thyroid)	C32.3	C78.39	D02.0	D14.1	D38.0	D49.1
commissure (anterior) (posterior)	C32.0	C78.39	D02.0	D14.1	D38.0	D49.1
extrinsic NEC	C32.1	C78.39	D02.0	D14.1	D38.0	D49.1
meaning hypopharynx	C13.9	C79.89	D00.08	D10.7	D37.05	D49.0
interarytenoid fold	C32.1	C78.39	D02.0	D14.1	D38.0	D49.1
intrinsic	C32.0	C78.39	D02.0	D14.1	D38.0	D49.1

◀ New ⇐ Revised ~~deleted~~ Deleted

	Malignant Primary	Malignant Secondary	Ca in situ	Benign	Uncertain Behavior	Unspecified Behavior
larynx, laryngeal NEC *(Continued)*						
overlapping lesion	C32.8	—	—	—	—	—
ventricular band	C32.1	C78.39	D02.0	D14.1	D38.0	D49.1
leg NEC	C76.5-	C79.89	D04.7-	D36.7	D48.7	D49.89
lens, crystalline	C69.4-	C79.49	D09.2-	D31.4-	D48.7	D49.89
lid (lower) (upper)	C44.10-	C79.2	D04.1-	D23.1-	D48.5	D49.2
basal cell carcinoma	C44.11-	—	—	—	—	—
specified type NEC	C44.19-	—	—	—	—	—
squamous cell carcinoma	C44.12-	—	—	—	—	—
ligament — *see also Neoplasm, connective tissue*						
broad	C57.1	C79.82	D07.39	D28.2	D39.8	D49.59
Mackenrodt's	C57.7	C79.82	D07.39	D28.7	D39.8	D49.59
non-uterine — *see Neoplasm, connective tissue*						
round	C57.2	C79.82	—	D28.2	D39.8	D49.59
sacro-uterine	C57.3	C79.82	—	D28.2	D39.8	D49.59
uterine	C57.3	C79.82	—	D28.2	D39.8	D49.59
utero-ovarian	C57.7	C79.82	D07.39	D28.2	D39.8	D49.59
uterosacral	C57.3	C79.82	—	D28.2	D39.8	D49.59
limb	C76.8	C79.89	D04.8	D36.7	D48.7	D49.89
lower	C76.5-	C79.89	D04.7-	D36.7	D48.7	D49.89
upper	C76.4-	C79.89	D04.6-	D36.7	D48.7	D49.89
limbus of cornea	C69.1-	C79.49	D09.2-	D31.1-	D48.7	D49.89
lingual NEC — *see also Neoplasm, tongue*	C02.9	C79.89	D00.07	D10.1	D37.02	D49.0
lingula, lung	C34.1-	C78.0-	D02.2-	D14.3-	D38.1	D49.1
lip	C00.9	C79.89	D00.01	D10.0	D37.01	D49.0
buccal aspect — *see Neoplasm, lip, internal*						
commissure	C00.6	C79.89	D00.01	D10.0	D37.01	D49.0
external	C00.2	C79.89	D00.01	D10.0	D37.01	D49.0
lower	C00.1	C79.89	D00.01	D10.0	D37.01	D49.0
upper	C00.0	C79.89	D00.01	D10.0	D37.01	D49.0
frenulum — *see Neoplasm, lip, internal*						
inner aspect — *see Neoplasm, lip, internal*						
internal	C00.5	C79.89	D00.01	D10.0	D37.01	D49.0
lower	C00.4	C79.89	D00.01	D10.0	D37.01	D49.0
upper	C00.3	C79.89	D00.01	D10.0	D37.01	D49.0
lipstick area	C00.2	C79.89	D00.01	D10.0	D37.01	D49.0
lower	C00.1	C79.89	D00.01	D10.0	D37.01	D49.0
upper	C00.0	C79.89	D00.01	D10.0	D37.01	D49.0

	Malignant Primary	Malignant Secondary	Ca in situ	Benign	Uncertain Behavior	Unspecified Behavior
lip *(Continued)*						
lower	C00.1	C79.89	D00.01	D10.0	D37.01	D49.0
internal	C00.4	C79.89	D00.01	D10.0	D37.01	D49.0
mucosa — *see Neoplasm, lip, internal*						
oral aspect — *see Neoplasm, lip, internal*						
overlapping lesion	C00.8	—	—	—	—	—
with oral cavity or pharynx	C14.8	—	—	—	—	—
skin (commissure) (lower) (upper)	C44.00	C79.2	D04.0	D23.0	D48.5	D49.2
basal cell carcinoma	C44.01	—	—	—	—	—
specified type NEC	C44.09	—	—	—	—	—
squamous cell carcinoma	C44.02	—	—	—	—	—
upper	C00.0	C79.89	D00.01	D10.0	D37.01	D49.0
internal	C00.3	C79.89	D00.01	D10.0	D37.01	D49.0
vermilion border	C00.2	C79.89	D00.01	D10.0	D37.01	D49.0
lower	C00.1	C79.89	D00.01	D10.0	D37.01	D49.0
upper	C00.0	C79.89	D00.01	D10.0	D37.01	D49.0
lipomatous — *see Lipoma, by site*						
liver — *see also Index to disease, by histology*	C22.9	C78.7	D01.5	D13.4	D37.6	D49.0
primary	C22.8	C78.7	D01.5	D13.4	D37.6	D49.0
lumbosacral plexus	C47.5	C79.89	—	D36.16	D48.2	D49.2
lung	C34.9-	C78.0-	D02.2-	D14.3-	D38.1	D49.1
azygos lobe	C34.1-	C78.0-	D02.2-	D14.3-	D38.1	D49.1
carina	C34.0-	C78.0-	D02.2-	D14.3-	D38.1	D49.1
hilus	C34.0-	C78.0-	D02.2-	D14.3-	D38.1	D49.1
linqula	C34.1-	C78.0-	D02.2-	D14.3-	D38.1	D49.1
lobe NEC	C34.9-	C78.0-	D02.2-	D14.3-	D38.1	D49.1
lower lobe	C34.3-	C78.0-	D02.2-	D14.3-	D38.1	D49.1
main bronchus	C34.0-	C78.0-	D02.2-	D14.3-	D38.1	D49.1
mesothelioma — *see Mesothelioma*						
middle lobe	C34.2	C78.0-	D02.21	D14.31	D38.1	D49.1
overlapping lesion	C34.8-	—	—	—	—	—
upper lobe	C34.1-	C78.0-	D02.2-	D14.3-	D38.1	D49.1
lymph, lymphatic channel NEC	C49.9	C79.89	—	D21.9	D48.1	D49.2
gland (secondary)	—	C77.9	—	D36.0	D48.7	D49.89
abdominal	—	C77.2	—	D36.0	D48.7	D49.89
aortic	—	C77.2	—	D36.0	D48.7	D49.89
arm	—	C77.3	—	D36.0	D48.7	D49.89
auricular (anterior) (posterior)	—	C77.0	—	D36.0	D48.7	D49.89

◀ New ⇐ Revised ~~deleted~~ Deleted

	Malignant Primary	Malignant Secondary	Ca in situ	Benign	Uncertain Behavior	Unspecified Behavior
lymph, lymphatic channel NEC *(Continued)* gland *(Continued)*						
axilla, axillary	—	C77.3	—	D36.0	D48.7	D49.89
brachial	—	C77.3	—	D36.0	D48.7	D49.89
bronchial	—	C77.1	—	D36.0	D48.7	D49.89
bronchopulmonary	—	C77.1	—	D36.0	D48.7	D49.89
celiac	—	C77.2	—	D36.0	D48.7	D49.89
cervical	—	C77.0	—	D36.0	D48.7	D49.89
cervicofacial	—	C77.0	—	D36.0	D48.7	D49.89
Cloquet	—	C77.4	—	D36.0	D48.7	D49.89
colic	—	C77.2	—	D36.0	D48.7	D49.89
common duct	—	C77.2	—	D36.0	D48.7	D49.89
cubital	—	C77.3	—	D36.0	D48.7	D49.89
diaphragmatic	—	C77.1	—	D36.0	D48.7	D49.89
epigastric, inferior	—	C77.1	—	D36.0	D48.7	D49.89
epitrochlear	—	C77.3	—	D36.0	D48.7	D49.89
esophageal	—	C77.1	—	D36.0	D48.7	D49.89
face	—	C77.0	—	D36.0	D48.7	D49.89
femoral	—	C77.4	—	D36.0	D48.7	D49.89
gastric	—	C77.2	—	D36.0	D48.7	D49.89
groin	—	C77.4	—	D36.0	D48.7	D49.89
head	—	C77.0	—	D36.0	D48.7	D49.89
hepatic	—	C77.2	—	D36.0	D48.7	D49.89
hilar (pulmonary)	—	C77.1	—	D36.0	D48.7	D49.89
splenic	—	C77.2	—	D36.0	D48.7	D49.89
hypogastric	—	C77.5	—	D36.0	D48.7	D49.89
ileocolic	—	C77.2	—	D36.0	D48.7	D49.89
iliac	—	C77.5	—	D36.0	D48.7	D49.89
infraclavicular	—	C77.3	—	D36.0	D48.7	D49.89
inguina, inguinal	—	C77.4	—	D36.0	D48.7	D49.89
innominate	—	C77.1	—	D36.0	D48.7	D49.89
intercostal	—	C77.1	—	D36.0	D48.7	D49.89
intestinal	—	C77.2	—	D36.0	D48.7	D49.89
intrabdominal	—	C77.2	—	D36.0	D48.7	D49.89
intrapelvic	—	C77.5	—	D36.0	D48.7	D49.89
intrathoracic	—	C77.1	—	D36.0	D48.7	D49.89
jugular	—	C77.0	—	D36.0	D48.7	D49.89
leg	—	C77.4	—	D36.0	D48.7	D49.89
limb						
lower	—	C77.4	—	D36.0	D48.7	D49.89
upper	—	C77.3	—	D36.0	D48.7	D49.89
lower limb	—	C77.4	—	D36.0	D48.7	D49.89
lumbar	—	C77.2	—	D36.0	D48.7	D49.89

	Malignant Primary	Malignant Secondary	Ca in situ	Benign	Uncertain Behavior	Unspecified Behavior
lymph, lymphatic channel NEC *(Continued)* gland *(Continued)*						
mandibular	—	C77.0	—	D36.0	D48.7	D49.89
mediastinal	—	C77.1	—	D36.0	D48.7	D49.89
mesenteric (inferior) (superior)	—	C77.2	—	D36.0	D48.7	D49.89
midcolic	—	C77.2	—	D36.0	D48.7	D49.89
multiple sites in categories C77.0 - C77.5	—	C77.8	—	D36.0	D48.7	D49.89
neck	—	C77.0	—	D36.0	D48.7	D49.89
obturator	—	C77.5	—	D36.0	D48.7	D49.89
occipital	—	C77.0	—	D36.0	D48.7	D49.89
pancreatic	—	C77.2	—	D36.0	D48.7	D49.89
para-aortic	—	C77.2	—	D36.0	D48.7	D49.89
paracervical	—	C77.5	—	D36.0	D48.7	D49.89
parametrial	—	C77.5	—	D36.0	D48.7	D49.89
parasternal	—	C77.1	—	D36.0	D48.7	D49.89
parotid	—	C77.0	—	D36.0	D48.7	D49.89
pectoral	—	C77.3	—	D36.0	D48.7	D49.89
pelvic	—	C77.5	—	D36.0	D48.7	D49.89
peri-aortic	—	C77.2	—	D36.0	D48.7	D49.89
peripancreatic	—	C77.2	—	D36.0	D48.7	D49.89
popliteal	—	C77.4	—	D36.0	D48.7	D49.89
porta hepatis	—	C77.2	—	D36.0	D48.7	D49.89
portal	—	C77.2	—	D36.0	D48.7	D49.89
preauricular	—	C77.0	—	D36.0	D48.7	D49.89
prelaryngeal	—	C77.0	—	D36.0	D48.7	D49.89
presymphysial	—	C77.5	—	D36.0	D48.7	D49.89
pretracheal	—	C77.0	—	D36.0	D48.7	D49.89
primary (any site) NEC	C96.9	—	—	—	—	—
pulmonary (hiler)	—	C77.1	—	D36.0	D48.7	D49.89
pyloric	—	C77.2	—	D36.0	D48.7	D49.89
retroperitoneal	—	C77.2	—	D36.0	D48.7	D49.89
retropharyngeal	—	C77.0	—	D36.0	D48.7	D49.89
Rosenmuller's	—	C77.4	—	D36.0	D48.7	D49.89
sacral	—	C77.5	—	D36.0	D48.7	D49.89
scalene	—	C77.0	—	D36.0	D48.7	D49.89
site NEC	—	C77.9	—	D36.0	D48.7	D49.89
splenic (hilar)	—	C77.2	—	D36.0	D48.7	D49.89
subclavicular	—	C77.3	—	D36.0	D48.7	D49.89
subinguinal	—	C77.4	—	D36.0	D48.7	D49.89
sublingual	—	C77.0	—	D36.0	D48.7	D49.89
submandibular	—	C77.0	—	D36.0	D48.7	D49.89

	Malignant Primary	Malignant Secondary	Ca in situ	Benign	Uncertain Behavior	Unspecified Behavior
lymph, lymphatic channel NEC *(Continued)*						
gland *(Continued)*						
submaxillary	—	C77.0	—	D36.0	D48.7	D49.89
submental	—	C77.0	—	D36.0	D48.7	D49.89
subscapular	—	C77.3	—	D36.0	D48.7	D49.89
supraclavicular	—	C77.0	—	D36.0	D48.7	D49.89
thoracic	—	C77.1	—	D36.0	D48.7	D49.89
tibial	—	C77.4	—	D36.0	D48.7	D49.89
tracheal	—	C77.1	—	D36.0	D48.7	D49.89
tracheobronchial	—	C77.1	—	D36.0	D48.7	D49.89
upper limb	—	C77.3	—	D36.0	D48.7	D49.89
Virchow's	—	C77.0	—	D36.0	D48.7	D49.89
node — *see also Neoplasm, lymph gland*						
primary NEC	C96.9	—	—	—	—	—
vessel — *see also Neoplasm, connective tissue*	C49.9	C79.89	—	D21.9	D48.1	D49.2
Mackenrodt's ligament	C57.7	C79.82	D07.39	D28.7	D39.8	D49.59
malar	C41.0	C79.51	—	D16.4-	D48.0	D49.2
region — *see Neoplasm, cheek*						
mammary gland — *see Neoplasm, breast*						
mandible	C41.1	C79.51	—	D16.5-	D48.0	D49.2
alveolar						
mucosa (carcinoma)	C03.1	C79.89	D00.03	D10.39	D37.09	D49.0
ridge or process	C41.1	C79.51	—	D16.5-	D48.0	D49.2
marrow (bone) NEC	C96.9	C79.52	—	—	D47.9	D49.89
mastectomy site (skin) — *see also Neoplasm, breast, skin*	C44.501	C79.2	—	—	—	—
specified as breast tissue	C50.8-	C79.81	—	—	—	—
mastoid (air cells) (antrum) (cavity)	C30.1	C78.39	D02.3	D14.0	D38.5	D49.1
bone or process	C41.0	C79.51	—	D16.4-	D48.0	D49.2
maxilla, maxillary (superior)	C41.0	C79.51	—	D16.4-	D48.0	D49.2
alveolar						
mucosa	C03.0	C79.89	D00.03	D10.39	D37.09	D49.0
ridge or process (carcinoma)	C41.0	C79.51	—	D16.4-	D48.0	D49.2
antrum	C31.0	C78.39	D02.3	D14.0	D38.5	D49.1
carcinoma	C03.0	C79.51	—	—	—	—
inferior — *see Neoplasm, mandible*						
sinus	C31.0	C78.39	D02.3	D14.0	D38.5	D49.1
meatus external (ear) — *see also Neoplasm, skin, ear*	C44.20-	C79.2	D04.2-	D23.2-	D48.5	D49.2
Meckel diverticulum, malignant	C17.3	C78.4	D01.49	D13.39	D37.2	D49.0

	Malignant Primary	Malignant Secondary	Ca in situ	Benign	Uncertain Behavior	Unspecified Behavior
mediastinum, mediastinal	C38.3	C78.1	—	D15.2	D38.3	D49.89
anterior	C38.1	C78.1	—	D15.2	D38.3	D49.89
posterior	C38.2	C78.1	—	D15.2	D38.3	D49.89
medulla						
adrenal	C74.1-	C79.7-	D09.3	D35.0-	D44.1-	D49.7
oblongata	C71.7	C79.31	—	D33.1	D43.1	D49.6
meibomian gland	C44.10-	C79.2	D04.1-	D23.1-	D48.5	D49.2
basal cell carcinoma	C44.11-	—	—	—	—	—
specified type NEC	C44.19-	—	—	—	—	—
squamous cell carcinoma	C44.12-	—	—	—	—	—
melanoma — *see Melanoma*						
meninges	C70.9	C79.49	—	D32.9	D42.9	D49.7
brain	C70.0	C79.32	—	D32.0	D42.0	D49.7
cerebral	C70.0	C79.32	—	D32.0	D42.0	D49.7
crainial	C70.0	C79.32	—	D32.0	D42.0	D49.7
intracranial	C70.0	C79.32	—	D32.0	D42.0	D49.7
spinal (cord)	C70.1	C79.49	—	D32.1	D42.1	D49.7
meniscus, knee joint (lateral) (medial)	C40.2-	C79.51	—	D16.2-	D48.0	D49.2
Merkel cell — *see Carcinoma, Merkel cell*						
mesentery, mesenteric	C48.1	C78.6	—	D20.1	D48.4	D49.0
mesoappendix	C48.1	C78.6	—	D20.1	D48.4	D49.0
mesocolon	C48.1	C78.6	—	D20.1	D48.4	D49.0
mesopharynx — *see Neoplasm, oropharynx*						
mesosalpinx	C57.1	C79.82	D07.39	D28.2	D39.8	D49.59
mesothelial tissue — *see Mesothelioma*						
mesothelioma — *see Mesothelioma*						
mesovarium	C57.1	C79.82	D07.39	D28.2	D39.8	D49.59
metacarpus (any bone)	C40.1-	C79.51	—	D16.1-	—	—
metastatic NEC — *see also Neoplasm, by site, secondary*	—	C79.9	—	—	—	—
metatarsus (any bone)	C40.3-	C79.51	—	D16.3-	—	—
midbrain	C71.7	C79.31	—	D33.1	D43.1	D49.6
milk duct — *see Neoplasm, breast*						
mons						
pubis	C51.9	C79.82	D07.1	D28.0	D39.8	D49.59
veneris	C51.9	C79.82	D07.1	D28.0	D39.8	D49.59
motor tract	C72.9	C79.49	—	D33.9	D43.9	D49.7
brain	C71.9	C79.31	—	D33.2	D43.2	D49.6
cauda equina	C72.1	C79.49	—	D33.4	D43.4	D49.7
spinal	C72.0	C79.49	—	D33.4	D43.4	D49.7

◀ New ⇐ Revised ~~deleted~~ Deleted

	Malignant Primary	Malignant Secondary	Ca in situ	Benign	Uncertain Behavior	Unspecified Behavior
mouth	C06.9	C79.89	D00.00	D10.30	D37.09	D49.0
book-leaf	C06.89	C79.89	—	—	—	—
floor	C04.9	C79.89	D00.06	D10.2	D37.09	D49.0
anterior portion	C04.0	C79.89	D00.06	D10.2	D37.09	D49.0
lateral portion	C04.1	C79.89	D00.06	D10.2	D37.09	D49.0
overlapping lesion	C04.8	—	—	—	—	—
overlapping NEC	C06.80	—	—	—	—	—
roof	C05.9	C79.89	D00.00	D10.39	D37.09	D49.0
specified part NEC	C06.89	C79.89	D00.00	D10.39	D37.09	D49.0
vestibule	C06.1	C79.89	D00.00	D10.39	D37.09	D49.0
mucosa						
alveolar (ridge or process)	C03.9	C79.89	D00.03	D10.39	D37.09	D49.0
lower	C03.1	C79.89	D00.03	D10.39	D37.09	D49.0
upper	C03.0	C79.89	D00.03	D10.39	D37.09	D49.0
buccal	C06.0	C79.89	D00.02	D10.39	D37.09	D49.0
cheek	C06.0	C79.89	D00.02	D10.39	D37.09	D49.0
lip — *see Neoplasm, lip, internal*						
nasal	C30.0	C78.39	D02.3	D14.0	D38.5	D49.1
oral	C06.0	C79.89	D00.02	D10.39	D37.09	D49.0
Mullerian duct						
female	C57.7	C79.82	D07.39	D28.7	D39.8	D49.59
male	C63.7	C79.82	D07.69	D29.8	D40.8	D49.59
muscle — *see also Neoplasm, connective tissue*						
extraocular	C69.6-	C79.49	D09.2-	D31.6-	D48.7	D49.89
myocardium	C38.0	C79.89	—	D15.1	D48.7	D49.89
myometrium	C54.2	C79.82	D07.0	D26.1	D39.0	D49.59
myopericardium	C38.0	C79.89	—	D15.1	D48.7	D49.89
nabothian gland (follicle)	C53.0	C79.82	D06.0	D26.0	D39.0	D49.59
nail — *see also Neoplasm, skin, limb*	C44.90	C79.2	D04.9	D23.9	D48.5	D49.2
finger — *see also Neoplasm, skin, limb, upper*	C44.60-	C79.2	D04.6-	D23.6-	D48.5	D49.2
toe — *see also Neoplasm, skin, limb, lower*	C44.70-	C79.2	D04.7-	D23.7-	D48.5	D49.2
nares, naris (anterior) (posterior)	C30.0	C78.39	D02.3	D14.0	D38.5	D49.1
nasal — *see Neoplasm, nose*						
nasolabial groove — *see also Neoplasm, skin, face*	C44.309	C79.2	D04.39	D23.39	D48.5	D49.2
nasolacrimal duct	C69.5-	C79.49	D09.2-	D31.5-	D48.7	D49.89
nasopharynx, nasopharyngeal	C11.9	C79.89	D00.08	D10.6	D37.05	D49.0
floor	C11.3	C79.89	D00.08	D10.6	D37.05	D49.0
overlapping lesion	C11.8	—	—	—	—	—
roof	C11.0	C79.89	D00.08	D10.6	D37.05	D49.0

	Malignant Primary	Malignant Secondary	Ca in situ	Benign	Uncertain Behavior	Unspecified Behavior
nasopharynx, nasopharyngeal *(Continued)*						
wall	C11.9	C79.89	D00.08	D10.6	D37.05	D49.0
anterior	C11.3	C79.89	D00.08	D10.6	D37.05	D49.0
lateral	C11.2	C79.89	D00.08	D10.6	D37.05	D49.0
posterior	C11.1	C79.89	D00.08	D10.6	D37.05	D49.0
superior	C11.0	C79.89	D00.08	D10.6	D37.05	D49.0
nates — *see also Neoplasm, skin, trunk*	C44.509	C79.2	D04.5	D23.5	D48.5	D49.2
neck NEC	C76.0	C79.89	D09.8	D36.7	D48.7	D49.89
skin	C44.40	—	—	—	—	—
basal cell carcinoma	C44.41	—	—	—	—	—
specified type NEC	C44.49	—	—	—	—	—
squamous cell carcinoma	C44.42	—	—	—	—	—
nerve (ganglion)	C47.9	C79.89	—	D36.10	D48.2	D49.2
abducens	C72.59	C79.49	—	D33.3	D43.3	D49.7
accessory (spinal)	C72.59	C79.49	—	D33.3	D43.3	D49.7
acoustic	C72.4-	C79.49	—	D33.3	D43.3	D49.7
auditory	C72.4-	C79.49	—	D33.3	D43.3	D49.7
autonomic NEC — *see also Neoplasm, nerve, peripheral*	C47.9	C79.89	—	D36.10	D48.2	D49.2
brachial	C47.1-	C79.89	—	D36.12	D48.2	D49.2
cranial	C72.50	C79.49	—	D33.3	D43.3	D49.7
specified NEC	C72.59	C79.49	—	D33.3	D43.3	D49.7
facial	C72.59	C79.49	—	D33.3	D43.3	D49.7
femoral	C47.2-	C79.89	—	D36.13	D48.2	D49.2
ganglion NEC — *see also Neoplasm, nerve, peripheral*	C47.9	C79.89	—	D36.10	D48.2	D49.2
glossopharyngeal	C72.59	C79.49	—	D33.3	D43.3	D49.7
hypoglossal	C72.59	C79.49	—	D33.3	D43.3	D49.7
intercostal	C47.3	C79.89	—	D36.14	D48.2	D49.2
lumbar	C47.6	C79.89	—	D36.17	D48.2	D49.2
median	C47.1-	C79.89	—	D36.12	D48.2	D49.2
obturator	C47.2-	C79.89	—	D36.13	D48.2	D49.2
oculomotor	C72.59	C79.49	—	D33.3	D43.3	D49.7
olfactory	C47.2-	C79.49	—	D33.3	D43.3	D49.7
optic	C72.3-	C79.49	—	D33.3	D43.3	D49.7
parasympathetic NEC	C47.9	C79.89	—	D36.10	D48.2	D49.2
peripheral NEC	C47.9	C79.89	—	D36.10	D48.2	D49.2
abdomen	C47.4	C79.89	—	D36.15	D48.2	D49.2
abdominal wall	C47.4	C79.89	—	D36.15	D48.2	D49.2
ankle	C47.2-	C79.89	—	D36.13	D48.2	D49.2

◀ New ◀ Revised ~~deleted~~ Deleted

	Malignant Primary	Malignant Secondary	Ca in situ	Benign	Uncertain Behavior	Unspecified Behavior
nerve *(Continued)*						
peripheral NEC *(Continued)*						
antecubital fossa or space	C47.1-	C79.89	—	D36.12	D48.2	D49.2
arm	C47.1-	C79.89	—	D36.12	D48.2	D49.2
auricle (ear)	C47.0	C79.89	—	D36.11	D48.2	D49.2
axilla	C47.3	C79.89	—	D36.12	D48.2	D49.2
back	C47.6	C79.89	—	D36.17	D48.2	D49.2
buttock	C47.5	C79.89	—	D36.16	D48.2	D49.2
calf	C47.2-	C79.89	—	D36.13	D48.2	D49.2
cervical region	C47.0	C79.89	—	D36.11	D48.2	D49.2
cheek	C47.0	C79.89	—	D36.11	D48.2	D49.2
chest (wall)	C47.3	C79.89	—	D36.14	D48.2	D49.2
chin	C47.0	C79.89	—	D36.11	D48.2	D49.2
ear (external)	C47.0	C79.89	—	D36.11	D48.2	D49.2
elbow	C47.1-	C79.89	—	D36.12	D48.2	D49.2
extrarectal	C47.5	C79.89	—	D36.16	D48.2	D49.2
extremity	C47.9	C79.89	—	D36.10	D48.2	D49.2
lower	C47.2-	C79.89	—	D36.13	D48.2	D49.2
upper	C47.1-	C79.89	—	D36.12	D48.2	D49.2
eyelid	C47.0	C79.89	—	D36.11	D48.2	D49.2
face	C47.0	C79.89	—	D36.11	D48.2	D49.2
finger	C47.1-	C79.89	—	D36.12	D48.2	D49.2
flank	C47.6	C79.89	—	D36.17	D48.2	D49.2
foot	C47.2-	C79.89	—	D36.13	D48.2	D49.2
forearm	C47.1-	C79.89	—	D36.12	D48.2	D49.2
forehead	C47.0	C79.89	—	D36.11	D48.2	D49.2
gluteal region	C47.5	C79.89	—	D36.16	D48.2	D49.2
groin	C47.5	C79.89	—	D36.16	D48.2	D49.2
hand	C47.1-	C79.89	—	D36.12	D48.2	D49.2
head	C47.0	C79.89	—	D36.11	D48.2	D49.2
heel	C47.2-	C79.89	—	D36.13	D48.2	D49.2
hip	C47.2-	C79.89	—	D36.13	D48.2	D49.2
infraclavicular region	C47.3	C79.89	—	D36.14	D48.2	D49.2
inguinal (canal) (region)	C47.5	C79.89	—	D36.16	D48.2	D49.2
intrathoracic	C47.3	C79.89	—	D36.14	D48.2	D49.2
ischiorectal fossa	C47.5	C79.89	—	D36.16	D48.2	D49.2
knee	C47.2-	C79.89	—	D36.13	D48.2	D49.2
leg	C47.2-	C79.89	—	D36.13	D48.2	D49.2
limb NEC	C47.9	C79.89	—	D36.10	D48.2	D49.2
lower	C47.2-	C79.89	—	D36.13	D48.2	D49.2
upper	C47.1-	C79.89	—	D36.12	D48.2	D49.2
nates	C47.5	C79.89	—	D36.16	D48.2	D49.2
neck	C47.0	C79.89	—	D36.11	D48.2	D49.2
orbit	C69.6-	C79.49	—	D31.6-	D48.7	D49.2

	Malignant Primary	Malignant Secondary	Ca in situ	Benign	Uncertain Behavior	Unspecified Behavior
nerve *(Continued)*						
peripheral NEC *(Continued)*						
pararectal	C47.5	C79.89	—	D36.16	D48.2	D49.2
paraurethral	C47.5	C79.89	—	D36.16	D48.2	D49.2
paravaginal	C47.5	C79.89	—	D36.16	D48.2	D49.2
pelvis (floor)	C47.5	C79.89	—	D36.16	D48.2	D49.2
pelvoabdominal	C47.8	C79.89	—	D36.17	D48.2	D49.2
perineum	C47.5	C79.89	—	D36.16	D48.2	D49.2
perirectal (tissue)	C47.5	C79.89	—	D36.16	D48.2	D49.2
periurethral (tissue)	C47.5	C79.89	—	D36.16	D48.2	D49.2
popliteal fossa or space	C47.2-	C79.89	—	D36.13	D48.2	D49.2
presacral	C47.5	C79.89	—	D36.16	D48.2	D49.2
pterygoid fossa	C47.0	C79.89	—	D36.11	D48.2	D49.2
rectovaginal septum or wall	C47.5	C79.89	—	D36.16	D48.2	D49.2
rectovesical	C47.5	C79.89	—	D36.16	D48.2	D49.2
sacrococcygeal region	C47.5	C79.89	—	D36.16	D48.2	D49.2
scalp	C47.0	C79.89	—	D36.11	D48.2	D49.2
scapular region	C47.3	C79.89	—	D36.14	D48.2	D49.2
shoulder	C47.1-	C79.89	—	D36.12	D48.2	D49.2
submental	C47.0	C79.89	—	D36.11	D48.2	D49.2
supraclavicular region	C47.0	C79.89	—	D36.11	D48.2	D49.2
temple	C47.0	C79.89	—	D36.11	D48.2	D49.2
temporal region	C47.0	C79.89	—	D36.11	D48.2	D49.2
thigh	C47.2-	C79.89	—	D36.13	D48.2	D49.2
thoracic (duct) (wall)	C47.3	C79.89	—	D36.14	D48.2	D49.2
thorax	C47.3	C79.89	—	D36.14	D48.2	D49.2
thumb	C47.1-	C79.89	—	D36.12	D48.2	D49.2
toe	C47.2-	C79.89	—	D36.13	D48.2	D49.2
trunk	C47.6	C79.89	—	D36.17	D48.2	D49.2
umbilicus	C47.4	C79.89	—	D36.15	D48.2	D49.2
vesicorectal	C47.5	C79.89	—	D36.16	D48.2	D49.2
wrist	C47.1-	C79.89	—	D36.12	D48.2	D49.2
radial	C47.1-	C79.89	—	D36.12	D48.2	D49.2
sacral	C47.5	C79.89	—	D36.16	D48.2	D49.2
sciatic	C47.2-	C79.89	—	D36.13	D48.2	D49.2
spinal NEC	C47.9	C79.89	—	D36.10	D48.2	D49.2
accessory	C72.59	C79.49	—	D33.3	D43.3	D49.7
sympathetic NEC—*see also Neoplasm, nerve, peripheral*	C47.9	C79.89	—	D36.10	D48.2	D49.2
trigeminal	C72.59	C79.49	—	D33.3	D43.3	D49.7
trochlear	C72.59	C79.49	—	D33.3	D43.3	D49.7
ulnar	C47.1-	C79.89	—	D36.12	D48.2	D49.2
vagus	C72.59	C79.49	—	D33.3	D43.3	D49.7

	Malignant Primary	Malignant Secondary	Ca in situ	Benign	Uncertain Behavior	Unspecified Behavior
nervous system (central)	C72.9	C79.40	—	D33.9	D43.9	D49.7
autonomic — *see Neoplasm, nerve, peripheral*						
parasympathetic — *see Neoplasm, nerve, peripheral*						
specified site NEC	—	C79.49	—	D33.7	D43.8	—
sympathetic — *see Neoplasm, nerve, peripheral*						
nevus — *see Nevus*						
nipple	C50.0-	C79.81	D05.-	D24.-	—	—
nose, nasal	C76.0	C79.89	D09.8	D36.7	D48.7	D49.89
ala (external) (nasi) — *see also Neoplasm, nose, skin*	C44.301	C79.2	D04.39	D23.39	D48.5	D49.2
bone	C41.0	C79.51	—	D16.4-	D48.0	D49.2
cartilage	C30.0	C78.39	D02.3	D14.0	D38.5	D49.1
cavity	C30.0	C78.39	D02.3	D14.0	D38.5	D49.1
choana	C11.3	C79.89	D00.08	D10.6	D37.05	D49.0
external (skin) — *see also Neoplasm, nose, skin*	C44.301	C79.2	D04.39	D23.39	D48.5	D49.2
fossa	C30.0	C78.39	D02.3	D14.0	D38.5	D49.1
internal	C30.0	C78.39	D02.3	D14.0	D38.5	D49.1
mucosa	C30.0	C78.39	D02.3	D14.0	D38.5	D49.1
septum	C30.0	C78.39	D02.3	D14.0	D38.5	D49.1
posterior margin	C11.3	C79.89	D00.08	D10.6	D37.05	D49.0
sinus — *see Neoplasm, sinus*						
skin	C44.301	C79.2	D04.39	D23.39	D48.5	D49.2
basal cell carcinoma	C44.311	—	—	—	—	—
specified type NEC	C44.391	—	—	—	—	—
squamous cell carcinoma	C44.321	—	—	—	—	—
turbinate (mucosa)	C30.0	C78.39	D02.3	D14.0	D38.5	D49.1
bone	C41.0	C79.51	—	D16.4-	D48.0	D49.2
vestibule	C30.0	C78.39	D02.3	D14.0	D38.5	D49.1
nostril	C30.0	C78.39	D02.3	D14.0	D38.5	D49.1
nucleus pulposus	C41.2	C79.51	—	D16.6	D48.0	D49.2
occipital						
bone	C41.0	C79.51	—	D16.4-	D48.0	D49.2
lobe or pole, brain	C71.4	C79.31	—	D33.0	D43.0	D49.6
odontogenic — *see Neoplasm, jaw bone*						
olfactory nerve or bulb	C72.2-	C79.49	—	D33.3	D43.3	D49.7
olive (brain)	C71.7	C79.31	—	D33.1	D43.1	D49.6
omentum	C48.1	C78.6	—	D20.1	D48.4	D49.0
operculum (brain)	C71.0	C79.31	—	D33.0	D43.0	D49.6

	Malignant Primary	Malignant Secondary	Ca in situ	Benign	Uncertain Behavior	Unspecified Behavior
optic nerve, chiasm, or tract	C72.3-	C79.49	—	D33.3	D43.3	D49.7
oral (cavity)	C06.9	C79.89	D00.00	D10.30	D37.09	D49.0
ill-defined	C14.8	C79.89	D00.00	D10.30	D37.09	D49.0
mucosa	C06.0	C79.89	D00.02	D10.39	D37.09	D49.0
orbit	C69.6-	C79.49	D09.2-	D31.6-	D48.7	D49.89
autonomic nerve	C69.6-	C79.49	—	D31.6-	D48.7	D49.2
bone	C41.0	C79.51	—	D16.4-	D48.0	D49.2
eye	C69.6-	C79.49	D09.2-	D31.6-	D48.7	D49.89
peripheral nerves	C69.6-	C79.49	—	D31.6-	D48.7	D49.2
soft parts	C69.6-	C79.49	D09.2-	D31.6-	D48.7	D49.89
organ of Zuckerkandl	C75.5	C79.89	—	D35.6	D44.7	D49.7
oropharynx	C10.9	C79.89	D00.08	D10.5	D37.05	D49.0
branchial cleft (vestige)	C10.4	C79.89	D00.08	D10.5	D37.05	D49.0
junctional region	C10.8	C79.89	D00.08	D10.5	D37.05	D49.0
lateral wall	C10.2	C79.89	D00.08	D10.5	D37.05	D49.0
overlapping lesion	C10.8	—	—	—	—	—
pillars or fauces	C09.1	C79.89	D00.08	D10.5	D37.05	D49.0
posterior wall	C10.3	C79.89	D00.08	D10.5	D37.05	D49.0
vallecula	C10.0	C79.89	D00.08	D10.5	D37.05	D49.0
os						
external	C53.1	C79.82	D06.1	D26.0	D39.0	D49.59 ◀
internal	C53.0	C79.82	D06.0	D26.0	D39.0	D49.59 ◀
ovary	C56.-	C79.6-	D07.39	D27.-	D39.1-	D49.59 ◀
oviduct	C57.0-	C79.82	D07.39	D28.2	D39.8	D49.59 ◀
palate	C05.9	C79.89	D00.00	D10.39	D37.09	D49.0
hard	C05.0	C79.89	D00.05	D10.39	D37.09	D49.0
junction of hard and soft palate	C05.9	C79.89	D00.00	D10.39	D37.09	D49.0
overlapping lesions	C05.8	—	—	—	—	—
soft	C05.1	C79.89	D00.04	D10.39	D37.09	D49.0
nasopharyngeal surface	C11.3	C79.89	D00.08	D10.6	D37.05	D49.0
posterior surface	C11.3	C79.89	D00.08	D10.6	D37.05	D49.0
superior surface	C11.3	C79.89	D00.08	D10.6	D37.05	D49.0
palatoglossal arch	C09.1	C79.89	D00.00	D10.5	D37.09	D49.0
palatopharyngeal arch	C09.1	C79.89	D00.00	D10.5	D37.09	D49.0
pallium	C71.0	C79.31	—	D33.0	D43.0	D49.6
palpebra	C44.10-	C79.2	D04.1-	D23.1-	D48.5	D49.2
basal cell carcinoma	C44.11-	—	—	—	—	—
specified type NEC	C44.19-	—	—	—	—	—
squamous cell carcinoma	C44.12-	—	—	—	—	—
pancreas	C25.9	C78.89	D01.7	D13.6	D37.8	D49.0
body	C25.1	C78.89	D01.7	D13.6	D37.8	D49.0
duct (of Santorini) (of Wirsung)	C25.3	C78.89	D01.7	D13.6	D37.8	D49.0
ectopic tissue	C25.7	C78.89	—	D13.6	D37.8	D49.0
head	C25.0	C78.89	D01.7	D13.6	D37.8	D49.0

◀ New ◀ Revised ~~deleted~~ Deleted

	Malignant Primary	Malignant Secondary	Ca in situ	Benign	Uncertain Behavior	Unspecified Behavior
pancreas *(Continued)*						
islet cells	C25.4	C78.89	D01.7	D13.7	D37.8	D49.0
neck	C25.7	C78.89	D01.7	D13.6	D37.8	D49.0
overlapping lesion	C25.8	—	—	—	—	—
tail	C25.2	C78.89	D01.7	D13.6	D37.8	D49.0
para-aortic body	C75.5	C79.89	—	D35.6	D44.7	D49.7
paraganglion NEC	C75.5	C79.89	—	D35.6	D44.7	D49.7
parametrium	C57.3	C79.82	—	D28.2	D39.8	D49.59
paranephric	C48.0	C78.6	—	D20.0	D48.3	D49.0
pararectal	C76.3	C79.89	—	D36.7	D48.7	D49.89
parasagittal (region)	C76.0	C79.89	D09.8	D36.7	D48.7	D49.89
parasellar	C72.9	C79.49	—	D33.9	D43.8	D49.7
parathyroid (gland)	C75.0	C79.89	D09.3	D35.1	D44.2	D49.7
paraurethral	C76.3	C79.89	—	D36.7	D48.7	D49.89
gland	C68.1	C79.19	D09.19	D30.8	D41.8	D49.59
paravaginal	C76.3	C79.89	—	D36.7	D48.7	D49.89
parenchyma, kidney	C64.-	C79.0-	D09.19	D30.0-	D41.0-	D49.51-
parietal						
bone	C41.0	C79.51	—	D16.4-	D48.0	D49.2
lobe, brain	C71.3	C79.31	—	D33.0	D43.0	D49.6
paroophoron	C57.1	C79.82	D07.39	D28.2	D39.8	D49.59
parotid (duct) (gland)	C07	C79.89	D00.00	D11.0	D37.030	D49.0
parovarium	C57.1	C79.82	D07.39	D28.2	D39.8	D49.59
patella	C40.20	C79.51	—	—	—	—
peduncle, cerebral	C71.7	C79.31	—	D33.1	D43.1	D49.6
pelvirectal junction	C19	C78.5	D01.1	D12.7	D37.5	D49.0
pelvis, pelvic	C76.3	C79.89	D09.8	D36.7	D48.7	D49.89
bone	C41.4	C79.51	—	D16.8	D48.0	D49.2
floor	C76.3	C79.89	D09.8	D36.7	D48.7	D49.89
renal	C65.-	C79.0-	D09.19	D30.1-	D41.1-	D49.51-
viscera	C76.3	C79.89	D09.8	D36.7	D48.7	D49.89
wall	C76.3	C79.89	D09.8	D36.7	D48.7	D49.89
pelvo-abdominal	C76.8	C79.89	D09.8	D36.7	D48.7	D49.89
penis	C60.9	C79.82	D07.4	D29.0	D40.8	D49.59
body	C60.2	C79.82	D07.4	D29.0	D40.8	D49.59
corpus (cavernosum)	C60.2	C79.82	D07.4	D29.0	D40.8	D49.59
glans	C60.1	C79.82	D07.4	D29.0	D40.8	D49.59
overlapping sites	C60.8	—	—	—	—	—
skin NEC	C60.9	C79.82	D07.4	D29.0	D40.8	D49.59
periadrenal (tissue)	C48.0	C78.6	—	D20.0	D48.3	D49.0
perianal (skin) — *see also Neoplasm, anus, skin*	C44.500	C79.2	D04.5	D23.5	D48.5	D49.2
pericardium	C38.0	C79.89	—	D15.1	D48.7	D49.89
perinephric	C48.0	C78.6	—	D20.0	D48.3	D49.0

	Malignant Primary	Malignant Secondary	Ca in situ	Benign	Uncertain Behavior	Unspecified Behavior
perineum	C76.3	C79.89	D09.8	D36.7	D48.7	D49.89
periodontal tissue NEC	C03.9	C79.89	D00.03	D10.39	D37.09	D49.0
periosteum — *see Neoplasm, bone*						
peripancreatic	C48.0	C78.6	—	D20.0	D48.3	D49.0
peripheral nerve NEC	C47.9	C79.89	—	D36.10	D48.2	D49.2
perirectal (tissue)	C76.3	C79.89	—	D36.7	D48.7	D49.89
perirenal (tissue)	C48.0	C78.6	—	D20.0	D48.3	D49.0
peritoneum, peritoneal (cavity)	C48.2	C78.6	—	D20.1	D48.4	D49.0
benign mesothelial tissue — *see Mesothelioma, benign*						
overlapping lesion	C48.8	—	—	—	—	—
with digestive organs	C26.9	—	—	—	—	—
parietal	C48.1	C78.6	—	D20.1	D48.4	D49.0
pelvic	C48.1	C78.6	—	D20.1	D48.4	D49.0
specified part NEC	C48.1	C78.6	—	D20.1	D48.4	D49.0
peritonsillar (tissue)	C76.0	C79.89	D09.8	D36.7	D48.7	D49.89
periurethral tissue	C76.3	C79.89	—	D36.7	D48.7	D49.89
phalanges						
foot	C40.3-	C79.51	—	D16.3-	—	—
hand	C40.1-	C79.51	—	D16.1-	—	—
pharynx, pharyngeal	C14.0	C79.89	D00.08	D10.9	D37.05	D49.0
bursa	C11.1	C79.89	D00.08	D10.6	D37.05	D49.0
fornix	C11.3	C79.89	D00.08	D10.6	D37.05	D49.0
recess	C11.2	C79.89	D00.08	D10.6	D37.05	D49.0
region	C14.0	C79.89	D00.08	D10.9	D37.05	D49.0
tonsil	C11.1	C79.89	D00.08	D10.6	D37.05	D49.0
wall (lateral) (posterior)	C14.0	C79.89	D00.08	D10.9	D37.05	D49.0
pia mater	C70.9	C79.40	—	D32.9	D42.9	D49.7
cerebral	C70.0	C79.32	—	D32.0	D42.0	D49.7
cranial	C70.0	C79.32	—	D32.0	D42.0	D49.7
spinal	C70.1	C79.49	—	D32.1	D42.1	D49.7
pillars of fauces	C09.1	C79.89	D00.08	D10.5	D37.05	D49.0
pineal (body) (gland)	C75.3	C79.89	D09.3	D35.4	D44.5	D49.7
pinna (ear) NEC — *see also Neoplasm, skin, ear*	C44.20-	C79.2	D04.2-	D23.2-	D48.5	D49.2
piriform fossa or sinus	C12	C79.89	D00.08	D10.7	D37.05	D49.0
pituitary (body) (fossa) (gland) (lobe)	C75.1	C79.89	D09.3	D35.2	D44.3	D49.7
placenta	C58	C79.82	D07.0	D26.7	D39.2	D49.59
pleura, pleural (cavity)	C38.4	C78.2	—	D19.0	D38.2	D49.1
overlapping lesion with heart or mediastinum	C38.8	—	—	—	—	—
parietal	C38.4	C78.2	—	D19.0	D38.2	D49.1
visceral	C38.4	C78.2	—	D19.0	D38.2	D49.1

◀ New ⇐ Revised ~~deleted~~ Deleted

	Malignant Primary	Malignant Secondary	Ca in situ	Benign	Uncertain Behavior	Unspecified Behavior
plexus						
brachial	C47.1-	C79.89	—	D36.12	D48.2	D49.2
cervical	C47.0	C79.89	—	D36.11	D48.2	D49.2
choroid	C71.5	C79.31	—	D33.0	D43.0	D49.6
lumbosacral	C47.5	C79.89	—	D36.16	D48.2	D49.2
sacral	C47.5	C79.89	—	D36.16	D48.2	D49.2
pluriendocrine	C75.8	C79.89	D09.3	D35.7	D44.9	D49.7
pole						
frontal	C71.1	C79.31	—	D33.0	D43.0	D49.6
occipital	C71.4	C79.31	—	D33.0	D43.0	D49.6
pons (varolii)	C71.7	C79.31	—	D33.1	D43.1	D49.6
popliteal fossa or space	C76.5-	C79.89	D04.7-	D36.7	D48.7	D49.89
postcricoid (region)	C13.0	C79.89	D00.08	D10.7	D37.05	D49.0
posterior fossa (cranial)	C71.9	C79.31	—	D33.2	D43.2	D49.6
postnasal space	C11.9	C79.89	D00.08	D10.6	D37.05	D49.0
prepuce	C60.0	C79.82	D07.4	D29.0	D40.8	D49.59
prepylorus	C16.4	C78.89	D00.2	D13.1	D37.1	D49.0
presacral (region)	C76.3	C79.89	—	D36.7	D48.7	D49.89
prostate (gland)	C61	C79.82	D07.5	D29.1	D40.0	D49.59
utricle	C68.0	C79.19	D09.19	D30.4	D41.3	D49.59
pterygoid fossa	C49.0	C79.89	—	D21.0	D48.1	D49.2
pubic bone	C41.4	C79.51	—	D16.8	D48.0	D49.2
pudenda, pudendum (femaie)	C51.9	C79.82	D07.1	D28.0	D39.8	D49.59
pulmonary — *see also Neoplasm, lung*	C34.9-	C78.0-	D02.2-	D14.3-	D38.1	D49.1
putamen	C71.0	C79.31	—	D33.0	D43.0	D49.6
pyloric						
antrum	C16.3	C78.89	D00.2	D13.1	D37.1	D49.0
canal	C16.4	C78.89	D00.2	D13.1	D37.1	D49.0
pylorus	C16.4	C78.89	D00.2	D13.1	D37.1	D49.0
pyramid (brain)	C71.7	C79.31	—	D33.1	D43.1	D49.6
pyriform fossa or sinus	C12	C79.89	D00.08	D10.7	D37.05	D49.0
radius (any part)	C40.0-	C79.51	—	D16.0-	—	—
Rathke's pouch	C75.1	C79.89	D09.3	D35.2	D44.3	D49.7
rectosigmoid (junction)	C19	C78.5	D01.1	D12.7	D37.5	D49.0
overlapping lesion with anus or rectum	C21.8	—	—	—	—	—
rectouterine pouch	C48.1	C78.6	—	D20.1	D48.4	D49.0
rectovaginal septum or wall	C76.3	C79.89	D09.8	D36.7	D48.7	D49.89
rectovesical septum	C76.3	C79.89	D09.8	D36.7	D48.7	D49.89
rectum (ampulla)	C20	C78.5	D01.2	D12.8	D37.5	D49.0
and colon	C19	C78.5	D01.1	D12.7	D37.5	D49.0
overlapping lesion with anus or rectosigmoid junction	C21.8	—	—	—	—	—

	Malignant Primary	Malignant Secondary	Ca in situ	Benign	Uncertain Behavior	Unspecified Behavior
renal	C64.-	C79.0-	D09.19	D30.0-	D41.0-	D49.51-
calyx	C65.-	C79.0-	D09.19	D30.1-	D41.1-	D49.51-
hilus	C65.-	C79.0-	D09.19	D30.1-	D41.1-	D49.51-
parenchyma	C64.-	C79.0-	D09.19	D30.0-	D41.0-	D49.51-
pelvis	C65.-	C79.0-	D09.19	D30.1-	D41.1-	D49.51-
respiratory						
organs or system NEC	C39.9	C78.30	D02.4	D14.4	D38.6	D49.1
tract NEC	C39.9	C78.30	D02.4	D14.4	D38.5	D49.1
upper	C39.0	C78.30	D02.4	D14.4	D38.5	D49.1
retina	C69.2-	C79.49	D09.2-	D31.2-	D48.7	D49.81
retrobulbar	C69.6-	C79.49	—	D31.6-	D48.7	D49.89
retrocecal	C48.0	C78.6	—	D20.0	D48.3	D49.0
retromolar (area) (triangle) (trigone)	C06.2	C79.89	D00.00	D10.39	D37.09	D49.0
retro-orbital	C76.0	C79.89	D09.8	D36.7	D48.7	D49.89
retroperitoneal (space) (tissue)	C48.0	C78.6	—	D20.0	D48.3	D49.0
retroperitoneum	C48.0	C78.6	—	D20.0	D48.3	D49.0
retropharyngeal	C14.0	C79.89	D00.08	D10.9	D37.05	D49.0
retrovesical (septum)	C76.3	C79.89	D09.8	D36.7	D48.7	D49.89
rhinencephalon	C71.0	C79.31	—	D33.0	D43.0	D49.6
rib	C41.3	C79.51	—	D16.7	D48.0	D49.2
Rosenmuller's fossa	C11.2	C79.89	D00.08	D10.6	D37.05	D49.0
round ligament	C57.2	C79.82	—	D28.2	D39.8	D49.59
sacrococcyx, sacrococcygeal	C41.4	C79.51	—	D16.8	D48.0	D49.2
region	C76.3	C79.89	D09.8	D36.7	D48.7	D49.89
sacrouterine ligament	C57.3	C79.82	—	D28.2	D39.8	D49.59
sacrum, sacral (vertebra)	C41.4	C79.51	—	D16.8	D48.0	D49.2
salivary gland or duct (major)	C08.9	C79.89	D00.00	D11.9	D37.039	D49.0
minor NEC	C06.9	C79.89	D00.00	D10.39	D37.04	D49.0
overlapping lesion	C08.9	—	—	—	—	—
parotid	C07	C79.89	D00.00	D11.0	D37.030	D49.0
pluriglandular	C08.9	C79.89	D00.00	D11.9	D37.039	D49.0
sublingual	C08.1	C79.89	D00.00	D11.7	D37.031	D49.0
submandibular	C08.0	C79.89	D00.00	D11.7	D37.032	D49.0
submaxillary	C08.0	C79.89	D00.00	D11.7	D37.032	D49.0
salpinx (uterine)	C57.0-	C79.82	D07.39	D28.2	D39.8	D49.59
Santorini's duct	C25.3	C78.89	D01.7	D13.6	D37.8	D49.0
scalp	C44.40	C79.2	D04.4	D23.4	D48.5	D49.2
basal cell carcinoma	C44.41	—	—	—	—	—
specified type NEC	C44.49	—	—	—	—	—
squamous cell carcinoma	C44.42	—	—	—	—	—
scapula (any part)	C40.0-	C79.51	—	D16.0-	—	—
scapular region	C76.1	C79.89	D09.8	D36.7	D48.7	D49.89

◀ New ⇐ Revised ~~deleted~~ Deleted

	Malignant Primary	Malignant Secondary	Ca in situ	Benign	Uncertain Behavior	Unspecified Behavior
scar NEC — *see also Neoplasm, skin, by site*	C44.90	C79.2	D04.9	D23.9	D48.5	D49.2
sciatic nerve	C47.2-	C79.89	—	D36.13	D48.2	D49.2
sclera	C69.4-	C79.49	D09.2-	D31.4-	D48.7	D49.89
scrotum (skin)	C63.2	C79.82	D07.61	D29.4	D40.8	D49.59
sebaceous gland — *see Neoplasm, skin*						
sella turcica	C75.1	C79.89	D09.3	D35.2	D44.3	D49.7
bone	C41.0	C79.51	—	D16.4-	D48.0	D49.2
semilunar cartilage (knee)	C40.2-	C79.51	—	D16.2-	D48.0	D49.2
seminal vesicle	C63.7	C79.82	D07.69	D29.8	D40.8	D49.59
septum						
nasal	C30.0	C78.39	D02.3	D14.0	D38.5	D49.1
posterior margin	C11.3	C79.89	D00.08	D10.6	D37.05	D49.0
rectovaginal	C76.3	C79.89	D09.8	D36.7	D48.7	D49.89
rectovesical	C76.3	C79.89	D09.8	D36.7	D48.7	D49.89
urethrovaginal	C57.9	C79.82	D07.30	D28.9	D39.9	D49.59
vesicovaginal	C57.9	C79.82	D07.30	D28.9	D39.9	D49.59
shoulder NEC	C76.4-	C79.89	D04.6-	D36.7	D48.7	D49.89
sigmoid flexure (lower) (upper)	C18.7	C78.5	D01.0	D12.5	D37.4	D49.0
sinus (accessory)	C31.9	C78.39	D02.3	D14.0	D38.5	D49.1
bone (any)	C41.0	C79.51	—	D16.4-	D48.0	D49.2
ethmoidal	C31.1	C78.39	D02.3	D14.0	D38.5	D49.1
frontal	C31.2	C78.39	D02.3	D14.0	D38.5	D49.1
maxillary	C31.0	C78.39	D02.3	D14.0	D38.5	D49.1
nasal, paranasal NEC	C31.9	C78.39	D02.3	D14.0	D38.5	D49.1
overlapping lesion	C31.8	—	—	—	—	—
pyriform	C12	C79.89	D00.08	D10.7	D37.05	D49.0
sphenoid	C31.3	C78.39	D02.3	D14.0	D38.5	D49.1
skeleton, skeletal NEC	C41.9	C79.51	—	D16.9-	D48.0	D49.2
Skene's gland	C68.1	C79.19	D09.19	D30.8	D41.8	D49.59
skin NOS	C44.90	C79.2	D04.9	D23.9	D48.5	D49.2
abdominal wall	C44.509	C79.2	D04.5	D23.5	D48.5	D49.2
basal cell carcinoma	C44.519	—	—	—	—	—
specified type NEC	C44.599	—	—	—	—	—
squamous cell carcinoma	C44.529	—	—	—	—	—
ala nasi — *see also Neoplasm, nose, skin*	C44.301	C79.2	D04.39	D23.39	D48.5	D49.2
ankle — *see also Neoplasm, skin, limb, lower*	C44.70-	C79.2	D04.7-	D23.7-	D48.5	D49.2
antecubital space — *see also Neoplasm, skin, limb, upper*	C44.60-	C79.2	D04.6-	D23.6-	D48.5	D49.2

	Malignant Primary	Malignant Secondary	Ca in situ	Benign	Uncertain Behavior	Unspecified Behavior
skin NOS *(Continued)*						
anus	C44.500	C79.2	D04.5	D23.5	D48.5	D49.2
basal cell carcinoma	C44.510	—	—	—	—	—
specified type NEC	C44.590	—	—	—	—	—
squamous cell carcinoma	C44.520	—	—	—	—	—
arm — *see also Neoplasm, skin, limb, upper*	C44.60-	C79.2	D04.6-	D23.6-	D48.5	D49.2
auditory canal (external) — *see also Neoplasm, skin, ear*	C44.20-	C79.2	D04.2-	D23.2-	D48.5	D49.2
auricle (ear) — *see also Neoplasm, skin, ear*	C44.20-	C79.2	D04.2-	D23.2-	D48.5	D49.2
auricular canal (external) — *see also Neoplasm, skin, ear*	C44.20-	C79.2	D04.2-	D23.2-	D48.5	D49.2
axilla, axillary fold — *see also Neoplasm, skin, trunk*	C44.509	C79.2	D04.5	D23.5	D48.5	D49.2
back — *see also Neoplasm, skin, trunk*	C44.509	C79.2	D04.5	D23.5	D48.5	D49.2
basal cell carcinoma	C44.91					
breast	C44.501	C79.2	D04.5	D23.5	D48.5	D49.2
basal cell carcinoma	C44.511	—	—	—	—	—
specified type NEC	C44.591	—	—	—	—	—
squamous cell carcinoma	C44.521	—	—	—	—	—
brow — *see also Neoplasm, skin, face*	C44.309	C79.2	D04.39	D23.39	D48.5	D49.2
buttock — *see also Neoplasm, skin, trunk*	C44.509	C79.2	D04.5	D23.5	D48.5	D49.2
calf — *see also Neoplasm, skin, limb, lower*	C44.70-	C79.2	D04.7-	D23.7-	D48.5	D49.2
canthus (eye) (inner) (outer)	C44.10-	C79.2	D04.1-	D23.1-	D48.5	D49.2
basal cell carcinoma	C44.11-	—	—	—	—	—
specified type NEC	C44.19-	—	—	—	—	—
squamous cell carcinoma	C44.12-	—	—	—	—	—
cervical region — *see also Neoplasm, skin, neck*	C44.40	C79.2	D04.4	D23.4	D48.5	D49.2
cheek (external) — *see also Neoplasm, skin, face*	C44.309	C79.2	D04.39	D23.39	D48.5	D49.2
chest (wall) — *see also Neoplasm, skin, trunk*	C44.509	C79.2	D04.5	D23.5	D48.5	D49.2
chin — *see also Neoplasm, skin, face*	C44.309	C79.2	D04.39	D23.39	D48.5	D49.2
clavicular area — *see also Neoplasm, skin, trunk*	C44.509	C79.2	D04.5	D23.5	D48.5	D49.2
clitoris	C51.2	C79.82	D07.1	D28.0	D39.8	D49.59
columnella — *see also Neoplasm, skin, face*	C44.309	C79.2	D04.39	D23.39	D48.5	D49.2

◀ New ◀ Revised ~~deleted~~ Deleted

	Malignant Primary	Malignant Secondary	Ca in situ	Benign	Uncertain Behavior	Unspecified Behavior
skin NOS *(Continued)*						
concha — *see also Neoplasm, skin, ear*	C44.20-	C79.2	D04.2-	D23.2-	D48.5	D49.2
ear (external)	C44.20-	C79.2	D04.2-	D23.2-	D48.5	D49.2
basal cell carcinoma	C44.21-	—	—	—	—	—
specified type NEC	C44.29-	—	—	—	—	—
squamous cell carcinoma	C44.22-	—	—	—	—	—
elbow — *see also Neoplasm, skin, limb, upper*	C44.60-	C79.2	D04.6-	D23.6-	D48.5	D49.2
eyebrow — *see also Neoplasm, skin, face*	C44.309	C79.2	D04.39	D23.39	D48.5	D49.2
eyelid	C44.10-	C79.2	D04.1-	D23.1-	D48.5	D49.2
basal cell carcinoma	C44.11-	—	—	—	—	—
specified type NEC	C44.19-	—	—	—	—	—
squamous cell carcinoma	C44.12-	—	—	—	—	—
face NOS	C44.300	C79.2	D04.30	D23.30	D48.5	D49.2
basal cell carcinoma	C44.310	—	—	—	—	—
specified type NEC	C44.390	—	—	—	—	—
squamous cell carcinoma	C44.320	—	—	—	—	—
female genital organs (external)	C51.9	C79.82	D07.1	D28.0	D39.8	D49.59
clitoris	C51.2	C79.82	D07.1	D28.0	D39.8	D49.59
labium NEC	C51.9	C79.82	D07.1	D28.0	D39.8	D49.59
majus	C51.0	C79.82	D07.1	D28.0	D39.8	D49.59
minus	C51.1	C79.82	D07.1	D28.0	D39.8	D49.59
pudendum	C51.9	C79.82	D07.1	D28.0	D39.8	D49.59
vulva	C51.9	C79.82	D07.1	D28.0	D39.8	D49.59
finger — *see also Neoplasm, skin, limb, upper*	C44.60-	C79.2	D04.6-	D23.6-	D48.5	D49.2
flank — *see also Neoplasm, skin, trunk*	C44.509	C79.2	D04.5	D23.5	D48.5	D49.2
foot — *see also Neoplasm, skin, limb, lower*	C44.70-	C79.2	D04.7-	D23.7-	D48.5	D49.2
forearm — *see also Neoplasm, skin, limb, upper*	C44.60-	C79.2	D04.6-	D23.6-	D48.5	D49.2
forehead — *see also Neoplasm, skin, face*	C44.309	C79.2	D04.39	D23.39	D48.5	D49.2
glabella — *see also Neoplasm, skin, face*	C44.309	C79.2	D04.39	D23.39	D48.5	D49.2
gluteal region — *see also Neoplasm, skin, trunk*	C44.509	C79.2	D04.5	D23.5	D48.5	D49.2
groin — *see also Neoplasm, skin, trunk*	C44.509	C79.2	D04.5	D23.5	D48.5	D49.2
hand — *see also Neoplasm, skin, limb, upper*	C44.60-	C79.2	D04.6-	D23.6-	D48.5	D49.2

	Malignant Primary	Malignant Secondary	Ca in situ	Benign	Uncertain Behavior	Unspecified Behavior
skin NOS *(Continued)*						
head NEC — *see also Neoplasm, skin, scalp*	C44.40	C79.2	D04.4	D23.4	D48.5	D49.2
heel — *see also Neoplasm, skin, limb, lower*	C44.70-	C79.2	D04.7-	D23.7-	D48.5	D49.2
helix — *see also Neoplasm, skin, ear*	C44.20-	C79.2	D04.2-	D23.2-	D48.5	D49.2
hip — *see also Neoplasm, skin, limb, lower*	C44.70-	C79.2	D04.7-	D23.7-	D48.5	D49.2
infraclavicular region — *see also Neoplasm, skin, trunk*	C44.509	C79.2	D04.5	D23.5	D48.5	D49.2
inguinal region — *see also Neoplasm, skin, trunk*	C44.509	C79.2	D04.5	D23.5	D48.5	D49.2
jaw — *see also Neoplasm, skin, face*	C44.309	C79.2	D04.39	D23.39	D48.5	D49.2
Kaposi's sarcoma — *see Kaposi's, sarcoma, skin*						
knee — *see also Neoplasm, skin, limb, lower*	C44.70-	C79.2	D04.7-	D23.7-	D48.5	D49.2
labia						
majora	C51.0	C79.82	D07.1	D28.0	D39.8	D49.59
minora	C51.1	C79.82	D07.1	D28.0	D39.8	D49.59
leg — *see also Neoplasm, skin, limb, lower*	C44.70-	C79.2	D04.7-	D23.7-	D48.5	D49.2
lid (lower) (upper)	C44.10-	C79.2	D04.1-	D23.1-	D48.5	D49.2
basal cell carcinoma	C44.11-	—	—	—	—	—
specified type NEC	C44.19-	—	—	—	—	—
squamous cell carcinoma	C44.12-	—	—	—	—	—
limb NEC	C44.90	C79.2	D04.9	D23.9	D48.5	D49.2
basal cell carcinoma	C44.91					
lower	C44.70-	C79.2	D04.7-	D23.7-	D48.5	D49.2
basal cell carcinoma	C44.71-	—	—	—	—	—
specified type NEC	C44.79-	—	—	—	—	—
squamous cell carcinoma	C44.72-	—	—	—	—	—
upper	C44.60-	C79.2	D04.6-	D23.6-	D48.5	D49.2
basal cell carcinoma	C44.61-	—	—	—	—	—
specified type NEC	C44.69-	—	—	—	—	—
squamous cell carcinoma	C44.62-	—	—	—	—	—
lip (lower) (upper)	C44.00	C79.2	D04.0	D23.0	D48.5	D49.2
basal cell carcinoma	C44.01	—	—	—	—	—
specified type NEC	C44.09	—	—	—	—	—
squamous cell carcinoma	C44.02	—	—	—	—	—

◀ New ⇐ Revised ~~deleted~~ Deleted

	Malignant Primary	Malignant Secondary	Ca in situ	Benign	Uncertain Behavior	Unspecified Behavior
skin NOS *(Continued)*						
male genital organs	C63.9	C79.82	D07.60	D29.9	D40.8	D49.59
penis	C60.9	C79.82	D07.4	D29.0	D40.8	D49.59
prepuce	C60.0	C79.82	D07.4	D29.0	D40.8	D49.59
scrotum	C63.2	C79.82	D07.61	D29.4	D40.8	D49.59
mastectomy site (skin) — *see also Neoplasm, skin, breast*	C44.501	C79.2	—	—	—	—
specified as breast tissue	C50.8-	C79.81	—	—	—	—
meatus, acoustic (external) — *see also Neoplasm, skin, ear*	C44.20-	C79.2	D04.2-	D23.2-	D48.5	D49.2
melanotic — *see Melanoma*						
Merkel cell — *see Carcinoma, Merkel cell*						
nates — *see also Neoplasm, skin, trunk*	C44.509	C79.2	D04.5	D23.5	D48.5	D49.2
neck	C44.40	C79.2	D04.4	D23.4	D48.5	D49.2
basal cell carcinoma	C44.41	—	—	—	—	—
specified type NEC	C44.49	—	—	—	—	—
squamous cell carcinoma	C44.42	—	—	—	—	—
nevus — *see Nevus, skin*						
nose (external) — *see also Neoplasm, nose, skin*	C44.301	C79.2	D04.39	D23.39	D48.5	D49.2
overlapping lesion	C44.80	—	—	—	—	—
basal cell carcinoma	C44.81	—	—	—	—	—
specified type NEC	C44.89	—	—	—	—	—
squamous cell carcinoma	C44.82	—	—	—	—	—
palm — *see also Neoplasm, skin, limb, upper*	C44.60-	C79.2	D04.6-	D23.6-	D48.5	D49.2
palpebra	C44.10-	C79.2	D04.1-	D23.1-	D48.5	D49.2
basal cell carcinoma	C44.11-	—	—	—	—	—
specified type NEC	C44.19-	—	—	—	—	—
squamous cell carcinoma	C44.12-	—	—	—	—	—
penis NEC	C60.9	C79.82	D07.4	D29.0	D40.8	D49.59
perianal — *see also Neoplasm, skin, anus*	C44.500	C79.2	D04.5	D23.5	D48.5	D49.2
perineum — *see also Neoplasm, skin, anus*	C44.500	C79.2	D04.5	D23.5	D48.5	D49.2
pinna — *see also Neoplasm, skin, ear*	C44.20-	C79.2	D04.2-	D23.2-	D48.5	D49.2
plantar — *see also Neoplasm, skin, limb, lower*	C44.70-	C79.2	D04.7-	D23.7-	D48.5	D49.2
popliteal fossa or space — *see also Neoplasm, skin, limb, lower*	C44.70-	C79.2	D04.7-	D23.7-	D48.5	D49.2
prepuce	C60.0	C79.82	D07.4	D29.0	D40.8	D49.59

	Malignant Primary	Malignant Secondary	Ca in situ	Benign	Uncertain Behavior	Unspecified Behavior
skin NOS *(Continued)*						
pubes — *see also Neoplasm, skin, trunk*	C44.509	C79.2	D04.5	D23.5	D48.5	D49.2
sacrococcygeal region — *see also Neoplasm, skin, trunk*	C44.509	C79.2	D04.5	D23.5	D48.5	D49.2
scalp	C44.40	C79.2	D04.4	D23.4	D48.5	D49.2
basal cell carcinoma	C44.41	—	—	—	—	—
specified type NEC	C44.49	—	—	—	—	—
squamous cell carcinoma	C44.42	—	—	—	—	—
scapular region — *see also Neoplasm, skin, trunk*	C44.509	C79.2	D04.5	D23.5	D48.5	D49.2
scrotum	C63.2	C79.82	D07.61	D29.4	D40.8	D49.59
shoulder — *see also Neoplasm, skin, limb, upper*	C44.60-	C79.2	D04.6-	D23.6-	D48.5	D49.2
sole (foot) — *see also Neoplasm, skin, limb, lower*	C44.70-	C79.2	D04.7-	D23.7-	D48.5	D49.2
specified sites NEC	C44.80	C79.2	D04.8	D23.9	D48.5	D49.2
basal cell carcinoma	C44.81	—	—	—	—	—
specified type NEC	C44.89	—	—	—	—	—
squamous cell carcinoma	C44.82	—	—	—	—	—
specified type NEC	C44.99	—	—	—	—	—
squamous cell carcinoma	C44.92	—	—	—	—	—
submammary fold — *see also Neoplasm, skin, trunk*	C44.509	C79.2	D04.5	D23.5	D48.5	D49.2
supraclavicular region — *see also Neoplasm, skin, neck*	C44.40	C79.2	D04.4	D23.4	D48.5	D49.2
temple — *see also Neoplasm, skin, face*	C44.309	C79.2	D04.39	D23.39	D48.5	D49.2
thigh — *see also Neoplasm, skin, limb, lower*	C44.70-	C79.2	D04.7-	D23.7-	D48.5	D49.2
thoracic wall — *see also Neoplasm, skin, trunk*	C44.509	C79.2	D04.5	D23.5	D48.5	D49.2
thumb — *see also Neoplasm, skin, limb, upper*	C44.60-	C79.2	D04.6-	D23.6-	D48.5	D49.2
toe — *see also Neoplasm, skin, limb, lower*	C44.70-	C79.2	D04.7-	D23.7-	D48.5	D49.2
tragus — *see also Neoplasm, skin, ear*	C44.20-	C79.2	D04.2-	D23.2-	D48.5	D49.2
trunk	C44.509	C79.2	D04.5	D23.5	D48.5	D49.2
basal cell carcinoma	C44.519	—	—	—	—	—
specified type NEC	C44.599	—	—	—	—	—
squamous cell carcinoma	C44.529	—	—	—	—	—
umbilicus — *see also Neoplasm, skin, trunk*	C44.509	C79.2	D04.5	D23.5	D48.5	D49.2

◀ New ⇐ Revised ~~deleted~~ Deleted

	Malignant Primary	Malignant Secondary	Ca in situ	Benign	Uncertain Behavior	Unspecified Behavior
skin NOS *(Continued)*						
vulva	C51.9	C79.82	D07.1	D28.0	D39.8	D49.59
overlapping lesion	C51.8	—	—	—	—	—
wrist — *see also Neoplasm, skin, limb, upper*	C44.60-	C79.2	D04.6-	D23.6-	D48.5	D49.2
skull	C41.0	C79.51	—	D16.4-	D48.0	D49.2
soft parts or tissues — *see Neoplasm, connective tissue*						
specified site NEC	C76.8	C79.89	D09.8	D36.7	D48.7	D49.89
spermatic cord	C63.1-	C79.82	D07.69	D29.8	D40.8	D49.59
sphenoid	C31.3	C78.39	D02.3	D14.0	D38.5	D49.1
bone	C41.0	C79.51	—	D16.4-	D48.0	D49.2
sinus	C31.3	C78.39	D02.3	D14.0	D38.5	D49.1
sphincter						
anal	C21.1	C78.5	D01.3	D12.9	D37.8	D49.0
of Oddi	C24.0	C78.89	D01.5	D13.5	D37.6	D49.0
spine, spinal (column)	C41.2	C79.51	—	D16.6	D48.0	D49.2
bulb	C71.7	C79.31	—	D33.1	D43.1	D49.6
coccyx	C41.4	C79.51	—	D16.8	D48.0	D49.2
cord (cervical) (lumbar) (sacral) (thoracic)	C72.0	C79.49	—	D33.4	D43.4	D49.7
dura mater	C70.1	C79.49	—	D32.1	D42.1	D49.7
lumbosacral	C41.2	C79.51	—	D16.6	D48.0	D49.2
marrow NEC	C96.9	C79.52	—	—	D47.9	D49.89
membrane	C70.1	C79.49	—	D32.1	D42.1	D49.7
meninges	C70.1	C79.49	—	D32.1	D42.1	D49.7
nerve (root)	C47.9	C79.89	—	D36.10	D48.2	D49.2
pia mater	C70.1	C79.49	—	D32.1	D42.1	D49.7
root	C47.9	C79.89	—	D36.10	D48.2	D49.2
sacrum	C41.4	C79.51	—	D16.8	D48.0	D49.2
spleen, splenic NEC	C26.1	C78.89	D01.7	D13.9	D37.8	D49.0
flexure (colon)	C18.5	C78.5	D01.0	D12.3	D37.4	D49.0
stem, brain	C71.7	C79.31	—	D33.1	D43.1	D49.6
Stensen's duct	C07	C79.89	D00.00	D11.0	D37.030	D49.0
sternum	C41.3	C79.51	—	D16.7	D48.0	D49.2
stomach	C16.9	C78.89	D00.2	D13.1	D37.1	D49.0
antrum (pyloric)	C16.3	C78.89	D00.2	D13.1	D37.1	D49.0
body	C16.2	C78.89	D00.2	D13.1	D37.1	D49.0
cardia	C16.0	C78.89	D00.2	D13.1	D37.1	D49.0
cardiac orifice	C16.0	C78.89	D00.2	D13.1	D37.1	D49.0
corpus	C16.2	C78.89	D00.2	D13.1	D37.1	D49.0
fundus	C16.1	C78.89	D00.2	D13.1	D37.1	D49.0
greater curvature NEC	C16.6	C78.89	D00.2	D13.1	D37.1	D49.0
lesser curvature NEC	C16.5	C78.89	D00.2	D13.1	D37.1	D49.0

	Malignant Primary	Malignant Secondary	Ca in situ	Benign	Uncertain Behavior	Unspecified Behavior
stomach *(Continued)*						
overlapping lesion	C16.8	—	—	—	—	—
prepylorus	C16.4	C78.89	D00.2	D13.1	D37.1	D49.0
pylorus	C16.4	C78.89	D00.2	D13.1	D37.1	D49.0
wall NEC	C16.9	C78.89	D00.2	D13.1	D37.1	D49.0
anterior NEC	C16.8	C78.89	D00.2	D13.1	D37.1	D49.0
posterior NEC	C16.8	C78.89	D00.2	D13.1	D37.1	D49.0
stroma, endometrial	C54.1	C79.82	D07.0	D26.1	D39.0	D49.59
stump, cervical	C53.8	C79.82	D06.7	D26.0	D39.0	D49.59
subcutaneous (nodule) (tissue) NEC — *see Neoplasm, connective tissue*						
subdural	C70.9	C79.32	—	D32.9	D42.9	D49.7
subglottis, subglottic	C32.2	C78.39	D02.0	D14.1	D38.0	D49.1
sublingual	C04.9	C79.89	D00.06	D10.2	D37.09	D49.0
gland or duct	C08.1	C79.89	D00.00	D11.7	D37.031	D49.0
submandibular gland	C08.0	C79.89	D00.00	D11.7	D37.032	D49.0
submaxillary gland or duct	C08.0	C79.89	D00.00	D11.7	D37.032	D49.0
submental	C76.0	C79.89	D09.8	D36.7	D48.7	D49.89
subpleural	C34.9-	C78.0-	D02.2-	D14.3-	D38.1	D49.1
substernal	C38.1	C78.1	—	D15.2	D38.3	D49.89
sudoriferous, sudoriparous gland, site unspecified	C44.90	C79.2	D04.9	D23.9	D48.5	D49.2
specified site — *see Neoplasm, skin*						
supraclavicular region	C76.0	C79.89	D09.8	D36.7	D48.7	D49.89
supraglottis	C32.1	C78.39	D02.0	D14.1	D38.0	D49.1
suprarenal	C74.9-	C79.7-	D09.3	D35.0-	D44.1-	D49.7
capsule	C74.9-	C79.7-	D09.3	D35.0-	D44.1-	D49.7
cortex	C74.0-	C79.7-	D09.3	D35.0-	D44.1-	D49.7
gland	C74.9-	C79.7-	D09.3	D35.0-	D44.1-	D49.7
medulla	C74.1-	C79.7-	D09.3	D35.0-	D44.1-	D49.7
suprasellar (region)	C71.9	C79.31	—	D33.2	D43.2	D49.6
supratentorial (brain) NEC	C71.0	C79.31	—	D33.0	D43.0	D49.6
sweat gland (apocrine) (eccrine), site unspecified	C44.90	C79.2	D04.9	D23.9	D48.5	D49.2
specified site — *see Neoplasm, skin*						
sympathetic nerve or nervous system NEC	C47.9	C79.89	—	D36.10	D48.2	D49.2
symphysis pubis	C41.4	C79.51	—	D16.8	D48.0	D49.2
synovial membrane — *see Neoplasm, connective tissue*						
tapetum, brain	C71.8	C79.31	—	D33.2	D43.2	D49.6

◀ New ⇐ Revised ~~deleted~~ Deleted

	Malignant Primary	Malignant Secondary	Ca in situ	Benign	Uncertain Behavior	Unspecified Behavior
tarsus (any bone)	C40.3-	C79.51	—	D16.3-	—	—
temple (skin) — *see also Neoplasm, skin, face*	C44.309	C79.2	D04.39	D23.39	D48.5	D49.2
temporal						
bone	C41.0	C79.51	—	D16.4-	D48.0	D49.2
lobe or pole	C71.2	C79.31	—	D33.0	D43.0	D49.6
region	C76.0	C79.89	D09.8	D36.7	D48.7	D49.89
skin — *see also Neoplasm, skin, face*	C44.309	C79.2	D04.39	D23.39	D48.5	D49.2
tendon (sheath) — *see Neoplasm, connective tissue*						
tentorium (cerebelli)	C70.0	C79.32	—	D32.0	D42.0	D49.7
testis, testes	C62.9-	C79.82	D07.69	D29.2-	D40.1-	D49.59 ⇐
descended	C62.1-	C79.82	D07.69	D29.2-	D40.1-	D49.59 ⇐
ectopic	C62.0-	C79.82	D07.69	D29.2-	D40.1-	D49.59 ⇐
retained	C62.0-	C79.82	D07.69	D29.2-	D40.1-	D49.59 ⇐
scrotal	C62.1-	C79.82	D07.69	D29.2-	D40.1-	D49.59 ⇐
undescended	C62.0-	C79.82	D07.69	D29.2-	D40.1-	D49.59 ⇐
unspecified whether descended or undescended	C62.9-	C79.82	D07.69	D29.2-	D40.1-	D49.59 ⇐
thalamus	C71.0	C79.31	—	D33.0	D43.0	D49.6
thigh NEC	C76.5-	C79.89	D04.7-	D36.7	D48.7	D49.89
thorax, thoracic (cavity) (organs NEC)	C76.1	C79.89	D09.8	D36.7	D48.7	D49.89
duct	C49.3	C79.89	—	D21.3	D48.1	D49.2
wall NEC	C76.1	C79.89	D09.8	D36.7	D48.7	D49.89
throat	C14.0	C79.89	D00.08	D10.9	D37.05	D49.0
thumb NEC	C76.4-	C79.89	D04.6-	D36.7	D48.7	D49.89
thymus (gland)	C37	C79.89	D09.3	D15.0	D38.4	D49.89
thyroglossal duct	C73	C79.89	D09.3	D34	D44.0	D49.7
thyroid (gland)	C73	C79.89	D09.3	D34	D44.0	D49.7
cartilage	C32.3	C78.39	D02.0	D14.1	D38.0	D49.1
tibia (any part)	C40.2-	C79.51	—	D16.2-	—	—
toe NEC	C76.5-	C79.89	D04.7-	D36.7	D48.7	D49.89
tongue	C02.9	C79.89	D00.07	D10.1	D37.02	D49.0
anterior (two-thirds) NEC	C02.3	C79.89	D00.07	D10.1	D37.02	D49.0
dorsal surface	C02.0	C79.89	D00.07	D10.1	D37.02	D49.0
ventral surface	C02.2	C79.89	D00.07	D10.1	D37.02	D49.0
base (dorsal surface)	C01	C79.89	D00.07	D10.1	D37.02	D49.0
border (lateral)	C02.1	C79.89	D00.07	D10.1	D37.02	D49.0
dorsal surface NEC	C02.0	C79.89	D00.07	D10.1	D37.02	D49.0
fixed part NEC	C01	C79.89	D00.07	D10.1	D37.02	D49.0
foreamen cecum	C02.0	C79.89	D00.07	D10.1	D37.02	D49.0
frenulum linguae	C02.2	C79.89	D00.07	D10.1	D37.02	D49.0

	Malignant Primary	Malignant Secondary	Ca in situ	Benign	Uncertain Behavior	Unspecified Behavior
tongue *(Continued)*						
junctional zone	C02.8	C79.89	D00.07	D10.1	D37.02	D49.0
margin (lateral)	C02.1	C79.89	D00.07	D10.1	D37.02	D49.0
midline NEC	C02.0	C79.89	D00.07	D10.1	D37.02	D49.0
mobile part NEC	C02.3	C79.89	D00.07	D10.1	D37.02	D49.0
overlapping lesion	C02.8	—	—	—	—	—
posterior (third)	C01	C79.89	D00.07	D10.1	D37.02	D49.0
root	C01	C79.89	D00.07	D10.1	D37.02	D49.0
surface (dorsal)	C02.0	C79.89	D00.07	D10.1	D37.02	D49.0
base	C01	C79.89	D00.07	D10.1	D37.02	D49.0
ventral	C02.2	C79.89	D00.07	D10.1	D37.02	D49.0
tip	C02.1	C79.89	D00.07	D10.1	D37.02	D49.0
tonsil	C02.4	C79.89	D00.07	D10.1	D37.02	D49.0
tonsil	C09.9	C79.89	D00.08	D10.4	D37.05	D49.0
fauces, faucial	C09.9	C79.89	D00.08	D10.4	D37.05	D49.0
lingual	C02.4	C79.89	D00.07	D10.1	D37.02	D49.0
overlapping sites	C09.8	—	—	—	—	—
palatine	C09.9	C79.89	D00.08	D10.4	D37.05	D49.0
pharyngeal	C11.1	C79.89	D00.08	D10.6	D37.05	D49.0
pillar (anterior) (posterior)	C09.1	C79.89	D00.08	D10.5	D37.05	D49.0
tonsillar fossa	C09.0	C79.89	D00.08	D10.5	D37.05	D49.0
tooth socket NEC	C03.9	C79.89	D00.03	D10.39	D37.09	D49.0
trachea (cartilage) (mucosa)	C33	C78.39	D02.1	D14.2	D38.1	D49.1
overlapping lesion with bronchus or lung	C34.8-	—	—	—	—	—
tracheobronchial	C34.8-	C78.39	D02.1	D14.2	D38.1	D49.1
overlapping lesion with lung	C34.8-	—	—	—	—	—
tragus — *see also Neoplasm, skin, ear*	C44.20-	C79.2	D04.2-	D23.2-	D48.5	D49.2
trunk NEC	C76.8	C79.89	D04.5	D36.7	D48.7	D49.89
tubo-ovarian	C57.8	C79.82	D07.39	D28.7	D39.8	D49.59 ⇐
tunica vaginalis	C63.7	C79.82	D07.69	D29.8	D40.8	D49.59 ⇐
turbinate (bone)	C41.0	C79.51	—	D16.4-	D48.0	D49.2
nasal	C30.0	C78.39	D02.3	D14.0	D38.5	D49.1
tympanic cavity	C30.1	C78.39	D02.3	D14.0	D38.5	D49.1
ulna (any part)	C40.0-	C79.51	—	D16.0-	—	—
umbilicus, umbilical — *see also Neoplasm, skin, trunk*	C44.509	C79.2	D04.5	D23.5	D48.5	D49.2
uncus, brain	C71.2	C79.31	—	D33.0	D43.0	D49.6
unknown site or unspecified	C80.1	C79.9	D09.9	D36.9	D48.9	D49.9
urachus	C67.7	C79.11	D09.0	D30.3	D41.4	D49.4
ureter, ureteral	C66.-	C79.19	D09.19	D30.2-	D41.2-	D49.59 ⇐
orifice (bladder)	C67.6	C79.11	D09.0	D30.3	D41.4	D49.4
ureter-bladder (junction)	C67.6	C79.11	D09.0	D30.3	D41.4	D49.4

◀ New ⇐ Revised ~~deleted~~ Deleted

	Malignant Primary	Malignant Secondary	Ca in situ	Benign	Uncertain Behavior	Unspecified Behavior
urethra, urethral (gland)	C68.0	C79.19	D09.19	D30.4	D41.3	D49.59
orifice, internal	C67.5	C79.11	D09.0	D30.3	D41.4	D49.4
urethrovaginal (septum)	C57.9	C79.82	D07.30	D28.9	D39.8	D49.59
urinary organ or system	C68.9	C79.10	D09.10	D30.9	D41.9	D49.59
bladder — *see Neoplasm, bladder*						
overlapping lesion	C68.8	—	—	—	—	—
specified sites NEC	C68.8	C79.19	D09.19	D30.8	D41.8	D49.59
utero-ovarian	C57.8	C79.82	D07.39	D28.7	D39.8	D49.59
ligament	C57.1	C79.82	D07.39	D28.2	D39.8	D49.59
uterosacral ligament	C57.3	C79.82	—	D28.2	D39.8	D49.59
uterus, uteri, uterine	C55	C79.82	D07.0	D26.9	D39.0	D49.59
adnexa NEC	C57.4	C79.82	D07.39	D28.7	D39.8	D49.59
body	C54.9	C79.82	D07.0	D26.1	D39.0	D49.59
cervix	C53.9	C79.82	D06.9	D26.0	D39.0	D49.59
cornu	C54.9	C79.82	D07.0	D26.1	D39.0	D49.59
corpus	C54.9	C79.82	D07.0	D26.1	D39.0	D49.59
endocervix (canal) (gland)	C53.0	C79.82	D06.0	D26.0	D39.0	D49.59
endometrium	C54.1	C79.82	D07.0	D26.1	D39.0	D49.59
exocervix	C53.1	C79.82	D06.1	D26.0	D39.0	D49.59
external os	C53.1	C79.82	D06.1	D26.0	D39.0	D49.59
fundus	C54.3	C79.82	D07.0	D26.1	D39.0	D49.59
internal os	C53.0	C79.82	D06.0	D26.0	D39.0	D49.59
isthmus	C54.0	C79.82	D07.0	D26.1	D39.0	D49.59
ligament	C57.3	C79.82	—	D28.2	D39.8	D49.59
broad	C57.1	C79.82	D07.39	D28.2	D39.8	D49.59
round	C57.2	C79.82	—	D28.2	D39.8	D49.59
lower segment	C54.0	C79.82	D07.0	D26.1	D39.0	D49.59
myometrium	C54.2	C79.82	D07.0	D26.1	D39.0	D49.59
overlapping sites	C54.8	—	—	—	—	—
squamocolumnar junction	C53.8	C79.82	D06.7	D26.0	D39.0	D49.59
tube	C57.0-	C79.82	D07.39	D28.2	D39.8	D49.59
utricle, prostatic	C68.0	C79.19	D09.19	D30.4	D41.3	D49.59
uveal tract	C69.4-	C79.49	D09.2-	D31.4-	D48.7	D49.89
uvula	C05.2	C79.89	D00.04	D10.39	D37.09	D49.0
vagina, vaginal (fornix) (vault) (wall)	C52	C79.82	D07.2	D28.1	D39.8	D49.59
vaginovesical	C57.9	C79.82	D07.30	D28.9	D39.9	D49.59
septum	C57.9	C79.82	D07.30	D28.9	D39.9	D49.59
vallecula (epigiottis)	C10.0	C79.89	D00.08	D10.5	D37.05	D49.0
vas deferens	C63.1-	C79.82	D07.69	D29.8	D40.8	D49.59
vascular — *see Neoplasm, connective tissue*						

	Malignant Primary	Malignant Secondary	Ca in situ	Benign	Uncertain Behavior	Unspecified Behavior
Vater's ampulla	C24.1	C78.89	D01.5	D13.5	D37.6	D49.0
vein, venous — *see Neoplasm, connective tissue*						
vena cava (abdominal) (inferior)	C49.4	C79.89	—	D21.4	D48.1	D49.2
superior	C49.3	C79.89	—	D21.3	D48.1	D49.2
ventricle (cerebral) (floor) (lateral) (third)	C71.5	C79.31	—	D33.0	D43.0	D49.6
cardiac (left) (right)	C38.0	C79.89	—	D15.1	D48.7	D49.89
fourth	C71.7	C79.31	—	D33.1	D43.1	D49.6
ventricular band of larynx	C32.1	C78.39	D02.0	D14.1	D38.0	D49.1
ventriculus — *see Neoplasm, stomach*						
vermillion border — *see Neoplasm, lip*						
vermis, cerebellum	C71.6	C79.31	—	D33.1	D43.1	D49.6
vertebra (column)	C41.2	C79.51	—	D16.6	D48.0	D49.2
coccyx	C41.4	C79.51	—	D16.8-	D48.0	D49.2
marrow NEC	C96.9	C79.52	—	—	D47.9	D49.89
sacrum	C41.4	C79.51	—	D16.8-	D48.0	D49.2
vesical — *see Neoplasm, bladder*						
vesicle, seminal	C63.7	C79.82	D07.69	D29.8	D40.8	D49.59
vesicocervical tissue	C57.9	C79.82	D07.30	D28.9	D39.9	D49.59
vesicorectal	C76.3	C79.82	D09.8	D36.7	D48.7	D49.89
vesicovaginal	C57.9	C79.82	D07.30	D28.9	D39.9	D49.59
septum	C57.9	C79.82	D07.30	D28.9	D39.8	D49.59
vessel (blood) — *see Neoplasm, connective tissue*						
vestibular gland, greater	C51.0	C79.82	D07.1	D28.0	D39.8	D49.59
vestibule						
mouth	C06.1	C79.89	D00.00	D10.39	D37.09	D49.0
nose	C30.0	C78.39	D02.3	D14.0	D38.5	D49.1
Virchow's gland	C77.0	C77.0	—	D36.0	D48.7	D49.89
viscera NEC	C76.8	C79.89	D09.8	D36.7	D48.7	D49.89
vocal cords (true)	C32.0	C78.39	D02.0	D14.1	D38.0	D49.1
false	C32.1	C78.39	D02.0	D14.1	D38.0	D49.1
vomer	C41.0	C79.51	—	D16.4-	D48.0	D49.2
vulva	C51.9	C79.82	D07.1	D28.0	D39.8	D49.59
vulvovaginal gland	C51.0	C79.82	D07.1	D28.0	D39.8	D49.59
Waldeyer's ring	C14.2	C79.89	D00.08	D10.9	D37.05	D49.0
Wharton's duct	C08.0	C79.89	D00.00	D11.7	D37.032	D49.0
white matter (central) (cerebral)	C71.0	C79.31	—	D33.0	D43.0	D49.6
windpipe	C33	C78.39	D02.1	D14.2	D38.1	D49.1

◀ New ⇐ Revised ~~deleted~~ Deleted

	Malignant Primary	Malignant Secondary	Ca in situ	Benign	Uncertain Behavior	Unspecified Behavior
Wirsung's duct	C25.3	C78.89	D01.7	D13.6	D37.8	D49.0
wolffian (body) (duct)						
female	C57.7	C79.82	D07.39	D28.7	D39.8	D49.59
male	C63.7	C79.82	D07.69	D29.8	D40.8	D49.59

	Malignant Primary	Malignant Secondary	Ca in situ	Benign	Uncertain Behavior	Unspecified Behavior
womb — *see Neoplasm, uterus*						
wrist NEC	C76.4-	C79.89	D04.6-	D36.7	D48.7	D49.89
xiphoid process	C41.3	C79.51	—	D16.7	D48.0	D49.2
Zuckerkandl organ	C75.5	C79.89	—	D35.6	D44.7	D49.7

◀ New ⇐ Revised ~~deleted~~ Deleted

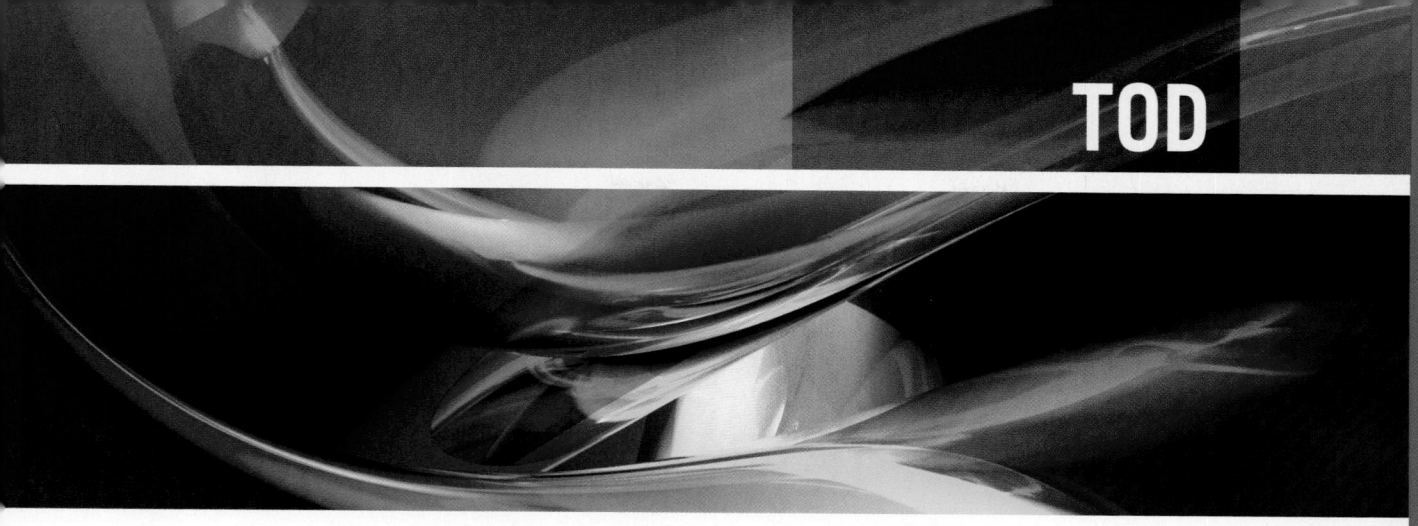

ICD-10-CM
Table of Drugs and Chemicals

Substance	External Cause (T-Code)					
	Poisoning, Accidental (Unintentional)	Poisoning, Intentional Self-Harm	Poisoning, Assault	Poisoning, Undetermined	Adverse Effect	Underdosing
#						
1-propanol	T51.3X1	T51.3X2	T51.3X3	T51.3X4	—	—
2-propanol	T51.2X1	T51.2X2	T51.2X3	T51.2X4	—	—
2,4-D (dichlorophen-oxyacetic acid)	T60.3X1	T60.3X2	T60.3X3	T60.3X4	—	—
2,4-toluene diisocyanate	T65.0X1	T65.0X2	T65.0X3	T65.0X4	—	—
2,4,5-T (trichloro-phenoxyacetic acid)	T60.1X1	T60.1X2	T60.1X3	T60.1X4	—	—
14-hydroxydihydro-morphinone	T40.2X1	T40.2X2	T40.2X3	T40.2X4	T40.2X5	T40.2X6
A						
ABOB	T37.5X1	T37.5X2	T37.5X3	T37.5X4	T37.5X5	T37.5X6
Abrine	T62.2X1	T62.2X2	T62.2X3	T62.2X4	—	—
Abrus (seed)	T62.2X1	T62.2X2	T62.2X3	T62.2X4	—	—
Absinthe	T51.0X1	T51.0X2	T51.0X3	T51.0X4	—	—
beverage	T51.0X1	T51.0X2	T51.0X3	T51.0X4	—	—
Acaricide	T60.8X1	T60.8X2	T60.8X3	T60.8X4	—	—
Acebutolol	T44.7X1	T44.7X2	T44.7X3	T44.7X4	T44.7X5	T44.7X6
Acecarbromal	T42.6X1	T42.6X2	T42.6X3	T42.6X4	T42.6X5	T42.6X6
Aceclidine	T44.1X1	T44.1X2	T44.1X3	T44.1X4	T44.1X5	T44.1X6
Acedapsone	T37.0X1	T37.0X2	T37.0X3	T37.0X4	T37.0X5	T37.0X6
Acefylline piperazine	T48.6X1	T48.6X2	T48.6X3	T48.6X4	T48.6X5	T48.6X6
Acemorphan	T40.2X1	T40.2X2	T40.2X3	T40.2X4	T40.2X5	T40.2X6
Acenocoumarin	T45.511	T45.512	T45.513	T45.514	T45.515	T45.516
Acenocoumarol	T45.511	T45.512	T45.513	T45.514	T45.515	T45.516
Acepifylline	T48.6X1	T48.6X2	T48.6X3	T48.6X4	T48.6X5	T48.6X6
Acepromazine	T43.3X1	T43.3X2	T43.3X3	T43.3X4	T43.3X5	T43.3X6
Acesulfamethoxypyridazine	T37.0X1	T37.0X2	T37.0X3	T37.0X4	T37.0X5	T37.0X6
Acetal	T52.8X1	T52.8X2	T52.8X3	T52.8X4	—	—
Acetaldehyde (vapor)	T52.8X1	T52.8X2	T52.8X3	T52.8X4	—	—
liquid	T65.891	T65.892	T65.893	T65.894	—	—
P-Acetamidophenol	T39.1X1	T39.1X2	T39.1X3	T39.1X4	T39.1X5	T39.1X6
Acetaminophen	T39.1X1	T39.1X2	T39.1X3	T39.1X4	T39.1X5	T39.1X6
Acetaminosalol	T39.1X1	T39.1X2	T39.1X3	T39.1X4	T39.1X5	T39.1X6
Acetanilide	T39.1X1	T39.1X2	T39.1X3	T39.1X4	T39.1X5	T39.1X6
Acetarsol	T37.3X1	T37.3X2	T37.3X3	T37.3X4	T37.3X5	T37.3X6
Acetazolamide	T50.2X1	T50.2X2	T50.2X3	T50.2X4	T50.2X5	T50.2X6
Acetiamine	T45.2X1	T45.2X2	T45.2X3	T45.2X4	T45.2X5	T45.2X6
Acetic						
acid	T54.2X1	T54.2X2	T54.2X3	T54.2X4	—	—
with sodium acetate (ointment)	T49.3X1	T49.3X2	T49.3X3	T49.3X4	T49.3X5	T49.3X6

Substance	External Cause (T-Code)					
	Poisoning, Accidental (Unintentional)	Poisoning, Intentional Self-Harm	Poisoning, Assault	Poisoning, Undetermined	Adverse Effect	Underdosing
Acetic *(Continued)*						
acid *(Continued)*						
ester (solvent) (vapor)	T52.8X1	T52.8X2	T52.8X3	T52.8X4	—	—
irrigating solution	T50.3X1	T50.3X2	T50.3X3	T50.3X4	T50.3X5	T50.3X6
medicinal (lotion)	T49.2X1	T49.2X2	T49.2X3	T49.2X4	T49.2X5	T49.2X6
anhydride	T65.891	T65.892	T65.893	T65.894	—	—
ether (vapor)	T52.8X1	T52.8X2	T52.8X3	T52.8X4	—	—
Acetohexamide	T38.3X1	T38.3X2	T38.3X3	T38.3X4	T38.3X5	T38.3X6
Acetohydroxamic acid	T50.991	T50.992	T50.993	T50.994	T50.995	T50.996
Acetomenaphthone	T45.7X1	T45.7X2	T45.7X3	T45.7X4	T45.7X5	T45.7X6
Acetomorphine	T40.1X1	T40.1X2	T40.1X3	T40.1X4	—	—
Acetone (oils)	T52.4X1	T52.4X2	T52.4X3	T52.4X4	—	—
chlorinated	T52.4X1	T52.4X2	T52.4X3	T52.4X4	—	—
vapor	T52.4X1	T52.4X2	T52.4X3	T52.4X4	—	—
Acetonitrile	T52.8X1	T52.8X2	T52.8X3	T52.8X4	—	—
Acetophenazine	T43.3X1	T43.3X2	T43.3X3	T43.3X4	T43.3X5	T43.3X6
Acetophenetedin	T39.1X1	T39.1X2	T39.1X3	T39.1X4	T39.1X5	T39.1X6
Acetophenone	T52.4X1	T52.4X2	T52.4X3	T52.4X4	—	—
Acetorphine	T40.2X1	T40.2X2	T40.2X3	T40.2X4	—	—
Acetosulfone (sodium)	T37.1X1	T37.1X2	T37.1X3	T37.1X4	T37.1X5	T37.1X6
Acetrizoate (sodium)	T50.8X1	T50.8X2	T50.8X3	T50.8X4	T50.8X5	T50.8X6
Acetylcarbromal	T42.6X1	T42.6X2	T42.6X3	T42.6X4	T42.6X5	T42.6X6
Acetrizoic acid	T50.8X1	T50.8X2	T50.8X3	T50.8X4	T50.8X5	T50.8X6
Acetyl						
bromide	T53.6X1	T53.6X2	T53.6X3	T53.6X4	—	—
chloride	T53.6X1	T53.6X2	T53.6X3	T53.6X4	—	—
Acetylcholine						
chloride	T44.1X1	T44.1X2	T44.1X3	T44.1X4	T44.1X5	T44.1X6
derivative	T44.1X1	T44.1X2	T44.1X3	T44.1X4	T44.1X5	T44.1X6
Acetylcysteine	T48.4X1	T48.4X2	T48.4X3	T48.4X4	T48.4X5	T48.4X6
Acetyldigitoxin	T46.0X1	T46.0X2	T46.0X3	T46.0X4	T46.0X5	T46.0X6
Acetyldigoxin	T46.0X1	T46.0X2	T46.0X3	T46.0X4	T46.0X5	T46.0X6
Acetyldihydrocodeine	T40.2X1	T40.2X2	T40.2X3	T40.2X4	—	—
Acetyldihydrocodeinone	T40.2X1	T40.2X2	T40.2X3	T40.2X4	—	—
Acetylene (gas)	T59.891	T59.892	T59.893	T59.894	—	—
dichloride	T53.6X1	T53.6X2	T53.6X3	T53.6X4	—	—
incomplete combustion of	T58.11	T58.12	T58.13	T58.14	—	—
industrial	T59.891	T59.892	T59.893	T59.894	—	—
tetrachloride	T53.6X1	T53.6X2	T53.6X3	T53.6X4	—	—
vapor	T53.6X1	T53.6X2	T53.6X3	T53.6X4	—	—
Acetylphenylhydrazine	T39.8X1	T39.8X2	T39.8X3	T39.8X4	T39.8X5	T39.8X6
Acetylpheneturide	T42.6X1	T42.6X2	T42.6X3	T42.6X4	T42.6X5	T42.6X6

Substance	Poisoning, Accidental (Unintentional)	Poisoning, Intentional Self-Harm	Poisoning, Assault	Poisoning, Undetermined	Adverse Effect	Underdosing
	External Cause (T-Code)					
Acetylsalicylic acid (salts)	T39.011	T39.012	T39.013	T39.014	T39.015	T39.016
enteric coated	T39.011	T39.012	T39.013	T39.014	T39.015	T39.016
Acetylsulfamethoxypyridazine	T37.0X1	T37.0X2	T37.0X3	T37.0X4	T37.0X5	T37.0X6
Achromycin	T36.4X1	T36.4X2	T36.4X3	T36.4X4	T36.4X5	T36.4X6
ophthalmic preparation	T49.5X1	T49.5X2	T49.5X3	T49.5X4	T49.5X5	T49.5X6
topical NEC	T49.0X1	T49.0X2	T49.0X3	T49.0X4	T49.0X5	T49.0X6
Aciclovir	T37.5X1	T37.5X2	T37.5X3	T37.5X4	T37.5X5	T37.5X6
Acid (corrosive) NEC	T54.2X1	T54.2X2	T54.2X3	T54.2X4	—	—
Acidifying agent NEC	T50.901	T50.902	T50.903	T50.904	T50.905	T50.906
Acipimox	T46.6X1	T46.6X2	T46.6X3	T46.6X4	T46.6X5	T46.6X6
Acitretin	T50.991	T50.992	T50.993	T50.994	T50.995	T50.996
Aclarubicin	T45.1X1	T45.1X2	T45.1X3	T45.1X4	T45.1X5	T45.1X6
Aclatonium napadisilate	T48.1X1	T48.1X2	T48.1X3	T48.1X4	T48.1X5	T48.1X6
Aconite (wild)	T46.991	T46.992	T46.993	T46.994	T46.995	T46.996
Aconitine	T46.991	T46.992	T46.993	T46.994	T46.995	T46.996
Aconitum ferox	T46.991	T46.992	T46.993	T46.994	T46.995	T46.996
Acridine	T65.6X1	T65.6X2	T65.6X3	T65.6X4	—	—
vapor	T59.891	T59.892	T59.893	T59.894	—	—
Acriflavine	T37.91	T37.92	T37.93	T37.94	T37.95	T37.96
Acriflavinium chloride	T49.0X1	T49.0X2	T49.0X3	T49.0X4	T49.0X5	T49.0X6
Acrinol	T49.0X1	T49.0X2	T49.0X3	T49.0X4	T49.0X5	T49.0X6
Acrisorcin	T49.0X1	T49.0X2	T49.0X3	T49.0X4	T49.0X5	T49.0X6
Acrivastine	T45.0X1	T45.0X2	T45.0X3	T45.0X4	T45.0X5	T45.0X6
Acrolein (gas)	T59.891	T59.892	T59.893	T59.894	—	—
liquid	T54.1X1	T54.1X2	T54.1X3	T54.1X4	—	—
Acrylamide	T65.891	T65.892	T65.893	T65.894	—	—
Acrylic resin	T49.3X1	T49.3X2	T49.3X3	T49.3X4	T49.3X5	T49.3X6
Acrylonitrile	T65.891	T65.892	T65.893	T65.894	—	—
Actaea spicata	T62.2X1	T62.2X2	T62.2X3	T62.2X4	—	—
berry	T62.1X1	T62.1X2	T62.1X3	T62.1X4	—	—
Acterol	T37.3X1	T37.3X2	T37.3X3	T37.3X4	T37.3X5	T37.3X6
ACTH	T38.811	T38.812	T38.813	T38.814	T38.815	T38.816
Actinomycin C	T45.1X1	T45.1X2	T45.1X3	T45.1X4	T45.1X5	T45.1X6
Actinomycin D	T45.1X1	T45.1X2	T45.1X3	T45.1X4	T45.1X5	T45.1X6
Activated charcoal — *see also Charcoal, medicinal*	T47.6X1	T47.6X2	T47.6X3	T47.6X4	T47.6X5	T47.6X6
Acyclovir	T37.5X1	T37.5X2	T37.5X3	T37.5X4	T37.5X5	T37.5X6
Adenine	T45.2X1	T45.2X2	T45.2X3	T45.2X4	T45.2X5	T45.2X6
arabinoside	T37.5X1	T37.5X2	T37.5X3	T37.5X4	T37.5X5	T37.5X6
Adenosine (phosphate)	T46.2X1	T46.2X2	T46.2X3	T46.2X4	T46.2X5	T46.2X6
ADH	T38.891	T38.892	T38.893	T38.894	T38.895	T38.896
Adhesive NEC	T65.891	T65.892	T65.893	T65.894	—	—

Substance	Poisoning, Accidental (Unintentional)	Poisoning, Intentional Self-Harm	Poisoning, Assault	Poisoning, Undetermined	Adverse Effect	Underdosing
	External Cause (T-Code)					
Adicillin	T36.0X1	T36.0X2	T36.0X3	T36.0X4	T36.0X5	T36.0X6
Adiphenine	T44.3X1	T44.3X2	T44.3X3	T44.3X4	T44.3X5	T44.3X6
Adipiodone	T50.8X1	T50.8X2	T50.8X3	T50.8X4	T50.8X5	T50.8X6
Adjunct, pharmaceutical	T50.901	T50.902	T50.903	T50.904	T50.905	T50.906
Adrenal (extract, cortex or medulla) (glucocorticoids) (hormones) (mineralo corticoids)	T38.0X1	T38.0X2	T38.0X3	T38.0X4	T38.0X5	T38.0X6
ENT agent	T49.6X1	T49.6X2	T49.6X3	T49.6X4	T49.6X5	T49.6X6
ophthalmic preparation	T49.5X1	T49.5X2	T49.5X3	T49.5X4	T49.5X5	T49.5X6
topical NEC	T49.0X1	T49.0X2	T49.0X3	T49.0X4	T49.0X5	T49.0X6
Adrenaline	T44.5X1	T44.5X2	T44.5X3	T44.5X4	T44.5X5	T44.5X6
Adrenalin — *see Adrenaline*						
Adrenergic NEC	T44.901	T44.902	T44.903	T44.904	T44.905	T44.906
blocking agent NEC	T44.8X1	T44.8X2	T44.8X3	T44.8X4	T44.8X5	T44.8X6
beta, heart	T44.7X1	T44.7X2	T44.7X3	T44.7X4	T44.7X5	T44.7X6
specified NEC	T44.991	T44.992	T44.993	T44.994	T44.995	T44.996
Adrenochrome						
(mono) semicarbazone	T46.991	T46.992	T46.993	T46.994	T46.995	T46.996
derivative	T46.991	T46.992	T46.993	T46.994	T46.995	T46.996
Adrenocorticotrophic hormone	T38.811	T38.812	T38.813	T38.814	T38.815	T38.816
Adrenocorticotrophin	T38.811	T38.812	T38.813	T38.814	T38.815	T38.816
Adriamycin	T45.1X1	T45.1X2	T45.1X3	T45.1X4	T45.1X5	T45.1X6
Aerosol spray NEC	T65.91	T65.92	T65.93	T65.94	—	—
Aerosporin	T36.8X1	T36.8X2	T36.8X3	T36.8X4	T36.8X5	T36.8X6
ENT agent	T49.6X1	T49.6X2	T49.6X3	T49.6X4	T49.6X5	T49.6X6
ophthalmic preparation	T49.5X1	T49.5X2	T49.5X3	T49.5X4	T49.5X5	T49.5X6
topical NEC	T49.0X1	T49.0X2	T49.0X3	T49.0X4	T49.0X5	T49.0X6
Aethusa cynapium	T62.2X1	T62.2X2	T62.2X3	T62.2X4	—	—
Afghanistan black	T40.7X1	T40.7X2	T40.7X3	T40.7X4	T40.7X5	T40.7X6
Aflatoxin	T64.01	T64.02	T64.03	T64.04	—	—
Afloqualone	T42.8X1	T42.8X2	T42.8X3	T42.8X4	T42.8X5	T42.8X6
African boxwood	T62.2X1	T62.2X2	T62.2X3	T62.2X4	—	—
Agar	T47.4X1	T47.4X2	T47.4X3	T47.4X4	T47.4X5	T47.4X6
Agonist						
predominantly						
alpha-adrenoreceptor	T44.4X1	T44.4X2	T44.4X3	T44.4X4	T44.4X5	T44.4X6
beta-adrenoreceptor	T44.5X1	T44.5X2	T44.5X3	T44.5X4	T44.5X5	T44.5X6
Agricultural agent NEC	T65.91	T65.92	T65.93	T65.94	—	—
Agrypnal	T42.3X1	T42.3X2	T42.3X3	T42.3X4	T42.3X5	T42.3X6
AHLG	T50.Z11	T50.Z12	T50.Z13	T50.Z14	T50.Z15	T50.Z16
Air contaminant(s), source/type NOS	T65.91	T65.92	T65.93	T65.94	—	—

◀ New ◀ Revised ~~deleted~~ Deleted

Substance	External Cause (T-Code)					
	Poisoning, Accidental (Unintentional)	Poisoning, Intentional Self-Harm	Poisoning, Assault	Poisoning, Undetermined	Adverse Effect	Underdosing
Ajmaline	T46.2X1	T46.2X2	T46.2X3	T46.2X4	T46.2X5	T46.2X6
Akritoin	T37.8X1	T37.8X2	T37.8X3	T37.8X4	T37.8X5	T37.8X6
Akee	T62.1X1	T62.1X2	T62.1X3	T62.1X4	—	—
Akrinol	T49.0X1	T49.0X2	T49.0X3	T49.0X4	T49.0X5	T49.0X6
Alacepril	T46.4X1	T46.4X2	T46.4X3	T46.4X4	T46.4X5	T46.4X6
Alantolactone	T37.4X1	T37.4X2	T37.4X3	T37.4X4	T37.4X5	T37.4X6
Albamycin	T36.8X1	T36.8X2	T36.8X3	T36.8X4	T36.8X5	T36.8X6
Albendazole	T37.4X1	T37.4X2	T37.4X3	T37.4X4	T37.4X5	T37.4X6
Albumin						
bovine	T45.8X1	T45.8X2	T45.8X3	T45.8X4	T45.8X5	T45.8X6
human serum	T45.8X1	T45.8X2	T45.8X3	T45.8X4	T45.8X5	T45.8X6
salt-poor	T45.8X1	T45.8X2	T45.8X3	T45.8X4	T45.8X5	T45.8X6
normal human serum	T45.8X1	T45.8X2	T45.8X3	T45.8X4	T45.8X5	T45.8X6
Albuterol	T48.6X1	T48.6X2	T48.6X3	T48.6X4	T48.6X5	T48.6X6
Albutoin	T42.0X1	T42.0X2	T42.0X3	T42.0X4	T42.0X5	T42.0X6
Alclometasone	T49.0X1	T49.0X2	T49.0X3	T49.0X4	T49.0X5	T49.0X6
Alcohol	T51.91	T51.92	T51.93	T51.94	—	—
absolute	T51.0X1	T51.0X2	T51.0X3	T51.0X4	—	—
beverage	T51.0X1	T51.0X2	T51.0X3	T51.0X4	—	—
allyl	T51.8X1	T51.8X2	T51.8X3	T51.8X4	—	—
amyl	T51.3X1	T51.3X2	T51.3X3	T51.3X4	—	—
antifreeze	T51.1X1	T51.1X2	T51.1X3	T51.1X4	—	—
beverage	T51.0X1	T51.0X2	T51.0X3	T51.0X4	—	—
butyl	T51.3X1	T51.3X2	T51.3X3	T51.3X4	—	—
dehydrated	T51.0X1	T51.0X2	T51.0X3	T51.0X4	—	—
beverage	T51.0X1	T51.0X2	T51.0X3	T51.0X4	—	—
denatured	T51.0X1	T51.0X2	T51.0X3	T51.0X4	—	—
deterrent NEC	T50.6X1	T50.6X2	T50.6X3	T50.6X4	T50.6X5	T50.6X6
diagnostic (gastric function)	T50.8X1	T50.8X2	T50.8X3	T50.8X4	T50.8X5	T50.8X6
ethyl	T51.0X1	T51.0X2	T51.0X3	T51.0X4	—	—
beverage	T51.0X1	T51.0X2	T51.0X3	T51.0X4	—	—
grain	T51.0X1	T51.0X2	T51.0X3	T51.0X4	—	—
beverage	T51.0X1	T51.0X2	T51.0X3	T51.0X4	—	—
industrial	T51.0X1	T51.0X2	T51.0X3	T51.0X4	—	—
isopropyl	T51.2X1	T51.2X2	T51.2X3	T51.2X4	—	—
methyl	T51.1X1	T51.1X2	T51.1X3	T51.1X4	—	—
preparation for consumption	T51.0X1	T51.0X2	T51.0X3	T51.0X4	—	—
propyl	T51.3X1	T51.3X2	T51.3X3	T51.3X4	—	—
secondary	T51.2X1	T51.2X2	T51.2X3	T51.2X4	—	—
radiator	T51.1X1	T51.1X2	T51.1X3	T51.1X4	—	—
rubbing	T51.2X1	T51.2X2	T51.2X3	T51.2X4	—	—
specified type NEC	T51.8X1	T51.8X2	T51.8X3	T51.8X4	—	—

Substance	External Cause (T-Code)					
	Poisoning, Accidental (Unintentional)	Poisoning, Intentional Self-Harm	Poisoning, Assault	Poisoning, Undetermined	Adverse Effect	Underdosing
Alcohol *(Continued)*						
surgical	T51.0X1	T51.0X2	T51.0X3	T51.0X4	—	—
vapor (from any type of Alcohol)	T59.891	T59.892	T59.893	T59.894	—	—
wood	T51.1X1	T51.1X2	T51.1X3	T51.1X4	—	—
Alcuronium (chloride)	T48.1X1	T48.1X2	T48.1X3	T48.1X4	T48.1X5	T48.1X6
Aldactone	T50.0X1	T50.0X2	T50.0X3	T50.0X4	T50.0X5	T50.0X6
Aldesulfone sodium	T37.1X1	T37.1X2	T37.1X3	T37.1X4	T37.1X5	T37.1X6
Aldicarb	T60.0X1	T60.0X2	T60.0X3	T60.0X4	—	—
Aldomet	T46.5X1	T46.5X2	T46.5X3	T46.5X4	T46.5X5	T46.5X6
Aldosterone	T50.0X1	T50.0X2	T50.0X3	T50.0X4	T50.0X5	T50.0X6
Aldrin (dust)	T60.1X1	T60.1X2	T60.1X3	T60.1X4	—	—
Aleve — *see Naproxen*						
Alexitol sodium	T47.1X1	T47.1X2	T47.1X3	T47.1X4	T47.1X5	T47.1X6
Alfacalcidol	T45.2X1	T45.2X2	T45.2X3	T45.2X4	T45.2X5	T45.2X6
Alfadolone	T41.1X1	T41.1X2	T41.1X3	T41.1X4	T41.1X5	T41.1X6
Alfaxalone	T41.1X1	T41.1X2	T41.1X3	T41.1X4	T41.1X5	T41.1X6
Alfentanil	T40.4X1	T40.4X2	T40.4X3	T40.4X4	T40.4X5	T40.4X6
Alfuzosin (hydrochloride)	T44.8X1	T44.8X2	T44.8X3	T44.8X4	T44.8X5	T44.8X6
Algae (harmful) (toxin)	T65.821	T65.822	T65.823	T65.824	—	—
Algeldrate	T47.1X1	T47.1X2	T47.1X3	T47.1X4	T47.1X5	T47.1X6
Algin	T47.8X1	T47.8X2	T47.8X3	T47.8X4	T47.8X5	T47.8X6
Alglucerase	T45.3X1	T45.3X2	T45.3X3	T45.3X4	T45.3X5	T45.3X6
Alidase	T45.3X1	T45.3X2	T45.3X3	T45.3X4	T45.3X5	T45.3X6
Alimemazine	T43.3X1	T43.3X2	T43.3X3	T43.3X4	T43.3X5	T43.3X6
Aliphatic thiocyanates	T65.0X1	T65.0X2	T65.0X3	T65.0X4	—	—
Alizapride	T45.0X1	T45.0X2	T45.0X3	T45.0X4	T45.0X5	T45.0X6
Alkali (caustic)	T54.3X1	T54.3X2	T54.3X3	T54.3X4	—	—
Alkalizing agent NEC	T50.901	T50.902	T50.903	T50.904	T50.905	T50.906
Alkaline antiseptic solution (aromatic)	T49.6X1	T49.6X2	T49.6X3	T49.6X4	T49.6X5	T49.6X6
Alkalinizing agents (medicinal)	T50.901	T50.902	T50.903	T50.904	T50.905	T50.906
Alka-seltzer	T39.011	T39.012	T39.013	T39.014	T39.015	T39.016
Alkavervir	T46.5X1	T46.5X2	T46.5X3	T46.5X4	T46.5X5	T46.5X6
Alkonium (bromide)	T49.0X1	T49.0X2	T49.0X3	T49.0X4	T49.0X5	T49.0X6
Alkylating drug NEC	T45.1X1	T45.1X2	T45.1X3	T45.1X4	T45.1X5	T45.1X6
antimyeloproliferative	T45.1X1	T45.1X2	T45.1X3	T45.1X4	T45.1X5	T45.1X6
lymphatic	T45.1X1	T45.1X2	T45.1X3	T45.1X4	T45.1X5	T45.1X6
Alkylisocyanate	T65.0X1	T65.0X2	T65.0X3	T65.0X4	—	—
Allantoin	T49.411	T49.412	T49.413	T49.414	T49.415	T49.416
Allegron	T43.0X1	T43.0X2	T43.0X3	T43.0X4	T43.0X5	T43.0X6
Allethrin	T49.0X1	T49.0X2	T49.0X3	T49.0X4	T49.0X5	T49.0X6
Allobarbital	T42.3X1	T42.3X2	T42.3X3	T42.3X4	T42.3X5	T42.3X6

◀ New ◀ Revised ~~deleted~~ Deleted

Substance	External Cause (T-Code)					
	Poisoning, Accidental (Unintentional)	Poisoning, Intentional Self-Harm	Poisoning, Assault	Poisoning, Undetermined	Adverse Effect	Underdosing
Allopurinol	T50.4X1	T50.4X2	T50.4X3	T50.4X4	T50.4X5	T50.4X6
Allyl						
alcohol	T51.8X1	T51.8X2	T51.8X3	T51.8X4	—	—
disulfide	T46.6X1	T46.6X2	T46.6X3	T46.6X4	T46.6X5	T46.6X6
Allylestrenol	T38.5X1	T38.5X2	T38.5X3	T38.5X4	T38.5X5	T38.5X6
Allylisopropylacetylurea	T42.6X1	T42.6X2	T42.6X3	T42.6X4	T42.6X5	T42.6X6
Allylisopropylmalonylurea	T42.3X1	T42.3X2	T42.3X3	T42.3X4	T42.3X5	T42.3X6
Allylthiourea	T49.3X1	T49.3X2	T49.3X3	T49.3X4	T49.3X5	T49.3X6
Allyltribromide	T42.6X1	T42.6X2	T42.6X3	T42.6X4	T42.6X5	T42.6X6
Allypropymal	T42.3X1	T42.3X2	T42.3X3	T42.3X4	T42.3X5	T42.3X6
Almagate	T47.1X1	T47.1X2	T47.1X3	T47.1X4	T47.1X5	T47.1X6
Almasilate	T47.1X1	T47.1X2	T47.1X3	T47.1X4	T47.1X5	T47.1X6
Almitrine	T50.7X1	T50.7X2	T50.7X3	T50.7X4	T50.7X5	T50.7X6
Aloes	T47.2X1	T47.2X2	T47.2X3	T47.2X4	T47.2X5	T47.2X6
Aloglutamol	T47.1X1	T47.1X2	T47.1X3	T47.1X4	T47.1X5	T47.1X6
Aloin	T47.2X1	T47.2X2	T47.2X3	T47.2X4	T47.2X5	T47.2X6
Aloxidone	T42.2X1	T42.2X2	T42.2X3	T42.2X4	T42.2X5	T42.2X6
Alpha						
acetyldigoxin	T46.0X1	T46.0X2	T46.0X3	T46.0X4	T46.0X5	T46.0X6
adrenergic blocking drug	T44.6X1	T44.6X2	T44.6X3	T44.6X4	T44.6X5	T44.6X6
amylase	T45.3X1	T45.3X2	T45.3X3	T45.3X4	T45.3X5	T45.3X6
tocoferol (acetate)	T45.2X1	T45.2X2	T45.2X3	T45.2X4	T45.2X5	T45.2X6
tocopherol	T45.2X1	T45.2X2	T45.2X3	T45.2X4	T45.2X5	T45.2X6
Alphadolone	T41.1X1	T41.1X2	T41.1X3	T41.1X4	T41.1X5	T41.1X6
Alphaprodine	T40.4X1	T40.4X2	T40.4X3	T40.4X4	T40.4X5	T40.4X6
Alphaxalone	T41.1X1	T41.1X2	T41.1X3	T41.1X4	T41.1X5	T41.1X6
Alprazolam	T42.4X1	T42.4X2	T42.4X3	T42.4X4	T42.4X5	T42.4X6
Alprenolol	T44.7X1	T44.7X2	T44.7X3	T44.7X4	T44.7X5	T44.7X6
Alprostadil	T46.7X1	T46.7X2	T46.7X3	T46.7X4	T46.7X5	T46.7X6
Alsactide	T38.811	T38.812	T38.813	T38.814	T38.815	T38.816
Alseroxylon	T46.5X1	T46.5X2	T46.5X3	T46.5X4	T46.5X5	T46.5X6
Alteplase	T45.611	T45.612	T45.613	T45.614	T45.615	T45.616
Altizide	T50.2X1	T50.2X2	T50.2X3	T50.2X4	T50.2X5	T50.2X6
Altretamine	T45.1X1	T45.1X2	T45.1X3	T45.1X4	T45.1X5	T45.1X6
Alum (medicinal)	T49.4X1	T49.4X2	T49.4X3	T49.4X4	T49.4X5	T49.4X6
nonmedicinal (ammonium) (potassium)	T56.891	T56.892	T56.893	T56.894	—	—
Aluminium, aluminum						
acetate	T49.2X1	T49.2X2	T49.2X3	T49.2X4	T49.2X5	T49.2X6
solution	T49.0X1	T49.0X2	T49.0X3	T49.0X4	T49.0X5	T49.0X6
aspirin	T39.011	T39.012	T39.013	T39.014	T39.015	T39.016
bis (acetylsalicylate)	T39.011	T39.012	T39.013	T39.014	T39.015	T39.016

Substance	External Cause (T-Code)					
	Poisoning, Accidental (Unintentional)	Poisoning, Intentional Self-Harm	Poisoning, Assault	Poisoning, Undetermined	Adverse Effect	Underdosing
Aluminium, aluminum *(Continued)*						
carbonate (gel, basic)	T47.1X1	T47.1X2	T47.1X3	T47.1X4	T47.1X5	T47.1X6
chlorhydroxide-complex	T47.1X1	T47.1X2	T47.1X3	T47.1X4	T47.1X5	T47.1X6
chloride	T49.2X1	T49.2X2	T49.2X3	T49.2X4	T49.2X5	T49.2X6
clofibrate	T46.6X1	T46.6X2	T46.6X3	T46.6X4	T46.6X5	T46.6X6
diacetate	T49.2X1	T49.2X2	T49.2X3	T49.2X4	T49.2X5	T49.2X6
glycinate	T47.1X1	T47.1X2	T47.1X3	T47.1X4	T47.1X5	T47.1X6
hydroxide (gel)	T47.1X1	T47.1X2	T47.1X3	T47.1X4	T47.1X5	T47.1X6
hydroxide-magnesium carb. gel	T47.1X1	T47.1X2	T47.1X3	T47.1X4	T47.1X5	T47.1X6
magnesium silicate	T47.1X1	T47.1X2	T47.1X3	T47.1X4	T47.1X5	T47.1X6
nicotinate	T46.7X1	T46.7X2	T46.7X3	T46.7X4	T46.7X5	T46.7X6
ointment (surgical) (topical)	T49.3X1	T49.3X2	T49.3X3	T49.3X4	T49.3X5	T49.3X6
phosphate	T47.1X1	T47.1X2	T47.1X3	T47.1X4	T47.1X5	T47.1X6
salicylate	T39.091	T39.092	T39.093	T39.094	T39.095	T39.096
silicate	T47.1X1	T47.1X2	T47.1X3	T47.1X4	T47.1X5	T47.1X6
sodium silicate	T47.1X1	T47.1X2	T47.1X3	T47.1X4	T47.1X5	T47.1X6
subacetate	T49.2X1	T49.2X2	T49.2X3	T49.2X4	T49.2X5	T49.2X6
sulfate	T49.0X1	T49.0X2	T49.0X3	T49.0X4	T49.0X5	T49.0X6
tannate	T47.6X1	T47.6X2	T47.6X3	T47.6X4	T47.6X5	T47.6X6
topical NEC	T49.3X1	T49.3X2	T49.3X3	T49.3X4	T49.3X5	T49.3X6
Alurate	T42.3X1	T42.3X2	T42.3X3	T42.3X4	T42.3X5	T42.3X6
Alverine	T44.3X1	T44.3X2	T44.3X3	T44.3X4	T44.3X5	T44.3X6
Alvodine	T40.2X1	T40.2X2	T40.2X3	T40.2X4	T40.2X5	T40.2X6
Amanita phalloides	T62.0X1	T62.0X2	T62.0X3	T62.0X4	—	—
Amanitine	T62.0X1	T62.0X2	T62.0X3	T62.0X4	—	—
Amantadine	T42.8X1	T42.8X2	T42.8X3	T42.8X4	T42.8X5	T42.8X6
Ambazone	T49.6X1	T49.6X2	T49.6X3	T49.6X4	T49.6X5	T49.6X6
Ambenonium (chloride)	T44.0X1	T44.0X2	T44.0X3	T44.0X4	T44.0X5	T44.0X6
Ambroxol	T48.4X1	T48.4X2	T48.4X3	T48.4X4	T48.4X5	T48.4X6
Ambuphylline	T48.6X1	T48.6X2	T48.6X3	T48.6X4	T48.6X5	T48.6X6
Ambutonium bromide	T44.3X1	T44.3X2	T44.3X3	T44.3X4	T44.3X5	T44.3X6
Amcinonide	T49.0X1	T49.0X2	T49.0X3	T49.0X4	T49.0X5	T49.0X6
Amdinocilline	T36.0X1	T36.0X2	T36.0X3	T36.0X4	T36.0X5	T36.0X6
Ametazole	T50.8X1	T50.8X2	T50.8X3	T50.8X4	T50.8X5	T50.8X6
Amethocaine	T41.3X1	T41.3X2	T41.3X3	T41.3X4	T41.3X5	T41.3X6
regional	T41.3X1	T41.3X2	T41.3X3	T41.3X4	T41.3X5	T41.3X6
spinal	T41.3X1	T41.3X2	T41.3X3	T41.3X4	T41.3X5	T41.3X6
Amethopterin	T45.1X1	T45.1X2	T45.1X3	T45.1X4	T45.1X5	T45.1X6
Amezinium metilsulfate	T44.991	T44.992	T44.993	T44.994	T44.995	T44.996
Amfebutamone	T43.291	T43.292	T43.293	T43.294	T43.295	T43.296
Amfepramone	T50.5X1	T50.5X2	T50.5X3	T50.5X4	T50.5X5	T50.5X6

◀ New ◀ Revised ~~deleted~~ Deleted

Substance	External Cause (T-Code)					
	Poisoning, Accidental (Unintentional)	Poisoning, Intentional Self-Harm	Poisoning, Assault	Poisoning, Undetermined	Adverse Effect	Underdosing
Amfetamine	T43.621	T43.622	T43.623	T43.624	T43.625	T43.626
Amfetaminil	T43.621	T43.622	T43.623	T43.624	T43.625	T43.626
Amfomycin	T36.8X1	T36.8X2	T36.8X3	T36.8X4	T36.8X5	T36.8X6
Amidefrine mesilate	T48.5X1	T48.5X2	T48.5X3	T48.5X4	T48.5X5	T48.5X6
Amidone	T40.3X1	T40.3X2	T40.3X3	T40.3X4	T40.3X5	T40.3X6
Amidopyrine	T39.2X1	T39.2X2	T39.2X3	T39.2X4	T39.2X5	T39.2X6
Amidotrizoate	T50.8X1	T50.8X2	T50.8X3	T50.8X4	T50.8X5	T50.8X6
Amiflamine	T43.1X1	T43.1X2	T43.1X3	T43.1X4	T43.1X5	T43.1X6
Amikacin	T36.5X1	T36.5X2	T36.5X3	T36.5X4	T36.5X5	T36.5X6
Amikhelline	T46.3X1	T46.3X2	T46.3X3	T46.3X4	T46.3X5	T46.3X6
Amiloride	T50.2X1	T50.2X2	T50.2X3	T50.2X4	T50.2X5	T50.2X6
Aminacrine	T49.0X1	T49.0X2	T49.0X3	T49.0X4	T49.0X5	T49.0X6
Amineptine	T43.011	T43.012	T43.013	T43.014	T43.015	T43.016
Aminitrozole	T37.3X1	T37.3X2	T37.3X3	T37.3X4	T37.3X5	T37.3X6
Aminoacetic acid (derivatives)	T50.3X1	T50.3X2	T50.3X3	T50.3X4	T50.3X5	T50.3X6
Amino acids	T50.3X1	T50.3X2	T50.3X3	T50.3X4	T50.3X5	T50.3X6
Aminoacridine	T49.0X1	T49.0X2	T49.0X3	T49.0X4	T49.0X5	T49.0X6
Aminobenzoic acid (-p)	T49.3X1	T49.3X2	T49.3X3	T49.3X4	T49.3X5	T49.3X6
4-Aminobutyric acid	T43.8X1	T43.8X2	T43.8X3	T43.8X4	T43.8X5	T43.8X6
Aminocaproic acid	T45.621	T45.622	T45.623	T45.624	T45.625	T45.626
Aminofenazone	T39.2X1	T39.2X2	T39.2X3	T39.2X4	T39.2X5	T39.2X6
Aminoethylisothiourium	T45.8X1	T45.8X2	T45.8X3	T45.8X4	T45.8X5	T45.8X6
Aminoglutethimide	T45.1X1	T45.1X2	T45.1X3	T45.1X4	T45.1X5	T45.1X6
Aminohippuric acid	T50.8X1	T50.8X2	T50.8X3	T50.8X4	T50.8X5	T50.8X6
Aminomethylbenzoic acid	T45.691	T45.692	T45.693	T45.694	T45.695	T45.696
Aminometradine	T50.2X1	T50.2X2	T50.2X3	T50.2X4	T50.2X5	T50.2X6
Aminopentamide	T44.3X1	T44.3X2	T44.3X3	T44.3X4	T44.3X5	T44.3X6
Aminophenazone	T39.2X1	T39.2X2	T39.2X3	T39.2X4	T39.2X5	T39.2X6
Aminophenol	T54.0X1	T54.0X2	T54.0X3	T54.0X4	—	—
4-Aminophenol derivatives	T39.1X1	T39.1X2	T39.1X3	T39.1X4	T39.1X5	T39.1X6
Aminophenylpyridone	T43.591	T43.592	T43.593	T43.594	T43.595	T43.596
Aminophylline	T48.6X1	T48.6X2	T48.6X3	T48.6X4	T48.6X5	T48.6X6
Aminopterin sodium	T45.1X1	T45.1X2	T45.1X3	T45.1X4	T45.1X5	T45.1X6
Aminopyrine	T39.2X1	T39.2X2	T39.2X3	T39.2X4	T39.2X5	T39.2X6
8-Aminoquinoline drugs	T37.2X1	T37.2X2	T37.2X3	T37.2X4	T37.2X5	T37.2X6
Aminorex	T50.5X1	T50.5X2	T50.5X3	T50.5X4	T50.5X5	T50.5X6
Aminosalicylic acid	T37.1X1	T37.1X2	T37.1X3	T37.1X4	T37.1X5	T37.1X6
Aminosalylum	T37.1X1	T37.1X2	T37.1X3	T37.1X4	T37.1X5	T37.1X6
Amiodarone	T46.2X1	T46.2X2	T46.2X3	T46.2X4	T46.2X5	T46.2X6
Amiphenazole	T50.7X1	T50.7X2	T50.7X3	T50.7X4	T50.7X5	T50.7X6
Amiquinsin	T46.5X1	T46.5X2	T46.5X3	T46.5X4	T46.5X5	T46.5X6
Amisometradine	T50.2X1	T50.2X2	T50.2X3	T50.2X4	T50.2X5	T50.2X6

Substance	External Cause (T-Code)					
	Poisoning, Accidental (Unintentional)	Poisoning, Intentional Self-Harm	Poisoning, Assault	Poisoning, Undetermined	Adverse Effect	Underdosing
Amisulpride	T43.591	T43.592	T43.593	T43.594	T43.595	T43.596
Amitriptyline	T43.021	T43.022	T43.023	T43.024	T43.025	T43.026
Amitriptylinoxide	T43.021	T43.022	T43.023	T43.024	T43.025	T43.026
Amlexanox	T48.6X1	T48.6X2	T48.6X3	T48.6X4	T48.6X5	T48.6X6
Ammonia (fumes) (gas) (vapor)	T59.891	T59.892	T59.893	T59.894	—	—
aromatic spirit	T48.991	T48.992	T48.993	T48.994	T48.995	T48.996
liquid (household)	T54.3X1	T54.3X2	T54.3X3	T54.3X4	—	—
Ammoniated mercury	T49.0X1	T49.0X2	T49.0X3	T49.0X4	T49.0X5	T49.0X6
Ammonium						
acid tartrate	T49.5X1	T49.5X2	T49.5X3	T49.5X4	T49.5X5	T49.5X6
bromide	T42.6X1	T42.6X2	T42.6X3	T42.6X4	T42.6X5	T42.6X6
carbonate	T54.3X1	T54.3X2	T54.3X3	T54.3X4	—	—
chloride	T50.991	T50.992	T50.993	T50.994	T50.995	T50.996
expectorant	T48.4X1	T48.4X2	T48.4X3	T48.4X4	T48.4X5	T48.4X6
compounds (household) NEC	T54.3X1	T54.3X2	T54.3X3	T54.3X4	—	—
fumes (any usage)	T59.891	T59.892	T59.893	T59.894	—	—
industrial	T54.3X1	T54.3X2	T54.3X3	T54.3X4	—	—
ichthyosulronate	T49.4X1	T49.4X2	T49.4X3	T49.4X4	T49.4X5	T49.4X6
mandelate	T37.91	T37.92	T37.93	T37.94	T37.95	T37.96
sulfamate	T60.3X1	T60.3X2	T60.3X3	T60.3X4	—	—
sulfonate resin	T47.8X1	T47.8X2	T47.8X3	T47.8X4	T47.8X5	T47.8X6
Amobarbital (sodium)	T42.3X1	T42.3X2	T42.3X3	T42.3X4	T42.3X5	T42.3X6
Amodiaquine	T37.2X1	T37.2X2	T37.2X3	T37.2X4	T37.2X5	T37.2X6
Amopyroquin(e)	T37.2X1	T37.2X2	T37.2X3	T37.2X4	T37.2X5	T37.2X6
Amoxapine	T43.011	T43.012	T43.013	T43.014	T43.015	T43.016
Amoxicillin	T36.0X1	T36.0X2	T36.0X3	T36.0X4	T36.0X5	T36.0X6
Amperozide	T43.591	T43.592	T43.593	T43.594	T43.595	T43.596
Amphenidone	T43.591	T43.592	T43.593	T43.594	T43.595	T43.596
Amphetamine NEC	T43.621	T43.622	T43.623	T43.624	T43.625	T43.626
Amphomycin	T36.8X1	T36.8X2	T36.8X3	T36.8X4	T36.8X5	T36.8X6
Amphotalide	T37.4X1	T37.4X2	T37.4X3	T37.4X4	T37.4X5	T37.4X6
Amphotericin B	T36.7X1	T36.7X2	T36.7X3	T36.7X4	T36.7X5	T36.7X6
topical	T49.0X1	T49.0X2	T49.0X3	T49.0X4	T49.0X5	T49.0X6
Ampicillin	T36.0X1	T36.0X2	T36.0X3	T36.0X4	T36.0X5	T36.0X6
Amprotropine	T44.3X1	T44.3X2	T44.3X3	T44.3X4	T44.3X5	T44.3X6
Amsacrine	T45.1X1	T45.1X2	T45.1X3	T45.1X4	T45.1X5	T45.1X6
Amygdaline	T62.2X1	T62.2X2	T62.2X3	T62.2X4	—	—
Amyl						
acetate	T52.8X1	T52.8X2	T52.8X3	T52.8X4	—	—
vapor	T59.891	T59.892	T59.893	T59.894	—	—
alcohol	T51.3X1	T51.3X2	T51.3X3	T51.3X4	—	—
chloride	T53.6X1	T53.6X2	T53.6X3	T53.6X4	—	—

Substance	External Cause (T-Code)					
	Poisoning, Accidental (Unintentional)	Poisoning, Intentional Self-Harm	Poisoning, Assault	Poisoning, Undetermined	Adverse Effect	Underdosing
Amyl *(Continued)*						
formate	T52.8X1	T52.8X2	T52.8X3	T52.8X4	—	—
nitrite	T46.3X1	T46.3X2	T46.3X3	T46.3X4	T46.3X5	T46.3X6
propionate	T65.891	T65.892	T65.893	T65.894	—	—
Amylase	T47.5X1	T47.5X2	T47.5X3	T47.5X4	T47.5X5	T47.5X6
Amyleine, regional	T41.3X1	T41.3X2	T41.3X3	T41.3X4	T41.3X5	T41.3X6
Amylene						
dichloride	T53.6X1	T53.6X2	T53.6X3	T53.6X4	—	—
hydrate	T51.3X1	T51.3X2	T51.3X3	T51.3X4	—	—
Amylmetacresol	T49.6X1	T49.6X2	T49.6X3	T49.6X4	T49.6X5	T49.6X6
Amylobarbitone	T42.3X1	T42.3X2	T42.3X3	T42.3X4	T42.3X5	T42.3X6
Amylocaine, regional	T41.3X1	T41.3X2	T41.3X3	T41.3X4	T41.3X5	T41.3X6
infiltration (subcutaneous)	T41.3X1	T41.3X2	T41.3X3	T41.3X4	T41.3X5	T41.3X6
nerve block (peripheral) (plexus)	T41.3X1	T41.3X2	T41.3X3	T41.3X4	T41.3X5	T41.3X6
spinal	T41.3X1	T41.3X2	T41.3X3	T41.3X4	T41.3X5	T41.3X6
topical (surface)	T41.3X1	T41.3X2	T41.3X3	T41.3X4	T41.3X5	T41.3X6
Amylopectin	T47.6X1	T47.6X2	T47.6X3	T47.6X4	T47.6X5	T47.6X6
Amytal (sodium)	T42.3X1	T42.3X2	T42.3X3	T42.3X4	T42.3X5	T42.3X6
Anabolic steroid	T38.7X1	T38.7X2	T38.7X3	T38.7X4	T38.7X5	T38.7X6
Analeptic NEC	T50.7X1	T50.7X2	T50.7X3	T50.7X4	T50.7X5	T50.7X6
Analgesic	T39.91	T39.92	T39.93	T39.94	T39.95	T39.96
anti-inflammatory NEC	T39.91	T39.92	T39.93	T39.94	T39.95	T39.96
propionic acid derivative	T39.311	T39.312	T39.313	T39.314	T39.315	T39.316
antirheumatic NEC	T39.4X1	T39.4X2	T39.4X3	T39.4X4	T39.4X5	T39.4X6
aromatic NEC	T39.1X1	T39.1X2	T39.1X3	T39.1X4	T39.1X5	T39.1X6
narcotic NEC	T40.601	T40.602	T40.603	T40.604	T40.605	T40.606
combination	T40.601	T40.602	T40.603	T40.604	T40.605	T40.606
obstetric	T40.601	T40.602	T40.603	T40.604	T40.605	T40.606
non-narcotic NEC	T39.91	T39.92	T39.93	T39.94	T39.95	T39.96
combination	T39.91	T39.92	T39.93	T39.94	T39.95	T39.96
pyrazole	T39.2X1	T39.2X2	T39.2X3	T39.2X4	T39.2X5	T39.2X6
specified NEC	T39.8X1	T39.8X2	T39.8X3	T39.8X4	T39.8X5	T39.8X6
Analgin	T39.2X1	T39.2X2	T39.2X3	T39.2X4	T39.2X5	T39.2X6
Anamirta cocculus	T62.1X1	T62.1X2	T62.1X3	T62.1X4	—	—
Ancillin	T36.0X1	T36.0X2	T36.0X3	T36.0X4	T36.0X5	T36.0X6
Ancrod	T45.691	T45.692	T45.693	T45.694	T45.695	T45.696
Androgen	T38.7X1	T38.7X2	T38.7X3	T38.7X4	T38.7X5	T38.7X6
Androgen-estrogen mixture	T38.7X1	T38.7X2	T38.7X3	T38.7X4	T38.7X5	T38.7X6
Androstalone	T38.7X1	T38.7X2	T38.7X3	T38.7X4	T38.7X5	T38.7X6
Androstanolone	T38.7X1	T38.7X2	T38.7X3	T38.7X4	T38.7X5	T38.7X6
Androsterone	T38.7X1	T38.7X2	T38.7X3	T38.7X4	T38.7X5	T38.7X6

Substance	External Cause (T-Code)					
	Poisoning, Accidental (Unintentional)	Poisoning, Intentional Self-Harm	Poisoning, Assault	Poisoning, Undetermined	Adverse Effect	Underdosing
Anemone pulsatilla	T62.2X1	T62.2X2	T62.2X3	T62.2X4	—	—
Anesthesia						
caudal	T41.3X1	T41.3X2	T41.3X3	T41.3X4	T41.3X5	T41.3X6
endotracheal	T41.0X1	T41.0X2	T41.0X3	T41.0X4	T41.0X5	T41.0X6
epidural	T41.3X1	T41.3X2	T41.3X3	T41.3X4	T41.3X5	T41.3X6
inhalation	T41.0X1	T41.0X2	T41.0X3	T41.0X4	T41.0X5	T41.0X6
local	T41.3X1	T41.3X2	T41.3X3	T41.3X4	T41.3X5	T41.3X6
mucosal	T41.3X1	T41.3X2	T41.3X3	T41.3X4	T41.3X5	T41.3X6
muscle relaxation	T48.1X1	T48.1X2	T48.1X3	T48.1X4	T48.1X5	T48.1X6
nerve blocking	T41.3X1	T41.3X2	T41.3X3	T41.3X4	T41.3X5	T41.3X6
plexus blocking	T41.3X1	T41.3X2	T41.3X3	T41.3X4	T41.3X5	T41.3X6
potentiated	T41.201	T41.202	T41.203	T41.204	T41.205	T41.206
rectal	T41.201	T41.202	T41.203	T41.204	T41.205	T41.206
general	T41.201	T41.202	T41.203	T41.204	T41.205	T41.206
local	T41.3X1	T41.3X2	T41.3X3	T41.3X4	T41.3X5	T41.3X6
regional	T41.3X1	T41.3X2	T41.3X3	T41.3X4	T41.3X5	T41.3X6
surface	T41.3X1	T41.3X2	T41.3X3	T41.3X4	T41.3X5	T41.3X6
Anesthetic NEC—*see also Anesthesia*	T41.41	T41.42	T41.43	T41.44	T41.45	T41.46
with muscle relaxant	T41.201	T41.202	T41.203	T41.204	T41.205	T41.206
general	T41.201	T41.202	T41.203	T41.204	T41.205	T41.206
local	T41.3X1	T41.3X2	T41.3X3	T41.3X4	T41.3X5	T41.3X6
gaseous NEC	T41.0X1	T41.0X2	T41.0X3	T41.0X4	T41.0X5	T41.0X6
general NEC	T41.201	T41.202	T41.203	T41.204	T41.205	T41.206
halogenated hydrocarbon derivatives NEC	T41.0X1	T41.0X2	T41.0X3	T41.0X4	T41.0X5	T41.0X6
infiltration NEC	T41.3X1	T41.3X2	T41.3X3	T41.3X4	T41.3X5	T41.3X6
intravenous NEC	T41.1X1	T41.1X2	T41.1X3	T41.1X4	T41.1X5	T41.1X6
local NEC	T41.3X1	T41.3X2	T41.3X3	T41.3X4	T41.3X5	T41.3X6
rectal	T41.201	T41.202	T41.203	T41.204	T41.205	T41.206
general	T41.201	T41.202	T41.203	T41.204	T41.205	T41.206
local	T41.3X1	T41.3X2	T41.3X3	T41.3X4	T41.3X5	T41.3X6
regional NEC	T41.3X1	T41.3X2	T41.3X3	T41.3X4	T41.3X5	T41.3X6
spinal NEC	T41.3X1	T41.3X2	T41.3X3	T41.3X4	T41.3X5	T41.3X6
thiobarbiturate	T41.1X1	T41.1X2	T41.1X3	T41.1X4	T41.1X5	T41.1X6
topical	T41.3X1	T41.3X2	T41.3X3	T41.3X4	T41.3X5	T41.3X6
Aneurine	T45.2X1	T45.2X2	T45.2X3	T45.2X4	T45.2X5	T45.2X6
Angio-Conray	T50.8X1	T50.8X2	T50.8X3	T50.8X4	T50.8X5	T50.8X6
Angiotensin	T44.5X1	T44.5X2	T44.5X3	T44.5X4	T44.5X5	T44.5X6
Angiotensinamide	T44.991	T44.992	T44.993	T44.994	T44.995	T44.996
Anhydrohydroxy-progesterone	T38.5X1	T38.5X2	T38.5X3	T38.5X4	T38.5X5	T38.5X6
Anhydron	T50.2X1	T50.2X2	T50.2X3	T50.2X4	T50.2X5	T50.2X6
Anileridine	T40.4X1	T40.4X2	T40.4X3	T40.4X4	T40.4X5	T40.4X6

◀ New ◀ Revised ~~deleted~~ Deleted

Substance	External Cause (T-Code)					
	Poisoning, Accidental (Unintentional)	Poisoning, Intentional Self-Harm	Poisoning, Assault	Poisoning, Undetermined	Adverse Effect	Underdosing
Aniline (dye) (liquid)	T65.3X1	T65.3X2	T65.3X3	T65.3X4	—	—
analgesic	T39.1X1	T39.1X2	T39.1X3	T39.1X4	T39.1X5	T39.1X6
derivatives, therapeutic NEC	T39.1X1	T39.1X2	T39.1X3	T39.1X4	T39.1X5	T39.1X6
vapor	T65.3X1	T65.3X2	T65.3X3	T65.3X4	—	—
Anise oil	T47.5X1	T47.5X2	T47.5X3	T47.5X4	T47.5X5	T47.5X6
Aniscoropine	T44.3X1	T44.3X2	T44.3X3	T44.3X4	T44.3X5	T44.3X6
Anisidine	T65.3X1	T65.3X2	T65.3X3	T65.3X4	—	—
Anisindione	T45.511	T45.512	T45.513	T45.514	T45.515	T45.516
Anisotropine methyl-bromide	T44.3X1	T44.3X2	T44.3X3	T44.3X4	T44.3X5	T44.3X6
Anistreplase	T45.611	T45.612	T45.613	T45.614	T45.615	T45.616
Anorexiant (central)	T50.5X1	T50.5X2	T50.5X3	T50.5X4	T50.5X5	T50.5X6
Anorexic agents	T50.5X1	T50.5X2	T50.5X3	T50.5X4	T50.5X5	T50.5X6
Ansamycin	T36.6X1	T36.6X2	T36.6X3	T36.6X4	T36.6X5	T36.6X6
Ant (bite) (sting)	T63.421	T63.422	T63.423	T63.424	—	—
Antabuse	T50.6X1	T50.6X2	T50.6X3	T50.6X4	T50.6X5	T50.6X6
Ant poison — *see Insecticide*						
Antacid NEC	T47.1X1	T47.1X2	T47.1X3	T47.1X4	T47.1X5	T47.1X6
Antagonist						
Aldosterone	T50.0X1	T50.0X2	T50.0X3	T50.0X4	T50.0X5	T50.0X6
alpha-adrenoreceptor	T44.6X1	T44.6X2	T44.6X3	T44.6X4	T44.6X5	T44.6X6
anticoagulant	T45.7X1	T45.7X2	T45.7X3	T45.7X4	T45.7X5	T45.7X6
beta-adrenoreceptor	T44.7X1	T44.7X2	T44.7X3	T44.7X4	T44.7X5	T44.7X6
extrapyramidal NEC	T44.3X1	T44.3X2	T44.3X3	T44.3X4	T44.3X5	T44.3X6
folic acid	T45.1X1	T45.1X2	T45.1X3	T45.1X4	T45.1X5	T45.1X6
H2 receptor	T47.0X1	T47.0X2	T47.0X3	T47.0X4	T47.0X5	T47.0X6
heavy metal	T45.8X1	T45.8X2	T45.8X3	T45.8X4	T45.8X5	T45.8X6
narcotic analgesic	T50.7X1	T50.7X2	T50.7X3	T50.7X4	T50.7X5	T50.7X6
opiate	T50.7X1	T50.7X2	T50.7X3	T50.7X4	T50.7X5	T50.7X6
pyrimidine	T45.1X1	T45.1X2	T45.1X3	T45.1X4	T45.1X5	T45.1X6
serotonin	T46.5X1	T46.5X2	T46.5X3	T46.5X4	T46.5X5	T46.5X6
Antazolin(e)	T45.0X1	T45.0X2	T45.0X3	T45.0X4	T45.0X5	T45.0X6
Anterior pituitary hormone NEC	T38.811	T38.812	T38.813	T38.814	T38.815	T38.816
Anthelmintic NEC	T37.4X1	T37.4X2	T37.4X3	T37.4X4	T37.4X5	T37.4X6
Anthiolimine	T37.4X1	T37.4X2	T37.4X3	T37.4X4	T37.4X5	T37.4X6
Anthralin	T49.4X1	T49.4X2	T49.4X3	T49.4X4	T49.4X5	T49.4X6
Anthramycin	T45.1X1	T45.1X2	T45.1X3	T45.1X4	T45.1X5	T45.1X6
Antiadrenergic NEC	T44.8X1	T44.8X2	T44.8X3	T44.8X4	T44.8X5	T44.8X6
Antiallergic NEC	T45.0X1	T45.0X2	T45.0X3	T45.0X4	T45.0X5	T45.0X6
Anti-anemic (drug) (preparation)	T45.8X1	T45.8X2	T45.8X3	T45.8X4	T45.8X5	T45.8X6
Antiandrogen NEC	T38.6X1	T38.6X2	T38.6X3	T38.6X4	T38.6X5	T38.6X6
Antianxiety drug NEC	T43.501	T43.502	T43.503	T43.504	T43.505	T43.506
Antiaris toxicaria	T65.891	T65.892	T65.893	T65.894	—	—

Substance	External Cause (T-Code)					
	Poisoning, Accidental (Unintentional)	Poisoning, Intentional Self-Harm	Poisoning, Assault	Poisoning, Undetermined	Adverse Effect	Underdosing
Antiarteriosclerotic drug	T46.6X1	T46.6X2	T46.6X3	T46.6X4	T46.6X5	T46.6X6
Antiasthmatic drug NEC	T48.6X1	T48.6X2	T48.6X3	T48.6X4	T48.6X5	T48.6X6
Antibiotic NEC	T36.91	T36.92	T36.93	T36.94	T36.95	T36.96
aminoglycoside	T36.5X1	T36.5X2	T36.5X3	T36.5X4	T36.5X5	T36.5X6
anticancer	T45.1X1	T45.1X2	T45.1X3	T45.1X4	T45.1X5	T45.1X6
antifungal	T36.7X1	T36.7X2	T36.7X3	T36.7X4	T36.7X5	T36.7X6
antimycobacterial	T36.5X1	T36.5X2	T36.5X3	T36.5X4	T36.5X5	T36.5X6
antineoplastic	T45.1X1	T45.1X2	T45.1X3	T45.1X4	T45.1X5	T45.1X6
cephalosporin (group)	T36.1X1	T36.1X2	T36.1X3	T36.1X4	T36.1X5	T36.1X6
chloramphenicol (group)	T36.2X1	T36.2X2	T36.2X3	T36.2X4	T36.2X5	T36.2X6
ENT	T49.6X1	T49.6X2	T49.6X3	T49.6X4	T49.6X5	T49.6X6
eye	T49.5X1	T49.5X2	T49.5X3	T49.5X4	T49.5X5	T49.5X6
fungicidal (local)	T49.0X1	T49.0X2	T49.0X3	T49.0X4	T49.0X5	T49.0X6
intestinal	T36.8X1	T36.8X2	T36.8X3	T36.8X4	T36.8X5	T36.8X6
b-lactam NEC	T36.1X1	T36.1X2	T36.1X3	T36.1X4	T36.1X5	T36.1X6
local	T49.0X1	T49.0X2	T49.0X3	T49.0X4	T49.0X5	T49.0X6
macrolides	T36.3X1	T36.3X2	T36.3X3	T36.3X4	T36.3X5	T36.3X6
polypeptide	T36.8X1	T36.8X2	T36.8X3	T36.8X4	T36.8X5	T36.8X6
specified NEC	T36.8X1	T36.8X2	T36.8X3	T36.8X4	T36.8X5	T36.8X6
tetracycline (group)	T36.4X1	T36.4X2	T36.4X3	T36.4X4	T36.4X5	T36.4X6
throat	T49.6X1	T49.6X2	T49.6X3	T49.6X4	T49.6X5	T49.6X6
Anticancer agents NEC	T45.1X1	T45.1X2	T45.1X3	T45.1X4	T45.1X5	T45.1X6
Anticholesterolemic drug NEC	T46.6X1	T46.6X2	T46.6X3	T46.6X4	T46.6X5	T46.6X6
Anticholinergic NEC	T44.3X1	T44.3X2	T44.3X3	T44.3X4	T44.3X5	T44.3X6
Anticholinesterase	T44.0X1	T44.0X2	T44.0X3	T44.0X4	T44.0X5	T44.0X6
organophosphorus	T44.0X1	T44.0X2	T44.0X3	T44.0X4	T44.0X5	T44.0X6
insecticide	T60.0X1	T60.0X2	T60.0X3	T60.0X4	—	—
nerve gas	T59.891	T59.892	T59.893	T59.894	—	—
reversible	T44.0X1	T44.0X2	T44.0X3	T44.0X4	T44.0X5	T44.0X6
ophthalmological	T49.5X1	T49.5X2	T49.5X3	T49.5X4	T49.5X5	T49.5X6
Anticoagulant NEC	T45.511	T45.512	T45.513	T45.514	T45.515	T45.516
Antagonist	T45.7X1	T45.7X2	T45.7X3	T45.7X4	T45.7X5	T45.7X6
Anti-common-cold drug NEC	T48.5X1	T48.5X2	T48.5X3	T48.5X4	T48.5X5	T48.5X6
Anticonvulsant	T42.71	T42.72	T42.73	T42.74	T42.75	T42.76
barbiturate	T42.3X1	T42.3X2	T42.3X3	T42.3X4	T42.3X5	T42.3X6
combination (with barbiturate)	T42.3X1	T42.3X2	T42.3X3	T42.3X4	T42.3X5	T42.3X6
hydantoin	T42.0X1	T42.0X2	T42.0X3	T42.0X4	T42.0X5	T42.0X6
hypnotic NEC	T42.6X1	T42.6X2	T42.6X3	T42.6X4	T42.6X5	T42.6X6
oxazolidinedione	T42.2X1	T42.2X2	T42.2X3	T42.2X4	T42.2X5	T42.2X6
pyrimidinedione	T42.6X1	T42.6X2	T42.6X3	T42.6X4	T42.6X5	T42.6X6
specified NEC	T42.6X1	T42.6X2	T42.6X3	T42.6X4	T42.6X5	T42.6X6
succinimide	T42.2X1	T42.2X2	T42.2X3	T42.2X4	T42.2X5	T42.2X6

Substance	External Cause (T-Code)					
	Poisoning, Accidental (Unintentional)	Poisoning, Intentional Self-Harm	Poisoning, Assault	Poisoning, Undetermined	Adverse Effect	Underdosing
Anti-D immunoglobulin (human)	T50.Z11	T50.Z12	T50.Z13	T50.Z14	T50.Z15	T50.Z16
Antidepressant NEC	T43.201	T43.202	T43.203	T43.204	T43.205	T43.206
monoamine oxidase inhibitor	T43.1X1	T43.1X2	T43.1X3	T43.1X4	T43.1X5	T43.1X6
selective serotonin norepinephrine reuptake inhibitor	T43.211	T43.212	T43.213	T43.214	T43.215	T43.216
selective serotonin reuptake inhibitor	T43.221	T43.222	T43.223	T43.224	T43.225	T43.226
specified NEC	T43.291	T43.292	T43.293	T43.294	T43.295	T43.296
tetracyclic	T43.021	T43.022	T43.023	T43.024	T43.025	T43.026
triazolopyridine	T43.221	T43.222	T43.223	T43.224	T43.225	T43.226
tricyclic	T43.011	T43.012	T43.013	T43.014	T43.015	T43.016
Antidiabetic NEC	T38.3X1	T38.3X2	T38.3X3	T38.3X4	T38.3X5	T38.3X6
biguanide	T38.3X1	T38.3X2	T38.3X3	T38.3X4	T38.3X5	T38.3X6
and sulfonyl combined	T38.3X1	T38.3X2	T38.3X3	T38.3X4	T38.3X5	T38.3X6
combined	T38.3X1	T38.3X2	T38.3X3	T38.3X4	T38.3X5	T38.3X6
sulfonylurea	T38.3X1	T38.3X2	T38.3X3	T38.3X4	T38.3X5	T38.3X6
Antidiarrheal drug NEC	T47.6X1	T47.6X2	T47.6X3	T47.6X4	T47.6X5	T47.6X6
absorbent	T47.6X1	T47.6X2	T47.6X3	T47.6X4	T47.6X5	T47.6X6
Antidiphtheria serum	T50.Z11	T50.Z12	T50.Z13	T50.Z14	T50.Z15	T50.Z16
Antidiuretic hormone	T38.891	T38.892	T38.893	T38.894	T38.895	T38.896
Antidote NEC	T50.6X1	T50.6X2	T50.6X3	T50.6X4	T50.6X5	T50.6X6
heavy metal	T45.8X1	T45.8X2	T45.8X3	T45.8X4	T45.8X5	T45.8X6
Antidysrhythmic NEC	T46.2X1	T46.2X2	T46.2X3	T46.2X4	T46.2X5	T46.2X6
Antiemetic drug	T45.0X1	T45.0X2	T45.0X3	T45.0X4	T45.0X5	T45.0X6
Antiepilepsy agent	T42.71	T42.72	T42.73	T42.74	T42.75	T42.76
combination	T42.5X1	T42.5X2	T42.5X3	T42.5X4	T42.5X5	T42.5X6
mixed	T42.5X1	T42.5X2	T42.5X3	T42.5X4	T42.5X5	T42.5X6
specified, NEC	T42.6X1	T42.6X2	T42.6X3	T42.6X4	T42.6X5	T42.6X6
Antiestrogen NEC	T38.6X1	T38.6X2	T38.6X3	T38.6X4	T38.6X5	T38.6X6
Antifertility pill	T38.4X1	T38.4X2	T38.4X3	T38.4X4	T38.4X5	T38.4X6
Antifibrinolytic drug	T45.621	T45.622	T45.623	T45.624	T45.625	T45.626
Antifilarial drug	T37.4X1	T37.4X2	T37.4X3	T37.4X4	T37.4X5	T37.4X6
Antiflatulent	T47.5X1	T47.5X2	T47.5X3	T47.5X4	T47.5X5	T47.5X6
Antifreeze	T65.91	T65.92	T65.93	T65.94	—	—
alcohol	T51.1X1	T51.1X2	T51.1X3	T51.1X4	—	—
ethylene glycol	T51.8X1	T51.8X2	T51.8X3	T51.8X4	—	—
Antifungal						
antibiotic (systemic)	T36.7X1	T36.7X2	T36.7X3	T36.7X4	T36.7X5	T36.7X6
anti-infective NEC	T37.91	T37.92	T37.93	T37.94	T37.95	T37.96
disinfectant, local	T49.0X1	T49.0X2	T49.0X3	T49.0X4	T49.0X5	T49.0X6
nonmedicinal (spray)	T60.3X1	T60.3X2	T60.3X3	T60.3X4	—	—
topical	T49.0X1	T49.0X2	T49.0X3	T49.0X4	T49.0X5	T49.0X6

Substance	External Cause (T-Code)					
	Poisoning, Accidental (Unintentional)	Poisoning, Intentional Self-Harm	Poisoning, Assault	Poisoning, Undetermined	Adverse Effect	Underdosing
Anti-gastric-secretion drug NEC	T47.1X1	T47.1X2	T47.1X3	T47.1X4	T47.1X5	T47.1X6
Antigonadotrophin NEC	T38.6X1	T38.6X2	T38.6X3	T38.6X4	T38.6X5	T38.6X6
Antihallucinogen	T43.501	T43.502	T43.503	T43.504	T43.505	T43.506
Antihelmintics	T37.4X1	T37.4X2	T37.4X3	T37.4X4	T37.4X5	T37.4X6
Antihemophilic						
factor	T45.8X1	T45.8X2	T45.8X3	T45.8X4	T45.8X5	T45.8X6
fraction	T45.8X1	T45.8X2	T45.8X3	T45.8X4	T45.8X5	T45.8X6
globulin concentrate	T45.7X1	T45.7X2	T45.7X3	T45.7X4	T45.7X5	T45.7X6
human plasma	T45.8X1	T45.8X2	T45.8X3	T45.8X4	T45.8X5	T45.8X6
plasma, dried	T45.7X1	T45.7X2	T45.7X3	T45.7X4	T45.7X5	T45.7X6
Antihemorrhoidal preparation	T49.2X1	T49.2X2	T49.2X3	T49.2X4	T49.2X5	T49.2X6
Antiheparin drug	T45.7X1	T45.7X2	T45.7X3	T45.7X4	T45.7X5	T45.7X6
Antihistamine	T45.0X1	T45.0X2	T45.0X3	T45.0X4	T45.0X5	T45.0X6
Antihookworm drug	T37.4X1	T37.4X2	T37.4X3	T37.4X4	T37.4X5	T37.4X6
Anti-human lymphocytic globulin	T50.Z11	T50.Z12	T50.Z13	T50.Z14	T50.Z15	T50.Z16
Antihyperlipidemic drug	T46.6X1	T46.6X2	T46.6X3	T46.6X4	T46.6X5	T46.6X6
Antihypertensive drug NEC	T46.5X1	T46.5X2	T46.5X3	T46.5X4	T46.5X5	T46.5X6
Anti-infective NEC	T37.91	T37.92	T37.93	T37.94	T37.95	T37.96
anthelmintic	T37.4X1	T37.4X2	T37.4X3	T37.4X4	T37.4X5	T37.4X6
antibiotics	T36.91	T36.92	T36.93	T36.94	T36.95	T36.96
specified NEC	T36.8X1	T36.8X2	T36.8X3	T36.8X4	T36.8X5	T36.8X6
antimalarial	T37.2X1	T37.2X2	T37.2X3	T37.2X4	T37.2X5	T37.2X6
antimycobacterial NEC	T37.1X1	T37.1X2	T37.1X3	T37.1X4	T37.1X5	T37.1X6
antibiotics	T36.5X1	T36.5X2	T36.5X3	T36.5X4	T36.5X5	T36.5X6
antiprotozoal NEC	T37.3X1	T37.3X2	T37.3X3	T37.3X4	T37.3X5	T37.3X6
blood	T37.2X1	T37.2X2	T37.2X3	T37.2X4	T37.2X5	T37.2X6
antiviral	T37.5X1	T37.5X2	T37.5X3	T37.5X4	T37.5X5	T37.5X6
arsenical	T37.8X1	T37.8X2	T37.8X3	T37.8X4	T37.8X5	T37.8X6
bismuth, local	T49.0X1	T49.0X2	T49.0X3	T49.0X4	T49.0X5	T49.0X6
ENT	T49.6X1	T49.6X2	T49.6X3	T49.6X4	T49.6X5	T49.6X6
eye NEC	T49.5X1	T49.5X2	T49.5X3	T49.5X4	T49.5X5	T49.5X6
heavy metals NEC	T37.8X1	T37.8X2	T37.8X3	T37.8X4	T37.8X5	T37.8X6
local NEC	T49.0X1	T49.0X2	T49.0X3	T49.0X4	T49.0X5	T49.0X6
specified NEC	T49.0X1	T49.0X2	T49.0X3	T49.0X4	T49.0X5	T49.0X6
mixed	T37.91	T37.92	T37.93	T37.94	T37.95	T37.96
ophthalmic preparation	T49.5X1	T49.5X2	T49.5X3	T49.5X4	T49.5X5	T49.5X6
topical NEC	T49.0X1	T49.0X2	T49.0X3	T49.0X4	T49.0X5	T49.0X6
Anti-inflammatory drug NEC	T49.0X1	T49.0X2	T49.0X3	T49.0X4	T49.0X5	T49.0X6
local	T49.0X1	T49.0X2	T49.0X3	T49.0X4	T49.0X5	T49.0X6
nonsteroidal NEC	T39.391	T39.392	T39.393	T39.394	T39.395	T39.396
propionic acid derivative	T39.311	T39.312	T39.313	T39.314	T39.315	T39.316
specified NEC	T39.391	T39.392	T39.393	T39.394	T39.395	T39.396

◀ New ◀ Revised ~~deleted~~ Deleted

Substance	External Cause (T-Code)					
	Poisoning, Accidental (Unintentional)	Poisoning, Intentional Self-Harm	Poisoning, Assault	Poisoning, Undetermined	Adverse Effect	Underdosing
Antikaluretic	T50.3X1	T50.3X2	T50.3X3	T50.3X4	T50.3X5	T50.3X6
Antiknock (tetraethyl lead)	T56.0X1	T56.0X2	T56.0X3	T56.0X4	—	—
Antilipemic drug NEC	T46.6X1	T46.6X2	T46.6X3	T46.6X4	T46.6X5	T46.6X6
Antimalarial	T37.2X1	T37.2X2	T37.2X3	T37.2X4	T37.2X5	T37.2X6
prophylactic NEC	T37.2X1	T37.2X2	T37.2X3	T37.2X4	T37.2X5	T37.2X6
pyrimidine derivative	T37.2X1	T37.2X2	T37.2X3	T37.2X4	T37.2X5	T37.2X6
Antimetabolite	T45.1X1	T45.1X2	T45.1X3	T45.1X4	T45.1X5	T45.1X6
Antimitotic agent	T45.1X1	T45.1X2	T45.1X3	T45.1X4	T45.1X5	T45.1X6
Antimony (compounds) (vapor) NEC	T56.891	T56.892	T56.893	T56.894	—	—
anti-infectives	T37.8X1	T37.8X2	T37.8X3	T37.8X4	T37.8X5	T37.8X6
dimercaptosuccinate	T37.3X1	T37.3X2	T37.3X3	T37.3X4	T37.3X5	T37.3X6
hydride	T56.891	T56.892	T56.893	T56.894	—	—
pesticide (vapor)	T60.8X1	T60.8X2	T60.8X3	T60.8X4	—	—
potassium (sodium) tartrate	T37.8X1	T37.8X2	T37.8X3	T37.8X4	T37.8X5	T37.8X6
sodium dimercaptosuccinate	T37.3X1	T37.3X2	T37.3X3	T37.3X4	T37.3X5	T37.3X6
tartrated	T37.8X1	T37.8X2	T37.8X3	T37.8X4	T37.8X5	T37.8X6
Antimuscarinic NEC	T44.3X1	T44.3X2	T44.3X3	T44.3X4	T44.3X5	T44.3X6
Antimycobacterial drug NEC	T37.1X1	T37.1X2	T37.1X3	T37.1X4	T37.1X5	T37.1X6
antibiotics	T36.5X1	T36.5X2	T36.5X3	T36.5X4	T36.5X5	T36.5X6
combination	T37.1X1	T37.1X2	T37.1X3	T37.1X4	T37.1X5	T37.1X6
Antinausea drug	T45.0X1	T45.0X2	T45.0X3	T45.0X4	T45.0X5	T45.0X6
Antinematode drug	T37.4X1	T37.4X2	T37.4X3	T37.4X4	T37.4X5	T37.4X6
Antineoplastic NEC	T45.1X1	T45.1X2	T45.1X3	T45.1X4	T45.1X5	T45.1X6
alkaloidal	T45.1X1	T45.1X2	T45.1X3	T45.1X4	T45.1X5	T45.1X6
antibiotics	T45.1X1	T45.1X2	T45.1X3	T45.1X4	T45.1X5	T45.1X6
combination	T45.1X1	T45.1X2	T45.1X3	T45.1X4	T45.1X5	T45.1X6
estrogen	T38.5X1	T38.5X2	T38.5X3	T38.5X4	T38.5X5	T38.5X6
steroid	T38.7X1	T38.7X2	T38.7X3	T38.7X4	T38.7X5	T38.7X6
Antiparasitic drug (systemic)	T37.91	T37.92	T37.93	T37.94	T37.95	T37.96
local	T49.0X1	T49.0X2	T49.0X3	T49.0X4	T49.0X5	T49.0X6
specified NEC	T37.8X1	T37.8X2	T37.8X3	T37.8X4	T37.8X5	T37.8X6
Antiparkinsonism drug NEC	T42.8X1	T42.8X2	T42.8X3	T42.8X4	T42.8X5	T42.8X6
Antiperspirant NEC	T49.2X1	T49.2X2	T49.2X3	T49.2X4	T49.2X5	T49.2X6
Antiphlogistic NEC	T39.4X1	T39.4X2	T39.4X3	T39.4X4	T39.4X5	T39.4X6
Antiplatyhelmintic drug	T37.4X1	T37.4X2	T37.4X3	T37.4X4	T37.4X5	T37.4X6
Antiprotozoal drug NEC	T37.3X1	T37.3X2	T37.3X3	T37.3X4	T37.3X5	T37.3X6
blood	T37.2X1	T37.2X2	T37.2X3	T37.2X4	T37.2X5	T37.2X6
local	T49.0X1	T49.0X2	T49.0X3	T49.0X4	T49.0X5	T49.0X6
Antipruritic drug NEC	T49.1X1	T49.1X2	T49.1X3	T49.1X4	T49.1X5	T49.1X6
Antipsychotic drug	T43.501	T43.502	T43.503	T43.504	T43.505	T43.506
specified NEC	T43.591	T43.592	T43.593	T43.594	T43.595	T43.596

Substance	External Cause (T-Code)					
	Poisoning, Accidental (Unintentional)	Poisoning, Intentional Self-Harm	Poisoning, Assault	Poisoning, Undetermined	Adverse Effect	Underdosing
Antipyretic	T39.91	T39.92	T39.93	T39.94	T39.95	T39.96
specified NEC	T39.8X1	T39.8X2	T39.8X3	T39.8X4	T39.8X5	T39.8X6
Antipyrine	T39.2X1	T39.2X2	T39.2X3	T39.2X4	T39.2X5	T39.2X6
Antirabies hyperimmune serum	T50.Z11	T50.Z12	T50.Z13	T50.Z14	T50.Z15	T50.Z16
Antirheumatic NEC	T39.4X1	T39.4X2	T39.4X3	T39.4X4	T39.4X5	T39.4X6
Antirigidity drug NEC	T42.8X1	T42.8X2	T42.8X3	T42.8X4	T42.8X5	T42.8X6
Antischistosomal drug	T37.4X1	T37.4X2	T37.4X3	T37.4X4	T37.4X5	T37.4X6
Antiscorpion sera	T50.Z11	T50.Z12	T50.Z13	T50.Z14	T50.Z15	T50.Z16
Antiseborrheics	T49.4X1	T49.4X2	T49.4X3	T49.4X4	T49.4X5	T49.4X6
Antiseptics (external) (medicinal)	T49.0X1	T49.0X2	T49.0X3	T49.0X4	T49.0X5	T49.0X6
Antistine	T45.0X1	T45.0X2	T45.0X3	T45.0X4	T45.0X5	T45.0X6
Antitapeworm drug	T37.4X1	T37.4X2	T37.4X3	T37.4X4	T37.4X5	T37.4X6
Antitetanus immunoglobulin	T50.Z11	T50.Z12	T50.Z13	T50.Z14	T50.Z15	T50.Z16
Antithyroid drug NEC	T38.2X1	T38.2X2	T38.2X3	T38.2X4	T38.2X5	T38.2X6
Antitoxin	T50.Z11	T50.Z12	T50.Z13	T50.Z14	T50.Z15	T50.Z16
diphtheria	T50.Z11	T50.Z12	T50.Z13	T50.Z14	T50.Z15	T50.Z16
gas gangrene	T50.Z11	T50.Z12	T50.Z13	T50.Z14	T50.Z15	T50.Z16
tetanus	T50.Z11	T50.Z12	T50.Z13	T50.Z14	T50.Z15	T50.Z16
Antitoxin, any	T50.901	T50.902	T50.903	T50.904	T50.905	T50.906
Antitrichomonal drug	T37.3X1	T37.3X2	T37.3X3	T37.3X4	T37.3X5	T37.3X6
Antituberculars	T37.1X1	T37.1X2	T37.1X3	T37.1X4	T37.1X5	T37.1X6
antibiotics	T36.5X1	T36.5X2	T36.5X3	T36.5X4	T36.5X5	T36.5X6
Antitussive NEC	T48.3X1	T48.3X2	T48.3X3	T48.3X4	T48.3X5	T48.3X6
codeine mixture	T40.2X1	T40.2X2	T40.2X3	T40.2X4	T40.2X5	T40.2X6
opiate	T40.2X1	T40.2X2	T40.2X3	T40.2X4	T40.2X5	T40.2X6
Antivaricose drug	T46.8X1	T46.8X2	T46.8X3	T46.8X4	T46.8X5	T46.8X6
Antivenin, antivenom (sera)	T50.Z11	T50.Z12	T50.Z13	T50.Z14	T50.Z15	T50.Z16
crotaline	T50.Z11	T50.Z12	T50.Z13	T50.Z14	T50.Z15	T50.Z16
spider bite	T50.Z11	T50.Z12	T50.Z13	T50.Z14	T50.Z15	T50.Z16
Antivertigo drug	T45.0X1	T45.0X2	T45.0X3	T45.0X4	T45.0X5	T45.0X6
Antiviral drug NEC	T37.5X1	T37.5X2	T37.5X3	T37.5X4	T37.5X5	T37.5X6
eye	T49.5X1	T49.5X2	T49.5X3	T49.5X4	T49.5X5	T49.5X6
Antiwhipworm drug	T37.4X1	T37.4X2	T37.4X3	T37.4X4	T37.4X5	T37.4X6
Ant poisons — *see Pesticides*						
Antrol — *see also by specific chemical substance*	T60.91	T60.92	T60.93	T60.94	—	—
fungicide	T60.91	T60.92	T60.93	T60.94	—	—
ANTU (alpha naphthylthiourea)	T60.4X1	T60.4X2	T60.4X3	T60.4X4	—	—
Apalcillin	T36.0X1	T36.0X2	T36.0X3	T36.0X4	T36.0X5	T36.0X6
APC	T48.5X1	T48.5X2	T48.5X3	T48.5X4	T48.5X5	T48.5X6
Aplonidine	T44.4X1	T44.4X2	T44.4X3	T44.4X4	T44.4X5	T44.4X6
Apomorphine	T47.7X1	T47.7X2	T47.7X3	T47.7X4	T47.7X5	T47.7X6

Substance	Poisoning, Accidental (Unintentional)	External Cause (T-Code): Poisoning, Intentional Self-Harm	Poisoning, Assault	Poisoning, Undetermined	Adverse Effect	Underdosing
Appetite depressants, central	T50.5X1	T50.5X2	T50.5X3	T50.5X4	T50.5X5	T50.5X6
Apraclonidine (hydrochloride)	T44.4X1	T44.4X2	T44.4X3	T44.4X4	T44.4X5	T44.4X6
Apresoline	T46.5X1	T46.5X2	T46.5X3	T46.5X4	T46.5X5	T46.5X6
Aprindine	T46.2X1	T46.2X2	T46.2X3	T46.2X4	T46.2X5	T46.2X6
Aprobarbital	T42.3X1	T42.3X2	T42.3X3	T42.3X4	T42.3X5	T42.3X6
Apronalide	T42.6X1	T42.6X2	T42.6X3	T42.6X4	T42.6X5	T42.6X6
Aprotinin	T45.621	T45.622	T45.623	T45.624	T45.625	T45.626
Aptocaine	T41.3X1	T41.3X2	T41.3X3	T41.3X4	T41.3X5	T41.3X6
Aqua fortis	T54.2X1	T54.2X2	T54.2X3	T54.2X4	—	—
Ara-A	T37.5X1	T37.5X2	T37.5X3	T37.5X4	T37.5X5	T37.5X6
Ara-C	T45.1X1	T45.1X2	T45.1X3	T45.1X4	T45.1X5	T45.1X6
Arachis oil	T49.3X1	T49.3X2	T49.3X3	T49.3X4	T49.3X5	T49.3X6
cathartic	T47.4X1	T47.4X2	T47.4X3	T47.4X4	T47.4X5	T47.4X6
Aralen	T37.2X1	T37.2X2	T37.2X3	T37.2X4	T37.2X5	T37.2X6
Arecoline	T44.1X1	T44.1X2	T44.1X3	T44.1X4	T44.1X5	T44.1X6
Arginine	T50.991	T50.992	T50.993	T50.994	T50.995	T50.996
glutamate	T50.991	T50.992	T50.993	T50.994	T50.995	T50.996
Argyrol	T49.0X1	T49.0X2	T49.0X3	T49.0X4	T49.0X5	T49.0X6
ENT agent	T49.6X1	T49.6X2	T49.6X3	T49.6X4	T49.6X5	T49.6X6
ophthalmic preparation	T49.5X1	T49.5X2	T49.5X3	T49.5X4	T49.5X5	T49.5X6
Aristocort	T38.0X1	T38.0X2	T38.0X3	T38.0X4	T38.0X5	T38.0X6
ENT agent	T49.6X1	T49.6X2	T49.6X3	T49.6X4	T49.6X5	T49.6X6
ophthalmic preparation	T49.5X1	T49.5X2	T49.5X3	T49.5X4	T49.5X5	T49.5X6
topical NEC	T49.0X1	T49.0X2	T49.0X3	T49.0X4	T49.0X5	T49.0X6
Aromatics, corrosive	T54.1X1	T54.1X2	T54.1X3	T54.1X4	—	—
disinfectants	T54.1X1	T54.1X2	T54.1X3	T54.1X4	—	—
Arsenate of lead	T57.0X1	T57.0X2	T57.0X3	T57.0X4	—	—
herbicide	T57.0X1	T57.0X2	T57.0X3	T57.0X4	—	—
Arsenic, arsenicals (compounds) (dust) (vapor) NEC	T57.0X1	T57.0X2	T57.0X3	T57.0X4	—	—
anti-infectives	T37.8X1	T37.8X2	T37.8X3	T37.8X4	T37.8X5	T37.8X6
pesticide (dust) (fumes)	T57.0X1	T57.0X2	T57.0X3	T57.0X4	—	—
Arsine (gas)	T57.0X1	T57.0X2	T57.0X3	T57.0X4	—	—
Arsphenamine (silver)	T37.8X1	T37.8X2	T37.8X3	T37.8X4	T37.8X5	T37.8X6
Arsthinol	T37.3X1	T37.3X2	T37.3X3	T37.3X4	T37.3X5	T37.3X6
Artane	T44.3X1	T44.3X2	T44.3X3	T44.3X4	T44.3X5	T44.3X6
Arthropod (venomous) NEC	T63.481	T63.482	T63.483	T63.484	—	—
Articaine	T41.3X1	T41.3X2	T41.3X3	T41.3X4	T41.3X5	T41.3X6
Asbestos	T57.8X1	T57.8X2	T57.8X3	T57.8X4	—	—
Ascaridole	T37.4X1	T37.4X2	T37.4X3	T37.4X4	T37.4X5	T37.4X6
Ascorbic acid	T45.2X1	T45.2X2	T45.2X3	T45.2X4	T45.2X5	T45.2X6
Asiaticoside	T49.0X1	T49.0X2	T49.0X3	T49.0X4	T49.0X5	T49.0X6

Substance	Poisoning, Accidental (Unintentional)	External Cause (T-Code): Poisoning, Intentional Self-Harm	Poisoning, Assault	Poisoning, Undetermined	Adverse Effect	Underdosing
Asparaginase	T45.1X1	T45.1X2	T45.1X3	T45.1X4	T45.1X5	T45.1X6
Aspidium (oleoresin)	T37.4X1	T37.4X2	T37.4X3	T37.4X4	T37.4X5	T37.4X6
Aspirin (aluminum) (soluble)	T39.011	T39.012	T39.013	T39.014	T39.015	T39.016
Aspoxicillin	T36.0X1	T36.0X2	T36.0X3	T36.0X4	T36.0X5	T36.0X6
Astemizole	T45.0X1	T45.0X2	T45.0X3	T45.0X4	T45.0X5	T45.0X6
Astringent (local)	T49.2X1	T49.2X2	T49.2X3	T49.2X4	T49.2X5	T49.2X6
specified NEC	T49.2X1	T49.2X2	T49.2X3	T49.2X4	T49.2X5	T49.2X6
Astromicin	T36.5X1	T36.5X2	T36.5X3	T36.5X4	T36.5X5	T36.5X6
Ataractic drug NEC	T43.501	T43.502	T43.503	T43.504	T43.505	T43.506
Atenolol	T44.7X1	T44.7X2	T44.7X3	T44.7X4	T44.7X5	T44.7X6
Atonia drug, intestinal	T47.4X1	T47.4X2	T47.4X3	T47.4X4	T47.4X5	T47.4X6
Atophan	T50.4X1	T50.4X2	T50.4X3	T50.4X4	T50.4X5	T50.4X6
Atracurium besilate	T48.1X1	T48.1X2	T48.1X3	T48.1X4	T48.1X5	T48.1X6
Atropine	T44.3X1	T44.3X2	T44.3X3	T44.3X4	T44.3X5	T44.3X6
derivative	T44.3X1	T44.3X2	T44.3X3	T44.3X4	T44.3X5	T44.3X6
methonitrate	T44.3X1	T44.3X2	T44.3X3	T44.3X4	T44.3X5	T44.3X6
Attapulgite	T47.6X1	T47.6X2	T47.6X3	T47.6X4	T47.6X5	T47.6X6
Attenuvax	T50.991	T50.992	T50.993	T50.994	T50.995	T50.996
Auramine	T65.891	T65.892	T65.893	T65.894	—	—
dye	T65.6X1	T65.6X2	T65.6X3	T65.6X4	—	—
fungicide	T60.3X1	T60.3X2	T60.3X3	T60.3X4	—	—
Auranofin	T39.4X1	T39.4X2	T39.4X3	T39.4X4	T39.4X5	T39.4X6
Aurantiin	T46.991	T46.992	T46.993	T46.994	T46.995	T46.996
Aureomycin	T36.4X1	T36.4X2	T36.4X3	T36.4X4	T36.4X5	T36.4X6
ophthalmic preparation	T49.5X1	T49.5X2	T49.5X3	T49.5X4	T49.5X5	T49.5X6
topical NEC	T49.0X1	T49.0X2	T49.0X3	T49.0X4	T49.0X5	T49.0X6
Aurothioglucose	T39.4X1	T39.4X2	T39.4X3	T39.4X4	T39.4X5	T39.4X6
Aurothioglycanide	T39.4X1	T39.4X2	T39.4X3	T39.4X4	T39.4X5	T39.4X6
Aurothiomalate sodium	T39.4X1	T39.4X2	T39.4X3	T39.4X4	T39.4X5	T39.4X6
Aurotioprol	T39.4X1	T39.4X2	T39.4X3	T39.4X4	T39.4X5	T39.4X6
Automobile fuel	T52.0X1	T52.0X2	T52.0X3	T52.0X4	—	—
Autonomic nervous system agent NEC	T44.901	T44.902	T44.903	T44.904	T44.905	T44.906
Avlosulfon	T37.1X1	T37.1X2	T37.1X3	T37.1X4	T37.1X5	T37.1X6
Avomine	T42.6X1	T42.6X2	T42.6X3	T42.6X4	T42.6X5	T42.6X6
Axerophthol	T45.2X1	T45.2X2	T45.2X3	T45.2X4	T45.2X5	T45.2X6
Azacitidine	T45.1X1	T45.1X2	T45.1X3	T45.1X4	T45.1X5	T45.1X6
Azacyclonol	T43.591	T43.592	T43.593	T43.594	T43.595	T43.596
Azadirachta	T60.2X1	T60.2X2	T60.2X3	T60.2X4	—	—
Azanidazole	T37.3X1	T37.3X2	T37.3X3	T37.3X4	T37.3X5	T37.3X6
Azapetine	T46.7X1	T46.7X2	T46.7X3	T46.7X4	T46.7X5	T46.7X6
Azapropazone	T39.2X1	T39.2X2	T39.2X3	T39.2X4	T39.2X5	T39.2X6

◀ New ◀ Revised ~~deleted~~ Deleted

Substance	External Cause (T-Code)					
	Poisoning, Accidental (Unintentional)	Poisoning, Intentional Self-Harm	Poisoning, Assault	Poisoning, Undetermined	Adverse Effect	Underdosing
Azaribine	T45.1X1	T45.1X2	T45.1X3	T45.1X4	T45.1X5	T45.1X6
Azaserine	T45.1X1	T45.1X2	T45.1X3	T45.1X4	T45.1X5	T45.1X6
Azatadine	T45.0X1	T45.0X2	T45.0X3	T45.0X4	T45.0X5	T45.0X6
Azatepa	T45.1X1	T45.1X2	T45.1X3	T45.1X4	T45.1X5	T45.1X6
Azathioprine	T45.1X1	T45.1X2	T45.1X3	T45.1X4	T45.1X5	T45.1X6
Azelaic acid	T49.0X1	T49.0X2	T49.0X3	T49.0X4	T49.0X5	T49.0X6
Azelastine	T45.0X1	T45.0X2	T45.0X3	T45.0X4	T45.0X5	T45.0X6
Azidocillin	T36.0X1	T36.0X2	T36.0X3	T36.0X4	T36.0X5	T36.0X6
Azidothymidine	T37.5X1	T37.5X2	T37.5X3	T37.5X4	T37.5X5	T37.5X6
Azinphos (ethyl) (methyl)	T60.0X1	T60.0X2	T60.0X3	T60.0X4	—	—
Aziridine (chelating)	T54.1X1	T54.1X2	T54.1X3	T54.1X4	—	—
Azithromycin	T36.3X1	T36.3X2	T36.3X3	T36.3X4	T36.3X5	T36.3X6
Azlocillin	T36.01	T36.02	T36.03	T36.04	T36.05	T36.06
Azobenzene smoke	T65.3X1	T65.3X2	T65.3X3	T65.3X4	—	—
acaricide	T60.8X1	T60.8X2	T60.8X3	T60.8X4	—	—
Azosulfamide	T37.0X1	T37.0X2	T37.0X3	T37.0X4	T37.0X5	T37.0X6
AZT	T37.5X1	T37.5X2	T37.5X3	T37.5X4	T37.5X5	T37.5X6
Aztreonam	T36.1X1	T36.1X2	T36.1X3	T36.1X4	T36.1X5	T36.1X6
Azulfidine	T37.0X1	T37.0X2	T37.0X3	T37.0X4	T37.0X5	T37.0X6
Azuresin	T50.8X1	T50.8X2	T50.8X3	T50.8X4	T50.8X5	T50.8X6
B						
Bacampicillin	T36.0X1	T36.0X2	T36.0X3	T36.0X4	T36.0X5	T36.0X6
Bacillus						
lactobacillus	T47.8X1	T47.8X2	T47.8X3	T47.8X4	T47.8X5	T47.8X6
subtilis	T47.6X1	T47.6X2	T47.6X3	T47.6X4	T47.6X5	T47.6X6
Bacimycin	T49.0X1	T49.0X2	T49.0X3	T49.0X4	T49.0X5	T49.0X6
ophthalmic preparation	T49.5X1	T49.5X2	T49.5X3	T49.5X4	T49.5X5	T49.5X6
Bacitracin zinc	T49.0X1	T49.0X2	T49.0X3	T49.0X4	T49.0X5	T49.0X6
with neomycin	T49.0X1	T49.0X2	T49.0X3	T49.0X4	T49.0X5	T49.0X6
ENT agent	T49.6X1	T49.6X2	T49.6X3	T49.6X4	T49.6X5	T49.6X6
ophthalmic preparation	T49.5X1	T49.5X2	T49.5X3	T49.5X4	T49.5X5	T49.5X6
topical NEC	T49.0X1	T49.0X2	T49.0X3	T49.0X4	T49.0X5	T49.0X6
Baclofen	T42.8X1	T42.8X2	T42.8X3	T42.8X4	T42.8X5	T42.8X6
Baking soda	T50.991	T50.992	T50.993	T50.994	T50.995	T50.996
BAL	T45.8X1	T45.8X2	T45.8X3	T45.8X4	T45.8X5	T45.8X6
Bambuterol	T48.6X1	T48.6X2	T48.6X3	T48.6X4	T48.6X5	T48.6X6
Bamethan (sulfate)	T46.7X1	T46.7X2	T46.7X3	T46.7X4	T46.7X5	T46.7X6
Bamifylline	T48.6X1	T48.6X2	T48.6X3	T48.6X4	T48.6X5	T48.6X6
Bamipine	T45.0X1	T45.0X2	T45.0X3	T45.0X4	T45.0X5	T45.0X6
Baneberry — *see Actaea spicata*						
Banewort — *see Belladonna*						

Substance	External Cause (T-Code)					
	Poisoning, Accidental (Unintentional)	Poisoning, Intentional Self-Harm	Poisoning, Assault	Poisoning, Undetermined	Adverse Effect	Underdosing
Barbenyl	T42.3X1	T42.3X2	T42.3X3	T42.3X4	T42.3X5	T42.3X6
Barbexaclone	T42.6X1	T42.6X2	T42.6X3	T42.6X4	T42.6X5	T42.6X6
Barbital	T42.3X1	T42.3X2	T42.3X3	T42.3X4	T42.3X5	T42.3X6
sodium	T42.3X1	T42.3X2	T42.3X3	T42.3X4	T42.3X5	T42.3X6
Barbitone	T42.3X1	T42.3X2	T42.3X3	T42.3X4	T42.3X5	T42.3X6
Barbiturate NEC	T42.3X1	T42.3X2	T42.3X3	T42.3X4	T42.3X5	T42.3X6
with tranquilizer	T42.3X1	T42.3X2	T42.3X3	T42.3X4	T42.3X5	T42.3X6
anesthetic (intravenous)	T41.1X1	T41.1X2	T41.1X3	T41.1X4	T41.1X5	T41.1X6
Barium (carbonate) (chloride) (sulfite)	T57.8X1	T57.8X2	T57.8X3	T57.8X4	—	—
diagnostic agent	T50.8X1	T50.8X2	T50.8X3	T50.8X4	T50.8X5	T50.8X6
pesticide	T60.4X1	T60.4X2	T60.4X3	T60.4X4	—	—
rodenticide	T60.4X1	T60.4X2	T60.4X3	T60.4X4	—	—
sulfate (medicinal)	T50.8X1	T50.8X2	T50.8X3	T50.8X4	T50.8X5	T50.8X6
Barrier cream	T49.3X1	T49.3X2	T49.3X3	T49.3X4	T49.3X5	T49.3X6
Basic fuchsin	T49.0X1	T49.0X2	T49.0X3	T49.0X4	T49.0X5	T49.0X6
Battery acid or fluid	T54.2X1	T54.2X2	T54.2X3	T54.2X4	—	—
Bay rum	T51.8X1	T51.8X2	T51.8X3	T51.8X4	—	—
BCG (vaccine)	T50.A91	T50.A92	T50.A93	T50.A94	T50.A95	T50.A96
BCNU	T45.1X1	T45.1X2	T45.1X3	T45.1X4	T45.1X5	T45.1X6
Bearsfoot	T62.2X1	T62.2X2	T62.2X3	T62.2X4	—	—
Beclamide	T42.6X1	T42.6X2	T42.6X3	T42.6X4	T42.6X5	T42.6X6
Beclomethasone	T44.5X1	T44.5X2	T44.5X3	T44.5X4	T44.5X5	T44.5X6
Bee (sting) (venom)	T63.441	T63.442	T63.443	T63.444	—	—
Befunolol	T49.5X1	T49.5X2	T49.5X3	T49.5X4	T49.5X5	T49.5X6
Bekanamycin	T36.5X1	T36.5X2	T36.5X3	T36.5X4	T36.5X5	T36.5X6
Belladonna — *see also Nightshade*						
alkaloids	T44.3X1	T44.3X2	T44.3X3	T44.3X4	T44.3X5	T44.3X6
extract	T44.3X1	T44.3X2	T44.3X3	T44.3X4	T44.3X5	T44.3X6
herb	T44.3X1	T44.3X2	T44.3X3	T44.3X4	T44.3X5	T44.3X6
Bemegride	T50.7X1	T50.7X2	T50.7X3	T50.7X4	T50.7X5	T50.7X6
Benactyzine	T44.3X1	T44.3X2	T44.3X3	T44.3X4	T44.3X5	T44.3X6
Benadryl	T45.0X1	T45.0X2	T45.0X3	T45.0X4	T45.0X5	T45.0X6
Benaprizine	T44.3X1	T44.3X2	T44.3X3	T44.3X4	T44.3X5	T44.3X6
Benazepril	T46.4X1	T46.4X2	T46.4X3	T46.4X4	T46.4X5	T46.4X6
Bencyclane	T46.7X1	T46.7X2	T46.7X3	T46.7X4	T46.7X5	T46.7X6
Bendazol	T46.3X1	T46.3X2	T46.3X3	T46.3X4	T46.3X5	T46.3X6
Bendrofluazide	T50.2X1	T50.2X2	T50.2X3	T50.2X4	T50.2X5	T50.2X6
Bendroflumethiazide	T50.2X1	T50.2X2	T50.2X3	T50.2X4	T50.2X5	T50.2X6
Benemid	T50.4X1	T50.4X2	T50.4X3	T50.4X4	T50.4X5	T50.4X6
Benethamine penicillin	T36.0X1	T36.0X2	T36.0X3	T36.0X4	T36.0X5	T36.0X6
Benisone	T49.0X1	T49.0X2	T49.0X3	T49.0X4	T49.0X5	T49.0X6

Substance	External Cause (T-Code)					
	Poisoning, Accidental (Unintentional)	Poisoning, Intentional Self-Harm	Poisoning, Assault	Poisoning, Undetermined	Adverse Effect	Underdosing
Benexate	T47.1X1	T47.1X2	T47.1X3	T47.1X4	T47.1X5	T47.1X6
Benfluorex	T46.6X1	T46.6X2	T46.6X3	T46.6X4	T46.6X5	T46.6X6
Benfotiamine	T45.2X1	T45.2X2	T45.2X3	T45.2X4	T45.2X5	T45.2X6
Benomyl	T60.0X1	T60.0X2	T60.0X3	T60.0X4	—	—
Benoquin	T49.8X1	T49.8X2	T49.8X3	T49.8X4	T49.8X5	T49.8X6
Benoxinate	T41.3X1	T41.3X2	T41.3X3	T41.3X4	T41.3X5	T41.3X6
Benperidol	T43.4X1	T43.4X2	T43.4X3	T43.4X4	T43.4X5	T43.4X6
Benproperine	T48.3X1	T48.3X2	T48.3X3	T48.3X4	T48.3X5	T48.3X6
Benserazide	T42.8X1	T42.8X2	T42.8X3	T42.8X4	T42.8X5	T42.8X6
Bentazepam	T42.4X1	T42.4X2	T42.4X3	T42.4X4	T42.4X5	T42.4X6
Bentiromide	T50.8X1	T50.8X2	T50.8X3	T50.8X4	T50.8X5	T50.8X6
Bentonite	T49.3X1	T49.3X2	T49.3X3	T49.3X4	T49.3X5	T49.3X6
Benzalbutyramide	T46.6X1	T46.6X2	T46.6X3	T46.6X4	T46.6X5	T46.6X6
Benzalkonium (chloride)	T49.0X1	T49.0X2	T49.0X3	T49.0X4	T49.0X5	T49.0X6
ophthalmic preparation	T49.5X1	T49.5X2	T49.5X3	T49.5X4	T49.5X5	T49.5X6
Benzamine	T41.3X1	T41.3X2	T41.3X3	T41.3X4	T41.3X5	T41.3X6
lactate	T49.1X1	T49.1X2	T49.1X3	T49.1X4	T49.1X5	T49.1X6
Benzamidosalicylate (calcium)	T37.1X1	T37.1X2	T37.1X3	T37.1X4	T37.1X5	T37.1X6
Benzamphetamine	T50.5X1	T50.5X2	T50.5X3	T50.5X4	T50.5X5	T50.5X6
Benzapril hydrochloride	T46.5X1	T46.5X2	T46.5X3	T46.5X4	T46.5X5	T46.5X6
Benzathine benzylpenicillin	T36.0X1	T36.0X2	T36.0X3	T36.0X4	T36.0X5	T36.0X6
Benzathine penicillin	T36.0X1	T36.0X2	T36.0X3	T36.0X4	T36.0X5	T36.0X6
Benzatropine	T42.8X1	T42.8X2	T42.8X3	T42.8X4	T42.8X5	T42.8X6
Benzbromarone	T50.4X1	T50.4X2	T50.4X3	T50.4X4	T50.4X5	T50.4X6
Benzcarbimine	T45.1X1	T45.1X2	T45.1X3	T45.1X4	T45.1X5	T45.1X6
Benzedrex	T44.991	T44.992	T44.993	T44.994	T44.995	T44.996
Benzedrine (amphetamine)	T43.621	T43.622	T43.623	T43.624	T43.625	T43.626
Benzenamine	T65.3X1	T65.3X2	T65.3X3	T65.3X4	—	—
Benzene	T52.1X1	T52.1X2	T52.1X3	T52.1X4	—	—
homologues (acetyl) (dimethyl) (methyl) (solvent)	T52.2X1	T52.2X2	T52.2X3	T52.2X4	—	—
Benzethonium (chloride)	T49.0X1	T49.0X2	T49.0X3	T49.0X4	T49.0X5	T49.0X6
Benzfetamine	T50.5X1	T50.5X2	T50.5X3	T50.5X4	T50.5X5	T50.5X6
Benzhexol	T44.3X1	T44.3X2	T44.3X3	T44.3X4	T44.3X5	T44.3X6
Benzhydramine (chloride)	T45.0X1	T45.0X2	T45.0X3	T45.0X4	T45.0X5	T45.0X6
Benzidine	T65.891	T65.892	T65.893	T65.894	—	—
Benzilonium bromide	T44.3X1	T44.3X2	T44.3X3	T44.3X4	T44.3X5	T44.3X6
Benzimidazole	T60.3X1	T60.3X2	T60.3X3	T60.3X4	—	—
Benzin(e) — *see Ligroin*						
Benziodarone	T46.3X1	T46.3X2	T46.3X3	T46.3X4	T46.3X5	T46.3X6
Benznidazole	T37.3X1	T37.3X2	T37.3X3	T37.3X4	T37.3X5	T37.3X6
Benzocaine	T41.3X1	T41.3X2	T41.3X3	T41.3X4	T41.3X5	T41.3X6

Substance	External Cause (T-Code)					
	Poisoning, Accidental (Unintentional)	Poisoning, Intentional Self-Harm	Poisoning, Assault	Poisoning, Undetermined	Adverse Effect	Underdosing
Benzoctamine	T43.0X1	T43.0X2	T43.0X3	T43.0X4	T43.0X5	T43.0X6
Benzodiapin	T42.4X1	T42.4X2	T42.4X3	T42.4X4	T42.4X5	T42.4X6
Benzodiazepine NEC	T42.4X1	T42.4X2	T42.4X3	T42.4X4	T42.4X5	T42.4X6
Benzoic acid	T49.0X1	T49.0X2	T49.0X3	T49.0X4	T49.0X5	T49.0X6
with salicylic acid	T49.0X1	T49.0X2	T49.0X3	T49.0X4	T49.0X5	T49.0X6
Benzoin (tincture)	T48.5X1	T48.5X2	T48.5X3	T48.5X4	T48.5X5	T48.5X6
Benzol (benzene)	T52.1X1	T52.1X2	T52.1X3	T52.1X4	—	—
vapor	T52.0X1	T52.0X2	T52.0X3	T52.0X4	—	—
Benzomorphan	T40.2X1	T40.2X2	T40.2X3	T40.2X4	T40.2X5	T40.2X6
Benzonatate	T48.3X1	T48.3X2	T48.3X3	T48.3X4	T48.3X5	T48.3X6
Benzophenones	T49.3X1	T49.3X2	T49.3X3	T49.3X4	T49.3X5	T49.3X6
Benzopyrone	T46.991	T46.992	T46.993	T46.994	T46.995	T46.996
Benzothiadiazides	T50.2X1	T50.2X2	T50.2X3	T50.2X4	T50.2X5	T50.2X6
Benzoxonium chloride	T49.0X1	T49.0X2	T49.0X3	T49.0X4	T49.0X5	T49.0X6
Benzoyl peroxide	T49.0X1	T49.0X2	T49.0X3	T49.0X4	T49.0X5	T49.0X6
Benzoylpas calcium	T37.1X1	T37.1X2	T37.1X3	T37.1X4	T37.1X5	T37.1X6
Benzperidin	T43.591	T43.592	T43.593	T43.594	T43.595	T43.596
Benzperidol	T43.591	T43.592	T43.593	T43.594	T43.595	T43.596
Benzphetamine	T50.5X1	T50.5X2	T50.5X3	T50.5X4	T50.5X5	T50.5X6
Benzpyrinium bromide	T44.1X1	T44.1X2	T44.1X3	T44.1X4	T44.1X5	T44.1X6
Benzquinamide	T45.0X1	T45.0X2	T45.0X3	T45.0X4	T45.0X5	T45.0X6
Benzthiazide	T50.2X1	T50.2X2	T50.2X3	T50.2X4	T50.2X5	T50.2X6
Benztropine						
anticholinergic	T44.3X1	T44.3X2	T44.3X3	T44.3X4	T44.3X5	T44.3X6
antiparkinson	T42.8X1	T42.8X2	T42.8X3	T42.8X4	T42.8X5	T42.8X6
Benzydamine	T49.0X1	T49.0X2	T49.0X3	T49.0X4	T49.0X5	T49.0X6
Benzyl						
acetate	T52.8X1	T52.8X2	T52.8X3	T52.8X4	—	—
alcohol	T49.0X1	T49.0X2	T49.0X3	T49.0X4	T49.0X5	T49.0X6
benzoate	T49.0X1	T49.0X2	T49.0X3	T49.0X4	T49.0X5	T49.0X6
Benzoic acid	T49.0X1	T49.0X2	T49.0X3	T49.0X4	T49.0X5	T49.0X6
morphine	T40.2X1	T40.2X2	T40.2X3	T40.2X4	—	—
nicotinate	T46.6X1	T46.6X2	T46.6X3	T46.6X4	T46.6X5	T46.6X6
penicillin	T36.0X1	T36.0X2	T36.0X3	T36.0X4	T36.0X5	T36.0X6
Benzylhydrochlorthia-zide	T50.2X1	T50.2X2	T50.2X3	T50.2X4	T50.2X5	T50.2X6
Benzylpenicillin	T36.0X1	T36.0X2	T36.0X3	T36.0X4	T36.0X5	T36.0X6
Benzylthiouracil	T38.2X1	T38.2X2	T38.2X3	T38.2X4	T38.2X5	T38.2X6
Bephenium hydroxy-naphthoate	T37.4X1	T37.4X2	T37.4X3	T37.4X4	T37.4X5	T37.4X6
Bepridil	T46.1X1	T46.1X2	T46.1X3	T46.1X4	T46.1X5	T46.1X6
Bergamot oil	T65.891	T65.892	T65.893	T65.894	—	—
Bergapten	T50.991	T50.992	T50.993	T50.994	T50.995	T50.996
Berries, poisonous	T62.1X1	T62.1X2	T62.1X3	T62.1X4	—	—

Substance	External Cause (T-Code)					
	Poisoning, Accidental (Unintentional)	Poisoning, Intentional Self-Harm	Poisoning, Assault	Poisoning, Undetermined	Adverse Effect	Underdosing
Beryllium (compounds)	T56.7X1	T56.7X2	T56.7X3	T56.7X4	—	—
b-acetyldigoxin	T46.0X1	T46.0X2	T46.0X3	T46.0X4	T46.0X5	T46.0X6
beta adrenergic blocking agent, heart	T44.7X1	T44.7X2	T44.7X3	T44.7X4	T44.7X5	T44.7X6
b-benzalbutyramide	T46.6X1	T46.6X2	T46.6X3	T46.6X4	T46.6X5	T46.6X6
Betacarotene	T45.2X1	T45.2X2	T45.2X3	T45.2X4	T45.2X5	T45.2X6
b-eucaine	T49.1X1	T49.1X2	T49.1X3	T49.1X4	T49.1X5	T49.1X6
Beta-Chlor	T42.6X1	T42.6X2	T42.6X3	T42.6X4	T42.6X5	T42.6X6
b-galactosidase	T47.5X1	T47.5X2	T47.5X3	T47.5X4	T47.5X5	T47.5X6
Betahistine	T46.7X1	T46.7X2	T46.7X3	T46.7X4	T46.7X5	T46.7X6
Betaine	T47.5X1	T47.5X2	T47.5X3	T47.5X4	T47.5X5	T47.5X6
Betamethasone	T49.0X1	T49.0X2	T49.0X3	T49.0X4	T49.0X5	T49.0X6
topical	T49.0X1	T49.0X2	T49.0X3	T49.0X4	T49.0X5	T49.0X6
Betamicin	T36.8X1	T36.8X2	T36.8X3	T36.8X4	T36.8X5	T36.8X6
Betanidine	T46.5X1	T46.5X2	T46.5X3	T46.5X4	T46.5X5	T46.5X6
b-sitosterol(s)	T46.6X1	T46.6X2	T46.6X3	T46.6X4	T46.6X5	T46.6X6
Betaxolol	T44.7X1	T44.7X2	T44.7X3	T44.7X4	T44.7X5	T44.7X6
Betazole	T50.8X1	T50.8X2	T50.8X3	T50.8X4	T50.8X5	T50.8X6
Bethanechol	T44.1X1	T44.1X2	T44.1X3	T44.1X4	T44.1X5	T44.1X6
chloride	T44.1X1	T44.1X2	T44.1X3	T44.1X4	T44.1X5	T44.1X6
Bethanidine	T46.5X1	T46.5X2	T46.5X3	T46.5X4	T46.5X5	T46.5X6
Betoxycaine	T41.3X1	T41.3X2	T41.3X3	T41.3X4	T41.3X5	T41.3X6
Betula oil	T49.3X1	T49.3X2	T49.3X3	T49.3X4	T49.3X5	T49.3X6
Bevantolol	T44.7X1	T44.7X2	T44.7X3	T44.7X4	T44.7X5	T44.7X6
Bevonium metilsulfate	T44.3X1	T44.3X2	T44.3X3	T44.3X4	T44.3X5	T44.3X6
Bezafibrate	T46.6X1	T46.6X2	T46.6X3	T46.6X4	T46.6X5	T46.6X6
Bezitramide	T40.4X1	T40.4X2	T40.4X3	T40.4X4	T40.4X5	T40.4X6
BHA	T50.991	T50.992	T50.993	T50.994	T50.995	T50.996
Bhang	T40.7X1	T40.7X2	T40.7X3	T40.7X4	T40.7X5	T40.7X6
BHC (medicinal)	T49.0X1	T49.0X2	T49.0X3	T49.0X4	T49.0X5	T49.0X6
nonmedicinal (vapor)	T53.6X1	T53.6X2	T53.6X3	T53.6X4	—	—
Bialamicol	T37.3X1	T37.3X2	T37.3X3	T37.3X4	T37.3X5	T37.3X6
Bibenzonium bromide	T48.3X1	T48.3X2	T48.3X3	T48.3X4	T48.3X5	T48.3X6
Bibrocathol	T49.5X1	T49.5X2	T49.5X3	T49.5X4	T49.5X5	T49.5X6
Bichloride of mercury—*see Mercury, chloride*						
Bichromates (calcium) (potassium) (sodium) (crystals)	T57.8X1	T57.8X2	T57.8X3	T57.8X4	—	—
fumes	T56.2X1	T56.2X2	T56.2X3	T56.2X4	—	—
Biclotymol	T49.6X1	T49.6X2	T49.6X3	T49.6X4	T49.6X5	T49.6X6
Bicucculine	T50.7X1	T50.7X2	T50.7X3	T50.7X4	T50.7X5	T50.7X6
Bifemelane	T43.291	T43.292	T43.293	T43.294	T43.295	T43.296
Biguanide derivatives, oral	T38.3X1	T38.3X2	T38.3X3	T38.3X4	T38.3X5	T38.3X6

Substance	External Cause (T-Code)					
	Poisoning, Accidental (Unintentional)	Poisoning, Intentional Self-Harm	Poisoning, Assault	Poisoning, Undetermined	Adverse Effect	Underdosing
Biligrafin	T50.8X1	T50.8X2	T50.8X3	T50.8X4	T50.8X5	T50.8X6
Bile salts	T47.5X1	T47.5X2	T47.5X3	T47.5X4	T47.5X5	T47.5X6
Bilopaque	T50.8X1	T50.8X2	T50.8X3	T50.8X4	T50.8X5	T50.8X6
Binifibrate	T46.6X1	T46.6X2	T46.6X3	T46.6X4	T46.6X5	T46.6X6
Binitrobenzol	T65.3X1	T65.3X2	T65.3X3	T65.3X4	—	—
Bioflavonoid(s)	T46.991	T46.992	T46.993	T46.994	T46.995	T46.996
Biological substance NEC	T50.901	T50.902	T50.903	T50.904	T50.905	T50.906
Biotin	T45.2X1	T45.2X2	T45.2X3	T45.2X4	T45.2X5	T45.2X6
Biperiden	T44.3X1	T44.3X2	T44.3X3	T44.3X4	T44.3X5	T44.3X6
Bisacodyl	T47.2X1	T47.2X2	T47.2X3	T47.2X4	T47.2X5	T47.2X6
Bisbentiamine	T45.2X1	T45.2X2	T45.2X3	T45.2X4	T45.2X5	T45.2X6
Bisbutiamine	T45.2X1	T45.2X2	T45.2X3	T45.2X4	T45.2X5	T45.2X6
Bisdequalinium (salts) (diacetate)	T49.6X1	T49.6X2	T49.6X3	T49.6X4	T49.6X5	T49.6X6
Bishydroxycoumarin	T45.511	T45.512	T45.513	T45.514	T45.515	T45.516
Bismarsen	T37.8X1	T37.8X2	T37.8X3	T37.8X4	T37.8X5	T37.8X6
Bismuth salts	T47.6X1	T47.6X2	T47.6X3	T47.6X4	T47.6X5	T47.6X6
aluminate	T47.1X1	T47.1X2	T47.1X3	T47.1X4	T47.1X5	T47.1X6
anti-infectives	T37.8X1	T37.8X2	T37.8X3	T37.8X4	T37.8X5	T37.8X6
formic iodide	T49.0X1	T49.0X2	T49.0X3	T49.0X4	T49.0X5	T49.0X6
glycolylarsenate	T49.0X1	T49.0X2	T49.0X3	T49.0X4	T49.0X5	T49.0X6
nonmedicinal (compounds) NEC	T65.91	T65.92	T65.93	T65.94	—	—
subcarbonate	T47.6X1	T47.6X2	T47.6X3	T47.6X4	T47.6X5	T47.6X6
subsalicylate	T37.8X1	T37.8X2	T37.8X3	T37.8X4	T37.8X5	T37.8X6
sulfarsphenamine	T37.8X1	T37.8X2	T37.8X3	T37.8X4	T37.8X5	T37.8X6
Bisoprolol	T44.7X1	T44.7X2	T44.7X3	T44.7X4	T44.7X5	T44.7X6
Bisoxatin	T47.2X1	T47.2X2	T47.2X3	T47.2X4	T47.2X5	T47.2X6
Bisulepin (hydrochloride)	T45.0X1	T45.0X2	T45.0X3	T45.0X4	T45.0X5	T45.0X6
Bithionol	T37.8X1	T37.8X2	T37.8X3	T37.8X4	T37.8X5	T37.8X6
anthelminthic	T37.4X1	T37.4X2	T37.4X3	T37.4X4	T37.4X5	T37.4X6
Bitolterol	T48.6X1	T48.6X2	T48.6X3	T48.6X4	T48.6X5	T48.6X6
Bitoscanate	T37.4X1	T37.4X2	T37.4X3	T37.4X4	T37.4X5	T37.4X6
Bitter almond oil	T62.8X1	T62.8X2	T62.8X3	T62.8X4	—	—
Bittersweet	T62.2X1	T62.2X2	T62.2X3	T62.2X4	—	—
Black						
flag	T60.91	T60.92	T60.93	T60.94	—	—
henbane	T62.2X1	T62.2X2	T62.2X3	T62.2X4	—	—
leaf (40)	T60.91	T60.92	T60.93	T60.94	—	—
widow spider (bite)	T63.311	T63.312	T63.313	T63.314	—	—
antivenin	T50.Z11	T50.Z12	T50.Z13	T50.Z14	T50.Z15	T50.Z16
Blast furnace gas (carbon monoxide from)	T58.8X1	T58.8X2	T58.8X3	T58.8X4	—	—
Bleach	T54.91	T54.92	T54.93	T54.94	—	—

Substance	External Cause (T-Code)					
	Poisoning, Accidental (Unintentional)	Poisoning, Intentional Self-Harm	Poisoning, Assault	Poisoning, Undetermined	Adverse Effect	Underdosing
Bleaching agent (medicinal)	T49.4X1	T49.4X2	T49.4X3	T49.4X4	T49.4X5	T49.4X6
Bleomycin	T45.1X1	T45.1X2	T45.1X3	T45.1X4	T45.1X5	T45.1X6
Blockain	T41.3X1	T41.3X2	T41.3X3	T41.3X4	T41.3X5	T41.3X6
infiltration (subcutaneous)	T41.3X1	T41.3X2	T41.3X3	T41.3X4	T41.3X5	T41.3X6
nerve block (peripheral) (plexus)	T41.3X1	T41.3X2	T41.3X3	T41.3X4	T41.3X5	T41.3X6
topical (surface)	T41.3X1	T41.3X2	T41.3X3	T41.3X4	T41.3X5	T41.3X6
Blockers, calcium channel	T46.1X1	T46.1X2	T46.1X3	T46.1X4	T46.1X5	T46.1X6
Blood (derivatives) (natural) (plasma) (whole)	T45.8X1	T45.8X2	T45.8X3	T45.8X4	T45.8X5	T45.8X6
dried	T45.8X1	T45.8X2	T45.8X3	T45.8X4	T45.8X5	T45.8X6
drug affecting NEC	T45.91	T45.92	T45.93	T45.94	T45.95	T45.96
expander NEC	T45.8X1	T45.8X2	T45.8X3	T45.8X4	T45.8X5	T45.8X6
fraction NEC	T45.8X1	T45.8X2	T45.8X3	T45.8X4	T45.8X5	T45.8X6
substitute (macromolecular)	T45.8X1	T45.8X2	T45.8X3	T45.8X4	T45.8X5	T45.8X6
Blue velvet	T40.2X1	T40.2X2	T40.2X3	T40.2X4	—	—
Bone meal	T62.8X1	T62.8X2	T62.8X3	T62.8X4	—	—
Bonine	T45.0X1	T45.0X2	T45.0X3	T45.0X4	T45.0X5	T45.0X6
Bopindolol	T44.7X1	T44.7X2	T44.7X3	T44.7X4	T44.7X5	T44.7X6
Boracic acid	T49.0X1	T49.0X2	T49.0X3	T49.0X4	T49.0X5	T49.0X6
ENT agent	T49.6X1	T49.6X2	T49.6X3	T49.6X4	T49.6X5	T49.6X6
ophthalmic preparation	T49.5X1	T49.5X2	T49.5X3	T49.5X4	T49.5X5	T49.5X6
Borane complex	T57.8X1	T57.8X2	T57.8X3	T57.8X4	—	—
Borate(s)	T57.8X1	T57.8X2	T57.8X3	T57.8X4	—	—
buffer	T50.991	T50.992	T50.993	T50.994	T50.995	T50.996
cleanser	T54.91	T54.92	T54.93	T54.94	—	—
sodium	T57.8X1	T57.8X2	T57.8X3	T57.8X4	—	—
Borax (cleanser)	T54.91	T54.92	T54.93	T54.94	—	—
Bordeaux mixture	T60.3X1	T60.3X2	T60.3X3	T60.3X4	—	—
Boric acid	T49.0X1	T49.0X2	T49.0X3	T49.0X4	T49.0X5	T49.0X6
ENT agent	T49.6X1	T49.6X2	T49.6X3	T49.6X4	T49.6X5	T49.6X6
ophthalmic preparation	T49.5X1	T49.5X2	T49.5X3	T49.5X4	T49.5X5	T49.5X6
Bornaprine	T44.3X1	T44.3X2	T44.3X3	T44.3X4	T44.3X5	T44.3X6
Boron	T57.8X1	T57.8X2	T57.8X3	T57.8X4	—	—
hydride NEC	T57.8X1	T57.8X2	T57.8X3	T57.8X4	—	—
fumes or gas	T57.8X1	T57.8X2	T57.8X3	T57.8X4	—	—
trifluoride	T59.891	T59.892	T59.893	T59.894	—	—
Botox	T48.291	T48.292	T48.293	T48.294	T48.295	T48.296
Botulinus anti-toxin (type A, B)	T50.Z11	T50.Z12	T50.Z13	T50.Z14	T50.Z15	T50.Z16
Brake fluid vapor	T59.891	T59.892	T59.893	T59.894	—	—
Brallobarbital	T42.3X1	T42.3X2	T42.3X3	T42.3X4	T42.3X5	T42.3X6
Bran (wheat)	T47.4X1	T47.4X2	T47.4X3	T47.4X4	T47.4X5	T47.4X6
Brass (fumes)	T56.891	T56.892	T56.893	T56.894	—	—

Substance	External Cause (T-Code)					
	Poisoning, Accidental (Unintentional)	Poisoning, Intentional Self-Harm	Poisoning, Assault	Poisoning, Undetermined	Adverse Effect	Underdosing
Brasso	T52.0X1	T52.0X2	T52.0X3	T52.0X4	—	—
Bretylium tosilate	T46.2X1	T46.2X2	T46.2X3	T46.2X4	T46.2X5	T46.2X6
Brevital (sodium)	T41.1X1	T41.1X2	T41.1X3	T41.1X4	T41.1X5	T41.1X6
Brinase	T45.3X1	T45.3X2	T45.3X3	T45.3X4	T45.3X5	T45.3X6
British antilewisite	T45.8X1	T45.8X2	T45.8X3	T45.8X4	T45.8X5	T45.8X6
Brodifacoum	T60.4X1	T60.4X2	T60.4X3	T60.4X4	—	—
Bromal (hydrate)	T42.6X1	T42.6X2	T42.6X3	T42.6X4	T42.6X5	T42.6X6
Bromazepam	T42.4X1	T42.4X2	T42.4X3	T42.4X4	T42.4X5	T42.4X6
Bromazine	T45.0X1	T45.0X2	T45.0X3	T45.0X4	T45.0X5	T45.0X6
Brombenzylcyanide	T59.3X1	T59.3X2	T59.3X3	T59.3X4	—	—
Bromelains	T45.3X1	T45.3X2	T45.3X3	T45.3X4	T45.3X5	T45.3X6
Bromethalin	T60.4X1	T60.4X2	T60.4X3	T60.4X4	—	—
Bromhexine	T48.4X1	T48.4X2	T48.4X3	T48.4X4	T48.4X5	T48.4X6
Bromide salts	T42.6X1	T42.6X2	T42.6X3	T42.6X4	T42.6X5	T42.6X6
Bromindione	T45.511	T45.512	T45.513	T45.514	T45.515	T45.516
Bromine						
compounds (medicinal)	T42.6X1	T42.6X2	T42.6X3	T42.6X4	T42.6X5	T42.6X6
sedative	T42.6X1	T42.6X2	T42.6X3	T42.6X4	T42.6X5	T42.6X6
vapor	T59.891	T59.892	T59.893	T59.894	—	—
Bromisovalum	T42.6X1	T42.6X2	T42.6X3	T42.6X4	T42.6X5	T42.6X6
Bromisoval	T42.6X1	T42.6X2	T42.6X3	T42.6X4	T42.6X5	T42.6X6
Bromobenzylcyanide	T59.3X1	T59.3X2	T59.3X3	T59.3X4	—	—
Bromochlorosalicylani-lide	T49.0X1	T49.0X2	T49.0X3	T49.0X4	T49.0X5	T49.0X6
Bromocriptine	T42.8X1	T42.8X2	T42.8X3	T42.8X4	T42.8X5	T42.8X6
Bromodiphenhydramine	T45.0X1	T45.0X2	T45.0X3	T45.0X4	T45.0X5	T45.0X6
Bromoform	T42.6X1	T42.6X2	T42.6X3	T42.6X4	T42.6X5	T42.6X6
Bromophenol blue reagent	T50.991	T50.992	T50.993	T50.994	T50.995	T50.996
Bromopride	T47.8X1	T47.8X2	T47.8X3	T47.8X4	T47.8X5	T47.8X6
Bromosalicylchloranitide	T49.0X1	T49.0X2	T49.0X3	T49.0X4	T49.0X5	T49.0X6
Bromosalicylhydroxamic acid	T37.1X1	T37.1X2	T37.1X3	T37.1X4	T37.1X5	T37.1X6
Bromo-seltzer	T39.1X1	T39.1X2	T39.1X3	T39.1X4	T39.1X5	T39.1X6
Bromoxynil	T60.3X1	T60.3X2	T60.3X3	T60.3X4	—	—
Bromperidol	T43.4X1	T43.4X2	T43.4X3	T43.4X4	T43.4X5	T43.4X6
Brompheniramine	T45.0X1	T45.0X2	T45.0X3	T45.0X4	T45.0X5	T45.0X6
Bromsulfophthalein	T50.8X1	T50.8X2	T50.8X3	T50.8X4	T50.8X5	T50.8X6
Bromural	T42.6X1	T42.6X2	T42.6X3	T42.6X4	T42.6X5	T42.6X6
Bromvaletone	T42.6X1	T42.6X2	T42.6X3	T42.6X4	T42.6X5	T42.6X6
Bronchodilator NEC	T48.6X1	T48.6X2	T48.6X3	T48.6X4	T48.6X5	T48.6X6
Brotizolam	T42.4X1	T42.4X2	T42.4X3	T42.4X4	T42.4X5	T42.4X6
Brovincamine	T46.7X1	T46.7X2	T46.7X3	T46.7X4	T46.7X5	T46.7X6
Brown spider (bite) (venom)	T63.391	T63.392	T63.393	T63.394	—	—

◀ New ◀ Revised ~~deleted~~ Deleted

Substance	External Cause (T-Code)					
	Poisoning, Accidental (Unintentional)	Poisoning, Intentional Self-Harm	Poisoning, Assault	Poisoning, Undetermined	Adverse Effect	Underdosing
Brown recluse spider (bite) (venom)	T63.331	T63.332	T63.333	T63.334	—	—
Broxaterol	T48.6X1	T48.6X2	T48.6X3	T48.6X4	T48.6X5	T48.6X6
Broxuridine	T45.1X1	T45.1X2	T45.1X3	T45.1X4	T45.1X5	T45.1X6
Broxyquinoline	T37.8X1	T37.8X2	T37.8X3	T37.8X4	T37.8X5	T37.8X6
Bruceine	T48.291	T48.292	T48.293	T48.294	T48.295	T48.296
Brucia	T62.2X1	T62.2X2	T62.2X3	T62.2X4	—	—
Brucine	T65.1X1	T65.1X2	T65.1X3	T65.1X4	—	—
Brunswick green — *see Copper*						
Bruten — *see Ibuprofen*						
Bryonia	T47.2X1	T47.2X2	T47.2X3	T47.2X4	T47.2X5	T47.2X6
Buclizine	T45.0X1	T45.0X2	T45.0X3	T45.0X4	T45.0X5	T45.0X6
Buclosamide	T49.0X1	T49.0X2	T49.0X3	T49.0X4	T49.0X5	T49.0X6
Budesonide	T44.5X1	T44.5X2	T44.5X3	T44.5X4	T44.5X5	T44.5X6
Budralazine	T46.5X1	T46.5X2	T46.5X3	T46.5X4	T46.5X5	T46.5X6
Bufferin	T39.011	T39.012	T39.013	T39.014	T39.015	T39.016
Buflomedil	T46.7X1	T46.7X2	T46.7X3	T46.7X4	T46.7X5	T46.7X6
Buformin	T38.3X1	T38.3X2	T38.3X3	T38.3X4	T38.3X5	T38.3X6
Bufotenine	T40.991	T40.992	T40.993	T40.994	—	—
Bufrolin	T48.6X1	T48.6X2	T48.6X3	T48.6X4	T48.6X5	T48.6X6
Bufylline	T48.6X1	T48.6X2	T48.6X3	T48.6X4	T48.6X5	T48.6X6
Bulk filler	T50.5X1	T50.5X2	T50.5X3	T50.5X4	T50.5X5	T50.5X6
cathartic	T47.4X1	T47.4X2	T47.4X3	T47.4X4	T47.4X5	T47.4X6
Bumetanide	T50.1X1	T50.1X2	T50.1X3	T50.1X4	T50.1X5	T50.1X6
Bunaftine	T46.2X1	T46.2X2	T46.2X3	T46.2X4	T46.2X5	T46.2X6
Bunamiodyl	T50.8X1	T50.8X2	T50.8X3	T50.8X4	T50.8X5	T50.8X6
Bunazosin	T44.6X1	T44.6X2	T44.6X3	T44.6X4	T44.6X5	T44.6X6
Bunitrolol	T44.7X1	T44.7X2	T44.7X3	T44.7X4	T44.7X5	T44.7X6
Buphenine	T46.7X1	T46.7X2	T46.7X3	T46.7X4	T46.7X5	T46.7X6
Bupivacaine	T41.3X1	T41.3X2	T41.3X3	T41.3X4	T41.3X5	T41.3X6
infiltration (subcutaneous)	T41.3X1	T41.3X2	T41.3X3	T41.3X4	T41.3X5	T41.3X6
nerve block (peripheral) (plexus)	T41.3X1	T41.3X2	T41.3X3	T41.3X4	T41.3X5	T41.3X6
spinal	T41.3X1	T41.3X2	T41.3X3	T41.3X4	T41.3X5	T41.3X6
Bupranolol	T44.7X1	T44.7X2	T44.7X3	T44.7X4	T44.7X5	T44.7X6
Buprenorphine	T40.4X1	T40.4X2	T40.4X3	T40.4X4	T40.4X5	T40.4X6
Bupropion	T43.291	T43.292	T43.293	T43.294	T43.295	T43.296
Burimamide	T47.1X1	T47.1X2	T47.1X3	T47.1X4	T47.1X5	T47.1X6
Buserelin	T38.891	T38.892	T38.893	T38.894	T38.895	T38.896
Buspirone	T43.591	T43.592	T43.593	T43.594	T43.595	T43.596
Busulfan, busulphan	T45.1X1	T45.1X2	T45.1X3	T45.1X4	T45.1X5	T45.1X6
Butabarbital (sodium)	T42.3X1	T42.3X2	T42.3X3	T42.3X4	T42.3X5	T42.3X6
Butabarbitone	T42.3X1	T42.3X2	T42.3X3	T42.3X4	T42.3X5	T42.3X6

Substance	External Cause (T-Code)					
	Poisoning, Accidental (Unintentional)	Poisoning, Intentional Self-Harm	Poisoning, Assault	Poisoning, Undetermined	Adverse Effect	Underdosing
Butabarpal	T42.3X1	T42.3X2	T42.3X3	T42.3X4	T42.3X5	T42.3X6
Butacaine	T41.3X1	T41.3X2	T41.3X3	T41.3X4	T41.3X5	T41.3X6
Butalamine	T46.7X1	T46.7X2	T46.7X3	T46.7X4	T46.7X5	T46.7X6
Butalbital	T42.3X1	T42.3X2	T42.3X3	T42.3X4	T42.3X5	T42.3X6
Butallylonal	T42.3X1	T42.3X2	T42.3X3	T42.3X4	T42.3X5	T42.3X6
Butamben	T41.3X1	T41.3X2	T41.3X3	T41.3X4	T41.3X5	T41.3X6
Butamirate	T48.3X1	T48.3X2	T48.3X3	T48.3X4	T48.3X5	T48.3X6
Butane (distributed in mobile container)	T59.891	T59.892	T59.893	T59.894	—	—
distributed through pipes	T59.891	T59.892	T59.893	T59.894	—	—
incomplete combustion	T58.11	T58.12	T58.13	T58.14	—	—
Butanilicaine	T41.3X1	T41.3X2	T41.3X3	T41.3X4	T41.3X5	T41.3X6
Butanol	T51.3X1	T51.3X2	T51.3X3	T51.3X4	—	—
Butanone, 2-butanone	T52.4X1	T52.4X2	T52.4X3	T52.4X4	—	—
Butantrone	T49.4X1	T49.4X2	T49.4X3	T49.4X4	T49.4X5	T49.4X6
Butaperazine	T43.3X1	T43.3X2	T43.3X3	T43.3X4	T43.3X5	T43.3X6
Butazolidin	T39.2X1	T39.2X2	T39.2X3	T39.2X4	T39.2X5	T39.2X6
Butetamate	T48.6X1	T48.6X2	T48.6X3	T48.6X4	T48.6X5	T48.6X6
Butethal	T42.3X1	T42.3X2	T42.3X3	T42.3X4	T42.3X5	T42.3X6
Butethamate	T44.3X1	T44.3X2	T44.3X3	T44.3X4	T44.3X5	T44.3X6
Buthalitone (sodium)	T41.1X1	T41.1X2	T41.1X3	T41.1X4	T41.1X5	T41.1X6
Butisol (sodium)	T42.3X1	T42.3X2	T42.3X3	T42.3X4	T42.3X5	T42.3X6
Butizide	T50.2X1	T50.2X2	T50.2X3	T50.2X4	T50.2X5	T50.2X6
Butobarbital	T42.3X1	T42.3X2	T42.3X3	T42.3X4	T42.3X5	T42.3X6
sodium	T42.3X1	T42.3X2	T42.3X3	T42.3X4	T42.3X5	T42.3X6
Butobarbitone	T42.3X1	T42.3X2	T42.3X3	T42.3X4	T42.3X5	T42.3X6
Butoconazole (nitrate)	T49.0X1	T49.0X2	T49.0X3	T49.0X4	T49.0X5	T49.0X6
Butorphanol	T40.4X1	T40.4X2	T40.4X3	T40.4X4	T40.4X5	T40.4X6
Butriptyline	T43.011	T43.012	T43.013	T43.014	T43.015	T43.016
Butropium bromide	T44.3X1	T44.3X2	T44.3X3	T44.3X4	T44.3X5	T44.3X6
Buttercups	T62.2X1	T62.2X2	T62.2X3	T62.2X4	—	—
Butter of antimony — *see Antimony*						
Butyl						
acetate (secondary)	T52.8X1	T52.8X2	T52.8X3	T52.8X4	—	—
alcohol	T51.3X1	T51.3X2	T51.3X3	T51.3X4	—	—
aminobenzoate	T41.3X1	T41.3X2	T41.3X3	T41.3X4	T41.3X5	T41.3X6
butyrate	T52.8X1	T52.8X2	T52.8X3	T52.8X4	—	—
carbinol	T51.3X1	T51.3X2	T51.3X3	T51.3X4	—	—
carbitol	T52.3X1	T52.3X2	T52.3X3	T52.3X4	—	—
cellosolve	T52.3X1	T52.3X2	T52.3X3	T52.3X4	—	—
chloral (hydrate)	T42.6X1	T42.6X2	T42.6X3	T42.6X4	T42.6X5	T42.6X6
formate	T52.8X1	T52.8X2	T52.8X3	T52.8X4	—	—

Substance	Poisoning, Accidental (Unintentional)	Poisoning, Intentional Self-Harm	Poisoning, Assault	Poisoning, Undetermined	Adverse Effect	Underdosing
	External Cause (T-Code)					
Butyl *(Continued)*						
lactate	T52.8X1	T52.8X2	T52.8X3	T52.8X4	—	—
propionate	T52.8X1	T52.8X2	T52.8X3	T52.8X4	—	—
scopolamine bromide	T44.3X1	T44.3X2	T44.3X3	T44.3X4	T44.3X5	T44.3X6
thiobarbital sodium	T41.1X1	T41.1X2	T41.1X3	T41.1X4	T41.1X5	T41.1X6
Butylated hydroxy-anisole	T50.991	T50.992	T50.993	T50.994	T50.995	T50.996
Butylchloral hydrate	T42.6X1	T42.6X2	T42.6X3	T42.6X4	T42.6X5	T42.6X6
Butyltoluene	T52.2X1	T52.2X2	T52.2X3	T52.2X4	—	—
Butyn	T41.3X1	T41.3X2	T41.3X3	T41.3X4	T41.3X5	T41.3X6
Butyrophenone (-based tranquilizers)	T43.4X1	T43.4X2	T43.4X3	T43.4X4	T43.4X5	T43.4X6
C						
Cabergoline	T42.8X1	T42.8X2	T42.8X3	T42.8X4	T42.8X5	T42.8X6
Cacodyl, cacodylic acid	T57.0X1	T57.0X2	T57.0X3	T57.0X4	—	—
Cactinomycin	T45.1X1	T45.1X2	T45.1X3	T45.1X4	T45.1X5	T45.1X6
Cade oil	T49.4X1	T49.4X2	T49.4X3	T49.4X4	T49.4X5	T49.4X6
Cadexomer iodine	T49.0X1	T49.0X2	T49.0X3	T49.0X4	T49.0X5	T49.0X6
Cadmium (chloride) (fumes) (oxide)	T56.3X1	T56.3X2	T56.3X3	T56.3X4	—	—
sulfide (medicinal) NEC	T49.4X1	T49.4X2	T49.4X3	T49.4X4	T49.4X5	T49.4X6
Cadralazine	T46.5X1	T46.5X2	T46.5X3	T46.5X4	T46.5X5	T46.5X6
Caffeine	T43.611	T43.612	T43.613	T43.614	T43.615	T43.616
Calabar bean	T62.2X1	T62.2X2	T62.2X3	T62.2X4	—	—
Caladium seguinum	T62.2X1	T62.2X2	T62.2X3	T62.2X4	—	—
Calamine (lotion)	T49.3X1	T49.3X2	T49.3X3	T49.3X4	T49.3X5	T49.3X6
Calcifediol	T45.2X1	T45.2X2	T45.2X3	T45.2X4	T45.2X5	T45.2X6
Calciferol	T45.2X1	T45.2X2	T45.2X3	T45.2X4	T45.2X5	T45.2X6
Calcitonin	T50.991	T50.992	T50.993	T50.994	T50.995	T50.996
Calcitriol	T45.2X1	T45.2X2	T45.2X3	T45.2X4	T45.2X5	T45.2X6
Calcium	T50.3X1	T50.3X2	T50.3X3	T50.3X4	T50.3X5	T50.3X6
actylsalicylate	T39.011	T39.012	T39.013	T39.014	T39.015	T39.016
benzamidosalicylate	T37.1X1	T37.1X2	T37.1X3	T37.1X4	T37.1X5	T37.1X6
bromide	T42.6X1	T42.6X2	T42.6X3	T42.6X4	T42.6X5	T42.6X6
bromolactobionate	T42.6X1	T42.6X2	T42.6X3	T42.6X4	T42.6X5	T42.6X6
carbaspirin	T39.011	T39.012	T39.013	T39.014	T39.015	T39.016
carbimide	T50.6X1	T50.6X2	T50.6X3	T50.6X4	T50.6X5	T50.6X6
carbonate	T47.1X1	T47.1X2	T47.1X3	T47.1X4	T47.1X5	T47.1X6
chloride	T50.991	T50.992	T50.993	T50.994	T50.995	T50.996
anhydrous	T50.991	T50.992	T50.993	T50.994	T50.995	T50.996
cyanide	T57.8X1	T57.8X2	T57.8X3	T57.8X4	—	—
dioctyl sulfosuccinate	T47.4X1	T47.4X2	T47.4X3	T47.4X4	T47.4X5	T47.4X6
disodium edathamil	T45.8X1	T45.8X2	T45.8X3	T45.8X4	T45.8X5	T45.8X6

Substance	Poisoning, Accidental (Unintentional)	Poisoning, Intentional Self-Harm	Poisoning, Assault	Poisoning, Undetermined	Adverse Effect	Underdosing
	External Cause (T-Code)					
Calcium *(Continued)*						
disodium edetate	T45.8X1	T45.8X2	T45.8X3	T45.8X4	T45.8X5	T45.8X6
dobesilate	T46.991	T46.992	T46.993	T46.994	T46.995	T46.996
EDTA	T45.8X1	T45.8X2	T45.8X3	T45.8X4	T45.8X5	T45.8X6
ferrous citrate	T45.4X1	T45.4X2	T45.4X3	T45.4X4	T45.4X5	T45.4X6
folinate	T45.8X1	T45.8X2	T45.8X3	T45.8X4	T45.8X5	T45.8X6
glubionate	T50.3X1	T50.3X2	T50.3X3	T50.3X4	T50.3X5	T50.3X6
gluconate	T50.3X1	T50.3X2	T50.3X3	T50.3X4	T50.3X5	T50.3X6
gluconogalactogluconate	T50.3X1	T50.3X2	T50.3X3	T50.3X4	T50.3X5	T50.3X6
hydrate, hydroxide	T54.3X1	T54.3X2	T54.3X3	T54.3X4	—	—
hypochlorite	T54.3X1	T54.3X2	T54.3X3	T54.3X4	—	—
iodide	T48.4X1	T48.4X2	T48.4X3	T48.4X4	T48.4X5	T48.4X6
ipodate	T50.8X1	T50.8X2	T50.8X3	T50.8X4	T50.8X5	T50.8X6
lactate	T50.3X1	T50.3X2	T50.3X3	T50.3X4	T50.3X5	T50.3X6
leucovorin	T45.8X1	T45.8X2	T45.8X3	T45.8X4	T45.8X5	T45.8X6
mandelate	T37.91	T37.92	T37.93	T37.94	T37.95	T37.96
oxide	T54.3X1	T54.3X2	T54.3X3	T54.3X4	—	—
pantothenate	T45.2X1	T45.2X2	T45.2X3	T45.2X4	T45.2X5	T45.2X6
phosphate	T50.3X1	T50.3X2	T50.3X3	T50.3X4	T50.3X5	T50.3X6
salicylate	T39.091	T39.092	T39.093	T39.094	T39.095	T39.096
salts	T50.3X1	T50.3X2	T50.3X3	T50.3X4	T50.3X5	T50.3X6
Calculus-dissolving drug	T50.991	T50.992	T50.993	T50.994	T50.995	T50.996
Calomel	T49.0X1	T49.0X2	T49.0X3	T49.0X4	T49.0X5	T49.0X6
Caloric agent	T50.3X1	T50.3X2	T50.3X3	T50.3X4	T50.3X5	T50.3X6
Calusterone	T38.7X1	T38.7X2	T38.7X3	T38.7X4	T38.7X5	T38.7X6
Camazepam	T42.4X1	T42.4X2	T42.4X3	T42.4X4	T42.4X5	T42.4X6
Camomile	T49.0X1	T49.0X2	T49.0X3	T49.0X4	T49.0X5	T49.0X6
Camoquin	T37.2X1	T37.2X2	T37.2X3	T37.2X4	T37.2X5	T37.2X6
Camphor						
insecticide	T60.2X1	T60.2X2	T60.2X3	T60.2X4	—	—
medicinal	T49.8X1	T49.8X2	T49.8X3	T49.8X4	T49.8X5	T49.8X6
Camylofin	T44.3X1	T44.3X2	T44.3X3	T44.3X4	T44.3X5	T44.3X6
Cancer chemotherapy drug regimen	T45.1X1	T45.1X2	T45.1X3	T45.1X4	T45.1X5	T45.1X6
Candeptin	T49.0X1	T49.0X2	T49.0X3	T49.0X4	T49.0X5	T49.0X6
Candicidin	T49.0X1	T49.0X2	T49.0X3	T49.0X4	T49.0X5	T49.0X6
Cannabinol	T40.7X1	T40.7X2	T40.7X3	T40.7X4	T40.7X5	T40.7X6
Cannabis (derivatives)	T40.7X1	T40.7X2	T40.7X3	T40.7X4	T40.7X5	T40.7X6
Canned heat	T51.1X1	T51.1X2	T51.1X3	T51.1X4	—	—
Canrenoic acid	T50.0X1	T50.0X2	T50.0X3	T50.0X4	T50.0X5	T50.0X6
Canrenone	T50.0X1	T50.0X2	T50.0X3	T50.0X4	T50.0X5	T50.0X6
Cantharides, cantharidin, cantharis	T49.8X1	T49.8X2	T49.8X3	T49.8X4	T49.8X5	T49.8X6

◀ New ⇐ Revised ~~deleted~~ Deleted

Substance	External Cause (T-Code)					
	Poisoning, Accidental (Unintentional)	Poisoning, Intentional Self-Harm	Poisoning, Assault	Poisoning, Undetermined	Adverse Effect	Underdosing
Canthaxanthin	T50.991	T50.992	T50.993	T50.994	T50.995	T50.996
Capillary-active drug NEC	T46.901	T46.902	T46.903	T46.904	T46.905	T46.906
Capreomycin	T36.8X1	T36.8X2	T36.8X3	T36.8X4	T36.8X5	T36.8X6
Capsicum	T49.4X1	T49.4X2	T49.4X3	T49.4X4	T49.4X5	T49.4X6
Captafol	T60.3X1	T60.3X2	T60.3X3	T60.3X4	—	—
Captan	T60.3X1	T60.3X2	T60.3X3	T60.3X4	—	—
Captodiame, captodiamine	T43.591	T43.592	T43.593	T43.594	T43.595	T43.596
Captopril	T46.4X1	T46.4X2	T46.4X3	T46.4X4	T46.4X5	T46.4X6
Caramiphen	T44.3X1	T44.3X2	T44.3X3	T44.3X4	T44.3X5	T44.3X6
Carazolol	T44.7X1	T44.7X2	T44.7X3	T44.7X4	T44.7X5	T44.7X6
Carbachol	T44.1X1	T44.1X2	T44.1X3	T44.1X4	T44.1X5	T44.1X6
Carbacrylamine (resin)	T50.3X1	T50.3X2	T50.3X3	T50.3X4	T50.3X5	T50.3X6
Carbamate (insecticide)	T60.0X1	T60.0X2	T60.0X3	T60.0X4	—	—
Carbamate (sedative)	T42.6X1	T42.6X2	T42.6X3	T42.6X4	T42.6X5	T42.6X6
herbicide	T60.0X1	T60.0X2	T60.0X3	T60.0X4	—	—
insecticide	T60.0X1	T60.0X2	T60.0X3	T60.0X4	—	—
Carbamazepine	T42.1X1	T42.1X2	T42.1X3	T42.1X4	T42.1X5	T42.1X6
Carbamide	T47.3X1	T47.3X2	T47.3X3	T47.3X4	T47.3X5	T47.3X6
peroxide	T49.0X1	T49.0X2	T49.0X3	T49.0X4	T49.0X5	T49.0X6
topical	T49.8X1	T49.8X2	T49.8X3	T49.8X4	T49.8X5	T49.8X6
Carbamylcholine chloride	T44.1X1	T44.1X2	T44.1X3	T44.1X4	T44.1X5	T44.1X6
Carbaril	T60.0X1	T60.0X2	T60.0X3	T60.0X4	—	—
Carbarsone	T37.3X1	T37.3X2	T37.3X3	T37.3X4	T37.3X5	T37.3X6
Carbaryl	T60.0X1	T60.0X2	T60.0X3	T60.0X4	—	—
Carbaspirin	T39.011	T39.012	T39.013	T39.014	T39.015	T39.016
Carbazochrome (salicylate) (sodium sulfonate)	T49.4X1	T49.4X2	T49.4X3	T49.4X4	T49.4X5	T49.4X6
Carbenicillin	T36.0X1	T36.0X2	T36.0X3	T36.0X4	T36.0X5	T36.0X6
Carbenoxolone	T47.1X1	T47.1X2	T47.1X3	T47.1X4	T47.1X5	T47.1X6
Carbetapentane	T48.3X1	T48.3X2	T48.3X3	T48.3X4	T48.3X5	T48.3X6
Carbethyl salicylate	T39.091	T39.092	T39.093	T39.094	T39.095	T39.096
Carbidopa (with levodopa)	T42.8X1	T42.8X2	T42.8X3	T42.8X4	T42.8X5	T42.8X6
Carbimazole	T38.2X1	T38.2X2	T38.2X3	T38.2X4	T38.2X5	T38.2X6
Carbinol	T51.1X1	T51.1X2	T51.1X3	T51.1X4	—	—
Carbinoxamine	T45.0X1	T45.0X2	T45.0X3	T45.0X4	T45.0X5	T45.0X6
Carbiphene	T39.8X1	T39.8X2	T39.8X3	T39.8X4	T39.8X5	T39.8X6
Carbitol	T52.3X1	T52.3X2	T52.3X3	T52.3X4	—	—
Carbocaine	T41.3X1	T41.3X2	T41.3X3	T41.3X4	T41.3X5	T41.3X6
infiltration (subcutaneous)	T41.3X1	T41.3X2	T41.3X3	T41.3X4	T41.3X5	T41.3X6
nerve block (peripheral) (plexus)	T41.3X1	T41.3X2	T41.3X3	T41.3X4	T41.3X5	T41.3X6
topical (surface)	T41.3X1	T41.3X2	T41.3X3	T41.3X4	T41.3X5	T41.3X6
Carbo medicinalis	T47.6X1	T47.6X2	T47.6X3	T47.6X4	T47.6X5	T47.6X6

Substance	External Cause (T-Code)					
	Poisoning, Accidental (Unintentional)	Poisoning, Intentional Self-Harm	Poisoning, Assault	Poisoning, Undetermined	Adverse Effect	Underdosing
Carbomycin	T36.8X1	T36.8X2	T36.8X3	T36.8X4	T36.8X5	T36.8X6
Carbocisteine	T48.4X1	T48.4X2	T48.4X3	T48.4X4	T48.4X5	T48.4X6
Carbocromen	T46.3X1	T46.3X2	T46.3X3	T46.3X4	T46.3X5	T46.3X6
Carbol fuchsin	T49.0X1	T49.0X2	T49.0X3	T49.0X4	T49.0X5	T49.0X6
Carbolic acid — *see also Phenol*	T54.0X1	T54.0X2	T54.0X3	T54.0X4	—	—
Carbolonium (bromide)	T48.1X1	T48.1X2	T48.1X3	T48.1X4	T48.1X5	T48.1X6
Carbon						
bisulfide (liquid)	T65.4X1	T65.4X2	T65.4X3	T65.4X4	—	—
vapor	T65.4X1	T65.4X2	T65.4X3	T65.4X4	—	—
dioxide (gas)	T59.7X1	T59.7X2	T59.7X3	T59.7X4	—	—
medicinal	T41.5X1	T41.5X2	T41.5X3	T41.5X4	T41.5X5	T41.5X6
nonmedicinal	T59.7X1	T59.7X2	T59.7X3	T59.7X4	—	—
snow	T49.4X1	T49.4X2	T49.4X3	T49.4X4	T49.4X5	T49.4X6
disulfide (liquid)	T65.4X1	T65.4X2	T65.4X3	T65.4X4	—	—
vapor	T65.4X1	T65.4X2	T65.4X3	T65.4X4	—	—
monoxide (from incomplete combustion)	T58.91	T58.92	T58.93	T58.94	—	—
blast furnace gas	T58.8X1	T58.8X2	T58.8X3	T58.8X4	—	—
butane (distributed in mobile container)	T58.11	T58.12	T58.13	T58.14	—	—
distributed through pipes	T58.11	T58.12	T58.13	T58.14	—	—
charcoal fumes	T58.2X1	T58.2X2	T58.2X3	T58.2X4	—	—
coal	T58.2X1	T58.2X2	T58.2X3	T58.2X4		
coke (in domestic stoves, fireplaces)	T58.2X1	T58.2X2	T58.2X3	T58.2X4	—	—
gas (piped)	T58.11	T58.12	T58.13	T58.14	—	—
solid (in domestic stoves, fireplaces)	T58.2X1	T58.2X2	T58.2X3	T58.2X4	—	—
exhaust gas (motor) not in transit	T58.01	T58.02	T58.03	T58.04	—	—
combustion engine, any not in watercraft	T58.01	T58.02	T58.03	T58.04	—	—
farm tractor, not in transit	T58.01	T58.02	T58.03	T58.04	—	—
gas engine	T58.01	T58.02	T58.03	T58.04	—	—
motor pump	T58.01	T58.02	T58.03	T58.04	—	—
motor vehicle, not in transit	T58.01	T58.02	T58.03	T58.04	—	—
fuel (in domestic use)	T58.2X1	T58.2X2	T58.2X3	T58.2X4	—	—
gas (piped)	T58.11	T58.12	T58.13	T58.14	—	—
in mobile container	T58.11	T58.12	T58.13	T58.14	—	—
utility	T58.11	T58.12	T58.13	T58.14	—	—
in mobile container	T58.11	T58.12	T58.13	T58.14	—	—
piped (natural)	T58.11	T58.12	T58.13	T58.14	—	—

Substance	External Cause (T-Code)					
	Poisoning, Accidental (Unintentional)	Poisoning, Intentional Self-Harm	Poisoning, Assault	Poisoning, Undetermined	Adverse Effect	Underdosing
Carbon *(Continued)*						
monoxide *(Continued)*						
illuminating gas	T58.11	T58.12	T58.13	T58.14	—	—
industrial fuels or gases, any	T58.8X1	T58.8X2	T58.8X3	T58.8X4	—	—
kerosene (in domestic stoves, fireplaces)	T58.2X1	T58.2X2	T58.2X3	T58.2X4	—	—
kiln gas or vapor	T58.8X1	T58.8X2	T58.8X3	T58.8X4	—	—
motor exhaust gas, not in transit	T58.01	T58.02	T58.03	T58.04	—	—
piped gas (manufactured) (natural)	T58.11	T58.12	T58.13	T58.14	—	—
producer gas	T58.8X1	T58.8X2	T58.8X3	T58.8X4	—	—
propane (distributed in mobile container)	T58.11	T58.12	T58.13	T58.14	—	—
distributed through pipes	T58.11	T58.12	T58.13	T58.14	—	—
specified source NEC	T58.8X1	T58.8X2	T58.8X3	T58.8X4	—	—
stove gas	T58.11	T58.12	T58.13	T58.14	—	—
piped	T58.11	T58.12	T58.13	T58.14	—	—
utility gas	T58.11	T58.12	T58.13	T58.14	—	—
piped	T58.11	T58.12	T58.13	T58.14	—	—
water gas	T58.11	T58.12	T58.13	T58.14	—	—
wood (in domestic stoves, fireplaces)	T58.2X1	T58.2X2	T58.2X3	T58.2X4	—	—
tetrachloride (vapor) NEC	T53.0X1	T53.0X2	T53.0X3	T53.0X4	—	—
liquid (cleansing agent) NEC	T53.0X1	T53.0X2	T53.0X3	T53.0X4	—	—
solvent	T53.0X1	T53.0X2	T53.0X3	T53.0X4	—	—
Carbonic acid gas	T59.7X1	T59.7X2	T59.7X3	T59.7X4	—	—
anhydrase inhibitor NEC	T50.2X1	T50.2X2	T50.2X3	T50.2X4	T50.2X5	T50.2X6
Carbophenothion	T60.0X1	T60.0X2	T60.0X3	T60.0X4	—	—
Carboplatin	T45.1X1	T45.1X2	T45.1X3	T45.1X4	T45.1X5	T45.1X6
Carboprost	T48.0X1	T48.0X2	T48.0X3	T48.0X4	T48.0X5	T48.0X6
Carboquone	T45.1X1	T45.1X2	T45.1X3	T45.1X4	T45.1X5	T45.1X6
Carbowax	T49.3X1	T49.3X2	T49.3X3	T49.3X4	T49.3X5	T49.3X6
Carboxymethyl-cellulose	T47.4X1	T47.4X2	T47.4X3	T47.4X4	T47.4X5	T47.4X6
S-Carboxymethyl-cysteine	T48.4X1	T48.4X2	T48.4X3	T48.4X4	T48.4X5	T48.4X6
Carbrital	T42.3X1	T42.3X2	T42.3X3	T42.3X4	T42.3X5	T42.3X6
Carbromal	T42.6X1	T42.6X2	T42.6X3	T42.6X4	T42.6X5	T42.6X6
Carbutamide	T38.3X1	T38.3X2	T38.3X3	T38.3X4	T38.3X5	T38.3X6
Carbuterol	T48.6X1	T48.6X2	T48.6X3	T48.6X4	T48.6X5	T48.6X6
Cardiac						
depressants	T46.2X1	T46.2X2	T46.2X3	T46.2X4	T46.2X5	T46.2X6
rhythm regulator	T46.2X1	T46.2X2	T46.2X3	T46.2X4	T46.2X5	T46.2X6
specified NEC	T46.2X1	T46.2X2	T46.2X3	T46.2X4	T46.2X5	T46.2X6

Substance	External Cause (T-Code)					
	Poisoning, Accidental (Unintentional)	Poisoning, Intentional Self-Harm	Poisoning, Assault	Poisoning, Undetermined	Adverse Effect	Underdosing
Cardiografin	T50.8X1	T50.8X2	T50.8X3	T50.8X4	T50.8X5	T50.8X6
Cardio-green	T50.8X1	T50.8X2	T50.8X3	T50.8X4	T50.8X5	T50.8X6
Cardiotonic (glycoside) NEC	T46.0X1	T46.0X2	T46.0X3	T46.0X4	T46.0X5	T46.0X6
Cardiovascular drug NEC	T46.901	T46.902	T46.903	T46.904	T46.905	T46.906
Cardrase	T50.2X1	T50.2X2	T50.2X3	T50.2X4	T50.2X5	T50.2X6
Carfusin	T49.0X1	T49.0X2	T49.0X3	T49.0X4	T49.0X5	T49.0X6
Carfecillin	T36.0X1	T36.0X2	T36.0X3	T36.0X4	T36.0X5	T36.0X6
Carfenazine	T43.3X1	T43.3X2	T43.3X3	T43.3X4	T43.3X5	T43.3X6
Carindacillin	T36.0X1	T36.0X2	T36.0X3	T36.0X4	T36.0X5	T36.0X6
Carisoprodol	T42.8X1	T42.8X2	T42.8X3	T42.8X4	T42.8X5	T42.8X6
Carmellose	T47.4X1	T47.4X2	T47.4X3	T47.4X4	T47.4X5	T47.4X6
Carminative	T47.5X1	T47.5X2	T47.5X3	T47.5X4	T47.5X5	T47.5X6
Carmofur	T45.1X1	T45.1X2	T45.1X3	T45.1X4	T45.1X5	T45.1X6
Carmustine	T45.1X1	T45.1X2	T45.1X3	T45.1X4	T45.1X5	T45.1X6
Carotene	T45.2X1	T45.2X2	T45.2X3	T45.2X4	T45.2X5	T45.2X6
Carphenazine	T43.3X1	T43.3X2	T43.3X3	T43.3X4	T43.3X5	T43.3X6
Carpipramine	T42.4X1	T42.4X2	T42.4X3	T42.4X4	T42.4X5	T42.4X6
Carprofen	T39.311	T39.312	T39.313	T39.314	T39.315	T39.316
Carpronium chloride	T44.3X1	T44.3X2	T44.3X3	T44.3X4	T44.3X5	T44.3X6
Carrageenan	T47.8X1	T47.8X2	T47.8X3	T47.8X4	T47.8X5	T47.8X6
Carteolol	T44.7X1	T44.7X2	T44.7X3	T44.7X4	T44.7X5	T44.7X6
Carter's Little Pills	T47.2X1	T47.2X2	T47.2X3	T47.2X4	T47.2X5	T47.2X6
Cascara (sagrada)	T47.2X1	T47.2X2	T47.2X3	T47.2X4	T47.2X5	T47.2X6
Cassava	T62.2X1	T62.2X2	T62.2X3	T62.2X4	—	—
Castellani's paint	T49.0X1	T49.0X2	T49.0X3	T49.0X4	T49.0X5	T49.0X6
Castor						
bean	T62.2X1	T62.2X2	T62.2X3	T62.2X4	—	—
oil	T47.2X1	T47.2X2	T47.2X3	T47.2X4	T47.2X5	T47.2X6
Catalase	T45.3X1	T45.3X2	T45.3X3	T45.3X4	T45.3X5	T45.3X6
Caterpillar (sting)	T63.431	T63.432	T63.433	T63.434	—	—
Catha (edulis) (tea)	T43.691	T43.692	T43.693	T43.694	—	—
Cathartic NEC	T47.4X1	T47.4X2	T47.4X3	T47.4X4	T47.4X5	T47.4X6
anthacene derivative	T47.2X1	T47.2X2	T47.2X3	T47.2X4	T47.2X5	T47.2X6
bulk	T47.4X1	T47.4X2	T47.4X3	T47.4X4	T47.4X5	T47.4X6
contact	T47.2X1	T47.2X2	T47.2X3	T47.2X4	T47.2X5	T47.2X6
emollient NEC	T47.4X1	T47.4X2	T47.4X3	T47.4X4	T47.4X5	T47.4X6
irritant NEC	T47.2X1	T47.2X2	T47.2X3	T47.2X4	T47.2X5	T47.2X6
mucilage	T47.4X1	T47.4X2	T47.4X3	T47.4X4	T47.4X5	T47.4X6
saline	T47.3X1	T47.3X2	T47.3X3	T47.3X4	T47.3X5	T47.3X6
vegetable	T47.2X1	T47.2X2	T47.2X3	T47.2X4	T47.2X5	T47.2X6
Cathine	T50.5X1	T50.5X2	T50.5X3	T50.5X4	T50.5X5	T50.5X6
Cathomycin	T36.8X1	T36.8X2	T36.8X3	T36.8X4	T36.8X5	T36.8X6

Substance	External Cause (T-Code)					
	Poisoning, Accidental (Unintentional)	Poisoning, Intentional Self-Harm	Poisoning, Assault	Poisoning, Undetermined	Adverse Effect	Underdosing
Cation exchange resin	T50.3X1	T50.3X2	T50.3X3	T50.3X4	T50.3X5	T50.3X6
Caustic(s) NEC	T54.91	T54.92	T54.93	T54.94	—	—
alkali	T54.3X1	T54.3X2	T54.3X3	T54.3X4	—	—
hydroxide	T54.3X1	T54.3X2	T54.3X3	T54.3X4	—	—
potash	T54.3X1	T54.3X2	T54.3X3	T54.3X4	—	—
soda	T54.3X1	T54.3X2	T54.3X3	T54.3X4	—	—
specified NEC	T54.91	T54.92	T54.93	T54.94	—	—
Ceepryn	T49.0X1	T49.0X2	T49.0X3	T49.0X4	T49.0X5	T49.0X6
ENT agent	T49.6X1	T49.6X2	T49.6X3	T49.6X4	T49.6X5	T49.6X6
lozenges	T49.6X1	T49.6X2	T49.6X3	T49.6X4	T49.6X5	T49.6X6
Cefacetrile	T36.1X1	T36.1X2	T36.1X3	T36.1X4	T36.1X5	T36.1X6
Cefaclor	T36.1X1	T36.1X2	T36.1X3	T36.1X4	T36.1X5	T36.1X6
Cefadroxil	T36.1X1	T36.1X2	T36.1X3	T36.1X4	T36.1X5	T36.1X6
Cefalexin	T36.1X1	T36.1X2	T36.1X3	T36.1X4	T36.1X5	T36.1X6
Cefaloglycin	T36.1X1	T36.1X2	T36.1X3	T36.1X4	T36.1X5	T36.1X6
Cefaloridine	T36.1X1	T36.1X2	T36.1X3	T36.1X4	T36.1X5	T36.1X6
Cefalosporins	T36.1X1	T36.1X2	T36.1X3	T36.1X4	T36.1X5	T36.1X6
Cefalotin	T36.1X1	T36.1X2	T36.1X3	T36.1X4	T36.1X5	T36.1X6
Cefamandole	T36.1X1	T36.1X2	T36.1X3	T36.1X4	T36.1X5	T36.1X6
Cefamycin antibiotic	T36.1X1	T36.1X2	T36.1X3	T36.1X4	T36.1X5	T36.1X6
Cefapirin	T36.1X1	T36.1X2	T36.1X3	T36.1X4	T36.1X5	T36.1X6
Cefatrizine	T36.1X1	T36.1X2	T36.1X3	T36.1X4	T36.1X5	T36.1X6
Cefazedone	T36.1X1	T36.1X2	T36.1X3	T36.1X4	T36.1X5	T36.1X6
Cefazolin	T36.1X1	T36.1X2	T36.1X3	T36.1X4	T36.1X5	T36.1X6
Cefbuperazone	T36.1X1	T36.1X2	T36.1X3	T36.1X4	T36.1X5	T36.1X6
Cefetamet	T36.1X1	T36.1X2	T36.1X3	T36.1X4	T36.1X5	T36.1X6
Cefixime	T36.1X1	T36.1X2	T36.1X3	T36.1X4	T36.1X5	T36.1X6
Cefmenoxime	T36.1X1	T36.1X2	T36.1X3	T36.1X4	T36.1X5	T36.1X6
Cefmetazole	T36.1X1	T36.1X2	T36.1X3	T36.1X4	T36.1X5	T36.1X6
Cefminox	T36.1X1	T36.1X2	T36.1X3	T36.1X4	T36.1X5	T36.1X6
Cefonicid	T36.1X1	T36.1X2	T36.1X3	T36.1X4	T36.1X5	T36.1X6
Cefoperazone	T36.1X1	T36.1X2	T36.1X3	T36.1X4	T36.1X5	T36.1X6
Ceforanide	T36.1X1	T36.1X2	T36.1X3	T36.1X4	T36.1X5	T36.1X6
Cefotaxime	T36.1X1	T36.1X2	T36.1X3	T36.1X4	T36.1X5	T36.1X6
Cefotetan	T36.1X1	T36.1X2	T36.1X3	T36.1X4	T36.1X5	T36.1X6
Cefotiam	T36.1X1	T36.1X2	T36.1X3	T36.1X4	T36.1X5	T36.1X6
Cefoxitin	T36.1X1	T36.1X2	T36.1X3	T36.1X4	T36.1X5	T36.1X6
Cefpimizole	T36.1X1	T36.1X2	T36.1X3	T36.1X4	T36.1X5	T36.1X6
Cefpiramide	T36.1X1	T36.1X2	T36.1X3	T36.1X4	T36.1X5	T36.1X6
Cefradine	T36.1X1	T36.1X2	T36.1X3	T36.1X4	T36.1X5	T36.1X6
Cefroxadine	T36.1X1	T36.1X2	T36.1X3	T36.1X4	T36.1X5	T36.1X6
Cefsulodin	T36.1X1	T36.1X2	T36.1X3	T36.1X4	T36.1X5	T36.1X6

Substance	External Cause (T-Code)					
	Poisoning, Accidental (Unintentional)	Poisoning, Intentional Self-Harm	Poisoning, Assault	Poisoning, Undetermined	Adverse Effect	Underdosing
Ceftazidime	T36.1X1	T36.1X2	T36.1X3	T36.1X4	T36.1X5	T36.1X6
Cefteram	T36.1X1	T36.1X2	T36.1X3	T36.1X4	T36.1X5	T36.1X6
Ceftezole	T36.1X1	T36.1X2	T36.1X3	T36.1X4	T36.1X5	T36.1X6
Ceftizoxime	T36.1X1	T36.1X2	T36.1X3	T36.1X4	T36.1X5	T36.1X6
Ceftriaxone	T36.1X1	T36.1X2	T36.1X3	T36.1X4	T36.1X5	T36.1X6
Cefuroxime	T36.1X1	T36.1X2	T36.1X3	T36.1X4	T36.1X5	T36.1X6
Cefuzonam	T36.1X1	T36.1X2	T36.1X3	T36.1X4	T36.1X5	T36.1X6
Celestone	T38.0X1	T38.0X2	T38.0X3	T38.0X4	T38.0X5	T38.0X6
topical	T49.0X1	T49.0X2	T49.0X3	T49.0X4	T49.0X5	T49.0X6
Celiprolol	T44.7X1	T44.7X2	T44.7X3	T44.7X4	T44.7X5	T44.7X6
Cellosolve	T52.91	T52.92	T52.93	T52.94	—	—
Cell stimulants and proliferants	T49.8X1	T49.8X2	T49.8X3	T49.8X4	T49.8X5	T49.8X6
Cellulose						
cathartic	T47.4X1	T47.4X2	T47.4X3	T47.4X4	T47.4X5	T47.4X6
hydroxyethyl	T47.4X1	T47.4X2	T47.4X3	T47.4X4	T47.4X5	T47.4X6
nitrates (topical)	T49.3X1	T49.3X2	T49.3X3	T49.3X4	T49.3X5	T49.3X6
oxidized	T49.4X1	T49.4X2	T49.4X3	T49.4X4	T49.4X5	T49.4X6
Centipede (bite)	T63.411	T63.412	T63.413	T63.414	—	—
Central nervous system						
depressants	T42.71	T42.72	T42.73	T42.74	T42.75	T42.76
anesthetic (general) NEC	T41.201	T41.202	T41.203	T41.204	T41.205	T41.206
gases NEC	T41.0X1	T41.0X2	T41.0X3	T41.0X4	T41.0X5	T41.0X6
intravenous	T41.1X1	T41.1X2	T41.1X3	T41.1X4	T41.1X5	T41.1X6
barbiturates	T42.3X1	T42.3X2	T42.3X3	T42.3X4	T42.3X5	T42.3X6
benzodiazepines	T42.4X1	T42.4X2	T42.4X3	T42.4X4	T42.4X5	T42.4X6
bromides	T42.6X1	T42.6X2	T42.6X3	T42.6X4	T42.6X5	T42.6X6
cannabis sativa	T40.7X1	T40.7X2	T40.7X3	T40.7X4	T40.7X5	T40.7X6
chloral hydrate	T42.6X1	T42.6X2	T42.6X3	T42.6X4	T42.6X5	T42.6X6
ethanol	T51.0X1	T51.0X2	T51.0X3	T51.0X4	—	—
hallucinogenics	T40.901	T40.902	T40.903	T40.904	T40.905	T40.906
hypnotics	T42.71	T42.72	T42.73	T42.74	T42.75	T42.76
specified NEC	T42.6X1	T42.6X2	T42.6X3	T42.6X4	T42.6X5	T42.6X6
muscle relaxants	T42.8X1	T42.8X2	T42.8X3	T42.8X4	T42.8X5	T42.8X6
paraldehyde	T42.6X1	T42.6X2	T42.6X3	T42.6X4	T42.6X5	T42.6X6
sedatives; sedative-hypnotics	T42.71	T42.72	T42.73	T42.74	T42.75	T42.76
mixed NEC	T42.6X1	T42.6X2	T42.6X3	T42.6X4	T42.6X5	T42.6X6
specified NEC	T42.6X1	T42.6X2	T42.6X3	T42.6X4	T42.6X5	T42.6X6
muscle-tone depressants	T42.8X1	T42.8X2	T42.8X3	T42.8X4	T42.8X5	T42.8X6
stimulants	T43.601	T43.602	T43.603	T43.604	T43.605	T43.606
amphetamines	T43.621	T43.622	T43.623	T43.624	T43.625	T43.626
analeptics	T50.7X1	T50.7X2	T50.7X3	T50.7X4	T50.7X5	T50.7X6

Substance	External Cause (T-Code)					
	Poisoning, Accidental (Unintentional)	Poisoning, Intentional Self-Harm	Poisoning, Assault	Poisoning, Undetermined	Adverse Effect	Underdosing
Central nervous system *(Continued)*						
stimulants *(Continued)*						
antidepressants	T43.201	T43.202	T43.203	T43.204	T43.205	T43.206
opiate antagonists	T50.7X1	T50.7X2	T50.7X3	T50.7X4	T50.7X5	T50.7X6
specified NEC	T43.691	T43.692	T43.693	T43.694	T43.695	T43.696
Cephalexin	T36.1X1	T36.1X2	T36.1X3	T36.1X4	T36.1X5	T36.1X6
Cephaloglycin	T36.1X1	T36.1X2	T36.1X3	T36.1X4	T36.1X5	T36.1X6
Cephaloridine	T36.1X1	T36.1X2	T36.1X3	T36.1X4	T36.1X5	T36.1X6
Cephalosporins	T36.1X1	T36.1X2	T36.1X3	T36.1X4	T36.1X5	T36.1X6
N (adicillin)	T36.0X1	T36.0X2	T36.0X3	T36.0X4	T36.0X5	T36.0X6
Cephalothin	T36.1X1	T36.1X2	T36.1X3	T36.1X4	T36.1X5	T36.1X6
Cephalotin	T36.1X1	T36.1X2	T36.1X3	T36.1X4	T36.1X5	T36.1X6
Cephradine	T36.1X1	T36.1X2	T36.1X3	T36.1X4	T36.1X5	T36.1X6
Cerbera (odallam)	T62.2X1	T62.2X2	T62.2X3	T62.2X4	—	—
Cerberin	T46.0X1	T46.0X2	T46.0X3	T46.0X4	T46.0X5	T46.0X6
Cerebral stimulants	T43.601	T43.602	T43.603	T43.604	T43.605	T43.606
psychotherapeutic	T43.601	T43.602	T43.603	T43.604	T43.605	T43.606
specified NEC	T43.691	T43.692	T43.693	T43.694	T43.695	T43.696
Cerium oxalate	T45.0X1	T45.0X2	T45.0X3	T45.0X4	T45.0X5	T45.0X6
Cerous oxalate	T45.0X1	T45.0X2	T45.0X3	T45.0X4	T45.0X5	T45.0X6
Ceruletide	T50.8X1	T50.8X2	T50.8X3	T50.8X4	T50.8X5	T50.8X6
Cetalkonium (chloride)	T49.0X1	T49.0X2	T49.0X3	T49.0X4	T49.0X5	T49.0X6
Cethexonium chloride	T49.0X1	T49.0X2	T49.0X3	T49.0X4	T49.0X5	T49.0X6
Cetiedil	T46.7X1	T46.7X2	T46.7X3	T46.7X4	T46.7X5	T46.7X6
Cetirizine	T45.0X1	T45.0X2	T45.0X3	T45.0X4	T45.0X5	T45.0X6
Cetomacrogol	T50.991	T50.992	T50.993	T50.994	T50.995	T50.996
Cetotiamine	T45.2X1	T45.2X2	T45.2X3	T45.2X4	T45.2X5	T45.2X6
Cetoxime	T45.0X1	T45.0X2	T45.0X3	T45.0X4	T45.0X5	T45.0X6
Cetraxate	T47.1X1	T47.1X2	T47.1X3	T47.1X4	T47.1X5	T47.1X6
Cetrimide	T49.0X1	T49.0X2	T49.0X3	T49.0X4	T49.0X5	T49.0X6
Cetrimonium (bromide)	T49.0X1	T49.0X2	T49.0X3	T49.0X4	T49.0X5	T49.0X6
Cetylpyridinium chloride	T49.0X1	T49.0X2	T49.0X3	T49.0X4	T49.0X5	T49.0X6
ENT agent	T49.6X1	T49.6X2	T49.6X3	T49.6X4	T49.6X5	T49.6X6
lozenges	T49.6X1	T49.6X2	T49.6X3	T49.6X4	T49.6X5	T49.6X6
Cevadillasee Sabadilla						
Cevitamic acid	T45.2X1	T45.2X2	T45.2X3	T45.2X4	T45.2X5	T45.2X6
Chalk, precipitated	T47.1X1	T47.1X2	T47.1X3	T47.1X4	T47.1X5	T47.1X6
Chamomile	T49.0X1	T49.0X2	T49.0X3	T49.0X4	T49.0X5	T49.0X6
Ch'an su	T46.0X1	T46.0X2	T46.0X3	T46.0X4	T46.0X5	T46.0X6
Charcoal	T47.6X1	T47.6X2	T47.6X3	T47.6X4	T47.6X5	T47.6X6
activated — *see also Charcoal, medicinal*	T47.6X1	T47.6X2	T47.6X3	T47.6X4	T47.6X5	T47.6X6

Substance	External Cause (T-Code)					
	Poisoning, Accidental (Unintentional)	Poisoning, Intentional Self-Harm	Poisoning, Assault	Poisoning, Undetermined	Adverse Effect	Underdosing
Charcoal *(Continued)*						
fumes (Carbon monoxide)	T58.2X1	T58.2X2	T58.2X3	T58.2X4	—	—
industrial	T58.8X1	T58.8X2	T58.8X3	T58.8X4	—	—
medicinal (activated)	T47.6X1	T47.6X2	T47.6X3	T47.6X4	T47.6X5	T47.6X6
antidiarrheal	T47.6X1	T47.6X2	T47.6X3	T47.6X4	T47.6X5	T47.6X6
poison control	T47.8X1	T47.8X2	T47.8X3	T47.8X4	T47.8X5	T47.8X6
specified use other than for diarrhea	T47.8X1	T47.8X2	T47.8X3	T47.8X4	T47.8X5	T47.8X6
topical	T49.8X1	T49.8X2	T49.8X3	T49.8X4	T49.8X5	T49.8X6
Chaulmosulfone	T37.1X1	T37.1X2	T37.1X3	T37.1X4	T37.1X5	T37.1X6
Chelating agent NEC	T50.6X1	T50.6X2	T50.6X3	T50.6X4	T50.6X5	T50.6X6
Chelidonium majus	T62.2X1	T62.2X2	T62.2X3	T62.2X4	—	—
Chemical substance NEC	T65.91	T65.92	T65.93	T65.94	—	—
Chenodeoxycholic acid	T47.5X1	T47.5X2	T47.5X3	T47.5X4	T47.5X5	T47.5X6
Chenodiol	T47.5X1	T47.5X2	T47.5X3	T47.5X4	T47.5X5	T47.5X6
Chenopodium	T37.4X1	T37.4X2	T37.4X3	T37.4X4	T37.4X5	T37.4X6
Cherry laurel	T62.2X1	T62.2X2	T62.2X3	T62.2X4	—	—
Chinidin(e)	T46.2X1	T46.2X2	T46.2X3	T46.2X4	T46.2X5	T46.2X6
Chiniofon	T37.8X1	T37.8X2	T37.8X3	T37.8X4	T37.8X5	T37.8X6
Chlophedianol	T48.3X1	T48.3X2	T48.3X3	T48.3X4	T48.3X5	T48.3X6
Chloral	T42.6X1	T42.6X2	T42.6X3	T42.6X4	T42.6X5	T42.6X6
derivative	T42.6X1	T42.6X2	T42.6X3	T42.6X4	T42.6X5	T42.6X6
hydrate	T42.6X1	T42.6X2	T42.6X3	T42.6X4	T42.6X5	T42.6X6
Chloralamide	T42.6X1	T42.6X2	T42.6X3	T42.6X4	T42.6X5	T42.6X6
Chloralodol	T42.6X1	T42.6X2	T42.6X3	T42.6X4	T42.6X5	T42.6X6
Chloralose	T60.4X1	T60.4X2	T60.4X3	T60.4X4	—	—
Chlorambucil	T45.1X1	T45.1X2	T45.1X3	T45.1X4	T45.1X5	T45.1X6
Chloramine	T57.8X1	T57.8X2	T57.8X3	T57.8X4	—	—
T	T49.0X1	T49.0X2	T49.0X3	T49.0X4	T49.0X5	T49.0X6
topical	T49.0X1	T49.0X2	T49.0X3	T49.0X4	T49.0X5	T49.0X6
Chloramphenicol	T36.2X1	T36.2X2	T36.2X3	T36.2X4	T36.2X5	T36.2X6
ENT agent	T49.6X1	T49.6X2	T49.6X3	T49.6X4	T49.6X5	T49.6X6
ophthalmic preparation	T49.5X1	T49.5X2	T49.5X3	T49.5X4	T49.5X5	T49.5X6
topical NEC	T49.0X1	T49.0X2	T49.0X3	T49.0X4	T49.0X5	T49.0X6
Chlorate (potassium) (sodium) NEC	T60.3X1	T60.3X2	T60.3X3	T60.3X4	—	—
herbicide	T60.3X1	T60.3X2	T60.3X3	T60.3X4	—	—
Chlorazanil	T50.2X1	T50.2X2	T50.2X3	T50.2X4	T50.2X5	T50.2X6
Chlorbenzene, chlorbenzol	T53.7X1	T53.7X2	T53.7X3	T53.7X4	—	—
Chlorbenzoxamine	T44.3X1	T44.3X2	T44.3X3	T44.3X4	T44.3X5	T44.3X6
Chlorbutol	T42.6X1	T42.6X2	T42.6X3	T42.6X4	T42.6X5	T42.6X6
Chlorcyclizine	T45.0X1	T45.0X2	T45.0X3	T45.0X4	T45.0X5	T45.0X6

◀ New ◀ Revised ~~deleted~~ Deleted

Substance	External Cause (T-Code)					
	Poisoning, Accidental (Unintentional)	Poisoning, Intentional Self-Harm	Poisoning, Assault	Poisoning, Undetermined	Adverse Effect	Underdosing
Chlordan(e) (dust)	T60.1X1	T60.1X2	T60.1X3	T60.1X4	—	—
Chlordantoin	T49.0X1	T49.0X2	T49.0X3	T49.0X4	T49.0X5	T49.0X6
Chlordiazepoxide	T42.4X1	T42.4X2	T42.4X3	T42.4X4	T42.4X5	T42.4X6
Chlordiethyl benzamide	T49.3X1	T49.3X2	T49.3X3	T49.3X4	T49.3X5	T49.3X6
Chloresium	T49.8X1	T49.8X2	T49.8X3	T49.8X4	T49.8X5	T49.8X6
Chlorethiazol	T42.6X1	T42.6X2	T42.6X3	T42.6X4	T42.6X5	T42.6X6
Chlorethyl — *see Ethyl chloride*						
Chloretone	T42.6X1	T42.6X2	T42.6X3	T42.6X4	T42.6X5	T42.6X6
Chlorex	T53.6X1	T53.6X2	T53.6X3	T53.6X4	—	—
insecticide	T60.1X1	T60.1X2	T60.1X3	T60.1X4	—	—
Chlorfenvinphos	T60.0X1	T60.0X2	T60.0X3	T60.0X4	—	—
Chlorhexadol	T42.6X1	T42.6X2	T42.6X3	T42.6X4	T42.6X5	T42.6X6
Chlorhexamide	T45.1X1	T45.1X2	T45.1X3	T45.1X4	T45.1X5	T45.1X6
Chlorhexidine	T49.0X1	T49.0X2	T49.0X3	T49.0X4	T49.0X5	T49.0X6
Chlorhydroxyquinolin	T49.0X1	T49.0X2	T49.0X3	T49.0X4	T49.0X5	T49.0X6
Chloride of lime (bleach)	T54.3X1	T54.3X2	T54.3X3	T54.3X4	—	—
Chlorimipramine	T43.011	T43.012	T43.013	T43.014	T43.015	T43.016
Chlorinated						
camphene	T53.6X1	T53.6X2	T53.6X3	T53.6X4	—	—
diphenyl	T53.7X1	T53.7X2	T53.7X3	T53.7X4	—	—
hydrocarbons NEC	T53.91	T53.92	T53.93	T53.94	—	—
solvents	T53.91	T53.92	T53.93	T53.94	—	—
lime (bleach)	T54.3X1	T54.3X2	T54.3X3	T54.3X4	—	—
and boric acid solution	T49.0X1	T49.0X2	T49.0X3	T49.0X4	T49.0X5	T49.0X6
naphthalene (insecticide)	T60.1X1	T60.1X2	T60.1X3	T60.1X4	—	—
industrial (non-pesticide)	T53.7X1	T53.7X2	T53.7X3	T53.7X4	—	—
pesticide NEC	T60.8X1	T60.8X2	T60.8X3	T60.8X4	—	—
soda — *see also sodium hypochlorite*						
solution	T49.0X1	T49.0X2	T49.0X3	T49.0X4	T49.0X5	T49.0X6
Chlorine (fumes) (gas)	T59.4X1	T59.4X2	T59.4X3	T59.4X4	—	—
bleach	T54.3X1	T54.3X2	T54.3X3	T54.3X4	—	—
compound gas NEC	T59.4X1	T59.4X2	T59.4X3	T59.4X4	—	—
disinfectant	T59.4X1	T59.4X2	T59.4X3	T59.4X4	—	—
releasing agents NEC	T59.4X1	T59.4X2	T59.4X3	T59.4X4	—	—
Chlorisondamine chloride	T46.991	T46.992	T46.993	T46.994	T46.995	T46.996
Chlormadinone	T38.5X1	T38.5X2	T38.5X3	T38.5X4	T38.5X5	T38.5X6
Chlormephos	T60.0X1	T60.0X2	T60.0X3	T60.0X4	—	—
Chlormerodrin	T50.2X1	T50.2X2	T50.2X3	T50.2X4	T50.2X5	T50.2X6
Chlormethiazole	T42.6X1	T42.6X2	T42.6X3	T42.6X4	T42.6X5	T42.6X6
Chlormethine	T45.1X1	T45.1X2	T45.1X3	T45.1X4	T45.1X5	T45.1X6
Chlormethylenecycline	T36.4X1	T36.4X2	T36.4X3	T36.4X4	T36.4X5	T36.4X6

Substance	External Cause (T-Code)					
	Poisoning, Accidental (Unintentional)	Poisoning, Intentional Self-Harm	Poisoning, Assault	Poisoning, Undetermined	Adverse Effect	Underdosing
Chlormezanone	T42.6X1	T42.6X2	T42.6X3	T42.6X4	T42.6X5	T42.6X6
Chloroacetic acid	T60.3X1	T60.3X2	T60.3X3	T60.3X4	—	—
Chloroacetone	T59.3X1	T59.3X2	T59.3X3	T59.3X4	—	—
Chloroacetophenone	T59.3X1	T59.3X2	T59.3X3	T59.3X4	—	—
Chloroaniline	T53.7X1	T53.7X2	T53.7X3	T53.7X4	—	—
Chlorobenzene, chlorobenzol	T53.7X1	T53.7X2	T53.7X3	T53.7X4	—	—
Chlorobromomethane (fire extinguisher)	T53.6X1	T53.6X2	T53.6X3	T53.6X4	—	—
Chlorobutanol	T49.0X1	T49.0X2	T49.0X3	T49.0X4	T49.0X5	T49.0X6
Chlorocresol	T49.0X1	T49.0X2	T49.0X3	T49.0X4	T49.0X5	T49.0X6
Chlorodehydro-methyltestosterone	T38.7X1	T38.7X2	T38.7X3	T38.7X4	T38.7X5	T38.7X6
Chlorodinitrobenzene	T53.7X1	T53.7X2	T53.7X3	T53.7X4	—	—
dust or vapor	T53.7X1	T53.7X2	T53.7X3	T53.7X4	—	—
Chlorodiphenyl	T53.7X1	T53.7X2	T53.7X3	T53.7X4	—	—
Chloroethane — *see Ethyl chloride*						
Chloroethylene	T53.6X1	T53.6X2	T53.6X3	T53.6X4	—	—
Chlorofluorocarbons	T53.5X1	T53.5X2	T53.5X3	T53.5X4	—	—
Chloroform (fumes) (vapor)	T53.1X1	T53.1X2	T53.1X3	T53.1X4	—	—
anesthetic	T41.0X1	T41.0X2	T41.0X3	T41.0X4	T41.0X5	T41.0X6
solvent	T53.1X1	T53.1X2	T53.1X3	T53.1X4	—	—
water, concentrated	T41.0X1	T41.0X2	T41.0X3	T41.0X4	T41.0X5	T41.0X6
Chloroguanide	T37.2X1	T37.2X2	T37.2X3	T37.2X4	T37.2X5	T37.2X6
Chloromycetin	T36.2X1	T36.2X2	T36.2X3	T36.2X4	T36.2X5	T36.2X6
ENT agent	T49.6X1	T49.6X2	T49.6X3	T49.6X4	T49.6X5	T49.6X6
ophthalmic preparation	T49.5X1	T49.5X2	T49.5X3	T49.5X4	T49.5X5	T49.5X6
otic solution	T49.6X1	T49.6X2	T49.6X3	T49.6X4	T49.6X5	T49.6X6
topical NEC	T49.0X1	T49.0X2	T49.0X3	T49.0X4	T49.0X5	T49.0X6
Chloronitrobenzene	T53.7X1	T53.7X2	T53.7X3	T53.7X4	—	—
dust or vapor	T53.7X1	T53.7X2	T53.7X3	T53.7X4	—	—
Chlorophacinone	T60.4X1	T60.4X2	T60.4X3	T60.4X4	—	—
Chlorophenol	T53.7X1	T53.7X2	T53.7X3	T53.7X4	—	—
Chlorophenothane	T60.1X1	T60.1X2	T60.1X3	T60.1X4	—	—
Chlorophyll	T50.991	T50.992	T50.993	T50.994	T50.995	T50.996
Chloropicrin (fumes)	T53.6X1	T53.6X2	T53.6X3	T53.6X4	—	—
fumigant	T60.8X1	T60.8X2	T60.8X3	T60.8X4	—	—
fungicide	T60.3X1	T60.3X2	T60.3X3	T60.3X4	—	—
pesticide	T60.8X1	T60.8X2	T60.8X3	T60.8X4	—	—
Chloroprocaine	T41.3X1	T41.3X2	T41.3X3	T41.3X4	T41.3X5	T41.3X6
infiltration (subcutaneous)	T41.3X1	T41.3X2	T41.3X3	T41.3X4	T41.3X5	T41.3X6
nerve block (peripheral) (plexus)	T41.3X1	T41.3X2	T41.3X3	T41.3X4	T41.3X5	T41.3X6
spinal	T41.3X1	T41.3X2	T41.3X3	T41.3X4	T41.3X5	T41.3X6

Substance	External Cause (T-Code)					
	Poisoning, Accidental (Unintentional)	Poisoning, Intentional Self-Harm	Poisoning, Assault	Poisoning, Undetermined	Adverse Effect	Underdosing
Chloroptic	T49.5X1	T49.5X2	T49.5X3	T49.5X4	T49.5X5	T49.5X6
Chloropurine	T45.1X1	T45.1X2	T45.1X3	T45.1X4	T45.1X5	T45.1X6
Chloropyramine	T45.0X1	T45.0X2	T45.0X3	T45.0X4	T45.0X5	T45.0X6
Chloropyrifos	T60.0X1	T60.0X2	T60.0X3	T60.0X4	—	—
Chloropyrilene	T45.0X1	T45.0X2	T45.0X3	T45.0X4	T45.0X5	T45.0X6
Chloroquine	T37.2X1	T37.2X2	T37.2X3	T37.2X4	T37.2X5	T37.2X6
Chlorothalonil	T60.3X1	T60.3X2	T60.3X3	T60.3X4	—	—
Chlorothen	T45.0X1	T45.0X2	T45.0X3	T45.0X4	T45.0X5	T45.0X6
Chlorothiazide	T50.2X1	T50.2X2	T50.2X3	T50.2X4	T50.2X5	T50.2X6
Chlorothymol	T49.4X1	T49.4X2	T49.4X3	T49.4X4	T49.4X5	T49.4X6
Chlorotrianisene	T38.5X1	T38.5X2	T38.5X3	T38.5X4	T38.5X5	T38.5X6
Chlorovinyldichloro-arsine, not in war	T57.0X1	T57.0X2	T57.0X3	T57.0X4	—	—
Chloroxine	T49.4X1	T49.4X2	T49.4X3	T49.4X4	T49.4X5	T49.4X6
Chloroxylenol	T49.0X1	T49.0X2	T49.0X3	T49.0X4	T49.0X5	T49.0X6
Chlorphenamine	T45.0X1	T45.0X2	T45.0X3	T45.0X4	T45.0X5	T45.0X6
Chlorphenesin	T42.8X1	T42.8X2	T42.8X3	T42.8X4	T42.8X5	T42.8X6
topical (antifungal)	T49.0X1	T49.0X2	T49.0X3	T49.0X4	T49.0X5	T49.0X6
Chlorpheniramine	T45.0X1	T45.0X2	T45.0X3	T45.0X4	T45.0X5	T45.0X6
Chlorphenoxamine	T45.0X1	T45.0X2	T45.0X3	T45.0X4	T45.0X5	T45.0X6
Chlorphentermine	T50.5X1	T50.5X2	T50.5X3	T50.5X4	T50.5X5	T50.5X6
Chlorprocaine — *see Chloroprocaine*						
Chlorproguanil	T37.2X1	T37.2X2	T37.2X3	T37.2X4	T37.2X5	T37.2X6
Chlorpromazine	T43.3X1	T43.3X2	T43.3X3	T43.3X4	T43.3X5	T43.3X6
Chlorpropamide	T38.3X1	T38.3X2	T38.3X3	T38.3X4	T38.3X5	T38.3X6
Chlorprothixene	T43.4X1	T43.4X2	T43.4X3	T43.4X4	T43.4X5	T43.4X6
Chlorquinaldol	T49.0X1	T49.0X2	T49.0X3	T49.0X4	T49.0X5	T49.0X6
Chlorquinol	T49.0X1	T49.0X2	T49.0X3	T49.0X4	T49.0X5	T49.0X6
Chlortalidone	T50.2X1	T50.2X2	T50.2X3	T50.2X4	T50.2X5	T50.2X6
Chlortetracycline	T36.4X1	T36.4X2	T36.4X3	T36.4X4	T36.4X5	T36.4X6
Chlorthalidone	T50.2X1	T50.2X2	T50.2X3	T50.2X4	T50.2X5	T50.2X6
Chlorthiophos	T60.0X1	T60.0X2	T60.0X3	T60.0X4	—	—
Chlorotrianisene	T38.5X1	T38.5X2	T38.5X3	T38.5X4	T38.5X5	T38.5X6
Chlor-Trimeton	T45.0X1	T45.0X2	T45.0X3	T45.0X4	T45.0X5	T45.0X6
Chlorthion	T60.0X1	T60.0X2	T60.0X3	T60.0X4	—	—
Chlorzoxazone	T42.8X1	T42.8X2	T42.8X3	T42.8X4	T42.8X5	T42.8X6
Choke damp	T59.7X1	T59.7X2	T59.7X3	T59.7X4	—	—
Cholagogues	T47.5X1	T47.5X2	T47.5X3	T47.5X4	T47.5X5	T47.5X6
Cholebrine	T50.8X1	T50.8X2	T50.8X3	T50.8X4	T50.8X5	T50.8X6
Cholecalciferol	T45.2X1	T45.2X2	T45.2X3	T45.2X4	T45.2X5	T45.2X6
Cholecystokinin	T50.8X1	T50.8X2	T50.8X3	T50.8X4	T50.8X5	T50.8X6
Cholera vaccine	T50.A91	T50.A92	T50.A93	T50.A94	T50.A95	T50.A96

Substance	External Cause (T-Code)					
	Poisoning, Accidental (Unintentional)	Poisoning, Intentional Self-Harm	Poisoning, Assault	Poisoning, Undetermined	Adverse Effect	Underdosing
Choleretic	T47.5X1	T47.5X2	T47.5X3	T47.5X4	T47.5X5	T47.5X6
Cholesterol-lowering agents	T46.6X1	T46.6X2	T46.6X3	T46.6X4	T46.6X5	T46.6X6
Cholestyramine (resin)	T46.6X1	T46.6X2	T46.6X3	T46.6X4	T46.6X5	T46.6X6
Cholic acid	T47.5X1	T47.5X2	T47.5X3	T47.5X4	T47.5X5	T47.5X6
Choline	T48.6X1	T48.6X2	T48.6X3	T48.6X4	T48.6X5	T48.6X6
chloride	T50.991	T50.992	T50.993	T50.994	T50.995	T50.996
dihydrogen citrate	T50.991	T50.992	T50.993	T50.994	T50.995	T50.996
salicylate	T39.091	T39.092	T39.093	T39.094	T39.095	T39.096
theophyllinate	T48.6X1	T48.6X2	T48.6X3	T48.6X4	T48.6X5	T48.6X6
Cholinergic (drug) NEC	T44.1X1	T44.1X2	T44.1X3	T44.1X4	T44.1X5	T44.1X6
muscle tone enhancer	T44.1X1	T44.1X2	T44.1X3	T44.1X4	T44.1X5	T44.1X6
organophosphorus	T44.0X1	T44.0X2	T44.0X3	T44.0X4	T44.0X5	T44.0X6
insecticide	T60.0X1	T60.0X2	T60.0X3	T60.0X4	—	—
nerve gas	T59.891	T59.892	T59.893	T59.894	—	—
trimethyl ammonium propanediol	T44.1X1	T44.1X2	T44.1X3	T44.1X4	T44.1X5	T44.1X6
Cholinesterase reactivator	T50.6X1	T50.6X2	T50.6X3	T50.6X4	T50.6X5	T50.6X6
Cholografin	T50.8X1	T50.8X2	T50.8X3	T50.8X4	T50.8X5	T50.8X6
Chorionic gonadotropin	T38.891	T38.892	T38.893	T38.894	T38.895	T38.896
Chromate	T56.2X1	T56.2X2	T56.2X3	T56.2X4	—	—
dust or mist	T56.2X1	T56.2X2	T56.2X3	T56.2X4	—	—
lead — *see also lead*	T56.0X1	T56.0X2	T56.0X3	T56.0X4	—	—
paint	T56.0X1	T56.0X2	T56.0X3	T56.0X4	—	—
Chromic						
acid	T56.2X1	T56.2X2	T56.2X3	T56.2X4	—	—
dust or mist	T56.2X1	T56.2X2	T56.2X3	T56.2X4	—	—
phosphate 32P	T45.1X1	T45.1X2	T45.1X3	T45.1X4	T45.1X5	T45.1X6
Chromium	T56.2X1	T56.2X2	T56.2X3	T56.2X4	—	—
compounds — *see Chromate*						
sesquioxide	T50.8X1	T50.8X2	T50.8X3	T50.8X4	T50.8X5	T50.8X6
Chromomycin A3	T45.1X1	T45.1X2	T45.1X3	T45.1X4	T45.1X5	T45.1X6
Chromonar	T46.3X1	T46.3X2	T46.3X3	T46.3X4	T46.3X5	T46.3X6
Chromyl chloride	T56.2X1	T56.2X2	T56.2X3	T56.2X4	—	—
Chrysarobin	T49.4X1	T49.4X2	T49.4X3	T49.4X4	T49.4X5	T49.4X6
Chrysazin	T47.2X1	T47.2X2	T47.2X3	T47.2X4	T47.2X5	T47.2X6
Chymar	T45.3X1	T45.3X2	T45.3X3	T45.3X4	T45.3X5	T45.3X6
ophthalmic preparation	T49.5X1	T49.5X2	T49.5X3	T49.5X4	T49.5X5	T49.5X6
Chymopapain	T45.3X1	T45.3X2	T45.3X3	T45.3X4	T45.3X5	T45.3X6
Chymotrypsin	T45.3X1	T45.3X2	T45.3X3	T45.3X4	T45.3X5	T45.3X6
ophthalmic preparation	T49.5X1	T49.5X2	T49.5X3	T49.5X4	T49.5X5	T49.5X6
Cianidanol	T50.991	T50.992	T50.993	T50.994	T50.995	T50.996
Cianopramine	T43.011	T43.012	T43.013	T43.014	T43.015	T43.016
Cibenzoline	T46.2X1	T46.2X2	T46.2X3	T46.2X4	T46.2X5	T46.2X6

◀ New ⇐ Revised ~~deleted~~ Deleted

Substance	External Cause (T-Code)					
	Poisoning, Accidental (Unintentional)	Poisoning, Intentional Self-Harm	Poisoning, Assault	Poisoning, Undetermined	Adverse Effect	Underdosing
Ciclacillin	T36.0X1	T36.0X2	T36.0X3	T36.0X4	T36.0X5	T36.0X6
Ciclobarbital — *see Hexobarbital*						
Ciclonicate	T46.7X1	T46.7X2	T46.7X3	T46.7X4	T46.7X5	T46.7X6
Ciclopirox (olamine)	T49.0X1	T49.0X2	T49.0X3	T49.0X4	T49.0X5	T49.0X6
Ciclosporin	T45.1X1	T45.1X2	T45.1X3	T45.1X4	T45.1X5	T45.1X6
Cicuta maculata or virosa	T62.2X1	T62.2X2	T62.2X3	T62.2X4	—	—
Cicutoxin	T62.2X1	T62.2X2	T62.2X3	T62.2X4	—	—
Cigarette lighter fluid	T52.0X1	T52.0X2	T52.0X3	T52.0X4	—	—
Cigarettes (tobacco)	T65.221	T65.222	T65.223	T65.224	—	—
Ciguatoxin	T61.01	T61.02	T61.03	T61.04	—	—
Cilazapril	T46.4X1	T46.4X2	T46.4X3	T46.4X4	T46.4X5	T46.4X6
Cimetidine	T47.0X1	T47.0X2	T47.0X3	T47.0X4	T47.0X5	T47.0X6
Cimetropium bromide	T44.3X1	T44.3X2	T44.3X3	T44.3X4	T44.3X5	T44.3X6
Cinchocaine	T41.3X1	T41.3X2	T41.3X3	T41.3X4	T41.3X5	T41.3X6
topical (surface)	T41.3X1	T41.3X2	T41.3X3	T41.3X4	T41.3X5	T41.3X6
Cinchona	T37.2X1	T37.2X2	T37.2X3	T37.2X4	T37.2X5	T37.2X6
Cinchonine alkaloids	T37.2X1	T37.2X2	T37.2X3	T37.2X4	T37.2X5	T37.2X6
Cinchophen	T50.4X1	T50.4X2	T50.4X3	T50.4X4	T50.4X5	T50.4X6
Cinepazide	T46.7X1	T46.7X2	T46.7X3	T46.7X4	T46.7X5	T46.7X6
Cinnamedrine	T48.5X1	T48.5X2	T48.5X3	T48.5X4	T48.5X5	T48.5X6
Cinnarizine	T45.0X1	T45.0X2	T45.0X3	T45.0X4	T45.0X5	T45.0X6
Cinoxacin	T37.8X1	T37.8X2	T37.8X3	T37.8X4	T37.8X5	T37.8X6
Ciprofibrate	T46.6X1	T46.6X2	T46.6X3	T46.6X4	T46.6X5	T46.6X6
Ciprofloxacin	T36.8X1	T36.8X2	T36.8X3	T36.8X4	T36.8X5	T36.8X6
Cisapride	T47.8X1	T47.8X2	T47.8X3	T47.8X4	T47.8X5	T47.8X6
Cisplatin	T45.1X1	T45.1X2	T45.1X3	T45.1X4	T45.1X5	T45.1X6
Citalopram	T43.221	T43.222	T43.223	T43.224	T43.225	T43.226
Citanest	T41.3X1	T41.3X2	T41.3X3	T41.3X4	T41.3X5	T41.3X6
infiltration (subcutaneous)	T41.3X1	T41.3X2	T41.3X3	T41.3X4	T41.3X5	T41.3X6
nerve block (peripheral) (plexus)	T41.3X1	T41.3X2	T41.3X3	T41.3X4	T41.3X5	T41.3X6
Citric acid	T47.5X1	T47.5X2	T47.5X3	T47.5X4	T47.5X5	T47.5X6
Citrovorum (factor)	T45.8X1	T45.8X2	T45.8X3	T45.8X4	T45.8X5	T45.8X6
Claviceps purpurea	T62.2X1	T62.2X2	T62.2X3	T62.2X4	—	—
Clavulanic acid	T36.1X1	T36.1X2	T36.1X3	T36.1X4	T36.1X5	T36.1X6
Cleaner, cleansing agent, type not specified	T65.891	T65.892	T65.893	T65.894	—	—
of paint or varnish	T52.91	T52.92	T52.93	T52.94	—	—
specified type NEC	T65.891	T65.892	T65.893	T65.894	—	—
Clebopride	T47.8X1	T47.8X2	T47.8X3	T47.8X4	T47.8X5	T47.8X6
Clefamide	T37.3X1	T37.3X2	T37.3X3	T37.3X4	T37.3X5	T37.3X6
Clemastine	T45.0X1	T45.0X2	T45.0X3	T45.0X4	T45.0X5	T45.0X6
Clematis vitalba	T62.2X1	T62.2X2	T62.2X3	T62.2X4	—	—

Substance	External Cause (T-Code)					
	Poisoning, Accidental (Unintentional)	Poisoning, Intentional Self-Harm	Poisoning, Assault	Poisoning, Undetermined	Adverse Effect	Underdosing
Clemizole	T45.0X1	T45.0X2	T45.0X3	T45.0X4	T45.0X5	T45.0X6
penicillin	T36.0X1	T36.0X2	T36.0X3	T36.0X4	T36.0X5	T36.0X6
Clenbuterol	T48.6X1	T48.6X2	T48.6X3	T48.6X4	T48.6X5	T48.6X6
Clidinium bromide	T44.3X1	T44.3X2	T44.3X3	T44.3X4	T44.3X5	T44.3X6
Clindamycin	T36.8X1	T36.8X2	T36.8X3	T36.8X4	T36.8X5	T36.8X6
Clinofibrate	T46.6X1	T46.6X2	T46.6X3	T46.6X4	T46.6X5	T46.6X6
Clioquinol	T37.8X1	T37.8X2	T37.8X3	T37.8X4	T37.8X5	T37.8X6
Cliradon	T40.2X1	T40.2X2	T40.2X3	T40.2X4	—	—
Clobazam	T42.4X1	T42.4X2	T42.4X3	T42.4X4	T42.4X5	T42.4X6
Clobenzorex	T50.5X1	T50.5X2	T50.5X3	T50.5X4	T50.5X5	T50.5X6
Clobetasol	T49.0X1	T49.0X2	T49.0X3	T49.0X4	T49.0X5	T49.0X6
Clobetasone	T49.0X1	T49.0X2	T49.0X3	T49.0X4	T49.0X5	T49.0X6
Clobutinol	T48.3X1	T48.3X2	T48.3X3	T48.3X4	T48.3X5	T48.3X6
Clocapramine	T43.0X1	T43.0X2	T43.0X3	T43.0X4	T43.0X5	T43.0X6
Clocortolone	T38.0X1	T38.0X2	T38.0X3	T38.0X4	T38.0X5	T38.0X6
Clodantoin	T49.0X1	T49.0X2	T49.0X3	T49.0X4	T49.0X5	T49.0X6
Clodronic acid	T50.991	T50.992	T50.993	T50.994	T50.995	T50.996
Clofazimine	T37.1X1	T37.1X2	T37.1X3	T37.1X4	T37.1X5	T37.1X6
Clofedanol	T48.3X1	T48.3X2	T48.3X3	T48.3X4	T48.3X5	T48.3X6
Clofenamide	T50.2X1	T50.2X2	T50.2X3	T50.2X4	T50.2X5	T50.2X6
Clofenotane	T49.0X1	T49.0X2	T49.0X3	T49.0X4	T49.0X5	T49.0X6
Clofezone	T39.2X1	T39.2X2	T39.2X3	T39.2X4	T39.2X5	T39.2X6
Clofibrate	T46.6X1	T46.6X2	T46.6X3	T46.6X4	T46.6X5	T46.6X6
Clofibride	T46.6X1	T46.6X2	T46.6X3	T46.6X4	T46.6X5	T46.6X6
Cloforex	T50.5X1	T50.5X2	T50.5X3	T50.5X4	T50.5X5	T50.5X6
Clomacran	T43.0X1	T43.0X2	T43.0X3	T43.0X4	T43.0X5	T43.0X6
Clomethiazole	T42.6X1	T42.6X2	T42.6X3	T42.6X4	T42.6X5	T42.6X6
Clometocillin	T36.0X1	T36.0X2	T36.0X3	T36.0X4	T36.0X5	T36.0X6
Clomifene	T38.5X1	T38.5X2	T38.5X3	T38.5X4	T38.5X5	T38.5X6
Clomiphene	T38.5X1	T38.5X2	T38.5X3	T38.5X4	T38.5X5	T38.5X6
Clomipramine	T43.011	T43.012	T43.013	T43.014	T43.015	T43.016
Clomocycline	T36.4X1	T36.4X2	T36.4X3	T36.4X4	T36.4X5	T36.4X6
Clonazepam	T42.4X1	T42.4X2	T42.4X3	T42.4X4	T42.4X5	T42.4X6
Clonidine	T46.5X1	T46.5X2	T46.5X3	T46.5X4	T46.5X5	T46.5X6
Clonixin	T39.8X1	T39.8X2	T39.8X3	T39.8X4	T39.8X5	T39.8X6
Clopamide	T50.2X1	T50.2X2	T50.2X3	T50.2X4	T50.2X5	T50.2X6
Clopenthixol	T43.4X1	T43.4X2	T43.4X3	T43.4X4	T43.4X5	T43.4X6
Cloperastine	T48.3X1	T48.3X2	T48.3X3	T48.3X4	T48.3X5	T48.3X6
Clophedianol	T48.3X1	T48.3X2	T48.3X3	T48.3X4	T48.3X5	T48.3X6
Cloponone	T36.2X1	T36.2X2	T36.2X3	T36.2X4	T36.2X5	T36.2X6
Cloprednol	T38.0X1	T38.0X2	T38.0X3	T38.0X4	T38.0X5	T38.0X6
Cloral betaine	T42.6X1	T42.6X2	T42.6X3	T42.6X4	T42.6X5	T42.6X6

Substance	Poisoning, Accidental (Unintentional)	Poisoning, Intentional Self-Harm	Poisoning, Assault	Poisoning, Undetermined	Adverse Effect	Underdosing
	External Cause (T-Code)					
Cloramfenicol	T36.2X1	T36.2X2	T36.2X3	T36.2X4	T36.2X5	T36.2X6
Clorazepate (dipotassium)	T42.4X1	T42.4X2	T42.4X3	T42.4X4	T42.4X5	T42.4X6
Clorexolone	T50.2X1	T50.2X2	T50.2X3	T50.2X4	T50.2X5	T50.2X6
Clorox (bleach)	T54.91	T54.92	T54.93	T54.94	—	—
Clorfenamine	T45.0X1	T45.0X2	T45.0X3	T45.0X4	T45.0X5	T45.0X6
Clorgiline	T43.1X1	T43.1X2	T43.1X3	T43.1X4	T43.1X5	T43.1X6
Clorotepine	T44.3X1	T44.3X2	T44.3X3	T44.3X4	T44.3X5	T44.3X6
Clorprenaline	T48.6X1	T48.6X2	T48.6X3	T48.6X4	T48.6X5	T48.6X6
Clortermine	T50.5X1	T50.5X2	T50.5X3	T50.5X4	T50.5X5	T50.5X6
Clotiapine	T43.591	T43.592	T43.593	T43.594	T43.595	T43.596
Clotiazepam	T42.4X1	T42.4X2	T42.4X3	T42.4X4	T42.4X5	T42.4X6
Clotibric acid	T46.6X1	T46.6X2	T46.6X3	T46.6X4	T46.6X5	T46.6X6
Clotrimazole	T49.0X1	T49.0X2	T49.0X3	T49.0X4	T49.0X5	T49.0X6
Cloxacillin	T36.0X1	T36.0X2	T36.0X3	T36.0X4	T36.0X5	T36.0X6
Cloxazolam	T42.4X1	T42.4X2	T42.4X3	T42.4X4	T42.4X5	T42.4X6
Cloxiquine	T49.0X1	T49.0X2	T49.0X3	T49.0X4	T49.0X5	T49.0X6
Clozapine	T42.4X1	T42.4X2	T42.4X3	T42.4X4	T42.4X5	T42.4X6
Coagulant NEC	T45.7X1	T45.7X2	T45.7X3	T45.7X4	T45.7X5	T45.7X6
Coal (carbon monoxide from) — *see also Carbon, monoxide, coal*	T58.2X1	T58.2X2	T58.2X3	T58.2X4	—	—
oil — *see Kerosene*						
tar	T49.1X1	T49.1X2	T49.1X3	T49.1X4	T49.1X5	T49.1X6
fumes	T59.891	T59.892	T59.893	T59.894	—	—
medicinal (ointment)	T49.4X1	T49.4X2	T49.4X3	T49.4X4	T49.4X5	T49.4X6
analgesics NEC	T39.2X1	T39.2X2	T39.2X3	T39.2X4	T39.2X5	T39.2X6
naphtha (solvent)	T52.0X1	T52.0X2	T52.0X3	T52.0X4		
Cobalamine	T45.2X1	T45.2X2	T45.2X3	T45.2X4	T45.2X5	T45.2X6
Cobalt (nonmedicinal) (fumes) (industrial)	T56.891	T56.892	T56.893	T56.894		
medicinal (trace) (chloride)	T45.8X1	T45.8X2	T45.8X3	T45.8X4	T45.8X5	T45.8X6
Cobra (venom)	T63.041	T63.042	T63.043	T63.044		
Coca (leaf)	T40.5X1	T40.5X2	T40.5X3	T40.5X4	T40.5X5	T40.5X6
Cocaine	T40.5X1	T40.5X2	T40.5X3	T40.5X4	T40.5X5	T40.5X6
topical anesthetic	T41.3X1	T41.3X2	T41.3X3	T41.3X4	T41.3X5	T41.3X6
Cocarboxylase	T45.3X1	T45.3X2	T45.3X3	T45.3X4	T45.3X5	T45.3X6
Coccidioidin	T50.8X1	T50.8X2	T50.8X3	T50.8X4	T50.8X5	T50.8X6
Cocculus indicus	T62.1X1	T62.1X2	T62.1X3	T62.1X4		
Cochineal	T65.6X1	T65.6X2	T65.6X3	T65.6X4		
medicinal products	T50.991	T50.992	T50.993	T50.994	T50.995	T50.996
Codeine	T40.2X1	T40.2X2	T40.2X3	T40.2X4	T40.2X5	T40.2X6
Cod-liver oil	T45.2X1	T45.2X2	T45.2X3	T45.2X4	T45.2X5	T45.2X6

Substance	Poisoning, Accidental (Unintentional)	Poisoning, Intentional Self-Harm	Poisoning, Assault	Poisoning, Undetermined	Adverse Effect	Underdosing
	External Cause (T-Code)					
Coenzyme A	T50.991	T50.992	T50.993	T50.994	T50.995	T50.996
Coffee	T62.8X1	T62.8X2	T62.8X3	T62.8X4	—	—
Cogalactoisomerase	T50.991	T50.992	T50.993	T50.994	T50.995	T50.996
Cogentin	T44.3X1	T44.3X2	T44.3X3	T44.3X4	T44.3X5	T44.3X6
Coke fumes or gas (carbon monoxide)	T58.2X1	T58.2X2	T58.2X3	T58.2X4	—	—
industrial use	T58.8X1	T58.8X2	T58.8X3	T58.8X4	—	—
Colace	T47.4X1	T47.4X2	T47.4X3	T47.4X4	T47.4X5	T47.4X6
Colaspase	T45.1X1	T45.1X2	T45.1X3	T45.1X4	T45.1X5	T45.1X6
Colchicine	T50.4X1	T50.4X2	T50.4X3	T50.4X4	T50.4X5	T50.4X6
Colchicum	T62.2X1	T62.2X2	T62.2X3	T62.2X4	—	—
Cold cream	T49.3X1	T49.3X2	T49.3X3	T49.3X4	T49.3X5	T49.3X6
Colecalciferol	T45.2X1	T45.2X2	T45.2X3	T45.2X4	T45.2X5	T45.2X6
Colestipol	T46.6X1	T46.6X2	T46.6X3	T46.6X4	T46.6X5	T46.6X6
Colestyramine	T46.6X1	T46.6X2	T46.6X3	T46.6X4	T46.6X5	T46.6X6
Colimycin	T36.8X1	T36.8X2	T36.8X3	T36.8X4	T36.8X5	T36.8X6
Colistimethate	T36.8X1	T36.8X2	T36.8X3	T36.8X4	T36.8X5	T36.8X6
Colistin	T36.8X1	T36.8X2	T36.8X3	T36.8X4	T36.8X5	T36.8X6
sulfate (eye preparation)	T49.5X1	T49.5X2	T49.5X3	T49.5X4	T49.5X5	T49.5X6
Collagen	T50.991	T50.992	T50.993	T50.994	T50.995	T50.996
Collagenase	T49.4X1	T49.4X2	T49.4X3	T49.4X4	T49.4X5	T49.4X6
Collodion	T49.3X1	T49.3X2	T49.3X3	T49.3X4	T49.3X5	T49.3X6
Colocynth	T47.2X1	T47.2X2	T47.2X3	T47.2X4	T47.2X5	T47.2X6
Colophony adhesive	T49.3X1	T49.3X2	T49.3X3	T49.3X4	T49.3X5	T49.3X6
Colorant — *see also Dye*	T50.991	T50.992	T50.993	T50.994	T50.995	T50.996
Coloring matter — *see Dye(s)*						
Combustion gas (after combustion) — *see Carbon, monoxide*						
prior to combustion	T59.891	T59.892	T59.893	T59.894	—	—
Compazine	T43.3X1	T43.3X2	T43.3X3	T43.3X4	T43.3X5	T43.3X6
Compound						
42 (warfarin)	T60.4X1	T60.4X2	T60.4X3	T60.4X4	—	—
269 (endrin)	T60.1X1	T60.1X2	T60.1X3	T60.1X4	—	—
497 (dieldrin)	T60.1X1	T60.1X2	T60.1X3	T60.1X4	—	—
1080 (sodium fluoroacetate)	T60.4X1	T60.4X2	T60.4X3	T60.4X4	—	—
3422 (parathion)	T60.0X1	T60.0X2	T60.0X3	T60.0X4	—	—
3911 (phorate)	T60.0X1	T60.0X2	T60.0X3	T60.0X4	—	—
3956 (toxaphene)	T60.1X1	T60.1X2	T60.1X3	T60.1X4	—	—
4049 (malathion)	T60.0X1	T60.0X2	T60.0X3	T60.0X4	—	—
4069 (malathion)	T60.0X1	T60.0X2	T60.0X3	T60.0X4	—	—
4124 (dicapthon)	T60.0X1	T60.0X2	T60.0X3	T60.0X4	—	—

◀ New ◀ Revised ~~deleted~~ Deleted

Substance	External Cause (T-Code)					
	Poisoning, Accidental (Unintentional)	Poisoning, Intentional Self-Harm	Poisoning, Assault	Poisoning, Undetermined	Adverse Effect	Underdosing
Compound *(Continued)*						
E (cortisone)	T38.0X1	T38.0X2	T38.0X3	T38.0X4	T38.0X5	T38.0X6
F (hydrocortisone)	T38.0X1	T38.0X2	T38.0X3	T38.0X4	T38.0X5	T38.0X6
Congener, anabolic	T38.7X1	T38.7X2	T38.7X3	T38.7X4	T38.7X5	T38.7X6
Congo red	T50.8X1	T50.8X2	T50.8X3	T50.8X4	T50.8X5	T50.8X6
Coniine, conine	T62.2X1	T62.2X2	T62.2X3	T62.2X4	—	—
Conium (maculatum)	T62.2X1	T62.2X2	T62.2X3	T62.2X4	—	—
Conjugated estrogenic substances	T38.5X1	T38.5X2	T38.5X3	T38.5X4	T38.5X5	T38.5X6
Contac	T48.5X1	T48.5X2	T48.5X3	T48.5X4	T48.5X5	T48.5X6
Contact lens solution	T49.5X1	T49.5X2	T49.5X3	T49.5X4	T49.5X5	T49.5X6
Contraceptive (oral)	T38.4X1	T38.4X2	T38.4X3	T38.4X4	T38.4X5	T38.4X6
vaginal	T49.8X1	T49.8X2	T49.8X3	T49.8X4	T49.8X5	T49.8X6
Contrast medium, radiography	T50.8X1	T50.8X2	T50.8X3	T50.8X4	T50.8X5	T50.8X6
Convallaria glycosides	T46.0X1	T46.0X2	T46.0X3	T46.0X4	T46.0X5	T46.0X6
Convallaria majalis	T62.2X1	T62.2X2	T62.2X3	T62.2X4	—	—
berry	T62.1X1	T62.1X2	T62.1X3	T62.1X4	—	—
Copper (dust) (fumes) (nonmedicinal) NEC	T56.4X1	T56.4X2	T56.4X3	T56.4X4	—	—
arsenate, arsenite	T57.0X1	T57.0X2	T57.0X3	T57.0X4	—	—
insecticide	T60.2X1	T60.2X2	T60.2X3	T60.2X4	—	—
emetic	T47.7X1	T47.7X2	T47.7X3	T47.7X4	T47.7X5	T47.7X6
fungicide	T60.3X1	T60.3X2	T60.3X3	T60.3X4	—	—
gluconate	T49.0X1	T49.0X2	T49.0X3	T49.0X4	T49.0X5	T49.0X6
insecticide	T60.2X1	T60.2X2	T60.2X3	T60.2X4	—	—
medicinal (trace)	T45.8X1	T45.8X2	T45.8X3	T45.8X4	T45.8X5	T45.8X6
oleate	T49.0X1	T49.0X2	T49.0X3	T49.0X4	T49.0X5	T49.0X6
sulfate	T56.4X1	T56.4X2	T56.4X3	T56.4X4	—	—
cupric	T56.4X1	T56.4X2	T56.4X3	T56.4X4	—	—
fungicide	T60.3X1	T60.3X2	T60.3X3	T60.3X4	—	—
medicinal						
ear	T49.6X1	T49.6X2	T49.6X3	T49.6X4	T49.6X5	T49.6X6
emetic	T47.7X1	T47.7X2	T47.7X3	T47.7X4	T47.7X5	T47.7X6
eye	T49.5X1	T49.5X2	T49.5X3	T49.5X4	T49.5X5	T49.5X6
cuprous	T56.4X1	T56.4X2	T56.4X3	T56.4X4	—	—
fungicide	T60.3X1	T60.3X2	T60.3X3	T60.3X4	—	—
medicinal						
ear	T49.6X1	T49.6X2	T49.6X3	T49.6X4	T49.6X5	T49.6X6
emetic	T47.7X1	T47.7X2	T47.7X3	T47.7X4	T47.7X5	T47.7X6
eye	T49.5X1	T49.5X2	T49.5X3	T49.5X4	T49.5X5	T49.5X6
Copperhead snake (bite) (venom)	T63.061	T63.062	T63.063	T63.064	—	—
Coral (sting)	T63.691	T63.692	T63.693	T63.694	—	—
snake (bite) (venom)	T63.021	T63.022	T63.023	T63.024	—	—

Substance	External Cause (T-Code)					
	Poisoning, Accidental (Unintentional)	Poisoning, Intentional Self-Harm	Poisoning, Assault	Poisoning, Undetermined	Adverse Effect	Underdosing
Corbadrine	T49.6X1	T49.6X2	T49.6X3	T49.6X4	T49.6X5	T49.6X6
Cordran	T49.0X1	T49.0X2	T49.0X3	T49.0X4	T49.0X5	T49.0X6
Cordite	T65.891	T65.892	T65.893	T65.894	—	—
vapor	T59.891	T59.892	T59.893	T59.894	—	—
Corn cures	T49.4X1	T49.4X2	T49.4X3	T49.4X4	T49.4X5	T49.4X6
Cornhusker's lotion	T49.3X1	T49.3X2	T49.3X3	T49.3X4	T49.3X5	T49.3X6
Corn starch	T49.3X1	T49.3X2	T49.3X3	T49.3X4	T49.3X5	T49.3X6
Coronary vasodilator NEC	T46.3X1	T46.3X2	T46.3X3	T46.3X4	T46.3X5	T46.3X6
Corrosive NEC	T54.91	T54.92	T54.93	T54.94	—	—
acid NEC	T54.2X1	T54.2X2	T54.2X3	T54.2X4	—	—
aromatics	T54.1X1	T54.1X2	T54.1X3	T54.1X4	—	—
disinfectant	T54.1X1	T54.1X2	T54.1X3	T54.1X4	—	—
fumes NEC	T54.91	T54.92	T54.93	T54.94	—	—
specified NEC	T54.91	T54.92	T54.93	T54.94	—	—
sublimate	T56.1X1	T56.1X2	T56.1X3	T56.1X4	—	—
Cortate	T38.0X1	T38.0X2	T38.0X3	T38.0X4	T38.0X5	T38.0X6
Cort-Dome	T38.0X1	T38.0X2	T38.0X3	T38.0X4	T38.0X5	T38.0X6
ENT agent	T49.6X1	T49.6X2	T49.6X3	T49.6X4	T49.6X5	T49.6X6
ophthalmic preparation	T49.5X1	T49.5X2	T49.5X3	T49.5X4	T49.5X5	T49.5X6
topical NEC	T49.0X1	T49.0X2	T49.0X3	T49.0X4	T49.0X5	T49.0X6
Cortef	T38.0X1	T38.0X2	T38.0X3	T38.0X4	T38.0X5	T38.0X6
ENT agent	T49.6X1	T49.6X2	T49.6X3	T49.6X4	T49.6X5	T49.6X6
ophthalmic preparation	T49.5X1	T49.5X2	T49.5X3	T49.5X4	T49.5X5	T49.5X6
topical NEC	T49.0X1	T49.0X2	T49.0X3	T49.0X4	T49.0X5	T49.0X6
Corticosteroid	T38.0X1	T38.0X2	T38.0X3	T38.0X4	T38.0X5	T38.0X6
ENT agent	T49.6X1	T49.6X2	T49.6X3	T49.6X4	T49.6X5	T49.6X6
mineral	T50.0X1	T50.0X2	T50.0X3	T50.0X4	T50.0X5	T50.0X6
ophthalmic	T49.5X1	T49.5X2	T49.5X3	T49.5X4	T49.5X5	T49.5X6
topical NEC	T49.0X1	T49.0X2	T49.0X3	T49.0X4	T49.0X5	T49.0X6
Corticotropin	T38.811	T38.812	T38.813	T38.814	T38.815	T38.816
Cortisol	T49.0X1	T49.0X2	T49.0X3	T49.0X4	T49.0X5	T49.0X6
ENT agent	T49.6X1	T49.6X2	T49.6X3	T49.6X4	T49.6X5	T49.6X6
ophthalmic preparation	T49.5X1	T49.5X2	T49.5X3	T49.5X4	T49.5X5	T49.5X6
topical NEC	T49.0X1	T49.0X2	T49.0X3	T49.0X4	T49.0X5	T49.0X6
Cortisone (acetate)	T38.0X1	T38.0X2	T38.0X3	T38.0X4	T38.0X5	T38.0X6
ENT agent	T49.6X1	T49.6X2	T49.6X3	T49.6X4	T49.6X5	T49.6X6
ophthalmic preparation	T49.5X1	T49.5X2	T49.5X3	T49.5X4	T49.5X5	T49.5X6
topical NEC	T49.0X1	T49.0X2	T49.0X3	T49.0X4	T49.0X5	T49.0X6
Cortivazol	T38.0X1	T38.0X2	T38.0X3	T38.0X4	T38.0X5	T38.0X6
Cortogen	T38.0X1	T38.0X2	T38.0X3	T38.0X4	T38.0X5	T38.0X6
ENT agent	T49.6X1	T49.6X2	T49.6X3	T49.6X4	T49.6X5	T49.6X6
ophthalmic preparation	T49.5X1	T49.5X2	T49.5X3	T49.5X4	T49.5X5	T49.5X6

◀ New ◀ Revised ~~deleted~~ Deleted

Substance	External Cause (T-Code)					
	Poisoning, Accidental (Unintentional)	Poisoning, Intentional Self-Harm	Poisoning, Assault	Poisoning, Undetermined	Adverse Effect	Underdosing
Cortone	T38.0X1	T38.0X2	T38.0X3	T38.0X4	T38.0X5	T38.0X6
ENT agent	T49.6X1	T49.6X2	T49.6X3	T49.6X4	T49.6X5	T49.6X6
ophthalmic preparation	T49.5X1	T49.5X2	T49.5X3	T49.5X4	T49.5X5	T49.5X6
Cortril	T38.0X1	T38.0X2	T38.0X3	T38.0X4	T38.0X5	T38.0X6
ENT agent	T49.6X1	T49.6X2	T49.6X3	T49.6X4	T49.6X5	T49.6X6
ophthalmic preparation	T49.5X1	T49.5X2	T49.5X3	T49.5X4	T49.5X5	T49.5X6
topical NEC	T49.0X1	T49.0X2	T49.0X3	T49.0X4	T49.0X5	T49.0X6
Corynebacterium parvum	T45.1X1	T45.1X2	T45.1X3	T45.1X4	T45.1X5	T45.1X6
Cosmetic preparation	T49.8X1	T49.8X2	T49.8X3	T49.8X4	T49.8X5	T49.8X6
Cosmetics	T49.8X1	T49.8X2	T49.8X3	T49.8X4	T49.8X5	T49.8X6
Cosyntropin	T38.811	T38.812	T38.813	T38.814	T38.815	T38.816
Cotarnine	T45.7X1	T45.7X2	T45.7X3	T45.7X4	T45.7X5	T45.7X6
Co-trimoxazole	T36.8X1	T36.8X2	T36.8X3	T36.8X4	T36.8X5	T36.8X6
Cottonseed oil	T49.3X1	T49.3X2	T49.3X3	T49.3X4	T49.3X5	T49.3X6
Cough mixture (syrup)	T48.4X1	T48.4X2	T48.4X3	T48.4X4	T48.4X5	T48.4X6
containing opiates	T40.2X1	T40.2X2	T40.2X3	T40.2X4	T40.2X5	T40.2X6
expectorants	T48.4X1	T48.4X2	T48.4X3	T48.4X4	T48.4X5	T48.4X6
Coumadin	T45.511	T45.512	T45.513	T45.514	T45.515	T45.516
rodenticide	T60.4X1	T60.4X2	T60.4X3	T60.4X4	—	—
Coumaphos	T60.0X1	T60.0X2	T60.0X3	T60.0X4	—	—
Coumarin	T45.511	T45.512	T45.513	T45.514	T45.515	T45.516
Coumetarol	T45.511	T45.512	T45.513	T45.514	T45.515	T45.516
Cowbane	T62.2X1	T62.2X2	T62.2X3	T62.2X4	—	—
Cozyme	T45.2X1	T45.2X2	T45.2X3	T45.2X4	T45.2X5	T45.2X6
Crack	T40.5X1	T40.5X2	T40.5X3	T40.5X4	—	—
Crataegus extract	T46.0X1	T46.0X2	T46.0X3	T46.0X4	T46.0X5	T46.0X6
Creolin	T54.1X1	T54.1X2	T54.1X3	T54.1X4	—	—
disinfectant	T54.1X1	T54.1X2	T54.1X3	T54.1X4	—	—
Creosol (compound)	T49.0X1	T49.0X2	T49.0X3	T49.0X4	T49.0X5	T49.0X6
Creosote (coal tar) (beechwood)	T49.0X1	T49.0X2	T49.0X3	T49.0X4	T49.0X5	T49.0X6
medicinal (expectorant)	T48.4X1	T48.4X2	T48.4X3	T48.4X4	T48.4X5	T48.4X6
syrup	T48.4X1	T48.4X2	T48.4X3	T48.4X4	T48.4X5	T48.4X6
Cresol(s)	T49.0X1	T49.0X2	T49.0X3	T49.0X4	T49.0X5	T49.0X6
and soap solution	T49.0X1	T49.0X2	T49.0X3	T49.0X4	T49.0X5	T49.0X6
Cresyl acetate	T49.0X1	T49.0X2	T49.0X3	T49.0X4	T49.0X5	T49.0X6
Cresylic acid	T49.0X1	T49.0X2	T49.0X3	T49.0X4	T49.0X5	T49.0X6
Crimidine	T60.4X1	T60.4X2	T60.4X3	T60.4X4	—	—
Croconazole	T37.8X1	T37.8X2	T37.8X3	T37.8X4	T37.8X5	T37.8X6
Cromoglicic acid	T48.6X1	T48.6X2	T48.6X3	T48.6X4	T48.6X5	T48.6X6
Cromolyn	T48.6X1	T48.6X2	T48.6X3	T48.6X4	T48.6X5	T48.6X6
Cromonar	T46.3X1	T46.3X2	T46.3X3	T46.3X4	T46.3X5	T46.3X6

Substance	External Cause (T-Code)					
	Poisoning, Accidental (Unintentional)	Poisoning, Intentional Self-Harm	Poisoning, Assault	Poisoning, Undetermined	Adverse Effect	Underdosing
Cropropamide	T39.8X1	T39.8X2	T39.8X3	T39.8X4	T39.8X5	T39.8X6
with crotethamide	T50.7X1	T50.7X2	T50.7X3	T50.7X4	T50.7X5	T50.7X6
Crotamiton	T49.0X1	T49.0X2	T49.0X3	T49.0X4	T49.0X5	T49.0X6
Crotethamide	T39.8X1	T39.8X2	T39.8X3	T39.8X4	T39.8X5	T39.8X6
with cropropamide	T50.7X1	T50.7X2	T50.7X3	T50.7X4	T50.7X5	T50.7X6
Croton (oil)	T47.2X1	T47.2X2	T47.2X3	T47.2X4	T47.2X5	T47.2X6
chloral	T42.6X1	T42.6X2	T42.6X3	T42.6X4	T42.6X5	T42.6X6
Crude oil	T52.0X1	T52.0X2	T52.0X3	T52.0X4	—	—
Cryogenine	T39.8X1	T39.8X2	T39.8X3	T39.8X4	T39.8X5	T39.8X6
Cryolite (vapor)	T60.1X1	T60.1X2	T60.1X3	T60.1X4	—	—
insecticide	T60.1X1	T60.1X2	T60.1X3	T60.1X4	—	—
Cryptenamine (tannates)	T46.5X1	T46.5X2	T46.5X3	T46.5X4	T46.5X5	T46.5X6
Crystal violet	T49.0X1	T49.0X2	T49.0X3	T49.0X4	T49.0X5	T49.0X6
Cuckoopint	T62.2X1	T62.2X2	T62.2X3	T62.2X4	—	—
Cumetharol	T45.511	T45.512	T45.513	T45.514	T45.515	T45.516
Cupric						
acetate	T60.3X1	T60.3X2	T60.3X3	T60.3X4	—	—
acetoarsenite	T57.0X1	T57.0X2	T57.0X3	T57.0X4	—	—
arsenate	T57.0X1	T57.0X2	T57.0X3	T57.0X4	—	—
gluconate	T49.0X1	T49.0X2	T49.0X3	T49.0X4	T49.0X5	T49.0X6
oleate	T49.0X1	T49.0X2	T49.0X3	T49.0X4	T49.0X5	T49.0X6
sulfate	T56.4X1	T56.4X2	T56.4X3	T56.4X4	—	—
Cuprous sulfate — *see also Copper sulfate*	T56.4X1	T56.4X2	T56.4X3	T56.4X4	—	—
Curare, curarine	T48.1X1	T48.1X2	T48.1X3	T48.1X4	T48.1X5	T48.1X6
Cyamemazine	T43.3X1	T43.3X2	T43.3X3	T43.3X4	T43.3X5	T43.3X6
Cyamopsis tetragono-loba	T46.6X1	T46.6X2	T46.6X3	T46.6X4	T46.6X5	T46.6X6
Cyanacetyl hydrazide	T37.1X1	T37.1X2	T37.1X3	T37.1X4	T37.1X5	T37.1X6
Cyanic acid (gas)	T59.891	T59.892	T59.893	T59.894	—	—
Cyanide(s) (compounds) (potassium) (sodium) NEC	T65.0X1	T65.0X2	T65.0X3	T65.0X4	—	—
dust or gas (inhalation) NEC	T57.3X1	T57.3X2	T57.3X3	T57.3X4	—	—
fumigant	T65.0X1	T65.0X2	T65.0X3	T65.0X4	—	—
hydrogen	T57.3X1	T57.3X2	T57.3X3	T57.3X4	—	—
mercuric — *see Mercury*						
pesticide (dust) (fumes)	T65.0X1	T65.0X2	T65.0X3	T65.0X4	—	—
Cyanoacrylate adhesive	T49.3X1	T49.3X2	T49.3X3	T49.3X4	T49.3X5	T49.3X6
Cyanocobalamin	T45.8X1	T45.8X2	T45.8X3	T45.8X4	T45.8X5	T45.8X6
Cyanogen (chloride) (gas) NEC	T59.891	T59.892	T59.893	T59.894	—	—
Cyclacillin	T36.0X1	T36.0X2	T36.0X3	T36.0X4	T36.0X5	T36.0X6
Cyclaine	T41.3X1	T41.3X2	T41.3X3	T41.3X4	T41.3X5	T41.3X6
Cyclamate	T50.991	T50.992	T50.993	T50.994	T50.995	T50.996

◀ New ◀ Revised ~~deleted~~ Deleted

Substance	External Cause (T-Code)					
	Poisoning, Accidental (Unintentional)	Poisoning, Intentional Self-Harm	Poisoning, Assault	Poisoning, Undetermined	Adverse Effect	Underdosing
Cyclamen europaeum	T62.2X1	T62.2X2	T62.2X3	T62.2X4	—	—
Cyclandelate	T46.7X1	T46.7X2	T46.7X3	T46.7X4	T46.7X5	T46.7X6
Cyclazocine	T50.7X1	T50.7X2	T50.7X3	T50.7X4	T50.7X5	T50.7X6
Cyclizine	T45.0X1	T45.0X2	T45.0X3	T45.0X4	T45.0X5	T45.0X6
Cyclobarbital	T42.3X1	T42.3X2	T42.3X3	T42.3X4	T42.3X5	T42.3X6
Cyclobarbitone	T42.3X1	T42.3X2	T42.3X3	T42.3X4	T42.3X5	T42.3X6
Cyclobenzaprine	T48.1X1	T48.1X2	T48.1X3	T48.1X4	T48.1X5	T48.1X6
Cyclodrine	T44.3X1	T44.3X2	T44.3X3	T44.3X4	T44.3X5	T44.3X6
Cycloguanil embonate	T37.2X1	T37.2X2	T37.2X3	T37.2X4	T37.2X5	T37.2X6
Cycloheptadiene	T43.291	T43.292	T43.293	T43.294	T43.295	T43.296
Cyclohexane	T52.8X1	T52.8X2	T52.8X3	T52.8X4	—	—
Cyclohexanol	T51.8X1	T51.8X2	T51.8X3	T51.8X4	—	—
Cyclohexanone	T52.4X1	T52.4X2	T52.4X3	T52.4X4	—	—
Cycloheximide	T60.3X1	T60.3X2	T60.3X3	T60.3X4	—	—
Cyclohexyl acetate	T52.8X1	T52.8X2	T52.8X3	T52.8X4	—	—
Cycloleucin	T45.1X1	T45.1X2	T45.1X3	T45.1X4	T45.1X5	T45.1X6
Cyclomethycaine	T41.3X1	T41.3X2	T41.3X3	T41.3X4	T41.3X5	T41.3X6
Cyclopentamine	T44.4X1	T44.4X2	T44.4X3	T44.4X4	T44.4X5	T44.4X6
Cyclopenthiazide	T50.2X1	T50.2X2	T50.2X3	T50.2X4	T50.2X5	T50.2X6
Cyclopentolate	T44.3X1	T44.3X2	T44.3X3	T44.3X4	T44.3X5	T44.3X6
Cyclophosphamide	T45.1X1	T45.1X2	T45.1X3	T45.1X4	T45.1X5	T45.1X6
Cycloplegic drug	T49.5X1	T49.5X2	T49.5X3	T49.5X4	T49.5X5	T49.5X6
Cyclopropane	T41.291	T41.292	T41.293	T41.294	T41.295	T41.296
Cyclopyrabital	T39.8X1	T39.8X2	T39.8X3	T39.8X4	T39.8X5	T39.8X6
Cycloserine	T37.1X1	T37.1X2	T37.1X3	T37.1X4	T37.1X5	T37.1X6
Cyclosporin	T45.1X1	T45.1X2	T45.1X3	T45.1X4	T45.1X5	T45.1X6
Cyclothiazide	T50.2X1	T50.2X2	T50.2X3	T50.2X4	T50.2X5	T50.2X6
Cycrimine	T44.3X1	T44.3X2	T44.3X3	T44.3X4	T44.3X5	T44.3X6
Cyhalothrin	T60.1X1	T60.1X2	T60.1X3	T60.1X4	—	—
Cymarin	T46.0X1	T46.0X2	T46.0X3	T46.0X4	T46.0X5	T46.0X6
Cypermethrin	T60.1X1	T60.1X2	T60.1X3	T60.1X4	—	—
Cyphenothrin	T60.2X1	T60.2X2	T60.2X3	T60.2X4	—	—
Cyproheptadine	T45.0X1	T45.0X2	T45.0X3	T45.0X4	T45.0X5	T45.0X6
Cyprolidol	T43.291	T43.292	T43.293	T43.294	T43.295	T43.296
Cyproterone	T38.6X1	T38.6X2	T38.6X3	T38.6X4	T38.6X5	T38.6X6
Cysteamine	T50.6X1	T50.6X2	T50.6X3	T50.6X4	T50.6X5	T50.6X6
Cytarabine	T45.1X1	T45.1X2	T45.1X3	T45.1X4	T45.1X5	T45.1X6
Cytisus						
laburnum	T62.2X1	T62.2X2	T62.2X3	T62.2X4	—	—
scoparius	T62.2X1	T62.2X2	T62.2X3	T62.2X4	—	—
Cytochrome C	T47.5X1	T47.5X2	T47.5X3	T47.5X4	T47.5X5	T47.5X6
Cytomel	T38.1X1	T38.1X2	T38.1X3	T38.1X4	T38.1X5	T38.1X6

Substance	External Cause (T-Code)					
	Poisoning, Accidental (Unintentional)	Poisoning, Intentional Self-Harm	Poisoning, Assault	Poisoning, Undetermined	Adverse Effect	Underdosing
Cytosine arabinoside	T45.1X1	T45.1X2	T45.1X3	T45.1X4	T45.1X5	T45.1X6
Cytoxan	T45.1X1	T45.1X2	T45.1X3	T45.1X4	T45.1X5	T45.1X6
Cytozyme	T45.7X1	T45.7X2	T45.7X3	T45.7X4	T45.7X5	T45.7X6
2,4-D	T60.3X1	T60.3X2	T60.3X3	T60.3X4	—	—
D						
Dacarbazine	T45.1X1	T45.1X2	T45.1X3	T45.1X4	T45.1X5	T45.1X6
Dactinomycin	T45.1X1	T45.1X2	T45.1X3	T45.1X4	T45.1X5	T45.1X6
DADPS	T37.1X1	T37.1X2	T37.1X3	T37.1X4	T37.1X5	T37.1X6
Dakin's solution	T49.0X1	T49.0X2	T49.0X3	T49.0X4	T49.0X5	T49.0X6
Dalapon (sodium)	T60.3X1	T60.3X2	T60.3X3	T60.3X4	—	—
Dalmane	T42.4X1	T42.4X2	T42.4X3	T42.4X4	T42.4X5	T42.4X6
Danazol	T38.6X1	T38.6X2	T38.6X3	T38.6X4	T38.6X5	T38.6X6
Danilone	T45.511	T45.512	T45.513	T45.514	T45.515	T45.516
Danthron	T47.2X1	T47.2X2	T47.2X3	T47.2X4	T47.2X5	T47.2X6
Dantrolene	T42.8X1	T42.8X2	T42.8X3	T42.8X4	T42.8X5	T42.8X6
Dantron	T47.2X1	T47.2X2	T47.2X3	T47.2X4	T47.2X5	T47.2X6
Daphne (gnidium) (mezereum)	T62.2X1	T62.2X2	T62.2X3	T62.2X4	—	—
berry	T62.1X1	T62.1X2	T62.1X3	T62.1X4	—	—
Dapsone	T37.1X1	T37.1X2	T37.1X3	T37.1X4	T37.1X5	T37.1X6
Daraprim	T37.2X1	T37.2X2	T37.2X3	T37.2X4	T37.2X5	T37.2X6
Darnel	T62.2X1	T62.2X2	T62.2X3	T62.2X4	—	—
Darvon	T39.8X1	T39.8X2	T39.8X3	T39.8X4	T39.8X5	T39.8X6
Daunomycin	T45.1X1	T45.1X2	T45.1X3	T45.1X4	T45.1X5	T45.1X6
Daunorubicin	T45.1X1	T45.1X2	T45.1X3	T45.1X4	T45.1X5	T45.1X6
DBI	T38.3X1	T38.3X2	T38.3X3	T38.3X4	T38.3X5	T38.3X6
D-Con	T60.91	T60.92	T60.93	T60.94	—	—
insecticide	T60.2X1	T60.2X2	T60.2X3	T60.2X4	—	—
rodenticide	T60.4X1	T60.4X2	T60.4X3	T60.4X4	—	—
DDAVP	T38.891	T38.892	T38.893	T38.894	T38.895	T38.896
DDE (bis(chlorophenyl)-dichloroethylene)	T60.2X1	T60.2X2	T60.2X3	T60.2X4	—	—
DDS	T37.1X1	T37.1X2	T37.1X3	T37.1X4	T37.1X5	T37.1X6
DDT (dust)	T60.1X1	T60.1X2	T60.1X3	T60.1X4	—	—
Deadly nightshade — *see also Belladonna*	T62.2X1	T62.2X2	T62.2X3	T62.2X4	—	—
berry	T62.1X1	T62.1X2	T62.1X3	T62.1X4	—	—
Deamino-D-arginine vasopressin	T38.891	T38.892	T38.893	T38.894	T38.895	T38.896
Deanol (aceglumate)	T50.991	T50.992	T50.993	T50.994	T50.995	T50.996
Debrisoquine	T46.5X1	T46.5X2	T46.5X3	T46.5X4	T46.5X5	T46.5X6
Decaborane	T57.8X1	T57.8X2	T57.8X3	T57.8X4	—	—
fumes	T59.891	T59.892	T59.893	T59.894	—	—

Substance	External Cause (T-Code)					
	Poisoning, Accidental (Unintentional)	Poisoning, Intentional Self-Harm	Poisoning, Assault	Poisoning, Undetermined	Adverse Effect	Underdosing
Decadron	T38.0X1	T38.0X2	T38.0X3	T38.0X4	T38.0X5	T38.0X6
ENT agent	T49.6X1	T49.6X2	T49.6X3	T49.6X4	T49.6X5	T49.6X6
ophthalmic preparation	T49.5X1	T49.5X2	T49.5X3	T49.5X4	T49.5X5	T49.5X6
topical NEC	T49.0X1	T49.0X2	T49.0X3	T49.0X4	T49.0X5	T49.0X6
Decahydronaphthalene	T52.8X1	T52.8X2	T52.8X3	T52.8X4	—	—
Decalin	T52.8X1	T52.8X2	T52.8X3	T52.8X4	—	—
Decamethonium (bromide)	T48.1X1	T48.1X2	T48.1X3	T48.1X4	T48.1X5	T48.1X6
Decholin	T47.5X1	T47.5X2	T47.5X3	T47.5X4	T47.5X5	T47.5X6
Declomycin	T36.4X1	T36.4X2	T36.4X3	T36.4X4	T36.4X5	T36.4X6
Decongestant, nasal (mucosa)	T48.5X1	T48.5X2	T48.5X3	T48.5X4	T48.5X5	T48.5X6
combination	T48.5X1	T48.5X2	T48.5X3	T48.5X4	T48.5X5	T48.5X6
Deet	T60.8X1	T60.8X2	T60.8X3	T60.8X4	—	—
Deferoxamine	T45.8X1	T45.8X2	T45.8X3	T45.8X4	T45.8X5	T45.8X6
Deflazacort	T38.0X1	T38.0X2	T38.0X3	T38.0X4	T38.0X5	T38.0X6
Deglycyrrhizinized extract of licorice	T48.4X1	T48.4X2	T48.4X3	T48.4X4	T48.4X5	T48.4X6
Dehydrocholic acid	T47.5X1	T47.5X2	T47.5X3	T47.5X4	T47.5X5	T47.5X6
Dehydroemetine	T37.3X1	T37.3X2	T37.3X3	T37.3X4	T37.3X5	T37.3X6
Dekalin	T52.8X1	T52.8X2	T52.8X3	T52.8X4	—	—
Delalutin	T38.5X1	T38.5X2	T38.5X3	T38.5X4	T38.5X5	T38.5X6
Delphinium	T62.2X1	T62.2X2	T62.2X3	T62.2X4	—	—
Deltasone	T38.0X1	T38.0X2	T38.0X3	T38.0X4	T38.0X5	T38.0X6
Deltra	T38.0X1	T38.0X2	T38.0X3	T38.0X4	T38.0X5	T38.0X6
Delvinal	T42.3X1	T42.3X2	T42.3X3	T42.3X4	T42.3X5	T42.3X6
Delorazepam	T42.4X1	T42.4X2	T42.4X3	T42.4X4	T42.4X5	T42.4X6
Deltamethrin	T60.1X1	T60.1X2	T60.1X3	T60.1X4	—	—
Demecarium (bromide)	T49.5X1	T49.5X2	T49.5X3	T49.5X4	T49.5X5	T49.5X6
Demeclocycline	T36.4X1	T36.4X2	T36.4X3	T36.4X4	T36.4X5	T36.4X6
Demecolcine	T45.1X1	T45.1X2	T45.1X3	T45.1X4	T45.1X5	T45.1X6
Demegestone	T38.5X1	T38.5X2	T38.5X3	T38.5X4	T38.5X5	T38.5X6
Demelanizing agents	T49.8X1	T49.8X2	T49.8X3	T49.8X4	T49.8X5	T49.8X6
Demephion -O and -S	T60.0X1	T60.0X2	T60.0X3	T60.0X4	—	—
Demerol	T40.2X1	T40.2X2	T40.2X3	T40.2X4	T40.2X5	T40.2X6
Demethylchlortetracycline	T36.4X1	T36.4X2	T36.4X3	T36.4X4	T36.4X5	T36.4X6
Demethyltetracycline	T36.4X1	T36.4X2	T36.4X3	T36.4X4	T36.4X5	T36.4X6
Demeton -O and -S	T60.0X1	T60.0X2	T60.0X3	T60.0X4	—	—
Demulcent (external)	T49.3X1	T49.3X2	T49.3X3	T49.3X4	T49.3X5	T49.3X6
specified NEC	T49.3X1	T49.3X2	T49.3X3	T49.3X4	T49.3X5	T49.3X6
Demulen	T38.4X1	T38.4X2	T38.4X3	T38.4X4	T38.4X5	T38.4X6
Denatured alcohol	T51.0X1	T51.0X2	T51.0X3	T51.0X4	—	—
Dendrid	T49.5X1	T49.5X2	T49.5X3	T49.5X4	T49.5X5	T49.5X6
Dental drug, topical application NEC	T49.7X1	T49.7X2	T49.7X3	T49.7X4	T49.7X5	T49.7X6

Substance	External Cause (T-Code)					
	Poisoning, Accidental (Unintentional)	Poisoning, Intentional Self-Harm	Poisoning, Assault	Poisoning, Undetermined	Adverse Effect	Underdosing
Dentifrice	T49.7X1	T49.7X2	T49.7X3	T49.7X4	T49.7X5	T49.7X6
Deodorant spray (feminine hygiene)	T49.8X1	T49.8X2	T49.8X3	T49.8X4	T49.8X5	T49.8X6
Deoxycortone	T50.0X1	T50.0X2	T50.0X3	T50.0X4	T50.0X5	T50.0X6
2-Deoxy-5-fluorouridine	T45.1X1	T45.1X2	T45.1X3	T45.1X4	T45.1X5	T45.1X6
5-Deoxy-5-fluorouridine	T45.1X1	T45.1X2	T45.1X3	T45.1X4	T45.1X5	T45.1X6
Deoxyribonuclease (pancreatic)	T45.3X1	T45.3X2	T45.3X3	T45.3X4	T45.3X5	T45.3X6
Depilatory	T49.4X1	T49.4X2	T49.4X3	T49.4X4	T49.4X5	T49.4X6
Deprenalin	T42.8X1	T42.8X2	T42.8X3	T42.8X4	T42.8X5	T42.8X6
Deprenyl	T42.8X1	T42.8X2	T42.8X3	T42.8X4	T42.8X5	T42.8X6
Depressant, appetite	T50.5X1	T50.5X2	T50.5X3	T50.5X4	T50.5X5	T50.5X6
Depressant						
appetite, central	T50.5X1	T50.5X2	T50.5X3	T50.5X4	T50.5X5	T50.5X6
cardiac	T46.2X1	T46.2X2	T46.2X3	T46.2X4	T46.2X5	T46.2X6
central nervous system (anesthetic) — *see also Central nervous system, depressants*	T42.71	T42.72	T42.73	T42.74	T42.75	T42.76
general anesthetic	T41.201	T41.202	T41.203	T41.204	T41.205	T41.206
muscle tone	T42.8X1	T42.8X2	T42.8X3	T42.8X4	T42.8X5	T42.8X6
muscle tone, central	T42.8X1	T42.8X2	T42.8X3	T42.8X4	T42.8X5	T42.8X6
psychotherapeutic	T43.501	T43.502	T43.503	T43.504	T43.505	T43.506
Deptropine	T45.0X1	T45.0X2	T45.0X3	T45.0X4	T45.0X5	T45.0X6
Dequalinium (chloride)	T49.0X1	T49.0X2	T49.0X3	T49.0X4	T49.0X5	T49.0X6
Derris root	T60.2X1	T60.2X2	T60.2X3	T60.2X4	—	—
Deserpidine	T43.011	T43.012	T43.013	T43.014	T43.015	T43.016
Desferrioxamine	T45.8X1	T45.8X2	T45.8X3	T45.8X4	T45.8X5	T45.8X6
Desipramine	T43.0X1	T43.0X2	T43.0X3	T43.0X4	T43.0X5	T43.0X6
Deslanoside	T46.0X1	T46.0X2	T46.0X3	T46.0X4	T46.0X5	T46.0X6
Desloughing agent	T49.4X1	T49.4X2	T49.4X3	T49.4X4	T49.4X5	T49.4X6
Desmethylimipramine	T43.011	T43.012	T43.013	T43.014	T43.015	T43.016
Desmopressin	T38.891	T38.892	T38.893	T38.894	T38.895	T38.896
Desocodeine	T40.2X1	T40.2X2	T40.2X3	T40.2X4	T40.2X5	T40.2X6
Desogestrel	T38.5X1	T38.5X2	T38.5X3	T38.5X4	T38.5X5	T38.5X6
Desomorphine	T40.2X1	T40.2X2	T40.2X3	T40.2X4	—	—
Desonide	T49.0X1	T49.0X2	T49.0X3	T49.0X4	T49.0X5	T49.0X6
Desoximetasone	T49.0X1	T49.0X2	T49.0X3	T49.0X4	T49.0X5	T49.0X6
Desoxycorticosteroid	T50.0X1	T50.0X2	T50.0X3	T50.0X4	T50.0X5	T50.0X6
Desoxycortone	T50.0X1	T50.0X2	T50.0X3	T50.0X4	T50.0X5	T50.0X6
Desoxyephedrine	T43.621	T43.622	T43.623	T43.624	T43.625	T43.626
Detaxtran	T46.6X1	T46.6X2	T46.6X3	T46.6X4	T46.6X5	T46.6X6
Detergent	T49.2X1	T49.2X2	T49.2X3	T49.2X4	T49.2X5	T49.2X6
external medication	T49.2X1	T49.2X2	T49.2X3	T49.2X4	T49.2X5	T49.2X6
local	T49.2X1	T49.2X2	T49.2X3	T49.2X4	T49.2X5	T49.2X6

Substance	External Cause (T-Code)					
	Poisoning, Accidental (Unintentional)	Poisoning, Intentional Self-Harm	Poisoning, Assault	Poisoning, Undetermined	Adverse Effect	Underdosing
Detergent *(Continued)*						
medicinal	T49.2X1	T49.2X2	T49.2X3	T49.2X4	T49.2X5	T49.2X6
nonmedicinal	T55.1X1	T55.1X2	T55.1X3	T55.1X4	—	—
specified NEC	T55.1X1	T55.1X2	T55.1X3	T55.1X4	T55.1X5	T55.1X6
Deterrent, alcohol	T50.6X1	T50.6X2	T50.6X3	T50.6X4	T50.6X5	T50.6X6
Detoxifying agent	T50.6X1	T50.6X2	T50.6X3	T50.6X4	T50.6X5	T50.6X6
Detrothyronine	T38.1X1	T38.1X2	T38.1X3	T38.1X4	T38.1X5	T38.1X6
Dettol (external medication)	T49.0X1	T49.0X2	T49.0X3	T49.0X4	T49.0X5	T49.0X6
Dexamethasone	T38.0X1	T38.0X2	T38.0X3	T38.0X4	T38.0X5	T38.0X6
ENT agent	T49.6X1	T49.6X2	T49.6X3	T49.6X4	T49.6X5	T49.6X6
ophthalmic preparation	T49.5X1	T49.5X2	T49.5X3	T49.5X4	T49.5X5	T49.5X6
topical NEC	T49.0X1	T49.0X2	T49.0X3	T49.0X4	T49.0X5	T49.0X6
Dexamfetamine	T43.621	T43.622	T43.623	T43.624	T43.625	T43.626
Dexamphetamine	T43.621	T43.622	T43.623	T43.624	T43.625	T43.626
Dexbrompheniramine	T45.0X1	T45.0X2	T45.0X3	T45.0X4	T45.0X5	T45.0X6
Dexchlorpheniramine	T45.0X1	T45.0X2	T45.0X3	T45.0X4	T45.0X5	T45.0X6
Dexedrine	T43.621	T43.622	T43.623	T43.624	T43.625	T43.626
Dexetimide	T44.3X1	T44.3X2	T44.3X3	T44.3X4	T44.3X5	T44.3X6
Dexfenfluramine	T50.5X1	T50.5X2	T50.5X3	T50.5X4	T50.5X5	T50.5X6
Dexpanthenol	T45.2X1	T45.2X2	T45.2X3	T45.2X4	T45.2X5	T45.2X6
Dextran (40) (70) (150)	T45.8X1	T45.8X2	T45.8X3	T45.8X4	T45.8X5	T45.8X6
Dextriferron	T45.4X1	T45.4X2	T45.4X3	T45.4X4	T45.4X5	T45.4X6
Dextroamphetamine	T43.621	T43.622	T43.623	T43.624	T43.625	T43.626
Dextro calcium pantothenate	T45.2X1	T45.2X2	T45.2X3	T45.2X4	T45.2X5	T45.2X6
Dextromethorphan	T48.3X1	T48.3X2	T48.3X3	T48.3X4	T48.3X5	T48.3X6
Dextromoramide	T40.4X1	T40.4X2	T40.4X3	T40.4X4	—	—
topical	T49.8X1	T49.8X2	T49.8X3	T49.8X4	T49.8X5	T49.8X6
Dextro pantothenyl alcohol	T45.2X1	T45.2X2	T45.2X3	T45.2X4	T45.2X5	T45.2X6
Dextropropoxyphene	T40.4X1	T40.4X2	T40.4X3	T40.4X4	T40.4X5	T40.4X6
Dextrorphan	T40.2X1	T40.2X2	T40.2X3	T40.2X4	T40.2X5	T40.2X6
Dextrose	T50.3X1	T50.3X2	T50.3X3	T50.3X4	T50.3X5	T50.3X6
concentrated solution, intravenous	T46.8X1	T46.8X2	T46.8X3	T46.8X4	T46.8X5	T46.8X6
Dextrothyroxin	T38.1X1	T38.1X2	T38.1X3	T38.1X4	T38.1X5	T38.1X6
Dextrothyroxine sodium	T38.1X1	T38.1X2	T38.1X3	T38.1X4	T38.1X5	T38.1X6
DFP	T44.0X1	T44.0X2	T44.0X3	T44.0X4	T44.0X5	T44.0X6
DHE	T37.3X1	T37.3X2	T37.3X3	T37.3X4	T37.3X5	T37.3X6
45	T46.5X1	T46.5X2	T46.5X3	T46.5X4	T46.5X5	T46.5X6
Diabinese	T38.3X1	T38.3X2	T38.3X3	T38.3X4	T38.3X5	T38.3X6
Diacetone alcohol	T52.4X1	T52.4X2	T52.4X3	T52.4X4	—	—
Diacetyl monoxime	T50.991	T50.992	T50.993	T50.994	—	—
Diacetylmorphine	T40.1X1	T40.1X2	T40.1X3	T40.1X4	—	—

Substance	External Cause (T-Code)					
	Poisoning, Accidental (Unintentional)	Poisoning, Intentional Self-Harm	Poisoning, Assault	Poisoning, Undetermined	Adverse Effect	Underdosing
Diachylon plaster	T49.4X1	T49.4X2	T49.4X3	T49.4X4	T49.4X5	T49.4X6
Diaethylstilboestrolum	T38.5X1	T38.5X2	T38.5X3	T38.5X4	T38.5X5	T38.5X6
Diagnostic agent NEC	T50.8X1	T50.8X2	T50.8X3	T50.8X4	T50.8X5	T50.8X6
Dial (soap)	T49.2X1	T49.2X2	T49.2X3	T49.2X4	T49.2X5	T49.2X6
sedative	T42.3X1	T42.3X2	T42.3X3	T42.3X4	T42.3X5	T42.3X6
Dialkyl carbonate	T52.91	T52.92	T52.93	T52.94	—	—
Diallylbarbituric acid	T42.3X1	T42.3X2	T42.3X3	T42.3X4	T42.3X5	T42.3X6
Diallymal	T42.3X1	T42.3X2	T42.3X3	T42.3X4	T42.3X5	T42.3X6
Dialysis solution (intraperitoneal)	T50.3X1	T50.3X2	T50.3X3	T50.3X4	T50.3X5	T50.3X6
Diaminodiphenylsulfone	T37.1X1	T37.1X2	T37.1X3	T37.1X4	T37.1X5	T37.1X6
Diamorphine	T40.1X1	T40.1X2	T40.1X3	T40.1X4	—	—
Diamox	T50.2X1	T50.2X2	T50.2X3	T50.2X4	T50.2X5	T50.2X6
Diamthazole	T49.0X1	T49.0X2	T49.0X3	T49.0X4	T49.0X5	T49.0X6
Dianthone	T47.2X1	T47.2X2	T47.2X3	T47.2X4	T47.2X5	T47.2X6
Diaphenylsulfone	T37.0X1	T37.0X2	T37.0X3	T37.0X4	T37.0X5	T37.0X6
Diasone (sodium)	T37.1X1	T37.1X2	T37.1X3	T37.1X4	T37.1X5	T37.1X6
Diastase	T47.5X1	T47.5X2	T47.5X3	T47.5X4	T47.5X5	T47.5X6
Diatrizoate	T50.8X1	T50.8X2	T50.8X3	T50.8X4	T50.8X5	T50.8X6
Diazepam	T42.4X1	T42.4X2	T42.4X3	T42.4X4	T42.4X5	T42.4X6
Diazinon	T60.0X1	T60.0X2	T60.0X3	T60.0X4	—	—
Diazomethane (gas)	T59.891	T59.892	T59.893	T59.894	—	—
Diazoxide	T46.5X1	T46.5X2	T46.5X3	T46.5X4	T46.5X5	T46.5X6
Dibekacin	T36.5X1	T36.5X2	T36.5X3	T36.5X4	T36.5X5	T36.5X6
Dibenamine	T44.6X1	T44.6X2	T44.6X3	T44.6X4	T44.6X5	T44.6X6
Dibenzepin	T43.011	T43.012	T43.013	T43.014	T43.015	T43.016
Dibenzheptropine	T45.0X1	T45.0X2	T45.0X3	T45.0X4	T45.0X5	T45.0X6
Dibenzyline	T44.6X1	T44.6X2	T44.6X3	T44.6X4	T44.6X5	T44.6X6
Diborane (gas)	T59.891	T59.892	T59.893	T59.894	—	—
Dibromochloropropane	T60.8X1	T60.8X2	T60.8X3	T60.8X4	—	—
Dibromodulcitol	T45.1X1	T45.1X2	T45.1X3	T45.1X4	T45.1X5	T45.1X6
Dibromoethane	T53.6X1	T53.6X2	T53.6X3	T53.6X4	—	—
Dibromomannitol	T45.1X1	T45.1X2	T45.1X3	T45.1X4	T45.1X5	T45.1X6
Dibromopropamidine isethionate	T49.0X1	T49.0X2	T49.0X3	T49.0X4	T49.0X5	T49.0X6
Dibrompropamidine	T49.0X1	T49.0X2	T49.0X3	T49.0X4	T49.0X5	T49.0X6
Dibucaine	T41.3X1	T41.3X2	T41.3X3	T41.3X4	T41.3X5	T41.3X6
topical (surface)	T41.3X1	T41.3X2	T41.3X3	T41.3X4	T41.3X5	T41.3X6
Dibunate sodium	T48.3X1	T48.3X2	T48.3X3	T48.3X4	T48.3X5	T48.3X6
Dibutoline sulfate	T44.3X1	T44.3X2	T44.3X3	T44.3X4	T44.3X5	T44.3X6
Dicamba	T60.3X1	T60.3X2	T60.3X3	T60.3X4	—	—
Dicapthon	T60.0X1	T60.0X2	T60.0X3	T60.0X4	—	—
Dichlobenil	T60.3X1	T60.3X2	T60.3X3	T60.3X4	—	—
Dichlone	T60.3X1	T60.3X2	T60.3X3	T60.3X4	—	—

Substance	External Cause (T-Code)					
	Poisoning, Accidental (Unintentional)	Poisoning, Intentional Self-Harm	Poisoning, Assault	Poisoning, Undetermined	Adverse Effect	Underdosing
Dichloralphenozone	T42.6X1	T42.6X2	T42.6X3	T42.6X4	T42.6X5	T42.6X6
Dichlorbenzidine	T65.3X1	T65.3X2	T65.3X3	T65.3X4	—	—
Dichlorhydrin	T52.8X1	T52.8X2	T52.8X3	T52.8X4	—	—
Dichlorhydroxyquinoline	T37.8X1	T37.8X2	T37.8X3	T37.8X4	T37.8X5	T37.8X6
Dichlorobenzene	T53.7X1	T53.7X2	T53.7X3	T53.7X4	—	—
Dichlorobenzyl alcohol	T49.6X1	T49.6X2	T49.6X3	T49.6X4	T49.6X5	T49.6X6
Dichlorodifluoromethane	T53.5X1	T53.5X2	T53.5X3	T53.5X4	—	—
Dichloroethane	T52.8X1	T52.8X2	T52.8X3	T52.8X4	—	—
Sym-Dichloroethyl ether	T53.6X1	T53.6X2	T53.6X3	T53.6X4	—	—
Dichloroethyl sulfide, not in war	T59.891	T59.892	T59.893	T59.894	—	—
Dichloroethylene	T53.6X1	T53.6X2	T53.6X3	T53.6X4	—	—
Dichloroformoxine, not in war	T59.891	T59.892	T59.893	T59.894	—	—
Dichlorohydrin, alpha-dichlorohydrin	T52.8X1	T52.8X2	T52.8X3	T52.8X4	—	—
Dichloromethane (solvent)	T53.4X1	T53.4X2	T53.4X3	T53.4X4	—	—
vapor	T53.4X1	T53.4X2	T53.4X3	T53.4X4	—	—
Dichloronaphthoquinone	T60.3X1	T60.3X2	T60.3X3	T60.3X4	—	—
Dichlorophen	T37.4X1	T37.4X2	T37.4X3	T37.4X4	T37.4X5	T37.4X6
2,4-Dichlorophenoxy-acetic acid	T60.3X1	T60.3X2	T60.3X3	T60.3X4	—	—
Dichloropropene	T60.3X1	T60.3X2	T60.3X3	T60.3X4	—	—
Dichloropropionic acid	T60.3X1	T60.3X2	T60.3X3	T60.3X4	—	—
Dichlorphenamide	T50.2X1	T50.2X2	T50.2X3	T50.2X4	T50.2X5	T50.2X6
Dichlorvos	T60.0X1	T60.0X2	T60.0X3	T60.0X4	—	—
Diclofenac	T39.391	T39.392	T39.393	T39.394	T39.395	T39.396
Diclofenamide	T50.2X1	T50.2X2	T50.2X3	T50.2X4	T50.2X5	T50.2X6
Diclofensine	T43.291	T43.292	T43.293	T43.294	T43.295	T43.296
Diclonixine	T39.8X1	T39.8X2	T39.8X3	T39.8X4	T39.8X5	T39.8X6
Dicloxacillin	T36.0X1	T36.0X2	T36.0X3	T36.0X4	T36.0X5	T36.0X6
Dicophane	T49.0X1	T49.0X2	T49.0X3	T49.0X4	T49.0X5	T49.0X6
Dicoumarol, dicoumarin, dicumarol	T45.511	T45.512	T45.513	T45.514	T45.515	T45.516
Dicrotophos	T60.0X1	T60.0X2	T60.0X3	T60.0X4	—	—
Dicyanogen (gas)	T65.0X1	T65.0X2	T65.0X3	T65.0X4	—	—
Dicyclomine	T44.3X1	T44.3X2	T44.3X3	T44.3X4	T44.3X5	T44.3X6
Dicycloverine	T44.3X1	T44.3X2	T44.3X3	T44.3X4	T44.3X5	T44.3X6
Dideoxycytidine	T37.5X1	T37.5X2	T37.5X3	T37.5X4	T37.5X5	T37.5X6
Dideoxyinosine	T37.5X1	T37.5X2	T37.5X3	T37.5X4	T37.5X5	T37.5X6
Dieldrin (vapor)	T60.1X1	T60.1X2	T60.1X3	T60.1X4	—	—
Diemal	T42.3X1	T42.3X2	T42.3X3	T42.3X4	T42.3X5	T42.3X6
Dienestrol	T38.5X1	T38.5X2	T38.5X3	T38.5X4	T38.5X5	T38.5X6
Dienoestrol	T38.5X1	T38.5X2	T38.5X3	T38.5X4	T38.5X5	T38.5X6
Dietetic drug NEC	T50.901	T50.902	T50.903	T50.904	T50.905	T50.906
Diethazine	T42.8X1	T42.8X2	T42.8X3	T42.8X4	T42.8X5	T42.8X6

Substance	External Cause (T-Code)					
	Poisoning, Accidental (Unintentional)	Poisoning, Intentional Self-Harm	Poisoning, Assault	Poisoning, Undetermined	Adverse Effect	Underdosing
Diethyl						
barbituric acid	T42.3X1	T42.3X2	T42.3X3	T42.3X4	T42.3X5	T42.3X6
carbamazine	T37.4X1	T37.4X2	T37.4X3	T37.4X4	T37.4X5	T37.4X6
carbinol	T51.3X1	T51.3X2	T51.3X3	T51.3X4	—	—
carbonate	T52.8X1	T52.8X2	T52.8X3	T52.8X4	—	—
ether (vapor)—*see also ether*	T41.0X1	T41.0X2	T41.0X3	T41.0X4	T41.0X5	T41.0X6
oxide	T52.8X1	T52.8X2	T52.8X3	T52.8X4	—	—
propion	T50.5X1	T50.5X2	T50.5X3	T50.5X4	T50.5X5	T50.5X6
stilbestrol	T38.5X1	T38.5X2	T38.5X3	T38.5X4	T38.5X5	T38.5X6
toluamide (nonmedicinal)	T60.8X1	T60.8X2	T60.8X3	T60.8X4	—	—
medicinal	T49.3X1	T49.3X2	T49.3X3	T49.3X4	T49.3X5	T49.3X6
Diethylcarbamazine	T37.4X1	T37.4X2	T37.4X3	T37.4X4	T37.4X5	T37.4X6
Diethylene						
dioxide	T52.8X1	T52.8X2	T52.8X3	T52.8X4	—	—
glycol (monoacetate) (monobutyl ether) (monoethyl ether)	T52.3X1	T52.3X2	T52.3X3	T52.3X4	—	—
Diethylhexylphthalate	T65.891	T65.892	T65.893	T65.894	—	—
Diethylpropion	T50.5X1	T50.5X2	T50.5X3	T50.5X4	T50.5X5	T50.5X6
Diethylstilbestrol	T38.5X1	T38.5X2	T38.5X3	T38.5X4	T38.5X5	T38.5X6
Diethylstilboestrol	T38.5X1	T38.5X2	T38.5X3	T38.5X4	T38.5X5	T38.5X6
Diethylsulfone-diethylmethane	T42.6X1	T42.6X2	T42.6X3	T42.6X4	T42.6X5	T42.6X6
Diethyltoluamide	T49.0X1	T49.0X2	T49.0X3	T49.0X4	T49.0X5	T49.0X6
Diethyltryptamine (DET)	T40.991	T40.992	T40.993	T40.994	—	—
Difebarbamate	T42.3X1	T42.3X2	T42.3X3	T42.3X4	T42.3X5	T42.3X6
Difencloxazine	T40.2X1	T40.2X2	T40.2X3	T40.2X4	T40.2X5	T40.2X6
Difenidol	T45.0X1	T45.0X2	T45.0X3	T45.0X4	T45.0X5	T45.0X6
Difenoxin	T47.6X1	T47.6X2	T47.6X3	T47.6X4	T47.6X5	T47.6X6
Difetarsone	T37.3X1	T37.3X2	T37.3X3	T37.3X4	T37.3X5	T37.3X6
Diffusin	T45.3X1	T45.3X2	T45.3X3	T45.3X4	T45.3X5	T45.3X6
Diflorasone	T49.0X1	T49.0X2	T49.0X3	T49.0X4	T49.0X5	T49.0X6
Diflubenzuron	T60.1X1	T60.1X2	T60.1X3	T60.1X4	—	—
Diflos	T44.0X1	T44.0X2	T44.0X3	T44.0X4	T44.0X5	T44.0X6
Diflucortolone	T49.0X1	T49.0X2	T49.0X3	T49.0X4	T49.0X5	T49.0X6
Diflunisal	T39.091	T39.092	T39.093	T39.094	T39.095	T39.096
Difluoromethyldopa	T42.8X1	T42.8X2	T42.8X3	T42.8X4	T42.8X5	T42.8X6
Difluorophate	T44.0X1	T44.0X2	T44.0X3	T44.0X4	T44.0X5	T44.0X6
Digestant NEC	T47.5X1	T47.5X2	T47.5X3	T47.5X4	T47.5X5	T47.5X6
Digitalin(e)	T46.0X1	T46.0X2	T46.0X3	T46.0X4	T46.0X5	T46.0X6
Digitalis (leaf) (glycoside)	T46.0X1	T46.0X2	T46.0X3	T46.0X4	T46.0X5	T46.0X6
lanata	T46.0X1	T46.0X2	T46.0X3	T46.0X4	T46.0X5	T46.0X6
purpurea	T46.0X1	T46.0X2	T46.0X3	T46.0X4	T46.0X5	T46.0X6
Digitoxin	T46.0X1	T46.0X2	T46.0X3	T46.0X4	T46.0X5	T46.0X6

Substance	External Cause (T-Code)					
	Poisoning, Accidental (Unintentional)	Poisoning, Intentional Self-Harm	Poisoning, Assault	Poisoning, Undetermined	Adverse Effect	Underdosing
Digitoxose	T46.0X1	T46.0X2	T46.0X3	T46.0X4	T46.0X5	T46.0X6
Digoxin	T46.0X1	T46.0X2	T46.0X3	T46.0X4	T46.0X5	T46.0X6
Digoxine	T46.0X1	T46.0X2	T46.0X3	T46.0X4	T46.0X5	T46.0X6
Dihydralazine	T46.5X1	T46.5X2	T46.5X3	T46.5X4	T46.5X5	T46.5X6
Dihydrazine	T46.5X1	T46.5X2	T46.5X3	T46.5X4	T46.5X5	T46.5X6
Dihydrocodeinone	T40.2X1	T40.2X2	T40.2X3	T40.2X4	T40.2X5	T40.2X6
Dihydroergocornine	T46.7X1	T46.7X2	T46.7X3	T46.7X4	T46.7X5	T46.7X6
Dihydroergocristine (mesilate)	T46.7X1	T46.7X2	T46.7X3	T46.7X4	T46.7X5	T46.7X6
Dihydroergokryptine	T46.7X1	T46.7X2	T46.7X3	T46.7X4	T46.7X5	T46.7X6
Dihydroergotamine	T46.5X1	T46.5X2	T46.5X3	T46.5X4	T46.5X5	T46.5X6
Dihydroergotoxine	T46.7X1	T46.7X2	T46.7X3	T46.7X4	T46.7X5	T46.7X6
mesilate	T46.7X1	T46.7X2	T46.7X3	T46.7X4	T46.7X5	T46.7X6
Dihydrohydroxycodein-one	T40.2X1	T40.2X2	T40.2X3	T40.2X4	T40.2X5	T40.2X6
Dihydrohydroxymorphinone	T40.2X1	T40.2X2	T40.2X3	T40.2X4	T40.2X5	T40.2X6
Dihydroisocodeine	T40.2X1	T40.2X2	T40.2X3	T40.2X4	T40.2X5	T40.2X6
Dihydromorphine	T40.2X1	T40.2X2	T40.2X3	T40.2X4	—	—
Dihydromorphinone	T40.2X1	T40.2X2	T40.2X3	T40.2X4	T40.2X5	T40.2X6
Dihydrostreptomycin	T36.5X1	T36.5X2	T36.5X3	T36.5X4	T36.5X5	T36.5X6
Dihydrotachysterol	T45.2X1	T45.2X2	T45.2X3	T45.2X4	T45.2X5	T45.2X6
Dihydroxyaluminum aminoacetate	T47.1X1	T47.1X2	T47.1X3	T47.1X4	T47.1X5	T47.1X6
Dihydroxyaluminum sodium carbonate	T47.1X1	T47.1X2	T47.1X3	T47.1X4	T47.1X5	T47.1X6
Dihydroxyanthraquinone	T47.2X1	T47.2X2	T47.2X3	T47.2X4	T47.2X5	T47.2X6
Dihydroxycodeinone	T40.2X1	T40.2X2	T40.2X3	T40.2X4	T40.2X5	T40.2X6
Dihydroxypropyl theophylline	T50.2X1	T50.2X2	T50.2X3	T50.2X4	T50.2X5	T50.2X6
Diiodohydroxyquin	T37.8X1	T37.8X2	T37.8X3	T37.8X4	T37.8X5	T37.8X6
topical	T49.0X1	T49.0X2	T49.0X3	T49.0X4	T49.0X5	T49.0X6
Diiodohydroxyquinoline	T37.8X1	T37.8X2	T37.8X3	T37.8X4	T37.8X5	T37.8X6
Diiodotyrosine	T38.2X1	T38.2X2	T38.2X3	T38.2X4	T38.2X5	T38.2X6
Diisopromine	T44.3X1	T44.3X2	T44.3X3	T44.3X4	T44.3X5	T44.3X6
Diisopropylamine	T46.3X1	T46.3X2	T46.3X3	T46.3X4	T46.3X5	T46.3X6
Diisopropylfluorophosphonate	T44.0X1	T44.0X2	T44.0X3	T44.0X4	T44.0X5	T44.0X6
Dilantin	T42.0X1	T42.0X2	T42.0X3	T42.0X4	T42.0X5	T42.0X6
Dilaudid	T40.2X1	T40.2X2	T40.2X3	T40.2X4	T40.2X5	T40.2X6
Dilazep	T46.3X1	T46.3X2	T46.3X3	T46.3X4	T46.3X5	T46.3X6
Dill	T47.5X1	T47.5X2	T47.5X3	T47.5X4	T47.5X5	T47.5X6
Diloxanide	T37.3X1	T37.3X2	T37.3X3	T37.3X4	T37.3X5	T37.3X6
Diltiazem	T46.1X1	T46.1X2	T46.1X3	T46.1X4	T46.1X5	T46.1X6
Dimazole	T49.0X1	T49.0X2	T49.0X3	T49.0X4	T49.0X5	T49.0X6
Dimefline	T50.7X1	T50.7X2	T50.7X3	T50.7X4	T50.7X5	T50.7X6
Dimefox	T60.0X1	T60.0X2	T60.0X3	T60.0X4	—	—

Substance	External Cause (T-Code)					
	Poisoning, Accidental (Unintentional)	Poisoning, Intentional Self-Harm	Poisoning, Assault	Poisoning, Undetermined	Adverse Effect	Underdosing
Dimemorfan	T48.3X1	T48.3X2	T48.3X3	T48.3X4	T48.3X5	T48.3X6
Dimenhydrinate	T45.0X1	T45.0X2	T45.0X3	T45.0X4	T45.0X5	T45.0X6
Dimercaprol (British anti-lewisite)	T45.8X1	T45.8X2	T45.8X3	T45.8X4	T45.8X5	T45.8X6
Dimercaptopropanol	T45.8X1	T45.8X2	T45.8X3	T45.8X4	T45.8X5	T45.8X6
Dimestrol	T38.5X1	T38.5X2	T38.5X3	T38.5X4	T38.5X5	T38.5X6
Dimetane	T45.0X1	T45.0X2	T45.0X3	T45.0X4	T45.0X5	T45.0X6
Dimethicone	T47.1X1	T47.1X2	T47.1X3	T47.1X4	T47.1X5	T47.1X6
Dimethindene	T45.0X1	T45.0X2	T45.0X3	T45.0X4	T45.0X5	T45.0X6
Dimethisoquin	T49.1X1	T49.1X2	T49.1X3	T49.1X4	T49.1X5	T49.1X6
Dimethisterone	T38.5X1	T38.5X2	T38.5X3	T38.5X4	T38.5X5	T38.5X6
Dimethoate	T60.0X1	T60.0X2	T60.0X3	T60.0X4	—	—
Dimethocaine	T41.3X1	T41.3X2	T41.3X3	T41.3X4	T41.3X5	T41.3X6
Dimethoxanate	T48.3X1	T48.3X2	T48.3X3	T48.3X4	T48.3X5	T48.3X6
Dimethyl						
arsine, arsinic acid	T57.0X1	T57.0X2	T57.0X3	T57.0X4	—	—
carbinol	T51.2X1	T51.2X2	T51.2X3	T51.2X4	—	—
carbonate	T52.8X1	T52.8X2	T52.8X3	T52.8X4	—	—
diguanide	T38.3X1	T38.3X2	T38.3X3	T38.3X4	T38.3X5	T38.3X6
ketone	T52.4X1	T52.4X2	T52.4X3	T52.4X4	—	—
vapor	T52.4X1	T52.4X2	T52.4X3	T52.4X4	—	—
meperidine	T40.2X1	T40.2X2	T40.2X3	T40.2X4	T40.2X5	T40.2X6
parathion	T60.0X1	T60.0X2	T60.0X3	T60.0X4	—	—
phthlate	T49.3X1	T49.3X2	T49.3X3	T49.3X4	T49.3X5	T49.3X6
polysiloxane	T47.8X1	T47.8X2	T47.8X3	T47.8X4	T47.8X5	T47.8X6
sulfate (fumes)	T59.891	T59.892	T59.893	T59.894	—	—
liquid	T65.891	T65.892	T65.893	T65.894	—	—
sulfoxide (nonmedicinal)	T52.8X1	T52.8X2	T52.8X3	T52.8X4	—	—
medicinal	T49.4X1	T49.4X2	T49.4X3	T49.4X4	T49.4X5	T49.4X6
tryptamine	T40.991	T40.992	T40.993	T40.994	—	—
tubocurarine	T48.1X1	T48.1X2	T48.1X3	T48.1X4	T48.1X5	T48.1X6
Dimethylamine sulfate	T49.4X1	T49.4X2	T49.4X3	T49.4X4	T49.4X5	T49.4X6
Dimethylformamide	T52.8X1	T52.8X2	T52.8X3	T52.8X4	—	—
Dimethyltubocurarinium chloride	T48.1X1	T48.1X2	T48.1X3	T48.1X4	T48.1X5	T48.1X6
Dimeticone	T47.1X1	T47.1X2	T47.1X3	T47.1X4	T47.1X5	T47.1X6
Dimetilan	T60.0X1	T60.0X2	T60.0X3	T60.0X4	—	—
Dimetindene	T45.0X1	T45.0X2	T45.0X3	T45.0X4	T45.0X5	T45.0X6
Dimetotiazine	T43.3X1	T43.3X2	T43.3X3	T43.3X4	T43.3X5	T43.3X6
Dimorpholamine	T50.7X1	T50.7X2	T50.7X3	T50.7X4	T50.7X5	T50.7X6
Dimoxyline	T46.3X1	T46.3X2	T46.3X3	T46.3X4	T46.3X5	T46.3X6
Dinitrobenzene	T65.3X1	T65.3X2	T65.3X3	T65.3X4	—	—
vapor	T59.891	T59.892	T59.893	T59.894	—	—

Substance	External Cause (T-Code)					
	Poisoning, Accidental (Unintentional)	Poisoning, Intentional Self-Harm	Poisoning, Assault	Poisoning, Undetermined	Adverse Effect	Underdosing
Dinitrobenzol	T65.3X1	T65.3X2	T65.3X3	T65.3X4	—	—
vapor	T59.891	T59.892	T59.893	T59.894	—	—
Dinitrobutylphenol	T65.3X1	T65.3X2	T65.3X3	T65.3X4	—	—
Dinitro (-ortho-)cresol (pesticide) (spray)	T65.3X1	T65.3X2	T65.3X3	T65.3X4	—	—
Dinitrocyclohexylphenol	T65.3X1	T65.3X2	T65.3X3	T65.3X4	—	—
Dinitrophenol	T65.3X1	T65.3X2	T65.3X3	T65.3X4	—	—
Dinoprost	T48.0X1	T48.0X2	T48.0X3	T48.0X4	T48.0X5	T48.0X6
Dinoprostone	T48.0X1	T48.0X2	T48.0X3	T48.0X4	T48.0X5	T48.0X6
Dinoseb	T60.3X1	T60.3X2	T60.3X3	T60.3X4	—	—
Dioctyl sulfosuccinate (calcium) (sodium)	T47.4X1	T47.4X2	T47.4X3	T47.4X4	T47.4X5	T47.4X6
Diodone	T50.8X1	T50.8X2	T50.8X3	T50.8X4	T50.8X5	T50.8X6
Diodoquin	T37.8X1	T37.8X2	T37.8X3	T37.8X4	T37.8X5	T37.8X6
Dionin	T40.2X1	T40.2X2	T40.2X3	T40.2X4	T40.2X5	T40.2X6
Diosmin	T46.991	T46.992	T46.993	T46.994	T46.995	T46.996
Dioxane	T52.8X1	T52.8X2	T52.8X3	T52.8X4	—	—
Dioxathion	T60.0X1	T60.0X2	T60.0X3	T60.0X4	—	—
Dioxin	T53.7X1	T53.7X2	T53.7X3	T53.7X4	—	—
Dioxopromethazine	T43.3X1	T43.3X2	T43.3X3	T43.3X4	T43.3X5	T43.3X6
Dioxyline	T46.3X1	T46.3X2	T46.3X3	T46.3X4	T46.3X5	T46.3X6
Dipentene	T52.8X1	T52.8X2	T52.8X3	T52.8X4	—	—
Diperodon	T41.3X1	T41.3X2	T41.3X3	T41.3X4	T41.3X5	T41.3X6
Diphacinone	T60.4X1	T60.4X2	T60.4X3	T60.4X4	—	—
Diphemanil	T44.3X1	T44.3X2	T44.3X3	T44.3X4	T44.3X5	T44.3X6
metilsulfate	T44.3X1	T44.3X2	T44.3X3	T44.3X4	T44.3X5	T44.3X6
Diphenadione	T45.511	T45.512	T45.513	T45.514	T45.515	T45.516
rodenticide	T60.4X1	T60.4X2	T60.4X3	T60.4X4	—	—
Diphenhydramine	T45.0X1	T45.0X2	T45.0X3	T45.0X4	T45.0X5	T45.0X6
Diphenidol	T45.0X1	T45.0X2	T45.0X3	T45.0X4	T45.0X5	T45.0X6
Diphenoxylate	T47.6X1	T47.6X2	T47.6X3	T47.6X4	T47.6X5	T47.6X6
Diphenylamine	T65.3X1	T65.3X2	T65.3X3	T65.3X4	—	—
Diphenylbutazone	T39.2X1	T39.2X2	T39.2X3	T39.2X4	T39.2X5	T39.2X6
Diphenylchloroarsine, not in war	T57.0X1	T57.0X2	T57.0X3	T57.0X4	—	—
Diphenylhydantoin	T42.0X1	T42.0X2	T42.0X3	T42.0X4	T42.0X5	T42.0X6
Diphenylmethane dye	T52.1X1	T52.1X2	T52.1X3	T52.1X4	—	—
Diphenylpyraline	T45.0X1	T45.0X2	T45.0X3	T45.0X4	T45.0X5	T45.0X6
Diphtheria						
antitoxin	T50.Z11	T50.Z12	T50.Z13	T50.Z14	T50.Z15	T50.Z16
toxoid	T50.A91	T50.A92	T50.A93	T50.A94	T50.A95	T50.A96
with tetanus toxoid	T50.A21	T50.A22	T50.A23	T50.A24	T50.A25	T50.A26
with pertussis component	T50.A11	T50.A12	T50.A13	T50.A14	T50.A15	T50.A16

Substance	External Cause (T-Code)					
	Poisoning, Accidental (Unintentional)	Poisoning, Intentional Self-Harm	Poisoning, Assault	Poisoning, Undetermined	Adverse Effect	Underdosing
Diphtheria *(Continued)*						
vaccine (combination)	T50.A91	T50.A92	T50.A93	T50.A94	T50.A95	T50.A96
combination						
including pertussis	T50.A11	T50.A12	T50.A13	T50.A14	T50.A15	T50.A16
without pertussis	T50.A21	T50.A22	T50.A23	T50.A24	T50.A25	T50.A26
Diphylline	T50.2X1	T50.2X2	T50.2X3	T50.2X4	T50.2X5	T50.2X6
Dipipanone	T40.4X1	T40.4X2	T40.4X3	T40.4X4	—	—
Dipivefrine	T49.5X1	T49.5X2	T49.5X3	T49.5X4	T49.5X5	T49.5X6
Diplovax	T50.B91	T50.B92	T50.B93	T50.B94	T50.B95	T50.B96
Diprophylline	T50.2X1	T50.2X2	T50.2X3	T50.2X4	T50.2X5	T50.2X6
Dipropyline	T48.291	T48.292	T48.293	T48.294	T48.295	T48.296
Dipyridamole	T46.3X1	T46.3X2	T46.3X3	T46.3X4	T46.3X5	T46.3X6
Dipyrone	T39.2X1	T39.2X2	T39.2X3	T39.2X4	T39.2X5	T39.2X6
Diquat (dibromide)	T60.3X1	T60.3X2	T60.3X3	T60.3X4	—	—
Disinfectant	T65.891	T65.892	T65.893	T65.894	—	—
alkaline	T54.3X1	T54.3X2	T54.3X3	T54.3X4	—	—
aromatic	T54.1X1	T54.1X2	T54.1X3	T54.1X4	—	—
intestinal	T37.8X1	T37.8X2	T37.8X3	T37.8X4	T37.8X5	T37.8X6
Disipal	T42.8X1	T42.8X2	T42.8X3	T42.8X4	T42.8X5	T42.8X6
Disodium edetate	T50.6X1	T50.6X2	T50.6X3	T50.6X4	T50.6X5	T50.6X6
Disoprofol	T41.291	T41.292	T41.293	T41.294	T41.295	T41.296
Disopyramide	T46.2X1	T46.2X2	T46.2X3	T46.2X4	T46.2X5	T46.2X6
Distigmine (bromide)	T44.0X1	T44.0X2	T44.0X3	T44.0X4	T44.0X5	T44.0X6
Disulfamide	T50.2X1	T50.2X2	T50.2X3	T50.2X4	T50.2X5	T50.2X6
Disulfanilamide	T37.0X1	T37.0X2	T37.0X3	T37.0X4	T37.0X5	T37.0X6
Disulfiram	T50.6X1	T50.6X2	T50.6X3	T50.6X4	T50.6X5	T50.6X6
Disulfoton	T60.0X1	T60.0X2	T60.0X3	T60.0X4	—	—
Dithiazanine iodide	T37.4X1	T37.4X2	T37.4X3	T37.4X4	T37.4X5	T37.4X6
Dithiocarbamate	T60.0X1	T60.0X2	T60.0X3	T60.0X4	—	—
Dithranol	T49.4X1	T49.4X2	T49.4X3	T49.4X4	T49.4X5	T49.4X6
Diucardin	T50.2X1	T50.2X2	T50.2X3	T50.2X4	T50.2X5	T50.2X6
Diupres	T50.2X1	T50.2X2	T50.2X3	T50.2X4	T50.2X5	T50.2X6
Diuretic NEC	T50.2X1	T50.2X2	T50.2X3	T50.2X4	T50.2X5	T50.2X6
benzothiadiazine	T50.2X1	T50.2X2	T50.2X3	T50.2X4	T50.2X5	T50.2X6
carbonic acid anhydrase inhibitors	T50.2X1	T50.2X2	T50.2X3	T50.2X4	T50.2X5	T50.2X6
furfuryl NEC	T50.2X1	T50.2X2	T50.2X3	T50.2X4	T50.2X5	T50.2X6
loop (high-ceiling)	T50.1X1	T50.1X2	T50.1X3	T50.1X4	T50.1X5	T50.1X6
mercurial NEC	T50.2X1	T50.2X2	T50.2X3	T50.2X4	T50.2X5	T50.2X6
osmotic	T50.2X1	T50.2X2	T50.2X3	T50.2X4	T50.2X5	T50.2X6
purine NEC	T50.2X1	T50.2X2	T50.2X3	T50.2X4	T50.2X5	T50.2X6
saluretic NEC	T50.2X1	T50.2X2	T50.2X3	T50.2X4	T50.2X5	T50.2X6

◀ New ⇐ Revised ~~deleted~~ Deleted

Substance	External Cause (T-Code)					
	Poisoning, Accidental (Unintentional)	Poisoning, Intentional Self-Harm	Poisoning, Assault	Poisoning, Undetermined	Adverse Effect	Underdosing
Diuretic NEC *(Continued)*						
sulfonamide	T50.2X1	T50.2X2	T50.2X3	T50.2X4	T50.2X5	T50.2X6
thiazide NEC	T50.2X1	T50.2X2	T50.2X3	T50.2X4	T50.2X5	T50.2X6
xanthine	T50.2X1	T50.2X2	T50.2X3	T50.2X4	T50.2X5	T50.2X6
Diurgin	T50.2X1	T50.2X2	T50.2X3	T50.2X4	T50.2X5	T50.2X6
Diuril	T50.2X1	T50.2X2	T50.2X3	T50.2X4	T50.2X5	T50.2X6
Diuron	T60.3X1	T60.3X2	T60.3X3	T60.3X4	—	—
Divalproex	T42.6X1	T42.6X2	T42.6X3	T42.6X4	T42.6X5	T42.6X6
Divinyl ether	T41.0X1	T41.0X2	T41.0X3	T41.0X4	T41.0X5	T41.0X6
Dixanthogen	T49.0X1	T49.0X2	T49.0X3	T49.0X4	T49.0X5	T49.0X6
Dixyrazine	T43.3X1	T43.3X2	T43.3X3	T43.3X4	T43.3X5	T43.3X6
D-lysergic acid diethylamide	T40.8X1	T40.8X2	T40.8X3	T40.8X4	—	—
DMCT	T36.4X1	T36.4X2	T36.4X3	T36.4X4	T36.4X5	T36.4X6
DMSO — *see Dimethyl sulfoxide*						
DNBP	T60.3X1	T60.3X2	T60.3X3	T60.3X4	—	—
DNOC	T65.3X1	T65.3X2	T65.3X3	T65.3X4	—	—
DOCA	T38.0X1	T38.0X2	T38.0X3	T38.0X4	T38.0X5	T38.0X6
Dobutamine	T44.5X1	T44.5X2	T44.5X3	T44.5X4	T44.5X5	T44.5X6
Docusate sodium	T47.4X1	T47.4X2	T47.4X3	T47.4X4	T47.4X5	T47.4X6
Dodicin	T49.0X1	T49.0X2	T49.0X3	T49.0X4	T49.0X5	T49.0X6
Dofamium chloride	T49.0X1	T49.0X2	T49.0X3	T49.0X4	T49.0X5	T49.0X6
Dolophine	T40.3X1	T40.3X2	T40.3X3	T40.3X4	T40.3X5	T40.3X6
Doloxene	T39.8X1	T39.8X2	T39.8X3	T39.8X4	T39.8X5	T39.8X6
Domestic gas (after combustion) — *see Gas, utility*						
prior to combustion	T59.891	T59.892	T59.893	T59.894	—	—
Domiodol	T48.4X1	T48.4X2	T48.4X3	T48.4X4	T48.4X5	T48.4X6
Domiphen (bromide)	T49.0X1	T49.0X2	T49.0X3	T49.0X4	T49.0X5	T49.0X6
Domperidone	T45.0X1	T45.0X2	T45.0X3	T45.0X4	T45.0X5	T45.0X6
Dopa	T42.8X1	T42.8X2	T42.8X3	T42.8X4	T42.8X5	T42.8X6
Dopamine	T44.991	T44.992	T44.993	T44.994	T44.995	T44.996
Doriden	T42.6X1	T42.6X2	T42.6X3	T42.6X4	T42.6X5	T42.6X6
Dormiral	T42.3X1	T42.3X2	T42.3X3	T42.3X4	T42.3X5	T42.3X6
Dormison	T42.6X1	T42.6X2	T42.6X3	T42.6X4	T42.6X5	T42.6X6
Dornase	T48.4X1	T48.4X2	T48.4X3	T48.4X4	T48.4X5	T48.4X6
Dorsacaine	T41.3X1	T41.3X2	T41.3X3	T41.3X4	T41.3X5	T41.3X6
Dosulepin	T43.011	T43.012	T43.013	T43.014	T43.015	T43.016
Dothiepin	T43.011	T43.012	T43.013	T43.014	T43.015	T43.016
Doxantrazole	T48.6X1	T48.6X2	T48.6X3	T48.6X4	T48.6X5	T48.6X6
Doxapram	T50.7X1	T50.7X2	T50.7X3	T50.7X4	T50.7X5	T50.7X6
Doxazosin	T44.6X1	T44.6X2	T44.6X3	T44.6X4	T44.6X5	T44.6X6
Doxepin	T43.011	T43.012	T43.013	T43.014	T43.015	T43.016

Substance	External Cause (T-Code)					
	Poisoning, Accidental (Unintentional)	Poisoning, Intentional Self-Harm	Poisoning, Assault	Poisoning, Undetermined	Adverse Effect	Underdosing
Doxifluridine	T45.1X1	T45.1X2	T45.1X3	T45.1X4	T45.1X5	T45.1X6
Doxorubicin	T45.1X1	T45.1X2	T45.1X3	T45.1X4	T45.1X5	T45.1X6
Doxycycline	T36.4X1	T36.4X2	T36.4X3	T36.4X4	T36.4X5	T36.4X6
Doxylamine	T45.0X1	T45.0X2	T45.0X3	T45.0X4	T45.0X5	T45.0X6
Dramamine	T45.0X1	T45.0X2	T45.0X3	T45.0X4	T45.0X5	T45.0X6
Drano (drain cleaner)	T54.3X1	T54.3X2	T54.3X3	T54.3X4	—	—
Dressing, live pulp	T49.7X1	T49.7X2	T49.7X3	T49.7X4	T49.7X5	T49.7X6
Drocode	T40.2X1	T40.2X2	T40.2X3	T40.2X4	T40.2X5	T40.2X6
Dromoran	T40.2X1	T40.2X2	T40.2X3	T40.2X4	T40.2X5	T40.2X6
Dromostanolone	T38.7X1	T38.7X2	T38.7X3	T38.7X4	T38.7X5	T38.7X6
Dronabinol	T40.7X1	T40.7X2	T40.7X3	T40.7X4	T40.7X5	T40.7X6
Droperidol	T43.591	T43.592	T43.593	T43.594	T43.595	T43.596
Dropropizine	T48.3X1	T48.3X2	T48.3X3	T48.3X4	T48.3X5	T48.3X6
Drostanolone	T38.7X1	T38.7X2	T38.7X3	T38.7X4	T38.7X5	T38.7X6
Drotaverine	T44.3X1	T44.3X2	T44.3X3	T44.3X4	T44.3X5	T44.3X6
Drotrecogin alfa	T45.511	T45.512	T45.513	T45.514	T45.515	T45.516
Drug NEC	T50.901	T50.902	T50.903	T50.904	T50.905	T50.906
specified NEC	T50.991	T50.992	T50.993	T50.994	T50.995	T50.996
DTIC	T45.1X1	T45.1X2	T45.1X3	T45.1X4	T45.1X5	T45.1X6
Duboisine	T44.3X1	T44.3X2	T44.3X3	T44.3X4	T44.3X5	T44.3X6
Dulcolax	T47.2X1	T47.2X2	T47.2X3	T47.2X4	T47.2X5	T47.2X6
Duponol (C) (EP)	T49.2X1	T49.2X2	T49.2X3	T49.2X4	T49.2X5	T49.2X6
Durabolin	T38.7X1	T38.7X2	T38.7X3	T38.7X4	T38.7X5	T38.7X6
Dyclone	T41.3X1	T41.3X2	T41.3X3	T41.3X4	T41.3X5	T41.3X6
Dyclonine	T41.3X1	T41.3X2	T41.3X3	T41.3X4	T41.3X5	T41.3X6
Dydrogesterone	T38.5X1	T38.5X2	T38.5X3	T38.5X4	T38.5X5	T38.5X6
Dye NEC	T65.6X1	T65.6X2	T65.6X3	T65.6X4	—	—
antiseptic	T49.0X1	T49.0X2	T49.0X3	T49.0X4	T49.0X5	T49.0X6
diagnostic agents	T50.8X1	T50.8X2	T50.8X3	T50.8X4	T50.8X5	T50.8X6
pharmaceutical NEC	T50.901	T50.902	T50.903	T50.904	T50.905	T50.906
Dyflos	T44.0X1	T44.0X2	T44.0X3	T44.0X4	T44.0X5	T44.0X6
Dymelor	T38.3X1	T38.3X2	T38.3X3	T38.3X4	T38.3X5	T38.3X6
Dynamite	T65.3X1	T65.3X2	T65.3X3	T65.3X4	—	—
fumes	T59.891	T59.892	T59.893	T59.894	—	—
Dyphylline	T44.3X1	T44.3X2	T44.3X3	T44.3X4	T44.3X5	T44.3X6
E						
Ear drug NEC	T49.6X1	T49.6X2	T49.6X3	T49.6X4	T49.6X5	T49.6X6
Ear preparations	T49.6X1	T49.6X2	T49.6X3	T49.6X4	T49.6X5	T49.6X6
Econazole	T49.0X1	T49.0X2	T49.0X3	T49.0X4	T49.0X5	T49.0X6
Ecothiopate iodide	T49.5X1	T49.5X2	T49.5X3	T49.5X4	T49.5X5	T49.5X6
Echothiophate, echothiopate, ecothiopate	T49.5X1	T49.5X2	T49.5X3	T49.5X4	T49.5X5	T49.5X6

Substance	External Cause (T-Code)					
	Poisoning, Accidental (Unintentional)	Poisoning, Intentional Self-Harm	Poisoning, Assault	Poisoning, Undetermined	Adverse Effect	Underdosing
Ecstasy	T43.621	T43.622	T43.623	T43.624	T43.625	T43.626
Ectylurea	T42.6X1	T42.6X2	T42.6X3	T42.6X4	T42.6X5	T42.6X6
Edathamil disodium	T45.8X1	T45.8X2	T45.8X3	T45.8X4	T45.8X5	T45.8X6
Edecrin	T50.1X1	T50.1X2	T50.1X3	T50.1X4	T50.1X5	T50.1X6
Edetate, disodium (calcium)	T45.8X1	T45.8X2	T45.8X3	T45.8X4	T45.8X5	T45.8X6
Edoxudine	T49.5X1	T49.5X2	T49.5X3	T49.5X4	T49.5X5	T49.5X6
Edrophonium	T44.0X1	T44.0X2	T44.0X3	T44.0X4	T44.0X5	T44.0X6
chloride	T44.0X1	T44.0X2	T44.0X3	T44.0X4	T44.0X5	T44.0X6
EDTA	T50.6X1	T50.6X2	T50.6X3	T50.6X4	T50.6X5	T50.6X6
Eflornithine	T37.2X1	T37.2X2	T37.2X3	T37.2X4	T37.2X5	T37.2X6
Efloxate	T46.3X1	T46.3X2	T46.3X3	T46.3X4	T46.3X5	T46.3X6
Elase	T49.8X1	T49.8X2	T49.8X3	T49.8X4	T49.8X5	T49.8X6
Elastase	T47.5X1	T47.5X2	T47.5X3	T47.5X4	T47.5X5	T47.5X6
Elaterium	T47.2X1	T47.2X2	T47.2X3	T47.2X4	T47.2X5	T47.2X6
Elcatonin	T50.991	T50.992	T50.993	T50.994	T50.995	T50.996
Elder	T62.2X1	T62.2X2	T62.2X3	T62.2X4	—	—
berry (unripe)	T62.1X1	T62.1X2	T62.1X3	T62.1X4	—	—
Electrolyte balance drug	T50.3X1	T50.3X2	T50.3X3	T50.3X4	T50.3X5	T50.3X6
Electrolytes NEC	T50.3X1	T50.3X2	T50.3X3	T50.3X4	T50.3X5	T50.3X6
Electrolytic agent NEC	T50.3X1	T50.3X2	T50.3X3	T50.3X4	T50.3X5	T50.3X6
Elemental diet	T50.901	T50.902	T50.903	T50.904	T50.905	T50.906
Elliptinium acetate	T45.1X1	T45.1X2	T45.1X3	T45.1X4	T45.1X5	T45.1X6
Embramine	T45.0X1	T45.0X2	T45.0X3	T45.0X4	T45.0X5	T45.0X6
Emepronium (salts)	T44.3X1	T44.3X2	T44.3X3	T44.3X4	T44.3X5	T44.3X6
bromide	T44.3X1	T44.3X2	T44.3X3	T44.3X4	T44.3X5	T44.3X6
Emetic NEC	T47.7X1	T47.7X2	T47.7X3	T47.7X4	T47.7X5	T47.7X6
Emetine	T37.3X1	T37.3X2	T37.3X3	T37.3X4	T37.3X5	T37.3X6
Emollient NEC	T49.3X1	T49.3X2	T49.3X3	T49.3X4	T49.3X5	T49.3X6
Emorfazone	T39.8X1	T39.8X2	T39.8X3	T39.8X4	T39.8X5	T39.8X6
Emylcamate	T43.591	T43.592	T43.593	T43.594	T43.595	T43.596
Enalapril	T46.4X1	T46.4X2	T46.4X3	T46.4X4	T46.4X5	T46.4X6
Enalaprilat	T46.4X1	T46.4X2	T46.4X3	T46.4X4	T46.4X5	T46.4X6
Encainide	T46.2X1	T46.2X2	T46.2X3	T46.2X4	T46.2X5	T46.2X6
Endocaine	T41.3X1	T41.3X2	T41.3X3	T41.3X4	T41.3X5	T41.3X6
Endosulfan	T60.2X1	T60.2X2	T60.2X3	T60.2X4	—	—
Endothall	T60.3X1	T60.3X2	T60.3X3	T60.3X4	—	—
Endralazine	T46.5X1	T46.5X2	T46.5X3	T46.5X4	T46.5X5	T46.5X6
Endrin	T60.1X1	T60.1X2	T60.1X3	T60.1X4	—	—
Enflurane	T41.0X1	T41.0X2	T41.0X3	T41.0X4	T41.0X5	T41.0X6
Enhexymal	T42.3X1	T42.3X2	T42.3X3	T42.3X4	T42.3X5	T42.3X6
Enocitabine	T45.1X1	T45.1X2	T45.1X3	T45.1X4	T45.1X5	T45.1X6
Enovid	T38.4X1	T38.4X2	T38.4X3	T38.4X4	T38.4X5	T38.4X6

Substance	External Cause (T-Code)					
	Poisoning, Accidental (Unintentional)	Poisoning, Intentional Self-Harm	Poisoning, Assault	Poisoning, Undetermined	Adverse Effect	Underdosing
Enoxacin	T36.8X1	T36.8X2	T36.8X3	T36.8X4	T36.8X5	T36.8X6
Enoxaparin (sodium)	T45.511	T45.512	T45.513	T45.514	T45.515	T45.516
Enpiprazole	T43.591	T43.592	T43.593	T43.594	T43.595	T43.596
Enprofylline	T48.6X1	T48.6X2	T48.6X3	T48.6X4	T48.6X5	T48.6X6
Enprostil	T47.1X1	T47.1X2	T47.1X3	T47.1X4	T47.1X5	T47.1X6
ENT preparations (anti-infectives)	T49.6X1	T49.6X2	T49.6X3	T49.6X4	T49.6X5	T49.6X6
Enviomycin	T36.8X1	T36.8X2	T36.8X3	T36.8X4	T36.8X5	T36.8X6
Enzodase	T45.3X1	T45.3X2	T45.3X3	T45.3X4	T45.3X5	T45.3X6
Enzyme NEC	T45.3X1	T45.3X2	T45.3X3	T45.3X4	T45.3X5	T45.3X6
depolymerizing	T49.8X1	T49.8X2	T49.8X3	T49.8X4	T49.8X5	T49.8X6
fibrolytic	T45.3X1	T45.3X2	T45.3X3	T45.3X4	T45.3X5	T45.3X6
gastric	T47.5X1	T47.5X2	T47.5X3	T47.5X4	T47.5X5	T47.5X6
intestinal	T47.5X1	T47.5X2	T47.5X3	T47.5X4	T47.5X5	T47.5X6
local action	T49.4X1	T49.4X2	T49.4X3	T49.4X4	T49.4X5	T49.4X6
proteolytic	T49.4X1	T49.4X2	T49.4X3	T49.4X4	T49.4X5	T49.4X6
thrombolytic	T45.3X1	T45.3X2	T45.3X3	T45.3X4	T45.3X5	T45.3X6
EPAB	T41.3X1	T41.3X2	T41.3X3	T41.3X4	T41.3X5	T41.3X6
Epanutin	T42.0X1	T42.0X2	T42.0X3	T42.0X4	T42.0X5	T42.0X6
Ephedra	T44.991	T44.992	T44.993	T44.994	T44.995	T44.996
Ephedrine	T44.991	T44.992	T44.993	T44.994	T44.995	T44.996
Epichlorhydrin, epichlorohydrin	T52.8X1	T52.8X2	T52.8X3	T52.8X4	—	—
Epicillin	T36.0X1	T36.0X2	T36.0X3	T36.0X4	T36.0X5	T36.0X6
Epiestriol	T38.5X1	T38.5X2	T38.5X3	T38.5X4	T38.5X5	T38.5X6
Epilim — *see Sodium valproate*						
Epimestrol	T38.5X1	T38.5X2	T38.5X3	T38.5X4	T38.5X5	T38.5X6
Epinephrine	T44.5X1	T44.5X2	T44.5X3	T44.5X4	T44.5X5	T44.5X6
Epirubicin	T45.1X1	T45.1X2	T45.1X3	T45.1X4	T45.1X5	T45.1X6
Epitiostanol	T38.7X1	T38.7X2	T38.7X3	T38.7X4	T38.7X5	T38.7X6
Epitizide	T50.2X1	T50.2X2	T50.2X3	T50.2X4	T50.2X5	T50.2X6
EPN	T60.0X1	T60.0X2	T60.0X3	T60.0X4	—	—
EPO	T45.8X1	T45.8X2	T45.8X3	T45.8X4	T45.8X5	T45.8X6
Epoetin alpha	T45.8X1	T45.8X2	T45.8X3	T45.8X4	T45.8X5	T45.8X6
Epomediol	T50.991	T50.992	T50.993	T50.994	T50.995	T50.996
Epoprostenol	T45.521	T45.522	T45.523	T45.524	T45.525	T45.526
Epoxy resin	T65.891	T65.892	T65.893	T65.894	—	—
Eprazinone	T48.4X1	T48.4X2	T48.4X3	T48.4X4	T48.4X5	T48.4X6
Epsilon amino-caproic acid	T45.621	T45.622	T45.623	T45.624	T45.625	T45.626
Epsom salt	T47.3X1	T47.3X2	T47.3X3	T47.3X4	T47.3X5	T47.3X6
Eptazocine	T40.4X1	T40.4X2	T40.4X3	T40.4X4	T40.4X5	T40.4X6
Equanil	T43.591	T43.592	T43.593	T43.594	T43.595	T43.596
Equisetum	T62.2X1	T62.2X2	T62.2X3	T62.2X4	—	—
diuretic	T50.2X1	T50.2X2	T50.2X3	T50.2X4	T50.2X5	T50.2X6

◀ New ⇐ Revised ~~deleted~~ Deleted

Substance	External Cause (T-Code)					
	Poisoning, Accidental (Unintentional)	Poisoning, Intentional Self-Harm	Poisoning, Assault	Poisoning, Undetermined	Adverse Effect	Underdosing
Ergobasine	T48.0X1	T48.0X2	T48.0X3	T48.0X4	T48.0X5	T48.0X6
Ergocalciferol	T45.2X1	T45.2X2	T45.2X3	T45.2X4	T45.2X5	T45.2X6
Ergoloid mesylates	T46.7X1	T46.7X2	T46.7X3	T46.7X4	T46.7X5	T46.7X6
Ergometrine	T48.0X1	T48.0X2	T48.0X3	T48.0X4	T48.0X5	T48.0X6
Ergonovine	T48.0X1	T48.0X2	T48.0X3	T48.0X4	T48.0X5	T48.0X6
Ergot NEC	T64.81	T64.82	T64.83	T64.84	—	—
derivative	T48.0X1	T48.0X2	T48.0X3	T48.0X4	T48.0X5	T48.0X6
medicinal (alkaloids)	T48.0X1	T48.0X2	T48.0X3	T48.0X4	T48.0X5	T48.0X6
prepared	T48.0X1	T48.0X2	T48.0X3	T48.0X4	T48.0X5	T48.0X6
Ergotamine	T46.5X1	T46.5X2	T46.5X3	T46.5X4	T46.5X5	T46.5X6
Ergotocine	T48.0X1	T48.0X2	T48.0X3	T48.0X4	T48.0X5	T48.0X6
Ergotrate	T48.0X1	T48.0X2	T48.0X3	T48.0X4	T48.0X5	T48.0X6
Eritrityl tetranitrate	T46.3X1	T46.3X2	T46.3X3	T46.3X4	T46.3X5	T46.3X6
Erythrityl tetranitrate	T46.3X1	T46.3X2	T46.3X3	T46.3X4	T46.3X5	T46.3X6
Erythrol tetranitrate	T46.3X1	T46.3X2	T46.3X3	T46.3X4	T46.3X5	T46.3X6
Erythromycin (salts)	T36.3X1	T36.3X2	T36.3X3	T36.3X4	T36.3X5	T36.3X6
ophthalmic preparation	T49.5X1	T49.5X2	T49.5X3	T49.5X4	T49.5X5	T49.5X6
topical NEC	T49.0X1	T49.0X2	T49.0X3	T49.0X4	T49.0X5	T49.0X6
Erythropoietin	T45.8X1	T45.8X2	T45.8X3	T45.8X4	T45.8X5	T45.8X6
human	T45.8X1	T45.8X2	T45.8X3	T45.8X4	T45.8X5	T45.8X6
Escin	T46.991	T46.992	T46.993	T46.994	T46.995	T46.996
Esculin	T45.2X1	T45.2X2	T45.2X3	T45.2X4	T45.2X5	T45.2X6
Esculoside	T45.2X1	T45.2X2	T45.2X3	T45.2X4	T45.2X5	T45.2X6
ESDT (ether-soluble tar distillate)	T49.1X1	T49.1X2	T49.1X3	T49.1X4	T49.1X5	T49.1X6
Eserine	T49.5X1	T49.5X2	T49.5X3	T49.5X4	T49.5X5	T49.5X6
Esflurbiprofen	T39.311	T39.312	T39.313	T39.314	T39.315	T39.316
Eskabarb	T42.3X1	T42.3X2	T42.3X3	T42.3X4	T42.3X5	T42.3X6
Eskalith	T43.8X1	T43.8X2	T43.8X3	T43.8X4	T43.8X5	T43.8X6
Esmolol	T44.7X1	T44.7X2	T44.7X3	T44.7X4	T44.7X5	T44.7X6
Estanozolol	T38.7X1	T38.7X2	T38.7X3	T38.7X4	T38.7X5	T38.7X6
Estazolam	T42.4X1	T42.4X2	T42.4X3	T42.4X4	T42.4X5	T42.4X6
Estradiol	T38.5X1	T38.5X2	T38.5X3	T38.5X4	T38.5X5	T38.5X6
with testosterone	T38.7X1	T38.7X2	T38.7X3	T38.7X4	T38.7X5	T38.7X6
benzoate	T38.5X1	T38.5X2	T38.5X3	T38.5X4	T38.5X5	T38.5X6
Estramustine	T45.1X1	T45.1X2	T45.1X3	T45.1X4	T45.1X5	T45.1X6
Estriol	T38.5X1	T38.5X2	T38.5X3	T38.5X4	T38.5X5	T38.5X6
Estrogen	T38.5X1	T38.5X2	T38.5X3	T38.5X4	T38.5X5	T38.5X6
with progesterone	T38.5X1	T38.5X2	T38.5X3	T38.5X4	T38.5X5	T38.5X6
conjugated	T38.5X1	T38.5X2	T38.5X3	T38.5X4	T38.5X5	T38.5X6
Estrone	T38.5X1	T38.5X2	T38.5X3	T38.5X4	T38.5X5	T38.5X6
Estropipate	T38.5X1	T38.5X2	T38.5X3	T38.5X4	T38.5X5	T38.5X6

Substance	External Cause (T-Code)					
	Poisoning, Accidental (Unintentional)	Poisoning, Intentional Self-Harm	Poisoning, Assault	Poisoning, Undetermined	Adverse Effect	Underdosing
Etacrynate sodium	T50.1X1	T50.1X2	T50.1X3	T50.1X4	T50.1X5	T50.1X6
Etacrynic acid	T50.1X1	T50.1X2	T50.1X3	T50.1X4	T50.1X5	T50.1X6
Etafedrine	T48.6X1	T48.6X2	T48.6X3	T48.6X4	T48.6X5	T48.6X6
Etafenone	T46.3X1	T46.3X2	T46.3X3	T46.3X4	T46.3X5	T46.3X6
Etambutol	T37.1X1	T37.1X2	T37.1X3	T37.1X4	T37.1X5	T37.1X6
Etamiphyllin	T48.6X1	T48.6X2	T48.6X3	T48.6X4	T48.6X5	T48.6X6
Etamivan	T50.7X1	T50.7X2	T50.7X3	T50.7X4	T50.7X5	T50.7X6
Etamsylate	T45.7X1	T45.7X2	T45.7X3	T45.7X4	T45.7X5	T45.7X6
Etebenecid	T50.4X1	T50.4X2	T50.4X3	T50.4X4	T50.4X5	T50.4X6
Ethacridine	T49.0X1	T49.0X2	T49.0X3	T49.0X4	T49.0X5	T49.0X6
Ethacrynic acid	T50.1X1	T50.1X2	T50.1X3	T50.1X4	T50.1X5	T50.1X6
Ethadione	T42.2X1	T42.2X2	T42.2X3	T42.2X4	T42.2X5	T42.2X6
Ethambutol	T37.1X1	T37.1X2	T37.1X3	T37.1X4	T37.1X5	T37.1X6
Ethamide	T50.2X1	T50.2X2	T50.2X3	T50.2X4	T50.2X5	T50.2X6
Ethamivan	T50.7X1	T50.7X2	T50.7X3	T50.7X4	T50.7X5	T50.7X6
Ethamsylate	T45.7X1	T45.7X2	T45.7X3	T45.7X4	T45.7X5	T45.7X6
Ethanol	T51.0X1	T51.0X2	T51.0X3	T51.0X4	—	—
beverage	T51.0X1	T51.0X2	T51.0X3	T51.0X4	—	—
Ethanolamine oleate	T46.8X1	T46.8X2	T46.8X3	T46.8X4	T46.8X5	T46.8X6
Ethaverine	T44.3X1	T44.3X2	T44.3X3	T44.3X4	T44.3X5	T44.3X6
Ethchlorvynol	T42.6X1	T42.6X2	T42.6X3	T42.6X4	T42.6X5	T42.6X6
Ethebenecid	T50.4X1	T50.4X2	T50.4X3	T50.4X4	T50.4X5	T50.4X6
Ether (vapor)	T41.0X1	T41.0X2	T41.0X3	T41.0X4	T41.0X5	T41.0X6
anesthetic	T41.0X1	T41.0X2	T41.0X3	T41.0X4	T41.0X5	T41.0X6
divinyl	T41.0X1	T41.0X2	T41.0X3	T41.0X4	T41.0X5	T41.0X6
ethyl (medicinal)	T41.0X1	T41.0X2	T41.0X3	T41.0X4	T41.0X5	T41.0X6
nonmedicinal	T52.8X1	T52.8X2	T52.8X3	T52.8X4	—	—
petroleum — *see Ligroin*						
solvent	T52.8X1	T52.8X2	T52.8X3	T52.8X4	—	—
Ethiazide	T50.2X1	T50.2X2	T50.2X3	T50.2X4	T50.2X5	T50.2X6
Ethidium chloride (vapor)	T59.891	T59.892	T59.893	T59.894	—	—
Ethinamate	T42.6X1	T42.6X2	T42.6X3	T42.6X4	T42.6X5	T42.6X6
Ethinylestradiol, ethinyloestradiol	T38.5X1	T38.5X2	T38.5X3	T38.5X4	T38.5X5	T38.5X6
with						
levonorgestrel	T38.4X1	T38.4X2	T38.4X3	T38.4X4	T38.4X5	T38.4X6
norethisterone	T38.4X1	T38.4X2	T38.4X3	T38.4X4	T38.4X5	T38.4X6
Ethiodized oil (131 I)	T50.8X1	T50.8X2	T50.8X3	T50.8X4	T50.8X5	T50.8X6
Ethion	T60.0X1	T60.0X2	T60.0X3	T60.0X4	—	—
Ethionamide	T37.1X1	T37.1X2	T37.1X3	T37.1X4	T37.1X5	T37.1X6
Ethioniamide	T37.1X1	T37.1X2	T37.1X3	T37.1X4	T37.1X5	T37.1X6
Ethisterone	T38.5X1	T38.5X2	T38.5X3	T38.5X4	T38.5X5	T38.5X6
Ethobral	T42.3X1	T42.3X2	T42.3X3	T42.3X4	T42.3X5	T42.3X6

Substance	External Cause (T-Code)					
	Poisoning, Accidental (Unintentional)	Poisoning, Intentional Self-Harm	Poisoning, Assault	Poisoning, Undetermined	Adverse Effect	Underdosing
Ethocaine (infiltration) (topical)	T41.3X1	T41.3X2	T41.3X3	T41.3X4	T41.3X5	T41.3X6
nerve block (peripheral) (plexus)	T41.3X1	T41.3X2	T41.3X3	T41.3X4	T41.3X5	T41.3X6
spinal	T41.3X1	T41.3X2	T41.3X3	T41.3X4	T41.3X5	T41.3X6
Ethoheptazine	T40.4X1	T40.4X2	T40.4X3	T40.4X4	T40.4X5	T40.4X6
Ethopropazine	T44.3X1	T44.3X2	T44.3X3	T44.3X4	T44.3X5	T44.3X6
Ethosuximide	T42.2X1	T42.2X2	T42.2X3	T42.2X4	T42.2X5	T42.2X6
Ethotoin	T42.0X1	T42.0X2	T42.0X3	T42.0X4	T42.0X5	T42.0X6
Ethoxazene	T37.91	T37.92	T37.93	T37.94	T37.95	T37.96
Ethoxazorutoside	T46.991	T46.992	T46.993	T46.994	T46.995	T46.996
2-Ethoxyethanol	T52.3X1	T52.3X2	T52.3X3	T52.3X4	—	—
Ethoxzolamide	T50.2X1	T50.2X2	T50.2X3	T50.2X4	T50.2X5	T50.2X6
Ethyl						
acetate	T52.8X1	T52.8X2	T52.8X3	T52.8X4	—	—
alcohol	T51.0X1	T51.0X2	T51.0X3	T51.0X4	—	—
beverage	T51.0X1	T51.0X2	T51.0X3	T51.0X4	—	—
aldehyde (vapor)	T59.891	T59.892	T59.893	T59.894	—	—
liquid	T52.8X1	T52.8X2	T52.8X3	T52.8X4	—	—
aminobenzoate	T41.3X1	T41.3X2	T41.3X3	T41.3X4	T41.3X5	T41.3X6
aminophenothiazine	T43.3X1	T43.3X2	T43.3X3	T43.3X4	T43.3X5	T43.3X6
benzoate	T52.8X1	T52.8X2	T52.8X3	T52.8X4	—	—
biscoumacetate	T45.511	T45.512	T45.513	T45.514	T45.515	T45.516
bromide (anesthetic)	T41.0X1	T41.0X2	T41.0X3	T41.0X4	T41.0X5	T41.0X6
carbamate	T45.1X1	T45.1X2	T45.1X3	T45.1X4	T45.1X5	T45.1X6
carbinol	T51.3X1	T51.3X2	T51.3X3	T51.3X4	—	—
carbonate	T52.8X1	T52.8X2	T52.8X3	T52.8X4	—	—
chaulmoograte	T37.1X1	T37.1X2	T37.1X3	T37.1X4	T37.1X5	T37.1X6
chloride (anesthetic)	T41.0X1	T41.0X2	T41.0X3	T41.0X4	T41.0X5	T41.0X6
anesthetic (local)	T41.3X1	T41.3X2	T41.3X3	T41.3X4	T41.3X5	T41.3X6
inhaled	T41.0X1	T41.0X2	T41.0X3	T41.0X4	T41.0X5	T41.0X6
local	T49.4X1	T49.4X2	T49.4X3	T49.4X4	T49.4X5	T49.4X6
solvent	T53.6X1	T53.6X2	T53.6X3	T53.6X4	—	—
dibunate	T48.3X1	T48.3X2	T48.3X3	T48.3X4	T48.3X5	T48.3X6
dichloroarsine (vapor)	T57.0X1	T57.0X2	T57.0X3	T57.0X4	—	—
estranol	T38.7X1	T38.7X2	T38.7X3	T38.7X4	T38.7X5	T38.7X6
ether — *see also ether*	T52.8X1	T52.8X2	T52.8X3	T52.8X4	—	—
formate NEC (solvent)	T52.0X1	T52.0X2	T52.0X3	T52.0X4	—	—
fumarate	T49.4X1	T49.4X2	T49.4X3	T49.4X4	T49.4X5	T49.4X6
hydroxyisobutyrate NEC (solvent)	T52.8X1	T52.8X2	T52.8X3	T52.8X4	—	—
iodoacetate	T59.3X1	T59.3X2	T59.3X3	T59.3X4	—	—
lactate NEC (solvent)	T52.8X1	T52.8X2	T52.8X3	T52.8X4	—	—
loflazepate	T42.4X1	T42.4X2	T42.4X3	T42.4X4	T42.4X5	T42.4X6

Substance	External Cause (T-Code)					
	Poisoning, Accidental (Unintentional)	Poisoning, Intentional Self-Harm	Poisoning, Assault	Poisoning, Undetermined	Adverse Effect	Underdosing
Ethyl *(Continued)*						
mercuric chloride	T56.1X1	T56.1X2	T56.1X3	T56.1X4	—	—
methylcarbinol	T51.8X1	T51.8X2	T51.8X3	T51.8X4	—	—
morphine	T40.2X1	T40.2X2	T40.2X3	T40.2X4	T40.2X5	T40.2X6
noradrenaline	T48.6X1	T48.6X2	T48.6X3	T48.6X4	T48.6X5	T48.6X6
oxybutyrate NEC (solvent)	T52.8X1	T52.8X2	T52.8X3	T52.8X4	—	—
Ethylene (gas)	T59.891	T59.892	T59.893	T59.894	—	—
anesthetic (general)	T41.0X1	T41.0X2	T41.0X3	T41.0X4	T41.0X5	T41.0X6
chlorohydrin	T52.8X1	T52.8X2	T52.8X3	T52.8X4	—	—
vapor	T53.6X1	T53.6X2	T53.6X3	T53.6X4	—	—
dichloride	T52.8X1	T52.8X2	T52.8X3	T52.8X4	—	—
vapor	T53.6X1	T53.6X2	T53.6X3	T53.6X4	—	—
dinitrate	T52.3X1	T52.3X2	T52.3X3	T52.3X4	—	—
glycol(s)	T52.8X1	T52.8X2	T52.8X3	T52.8X4	—	—
dinitrate	T52.3X1	T52.3X2	T52.3X3	T52.3X4	—	—
monobutyl ether	T52.3X1	T52.3X2	T52.3X3	T52.3X4	—	—
imine	T54.1X1	T54.1X2	T54.1X3	T54.1X4	—	—
oxide (fumigant) (nonmedicinal)	T59.891	T59.892	T59.893	T59.894	—	—
medicinal	T49.0X1	T49.0X2	T49.0X3	T49.0X4	T49.0X5	T49.0X6
Ethylenediamine theophylline	T48.6X1	T48.6X2	T48.6X3	T48.6X4	T48.6X5	T48.6X6
Ethylenediaminetetra-acetic acid	T50.6X1	T50.6X2	T50.6X3	T50.6X4	T50.6X5	T50.6X6
Ethylenedinitrilotetra-acetate	T50.6X1	T50.6X2	T50.6X3	T50.6X4	T50.6X5	T50.6X6
Ethylestrenol	T38.7X1	T38.7X2	T38.7X3	T38.7X4	T38.7X5	T38.7X6
Ethylhydroxycellulose	T47.4X1	T47.4X2	T47.4X3	T47.4X4	T47.4X5	T47.4X6
Ethylidene						
chloride NEC	T53.6X1	T53.6X2	T53.6X3	T53.6X4	—	—
diacetate	T60.3X1	T60.3X2	T60.3X3	T60.3X4	—	—
dicoumarin	T45.511	T45.512	T45.513	T45.514	T45.515	T45.516
dicoumarol	T45.511	T45.512	T45.513	T45.514	T45.515	T45.516
diethyl ether	T52.0X1	T52.0X2	T52.0X3	T52.0X4	—	—
Ethylmorphine	T40.2X1	T40.2X2	T40.2X3	T40.2X4	T40.2X5	T40.2X6
Ethylnorepinephrine	T48.6X1	T48.6X2	T48.6X3	T48.6X4	T48.6X5	T48.6X6
Ethylparachlorophen-oxyisobutyrate	T46.6X1	T46.6X2	T46.6X3	T46.6X4	T46.6X5	T46.6X6
Ethynodiol	T38.4X1	T38.4X2	T38.4X3	T38.4X4	T38.4X5	T38.4X6
with mestranol diacetate	T38.4X1	T38.4X2	T38.4X3	T38.4X4	T38.4X5	T38.4X6
Etidocaine	T41.3X1	T41.3X2	T41.3X3	T41.3X4	T41.3X5	T41.3X6
infiltration (subcutaneous)	T41.3X1	T41.3X2	T41.3X3	T41.3X4	T41.3X5	T41.3X6
nerve (peripheral) (plexus)	T41.3X1	T41.3X2	T41.3X3	T41.3X4	T41.3X5	T41.3X6
Etidronate	T50.991	T50.992	T50.993	T50.994	T50.995	T50.996
Etidronic acid (disodium salt)	T50.991	T50.992	T50.993	T50.994	T50.995	T50.996
Etifoxine	T42.6X1	T42.6X2	T42.6X3	T42.6X4	T42.6X5	T42.6X6

◀ New ◀ Revised ~~deleted~~ Deleted

Substance	External Cause (T-Code)					
	Poisoning, Accidental (Unintentional)	Poisoning, Intentional Self-Harm	Poisoning, Assault	Poisoning, Undetermined	Adverse Effect	Underdosing
Etilefrine	T44.4X1	T44.4X2	T44.4X3	T44.4X4	T44.4X5	T44.4X6
Etilfen	T42.3X1	T42.3X2	T42.3X3	T42.3X4	T42.3X5	T42.3X6
Etinodiol	T38.4X1	T38.4X2	T38.4X3	T38.4X4	T38.4X5	T38.4X6
Etiroxate	T46.6X1	T46.6X2	T46.6X3	T46.6X4	T46.6X5	T46.6X6
Etizolam	T42.4X1	T42.4X2	T42.4X3	T42.4X4	T42.4X5	T42.4X6
Etodolac	T39.391	T39.392	T39.393	T39.394	T39.395	T39.396
Etofamide	T37.3X1	T37.3X2	T37.3X3	T37.3X4	T37.3X5	T37.3X6
Etofibrate	T46.6X1	T46.6X2	T46.6X3	T46.6X4	T46.6X5	T46.6X6
Etofylline	T46.7X1	T46.7X2	T46.7X3	T46.7X4	T46.7X5	T46.7X6
clofibrate	T46.6X1	T46.6X2	T46.6X3	T46.6X4	T46.6X5	T46.6X6
Etoglucid	T45.1X1	T45.1X2	T45.1X3	T45.1X4	T45.1X5	T45.1X6
Etomidate	T41.1X1	T41.1X2	T41.1X3	T41.1X4	T41.1X5	T41.1X6
Etomide	T39.8X1	T39.8X2	T39.8X3	T39.8X4	T39.8X5	T39.8X6
Etomidoline	T44.3X1	T44.3X2	T44.3X3	T44.3X4	T44.3X5	T44.3X6
Etoposide	T45.1X1	T45.1X2	T45.1X3	T45.1X4	T45.1X5	T45.1X6
Etorphine	T40.2X1	T40.2X2	T40.2X3	T40.2X4	T40.2X5	T40.2X6
Etoval	T42.3X1	T42.3X2	T42.3X3	T42.3X4	T42.3X5	T42.3X6
Etozolin	T50.1X1	T50.1X2	T50.1X3	T50.1X4	T50.1X5	T50.1X6
Etretinate	T50.991	T50.992	T50.993	T50.994	T50.995	T50.996
Etryptamine	T43.691	T43.692	T43.693	T43.694	T43.695	T43.696
Etybenzatropine	T44.3X1	T44.3X2	T44.3X3	T44.3X4	T44.3X5	T44.3X6
Etynodiol	T38.4X1	T38.4X2	T38.4X3	T38.4X4	T38.4X5	T38.4X6
Eucaine	T41.3X1	T41.3X2	T41.3X3	T41.3X4	T41.3X5	T41.3X6
Eucalyptus oil	T49.7X1	T49.7X2	T49.7X3	T49.7X4	T49.7X5	T49.7X6
Eucatropine	T49.5X1	T49.5X2	T49.5X3	T49.5X4	T49.5X5	T49.5X6
Eucodal	T40.2X1	T40.2X2	T40.2X3	T40.2X4	T40.2X5	T40.2X6
Euneryl	T42.3X1	T42.3X2	T42.3X3	T42.3X4	T42.3X5	T42.3X6
Euphthalmine	T44.3X1	T44.3X2	T44.3X3	T44.3X4	T44.3X5	T44.3X6
Eurax	T49.0X1	T49.0X2	T49.0X3	T49.0X4	T49.0X5	T49.0X6
Euresol	T49.4X1	T49.4X2	T49.4X3	T49.4X4	T49.4X5	T49.4X6
Euthroid	T38.1X1	T38.1X2	T38.1X3	T38.1X4	T38.1X5	T38.1X6
Evans blue	T50.8X1	T50.8X2	T50.8X3	T50.8X4	T50.8X5	T50.8X6
Evipal	T42.3X1	T42.3X2	T42.3X3	T42.3X4	T42.3X5	T42.3X6
sodium	T41.1X1	T41.1X2	T41.1X3	T41.1X4	T41.1X5	T41.1X6
Evipan	T42.3X1	T42.3X2	T42.3X3	T42.3X4	T42.3X5	T42.3X6
sodium	T41.1X1	T41.1X2	T41.1X3	T41.1X4	T41.1X5	T41.1X6
Exalamide	T49.0X1	T49.0X2	T49.0X3	T49.0X4	T49.0X5	T49.0X6
Exalgin	T39.1X1	T39.1X2	T39.1X3	T39.1X4	T39.1X5	T39.1X6
Excipients, pharmaceutical	T50.901	T50.902	T50.903	T50.904	T50.905	T50.906
Exhaust gas (engine) (motor vehicle)	T58.01	T58.02	T58.03	T58.04	—	—
Ex-Lax (phenolphthalein)	T47.2X1	T47.2X2	T47.2X3	T47.2X4	T47.2X5	T47.2X6
Expectorant NEC	T48.4X1	T48.4X2	T48.4X3	T48.4X4	T48.4X5	T48.4X6

Substance	External Cause (T-Code)					
	Poisoning, Accidental (Unintentional)	Poisoning, Intentional Self-Harm	Poisoning, Assault	Poisoning, Undetermined	Adverse Effect	Underdosing
Extended insulin zinc suspension	T38.3X1	T38.3X2	T38.3X3	T38.3X4	T38.3X5	T38.3X6
External medications (skin) (mucous membrane)	T49.91	T49.92	T49.93	T49.94	T49.95	T49.96
dental agent	T49.7X1	T49.7X2	T49.7X3	T49.7X4	T49.7X5	T49.7X6
ENT agent	T49.6X1	T49.6X2	T49.6X3	T49.6X4	T49.6X5	T49.6X6
ophthalmic preparation	T49.5X1	T49.5X2	T49.5X3	T49.5X4	T49.5X5	T49.5X6
specified NEC	T49.8X1	T49.8X2	T49.8X3	T49.8X4	T49.8X5	T49.8X6
Extrapyramidal antagonist NEC	T44.3X1	T44.3X2	T44.3X3	T44.3X4	T44.3X5	T44.3X6
Eye agents (anti-infective)	T49.5X1	T49.5X2	T49.5X3	T49.5X4	T49.5X5	T49.5X6
Eye drug NEC	T49.5X1	T49.5X2	T49.5X3	T49.5X4	T49.5X5	T49.5X6
F						
FAC (fluorouracil + doxorubicin + cyclophosphamide)	T45.1X1	T45.1X2	T45.1X3	T45.1X4	T45.1X5	T45.1X6
Factor						
I (fibrinogen)	T45.8X1	T45.8X2	T45.8X3	T45.8X4	T45.8X5	T45.8X6
III (thromboplastin)	T45.8X1	T45.8X2	T45.8X3	T45.8X4	T45.8X5	T45.8X6
VIII (antihemophilic Factor) (Concentrate)	T45.8X1	T45.8X2	T45.8X3	T45.8X4	T45.8X5	T45.8X6
IX complex	T45.7X1	T45.7X2	T45.7X3	T45.7X4	T45.7X5	T45.7X6
human	T45.8X1	T45.8X2	T45.8X3	T45.8X4	T45.8X5	T45.8X6
Famotidine	T47.0X1	T47.0X2	T47.0X3	T47.0X4	T47.0X5	T47.0X6
Fat suspension, intravenous	T50.991	T50.992	T50.993	T50.994	T50.995	T50.996
Fazadinium bromide	T48.1X1	T48.1X2	T48.1X3	T48.1X4	T48.1X5	T48.1X6
Febarbamate	T42.3X1	T42.3X2	T42.3X3	T42.3X4	T42.3X5	T42.3X6
Fecal softener	T47.4X1	T47.4X2	T47.4X3	T47.4X4	T47.4X5	T47.4X6
Fedrilate	T48.3X1	T48.3X2	T48.3X3	T48.3X4	T48.3X5	T48.3X6
Felodipine	T46.1X1	T46.1X2	T46.1X3	T46.1X4	T46.1X5	T46.1X6
Felypressin	T38.891	T38.892	T38.893	T38.894	T38.895	T38.896
Femoxetine	T43.221	T43.222	T43.223	T43.224	T43.225	T43.226
Fenalcomine	T46.3X1	T46.3X2	T46.3X3	T46.3X4	T46.3X5	T46.3X6
Fenamisal	T37.1X1	T37.1X2	T37.1X3	T37.1X4	T37.1X5	T37.1X6
Fenazone	T39.2X1	T39.2X2	T39.2X3	T39.2X4	T39.2X5	T39.2X6
Fenbendazole	T37.4X1	T37.4X2	T37.4X3	T37.4X4	T37.4X5	T37.4X6
Fenbutrazate	T50.5X1	T50.5X2	T50.5X3	T50.5X4	T50.5X5	T50.5X6
Fencamfamine	T43.691	T43.692	T43.693	T43.694	T43.695	T43.696
Fendiline	T46.1X1	T46.1X2	T46.1X3	T46.1X4	T46.1X5	T46.1X6
Fenetylline	T43.691	T43.692	T43.693	T43.694	T43.695	T43.696
Fenflumizole	T39.391	T39.392	T39.393	T39.394	T39.395	T39.396
Fenfluramine	T50.5X1	T50.5X2	T50.5X3	T50.5X4	T50.5X5	T50.5X6
Fenobarbital	T42.3X1	T42.3X2	T42.3X3	T42.3X4	T42.3X5	T42.3X6
Fenofibrate	T46.6X1	T46.6X2	T46.6X3	T46.6X4	T46.6X5	T46.6X6
Fenoprofen	T39.311	T39.312	T39.313	T39.314	T39.315	T39.316
Fenoterol	T48.6X1	T48.6X2	T48.6X3	T48.6X4	T48.6X5	T48.6X6

Substance	External Cause (T-Code)					
	Poisoning, Accidental (Unintentional)	Poisoning, Intentional Self-Harm	Poisoning, Assault	Poisoning, Undetermined	Adverse Effect	Underdosing
Fenoverine	T44.3X1	T44.3X2	T44.3X3	T44.3X4	T44.3X5	T44.3X6
Fenoxazoline	T48.5X1	T48.5X2	T48.5X3	T48.5X4	T48.5X5	T48.5X6
Fenproporex	T50.5X1	T50.5X2	T50.5X3	T50.5X4	T50.5X5	T50.5X6
Fenquizone	T50.2X1	T50.2X2	T50.2X3	T50.2X4	T50.2X5	T50.2X6
Fentanyl	T40.4X1	T40.4X2	T40.4X3	T40.4X4	T40.4X5	T40.4X6
Fentazin	T43.3X1	T43.3X2	T43.3X3	T43.3X4	T43.3X5	T43.3X6
Fenthion	T60.0X1	T60.0X2	T60.0X3	T60.0X4	—	—
Fenticlor	T49.0X1	T49.0X2	T49.0X3	T49.0X4	T49.0X5	T49.0X6
Fenylbutazone	T39.2X1	T39.2X2	T39.2X3	T39.2X4	T39.2X5	T39.2X6
Feprazone	T39.2X1	T39.2X2	T39.2X3	T39.2X4	T39.2X5	T39.2X6
Fer de lance (bite) (venom)	T63.061	T63.062	T63.063	T63.064	—	—
Ferric—*see also Iron*						
chloride	T45.4X1	T45.4X2	T45.4X3	T45.4X4	T45.4X5	T45.4X6
citrate	T45.4X1	T45.4X2	T45.4X3	T45.4X4	T45.4X5	T45.4X6
hydroxide						
colloidal	T45.4X1	T45.4X2	T45.4X3	T45.4X4	T45.4X5	T45.4X6
polymaltose	T45.4X1	T45.4X2	T45.4X3	T45.4X4	T45.4X5	T45.4X6
pyrophosphate	T45.4X1	T45.4X2	T45.4X3	T45.4X4	T45.4X5	T45.4X6
Ferritin	T45.4X1	T45.4X2	T45.4X3	T45.4X4	T45.4X5	T45.4X6
Ferrocholinate	T45.4X1	T45.4X2	T45.4X3	T45.4X4	T45.4X5	T45.4X6
Ferrodextrane	T45.4X1	T45.4X2	T45.4X3	T45.4X4	T45.4X5	T45.4X6
Ferropolimaler	T45.4X1	T45.4X2	T45.4X3	T45.4X4	T45.4X5	T45.4X6
Ferrous—*see also Iron*						
phosphate	T45.4X1	T45.4X2	T45.4X3	T45.4X4	T45.4X5	T45.4X6
salt	T45.4X1	T45.4X2	T45.4X3	T45.4X4	T45.4X5	T45.4X6
with folic acid	T45.4X1	T45.4X2	T45.4X3	T45.4X4	T45.4X5	T45.4X6
Ferrous fumerate, gluconate, lactate, salt NEC, sulfate (medicinal)	T45.4X1	T45.4X2	T45.4X3	T45.4X4	T45.4X5	T45.4X6
Ferrovanadium (fumes)	T59.891	T59.892	T59.893	T59.894	—	—
Ferrum—*see Iron*						
Fertilizers NEC	T65.891	T65.892	T65.893	T65.894	—	—
with herbicide mixture	T60.3X1	T60.3X2	T60.3X3	T60.3X4	—	—
Fetoxilate	T47.6X1	T47.6X2	T47.6X3	T47.6X4	T47.6X5	T47.6X6
Fiber, dietary	T47.4X1	T47.4X2	T47.4X3	T47.4X4	T47.4X5	T47.4X6
Fibrinogen (human)	T45.8X1	T45.8X2	T45.8X3	T45.8X4	T45.8X5	T45.8X6
Fibrinolysin (human)	T45.691	T45.692	T45.693	T45.694	T45.695	T45.696
Fibrinolysis						
affecting drug	T45.601	T45.602	T45.603	T45.604	T45.605	T45.606
inhibitor NEC	T45.621	T45.622	T45.623	T45.624	T45.625	T45.626
Fibrinolytic drug	T45.611	T45.612	T45.613	T45.614	T45.615	T45.616
Filix mas	T37.4X1	T37.4X2	T37.4X3	T37.4X4	T37.4X5	T37.4X6
Filtering cream	T49.3X1	T49.3X2	T49.3X3	T49.3X4	T49.3X5	T49.3X6

Substance	External Cause (T-Code)					
	Poisoning, Accidental (Unintentional)	Poisoning, Intentional Self-Harm	Poisoning, Assault	Poisoning, Undetermined	Adverse Effect	Underdosing
Fiorinal	T39.011	T39.012	T39.013	T39.014	T39.015	T39.016
Firedamp	T59.891	T59.892	T59.893	T59.894	—	—
Fish, noxious, nonbacterial	T61.91	T61.92	T61.93	T61.94	—	—
ciguatera	T61.01	T61.02	T61.03	T61.04	—	—
scombroid	T61.11	T61.12	T61.13	T61.14	—	—
shell	T61.781	T61.782	T61.783	T61.784	—	—
specified NEC	T61.771	T61.772	T61.773	T61.774	—	—
Flagyl	T37.3X1	T37.3X2	T37.3X3	T37.3X4	T37.3X5	T37.3X6
Flavine adenine dinucleotide	T45.2X1	T45.2X2	T45.2X3	T45.2X4	T45.2X5	T45.2X6
Flavodic acid	T46.991	T46.992	T46.993	T46.994	T46.995	T46.996
Flavoxate	T44.3X1	T44.3X2	T44.3X3	T44.3X4	T44.3X5	T44.3X6
Flaxedil	T48.1X1	T48.1X2	T48.1X3	T48.1X4	T48.1X5	T48.1X6
Flaxseed (medicinal)	T49.3X1	T49.3X2	T49.3X3	T49.3X4	T49.3X5	T49.3X6
Flecainide	T46.2X1	T46.2X2	T46.2X3	T46.2X4	T46.2X5	T46.2X6
Fleroxacin	T36.8X1	T36.8X2	T36.8X3	T36.8X4	T36.8X5	T36.8X6
Floctafenine	T39.8X1	T39.8X2	T39.8X3	T39.8X4	T39.8X5	T39.8X6
Flomax	T44.6X1	T44.6X2	T44.6X3	T44.6X4	T44.6X5	T44.6X6
Flomoxef	T36.1X1	T36.1X2	T36.1X3	T36.1X4	T36.1X5	T36.1X6
Flopropione	T44.3X1	T44.3X2	T44.3X3	T44.3X4	T44.3X5	T44.3X6
Florantyrone	T47.5X1	T47.5X2	T47.5X3	T47.5X4	T47.5X5	T47.5X6
Floraquin	T37.8X1	T37.8X2	T37.8X3	T37.8X4	T37.8X5	T37.8X6
Florinef	T38.0X1	T38.0X2	T38.0X3	T38.0X4	T38.0X5	T38.0X6
ENT agent	T49.6X1	T49.6X2	T49.6X3	T49.6X4	T49.6X5	T49.6X6
ophthalmic preparation	T49.5X1	T49.5X2	T49.5X3	T49.5X4	T49.5X5	T49.5X6
topical NEC	T49.0X1	T49.0X2	T49.0X3	T49.0X4	T49.0X5	T49.0X6
Flowers of sulfur	T49.4X1	T49.4X2	T49.4X3	T49.4X4	T49.4X5	T49.4X6
Floxuridine	T45.1X1	T45.1X2	T45.1X3	T45.1X4	T45.1X5	T45.1X6
Fluanisone	T43.4X1	T43.4X2	T43.4X3	T43.4X4	T43.4X5	T43.4X6
Flubendazole	T37.4X1	T37.4X2	T37.4X3	T37.4X4	T37.4X5	T37.4X6
Fluclorolone acetonide	T49.0X1	T49.0X2	T49.0X3	T49.0X4	T49.0X5	T49.0X6
Flucloxacillin	T36.0X1	T36.0X2	T36.0X3	T36.0X4	T36.0X5	T36.0X6
Fluconazole	T37.8X1	T37.8X2	T37.8X3	T37.8X4	T37.8X5	T37.8X6
Flucytosine	T37.8X1	T37.8X2	T37.8X3	T37.8X4	T37.8X5	T37.8X6
Fludeoxyglucose (18F)	T50.8X1	T50.8X2	T50.8X3	T50.8X4	T50.8X5	T50.8X6
Fludiazepam	T42.4X1	T42.4X2	T42.4X3	T42.4X4	T42.4X5	T42.4X6
Fludrocortisone	T50.0X1	T50.0X2	T50.0X3	T50.0X4	T50.0X5	T50.0X6
ENT agent	T49.6X1	T49.6X2	T49.6X3	T49.6X4	T49.6X5	T49.6X6
ophthalmic preparation	T49.5X1	T49.5X2	T49.5X3	T49.5X4	T49.5X5	T49.5X6
topical NEC	T49.0X1	T49.0X2	T49.0X3	T49.0X4	T49.0X5	T49.0X6
Fludroxycortide	T49.0X1	T49.0X2	T49.0X3	T49.0X4	T49.0X5	T49.0X6
Flufenamic acid	T39.391	T39.392	T39.393	T39.394	T39.395	T39.396
Fluindione	T45.511	T45.512	T45.513	T45.514	T45.515	T45.516

Substance	External Cause (T-Code)					
	Poisoning, Accidental (Unintentional)	Poisoning, Intentional Self-Harm	Poisoning, Assault	Poisoning, Undetermined	Adverse Effect	Underdosing
Flumequine	T37.8X1	T37.8X2	T37.8X3	T37.8X4	T37.8X5	T37.8X6
Flumethasone	T49.0X1	T49.0X2	T49.0X3	T49.0X4	T49.0X5	T49.0X6
Flumethiazide	T50.2X1	T50.2X2	T50.2X3	T50.2X4	T50.2X5	T50.2X6
Flumidin	T37.5X1	T37.5X2	T37.5X3	T37.5X4	T37.5X5	T37.5X6
Flunarizine	T46.7X1	T46.7X2	T46.7X3	T46.7X4	T46.7X5	T46.7X6
Flunidazole	T37.8X1	T37.8X2	T37.8X3	T37.8X4	T37.8X5	T37.8X6
Flunisolide	T48.6X1	T48.6X2	T48.6X3	T48.6X4	T48.6X5	T48.6X6
Flunitrazepam	T42.4X1	T42.4X2	T42.4X3	T42.4X4	T42.4X5	T42.4X6
Fluocinolone (acetonide)	T49.0X1	T49.0X2	T49.0X3	T49.0X4	T49.0X5	T49.0X6
Fluocinonide	T49.0X1	T49.0X2	T49.0X3	T49.0X4	T49.0X5	T49.0X6
Fluocortin (butyl)	T49.0X1	T49.0X2	T49.0X3	T49.0X4	T49.0X5	T49.0X6
Fluocortolone	T49.0X1	T49.0X2	T49.0X3	T49.0X4	T49.0X5	T49.0X6
Fluohydrocortisone	T38.0X1	T38.0X2	T38.0X3	T38.0X4	T38.0X5	T38.0X6
ENT agent	T49.6X1	T49.6X2	T49.6X3	T49.6X4	T49.6X5	T49.6X6
ophthalmic preparation	T49.5X1	T49.5X2	T49.5X3	T49.5X4	T49.5X5	T49.5X6
topical NEC	T49.0X1	T49.0X2	T49.0X3	T49.0X4	T49.0X5	T49.0X6
Fluonid	T49.0X1	T49.0X2	T49.0X3	T49.0X4	T49.0X5	T49.0X6
Fluopromazine	T43.3X1	T43.3X2	T43.3X3	T43.3X4	T43.3X5	T43.3X6
Fluoroacetate	T60.8X1	T60.8X2	T60.8X3	T60.8X4	—	—
Fluorescein	T50.8X1	T50.8X2	T50.8X3	T50.8X4	T50.8X5	T50.8X6
Fluorhydrocortisone	T50.0X1	T50.0X2	T50.0X3	T50.0X4	T50.0X5	T50.0X6
Fluoride (nonmedicinal) (pesticide) (sodium) NEC	T60.8X1	T60.8X2	T60.8X3	T60.8X4	—	—
hydrogen — *see Hydrofluoric acid*						
medicinal NEC	T50.991	T50.992	T50.993	T50.994	T50.995	T50.996
dental use	T49.7X1	T49.7X2	T49.7X3	T49.7X4	T49.7X5	T49.7X6
not pesticide NEC	T54.91	T54.92	T54.93	T54.94	—	—
stannous	T49.7X1	T49.7X2	T49.7X3	T49.7X4	T49.7X5	T49.7X6
Fluorinated corticosteroids	T38.0X1	T38.0X2	T38.0X3	T38.0X4	T38.0X5	T38.0X6
Fluorine (gas)	T59.5X1	T59.5X2	T59.5X3	T59.5X4	—	—
salt — *see Fluoride(s)*						
Fluoristan	T49.7X1	T49.7X2	T49.7X3	T49.7X4	T49.7X5	T49.7X6
Fluormetholone	T49.0X1	T49.0X2	T49.0X3	T49.0X4	T49.0X5	T49.0X6
Fluoroacetate	T60.8X1	T60.8X2	T60.8X3	T60.8X4	—	—
Fluorocarbon monomer	T53.6X1	T53.6X2	T53.6X3	T53.6X4	—	—
Fluorocytosine	T37.8X1	T37.8X2	T37.8X3	T37.8X4	T37.8X5	T37.8X6
Fluorodeoxyuridine	T45.1X1	T45.1X2	T45.1X3	T45.1X4	T45.1X5	T45.1X6
Fluorometholone	T49.0X1	T49.0X2	T49.0X3	T49.0X4	T49.0X5	T49.0X6
ophthalmic preparation	T49.5X1	T49.5X2	T49.5X3	T49.5X4	T49.5X5	T49.5X6
Fluorophosphate insecticide	T60.0X1	T60.0X2	T60.0X3	T60.0X4	—	—
Fluorosol	T46.3X1	T46.3X2	T46.3X3	T46.3X4	T46.3X5	T46.3X6
Fluorouracil	T45.1X1	T45.1X2	T45.1X3	T45.1X4	T45.1X5	T45.1X6

Substance	External Cause (T-Code)					
	Poisoning, Accidental (Unintentional)	Poisoning, Intentional Self-Harm	Poisoning, Assault	Poisoning, Undetermined	Adverse Effect	Underdosing
Fluorphenylalanine	T49.5X1	T49.5X2	T49.5X3	T49.5X4	T49.5X5	T49.5X6
Fluothane	T41.0X1	T41.0X2	T41.0X3	T41.0X4	T41.0X5	T41.0X6
Fluoxetine	T43.221	T43.222	T43.223	T43.224	T43.225	T43.226
Fluoxymesterone	T38.7X1	T38.7X2	T38.7X3	T38.7X4	T38.7X5	T38.7X6
Flupenthixol	T43.4X1	T43.4X2	T43.4X3	T43.4X4	T43.4X5	T43.4X6
Flupentixol	T43.4X1	T43.4X2	T43.4X3	T43.4X4	T43.4X5	T43.4X6
Fluphenazine	T43.3X1	T43.3X2	T43.3X3	T43.3X4	T43.3X5	T43.3X6
Fluprednidene	T49.0X1	T49.0X2	T49.0X3	T49.0X4	T49.0X5	T49.0X6
Fluprednisolone	T38.0X1	T38.0X2	T38.0X3	T38.0X4	T38.0X5	T38.0X6
Fluradoline	T39.8X1	T39.8X2	T39.8X3	T39.8X4	T39.8X5	T39.8X6
Flurandrenolide	T49.0X1	T49.0X2	T49.0X3	T49.0X4	T49.0X5	T49.0X6
Flurandrenolone	T49.0X1	T49.0X2	T49.0X3	T49.0X4	T49.0X5	T49.0X6
Flurazepam	T42.4X1	T42.4X2	T42.4X3	T42.4X4	T42.4X5	T42.4X6
Flurbiprofen	T39.311	T39.312	T39.313	T39.314	T39.315	T39.316
Flurobate	T49.0X1	T49.0X2	T49.0X3	T49.0X4	T49.0X5	T49.0X6
Flurotyl	T43.291	T43.292	T43.293	T43.294	T43.295	T43.296
Fluroxene	T41.0X1	T41.0X2	T41.0X3	T41.0X4	T41.0X5	T41.0X6
Fluspirilene	T43.591	T43.592	T43.593	T43.594	T43.595	T43.596
Flutamide	T38.6X1	T38.6X2	T38.6X3	T38.6X4	T38.6X5	T38.6X6
Flutazolam	T42.4X1	T42.4X2	T42.4X3	T42.4X4	T42.4X5	T42.4X6
Fluticasone propionate	T49.1X1	T49.1X2	T49.1X3	T49.1X4	T49.1X5	T49.1X6
Flutoprazepam	T42.4X1	T42.4X2	T42.4X3	T42.4X4	T42.4X5	T42.4X6
Flutropium bromide	T48.6X1	T48.6X2	T48.6X3	T48.6X4	T48.6X5	T48.6X6
Fluvoxamine	T43.221	T43.222	T43.223	T43.224	T43.225	T43.226
Folacin	T45.8X1	T45.8X2	T45.8X3	T45.8X4	T45.8X5	T45.8X6
Folic acid	T45.8X1	T45.8X2	T45.8X3	T45.8X4	T45.8X5	T45.8X6
with ferrous salt	T45.2X1	T45.2X2	T45.2X3	T45.2X4	T45.2X5	T45.2X6
antagonist	T45.1X1	T45.1X2	T45.1X3	T45.1X4	T45.1X5	T45.1X6
Folinic acid	T45.8X1	T45.8X2	T45.8X3	T45.8X4	T45.8X5	T45.8X6
Folium stramoniae	T48.6X1	T48.6X2	T48.6X3	T48.6X4	T48.6X5	T48.6X6
Follicle-stimulating hormone, human	T38.811	T38.812	T38.813	T38.814	T38.815	T38.816
Folpet	T60.3X1	T60.3X2	T60.3X3	T60.3X4	—	—
Fominoben	T48.3X1	T48.3X2	T48.3X3	T48.3X4	T48.3X5	T48.3X6
Food, foodstuffs, noxious, nonbacterial, NEC	T62.91	T62.92	T62.93	T62.94	—	—
berries	T62.1X1	T62.1X2	T62.1X3	T62.1X4	—	—
fish — *see also Fish*	T61.91	T61.92	T61.93	T61.94	—	—
mushrooms	T62.0X1	T62.0X2	T62.0X3	T62.0X4	—	—
plants	T62.2X1	T62.2X2	T62.2X3	T62.2X4	—	—
seafood	T61.91	T61.92	T61.93	T61.94	—	—
specified NEC	T61.8X1	T61.8X2	T61.8X3	T61.8X4	—	—
seeds	T62.2X1	T62.2X2	T62.2X3	T62.2X4	—	—

Substance	External Cause (T-Code)					
	Poisoning, Accidental (Unintentional)	Poisoning, Intentional Self-Harm	Poisoning, Assault	Poisoning, Undetermined	Adverse Effect	Underdosing
Food, foodstuffs, noxious, nonbacterial, NEC *(Continued)*						
shellfish	T61.781	T61.782	T61.783	T61.784	—	—
specified NEC	T62.8X1	T62.8X2	T62.8X3	T62.8X4	—	—
Fool's parsley	T62.2X1	T62.2X2	T62.2X3	T62.2X4	—	—
Formaldehyde (solution), gas or vapor	T59.2X1	T59.2X2	T59.2X3	T59.2X4	—	—
fungicide	T60.3X1	T60.3X2	T60.3X3	T60.3X4	—	—
Formalin	T59.2X1	T59.2X2	T59.2X3	T59.2X4	—	—
fungicide	T60.3X1	T60.3X2	T60.3X3	T60.3X4	—	—
vapor	T59.2X1	T59.2X2	T59.2X3	T59.2X4	—	—
Formic acid	T54.2X1	T54.2X2	T54.2X3	T54.2X4	—	—
vapor	T59.891	T59.892	T59.893	T59.894	—	—
Foscarnet sodium	T37.5X1	T37.5X2	T37.5X3	T37.5X4	T37.5X5	T37.5X6
Fosfestrol	T38.5X1	T38.5X2	T38.5X3	T38.5X4	T38.5X5	T38.5X6
Fosfomycin	T36.8X1	T36.8X2	T36.8X3	T36.8X4	T36.8X5	T36.8X6
Fosfonet sodium	T37.5X1	T37.5X2	T37.5X3	T37.5X4	T37.5X5	T37.5X6
Fosinopril	T46.4X1	T46.4X2	T46.4X3	T46.4X4	T46.4X5	T46.4X6
sodium	T46.4X1	T46.4X2	T46.4X3	T46.4X4	T46.4X5	T46.4X6
Fowler's solution	T57.0X1	T57.0X2	T57.0X3	T57.0X4	—	—
Foxglove	T62.2X1	T62.2X2	T62.2X3	T62.2X4	—	—
Framycetin	T36.5X1	T36.5X2	T36.5X3	T36.5X4	T36.5X5	T36.5X6
Frangula	T47.2X1	T47.2X2	T47.2X3	T47.2X4	T47.2X5	T47.2X6
extract	T47.2X1	T47.2X2	T47.2X3	T47.2X4	T47.2X5	T47.2X6
Frei antigen	T50.8X1	T50.8X2	T50.8X3	T50.8X4	T50.8X5	T50.8X6
Freon	T53.5X1	T53.5X2	T53.5X3	T53.5X4	—	—
Fructose	T50.3X1	T50.3X2	T50.3X3	T50.3X4	T50.3X5	T50.3X6
Frusemide	T50.1X1	T50.1X2	T50.1X3	T50.1X4	T50.1X5	T50.1X6
FSH	T38.811	T38.812	T38.813	T38.814	T38.815	T38.816
Ftorafur	T45.1X1	T45.1X2	T45.1X3	T45.1X4	T45.1X5	T45.1X6
Fuel						
automobile	T52.0X1	T52.0X2	T52.0X3	T52.0X4	—	—
exhaust gas, not in transit	T58.01	T58.02	T58.03	T58.04	—	—
vapor NEC	T52.0X1	T52.0X2	T52.0X3	T52.0X4	—	—
gas (domestic use) — *see also Carbon, monoxide, fuel, utility*	T59.891	T59.892	T59.893	T59.894	—	—
utility	T59.891	T59.892	T59.893	T59.894	—	—
in mobile container	T59.891	T59.892	T59.893	T59.894	—	—
incomplete combustion of — *see Carbon, monoxide, fuel, utility*						
piped (natural)	T59.891	T59.892	T59.893	T59.894	—	—
industrial, incomplete combustion	T58.8X1	T58.8X2	T58.8X3	T58.8X4	—	—

Substance	External Cause (T-Code)					
	Poisoning, Accidental (Unintentional)	Poisoning, Intentional Self-Harm	Poisoning, Assault	Poisoning, Undetermined	Adverse Effect	Underdosing
Fugillin	T36.8X1	T36.8X2	T36.8X3	T36.8X4	T36.8X5	T36.8X6
Fulminate of mercury	T56.1X1	T56.1X2	T56.1X3	T56.1X4	—	—
Fulvicin	T36.7X1	T36.7X2	T36.7X3	T36.7X4	T36.7X5	T36.7X6
Fumadil	T36.8X1	T36.8X2	T36.8X3	T36.8X4	T36.8X5	T36.8X6
Fumagillin	T36.8X1	T36.8X2	T36.8X3	T36.8X4	T36.8X5	T36.8X6
Fumaric acid	T49.4X1	T49.4X2	T49.4X3	T49.4X4	T49.4X5	T49.4X6
Fumes (from)	T59.91	T59.92	T59.93	T59.94	—	—
carbon monoxide — *see Carbon, monoxide*						
charcoal (domestic use) — *see Charcoal, fumes*						
chloroform — *see Chloroform*						
coke (in domestic stoves, fireplaces) — *see Coke, fumes*						
corrosive NEC	T54.91	T54.92	T54.93	T54.94	—	—
ether — *see ether*						
freons	T53.5X1	T53.5X2	T53.5X3	T53.5X4	—	—
hydrocarbons	T59.891	T59.892	T59.893	T59.894	—	—
petroleum (liquefied)	T59.891	T59.892	T59.893	T59.894	—	—
distributed through pipes (pure or mixed with air)	T59.891	T59.892	T59.893	T59.894	—	—
lead — *see lead*						
metal — *see Metals, or the specified metal*						
nitrogen dioxide	T59.0X1	T59.0X2	T59.0X3	T59.0X4	—	—
pesticides — *see Pesticides*						
petroleum (liquefied)	T59.891	T59.892	T59.893	T59.894	—	—
distributed through pipes (pure or mixed with air)	T59.891	T59.892	T59.893	T59.894	—	—
polyester	T59.891	T59.892	T59.893	T59.894	—	—
specified source NEC — *see also substance specified*	T59.891	T59.892	T59.893	T59.894	—	—
sulfur dioxide	T59.1X1	T59.1X2	T59.1X3	T59.1X4	—	—
Fumigant NEC	T60.91	T60.92	T60.93	T60.94	—	—
Fungi, noxious, used as food	T62.0X1	T62.0X2	T62.0X3	T62.0X4	—	—
Fungicide NEC (nonmedicinal)	T60.3X1	T60.3X2	T60.3X3	T60.3X4	—	—
Fungizone	T36.7X1	T36.7X2	T36.7X3	T36.7X4	T36.7X5	T36.7X6
topical	T49.0X1	T49.0X2	T49.0X3	T49.0X4	T49.0X5	T49.0X6
Furacin	T49.0X1	T49.0X2	T49.0X3	T49.0X4	T49.0X5	T49.0X6
Furadantin	T37.91	T37.92	T37.93	T37.94	T37.95	T37.96
Furazolidone	T37.8X1	T37.8X2	T37.8X3	T37.8X4	T37.8X5	T37.8X6
Furazolium chloride	T49.0X1	T49.0X2	T49.0X3	T49.0X4	T49.0X5	T49.0X6
Furfural	T52.8X1	T52.8X2	T52.8X3	T52.8X4	—	—

Substance	External Cause (T-Code)					
	Poisoning, Accidental (Unintentional)	Poisoning, Intentional Self-Harm	Poisoning, Assault	Poisoning, Undetermined	Adverse Effect	Underdosing
Furnace (coal burning) (domestic), gas from industrial	T58.2X1	T58.2X2	T58.2X3	T58.2X4	—	—
industrial	T58.8X1	T58.8X2	T58.8X3	T58.8X4	—	—
Furniture polish	T65.891	T65.892	T65.893	T65.894	—	—
Furosemide	T50.1X1	T50.1X2	T50.1X3	T50.1X4	T50.1X5	T50.1X6
Furoxone	T37.91	T37.92	T37.93	T37.94	T37.95	T37.96
Fursultiamine	T45.2X1	T45.2X2	T45.2X3	T45.2X4	T45.2X5	T45.2X6
Fusafungine	T36.8X1	T36.8X2	T36.8X3	T36.8X4	T36.8X5	T36.8X6
Fusel oil (any) (amyl) (butyl) (propyl), vapor	T51.3X1	T51.3X2	T51.3X3	T51.3X4	—	—
Fusidate (ethanolamine) (sodium)	T36.8X1	T36.8X2	T36.8X3	T36.8X4	T36.8X5	T36.8X6
Fusidic acid	T36.8X1	T36.8X2	T36.8X3	T36.8X4	T36.8X5	T36.8X6
Fytic acid, nonasodium	T50.6X1	T50.6X2	T50.6X3	T50.6X4	T50.6X5	T50.6X6
G						
GABA	T43.8X1	T43.8X2	T43.8X3	T43.8X4	T43.8X5	T43.8X6
Gadopentetic acid	T50.8X1	T50.8X2	T50.8X3	T50.8X4	T50.8X5	T50.8X6
Galactose	T50.3X1	T50.3X2	T50.3X3	T50.3X4	T50.3X5	T50.3X6
b-Galactosidase	T47.5X1	T47.5X2	T47.5X3	T47.5X4	T47.5X5	T47.5X6
Galantamine	T44.0X1	T44.0X2	T44.0X3	T44.0X4	T44.0X5	T44.0X6
Gallamine (triethiodide)	T48.1X1	T48.1X2	T48.1X3	T48.1X4	T48.1X5	T48.1X6
Gallium citrate	T50.991	T50.992	T50.993	T50.994	T50.995	T50.996
Gallopamil	T46.1X1	T46.1X2	T46.1X3	T46.1X4	T46.1X5	T46.1X6
Gamboge	T47.2X1	T47.2X2	T47.2X3	T47.2X4	T47.2X5	T47.2X6
Gamimune	T50.Z11	T50.Z12	T50.Z13	T50.Z14	T50.Z15	T50.Z16
Gamma-aminobutyric acid	T43.8X1	T43.8X2	T43.8X3	T43.8X4	T43.8X5	T43.8X6
Gamma-benzene hexachloride (medicinal)	T49.0X1	T49.0X2	T49.0X3	T49.0X4	T49.0X5	T49.0X6
nonmedicinal, vapor	T53.6X1	T53.6X2	T53.6X3	T53.6X4	—	—
Gamma-BHC (medicinal) — *see also Gamma-benzene hexachloride*	T49.0X1	T49.0X2	T49.0X3	T49.0X4	T49.0X5	T49.0X6
Gamma globulin	T50.Z11	T50.Z12	T50.Z13	T50.Z14	T50.Z15	T50.Z16
Gamulin	T50.Z11	T50.Z12	T50.Z13	T50.Z14	T50.Z15	T50.Z16
Ganciclovir (sodium)	T37.5X1	T37.5X2	T37.5X3	T37.5X4	T37.5X5	T37.5X6
Ganglionic blocking drug NEC	T44.2X1	T44.2X2	T44.2X3	T44.2X4	T44.2X5	T44.2X6
specified NEC	T44.2X1	T44.2X2	T44.2X3	T44.2X4	T44.2X5	T44.2X6
Ganja	T40.7X1	T40.7X2	T40.7X3	T40.7X4	T40.7X5	T40.7X6
Garamycin	T36.5X1	T36.5X2	T36.5X3	T36.5X4	T36.5X5	T36.5X6
ophthalmic preparation	T49.5X1	T49.5X2	T49.5X3	T49.5X4	T49.5X5	T49.5X6
topical NEC	T49.0X1	T49.0X2	T49.0X3	T49.0X4	T49.0X5	T49.0X6
Gardenal	T42.3X1	T42.3X2	T42.3X3	T42.3X4	T42.3X5	T42.3X6
Gardepanyl	T42.3X1	T42.3X2	T42.3X3	T42.3X4	T42.3X5	T42.3X6

Substance	External Cause (T-Code)					
	Poisoning, Accidental (Unintentional)	Poisoning, Intentional Self-Harm	Poisoning, Assault	Poisoning, Undetermined	Adverse Effect	Underdosing
Gas	T59.91	T59.92	T59.93	T59.94	—	—
acetylene	T59.891	T59.892	T59.893	T59.894	—	—
incomplete combustion of	T58.11	T58.12	T58.13	T58.14	—	—
air contaminants, source or type not specified	T59.91	T59.92	T59.93	T59.94	—	—
anesthetic	T41.0X1	T41.0X2	T41.0X3	T41.0X4	T41.0X5	T41.0X6
blast furnace	T58.8X1	T58.8X2	T58.8X3	T58.8X4	—	—
butane — *see butane*						
carbon monoxide — *see Carbon, monoxide*						
chlorine	T59.4X1	T59.4X2	T59.4X3	T59.4X4	—	—
coal	T58.2X1	T58.2X2	T58.2X3	T58.2X4	—	—
cyanide	T57.3X1	T57.3X2	T57.3X3	T57.3X4	—	—
dicyanogen	T65.0X1	T65.0X2	T65.0X3	T65.0X4	—	—
domestic — *see Domestic gas*	T57.91	T57.92	T57.93	T57.94	—	—
exhaust	T57.91	T57.92	T57.93	T57.94	—	—
from utility (for cooking, heating, or lighting) (after combustion) — *see Carbon, monoxide, fuel, utility*						
prior to combustion	T59.891	T59.892	T59.893	T59.894	—	—
from wood or coal-burning stove or fireplace	T57.91	T57.92	T57.93	T57.94	—	—
fuel (domestic use) (after combustion) — *see also Carbon, monoxide, fuel*	T57.91	T57.92	T57.93	T57.94	—	—
industrial use	T58.8X1	T58.8X2	T58.8X3	T58.8X4	—	—
prior to combustion	T59.891	T59.892	T59.893	T59.894	—	—
utility	T59.891	T59.892	T59.893	T59.894	—	—
in mobile container	T59.891	T59.892	T59.893	T59.894	—	—
incomplete combustion of — *see Carbon, monoxide, fuel, utility*						
piped (natural)	T59.891	T59.892	T59.893	T59.894	—	—
garage	T58.01	T58.02	T58.03	T58.04	—	—
hydrocarbon NEC	T59.891	T59.892	T59.893	T59.894	—	—
incomplete combustion of — *see Carbon, monoxide, fuel, utility*						
liquefied — *see butane*						
piped	T59.891	T59.892	T59.893	T59.894	—	—
hydrocyanic acid	T65.0X1	T65.0X2	T65.0X3	T65.0X4	—	—

Substance	External Cause (T-Code)					
	Poisoning, Accidental (Unintentional)	Poisoning, Intentional Self-Harm	Poisoning, Assault	Poisoning, Undetermined	Adverse Effect	Underdosing
Gas *(Continued)*						
illuminating (after combustion)	T58.11	T58.12	T58.13	T58.14	—	—
prior to combustion	T59.891	T59.892	T59.893	T59.894	—	—
incomplete combustion, any — *see Carbon, monoxide*						
kiln	T58.8X1	T58.8X2	T58.8X3	T58.8X4	—	—
lacrimogenic	T59.3X1	T59.3X2	T59.3X3	T59.3X4	—	—
liquefied petroleum — *see butane*						
marsh	T59.891	T59.892	T59.893	T59.894	—	—
motor exhaust, not in transit	T58.01	T58.02	T58.03	T58.04	—	—
mustard, not in war	T59.891	T59.892	T59.893	T59.894	—	—
natural	T59.891	T59.892	T59.893	T59.894	—	—
nerve, not in war	T59.91	T59.92	T59.93	T59.94	—	—
oil	T52.0X1	T52.0X2	T52.0X3	T52.0X4	—	—
petroleum (liquefied) (distributed in mobile containers)	T59.891	T59.892	T59.893	T59.894	—	—
piped (pure or mixed with air)	T59.891	T59.892	T59.893	T59.894	—	—
piped (manufactured) (natural) NEC	T59.891	T59.892	T59.893	T59.894	—	—
producer	T58.8X1	T58.8X2	T58.8X3	T58.8X4	—	—
propane — *see propane*						
refrigerant (chlorofluoro-carbon)	T53.5X1	T53.5X2	T53.5X3	T53.5X4	—	—
not chlorofluoro-carbon	T59.891	T59.892	T59.893	T59.894	—	—
sewer	T59.91	T59.92	T59.93	T59.94	—	—
specified source NEC	T59.91	T59.92	T59.93	T59.94	—	—
stove (after combustion)	T58.11	T58.12	T58.13	T58.14	—	—
tear	T59.3X1	T59.3X2	T59.3X3	T59.3X4	—	—
therapeutic	T41.5X1	T41.5X2	T41.5X3	T41.5X4	T41.5X5	T41.5X6
utility (for cooking, heating, or lighting) (piped) NEC	T59.891	T59.892	T59.893	T59.894	—	—
in mobile container	T59.891	T59.892	T59.893	T59.894	—	—
incomplete combustion of — *see Carbon, monoxide, fuel, utilty*						
piped (natural)	T59.891	T59.892	T59.893	T59.894	—	—
water	T58.11	T58.12	T58.13	T58.14	—	—
incomplete combustion of — *see Carbon, monoxide,* fuel, utility						

Substance	External Cause (T-Code)					
	Poisoning, Accidental (Unintentional)	Poisoning, Intentional Self-Harm	Poisoning, Assault	Poisoning, Undetermined	Adverse Effect	Underdosing
Gaseous substance — *see Gas*						
Gasoline	T52.0X1	T52.0X2	T52.0X3	T52.0X4	—	—
vapor	T52.0X1	T52.0X2	T52.0X3	T52.0X4	—	—
Gastric enzymes	T47.5X1	T47.5X2	T47.5X3	T47.5X4	T47.5X5	T47.5X6
Gastrografin	T50.8X1	T50.8X2	T50.8X3	T50.8X4	T50.8X5	T50.8X6
Gastrointestinal drug	T47.91	T47.92	T47.93	T47.94	T47.95	T47.96
biological	T47.8X1	T47.8X2	T47.8X3	T47.8X4	T47.8X5	T47.8X6
specified NEC	T47.8X1	T47.8X2	T47.8X3	T47.8X4	T47.8X5	T47.8X6
Gaultheria procumbens	T62.2X1	T62.2X2	T62.2X3	T62.2X4	—	—
Gelatin (intravenous)	T45.8X1	T45.8X2	T45.8X3	T45.8X4	T45.8X5	T45.8X6
absorbable (sponge)	T45.7X1	T45.7X2	T45.7X3	T45.7X4	T45.7X5	T45.7X6
Gefarnate	T44.3X1	T44.3X2	T44.3X3	T44.3X4	T44.3X5	T44.3X6
Gelfilm	T49.8X1	T49.8X2	T49.8X3	T49.8X4	T49.8X5	T49.8X6
Gelfoam	T45.7X1	T45.7X2	T45.7X3	T45.7X4	T45.7X5	T45.7X6
Gelsemine	T50.991	T50.992	T50.993	T50.994	T50.995	T50.996
Gelsemium (sempervirens)	T62.2X1	T62.2X2	T62.2X3	T62.2X4	—	—
Gemeprost	T48.0X1	T48.0X2	T48.0X3	T48.0X4	T48.0X5	T48.0X6
Gemfibrozil	T46.6X1	T46.6X2	T46.6X3	T46.6X4	T46.6X5	T46.6X6
Gemonil	T42.3X1	T42.3X2	T42.3X3	T42.3X4	T42.3X5	T42.3X6
Gentamicin	T36.5X1	T36.5X2	T36.5X3	T36.5X4	T36.5X5	T36.5X6
ophthalmic preparation	T49.5X1	T49.5X2	T49.5X3	T49.5X4	T49.5X5	T49.5X6
topical NEC	T49.0X1	T49.0X2	T49.0X3	T49.0X4	T49.0X5	T49.0X6
Gentian	T47.5X1	T47.5X2	T47.5X3	T47.5X4	T47.5X5	T47.5X6
violet	T49.0X1	T49.0X2	T49.0X3	T49.0X4	T49.0X5	T49.0X6
Gepefrine	T44.4X1	T44.4X2	T44.4X3	T44.4X4	T44.4X5	T44.4X6
Gestonorone caproate	T38.5X1	T38.5X2	T38.5X3	T38.5X4	T38.5X5	T38.5X6
Gexane	T49.0X1	T49.0X2	T49.0X3	T49.0X4	T49.0X5	T49.0X6
Gila monster (venom)	T63.111	T63.112	T63.113	T63.114	—	—
Ginger	T47.5X1	T47.5X2	T47.5X3	T47.5X4	T47.5X5	T47.5X6
Jamaica — *see Jamaica, ginger*						
Gitalin	T46.0X1	T46.0X2	T46.0X3	T46.0X4	T46.0X5	T46.0X6
amorphous	T46.0X1	T46.0X2	T46.0X3	T46.0X4	T46.0X5	T46.0X6
Gitaloxin	T46.0X1	T46.0X2	T46.0X3	T46.0X4	T46.0X5	T46.0X6
Gitoxin	T46.0X1	T46.0X2	T46.0X3	T46.0X4	T46.0X5	T46.0X6
Glafenine	T39.8X1	T39.8X2	T39.8X3	T39.8X4	T39.8X5	T39.8X6
Glandular extract (medicinal) NEC	T50.Z91	T50.Z92	T50.Z93	T50.Z94	T50.Z95	T50.Z96
Glaucarubin	T37.3X1	T37.3X2	T37.3X3	T37.3X4	T37.3X5	T37.3X6
Glibenclamide	T38.3X1	T38.3X2	T38.3X3	T38.3X4	T38.3X5	T38.3X6
Glibornuride	T38.3X1	T38.3X2	T38.3X3	T38.3X4	T38.3X5	T38.3X6
Gliclazide	T38.3X1	T38.3X2	T38.3X3	T38.3X4	T38.3X5	T38.3X6
Glimidine	T38.3X1	T38.3X2	T38.3X3	T38.3X4	T38.3X5	T38.3X6

◀ New ⇐ Revised ~~deleted~~ Deleted

Substance	External Cause (T-Code)					
	Poisoning, Accidental (Unintentional)	Poisoning, Intentional Self-Harm	Poisoning, Assault	Poisoning, Undetermined	Adverse Effect	Underdosing
Glipizide	T38.3X1	T38.3X2	T38.3X3	T38.3X4	T38.3X5	T38.3X6
Gliquidone	T38.3X1	T38.3X2	T38.3X3	T38.3X4	T38.3X5	T38.3X6
Glisolamide	T38.3X1	T38.3X2	T38.3X3	T38.3X4	T38.3X5	T38.3X6
Glisoxepide	T38.3X1	T38.3X2	T38.3X3	T38.3X4	T38.3X5	T38.3X6
Globin zinc insulin	T38.3X1	T38.3X2	T38.3X3	T38.3X4	T38.3X5	T38.3X6
Globulin						
antilymphocytic	T50.Z11	T50.Z12	T50.Z13	T50.Z14	T50.Z15	T50.Z16
antirhesus	T50.Z11	T50.Z12	T50.Z13	T50.Z14	T50.Z15	T50.Z16
antivenin	T50.Z11	T50.Z12	T50.Z13	T50.Z14	T50.Z15	T50.Z16
antiviral	T50.Z11	T50.Z12	T50.Z13	T50.Z14	T50.Z15	T50.Z16
Glucagon	T38.3X1	T38.3X2	T38.3X3	T38.3X4	T38.3X5	T38.3X6
Glucocorticoids	T38.0X1	T38.0X2	T38.0X3	T38.0X4	T38.0X5	T38.0X6
Glucocorticosteroid	T38.0X1	T38.0X2	T38.0X3	T38.0X4	T38.0X5	T38.0X6
Gluconic acid	T50.991	T50.992	T50.993	T50.994	T50.995	T50.996
Glucosamine sulfate	T39.4X1	T39.4X2	T39.4X3	T39.4X4	T39.4X5	T39.4X6
Glucose	T50.3X1	T50.3X2	T50.3X3	T50.3X4	T50.3X5	T50.3X6
with sodium chloride	T50.3X1	T50.3X2	T50.3X3	T50.3X4	T50.3X5	T50.3X6
Glucosulfone sodium	T37.1X1	T37.1X2	T37.1X3	T37.1X4	T37.1X5	T37.1X6
Glucurolactone	T47.8X1	T47.8X2	T47.8X3	T47.8X4	T47.8X5	T47.8X6
Glue NEC	T52.8X1	T52.8X2	T52.8X3	T52.8X4	—	—
Glutamic acid	T47.5X1	T47.5X2	T47.5X3	T47.5X4	T47.5X5	T47.5X6
Glutaral (medicinal)	T49.0X1	T49.0X2	T49.0X3	T49.0X4	T49.0X5	T49.0X6
nonmedicinal	T65.891	T65.892	T65.893	T65.894	—	—
Glutaraldehyde (nonmedicinal)	T65.891	T65.892	T65.893	T65.894	—	—
medicinal	T49.0X1	T49.0X2	T49.0X3	T49.0X4	T49.0X5	T49.0X6
Glutathione	T50.6X1	T50.6X2	T50.6X3	T50.6X4	T50.6X5	T50.6X6
Glutethimide	T42.6X1	T42.6X2	T42.6X3	T42.6X4	T42.6X5	T42.6X6
Glyburide	T38.3X1	T38.3X2	T38.3X3	T38.3X4	T38.3X5	T38.3X6
Glycerin	T47.4X1	T47.4X2	T47.4X3	T47.4X4	T47.4X5	T47.4X6
Glycerol	T47.4X1	T47.4X2	T47.4X3	T47.4X4	T47.4X5	T47.4X6
borax	T49.6X1	T49.6X2	T49.6X3	T49.6X4	T49.6X5	T49.6X6
intravenous	T50.3X1	T50.3X2	T50.3X3	T50.3X4	T50.3X5	T50.3X6
iodinated	T48.4X1	T48.4X2	T48.4X3	T48.4X4	T48.4X5	T48.4X6
Glycerophosphate	T50.991	T50.992	T50.993	T50.994	T50.995	T50.996
Glyceryl						
gualacolate	T48.4X1	T48.4X2	T48.4X3	T48.4X4	T48.4X5	T48.4X6
nitrate	T46.3X1	T46.3X2	T46.3X3	T46.3X4	T46.3X5	T46.3X6
triacetate (topical)	T49.0X1	T49.0X2	T49.0X3	T49.0X4	T49.0X5	T49.0X6
trinitrate	T46.3X1	T46.3X2	T46.3X3	T46.3X4	T46.3X5	T46.3X6
Glycine	T50.3X1	T50.3X2	T50.3X3	T50.3X4	T50.3X5	T50.3X6
Glyclopyramide	T38.3X1	T38.3X2	T38.3X3	T38.3X4	T38.3X5	T38.3X6
Glycobiarsol	T37.3X1	T37.3X2	T37.3X3	T37.3X4	T37.3X5	T37.3X6

Substance	External Cause (T-Code)					
	Poisoning, Accidental (Unintentional)	Poisoning, Intentional Self-Harm	Poisoning, Assault	Poisoning, Undetermined	Adverse Effect	Underdosing
Glycols (ether)	T52.3X1	T52.3X2	T52.3X3	T52.3X4	—	—
Glyconiazide	T37.1X1	T37.1X2	T37.1X3	T37.1X4	T37.1X5	T37.1X6
Glycopyrrolate	T44.3X1	T44.3X2	T44.3X3	T44.3X4	T44.3X5	T44.3X6
Glycopyrronium	T44.3X1	T44.3X2	T44.3X3	T44.3X4	T44.3X5	T44.3X6
bromide	T44.3X1	T44.3X2	T44.3X3	T44.3X4	T44.3X5	T44.3X6
Glycoside, cardiac (stimulant)	T46.0X1	T46.0X2	T46.0X3	T46.0X4	T46.0X5	T46.0X6
Glycyclamide	T38.3X1	T38.3X2	T38.3X3	T38.3X4	T38.3X5	T38.3X6
Glycyrrhiza extract	T48.4X1	T48.4X2	T48.4X3	T48.4X4	T48.4X5	T48.4X6
Glycyrrhizic acid	T48.4X1	T48.4X2	T48.4X3	T48.4X4	T48.4X5	T48.4X6
Glycyrrhizinate potassium	T48.4X1	T48.4X2	T48.4X3	T48.4X4	T48.4X5	T48.4X6
Glymidine sodium	T38.3X1	T38.3X2	T38.3X3	T38.3X4	T38.3X5	T38.3X6
Glyphosate	T60.3X1	T60.3X2	T60.3X3	T60.3X4	—	—
Glyphylline	T48.6X1	T48.6X2	T48.6X3	T48.6X4	T48.6X5	T48.6X6
Gold						
colloidal (I98Au)	T45.1X1	T45.1X2	T45.1X3	T45.1X4	T45.1X5	T45.1X6
salts	T39.4X1	T39.4X2	T39.4X3	T39.4X4	T39.4X5	T39.4X6
Golden sulfide of antimony	T56.891	T56.892	T56.893	T56.894	—	—
Goldylocks	T62.2X1	T62.2X2	T62.2X3	T62.2X4	—	—
Gonadal tissue extract	T38.901	T38.902	T38.903	T38.904	T38.905	T38.906
female	T38.5X1	T38.5X2	T38.5X3	T38.5X4	T38.5X5	T38.5X6
male	T38.7X1	T38.7X2	T38.7X3	T38.7X4	T38.7X5	T38.7X6
Gonadorelin	T38.891	T38.892	T38.893	T38.894	T38.895	T38.896
Gonadotropin	T38.891	T38.892	T38.893	T38.894	T38.895	T38.896
chorionic	T38.891	T38.892	T38.893	T38.894	T38.895	T38.896
pituitary	T38.811	T38.812	T38.813	T38.814	T38.815	T38.816
Goserelin	T45.1X1	T45.1X2	T45.1X3	T45.1X4	T45.1X5	T45.1X6
Grain alcohol	T51.0X1	T51.0X2	T51.0X3	T51.0X4	—	—
Gramicidin	T49.0X1	T49.0X2	T49.0X3	T49.0X4	T49.0X5	T49.0X6
Granisetron	T45.0X1	T45.0X2	T45.0X3	T45.0X4	T45.0X5	T45.0X6
Gratiola officinalis	T62.2X1	T62.2X2	T62.2X3	T62.2X4	—	—
Grease	T65.891	T65.892	T65.893	T65.894	—	—
Green hellebore	T62.2X1	T62.2X2	T62.2X3	T62.2X4	—	—
Green soap	T49.2X1	T49.2X2	T49.2X3	T49.2X4	T49.2X5	T49.2X6
Grifulvin	T36.7X1	T36.7X2	T36.7X3	T36.7X4	T36.7X5	T36.7X6
Griseofulvin	T36.7X1	T36.7X2	T36.7X3	T36.7X4	T36.7X5	T36.7X6
Growth hormone	T38.811	T38.812	T38.813	T38.814	T38.815	T38.816
Guaiacol derivatives	T48.4X1	T48.4X2	T48.4X3	T48.4X4	T48.4X5	T48.4X6
Guaiac reagent	T50.991	T50.992	T50.993	T50.994	T50.995	T50.996
Guaifenesin	T48.4X1	T48.4X2	T48.4X3	T48.4X4	T48.4X5	T48.4X6
Guaimesal	T48.4X1	T48.4X2	T48.4X3	T48.4X4	T48.4X5	T48.4X6
Guaiphenesin	T48.4X1	T48.4X2	T48.4X3	T48.4X4	T48.4X5	T48.4X6
Guamecycline	T36.4X1	T36.4X2	T36.4X3	T36.4X4	T36.4X5	T36.4X6

Substance	Poisoning, Accidental (Unintentional)	Poisoning, Intentional Self-Harm	Poisoning, Assault	Poisoning, Undetermined	Adverse Effect	Underdosing
	External Cause (T-Code)					
Guanabenz	T46.5X1	T46.5X2	T46.5X3	T46.5X4	T46.5X5	T46.5X6
Guanacline	T46.5X1	T46.5X2	T46.5X3	T46.5X4	T46.5X5	T46.5X6
Guanadrel	T46.5X1	T46.5X2	T46.5X3	T46.5X4	T46.5X5	T46.5X6
Guanatol	T37.2X1	T37.2X2	T37.2X3	T37.2X4	T37.2X5	T37.2X6
Guanethidine	T46.5X1	T46.5X2	T46.5X3	T46.5X4	T46.5X5	T46.5X6
Guanfacine	T46.5X1	T46.5X2	T46.5X3	T46.5X4	T46.5X5	T46.5X6
Guano	T65.891	T65.892	T65.893	T65.894	—	—
Guanochlor	T46.5X1	T46.5X2	T46.5X3	T46.5X4	T46.5X5	T46.5X6
Guanoclor	T46.5X1	T46.5X2	T46.5X3	T46.5X4	T46.5X5	T46.5X6
Guanoctine	T46.5X1	T46.5X2	T46.5X3	T46.5X4	T46.5X5	T46.5X6
Guanoxabenz	T46.5X1	T46.5X2	T46.5X3	T46.5X4	T46.5X5	T46.5X6
Guanoxan	T46.5X1	T46.5X2	T46.5X3	T46.5X4	T46.5X5	T46.5X6
Guar gum (medicinal)	T46.6X1	T46.6X2	T46.6X3	T46.6X4	T46.6X5	T46.6X6
H						
Hachimycin	T36.7X1	T36.7X2	T36.7X3	T36.7X4	T36.7X5	T36.7X6
Hair						
dye	T49.4X1	T49.4X2	T49.4X3	T49.4X4	T49.4X5	T49.4X6
preparation NEC	T49.4X1	T49.4X2	T49.4X3	T49.4X4	T49.4X5	T49.4X6
Halazepam	T42.4X1	T42.4X2	T42.4X3	T42.4X4	T42.4X5	T42.4X6
Halcinolone	T49.0X1	T49.0X2	T49.0X3	T49.0X4	T49.0X5	T49.0X6
Halcinonide	T49.0X1	T49.0X2	T49.0X3	T49.0X4	T49.0X5	T49.0X6
Halethazole	T49.0X1	T49.0X2	T49.0X3	T49.0X4	T49.0X5	T49.0X6
Hallucinogen NEC	T40.901	T40.902	T40.903	T40.904	T40.905	T40.906
Halofantrine	T37.2X1	T37.2X2	T37.2X3	T37.2X4	T37.2X5	T37.2X6
Halofenate	T46.6X1	T46.6X2	T46.6X3	T46.6X4	T46.6X5	T46.6X6
Halometasone	T49.0X1	T49.0X2	T49.0X3	T49.0X4	T49.0X5	T49.0X6
Haloperidol	T43.4X1	T43.4X2	T43.4X3	T43.4X4	T43.4X5	T43.4X6
Haloprogin	T49.0X1	T49.0X2	T49.0X3	T49.0X4	T49.0X5	T49.0X6
Halotex	T49.0X1	T49.0X2	T49.0X3	T49.0X4	T49.0X5	T49.0X6
Halothane	T41.0X1	T41.0X2	T41.0X3	T41.0X4	T41.0X5	T41.0X6
Haloxazolam	T42.4X1	T42.4X2	T42.4X3	T42.4X4	T42.4X5	T42.4X6
Halquinols	T49.0X1	T49.0X2	T49.0X3	T49.0X4	T49.0X5	T49.0X6
Hamamelis	T49.2X1	T49.2X2	T49.2X3	T49.2X4	T49.2X5	T49.2X6
Haptendextran	T45.8X1	T45.8X2	T45.8X3	T45.8X4	T45.8X5	T45.8X6
Harmonyl	T46.5X1	T46.5X2	T46.5X3	T46.5X4	T46.5X5	T46.5X6
Hartmann's solution	T50.3X1	T50.3X2	T50.3X3	T50.3X4	T50.3X5	T50.3X6
Hashish	T40.7X1	T40.7X2	T40.7X3	T40.7X4	T40.7X5	T40.7X6
Hawaiian Woodrose seeds	T40.991	T40.992	T40.993	T40.994	—	—
HCB	T60.3X1	T60.3X2	T60.3X3	T60.3X4	—	—
HCH	T53.6X1	T53.6X2	T53.6X3	T53.6X4	—	—
medicinal	T49.0X1	T49.0X2	T49.0X3	T49.0X4	T49.0X5	T49.0X6

Substance	Poisoning, Accidental (Unintentional)	Poisoning, Intentional Self-Harm	Poisoning, Assault	Poisoning, Undetermined	Adverse Effect	Underdosing
	External Cause (T-Code)					
HCN	T57.3X1	T57.3X2	T57.3X3	T57.3X4	—	—
Headache cures, drugs, powders NEC	T50.901	T50.902	T50.903	T50.904	T50.905	T50.906
Heavenly Blue (morning glory)	T40.991	T40.992	T40.993	T40.994	—	—
Heavy metal antidote	T45.8X1	T45.8X2	T45.8X3	T45.8X4	T45.8X5	T45.8X6
Hedaquinium	T49.0X1	T49.0X2	T49.0X3	T49.0X4	T49.0X5	T49.0X6
Hedge hyssop	T62.2X1	T62.2X2	T62.2X3	T62.2X4	—	—
Heet	T49.8X1	T49.8X2	T49.8X3	T49.8X4	T49.8X5	T49.8X6
Helium	T48.991	T48.992	T48.993	T48.994	T48.995	T48.996
Helenin	T37.4X1	T37.4X2	T37.4X3	T37.4X4	T37.4X5	T37.4X6
Hellebore (black) (green) (white)	T62.2X1	T62.2X2	T62.2X3	T62.2X4	—	—
Helium (nonmedicinal) NEC	T59.891	T59.892	T59.893	T59.894	—	—
medicinal	T48.991	T48.992	T48.993	T48.994	T48.995	T48.996
Hematin	T45.8X1	T45.8X2	T45.8X3	T45.8X4	T45.8X5	T45.8X6
Hematinic preparation	T45.8X1	T45.8X2	T45.8X3	T45.8X4	T45.8X5	T45.8X6
Hemlock	T62.2X1	T62.2X2	T62.2X3	T62.2X4	—	—
Hemostatic	T45.621	T45.622	T45.623	T45.624	T45.625	T45.626
drug, systemic	T45.621	T45.622	T45.623	T45.624	T45.625	T45.626
Hemostyptic	T49.4X1	T49.4X2	T49.4X3	T49.4X4	T49.4X5	T49.4X6
Henbane	T62.2X1	T62.2X2	T62.2X3	T62.2X4	—	—
Heparin (sodium)	T45.511	T45.512	T45.513	T45.514	T45.515	T45.516
action reverser	T45.7X1	T45.7X2	T45.7X3	T45.7X4	T45.7X5	T45.7X6
Heparin-fraction	T45.511	T45.512	T45.513	T45.514	T45.515	T45.516
Heparinoid (systemic)	T45.511	T45.512	T45.513	T45.514	T45.515	T45.516
Hepatic secretion stimulant	T47.8X1	T47.8X2	T47.8X3	T47.8X4	T47.8X5	T47.8X6
Hepatitis B						
immune globulin	T50.Z11	T50.Z12	T50.Z13	T50.Z14	T50.Z15	T50.Z16
vaccine	T50.B91	T50.B92	T50.B93	T50.B94	T50.B95	T50.B96
Hepronicate	T46.7X1	T46.7X2	T46.7X3	T46.7X4	T46.7X5	T46.7X6
Heptabarb	T42.3X1	T42.3X2	T42.3X3	T42.3X4	T42.3X5	T42.3X6
Heptabarbitone	T42.3X1	T42.3X2	T42.3X3	T42.3X4	T42.3X5	T42.3X6
Heptabarbital	T42.3X1	T42.3X2	T42.3X3	T42.3X4	T42.3X5	T42.3X6
Heptachlor	T60.1X1	T60.1X2	T60.1X3	T60.1X4	—	—
Heptalgin	T40.2X1	T40.2X2	T40.2X3	T40.2X4	T40.2X5	T40.2X6
Heptaminol	T46.3X1	T46.3X2	T46.3X3	T46.3X4	T46.3X5	T46.3X6
Herbicide NEC	T60.3X1	T60.3X2	T60.3X3	T60.3X4	—	—
Heroin	T40.1X1	T40.1X2	T40.1X3	T40.1X4	—	—
Herplex	T49.5X1	T49.5X2	T49.5X3	T49.5X4	T49.5X5	T49.5X6
HES	T45.8X1	T45.8X2	T45.8X3	T45.8X4	T45.8X5	T45.8X6
Hesperidin	T46.991	T46.992	T46.993	T46.994	T46.995	T46.996
Hetacillin	T36.0X1	T36.0X2	T36.0X3	T36.0X4	T36.0X5	T36.0X6

Substance	External Cause (T-Code)					
	Poisoning, Accidental (Unintentional)	Poisoning, Intentional Self-Harm	Poisoning, Assault	Poisoning, Undetermined	Adverse Effect	Underdosing
Hetastarch	T45.8X1	T45.8X2	T45.8X3	T45.8X4	T45.8X5	T45.8X6
HETP	T60.0X1	T60.0X2	T60.0X3	T60.0X4	—	—
Hexachlorobenzene (vapor)	T60.3X1	T60.3X2	T60.3X3	T60.3X4	—	—
Hexachlorocyclohexane	T53.6X1	T53.6X2	T53.6X3	T53.6X4	—	—
Hexachlorophene	T49.0X1	T49.0X2	T49.0X3	T49.0X4	T49.0X5	T49.0X6
Hexadiline	T46.3X1	T46.3X2	T46.3X3	T46.3X4	T46.3X5	T46.3X6
Hexadimethrine (bromide)	T45.7X1	T45.7X2	T45.7X3	T45.7X4	T45.7X5	T45.7X6
Hexadylamine	T46.3X1	T46.3X2	T46.3X3	T46.3X4	T46.3X5	T46.3X6
Hexaethyl tetraphosphate	T60.0X1	T60.0X2	T60.0X3	T60.0X4	—	—
Hexafluorenium bromide	T48.1X1	T48.1X2	T48.1X3	T48.1X4	T48.1X5	T48.1X6
Hexafluorodiethyl ether	T43.291	T43.292	T43.293	T43.294	T43.295	T43.296
Hexafluronium (bromide)	T48.1X1	T48.1X2	T48.1X3	T48.1X4	T48.1X5	T48.1X6
Hexahydrobenzol	T52.8X1	T52.8X2	T52.8X3	T52.8X4	—	—
Hexahydrocresol(s)	T51.8X1	T51.8X2	T51.8X3	T51.8X4	—	—
arsenide	T57.0X1	T57.0X2	T57.0X3	T57.0X4	—	—
arseniurated	T57.0X1	T57.0X2	T57.0X3	T57.0X4	—	—
cyanide	T57.3X1	T57.3X2	T57.3X3	T57.3X4	—	—
gas	T59.891	T59.892	T59.893	T59.894	—	—
Fluoride (liquid)	T57.8X1	T57.8X2	T57.8X3	T57.8X4	—	—
vapor	T59.891	T59.892	T59.893	T59.894	—	—
phophorated	T60.0X1	T60.0X2	T60.0X3	T60.0X4	—	—
sulfate	T57.8X1	T57.8X2	T57.8X3	T57.8X4	—	—
sulfide (gas)	T59.6X1	T59.6X2	T59.6X3	T59.6X4	—	—
arseniurated	T57.0X1	T57.0X2	T57.0X3	T57.0X4	—	—
sulfurated	T57.8X1	T57.8X2	T57.8X3	T57.8X4	—	—
Hexahydrophenol	T51.8X1	T51.8X2	T51.8X3	T51.8X4	—	—
Hexa-germ	T49.2X1	T49.2X2	T49.2X3	T49.2X4	T49.2X5	T49.2X6
Hexalen	T51.8X1	T51.8X2	T51.8X3	T51.8X4	—	—
Hexamethonium bromide	T44.2X1	T44.2X2	T44.2X3	T44.2X4	T44.2X5	T44.2X6
Hexamethylene	T52.8X1	T52.8X2	T52.8X3	T52.8X4	—	—
Hexamethylmelamine	T45.1X1	T45.1X2	T45.1X3	T45.1X4	T45.1X5	T45.1X6
Hexamidine	T49.0X1	T49.0X2	T49.0X3	T49.0X4	T49.0X5	T49.0X6
Hexamine (mandelate)	T37.8X1	T37.8X2	T37.8X3	T37.8X4	T37.8X5	T37.8X6
Hexanone, 2-hexanone	T52.4X1	T52.4X2	T52.4X3	T52.4X4	—	—
Hexanuorenium	T48.1X1	T48.1X2	T48.1X3	T48.1X4	T48.1X5	T48.1X6
Hexapropymate	T42.6X1	T42.6X2	T42.6X3	T42.6X4	T42.6X5	T42.6X6
Hexasonium iodide	T44.3X1	T44.3X2	T44.3X3	T44.3X4	T44.3X5	T44.3X6
Hexcarbacholine bromide	T48.1X1	T48.1X2	T48.1X3	T48.1X4	T48.1X5	T48.1X6
Hexemal	T42.3X1	T42.3X2	T42.3X3	T42.3X4	T42.3X5	T42.3X6
Hexestrol	T38.5X1	T38.5X2	T38.5X3	T38.5X4	T38.5X5	T38.5X6
Hexethal (sodium)	T42.3X1	T42.3X2	T42.3X3	T42.3X4	T42.3X5	T42.3X6
Hexetidine	T37.8X1	T37.8X2	T37.8X3	T37.8X4	T37.8X5	T37.8X6

Substance	External Cause (T-Code)					
	Poisoning, Accidental (Unintentional)	Poisoning, Intentional Self-Harm	Poisoning, Assault	Poisoning, Undetermined	Adverse Effect	Underdosing
Hexobarbital	T42.3X1	T42.3X2	T42.3X3	T42.3X4	T42.3X5	T42.3X6
rectal	T41.291	T41.292	T41.293	T41.294	T41.295	T41.296
sodium	T41.1X1	T41.1X2	T41.1X3	T41.1X4	T41.1X5	T41.1X6
Hexobendine	T46.3X1	T46.3X2	T46.3X3	T46.3X4	T46.3X5	T46.3X6
Hexocyclium	T44.3X1	T44.3X2	T44.3X3	T44.3X4	T44.3X5	T44.3X6
metilsulfate	T44.3X1	T44.3X2	T44.3X3	T44.3X4	T44.3X5	T44.3X6
Hexoestrol	T38.5X1	T38.5X2	T38.5X3	T38.5X4	T38.5X5	T38.5X6
Hexone	T52.4X1	T52.4X2	T52.4X3	T52.4X4	—	—
Hexoprenaline	T48.6X1	T48.6X2	T48.6X3	T48.6X4	T48.6X5	T48.6X6
Hexylcaine	T41.3X1	T41.3X2	T41.3X3	T41.3X4	T41.3X5	T41.3X6
Hexylresorcinol	T52.2X1	T52.2X2	T52.2X3	T52.2X4	—	—
HGH (human growth hormone)	T38.811	T38.812	T38.813	T38.814	T38.815	T38.816
Hinkle's pills	T47.2X1	T47.2X2	T47.2X3	T47.2X4	T47.2X5	T47.2X6
Histalog	T50.8X1	T50.8X2	T50.8X3	T50.8X4	T50.8X5	T50.8X6
Histamine (phosphate)	T50.8X1	T50.8X2	T50.8X3	T50.8X4	T50.8X5	T50.8X6
Histoplasmin	T50.8X1	T50.8X2	T50.8X3	T50.8X4	T50.8X5	T50.8X6
Holly berries	T62.2X1	T62.2X2	T62.2X3	T62.2X4	—	—
Homatropine	T44.3X1	T44.3X2	T44.3X3	T44.3X4	T44.3X5	T44.3X6
methylbromide	T44.3X1	T44.3X2	T44.3X3	T44.3X4	T44.3X5	T44.3X6
Homochlorcyclizine	T45.0X1	T45.0X2	T45.0X3	T45.0X4	T45.0X5	T45.0X6
Homosalate	T49.3X1	T49.3X2	T49.3X3	T49.3X4	T49.3X5	T49.3X6
Homo-tet	T50.Z11	T50.Z12	T50.Z13	T50.Z14	T50.Z15	T50.Z16
Hormone	T38.801	T38.802	T38.803	T38.804	T38.805	T38.806
adrenal cortical steroids	T38.0X1	T38.0X2	T38.0X3	T38.0X4	T38.0X5	T38.0X6
androgenic	T38.7X1	T38.7X2	T38.7X3	T38.7X4	T38.7X5	T38.7X6
anterior pituitary NEC	T38.811	T38.812	T38.813	T38.814	T38.815	T38.816
antidiabetic agents	T38.3X1	T38.3X2	T38.3X3	T38.3X4	T38.3X5	T38.3X6
antidiuretic	T38.891	T38.892	T38.893	T38.894	T38.895	T38.896
cancer therapy	T45.1X1	T45.1X2	T45.1X3	T45.1X4	T45.1X5	T45.1X6
follicle stimulating	T38.811	T38.812	T38.813	T38.814	T38.815	T38.816
gonadotropic	T38.891	T38.892	T38.893	T38.894	T38.895	T38.896
pituitary	T38.811	T38.812	T38.813	T38.814	T38.815	T38.816
growth	T38.811	T38.812	T38.813	T38.814	T38.815	T38.816
luteinizing	T38.811	T38.812	T38.813	T38.814	T38.815	T38.816
ovarian	T38.5X1	T38.5X2	T38.5X3	T38.5X4	T38.5X5	T38.5X6
oxytocic	T48.0X1	T48.0X2	T48.0X3	T48.0X4	T48.0X5	T48.0X6
parathyroid (derivatives)	T50.991	T50.992	T50.993	T50.994	T50.995	T50.996
pituitary (posterior) NEC	T38.891	T38.892	T38.893	T38.894	T38.895	T38.896
anterior	T38.811	T38.812	T38.813	T38.814	T38.815	T38.816
specified, NEC	T38.891	T38.892	T38.893	T38.894	T38.895	T38.896
thyroid	T38.1X1	T38.1X2	T38.1X3	T38.1X4	T38.1X5	T38.1X6
Hornet (sting)	T63.451	T63.452	T63.453	T63.454	—	—

◀ New ◀ Revised ~~deleted~~ Deleted

Substance	External Cause (T-Code)					
	Poisoning, Accidental (Unintentional)	Poisoning, Intentional Self-Harm	Poisoning, Assault	Poisoning, Undetermined	Adverse Effect	Underdosing
Horse anti-human lymphocytic serum	T50.Z11	T50.Z12	T50.Z13	T50.Z14	T50.Z15	T50.Z16
Horticulture agent NEC	T65.91	T65.92	T65.93	T65.94	—	—
with pesticide	T60.91	T60.92	T60.93	T60.94	—	—
Human						
albumin	T45.8X1	T45.8X2	T45.8X3	T45.8X4	T45.8X5	T45.8X6
growth hormone (HGH)	T38.811	T38.812	T38.813	T38.814	T38.815	T38.816
immune serum	T50.Z11	T50.Z12	T50.Z13	T50.Z14	T50.Z15	T50.Z16
Hyaluronidase	T45.3X1	T45.3X2	T45.3X3	T45.3X4	T45.3X5	T45.3X6
Hyazyme	T45.3X1	T45.3X2	T45.3X3	T45.3X4	T45.3X5	T45.3X6
Hycodan	T40.2X1	T40.2X2	T40.2X3	T40.2X4	T40.2X5	T40.2X6
Hydantoin derivative NEC	T42.0X1	T42.0X2	T42.0X3	T42.0X4	T42.0X5	T42.0X6
Hydeltra	T38.0X1	T38.0X2	T38.0X3	T38.0X4	T38.0X5	T38.0X6
Hydergine	T44.6X1	T44.6X2	T44.6X3	T44.6X4	T44.6X5	T44.6X6
Hydrabamine penicillin	T36.0X1	T36.0X2	T36.0X3	T36.0X4	T36.0X5	T36.0X6
Hydralazine	T46.5X1	T46.5X2	T46.5X3	T46.5X4	T46.5X5	T46.5X6
Hydrargaphen	T49.0X1	T49.0X2	T49.0X3	T49.0X4	T49.0X5	T49.0X6
Hydrargyri amino-chloridum	T49.0X1	T49.0X2	T49.0X3	T49.0X4	T49.0X5	T49.0X6
Hydrastine	T48.291	T48.292	T48.293	T48.294	T48.295	T48.296
Hydrazine	T54.1X1	T54.1X2	T54.1X3	T54.1X4	—	—
monoamine oxidase inhibitors	T43.1X1	T43.1X2	T43.1X3	T43.1X4	T43.1X5	T43.1X6
Hydrazoic acid, azides	T54.2X1	T54.2X2	T54.2X3	T54.2X4	—	—
Hydriodic acid	T48.4X1	T48.4X2	T48.4X3	T48.4X4	T48.4X5	T48.4X6
Hydrocarbon gas	T59.891	T59.892	T59.893	T59.894	—	—
incomplete combustion of— *see Carbon, monoxide, fuel, utility*						
liquefied (mobile container)	T59.891	T59.892	T59.893	T59.894	—	—
piped (natural)	T59.891	T59.892	T59.893	T59.894	—	—
Hydrochloric acid (liquid)	T54.2X1	T54.2X2	T54.2X3	T54.2X4	—	—
medicinal (digestant)	T47.5X1	T47.5X2	T47.5X3	T47.5X4	T47.5X5	T47.5X6
vapor	T59.891	T59.892	T59.893	T59.894	—	—
Hydrochlorothiazide	T50.2X1	T50.2X2	T50.2X3	T50.2X4	T50.2X5	T50.2X6
Hydrocodone	T40.2X1	T40.2X2	T40.2X3	T40.2X4	T40.2X5	T40.2X6
Hydrocortisone (derivatives)	T38.0X1	T38.0X2	T38.0X3	T38.0X4	T38.0X5	T38.0X6
aceponate	T49.0X1	T49.0X2	T49.0X3	T49.0X4	T49.0X5	T49.0X6
ENT agent	T49.6X1	T49.6X2	T49.6X3	T49.6X4	T49.6X5	T49.6X6
ophthalmic preparation	T49.5X1	T49.5X2	T49.5X3	T49.5X4	T49.5X5	T49.5X6
topical NEC	T49.0X1	T49.0X2	T49.0X3	T49.0X4	T49.0X5	T49.0X6
Hydrocortone	T38.0X1	T38.0X2	T38.0X3	T38.0X4	T38.0X5	T38.0X6
ENT agent	T49.6X1	T49.6X2	T49.6X3	T49.6X4	T49.6X5	T49.6X6
ophthalmic preparation	T49.5X1	T49.5X2	T49.5X3	T49.5X4	T49.5X5	T49.5X6
topical NEC	T49.0X1	T49.0X2	T49.0X3	T49.0X4	T49.0X5	T49.0X6

Substance	External Cause (T-Code)					
	Poisoning, Accidental (Unintentional)	Poisoning, Intentional Self-Harm	Poisoning, Assault	Poisoning, Undetermined	Adverse Effect	Underdosing
Hydrocyanic acid (liquid)	T57.3X1	T57.3X2	T57.3X3	T57.3X4	—	—
gas	T65.0X1	T65.0X2	T65.0X3	T65.0X4	—	—
Hydroflumethiazide	T50.2X1	T50.2X2	T50.2X3	T50.2X4	T50.2X5	T50.2X6
Hydrofluoric acid (liquid)	T54.2X1	T54.2X2	T54.2X3	T54.2X4	—	—
vapor	T59.891	T59.892	T59.893	T59.894	—	—
Hydrogen	T59.891	T59.892	T59.893	T59.894	—	—
arsenide	T57.0X1	T57.0X2	T57.0X3	T57.0X4	—	—
arseniureted	T57.0X1	T57.0X2	T57.0X3	T57.0X4	—	—
chloride	T57.8X1	T57.8X2	T57.8X3	T57.8X4	—	—
cyanide (salts)	T57.3X1	T57.3X2	T57.3X3	T57.3X4	—	—
gas	T57.3X1	T57.3X2	T57.3X3	T57.3X4	—	—
Fluoride	T59.5X1	T59.5X2	T59.5X3	T59.5X4	—	—
vapor	T59.5X1	T59.5X2	T59.5X3	T59.5X4	—	—
peroxide	T49.0X1	T49.0X2	T49.0X3	T49.0X4	T49.0X5	T49.0X6
phosphureted	T57.1X1	T57.1X2	T57.1X3	T57.1X4	—	—
sulfide	T59.6X1	T59.6X2	T59.6X3	T59.6X4	—	—
arseniureted	T57.0X1	T57.0X2	T57.0X3	T57.0X4	—	—
sulfureted	T59.6X1	T59.6X2	T59.6X3	T59.6X4	—	—
Hydromethylpyridine	T46.7X1	T46.7X2	T46.7X3	T46.7X4	T46.7X5	T46.7X6
Hydromorphinol	T40.2X1	T40.2X2	T40.2X3	T40.2X4	—	—
Hydromorphinone	T40.2X1	T40.2X2	T40.2X3	T40.2X4	T40.2X5	T40.2X6
Hydromorphone	T40.2X1	T40.2X2	T40.2X3	T40.2X4	T40.2X5	T40.2X6
Hydromox	T50.2X1	T50.2X2	T50.2X3	T50.2X4	T50.2X5	T50.2X6
Hydrophilic lotion	T49.3X1	T49.3X2	T49.3X3	T49.3X4	T49.3X5	T49.3X6
Hydroquinidine	T46.2X1	T46.2X2	T46.2X3	T46.2X4	T46.2X5	T46.2X6
Hydroquinone	T52.2X1	T52.2X2	T52.2X3	T52.2X4	—	—
vapor	T59.891	T59.892	T59.893	T59.894	—	—
Hydrosulfuric acid (gas)	T59.6X1	T59.6X2	T59.6X3	T59.6X4	—	—
Hydrotalcite	T47.1X1	T47.1X2	T47.1X3	T47.1X4	T47.1X5	T47.1X6
Hydrous wool fat	T49.3X1	T49.3X2	T49.3X3	T49.3X4	T49.3X5	T49.3X6
Hydroxide, caustic	T54.3X1	T54.3X2	T54.3X3	T54.3X4	—	—
Hydroxocobalamin	T45.8X1	T45.8X2	T45.8X3	T45.8X4	T45.8X5	T45.8X6
Hydroxyamphetamine	T49.5X1	T49.5X2	T49.5X3	T49.5X4	T49.5X5	T49.5X6
Hydroxycarbamide	T45.1X1	T45.1X2	T45.1X3	T45.1X4	T45.1X5	T45.1X6
Hydroxychloroquine	T37.8X1	T37.8X2	T37.8X3	T37.8X4	T37.8X5	T37.8X6
Hydroxydihydrocodeinone	T40.2X1	T40.2X2	T40.2X3	T40.2X4	T40.2X5	T40.2X6
Hydroxyestrone	T38.5X1	T38.5X2	T38.5X3	T38.5X4	T38.5X5	T38.5X6
Hydroxyethyl starch	T45.8X1	T45.8X2	T45.8X3	T45.8X4	T45.8X5	T45.8X6
Hydroxymethylpentanone	T52.4X1	T52.4X2	T52.4X3	T52.4X4	—	—
Hydroxyphenamate	T43.591	T43.592	T43.593	T43.594	T43.595	T43.596
Hydroxyphenylbutazone	T39.2X1	T39.2X2	T39.2X3	T39.2X4	T39.2X5	T39.2X6

◀ New ⇐ Revised ~~deleted~~ Deleted

Substance	External Cause (T-Code)					
	Poisoning, Accidental (Unintentional)	Poisoning, Intentional Self-Harm	Poisoning, Assault	Poisoning, Undetermined	Adverse Effect	Underdosing
Hydroxyprogesterone	T38.5X1	T38.5X2	T38.5X3	T38.5X4	T38.5X5	T38.5X6
caproate	T38.5X1	T38.5X2	T38.5X3	T38.5X4	T38.5X5	T38.5X6
Hydroxyquinoline (derivatives) NEC	T37.8X1	T37.8X2	T37.8X3	T37.8X4	T37.8X5	T37.8X6
Hydroxystilbamidine	T37.3X1	T37.3X2	T37.3X3	T37.3X4	T37.3X5	T37.3X6
Hydroxytoluene (nonmedicinal)	T54.0X1	T54.0X2	T54.0X3	T54.0X4	—	—
medicinal	T49.0X1	T49.0X2	T49.0X3	T49.0X4	T49.0X5	T49.0X6
Hydroxyurea	T45.1X1	T45.1X2	T45.1X3	T45.1X4	T45.1X5	T45.1X6
Hydroxyzine	T43.591	T43.592	T43.593	T43.594	T43.595	T43.596
Hyoscine	T44.3X1	T44.3X2	T44.3X3	T44.3X4	T44.3X5	T44.3X6
Hyoscyamine	T44.3X1	T44.3X2	T44.3X3	T44.3X4	T44.3X5	T44.3X6
Hyoscyamus	T44.3X1	T44.3X2	T44.3X3	T44.3X4	T44.3X5	T44.3X6
dry extract	T44.3X1	T44.3X2	T44.3X3	T44.3X4	T44.3X5	T44.3X6
Hypaque	T50.8X1	T50.8X2	T50.8X3	T50.8X4	T50.8X5	T50.8X6
Hypertussis	T50.Z11	T50.Z12	T50.Z13	T50.Z14	T50.Z15	T50.Z16
Hypnotic	T42.71	T42.72	T42.73	T42.74	T42.75	T42.76
anticonvulsant	T42.71	T42.72	T42.73	T42.74	T42.75	T42.76
specified NEC	T42.6X1	T42.6X2	T42.6X3	T42.6X4	T42.6X5	T42.6X6
Hypochlorite	T49.0X1	T49.0X2	T49.0X3	T49.0X4	T49.0X5	T49.0X6
Hypophysis, posterior	T38.891	T38.892	T38.893	T38.894	T38.895	T38.896
Hypotensive NEC	T46.5X1	T46.5X2	T46.5X3	T46.5X4	T46.5X5	T46.5X6
Hypromellose	T49.5X1	T49.5X2	T49.5X3	T49.5X4	T49.5X5	T49.5X6
I						
Ibacitabine	T37.5X1	T37.5X2	T37.5X3	T37.5X4	T37.5X5	T37.5X6
Ibopamine	T44.991	T44.992	T44.993	T44.994	T44.995	T44.996
Ibufenac	T39.311	T39.312	T39.313	T39.314	T39.315	T39.316
Ibuprofen	T39.311	T39.312	T39.313	T39.314	T39.315	T39.316
Ibuproxam	T39.311	T39.312	T39.313	T39.314	T39.315	T39.316
Ibuterol	T48.6X1	T48.6X2	T48.6X3	T48.6X4	T48.6X5	T48.6X6
Ichthammol	T49.0X1	T49.0X2	T49.0X3	T49.0X4	T49.0X5	T49.0X6
Ichthyol	T49.4X1	T49.4X2	T49.4X3	T49.4X4	T49.4X5	T49.4X6
Idarubicin	T45.1X1	T45.1X2	T45.1X3	T45.1X4	T45.1X5	T45.1X6
Idrocilamide	T42.8X1	T42.8X2	T42.8X3	T42.8X4	T42.8X5	T42.8X6
Ifenprodil	T46.7X1	T46.7X2	T46.7X3	T46.7X4	T46.7X5	T46.7X6
Ifosfamide	T45.1X1	T45.1X2	T45.1X3	T45.1X4	T45.1X5	T45.1X6
Iletin	T38.3X1	T38.3X2	T38.3X3	T38.3X4	T38.3X5	T38.3X6
Ilex	T62.2X1	T62.2X2	T62.2X3	T62.2X4	—	—
Illuminating gas (after combustion)	T58.11	T58.12	T58.13	T58.14	—	—
prior to combustion	T59.891	T59.892	T59.893	T59.894	—	—
Ilopan	T45.2X1	T45.2X2	T45.2X3	T45.2X4	T45.2X5	T45.2X6
Iloprost	T46.7X1	T46.7X2	T46.7X3	T46.7X4	T46.7X5	T46.7X6

Substance	External Cause (T-Code)					
	Poisoning, Accidental (Unintentional)	Poisoning, Intentional Self-Harm	Poisoning, Assault	Poisoning, Undetermined	Adverse Effect	Underdosing
Ilotycin	T36.3X1	T36.3X2	T36.3X3	T36.3X4	T36.3X5	T36.3X6
ophthalmic preparation	T49.5X1	T49.5X2	T49.5X3	T49.5X4	T49.5X5	T49.5X6
topical NEC	T49.0X1	T49.0X2	T49.0X3	T49.0X4	T49.0X5	T49.0X6
Imidazole-4-carboxamide	T45.1X1	T45.1X2	T45.1X3	T45.1X4	T45.1X5	T45.1X6
Imipenem	T36.0X1	T36.0X2	T36.0X3	T36.0X4	T36.0X5	T36.0X6
Imipramine	T43.011	T43.012	T43.013	T43.014	T43.015	T43.016
Iminostilbene	T42.1X1	T42.1X2	T42.1X3	T42.1X4	T42.1X5	T42.1X6
Immu-G	T50.Z11	T50.Z12	T50.Z13	T50.Z14	T50.Z15	T50.Z16
Immuglobin	T50.Z11	T50.Z12	T50.Z13	T50.Z14	T50.Z15	T50.Z16
Immune						
globulin	T50.Z11	T50.Z12	T50.Z13	T50.Z14	T50.Z15	T50.Z16
serum globulin	T50.Z11	T50.Z12	T50.Z13	T50.Z14	T50.Z15	T50.Z16
Immunoglobin human (intravenous) (normal)	T50.Z11	T50.Z12	T50.Z13	T50.Z14	T50.Z15	T50.Z16
unmodified	T50.Z11	T50.Z12	T50.Z13	T50.Z14	T50.Z15	T50.Z16
Immunosuppressive drug	T45.1X1	T45.1X2	T45.1X3	T45.1X4	T45.1X5	T45.1X6
Immu-tetanus	T50.Z11	T50.Z12	T50.Z13	T50.Z14	T50.Z15	T50.Z16
Indalpine	T43.221	T43.222	T43.223	T43.224	T43.225	T43.226
Indanazoline	T48.5X1	T48.5X2	T48.5X3	T48.5X4	T48.5X5	T48.5X6
Indandione (derivatives)	T45.511	T45.512	T45.513	T45.514	T45.515	T45.516
Indapamide	T46.5X1	T46.5X2	T46.5X3	T46.5X4	T46.5X5	T46.5X6
Indendione (derivatives)	T45.511	T45.512	T45.513	T45.514	T45.515	T45.516
Indenolol	T44.7X1	T44.7X2	T44.7X3	T44.7X4	T44.7X5	T44.7X6
Inderal	T44.7X1	T44.7X2	T44.7X3	T44.7X4	T44.7X5	T44.7X6
Indian						
hemp	T40.7X1	T40.7X2	T40.7X3	T40.7X4	T40.7X5	T40.7X6
tobacco	T62.2X1	T62.2X2	T62.2X3	T62.2X4	—	—
Indigo carmine	T50.8X1	T50.8X2	T50.8X3	T50.8X4	T50.8X5	T50.8X6
Indobufen	T45.521	T45.522	T45.523	T45.524	T45.525	T45.526
Indocin	T39.2X1	T39.2X2	T39.2X3	T39.2X4	T39.2X5	T39.2X6
Indocyanine green	T50.8X1	T50.8X2	T50.8X3	T50.8X4	T50.8X5	T50.8X6
Indometacin	T39.391	T39.392	T39.393	T39.394	T39.395	T39.396
Indomethacin	T39.391	T39.392	T39.393	T39.394	T39.395	T39.396
farnesil	T39.4X1	T39.4X2	T39.4X3	T39.4X4	T39.4X5	T39.4X6
Indoramin	T44.6X1	T44.6X2	T44.6X3	T44.6X4	T44.6X5	T44.6X6
Industrial						
alcohol	T51.0X1	T51.0X2	T51.0X3	T51.0X4	—	—
fumes	T59.891	T59.892	T59.893	T59.894	—	—
solvents (fumes) (vapors)	T52.91	T52.92	T52.93	T52.94	—	—
Influenza vaccine	T50.B91	T50.B92	T50.B93	T50.B94	T50.B95	T50.B96
Ingested substance NEC	T65.91	T65.92	T65.93	T65.94	—	—
INH	T37.1X1	T37.1X2	T37.1X3	T37.1X4	T37.1X5	T37.1X6

Substance	External Cause (T-Code)					
	Poisoning, Accidental (Unintentional)	Poisoning, Intentional Self-Harm	Poisoning, Assault	Poisoning, Undetermined	Adverse Effect	Underdosing
Inhalation, gas (noxious) — *see Gas*						
Inhibitor						
angiotensin-converting enzyme	T46.4X1	T46.4X2	T46.4X3	T46.4X4	T46.4X5	T46.4X6
carbonic anhydrase	T50.2X1	T50.2X2	T50.2X3	T50.2X4	T50.2X5	T50.2X6
fibrinolysis	T45.621	T45.622	T45.623	T45.624	T45.625	T45.626
monoamine oxidase NEC	T43.1X1	T43.1X2	T43.1X3	T43.1X4	T43.1X5	T43.1X6
hydrazine	T43.1X1	T43.1X2	T43.1X3	T43.1X4	T43.1X5	T43.1X6
postsynaptic	T43.8X1	T43.8X2	T43.8X3	T43.8X4	T43.8X5	T43.8X6
prothrombin synthesis	T45.511	T45.512	T45.513	T45.514	T45.515	T45.516
Ink	T65.891	T65.892	T65.893	T65.894	—	—
Inorganic substance NEC	T57.91	T57.92	T57.93	T57.94	—	—
Inosine pranobex	T37.5X1	T37.5X2	T37.5X3	T37.5X4	T37.5X5	T37.5X6
Inositol	T50.991	T50.992	T50.993	T50.994	T50.995	T50.996
nicotinate	T46.7X1	T46.7X2	T46.7X3	T46.7X4	T46.7X5	T46.7X6
Inproquone	T45.1X1	T45.1X2	T45.1X3	T45.1X4	T45.1X5	T45.1X6
Insect (sting), venomous	T63.481	T63.482	T63.483	T63.484	—	—
ant	T63.421	T63.422	T63.423	T63.424	—	—
bee	T63.441	T63.442	T63.443	T63.444	—	—
caterpillar	T63.431	T63.432	T63.433	T63.434	—	—
hornet	T63.451	T63.452	T63.453	T63.454	—	—
wasp	T63.461	T63.462	T63.463	T63.464	—	—
Insecticide NEC	T60.91	T60.92	T60.93	T60.94	—	—
carbamate	T60.0X1	T60.0X2	T60.0X3	T60.0X4	—	—
chlorinated	T60.1X1	T60.1X2	T60.1X3	T60.1X4	—	—
mixed	T60.91	T60.92	T60.93	T60.94	—	—
organochlorine	T60.1X1	T60.1X2	T60.1X3	T60.1X4	—	—
organophosphorus	T60.0X1	T60.0X2	T60.0X3	T60.0X4	—	—
Insular tissue extract	T38.3X1	T38.3X2	T38.3X3	T38.3X4	T38.3X5	T38.3X6
Insulin (amorphous) (globin) (isophane) (Lente) (NPH) (Semilente) (Ultralente)	T38.3X1	T38.3X2	T38.3X3	T38.3X4	T38.3X5	T38.3X6
defalan	T38.3X1	T38.3X2	T38.3X3	T38.3X4	T38.3X5	T38.3X6
human	T38.3X1	T38.3X2	T38.3X3	T38.3X4	T38.3X5	T38.3X6
injection, soluble	T38.3X1	T38.3X2	T38.3X3	T38.3X4	T38.3X5	T38.3X6
biphasic	T38.3X1	T38.3X2	T38.3X3	T38.3X4	T38.3X5	T38.3X6
intermediate acting	T38.3X1	T38.3X2	T38.3X3	T38.3X4	T38.3X5	T38.3X6
protamine zinc	T38.3X1	T38.3X2	T38.3X3	T38.3X4	T38.3X5	T38.3X6
slow acting	T38.3X1	T38.3X2	T38.3X3	T38.3X4	T38.3X5	T38.3X6
zinc						
protamine injection	T38.3X1	T38.3X2	T38.3X3	T38.3X4	T38.3X5	T38.3X6
suspension (amorphous) (crystalline)	T38.3X1	T38.3X2	T38.3X3	T38.3X4	T38.3X5	T38.3X6

Substance	External Cause (T-Code)					
	Poisoning, Accidental (Unintentional)	Poisoning, Intentional Self-Harm	Poisoning, Assault	Poisoning, Undetermined	Adverse Effect	Underdosing
Interferon (alpha) (beta) (gamma)	T37.5X1	T37.5X2	T37.5X3	T37.5X4	T37.5X5	T37.5X6
Intestinal motility control drug	T47.6X1	T47.6X2	T47.6X3	T47.6X4	T47.6X5	T47.6X6
biological	T47.8X1	T47.8X2	T47.8X3	T47.8X4	T47.8X5	T47.8X6
Intranarcon	T41.1X1	T41.1X2	T41.1X3	T41.1X4	T41.1X5	T41.1X6
Intravenous						
amino acids	T50.991	T50.992	T50.993	T50.994	T50.995	T50.996
fat suspension	T50.991	T50.992	T50.993	T50.994	T50.995	T50.996
Inulin	T50.8X1	T50.8X2	T50.8X3	T50.8X4	T50.8X5	T50.8X6
Invert sugar	T50.3X1	T50.3X2	T50.3X3	T50.3X4	T50.3X5	T50.3X6
Inza — *see Naproxen*						
Iobenzamic acid	T50.8X1	T50.8X2	T50.8X3	T50.8X4	T50.8X5	T50.8X6
Iocarmic acid	T50.8X1	T50.8X2	T50.8X3	T50.8X4	T50.8X5	T50.8X6
Iocetamic acid	T50.8X1	T50.8X2	T50.8X3	T50.8X4	T50.8X5	T50.8X6
Iodamide	T50.8X1	T50.8X2	T50.8X3	T50.8X4	T50.8X5	T50.8X6
Iodide NEC — *see also Iodine*	T49.0X1	T49.0X2	T49.0X3	T49.0X4	T49.0X5	T49.0X6
mercury (ointment)	T49.0X1	T49.0X2	T49.0X3	T49.0X4	T49.0X5	T49.0X6
methylate	T49.0X1	T49.0X2	T49.0X3	T49.0X4	T49.0X5	T49.0X6
potassium (expectorant) NEC	T48.4X1	T48.4X2	T48.4X3	T48.4X4	T48.4X5	T48.4X6
Iodinated						
contrast medium	T50.8X1	T50.8X2	T50.8X3	T50.8X4	T50.8X5	T50.8X6
glycerol	T48.4X1	T48.4X2	T48.4X3	T48.4X4	T48.4X5	T48.4X6
human serum albumin (131I)	T50.8X1	T50.8X2	T50.8X3	T50.8X4	T50.8X5	T50.8X6
Iodine (antiseptic, external) (tincture) NEC	T49.0X1	T49.0X2	T49.0X3	T49.0X4	T49.0X5	T49.0X6
125 — *see also Radiation sickness, and Exposure to radioactivce isotopes*	T50.8X1	T50.8X2	T50.8X3	T50.8X4	T50.8X5	T50.8X6
therapeutic	T50.991	T50.992	T50.993	T50.994	T50.995	T50.996
131 — *see also Radiation sickness, and Exposure to radioactivce isotopes*	T50.8X1	T50.8X2	T50.8X3	T50.8X4	T50.8X5	T50.8X6
therapeutic	T38.2X1	T38.2X2	T38.2X3	T38.2X4	T38.2X5	T38.2X6
diagnostic	T50.8X1	T50.8X2	T50.8X3	T50.8X4	T50.8X5	T50.8X6
for thyroid conditions (antithyroid)	T38.2X1	T38.2X2	T38.2X3	T38.2X4	T38.2X5	T38.2X6
solution	T49.0X1	T49.0X2	T49.0X3	T49.0X4	T49.0X5	T49.0X6
vapor	T59.891	T59.892	T59.893	T59.894	—	—
Iodipamide	T50.8X1	T50.8X2	T50.8X3	T50.8X4	T50.8X5	T50.8X6
Iodized (poppy seed) oil	T50.8X1	T50.8X2	T50.8X3	T50.8X4	T50.8X5	T50.8X6
Iodobismitol	T37.8X1	T37.8X2	T37.8X3	T37.8X4	T37.8X5	T37.8X6
Iodochlorhydroxyquin	T37.8X1	T37.8X2	T37.8X3	T37.8X4	T37.8X5	T37.8X6
topical	T49.0X1	T49.0X2	T49.0X3	T49.0X4	T49.0X5	T49.0X6
Iodochlorhydroxyquino-line	T37.8X1	T37.8X2	T37.8X3	T37.8X4	T37.8X5	T37.8X6
Iodocholesterol (131I)	T50.8X1	T50.8X2	T50.8X3	T50.8X4	T50.8X5	T50.8X6

◀ New ◀ Revised ~~deleted~~ Deleted

Substance	External Cause (T-Code)					
	Poisoning, Accidental (Unintentional)	Poisoning, Intentional Self-Harm	Poisoning, Assault	Poisoning, Undetermined	Adverse Effect	Underdosing
Iodoform	T49.0X1	T49.0X2	T49.0X3	T49.0X4	T49.0X5	T49.0X6
Iodohippuric acid	T50.8X1	T50.8X2	T50.8X3	T50.8X4	T50.8X5	T50.8X6
Iodopanoic acid	T50.8X1	T50.8X2	T50.8X3	T50.8X4	T50.8X5	T50.8X6
Iodophthalein (sodium)	T50.8X1	T50.8X2	T50.8X3	T50.8X4	T50.8X5	T50.8X6
Iodopyracet	T50.8X1	T50.8X2	T50.8X3	T50.8X4	T50.8X5	T50.8X6
Iodoquinol	T37.8X1	T37.8X2	T37.8X3	T37.8X4	T37.8X5	T37.8X6
Iodoxamic acid	T50.8X1	T50.8X2	T50.8X3	T50.8X4	T50.8X5	T50.8X6
Iofendylate	T50.8X1	T50.8X2	T50.8X3	T50.8X4	T50.8X5	T50.8X6
Ioglycamic acid	T50.8X1	T50.8X2	T50.8X3	T50.8X4	T50.8X5	T50.8X6
Iohexol	T50.8X1	T50.8X2	T50.8X3	T50.8X4	T50.8X5	T50.8X6
Ion exchange resin						
anion	T47.8X1	T47.8X2	T47.8X3	T47.8X4	T47.8X5	T47.8X6
cation	T50.3X1	T50.3X2	T50.3X3	T50.3X4	T50.3X5	T50.3X6
cholestyramine	T46.6X1	T46.6X2	T46.6X3	T46.6X4	T46.6X5	T46.6X6
intestinal	T47.8X1	T47.8X2	T47.8X3	T47.8X4	T47.8X5	T47.8X6
Iopamidol	T50.8X1	T50.8X2	T50.8X3	T50.8X4	T50.8X5	T50.8X6
Iopanoic acid	T50.8X1	T50.8X2	T50.8X3	T50.8X4	T50.8X5	T50.8X6
Iophenoic acid	T50.8X1	T50.8X2	T50.8X3	T50.8X4	T50.8X5	T50.8X6
Iopodate, sodium	T50.8X1	T50.8X2	T50.8X3	T50.8X4	T50.8X5	T50.8X6
Iopodic acid	T50.8X1	T50.8X2	T50.8X3	T50.8X4	T50.8X5	T50.8X6
Iopromide	T50.8X1	T50.8X2	T50.8X3	T50.8X4	T50.8X5	T50.8X6
Iopydol	T50.8X1	T50.8X2	T50.8X3	T50.8X4	T50.8X5	T50.8X6
Iotalamic acid	T50.8X1	T50.8X2	T50.8X3	T50.8X4	T50.8X5	T50.8X6
Iothalamate	T50.8X1	T50.8X2	T50.8X3	T50.8X4	T50.8X5	T50.8X6
Iothiouracil	T38.2X1	T38.2X2	T38.2X3	T38.2X4	T38.2X5	T38.2X6
Iotrol	T50.8X1	T50.8X2	T50.8X3	T50.8X4	T50.8X5	T50.8X6
Iotrolan	T50.8X1	T50.8X2	T50.8X3	T50.8X4	T50.8X5	T50.8X6
Iotroxate	T50.8X1	T50.8X2	T50.8X3	T50.8X4	T50.8X5	T50.8X6
Iotroxic acid	T50.8X1	T50.8X2	T50.8X3	T50.8X4	T50.8X5	T50.8X6
Ioversol	T50.8X1	T50.8X2	T50.8X3	T50.8X4	T50.8X5	T50.8X6
Ioxaglate	T50.8X1	T50.8X2	T50.8X3	T50.8X4	T50.8X5	T50.8X6
Ioxaglic acid	T50.8X1	T50.8X2	T50.8X3	T50.8X4	T50.8X5	T50.8X6
Ioxitalamic acid	T50.8X1	T50.8X2	T50.8X3	T50.8X4	T50.8X5	T50.8X6
Ipecac	T47.7X1	T47.7X2	T47.7X3	T47.7X4	T47.7X5	T47.7X6
Ipecacuanha	T48.4X1	T48.4X2	T48.4X3	T48.4X4	T48.4X5	T48.4X6
Ipodate, calcium	T50.8X1	T50.8X2	T50.8X3	T50.8X4	T50.8X5	T50.8X6
Ipral	T42.3X1	T42.3X2	T42.3X3	T42.3X4	T42.3X5	T42.3X6
Ipratropium (bromide)	T48.6X1	T48.6X2	T48.6X3	T48.6X4	T48.6X5	T48.6X6
Ipriflavone	T46.3X1	T46.3X2	T46.3X3	T46.3X4	T46.3X5	T46.3X6
Iprindole	T43.011	T43.012	T43.013	T43.014	T43.015	T43.016
Iproclozide	T43.1X1	T43.1X2	T43.1X3	T43.1X4	T43.1X5	T43.1X6
Iprofenin	T50.8X1	T50.8X2	T50.8X3	T50.8X4	T50.8X5	T50.8X6

Substance	External Cause (T-Code)					
	Poisoning, Accidental (Unintentional)	Poisoning, Intentional Self-Harm	Poisoning, Assault	Poisoning, Undetermined	Adverse Effect	Underdosing
Iproheptine	T49.2X1	T49.2X2	T49.2X3	T49.2X4	T49.2X5	T49.2X6
Iproniazid	T43.1X1	T43.1X2	T43.1X3	T43.1X4	T43.1X5	T43.1X6
Iproplatin	T45.1X1	T45.1X2	T45.1X3	T45.1X4	T45.1X5	T45.1X6
Iproveratril	T46.1X1	T46.1X2	T46.1X3	T46.1X4	T46.1X5	T46.1X6
Iron (compounds) (medicinal) NEC	T45.4X1	T45.4X2	T45.4X3	T45.4X4	T45.4X5	T45.4X6
ammonium	T45.4X1	T45.4X2	T45.4X3	T45.4X4	T45.4X5	T45.4X6
dextran injection	T45.4X1	T45.4X2	T45.4X3	T45.4X4	T45.4X5	T45.4X6
nonmedicinal	T56.891	T56.892	T56.893	T56.894	—	—
salts	T45.4X1	T45.4X2	T45.4X3	T45.4X4	T45.4X5	T45.4X6
sorbitex	T45.4X1	T45.4X2	T45.4X3	T45.4X4	T45.4X5	T45.4X6
sorbitol citric acid complex	T45.4X1	T45.4X2	T45.4X3	T45.4X4	T45.4X5	T45.4X6
Irrigating fluid (vaginal)	T49.8X1	T49.8X2	T49.8X3	T49.8X4	T49.8X5	T49.8X6
eye	T49.5X1	T49.5X2	T49.5X3	T49.5X4	T49.5X5	T49.5X6
Isepamicin	T36.5X1	T36.5X2	T36.5X3	T36.5X4	T36.5X5	T36.5X6
Isoaminile (citrate)	T48.3X1	T48.3X2	T48.3X3	T48.3X4	T48.3X5	T48.3X6
Isoamyl nitrite	T46.3X1	T46.3X2	T46.3X3	T46.3X4	T46.3X5	T46.3X6
Isobenzan	T60.1X1	T60.1X2	T60.1X3	T60.1X4	—	—
Isobutyl acetate	T52.8X1	T52.8X2	T52.8X3	T52.8X4	—	—
Isocarboxazid	T43.1X1	T43.1X2	T43.1X3	T43.1X4	T43.1X5	T43.1X6
Isoconazole	T49.0X1	T49.0X2	T49.0X3	T49.0X4	T49.0X5	T49.0X6
Isocyanate	T65.0X1	T65.0X2	T65.0X3	T65.0X4	—	—
Isoephedrine	T44.991	T44.992	T44.993	T44.994	T44.995	T44.996
Isoetarine	T48.6X1	T48.6X2	T48.6X3	T48.6X4	T48.6X5	T48.6X6
Isoethadione	T42.2X1	T42.2X2	T42.2X3	T42.2X4	T42.2X5	T42.2X6
Isoetharine	T44.5X1	T44.5X2	T44.5X3	T44.5X4	T44.5X5	T44.5X6
Isoflurane	T41.0X1	T41.0X2	T41.0X3	T41.0X4	T41.0X5	T41.0X6
Isoflurophate	T44.0X1	T44.0X2	T44.0X3	T44.0X4	T44.0X5	T44.0X6
Isomaltose, ferric complex	T45.4X1	T45.4X2	T45.4X3	T45.4X4	T45.4X5	T45.4X6
Isometheptene	T44.3X1	T44.3X2	T44.3X3	T44.3X4	T44.3X5	T44.3X6
Isoniazid	T37.1X1	T37.1X2	T37.1X3	T37.1X4	T37.1X5	T37.1X6
with						
rifampicin	T36.6X1	T36.6X2	T36.6X3	T36.6X4	T36.6X5	T36.6X6
thioacetazone	T37.1X1	T37.1X2	T37.1X3	T37.1X4	T37.1X5	T37.1X6
Isonicotinic acid hydrazide	T37.1X1	T37.1X2	T37.1X3	T37.1X4	T37.1X5	T37.1X6
Isonipecaine	T40.4X1	T40.4X2	T40.4X3	T40.4X4	T40.4X5	T40.4X6
Isopentaquine	T37.2X1	T37.2X2	T37.2X3	T37.2X4	T37.2X5	T37.2X6
Isophane insulin	T38.3X1	T38.3X2	T38.3X3	T38.3X4	T38.3X5	T38.3X6
Isophorone	T65.891	T65.892	T65.893	T65.894	—	—
Isophosphamide	T45.1X1	T45.1X2	T45.1X3	T45.1X4	T45.1X5	T45.1X6
Isopregnenone	T38.5X1	T38.5X2	T38.5X3	T38.5X4	T38.5X5	T38.5X6
Isoprenaline	T48.6X1	T48.6X2	T48.6X3	T48.6X4	T48.6X5	T48.6X6
Isopromethazine	T43.3X1	T43.3X2	T43.3X3	T43.3X4	T43.3X5	T43.3X6

Substance	External Cause (T-Code)					
	Poisoning, Accidental (Unintentional)	Poisoning, Intentional Self-Harm	Poisoning, Assault	Poisoning, Undetermined	Adverse Effect	Underdosing
Isopropamide	T44.3X1	T44.3X2	T44.3X3	T44.3X4	T44.3X5	T44.3X6
iodide	T44.3X1	T44.3X2	T44.3X3	T44.3X4	T44.3X5	T44.3X6
Isopropanol	T51.2X1	T51.2X2	T51.2X3	T51.2X4	—	—
Isopropyl						
acetate	T52.8X1	T52.8X2	T52.8X3	T52.8X4	—	—
alcohol	T51.2X1	T51.2X2	T51.2X3	T51.2X4	—	—
medicinal	T49.4X1	T49.4X2	T49.4X3	T49.4X4	T49.4X5	T49.4X6
ether	T52.8X1	T52.8X2	T52.8X3	T52.8X4	—	—
Isopropylaminophena-zone	T39.2X1	T39.2X2	T39.2X3	T39.2X4	T39.2X5	T39.2X6
Isoproterenol	T48.6X1	T48.6X2	T48.6X3	T48.6X4	T48.6X5	T48.6X6
Isosorbide dinitrate	T46.3X1	T46.3X2	T46.3X3	T46.3X4	T46.3X5	T46.3X6
Isothipendyl	T45.0X1	T45.0X2	T45.0X3	T45.0X4	T45.0X5	T45.0X6
Isotretinoin	T50.991	T50.992	T50.993	T50.994	T50.995	T50.996
Isoxazolyl penicillin	T36.0X1	T36.0X2	T36.0X3	T36.0X4	T36.0X5	T36.0X6
Isoxicam	T39.391	T39.392	T39.393	T39.394	T39.395	T39.396
Isoxsuprine	T46.7X1	T46.7X2	T46.7X3	T46.7X4	T46.7X5	T46.7X6
Ispagula	T47.4X1	T47.4X2	T47.4X3	T47.4X4	T47.4X5	T47.4X6
husk	T47.4X1	T47.4X2	T47.4X3	T47.4X4	T47.4X5	T47.4X6
Isradipine	T46.1X1	T46.1X2	T46.1X3	T46.1X4	T46.1X5	T46.1X6
l-thyroxine sodium	T38.1X1	T38.1X2	T38.1X3	T38.1X4	T38.1X5	T38.1X6
Itraconazole	T37.8X1	T37.8X2	T37.8X3	T37.8X4	T37.8X5	T37.8X6
Itramin tosilate	T46.3X1	T46.3X2	T46.3X3	T46.3X4	T46.3X5	T46.3X6
Ivermectin	T37.4X1	T37.4X2	T37.4X3	T37.4X4	T37.4X5	T37.4X6
Izoniazid	T37.1X1	T37.1X2	T37.1X3	T37.1X4	T37.1X5	T37.1X6
with thioacetazone	T37.1X1	T37.1X2	T37.1X3	T37.1X4	T37.1X5	T37.1X6
J						
Jalap	T47.2X1	T47.2X2	T47.2X3	T47.2X4	T47.2X5	T47.2X6
Jamaica						
dogwood (bark)	T39.8X1	T39.8X2	T39.8X3	T39.8X4	T39.8X5	T39.8X6
ginger	T65.891	T65.892	T65.893	T65.894	—	—
root	T62.2X1	T62.2X2	T62.2X3	T62.2X4	—	—
Jatropha	T62.2X1	T62.2X2	T62.2X3	T62.2X4	—	—
curcas	T62.2X1	T62.2X2	T62.2X3	T62.2X4	—	—
Jectofer	T45.4X1	T45.4X2	T45.4X3	T45.4X4	T45.4X5	T45.4X6
Jellyfish (sting)	T63.621	T63.622	T63.623	T63.624	—	—
Jequirity (bean)	T62.2X1	T62.2X2	T62.2X3	T62.2X4	—	—
Jimson weed (stramonium)	T62.2X1	T62.2X2	T62.2X3	T62.2X4	—	—
seeds	T62.2X1	T62.2X2	T62.2X3	T62.2X4	—	—
Josamycin	T36.3X1	T36.3X2	T36.3X3	T36.3X4	T36.3X5	T36.3X6
Juniper tar	T49.1X1	T49.1X2	T49.1X3	T49.1X4	T49.1X5	T49.1X6

Substance	External Cause (T-Code)					
	Poisoning, Accidental (Unintentional)	Poisoning, Intentional Self-Harm	Poisoning, Assault	Poisoning, Undetermined	Adverse Effect	Underdosing
K						
Kallidinogenase	T46.7X1	T46.7X2	T46.7X3	T46.7X4	T46.7X5	T46.7X6
Kallikrein	T46.7X1	T46.7X2	T46.7X3	T46.7X4	T46.7X5	T46.7X6
Kanamycin	T36.5X1	T36.5X2	T36.5X3	T36.5X4	T36.5X5	T36.5X6
Kantrex	T36.5X1	T36.5X2	T36.5X3	T36.5X4	T36.5X5	T36.5X6
Kaolin	T47.6X1	T47.6X2	T47.6X3	T47.6X4	T47.6X5	T47.6X6
light	T47.6X1	T47.6X2	T47.6X3	T47.6X4	T47.6X5	T47.6X6
Karaya (gum)	T47.4X1	T47.4X2	T47.4X3	T47.4X4	T47.4X5	T47.4X6
Kebuzone	T39.2X1	T39.2X2	T39.2X3	T39.2X4	T39.2X5	T39.2X6
Kelevan	T60.1X1	T60.1X2	T60.1X3	T60.1X4	—	—
Kemithal	T41.1X1	T41.1X2	T41.1X3	T41.1X4	T41.1X5	T41.1X6
Kenacort	T38.0X1	T38.0X2	T38.0X3	T38.0X4	T38.0X5	T38.0X6
Keratolytic drug NEC	T49.4X1	T49.4X2	T49.4X3	T49.4X4	T49.4X5	T49.4X6
anthracene	T49.4X1	T49.4X2	T49.4X3	T49.4X4	T49.4X5	T49.4X6
Keratoplastic NEC	T49.4X1	T49.4X2	T49.4X3	T49.4X4	T49.4X5	T49.4X6
Kerosene, kerosine (fuel) (solvent) NEC	T52.0X1	T52.0X2	T52.0X3	T52.0X4	—	—
insecticide	T52.0X1	T52.0X2	T52.0X3	T52.0X4	—	—
vapor	T52.0X1	T52.0X2	T52.0X3	T52.0X4	—	—
Ketamine	T41.291	T41.292	T41.293	T41.294	T41.295	T41.296
Ketazolam	T42.4X1	T42.4X2	T42.4X3	T42.4X4	T42.4X5	T42.4X6
Ketazon	T39.2X1	T39.2X2	T39.2X3	T39.2X4	T39.2X5	T39.2X6
Ketobemidone	T40.4X1	T40.4X2	T40.4X3	T40.4X4	—	—
Ketoconazole	T49.0X1	T49.0X2	T49.0X3	T49.0X4	T49.0X5	T49.0X6
Ketols	T52.4X1	T52.4X2	T52.4X3	T52.4X4	—	—
Ketone oils	T52.4X1	T52.4X2	T52.4X3	T52.4X4	—	—
Ketoprofen	T39.311	T39.312	T39.313	T39.314	T39.315	T39.316
Ketorolac	T39.8X1	T39.8X2	T39.8X3	T39.8X4	T39.8X5	T39.8X6
Ketotifen	T45.0X1	T45.0X2	T45.0X3	T45.0X4	T45.0X5	T45.0X6
Khat	T43.691	T43.692	T43.693	T43.694	—	—
Khellin	T46.3X1	T46.3X2	T46.3X3	T46.3X4	T46.3X5	T46.3X6
Khelloside	T46.3X1	T46.3X2	T46.3X3	T46.3X4	T46.3X5	T46.3X6
Kiln gas or vapor (carbon monoxide)	T58.8X1	T58.8X2	T58.8X3	T58.8X4	—	—
Kitasamycin	T36.3X1	T36.3X2	T36.3X3	T36.3X4	T36.3X5	T36.3X6
Konsyl	T47.4X1	T47.4X2	T47.4X3	T47.4X4	T47.4X5	T47.4X6
Kosam seed	T62.2X1	T62.2X2	T62.2X3	T62.2X4	—	—
Krait (venom)	T63.091	T63.092	T63.093	T63.094	—	—
Kwell (insecticide)	T60.1X1	T60.1X2	T60.1X3	T60.1X4	—	—
anti-infective (topical)	T49.0X1	T49.0X2	T49.0X3	T49.0X4	T49.0X5	T49.0X6

◀ New ◀ Revised ~~deleted~~ Deleted

Substance	Poisoning, Accidental (Unintentional)	Poisoning, Intentional Self-Harm	Poisoning, Assault	Poisoning, Undetermined	Adverse Effect	Underdosing
	External Cause (T-Code)					
L						
Labetalol	T44.8X1	T44.8X2	T44.8X3	T44.8X4	T44.8X5	T44.8X6
Laburnum (seeds)	T62.2X1	T62.2X2	T62.2X3	T62.2X4	—	—
leaves	T62.2X1	T62.2X2	T62.2X3	T62.2X4	—	—
Lachesine	T49.5X1	T49.5X2	T49.5X3	T49.5X4	T49.5X5	T49.5X6
Lacidipine	T46.5X1	T46.5X2	T46.5X3	T46.5X4	T46.5X5	T46.5X6
Lacquer	T65.6X1	T65.6X2	T65.6X3	T65.6X4	—	—
Lacrimogenic gas	T59.3X1	T59.3X2	T59.3X3	T59.3X4	—	—
Lactated potassic saline	T50.3X1	T50.3X2	T50.3X3	T50.3X4	T50.3X5	T50.3X6
Lactic acid	T49.8X1	T49.8X2	T49.8X3	T49.8X4	T49.8X5	T49.8X6
Lactobacillus						
acidophilus	T47.6X1	T47.6X2	T47.6X3	T47.6X4	T47.6X5	T47.6X6
compound	T47.6X1	T47.6X2	T47.6X3	T47.6X4	T47.6X5	T47.6X6
bifidus, lyophilized	T47.6X1	T47.6X2	T47.6X3	T47.6X4	T47.6X5	T47.6X6
bulgaricus	T47.6X1	T47.6X2	T47.6X3	T47.6X4	T47.6X5	T47.6X6
sporogenes	T47.6X1	T47.6X2	T47.6X3	T47.6X4	T47.6X5	T47.6X6
Lactoflavin	T45.2X1	T45.2X2	T45.2X3	T45.2X4	T45.2X5	T45.2X6
Lactose (as excipient)	T50.901	T50.902	T50.903	T50.904	T50.905	T50.906
Lactuca (virosa) (extract)	T42.6X1	T42.6X2	T42.6X3	T42.6X4	T42.6X5	T42.6X6
Lactucarium	T42.6X1	T42.6X2	T42.6X3	T42.6X4	T42.6X5	T42.6X6
Lactulose	T47.3X1	T47.3X2	T47.3X3	T47.3X4	T47.3X5	T47.3X6
Laevo — *see Levo-*						
Lanatosides	T46.0X1	T46.0X2	T46.0X3	T46.0X4	T46.0X5	T46.0X6
Lanolin	T49.3X1	T49.3X2	T49.3X3	T49.3X4	T49.3X5	T49.3X6
Largactil	T43.3X1	T43.3X2	T43.3X3	T43.3X4	T43.3X5	T43.3X6
Larkspur	T62.2X1	T62.2X2	T62.2X3	T62.2X4	—	—
Laroxyl	T43.011	T43.012	T43.013	T43.014	T43.015	T43.016
Lassar's paste	T49.4X1	T49.4X2	T49.4X3	T49.4X4	T49.4X5	T49.4X6
Lasix	T50.1X1	T50.1X2	T50.1X3	T50.1X4	T50.1X5	T50.1X6
Latamoxef	T36.1X1	T36.1X2	T36.1X3	T36.1X4	T36.1X5	T36.1X6
Latex	T65.811	T65.812	T65.813	T65.814	—	—
Lathyrus (seed)	T62.2X1	T62.2X2	T62.2X3	T62.2X4	—	—
Laudanum	T40.0X1	T40.0X2	T40.0X3	T40.0X4	T40.0X5	T40.0X6
Laudexium	T48.1X1	T48.1X2	T48.1X3	T48.1X4	T48.1X5	T48.1X6
Laughing gas	T41.0X1	T41.0X2	T41.0X3	T41.0X4	T41.0X5	T41.0X6
Laurel, black or cherry	T62.2X1	T62.2X2	T62.2X3	T62.2X4	—	—
Laurolinium	T49.0X1	T49.0X2	T49.0X3	T49.0X4	T49.0X5	T49.0X6
Lauryl sulfoacetate	T49.2X1	T49.2X2	T49.2X3	T49.2X4	T49.2X5	T49.2X6

Substance	Poisoning, Accidental (Unintentional)	Poisoning, Intentional Self-Harm	Poisoning, Assault	Poisoning, Undetermined	Adverse Effect	Underdosing
	External Cause (T-Code)					
Laxative NEC	T47.4X1	T47.4X2	T47.4X3	T47.4X4	T47.4X5	T47.4X6
osmotic	T47.3X1	T47.3X2	T47.3X3	T47.3X4	T47.3X5	T47.3X6
saline	T47.3X1	T47.3X2	T47.3X3	T47.3X4	T47.3X5	T47.3X6
stimulant	T47.2X1	T47.2X2	T47.2X3	T47.2X4	T47.2X5	T47.2X6
L-dopa	T42.8X1	T42.8X2	T42.8X3	T42.8X4	T42.8X5	T42.8X6
Lead (dust) (fumes) (vapor) NEC	T56.0X1	T56.0X2	T56.0X3	T56.0X4	—	—
acetate	T49.2X1	T49.2X2	T49.2X3	T49.2X4	T49.2X5	T49.2X6
alkyl (fuel additive)	T56.0X1	T56.0X2	T56.0X3	T56.0X4	—	—
anti-infectives	T37.8X1	T37.8X2	T37.8X3	T37.8X4	T37.8X5	T37.8X6
antiknock compound (tetraethyl)	T56.0X1	T56.0X2	T56.0X3	T56.0X4	—	—
arsenate, arsenite (dust) (herbicide) (insecticide) (vapor)	T57.0X1	T57.0X2	T57.0X3	T57.0X4	—	—
carbonate	T56.0X1	T56.0X2	T56.0X3	T56.0X4	—	—
paint	T56.0X1	T56.0X2	T56.0X3	T56.0X4	—	—
chromate	T56.0X1	T56.0X2	T56.0X3	T56.0X4	—	—
paint	T56.0X1	T56.0X2	T56.0X3	T56.0X4	—	—
dioxide	T56.0X1	T56.0X2	T56.0X3	T56.0X4	—	—
inorganic	T56.0X1	T56.0X2	T56.0X3	T56.0X4	—	—
iodide	T56.0X1	T56.0X2	T56.0X3	T56.0X4	—	—
pigment (paint)	T56.0X1	T56.0X2	T56.0X3	T56.0X4	—	—
monoxide (dust)	T56.0X1	T56.0X2	T56.0X3	T56.0X4	—	—
paint	T56.0X1	T56.0X2	T56.0X3	T56.0X4	—	—
organic	T56.0X1	T56.0X2	T56.0X3	T56.0X4	—	—
oxide	T56.0X1	T56.0X2	T56.0X3	T56.0X4	—	—
paint	T56.0X1	T56.0X2	T56.0X3	T56.0X4	—	—
paint	T56.0X1	T56.0X2	T56.0X3	T56.0X4	—	—
salts	T56.0X1	T56.0X2	T56.0X3	T56.0X4	—	—
specified compound NEC	T56.0X1	T56.0X2	T56.0X3	T56.0X4	—	—
tetra-ethyl	T56.0X1	T56.0X2	T56.0X3	T56.0X4	—	—
Lebanese red	T40.7X1	T40.7X2	T40.7X3	T40.7X4	T40.7X5	T40.7X6
Lefetamine	T39.8X1	T39.8X2	T39.8X3	T39.8X4	T39.8X5	T39.8X6
Lenperone	T43.4X1	T43.4X2	T43.4X3	T43.4X4	T43.4X5	T43.4X6
Lente lietin (insulin)	T38.3X1	T38.3X2	T38.3X3	T38.3X4	T38.3X5	T38.3X6
Leptazol	T50.7X1	T50.7X2	T50.7X3	T50.7X4	T50.7X5	T50.7X6
Leptophos	T60.0X1	T60.0X2	T60.0X3	T60.0X4	—	—
Leritine	T40.2X1	T40.2X2	T40.2X3	T40.2X4	T40.2X5	T40.2X6
Letosteine	T48.4X1	T48.4X2	T48.4X3	T48.4X4	T48.4X5	T48.4X6
Letter	T38.1X1	T38.1X2	T38.1X3	T38.1X4	T38.1X5	T38.1X6
Lettuce opium	T42.6X1	T42.6X2	T42.6X3	T42.6X4	T42.6X5	T42.6X6
Leucinocaine	T41.3X1	T41.3X2	T41.3X3	T41.3X4	T41.3X5	T41.3X6

Substance	Poisoning, Accidental (Unintentional)	Poisoning, Intentional Self-Harm	Poisoning, Assault	Poisoning, Undetermined	Adverse Effect	Underdosing
		External Cause (T-Code)				
Leucocianidol	T46.991	T46.992	T46.993	T46.994	T46.995	T46.996
Leucovorin (factor)	T45.8X1	T45.8X2	T45.8X3	T45.8X4	T45.8X5	T45.8X6
Leukeran	T45.1X1	T45.1X2	T45.1X3	T45.1X4	T45.1X5	T45.1X6
Leuprolide	T38.891	T38.892	T38.893	T38.894	T38.895	T38.896
Levalbuterol	T48.6X1	T48.6X2	T48.6X3	T48.6X4	T48.6X5	T48.6X6
Levallorphan	T50.7X1	T50.7X2	T50.7X3	T50.7X4	T50.7X5	T50.7X6
Levamisole	T37.4X1	T37.4X2	T37.4X3	T37.4X4	T37.4X5	T37.4X6
Levanil	T42.6X1	T42.6X2	T42.6X3	T42.6X4	T42.6X5	T42.6X6
Levarterenol	T44.4X1	T44.4X2	T44.4X3	T44.4X4	T44.4X5	T44.4X6
Levdropropizine	T48.3X1	T48.3X2	T48.3X3	T48.3X4	T48.3X5	T48.3X6
Levobunolol	T49.5X1	T49.5X2	T49.5X3	T49.5X4	T49.5X5	T49.5X6
Levocabastine (hydrochloride)	T45.0X1	T45.0X2	T45.0X3	T45.0X4	T45.0X5	T45.0X6
Levocarnitine	T50.991	T50.992	T50.993	T50.994	T50.995	T50.996
Levodopa	T42.8X1	T42.8X2	T42.8X3	T42.8X4	T42.8X5	T42.8X6
with carbidopa	T42.8X1	T42.8X2	T42.8X3	T42.8X4	T42.8X5	T42.8X6
Levo-dromoran	T40.2X1	T40.2X2	T40.2X3	T40.2X4	T40.2X5	T40.2X6
Levoglutamide	T50.991	T50.992	T50.993	T50.994	T50.995	T50.996
Levoid	T38.1X1	T38.1X2	T38.1X3	T38.1X4	T38.1X5	T38.1X6
Levo-iso-methadone	T40.3X1	T40.3X2	T40.3X3	T40.3X4	T40.3X5	T40.3X6
Levomepromazine	T43.3X1	T43.3X2	T43.3X3	T43.3X4	T43.3X5	T43.3X6
Levonordefrin	T49.6X1	T49.6X2	T49.6X3	T49.6X4	T49.6X5	T49.6X6
Levonorgestrel	T38.4X1	T38.4X2	T38.4X3	T38.4X4	T38.4X5	T38.4X6
with ethinylestradiol	T38.5X1	T38.5X2	T38.5X3	T38.5X4	T38.5X5	T38.5X6
Levopromazine	T43.3X1	T43.3X2	T43.3X3	T43.3X4	T43.3X5	T43.3X6
Levoprome	T42.6X1	T42.6X2	T42.6X3	T42.6X4	T42.6X5	T42.6X6
Levopropoxyphene	T40.4X1	T40.4X2	T40.4X3	T40.4X4	T40.4X5	T40.4X6
Levopropylhexedrine	T50.5X1	T50.5X2	T50.5X3	T50.5X4	T50.5X5	T50.5X6
Levoproxyphylline	T48.6X1	T48.6X2	T48.6X3	T48.6X4	T48.6X5	T48.6X6
Levorphanol	T40.4X1	T40.4X2	T40.4X3	T40.4X4	T40.4X5	T40.4X6
Levothyroxine	T38.1X1	T38.1X2	T38.1X3	T38.1X4	T38.1X5	T38.1X6
sodium	T38.1X1	T38.1X2	T38.1X3	T38.1X4	T38.1X5	T38.1X6
Levsin	T44.3X1	T44.3X2	T44.3X3	T44.3X4	T44.3X5	T44.3X6
Levulose	T50.3X1	T50.3X2	T50.3X3	T50.3X4	T50.3X5	T50.3X6
Lewisite (gas), not in war	T57.0X1	T57.0X2	T57.0X3	T57.0X4	—	—
Librium	T42.4X1	T42.4X2	T42.4X3	T42.4X4	T42.4X5	T42.4X6
Lidex	T49.0X1	T49.0X2	T49.0X3	T49.0X4	T49.0X5	T49.0X6
Lidocaine	T41.3X1	T41.3X2	T41.3X3	T41.3X4	T41.3X5	T41.3X6
regional	T41.3X1	T41.3X2	T41.3X3	T41.3X4	T41.3X5	T41.3X6
spinal	T41.3X1	T41.3X2	T41.3X3	T41.3X4	T41.3X5	T41.3X6
Lidofenin	T50.8X1	T50.8X2	T50.8X3	T50.8X4	T50.8X5	T50.8X6
Lidoflazine	T46.1X1	T46.1X2	T46.1X3	T46.1X4	T46.1X5	T46.1X6
Lighter fluid	T52.0X1	T52.0X2	T52.0X3	T52.0X4	—	—

Substance	Poisoning, Accidental (Unintentional)	Poisoning, Intentional Self-Harm	Poisoning, Assault	Poisoning, Undetermined	Adverse Effect	Underdosing
		External Cause (T-Code)				
Lignin hemicellulose	T47.6X1	T47.6X2	T47.6X3	T47.6X4	T47.6X5	T47.6X6
Lignocaine	T41.3X1	T41.3X2	T41.3X3	T41.3X4	T41.3X5	T41.3X6
regional	T41.3X1	T41.3X2	T41.3X3	T41.3X4	T41.3X5	T41.3X6
spinal	T41.3X1	T41.3X2	T41.3X3	T41.3X4	T41.3X5	T41.3X6
Ligroin(e) (solvent)	T52.0X1	T52.0X2	T52.0X3	T52.0X4	—	—
vapor	T59.891	T59.892	T59.893	T59.894	—	—
Ligustrum vulgare	T62.2X1	T62.2X2	T62.2X3	T62.2X4	—	—
Lily of the valley	T62.2X1	T62.2X2	T62.2X3	T62.2X4	—	—
Lime (chloride)	T54.3X1	T54.3X2	T54.3X3	T54.3X4	—	—
Limonene	T52.8X1	T52.8X2	T52.8X3	T52.8X4	—	—
Lincomycin	T36.8X1	T36.8X2	T36.8X3	T36.8X4	T36.8X5	T36.8X6
Lindane (insecticide) (nonmedicinal) (vapor)	T53.6X1	T53.6X2	T53.6X3	T53.6X4	—	—
medicinal	T49.0X1	T49.0X2	T49.0X3	T49.0X4	T49.0X5	T49.0X6
Liniments NEC	T49.91	T49.92	T49.93	T49.94	T49.95	T49.96
Linoleic acid	T46.6X1	T46.6X2	T46.6X3	T46.6X4	T46.6X5	T46.6X6
Linolenic acid	T46.6X1	T46.6X2	T46.6X3	T46.6X4	T46.6X5	T46.6X6
Linseed	T47.4X1	T47.4X2	T47.4X3	T47.4X4	T47.4X5	T47.4X6
Liothyronine	T38.1X1	T38.1X2	T38.1X3	T38.1X4	T38.1X5	T38.1X6
Liotrix	T38.1X1	T38.1X2	T38.1X3	T38.1X4	T38.1X5	T38.1X6
Lipancreatin	T47.5X1	T47.5X2	T47.5X3	T47.5X4	T47.5X5	T47.5X6
Lipo-alprostadil	T46.7X1	T46.7X2	T46.7X3	T46.7X4	T46.7X5	T46.7X6
Lipo-Lutin	T38.5X1	T38.5X2	T38.5X3	T38.5X4	T38.5X5	T38.5X6
Lipotropic drug NEC	T50.901	T50.902	T50.903	T50.904	T50.905	T50.906
Liquefied petroleum gases	T59.891	T59.892	T59.893	T59.894	—	—
piped (pure or mixed with air)	T59.891	T59.892	T59.893	T59.894	—	—
Liquid						
paraffin	T47.4X1	T47.4X2	T47.4X3	T47.4X4	T47.4X5	T47.4X6
petrolatum	T47.4X1	T47.4X2	T47.4X3	T47.4X4	T47.4X5	T47.4X6
topical	T49.3X1	T49.3X2	T49.3X3	T49.3X4	T49.3X5	T49.3X6
specified NEC	T65.891	T65.892	T65.893	T65.894	—	—
substance	T65.91	T65.92	T65.93	T65.94	—	—
Liquor creosolis compositus	T65.891	T65.892	T65.893	T65.894	—	—
Liquorice	T48.4X1	T48.4X2	T48.4X3	T48.4X4	T48.4X5	T48.4X6
extract	T47.8X1	T47.8X2	T47.8X3	T47.8X4	T47.8X5	T47.8X6
Lirugen	T50.991	T50.992	T50.993	T50.994	T50.995	T50.996
Lisinopril	T46.4X1	T46.4X2	T46.4X3	T46.4X4	T46.4X5	T46.4X6
Lisuride	T42.8X1	T42.8X2	T42.8X3	T42.8X4	T42.8X5	T42.8X6
Lithane	T43.8X1	T43.8X2	T43.8X3	T43.8X4	T43.8X5	T43.8X6
Lithium	T56.891	T56.892	T56.893	T56.894	—	—
gluconate	T43.591	T43.592	T43.593	T43.594	T43.595	T43.596
salts (carbonate)	T43.591	T43.592	T43.593	T43.594	T43.595	T43.596

◀ New ◀ Revised ~~deleted~~ Deleted

Substance	External Cause (T-Code)					
	Poisoning, Accidental (Unintentional)	Poisoning, Intentional Self-Harm	Poisoning, Assault	Poisoning, Undetermined	Adverse Effect	Underdosing
Lithonate	T43.8X1	T43.8X2	T43.8X3	T43.8X4	T43.8X5	T43.8X6
Liver						
extract	T45.8X1	T45.8X2	T45.8X3	T45.8X4	T45.8X5	T45.8X6
for parenteral use	T45.8X1	T45.8X2	T45.8X3	T45.8X4	T45.8X5	T45.8X6
fraction 1	T45.8X1	T45.8X2	T45.8X3	T45.8X4	T45.8X5	T45.8X6
hydrolysate	T45.8X1	T45.8X2	T45.8X3	T45.8X4	T45.8X5	T45.8X6
Lizard (bite) (venom)	T63.121	T63.122	T63.123	T63.124	—	—
LMD	T45.8X1	T45.8X2	T45.8X3	T45.8X4	T45.8X5	T45.8X6
Lobelia	T62.2X1	T62.2X2	T62.2X3	T62.2X4	—	—
Lobeline	T50.7X1	T50.7X2	T50.7X3	T50.7X4	T50.7X5	T50.7X6
Local action drug NEC	T49.8X1	T49.8X2	T49.8X3	T49.8X4	T49.8X5	T49.8X6
Locorten	T49.0X1	T49.0X2	T49.0X3	T49.0X4	T49.0X5	T49.0X6
Lofepramine	T43.011	T43.012	T43.013	T43.014	T43.015	T43.016
Lolium temulentum	T62.2X1	T62.2X2	T62.2X3	T62.2X4	—	—
Lomotil	T47.6X1	T47.6X2	T47.6X3	T47.6X4	T47.6X5	T47.6X6
Lomustine	T45.1X1	T45.1X2	T45.1X3	T45.1X4	T45.1X5	T45.1X6
Lonidamine	T45.1X1	T45.1X2	T45.1X3	T45.1X4	T45.1X5	T45.1X6
Loperamide	T47.6X1	T47.6X2	T47.6X3	T47.6X4	T47.6X5	T47.6X6
Loprazolam	T42.4X1	T42.4X2	T42.4X3	T42.4X4	T42.4X5	T42.4X6
Lorajmine	T46.2X1	T46.2X2	T46.2X3	T46.2X4	T46.2X5	T46.2X6
Loratidine	T45.0X1	T45.0X2	T45.0X3	T45.0X4	T45.0X5	T45.0X6
Lorazepam	T42.4X1	T42.4X2	T42.4X3	T42.4X4	T42.4X5	T42.4X6
Lorcainide	T46.2X1	T46.2X2	T46.2X3	T46.2X4	T46.2X5	T46.2X6
Lormetazepam	T42.4X1	T42.4X2	T42.4X3	T42.4X4	T42.4X5	T42.4X6
Lotions NEC	T49.91	T49.92	T49.93	T49.94	T49.95	T49.96
Lotusate	T42.3X1	T42.3X2	T42.3X3	T42.3X4	T42.3X5	T42.3X6
Lovastatin	T46.6X1	T46.6X2	T46.6X3	T46.6X4	T46.6X5	T46.6X6
Loxapine	T43.591	T43.592	T43.593	T43.594	T43.595	T43.596
Lowila	T49.2X1	T49.2X2	T49.2X3	T49.2X4	T49.2X5	T49.2X6
Lozenges (throat)	T49.6X1	T49.6X2	T49.6X3	T49.6X4	T49.6X5	T49.6X6
LSD	T40.8X1	T40.8X2	T40.8X3	T40.8X4	—	—
L-Tryptophan — *see amino acid*						
Lubricant, eye	T49.5X1	T49.5X2	T49.5X3	T49.5X4	T49.5X5	T49.5X6
Lubricating oil NEC	T52.0X1	T52.0X2	T52.0X3	T52.0X4	—	—
Lucanthone	T37.4X1	T37.4X2	T37.4X3	T37.4X4	T37.4X5	T37.4X6
Luminal	T42.3X1	T42.3X2	T42.3X3	T42.3X4	T42.3X5	T42.3X6
Lung irritant (gas) NEC	T59.91	T59.92	T59.93	T59.94	—	—
Luteinizing hormone	T38.811	T38.812	T38.813	T38.814	T38.815	T38.816
Lutocylol	T38.5X1	T38.5X2	T38.5X3	T38.5X4	T38.5X5	T38.5X6
Lutromone	T38.5X1	T38.5X2	T38.5X3	T38.5X4	T38.5X5	T38.5X6
Lututrin	T48.291	T48.292	T48.293	T48.294	T48.295	T48.296
Lye (Concentrated)	T54.3X1	T54.3X2	T54.3X3	T54.3X4	—	—

Substance	External Cause (T-Code)					
	Poisoning, Accidental (Unintentional)	Poisoning, Intentional Self-Harm	Poisoning, Assault	Poisoning, Undetermined	Adverse Effect	Underdosing
Lygranum (skin test)	T50.8X1	T50.8X2	T50.8X3	T50.8X4	T50.8X5	T50.8X6
Lymecycline	T36.4X1	T36.4X2	T36.4X3	T36.4X4	T36.4X5	T36.4X6
Lymphogranuloma venereum antigen	T50.8X1	T50.8X2	T50.8X3	T50.8X4	T50.8X5	T50.8X6
Lynestrenol	T38.4X1	T38.4X2	T38.4X3	T38.4X4	T38.4X5	T38.4X6
Lypressin	T38.891	T38.892	T38.893	T38.894	T38.895	T38.896
Lyovac Sodium Edecrin	T50.1X1	T50.1X2	T50.1X3	T50.1X4	T50.1X5	T50.1X6
Lysergic acid diethylamide	T40.8X1	T40.8X2	T40.8X3	T40.8X4	—	—
Lysergide	T40.8X1	T40.8X2	T40.8X3	T40.8X4	—	—
Lysine vasopressin	T38.891	T38.892	T38.893	T38.894	T38.895	T38.896
Lysol	T54.1X1	T54.1X2	T54.1X3	T54.1X4	—	—
Lysozyme	T49.0X1	T49.0X2	T49.0X3	T49.0X4	T49.0X5	T49.0X6
Lytta (vitatta)	T49.8X1	T49.8X2	T49.8X3	T49.8X4	T49.8X5	T49.8X6
M						
Mace	T59.3X1	T59.3X2	T59.3X3	T59.3X4	—	—
Macrogol	T50.991	T50.992	T50.993	T50.994	T50.995	T50.996
Macrolide						
anabolic drug	T38.7X1	T38.7X2	T38.7X3	T38.7X4	T38.7X5	T38.7X6
antibiotic	T36.3X1	T36.3X2	T36.3X3	T36.3X4	T36.3X5	T36.3X6
Mafenide	T49.0X1	T49.0X2	T49.0X3	T49.0X4	T49.0X5	T49.0X6
Magaldrate	T47.1X1	T47.1X2	T47.1X3	T47.1X4	T47.1X5	T47.1X6
Magic mushroom	T40.991	T40.992	T40.993	T40.994	—	—
Magnamycin	T36.8X1	T36.8X2	T36.8X3	T36.8X4	T36.8X5	T36.8X6
Magnesia magma	T47.1X1	T47.1X2	T47.1X3	T47.1X4	T47.1X5	T47.1X6
Magnesium NEC	T56.891	T56.892	T56.893	T56.894	—	—
carbonate	T47.1X1	T47.1X2	T47.1X3	T47.1X4	T47.1X5	T47.1X6
citrate	T47.4X1	T47.4X2	T47.4X3	T47.4X4	T47.4X5	T47.4X6
hydroxide	T47.1X1	T47.1X2	T47.1X3	T47.1X4	T47.1X5	T47.1X6
oxide	T47.1X1	T47.1X2	T47.1X3	T47.1X4	T47.1X5	T47.1X6
peroxide	T49.0X1	T49.0X2	T49.0X3	T49.0X4	T49.0X5	T49.0X6
salicylate	T39.091	T39.092	T39.093	T39.094	T39.095	T39.096
silicofluoride	T50.3X1	T50.3X2	T50.3X3	T50.3X4	T50.3X5	T50.3X6
sulfate	T47.4X1	T47.4X2	T47.4X3	T47.4X4	T47.4X5	T47.4X6
thiosulfate	T45.0X1	T45.0X2	T45.0X3	T45.0X4	T45.0X5	T45.0X6
trisilicate	T47.1X1	T47.1X2	T47.1X3	T47.1X4	T47.1X5	T47.1X6
Malathion (medicinal)	T49.0X1	T49.0X2	T49.0X3	T49.0X4	T49.0X5	T49.0X6
insecticide	T60.0X1	T60.0X2	T60.0X3	T60.0X4	—	—
Male fern extract	T37.4X1	T37.4X2	T37.4X3	T37.4X4	T37.4X5	T37.4X6
M-AMSA	T45.1X1	T45.1X2	T45.1X3	T45.1X4	T45.1X5	T45.1X6
Mandelic acid	T37.8X1	T37.8X2	T37.8X3	T37.8X4	T37.8X5	T37.8X6
Manganese (dioxide) (salts)	T57.2X1	T57.2X2	T57.2X3	T57.2X4	—	—
medicinal	T50.991	T50.992	T50.993	T50.994	T50.995	T50.996

Substance	External Cause (T-Code)					
	Poisoning, Accidental (Unintentional)	Poisoning, Intentional Self-Harm	Poisoning, Assault	Poisoning, Undetermined	Adverse Effect	Underdosing
Mannitol	T47.3X1	T47.3X2	T47.3X3	T47.3X4	T47.3X5	T47.3X6
hexanitrate	T46.3X1	T46.3X2	T46.3X3	T46.3X4	T46.3X5	T46.3X6
Mannomustine	T45.1X1	T45.1X2	T45.1X3	T45.1X4	T45.1X5	T45.1X6
MAO inhibitors	T43.1X1	T43.1X2	T43.1X3	T43.1X4	T43.1X5	T43.1X6
Mapharsen	T37.8X1	T37.8X2	T37.8X3	T37.8X4	T37.8X5	T37.8X6
Maphenide	T49.0X1	T49.0X2	T49.0X3	T49.0X4	T49.0X5	T49.0X6
Maprotiline	T43.021	T43.022	T43.023	T43.024	T43.025	T43.026
Marcaine	T41.3X1	T41.3X2	T41.3X3	T41.3X4	T41.3X5	T41.3X6
infiltration (subcutaneous)	T41.3X1	T41.3X2	T41.3X3	T41.3X4	T41.3X5	T41.3X6
nerve block (peripheral) (plexus)	T41.3X1	T41.3X2	T41.3X3	T41.3X4	T41.3X5	T41.3X6
Marezine	T45.0X1	T45.0X2	T45.0X3	T45.0X4	T45.0X5	T45.0X6
Marihuana	T40.7X1	T40.7X2	T40.7X3	T40.7X4	T40.7X5	T40.7X6
Marijuana	T40.7X1	T40.7X2	T40.7X3	T40.7X4	T40.7X5	T40.7X6
Marine (sting)	T63.691	T63.692	T63.693	T63.694	—	—
animals (sting)	T63.691	T63.692	T63.693	T63.694	—	—
plants (sting)	T63.711	T63.712	T63.713	T63.714	—	—
Marplan	T43.1X1	T43.1X2	T43.1X3	T43.1X4	T43.1X5	T43.1X6
Marsh gas	T59.891	T59.892	T59.893	T59.894	—	—
Marsilid	T43.1X1	T43.1X2	T43.1X3	T43.1X4	T43.1X5	T43.1X6
Matulane	T45.1X1	T45.1X2	T45.1X3	T45.1X4	T45.1X5	T45.1X6
Mazindol	T50.5X1	T50.5X2	T50.5X3	T50.5X4	T50.5X5	T50.5X6
MCPA	T60.3X1	T60.3X2	T60.3X3	T60.3X4	—	—
MDMA	T43.621	T43.622	T43.623	T43.624	T43.625	T43.626
Meadow saffron	T62.2X1	T62.2X2	T62.2X3	T62.2X4	—	—
Measles virus vaccine (attenuated)	T50.B91	T50.B92	T50.B93	T50.B94	T50.B95	T50.B96
Meat, noxious	T62.8X1	T62.8X2	T62.8X3	T62.8X4	—	—
Meballymal	T42.3X1	T42.3X2	T42.3X3	T42.3X4	T42.3X5	T42.3X6
Mebanazine	T43.1X1	T43.1X2	T43.1X3	T43.1X4	T43.1X5	T43.1X6
Mebaral	T42.3X1	T42.3X2	T42.3X3	T42.3X4	T42.3X5	T42.3X6
Mebendazole	T37.4X1	T37.4X2	T37.4X3	T37.4X4	T37.4X5	T37.4X6
Mebeverine	T44.3X1	T44.3X2	T44.3X3	T44.3X4	T44.3X5	T44.3X6
Mebhydrolin	T45.0X1	T45.0X2	T45.0X3	T45.0X4	T45.0X5	T45.0X6
Mebumal	T42.3X1	T42.3X2	T42.3X3	T42.3X4	T42.3X5	T42.3X6
Mebutamate	T43.591	T43.592	T43.593	T43.594	T43.595	T43.596
Mecamylamine	T44.2X1	T44.2X2	T44.2X3	T44.2X4	T44.2X5	T44.2X6
Mechlorethamine	T45.1X1	T45.1X2	T45.1X3	T45.1X4	T45.1X5	T45.1X6
Mecillinam	T36.0X1	T36.0X2	T36.0X3	T36.0X4	T36.0X5	T36.0X6
Meclizine (hydrochloride)	T45.0X1	T45.0X2	T45.0X3	T45.0X4	T45.0X5	T45.0X6
Meclocycline	T36.4X1	T36.4X2	T36.4X3	T36.4X4	T36.4X5	T36.4X6
Meclofenamate	T39.391	T39.392	T39.393	T39.394	T39.395	T39.396
Meclofenamic acid	T39.391	T39.392	T39.393	T39.394	T39.395	T39.396

Substance	External Cause (T-Code)					
	Poisoning, Accidental (Unintentional)	Poisoning, Intentional Self-Harm	Poisoning, Assault	Poisoning, Undetermined	Adverse Effect	Underdosing
Meclofenoxate	T43.691	T43.692	T43.693	T43.694	T43.695	T43.696
Meclozine	T45.0X1	T45.0X2	T45.0X3	T45.0X4	T45.0X5	T45.0X6
Mecobalamin	T45.8X1	T45.8X2	T45.8X3	T45.8X4	T45.8X5	T45.8X6
Mecoprop	T60.3X1	T60.3X2	T60.3X3	T60.3X4	—	—
Mecrilate	T49.3X1	T49.3X2	T49.3X3	T49.3X4	T49.3X5	T49.3X6
Mecysteine	T48.4X1	T48.4X2	T48.4X3	T48.4X4	T48.4X5	T48.4X6
Medazepam	T42.4X1	T42.4X2	T42.4X3	T42.4X4	T42.4X5	T42.4X6
Medicament NEC	T50.901	T50.902	T50.903	T50.904	T50.905	T50.906
Medinal	T42.3X1	T42.3X2	T42.3X3	T42.3X4	T42.3X5	T42.3X6
Medomin	T42.3X1	T42.3X2	T42.3X3	T42.3X4	T42.3X5	T42.3X6
Medrogestone	T38.5X1	T38.5X2	T38.5X3	T38.5X4	T38.5X5	T38.5X6
Medroxalol	T44.8X1	T44.8X2	T44.8X3	T44.8X4	T44.8X5	T44.8X6
Medroxyprogesterone acetate (depot)	T38.5X1	T38.5X2	T38.5X3	T38.5X4	T38.5X5	T38.5X6
Medrysone	T49.0X1	T49.0X2	T49.0X3	T49.0X4	T49.0X5	T49.0X6
Mefenamic acid	T39.391	T39.392	T39.393	T39.394	T39.395	T39.396
Mefenorex	T50.5X1	T50.5X2	T50.5X3	T50.5X4	T50.5X5	T50.5X6
Mefloquine	T37.2X1	T37.2X2	T37.2X3	T37.2X4	T37.2X5	T37.2X6
Mefruside	T50.2X1	T50.2X2	T50.2X3	T50.2X4	T50.2X5	T50.2X6
Megahallucinogen	T40.901	T40.902	T40.903	T40.904	T40.905	T40.906
Megestrol	T38.5X1	T38.5X2	T38.5X3	T38.5X4	T38.5X5	T38.5X6
Meglumine						
antimoniate	T37.8X1	T37.8X2	T37.8X3	T37.8X4	T37.8X5	T37.8X6
diatrizoate	T50.8X1	T50.8X2	T50.8X3	T50.8X4	T50.8X5	T50.8X6
iodipamide	T50.8X1	T50.8X2	T50.8X3	T50.8X4	T50.8X5	T50.8X6
iotroxate	T50.8X1	T50.8X2	T50.8X3	T50.8X4	T50.8X5	T50.8X6
MEK (methyl ethyl ketone)	T52.4X1	T52.4X2	T52.4X3	T52.4X4	—	—
Meladrazine	T44.3X1	T44.3X2	T44.3X3	T44.3X4	T44.3X5	T44.3X6
Meladinin	T49.3X1	T49.3X2	T49.3X3	T49.3X4	T49.3X5	T49.3X6
Melaleuca alternifolia oil	T49.0X1	T49.0X2	T49.0X3	T49.0X4	T49.0X5	T49.0X6
Melanizing agents	T49.3X1	T49.3X2	T49.3X3	T49.3X4	T49.3X5	T49.3X6
Melanocyte-stimulating hormone	T38.891	T38.892	T38.893	T38.894	T38.895	T38.896
Melarsonyl potassium	T37.3X1	T37.3X2	T37.3X3	T37.3X4	T37.3X5	T37.3X6
Melarsoprol	T37.3X1	T37.3X2	T37.3X3	T37.3X4	T37.3X5	T37.3X6
Melia azedarach	T62.2X1	T62.2X2	T62.2X3	T62.2X4	—	—
Melitracen	T43.011	T43.012	T43.013	T43.014	T43.015	T43.016
Mellaril	T43.3X1	T43.3X2	T43.3X3	T43.3X4	T43.3X5	T43.3X6
Meloxine	T49.3X1	T49.3X2	T49.3X3	T49.3X4	T49.3X5	T49.3X6
Melperone	T43.4X1	T43.4X2	T43.4X3	T43.4X4	T43.4X5	T43.4X6
Melphalan	T45.1X1	T45.1X2	T45.1X3	T45.1X4	T45.1X5	T45.1X6
Memantine	T43.8X1	T43.8X2	T43.8X3	T43.8X4	T43.8X5	T43.8X6

◀ New ◀ Revised ~~deleted~~ Deleted

Substance	External Cause (T-Code)					
	Poisoning, Accidental (Unintentional)	Poisoning, Intentional Self-Harm	Poisoning, Assault	Poisoning, Undetermined	Adverse Effect	Underdosing
Menadiol	T45.7X1	T45.7X2	T45.7X3	T45.7X4	T45.7X5	T45.7X6
sodium sulfate	T45.7X1	T45.7X2	T45.7X3	T45.7X4	T45.7X5	T45.7X6
Menadione	T45.7X1	T45.7X2	T45.7X3	T45.7X4	T45.7X5	T45.7X6
sodium bisulfite	T45.7X1	T45.7X2	T45.7X3	T45.7X4	T45.7X5	T45.7X6
Menaphthone	T45.7X1	T45.7X2	T45.7X3	T45.7X4	T45.7X5	T45.7X6
Menaquinone	T45.7X1	T45.7X2	T45.7X3	T45.7X4	T45.7X5	T45.7X6
Menatetrenone	T45.7X1	T45.7X2	T45.7X3	T45.7X4	T45.7X5	T45.7X6
Meningococcal vaccine	T50.A91	T50.A92	T50.A93	T50.A94	T50.A95	T50.A96
Menningovax (-AC) (-C)	T50.A91	T50.A92	T50.A93	T50.A94	T50.A95	T50.A96
Menotropins	T38.811	T38.812	T38.813	T38.814	T38.815	T38.816
Menthol	T48.5X1	T48.5X2	T48.5X3	T48.5X4	T48.5X5	T48.5X6
Mepacrine	T37.2X1	T37.2X2	T37.2X3	T37.2X4	T37.2X5	T37.2X6
Meparfynol	T42.6X1	T42.6X2	T42.6X3	T42.6X4	T42.6X5	T42.6X6
Mepartricin	T36.7X1	T36.7X2	T36.7X3	T36.7X4	T36.7X5	T36.7X6
Mepazine	T43.3X1	T43.3X2	T43.3X3	T43.3X4	T43.3X5	T43.3X6
Mepenzolate	T44.3X1	T44.3X2	T44.3X3	T44.3X4	T44.3X5	T44.3X6
bromide	T44.3X1	T44.3X2	T44.3X3	T44.3X4	T44.3X5	T44.3X6
Meperidine	T40.4X1	T40.4X2	T40.4X3	T40.4X4	T40.4X5	T40.4X6
Mephebarbital	T42.3X1	T42.3X2	T42.3X3	T42.3X4	T42.3X5	T42.3X6
Mephenamin(e)	T42.8X1	T42.8X2	T42.8X3	T42.8X4	T42.8X5	T42.8X6
Mephenesin	T42.8X1	T42.8X2	T42.8X3	T42.8X4	T42.8X5	T42.8X6
Mephenhydramine	T45.0X1	T45.0X2	T45.0X3	T45.0X4	T45.0X5	T45.0X6
Mephenoxalone	T42.8X1	T42.8X2	T42.8X3	T42.8X4	T42.8X5	T42.8X6
Mephentermine	T44.991	T44.992	T44.993	T44.994	T44.995	T44.996
Mephenytoin	T42.0X1	T42.0X2	T42.0X3	T42.0X4	T42.0X5	T42.0X6
with phenobarbital	T42.3X1	T42.3X2	T42.3X3	T42.3X4	T42.3X5	T42.3X6
Mephobarbital	T42.3X1	T42.3X2	T42.3X3	T42.3X4	T42.3X5	T42.3X6
Mephosfolan	T60.0X1	T60.0X2	T60.0X3	T60.0X4	—	—
Mepindolol	T44.7X1	T44.7X2	T44.7X3	T44.7X4	T44.7X5	T44.7X6
Mepiperphenidol	T44.3X1	T44.3X2	T44.3X3	T44.3X4	T44.3X5	T44.3X6
Mepitiostane	T38.7X1	T38.7X2	T38.7X3	T38.7X4	T38.7X5	T38.7X6
Mepivacaine	T41.3X1	T41.3X2	T41.3X3	T41.3X4	T41.3X5	T41.3X6
epidural	T41.3X1	T41.3X2	T41.3X3	T41.3X4	T41.3X5	T41.3X6
Meprednisone	T38.0X1	T38.0X2	T38.0X3	T38.0X4	T38.0X5	T38.0X6
Meprobam	T43.591	T43.592	T43.593	T43.594	T43.595	T43.596
Meprobamate	T43.591	T43.592	T43.593	T43.594	T43.595	T43.596
Meproscillarin	T46.0X1	T46.0X2	T46.0X3	T46.0X4	T46.0X5	T46.0X6
Meprylcaine	T41.3X1	T41.3X2	T41.3X3	T41.3X4	T41.3X5	T41.3X6
Meptazinol	T39.8X1	T39.8X2	T39.8X3	T39.8X4	T39.8X5	T39.8X6
Mepyramine	T45.0X1	T45.0X2	T45.0X3	T45.0X4	T45.0X5	T45.0X6
Mequitazine	T43.3X1	T43.3X2	T43.3X3	T43.3X4	T43.3X5	T43.3X6
Meralluride	T50.2X1	T50.2X2	T50.2X3	T50.2X4	T50.2X5	T50.2X6

Substance	External Cause (T-Code)					
	Poisoning, Accidental (Unintentional)	Poisoning, Intentional Self-Harm	Poisoning, Assault	Poisoning, Undetermined	Adverse Effect	Underdosing
Merbaphen	T50.2X1	T50.2X2	T50.2X3	T50.2X4	T50.2X5	T50.2X6
Merbromin	T49.0X1	T49.0X2	T49.0X3	T49.0X4	T49.0X5	T49.0X6
Mercaptobenzothiazole salts	T49.0X1	T49.0X2	T49.0X3	T49.0X4	T49.0X5	T49.0X6
Mercaptomerin	T50.2X1	T50.2X2	T50.2X3	T50.2X4	T50.2X5	T50.2X6
Mercaptopurine	T45.1X1	T45.1X2	T45.1X3	T45.1X4	T45.1X5	T45.1X6
Mercumatilin	T50.2X1	T50.2X2	T50.2X3	T50.2X4	T50.2X5	T50.2X6
Mercuramide	T50.2X1	T50.2X2	T50.2X3	T50.2X4	T50.2X5	T50.2X6
Mercurochrome	T49.0X1	T49.0X2	T49.0X3	T49.0X4	T49.0X5	T49.0X6
Mercurophylline	T50.2X1	T50.2X2	T50.2X3	T50.2X4	T50.2X5	T50.2X6
Mercury, mercurial, mercuric, mercurous (compounds) (cyanide) (fumes) (nonmedicinal) (vapor) NEC	T56.1X1	T56.1X2	T56.1X3	T56.1X4	—	—
ammoniated	T49.0X1	T49.0X2	T49.0X3	T49.0X4	T49.0X5	T49.0X6
anti-infective						
local	T49.0X1	T49.0X2	T49.0X3	T49.0X4	T49.0X5	T49.0X6
systemic	T37.8X1	T37.8X2	T37.8X3	T37.8X4	T37.8X5	T37.8X6
topical	T49.0X1	T49.0X2	T49.0X3	T49.0X4	T49.0X5	T49.0X6
chloride (ammoniated)	T49.0X1	T49.0X2	T49.0X3	T49.0X4	T49.0X5	T49.0X6
fungicide	T56.1X1	T56.1X2	T56.1X3	T56.1X4	—	—
diuretic NEC	T50.2X1	T50.2X2	T50.2X3	T50.2X4	T50.2X5	T50.2X6
fungicide	T56.1X1	T56.1X2	T56.1X3	T56.1X4	—	—
organic (fungicide)	T56.1X1	T56.1X2	T56.1X3	T56.1X4	—	—
oxide, yellow	T49.0X1	T49.0X2	T49.0X3	T49.0X4	T49.0X5	T49.0X6
Mersalyl	T50.2X1	T50.2X2	T50.2X3	T50.2X4	T50.2X5	T50.2X6
Merthiolate	T49.0X1	T49.0X2	T49.0X3	T49.0X4	T49.0X5	T49.0X6
ophthalmic preparation	T49.5X1	T49.5X2	T49.5X3	T49.5X4	T49.5X5	T49.5X6
Meruvax	T50.B91	T50.B92	T50.B93	T50.B94	T50.B95	T50.B96
Mesalazine	T47.8X1	T47.8X2	T47.8X3	T47.8X4	T47.8X5	T47.8X6
Mescal buttons	T40.991	T40.992	T40.993	T40.994	—	—
Mescaline	T40.991	T40.992	T40.993	T40.994	—	—
Mesna	T48.4X1	T48.4X2	T48.4X3	T48.4X4	T48.4X5	T48.4X6
Mesoglycan	T46.6X1	T46.6X2	T46.6X3	T46.6X4	T46.6X5	T46.6X6
Mesoridazine	T43.3X1	T43.3X2	T43.3X3	T43.3X4	T43.3X5	T43.3X6
Mestanolone	T38.7X1	T38.7X2	T38.7X3	T38.7X4	T38.7X5	T38.7X6
Mesterolone	T38.7X1	T38.7X2	T38.7X3	T38.7X4	T38.7X5	T38.7X6
Mestranol	T38.5X1	T38.5X2	T38.5X3	T38.5X4	T38.5X5	T38.5X6
Mesulergine	T42.8X1	T42.8X2	T42.8X3	T42.8X4	T42.8X5	T42.8X6
Mesulfen	T49.0X1	T49.0X2	T49.0X3	T49.0X4	T49.0X5	T49.0X6
Mesuximide	T42.2X1	T42.2X2	T42.2X3	T42.2X4	T42.2X5	T42.2X6
Metabutethamine	T41.3X1	T41.3X2	T41.3X3	T41.3X4	T41.3X5	T41.3X6
Metactesylacetate	T49.0X1	T49.0X2	T49.0X3	T49.0X4	T49.0X5	T49.0X6

Substance	External Cause (T-Code)					
	Poisoning, Accidental (Unintentional)	Poisoning, Intentional Self-Harm	Poisoning, Assault	Poisoning, Undetermined	Adverse Effect	Underdosing
Metacycline	T36.4X1	T36.4X2	T36.4X3	T36.4X4	T36.4X5	T36.4X6
Metaldehyde (snail killer) NEC	T60.8X1	T60.8X2	T60.8X3	T60.8X4	—	—
Metals (heavy) (nonmedicinal)	T56.91	T56.92	T56.93	T56.94	—	—
dust, fumes, or vapor NEC	T56.91	T56.92	T56.93	T56.94	—	—
light NEC	T56.91	T56.92	T56.93	T56.94	—	—
dust, fumes, or vapor NEC	T56.91	T56.92	T56.93	T56.94	—	—
specified NEC	T56.891	T56.892	T56.893	T56.894	—	—
thallium	T56.811	T56.812	T56.813	T56.814	—	—
Metamfetamine	T43.621	T43.622	T43.623	T43.624	T43.625	T43.626
Metamizole sodium	T39.2X1	T39.2X2	T39.2X3	T39.2X4	T39.2X5	T39.2X6
Metampicillin	T36.0X1	T36.0X2	T36.0X3	T36.0X4	T36.0X5	T36.0X6
Metamucil	T47.4X1	T47.4X2	T47.4X3	T47.4X4	T47.4X5	T47.4X6
Metaphen	T49.0X1	T49.0X2	T49.0X3	T49.0X4	T49.0X5	T49.0X6
Metandienone	T38.7X1	T38.7X2	T38.7X3	T38.7X4	T38.7X5	T38.7X6
Metandrostenolone	T38.7X1	T38.7X2	T38.7X3	T38.7X4	T38.7X5	T38.7X6
Metaphos	T60.0X1	T60.0X2	T60.0X3	T60.0X4	—	—
Metapramine	T43.011	T43.012	T43.013	T43.014	T43.015	T43.016
Metaproterenol	T48.291	T48.292	T48.293	T48.294	T48.295	T48.296
Metaraminol	T44.4X1	T44.4X2	T44.4X3	T44.4X4	T44.4X5	T44.4X6
Metaxalone	T42.8X1	T42.8X2	T42.8X3	T42.8X4	T42.8X5	T42.8X6
Metenolone	T38.7X1	T38.7X2	T38.7X3	T38.7X4	T38.7X5	T38.7X6
Metergoline	T42.8X1	T42.8X2	T42.8X3	T42.8X4	T42.8X5	T42.8X6
Metescufylline	T46.991	T46.992	T46.993	T46.994	T46.995	T46.996
Metetoin	T42.0X1	T42.0X2	T42.0X3	T42.0X4	T42.0X5	T42.0X6
Metformin	T38.3X1	T38.3X2	T38.3X3	T38.3X4	T38.3X5	T38.3X6
Methacholine	T44.1X1	T44.1X2	T44.1X3	T44.1X4	T44.1X5	T44.1X6
Methacycline	T36.4X1	T36.4X2	T36.4X3	T36.4X4	T36.4X5	T36.4X6
Methadone	T40.3X1	T40.3X2	T40.3X3	T40.3X4	T40.3X5	T40.3X6
Methallenestril	T38.5X1	T38.5X2	T38.5X3	T38.5X4	T38.5X5	T38.5X6
Methallenoestril	T38.5X1	T38.5X2	T38.5X3	T38.5X4	T38.5X5	T38.5X6
Methamphetamine	T43.621	T43.622	T43.623	T43.624	T43.625	T43.626
Methampyrone	T39.2X1	T39.2X2	T39.2X3	T39.2X4	T39.2X5	T39.2X6
Methandienone	T38.7X1	T38.7X2	T38.7X3	T38.7X4	T38.7X5	T38.7X6
Methandriol	T38.7X1	T38.7X2	T38.7X3	T38.7X4	T38.7X5	T38.7X6
Methandrostenolone	T38.7X1	T38.7X2	T38.7X3	T38.7X4	T38.7X5	T38.7X6
Methane	T59.891	T59.892	T59.893	T59.894	—	—
Methanethiol	T59.891	T59.892	T59.893	T59.894	—	—
Methaniazide	T37.1X1	T37.1X2	T37.1X3	T37.1X4	T37.1X5	T37.1X6
Methanol (vapor)	T51.1X1	T51.1X2	T51.1X3	T51.1X4	—	—
Methantheline	T44.3X1	T44.3X2	T44.3X3	T44.3X4	T44.3X5	T44.3X6
Methanthelinium bromide	T44.3X1	T44.3X2	T44.3X3	T44.3X4	T44.3X5	T44.3X6
Methaphenilene	T45.0X1	T45.0X2	T45.0X3	T45.0X4	T45.0X5	T45.0X6

Substance	External Cause (T-Code)					
	Poisoning, Accidental (Unintentional)	Poisoning, Intentional Self-Harm	Poisoning, Assault	Poisoning, Undetermined	Adverse Effect	Underdosing
Methapyrilene	T45.0X1	T45.0X2	T45.0X3	T45.0X4	T45.0X5	T45.0X6
Methaqualone (compound)	T42.6X1	T42.6X2	T42.6X3	T42.6X4	T42.6X5	T42.6X6
Metharbital	T42.3X1	T42.3X2	T42.3X3	T42.3X4	T42.3X5	T42.3X6
Methazolamide	T50.2X1	T50.2X2	T50.2X3	T50.2X4	T50.2X5	T50.2X6
Methdilazine	T43.3X1	T43.3X2	T43.3X3	T43.3X4	T43.3X5	T43.3X6
Methedrine	T43.621	T43.622	T43.623	T43.624	T43.625	T43.626
Methenamine (mandelate)	T37.8X1	T37.8X2	T37.8X3	T37.8X4	T37.8X5	T37.8X6
Methenolone	T38.7X1	T38.7X2	T38.7X3	T38.7X4	T38.7X5	T38.7X6
Methergine	T48.0X1	T48.0X2	T48.0X3	T48.0X4	T48.0X5	T48.0X6
Methetoin	T42.0X1	T42.0X2	T42.0X3	T42.0X4	T42.0X5	T42.0X6
Methiacil	T38.2X1	T38.2X2	T38.2X3	T38.2X4	T38.2X5	T38.2X6
Methicillin	T36.0X1	T36.0X2	T36.0X3	T36.0X4	T36.0X5	T36.0X6
Methimazole	T38.2X1	T38.2X2	T38.2X3	T38.2X4	T38.2X5	T38.2X6
Methiodal sodium	T50.8X1	T50.8X2	T50.8X3	T50.8X4	T50.8X5	T50.8X6
Methionine	T50.991	T50.992	T50.993	T50.994	T50.995	T50.996
Methisazone	T37.5X1	T37.5X2	T37.5X3	T37.5X4	T37.5X5	T37.5X6
Methisoprinol	T37.5X1	T37.5X2	T37.5X3	T37.5X4	T37.5X5	T37.5X6
Methitural	T42.3X1	T42.3X2	T42.3X3	T42.3X4	T42.3X5	T42.3X6
Methixene	T44.3X1	T44.3X2	T44.3X3	T44.3X4	T44.3X5	T44.3X6
Methobarbital, methobarbitone	T42.3X1	T42.3X2	T42.3X3	T42.3X4	T42.3X5	T42.3X6
Methocarbamol	T42.8X1	T42.8X2	T42.8X3	T42.8X4	T42.8X5	T42.8X6
skeletal muscle relaxant	T48.1X1	T48.1X2	T48.1X3	T48.1X4	T48.1X5	T48.1X6
Methohexital	T41.1X1	T41.1X2	T41.1X3	T41.1X4	T41.1X5	T41.1X6
Methohexitone	T41.1X1	T41.1X2	T41.1X3	T41.1X4	T41.1X5	T41.1X6
Methoin	T42.0X1	T42.0X2	T42.0X3	T42.0X4	T42.0X5	T42.0X6
Methopholine	T39.8X1	T39.8X2	T39.8X3	T39.8X4	T39.8X5	T39.8X6
Methopromazine	T43.3X1	T43.3X2	T43.3X3	T43.3X4	T43.3X5	T43.3X6
Methorate	T48.3X1	T48.3X2	T48.3X3	T48.3X4	T48.3X5	T48.3X6
Methoserpidine	T46.5X1	T46.5X2	T46.5X3	T46.5X4	T46.5X5	T46.5X6
Methotrexate	T45.1X1	T45.1X2	T45.1X3	T45.1X4	T45.1X5	T45.1X6
Methotrimeprazine	T43.3X1	T43.3X2	T43.3X3	T43.3X4	T43.3X5	T43.3X6
Methoxa-Dome	T49.3X1	T49.3X2	T49.3X3	T49.3X4	T49.3X5	T49.3X6
Methoxamine	T44.4X1	T44.4X2	T44.4X3	T44.4X4	T44.4X5	T44.4X6
Methoxsalen	T50.991	T50.992	T50.993	T50.994	T50.995	T50.996
Methoxyaniline	T65.3X1	T65.3X2	T65.3X3	T65.3X4	—	—
Methoxybenzyl penicillin	T36.0X1	T36.0X2	T36.0X3	T36.0X4	T36.0X5	T36.0X6
Methoxychlor	T53.7X1	T53.7X2	T53.7X3	T53.7X4	—	—
Methoxy-DDT	T53.7X1	T53.7X2	T53.7X3	T53.7X4	—	—
2-Methoxyethanol	T52.3X1	T52.3X2	T52.3X3	T52.3X4	—	—
Methoxyflurane	T41.0X1	T41.0X2	T41.0X3	T41.0X4	T41.0X5	T41.0X6
Methoxyphenamine	T48.6X1	T48.6X2	T48.6X3	T48.6X4	T48.6X5	T48.6X6
Methoxypromazine	T43.3X1	T43.3X2	T43.3X3	T43.3X4	T43.3X5	T43.3X6

◀ New ◀ Revised ~~deleted~~ Deleted

Substance	External Cause (T-Code)					
	Poisoning, Accidental (Unintentional)	Poisoning, Intentional Self-Harm	Poisoning, Assault	Poisoning, Undetermined	Adverse Effect	Underdosing
5-Methoxypsoralen (5-MOP)	T50.991	T50.992	T50.993	T50.994	T50.995	T50.996
8-Methoxypsoralen (8-MOP)	T50.991	T50.992	T50.993	T50.994	T50.995	T50.996
Methscopolamine bromide	T44.3X1	T44.3X2	T44.3X3	T44.3X4	T44.3X5	T44.3X6
Methsuximide	T42.2X1	T42.2X2	T42.2X3	T42.2X4	T42.2X5	T42.2X6
Methyclothiazide	T50.2X1	T50.2X2	T50.2X3	T50.2X4	T50.2X5	T50.2X6
Methyl						
acetate	T52.4X1	T52.4X2	T52.4X3	T52.4X4	—	—
acetone	T52.4X1	T52.4X2	T52.4X3	T52.4X4	—	—
acrylate	T65.891	T65.892	T65.893	T65.894	—	—
alcohol	T51.1X1	T51.1X2	T51.1X3	T51.1X4	—	—
aminophenol	T65.3X1	T65.3X2	T65.3X3	T65.3X4	—	—
amphetamine	T43.621	T43.622	T43.623	T43.624	T43.625	T43.626
androstanolone	T38.7X1	T38.7X2	T38.7X3	T38.7X4	T38.7X5	T38.7X6
atropine	T44.3X1	T44.3X2	T44.3X3	T44.3X4	T44.3X5	T44.3X6
benzene	T52.2X1	T52.2X2	T52.2X3	T52.2X4	—	—
benzoate	T52.8X1	T52.8X2	T52.8X3	T52.8X4	—	—
benzol	T52.2X1	T52.2X2	T52.2X3	T52.2X4	—	—
bromide (gas)	T59.891	T59.892	T59.893	T59.894	—	—
fumigant	T60.8X1	T60.8X2	T60.8X3	T60.8X4	—	—
butanol	T51.3X1	T51.3X2	T51.3X3	T51.3X4	—	—
carbinol	T51.1X1	T51.1X2	T51.1X3	T51.1X4	—	—
carbonate	T52.8X1	T52.8X2	T52.8X3	T52.8X4	—	—
CCNU	T45.1X1	T45.1X2	T45.1X3	T45.1X4	T45.1X5	T45.1X6
cellosolve	T52.91	T52.92	T52.93	T52.94	—	—
cellulose	T47.4X1	T47.4X2	T47.4X3	T47.4X4	T47.4X5	T47.4X6
chloride (gas)	T59.891	T59.892	T59.893	T59.894	—	—
chloroformate	T59.3X1	T59.3X2	T59.3X3	T59.3X4	—	—
cyclohexane	T52.8X1	T52.8X2	T52.8X3	T52.8X4	—	—
cyclohexanol	T51.8X1	T51.8X2	T51.8X3	T51.8X4	—	—
cyclohexanone	T52.8X1	T52.8X2	T52.8X3	T52.8X4	—	—
cyclohexyl acetate	T52.8X1	T52.8X2	T52.8X3	T52.8X4	—	—
demeton	T60.0X1	T60.0X2	T60.0X3	T60.0X4	—	—
dihydromorphinone	T40.2X1	T40.2X2	T40.2X3	T40.2X4	T40.2X5	T40.2X6
ergometrine	T48.0X1	T48.0X2	T48.0X3	T48.0X4	T48.0X5	T48.0X6
ergonovine	T48.0X1	T48.0X2	T48.0X3	T48.0X4	T48.0X5	T48.0X6
ethyl ketone	T52.4X1	T52.4X2	T52.4X3	T52.4X4	—	—
glucamine antimonate	T37.8X1	T37.8X2	T37.8X3	T37.8X4	T37.8X5	T37.8X6
hydrazine	T65.891	T65.892	T65.893	T65.894	—	—
iodide	T65.891	T65.892	T65.893	T65.894	—	—
isobutyl ketone	T52.4X1	T52.4X2	T52.4X3	T52.4X4	—	—
isothiocyanate	T60.3X1	T60.3X2	T60.3X3	T60.3X4	—	—
mercaptan	T59.891	T59.892	T59.893	T59.894	—	—

Substance	External Cause (T-Code)					
	Poisoning, Accidental (Unintentional)	Poisoning, Intentional Self-Harm	Poisoning, Assault	Poisoning, Undetermined	Adverse Effect	Underdosing
Methyl *(Continued)*						
morphine NEC	T40.2X1	T40.2X2	T40.2X3	T40.2X4	T40.2X5	T40.2X6
nicotinate	T49.4X1	T49.4X2	T49.4X3	T49.4X4	T49.4X5	T49.4X6
paraben	T49.0X1	T49.0X2	T49.0X3	T49.0X4	T49.0X5	T49.0X6
parafynol	T42.6X1	T42.6X2	T42.6X3	T42.6X4	T42.6X5	T42.6X6
parathion	T60.0X1	T60.0X2	T60.0X3	T60.0X4	—	—
peridol	T43.4X1	T43.4X2	T43.4X3	T43.4X4	T43.4X5	T43.4X6
phenidate	T43.631	T43.632	T43.633	T43.634	T43.635	T43.636
prednisolone	T38.0X1	T38.0X2	T38.0X3	T38.0X4	T38.0X5	T38.0X6
ENT agent	T49.6X1	T49.6X2	T49.6X3	T49.6X4	T49.6X5	T49.6X6
ophthalmic preparation	T49.5X1	T49.5X2	T49.5X3	T49.5X4	T49.5X5	T49.5X6
topical NEC	T49.0X1	T49.0X2	T49.0X3	T49.0X4	T49.0X5	T49.0X6
propylcarbinol	T51.3X1	T51.3X2	T51.3X3	T51.3X4	—	—
rosaniline NEC	T49.0X1	T49.0X2	T49.0X3	T49.0X4	T49.0X5	T49.0X6
salicylate	T49.2X1	T49.2X2	T49.2X3	T49.2X4	T49.2X5	T49.2X6
sulfate (fumes)	T59.891	T59.892	T59.893	T59.894	—	—
liquid	T52.8X1	T52.8X2	T52.8X3	T52.8X4	—	—
sulfonal	T42.6X1	T42.6X2	T42.6X3	T42.6X4	T42.6X5	T42.6X6
testosterone	T38.7X1	T38.7X2	T38.7X3	T38.7X4	T38.7X5	T38.7X6
thiouracil	T38.2X1	T38.2X2	T38.2X3	T38.2X4	T38.2X5	T38.2X6
Methylamphetamine	T43.621	T43.622	T43.623	T43.624	T43.625	T43.626
Methylated spirit	T51.1X1	T51.1X2	T51.1X3	T51.1X4	—	—
Methylatropine nitrate	T44.3X1	T44.3X2	T44.3X3	T44.3X4	T44.3X5	T44.3X6
Methylbenactyzium bromide	T44.3X1	T44.3X2	T44.3X3	T44.3X4	T44.3X5	T44.3X6
Methylbenzethonium chloride	T49.0X1	T49.0X2	T49.0X3	T49.0X4	T49.0X5	T49.0X6
Methylcellulose	T47.4X1	T47.4X2	T47.4X3	T47.4X4	T47.4X5	T47.4X6
laxative	T47.4X1	T47.4X2	T47.4X3	T47.4X4	T47.4X5	T47.4X6
Methylchlorophenoxy-acetic acid	T60.3X1	T60.3X2	T60.3X3	T60.3X4	—	—
Methyldopa	T46.5X1	T46.5X2	T46.5X3	T46.5X4	T46.5X5	T46.5X6
Methyldopate	T46.5X1	T46.5X2	T46.5X3	T46.5X4	T46.5X5	T46.5X6
Methylene						
blue	T50.6X1	T50.6X2	T50.6X3	T50.6X4	T50.6X5	T50.6X6
chloride or dichloride (solvent) NEC	T53.4X1	T53.4X2	T53.4X3	T53.4X4	—	—
Methylenedioxyamphet-amine	T43.621	T43.622	T43.623	T43.624	T43.625	T43.626
Methylenedioxymethamphetamine	T43.621	T43.622	T43.623	T43.624	T43.625	T43.626
Methylergometrine	T48.0X1	T48.0X2	T48.0X3	T48.0X4	T48.0X5	T48.0X6
Methylergonovine	T48.0X1	T48.0X2	T48.0X3	T48.0X4	T48.0X5	T48.0X6
Methylestrenolone	T38.5X1	T38.5X2	T38.5X3	T38.5X4	T38.5X5	T38.5X6
Methylethyl cellulose	T50.991	T50.992	T50.993	T50.994	T50.995	T50.996
Methylhexabital	T42.3X1	T42.3X2	T42.3X3	T42.3X4	T42.3X5	T42.3X6
Methylmorphine	T40.2X1	T40.2X2	T40.2X3	T40.2X4	T40.2X5	T40.2X6

Substance	External Cause (T-Code)					
	Poisoning, Accidental (Unintentional)	Poisoning, Intentional Self-Harm	Poisoning, Assault	Poisoning, Undetermined	Adverse Effect	Underdosing
Methylparaben (ophthalmic)	T49.5X1	T49.5X2	T49.5X3	T49.5X4	T49.5X5	T49.5X6
Methylparafynol	T42.6X1	T42.6X2	T42.6X3	T42.6X4	T42.6X5	T42.6X6
Methylpentynol, methylpenthynol	T42.6X1	T42.6X2	T42.6X3	T42.6X4	T42.6X5	T42.6X6
Methylphenidate	T43.631	T43.632	T43.633	T43.634	T43.635	T43.636
Methylphenobarbital	T42.3X1	T42.3X2	T42.3X3	T42.3X4	T42.3X5	T42.3X6
Methylpolysiloxane	T47.1X1	T47.1X2	T47.1X3	T47.1X4	T47.1X5	T47.1X6
Methylprednisolone — *see Methyl, prednisolone*						
Methylrosaniline	T49.0X1	T49.0X2	T49.0X3	T49.0X4	T49.0X5	T49.0X6
Methylrosanilinium chloride	T49.0X1	T49.0X2	T49.0X3	T49.0X4	T49.0X5	T49.0X6
Methyltestosterone	T38.7X1	T38.7X2	T38.7X3	T38.7X4	T38.7X5	T38.7X6
Methylthionine chloride	T50.6X1	T50.6X2	T50.6X3	T50.6X4	T50.6X5	T50.6X6
Methylthioninium chloride	T50.6X1	T50.6X2	T50.6X3	T50.6X4	T50.6X5	T50.6X6
Methylthiouracil	T38.2X1	T38.2X2	T38.2X3	T38.2X4	T38.2X5	T38.2X6
Methyprylon	T42.6X1	T42.6X2	T42.6X3	T42.6X4	T42.6X5	T42.6X6
Methysergide	T46.5X1	T46.5X2	T46.5X3	T46.5X4	T46.5X5	T46.5X6
Metiamide	T47.1X1	T47.1X2	T47.1X3	T47.1X4	T47.1X5	T47.1X6
Meticillin	T36.0X1	T36.0X2	T36.0X3	T36.0X4	T36.0X5	T36.0X6
Meticrane	T50.2X1	T50.2X2	T50.2X3	T50.2X4	T50.2X5	T50.2X6
Metildigoxin	T46.0X1	T46.0X2	T46.0X3	T46.0X4	T46.0X5	T46.0X6
Metipranolol	T49.5X1	T49.5X2	T49.5X3	T49.5X4	T49.5X5	T49.5X6
Metirosine	T46.5X1	T46.5X2	T46.5X3	T46.5X4	T46.5X5	T46.5X6
Metisazone	T37.5X1	T37.5X2	T37.5X3	T37.5X4	T37.5X5	T37.5X6
Metixene	T44.3X1	T44.3X2	T44.3X3	T44.3X4	T44.3X5	T44.3X6
Metizoline	T48.5X1	T48.5X2	T48.5X3	T48.5X4	T48.5X5	T48.5X6
Metoclopramide	T45.0X1	T45.0X2	T45.0X3	T45.0X4	T45.0X5	T45.0X6
Metofenazate	T43.3X1	T43.3X2	T43.3X3	T43.3X4	T43.3X5	T43.3X6
Metofoline	T39.8X1	T39.8X2	T39.8X3	T39.8X4	T39.8X5	T39.8X6
Metolazone	T50.2X1	T50.2X2	T50.2X3	T50.2X4	T50.2X5	T50.2X6
Metopon	T40.2X1	T40.2X2	T40.2X3	T40.2X4	T40.2X5	T40.2X6
Metoprine	T45.1X1	T45.1X2	T45.1X3	T45.1X4	T45.1X5	T45.1X6
Metoprolol	T44.7X1	T44.7X2	T44.7X3	T44.7X4	T44.7X5	T44.7X6
Metrifonate	T60.0X1	T60.0X2	T60.0X3	T60.0X4	—	—
Metrizamide	T50.8X1	T50.8X2	T50.8X3	T50.8X4	T50.8X5	T50.8X6
Metrizoic acid	T50.8X1	T50.8X2	T50.8X3	T50.8X4	T50.8X5	T50.8X6
Metronidazole	T37.8X1	T37.8X2	T37.8X3	T37.8X4	T37.8X5	T37.8X6
Metycaine	T41.3X1	T41.3X2	T41.3X3	T41.3X4	T41.3X5	T41.3X6
infiltration (subcutaneous)	T41.3X1	T41.3X2	T41.3X3	T41.3X4	T41.3X5	T41.3X6
nerve block (peripheral) (plexus)	T41.3X1	T41.3X2	T41.3X3	T41.3X4	T41.3X5	T41.3X6
topical (surface)	T41.3X1	T41.3X2	T41.3X3	T41.3X4	T41.3X5	T41.3X6
Metyrapone	T50.8X1	T50.8X2	T50.8X3	T50.8X4	T50.8X5	T50.8X6
Mevinphos	T60.0X1	T60.0X2	T60.0X3	T60.0X4	—	—

Substance	External Cause (T-Code)					
	Poisoning, Accidental (Unintentional)	Poisoning, Intentional Self-Harm	Poisoning, Assault	Poisoning, Undetermined	Adverse Effect	Underdosing
Mexazolam	T42.4X1	T42.4X2	T42.4X3	T42.4X4	T42.4X5	T42.4X6
Mexenone	T49.3X1	T49.3X2	T49.3X3	T49.3X4	T49.3X5	T49.3X6
Mexiletine	T46.2X1	T46.2X2	T46.2X3	T46.2X4	T46.2X5	T46.2X6
Mezereon	T62.2X1	T62.2X2	T62.2X3	T62.2X4	—	—
berries	T62.1X1	T62.1X2	T62.1X3	T62.1X4	—	—
Mezlocillin	T36.0X1	T36.0X2	T36.0X3	T36.0X4	T36.0X5	T36.0X6
Mianserin	T43.021	T43.022	T43.023	T43.024	T43.025	T43.026
Micatin	T49.0X1	T49.0X2	T49.0X3	T49.0X4	T49.0X5	T49.0X6
Miconazole	T49.0X1	T49.0X2	T49.0X3	T49.0X4	T49.0X5	T49.0X6
Micronomicin	T36.5X1	T36.5X2	T36.5X3	T36.5X4	T36.5X5	T36.5X6
Midazolam	T42.4X1	T42.4X2	T42.4X3	T42.4X4	T42.4X5	T42.4X6
Midecamycin	T36.3X1	T36.3X2	T36.3X3	T36.3X4	T36.3X5	T36.3X6
Mifepristone	T38.6X1	T38.6X2	T38.6X3	T38.6X4	T38.6X5	T38.6X6
Milk of magnesia	T47.1X1	T47.1X2	T47.1X3	T47.1X4	T47.1X5	T47.1X6
Millipede (tropical) (venomous)	T63.411	T63.412	T63.413	T63.414	—	—
Miltown	T43.591	T43.592	T43.593	T43.594	T43.595	T43.596
Milverine	T44.3X1	T44.3X2	T44.3X3	T44.3X4	T44.3X5	T44.3X6
Minaprine	T43.291	T43.292	T43.293	T43.294	T43.295	T43.296
Minaxolone	T41.291	T41.292	T41.293	T41.294	T41.295	T41.296
Mineral						
acids	T54.2X1	T54.2X2	T54.2X3	T54.2X4	—	—
oil (laxative) (medicinal)	T47.4X1	T47.4X2	T47.4X3	T47.4X4	T47.4X5	T47.4X6
emulsion	T47.2X1	T47.2X2	T47.2X3	T47.2X4	T47.2X5	T47.2X6
nonmedicinal	T52.0X1	T52.0X2	T52.0X3	T52.0X4	—	—
topical	T49.3X1	T49.3X2	T49.3X3	T49.3X4	T49.3X5	T49.3X6
salt NEC	T50.3X1	T50.3X2	T50.3X3	T50.3X4	T50.3X5	T50.3X6
spirits	T52.0X1	T52.0X2	T52.0X3	T52.0X4	—	—
Mineralocorticosteroid	T50.0X1	T50.0X2	T50.0X3	T50.0X4	T50.0X5	T50.0X6
Minocycline	T36.4X1	T36.4X2	T36.4X3	T36.4X4	T36.4X5	T36.4X6
Minoxidil	T46.7X1	T46.7X2	T46.7X3	T46.7X4	T46.7X5	T46.7X6
Miokamycin	T36.3X1	T36.3X2	T36.3X3	T36.3X4	T36.3X5	T36.3X6
Miotic drug	T49.5X1	T49.5X2	T49.5X3	T49.5X4	T49.5X5	T49.5X6
Mipafox	T60.0X1	T60.0X2	T60.0X3	T60.0X4	—	—
Mirex	T60.1X1	T60.1X2	T60.1X3	T60.1X4	—	—
Mirtazapine	T43.021	T43.022	T43.023	T43.024	T43.025	T43.026
Misonidazole	T37.3X1	T37.3X2	T37.3X3	T37.3X4	T37.3X5	T37.3X6
Misoprostol	T47.1X1	T47.1X2	T47.1X3	T47.1X4	T47.1X5	T47.1X6
Mithramycin	T45.1X1	T45.1X2	T45.1X3	T45.1X4	T45.1X5	T45.1X6
Mitobronitol	T45.1X1	T45.1X2	T45.1X3	T45.1X4	T45.1X5	T45.1X6
Mitoguazone	T45.1X1	T45.1X2	T45.1X3	T45.1X4	T45.1X5	T45.1X6
Mitolactol	T45.1X1	T45.1X2	T45.1X3	T45.1X4	T45.1X5	T45.1X6
Mitomycin	T45.1X1	T45.1X2	T45.1X3	T45.1X4	T45.1X5	T45.1X6

Substance	External Cause (T-Code)					
	Poisoning, Accidental (Unintentional)	Poisoning, Intentional Self-Harm	Poisoning, Assault	Poisoning, Undetermined	Adverse Effect	Underdosing
Mitopodozide	T45.1X1	T45.1X2	T45.1X3	T45.1X4	T45.1X5	T45.1X6
Mitotane	T45.1X1	T45.1X2	T45.1X3	T45.1X4	T45.1X5	T45.1X6
Mitoxantrone	T45.1X1	T45.1X2	T45.1X3	T45.1X4	T45.1X5	T45.1X6
Mivacurium chloride	T48.1X1	T48.1X2	T48.1X3	T48.1X4	T48.1X5	T48.1X6
Miyari bacteria	T47.6X1	T47.6X2	T47.6X3	T47.6X4	T47.6X5	T47.6X6
Moclobemide	T43.1X1	T43.1X2	T43.1X3	T43.1X4	T43.1X5	T43.1X6
Moderil	T46.5X1	T46.5X2	T46.5X3	T46.5X4	T46.5X5	T46.5X6
Mofebutazone	T39.2X1	T39.2X2	T39.2X3	T39.2X4	T39.2X5	T39.2X6
Mogadon — *see Nitrazepam*						
Molindone	T43.591	T43.592	T43.593	T43.594	T43.595	T43.596
Molsidomine	T46.3X1	T46.3X2	T46.3X3	T46.3X4	T46.3X5	T46.3X6
Mometasone	T49.0X1	T49.0X2	T49.0X3	T49.0X4	T49.0X5	T49.0X6
Monistat	T49.0X1	T49.0X2	T49.0X3	T49.0X4	T49.0X5	T49.0X6
Monkshood	T62.2X1	T62.2X2	T62.2X3	T62.2X4	—	—
Monoamine oxidase inhibitor NEC	T43.1X1	T43.1X2	T43.1X3	T43.1X4	T43.1X5	T43.1X6
hydrazine	T43.1X1	T43.1X2	T43.1X3	T43.1X4	T43.1X5	T43.1X6
Monobenzone	T49.4X1	T49.4X2	T49.4X3	T49.4X4	T49.4X5	T49.4X6
Monochloroacetic acid	T60.3X1	T60.3X2	T60.3X3	T60.3X4	—	—
Monochlorobenzene	T53.7X1	T53.7X2	T53.7X3	T53.7X4	—	—
Monoethanolamine	T46.8X1	T46.8X2	T46.8X3	T46.8X4	T46.8X5	T46.8X6
oleate	T46.8X1	T46.8X2	T46.8X3	T46.8X4	T46.8X5	T46.8X6
Monooctanoin	T50.991	T50.992	T50.993	T50.994	T50.995	T50.996
Monophenylbutazone	T39.2X1	T39.2X2	T39.2X3	T39.2X4	T39.2X5	T39.2X6
Monosodium glutamate	T65.891	T65.892	T65.893	T65.894	—	—
Monosulfiram	T49.0X1	T49.0X2	T49.0X3	T49.0X4	T49.0X5	T49.0X6
Monoxide, carbon — *see Carbon, monoxide*	T57.91	T57.92	T57.93	T57.94	—	—
Monoxidine hydrochloride	T46.1X1	T46.1X2	T46.1X3	T46.1X4	T46.1X5	T46.1X6
Monuron	T60.3X1	T60.3X2	T60.3X3	T60.3X4	—	—
Moperone	T43.4X1	T43.4X2	T43.4X3	T43.4X4	T43.4X5	T43.4X6
Mopidamol	T45.1X1	T45.1X2	T45.1X3	T45.1X4	T45.1X5	T45.1X6
MOPP (mechlorethamine + vincristine + prednisone + procarbazine)	T45.1X1	T45.1X2	T45.1X3	T45.1X4	T45.1X5	T45.1X6
Morfin	T40.2X1	T40.2X2	T40.2X3	T40.2X4	T40.2X5	T40.2X6
Morinamide	T37.1X1	T37.1X2	T37.1X3	T37.1X4	T37.1X5	T37.1X6
Morning glory seeds	T40.991	T40.992	T40.993	T40.994	—	—
Moroxydine	T37.5X1	T37.5X2	T37.5X3	T37.5X4	T37.5X5	T37.5X6
Morphazinamide	T37.1X1	T37.1X2	T37.1X3	T37.1X4	T37.1X5	T37.1X6
Morphine	T40.2X1	T40.2X2	T40.2X3	T40.2X4	T40.2X5	T40.2X6
antagonist	T50.7X1	T50.7X2	T50.7X3	T50.7X4	T50.7X5	T50.7X6
Morpholinylethylmorphine	T40.2X1	T40.2X2	T40.2X3	T40.2X4	—	—
Morsuximide	T42.2X1	T42.2X2	T42.2X3	T42.2X4	T42.2X5	T42.2X6

Substance	External Cause (T-Code)					
	Poisoning, Accidental (Unintentional)	Poisoning, Intentional Self-Harm	Poisoning, Assault	Poisoning, Undetermined	Adverse Effect	Underdosing
Mosapramine	T43.591	T43.592	T43.593	T43.594	T43.595	T43.596
Moth balls — *see also Pesticides*	T60.2X1	T60.2X2	T60.2X3	T60.2X4	—	—
naphthalene	T60.2X1	T60.2X2	T60.2X3	T60.2X4	—	—
paradichlorobenzene	T60.1X1	T60.1X2	T60.1X3	T60.1X4	—	—
Motor exhaust gas	T58.01	T58.02	T58.03	T58.04	—	—
Mouthwash (antiseptic) (zinc chloride)	T49.6X1	T49.6X2	T49.6X3	T49.6X4	T49.6X5	T49.6X6
Moxastine	T45.0X1	T45.0X2	T45.0X3	T45.0X4	T45.0X5	T45.0X6
Moxaverine	T44.3X1	T44.3X2	T44.3X3	T44.3X4	T44.3X5	T44.3X6
Moxifensine	T43.291	T43.292	T43.293	T43.294	T43.295	T43.296
Moxisylyte	T46.7X1	T46.7X2	T46.7X3	T46.7X4	T46.7X5	T46.7X6
Mucilage, plant	T47.4X1	T47.4X2	T47.4X3	T47.4X4	T47.4X5	T47.4X6
Mucolytic drug	T48.4X1	T48.4X2	T48.4X3	T48.4X4	T48.4X5	T48.4X6
Mucomyst	T48.4X1	T48.4X2	T48.4X3	T48.4X4	T48.4X5	T48.4X6
Mucous membrane agents (external)	T49.91	T49.92	T49.93	T49.94	T49.95	T49.96
specified NEC	T49.8X1	T49.8X2	T49.8X3	T49.8X4	T49.8X5	T49.8X6
Mumps						
immune globulin (human)	T50.Z11	T50.Z12	T50.Z13	T50.Z14	T50.Z15	T50.Z16
skin test antigen	T50.8X1	T50.8X2	T50.8X3	T50.8X4	T50.8X5	T50.8X6
vaccine	T50.B91	T50.B92	T50.B93	T50.B94	T50.B95	T50.B96
Mumpsvax	T50.B91	T50.B92	T50.B93	T50.B94	T50.B95	T50.B96
Mupirocin	T49.0X1	T49.0X2	T49.0X3	T49.0X4	T49.0X5	T49.0X6
Muriatic acid — *see Hydrochloric acid*						
Muromonab-CD3	T45.1X1	T45.1X2	T45.1X3	T45.1X4	T45.1X5	T45.1X6
Muscle relaxant — *see Relaxant, muscle*						
Muscle-action drug NEC	T48.201	T48.202	T48.203	T48.204	T48.205	T48.206
Muscle affecting agents NEC	T48.201	T48.202	T48.203	T48.204	T48.205	T48.206
oxytocic	T48.0X1	T48.0X2	T48.0X3	T48.0X4	T48.0X5	T48.0X6
relaxants	T48.201	T48.202	T48.203	T48.204	T48.205	T48.206
central nervous system	T42.8X1	T42.8X2	T42.8X3	T42.8X4	T42.8X5	T42.8X6
skeletal	T48.1X1	T48.1X2	T48.1X3	T48.1X4	T48.1X5	T48.1X6
smooth	T44.3X1	T44.3X2	T44.3X3	T44.3X4	T44.3X5	T44.3X6
Muscle-tone depressant, central NEC	T42.8X1	T42.8X2	T42.8X3	T42.8X4	T42.8X5	T42.8X6
specified NEC	T42.8X1	T42.8X2	T42.8X3	T42.8X4	T42.8X5	T42.8X6
Mushroom, noxious	T62.0X1	T62.0X2	T62.0X3	T62.0X4	—	—
Mussel, noxious	T61.781	T61.782	T61.783	T61.784	—	—
Mustard (emetic)	T47.7X1	T47.7X2	T47.7X3	T47.7X4	T47.7X5	T47.7X6
black	T47.7X1	T47.7X2	T47.7X3	T47.7X4	T47.7X5	T47.7X6
gas, not in war	T59.91	T59.92	T59.93	T59.94	—	—
nitrogen	T45.1X1	T45.1X2	T45.1X3	T45.1X4	T45.1X5	T45.1X6

Substance	External Cause (T-Code)					
	Poisoning, Accidental (Unintentional)	Poisoning, Intentional Self-Harm	Poisoning, Assault	Poisoning, Undetermined	Adverse Effect	Underdosing
Mustine	T45.1X1	T45.1X2	T45.1X3	T45.1X4	T45.1X5	T45.1X6
M-vac	T45.1X1	T45.1X2	T45.1X3	T45.1X4	T45.1X5	T45.1X6
Mycifradin	T36.5X1	T36.5X2	T36.5X3	T36.5X4	T36.5X5	T36.5X6
topical	T49.0X1	T49.0X2	T49.0X3	T49.0X4	T49.0X5	T49.0X6
Mycitracin	T36.8X1	T36.8X2	T36.8X3	T36.8X4	T36.8X5	T36.8X6
ophthalmic preparation	T49.5X1	T49.5X2	T49.5X3	T49.5X4	T49.5X5	T49.5X6
Mycostatin	T36.7X1	T36.7X2	T36.7X3	T36.7X4	T36.7X5	T36.7X6
topical	T49.0X1	T49.0X2	T49.0X3	T49.0X4	T49.0X5	T49.0X6
Mycotoxins	T64.81	T64.82	T64.83	T64.84	—	—
aflatoxin	T64.01	T64.02	T64.03	T64.04	—	—
specified NEC	T64.81	T64.82	T64.83	T64.84	—	—
Mydriacyl	T44.3X1	T44.3X2	T44.3X3	T44.3X4	T44.3X5	T44.3X6
Mydriatic drug	T49.5X1	T49.5X2	T49.5X3	T49.5X4	T49.5X5	T49.5X6
Myelobromal	T45.1X1	T45.1X2	T45.1X3	T45.1X4	T45.1X5	T45.1X6
Myleran	T45.1X1	T45.1X2	T45.1X3	T45.1X4	T45.1X5	T45.1X6
Myochrysin(e)	T39.2X1	T39.2X2	T39.2X3	T39.2X4	T39.2X5	T39.2X6
Myoneural blocking agents	T48.1X1	T48.1X2	T48.1X3	T48.1X4	T48.1X5	T48.1X6
Myralact	T49.0X1	T49.0X2	T49.0X3	T49.0X4	T49.0X5	T49.0X6
Myristica fragrans	T62.2X1	T62.2X2	T62.2X3	T62.2X4	—	—
Myristicin	T65.891	T65.892	T65.893	T65.894	—	—
Mysoline	T42.3X1	T42.3X2	T42.3X3	T42.3X4	T42.3X5	T42.3X6
N						
Nabilone	T40.7X1	T40.7X2	T40.7X3	T40.7X4	T40.7X5	T40.7X6
Nabumetone	T39.391	T39.392	T39.393	T39.394	T39.395	T39.396
Nadolol	T44.7X1	T44.7X2	T44.7X3	T44.7X4	T44.7X5	T44.7X6
Nafcillin	T36.0X1	T36.0X2	T36.0X3	T36.0X4	T36.0X5	T36.0X6
Nafoxidine	T38.6X1	T38.6X2	T38.6X3	T38.6X4	T38.6X5	T38.6X6
Naftazone	T46.991	T46.992	T46.993	T46.994	T46.995	T46.996
Naftidrofuryl (oxalate)	T46.7X1	T46.7X2	T46.7X3	T46.7X4	T46.7X5	T46.7X6
Naftifine	T49.0X1	T49.0X2	T49.0X3	T49.0X4	T49.0X5	T49.0X6
Nail polish remover	T52.91	T52.92	T52.93	T52.94	—	—
Nalbuphine	T40.4X1	T40.4X2	T40.4X3	T40.4X4	T40.4X5	T40.4X6
Naled	T60.0X1	T60.0X2	T60.0X3	T60.0X4	—	—
Nalidixic acid	T37.8X1	T37.8X2	T37.8X3	T37.8X4	T37.8X5	T37.8X6
Nalorphine	T50.7X1	T50.7X2	T50.7X3	T50.7X4	T50.7X5	T50.7X6
Naloxone	T50.7X1	T50.7X2	T50.7X3	T50.7X4	T50.7X5	T50.7X6
Naltrexone	T50.7X1	T50.7X2	T50.7X3	T50.7X4	T50.7X5	T50.7X6
Namenda	T43.8X1	T43.8X2	T43.8X3	T43.8X4	T43.8X5	T43.8X6
Nandrolone	T38.7X1	T38.7X2	T38.7X3	T38.7X4	T38.7X5	T38.7X6
Naphazoline	T48.5X1	T48.5X2	T48.5X3	T48.5X4	T48.5X5	T48.5X6

Substance	External Cause (T-Code)					
	Poisoning, Accidental (Unintentional)	Poisoning, Intentional Self-Harm	Poisoning, Assault	Poisoning, Undetermined	Adverse Effect	Underdosing
Naphtha (painters') (petroleum)	T52.0X1	T52.0X2	T52.0X3	T52.0X4	—	—
solvent	T52.0X1	T52.0X2	T52.0X3	T52.0X4	—	—
vapor	T52.0X1	T52.0X2	T52.0X3	T52.0X4	—	—
Naphthalene (non-chlorinated)	T60.2X1	T60.2X2	T60.2X3	T60.2X4	—	—
chlorinated	T60.1X1	T60.1X2	T60.1X3	T60.1X4	—	—
vapor	T60.1X1	T60.1X2	T60.1X3	T60.1X4	—	—
insecticide or moth repellent	T60.2X1	T60.2X2	T60.2X3	T60.2X4	—	—
chlorinated	T60.1X1	T60.1X2	T60.1X3	T60.1X4	—	—
vapor	T60.2X1	T60.2X2	T60.2X3	T60.2X4	—	—
chlorinated	T60.1X1	T60.1X2	T60.1X3	T60.1X4	—	—
Naphthol	T65.891	T65.892	T65.893	T65.894	—	—
Naphthylamine	T65.891	T65.892	T65.893	T65.894	—	—
Naphthylthiourea (ANTU)	T60.4X1	T60.4X2	T60.4X3	T60.4X4	—	—
Naprosyn — *see Naproxen*						
Naproxen	T39.311	T39.312	T39.313	T39.314	T39.315	T39.316
Narcotic (drug)	T40.601	T40.602	T40.603	T40.604	T40.605	T40.606
analgesic NEC	T40.601	T40.602	T40.603	T40.604	T40.605	T40.606
antagonist	T50.7X1	T50.7X2	T50.7X3	T50.7X4	T50.7X5	T50.7X6
specified NEC	T40.691	T40.692	T40.693	T40.694	T40.695	T40.696
synthetic	T40.4X1	T40.4X2	T40.4X3	T40.4X4	T40.4X5	T40.4X6
Narcotine	T48.3X1	T48.3X2	T48.3X3	T48.3X4	T48.3X5	T48.3X6
Nardil	T43.1X1	T43.1X2	T43.1X3	T43.1X4	T43.1X5	T43.1X6
Nasal drug NEC	T49.6X1	T49.6X2	T49.6X3	T49.6X4	T49.6X5	T49.6X6
Natamycin	T49.0X1	T49.0X2	T49.0X3	T49.0X4	T49.0X5	T49.0X6
Natrium cyanide — *see Cyanide(s)*						
Natural gas	T59.891	T59.892	T59.893	T59.894	—	—
incomplete combustion	T57.91	T57.92	T57.93	T57.94	—	—
Natural						
blood (product)	T45.8X1	T45.8X2	T45.8X3	T45.8X4	T45.8X5	T45.8X6
gas (piped)	T59.891	T59.892	T59.893	T59.894	—	—
incomplete combustion	T58.11	T58.12	T58.13	T58.14	—	—
Nealbarbital	T42.3X1	T42.3X2	T42.3X3	T42.3X4	T42.3X5	T42.3X6
Nectadon	T48.3X1	T48.3X2	T48.3X3	T48.3X4	T48.3X5	T48.3X6
Nedocromil	T48.6X1	T48.6X2	T48.6X3	T48.6X4	T48.6X5	T48.6X6
Nefopam	T39.8X1	T39.8X2	T39.8X3	T39.8X4	T39.8X5	T39.8X6
Nematocyst (sting)	T63.691	T63.692	T63.693	T63.694	—	—
Nembutal	T42.3X1	T42.3X2	T42.3X3	T42.3X4	T42.3X5	T42.3X6
Nemonapride	T43.591	T43.592	T43.593	T43.594	T43.595	T43.596
Neoarsphenamine	T37.8X1	T37.8X2	T37.8X3	T37.8X4	T37.8X5	T37.8X6

Substance	External Cause (T-Code)					
	Poisoning, Accidental (Unintentional)	Poisoning, Intentional Self-Harm	Poisoning, Assault	Poisoning, Undetermined	Adverse Effect	Underdosing
Neocinchophen	T50.4X1	T50.4X2	T50.4X3	T50.4X4	T50.4X5	T50.4X6
Neomycin (derivatives)	T36.5X1	T36.5X2	T36.5X3	T36.5X4	T36.5X5	T36.5X6
with						
bacitracin	T49.0X1	T49.0X2	T49.0X3	T49.0X4	T49.0X5	T49.0X6
neostigmine	T44.0X1	T44.0X2	T44.0X3	T44.0X4	T44.0X5	T44.0X6
ENT agent	T49.6X1	T49.6X2	T49.6X3	T49.6X4	T49.6X5	T49.6X6
ophthalmic preparation	T49.5X1	T49.5X2	T49.5X3	T49.5X4	T49.5X5	T49.5X6
topical NEC	T49.0X1	T49.0X2	T49.0X3	T49.0X4	T49.0X5	T49.0X6
Neonal	T42.3X1	T42.3X2	T42.3X3	T42.3X4	T42.3X5	T42.3X6
Neoprontosil	T37.0X1	T37.0X2	T37.0X3	T37.0X4	T37.0X5	T37.0X6
Neosalvarsan	T37.8X1	T37.8X2	T37.8X3	T37.8X4	T37.8X5	T37.8X6
Neosilversalvarsan	T37.8X1	T37.8X2	T37.8X3	T37.8X4	T37.8X5	T37.8X6
Neosporin	T36.8X1	T36.8X2	T36.8X3	T36.8X4	T36.8X5	T36.8X6
ENT agent	T49.6X1	T49.6X2	T49.6X3	T49.6X4	T49.6X5	T49.6X6
opthalmic preparation	T49.5X1	T49.5X2	T49.5X3	T49.5X4	T49.5X5	T49.5X6
topical NEC	T49.0X1	T49.0X2	T49.0X3	T49.0X4	T49.0X5	T49.0X6
Neostigmine bromide	T44.0X1	T44.0X2	T44.0X3	T44.0X4	T44.0X5	T44.0X6
Neraval	T42.3X1	T42.3X2	T42.3X3	T42.3X4	T42.3X5	T42.3X6
Neravan	T42.3X1	T42.3X2	T42.3X3	T42.3X4	T42.3X5	T42.3X6
Nerium oleander	T62.2X1	T62.2X2	T62.2X3	T62.2X4	—	—
Nerve gas, not in war	T59.91	T59.92	T59.93	T59.94	—	—
Nesacaine	T41.3X1	T41.3X2	T41.3X3	T41.3X4	T41.3X5	T41.3X6
infiltration (subcutaneous)	T41.3X1	T41.3X2	T41.3X3	T41.3X4	T41.3X5	T41.3X6
nerve block (peripheral) (plexus)	T41.3X1	T41.3X2	T41.3X3	T41.3X4	T41.3X5	T41.3X6
Netilmicin	T36.5X1	T36.5X2	T36.5X3	T36.5X4	T36.5X5	T36.5X6
Neurobarb	T42.3X1	T42.3X2	T42.3X3	T42.3X4	T42.3X5	T42.3X6
Neuroleptic drug NEC	T43.501	T43.502	T43.503	T43.504	T43.505	T43.506
Neuromuscular blocking drug	T48.1X1	T48.1X2	T48.1X3	T48.1X4	T48.1X5	T48.1X6
Neutral insulin injection	T38.3X1	T38.3X2	T38.3X3	T38.3X4	T38.3X5	T38.3X6
Neutral spirits	T51.0X1	T51.0X2	T51.0X3	T51.0X4	—	—
beverage	T51.0X1	T51.0X2	T51.0X3	T51.0X4	—	—
Niacin	T46.7X1	T46.7X2	T46.7X3	T46.7X4	T46.7X5	T46.7X6
Niacinamide	T45.2X1	T45.2X2	T45.2X3	T45.2X4	T45.2X5	T45.2X6
Nialamide	T43.1X1	T43.1X2	T43.1X3	T43.1X4	T43.1X5	T43.1X6
Niaprazine	T42.6X1	T42.6X2	T42.6X3	T42.6X4	T42.6X5	T42.6X6
Nicametate	T46.7X1	T46.7X2	T46.7X3	T46.7X4	T46.7X5	T46.7X6
Nicardipine	T46.1X1	T46.1X2	T46.1X3	T46.1X4	T46.1X5	T46.1X6
Nicergoline	T46.7X1	T46.7X2	T46.7X3	T46.7X4	T46.7X5	T46.7X6
Nickel (carbonyl) (tetra-carbonyl) (fumes) (vapor)	T56.891	T56.892	T56.893	T56.894	—	—

Substance	External Cause (T-Code)					
	Poisoning, Accidental (Unintentional)	Poisoning, Intentional Self-Harm	Poisoning, Assault	Poisoning, Undetermined	Adverse Effect	Underdosing
Nickelocene	T56.891	T56.892	T56.893	T56.894	—	—
Niclosamide	T37.4X1	T37.4X2	T37.4X3	T37.4X4	T37.4X5	T37.4X6
Nicofuranose	T46.7X1	T46.7X2	T46.7X3	T46.7X4	T46.7X5	T46.7X6
Nicomorphine	T40.2X1	T40.2X2	T40.2X3	T40.2X4	—	—
Nicorandil	T46.3X1	T46.3X2	T46.3X3	T46.3X4	T46.3X5	T46.3X6
Nicotiana (plant)	T62.2X1	T62.2X2	T62.2X3	T62.2X4	—	—
Nicotinamide	T45.2X1	T45.2X2	T45.2X3	T45.2X4	T45.2X5	T45.2X6
Nicotine (insecticide) (spray) (sulfate) NEC	T60.2X1	T60.2X2	T60.2X3	T60.2X4	—	—
from tobacco	T65.291	T65.292	T65.293	T65.294	—	—
cigarettes	T65.221	T65.222	T65.223	T65.224	—	—
not insecticide	T65.291	T65.292	T65.293	T65.294	—	—
Nicotinic acid	T46.7X1	T46.7X2	T46.7X3	T46.7X4	T46.7X5	T46.7X6
Nicotinyl alcohol	T46.7X1	T46.7X2	T46.7X3	T46.7X4	T46.7X5	T46.7X6
Nicoumalone	T45.511	T45.512	T45.513	T45.514	T45.515	T45.516
Nifedipine	T46.1X1	T46.1X2	T46.1X3	T46.1X4	T46.1X5	T46.1X6
Nifenazone	T39.2X1	T39.2X2	T39.2X3	T39.2X4	T39.2X5	T39.2X6
Nifuraldezone	T37.91	T37.92	T37.93	T37.94	T37.95	T37.96
Nifuratel	T37.8X1	T37.8X2	T37.8X3	T37.8X4	T37.8X5	T37.8X6
Nifurtimox	T37.3X1	T37.3X2	T37.3X3	T37.3X4	T37.3X5	T37.3X6
Nifurtoinol	T37.8X1	T37.8X2	T37.8X3	T37.8X4	T37.8X5	T37.8X6
Nightshade, deadly (solanum)—*see also Belladonna*	T62.2X1	T62.2X2	T62.2X3	T62.2X4	—	—
berry	T62.1X1	T62.1X2	T62.1X3	T62.1X4	—	—
Nikethamide	T50.7X1	T50.7X2	T50.7X3	T50.7X4	T50.7X5	T50.7X6
Nilstat	T36.7X1	T36.7X2	T36.7X3	T36.7X4	T36.7X5	T36.7X6
topical	T49.0X1	T49.0X2	T49.0X3	T49.0X4	T49.0X5	T49.0X6
Nilutamide	T38.6X1	T38.6X2	T38.6X3	T38.6X4	T38.6X5	T38.6X6
Nimesulide	T39.391	T39.392	T39.393	T39.394	T39.395	T39.396
Nimetazepam	T42.4X1	T42.4X2	T42.4X3	T42.4X4	T42.4X5	T42.4X6
Nimodipine	T46.1X1	T46.1X2	T46.1X3	T46.1X4	T46.1X5	T46.1X6
Nimorazole	T37.3X1	T37.3X2	T37.3X3	T37.3X4	T37.3X5	T37.3X6
Nimustine	T45.1X1	T45.1X2	T45.1X3	T45.1X4	T45.1X5	T45.1X6
Niridazole	T37.4X1	T37.4X2	T37.4X3	T37.4X4	T37.4X5	T37.4X6
Nisentil	T40.2X1	T40.2X2	T40.2X3	T40.2X4	T40.2X5	T40.2X6
Nisoldipine	T46.1X1	T46.1X2	T46.1X3	T46.1X4	T46.1X5	T46.1X6
Nitramine	T65.3X1	T65.3X2	T65.3X3	T65.3X4	—	—
Nitrate, organic	T46.3X1	T46.3X2	T46.3X3	T46.3X4	T46.3X5	T46.3X6
Nitrazepam	T42.4X1	T42.4X2	T42.4X3	T42.4X4	T42.4X5	T42.4X6
Nitrefazole	T50.6X1	T50.6X2	T50.6X3	T50.6X4	T50.6X5	T50.6X6
Nitrendipine	T46.1X1	T46.1X2	T46.1X3	T46.1X4	T46.1X5	T46.1X6

Substance	External Cause (T-Code)					
	Poisoning, Accidental (Unintentional)	Poisoning, Intentional Self-Harm	Poisoning, Assault	Poisoning, Undetermined	Adverse Effect	Underdosing
Nitric						
acid (liquid)	T54.2X1	T54.2X2	T54.2X3	T54.2X4	—	—
vapor	T59.891	T59.892	T59.893	T59.894	—	—
oxide (gas)	T59.0X1	T59.0X2	T59.0X3	T59.0X4	—	—
Nitrimidazine	T37.3X1	T37.3X2	T37.3X3	T37.3X4	T37.3X5	T37.3X6
Nitrite, amyl (medicinal) (vapor)	T46.3X1	T46.3X2	T46.3X3	T46.3X4	T46.3X5	T46.3X6
Nitroaniline	T65.3X1	T65.3X2	T65.3X3	T65.3X4	—	—
vapor	T59.891	T59.892	T59.893	T59.894	—	—
Nitrobenzene, nitrobenzol	T65.3X1	T65.3X2	T65.3X3	T65.3X4	—	—
vapor	T65.3X1	T65.3X2	T65.3X3	T65.3X4	—	—
Nitrocellulose	T65.891	T65.892	T65.893	T65.894	—	—
lacquer	T65.891	T65.892	T65.893	T65.894	—	—
Nitrodiphenyl	T65.3X1	T65.3X2	T65.3X3	T65.3X4	—	—
Nitrofural	T49.0X1	T49.0X2	T49.0X3	T49.0X4	T49.0X5	T49.0X6
Nitrofurantoin	T37.8X1	T37.8X2	T37.8X3	T37.8X4	T37.8X5	T37.8X6
Nitrofurazone	T49.0X1	T49.0X2	T49.0X3	T49.0X4	T49.0X5	T49.0X6
Nitrogen	T59.0X1	T59.0X2	T59.0X3	T59.0X4	—	—
mustard	T45.1X1	T45.1X2	T45.1X3	T45.1X4	T45.1X5	T45.1X6
Nitroglycerin, nitro-glycerol (medicinal)	T46.3X1	T46.3X2	T46.3X3	T46.3X4	T46.3X5	T46.3X6
nonmedicinal	T65.5X1	T65.5X2	T65.5X3	T65.5X4	—	—
fumes	T65.5X1	T65.5X2	T65.5X3	T65.5X4	—	—
Nitroglycol	T52.3X1	T52.3X2	T52.3X3	T52.3X4	—	—
Nitrohydrochloric acid	T54.2X1	T54.2X2	T54.2X3	T54.2X4	—	—
Nitromersol	T49.0X1	T49.0X2	T49.0X3	T49.0X4	T49.0X5	T49.0X6
Nitronaphthalene	T65.891	T65.892	T65.893	T65.894	—	—
Nitrophenol	T54.0X1	T54.0X2	T54.0X3	T54.0X4	—	—
Nitropropane	T52.8X1	T52.8X2	T52.8X3	T52.8X4	—	—
Nitroprusside	T46.5X1	T46.5X2	T46.5X3	T46.5X4	T46.5X5	T46.5X6
Nitrosodimethylamine	T65.3X1	T65.3X2	T65.3X3	T65.3X4	—	—
Nitrothiazol	T37.4X1	T37.4X2	T37.4X3	T37.4X4	T37.4X5	T37.4X6
Nitrotoluene, nitrotoluol	T65.3X1	T65.3X2	T65.3X3	T65.3X4	—	—
vapor	T65.3X1	T65.3X2	T65.3X3	T65.3X4	—	—
Nitrous						
acid (liquid)	T54.2X1	T54.2X2	T54.2X3	T54.2X4	—	—
fumes	T59.891	T59.892	T59.893	T59.894	—	—
ether spirit	T46.3X1	T46.3X2	T46.3X3	T46.3X4	T46.3X5	T46.3X6
oxide	T41.0X1	T41.0X2	T41.0X3	T41.0X4	T41.0X5	T41.0X6
Nitroxoline	T37.8X1	T37.8X2	T37.8X3	T37.8X4	T37.8X5	T37.8X6
Nitrozone	T49.0X1	T49.0X2	T49.0X3	T49.0X4	T49.0X5	T49.0X6
Nizatidine	T47.0X1	T47.0X2	T47.0X3	T47.0X4	T47.0X5	T47.0X6

Substance	External Cause (T-Code)					
	Poisoning, Accidental (Unintentional)	Poisoning, Intentional Self-Harm	Poisoning, Assault	Poisoning, Undetermined	Adverse Effect	Underdosing
Nizofenone	T43.8X1	T43.8X2	T43.8X3	T43.8X4	T43.8X5	T43.8X6
Noctec	T42.6X1	T42.6X2	T42.6X3	T42.6X4	T42.6X5	T42.6X6
Noludar	T42.6X1	T42.6X2	T42.6X3	T42.6X4	T42.6X5	T42.6X6
Noptil	T42.3X1	T42.3X2	T42.3X3	T42.3X4	T42.3X5	T42.3X6
Nomegestrol	T38.5X1	T38.5X2	T38.5X3	T38.5X4	T38.5X5	T38.5X6
Nomifensine	T43.291	T43.292	T43.293	T43.294	T43.295	T43.296
Nonoxinol	T49.8X1	T49.8X2	T49.8X3	T49.8X4	T49.8X5	T49.8X6
Nonylphenoxy (polyethoxy-ethanol)	T49.8X1	T49.8X2	T49.8X3	T49.8X4	T49.8X5	T49.8X6
Noptil	T42.3X1	T42.3X2	T42.3X3	T42.3X4	T42.3X5	T42.3X6
Noradrenaline	T44.4X1	T44.4X2	T44.4X3	T44.4X4	T44.4X5	T44.4X6
Noramidopyrine	T39.2X1	T39.2X2	T39.2X3	T39.2X4	T39.2X5	T39.2X6
methanesulfonate sodium	T39.2X1	T39.2X2	T39.2X3	T39.2X4	T39.2X5	T39.2X6
Norbormide	T60.4X1	T60.4X2	T60.4X3	T60.4X4	—	—
Nordazepam	T42.4X1	T42.4X2	T42.4X3	T42.4X4	T42.4X5	T42.4X6
Norepinephrine	T44.4X1	T44.4X2	T44.4X3	T44.4X4	T44.4X5	T44.4X6
Norethandrolone	T38.7X1	T38.7X2	T38.7X3	T38.7X4	T38.7X5	T38.7X6
Norethindrone	T38.4X1	T38.4X2	T38.4X3	T38.4X4	T38.4X5	T38.4X6
Norethisterone (acetate) (enantate)	T38.4X1	T38.4X2	T38.4X3	T38.4X4	T38.4X5	T38.4X6
with ethinylestradiol	T38.5X1	T38.5X2	T38.5X3	T38.5X4	T38.5X5	T38.5X6
Noretynodrel	T38.5X1	T38.5X2	T38.5X3	T38.5X4	T38.5X5	T38.5X6
Norfenefrine	T44.4X1	T44.4X2	T44.4X3	T44.4X4	T44.4X5	T44.4X6
Norfloxacin	T36.8X1	T36.8X2	T36.8X3	T36.8X4	T36.8X5	T36.8X6
Norgestrel	T38.4X1	T38.4X2	T38.4X3	T38.4X4	T38.4X5	T38.4X6
Norgestrienone	T38.4X1	T38.4X2	T38.4X3	T38.4X4	T38.4X5	T38.4X6
Norlestrin	T38.4X1	T38.4X2	T38.4X3	T38.4X4	T38.4X5	T38.4X6
Norlutin	T38.4X1	T38.4X2	T38.4X3	T38.4X4	T38.4X5	T38.4X6
Normal serum albumin (human), salt-poor	T45.8X1	T45.8X2	T45.8X3	T45.8X4	T45.8X5	T45.8X6
Normethandrone	T38.5X1	T38.5X2	T38.5X3	T38.5X4	T38.5X5	T38.5X6
Normison — *see Benzodiazepines*						
Normorphine	T40.2X1	T40.2X2	T40.2X3	T40.2X4	—	—
Norpseudoephedrine	T50.5X1	T50.5X2	T50.5X3	T50.5X4	T50.5X5	T50.5X6
Nortestosterone (furanpropionate)	T38.7X1	T38.7X2	T38.7X3	T38.7X4	T38.7X5	T38.7X6
Nortriptyline	T43.011	T43.012	T43.013	T43.014	T43.015	T43.016
Noscapine	T48.3X1	T48.3X2	T48.3X3	T48.3X4	T48.3X5	T48.3X6
Nose preparations	T49.6X1	T49.6X2	T49.6X3	T49.6X4	T49.6X5	T49.6X6
Novobiocin	T36.5X1	T36.5X2	T36.5X3	T36.5X4	T36.5X5	T36.5X6
Novocain (infiltration) (topical)	T41.3X1	T41.3X2	T41.3X3	T41.3X4	T41.3X5	T41.3X6
nerve block (peripheral) (plexus)	T41.3X1	T41.3X2	T41.3X3	T41.3X4	T41.3X5	T41.3X6
spinal	T41.3X1	T41.3X2	T41.3X3	T41.3X4	T41.3X5	T41.3X6

◀ New ◀ Revised ~~deleted~~ Deleted

Substance	External Cause (T-Code)					
	Poisoning, Accidental (Unintentional)	Poisoning, Intentional Self-Harm	Poisoning, Assault	Poisoning, Undetermined	Adverse Effect	Underdosing
Noxious foodstuff	T62.91	T62.92	T62.93	T62.94	—	—
specified NEC	T62.8X1	T62.8X2	T62.8X3	T62.8X4	—	—
Noxiptiline	T43.011	T43.012	T43.013	T43.014	T43.015	T43.016
Noxytiolin	T49.0X1	T49.0X2	T49.0X3	T49.0X4	T49.0X5	T49.0X6
NPH Iletin (insulin)	T38.3X1	T38.3X2	T38.3X3	T38.3X4	T38.3X5	T38.3X6
Numorphan	T40.2X1	T40.2X2	T40.2X3	T40.2X4	T40.2X5	T40.2X6
Nunol	T42.3X1	T42.3X2	T42.3X3	T42.3X4	T42.3X5	T42.3X6
Nupercaine (spinal anesthetic)	T41.3X1	T41.3X2	T41.3X3	T41.3X4	T41.3X5	T41.3X6
topical (surface)	T41.3X1	T41.3X2	T41.3X3	T41.3X4	T41.3X5	T41.3X6
Nutmeg oil (liniment)	T49.3X1	T49.3X2	T49.3X3	T49.3X4	T49.3X5	T49.3X6
Nutritional supplement	T50.901	T50.902	T50.903	T50.904	T50.905	T50.906
Nux vomica	T65.1X1	T65.1X2	T65.1X3	T65.1X4	—	—
Nydrazid	T37.1X1	T37.1X2	T37.1X3	T37.1X4	T37.1X5	T37.1X6
Nylidrin	T46.7X1	T46.7X2	T46.7X3	T46.7X4	T46.7X5	T46.7X6
Nystatin	T36.7X1	T36.7X2	T36.7X3	T36.7X4	T36.7X5	T36.7X6
topical	T49.0X1	T49.0X2	T49.0X3	T49.0X4	T49.0X5	T49.0X6
Nytol	T45.0X1	T45.0X2	T45.0X3	T45.0X4	T45.0X5	T45.0X6
O						
Obidoxime chloride	T50.6X1	T50.6X2	T50.6X3	T50.6X4	T50.6X5	T50.6X6
Octafonium (chloride)	T49.3X1	T49.3X2	T49.3X3	T49.3X4	T49.3X5	T49.3X6
Octamethyl pyrophosphoramide	T60.0X1	T60.0X2	T60.0X3	T60.0X4	—	—
Octanoin	T50.991	T50.992	T50.993	T50.994	T50.995	T50.996
Octatropine methylbromide	T44.3X1	T44.3X2	T44.3X3	T44.3X4	T44.3X5	T44.3X6
Octotiamine	T45.2X1	T45.2X2	T45.2X3	T45.2X4	T45.2X5	T45.2X6
Octoxinol (9)	T49.8X1	T49.8X2	T49.8X3	T49.8X4	T49.8X5	T49.8X6
Octreotide	T38.991	T38.992	T38.993	T38.994	T38.995	T38.996
Octyl nitrite	T46.3X1	T46.3X2	T46.3X3	T46.3X4	T46.3X5	T46.3X6
Oestradiol	T38.5X1	T38.5X2	T38.5X3	T38.5X4	T38.5X5	T38.5X6
Oestriol	T38.5X1	T38.5X2	T38.5X3	T38.5X4	T38.5X5	T38.5X6
Oestrogen	T38.5X1	T38.5X2	T38.5X3	T38.5X4	T38.5X5	T38.5X6
Oestrone	T38.5X1	T38.5X2	T38.5X3	T38.5X4	T38.5X5	T38.5X6
Ofloxacin	T36.8X1	T36.8X2	T36.8X3	T36.8X4	T36.8X5	T36.8X6
Oil (of)	T65.891	T65.892	T65.893	T65.894	—	—
bitter almond	T62.8X1	T62.8X2	T62.8X3	T62.8X4	—	—
cloves	T49.7X1	T49.7X2	T49.7X3	T49.7X4	T49.7X5	T49.7X6
colors	T65.6X1	T65.6X2	T65.6X3	T65.6X4	—	—
fumes	T59.891	T59.892	T59.893	T59.894	—	—
lubricating	T52.0X1	T52.0X2	T52.0X3	T52.0X4	—	—
Niobe	T52.8X1	T52.8X2	T52.8X3	T52.8X4	—	—

Substance	External Cause (T-Code)					
	Poisoning, Accidental (Unintentional)	Poisoning, Intentional Self-Harm	Poisoning, Assault	Poisoning, Undetermined	Adverse Effect	Underdosing
Oil (of) *(Continued)*						
vitriol (liquid)	T54.2X1	T54.2X2	T54.2X3	T54.2X4	—	—
fumes	T54.2X1	T54.2X2	T54.2X3	T54.2X4	—	—
wintergreen (bitter) NEC	T49.3X1	T49.3X2	T49.3X3	T49.3X4	T49.3X5	T49.3X6
Oily preparation (for skin)	T49.3X1	T49.3X2	T49.3X3	T49.3X4	T49.3X5	T49.3X6
Ointment NEC	T49.3X1	T49.3X2	T49.3X3	T49.3X4	T49.3X5	T49.3X6
Olanzapine	T43.591	T43.592	T43.593	T43.594	T43.595	T43.596
Oleander	T62.2X1	T62.2X2	T62.2X3	T62.2X4	—	—
Oleandomycin	T36.3X1	T36.3X2	T36.3X3	T36.3X4	T36.3X5	T36.3X6
Oleandrin	T46.0X1	T46.0X2	T46.0X3	T46.0X4	T46.0X5	T46.0X6
Oleic acid	T46.6X1	T46.6X2	T46.6X3	T46.6X4	T46.6X5	T46.6X6
Oleovitamin A	T45.2X1	T45.2X2	T45.2X3	T45.2X4	T45.2X5	T45.2X6
Oleum ricini	T47.2X1	T47.2X2	T47.2X3	T47.2X4	T47.2X5	T47.2X6
Olive oil (medicinal) NEC	T47.4X1	T47.4X2	T47.4X3	T47.4X4	T47.4X5	T47.4X6
Olivomycin	T45.1X1	T45.1X2	T45.1X3	T45.1X4	T45.1X5	T45.1X6
Olsalazine	T47.8X1	T47.8X2	T47.8X3	T47.8X4	T47.8X5	T47.8X6
Omeprazole	T47.1X1	T47.1X2	T47.1X3	T47.1X4	T47.1X5	T47.1X6
OMPA	T60.0X1	T60.0X2	T60.0X3	T60.0X4	—	—
Ondansetron	T45.0X1	T45.0X2	T45.0X3	T45.0X4	T45.0X5	T45.0X6
Oncovin	T45.1X1	T45.1X2	T45.1X3	T45.1X4	T45.1X5	T45.1X6
Ophthaine	T41.3X1	T41.3X2	T41.3X3	T41.3X4	T41.3X5	T41.3X6
Ophthetic	T41.3X1	T41.3X2	T41.3X3	T41.3X4	T41.3X5	T41.3X6
Opiate NEC	T40.601	T40.602	T40.603	T40.604	T40.605	T40.606
antagonists	T50.7X1	T50.7X2	T50.7X3	T50.7X4	T50.7X5	T50.7X6
Opioid NEC	T40.2X1	T40.2X2	T40.2X3	T40.2X4	T40.2X5	T40.2X6
Opipramol	T43.011	T43.012	T43.013	T43.014	T43.015	T43.016
Opium alkaloids (total)	T40.0X1	T40.0X2	T40.0X3	T40.0X4	T40.0X5	T40.0X6
standardized powdered	T40.0X1	T40.0X2	T40.0X3	T40.0X4	T40.0X5	T40.0X6
tincture (camphorated)	T40.0X1	T40.0X2	T40.0X3	T40.0X4	T40.0X5	T40.0X6
Oracon	T38.4X1	T38.4X2	T38.4X3	T38.4X4	T38.4X5	T38.4X6
Oragrafin	T50.8X1	T50.8X2	T50.8X3	T50.8X4	T50.8X5	T50.8X6
Oral contraceptives	T38.4X1	T38.4X2	T38.4X3	T38.4X4	T38.4X5	T38.4X6
Oral rehydration salts	T50.3X1	T50.3X2	T50.3X3	T50.3X4	T50.3X5	T50.3X6
Orazamide	T50.991	T50.992	T50.993	T50.994	T50.995	T50.996
Orciprenaline	T48.291	T48.292	T48.293	T48.294	T48.295	T48.296
Organidin	T48.4X1	T48.4X2	T48.4X3	T48.4X4	T48.4X5	T48.4X6
Organonitrate NEC	T46.3X1	T46.3X2	T46.3X3	T46.3X4	T46.3X5	T46.3X6
Organophosphates	T60.0X1	T60.0X2	T60.0X3	T60.0X4	—	—
Orimune	T50.B91	T50.B92	T50.B93	T50.B94	T50.B95	T50.B96
Orinase	T38.3X1	T38.3X2	T38.3X3	T38.3X4	T38.3X5	T38.3X6
Ormeloxifene	T38.6X1	T38.6X2	T38.6X3	T38.6X4	T38.6X5	T38.6X6

Substance	Poisoning, Accidental (Unintentional)	Poisoning, Intentional Self-Harm	Poisoning, Assault	Poisoning, Undetermined	Adverse Effect	Underdosing
	External Cause (T-Code)					
Ornidazole	T37.3X1	T37.3X2	T37.3X3	T37.3X4	T37.3X5	T37.3X6
Ornithine aspartate	T50.991	T50.992	T50.993	T50.994	T50.995	T50.996
Ornoprostil	T47.1X1	T47.1X2	T47.1X3	T47.1X4	T47.1X5	T47.1X6
Orphenadrine (hydrochloride)	T42.8X1	T42.8X2	T42.8X3	T42.8X4	T42.8X5	T42.8X6
Ortal (sodium)	T42.3X1	T42.3X2	T42.3X3	T42.3X4	T42.3X5	T42.3X6
Orthoboric acid	T49.0X1	T49.0X2	T49.0X3	T49.0X4	T49.0X5	T49.0X6
ENT agent	T49.6X1	T49.6X2	T49.6X3	T49.6X4	T49.6X5	T49.6X6
ophthalmic preparation	T49.5X1	T49.5X2	T49.5X3	T49.5X4	T49.5X5	T49.5X6
Orthocaine	T41.3X1	T41.3X2	T41.3X3	T41.3X4	T41.3X5	T41.3X6
Orthodichlorobenzene	T53.7X1	T53.7X2	T53.7X3	T53.7X4	—	—
Ortho-Novum	T38.4X1	T38.4X2	T38.4X3	T38.4X4	T38.4X5	T38.4X6
Orthotolidine (reagent)	T54.2X1	T54.2X2	T54.2X3	T54.2X4	—	—
Osmic acid (liquid)	T54.2X1	T54.2X2	T54.2X3	T54.2X4	—	—
fumes	T54.2X1	T54.2X2	T54.2X3	T54.2X4	—	—
Osmotic diuretics	T50.2X1	T50.2X2	T50.2X3	T50.2X4	T50.2X5	T50.2X6
Otilonium bromide	T44.3X1	T44.3X2	T44.3X3	T44.3X4	T44.3X5	T44.3X6
Otorhinolaryngological drug NEC	T49.6X1	T49.6X2	T49.6X3	T49.6X4	T49.6X5	T49.6X6
Ouabain(e)	T46.0X1	T46.0X2	T46.0X3	T46.0X4	T46.0X5	T46.0X6
Ovarian						
hormone	T38.5X1	T38.5X2	T38.5X3	T38.5X4	T38.5X5	T38.5X6
stimulant	T38.5X1	T38.5X2	T38.5X3	T38.5X4	T38.5X5	T38.5X6
Ovral	T38.4X1	T38.4X2	T38.4X3	T38.4X4	T38.4X5	T38.4X6
Ovulen	T38.4X1	T38.4X2	T38.4X3	T38.4X4	T38.4X5	T38.4X6
Oxacillin	T36.0X1	T36.0X2	T36.0X3	T36.0X4	T36.0X5	T36.0X6
Oxalic acid	T54.2X1	T54.2X2	T54.2X3	T54.2X4	—	—
ammonium salt	T50.991	T50.992	T50.993	T50.994	T50.995	T50.996
Oxamniquine	T37.4X1	T37.4X2	T37.4X3	T37.4X4	T37.4X5	T37.4X6
Oxanamide	T43.591	T43.592	T43.593	T43.594	T43.595	T43.596
Oxandrolone	T38.7X1	T38.7X2	T38.7X3	T38.7X4	T38.7X5	T38.7X6
Oxantel	T37.4X1	T37.4X2	T37.4X3	T37.4X4	T37.4X5	T37.4X6
Oxapium iodide	T44.3X1	T44.3X2	T44.3X3	T44.3X4	T44.3X5	T44.3X6
Oxaprotiline	T43.021	T43.022	T43.023	T43.024	T43.025	T43.026
Oxaprozin	T39.311	T39.312	T39.313	T39.314	T39.315	T39.316
Oxatomide	T45.0X1	T45.0X2	T45.0X3	T45.0X4	T45.0X5	T45.0X6
Oxazepam	T42.4X1	T42.4X2	T42.4X3	T42.4X4	T42.4X5	T42.4X6
Oxazimedrine	T50.5X1	T50.5X2	T50.5X3	T50.5X4	T50.5X5	T50.5X6
Oxazolam	T42.4X1	T42.4X2	T42.4X3	T42.4X4	T42.4X5	T42.4X6
Oxazolidine derivatives	T42.2X1	T42.2X2	T42.2X3	T42.2X4	T42.2X5	T42.2X6
Oxazolidinedione (derivative)	T42.2X1	T42.2X2	T42.2X3	T42.2X4	T42.2X5	T42.2X6
Ox bile extract	T47.5X1	T47.5X2	T47.5X3	T47.5X4	T47.5X5	T47.5X6
Oxcarbazepine	T42.1X1	T42.1X2	T42.1X3	T42.1X4	T42.1X5	T42.1X6
Oxedrine	T44.4X1	T44.4X2	T44.4X3	T44.4X4	T44.4X5	T44.4X6

Substance	Poisoning, Accidental (Unintentional)	Poisoning, Intentional Self-Harm	Poisoning, Assault	Poisoning, Undetermined	Adverse Effect	Underdosing
	External Cause (T-Code)					
Oxeladin (citrate)	T48.3X1	T48.3X2	T48.3X3	T48.3X4	T48.3X5	T48.3X6
Oxendolone	T38.5X1	T38.5X2	T38.5X3	T38.5X4	T38.5X5	T38.5X6
Oxetacaine	T41.3X1	T41.3X2	T41.3X3	T41.3X4	T41.3X5	T41.3X6
Oxethazine	T41.3X1	T41.3X2	T41.3X3	T41.3X4	T41.3X5	T41.3X6
Oxetorone	T39.8X1	T39.8X2	T39.8X3	T39.8X4	T39.8X5	T39.8X6
Oxiconazole	T49.0X1	T49.0X2	T49.0X3	T49.0X4	T49.0X5	T49.0X6
Oxidizing agent NEC	T54.91	T54.92	T54.93	T54.94	—	—
Oxipurinol	T50.4X1	T50.4X2	T50.4X3	T50.4X4	T50.4X5	T50.4X6
Oxitriptan	T43.291	T43.292	T43.293	T43.294	T43.295	T43.296
Oxitropium bromide	T48.6X1	T48.6X2	T48.6X3	T48.6X4	T48.6X5	T48.6X6
Oxodipine	T46.1X1	T46.1X2	T46.1X3	T46.1X4	T46.1X5	T46.1X6
Oxolamine	T48.3X1	T48.3X2	T48.3X3	T48.3X4	T48.3X5	T48.3X6
Oxolinic acid	T37.8X1	T37.8X2	T37.8X3	T37.8X4	T37.8X5	T37.8X6
Oxomemazine	T43.3X1	T43.3X2	T43.3X3	T43.3X4	T43.3X5	T43.3X6
Oxophenarsine	T37.3X1	T37.3X2	T37.3X3	T37.3X4	T37.3X5	T37.3X6
Oxprenolol	T44.7X1	T44.7X2	T44.7X3	T44.7X4	T44.7X5	T44.7X6
Oxsoralen	T49.3X1	T49.3X2	T49.3X3	T49.3X4	T49.3X5	T49.3X6
Oxtriphylline	T48.6X1	T48.6X2	T48.6X3	T48.6X4	T48.6X5	T48.6X6
Oxybate sodium	T41.291	T41.292	T41.293	T41.294	T41.295	T41.296
Oxybuprocaine	T41.3X1	T41.3X2	T41.3X3	T41.3X4	T41.3X5	T41.3X6
Oxybutynin	T44.3X1	T44.3X2	T44.3X3	T44.3X4	T44.3X5	T44.3X6
Oxychlorosene	T49.0X1	T49.0X2	T49.0X3	T49.0X4	T49.0X5	T49.0X6
Oxycodone	T40.2X1	T40.2X2	T40.2X3	T40.2X4	T40.2X5	T40.2X6
Oxyfedrine	T46.3X1	T46.3X2	T46.3X3	T46.3X4	T46.3X5	T46.3X6
Oxygen	T41.5X1	T41.5X2	T41.5X3	T41.5X4	T41.5X5	T41.5X6
Oxylone	T49.0X1	T49.0X2	T49.0X3	T49.0X4	T49.0X5	T49.0X6
ophthalmic preparation	T49.5X1	T49.5X2	T49.5X3	T49.5X4	T49.5X5	T49.5X6
Oxymesterone	T38.7X1	T38.7X2	T38.7X3	T38.7X4	T38.7X5	T38.7X6
Oxymetazoline	T48.5X1	T48.5X2	T48.5X3	T48.5X4	T48.5X5	T48.5X6
Oxymetholone	T38.7X1	T38.7X2	T38.7X3	T38.7X4	T38.7X5	T38.7X6
Oxymorphone	T40.2X1	T40.2X2	T40.2X3	T40.2X4	T40.2X5	T40.2X6
Oxypertine	T43.591	T43.592	T43.593	T43.594	T43.595	T43.596
Oxyphenbutazone	T39.2X1	T39.2X2	T39.2X3	T39.2X4	T39.2X5	T39.2X6
Oxyphencyclimine	T44.3X1	T44.3X2	T44.3X3	T44.3X4	T44.3X5	T44.3X6
Oxyphenisatine	T47.2X1	T47.2X2	T47.2X3	T47.2X4	T47.2X5	T47.2X6
Oxyphenonium bromide	T44.3X1	T44.3X2	T44.3X3	T44.3X4	T44.3X5	T44.3X6
Oxypolygelatin	T45.8X1	T45.8X2	T45.8X3	T45.8X4	T45.8X5	T45.8X6
Oxyquinoline (derivatives)	T37.8X1	T37.8X2	T37.8X3	T37.8X4	T37.8X5	T37.8X6
Oxytetracycline	T36.4X1	T36.4X2	T36.4X3	T36.4X4	T36.4X5	T36.4X6
Oxytocic drug NEC	T48.0X1	T48.0X2	T48.0X3	T48.0X4	T48.0X5	T48.0X6
Oxytocin (synthetic)	T48.0X1	T48.0X2	T48.0X3	T48.0X4	T48.0X5	T48.0X6
Ozone	T59.891	T59.892	T59.893	T59.894	—	—

Substance	Poisoning, Accidental (Unintentional)	Poisoning, Intentional Self-Harm	Poisoning, Assault	Poisoning, Undetermined	Adverse Effect	Underdosing
	External Cause (T-Code)					
P						
PABA	T49.3X1	T49.3X2	T49.3X3	T49.3X4	T49.3X5	T49.3X6
Packed red cells	T45.8X1	T45.8X2	T45.8X3	T45.8X4	T45.8X5	T45.8X6
Padimate	T49.3X1	T49.3X2	T49.3X3	T49.3X4	T49.3X5	T49.3X6
Paint NEC	T65.6X1	T65.6X2	T65.6X3	T65.6X4	—	—
cleaner	T52.91	T52.92	T52.93	T52.94	—	—
fumes NEC	T59.891	T59.892	T59.893	T59.894	—	—
lead (fumes)	T56.0X1	T56.0X2	T56.0X3	T56.0X4	—	—
solvent NEC	T52.8X1	T52.8X2	T52.8X3	T52.8X4	—	—
stripper	T52.8X1	T52.8X2	T52.8X3	T52.8X4	—	—
Palfium	T40.2X1	T40.2X2	T40.2X3	T40.2X4	—	—
Palm kernel oil	T50.991	T50.992	T50.993	T50.994	T50.995	T50.996
Paludrine	T37.2X1	T37.2X2	T37.2X3	T37.2X4	T37.2X5	T37.2X6
PAM (pralidoxime)	T50.6X1	T50.6X2	T50.6X3	T50.6X4	T50.6X5	T50.6X6
Pamaquine (naphthoute)	T37.2X1	T37.2X2	T37.2X3	T37.2X4	T37.2X5	T37.2X6
Panadol	T39.1X1	T39.1X2	T39.1X3	T39.1X4	T39.1X5	T39.1X6
Pancreatic						
digestive secretion stimulant	T47.8X1	T47.8X2	T47.8X3	T47.8X4	T47.8X5	T47.8X6
dornase	T45.3X1	T45.3X2	T45.3X3	T45.3X4	T45.3X5	T45.3X6
Pancreatin	T47.5X1	T47.5X2	T47.5X3	T47.5X4	T47.5X5	T47.5X6
Pancrelipase	T47.5X1	T47.5X2	T47.5X3	T47.5X4	T47.5X5	T47.5X6
Pancuronium (bromide)	T48.1X1	T48.1X2	T48.1X3	T48.1X4	T48.1X5	T48.1X6
Pangamic acid	T45.2X1	T45.2X2	T45.2X3	T45.2X4	T45.2X5	T45.2X6
Panthenol	T45.2X1	T45.2X2	T45.2X3	T45.2X4	T45.2X5	T45.2X6
topical	T49.8X1	T49.8X2	T49.8X3	T49.8X4	T49.8X5	T49.8X6
Pantopon	T40.0X1	T40.0X2	T40.0X3	T40.0X4	T40.0X5	T40.0X6
Pantothenic acid	T45.2X1	T45.2X2	T45.2X3	T45.2X4	T45.2X5	T45.2X6
Panwarfin	T45.511	T45.512	T45.513	T45.514	T45.515	T45.516
Papain	T47.5X1	T47.5X2	T47.5X3	T47.5X4	T47.5X5	T47.5X6
digestant	T47.5X1	T47.5X2	T47.5X3	T47.5X4	T47.5X5	T47.5X6
Papaveretum	T40.0X1	T40.0X2	T40.0X3	T40.0X4	T40.0X5	T40.0X6
Papaverine	T44.3X1	T44.3X2	T44.3X3	T44.3X4	T44.3X5	T44.3X6
Para-acetamidophenol	T39.1X1	T39.1X2	T39.1X3	T39.1X4	T39.1X5	T39.1X6
Para-aminobenzoic acid	T49.3X1	T49.3X2	T49.3X3	T49.3X4	T49.3X5	T49.3X6
Para-aminophenol derivatives	T39.1X1	T39.1X2	T39.1X3	T39.1X4	T39.1X5	T39.1X6
Para-aminosalicylic acid	T37.1X1	T37.1X2	T37.1X3	T37.1X4	T37.1X5	T37.1X6
Paracetaldehyde	T42.6X1	T42.6X2	T42.6X3	T42.6X4	T42.6X5	T42.6X6
Paracetamol	T39.1X1	T39.1X2	T39.1X3	T39.1X4	T39.1X5	T39.1X6
Parachlorophenol (camphorated)	T49.0X1	T49.0X2	T49.0X3	T49.0X4	T49.0X5	T49.0X6
Paracodin	T40.2X1	T40.2X2	T40.2X3	T40.2X4	T40.2X5	T40.2X6
Paradione	T42.2X1	T42.2X2	T42.2X3	T42.2X4	T42.2X5	T42.2X6

Substance	Poisoning, Accidental (Unintentional)	Poisoning, Intentional Self-Harm	Poisoning, Assault	Poisoning, Undetermined	Adverse Effect	Underdosing
	External Cause (T-Code)					
Paraffin(s) (wax)	T52.0X1	T52.0X2	T52.0X3	T52.0X4	—	—
liquid (medicinal)	T47.4X1	T47.4X2	T47.4X3	T47.4X4	T47.4X5	T47.4X6
nonmedicinal	T52.0X1	T52.0X2	T52.0X3	T52.0X4	—	—
Paraformaldehyde	T60.3X1	T60.3X2	T60.3X3	T60.3X4	—	—
Paraldehyde	T42.6X1	T42.6X2	T42.6X3	T42.6X4	T42.6X5	T42.6X6
Paramethadione	T42.2X1	T42.2X2	T42.2X3	T42.2X4	T42.2X5	T42.2X6
Paramethasone	T38.0X1	T38.0X2	T38.0X3	T38.0X4	T38.0X5	T38.0X6
acetate	T49.0X1	T49.0X2	T49.0X3	T49.0X4	T49.0X5	T49.0X6
Paraoxon	T60.0X1	T60.0X2	T60.0X3	T60.0X4	—	—
Paraquat	T60.3X1	T60.3X2	T60.3X3	T60.3X4	—	—
Parasympatholytic NEC	T44.3X1	T44.3X2	T44.3X3	T44.3X4	T44.3X5	T44.3X6
Parasympathomimetic drug NEC	T44.1X1	T44.1X2	T44.1X3	T44.1X4	T44.1X5	T44.1X6
Parathion	T60.0X1	T60.0X2	T60.0X3	T60.0X4	—	—
Parathormone	T50.991	T50.992	T50.993	T50.994	T50.995	T50.996
Parathyroid extract	T50.991	T50.992	T50.993	T50.994	T50.995	T50.996
Paratyphoid vaccine	T50.A91	T50.A92	T50.A93	T50.A94	T50.A95	T50.A96
Paredrine	T44.4X1	T44.4X2	T44.4X3	T44.4X4	T44.4X5	T44.4X6
Paregoric	T40.0X1	T40.0X2	T40.0X3	T40.0X4	T40.0X5	T40.0X6
Pargyline	T46.5X1	T46.5X2	T46.5X3	T46.5X4	T46.5X5	T46.5X6
Paris green	T57.0X1	T57.0X2	T57.0X3	T57.0X4	—	—
insecticide	T57.0X1	T57.0X2	T57.0X3	T57.0X4	—	—
Parnate	T43.1X1	T43.1X2	T43.1X3	T43.1X4	T43.1X5	T43.1X6
Paromomycin	T36.5X1	T36.5X2	T36.5X3	T36.5X4	T36.5X5	T36.5X6
Paroxypropione	T45.1X1	T45.1X2	T45.1X3	T45.1X4	T45.1X5	T45.1X6
Parzone	T40.2X1	T40.2X2	T40.2X3	T40.2X4	T40.2X5	T40.2X6
PAS	T37.1X1	T37.1X2	T37.1X3	T37.1X4	T37.1X5	T37.1X6
Pasiniazid	T37.1X1	T37.1X2	T37.1X3	T37.1X4	T37.1X5	T37.1X6
PBB (polybrominated biphenyls)	T65.891	T65.892	T65.893	T65.894	—	—
PCB	T65.891	T65.892	T65.893	T65.894	—	—
PCP						
meaning pentachlorophenol	T60.1X1	T60.1X2	T60.1X3	T60.1X4	—	—
fungicide	T60.3X1	T60.3X2	T60.3X3	T60.3X4	—	—
herbicide	T60.3X1	T60.3X2	T60.3X3	T60.3X4	—	—
insecticide	T60.1X1	T60.1X2	T60.1X3	T60.1X4	—	—
meaning phencyclidine	T40.991	T40.992	T40.993	T40.994	—	—
Peach kernel oil (emulsion)	T47.4X1	T47.4X2	T47.4X3	T47.4X4	T47.4X5	T47.4X6
Peanut oil (emulsion) NEC	T47.4X1	T47.4X2	T47.4X3	T47.4X4	T47.4X5	T47.4X6
topical	T49.3X1	T49.3X2	T49.3X3	T49.3X4	T49.3X5	T49.3X6
Pearly Gates (morning glory seeds)	T40.991	T40.992	T40.993	T40.994	—	—
Pecazine	T43.3X1	T43.3X2	T43.3X3	T43.3X4	T43.3X5	T43.3X6
Pectin	T47.6X1	T47.6X2	T47.6X3	T47.6X4	T47.6X5	T47.6X6

Substance	Poisoning, Accidental (Unintentional)	Poisoning, Intentional Self-Harm	Poisoning, Assault	Poisoning, Undetermined	Adverse Effect	Underdosing
	External Cause (T-Code)					
Pefloxacin	T37.8X1	T37.8X2	T37.8X3	T37.8X4	T37.8X5	T37.8X6
Pegademase, bovine	T50.Z91	T50.Z92	T50.Z93	T50.Z94	T50.Z95	T50.Z96
Pelletierine tannate	T37.4X1	T37.4X2	T37.4X3	T37.4X4	T37.4X5	T37.4X6
Pemirolast (potassium)	T48.6X1	T48.6X2	T48.6X3	T48.6X4	T48.6X5	T48.6X6
Pemoline	T50.7X1	T50.7X2	T50.7X3	T50.7X4	T50.7X5	T50.7X6
Pempidine	T44.2X1	T44.2X2	T44.2X3	T44.2X4	T44.2X5	T44.2X6
Penamecillin	T36.0X1	T36.0X2	T36.0X3	T36.0X4	T36.0X5	T36.0X6
Penbutolol	T44.7X1	T44.7X2	T44.7X3	T44.7X4	T44.7X5	T44.7X6
Penethamate	T36.0X1	T36.0X2	T36.0X3	T36.0X4	T36.0X5	T36.0X6
Penfluridol	T43.591	T43.592	T43.593	T43.594	T43.595	T43.596
Penflutizide	T50.2X1	T50.2X2	T50.2X3	T50.2X4	T50.2X5	T50.2X6
Pengitoxin	T46.0X1	T46.0X2	T46.0X3	T46.0X4	T46.0X5	T46.0X6
Penicillamine	T50.6X1	T50.6X2	T50.6X3	T50.6X4	T50.6X5	T50.6X6
Penicillin (any)	T36.0X1	T36.0X2	T36.0X3	T36.0X4	T36.0X5	T36.0X6
Penicillinase	T45.3X1	T45.3X2	T45.3X3	T45.3X4	T45.3X5	T45.3X6
Penicilloyl polylysine	T50.8X1	T50.8X2	T50.8X3	T50.8X4	T50.8X5	T50.8X6
Penimepicycline	T36.4X1	T36.4X2	T36.4X3	T36.4X4	T36.4X5	T36.4X6
Pentachloroethane	T53.6X1	T53.6X2	T53.6X3	T53.6X4	—	—
Pentachloronaphthalene	T53.7X1	T53.7X2	T53.7X3	T53.7X4	—	—
Pentachlorophenol (pesticide)	T60.1X1	T60.1X2	T60.1X3	T60.1X4	—	—
fungicide	T60.3X1	T60.3X2	T60.3X3	T60.3X4	—	—
herbicide	T60.3X1	T60.3X2	T60.3X3	T60.3X4	—	—
insecticide	T60.1X1	T60.1X2	T60.1X3	T60.1X4	—	—
Pentaerythritol tetranitrate	T46.3X1	T46.3X2	T46.3X3	T46.3X4	T46.3X5	T46.3X6
Pentaerythritol	T46.3X1	T46.3X2	T46.3X3	T46.3X4	T46.3X5	T46.3X6
chloral	T42.6X1	T42.6X2	T42.6X3	T42.6X4	T42.6X5	T42.6X6
tetranitrate NEC	T46.3X1	T46.3X2	T46.3X3	T46.3X4	T46.3X5	T46.3X6
Pentagastrin	T50.8X1	T50.8X2	T50.8X3	T50.8X4	T50.8X5	T50.8X6
Pentalin	T53.6X1	T53.6X2	T53.6X3	T53.6X4	—	—
Pentamethonium bromide	T44.2X1	T44.2X2	T44.2X3	T44.2X4	T44.2X5	T44.2X6
Pentamidine	T37.3X1	T37.3X2	T37.3X3	T37.3X4	T37.3X5	T37.3X6
Pentanol	T51.3X1	T51.3X2	T51.3X3	T51.3X4	—	—
Pentapyrrolinium (bitartrate)	T44.2X1	T44.2X2	T44.2X3	T44.2X4	T44.2X5	T44.2X6
Pentaquine	T37.2X1	T37.2X2	T37.2X3	T37.2X4	T37.2X5	T37.2X6
Pentazocine	T40.4X1	T40.4X2	T40.4X3	T40.4X4	T40.4X5	T40.4X6
Pentetrazole	T50.7X1	T50.7X2	T50.7X3	T50.7X4	T50.7X5	T50.7X6
Penthienate bromide	T44.3X1	T44.3X2	T44.3X3	T44.3X4	T44.3X5	T44.3X6
Pentifylline	T46.7X1	T46.7X2	T46.7X3	T46.7X4	T46.7X5	T46.7X6
Pentobarbital	T42.3X1	T42.3X2	T42.3X3	T42.3X4	T42.3X5	T42.3X6
sodium	T42.3X1	T42.3X2	T42.3X3	T42.3X4	T42.3X5	T42.3X6
Pentobarbitone	T42.3X1	T42.3X2	T42.3X3	T42.3X4	T42.3X5	T42.3X6
Pentolonium tartrate	T44.2X1	T44.2X2	T44.2X3	T44.2X4	T44.2X5	T44.2X6

Substance	Poisoning, Accidental (Unintentional)	Poisoning, Intentional Self-Harm	Poisoning, Assault	Poisoning, Undetermined	Adverse Effect	Underdosing
	External Cause (T-Code)					
Pentosan polysulfate (sodium)	T39.8X1	T39.8X2	T39.8X3	T39.8X4	T39.8X5	T39.8X6
Pentostatin	T45.1X1	T45.1X2	T45.1X3	T45.1X4	T45.1X5	T45.1X6
Pentothal	T41.1X1	T41.1X2	T41.1X3	T41.1X4	T41.1X5	T41.1X6
Pentoxifylline	T46.7X1	T46.7X2	T46.7X3	T46.7X4	T46.7X5	T46.7X6
Pentoxyverine	T48.3X1	T48.3X2	T48.3X3	T48.3X4	T48.3X5	T48.3X6
Pentrinat	T46.3X1	T46.3X2	T46.3X3	T46.3X4	T46.3X5	T46.3X6
Pentylenetetrazole	T50.7X1	T50.7X2	T50.7X3	T50.7X4	T50.7X5	T50.7X6
Pentylsalicylamide	T37.1X1	T37.1X2	T37.1X3	T37.1X4	T37.1X5	T37.1X6
Pentymal	T42.3X1	T42.3X2	T42.3X3	T42.3X4	T42.3X5	T42.3X6
Peplomycin	T45.1X1	T45.1X2	T45.1X3	T45.1X4	T45.1X5	T45.1X6
Peppermint (oil)	T47.5X1	T47.5X2	T47.5X3	T47.5X4	T47.5X5	T47.5X6
Pepsin	T47.5X1	T47.5X2	T47.5X3	T47.5X4	T47.5X5	T47.5X6
digestant	T47.5X1	T47.5X2	T47.5X3	T47.5X4	T47.5X5	T47.5X6
Pepstatin	T47.1X1	T47.1X2	T47.1X3	T47.1X4	T47.1X5	T47.1X6
Peptavlon	T50.8X1	T50.8X2	T50.8X3	T50.8X4	T50.8X5	T50.8X6
Perazine	T43.3X1	T43.3X2	T43.3X3	T43.3X4	T43.3X5	T43.3X6
Percaine (spinal)	T41.3X1	T41.3X2	T41.3X3	T41.3X4	T41.3X5	T41.3X6
topical (surface)	T41.3X1	T41.3X2	T41.3X3	T41.3X4	T41.3X5	T41.3X6
Perchloroethylene	T53.3X1	T53.3X2	T53.3X3	T53.3X4	—	—
medicinal	T37.4X1	T37.4X2	T37.4X3	T37.4X4	T37.4X5	T37.4X6
vapor	T53.3X1	T53.3X2	T53.3X3	T53.3X4	—	—
Percodan	T40.2X1	T40.2X2	T40.2X3	T40.2X4	T40.2X5	T40.2X6
Percogesic — *see also acetaminophen*	T45.0X1	T45.0X2	T45.0X3	T45.0X4	T45.0X5	T45.0X6
Percorten	T38.0X1	T38.0X2	T38.0X3	T38.0X4	T38.0X5	T38.0X6
Pergolide	T42.8X1	T42.8X2	T42.8X3	T42.8X4	T42.8X5	T42.8X6
Pergonal	T38.811	T38.812	T38.813	T38.814	T38.815	T38.816
Perhexilene	T46.3X1	T46.3X2	T46.3X3	T46.3X4	T46.3X5	T46.3X6
Perhexiline (maleate)	T46.3X1	T46.3X2	T46.3X3	T46.3X4	T46.3X5	T46.3X6
Periactin	T45.0X1	T45.0X2	T45.0X3	T45.0X4	T45.0X5	T45.0X6
Periciazine	T43.3X1	T43.3X2	T43.3X3	T43.3X4	T43.3X5	T43.3X6
Periclor	T42.6X1	T42.6X2	T42.6X3	T42.6X4	T42.6X5	T42.6X6
Perindopril	T46.4X1	T46.4X2	T46.4X3	T46.4X4	T46.4X5	T46.4X6
Perisoxal	T39.8X1	T39.8X2	T39.8X3	T39.8X4	T39.8X5	T39.8X6
Peritrate	T46.3X1	T46.3X2	T46.3X3	T46.3X4	T46.3X5	T46.3X6
Peritoneal dialysis solution	T50.3X1	T50.3X2	T50.3X3	T50.3X4	T50.3X5	T50.3X6
Perlapine	T42.4X1	T42.4X2	T42.4X3	T42.4X4	T42.4X5	T42.4X6
Permanganate	T65.891	T65.892	T65.893	T65.894	—	—
Permethrin	T60.1X1	T60.1X2	T60.1X3	T60.1X4	—	—
Pernocton	T42.3X1	T42.3X2	T42.3X3	T42.3X4	T42.3X5	T42.3X6
Pernoston	T42.3X1	T42.3X2	T42.3X3	T42.3X4	T42.3X5	T42.3X6
Peronine	T40.2X1	T40.2X2	T40.2X3	T40.2X4	—	—
Perphenazine	T43.3X1	T43.3X2	T43.3X3	T43.3X4	T43.3X5	T43.3X6

◀ New ◀ Revised ~~deleted~~ Deleted

Substance	External Cause (T-Code)					
	Poisoning, Accidental (Unintentional)	Poisoning, Intentional Self-Harm	Poisoning, Assault	Poisoning, Undetermined	Adverse Effect	Underdosing
Pertofrane	T43.011	T43.012	T43.013	T43.014	T43.015	T43.016
Pertussis						
immune serum (human)	T50.Z11	T50.Z12	T50.Z13	T50.Z14	T50.Z15	T50.Z16
vaccine (with diphtheria toxoid) (with tetanus toxoid)	T50.A11	T50.A12	T50.A13	T50.A14	T50.A15	T50.A16
Peruvian balsam	T49.0X1	T49.0X2	T49.0X3	T49.0X4	T49.0X5	T49.0X6
Peruvoside	T46.0X1	T46.0X2	T46.0X3	T46.0X4	T46.0X5	T46.0X6
Pesticide (dust) (fumes) (vapor) NEC	T60.91	T60.92	T60.93	T60.94	—	—
arsenic	T57.0X1	T57.0X2	T57.0X3	T57.0X4	—	—
chlorinated	T60.1X1	T60.1X2	T60.1X3	T60.1X4	—	—
cyanide	T65.0X1	T65.0X2	T65.0X3	T65.0X4	—	—
kerosene	T52.0X1	T52.0X2	T52.0X3	T52.0X4	—	—
mixture (of compounds)	T60.91	T60.92	T60.93	T60.94	—	—
naphthalene	T60.2X1	T60.2X2	T60.2X3	T60.2X4	—	—
organochlorine (compounds)	T60.1X1	T60.1X2	T60.1X3	T60.1X4	—	—
petroleum (distillate) (products) NEC	T60.8X1	T60.8X2	T60.8X3	T60.8X4	—	—
specified ingredient NEC	T60.8X1	T60.8X2	T60.8X3	T60.8X4	—	—
strychnine	T65.1X1	T65.1X2	T65.1X3	T65.1X4	—	—
thallium	T60.4X1	T60.4X2	T60.4X3	T60.4X4	—	—
Pethidine	T40.4X1	T40.4X2	T40.4X3	T40.4X4	T40.4X5	T40.4X6
Petrichloral	T42.6X1	T42.6X2	T42.6X3	T42.6X4	T42.6X5	T42.6X6
Petrol	T52.0X1	T52.0X2	T52.0X3	T52.0X4	—	—
vapor	T52.0X1	T52.0X2	T52.0X3	T52.0X4	—	—
Petrolatum	T49.3X1	T49.3X2	T49.3X3	T49.3X4	T49.3X5	T49.3X6
hydrophilic	T49.3X1	T49.3X2	T49.3X3	T49.3X4	T49.3X5	T49.3X6
liquid	T47.4X1	T47.4X2	T47.4X3	T47.4X4	T47.4X5	T47.4X6
topical	T49.3X1	T49.3X2	T49.3X3	T49.3X4	T49.3X5	T49.3X6
nonmedicinal	T52.0X1	T52.0X2	T52.0X3	T52.0X4	—	—
red veterinary	T49.3X1	T49.3X2	T49.3X3	T49.3X4	T49.3X5	T49.3X6
white	T49.3X1	T49.3X2	T49.3X3	T49.3X4	T49.3X5	T49.3X6
Petroleum (products) NEC	T52.0X1	T52.0X2	T52.0X3	T52.0X4	—	—
benzine(s) — *see Ligroin*						
ether — *see Ligroin*						
jelly — *see Petrolatum*						
naphtha — *see Ligroin*						
pesticide	T60.8X1	T60.8X2	T60.8X3	T60.8X4	—	—
solids	T52.0X1	T52.0X2	T52.0X3	T52.0X4	—	—
solvents	T52.0X1	T52.0X2	T52.0X3	T52.0X4	—	—
vapor	T52.0X1	T52.0X2	T52.0X3	T52.0X4	—	—
Peyote	T40.991	T40.992	T40.993	T40.994	—	—
Phanodorm, phanodorn	T42.3X1	T42.3X2	T42.3X3	T42.3X4	T42.3X5	T42.3X6

Substance	External Cause (T-Code)					
	Poisoning, Accidental (Unintentional)	Poisoning, Intentional Self-Harm	Poisoning, Assault	Poisoning, Undetermined	Adverse Effect	Underdosing
Phanquinone	T37.3X1	T37.3X2	T37.3X3	T37.3X4	T37.3X5	T37.3X6
Phanquone	T37.3X1	T37.3X2	T37.3X3	T37.3X4	T37.3X5	T37.3X6
Pharmaceutical						
adjunct NEC	T50.901	T50.902	T50.903	T50.904	T50.905	T50.906
excipient NEC	T50.901	T50.902	T50.903	T50.904	T50.905	T50.906
sweetener	T50.901	T50.902	T50.903	T50.904	T50.905	T50.906
viscous agent	T50.901	T50.902	T50.903	T50.904	T50.905	T50.906
Phemitone	T42.3X1	T42.3X2	T42.3X3	T42.3X4	T42.3X5	T42.3X6
Phenacaine	T41.3X1	T41.3X2	T41.3X3	T41.3X4	T41.3X5	T41.3X6
Phenacemide	T42.6X1	T42.6X2	T42.6X3	T42.6X4	T42.6X5	T42.6X6
Phenacetin	T39.1X1	T39.1X2	T39.1X3	T39.1X4	T39.1X5	T39.1X6
Phenadoxone	T40.2X1	T40.2X2	T40.2X3	T40.2X4	—	—
Phenaglycodol	T43.591	T43.592	T43.593	T43.594	T43.595	T43.596
Phenantoin	T42.0X1	T42.0X2	T42.0X3	T42.0X4	T42.0X5	T42.0X6
Phenaphthazine reagent	T50.991	T50.992	T50.993	T50.994	T50.995	T50.996
Phenazocine	T40.4X1	T40.4X2	T40.4X3	T40.4X4	T40.4X5	T40.4X6
Phenazone	T39.2X1	T39.2X2	T39.2X3	T39.2X4	T39.2X5	T39.2X6
Phenazopyridine	T39.8X1	T39.8X2	T39.8X3	T39.8X4	T39.8X5	T39.8X6
Phenbenicillin	T36.0X1	T36.0X2	T36.0X3	T36.0X4	T36.0X5	T36.0X6
Phenbutrazate	T50.5X1	T50.5X2	T50.5X3	T50.5X4	T50.5X5	T50.5X6
Phencyclidine	T40.991	T40.992	T40.993	T40.994	T40.995	T40.996
Phendimetrazine	T50.5X1	T50.5X2	T50.5X3	T50.5X4	T50.5X5	T50.5X6
Phenelzine	T43.1X1	T43.1X2	T43.1X3	T43.1X4	T43.1X5	T43.1X6
Phenemal	T42.3X1	T42.3X2	T42.3X3	T42.3X4	T42.3X5	T42.3X6
Phenergan	T42.6X1	T42.6X2	T42.6X3	T42.6X4	T42.6X5	T42.6X6
Pheneticillin	T36.0X1	T36.0X2	T36.0X3	T36.0X4	T36.0X5	T36.0X6
Pheneturide	T42.6X1	T42.6X2	T42.6X3	T42.6X4	T42.6X5	T42.6X6
Phenformin	T38.3X1	T38.3X2	T38.3X3	T38.3X4	T38.3X5	T38.3X6
Phenglutarimide	T44.3X1	T44.3X2	T44.3X3	T44.3X4	T44.3X5	T44.3X6
Phenicarbazide	T39.8X1	T39.8X2	T39.8X3	T39.8X4	T39.8X5	T39.8X6
Phenindamine	T45.0X1	T45.0X2	T45.0X3	T45.0X4	T45.0X5	T45.0X6
Phenindione	T45.511	T45.512	T45.513	T45.514	T45.515	T45.516
Pheniprazine	T43.1X1	T43.1X2	T43.1X3	T43.1X4	T43.1X5	T43.1X6
Pheniramine	T45.0X1	T45.0X2	T45.0X3	T45.0X4	T45.0X5	T45.0X6
Phenisatin	T47.2X1	T47.2X2	T47.2X3	T47.2X4	T47.2X5	T47.2X6
Phenmetrazine	T50.5X1	T50.5X2	T50.5X3	T50.5X4	T50.5X5	T50.5X6
Phenobal	T42.3X1	T42.3X2	T42.3X3	T42.3X4	T42.3X5	T42.3X6
Phenobarbital	T42.3X1	T42.3X2	T42.3X3	T42.3X4	T42.3X5	T42.3X6
with						
mephenytoin	T42.3X1	T42.3X2	T42.3X3	T42.3X4	T42.3X5	T42.3X6
phenytoin	T42.3X1	T42.3X2	T42.3X3	T42.3X4	T42.3X5	T42.3X6
sodium	T42.3X1	T42.3X2	T42.3X3	T42.3X4	T42.3X5	T42.3X6

◀ New ◀ Revised ~~deleted~~ Deleted

Substance	External Cause (T-Code)					
	Poisoning, Accidental (Unintentional)	Poisoning, Intentional Self-Harm	Poisoning, Assault	Poisoning, Undetermined	Adverse Effect	Underdosing
Phenobarbitone	T42.3X1	T42.3X2	T42.3X3	T42.3X4	T42.3X5	T42.3X6
Phenobutiodil	T50.8X1	T50.8X2	T50.8X3	T50.8X4	T50.8X5	T50.8X6
Phenoctide	T49.0X1	T49.0X2	T49.0X3	T49.0X4	T49.0X5	T49.0X6
Phenol	T49.0X1	T49.0X2	T49.0X3	T49.0X4	T49.0X5	T49.0X6
disinfectant	T54.0X1	T54.0X2	T54.0X3	T54.0X4	—	—
in oil injection	T46.8X1	T46.8X2	T46.8X3	T46.8X4	T46.8X5	T46.8X6
medicinal	T49.1X1	T49.1X2	T49.1X3	T49.1X4	T49.1X5	T49.1X6
nonmedicinal NEC	T54.0X1	T54.0X2	T54.0X3	T54.0X4	—	—
pesticide	T60.8X1	T60.8X2	T60.8X3	T60.8X4	—	—
red	T50.8X1	T50.8X2	T50.8X3	T50.8X4	T50.8X5	T50.8X6
Phenolic preparation	T49.1X1	T49.1X2	T49.1X3	T49.1X4	T49.1X5	T49.1X6
Phenolphthalein	T47.2X1	T47.2X2	T47.2X3	T47.2X4	T47.2X5	T47.2X6
Phenolsulfonphthalein	T50.8X1	T50.8X2	T50.8X3	T50.8X4	T50.8X5	T50.8X6
Phenomorphan	T40.2X1	T40.2X2	T40.2X3	T40.2X4	—	—
Phenonyl	T42.3X1	T42.3X2	T42.3X3	T42.3X4	T42.3X5	T42.3X6
Phenoperidine	T40.4X1	T40.4X2	T40.4X3	T40.4X4	—	—
Phenopyrazone	T46.991	T46.992	T46.993	T46.994	T46.995	T46.996
Phenoquin	T50.4X1	T50.4X2	T50.4X3	T50.4X4	T50.4X5	T50.4X6
Phenothiazine (psychotropic) NEC	T43.3X1	T43.3X2	T43.3X3	T43.3X4	T43.3X5	T43.3X6
insecticide	T60.2X1	T60.2X2	T60.2X3	T60.2X4	—	—
Phenothrin	T49.0X1	T49.0X2	T49.0X3	T49.0X4	T49.0X5	T49.0X6
Phenoxybenzamine	T46.7X1	T46.7X2	T46.7X3	T46.7X4	T46.7X5	T46.7X6
Phenoxyethanol	T49.0X1	T49.0X2	T49.0X3	T49.0X4	T49.0X5	T49.0X6
Phenoxymethyl penicillin	T36.0X1	T36.0X2	T36.0X3	T36.0X4	T36.0X5	T36.0X6
Phenprobamate	T42.8X1	T42.8X2	T42.8X3	T42.8X4	T42.8X5	T42.8X6
Phenprocoumon	T45.511	T45.512	T45.513	T45.514	T45.515	T45.516
Phensuximide	T42.2X1	T42.2X2	T42.2X3	T42.2X4	T42.2X5	T42.2X6
Phentermine	T50.5X1	T50.5X2	T50.5X3	T50.5X4	T50.5X5	T50.5X6
Phenthicillin	T36.0X1	T36.0X2	T36.0X3	T36.0X4	T36.0X5	T36.0X6
Phentolamine	T46.7X1	T46.7X2	T46.7X3	T46.7X4	T46.7X5	T46.7X6
Phenyl						
butazone	T39.2X1	T39.2X2	T39.2X3	T39.2X4	T39.2X5	T39.2X6
enediamine	T65.3X1	T65.3X2	T65.3X3	T65.3X4	—	—
hydrazine	T65.3X1	T65.3X2	T65.3X3	T65.3X4	—	—
antineoplastic	T45.1X1	T45.1X2	T45.1X3	T45.1X4	T45.1X5	T45.1X6
mercuric compounds — *see Mercury*						
salicylate	T49.3X1	T49.3X2	T49.3X3	T49.3X4	T49.3X5	T49.3X6
Phenylalanine mustard	T45.1X1	T45.1X2	T45.1X3	T45.1X4	T45.1X5	T45.1X6
Phenylbutazone	T39.2X1	T39.2X2	T39.2X3	T39.2X4	T39.2X5	T39.2X6
Phenylenediamine	T65.3X1	T65.3X2	T65.3X3	T65.3X4	—	—
Phenylephrine	T44.4X1	T44.4X2	T44.4X3	T44.4X4	T44.4X5	T44.4X6

Substance	External Cause (T-Code)					
	Poisoning, Accidental (Unintentional)	Poisoning, Intentional Self-Harm	Poisoning, Assault	Poisoning, Undetermined	Adverse Effect	Underdosing
Phenylethylbiguanide	T38.3X1	T38.3X2	T38.3X3	T38.3X4	T38.3X5	T38.3X6
Phenylmercuric						
acetate	T49.0X1	T49.0X2	T49.0X3	T49.0X4	T49.0X5	T49.0X6
borate	T49.0X1	T49.0X2	T49.0X3	T49.0X4	T49.0X5	T49.0X6
nitrate	T49.0X1	T49.0X2	T49.0X3	T49.0X4	T49.0X5	T49.0X6
Phenylmethylbarbitone	T42.3X1	T42.3X2	T42.3X3	T42.3X4	T42.3X5	T42.3X6
Phenylpropanol	T47.5X1	T47.5X2	T47.5X3	T47.5X4	T47.5X5	T47.5X6
Phenylpropanolamine	T44.991	T44.992	T44.993	T44.994	T44.995	T44.996
Phenylsulfthion	T60.0X1	T60.0X2	T60.0X3	T60.0X4	—	—
Phenyltoloxamine	T45.0X1	T45.0X2	T45.0X3	T45.0X4	T45.0X5	T45.0X6
Phenyramidol, phenyramidon	T39.8X1	T39.8X2	T39.8X3	T39.8X4	T39.8X5	T39.8X6
Phenytoin	T42.0X1	T42.0X2	T42.0X3	T42.0X4	T42.0X5	T42.0X6
with Phenobarbital	T42.3X1	T42.3X2	T42.3X3	T42.3X4	T42.3X5	T42.3X6
pHisoHex	T49.2X1	T49.2X2	T49.2X3	T49.2X4	T49.2X5	T49.2X6
Pholcodine	T48.3X1	T48.3X2	T48.3X3	T48.3X4	T48.3X5	T48.3X6
Pholedrine	T46.991	T46.992	T46.993	T46.994	T46.995	T46.996
Phorate	T60.0X1	T60.0X2	T60.0X3	T60.0X4	—	—
Phosdrin	T60.0X1	T60.0X2	T60.0X3	T60.0X4	—	—
Phosfolan	T60.0X1	T60.0X2	T60.0X3	T60.0X4	—	—
Phosgene (gas)	T59.891	T59.892	T59.893	T59.894	—	—
Phosphamidon	T60.0X1	T60.0X2	T60.0X3	T60.0X4	—	—
Phosphate	T65.891	T65.892	T65.893	T65.894	—	—
laxative	T47.4X1	T47.4X2	T47.4X3	T47.4X4	T47.4X5	T47.4X6
organic	T60.0X1	T60.0X2	T60.0X3	T60.0X4	—	—
solvent	T52.91	T52.92	T52.93	T52.94	—	—
tricresyl	T65.891	T65.892	T65.893	T65.894	—	—
Phosphine	T57.1X1	T57.1X2	T57.1X3	T57.1X4	—	—
fumigant	T57.1X1	T57.1X2	T57.1X3	T57.1X4	—	—
Phospholine	T49.5X1	T49.5X2	T49.5X3	T49.5X4	T49.5X5	T49.5X6
Phosphoric acid	T54.2X1	T54.2X2	T54.2X3	T54.2X4	—	—
Phosphorus (compound) NEC	T57.1X1	T57.1X2	T57.1X3	T57.1X4	—	—
pesticide	T60.0X1	T60.0X2	T60.0X3	T60.0X4	—	—
Phthalates	T65.891	T65.892	T65.893	T65.894	—	—
Phthalic anhydride	T65.891	T65.892	T65.893	T65.894	—	—
Phthalimidoglutarimide	T42.6X1	T42.6X2	T42.6X3	T42.6X4	T42.6X5	T42.6X6
Phthalylsulfathiazole	T37.0X1	T37.0X2	T37.0X3	T37.0X4	T37.0X5	T37.0X6
Phylloquinone	T45.7X1	T45.7X2	T45.7X3	T45.7X4	T45.7X5	T45.7X6
Physeptone	T40.3X1	T40.3X2	T40.3X3	T40.3X4	T40.3X5	T40.3X6
Physostigma venenosum	T62.2X1	T62.2X2	T62.2X3	T62.2X4	—	—
Physostigmine	T49.5X1	T49.5X2	T49.5X3	T49.5X4	T49.5X5	T49.5X6
Phytolacca decandra	T62.2X1	T62.2X2	T62.2X3	T62.2X4	—	—
berries	T62.1X1	T62.1X2	T62.1X3	T62.1X4	—	—

Substance	External Cause (T-Code)					
	Poisoning, Accidental (Unintentional)	Poisoning, Intentional Self-Harm	Poisoning, Assault	Poisoning, Undetermined	Adverse Effect	Underdosing
Phytomenadione	T45.7X1	T45.7X2	T45.7X3	T45.7X4	T45.7X5	T45.7X6
Phytonadione	T45.7X1	T45.7X2	T45.7X3	T45.7X4	T45.7X5	T45.7X6
Picoperine	T48.3X1	T48.3X2	T48.3X3	T48.3X4	T48.3X5	T48.3X6
Picosulfate (sodium)	T47.2X1	T47.2X2	T47.2X3	T47.2X4	T47.2X5	T47.2X6
Picric (acid)	T54.2X1	T54.2X2	T54.2X3	T54.2X4	—	—
Picrotoxin	T50.7X1	T50.7X2	T50.7X3	T50.7X4	T50.7X5	T50.7X6
Piketoprofen	T49.0X1	T49.0X2	T49.0X3	T49.0X4	T49.0X5	T49.0X6
Pilocarpine	T44.1X1	T44.1X2	T44.1X3	T44.1X4	T44.1X5	T44.1X6
Pilocarpus (jaborandi) extract	T44.1X1	T44.1X2	T44.1X3	T44.1X4	T44.1X5	T44.1X6
Pilsicainide (hydrochloride)	T46.2X1	T46.2X2	T46.2X3	T46.2X4	T46.2X5	T46.2X6
Pimaricin	T36.7X1	T36.7X2	T36.7X3	T36.7X4	T36.7X5	T36.7X6
Pimeclone	T50.7X1	T50.7X2	T50.7X3	T50.7X4	T50.7X5	T50.7X6
Pimelic ketone	T52.8X1	T52.8X2	T52.8X3	T52.8X4	—	—
Pimethixene	T45.0X1	T45.0X2	T45.0X3	T45.0X4	T45.0X5	T45.0X6
Piminodine	T40.2X1	T40.2X2	T40.2X3	T40.2X4	T40.2X5	T40.2X6
Pimozide	T43.591	T43.592	T43.593	T43.594	T43.595	T43.596
Pinacidil	T46.5X1	T46.5X2	T46.5X3	T46.5X4	T46.5X5	T46.5X6
Pinaverium bromide	T44.3X1	T44.3X2	T44.3X3	T44.3X4	T44.3X5	T44.3X6
Pinazepam	T42.4X1	T42.4X2	T42.4X3	T42.4X4	T42.4X5	T42.4X6
Pindolol	T44.7X1	T44.7X2	T44.7X3	T44.7X4	T44.7X5	T44.7X6
Pindone	T60.4X1	T60.4X2	T60.4X3	T60.4X4	—	—
Pine oil (disinfectant)	T65.891	T65.892	T65.893	T65.894	—	—
Pinkroot	T37.4X1	T37.4X2	T37.4X3	T37.4X4	T37.4X5	T37.4X6
Pipadone	T40.2X1	T40.2X2	T40.2X3	T40.2X4	—	—
Pipamazine	T45.0X1	T45.0X2	T45.0X3	T45.0X4	T45.0X5	T45.0X6
Pipamperone	T43.4X1	T43.4X2	T43.4X3	T43.4X4	T43.4X5	T43.4X6
Pipazetate	T48.3X1	T48.3X2	T48.3X3	T48.3X4	T48.3X5	T48.3X6
Pipemidic acid	T37.8X1	T37.8X2	T37.8X3	T37.8X4	T37.8X5	T37.8X6
Pipenzolate bromide	T44.3X1	T44.3X2	T44.3X3	T44.3X4	T44.3X5	T44.3X6
Piperacetazine	T43.3X1	T43.3X2	T43.3X3	T43.3X4	T43.3X5	T43.3X6
Piperacillin	T36.0X1	T36.0X2	T36.0X3	T36.0X4	T36.0X5	T36.0X6
Piperazine	T37.4X1	T37.4X2	T37.4X3	T37.4X4	T37.4X5	T37.4X6
estrone sulfate	T38.5X1	T38.5X2	T38.5X3	T38.5X4	T38.5X5	T38.5X6
Piper cubeba	T62.2X1	T62.2X2	T62.2X3	T62.2X4	—	—
Piperidione	T48.3X1	T48.3X2	T48.3X3	T48.3X4	—	—
Piperidolate	T44.3X1	T44.3X2	T44.3X3	T44.3X4	T44.3X5	T44.3X6
Piperocaine	T41.3X1	T41.3X2	T41.3X3	T41.3X4	T41.3X5	T41.3X6
infiltration (subcutaneous)	T41.3X1	T41.3X2	T41.3X3	T41.3X4	T41.3X5	T41.3X6
nerve block (peripheral) (plexus)	T41.3X1	T41.3X2	T41.3X3	T41.3X4	T41.3X5	T41.3X6
topical (surface)	T41.3X1	T41.3X2	T41.3X3	T41.3X4	T41.3X5	T41.3X6
Piperonyl butoxide	T60.8X1	T60.8X2	T60.8X3	T60.8X4	—	—
Pipethanate	T44.3X1	T44.3X2	T44.3X3	T44.3X4	T44.3X5	T44.3X6

Substance	External Cause (T-Code)					
	Poisoning, Accidental (Unintentional)	Poisoning, Intentional Self-Harm	Poisoning, Assault	Poisoning, Undetermined	Adverse Effect	Underdosing
Pipobroman	T45.1X1	T45.1X2	T45.1X3	T45.1X4	T45.1X5	T45.1X6
Pipofezine	T43.0X1	T43.0X2	T43.0X3	T43.0X4	T43.0X5	T43.0X6
Pipotiazine	T43.3X1	T43.3X2	T43.3X3	T43.3X4	T43.3X5	T43.3X6
Pipoxizine	T45.0X1	T45.0X2	T45.0X3	T45.0X4	T45.0X5	T45.0X6
Pipradrol	T43.691	T43.692	T43.693	T43.694	T43.695	T43.696
Piprinhydrinate	T45.0X1	T45.0X2	T45.0X3	T45.0X4	T45.0X5	T45.0X6
Pirarubicin	T45.1X1	T45.1X2	T45.1X3	T45.1X4	T45.1X5	T45.1X6
Pirazinamide	T37.1X1	T37.1X2	T37.1X3	T37.1X4	T37.1X5	T37.1X6
Pirbuterol	T48.6X1	T48.6X2	T48.6X3	T48.6X4	T48.6X5	T48.6X6
Pirenzepine	T47.1X1	T47.1X2	T47.1X3	T47.1X4	T47.1X5	T47.1X6
Piretanide	T50.1X1	T50.1X2	T50.1X3	T50.1X4	T50.1X5	T50.1X6
Piribedil	T42.8X1	T42.8X2	T42.8X3	T42.8X4	T42.8X5	T42.8X6
Piridoxilate	T46.3X1	T46.3X2	T46.3X3	T46.3X4	T46.3X5	T46.3X6
Piritramide	T40.4X1	T40.4X2	T40.4X3	T40.4X4	—	—
Pirlindole	T43.0X1	T43.0X2	T43.0X3	T43.0X4	T43.0X5	T43.0X6
Piromidic acid	T37.8X1	T37.8X2	T37.8X3	T37.8X4	T37.8X5	T37.8X6
Piroxicam	T39.391	T39.392	T39.393	T39.394	T39.395	T39.396
beta-cyclodextrin complex	T39.8X1	T39.8X2	T39.8X3	T39.8X4	T39.8X5	T39.8X6
Pirozadil	T46.6X1	T46.6X2	T46.6X3	T46.6X4	T46.6X5	T46.6X6
Piscidia (bark) (erythrina)	T39.8X1	T39.8X2	T39.8X3	T39.8X4	T39.8X5	T39.8X6
Pitch	T65.891	T65.892	T65.893	T65.894	—	—
Pitkin's solution	T41.3X1	T41.3X2	T41.3X3	T41.3X4	T41.3X5	T41.3X6
Pitocin	T48.0X1	T48.0X2	T48.0X3	T48.0X4	T48.0X5	T48.0X6
Pitressin (tannate)	T38.891	T38.892	T38.893	T38.894	T38.895	T38.896
Pituitary extracts (posterior)	T38.891	T38.892	T38.893	T38.894	T38.895	T38.896
anterior	T38.811	T38.812	T38.813	T38.814	T38.815	T38.816
Pituitrin	T38.891	T38.892	T38.893	T38.894	T38.895	T38.896
Pivampicillin	T36.0X1	T36.0X2	T36.0X3	T36.0X4	T36.0X5	T36.0X6
Pivmecillinam	T36.0X1	T36.0X2	T36.0X3	T36.0X4	T36.0X5	T36.0X6
Placental hormone	T38.891	T38.892	T38.893	T38.894	T38.895	T38.896
Placidyl	T42.6X1	T42.6X2	T42.6X3	T42.6X4	T42.6X5	T42.6X6
Plague vaccine	T50.A91	T50.A92	T50.A93	T50.A94	T50.A95	T50.A96
Plant						
food or fertilizer NEC	T65.891	T65.892	T65.893	T65.894	—	—
containing herbicide	T60.3X1	T60.3X2	T60.3X3	T60.3X4	—	—
noxious, used as food	T62.2X1	T62.2X2	T62.2X3	T62.2X4	—	—
berries	T62.1X1	T62.1X2	T62.1X3	T62.1X4	—	—
seeds	T62.2X1	T62.2X2	T62.2X3	T62.2X4	—	—
specified type NEC	T62.2X1	T62.2X2	T62.2X3	T62.2X4	—	—
Plasma	T45.8X1	T45.8X2	T45.8X3	T45.8X4	T45.8X5	T45.8X6
expander NEC	T45.8X1	T45.8X2	T45.8X3	T45.8X4	T45.8X5	T45.8X6
protein fraction (human)	T45.8X1	T45.8X2	T45.8X3	T45.8X4	T45.8X5	T45.8X6

Substance	External Cause (T-Code)					
	Poisoning, Accidental (Unintentional)	Poisoning, Intentional Self-Harm	Poisoning, Assault	Poisoning, Undetermined	Adverse Effect	Underdosing
Plasmanate	T45.8X1	T45.8X2	T45.8X3	T45.8X4	T45.8X5	T45.8X6
Plasminogen (tissue) activator	T45.611	T45.612	T45.613	T45.614	T45.615	T45.616
Plaster dressing	T49.3X1	T49.3X2	T49.3X3	T49.3X4	T49.3X5	T49.3X6
Plastic dressing	T49.3X1	T49.3X2	T49.3X3	T49.3X4	T49.3X5	T49.3X6
Plegicil	T43.3X1	T43.3X2	T43.3X3	T43.3X4	T43.3X5	T43.3X6
Plicamycin	T45.1X1	T45.1X2	T45.1X3	T45.1X4	T45.1X5	T45.1X6
Podophyllotoxin	T49.8X1	T49.8X2	T49.8X3	T49.8X4	T49.8X5	T49.8X6
Podophyllum (resin)	T49.4X1	T49.4X2	T49.4X3	T49.4X4	T49.4X5	T49.4X6
Poison NEC	T65.91	T65.92	T65.93	T65.94	—	—
Poisonous berries	T62.1X1	T62.1X2	T62.1X3	T62.1X4	—	—
Pokeweed (any part)	T62.2X1	T62.2X2	T62.2X3	T62.2X4	—	—
Poldine metilsulfate	T44.3X1	T44.3X2	T44.3X3	T44.3X4	T44.3X5	T44.3X6
Polidexide (sulfate)	T46.6X1	T46.6X2	T46.6X3	T46.6X4	T46.6X5	T46.6X6
Polidocanol	T46.8X1	T46.8X2	T46.8X3	T46.8X4	T46.8X5	T46.8X6
Poliomyelitis vaccine	T50.B91	T50.B92	T50.B93	T50.B94	T50.B95	T50.B96
Polish (car) (floor) (furniture) (metal) (porcelain) (silver)	T65.891	T65.892	T65.893	T65.894	—	—
abrasive	T65.891	T65.892	T65.893	T65.894	—	—
porcelain	T65.891	T65.892	T65.893	T65.894	—	—
Poloxalkol	T47.4X1	T47.4X2	T47.4X3	T47.4X4	T47.4X5	T47.4X6
Poloxamer	T47.4X1	T47.4X2	T47.4X3	T47.4X4	T47.4X5	T47.4X6
Polyaminostyrene resins	T50.3X1	T50.3X2	T50.3X3	T50.3X4	T50.3X5	T50.3X6
Polycarbophil	T47.4X1	T47.4X2	T47.4X3	T47.4X4	T47.4X5	T47.4X6
Polychlorinated biphenyl	T65.891	T65.892	T65.893	T65.894	—	—
Polycycline	T36.4X1	T36.4X2	T36.4X3	T36.4X4	T36.4X5	T36.4X6
Polyester fumes	T59.891	T59.892	T59.893	T59.894	—	—
Polyester resin hardener	T52.91	T52.92	T52.93	T52.94	—	—
fumes	T59.891	T59.892	T59.893	T59.894	—	—
Polyestradiol phosphate	T38.5X1	T38.5X2	T38.5X3	T38.5X4	T38.5X5	T38.5X6
Polyethanolamine alkyl sulfate	T49.2X1	T49.2X2	T49.2X3	T49.2X4	T49.2X5	T49.2X6
Polyethylene adhesive	T49.3X1	T49.3X2	T49.3X3	T49.3X4	T49.3X5	T49.3X6
Polyferose	T45.4X1	T45.4X2	T45.4X3	T45.4X4	T45.4X5	T45.4X6
Polygeline	T45.8X1	T45.8X2	T45.8X3	T45.8X4	T45.8X5	T45.8X6
Polymyxin	T36.8X1	T36.8X2	T36.8X3	T36.8X4	T36.8X5	T36.8X6
B	T36.8X1	T36.8X2	T36.8X3	T36.8X4	T36.8X5	T36.8X6
ENT agent	T49.6X1	T49.6X2	T49.6X3	T49.6X4	T49.6X5	T49.6X6
ophthalmic preparation	T49.5X1	T49.5X2	T49.5X3	T49.5X4	T49.5X5	T49.5X6
topical NEC	T49.0X1	T49.0X2	T49.0X3	T49.0X4	T49.0X5	T49.0X6
E sulfate (eye preparation)	T49.5X1	T49.5X2	T49.5X3	T49.5X4	T49.5X5	T49.5X6
Polynoxylin	T49.0X1	T49.0X2	T49.0X3	T49.0X4	T49.0X5	T49.0X6
Polyoestradiol phosphate	T38.5X1	T38.5X2	T38.5X3	T38.5X4	T38.5X5	T38.5X6
Polyoxymethyleneurea	T49.0X1	T49.0X2	T49.0X3	T49.0X4	T49.0X5	T49.0X6

Substance	External Cause (T-Code)					
	Poisoning, Accidental (Unintentional)	Poisoning, Intentional Self-Harm	Poisoning, Assault	Poisoning, Undetermined	Adverse Effect	Underdosing
Polysilane	T47.8X1	T47.8X2	T47.8X3	T47.8X4	T47.8X5	T47.8X6
Polytetrafluoroethylene (inhaled)	T59.891	T59.892	T59.893	T59.894	—	—
Polythiazide	T50.2X1	T50.2X2	T50.2X3	T50.2X4	T50.2X5	T50.2X6
Polyvidone	T45.8X1	T45.8X2	T45.8X3	T45.8X4	T45.8X5	T45.8X6
Polyvinylpyrrolidone	T45.8X1	T45.8X2	T45.8X3	T45.8X4	T45.8X5	T45.8X6
Pontocaine (hydrochloride) (infiltration) (topical)	T41.3X1	T41.3X2	T41.3X3	T41.3X4	T41.3X5	T41.3X6
nerve block (peripheral) (plexus)	T41.3X1	T41.3X2	T41.3X3	T41.3X4	T41.3X5	T41.3X6
spinal	T41.3X1	T41.3X2	T41.3X3	T41.3X4	T41.3X5	T41.3X6
Porfiromycin	T45.1X1	T45.1X2	T45.1X3	T45.1X4	T45.1X5	T45.1X6
Posterior pituitary hormone NEC	T38.891	T38.892	T38.893	T38.894	T38.895	T38.896
Pot	T40.7X1	T40.7X2	T40.7X3	T40.7X4	T40.7X5	T40.7X6
Potash (caustic)	T54.3X1	T54.3X2	T54.3X3	T54.3X4	—	—
Potassic saline injection (lactated)	T50.3X1	T50.3X2	T50.3X3	T50.3X4	T50.3X5	T50.3X6
Potassium (salts) NEC	T50.3X1	T50.3X2	T50.3X3	T50.3X4	T50.3X5	T50.3X6
aminobenzoate	T45.8X1	T45.8X2	T45.8X3	T45.8X4	T45.8X5	T45.8X6
aminosalicylate	T37.1X1	T37.1X2	T37.1X3	T37.1X4	T37.1X5	T37.1X6
antimony 'tartrate'	T37.8X1	T37.8X2	T37.8X3	T37.8X4	T37.8X5	T37.8X6
arsenite (solution)	T57.0X1	T57.0X2	T57.0X3	T57.0X4	—	—
bichromate	T56.2X1	T56.2X2	T56.2X3	T56.2X4	—	—
bisulfate	T47.3X1	T47.3X2	T47.3X3	T47.3X4	T47.3X5	T47.3X6
bromide	T42.6X1	T42.6X2	T42.6X3	T42.6X4	T42.6X5	T42.6X6
canrenoate	T50.0X1	T50.0X2	T50.0X3	T50.0X4	T50.0X5	T50.0X6
carbonate	T54.3X1	T54.3X2	T54.3X3	T54.3X4	—	—
chlorate NEC	T65.891	T65.892	T65.893	T65.894	—	—
chloride	T50.3X1	T50.3X2	T50.3X3	T50.3X4	T50.3X5	T50.3X6
citrate	T50.991	T50.992	T50.993	T50.994	T50.995	T50.996
cyanide	T65.0X1	T65.0X2	T65.0X3	T65.0X4	—	—
ferric hexacyanoferrate (medicinal)	T50.6X1	T50.6X2	T50.6X3	T50.6X4	T50.6X5	T50.6X6
nonmedicinal	T65.891	T65.892	T65.893	T65.894	—	—
Fluoride	T57.8X1	T57.8X2	T57.8X3	T57.8X4	—	—
glucaldrate	T47.1X1	T47.1X2	T47.1X3	T47.1X4	T47.1X5	T47.1X6
hydroxide	T54.3X1	T54.3X2	T54.3X3	T54.3X4	—	—
iodate	T49.0X1	T49.0X2	T49.0X3	T49.0X4	T49.0X5	T49.0X6
iodide	T48.4X1	T48.4X2	T48.4X3	T48.4X4	T48.4X5	T48.4X6
nitrate	T57.8X1	T57.8X2	T57.8X3	T57.8X4	—	—
oxalate	T65.891	T65.892	T65.893	T65.894	—	—
perchlorate (nonmedicinal) NEC	T65.891	T65.892	T65.893	T65.894	—	—
antithyroid	T38.2X1	T38.2X2	T38.2X3	T38.2X4	T38.2X5	T38.2X6
medicinal	T38.2X1	T38.2X2	T38.2X3	T38.2X4	T38.2X5	T38.2X6

Substance	External Cause (T-Code)					
	Poisoning, Accidental (Unintentional)	Poisoning, Intentional Self-Harm	Poisoning, Assault	Poisoning, Undetermined	Adverse Effect	Underdosing
Permanganate (nonmedicinal)	T65.891	T65.892	T65.893	T65.894	—	—
medicinal	T49.0X1	T49.0X2	T49.0X3	T49.0X4	T49.0X5	T49.0X6
sulfate	T47.2X1	T47.2X2	T47.2X3	T47.2X4	T47.2X5	T47.2X6
Potassium-removing resin	T50.3X1	T50.3X2	T50.3X3	T50.3X4	T50.3X5	T50.3X6
Potassium-retaining drug	T50.3X1	T50.3X2	T50.3X3	T50.3X4	T50.3X5	T50.3X6
Povidone	T45.8X1	T45.8X2	T45.8X3	T45.8X4	T45.8X5	T45.8X6
iodine	T49.0X1	T49.0X2	T49.0X3	T49.0X4	T49.0X5	T49.0X6
Practolol	T44.7X1	T44.7X2	T44.7X3	T44.7X4	T44.7X5	T44.7X6
Prajmalium bitartrate	T46.2X1	T46.2X2	T46.2X3	T46.2X4	T46.2X5	T46.2X6
Pralidoxime (iodide)	T50.6X1	T50.6X2	T50.6X3	T50.6X4	T50.6X5	T50.6X6
chloride	T50.6X1	T50.6X2	T50.6X3	T50.6X4	T50.6X5	T50.6X6
Pramiverine	T44.3X1	T44.3X2	T44.3X3	T44.3X4	T44.3X5	T44.3X6
Pramocaine	T49.1X1	T49.1X2	T49.1X3	T49.1X4	T49.1X5	T49.1X6
Pramoxine	T49.1X1	T49.1X2	T49.1X3	T49.1X4	T49.1X5	T49.1X6
Prasterone	T38.7X1	T38.7X2	T38.7X3	T38.7X4	T38.7X5	T38.7X6
Pravastatin	T46.6X1	T46.6X2	T46.6X3	T46.6X4	T46.6X5	T46.6X6
Prazepam	T42.4X1	T42.4X2	T42.4X3	T42.4X4	T42.4X5	T42.4X6
Praziquantel	T37.4X1	T37.4X2	T37.4X3	T37.4X4	T37.4X5	T37.4X6
Prazitone	T43.291	T43.292	T43.293	T43.294	T43.295	T43.296
Prazosin	T44.6X1	T44.6X2	T44.6X3	T44.6X4	T44.6X5	T44.6X6
Prednicarbate	T49.0X1	T49.0X2	T49.0X3	T49.0X4	T49.0X5	T49.0X6
Prednimustine	T45.1X1	T45.1X2	T45.1X3	T45.1X4	T45.1X5	T45.1X6
Prednisolone	T38.0X1	T38.0X2	T38.0X3	T38.0X4	T38.0X5	T38.0X6
ENT agent	T49.6X1	T49.6X2	T49.6X3	T49.6X4	T49.6X5	T49.6X6
ophthalmic preparation	T49.5X1	T49.5X2	T49.5X3	T49.5X4	T49.5X5	T49.5X6
steaglate	T49.0X1	T49.0X2	T49.0X3	T49.0X4	T49.0X5	T49.0X6
topical NEC	T49.0X1	T49.0X2	T49.0X3	T49.0X4	T49.0X5	T49.0X6
Prednisone	T38.0X1	T38.0X2	T38.0X3	T38.0X4	T38.0X5	T38.0X6
Prednylidene	T38.0X1	T38.0X2	T38.0X3	T38.0X4	T38.0X5	T38.0X6
Pregnandiol	T38.5X1	T38.5X2	T38.5X3	T38.5X4	T38.5X5	T38.5X6
Pregneninolone	T38.5X1	T38.5X2	T38.5X3	T38.5X4	T38.5X5	T38.5X6
Preludin	T43.691	T43.692	T43.693	T43.694	T43.695	T43.696
Premarin	T38.5X1	T38.5X2	T38.5X3	T38.5X4	T38.5X5	T38.5X6
Premedication anesthetic	T41.201	T41.202	T41.203	T41.204	T41.205	T41.206
Prenalterol	T44.5X1	T44.5X2	T44.5X3	T44.5X4	T44.5X5	T44.5X6
Prenoxdiazine	T48.3X1	T48.3X2	T48.3X3	T48.3X4	T48.3X5	T48.3X6
Prenylamine	T46.3X1	T46.3X2	T46.3X3	T46.3X4	T46.3X5	T46.3X6
Preparation, local	T49.4X1	T49.4X2	T49.4X3	T49.4X4	T49.4X5	T49.4X6
Preparation H	T49.8X1	T49.8X2	T49.8X3	T49.8X4	T49.8X5	T49.8X6
Preservative (nonmedicinal)	T65.891	T65.892	T65.893	T65.894	—	—
medicinal	T50.901	T50.902	T50.903	T50.904	T50.905	T50.906
wood	T60.91	T60.92	T60.93	T60.94	—	—

Substance	External Cause (T-Code)					
	Poisoning, Accidental (Unintentional)	Poisoning, Intentional Self-Harm	Poisoning, Assault	Poisoning, Undetermined	Adverse Effect	Underdosing
Prethcamide	T50.7X1	T50.7X2	T50.7X3	T50.7X4	T50.7X5	T50.7X6
Pride of China	T62.2X1	T62.2X2	T62.2X3	T62.2X4	—	—
Pridinol	T44.3X1	T44.3X2	T44.3X3	T44.3X4	T44.3X5	T44.3X6
Prifinium bromide	T44.3X1	T44.3X2	T44.3X3	T44.3X4	T44.3X5	T44.3X6
Prilocaine	T41.3X1	T41.3X2	T41.3X3	T41.3X4	T41.3X5	T41.3X6
infiltration (subcutaneous)	T41.3X1	T41.3X2	T41.3X3	T41.3X4	T41.3X5	T41.3X6
nerve block (peripheral) (plexus)	T41.3X1	T41.3X2	T41.3X3	T41.3X4	T41.3X5	T41.3X6
regional	T41.3X1	T41.3X2	T41.3X3	T41.3X4	T41.3X5	T41.3X6
Primaquine	T37.2X1	T37.2X2	T37.2X3	T37.2X4	T37.2X5	T37.2X6
Primidone	T42.6X1	T42.6X2	T42.6X3	T42.6X4	T42.6X5	T42.6X6
Primula (veris)	T62.2X1	T62.2X2	T62.2X3	T62.2X4	—	—
Prinadol	T40.2X1	T40.2X2	T40.2X3	T40.2X4	T40.2X5	T40.2X6
Priscol, Priscoline	T44.6X1	T44.6X2	T44.6X3	T44.6X4	T44.6X5	T44.6X6
Pristinamycin	T36.3X1	T36.3X2	T36.3X3	T36.3X4	T36.3X5	T36.3X6
Privet	T62.2X1	T62.2X2	T62.2X3	T62.2X4	—	—
berries	T62.1X1	T62.1X2	T62.1X3	T62.1X4	—	—
Privine	T44.4X1	T44.4X2	T44.4X3	T44.4X4	T44.4X5	T44.4X6
Pro-Banthine	T44.3X1	T44.3X2	T44.3X3	T44.3X4	T44.3X5	T44.3X6
Probarbital	T42.3X1	T42.3X2	T42.3X3	T42.3X4	T42.3X5	T42.3X6
Probenecid	T50.4X1	T50.4X2	T50.4X3	T50.4X4	T50.4X5	T50.4X6
Probucol	T46.6X1	T46.6X2	T46.6X3	T46.6X4	T46.6X5	T46.6X6
Procainamide	T46.2X1	T46.2X2	T46.2X3	T46.2X4	T46.2X5	T46.2X6
Procaine	T41.3X1	T41.3X2	T41.3X3	T41.3X4	T41.3X5	T41.3X6
benzylpenicillin	T36.0X1	T36.0X2	T36.0X3	T36.0X4	T36.0X5	T36.0X6
nerve block (periphreal) (plexus)	T41.3X1	T41.3X2	T41.3X3	T41.3X4	T41.3X5	T41.3X6
penicillin G	T36.0X1	T36.0X2	T36.0X3	T36.0X4	T36.0X5	T36.0X6
regional	T41.3X1	T41.3X2	T41.3X3	T41.3X4	T41.3X5	T41.3X6
spinal	T41.3X1	T41.3X2	T41.3X3	T41.3X4	T41.3X5	T41.3X6
Procalmidol	T43.591	T43.592	T43.593	T43.594	T43.595	T43.596
Procarbazine	T45.1X1	T45.1X2	T45.1X3	T45.1X4	T45.1X5	T45.1X6
Procaterol	T44.5X1	T44.5X2	T44.5X3	T44.5X4	T44.5X5	T44.5X6
Prochlorperazine	T43.3X1	T43.3X2	T43.3X3	T43.3X4	T43.3X5	T43.3X6
Procyclidine	T44.3X1	T44.3X2	T44.3X3	T44.3X4	T44.3X5	T44.3X6
Producer gas	T58.8X1	T58.8X2	T58.8X3	T58.8X4	—	—
Profadol	T40.4X1	T40.4X2	T40.4X3	T40.4X4	T40.4X5	T40.4X6
Profenamine	T44.3X1	T44.3X2	T44.3X3	T44.3X4	T44.3X5	T44.3X6
Profenil	T44.3X1	T44.3X2	T44.3X3	T44.3X4	T44.3X5	T44.3X6
Proflavine	T49.0X1	T49.0X2	T49.0X3	T49.0X4	T49.0X5	T49.0X6
Progabide	T42.6X1	T42.6X2	T42.6X3	T42.6X4	T42.6X5	T42.6X6
Progestin	T38.5X1	T38.5X2	T38.5X3	T38.5X4	T38.5X5	T38.5X6
oral contraceptive	T38.4X1	T38.4X2	T38.4X3	T38.4X4	T38.4X5	T38.4X6

◀ New ⇐ Revised ~~deleted~~ Deleted

Substance	External Cause (T-Code)					
	Poisoning, Accidental (Unintentional)	Poisoning, Intentional Self-Harm	Poisoning, Assault	Poisoning, Undetermined	Adverse Effect	Underdosing
Progesterone	T38.5X1	T38.5X2	T38.5X3	T38.5X4	T38.5X5	T38.5X6
Progestogen NEC	T38.5X1	T38.5X2	T38.5X3	T38.5X4	T38.5X5	T38.5X6
Progestone	T38.5X1	T38.5X2	T38.5X3	T38.5X4	T38.5X5	T38.5X6
Proglumide	T47.1X1	T47.1X2	T47.1X3	T47.1X4	T47.1X5	T47.1X6
Proguanil	T37.2X1	T37.2X2	T37.2X3	T37.2X4	T37.2X5	T37.2X6
Prolactin	T38.811	T38.812	T38.813	T38.814	T38.815	T38.816
Prolintane	T43.691	T43.692	T43.693	T43.694	T43.695	T43.696
Proloid	T38.1X1	T38.1X2	T38.1X3	T38.1X4	T38.1X5	T38.1X6
Proluton	T38.5X1	T38.5X2	T38.5X3	T38.5X4	T38.5X5	T38.5X6
Promacetin	T37.1X1	T37.1X2	T37.1X3	T37.1X4	T37.1X5	T37.1X6
Promazine	T43.3X1	T43.3X2	T43.3X3	T43.3X4	T43.3X5	T43.3X6
Promedol	T40.2X1	T40.2X2	T40.2X3	T40.2X4	—	—
Promegestone	T38.5X1	T38.5X2	T38.5X3	T38.5X4	T38.5X5	T38.5X6
Promethazine (teoclate)	T43.3X1	T43.3X2	T43.3X3	T43.3X4	T43.3X5	T43.3X6
Promin	T37.1X1	T37.1X2	T37.1X3	T37.1X4	T37.1X5	T37.1X6
Pronase	T45.3X1	T45.3X2	T45.3X3	T45.3X4	T45.3X5	T45.3X6
Pronestyl (hydrochloride)	T46.2X1	T46.2X2	T46.2X3	T46.2X4	T46.2X5	T46.2X6
Pronetalol	T44.7X1	T44.7X2	T44.7X3	T44.7X4	T44.7X5	T44.7X6
Prontosil	T37.0X1	T37.0X2	T37.0X3	T37.0X4	T37.0X5	T37.0X6
Propachlor	T60.3X1	T60.3X2	T60.3X3	T60.3X4	—	—
Propafenone	T46.2X1	T46.2X2	T46.2X3	T46.2X4	T46.2X5	T46.2X6
Propallylonal	T42.3X1	T42.3X2	T42.3X3	T42.3X4	T42.3X5	T42.3X6
Propamidine	T49.0X1	T49.0X2	T49.0X3	T49.0X4	T49.0X5	T49.0X6
Propane (distributed in mobile container)	T59.891	T59.892	T59.893	T59.894	—	—
distributed through pipes	T59.891	T59.892	T59.893	T59.894	—	—
incomplete combustion	T57.11	T57.12	T57.13	T57.14	—	—
Propanidid	T41.291	T41.292	T41.293	T41.294	T41.295	T41.296
Propanil	T60.3X1	T60.3X2	T60.3X3	T60.3X4	—	—
1-Propanol	T51.3X1	T51.3X2	T51.3X3	T51.3X4	—	—
2-Propanol	T51.2X1	T51.2X2	T51.2X3	T51.2X4	—	—
Propantheline	T44.3X1	T44.3X2	T44.3X3	T44.3X4	T44.3X5	T44.3X6
bromide	T44.3X1	T44.3X2	T44.3X3	T44.3X4	T44.3X5	T44.3X6
Proparacaine	T41.3X1	T41.3X2	T41.3X3	T41.3X4	T41.3X5	T41.3X6
Propatylnitrate	T46.3X1	T46.3X2	T46.3X3	T46.3X4	T46.3X5	T46.3X6
Propicillin	T36.0X1	T36.0X2	T36.0X3	T36.0X4	T36.0X5	T36.0X6
Propiolactone	T49.0X1	T49.0X2	T49.0X3	T49.0X4	T49.0X5	T49.0X6
Propiomazine	T45.0X1	T45.0X2	T45.0X3	T45.0X4	T45.0X5	T45.0X6
~~Propionaldehyde (medicinal)~~	~~T42.6X1~~	~~T42.6X2~~	~~T42.6X3~~	~~T42.6X4~~	~~T42.6X5~~	~~T42.6X6~~
Propionaldehyde (medicinal)	T42.6X1	T42.6X2	T42.6X3	T42.6X4	T42.6X5	T42.6X6 ◀
Propionate (calcium) (sodium)	T49.0X1	T49.0X2	T49.0X3	T49.0X4	T49.0X5	T49.0X6
Propion gel	T49.0X1	T49.0X2	T49.0X3	T49.0X4	T49.0X5	T49.0X6

Substance	External Cause (T-Code)					
	Poisoning, Accidental (Unintentional)	Poisoning, Intentional Self-Harm	Poisoning, Assault	Poisoning, Undetermined	Adverse Effect	Underdosing
Propitocaine	T41.3X1	T41.3X2	T41.3X3	T41.3X4	T41.3X5	T41.3X6
infiltration (subcutaneous)	T41.3X1	T41.3X2	T41.3X3	T41.3X4	T41.3X5	T41.3X6
nerve block (peripheral) (plexus)	T41.3X1	T41.3X2	T41.3X3	T41.3X4	T41.3X5	T41.3X6
Propofol	T41.291	T41.292	T41.293	T41.294	T41.295	T41.296
Propoxur	T60.0X1	T60.0X2	T60.0X3	T60.0X4	—	—
Propoxycaine	T41.3X1	T41.3X2	T41.3X3	T41.3X4	T41.3X5	T41.3X6
infiltration (subcutaneous)	T41.3X1	T41.3X2	T41.3X3	T41.3X4	T41.3X5	T41.3X6
nerve block (peripheral) (plexus)	T41.3X1	T41.3X2	T41.3X3	T41.3X4	T41.3X5	T41.3X6
topical (surface)	T41.3X1	T41.3X2	T41.3X3	T41.3X4	T41.3X5	T41.3X6
Propoxyphene	T40.4X1	T40.4X2	T40.4X3	T40.4X4	T40.4X5	T40.4X6
Propranolol	T44.7X1	T44.7X2	T44.7X3	T44.7X4	T44.7X5	T44.7X6
Propyl						
alcohol	T51.3X1	T51.3X2	T51.3X3	T51.3X4	—	—
carbinol	T51.3X1	T51.3X2	T51.3X3	T51.3X4	—	—
hexadrine	T44.4X1	T44.4X2	T44.4X3	T44.4X4	T44.4X5	T44.4X6
iodone	T50.8X1	T50.8X2	T50.8X3	T50.8X4	T50.8X5	T50.8X6
thiouracil	T38.2X1	T38.2X2	T38.2X3	T38.2X4	T38.2X5	T38.2X6
Propylaminophenothiazine	T43.3X1	T43.3X2	T43.3X3	T43.3X4	T43.3X5	T43.3X6
Propylene	T59.891	T59.892	T59.893	T59.894	—	—
Propylhexedrine	T48.5X1	T48.5X2	T48.5X3	T48.5X4	T48.5X5	T48.5X6
Propyliodone	T50.8X1	T50.8X2	T50.8X3	T50.8X4	T50.8X5	T50.8X6
Propylthiouracil	T38.2X1	T38.2X2	T38.2X3	T38.2X4	T38.2X5	T38.2X6
Propylparaben (ophthalmic)	T49.5X1	T49.5X2	T49.5X3	T49.5X4	T49.5X5	T49.5X6
Propyphenazone	T39.2X1	T39.2X2	T39.2X3	T39.2X4	T39.2X5	T39.2X6
Proquazone	T39.391	T39.392	T39.393	T39.394	T39.395	T39.396
Proscillaridin	T46.0X1	T46.0X2	T46.0X3	T46.0X4	T46.0X5	T46.0X6
Prostacyclin	T45.521	T45.522	T45.523	T45.524	T45.525	T45.526
Prostaglandin (I2)	T45.521	T45.522	T45.523	T45.524	T45.525	T45.526
E1	T46.7X1	T46.7X2	T46.7X3	T46.7X4	T46.7X5	T46.7X6
E2	T48.0X1	T48.0X2	T48.0X3	T48.0X4	T48.0X5	T48.0X6
F2 alpha	T48.0X1	T48.0X2	T48.0X3	T48.0X4	T48.0X5	T48.0X6
Prostigmin	T44.0X1	T44.0X2	T44.0X3	T44.0X4	T44.0X5	T44.0X6
Prosultiamine	T45.2X1	T45.2X2	T45.2X3	T45.2X4	T45.2X5	T45.2X6
Protamine sulfate	T45.7X1	T45.7X2	T45.7X3	T45.7X4	T45.7X5	T45.7X6
zinc insulin	T38.3X1	T38.3X2	T38.3X3	T38.3X4	T38.3X5	T38.3X6
Protease	T47.5X1	T47.5X2	T47.5X3	T47.5X4	T47.5X5	T47.5X6
Protectant, skin NEC	T49.3X1	T49.3X2	T49.3X3	T49.3X4	T49.3X5	T49.3X6
Protein hydrolysate	T50.991	T50.992	T50.993	T50.994	T50.995	T50.996
Prothiaden — *see Dothiepin hydrochloride*						
Prothionamide	T37.1X1	T37.1X2	T37.1X3	T37.1X4	T37.1X5	T37.1X6

◀ New ⇐ Revised ~~deleted~~ Deleted

Substance	External Cause (T-Code)					
	Poisoning, Accidental (Unintentional)	Poisoning, Intentional Self-Harm	Poisoning, Assault	Poisoning, Undetermined	Adverse Effect	Underdosing
Prothipendyl	T43.591	T43.592	T43.593	T43.594	T43.595	T43.596
Prothoate	T60.0X1	T60.0X2	T60.0X3	T60.0X4	—	—
Prothrombin						
activator	T45.7X1	T45.7X2	T45.7X3	T45.7X4	T45.7X5	T45.7X6
synthesis inhibitor	T45.511	T45.512	T45.513	T45.514	T45.515	T45.516
Protionamide	T37.1X1	T37.1X2	T37.1X3	T37.1X4	T37.1X5	T37.1X6
Protirelin	T38.891	T38.892	T38.893	T38.894	T38.895	T38.896
Protokylol	T48.6X1	T48.6X2	T48.6X3	T48.6X4	T48.6X5	T48.6X6
Protopam	T50.6X1	T50.6X2	T50.6X3	T50.6X4	T50.6X5	T50.6X6
Protoveratrine(s) (A) (B)	T46.5X1	T46.5X2	T46.5X3	T46.5X4	T46.5X5	T46.5X6
Protriptyline	T43.011	T43.012	T43.013	T43.014	T43.015	T43.016
Provera	T38.5X1	T38.5X2	T38.5X3	T38.5X4	T38.5X5	T38.5X6
Provitamin A	T45.2X1	T45.2X2	T45.2X3	T45.2X4	T45.2X5	T45.2X6
Proxibarbal	T42.3X1	T42.3X2	T42.3X3	T42.3X4	T42.3X5	T42.3X6
Proxymetacaine	T41.3X1	T41.3X2	T41.3X3	T41.3X4	T41.3X5	T41.3X6
Proxyphylline	T48.6X1	T48.6X2	T48.6X3	T48.6X4	T48.6X5	T48.6X6
Prozac — *see Fluoxetine hydrochloride*						
Prunus						
laurocerasus	T62.2X1	T62.2X2	T62.2X3	T62.2X4	—	—
virginiana	T62.2X1	T62.2X2	T62.2X3	T62.2X4	—	—
Prussian blue						
commercial	T65.891	T65.892	T65.893	T65.894	—	—
therapeutic	T50.6X1	T50.6X2	T50.6X3	T50.6X4	T50.6X5	T50.6X6
Prussic acid	T65.0X1	T65.0X2	T65.0X3	T65.0X4	—	—
vapor	T57.3X1	T57.3X2	T57.3X3	T57.3X4	—	—
Pseudoephedrine	T44.991	T44.992	T44.993	T44.994	T44.995	T44.996
Psilocin	T40.991	T40.992	T40.993	T40.994	—	—
Psilocybin	T40.991	T40.992	T40.993	T40.994	—	—
Psilocybine	T40.991	T40.992	T40.993	T40.994	—	—
Psoralene (nonmedicinal)	T65.891	T65.892	T65.893	T65.894	—	—
Psoralens (medicinal)	T50.991	T50.992	T50.993	T50.994	T50.995	T50.996
PSP (phenolsulfonphthalein)	T50.8X1	T50.8X2	T50.8X3	T50.8X4	T50.8X5	T50.8X6
Psychodysleptic drug NEC	T40.901	T40.902	T40.903	T40.904	T40.905	T40.906
Psychostimulant	T43.601	T43.602	T43.603	T43.604	T43.605	T43.606
amphetamine	T43.621	T43.622	T43.623	T43.624	T43.625	T43.626
caffeine	T43.611	T43.612	T43.613	T43.614	T43.615	T43.616
methylphenidate	T43.631	T43.632	T43.633	T43.634	T43.635	T43.636
specified NEC	T43.691	T43.692	T43.693	T43.694	T43.695	T43.696
Psychotherapeutic drug NEC	T43.91	T43.92	T43.93	T43.94	T43.95	T43.96
antidepressants — *see also Antidepressant*	T43.201	T43.202	T43.203	T43.204	T43.205	T43.206

Substance	External Cause (T-Code)					
	Poisoning, Accidental (Unintentional)	Poisoning, Intentional Self-Harm	Poisoning, Assault	Poisoning, Undetermined	Adverse Effect	Underdosing
Psychotherapeutic drug NEC *(Continued)*						
specified NEC	T43.8X1	T43.8X2	T43.8X3	T43.8X4	T43.8X5	T43.8X6
tranquilizers NEC	T43.501	T43.502	T43.503	T43.504	T43.505	T43.506
Psychotomimetic agents	T40.901	T40.902	T40.903	T40.904	T40.905	T40.906
Psychotropic drug NEC	T43.91	T43.92	T43.93	T43.94	T43.95	T43.96
specified NEC	T43.8X1	T43.8X2	T43.8X3	T43.8X4	T43.8X5	T43.8X6
Psyllium hydrophilic mucilloid	T47.4X1	T47.4X2	T47.4X3	T47.4X4	T47.4X5	T47.4X6
Pteroylglutamic acid	T45.8X1	T45.8X2	T45.8X3	T45.8X4	T45.8X5	T45.8X6
Pteroyltriglutamate	T45.1X1	T45.1X2	T45.1X3	T45.1X4	T45.1X5	T45.1X6
PTFE — *see Polytetrafluoroethylene*						
Pulp						
devitalizing paste	T49.7X1	T49.7X2	T49.7X3	T49.7X4	T49.7X5	T49.7X6
dressing	T49.7X1	T49.7X2	T49.7X3	T49.7X4	T49.7X5	T49.7X6
Pulsatilla	T62.2X1	T62.2X2	T62.2X3	T62.2X4	—	—
Pumpkin seed extract	T37.4X1	T37.4X2	T37.4X3	T37.4X4	T37.4X5	T37.4X6
Purex (bleach)	T54.91	T54.92	T54.93	T54.94	—	—
Purgative NEC — *see also Cathartic*	T47.4X1	T47.4X2	T47.4X3	T47.4X4	T47.4X5	T47.4X6
Purine analogue (antineoplastic)	T45.1X1	T45.1X2	T45.1X3	T45.1X4	T45.1X5	T45.1X6
Purine diuretics	T50.2X1	T50.2X2	T50.2X3	T50.2X4	T50.2X5	T50.2X6
Purinethol	T45.1X1	T45.1X2	T45.1X3	T45.1X4	T45.1X5	T45.1X6
PVP	T45.8X1	T45.8X2	T45.8X3	T45.8X4	T45.8X5	T45.8X6
Pyrabital	T39.8X1	T39.8X2	T39.8X3	T39.8X4	T39.8X5	T39.8X6
Pyramidon	T39.2X1	T39.2X2	T39.2X3	T39.2X4	T39.2X5	T39.2X6
Pyrantel	T37.4X1	T37.4X2	T37.4X3	T37.4X4	T37.4X5	T37.4X6
Pyrathiazine	T45.0X1	T45.0X2	T45.0X3	T45.0X4	T45.0X5	T45.0X6
Pyrazinamide	T37.1X1	T37.1X2	T37.1X3	T37.1X4	T37.1X5	T37.1X6
Pyrazinoic acid (amide)	T37.1X1	T37.1X2	T37.1X3	T37.1X4	T37.1X5	T37.1X6
Pyrazole (derivatives)	T39.2X1	T39.2X2	T39.2X3	T39.2X4	T39.2X5	T39.2X6
Pyrazolone analgesic NEC	T39.2X1	T39.2X2	T39.2X3	T39.2X4	T39.2X5	T39.2X6
Pyrethrin, pyrethrum (nonmedicinal)	T60.2X1	T60.2X2	T60.2X3	T60.2X4	—	—
Pyrethrum extract	T49.0X1	T49.0X2	T49.0X3	T49.0X4	T49.0X5	T49.0X6
Pyribenzamine	T45.0X1	T45.0X2	T45.0X3	T45.0X4	T45.0X5	T45.0X6
Pyridine	T52.8X1	T52.8X2	T52.8X3	T52.8X4	—	—
aldoxime methiodide	T50.6X1	T50.6X2	T50.6X3	T50.6X4	T50.6X5	T50.6X6
aldoxime methyl chloride	T50.6X1	T50.6X2	T50.6X3	T50.6X4	T50.6X5	T50.6X6
vapor	T59.891	T59.892	T59.893	T59.894	—	—
Pyridium	T39.8X1	T39.8X2	T39.8X3	T39.8X4	T39.8X5	T39.8X6
Pyridostigmine bromide	T44.0X1	T44.0X2	T44.0X3	T44.0X4	T44.0X5	T44.0X6
Pyridoxal phosphate	T45.2X1	T45.2X2	T45.2X3	T45.2X4	T45.2X5	T45.2X6

Substance	Poisoning, Accidental (Unintentional)	Poisoning, Intentional Self-Harm	Poisoning, Assault	Poisoning, Undetermined	Adverse Effect	Underdosing
	External Cause (T-Code)					
Pyridoxine	T45.2X1	T45.2X2	T45.2X3	T45.2X4	T45.2X5	T45.2X6
Pyrilamine	T45.0X1	T45.0X2	T45.0X3	T45.0X4	T45.0X5	T45.0X6
Pyrimethamine	T37.2X1	T37.2X2	T37.2X3	T37.2X4	T37.2X5	T37.2X6
with sulfadoxine	T37.2X1	T37.2X2	T37.2X3	T37.2X4	T37.2X5	T37.2X6
Pyrimidine antagonist	T45.1X1	T45.1X2	T45.1X3	T45.1X4	T45.1X5	T45.1X6
Pyriminil	T60.4X1	T60.4X2	T60.4X3	T60.4X4	—	—
Pyrithione zinc	T49.4X1	T49.4X2	T49.4X3	T49.4X4	T49.4X5	T49.4X6
Pyrithyldione	T42.6X1	T42.6X2	T42.6X3	T42.6X4	T42.6X5	T42.6X6
Pyrogallic acid	T49.0X1	T49.0X2	T49.0X3	T49.0X4	T49.0X5	T49.0X6
Pyrogallol	T49.0X1	T49.0X2	T49.0X3	T49.0X4	T49.0X5	T49.0X6
Pyroxylin	T49.3X1	T49.3X2	T49.3X3	T49.3X4	T49.3X5	T49.3X6
Pyrrobutamine	T45.0X1	T45.0X2	T45.0X3	T45.0X4	T45.0X5	T45.0X6
Pyrrolizidine alkaloids	T62.8X1	T62.8X2	T62.8X3	T62.8X4	—	—
Pyrvinium chloride	T37.4X1	T37.4X2	T37.4X3	T37.4X4	T37.4X5	T37.4X6
PZI	T38.3X1	T38.3X2	T38.3X3	T38.3X4	T38.3X5	T38.3X6
Q						
Quaalude	T42.6X1	T42.6X2	T42.6X3	T42.6X4	T42.6X5	T42.6X6
Quarternary ammonium						
anti-infective	T49.0X1	T49.0X2	T49.0X3	T49.0X4	T49.0X5	T49.0X6
ganglion blocking	T44.2X1	T44.2X2	T44.2X3	T44.2X4	T44.2X5	T44.2X6
parasympatholytic	T44.3X1	T44.3X2	T44.3X3	T44.3X4	T44.3X5	T44.3X6
Quazepam	T42.4X1	T42.4X2	T42.4X3	T42.4X4	T42.4X5	T42.4X6
Quicklime	T54.3X1	T54.3X2	T54.3X3	T54.3X4	—	—
Quillaja extract	T48.4X1	T48.4X2	T48.4X3	T48.4X4	T48.4X5	T48.4X6
Quinacrine	T37.2X1	T37.2X2	T37.2X3	T37.2X4	T37.2X5	T37.2X6
Quinaglute	T46.2X1	T46.2X2	T46.2X3	T46.2X4	T46.2X5	T46.2X6
Quinalbarbital	T42.3X1	T42.3X2	T42.3X3	T42.3X4	T42.3X5	T42.3X6
Quinalbarbitone sodium	T42.3X1	T42.3X2	T42.3X3	T42.3X4	T42.3X5	T42.3X6
Quinalphos	T60.0X1	T60.0X2	T60.0X3	T60.0X4	—	—
Quinapril	T46.4X1	T46.4X2	T46.4X3	T46.4X4	T46.4X5	T46.4X6
Quinestradiol	T38.5X1	T38.5X2	T38.5X3	T38.5X4	T38.5X5	T38.5X6
Quinestradol	T38.5X1	T38.5X2	T38.5X3	T38.5X4	T38.5X5	T38.5X6
Quinestrol	T38.5X1	T38.5X2	T38.5X3	T38.5X4	T38.5X5	T38.5X6
Quinethazone	T50.2X1	T50.2X2	T50.2X3	T50.2X4	T50.2X5	T50.2X6
Quingestanol	T38.4X1	T38.4X2	T38.4X3	T38.4X4	T38.4X5	T38.4X6
Quinidine	T46.2X1	T46.2X2	T46.2X3	T46.2X4	T46.2X5	T46.2X6
Quinine	T37.2X1	T37.2X2	T37.2X3	T37.2X4	T37.2X5	T37.2X6
Quiniobine	T37.8X1	T37.8X2	T37.8X3	T37.8X4	T37.8X5	T37.8X6
Quinisocaine	T49.1X1	T49.1X2	T49.1X3	T49.1X4	T49.1X5	T49.1X6
Quinocide	T37.2X1	T37.2X2	T37.2X3	T37.2X4	T37.2X5	T37.2X6
Quinoline (derivatives) NEC	T37.8X1	T37.8X2	T37.8X3	T37.8X4	T37.8X5	T37.8X6

Substance	Poisoning, Accidental (Unintentional)	Poisoning, Intentional Self-Harm	Poisoning, Assault	Poisoning, Undetermined	Adverse Effect	Underdosing
	External Cause (T-Code)					
Quinupramine	T43.011	T43.012	T43.013	T43.014	T43.015	T43.016
Quotane	T41.3X1	T41.3X2	T41.3X3	T41.3X4	T41.3X5	T41.3X6
R						
Rabies						
immune globulin (human)	T50.Z11	T50.Z12	T50.Z13	T50.Z14	T50.Z15	T50.Z16
vaccine	T50.B91	T50.B92	T50.B93	T50.B94	T50.B95	T50.B96
Racemoramide	T40.2X1	T40.2X2	T40.2X3	T40.2X4	—	—
Racemorphan	T40.2X1	T40.2X2	T40.2X3	T40.2X4	T40.2X5	T40.2X6
Racepinefrin	T44.5X1	T44.5X2	T44.5X3	T44.5X4	T44.5X5	T44.5X6
Raclopride	T43.591	T43.592	T43.593	T43.594	T43.595	T43.596
Radiator alcohol	T51.1X1	T51.1X2	T51.1X3	T51.1X4	—	—
Radioactive drug NEC	T50.8X1	T50.8X2	T50.8X3	T50.8X4	T50.8X5	T50.8X6
Radio-opaque (drugs) (materials)	T50.8X1	T50.8X2	T50.8X3	T50.8X4	T50.8X5	T50.8X6
Ramifenazone	T39.2X1	T39.2X2	T39.2X3	T39.2X4	T39.2X5	T39.2X6
Ramipril	T46.4X1	T46.4X2	T46.4X3	T46.4X4	T46.4X5	T46.4X6
Ranitidine	T47.0X1	T47.0X2	T47.0X3	T47.0X4	T47.0X5	T47.0X6
Ranunculus	T62.2X1	T62.2X2	T62.2X3	T62.2X4	—	—
Rat poison NEC	T60.4X1	T60.4X2	T60.4X3	T60.4X4	—	—
Rattlesnake (venom)	T63.011	T63.012	T63.013	T63.014	—	—
Raubasine	T46.7X1	T46.7X2	T46.7X3	T46.7X4	T46.7X5	T46.7X6
Raudixin	T46.5X1	T46.5X2	T46.5X3	T46.5X4	T46.5X5	T46.5X6
Rautensin	T46.5X1	T46.5X2	T46.5X3	T46.5X4	T46.5X5	T46.5X6
Rautina	T46.5X1	T46.5X2	T46.5X3	T46.5X4	T46.5X5	T46.5X6
Rautotal	T46.5X1	T46.5X2	T46.5X3	T46.5X4	T46.5X5	T46.5X6
Rauwiloid	T46.5X1	T46.5X2	T46.5X3	T46.5X4	T46.5X5	T46.5X6
Rauwoldin	T46.5X1	T46.5X2	T46.5X3	T46.5X4	T46.5X5	T46.5X6
Rauwolfia (alkaloids)	T46.5X1	T46.5X2	T46.5X3	T46.5X4	T46.5X5	T46.5X6
Razoxane	T45.1X1	T45.1X2	T45.1X3	T45.1X4	T45.1X5	T45.1X6
Realgar	T57.0X1	T57.0X2	T57.0X3	T57.0X4	—	—
Recombinant (R)—*see specific protein*						
Red blood cells, packed	T45.8X1	T45.8X2	T45.8X3	T45.8X4	T45.8X5	T45.8X6
Red squill (scilliroside)	T60.4X1	T60.4X2	T60.4X3	T60.4X4	—	—
Reducing agent, industrial NEC	T65.891	T65.892	T65.893	T65.894	—	—
Refrigerant gas (chlorofluoro-carbon)	T53.5X1	T53.5X2	T53.5X3	T53.5X4	—	—
not chlorofluoro-carbon	T59.891	T59.892	T59.893	T59.894	—	—
Regroton	T50.2X1	T50.2X2	T50.2X3	T50.2X4	T50.2X5	T50.2X6
Rehydration salts (oral)	T50.3X1	T50.3X2	T50.3X3	T50.3X4	T50.3X5	T50.3X6
Rela	T42.8X1	T42.8X2	T42.8X3	T42.8X4	T42.8X5	T42.8X6

Substance	External Cause (T-Code)					
	Poisoning, Accidental (Unintentional)	Poisoning, Intentional Self-Harm	Poisoning, Assault	Poisoning, Undetermined	Adverse Effect	Underdosing
Relaxant, muscle						
anesthetic	T48.1X1	T48.1X2	T48.1X3	T48.1X4	T48.1X5	T48.1X6
central nervous system	T42.8X1	T42.8X2	T42.8X3	T42.8X4	T42.8X5	T42.8X6
skeletal NEC	T48.1X1	T48.1X2	T48.1X3	T48.1X4	T48.1X5	T48.1X6
smooth NEC	T44.3X1	T44.3X2	T44.3X3	T44.3X4	T44.3X5	T44.3X6
Remoxipride	T43.591	T43.592	T43.593	T43.594	T43.595	T43.596
Renese	T50.2X1	T50.2X2	T50.2X3	T50.2X4	T50.2X5	T50.2X6
Renografin	T50.8X1	T50.8X2	T50.8X3	T50.8X4	T50.8X5	T50.8X6
Replacement solution	T50.3X1	T50.3X2	T50.3X3	T50.3X4	T50.3X5	T50.3X6
Reproterol	T48.6X1	T48.6X2	T48.6X3	T48.6X4	T48.6X5	T48.6X6
Rescinnamine	T46.5X1	T46.5X2	T46.5X3	T46.5X4	T46.5X5	T46.5X6
Reserpin(e)	T46.5X1	T46.5X2	T46.5X3	T46.5X4	T46.5X5	T46.5X6
Resorcin, resorcinol (nonmedicinal)	T65.891	T65.892	T65.893	T65.894	—	—
medicinal	T49.4X1	T49.4X2	T49.4X3	T49.4X4	T49.4X5	T49.4X6
Respaire	T48.4X1	T48.4X2	T48.4X3	T48.4X4	T48.4X5	T48.4X6
Respiratory drug NEC	T48.901	T48.902	T48.903	T48.904	T48.905	T48.906
antiasthmatic NEC	T48.6X1	T48.6X2	T48.6X3	T48.6X4	T48.6X5	T48.6X6
anti-common-cold NEC	T48.5X1	T48.5X2	T48.5X3	T48.5X4	T48.5X5	T48.5X6
expectorant NEC	T48.4X1	T48.4X2	T48.4X3	T48.4X4	T48.4X5	T48.4X6
stimulant	T48.901	T48.902	T48.903	T48.904	T48.905	T48.906
Retinoic acid	T49.0X1	T49.0X2	T49.0X3	T49.0X4	T49.0X5	T49.0X6
Retinol	T45.2X1	T45.2X2	T45.2X3	T45.2X4	T45.2X5	T45.2X6
Rh (D) immune globulin (human)	T50.Z11	T50.Z12	T50.Z13	T50.Z14	T50.Z15	T50.Z16
Rhodine	T39.011	T39.012	T39.013	T39.014	T39.015	T39.016
RhoGAM	T50.Z11	T50.Z12	T50.Z13	T50.Z14	T50.Z15	T50.Z16
Rhubarb						
dry extract	T47.2X1	T47.2X2	T47.2X3	T47.2X4	T47.2X5	T47.2X6
tincture, compound	T47.2X1	T47.2X2	T47.2X3	T47.2X4	T47.2X5	T47.2X6
Ribavirin	T37.5X1	T37.5X2	T37.5X3	T37.5X4	T37.5X5	T37.5X6
Riboflavin	T45.2X1	T45.2X2	T45.2X3	T45.2X4	T45.2X5	T45.2X6
Ribostamycin	T36.5X1	T36.5X2	T36.5X3	T36.5X4	T36.5X5	T36.5X6
Ricin	T62.2X1	T62.2X2	T62.2X3	T62.2X4	—	—
Ricinus communis	T62.2X1	T62.2X2	T62.2X3	T62.2X4	—	—
Rickettsial vaccine NEC	T50.A91	T50.A92	T50.A93	T50.A94	T50.A95	T50.A96
Rifabutin	T36.6X1	T36.6X2	T36.6X3	T36.6X4	T36.6X5	T36.6X6
Rifamide	T36.6X1	T36.6X2	T36.6X3	T36.6X4	T36.6X5	T36.6X6
Rifampicin	T36.6X1	T36.6X2	T36.6X3	T36.6X4	T36.6X5	T36.6X6
with isoniazid	T37.1X1	T37.1X2	T37.1X3	T37.1X4	T37.1X5	T37.1X6
Rifampin	T36.6X1	T36.6X2	T36.6X3	T36.6X4	T36.6X5	T36.6X6
Rifamycin	T36.6X1	T36.6X2	T36.6X3	T36.6X4	T36.6X5	T36.6X6
Rifaximin	T36.6X1	T36.6X2	T36.6X3	T36.6X4	T36.6X5	T36.6X6

Substance	External Cause (T-Code)					
	Poisoning, Accidental (Unintentional)	Poisoning, Intentional Self-Harm	Poisoning, Assault	Poisoning, Undetermined	Adverse Effect	Underdosing
Rimantadine	T37.5X1	T37.5X2	T37.5X3	T37.5X4	T37.5X5	T37.5X6
Rimazolium metilsulfate	T39.8X1	T39.8X2	T39.8X3	T39.8X4	T39.8X5	T39.8X6
Rimifon	T37.1X1	T37.1X2	T37.1X3	T37.1X4	T37.1X5	T37.1X6
Rimiterol	T48.6X1	T48.6X2	T48.6X3	T48.6X4	T48.6X5	T48.6X6
Ringer (lactate) solution	T50.3X1	T50.3X2	T50.3X3	T50.3X4	T50.3X5	T50.3X6
Ristocetin	T36.8X1	T36.8X2	T36.8X3	T36.8X4	T36.8X5	T36.8X6
Ritalin	T43.631	T43.632	T43.633	T43.634	T43.635	T43.636
Ritodrine	T44.5X1	T44.5X2	T44.5X3	T44.5X4	T44.5X5	T44.5X6
Roach killer — *see Insecticide*						
Rociverine	T44.3X1	T44.3X2	T44.3X3	T44.3X4	T44.3X5	T44.3X6
Rocky Mountain spotted fever vaccine	T50.A91	T50.A92	T50.A93	T50.A94	T50.A95	T50.A96
Rodenticide NEC	T60.4X1	T60.4X2	T60.4X3	T60.4X4	—	—
Rohypnol	T42.4X1	T42.4X2	T42.4X3	T42.4X4	T42.4X5	T42.4X6
Rokitamycin	T36.3X1	T36.3X2	T36.3X3	T36.3X4	T36.3X5	T36.3X6
Rolaids	T47.1X1	T47.1X2	T47.1X3	T47.1X4	T47.1X5	T47.1X6
Rolitetracycline	T36.4X1	T36.4X2	T36.4X3	T36.4X4	T36.4X5	T36.4X6
Romilar	T48.3X1	T48.3X2	T48.3X3	T48.3X4	T48.3X5	T48.3X6
Ronifibrate	T46.6X1	T46.6X2	T46.6X3	T46.6X4	T46.6X5	T46.6X6
Rosaprostol	T47.1X1	T47.1X2	T47.1X3	T47.1X4	T47.1X5	T47.1X6
Rose bengal sodium (131I)	T50.8X1	T50.8X2	T50.8X3	T50.8X4	T50.8X5	T50.8X6
Rose water ointment	T49.3X1	T49.3X2	T49.3X3	T49.3X4	T49.3X5	T49.3X6
Rosoxacin	T37.8X1	T37.8X2	T37.8X3	T37.8X4	T37.8X5	T37.8X6
Rotenone	T60.2X1	T60.2X2	T60.2X3	T60.2X4	—	—
Rotoxamine	T45.0X1	T45.0X2	T45.0X3	T45.0X4	T45.0X5	T45.0X6
Rough-on-rats	T60.4X1	T60.4X2	T60.4X3	T60.4X4	—	—
Roxatidine	T47.0X1	T47.0X2	T47.0X3	T47.0X4	T47.0X5	T47.0X6
Roxithromycin	T36.3X1	T36.3X2	T36.3X3	T36.3X4	T36.3X5	T36.3X6
Rt-PA	T45.611	T45.612	T45.613	T45.614	T45.615	T45.616
Rubbing alcohol	T51.2X1	T51.2X2	T51.2X3	T51.2X4	—	—
Rubefacient	T49.4X1	T49.4X2	T49.4X3	T49.4X4	T49.4X5	T49.4X6
Rubella vaccine	T50.B91	T50.B92	T50.B93	T50.B94	T50.B95	T50.B96
Rubelogen	T50.B91	T50.B92	T50.B93	T50.B94	T50.B95	T50.B96
Rubeovax	T50.991	T50.992	T50.993	T50.994	T50.995	T50.996
Rubidium chloride Rb82	T50.8X1	T50.8X2	T50.8X3	T50.8X4	T50.8X5	T50.8X6
Rubidomycin	T45.1X1	T45.1X2	T45.1X3	T45.1X4	T45.1X5	T45.1X6
Rue	T62.2X1	T62.2X2	T62.2X3	T62.2X4	—	—
Rufocromomycin	T45.1X1	T45.1X2	T45.1X3	T45.1X4	T45.1X5	T45.1X6
Russel's viper venin	T45.7X1	T45.7X2	T45.7X3	T45.7X4	T45.7X5	T45.7X6
Ruta (graveolens)	T62.2X1	T62.2X2	T62.2X3	T62.2X4	—	—
Rutinum	T46.991	T46.992	T46.993	T46.994	T46.995	T46.996
Rutoside	T46.991	T46.992	T46.993	T46.994	T46.995	T46.996

Substance	Poisoning, Accidental (Unintentional)	External Cause (T-Code): Poisoning, Intentional Self-Harm	Poisoning, Assault	Poisoning, Undetermined	Adverse Effect	Underdosing
S						
Sabadilla (plant)	T62.2X1	T62.2X2	T62.2X3	T62.2X4	—	—
pesticide	T60.2X1	T60.2X2	T60.2X3	T60.2X4	—	—
Saccharated iron oxide	T45.8X1	T45.8X2	T45.8X3	T45.8X4	T45.8X5	T45.8X6
Saccharin	T50.901	T50.902	T50.903	T50.904	T50.905	T50.906
Saccharomyces boulardii	T47.6X1	T47.6X2	T47.6X3	T47.6X4	T47.6X5	T47.6X6
Safflower oil	T46.6X1	T46.6X2	T46.6X3	T46.6X4	T46.6X5	T46.6X6
Safrazine	T43.1X1	T43.1X2	T43.1X3	T43.1X4	T43.1X5	T43.1X6
Salazosulfapyridine	T37.0X1	T37.0X2	T37.0X3	T37.0X4	T37.0X5	T37.0X6
Salbutamol	T48.6X1	T48.6X2	T48.6X3	T48.6X4	T48.6X5	T48.6X6
Salicylamide	T39.091	T39.092	T39.093	T39.094	T39.095	T39.096
Salicylate NEC	T39.091	T39.092	T39.093	T39.094	T39.095	T39.096
methyl	T49.3X1	T49.3X2	T49.3X3	T49.3X4	T49.3X5	T49.3X6
theobromine calcium	T50.2X1	T50.2X2	T50.2X3	T50.2X4	T50.2X5	T50.2X6
Salicylazosulfapyridine	T37.0X1	T37.0X2	T37.0X3	T37.0X4	T37.0X5	T37.0X6
Salicylhydroxamic acid	T49.0X1	T49.0X2	T49.0X3	T49.0X4	T49.0X5	T49.0X6
Salicylic acid	T49.4X1	T49.4X2	T49.4X3	T49.4X4	T49.4X5	T49.4X6
with benzoic acid	T49.4X1	T49.4X2	T49.4X3	T49.4X4	T49.4X5	T49.4X6
congeners	T39.091	T39.092	T39.093	T39.094	T39.095	T39.096
derivative	T39.091	T39.092	T39.093	T39.094	T39.095	T39.096
salts	T39.091	T39.092	T39.093	T39.094	T39.095	T39.096
Salinazid	T37.1X1	T37.1X2	T37.1X3	T37.1X4	T37.1X5	T37.1X6
Salmeterol	T48.6X1	T48.6X2	T48.6X3	T48.6X4	T48.6X5	T48.6X6
Salol	T49.3X1	T49.3X2	T49.3X3	T49.3X4	T49.3X5	T49.3X6
Salsalate	T39.091	T39.092	T39.093	T39.094	T39.095	T39.096
Salt substitute	T50.901	T50.902	T50.903	T50.904	T50.905	T50.906
Salt-replacing drug	T50.901	T50.902	T50.903	T50.904	T50.905	T50.906
Salt-retaining mineralocorticoid	T50.0X1	T50.0X2	T50.0X3	T50.0X4	T50.0X5	T50.0X6
Saluretic NEC	T50.2X1	T50.2X2	T50.2X3	T50.2X4	T50.2X5	T50.2X6
Saluron	T50.2X1	T50.2X2	T50.2X3	T50.2X4	T50.2X5	T50.2X6
Salvarsan 606 (neosilver) (silver)	T37.8X1	T37.8X2	T37.8X3	T37.8X4	T37.8X5	T37.8X6
Sambucus canadensis	T62.2X1	T62.2X2	T62.2X3	T62.2X4	—	—
berry	T62.1X1	T62.1X2	T62.1X3	T62.1X4	—	—
Sandril	T46.5X1	T46.5X2	T46.5X3	T46.5X4	T46.5X5	T46.5X6
Sanguinaria canadensis	T62.2X1	T62.2X2	T62.2X3	T62.2X4	—	—
Saniflush (cleaner)	T54.2X1	T54.2X2	T54.2X3	T54.2X4	—	—
Santonin	T37.4X1	T37.4X2	T37.4X3	T37.4X4	T37.4X5	T37.4X6
Santyl	T49.8X1	T49.8X2	T49.8X3	T49.8X4	T49.8X5	T49.8X6
Saralasin	T46.5X1	T46.5X2	T46.5X3	T46.5X4	T46.5X5	T46.5X6
Sarcolysin	T45.1X1	T45.1X2	T45.1X3	T45.1X4	T45.1X5	T45.1X6
Sarkomycin	T45.1X1	T45.1X2	T45.1X3	T45.1X4	T45.1X5	T45.1X6
Saroten	T43.011	T43.012	T43.013	T43.014	T43.015	T43.016

Substance	Poisoning, Accidental (Unintentional)	External Cause (T-Code): Poisoning, Intentional Self-Harm	Poisoning, Assault	Poisoning, Undetermined	Adverse Effect	Underdosing
Saturnine — *see Lead*						
Savin (oil)	T49.4X1	T49.4X2	T49.4X3	T49.4X4	T49.4X5	T49.4X6
Scammony	T47.2X1	T47.2X2	T47.2X3	T47.2X4	T47.2X5	T47.2X6
Scarlet red	T49.8X1	T49.8X2	T49.8X3	T49.8X4	T49.8X5	T49.8X6
Scheele's green	T57.0X1	T57.0X2	T57.0X3	T57.0X4	—	—
insecticide	T57.0X1	T57.0X2	T57.0X3	T57.0X4	—	—
Schizontozide (blood) (tissue)	T37.2X1	T37.2X2	T37.2X3	T37.2X4	T37.2X5	T37.2X6
Schradan	T60.0X1	T60.0X2	T60.0X3	T60.0X4	—	—
Schweinfurth green	T57.0X1	T57.0X2	T57.0X3	T57.0X4	—	—
insecticide	T57.0X1	T57.0X2	T57.0X3	T57.0X4	—	—
Scilla, rat poison	T60.4X1	T60.4X2	T60.4X3	T60.4X4	—	—
Scillaren	T60.4X1	T60.4X2	T60.4X3	T60.4X4	—	—
Sclerosing agent	T46.8X1	T46.8X2	T46.8X3	T46.8X4	T46.8X5	T46.8X6
Scombrotoxin	T61.11	T61.12	T61.13	T61.14	—	—
Scopolamine	T44.3X1	T44.3X2	T44.3X3	T44.3X4	T44.3X5	T44.3X6
Scopolia extract	T44.3X1	T44.3X2	T44.3X3	T44.3X4	T44.3X5	T44.3X6
Scouring powder	T65.891	T65.892	T65.893	T65.894	—	—
Sea						
anemone (sting)	T63.631	T63.632	T63.633	T63.634	—	—
cucumber (sting)	T63.691	T63.692	T63.693	T63.694	—	—
snake (bite) (venom)	T63.091	T63.092	T63.093	T63.094	—	—
urchin spine (puncture)	T63.691	T63.692	T63.693	T63.694	—	—
Seafood	T61.91	T61.92	T61.93	T61.94	—	—
specified NEC	T61.8X1	T61.8X2	T61.8X3	T61.8X4	—	—
Secbutabarbital	T42.3X1	T42.3X2	T42.3X3	T42.3X4	T42.3X5	T42.3X6
Secbutabarbitone	T42.3X1	T42.3X2	T42.3X3	T42.3X4	T42.3X5	T42.3X6
Secnidazole	T37.3X1	T37.3X2	T37.3X3	T37.3X4	T37.3X5	T37.3X6
Secobarbital	T42.3X1	T42.3X2	T42.3X3	T42.3X4	T42.3X5	T42.3X6
Seconal	T42.3X1	T42.3X2	T42.3X3	T42.3X4	T42.3X5	T42.3X6
Secretin	T50.8X1	T50.8X2	T50.8X3	T50.8X4	T50.8X5	T50.8X6
Sedative NEC	T42.71	T42.72	T42.73	T42.74	T42.75	T42.76
mixed NEC	T42.6X1	T42.6X2	T42.6X3	T42.6X4	T42.6X5	T42.6X6
Sedormid	T42.6X1	T42.6X2	T42.6X3	T42.6X4	T42.6X5	T42.6X6
Seed disinfectant or dressing	T60.8X1	T60.8X2	T60.8X3	T60.8X4	—	—
Seeds (poisonous)	T62.2X1	T62.2X2	T62.2X3	T62.2X4	—	—
Selegiline	T42.8X1	T42.8X2	T42.8X3	T42.8X4	T42.8X5	T42.8X6
Selenium NEC	T56.891	T56.892	T56.893	T56.894	—	—
disulfide or sulfide	T49.4X1	T49.4X2	T49.4X3	T49.4X4	T49.4X5	T49.4X6
fumes	T59.891	T59.892	T59.893	T59.894	—	—
sulfide	T49.4X1	T49.4X2	T49.4X3	T49.4X4	T49.4X5	T49.4X6
Selenomethionine (75Se)	T50.8X1	T50.8X2	T50.8X3	T50.8X4	T50.8X5	T50.8X6
Selsun	T49.4X1	T49.4X2	T49.4X3	T49.4X4	T49.4X5	T49.4X6

Substance	External Cause (T-Code)					
	Poisoning, Accidental (Unintentional)	Poisoning, Intentional Self-Harm	Poisoning, Assault	Poisoning, Undetermined	Adverse Effect	Underdosing
Semustine	T45.1X1	T45.1X2	T45.1X3	T45.1X4	T45.1X5	T45.1X6
Senega syrup	T48.4X1	T48.4X2	T48.4X3	T48.4X4	T48.4X5	T48.4X6
Senna	T47.2X1	T47.2X2	T47.2X3	T47.2X4	T47.2X5	T47.2X6
Sennoside A+B	T47.2X1	T47.2X2	T47.2X3	T47.2X4	T47.2X5	T47.2X6
Septisol	T49.2X1	T49.2X2	T49.2X3	T49.2X4	T49.2X5	T49.2X6
Seractide	T38.811	T38.812	T38.813	T38.814	T38.815	T38.816
Serax	T42.4X1	T42.4X2	T42.4X3	T42.4X4	T42.4X5	T42.4X6
Serenesil	T42.6X1	T42.6X2	T42.6X3	T42.6X4	T42.6X5	T42.6X6
Serenium (hydrochloride)	T37.91	T37.92	T37.93	T37.94	T37.95	T37.96
Serepax — *see Oxazepam*						
Sermorelin	T38.891	T38.892	T38.893	T38.894	T38.895	T38.896
Sernyl	T41.1X1	T41.1X2	T41.1X3	T41.1X4	T41.1X5	T41.1X6
Serotonin	T50.991	T50.992	T50.993	T50.994	T50.995	T50.996
Serpasil	T46.5X1	T46.5X2	T46.5X3	T46.5X4	T46.5X5	T46.5X6
Serrapeptase	T45.3X1	T45.3X2	T45.3X3	T45.3X4	T45.3X5	T45.3X6
Serum						
antibotulinus	T50.Z11	T50.Z12	T50.Z13	T50.Z14	T50.Z15	T50.Z16
anticytotoxic	T50.Z11	T50.Z12	T50.Z13	T50.Z14	T50.Z15	T50.Z16
antidiphtheria	T50.Z11	T50.Z12	T50.Z13	T50.Z14	T50.Z15	T50.Z16
antimeningococcus	T50.Z11	T50.Z12	T50.Z13	T50.Z14	T50.Z15	T50.Z16
anti-Rh	T50.Z11	T50.Z12	T50.Z13	T50.Z14	T50.Z15	T50.Z16
anti-snake-bite	T50.Z11	T50.Z12	T50.Z13	T50.Z14	T50.Z15	T50.Z16
antitetanic	T50.Z11	T50.Z12	T50.Z13	T50.Z14	T50.Z15	T50.Z16
antitoxic	T50.Z11	T50.Z12	T50.Z13	T50.Z14	T50.Z15	T50.Z16
complement (inhibitor)	T45.8X1	T45.8X2	T45.8X3	T45.8X4	T45.8X5	T45.8X6
convalescent	T50.Z11	T50.Z12	T50.Z13	T50.Z14	T50.Z15	T50.Z16
hemolytic complement	T45.8X1	T45.8X2	T45.8X3	T45.8X4	T45.8X5	T45.8X6
immune (human)	T50.Z11	T50.Z12	T50.Z13	T50.Z14	T50.Z15	T50.Z16
protective NEC	T50.Z11	T50.Z12	T50.Z13	T50.Z14	T50.Z15	T50.Z16
Setastine	T45.0X1	T45.0X2	T45.0X3	T45.0X4	T45.0X5	T45.0X6
Setoperone	T43.591	T43.592	T43.593	T43.594	T43.595	T43.596
Sewer gas	T59.91	T59.92	T59.93	T59.94	—	—
Shampoo	T55.0X1	T55.0X2	T55.0X3	T55.0X4	—	—
Shellfish, noxious, nonbacterial	T61.781	T61.782	T61.783	T61.784	—	—
Sildenafil	T46.7X1	T46.7X2	T46.7X3	T46.7X4	T46.7X5	T46.7X6
Silibinin	T50.991	T50.992	T50.993	T50.994	T50.995	T50.996
Silicone NEC	T65.891	T65.892	T65.893	T65.894	—	—
medicinal	T49.3X1	T49.3X2	T49.3X3	T49.3X4	T49.3X5	T49.3X6
Silvadene	T49.0X1	T49.0X2	T49.0X3	T49.0X4	T49.0X5	T49.0X6
Silver	T49.0X1	T49.0X2	T49.0X3	T49.0X4	T49.0X5	T49.0X6
anti-infectives	T49.0X1	T49.0X2	T49.0X3	T49.0X4	T49.0X5	T49.0X6
arsphenamine	T37.8X1	T37.8X2	T37.8X3	T37.8X4	T37.8X5	T37.8X6

Substance	External Cause (T-Code)					
	Poisoning, Accidental (Unintentional)	Poisoning, Intentional Self-Harm	Poisoning, Assault	Poisoning, Undetermined	Adverse Effect	Underdosing
Silver *(Continued)*						
colloidal	T49.0X1	T49.0X2	T49.0X3	T49.0X4	T49.0X5	T49.0X6
nitrate	T49.0X1	T49.0X2	T49.0X3	T49.0X4	T49.0X5	T49.0X6
ophthalmic preparation	T49.5X1	T49.5X2	T49.5X3	T49.5X4	T49.5X5	T49.5X6
toughened (keratolytic)	T49.4X1	T49.4X2	T49.4X3	T49.4X4	T49.4X5	T49.4X6
nonmedicinal (dust)	T56.891	T56.892	T56.893	T56.894	—	—
protein	T49.5X1	T49.5X2	T49.5X3	T49.5X4	T49.5X5	T49.5X6
salvarsan	T37.8X1	T37.8X2	T37.8X3	T37.8X4	T37.8X5	T37.8X6
sulfadiazine	T49.4X1	T49.4X2	T49.4X3	T49.4X4	T49.4X5	T49.4X6
Silymarin	T50.991	T50.992	T50.993	T50.994	T50.995	T50.996
Simaldrate	T47.1X1	T47.1X2	T47.1X3	T47.1X4	T47.1X5	T47.1X6
Simazine	T60.3X1	T60.3X2	T60.3X3	T60.3X4	—	—
Simethicone	T47.1X1	T47.1X2	T47.1X3	T47.1X4	T47.1X5	T47.1X6
Simfibrate	T46.6X1	T46.6X2	T46.6X3	T46.6X4	T46.6X5	T46.6X6
Simvastatin	T46.6X1	T46.6X2	T46.6X3	T46.6X4	T46.6X5	T46.6X6
Sincalide	T50.8X1	T50.8X2	T50.8X3	T50.8X4	T50.8X5	T50.8X6
Sinequan	T43.011	T43.012	T43.013	T43.014	T43.015	T43.016
Singoserp	T46.5X1	T46.5X2	T46.5X3	T46.5X4	T46.5X5	T46.5X6
Sintrom	T45.511	T45.512	T45.513	T45.514	T45.515	T45.516
Sisomicin	T36.5X1	T36.5X2	T36.5X3	T36.5X4	T36.5X5	T36.5X6
Sitosterols	T46.6X1	T46.6X2	T46.6X3	T46.6X4	T46.6X5	T46.6X6
Skeletal muscle relaxants	T48.1X1	T48.1X2	T48.1X3	T48.1X4	T48.1X5	T48.1X6
Skin						
agents (external)	T49.91	T49.92	T49.93	T49.94	T49.95	T49.96
specified NEC	T49.8X1	T49.8X2	T49.8X3	T49.8X4	T49.8X5	T49.8X6
test antigen	T50.8X1	T50.8X2	T50.8X3	T50.8X4	T50.8X5	T50.8X6
Sleep-eze	T45.0X1	T45.0X2	T45.0X3	T45.0X4	T45.0X5	T45.0X6
Sleeping draught, pill	T42.71	T42.72	T42.73	T42.74	T42.75	T42.76
Smallpox vaccine	T50.B11	T50.B12	T50.B13	T50.B14	T50.B15	T50.B16
Smelter fumes NEC	T56.91	T56.92	T56.93	T56.94	—	—
Smog	T59.1X1	T59.1X2	T59.1X3	T59.1X4	—	—
Smoke NEC	T59.811	T59.812	T59.813	T59.814	—	—
Smooth muscle relaxant	T44.3X1	T44.3X2	T44.3X3	T44.3X4	T44.3X5	T44.3X6
Snail killer NEC	T60.8X1	T60.8X2	T60.8X3	T60.8X4	—	—
Snake venom or bite	T63.001	T63.002	T63.003	T63.004	—	—
hemocoagulase	T45.7X1	T45.7X2	T45.7X3	T45.7X4	T45.7X5	T45.7X6
Snuff	T65.211	T65.212	T65.213	T65.214	—	—
Soap (powder) (product)	T55.0X1	T55.0X2	T55.0X3	T55.0X4	—	—
enema	T47.4X1	T47.4X2	T47.4X3	T47.4X4	T47.4X5	T47.4X6
medicinal, soft	T49.2X1	T49.2X2	T49.2X3	T49.2X4	T49.2X5	T49.2X6
superfatted	T49.2X1	T49.2X2	T49.2X3	T49.2X4	T49.2X5	T49.2X6
Sobrerol	T48.4X1	T48.4X2	T48.4X3	T48.4X4	T48.4X5	T48.4X6

Substance	Poisoning, Accidental (Unintentional)	Poisoning, Intentional Self-Harm	Poisoning, Assault	Poisoning, Undetermined	Adverse Effect	Underdosing
	External Cause (T-Code)					
Soda (caustic)	T54.3X1	T54.3X2	T54.3X3	T54.3X4	—	—
bicarb	T47.1X1	T47.1X2	T47.1X3	T47.1X4	T47.1X5	T47.1X6
chlorinated — *see Sodium, hypochlorite*						
Sodium						
acetosulfone	T37.1X1	T37.1X2	T37.1X3	T37.1X4	T37.1X5	T37.1X6
acetrizoate	T50.8X1	T50.8X2	T50.8X3	T50.8X4	T50.8X5	T50.8X6
acid phosphate	T50.3X1	T50.3X2	T50.3X3	T50.3X4	T50.3X5	T50.3X6
alginate	T47.8X1	T47.8X2	T47.8X3	T47.8X4	T47.8X5	T47.8X6
amidotrizoate	T50.8X1	T50.8X2	T50.8X3	T50.8X4	T50.8X5	T50.8X6
aminopterin	T45.1X1	T45.1X2	T45.1X3	T45.1X4	T45.1X5	T45.1X6
amylosulfate	T47.8X1	T47.8X2	T47.8X3	T47.8X4	T47.8X5	T47.8X6
amytal	T42.3X1	T42.3X2	T42.3X3	T42.3X4	T42.3X5	T42.3X6
antimony gluconate	T37.3X1	T37.3X2	T37.3X3	T37.3X4	T37.3X5	T37.3X6
arsenate	T57.0X1	T57.0X2	T57.0X3	T57.0X4	—	—
aurothiomalate	T39.4X1	T39.4X2	T39.4X3	T39.4X4	T39.4X5	T39.4X6
aurothiosulfate	T39.4X1	T39.4X2	T39.4X3	T39.4X4	T39.4X5	T39.4X6
barbiturate	T42.3X1	T42.3X2	T42.3X3	T42.3X4	T42.3X5	T42.3X6
basic phosphate	T47.4X1	T47.4X2	T47.4X3	T47.4X4	T47.4X5	T47.4X6
bicarbonate	T47.1X1	T47.1X2	T47.1X3	T47.1X4	T47.1X5	T47.1X6
bichromate	T57.8X1	T57.8X2	T57.8X3	T57.8X4	—	—
biphosphate	T50.3X1	T50.3X2	T50.3X3	T50.3X4	T50.3X5	T50.3X6
bisulfate	T65.891	T65.892	T65.893	T65.894	—	—
borate						
cleanser	T57.8X1	T57.8X2	T57.8X3	T57.8X4	—	—
eye	T49.5X1	T49.5X2	T49.5X3	T49.5X4	T49.5X5	T49.5X6
therapeutic	T49.8X1	T49.8X2	T49.8X3	T49.8X4	T49.8X5	T49.8X6
bromide	T42.6X1	T42.6X2	T42.6X3	T42.6X4	T42.6X5	T42.6X6
cacodylate (nonmedicinal) NEC	T50.8X1	T50.8X2	T50.8X3	T50.8X4	T50.8X5	T50.8X6
anti-infective	T37.8X1	T37.8X2	T37.8X3	T37.8X4	T37.8X5	T37.8X6
herbicide	T60.3X1	T60.3X2	T60.3X3	T60.3X4	—	—
calcium edetate	T45.8X1	T45.8X2	T45.8X3	T45.8X4	T45.8X5	T45.8X6
carbonate NEC	T54.3X1	T54.3X2	T54.3X3	T54.3X4	—	—
chlorate NEC	T65.891	T65.892	T65.893	T65.894	—	—
herbicide	T54.91	T54.92	T54.93	T54.94	—	—
chloride	T50.3X1	T50.3X2	T50.3X3	T50.3X4	T50.3X5	T50.3X6
with glucose	T50.3X1	T50.3X2	T50.3X3	T50.3X4	T50.3X5	T50.3X6
chromate	T65.891	T65.892	T65.893	T65.894	—	—
citrate	T50.991	T50.992	T50.993	T50.994	T50.995	T50.996
cromoglicate	T48.6X1	T48.6X2	T48.6X3	T48.6X4	T48.6X5	T48.6X6
cyanide	T65.0X1	T65.0X2	T65.0X3	T65.0X4	—	—
cyclamate	T50.3X1	T50.3X2	T50.3X3	T50.3X4	T50.3X5	T50.3X6

Substance	Poisoning, Accidental (Unintentional)	Poisoning, Intentional Self-Harm	Poisoning, Assault	Poisoning, Undetermined	Adverse Effect	Underdosing
	External Cause (T-Code)					
Sodium *(Continued)*						
dehydrocholate	T45.8X1	T45.8X2	T45.8X3	T45.8X4	T45.8X5	T45.8X6
diatrizoate	T50.8X1	T50.8X2	T50.8X3	T50.8X4	T50.8X5	T50.8X6
dibunate	T48.4X1	T48.4X2	T48.4X3	T48.4X4	T48.4X5	T48.4X6
dioctyl sulfosuccinate	T47.4X1	T47.4X2	T47.4X3	T47.4X4	T47.4X5	T47.4X6
dipantoyl ferrate	T45.8X1	T45.8X2	T45.8X3	T45.8X4	T45.8X5	T45.8X6
edetate	T45.8X1	T45.8X2	T45.8X3	T45.8X4	T45.8X5	T45.8X6
ethacrynate	T50.1X1	T50.1X2	T50.1X3	T50.1X4	T50.1X5	T50.1X6
feredetate	T45.8X1	T45.8X2	T45.8X3	T45.8X4	T45.8X5	T45.8X6
Fluoride — *see Fluoride*						
fluoroacetate (dust) (pesticide)	T60.4X1	T60.4X2	T60.4X3	T60.4X4	—	—
free salt	T50.3X1	T50.3X2	T50.3X3	T50.3X4	T50.3X5	T50.3X6
fusidate	T36.8X1	T36.8X2	T36.8X3	T36.8X4	T36.8X5	T36.8X6
glucaldrate	T47.1X1	T47.1X2	T47.1X3	T47.1X4	T47.1X5	T47.1X6
glucosulfone	T37.1X1	T37.1X2	T37.1X3	T37.1X4	T37.1X5	T37.1X6
glutamate	T45.8X1	T45.8X2	T45.8X3	T45.8X4	T45.8X5	T45.8X6
hydrogen carbonate	T50.3X1	T50.3X2	T50.3X3	T50.3X4	T50.3X5	T50.3X6
hydroxide	T54.3X1	T54.3X2	T54.3X3	T54.3X4	—	—
hypochlorite (bleach) NEC	T54.3X1	T54.3X2	T54.3X3	T54.3X4	—	—
disinfectant	T54.3X1	T54.3X2	T54.3X3	T54.3X4	—	—
medicinal (anti-infective) (external)	T49.0X1	T49.0X2	T49.0X3	T49.0X4	T49.0X5	T49.0X6
vapor	T54.3X1	T54.3X2	T54.3X3	T54.3X4	—	—
hyposulfite	T49.0X1	T49.0X2	T49.0X3	T49.0X4	T49.0X5	T49.0X6
indigotin disulfonate	T50.8X1	T50.8X2	T50.8X3	T50.8X4	T50.8X5	T50.8X6
iodide	T50.991	T50.992	T50.993	T50.994	T50.995	T50.996
I-131	T50.8X1	T50.8X2	T50.8X3	T50.8X4	T50.8X5	T50.8X6
therapeutic	T38.2X1	T38.2X2	T38.2X3	T38.2X4	T38.2X5	T38.2X6
iodohippurate (131I)	T50.8X1	T50.8X2	T50.8X3	T50.8X4	T50.8X5	T50.8X6
iopodate	T50.8X1	T50.8X2	T50.8X3	T50.8X4	T50.8X5	T50.8X6
iothalamate	T50.8X1	T50.8X2	T50.8X3	T50.8X4	T50.8X5	T50.8X6
iron edetate	T45.4X1	T45.4X2	T45.4X3	T45.4X4	T45.4X5	T45.4X6
lactate (compound solution)	T45.8X1	T45.8X2	T45.8X3	T45.8X4	T45.8X5	T45.8X6
lauryl (sulfate)	T49.2X1	T49.2X2	T49.2X3	T49.2X4	T49.2X5	T49.2X6
(L)-triiodothyronine	T38.1X1	T38.1X2	T38.1X3	T38.1X4	T38.1X5	T38.1X6
magnesium citrate	T50.991	T50.992	T50.993	T50.994	T50.995	T50.996
mersalate	T50.2X1	T50.2X2	T50.2X3	T50.2X4	T50.2X5	T50.2X6
metasilicate	T65.891	T65.892	T65.893	T65.894	—	—
metrizoate	T50.8X1	T50.8X2	T50.8X3	T50.8X4	T50.8X5	T50.8X6
monofluoroacetate (pesticide)	T60.1X1	T60.1X2	T60.1X3	T60.1X4	—	—
morrhuate	T46.8X1	T46.8X2	T46.8X3	T46.8X4	T46.8X5	T46.8X6
nafcillin	T36.0X1	T36.0X2	T36.0X3	T36.0X4	T36.0X5	T36.0X6

◀ New ◀ Revised ~~deleted~~ Deleted

Substance	External Cause (T-Code)					
	Poisoning, Accidental (Unintentional)	Poisoning, Intentional Self-Harm	Poisoning, Assault	Poisoning, Undetermined	Adverse Effect	Underdosing
Sodium *(Continued)*						
nitrate (oxidizing agent)	T65.891	T65.892	T65.893	T65.894	—	—
nitrite	T50.6X1	T50.6X2	T50.6X3	T50.6X4	T50.6X5	T50.6X6
nitroferricyanide	T46.5X1	T46.5X2	T46.5X3	T46.5X4	T46.5X5	T46.5X6
nitroprusside	T46.5X1	T46.5X2	T46.5X3	T46.5X4	T46.5X5	T46.5X6
oxalate	T65.891	T65.892	T65.893	T65.894	—	—
oxide/peroxide	T65.891	T65.892	T65.893	T65.894	—	—
oxybate	T41.291	T41.292	T41.293	T41.294	T41.295	T41.296
para-aminohippurate	T50.8X1	T50.8X2	T50.8X3	T50.8X4	T50.8X5	T50.8X6
perborate (nonmedicinal) NEC	T65.891	T65.892	T65.893	T65.894	—	—
medicinal	T49.0X1	T49.0X2	T49.0X3	T49.0X4	T49.0X5	T49.0X6
soap	T55.0X1	T55.0X2	T55.0X3	T55.0X4	—	—
percarbonate — *see Sodium, perborate*						
pertechnetate Tc99m	T50.8X1	T50.8X2	T50.8X3	T50.8X4	T50.8X5	T50.8X6
phosphate						
cellulose	T45.8X1	T45.8X2	T45.8X3	T45.8X4	T45.8X5	T45.8X6
dibasic	T47.2X1	T47.2X2	T47.2X3	T47.2X4	T47.2X5	T47.2X6
monobasic	T47.2X1	T47.2X2	T47.2X3	T47.2X4	T47.2X5	T47.2X6
phytate	T50.6X1	T50.6X2	T50.6X3	T50.6X4	T50.6X5	T50.6X6
picosulfate	T47.2X1	T47.2X2	T47.2X3	T47.2X4	T47.2X5	T47.2X6
polyhydroxyaluminium monocarbonate	T47.1X1	T47.1X2	T47.1X3	T47.1X4	T47.1X5	T47.1X6
polystyrene sulfonate	T50.3X1	T50.3X2	T50.3X3	T50.3X4	T50.3X5	T50.3X6
propionate	T49.0X1	T49.0X2	T49.0X3	T49.0X4	T49.0X5	T49.0X6
propyl hydroxybenzoate	T50.991	T50.992	T50.993	T50.994	T50.995	T50.996
psylliate	T46.8X1	T46.8X2	T46.8X3	T46.8X4	T46.8X5	T46.8X6
removing resins	T50.3X1	T50.3X2	T50.3X3	T50.3X4	T50.3X5	T50.3X6
salicylate	T39.091	T39.092	T39.093	T39.094	T39.095	T39.096
salt NEC	T50.3X1	T50.3X2	T50.3X3	T50.3X4	T50.3X5	T50.3X6
selenate	T60.2X1	T60.2X2	T60.2X3	T60.2X4	—	—
stibogluconate	T37.3X1	T37.3X2	T37.3X3	T37.3X4	T37.3X5	T37.3X6
sulfate	T47.4X1	T47.4X2	T47.4X3	T47.4X4	T47.4X5	T47.4X6
sulfoxone	T37.1X1	T37.1X2	T37.1X3	T37.1X4	T37.1X5	T37.1X6
tetradecyl sulfate	T46.8X1	T46.8X2	T46.8X3	T46.8X4	T46.8X5	T46.8X6
thiopental	T41.1X1	T41.1X2	T41.1X3	T41.1X4	T41.1X5	T41.1X6
thiosalicylate	T39.091	T39.092	T39.093	T39.094	T39.095	T39.096
thiosulfate	T50.6X1	T50.6X2	T50.6X3	T50.6X4	T50.6X5	T50.6X6
tolbutamide	T38.3X1	T38.3X2	T38.3X3	T38.3X4	T38.3X5	T38.3X6
l-triiodothyronine	T38.1X1	T38.1X2	T38.1X3	T38.1X4	T38.1X5	T38.1X6
tyropanoate	T50.8X1	T50.8X2	T50.8X3	T50.8X4	T50.8X5	T50.8X6
valproate	T42.6X1	T42.6X2	T42.6X3	T42.6X4	T42.6X5	T42.6X6
versenate	T50.6X1	T50.6X2	T50.6X3	T50.6X4	T50.6X5	T50.6X6

Substance	External Cause (T-Code)					
	Poisoning, Accidental (Unintentional)	Poisoning, Intentional Self-Harm	Poisoning, Assault	Poisoning, Undetermined	Adverse Effect	Underdosing
Sodium-free salt	T50.901	T50.902	T50.903	T50.904	T50.905	T50.906
Sodium-removing resin	T50.3X1	T50.3X2	T50.3X3	T50.3X4	T50.3X5	T50.3X6
Soft soap	T55.0X1	T55.0X2	T55.0X3	T55.0X4	—	—
Solanine	T62.2X1	T62.2X2	T62.2X3	T62.2X4	—	—
berries	T62.1X1	T62.1X2	T62.1X3	T62.1X4	—	—
Solanum dulcamara	T62.2X1	T62.2X2	T62.2X3	T62.2X4	—	—
berries	T62.1X1	T62.1X2	T62.1X3	T62.1X4	—	—
Solapsone	T37.1X1	T37.1X2	T37.1X3	T37.1X4	T37.1X5	T37.1X6
Solar lotion	T49.3X1	T49.3X2	T49.3X3	T49.3X4	T49.3X5	T49.3X6
Solasulfone	T37.1X1	T37.1X2	T37.1X3	T37.1X4	T37.1X5	T37.1X6
Soldering fluid	T65.891	T65.892	T65.893	T65.894	—	—
Solid substance	T65.91	T65.92	T65.93	T65.94	—	—
specified NEC	T65.891	T65.892	T65.893	T65.894	—	—
Solvent, industrial NEC	T52.91	T52.92	T52.93	T52.94	—	—
naphtha	T52.0X1	T52.0X2	T52.0X3	T52.0X4	—	—
petroleum	T52.0X1	T52.0X2	T52.0X3	T52.0X4	—	—
specified NEC	T52.8X1	T52.8X2	T52.8X3	T52.8X4	—	—
Soma	T42.8X1	T42.8X2	T42.8X3	T42.8X4	T42.8X5	T42.8X6
Somatorelin	T38.891	T38.892	T38.893	T38.894	T38.895	T38.896
Somatostatin	T38.991	T38.992	T38.993	T38.994	T38.995	T38.996
Somatotropin	T38.811	T38.812	T38.813	T38.814	T38.815	T38.816
Somatrem	T38.811	T38.812	T38.813	T38.814	T38.815	T38.816
Somatropin	T38.811	T38.812	T38.813	T38.814	T38.815	T38.816
Sominex	T45.0X1	T45.0X2	T45.0X3	T45.0X4	T45.0X5	T45.0X6
Somnos	T42.6X1	T42.6X2	T42.6X3	T42.6X4	T42.6X5	T42.6X6
Somonal	T42.3X1	T42.3X2	T42.3X3	T42.3X4	T42.3X5	T42.3X6
Soneryl	T42.3X1	T42.3X2	T42.3X3	T42.3X4	T42.3X5	T42.3X6
Soothing syrup	T50.901	T50.902	T50.903	T50.904	T50.905	T50.906
Sopor	T42.6X1	T42.6X2	T42.6X3	T42.6X4	T42.6X5	T42.6X6
Soporific	T42.71	T42.72	T42.73	T42.74	T42.75	T42.76
Soporific drug	T42.71	T42.72	T42.73	T42.74	T42.75	T42.76
specified type NEC	T42.6X1	T42.6X2	T42.6X3	T42.6X4	T42.6X5	T42.6X6
Sorbide nitrate	T46.3X1	T46.3X2	T46.3X3	T46.3X4	T46.3X5	T46.3X6
Sorbitol	T47.4X1	T47.4X2	T47.4X3	T47.4X4	T47.4X5	T47.4X6
Sotalol	T44.7X1	T44.7X2	T44.7X3	T44.7X4	T44.7X5	T44.7X6
Sotradecol	T46.8X1	T46.8X2	T46.8X3	T46.8X4	T46.8X5	T46.8X6
Soysterol	T46.6X1	T46.6X2	T46.6X3	T46.6X4	T46.6X5	T46.6X6
Spacoline	T44.3X1	T44.3X2	T44.3X3	T44.3X4	T44.3X5	T44.3X6
Spanish fly	T49.8X1	T49.8X2	T49.8X3	T49.8X4	T49.8X5	T49.8X6
Sparine	T43.3X1	T43.3X2	T43.3X3	T43.3X4	T43.3X5	T43.3X6
Sparteine	T48.0X1	T48.0X2	T48.0X3	T48.0X4	T48.0X5	T48.0X6

Substance	External Cause (T-Code)					
	Poisoning, Accidental (Unintentional)	Poisoning, Intentional Self-Harm	Poisoning, Assault	Poisoning, Undetermined	Adverse Effect	Underdosing
Spasmolytic						
anticholinergics	T44.3X1	T44.3X2	T44.3X3	T44.3X4	T44.3X5	T44.3X6
autonomic	T44.3X1	T44.3X2	T44.3X3	T44.3X4	T44.3X5	T44.3X6
bronchial NEC	T48.6X1	T48.6X2	T48.6X3	T48.6X4	T48.6X5	T48.6X6
quaternary ammonium	T44.3X1	T44.3X2	T44.3X3	T44.3X4	T44.3X5	T44.3X6
skeletal muscle NEC	T48.1X1	T48.1X2	T48.1X3	T48.1X4	T48.1X5	T48.1X6
Spectinomycin	T36.5X1	T36.5X2	T36.5X3	T36.5X4	T36.5X5	T36.5X6
Speed	T43.621	T43.622	T43.623	T43.624	T43.625	T43.626
Spermicide	T49.8X1	T49.8X2	T49.8X3	T49.8X4	T49.8X5	T49.8X6
Spider (bite) (venom)	T63.391	T63.392	T63.393	T63.394	—	—
antivenin	T50.Z11	T50.Z12	T50.Z13	T50.Z14	T50.Z15	T50.Z16
Spigelia (root)	T37.4X1	T37.4X2	T37.4X3	T37.4X4	T37.4X5	T37.4X6
Spindle inactivator	T50.4X1	T50.4X2	T50.4X3	T50.4X4	T50.4X5	T50.4X6
Spiperone	T43.4X1	T43.4X2	T43.4X3	T43.4X4	T43.4X5	T43.4X6
Spiramycin	T36.3X1	T36.3X2	T36.3X3	T36.3X4	T36.3X5	T36.3X6
Spirapril	T46.4X1	T46.4X2	T46.4X3	T46.4X4	T46.4X5	T46.4X6
Spirilene	T43.591	T43.592	T43.593	T43.594	T43.595	T43.596
Spirit(s) (neutral) NEC	T51.0X1	T51.0X2	T51.0X3	T51.0X4	—	—
beverage	T51.0X1	T51.0X2	T51.0X3	T51.0X4	—	—
industrial	T51.0X1	T51.0X2	T51.0X3	T51.0X4	—	—
mineral	T52.0X1	T52.0X2	T52.0X3	T52.0X4	—	—
of salt — *see Hydrochloric acid*						
surgical	T51.0X1	T51.0X2	T51.0X3	T51.0X4	—	—
Spironolactone	T50.0X1	T50.0X2	T50.0X3	T50.0X4	T50.0X5	T50.0X6
Spiroperidol	T43.4X1	T43.4X2	T43.4X3	T43.4X4	T43.4X5	T43.4X6
Sponge, absorbable (gelatin)	T45.7X1	T45.7X2	T45.7X3	T45.7X4	T45.7X5	T45.7X6
Sporostacin	T49.0X1	T49.0X2	T49.0X3	T49.0X4	T49.0X5	T49.0X6
Spray (aerosol)	T65.91	T65.92	T65.93	T65.94	—	—
cosmetic	T65.891	T65.892	T65.893	T65.894	—	—
medicinal NEC	T50.901	T50.902	T50.903	T50.904	T50.905	T50.906
pesticides — *see Pesticides*						
specified content — *see specific substance*						
Spurge flax	T62.2X1	T62.2X2	T62.2X3	T62.2X4	—	—
Spurges	T62.2X1	T62.2X2	T62.2X3	T62.2X4	—	—
Sputum viscosity-lowering drug	T48.4X1	T48.4X2	T48.4X3	T48.4X4	T48.4X5	T48.4X6
Squill	T46.0X1	T46.0X2	T46.0X3	T46.0X4	T46.0X5	T46.0X6
rat poison	T60.4X1	T60.4X2	T60.4X3	T60.4X4	—	—
Squirting cucumber (cathartic)	T47.2X1	T47.2X2	T47.2X3	T47.2X4	T47.2X5	T47.2X6
Stains	T65.6X1	T65.6X2	T65.6X3	T65.6X4	—	—
Stannous fluoride	T49.7X1	T49.7X2	T49.7X3	T49.7X4	T49.7X5	T49.7X6
Stanolone	T38.7X1	T38.7X2	T38.7X3	T38.7X4	T38.7X5	T38.7X6

Substance	External Cause (T-Code)					
	Poisoning, Accidental (Unintentional)	Poisoning, Intentional Self-Harm	Poisoning, Assault	Poisoning, Undetermined	Adverse Effect	Underdosing
Stanozolol	T38.7X1	T38.7X2	T38.7X3	T38.7X4	T38.7X5	T38.7X6
Staphisagria or stavesacre (pediculicide)	T49.0X1	T49.0X2	T49.0X3	T49.0X4	T49.0X5	T49.0X6
Starch	T50.901	T50.902	T50.903	T50.904	T50.905	T50.906
Stelazine	T43.3X1	T43.3X2	T43.3X3	T43.3X4	T43.3X5	T43.3X6
Stemetil	T43.3X1	T43.3X2	T43.3X3	T43.3X4	T43.3X5	T43.3X6
Stepronin	T48.4X1	T48.4X2	T48.4X3	T48.4X4	T48.4X5	T48.4X6
Sterculia	T47.4X1	T47.4X2	T47.4X3	T47.4X4	T47.4X5	T47.4X6
Sternutator gas	T59.891	T59.892	T59.893	T59.894	—	—
Steroid	T38.0X1	T38.0X2	T38.0X3	T38.0X4	T38.0X5	T38.0X6
anabolic	T38.7X1	T38.7X2	T38.7X3	T38.7X4	T38.7X5	T38.7X6
androgenic	T38.7X1	T38.7X2	T38.7X3	T38.7X4	T38.7X5	T38.7X6
antineoplastic, hormone	T38.7X1	T38.7X2	T38.7X3	T38.7X4	T38.7X5	T38.7X6
estrogen	T38.5X1	T38.5X2	T38.5X3	T38.5X4	T38.5X5	T38.5X6
ENT agent	T49.6X1	T49.6X2	T49.6X3	T49.6X4	T49.6X5	T49.6X6
ophthalmic preparation	T49.5X1	T49.5X2	T49.5X3	T49.5X4	T49.5X5	T49.5X6
topical NEC	T49.0X1	T49.0X2	T49.0X3	T49.0X4	T49.0X5	T49.0X6
Stibine	T56.891	T56.892	T56.893	T56.894	—	—
Stibogluconate	T37.3X1	T37.3X2	T37.3X3	T37.3X4	T37.3X5	T37.3X6
Stibophen	T37.4X1	T37.4X2	T37.4X3	T37.4X4	T37.4X5	T37.4X6
Stilbamidine (isetionate)	T37.3X1	T37.3X2	T37.3X3	T37.3X4	T37.3X5	T37.3X6
Stilbestrol	T38.5X1	T38.5X2	T38.5X3	T38.5X4	T38.5X5	T38.5X6
Stilboestrol	T38.5X1	T38.5X2	T38.5X3	T38.5X4	T38.5X5	T38.5X6
Stimulant						
central nervous system — *see also Psychostimulant*	T43.601	T43.602	T43.603	T43.604	T43.605	T43.606
analeptics	T50.7X1	T50.7X2	T50.7X3	T50.7X4	T50.7X5	T50.7X6
opiate antagonist	T50.7X1	T50.7X2	T50.7X3	T50.7X4	T50.7X5	T50.7X6
psychotherapeutic NEC — *see also Psychotherapeutic drug*	T43.601	T43.602	T43.603	T43.604	T43.605	T43.606
specified NEC	T43.691	T43.692	T43.693	T43.694	T43.695	T43.696
respiratory	T48.901	T48.902	T48.903	T48.904	T48.905	T48.906
Stone-dissolving drug	T50.901	T50.902	T50.903	T50.904	T50.905	T50.906
Storage battery (cells) (acid)	T54.2X1	T54.2X2	T54.2X3	T54.2X4	—	—
Stovaine	T41.3X1	T41.3X2	T41.3X3	T41.3X4	T41.3X5	T41.3X6
infiltration (subcutaneous)	T41.3X1	T41.3X2	T41.3X3	T41.3X4	T41.3X5	T41.3X6
nerve block (peripheral) (plexus)	T41.3X1	T41.3X2	T41.3X3	T41.3X4	T41.3X5	T41.3X6
spinal	T41.3X1	T41.3X2	T41.3X3	T41.3X4	T41.3X5	T41.3X6
topical (surface)	T41.3X1	T41.3X2	T41.3X3	T41.3X4	T41.3X5	T41.3X6
Stovarsal	T37.8X1	T37.8X2	T37.8X3	T37.8X4	T37.8X5	T37.8X6
Stove gas — *see Gas, stove*	T57.91	T57.92	T57.93	T57.94	—	—

◀ New ◀ Revised ~~deleted~~ Deleted

Substance	External Cause (T-Code)					
	Poisoning, Accidental (Unintentional)	Poisoning, Intentional Self-Harm	Poisoning, Assault	Poisoning, Undetermined	Adverse Effect	Underdosing
Stoxil	T49.5X1	T49.5X2	T49.5X3	T49.5X4	T49.5X5	T49.5X6
Stramonium	T48.6X1	T48.6X2	T48.6X3	T48.6X4	T48.6X5	T48.6X6
natural state	T62.2X1	T62.2X2	T62.2X3	T62.2X4	—	—
Streptodornase	T45.3X1	T45.3X2	T45.3X3	T45.3X4	T45.3X5	T45.3X6
Streptoduocin	T36.5X1	T36.5X2	T36.5X3	T36.5X4	T36.5X5	T36.5X6
Streptokinase	T45.611	T45.612	T45.613	T45.614	T45.615	T45.616
Streptomycin (derivative)	T36.5X1	T36.5X2	T36.5X3	T36.5X4	T36.5X5	T36.5X6
Streptonivicin	T36.5X1	T36.5X2	T36.5X3	T36.5X4	T36.5X5	T36.5X6
Streptovarycin	T36.5X1	T36.5X2	T36.5X3	T36.5X4	T36.5X5	T36.5X6
Streptozocin	T45.1X1	T45.1X2	T45.1X3	T45.1X4	T45.1X5	T45.1X6
Streptozotocin	T45.1X1	T45.1X2	T45.1X3	T45.1X4	T45.1X5	T45.1X6
Stripper (paint) (solvent)	T52.8X1	T52.8X2	T52.8X3	T52.8X4	—	—
Strobane	T60.1X1	T60.1X2	T60.1X3	T60.1X4	—	—
Strofantina	T46.0X1	T46.0X2	T46.0X3	T46.0X4	T46.0X5	T46.0X6
Strophanthin (g) (k)	T46.0X1	T46.0X2	T46.0X3	T46.0X4	T46.0X5	T46.0X6
Strophanthus	T46.0X1	T46.0X2	T46.0X3	T46.0X4	T46.0X5	T46.0X6
Strophantin	T46.0X1	T46.0X2	T46.0X3	T46.0X4	T46.0X5	T46.0X6
Strophantin-g	T46.0X1	T46.0X2	T46.0X3	T46.0X4	T46.0X5	T46.0X6
Strychnine (nonmedicinal) (pesticide) (salts)	T65.1X1	T65.1X2	T65.1X3	T65.1X4	—	—
medicinal	T48.291	T48.292	T48.293	T48.294	T48.295	T48.296
Strychnos (ignatii) — *see Strychnine*						
Styramate	T42.8X1	T42.8X2	T42.8X3	T42.8X4	T42.8X5	T42.8X6
Styrene	T65.891	T65.892	T65.893	T65.894	—	—
Succinimide, antiepileptic or anticonvulsant	T42.2X1	T42.2X2	T42.2X3	T42.2X4	T42.2X5	T42.2X6
mercuric — *see Mercury*						
Succinylcholine	T48.1X1	T48.1X2	T48.1X3	T48.1X4	T48.1X5	T48.1X6
Succinylsulfathiazole	T37.0X1	T37.0X2	T37.0X3	T37.0X4	T37.0X5	T37.0X6
Sucralfate	T47.1X1	T47.1X2	T47.1X3	T47.1X4	T47.1X5	T47.1X6
Sucrose	T50.3X1	T50.3X2	T50.3X3	T50.3X4	T50.3X5	T50.3X6
Sufentanil	T40.4X1	T40.4X2	T40.4X3	T40.4X4	T40.4X5	T40.4X6
Sulbactam	T36.0X1	T36.0X2	T36.0X3	T36.0X4	T36.0X5	T36.0X6
Sulbenicillin	T36.0X1	T36.0X2	T36.0X3	T36.0X4	T36.0X5	T36.0X6
Sulbentine	T49.0X1	T49.0X2	T49.0X3	T49.0X4	T49.0X5	T49.0X6
Sulfacetamide	T49.0X1	T49.0X2	T49.0X3	T49.0X4	T49.0X5	T49.0X6
ophthalmic preparation	T49.5X1	T49.5X2	T49.5X3	T49.5X4	T49.5X5	T49.5X6
Sulfachlorpyridazine	T37.0X1	T37.0X2	T37.0X3	T37.0X4	T37.0X5	T37.0X6
Sulfacitine	T37.0X1	T37.0X2	T37.0X3	T37.0X4	T37.0X5	T37.0X6
Sulfadiasulfone sodium	T37.0X1	T37.0X2	T37.0X3	T37.0X4	T37.0X5	T37.0X6
Sulfadiazine	T37.0X1	T37.0X2	T37.0X3	T37.0X4	T37.0X5	T37.0X6
silver (topical)	T49.0X1	T49.0X2	T49.0X3	T49.0X4	T49.0X5	T49.0X6

Substance	External Cause (T-Code)					
	Poisoning, Accidental (Unintentional)	Poisoning, Intentional Self-Harm	Poisoning, Assault	Poisoning, Undetermined	Adverse Effect	Underdosing
Sulfadimethoxine	T37.0X1	T37.0X2	T37.0X3	T37.0X4	T37.0X5	T37.0X6
Sulfadimidine	T37.0X1	T37.0X2	T37.0X3	T37.0X4	T37.0X5	T37.0X6
Sulfadoxine	T37.0X1	T37.0X2	T37.0X3	T37.0X4	T37.0X5	T37.0X6
with pyrimethamine	T37.2X1	T37.2X2	T37.2X3	T37.2X4	T37.2X5	T37.2X6
Sulfaethidole	T37.0X1	T37.0X2	T37.0X3	T37.0X4	T37.0X5	T37.0X6
Sulfafurazole	T37.0X1	T37.0X2	T37.0X3	T37.0X4	T37.0X5	T37.0X6
Sulfaguanidine	T37.0X1	T37.0X2	T37.0X3	T37.0X4	T37.0X5	T37.0X6
Sulfalene	T37.0X1	T37.0X2	T37.0X3	T37.0X4	T37.0X5	T37.0X6
Sulfaloxate	T37.0X1	T37.0X2	T37.0X3	T37.0X4	T37.0X5	T37.0X6
Sulfaloxic acid	T37.0X1	T37.0X2	T37.0X3	T37.0X4	T37.0X5	T37.0X6
Sulfamazone	T39.2X1	T39.2X2	T39.2X3	T39.2X4	T39.2X5	T39.2X6
Sulfamerazine	T37.0X1	T37.0X2	T37.0X3	T37.0X4	T37.0X5	T37.0X6
Sulfameter	T37.0X1	T37.0X2	T37.0X3	T37.0X4	T37.0X5	T37.0X6
Sulfamethazine	T37.0X1	T37.0X2	T37.0X3	T37.0X4	T37.0X5	T37.0X6
Sulfamethizole	T37.0X1	T37.0X2	T37.0X3	T37.0X4	T37.0X5	T37.0X6
Sulfamethoxazole	T37.0X1	T37.0X2	T37.0X3	T37.0X4	T37.0X5	T37.0X6
with trimethoprim	T36.8X1	T36.8X2	T36.8X3	T36.8X4	T36.8X5	T36.8X6
Sulfamethoxydiazine	T37.0X1	T37.0X2	T37.0X3	T37.0X4	T37.0X5	T37.0X6
Sulfamethoxypyridazine	T37.0X1	T37.0X2	T37.0X3	T37.0X4	T37.0X5	T37.0X6
Sulfamethylthiazole	T37.0X1	T37.0X2	T37.0X3	T37.0X4	T37.0X5	T37.0X6
Sulfametoxydiazine	T37.0X1	T37.0X2	T37.0X3	T37.0X4	T37.0X5	T37.0X6
Sulfamidopyrine	T39.2X1	T39.2X2	T39.2X3	T39.2X4	T39.2X5	T39.2X6
Sulfamonomethoxine	T37.0X1	T37.0X2	T37.0X3	T37.0X4	T37.0X5	T37.0X6
Sulfamoxole	T37.0X1	T37.0X2	T37.0X3	T37.0X4	T37.0X5	T37.0X6
Sulfamylon	T49.0X1	T49.0X2	T49.0X3	T49.0X4	T49.0X5	T49.0X6
Sulfan blue (diagnostic dye)	T50.8X1	T50.8X2	T50.8X3	T50.8X4	T50.8X5	T50.8X6
Sulfanilamide	T37.0X1	T37.0X2	T37.0X3	T37.0X4	T37.0X5	T37.0X6
Sulfanilylguanidine	T37.0X1	T37.0X2	T37.0X3	T37.0X4	T37.0X5	T37.0X6
Sulfaperin	T37.0X1	T37.0X2	T37.0X3	T37.0X4	T37.0X5	T37.0X6
Sulfaphenazole	T37.0X1	T37.0X2	T37.0X3	T37.0X4	T37.0X5	T37.0X6
Sulfaphenylthiazole	T37.0X1	T37.0X2	T37.0X3	T37.0X4	T37.0X5	T37.0X6
Sulfaproxyline	T37.0X1	T37.0X2	T37.0X3	T37.0X4	T37.0X5	T37.0X6
Sulfapyridine	T37.0X1	T37.0X2	T37.0X3	T37.0X4	T37.0X5	T37.0X6
Sulfapyrimidine	T37.0X1	T37.0X2	T37.0X3	T37.0X4	T37.0X5	T37.0X6
Sulfarsphenamine	T37.8X1	T37.8X2	T37.8X3	T37.8X4	T37.8X5	T37.8X6
Sulfasalazine	T37.0X1	T37.0X2	T37.0X3	T37.0X4	T37.0X5	T37.0X6
Sulfasuxidine	T37.0X1	T37.0X2	T37.0X3	T37.0X4	T37.0X5	T37.0X6
Sulfasymazine	T37.0X1	T37.0X2	T37.0X3	T37.0X4	T37.0X5	T37.0X6
Sulfated amylopectin	T47.8X1	T47.8X2	T47.8X3	T47.8X4	T47.8X5	T47.8X6
Sulfathiazole	T37.0X1	T37.0X2	T37.0X3	T37.0X4	T37.0X5	T37.0X6
Sulfatostearate	T49.2X1	T49.2X2	T49.2X3	T49.2X4	T49.2X5	T49.2X6
Sulfinpyrazone	T50.4X1	T50.4X2	T50.4X3	T50.4X4	T50.4X5	T50.4X6

Substance	External Cause (T-Code)					
	Poisoning, Accidental (Unintentional)	Poisoning, Intentional Self-Harm	Poisoning, Assault	Poisoning, Undetermined	Adverse Effect	Underdosing
Sulfiram	T49.0X1	T49.0X2	T49.0X3	T49.0X4	T49.0X5	T49.0X6
Sulfisomidine	T37.0X1	T37.0X2	T37.0X3	T37.0X4	T37.0X5	T37.0X6
Sulfisoxazole	T37.0X1	T37.0X2	T37.0X3	T37.0X4	T37.0X5	T37.0X6
ophthalmic preparation	T49.5X1	T49.5X2	T49.5X3	T49.5X4	T49.5X5	T49.5X6
Sulfobromophthalein (sodium)	T50.8X1	T50.8X2	T50.8X3	T50.8X4	T50.8X5	T50.8X6
Sulfobromphthalein	T50.8X1	T50.8X2	T50.8X3	T50.8X4	T50.8X5	T50.8X6
Sulfogaiacol	T48.4X1	T48.4X2	T48.4X3	T48.4X4	T48.4X5	T48.4X6
Sulfomyxin	T36.8X1	T36.8X2	T36.8X3	T36.8X4	T36.8X5	T36.8X6
Sulfonal	T42.6X1	T42.6X2	T42.6X3	T42.6X4	T42.6X5	T42.6X6
Sulfonamide NEC	T37.0X1	T37.0X2	T37.0X3	T37.0X4	T37.0X5	T37.0X6
eye	T49.5X1	T49.5X2	T49.5X3	T49.5X4	T49.5X5	T49.5X6
Sulfonazide	T37.1X1	T37.1X2	T37.1X3	T37.1X4	T37.1X5	T37.1X6
Sulfones	T37.1X1	T37.1X2	T37.1X3	T37.1X4	T37.1X5	T37.1X6
Sulfonethylmethane	T42.6X1	T42.6X2	T42.6X3	T42.6X4	T42.6X5	T42.6X6
Sulfonmethane	T42.6X1	T42.6X2	T42.6X3	T42.6X4	T42.6X5	T42.6X6
Sulfonphthal, sulfonphthol	T50.8X1	T50.8X2	T50.8X3	T50.8X4	T50.8X5	T50.8X6
Sulfonylurea derivatives, oral	T38.3X1	T38.3X2	T38.3X3	T38.3X4	T38.3X5	T38.3X6
Sulforidazine	T43.3X1	T43.3X2	T43.3X3	T43.3X4	T43.3X5	T43.3X6
Sulfoxone	T37.1X1	T37.1X2	T37.1X3	T37.1X4	T37.1X5	T37.1X6
Sulfur, sulfurated, sulfuric, sulfurous, sulfuryl (compounds NEC) (medicinal)	T49.4X1	T49.4X2	T49.4X3	T49.4X4	T49.4X5	T49.4X6
acid	T54.2X1	T54.2X2	T54.2X3	T54.2X4	—	—
dioxide (gas)	T59.1X1	T59.1X2	T59.1X3	T59.1X4	—	—
ether — *see Ether(s)*						
hydrogen	T59.6X1	T59.6X2	T59.6X3	T59.6X4	—	—
medicinal (keratolytic) (ointment) NEC	T49.4X1	T49.4X2	T49.4X3	T49.4X4	T49.4X5	T49.4X6
ointment	T49.0X1	T49.0X2	T49.0X3	T49.0X4	T49.0X5	T49.0X6
pesticide (vapor)	T60.91	T60.92	T60.93	T60.94	—	—
vapor NEC	T59.891	T59.892	T59.893	T59.894	—	—
Sulfuric acid	T54.2X1	T54.2X2	T54.2X3	T54.2X4	—	—
Sulglicotide	T47.1X1	T47.1X2	T47.1X3	T47.1X4	T47.1X5	T47.1X6
Sulindac	T39.391	T39.392	T39.393	T39.394	T39.395	T39.396
Sulisatin	T47.2X1	T47.2X2	T47.2X3	T47.2X4	T47.2X5	T47.2X6
Sulisobenzone	T49.3X1	T49.3X2	T49.3X3	T49.3X4	T49.3X5	T49.3X6
Sulkowitch's reagent	T50.8X1	T50.8X2	T50.8X3	T50.8X4	T50.8X5	T50.8X6
Sulmetozine	T44.3X1	T44.3X2	T44.3X3	T44.3X4	T44.3X5	T44.3X6
Suloctidil	T46.7X1	T46.7X2	T46.7X3	T46.7X4	T46.7X5	T46.7X6
Sulph — *see also Sulf-*						
Sulphadiazine	T37.0X1	T37.0X2	T37.0X3	T37.0X4	T37.0X5	T37.0X6

Substance	External Cause (T-Code)					
	Poisoning, Accidental (Unintentional)	Poisoning, Intentional Self-Harm	Poisoning, Assault	Poisoning, Undetermined	Adverse Effect	Underdosing
Sulphadimethoxine	T37.0X1	T37.0X2	T37.0X3	T37.0X4	T37.0X5	T37.0X6
Sulphadimidine	T37.0X1	T37.0X2	T37.0X3	T37.0X4	T37.0X5	T37.0X6
Sulphadione	T37.1X1	T37.1X2	T37.1X3	T37.1X4	T37.1X5	T37.1X6
Sulphafurazole	T37.0X1	T37.0X2	T37.0X3	T37.0X4	T37.0X5	T37.0X6
Sulphamethizole	T37.0X1	T37.0X2	T37.0X3	T37.0X4	T37.0X5	T37.0X6
Sulphamethoxazole	T37.0X1	T37.0X2	T37.0X3	T37.0X4	T37.0X5	T37.0X6
Sulphan blue	T50.8X1	T50.8X2	T50.8X3	T50.8X4	T50.8X5	T50.8X6
Sulphaphenazole	T37.0X1	T37.0X2	T37.0X3	T37.0X4	T37.0X5	T37.0X6
Sulphapyridine	T37.0X1	T37.0X2	T37.0X3	T37.0X4	T37.0X5	T37.0X6
Sulphasalazine	T37.0X1	T37.0X2	T37.0X3	T37.0X4	T37.0X5	T37.0X6
Sulphinpyrazone	T50.4X1	T50.4X2	T50.4X3	T50.4X4	T50.4X5	T50.4X6
Sulpiride	T43.591	T43.592	T43.593	T43.594	T43.595	T43.596
Sulprostone	T48.0X1	T48.0X2	T48.0X3	T48.0X4	T48.0X5	T48.0X6
Sulpyrine	T39.2X1	T39.2X2	T39.2X3	T39.2X4	T39.2X5	T39.2X6
Sultamicillin	T36.0X1	T36.0X2	T36.0X3	T36.0X4	T36.0X5	T36.0X6
Sulthiame	T42.6X1	T42.6X2	T42.6X3	T42.6X4	T42.6X5	T42.6X6
Sultiame	T42.6X1	T42.6X2	T42.6X3	T42.6X4	T42.6X5	T42.6X6
Sultopride	T43.591	T43.592	T43.593	T43.594	T43.595	T43.596
Sumatriptan	T39.8X1	T39.8X2	T39.8X3	T39.8X4	T39.8X5	T39.8X6
Sunflower seed oil	T46.6X1	T46.6X2	T46.6X3	T46.6X4	T46.6X5	T46.6X6
Superinone	T48.4X1	T48.4X2	T48.4X3	T48.4X4	T48.4X5	T48.4X6
Suprofen	T39.311	T39.312	T39.313	T39.314	T39.315	T39.316
Suramin (sodium)	T37.4X1	T37.4X2	T37.4X3	T37.4X4	T37.4X5	T37.4X6
Surfacaine	T41.3X1	T41.3X2	T41.3X3	T41.3X4	T41.3X5	T41.3X6
Surital	T41.1X1	T41.1X2	T41.1X3	T41.1X4	T41.1X5	T41.1X6
Sutilains	T45.3X1	T45.3X2	T45.3X3	T45.3X4	T45.3X5	T45.3X6
Suxamethonium (chloride)	T48.1X1	T48.1X2	T48.1X3	T48.1X4	T48.1X5	T48.1X6
Suxethonium (chloride)	T48.1X1	T48.1X2	T48.1X3	T48.1X4	T48.1X5	T48.1X6
Suxibuzone	T39.2X1	T39.2X2	T39.2X3	T39.2X4	T39.2X5	T39.2X6
Sweet oil (birch)	T49.3X1	T49.3X2	T49.3X3	T49.3X4	T49.3X5	T49.3X6
Sweet niter spirit	T46.3X1	T46.3X2	T46.3X3	T46.3X4	T46.3X5	T46.3X6
Sweetener	T50.901	T50.902	T50.903	T50.904	T50.905	T50.906
Sym-dichloroethyl ether	T53.6X1	T53.6X2	T53.6X3	T53.6X4	—	—
Sympatholytic NEC	T44.8X1	T44.8X2	T44.8X3	T44.8X4	T44.8X5	T44.8X6
haloalkylamine	T44.8X1	T44.8X2	T44.8X3	T44.8X4	T44.8X5	T44.8X6
Sympathomimetic NEC	T44.901	T44.902	T44.903	T44.904	T44.905	T44.906
anti-common-cold	T48.5X1	T48.5X2	T48.5X3	T48.5X4	T48.5X5	T48.5X6
bronchodilator	T48.6X1	T48.6X2	T48.6X3	T48.6X4	T48.6X5	T48.6X6
specified NEC	T44.991	T44.992	T44.993	T44.994	T44.995	T44.996
Synagis	T50.B91	T50.B92	T50.B93	T50.B94	T50.B95	T50.B96
Synalar	T49.0X1	T49.0X2	T49.0X3	T49.0X4	T49.0X5	T49.0X6
Synthroid	T38.1X1	T38.1X2	T38.1X3	T38.1X4	T38.1X5	T38.1X6

Substance	External Cause (T-Code)					
	Poisoning, Accidental (Unintentional)	Poisoning, Intentional Self-Harm	Poisoning, Assault	Poisoning, Undetermined	Adverse Effect	Underdosing
Syntocinon	T48.0X1	T48.0X2	T48.0X3	T48.0X4	T48.0X5	T48.0X6
Syrosingopine	T46.5X1	T46.5X2	T46.5X3	T46.5X4	T46.5X5	T46.5X6
Systemic drug	T45.91	T45.92	T45.93	T45.94	T45.95	T45.96
specified NEC	T45.8X1	T45.8X2	T45.8X3	T45.8X4	T45.8X5	T45.8X6
2,4,5-T	T60.3X1	T60.3X2	T60.3X3	T60.3X4	—	—
T						
Tablets — *see also specified substance*	T50.901	T50.902	T50.903	T50.904	T50.905	T50.906
Tace	T38.5X1	T38.5X2	T38.5X3	T38.5X4	T38.5X5	T38.5X6
Tacrine	T44.0X1	T44.0X2	T44.0X3	T44.0X4	T44.0X5	T44.0X6
Tadalafil	T46.7X1	T46.7X2	T46.7X3	T46.7X4	T46.7X5	T46.7X6
Talampicillin	T36.0X1	T36.0X2	T36.0X3	T36.0X4	T36.0X5	T36.0X6
Talbutal	T42.3X1	T42.3X2	T42.3X3	T42.3X4	T42.3X5	T42.3X6
Talc powder	T49.3X1	T49.3X2	T49.3X3	T49.3X4	T49.3X5	T49.3X6
Talcum	T49.3X1	T49.3X2	T49.3X3	T49.3X4	T49.3X5	T49.3X6
Taleranol	T38.6X1	T38.6X2	T38.6X3	T38.6X4	T38.6X5	T38.6X6
Tamoxifen	T38.6X1	T38.6X2	T38.6X3	T38.6X4	T38.6X5	T38.6X6
Tamsulosin	T44.6X1	T44.6X2	T44.6X3	T44.6X4	T44.6X5	T44.6X6
Tandearil, tanderil	T39.2X1	T39.2X2	T39.2X3	T39.2X4	T39.2X5	T39.2X6
Tannic acid	T49.2X1	T49.2X2	T49.2X3	T49.2X4	T49.2X5	T49.2X6
medicinal (astringent)	T49.2X1	T49.2X2	T49.2X3	T49.2X4	T49.2X5	T49.2X6
Tannin — *see Tannic acid*						
Tansy	T62.2X1	T62.2X2	T62.2X3	T62.2X4	—	—
TAO	T36.3X1	T36.3X2	T36.3X3	T36.3X4	T36.3X5	T36.3X6
Tapazole	T38.2X1	T38.2X2	T38.2X3	T38.2X4	T38.2X5	T38.2X6
Tar NEC	T52.0X1	T52.0X2	T52.0X3	T52.0X4	—	—
camphor	T60.1X1	T60.1X2	T60.1X3	T60.1X4	—	—
distillate	T49.1X1	T49.1X2	T49.1X3	T49.1X4	T49.1X5	T49.1X6
fumes	T59.891	T59.892	T59.893	T59.894	—	—
medicinal	T49.1X1	T49.1X2	T49.1X3	T49.1X4	T49.1X5	T49.1X6
ointment	T49.1X1	T49.1X2	T49.1X3	T49.1X4	T49.1X5	T49.1X6
Taractan	T43.591	T43.592	T43.593	T43.594	T43.595	T43.596
Tarantula (venomous)	T63.321	T63.322	T63.323	T63.324	—	—
Tartar emetic	T37.8X1	T37.8X2	T37.8X3	T37.8X4	T37.8X5	T37.8X6
Tartaric acid	T65.891	T65.892	T65.893	T65.894	—	—
Tartrated antimony (anti-infective)	T37.8X1	T37.8X2	T37.8X3	T37.8X4	T37.8X5	T37.8X6
Tartrate, laxative	T47.4X1	T47.4X2	T47.4X3	T47.4X4	T47.4X5	T47.4X6
Tauromustine	T45.1X1	T45.1X2	T45.1X3	T45.1X4	T45.1X5	T45.1X6
TCA — *see Trichloroacetic acid*						
TCDD	T53.7X1	T53.7X2	T53.7X3	T53.7X4	—	—
TDI (vapor)	T65.0X1	T65.0X2	T65.0X3	T65.0X4	—	—

Substance	External Cause (T-Code)					
	Poisoning, Accidental (Unintentional)	Poisoning, Intentional Self-Harm	Poisoning, Assault	Poisoning, Undetermined	Adverse Effect	Underdosing
Tear						
gas	T59.3X1	T59.3X2	T59.3X3	T59.3X4	—	—
solution	T49.5X1	T49.5X2	T49.5X3	T49.5X4	T49.5X5	T49.5X6
Teclothiazide	T50.2X1	T50.2X2	T50.2X3	T50.2X4	T50.2X5	T50.2X6
Teclozan	T37.3X1	T37.3X2	T37.3X3	T37.3X4	T37.3X5	T37.3X6
Tegafur	T45.1X1	T45.1X2	T45.1X3	T45.1X4	T45.1X5	T45.1X6
Tegretol	T42.1X1	T42.1X2	T42.1X3	T42.1X4	T42.1X5	T42.1X6
Teicoplanin	T36.8X1	T36.8X2	T36.8X3	T36.8X4	T36.8X5	T36.8X6
Telepaque	T50.8X1	T50.8X2	T50.8X3	T50.8X4	T50.8X5	T50.8X6
Tellurium	T56.891	T56.892	T56.893	T56.894	—	—
fumes	T56.891	T56.892	T56.893	T56.894	—	—
TEM	T45.1X1	T45.1X2	T45.1X3	T45.1X4	T45.1X5	T45.1X6
Temazepam	T42.4X1	T42.4X2	T42.4X3	T42.4X4	T42.4X5	T42.4X6
Temocillin	T36.0X1	T36.0X2	T36.0X3	T36.0X4	T36.0X5	T36.0X6
Tenamfetamine	T43.621	T43.622	T43.623	T43.624	T43.625	T43.626
Teniposide	T45.1X1	T45.1X2	T45.1X3	T45.1X4	T45.1X5	T45.1X6
Tenitramine	T46.3X1	T46.3X2	T46.3X3	T46.3X4	T46.3X5	T46.3X6
Tenoglicin	T48.4X1	T48.4X2	T48.4X3	T48.4X4	T48.4X5	T48.4X6
Tenonitrozole	T37.3X1	T37.3X2	T37.3X3	T37.3X4	T37.3X5	T37.3X6
Tenoxicam	T39.391	T39.392	T39.393	T39.394	T39.395	T39.396
TEPA	T45.1X1	T45.1X2	T45.1X3	T45.1X4	T45.1X5	T45.1X6
TEPP	T60.0X1	T60.0X2	T60.0X3	T60.0X4	—	—
Teprotide	T46.5X1	T46.5X2	T46.5X3	T46.5X4	T46.5X5	T46.5X6
Terazosin	T44.6X1	T44.6X2	T44.6X3	T44.6X4	T44.6X5	T44.6X6
Terbufos	T60.0X1	T60.0X2	T60.0X3	T60.0X4	—	—
Terbutaline	T48.6X1	T48.6X2	T48.6X3	T48.6X4	T48.6X5	T48.6X6
Terconazole	T49.0X1	T49.0X2	T49.0X3	T49.0X4	T49.0X5	T49.0X6
Terfenadine	T45.0X1	T45.0X2	T45.0X3	T45.0X4	T45.0X5	T45.0X6
Teriparatide (acetate)	T50.991	T50.992	T50.993	T50.994	T50.995	T50.996
Terizidone	T37.1X1	T37.1X2	T37.1X3	T37.1X4	T37.1X5	T37.1X6
Terlipressin	T38.891	T38.892	T38.893	T38.894	T38.895	T38.896
Terodiline	T46.3X1	T46.3X2	T46.3X3	T46.3X4	T46.3X5	T46.3X6
Teroxalene	T37.4X1	T37.4X2	T37.4X3	T37.4X4	T37.4X5	T37.4X6
Terpin(cis) hydrate	T48.4X1	T48.4X2	T48.4X3	T48.4X4	T48.4X5	T48.4X6
Terramycin	T36.4X1	T36.4X2	T36.4X3	T36.4X4	T36.4X5	T36.4X6
Tertatolol	T44.7X1	T44.7X2	T44.7X3	T44.7X4	T44.7X5	T44.7X6
Tessalon	T48.3X1	T48.3X2	T48.3X3	T48.3X4	T48.3X5	T48.3X6
Testolactone	T38.7X1	T38.7X2	T38.7X3	T38.7X4	T38.7X5	T38.7X6
Testosterone	T38.7X1	T38.7X2	T38.7X3	T38.7X4	T38.7X5	T38.7X6
Tetanus toxoid or vaccine	T50.A91	T50.A92	T50.A93	T50.A94	T50.A95	T50.A96
antitoxin	T50.Z11	T50.Z12	T50.Z13	T50.Z14	T50.Z15	T50.Z16
immune globulin (human)	T50.Z11	T50.Z12	T50.Z13	T50.Z14	T50.Z15	T50.Z16

Substance	External Cause (T-Code)					
	Poisoning, Accidental (Unintentional)	Poisoning, Intentional Self-Harm	Poisoning, Assault	Poisoning, Undetermined	Adverse Effect	Underdosing
Tetanus toxoid or vaccine *(Continued)*						
toxoid	T50.A91	T50.A92	T50.A93	T50.A94	T50.A95	T50.A96
with diphtheria toxoid	T50.A21	T50.A22	T50.A23	T50.A24	T50.A25	T50.A26
with pertussis	T50.A11	T50.A12	T50.A13	T50.A14	T50.A15	T50.A16
Tetrabenazine	T43.591	T43.592	T43.593	T43.594	T43.595	T43.596
Tetracaine	T41.3X1	T41.3X2	T41.3X3	T41.3X4	T41.3X5	T41.3X6
nerve block (peripheral) (plexus)	T41.3X1	T41.3X2	T41.3X3	T41.3X4	T41.3X5	T41.3X6
regional	T41.3X1	T41.3X2	T41.3X3	T41.3X4	T41.3X5	T41.3X6
spinal	T41.3X1	T41.3X2	T41.3X3	T41.3X4	T41.3X5	T41.3X6
Tetrachlorethylene — *see Tetrachloroethylene*						
Tetrachlormethiazide	T50.2X1	T50.2X2	T50.2X3	T50.2X4	T50.2X5	T50.2X6
2,3,7,8-Tetrachlorodibenzo-p-dioxin	T53.7X1	T53.7X2	T53.7X3	T53.7X4	—	—
Tetrachloroethane	T53.6X1	T53.6X2	T53.6X3	T53.6X4	—	—
vapor	T53.6X1	T53.6X2	T53.6X3	T53.6X4	—	—
paint or varnish	T53.6X1	T53.6X2	T53.6X3	T53.6X4	—	—
Tetrachloroethylene (liquid)	T53.3X1	T53.3X2	T53.3X3	T53.3X4	—	—
medicinal	T37.4X1	T37.4X2	T37.4X3	T37.4X4	T37.4X5	T37.4X6
vapor	T53.3X1	T53.3X2	T53.3X3	T53.3X4	—	—
Tetrachloromethane — *see Carbon tetrachloride*						
Tetracosactide	T38.811	T38.812	T38.813	T38.814	T38.815	T38.816
Tetracosactrin	T38.811	T38.812	T38.813	T38.814	T38.815	T38.816
Tetracycline	T36.4X1	T36.4X2	T36.4X3	T36.4X4	T36.4X5	T36.4X6
ophthalmic preparation	T49.5X1	T49.5X2	T49.5X3	T49.5X4	T49.5X5	T49.5X6
topical NEC	T49.0X1	T49.0X2	T49.0X3	T49.0X4	T49.0X5	T49.0X6
Tetradifon	T60.8X1	T60.8X2	T60.8X3	T60.8X4	—	—
Tetradotoxin	T61.771	T61.772	T61.773	T61.774	—	—
Tetraethyl						
lead	T56.0X1	T56.0X2	T56.0X3	T56.0X4	—	—
pyrophosphate	T60.0X1	T60.0X2	T60.0X3	T60.0X4	—	—
Tetraethylammonium chloride	T44.2X1	T44.2X2	T44.2X3	T44.2X4	T44.2X5	T44.2X6
Tetraethylthiuram disulfide	T50.6X1	T50.6X2	T50.6X3	T50.6X4	T50.6X5	T50.6X6
Tetrahydroaminoacridine	T44.0X1	T44.0X2	T44.0X3	T44.0X4	T44.0X5	T44.0X6
Tetrahydrocannabinol	T40.7X1	T40.7X2	T40.7X3	T40.7X4	T40.7X5	T40.7X6
Tetrahydrofuran	T52.8X1	T52.8X2	T52.8X3	T52.8X4	—	—
Tetrahydronaphthalene	T52.8X1	T52.8X2	T52.8X3	T52.8X4	—	—
Tetrahydrozoline	T49.5X1	T49.5X2	T49.5X3	T49.5X4	T49.5X5	T49.5X6
Tetralin	T52.8X1	T52.8X2	T52.8X3	T52.8X4	—	—
Tetramethrin	T60.2X1	T60.2X2	T60.2X3	T60.2X4	—	—

Substance	External Cause (T-Code)					
	Poisoning, Accidental (Unintentional)	Poisoning, Intentional Self-Harm	Poisoning, Assault	Poisoning, Undetermined	Adverse Effect	Underdosing
Tetramethylthiuram (disulfide) NEC	T60.3X1	T60.3X2	T60.3X3	T60.3X4	—	—
medicinal	T49.0X1	T49.0X2	T49.0X3	T49.0X4	T49.0X5	T49.0X6
Tetramisole	T37.4X1	T37.4X2	T37.4X3	T37.4X4	T37.4X5	T37.4X6
Tetranicotinoyl fructose	T46.7X1	T46.7X2	T46.7X3	T46.7X4	T46.7X5	T46.7X6
Tetronal	T42.6X1	T42.6X2	T42.6X3	T42.6X4	T42.6X5	T42.6X6
Tetrazepam	T42.4X1	T42.4X2	T42.4X3	T42.4X4	T42.4X5	T42.4X6
Tetryl	T65.3X1	T65.3X2	T65.3X3	T65.3X4	—	—
Tetrylammonium chloride	T44.2X1	T44.2X2	T44.2X3	T44.2X4	T44.2X5	T44.2X6
Tetryzoline	T49.5X1	T49.5X2	T49.5X3	T49.5X4	T49.5X5	T49.5X6
Thalidomide	T45.1X1	T45.1X2	T45.1X3	T45.1X4	T45.1X5	T45.1X6
Thallium (compounds) (dust) NEC	T56.811	T56.812	T56.813	T56.814	—	—
pesticide	T60.4X1	T60.4X2	T60.4X3	T60.4X4	—	—
THC	T40.7X1	T40.7X2	T40.7X3	T40.7X4	T40.7X5	T40.7X6
Thebacon	T48.3X1	T48.3X2	T48.3X3	T48.3X4	T48.3X5	T48.3X6
Thebaine	T40.2X1	T40.2X2	T40.2X3	T40.2X4	T40.2X5	T40.2X6
Thenoic acid	T49.6X1	T49.6X2	T49.6X3	T49.6X4	T49.6X5	T49.6X6
Thenyldiamine	T45.0X1	T45.0X2	T45.0X3	T45.0X4	T45.0X5	T45.0X6
Theobromine (calcium salicylate)	T48.6X1	T48.6X2	T48.6X3	T48.6X4	T48.6X5	T48.6X6
sodium salicylate	T48.6X1	T48.6X2	T48.6X3	T48.6X4	T48.6X5	T48.6X6
Theophyllamine	T48.6X1	T48.6X2	T48.6X3	T48.6X4	T48.6X5	T48.6X6
Theophylline	T48.6X1	T48.6X2	T48.6X3	T48.6X4	T48.6X5	T48.6X6
aminobenzoic acid	T48.6X1	T48.6X2	T48.6X3	T48.6X4	T48.6X5	T48.6X6
ethylenediamine	T48.6X1	T48.6X2	T48.6X3	T48.6X4	T48.6X5	T48.6X6
piperazine p-amino-benzoate	T48.6X1	T48.6X2	T48.6X3	T48.6X4	T48.6X5	T48.6X6
Thiabendazole	T37.4X1	T37.4X2	T37.4X3	T37.4X4	T37.4X5	T37.4X6
Thialbarbital	T41.1X1	T41.1X2	T41.1X3	T41.1X4	T41.1X5	T41.1X6
Thiamazole	T38.2X1	T38.2X2	T38.2X3	T38.2X4	T38.2X5	T38.2X6
Thiambutosine	T37.1X1	T37.1X2	T37.1X3	T37.1X4	T37.1X5	T37.1X6
Thiamine	T45.2X1	T45.2X2	T45.2X3	T45.2X4	T45.2X5	T45.2X6
Thiamphenicol	T36.2X1	T36.2X2	T36.2X3	T36.2X4	T36.2X5	T36.2X6
Thiamylal	T41.1X1	T41.1X2	T41.1X3	T41.1X4	T41.1X5	T41.1X6
sodium	T41.1X1	T41.1X2	T41.1X3	T41.1X4	T41.1X5	T41.1X6
Thiazesim	T43.291	T43.292	T43.293	T43.294	T43.295	T43.296
Thiazides (diuretics)	T50.2X1	T50.2X2	T50.2X3	T50.2X4	T50.2X5	T50.2X6
Thiazinamium metilsulfate	T43.3X1	T43.3X2	T43.3X3	T43.3X4	T43.3X5	T43.3X6
Thiethylperazine	T43.3X1	T43.3X2	T43.3X3	T43.3X4	T43.3X5	T43.3X6
Thimerosal	T49.0X1	T49.0X2	T49.0X3	T49.0X4	T49.0X5	T49.0X6
ophthalmic preparation	T49.5X1	T49.5X2	T49.5X3	T49.5X4	T49.5X5	T49.5X6
Thioacetazone	T37.1X1	T37.1X2	T37.1X3	T37.1X4	T37.1X5	T37.1X6
with isoniazid	T37.1X1	T37.1X2	T37.1X3	T37.1X4	T37.1X5	T37.1X6
Thiobarbital sodium	T41.1X1	T41.1X2	T41.1X3	T41.1X4	T41.1X5	T41.1X6

◀ New ⟸ Revised ~~deleted~~ Deleted

Substance	External Cause (T-Code)					
	Poisoning, Accidental (Unintentional)	Poisoning, Intentional Self-Harm	Poisoning, Assault	Poisoning, Undetermined	Adverse Effect	Underdosing
Thiobarbiturate anesthetic	T41.1X1	T41.1X2	T41.1X3	T41.1X4	T41.1X5	T41.1X6
Thiobismol	T37.8X1	T37.8X2	T37.8X3	T37.8X4	T37.8X5	T37.8X6
Thiobutabarbital sodium	T41.1X1	T41.1X2	T41.1X3	T41.1X4	T41.1X5	T41.1X6
Thiocarbamate (insecticide)	T60.0X1	T60.0X2	T60.0X3	T60.0X4	—	—
Thiocarbamide	T38.2X1	T38.2X2	T38.2X3	T38.2X4	T38.2X5	T38.2X6
Thiocarbarsone	T37.8X1	T37.8X2	T37.8X3	T37.8X4	T37.8X5	T37.8X6
Thiocarlide	T37.1X1	T37.1X2	T37.1X3	T37.1X4	T37.1X5	T37.1X6
Thioctamide	T50.991	T50.992	T50.993	T50.994	T50.995	T50.996
Thioctic acid	T50.991	T50.992	T50.993	T50.994	T50.995	T50.996
Thiofos	T60.0X1	T60.0X2	T60.0X3	T60.0X4	—	—
Thioglycolate	T49.4X1	T49.4X2	T49.4X3	T49.4X4	T49.4X5	T49.4X6
Thioglycolic acid	T65.891	T65.892	T65.893	T65.894	—	—
Thioguanine	T45.1X1	T45.1X2	T45.1X3	T45.1X4	T45.1X5	T45.1X6
Thiomercaptomerin	T50.2X1	T50.2X2	T50.2X3	T50.2X4	T50.2X5	T50.2X6
Thiomerin	T50.2X1	T50.2X2	T50.2X3	T50.2X4	T50.2X5	T50.2X6
Thiomersal	T49.0X1	T49.0X2	T49.0X3	T49.0X4	T49.0X5	T49.0X6
Thionazin	T60.0X1	T60.0X2	T60.0X3	T60.0X4	—	—
Thiopental (sodium)	T41.1X1	T41.1X2	T41.1X3	T41.1X4	T41.1X5	T41.1X6
Thiopentone (sodium)	T41.1X1	T41.1X2	T41.1X3	T41.1X4	T41.1X5	T41.1X6
Thiopropazate	T43.3X1	T43.3X2	T43.3X3	T43.3X4	T43.3X5	T43.3X6
Thioproperazine	T43.3X1	T43.3X2	T43.3X3	T43.3X4	T43.3X5	T43.3X6
Thioridazine	T43.3X1	T43.3X2	T43.3X3	T43.3X4	T43.3X5	T43.3X6
Thiosinamine	T49.3X1	T49.3X2	T49.3X3	T49.3X4	T49.3X5	T49.3X6
Thiotepa	T45.1X1	T45.1X2	T45.1X3	T45.1X4	T45.1X5	T45.1X6
Thiothixene	T43.4X1	T43.4X2	T43.4X3	T43.4X4	T43.4X5	T43.4X6
Thiouracil (benzyl) (methyl) (propyl)	T38.2X1	T38.2X2	T38.2X3	T38.2X4	T38.2X5	T38.2X6
Thiourea	T38.2X1	T38.2X2	T38.2X3	T38.2X4	T38.2X5	T38.2X6
Thiphenamil	T44.3X1	T44.3X2	T44.3X3	T44.3X4	T44.3X5	T44.3X6
Thiram	T60.3X1	T60.3X2	T60.3X3	T60.3X4	—	—
medicinal	T49.2X1	T49.2X2	T49.2X3	T49.2X4	T49.2X5	T49.2X6
Thonzylamine (systemic)	T45.0X1	T45.0X2	T45.0X3	T45.0X4	T45.0X5	T45.0X6
mucosal decongestant	T48.5X1	T48.5X2	T48.5X3	T48.5X4	T48.5X5	T48.5X6
Thorazine	T43.3X1	T43.3X2	T43.3X3	T43.3X4	T43.3X5	T43.3X6
Thorium dioxide suspension	T50.8X1	T50.8X2	T50.8X3	T50.8X4	T50.8X5	T50.8X6
Thornapple	T62.2X1	T62.2X2	T62.2X3	T62.2X4	—	—
Throat drug NEC	T49.6X1	T49.6X2	T49.6X3	T49.6X4	T49.6X5	T49.6X6
Thrombin	T45.7X1	T45.7X2	T45.7X3	T45.7X4	T45.7X5	T45.7X6
Thrombolysin	T45.611	T45.612	T45.613	T45.614	T45.615	T45.616
Thromboplastin	T45.7X1	T45.7X2	T45.7X3	T45.7X4	T45.7X5	T45.7X6
Thurfyl nicotinate	T46.7X1	T46.7X2	T46.7X3	T46.7X4	T46.7X5	T46.7X6
Thymol	T49.0X1	T49.0X2	T49.0X3	T49.0X4	T49.0X5	T49.0X6

Substance	External Cause (T-Code)					
	Poisoning, Accidental (Unintentional)	Poisoning, Intentional Self-Harm	Poisoning, Assault	Poisoning, Undetermined	Adverse Effect	Underdosing
Thymopentin	T37.5X1	T37.5X2	T37.5X3	T37.5X4	T37.5X5	T37.5X6
Thymoxamine	T46.7X1	T46.7X2	T46.7X3	T46.7X4	T46.7X5	T46.7X6
Thymus extract	T38.891	T38.892	T38.893	T38.894	T38.895	T38.896
Thyreotrophic hormone	T38.811	T38.812	T38.813	T38.814	T38.815	T38.816
Thyroglobulin	T38.1X1	T38.1X2	T38.1X3	T38.1X4	T38.1X5	T38.1X6
Thyroid (hormone)	T38.1X1	T38.1X2	T38.1X3	T38.1X4	T38.1X5	T38.1X6
Thyrolar	T38.1X1	T38.1X2	T38.1X3	T38.1X4	T38.1X5	T38.1X6
Thyrotrophin	T38.811	T38.812	T38.813	T38.814	T38.815	T38.816
Thyrotropic hormone	T38.811	T38.812	T38.813	T38.814	T38.815	T38.816
Thyroxine	T38.1X1	T38.1X2	T38.1X3	T38.1X4	T38.1X5	T38.1X6
Tiabendazole	T37.4X1	T37.4X2	T37.4X3	T37.4X4	T37.4X5	T37.4X6
Tiamizide	T50.2X1	T50.2X2	T50.2X3	T50.2X4	T50.2X5	T50.2X6
Tianeptine	T43.291	T43.292	T43.293	T43.294	T43.295	T43.296
Tiapamil	T46.1X1	T46.1X2	T46.1X3	T46.1X4	T46.1X5	T46.1X6
Tiapride	T43.591	T43.592	T43.593	T43.594	T43.595	T43.596
Tiaprofenic acid	T39.311	T39.312	T39.313	T39.314	T39.315	T39.316
Tiaramide	T39.8X1	T39.8X2	T39.8X3	T39.8X4	T39.8X5	T39.8X6
Ticarcillin	T36.0X1	T36.0X2	T36.0X3	T36.0X4	T36.0X5	T36.0X6
Ticlatone	T49.0X1	T49.0X2	T49.0X3	T49.0X4	T49.0X5	T49.0X6
Ticlopidine	T45.521	T45.522	T45.523	T45.524	T45.525	T45.526
Ticrynafen	T50.1X1	T50.1X2	T50.1X3	T50.1X4	T50.1X5	T50.1X6
Tidiacic	T50.991	T50.992	T50.993	T50.994	T50.995	T50.996
Tiemonium	T44.3X1	T44.3X2	T44.3X3	T44.3X4	T44.3X5	T44.3X6
iodide	T44.3X1	T44.3X2	T44.3X3	T44.3X4	T44.3X5	T44.3X6
Tienilic acid	T50.1X1	T50.1X2	T50.1X3	T50.1X4	T50.1X5	T50.1X6
Tifenamil	T44.3X1	T44.3X2	T44.3X3	T44.3X4	T44.3X5	T44.3X6
Tigan	T45.0X1	T45.0X2	T45.0X3	T45.0X4	T45.0X5	T45.0X6
Tigloidine	T44.3X1	T44.3X2	T44.3X3	T44.3X4	T44.3X5	T44.3X6
Tilactase	T47.5X1	T47.5X2	T47.5X3	T47.5X4	T47.5X5	T47.5X6
Tiletamine	T41.291	T41.292	T41.293	T41.294	T41.295	T41.296
Tilidine	T40.4X1	T40.4X2	T40.4X3	T40.4X4	—	—
Timepidium bromide	T44.3X1	T44.3X2	T44.3X3	T44.3X4	T44.3X5	T44.3X6
Timiperone	T43.4X1	T43.4X2	T43.4X3	T43.4X4	T43.4X5	T43.4X6
Timolol	T44.7X1	T44.7X2	T44.7X3	T44.7X4	T44.7X5	T44.7X6
Tin (chloride) (dust) (oxide) NEC	T56.6X1	T56.6X2	T56.6X3	T56.6X4	—	—
anti-infectives	T37.8X1	T37.8X2	T37.8X3	T37.8X4	T37.8X5	T37.8X6
Tincture, iodine — *see Iodine*						
Tindal	T43.3X1	T43.3X2	T43.3X3	T43.3X4	T43.3X5	T43.3X6
Tinidazole	T37.3X1	T37.3X2	T37.3X3	T37.3X4	T37.3X5	T37.3X6
Tinoridine	T39.8X1	T39.8X2	T39.8X3	T39.8X4	T39.8X5	T39.8X6
Tiocarlide	T37.1X1	T37.1X2	T37.1X3	T37.1X4	T37.1X5	T37.1X6
Tioclomarol	T45.511	T45.512	T45.513	T45.514	T45.515	T45.516

◀ New ◀ Revised ~~deleted~~ Deleted

Substance	Poisoning, Accidental (Unintentional)	Poisoning, Intentional Self-Harm	Poisoning, Assault	Poisoning, Undetermined	Adverse Effect	Underdosing
	External Cause (T-Code)					
Tioconazole	T49.0X1	T49.0X2	T49.0X3	T49.0X4	T49.0X5	T49.0X6
Tioguanine	T45.1X1	T45.1X2	T45.1X3	T45.1X4	T45.1X5	T45.1X6
Tiopronin	T50.991	T50.992	T50.993	T50.994	T50.995	T50.996
Tiotixene	T43.4X1	T43.4X2	T43.4X3	T43.4X4	T43.4X5	T43.4X6
Tioxolone	T49.4X1	T49.4X2	T49.4X3	T49.4X4	T49.4X5	T49.4X6
Tipepidine	T48.3X1	T48.3X2	T48.3X3	T48.3X4	T48.3X5	T48.3X6
Tiquizium bromide	T44.3X1	T44.3X2	T44.3X3	T44.3X4	T44.3X5	T44.3X6
Tiratricol	T38.1X1	T38.1X2	T38.1X3	T38.1X4	T38.1X5	T38.1X6
Tisopurine	T50.4X1	T50.4X2	T50.4X3	T50.4X4	T50.4X5	T50.4X6
Titanium (compounds) (vapor)	T56.891	T56.892	T56.893	T56.894	—	—
dioxide	T49.3X1	T49.3X2	T49.3X3	T49.3X4	T49.3X5	T49.3X6
ointment	T49.3X1	T49.3X2	T49.3X3	T49.3X4	T49.3X5	T49.3X6
oxide	T49.3X1	T49.3X2	T49.3X3	T49.3X4	T49.3X5	T49.3X6
tetrachloride	T56.891	T56.892	T56.893	T56.894	—	—
Titanocene	T56.891	T56.892	T56.893	T56.894	—	—
Titroid	T38.1X1	T38.1X2	T38.1X3	T38.1X4	T38.1X5	T38.1X6
Tizanidine	T42.8X1	T42.8X2	T42.8X3	T42.8X4	T42.8X5	T42.8X6
TMTD	T60.3X1	T60.3X2	T60.3X3	T60.3X4	—	—
TNT (fumes)	T65.3X1	T65.3X2	T65.3X3	T65.3X4	—	—
Toadstool	T62.0X1	T62.0X2	T62.0X3	T62.0X4	—	—
Tobacco NEC	T65.291	T65.292	T65.293	T65.294	—	—
cigarettes	T65.221	T65.222	T65.223	T65.224	—	—
Indian	T62.2X1	T62.2X2	T62.2X3	T62.2X4	—	—
smoke, second-hand	T65.221	T65.222	T65.223	T65.224	—	—
Tobramycin	T36.5X1	T36.5X2	T36.5X3	T36.5X4	T36.5X5	T36.5X6
Tocainide	T46.2X1	T46.2X2	T46.2X3	T46.2X4	T46.2X5	T46.2X6
Tocoferol	T45.2X1	T45.2X2	T45.2X3	T45.2X4	T45.2X5	T45.2X6
Tocopherol	T45.2X1	T45.2X2	T45.2X3	T45.2X4	T45.2X5	T45.2X6
acetate	T45.2X1	T45.2X2	T45.2X3	T45.2X4	T45.2X5	T45.2X6
Tocosamine	T48.0X1	T48.0X2	T48.0X3	T48.0X4	T48.0X5	T48.0X6
Todralazine	T46.5X1	T46.5X2	T46.5X3	T46.5X4	T46.5X5	T46.5X6
Tofisopam	T42.4X1	T42.4X2	T42.4X3	T42.4X4	T42.4X5	T42.4X6
Tofranil	T43.011	T43.012	T43.013	T43.014	T43.015	T43.016
Toilet deodorizer	T65.891	T65.892	T65.893	T65.894	—	—
Tolamolol	T44.7X1	T44.7X2	T44.7X3	T44.7X4	T44.7X5	T44.7X6
Tolazamide	T38.3X1	T38.3X2	T38.3X3	T38.3X4	T38.3X5	T38.3X6
Tolazoline	T46.7X1	T46.7X2	T46.7X3	T46.7X4	T46.7X5	T46.7X6
Tolbutamide (sodium)	T38.3X1	T38.3X2	T38.3X3	T38.3X4	T38.3X5	T38.3X6
Tolciclate	T49.0X1	T49.0X2	T49.0X3	T49.0X4	T49.0X5	T49.0X6
Tolmetin	T39.391	T39.392	T39.393	T39.394	T39.395	T39.396
Tolnaftate	T49.0X1	T49.0X2	T49.0X3	T49.0X4	T49.0X5	T49.0X6
Tolonidine	T46.5X1	T46.5X2	T46.5X3	T46.5X4	T46.5X5	T46.5X6

Substance	Poisoning, Accidental (Unintentional)	Poisoning, Intentional Self-Harm	Poisoning, Assault	Poisoning, Undetermined	Adverse Effect	Underdosing
	External Cause (T-Code)					
Toloxatone	T42.6X1	T42.6X2	T42.6X3	T42.6X4	T42.6X5	T42.6X6
Tolperisone	T44.3X1	T44.3X2	T44.3X3	T44.3X4	T44.3X5	T44.3X6
Tolserol	T42.8X1	T42.8X2	T42.8X3	T42.8X4	T42.8X5	T42.8X6
Toluene (liquid)	T52.2X1	T52.2X2	T52.2X3	T52.2X4	—	—
diisocyanate	T65.0X1	T65.0X2	T65.0X3	T65.0X4	—	—
Toluidine	T65.891	T65.892	T65.893	T65.894	—	—
vapor	T59.891	T59.892	T59.893	T59.894	—	—
Toluol (liquid)	T52.2X1	T52.2X2	T52.2X3	T52.2X4	—	—
vapor	T52.2X1	T52.2X2	T52.2X3	T52.2X4	—	—
Toluylenediamine	T65.3X1	T65.3X2	T65.3X3	T65.3X4	—	—
Tolylene-2,4-diisocyanate	T65.0X1	T65.0X2	T65.0X3	T65.0X4	—	—
Tonic NEC	T50.901	T50.902	T50.903	T50.904	T50.905	T50.906
Topical action drug NEC	T49.91	T49.92	T49.93	T49.94	T49.95	T49.96
ear, nose or throat	T49.6X1	T49.6X2	T49.6X3	T49.6X4	T49.6X5	T49.6X6
eye	T49.5X1	T49.5X2	T49.5X3	T49.5X4	T49.5X5	T49.5X6
skin	T49.91	T49.92	T49.93	T49.94	T49.95	T49.96
specified NEC	T49.8X1	T49.8X2	T49.8X3	T49.8X4	T49.8X5	T49.8X6
Toquizine	T44.3X1	T44.3X2	T44.3X3	T44.3X4	T44.3X5	T44.3X6
Toremifene	T38.6X1	T38.6X2	T38.6X3	T38.6X4	T38.6X5	T38.6X6
Tosylchloramide sodium	T49.8X1	T49.8X2	T49.8X3	T49.8X4	T49.8X5	T49.8X6
Toxaphene (dust) (spray)	T60.1X1	T60.1X2	T60.1X3	T60.1X4	—	—
Toxin, diphtheria (Schick Test)	T50.8X1	T50.8X2	T50.8X3	T50.8X4	T50.8X5	T50.8X6
Toxoid						
combined	T50.A21	T50.A22	T50.A23	T50.A24	T50.A25	T50.A26
diphtheria	T50.A91	T50.A92	T50.A93	T50.A94	T50.A95	T50.A96
tetanus	T50.A91	T50.A92	T50.A93	T50.A94	T50.A95	T50.A96
Trace element NEC	T45.8X1	T45.8X2	T45.8X3	T45.8X4	T45.8X5	T45.8X6
Tractor fuel NEC	T52.0X1	T52.0X2	T52.0X3	T52.0X4	—	—
Tragacanth	T50.991	T50.992	T50.993	T50.994	T50.995	T50.996
Tramadol	T40.4X1	T40.4X2	T40.4X3	T40.4X4	T40.4X5	T40.4X6
Tramazoline	T48.5X1	T48.5X2	T48.5X3	T48.5X4	T48.5X5	T48.5X6
Tranexamic acid	T45.621	T45.622	T45.623	T45.624	T45.625	T45.626
Tranilast	T45.0X1	T45.0X2	T45.0X3	T45.0X4	T45.0X5	T45.0X6
Tranquilizer NEC	T43.501	T43.502	T43.503	T43.504	T43.505	T43.506
with hypnotic or sedative	T42.6X1	T42.6X2	T42.6X3	T42.6X4	T42.6X5	T42.6X6
benzodiazepine NEC	T42.4X1	T42.4X2	T42.4X3	T42.4X4	T42.4X5	T42.4X6
butyrophenone NEC	T43.4X1	T43.4X2	T43.4X3	T43.4X4	T43.4X5	T43.4X6
carbamate	T43.591	T43.592	T43.593	T43.594	T43.595	T43.596
dimethylamine	T43.3X1	T43.3X2	T43.3X3	T43.3X4	T43.3X5	T43.3X6
ethylamine	T43.3X1	T43.3X2	T43.3X3	T43.3X4	T43.3X5	T43.3X6
hydroxyzine	T43.591	T43.592	T43.593	T43.594	T43.595	T43.596
major NEC	T43.501	T43.502	T43.503	T43.504	T43.505	T43.506

◀ New ◀ Revised ~~deleted~~ Deleted

Substance	External Cause (T-Code)					
	Poisoning, Accidental (Unintentional)	Poisoning, Intentional Self-Harm	Poisoning, Assault	Poisoning, Undetermined	Adverse Effect	Underdosing
Tranquilizer NEC *(Continued)*						
penothiazine NEC	T43.3X1	T43.3X2	T43.3X3	T43.3X4	T43.3X5	T43.3X6
phenothiazine-based	T43.3X1	T43.3X2	T43.3X3	T43.3X4	T43.3X5	T43.3X6
piperazine NEC	T43.3X1	T43.3X2	T43.3X3	T43.3X4	T43.3X5	T43.3X6
piperidine	T43.3X1	T43.3X2	T43.3X3	T43.3X4	T43.3X5	T43.3X6
propylamine	T43.3X1	T43.3X2	T43.3X3	T43.3X4	T43.3X5	T43.3X6
specified NEC	T43.591	T43.592	T43.593	T43.594	T43.595	T43.596
thioxanthene NEC	T43.591	T43.592	T43.593	T43.594	T43.595	T43.596
Tranxene	T42.4X1	T42.4X2	T42.4X3	T42.4X4	T42.4X5	T42.4X6
Tranylcypromine	T43.1X1	T43.1X2	T43.1X3	T43.1X4	T43.1X5	T43.1X6
Trapidil	T46.3X1	T46.3X2	T46.3X3	T46.3X4	T46.3X5	T46.3X6
Trasentine	T44.3X1	T44.3X2	T44.3X3	T44.3X4	T44.3X5	T44.3X6
Travert	T50.3X1	T50.3X2	T50.3X3	T50.3X4	T50.3X5	T50.3X6
Trazodone	T43.211	T43.212	T43.213	T43.214	T43.215	T43.216
Trecator	T37.1X1	T37.1X2	T37.1X3	T37.1X4	T37.1X5	T37.1X6
Treosulfan	T45.1X1	T45.1X2	T45.1X3	T45.1X4	T45.1X5	T45.1X6
Tretamine	T45.1X1	T45.1X2	T45.1X3	T45.1X4	T45.1X5	T45.1X6
Tretinoin	T49.0X1	T49.0X2	T49.0X3	T49.0X4	T49.0X5	T49.0X6
Tretoquinol	T48.6X1	T48.6X2	T48.6X3	T48.6X4	T48.6X5	T48.6X6
Triacetin	T49.0X1	T49.0X2	T49.0X3	T49.0X4	T49.0X5	T49.0X6
Triacetoxyanthracene	T49.4X1	T49.4X2	T49.4X3	T49.4X4	T49.4X5	T49.4X6
Triacetyloleandomycin	T36.3X1	T36.3X2	T36.3X3	T36.3X4	T36.3X5	T36.3X6
Triamcinolone	T49.0X1	T49.0X2	T49.0X3	T49.0X4	T49.0X5	T49.0X6
ENT agent	T49.6X1	T49.6X2	T49.6X3	T49.6X4	T49.6X5	T49.6X6
hexacetonide	T49.0X1	T49.0X2	T49.0X3	T49.0X4	T49.0X5	T49.0X6
ophthalmic preparation	T49.5X1	T49.5X2	T49.5X3	T49.5X4	T49.5X5	T49.5X6
topical NEC	T49.0X1	T49.0X2	T49.0X3	T49.0X4	T49.0X5	T49.0X6
Triampyzine	T44.3X1	T44.3X2	T44.3X3	T44.3X4	T44.3X5	T44.3X6
Triamterene	T50.2X1	T50.2X2	T50.2X3	T50.2X4	T50.2X5	T50.2X6
Triazine (herbicide)	T60.3X1	T60.3X2	T60.3X3	T60.3X4	—	—
Triaziquone	T45.1X1	T45.1X2	T45.1X3	T45.1X4	T45.1X5	T45.1X6
Triazolam	T42.4X1	T42.4X2	T42.4X3	T42.4X4	T42.4X5	T42.4X6
Triazole (herbicide)	T60.3X1	T60.3X2	T60.3X3	T60.3X4	—	—
Tribenoside	T46.991	T46.992	T46.993	T46.994	T46.995	T46.996
Tribromacetaldehyde	T42.6X1	T42.6X2	T42.6X3	T42.6X4	T42.6X5	T42.6X6
Tribromoethanol, rectal	T41.291	T41.292	T41.293	T41.294	T41.295	T41.296
Tribromomethane	T42.6X1	T42.6X2	T42.6X3	T42.6X4	T42.6X5	T42.6X6
Trichlorethane	T53.2X1	T53.2X2	T53.2X3	T53.2X4	—	—
Trichlorethylene	T53.2X1	T53.2X2	T53.2X3	T53.2X4	—	—
Trichlorfon	T60.0X1	T60.0X2	T60.0X3	T60.0X4	—	—
Trichlormethiazide	T50.2X1	T50.2X2	T50.2X3	T50.2X4	T50.2X5	T50.2X6
Trichlormethine	T45.1X1	T45.1X2	T45.1X3	T45.1X4	T45.1X5	T45.1X6

Substance	External Cause (T-Code)					
	Poisoning, Accidental (Unintentional)	Poisoning, Intentional Self-Harm	Poisoning, Assault	Poisoning, Undetermined	Adverse Effect	Underdosing
Trichloroacetic acid, Trichloracetic acid	T54.2X1	T54.2X2	T54.2X3	T54.2X4	—	—
medicinal	T49.4X1	T49.4X2	T49.4X3	T49.4X4	T49.4X5	T49.4X6
Trichloroethane	T53.2X1	T53.2X2	T53.2X3	T53.2X4	—	—
Trichloroethanol	T42.6X1	T42.6X2	T42.6X3	T42.6X4	T42.6X5	T42.6X6
Trichloroethylene (liquid) (vapor)	T53.2X1	T53.2X2	T53.2X3	T53.2X4	—	—
anesthetic (gas)	T41.0X1	T41.0X2	T41.0X3	T41.0X4	T41.0X5	T41.0X6
vapor NEC	T53.2X1	T53.2X2	T53.2X3	T53.2X4	—	—
Trichloroethyl phosphate	T42.6X1	T42.6X2	T42.6X3	T42.6X4	T42.6X5	T42.6X6
Trichlorofluoromethane NEC	T53.5X1	T53.5X2	T53.5X3	T53.5X4	—	—
Trichloronate	T60.0X1	T60.0X2	T60.0X3	T60.0X4	—	—
2,4,5-Trichlorophen-oxyacetic acid	T60.3X1	T60.3X2	T60.3X3	T60.3X4	—	—
Trichloropropane	T53.6X1	T53.6X2	T53.6X3	T53.6X4	—	—
Trichlorotriethylamine	T45.1X1	T45.1X2	T45.1X3	T45.1X4	T45.1X5	T45.1X6
Trichomonacides NEC	T37.3X1	T37.3X2	T37.3X3	T37.3X4	T37.3X5	T37.3X6
Trichomycin	T36.7X1	T36.7X2	T36.7X3	T36.7X4	T36.7X5	T36.7X6
Triclobisonium chloride	T49.0X1	T49.0X2	T49.0X3	T49.0X4	T49.0X5	T49.0X6
Triclocarban	T49.0X1	T49.0X2	T49.0X3	T49.0X4	T49.0X5	T49.0X6
Triclofos	T42.6X1	T42.6X2	T42.6X3	T42.6X4	T42.6X5	T42.6X6
Triclosan	T49.0X1	T49.0X2	T49.0X3	T49.0X4	T49.0X5	T49.0X6
Tricresyl phosphate	T65.891	T65.892	T65.893	T65.894	—	—
solvent	T52.91	T52.92	T52.93	T52.94	—	—
Tricyclamol chloride	T44.3X1	T44.3X2	T44.3X3	T44.3X4	T44.3X5	T44.3X6
Tridesilon	T49.0X1	T49.0X2	T49.0X3	T49.0X4	T49.0X5	T49.0X6
Tridihexethyl iodide	T44.3X1	T44.3X2	T44.3X3	T44.3X4	T44.3X5	T44.3X6
Tridione	T42.2X1	T42.2X2	T42.2X3	T42.2X4	T42.2X5	T42.2X6
Trientine	T45.8X1	T45.8X2	T45.8X3	T45.8X4	T45.8X5	T45.8X6
Triethanolamine NEC	T54.3X1	T54.3X2	T54.3X3	T54.3X4	—	—
detergent	T54.3X1	T54.3X2	T54.3X3	T54.3X4	—	—
trinitrate (biphosphate)	T46.3X1	T46.3X2	T46.3X3	T46.3X4	T46.3X5	T46.3X6
Triethanomelamine	T45.1X1	T45.1X2	T45.1X3	T45.1X4	T45.1X5	T45.1X6
Triethylenemelamine	T45.1X1	T45.1X2	T45.1X3	T45.1X4	T45.1X5	T45.1X6
Triethylenephosphoramide	T45.1X1	T45.1X2	T45.1X3	T45.1X4	T45.1X5	T45.1X6
Triethylenethiophosphoramide	T45.1X1	T45.1X2	T45.1X3	T45.1X4	T45.1X5	T45.1X6
Trifluoperazine	T43.3X1	T43.3X2	T43.3X3	T43.3X4	T43.3X5	T43.3X6
Trifluoroethyl vinyl ether	T41.0X1	T41.0X2	T41.0X3	T41.0X4	T41.0X5	T41.0X6
Trifluperidol	T43.4X1	T43.4X2	T43.4X3	T43.4X4	T43.4X5	T43.4X6
Triflupromazine	T43.3X1	T43.3X2	T43.3X3	T43.3X4	T43.3X5	T43.3X6
Trifluridine	T37.5X1	T37.5X2	T37.5X3	T37.5X4	T37.5X5	T37.5X6
Triflusal	T45.521	T45.522	T45.523	T45.524	T45.525	T45.526
Trihexyphenidyl	T44.3X1	T44.3X2	T44.3X3	T44.3X4	T44.3X5	T44.3X6
Triiodothyronine	T38.1X1	T38.1X2	T38.1X3	T38.1X4	T38.1X5	T38.1X6

◀ New ◀ Revised ~~deleted~~ Deleted

Substance	Poisoning, Accidental (Unintentional)	Poisoning, Intentional Self-Harm	Poisoning, Assault	Poisoning, Undetermined	Adverse Effect	Underdosing
	External Cause (T-Code)					
Trilene	T41.0X1	T41.0X2	T41.0X3	T41.0X4	T41.0X5	T41.0X6
Trilostane	T38.991	T38.992	T38.993	T38.994	T38.995	T38.996
Trimebutine	T44.3X1	T44.3X2	T44.3X3	T44.3X4	T44.3X5	T44.3X6
Trimecaine	T41.3X1	T41.3X2	T41.3X3	T41.3X4	T41.3X5	T41.3X6
Trimeprazine (tartrate)	T44.3X1	T44.3X2	T44.3X3	T44.3X4	T44.3X5	T44.3X6
Trimetaphan camsilate	T44.2X1	T44.2X2	T44.2X3	T44.2X4	T44.2X5	T44.2X6
Trimetazidine	T46.7X1	T46.7X2	T46.7X3	T46.7X4	T46.7X5	T46.7X6
Trimethadione	T42.2X1	T42.2X2	T42.2X3	T42.2X4	T42.2X5	T42.2X6
Trimethaphan	T44.2X1	T44.2X2	T44.2X3	T44.2X4	T44.2X5	T44.2X6
Trimethidinium	T44.2X1	T44.2X2	T44.2X3	T44.2X4	T44.2X5	T44.2X6
Trimethobenzamide	T45.0X1	T45.0X2	T45.0X3	T45.0X4	T45.0X5	T45.0X6
Trimethoprim	T37.8X1	T37.8X2	T37.8X3	T37.8X4	T37.8X5	T37.8X6
with sulfamethoxazole	T36.8X1	T36.8X2	T36.8X3	T36.8X4	T36.8X5	T36.8X6
Trimethylcarbinol	T51.3X1	T51.3X2	T51.3X3	T51.3X4	—	—
Trimethylpsoralen	T49.3X1	T49.3X2	T49.3X3	T49.3X4	T49.3X5	T49.3X6
Trimeton	T45.0X1	T45.0X2	T45.0X3	T45.0X4	T45.0X5	T45.0X6
Trimetrexate	T45.1X1	T45.1X2	T45.1X3	T45.1X4	T45.1X5	T45.1X6
Trimipramine	T43.011	T43.012	T43.013	T43.014	T43.015	T43.016
Trimustine	T45.1X1	T45.1X2	T45.1X3	T45.1X4	T45.1X5	T45.1X6
Trinitrine	T46.3X1	T46.3X2	T46.3X3	T46.3X4	T46.3X5	T46.3X6
Trinitrobenzol	T65.3X1	T65.3X2	T65.3X3	T65.3X4	—	—
Trinitrophenol	T65.3X1	T65.3X2	T65.3X3	T65.3X4	—	—
Trinitrotoluene (fumes)	T65.3X1	T65.3X2	T65.3X3	T65.3X4	—	—
Trional	T42.6X1	T42.6X2	T42.6X3	T42.6X4	T42.6X5	T42.6X6
Triorthocresyl phosphate	T65.891	T65.892	T65.893	T65.894	—	—
Trioxide of arsenic	T57.0X1	T57.0X2	T57.0X3	T57.0X4	—	—
Trioxysalen	T49.4X1	T49.4X2	T49.4X3	T49.4X4	T49.4X5	T49.4X6
Tripamide	T50.2X1	T50.2X2	T50.2X3	T50.2X4	T50.2X5	T50.2X6
Triparanol	T46.6X1	T46.6X2	T46.6X3	T46.6X4	T46.6X5	T46.6X6
Tripelennamine	T45.0X1	T45.0X2	T45.0X3	T45.0X4	T45.0X5	T45.0X6
Triperiden	T44.3X1	T44.3X2	T44.3X3	T44.3X4	T44.3X5	T44.3X6
Triperidol	T43.4X1	T43.4X2	T43.4X3	T43.4X4	T43.4X5	T43.4X6
Triphenylphosphate	T65.891	T65.892	T65.893	T65.894	—	—
Triple						
bromides	T42.6X1	T42.6X2	T42.6X3	T42.6X4	T42.6X5	T42.6X6
carbonate	T47.1X1	T47.1X2	T47.1X3	T47.1X4	T47.1X5	T47.1X6
vaccine						
DPT	T50.A11	T50.A12	T50.A13	T50.A14	T50.A15	T50.A16
including pertussis	T50.A11	T50.A12	T50.A13	T50.A14	T50.A15	T50.A16
MMR	T50.B91	T50.B92	—	—	—	—
Triprolidine	T45.0X1	T45.0X2	T45.0X3	T45.0X4	T45.0X5	T45.0X6
Trisodium hydrogen edetate	T50.6X1	T50.6X2	T50.6X3	T50.6X4	T50.6X5	T50.6X6

Substance	Poisoning, Accidental (Unintentional)	Poisoning, Intentional Self-Harm	Poisoning, Assault	Poisoning, Undetermined	Adverse Effect	Underdosing
	External Cause (T-Code)					
Trisoralen	T49.3X1	T49.3X2	T49.3X3	T49.3X4	T49.3X5	T49.3X6
Trisulfapyrimidines	T37.0X1	T37.0X2	T37.0X3	T37.0X4	T37.0X5	T37.0X6
Trithiozine	T44.3X1	T44.3X2	T44.3X3	T44.3X4	T44.3X5	T44.3X6
Tritiozine	T44.3X1	T44.3X2	T44.3X3	T44.3X4	T44.3X5	T44.3X6
Tritoqualine	T45.0X1	T45.0X2	T45.0X3	T45.0X4	T45.0X5	T45.0X6
Trofosfamide	T45.1X1	T45.1X2	T45.1X3	T45.1X4	T45.1X5	T45.1X6
Troleandomycin	T36.3X1	T36.3X2	T36.3X3	T36.3X4	T36.3X5	T36.3X6
Trolnitrate (phosphate)	T46.3X1	T46.3X2	T46.3X3	T46.3X4	T46.3X5	T46.3X6
Tromantadine	T37.5X1	T37.5X2	T37.5X3	T37.5X4	T37.5X5	T37.5X6
Trometamol	T50.2X1	T50.2X2	T50.2X3	T50.2X4	T50.2X5	T50.2X6
Tromethamine	T50.2X1	T50.2X2	T50.2X3	T50.2X4	T50.2X5	T50.2X6
Tronothane	T41.3X1	T41.3X2	T41.3X3	T41.3X4	T41.3X5	T41.3X6
Tropacine	T44.3X1	T44.3X2	T44.3X3	T44.3X4	T44.3X5	T44.3X6
Tropatepine	T44.3X1	T44.3X2	T44.3X3	T44.3X4	T44.3X5	T44.3X6
Tropicamide	T44.3X1	T44.3X2	T44.3X3	T44.3X4	T44.3X5	T44.3X6
Trospium chloride	T44.3X1	T44.3X2	T44.3X3	T44.3X4	T44.3X5	T44.3X6
Troxerutin	T46.991	T46.992	T46.993	T46.994	T46.995	T46.996
Troxidone	T42.2X1	T42.2X2	T42.2X3	T42.2X4	T42.2X5	T42.2X6
Tryparsamide	T37.3X1	T37.3X2	T37.3X3	T37.3X4	T37.3X5	T37.3X6
Trypsin	T45.3X1	T45.3X2	T45.3X3	T45.3X4	T45.3X5	T45.3X6
Tryptizol	T43.011	T43.012	T43.013	T43.014	T43.015	T43.016
TSH	T38.811	T38.812	T38.813	T38.814	T38.815	T38.816
Tuaminoheptane	T48.5X1	T48.5X2	T48.5X3	T48.5X4	T48.5X5	T48.5X6
Tuberculin, purified protein derivative (PPD)	T50.8X1	T50.8X2	T50.8X3	T50.8X4	T50.8X5	T50.8X6
Tubocurare	T48.1X1	T48.1X2	T48.1X3	T48.1X4	T48.1X5	T48.1X6
Tubocurarine (chloride)	T48.1X1	T48.1X2	T48.1X3	T48.1X4	T48.1X5	T48.1X6
Tulobuterol	T48.6X1	T48.6X2	T48.6X3	T48.6X4	T48.6X5	T48.6X6
Turpentine (spirits of)	T52.8X1	T52.8X2	T52.8X3	T52.8X4	—	—
vapor	T52.8X1	T52.8X2	T52.8X3	T52.8X4	—	—
Tybamate	T43.591	T43.592	T43.593	T43.594	T43.595	T43.596
Tyloxapol	T48.4X1	T48.4X2	T48.4X3	T48.4X4	T48.4X5	T48.4X6
Tymazoline	T48.5X1	T48.5X2	T48.5X3	T48.5X4	T48.5X5	T48.5X6
Typhoid-paratyphoid vaccine	T50.A91	T50.A92	T50.A93	T50.A94	T50.A95	T50.A96
Typhus vaccine	T50.A91	T50.A92	T50.A93	T50.A94	T50.A95	T50.A96
Tyropanoate	T50.8X1	T50.8X2	T50.8X3	T50.8X4	T50.8X5	T50.8X6
Tyrothricin	T49.6X1	T49.6X2	T49.6X3	T49.6X4	T49.6X5	T49.6X6
ENT agent	T49.6X1	T49.6X2	T49.6X3	T49.6X4	T49.6X5	T49.6X6
ophthalmic preparation	T49.5X1	T49.5X2	T49.5X3	T49.5X4	T49.5X5	T49.5X6
U						
Ufenamate	T39.391	T39.392	T39.393	T39.394	T39.395	T39.396
Ultraviolet light protectant	T49.3X1	T49.3X2	T49.3X3	T49.3X4	T49.3X5	T49.3X6

◀ New ◀ Revised ~~deleted~~ Deleted

Substance	External Cause (T-Code)					
	Poisoning, Accidental (Unintentional)	Poisoning, Intentional Self-Harm	Poisoning, Assault	Poisoning, Undetermined	Adverse Effect	Underdosing
Undecenoic acid	T49.0X1	T49.0X2	T49.0X3	T49.0X4	T49.0X5	T49.0X6
Undecoylium	T49.0X1	T49.0X2	T49.0X3	T49.0X4	T49.0X5	T49.0X6
Undecylenic acid (derivatives)	T49.0X1	T49.0X2	T49.0X3	T49.0X4	T49.0X5	T49.0X6
Unna's boot	T49.3X1	T49.3X2	T49.3X3	T49.3X4	T49.3X5	T49.3X6
Unsaturated fatty acid	T46.6X1	T46.6X2	T46.6X3	T46.6X4	T46.6X5	T46.6X6
Uracil mustard	T45.1X1	T45.1X2	T45.1X3	T45.1X4	T45.1X5	T45.1X6
Uramustine	T45.1X1	T45.1X2	T45.1X3	T45.1X4	T45.1X5	T45.1X6
Urapidil	T46.5X1	T46.5X2	T46.5X3	T46.5X4	T46.5X5	T46.5X6
Urari	T48.1X1	T48.1X2	T48.1X3	T48.1X4	T48.1X5	T48.1X6
Urate oxidase	T50.4X1	T50.4X2	T50.4X3	T50.4X4	T50.4X5	T50.4X6
Urea	T47.3X1	T47.3X2	T47.3X3	T47.3X4	T47.3X5	T47.3X6
peroxide	T49.0X1	T49.0X2	T49.0X3	T49.0X4	T49.0X5	T49.0X6
stibamine	T37.4X1	T37.4X2	T37.4X3	T37.4X4	T37.4X5	T37.4X6
topical	T49.8X1	T49.8X2	T49.8X3	T49.8X4	T49.8X5	T49.8X6
Urethane	T45.1X1	T45.1X2	T45.1X3	T45.1X4	T45.1X5	T45.1X6
Urginea (maritima) (scilla) — *see Squill*						
Uric acid metabolism drug NEC	T50.4X1	T50.4X2	T50.4X3	T50.4X4	T50.4X5	T50.4X6
Uricosuric agent	T50.4X1	T50.4X2	T50.4X3	T50.4X4	T50.4X5	T50.4X6
Urinary anti-infective	T37.8X1	T37.8X2	T37.8X3	T37.8X4	T37.8X5	T37.8X6
Urofollitropin	T38.811	T38.812	T38.813	T38.814	T38.815	T38.816
Urokinase	T45.611	T45.612	T45.613	T45.614	T45.615	T45.616
Urokon	T50.8X1	T50.8X2	T50.8X3	T50.8X4	T50.8X5	T50.8X6
Ursodeoxycholic acid	T50.991	T50.992	T50.993	T50.994	T50.995	T50.996
Ursodiol	T50.991	T50.992	T50.993	T50.994	T50.995	T50.996
Urtica	T62.2X1	T62.2X2	T62.2X3	T62.2X4	—	—
Utility gas — *see Gas, utility*						
V						
Vaccine NEC	T50.Z91	T50.Z92	T50.Z93	T50.Z94	T50.Z95	T50.Z96
antineoplastic	T50.Z91	T50.Z92	T50.Z93	T50.Z94	T50.Z95	T50.Z96
bacterial NEC	T50.A91	T50.A92	T50.A93	T50.A94	T50.A95	T50.A96
with						
other bacterial component	T50.A91	T50.A92	T50.A93	T50.A94	T50.A95	T50.A96
pertussis component	T50.A91	T50.A92	T50.A93	T50.A94	T50.A95	T50.A96
viral-rickettsial component	T50.A91	T50.A92	T50.A93	T50.A94	T50.A95	T50.A96
mixed NEC	T50.A91	T50.A92	T50.A93	T50.A94	T50.A95	T50.A96
BCG	T50.A91	T50.A92	T50.A93	T50.A94	T50.A95	T50.A96
cholera	T50.A91	T50.A92	T50.A93	T50.A94	T50.A95	T50.A96
diphtheria	T50.A91	T50.A92	T50.A93	T50.A94	T50.A95	T50.A96
with tetanus	T50.A21	T50.A22	T50.A23	T50.A24	T50.A25	T50.A26
and pertussis	T50.A11	T50.A12	T50.A13	T50.A14	T50.A15	T50.A16

Substance	External Cause (T-Code)					
	Poisoning, Accidental (Unintentional)	Poisoning, Intentional Self-Harm	Poisoning, Assault	Poisoning, Undetermined	Adverse Effect	Underdosing
Vaccine NEC *(Continued)*						
influenza	T50.B91	T50.B92	T50.B93	T50.B94	T50.B95	T50.B96
measles	T50.B91	T50.B92	T50.B93	T50.B94	T50.B95	T50.B96
with mumps and rubella	T50.B91	T50.B92	T50.B93	T50.B94	T50.B95	T50.B96
meningococcal	T50.A91	T50.A92	T50.A93	T50.A94	T50.A95	T50.A96
mumps	T50.B91	T50.B92	T50.B93	T50.B94	T50.B95	T50.B96
paratyphoid	T50.A91	T50.A92	T50.A93	T50.A94	T50.A95	T50.A96
pertussis	T50.A11	T50.A12	T50.A13	T50.A14	T50.A15	T50.A16
with diphtheria	T50.A11	T50.A12	T50.A13	T50.A14	T50.A15	T50.A16
and tetanus	T50.A11	T50.A12	T50.A13	T50.A14	T50.A15	T50.A16
plague	T50.A91	T50.A92	T50.A93	T50.A94	T50.A95	T50.A96
poliomyelitis	T50.B91	T50.B92	T50.B93	T50.B94	T50.B95	T50.B96
poliovirus	T50.B91	T50.B92	T50.B93	T50.B94	T50.B95	T50.B96
rabies	T50.B91	T50.B92	T50.B93	T50.B94	T50.B95	T50.B96
respiratory syncytial virus	T50.B91	T50.B92	T50.B93	T50.B94	T50.B95	T50.B96
rickettsial NEC	T50.A91	T50.A92	T50.A93	T50.A94	T50.A95	T50.A96
with						
bacterial component	T50.A21	T50.A22	T50.A23	T50.A24	T50.A25	T50.A26
Rocky Mountain spotted fever	T50.A91	T50.A92	T50.A93	T50.A94	T50.A95	T50.A96
rubella	T50.B91	T50.B92	T50.B93	T50.B94	T50.B95	T50.B96
sabin oral	T50.B91	T50.B92	T50.B93	T50.B94	T50.B95	T50.B96
smallpox	T50.B11	T50.B12	T50.B13	T50.B14	T50.B15	T50.B16
TAB	T50.A91	T50.A92	T50.A93	T50.A94	T50.A95	T50.A96
tetanus	T50.A91	T50.A92	T50.A93	T50.A94	T50.A95	T50.A96
typhoid	T50.A91	T50.A92	T50.A93	T50.A94	T50.A95	T50.A96
typhus	T50.A91	T50.A92	T50.A93	T50.A94	T50.A95	T50.A96
viral NEC	T50.B91	T50.B92	T50.B93	T50.B94	T50.B95	T50.B96
yellow fever	T50.B91	T50.B92	T50.B93	T50.B94	T50.B95	T50.B96
Vaccinia immune globulin	T50.Z11	T50.Z12	T50.Z13	T50.Z14	T50.Z15	T50.Z16
Vaginal contraceptives	T49.8X1	T49.8X2	T49.8X3	T49.8X4	T49.8X5	T49.8X6
Valerian						
root	T42.6X1	T42.6X2	T42.6X3	T42.6X4	T42.6X5	T42.6X6
tincture	T42.6X1	T42.6X2	T42.6X3	T42.6X4	T42.6X5	T42.6X6
Valethamate bromide	T44.3X1	T44.3X2	T44.3X3	T44.3X4	T44.3X5	T44.3X6
Valisone	T49.0X1	T49.0X2	T49.0X3	T49.0X4	T49.0X5	T49.0X6
Valium	T42.4X1	T42.4X2	T42.4X3	T42.4X4	T42.4X5	T42.4X6
Valmid	T42.6X1	T42.6X2	T42.6X3	T42.6X4	T42.6X5	T42.6X6
Valnoctamide	T42.6X1	T42.6X2	T42.6X3	T42.6X4	T42.6X5	T42.6X6
Valproate (sodium)	T42.6X1	T42.6X2	T42.6X3	T42.6X4	T42.6X5	T42.6X6
Valproic acid	T42.6X1	T42.6X2	T42.6X3	T42.6X4	T42.6X5	T42.6X6
Valpromide	T42.6X1	T42.6X2	T42.6X3	T42.6X4	T42.6X5	T42.6X6
Vanadium	T56.891	T56.892	T56.893	T56.894	—	—

Substance	External Cause (T-Code)					
	Poisoning, Accidental (Unintentional)	Poisoning, Intentional Self-Harm	Poisoning, Assault	Poisoning, Undetermined	Adverse Effect	Underdosing
Vancomycin	T36.8X1	T36.8X2	T36.8X3	T36.8X4	T36.8X5	T36.8X6
Vapor — *see also Gas*	T59.91	T59.92	T59.93	T59.94	—	—
kiln (carbon monoxide)	T58.8X1	T58.8X2	T58.8X3	T58.8X4	—	—
lead — *see lead*						
specified source NEC	T59.891	T59.892	T59.893	T59.894	—	—
Vardenafil	T46.7X1	T46.7X2	T46.7X3	T46.7X4	T46.7X5	T46.7X6
Varicose reduction drug	T46.8X1	T46.8X2	T46.8X3	T46.8X4	T46.8X5	T46.8X6
Varnish	T65.4X1	T65.4X2	T65.4X3	T65.4X4	—	—
cleaner	T52.91	T52.92	T52.93	T52.94	—	—
Vaseline	T49.3X1	T49.3X2	T49.3X3	T49.3X4	T49.3X5	T49.3X6
Vasodilan	T46.7X1	T46.7X2	T46.7X3	T46.7X4	T46.7X5	T46.7X6
Vasodilator						
coronary NEC	T46.3X1	T46.3X2	T46.3X3	T46.3X4	T46.3X5	T46.3X6
peripheral NEC	T46.7X1	T46.7X2	T46.7X3	T46.7X4	T46.7X5	T46.7X6
Vasopressin	T38.891	T38.892	T38.893	T38.894	T38.895	T38.896
Vasopressor drugs	T38.891	T38.892	T38.893	T38.894	T38.895	T38.896
Vecuronium bromide	T48.1X1	T48.1X2	T48.1X3	T48.1X4	T48.1X5	T48.1X6
Vegetable extract, astringent	T49.2X1	T49.2X2	T49.2X3	T49.2X4	T49.2X5	T49.2X6
Venlafaxine	T43.211	T43.212	T43.213	T43.214	T43.215	T43.216
Venom, venomous (bite) (sting)	T63.91	T63.92	T63.93	T63.94	—	—
amphibian NEC	T63.831	T63.832	T63.833	T63.834	—	—
animal NEC	T63.891	T63.892	T63.893	T63.894	—	—
ant	T63.421	T63.422	T63.423	T63.424	—	—
arthropod NEC	T63.481	T63.482	T63.483	T63.484	—	—
bee	T63.441	T63.442	T63.443	T63.444	—	—
centipede	T63.411	T63.412	T63.413	T63.414	—	—
fish	T63.591	T63.592	T63.593	T63.594	—	—
frog	T63.811	T63.812	T63.813	T63.814	—	—
hornet	T63.451	T63.452	T63.453	T63.454	—	—
insect NEC	T63.481	T63.482	T63.483	T63.484	—	—
lizard	T63.121	T63.122	T63.123	T63.124	—	—
marine						
animals	T63.691	T63.692	T63.693	T63.694	—	—
bluebottle	T63.611	T63.612	T63.613	T63.614	—	—
jellyfish NEC	T63.621	T63.622	T63.623	T63.624	—	—
Portugese Man-o-war	T63.611	T63.612	T63.613	T63.614	—	—
sea anemone	T63.631	T63.632	T63.633	T63.634	—	—
specified NEC	T63.691	T63.692	T63.693	T63.694	—	—
fish	T63.591	T63.592	T63.593	T63.594	—	—
plants	T63.711	T63.712	T63.713	T63.714	—	—
sting ray	T63.511	T63.512	T63.513	T63.514	—	—

Substance	External Cause (T-Code)					
	Poisoning, Accidental (Unintentional)	Poisoning, Intentional Self-Harm	Poisoning, Assault	Poisoning, Undetermined	Adverse Effect	Underdosing
Venom, venomous *(Continued)*						
millipede (tropical)	T63.411	T63.412	T63.413	T63.414	—	—
plant NEC	T63.791	T63.792	T63.793	T63.794	—	—
marine	T63.711	T63.712	T63.713	T63.714	—	—
reptile	T63.191	T63.192	T63.193	T63.194	—	—
gila monster	T63.111	T63.112	T63.113	T63.114	—	—
lizard NEC	T63.121	T63.122	T63.123	T63.124	—	—
scorpion	T63.2X1	T63.2X2	T63.2X3	T63.2X4	—	—
snake	T63.001	T63.002	T63.003	T63.004	—	—
African NEC	T63.081	T63.082	T63.083	T63.084	—	—
American (North) (South) NEC	T63.061	T63.062	T63.063	T63.064	—	—
Asian	T63.081	T63.082	T63.083	T63.084	—	—
Australian	T63.071	T63.072	T63.073	T63.074	—	—
cobra	T63.041	T63.042	T63.043	T63.044	—	—
coral snake	T63.021	T63.022	T63.023	T63.024	—	—
rattlesnake	T63.011	T63.012	T63.013	T63.014	—	—
specified NEC	T63.091	T63.092	T63.093	T63.094	—	—
taipan	T63.031	T63.032	T63.033	T63.034	—	—
specified NEC	T63.891	T63.892	T63.893	T63.894	—	—
spider	T63.301	T63.302	T63.303	T63.304	—	—
black widow	T63.311	T63.312	T63.313	T63.314	—	—
brown recluse	T63.331	T63.332	T63.333	T63.334	—	—
specified NEC	T63.391	T63.392	T63.393	T63.394	—	—
tarantula	T63.321	T63.322	T63.323	T63.324	—	—
sting ray	T63.511	T63.512	T63.513	T63.514	—	—
toad	T63.821	T63.822	T63.823	T63.824	—	—
wasp	T63.461	T63.462	T63.463	T63.464	—	—
Venous sclerosing drug NEC	T46.8X1	T46.8X2	T46.8X3	T46.8X4	T46.8X5	T46.8X6
Ventolin — *see Albuterol*						
Verapamil	T46.1X1	T46.1X2	T46.1X3	T46.1X4	T46.1X5	T46.1X6
Veramon	T42.3X1	T42.3X2	T42.3X3	T42.3X4	T42.3X5	T42.3X6
Veratrine	T46.5X1	T46.5X2	T46.5X3	T46.5X4	T46.5X5	T46.5X6
Veratrum						
album	T62.2X1	T62.2X2	T62.2X3	T62.2X4	—	—
alkaloids	T46.5X1	T46.5X2	T46.5X3	T46.5X4	T46.5X5	T46.5X6
viride	T62.2X1	T62.2X2	T62.2X3	T62.2X4	—	—
Verdigris	T60.3X1	T60.3X2	T60.3X3	T60.3X4	—	—
Veronal	T42.3X1	T42.3X2	T42.3X3	T42.3X4	T42.3X5	T42.3X6
Veroxil	T37.4X1	T37.4X2	T37.4X3	T37.4X4	T37.4X5	T37.4X6
Versenate	T50.6X1	T50.6X2	T50.6X3	T50.6X4	T50.6X5	T50.6X6

Substance	External Cause (T-Code)					
	Poisoning, Accidental (Unintentional)	Poisoning, Intentional Self-Harm	Poisoning, Assault	Poisoning, Undetermined	Adverse Effect	Underdosing
Versidyne	T39.8X1	T39.8X2	T39.8X3	T39.8X4	T39.8X5	T39.8X6
Vetrabutine	T48.0X1	T48.0X2	T48.0X3	T48.0X4	T48.0X5	T48.0X6
Vidarabine	T37.5X1	T37.5X2	T37.5X3	T37.5X4	T37.5X5	T37.5X6
Vienna						
green	T57.0X1	T57.0X2	T57.0X3	T57.0X4	—	—
insecticide	T60.2X1	T60.2X2	T60.2X3	T60.2X4	—	—
red	T57.0X1	T57.0X2	T57.0X3	T57.0X4	—	—
pharmaceutical dye	T50.991	T50.992	T50.993	T50.994	T50.995	T50.996
Vigabatrin	T42.6X1	T42.6X2	T42.6X3	T42.6X4	T42.6X5	T42.6X6
Viloxazine	T43.291	T43.292	T43.293	T43.294	T43.295	T43.296
Viminol	T39.8X1	T39.8X2	T39.8X3	T39.8X4	T39.8X5	T39.8X6
Vinbarbital, vinbarbitone	T42.3X1	T42.3X2	T42.3X3	T42.3X4	T42.3X5	T42.3X6
Vinblastine	T45.1X1	T45.1X2	T45.1X3	T45.1X4	T45.1X5	T45.1X6
Vinburnine	T46.7X1	T46.7X2	T46.7X3	T46.7X4	T46.7X5	T46.7X6
Vincamine	T45.1X1	T45.1X2	T45.1X3	T45.1X4	T45.1X5	T45.1X6
Vincristine	T45.1X1	T45.1X2	T45.1X3	T45.1X4	T45.1X5	T45.1X6
Vindesine	T45.1X1	T45.1X2	T45.1X3	T45.1X4	T45.1X5	T45.1X6
Vinesthene, vinethene	T41.0X1	T41.0X2	T41.0X3	T41.0X4	T41.0X5	T41.0X6
Vinorelbine tartrate	T45.1X1	T45.1X2	T45.1X3	T45.1X4	T45.1X5	T45.1X6
Vinpocetine	T46.7X1	T46.7X2	T46.7X3	T46.7X4	T46.7X5	T46.7X6
Vinyl						
acetate	T65.891	T65.892	T65.893	T65.894	—	—
bital	T42.3X1	T42.3X2	T42.3X3	T42.3X4	T42.3X5	T42.3X6
bromide	T65.891	T65.892	T65.893	T65.894	—	—
chloride	T59.891	T59.892	T59.893	T59.894	—	—
ether	T41.0X1	T41.0X2	T41.0X3	T41.0X4	T41.0X5	T41.0X6
Vinylbital	T42.3X1	T42.3X2	T42.3X3	T42.3X4	T42.3X5	T42.3X6
Vinylidene chloride	T65.891	T65.892	T65.893	T65.894	—	—
Vioform	T37.8X1	T37.8X2	T37.8X3	T37.8X4	T37.8X5	T37.8X6
topical	T49.0X1	T49.0X2	T49.0X3	T49.0X4	T49.0X5	T49.0X6
Viomycin	T36.8X1	T36.8X2	T36.8X3	T36.8X4	T36.8X5	T36.8X6
Viosterol	T45.2X1	T45.2X2	T45.2X3	T45.2X4	T45.2X5	T45.2X6
Viper (venom)	T63.091	T63.092	T63.093	T63.094	—	—
Viprynium	T37.4X1	T37.4X2	T37.4X3	T37.4X4	T37.4X5	T37.4X6
Viquidil	T46.7X1	T46.7X2	T46.7X3	T46.7X4	T46.7X5	T46.7X6
Viral vaccine NEC	T50.B91	T50.B92	T50.B93	T50.B94	T50.B95	T50.B96
Virginiamycin	T36.8X1	T36.8X2	T36.8X3	T36.8X4	T36.8X5	T36.8X6
Virugon	T37.5X1	T37.5X2	T37.5X3	T37.5X4	T37.5X5	T37.5X6
Viscous agent	T50.901	T50.902	T50.903	T50.904	T50.905	T50.906
Visine	T49.5X1	T49.5X2	T49.5X3	T49.5X4	T49.5X5	T49.5X6
Visnadine	T46.3X1	T46.3X2	T46.3X3	T46.3X4	T46.3X5	T46.3X6

Substance	External Cause (T-Code)					
	Poisoning, Accidental (Unintentional)	Poisoning, Intentional Self-Harm	Poisoning, Assault	Poisoning, Undetermined	Adverse Effect	Underdosing
Vitamin NEC	T45.2X1	T45.2X2	T45.2X3	T45.2X4	T45.2X5	T45.2X6
A	T45.2X1	T45.2X2	T45.2X3	T45.2X4	T45.2X5	T45.2X6
B NEC	T45.2X1	T45.2X2	T45.2X3	T45.2X4	T45.2X5	T45.2X6
nicotinic acid	T46.7X1	T46.7X2	T46.7X3	T46.7X4	T46.7X5	T46.7X6
B1	T45.2X1	T45.2X2	T45.2X3	T45.2X4	T45.2X5	T45.2X6
B2	T45.2X1	T45.2X2	T45.2X3	T45.2X4	T45.2X5	T45.2X6
B6	T45.2X1	T45.2X2	T45.2X3	T45.2X4	T45.2X5	T45.2X6
B12	T45.2X1	T45.2X2	T45.2X3	T45.2X4	T45.2X5	T45.2X6
B15	T45.2X1	T45.2X2	T45.2X3	T45.2X4	T45.2X5	T45.2X6
C	T45.2X1	T45.2X2	T45.2X3	T45.2X4	T45.2X5	T45.2X6
D	T45.2X1	T45.2X2	T45.2X3	T45.2X4	T45.2X5	T45.2X6
D2	T45.2X1	T45.2X2	T45.2X3	T45.2X4	T45.2X5	T45.2X6
D3	T45.2X1	T45.2X2	T45.2X3	T45.2X4	T45.2X5	T45.2X6
E	T45.2X1	T45.2X2	T45.2X3	T45.2X4	T45.2X5	T45.2X6
E acetate	T45.2X1	T45.2X2	T45.2X3	T45.2X4	T45.2X5	T45.2X6
hematopoietic	T45.8X1	T45.8X2	T45.8X3	T45.8X4	T45.8X5	T45.8X6
K NEC	T45.7X1	T45.7X2	T45.7X3	T45.7X4	T45.7X5	T45.7X6
K1	T45.7X1	T45.7X2	T45.7X3	T45.7X4	T45.7X5	T45.7X6
K2	T45.7X1	T45.7X2	T45.7X3	T45.7X4	T45.7X5	T45.7X6
PP	T45.2X1	T45.2X2	T45.2X3	T45.2X4	T45.2X5	T45.2X6
ulceroprotectant	T47.1X1	T47.1X2	T47.1X3	T47.1X4	T47.1X5	T47.1X6
Vleminckx's solution	T49.4X1	T49.4X2	T49.4X3	T49.4X4	T49.4X5	T49.4X6
Voltaren — *see Diclofenac sodium*						
W						
Warfarin	T45.511	T45.512	T45.513	T45.514	T45.515	T45.516
rodenticide	T60.4X1	T60.4X2	T60.4X3	T60.4X4	—	—
sodium	T60.4X1	T60.4X2	T60.4X3	T60.4X4	—	—
Wasp (sting)	T63.461	T63.462	T63.463	T63.464	—	—
Water						
balance drug	T50.3X1	T50.3X2	T50.3X3	T50.3X4	T50.3X5	T50.3X6
distilled	T50.3X1	T50.3X2	T50.3X3	T50.3X4	T50.3X5	T50.3X6
gas — *see Gas, water*						
incomplete combustion of — *see Carbon, monoxide, fuel, utility*						
hemlock	T62.2X1	T62.2X2	T62.2X3	T62.2X4	—	—
moccasin (venom)	T63.061	T63.062	T63.063	T63.064	—	—
purified	T50.3X1	T50.3X2	T50.3X3	T50.3X4	T50.3X5	T50.3X6
Wax (paraffin) (petroleum)	T52.0X1	T52.0X2	T52.0X3	T52.0X4	—	—
automobile	T65.891	T65.892	T65.893	T65.894	—	—
floor	T52.0X1	T52.0X2	T52.0X3	T52.0X4	—	—

◀ New ◀ Revised ~~deleted~~ Deleted

Substance	External Cause (T-Code)					
	Poisoning, Accidental (Unintentional)	Poisoning, Intentional Self-Harm	Poisoning, Assault	Poisoning, Undetermined	Adverse Effect	Underdosing
Weed killers NEC	T60.3X1	T60.3X2	T60.3X3	T60.3X4	—	—
Welldorm	T42.6X1	T42.6X2	T42.6X3	T42.6X4	T42.6X5	T42.6X6
White						
arsenic	T57.0X1	T57.0X2	T57.0X3	T57.0X4	—	—
hellebore	T62.2X1	T62.2X2	T62.2X3	T62.2X4	—	—
lotion (keratolytic)	T49.4X1	T49.4X2	T49.4X3	T49.4X4	T49.4X5	T49.4X6
spirit	T52.0X1	T52.0X2	T52.0X3	T52.0X4	—	—
Whitewash	T65.891	T65.892	T65.893	T65.894	—	—
Whole blood (human)	T45.8X1	T45.8X2	T45.8X3	T45.8X4	T45.8X5	T45.8X6
Wild						
black cherry	T62.2X1	T62.2X2	T62.2X3	T62.2X4	—	—
poisonous plants NEC	T62.2X1	T62.2X2	T62.2X3	T62.2X4	—	—
Window cleaning fluid	T65.891	T65.892	T65.893	T65.894	—	—
Wintergreen (oil)	T49.3X1	T49.3X2	T49.3X3	T49.3X4	T49.3X5	T49.3X6
Wisterine	T62.2X1	T62.2X2	T62.2X3	T62.2X4	—	—
Witch hazel	T49.2X1	T49.2X2	T49.2X3	T49.2X4	T49.2X5	T49.2X6
Wood alcohol or spirit	T51.1X1	T51.1X2	T51.1X3	T51.1X4	—	—
Wool fat (hydrous)	T49.3X1	T49.3X2	T49.3X3	T49.3X4	T49.3X5	T49.3X6
Woorali	T48.1X1	T48.1X2	T48.1X3	T48.1X4	T48.1X5	T48.1X6
Wormseed, American	T37.4X1	T37.4X2	T37.4X3	T37.4X4	T37.4X5	T37.4X6
X						
Xamoterol	T44.5X1	T44.5X2	T44.5X3	T44.5X4	T44.5X5	T44.5X6
Xanthine diuretics	T50.2X1	T50.2X2	T50.2X3	T50.2X4	T50.2X5	T50.2X6
Xanthinol nicotinate	T46.7X1	T46.7X2	T46.7X3	T46.7X4	T46.7X5	T46.7X6
Xanthotoxin	T49.3X1	T49.3X2	T49.3X3	T49.3X4	T49.3X5	T49.3X6
Xantinol nicotinate	T46.7X1	T46.7X2	T46.7X3	T46.7X4	T46.7X5	T46.7X6
Xantocillin	T36.0X1	T36.0X2	T36.0X3	T36.0X4	T36.0X5	T36.0X6
Xenon (127Xe) (133Xe)	T50.8X1	T50.8X2	T50.8X3	T50.8X4	T50.8X5	T50.8X6
Xenysalate	T49.4X1	T49.4X2	T49.4X3	T49.4X4	T49.4X5	T49.4X6
Xibornol	T37.8X1	T37.8X2	T37.8X3	T37.8X4	T37.8X5	T37.8X6
Xigris	T45.511	T45.512	T45.513	T45.514	T45.515	T45.516
Xipamide	T50.2X1	T50.2X2	T50.2X3	T50.2X4	T50.2X5	T50.2X6
Xylene (vapor)	T52.2X1	T52.2X2	T52.2X3	T52.2X4	—	—
Xylocaine (infiltration) (topical)	T41.3X1	T41.3X2	T41.3X3	T41.3X4	T41.3X5	T41.3X6
nerve block (peripheral) (plexus)	T41.3X1	T41.3X2	T41.3X3	T41.3X4	T41.3X5	T41.3X6
spinal	T41.3X1	T41.3X2	T41.3X3	T41.3X4	T41.3X5	T41.3X6
Xylol (vapor)	T52.2X1	T52.2X2	T52.2X3	T52.2X4	—	—
Xylometazoline	T48.5X1	T48.5X2	T48.5X3	T48.5X4	T48.5X5	T48.5X6

Substance	External Cause (T-Code)					
	Poisoning, Accidental (Unintentional)	Poisoning, Intentional Self-Harm	Poisoning, Assault	Poisoning, Undetermined	Adverse Effect	Underdosing
Y						
Yeast	T45.2X1	T45.2X2	T45.2X3	T45.2X4	T45.2X5	T45.2X6
dried	T45.2X1	T45.2X2	T45.2X3	T45.2X4	T45.2X5	T45.2X6
Yellow						
fever vaccine	T50.B91	T50.B92	T50.B93	T50.B94	T50.B95	T50.B96
jasmine	T62.2X1	T62.2X2	T62.2X3	T62.2X4	—	—
phenolphthalein	T47.2X1	T47.2X2	T47.2X3	T47.2X4	T47.2X5	T47.2X6
Yew	T62.2X1	T62.2X2	T62.2X3	T62.2X4	—	—
Yohimbic acid	T40.991	T40.992	T40.993	T40.994	T40.995	T40.996
Z						
Zactane	T39.8X1	T39.8X2	T39.8X3	T39.8X4	T39.8X5	T39.8X6
Zalcitabine	T37.5X1	T37.5X2	T37.5X3	T37.5X4	T37.5X5	T37.5X6
Zaroxolyn	T50.2X1	T50.2X2	T50.2X3	T50.2X4	T50.2X5	T50.2X6
Zephiran (topical)	T49.0X1	T49.0X2	T49.0X3	T49.0X4	T49.0X5	T49.0X6
ophthalmic preparation	T49.5X1	T49.5X2	T49.5X3	T49.5X4	T49.5X5	T49.5X6
Zeranol	T38.7X1	T38.7X2	T38.7X3	T38.7X4	T38.7X5	T38.7X6
Zerone	T51.1X1	T51.1X2	T51.1X3	T51.1X4	—	—
Zidovudine	T37.5X1	T37.5X2	T37.5X3	T37.5X4	T37.5X5	T37.5X6
Zimeldine	T43.221	T43.222	T43.223	T43.224	T43.225	T43.226
Zinc (compounds) (fumes) (vapor) NEC	T56.5X1	T56.5X2	T56.5X3	T56.5X4	—	—
anti-infectives	T49.0X1	T49.0X2	T49.0X3	T49.0X4	T49.0X5	T49.0X6
antivaricose	T46.8X1	T46.8X2	T46.8X3	T46.8X4	T46.8X5	T46.8X6
bacitracin	T49.0X1	T49.0X2	T49.0X3	T49.0X4	T49.0X5	T49.0X6
chloride (mouthwash)	T49.6X1	T49.6X2	T49.6X3	T49.6X4	T49.6X5	T49.6X6
chromate	T56.5X1	T56.5X2	T56.5X3	T56.5X4	—	—
gelatin	T49.3X1	T49.3X2	T49.3X3	T49.3X4	T49.3X5	T49.3X6
oxide	T49.3X1	T49.3X2	T49.3X3	T49.3X4	T49.3X5	T49.3X6
plaster	T49.3X1	T49.3X2	T49.3X3	T49.3X4	T49.3X5	T49.3X6
peroxide	T49.0X1	T49.0X2	T49.0X3	T49.0X4	T49.0X5	T49.0X6
pesticides	T56.5X1	T56.5X2	T56.5X3	T56.5X4	—	—
phosphide	T60.4X1	T60.4X2	T60.4X3	T60.4X4	—	—
pyrithionate	T49.4X1	T49.4X2	T49.4X3	T49.4X4	T49.4X5	T49.4X6
stearate	T49.3X1	T49.3X2	T49.3X3	T49.3X4	T49.3X5	T49.3X6
sulfate	T49.5X1	T49.5X2	T49.5X3	T49.5X4	T49.5X5	T49.5X6
ENT agent	T49.6X1	T49.6X2	T49.6X3	T49.6X4	T49.6X5	T49.6X6
ophthalmic solution	T49.5X1	T49.5X2	T49.5X3	T49.5X4	T49.5X5	T49.5X6
topical NEC	T49.0X1	T49.0X2	T49.0X3	T49.0X4	T49.0X5	T49.0X6
undecylenate	T49.0X1	T49.0X2	T49.0X3	T49.0X4	T49.0X5	T49.0X6

◀ New ◀ Revised ~~deleted~~ Deleted

Substance	External Cause (T-Code)					
	Poisoning, Accidental (Unintentional)	Poisoning, Intentional Self-Harm	Poisoning, Assault	Poisoning, Undetermined	Adverse Effect	Underdosing
Zineb	T60.0X1	T60.0X2	T60.0X3	T60.0X4	—	—
Zinostatin	T45.1X1	T45.1X2	T45.1X3	T45.1X4	T45.1X5	T45.1X6
Zipeprol	T48.3X1	T48.3X2	T48.3X3	T48.3X4	T48.3X5	T48.3X6
Zofenopril	T46.4X1	T46.4X2	T46.4X3	T46.4X4	T46.4X5	T46.4X6
Zolpidem	T42.6X1	T42.6X2	T42.6X3	T42.6X4	T42.6X5	T42.6X6
Zomepirac	T39.391	T39.392	T39.393	T39.394	T39.395	T39.396
Zopiclone	T42.6X1	T42.6X2	T42.6X3	T42.6X4	T42.6X5	T42.6X6

Substance	External Cause (T-Code)					
	Poisoning, Accidental (Unintentional)	Poisoning, Intentional Self-Harm	Poisoning, Assault	Poisoning, Undetermined	Adverse Effect	Underdosing
Zorubicin	T45.1X1	T45.1X2	T45.1X3	T45.1X4	T45.1X5	T45.1X6
Zotepine	T43.591	T43.592	T43.593	T43.594	T43.595	T43.596
Zovant	T45.511	T45.512	T45.513	T45.514	T45.515	T45.516
Zoxazolamine	T42.8X1	T42.8X2	T42.8X3	T42.8X4	T42.8X5	T42.8X6
Zuclopenthixol	T43.4X1	T43.4X2	T43.4X3	T43.4X4	T43.4X5	T43.4X6
Zygadenus (venenosus)	T62.2X1	T62.2X2	T62.2X3	T62.2X4	—	—
Zyprexa	T43.591	T43.592	T43.593	T43.594	T43.595	T43.596

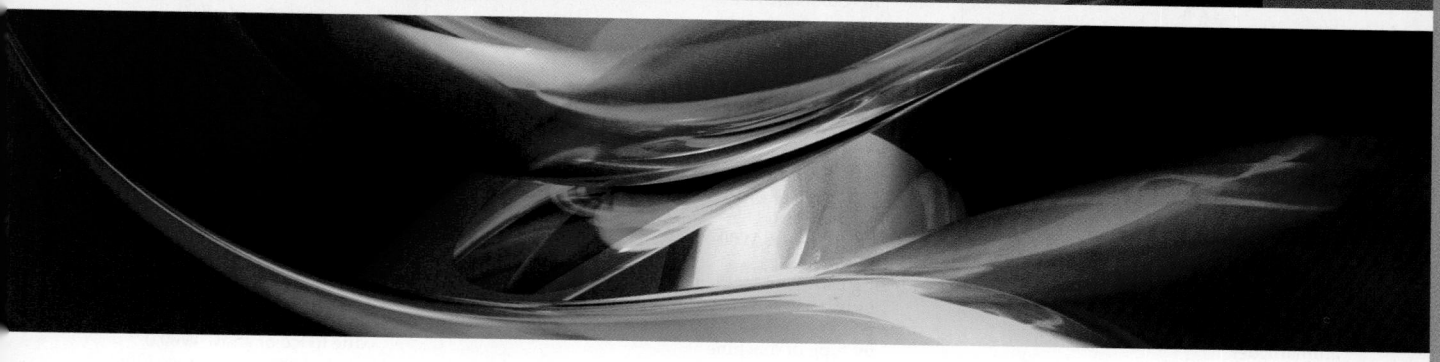

External Cause of Injuries Index

A

Abandonment (causing exposure to weather conditions) (with intent to injure or kill) NEC X58
Abuse (adult) (child) (mental) (physical) (sexual) X58
Accident (to) X58
aircraft (in transit) (powered) —*see also* Accident, transport, aircraft
due to, caused by cataclysm —*see* Forces of nature, by type
animal-drawn vehicle —*see* Accident, transport, animal-drawn vehicle occupant
animal-rider —*see* Accident, transport, animal-rider
automobile —*see* Accident, transport, car occupant
bare foot water skiier V94.4
boat, boating —*see also* Accident, watercraft
striking swimmer
powered V94.11
unpowered V94.12
bus —*see* Accident, transport, bus occupant
cable car, not on rails V98.0
on rails —*see* Accident, transport, streetcar occupant
car —*see* Accident, transport, car occupant
caused by, due to
animal NEC W64
chain hoist W24.0
cold (excessive) —*see* Exposure, cold
corrosive liquid, substance —*see* Table of Drugs and Chemicals ◄
cutting or piercing instrument —*see* Contact, with, by type of instrument
drive belt W24.0
electric
current —*see* Exposure, electric current
motor —*see also* Contact, with, by type of machine W31.3
current (of) W86.8
environmental factor NEC X58
explosive material —*see* Explosion
fire, flames —*see* Exposure, fire
firearm missile —*see* Discharge, firearm by type
heat (excessive) —*see* Heat
hot —*see* Contact, with, hot
ignition —*see* Ignition
lifting device W24.0
lightning —*see* subcategory T75.0
causing fire —*see* Exposure, fire
machine, machinery —*see* Contact, with, by type of machine
natural factor NEC X58
pulley (block) W24.0
radiation —*see* Radiation
steam X13.1
inhalation X13.0
pipe X16
thunderbolt —*see* subcategory T75.0
causing fire —*see* Exposure, fire
transmission device W24.1
coach —*see* Accident, transport, bus occupant
coal car —*see* Accident, transport, industrial vehicle occupant
diving —*see also* Fall, into, water
with
drowning or submersion —*see* Drowning
forklift —*see* Accident, transport, industrial vehicle occupant
heavy transport vehicle NOS —*see* Accident, transport, truck occupant
ice yacht V98.2

Accident *(Continued)*
in
medical, surgical procedure
as, or due to misadventure —*see* Misadventure
causing an abnormal reaction or later complication without mention of misadventure —*see also* Complication of or following, by type of procedure Y84.9
land yacht V98.1
late effect of —*see* W00-X58 with 7th character S
logging car —*see* Accident, transport, industrial vehicle occupant
machine, machinery —*see also* Contact, with, by type of machine
on board watercraft V93.69
explosion —*see* Explosion, in, watercraft
fire —*see* Burn, on board watercraft
powered craft V93.63
ferry boat V93.61
fishing boat V93.62
jetskis V93.63
liner V93.61
merchant ship V93.60
passenger ship V93.61
sailboat V93.64
mine tram —*see* Accident, transport, industrial vehicle occupant
mobility scooter (motorized) —*see* Accident, transport, pedestrian, conveyance, specified type NEC
motor scooter —*see* Accident, transport, motorcyclist
motor vehicle NOS (traffic) —*see also* Accident, transport V89.2
nontraffic V89.0
three-wheeled NOS —*see* Accident, transport, three-wheeled motor vehicle occupant
motorcycle NOS —*see* Accident, transport, motorcyclist
nonmotor vehicle NOS (nontraffic) —*see also* Accident, transport V89.1
traffic NOS V89.3
nontraffic (victim's mode of transport NOS) V88.9
collision (between) V88.7
bus and truck V88.5
car and:
bus V88.3
pickup V88.2
three-wheeled motor vehicle V88.0
train V88.6
truck V88.4
two-wheeled motor vehicle V88.0
van V88.2
specified vehicle NEC and:
three-wheeled motor vehicle V88.1
two-wheeled motor vehicle V88.1
known mode of transport —*see* Accident, transport, by type of vehicle
noncollision V88.8
on board watercraft V93.89
powered craft V93.83
ferry boat V93.81
fishing boat V93.82
jetskis V93.83
liner V93.81
merchant ship V93.80
passenger ship V93.81
unpowered craft V93.88
canoe V93.85
inflatable V93.86
in tow
recreational V94.31
specified NEC V94.32
kayak V93.85

Accident *(Continued)*
on board watercraft *(Continued)*
unpowered craft *(Continued)*
sailboat V93.84
surf-board V93.88
water skis V93.87
windsurfer V93.88
parachutist V97.29
entangled in object V97.21
injured on landing V97.22
pedal cycle —*see* Accident, transport, pedal cyclist
pedestrian (on foot)
with
another pedestrian W51
with fall W03
due to ice or snow W00.0
on pedestrian conveyance NEC V00.09
roller skater (in-line) V00.01
skate boarder V00.02
transport vehicle —*see* Accident, transport
on pedestrian conveyance —*see* Accident, transport, pedestrian, conveyance
pick-up truck or van —*see* Accident, transport, pickup truck occupant
quarry truck —*see* Accident, transport, industrial vehicle occupant
railway vehicle (any) (in motion) —*see* Accident, transport, railway vehicle occupant
due to cataclysm —*see* Forces of nature, by type
scooter (non-motorized) —*see* Accident, transport, pedestrian, conveyance, scooter
sequelae of —*see* W00-X58 with 7th character S
skateboard —*see* Accident, transport, pedestrian, conveyance, skateboard
ski (ing) —*see* Accident, transport, pedestrian, conveyance
lift V98.3
specified cause NEC X58
streetcar —*see* Accident, transport, streetcar occupant
traffic (victim's mode of transport NOS) V87.9
collision (between) V87.7
bus and truck V87.5
car and:
bus V87.3
pickup V87.2
three-wheeled motor vehicle V87.0
train V87.6
truck V87.4
two-wheeled motor vehicle V87.0
van V87.2
specified vehicle NEC and:
three-wheeled motor vehicle V87.1
two-wheeled motor vehicle V87.1
known mode of transport —*see* Accident, transport, by type of vehicle
noncollision V87.8
transport (involving injury to) V99
18 wheeler —*see* Accident, transport, truck occupant
agricultural vehicle occupant (nontraffic) V84.9
driver V84.5
hanger-on V84.7
passenger V84.6
traffic V84.3
driver V84.0
hanger-on V84.2
passenger V84.1
while boarding or alighting V84.4

◄ New ⇐ Revised ~~deleted~~ Deleted

Accident *(Continued)*
transport *(Continued)*
aircraft NEC V97.89
military NEC V97.818
with civilian aircraft V97.810
civilian injured by V97.811
occupant injured (in)
nonpowered craft accident V96.9
balloon V96.00
collision V96.03
crash V96.01
explosion V96.05
fire V96.04
forced landing V96.02
specified type NEC V96.09
glider V96.20
collision V96.23
crash V96.21
explosion V96.25
fire V96.24
forced landing V96.22
specified type NEC V96.29
hang glider V96.10
collision V96.13
crash V96.11
explosion V96.15
fire V96.14
forced landing V96.12
specified type NEC V96.19
specified craft NEC V96.8
powered craft accident V95.9
fixed wing NEC
commercial V95.30
collision V95.33
crash V95.31
explosion V95.35
fire V95.34
forced landing V95.32
specified type NEC V95.39
private V95.20
collision V95.23
crash V95.21
explosion V95.25
fire V95.24
forced landing V95.22
specified type NEC V95.29
glider V95.10
collision V95.13
crash V95.11
explosion V95.15
fire V95.14
forced landing V95.12
specified type NEC V95.19
helicopter V95.00
collision V95.03
crash V95.01
explosion V95.05
fire V95.04
forced landing V95.02
specified type NEC V95.09
spacecraft V95.40
collision V95.43
crash V95.41
explosion V95.45
fire V95.44
forced landing V95.42
specified type NEC V95.49
specified craft NEC V95.8
ultralight V95.10
collision V95.13
crash V95.11
explosion V95.15
fire V95.14
forced landing V95.12
specified type NEC V95.19
specified accident NEC V97.0
while boarding or alighting V97.1

Accident *(Continued)*
transport *(Continued)*
aircraft NEC *(Continued)*
person (injured by)
falling from, in or on aircraft V97.0
machinery on aircraft V97.89
on ground with aircraft involvement V97.39
rotating propeller V97.32
struck by object falling from aircraft V97.31
sucked into aircraft jet V97.33
while boarding or alighting aircraft V97.1
airport (battery-powered) passenger vehicle —*see* Accident, transport, industrial vehicle occupant
all-terrain vehicle occupant (nontraffic) V86.99
driver V86.59
dune buggy —*see* Accident, transport, dune buggy occupant
hanger-on V86.79
passenger V86.69
snowmobile —*see* Accident, transport, snowmobile occupant
traffic V86.39
driver V86.09
hanger-on V86.29
passenger V86.19
while boarding or alighting V86.49
ambulance occupant (traffic) V86.31
driver V86.01
hanger-on V86.21
nontraffic V86.91
driver V86.51
hanger-on V86.71
passenger V86.61
passenger V86.11
while boarding or alighting V86.41
animal-drawn vehicle occupant (in) V80.929
collision (with)
animal V80.12
being ridden V80.711
animal-drawn vehicle V80.721
bus V80.42
car V80.42
fixed or stationary object V80.82
military vehicle V80.920
nonmotor vehicle V80.791
pedal cycle V80.22
pedestrian V80.12
pickup V80.42
railway train or vehicle V80.62
specified motor vehicle NEC V80.52
streetcar V80.731
truck V80.42
two-or three-wheeled motor vehicle V80.32
van V80.42
noncollision V80.02
specified circumstance NEC V80. 928
animal-rider V80.919
collision (with)
animal V80.11
being ridden V80.710
animal-drawn vehicle V80.720
bus V80.41
car V80.41
fixed or stationary object V80.81
military vehicle V80.910
nonmotor vehicle V80.790
pedal cycle V80.21
pedestrian V80.11
pickup V80.41
railway train or vehicle V80.61
specified motor vehicle NEC V80.51
streetcar V80.730
truck V80.41

Accident *(Continued)*
transport *(Continued)*
animal-rider *(Continued)*
collision *(Continued)*
two- or three-wheeled motor vehicle V80.31
van V80.41
noncollision V80.018
specified as horse rider V80.010
specified circumstance NEC V80.918
armored car —*see* Accident, transport, truck occupant
battery-powered truck (baggage) (mail) —*see* Accident, transport, industrial vehicle occupant
bus occupant V79.9
collision (with)
animal (traffic) V70.9
being ridden (traffic) V76.9
nontraffic V76.3
while boarding or alighting V76.4
nontraffic V70.3
while boarding or alighting V70.4
animal-drawn vehicle (traffic) V76.9
nontraffic V76.3
while boarding or alighting V76.4
bus (traffic) V74.9
nontraffic V74.3
while boarding or alighting V74.4
car (traffic) V73.9
nontraffic V73.3
while boarding or alighting V73.4
motor vehicle NOS (traffic) V79.60
nontraffic V79.20
specified type NEC (traffic) V79.69
nontraffic V79.29
pedal cycle (traffic) V71.9
nontraffic V71.3
while boarding or alighting V71.4
pickup truck (traffic) V73.9
nontraffic V73.3
while boarding or alighting V73.4
railway vehicle (traffic) V75.9
nontraffic V75.3
while boarding or alighting V75.4
specified vehicle NEC (traffic) V76.9
nontraffic V76.3
while boarding or alighting V76.4
stationary object (traffic) V77.9
nontraffic V77.3
while boarding or alighting V77.4
streetcar (traffic) V76.9
nontraffic V76.3
while boarding or alighting V76.4
three wheeled motor vehicle (traffic) V72.9
nontraffic V72.3
while boarding or alighting V72.4
truck (traffic) V74.9
nontraffic V74.3
while boarding or alighting V74.4
two wheeled motor vehicle (traffic) V72.9
nontraffic V72.3
while boarding or alighting V72.4
van (traffic) V73.9
nontraffic V73.3
while boarding or alighting V73.4
driver
collision (with)
animal (traffic) V70.5
being ridden (traffic) V76.5
nontraffic V76.0
nontraffic V70.0
animal-drawn vehicle (traffic) V76.5
nontraffic V76.0
bus (traffic) V74.5
nontraffic V74.0
car (traffic) V73.5
nontraffic V73.0

A

Accident *(Continued)*
transport *(Continued)*
bus occupant *(Continued)*
driver *(Continued)*
collision *(Continued)*
motor vehicle NOS (traffic) V79.40
nontraffic V79.00
specified type NEC (traffic) V79.49
nontraffic V79.09
pedal cycle (traffic) V71.5
nontraffic V71.0
pickup truck (traffic) V73.5
nontraffic V73.0
railway vehicle (traffic) V75.5
nontraffic V75.0
specified vehicle NEC (traffic) V76.5
nontraffic V76.0
stationary object (traffic) V77.5
nontraffic V77.0
streetcar (traffic) V76.5
nontraffic V76.0
three wheeled motor vehicle (traffic) V72.5
nontraffic V72.0
truck (traffic) V74.5
nontraffic V74.0
two wheeled motor vehicle (traffic) V72.5
nontraffic V72.0
van (traffic) V73.5
nontraffic V73.0
noncollision accident (traffic) V78.5
nontraffic V78.0
hanger-on
collision (with)
animal (traffic) V70.7
being ridden (traffic) V76.7
nontraffic V76.2
nontraffic V70.2
animal-drawn vehicle (traffic) V76.7
nontraffic V76.2
bus (traffic) V74.7
nontraffic V74.2
car (traffic) V73.7
nontraffic V73.2
pedal cycle (traffic) V71.7
nontraffic V71.2
pickup truck (traffic) V73.7
nontraffic V73.2
railway vehicle (traffic) V75.7
nontraffic V75.2
specified vehicle NEC (traffic) V76.7
nontraffic V76.2
stationary object (traffic) V77.7
nontraffic V77.2
streetcar (traffic) V76.7
nontraffic V76.2
three wheeled motor vehicle (traffic) V72.7
nontraffic V72.2
truck (traffic) V74.7
nontraffic V74.2
two wheeled motor vehicle (traffic) V72.7
nontraffic V72.2
van (traffic) V73.7
nontraffic V73.2
noncollision accident (traffic) V78.7
nontraffic V78.2
noncollision accident (traffic) V78.9
nontraffic V78.3
while boarding or alighting V78.4
nontraffic V79.3
passenger
collision (with)
animal (traffic) V70.6
being ridden (traffic) V76.6
nontraffic V76.1
nontraffic V70.1

Accident *(Continued)*
transport *(Continued)*
bus occupant *(Continued)*
passenger *(Continued)*
collision *(Continued)*
animal-drawn vehicle (traffic) V76.6
nontraffic V76.1
bus (traffic) V74.6
nontraffic V74.1
car (traffic) V73.6
nontraffic V73.1
motor vehicle NOS (traffic) V79.50
nontraffic V79.10
specified type NEC (traffic) V79.59
nontraffic V79.19
pedal cycle (traffic) V71.6
nontraffic V71.1
pickup truck (traffic) V73.6
nontraffic V73.1
railway vehicle (traffic) V75.6
nontraffic V75.1
specified vehicle NEC (traffic) V76.6
nontraffic V76.1
stationary object (traffic) V77.6
nontraffic V77.1
streetcar (traffic) V76.6
nontraffic V76.1
three wheeled motor vehicle (traffic) V72.6
nontraffic V72.1
truck (traffic) V74.6
nontraffic V74.1
two wheeled motor vehicle (traffic) V72.6
nontraffic V72.1
van (traffic) V73.6
nontraffic V73.1
noncollision accident (traffic) V78.6
nontraffic V78.1
specified type NEC V79.88
military vehicle V79.81
cable car, not on rails V98.0
on rails —*see* Accident, transport, streetcar occupant
car occupant V49.9
ambulance occupant —*see* Accident, transport, ambulance occupant
collision (with)
animal (traffic) V40.9
being ridden (traffic) V46.9
nontraffic V46.3
while boarding or alighting V46.4
nontraffic V40.3
while boarding or alighting V40.4
animal-drawn vehicle (traffic) V46.9
nontraffic V46.3
while boarding or alighting V46.4
bus (traffic) V44.9
nontraffic V44.3
while boarding or alighting V44.4
car (traffic) V43.92
nontraffic V43.32
while boarding or alighting V43.42
motor vehicle NOS (traffic) V49.60
nontraffic V49.20
specified type NEC (traffic) V49.69
nontraffic V49.29
pedal cycle (traffic) V41.9
nontraffic V41.3
while boarding or alighting V41.4
pickup truck (traffic) V43.93
nontraffic V43.33
while boarding or alighting V43.43
railway vehicle (traffic) V45.9
nontraffic V45.3
while boarding or alighting V45.4
specified vehicle NEC (traffic) V46.9
nontraffic V46.3
while boarding or alighting V46.4

Accident *(Continued)*
transport *(Continued)*
car occupant *(Continued)*
collision *(Continued)*
sport utility vehicle (traffic) V43.91
nontraffic V43.31
while boarding or alighting V43.41
stationary object (traffic) V47.92
nontraffic V47.32
while boarding or alighting V47.4
streetcar (traffic) V46.9
nontraffic V46.3
while boarding or alighting V46.4
three wheeled motor vehicle (traffic) V42.9
nontraffic V42.3
while boarding or alighting V42.4
truck (traffic) V44.9
nontraffic V44.3
while boarding or alighting V44.4
two wheeled motor vehicle (traffic) V42.9
nontraffic V42.3
while boarding or alighting V42.4
van (traffic) V43.94
nontraffic V43.34
while boarding or alighting V43.44
driver
collision (with)
animal (traffic) V40.5
being ridden (traffic) V46.5
nontraffic V46.0
nontraffic V40.0
animal-drawn vehicle (traffic) V46.5
nontraffic V46.0
bus (traffic) V44.5
nontraffic V44.0
car (traffic) V43.52
nontraffic V43.02
motor vehicle NOS (traffic) V49.40
nontraffic V49.00
specified type NEC (traffic) V49.49
nontraffic V49.09
pedal cycle (traffic) V41.5
nontraffic V41.0
pickup truck (traffic) V43.53
nontraffic V43.03
railway vehicle (traffic) V45.5
nontraffic V45.0
specified vehicle NEC (traffic) V46.5
nontraffic V46.0
sport utility vehicle (traffic) V43.51
nontraffic V43.01
stationary object (traffic) V47.52
nontraffic V47.02
streetcar (traffic) V46.5
nontraffic V46.0
three wheeled motor vehicle (traffic) V42.5
nontraffic V42.0
truck (traffic) V44.5
nontraffic V44.0
two wheeled motor vehicle (traffic) V42.5
nontraffic V42.0
van (traffic) V43.54
nontraffic V43.04
noncollision accident (traffic) V48.5
nontraffic V48.0
hanger-on
collision (with)
animal (traffic) V40.7
being ridden (traffic) V46.7
nontraffic V46.2
nontraffic V40.2
animal-drawn vehicle (traffic) V46.7
nontraffic V46.2
bus (traffic) V44.7
nontraffic V44.2

Accident *(Continued)*
transport *(Continued)*
car occupant *(Continued)*
hanger-on *(Continued)*
collision *(Continued)*
car (traffic) V43.72
nontraffic V43.22
pedal cycle (traffic) V41.7
nontraffic V41.2
pickup truck (traffic) V43.73
nontraffic V43.23
railway vehicle (traffic) V45.7
nontraffic V45.2
specified vehicle NEC (traffic) V46.7
nontraffic V46.2
sport utility vehicle (traffic) V43.71
nontraffic V43.21
stationary object (traffic) V47.7
nontraffic V47.2
streetcar (traffic) V46.7
nontraffic V46.2
three wheeled motor vehicle (traffic) V42.7
nontraffic V42.2
truck (traffic) V44.7
nontraffic V44.2
two wheeled motor vehicle (traffic) V42.7
nontraffic V42.2
van (traffic) V43.74
nontraffic V43.24
noncollision accident (traffic) V48.7
nontraffic V48.2
noncollision accident (traffic) V48.9
nontraffic V48.3
while boarding or alighting V48.4
nontraffic V49.3
passenger
collision (with)
animal (traffic) V40.6
being ridden (traffic) V46.6
nontraffic V46.1
nontraffic V40.1
animal-drawn vehicle (traffic) V46.6
nontraffic V46.1
bus (traffic) V44.6
nontraffic V44.1
car (traffic) V43.62
nontraffic V43.12
motor vehicle NOS (traffic) V49.50
nontraffic V49.10
specified type NEC (traffic) V49.59
nontraffic V49.19
pedal cycle (traffic) V41.6
nontraffic V41.1
pickup truck (traffic) V43.63
nontraffic V43.13
railway vehicle (traffic) V45.6
nontraffic V45.1
specified vehicle NEC (traffic) V46.6
nontraffic V46.1
sport utility vehicle (traffic) V43.61
nontraffic V43.11
stationary object (traffic) V47.62
nontraffic V47.12
streetcar (traffic) V46.6
nontraffic V46.1
three wheeled motor vehicle (traffic) V42.6
nontraffic V42.1
truck (traffic) V44.6
nontraffic V44.1
two wheeled motor vehicle (traffic) V42.6
nontraffic V42.1
van (traffic) V43.64
nontraffic V43.14
noncollision accident (traffic) V48.6
nontraffic V48.1
specified type NEC V49.88
military vehicle V49.81

Accident *(Continued)*
transport *(Continued)*
coal car —*see* Accident, transport, industrial vehicle occupant
construction vehicle occupant (nontraffic) V85.9
driver V85.5
hanger-on V85.7
passenger V85.6
traffic V85.3
driver V85.0
hanger-on V85.2
passenger V85.1
while boarding or alighting V85.4
dirt bike rider —*see* Accident, transport, all-terrain vehicle occupant
due to cataclysm —*see* Forces of nature, by type
dune buggy occupant (nontraffic) V86.93
driver V86.53
hanger-on V86.73
passenger V86.63
traffic V86.33
driver V86.03
hanger-on V86.23
passenger V86.13
while boarding or alighting V86.43
forklift —*see* Accident, transport, industrial vehicle occupant
go cart —*see* Accident, transport, all-terrain vehicle occupant
golf cart —*see* Accident, transport, all-terrain vehicle occupant
heavy transport vehicle occupant —*see* Accident, transport, truck occupant
ice yacht V98.2
industrial vehicle occupant (nontraffic) V83.9
driver V83.5
hanger-on V83.7
passenger V83.6
traffic V83.3
driver V83.0
hanger-on V83.2
passenger V83.1
while boarding or alighting V83.4
interurban electric car —*see* Accident, transport, streetcar
land yacht V98.1
logging car —*see* Accident, transport, industrial vehicle occupant
military vehicle occupant (traffic) V86.34
driver V86.04
hanger-on V86.24
nontraffic V86.94
driver V86.54
hanger-on V86.74
passenger V86.64
passenger V86.14
while boarding or alighting V86.44
mine tram —*see* Accident, transport, industrial vehicle occupant
motor vehicle NEC occupant (traffic) V89.2 ◄
~~driver V86.09~~
~~hanger-on V86.29~~
~~nontraffic V86.99~~
~~driver V86.59~~
~~hanger-on V86.79~~
~~passenger V86.69~~
~~passenger V86.19~~
~~while boarding or alighting V86.49~~
motorcoach —*see* Accident, transport, bus occupant
motorcyclist V29.9
collision (with)
animal (traffic) V20.9
being ridden (traffic) V26.9
nontraffic V26.2
while boarding or alighting V26.3
nontraffic V20.2
while boarding or alighting V20.3

Accident *(Continued)*
transport *(Continued)*
motorcyclist *(Continued)*
collision *(Continued)*
animal-drawn vehicle (traffic) V26.9
nontraffic V26.2
while boarding or alighting V26.3
bus (traffic) V24.9
nontraffic V24.2
while boarding or alighting V24.3
car (traffic) V23.9
nontraffic V23.2
while boarding or alighting V23.3
motor vehicle NOS (traffic) V29.60
nontraffic V29.20
specified type NEC (traffic) V29.69
nontraffic V29.29
pedal cycle (traffic) V21.9
nontraffic V21.2
while boarding or alighting V21.3
pickup truck (traffic) V23.9
nontraffic V23.2
while boarding or alighting V23.3
railway vehicle (traffic) V25.9
nontraffic V25.2
while boarding or alighting V25.3
specified vehicle NEC (traffic) V26.9
nontraffic V26.2
while boarding or alighting V26.3
stationary object (traffic) V27.9
nontraffic V27.2
while boarding or alighting V27.3
streetcar (traffic) V26.9
nontraffic V26.2
while boarding or alighting V26.3
three wheeled motor vehicle (traffic) V22.9
nontraffic V22.2
while boarding or alighting V22.3
truck (traffic) V24.9
nontraffic V24.2
while boarding or alighting V24.3
two wheeled motor vehicle (traffic) V22.9
nontraffic V22.2
while boarding or alighting V22.3
van (traffic) V23.9
nontraffic V23.2
while boarding or alighting V23.3
driver
collision (with)
animal (traffic) V20.4
being ridden (traffic) V26.4
nontraffic V26.0
nontraffic V20.0
animal-drawn vehicle (traffic) V26.4
nontraffic V26.0
bus (traffic) V24.4
nontraffic V24.0
car (traffic) V23.4
nontraffic V23.0
motor vehicle NOS (traffic) V29.40
nontraffic V29.00
specified type NEC (traffic) V29.49
nontraffic V29.09
pedal cycle (traffic) V21.4
nontraffic V21.0
pickup truck (traffic) V23.4
nontraffic V23.0
railway vehicle (traffic) V25.4
nontraffic V25.0
specified vehicle NEC (traffic) V26.4
nontraffic V26.0
stationary object (traffic) V27.4
nontraffic V27.0
streetcar (traffic) V26.4
nontraffic V26.0
three wheeled motor vehicle (traffic) V22.4
nontraffic V22.0

A

Accident *(Continued)*
transport *(Continued)*
motorcyclist *(Continued)*
driver *(Continued)*
collision *(Continued)*
truck (traffic) V24.4
nontraffic V24.0
two wheeled motor vehicle (traffic) V22.4
nontraffic V22.0
van (traffic) V23.4
nontraffic V23.0
noncollision accident (traffic) V28.4
nontraffic V28.0
noncollision accident (traffic) V28.9
nontraffic V28.2
while boarding or alighting V28.3
nontraffic V29.3
passenger
collision (with)
animal (traffic) V20.5
being ridden (traffic) V26.5
nontraffic V26.1
nontraffic V20.1
animal-drawn vehicle (traffic) V26.5
nontraffic V26.1
bus (traffic) V24.5
nontraffic V24.1
car (traffic) V23.5
nontraffic V23.1
motor vehicle NOS (traffic) V29.50
nontraffic V29.10
specified type NEC (traffic) V29.59
nontraffic V29.19
pedal cycle (traffic) V21.5
nontraffic V21.1
pickup truck (traffic) V23.5
nontraffic V23.1
railway vehicle (traffic) V25.5
nontraffic V25.1
specified vehicle NEC (traffic) V26.5
nontraffic V26.1
stationary object (traffic) V27.5
nontraffic V27.1
streetcar (traffic) V26.5
nontraffic V26.1
three wheeled motor vehicle (traffic) V22.5
nontraffic V22.1
truck (traffic) V24.5
nontraffic V24.1
two wheeled motor vehicle (traffic) V22.5
nontraffic V22.1
van (traffic) V23.5
nontraffic V23.1
noncollision accident (traffic) V28.5
nontraffic V28.1
specified type NEC V29.88
military vehicle V29.81
occupant (of)
aircraft (powered) V95.9
fixed wing
commercial —*see* Accident, transport, aircraft, occupant, powered, fixed wing, commercial
private —*see* Accident, transport, aircraft, occupant, powered, fixed wing, private
nonpowered V96.9
specified NEC V95.8
airport battery-powered vehicle —*see* Accident, transport, industrial vehicle occupant
all-terrain vehicle (ATV) —*see* Accident, transport, all-terrain vehicle occupant

Accident *(Continued)*
transport *(Continued)*
occupant *(Continued)*
animal-drawn vehicle —*see* Accident, transport, animal-drawn vehicle occupant
automobile —*see* Accident, transport, car occupant
balloon V96.00
battery-powered vehicle —*see* Accident, transport, industrial vehicle occupant
bicycle —*see* Accident, transport, pedal cyclist
motorized —*see* Accident, transport, motorcycle rider
boat NEC —*see* Accident, watercraft
bulldozer —*see* Accident, transport, construction vehicle occupant
bus —*see* Accident, transport, bus occupant
cable car (on rails) —*see also* Accident, transport, streetcar occupant
not on rails V98.0
car —*see also* Accident, transport, car occupant
cable (on rails) —*see also* Accident, transport, streetcar occupant
not on rails V98.0
coach —*see* Accident, transport, bus occupant
coal-car —*see* Accident, transport, industrial vehicle occupant
digger —*see* Accident, transport, construction vehicle occupant
dump truck —*see* Accident, transport, construction vehicle occupant
earth-leveler —*see* Accident, transport, construction vehicle occupant
farm machinery (self-propelled) —*see* Accident, transport, agricultural vehicle occupant
forklift —*see* Accident, transport, industrial vehicle occupant
glider (unpowered) V96.20
hang V96.10
powered (microlight) (ultralight) —*see* Accident, transport, aircraft, occupant, powered, glider
glider (unpowered) NEC V96.20
hang-glider V96.10
harvester —*see* Accident, transport, agricultural vehicle occupant
heavy (transport) vehicle —*see* Accident, transport, truck occupant
helicopter —*see* Accident, transport, aircraft, occupant, helicopter
ice-yacht V98.2
kite (carrying person) V96.8
land-yacht V98.1
logging car —*see* Accident, transport, industrial vehicle occupant
mechanical shovel —*see* Accident, transport, construction vehicle occupant
microlight —*see* Accident, transport, aircraft, occupant, powered, glider
minibus —*see* Accident, transport, pickup truck occupant
minivan —*see* Accident, transport, pickup truck occupant
moped —*see* Accident, transport, motorcycle
motor scooter —*see* Accident, transport, motorcycle
motorcycle (with sidecar) —*see* Accident, transport, motorcycle
pedal cycle —*see also* Accident, transport, pedal cyclist
pick-up (truck) —*see* Accident, transport, pickup truck occupant

Accident *(Continued)*
transport *(Continued)*
occupant *(Continued)*
railway (train) (vehicle) (subterranean) (elevated) —*see* Accident, transport, railway vehicle occupant
rickshaw —*see* Accident, transport, pedal cycle
pedal driven —*see* Accident, transport, pedal cyclist
road-roller —*see* Accident, transport, construction vehicle occupant
ship NOS V94.9
ski-lift (chair) (gondola) V98.3
snowmobile —*see* Accident, transport, snowmobile occupant
spacecraft, spaceship —*see* Accident, transport, aircraft, occupant, spacecraft
sport utility vehicle —*see* Accident, transport, pickup truck occupant
streetcar (interurban) (operating on public street or highway) —*see* Accident, transport, streetcar occupant
SUV —*see* Accident, transport, pickup truck occupant
téléférique V98.0
three-wheeled vehicle (motorized) —*see also* Accident, transport, three-wheeled motor vehicle occupant
nonmotorized —*see* Accident, transport, pedal cycle
tractor (farm) (and trailer) —*see* Accident, transport, agricultural vehicle occupant
train —*see* Accident, transport, railway vehicle occupant
tram —*see* Accident, transport, streetcar occupant
in mine or quarry —*see* Accident, transport, industrial vehicle occupant
tricycle —*see* Accident, transport, pedal cycle
motorized —*see* Accident, transport, three-wheeled motor vehicle
trolley —*see* Accident, transport, streetcar occupant
in mine or quarry —*see* Accident, transport, industrial vehicle occupant
tub, in mine or quarry —*see* Accident, transport, industrial vehicle occupant
ultralight —*see* Accident, transport, aircraft, occupant, powered, glider
van —*see* Accident, transport, van occupant
vehicle NEC V89.9
heavy transport —*see* Accident, transport, truck occupant
motor (traffic) NEC V89.2
nontraffic NEC V89.0
watercraft NOS V94.9
causing drowning —*see* Drowning, resulting from accident to boat
parachutist V97.29
after accident to aircraft —*see* Accident, transport, aircraft
entangled in object V97.21
injured on landing V97.22
pedal cyclist V19.9
collision (with)
animal (traffic) V10.9
being ridden (traffic) V16.9
nontraffic V16.2
while boarding or alighting V16.3
nontraffic V10.2
while boarding or alighting V10.3

◀ New ⇐ Revised ~~deleted~~ Deleted

Accident *(Continued)*
transport *(Continued)*
pedal cyclist *(Continued)*
collision *(Continued)*
animal-drawn vehicle (traffic) V16.9
nontraffic V16.2
while boarding or alighting V16.3
bus (traffic) V14.9
nontraffic V14.2
while boarding or alighting V14.3
car (traffic) V13.9
nontraffic V13.2
while boarding or alighting V13.3
motor vehicle NOS (traffic) V19.60
nontraffic V19.20
specified type NEC (traffic) V19.69
nontraffic V19.29
pedal cycle (traffic) V11.9
nontraffic V11.2
while boarding or alighting V11.3
pickup truck (traffic) V13.9
nontraffic V13.2
while boarding or alighting V13.3
railway vehicle (traffic) V15.9
nontraffic V15.2
while boarding or alighting V15.3
specified vehicle NEC (traffic) V16.9
nontraffic V16.2
while boarding or alighting V16.3
stationary object (traffic) V17.9
nontraffic V17.2
while boarding or alighting V17.3
streetcar (traffic) V16.9
nontraffic V16.2
while boarding or alighting V16.3
three wheeled motor vehicle (traffic) V12.9
nontraffic V12.2
while boarding or alighting V12.3
truck (traffic) V14.9
nontraffic V14.2
while boarding or alighting V14.3
two wheeled motor vehicle (traffic) V12.9
nontraffic V12.2
while boarding or alighting V12.3
van (traffic) V13.9
nontraffic V13.2
while boarding or alighting V13.3
driver
collision (with)
animal (traffic) V10.4
being ridden (traffic) V16.4
nontraffic V16.0
nontraffic V10.0
animal-drawn vehicle (traffic) V16.4
nontraffic V16.0
bus (traffic) V14.4
nontraffic V14.0
car (traffic) V13.4
nontraffic V13.0
motor vehicle NOS (traffic) V19.40
nontraffic V19.00
specified type NEC (traffic) V19.49
nontraffic V19.09
pedal cycle (traffic) V11.4
nontraffic V11.0
pickup truck (traffic) V13.4
nontraffic V13.0
railway vehicle (traffic) V15.4
nontraffic V15.0
specified vehicle NEC (traffic) V16.4
nontraffic V16.0
stationary object (traffic) V17.4
nontraffic V17.0
streetcar (traffic) V16.4
nontraffic V16.0
three wheeled motor vehicle (traffic) V12.4
nontraffic V12.0

Accident *(Continued)*
transport *(Continued)*
pedal cyclist *(Continued)*
driver *(Continued)*
collision *(Continued)*
truck (traffic) V14.4
nontraffic V14.0
two wheeled motor vehicle (traffic) V12.4
nontraffic V12.0
van (traffic) V13.4
nontraffic V13.0
noncollision accident (traffic) V18.4
nontraffic V18.0
noncollision accident (traffic) V18.9
nontraffic V18.2
while boarding or alighting V18.3
nontraffic V19.3
passenger
collision (with)
animal (traffic) V10.5
being ridden (traffic) V16.5
nontraffic V16.1
nontraffic V10.1
animal-drawn vehicle (traffic) V16.5
nontraffic V16.1
bus (traffic) V14.5
nontraffic V14.1
car (traffic) V13.5
nontraffic V13.1
motor vehicle NOS (traffic) V19.50
nontraffic V19.10
specified type NEC (traffic) V19.59
nontraffic V19.19
pedal cycle (traffic) V11.5
nontraffic V11.1
pickup truck (traffic) V13.5
nontraffic V13.1
railway vehicle (traffic) V15.5
nontraffic V15.1
specified vehicle NEC (traffic) V16.5
nontraffic V16.1
stationary object (traffic) V17.5
nontraffic V17.1
streetcar (traffic) V16.5
nontraffic V16.1
three wheeled motor vehicle (traffic) V12.5
nontraffic V12.1
truck (traffic) V14.5
nontraffic V14.1
two wheeled motor vehicle (traffic) V12.5
nontraffic V12.1
van (traffic) V13.5
nontraffic V13.1
noncollision accident (traffic) V18.5
nontraffic V18.1
specified type NEC V19.88
military vehicle V19.81
pedestrian
conveyance (occupant) V09.9
babystroller V00.828
collision (with) V09.9
animal being ridden or animal drawn vehicle V06.99
nontraffic V06.09
traffic V06.19
bus or heavy transport V04.99
nontraffic V04.09
traffic V04.19
car V03.99
nontraffic V03.09
traffic V03.19
pedal cycle V01.99
nontraffic V01.09
traffic V01.19
pick-up truck or van V03.99
nontraffic V03.09
traffic V03.19

Accident *(Continued)*
transport *(Continued)*
pedestrian *(Continued)*
conveyance *(Continued)*
babystroller *(Continued)*
collision *(Continued)*
railway (train) (vehicle) V05.99
nontraffic V05.09
traffic V05.19
stationary object V00.822
streetcar V06.99
nontraffic V06.09
traffic V06.19
two- or three-wheeled motor vehicle V02.99
nontraffic V02.09
traffic V02.19
vehicle V09.9
animal-drawn V06.99
nontraffic V06.09
traffic V06.19
motor
nontraffic V09.00
traffic V09.20
fall V00.821
nontraffic V09.1
involving motor vehicle NEC V09.00
traffic V09.3
involving motor vehicle NEC V09.20
flat-bottomed NEC V00.388
collision (with) V09.9
animal being ridden or animal drawn vehicle V06.99
nontraffic V06.09
traffic V06.19
bus or heavy transport V04.99
nontraffic V04.09
traffic V04.19
car V03.99
nontraffic V03.09
traffic V03.19
pedal cycle V01.99
nontraffic V01.09
traffic V01.19
pick-up truck or van V03.99
nontraffic V03.09
traffic V03.19
railway (train) (vehicle) V05.99
nontraffic V05.09
traffic V05.19
stationary object V00.382
streetcar V06.99
nontraffic V06.09
traffic V06.19
two-or three-wheeled motor vehicle V02.99
nontraffic V02.09
traffic V02.19
vehicle V09.9
animal-drawn V06.99
nontraffic V06.09
traffic V06.19
motor
nontraffic V09.00
traffic V09.20
fall V00.381
nontraffic V09.1
involving motor vehicle NEC V09.00
snow
board —*see* Accident, transport, pedestrian, conveyance, snow board
ski —*see* Accident, transport, pedestrian, conveyance, skis (snow)
traffic V09.3
involving motor vehicle NEC V09.20

Accident *(Continued)*
transport *(Continued)*
pedestrian *(Continued)*
conveyance *(Continued)*
gliding type NEC V00.288
collision (with) V09.9
animal being ridden or animal drawn vehicle V06.99
nontraffic V06.09
traffic V06.19
bus or heavy transport V04.99
nontraffic V04.09
traffic V04.19
car V03.99
nontraffic V03.09
traffic V03.19
pedal cycle V01.99
nontraffic V01.09
traffic V01.19
pick-up truck or van V03.99
nontraffic V03.09
traffic V03.19
railway (train) (vehicle) V05.99
nontraffic V05.09
traffic V05.19
stationary object V00.282
streetcar V06.99
nontraffic V06.09
traffic V06.19
two- or three-wheeled motor vehicle V02.99
nontraffic V02.09
traffic V02.19
vehicle V09.9
animal-drawn V06.99
nontraffic V06.09
traffic V06.19
motor
nontraffic V09.00
traffic V09.20
fall V00.281
heelies —*see* Accident, transport, pedestrian, conveyance, heelies
ice skate —*see* Accident, transport, pedestrian, conveyance, ice skate
nontraffic V09.1
involving motor vehicle NEC V09.00
sled —*see* Accident, transport, pedestrian, conveyance, sled
traffic V09.3
involving motor vehicle NEC V09.20
wheelies —*see* Accident, transport, pedestrian, conveyance, heelies
heelies V00.158
colliding with stationary object V00.152
fall V00.151
ice skates V00.218
collision (with) V09.9
animal being ridden or animal drawn vehicle V06.99
nontraffic V06.09
traffic V06.19
bus or heavy transport V04.99
nontraffic V04.09
traffic V04.19
car V03.99
nontraffic V03.09
traffic V03.19
pedal cycle V01.99
nontraffic V01.09
traffic V01.19
pick-up truck or van V03.99
nontraffic V03.09
traffic V03.19

Accident *(Continued)*
transport *(Continued)*
pedestrian *(Continued)*
conveyance *(Continued)*
ice skates *(Continued)*
collision *(Continued)*
railway (train) (vehicle) V05.99
nontraffic V05.09
traffic V05.19
stationary object V00.212
streetcar V06.99
nontraffic V06.09
traffic V06.19
two- or three-wheeled motor vehicle V02.99
nontraffic V02.09
traffic V02.19
vehicle V09.9
animal-drawn V06.99
nontraffic V06.09
traffic V06.19
motor
nontraffic V09.00
traffic V09.20
fall V00.211
nontraffic V09.1
involving motor vehicle NEC V09.00
traffic V09.3
involving motor vehicle NEC V09.20
motorized mobility scooter V00.838
collision with stationary object V00.832
fall from V00.831
nontraffic V09.1
involving motor vehicle V09.00
military V09.01
specified type NEC V09.09
roller skates (non in-line) V00.128
collision (with) V09.9
animal being ridden or animal drawn vehicle V06.91
nontraffic V06.01
traffic V06.11
bus or heavy transport V04.91
nontraffic V04.01
traffic V04.11
car V03.91
nontraffic V03.01
traffic V03.11
pedal cycle V01.91
nontraffic V01.01
traffic V01.11
pick-up truck or van V03.91
nontraffic V03.01
traffic V03.11
railway (train) (vehicle) V05.91
nontraffic V05.01
traffic V05.11
stationary object V00.122
streetcar V06.91
nontraffic V06.01
traffic V06.11
two- or three-wheeled motor vehicle V02.91
nontraffic V02.01
traffic V02.11
vehicle V09.9
animal-drawn V06.91
nontraffic V06.01
traffic V06.11
motor
nontraffic V09.00
traffic V09.20
fall V00.121

Accident *(Continued)*
transport *(Continued)*
pedestrian *(Continued)*
conveyance *(Continued)*
roller skates *(Continued)*
in-line V00.118
collision —*see also* Accident, transport, pedestrian, conveyance occupant, roller skates, collision
with stationary object V00.112
fall V00.111
nontraffic V09.1
involving motor vehicle NEC V09.00
traffic V09.3
involving motor vehicle NEC V09.20
rolling shoes V00.158
colliding with stationary object V00.152
fall V00.151
rolling type NEC V00.188
collision (with) V09.9
animal being ridden or animal drawn vehicle V06.99
nontraffic V06.09
traffic V06.19
bus or heavy transport V04.99
nontraffic V04.09
traffic V04.19
car V03.99
nontraffic V03.09
traffic V03.19
pedal cycle V01.99
nontraffic V01.09
traffic V01.19
pick-up truck or van V03.99
nontraffic V03.09
traffic V03.19
railway (train) (vehicle) V05.99
nontraffic V05.09
traffic V05.19
stationary object V00.182
streetcar V06.99
nontraffic V06.09
traffic V06.19
two- or three-wheeled motor vehicle V02.99
nontraffic V02.09
traffic V02.19
vehicle V09.9
animal-drawn V06.99
nontraffic V06.09
traffic V06.19
motor
nontraffic V09.00
traffic V09.20
fall V00.181
in-line roller skate —*see* Accident, transport, pedestrian, conveyance, roller skate, in-line
nontraffic V09.1
involving motor vehicle NEC V09.00
roller skate —*see* Accident, transport, pedestrian, conveyance, roller skate
scooter (non-motorized) —*see* Accident, transport, pedestrian, conveyance, scooter
skateboard —*see* Accident, transport, pedestrian, conveyance, skateboard
traffic V09.3
involving motor vehicle NEC V09.20

Accident *(Continued)*
transport *(Continued)*
pedestrian *(Continued)*
conveyance *(Continued)*
scooter (non-motorized) V00.148
collision (with) V09.9
animal being ridden or animal drawn vehicle V06.99
nontraffic V06.09
traffic V06.19
bus or heavy transport V04.99
nontraffic V04.09
traffic V04.19
car V03.99
nontraffic V03.09
traffic V03.19
pedal cycle V01.99
nontraffic V01.09
traffic V01.19
pick-up truck or van V03.99
nontraffic V03.09
traffic V03.19
railway (train) (vehicle) V05.99
nontraffic V05.09
traffic V05.19
stationary object V00.142
streetcar V06.99
nontraffic V06.09
traffic V06.19
two- or three-wheeled motor vehicle V02.99
nontraffic V02.09
traffic V02.19
vehicle V09.9
animal-drawn V06.99
nontraffic V06.09
traffic V06.19
motor
nontraffic V09.00
traffic V09.20
fall V00.141
nontraffic V09.1
involving motor vehicle NEC V09.00
traffic V09.3
involving motor vehicle NEC V09.20
skate board V00.138
collision (with) V09.9
animal being ridden or animal drawn vehicle V06.92
nontraffic V06.02
traffic V06.12
bus or heavy transport V04.92
nontraffic V04.02
traffic V04.12
car V03.92
nontraffic V03.02
traffic V03.12
pedal cycle V01.92
nontraffic V01.02
traffic V01.12
pick-up truck or van V03.92
nontraffic V03.02
traffic V03.12
railway (train) (vehicle) V05.92
nontraffic V05.02
traffic V05.12
stationary object V00.132
streetcar V06.92
nontraffic V06.02
traffic V06.12
two- or three-wheeled motor vehicle V02.92
nontraffic V02.02
traffic V02.12

Accident *(Continued)*
transport *(Continued)*
pedestrian *(Continued)*
conveyance *(Continued)*
skate board *(Continued)*
collision *(Continued)*
vehicle V09.9
animal-drawn V06.92
nontraffic V06.02
traffic V06.12
motor
nontraffic V09.00
traffic V09.20
fall V00.131
nontraffic V09.1
involving motor vehicle NEC V09.00
traffic V09.3
involving motor vehicle NEC V09.20
skis (snow) V00.328
collision (with) V09.9
animal being ridden or animal drawn vehicle V06.99
nontraffic V06.09
traffic V06.19
bus or heavy transport V04.99
nontraffic V04.09
traffic V04.19
car V03.99
nontraffic V03.09
traffic V03.19
pedal cycle V01.99
nontraffic V01.09
traffic V01.19
pick-up truck or van V03.99
nontraffic V03.09
traffic V03.19
railway (train) (vehicle) V05.99
nontraffic V05.09
traffic V05.19
stationary object V00.322
streetcar V06.99
nontraffic V06.09
traffic V06.19
two- or three-wheeled motor vehicle V02.99
nontraffic V02.09
traffic V02.19
vehicle V09.9
animal-drawn V06.99
nontraffic V06.09
traffic V06.19
motor
nontraffic V09.00
traffic V09.20
fall V00.321
nontraffic V09.1
involving motor vehicle NEC V09.00
traffic V09.3
involving motor vehicle NEC V09.20
sled V00.228
collision (with) V09.9
animal being ridden or animal drawn vehicle V06.99
nontraffic V06.09
traffic V06.19
bus or heavy transport V04.99
nontraffic V04.09
traffic V04.19
car V03.99
nontraffic V03.09
traffic V03.19
pedal cycle V01.99
nontraffic V01.09
traffic V01.19
pick-up truck or van V03.99
nontraffic V03.09
traffic V03.19

Accident *(Continued)*
transport *(Continued)*
pedestrian *(Continued)*
conveyance *(Continued)*
sled *(Continued)*
collision *(Continued)*
railway (train) (vehicle) V05.99
nontraffic V05.09
traffic V05.19
stationary object V00.222
streetcar V06.99
nontraffic V06.09
traffic V06.19
two- or three-wheeled motor vehicle V02.99
nontraffic V02.09
traffic V02.19
vehicle V09.9
animal-drawn V06.99
nontraffic V06.09
traffic V06.19
motor
nontraffic V09.00
traffic V09.20
fall V00.221
nontraffic V09.1
involving motor vehicle NEC V09.00
traffic V09.3
involving motor vehicle NEC V09.20
snow board V00.318
collision (with) V09.9
animal being ridden or animal drawn vehicle V06.99
nontraffic V06.09
traffic V06.19
bus or heavy transport V04.99
nontraffic V04.09
traffic V04.19
car V03.99
nontraffic V03.09
traffic V03.19
pedal cycle V01.99
nontraffic V01.09
traffic V01.19
pick-up truck or van V03.99
nontraffic V03.09
traffic V03.19
railway (train) (vehicle) V05.99
nontraffic V05.09
traffic V05.19
stationary object V00.312
streetcar V06.99
nontraffic V06.09
traffic V06.19
two- or three-wheeled motor vehicle V02.99
nontraffic V02.09
traffic V02.19
vehicle V09.9
animal-drawn V06.99
nontraffic V06.09
traffic V06.19
motor
nontraffic V09.00
traffic V09.20
fall V00.311
nontraffic V09.1
involving motor vehicle NEC V09.00
traffic V09.3
involving motor vehicle NEC V09.20
specified type NEC V00.898
collision (with) V09.9
animal being ridden or animal drawn vehicle V06.99
nontraffic V06.09
traffic V06.19

A

Accident *(Continued)*
transport *(Continued)*
pedestrian *(Continued)*
conveyance *(Continued)*
specified type NEC *(Continued)*
collision *(Continued)*
bus or heavy transport V04.99
nontraffic V04.09
traffic V04.19
car V03.99
nontraffic V03.09
traffic V03.19
pedal cycle V01.99
nontraffic V01.09
traffic V01.19
pick-up truck or van V03.99
nontraffic V03.09
traffic V03.19
railway (train) (vehicle) V05.99
nontraffic V05.09
traffic V05.19
stationary object V00.892
streetcar V06.99
nontraffic V06.09
traffic V06.19
two- or three-wheeled motor vehicle V02.99
nontraffic V02.09
traffic V02.19
vehicle V09.9
animal-drawn V06.99
nontraffic V06.09
traffic V06.19
motor
nontraffic V09.00
traffic V09.20
fall V00.891
nontraffic V09.1
involving motor vehicle NEC V09.00
traffic V09.3
involving motor vehicle NEC V09.20
traffic V09.3
involving motor vehicle V09.20
military V09.21
specified type NEC V09.29
wheelchair (powered) V00.818
collision (with) V09.9
animal being ridden or animal drawn vehicle V06.99
nontraffic V06.09
traffic V06.19
bus or heavy transport V04.99
nontraffic V04.09
traffic V04.19
car V03.99
nontraffic V03.09
traffic V03.19
pedal cycle V01.99
nontraffic V01.09
traffic V01.19
pick-up truck or van V03.99
nontraffic V03.09
traffic V03.19
railway (train) (vehicle) V05.99
nontraffic V05.09
traffic V05.19
stationary object V00.812
streetcar V06.99
nontraffic V06.09
traffic V06.19
two- or three-wheeled motor vehicle V02.99
nontraffic V02.09
traffic V02.19

Accident *(Continued)*
transport *(Continued)*
pedestrian *(Continued)*
conveyance *(Continued)*
wheelchair *(Continued)*
collision *(Continued)*
vehicle V09.9
animal-drawn V06.99
nontraffic V06.09
traffic V06.19
motor
nontraffic V09.00
traffic V09.20
fall V00.811
nontraffic V09.1
involving motor vehicle NEC V09.00
traffic V09.3
involving motor vehicle NEC V09.20
wheeled shoe V00.158
colliding with stationary object V00.152
fall V00.151
on foot —*see also* Accident, pedestrian
collision (with)
animal being ridden or animal drawn vehicle V06.90
nontraffic V06.00
traffic V06.10
bus or heavy transport V04.90
nontraffic V04.00
traffic V04.10
car V03.90
nontraffic V03.00
traffic V03.10
pedal cycle V01.90
nontraffic V01.00
traffic V01.10
pick-up truck or van V03.90
nontraffic V03.00
traffic V03.10
railway (train) (vehicle) V05.90
nontraffic V05.00
traffic V05.10
streetcar V06.90
nontraffic V06.00
traffic V06.10
two- or three-wheeled motor vehicle V02.90
nontraffic V02.00
traffic V02.10
vehicle V09.9
animal-drawn V06.90
nontraffic V06.00
traffic V06.10
motor
nontraffic V09.00
traffic V09.20
nontraffic V09.1
involving motor vehicle V09.00
military V09.01
specified type NEC V09.09
traffic V09.3
involving motor vehicle V09.20
military V09.21
specified type NEC V09.29
person NEC (unknown way or transportation) V99
collision (between)
bus (with)
heavy transport vehicle (traffic) V87.5
nontraffic V88.5
car (with)
nontraffic V88.5
bus (traffic) V87.3
nontraffic V88.3
heavy transport vehicle (traffic) V87.4
nontraffic V88.4

Accident *(Continued)*
transport *(Continued)*
person NEC *(Continued)*
collision *(Continued)*
car *(Continued)*
pick-up truck or van (traffic) V87.2
nontraffic V88.2
train or railway vehicle (traffic) V87.6
nontraffic V88.6
two- or three-wheeled motor vehicle (traffic) V87.0
nontraffic V88.0
motor vehicle (traffic) NEC V87.7
nontraffic V88.7
two- or three-wheeled vehicle (with) (traffic)
motor vehicle NEC V87.1
nontraffic V88.1
nonmotor vehicle (collision) (noncollision) (traffic) V87.9
nontraffic V88.9
pickup truck occupant V59.9
collision (with)
animal (traffic) V50.9
being ridden (traffic) V56.9
nontraffic V56.3
while boarding or alighting V56.4
nontraffic V50.3
while boarding or alighting V50.4
animal-drawn vehicle (traffic) V56.9
nontraffic V56.3
while boarding or alighting V56.4
bus (traffic) V54.9
nontraffic V54.3
while boarding or alighting V54.4
car (traffic) V53.9
nontraffic V53.3
while boarding or alighting V53.4
motor vehicle NOS (traffic) V59.60
nontraffic V59.20
specified type NEC (traffic) V59.69
nontraffic V59.29
pedal cycle (traffic) V51.9
nontraffic V51.3
while boarding or alighting V51.4
pickup truck (traffic) V53.9
nontraffic V53.3
while boarding or alighting V53.4
railway vehicle (traffic) V55.9
nontraffic V55.3
while boarding or alighting V55.4
specified vehicle NEC (traffic) V56.9
nontraffic V56.3
while boarding or alighting V56.4
stationary object (traffic) V57.9
nontraffic V57.3
while boarding or alighting V57.4
streetcar (traffic) V56.9
nontraffic V56.3
while boarding or alighting V56.4
three wheeled motor vehicle (traffic) V52.9
nontraffic V52.3
while boarding or alighting V52.4
truck (traffic) V54.9
nontraffic V54.3
while boarding or alighting V54.4
two wheeled motor vehicle (traffic) V52.9
nontraffic V52.3
while boarding or alighting V52.4
van (traffic) V53.9
nontraffic V53.3
while boarding or alighting V53.4
driver
collision (with)
animal (traffic) V50.5
being ridden (traffic) V56.5
nontraffic V56.0
nontraffic V50.0

A

◀ New ◀ Revised ~~deleted~~ Deleted

Accident *(Continued)*
transport *(Continued)*
pickup truck occupant *(Continued)*
driver *(Continued)*
collision *(Continued)*
animal-drawn vehicle (traffic) V56.5
nontraffic V56.0
bus (traffic) V54.5
nontraffic V54.0
car (traffic) V53.5
nontraffic V53.0
motor vehicle NOS (traffic) V59.40
nontraffic V59.00
specified type NEC (traffic) V59.49
nontraffic V59.09
pedal cycle (traffic) V51.5
nontraffic V51.0
pickup truck (traffic) V53.5
nontraffic V53.0
railway vehicle (traffic) V55.5
nontraffic V55.0
specified vehicle NEC (traffic) V56.5
nontraffic V56.0
stationary object (traffic) V57.5
nontraffic V57.0
streetcar (traffic) V56.5
nontraffic V56.0
three wheeled motor vehicle (traffic) V52.5
nontraffic V52.0
truck (traffic) V54.5
nontraffic V54.0
two wheeled motor vehicle (traffic) V52.5
nontraffic V52.0
van (traffic) V53.5
nontraffic V53.0
noncollision accident (traffic) V58.5
nontraffic V58.0
hanger-on
collision (with)
animal (traffic) V50.7
being ridden (traffic) V56.7
nontraffic V56.2
nontraffic V50.2
animal-drawn vehicle (traffic) V56.7
nontraffic V56.2
bus (traffic) V54.7
nontraffic V54.2
car (traffic) V53.7
nontraffic V53.2
pedal cycle (traffic) V51.7
nontraffic V51.2
pickup truck (traffic) V53.7
nontraffic V53.2
railway vehicle (traffic) V55.7
nontraffic V55.2
specified vehicle NEC (traffic) V56.7
nontraffic V56.2
stationary object (traffic) V57.7
nontraffic V57.2
streetcar (traffic) V56.7
nontraffic V56.2
three wheeled motor vehicle (traffic) V52.7
nontraffic V52.2
truck (traffic) V54.7
nontraffic V54.2
two wheeled motor vehicle (traffic) V52.7
nontraffic V52.2
van (traffic) V53.7
nontraffic V53.2
noncollision accident (traffic) V58.7
nontraffic V58.2
noncollision accident (traffic) V58.9
nontraffic V58.3
while boarding or alighting V58.4
nontraffic V59.3

Accident *(Continued)*
transport *(Continued)*
pickup truck occupant *(Continued)*
passenger
collision (with)
animal (traffic) V50.6
being ridden (traffic) V56.6
nontraffic V56.1
nontraffic V50.1
animal-drawn vehicle (traffic) V56.6
nontraffic V56.1
bus (traffic) V54.6
nontraffic V54.1
car (traffic) V53.6
nontraffic V53.1
motor vehicle NOS (traffic) V59.50
nontraffic V59.10
specified type NEC (traffic) V59.59
nontraffic V59.19
pedal cycle (traffic) V51.6
nontraffic V51.1
pickup truck (traffic) V53.6
nontraffic V53.1
railway vehicle (traffic) V55.6
nontraffic V55.1
specified vehicle NEC (traffic) V56.6
nontraffic V56.1
stationary object (traffic) V57.6
nontraffic V57.1
streetcar (traffic) V56.6
nontraffic V56.1
three wheeled motor vehicle (traffic) V52.6
nontraffic V52.1
truck (traffic) V54.6
nontraffic V54.1
two wheeled motor vehicle (traffic) V52.6
nontraffic V52.1
van (traffic) V53.6
nontraffic V53.1
noncollision accident (traffic) V58.6
nontraffic V58.1
specified type NEC V59.88
military vehicle V59.81
quarry truck —*see* Accident, transport, industrial vehicle occupant
race car —*see* Accident, transport, motor vehicle NEC occupant
railway vehicle occupant V81.9
collision (with) V81.3
motor vehicle (non-military) (traffic) V81.1
military V81.83
nontraffic V81.0
rolling stock V81.2
specified object NEC V81.3
during derailment V81.7
with antecedent collision —*see* Accident, transport, railway vehicle occupant, collision ◀
explosion V81.81
fall (in railway vehicle) V81.5
during derailment V81.7
with antecedent collision —*see* Accident, transport, railway vehicle occupant, collision ◀
from railway vehicle V81.6
during derailment V81.7
with antecedent collision —*see* Accident, transport, railway vehicle occupant, collision ◀
while boarding or alighting V81.4
fire V81.81
object falling onto train V81.82
specified type NEC V81.89
while boarding or alighting V81.4
ski lift V98.3

Accident *(Continued)*
transport *(Continued)*
snowmobile occupant (nontraffic) V86.92
driver V86.52
hanger-on V86.72
passenger V86.62
traffic V86.32
driver V86.02
hanger-on V86.22
passenger V86.12
while boarding or alighting V86.42
specified NEC V98.8
sport utility vehicle occupant —*see also* Accident, transport, pickup truck occupant ⇐
~~collision (with)~~
~~stationary object (traffic) V47.91~~
~~nontraffic V47.31~~
~~driver~~
~~collision (with)~~
~~stationary object (traffic) V47.51~~
~~nontraffic V47.01~~
~~passenger~~
~~collision (with)~~
~~stationary object (traffic) V47.61~~
~~nontraffic V47.11~~
streetcar occupant V82.9
collision (with) V82.3
motor vehicle (traffic) V82.1
nontraffic V82.0
rolling stock V82.2
during derailment V82.7
with antecedent collision —*see* Accident, transport, streetcar occupant, collision ◀
fall (in streetcar) V82.5
during derailment V82.7
with antecedent collision —*see* Accident, transport, streetcar occupant, collision ◀
from streetcar V82.6
during derailment V82.7
with antecedent collision —*see* Accident, transport, streetcar occupant, collision ◀
while boarding or alighting V82.4
while boarding or alighting V82.4
specified type NEC V82.8
while boarding or alighting V82.4
three-wheeled motor vehicle occupant V39.9
collision (with)
animal (traffic) V30.9
being ridden (traffic) V36.9
nontraffic V36.3
while boarding or alighting V36.4
nontraffic V30.3
while boarding or alighting V30.4
animal-drawn vehicle (traffic) V36.9
nontraffic V36.3
while boarding or alighting V36.4
bus (traffic) V34.9
nontraffic V34.3
while boarding or alighting V34.4
car (traffic) V33.9
nontraffic V33.3
while boarding or alighting V33.4
motor vehicle NOS (traffic) V39.60
nontraffic V39.20
specified type NEC (traffic) V39.69
nontraffic V39.29
pedal cycle (traffic) V31.9
nontraffic V31.3
while boarding or alighting V31.4
pickup truck (traffic) V33.9
nontraffic V33.3
while boarding or alighting V33.4
railway vehicle (traffic) V35.9
nontraffic V35.3
while boarding or alighting V35.4

Accident *(Continued)*
transport *(Continued)*
three-wheeled motor vehicle occupant *(Continued)*
collision *(Continued)*
specified vehicle NEC (traffic) V36.9
nontraffic V36.3
while boarding or alighting V36.4
stationary object (traffic) V37.9
nontraffic V37.3
while boarding or alighting V37.4
streetcar (traffic) V36.9
nontraffic V36.3
while boarding or alighting V36.4
three wheeled motor vehicle (traffic) V32.9
nontraffic V32.3
while boarding or alighting V32.4
truck (traffic) V34.9
nontraffic V34.3
while boarding or alighting V34.4
two wheeled motor vehicle (traffic) V32.9
nontraffic V32.3
while boarding or alighting V32.4
van (traffic) V33.9
nontraffic V33.3
while boarding or alighting V33.4
driver
collision (with)
animal (traffic) V30.5
being ridden (traffic) V36.5
nontraffic V36.0
nontraffic V30.0
animal-drawn vehicle (traffic) V36.5
nontraffic V36.0
bus (traffic) V34.5
nontraffic V34.0
car (traffic) V33.5
nontraffic V33.0
motor vehicle NOS (traffic) V39.40
nontraffic V39.00
specified type NEC (traffic) V39.49
nontraffic V39.09
pedal cycle (traffic) V31.5
nontraffic V31.0
pickup truck (traffic) V33.5
nontraffic V33.0
railway vehicle (traffic) V35.5
nontraffic V35.0
specified vehicle NEC (traffic) V36.5
nontraffic V36.0
stationary object (traffic) V37.5
nontraffic V37.0
streetcar (traffic) V36.5
nontraffic V36.0
three wheeled motor vehicle (traffic) V32.5
nontraffic V32.0
truck (traffic) V34.5
nontraffic V34.0
two wheeled motor vehicle (traffic) V32.5
nontraffic V32.0
van (traffic) V33.5
nontraffic V33.0
noncollision accident (traffic) V38.5
nontraffic V38.0
hanger-on
collision (with)
animal (traffic) V30.7
being ridden (traffic) V36.7
nontraffic V36.2
nontraffic V30.2
animal-drawn vehicle (traffic) V36.7
nontraffic V36.2
bus (traffic) V34.7
nontraffic V34.2
car (traffic) V33.7
nontraffic V33.2

Accident *(Continued)*
transport *(Continued)*
three-wheeled motor vehicle occupant *(Continued)*
hanger-on *(Continued)*
collision *(Continued)*
pedal cycle (traffic) V31.7
nontraffic V31.2
pickup truck (traffic) V33.7
nontraffic V33.2
railway vehicle (traffic) V35.7
nontraffic V35.2
specified vehicle NEC (traffic) V36.7
nontraffic V36.2
stationary object (traffic) V37.7
nontraffic V37.2
streetcar (traffic) V36.7
nontraffic V36.2
three wheeled motor vehicle (traffic) V32.7
nontraffic V32.2
truck (traffic) V34.7
nontraffic V34.2
two wheeled motor vehicle (traffic) V32.7
nontraffic V32.2
van (traffic) V33.7
nontraffic V33.2
noncollision accident (traffic) V38.7
nontraffic V38.2
noncollision accident (traffic) V38.9
nontraffic V38.3
while boarding or alighting V38.4
nontraffic V39.3
passenger
collision (with)
animal (traffic) V30.6
being ridden (traffic) V36.6
nontraffic V36.1
nontraffic V30.1
animal-drawn vehicle (traffic) V36.6
nontraffic V36.1
bus (traffic) V34.6
nontraffic V34.1
car (traffic) V33.6
nontraffic V33.1
motor vehicle NOS (traffic) V39.50
nontraffic V39.10
specified type NEC (traffic) V39.59
nontraffic V39.19
pedal cycle (traffic) V31.6
nontraffic V31.1
pickup truck (traffic) V33.6
nontraffic V33.1
railway vehicle (traffic) V35.6
nontraffic V35.1
specified vehicle NEC (traffic) V36.6
nontraffic V36.1
stationary object (traffic) V37.6
nontraffic V37.1
streetcar (traffic) V36.6
nontraffic V36.1
three wheeled motor vehicle (traffic) V32.6
nontraffic V32.1
truck (traffic) V34.6
nontraffic V34.1
two wheeled motor vehicle (traffic) V32.6
nontraffic V32.1
van (traffic) V33.6
nontraffic V33.1
noncollision accident (traffic) V38.6
nontraffic V38.1
specified type NEC V39.89
military vehicle V39.81
tractor (farm) (and trailer) —*see* Accident, transport, agricultural vehicle occupant

Accident *(Continued)*
transport *(Continued)*
tram —*see* Accident, transport, streetcar
in mine or quarry —*see* Accident, transport, industrial vehicle occupant
trolley —*see* Accident, transport, streetcar
in mine or quarry —*see* Accident, transport, industrial vehicle occupant
truck (heavy) occupant V69.9
collision (with)
animal (traffic) V60.9
being ridden (traffic) V66.9
nontraffic V66.3
while boarding or alighting V66.4
nontraffic V60.3
while boarding or alighting V60.4
animal-drawn vehicle (traffic) V66.9
nontraffic V66.3
while boarding or alighting V66.4
bus (traffic) V64.9
nontraffic V64.3
while boarding or alighting V64.4
car (traffic) V63.9
nontraffic V63.3
while boarding or alighting V63.4
motor vehicle NOS (traffic) V69.60
nontraffic V69.20
specified type NEC (traffic) V69.69
nontraffic V69.29
pedal cycle (traffic) V61.9
nontraffic V61.3
while boarding or alighting V61.4
pickup truck (traffic) V63.9
nontraffic V63.3
while boarding or alighting V63.4
railway vehicle (traffic) V65.9
nontraffic V65.3
while boarding or alighting V65.4
specified vehicle NEC (traffic) V66.9
nontraffic V66.3
while boarding or alighting V66.4
stationary object (traffic) V67.9
nontraffic V67.3
while boarding or alighting V67.4
streetcar (traffic) V66.9
nontraffic V66.3
while boarding or alighting V66.4
three wheeled motor vehicle (traffic) V62.9
nontraffic V62.3
while boarding or alighting V62.4
truck (traffic) V64.9
nontraffic V64.3
while boarding or alighting V64.4
two wheeled motor vehicle (traffic) V62.9
nontraffic V62.3
while boarding or alighting V62.4
van (traffic) V63.9
nontraffic V63.3
while boarding or alighting V63.4
driver
collision (with)
animal (traffic) V60.5
being ridden (traffic) V66.5
nontraffic V66.0
nontraffic V60.0
animal-drawn vehicle (traffic) V66.5
nontraffic V66.0
bus (traffic) V64.5
nontraffic V64.0
car (traffic) V63.5
nontraffic V63.0
motor vehicle NOS (traffic) V69.40
nontraffic V69.00
specified type NEC (traffic) V69.49
nontraffic V69.09

A

◀ New ◀ Revised ~~deleted~~ Deleted

Accident *(Continued)*
transport *(Continued)*
truck occupant *(Continued)*
driver *(Continued)*
collision *(Continued)*
pedal cycle (traffic) V61.5
nontraffic V61.0
pickup truck (traffic) V63.5
nontraffic V63.0
railway vehicle (traffic) V65.5
nontraffic V65.0
specified vehicle NEC (traffic) V66.5
nontraffic V66.0
stationary object (traffic) V67.5
nontraffic V67.0
streetcar (traffic) V66.5
nontraffic V66.0
three wheeled motor vehicle (traffic) V62.5
nontraffic V62.0
truck (traffic) V64.5
nontraffic V64.0
two wheeled motor vehicle (traffic) V62.5
nontraffic V62.0
van (traffic) V63.5
nontraffic V63.0
noncollision accident (traffic) V68.5
nontraffic V68.0
dump —*see* Accident, transport, construction vehicle occupant
hanger-on
collision (with)
animal (traffic) V60.7
being ridden (traffic) V66.7
nontraffic V66.2
nontraffic V60.2
animal-drawn vehicle (traffic) V66.7
nontraffic V66.2
bus (traffic) V64.7
nontraffic V64.2
car (traffic) V63.7
nontraffic V63.2
pedal cycle (traffic) V61.7
nontraffic V61.2
pickup truck (traffic) V63.7
nontraffic V63.2
railway vehicle (traffic) V65.7
nontraffic V65.2
specified vehicle NEC (traffic) V66.7
nontraffic V66.2
stationary object (traffic) V67.7
nontraffic V67.2
streetcar (traffic) V66.7
nontraffic V66.2
three wheeled motor vehicle (traffic) V62.7
nontraffic V62.2
truck (traffic) V64.7
nontraffic V64.2
two wheeled motor vehicle (traffic) V62.7
nontraffic V62.2
van (traffic) V63.7
nontraffic V63.2
noncollision accident (traffic) V68.7
nontraffic V68.2
noncollision accident (traffic) V68.9
nontraffic V68.3
while boarding or alighting V68.4
nontraffic V69.3
passenger
collision (with)
animal (traffic) V60.6
being ridden (traffic) V66.6
nontraffic V66.1
nontraffic V60.1
animal-drawn vehicle (traffic) V66.6
nontraffic V66.1
bus (traffic) V64.6
nontraffic V64.1

Accident *(Continued)*
transport *(Continued)*
truck occupant *(Continued)*
passenger *(Continued)*
collision *(Continued)*
car (traffic) V63.6
nontraffic V63.1
motor vehicle NOS (traffic) V69.50
nontraffic V69.10
specified type NEC (traffic) V69.59
nontraffic V69.19
pedal cycle (traffic) V61.6
nontraffic V61.1
pickup truck (traffic) V63.6
nontraffic V63.1
railway vehicle (traffic) V65.6
nontraffic V65.1
specified vehicle NEC (traffic) V66.6
nontraffic V66.1
stationary object (traffic) V67.6
nontraffic V67.1
streetcar (traffic) V66.6
nontraffic V66.1
three wheeled motor vehicle (traffic) V62.6
nontraffic V62.1
truck (traffic) V64.6
nontraffic V64.1
two wheeled motor vehicle (traffic) V62.6
nontraffic V62.1
van (traffic) V63.6
nontraffic V63.1
noncollision accident (traffic) V68.6
nontraffic V68.1
pickup —*see* Accident, transport, pickup truck occupant
specified type NEC V69.88
military vehicle V69.81
van occupant V59.9
collision (with)
animal (traffic) V50.9
being ridden (traffic) V56.9
nontraffic V56.3
while boarding or alighting V56.4
nontraffic V50.3
while boarding or alighting V50.4
animal-drawn vehicle (traffic) V56.9
nontraffic V56.3
while boarding or alighting V56.4
bus (traffic) V54.9
nontraffic V54.3
while boarding or alighting V54.4
car (traffic) V53.9
nontraffic V53.3
while boarding or alighting V53.4
motor vehicle NOS (traffic) V59.60
nontraffic V59.20
specified type NEC (traffic) V59.69
nontraffic V59.29
pedal cycle (traffic) V51.9
nontraffic V51.3
while boarding or alighting V51.4
pickup truck (traffic) V53.9
nontraffic V53.3
while boarding or alighting V53.4
railway vehicle (traffic) V55.9
nontraffic V55.3
while boarding or alighting V55.4
specified vehicle NEC (traffic) V56.9
nontraffic V56.3
while boarding or alighting V56.4
stationary object (traffic) V57.9
nontraffic V57.3
while boarding or alighting V57.4
streetcar (traffic) V56.9
nontraffic V56.3
while boarding or alighting V56.4

Accident *(Continued)*
transport *(Continued)*
van occupant *(Continued)*
collision *(Continued)*
three wheeled motor vehicle (traffic) V52.9
nontraffic V52.3
while boarding or alighting V52.4
truck (traffic) V54.9
nontraffic V54.3
while boarding or alighting V54.4
two wheeled motor vehicle (traffic) V52.9
nontraffic V52.3
while boarding or alighting V52.4
van (traffic) V53.9
nontraffic V53.3
while boarding or alighting V53.4
driver
collision (with)
animal (traffic) V50.5
being ridden (traffic) V56.5
nontraffic V56.0
nontraffic V50.0
animal-drawn vehicle (traffic) V56.5
nontraffic V56.0
bus (traffic) V54.5
nontraffic V54.0
car (traffic) V53.5
nontraffic V53.0
motor vehicle NOS (traffic) V59.40
nontraffic V59.00
specified type NEC (traffic) V59.49
nontraffic V59.09
pedal cycle (traffic) V51.5
nontraffic V51.0
pickup truck (traffic) V53.5
nontraffic V53.0
railway vehicle (traffic) V55.5
nontraffic V55.0
specified vehicle NEC (traffic) V56.5
nontraffic V56.0
stationary object (traffic) V57.5
nontraffic V57.0
streetcar (traffic) V56.5
nontraffic V56.0
three wheeled motor vehicle (traffic) V52.5
nontraffic V52.0
truck (traffic) V54.5
nontraffic V54.0
two wheeled motor vehicle (traffic) V52.5
nontraffic V52.0
van (traffic) V53.5
nontraffic V53.0
noncollision accident (traffic) V58.5
nontraffic V58.0
hanger-on
collision (with)
animal (traffic) V50.7
being ridden (traffic) V56.7
nontraffic V56.2
nontraffic V50.2
animal-drawn vehicle (traffic) V56.7
nontraffic V56.2
bus (traffic) V54.7
nontraffic V54.2
car (traffic) V53.7
nontraffic V53.2
pedal cycle (traffic) V51.7
nontraffic V51.2
pickup truck (traffic) V53.7
nontraffic V53.2
railway vehicle (traffic) V55.7
nontraffic V55.2
specified vehicle NEC (traffic) V56.7
nontraffic V56.2
stationary object (traffic) V57.7
nontraffic V57.2

A

Accident *(Continued)*
transport *(Continued)*
van occupant *(Continued)*
hanger-on *(Continued)*
collision *(Continued)*
streetcar (traffic) V56.7
nontraffic V56.2
three wheeled motor vehicle (traffic) V52.7
nontraffic V52.2
truck (traffic) V54.7
nontraffic V54.2
two wheeled motor vehicle (traffic) V52.7
nontraffic V52.2
van (traffic) V53.7
nontraffic V53.2
noncollision accident (traffic) V58.7
nontraffic V58.2
noncollision accident (traffic) V58.9
nontraffic V58.3
while boarding or alighting V58.4
nontraffic V59.3
passenger
collision (with)
animal (traffic) V50.6
being ridden (traffic) V56.6
nontraffic V56.1
nontraffic V50.1
animal-drawn vehicle (traffic) V56.6
nontraffic V56.1
bus (traffic) V54.6
nontraffic V54.1
car (traffic) V53.6
nontraffic V53.1
motor vehicle NOS (traffic) V59.50
nontraffic V59.10
specified type NEC (traffic) V59.59
nontraffic V59.19
pedal cycle (traffic) V51.6
nontraffic V51.1
pickup truck (traffic) V53.6
nontraffic V53.1
railway vehicle (traffic) V55.6
nontraffic V55.1
specified vehicle NEC (traffic) V56.6
nontraffic V56.1
stationary object (traffic) V57.6
nontraffic V57.1
streetcar (traffic) V56.6
nontraffic V56.1
three wheeled motor vehicle (traffic) V52.6
nontraffic V52.1
truck (traffic) V54.6
nontraffic V54.1
two wheeled motor vehicle (traffic) V52.6
nontraffic V52.1
van (traffic) V53.6
nontraffic V53.1
noncollision accident (traffic) V58.6
nontraffic V58.1
specified type NEC V59.88
military vehicle V59.81
watercraft occupant —*see* Accident, watercraft
vehicle NEC V89.9
animal-drawn NEC —*see* Accident, transport, animal-drawn vehicle occupant
special
agricultural —*see* Accident, transport, agricultural vehicle occupant
construction —*see* Accident, transport, construction vehicle occupant
industrial —*see* Accident, transport, industrial vehicle occupant
three-wheeled NEC (motorized) —*see* Accident, transport, three-wheeled motor vehicle occupant

Accident *(Continued)*
watercraft V94.9
causing
drowning —*see* Drowning, due to, accident to, watercraft ◀
injury NEC V91.89
crushed between craft and object V91.19
powered craft V91.13
ferry boat V91.11
fishing boat V91.12
jetskis V91.13
liner V91.11
merchant ship V91.10
passenger ship V91.11
unpowered craft V91.18
canoe V91.15
inflatable V91.16
kayak V91.15
sailboat V91.14
surf-board V91.18
windsurfer V91.18
fall on board V91.29
powered craft V91.23
ferry boat V91.21
fishing boat V91.22
jetskis V91.23
liner V91.21
merchant ship V91.20
passenger ship V91.21
unpowered craft
canoe V91.25
inflatable V91.26
kayak V91.25
sailboat V91.24
fire on board causing burn V91.09
powered craft V91.03
ferry boat V91.01
fishing boat V91.02
jetskis V91.03
liner V91.01
merchant ship V91.00
passenger ship V91.01
unpowered craft V91.08
canoe V91.05
inflatable V91.06
kayak V91.05
sailboat V91.04
surf-board V91.08
water skis V91.07
windsurfer V91.08
hit by falling object V91.39
powered craft V91.33
ferry boat V91.31
fishing boat V91.32
jetskis V91.33
liner V91.31
merchant ship V91.30
passenger ship V91.31
unpowered craft V91.38
canoe V91.35
inflatable V91.36
kayak V91.35
sailboat V91.34
surf-board V91.38
water skis V91.37
windsurfer V91.38
specified type NEC V91.89
powered craft V91.83
ferry boat V91.81
fishing boat V91.82
jetskis V91.83
liner V91.81
merchant ship V91.80
passenger ship V91.81
unpowered craft V91.88
canoe V91.85
inflatable V91.86
kayak V91.85
sailboat V91.84
surf-board V91.88

Accident *(Continued)*
watercraft *(Continued)*
causing *(Continued)*
injury NEC *(Continued)*
specified type NEC *(Continued)*
unpowered craft *(Continued)*
water skis V91.87
windsurfer V91.88
due to, caused by cataclysm —*see* Forces of nature, by type
military NEC V94.818
with civilian watercraft V94.810
civilian in water injured by V94.811
nonpowered, struck by
nonpowered vessel V94.22
powered vessel V94.21
specified type NEC V94.89
striking swimmer
powered V94.11
unpowered V94.12
Acid throwing (assault) Y08.89
Activity (involving) (of victim at time of event) Y93.9
aerobic and step exercise (class) Y93.A3
alpine skiing Y93.23
animal care NEC Y93.K9
arts and handcrafts NEC Y93.D9
athletics NEC Y93.79
athletics played as a team or group NEC Y93.69
athletics played individually NEC Y93.59
baking Y93.G3
ballet Y93.41
barbells Y93.B3
BASE (Building, Antenna, Span, Earth) jumping Y93.33
baseball Y93.64
basketball Y93.67
bathing (personal) Y93.E1
beach volleyball Y93.68
bike riding Y93.55
blackout game Y93.85 ◀
boogie boarding Y93.18
bowling Y93.54
boxing Y93.71
brass instrument playing Y93.J4
building construction Y93.H3
bungee jumping Y93.34
calisthenics Y93.A2
canoeing (in calm and turbulent water) Y93.16
capture the flag Y93.6A
cardiorespiratory exercise NEC Y93.A9
caregiving (providing) NEC Y93.F9
bathing Y93.F1
lifting Y93.F2
cellular
communication device Y93.C2
telephone Y93.C2
challenge course Y93.A5
cheerleading Y93.45
choking game Y93.85 ◀
circuit training Y93.A4
cleaning
floor Y93.E5
climbing NEC Y93.39
mountain Y93.31
rock Y93.31
wall Y93.31
clothing care and maintenance NEC Y93.E9
combatives Y93.75
computer
keyboarding Y93.C1
technology NEC Y93.C9
confidence course Y93.A5
construction (building) Y93.H3
cooking and baking Y93.G3
cool down exercises Y93.A2
cricket Y93.69
crocheting Y93.D1
cross country skiing Y93.24
dancing (all types) Y93.41

◀ New ⇐ Revised ~~deleted~~ Deleted

Activity *(Continued)*
digging
dirt Y93.H1
dirt digging Y93.H1
dishwashing Y93.G1
diving (platform) (springboard) Y93.12
underwater Y93.15
dodge ball Y93.6A
downhill skiing Y93.23
drum playing Y93.J2
dumbbells Y93.B3
electronic
devices NEC Y93.C9
hand held interactive Y93.C2
game playing (using) (with)
interactive device Y93.C2
keyboard or other stationary device Y93.C1
elliptical machine Y93.A1
exercise (s)
machines ((primarily) for)
cardiorespiratory conditioning Y93.A1
muscle strengthening Y93.B1
muscle strengthening (non-machine) NEC Y93.B9
external motion NEC Y93.I9
rollercoaster Y93.I1
fainting game Y93.85 ◀
field hockey Y93.65
figure skating (pairs) (singles) Y93.21
flag football Y93.62
floor mopping and cleaning Y93.E5
food preparation and clean up Y93.G1
football (American) NOS Y93.61
flag Y93.62
tackle Y93.61
touch Y93.62
four square Y93.6A
free weights Y93.B3
frisbee (ultimate) Y93.74
furniture
building Y93.D3
finishing Y93.D3
repair Y93.D3
game playing (electronic)
using interactive device Y93.C2
using keyboard or other stationary device Y93.C1
gardening Y93.H2
golf Y93.53
grass drills Y93.A6
grilling and smoking food Y93.G2
grooming and shearing an animal Y93.K3
guerilla drills Y93.A6
gymnastics (rhythmic) Y93.43
hand held interactive electronic device Y93.C2
handball Y93.73
handcrafts NEC Y93.D9
hang gliding Y93.35
hiking (on level or elevated terrain) Y93.01
hockey (ice) Y93.22
field Y93.65
horseback riding Y93.52
household (interior) maintenance NEC Y93.E9
ice NEC Y93.29
dancing Y93.21
hockey Y93.22
skating Y93.21
inline roller skating Y93.51
ironing Y93.E4
judo Y93.75
jumping (off) NEC Y93.39
BASE (Building, Antenna, Span, Earth) Y93.33
bungee Y93.34
jacks Y93.A2
rope Y93.56
jumping jacks Y93.A2
jumping rope Y93.56
karate Y93.75

Activity *(Continued)*
kayaking (in calm and turbulent water) Y93.16
keyboarding (computer) Y93.C1
kickball Y93.6A
knitting Y93.D1
lacrosse Y93.65
land maintenance NEC Y93.H9
landscaping Y93.H2
laundry Y93.E2
machines (exercise)
primarily for cardiorespiratory conditioning Y93.A1
primarily for muscle strengthening Y93.B1
maintenance
exterior building NEC Y93.H9
household (interior) NEC Y93.E9
land Y93.H9
property Y93.H9
marching (on level or elevated terrain) Y93.01
martial arts Y93.75
microwave oven Y93.G3
milking an animal Y93.K2
mopping (floor) Y93.E5
mountain climbing Y93.31
muscle strengthening
exercises (non-machine) NEC Y93.B9
machines Y93.B1
musical keyboard (electronic) playing Y93.J1
nordic skiing Y93.24
obstacle course Y93.A5
oven (microwave) Y93.G3
packing up and unpacking in moving to a new residence Y93.E6
parasailing Y93.19
pass out game Y93.85 ◀
percussion instrument playing NEC Y93.J2
personal
bathing and showering Y93.E1
hygiene NEC Y93.E8
showering Y93.E1
physical games generally associated with school recess, summer camp and children Y93.6A
physical training NEC Y93.A9
piano playing Y93.J1
pilates Y93.B4
platform diving Y93.12
playing musical instrument
brass instrument Y93.J4
drum Y93.J2
musical keyboard (electronic) Y93.J1
percussion instrument NEC Y93.J2
piano Y93.J1
string instrument Y93.J3
winds instrument Y93.J4
property maintenance
exterior NEC Y93.H9
interior NEC Y93.E9
pruning (garden and lawn) Y93.H2
pull-ups Y93.B2
push-ups Y93.B2
racquetball Y93.73
rafting (in calm and turbulent water) Y93.16
raking (leaves) Y93.H1
rappelling Y93.32
refereeing a sports activity Y93.81
residential relocation Y93.E6
rhythmic gymnastics Y93.43
rhythmic movement NEC Y93.49
riding
horseback Y93.52
rollercoaster Y93.I1
rock climbing Y93.31
roller skating (inline) Y93.51
rollercoaster riding Y93.I1
rough housing and horseplay Y93.83
rowing (in calm and turbulent water) Y93.16
rugby Y93.63
SCUBA diving Y93.15
sewing Y93.D2

Activity *(Continued)*
shoveling Y93.H1
dirt Y93.H1
snow Y93.H1
showering (personal) Y93.E1
sit-ups Y93.B2
skateboarding Y93.51
skating (ice) Y93.21
roller Y93.51
skiing (alpine) (downhill) Y93.23
cross country Y93.24
nordic Y93.24
water Y93.17
sledding (snow) Y93.23
sleeping (sleep) Y93.84
smoking and grilling food Y93.G2
snorkeling Y93.15
snow NEC Y93.29
boarding Y93.23
shoveling Y93.H1
sledding Y93.23
tubing Y93.23
soccer Y93.66
softball Y93.64
specified NEC Y93.89
spectator at an event Y93.82
sports NEC Y93.79
sports played as a team or group NEC Y93.69
sports played individually NEC Y93.59
springboard diving Y93.12
squash Y93.73
stationary bike Y93.A1
step (stepping) exercise (class) Y93.A3
stepper machine Y93.A1
stove Y93.G3
string instrument playing Y93.J3
surfing Y93.18
wind Y93.18
swimming Y93.11
tackle football Y93.61
tap dancing Y93.41
tennis Y93.73
tobogganing Y93.23
touch football Y93.62
track and field events (non-running) Y93.57
running Y93.02
trampoline Y93.44
treadmill Y93.A1
trimming shrubs Y93.H2
tubing (in calm and turbulent water) Y93.16
snow Y93.23
ultimate frisbee Y93.74
underwater diving Y93.15
unpacking in moving to a new residence Y93.E6
use of stove, oven and microwave oven Y93.G3
vacuuming Y93.E3
volleyball (beach) (court) Y93.68
wake boarding Y93.17
walking (on level or elevated terrain) Y93.01
an animal Y93.K1
walking an animal Y93.K1
wall climbing Y93.31
warm up and cool down exercises Y93.A2
water NEC Y93.19
aerobics Y93.14
craft NEC Y93.19
exercise Y93.14
polo Y93.13
skiing Y93.17
sliding Y93.18
survival training and testing Y93.19
weeding (garden and lawn) Y93.H2
wind instrument playing Y93.J4
windsurfing Y93.18
wrestling Y93.72
yoga Y93.42

Adverse effect of drugs —*see* Table of Drugs and Chemicals

A

Aerosinusitis —*see* Air, pressure
After-effect, late —*see* Sequelae
Air
blast in war operations —*see* War operations, air blast
pressure
change, rapid
during
ascent W94.29
while (in) (surfacing from)
aircraft W94.23
deep water diving W94.21
underground W94.22
descent W94.39
in
aircraft W94.31
water W94.32
high, prolonged W94.0
low, prolonged W94.12
due to residence or long visit at high altitude W94.11
Alpine sickness W94.11
Altitude sickness W94.11
Anaphylactic shock, anaphylaxis —*see* Table of Drugs and Chemicals ◀
Andes disease W94.11
Arachnidism, arachnoidism X58
Arson (with intent to injure or kill) X97
Asphyxia, asphyxiation
by
food (bone) (seed) —*see* categories T17 and T18
gas —*see also* Table of Drugs and Chemicals ◀
legal
execution —*see* Legal, intervention, gas
intervention —*see* Legal, intervention, gas
from
fire —*see also* Exposure, fire
in war operations —*see* War operations, fire
ignition —*see* Ignition
vomitus T17.81
in war operations —*see* War operations, restriction of airway
Aspiration
food (any type) (into respiratory tract) (with asphyxia, obstruction respiratory tract, suffocation) —*see* categories T17 and T18
foreign body —*see* Foreign body, aspiration
vomitus (with asphyxia, obstruction respiratory tract, suffocation) T17.81
Assassination (attempt) —*see* Assault
Assault (homicidal) (by) (in) Y09
arson X97
bite (of human being) Y04.1
bodily force Y04.8
bite Y04.1
bumping into Y04.2
sexual —*see* subcategories T74.0, T76.0
unarmed fight Y04.0

Assault *(Continued)*
bomb X96.9
antipersonnel X96.0
fertilizer X96.3
gasoline X96.1
letter X96.2
petrol X96.1
pipe X96.3
specified NEC X96.8
brawl (hand) (fists) (foot) (unarmed) Y04.0
burning, burns (by fire) NEC X97
acid Y08.89
caustic, corrosive substance Y08.89
chemical from swallowing caustic, corrosive substance —*see* Table of Drugs and Chemicals ◀
cigarette(s) X97
hot object X98.9
fluid NEC X98.2
household appliance X98.3
specified NEC X98.8
steam X98.0
tap water X98.1
vapors X98.0
scalding —*see* Assault, burning
steam X98.0
vitriol Y08.89
caustic, corrosive substance (gas) Y08.89
crashing of
aircraft Y08.81
motor vehicle Y03.8
pushed in front of Y02.0
run over Y03.0
specified NEC Y03.8
cutting or piercing instrument X99.9
dagger X99.2
glass X99.0
knife X99.1
specified NEC X99.8
sword X99.2
dagger X99.2
drowning (in) X92.9
bathtub X92.0
natural water X92.3
specified NEC X92.8
swimming pool X92.1
following fall X92.2
dynamite X96.8
explosive (s) (material) X96.9
fight (hand) (fists) (foot) (unarmed) Y04.0
with weapon —*see* Assault, by type of weapon
fire X97
firearm X95.9
airgun X95.01
handgun X93
hunting rifle X94.1
larger X94.9
specified NEC X94.8
machine gun X94.2
shotgun X94.0
specified NEC X95.8

Assault *(Continued)*
from high place Y01
gunshot (wound) NEC —*see* Assault, firearm, by type
incendiary device X97
injury Y09
to child due to criminal abortion attempt NEC Y08.89
knife X99.1
late effect of —*see* X92-Y08 with 7th character S
placing before moving object NEC Y02.8
motor vehicle Y02.0
poisoning —*see* categories T36-T65 with 7th character S
puncture, any part of body —*see* Assault, cutting or piercing instrument
pushing
before moving object NEC Y02.8
motor vehicle Y02.0
subway train Y02.1
train Y02.1
rape T74.2-
scalding —*see* Assault, burning
sequelae of —*see* X92-Y08 with 7th character S
sexual (by bodily force) T74.2-
shooting —*see* Assault, firearm
specified means NEC Y08.89
stab, any part of body —*see* Assault, cutting or piercing instrument
steam X98.0
striking against
other person Y04.2
sports equipment Y08.09
baseball bat Y08.02
hockey stick Y08.01
struck by
sports equipment Y08.09
baseball bat Y08.02
hockey stick Y08.01
submersion —*see* Assault, drowning
violence Y09
weapon Y09
blunt Y00
cutting or piercing —*see* Assault, cutting or piercing instrument
firearm —*see* Assault, firearm
wound Y09
cutting —*see* Assault, cutting or piercing instrument
gunshot —*see* Assault, firearm
knife X99.1
piercing —*see* Assault, cutting or piercing instrument
puncture —*see* Assault, cutting or piercing instrument
stab —*see* Assault, cutting or piercing instrument
Attack by mammals NEC W55.89
Avalanche —*see* Landslide ◀
Aviator's disease —*see* Air, pressure

A

◀ New ◀ Revised ~~deleted~~ Deleted

B

Barotitis, barodontalgia, barosinusitis, barotrauma (otitic) (sinus) —*see* Air, pressure
Battered (baby) (child) (person) (syndrome) X58
Bayonet wound W26.1
  in
    legal intervention —*see* Legal, intervention, sharp object, bayonet
    war operations —*see* War operations, combat
  stated as undetermined whether accidental or intentional Y28.8
  suicide (attempt) X78.2
Bean in nose —*see* categories T17 and T18
Bed set on fire NEC —*see* Exposure, fire, uncontrolled, building, bed
Beheading (by guillotine)
  homicide X99.9
  legal execution —*see* Legal, intervention
Bending, injury in (prolonged) (static) X50.1 ⇐
Bends —*see* Air, pressure, change
Bite, bitten by
  alligator W58.01
  arthropod (nonvenomous) NEC W57
  bull W55.21
  cat W55.01
  cow W55.21
  crocodile W58.11
  dog W54.0
  goat W55.31
  hoof stock NEC W55.31
  horse W55.11
  human being (accidentally) W50.3
    with intent to injure or kill Y04.1
    as, or caused by, a crowd or human stampede (with fall) W52
    assault Y04.1
    homicide (attempt) Y04.1
    in
      fight Y04.1
  insect (nonvenomous) W57
  lizard (nonvenomous) W59.01
  mammal NEC W55.81
    marine W56.31 ◀
  marine animal (nonvenomous) W56.81
  millipede W57
  moray eel W56.51
  mouse W53.01
  person (s) (accidentally) W50.3
    with intent to injure or kill Y04.1
    as, or caused by, a crowd or human stampede (with fall) W52
    assault Y04.1
    homicide (attempt) Y04.1
    in
      fight Y04.1
  pig W55.41
  raccoon W55.51
  rat W53.11
  reptile W59.81
    lizard W59.01
    snake W59.11
    turtle W59.21
      terrestrial W59.81
  rodent W53.81
    mouse W53.01
    rat W53.11
    specified NEC W53.81
    squirrel W53.21
  shark W56.41
  sheep W55.31
  snake (nonvenomous) W59.11
  spider (nonvenomous) W57
  squirrel W53.21
Blast (air) **in war operations** —*see* War operations, blast
Blizzard X37.2
Blood alcohol level Y90.9
  20-39mg/100ml Y90.1
  40-59mg/100ml Y90.2
  60-79mg/100ml Y90.3
  80-99mg/100ml Y90.4
  100-119mg/100ml Y90.5
  120-199mg/100ml Y90.6
  200-239mg/100ml Y90.7
  less than 20mg/100ml Y90.0
  presence in blood, level not specified Y90.9
Blow X58
  by law-enforcing agent, police (on duty) —*see* Legal, intervention, manhandling
    blunt object —*see* Legal, intervention, blunt object
Blowing up —*see* Explosion
Brawl (hand) (fists) (foot) Y04.0
Breakage (accidental) (part of)
  ladder (causing fall) W11
  scaffolding (causing fall) W12
Broken
  glass, contact with —*see* Contact, with, glass
  power line (causing electric shock) W85
Bumping against, into (accidentally)
  object NEC W22.8
    with fall —*see* Fall, due to, bumping against, object
    caused by crowd or human stampede (with fall) W52
    sports equipment W21.9
  person (s) W51
    with fall W03
      due to ice or snow W00.0
    assault Y04.2
    caused by, a crowd or human stampede (with fall) W52
    homicide (attempt) Y04.2
  sports equipment W21.9
Burn, burned, burning (accidental) (by) (from) (on)
  acid NEC —*see* Table of Drugs and Chemicals ⇐
  bed linen —*see* Exposure, fire, uncontrolled, in building, bed
  blowtorch X08.8
    with ignition of clothing NEC X06.2
      nightwear X05
  bonfire, campfire (controlled) —*see also* Exposure, fire, controlled, not in building
    uncontrolled —*see* Exposure, fire, uncontrolled, not in building
  candle X08.8
    with ignition of clothing NEC X06.2
      nightwear X05
  caustic liquid, substance (external) (internal) NEC —*see* Table of Drugs and Chemicals ⇐
  chemical (external) (internal) —*see also* Table of Drugs and Chemicals ⇐
    in war operations —*see* War operations, fire
  cigar (s) or cigarette (s) X08.8
    with ignition of clothing NEC X06.2
      nightwear X05
  clothes, clothing NEC (from controlled fire) X06.2
    with conflagration —*see* Exposure, fire, uncontrolled, building
      not in building or structure —*see* Exposure, fire, uncontrolled, not in building
  cooker (hot) X15.8
    stated as undetermined whether accidental or intentional Y27.3
    suicide (attempt) X77.3
  electric blanket X16
  engine (hot) X17
  fire, flames —*see* Exposure, fire
  flare, Very pistol —*see* Discharge, firearm NEC
Burn, burned, burning *(Continued)*
  heat
    from appliance (electrical) (household) X15.8
      cooker X15.8
      hotplate X15.2
      kettle X15.8
      light bulb X15.8
      saucepan X15.3
      skillet X15.3
      stated as undetermined whether accidental or intentional Y27.3
      stove X15.0
      suicide (attempt) X77.3
      toaster X15.1
    in local application or packing during medical or surgical procedure Y63.5
  heating
    appliance, radiator or pipe X16
  homicide (attempt) —*see* Assault, burning
  hot
    air X14.1
    cooker X15.8
    drink X10.0
    engine X17
    fat X10.2
    fluid NEC X12
    food X10.1
    gases X14.1
    heating appliance X16
    household appliance NEC X15.8
    kettle X15.8
    liquid NEC X12
    machinery X17
    metal (molten) (liquid) NEC X18
    object (not producing fire or flames) NEC X19
    oil (cooking) X10.2
    pipe (s) X16
    radiator X16
    saucepan (glass) (metal) X15.3
    stove (kitchen) X15.0
    substance NEC X19
      caustic or corrosive NEC —*see* Table of Drugs and Chemicals ⇐
    toaster X15.1
    tool X17
    vapor X13.1
    water (tap) —*see* Contact, with, hot, tap water
  hotplate X15.2
    suicide (attempt) X77.3
  ignition —*see* Ignition
  in war operations —*see* War operations, fire
  inflicted by other person X97
    by hot objects, hot vapor, and steam —*see* Assault, burning, hot object
  internal, from swallowed caustic, corrosive liquid, substance —*see* Table of Drugs and Chemicals ⇐
  iron (hot) X15.8
    stated as undetermined whether accidental or intentional Y27.3
    suicide (attempt) X77.3
  kettle (hot) X15.8
    stated as undetermined whether accidental or intentional Y27.3
    suicide (attempt) X77.3
  lamp (flame) X08.8
    with ignition of clothing NEC X06.2
      nightwear X05
  lighter (cigar) (cigarette) X08.8
    with ignition of clothing NEC X06.2
      nightwear X05
  lightning —*see* subcategory T75.0
    causing fire —*see* Exposure, fire
  liquid (boiling) (hot) NEC X12
    stated as undetermined whether accidental or intentional Y27.2
    suicide (attempt) X77.2

Burn, burned, burning *(Continued)*
local application of externally applied substance in medical or surgical care Y63.5
machinery (hot) X17
matches X08.8
with ignition of clothing NEC X06.2
nightwear X05
mattress —*see* Exposure, fire, uncontrolled, building, bed
medicament, externally applied Y63.5
metal (hot) (liquid) (molten) NEC X18
nightwear (nightclothes, nightdress, gown, pajamas, robe) X05
object (hot) NEC X19
on board watercraft
due to
accident to watercraft V91.09
powered craft V91.03
ferry boat V91.01
fishing boat V91.02
jetskis V91.03
liner V91.01
merchant ship V91.00
passenger ship V91.01
unpowered craft V91.08
canoe V91.05
inflatable V91.06
kayak V91.05
sailboat V91.04
surf-board V91.08
water skis V91.07
windsurfer V91.08
fire on board V93.09
ferry boat V93.01
fishing boat V93.02
jetskis V93.03
liner V93.01
merchant ship V93.00
passenger ship V93.01
powered craft NEC V93.03
sailboat V93.04

Burn, burned, burning *(Continued)*
on board watercraft *(Continued)*
due to *(Continued)*
specified heat source NEC on board V93.19
ferry boat V93.11
fishing boat V93.12
jetskis V93.13
liner V93.11
merchant ship V93.10
passenger ship V93.11
powered craft NEC V93.13
sailboat V93.14
pipe (hot) X16
smoking X08.8
with ignition of clothing NEC X06.2
nightwear X05
powder —*see* Powder burn
radiator (hot) X16
saucepan (hot) (glass) (metal) X15.3
stated as undetermined whether accidental or intentional Y27.3
suicide (attempt) X77.3
self-inflicted X76
stated as undetermined whether accidental or intentional Y26
stated as undetermined whether accidental or intentional Y27.0
steam X13.1
pipe X16
stated as undetermined whether accidental or intentional Y27.8
stated as undetermined whether accidental or intentional Y27.0
suicide (attempt) X77.0
stove (hot) (kitchen) X15.0
stated as undetermined whether accidental or intentional Y27.3
suicide (attempt) X77.3

Burn, burned, burning *(Continued)*
substance (hot) NEC X19
boiling X12
stated as undetermined whether accidental or intentional Y27.2
suicide (attempt) X77.2
molten (metal) X18
suicide (attempt) NEC X76
hot
household appliance X77.3
object X77.9
stated as undetermined whether accidental or intentional Y27.0
therapeutic misadventure
heat in local application or packing during medical or surgical procedure Y63.5
overdose of radiation Y63.2
toaster (hot) X15.1
stated as undetermined whether accidental or intentional Y27.3
suicide (attempt) X77.3
tool (hot) X17
torch, welding X08.8
with ignition of clothing NEC X06.2
nightwear X05
trash fire (controlled) —*see* Exposure, fire, controlled, not in building
uncontrolled —*see* Exposure, fire, uncontrolled, not in building
vapor (hot) X13.1
stated as undetermined whether accidental or intentional Y27.0
suicide (attempt) X77.0
Very pistol —*see* Discharge, firearm NEC
Butted by animal W55.82
bull W55.22
cow W55.22
goat W55.32
horse W55.12
pig W55.42
sheep W55.32

B

C

Caisson disease —*see* Air, pressure, change
Campfire (exposure to) (controlled) —*see also* Exposure, fire, controlled, not in building
  uncontrolled —*see* Exposure, fire, uncontrolled, not in building
Capital punishment (any means) —*see* Legal, intervention
Car sickness T75.3
Casualty (not due to war) NEC X58
  war —*see* War operations
Cat
  bite W55.01
  scratch W55.03
Cataclysm, cataclysmic (any injury) NEC —*see* Forces of nature
Catching fire —*see* Exposure, fire
Caught
  between
    folding object W23.0
    objects (moving) (stationary and moving) W23.0
      and machinery —*see* Contact, with, by type of machine
      stationary W23.1
    sliding door and door frame W23.0
  by, in
    machinery (moving parts of) —*see* Contact, with, by type of machine
    washing-machine wringer W23.0
  under packing crate (due to losing grip) W23.1
Cave-in caused by cataclysmic earth surface movement or eruption —*see* Landslide
Change(s) **in air pressure** —*see* Air, pressure, change
Choked, choking (on) (any object except food or vomitus)
  food (bone) (seed) —*see* categories T17 and T18
  vomitus T17.81-
Civil insurrection —*see* War operations
Cloudburst (any injury) X37.8
Cold, exposure to (accidental) (excessive) (extreme) (natural) (place) **NEC** —*see* Exposure, cold
Collapse
  building W20.1
    burning (uncontrolled fire) X00.2
  dam or man-made structure (causing earth movement) X36.0
  machinery —*see* Contact, with, by type of machine
  structure W20.1
    burning (uncontrolled fire) X00.2
Collision (accidental) **NEC** —*see also* Accident, transport V89.9
  pedestrian W51
    with fall W03
      due to ice or snow W00.0
      involving pedestrian conveyance —*see* Accident, transport, pedestrian, conveyance
    and
      crowd or human stampede (with fall) W52
      object W22.8
        with fall —*see* Fall, due to, bumping against, object
  person (s) —*see* Collision, pedestrian
  transport vehicle NEC V89.9
    and
      avalanche, fallen or not moving —*see* Accident, transport
        falling or moving —*see* Landslide ◀
      landslide, fallen or not moving —*see* Accident, transport
        falling or moving —*see* Landslide
Collision NEC *(Continued)*
  transport vehicle NEC *(Continued)*
    due to cataclysm —*see* Forces of nature, by type
    intentional, purposeful suicide (attempt) —*see* Suicide, collision
Combustion, spontaneous —*see* Ignition
Complication (delayed) **of or following** (medical or surgical procedure) Y84.9
  with misadventure —*see* Misadventure
  amputation of limb (s) Y83.5
  anastomosis (arteriovenous) (blood vessel) (gastrojejunal) (tendon) (natural or artificial material) Y83.2
  aspiration (of fluid) Y84.4
    tissue Y84.8
  biopsy Y84.8
  blood
    sampling Y84.7
    transfusion
      procedure Y84.8
  bypass Y83.2
  catheterization (urinary) Y84.6
    cardiac Y84.0
  colostomy Y83.3
  cystostomy Y83.3
  dialysis (kidney) Y84.1
  drug —*see* Table of Drugs and Chemicals ⇐
  due to misadventure —*see* Misadventure
  duodenostomy Y83.3
  electroshock therapy Y84.3
  external stoma, creation of Y83.3
  formation of external stoma Y83.3
  gastrostomy Y83.3
  graft Y83.2
  hypothermia (medically-induced) Y84.8
  implant, implantation (of)
    artificial
      internal device (cardiac pacemaker) (electrodes in brain) (heart valve prosthesis) (orthopedic) Y83.1
      material or tissue (for anastomosis or bypass) Y83.2
        with creation of external stoma Y83.3
    natural tissues (for anastomosis or bypass) Y83.2
      with creation of external stoma Y83.3
  infusion
    procedure Y84.8
  injection —*see* Table of Drugs and Chemicals ⇐
    procedure Y84.8
  insertion of gastric or duodenal sound Y84.5
  insulin-shock therapy Y84.3
  paracentesis (abdominal) (thoracic) (aspirative) Y84.4
  procedures other than surgical operation —*see* Complication of or following, by type of procedure
  radiological procedure or therapy Y84.2
  removal of organ (partial) (total) NEC Y83.6
  sampling
    blood Y84.7
    fluid NEC Y84.4
    tissue Y84.8
  shock therapy Y84.3
  surgical operation NEC —*see also* Complication of or following, by type of operation Y83.9
    reconstructive NEC Y83.4
      with
        anastomosis, bypass or graft Y83.2
        formation of external stoma Y83.3
    specified NEC Y83.8
  transfusion —*see also* Table of Drugs and Chemicals ⇐
    procedure Y84.8
  transplant, transplantation (heart) (kidney) (liver) (whole organ, any) Y83.0
    partial organ Y83.4
  ureterostomy Y83.3
Complication of or following *(Continued)*
  vaccination —*see also* Table of Drugs and Chemicals ⇐
    procedure Y84.8
Compression
  divers' squeeze —*see* Air, pressure, change
  trachea by
    food (lodged in esophagus) —*see* categories T17 and T18
    vomitus (lodged in esophagus) T17.81-
Conflagration —*see* Exposure, fire, uncontrolled
Constriction (external)
  hair W49.01
  jewelry W49.04
  ring W49.04
  rubber band W49.03
  specified item NEC W49.09
  string W49.02
  thread W49.02
Contact (accidental)
  with
    abrasive wheel (metalworking) W31.1
    alligator W58.09
      bite W58.01
      crushing W58.03
      strike W58.02
    amphibian W62.9
      frog W62.0
      toad W62.1
    animal (nonvenomous) NEC W64
      marine W56.89
        bite W56.81
        dolphin —*see* Contact, with, dolphin
        fish NEC —*see* Contact, with, fish
        mammal —*see* Contact, with, mammal, marine
        orca —*see* Contact, with, orca
        sea lion —*see* Contact, with, sea lion
        shark —*see* Contact, with, shark
        strike W56.82
    animate mechanical force NEC W64
    arrow W21.89
      not thrown, projected or falling W45.8
    arthropods (nonvenomous) W57
    axe W27.0
    band-saw (industrial) W31.2
    bayonet —*see* Bayonet wound
    bee (s) X58
    bench-saw (industrial) W31.2
    bird W61.99
      bite W61.91
      chicken —*see* Contact, with, chicken
      duck —*see* Contact, with, duck
      goose —*see* Contact, with, goose
      macaw —*see* Contact, with, macaw
      parrot —*see* Contact, with, parrot
      psittacine —*see* Contact, with, psittacine
      strike W61.92
      turkey —*see* Contact, with, turkey
    blender W29.0
    boiling water X12
      stated as undetermined whether accidental or intentional Y27.2
      suicide (attempt) X77.2
    bore, earth-drilling or mining (land) (seabed) W31.0
    buffalo —*see* Contact, with, hoof stock NEC
    bull W55.29
      bite W55.21
      gored W55.22
      strike W55.22
    bumper cars W31.81
    camel —*see* Contact, with, hoof stock NEC
    can
      lid W26.8 ⇐
      opener W27.4
        powered W29.0
    cat W55.09
      bite W55.01
      scratch W55.03
    caterpillar (venomous) X58

Contact *(Continued)*
with *(Continued)*
centipede (venomous) X58
chain
hoist W24.0
agricultural operations W30.89
saw W29.3
chicken W61.39
peck W61.33
strike W61.32
chisel W27.0
circular saw W31.2
cobra X58
combine (harvester) W30.0
conveyer belt W24.1
cooker (hot) X15.8
stated as undetermined whether accidental or intentional Y27.3
suicide (attempt) X77.3
coral X58
cotton gin W31.82
cow W55.29
bite W55.21
strike W55.22
crane W24.0
agricultural operations W30.89
crocodile W58.19
bite W58.11
crushing W58.13
strike W58.12
dagger W26.1
stated as undetermined whether accidental or intentional Y28.2
suicide (attempt) X78.2
dairy equipment W31.82
dart W21.89
not thrown, projected or falling W45.8
deer —*see* Contact, with, hoof stock NEC
derrick W24.0
agricultural operations W30.89
hay W30.2
dog W54.8
bite W54.0
strike W54.1
dolphin W56.09
bite W56.01
strike W56.02
donkey —*see* Contact, with, hoof stock NEC
drill (powered) W29.8
earth (land) (seabed) W31.0
nonpowered W27.8
drive belt W24.0
agricultural operations W30.89
dry ice —*see* Exposure, cold, man-made
dryer (clothes) (powered) (spin) W29.2
duck W61.69
bite W61.61
strike W61.62
earth(-)
drilling machine (industrial) W31.0
scraping machine in stationary use W31.83
edge of stiff paper W26.2
electric
beater W29.0
blanket X16
fan W29.2
commercial W31.82
knife W29.1
mixer W29.0
elevator (building) W24.0
agricultural operations W30.89
grain W30.3
engine (s), hot NEC X17
excavating machine W31.0
farm machine W30.9
feces —*see* Contact, with, by type of animal
fer de lance X58

Contact *(Continued)*
with *(Continued)*
fish W56.59
bite W56.51
shark —*see* Contact, with, shark
strike W56.52
flying horses W31.81
forging (metalworking) machine W31.1
fork W27.4
forklift (truck) W24.0
agricultural operations W30.89
frog W62.0
garden
cultivator (powered) W29.3
riding W30.89
fork W27.1
gas turbine W31.3
Gila monster X58
giraffe —*see* Contact, with, hoof stock NEC
glass (sharp) (broken) W25
with subsequent fall W18.02
assault X99.0
due to fall —*see* Fall, by type
stated as undetermined whether accidental or intentional Y28. 0
suicide (attempt) X78.0
goat W55.39
bite W55.31
strike W55.32
goose W61.59
bite W61.51
strike W61.52
hand
saw W27.0
tool (not powered) NEC W27.8
powered W29.8
harvester W30.0
hay-derrick W30.2
heat NEC X19
from appliance (electrical) (household) —*see* Contact, with, hot, household appliance
heating appliance X16
heating
appliance (hot) X16
pad (electric) X16
hedge-trimmer (powered) W29.3
hoe W27.1
hoist (chain) (shaft) NEC W24.0
agricultural W30.89
hoof stock NEC W55.39
bite W55.31
strike W55.32
hornet (s) X58
horse W55.19
bite W55.11
strike W55.12
hot
air X14.1
inhalation X14.0
cooker X15.8
drinks X10.0
engine X17
fats X10.2
fluids NEC X12
assault X98.2
suicide (attempt) X77.2
undetermined whether accidental or intentional Y27.2
food X10.1
gases X14.1
inhalation X14.0
heating appliance X16
household appliance X15.8
assault X98.3
cooker X15.8
hotplate X15.2
kettle X15.8
light bulb X15.8

Contact *(Continued)*
with *(Continued)*
hot *(Continued)*
household appliance *(Continued)*
object NEC X19
assault X98.8
stated as undetermined whether accidental or intentional Y27.9
suicide (attempt) X77.8
saucepan X15.3
skillet X15.3
stated as undetermined whether accidental or intentional Y27.3
stove X15.0
suicide (attempt) X77.3
toaster X15.1
kettle X15.8
light bulb X15.8
liquid NEC —*see also* Burn X12
drinks X10.0
stated as undetermined whether accidental or intentional Y27.2
suicide (attempt) X77.2
tap water X11.8
stated as undetermined whether accidental or intentional Y27.1
suicide (attempt) X77.1
machinery X17
metal (molten) (liquid) NEC X18
object (not producing fire or flames) NEC X19
oil (cooking) X10.2
pipe X16
plate X15.2
radiator X16
saucepan (glass) (metal) X15.3
skillet X15.3
stove (kitchen) X15.0
substance NEC X19
tap-water X11.8
assault X98.1
heated on stove X12
stated as undetermined whether accidental or intentional Y27.2
suicide (attempt) X77.2
in bathtub X11.0
running X11.1
stated as undetermined whether accidental or intentional Y27.1
suicide (attempt) X77.1
toaster X15.1
tool X17
vapors X13.1
inhalation X13.0
water (tap) X11.8
boiling X12
stated as undetermined whether accidental or intentional Y27.2
suicide (attempt) X77.2
heated on stove X12
stated as undetermined whether accidental or intentional Y27.2
suicide (attempt) X77.2
in bathtub X11.0
running X11.1
stated as undetermined whether accidental or intentional Y27.1
suicide (attempt) X77.1
hotplate X15.2
ice-pick W27.4
insect (nonvenomous) NEC W57
kettle (hot) X15.8
knife W26.0
assault X99.1
electric W29.1
stated as undetermined whether accidental or intentional Y28.1
suicide (attempt) X78.1
lathe (metalworking) W31.1
turnings W45.8
woodworking W31.2

Contact *(Continued)*
with *(Continued)*
lawnmower (powered) (ridden) W28
causing electrocution W86.8
suicide (attempt) X83.1
unpowered W27.1
lift, lifting (devices) W24.0
agricultural operations W30.89
shaft W24.0
liquefied gas —*see* Exposure, cold, man-made
liquid air, hydrogen, nitrogen —*see* Exposure, cold, man-made
lizard (nonvenomous) W59.09
bite W59.01
strike W59.02
llama —*see* Contact, with, hoof stock NEC
macaw W61.19
bite W61.11
strike W61.12
machine, machinery W31.9
abrasive wheel W31.1
agricultural including animal-powered W30.9
combine harvester W30.0
grain storage elevator W30.3
hay derrick W30.2
power take-off device W30.1
reaper W30.0
specified NEC W30.89
thresher W30.0
transport vehicle, stationary W30.81
band saw W31.2
bench saw W31.2
circular saw W31.2
commercial NEC W31.82
drilling, metal (industrial) W31.1
earth-drilling W31.0
earthmoving or scraping W31.89
excavating W31.89
forging machine W31.1
gas turbine W31.3
hot X17
internal combustion engine W31.3
land drill W31.0
lathe W31.1
lifting (devices) W24.0
metal drill W31.1
metalworking (industrial) W31.1
milling, metal W31.1
mining W31.0
molding W31.2
overhead plane W31.2
power press, metal W31.1
prime mover W31.3
printing W31.89
radial saw W31.2
recreational W31.81
roller-coaster W31.81
rolling mill, metal W31.1
sander W31.2
seabed drill W31.0
shaft
hoist W31.0
lift W31.0
specified NEC W31.89
spinning W31.89
steam engine W31.3
transmission W24.1
undercutter W31.0
water driven turbine W31.3
weaving W31.89
woodworking or forming (industrial) W31.2
mammal (feces) (urine) W55.89
bull —*see* Contact, with, bull
cat —*see* Contact, with, cat
cow —*see* Contact, with, cow
goat —*see* Contact, with, goat
hoof stock —*see* Contact, with, hoof stock

Contact *(Continued)*
with *(Continued)*
mammal *(Continued)*
horse —*see* Contact, with, horse
marine W56.39
dolphin —*see* Contact, with, dolphin
orca —*see* Contact, with, orca
sea lion —*see* Contact, with, sea lion
specified NEC W56.39
bite W56.31
strike W56.32
pig —*see* Contact, with, pig
raccoon —*see* Contact, with, raccoon
rodent —*see* Contact, with, rodent
sheep —*see* Contact, with, sheep
specified NEC W55.89
bite W55.81
strike W55.82
marine
animal W56.89
bite W56.81
dolphin —*see* Contact, with, dolphin
fish NEC —*see* Contact, with, fish
mammal —*see* Contact, with, mammal, marine
orca —*see* Contact, with, orca
sea lion —*see* Contact, with, sea lion
shark —*see* Contact, with, shark
strike W56.82
meat
grinder (domestic) W29.0
industrial W31.82
nonpowered W27.4
slicer (domestic) W29.0
industrial W31.82
merry go round W31.81
metal, (hot) (liquid) (molten) NEC X18
millipede W57
nail W45.0
gun W29.4
needle (sewing) W27.3
hypodermic W46.0
contaminated W46.1
object (blunt) NEC
hot NEC X19
legal intervention —*see* Legal, intervention, blunt object
sharp NEC W45.8
inflicted by other person NEC W45.8
stated as
intentional homicide (attempt) —*see* Assault, cutting or piercing instrument
legal intervention —*see* Legal, intervention, sharp object
self-inflicted X78.9
orca W56.29
bite W56.21
strike W56.22
overhead plane W31.2
paper (as sharp object) W26.2 ⟸
paper-cutter W27.5
parrot W61.09
bite W61.01
strike W61.02
pig W55.49
bite W55.41
strike W55.42
pipe, hot X16
pitchfork W27.1
plane (metal) (wood) W27.0
overhead W31.2
plant thorns, spines, sharp leaves or other mechanisms W60
powered
garden cultivator W29.3
household appliance, implement, or machine W29.8
saw (industrial) W31.2
hand W29.8
printing machine W31.89

Contact *(Continued)*
with *(Continued)*
psittacine bird W61.29
bite W61.21
macaw —*see* Contact, with, macaw ⟸
parrot —*see* Contact, with, parrot
strike W61.22
pulley (block) (transmission) W24.0
agricultural operations W30.89
raccoon W55.59
bite W55.51
strike W55.52
radial-saw (industrial) W31.2
radiator (hot) X16
rake W27.1
rattlesnake X58
reaper W30.0
reptile W59.89
lizard —*see* Contact, with, lizard
snake —*see* Contact, with, snake
specified NEC W59.89
bite W59.81
crushing W59.83
strike W59.82
turtle —*see* Contact, with, turtle
rivet gun (powered) W29.4
road scraper —*see* Accident, transport, construction vehicle
rodent (feces) (urine) W53.89
bite W53.81
mouse W53.09
bite W53.01
rat W53.19
bite W53.11
specified NEC W53.89
bite W53.81
squirrel W53.29
bite W53.21
roller coaster W31.81
rope NEC W24.0
agricultural operations W30.89
saliva —*see* Contact, with, by type of animal
sander W29.8
industrial W31.2
saucepan (hot) (glass) (metal) X15.3
saw W27.0
band (industrial) W31.2
bench (industrial) W31.2
chain W29.3
hand W27.0
sawing machine, metal W31.1
scissors W27.2
scorpion X58
screwdriver W27.0
powered W29.8
sea
anemone, cucumber or urchin (spine) X58
lion W56.19
bite W56.11
strike W56.12
serpent —*see* Contact, with, snake, by type
sewing-machine (electric) (powered) W29.2
not powered W27.8
shaft (hoist) (lift) (transmission) NEC W24.0
agricultural W30.89
shark W56.49
bite W56.41
strike W56.42
sharp object(s) W26.9 ◀
specified NEC W26.8 ◀
shears (hand) W27.2
powered (industrial) W31.1
domestic W29.2
sheep W55.39
bite W55.31
strike W55.32
shovel W27.8
steam —*see* Accident, transport, construction vehicle

◀ New ⟸ Revised ~~deleted~~ Deleted

Contact *(Continued)*
with *(Continued)*
snake (nonvenomous) W59.19
bite W59.11
crushing W59.13
strike W59.12
spade W27.1
spider (venomous) X58
spin-drier W29.2
spinning machine W31.89
splinter W45.8
sports equipment W21.9
staple gun (powered) W29.8
steam X13.1
engine W31.3
inhalation X13.0
pipe X16
shovel W31.89
stove (hot) (kitchen) X15.0
substance, hot NEC X19
molten (metal) X18
sword W26.1
assault X99.2
stated as undetermined whether accidental or intentional Y28.2
suicide (attempt) X78.2
tarantula X58
thresher W30.0
tin can lid W26.8 ⇐
toad W62.1
toaster (hot) X15.1
tool W27.8
hand (not powered) W27.8
auger W27.0
axe W27.0
can opener W27.4
chisel W27.0
fork W27.4
garden W27.1
handsaw W27.0
hoe W27.1
ice-pick W27.4
kitchen utensil W27.4
manual
lawn mower W27.1
sewing machine W27.8
meat grinder W27.4
needle (sewing) W27.3
hypodermic W46.0
contaminated W46.1
paper cutter W27.5
pitchfork W27.1
rake W27.1
scissors W27.2
screwdriver W27.0
specified NEC W27.8
workbench W27.0
hot X17
powered W29.8
blender W29.0
commercial W31.82
can opener W29.0
commercial W31.82
chainsaw W29.3
clothes dryer W29.2
commercial W31.82
dishwasher W29.2
commercial W31.82
edger W29.3
electric fan W29.2
commercial W31.82
electric knife W29.1
food processor W29.0
commercial W31.82
garbage disposal W29.0
commercial W31.82

Contact *(Continued)*
with *(Continued)*
tool *(Continued)*
powered *(Continued)*
garden tool W29.3
hedge trimmer W29.3
ice maker W29.0
commercial W31.82
kitchen appliance W29.0
commercial W31.82
lawn mower W28
meat grinder W29.0
commercial W31.82
mixer W29.0
commercial W31.82
rototiller W29.3
sewing machine W29.2
commercial W31.82
washing machine W29.2
commercial W31.82
transmission device (belt, cable, chain, gear, pinion, shaft) W24.1
agricultural operations W30.89
turbine (gas) (water-driven) W31.3
turkey W61.49
peck W61.43
strike W61.42
turtle (nonvenomous) W59.29
bite W59.21
strike W59.22
terrestrial W59.89
bite W59.81
crushing W59.83
strike W59.82
under-cutter W31.0
urine —*see* Contact, with, by type of animal
vehicle
agricultural use (transport) —*see* Accident, transport, agricultural vehicle
not on public highway W30.81
industrial use (transport) —*see* Accident, transport, industrial vehicle
not on public highway W31.83
off-road use (transport) —*see* Accident, transport, all-terrain or off-road vehicle
not on public highway W31.83
special construction use (transport) —*see* Accident, transport, construction vehicle
not on public highway W31.83
venomous
animal X58
arthropods X58
lizard X58
marine animal NEC X58
marine plant NEC X58
millipedes (tropical) X58
plant (s) X58
snake X58
spider X58
viper X58
washing-machine (powered) W29.2
wasp X58
weaving-machine W31.89
winch W24.0
agricultural operations W30.89
wire NEC W24.0
agricultural operations W30.89
wood slivers W45.8
yellow jacket X58
zebra —*see* Contact, with, hoof stock NEC
pressure X50.9 ◀
stress X50.9 ◀
Coup de soleil X32

Crash
aircraft (in transit) (powered) V95.9
balloon V96.01
fixed wing NEC (private) V95.21
commercial V95.31
glider V96.21
hang V96.11
powered V95.11
helicopter V95.01
in war operations —*see* War operations, destruction of aircraft
microlight V95.11
nonpowered V96.9
specified NEC V96.8
powered NEC V95.8
stated as
homicide (attempt) Y08.81
suicide (attempt) X83.0
ultralight V95.11
spacecraft V95.41
transport vehicle NEC —*see also* Accident, transport V89.9
homicide (attempt) Y03.8
motor NEC (traffic) V89.2
homicide (attempt) Y03.8
suicide (attempt) —*see* Suicide, collision
Cruelty (mental) (physical) (sexual) X58
Crushed (accidentally) X58
between objects (moving) (stationary and moving) W23.0
stationary W23.1
by
alligator W58.03
avalanche NEC —*see* Landslide ◀
cave-in W20.0
caused by cataclysmic earth surface movement —*see* Landslide ◀
crocodile W58.13
crowd or human stampede W52
falling
aircraft V97.39
in war operations —*see* War operations, destruction of aircraft
earth, material W20.0
caused by cataclysmic earth surface movement —*see* Landslide
object NEC W20.8
landslide NEC —*see* Landslide ◀
lizard (nonvenomous) W59.09
machinery —*see* Contact, with, by type of machine
reptile NEC W59.89
snake (nonvenomous) W59.13
in
machinery —*see* Contact, with, by type of machine
Cut, cutting (any part of body) (accidental) —*see also* Contact, with, by object or machine
during medical or surgical treatment as misadventure —*see* Index to Diseases and Injuries, Complications ⇐
homicide (attempt) —*see* Assault, cutting or piercing instrument
inflicted by other person —*see* Assault, cutting or piercing instrument
legal
execution —*see* Legal, intervention
intervention —*see* Legal, intervention, sharp object
machine NEC —*see also* Contact, with, by type of machine W31.9
self-inflicted —*see* Suicide, cutting or piercing instrument
suicide (attempt) —*see* Suicide, cutting or piercing instrument
Cyclone (any injury) X37.1

◀ New ⇐ Revised ~~deleted~~ Deleted

D

Decapitation (accidental circumstances) NEC X58
homicide X99.9
legal execution —*see* Legal, intervention
Dehydration from lack of water X58
Deprivation X58
Derailment (accidental)
railway (rolling stock) (train) (vehicle) (without antecedent collision) V81.7
with antecedent collision —*see* Accident, transport, railway vehicle occupant
streetcar (without antecedent collision) V82.7
with antecedent collision —*see* Accident, transport, streetcar occupant
Descent
parachute (voluntary) (without accident to aircraft) V97.29
due to accident to aircraft —*see* Accident, transport, aircraft
Desertion X58
Destitution X58
Disability, late effect or sequela of injury —*see* Sequelae
Discharge (accidental)
airgun W34.010
assault X95.01
homicide (attempt) X95.01
stated as undetermined whether accidental or intentional Y24.0
suicide (attempt) X74.01
BB gun —*see* Discharge, airgun
firearm (accidental) W34.00
assault X95.9
handgun (pistol) (revolver) W32.0
assault X93
homicide (attempt) X93
legal intervention —*see* Legal, intervention, firearm, handgun
stated as undetermined whether accidental or intentional Y22
suicide (attempt) X72
homicide (attempt) X95.9
hunting rifle W33.02
assault X94.1
homicide (attempt) X94.1
legal intervention
injuring
bystander Y35.032
law enforcement personnel Y35.031
suspect Y35.033
stated as undetermined whether accidental or intentional Y23.1
suicide (attempt) X73.1
larger W33.00
assault X94.9
homicide (attempt) X94.9
hunting rifle —*see* Discharge, firearm, hunting rifle
legal intervention —*see* Legal, intervention, firearm by type of firearm
machine gun —*see* Discharge, firearm, machine gun
shotgun —*see* Discharge, firearm, shotgun
specified NEC W33.09
assault X94.8
homicide (attempt) X94.8
legal intervention
injuring
bystander Y35.092
law enforcement personnel Y35.091
suspect Y35.093
stated as undetermined whether accidental or intentional Y23.8
suicide (attempt) X73.8
Discharge *(Continued)*
firearm *(Continued)*
larger *(Continued)*
stated as undetermined whether accidental or intentional Y23.9
suicide (attempt) X73.9
legal intervention
injuring
bystander Y35.002
law enforcement personnel Y35.001
suspect Y35.03
using rubber bullet
injuring
bystander Y35.042
law enforcement personnel Y35.041
suspect Y35.043
machine gun W33.03
assault X94.2
homicide (attempt) X94.2
legal intervention —*see* Legal, intervention, firearm, machine gun
stated as undetermined whether accidental or intentional Y23.3
suicide (attempt) X73.2
pellet gun —*see* Discharge, airgun
shotgun W33.01
assault X94.0
homicide (attempt) X94.0
legal intervention —*see* Legal, intervention, firearm, specified NEC
stated as undetermined whether accidental or intentional Y23.0
suicide (attempt) X73.0
specified NEC W34.09
assault X95.8
homicide (attempt) X95.8
legal intervention —*see* Legal, intervention, firearm, specified NEC
stated as undetermined whether accidental or intentional Y24.8
suicide (attempt) X74.8
stated as undetermined whether accidental or intentional Y24.9
suicide (attempt) X74.9
Very pistol W34.09
assault X95.8
homicide (attempt) X95.8
stated as undetermined whether accidental or intentional Y24.8
suicide (attempt) X74.8
firework (s) W39
stated as undetermined whether accidental or intentional Y25
gas-operated gun NEC W34.018
airgun —*see* Discharge, airgun
assault X95.09
homicide (attempt) X95.09
paintball gun —*see* Discharge, paintball gun
stated as undetermined whether accidental or intentional Y24.8
suicide (attempt) X74.09
gun NEC —*see also* Discharge, firearm NEC
air —*see* Discharge, airgun
BB —*see* Discharge, airgun
for single hand use —*see* Discharge, firearm, handgun
hand —*see* Discharge, firearm, handgun
machine —*see* Discharge, firearm, machine gun
other specified —*see* Discharge, firearm NEC
paintball —*see* Discharge, paintball gun
pellet —*see* Discharge, airgun
handgun —*see* Discharge, firearm, handgun
machine gun —*see* Discharge, firearm, machine gun
paintball gun W34.011
assault X95.02
homicide (attempt) X95.02
Discharge *(Continued)*
paintball gun *(Continued)*
stated as undetermined whether accidental or intentional Y24.8
suicide (attempt) X74.02
pistol —*see* Discharge, firearm, handgun
flare —*see* Discharge, firearm, Very pistol
pellet —*see* Discharge, airgun
Very —*see* Discharge, firearm, Very pistol
revolver —*see* Discharge, firearm, handgun
rifle (hunting) —*see* Discharge, firearm, hunting rifle
shotgun —*see* Discharge, firearm, shotgun
spring-operated gun NEC W34.018
assault X95.09
homicide (attempt) X95.09
stated as undetermined whether accidental or intentional Y24.8
suicide (attempt) X74.09
Disease
Andes W94.11
aviator's —*see* Air, pressure
range W94.11
Diver's disease, palsy, paralysis, squeeze —*see* Air, pressure
Diving (into water) —*see* Accident, diving
Dog bite W54.0
Dragged by transport vehicle NEC —*see also* Accident, transport V09.9
Drinking poison (accidental) —*see* Table of Drugs and Chemicals
Dropped (accidentally) **while being carried or supported by other person** W04
Drowning (accidental) W74
assault X92.9
due to
accident (to)
machinery —*see* Contact, with, by type of machine
watercraft V90.89
burning V90.29
powered V90.23
fishing boat V90.22
jetskis V90.23
merchant ship V90.20
passenger ship V90.21
unpowered V90.28
canoe V90.25
inflatable V90.26
kayak V90.25
sailboat V90.24
water skis V90.27
crushed V90.39
powered V90.33
fishing boat V90.32
jetskis V90.33
merchant ship V90.30
passenger ship V90.31
unpowered V90.38
canoe V90.35
inflatable V90.36
kayak V90.35
sailboat V90.34
water skis V90.37
overturning V90.09
powered V90.03
fishing boat V90.02
jetskis V90.03
merchant ship V90.00
passenger ship V90.01
unpowered V90.08
canoe V90.05
inflatable V90.06
kayak V90.05
sailboat V90.04
sinking V90.19
powered V90.13
fishing boat V90.12
jetskis V90.13
merchant ship V90.10
passenger ship V90.11

Drowning *(Continued)*
due to *(Continued)*
accident *(Continued)*
watercraft *(Continued)*
sinking *(Continued)*
unpowered V90.18
canoe V90.15
inflatable V90.16
kayak V90.15
sailboat V90.14
specified type NEC V90.89
powered V90.83
fishing boat V90.82
jetskis V90.83
merchant ship V90.80
passenger ship V90.81
unpowered V90.88
canoe V90.85
inflatable V90.86
kayak V90.85
sailboat V90.84
water skis V90.87
avalanche —*see* Landslide ◀
cataclysmic
earth surface movement NEC —*see* Forces of nature, earth movement ◀
storm —*see* Forces of nature, cataclysmic storm ◀
cloudburst X37.8
cyclone X37.1
fall overboard (from) V92.09
powered craft V92.03
ferry boat V92.01
fishing boat V92.02
jetskis V92.03
liner V92.01
merchant ship V92.00
passenger ship V92.01
resulting from
accident to watercraft —*see* Drowning, due to, accident to, watercraft
being washed overboard (from) V92.29
powered craft V92.23
ferry boat V92.21
fishing boat V92.22
jetskis V92.23
liner V92.21
merchant ship V92.20
passenger ship V92.21
unpowered craft V92.28
canoe V92.25
inflatable V92.26
kayak V92.25
sailboat V92.24
surf-board V92.28
water skis V92.27
windsurfer V92.28
motion of watercraft V92.19
powered craft V92.13
ferry boat V92.11
fishing boat V92.12
jetskis V92.13
liner V92.11
merchant ship V92.10
passenger ship V92.11
unpowered craft
canoe V92.15
inflatable V92.16
kayak V92.15
sailboat V92.14
unpowered craft V92.08
canoe V92.05
inflatable V92.06
kayak V92.05

Drowning *(Continued)*
due to *(Continued)*
fall overboard *(Continued)*
unpowered craft *(Continued)*
sailboat V92.04
surf-board V92.08
water skis V92.07
windsurfer V92.08
hurricane X37.0
jumping into water from watercraft (involved in accident) —*see also* Drowning, due to, accident to, watercraft
without accident to or on watercraft W16.711
tidal wave NEC —*see* Forces of nature, tidal wave ◀
torrential rain X37.8
following
fall
into
bathtub W16.211
bucket W16.221
fountain —*see* Drowning, following, fall, into, water, specified NEC
quarry —*see* Drowning, following, fall, into, water, specified NEC
reservoir —*see* Drowning, following, fall, into, water, specified NEC
swimming-pool W16.011
stated as undetermined whether accidental or intentional Y21.3
striking
bottom W16.021
wall W16.031
suicide (attempt) X71.2
water NOS W16.41
natural (lake) (open sea) (river) (stream) (pond) W16.111
striking
bottom W16.121
side W16.131
specified NEC W16.311
striking
bottom W16.321
wall W16.331
overboard NEC —*see* Drowning, due to, fall overboard
jump or dive
from boat W16.711
striking bottom W16.721
into
fountain —*see* Drowning, following, jump or dive, into, water, specified NEC
quarry —*see* Drowning, following, jump or dive, into, water, specified NEC
reservoir —*see* Drowning, following, jump or dive, into, water, specified NEC
swimming-pool W16.511
striking
bottom W16.521
wall W16.531
suicide (attempt) X71.2
water NOS W16.91
natural (lake) (open sea) (river) (stream) (pond) W16.611
specified NEC W16.811
striking
bottom W16.821
wall W16.831
striking bottom W16.621

Drowning *(Continued)*
homicide (attempt) X92.9
in
bathtub (accidental) W65
assault X92.0
following fall W16.211
stated as undetermined whether accidental or intentional Y21.1
stated as undetermined whether accidental or intentional Y21.0
suicide (attempt) X71.0
lake —*see* Drowning, in, natural water
natural water (lake) (open sea) (river) (stream) (pond) W69
assault X92.3
following
dive or jump W16.611
striking bottom W16.621
fall W16.111
striking
bottom W16.121
side W16.131
stated as undetermined whether accidental or intentional Y21.4
suicide (attempt) X71.3
quarry —*see* Drowning, in, specified place NEC
quenching tank —*see* Drowning, in, specified place NEC
reservoir —*see* Drowning, in, specified place NEC
river —*see* Drowning, in, natural water
sea —*see* Drowning, in, natural water
specified place NEC W73
assault X92.8
following
dive or jump W16.811
striking
bottom W16.821
wall W16.831
fall W16.311
striking
bottom W16.321
wall W16.331
stated as undetermined whether accidental or intentional Y21.8
suicide (attempt) X71.8
stream —*see* Drowning, in, natural water
swimming-pool W67
assault X92.1
following fall X92.2
following
dive or jump W16.511
striking
bottom W16.521
wall W16.531
fall W16.011
striking
bottom W16.021
wall W16.031
stated as undetermined whether accidental or intentional Y21.2
following fall Y21.3
suicide (attempt) X71.1
following fall X71.2
war operations —*see* War operations, restriction of airway
resulting from accident to watercraft —*see* Drowning, due to, accident, watercraft
self-inflicted X71.9
stated as undetermined whether accidental or intentional Y21.9
suicide (attempt) X71.9

◀ New ◀ Revised ~~deleted~~ Deleted

E

Earth (surface) movement NEC —*see* Forces of nature, earth movement ⬅
Earth falling (on) W20.0
caused by cataclysmic earth surface movement or eruption —*see* Landslide ◀
Earthquake (any injury) X34
Effect (s) (adverse) of
air pressure (any) —*see* Air, pressure
cold, excessive (exposure to) —*see* Exposure, cold
heat (excessive) —*see* Heat
hot place (weather) —*see* Heat ⬅
insolation X30
late —*see* Sequelae
motion —*see* Motion
nuclear explosion or weapon in war operations —*see* War operations, nuclear weapon
radiation —*see* Radiation
travel —*see* Travel
Electric shock (accidental) (by) (in) —*see* Exposure, electric current
Electrocution (accidental) —*see* Exposure, electric current
Endotracheal tube wrongly placed during anesthetic procedure Y65.3
Entanglement
in
bed linen, causing suffocation —*see* category T71
wheel of pedal cycle V19.88
Entry of foreign body or material —*see* Foreign body
Environmental pollution related condition —*see* Z57
Execution, legal (any method) —*see* Legal, intervention
Exhaustion
cold —*see* Exposure, cold
due to excessive exertion —*see also* Overexertion X50.9 ⬅
heat —*see* Heat
Explosion (accidental) (of) (with secondary fire) W40.9
acetylene W40.1
aerosol can W36.1
air tank (compressed) (in machinery) W36.2
aircraft (in transit) (powered) NEC V95.9
balloon V96.05
fixed wing NEC (private) V95.25
commercial V95.35
glider V96.25
hang V96.15
powered V95.15
helicopter V95.05
in war operations —*see* War operations, destruction of aircraft
microlight V95.15
nonpowered V96.9
specified NEC V96.8
powered NEC V95.8
stated as
homicide (attempt) Y03.8
suicide (attempt) X83.0
ultralight V95.15
anesthetic gas in operating room W40.1
antipersonnel bomb W40.8
assault X96.0
homicide (attempt) X96.0
suicide (attempt) X75
assault X96.9
bicycle tire W37.0
blasting (cap) (materials) W40.0
boiler (machinery), not on transport vehicle W35
on watercraft —*see* Explosion, in, watercraft
butane W40.1
caused by other person X96.9
coal gas W40.1

Explosion *(Continued)*
detonator W40.0
dump (munitions) W40.8
dynamite W40.0
in
assault X96.8
homicide (attempt) X96.8
legal intervention
injuring
bystander Y35.112
law enforcement personnel Y35.111
suspect Y35.113
suicide (attempt) X75
explosive (material) W40.9
gas W40.1
in blasting operation W40.0
specified NEC W40.8
in
assault X96.8
homicide (attempt) X96.8
legal intervention
injuring
bystander Y35.192
law enforcement personnel Y35.191
suspect Y35.193
suicide (attempt) X75
factory (munitions) W40.8
fertilizer bomb W40.8
assault X96.3
homicide (attempt) X96.3
suicide (attempt) X75
fire-damp W40.1
firearm (parts) NEC W34.19
airgun W34.110
BB gun W34.110
gas, air or spring-operated gun NEC W34.118
handgun W32.1
hunting rifle W33.12
larger firearm W33.10
specified NEC W33.19
machine gun W33.13
paintball gun W34.111
pellet gun W34.110
shotgun W33.11
Very pistol [flare] W34.19
fireworks W39
gas (coal) (explosive) W40.1
cylinder W36.9
aerosol can W36.1
air tank W36.2
pressurized W36.3
specified NEC W36.8
gasoline (fumes) (tank) not in moving motor vehicle W40.1
bomb W40.8
assault X96.1
homicide (attempt) X96.1
suicide (attempt) X75
in motor vehicle —*see* Accident, transport, by type of vehicle
grain store W40.8
grenade W40.8
in
assault X96.8
homicide (attempt) X96.8
legal intervention
injuring
bystander Y35.192
law enforcement personnel Y35.191
suspect Y35.193
suicide (attempt) X75
handgun (parts) —*see* Explosion, firearm, handgun (parts)
homicide (attempt) X96.9
antipersonnel bomb —*see* Explosion, antipersonnel bomb
fertilizer bomb —*see* Explosion, fertilizer bomb

Explosion *(Continued)*
homicide *(Continued)*
gasoline bomb —*see* Explosion, gasoline bomb
letter bomb —*see* Explosion, letter bomb
pipe bomb —*see* Explosion, pipe bomb
specified NEC X96.8
hose, pressurized W37.8
hot water heater, tank (in machinery) W35
on watercraft —*see* Explosion, in, watercraft
in, on
dump W40.8
factory W40.8
mine (of explosive gases) NEC W40.1
watercraft V93.59
powered craft V93.53
ferry boat V93.51
fishing boat V93.52
jetskis V93.53
liner V93.51
merchant ship V93.50
passenger ship V93.51
sailboat V93.54
letter bomb W40.8
assault X96.2
homicide (attempt) X96.2
suicide (attempt) X75
machinery —*see also* Contact, with, by type of machine
on board watercraft —*see* Explosion, in, watercraft
pressure vessel —*see* Explosion, by type of vessel
methane W40.1
mine W40.1
missile NEC W40.8
mortar bomb W40.8
in
assault X96.8
homicide (attempt) X96.8
legal intervention
injuring
bystander Y35.192
law enforcement personnel Y35.191
suspect Y35.193
suicide (attempt) X75
munitions (dump) (factory) W40.8
pipe, pressurized W37.8
bomb W40.8
assault X96.4
homicide (attempt) X96.4
suicide (attempt) X75
pressure, pressurized
cooker W38
gas tank (in machinery) W36.3
hose W37.8
pipe W37.8
specified device NEC W38
tire W37.8
bicycle W37.0
vessel (in machinery) W38
propane W40.1
self-inflicted X75
shell (artillery) NEC W40.8
during war operations —*see* War operations, explosion
in
legal intervention
injuring
bystander Y35.122
law enforcement personnel Y35.121
suspect Y35.123
war —*see* War operations, explosion
spacecraft V95.45
stated as undetermined whether accidental or intentional Y25
steam or water lines (in machinery) W37.8
stove W40.9
suicide (attempt) X75

E

Explosion *(Continued)*
tire, pressurized W37.8
bicycle W37.0
undetermined whether accidental or intentional Y25
vehicle tire NEC W37.8
bicycle W37.0
war operations —*see* War operations, explosion
Exposure (to) X58
air pressure change —*see* Air, pressure
cold (accidental) (excessive) (extreme) (natural) (place) X31
assault Y08.89
due to
man-made conditions W93.8
dry ice (contact) W93.01
inhalation W93.02
liquid air (contact) (hydrogen) (nitrogen) W93.11
inhalation W93.12
refrigeration unit (deep freeze) W93.2
suicide (attempt) X83.2
weather (conditions) X31
homicide (attempt) Y08.89
self-inflicted X83.2
due to abandonment or neglect X58
electric current W86.8
appliance (faulty) W86.8
domestic W86.0
caused by other person Y08.89
conductor (faulty) W86.1
control apparatus (faulty) W86.1
electric power generating plant, distribution station W86.1
electroshock gun —*see* Exposure, electric current, taser
high-voltage cable W85
homicide (attempt) Y08.89
legal execution —*see* Legal, intervention, specified means NEC
lightning —*see* subcategory T75.0
live rail W86.8
misadventure in medical or surgical procedure in electroshock therapy Y63.4
motor (electric) (faulty) W86.8
domestic W86.0
self-inflicted X83.1
specified NEC W86.8
domestic W86.0
stun gun —*see* Exposure, electric current, taser
suicide (attempt) X83.1
taser W86.8
assault Y08.89
legal intervention —*see* category Y35
self-harm (intentional) X83.8
undetermined intent Y33
third rail W86.8
transformer (faulty) W86.1
transmission lines W85
environmental tobacco smoke X58
excessive
cold —*see* Exposure, cold
heat (natural) NEC X30
man-made W92
factor (s) NOS X58
environmental NEC X58
man-made NEC W99
natural NEC —*see* Forces of nature ◀
specified NEC X58
fire, flames (accidental) X08.8
assault X97
campfire —*see* Exposure, fire, controlled, not in building
controlled (in)
with ignition (of) clothing —*see also* Ignition, clothes X06.2
nightwear X05
Exposure *(Continued)*
fire, flames *(Continued)*
controlled *(Continued)*
bonfire —*see* Exposure, fire, controlled, not in building
brazier (in building or structure) —*see also* Exposure, fire, controlled, building
not in building or structure —*see* Exposure, fire, controlled, not in building
building or structure X02.0
with
fall from building X02.3
from building X02.5
injury due to building collapse X02.2
smoke inhalation X02.1
hit by object from building X02.4
specified mode of injury NEC X02.8
fireplace, furnace or stove —*see* Exposure, fire, controlled, building
not in building or structure X03.0
with
fall X03.3
smoke inhalation X03.1
hit by object X03.4
specified mode of injury NEC X03.8
trash —*see* Exposure, fire, controlled, not in building
fireplace —*see* Exposure, fire, controlled, building
fittings or furniture (in building or structure) (uncontrolled) —*see* Exposure, fire, uncontrolled, building
forest (uncontrolled) —*see* Exposure, fire, uncontrolled, not in building
grass (uncontrolled) —*see* Exposure, fire, uncontrolled, not in building
hay (uncontrolled) —*see* Exposure, fire, uncontrolled, not in building
homicide (attempt) X97
ignition of highly flammable material X04
in, of, on, starting in
machinery —*see* Contact, with, by type of machine
motor vehicle (in motion) —*see also* Accident, transport, occupant by type of vehicle V87.8
with collision —*see* Collision
railway rolling stock, train, vehicle V81.81
with collision —*see* Accident, transport, railway vehicle occupant
street car (in motion) V82.8
with collision —*see* Accident, transport, streetcar occupant
transport vehicle NEC —*see also* Accident, transport
with collision —*see* Collision
war operations —*see also* War operations, fire
from nuclear explosion —*see* War operations, nuclear weapons
watercraft (in transit) (not in transit) V91.09
localized —*see* Burn, on board watercraft, due to, fire on board
powered craft V91.03
ferry boat V91.01
fishing boat V91.02
jet skis V91.03
liner V91.01
merchant ship V91.00
passenger ship V91.01
unpowered craft V91.08
canoe V91.05
inflatable V91.06
kayak V91.05
sailboat V91.04
Exposure *(Continued)*
fire, flames *(Continued)*
in, of, on, starting in *(Continued)*
watercraft *(Continued)*
unpowered craft *(Continued)*
surf-board V91.08
waterskis V91.07
windsurfer V91.08
lumber (uncontrolled) —*see* Exposure, fire, uncontrolled, not in building
mine (uncontrolled) —*see* Exposure, fire, uncontrolled, not in building
prairie (uncontrolled) —*see* Exposure, fire, uncontrolled, not in building
resulting from
explosion —*see* Explosion
lightning X08.8
self-inflicted X76
specified NEC X08.8
started by other person X97
stated as undetermined whether accidental or intentional Y26
stove —*see* Exposure, fire, controlled, building
suicide (attempt) X76
tunnel (uncontrolled) —*see* Exposure, fire, uncontrolled, not in building
uncontrolled
in building or structure X00.0
with
fall from building X00.3
injury due to building collapse X00.2
jump from building X00.5
smoke inhalation X00.1
bed X08.00
due to
cigarette X08.01
specified material NEC X08.09
furniture NEC X08.20
due to
cigarette X08.21
specified material NEC X08.29
hit by object from building X00.4
sofa X08.10
due to
cigarette X08.11
specified material NEC X08.19
specified mode of injury NEC X00.8
not in building or structure (any) X01.0
with
fall X01.3
smoke inhalation X01.1
hit by object X01.4
specified mode of injury NEC X01.8
undetermined whether accidental or intentional Y26
forces of nature NEC —*see* Forces of nature ◀
G-forces (abnormal) W49.9
gravitational forces (abnormal) W49.9
heat (natural) NEC —*see* Heat
high-pressure jet (hydraulic) (pneumatic) W49.9
hydraulic jet W49.9
inanimate mechanical force W49.9
jet, high-pressure (hydraulic) (pneumatic) W49.9
lightning —*see* subcategory T75.0
causing fire —*see* Exposure, fire
mechanical forces NEC W49.9
animate NEC W64
inanimate NEC W49.9
noise W42.9
supersonic W42.0
noxious substance —*see* Table of Drugs and Chemicals ⇐
pneumatic jet W49.9

◀ New ⇐ Revised ~~deleted~~ Deleted

Exposure *(Continued)*
prolonged in deep-freeze unit or refrigerator W93.2
radiation —*see* Radiation
smoke —*see also* Exposure, fire
tobacco, second hand Z77.22
specified factors NEC X58
sunlight X32
man-made (sun lamp) W89.8
tanning bed W89.1
supersonic waves W42.0
transmission line (s), electric W85
vibration W49.9

Exposure *(Continued)*
waves
infrasound W49.9
sound W42.9
supersonic W42.0
weather NEC —*see* Forces of nature ◀

External cause status Y99.9
child assisting in compensated work for family Y99.8
civilian activity done for financial or other compensation Y99.0
civilian activity done for income or pay Y99.0

External cause status *(Continued)*
family member assisting in compensated work for other family member Y99.8
hobby not done for income Y99.8
leisure activity Y99.8
military activity Y99.1
off-duty activity of military personnel Y99.8
recreation or sport not for income or while a student Y99.8
specified NEC Y99.8
student activity Y99.8
volunteer activity Y99.2

E

F

Factors, supplemental
alcohol
blood level
less than 20mg/100ml Y90.0
presence in blood, level not specified Y90.9
20-39mg/100ml Y90.1
40-59mg/100ml Y90.2
60-79mg/100ml Y90.3
80-99mg/100ml Y90.4
100-119mg/100ml Y90.5
120-199mg/100ml Y90.6
200-239mg/100ml Y90.7
240mg/100ml or more Y90.8
presence in blood, but level not specified Y90.9
environmental-pollution-related condition —*see* Z57
nosocomial condition Y95
work-related condition Y99.0
Failure
in suture or ligature during surgical procedure Y65.2
mechanical, of instrument or apparatus (any) (during any medical or surgical procedure) Y65.8
sterile precautions (during medical and surgical care) —*see* Misadventure, failure, sterile precautions, by type of procedure
to
introduce tube or instrument Y65.4
endotracheal tube during anesthesia Y65.3
make curve (transport vehicle) NEC —*see* Accident, transport
remove tube or instrument Y65.4
Fall, falling (accidental) W19
building W20.1
burning (uncontrolled fire) X00.3
down
embankment W17.81
escalator W10.0
hill W17.81
ladder W11
ramp W10.2
stairs, steps W10.9
due to
bumping against
object W18.00
sharp glass W18.02
specified NEC W18.09
sports equipment W18.01
person W03
due to ice or snow W00.0
on pedestrian conveyance —*see* Accident, transport, pedestrian, conveyance
collision with another person W03
due to ice or snow W00.0
involving pedestrian conveyance —*see* Accident, transport, pedestrian, conveyance
grocery cart tipping over W17.82
ice or snow W00.9
from one level to another W00.2
on stairs or steps W00.1
involving pedestrian conveyance —*see* Accident, transport, pedestrian, conveyance
on same level W00.0
slipping (on moving sidewalk) W01.0
with subsequent striking against object W01.10
furniture W01.190
sharp object W01.119
glass W01.110
power tool or machine W01.111
specified NEC W01.118
specified NEC W01.198
Fall, falling *(Continued)*
due to *(Continued)*
striking against
object W18.00
sharp glass W18.02
specified NEC W18.09
sports equipment W18.01
person W03
due to ice or snow W00.0
on pedestrian conveyance —*see* Accident, transport, pedestrian, conveyance
earth (with asphyxia or suffocation (by pressure)) —*see* Earth, falling
from, off, out of
aircraft NEC (with accident to aircraft NEC) V97.0
while boarding or alighting V97.1
balcony W13.0
bed W06
boat, ship, watercraft NEC (with drowning or submersion) —*see* Drowning, due to, fall overboard
with hitting bottom or object V94.0
bridge W13.1
building W13.9
burning (uncontrolled fire) X00.3
cavity W17.2
chair W07
cherry picker W17.89
cliff W15
dock W17.4
embankment W17.81
escalator W10.0
flagpole W13.8
furniture NEC W08
grocery cart W17.82
haystack W17.89
high place NEC W17.89
stated as undetermined whether accidental or intentional Y30
hole W17.2
incline W10.2
ladder W11
lifting device W17.89
machine, machinery —*see also* Contact, with, by type of machine
not in operation W17.89
manhole W17.1
mobile elevated work platform [MEWP] W17.89
motorized mobility scooter W05.2
one level to another NEC W17.89
intentional, purposeful, suicide (attempt) X80
stated as undetermined whether accidental or intentional Y30
pit W17.2
playground equipment W09.8
jungle gym W09.2
slide W09.0
swing W09.1
quarry W17.89
railing W13.9
ramp W10.2
roof W13.2
scaffolding W12
scooter (nonmotorized) W05.1
motorized mobility W05.2
sky lift W17.89
stairs, steps W10.9
curb W10.1
due to ice or snow W00.1
escalator W10.0
incline W10.2
ramp W10.2
sidewalk curb W10.1
specified NEC W10.8
stepladder W11
storm drain W17.1
Fall, falling *(Continued)*
from, off, out of *(Continued)*
streetcar NEC V82.6
with antecedent collision —*see* Accident, transport, streetcar occupant
while boarding or alighting V82.4
structure NEC W13.8
burning (uncontrolled fire) X00.3
table W08
toilet W18.11
with subsequent striking against object W18.12
train NEC V81.6
during derailment (without antecedent collision) V81.7
with antecedent collision —*see* Accident, transport, railway vehicle occupant
while boarding or alighting V81.4
transport vehicle after collision —*see* Accident, transport, by type of vehicle, collision
tree W14
vehicle (in motion) NEC —*see also* Accident, transport V89.9
motor NEC —*see also* Accident, transport, occupant, by type of vehicle V87.8
stationary W17.89
while boarding or alighting —*see* Accident, transport, by type of vehicle, while boarding or alighting ◀
viaduct W13.8
wall W13.8
watercraft —*see also* Drowning, due to, fall overboard
with hitting bottom or object V94.0
well W17.0
wheelchair, non-moving W05.0
powered —*see* Accident, transport, pedestrian, conveyance occupant, specified type NEC
window W13.4
in, on
aircraft NEC V97.0
with accident to aircraft V97.0
while boarding or alighting V97.1
bathtub (empty) W18.2
filled W16.212
causing drowning W16.211
escalator W10.0
incline W10.2
ladder W11
machine, machinery —*see* Contact, with, by type of machine
object, edged, pointed or sharp (with cut) —*see* Fall, by type
playground equipment W09.8
jungle gym W09.2
slide W09.0
swing W09.1
ramp W10.2
scaffolding W12
shower W18.2
causing drowning W16.211
staircase, stairs, steps W10.9
curb W10.1
due to ice or snow W00.1
escalator W10.0
incline W10.2
specified NEC W10.8
streetcar (without antecedent collision) V82.5
with antecedent collision —*see* Accident, transport, streetcar occupant
while boarding or alighting V82.4

◀ New ⇐ Revised ~~deleted~~ Deleted

Fall, falling *(Continued)*
in, on *(Continued)*
train (without antecedent collision) V81.5
with antecedent collision —*see* Accident, transport, railway vehicle occupant
during derailment (without antecedent collision) V81.7
with antecedent collision —*see* Accident, transport, railway vehicle occupant
while boarding or alighting V81.4
transport vehicle after collision —*see* Accident, transport, by type of vehicle, collision
watercraft V93.39
due to
accident to craft V91.29
powered craft V91.23
ferry boat V91.21
fishing boat V91.22
jetskis V91.23
liner V91.21
merchant ship V91.20
passenger ship V91.21
unpowered craft
canoe V91.25
inflatable V91.26
kayak V91.25
sailboat V91.24
powered craft V93.33
ferry boat V93.31
fishing boat V93.32
jetskis V93.33
liner V93.31
merchant ship V93.30
passenger ship V93.31
unpowered craft V93.38
canoe V93.35
inflatable V93.36
kayak V93.35
sailboat V93.34
surf-board V93.38
windsurfer V93.38
into
cavity W17.2
dock W17.4
fire —*see* Exposure, fire, by type
haystack W17.89
hole W17.2
~~lake —see Fall, into, water~~
manhole W17.1
moving part of machinery —*see* Contact, with, by type of machine
ocean —*see* Fall, into, water
opening in surface NEC W17.89
pit W17.2
pond —*see* Fall, into, water
quarry W17.89
river —*see* Fall, into, water
shaft W17.89
storm drain W17.1
stream —*see* Fall, into, water
swimming pool —*see also* Fall, into, water, in, swimming pool
empty W17.3
tank W17.89
water W16.42
causing drowning W16.41
from watercraft —*see* Drowning, due to, fall overboard
hitting diving board W21.4
in
bathtub W16.212
causing drowning W16.211
bucket W16.222
causing drowning W16.221
natural body of water W16.112
causing drowning W16.111
striking
bottom W16.122
causing drowning W16.121

Fall, falling *(Continued)*
into *(Continued)*
water *(Continued)*
in *(Continued)*
natural body of water *(Continued)*
striking *(Continued)*
side W16.132
causing drowning W16.131
specified water NEC W16.312
causing drowning W16.311
striking
bottom W16.322
causing drowning W16.321
wall W16.332
causing drowning W16.331
swimming pool W16.012
causing drowning W16.011
striking
bottom W16.022
causing drowning W16.021
wall W16.032
causing drowning W16.031
utility bucket W16.222
causing drowning W16.221
well W17.0
involving
bed W06
chair W07
furniture NEC W08
glass —*see* Fall, by type
playground equipment W09.8
jungle gym W09.2
slide W09.0
swing W09.1
roller blades —*see* Accident, transport, pedestrian, conveyance
skateboard (s) —*see* Accident, transport, pedestrian, conveyance
skates (ice) (in line) (roller) —*see* Accident, transport, pedestrian, conveyance
skis —*see* Accident, transport, pedestrian, conveyance
table W08
wheelchair, non-moving W05.0
powered —*see* Accident, transport, pedestrian, conveyance, specified type NEC
object —*see* Struck by, object, falling
off
toilet W18.11
with subsequent striking against object W18.12
on same level W18.30
due to
specified NEC W18.39
stepping on an object W18.31
out of
bed W06
building NEC W13.8
chair W07
furniture NEC W08
wheelchair, non-moving W05.0
powered —*see* Accident, transport, pedestrian, conveyance, specified type NEC
window W13.4
over
animal W01.0
cliff W15
embankment W17.81
small object W01.0
rock W20.8
same level W18.30
from
being crushed, pushed, or stepped on by a crowd or human stampede W52
collision, pushing, shoving, by or with other person W03
slipping, stumbling, tripping W01.0

Fall, falling *(Continued)*
same level *(Continued)*
involving ice or snow W00.0
involving skates (ice) (roller), skateboard, skis —*see* Accident, transport, pedestrian, conveyance
snowslide (avalanche) —*see* Landslide ◀
stone W20.8
structure W20.1
burning (uncontrolled fire) X00.3
through
bridge W13.1
floor W13.3
roof W13.2
wall W13.8
window W13.4
timber W20.8
tree (caused by lightning) W20.8
while being carried or supported by other person (s) W04
Fallen on by
animal (not being ridden) NEC W55.89
Felo-de-se —*see* Suicide
Fight (hand) (fists) (foot) —*see* Assault, fight
Fire (accidental) —*see* Exposure, fire
Firearm discharge —*see* Discharge, firearm
Fireball effects from nuclear explosion in war operations —*see* War operations, nuclear weapons
Fireworks (explosion) W39
Flash burns from explosion —*see* Explosion
Flood (any injury) (caused by) X38
collapse of man-made structure causing earth movement X36.0
tidal wave —*see* Forces of nature, tidal wave
Food (any type) in
air passages (with asphyxia, obstruction, or suffocation) —*see* categories T17 and T18
alimentary tract causing asphyxia (due to compression of trachea) —*see* categories T17 and T18
Forces of nature X39.8
avalanche X36.1
causing transport accident —*see* Accident, transport, by type of vehicle
blizzard X37.2
cataclysmic storm X37.9
with flood X38
blizzard X37.2
cloudburst X37.8
cyclone X37.1
dust storm X37.3
hurricane X37.0
specified storm NEC X37.8
storm surge X37.0
tornado X37.1
twister X37.1
typhoon X37.0
cloudburst X37.8
cold (natural) X31
cyclone X37.1
dam collapse causing earth movement X36.0
dust storm X37.3
earth movement X36.1
caused by dam or structure collapse X36.0
earthquake X34
earthquake X34
flood (caused by) X38
dam collapse X36.0
tidal wave —*see* Forces of nature, tidal wave ◀
heat (natural) X30
hurricane X37.0
landslide X36.1
causing transport accident —*see* Accident, transport, by type of vehicle
lightning —*see* subcategory T75.0
causing fire —*see* Exposure, fire
mudslide X36.1
causing transport accident —*see* Accident, transport, by type of vehicle

F

Forces of nature *(Continued)*
radiation (natural) X39.08
radon X39.01
radon X39.01
specified force NEC X39.8
storm surge X37.0
structure collapse causing
earth movement
X36.0
sunlight X32
tidal wave X37.41
due to
earthquake X37.41
landslide X37.43
storm X37.42
volcanic eruption X37.41
tornado X37.1

Forces of nature *(Continued)*
tsunami X37.41
twister X37.1
typhoon X37.0
volcanic eruption X35
Foreign body ◀
aspiration - *see* Index to Diseases and Injuries, Foreign body, respitory tract ◀
embedded in skin W45 ◀
entering through skin W45.8 ◀
can lid W26.2 ◀
nail W45.0 ◀
paper W26.2 ◀
specified NEC 45.8 ◀
splinter W45.8 ◀

Forest fire (exposure to) —*see* Exposure, fire, uncontrolled, not in building
Found injured X58
from exposure (to) —*see* Exposure
on
highway, road(way), street V89.9
railway right of way V81.9
Fracture (circumstances unknown or unspecified) X58
due to specified cause NEC X58
Freezing —*see* Exposure, cold
Frostbite X31
due to man-made conditions —*see* Exposure, cold, man-made
Frozen —*see* Exposure, cold

G

Gored by bull W55.22
Gunshot wound W34.00

H

Hailstones, injured by X39.8
Hanged herself or himself —*see* Hanging, self-inflicted
Hanging (accidental) —*see also* category T71
legal execution —*see* Legal, intervention, specified means NEC
Heat (effects of) (excessive) X30
due to
man-made conditions W92
on board watercraft V93.29
fishing boat V93.22
merchant ship V93.20
passenger ship V93.21
sailboat V93.24
specified powered craft NEC V93.23
weather (conditions) X30

Heat *(Continued)*
from
electric heating apparatus causing burning X16
nuclear explosion in war operations —*see* War operations, nuclear weapons
inappropriate in local application or packing in medical or surgical procedure Y63.5
Hemorrhage
delayed following medical or surgical treatment without mention of misadventure —*see* Index to Diseases and Injuries, Complication(s) ⇐
during medical or surgical treatment as misadventure —*see* Index to Diseases and Injuries, Complication(s) ⇐

High
altitude (effects) —*see* Air, pressure, low
level of radioactivity, effects —*see* Radiation
pressure (effects) —*see* Air, pressure, high
temperature, effects —*see* Heat
Hit, hitting (accidental) by —*see* Struck by
Hitting against —*see* Striking against
Homicide (attempt) (justifiable) —*see* Assault
Hot
place, effects —*see also* Heat
weather, effects X30
House fire (uncontrolled) —*see* Exposure, fire, uncontrolled, building
Humidity, causing problem X39.8
Hunger X58
Hurricane (any injury) X37.0
Hypobarism, hypobaropathy —*see* Air, pressure, low

◀ New ⇐ Revised ~~deleted~~ Deleted

I

Ictus
caloris —*see also* Heat
solaris X30
Ignition (accidental) —*see also* Exposure, fire X08.8
anesthetic gas in operating room W40.1
apparel X06.2
from highly flammable material X04
nightwear X05
bed linen (sheets) (spreads) (pillows) (mattress) —*see* Exposure, fire, uncontrolled, building, bed
benzine X04
clothes, clothing NEC (from controlled fire) X06.2
from
highly flammable material X04
ether X04
in operating room W40.1
explosive material —*see* Explosion
gasoline X04
jewelry (plastic) (any) X06.0
kerosene X04
material
explosive —*see* Explosion
highly flammable with secondary explosion X04
nightwear X05
paraffin X04
petrol X04
Immersion (accidental) —*see also* Drowning
hand or foot due to cold (excessive) X31
Implantation of quills of porcupine W55.89
Inanition (from) (hunger) X58
thirst X58.8
Inappropriate operation performed
correct operation on wrong side or body part (wrong side) (wrong site) Y65.53
operation intended for another patient done on wrong patient Y65.52
wrong operation performed on correct patient Y65.51
Inattention after, at birth (homicidal intent) (infanticidal intent) X58
Incident, adverse
device
anesthesiology Y70.8
accessory Y70.2
diagnostic Y70.0
miscellaneous Y70.8
monitoring Y70.0
prosthetic Y70.2
rehabilitative Y70.1
surgical Y70.3
therapeutic Y70.1
cardiovascular Y71.8
accessory Y71.2
diagnostic Y71.0
miscellaneous Y71.8
monitoring Y71.0
prosthetic Y71.2
rehabilitative Y71.1
surgical Y71.3
therapeutic Y71.1
gastroenterology Y73.8
accessory Y73.2
diagnostic Y73.0
miscellaneous Y73.8
monitoring Y73.0
prosthetic Y73.2
rehabilitative Y73.1
surgical Y73.3
therapeutic Y73.1
general
hospital Y74.8
accessory Y74.2
diagnostic Y74.0
Incident, adverse *(Continued)*
device *(Continued)*
general *(Continued)*
hospital *(Continued)*
miscellaneous Y74.8
monitoring Y74.0
prosthetic Y74.2
rehabilitative Y74.1
surgical Y74.3
therapeutic Y74.1
surgical Y81.8
accessory Y81.2
diagnostic Y81.0
miscellaneous Y81.8
monitoring Y81.0
prosthetic Y81.2
rehabilitative Y81.1
surgical Y81.3
therapeutic Y81.1
gynecological Y76.8
accessory Y76.2
diagnostic Y76.0
miscellaneous Y76.8
monitoring Y76.0
prosthetic Y76.2
rehabilitative Y76.1
surgical Y76.3
therapeutic Y76.1
medical Y82.9
specified type NEC Y82.8
neurological Y75.8
accessory Y75.2
diagnostic Y75.0
miscellaneous Y75.8
monitoring Y75.0
prosthetic Y75.2
rehabilitative Y75.1
surgical Y75.3
therapeutic Y75.1
obstetrical Y76.8
accessory Y76.2
diagnostic Y76.0
miscellaneous Y76.8
monitoring Y76.0
prosthetic Y76.2
rehabilitative Y76.1
surgical Y76.3
therapeutic Y76.1
ophthalmic Y77.8
accessory Y77.2
diagnostic Y77.0
miscellaneous Y77.8
monitoring Y77.0
prosthetic Y77.2
rehabilitative Y77.1
surgical Y77.3
therapeutic Y77.1
orthopedic Y79.8
accessory Y79.2
diagnostic Y79.0
miscellaneous Y79.8
monitoring Y79.0
prosthetic Y79.2
rehabilitative Y79.1
surgical Y79.3
therapeutic Y79.1
otorhinolaryngological Y72.8
accessory Y72.2
diagnostic Y72.0
miscellaneous Y72.8
monitoring Y72.0
prosthetic Y72.2
rehabilitative Y72.1
surgical Y72.3
therapeutic Y72.1
personal use Y74.8
accessory Y74.2
diagnostic Y74.0
miscellaneous Y74.8
monitoring Y74.0
prosthetic Y74.2
Incident, adverse *(Continued)*
device *(Continued)*
personal use *(Continued)*
rehabilitative Y74.1
surgical Y74.3
therapeutic Y74.1
physical medicine Y80.8
accessory Y80.2
diagnostic Y80.0
miscellaneous Y80.8
monitoring Y80.0
prosthetic Y80.2
rehabilitative Y80.1
surgical Y80.3
therapeutic Y80.1
plastic surgical Y81.8
accessory Y81.2
diagnostic Y81.0
miscellaneous Y81.8
monitoring Y81.0
prosthetic Y81.2
rehabilitative Y81.1
surgical Y81.3
therapeutic Y81.1
radiological Y78.8
accessory Y78.2
diagnostic Y78.0
miscellaneous Y78.8
monitoring Y78.0
prosthetic Y78.2
rehabilitative Y78.1
surgical Y78.3
therapeutic Y78.1
urology Y73.8
accessory Y73.2
diagnostic Y73.0
miscellaneous Y73.8
monitoring Y73.0
prosthetic Y73.2
rehabilitative Y73.1
surgical Y73.3
therapeutic Y73.1
Incineration (accidental) —*see* Exposure, fire
Infanticide —*see* Assault
Infrasound waves (causing injury) W49.9
Ingestion
foreign body (causing injury) (with obstruction) —*see* Foreign body, alimentary canal
poisonous
plant (s) X58
substance NEC —*see* Table of Drugs and Chemicals ⇐
Inhalation
excessively cold substance, man-made —*see* Exposure, cold, man-made
food (any type) (into respiratory tract) (with asphyxia, obstruction respiratory tract, suffocation) —*see* categories T17 and T18
foreign body —*see* Foreign body, aspiration
gastric contents (with asphyxia, obstruction respiratory passage, suffocation) T17.81-
hot air or gases X14.0
liquid air, hydrogen, nitrogen W93.12
suicide (attempt) X83.2
steam X13.0
assault X98.0
stated as undetermined whether accidental or intentional Y27.0
suicide (attempt) X77.0
toxic gas —*see* Table of Drugs and Chemicals ⇐
vomitus (with asphyxia, obstruction respiratory passage, suffocation)T17.81-
Injury, injured (accidental(ly)) **NOS** X58
by, caused by, from
assault —*see* Assault
law-enforcing agent, police, in course of legal intervention —*see* Legal intervention
suicide (attempt) X83.8

Injury, injured NOS *(Continued)*
due to, in
civil insurrection —*see* War operations
fight —*see also* Assault, fight Y04.0
war operations —*see* War operations
homicide —*see also* Assault Y09
inflicted (by)
in course of arrest (attempted), suppression of disturbance, maintenance of order, by law-enforcing agents —*see* Legal intervention

Injury, injured NOS *(Continued)*
inflicted *(Continued)*
other person
stated as
accidental X58
intentional, homicide (attempt) —*see* Assault
undetermined whether accidental or intentional Y33
purposely (inflicted) by other person (s) —*see* Assault
self-inflicted X83.8
stated as accidental X58
specified cause NEC X58

Injury, injured NOS *(Continued)*
undetermined whether accidental or intentional Y33
Insolation, effects X30
Insufficient nourishment X58
Interruption of respiration (by)
food (lodged in esophagus) —*see* categories T17 and T18
vomitus (lodged in esophagus) T17.81-
Intervention, legal —*see* Legal intervention
Intoxication
drug —*see* Table of Drugs and Chemicals ⇐
poison —*see* Table of Drugs and Chemicals ⇐

J

Jammed (accidentally)
between objects (moving) (stationary and moving) W23.0
stationary W23.1
Jumped, jumping
before moving object NEC X81.8
motor vehicle X81.0
subway train X81.1
train X81.1
undetermined whether accidental or intentional Y31
from
boat (into water) voluntarily, without accident (to or on boat) W16.712
with
accident to or on boat —*see* Accident, watercraft
drowning or submersion W16.711
suicide (attempt) X71.3

Jumped, jumping *(Continued)*
from *(Continued)*
boat voluntarily, without accident *(Continued)*
striking bottom W16.722
causing drowning W16.721
building —*see also* Jumped, from, high place W13.9
burning (uncontrolled fire) X00.5
high place NEC W17.89
suicide (attempt) X80
undetermined whether accidental or intentional Y30
structure —*see also* Jumped, from, high place W13.9
burning (uncontrolled fire) X00.5
into water W16.92
causing drowning W16.91
from, off watercraft —*see* Jumped, from, boat

Jumped, jumping *(Continued)*
into water *(Continued)*
in
natural body W16.612
causing drowning W16.611
striking bottom W16.622
causing drowning W16.621
specified place NEC W16.812
causing drowning W16.811
striking
bottom W16.822
causing drowning W16.821
wall W16.832
causing drowning W16.831
swimming pool W16.512
causing drowning W16.511
striking
bottom W16.522
causing drowning W16.521
wall W16.532
causing drowning W16.531
suicide (attempt) X71.3

K

Kicked by
animal NEC W55.82
person (s) (accidentally) W50.1
with intent to injure or kill Y04.0
as, or caused by, a crowd or human stampede (with fall) W52
assault Y04.0
homicide (attempt) Y04.0
in
fight Y04.0
legal intervention
injuring
bystander Y35.812
law enforcement personnel Y35.811
suspect Y35.813
~~Kicking against~~
~~object W22.8~~
~~sports equipment W21.9~~
~~stationary W22.09~~
~~sports equipment W21.89~~
~~person —see Striking against, person~~
~~sports equipment W21.9~~

Kicking ◀
against ◀
object W22.8 ◀
sports equipment W21.9 ◀
stationary W22.09 ◀
sports equipment W21.89 ◀
person —*see* Striking against, person ◀
sports equipment W21.9 ◀
carpet stretcher with knee X50.3 ◀
Killed, killing (accidentally) **NOS** —*see also* Injury X58
in
action —*see* War operations
brawl, fight (hand) (fists) (foot) Y04.0
by weapon —*see also* Assault
cutting, piercing —*see* Assault, cutting or piercing instrument
firearm —*see* Discharge, firearm, by type, homicide

Killed, killing NOS *(Continued)*
self
stated as
accident NOS X58
suicide —*see* Suicide
undetermined whether accidental or intentional Y33
Kneeling (prolonged) (static) X50.1 ◀
Knocked down (accidentally) (by) **NOS** X58
animal (not being ridden) NEC —*see also* Struck by, by type of animal
crowd or human stampede W52
person W51
in brawl, fight Y04.0
transport vehicle NEC —*see also* Accident, transport V09.9

◀ New ⇐ Revised ~~deleted~~ Deleted

L

Laceration NEC —*see* Injury
Lack of
care (helpless person) (infant) (newborn) X58
food except as result of abandonment or neglect X58
due to abandonment or neglect X58
water except as result of transport accident X58
due to transport accident —*see* Accident, transport, by type ◀
helpless person, infant, newborn X58
Landslide (falling on transport vehicle) X36.1
caused by collapse of man-made structure X36.0
Late effect —*see* Sequelae
Legal
execution (any method) —*see* Legal, intervention
intervention (by)
baton —*see* Legal, intervention, blunt object, baton
bayonet —*see* Legal, intervention, sharp object, bayonet
blow —*see* Legal, intervention, manhandling
blunt object
baton
injuring
bystander Y35.312
law enforcement personnel Y35.311
suspect Y35.313
injuring
bystander Y35.302
law enforcement personnel Y35.301
suspect Y35.303
specified NEC
injuring
bystander Y35.392
law enforcement personnel Y35.391
suspect Y35.393
stave
injuring
bystander Y35.392
law enforcement personnel Y35.391
suspect Y35.393
bomb —*see* Legal, intervention, explosive
cutting or piercing instrument —*see* Legal, intervention, sharp object
dynamite —*see* Legal, intervention, explosive, dynamite
explosive (s)
dynamite
injuring
bystander Y35.112
law enforcement personnel Y35.111
suspect Y35.113
grenade
injuring
bystander Y35.192
law enforcement personnel Y35.191
suspect Y35.193
injuring
bystander Y35.102
law enforcement personnel Y35.101
suspect Y35.103
Legal *(Continued)*
intervention *(Continued)*
explosive *(Continued)*
mortar bomb
injuring
bystander Y35.192
law enforcement personnel Y35.191
suspect Y35.193
shell
injuring
bystander Y35.122
law enforcement personnel Y35.121
suspect Y35.123
specified NEC
injuring
bystander Y35.192
law enforcement personnel Y35.191
suspect Y35.193
firearm (s) (discharge)
handgun
injuring
bystander Y35.022
law enforcement personnel Y35.021
suspect Y35.023
injuring
bystander Y35.002
law enforcement personnel Y35.001
suspect Y35.003
machine gun
injuring
bystander Y35.012
law enforcement personnel Y35.011
suspect Y35.013
rifle pellet
injuring
bystander Y35.032
law enforcement personnel Y35.031
suspect Y35.033
rubber bullet
injuring
bystander Y35.042
law enforcement personnel Y35.041
suspect Y35.043
shotgun —*see* Legal, intervention, firearm, specified NEC
specified NEC
injuring
bystander Y35.092
law enforcement personnel Y35.091
suspect Y35.093
gas (asphyxiation) (poisoning)
injuring
bystander Y35.202
law enforcement personnel Y35.201
suspect Y35.203
specified NEC
injuring
bystander Y35.292
law enforcement personnel Y35.291
suspect Y35.293
tear gas
injuring
bystander Y35.212
law enforcement personnel Y35.211
suspect Y35.213
Legal *(Continued)*
intervention *(Continued)*
grenade —*see* Legal, intervention, explosive, grenade
injuring
bystander Y35.92
law enforcement personnel Y35.91
suspect Y35.93
late effect (of) —*see* with 7th character S Y35
manhandling
injuring
bystander Y35.812
law enforcement personnel Y35.811
suspect Y35.813
sequelae (of) —*see* with 7th character S Y35
sharp objects
bayonet
injuring
bystander Y35.412
law enforcement personnel Y35.411
suspect Y35.413
injuring
bystander Y35.402
law enforcement personnel Y35.401
suspect Y35.403
specified NEC
injuring
bystander Y35.492
law enforcement personnel Y35.491
suspect Y35.493
specified means NEC
injuring
bystander Y35.892
law enforcement personnel Y35.891
suspect Y35.893
stabbing —*see* Legal, intervention, sharp object
stave —*see* Legal, intervention, blunt object, stave
tear gas —*see* Legal, intervention, gas, tear gas
truncheon —*see* Legal, intervention, blunt object, stave
Lifting —*see also* Overexertion ◀
heavy objects X50.0 ◀
weights X50.0 ◀
Lightning (shock) (stroke) (struck by) —*see* subcategory T75.0
causing fire —*see* Exposure, fire
Loss of control (transport vehicle) **NEC** —*see* Accident, transport
Lost at sea NOS —*see* Drowning, due to, fall overboard
Low
pressure (effects) —*see* Air, pressure, low
temperature (effects) —*see* Exposure, cold
Lying before train, vehicle or other moving object X81.8
subway train X81.1
train X81.1
undetermined whether accidental or intentional Y31
Lynching —*see* Assault

L

M

Malfunction (mechanism or component) (of)
firearm
airgun W34.10
BB gun W34.110
gas, air or spring-operated gun NEC W34.118
handgun W32.1
hunting rifle W33.12
larger firearm W33.10
specified NEC W33.19
machine gun W33.13
paintball gun W34.111
pellet gun W34.110
shotgun W33.11
specified NEC W34.19
Very pistol [flare] W34.19
handgun —*see* Malfunction, firearm, handgun
Maltreatment —*see* Perpetrator
Mangled (accidentally) **NOS** X58
Manhandling (in brawl, fight) Y04.0
legal intervention —*see* Legal, intervention, manhandling
Manslaughter (nonaccidental) —*see* Assault
Mauled by animal NEC W55.89
Medical procedure, complication of (delayed or as an abnormal reaction without mention of misadventure) —*see* Complication of or following, by specified type of procedure
due to or as a result of misadventure —*see* Misadventure
Melting (due to fire) —*see also* Exposure, fire
apparel NEC X06.3
clothes, clothing NEC X06.3
nightwear X05
fittings or furniture (burning building) (uncontrolled fire) X00.8
nightwear X05
plastic jewelry X06.1
Mental cruelty X58
Military operations (injuries to military and civilians occuring during peacetime on military property and during routine military exercises and operations) (by) (from) (involving) Y37.90-
air blast Y37.20-
aircraft
destruction —*see* Military operations, destruction of aircraft
airway restriction —*see* Military operations, restriction of airways
asphyxiation —*see* Military operations, restriction of airways
biological weapons Y37.6X-
blast Y37.20-
blast fragments Y37.20-
blast wave Y37.20-
blast wind Y37.20-
bomb Y37.20-
dirty Y37.50-
gasoline Y37.31-
incendiary Y37.31-
petrol Y37.31-
bullet Y37.43-
incendiary Y37.32-
rubber Y37.41-
chemical weapons Y37.7X-
combat
hand to hand (unarmed) combat Y37.44-
using blunt or piercing object Y37.45-
conflagration —*see* Military operations, fire
conventional warfare NEC Y37.49-
depth-charge Y37.01-
destruction of aircraft Y37.10-
due to
air to air missile Y37.11-
collision with other aircraft Y37.12-

Military operations *(Continued)*
destruction of aircraft *(Continued)*
due to *(Continued)*
detonation (accidental) of onboard munitions and explosives Y37.14-
enemy fire or explosives Y37.11-
explosive placed on aircraft Y37.11-
onboard fire Y37.13-
rocket propelled grenade [RPG] Y37.11-
small arms fire Y37.11-
surface to air missile Y37.11-
specified NEC Y37.19-
detonation (accidental) of
onboard marine weapons Y37.05-
own munitions or munitions launch device Y37.24-
dirty bomb Y37.50-
explosion (of) Y37.20-
aerial bomb Y37.21-
bomb NOS —*see also* Military operations, bomb (s) Y37.20-
fragments Y37.20-
grenade Y37.29-
guided missile Y37.22-
improvised explosive device [IED] (person-borne) (roadside) (vehicle-borne) Y37.23-
land mine Y37.29-
marine mine (at sea) (in harbor) Y37.02-
marine weapon Y37.00-
specified NEC Y37.09-
own munitions or munitions launch device (accidental) Y37.24-
sea-based artillery shell Y37.03-
specified NEC Y37.29-
torpedo Y37.04-
fire Y37.30-
specified NEC Y37.39-
firearms
discharge Y37.43-
pellets Y37.42-
flamethrower Y37.33-
fragments (from) (of)
improvised explosive device [IED] (person-borne) (roadside) (vehicle-borne) Y37.26-
munitions Y37.25-
specified NEC Y37.29-
weapons Y37.27-
friendly fire Y37.92-
hand to hand (unarmed) combat Y37.44-
hot substances —*see* Military operations, fire
incendiary bullet Y37.32-
nuclear weapon (effects of) Y37.50-
acute radiation exposure Y37.54-
blast pressure Y37.51-
direct blast Y37.51-
direct heat Y37.53-
fallout exposure Y37.54-
fireball Y37.53-
indirect blast (struck or crushed by blast debris) (being thrown by blast) Y37.52-
ionizing radiation (immediate exposure) Y37.54-
nuclear radiation Y37.54-
radiation
ionizing (immediate exposure) Y37.54-
nuclear Y37.54-
thermal Y37.53-
secondary effects Y37.54-
specified NEC Y37.59-
thermal radiation Y37.53-
restriction of air (airway)
intentional Y37.46-
unintentional Y37.47-
rubber bullets Y37.41-
shrapnel NOS Y37.29-
suffocation —*see* Military operations, restriction of airways
unconventional warfare NEC Y37.7X-

Military operations *(Continued)*
underwater blast NOS Y37.00-
warfare
conventional NEC Y37.49-
unconventional NEC Y37.7X-
weapon of mass destruction [WMD] Y37.91-
weapons
biological weapons Y37.6X-
chemical Y37.7X-
nuclear (effects of) Y37.50-
acute radiation exposure Y37.54-
blast pressure Y37.51-
direct blast Y37.51-
direct heat Y37.53-
fallout exposure Y37.54-
fireball Y37.53-
~~indirect blast (struck or crushed by blast debris) (being thrown by blast) Y37.52-~~
radiation
ionizing (immediate exposure) Y37.54-
nuclear Y37.54-
thermal Y37.53-
secondary effects Y37.54-
specified NEC Y37.59-
of mass destruction [WMD] Y37.91-
Misadventure (s) to patient (s) during surgical or medical care Y69
contaminated medical or biological substance (blood, drug, fluid) Y64.9
administered (by) NEC Y64.9
immunization Y64.1
infusion Y64.0
injection Y64.1
specified means NEC Y64.8
transfusion Y64.0
vaccination Y64.1
excessive amount of blood or other fluid during transfusion or infusion Y63.0
failure
in dosage Y63.9
electroshock therapy Y63.4
inappropriate temperature (too hot or too cold) in local application and packing Y63.5
infusion
excessive amount of fluid Y63.0
incorrect dilution of fluid Y63.1
insulin-shock therapy Y63.4
nonadministration of necessary drug or biological substance Y63.6 ◄
overdose —*see* Table of Drugs and Chemicals ◄
radiation, in therapy Y63.2
radiation
overdose Y63.2
specified procedure NEC Y63.8
transfusion
excessive amount of blood Y63.0
mechanical, of instrument or apparatus (any) (during any procedure) Y65.8
sterile precautions (during procedure) Y62.9
aspiration of fluid or tissue (by puncture or catheterization, except heart) Y62.6
biopsy (except needle aspiration) Y62.8
needle (aspirating) Y62.6
blood sampling Y62.6
catheterization Y62.6
heart Y62.5
dialysis (kidney) Y62.2
endoscopic examination Y62.4
enema Y62.8
immunization Y62.3
infusion Y62.1
injection Y62.3
needle biopsy Y62.6
paracentesis (abdominal) (thoracic) Y62.6
perfusion Y62.2

◄ New ◄ Revised ~~deleted~~ Deleted

Misadventure (s) to patient (s) during surgical or medical care *(Continued)*
failure *(Continued)*
sterile precautions *(Continued)*
puncture (lumbar) Y62.6
removal of catheter or packing Y62.8
specified procedure NEC Y62.8
surgical operation Y62.0
transfusion Y62.1
vaccination Y62.3
suture or ligature during surgical procedure Y65.2
to introduce or to remove tube or instrument —*see* Failure, to ◀
hemorrhage —*see* Index to Diseases and Injuries, Complication(s) ⇐
inadvertent exposure of patient to radiation Y63.3
inappropriate
operation performed —*see* Inappropriate operation performed
temperature (too hot or too cold) in local application or packing Y63.5

Misadventure (s) to patient (s) during surgical or medical care *(Continued)*
infusion —*see also* Misadventure, by type, infusion Y69
excessive amount of fluid Y63.0
incorrect dilution of fluid Y63.1
wrong fluid Y65.1
mismatched blood in transfusion Y65.0
nonadministration of necessary drug or biological substance Y63.6 ⇐
overdose —*see* Table of Drugs and Chemicals ⇐
radiation (in therapy) Y63.2
perforation —*see* Index to Diseases and Injuries, Complication(s) ⇐
performance of inappropriate operation —*see* Inappropriate operation performed
puncture —*see* Index to Diseases and Injuries, Complication(s) ⇐
specified type NEC Y65.8
failure
suture or ligature during surgical operation Y65.2
to introduce or to remove tube or instrument —*see* Failure, to ◀
infusion of wrong fluid Y65.1

Misadventure (s) to patient (s) during surgical or medical care *(Continued)*
specified type NEC *(Continued)*
performance of inappropriate operation —*see* Inappropriate operation performed
transfusion of mismatched blood Y65.0
wrong
fluid in infusion Y65.1
placement of endotracheal tube during anesthetic procedure Y65.3
transfusion —*see* Misadventure, by type, transfusion
excessive amount of blood Y63.0
mismatched blood Y65.0
wrong
drug given in error —*see* Table of Drugs and Chemicals ⇐
fluid in infusion Y65.1
placement of endotracheal tube during anesthetic procedure Y65.3
Mismatched blood in transfusion Y65.0
Motion sickness T75.3
Mountain sickness W94.11
Mudslide (of cataclysmic nature) —*see* Landslide
Murder (attempt) —*see* Assault

N

Nail ◀
contact with W45.0 ◀
gun W29.4 ◀
embedded in skin W45.0 ◀
~~Nail, contact with W45.0~~
~~gun W29.4~~

Neglect (criminal) (homicidal intent) X58
Noise (causing injury) (pollution) W42.9
supersonic W42.0
Nonadministration (of)
drug or biological substance (necessary) Y63.6 ⇐
surgical and medical care Y66
Nosocomial condition Y95

O

Object
falling
from, in, on, hitting
machinery —*see* Contact, with, by type of machine
set in motion by
accidental explosion or rupture of pressure vessel W38
firearm —*see* Discharge, firearm, by type
machine (ry) —*see* Contact, with, by type of machine
Overdose (drug) —*see* Table of Drugs and Chemicals ⇐
radiation Y63.2

Overexertion X50.9 ⇐
from ◀
prolonged static or awkward postures X50.1 ◀
repetitive movements X50.3 ◀
specified strenuous movements or postures NEC X50.9 ◀
strenuous movement or load X50.0 ◀
Overexposure (accidental) (to)
cold —*see also* Exposure, cold X31
due to man-made conditions —*see* Exposure, cold, man-made
heat —*see also* Heat X30
radiation —*see* Radiation
radioactivity W88.0
sun (sunburn) X32

Overexposure *(Continued)*
weather NEC —*see* Forces of nature ◀
wind NEC —*see* Forces of nature ◀
Overheated —*see* Heat
Overturning (accidental)
machinery —*see* Contact, with, by type of machine
transport vehicle NEC —*see also* Accident, transport V89.9
watercraft (causing drowning, submersion) —*see also* Drowning, due to, accident to, watercraft, overturning
causing injury except drowning or submersion —*see* Accident, watercraft, causing, injury NEC ◀

P

Parachute descent (voluntary) (without accident to aircraft) V97.29
due to accident to aircraft —*see* Accident, transport, aircraft
Pecked by bird W61.99
Perforation during medical or surgical treatment as misadventure —*see* Index to Diseases and Injuries, Complication(s) ◀
Perpetrator, perpetration, of assault, maltreatment and neglect (by) Y07.9
boyfriend Y07.03
brother Y07.410
stepbrother Y07.435
coach Y07.53
cousin
female Y07.491
male Y07.490
daycare provider Y07.519
at-home
adult care Y07.512
childcare Y07.510
care center
adult care Y07.513
childcare Y07.511
family member NEC Y07.499
father Y07.11
adoptive Y07.13
foster Y07.420
stepfather Y07.430
foster father Y07.420
foster mother Y07.421
girl friend Y07.04
healthcare provider Y07.529
mental health Y07.521
specified NEC Y07.528
husband Y07.01
instructor Y07.53
mother Y07.12
adoptive Y07.14
foster Y07.421
stepmother Y07.433
nonfamily member Y07.50
specified NEC Y07.59
nurse Y07.528
occupational therapist Y07.528
partner of parent
female Y07.434
male Y07.432
physical therapist Y07.528
sister Y07.411
speech therapist Y07.528
stepbrother Y07.435
stepfather Y07.430
stepmother Y07.433
stepsister Y07.436
teacher Y07.53
wife Y07.02
Piercing —*see* Contact, with, by type of object or machine
Pinched
between objects (moving) (stationary and moving) W23.0
stationary W23.1
Pinned under machine (ry) —*see* Contact, with, by type of machine
Place of occurrence Y92.9
abandoned house Y92.89
airplane Y92.813
airport Y92.520
ambulatory health services establishment NEC Y92.538
ambulatory surgery center Y92.530
amusement park Y92.831
apartment (co-op) —*see* Place of occurrence, residence, apartment
assembly hall Y92.29
bank Y92.510
barn Y92.71
baseball field Y92.320

Place of occurrence *(Continued)*
basketball court Y92.310
beach Y92.832
boarding house —*see* Place of occurrence, residence, boarding house
boat Y92.814
bowling alley Y92.39
bridge Y92.89
building under construction Y92.61
bus Y92.811
station Y92.521
cafe Y92.511
campsite Y92.833
campus —*see* Place of occurrence, school
canal Y92.89
car Y92.810
casino Y92.59
children's home —*see* Place of occurrence, residence, institutional, orphanage
church Y92.22
cinema Y92.26
clubhouse Y92.29
coal pit Y92.64
college (community) Y92.214
condominium —*see* Place of occurrence, residence, apartment
construction area —*see* Place of occurrence, industrial and construction area
convalescent home —*see* Place of occurrence, residence, institutional, nursing home
court-house Y92.240
cricket ground Y92.328
cultural building Y92.258
art gallery Y92.250
museum Y92.251
music hall Y92.252
opera house Y92.253
specified NEC Y92.258
theater Y92.254
dancehall Y92.252
day nursery Y92.210
dentist office Y92.531
derelict house Y92.89
desert Y92.820
dock NOS Y92.89
dockyard Y92.62
doctor's office Y92.531
dormitory —*see* Place of occurrence, residence, institutional, school dormitory
dry dock Y92.62
factory (building) (premises) Y92.63
farm (land under cultivation) (outbuildings) Y92.79
barn Y92.71
chicken coop Y92.72
field Y92.73
hen house Y92.72
house —*see* Place of occurrence, residence, house
orchard Y92.74
specified NEC Y92.79
football field Y92.321
forest Y92.821
freeway Y92.411
gallery Y92.250
garage (commercial) Y92.59
boarding house Y92.044
military base Y92.135
mobile home Y92.025
nursing home Y92.124
orphanage Y92.114
private house Y92.015
reform school Y92.155
gas station Y92.524
gasworks Y92.69
golf course Y92.39
gravel pit Y92.64
grocery Y92.512
gymnasium Y92.39
handball court Y92.318
harbor Y92.89

Place of occurrence *(Continued)*
harness racing course Y92.39
healthcare provider office Y92.531
highway (interstate) Y92.411
hill Y92.828
hockey rink Y92.330
home —*see* Place of occurrence, residence
hospice —*see* Place of occurrence, residence, institutional, nursing home
hospital Y92.239
cafeteria Y92.233
corridor Y92.232
operating room Y92.234
patient
bathroom Y92.231
room Y92.230
specified NEC Y92.238
hotel Y92.59
house —*see also* Place of occurrence, residence
abandoned Y92.89
under construction Y92.61
industrial and construction area (yard) Y92.69
building under construction Y92.61
dock Y92.62
dry dock Y92.62
factory Y92.63
gasworks Y92.69
mine Y92.64
oil rig Y92.65
pit Y92.64
power station Y92.69
shipyard Y92.62
specified NEC Y92.69
tunnel under construction Y92.69
workshop Y92.69
kindergarten Y92.211
lacrosse field Y92.328
lake Y92.828
library Y92.241
mall Y92.59
market Y92.512
marsh Y92.828
military
base —*see* Place of occurrence, residence, institutional, military base
training ground Y92.84
mine Y92.64
mosque Y92.22
motel Y92.59
motorway (interstate) Y92.411
mountain Y92.828
movie-house Y92.26
museum Y92.251
music-hall Y92.252
not applicable Y92.9
nuclear power station Y92.69
nursing home —*see* Place of occurrence, residence, institutional, nursing home
office building Y92.59
offshore installation Y92.65
oil rig Y92.65
old people's home —*see* Place of occurrence, residence, institutional, specified NEC
opera-house Y92.253
orphanage —*see* Place of occurrence, residence, institutional, orphanage
outpatient surgery center Y92.530
park (public) Y92.830
amusement Y92.831
parking garage Y92.89
lot Y92.481
pavement Y92.480
physician office Y92.531
polo field Y92.328
pond Y92.828
post office Y92.242
power station Y92.69
prairie Y92.828
prison —*see* Place of occurrence, residence, institutional, prison

◀ New ◀ Revised ~~deleted~~ Deleted

Place of occurrence *(Continued)*
public
administration building Y92.248
city hall Y92.243
courthouse Y92.240
library Y92.241
post office Y92.242
specified NEC Y92.248
building NEC Y92.29
hall Y92.29
place NOS Y92.89
race course Y92.39
radio station Y92.59
railway line (bridge) Y92.85
ranch (outbuildings) —*see* Place of occurrence, farm
recreation area Y92.838
amusement park Y92.831
beach Y92.832
campsite Y92.833
park (public) Y92.830
seashore Y92.832
specified NEC Y92.838
reform school —*see* Place of occurrence, residence, institutional, reform school
religious institution Y92.22
residence (non-institutional) (private) Y92.009
apartment Y92.039
bathroom Y92.031
bedroom Y92.032
kitchen Y92.030
specified NEC Y92.038
bathroom Y92.002
bedroom Y92.003
boarding house Y92.049
bathroom Y92.041
bedroom Y92.042
driveway Y92.043
garage Y92.044
garden Y92.046
kitchen Y92.040
specified NEC Y92.048
swimming pool Y92.045
yard Y92.046
dining room Y92.001
garden Y92.007
home Y92.009
house, single family Y92.019
bathroom Y92.012
bedroom Y92.013
dining room Y92.011
driveway Y92.014
garage Y92.015
garden Y92.017
kitchen Y92.010
specified NEC Y92.018
swimming pool Y92.016
yard Y92.017
institutional Y92.10
children's home —*see* Place of occurrence, residence, institutional, orphanage
hospice —*see* Place of occurrence, residence, institutional, nursing home
military base Y92.139
barracks Y92.133
garage Y92.135
garden Y92.137
kitchen Y92.130
mess hall Y92.131
specified NEC Y92.138
swimming pool Y92.136
yard Y92.137
nursing home Y92.129
bathroom Y92.121
bedroom Y92.122
driveway Y92.123
garage Y92.124
garden Y92.126
kitchen Y92.120

Place of occurrence *(Continued)*
residence *(Continued)*
institutional *(Continued)*
nursing home *(Continued)*
specified NEC Y92.128
swimming pool Y92.125
yard Y92.126
orphanage Y92.119
bathroom Y92.111
bedroom Y92.112
driveway Y92.113
garage Y92.114
garden Y92.116
kitchen Y92.110
specified NEC Y92.118
swimming pool Y92.115
yard Y92.116
prison Y92.149
bathroom Y92.142
cell Y92.143
courtyard Y92.147
dining room Y92.141
kitchen Y92.140
specified NEC Y92.148
swimming pool Y92.146
reform school Y92.159
bathroom Y92.152
bedroom Y92.153
dining room Y92.151
driveway Y92.154
garage Y92.155
garden Y92.157
kitchen Y92.150
specified NEC Y92.158
swimming pool Y92.156
yard Y92.157
school dormitory Y92.169
bathroom Y92.162
bedroom Y92.163
dining room Y92.161
kitchen Y92.160
specified NEC Y92.168
specified NEC Y92.199
bathroom Y92.192
bedroom Y92.193
dining room Y92.191
driveway Y92.194
garage Y92.195
garden Y92.197
kitchen Y92.190
specified NEC Y92.198
swimming pool Y92.196
yard Y92.197
kitchen Y92.000
mobile home Y92.029
bathroom Y92.022
bedroom Y92.023
dining room Y92.021
driveway Y92.024
garage Y92.025
garden Y92.027
kitchen Y92.020
specified NEC Y92.028
swimming pool Y92.026
yard Y92.027
specified place in residence NEC Y92.008 ◄
specified residence type NEC Y92.099
bathroom Y92.091
bedroom Y92.092
driveway Y92.093
garage Y92.094
garden Y92.096
kitchen Y92.090
specified NEC Y92.098
swimming pool Y92.095
yard Y92.096
restaurant Y92.511
riding school Y92.39
river Y92.828
road Y92.488
rodeo ring Y92.39

Place of occurrence *(Continued)*
rugby field Y92.328
same day surgery center Y92.530
sand pit Y92.64
school (private) (public) (state) Y92.219
college Y92.214
daycare center Y92.210
elementary school Y92.211
high school Y92.213
kindergarten Y92.211
middle school Y92.212
specified NEC Y92.218
trace school Y92.215
university Y92.214
vocational school Y92.215
sea (shore) Y92.832
senior citizen center Y92.29
service area
airport Y92.520
bus station Y92.521
gas station Y92.524
highway rest stop Y92.523
railway station Y92.522
shipyard Y92.62
shop(commercial) Y92.513
sidewalk Y92.480
silo Y92.79
skating rink (roller) Y92.331
ice Y92.330
slaughter house Y92.86
soccer field Y92.322
specified place NEC Y92.89
sports area Y92.39
athletic
court Y92.318
basketball Y92.310
specified NEC Y92.318
squash Y92.311
tennis Y92.312
field Y92.328
baseball Y92.320
cricket ground Y92.328
football Y92.321
hockey Y92.328
soccer Y92.322
specified NEC Y92.328
golf course Y92.39
gymnasium Y92.39
riding school Y92.39
skating rink (roller) Y92.331
ice Y92.330
stadium Y92.39
swimming pool Y92.34
squash court Y92.311
stadium Y92.39
steeplechasing course Y92.39
store Y92.512
stream Y92.828
street and highway Y92.410
bike path Y92.482
freeway Y92.411
highway ramp Y92.415
interstate highway Y92.411
local residential or business street Y92.414
motorway Y92.411
parking lot Y92.481
parkway Y92.412
sidewalk Y92.480
specified NEC Y92.488
state road Y92.413
subway car Y92.816
supermarket Y92.512
swamp Y92.828
swimming pool (public) Y92.34
private (at) Y92.095
boarding house Y92.045
military base Y92.136
mobile home Y92.026
nursing home Y92.125
orphanage Y92.115

Place of occurrence *(Continued)*
swimming pool *(Continued)*
private *(Continued)*
prison Y92.146
reform school Y92.156
single family residence Y92.016
synagogue Y92.22
television station Y92.59
tennis court Y92.312
theater Y92.254
trade area Y92.59
bank Y92.510
cafe Y92.511
casino Y92.59
garage Y92.59
hotel Y92.59
market Y92.512
office building Y92.59
radio station Y92.59
restaurant Y92.511
shop Y92.513
shopping mall Y92.59
store Y92.512
supermarket Y92.512
television station Y92.59
warehouse Y92.59
trailer park, residential —*see* Place of occurrence, residence, mobile home
trailer site NOS Y92.89
train Y92.815
station Y92.522
truck Y92.812
tunnel under construction Y92. 69
university Y92.214
urgent (health) care center Y92.532
vehicle (transport) Y92.818
airplane Y92.813
boat Y92.814
bus Y92.811
car Y92.810
specified NEC Y92.818
subway car Y92.816
train Y92.815
truck Y92.812
warehouse Y92.59
water reservoir Y92.89
wilderness area Y92.828
desert Y92.820
forest Y92.821
marsh Y92.828
mountain Y92.828
prairie Y92.828
specified NEC Y92.828
swamp Y92.828
workshop Y92.69
yard, private Y92.096
boarding house Y92.046
mobile home Y92.027
single family house Y92.017

Place of occurrence *(Continued)*
youth center Y92.29
zoo (zoological garden) Y92.834
Plumbism —*see* Table of Drugs and Chemicals, lead ⇐
Poisoning (accidental) (by) —*see also* Table of Drugs and Chemicals ⇐
by plant, thorns, spines, sharp leaves or other mechanisms NEC X58
carbon monoxide
generated by
motor vehicle —*see* Accident, transport
watercraft (in transit) (not in transit) V93.89
ferry boat V93.81
fishing boat V93.82
jet skis V93.83
liner V93.81
merchant ship V93.80
passenger ship V93.81
powered craft NEC V93.83
caused by injection of poisons into skin by plant thorns, spines, sharp leaves X58
marine or sea plants (venomous) X58
exhaust gas
generated by
motor vehicle —*see* Accident, transport
watercraft (in transit) (not in transit) V93.89
ferry boat V93.81
fishing boat V93.82
jet skis V93.83
liner V93.81
merchant ship V93.80
passenger ship V93.81
powered craft NEC V93.83
fumes or smoke due to
explosion —*see also* Explosion W40.9
fire —*see* Exposure, fire
ignition —*see* Ignition
gas
in legal intervention —*see* Legal, intervention, gas
legal execution —*see* Legal, intervention, gas
in war operations —*see* War operations
legal
execution —*see* Legal, intervention, gas
intervention
by gas —*see* Legal, intervention, gas
other specified means —*see* Legal, intervention, specified means NEC
Powder burn (by) (from)
airgun W34.110
BB gun W34.110
firearm NEC W34.19
gas, air or spring-operated gun NEC W34.118
handgun W32.1
hunting rifle W33.12

Powder burn *(Continued)*
larger firearm W33.10
specified NEC W33.19
machine gun W33.13
paintball gun W34.111
pellet gun W34.110
shotgun W33.11
Very pistol [flare] W34.19
Premature cessation (of) surgical and medical care Y66
Privation (food) (water) X58
Procedure (operation)
correct, on wrong side or body part (wrong side) (wrong site) Y65.53
intended for another patient done on wrong patient Y65.52
performed on patient not scheduled for surgery Y65.52
performed on wrong patient Y65.52
wrong, performed on correct patient Y65.51
Prolonged
sitting in transport vehicle —*see* Travel, by type of vehicle
stay in
high altitude as cause of anoxia, barodontalgia, barotitis or hypoxia W94.11
weightless environment X52
Pulling, excessive —*see also* Overexertion X50.9 ⇐
Puncture, puncturing —*see also* Contact, with, by type of object or machine
by
plant thorns, spines, sharp leaves or other mechanisms NEC W60
during medical or surgical treatment as misadventure —*see* Index to Diseases and Injuries, Complication(s) ⇐
Pushed, pushing (accidental) (injury in) ⇐
by other person (s) (accidental) W51
with fall W03
due to ice or snow W00.0
as, or caused by, a crowd or human stampede (with fall) W52
before moving object NEC Y02.8
motor vehicle Y02.0
subway train Y02.1
train Y02.1
from
high place NEC
in accidental circumstances W17.89
stated as
intentional, homicide (attempt) Y01
undetermined whether accidental or intentional Y30
transport vehicle NEC —*see also* Accident, transport V89.9
stated as
intentional, homicide (attempt) Y08.89
overexertion X50.9 ◀

◀ New ⇐ Revised ~~deleted~~ Deleted

R

Radiation (exposure to)
arc lamps W89.0
atomic power plant (malfunction) NEC W88.1
complication of or abnormal reaction to medical radiotherapy Y84.2
electromagnetic, ionizing W88.0
gamma rays W88.1
in
war operations (from or following nuclear explosion) —*see also* War operations
inadvertent exposure of patient (receiving test or therapy) Y63.3
infrared (heaters and lamps) W90.1
excessive heat from W92
ionized, ionizing (particles, artificially accelerated)
radioisotopes W88.1
specified NEC W88.8
x-rays W88.0
isotopes, radioactive —*see* Radiation, radioactive isotopes
laser (s) W90.2
in war operations —*see* War operations
misadventure in medical care Y63.2
light sources (man-made visible and ultraviolet) W89.9
natural X32
specified NEC W89.8
tanning bed W89.1
welding light W89.0
man-made visible light W89.9
specified NEC W89.8
tanning bed W89.1
welding light W89.0
microwave W90.8
misadventure in medical or surgical procedure Y63.2

Radiation *(Continued)*
natural NEC X39.08
radon X39.01
overdose (in medical or surgical procedure) Y63.2
radar W90.0
radioactive isotopes (any) W88.1
atomic power plant malfunction W88.1
misadventure in medical or surgical treatment Y63.2
radiofrequency W90.0
radium NEC W88.1
sun X32
ultraviolet (light) (man-made) W89.9
natural X32
specified NEC W89.8
tanning bed W89.1
welding light W89.0
welding arc, torch, or light W89.0
excessive heat from W92
x-rays (hard) (soft) W88.0
Range disease W94.11
Rape (attempted) T74.2-
Rat bite W53.11
Reaching (prolonged) (static) X50.1 ◀
Reaction, abnormal to medical procedure —*see also* Complication of or following, by type of procedure Y84.9
with misadventure —*see* Misadventure
biologicals —*see* Table of Drugs and Chemicals ⇐
drugs —*see* Table of Drugs and Chemicals ⇐
vaccine —*see* Table of Drugs and Chemicals ⇐
Recoil
airgun W34.110
BB gun W34.110
firearm NEC W34.19
gas, air or spring-operated gun NEC W34.118

Recoil *(Continued)*
handgun W32.1
hunting rifle W33.12
larger firearm W33.10
specified NEC W33.19
machine gun W33.13
paintball gun W34.111
pellet W34.110
shotgun W33.11
Very pistol [flare] W34.19
Reduction in
atmospheric pressure —*see* Air, pressure, change
Rock falling on or hitting (accidentally) (person) W20.8
in cave-in W20.0
Run over (accidentally) (by)
animal (not being ridden) NEC W55.89
machinery —*see* Contact, with, by specified type of machine
transport vehicle NEC —*see also* Accident, transport V09.9
intentional homicide (attempt) Y03.0
motor NEC V09.20
intentional homicide (attempt) Y03.0
Running
before moving object X81.8
motor vehicle X81.0
Running off, away
animal (being ridden) —*see also* Accident, transport V80.918
not being ridden W55.89
animal-drawn vehicle NEC —*see also* Accident, transport V80.928
highway, road(way), street
transport vehicle NEC —*see also* Accident, transport V89.9
Rupture pressurized devices —*see* Explosion, by type of device

R

S

Saturnism —*see* Table of Drugs and Chemicals, lead ⬅
Scald, scalding (accidental) (by) (from) (in) X19
air (hot) X14.1
gases (hot) X14.1
homicide (attempt) —*see* Assault, burning, hot object
inflicted by other person
stated as intentional, homicide (attempt) —*see* Assault, burning, hot object
liquid (boiling) (hot) NEC X12
stated as undetermined whether accidental or intentional Y27.2
suicide (attempt) X77.2
local application of externally applied substance in medical or surgical care Y63.5
metal (molten) (liquid) (hot) NEC X18
self-inflicted X77.9
stated as undetermined whether accidental or intentional Y27.8
steam X13.1
assault X98.0
stated as undetermined whether accidental or intentional Y27.0
suicide (attempt) X77.0
suicide (attempt) X77.9
vapor (hot) X13.1
assault X98.0
stated as undetermined whether accidental or intentional Y27.0
suicide (attempt) X77.0
Scratched by
cat W55.03
person (s) (accidentally) W50.4
with intent to injure or kill Y04.0
as, or caused by, a crowd or human stampede (with fall) W52
assault Y04.0
homicide (attempt) Y04.0
in
fight Y04.0
legal intervention
injuring
bystander Y35.892
law enforcement personnel Y35.891
suspect Y35.893
Seasickness T75.3
Self-harm NEC —*see also* External cause by type, undetermined whether accidental or intentional
intentional —*see* Suicide
poisoning NEC —*see* Table of drugs and biologicals, accident
Self-inflicted (injury) **NEC** —*see also* External cause by type, undetermined whether accidental or intentional
intentional —*see* Suicide
poisoning NEC —*see* Table of drugs and biologicals, accident
Sequelae (of)
accident NEC —*see* W00-X58 with 7th character S
assault (homicidal) (any means) —*see* X92-Y08 with 7th character S
homicide, attempt (any means) —*see* X92-Y08 with 7th character S
injury undetermined whether accidentally or purposely inflicted —*see* Y21-Y33 with 7th character S
intentional self-harm (classifiable to X71-X83) —*see* X71-X83 with 7th character S
legal intervention (*see* with 7th character S Y35)
motor vehicle accident —*see* V00-V99 with 7th character S
suicide, attempt (any means) —*see* X71-X83 with 7th character S
Sequelae *(Continued)*
transport accident —*see* V00-V99 with 7th character S
war operations —*see* War operations
Shock
electric —*see* Exposure, electric current
from electric appliance (any) (faulty) W86.8
domestic W86.0
suicide (attempt) X83.1
Shooting, shot (accidental (ly)) —*see also* Discharge, firearm, by type
herself or himself —*see* Discharge, firearm by type, self-inflicted
homicide (attempt) —*see* Discharge, firearm by type, homicide
in war operations —*see* War operations
inflicted by other person —*see* Discharge, firearm by type, homicide
accidental —*see* Discharge, firearm, by type of firearm
legal
execution —*see* Legal, intervention, firearm
intervention —*see* Legal, intervention, firearm
self-inflicted —*see* Discharge, firearm by type, suicide
accidental —*see* Discharge, firearm, by type of firearm
suicide (attempt) —*see* Discharge, firearm by type, suicide
Shoving (accidentally) **by other person** —*see* Pushed, by other person ⬅
Sickness
alpine W94.11
motion —*see* Motion
mountain W94.11
Sinking (accidental)
watercraft (causing drowning, submersion) —*see also* Drowning, due to, accident to, watercraft, sinking
causing injury except drowning or submersion —*see* Accident, watercraft, causing, injury NEC ◀
Siriasis X32
Sitting (prolonged) (static) X50.1 ◀
Slashed wrists —*see* Cut, self-inflicted
Slipping (accidental) (on same level) (with fall) W01.0
without fall W18.40
due to
specified NEC W18.49
stepping from one level to another W18.43
stepping into hole or opening W18.42
stepping on object W18.41
on
ice W00.0
with skates —*see* Accident, transport, pedestrian, conveyance
mud W01.0
oil W01.0
snow W00.0
with skis —*see* Accident, transport, pedestrian, conveyance
surface (slippery) (wet) NEC W01.0
Sliver, wood, contact with W45.8
Smoldering (due to fire) —*see* Exposure, fire
Sodomy (attempted) **by force** T74.2-
Sound waves (causing injury) W42.9
supersonic W42.0
Splinter, contact with W45.8
Stab, stabbing —*see* Cut ◀
Standing (prolonged) (static) X50.1 ◀
Starvation X58
Status of external cause Y99.9
child assisting in compensated work for family Y99.8
civilian activity done for financial or other compensation Y99.0
civilian activity done for income or pay Y99.0
Status of external cause *(Continued)*
family member assisting in compensated work for other family member Y99.8
hobby not done for income Y99.8
leisure activity Y99.8
military activity Y99.1
off-duty activity of military personnel Y99.8
recreation or sport not for income or while a student Y99.8
specified NEC Y99.8
student activity Y99.8
volunteer activity Y99.2
Stepped on
by
animal (not being ridden) NEC W55.89
crowd or human stampede W52
person W50.0
Stepping on
object W22.8
with fall W18.31
sports equipment W21.9
stationary W22.09
sports equipment W21.89
person W51
by crowd or human stampede W52
sports equipment W21.9
Sting
arthropod, nonvenomous W57
insect, nonvenomous W57
Storm (cataclysmic) —*see* Forces of nature, cataclysmic storm ⬅
Straining, excessive —*see also* Overexertion X50.9 ⬅
Strangling —*see* Strangulation
Strangulation (accidental) —*see* category T71
Strenuous movements —*see also* Overexertion X50.9 ⬅
Striking against
airbag (automobile) W22.10
driver side W22.11
front passenger side W22.12
specified NEC W22.19
bottom when
diving or jumping into water (in) W16.822
causing drowning W16.821
from boat W16.722
causing drowning W16.721
natural body W16.622
causing drowning W16.821
swimming pool W16.522
causing drowning W16.521
falling into water (in) W16.322
causing drowning W16.321
fountain —*see* Striking against, bottom when, falling into water, specified NEC
natural body W16.122
causing drowning W16.121
reservoir —*see* Striking against, bottom when, falling into water, specified NEC
specified NEC W16.322
causing drowning W16.321
swimming pool W16.022
causing drowning W16.021
diving board (swimming-pool) W21.4
object W22.8
with
drowning or submersion —*see* Drowning
fall —*see* Fall, due to, bumping against, object
caused by crowd or human stampede (with fall) W52
furniture W22.03
lamppost W22.02
sports equipment W21.9
stationary W22.09
sports equipment W21.89
wall W22.01

◀ New ⬅ Revised ~~deleted~~ Deleted

Striking against *(Continued)*
person (s) W51
with fall W03
due to ice or snow W00.0
as, or caused by, a crowd or human stampede (with fall) W52
assault Y04.2
homicide (attempt) Y04.2
sports equipment W21.9
wall (when) W22.01
diving or jumping into water (in) W16.832
causing drowning W16.831
swimming pool W16.532
causing drowning W16.531
falling into water (in) W16.332
causing drowning W16.331
fountain —*see* Striking against, wall when, falling into water, specified NEC
natural body W16.132
causing drowning W16.131
reservoir —*see* Striking against, wall when, falling into water, specified NEC
specified NEC W16.332
causing drowning W16.331
swimming pool W16.032
causing drowning W16.031
swimming pool (when) W22.042
causing drowning W22.041
diving or jumping into water W16.532
causing drowning W16.531
falling into water W16.032
causing drowning W16.031
Struck (accidentally) by
airbag (automobile) W22.10
driver side W22.11
front passenger side W22.12
specified NEC W22.19
alligator W58.02
animal (not being ridden) NEC W55.89
avalanche —*see* Landslide ◀
ball (hit) (thrown) W21.00
assault Y08.09
baseball W21.03
basketball W21.05
football W21.01
golf ball W21.04
football W21.01
soccer W21.02
softball W21.07
specified NEC W21.09
volleyball W21.06
bat or racquet
baseball bat W21.11
assault Y08.02
golf club W21.13
assault Y08.09
specified NEC W21.19
assault Y08.09
tennis racquet W21.12
assault Y08.09
bullet —*see also* Discharge, firearm by type
in war operations —*see* War operations
crocodile W58.12
dog W54.1
flare, Very pistol —*see* Discharge, firearm NEC
hailstones X39.8
hockey (ice)
field
puck W21.221
stick W21.211
puck W21.220
stick W21.210
assault Y08.01
landslide —*see* Landslide ◀
law-enforcement agent (on duty) —*see* Legal, intervention, manhandling
with blunt object —*see* Legal, intervention, blunt object

Struck by *(Continued)*
lightning —*see* subcategory T75.0
causing fire —*see* Exposure, fire
machine —*see* Contact, with, by type of machine
mammal NEC W55.89
marine W56.32
marine animal W56.82
missile
firearm —*see* Discharge, firearm by type
in war operations —*see* War operations, missile
object W22.8
blunt W22.8
assault Y00
suicide (attempt) X79
undetermined whether accidental or intentional Y29
falling W20.8
from, in, on
building W20.1
burning (uncontrolled fire) X00.4
cataclysmic
earth surface movement NEC —*see* Landslide ◀
storm —*see* Forces of nature, cataclysmic storm ◀
cave-in W20.0
earthquake X34
machine (in operation) —*see* Contact, with, by type of machine
structure W20.1
burning X00.4
transport vehicle (in motion) —*see* Accident, transport, by type of vehicle
watercraft V93.49
due to
accident to craft V91.39
powered craft V91.33
ferry boat V91.31
fishing boat V91.32
jetskis V91.33
liner V91.31
merchant ship V91.30
passenger ship V91.31
unpowered craft V91.38
canoe V91.35
inflatable V91.36
kayak V91.35
sailboat V91.34
surf-board V91.38
windsurfer V91.38
powered craft V93.43
ferry boat V93.41
fishing boat V93.42
jetskis V93.43
liner V93.41
merchant ship V93.40
passenger ship V93.41
unpowered craft V93.48
sailboat V93.44
surf-board V93.48
windsurfer V93.48
moving NEC W20.8
projected W20.8
assault Y00
in sports W21.9
assault Y08.09
ball W21.00
baseball W21.03
basketball W21.05
football W21.01
golf ball W21.04
soccer W21.02
softball W21.07
specified NEC W21.09
volleyball W21.06
bat or racquet
baseball bat W21.11
assault Y08.02

Struck by *(Continued)*
object *(Continued)*
projected *(Continued)*
in sports *(Continued)*
bat or racquet *(Continued)*
golf club W21.13
assault Y08.09-
specified NEC W21.19
assault Y08.09
tennis racquet W21.12
assault Y08.09
hockey (ice)
field
puck W21.221
stick W21.211
puck W21.220
stick W21.210
assault Y08.01
specified NEC W21.89
set in motion by explosion —*see* Explosion
thrown W20.8
assault Y00
in sports W21.9
assault Y08.09
ball W21.00
baseball W21.03
basketball W21.05
football W21.01
golf ball W21.04
soccer W21.02
soft ball W21.07
specified NEC W21.09
volleyball W21.06
bat or racquet
baseball bat W21.11
assault Y08.02
golf club W21.13
assault Y08.09
specified NEC W21.19
assault Y08.09
tennis racquet W21.12
assault Y08.09
hockey (ice)
field
puck W21.221
stick W21.211
puck W21.220
stick W21.210
assault Y08.01
specified NEC W21.89
other person (s) W50.0
with
blunt object W22.8
intentional, homicide (attempt) Y00
sports equipment W21.9
undetermined whether accidental or intentional Y29
fall W03
due to ice or snow W00.0
as, or caused by, a crowd or human stampede (with fall) W52
assault Y04.2
homicide (attempt) Y04.2
in legal intervention
injuring
bystander Y35.812
law enforcement personnel Y35.811
suspect Y35.813
sports equipment W21.9
police (on duty) —*see* Legal, intervention, manhandling
with blunt object —*see* Legal, intervention, blunt object
sports equipment W21.9
assault Y08.09
ball W21.00
baseball W21.03
basketball W21.05
football W21.01
golf ball W21.04
soccer W21.02

S

Struck by *(Continued)*
sports equipment *(Continued)*
ball *(Continued)*
soft ball W21.07
specified NEC W21.09
volleyball W21.06
bat or racquet
baseball bat W21.11
assault Y08.02
golf club W21.13
assault Y08.09
specified NEC W21.19
tennis racquet W21.12
assault Y08.09
cleats (shoe) W21.31
foot wear NEC W21.39
football helmet W21.81
hockey (ice)
field
puck W21.221
stick W21.211
puck W21.220
stick W21.210
assault Y08.01
skate blades W21.32
specified NEC W21.89
assault Y08.09
thunderbolt —*see* subcategory T75.0
causing fire —*see* Exposure, fire
transport vehicle NEC —*see also* Accident, transport V09.9
intentional, homicide (attempt) Y03.0
motor NEC —*see also* Accident, transport V09.20
homicide Y03.0
vehicle (transport) NEC —*see* Accident, transport, by type of vehicle
stationary (falling from jack, hydraulic lift, ramp) W20.8
Stumbling
without fall W18.40
due to
specified NEC W18.49
stepping from one level to another W18.43
stepping into hole or opening W18.42
stepping on object W18.41
over
animal NEC W01.0
with fall W18.09
carpet, rug or (small) object W22.8
with fall W18.09
person W51
with fall W03
due to ice or snow W00.0
Submersion (accidental) —*see* Drowning
Suffocation (accidental) (by external means) (by pressure) (mechanical) —*see also* category T71
due to, by
avalanche —*see* Landslide
explosion —*see* Explosion
fire —*see* Exposure, fire
food, any type (aspiration) (ingestion) (inhalation) —*see* categories T17 and T18
ignition —*see* Ignition
landslide —*see* Landslide
machine (ry) —*see* Contact, with, by type of machine
vomitus (aspiration) (inhalation) T17.81-
in
burning building X00.8
Suicide, suicidal (attempted) (by) X83.8
blunt object X79
burning, burns X76
hot object X77.9
fluid NEC X77.2
household appliance X77.3
specified NEC X77.8
steam X77.0
tap water X77.1
vapors X77.0
caustic substance —*see* Table of Drugs and Chemicals ⇐
cold, extreme X83.2
collision of motor vehicle with
motor vehicle X82.0
specified NEC X82.8
train X82.1
tree X82.2
crashing of aircraft X83.0
cut (any part of body) X78.9
cutting or piercing instrument X78.9
dagger X78.2
glass X78.0
knife X78.1
specified NEC X78.8
sword X78.2
drowning (in) X71.9
bathtub X71.0
natural water X71.3
specified NEC X71.8
swimming pool X71.1
following fall X71.2
electrocution X83.1
explosive (s) (material) X75
fire, flames X76
firearm X74.9
airgun X74.01
handgun X72
Suicide, suicidal *(Continued)*
firearm *(Continued)*
hunting rifle X73.1
larger X73.9
specified NEC X73.8
machine gun X73.2
shotgun X73.0
specified NEC X74.8
hanging X83.8
hot object —*see* Suicide, burning, hot object
jumping
before moving object X81.8
motor vehicle X81.0
subway train X81.1
train X81.1
from high place X80
late effect of attempt —*see* X71-X83 with 7th character S
lying before moving object, train, vehicle X81.8
poisoning —*see* Table of Drugs and Chemicals ⇐
puncture (any part of body) —*see* Suicide, cutting or piercing instrument
scald —*see* Suicide, burning, hot object
sequelae of attempt —*see* X71-X83 with 7th character S
sharp object (any) —*see* Suicide, cutting or piercing instrument
shooting —*see* Suicide, firearm
specified means NEC X83.8
stab (any part of body) —*see* Suicide, cutting or piercing instrument
steam, hot vapors X77.0
strangulation X83.8
submersion —*see* Suicide, drowning
suffocation X83.8
wound NEC X83.8
Sunstroke X32
Supersonic waves (causing injury) W42.0
Surgical procedure, complication of (delayed or as an abnormal reaction without mention of misadventure) —*see also* Complication of or following, by type of procedure
due to or as a result of misadventure —*see* Misadventure
Swallowed, swallowing
foreign body —*see* Foreign body, alimentary canal
poison —*see* Table of Drugs and Chemicals
substance
caustic or corrosive —*see* Table of Drugs and Chemicals
poisonous —*see* Table of Drugs and Chemicals

S

◀ New ⇐ Revised ~~deleted~~ Deleted

T

Tackle in sport W03
Terrorism (involving) Y38.80
biological weapons Y38.6X-
chemical weapons Y38.7X-
conflagration Y38.3X-
drowning and submersion Y38.89- ◀
explosion Y38.2X-
destruction of aircraft Y38.1X-
marine weapons Y38.0X-
fire Y38.3X-
firearms Y38.4X-
hot substances Y38.3X- ⇐
lasers Y38.89- ◀
nuclear weapons Y38.5X-
piercing or stabbing instruments Y38.89- ◀
secondary effects Y38.9X- ◀
specified method NEC Y38.89- ⇐
suicide bomber Y38.81- ◀
Thirst X58
Threat to breathing
aspiration —*see* Aspiration
due to cave-in, falling earth or substance NEC —*see* category T71
Thrown (accidentally)
against part (any) of or object in transport vehicle (in motion) NEC —*see also* Accident, transport
Thrown *(Continued)*
from
high place, homicide (attempt) Y01
machinery —*see* Contact, with, by type of machine
transport vehicle NEC —*see also* Accident, transport V89.9
off —*see* Thrown, from
Thunderbolt —*see* subcategory T75.0
causing fire —*see* Exposure, fire
Tidal wave (any injury) **NEC** —*see* Forces of nature, tidal wave ⇐
Took
overdose (drug) —*see* Table of Drugs and Chemicals ⇐
poison —*see* Table of Drugs and Chemicals ⇐
Tornado (any injury) X37.1
Torrential rain (any injury) X37.8
Torture X58
Trampled by animal NEC W55.89
Trapped (accidentally)
between objects (moving) (stationary and moving) —*see* Caught
by part (any) of
motorcycle V29.88
pedal cycle V19.88
transport vehicle NEC —*see also* Accident, transport V89.9
Travel (effects) (sickness) T75.3
Tree falling on or hitting (accidentally) (person) W20.8
Tripping
without fall W18.40
due to
specified NEC W18.49
stepping from one level to another W18.43
stepping into hole or opening W18.42
stepping on object W18.41
over
animal W01.0
with fall W01.0
carpet, rug or (small) object W22.8
with fall W18.09
person W51
with fall W03
due to ice or snow W00.0
Twisted by person (s) (accidentally) W50.2
with intent to injure or kill Y04.0
as, or caused by, a crowd or human stampede (with fall) W52
assault Y04.0
homicide (attempt) Y04.0
in
fight Y04.0
legal intervention —*see* Legal, intervention, manhandling
Twisting (prolonged) (static) X50.1 ◀

U

Underdosing of necessary drugs, medicaments or biological substances Y63.6 ⇐
Undetermined intent (contact) (exposure)
automobile collision Y32
blunt object Y29
drowning (submersion) (in) Y21.9
bathtub Y21.0
after fall Y21.1
natural water (lake) (ocean) (pond) (river) (stream) Y21.4
specified place NEC Y21.8
swimming pool Y21.2
after fall Y21.3
explosive material Y25
fall, jump or push from high place Y30
falling, lying or running before moving object Y31
fire Y26
Undetermined intent *(Continued)*
firearm discharge Y24.9
airgun (BB) (pellet) Y24.0
handgun (pistol) (revolver) Y22
hunting rifle Y23.1
larger Y23.9
hunting rifle Y23.1
machine gun Y23.3
military Y23.2
shotgun Y23.0
specified type NEC Y23.8
machine gun Y23.3
military Y23.2
shotgun Y23.0
specified type NEC Y24.8
Very pistol Y24.8
hot object Y27.9
fluid NEC Y27.2
household appliance Y27.3
specified object NEC Y27.8
Undetermined intent *(Continued)*
hot object *(Continued)*
steam Y27.0
tap water Y27.1
vapor Y27.0
jump, fall or push from high place Y30
lying, falling or running before moving object Y31
motor vehicle crash Y32
push, fall or jump from high place Y30
running, falling or lying before moving object Y31
sharp object Y28.9
dagger Y28.2
glass Y28.0
knife Y28.1
specified object NEC Y28.8
sword Y28.2
smoke Y26
specified event NEC Y33
Use of hand as hammer X50.3 ◀

V

Vibration (causing injury) W49.9
Victim (of)
avalanche —*see* Landslide ◀
earth movements NEC —*see* Forces of nature, earth movement ◀
earthquake X34
Victim *(Continued)*
flood —*see* Flood ◀
landslide —*see* Landslide ◀
lightning —*see* subcategory T75.0
causing fire —*see* Exposure, fire
storm (cataclysmic) NEC —*see* Forces of nature, cataclysmic storm ◀
volcanic eruption X35
Volcanic eruption (any injury) X35
Vomitus, gastric contents in air passages (with asphyxia, obstruction or suffocation) T17.81-

W

Walked into stationary object (any) W22.09
furniture W22.03
lamppost W22.02
wall W22.01
War operations (injuries to military personnel and civilians during war, civil insurrection and peacekeeping missions) (by) (from) (involving) Y36.90-
after cessation of hostilities Y36.89-
explosion (of)
bomb placed during war operations Y36.82-
mine placed during war operations Y36.81-
specified NEC Y36.88-
air blast Y36.20-
aircraft
destruction —*see* War operations, destruction of aircraft
airway restriction —*see* War operations, restriction of airways
asphyxiation —*see* War operations, restriction of airways
biological weapons Y36.6X-
blast Y36.20-
blast fragments Y36.20-
blast wave Y36.20-
blast wind Y36.20-
bomb Y36.20-
dirty Y36.50-
gasoline Y36.31-
incendiary Y36.31-
petrol Y36.31-
bullet Y36.43-
incendiary Y36.32-
rubber Y36.41-
chemical weapons Y36.7X-
combat
hand to hand (unarmed) combat Y36.44-
using blunt or piercing object Y36.45-
conflagration —*see* War operations, fire
conventional warfare NEC Y36.49-
depth-charge Y36.01-
destruction of aircraft Y36.10-
due to
air to air missile Y36.11-
collision with other aircraft Y36.12-
detonation (accidental) of onboard munitions and explosives Y36.14-
enemy fire or explosives Y36.11-
explosive placed on aircraft Y36.11-
onboard fire Y36.13-
rocket propelled grenade [RPG] Y36.11-
small arms fire Y36.11-
surface to air missile Y36.11-
specified NEC Y36.19-
detonation (accidental) of
onboard marine weapons Y36.05-
own munitions or munitions launch device Y36.24-

War operations *(Continued)*
dirty bomb Y36.50-
explosion (of) Y36.20-
aerial bomb Y36.21-
after cessation of hostilities
bomb placed during war operations Y36.82-
mine placed during war operations Y36.81-
bomb NOS —*see also* War operations, bomb (s) Y36.20-
fragments Y36.20-
grenade Y36.29-
guided missile Y36.22-
improvised explosive device [IED] (person-borne) (roadside) (vehicle-borne) Y36.23-
land mine Y36.29-
marine mine (at sea) (in harbor) Y36.02-
marine weapon Y36.00-
specified NEC Y36.09-
own munitions or munitions launch device (accidental) Y36.24-
sea-based artillery shell Y36.03-
specified NEC Y36.29-
torpedo Y36.04-
fire Y36.30-
specified NEC Y36.39-
firearms
discharge Y36.43-
pellets Y36.42-
flamethrower Y36.33-
fragments (from) (of)
improvised explosive device [IED] (person-borne) (roadside) (vehicle-borne) Y36.26-
munitions Y36.25-
specified NEC Y36.29-
weapons Y36.27-
friendly fire Y36.92
hand to hand (unarmed) combat Y36.44-
hot substances —*see* War operations, fire
incendiary bullet Y36.32-
nuclear weapon (effects of) Y36.50-
acute radiation exposure Y36.54-
blast pressure Y36.51-
direct blast Y36.51-
direct heat Y36.53-
fallout exposure Y36.54-
fireball Y36.53-
indirect blast (struck or crushed by blast debris) (being thrown by blast) Y36.52-
ionizing radiation (immediate exposure) Y36.54-
nuclear radiation Y36.54-
radiation
ionizing (immediate exposure) Y36.54-

War operations *(Continued)*
nuclear weapon *(Continued)*
radiation *(Continued)*
nuclear Y36.54-
thermal Y36.53-
secondary effects Y36.54-
specified NEC Y36.59-
thermal radiation Y36.53-
restriction of air (airway)
intentional Y36.46-
unintentional Y36.47-
rubber bullets Y36.41-
shrapnel NOS Y36.29-
suffocation —*see* War operations, restriction of airways
unconventional warfare NEC Y36.7X-
underwater blast NOS Y36.00-
warfare
conventional NEC Y36.49-
unconventional NEC Y36.7X-
weapon of mass destruction [WMD] Y36.91
weapons
biological weapons Y36.6X-
chemical Y36.7X-
nuclear (effects of) Y36.50-
acute radiation exposure Y36.54-
blast pressure Y36.51-
direct blast Y36.51-
direct heat Y36.53-
fallout exposure Y36.54-
fireball Y36.53-
~~indirect blast (struck or crushed by blast debris) (being thrown by blast) Y36.52-~~
radiation
ionizing (immediate exposure) Y36.54-
nuclear Y36.54-
thermal Y36.53-
secondary effects Y36.54-
specified NEC Y36.59-
of mass destruction [WMD] Y36.91-
Washed
away by flood —*see* Flood
off road by storm (transport vehicle) —*see* Forces of nature, cataclysmic storm
Weather exposure NEC —*see* Forces of nature
Weightlessness (causing injury) (effects of) (in spacecraft, real or simulated) X52
Work related condition Y99.0
Wound (accidental) **NEC** —*see also* Injury X58
battle —*see also* War operations Y36.90
gunshot —*see* Discharge, firearm by type
Wreck transport vehicle NEC —*see also* Accident, transport V89.9
Wrong
device implanted into correct surgical site Y65.51
fluid in infusion Y65.1
patient, procedure performed on Y65.52
procedure (operation) on correct patient Y65.51

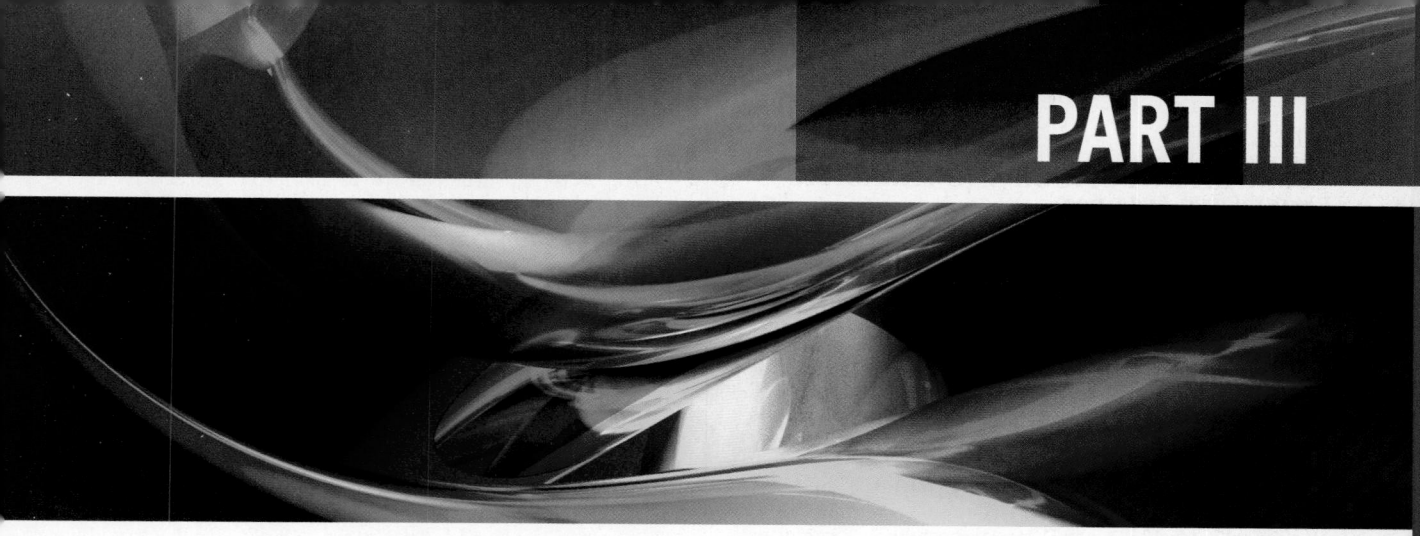

PART III

ICD-10-CM Tabular List of Diseases and Injuries

CHAPTER 1

CERTAIN INFECTIOUS AND PARASITIC DISEASES (A00-B99)

OGCR Chapter-Specific Coding Guidelines

1. Chapter 1: Certain Infectious and Parasitic Diseases (A00-B99)

a. Human Immunodeficiency Virus (HIV) Infections

1) Code only confirmed cases

Code only confirmed cases of HIV infection/illness. This is an exception to the hospital inpatient guideline Section II, H.

In this context, "confirmation" does not require documentation of positive serology or culture for HIV; the provider's diagnostic statement that the patient is HIV positive, or has an HIV-related illness is sufficient.

2) Selection and sequencing of HIV codes

(a) Patient admitted for HIV-related condition

If a patient is admitted for an HIV-related condition, the principal diagnosis should be B20, Human immunodeficiency virus [HIV] disease followed by additional diagnosis codes for all reported HIV-related conditions.

(b) Patient with HIV disease admitted for unrelated condition

If a patient with HIV disease is admitted for an unrelated condition (such as a traumatic injury), the code for the unrelated condition (e.g., the nature of injury code) should be the principal diagnosis. Other diagnoses would be B20 followed by additional diagnosis codes for all reported HIV-related conditions.

(c) Whether the patient is newly diagnosed

Whether the patient is newly diagnosed or has had previous admissions/encounters for HIV conditions is irrelevant to the sequencing decision.

(d) Asymptomatic human immunodeficiency virus

Z21, Asymptomatic human immunodeficiency virus [HIV] infection status, is to be applied when the patient without any documentation of symptoms is listed as being "HIV positive," "known HIV," "HIV test positive," or similar terminology. Do not use this code if the term "AIDS" is used or if the patient is treated for any HIV-related illness or is described as having any condition(s) resulting from his/her HIV positive status; use B20 in these cases.

(e) Patients with inconclusive HIV serology

Patients with inconclusive HIV serology, but no definitive diagnosis or manifestations of the illness, may be assigned code R75, Inconclusive laboratory evidence of human immunodeficiency virus [HIV].

(f) Previously diagnosed HIV-related illness

Patients with any known prior diagnosis of an HIV-related illness should be coded to B20. Once a patient has developed an HIV-related illness, the patient should always be assigned code B20 on every subsequent admission/encounter. Patients previously diagnosed with any HIV illness (B20) should never be assigned to R75 or Z21, Asymptomatic human immunodeficiency virus [HIV] infection status.

(g) HIV Infection in Pregnancy, Childbirth and the Puerperium

During pregnancy, childbirth or the puerperium, a patient admitted (or presenting for a health care encounter) because of an HIV-related illness should receive a principal diagnosis code of O98.7-, Human immunodeficiency [HIV] disease complicating pregnancy, childbirth and the puerperium, followed by B20 and the code(s) for the HIV-related illness(es). Codes from Chapter 15 always take sequencing priority.

Patients with asymptomatic HIV infection status admitted (or presenting for a health care encounter) during pregnancy, childbirth, or the puerperium should receive codes of O98.7- and Z21.

(h) Encounters for testing for HIV

If a patient is being seen to determine his/her HIV status, use code Z11.4, Encounter for screening for human immunodeficiency virus [HIV]. Use additional codes for any associated high risk behavior.

If a patient with signs or symptoms is being seen for HIV testing, code the signs and symptoms. An additional counseling code Z71.7, Human immunodeficiency virus [HIV] counseling, may be used if counseling is provided during the encounter for the test.

When a patient returns to be informed of his/her HIV test results and the test result is negative, use code Z71.7, Human immunodeficiency virus [HIV] counseling.

If the results are positive, see previous guidelines and assign codes as appropriate.

b. Infectious agents as the cause of diseases classified to other chapters

Certain infections are classified in chapters other than Chapter 1 and no organism is identified as part of the infection code. In these instances, it is necessary to use an additional code from Chapter 1 to identify the organism. A code from category B95, Streptococcus, Staphylococcus, and Enterococcus as the cause of diseases classified to other chapters, B96, Other bacterial agents as the cause of diseases classified to other chapters, or B97, Viral agents as the cause of diseases classified to other chapters, is to be used as an additional code to identify the organism. An instructional note will be found at the infection code advising that an additional organism code is required.

c. Infections resistant to antibiotics

Many bacterial infections are resistant to current antibiotics. It is necessary to identify all infections documented as antibiotic resistant. Assign a code from category Z16, Resistance to antimicrobial drugs, following the infection code only if the infection code does not identify drug resistance.

d. Sepsis, Severe Sepsis, and Septic Shock

1) Coding of Sepsis and Severe Sepsis

(a) Sepsis

For a diagnosis of sepsis, assign the appropriate code for the underlying systemic infection. If the type of infection or causal organism is not further specified, assign code A41.9, Sepsis, unspecified organism.

A code from subcategory R65.2, Severe sepsis, should not be assigned unless severe sepsis or an associated acute organ dysfunction is documented.

(i) Negative or inconclusive blood cultures and sepsis
Negative or inconclusive blood cultures do not preclude a diagnosis of sepsis in patients with clinical evidence of the condition, however, the provider should be queried.

(ii) Urosepsis
The term urosepsis is a nonspecific term. It is not to be considered synonymous with sepsis. It has no default code in the Alphabetic Index. Should a provider use this term, he/she must be queried for clarification.

(iii) Sepsis with organ dysfunction
If a patient has sepsis and associated acute organ dysfunction or multiple organ dysfunction (MOD), follow the instructions for coding severe sepsis.

(iv) Acute organ dysfunction that is not clearly associated with the sepsis
If a patient has sepsis and an acute organ dysfunction, but the medical record documentation indicates that the acute organ dysfunction is related to a medical condition other than the sepsis, do not assign a code from subcategory R65.2, Severe sepsis. An acute organ dysfunction must be associated with the sepsis in order to assign the severe sepsis code. If the documentation is not clear as to whether an acute organ dysfunction is related to the sepsis or another medical condition, query the provider.

(b) Severe sepsis

The coding of severe sepsis requires a minimum of 2 codes: first a code for the underlying systemic infection, followed by a code from subcategory R65.2, Severe sepsis. If the causal organism is not documented, assign code A41.9, Sepsis, unspecified organism, for the infection. Additional code(s) for the associated acute organ dysfunction are also required.

Due to the complex nature of severe sepsis, some cases may require querying the provider prior to assignment of the codes.

2) Septic shock

(a) Septic shock generally refers to circulatory failure associated with severe sepsis, and therefore, it represents a type of acute organ dysfunction.

For all cases of septic shock, the code for the systemic infection should be sequenced first, followed by code R65.21, Severe sepsis with septic shock or code T81.12, Postprocedural septic shock. Any additional codes for the other acute organ dysfunctions should also be assigned. As noted in the sequencing instructions in the Tabular List, the code for septic shock cannot be assigned as a principal diagnosis.

3) Sequencing of severe sepsis

If severe sepsis is present on admission, and meets the definition of principal diagnosis, the underlying systemic infection should be assigned as principal diagnosis followed by the appropriate code from subcategory R65.2 as required by the sequencing rules in the Tabular List. A code from subcategory R65.2 can never be assigned as a principal diagnosis.

When severe sepsis develops during an encounter (it was not present on admission) the underlying systemic infection and the appropriate code from subcategory R65.2 should be assigned as secondary diagnoses.

Severe sepsis may be present on admission but the diagnosis may not be confirmed until sometime after admission. If the documentation is not clear whether severe sepsis was present on admission, the provider should be queried.

4) Sepsis and severe sepsis with a localized infection

If the reason for admission is both sepsis or severe sepsis and a localized infection, such as pneumonia or cellulitis, a code(s) for the underlying systemic infection should be assigned first and the code for the localized infection should be assigned as a secondary diagnosis. If the patient has severe sepsis, a code from subcategory R65.2 should also be assigned as a secondary diagnosis. If the patient is admitted with a localized infection, such as pneumonia, and sepsis/severe sepsis doesn't develop until after admission, the localized infection should be assigned first, followed by the appropriate sepsis/severe sepsis codes.

5) Sepsis due to a postprocedural infection

(a) Documentation of causal relationship

As with all postprocedural complications, code assignment is based on the provider's documentation of the relationship between the infection and the procedure.

(b) Sepsis due to a postprocedural infection

For such cases, the postprocedural infection code, such as, T80.2, Infections following infusion, transfusion, and therapeutic injection, T81.4, Infection following a procedure, T88.0, Infection following immunization, or O86.0, Infection of obstetric surgical wound, should be coded first, followed by the code for the specific infection. If the patient has severe sepsis the appropriate code from subcategory R65.2 should also be assigned with the additional code(s) for any acute organ dysfunction.

(c) Postprocedural infection and postprocedural septic shock

In cases where a postprocedural infection has occurred and has resulted in severe sepsis the code for the precipitating complication such as code T81.4, Infection following a procedure, or O86.0, Infection of obstetrical surgical wound should be coded first followed by code R65.20, Severe sepsis without septic shock. A Code for the systemic infection should also be assigned.

If a postprocedural infection has resulted in postprocedural septic shock, the code for the precipitating complication such as code T81.4, Infection following a procedure, or O86.0, Infection of obstetrical surgical wound should be coded first followed by code T81.12-, Postprocedural septic shock. A code for the systemic infection should also be assigned.

6) Sepsis and severe sepsis associated with a noninfectious process (condition)

In some cases a noninfectious process (condition), such as trauma, may lead to an infection which can result in sepsis or severe sepsis. If sepsis or severe sepsis is documented as associated with a noninfectious condition, such as a burn or serious injury, and this condition meets the definition for principal diagnosis, the code for the noninfectious condition should be sequenced first, followed by the code for the resulting infection. If severe sepsis is present, a code from subcategory R65.2 should also be assigned with any associated organ dysfunction(s) codes. It is not necessary to assign a code from subcategory R65.1, Systemic inflammatory response syndrome (SIRS) of non-infectious origin, for these cases.

If the infection meets the definition of principal diagnosis it should be sequenced before the non-infectious condition. When both the associated non-infectious condition and the infection meet the definition of principal diagnosis either may be assigned as principal diagnosis.

Only one code from category R65, Symptoms and signs specifically associated with systemic inflammation and infection, should be assigned. Therefore, when a non-infectious condition leads to an infection resulting in severe sepsis, assign the appropriate code from subcategory R65.2, Severe sepsis. Do not additionally assign a code from subcategory R65.1, Systemic inflammatory response syndrome (SIRS) of non-infectious origin.

See Section I.C.18. SIRS due to non-infectious process

7) Sepsis and septic shock complicating abortion, pregnancy, childbirth, and the puerperium

See Section I.C.15. Sepsis and septic shock complicating abortion, pregnancy, childbirth and the puerperium

8) Newborn sepsis

See Section I.C.16. f. Bacterial sepsis of Newborn

e. Methicillin Resistant Staphylococcus aureus (MRSA) Conditions

1) Selection and sequencing of MRSA codes

(a) Combination codes for MRSA infection

When a patient is diagnosed with an infection that is due to methicillin resistant *Staphylococcus aureus* (MRSA), and that infection has a combination code that includes the causal organism (e.g., sepsis, pneumonia) assign the appropriate combination code for the condition (e.g., code A41.02, Sepsis due to Methicillin resistant Staphylococcus aureus or code J15.212, Pneumonia due to Methicillin resistant Staphylococcus aureus). Do not assign code B95.62, Methicillin resistant Staphylococcus aureus infection as the cause of diseases classified elsewhere, as an additional code because the combination code includes the type of infection and the MRSA organism. Do not assign a code from subcategory Z16.11, Resistance to penicillins, as an additional diagnosis.

See Section C.1. for instructions on coding and sequencing of sepsis and severe sepsis.

(b) Other codes for MRSA infection

When there is documentation of a current infection (e.g., wound infection, stitch abscess, urinary tract infection) due to MRSA, and that infection does not have a combination code that includes the causal organism, assign the appropriate code to identify the condition along with code B95.62, Methicillin resistant Staphylococcus aureus infection as the cause of diseases classified elsewhere for the MRSA infection. Do not assign a code from subcategory Z16.11, Resistance to penicillins.

(c) Methicillin susceptible Staphylococcus aureus (MSSA) and MRSA colonization

The condition or state of being colonized or carrying MSSA or MRSA is called colonization or carriage, while an individual person is described as being colonized or being a carrier. Colonization means that MSSA or MSRA is present on or in the body without necessarily causing illness. A positive MRSA colonization test might be documented by the provider as "MRSA screen positive" or "MRSA nasal swab positive".

Assign code Z22.322, Carrier or suspected carrier of Methicillin resistant Staphylococcus aureus, for patients documented as having MRSA colonization. Assign code Z22.321, Carrier or suspected carrier of Methicillin susceptible Staphylococcus aureus, for patient documented as having MSSA colonization. Colonization is not necessarily indicative of a disease process or as the cause of a specific condition the patient may have unless documented as such by the provider.

(d) MRSA colonization and infection

If a patient is documented as having both MRSA colonization and infection during a hospital admission, code Z22.322, Carrier or suspected carrier of Methicillin resistant Staphylococcus aureus, and a code for the MRSA infection may both be assigned.

f. Zika virus infections

1) Code only confirmed cases

Code only a confirmed diagnosis of Zika virus (A92.5, Zika virus disease) as documented by the provider. This is an exception to the hospital inpatient guideline Section II, H.

In this context, "confirmation" does not require documentation of the type of test performed; the physician's diagnostic statement that the condition is confirmed is sufficient. This code should be assigned regardless of the stated mode of transmission.

If the provider documents "suspected", "possible" or "probable" Zika, do not assign code A92.5. Assign a code(s) explaining the reason for encounter (such as fever, rash, or joint pain) or Z20.828, Contact with and (suspected) exposure to other viral communicable diseases.

CHAPTER 1

CERTAIN INFECTIOUS AND PARASITIC DISEASES (A00-B99)

Includes diseases generally recognized as communicable or transmissible

Use additional code to identify resistance to antimicrobial drugs (Z16.-)

Excludes1 certain localized infections - see body system-related chapters

Excludes2 carrier or suspected carrier of infectious disease (Z22.-)
infectious and parasitic diseases complicating pregnancy, childbirth and the puerperium (O98.-)
infectious and parasitic diseases specific to the perinatal period (P35-P39)
influenza and other acute respiratory infections (J00-J22)

This chapter contains the following blocks:

A00-A09	Intestinal infectious diseases
A15-A19	Tuberculosis
A20-A28	Certain zoonotic bacterial diseases
A30-A49	Other bacterial diseases
A50-A64	Infections with a predominantly sexual mode of transmission
A65-A69	Other spirochetal diseases
A70-A74	Other diseases caused by chlamydiae
A75-A79	Rickettsioses
A80-A89	Viral and prion infections of the central nervous system
A90-A99	Arthropod-borne viral fevers and viral hemorrhagic fevers
B00-B09	Viral infections characterized by skin and mucous membrane lesions
B10	Other human herpesviruses
B15-B19	Viral hepatitis
B20	Human immunodeficiency virus [HIV] disease
B25-B34	Other viral diseases
B35-B49	Mycoses
B50-B64	Protozoal diseases
B65-B83	Helminthiases
B85-B89	Pediculosis, acariasis and other infestations
B90-B94	Sequelae of infectious and parasitic diseases
B95-B97	Bacterial and viral infectious agents
B99	Other infectious diseases

INTESTINAL INFECTIOUS DISEASES (A00-A09)

A00 Cholera
A serious, often deadly, infectious disease of the small intestine
Ex: For category A00 CC codes: A00.0-A00.9

A00.0 Cholera due to Vibrio cholerae 01, biovar cholerae
Classical cholera

A00.1 Cholera due to Vibrio cholerae 01, biovar eltor
Cholera eltor

A00.9 Cholera, unspecified

A01 Typhoid and paratyphoid fevers
Caused by Salmonella typhi and Salmonella paratyphi A, B, and C bacteria
Ex: For category A01 CC codes: A01.00-A01.4

A01.0 Typhoid fever
Infection due to Salmonella typhi

A01.00 Typhoid fever, unspecified

A01.01 Typhoid meningitis

A01.02 Typhoid fever with heart involvement
Typhoid endocarditis
Typhoid myocarditis

A01.03 Typhoid pneumonia

A01.04 Typhoid arthritis

A01.05 Typhoid osteomyelitis

A01.09 Typhoid fever with other complications

A01.1 Paratyphoid fever A

A01.2 Paratyphoid fever B

A01.3 Paratyphoid fever C

A01.4 Paratyphoid fever, unspecified
Infection due to Salmonella paratyphi NOS

A02 Other salmonella infections
Includes infection or foodborne intoxication due to any Salmonella species other than S. typhi and S. paratyphi

A02.0 Salmonella enteritis
Salmonellosis
Ex: A01.00-A01.09, A01.4-A02.0, A03.9-A05.2, A07.4, A08.0-A09, A48.51-A48.52, K30, K52.1-K52.3, K52.82-K52.9, K58.0-K58.9, K65.0, K65.2, K65.8, K68.12-K68.9, P76.8-P77.9, P78.1, P78.3-P78.89

A02.1 Salmonella sepsis
Ex: A02.1, A20.7, A22.7, A26.7, A32.7, A39.2-A39.4, A40.0-A40.1, A40.8-A41.9, A42.7, A48.2-A48.4, A48.8-A49.9, A54.86, B00.7, B37.7, B92, B94.2-B96.89, P36.0-P36.9, P39.2, P39.4-P39.9, R65.10-R65.20, Z16.10-Z16.39

A02.2 Localized salmonella infections

A02.20 Localized salmonella infection, unspecified
Specified in the documentation as localized, but unspecified as to type

A02.21 Salmonella meningitis
Specified as localized in the meninges
Ex: A02.21, A17.0-A17.1, A27.81, A39.0, A50.41, A51.41, A52.13, A54.82, A54.84, A54.89-A54.9, A74.81-A74.9, A87.0-A87.9, A96.2, A98.3-A98.4, B26.1, B33.24, B33.4-B33.8, B34.1-B34.2, B34.4-B34.8, B37.5, B38.4, B45.1, B58.2, B92, B94.2-94.9, B97.10, B97.19, B97.29, B97.5-B97.6, B97.81-B97.89, G00.0-G03.9, G04.2, G32.89, G96.8-G96.9, G98.0-G98.8, G99.8

A02.22 Salmonella pneumonia
Specified as localized in the lungs
Ex: A02.22, A15.0-A15.6, A15.8-A15.9, A17.9, A18.82, A18.84, A18.89, A20.2, A21.1, A22.1, A31.0, A37.01, A37.11, A37.81, A37.91, A42.0, A43.0, A48.1, B25.0, B39.0-B39.2, B44.0, B58.3, B59, B67.1, J09.X1-J09.X2, J10.00-J10.1, J11.00-J11.1, J12.0-J12.3, J12.89-J18.1, J18.8-J18.9, J22, J60, J62.0-J67.7, J68.0-J70.4, J70.8-J70.9, J98.4, J98.8-J99, R91.1

A02.23 Salmonella arthritis
Specified as localized in the joints
Ex: A02.23, A18.02, A18.09, A39.83-A39.84, A54.40, A54.42-A54.43, A54.82, A54.84, A54.89-A54.9, B06.82, M00.00-M02.30, M02.319, M02.329, M02.339, M02.349, M02.359, M02.369, M02.379-M02.9, M05.40-M05.59, M05.70-M06.09, M06.20-M06.39, M06.80-M07.69, M11.00-M11.9, M12.10-M15.0, M15.3-M15.9, M16.2-M16.9, M17.2-M17.9, M18.2-M18.9, M19.111-M19.93, M24.10-M24.176, M25.00, M25.08-M25.18, M25.40-M25.676, M25.80-M25.9, M35.2, M36.1-M36.4, R29.4

A02.24 Salmonella osteomyelitis
Specified as localized in bone
Ex: A02.24, A18.03-A18.09, M46.20-M46.39, M86.00-M86.9

A02.25 Salmonella pyelonephritis
Salmonella tubulo-interstitial nephropathy
Ex: A02.25-A02.29

A02.29 Salmonella with other localized infection
Specified as localized (because it is still under localized heading) but does not assign into any of the above codes
Ex: A02.25-A02.29

Item 1-1 Salmonella is a bacterium that lives in the intestines of fowl and mammals and can spread to humans through improper food preparation and cooking. Salmonellosis is an infection with the bacterium. Symptoms include diarrhea, fever, and abdominal cramps 12 to 72 hours after infection. The illness usually lasts 4 to 7 days, and most persons recover without treatment. The diarrhea may be so severe that the patient needs to be hospitalized. Patients with immunocompromised systems in chronic, ill health are more likely to have the infection invade their bloodstream with life-threatening results. For example, patients with sickle cell disease are more prone to salmonella osteomyelitis than others.

◀ New ◀ Revised ~~deleted~~ Deleted Excludes 1 Excludes 2 Includes Use additional Code first Code also Unspecified
OGCR Official Guidelines ● Unacceptable Principal Diagnosis X Assign placeholder X ● Use Additional Character(s) ▶ Manifestation Code Coding Clinic

A02.8 Other specified salmonella infections
Any specified salmonella infection which does NOT assign into any of the above codes (not specified as localized)
Ex: A02.8

A02.9 Salmonella infection, unspecified
Unspecified in the documentation as to specific type of salmonella
Ex: A02.9

A03 Shigellosis
An infectious disease caused by bacteria (Shigella)

A03.0 Shigellosis due to Shigella dysenteriae
Group A shigellosis [Shiga-Kruse dysentery]
Ex: A00.1, A01.00-A01.09, A01.4-A02.0, A03.0, A03.9, A04.9-A05.2, A06.0-A06.2, A06.9, A07.1-A07.9, A08.4-A09, A18.32-A18.39, A18.83, A48.51-A48.52, B37.82, B82.9, J09.X3-J09.X9, J10.2-J10.89, J11.2-J11.89, K30, K31.84, K50.00-K51.919, K52.1-K52.3, K52.82-K55.1, K55.30-K55.33, K55.8-K55.9, K58.0-K58.9, P70.0-P70.4, P70.9-P71.9, P72.1, P72.9-P74.4, P74.9, P76.8-P77.9, P78.1, P78.3-P78.89, P94.0

A03.1 Shigellosis due to Shigella flexneri
Group B shigellosis

A03.2 Shigellosis due to Shigella boydii
Group C shigellosis

A03.3 Shigellosis due to Shigella sonnei
Group D shigellosis

A03.8 Other shigellosis

A03.9 Shigellosis, unspecified
Bacillary dysentery NOS

A04 Other bacterial intestinal infections
Excludes1 bacterial foodborne intoxications, NEC (A05.-)
tuberculous enteritis (A18.32)
Ex: **For category A04 CC codes A04.0-A04.4:** A02.0, A03.9-A05.0, A05.2, A07.4, A08.0-A09, J09.X3-J09.X9, J10.2-J10.89, J11.2-J11.89, K30, K31.84, K52.1-K52.3, K52.82-K52.9, K58.0-K58.9, K65.0, K65.2, K65.8, K68.12-K68.9, P76.8-P77.9, P78.1, P78.3-P78.89 **For category A04 CC codes A04.5-A04.8:** A00.1, A01.00-A01.09, A01.4-A02.0, A03.9, A04.0-A04.8, A04.9-A05.2, A06.0-A06.2, A06.9, A07.1-A09, A18.32-A18.39, A18.83, A48.51-A48.52, B37.82, B82.9, J09.X3-J09.X9, J10.2-J10.89, J11.2-J11.89, K30, K31.84, K50.00-K51.919, K52.1-K52.3, K52.82-K55.1, K55.30-K55.33, K55.8-K55.9, K58.0-K58.9, P70.0-P70.4, P70.9-P71.9, P72.1, P72.9-P74.4, P74.9, P76.8-P77.9, P78.1, P78.3-P78.89, P94.0

A04.0 Enteropathogenic Escherichia coli infection
Pertaining to or producing intestinal disease

A04.1 Enterotoxigenic Escherichia coli infection
Producing or containing intestinal toxin

A04.2 Enteroinvasive Escherichia coli infection
Capable of penetrating and spreading through intestinal mucosal epithelium

A04.3 Enterohemorrhagic Escherichia coli infection
Causing bloody diarrhea, resulting from microorganisms

A04.4 Other intestinal Escherichia coli infections
Escherichia coli enteritis NOS

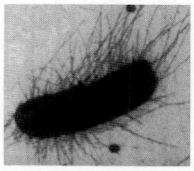

Figure 1-1 Electron micrograph of escherichia coli (E. coli) expressing P fimbriae. (From Mandell, Bennett, & Dolin: Principles and Practice of Infectious Diseases, ed 7, Churchill Livingstone, An Imprint of Elsevier, 2009)

Item 1–2 ***Escherichia coli [E. coli]*** is a gram-negative bacterium found in the intestinal tracts of humans and animals and is usually nonpathogenic. Pathogenic strains can cause diarrhea or pyogenic (pus-producing) infections. Can be a threat to food safety.

A04.5 Campylobacter enteritis
Spiral shaped bacterium

A04.6 Enteritis due to Yersinia enterocolitica
Excludes1 extraintestinal yersiniosis (A28.2)
Transmitted by infected food /water and person-to-person contact, affecting intestinal tract

A04.7 Enterocolitis due to Clostridium difficile
Foodborne intoxication by Clostridium difficile
Pseudomembraneous colitis
Marked by fibrinous deposit (false membrane) with enmeshed necrotic cells

A04.8 Other specified bacterial intestinal infections

A04.9 Bacterial intestinal infection, unspecified
Bacterial enteritis NOS
Ex: A00.1, A01.00-A01.09, A01.4-A02.0, A03.9-A05.0, A05.2, A06.0-A06.2, A06.9, A07.1-A09, A18.32-A18.39, A18.83, B37.82, B82.9, J09.X3-J09.X9, J10.2-J10.89, J11.2-J11.89, K30, K31.84, K52.1-K52.3, K52.82-K52.9, K58.0-K58.9, K65.0, K65.2, K65.8, K68.12-K68.9, P76.8-P77.9, P78.1, P78.3-P78.89

A05 Other bacterial foodborne intoxications, not elsewhere classified
Excludes1 Clostridium difficile foodborne intoxication and infection (A04.7)
Escherichia coli infection (A04.0-A04.4)
listeriosis (A32.-)
salmonella foodborne intoxication and infection (A02.-)
toxic effect of noxious foodstuffs (T61-T62)

A05.0 Foodborne staphylococcal intoxication
Ex: A00.0-A09, A48.51-A48.52

A05.1 Botulism food poisoning
Botulism NOS
Classical foodborne intoxication due to Clostridium botulinum
Excludes1 infant botulism (A48.51)
wound botulism (A48.52)
Ex: A04.7, A05.0-A05.2, A48.51-A48.52

A05.2 Foodborne Clostridium perfringens [Clostridium welchii] intoxication
Type A causes gas gangrene and necrotizing colitis; major cause of food poisoning in humans
Enteritis necroticans
Pig-bel
Ex: A02.0, A03.9-A05.2, A07.4, A08.0-A09, A48.51-A48.52, J09.X3-J09.X9, J10.2-J10.89, J11.2-J11.89, K30, K31.84, K52.1-K52.3, K52.82-K52.9, K58.0-K58.9, K65.0, K65.2, K65.8, K68.12-K68.9, P76.8-P77.9, P78.1, P78.3-P78.89

A05.3 Foodborne Vibrio parahaemolyticus intoxication
Organism that survives only in high salt environment (halophilic), major cause of gastroenteritis due to consumption of raw or improperly cooked fish/seafood
Ex: A00.0-A09, A48.51-A48.52

A05.4 Foodborne Bacillus cereus intoxication
Spore-forming species commonly found in soil, causes food poisoning from formation of intestinal toxins in contaminated foods
Ex: A00.0-A09, A48.51-A48.52

A05.5 Foodborne Vibrio vulnificus intoxication
Species that survives in high salt environment (halophilic) with infection by eating raw seafood causes septicemia and cellulitis
Ex: A00.0-A09, A48.51-A48.52

A05.8 Other specified bacterial foodborne intoxications
Ex: A00.0-A09, A48.51-A48.52

A05.9 Bacterial foodborne intoxication, unspecified

● **A06 Amebiasis**
An intestinal illness caused by the microscopic parasite Entamoeba histolytica
Includes infection due to Entamoeba histolytica
Excludes1 other protozoal intestinal diseases (A07.-)
Excludes2 acanthamebiasis (B60.1-)
Naegleriasis (B60.2)

A06.0 Acute amebic dysentery
Acute amebiasis
Intestinal amebiasis NOS
Ex: A06.0-A06.1, A07.4

A06.1 Chronic intestinal amebiasis
Ex: A06.0-A06.1, A07.4

A06.2 Amebic nondysenteric colitis
Pertaining to single cell microorganism
Ex: A02.0, A03.9-A05.0, A05.2, A06.0-A06.2, A06.9, A07.1-A09, B82.9, J09.X3-J09.X9, J10.2-J10.89, J11.2-J11.89, K30, K31.84, K50.00-K51.919, K52.1-K52.3, K52.82-K55.1, K55.30-K55.33, K55.8-K55.9, K58.0-K58.9, P76.8-P77.9, P78.1, P78.3, P78.81-P78.89

A06.3 Ameboma of intestine
Tumorlike mass produced by localized inflammation often in intestine
Ameboma NOS
Ex: A06.0-A06.6, A06.81-A06.89

A06.4 Amebic liver abscess
Hepatic amebiasis
Ex: A06.4, K75.0

A06.5 Amebic lung abscess
Amebic abscess of lung (and liver)
Ex: A06.5, J85.0-J85.2

A06.6 Amebic brain abscess
Amebic abscess of brain (and liver) (and lung)
Ex: A06.6, G06.0

A06.7 Cutaneous amebiasis

● **A06.8 Amebic infection of other sites**

A06.81 Amebic cystitis
Ex: A06.0-A06.6, A06.81-A06.89

A06.82 Other amebic genitourinary infections
Amebic balanitis
Amebic vesiculitis
Amebic vulvovaginitis
Ex: A06.0-A06.6, A06.81-A06.89

A06.89 Other amebic infections
Amebic appendicitis
Amebic splenic abscess
Ex: A06.0-A06.6, A06.81-A06.89

A06.9 Amebiasis, unspecified

● **A07 Other protozoal intestinal diseases**
Ex: **For category A07 CC codes unless otherwise indicated:** A02.0, A03.9-A05.0, A05.2, A06.0-A06.2, A06.9, A07.1-A09, B82.9, J09.X3-J09.X9, J10.2-J10.89, J11.2-J11.89, K30, K31.84, K52.1-K52.3, K52.82-K52.9, K58.0-K58.9

A07.0 Balantidiasis
Balantidial dysentery
Infection by protozoa that may cause diarrhea and dysentery, with ulceration of colonic mucous membranes

A07.1 Giardiasis [lambliasis]
Common infection in small intestine spread by contaminated food, water, or direct person-to-person contact

A07.2 Cryptosporidiosis
Human infection with protozoa usually seen as self-limited diarrhea in those who work with cattle

A07.3 Isosporiasis
Human intestinal disease caused by protozoa
Infection due to Isospora belli and Isospora hominis
Intestinal coccidiosis
Isosporosis

A07.4 Cyclosporiasis
Infection by protozoa with most common species infecting humans being C cayetanensis
Ex: A02.0, A03.9-A05.0, A05.2, A06.0-A06.2, A06.9, A07.1-A09, B82.9, J09.X3-J09.X9, J10.2-J10.89, J11.2-J11.89, K30, K31.84, K52.1-K52.3, K52.82-K52.9, K58.0-K58.9, K65.0, K65.2, K65.8, K68.12-K68.9

A07.8 Other specified protozoal intestinal diseases
Intestinal microsporidiosis
Intestinal trichomoniasis
Sarcocystosis
Sarcosporidiosis

A07.9 Protozoal intestinal disease, unspecified
Flagellate diarrhea
Protozoal colitis
Protozoal diarrhea
Protozoal dysentery

● **A08 Viral and other specified intestinal infections**
Excludes1 influenza with involvement of gastrointestinal tract (J09.X3, J10.2, J11.2)
Ex: **For category A08 CC codes:** A02.0, A03.9-A05.0, A05.2, A06.0-A06.2, A06.9, A07.1-A09, A18.32-A18.39, A18.83, B37.82, B82.9, J09.X3-J09.X9, J10.2-J10.89, J11.2-J11.89, K30, K31.84, K52.1-K52.3, K52.82-K52.9, K58.0-K58.9, K65.0, K65.2, K65.8, K68.12-K68.9, P76.8-P77.9, P78.1, P78.3-P78.89

A08.0 Rotaviral enteritis

● **A08.1 Acute gastroenteropathy due to Norwalk agent and other small round viruses**

A08.11 Acute gastroenteropathy due to Norwalk agent
Acute gastroenteropathy due to Norovirus
Acute gastroenteropathy due to Norwalk-like agent

A08.19 Acute gastroenteropathy due to other small round viruses
Acute gastroenteropathy due to small round virus [SRV] NOS

A08.2 Adenoviral enteritis

● **A08.3 Other viral enteritis**

A08.31 Calicivirus enteritis

A08.32 Astrovirus enteritis

A08.39 Other viral enteritis
Coxsackie virus enteritis
Echovirus enteritis
Enterovirus enteritis NEC
Torovirus enteritis

A08.4 Viral intestinal infection, unspecified
Viral enteritis NOS
Viral gastroenteritis NOS
Viral gastroenteropathy NOS

A08.8 Other specified intestinal infections

A09 Infectious gastroenteritis and colitis, unspecified
Infectious colitis NOS
Infectious enteritis NOS
Infectious gastroenteritis NOS
Excludes1 colitis NOS (K52.9)
diarrhea NOS (R19.7)
enteritis NOS (K52.9)
gastroenteritis NOS (K52.9)
noninfective gastroenteritis and colitis, unspecified (K52.9)
Ex: A00.0-A09, A48.51-A48.52

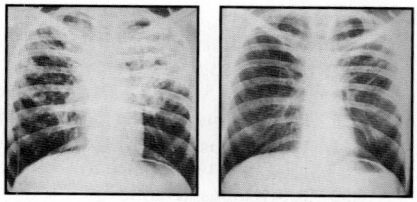

Figure 1-2 Far advanced bilateral pulmonary tuberculosis before and after 8 months of treatment with streptomycin, PAS, and isoniazid. (From Hinshaw HC, Garland LH: Diseases of the Chest, ed 4, Philadelphia, WB Saunders, 1980)

Item 1–3 Tuberculosis is a common and deadly infectious disease caused by the *Mycobacterium tuberculosis* organism. The first tuberculosis infection is called the **primary infection** and most commonly attacks the lungs but can affect the central nervous system, lymphatic system, circulatory system, genitourinary system, bones, joints, and even the skin. A **Ghon** lesion is the **initial lesion.** A **secondary lesion** occurs when the tubercle bacilli are carried to other areas.

Item 1–4 Although it primarily affects the lungs, the bacteria ***Mycobacterium tuberculosis*** can travel from the pulmonary circulation to virtually any organ in the body, much as a cancer metastasizes to a secondary site. If the immune system becomes compromised by age or disease, what would otherwise be a self-limiting primary tuberculosis in the lungs will develop in other organs. These are known as extrapulmonary sites.

TUBERCULOSIS (A15-A19)

Includes infections due to Mycobacterium tuberculosis and Mycobacterium bovis

Excludes1 congenital tuberculosis (P37.0)
nonspecific reaction to test for tuberculosis without active tuberculosis (R76.1-)
pneumoconiosis associated with tuberculosis, any type in A15 (J65)
positive PPD (R76.11)
positive tuberculin skin test without active tuberculosis (R76.11)
sequelae of tuberculosis (B90.-)
silicotuberculosis (J65)

● **A15 Respiratory tuberculosis**
Ex: For category A15 CC codes unless otherwise indicated: A15.0-A15.9, A17.9, A18.82, A18.84, A18.89-A19.9, A22.1, A31.0, A31.2-A31.9, A37.01, A37.11, A37.81, A37.91, A48.1, A49.3-A49.9, B25.0, B44.0, B90.9, B92, B94.2-B94.9, B96.0, B96.6-B96.89, J09.X1-J09.X2, J10.00-J10.1, J11.00-J11.1, J12.0-J12.3, J12.89-J18.1, J18.8-J18.9, J44.9, J47.0-J70.4, J70.8-J70.9, J98.4, R91.1

A15.0 Tuberculosis of lung
Tuberculous bronchiectasis
Chronic dilatation of bronchi
Tuberculous fibrosis of lung
Tuberculous pneumonia
Tuberculous pneumothorax

A15.4 Tuberculosis of intrathoracic lymph nodes
Tuberculosis of hilar lymph nodes
Tuberculosis of mediastinal lymph nodes
Tuberculosis of tracheobronchial lymph nodes
Excludes1 tuberculosis specified as primary (A15.7)

A15.5 Tuberculosis of larynx, trachea and bronchus
Tuberculosis of bronchus
Tuberculosis of glottis
Tuberculosis of larynx
Tuberculosis of trachea

A15.6 Tuberculous pleurisy
Tuberculosis of pleura
Tuberculous empyema
Excludes1 primary respiratory tuberculosis (A15.7)

A15.7 Primary respiratory tuberculosis
Ex: A15.0-A17.82, A17.89-A19.9

A15.8 Other respiratory tuberculosis
Mediastinal tuberculosis
Nasopharyngeal tuberculosis
Tuberculosis of nose
Tuberculosis of sinus [any nasal]
Ex: A15.0-A17.82, A17.89, A18.31-A18.39, A18.83, A19.0-A19.9

A15.9 Respiratory tuberculosis unspecified
Ex: A15.0-A17.82, A17.89, A18.31-A18.39, A18.83, A19.0-A19.9

● **A17 Tuberculosis of nervous system**

A17.0 Tuberculous meningitis
Tuberculosis of meninges (cerebral) (spinal)
Tuberculous leptomeningitis
Excludes1 tuberculous meningoencephalitis (A17.82)
Ex: A02.21, A17.0-A17.1, A17.89-A17.9, A18.82, A18.84, A18.89, A27.81, A31.2-A31.9, A39.0, A49.3-A49.9, A50.41, A51.41, A52.13, A54.82, A54.84, A54.89-A54.9, A87.0-A87.9, B00.3, B02.1, B26.1, B37.5, B38.4, B45.1, B58.2, B90.0, B92, B94.2-B94.9, B96.0, B96.6-B96.89, G00.0-G03.9, G04.2, G32.89, G61.0, G96.8-G96.9, G98.0-G98.8, G99.8

A17.1 Meningeal tuberculoma
Tuberculoma of meninges (cerebral) (spinal)
Excludes2 tuberculoma of brain and spinal cord (A17.81)
Ex: See A17.0

● **A17.8 Other tuberculosis of nervous system**

A17.81 Tuberculoma of brain and spinal cord
Tuberculous abscess of brain and spinal cord
Ex: A17.81-A17.82, A17.89-A17.9, A18.82, A18.84, A18.89, A31.2-A31.9, A49.3-A49.9, B90.0, B92, B94.2-B94.9, B96.0, B96.6-B96.89

A17.82 Tuberculous meningoencephalitis
Inflammation of brain and meninges; AKA cerebromeningitis and encephalomeningitis
Tuberculous myelitis
Ex: See A17.81

A17.83 Tuberculous neuritis
Tuberculous mononeuropathy
Ex: No exclusions

A17.89 Other tuberculosis of nervous system
Tuberculous polyneuropathy
Ex: A17.89-A17.9, A18.82, A18.84, A18.89, A31.2-A31.9, A49.3-A49.9, B90.0, B92, B94.2-B94.9, B96.0, B96.6-B96.89

A17.9 Tuberculosis of nervous system, unspecified
Ex: A17.9, A18.82, A18.84, A18.89, A31.2-A31.9, A49.3-A49.9, B92, B94.2-B94.9, B96.0, B96.6-B96.89

● **A18 Tuberculosis of other organs**

● **A18.0 Tuberculosis of bones and joints**

A18.01 Tuberculosis of spine
Pott's disease or curvature of spine
Tuberculous arthritis
Tuberculous osteomyelitis of spine
Tuberculous spondylitis
Ex: A18.01

A18.02 Tuberculous arthritis of other joints
Tuberculosis of hip (joint)
Tuberculosis of knee (joint)
Ex: A18.02

A18.03 Tuberculosis of other bones
Tuberculous mastoiditis
Tuberculous osteomyelitis
Ex: A18.01, A18.03

A18.09 Other musculoskeletal tuberculosis
Tuberculous myositis
Tuberculous synovitis
Tuberculous tenosynovitis
Ex: A18.01-A18.02, A18.09

● **A18.1 Tuberculosis of genitourinary system**

A18.10 Tuberculosis of genitourinary system, unspecified
Ex: A17.9, A18.10, A18.82, A18.84, A18.89, A31.2-A31.9, A49.3-A49.9, B90.1, B92, B94.2-B94.9, B96.0, B96.6-B96.89

A18.11 Tuberculosis of kidney and ureter
Ex: A17.9, A18.10-A18.13, A18.82, A18.84, A18.89, A31.2-A31.9, A49.3-A49.9, B90.1, B92, B94.2-B94.9, B96.0, B96.6-B96.89

A18.12 Tuberculosis of bladder
Ex: See A18.11

A18.13 Tuberculosis of other urinary organs
Tuberculous urethritis
Ex: See A18.11

A18.14 Tuberculosis of prostate ♂ A
Ex: A17.9, A18.10, A18.82, A18.84, A18.89, A31.2-A31.9, A49.3-A49.9, B90.1, B92, B94.2-B94.9, B96.0, B96.6-B96.89

A18.15 Tuberculosis of other male genital organs ♂
Ex: See A18.14

A18.16 Tuberculosis of cervix ♀
Ex: A17.9, A18.0, A18.16-A18.18, A18.82, A18.84, A18.89, A31.2-A31.9, A49.3-A49.9, B90.1, B92, B94.2-B94.9, B96.0, B96.6-B96.89

A18.17 Tuberculous female pelvic inflammatory disease ♀
Tuberculous endometritis
Tuberculous oophoritis and salpingitis
Oophoritis = inflammation of ovary
Salpingitis = inflammation of fallopian tube
Ex: See A18.16

A18.18 Tuberculosis of other female genital organs ♀
Tuberculous ulceration of vulva
Ex: See A18.16

A18.2 Tuberculous peripheral lymphadenopathy
Tuberculous adenitis
Excludes2 tuberculosis of bronchial and mediastinal lymph nodes (A15.4)
tuberculosis of mesenteric and retroperitoneal lymph nodes (A18.39)
tuberculous tracheobronchial adenopathy (A15.4)
Ex: A17.9, A18.2, A18.82, A18.84, A18.89, A31.2-A31.9, A49.3-A49.9, B92, B94.2-B94.9, B96.0, B96.6-B96.89

● **A18.3 Tuberculosis of intestines, peritoneum and mesenteric glands**
Ex: **For category A18.3 CC codes:** A17.9, A18.31-A18.39, A18.82-A18.84, A18.89, A31.2-A31.9, A49.3-A49.9, B92, B94.2-B94.9, B96.0, B96.6-B96.89

A18.31 Tuberculous peritonitis
Tuberculous ascites

A18.32 Tuberculous enteritis
Tuberculosis of anus and rectum
Tuberculosis of intestine (large) (small)

A18.39 Retroperitoneal tuberculosis
Tuberculosis of mesenteric glands
Tuberculosis of retroperitoneal (lymph glands)

A18.4 Tuberculosis of skin and subcutaneous tissue
Erythema induratum, tuberculous
Lupus excedens
Lupus vulgaris NOS
Lupus vulgaris of eyelid
Cutaneous tuberculosis characterized by reddish brown plaque on skin surrounded by papules and nodules
Scrofuloderma
Type of cutaneous tuberculosis, with direct extension of tuberculosis into skin from underlying structures; AKA tuberculosis colliquativa
Tuberculosis of external ear
Excludes2 lupus erythematosus (L93.-)
lupus NOS (M32.9)
systemic (M32.-)
Ex: A15.0-A17.82, A17.89-A19.9

● **A18.5 Tuberculosis of eye**
Excludes2 lupus vulgaris of eyelid (A18.4)
Ex: **For category A18.5 CC codes:** A17.9, A18.50-A18.59, A18.82, A18.84, A18.89, A31.2-A31.9, A49.3-A49.9, B92, B94.2-B94.9, B96.0, B96.6-B96.89

A18.50 Tuberculosis of eye, unspecified

A18.51 Tuberculous episcleritis
Inflammation of episclera and adjacent tissues

A18.52 Tuberculous keratitis
Tuberculous interstitial keratitis
Tuberculous keratoconjunctivitis (interstitial) (phlyctenular)
Inflammation of cornea and conjunctiva

A18.53 Tuberculous chorioretinitis
Inflammation of choroid and retina; retinochoroiditis

A18.54 Tuberculous iridocyclitis
Inflammation of iris and ciliary body

A18.59 Other tuberculosis of eye
Tuberculous conjunctivitis

A18.6 Tuberculosis of (inner) (middle) ear
Tuberculous otitis media
Excludes2 tuberculosis of external ear (A18.4)
tuberculous mastoiditis (A18.03)
Ex: A17.9, A18.6, A18.82, A18.84, A18.89, A31.2-A31.9, A49.3-A49.9, B92, B94.2-B94.9, B96.0, B96.6-B96.89

A18.7 Tuberculosis of adrenal glands
Tuberculous Addison's disease
Ex: A17.9, A18.7, A18.82, A18.84, A18.89, A31.2-A31.9, A49.3-A49.9, B92, B94.2-B94.9, B96.0, B96.6-B96.89

● **A18.8 Tuberculosis of other specified organs**

A18.81 Tuberculosis of thyroid gland
Ex: A17.9, A18.81-A18.82, A18.84, A18.89, A31.2-A31.9, A49.3-A49.9, B92, B94.2-B94.9, B96.0, B96.6-B96.89

A18.82 Tuberculosis of other endocrine glands
Tuberculosis of pituitary gland
Tuberculosis of thymus gland
Ex: See A17.9

A18.83 Tuberculosis of digestive tract organs, not elsewhere classified
Excludes1 tuberculosis of intestine (A18.32)
Ex: See A18.3

A18.84 Tuberculosis of heart
Tuberculous cardiomyopathy
Tuberculous endocarditis
Tuberculous myocarditis
Tuberculous pericarditis
Ex: See A17.9

A18.85 Tuberculosis of spleen
Ex: A17.9, A18.82, A18.84-A18.85 A18.89, A31.2-A31.9, A49.3-A49.9, B92, B94.2-B94.9, B96.0, B96.6-B96.89

A18.89 Tuberculosis of other sites
Tuberculosis of muscle
Tuberculous cerebral arteritis
Ex: See A17.9

● **A19 Miliary tuberculosis**
Includes disseminated tuberculosis
generalized tuberculosis
tuberculous polyserositis
Ex: **For category A19 CC codes:** A17.9, A18.82, A18.84, A18.89, A19.0-A19.9, A31.2-A31.9, A49.3-A49.9, B92, B94.2-B94.9, B96.0, B96.6-B96.89

A19.0 Acute miliary tuberculosis of a single specified site

A19.1 Acute miliary tuberculosis of multiple sites

A19.2 Acute miliary tuberculosis, unspecified

A19.8 Other miliary tuberculosis

A19.9 Miliary tuberculosis, unspecified

Item 1-5 Miliary tuberculosis can be a life-threatening condition. If a tuberculous lesion enters a blood vessel, immense dissemination of tuberculous organisms can occur if the immune system is weak. High-risk populations—children under 4 years of age, the elderly, or the immunocompromised—are particularly prone to this type of infection. The lesions will have a millet seedlike appearance on chest x-ray. Bronchial washings and biopsy may aid in diagnosis.

CERTAIN ZOONOTIC BACTERIAL DISEASES (A20-A28)

A20 Plague
Infectious disease caused by a Yersinia pestis bacterium, transmitted by a rodent flea bite or handling of infected animal
Includes infection due to Yersinia pestis

A20.0 Bubonic plague
Ex: A20.0-A20.9

A20.1 Cellulocutaneous plague
Skin and subcutaneous tissue plague
Ex: A20.0-A20.9

A20.2 Pneumonic plague
Ex: A20.2, J12.81

A20.3 Plague meningitis
Ex: A20.3, A20.8

A20.7 Septicemic plague
Ex: A02.1, A20.0-A20.9, A22.7, A26.7, A32.7, A40.0-A40.1, A40.8-A41.9, A42.7, A54.86, B37.7, P36.0-P36.9, P39.2, P39.4-P39.9, R65.10-R65.20

A20.8 Other forms of plague
Abortive plague
Asymptomatic plague
Pestis minor
Systemic bacterial disease
Ex: See A20.3

A20.9 Plague, unspecified
Ex: A20.9

A21 Tularemia
Caused by Francisella tularensis bacterium found in rodents, rabbits, and hares and transmitted to humans by contact with infected animal tissues or by ticks, biting flies, or mosquitoes
Includes deer-fly fever
infection due to Francisella tularensis
rabbit fever

A21.0 Ulceroglandular tularemia
Most common form of tularemia in humans is painful, swollen, erythematous papule at point of inoculation that ruptures to form shallow ulcer
Ex: A21.0

A21.1 Oculoglandular tularemia
Primary site of entry is conjunctival sac, results in granulomatous corneal lesions
Ophthalmic tularemia
Ex: A21.1, J12.81

A21.2 Pulmonary tularemia
Ex: A22.1, A37.01, A37.11, A37.81, A37.91, A48.1, B25.0, B44.0, J09.X1-J09.X2, J10.00-J10.1, J11.00-J11.1, J15.29, J15.5-J18.0, J18.8-J18.9, J22, J60-J70.4, J70.8-J70.9, J98.4, J98.8-J99, R91.1

A21.3 Gastrointestinal tularemia
Abdominal tularemia
Ex: A21.3

A21.7 Generalized tularemia
Ex: A21.0-A21.9

A21.8 Other forms of tularemia
Ex: A21.0-A21.9

A21.9 Tularemia, unspecified
Ex: A21.0-A21.9

Item 1-6 Brucellosis: An infectious disease caused by the bacterium Brucella. Humans are infected by contact with contaminated animals or animal products. In humans brucellosis symptoms that are similar to the flu include fever, sweats, headaches, back pains, and physical weakness. Severe infections of the central nervous system or lining of the heart may occur. Brucellosis can also cause chronic symptoms that include recurrent fevers, joint pain, and fatigue.

A22 Anthrax
An acute infectious disease caused by the spore-forming Bacillus anthracis; occurs in humans exposed to infected animals or tissue from infected animals
Includes infection due to Bacillus anthracis

A22.0 Cutaneous anthrax
Malignant carbuncle
Malignant pustule
Ex: A22.0

A22.1 Pulmonary anthrax
Inhalation anthrax
Ragpicker's disease
Woolsorter's disease
Ex: A15.0-A15.9, A17.9, A18.82, A18.84, A18.89, A20.2, A21.1-A21.2, A22.1, A31.0, A37.01, A37.11, A37.81, A37.91, A42.0, A43.0, A48.1, B25.0, B39.0-B39.2, B44.0, B58.3, B59, B67.1, J09.X1-J09.X2, J10.00-J10.1, J11.00-J11.1, J12.0-J12.3, J12.81-J18.1, J18.8-J18.9, J22, J44.9, J47.0-J70.4, J70.8-J70.9, J98.4, J98.8-J99, R91.1

A22.2 Gastrointestinal anthrax
Ex: A22.2

A22.7 Anthrax sepsis
Infectious bacterial disease
MCC when PDx is its own MCC
Ex: See A02.1

A22.8 Other forms of anthrax
Anthrax meningitis
Ex: A22.8

A22.9 Anthrax, unspecified
Ex: A22.0-A22.9

A23 Brucellosis
Includes Malta fever
Mediterranean fever
undulant fever

A23.0 Brucellosis due to Brucella melitensis
Resulting in flu-like symptoms that may lead to chronic symptoms that include recurrent fevers, joint pain, and fatigue

A23.1 Brucellosis due to Brucella abortus
Most common cause of brucellosis in humans; AKA Bang bacillus

A23.2 Brucellosis due to Brucella suis
Species found primarily in pigs, rabbits, and reindeer

A23.3 Brucellosis due to Brucella canis
Species that causes respiratory tract infection in humans

A23.8 Other brucellosis
Ex: A23.0-A23.9

A23.9 Brucellosis, unspecified
Ex: A23.0-A23.9

A24 Glanders and melioidosis
Infection, usually of rodents, which spreads to other animals and humans, caused by Burkholderia pseudomallei *through break in skin contaminated with infested soil or water*
Ex: **For category A24 CC codes unless otherwise indicated:** A24.1-A24.9

A24.0 Glanders
Infection due to Pseudomonas mallei
Malleus
Ex: A24.0

A24.1 Acute and fulminating melioidosis
Melioidosis pneumonia
Melioidosis sepsis

A24.2 Subacute and chronic melioidosis

A24.3 Other melioidosis

A24.9 Melioidosis, unspecified
Infection due to Pseudomonas pseudomallei NOS
Whitmore's disease

A25 Rat-bite fevers
RBF, infectious disease caused by Streptobacillus moniliformis or Spirillum minus.
Ex: For category A25 CC codes: A25.0-A25.9

A25.0 Spirillosis
Any disease condition caused by spirilla
Sodoku

A25.1 Streptobacillosis
Acute, febrile human illness caused by bacteria transmitted by rats in most cases, passed from rodent to human via rodent's urine or mucous secretions; AKA rat fever
Epidemic arthritic erythema
Haverhill fever
Streptobacillary rat-bite fever

A25.9 Rat-bite fever, unspecified

A26 Erysipeloid
Infection with Erysipelothrix rhusiopathiae, *occurring often as occupational disease resulting from handling infected fish, shellfish, meat, or poultry*

A26.0 Cutaneous erysipeloid
Erythema migrans

A26.7 Erysipelothrix sepsis
MCC when PDx is its own MCC
Ex: A02.1, A20.7, A22.7, A26.7, A32.7, A39.2-A39.4, A40.0-A40.1, A40.8-A41.9, A42.7, A48.2-A48.4, A48.8-A49.9, A54.86, B00.7, B3.77, B92, B94.2-B96.89, R65.10-R65.20, Z16.10-Z16.39

A26.8 Other forms of erysipeloid

A26.9 Erysipeloid, unspecified

A27 Leptospirosis
Occurs most commonly in the tropics
Ex: For category A27 CC codes unless otherwise indicated: A27.0-A27.9

A27.0 Leptospirosis icterohemorrhagica
Leptospiral or spirochetal jaundice (hemorrhagic)
Weil's disease

A27.8 Other forms of leptospirosis

A27.81 Aseptic meningitis in leptospirosis
Ex: A02.21, A17.0-A17.1, A27.0-A27.9, A39.0, A50.41, A51.41, A52.13, A54.82, A54.84, A54.89-A54.9, A74.81-A74.9, A87.0-A87.9, A96.2, A98.3-A98.4, B26.1, B33.24, B33.4-B33.8, B34.1-B34.2, B34.4-B34.8, B37.5, B38.4, B45.1, B58.2, B92, B94.2-B94.9, B97.10, B97.19, B97.29, B97.5-B97.6, B97.81-B97.89, G00.0-G03.9, G04.2, G32.89, G61.0, G96.8-G96.9, G98.0-G98.8, G99.8

A27.89 Other forms of leptospirosis

A27.9 Leptospirosis, unspecified

A28 Other zoonotic bacterial diseases, not elsewhere classified
Ex: For category A28 CC codes unless otherwise indicated: A26.0, A26.8-A26.9, A28.0, A28.2-A28.9, A32.0-A32.12, A32.81-A32.9

A28.0 Pasteurellosis
Infection of humans or other animals by species of Pasteurella

A28.1 Cat-scratch disease
Cat-scratch fever
Ex: A28.1, B97.21

A28.2 Extraintestinal yersiniosis
Infection from Yersinia enterocolitica; *AKA enteric yersiniosis, intestinal yersiniosis, Yersinia enteritis*
Excludes1 enteritis due to Yersinia enterocolitica (A04.6)
plague (A20.-)

A28.8 Other specified zoonotic bacterial diseases, not elsewhere classified

A28.9 Zoonotic bacterial disease, unspecified

OTHER BACTERIAL DISEASES (A30-A49)

A30 Leprosy [Hansen's disease]
Chronic infectious disease attacking the skin, peripheral nerves, and mucous membranes
Includes infection due to Mycobacterium leprae
Excludes1 sequelae of leprosy (B92)

A30.0 Indeterminate leprosy
I leprosy
Ex: A30.0

A30.1 Tuberculoid leprosy
TT leprosy
Ex: A30.1

A30.2 Borderline tuberculoid leprosy
BT leprosy
Ex: A30.2-A30.4

A30.3 Borderline leprosy
BB leprosy
Ex: A30.2-A30.4

A30.4 Borderline lepromatous leprosy
BL leprosy
Ex: A30.2-A30.4

A30.5 Lepromatous leprosy
LL leprosy
Ex: A30.5

A30.8 Other forms of leprosy
Ex: A30.8

A30.9 Leprosy, unspecified
Ex: A30.9

A31 Infection due to other mycobacteria
Excludes2 leprosy (A30.-)
tuberculosis (A15-A19)
Ex: For category A31 CC codes unless otherwise indicated: A31.0-A31.9

A31.0 Pulmonary mycobacterial infection
Infection due to Mycobacterium avium
Infection due to Mycobacterium intracellulare [Battey bacillus]
Infection due to Mycobacterium kansasii
Ex: A15.0-A15.9, A17.9, A18.82, A18.84, A18.89, A22.1, A31.0, A31.2-A31.9, A37.01, A37.11, A37.81, A37.91, A48.1, A49.3-A49.9, B25.0, B44.0, B90.0, B92, B94.2-B94.9, B96.0, B96.6-B96.89, J09.X1-J09.X2, J10.00-J10.1, J11.00-J11.1, J12.0-J12.3, J12.89-J18.1, J18.8-J18.9, J44.9, J47.0-J70.4, J70.8-J70.9, J98.4, R91.1

A31.1 Cutaneous mycobacterial infection
Buruli ulcer
Infection due to Mycobacterium marinum
Infection due to Mycobacterium ulcerans

A31.2 Disseminated mycobacterium avium-intracellulare complex (DMAC)
MAC sepsis

A31.8 Other mycobacterial infections

A31.9 Mycobacterial infection, unspecified
Atypical mycobacterial infection NOS
Mycobacteriosis NOS

A32 Listeriosis
Infection caused by Listeria monocytogenes
Includes listerial foodborne infection
Excludes1 neonatal (disseminated) listeriosis (P37.2)
Ex: For category A32 CC codes unless otherwise indicated: A26.0, A26.8-A26.9, A28.0, A28.2-A28.9, A32.0-A32.12, A32.81-A32.9

A32.0 Cutaneous listeriosis

A32.1 Listerial meningitis and meningoencephalitis

A32.11 Listerial meningitis

A32.12 Listerial meningoencephalitis

◀ New ◀ Revised ~~deleted~~ Deleted Excludes 1 Excludes 2 Includes Use additional Code first Code also Unspecified
OGCR Official Guidelines ● Unacceptable Principal Diagnosis X Assign placeholder X ● Use Additional Character(s) ▶ Manifestation Code Coding Clinic

A32.7 Listerial sepsis
MCC when PDx is its own MCC
Ex: See A26.7

A32.8 Other forms of listeriosis

A32.81 Oculoglandular listeriosis
Primary infection site is conjunctival sac, which if untreated may result in perforation of cornea and optic atrophy

A32.82 Listerial endocarditis
Exudative and proliferative inflammatory condition of endocardium caused by listeria bacteria

A32.89 Other forms of listeriosis
Listerial cerebral arteritis

A32.9 Listeriosis, unspecified

A33 Tetanus neonatorum N
Neonate = newborn
Ex: A33, P29.0-P29.2, P29.4, P29.89-P29.9, P94.1-P94.9, P96.0, P96.3-P96.5, P96.82-P96.89

A34 Obstetrical tetanus ♀ M
Ex: A34, O08.0, O08.2-O08.9, O11.4, O11.5, O12.04, O12.05, O12.14, O12.15, O12.24, O12.25, O13.4, O13.5, O14.04, O14.05, O14.14, O14.15, O14.24, O14.25, O14.94, O14.95, O16.4, O16.5, O20.0-O20.9, O25.10-O25.3, O26.10-O26.13, O26.30-O26.43, O26.63-O26.819, O26.841-O26.86, O26.891-O26.93, O29.011-O29.93, O35.7XX0-O35.7XX9, O44.00-O44.13, O44.20-O44.53, O45.8X1-O45.93, O75.4, O75.81, O75.89-O75.9, O80, O90.89, O99.111-O99.285, O99.330-O99.335, O99.350-O99.355, O99.511-O99.73, O99.820-O99.825, O99.840-O9A.53

A35 Other tetanus
Tetanus NOS
Excludes1 tetanus neonatorum (A33)
obstetrical tetanus (A34)
Ex: A35, B92, B94.2-B94.9

A36 Diphtheria
Ex: **For category A36 CC codes unless otherwise indicated:** A36.0-A36.9

A36.0 Pharyngeal diphtheria
Diphtheritic membranous angina
Tonsillar diphtheria

A36.1 Nasopharyngeal diphtheria

A36.2 Laryngeal diphtheria
Diphtheritic laryngotracheitis

A36.3 Cutaneous diphtheria
Excludes2 erythrasma (L08.1)

A36.8 Other diphtheria

A36.81 Diphtheritic cardiomyopathy
Diphtheritic myocarditis
Ex: A36.81, A52.06, B33.20-B33.22, I00, I01.2-I01.9, I09.0, I09.9, I23.0-I23.3, I23.6-I23.8, I40.0-I41, I51.0, I51.4, I87.8-I87.9, I99.8-I99.9

A36.82 Diphtheritic radiculomyelitis

A36.83 Diphtheritic polyneuritis

A36.84 Diphtheritic tubulo-interstitial nephropathy

A36.85 Diphtheritic cystitis

A36.86 Diphtheritic conjunctivitis

A36.89 Other diphtheritic complications
Diphtheritic peritonitis

A36.9 Diphtheria, unspecified

Item 1-7 Diptheria: A highly contagious bacterial disease that results in the formation of an adherent membrane in the throat that may lead to suffocation. In its most poisonous form, it attacks the heart and lungs. It is spread by direct physical contact or breathing the aerosolized secretions of infected individuals. The exact location is specified in the codes.

A37 Whooping cough
Pertussis is a highly contagious disease caused by the bacterium Bordetella pertussis and results in a whooping sounding cough.
Ex: **For category A37 CC codes A37.00, A37.10, A37.80, A37.90:** A37.00-A37.91
For category A37 CC codes A37.01, A37.11, A37.81, A37.91: A15.0-A15.9, A17.9, A18.82, A18.84, A18.89, A21.2, A22.1, A31.0, A37.00-A37.91, A42.0, A43.0, A48.1, B25.0, B39.0-B39.2, B44.0, B58.3, B59, B67.1, J09.X1-J09.X2, J10.00-J10.1, J11.00-J11.1, J12.0-J12.3, J12.89-J18.1, J18.8-J18.9, J22, J44.9, J47.0-J70.4, J70.8-J70.9, J98.4, J98.8-J98.9, Q33.4, R91.1

A37.0 Whooping cough due to Bordetella pertussis

A37.00 Whooping cough due to Bordetella pertussis without pneumonia

A37.01 Whooping cough due to Bordetella pertussis with pneumonia
MCC when PDx is its own MCC

A37.1 Whooping cough due to Bordetella parapertussis

A37.10 Whooping cough due to Bordetella parapertussis without pneumonia

A37.11 Whooping cough due to Bordetella parapertussis with pneumonia
MCC when PDx is its own MCC

A37.8 Whooping cough due to other Bordetella species

A37.80 Whooping cough due to other Bordetella species without pneumonia

A37.81 Whooping cough due to other Bordetella species with pneumonia
MCC when PDx is its own MCC

A37.9 Whooping cough, unspecified species

A37.90 Whooping cough, unspecified species without pneumonia

A37.91 Whooping cough, unspecified species with pneumonia
MCC when PDx is its own MCC

A38 Scarlet fever
Most commonly caused by the bacteria Streptococcus pneumoniae and Neisseria meningitides
Includes scarlatina
Excludes2 streptococcal sore throat (J02.0)
Ex: **For category A38 CC codes:** A38.0-A38.9, A46, J02.0, J03.00-J03.01

A38.0 Scarlet fever with otitis media

A38.1 Scarlet fever with myocarditis

A38.8 Scarlet fever with other complications

A38.9 Scarlet fever, uncomplicated
Scarlet fever, NOS

A39 Meningococcal infection
Most commonly caused by the bacteria Streptococcus pneumoniae and Neisseria meningitides

A39.0 Meningococcal meningitis
Ex: A02.21, A17.0-A17.1, A27.81, A39.0, A39.89-A39.9, A49.3-A49.9, A50.41, A51.41, A52.13, A54.82, A54.84, A54.89-A54.9, A87.0-A87.9, B00.3, B02.1, B26.1, B37.5, B38.4, B45.1, B58.2, B92, B94.2-B94.9, B96.0, B96.6-B96.89, G00.0-G03.9, G04.2, G32.89, G61.0, G96.8-G96.9, G98.0-G98.8, G99.8

A39.1 Waterhouse-Friderichsen syndrome
Fulminating complication of meningococcemia
Meningococcal hemorrhagic adrenalitis
Meningococcic adrenal syndrome
Ex: A39.1, A39.89-A39.9, A49.3-A49.9, B92, B94.2-B94.9, B96.0, B96.6-B96.89

A39.2 Acute meningococcemia
Ex: A02.1, A20.7, A22.7, A26.7, A32.7, A39.2-A39.4, A39.89-A41.9, A42.7, A49.3-A49.9, A54.86, B00.7, B37.7, B92, B94.2-B94.9, B96.0, B96.6-B96.89, R65.10-R65.20

A39.3 Chronic meningococcemia
Ex: See A39.2

A39.4 Meningococcemia, unspecified
Ex: See A39.2

● **A39.5 Meningococcal heart disease**

A39.50 Meningococcal carditis, unspecified
Ex: A39.50, A39.89-A39.9, A49.3-A49.9, B92, B94.2-B94.9, B96.0, B96.6-B96.89

A39.51 Meningococcal endocarditis
Ex: A39.51, A39.89-A39.9, A49.3-A49.9, B92, B94.2-B94.9, B96.0, B96.6-B96.89

A39.52 Meningococcal myocarditis
Ex: A39.52, A49.3-A49.9, B92, B94.2-B94.9, B96.0, B96.6-B96.89

A39.53 Meningococcal pericarditis
Ex: A39.53, A39.89-A39.9, A49.3-A49.9, B92, B94.2-B94.9, B96.0, B96.6-B96.89

● **A39.8 Other meningococcal infections**

A39.81 Meningococcal encephalitis
Ex: A39.81, A39.89-A39.9, A49.3-A49.9, B92, B94.2-B94.9, B96.0, B96.6-B96.89

A39.82 Meningococcal retrobulbar neuritis
Optic neuritis in portion of optic nerve posterior to eyeball; AKA postocular optic neuritis
Ex: A39.82, A39.89-A39.9, A49.3-A49.9, B92, B94.2-B94.9, B96.0, B96.6-B96.89

A39.83 Meningococcal arthritis
Ex: A39.83-A39.9, A49.3-A49.9, B92, B94.2-B94.9, B96.0, B96.6-B96.89

A39.84 Postmeningococcal arthritis
Ex: See A39.83

A39.89 Other meningococcal infections
Meningococcal conjunctivitis
Ex: A39.89-A39.9, A49.3-A49.9, B92, B94.2-B94.9, B96.0, B96.6-B96.89

A39.9 Meningococcal infection, unspecified
Meningococcal disease NOS
Ex: See A39.89

● **A40 Streptococcal sepsis**

Code first
postprocedural streptococcal sepsis (T81.4-)
streptococcal sepsis during labor (O75.3)
streptococcal sepsis following abortion or ectopic or molar pregnancy (O03-O07, O08.0)
streptococcal sepsis following immunization (T88.0)
streptococcal sepsis following infusion, transfusion or therapeutic injection (T80.2-)

Excludes1 neonatal (P36.0-P36.1)
puerperal sepsis (O85)
sepsis due to Streptococcus, group D (A41.81)

Ex: **For category A40 CC codes unless otherwise indicated:** A02.1, A20.7, A22.7, A26.7, A32.7, A39.2-A39.4, A40.0-A40.1, A40.8-A41.9, A42.7, A48.2-A48.4, A48.8-A49.9, A54.86, B00.7, B3.77, B92, B94.2-B96.89, R65.10-R65.20, Z16.10-Z16.39

A40.0 Sepsis due to streptococcus, group A

A40.1 Sepsis due to streptococcus, group B

A40.3 Sepsis due to Streptococcus pneumoniae
Pneumococcal sepsis
Ex: No exclusions

A40.8 Other streptococcal sepsis

A40.9 Streptococcal sepsis, unspecified

● **A41 Other sepsis**

Code first
postprocedural sepsis (T81.4-)
sepsis during labor (O75.3)
sepsis following abortion, ectopic or molar pregnancy (O03-O07, O08.0)
sepsis following immunization (T88.0)
sepsis following infusion, transfusion or therapeutic injection (T80.2-)

Excludes1 bacteremia NOS (R78.81)
neonatal (P36.-)
puerperal sepsis (O85)
~~sepsis NOS (A41.9)~~
streptococcal sepsis (A40.-)

Excludes2 sepsis (due to) (in) actinomycotic (A42.7)
sepsis (due to) (in) anthrax (A22.7)
sepsis (due to) (in) candidal (B37.7)
sepsis (due to) (in) Erysipelothrix (A26.7)
sepsis (due to) (in) extraintestinal yersiniosis (A28.2)
sepsis (due to) (in) gonococcal (A54.86)
sepsis (due to) (in) herpesviral (B00.7)
sepsis (due to) (in) listerial (A32.7)
sepsis (due to) (in) melioidosis (A24.1)
sepsis (due to) (in) meningococcal (A39.2-A39.4)
sepsis (due to) (in) plague (A20.7)
sepsis (due to) (in) tularemia (A21.7)
toxic shock syndrome (A48.3)

Ex: **For category A41 CC codes:** A02.1, A20.7, A22.7, A26.7, A32.7, A39.2-A39.4, A40.0-A40.1, A40.8-A41.9, A42.7, A48.2-A48.4, A48.8-A49.9, A54.86, B00.7, B3.77, B92, B94.2-B96.89, R65.10-R65.20, Z16.10-Z16.39

Coding Clinic: 2016, Q1, P39

● **A41.0 Sepsis due to Staphylococcus aureus**

A41.01 Sepsis due to Methicillin susceptible Staphylococcus aureus
MSSA sepsis
Staphylococcus aureus sepsis NOS

A41.02 Sepsis due to Methicillin resistant Staphylococcus aureus

A41.1 Sepsis due to other specified staphylococcus
Coagulase negative staphylococcus sepsis

A41.2 Sepsis due to unspecified staphylococcus

A41.3 Sepsis due to Hemophilus influenzae

A41.4 Sepsis due to anaerobes
Excludes1 gas gangrene (A48.0)

● **A41.5 Sepsis due to other Gram-negative organisms**

A41.50 Gram-negative sepsis, unspecified
Gram-negative sepsis NOS

A41.51 Sepsis due to Escherichia coli [E. coli]

A41.52 Sepsis due to Pseudomonas
Pseudomonas aeroginosa

A41.53 Sepsis due to Serratia

A41.59 Other Gram-negative sepsis

● **A41.8 Other specified sepsis**

A41.81 Sepsis due to Enterococcus

A41.89 Other specified sepsis

A41.9 Sepsis, unspecified organism
Septicemia NOS

A42 Actinomycosis
Excludes1 actinomycetoma (B47.1)
A42.0 Pulmonary actinomycosis
Ex: A42.0, A42.81-A43.0, A43.8-A43.9, B47.1, J12.81
A42.1 Abdominal actinomycosis
Ex: A42.1, A42.81-A42.9, A43.8-A43.9, B47.1
A42.2 Cervicofacial actinomycosis
Ex: A42.2, A42.81-A42.9, A43.8-A43.9, B47.1
A42.7 Actinomycotic sepsis
Ex: See A26.7
A42.8 Other forms of actinomycosis
Ex: **For category A42.8 CC codes:** A42.0-A42.2, A42.81-A43.9, B47.1-B47.9, L08.1
A42.81 Actinomycotic meningitis
A42.82 Actinomycotic encephalitis
A42.89 Other forms of actinomycosis
A42.9 Actinomycosis, unspecified
Ex: A42.0-A42.2, A42.81-A43.9, B47.1-B47.9, L08.1

A43 Nocardiosis
A43.0 Pulmonary nocardiosis
Ex: See A42.0
A43.1 Cutaneous nocardiosis
Ex: A42.81-A42.9, A43.1-A43.9, B47.1, L08.1
A43.8 Other forms of nocardiosis
Ex: See A42.9
A43.9 Nocardiosis, unspecified
Ex: See A42.9

A44 Bartonellosis
Ex: **For category A44 CC codes:** A44.0-A44.9, A68.0-A68.9, A69.20-A69.29, A75.0-A79.9, B55.0-B57.5, B60.0
A44.0 Systemic bartonellosis
Oroya fever
A44.1 Cutaneous and mucocutaneous bartonellosis
Verruga peruana
A44.8 Other forms of bartonellosis
A44.9 Bartonellosis, unspecified

A46 Erysipelas
Excludes1 postpartum or puerperal erysipelas (O86.89)

A48 Other bacterial diseases, not elsewhere classified
Excludes1 actinomycetoma (B47.1)
A48.0 Gas gangrene
Clostridial cellulitis
Clostridial myonecrosis
Ex: A48.0, B92, B94.2-B94.9
A48.1 Legionnaires' disease
Ex: A15.0-A15.9, A17.9, A18.82, A18.84, A18.89, A21.2, A22.1, A31.0, A37.01, A37.11, A37.81, A37.91, A42.0, A43.0, A48.1, B25.0, B39.0-B39.2, B44.0, B58.3, B59, B67.1, J09.X1-J09.X2, J10.00-J10.1, J11.00-J11.1, J12.0-J12.3, J12.89-J18.1, J18.8-J18.9, J22, J44.9, J47.0-J70.4, J70.8-J70.9, J98.4, J98.8-J98.9, Q33.4, R91.1
A48.2 Nonpneumonic Legionnaires' disease [Pontiac fever]
A48.3 Toxic shock syndrome
Use additional code to identify the organism (B95, B96)
Excludes1 endotoxic shock NOS (R57.8)
sepsis NOS (A41.9)
Ex: A48.3, G89.0-G89.4, R09.89, R29.700-R29.742, R41.0-R41.3, R41.82, R41.9, R44.8-R44.9, R45.83-R45.84, R46.0-R46.89, R52,R57.0-R57.9, R65.21, R68.0-R68.19, R68.81-R68.89, R69
A48.4 Brazilian purpuric fever
Systemic Hemophilus aegyptius infection

Item 1–8 Gas gangrene is a necrotizing subcutaneous infection that will cause tissue death. Patients with poor circulation (e.g., diabetes, peripheral nephropathy) will have low oxygen content in their tissues (hypoxia), which allows the Clostridium bacteria to flourish. Gas gangrene often occurs at the site of a surgical wound or trauma. Onset is sudden and dramatic. Treatment can include debridement, amputation, and/or hyperbaric oxygen treatments.

A48.5 Other specified botulism
Non-foodborne intoxication due to toxins of Clostridium botulinum [C. botulinum]
Excludes1 food poisoning due to toxins of Clostridium botulinum (A05.1)
A48.51 Infant botulism P
Ex: A04.7, A05.0-A05.2, A48.51-A48.52
A48.52 Wound botulism
Non-foodborne botulism NOS
Use additional code for associated wound
Ex: A04.7, A05.0-A05.2, A48.51-A48.52
A48.8 Other specified bacterial diseases

A49 Bacterial infection of unspecified site
Excludes1 bacterial agents as the cause of diseases classified elsewhere (B95-B96)
chlamydial infection NOS (A74.9)
meningococcal infection NOS (A39.9)
rickettsial infection NOS (A79.9)
spirochetal infection NOS (A69.9)
A49.0 Staphylococcal infection, unspecified site
A49.01 Methicillin susceptible Staphylococcus aureus infection, unspecified site
Methicillin susceptible Staphylococcus aureus (MSSA) infection
Staphylococcus aureus infection NOS
A49.02 Methicillin resistant Staphylococcus aureus infection, unspecified site
Methicillin resistant Staphylococcus aureus (MRSA) infection
A49.1 Streptococcal infection, unspecified site
A49.2 Hemophilus influenzae infection, unspecified site
Any of seven bacterium of genus Haemophilus
A49.3 Mycoplasma infection, unspecified site
Bacterium of class Mollicutes, unusual group of bacteria distinguished by absence of cell wall
A49.8 Other bacterial infections of unspecified site
A49.9 Bacterial infection, unspecified
Excludes1 bacteremia NOS (R78.81)

INFECTIONS WITH A PREDOMINANTLY SEXUAL MODE OF TRANSMISSION (A50-A64)

Excludes1 human immunodeficiency virus [HIV] disease (B20)
nonspecific and nongonococcal urethritis (N34.1)
Reiter's disease (M02.3-)

A50 Congenital syphilis
A50.0 Early congenital syphilis, symptomatic
Any congenital syphilitic condition specified as early or manifest less than two years after birth
Ex: **For category A50.0 CC codes:** A50.01-A51.46, A51.5-A53.9
A50.01 Early congenital syphilitic oculopathy
A50.02 Early congenital syphilitic osteochondropathy
A50.03 Early congenital syphilitic pharyngitis
Early congenital syphilitic laryngitis
A50.04 Early congenital syphilitic pneumonia
A50.05 Early congenital syphilitic rhinitis
A50.06 Early cutaneous congenital syphilis
A50.07 Early mucocutaneous congenital syphilis
A50.08 Early visceral congenital syphilis
A50.09 Other early congenital syphilis, symptomatic

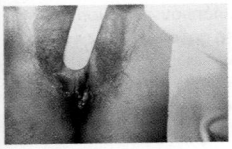

Figure 1-3 Chancre of primary syphilis. (From Mandell, Bennett, & Dolin: Principles and Practice of Infectious Diseases, ed 7, Churchill Livingstone, An Imprint of Elsevier, 2009)

Item 1–9 Syphilis, also known as lues, is the most serious of the venereal diseases caused by *Treponema pallidum*. The **primary** stage is characterized by an ulceration known as **chancre,** which usually appears on the genitals but can also develop on the anus, lips, tonsils, breasts, or fingers. Syphilis is easy to cure in its early stages. A single intramuscular injection of penicillin will usually cure a person who has had syphilis for less than a year.

The **secondary** stage is characterized by a rash that can affect any area of the body. **Latent** syphilis is divided into **early,** which is diagnosed within two years of infection, and **late,** which is diagnosed two years or more after infection. Additional doses of penicillin or another antibiotic are needed to treat someone who has had syphilis for longer than a year. For those allergic to penicillin, there are other antibiotic treatments. **Congenital** syphilis is also labeled **early** or **late** based on the time of diagnosis.

A50.1 Early congenital syphilis, latent
Congenital syphilis without clinical manifestations, with positive serological reaction and negative spinal fluid test, less than two years after birth

A50.2 Early congenital syphilis, unspecified
Congenital syphilis NOS less than two years after birth
Ex: A50.01-A51.46, A51.5-A54.85, A54.89-A58, A63.8, A64, B92, B94.2-B94.9, M02.30-M02.39, N34.1

● **A50.3 Late congenital syphilitic oculopathy**
Excludes1 Hutchinson's triad (A50.53)
Ex: For category A50.3 CC codes: A50.01-A51.46, A51.5-A53.9

A50.30 Late congenital syphilitic oculopathy, unspecified

A50.31 Late congenital syphilitic interstitial keratitis

A50.32 Late congenital syphilitic chorioretinitis

A50.39 Other late congenital syphilitic oculopathy

● **A50.4 Late congenital neurosyphilis [juvenile neurosyphilis]**
Use additional code to identify any associated mental disorder
Excludes1 Hutchinson's triad (A50.53)
Ex: For category A50.4 CC codes unless otherwise indicated: A50.01-A51.46, A51.5-A53.9, A56.00-A56.8, A63.8-A64, B92, B94.2-B94.9, N34.1

A50.40 Late congenital neurosyphilis, unspecified
Juvenile neurosyphilis NOS

A50.41 Late congenital syphilitic meningitis
Ex: A02.21, A17.0-A17.1, A27.81, A39.0, A50.01-A51.46, A51.5-A53.9, A54.82, A54.84, A54.89-A54.9, A56.00-A56.8, A63.8-A64, A87.0-A87.9, B00.3, B02.1, B26.1, B37.5, B38.4, B45.1, B58.2, B92, B94.2-B94.9, G00.0-G03.9, G04.2, G32.89, G61.0, G96.8-G96.9, G98.0-G98.8, G99.8, N34.1

A50.42 Late congenital syphilitic encephalitis

A50.43 Late congenital syphilitic polyneuropathy

A50.44 Late congenital syphilitic optic nerve atrophy
Ex: A50.01-A51.46, A51.5-A53.9

A50.45 Juvenile general paresis
Dementia paralytica juvenilis
Juvenile tabetoparetic neurosyphilis

A50.49 Other late congenital neurosyphilis
Juvenile tabes dorsalis

● **A50.5 Other late congenital syphilis, symptomatic**
Any congenital syphilitic condition specified as late or manifest two years or more after birth
Ex: For category A50.5 CC codes: A50.01-A51.46, A51.5-A53.9

A50.51 Clutton's joints

A50.52 Hutchinson's teeth

A50.53 Hutchinson's triad

A50.54 Late congenital cardiovascular syphilis

A50.55 Late congenital syphilitic arthropathy

A50.56 Late congenital syphilitic osteochondropathy

A50.57 Syphilitic saddle nose

A50.59 Other late congenital syphilis, symptomatic

A50.6 Late congenital syphilis, latent
Congenital syphilis without clinical manifestations, with positive serological reaction and negative spinal fluid test, two years or more after birth.

A50.7 Late congenital syphilis, unspecified
Congenital syphilis NOS two years or more after birth.

A50.9 Congenital syphilis, unspecified

● **A51 Early syphilis**

A51.0 Primary genital syphilis
Syphilitic chancre NOS

A51.1 Primary anal syphilis

A51.2 Primary syphilis of other sites

● **A51.3 Secondary syphilis of skin and mucous membranes**

A51.31 Condyloma latum
Ex: A50.01-A51.46, A51.5-A53.9

A51.32 Syphilitic alopecia
Ex: A50.01-A51.46, A51.5-A54.85, A54.89-A58, A63.8, A64, M02.30-M02.39, N34.1

A51.39 Other secondary syphilis of skin
Syphilitic leukoderma
Syphilitic mucous patch
Excludes1 late syphilitic leukoderma (A52.79)
Ex: A50.01-A51.46, A51.5-A53.9

● **A51.4 Other secondary syphilis**

A51.41 Secondary syphilitic meningitis
Ex: A02.21, A17.0-A17.1, A27.81, A39.0, A50.01-A51.46, A51.5-A54.49, A54.5-A54.85, A54.89-A58, A63.8-A64, A74.81-A74.9, A87.0-A87.9, A96.2, A98.3-A98.4, B26.1, B33.24, B33.4-B33.8, B34.1-B34.2, B34.4-B34.8, B37.5, B38.4, B45.1, B58.2, B92, B94.2-B94.9, B97.10, B97.19, B97.29, B97.5-B97.6, B97.81-B97.89, G00.0-G03.9, G04.2, G32.89, G61.0, G96.8-G96.9, G98.0-G98.8, G99.8, M02.30-M02.39, N34.1

A51.42 Secondary syphilitic female pelvic disease ♀
Ex: See A50.2

A51.43 Secondary syphilitic oculopathy
Secondary syphilitic chorioretinitis
Secondary syphilitic iridocyclitis, iritis
Secondary syphilitic uveitis
Ex: See A50.01-A51.46, A51.5-A53.9

A51.44 Secondary syphilitic nephritis
Ex: See A50.2

A51.45 Secondary syphilitic hepatitis
Ex: A50.01-A51.46, A51.5-A54.85, A54.89-A58, A63.8, A64, K71.0-K71.9, K73.1-K73.8, K74.0-K74.69, K75.2-K76.0, K76.4-K76.5, K76.89-K76.9, M02.30-M02.39, N34.1

A51.46 Secondary syphilitic osteopathy
Ex: A18.09, A50.01-A51.46, A51.5-A54.85, A54.89-A58, A63.8, A64, A66.6, M02.30-M02.39, M84.80-M84.9, M85.10-M85.19, M85.80-M85.89, M86.30-M86.8X9, M89.20-M89.39, M89.50-M89.59, M89.8X0-M89.8X9, M94.1, M94.351-M94.8X9, N34.1

A51.49 Other secondary syphilitic conditions
Secondary syphilitic lymphadenopathy
Secondary syphilitic myositis

A51.5 Early syphilis, latent
Syphilis (acquired) without clinical manifestations, with positive serological reaction and negative spinal fluid test, less than two years after infection.

A51.9 Early syphilis, unspecified

A52 Late syphilis

A52.0 Cardiovascular and cerebrovascular syphilis
Ex: **For category A52.0 CC codes:** A50.01-A51.46, A51.5-A53.9, A56.00-A56.8, A63.8-A64, B92, B94.2-B94.9, N34.1

A52.00 Cardiovascular syphilis, unspecified

A52.01 Syphilitic aneurysm of aorta

A52.02 Syphilitic aortitis

A52.03 Syphilitic endocarditis
Syphilitic aortic valve incompetence or stenosis
Syphilitic mitral valve stenosis
Syphilitic pulmonary valve regurgitation

A52.04 Syphilitic cerebral arteritis

A52.05 Other cerebrovascular syphilis
Syphilitic cerebral aneurysm (ruptured) (non-ruptured)
Syphilitic cerebral thrombosis

A52.06 Other syphilitic heart involvement
Syphilitic coronary artery disease
Syphilitic myocarditis
Syphilitic pericarditis

A52.09 Other cardiovascular syphilis

A52.1 Symptomatic neurosyphilis
Ex: **For category A52.1 CC codes unless otherwise indicated:** A50.01-A51.46, A51.5-A53.9, A56.00-A56.8, A63.8-A64, B92, B94.2-B94.9, N34.1

A52.10 Symptomatic neurosyphilis, unspecified

A52.11 Tabes dorsalis
Cognitive decline with progressive degeneration of posterior columns, roots, and ganglia of spinal cord, occur 15-20 years after initial infection of syphilis; AKA Duchenne disease
Locomotor ataxia (progressive)
Tabetic neurosyphilis

A52.12 Other cerebrospinal syphilis

A52.13 Late syphilitic meningitis
Ex: See A50.41

A52.14 Late syphilitic encephalitis

A52.15 Late syphilitic neuropathy
Late syphilitic acoustic neuritis
Late syphilitic optic (nerve) atrophy
Late syphilitic polyneuropathy
Late syphilitic retrobulbar neuritis

A52.16 Charcôt's arthropathy (tabetic)
Progressive musculoskeletal condition characterized by joint dislocation, fractures, and deformities, results in progressive destruction of bone and soft tissue of weight-bearing joints

A52.17 General paresis
Chronic meningoencephalitis results in loss of cortical function, or progressive dementia and generalized paralysis, occurring 10-20 years after initial infection of syphilis; AKA Bayle disease, dementia paralytica, paralytic dementiaparetic neurosyphilis, syphilitic meningoencephalitis
Dementia paralytica

A52.19 Other symptomatic neurosyphilis
Syphilitic parkinsonism

A52.2 Asymptomatic neurosyphilis
Ex: See A52.10

A52.3 Neurosyphilis, unspecified
Gumma (syphilitic)
Destructive lesions of syphilis
Syphilis (late)
Syphiloma
Ex: See A52.10

A52.7 Other symptomatic late syphilis
Ex: **For category A52.7 CC codes unless otherwise indicated:** A50.01-A51.46, A51.5-A54.85, A54.89-A58, A63.8, A64, M02.30-M02.39, N34.1

A52.71 Late syphilitic oculopathy
Late syphilitic chorioretinitis
Late syphilitic episcleritis
Ex: A18.50-A18.59, A50.01-A51.46, A51.5-A54.85, A54.89-A58, A63.8-A64, H15.001-H15.009, H15.091-H15.129, M02.30-M02.39, N34.1

A52.72 Syphilis of lung and bronchus

A52.73 Symptomatic late syphilis of other respiratory organs

A52.74 Syphilis of liver and other viscera
Late syphilitic peritonitis

A52.75 Syphilis of kidney and ureter
Syphilitic glomerular disease

A52.76 Other genitourinary symptomatic late syphilis
Late syphilitic female pelvic inflammatory disease

A52.77 Syphilis of bone and joint

A52.78 Syphilis of other musculoskeletal tissue
Late syphilitic bursitis
Syphilis [stage unspecified] of bursa
Syphilis [stage unspecified] of muscle
Syphilis [stage unspecified] of synovium
Syphilis [stage unspecified] of tendon

A52.79 Other symptomatic late syphilis
Late syphilitic leukoderma
Syphilis of adrenal gland
Syphilis of pituitary gland
Syphilis of thyroid gland
Syphilitic splenomegaly
Excludes1 syphilitic leukoderma (secondary) (A51.39)

A52.8 Late syphilis, latent
Syphilis (acquired) without clinical manifestations, with positive serological reaction and negative spinal fluid test, two years or more after infection

A52.9 Late syphilis, unspecified

● **A53 Other and unspecified syphilis**

A53.0 Latent syphilis, unspecified as early or late
Latent syphilis NOS
Positive serological reaction for syphilis

A53.9 Syphilis, unspecified
Infection due to Treponema pallidum NOS
Syphilis (acquired) NOS
Excludes1 syphilis NOS under two years of age (A50.2)

● **A54 Gonococcal infection**

● **A54.0 Gonococcal infection of lower genitourinary tract without periurethral or accessory gland abscess**
Excludes1 gonococcal infection with genitourinary gland abscess (A54.1)
gonococcal infection with periurethral abscess (A54.1)
Ex: **For category A54.0 CC codes:** A54.00-A54.29, A54.82, A54.84, A54.89, A54.9, A56.00-A56.8, A63.8-A64, B92, B94.-B94.9, N34.1

A54.00 Gonococcal infection of lower genitourinary tract, unspecified

A54.01 Gonococcal cystitis and urethritis, unspecified

A54.02 Gonococcal vulvovaginitis, unspecified ♀

A54.03 Gonococcal cervicitis, unspecified ♀

A54.09 Other gonococcal infection of lower genitourinary tract

A54.1 Gonococcal infection of lower genitourinary tract with periurethral and accessory gland abscess
Gonococcal Bartholin's gland abscess

● **A54.2 Gonococcal pelviperitonitis and other gonococcal genitourinary infection**
Ex: **For category A54.2 CC codes:** A54.00-A54.29, A54.82, A54.84, A54.89, A54.9, A56.00-A56.8, A63.8-A64, B92, B94.-B94.9, N34.1

A54.21 Gonococcal infection of kidney and ureter

A54.22 Gonococcal prostatitis ♂

A54.23 Gonococcal infection of other male genital organs ♂
Gonococcal epididymitis
Gonococcal orchitis

A54.24 Gonococcal female pelvic inflammatory disease ♀
Gonococcal pelviperitonitis
Excludes1 gonococcal peritonitis (A54.85)

A54.29 Other gonococcal genitourinary infections

● **A54.3 Gonococcal infection of eye**
Ex: **For category A54.3 CC codes:** A50.01-A51.46, A51.5-A54.85, A54.89-A58, A63.8, A64, M02.30-M02.39, N34.1

A54.30 Gonococcal infection of eye, unspecified

A54.31 Gonococcal conjunctivitis
Form of bacterial conjunctivitis contracted by newborns during delivery; AKA neonatal conjunctivitis
Ophthalmia neonatorum due to gonococcus

A54.32 Gonococcal iridocyclitis
Inflammation of iris and of ciliary body due to gonococcal infection

A54.33 Gonococcal keratitis
Inflammation of cornea due to gonococcal infection; AKA keratoconjunctivitis, keratopathy

A54.39 Other gonococcal eye infection
Gonococcal endophthalmia

● **A54.4 Gonococcal infection of musculoskeletal system**
Ex: **For category A54.4 CC codes:** A02.23, A17.9, A18.02, A18.09, A18.82, A18.84, A18.89, A39.83-A39.84, A50.01-A51.9, A52.00-A54.89, A54.9-A58, A63.8, A64, B06.82, M00.00-M02.9, M05.40-M05.59, M05.70-M06.09, M06.20-M06.39, M06.80-M07.69, M11.00-M11.9, M12.10-M15.0, M15.3-M15.9, M16.2-M16.9, M17.2-M17.9, M18.2-M18.9, M19.111-M19.93, M24.10-M24.176, M25.00, M25.08, M25.10-M25.18, M25.40-M25.676, M25.80-M25.9, M35.2, M36.1-M36.4, N34.1, R29.4

A54.40 Gonococcal infection of musculoskeletal system, unspecified

A54.41 Gonococcal spondylopathy
Disorder of vertebrae due to gonococcal infection; AKA rachiopathy

A54.42 Gonococcal arthritis
Excludes2 gonococcal infection of spine (A54.41)

A54.43 Gonococcal osteomyelitis
Excludes2 gonococcal infection of spine (A54.41)

A54.49 Gonococcal infection of other musculoskeletal tissue
Gonococcal bursitis
Gonococcal myositis
Gonococcal synovitis
Gonococcal tenosynovitis

A54.5 Gonococcal pharyngitis

A54.6 Gonococcal infection of anus and rectum

● **A54.8 Other gonococcal infections**

A54.81 Gonococcal meningitis
Ex: See A54.41

A54.82 Gonococcal brain abscess
Ex: A50.01-A51.46, A51.5-A54.85, A54.89-A58, A63.8, A64, M02.30-M02.39, N25.81-N25.89, N34.1

A54.83 Gonococcal heart infection
Gonococcal endocarditis
Gonococcal myocarditis
Gonococcal pericarditis
Ex: A01.00-A01.09, A39.51, A50.01-A58, A63.8-A64, A78, B33.20-B33.22, B37.6, B40.0-B40.9, I00, I01.1-I02.0, I05.0-I05.1, I05.2, I05.8-I08.3, I08.9-I09.1, I09.89-I09.9, I23.0-I23.3, I23.6-I23.8, I33.0-I41, I42.4, I51.0, I51.4, I87.8-I87.9, I99.8-I99.9, M00.00, M00.08-M00.10, M00.18-M00.20, M00.28-M00.80, M00.88-M00.9, M02.30-M02.39, N34.1, Q22.2, Q23.8, Q23.9, Q24.8, T82.6XX[A]

A54.84 Gonococcal pneumonia
Ex: See A54.82

A54.85 Gonococcal peritonitis
Excludes1 gonococcal pelviperitonitis (A54.24)
Ex: A18.31, A34, A50.01-A58, A63.8, A64, K35.2-K35.3, K63.4, K63.89-K63.9, K65.1, K65.3, K65.9, K67, K86.81-K86.89, K92.89-K92.9, M02.30-M02.39, N34.1, N73.3-N73.4, N73.6, O08.0, O08.82, O85, O86.12, O86.81, O86.89, P78.0, R11.13, T81.60X[A]-T81.69X[A]

A54.86 Gonococcal sepsis
MCC when PDx is its own MCC
Ex: A02.1, A20.7, A22.7, A26.7, A32.7, A39.2-A39.4, A40.0-A40.1, A40.8-A41.9, A42.7, A48.2-A48.4, A48.8-A49.9, A54.86, B00.7, B3.77, B92, B94.2-B96.89, R65.10-R65.20, Z16.10-Z16.39

A54.89 Other gonococcal infections
Gonococcal keratoderma
Gonococcal lymphadenitis
Ex: See A54.82

A54.9 Gonococcal infection, unspecified
Ex: See A54.82

A55 Chlamydial lymphogranuloma (venereum)
Climatic or tropical bubo
Durand-Nicolas-Favre disease
Esthiomene
Lymphogranuloma inguinale

Item 1-10 An STD (sexually transmitted disease) caused by **Neisseria gonorrhoeae** that flourishes in the warm, moist areas of the reproductive tract. Untreated gonorrhea spreads to other parts of the body, causing inflammation of the testes or prostate or pelvic inflammatory disease (PID).

A56 Other sexually transmitted chlamydial diseases

Includes sexually transmitted diseases due to Chlamydia trachomatis

Excludes1 neonatal chlamydial conjunctivitis (P39.1)
neonatal chlamydial pneumonia (P23.1)

Excludes2 chlamydial lymphogranuloma (A55)
conditions classified to A74.-

A56.0 Chlamydial infection of lower genitourinary tract

A56.00 Chlamydial infection of lower genitourinary tract, unspecified

A56.01 Chlamydial cystitis and urethritis

A56.02 Chlamydial vulvovaginitis ♀

A56.09 Other chlamydial infection of lower genitourinary tract
Chlamydial cervicitis

A56.1 Chlamydial infection of pelviperitoneum and other genitourinary organs

A56.11 Chlamydial female pelvic inflammatory disease ♀

A56.19 Other chlamydial genitourinary infection
Chlamydial epididymitis
Chlamydial orchitis

A56.2 Chlamydial infection of genitourinary tract, unspecified

A56.3 Chlamydial infection of anus and rectum

A56.4 Chlamydial infection of pharynx

A56.8 Sexually transmitted chlamydial infection of other sites

A57 Chancroid
Ulcus molle
Sexually transmitted infection caused by bacteria, Haemophilus ducreyi

A58 Granuloma inguinale
Chronic, progressive, ulcerative granulomatous disease
Donovanosis

A59 Trichomoniasis

Excludes2 intestinal trichomoniasis (A07.8)

A common STD caused by a parasite, Trichomonas vaginalis

A59.0 Urogenital trichomoniasis

A59.00 Urogenital trichomoniasis, unspecified
Fluor (vaginalis) due to Trichomonas
Leukorrhea (vaginalis) due to Trichomonas

A59.01 Trichomonal vulvovaginitis ♀

A59.02 Trichomonal prostatitis ♂

A59.03 Trichomonal cystitis and urethritis

A59.09 Other urogenital trichomoniasis
Common sexually transmitted disease (STD) caused by single-celled protozoan parasite; AKA trich
Trichomonas cervicitis

A59.8 Trichomoniasis of other sites

A59.9 Trichomoniasis, unspecified

A60 Anogenital herpesviral [herpes simplex] infections

A60.0 Herpesviral infection of genitalia and urogenital tract

A60.00 Herpesviral infection of urogenital system, unspecified

A60.01 Herpesviral infection of penis ♂

A60.02 Herpesviral infection of other male genital organs ♂

A60.03 Herpesviral cervicitis ♀

A60.04 Herpesviral vulvovaginitis ♀
Herpesviral [herpes simplex] ulceration
Herpesviral [herpes simplex] vaginitis
Herpesviral [herpes simplex] vulvitis

A60.09 Herpesviral infection of other urogenital tract

A60.1 Herpesviral infection of perianal skin and rectum

A60.9 Anogenital herpesviral infection, unspecified

A63 Other predominantly sexually transmitted diseases, not elsewhere classified

Excludes2 molluscum contagiosum (B08.1)
papilloma of cervix (D26.0)

A63.0 Anogenital (venereal) warts
Anogenital warts due to (human) papillomavirus [HPV]
Condyloma acuminatum

A63.8 Other specified predominantly sexually transmitted diseases

A64 Unspecified sexually transmitted disease

OTHER SPIROCHETAL DISEASES (A65-A69)

Excludes2 leptospirosis (A27.-)
syphilis (A50-A53)

A65 Nonvenereal syphilis
Bejel
Endemic syphilis
Njovera

A66 Yaws
Endemic, infectious, tropical disease caused by spirochete, spread by direct contact; AKA frambesia, framboesia, frambesia tropica

Includes bouba
frambesia (tropica)
pian

A66.0 Initial lesions of yaws
Chancre of yaws
Frambesia, initial or primary
Initial frambesial ulcer
Mother yaw

A66.1 Multiple papillomata and wet crab yaws
Frambesioma
Pianoma
Plantar or palmar papilloma of yaws

A66.2 Other early skin lesions of yaws
Cutaneous yaws, less than five years after infection
Early yaws (cutaneous)(macular)(maculopapular)(micropapular)(papular)
Frambeside of early yaws

A66.3 Hyperkeratosis of yaws
Hypertrophy of stratum corneum of skin in which there are small, hard, verrucous scales
Ghoul hand
Hyperkeratosis, palmar or plantar (early) (late) due to yaws
Worm-eaten soles

A66.4 Gummata and ulcers of yaws
Small, rubbery granuloma with necrotic center and inflamed characteristic of advanced stage of syphilis; AKA syphiloma
Gummatous frambeside
Nodular late yaws (ulcerated)

A66.5 Gangosa
Manifestation of yaws that develops in the soft palate and spreads eroding bone, cartilage, and soft tissue
Rhinopharyngitis mutilans

A66.6 Bone and joint lesions of yaws
Yaws ganglion
Yaws goundou
Yaws gumma, bone
Yaws gummatous osteitis or periostitis
Yaws hydrarthrosis
Yaws osteitis
Yaws periostitis (hypertrophic)

A66.7 Other manifestations of yaws
Juxta-articular nodules of yaws
Mucosal yaws

A66.8 Latent yaws
Yaws without clinical manifestations, with positive serology

A66.9 Yaws, unspecified

A67 Pinta [carate]
Group of nonvenereal diseases caused by Treponema species

A67.0 Primary lesions of pinta
Chancre (primary) of pinta
Papule (primary) of pinta

A67.1 Intermediate lesions of pinta
Erythematous plaques of pinta
Hyperchromic lesions of pinta
Hyperkeratosis of pinta
Pintids

A67.2 Late lesions of pinta
Achromic skin lesions of pinta
Cicatricial skin lesions of pinta
Dyschromic skin lesions of pinta

A67.3 Mixed lesions of pinta
Achromic with hyperchromic skin lesions of pinta [carate]

A67.9 Pinta, unspecified

A68 Relapsing fevers
Includes recurrent fever
Excludes2 Lyme disease (A69.2-)
Ex: **For category A68 CC codes:** A44.0-A44.9, A68.0-A68.9, A69.20-A69.29, A75.0-A79.9, B55.0-B57.5, B60.0

A68.0 Louse-borne relapsing fever
Relapsing fever due to Borrelia recurrentis

A68.1 Tick-borne relapsing fever
Relapsing fever due to any Borrelia species other than Borrelia recurrentis

A68.9 Relapsing fever, unspecified

A69 Other spirochetal infections

A69.0 Necrotizing ulcerative stomatitis
Cancrum oris
Fusospirochetal gangrene
Noma
Stomatitis gangrenosa

A69.1 Other Vincent's infections
Fusospirochetal pharyngitis
Necrotizing ulcerative (acute) gingivitis
Necrotizing ulcerative (acute) gingivostomatitis
Spirochetal stomatitis
Trench mouth
Vincent's angina
Vincent's gingivitis
Ex: A69.1

A69.2 Lyme disease
Erythema chronicum migrans due to Borrelia burgdorferi
Ex: **For category A69.2 CC codes:** See A68

A69.20 Lyme disease, unspecified

A69.21 Meningitis due to Lyme disease

A69.22 Other neurologic disorders in Lyme disease
Cranial neuritis
Meningoencephalitis
Polyneuropathy

A69.23 Arthritis due to Lyme disease

A69.29 Other conditions associated with Lyme disease
Myopericarditis due to Lyme disease

A69.8 Other specified spirochetal infections

A69.9 Spirochetal infection, unspecified

Item 1-11 Cancrum oris, also known as **noma** or **gangrenous stomatitis,** begins as an ulcer of the gingiva and results in a progressive gangrenous process.

OTHER DISEASES CAUSED BY CHLAMYDIAE (A70-A74)

Excludes1 sexually transmitted chlamydial diseases (A55-A56)

A70 Chlamydia psittaci infections
Ornithosis
Parrot fever
Psittacosis
Ex: A70

A71 Trachoma
Excludes1 sequelae of trachoma (B94.0)

A71.0 Initial stage of trachoma
Trachoma dubium

A71.1 Active stage of trachoma
Granular conjunctivitis (trachomatous)
Trachomatous follicular conjunctivitis
Trachomatous pannus

A71.9 Trachoma, unspecified

A74 Other diseases caused by chlamydiae
Excludes1 neonatal chlamydial conjunctivitis (P39.1)
neonatal chlamydial pneumonia (P23.1)
Reiter's disease (M02.3-)
sexually transmitted chlamydial diseases (A55-A56)
Excludes2 chlamydial pneumonia (J16.0)

A74.0 Chlamydial conjunctivitis
Paratrachoma

A74.8 Other chlamydial diseases

A74.81 Chlamydial peritonitis

A74.89 Other chlamydial diseases

A74.9 Chlamydial infection, unspecified
Chlamydiosis NOS

RICKETTSIOSES (A75-A79)

A75 Typhus fever
Excludes1 rickettsiosis due to Ehrlichia sennetsu (A79.81)
Ex: **For category A75 CC codes unless otherwise indicated:** See A68

A75.0 Epidemic louse-borne typhus fever due to Rickettsia prowazekii
Organisms transmitted between humans via louse
Classical typhus (fever)
Epidemic (louse-borne) typhus

A75.1 Recrudescent typhus [Brill's disease]
Brill-Zinsser disease

A75.2 Typhus fever due to Rickettsia typhi
Murine (flea-borne) typhus

A75.3 Typhus fever due to Rickettsia tsutsugamushi
Scrub (mite-borne) typhus
Tsutsugamushi fever

A75.9 Typhus fever, unspecified
Typhus (fever) NOS
Ex: A17.82, A44.0-A44.9, A50.42, A52.14, A68.0-A68.9, A69.20-A69.29, A75.0-A79.9, A81.1, A81.82-A81.89, A83.0-A85.8, A87.2, A88.0, A88.8, A92.1-A92.8, A93.0, B00.4, B00.82, B01.11-B01.12, B04, B06.01, B08.09, B08.20-B08.22, B08.60-B08.79, B09, B10.01-B10.09, B26.2, B33.1, B45.0, B45.2-B45.9, B50.9, B55.0-B57.5, B58.2, B60.0, B75, B97.10, B97.21, G04.00-G04.01, G04.31, G04.81-G05.4, G37.0, G37.4-G37.5, J09.X3-J09.X9, J10.2-J10.89, J11.2-J11.89, L44.4, M1A.10X0-M1A.19X1, P35.2-P35.9, P37.0-P37.4, P37.8-P37.9, T56.0X1-T56.0X4[A]

Item 1-12 Rickettsioses are diseases spread from ticks, lice, fleas, or mites to humans.

Typhus is spread to humans chiefly by the fleas of rats.

Endemic identifies a disease as being present in low numbers of humans at all times, whereas **epidemic** identifies a disease as being present in high numbers of humans at a specific time. Morbidity (death) is higher in epidemic diseases.

Brill's disease, also known as **Brill-Zinsser disease,** is spread from human to human by body lice and also from the lice of flying squirrels. **Scrub typhus** is spread in the same ways as Brill's disease.

Malaria is spread to humans by mosquitoes.

● **A77 Spotted fever [tick-borne rickettsioses]**
Ex: For category A77 CC codes: See A68

A77.0 Spotted fever due to Rickettsia rickettsii
Rocky Mountain spotted fever
Sao Paulo fever

A77.1 Spotted fever due to Rickettsia conorii
African tick typhus
Boutonneuse fever
India tick typhus
Kenya tick typhus
Marseilles fever
Mediterranean tick fever

A77.2 Spotted fever due to Rickettsia siberica
North Asian tick fever
Siberian tick typhus

A77.3 Spotted fever due to Rickettsia australis
Queensland tick typhus

● **A77.4 Ehrlichiosis**
Type of tick-borne fever caused by bacteria infection
Excludes1 Rickettsiosis due to Ehrlichia sennetsu (A79.81)

A77.40 Ehrlichiosis, unspecified

A77.41 Ehrlichiosis chafeensis [E. chafeensis]

A77.49 Other ehrlichiosis

A77.8 Other spotted fevers

A77.9 Spotted fever, unspecified
Tick-borne typhus NOS

A78 Q fever
Infection due to Coxiella burnetii
Nine Mile fever
Quadrilateral fever
Ex: See A68

● **A79 Other rickettsioses**
Ex: For category A79 CC codes unless otherwise indicated: A77.0-A79.9

A79.0 Trench fever
Quintan fever
Wolhynian fever
Ex: See A68

A79.1 Rickettsialpox due to Rickettsia akari
Kew Garden fever
Vesicular rickettsiosis

● **A79.8 Other specified rickettsioses**

A79.81 Rickettsiosis due to Ehrlichia sennetsu

A79.89 Other specified rickettsioses

A79.9 Rickettsiosis, unspecified
Rickettsial infection NOS

VIRAL AND PRION INFECTIONS OF THE CENTRAL NERVOUS SYSTEM (A80-A89)

Excludes1 postpolio syndrome (G14)
sequelae of poliomyelitis (B91)
sequelae of viral encephalitis (B94.1)

● **A80 Acute poliomyelitis**
Ex: For category A80 CC codes: A80.0-A80.39

A80.0 Acute paralytic poliomyelitis, vaccine-associated

A80.1 Acute paralytic poliomyelitis, wild virus, imported

A80.2 Acute paralytic poliomyelitis, wild virus, indigenous

● **A80.3 Acute paralytic poliomyelitis, other and unspecified**

A80.30 Acute paralytic poliomyelitis, unspecified

A80.39 Other acute paralytic poliomyelitis

A80.4 Acute nonparalytic poliomyelitis

A80.9 Acute poliomyelitis, unspecified

Item 1-13 Acute Poliomyelitis: Also called infantile paralysis and is caused by the poliovirus, which enters the body orally and infects the intestinal wall and then enters the blood stream and central nervous system, causing muscle weakness and paralysis. This disease has been nearly eradicated with the polio vaccine.

● **A81 Atypical virus infections of central nervous system**
Includes diseases of the central nervous system caused by prions
Use additional code to identify:
dementia with behavioral disturbance (F02.81)
dementia without behavioral disturbance (F02.80)

● **A81.0 Creutzfeldt-Jakob disease**
Ex: For category A81.0 CC codes: A17.82, A50.42, A52.14, A75.9, A79.9, A81.00-A81.9, A83.0-A85.8, A87.2, A88.0, A88.8, A92.1-A92.2, A92.4-A92.8, A93.0, B00.4, B00.82, B01.11-B01.12, B04, B06.01, B08.09, B08.20-B08.22, B08.60-B08.79, B09, B10.01-B10.09, B26.2, B33.1, B45.0, B45.2-B45.9, B58.2, B75, B97.10, G04.00-G04.01, G04.31, G04.81-G05.4, G37.0, G37.4-G37.5, I67.3, J09.X3-J09.X9, J10.2-J10.89, J11.2-J11.89, L44.4, M1A.10X0-M1A.19X1, P35.2-P35.9, P37.0-P37.4, P37.8-P37.9, T56.0X1-T56.0X4[A]

A81.00 Creutzfeldt-Jakob disease, unspecified
Jakob-Creutzfeldt disease, unspecified

A81.01 Variant Creutzfeldt-Jakob disease
vCJD

A81.09 Other Creutzfeldt-Jakob disease
CJD
Familial Creutzfeldt-Jakob disease
Iatrogenic Creutzfeldt-Jakob disease
Sporadic Creutzfeldt-Jakob disease
Subacute spongiform encephalopathy (with dementia)

A81.1 Subacute sclerosing panencephalitis
Type of viral encephalitis that causes parenchymatous lesions in gray and white matter of brain
Dawson's inclusion body encephalitis
Van Bogaert's sclerosing leukoencephalopathy
Ex: A81.1, B92, B94.2-B94.9

A81.2 Progressive multifocal leukoencephalopathy
Group of diseases affecting white matter of brain
Multifocal leukoencephalopathy NOS
Ex: A17.82, A50.42, A52.14, A75.9, A79.9, A81.00-A81.9, A83.0-A85.8, A87.2, A88.0, A88.8, A92.1-A92.2, A92.4-A92.8, A93.0, B00.4, B00.82, B01.11-B01.12, B04, B06.01, B08.09, B08.20-B08.22, B08.60-B08.79, B09, B10.01-B10.09, B26.2, B27.00-B27.99, B33.1, B45.0, B45.2-B45.9, B58.2, B75, G04.00-G04.01, G04.31, G04.81-G05.4, G37.0, G37.4-G37.5, I67.3, J09.X3-J09.X9, J10.2-J10.89, J11.2-J11.89, L44.4, M1A.10X0-M1A.19X1, P35.2-P35.9, P37.0-P37.4, P37.8-P37.9, T56.0X1-T56.0X4[A]

● **A81.8 Other atypical virus infections of central nervous system**
Ex: For category A81.8 CC codes unless otherwise indicated: A81.00-A81.9, A92.30-A92.39, B97.21, I67.3

A81.81 Kuru
Ex: A81.00-A81.9, I67.3

A81.82 Gerstmann-Sträussler-Scheinker syndrome
GSS syndrome

A81.83 Fatal familial insomnia
FFI

A81.89 Other atypical virus infections of central nervous system

A81.9 Atypical virus infection of central nervous system, unspecified
Prion diseases of the central nervous system NOS
Ex: A81.00-A81.9, I67.3

● **A82 Rabies**
Viral disease affecting the central nervous system and transmitted from infected mammals to man.
Ex: For category A82 CC codes: A82.0-A82.9

A82.0 Sylvatic rabies

A82.1 Urban rabies

A82.9 Rabies, unspecified

● **A83 Mosquito-borne viral encephalitis**
Inflammation of the brain caused most commonly by Herpes Simplex virus.
Includes mosquito-borne viral meningoencephalitis
Excludes2 Venezuelan equine encephalitis (A92.2)
West Nile fever (A92.3-)
West Nile virus (A92.3-)
Ex: **For category A83 CC codes:** A17.82, A50.42, A52.14, A75.9, A79.9, A81.1, A81.82-A81.89, A83.0-A85.8, A87.2, A88.0, A88.8, A92.1-A92.8, A93.0, B00.4, B00.82, B01.11-B01.12, B04, B06.01, B08.09, B08.20-B08.22, B08.60-B08.79, B09, B10.01-B10.09, B26.2, B27.00-B27.99, B33.1, B45.0, B45.2-B45.9, B58.2, B75, B97.10-B97.21, G04.00-G04.01, G04.31, G04.81-G04.91, G05.3-G05.4, G37.0, G37.4-G37.5, J09.X3-J09.X9, J10.2-J10.89, J11.2-J11.89, L44.4, M1A.10X0-M1A.19X1, P35.2-P35.9, P37.0-P37.9, T56.0X1-T56.0X4[A]

A83.0 Japanese encephalitis
A83.1 Western equine encephalitis
A83.2 Eastern equine encephalitis
A83.3 St. Louis encephalitis
A83.4 Australian encephalitis
Kunjin virus disease
A83.5 California encephalitis
California meningoencephalitis
La Crosse encephalitis
A83.6 Rocio virus disease
Mosquito-borne virus
A83.8 Other mosquito-borne viral encephalitis
A83.9 Mosquito-borne viral encephalitis, unspecified

● **A84 Tick-borne viral encephalitis**
Includes tick-borne viral meningoencephalitis
Ex: **For category A84 CC codes:** See A83

A84.0 Far Eastern tick-borne encephalitis [Russian spring-summer encephalitis]
A84.1 Central European tick-borne encephalitis
A84.8 Other tick-borne viral encephalitis
Louping ill
Powassan virus disease
A84.9 Tick-borne viral encephalitis, unspecified

● **A85 Other viral encephalitis, not elsewhere classified**
Includes specified viral encephalomyelitis NEC
specified viral meningoencephalitis NEC
Excludes1 benign myalgic encephalomyelitis (G93.3)
encephalitis due to cytomegalovirus (B25.8)
encephalitis due to herpesvirus NEC (B10.0-)
encephalitis due to herpesvirus [herpes simplex] (B00.4)
encephalitis due to measles virus (B05.0)
encephalitis due to mumps virus (B26.2)
encephalitis due to poliomyelitis virus (A80.-)
encephalitis due to zoster (B02.0)
lymphocytic choriomeningitis (A87.2)
Ex: **For category A85 CC codes unless otherwise indicated:** A17.82, A50.42, A52.14, A75.9, A79.9, A81.1, A81.82-A81.89, A83.0-A85.8, A87.2, A88.0, A88.8, A92.1-A92.8, A93.0, B00.4, B00.82, B01.11-B01.12, B04, B06.01, B08.09, B08.20-B08.22, B08.60-B08.79, B09, B10.01-B10.09, B26.2, B27.00-B27.99, B33.1, B45.0, B45.2-B45.9, B58.2, B75, B97.10-B97.21, G04.00-G04.01, G04.31, G04.81-G04.91, G05.3-G05.4, G37.0, G37.4-G37.5, H66.40-H66.43, J09.X3-J09.X9, J10.2-J10.89, J11.2-J11.89, L44.4, M1A.10X0-M1A.19X1, M32.0-M32.9, P35.2-P35.9, P37.0-P37.9, T56.0X1-T56.0X4[A]

A85.0 Enteroviral encephalitis
Enteroviral encephalomyelitis
A85.1 Adenoviral encephalitis
Adenoviral meningoencephalitis
A85.2 Arthropod-borne viral encephalitis, unspecified
Excludes1 West nile virus with encephalitis (A92.31)
Ex: See A83
A85.8 Other specified viral encephalitis
Encephalitis lethargica
Von Economo-Cruchet disease

Item 1-14 **Encephalitis** is an inflammation of the brain most often caused by a virus but may also be caused by a bacteria and most commonly transmitted by a mosquito. **Myelitis** is an inflammation of the spinal cord that may disrupt CNS function. Untreated myelitis may rapidly lead to permanent damage to the spinal cord. **Encephalomyelitis** is a general term for an inflammation of the brain and spinal cord.

A86 Unspecified viral encephalitis
Viral encephalomyelitis NOS
Viral meningoencephalitis NOS
Ex: A17.82, A50.42, A52.14, A75.9, A79.9, A81.1, A81.82-A81.89, A83.0-A86, A87.2, A88.0, A88.8-A89, A92.1-A92.2, A92.4-A92.8, A93.0, B00.4, B00.82, B01.11-B01.12, B04, B06.01, B08.09, B08.20-B08.22, B08.60-B08.79, B09, B10.01-B10.09, B26.2, B27.00-B27.99, B33.1, B45.0, B45.2-B45.9, B58.2, B75, B97.10, G04.00-G04.01, G04.31, G04.81-G04.91, G05.3-G05.4, G37.0, G37.4-G37.5, H66.40-H66.43, J09.X3-J09.X9, J10.2-J10.89, J11.2-J11.89, L44.4, M1A.10X0-M1A.19X1, M32.0-M32.9, P35.2-P35.9, P37.0-P37.9, T56.0X1-T56.0X4[A]

● **A87 Viral meningitis**
Excludes1 meningitis due to herpesvirus [herpes simplex] (B00.3)
meningitis due to measles virus (B05.1)
meningitis due to mumps virus (B26.1)
meningitis due to poliomyelitis virus (A80.-)
meningitis due to zoster (B02.1)
Ex: **For category A87 CC codes unless otherwise indicated:** A02.21, A17.0-A17.1, A27.81, A39.0, A50.41, A51.41, A52.13, A54.82-A54.84, A54.89-A54.9, A74.81-A74.9, A87.0-A87.9, A96.2, A98.3-A98.4, B26.1, B33.24, B33.4-B33.8, B34.1-B34.8, B37.5, B38.4, B45.1, B58.2, B92, B94.2-B94.9, B97.10, B97.19, B97.29, B97.5-B97.6, B97.81-B97.89, G00.0-G03.9, G04.2, G32.89, G61.0, G96.8-G96.9, G98.0-G98.8, G99.8

A87.0 Enteroviral meningitis
Group of common viruses responsible for the majority of viral meningitis
Coxsackievirus meningitis
Echovirus meningitis
A87.1 Adenoviral meningitis
A87.2 Lymphocytic choriomeningitis
Lymphocytic meningoencephalitis
Ex: A02.21, A17.0-A17.1, A27.81, A39.0, A50.41, A51.41, A52.13, A54.82-A54.84, A54.89-A54.9, A74.81-A74.9, A87.0-A87.9, A92-30-A92-39, A96.2, A98.3-A98.4, B26.1, B33.24, B33.4-B33.8, B34.1-B34.8, B37.5, B38.4, B45.1, B58.2, B92, B94.2-B94.9, B97.10, B97.19, B97.21-B97.29, B97.5-B97.6, B97.81-B97.89, G00.0-G03.9, G04.2, G32.89, G61.0, G96.8-G96.9, G98.0-G98.8, G99.8
A87.8 Other viral meningitis
A87.9 Viral meningitis, unspecified

● **A88 Other viral infections of central nervous system, not elsewhere classified**
Excludes1 viral encephalitis NOS (A86)
viral meningitis NOS (A87.9)
A88.0 Enteroviral exanthematous fever [Boston exanthem]
Infectious skin eruption
Ex: See A83
A88.1 Epidemic vertigo
A88.8 Other specified viral infections of central nervous system
Ex: See A85

A89 Unspecified viral infection of central nervous system
Ex: See A86

ARTHROPOD-BORNE VIRAL FEVERS AND VIRAL HEMORRHAGIC FEVERS (A90-A99)

A90 Dengue fever [classical dengue]
Acute, self-limited disease, characterized by fever, prostration, severe muscle pains, headache, rash, lymphadenopathy, and leukopenia, caused by dengue virus; AKA breakbone, dandy
Excludes1 dengue hemorrhagic fever (A91)
Ex: A90

A91 Dengue hemorrhagic fever
Serious follow-up to regular dengue, with symptoms of hemorrhage
Ex: A91, A92.0-A94, A98.0-A98.2, A98.8-A99, B33.1

● **A92 Other mosquito-borne viral fevers**
Excludes1 Ross River disease (B33.1)
A92.0 Chikungunya virus disease
Transmitted by mosquitoes
Chikungunya (hemorrhagic) fever
Ex: See A91

OGCR Section I. C.1.f.

Certain Infectious and Parasitic Diseases (A00-B99)

Zika virus infections

Code only confirmed cases

Code only a confirmed diagnosis of Zika virus (A92.5, Zika virus disease) as documented by the provider. This is an exception to the hospital inpatient guideline Section II, H.

In this context, "confirmation" does not require documentation of the type of test performed; the physician's diagnostic statement that the condition is confirmed is sufficient. This code should be assigned regardless of the stated mode of transmission.

If the provider documents "suspected", "possible" or "probable" Zika, do not assign code A92.5. Assign a code(s) explaining the reason for encounter (such as fever, rash, or joint pain) or Z20.828, Contact with and (suspected) exposure to other viral communicable diseases.

A92.1 O'nyong-nyong fever
Acute, nonfatal febrile disease transmitted by mosquitoes, which clinically resembles dengue and chikungunya
Ex: A17.82, A50.42, A52.14, A75.9, A79.9, A81.1, A81.82-A81.89, A83.0-A85.8, A87.2, A88.0, A88.8, A91-A94, A98.0-A98.2, A98.8-A99, B00.4, B00.82, B01.11-B01.12, B04, B06.01, B08.09, B08.20-B08.22, B08.60-B08.79, B09, B10.01-B10.09, B26.2, B27.00-B27.99, B33.1, B45.0, B45.2-B45.9, B58.2, B75, B97.10, B97.21, G04.00-G04.01, G04.31, G04.81-G04.91, G05.3-G05.4, G37.0, G37.4-G37.5, J09.X3-J09.X9, J10.2-J10.89, J11.2-J11.89, L44.4, M1A.10X0-M1A.19X1, P35.2-P35.9, P37.0-P37.9, T56.0X1-T56.0X4[A]

A92.2 Venezuelan equine fever
Venezuelan equine encephalitis
Venezuelan equine encephalomyelitis virus disease
Ex: See A92.1

● **A92.3 West Nile virus infection**
West Nile fever
Ex: **For category A92.3 CC codes:** A17.82, A50.42, A52.14, A75.9, A79.9, A81.1, A81.82-A81.89, A83.0-A85.8, A87.2, A88.0, A88.8, A91, A92.0-A92.2, A92.4-A94, A98.0-A98.2, A98.8-A99, B00.4, B00.82, B01.11-B01.12, B04, B06.01, B08.09, B08.20-B08.22, B08.60-B08.79, B09, B10.01-B10.09, B26.2, B27.00-B27.99, B33.1, B45.0, B45.2-B45.9, B58.2, B75, B97.10, G04.00-G04.01, G04.31, G04.81-G04.91, G05.3-G05.4, G37.0, G37.4-G37.5, J09.X3-J09.X9, J10.2-J10.89, J11.2-J11.89, L44.4, P35.2-P35.9, P37.0-P37.9

A92.30 West Nile virus infection, unspecified
West Nile fever NOS
West Nile fever without complications
West Nile virus NOS

A92.31 West Nile virus infection with encephalitis
West Nile encephalitis
West Nile encephalomyelitis

A92.32 West Nile virus infection with other neurologic manifestation
Use additional code to specify the neurologic manifestation

A92.39 West Nile virus infection with other complications
Use additional code to specify the other conditions

A92.4 Rift Valley fever
Ex: See A92.1

A92.5 Zika virus disease ◀
Zika virus fever ◀
Zika virus infection ◀
Zika NOS ◀
Ex: See A92.1

A92.8 Other specified mosquito-borne viral fevers
Ex: See A92.1

A92.9 Mosquito-borne viral fever, unspecified
Ex: See A91

● **A93 Other arthropod-borne viral fevers, not elsewhere classified**

A93.0 Oropouche virus disease
Tropical viral infection
Oropouche fever
Ex: See A92.1

A93.1 Sandfly fever
Pappataci fever
Phlebotomus fever
Ex: See A91

A93.2 Colorado tick fever
Ex: See A91

A93.8 Other specified arthropod-borne viral fevers
Piry virus disease
Vesicular stomatitis virus disease [Indiana fever]
Ex: See A91

A94 Unspecified arthropod-borne viral fever
Arboviral fever NOS
Arbovirus infection NOS
Ex: See A91

● **A95 Yellow fever**
Acute infectious disease transmitted by mosquitoes
Ex: **For category A95 CC codes:** A95.0-A95.9

A95.0 Sylvatic yellow fever
Jungle yellow fever

A95.1 Urban yellow fever

A95.9 Yellow fever, unspecified

● **A96 Arenaviral hemorrhagic fever**
Virus that causes various hemorrhagic fevers
Ex: **For category A96 CC codes:** A74.81-A74.9, A88.1, A96.0-A96.9, A98.3-A98.5, B25.8-B25.9, B33.24-B34.2, B34.4-B34.8, B97.0-B97.89

A96.0 Junin hemorrhagic fever
Argentinian hemorrhagic fever

A96.1 Machupo hemorrhagic fever
Transmitted by contact with infected rodents
Bolivian hemorrhagic fever

A96.2 Lassa fever
Acute type of hemorrhagic fever caused by contact with disease carrying mouse or person

A96.8 Other arenaviral hemorrhagic fevers

A96.9 Arenaviral hemorrhagic fever, unspecified

● **A98 Other viral hemorrhagic fevers, not elsewhere classified**
Excludes1 chikungunya hemorrhagic fever (A92.0)
dengue hemorrhagic fever (A91)
Ex: **For category A98 CC codes unless otherwise indicated:** See A91

A98.0 Crimean-Congo hemorrhagic fever
Virus transmitted by ticks and contact with blood, secretions, or fluids from infected humans or animals
Central Asian hemorrhagic fever

A98.1 Omsk hemorrhagic fever
Transmitted to humans by bites of infected ticks or contact with infected muskrats

A98.2 Kyasanur Forest disease
Transmitted via infected monkeys, voles, ticks

A98.3 Marburg virus disease
Rare, acute, often fatal type of hemorrhagic fever

A98.4 Ebola virus disease

A98.5 Hemorrhagic fever with renal syndrome
Epidemic hemorrhagic fever
Korean hemorrhagic fever
Russian hemorrhagic fever
Hantaan virus disease
Hantavirus disease with renal manifestations
Nephropathia epidemica
Songo fever
Excludes1 hantavirus (cardio)-pulmonary syndrome (B33.4)
Ex: A17.9, A18.10-A18.11, A18.13, A18.82, A18.84, A18.89, A54.21, A54.29, A54.82, A54.84, A54.89-A54.9, A59.00, A59.8-A59.9, A98.5, B37.41-B37.49, B97.21, E08.21-E08.29, E08.618-E08.638, E08.649-E08.8, E09.21-E09.29, E09.618-E09.638, E09.649-E09.8, E10.21-E10.29, E10.618-E10.638, E10.649, E10.69-E10.8, E11.21-E11.29, E11.618-E11.638, E11.649, E11.69-E11.8, E13.21-E13.29, E13.618-E13.638, E13.649-E13.8, M10.30-M10.39, N00.0-N11.0, N11.8-N13.39, N13.6, N14.0-N17.9, N19, N25.0-N26.1, N26.9-N27.9, N28.1-N29, N36.41-N36.43, N36.8-N36.9, N39.8-N39.9, R31.0-R31.9

A98.8 Other specified viral hemorrhagic fevers

A99 Unspecified viral hemorrhagic fever
Ex: See A91

VIRAL INFECTIONS CHARACTERIZED BY SKIN AND MUCOUS MEMBRANE LESIONS (B00-B09)

● **B00 Herpesviral [herpes simplex] infections**

Excludes1 congenital herpesviral infections (P35.2)

Excludes2 anogenital herpesviral infection (A60.-)
gammaherpesviral mononucleosis (B27.0-)
herpangina (B08.5)

B00.0 Eczema herpeticum
Cutaneous eruption caused by herpes simplex virus (HSV) type 1, HSV-2, coxsackievirus A16, or vaccinia virus
Kaposi's varicelliform eruption

B00.1 Herpesviral vesicular dermatitis
Vesicle formation; characteristics include formation of blisters and scabs on feet and legs
Herpes simplex facialis
Herpes simplex labialis
Herpes simplex otitis externa
Vesicular dermatitis of ear
Vesicular dermatitis of lip

B00.2 Herpesviral gingivostomatitis and pharyngotonsillitis CC
Inflammation involving both gingivae and oral mucosa
Herpesviral pharyngitis
Inflammation of pharynx and tonsils; AKA tonsillopharyngitis
Ex: B00.2

B00.3 Herpesviral meningitis MCC
Ex: A02.21, A17.0-A17.1, A27.81, A39.0, A50.41, A51.41, A52.13, A54.82, A54.84, A54.89-A54.9, A87.0-A87.9, B00.3, B00.82-B00.9, B02.1, B10.81-B10.89, B26.1, B37.5, B38.4, B45.1, B58.2, B92, B94.2-B94.9, G00.0-G03.9, G04.2, G32.89, G61.0, G96.8-G96.9, G98.0-G98.8, G99.8

B00.4 Herpesviral encephalitis MCC
Herpesviral meningoencephalitis
Simian B disease

Excludes1 herpesviral encephalitis due to herpesvirus 6 and 7 (B10.01, B10.09)
non-simplex herpesviral encephalitis (B10.0-)

Ex: B00.4, B00.82-B00.9, B10.01-B10.89, B92, B94.2-B94.9

● **B00.5 Herpesviral ocular disease**
Ex: **For category B00.5 CC codes:** B00.50-B00.59, B00.89-B00.9, B10.81-B10.89

B00.50 Herpesviral ocular disease, unspecified CC

B00.51 Herpesviral iridocyclitis CC
Herpesviral iritis
Herpesviral uveitis, anterior

B00.52 Herpesviral keratitis CC
Herpesviral keratoconjunctivitis

B00.53 Herpesviral conjunctivitis CC

B00.59 Other herpesviral disease of eye CC
Herpesviral dermatitis of eyelid

B00.7 Disseminated herpesviral disease MCC
Herpesviral sepsis
Ex: A02.1, A20.7, A22.7, A26.7, A32.7, A39.2-A39.4, A40.0-A41.9, A42.7, A54.86, B00.7, B00.82-B00.9, B10.81-B10.89, B37.7, B92, B94.2-B94.9, R65.10-R65.20

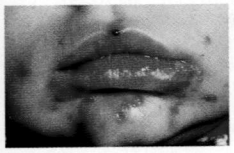

Figure 1-4 Primary herpes simplex in and around the mouth. The infection is usually acquired from siblings or parents and is readily transmitted to other direct contacts. (From Forbes, Jackson: Colour Atlas and Text of Clinical Medicine, International Edition, Mosby, 2002)

Item 1-15 Herpes is a viral disease for which there is no cure. There are two types of the herpes simplex virus: **Type I** causes **cold sores** or **fever blisters,** and **Type II** causes **genital herpes.** The virus can be spread from a sore on the lips to the genitals or from the genitals to the lips.

● **B00.8 Other forms of herpesviral infections**

B00.81 Herpesviral hepatitis CC
Ex: B00.3, B00.81-B00.9, B10.81-B10.89, B92, B94.2-B94.9

B00.82 Herpes simplex myelitis MCC
Ex: A74.81-A74.9, A96.2, A98.3-A98.4, B00.82-B00.9, B01.12, B02.24, B10.81-B10.89, B33.24, B33.4-B33.8, B34.1-B34.2, B34.4-B34.8, B92, B94.2-B94.9, B97.10, B97.19, B97.29, B97.5-B97.6, B97.81-B97.89, G04.00-G04.01, G04.31, G04.81-G04.89, G05.3-G05.4, G37.3

B00.89 Other herpesviral infection CC
Herpesviral whitlow
Ex: A74.81-A74.9, A96.2, A98.3-A98.4, B00.82-B00.9, B10.81-B10.89, B33.24, B33.4-B33.8, B34.1-B34.2, B34.4-B34.8, B92, B94.2-B94.9, B97.10, B97.19, B97.29, B97.5-B97.6, B97.81-B97.89

B00.9 Herpesviral infection, unspecified
Herpes simplex infection NOS

● **B01 Varicella [chickenpox]**
Very contagious disease caused by the varicella zoster virus that results in an itchy outbreak of skin blisters (varicella). The same virus causes shingles (zoster).

B01.0 Varicella meningitis CC
Ex: A74.81-A74.9, A96.2, A98.3-A98.4, B01.0, B01.12, B01.81-B01.9, B08.04, B33.24, B33.4-B33.8, B34.1-B34.2, B34.4-B34.8, B92, B94.2-B94.9, B97.10, B97.19, B97.29, B97.5-B97.6, B97.81-B97.89

● **B01.1 Varicella encephalitis, myelitis and encephalomyelitis**
Postchickenpox encephalitis, myelitis and encephalomyelitis

B01.11 Varicella encephalitis and encephalomyelitis MCC
Postchickenpox encephalitis and encephalomyelitis
Ex: A74.81-A74.9, A96.2, A98.3-A98.4, B01.0-B01.12, B01.81-B01.9, B08.04, B33.24, B33.4-B33.8, B34.1-B34.2, B34.4-B34.8, B92, B94.2-B94.9, B97.10, B97.19, B97.29, B97.5-B97.6, B97.81-B97.89

B01.12 Varicella myelitis MCC
Postchickenpox myelitis
Ex: A74.81-A74.9, A96.2, A98.3-A98.4, B00.82, B01.0, B01.12, B01.81-B01.9, B02.24, B08.04, B33.24, B33.4-B33.8, B34.1-B34.2, B34.4-B34.8, B92, B94.2-B94.9, B97.10, B97.19, B97.29, B97.5-B97.6, B97.81-B97.89, G04.00-G04.01, G04.31, G04.81-G04.89, G05.3-G05.4, G37.3

B01.2 Varicella pneumonia MCC
Ex: A74.81-A74.9, A96.2, A98.3-A98.4, B01.0, B01.12-B01.9, B08.04, B33.24, B33.4-B33.8, B34.1-B34.2, B34.4-B34.8, B92, B94.2-B94.9, B97.10, B97.19, B97.29, B97.5-B97.6, B97.81-B97.89

● **B01.8 Varicella with other complications**
Ex: **For category B01.8 CC codes:** See B01.0

B01.81 Varicella keratitis CC

B01.89 Other varicella complications CC

B01.9 Varicella without complication CC
Varicella NOS
Ex: See B01.0

● **B02 Zoster [herpes zoster]**

Includes shingles
zona

B02.0 Zoster encephalitis CC
Zoster meningoencephalitis
Ex: A74.81-A74.9, A96.2, A98.3-A98.4, B00.3, B00.82-B00.9, B02.0-B02.29, B02.7-B02.9, B10.81-B10.89, B33.24, B33.4-B33.8, B34.1-B34.2, B34.4-B34.8, B92, B94.2-B94.9, B97.10, B97.19, B97.29, B97.5-B97.6, B97.81-B97.89

B02.1 Zoster meningitis MCC
Ex: A02.21, A17.0-A17.1, A27.81, A39.0, A50.41, A51.41, A52.13, A54.82, A54.84, A54.89-A54.9, A74.81-A74.9, A87.0-A87.9, A96.2, A98.3-A98.4, B00.3, B00.82-B00.9, B02.0-B02.29, B02.7-B02.9, B10.81-B10.89, B26.1, B33.24, B33.4, B33.8, B34.1-B34.2, B34.4-B34.8, B37.5, B38.4, B45.1, B58.2, B92, B94.2-B94.9, B97.10, B97.19, B97.29, B97.5-B97.6, B97.81-B97.89, G00.0-G03.9, G04.2, G32.89, G61.0, G96.8-G96.9, G98.0-G98.8, G99.8

Item 1-16 Zoster: Also known as ***shingles*** and is caused by the same virus as chickenpox. After exposure, the virus lies dormant in nerve tissue and is activated by factors including aging, stress, suppression of the immune system, and certain medication. It begins as a unilateral rash that leads to blisters and sores on the skin. It may involve the nerve pathways of the eye, forehead, nose, and eyelids and may be very painful with long-term systemic effects.

B02.2 Zoster with other nervous system involvement
Exc For category B02.2 CC codes unless otherwise indicated: see B02.0

B02.21 Postherpetic geniculate ganglionitis

B02.22 Postherpetic trigeminal neuralgia

B02.23 Postherpetic polyneuropathy

B02.24 Postherpetic myelitis
Herpes zoster myelitis
Exc A74.81-A74.9, A96.2, A98.3-A98.4, B00.3, B00.82-B00.9, B01.12, B02.0-B02.29, B02.7-B02.9, B10.81-B10.89, B33.24, B33.4-B33.8, B34.1-B34.2, B34.4-B34.8, B92, B94.2-B94.9, B97.10, B97.19, B97.29, B97.5-B97.6, B97.81-B97.89, G04.00-G04.01, G04.31, G04.81-G04.89, G05.3-G05.4, G37.3

B02.29 Other postherpetic nervous system involvement
Postherpetic radiculopathy

B02.3 Zoster ocular disease
Exc For category B02.3 CC codes: B02.30-B02.39

B02.30 Zoster ocular disease, unspecified

B02.31 Zoster conjunctivitis

B02.32 Zoster iridocyclitis

B02.33 Zoster keratitis
Herpes zoster keratoconjunctivitis

B02.34 Zoster scleritis

B02.39 Other herpes zoster eye disease
Zoster blepharitis

B02.7 Disseminated zoster
Exc A60.00-A60.9, A74.81-A74.9, A96.2, A98.3-A98.4, B00.0-B00.2, B00.4-B00.9, B02.0-B02.9, B10.01-B10.89, B33.24, B33.4-B33.8, B34.1-B34.2, B34.4, B34.8, B92, B94.2-B94.9, B97.10, B97.19, B97.29, B97.5-B97.6, B97.81-B97.89

B02.8 Zoster with other complications
Herpes zoster otitis externa
Exc See B02.7

B02.9 Zoster without complications
Zoster NOS

B03 Smallpox

Note: In 1980 the 33rd World Health Assembly declared that smallpox had been eradicated. The classification is maintained for surveillance purposes.
Exc B01.0-B01.9, B03, B08.010-B08.04

B04 Monkeypox
Disease occurring in captive monkeys and other mammals that may be transmitted to humans, clinically similar to smallpox
Exc B04, B08.010-B08.011, B08.09, B08.3, B08.60-B08.79, B09, L44.4

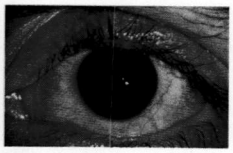

Figure 1-5 Photograph of eyelids with marginal blepharitis. (From Mandell, Bennett, & Dolin: Principles and Practice of Infectious Diseases, ed 7, Churchill Livingstone, An Imprint of Elsevier, 2009)

Item 1-17 Blepharitis is a common condition in which the eyelid is swollen and yellow scaling and conjunctivitis develop. Usually the hair on the scalp and brow is involved.

B05 Measles
Includes morbilli
Excludes1 subacute sclerosing panencephalitis (A81.1)

B05.0 Measles complicated by encephalitis
Postmeasles encephalitis
Exc A74.81-A74.9, A96.2, A98.3-A98.4, B05.0-B05.1, B05.4, B05.89-B05.9, B33.24, B33.4-B33.8, B34.1-B34.2, B34.4-B34.8, B92, B94.2-B94.9, B97.10, B97.19, B97.29, B97.5-B97.6, B97.81-B97.89

B05.1 Measles complicated by meningitis
Postmeasles meningitis
Exc A74.81-A74.9, A96.2, A98.3-A98.4, B05.1, B05.4, B05.89-B05.9, B33.24, B33.4-B33.8, B34.1-B34.2, B34.4-B34.8, B92, B94.2-B94.9, B97.10, B97.19, B97.29, B97.5-B97.6, B97.81-B97.89

B05.2 Measles complicated by pneumonia
Postmeasles pneumonia
Exc A74.81-A74.9, A96.2, A98.3-A98.4, B05.1-B05.2, B05.4, B05.89-B05.9, B33.24, B33.4-B33.8, B34.1-B34.2, B34.4-B34.8, B92, B94.2-B94.9, B97.10, B97.19, B97.29, B97.5-B97.6, B97.81-B97.89

B05.3 Measles complicated by otitis media
Postmeasles otitis media

B05.4 Measles with intestinal complications
Exc See B05.1

B05.8 Measles with other complications

B05.81 Measles keratitis and keratoconjunctivitis
Exc A74.81-A74.9, A96.2, A98.3-A98.4, B05.1, B05.4, B05.81-B05.9, B33.24, B33.4-B33.8, B34.1-B34.2, B34.4-B34.8, B92, B94.2-B94.9, B97.10, B97.19, B97.29, B97.5-B97.6, B97.81-B97.89

B05.89 Other measles complications
Exc See B05.1

B05.9 Measles without complication
Measles NOS

B06 Rubella [German measles]
Excludes1 congenital rubella (P35.0)

B06.0 Rubella with neurological complications
Exc For category B06.0 CC codes: A74.81-A74.9, A96.2, A98.3-A98.4, B05.1, B05.4, B05.81-B05.9, B06.00-B06.81, B06.89-B06.9, B33.24, B33.4-B33.8, B34.1-B34.2, B34.4-B34.8, B92, B94.2-B94.9, B97.10, B97.19, B97.29, B97.5-B97.6, B97.81-B97.89

B06.00 Rubella with neurological complication, unspecified

B06.01 Rubella encephalitis
Rubella meningoencephalitis

B06.02 Rubella meningitis

B06.09 Other neurological complications of rubella

B06.8 Rubella with other complications

B06.81 Rubella pneumonia
Exc See B06.0

B06.82 Rubella arthritis
Exc A74.81-A74.9, A96.2, A98.3-A98.4, B05.1, B05.4, B05.81-B05.9, B06.81-B06.82, B06.89-B06.9, B33.24, B33.4-B33.8, B34.1-B34.2, B34.4-B34.8, B92, B94.2-B94.9, B97.10, B97.19, B97.29, B97.5-B97.6, B97.81-B97.89

B06.89 Other rubella complications
Exc See B06.0

B06.9 Rubella without complication
Rubella NOS

● **B07 Viral warts**

Includes verruca simplex
verruca vulgaris
viral warts due to human papillomavirus

Excludes2 anogenital (venereal) warts (A63.0)
papilloma of bladder (D41.4)
papilloma of cervix (D26.0)
papilloma larynx (D14.1)

B07.0 Plantar wart
Verruca plantaris

B07.8 Other viral warts
Common wart
Flat wart
Verruca plana

B07.9 Viral wart, unspecified

● **B08 Other viral infections characterized by skin and mucous membrane lesions, not elsewhere classified**

Excludes1 vesicular stomatitis virus disease (A93.8)

● **B08.0 Other orthopoxvirus infections**

Excludes2 monkeypox (B04)

● **B08.01 Cowpox and vaccinia not from vaccine**

B08.010 Cowpox

B08.011 Vaccinia not from vaccine

Excludes1 vaccinia (from vaccination) (generalized) (T88.1)

B08.02 Orf virus disease
Contagious pustular dermatitis
Ecthyma contagiosum

B08.03 Pseudocowpox [milker's node]

B08.04 Paravaccinia, unspecified

B08.09 Other orthopoxvirus infections
Orthopoxvirus infection NOS

B08.1 Molluscum contagiosum
Various skin diseases characterized by soft, rounded, cutaneous lesions

● **B08.2 Exanthema subitum [sixth disease] Roseola infantum**
Acute, short-lived high fever in infants and young children followed by a rash mainly on the trunk, caused by human herpesvirus 6

B08.20 Exanthema subitum [sixth disease], unspecified Roseola infantum, unspecified P

B08.21 Exanthema subitum [sixth disease] due to human herpesvirus 6 Roseola infantum due to human herpesvirus 6 P
Virus results in sudden rash; infection results in lifelong persistence

B08.22 Exanthema subitum [sixth disease] due to human herpesvirus 7 Roseola infantum due to human herpesvirus 7 P

B08.3 Erythema infectiosum [fifth disease]
Moderately contagious, epidemic disease in children caused by B19 virus; onset of rash that begins as redness of cheeks, later there is rash on trunk and limbs; when this fades, there may be central clearing that leaves lacelike pattern
Ex: B08.3, B34.3

B08.4 Enteroviral vesicular stomatitis with exanthem
Hand, foot and mouth disease
Check your documentation—this code is HAND, foot, and mouth disease. Code B08.8 is foot and mouth disease.

B08.5 Enteroviral vesicular pharyngitis
Herpangina

● **B08.6 Parapoxvirus infections**

B08.60 Parapoxvirus infection, unspecified

B08.61 Bovine stomatitis

B08.62 Sealpox

B08.69 Other parapoxvirus infections

● **B08.7 Yatapoxvirus infections**

B08.70 Yatapoxvirus infection, unspecified

B08.71 Tanapox virus disease
Ex: B04, B08.010-B08.011, B08.09, B08.3, B08.60-B08.79, B09, L44.4

B08.72 Yaba pox virus disease
Yaba monkey tumor disease

B08.79 Other yatapoxvirus infections

B08.8 Other specified viral infections characterized by skin and mucous membrane lesions
Enteroviral lymphonodular pharyngitis
Foot-and-mouth disease
Check your documentation. Code B08.4 is for HAND, foot, and mouth disease.
Poxvirus NEC

B09 Unspecified viral infection characterized by skin and mucous membrane lesions
Viral enanthema NOS
Viral exanthema NOS

OTHER HUMAN HERPESVIRUSES (B10)

● **B10 Other human herpesviruses**

Excludes2 cytomegalovirus (B25.9)
Epstein-Barr virus (B27.0-)
herpes NOS (B00.9)
herpes simplex (B00.-)
herpes zoster (B02.-)
human herpesvirus NOS (B00.-)
human herpesvirus 1 and 2 (B00.-)
human herpesvirus 3 (B01.-, B02.-)
human herpesvirus 4 (B27.0-)
human herpesvirus 5 (B25.-)
varicella (B01.-)
zoster (B02.-)

● **B10.0 Other human herpesvirus encephalitis**

Excludes2 herpes encephalitis NOS (B00.4)
herpes simplex encephalitis (B00.4)
human herpesvirus encephalitis (B00.4)
simian B herpes virus encephalitis (B00.4)

Ex: **For category B10.0 CC codes:** B00.4, B00.82-B00.9, B10.01-B10.89, B92, B94.2-B94.9

B10.01 Human herpesvirus 6 encephalitis
Sudden rash or roseola

B10.09 Other human herpesvirus encephalitis
Human herpesvirus 7 encephalitis
Virus closely related to human herpesvirus 6, but not known to cause any disease

● **B10.8 Other human herpesvirus infection**

B10.81 Human herpesvirus 6 infection
Causative agent of exanthema subitum that results in sudden rash

B10.82 Human herpesvirus 7 infection
Closely related to human herpesvirus 6, but not known cause any disease

B10.89 Other human herpesvirus infection
Human herpesvirus 8 infection
May be the cause of Kaposi sarcoma, a malignant tumor
Kaposi's sarcoma-associated herpesvirus infection

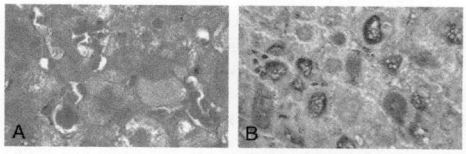

Figure 1-6 Hepatitis B viral infection. **A.** Liver parenchyma showing hepatocytes with diffuse granular cytoplasm, so-called ground glass hepatocytes (H&E). **B.** Immunoperoxidase stains from the same case, showing cytoplasmic inclusions of viral particles. (From Kumar: Robbins and Cotran: Pathologic Basis of Disease, ed 8, Saunders, An Imprint of Elsevier, 2009)

Item 1–18 Hepatitis A (HAV) was formerly called epidemic, infectious, short-incubation, or acute catarrhal jaundice hepatitis. The primary transmission mode is the oral–fecal route. **Hepatitis B (HBV)** was formerly called long-incubation period, serum, or homologous serum hepatitis. Transmission modes are through blood from infected persons and from body fluids of infected mother to neonate. **Hepatitis C (HCV),** caused by the hepatitis C virus, is primarily transfusion associated. **Hepatitis D (HDV),** also called delta hepatitis, is caused by the hepatitis D virus in patients formerly or currently infected with hepatitis B. **Hepatitis E (HEV)** is also called enterically transmitted non-A, non-B hepatitis. The primary transmission mode is the oral–fecal route, usually through contaminated water.

VIRAL HEPATITIS (B15-B19)

Excludes1 sequelae of viral hepatitis (B94.2)
Excludes2 cytomegaloviral hepatitis (B25.1)
herpesviral [herpes simplex] hepatitis (B00.81)

B15 Acute hepatitis A
Ex: For category B15 CC codes: A74.81-A74.9, A96.2, A98.3-A98.4, B15.0-B19.9, B33.24, B33.4-B33.8, B34.1-B34.2, B34.4-B34.8, B92, B94.2-B94.9, B97.10, B97.19, B97.29, B97.5-B97.6, B97.81-B97.89

B15.0 Hepatitis A with hepatic coma

B15.9 Hepatitis A without hepatic coma
Hepatitis A (acute) (viral) NOS

B16 Acute hepatitis B
Ex: For category B16 CC codes: see B15

B16.0 Acute hepatitis B with delta-agent with hepatic coma

B16.1 Acute hepatitis B with delta-agent without hepatic coma

B16.2 Acute hepatitis B without delta-agent with hepatic coma

B16.9 Acute hepatitis B without delta-agent and without hepatic coma
Hepatitis B (acute) (viral) NOS

B17 Other acute viral hepatitis
Ex: For category B17 CC codes: see B15

B17.0 Acute delta-(super) infection of hepatitis B carrier

B17.1 Acute hepatitis C

B17.10 Acute hepatitis C without hepatic coma
Acute hepatitis C NOS

B17.11 Acute hepatitis C with hepatic coma

B17.2 Acute hepatitis E

B17.8 Other specified acute viral hepatitis
Hepatitis non-A non-B (acute) (viral) NEC

B17.9 Acute viral hepatitis, unspecified
Acute hepatitis NOS
Acute infectious hepatitis NOS ◀

B18 Chronic viral hepatitis
Includes Carrier of viral hepatitis ◀
Ex: For category B18 CC codes: see B15

B18.0 Chronic viral hepatitis B with delta-agent

B18.1 Chronic viral hepatitis B without delta-agent
Carrier of viral hepatitis B ◀
Chronic (viral) hepatitis B

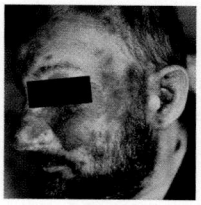

Figure 1-7 Kaposi's sarcoma. There are large confluent hyperpigmented patch-stage lesions with lymphedema. (From Cohen & Powderly: Infectious Diseases, ed 3, Mosby, An Imprint of Elsevier, 2010)

Item 1–19 AIDS (acquired immune deficiency syndrome) is caused by **HIV** (human immunodeficiency virus). HIV affects certain white blood cells (T-4 lymphocytes) and destroys the ability of the cells to fight infections, making patients susceptible to a host of infectious diseases (e.g., ***Pneumocystis carinii pneumonia (PCP), Kaposi's sarcoma,*** and ***lymphoma). AIDS-related complex (ARC)*** is an early stage of AIDS in which tests for HIV are positive but the symptoms are mild.

B18.2 Chronic viral hepatitis C
Carrier of viral hepatitis C ◀

B18.8 Other chronic viral hepatitis
Carrier of other viral hepatitis ◀

B18.9 Chronic viral hepatitis, unspecified
Carrier of unspecified viral hepatitis ◀

B19 Unspecified viral hepatitis
Ex: For category B19 CC codes: see B15

B19.0 Unspecified viral hepatitis with hepatic coma

B19.1 Unspecified viral hepatitis B

B19.10 Unspecified viral hepatitis B without hepatic coma
Unspecified viral hepatitis B NOS

B19.11 Unspecified viral hepatitis B with hepatic coma

B19.2 Unspecified viral hepatitis C

B19.20 Unspecified viral hepatitis C without hepatic coma
Viral hepatitis C NOS

B19.21 Unspecified viral hepatitis C with hepatic coma

B19.9 Unspecified viral hepatitis without hepatic coma
Viral hepatitis NOS

OGCR Section I. C.1.a

Certain Infectious and Parasitic Diseases (A00-B99)
a. Human Immunodeficiency Virus (HIV) Infections
1) Code only confirmed cases
Code only confirmed cases of HIV infection illness. This is an exception to the hospital inpatient guideline Section II, H.
In this context, "confirmation" does not require documentation of positive serology or culture for HIV; the provider's diagnostic statement that the patient is HIV positive, or has an HIV-related illness is sufficient.

HUMAN IMMUNODEFICIENCY VIRUS [HIV] DISEASE (B20)

B20 Human immunodeficiency virus [HIV] disease
Includes acquired immune deficiency syndrome [AIDS]
AIDS-related complex [ARC]
HIV infection, symptomatic
Code first Human immunodeficiency virus [HIV] disease complicating pregnancy, childbirth and the puerperium, if applicable (O98.7-)
Use additional code(s) to identify all manifestations of HIV infection
Excludes1 asymptomatic human immunodeficiency virus [HIV] infection status (Z21)
exposure to HIV virus (Z20.6)
inconclusive serologic evidence of HIV (R75)
Ex: B20, B92, B94.2-B94.9

OTHER VIRAL DISEASES (B25-B34)

B25 Cytomegaloviral disease
AKA: HCMV or Human Herpesvirus 5 (HHV-5)
Excludes1 congenital cytomegalovirus infection (P35.1)
cytomegaloviral mononucleosis (B27.1-)

B25.0 Cytomegaloviral pneumonitis
MCC when PDx is its own MCC
Ex: A15.0-A15.9, A17.9, A18.82, A18.84, A18.89, A21.2, A22.1, A31.0, A37.01, A37.11, A37.81, A37.91, A42.0, A43.0, A48.1, B25.0, B39.0-B39.2, B44.0, B58.3, B59, B67.1, J09.X1-J09.X2, J10.00-J10.1, J11.00-J11.1, J12.0-J12.3, J12.89-J18.1, J18.8-J18.9, J22, J44.9, J47.0-J70.4, J70.8-J70.9, J98.4, J98.8-J98.9, Q33.4, R91.1

B25.1 Cytomegaloviral hepatitis
CC when PDx is its own CC
Ex: No exclusions

B25.2 Cytomegaloviral pancreatitis
MCC when PDx is its own MCC
Ex: B25.2, K85.00-K86.1, K86.81-K86.9

B25.8 Other cytomegaloviral diseases
Cytomegaloviral encephalitis
Ex: A96.0-A96.9, A98.3-A98.5, B25.8-B25.9, B33.24-B34.2, B34.4-B34.8, B97.0-B97.32, B97.39, B97.5-B97.89

B25.9 Cytomegaloviral disease, unspecified
Ex: See B25.8

B26 Mumps
Includes epidemic parotitis
infectious parotitis
Acute, contagious, viral disease

B26.0 Mumps orchitis ♂
Ex: A74.81-A74.9, A96.2, A98.3-A98.4, B26.0, B26.82-B26.83, B26.85-B26.9, B33.24, B33.4-B33.8, B34.1-B34.8, B92, B94.2-B94.9, B97.10, B97.19, B97.29, B97.5-B97.6, B97.81-B97.89

B26.1 Mumps meningitis
Ex: A02.21, A17.0-A17.1, A27.81, A39.0, A50.41, A51.41, A52.13, A54.82, A54.84, A54.89-A54.9, A74.81-A74.9, A87.0-A87.9, A96.2, A98.3-A98.4, B00.3, B02.1, B26.1, B26.82-B26.83, B26.85-B26.9, B33.24, B33.4-B33.8, B34.1-B34.2, B34.4-B34.8, B37.5, B38.4, B45.1, B58.2, B92, B94.2, B94.8-B94.9, B97.10, B97.19, B97.29, B97.5-B97.6, B97.81-B97.89, G00.0-G03.9, G04.2, G32.89, G61.0, G96.8-G96.9, G98.0-G98.8, G99.8

B26.2 Mumps encephalitis
Ex: A74.81-A74.9, A96.2, A98.3-A98.4, B26.2, B26.82-B26.83, B26.85-B26.9, B33.24, B33.4, B33.8, B34.1-B34.2, B34.4-B34.8, B92, B94.2, B94.8-B94.9, B97.10, B97.19, B97.29, B97.5-B97.6, B97.81-B97.89

B26.3 Mumps pancreatitis
Ex: A74.81-A74.9, A96.2, A98.3-A98.4, B26.3, B26.82-B26.83, B26.85-B26.9, B33.24, B33.4, B33.8, B34.1-B34.2, B34.4-B34.8, B92, B94.2, B94.8-B94.9, B97.10, B97.19, B97.29, B97.5-B97.6, B97.81-B97.89

B26.8 Mumps with other complications
Ex: For category B26.8 CC codes unless otherwise indicated:
A74.81-A74.9, A96.2, A98.3-A98.4, B26.82-B26.83, B26.85-B26.9, B33.24, B33.4, B33.8, B34.1-B34.2, B34.4-B34.8, B92, B94.2, B94.8-B94.9, B97.10, B97.19, B97.29, B97.5-B97.6, B97.81-B97.89

B26.81 Mumps hepatitis
Ex: A74.81-A74.9, A96.2, A98.3-A98.4, B26.81-B26.83, B26.85-B26.9, B33.24, B33.4, B33.8, B34.1-B34.2, B34.4-B34.8, B92, B94.2, B94.8-B94.9, B97.10, B97.19, B97.29, B97.5-B97.6, B97.81-B97.89

B26.82 Mumps myocarditis

B26.83 Mumps nephritis

B26.84 Mumps polyneuropathy
Ex: A74.81-A74.9, A96.2, A98.3-A98.4, B26.82-B26.9, B33.24, B33.4, B33.8, B34.1-B34.2, B34.4-B34.8, B92, B94.2, B94.8-B94.9, B97.10, B97.19, B97.29, B97.5-B97.6, B97.81-B97.89

B26.85 Mumps arthritis

B26.89 Other mumps complications

B26.9 Mumps without complication
Mumps NOS
Mumps parotitis NOS

B27 Infectious mononucleosis
Includes glandular fever
monocytic angina
Pfeiffer's disease

B27.0 Gammaherpesviral mononucleosis
AKA: Pfeiffer's disease, infective mononucleosis
Mononucleosis due to Epstein-Barr virus

B27.00 Gammaherpesviral mononucleosis without complication
Infective mononucleosis

B27.01 Gammaherpesviral mononucleosis with polyneuropathy

B27.02 Gammaherpesviral mononucleosis with meningitis

B27.09 Gammaherpesviral mononucleosis with other complications
Hepatomegaly in gammaherpesviral mononucleosis

B27.1 Cytomegaloviral mononucleosis
Infectious disease resembling infectious mononucleosis

B27.10 Cytomegaloviral mononucleosis without complications

B27.11 Cytomegaloviral mononucleosis with polyneuropathy

B27.12 Cytomegaloviral mononucleosis with meningitis

B27.19 Cytomegaloviral mononucleosis with other complication
Hepatomegaly in cytomegaloviral mononucleosis

B27.8 Other infectious mononucleosis

B27.80 Other infectious mononucleosis without complication

B27.81 Other infectious mononucleosis with polyneuropathy

B27.82 Other infectious mononucleosis with meningitis

B27.89 Other infectious mononucleosis with other complication
Hepatomegaly in other infectious mononucleosis

B27.9 Infectious mononucleosis, unspecified

B27.90 Infectious mononucleosis, unspecified without complication

B27.91 Infectious mononucleosis, unspecified with polyneuropathy

B27.92 Infectious mononucleosis, unspecified with meningitis

B27.99 Infectious mononucleosis, unspecified with other complication
Hepatomegaly in unspecified infectious mononucleosis

B30 Viral conjunctivitis
Excludes1 herpesviral [herpes simplex] ocular disease (B00.5)
ocular zoster (B02.3)

B30.0 Keratoconjunctivitis due to adenovirus
Epidemic keratoconjunctivitis
Shipyard eye

B30.1 Conjunctivitis due to adenovirus
Acute adenoviral follicular conjunctivitis
Swimming-pool conjunctivitis

B30.2 Viral pharyngoconjunctivitis

B30.3 Acute epidemic hemorrhagic conjunctivitis (enteroviral)
Conjunctivitis due to coxsackievirus 24
Conjunctivitis due to enterovirus 70
Hemorrhagic conjunctivitis (acute)(epidemic)

B30.8 Other viral conjunctivitis
Newcastle conjunctivitis

B30.9 Viral conjunctivitis, unspecified

B33 Other viral diseases, not elsewhere classified

B33.0 Epidemic myalgia
Acute infectious disease, caused by group A coxsackie viruses or other enteroviruses with symptoms that include sudden pain in chest or upper abdomen with fever
Bornholm disease

B33.1 Ross River disease
Epidemic polyarthritis and exanthema
Ross River fever
Ex: See A92.1

B33.2 Viral carditis
Coxsackie (virus) carditis

B33.20 Viral carditis, unspecified
Ex: A52.06, B33.20-B33.22, I00, I01.2-I01.9, I09.0, I09.9, I23.0-I23.3, I23.6-I23.8, I40.0-I41, I51.0, I51.4, I87.8-I87.9, I99.8-I99.9

B33.21 Viral endocarditis
Ex: A01.00-A01.09, A39.51, A52.03, A78, B33.21, B37.6, B40.0-B40.9, I00, I01.1, I01.8-I02.0, I05.0-I07.9, I08.1-I08.3, I08.9, I09.1, I09.89-I09.9, I33.0-I39, I42.4, I87.8-I87.9, I99.8-I99.9, Q22.2, Q23.8-Q23.9, Q24.8, T82.6XXA

B33.22 Viral myocarditis
Ex: See B33.20

B33.23 Viral pericarditis
Ex: B33.23, I01.0, I09.2, I30.0-I30.9, I31.3-I32, I87.8-I87.9, I99.8-I99.9

B33.24 Viral cardiomyopathy

B33.3 Retrovirus infections, not elsewhere classified
Retrovirus infection NOS

B33.4 Hantavirus (cardio)-pulmonary syndrome [HPS] [HCPS]
Hantavirus disease with pulmonary manifestations
Sin nombre virus disease
Use additional code to identify any associated acute kidney failure (N17.9)
Excludes1 hantavirus disease with renal manifestations (A98.5)
hemorrhagic fever with renal manifestations (A98.5)
Ex: A74.81-A74.9, A88.1, A96.0-A96.9, A98.3-A98.5, B19.20-B19.21, B25.8-B25.9, B33.24, B33.3-B34.2, B34.4-B34.8, B97.0-B97.89

B33.8 Other specified viral diseases
Excludes1 anogenital human papillomavirus infection (A63.0)
viral warts due to human papillomavirus infection (B07)

B34 Viral infection of unspecified site
Excludes1 anogenital human papillomavirus infection (A63.0)
cytomegaloviral disease NOS (B25.9)
herpesvirus [herpes simplex] infection NOS (B00.9)
retrovirus infection NOS (B33.3)
viral agents as the cause of diseases classified elsewhere (B97.-)
viral warts due to human papillomavirus infection (B07)

B34.0 Adenovirus infection, unspecified

B34.1 Enterovirus infection, unspecified
Intestinal tract infection
Coxsackievirus infection NOS
Echovirus infection NOS

B34.2 Coronavirus infection, unspecified
Excludes1 pneumonia due to SARS-associated coronavirus (J12.81)

B34.3 Parvovirus infection, unspecified
Ex: B08.3, B34.3

B34.4 Papovavirus infection, unspecified

B34.8 Other viral infections of unspecified site

B34.9 Viral infection, unspecified
Viremia NOS

MYCOSES (B35-B49)

Excludes2 hypersensitivity pneumonitis due to organic dust (J67.-)
mycosis fungoides (C84.0-)

B35 Dermatophytosis
AKA tinea or ringworm
Includes favus
infections due to species of Epidermophyton, Micro-sporum and Trichophyton
tinea, any type except those in B36.-

B35.0 Tinea barbae and tinea capitis
Beard ringworm
Kerion
Scalp ringworm
Sycosis, mycotic

B35.1 Tinea unguium
White patches or pits on surface or edges of nails, followed by infection under nail plate
Dermatophytic onychia
Dermatophytosis of nail
Onychomycosis
Ringworm of nails

B35.2 Tinea manuum
Tinea of hands
Dermatophytosis of hand
Hand ringworm

B35.3 Tinea pedis
Tinea affecting feet
Athlete's foot
Dermatophytosis of foot
Foot ringworm

B35.4 Tinea corporis
Infecting skin areas other than hands
Ringworm of the body

B35.5 Tinea imbricata
Chronic tropical tinea corporis; AKA Oriental ringworm, tinea inguinalis, tinea cruris
Tokelau

B35.6 Tinea cruris
In groin or perineal area, spreading to adjacent regions; AKA jock itch, eczema marginatum, ringworm of groin, or t inguinalis
Dhobi itch
Groin ringworm
Jock itch

B35.8 Other dermatophytoses
Disseminated dermatophytosis
Granulomatous dermatophytosis

B35.9 Dermatophytosis, unspecified
Ringworm NOS

B36 Other superficial mycoses

B36.0 Pityriasis versicolor
Common, chronic, symptomless disorder that includes macular patches of various sizes and shapes; AKA liver spots
Tinea flava
Tinea versicolor

B36.1 Tinea nigra
Minor fungal infection, with dark lesions, usually on skin of hands
Keratomycosis nigricans palmaris
Microsporosis nigra
Pityriasis nigra

B36.2 White piedra
White to light brown nodules on hair of beard, axilla, or groin; AKA trichosporosis
Tinea blanca

B36.3 Black piedra
Characterized by small black or brown nodules on shafts of scalp hair

B36.8 Other specified superficial mycoses

B36.9 Superficial mycosis, unspecified

B37 Candidiasis
Includes candidosis
moniliasis
Excludes1 neonatal candidiasis (P37.5)

B37.0 Candidal stomatitis
Oral thrush
Ex: B37.0-B37.9, B48.3, B49, B92, B94.2-B94.9

B37.1 Pulmonary candidiasis
Candidal bronchitis
Candidal pneumonia
Ex: See B37.0

B37.2 Candidiasis of skin and nail
Candidal onychia
Candidal paronychia
Excludes2 diaper dermatitis (L22)

B37.3 Candidiasis of vulva and vagina ♀
Candidal vulvovaginitis
Monilial vulvovaginitis
Vaginal thrush

B37.4 Candidiasis of other urogenital sites
Ex: **For category B37.4 CC codes:** B37.1, B37.41-B37.82, B37.84-B37.9, N25.81-N25.89

B37.41 Candidal cystitis and urethritis

B37.42 Candidal balanitis
Male condition only

B37.49 Other urogenital candidiasis
Candidal pyelonephritis

B37.5 Candidal meningitis
Ex: A02.21, A17.0-A17.1, A27.81, A39.0, A50.41, A51.41, A52.13, A54.82, A54.84, A54.89-A54.9, A87.0-A87.9, B00.3, B02.1, B26.1, B37.0-B38.4, B45.1, B48.3, B49, B58.2, B92, B94.2-B94.9, G00.0-G03.9, G04.2, G32.89, G61.0, G96.8-G96.9, G98.0, G98.8-G99.8

B37.6 Candidal endocarditis
Ex: See B37.0

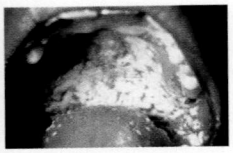

Figure 1-8 Oral candidiasis (thrush). *(Courtesy of Stephen Raffanti, MD, MPH.)* (From Mandell, Bennett, & Dolin: Principles and Practice of Infectious Diseases, ed 7, Churchill Livingstone, An Imprint of Elsevier, 2009)

Item 1-20 Candidiasis, also called oidiomycosis or moniliasis, is a fungal infection. It most often appears on moist cutaneous areas of the body but can also be responsible for a variety of systemic infections such as endocarditis, meningitis, arthritis, and myositis. Antifungal medications cure most yeast infections.

B37.7 Candidal sepsis
Disseminated candidiasis systemic candidiasis
MCC when PDx is its own MCC
Ex: A02.1, A20.7, A22.7, A26.7, A32.7, A39.2-A39.4, A40.0-A40.1, A40.8-A41.9, A42.7, A48.2-A48.4, A48.8-A49.9, A54.86, B00.7, B37.0-B37.9, B48.3, B49, B92, B94.2-B96.89, R65.10-R65.20, Z16.10-Z16.39

B37.8 Candidiasis of other sites
Ex: **For category B37.8 CC codes unless otherwise indicated:** B37.0-B37.9, B48.3, B49, B92, B94.2-B94.9

B37.81 Candidal esophagitis

B37.82 Candidal enteritis
Candidal proctitis

B37.83 Candidal cheilitis
Inflammation affecting lip

B37.84 Candidal otitis externa
Inflammation of external auditory canal

B37.89 Other sites of candidiasis
Infection manifested by invasive candidiasis
Candidal osteomyelitis
Ex: B37.1, B37.5-B37.82, B37.84-B37.9

B37.9 Candidiasis, unspecified
Thrush NOS

B38 Coccidioidomycosis
Fungal disease; AKA coccidioidosis, coccidioidal granuloma, Posadas, or Posadas-Wernicke disease

B38.0 Acute pulmonary coccidioidomycosis
Ex: B38.0-B38.2, B38.7, B38.89-B38.9, B48.3, B49, B92, B94.2-B94.9

B38.1 Chronic pulmonary coccidioidomycosis
Ex: B38.0-B39.9

B38.2 Pulmonary coccidioidomycosis, unspecified
Ex: See B38.1

B38.3 Cutaneous coccidioidomycosis
Ex: B38.0-B38.9

B38.4 Coccidioidomycosis meningitis
Ex: A02.21, A17.0-A17.1, A27.81, A39.0, A50.41, A51.41, A52.13, A54.82, A54.84, A54.89-A54.9, A87.0-A87.9, B00.3, B02.1, B26.1, B37.5, B38.4-B38.87, B38.89-B38.9, B45.1, B48.3, B49, B58.2, B92, B94.2-B94.9, G00.0-G03.9, G04.2, G32.89, G61.0, G96.8-G96.9, G98.0, G98.8-G99.8

B38.7 Disseminated coccidioidomycosis
Generalized coccidioidomycosis
Ex: B38.7, B38.89-B38.9, B48.3, B49, B92, B94.2-B94.9

B38.8 Other forms of coccidioidomycosis

B38.81 Prostatic coccidioidomycosis ♂
Ex: See B38.3

B38.89 Other forms of coccidioidomycosis
Ex: See B38.7

B38.9 Coccidioidomycosis, unspecified
Ex: See B38.7

B39 Histoplasmosis
Infection resulting from inhalation or ingestion of spores; AKA Darling disease
Code first associated AIDS (B20)
Use additional code for any associated manifestations, such as:
endocarditis (I39)
meningitis (G02)
pericarditis (I32)
retinitis (H32)

B39.0 Acute pulmonary histoplasmosis capsulati
Ex: A22.1, A37.01-A37.11, A37.81, A37.9, A48.1, B25.0, B39.0-B39.4, B39.9-B44.0, B48.3, B49, B92, B94.2-B94.9, J09.X1-J09.X2, J10.00-J10.1, J11.00-J11.1, J12.0-J12.3, J12.89-J18.1, J18.8-J18.9, J44.9, J47.0-J47.9, J60-J70.4, J70.8-J70.9, J98.4, R91.1

B39.1 Chronic pulmonary histoplasmosis capsulati
Ex: See B39.0

B39.2 Pulmonary histoplasmosis capsulati, unspecified
Ex: See B39.0

B39.3 Disseminated histoplasmosis capsulati
Generalized histoplasmosis capsulati
Ex: B38.0-B39.4

Item 1–21 Bird and bat droppings that fall into the soil give rise to a fungus that can spread airborne spores. When inhaled into the lungs, these spores divide and multiply into lesions. Histoplasmosis capsulatum takes three forms: primary (lodged in the lungs only), chronic (resembles TB), and disseminated (infection has moved to other organs). This is an opportunistic infection in immunosuppressed patients.

B39.4 Histoplasmosis capsulati, unspecified
American histoplasmosis

B39.5 Histoplasmosis duboisii
African histoplasmosis

B39.9 Histoplasmosis, unspecified

B40 Blastomycosis
Rare and potentially fatal infection caused by inhaling fungus found in moist soil in temperate climates.

Excludes1 Brazilian blastomycosis (B41.-)
keloidal blastomycosis (B48.0)

Ex: **For category B40 CC codes:** B40.0-B40.9, B48.3, B49, B92, B94.2-B94.9

B40.0 Acute pulmonary blastomycosis CC
B40.1 Chronic pulmonary blastomycosis CC
B40.2 Pulmonary blastomycosis, unspecified CC
B40.3 Cutaneous blastomycosis CC
B40.7 Disseminated blastomycosis CC
Generalized blastomycosis
B40.8 Other forms of blastomycosis
B40.81 Blastomycotic meningoencephalitis CC
Meningomyelitis due to blastomycosis
B40.89 Other forms of blastomycosis CC
B40.9 Blastomycosis, unspecified CC

B41 Paracoccidioidomycosis
Fungal infection usually chronic that begins in lungs, spreads to mucocutaneous areas which may extend to skin, tonsils, gastrointestinal lymphatics, liver, and spleen; AKA Almeida or Lutz-Splendore-Almeida disease, Brazilian or South American blastomycosis, or paracoccidioidal granuloma

Includes Brazilian blastomycosis
Lutz' disease

Ex: **For category B41 CC codes:** B41.0-B41.9, B48.3, B49, B92, B94.2-B94.9

B41.0 Pulmonary paracoccidioidomycosis CC
B41.7 Disseminated paracoccidioidomycosis CC
Generalized paracoccidioidomycosis
B41.8 Other forms of paracoccidioidomycosis CC
B41.9 Paracoccidioidomycosis, unspecified CC

B42 Sporotrichosis
Chronic fungal infection with nodular lesions
B42.0 Pulmonary sporotrichosis
B42.1 Lymphocutaneous sporotrichosis
B42.7 Disseminated sporotrichosis
Generalized sporotrichosis
B42.8 Other forms of sporotrichosis
B42.81 Cerebral sporotrichosis
Meningitis due to sporotrichosis
B42.82 Sporotrichosis arthritis
B42.89 Other forms of sporotrichosis
B42.9 Sporotrichosis, unspecified

B43 Chromomycosis and pheomycotic abscess
Chronic fungal infection of skin, initiated at site of puncture affecting lower limb or foot (mossy foot)
B43.0 Cutaneous chromomycosis
Dermatitis verrucosa
B43.1 Pheomycotic brain abscess
Cerebral chromomycosis
B43.2 Subcutaneous pheomycotic abscess and cyst
B43.8 Other forms of chromomycosis
B43.9 Chromomycosis, unspecified

B44 Aspergillosis
Infection marked by inflammatory lesions in skin, ear, orbit, nasal sinuses, lungs, and occasionally bones and meninges

Includes aspergilloma

Ex: **For category B44 CC codes unless otherwise indicated:** B44.1-B44.7, B44.89-B44.9, B48.3-B48.4, B49, B92, B94.2-B94.9

B44.0 Invasive pulmonary aspergillosis MCC
MCC when PDx is its own MCC
Ex: See B25.0
B44.1 Other pulmonary aspergillosis CC
B44.2 Tonsillar aspergillosis CC
B44.7 Disseminated aspergillosis CC
Generalized aspergillosis
B44.8 Other forms of aspergillosis
B44.81 Allergic bronchopulmonary aspergillosis CC
Ex: B44.81, J22, J98.8-J98.9
B44.89 Other forms of aspergillosis CC
B44.9 Aspergillosis, unspecified CC

B45 Cryptococcosis
Infection in the immunocompromised and fatal if left untreated; AKA torulosis, Buschke, or Busse-Buschke disease

Ex: **For category B45 CC codes unless otherwise indicated:** B45.0, B45.2-B45.9, B48.3, B49, B92, B94.2-B94.9

B45.0 Pulmonary cryptococcosis CC
B45.1 Cerebral cryptococcosis MCC
Cryptococcal meningitis
Cryptococcosis meningocerebralis
MCC when PDx is its own MCC
Ex: A02.21, A17.0-A17.1, A27.81, A39.0, A50.41, A51.41, A52.13, A54.82, A54.84, A54.89-A54.9, A87.0-A87.9, B00.3, B02.1, B26.1, B37.5, B38.4, B45.1, B58.2, E08.40-E08.49, E08.618-E08.638, E08.649-E08.8, E09.40-E09.49, E09.618-E09.638, E09.649-E09.8, E10.40-E10.49, E10.618-E10.638, E10.649, E10.69, E10.8, E11.40-E11.49, E11.618-E11.638, E11.649, E11.69-E11.8, E13.40-E13.49, E13.618-E13.638, E13.649-E13.69, E13.8, G00.0-G03.9, G04.2, G32.89, G61.0, G96.8-G96.9, G98.0-G98.8, G99.8
B45.2 Cutaneous cryptococcosis CC
B45.3 Osseous cryptococcosis CC
B45.7 Disseminated cryptococcosis CC
Generalized cryptococcosis
B45.8 Other forms of cryptococcosis CC
B45.9 Cryptococcosis, unspecified CC

B46 Zygomycosis
Fungal infections including subcutaneous lesions and infection of sinuses, brain, or lungs

Ex: **For category B46 CC codes:** B46.0-B46.9, B48.3, B49, B92, B94.2-B94.9

B46.0 Pulmonary mucormycosis MCC
Fungal infection affecting lung
B46.1 Rhinocerebral mucormycosis MCC
B46.2 Gastrointestinal mucormycosis MCC
B46.3 Cutaneous mucormycosis MCC
Subcutaneous mucormycosis
B46.4 Disseminated mucormycosis MCC
Generalized mucormycosis
B46.5 Mucormycosis, unspecified MCC
B46.8 Other zygomycoses MCC
Entomophthoromycosis
B46.9 Zygomycosis, unspecified MCC
Phycomycosis NOS

B47 Mycetoma
Slow progressive, destructive fungal infection of cutaneous and subcutaneous tissues, fascia, and bone, primarily seen in foot (Madura foot) or leg

B47.0 Eumycetoma
Madura foot, mycotic Maduromycosis
Ex: B47.0, B48.3, B49, B92, B94.2-B94.9

B47.1 Actinomycetoma
Ex: A42.0-A42.2, A42.81-A43.9, B47.1-B47.9, L08.1

B47.9 Mycetoma, unspecified
Madura foot NOS
Ex: A42.81-A42.9, A43.8-A43.9, B47.1-B47.9

B48 Other mycoses, not elsewhere classified

B48.0 Lobomycosis
Infection with symptoms of red, smooth, hard cutaneous nodules resembling keloids
Keloidal blastomycosis
Lobo's disease

B48.1 Rhinosporidiosis
Chronic, localized granulomatous fungal infection, affecting mucocutaneous tissues, usually of nose characterized by polyps, papillomas, and wartlike lesions

B48.2 Allescheriasis
Fungal infection
Infection due to Pseudallescheria boydii
Excludes1 eumycetoma (B47.0)
Ex: B48.2-B48.3, B49, B92, B94.2-B94.9

B48.3 Geotrichosis
Fungal infection usually of bronchi, lungs, mouth, or intestinal tract
Geotrichum stomatitis
Ex: B48.3, B49

B48.4 Penicillosis
Fungal infection
Ex: B44.1-B44.7, B44.89-B44.9, B48.3-B48.4, B49, B92, B94.2-B94.9

B48.8 Other specified mycoses
Adiaspiromycosis
Infection of tissue and organs by Alternaria
Infection of tissue and organs by Drechslera
Infection of tissue and organs by Fusarium
Infection of tissue and organs by saprophytic fungi NEC
Ex: B48.3, B48.8-B49, B92, B94.2-B94.9

B49 Unspecified mycosis
Fungemia NOS
Ex: B48.3, B49

PROTOZOAL DISEASES (B50-B64)

Excludes1 amebiasis (A06.-)
other protozoal intestinal diseases (A07.-)

B50 Plasmodium falciparum malaria
Severe form of malaria that can be fatal
Includes mixed infections of Plasmodium falciparum with any other Plasmodium species
Ex: For category B50 CC codes: B50.0-B57.5

B50.0 Plasmodium falciparum malaria with cerebral complications
Cerebral malaria NOS

B50.8 Other severe and complicated Plasmodium falciparum malaria
Severe or complicated Plasmodium falciparum malaria NOS

B50.9 Plasmodium falciparum malaria, unspecified

B51 Plasmodium vivax malaria
Includes mixed infections of Plasmodium vivax with other Plasmodium species, except Plasmodium falciparum
Excludes1 plasmodium vivav with Plasmodium falciparum (B50.-)
Ex: For category B51 CC codes unless otherwise indicated: B50.0-B57.5

B51.0 Plasmodium vivax malaria with rupture of spleen

B51.8 Plasmodium vivax malaria with other complications

B51.9 Plasmodium vivax malaria without complication
Plasmodium vivax malaria NOS
Ex: A44.0-A44.9, A68.0-A68.9, A69.20-A69.29, B50.0-B57.5, B60.0

B52 Plasmodium malariae malaria
Causes fever that recurs at approximately three-day intervals (quartan fever), longer than two-day (tertian) intervals of other malarial parasites
Includes mixed infections of Plasmodium malariae with other Plasmodium species, except Plasmodium falciparum and Plasmodium vivax
Excludes1 plasmodium falciparum (B50.-)
plasmodium vivax (B51.-)
Ex: For category B52 CC codes unless otherwise indicated: B50.0-B57.5

B52.0 Plasmodium malariae malaria with nephropathy
CC when PDx is its own CC
Ex: A17.9, A18.10-A18.13, A18.82, A18.84, A18.89, A54.21, A54.29, A54.82, A54.84, A54.89-A54.9, A59.00, A59.8-A59.9, B37.41-B37.49, B50.0-B57.5, E08.21-E08.29, E08.618, E08.620-E08.638, E08.649-E08.8, E09.21-E09.29, E09.618-E09.638, E09.649-E09.8, E10.21-E10.29, E10.618-E10.638, E10.649, E10.69-E10.8, E11.21-E11.29, E11.618-E11.638, E11.649, E11.69-E11.8, E13.21-E13.29, E13.618-E13.638, E13.649-E13.8, E88.3, M10.30-M10.39, N00.0-N11.0, N11.8-N13.39, N13.6, N14.0-N19, N25.0-N26.1, N26.9-N27.9, N28.1-N29, N36.41-N36.43, N36.8-N36.9, N39.8-N39.9, R31.0-R31.9

B52.8 Plasmodium malariae malaria with other complications

B52.9 Plasmodium malariae malaria without complication
Plasmodium malariae malaria NOS

B53 Other specified malaria
Ex: For category B53 CC codes unless otherwise indicated: B50.0-B57.5

B53.0 Plasmodium ovale malaria
Least diagnosed type of malaria spread by female mosquitoes of rare species
Excludes1 plasmodium ovale with Plasmodium falciparum (B50.-)
plasmodium ovale with Plasmodium malariae (B52.-)
plasmodium ovale with Plasmodium vivax (B51.-)

B53.1 Malaria due to simian plasmodia
Malaria-like disease (parasite infection)
Excludes1 malaria due to simian plasmodia with Plasmodium falciparum (B50.-)
malaria due to simian plasmodia with Plasmodium malariae (B52.-)
malaria due to simian plasmodia with Plasmodium ovale (B53.0)
malaria due to simian plasmodia with Plasmodium vivax (B51.-)

B53.8 Other malaria, not elsewhere classified

B54 Unspecified malaria
Ex: B50.0-B57.5, B97.21

B55 Leishmaniasis
Protozoal infection
Ex: For category B55 CC codes: A44.0-A44.9, A68.0-A68.9, A69.20-A69.29, A75.0-A79.9, B50.0-B57.5, B60.0

B55.0 Visceral leishmaniasis
Kala-azar
Post-kala-azar dermal leishmaniasis

B55.1 Cutaneous leishmaniasis

B55.2 Mucocutaneous leishmaniasis

B55.9 Leishmaniasis, unspecified

● **B56 African trypanosomiasis**
Human African trypanosomiasis (HAT) is transmitted by fly bites
Ex: **For category B56 CC codes:** A44.0-A44.9, A68.0-A68.9, A69.20-A69.29, A75.0-A79.9, B50.0-B57.5, B60.0

B56.0 Gambiense trypanosomiasis
Infection due to Trypanosoma brucei gambiense
West African sleeping sickness

B56.1 Rhodesiense trypanosomiasis
East African sleeping sickness
Infection due to Trypanosoma brucei rhodesiense

B56.9 African trypanosomiasis, unspecified
Sleeping sickness NOS

● **B57 Chagas' disease**
Tropical parasitic disease
Includes American trypanosomiasis
infection due to Trypanosoma cruzi

B57.0 Acute Chagas' disease with heart involvement
Acute Chagas' disease with myocarditis
Ex: B57.0, B57.2, B92, B94.2-B94.9

B57.1 Acute Chagas' disease without heart involvement
Acute Chagas' disease NOS
Ex: See B56

B57.2 Chagas' disease (chronic) with heart involvement
American trypanosomiasis NOS
Chagas' disease (chronic) NOS
Chagas' disease (chronic) with myocarditis
Trypanosomiasis NOS
Ex: See B57.0

● **B57.3 Chagas' disease (chronic) with digestive system involvement**
Ex: **For category B57.3 CC codes:** A44.0-A44.9, A68.0-A68.9, A69.20-A69.29, A75.0-A79.9, B50.0-B57.5, B60.0

B57.30 Chagas' disease with digestive system involvement, unspecified

B57.31 Megaesophagus in Chagas' disease

B57.32 Megacolon in Chagas' disease

B57.39 Other digestive system involvement in Chagas' disease

● **B57.4 Chagas' disease (chronic) with nervous system involvement**
Ex: **For category B57.4 CC codes:** A44.0-A44.9, A68.0-A68.9, A69.20-A69.29, A75.0-A79.9, B50.0-B57.5, B60.0

B57.40 Chagas' disease with nervous system involvement, unspecified

B57.41 Meningitis in Chagas' disease

B57.42 Meningoencephalitis in Chagas' disease

B57.49 Other nervous system involvement in Chagas' disease

B57.5 Chagas' disease (chronic) with other organ involvement
Ex: See B57.4

● **B58 Toxoplasmosis**
Infection by protozoon transmitted in cysts in feces of cats
Includes infection due to Toxoplasma gondii
Excludes1 congenital toxoplasmosis (P37.1)

● **B58.0 Toxoplasma oculopathy**

B58.00 Toxoplasma oculopathy, unspecified
Ex: B58.00, B58.82-B58.9, B92, B94.2-B94.9

B58.01 Toxoplasma chorioretinitis
Ex: B58.00-B58.01, B58.82-B58.9, B92, B94.2-B94.9

B58.09 Other toxoplasma oculopathy
Toxoplasma uveitis
Ex: B58.00, B58.09, B58.82-B58.9, B92, B94.2-B94.9

B58.1 Toxoplasma hepatitis
Ex: B58.00, B58.1, B58.82-B58.9, B92, B94.2-B94.9

B58.2 Toxoplasma meningoencephalitis
Ex: B58.00, B58.2, B58.82-B58.9, B92, B94.2-B94.9

Item 1–22 Toxoplasmosis is caused by the protozoa **Toxoplasma gondii,** of which the house cat can be a host. Human infection occurs when contact is made with materials containing the pathogen, such as feces, contaminated soil, or ingestion of infected lamb, goat, or pork. Of the infected, very few have symptoms because a healthy person's immune system keeps the parasite from causing illness. When the immune system is compromised, symptoms may occur. Clinical symptoms include flu-like symptoms, but the disease progresses to include the eyes and the brain in babies.

B58.3 Pulmonary toxoplasmosis
Ex: A22.1, A37.01, A37.11, A37.81, A37.91, A48.1, B25.0, B44.0, B58.00, B58.3, B58.82-B58.9, B92, B94.2-B94.9, J09.X1-J09.X2, J10.00-J10.1, J11.00-J11.1, J12.0-J12.3, J12.89-J18.1, J18.8-J18.9, J44.9, J47.0-J70.4, J70.8-J70.9, J98.4, R91.1

● **B58.8 Toxoplasmosis with other organ involvement**
Ex: **For category B58.8 CC codes unless otherwise indicated:** B58.00, B58.82-B58.9, B92, B94.2-B94.9

B58.81 Toxoplasma myocarditis
Ex: B58.00, B58.81-B58.9, B92, B94.2-B94.9

B58.82 Toxoplasma myositis

B58.83 Toxoplasma tubulo-interstitial nephropathy
Toxoplasma pyelonephritis

B58.89 Toxoplasmosis with other organ involvement

B58.9 Toxoplasmosis, unspecified
Ex: B58.9

B59 Pneumocystosis
Caused by fungus
Pneumonia due to Pneumocystis carinii
Pneumonia due to Pneumocystis jiroveci
Ex: A22.1, A37.01, A37.11, A37.81, A37.91, A48.1, B25.0, B44.0, B59, B92, B94.2-B94.9, J09.X1-J09.X2, J10.00-J10.1, J11.00-J11.1, J12.0-J12.3, J12.89-J15.20, J15.211-J18.1, J18.8-J18.9, J44.9, J47.0-J70.4, J70.8-J70.9, J98.4, R91.1

● **B60 Other protozoal diseases, not elsewhere classified**
Excludes1 cryptosporidiosis (A07.2)
intestinal microsporidiosis (A07.8)
isosporiasis (A07.3)

B60.0 Babesiosis
Tickborne disease caused by microscopic organisms
Piroplasmosis
Ex: A44.0-A44.9, A68.0-A68.9, A69.20-A69.29, A75.0-A79.9, B50.0-B57.5, B60.0

● **B60.1 Acanthamebiasis**
Ex: **For category B60.1 CC codes:** B59, B60.10-B60.11, B60.19-B64, B89, B99.8-B99.9, L94.6, M35.2

B60.10 Acanthamebiasis, unspecified

B60.11 Meningoencephalitis due to Acanthamoeba (culbertsoni)

B60.12 Conjunctivitis due to Acanthamoeba

● **B60.13 Keratoconjunctivitis due to Acanthamoeba**

B60.19 Other acanthamebic disease

B60.2 Naegleriasis
Infection with microscopic organisms
Primary amebic meningoencephalitis
Ex: B59, B60.10-B60.11, B60.19-B64, B89, B99.8-B99.9, L94.6, M35.2

B60.8 Other specified protozoal diseases
Microsporidiosis

B64 Unspecified protozoal disease

HELMINTHIASES (B65-B83)

Diseases or infestations caused by parasitic worms

● **B65 Schistosomiasis [bilharziasis]**
Infection with flukes (flat parasitic worms)
Includes snail fever
Ex: **For category B64 CC codes:** B65.0-B65.9

B65.0 Schistosomiasis due to Schistosoma haematobium [urinary schistosomiasis]

B65.1 Schistosomiasis due to Schistosoma mansoni [intestinal schistosomiasis]

B65.2 Schistosomiasis due to Schistosoma japonicum
Asiatic schistosomiasis

B65.3 Cercarial dermatitis
Swimmer's itch

B65.8 Other schistosomiasis
Infection due to Schistosoma intercalatum
Infection due to Schistosoma mattheei
Infection due to Schistosoma mekongi

B65.9 Schistosomiasis, unspecified

● **B66 Other fluke infections**
Trematode (parasitic worms)
Ex: For category B66 CC codes: B66.0-B66.9

B66.0 Opisthorchiasis
Infection due to cat liver fluke
Infection due to Opisthorchis (felineus)(viverrini)

B66.1 Clonorchiasis
Chinese liver fluke disease
Infection due to Clonorchis sinensis
Oriental liver fluke disease

B66.2 Dicroceliasis
Liver fluke
Infection due to Dicrocoelium dendriticum
Lancet fluke infection

B66.3 Fascioliasis
Infection due to Fasciola gigantica
Infection due to Fasciola hepatica
Infection due to Fasciola indica
Sheep liver fluke disease

B66.4 Paragonimiasis
Infection due to Paragonimus species
Lung fluke disease
Pulmonary distomiasis

B66.5 Fasciolopsiasis
Largest intestinal fluke in humans
Infection due to Fasciolopsis buski
Intestinal distomiasis

B66.8 Other specified fluke infections
Echinostomiasis
Heterophyiasis
Metagonimiasis
Nanophyetiasis
Watsoniasis

B66.9 Fluke infection, unspecified

● **B67 Echinococcosis**
Larval forms of tapeworms usually of liver or lungs
Includes hydatidosis

B67.0 Echinococcus granulosus infection of liver
Ex: B67.0, B67.8-B67.99

B67.1 Echinococcus granulosus infection of lung
Ex: B67.1, B67.8-B67.99, J12.81

B67.2 Echinococcus granulosus infection of bone
Ex: B67.2, B67.32-B67.39, B67.8-B67.99

● **B67.3 Echinococcus granulosus infection, other and multiple sites**

B67.31 Echinococcus granulosus infection, thyroid gland
Ex: B67.31, B67.8-B67.99

B67.32 Echinococcus granulosus infection, multiple sites
Ex: See B67.2

B67.39 Echinococcus granulosus infection, other sites
Ex: See B67.2

B67.4 Echinococcus granulosus infection, unspecified
Dog tapeworm (infection)
Ex: B67.4, B67.8-B67.99

B67.5 Echinococcus multilocularis infection of liver
Ex: B67.5, B67.8-B67.99

Item 1-23 Echinococcosis: Also known as hydatid disease; is caused by Echinococcus granulosus, E. multilocularis, and E. vogeli tapeworms; and is contracted from infected food. Found in southern South America, the Mediterranean, the Middle East, central Asia, and Africa and uncommon in the United States but has been reported in California, New Mexico, Arizona and Utah. The disease is treated with medication over a long course as it is resistive.

● **B67.6 Echinococcus multilocularis infection, other and multiple sites**
Ex: For category B67.6 CC codes: B67.61-B67.69, B67.8-B67.99

B67.61 Echinococcus multilocularis infection, multiple sites

B67.69 Echinococcus multilocularis infection, other sites

B67.7 Echinococcus multilocularis infection, unspecified
Ex: B67.7-B67.99

B67.8 Echinococcosis, unspecified, of liver
Ex: B67.8-B67.99

● **B67.9 Echinococcosis, other and unspecified**
Ex: For category B67.9 CC codes: B67.8-B67.99

B67.90 Echinococcosis, unspecified
Echinococcosis NOS

B67.99 Other echinococcosis

● **B68 Taeniasis**
Intestinal tapeworm (cestode) infection from raw or undercooked meat of infected animal
Excludes1 cysticercosis (B69.-)

B68.0 Taenia solium taeniasis
Pork tapeworm (infection)
Ex: A00.1, A01.00-A01.09, A01.4-A02.0, A03.9-A05.2, A06.0-A06.2, A06.9, A07.1-A09, A18.32-A18.39, A18.83, A48.51-A48.52, B37.82, B68.0-B71.9, B82.9, J09.X3-J09.X9, J10.2-J10.89, J11.2-J11.89, K30, K31.84, K52.1-K52.3, K52.82-K52.9, K58.0-K58.9, P76.8-P77.9, P78.1, P78.3-P78.89

B68.1 Taenia saginata taeniasis
Beef tapeworm (infection)
Infection due to adult tapeworm Taenia saginata
Ex: B68.0-B71.9

B68.9 Taeniasis, unspecified
Ex: B68.0-B71.9

● **B69 Cysticercosis**
Systemic illness caused by the larvae of pork tapeworm
Includes cysticerciasis infection due to larval form of Taenia solium
Ex: For category B69 CC codes: B68.0-B71.9

B69.0 Cysticercosis of central nervous system

B69.1 Cysticercosis of eye

● **B69.8 Cysticercosis of other sites**

B69.81 Myositis in cysticercosis

B69.89 Cysticercosis of other sites

B69.9 Cysticercosis, unspecified

● **B70 Diphyllobothriasis and sparganosis**
Infection with tapeworms seen most often from inadequately cooked fish
Ex: For category B70 CC codes: B68.0-B71.9

B70.0 Diphyllobothriasis
Diphyllobothrium (adult) (latum) (pacificum) infection
Fish tapeworm (infection)
Excludes2 larval diphyllobothriasis (B70.1)

B70.1 Sparganosis
Infection with migrating tapeworm larvae, which invade subcutaneous tissues, causing inflammation and fibrosis that resembles cellulitis
Infection due to Sparganum (mansoni) (proliferum)
Infection due to Spirometra larva
Larval diphyllobothriasis
Spirometrosis

B71 Other cestode infections
Ex: For category B71 CC codes: B68.0-B71.9

B71.0 Hymenolepiasis
Intestinal infestation with tapeworms
Dwarf tapeworm infection
Rat tapeworm (infection)

B71.1 Dipylidiasis
Infection with tapeworm common to dogs and cats and seen in children having close contact with infected pets

B71.8 Other specified cestode infections
Infection by the larval stage of a tapeworm, usually through fruit or vegetables
Coenurosis

B71.9 Cestode infection, unspecified
Tapeworm (infection) NOS

B72 Dracunculiasis
Infection with roundworms
Includes guinea worm infection
infection due to Dracunculus medinensis
Ex: B72-B74.9

B73 Onchocerciasis
Infection with parasitic worm
Includes onchocerca volvulus infection
onchocercosis
river blindness

B73.0 Onchocerciasis with eye disease
Ex: For category B73 CC codes: B72-B74.9

B73.00 Onchocerciasis with eye involvement, unspecified

B73.01 Onchocerciasis with endophthalmitis

B73.02 Onchocerciasis with glaucoma

B73.09 Onchocerciasis with other eye involvement
Infestation of eyelid due to onchocerciasis

B73.1 Onchocerciasis without eye disease

B74 Filariasis
Infestation with slender threadlike worms
Excludes2 onchocerciasis (B73)
tropical (pulmonary) eosinophilia NOS (J82)
Ex: For category B74 CC codes: B72-B74.9

B74.0 Filariasis due to Wuchereria bancrofti
Bancroftian elephantiasis
Bancroftian filariasis

B74.1 Filariasis due to Brugia malayi

B74.2 Filariasis due to Brugia timori

B74.3 Loiasis
Infection with round worms growing in subcutaneous connective tissue
Calabar swelling
Eyeworm disease of Africa
Loa loa infection

B74.4 Mansonelliasis
Infection with filarial parasite
Infection due to Mansonella ozzardi
Infection due to Mansonella perstans
Infection due to Mansonella streptocerca

B74.8 Other filariases
Dirofilariasis

B74.9 Filariasis, unspecified

B75 Trichinellosis
Infestation with parasitic roundworms ingested in undercooked contaminated meat
Includes infection due to Trichinella species trichiniasis
Ex: A17.82, A50.42, A52.14, A75.9, A79.9, A81.1, A81.82-A81.89, A83.0-A85.8, A87.2, A88.0, A88.8, A92.1-A92.8, A93.0, B00.4, B00.82, B01.11-B01.12, B04, B06.01, B08.09, B08.20-B08.22, B08.60-B08.79, B09, B10.01-B10.09, B26.2, B33.1, B45.0, B45.2-B45.9, B58.2, B75, B97.10, B97.21, G04.00-G04.01, G04.31, G04.81-G05.4, G37.0, G37.4-G37.5, J09.X3-J09.X9, J10.2-J10.89, J11.2-J11.89, L44.4, M1A.10X0-M1A.10X1, M1A.1110-M1A.19X1, P35.2-P35.9, P37.0-P37.4, P37.8-P37.9, T56.0X1-T56.0X4[A]

B76 Hookworm diseases
Occurs in hot, humid parts of world where larvae are soil borne, enter digestive tract through skin of feet/legs or in contaminated food/water; AKA ground itch
Includes uncinariasis
Ex: For category B76 CC codes: B76.0-B76.9

B76.0 Ancylostomiasis
Infection due to Ancylostoma species

B76.1 Necatoriasis
Infection due to Necator americanus

B76.8 Other hookworm diseases

B76.9 Hookworm disease, unspecified
Cutaneous larva migrans NOS

B77 Ascariasis
Infection by roundworm in small intestine
Includes ascaridiasis
roundworm infection

B77.0 Ascariasis with intestinal complications
Ex: B77.0-B78.0, B78.7-B82.0

B77.8 Ascariasis with other complications

B77.81 Ascariasis pneumonia
MCC when PDx is its own MCC
Ex: A15.0-A15.6, A15.8-A15.9, A17.9, A18.82, A18.84, A18.89, A21.2, A22.1, A31.0, A37.01, A37.11, A37.81, A37.91, A42.0, A43.0, A48.1, B25.0, B39.0-B39.2, B44.0, B58.3, B59, B67.1, B77.0-B78.0, B78.7-B82.0, J09.X1-J09.X2, J10.00-J10.1, J11.00-J11.1, J12.0-J12.3, J12.89-J18.1, J18.8-J18.9, J22, J44.9, J47.0-J70.4, J70.8-J70.9, J98.4, J98.8-J99, Q33.4, R91.1

B77.89 Ascariasis with other complications
Ex: See B77.0

B77.9 Ascariasis, unspecified
Ex: See B77.0

B78 Strongyloidiasis
Infection with adult female roundworms
Excludes1 trichostrongyliasis (B81.2)
Ex: For category B78 CC codes: B77.0-B78.0, B78.7-B82.0

B78.0 Intestinal strongyloidiasis

B78.1 Cutaneous strongyloidiasis

B78.7 Disseminated strongyloidiasis

B78.9 Strongyloidiasis, unspecified

B79 Trichuriasis
Intestinal infection with roundworms
Includes trichocephaliasis
whipworm (disease)(infection)
Ex: See B78

B80 Enterobiasis
Intestinal infection with pinworms
Includes oxyuriasis
pinworm infection
threadworm infection
Ex: See B78

B81 Other intestinal helminthiases, not elsewhere classified
Diseases or infestations caused by parasitic worms
Excludes1 angiostrongyliasis due to Parastrongylus cantonensis (B83.2)
Ex: For category B81 CC codes B81.0-B81.2: B77.0-B78.0, B78.7-B82.0 For category B81 CC codes B81.3-B81.8: B77.0-B78.0, B78.7-B83.3, B83.8-B83.9

B81.0 Anisakiasis
Roundworm infection via contaminated undercooked infected fish or marine mammals
Infection due to Anisakis larva

B81.1 Intestinal capillariasis
Infestation with of parasites (nematodes)
Capillariasis NOS
Infection due to Capillaria philippinensis
Excludes2 hepatic capillariasis (B83.8)

B81.2 Trichostrongyliasis

B81.3 Intestinal angiostrongyliasis
Angiostrongyliasis due to Parastrongylus costaricensis

B81.4 Mixed intestinal helminthiases
Infection due to intestinal helminths classified to more than one of the categories B65.0-B81.3 and B81.8
Mixed helminthiasis NOS

B81.8 Other specified intestinal helminthiases
Infection due to Oesophagostomum species [esophagostomiasis]
Infection due to Ternidens diminutus [ternidensiasis]

B82 Unspecified intestinal parasitism

B82.0 Intestinal helminthiasis, unspecified
Infected with worms
Ex: See B81.3

B82.9 Intestinal parasitism, unspecified

B83 Other helminthiases
Caused by parasitic worms
Excludes1 capillariasis NOS (B81.1)
Excludes2 intestinal capillariasis (B81.1)

B83.0 Visceral larva migrans
Prolonged migration of nematode larvae
Toxocariasis

B83.1 Gnathostomiasis
Infection with nematode occurring from ingested undercooked fish contaminated with larvae; larvae migrate to subcutaneous tissue or deeper tissues, results are abscesses
Wandering swelling

B83.2 Angiostrongyliasis due to Parastrongylus cantonensis
Nematode infection caused by eating contaminated raw snails, slugs, or paratenic hosts such as prawns or crabs; larval worms migrate to central nervous system resulting in eosinophilic meningitis
Eosinophilic meningoencephalitis due to Parastrongylus cantonensis
Excludes2 intestinal angiostrongyliasis (B81.3)

B83.3 Syngamiasis
Infestation with gapeworm from turkey, pheasant, guinea fowl, goose, and wild birds
Syngamosis

B83.4 Internal hirudiniasis
Infestation by leeches
Excludes2 external hirudiniasis (B88.3)

B83.8 Other specified helminthiases
Parasitic worm infestation
Acanthocephaliasis
Gongylonemiasis
Hepatic capillariasis
Metastrongyliasis
Thelaziasis

B83.9 Helminthiasis, unspecified
Worms NOS
Excludes1 intestinal helminthiasis NOS (B82.0)

PEDICULOSIS, ACARIASIS AND OTHER INFESTATIONS (B85-B89)

B85 Pediculosis and phthiriasis
Infestation of lice

B85.0 Pediculosis due to Pediculus humanus capitis
Head-louse infestation

B85.1 Pediculosis due to Pediculus humanus corporis
Body-louse infestation

B85.2 Pediculosis, unspecified

B85.3 Phthiriasis
Crab or pubic lice
Infestation by crab-louse
Infestation by Phthirus pubis

B85.4 Mixed pediculosis and phthiriasis
Infestation classifiable to more than one of the categories B85.0-B85.3

B86 Scabies
Sarcoptic itch
Contagious dermatitis caused by mites

B87 Myiasis
Infestation by fly maggots
Includes infestation by larva of flies

B87.0 Cutaneous myiasis
Creeping myiasis

B87.1 Wound myiasis
Traumatic myiasis

B87.2 Ocular myiasis

B87.3 Nasopharyngeal myiasis
Laryngeal myiasis

B87.4 Aural myiasis

B87.8 Myiasis of other sites

B87.81 Genitourinary myiasis

B87.82 Intestinal myiasis

B87.89 Myiasis of other sites

B87.9 Myiasis, unspecified

B88 Other infestations

B88.0 Other acariasis
Acarine dermatitis
Dermatitis due to Demodex species
Dermatitis due to Dermanyssus gallinae
Dermatitis due to Liponyssoides sanguineus
Trombiculosis
Excludes2 scabies (B86)

B88.1 Tungiasis [sandflea infestation]
Inflammatory skin disease caused by infestation of fleas

B88.2 Other arthropod infestations
Scarabiasis

B88.3 External hirudiniasis
Leech infestation NOS
Excludes2 internal hirudiniasis (B83.4)

B88.8 Other specified infestations
Infection of topical fresh water fish parasite
Ichthyoparasitism due to Vandellia cirrhosa
Linguatulosis
Porocephaliasis

B88.9 Infestation, unspecified
Infestation (skin) NOS
Infestation by mites NOS
Skin parasites NOS

B89 Unspecified parasitic disease

SEQUELAE OF INFECTIOUS AND PARASITIC DISEASES (B90-B94)

Note: Categories B90-B94 are to be used to indicate conditions in categories A00-B89 as the cause of sequelae, which are themselves classified elsewhere. The 'sequelae' include conditions specified as such; they also include residuals of diseases classifiable to the above categories if there is evidence that the disease itself is no longer present. Codes from these categories are not to be used for chronic infections. Code chronic current infections to active infectious disease as appropriate.

Code first condition resulting from (sequela) the infectious or parasitic disease

B90 Sequelae of tuberculosis
Condition resulting from tuberculosis

B90.0 Sequelae of central nervous system tuberculosis

B90.1 Sequelae of genitourinary tuberculosis

B90.2 Sequelae of tuberculosis of bones and joints

B90.8 Sequelae of tuberculosis of other organs
Excludes2 sequelae of respiratory tuberculosis (B90.9)

B90.9 Sequelae of respiratory and unspecified tuberculosis
Sequelae of tuberculosis NOS

B91 Sequelae of poliomyelitis

Excludes1 postpolio syndrome (G14)

B92 Sequelae of leprosy

● **B94 Sequelae of other and unspecified infectious and parasitic diseases**

B94.0 Sequelae of trachoma

B94.1 Sequelae of viral encephalitis

B94.2 Sequelae of viral hepatitis

B94.8 Sequelae of other specified infectious and parasitic diseases

B94.9 Sequelae of unspecified infectious and parasitic disease

OGCR Section I.C.1.b

Certain infectious and parasitic diseases

Infectious agents as the cause of diseases classified to other chapters

Certain infections are classified in chapters other than Chapter 1 and no organism is identified as part of the infection code. In these instances, it is necessary to use an additional code from Chapter 1 to identify the organism. A code from category B95, Streptococcus, Staphylococcus, and Enterococcus as the cause of diseases classified to other chapters, B96, Other bacterial agents as the cause of diseases classified to other chapters, or B97, Viral agents as the cause of diseases classified to other chapters, is to be used as an additional code to identify the organism. An instructional note will be found at the infection code advising that an additional organism code is required.

BACTERIAL AND VIRAL INFECTIOUS AGENTS (B95-B97)

Note: These categories are provided for use as supplementary or additional codes to identify the infectious agent(s) in diseases classified elsewhere.

Code the disease first, then the bacterium. Do not report codes from B95-B97 for sepsis.

● **B95 Streptococcus, Staphylococcus, and Enterococcus as the cause of diseases classified elsewhere**

B95.0 Streptococcus, group A, as the cause of diseases classified elsewhere

B95.1 Streptococcus, group B, as the cause of diseases classified elsewhere

B95.2 Enterococcus as the cause of diseases classified elsewhere

B95.3 Streptococcus pneumoniae as the cause of diseases classified elsewhere

B95.4 Other streptococcus as the cause of diseases classified elsewhere

B95.5 Unspecified streptococcus as the cause of diseases classified elsewhere

● **B95.6 Staphylococcus aureus as the cause of diseases classified elsewhere**

B95.61 Methicillin susceptible Staphylococcus aureus infection as the cause of diseases classified elsewhere

Methicillin susceptible Staphylococcus aureus (MSSA) infection as the cause of diseases classified elsewhere

Staphylococcus aureus infection NOS as the cause of diseases classified elsewhere

B95.62 Methicillin resistant Staphylococcus aureus infection as the cause of diseases classified elsewhere

Methicillin resistant staphylococcus aureus (MRSA) infection as the cause of diseases classified elsewhere

Coding Clinic: 2016, Q1, P13

B95.7 Other staphylococcus as the cause of diseases classified elsewhere

B95.8 Unspecified staphylococcus as the cause of diseases classified elsewhere

● **B96 Other bacterial agents as the cause of diseases classified elsewhere**

B96.0 Mycoplasma pneumoniae [M. pneumoniae] as the cause of diseases classified elsewhere

Pleuro-pneumonia-like-organism [PPLO]

B96.1 Klebsiella pneumoniae [K. pneumoniae] as the cause of diseases classified elsewhere

● **B96.2 Escherichia coli [E. coli] as the cause of diseases classified elsewhere**

B96.20 Unspecified Escherichia coli [E. coli] as the cause of diseases classified elsewhere

Escherichia coli [E. coli] NOS

B96.21 Shiga toxin-producing Escherichia coli [E. coli] (STEC) O157 as the cause of diseases classified elsewhere

E. coli O157:H- (nonmotile) with confirmation of Shiga toxin

E. coli O157 with confirmation of Shiga toxin when H antigen is unknown, or is not H7

O157:H7 Escherichia coli [E.coli] with or without confirmation of Shiga toxin-production

Shiga toxin-producing Escherichia coli [E.coli] O157:H7 with or without confirmation of Shiga toxin-production

STEC O157:H7 with or without confirmation of Shiga toxin-production

B96.22 Other specified Shiga toxin-producing Escherichia coli [E. coli] (STEC) as the cause of diseases classified elsewhere

Non-O157 Shiga toxin-producing Escherichia coli [E.coli]

Non-O157 Shiga toxin-producing Escherichia coli [E.coli] with known O group

B96.23 Unspecified Shiga toxin-producing Escherichia coli [E. coli] (STEC) as the cause of diseases classified elsewhere

Shiga toxin-producing Escherichia coli [E. coli] with unspecified O group

STEC NOS

B96.29 Other Escherichia coli [E. coli] as the cause of diseases classified elsewhere

Non-Shiga toxin-producing E. coli

B96.3 Hemophilus influenzae [H. influenzae] as the cause of diseases classified elsewhere

B96.4 Proteus (mirabilis) (morganii) as the cause of diseases classified elsewhere

B96.5 Pseudomonas (aeruginosa) (mallei) (pseudomallei) as the cause of diseases classified elsewhere

Coding Clinic: 2015, Q1, P18

B96.6 Bacteroides fragilis [B. fragilis] as the cause of diseases classified elsewhere

B96.7 Clostridium perfringens [C. perfringens] as the cause of diseases classified elsewhere

● **B96.8 Other specified bacterial agents as the cause of diseases classified elsewhere**

B96.81 Helicobacter pylori [H. pylori] as the cause of diseases classified elsewhere

B96.82 Vibrio vulnificus as the cause of diseases classified elsewhere

B96.89 Other specified bacterial agents as the cause of diseases classified elsewhere

● **B97 Viral agents as the cause of diseases classified elsewhere**

B97.0 Adenovirus as the cause of diseases classified elsewhere

● **B97.1 Enterovirus as the cause of diseases classified elsewhere**

B97.10 Unspecified enterovirus as the cause of diseases classified elsewhere

B97.11 Coxsackievirus as the cause of diseases classified elsewhere

B97.12 Echovirus as the cause of diseases classified elsewhere

B97.19 Other enterovirus as the cause of diseases classified elsewhere

● **B97.2 Coronavirus as the cause of diseases classified elsewhere**

B97.21 SARS-associated coronavirus as the cause of diseases classified elsewhere

Excludes1 pneumonia due to SARS-associated coronavirus (J12.81)

Ex: A15.0-A15.6, A15.8-A15.9, A17.9, A18.82, A18.84, A18.89, A21.2, A22.1, A31.0, A37.01, A37.11, A37.81, A37.91, A42.0, A43.0, A48.1, B25.0, B34.1-B34.2, B34.4-B34.8, B39.0-B39.2, B44.0, B58.3, B59, B67.1, B97.19-B97.29, B97.5-B97.6, B97.81-B97.89, J09.X1-J09.X2, J10.00-J10.1, J11.00-J11.1, J12.0-J12.3, J12.89-J15.20, J15.211-J18.1, J18.8-J18.9, J22, J44.9, J47.0-J70.4, J70.8-J70.9, J98.4, J98.8-J99, Q33.4, R91.1

B97.29 Other coronavirus as the cause of diseases classified elsewhere

● **B97.3 Retrovirus as the cause of diseases classified elsewhere**

Excludes1 human immunodeficiency virus [HIV] disease (B20)

B97.30 Unspecified retrovirus as the cause of diseases classified elsewhere

B97.31 Lentivirus as the cause of diseases classified elsewhere

B97.32 Oncovirus as the cause of diseases classified elsewhere

B97.33 Human T-cell lymphotrophic virus, type I [HTLV-I] as the cause of diseases classified elsewhere

Ex: A74.81, A74.9, B33.3-B33.4, B34.1-B34.2, B34.4-B34.8, B97.10, B97.19-B97.29, B97.31-B97.39, B97.5-B97.6, B97.81-B97.89

B97.34 Human T-cell lymphotrophic virus, type II [HTLV-II] as the cause of diseases classified elsewhere

Ex: A74.81, A74.9, B33.3-B33.4, B34.1-B34.2, B34.4-B34.8, B97.10, B97.19-B97.39, B97.5-B97.6, B97.81, B97.89

Item 1–24 **Retrovirus** develops by copying its RNA, genetic materials, into the DNA, which then produces new virus particles. It is from the Retroviridae virus family. **Human T-cell lymphotropic virus, Type I (HTLV-I)** is also called human T-cell leukemia virus, Type I, and is a retrovirus thought to cause T-cell leukemia/lymphoma. **Human T-cell lymphotropic virus, Type II (HTLV-II),** is also called human T-cell leukemia virus, Type II, and is a retrovirus associated with hematologic disorders.

HIV-2 is one of the serotypes of HIV and is usually confined to West Africa, whereas HIV-**1** is found worldwide.

B97.35 Human immunodeficiency virus, type 2 [HIV 2] as the cause of diseases classified elsewhere

Ex: A74.81, A74.9, B20, B33.3-B33.4, B34.1-B34.2, B34.4, B34.8, B97.10, B97.19-B97.39, B97.5-B97.6, B97.81, B97.89

B97.39 Other retrovirus as the cause of diseases classified elsewhere

B97.4 Respiratory syncytial virus as the cause of diseases classified elsewhere

B97.5 Reovirus as the cause of diseases classified elsewhere

B97.6 Parvovirus as the cause of diseases classified elsewhere

B97.7 Papillomavirus as the cause of diseases classified elsewhere

● **B97.8 Other viral agents as the cause of diseases classified elsewhere**

B97.81 Human metapneumovirus as the cause of diseases classified elsewhere

B97.89 Other viral agents as the cause of diseases classified elsewhere

OTHER INFECTIOUS DISEASES (B99)

● **B99 Other and unspecified infectious diseases**

B99.8 Other infectious disease

B99.9 Unspecified infectious disease

CHAPTER 2

NEOPLASMS (C00-D49)

OGCR Chapter-Specific Coding Guidelines

2. **Chapter 2: Neoplasms (C00-D49)**
General guidelines
Chapter 2 of the ICD-10-CM contains the codes for most benign and all malignant neoplasms. Certain benign neoplasms, such as prostatic adenomas, may be found in the specific body system chapters. To properly code a neoplasm it is necessary to determine from the record if the neoplasm is benign, in-situ, malignant, or of uncertain histologic behavior. If malignant, any secondary (metastatic) sites should also be determined.

Primary malignant neoplasms overlapping site boundaries
A primary malignant neoplasm that overlaps two or more contiguous (next to each other) sites should be classified to the subcategory/code .8 ('overlapping lesion'), unless the combination is specifically indexed elsewhere. For multiple neoplasms of the same site that are not contiguous such as tumors in different quadrants of the same breast, codes for each site should be assigned.

Malignant neoplasm of ectopic tissue
Malignant neoplasms of ectopic tissue are to be coded to the site of origin mentioned, e.g., ectopic pancreatic malignant neoplasms involving the stomach are coded to pancreas, unspecified (C25.9).

The neoplasm table in the Alphabetic Index should be referenced first. However, if the histological term is documented, that term should be referenced first, rather than going immediately to the Neoplasm Table, in order to determine which column in the Neoplasm Table is appropriate. For example, if the documentation indicates "adenoma," refer to the term in the Alphabetic Index to review the entries under this term and the instructional note to "see also neoplasm, by site, benign." The table provides the proper code based on the type of neoplasm and the site. It is important to select the proper column in the table that corresponds to the type of neoplasm. The Tabular List should then be referenced to verify that the correct code has been selected from the table and that a more specific site code does not exist.

See Section I.C.21. Factors influencing health status and contact with health services, Status, for information regarding Z15.0, codes for genetic susceptibility to cancer.

a. Treatment directed at the malignancy
If the treatment is directed at the malignancy, designate the malignancy as the principal diagnosis.

The only exception to this guideline is if a patient admission/encounter is solely for the administration of chemotherapy, immunotherapy or radiation therapy, assign the appropriate Z51.— code as the first-listed or principal diagnosis, and the diagnosis or problem for which the service is being performed as a secondary diagnosis.

b. Treatment of secondary site
When a patient is admitted because of a primary neoplasm with metastasis and treatment is directed toward the secondary site only, the secondary neoplasm is designated as the principal diagnosis even though the primary malignancy is still present.

c. Coding and sequencing of complications
Coding and sequencing of complications associated with the malignancies or with the therapy thereof are subject to the following guidelines:

1) Anemia associated with malignancy
When admission/encounter is for management of an anemia associated with the malignancy, and the treatment is only for anemia, the appropriate code for the malignancy is sequenced as the principal or first-listed diagnosis followed by the appropriate code for the anemia (such as code D63.0, Anemia in neoplastic disease).

2) Anemia associated with chemotherapy, immunotherapy and radiation therapy
When the admission/encounter is for management of an anemia associated with an adverse effect of the administration of chemotherapy or immunotherapy and the only treatment is for the anemia, the anemia code is sequenced first followed by the appropriate codes for the neoplasm and the adverse effect (T45.1X5, Adverse effect of antineoplastic and immunosuppressive drugs).

When the admission/encounter is for management of an anemia associated with an adverse effect of radiotherapy, the anemia code should be sequenced first, followed by the appropriate neoplasm code and code Y84.2, Radiological procedure and radiotherapy as the cause of abnormal reaction of the patient, or of later complication, without mention of misadventure at the time of the procedure.

3) Management of dehydration due to the malignancy
When the admission/encounter is for management of dehydration due to the malignancy and only the dehydration is being treated (intravenous rehydration), the dehydration is sequenced first, followed by the code(s) for the malignancy.

4) Treatment of a complication resulting from a surgical procedure
When the admission/encounter is for treatment of a complication resulting from a surgical procedure, designate the complication as the principal or first-listed diagnosis if treatment is directed at resolving the complication.

d. Primary malignancy previously excised
When a primary malignancy has been previously excised or eradicated from its site and there is no further treatment directed to that site and there is no evidence of any existing primary malignancy, a code from category Z85, Personal history of malignant neoplasm, should be used to indicate the former site of the malignancy. Any mention of extension, invasion, or metastasis to another site is coded as a secondary malignant neoplasm to that site. The secondary site may be the principal or first-listed with the Z85 code used as a secondary code.

e. Admissions/Encounters involving chemotherapy, immunotherapy and radiation therapy

1) Episode of care involves surgical removal of neoplasm
When an episode of care involves the surgical removal of a neoplasm, primary or secondary site, followed by adjunct chemotherapy or radiation treatment during the same episode of care, the code for the neoplasm should be assigned as principal or first-listed diagnosis.

2) Patient admission/encounter solely for administration of chemotherapy, immunotherapy and radiation therapy
If a patient admission/encounter is solely for the administration of chemotherapy, immunotherapy or radiation therapy assign code Z51.0, Encounter for antineoplastic radiation therapy, or Z51.11, Encounter for antineoplastic chemotherapy, or Z51.12, Encounter for antineoplastic immunotherapy as the first-listed or principal diagnosis. If a patient receives more than one of these therapies during the same admission more than one of these codes may be assigned, in any sequence.

The malignancy for which the therapy is being administered should be assigned as a secondary diagnosis.

3) Patient admitted for radiation therapy, chemotherapy or immunotherapy and develops complications
When a patient is admitted for the purpose of radiotherapy, immunotherapy or chemotherapy and develops complications such as uncontrolled nausea and vomiting or dehydration, the principal or first-listed diagnosis is Z51.0, Encounter for antineoplastic radiation therapy, or Z51.11, Encounter for antineoplastic chemotherapy, or Z51.12, Encounter for antineoplastic immunotherapy followed by any codes for the complications.

f. Admission/encounter to determine extent of malignancy
When the reason for admission/encounter is to determine the extent of the malignancy, or for a procedure such as paracentesis or thoracentesis, the primary malignancy or appropriate metastatic site is designated as the principal or first-listed diagnosis, even though chemotherapy or radiotherapy is administered.

g. Symptoms, signs, and abnormal findings listed in Chapter 18 associated with neoplasms
Symptoms, signs, and ill-defined conditions listed in Chapter 18 characteristic of, or associated with, an existing primary or secondary site malignancy cannot be used to replace the malignancy as principal or first-listed diagnosis, regardless of the number of admissions or encounters for treatment and care of the neoplasm.

See section I.C.21. Factors influencing health status and contact with health services, Encounter for prophylactic organ removal.

h. Admission/encounter for pain control/management
See Section I.C.6. for information on coding admission/encounter for pain control/management.

i. Malignancy in two or more noncontiguous sites
A patient may have more than one malignant tumor in the same organ. These tumors may represent different primaries or metastatic disease, depending on the site. Should the documentation be unclear, the provider should be queried as to the status of each tumor so that the correct codes can be assigned.

j. Disseminated malignant neoplasm, unspecified
Code C80.0, Disseminated malignant neoplasm, unspecified, is for use only in those cases where the patient has advanced metastatic disease and no known primary or secondary sites are specified. It should not be used in place of assigning codes for the primary site and all known secondary sites.

k. Malignant neoplasm without specification of site
Code C80.1, Malignant (primary) neoplasm, unspecified, equates to Cancer, unspecified. This code should only be used when no determination can be made as to the primary site of a malignancy. This code should rarely be used in the inpatient setting.

l. Sequencing of neoplasm codes

1) Encounter for treatment of primary malignancy
If the reason for the encounter is for treatment of a primary malignancy, assign the malignancy as the principal/first-listed diagnosis. The primary site is to be sequenced first, followed by any metastatic sites.

2) Encounter for treatment of secondary malignancy
When an encounter is for a primary malignancy with metastasis and treatment is directed toward the metastatic (secondary) site(s) only, the metastatic site(s) is designated as the principal/first-listed diagnosis. The primary malignancy is coded as an additional code.

3) Malignant neoplasm in a pregnant patient
When a pregnant woman has a malignant neoplasm, a code from subcategory O9A.1-, Malignant neoplasm complicating pregnancy, childbirth, and the puerperium, should be sequenced first, followed by the appropriate code from Chapter 2 to indicate the type of neoplasm.

4) Encounter for complication associated with a neoplasm
When an encounter is for management of a complication associated with a neoplasm, such as dehydration, and the treatment is only for the complication, the complication is coded first, followed by the appropriate code(s) for the neoplasm.

The exception to this guideline is anemia. When the admission/encounter is for management of an anemia associated with the malignancy, and the treatment is only for anemia, the appropriate code for the malignancy is sequenced as the principal or first-listed diagnosis followed by code D63.0, Anemia in neoplastic disease.

5) Complication from surgical procedure for treatment of a neoplasm
When an encounter is for treatment of a complication resulting from a surgical procedure performed for the treatment of the neoplasm, designate the complication as the principal/first-listed diagnosis. See guideline regarding the coding of a current malignancy versus personal history to determine if the code for the neoplasm should also be assigned.

6) Pathologic fracture due to a neoplasm
When an encounter is for a pathological fracture due to a neoplasm, and the focus of treatment is the fracture, a code from subcategory M84.5, Pathological fracture in neoplastic disease, should be sequenced first, followed by the code for the neoplasm.

If the focus of treatment is the neoplasm with an associated pathological fracture, the neoplasm code should be sequenced first, followed by a code from M84.5 for the pathological fracture.

m. Current malignancy versus personal history of malignancy
When a primary malignancy has been excised but further treatment, such as an additional surgery for the malignancy, radiation therapy or chemotherapy is directed to that site, the primary malignancy code should be used until treatment is completed.

When a primary malignancy has been previously excised or eradicated from its site, there is no further treatment (of the malignancy) directed to that site, and there is no evidence of any existing primary malignancy, a code from category Z85, Personal history of malignant neoplasm, should be used to indicate the former site of the malignancy.

See Section I.C.21. Factors influencing health status and contact with health services, History (of)

n. Leukemia, Multiple Myeloma, and Malignant Plasma Cell Neoplasms in remission versus personal history
The categories for leukemia, and category C90, Multiple myeloma and malignant plasma cell neoplasms, have codes indicating whether or not the leukemia has achieved remission. There are also codes Z85.6, Personal history of leukemia, and Z85.79, Personal history of other malignant neoplasms of lymphoid, hematopoietic and related tissues. If the documentation is unclear, as to whether the leukemia has achieved remission, the provider should be queried.

See Section I.C.21. Factors influencing health status and contact with health services, History (of)

o. Aftercare following surgery for neoplasm
See Section I.C.21. Factors influencing health status and contact with health services, Aftercare

p. Follow-up care for completed treatment of a malignancy
See Section I.C.21. Factors influencing health status and contact with health services, Follow-up

q. Prophylactic organ removal for prevention of malignancy
See Section I.C. 21, Factors influencing health status and contact with health services, Prophylactic organ removal

r. Malignant neoplasm associated with transplanted organ
A malignant neoplasm of a transplanted organ should be coded as a transplant complication. Assign first the appropriate code from category T86.-, Complications of transplanted organs and tissue, followed by code C80.2, Malignant neoplasm associated with transplanted organ. Use an additional code for the specific malignancy.

Item 2-1 Neoplasm: Neo = new, plasm = growth, development, formation. This new growth (mass, tumor) can be malignant or benign, which is confirmed by the pathology report. Do not assign a code to a neoplasm until you review the pathology report. Certain CPT codes will specify benign or malignant lesion, so be certain the diagnosis code supports the procedure code.

CHAPTER 2

NEOPLASMS (C00-D49)

This chapter contains the following blocks:

C00-C14	Malignant neoplasms of lip, oral cavity and pharynx
C15-C26	Malignant neoplasms of digestive organs
C30-C39	Malignant neoplasms of respiratory and intrathoracic organs
C40-C41	Malignant neoplasms of bone and articular cartilage
C43-C44	Melanoma and other malignant neoplasms of skin
C45-C49	Malignant neoplasms of mesothelial and soft tissue
C50	Malignant neoplasms of breast
C51-C58	Malignant neoplasms of female genital organs
C60-C63	Malignant neoplasms of male genital organs
C64-C68	Malignant neoplasms of urinary tract
C69-C72	Malignant neoplasms of eye, brain and other parts of central nervous system
C73-C75	Malignant neoplasms of thyroid and other endocrine glands
C7A	Malignant neuroendocrine tumors
C7B	Secondary neuroendocrine tumors
C76-C80	Malignant neoplasms of ill-defined, other secondary and unspecified sites
C81-C96	Malignant neoplasms of lymphoid, hematopoietic and related tissue
D00-D09	In situ neoplasms
D10-D36	Benign neoplasms, except benign neuroendocrine tumors
D3A	Benign neuroendocrine tumors
D37-D48	Neoplasms of uncertain behavior, polycythemia vera and myelodysplastic syndromes
D49	Neoplasms of unspecified behavior

Notes: Functional activity

All neoplasms are classified in this chapter, whether they are functionally active or not. An additional code from Chapter 4 may be used, to identify functional activity associated with any neoplasm.

Morphology [Histology]

Chapter 2 classifies neoplasms primarily by site (topography), with broad groupings for behavior, malignant, in situ, benign, etc. The Table of Neoplasms should be used to identify the correct topography code. In a few cases, such as for malignant melanoma and certain neuroendocrine tumors, the morphology (histologic type) is included in the category and codes.

Primary malignant neoplasms overlapping site boundaries

A primary malignant neoplasm that overlaps two or more contiguous (next to each other) sites should be classified to the subcategory/code .8 ('overlapping lesion'), unless the combination is specifically indexed elsewhere. For multiple neoplasms of the same site that are not contiguous, such as tumors in different quadrants of the same breast, codes for each site should be assigned.

Malignant neoplasm of ectopic tissue

Malignant neoplasms of ectopic tissue are to be coded to the site mentioned, e.g., ectopic pancreatic malignant neoplasms are coded to pancreas, unspecified (C25.9).

MALIGNANT NEOPLASMS (C00-C96)

MALIGNANT NEOPLASMS, STATED OR PRESUMED TO BE PRIMARY (OF SPECIFIED SITES), AND CERTAIN SPECIFIED HISTOLOGIES, EXCEPT NEUROENDOCRINE, AND OF LYMPHOID, HEMATOPOIETIC AND RELATED TISSUE (C00-C75)

MALIGNANT NEOPLASMS OF LIP, ORAL CAVITY AND PHARYNX (C00-C14)

C00 Malignant neoplasm of lip

Use additional code to identify:
alcohol abuse and dependence (F10.-)
history of tobacco dependence (Z87.891)
tobacco dependence (F17.-)
tobacco use (Z72.0)

Excludes1 malignant melanoma of lip (C43.0)
Merkel cell carcinoma of lip (C4A.0)
other and unspecified malignant neoplasm of skin of lip (C44.0-)

C00.0 Malignant neoplasm of external upper lip
Malignant neoplasm of lipstick area of upper lip
Malignant neoplasm of upper lip NOS
Malignant neoplasm of vermilion border of upper lip

C00.1 Malignant neoplasm of external lower lip
Malignant neoplasm of lower lip NOS
Malignant neoplasm of lipstick area of lower lip
Malignant neoplasm of vermilion border of lower lip

C00.2 Malignant neoplasm of external lip, unspecified
Malignant neoplasm of vermilion border of lip NOS

C00.3 Malignant neoplasm of upper lip, inner aspect
Malignant neoplasm of buccal aspect of upper lip
Malignant neoplasm of frenulum of upper lip
Malignant neoplasm of mucosa of upper lip
Malignant neoplasm of oral aspect of upper lip

C00.4 Malignant neoplasm of lower lip, inner aspect
Malignant neoplasm of buccal aspect of lower lip
Malignant neoplasm of frenulum of lower lip
Malignant neoplasm of mucosa of lower lip
Malignant neoplasm of oral aspect of lower lip

C00.5 Malignant neoplasm of lip, unspecified, inner aspect
Malignant neoplasm of buccal aspect of lip, unspecified
Malignant neoplasm of frenulum of lip, unspecified
Malignant neoplasm of mucosa of lip, unspecified
Malignant neoplasm of oral aspect of lip, unspecified

C00.6 Malignant neoplasm of commissure of lip, unspecified
Commissure: Site of union of corresponding parts

C00.8 Malignant neoplasm of overlapping sites of lip

C00.9 Malignant neoplasm of lip, unspecified

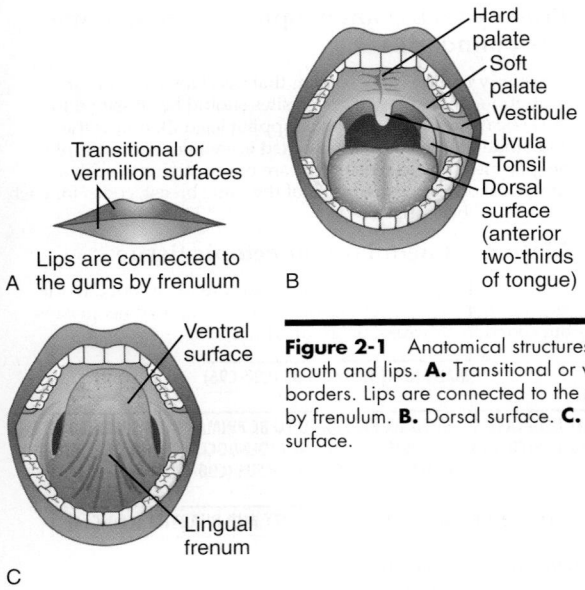

Figure 2-1 Anatomical structures of the mouth and lips. **A.** Transitional or vermilion borders. Lips are connected to the gums by frenulum. **B.** Dorsal surface. **C.** Ventral surface.

C01 Malignant neoplasm of base of tongue
Malignant neoplasm of dorsal surface of base of tongue
Malignant neoplasm of fixed part of tongue NOS
Malignant neoplasm of posterior third of tongue
Use additional code to identify:
alcohol abuse and dependence (F10.-)
history of tobacco dependence (Z87.891) ⇐
tobacco dependence (F17.-)
tobacco use (Z72.0)

● **C02 Malignant neoplasm of other and unspecified parts of tongue**
Use additional code to identify:
alcohol abuse and dependence (F10.-)
history of tobacco dependence (Z87.891) ⇐
tobacco dependence (F17.-)
tobacco use (Z72.0)

C02.0 Malignant neoplasm of dorsal surface of tongue
Malignant neoplasm of anterior two-thirds of tongue, dorsal surface
Excludes2 malignant neoplasm of dorsal surface of base of tongue (C01)

C02.1 Malignant neoplasm of border of tongue
Malignant neoplasm of tip of tongue

C02.2 Malignant neoplasm of ventral surface of tongue
Malignant neoplasm of anterior two-thirds of tongue, ventral surface
Malignant neoplasm of frenulum linguae

C02.3 Malignant neoplasm of anterior two-thirds of tongue, part unspecified
Malignant neoplasm of middle third of tongue NOS
Malignant neoplasm of mobile part of tongue NOS

C02.4 Malignant neoplasm of lingual tonsil
Lingual tonsil: Aggregation of lymph follicles at root of tongue
Excludes2 malignant neoplasm of tonsil NOS (C09.9)

C02.8 Malignant neoplasm of overlapping sites of tongue
Malignant neoplasm of two or more contiguous sites of tongue

C02.9 Malignant neoplasm of tongue, unspecified

● **C03 Malignant neoplasm of gum**
Includes malignant neoplasm of alveolar (ridge) mucosa
malignant neoplasm of gingiva
Use additional code to identify:
alcohol abuse and dependence (F10.-)
history of tobacco dependence (Z87.891) ⇐
tobacco dependence (F17.-)
tobacco use (Z72.0)
Excludes2 malignant odontogenic neoplasms (C41.0-C41.1)

C03.0 Malignant neoplasm of upper gum

C03.1 Malignant neoplasm of lower gum

C03.9 Malignant neoplasm of gum, unspecified

● **C04 Malignant neoplasm of floor of mouth**
Use additional code to identify:
alcohol abuse and dependence (F10.-)
history of tobacco dependence (Z87.891) ⇐
tobacco dependence (F17.-)
tobacco use (Z72.0)

C04.0 Malignant neoplasm of anterior floor of mouth
Malignant neoplasm of anterior to the premolar-canine junction

C04.1 Malignant neoplasm of lateral floor of mouth

C04.8 Malignant neoplasm of overlapping sites of floor of mouth

C04.9 Malignant neoplasm of floor of mouth, unspecified

● **C05 Malignant neoplasm of palate**
Use additional code to identify:
alcohol abuse and dependence (F10.-)
history of tobacco dependence (Z87.891) ⇐
tobacco dependence (F17.-)
tobacco use (Z72.0)
Excludes1 Kaposi's sarcoma of palate (C46.2)

C05.0 Malignant neoplasm of hard palate

C05.1 Malignant neoplasm of soft palate
Excludes2 malignant neoplasm of nasopharyngeal surface of soft palate (C11.3)

C05.2 Malignant neoplasm of uvula

C05.8 Malignant neoplasm of overlapping sites of palate

C05.9 Malignant neoplasm of palate, unspecified
Malignant neoplasm of roof of mouth

● **C06 Malignant neoplasm of other and unspecified parts of mouth**
Use additional code to identify:
alcohol abuse and dependence (F10.-)
history of tobacco dependence (Z87.891) ⇐
tobacco dependence (F17.-)
tobacco use (Z72.0)

C06.0 Malignant neoplasm of cheek mucosa
Malignant neoplasm of buccal mucosa NOS
Malignant neoplasm of internal cheek

C06.1 Malignant neoplasm of vestibule of mouth
Malignant neoplasm of buccal sulcus (upper) (lower)
Malignant neoplasm of labial sulcus (upper) (lower)

C06.2 Malignant neoplasm of retromolar area

● **C06.8 Malignant neoplasm of overlapping sites of other and unspecified parts of mouth**

C06.80 Malignant neoplasm of overlapping sites of unspecified parts of mouth

C06.89 Malignant neoplasm of overlapping sites of other parts of mouth 'book leaf' neoplasm [ventral surface of tongue and floor of mouth]

C06.9 Malignant neoplasm of mouth, unspecified
Malignant neoplasm of minor salivary gland, unspecified site
Malignant neoplasm of oral cavity NOS

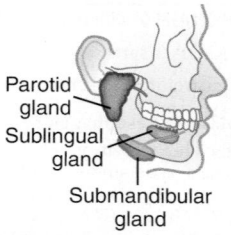

Figure 2-2 Major salivary glands.

C07 Malignant neoplasm of parotid gland
Use additional code to identify:
alcohol abuse and dependence (F10.-)
exposure to environmental tobacco smoke (Z77.22)
exposure to tobacco smoke in the perinatal period (P96.81)
history of tobacco dependence (Z87.891)
occupational exposure to environmental tobacco smoke (Z57.31)
tobacco dependence (F17.-)
tobacco use (Z72.0)

C08 Malignant neoplasm of other and unspecified major salivary glands
Includes malignant neoplasm of salivary ducts
Use additional code to identify:
alcohol abuse and dependence (F10.-)
exposure to environmental tobacco smoke (Z77.22)
exposure to tobacco smoke in the perinatal period (P96.81)
history of tobacco dependence (Z87.891)
occupational exposure to environmental tobacco smoke (Z57.31)
tobacco dependence (F17.-)
tobacco use (Z72.0)
Excludes1 malignant neoplasms of specified minor salivary glands which are classified according to their anatomical location
Excludes2 malignant neoplasms of minor salivary glands NOS (C06.9)
malignant neoplasm of parotid gland (C07)

C08.0 Malignant neoplasm of submandibular gland
Malignant neoplasm of submaxillary gland

C08.1 Malignant neoplasm of sublingual gland

C08.9 Malignant neoplasm of major salivary gland, unspecified
Malignant neoplasm of salivary gland (major) NOS

★**(See Plate 61 on page 73.)**

C09 Malignant neoplasm of tonsil
Use additional code to identify:
alcohol abuse and dependence (F10.-)
exposure to environmental tobacco smoke (Z77.22)
exposure to tobacco smoke in the perinatal period (P96.81)
history of tobacco dependence (Z87.891)
occupational exposure to environmental tobacco smoke (Z57.31)
tobacco dependence (F17.-)
tobacco use (Z72.0)
Excludes2 malignant neoplasm of lingual tonsil (C02.4)
malignant neoplasm of pharyngeal tonsil (C11.1)

C09.0 Malignant neoplasm of tonsillar fossa
Surface of palatine (two masses of lymphatic tissue on sides of throat) tonsils

C09.1 Malignant neoplasm of tonsillar pillar (anterior) (posterior)
Extension from palatine (two masses of lymphatic tissue on sides of throat) tonsils

C09.8 Malignant neoplasm of overlapping sites of tonsil

C09.9 Malignant neoplasm of tonsil, unspecified
Malignant neoplasm of tonsil NOS
Malignant neoplasm of faucial tonsils
Malignant neoplasm of palatine tonsils

C10 Malignant neoplasm of oropharynx
Area of throat at back of mouth
Use additional code to identify:
alcohol abuse and dependence (F10.-)
exposure to environmental tobacco smoke (Z77.22)
exposure to tobacco smoke in the perinatal period (P96.81)
history of tobacco dependence (Z87.891)
occupational exposure to environmental tobacco smoke (Z57.31)
tobacco dependence (F17.-)
tobacco use (Z72.0)
Excludes2 malignant neoplasm of tonsil (C09.-)

C10.0 Malignant neoplasm of vallecula
Vallecula, depression or furrow

C10.1 Malignant neoplasm of anterior surface of epiglottis
Malignant neoplasm of epiglottis, free border [margin]
Malignant neoplasm of glossoepiglottic fold(s)
Excludes2 malignant neoplasm of epiglottis (suprahyoid portion) NOS (C32.1)

C10.2 Malignant neoplasm of lateral wall of oropharynx

C10.3 Malignant neoplasm of posterior wall of oropharynx

C10.4 Malignant neoplasm of branchial cleft
Congenital slitlike openings formed between branchial arches pharyngeal groove
Malignant neoplasm of branchial cyst [site of neoplasm]

C10.8 Malignant neoplasm of overlapping sites of oropharynx
Malignant neoplasm of junctional region of oropharynx

C10.9 Malignant neoplasm of oropharynx, unspecified

C11 Malignant neoplasm of nasopharynx
Use additional code to identify:
exposure to environmental tobacco smoke (Z77.22)
exposure to tobacco smoke in the perinatal period (P96.81)
history of tobacco dependence (Z87.891)
occupational exposure to environmental tobacco smoke (Z57.31)
tobacco dependence (F17.-)
tobacco use (Z72.0)

C11.0 Malignant neoplasm of superior wall of nasopharynx
Part of pharynx that lies above soft palate
Malignant neoplasm of roof of nasopharynx

C11.1 Malignant neoplasm of posterior wall of nasopharynx
Malignant neoplasm of adenoid
Malignant neoplasm of pharyngeal tonsil

C11.2 Malignant neoplasm of lateral wall of nasopharynx
Malignant neoplasm of fossa of Rosenmüller
Malignant neoplasm of opening of auditory tube
Malignant neoplasm of pharyngeal recess

C11.3 Malignant neoplasm of anterior wall of nasopharynx
Malignant neoplasm of floor of nasopharynx
Malignant neoplasm of nasopharyngeal (anterior) (posterior) surface of soft palate
Malignant neoplasm of posterior margin of nasal choana
Malignant neoplasm of posterior margin of nasal septum

C11.8 Malignant neoplasm of overlapping sites of nasopharynx

C11.9 Malignant neoplasm of nasopharynx, unspecified
Malignant neoplasm of nasopharyngeal wall NOS

C12 Malignant neoplasm of pyriform sinus
Malignant neoplasm of pyriform fossa
Use additional code to identify:
exposure to environmental tobacco smoke (Z77.22)
exposure to tobacco smoke in the perinatal period (P96.81)
history of tobacco dependence (Z87.891)
occupational exposure to environmental tobacco smoke (Z57.31)
tobacco dependence (F17.-)
tobacco use (Z72.0)

● **C13 Malignant neoplasm of hypopharynx**

Use additional code to identify:
exposure to environmental tobacco smoke (Z77.22)
exposure to tobacco smoke in the perinatal period (P96.81)
history of tobacco dependence (Z87.891) ◀
occupational exposure to environmental tobacco smoke (Z57.31)
tobacco dependence (F17.-)
tobacco use (Z72.0)

Excludes2 malignant neoplasm of pyriform sinus (C12)

C13.0 Malignant neoplasm of postcricoid region
Behind the cricoid cartilage of neck

C13.1 Malignant neoplasm of aryepiglottic fold, hypopharyngeal aspect
Arytenoepiglottic fold, triangular opening between side of epiglottis and apex of arytenoid cartilage
Malignant neoplasm of aryepiglottic fold, marginal zone
Malignant neoplasm of aryepiglottic fold NOS
Malignant neoplasm of interarytenoid fold, marginal zone
Malignant neoplasm of interarytenoid fold NOS

Excludes2 malignant neoplasm of aryepiglottic fold or interarytenoid fold, laryngeal aspect (C32.1)

C13.2 Malignant neoplasm of posterior wall of hypopharynx

C13.8 Malignant neoplasm of overlapping sites of hypopharynx

C13.9 Malignant neoplasm of hypopharynx, unspecified
Malignant neoplasm of hypopharyngeal wall NOS

● **C14 Malignant neoplasm of other and ill-defined sites in the lip, oral cavity and pharynx**

Use additional code to identify:
alcohol abuse and dependence (F10.-)
exposure to environmental tobacco smoke (Z77.22)
exposure to tobacco smoke in the perinatal period (P96.81)
history of tobacco dependence (Z87.891) ◀
occupational exposure to environmental tobacco smoke (Z57.31)
tobacco dependence (F17.-)
tobacco use (Z72.0)

Excludes1 malignant neoplasm of oral cavity NOS (C06.9)

C14.0 Malignant neoplasm of pharynx, unspecified

C14.2 Malignant neoplasm of Waldeyer's ring

C14.8 Malignant neoplasm of overlapping sites of lip, oral cavity and pharynx
Primary malignant neoplasm of two or more contiguous sites of lip, oral cavity and pharynx

Excludes1 'book leaf' neoplasm [ventral surface of tongue and floor of mouth] (C06.89)

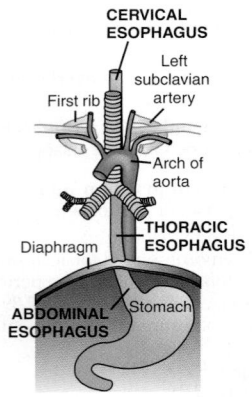

Figure 2-3 The esophagus is the muscular tube that connects the pharynx and the stomach. The 10 inch (25 cm) long esophagus is divided into three parts: **cervical, thoracic,** and **abdominal.**

MALIGNANT NEOPLASM OF DIGESTIVE ORGANS (C15-C26)

Excludes1 Kaposi's sarcoma of gastrointestinal sites (C46.4)

Excludes2 gastrointestinal stromal tumors (C49.A-) ◀

● **C15 Malignant neoplasms of esophagus**

Use additional code to identify:
alcohol abuse and dependence (F10.-)

Ex: **For category C15 CC codes:** C15.3-C15.9, C26.0, C26.9, C45.7-C45.9, C46.4, C76.8, C7A.00, C7A.098-C7B.00, C7B.1, C80.0-C80.2, D49.0, D49.81-D49.9

C15.3 Malignant neoplasm of upper third of esophagus

C15.4 Malignant neoplasm of middle third of esophagus

C15.5 Malignant neoplasm of lower third of esophagus

Excludes1 malignant neoplasm of cardio-esophageal junction (C16.0)

C15.8 Malignant neoplasm of overlapping sites of esophagus

C15.9 Malignant neoplasm of esophagus, unspecified

● **C16 Malignant neoplasm of stomach**

Use additional code to identify:
alcohol abuse and dependence (F10.-)

Excludes2 malignant carcinoid tumor of the stomach (C7A.092)

Ex: **For category C16 CC codes:** C16.0-C16.9, C26.0, C26.9, C45.7-C45.9, C46.4, C49.A2, C76.8, C7A.00, C7A.092, C7A.094-C7B.00, C7B.1, C80.0-C80.2, D49.0, D49.81-D49.9

C16.0 Malignant neoplasm of cardia
Malignant neoplasm of cardiac orifice
Malignant neoplasm of cardio-esophageal junction
Malignant neoplasm of esophagus and stomach
Malignant neoplasm of gastro-esophageal junction

C16.1 Malignant neoplasm of fundus of stomach

C16.2 Malignant neoplasm of body of stomach

C16.3 Malignant neoplasm of pyloric antrum
Malignant neoplasm of gastric antrum

C16.4 Malignant neoplasm of pylorus
Malignant neoplasm of prepylorus
Malignant neoplasm of pyloric canal

C16.5 Malignant neoplasm of lesser curvature of stomach, unspecified
Malignant neoplasm of lesser curvature of stomach, not classifiable to C16.1-C16.4

C16.6 Malignant neoplasm of greater curvature of stomach, unspecified
Malignant neoplasm of greater curvature of stomach, not classifiable to C16.0-C16.4

C16.8 Malignant neoplasm of overlapping sites of stomach

C16.9 Malignant neoplasm of stomach, unspecified
Gastric cancer NOS

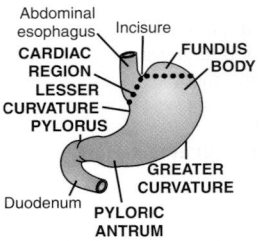

Figure 2-4 Parts of the stomach.

Item 2-2 The esophagus opens into the stomach through the **cardiac orifice,** also called the **cardioesophageal junction.** The **cardia** is adjacent to the cardiac orifice. The stomach widens into the **greater** and **lesser curvatures.** The **pyloric antrum** precedes the **pylorus,** which opens to the duodenum.

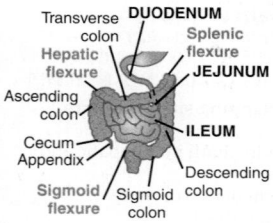

Figure 2-5 Small intestine and colon.

C17 Malignant neoplasm of small intestine

Excludes1 malignant carcinoid tumor of the small intestine (C7A.01)

C17.0 Malignant neoplasm of duodenum
First or proximal portion of small intestine, extending from pylorus to jejunum
Ex: C17.0, C17.8-C17.9, C26.0, C26.9, C45.7-C45.9, C46.4, C76.8, C7A.00-C7A.010, C7A.019, C7A.098-C7B.00, C7B.1, C80.0-C80.2, D49.0, D49.81-D49.9

C17.1 Malignant neoplasm of jejunum
Second section of small intestine, extending from duodenum to ileum
Ex: C17.1, C17.8-C17.9, C26.0, C26.9, C45.7-C45.9, C46.4, C76.8, C7A.00, C7A.011, C7A.019, C7A.098, C7A.1-C7B.00, C7B.1, C80.0-C80.2, D49.0, D49.81-D49.9

C17.2 Malignant neoplasm of ileum
Distal and longest portion of small intestine, extending from jejunum to cecum

Excludes1 malignant neoplasm of ileocecal valve (C18.0)

Ex: C17.2, C17.8-C17.9, C26.0, C26.9, C45.7-C45.9, C46.4, C76.8, C7A.00, C7A.012-C7A.019, C7A.098, C7A.1-C7B.00, C7B.1, C80.0-C80.2, D49.0, D49.81-D49.9

C17.3 Meckel's diverticulum, malignant
Appendage of ileum

Excludes1 Meckel's diverticulum, congenital (Q43.0)

Ex: C17.3-C17.9, C26.0, C26.9, C45.7-C45.9, C46.4, C76.8, C7A.00, C7A.019, C7A.098-C7B.00, C7B.1, C80.0-C80.2, D49.0, D49.81-D49.9

C17.8 Malignant neoplasm of overlapping sites of small intestine
Ex: C17.8-C17.9, C26.0, C26.9, C45.7-C45.9, C46.4, C76.8, C7A.00, C7A.019, C7A.098, C7A.1-C7B.00, C7B.1, C80.0-C80.2, D49.0, D49.81-D49.9

C17.9 Malignant neoplasm of small intestine, unspecified
Ex: See C17.8

C18 Malignant neoplasm of colon

Excludes1 malignant carcinoid tumors of the colon (C7A.02)

C18.0 Malignant neoplasm of cecum
First section of large intestine
Malignant neoplasm of ileocecal valve
Ex: C18.0, C18.8-C18.9, C26.0-C26.9, C45.7-C45.9, C46.4, C76.8, C7A.00, C7A.021, C7A.029, C7A.098-C7B.00, C7B.1, C80.0-C80.2, D49.0, D49.81-D49.9

C18.1 Malignant neoplasm of appendix
Blind ended tube connected to the cecum; AKA vermiform appendix
Ex: C18.1, C18.8-C18.9, C26.0, C26.9, C45.7-C45.9, C46.4, C76.8, C7A.00, C7A.020, C7A.029, C7A.098, C7A.1-C7B.00, C7B.1, C80.0-C80.2, D49.0, D49.81-D49.9

C18.2 Malignant neoplasm of ascending colon
Ascending colon is between cecum and right colic flexure
Ex: C18.2, C18.8-C18.9, C26.0, C26.9, C45.7-C45.9, C46.4, C76.8, C7A.00, C7A.022, C7A.029, C7A.098, C7A.1-C7B.00, C7B.1, C80.0-C80.2, D49.0, D49.81-D49.9

C18.3 Malignant neoplasm of hepatic flexure
A flexure is a bending in a structure or organ. Note the three flexures illustrated in Figure 2–5.
Ex: C18.3, C18.8-C18.9, C26.0, C26.9, C45.7-C45.9, C46.4, C76.8, C7A.00, C7A.029, C7A.098-C7B.00, C7B.1, C80.0-C80.2, D49.0, D49.81-D49.9

C18.4 Malignant neoplasm of transverse colon
Portion of colon that runs transversely across upper part of abdomen, between right and left colic flexures
Ex: C18.4, C18.8-C18.9, C26.0, C26.9, C45.7-C45.9, C46.4, C76.8, C7A.00, C7A.023, C7A.029, C7A.098, C7A.1-C7B.00, C7B.1, C80.0-C80.2, D49.0, D49.81-D49.9

C18.5 Malignant neoplasm of splenic flexure
Bend at junction of transverse and descending colon
Ex: C18.5, C18.8-C18.9, C26.0, C26.9, C45.7-C45.9, C46.4, C76.8, C7A.00, C7A.029, C7A.098-C7B.00, C7B.1, C80.0-C80.2, D49.0, D49.81-D49.9

C18.6 Malignant neoplasm of descending colon
Portion between left colic flexure and sigmoid colon at pelvic brim; AKA iliac colon
Ex: C18.6, C18.8-C18.9, C26.0, C26.9, C45.7-C45.9, C46.4, C76.8, C7A.00, C7A.024, C7A.029, C7A.098-C7B.00, C7B.1, C80.0-C80.2, D49.0, D49.81-D49.9

C18.7 Malignant neoplasm of sigmoid colon
S-shaped part of colon extending from pelvic brim to third segment of sacrum
Malignant neoplasm of sigmoid (flexure)

Excludes1 malignant neoplasm of rectosigmoid junction (C19)

Ex: C18.7-C18.9, C26.0, C26.9, C45.7-C45.9, C46.4, C76.8, C7A.00, C7A.025, C7A.029, C7A.098, C7A.1-C7B.00, C7B.1, C80.0-C80.2, D49.0, D49.81-D49.9

C18.8 Malignant neoplasm of overlapping sites of colon
Ex: C18.8-C18.9, C26.0, C26.9, C45.7-C45.9, C46.4, C76.8, C7A.00, C7A.029, C7A.098, C7A.1-C7B.00, C7B.1, C80.0-C80.2, D49.0, D49.81-D49.9

C18.9 Malignant neoplasm of colon, unspecified
Malignant neoplasm of large intestine NOS
Ex: See C18.8

C19 Malignant neoplasm of rectosigmoid junction
Malignant neoplasm of colon with rectum
Malignant neoplasm of rectosigmoid (colon)

Excludes1 malignant carcinoid tumors of the colon (C7A.02-)

Ex: C19, C21.2-C21.8, C26.0, C26.9, C45.7-C45.9, C46.4, C76.8, C7A.00, C7A.098, C7A.1-C7B.00, C7B.1, C80.0-C80.2, D49.0, D49.81-D49.9

C20 Malignant neoplasm of rectum
Malignant neoplasm of rectal ampulla

Excludes1 malignant carcinoid tumor of the rectum (C7A.026)

Ex: C20, C21.2-C21.8, C26.0, C26.9, C45.7-C45.9, C46.4, C76.8, C7A.00, C7A.026, C7A.098, C7A.1-C7B.00, C7B.1, C80.0-C80.2, D49.0, D49.81-D49.9

C21 Malignant neoplasm of anus and anal canal

Excludes2 malignant carcinoid tumors of the colon (C7A.02-)
malignant melanoma of anal margin (C43.51)
malignant melanoma of anal skin (C43.51)
malignant melanoma of perianal skin (C43.51)
other and unspecified malignant neoplasm of anal margin (C44.500, C44.510, C44.520, C44.590)
other and unspecified malignant neoplasm of anal skin (C44.500, C44.510, C44.520, C44.590)
other and unspecified malignant neoplasm of perianal skin (C44.500, C44.510, C44.520, C44.590)

Ex: **For category C21 CC codes C21.0-C21.1:** C21.0-C21.8, C26.0, C26.9, C45.7-C45.9, C46.4, C76.8, C7A.00, C7A.098, C7A.1-C7B.00, C7B.1, C80.0-C80.2, D49.0, D49.81-D49.9 **For category C21 CC codes C21.2-C21.8:** C21.2-C21.8, C26.0, C26.9, C45.7-C45.9, C46.4, C76.8, C7A.00, C7A.098, C7A.1-C7B.00, C7B.1, C80.0-C80.2, D49.0, D49.81-D49.9

C21.0 Malignant neoplasm of anus, unspecified

C21.1 Malignant neoplasm of anal canal
Terminal part of large intestine
Malignant neoplasm of anal sphincter

C21.2 Malignant neoplasm of cloacogenic zone

C21.8 Malignant neoplasm of overlapping sites of rectum, anus and anal canal
Malignant neoplasm of anorectal junction
Malignant neoplasm of anorectum
Primary malignant neoplasm of two or more contiguous sites of rectum, anus and anal canal

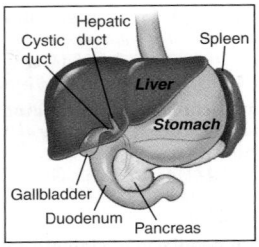

Figure 2-6 Diagram of liver, gallbladder, hepatic duct, pancreas, and spleen. (From Thibodeau and Patton: Anatomy and Physiology, ed 7, Mosby, 2010)

● **C22 Malignant neoplasm of liver and intrahepatic bile ducts**
Intrahepatic: Within liver
Use additional code to identify:
alcohol abuse and dependence (F10.-)
hepatitis B (B16.-, B18.0-B18.1) hepatitis C (B17.1-, B18.2)
Excludes1 malignant neoplasm of biliary tract NOS (C24.9)
secondary malignant neoplasm of liver and intrahepatic bile duct (C78.7)
Ex: **For catgory C22 CC codes:** C22.0-C22.9, C26.0, C26.9, C45.7-C45.9, C46.4, C76.8, C7A.00, C7A.098, C7A.1-C7B.00, C7B.1, C80.0-C80.2, D49.0, D49.81-D49.9

C22.0 Liver cell carcinoma
Hepatocellular carcinoma
Hepatoma

C22.1 Intrahepatic bile duct carcinoma
Cholangiocarcinoma
Adenocarcinoma (cancer that originates in glandular tissue) arising from epithelium of intrahepatic bile ducts
Excludes1 malignant neoplasm of hepatic duct (C24.0)

C22.2 Hepatoblastoma
Malignant intrahepatic tumor

C22.3 Angiosarcoma of liver
Kupffer cell sarcoma

C22.4 Other sarcomas of liver

C22.7 Other specified carcinomas of liver

C22.8 Malignant neoplasm of liver, primary, unspecified as to type

C22.9 Malignant neoplasm of liver, not specified as primary or secondary

C23 Malignant neoplasm of gallbladder
Ex: C23, C24.8-C24.9, C26.0, C26.9, C45.7-C45.9, C46.4, C76.8, C7A.00, C7A.098, C7A.1-C7B.00, C7B.1, C8.00-C8.02, D49.0, D49.81-D49.9

● **C24 Malignant neoplasm of other and unspecified parts of biliary tract**
Excludes1 malignant neoplasm of intrahepatic bile duct (C22.1)

C24.0 Malignant neoplasm of extrahepatic bile duct
Extrahepatic = outside the liver
Malignant neoplasm of biliary duct or passage NOS
Malignant neoplasm of common bile duct
Malignant neoplasm of cystic duct
Malignant neoplasm of hepatic duct
Ex: C24.0, C24.8-C24.9, C26.0, C26.9, C45.7-C45.9, C46.4, C76.8, C7A.00, C7A.098-C7B.00, C7B.1, C80.0-C80.2, D49.0, D49.81-D49.9

C24.1 Malignant neoplasm of ampulla of Vater
Union of pancreatic duct and common bile duct
Ex: C24.1, C24.8-C24.9, C26.0, C26.9, C45.7-C45.9, C46.4, C76.8, C7A.00, C7A.098, C7A.1, C7A.8, C7B.00, C7B.1, C80.0-C80.2, D49.0, D49.81-D49.9

C24.8 Malignant neoplasm of overlapping sites of biliary tract
Malignant neoplasm involving both intrahepatic and extrahepatic bile ducts
Primary malignant neoplasm of two or more contiguous sites of biliary tract
Ex: C24.8-C24.9, C26.0, C26.9, C45.7-C45.9, C46.4, C76.8, C7A.00, C7A.098-C7A.8, C7B.00, C7B.1, C80.0-C80.2, D49.0, D49.81-D49.9

C24.9 Malignant neoplasm of biliary tract, unspecified
Ex: See C24.8

● **C25 Malignant neoplasm of pancreas**
Check documentation for specific site.
Code also exocrine pancreatic insufficiency (K86.81) ◀
Use additional code to identify:
alcohol abuse and dependence (F10.-)
Ex: **For catgory C25 CC codes:** C25.0-C26.0, C26.9, C45.7-C45.9, C46.4, C76.8, C7A.00, C7A.098, C7A.1-C7B.00, C7B.1, C8.00-C80.2, D49.0, D49.81-D49.9

C25.0 Malignant neoplasm of head of pancreas

C25.1 Malignant neoplasm of body of pancreas

C25.2 Malignant neoplasm of tail of pancreas

C25.3 Malignant neoplasm of pancreatic duct

C25.4 Malignant neoplasm of endocrine pancreas
Malignant neoplasm of islets of Langerhans
That part of the pancreas that acts as endocrine gland and consists of islets of Langerhans
Use additional code to identify any functional activity.

C25.7 Malignant neoplasm of other parts of pancreas
Malignant neoplasm of neck of pancreas

C25.8 Malignant neoplasm of overlapping sites of pancreas

C25.9 Malignant neoplasm of pancreas, unspecified

● **C26 Malignant neoplasm of other and ill-defined digestive organs**
Excludes1 malignant neoplasm of peritoneum and retroperitoneum (C48.-)

C26.0 Malignant neoplasm of intestinal tract, part unspecified
Malignant neoplasm of intestine NOS

C26.1 Malignant neoplasm of spleen
Excludes1 Hodgkin lymphoma (C81.-)
non-Hodgkin lymphoma (C82-C85)

C26.9 Malignant neoplasm of ill-defined sites within the digestive system
Malignant neoplasm of alimentary canal or tract NOS
Malignant neoplasm of gastrointestinal tract NOS
Excludes1 malignant neoplasm of abdominal NOS (C76.2)
malignant neoplasm of intra-abdominal NOS (C76.2)

Item 2-3 Islets of Langerhans (endocrine producing cells comprising 1% to 2% of the pancreatic mass) make and secrete hormones that regulate the body's production of insulin, glucagon, and stomach acid. Breakdown of the insulin-producing cells can cause diabetes mellitus. Islet cell tumors can be benign or malignant and include glucagonomas, insulinomas, gastrinomas, and neuroendocrine tumor. The neoplasm table must be consulted for the correct neoplasm code.

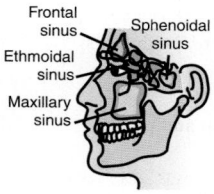

Figure 2-7 Paranasal sinuses. (From Buck CJ: Step-by-Step Medical Coding, ed 2016, St. Louis, Elsevier, 2016)

MALIGNANT NEOPLASMS OF RESPIRATORY AND INTRATHORACIC ORGANS (C30-C39)

Includes malignant neoplasm of middle ear
Excludes1 mesothelioma (C45.-)

C30 Malignant neoplasm of nasal cavity and middle ear

C30.0 Malignant neoplasm of nasal cavity
Malignant neoplasm of cartilage of nose
Malignant neoplasm of nasal concha
Malignant neoplasm of internal nose
Malignant neoplasm of septum of nose
Malignant neoplasm of vestibule of nose
Anterior part of nasal cavity
Excludes1 malignant neoplasm of nasal bone (C41.0)
malignant neoplasm of nose NOS (C76.0)
malignant neoplasm of olfactory bulb (C72.2-)
malignant neoplasm of posterior margin of nasal septum and choana (C11.3)
malignant melanoma of skin of nose (C43.31)
malignant neoplasm of turbinates (C41.0)
other and unspecified malignant neoplasm of skin of nose C44.301, C44.311, C44.321, C44.391)

C30.1 Malignant neoplasm of middle ear
Malignant neoplasm of antrum tympanicum
Bony cavity or chamber
Malignant neoplasm of auditory tube
Malignant neoplasm of eustachian tube
Malignant neoplasm of inner ear
Malignant neoplasm of mastoid air cells
Malignant neoplasm of tympanic cavity
Excludes1 malignant neoplasm of auricular canal (external) (C43.2-, C44.2-)
malignant neoplasm of bone of ear (meatus) (C41.0)
malignant neoplasm of cartilage of ear (C49.0)
malignant melanoma of skin of (external) ear (C43.2-)
other and unspecified malignant neoplasm of skin of (external) ear (C44.2-)

C31 Malignant neoplasm of accessory sinuses
Paired sinuses in bones of face

C31.0 Malignant neoplasm of maxillary sinus
Malignant neoplasm of antrum (Highmore) (maxillary)

C31.1 Malignant neoplasm of ethmoidal sinus

C31.2 Malignant neoplasm of frontal sinus

C31.3 Malignant neoplasm of sphenoid sinus

C31.8 Malignant neoplasm of overlapping sites of accessory sinuses

C31.9 Malignant neoplasm of accessory sinus, unspecified

C32 Malignant neoplasm of larynx
Use additional code to identify:
alcohol abuse and dependence (F10.-)
exposure to environmental tobacco smoke (Z77.22)
exposure to tobacco smoke in the perinatal period (P96.81)
history of tobacco dependence (Z87.891)
occupational exposure to environmental tobacco smoke (Z57.31)
tobacco dependence (F17.-)
tobacco use (Z72.0)

C32.0 Malignant neoplasm of glottis
Vocal apparatus of larynx, consisting of true vocal cords (plicae vocales) and opening between them (rima glottidis)
Malignant neoplasm of intrinsic larynx
Malignant neoplasm of laryngeal commissure (anterior) (posterior)
Malignant neoplasm of vocal cord (true) NOS
***True** vocal cords ("lower vocal folds") produce vocalization when air from the lungs passes between them. Check your documentation. Code C32.1 is for malignant neoplasm of the **false** vocal cords.*

C32.1 Malignant neoplasm of supraglottis
Area of pharynx above glottis
Malignant neoplasm of aryepiglottic fold or interarytenoid fold, laryngeal aspect
Malignant neoplasm of epiglottis (suprahyoid portion) NOS
Malignant neoplasm of extrinsic larynx
Malignant neoplasm of false vocal cord
***False** vocal cords ("upper vocal folds") are not involved in vocalization. Check your documentation. Code C32.0 is for true vocal cords.*
Malignant neoplasm of posterior (laryngeal) surface of epiglottis
Malignant neoplasm of ventricular bands
Excludes2 malignant neoplasm of anterior surface of epiglottis (C10.1)
malignant neoplasm of aryepiglottic fold or interarytenoid fold, hypopharyngeal aspect (C13.1)
malignant neoplasm of aryepiglottic fold or interarytenoid fold, marginal zone (C13.1)
malignant neoplasm of aryepiglottic fold or interarytenoid fold NOS (C13.1)

C32.2 Malignant neoplasm of subglottis
Lowest part of larynx from just below vocal cords down to top of trachea

C32.3 Malignant neoplasm of laryngeal cartilage
Cartilages of larynx, including cricoid, thyroid, and epiglottic, and two each of arytenoid, corniculate, and cuneiform

C32.8 Malignant neoplasm of overlapping sites of larynx

C32.9 Malignant neoplasm of larynx, unspecified

C33 Malignant neoplasm of trachea
Use additional code to identify:
exposure to environmental tobacco smoke (Z77.22)
exposure to tobacco smoke in the perinatal period (P96.81)
history of tobacco dependence (Z87.891)
occupational exposure to environmental tobacco smoke (Z57.31)
tobacco dependence (F17.-)
tobacco use (Z72.0)
Ex: C33, C34.00-C34.92, C39.9, C45.7-C45.9, C46.50-C46.52, C76.1, C76.8, C78.00-C78.1, C78.30-C78.39, C7A.00, C7A.090, C7A.098-C7B.00, C7B.1, C80.0-C80.2, D49.1, D49.81-D49.9

C34 Malignant neoplasm of bronchus and lung

Use additional code to identify:
exposure to environmental tobacco smoke (Z77.22)
exposure to tobacco smoke in the perinatal period (P96.81)
history of tobacco dependence (Z87.891)
occupational exposure to environmental tobacco smoke (Z57.31)
tobacco dependence (F17.-)
tobacco use (Z72.0)

Excludes1 Kaposi's sarcoma of lung (C46.5-)
malignant carcinoid tumor of the bronchus and lung (C7A.090)

C34.0 Malignant neoplasm of main bronchus
Malignant neoplasm of carina
Ridgelike structure
Malignant neoplasm of hilus (of lung)
Anatomic depression or pit
Ex: **For category C34.0 CC codes:** C34.00-C34.02, C34.80-C34.92, C39.9, C45.7-C45.9, C46.50-C46.52, C76.8, C7A.00, C7A.090, C7A.098, C7A.1-C7B.00, C7B.1, C80.0-C80.2, D49.1, D49.81-D49.9

C34.00 Malignant neoplasm of unspecified main bronchus

C34.01 Malignant neoplasm of right main bronchus

C34.02 Malignant neoplasm of left main bronchus

C34.1 Malignant neoplasm of upper lobe, bronchus or lung
Ex: **For category C34.1 CC codes:** C34.10-C34.12, C34.80-C34.92, C39.9, C45.7-C45.9, C46.50-C46.52, C76.8, C7A.00, C7A.090, C7A.098-C7B.00, C7B.1, C80.0-C80.2, D49.1, D49.81-D49.9

C34.10 Malignant neoplasm of unspecified bronchus or lung

C34.11 Malignant neoplasm of upper lobe, right bronchus or lung

C34.12 Malignant neoplasm of upper lobe, left bronchus or lung

C34.2 Malignant neoplasm of middle lobe, bronchus or lung
Ex: C34.2, C34.80-C34.92, C39.9, C45.7-C45.9, C46.50-C46.52, C76.8, C7A.00, C7A.090, C7A.098-C7B.00, C7B.1, C80.0-C80.2, D49.1, D49.81-D49.9

C34.3 Malignant neoplasm of lower lobe, bronchus or lung
Ex: **For category C34.4 CC codes:** C34.30-C34.92, C39.9, C45.7-C45.9, C46.50-C46.52, C76.8, C7A.00, C7A.090, C7A.098-C7B.00, C7B.1, C80.0-C80.2, D49.1, D49.81-D49.9

C34.30 Malignant neoplasm of lower lobe, unspecified bronchus or lung

C34.31 Malignant neoplasm of lower lobe, right bronchus or lung

C34.32 Malignant neoplasm of lower lobe, left bronchus or lung

C34.8 Malignant neoplasm of overlapping sites of bronchus and lung
Ex: **For category C34.8 CC codes:** C34.80-C34.92, C39.9, C45.7-C45.9, C46.50-C46.52, C76.8, C7A.00, C7A.090, C7A.098-C7B.00, C7B.1, C80.0-C80.2, D49.1, D49.81-D49.9

C34.80 Malignant neoplasm of overlapping sites of unspecified bronchus and lung

C34.81 Malignant neoplasm of overlapping sites of right bronchus and lung

C34.82 Malignant neoplasm of overlapping sites of left bronchus and lung

C34.9 Malignant neoplasm of unspecified part of bronchus or lung
Ex: **For category C34.9 CC codes:** See C34.8

C34.90 Malignant neoplasm of unspecified part of unspecified bronchus or lung
Lung cancer NOS

C34.91 Malignant neoplasm of unspecified part of right bronchus or lung

C34.92 Malignant neoplasm of unspecified part of left bronchus or lung

C37 Malignant neoplasm of thymus

Excludes1 malignant carcinoid tumor of the thymus (C7A.091)

Ex: C37, C7A.091

C38 Malignant neoplasm of heart, mediastinum and pleura

Excludes1 mesothelioma (C45.-)

Ex: **For category C38 CC codes unless otherwise indicated:** C38.1-C38.3, C38.8, C39.9, C45.7-C45.9, C76.8, C7A.00, C7A.098-C7B.00, C7B.1, C80.0-C80.2, D49.1, D49.81-D49.9

C38.0 Malignant neoplasm of heart
Malignant neoplasm of pericardium

Excludes1 malignant neoplasm of great vessels (C49.3)

Ex: C38.0, C45.2

C38.1 Malignant neoplasm of anterior mediastinum

C38.2 Malignant neoplasm of posterior mediastinum

C38.3 Malignant neoplasm of mediastinum, part unspecified

C38.4 Malignant neoplasm of pleura
Ex: C38.4, C39.9, C45.0, C45.7-C45.9, C76.8, C7A.00, C7A.098, C7A.1-C7B.00, C7B.1, C80.0-C80.2, D49.1, D49.81-D49.9

C38.8 Malignant neoplasm of overlapping sites of heart, mediastinum and pleura
Pleura are comprised of serous membrane that lines the thoracic cavity (parietal) and covers the lungs (visceral).

C39 Malignant neoplasm of other and ill-defined sites in the respiratory system and intrathoracic organs
Intrathoracic: within thorax/chest

Use additional code to identify:
exposure to environmental tobacco smoke (Z77.22)
exposure to tobacco smoke in the perinatal period (P96.81)
history of tobacco dependence (Z87.891)
occupational exposure to environmental tobacco smoke (Z57.31)
tobacco dependence (F17.-)
tobacco use (Z72.0)

Excludes1 intrathoracic malignant neoplasm NOS (C76.1)
thoracic malignant neoplasm NOS (C76.1)

C39.0 Malignant neoplasm of upper respiratory tract, part unspecified

C39.9 Malignant neoplasm of lower respiratory tract, part unspecified
Malignant neoplasm of respiratory tract NOS

MALIGNANT NEOPLASMS OF BONE AND ARTICULAR CARTILAGE (C40-C41)

Includes malignant neoplasm of cartilage (articular) (joint)
malignant neoplasm of periosteum

Excludes1 malignant neoplasm of bone marrow NOS (C96.9)
malignant neoplasm of synovia (C49.-)

C40 Malignant neoplasm of bone and articular cartilage of limbs

Use additional code to identify major osseous defect, if applicable (M89.7-)

C40.0 Malignant neoplasm of scapula and long bones of upper limb
Ex: **For category C40.0 CC codes:** C40.00-C40.02, C40.80-C40.92, C41.9, Z51.0

C40.00 Malignant neoplasm of scapula and long bones of unspecified upper limb

C40.01 Malignant neoplasm of scapula and long bones of right upper limb

C40.02 Malignant neoplasm of scapula and long bones of left upper limb

C40.1 Malignant neoplasm of short bones of upper limb
Ex: **For category C40.1 CC codes:** C40.10-C40.12, C40.80-C40.92, C41.9, Z51.0

C40.10 Malignant neoplasm of short bones of unspecified upper limb

C40.11 Malignant neoplasm of short bones of right upper limb

C40.12 Malignant neoplasm of short bones of left upper limb

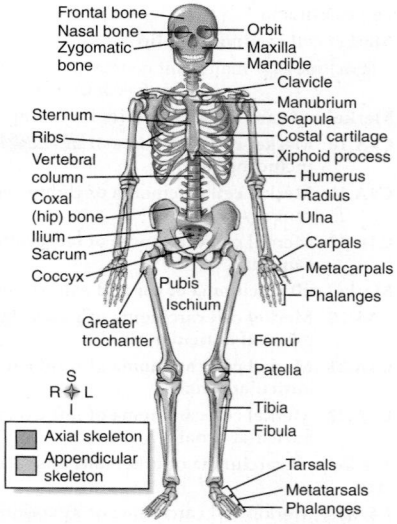

Figure 2-8 Diagram of skeleton of trunk and limbs with bones labeled. (From Thibodeau and Patton: Anatomy and Physiology, ed 7, Mosby, 2010)

● **C40.2 Malignant neoplasm of long bones of lower limb**
Ex: For catgory C40.2 CC codes: C40.20-C40.22, C40.80-C40.92, C41.9, Z51.0

C40.20 Malignant neoplasm of long bones of unspecified lower limb

C40.21 Malignant neoplasm of long bones of right lower limb

C40.22 Malignant neoplasm of long bones of left lower limb

● **C40.3 Malignant neoplasm of short bones of lower limb**
Ex: For catgory C40.3 CC codes: C40.30-C40.92, C41.9, Z51.0

C40.30 Malignant neoplasm of short bones of unspecified lower limb

C40.31 Malignant neoplasm of short bones of right lower limb

C40.32 Malignant neoplasm of short bones of left lower limb

● **C40.8 Malignant neoplasm of overlapping sites of bone and articular cartilage of limb**
Ex: For catgory C40.8 CC codes: C40.00-C41.9, Z51.0

C40.80 Malignant neoplasm of overlapping sites of bone and articular cartilage of unspecified limb

C40.81 Malignant neoplasm of overlapping sites of bone and articular cartilage of right limb

C40.82 Malignant neoplasm of overlapping sites of bone and articular cartilage of left limb

● **C40.9 Malignant neoplasm of unspecified bones and articular cartilage of limb**
Ex: For category C40.9 CC codes: See C40.8

C40.90 Malignant neoplasm of unspecified bones and articular cartilage of unspecified limb

C40.91 Malignant neoplasm of unspecified bones and articular cartilage of right limb

C40.92 Malignant neoplasm of unspecified bones and articular cartilage of left limb

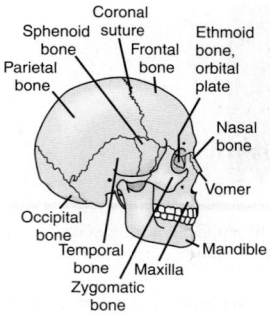

Figure 2-9 Bones of the skull.

● **C41 Malignant neoplasm of bone and articular cartilage of other and unspecified sites**
Excludes1 malignant neoplasm of bones of limbs (C40.-)
malignant neoplasm of cartilage of ear (C49.0)
malignant neoplasm of cartilage of eyelid (C49.0)
malignant neoplasm of cartilage of larynx (C32.3)
malignant neoplasm of cartilage of limbs (C40.-)
malignant neoplasm of cartilage of nose (C30.0)

C41.0 Malignant neoplasm of bones of skull and face
Malignant neoplasm of maxilla (superior)
Malignant neoplasm of orbital bone
Excludes2 carcinoma, any type except intraosseous or odontogenic of:
maxillary sinus (C31.0)
upper jaw (C03.0)
malignant neoplasm of jaw bone (lower) (C41.1)
Ex: C40.80-C41.0, C41.9, Z51.0

C41.1 Malignant neoplasm of mandible
Malignant neoplasm of inferior maxilla
Malignant neoplasm of lower jaw bone
Excludes2 carcinoma, any type except intraosseous or odontogenic of:
jaw NOS (C03.9)
lower (C03.1)
malignant neoplasm of upper jaw bone (C41.0)
Ex: C40.80-C40.92, C41.1, C41.9, Z51.0

C41.2 Malignant neoplasm of vertebral column
Excludes1 malignant neoplasm of sacrum and coccyx (C41.4)
Ex: C40.80-C40.9, C41.2, C41.9, Z51.0

C41.3 Malignant neoplasm of ribs, sternum and clavicle
Ex: C40.80-C40.92, C41.3, C41.9, Z51.0

C41.4 Malignant neoplasm of pelvic bones, sacrum and coccyx
Ex: C40.80-C40.92, C41.4-C41.9, Z51.0

C41.9 Malignant neoplasm of bone and articular cartilage, unspecified
Ex: See C40.8

MELANOMA AND OTHER MALIGNANT NEOPLASMS OF SKIN (C43-C44)

● **C43 Malignant melanoma of skin**
Excludes1 melanoma in situ (D03.-)
Excludes2 malignant melanoma of skin of genital organs (C51-C52, C60.-, C63.-)
Merkel cell carcinoma (C4A.-)
sites other than skin-code to malignant neoplasm of the site

C43.0 Malignant melanoma of lip
Excludes1 malignant neoplasm of vermilion border of lip (C00.0-C00.2)

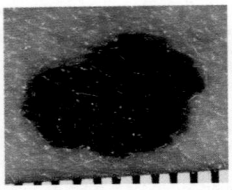

Figure 2-10 Malignant melanoma of skin. (From Goldman: Cecil Textbook of Medicine, ed 22, Saunders, 2004)

Item 2–4 Malignant melanoma is a serious form of skin cancer that affects the melanocytes (pigment-forming cells) and is caused by ultraviolet (UV) rays from the sun that damage skin. It is most commonly seen in the 40- to 60-year-olds with fair skin, blue or green eyes, and red or blond hair who sunburn easily.

Melanoma can spread very rapidly and is the most deadly form of skin cancer. It is less common than other types of skin cancer. The rate of melanoma is increasing and currently is the leading cause of death from skin disease.

● **C43.1 Malignant melanoma of eyelid, including canthus**
Canthus: Either corner of eye where upper and lower eyelids meet
- **C43.10 Malignant melanoma of unspecified eyelid, including canthus**
- **C43.11 Malignant melanoma of right eyelid, including canthus**
- **C43.12 Malignant melanoma of left eyelid, including canthus**

● **C43.2 Malignant melanoma of ear and external auricular canal**
- **C43.20 Malignant melanoma of unspecified ear and external auricular canal**
- **C43.21 Malignant melanoma of right ear and external auricular canal**
- **C43.22 Malignant melanoma of left ear and external auricular canal**

● **C43.3 Malignant melanoma of other and unspecified parts of face**
- **C43.30 Malignant melanoma of unspecified part of face**
- **C43.31 Malignant melanoma of nose**
- **C43.39 Malignant melanoma of other parts of face**

C43.4 Malignant melanoma of scalp and neck

● **C43.5 Malignant melanoma of trunk**
Excludes2 malignant neoplasm of anus NOS (C21.0)
malignant neoplasm of scrotum (C63.2)
- **C43.51 Malignant melanoma of anal skin**
Malignant melanoma of anal margin
Malignant melanoma of perianal skin
- **C43.52 Malignant melanoma of skin of breast**
- **C43.59 Malignant melanoma of other part of trunk**

● **C43.6 Malignant melanoma of upper limb, including shoulder**
- **C43.60 Malignant melanoma of upper limb, including shoulder, unspecified side**
- **C43.61 Malignant melanoma of right upper limb, including shoulder**
- **C43.62 Malignant melanoma of left upper limb, including shoulder**

● **C43.7 Malignant melanoma of lower limb, including hip**
- **C43.70 Malignant melanoma of unspecified lower limb, including hip**
- **C43.71 Malignant melanoma of right lower limb, including hip**
- **C43.72 Malignant melanoma of left lower limb, including hip**

C43.8 Malignant melanoma of overlapping sites of skin

C43.9 Malignant melanoma of skin, unspecified
Malignant melanoma of unspecified site of skin
Melanoma (malignant) NOS

● **C4A Merkel cell carcinoma**
- **C4A.0 Merkel cell carcinoma of lip**
Excludes1 malignant neoplasm of vermilion border of lip (C00.0-C00.2)

● **C4A.1 Merkel cell carcinoma of eyelid, including canthus**
- **C4A.10 Merkel cell carcinoma of unspecified eyelid, including canthus**
- **C4A.11 Merkel cell carcinoma of right eyelid, including canthus**
- **C4A.12 Merkel cell carcinoma of left eyelid, including canthus**

● **C4A.2 Merkel cell carcinoma of ear and external auricular canal**
- **C4A.20 Merkel cell carcinoma of unspecified ear and external auricular canal**
- **C4A.21 Merkel cell carcinoma of right ear and external auricular canal**
- **C4A.22 Merkel cell carcinoma of left ear and external auricular canal**

● **C4A.3 Merkel cell carcinoma of other and unspecified parts of face**
- **C4A.30 Merkel cell carcinoma of unspecified part of face**
- **C4A.31 Merkel cell carcinoma of nose**
- **C4A.39 Merkel cell carcinoma of other parts of face**

C4A.4 Merkel cell carcinoma of scalp and neck

● **C4A.5 Merkel cell carcinoma of trunk**
Excludes2 malignant neoplasm of anus NOS (C21.0)
malignant neoplasm of scrotum (C63.2)
- **C4A.51 Merkel cell carcinoma of anal skin**
Merkel cell carcinoma of anal margin
Merkel cell carcinoma of perianal skin
- **C4A.52 Merkel cell carcinoma of skin of breast**
- **C4A.59 Merkel cell carcinoma of other part of trunk**

● **C4A.6 Merkel cell carcinoma of upper limb, including shoulder**
- **C4A.60 Merkel cell carcinoma of unspecified upper limb, including shoulder**
- **C4A.61 Merkel cell carcinoma of right upper limb, including shoulder**
- **C4A.62 Merkel cell carcinoma of left upper limb, including shoulder**

● **C4A.7 Merkel cell carcinoma of lower limb, including hip**
- **C4A.70 Merkel cell carcinoma of unspecified lower limb, including hip**
- **C4A.71 Merkel cell carcinoma of right lower limb, including hip**
- **C4A.72 Merkel cell carcinoma of left lower limb, including hip**

C4A.8 Merkel cell carcinoma of overlapping sites

C4A.9 Merkel cell carcinoma, unspecified
Merkel cell carcinoma of unspecified site
Merkel cell carcinoma NOS

● **C44 Other and unspecified malignant neoplasm of skin**
Includes malignant neoplasm of sebaceous glands
malignant neoplasm of sweat glands
Excludes1 Kaposi's sarcoma of skin (C46.0)
malignant melanoma of skin (C43.-)
malignant neoplasm of skin of genital organs (C51-C52, C60.-, C63.2)
Merkel cell carcinoma (C4A.-)

● **C44.0 Other and unspecified malignant neoplasm of skin of lip**
Excludes1 malignant neoplasm of lip (C00.-)
- **C44.00 Unspecified malignant neoplasm of skin of lip**
- **C44.01 Basal cell carcinoma of skin of lip**
- **C44.02 Squamous cell carcinoma of skin of lip**
- **C44.09 Other specified malignant neoplasm of skin of lip**

- **C44.1** Other and unspecified malignant neoplasm of skin of eyelid, including canthus

  Excludes1 connective tissue of eyelid (C49.0)

  - **C44.10** Unspecified malignant neoplasm of skin of eyelid, including canthus
    - C44.101 Unspecified malignant neoplasm of skin of unspecified eyelid, including canthus
    - C44.102 Unspecified malignant neoplasm of skin of right eyelid, including canthus
    - C44.109 Unspecified malignant neoplasm of skin of left eyelid, including canthus
  - **C44.11** Basal cell carcinoma of skin of eyelid, including canthus
    - C44.111 Basal cell carcinoma of skin of unspecified eyelid, including canthus
    - C44.112 Basal cell carcinoma of skin of right eyelid, including canthus
    - C44.119 Basal cell carcinoma of skin of left eyelid, including canthus
  - **C44.12** Squamous cell carcinoma of skin of eyelid, including canthus
    - C44.121 Squamous cell carcinoma of skin of unspecified eyelid, including canthus
    - C44.122 Squamous cell carcinoma of skin of right eyelid, including canthus
    - C44.129 Squamous cell carcinoma of skin of left eyelid, including canthus
  - **C44.19** Other specified malignant neoplasm of skin of eyelid, including canthus
    - C44.191 Other specified malignant neoplasm of skin of unspecified eyelid, including canthus
    - C44.192 Other specified malignant neoplasm of skin of right eyelid, including canthus
    - C44.199 Other specified malignant neoplasm of skin of left eyelid, including canthus
- **C44.2** Other and unspecified malignant neoplasm of skin of ear and external auricular canal

  Excludes1 connective tissue of ear (C49.0)

  - **C44.20** Unspecified malignant neoplasm of skin of ear and external auricular canal
    - C44.201 Unspecified malignant neoplasm of skin of unspecified ear and external auricular canal
    - C44.202 Unspecified malignant neoplasm of skin of right ear and external auricular canal
    - C44.209 Unspecified malignant neoplasm of skin of left ear and external auricular canal
  - **C44.21** Basal cell carcinoma of skin of ear and external auricular canal
    - C44.211 Basal cell carcinoma of skin of unspecified ear and external auricular canal
    - C44.212 Basal cell carcinoma of skin of right ear and external auricular canal
    - C44.219 Basal cell carcinoma of skin of left ear and external auricular canal
  - **C44.22** Squamous cell carcinoma of skin of ear and external auricular canal
    - C44.221 Squamous cell carcinoma of skin of unspecified ear and external auricular canal
    - C44.222 Squamous cell carcinoma of skin of right ear and external auricular canal
    - C44.229 Squamous cell carcinoma of skin of left ear and external auricular canal
  - **C44.29** Other specified malignant neoplasm of skin of ear and external auricular canal
    - C44.291 Other specified malignant neoplasm of skin of unspecified ear and external auricular canal
    - C44.292 Other specified malignant neoplasm of skin of right ear and external auricular canal
    - C44.299 Other specified malignant neoplasm of skin of left ear and external auricular canal
- **C44.3** Other and unspecified malignant neoplasm of skin of other and unspecified parts of face
  - **C44.30** Unspecified malignant neoplasm of skin of other and unspecified parts of face
    - C44.300 Unspecified malignant neoplasm of skin of unspecified part of face
    - C44.301 Unspecified malignant neoplasm of skin of nose
    - C44.309 Unspecified malignant neoplasm of skin of other parts of face
  - **C44.31** Basal cell carcinoma of skin of other and unspecified parts of face
    - C44.310 Basal cell carcinoma of skin of unspecified parts of face
    - C44.311 Basal cell carcinoma of skin of nose
    - C44.319 Basal cell carcinoma of skin of other parts of face
  - **C44.32** Squamous cell carcinoma of skin of other and unspecified parts of face
    - C44.320 Squamous cell carcinoma of skin of unspecified parts of face
    - C44.321 Squamous cell carcinoma of skin of nose
    - C44.329 Squamous cell carcinoma of skin of other parts of face
  - **C44.39** Other specified malignant neoplasm of skin of other and unspecified parts of face
    - C44.390 Other specified malignant neoplasm of skin of unspecified parts of face
    - C44.391 Other specified malignant neoplasm of skin of nose
    - C44.399 Other specified malignant neoplasm of skin of other parts of face
- **C44.4** Other and unspecified malignant neoplasm of skin of scalp and neck
  - C44.40 Unspecified malignant neoplasm of skin of scalp and neck
  - C44.41 Basal cell carcinoma of skin of scalp and neck
  - C44.42 Squamous cell carcinoma of skin of scalp and neck
  - C44.49 Other specified malignant neoplasm of skin of scalp and neck

- **C44.5 Other and unspecified malignant neoplasm of skin of trunk**
  - **Excludes1** anus NOS (C21.0)
    scrotum (C63.2)
  - **C44.50 Unspecified malignant neoplasm of skin of trunk**
    - **C44.500 Unspecified malignant neoplasm of anal skin**
      - Unspecified malignant neoplasm of anal margin
      - Unspecified malignant neoplasm of perianal skin
    - **C44.501 Unspecified malignant neoplasm of skin of breast**
    - **C44.509 Unspecified malignant neoplasm of skin of other part of trunk**
  - **C44.51 Basal cell carcinoma of skin of trunk**
    - **C44.510 Basal cell carcinoma of anal skin**
      - Basal cell carcinoma of anal margin
      - Basal cell carcinoma of perianal skin
    - **C44.511 Basal cell carcinoma of skin of breast**
    - **C44.519 Basal cell carcinoma of skin of other part of trunk**
  - **C44.52 Squamous cell carcinoma of skin of trunk**
    - **C44.520 Squamous cell carcinoma of anal skin**
      - Squamous cell carcinoma of anal margin
      - Squamous cell carcinoma of perianal skin
    - **C44.521 Squamous cell carcinoma of skin of breast**
    - **C44.529 Squamous cell carcinoma of skin of other part of trunk**
  - **C44.59 Other specified malignant neoplasm of skin of trunk**
    - **C44.590 Other specified malignant neoplasm of anal skin**
      - Other specified malignant neoplasm of anal margin
      - Other specified malignant neoplasm of perianal skin
    - **C44.591 Other specified malignant neoplasm of skin of breast**
    - **C44.599 Other specified malignant neoplasm of skin of other part of trunk**
- **C44.6 Other and unspecified malignant neoplasm of skin of upper limb, including shoulder**
  - **C44.60 Unspecified malignant neoplasm of skin of upper limb, including shoulder**
    - **C44.601 Unspecified malignant neoplasm of skin of unspecified upper limb, including shoulder**
    - **C44.602 Unspecified malignant neoplasm of skin of right upper limb, including shoulder**
    - **C44.609 Unspecified malignant neoplasm of skin of left upper limb, including shoulder**
  - **C44.61 Basal cell carcinoma of skin of upper limb, including shoulder**
    - **C44.611 Basal cell carcinoma of skin of unspecified upper limb, including shoulder**
    - **C44.612 Basal cell carcinoma of skin of right upper limb, including shoulder**
    - **C44.619 Basal cell carcinoma of skin of left upper limb, including shoulder**
  - **C44.62 Squamous cell carcinoma of skin of upper limb, including shoulder**
    - **C44.621 Squamous cell carcinoma of skin of unspecified upper limb, including shoulder**
    - **C44.622 Squamous cell carcinoma of skin of right upper limb, including shoulder**
    - **C44.629 Squamous cell carcinoma of skin of left upper limb, including shoulder**
  - **C44.69 Other specified malignant neoplasm of skin of upper limb, including shoulder**
    - **C44.691 Other specified malignant neoplasm of skin of unspecified upper limb, including shoulder**
    - **C44.692 Other specified malignant neoplasm of skin of right upper limb, including shoulder**
    - **C44.699 Other specified malignant neoplasm of skin of left upper limb, including shoulder**
- **C44.7 Other and unspecified malignant neoplasm of skin of lower limb, including hip**
  - **C44.70 Unspecified malignant neoplasm of skin of lower limb, including hip**
    - **C44.701 Unspecified malignant neoplasm of skin of unspecified lower limb, including hip**
    - **C44.702 Unspecified malignant neoplasm of skin of right lower limb, including hip**
    - **C44.709 Unspecified malignant neoplasm of skin of left lower limb, including hip**
  - **C44.71 Basal cell carcinoma of skin of lower limb, including hip**
    - **C44.711 Basal cell carcinoma of skin of unspecified lower limb, including hip**
    - **C44.712 Basal cell carcinoma of skin of right lower limb, including hip**
    - **C44.719 Basal cell carcinoma of skin of left lower limb, including hip**
  - **C44.72 Squamous cell carcinoma of skin of lower limb, including hip**
    - **C44.721 Squamous cell carcinoma of skin of unspecified lower limb, including hip**
    - **C44.722 Squamous cell carcinoma of skin of right lower limb, including hip**
    - **C44.729 Squamous cell carcinoma of skin of left lower limb, including hip**
  - **C44.79 Other specified malignant neoplasm of skin of lower limb, including hip**
    - **C44.791 Other specified malignant neoplasm of skin of unspecified lower limb, including hip**
    - **C44.792 Other specified malignant neoplasm of skin of right lower limb, including hip**
    - **C44.799 Other specified malignant neoplasm of skin of left lower limb, including hip**
- **C44.8 Other and unspecified malignant neoplasm of overlapping sites of skin**
  - **C44.80 Unspecified malignant neoplasm of overlapping sites of skin**
  - **C44.81 Basal cell carcinoma of overlapping sites of skin**
  - **C44.82 Squamous cell carcinoma of overlapping sites of skin**
  - **C44.89 Other specified malignant neoplasm of overlapping sites of skin**

C44.9 Other and unspecified malignant neoplasm of skin, unspecified

C44.90 Unspecified malignant neoplasm of skin, unspecified
Malignant neoplasm of unspecified site of skin

C44.91 Basal cell carcinoma of skin, unspecified

C44.92 Squamous cell carcinoma of skin, unspecified

C44.99 Other specified malignant neoplasm of skin, unspecified

MALIGNANT NEOPLASMS OF MESOTHELIAL AND SOFT TISSUE (C45-C49)

C45 Mesothelioma
Malignant cells develop in protective lining that covers internal organs (mesothelium) caused by exposure to asbestos

C45.0 Mesothelioma of pleura
Excludes1 other malignant neoplasm of pleura (C38.4)
Ex: C38.4, C39.9, C45.0, C45.7-C45.9, C76.8, C7A.00, C7A.098, C7A.1-C7B.00, C7B.1, C80.0-C80.2, D49.1, D49.81-D49.9

C45.1 Mesothelioma of peritoneum
Mesothelioma of cul-de-sac
Mesothelioma of mesentery
Mesothelioma of mesocolon
Mesothelioma of omentum
Mesothelioma of peritoneum (parietal) (pelvic)
Excludes1 other malignant neoplasm of soft tissue of peritoneum (C48.-)
Ex: C45.1, C48.0-C48.8, Z51.0

C45.2 Mesothelioma of pericardium
Excludes1 other malignant neoplasm of pericardium (C38.0)
Ex: C38.0, C45.2

C45.7 Mesothelioma of other sites

C45.9 Mesothelioma, unspecified

C46 Kaposi's sarcoma
Code first any human immunodeficiency virus [HIV] disease (B20)

C46.0 Kaposi's sarcoma of skin
Ex: C46.0, C46.7-C46.9, Z51.0

C46.1 Kaposi's sarcoma of soft tissue
Kaposi's sarcoma of blood vessel
Kaposi's sarcoma of connective tissue
Kaposi's sarcoma of fascia
Kaposi's sarcoma of ligament
Kaposi's sarcoma of lymphatic(s) NEC
Kaposi's sarcoma of muscle
Excludes2 Kaposi's sarcoma of lymph glands and nodes (C46.3)
Ex: C46.1, C46.7-C46.9, Z51.0

C46.2 Kaposi's sarcoma of palate
Ex: C46.2, C46.7-C46.9, Z51.0

C46.3 Kaposi's sarcoma of lymph nodes
Ex: C45.7-C45.9, C46.3, C76.8-C77.9, C7A.00, C7A.098-C7B.01, C7B.1, C80.0-C80.2, D49.81-D49.9

C46.4 Kaposi's sarcoma of gastrointestinal sites
Ex: C46.4, C46.7-C46.9, Z51.0

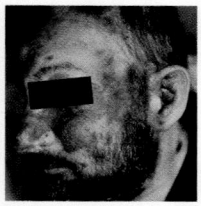

Figure 2-11 Kaposi's sarcoma. There are large confluent hyperpigmented patch-stage lesions with lymphedema. (From Cohen & Powderly: Infectious Diseases, ed 3, Mosby, An Imprint of Elsevier, 2010)

Item 2–5 Kaposi's sarcoma is a cancer that causes patches of abnormal tissue to grow under the skin; in the lining of the mouth, nose, and throat; or in other organs, often beginning and spreading to other organs. Patients who have had organ transplants or patients with AIDS are at high risk for this malignancy.

C46.5 Kaposi's sarcoma of lung
Ex: For catgory C46.5 CC codes: C34.80-C34.92, C39.9, C45.7-C45.9, C46.50-C46.52, C76.8, C7A.00, C7A.090, C7A.098-C7B.00, C7B.1, C80.0-C80.2, D49.1, D49.81-D49.9

C46.50 Kaposi's sarcoma of unspecified lung

C46.51 Kaposi's sarcoma of right lung

C46.52 Kaposi's sarcoma of left lung

C46.7 Kaposi's sarcoma of other sites
Ex: C46.0-C46.9, Z51.0

C46.9 Kaposi's sarcoma, unspecified
Kaposi's sarcoma of unspecified site
Ex: C45.7-C46.9, C51.0-C72.9, C76.0-C79.9, C7A.00, C7A.093, C7A.098-C7B.8, C80.0-C80.2, D00.00-D02.4, D04.0-D09.9, D37.01-D44.9, D48.0-D49.9, Z51.0

C47 Malignant neoplasm of peripheral nerves and autonomic nervous system
Includes malignant neoplasm of sympathetic and parasympathetic nerves and ganglia
Excludes1 Kaposi's sarcoma of soft tissue (C46.1)
Ex: For category C47 CC Codes: Z51.0

C47.0 Malignant neoplasm of peripheral nerves of head, face and neck
Excludes1 malignant neoplasm of peripheral nerves of orbit (C69.6-)

C47.1 Malignant neoplasm of peripheral nerves of upper limb, including shoulder

C47.10 Malignant neoplasm of peripheral nerves of unspecified upper limb, including shoulder

C47.11 Malignant neoplasm of peripheral nerves of right upper limb, including shoulder

C47.12 Malignant neoplasm of peripheral nerves of left upper limb, including shoulder

C47.2 Malignant neoplasm of peripheral nerves of lower limb, including hip

C47.20 Malignant neoplasm of peripheral nerves of unspecified lower limb, including hip

C47.21 Malignant neoplasm of peripheral nerves of right lower limb, including hip

C47.22 Malignant neoplasm of peripheral nerves of left lower limb, including hip

C47.3 Malignant neoplasm of peripheral nerves of thorax

C47.4 Malignant neoplasm of peripheral nerves of abdomen

C47.5 Malignant neoplasm of peripheral nerves of pelvis

C47.6 Malignant neoplasm of peripheral nerves of trunk, unspecified
Malignant neoplasm of peripheral nerves of unspecified part of trunk

C47.8 Malignant neoplasm of overlapping sites of peripheral nerves and autonomic nervous system

C47.9 Malignant neoplasm of peripheral nerves and autonomic nervous system, unspecified
Malignant neoplasm of unspecified site of peripheral nerves and autonomic nervous system

C48 Malignant neoplasm of retroperitoneum and peritoneum
Excludes1 Kaposi's sarcoma of connective tissue (C46.1) mesothelioma (C45.-)
Ex: For category C48 unless otherwise indicated: C45.1, C48.0-C48.8, Z51.0

C48.0 Malignant neoplasm of retroperitoneum
Behind/outside of peritoneum
Ex: C48.0, Z51.0

C48.1 Malignant neoplasm of specified parts of peritoneum
Serous membrane lining abdominopelvic walls and covering viscera
Malignant neoplasm of cul-de-sac
Malignant neoplasm of mesentery
Malignant neoplasm of mesocolon
Malignant neoplasm of omentum
Malignant neoplasm of parietal peritoneum
Malignant neoplasm of pelvic peritoneum

C48.2 Malignant neoplasm of peritoneum, unspecified

C48.8 Malignant neoplasm of overlapping sites of retroperitoneum and peritoneum

● **C49 Malignant neoplasm of other connective and soft tissue**

Includes malignant neoplasm of blood vessel
malignant neoplasm of bursa
malignant neoplasm of cartilage
malignant neoplasm of fascia
malignant neoplasm of fat
malignant neoplasm of ligament, except uterine
malignant neoplasm of lymphatic vessel
malignant neoplasm of muscle
malignant neoplasm of synovia
malignant neoplasm of tendon (sheath)

Excludes1 malignant neoplasm of cartilage (of):
articular (C40-C41)
larynx (C32.3)
nose (C30.0)
malignant neoplasm of connective tissue of breast (C50.-)

Excludes2 Kaposi's sarcoma of soft tissue (C46.1)
malignant neoplasm of heart (C38.0)
malignant neoplasm of peripheral nerves and autonomic nervous system (C47.-)
malignant neoplasm of peritoneum (C48.2)
malignant neoplasm of retroperitoneum (C48.0)
malignant neoplasm of uterine ligament (C57.3)
mesothelioma (C45.-)

Ex: For category C49 unless otherwise indicated: Z51.0

C49.0 Malignant neoplasm of connective and soft tissue of head, face and neck
Malignant neoplasm of connective tissue of ear
Malignant neoplasm of connective tissue of eyelid
Excludes1 connective tissue of orbit (C69.6-)

● **C49.1 Malignant neoplasm of connective and soft tissue of upper limb, including shoulder**
C49.10 Malignant neoplasm of connective and soft tissue of unspecified upper limb, including shoulder
C49.11 Malignant neoplasm of connective and soft tissue of right upper limb, including shoulder
C49.12 Malignant neoplasm of connective and soft tissue of left upper limb, including shoulder

● **C49.2 Malignant neoplasm of connective and soft tissue of lower limb, including hip**
C49.20 Malignant neoplasm of connective and soft tissue of unspecified lower limb, including hip
C49.21 Malignant neoplasm of connective and soft tissue of right lower limb, including hip
C49.22 Malignant neoplasm of connective and soft tissue of left lower limb, including hip

C49.3 Malignant neoplasm of connective and soft tissue of thorax
Malignant neoplasm of axilla
Malignant neoplasm of diaphragm
Malignant neoplasm of great vessels
Excludes1 malignant neoplasm of breast (C50.-)
malignant neoplasm of heart (C38.0)
malignant neoplasm of mediastinum (C38.1-C38.3)
malignant neoplasm of thymus (C37)
Coding Clinic: 2015, Q3, P19

C49.4 Malignant neoplasm of connective and soft tissue of abdomen
Malignant neoplasm of abdominal wall
Malignant neoplasm of hypochondrium

C49.5 Malignant neoplasm of connective and soft tissue of pelvis
Malignant neoplasm of buttock
Malignant neoplasm of groin
Malignant neoplasm of perineum

C49.6 Malignant neoplasm of connective and soft tissue of trunk, unspecified
Malignant neoplasm of back NOS

C49.8 Malignant neoplasm of overlapping sites of connective and soft tissue
Primary malignant neoplasm of two or more contiguous sites of connective and soft tissue

C49.9 Malignant neoplasm of connective and soft tissue, unspecified

● **C49.A Gastrointestinal stromal tumor** ◀
Ex: For category C49.A CC codes unless otherwise indicated: Z51.0
C49.A0 Gastrointestinal stromal tumor, unspecified site ◀
C49.A1 Gastrointestinal stromal tumor of esophagus ◀
C49.A2 Gastrointestinal stromal tumor of stomach ◀
Ex: D80.0, D80.3-D81.4, D81.6-D81.7, D81.89-D84.0, D84.8-D84.9, D89.3-D89.9
C49.A3 Gastrointestinal stromal tumor of small intestine ◀
C49.A4 Gastrointestinal stromal tumor of large intestine ◀
C49.A5 Gastrointestinal stromal tumor of rectum ◀
C49.A9 Gastrointestinal stromal tumor of other sites ◀

MALIGNANT NEOPLASMS OF BREAST (C50)

● **C50 Malignant neoplasm of breast**

Includes connective tissue of breast
Paget's disease of breast
Paget's disease of nipple
Intraductal carcinoma of breast characterized by eczema-like inflammatory skin changes

Use additional code to identify estrogen receptor status (Z17.0, Z17.1)

Excludes1 skin of breast (C44.501, C44.511, C44.521, C44.591)

● **C50.0 Malignant neoplasm of nipple and areola**
● **C50.01 Malignant neoplasm of nipple and areola, female**
C50.011 Malignant neoplasm of nipple and areola, right female breast ♀
C50.012 Malignant neoplasm of nipple and areola, left female breast ♀
C50.019 Malignant neoplasm of nipple and areola, unspecified female breast ♀
● **C50.02 Malignant neoplasm of nipple and areola, male**
C50.021 Malignant neoplasm of nipple and areola, right male breast ♂
C50.022 Malignant neoplasm of nipple and areola, left male breast ♂
C50.029 Malignant neoplasm of nipple and areola, unspecified male breast ♂

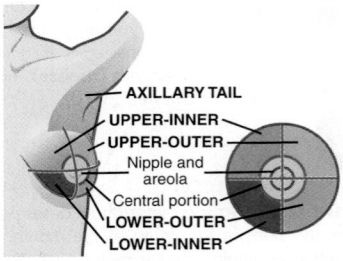

Figure 2-12 Female breast quadrants and axillary tail.

- **C50.1** Malignant neoplasm of central portion of breast
  - **C50.11** Malignant neoplasm of central portion of breast, female
    - C50.111 Malignant neoplasm of central portion of right female breast ♀
    - C50.112 Malignant neoplasm of central portion of left female breast ♀
    - C50.119 Malignant neoplasm of central portion of unspecified female breast ♀
  - **C50.12** Malignant neoplasm of central portion of breast, male
    - C50.121 Malignant neoplasm of central portion of right male breast ♂
    - C50.122 Malignant neoplasm of central portion of left male breast ♂
    - C50.129 Malignant neoplasm of central portion of unspecified male breast ♂
- **C50.2** Malignant neoplasm of upper-inner quadrant of breast
  - **C50.21** Malignant neoplasm of upper-inner quadrant of breast, female
    - C50.211 Malignant neoplasm of upper-inner quadrant of right female breast ♀
    - C50.212 Malignant neoplasm of upper-inner quadrant of left female breast ♀
    - C50.219 Malignant neoplasm of upper-inner quadrant of unspecified female breast ♀
  - **C50.22** Malignant neoplasm of upper-inner quadrant of breast, male
    - C50.221 Malignant neoplasm of upper-inner quadrant of right male breast ♂
    - C50.222 Malignant neoplasm of upper-inner quadrant of left male breast ♂
    - C50.229 Malignant neoplasm of upper-inner quadrant of unspecified male breast ♂
- **C50.3** Malignant neoplasm of lower-inner quadrant of breast
  - **C50.31** Malignant neoplasm of lower-inner quadrant of breast, female
    - C50.311 Malignant neoplasm of lower-inner quadrant of right female breast ♀
    - C50.312 Malignant neoplasm of lower-inner quadrant of left female breast ♀
    - C50.319 Malignant neoplasm of lower-inner quadrant of unspecified female breast ♀
  - **C50.32** Malignant neoplasm of lower-inner quadrant of breast, male
    - C50.321 Malignant neoplasm of lower-inner quadrant of right male breast ♂
    - C50.322 Malignant neoplasm of lower-inner quadrant of left male breast ♂
    - C50.329 Malignant neoplasm of lower-inner quadrant of unspecified male breast ♂
- **C50.4** Malignant neoplasm of upper-outer quadrant of breast
  - **C50.41** Malignant neoplasm of upper-outer quadrant of breast, female
    - C50.411 Malignant neoplasm of upper-outer quadrant of right female breast ♀
    - C50.412 Malignant neoplasm of upper-outer quadrant of left female breast ♀
    - C50.419 Malignant neoplasm of upper-outer quadrant of unspecified female breast ♀
  - **C50.42** Malignant neoplasm of upper-outer quadrant of breast, male
    - C50.421 Malignant neoplasm of upper-outer quadrant of right male breast ♂
    - C50.422 Malignant neoplasm of upper-outer quadrant of left male breast ♂
    - C50.429 Malignant neoplasm of upper-outer quadrant of unspecified male breast ♂
- **C50.5** Malignant neoplasm of lower-outer quadrant of breast
  - **C50.51** Malignant neoplasm of lower-outer quadrant of breast, female
    - C50.511 Malignant neoplasm of lower-outer quadrant of right female breast ♀
    - C50.512 Malignant neoplasm of lower-outer quadrant of left female breast ♀
    - C50.519 Malignant neoplasm of lower-outer quadrant of unspecified female breast ♀
  - **C50.52** Malignant neoplasm of lower-outer quadrant of breast, male
    - C50.521 Malignant neoplasm of lower-outer quadrant of right male breast ♂
    - C50.522 Malignant neoplasm of lower-outer quadrant of left male breast ♂
    - C50.529 Malignant neoplasm of lower-outer quadrant of unspecified male breast ♂
- **C50.6** Malignant neoplasm of axillary tail of breast
  - **C50.61** Malignant neoplasm of axillary tail of breast, female
    - C50.611 Malignant neoplasm of axillary tail of right female breast ♀
    - C50.612 Malignant neoplasm of axillary tail of left female breast ♀
    - C50.619 Malignant neoplasm of axillary tail of unspecified female breast ♀
  - **C50.62** Malignant neoplasm of axillary tail of breast, male
    - C50.621 Malignant neoplasm of axillary tail of right male breast ♂
    - C50.622 Malignant neoplasm of axillary tail of left male breast ♂
    - C50.629 Malignant neoplasm of axillary tail of unspecified male breast ♂
- **C50.8** Malignant neoplasm of overlapping sites of breast
  - **C50.81** Malignant neoplasm of overlapping sites of breast, female
    - C50.811 Malignant neoplasm of overlapping sites of right female breast ♀
    - C50.812 Malignant neoplasm of overlapping sites of left female breast ♀
    - C50.819 Malignant neoplasm of overlapping sites of unspecified female breast ♀
  - **C50.82** Malignant neoplasm of overlapping sites of breast, male
    - C50.821 Malignant neoplasm of overlapping sites of right male breast ♂
    - C50.822 Malignant neoplasm of overlapping sites of left male breast ♂
    - C50.829 Malignant neoplasm of overlapping sites of unspecified male breast ♂
- **C50.9** Malignant neoplasm of breast of unspecified site
  - **C50.91** Malignant neoplasm of breast of unspecified site, female
    - C50.911 Malignant neoplasm of unspecified site of right female breast ♀
    - C50.912 Malignant neoplasm of unspecified site of left female breast ♀
    - C50.919 Malignant neoplasm of unspecified site of unspecified female breast ♀

● **C50.92 Malignant neoplasm of breast of unspecified site, male**

C50.921 Malignant neoplasm of unspecified site of right male breast ♂

C50.922 Malignant neoplasm of unspecified site of left male breast ♂

C50.929 Malignant neoplasm of unspecified site of unspecified male breast ♂

MALIGNANT NEOPLASMS OF FEMALE GENITAL ORGANS (C51-C58)

Includes malignant neoplasm of skin of female genital organs

● **C51 Malignant neoplasm of vulva**

Excludes1 carcinoma in situ of vulva (D07.1)

C51.0 Malignant neoplasm of labium majus ♀
Outer folds of skin external female genitalia
Malignant neoplasm of Bartholin's [greater vestibular] gland

C51.1 Malignant neoplasm of labium minus ♀
Two inner folds surrounding vulva in female genitalia

C51.2 Malignant neoplasm of clitoris ♀

C51.8 Malignant neoplasm of overlapping sites of vulva ♀

C51.9 Malignant neoplasm of vulva, unspecified ♀
Malignant neoplasm of external female genitalia NOS
Malignant neoplasm of pudendum

C52 Malignant neoplasm of vagina ♀

Excludes1 carcinoma in situ of vagina (D07.2)

● **C53 Malignant neoplasm of cervix uteri**

Excludes1 carcinoma in situ of cervix uteri (D06.-)

C53.0 Malignant neoplasm of endocervix ♀
Inside the cervix

C53.1 Malignant neoplasm of exocervix ♀
Outside the cervix

C53.8 Malignant neoplasm of overlapping sites of cervix uteri ♀

C53.9 Malignant neoplasm of cervix uteri, unspecified ♀

● **C54 Malignant neoplasm of corpus uteri**

C54.0 Malignant neoplasm of isthmus uteri ♀
Constricted part of uterus between cervix and body
Malignant neoplasm of lower uterine segment

C54.1 Malignant neoplasm of endometrium ♀
Lining of uterus

C54.2 Malignant neoplasm of myometrium ♀
Middle layer of uterine wall consisting of smooth muscle supporting stromal and vascular tissue

C54.3 Malignant neoplasm of fundus uteri ♀
Top rounded portion of uterus

C54.8 Malignant neoplasm of overlapping sites of corpus uteri ♀
Main body of uterus

C54.9 Malignant neoplasm of corpus uteri, unspecified ♀

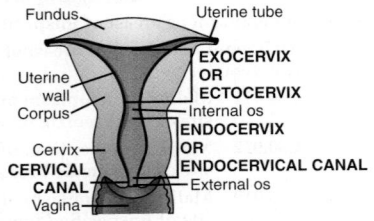

Figure 2-13 Cervix uteri.

C55 Malignant neoplasm of uterus, part unspecified ♀

● **C56 Malignant neoplasm of ovary**

Use additional code to identify any functional activity

Ex For category C56 CC Codes: C45.9, C56.1-C57.4, C76.3, C79.60-C79.62, C7A.00, C7A.098-C7B.00, C7B.1, C80.0-C80.2

C56.1 Malignant neoplasm of right ovary ♀

C56.2 Malignant neoplasm of left ovary ♀

C56.9 Malignant neoplasm of unspecified ovary ♀

● **C57 Malignant neoplasm of other and unspecified female genital organs**

● **C57.0 Malignant neoplasm of fallopian tube**
Malignant neoplasm of oviduct
Malignant neoplasm of uterine tube

C57.00 Malignant neoplasm of unspecified fallopian tube ♀

C57.01 Malignant neoplasm of right fallopian tube ♀

C57.02 Malignant neoplasm of left fallopian tube ♀

● **C57.1 Malignant neoplasm of broad ligament**

C57.10 Malignant neoplasm of unspecified broad ligament ♀

C57.11 Malignant neoplasm of right broad ligament ♀

C57.12 Malignant neoplasm of left broad ligament ♀

● **C57.2 Malignant neoplasm of round ligament**

C57.20 Malignant neoplasm of unspecified round ligament ♀

C57.21 Malignant neoplasm of right round ligament ♀

C57.22 Malignant neoplasm of left round ligament ♀

C57.3 Malignant neoplasm of parametrium ♀
Malignant neoplasm of uterine ligament NOS

C57.4 Malignant neoplasm of uterine adnexa, unspecified ♀

C57.7 Malignant neoplasm of other specified female genital organs ♀
Malignant neoplasm of wolffian body or duct

C57.8 Malignant neoplasm of overlapping sites of female genital organs ♀
Primary malignant neoplasm of two or more contiguous sites of the female genital organs whose point of origin cannot be determined
Primary tubo-ovarian malignant neoplasm whose point of origin cannot be determined
Primary utero-ovarian malignant neoplasm whose point of origin cannot be determined

C57.9 Malignant neoplasm of female genital organ, unspecified ♀
Malignant neoplasm of female genitourinary tract NOS

C58 Malignant neoplasm of placenta ♀ M

Includes choriocarcinoma NOS
chorionepithelioma NOS

Excludes1 chorioadenoma (destruens) (D39.2)
hydatidiform mole NOS (O01.9)
invasive hydatidiform mole (D39.2)
male choriocarcinoma NOS (C62.9-)
malignant hydatidiform mole (D39.2)

MALIGNANT NEOPLASMS OF MALE GENITAL ORGANS (C60-C63)

Includes malignant neoplasm of skin of male genital organs

● **C60 Malignant neoplasm of penis**

C60.0 Malignant neoplasm of prepuce ♂
Malignant neoplasm of foreskin

C60.1 Malignant neoplasm of glans penis ♂

C60.2 Malignant neoplasm of body of penis ♂
Malignant neoplasm of corpus cavernosum

C60.8 Malignant neoplasm of overlapping sites of penis ♂

C60.9 Malignant neoplasm of penis, unspecified ♂
Malignant neoplasm of skin of penis NOS

◀ New ⇐ Revised ~~deleted~~ Deleted Excludes 1 Excludes 2 Includes Use additional Code first Code also Unspecified
OGCR Official Guidelines ● Unacceptable Principal Diagnosis X Assign placeholder X ● Use Additional Character(s) ▶ Manifestation Code Coding Clinic

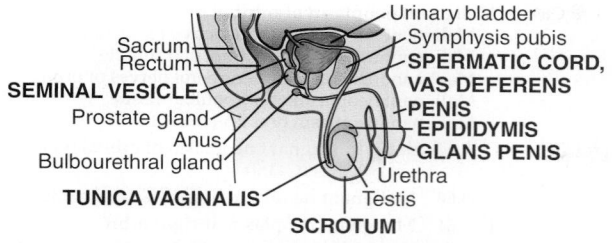

Figure 2-14 Penis and other male genital organs.

C61 Malignant neoplasm of prostate ♂
Use additional code to identify: ◀
hormone sensitivity status (Z19.1-Z19.2) ◀
rising PSA following treatment for malignant neoplasm of prostate (R97.21) ◀
Excludes1 malignant neoplasm of seminal vesicle (C63.7)

● **C62 Malignant neoplasm of testis**
Use additional code to identify any functional activity.

● **C62.0 Malignant neoplasm of undescended testis**
Malignant neoplasm of ectopic testis
Malignant neoplasm of retained testis

C62.00 Malignant neoplasm of unspecified undescended testis ♂

C62.01 Malignant neoplasm of undescended right testis ♂

C62.02 Malignant neoplasm of undescended left testis ♂

● **C62.1 Malignant neoplasm of descended testis**
Malignant neoplasm of scrotal testis

C62.10 Malignant neoplasm of unspecified descended testis, unspecified side ♂

C62.11 Malignant neoplasm of descended right testis ♂

C62.12 Malignant neoplasm of descended left testis ♂

● **C62.9 Malignant neoplasm of testis, unspecified whether descended or undescended**

C62.90 Malignant neoplasm of unspecified testis, unspecified whether descended or undescended ♂
Malignant neoplasm of testis NOS

C62.91 Malignant neoplasm of right testis, unspecified whether descended or undescended ♂

C62.92 Malignant neoplasm of left testis, unspecified whether descended or undescended ♂

● **C63 Malignant neoplasm of other and unspecified male genital organs**

● **C63.0 Malignant neoplasm of epididymis**

C63.00 Malignant neoplasm of unspecified epididymis ♂

C63.01 Malignant neoplasm of right epididymis ♂

C63.02 Malignant neoplasm of left epididymis ♂

● **C63.1 Malignant neoplasm of spermatic cord**

C63.10 Malignant neoplasm of unspecified spermatic cord ♂

C63.11 Malignant neoplasm of right spermatic cord ♂

C63.12 Malignant neoplasm of left spermatic cord ♂

C63.2 Malignant neoplasm of scrotum ♂
Malignant neoplasm of skin of scrotum

C63.7 Malignant neoplasm of other specified male genital organs ♂
Malignant neoplasm of seminal vesicle
Malignant neoplasm of tunica vaginalis

C63.8 Malignant neoplasm of overlapping sites of male genital organs ♂
Primary malignant neoplasm of two or more contiguous sites of male genital organs whose point of origin cannot be determined

C63.9 Malignant neoplasm of male genital organ, unspecified ♂
Malignant neoplasm of male genitourinary tract NOS

MALIGNANT NEOPLASMS OF URINARY TRACT (C64-C68)

● **C64 Malignant neoplasm of kidney, except renal pelvis**
Excludes1 malignant carcinoid tumor of the kidney (C7A.093)
malignant neoplasm of renal calyces (C65.-)
malignant neoplasm of renal pelvis (C65.-)
Ex: **For category C64 CC Codes:** C45.7-C45.9, C64.1-C65.9, C68.8-C68.9, C76.8, C7A.00, C7A.093, C7A.098-C7B.00, C7B.1, C80.0-C80.2, D49.511-D49.59, D49.81-D49.9

C64.1 Malignant neoplasm of right kidney, except renal pelvis

C64.2 Malignant neoplasm of left kidney, except renal pelvis

C64.9 Malignant neoplasm of unspecified kidney, except renal pelvis

● **C65 Malignant neoplasm of renal pelvis**
Includes malignant neoplasm of pelviureteric junction
malignant neoplasm of renal calyces
Ex: **For category C65 CC Codes:** See C64

C65.1 Malignant neoplasm of right renal pelvis

C65.2 Malignant neoplasm of left renal pelvis

C65.9 Malignant neoplasm of unspecified renal pelvis

● **C66 Malignant neoplasm of ureter**
Excludes1 malignant neoplasm of ureteric orifice of bladder (C67.6)
Ex: **For category C66 CC Codes:** C45.7-C45.9, C66.1-C66.9, C68.8-C68.9, C76.8, C7A.00, C7A.098, C7A.1-C7B.00, C7B.1, C80.0-C80.2, D49.511-D49.59, D49.81-D49.9

C66.1 Malignant neoplasm of right ureter

C66.2 Malignant neoplasm of left ureter

C66.9 Malignant neoplasm of unspecified ureter

● **C67 Malignant neoplasm of bladder**

C67.0 Malignant neoplasm of trigone of bladder
Triangular area formed by three openings in the floor of urinary bladder

C67.1 Malignant neoplasm of dome of bladder
Vaulted roof

C67.2 Malignant neoplasm of lateral wall of bladder
Side walls

C67.3 Malignant neoplasm of anterior wall of bladder
Front wall

C67.4 Malignant neoplasm of posterior wall of bladder
Back wall

C67.5 Malignant neoplasm of bladder neck
Joining of bladder and urethra
Malignant neoplasm of internal urethral orifice

C67.6 Malignant neoplasm of ureteric orifice
Opening from bladder to ureters

C67.7 Malignant neoplasm of urachus
Embryonic canal that connects the urinary bladder with the structure that forms the umbilical cord (allantois)

C67.8 Malignant neoplasm of overlapping sites of bladder

C67.9 Malignant neoplasm of bladder, unspecified
Coding Clinic: 2016, Q1, P19

● **C68 Malignant neoplasm of other and unspecified urinary organs**
Excludes1 malignant neoplasm of female genitourinary tract NOS (C57.9)
malignant neoplasm of male genitourinary tract NOS (C63.9)
Ex: **For category C68 CC codes C68.0-C68.1:** C68.0-C68.9, C79.82 **For category C68 CC codes C68.8-C68.9:** C6.41-C66.9, C68.0-C68.9, C76.3, C79.00-C79.19, C7A.093

C68.0 Malignant neoplasm of urethra
Excludes1 malignant neoplasm of urethral orifice of bladder (C67.5)

C68.1 Malignant neoplasm of paraurethral glands
Group of glands of female urethra drained by paraurethral ducts; AKA Skene glands, female prostate

C68.8 Malignant neoplasm of overlapping sites of urinary organs
Primary malignant neoplasm of two or more contiguous sites of urinary organs whose point of origin cannot be determined

C68.9 Malignant neoplasm of urinary organ, unspecified
Malignant neoplasm of urinary system NOS

MALIGNANT NEOPLASMS OF EYE, BRAIN AND OTHER PARTS OF CENTRAL NERVOUS SYSTEM (C69-C72)

C69 Malignant neoplasm of eye and adnexa
Excludes1 malignant neoplasm of connective tissue of eyelid (C49.0)
malignant neoplasm of eyelid (skin) (C43.1-, C44.1-)
malignant neoplasm of optic nerve (C72.3-)

C69.0 Malignant neoplasm of conjunctiva
C69.00 Malignant neoplasm of unspecified conjunctiva
C69.01 Malignant neoplasm of right conjunctiva
C69.02 Malignant neoplasm of left conjunctiva

C69.1 Malignant neoplasm of cornea
C69.10 Malignant neoplasm of unspecified cornea
C69.11 Malignant neoplasm of right cornea
C69.12 Malignant neoplasm of left cornea

C69.2 Malignant neoplasm of retina
Excludes1 dark area on retina (D49.81)
neoplasm of unspecified behavior of retina and choroid (D49.81)
retinal freckle (D49.81)
C69.20 Malignant neoplasm of unspecified retina
C69.21 Malignant neoplasm of right retina
C69.22 Malignant neoplasm of left retina

C69.3 Malignant neoplasm of choroid
C69.30 Malignant neoplasm of unspecified choroid
C69.31 Malignant neoplasm of right choroid
C69.32 Malignant neoplasm of left choroid

C69.4 Malignant neoplasm of ciliary body
C69.40 Malignant neoplasm of unspecified ciliary body
C69.41 Malignant neoplasm of right ciliary body
C69.42 Malignant neoplasm of left ciliary body

C69.5 Malignant neoplasm of lacrimal gland and duct
Malignant neoplasm of lacrimal sac
Malignant neoplasm of nasolacrimal duct
C69.50 Malignant neoplasm of unspecified lacrimal gland and duct
C69.51 Malignant neoplasm of right lacrimal gland and duct
C69.52 Malignant neoplasm of left lacrimal gland and duct

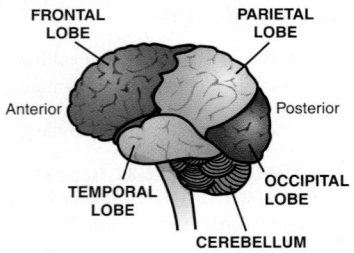

Figure 2-15 The brain.

C69.6 Malignant neoplasm of orbit
Malignant neoplasm of connective tissue of orbit
Malignant neoplasm of extraocular muscle
Malignant neoplasm of peripheral nerves of orbit
Malignant neoplasm of retrobulbar tissue
Malignant neoplasm of retro-ocular tissue
Excludes1 malignant neoplasm of orbital bone (C41.0)
C69.60 Malignant neoplasm of unspecified orbit
C69.61 Malignant neoplasm of right orbit
C69.62 Malignant neoplasm of left orbit

C69.8 Malignant neoplasm of overlapping sites of eye and adnexa
C69.80 Malignant neoplasm of overlapping sites of unspecified eye and adnexa
C69.81 Malignant neoplasm of overlapping sites of right eye and adnexa
C69.82 Malignant neoplasm of overlapping sites of left eye and adnexa

C69.9 Malignant neoplasm of unspecified site of eye
Malignant neoplasm of eyeball
C69.90 Malignant neoplasm of unspecified site of unspecified eye
C69.91 Malignant neoplasm of unspecified site of right eye
C69.92 Malignant neoplasm of unspecified site of left eye

C70 Malignant neoplasm of meninges
C70.0 Malignant neoplasm of cerebral meninges
Ex: C45.7-C45.9, C70.0, C70.9, C72.9, C76.8, C7A.00, C7A.098-C7B.00, C7B.1, C80.0-C80.2, D49.6-D49.9
C70.1 Malignant neoplasm of spinal meninges
Ex: C45.7-C45.9, C70.1, C72.9, C76.8, C7A.00, C7A.098-C7B.00, C7B.1, C80.0-C80.2, D49.6-D49.9
C70.9 Malignant neoplasm of meninges, unspecified
Ex: See C70.0

C71 Malignant neoplasm of brain
Excludes1 malignant neoplasm of cranial nerves (C72.2-C72.5)
retrobulbar malignant neoplasm (C69.6-)
Ex: For category C71 CC codes: C45.7-C45.9, C70.0, C70.9-C71.9, C72.20-C72.9, C76.8, C7A.00, C7A.098-C7B.00, C7B.1, C80.0-C80.2, D49.6-D49.9
C71.0 Malignant neoplasm of cerebrum, except lobes and ventricles
Malignant neoplasm of supratentorial NOS
C71.1 Malignant neoplasm of frontal lobe
C71.2 Malignant neoplasm of temporal lobe
C71.3 Malignant neoplasm of parietal lobe
C71.4 Malignant neoplasm of occipital lobe
C71.5 Malignant neoplasm of cerebral ventricle
Excludes1 malignant neoplasm of fourth cerebral ventricle (C71.7)
C71.6 Malignant neoplasm of cerebellum
C71.7 Malignant neoplasm of brain stem
Malignant neoplasm of fourth cerebral ventricle
Infratentorial malignant neoplasm NOS
C71.8 Malignant neoplasm of overlapping sites of brain
C71.9 Malignant neoplasm of brain, unspecified

C72 Malignant neoplasm of spinal cord, cranial nerves and other parts of central nervous system
Excludes1 malignant neoplasm of meninges (C70.-)
malignant neoplasm of peripheral nerves and autonomic nervous system (C47.-)
Ex: For category C72 unless otherwise indicated: C45.7-C45.9, C72.20-C72.9, C76.8, C7A.00, C7A.098-C7B.00, C7B.1, C80.0-C80.2, D49.6-D49.9
C72.0 Malignant neoplasm of spinal cord
Ex: C45.7-C45.9, C72.0-C72.1, C72.9, C76.8, C7A.00, C7A.098, C7A.1-C7B.00, C7B.1, C80.0-C80.2, D49.6-D49.9

C72.1 Malignant neoplasm of cauda equina
Lower end of spinal column
Ex: See C72.0

C72.2 Malignant neoplasm of olfactory nerve
Malignant neoplasm of olfactory bulb

C72.20 Malignant neoplasm of unspecified olfactory nerve

C72.21 Malignant neoplasm of right olfactory nerve

C72.22 Malignant neoplasm of left olfactory nerve

C72.3 Malignant neoplasm of optic nerve

C72.30 Malignant neoplasm of unspecified optic nerve

C72.31 Malignant neoplasm of right optic nerve

C72.32 Malignant neoplasm of left optic nerve

C72.4 Malignant neoplasm of acoustic nerve

C72.40 Malignant neoplasm of unspecified acoustic nerve

C72.41 Malignant neoplasm of right acoustic nerve

C72.42 Malignant neoplasm of left acoustic nerve

C72.5 Malignant neoplasm of other and unspecified cranial nerves

C72.50 Malignant neoplasm of unspecified cranial nerve
Malignant neoplasm of cranial nerve NOS

C72.59 Malignant neoplasm of other cranial nerves

C72.9 Malignant neoplasm of central nervous system, unspecified
Malignant neoplasm of unspecified site of central nervous system
Malignant neoplasm of nervous system NOS
Ex: C45.7-C45.9, C70.0-C72.9, C76.8, C79.31-C79.49, C7A.00, C7A.098-C7B.00, C7B.1, C80.0-C80.2, D49.6-D49.9

MALIGNANT NEOPLASMS OF THYROID AND OTHER ENDOCRINE GLANDS (C73-C75)

C73 Malignant neoplasm of thyroid gland
Use additional code to identify any functional activity

C74 Malignant neoplasm of adrenal gland
Ex: **For category C74 CC codes:** C45.7-C45.9, C74.00-C74.92, C75.9, C76.2, C76.8, C79.70-C79.72, C7A.00, C7A.098-C7B.00, C7B.1, C80.0-C80.2

C74.0 Malignant neoplasm of cortex of adrenal gland

C74.00 Malignant neoplasm of cortex of unspecified adrenal gland

C74.01 Malignant neoplasm of cortex of right adrenal gland

C74.02 Malignant neoplasm of cortex of left adrenal gland

C74.1 Malignant neoplasm of medulla of adrenal gland
Pair of glands situated on top of or above each kidney ("suprarenal")

C74.10 Malignant neoplasm of medulla of unspecified adrenal gland

C74.11 Malignant neoplasm of medulla of right adrenal gland

C74.12 Malignant neoplasm of medulla of left adrenal gland

C74.9 Malignant neoplasm of unspecified part of adrenal gland

C74.90 Malignant neoplasm of unspecified part of unspecified adrenal gland

C74.91 Malignant neoplasm of unspecified part of right adrenal gland

C74.92 Malignant neoplasm of unspecified part of left adrenal gland

C75 Malignant neoplasm of other endocrine glands and related structures

Excludes1 malignant carcinoid tumors (C7A.0-)
malignant neoplasm of adrenal gland (C74.-)
malignant neoplasm of endocrine pancreas (C25.4)
malignant neoplasm of islets of Langerhans (C25.4)
malignant neoplasm of ovary (C56.-)
malignant neoplasm of testis (C62.-)
malignant neoplasm of thymus (C37)
malignant neoplasm of thyroid gland (C73)
malignant neuroendocrine tumors (C7A.-)

C75.0 Malignant neoplasm of parathyroid gland
Ex: C75.0, C75.8-C75.9

C75.1 Malignant neoplasm of pituitary gland
Ex: C75.1-C75.2, Z51.0

C75.2 Malignant neoplasm of craniopharyngeal duct
Ex: See C75.1

C75.3 Malignant neoplasm of pineal gland
Ex: C75.3, Z51.0

C75.4 Malignant neoplasm of carotid body
Ex: C75.4, C75.8-C75.9

C75.5 Malignant neoplasm of aortic body and other paraganglia
Ex: C75.4-C75.9

C75.8 Malignant neoplasm with pluriglandular involvement, unspecified
Ex: C74.00-C75.9

C75.9 Malignant neoplasm of endocrine gland, unspecified
Ex: See C75.8

MALIGNANT NEUROENDOCRINE TUMORS (C7A)

C7A Malignant neuroendocrine tumors
Code also any associated multiple endocrine neoplasia [MEN] syndromes (E31.2-)
Use additional code to identify any associated endocrine syndrome, such as:
carcinoid syndrome (E34.0)

Excludes2 malignant pancreatic islet cell tumors (C25.4)
Merkel cell carcinoma (C4A.-)

C7A.0 Malignant carcinoid tumors

C7A.00 Malignant carcinoid tumor of unspecified site
Ex: C45.7-C45.9, C76.8, C79.89-C79.9, C7A.00-C7B.00, C7B.09-C7B.8, C80.0-C80.2, D49.81-D49.9

C7A.01 Malignant carcinoid tumors of the small intestine

C7A.010 Malignant carcinoid tumor of the duodenum
Ex: C17.0, C17.8-C17.9, C26.0, C26.9, C45.7-C45.9, C46.4, C76.8, C7A.00-C7B.00, C7B.1, C80.0-C80.2, D49.0, D49.81-D49.9

C7A.011 Malignant carcinoid tumor of the jejunum
Ex: C17.1, C17.8-C17.9, C26.0, C26.9, C45.7-C45.9, C46.4, C76.8, C7A.00-C7B.00, C7B.1, C80.0-C80.2, D49.0, D49.81-D49.9

C7A.012 Malignant carcinoid tumor of the ileum
Ex: C17.2, C17.8-C17.9, C26.0, C26.9, C45.7-C45.9, C46.4, C76.8, C7A.00-C7B.00, C7B.1, C80.0-C80.2, D49.0, D49.81-D49.9

C7A.019 Malignant carcinoid tumor of the small intestine, unspecified portion
Ex: C17.8-C17.9, C26.0, C26.9, C45.7-C45.9, C46.4, C76.8, C7A.00-C7B.00, C7B.1, C80.0-C80.2, D49.0, D49.81-D49.9

● **C7A.02 Malignant carcinoid tumors of the appendix, large intestine, and rectum**

C7A.020 Malignant carcinoid tumor of the appendix
Ex: C18.1, C18.8-C18.9, C26.0, C26.9, C45.7-C45.9, C46.4, C76.8, C7A.00-C7B.00, C7B.1, C80.0-C80.2, D49.0, D49.81-D49.9

C7A.021 Malignant carcinoid tumor of the cecum
Ex: C18.0, C18.8-C18.9, C26.0, C26.9, C45.7-C45.9, C46.4, C76.8, C7A.00-C7B.00, C7B.1, C80.0-C80.2, D49.0, D49.81-D49.9

C7A.022 Malignant carcinoid tumor of the ascending colon
Ex: C18.2, C18.8-C18.9, C26.0, C26.9, C45.7-C45.9, C46.4, C76.8, C7A.00-C7B.00, C7B.1, C80.0-C80.2, D49.0, D49.81-D49.9

C7A.023 Malignant carcinoid tumor of the transverse colon
Ex: C18.4, C18.8-C18.9, C26.0, C26.9, C45.7-C45.9, C46.4, C76.8, C7A.00-C7B.00, C7B.1, C80.0-C80.2, D49.0, D49.81-D49.9

C7A.024 Malignant carcinoid tumor of the descending colon
Ex: C18.6, C18.8-C18.9, C26.0, C26.9, C45.7-C45.9, C46.4, C76.8, C7A.00-C7B.00, C7B.1, C80.0-C80.2, D49.0, D49.81-D49.9

C7A.025 Malignant carcinoid tumor of the sigmoid colon
Ex: C18.7-C18.9, C26.0, C26.9, C45.7-C45.9, C46.4, C76.8, C7A.00-C7B.00, C7B.1, C80.0-C80.2, D49.0, D49.81-D49.9

C7A.026 Malignant carcinoid tumor of the rectum
Ex: C20, C21.2-C21.8, C26.0, C26.9, C45.7-C45.9, C46.4, C76.8, C7A.00-C7B.00, C7B.1, C80.0-C80.2, D49.0, D49.81-D49.9

C7A.029 Malignant carcinoid tumor of the large intestine, unspecified portion
Malignant carcinoid tumor of the colon NOS
Ex: C18.8-C18.9, C26.0, C26.9, C45.7-C45.9, C46.4, C76.8, C7A.00-C7B.00, C7B.1, C80.0-C80.2, D49.0, D49.81-D49.9

● **C7A.09 Malignant carcinoid tumors of other sites**
Ex: For category C7A.09 CC codes unless otherwise indicated: C16.0-C16.9, C26.0, C26.9, C45.7-C45.9, C46.4, C49.A2, C76.8, C7A.00-C7B.00, C7B.1, C80.0-C80.2, D49.0, D49.81-D49.9

C7A.090 Malignant carcinoid tumor of the bronchus and lung
Ex: C34.80-C34.92, C39.9, C45.7-C45.9, C46.50-C46.52, C76.8, C7A.00-C7B.00, C7B.1, C80.0-C80.2, D49.1, D49.81-D49.9

C7A.091 Malignant carcinoid tumor of the thymus
Ex: C37, C7A.00-C7A.8

C7A.092 Malignant carcinoid tumor of the stomach

C7A.093 Malignant carcinoid tumor of the kidney
Ex: C45.7-C45.9, C64.1-C65.9, C68.8-C68.9, C76.8, C7A.00-C7B.00, C7B.1, C80.0-C80.2, D49.511-D49.59, D49.81-D49.9

C7A.094 Malignant carcinoid tumor of the foregut unspecified ◄

C7A.095 Malignant carcinoid tumor of the midgut unspecified ◄

C7A.096 Malignant carcinoid tumor of the hindgut unspecified ◄

C7A.098 Malignant carcinoid tumors of other sites
Ex: C45.7-C45.9, C76.8, C79.89-C79.9, C7A.00-C7B.00, C7B.09-C7B.8, C80.0-C80.2, D49.81-D49.9

C7A.1 Malignant poorly differentiated neuroendocrine tumors
Malignant poorly differentiated neuroendocrine tumor NOS
Malignant poorly differentiated neuroendocrine carcinoma, any site
High grade neuroendocrine carcinoma, any site
Ex: See C7A.098

C7A.8 Other malignant neuroendocrine tumors
Secondary neuroendocrine tumors (C7B)
Ex: See C7A.098

SECONDARY NEUROENDOCRINE TUMORS (C7B)

● **C7B Secondary neuroendocrine tumors**
Use additional code to identify any functional activity

● **C7B.0 Secondary carcinoid tumors**

C7B.00 Secondary carcinoid tumors, unspecified site

C7B.01 Secondary carcinoid tumors of distant lymph nodes
Ex: C45.7-C45.9, C46.3, C76.8-C77.9, C7A.00, C7A.098-C7B.8, C80.0-C80.2, D49.81-D49.9

C7B.02 Secondary carcinoid tumors of liver
Ex: C45.7-C45.9, C76.8, C78.7-C78.89, C79.89-C79.9, C7A.00, C7A.098-C7B.8, C80.0-C80.2, D49.81-D49.9

C7B.03 Secondary carcinoid tumors of bone
Ex: C45.7-C45.9, C76.8, C79.51-C79.52, C79.89-C79.9, C7A.00, C7A.098-C7B.8, C80.0-C80.2, D49.81-D49.9

C7B.04 Secondary carcinoid tumors of peritoneum
Mesentary metastasis of carcinoid tumor
Ex: C45.7-C45.9, C76.8, C78.6, C78.80-C78.89, C79.89-C79.9, C7A.00, C7A.098-C7B.8, C80.0-C80.2, D49.81-D49.9

C7B.09 Secondary carcinoid tumors of other sites
Ex: C45.7-C45.9, C76.8, C79.89-C79.9, C7A.00, C7A.098-C7B.8, C80.0-C80.2, D49.81-D49.9

C7B.1 Secondary Merkel cell carcinoma
Merkel cell carcinoma nodal presentation
Merkel cell carcinoma visceral metastatic presentation

C7B.8 Other secondary neuroendocrine tumors
Ex: See C7B.09

MALIGNANT NEOPLASMS OF ILL-DEFINED, OTHER SECONDARY AND UNSPECIFIED SITES (C76-C80)

● **C76 Malignant neoplasm of other and ill-defined sites**
Excludes1 malignant neoplasm of female genitourinary tract NOS (C57.9)
malignant neoplasm of male genitourinary tract NOS (C63.9)
malignant neoplasm of lymphoid, hematopoietic and related tissue (C81-C96)
malignant neoplasm of skin (C44.-)
malignant neoplasm of unspecified site NOS (C80.1)

C76.0 Malignant neoplasm of head, face and neck
Malignant neoplasm of cheek NOS
Malignant neoplasm of nose NOS

C76.1 Malignant neoplasm of thorax
Intrathoracic malignant neoplasm NOS
Malignant neoplasm of axilla NOS
Thoracic malignant neoplasm NOS

C76.2 Malignant neoplasm of abdomen

C76.3 Malignant neoplasm of pelvis
Malignant neoplasm of groin NOS
Malignant neoplasm of sites overlapping systems within the pelvis
Rectovaginal (septum) malignant neoplasm
Between rectum and vagina
Rectovesical (septum) malignant neoplasm
Between rectum and urinary bladder; AKA vesicorectal

● **C76.4 Malignant neoplasm of upper limb**

C76.40 Malignant neoplasm of unspecified upper limb

C76.41 Malignant neoplasm of right upper limb

C76.42 Malignant neoplasm of left upper limb

C76.5 Malignant neoplasm of lower limb

C76.50 Malignant neoplasm of unspecified lower limb

C76.51 Malignant neoplasm of right lower limb

C76.52 Malignant neoplasm of left lower limb

C76.8 Malignant neoplasm of other specified ill-defined sites

Malignant neoplasm of overlapping ill-defined sites

C77 Secondary and unspecified malignant neoplasm of lymph nodes

Excludes1 malignant neoplasm of lymph nodes, specified as primary (C81-C86, C88, C96.-)
mesentary metastasis of carcinoid tumor (C7B.04)
secondary carcinoid tumors of distant lymph nodes (C7B.01)

Ex: **For category C77 CC codes:** C45.7-C45.9, C46.3, C76.8-C77.9, C7A.00, C7A.098-C7B.01, C7B.1, C80.0-C80.2, D49.81-D49.9

C77.0 Secondary and unspecified malignant neoplasm of lymph nodes of head, face and neck

Secondary and unspecified malignant neoplasm of supraclavicular lymph nodes

C77.1 Secondary and unspecified malignant neoplasm of intrathoracic lymph nodes

C77.2 Secondary and unspecified malignant neoplasm of intra-abdominal lymph nodes

C77.3 Secondary and unspecified malignant neoplasm of axilla and upper limb lymph nodes

Secondary and unspecified malignant neoplasm of pectoral lymph nodes

C77.4 Secondary and unspecified malignant neoplasm of inguinal and lower limb lymph nodes

C77.5 Secondary and unspecified malignant neoplasm of intrapelvic lymph nodes

C77.8 Secondary and unspecified malignant neoplasm of lymph nodes of multiple regions

C77.9 Secondary and unspecified malignant neoplasm of lymph node, unspecified

C78 Secondary malignant neoplasm of respiratory and digestive organs

Excludes1 secondary carcinoid tumors of liver (C7B.02)
secondary carcinoid tumors of peritoneum (C7B.04)

Excludes2 lymph node metastases (C77.0) ◀

C78.0 Secondary malignant neoplasm of lung

Ex: **For category C78.0 CC Codes:** C45.7-C45.9, C76.8, C78.00-C78.39, C79.89-C79.9, C7A.00, C7A.098-C7B.00, C7B.09-C7B.8, C80.0-C80.2, D49.81-D49.9

C78.00 Secondary malignant neoplasm of unspecified lung

C78.01 Secondary malignant neoplasm of right lung

C78.02 Secondary malignant neoplasm of left lung

C78.1 Secondary malignant neoplasm of mediastinum

Thoracic cavity between pleural cavities

Ex: C45.7-C45.9, C76.8, C78.1, C78.30-C78.39, C79.89-C79.9, C7A.00, C7A.098-C7B.00, C7B.09-C7B.8, C80.0-C80.2, D49.81-D49.9

C78.2 Secondary malignant neoplasm of pleura

Serous membrane covering lungs and lining thoracic cavity

Ex: C45.7-C45.9, C76.8, C78.2-C78.39, C79.89-C79.9, C7A.00, C7A.098-C7B.00, C7B.09-C7B.8, C80.0-C80.2, D49.81-D49.9, J91.0

C78.3 Secondary malignant neoplasm of other and unspecified respiratory organs

Ex: **For category C78.3 CC Codes:** C45.7-C45.9, C76.8, C78.00-C78.39, C79.89-C79.9, C7A.00, C7A.098-C7B.00, C7B.09-C7B.8, C80.0-C80.2, D49.81-D49.9

C78.30 Secondary malignant neoplasm of unspecified respiratory organ

C78.39 Secondary malignant neoplasm of other respiratory organs

C78.4 Secondary malignant neoplasm of small intestine

Ex: C45.7-C45.9, C76.8, C78.4, C78.80-C78.89, C79.89-C79.9, C7A.00, C7A.098-C7B.00, C7B.09-C7B.8, C80.0-C80.2, D49.81-D49.9

C78.5 Secondary malignant neoplasm of large intestine and rectum

Ex: C45.7-C45.9, C76.8, C78.5, C78.80-C78.89, C79.89-C79.9, C7A.00, C7A.098-C7B.00, C7B.09-C7B.8, C80.0-C80.2, D49.81-D49.9

C78.6 Secondary malignant neoplasm of retroperitoneum and peritoneum

Ex: C45.7-C45.9, C76.8, C78.6, C78.80-C78.89, C79.89-C79.9, C7A.00, C7A.098-C7B.00, C7B.04-C7B.8, C80.0-C80.2, D49.81-D49.9

C78.7 Secondary malignant neoplasm of liver and intrahepatic bile duct

Ex: C45.7-C45.9, C76.8, C78.7-C78.89, C79.89-C79.9, C7A.00, C7A.098-C7A.8, C7B.00, C7B.02, C7B.09-C7B.8, C80.0-C80.2, D49.81-D4.99

C78.8 Secondary malignant neoplasm of other and unspecified digestive organs

Ex: **For category C78.8 CC Codes:** C45.7-C45.9, C76.8, C78.4-C78.89, C79.89-C79.9, C7A.00, C7A.098-C7B.00, C7B.02, C7B.04-C7B.8, C80.0-C80.2, D49.81-D49.9

C78.80 Secondary malignant neoplasm of unspecified digestive organ

C78.89 Secondary malignant neoplasm of other digestive organs

Code also exocrine pancreatic insufficiency (K86.81) ◀

C79 Secondary malignant neoplasm of other and unspecified sites

Excludes1 secondary carcinoid tumors (C7B.-)
secondary neuroendocrine tumors (C7B.-)

Excludes2 lymph node metastases (C77.0) ◀

C79.0 Secondary malignant neoplasm of kidney and renal pelvis

Ex: **For category C79.0 CC Codes:** C45.7-C45.9, C76.8, C79.00-C79.19, C79.89-C79.9, C7A.00, C7A.098-C7B.00, C7B.09-C7B.8, C80.0-C80.2, D49.81-D49.9

C79.00 Secondary malignant neoplasm of unspecified kidney and renal pelvis

C79.01 Secondary malignant neoplasm of right kidney and renal pelvis

C79.02 Secondary malignant neoplasm of left kidney and renal pelvis

C79.1 Secondary malignant neoplasm of bladder and other and unspecified urinary organs

Ex: See C79.0

C79.10 Secondary malignant neoplasm of unspecified urinary organs

C79.11 Secondary malignant neoplasm of bladder

C79.19 Secondary malignant neoplasm of other urinary organs

C79.2 Secondary malignant neoplasm of skin

Excludes1 secondary Merkel cell carcinoma (C7B.1)

Ex: C45.7-C45.9, C76.8, C79.2, C79.89-C79.9, C7A.00, C7A.098-C7B.00, C7B.09-C7B.8, C80.0-C80.2, D49.81-D49.9

C79.3 Secondary malignant neoplasm of brain and cerebral meninges

C79.31 Secondary malignant neoplasm of brain

C45.7-C45.9, C76.8, C79.31, C79.89-C79.9, C7A.00, C7A.098-C7B.00, C7B.09-C7B.8, C80.0-C80.2, D49.81-D49.9

C79.32 Secondary malignant neoplasm of cerebral meninges

Ex: C45.7-C45.9, C76.8, C79.32-C79.49, C79.89-C79.9, C7A.00, C7A.098-C7B.00, C7B.09-C7B.8, C80.0-C80.2, D49.81-D49.9

C79.4 Secondary malignant neoplasm of other and unspecified parts of nervous system

Ex: **For category C79.4 CC codes:** See C79.32

C79.40 Secondary malignant neoplasm of unspecified part of nervous system

C79.49 Secondary malignant neoplasm of other parts of nervous system

Item 2–6 The adrenal glands are a pair of glands situated on top of or above each kidney ("suprarenal") and chiefly responsible for regulating the stress response through the synthesis of corticosteroids and catecholamines, including cortisol and adrenaline.

● **C79.5 Secondary malignant neoplasm of bone and bone marrow**

Excludes1 secondary carcinoid tumors of bone (C7B.03)

Ex: **For category C79.5 CC codes:** C45.7-C45.9, C76.8, C79.51-C79.52, C79.89-C79.9, C7A.00, C7A.098-C7B.00, C7B.03, C7B.09-C7B.8, C80.0-C80.2, D49.81-D49.9

C79.51 Secondary malignant neoplasm of bone

C79.52 Secondary malignant neoplasm of bone marrow

● **C79.6 Secondary malignant neoplasm of ovary**

Ex: **For category C79.6 CC codes:** C45.7-C45.9, C76.8, C79.60-C79.62, C79.89-C79.9, C7A.00, C7A.098-C7B.00, C7B.09-C7B.8, C80.0-C80.2, D49.81-D49.9

C79.60 Secondary malignant neoplasm of unspecified ovary ♀

C79.61 Secondary malignant neoplasm of right ovary ♀

C79.62 Secondary malignant neoplasm of left ovary ♀

● **C79.7 Secondary malignant neoplasm of adrenal gland**

Ex: **For category C79.7 CC codes:** C45.7-C45.9, C76.8, C79.70-C79.72, C79.89-C79.9, C7A.00, C7A.098-C7B.00, C7B.09-C7B.8, C80.0-C80.2, D49.81-D49.9

C79.70 Secondary malignant neoplasm of unspecified adrenal gland

C79.71 Secondary malignant neoplasm of right adrenal gland

C79.72 Secondary malignant neoplasm of left adrenal gland

● **C79.8 Secondary malignant neoplasm of other specified sites**

C79.81 Secondary malignant neoplasm of breast

Ex: C45.7-C45.9, C76.8, C79.81, C79.89-C79.9, C7A.00, C7A.098-C7B.00, C7B.09-C7B.8, C80.0-C80.2, D49.81-D49.9

C79.82 Secondary malignant neoplasm of genital organs

Ex: C45.7-C45.9, C76.8, C79.82-C79.9, C7A.00, C7A.098-C7B.00, C7B.09-C7B.8, C80.0-C80.2, D49.81-D49.9

C79.89 Secondary malignant neoplasm of other specified sites

Ex: C45.7-C45.9, C76.8, C79.89-C79.9, C7A.00, C7A.098-C7B.00, C7B.09, C7B.1-C7B.8, C80.0-C80.2, D49.81-D49.9

C79.9 Secondary malignant neoplasm of unspecified site

Metastatic cancer NOS
Metastatic disease NOS

Excludes1 carcinomatosis NOS (C80.0)
generalized cancer NOS (C80.0)
malignant (primary) neoplasm of unspecified site (C80.1)

Ex: See C79.89

OGCR Section I.C.2.j and k

Disseminated malignant neoplasm, unspecified

j. Code C80.0, Disseminated malignant neoplasm, unspecified, is for use only in those cases where the patient has advanced metastatic disease and no known primary or secondary sites are specified. It should not be used in place of assigning codes for the primary site and all known secondary sites.

Malignant neoplasm without specification of site

k. Code C80.1, Malignant (primary) neoplasm, unspecified, equates to Cancer, unspecified. This code should only be used when no determination can be made as to the primary site of a malignancy. This code should rarely be used in the inpatient setting.

● **C80 Malignant neoplasm without specification of site**

Excludes1 malignant carcinoid tumor of unspecified site (C7A.00)
malignant neoplasm of specified multiple sites-code to each site

C80.0 Disseminated malignant neoplasm, unspecified

Carcinomatosis NOS
Generalized cancer, unspecified site (primary) (secondary)
Generalized malignancy, unspecified site (primary) (secondary)

Ex: C45.7-C45.9, C76.8, C79.89-C79.9, C7A.00, C7A.098-C7B.00, C7B.09, C7B.1-C7B.8, C80.0-C80.2, D49.81-D49.9

C80.1 Malignant (primary) neoplasm, unspecified

Cancer NOS
Cancer unspecified site (primary)
Carcinoma unspecified site (primary)
Malignancy unspecified site (primary)

Excludes1 secondary malignant neoplasm of unspecified site (C79.9)

● **C80.2 Malignant neoplasm associated with transplanted organ**

Code first complication of transplanted organ (T86.-)

Use additional code to identify the specific malignancy

Ex: See C80.0

★ **(See Plate 315 on page 49.)**

MALIGNANT NEOPLASMS OF LYMPHOID, HEMATOPOIETIC AND RELATED TISSUE (C81-C96)

Excludes2 Kaposi's sarcoma of lymph nodes (C46.3)
secondary and unspecified neoplasm of lymph nodes (C77.-)
secondary neoplasm of bone marrow (C79.52)
secondary neoplasm of spleen (C78.89)

● **C81 Hodgkin lymphoma**

Form of malignant lymphoma with four types, nodular sclerosis, mixed cellularity, lymphocyte depleted, and lymphocyte predominant

Excludes1 personal history of Hodgkin lymphoma (Z85.71)

● **C81.0 Nodular lymphocyte predominant Hodgkin lymphoma**

Least aggressive, least common, typically no symptoms

Lymphocytic-histiocytic predominance Hodgkin's disease

C81.00 Nodular lymphocyte predominant Hodgkin lymphoma, unspecified site

Ex: C81.00-C81.09, C81.40-C81.49, C81.90, C81.98, D49.81-D49.9

C81.01 Nodular lymphocyte predominant Hodgkin lymphoma, lymph nodes of head, face, and neck

Ex: C81.00-C81.01, C81.08-C81.09, C81.40-C81.41, C81.48-C81.49, C81.90-C81.91, C81.98, D49.81-D49.9

C81.02 Nodular lymphocyte predominant Hodgkin lymphoma, intrathoracic lymph nodes

Ex: C81.00-C81.02, C81.08-C81.09, C81.40-C81.42, C81.48-C81.49, C81.90-C81.92, C81.98, D49.81-D49.9

C81.03 Nodular lymphocyte predominant Hodgkin lymphoma, intra-abdominal lymph nodes

Ex: C81.00, C81.03, C81.08-C81.09, C81.40, C81.43, C81.48-C81.49, C81.90, C81.93, C81.98, D49.81-D49.9

C81.04 Nodular lymphocyte predominant Hodgkin lymphoma, lymph nodes of axilla and upper limb

Ex: C81.00, C81.04, C81.08-C81.09, C81.40, C81.44, C81.48-C81.49, C81.90, C81.94, C81.98, D49.81-D49.9

C81.05 Nodular lymphocyte predominant Hodgkin lymphoma, lymph nodes of inguinal region and lower limb

Ex: C81.00, C81.05, C81.08-C81.09, C81.40, C81.45, C81.48-C81.49, C81.90, C81.95, C81.98, D49.81-D49.9

C81.06 **Nodular lymphocyte predominant Hodgkin lymphoma, intrapelvic lymph nodes**
Ex: C81.00, C81.06, C81.08-C81.09, C81.40, C81.46, C81.48-C81.49, C81.90, C81.96, C81.98, D49.81-D49.9

C81.07 **Nodular lymphocyte predominant Hodgkin lymphoma, spleen**
Ex: C81.00, C81.07-C81.09, C81.40, C81.47-C81.49, C81.90, C81.97-C81.98, D49.81-D49.9

C81.08 **Nodular lymphocyte predominant Hodgkin lymphoma, lymph nodes of multiple sites**
Ex: See C81.00

C81.09 **Nodular lymphocyte predominant Hodgkin lymphoma, extranodal and solid organ sites**
Ex: See C81.00

● **C81.1** **Nodular sclerosis Hodgkin lymphoma**
Nodular sclerosis classical Hodgkin lymphoma ◀
Moderately aggressive; most common in young adults

C81.10 **Nodular sclerosis Hodgkin lymphoma, unspecified site**
Ex: C81.10-C81.19, C81.90, C81.98, D49.81-D49.9

C81.11 **Nodular sclerosis Hodgkin lymphoma, lymph nodes of head, face, and neck**
Ex: C81.10-C81.11, C81.18-C81.19, C81.90-C81.91, C81.98, D49.81-D49.9

C81.12 **Nodular sclerosis Hodgkin lymphoma, intrathoracic lymph nodes**
Ex: C81.10, C81.12, C81.18-C81.19, C81.90, C81.92, C81.98, D49.81-D49.9

C81.13 **Nodular sclerosis Hodgkin lymphoma, intra-abdominal lymph nodes**
Ex: C81.10, C81.13, C81.18-C81.19, C81.90, C81.93, C81.98, D49.81-D49.9

C81.14 **Nodular sclerosis Hodgkin lymphoma, lymph nodes of axilla and upper limb**
Ex: C81.10, C81.14, C81.18-C81.19, C81.90, C81.94, C81.98, D49.81-D49.9

C81.15 **Nodular sclerosis Hodgkin lymphoma, lymph nodes of inguinal region and lower limb**
Ex: C81.10, C81.15, C81.18-C81.19, C81.90, C81.95, C81.98, D49.81-D49.9

C81.16 **Nodular sclerosis Hodgkin lymphoma, intrapelvic lymph nodes**
Ex: C81.10, C81.16, C81.18-C81.19, C81.90, C81.96, C81.98, D49.81-D49.9

C81.17 **Nodular sclerosis Hodgkin lymphoma, spleen**
Ex: C81.10, C81.17-C81.19, C81.90, C81.97-C81.98, D49.81-D49.9

C81.18 **Nodular sclerosis Hodgkin lymphoma, lymph nodes of multiple sites**
Ex: See C81.10

C81.19 **Nodular sclerosis Hodgkin lymphoma, extranodal and solid organ sites**
Ex: See C81.10

● **C81.2** **Mixed cellularity Hodgkin lymphoma**
Mixed cellularity classical Hodgkin lymphoma ◀
A type of Hodgkin's that is moderately aggressive with mixed cell types

C81.20 **Mixed cellularity Hodgkin lymphoma, unspecified site**
Ex: C81.20-C81.29, C81.90, C81.98, D49.81-D49.9

C81.21 **Mixed cellularity Hodgkin lymphoma, lymph nodes of head, face, and neck**
Ex: C81.20-C81.21, C81.28-C81.29, C81.90-C81.91, C81.98, D49.81-D49.9

C81.22 **Mixed cellularity Hodgkin lymphoma, intrathoracic lymph nodes**
Ex: C81.20, C81.22, C81.28-C81.29, C81.90, C81.92, C81.98, D49.81-D49.9

C81.23 **Mixed cellularity Hodgkin lymphoma, intra-abdominal lymph nodes**
Ex: C81.20, C81.23, C81.28-C81.29, C81.90, C81.93, C81.98, D49.81-D49.9

C81.24 **Mixed cellularity Hodgkin lymphoma, lymph nodes of axilla and upper limb**
Ex: C81.20, C81.24, C81.28-C81.29, C81.90, C81.94, C81.98, D49.81-D49.9

C81.25 **Mixed cellularity Hodgkin lymphoma, lymph nodes of inguinal region and lower limb**
Ex: C81.20, C81.25, C81.28-C81.29, C81.90, C81.95, C81.98, D49.81-D49.9

C81.26 **Mixed cellularity Hodgkin lymphoma, intrapelvic lymph nodes**
Ex: C81.20, C81.26, C81.28-C81.29, C81.90, C81.96, C81.98, D49.81-D49.9

C81.27 **Mixed cellularity Hodgkin lymphoma, spleen**
Ex: C81.20, C81.27, C81.28-C81.29, C81.90, C81.97, C81.98, D49.81-D49.9

C81.28 **Mixed cellularity Hodgkin lymphoma, lymph nodes of multiple sites**
Ex: See C81.20

C81.29 **Mixed cellularity Hodgkin lymphoma, extranodal and solid organ sites**
Ex: See C81.20

● **C81.3** **Lymphocyte depleted Hodgkin lymphoma**
Lymphocyte depleted classical Hodgkin lymphoma ◀
Most aggressive type with poor prognosis

C81.30 **Lymphocyte depleted Hodgkin lymphoma, unspecified site**
Ex: C81.30-C81.39, C81.90, C81.98, D49.81-D49.9

C81.31 **Lymphocyte depleted Hodgkin lymphoma, lymph nodes of head, face, and neck**
Ex: C81.30-C81.31, C81.38-C81.39, C81.90-C81.91, C81.98, D49.81-D49.9

C81.32 **Lymphocyte depleted Hodgkin lymphoma, intrathoracic lymph nodes**
Ex: C81.30, C81.32, C81.38-C81.39, C81.90, C81.92, C81.98, D49.81-D49.9

C81.33 **Lymphocyte depleted Hodgkin lymphoma, intra-abdominal lymph nodes**
Ex: C81.30, C81.33, C81.38-C81.39, C81.90, C81.93, C81.98, D49.81-D49.9

C81.34 **Lymphocyte depleted Hodgkin lymphoma, lymph nodes of axilla and upper limb**
Ex: C81.30, C81.34, C81.38-C81.39, C81.90, C81.94, C81.98, D49.81-D49.9

C81.35 **Lymphocyte depleted Hodgkin lymphoma, lymph nodes of inguinal region and lower limb**
Ex: C81.30, C81.35, C81.38-C81.39, C81.90, C81.95, C81.98, D49.81-D49.9

C81.36 **Lymphocyte depleted Hodgkin lymphoma, intrapelvic lymph nodes**
Ex: C81.30, C81.36, C81.38-C81.39, C81.90, C81.96, C81.98, D49.81-D49.9

C81.37 **Lymphocyte depleted Hodgkin lymphoma, spleen**
Ex: C81.30, C81.37, C81.38-C81.39, C81.90, C81.97, C81.98, D49.81-D49.9

C81.38 **Lymphocyte depleted Hodgkin lymphoma, lymph nodes of multiple sites**
Ex: C81.30-C81.39, C81.98, D49.81-D49.9

C81.39 **Lymphocyte depleted Hodgkin lymphoma, extranodal and solid organ sites**
Ex: See C81.30

● **C81.4 Lymphocyte-rich Hodgkin lymphoma**
Lymphocyte-rich classical Hodgkin lymphoma ◀
Excludes1 nodular lymphocyte predominant Hodgkin lymphoma (C81.0-)

C81.40 Lymphocyte-rich Hodgkin lymphoma, unspecified site
Ex: C81.00-C81.09, C81.40-C81.49, C81.90, C81.98, D49.81-D49.9

C81.41 Lymphocyte-rich Hodgkin lymphoma, lymph nodes of head, face, and neck
Ex: C81.00-C81.01, C81.08-C81.09, C81.40-C81.41, C81.48-C81.49, C81.90-C81.91, C81.98, D49.81-D49.9

C81.42 Lymphocyte-rich Hodgkin lymphoma, intrathoracic lymph nodes
Ex: C81.00-C81.02, C81.08-C81.09, C81.40-C81.42, C81.48-C81.49, C81.90-C81.92, C81.98, D49.81-D49.9

C81.43 Lymphocyte-rich Hodgkin lymphoma, intra-abdominal lymph nodes
Ex: C81.00, C81.03, C81.08-C81.09, C81.40, C81.43, C81.48-C81.49, C81.90, C81.93, C81.98, D49.81-D49.9

C81.44 Lymphocyte-rich Hodgkin lymphoma, lymph nodes of axilla and upper limb
Ex: C81.00, C81.04, C81.08-C81.09, C81.40, C81.44, C81.48-C81.49, C81.90, C81.94, C81.98, D49.81-D49.9

C81.45 Lymphocyte-rich Hodgkin lymphoma, lymph nodes of inguinal region and lower limb
Ex: C81.00, C81.05, C81.08-C81.09, C81.40, C81.45, C81.48-C81.49, C81.90, C81.95, C81.98, D49.81-D49.9

C81.46 Lymphocyte-rich Hodgkin lymphoma, intrapelvic lymph nodes
Ex: C81.00, C81.06, C81.08-C81.09, C81.40, C81.46, C81.48-C81.49, C81.90, C81.96, C81.98, D49.81-D49.9

C81.47 Lymphocyte-rich Hodgkin lymphoma, spleen
Ex: C81.00, C81.07-C81.09, C81.40, C81.47-C81.49, C81.90, C81.97-C81.98, D49.81-D49.9

C81.48 Lymphocyte-rich Hodgkin lymphoma, lymph nodes of multiple sites
Ex: See C81.40

C81.49 Lymphocyte-rich Hodgkin lymphoma, extranodal and solid organ sites
Ex: See C81.40

● **C81.7 Other Hodgkin lymphoma**
Classical Hodgkin lymphoma NOS
Other classical Hodgkin lymphoma ◀

C81.70 Other Hodgkin lymphoma, unspecified site
Ex: C81.70-C81.79, C81.90, C81.98, D49.81-D49.9

C81.71 Other Hodgkin lymphoma, lymph nodes of head, face, and neck
Ex: C81.70-C81.71, C81.78-C81.79, C81.90-C81.91, C81.98, D49.81-D49.9

C81.72 Other Hodgkin lymphoma, intrathoracic lymph nodes
Ex: C81.70, C81.72, C81.78-C81.79, C81.90, C81.92, C81.98, D49.81-D49.9

C81.73 Other Hodgkin lymphoma, intra-abdominal lymph nodes
Ex: C81.70, C81.73, C81.78-C81.79, C81.90, C81.93, C81.98, D49.81-D49.9

C81.74 Other Hodgkin lymphoma, lymph nodes of axilla and upper limb
Ex: C81.70, C81.74, C81.78-C81.79, C81.90, C81.94, C81.98, D49.81-D49.9

C81.75 Other Hodgkin lymphoma, lymph nodes of inguinal region and lower limb
Ex: C81.70, C81.75, C81.78-C81.79, C81.90, C81.95, C81.98, D49.81-D49.9

C81.76 Other Hodgkin lymphoma, intrapelvic lymph nodes
Ex: C81.70, C81.76, C81.78-C81.79, C81.90, C81.96, C81.98, D49.81-D49.9

C81.77 Other Hodgkin lymphoma, spleen
Ex: C81.70, C81.77, C81.78-C81.79, C81.90, C81.97, C81.98, D49.81-D49.9

C81.78 Other Hodgkin lymphoma, lymph nodes of multiple sites
Ex: See C81.70

C81.79 Other Hodgkin lymphoma, extranodal and solid organ sites
Ex: See C81.70

● **C81.9 Hodgkin lymphoma, unspecified**

C81.90 Hodgkin lymphoma, unspecified, unspecified site
Ex: C81.90-C81.98, D49.81-D49.9

C81.91 Hodgkin lymphoma, unspecified, lymph nodes of head, face, and neck
Ex: C81.90-C81.91, C81.98, D49.81-D49.9

C81.92 Hodgkin lymphoma, unspecified, intrathoracic lymph nodes
Ex: C81.90, C81.92, C81.98, D49.81-D49.9

C81.93 Hodgkin lymphoma, unspecified, intra-abdominal lymph nodes
Ex: C81.90, C81.93, C81.98, D49.81-D49.9

C81.94 Hodgkin lymphoma, unspecified, lymph nodes of axilla and upper limb
Ex: C81.90, C81.94, C81.98, D49.81-D49.9

C81.95 Hodgkin lymphoma, unspecified, lymph nodes of inguinal region and lower limb
Ex: C81.90, C81.95, C81.98, D49.81-D49.9

C81.96 Hodgkin lymphoma, unspecified, intrapelvic lymph nodes
Ex: C81.90, C81.96, C81.98, D49.81-D49.9

C81.97 Hodgkin lymphoma, unspecified, spleen
Ex: C81.90, C81.97-C81.98, D49.81-D49.9

C81.98 Hodgkin lymphoma, unspecified, lymph nodes of multiple sites
Ex: See C81.90

C81.99 Hodgkin lymphoma, unspecified, extranodal and solid organ sites
Ex: No exclusions

● **C82 Follicular lymphoma**
Group of malignant lymphomas
Includes follicular lymphoma with or without diffuse areas
Excludes1 mature T/NK-cell lymphomas (C84.-)
personal history of non-Hodgkin lymphoma (Z85.72)

● **C82.0 Follicular lymphoma grade I**

C82.00 Follicular lymphoma grade I, unspecified site
Ex: C82.00-C82.50, C82.59-C82.99, C83.10, C83.19, C84.40, C84.49, C84.60, C84.69-C84.70, C84.79, C84.A0, C84.A9, C84.Z0, C84.Z9, C84.90, C84.99-C85.10, C85.19-C85.20, C85.29-C85.80, C85.89-C85.90, C85.99, C86.4, C88.4, C96.4, C96.9, C96.Z,

C82.01 Follicular lymphoma grade I, lymph nodes of head, face, and neck
Ex: C82.00-C82.01, C82.08-C82.11, C82.18-C82.21, C82.28-C82.31, C82.38-C82.41, C82.48-C82.49, C82.51, C82.60-C82.61, C82.68-C82.81, C82.88-C82.91, C82.98-C82.99, C83.11, C84.41, C84.61, C84.71, C84.A1, C84.Z1, C84.91, C85.11, C85.21, C85.81, C85.91, C86.0, D49.81-D49.9

C82.02 Follicular lymphoma grade I, intrathoracic lymph nodes
Ex: C82.00, C82.02, C82.08-C82.10, C82.12, C82.18-C82.20, C82.22, C82.28-C82.30, C82.32, C82.38-C82.40, C82.42, C82.48-C82.49, C82.52, C82.60, C82.62, C82.68-C82.80, C82.82, C82.88-C82.90, C82.92, C82.98-C82.99, C83.12, C84.42, C84.62, C84.72, C84.92, C84.A2, C84.Z2, C85.12, C85.22, C85.82, C85.92, D49.81-D49.9

C82.03 Follicular lymphoma grade I, intra-abdominal lymph nodes
Ex: C82.00, C82.03, C82.08-C82.10, C82.13, C82.18-C82.20, C12.23, C82.28-C82.30, C82.33, C82.38-C82.40, C82.43, C82.48-C82.49, C82.53, C82.60, C82.63, C82.68-C82.80, C82.83, C82.88-C82.90, C82.93, C82.98-C82.99, C83.13, C84.43, C84.63, C84.73, C84.93, C84.A3, C84.Z3, C85.13, C85.23, C85.83, C85.93, C86.2, C86.3, D49.81-D49.9

C82.04 Follicular lymphoma grade I, lymph nodes of axilla and upper limb
Ex: C82.00, C82.04, C82.08-C82.10, C82.14, C82.18-C82.20, C82.24, C82.28-C82.30, C82.34, C82.38-C82.40, C82.44, C82.48-C82.49, C82.54, C82.60, C82.64, C82.68-C82.80, C82.84, C82.88-C82.90, C82.94, C82.98-C82.99, C83.14, C84.44, C84.64, C84.74, C84.94, C84.A4, C84.Z4, C85.14, C85.24, C85.84, C85.94, D49.81-D49.9

C82.05 Follicular lymphoma grade I, lymph nodes of inguinal region and lower limb
Ex: C82.00, C82.05, C82.08-C82.10, C82.15, C82.18-C82.20, C82.25, C82.28-C82.30, C82.35, C82.38-C82.40, C82.45, C82.48-C82.49, C82.55, C82.60, C82.65, C82.68-C82.80, C82.85, C82.88-C82.90, C82.95, C82.98-C82.99, C83.15, C84.45, C84.65, C84.75, C84.95, C84.A5, C84.Z5, C85.15, C85.25, C85.85, C85.95, D49.81-D49.9

C82.06 Follicular lymphoma grade I, intrapelvic lymph nodes
Ex: C82.00, C82.06, C82.08-C82.10, C82.16, C82.18-C82.20, C82.26, C82.28-C82.30, C82.36, C82.38-C82.40, C82.46, C82.48-C82.49, C82.56, C82.60, C82.66, C82.68-C82.80, C82.86, C82.88-C82.90, C82.96, C82.98-C82.99, C83.16, C84.46, C84.66, C84.76, C84.96, C84.A6, C84.Z6, C85.16, C85.26, C85.86, C85.96, D49.81-D49.9

C82.07 Follicular lymphoma grade I, spleen
Ex: C82.00, C82.07, C82.08-C82.10, C82.17-C82.20, C82.27-C82.30, C82.37-C82.40, C82.47-C82.49, C82.57, C82.60, C82.67-C82.80, C82.87-C82.90, C82.97-C82.99, C83.17, C84.47, C84.67, C84.77, C84.97, C84.A7, C84.Z7, C85.17, C85.27, C85.87, C85.97, C86.1, D49.81-D49.9

C82.08 Follicular lymphoma grade I, lymph nodes of multiple sites
Ex: C82.00-C82.49, C82.58, C82.60-C82.99, C83.18, C84.48, C84.68, C84.78, C84.98, C84.A8, C84.Z8, C85.18, C85.28, C85.88, C85.98, D49.81-D49.9

C82.09 Follicular lymphoma grade I, extranodal and solid organ sites
Ex: See C82.00

C82.1 Follicular lymphoma grade II

C82.10 Follicular lymphoma grade II, unspecified site
Ex: See C82.00

C82.11 Follicular lymphoma grade II, lymph nodes of head, face, and neck
Ex: See C82.01

C82.12 Follicular lymphoma grade II, intrathoracic lymph nodes
Ex: See C82.02

C82.13 Follicular lymphoma grade II, intra-abdominal lymph nodes
Ex: See C82.03

C82.14 Follicular lymphoma grade II, lymph nodes of axilla and upper limb
Ex: See C82.04

C82.15 Follicular lymphoma grade II, lymph nodes of inguinal region and lower limb
Ex: See C82.05

C82.16 Follicular lymphoma grade II, intrapelvic lymph nodes
Ex: See C82.06

C82.17 Follicular lymphoma grade II, spleen
Ex: See C82.07

C82.18 Follicular lymphoma grade II, lymph nodes of multiple sites
Ex: See C82.08

C82.19 Follicular lymphoma grade II, extranodal and solid organ sites
Ex: See C82.00

C82.2 Follicular lymphoma grade III, unspecified

C82.20 Follicular lymphoma grade III, unspecified, unspecified site
Ex: See C82.00

C82.21 Follicular lymphoma grade III, unspecified, lymph nodes of head, face, and neck
Ex: See C82.01

C82.22 Follicular lymphoma grade III, unspecified, intrathoracic lymph nodes
Ex: See C82.02

C82.23 Follicular lymphoma grade III, unspecified, intra-abdominal lymph nodes
Ex: See C82.03

C82.24 Follicular lymphoma grade III, unspecified, lymph nodes of axilla and upper limb
Ex: See C82.04

C82.25 Follicular lymphoma grade III, unspecified, lymph nodes of inguinal region and lower limb
Ex: See C82.05

C82.26 Follicular lymphoma grade III, unspecified, intrapelvic lymph nodes
Ex: See C82.06

C82.27 Follicular lymphoma grade III, unspecified, spleen
Ex: See C82.07

C82.28 Follicular lymphoma grade III, unspecified, lymph nodes of multiple sites
Ex: See C82.08

C82.29 Follicular lymphoma grade III, unspecified, extranodal and solid organ sites
Ex: See C82.00

C82.3 Follicular lymphoma grade IIIa

C82.30 Follicular lymphoma grade IIIa, unspecified site
Ex: See C82.00

C82.31 Follicular lymphoma grade IIIa, lymph nodes of head, face, and neck
Ex: See C82.01

C82.32 Follicular lymphoma grade IIIa, intrathoracic lymph nodes
Ex: See C82.02

C82.33 Follicular lymphoma grade IIIa, intra-abdominal lymph nodes
Ex: See C82.03

C82.34 Follicular lymphoma grade IIIa, lymph nodes of axilla and upper limb
Ex: See C82.04

C82.35 Follicular lymphoma grade IIIa, lymph nodes of inguinal region and lower limb
Ex: See C82.05

C82.36 Follicular lymphoma grade IIIa, intrapelvic lymph nodes
Ex: See C82.06

C82.37 Follicular lymphoma grade IIIa, spleen
Ex: See C82.07

C82.38 Follicular lymphoma grade IIIa, lymph nodes of multiple sites
Ex: See C82.08

C82.39 Follicular lymphoma grade IIIa, extranodal and solid organ sites
Ex: See C82.00

C82.4 Follicular lymphoma grade IIIb

C82.40 Follicular lymphoma grade IIIb, unspecified site
Ex: See C82.00

C82.41 Follicular lymphoma grade IIIb, lymph nodes of head, face, and neck
Ex: See C82.01

C82.42 Follicular lymphoma grade IIIb, intrathoracic lymph nodes
Ex: See C82.02

C82.43 Follicular lymphoma grade IIIb, intra-abdominal lymph nodes
Ex: See C82.03

C82.44 Follicular lymphoma grade IIIb, lymph nodes of axilla and upper limb
Ex: See C82.04

C82.45 Follicular lymphoma grade IIIb, lymph nodes of inguinal region and lower limb
Ex: See C82.05

C82.46 Follicular lymphoma grade IIIb, intrapelvic lymph nodes
Ex: See C82.06

C82.47 Follicular lymphoma grade IIIb, spleen
Ex: See C82.07

C82.48 Follicular lymphoma grade IIIb, lymph nodes of multiple sites
Ex: See C82.08

C82.49 Follicular lymphoma grade IIIb, extranodal and solid organ sites
Ex: See C82.00

● C82.5 Diffuse follicle center lymphoma

C82.50 Diffuse follicle center lymphoma, unspecified site
Ex: C82.50-C82.59, C83.10-C83.19, C84.40-C84.49, C84.60-C84.79, C84.90-C84.99, C84.A0-C84.Z9, C85.10-C86.4, C88.4, C96.4, C96.9, C96.Z, D49.81-D49.9

C82.51 Diffuse follicle center lymphoma, lymph nodes of head, face, and neck
Ex: C82.50-C82.51, C82.58-C82.59, C83.10-C83.11, C83.18-C83.19, C84.40-C84.41, C84.48-C84.61, C84.68-C84.71, C84.78-C84.79, C84.90-C84.91, C84.98-C84.99, C84.A0-C84.A1, C84.A8-C84.A9, C84.Z0-C84.Z1, C84.Z8-C84.Z9, C85.10-C85.11, C85.18-C85.21, C85.28-C85.81, C85.88-C85.91, C85.98-C85.99, C86.0, C86.4, C88.4, D49.81-D49.9

C82.52 Diffuse follicle center lymphoma, intrathoracic lymph nodes
Ex: C82.50, C82.52, C82.58-C82.59, C83.10, C83.12, C83.18-C83.19, C84.40, C84.42, C84.48-C84.60, C84.62, C84.68-C84.70, C84.72, C84.78-C84.79, C84.90, C84.92, C84.98-C84.99, C84.A0, C84.A2, C84.A8-C84.A9, C84.Z0, C84.Z2, C84.Z8-C84.Z9, C85.10, C85.12, C85.18-C85.20, C85.22, C85.28-C85.80, C85.82, C85.88-C85.90, C85.92, C85.98-C85.99, C86.4, C88.4, D49.81-D49.9

C82.53 Diffuse follicle center lymphoma, intra-abdominal lymph nodes
Ex: C82.50, C82.53, C82.58-C82.59, C83.10, C83.13, C83.18-C83.19, C84.40, C84.43, C84.48-C84.60, C84.63, C84.68-C84.70, C84.73, C84.78-C84.79, C84.90, C84.93, C84.98-C84.99, C84.A0, C84.A3, C84.A8-C84.A9, C84.Z0, C84.Z3, C84.Z8-C84.Z9, C85.10, C85.13, C85.18-C85.20, C85.22, C85.28-C85.80, C85.83, C85.88-C85.90, C85.93, C85.98-C85.99, C86.2-C86.4, C88.4, D49.81-D49.9

C82.54 Diffuse follicle center lymphoma, lymph nodes of axilla and upper limb
Ex: C82.50, C82.54, C82.58-C82.59, C83.10, C83.14, C83.18-C83.19, C84.40, C84.44, C84.48-C84.60, C84.64, C84.68-C84.70, C84.74, C84.78-C84.79, C84.90, C84.94, C84.98-C84.99, C84.A0, C84.A4, C84.A8-C84.A9, C84.Z0, C84.Z4, C84.Z8-C84.Z9, C85.10, C85.14, C85.18-C85.20, C85.24, C85.28-C85.80, C85.84, C85.88-C85.90, C85.94, C85.98-C85.99, C86.4, C88.4, D49.81-D49.9

C82.55 Diffuse follicle center lymphoma, lymph nodes of inguinal region and lower limb
Ex: C82.50, C82.55, C82.58-C82.59, C83.10, C83.15, C83.18-C83.19, C84.40, C84.45, C84.48-C84.60, C84.65, C84.68-C84.70, C84.75, C84.78-C84.79, C84.90, C84.95, C84.98-C84.99, C84.A0, C84.A5, C84.A8-C84.A9, C84.Z0, C84.Z5, C84.Z8-C84.Z9, C85.10, C85.15, C85.18-C85.20, C85.25, C85.28-C85.80, C85.85, C85.88-C85.90, C85.95, C85.98-C85.99, C86.4, C88.4, D49.81-D49.9

C82.56 Diffuse follicle center lymphoma, intrapelvic lymph nodes
Ex: C82.50, C82.56, C82.58-C82.59, C83.10, C83.16, C83.18-C83.19, C84.40, C84.46, C84.48-C84.60, C84.66, C84.68-C84.70, C84.76, C84.78-C84.79, C84.90, C84.96, C84.98-C84.99, C84.A0, C84.A6, C84.A8-C84.A9, C84.Z0, C84.Z6, C84.Z8-C84.Z9, C85.10, C85.16, C85.18-C85.20, C85.26, C85.28-C85.80, C85.86, C85.88-C85.90, C85.96, C85.98-C85.99, C86.4, C88.4, D49.81-D49.9

C82.57 Diffuse follicle center lymphoma, spleen
Ex: C82.50, C82.57, C82.58-C82.59, C83.10, C83.17, C83.18-C83.19, C84.40, C84.47-C84.49, C84.60, C84.67, C84.68-C84.69, C84.70, C84.77, C84.78-C84.79, C84.90, C84.97-C84.99, C84.A0, C84.A7-C84.A9, C84.Z0, C84.Z7, C84.Z8-C84.Z9, C85.10, C85.17-C85.20, C85.27-C85.29, C85.80, C85.87-C85.90, C85.97-C85.99, C86.1, C86.4, C88.4, D49.81-D49.9

C82.58 Diffuse follicle center lymphoma, lymph nodes of multiple sites
Ex: C82.50-C82.59, C83.10-C83.19, C84.40-C84.49, C84.60-C84.79, C84.90-C84.99, C84.A0-C84.Z9, C85.10-C86.4, C88.4, D49.81-D49.9

C82.59 Diffuse follicle center lymphoma, extranodal and solid organ sites
Ex: See C82.50

● C82.6 Cutaneous follicle center lymphoma

C82.60 Cutaneous follicle center lymphoma, unspecified site
Ex: See C82.00

C82.61 Cutaneous follicle center lymphoma, lymph nodes of head, face, and neck
Ex: See C82.01

C82.62 Cutaneous follicle center lymphoma, intrathoracic lymph nodes
Ex: See C82.02

C82.63 Cutaneous follicle center lymphoma, intra-abdominal lymph nodes
Ex: See C82.03

C82.64 Cutaneous follicle center lymphoma, lymph nodes of axilla and upper limb
Ex: See C82.04

C82.65 Cutaneous follicle center lymphoma, lymph nodes of inguinal region and lower limb
Ex: See C82.05

C82.66 Cutaneous follicle center lymphoma, intrapelvic lymph nodes
Ex: See C82.06

C82.67 Cutaneous follicle center lymphoma, spleen
Ex: See C82.07

C82.68 Cutaneous follicle center lymphoma, lymph nodes of multiple sites
Ex: See C82.08

C82.69 Cutaneous follicle center lymphoma, extranodal and solid organ sites
Ex: See C82.00

● C82.8 Other types of follicular lymphoma

C82.80 Other types of follicular lymphoma, unspecified site
Ex: See C82.00

C82.81 Other types of follicular lymphoma, lymph nodes of head, face, and neck
Ex: See C82.01

C82.82 Other types of follicular lymphoma, intrathoracic lymph nodes
Ex: See C82.02

C82.83 Other types of follicular lymphoma, intra-abdominal lymph nodes
Ex: See C82.03

C82.84 Other types of follicular lymphoma, lymph nodes of axilla and upper limb
Ex: See C82.04

C82.85 Other types of follicular lymphoma, lymph nodes of inguinal region and lower limb
Ex: See C82.05

C82.86 Other types of follicular lymphoma, intrapelvic lymph nodes
Ex: See C82.06

C82.87 Other types of follicular lymphoma, spleen
Ex: See C82.07

C82.88 Other types of follicular lymphoma, lymph nodes of multiple sites
Ex: See C82.08

C82.89 Other types of follicular lymphoma, extranodal and solid organ sites
Ex: See C82.00

C82.9 Follicular lymphoma, unspecified

C82.90 Follicular lymphoma, unspecified, unspecified site
Ex: See C82.00

C82.91 Follicular lymphoma, unspecified, lymph nodes of head, face, and neck
Ex: See C82.01

C82.92 Follicular lymphoma, unspecified, intrathoracic lymph nodes
Ex: See C82.02

C82.93 Follicular lymphoma, unspecified, intra-abdominal lymph nodes
Ex: See C82.03

C82.94 Follicular lymphoma, unspecified, lymph nodes of axilla and upper limb
Ex: See C82.04

C82.95 Follicular lymphoma, unspecified, lymph nodes of inguinal region and lower limb
Ex: See C82.05

C82.96 Follicular lymphoma, unspecified, intrapelvic lymph nodes
Ex: See C82.06

C82.97 Follicular lymphoma, unspecified, spleen
Ex: See C82.07

C82.98 Follicular lymphoma, unspecified, lymph nodes of multiple sites
Ex: See C82.08

C82.99 Follicular lymphoma, unspecified, extranodal and solid organ sites
Ex: See C82.00

C83 Non-follicular lymphoma

Excludes1 personal history of non-Hodgkin lymphoma (Z85.72)

C83.0 Small cell B-cell lymphoma
Lymphoplasmacytic lymphoma
Nodal marginal zone lymphoma
Non-leukemic variant of B-CLL
Splenic marginal zone lymphoma

Excludes1 chronic lymphocytic leukemia (C91.1)
mature T/NK-cell lymphomas (C84.-)
Waldenström macroglobulinemia (C88.0)

C83.00 Small cell B-cell lymphoma, unspecified site
Ex: C83.00-C83.09, C83.80-C83.99, C86.5-C86.6, D49.81-D49.9

C83.01 Small cell B-cell lymphoma, lymph nodes of head, face, and neck
Ex: C83.00-C83.01, C83.08-C83.09, C83.80-C83.81, C83.88-C83.91, C83.98-C83.99, C86.5-C86.6, D49.81-D49.9

C83.02 Small cell B-cell lymphoma, intrathoracic lymph nodes
Ex: C83.00, C83.02, C83.08-C83.09, C83.80, C83.82, C83.88-C83.89, C83.90, C83.92, C83.98-C83.99, C86.5-C86.6, D49.81-D49.9

C83.03 Small cell B-cell lymphoma, intra-abdominal lymph nodes
Ex: C83.00, C83.03, C83.08-C83.09, C83.80, C83.83, C83.88-C83.89, C83.90, C83.93, C83.98-C83.99, C86.5-C86.6, D49.81-D49.9

C83.04 Small cell B-cell lymphoma, lymph nodes of axilla and upper limb
Ex: C83.00, C83.04, C83.08-C83.09, C83.80, C83.84, C83.88-C83.89, C83.90, C83.94, C83.98-C83.99, C86.5-C86.6, D49.81-D49.9

C83.05 Small cell B-cell lymphoma, lymph nodes of inguinal region and lower limb
Ex: C83.00, C83.05, C83.08-C83.09, C83.80, C83.85, C83.88-C83.89, C83.90, C83.95, C83.98-C83.99, C86.5-C86.6, D49.81-D49.9

C83.06 Small cell B-cell lymphoma, intrapelvic lymph nodes
Ex: C83.00, C83.06, C83.08-C83.09, C83.80, C83.86, C83.88-C83.89, C83.90, C83.96, C83.98-C83.99, C86.5-C86.6, D49.81-D49.9

C83.07 Small cell B-cell lymphoma, spleen
Ex: C83.00, C83.07-C83.09, C83.80, C83.87-C83.89, C83.90, C83.97-C83.99, C86.5-C86.6, D49.81-D49.9

C83.08 Small cell B-cell lymphoma, lymph nodes of multiple sites
Ex: See C83.00

C83.09 Small cell B-cell lymphoma, extranodal and solid organ sites
Ex: See C83.00

C83.1 Mantle cell lymphoma
Centrocytic lymphoma
Malignant lymphomatous polyposis

C83.10 Mantle cell lymphoma, unspecified site
Ex: See C82.50

C83.11 Mantle cell lymphoma, lymph nodes of head, face, and neck
Ex: See C82.51

C83.12 Mantle cell lymphoma, intrathoracic lymph nodes
Ex: See C82.52

C83.13 Mantle cell lymphoma, intra-abdominal lymph nodes
Ex: See C82.53

C83.14 Mantle cell lymphoma, lymph nodes of axilla and upper limb
Ex: See C82.54

C83.15 Mantle cell lymphoma, lymph nodes of inguinal region and lower limb
Ex: See C82.55

C83.16 Mantle cell lymphoma, intrapelvic lymph nodes
Ex: See C82.56

C83.17 Mantle cell lymphoma, spleen
Ex: See C82.57

C83.18 Mantle cell lymphoma, lymph nodes of multiple sites
Ex: See C82.58

C83.19 Mantle cell lymphoma, extranodal and solid organ sites
Ex: See C82.50

C83.3 Diffuse large B-cell lymphoma
Anaplastic diffuse large B-cell lymphoma
CD30-positive diffuse large B-cell lymphoma
Centroblastic diffuse large B-cell lymphoma
Diffuse large B-cell lymphoma, subtype not specified
Immunoblastic diffuse large B-cell lymphoma
Plasmablastic diffuse large B-cell lymphoma
Diffuse large B-cell lymphoma, subtype not specified
T-cell rich diffuse large B-cell lymphoma

Excludes1 mediastinal (thymic) large B-cell lymphoma (C85.2-)
mature T/NK-cell lymphomas (C84.-)

C83.30 Diffuse large B-cell lymphoma, unspecified site
Ex: C83.30-C83.39, D49.81-D49.9

C83.31 Diffuse large B-cell lymphoma, lymph nodes of head, face, and neck
Ex: C83.30-C83.31, C83.38-C83.39, D49.81-D49.9

C83.32 Diffuse large B-cell lymphoma, intrathoracic lymph nodes
Ex: C83.30, C83.32, C83.38-C83.39, D49.81-D49.9

C83.33 Diffuse large B-cell lymphoma, intra-abdominal lymph nodes
Ex: C83.30, C83.33, C83.38-C83.39, D49.81-D49.9

C83.34 Diffuse large B-cell lymphoma, lymph nodes of axilla and upper limb
Ex: C83.30, C83.34, C83.38-C83.39, D49.81-D49.9

C83.35 Diffuse large B-cell lymphoma, lymph nodes of inguinal region and lower limb
Ex: C83.30, C83.35, C83.38-C83.39, D49.81-D49.9

C83.36 Diffuse large B-cell lymphoma, intrapelvic lymph nodes
Ex: C83.30, C83.36, C83.38-C83.39, D49.81-D49.9

C83.37 Diffuse large B-cell lymphoma, spleen
Ex: C83.30, C83.37-C83.39, D49.81-D49.9

C83.38 Diffuse large B-cell lymphoma, lymph nodes of multiple sites
Ex: See C83.30

C83.39 Diffuse large B-cell lymphoma, extranodal and solid organ sites
Ex: See C83.30

● **C83.5 Lymphoblastic (diffuse) lymphoma**
Highly malignant type of non-Hodgkin lymphoma with diffuse infiltration
B-precursor lymphoma
Lymphoblastic B-cell lymphoma
Lymphoblastic lymphoma NOS
Lymphoblastic T-cell lymphoma
T-precursor lymphoma

C83.50 Lymphoblastic (diffuse) lymphoma, unspecified site
Ex: C83.50-C83.59, D49.81-D49.9

C83.51 Lymphoblastic (diffuse) lymphoma, lymph nodes of head, face, and neck
Ex: C83.50-C83.51, C83.58-C83.59, D49.81-D49.9

C83.52 Lymphoblastic (diffuse) lymphoma, intrathoracic lymph nodes
Ex: C83.50, C83.52, C83.58-C83.59, D49.81-D49.9

C83.53 Lymphoblastic (diffuse) lymphoma, intra-abdominal lymph nodes
Ex: C83.50, C83.53, C83.58-C83.59, D49.81-D49.9

C83.54 Lymphoblastic (diffuse) lymphoma, lymph nodes of axilla and upper limb
Ex: C83.50, C83.54, C83.58-C83.59, D49.81-D49.9

C83.55 Lymphoblastic (diffuse) lymphoma, lymph nodes of inguinal region and lower limb
Ex: C83.50, C83.55, C83.58-C83.59, D49.81-D49.9

C83.56 Lymphoblastic (diffuse) lymphoma, intrapelvic lymph nodes
Ex: C83.50, C83.56, C83.58-C83.59, D49.81-D49.9

C83.57 Lymphoblastic (diffuse) lymphoma, spleen
Ex: C83.50, C83.57-C83.59, D49.81-D49.9

C83.58 Lymphoblastic (diffuse) lymphoma, lymph nodes of multiple sites
Ex: See C83.50

C83.59 Lymphoblastic (diffuse) lymphoma, extranodal and solid organ sites
Ex: See C83.50

● **C83.7 Burkitt lymphoma**
Form of small cell lymphoma
Atypical Burkitt lymphoma
Burkitt-like lymphoma
Excludes1 mature B-cell leukemia Burkitt type (C91.A-)

C83.70 Burkitt lymphoma, unspecified site
Ex: C83.70-C83.79, D49.81-D49.9

C83.71 Burkitt lymphoma, lymph nodes of head, face, and neck
Ex: C83.70-C83.71, C83.78-C83.79, D49.81-D49.9

C83.72 Burkitt lymphoma, intrathoracic lymph nodes
Ex: C83.70, C83.72, C83.78-C83.79, D49.81-D49.9

C83.73 Burkitt lymphoma, intra-abdominal lymph nodes
Ex: C83.70, C83.73, C83.78-C83.79, D49.81-D49.9

C83.74 Burkitt lymphoma, lymph nodes of axilla and upper limb
Ex: C83.70, C83.74, C83.78-C83.79, D49.81-D49.9

C83.75 Burkitt lymphoma, lymph nodes of inguinal region and lower limb
Ex: C83.70, C83.75, C83.78-C83.79, D49.81-D49.9

C83.76 Burkitt lymphoma, intrapelvic lymph nodes
Ex: C83.70, C83.76, C83.78-C83.79, D49.81-D49.9

C83.77 Burkitt lymphoma, spleen
Ex: C83.70, C83.77-C83.79, D49.81-D49.9

C83.78 Burkitt lymphoma, lymph nodes of multiple sites
Ex: See C83.70

C83.79 Burkitt lymphoma, extranodal and solid organ sites
Ex: See C83.70

● **C83.8 Other non-follicular lymphoma**
Intravascular large B-cell lymphoma
Lymphoid granulomatosis
Primary effusion B-cell lymphoma
Excludes1 mediastinal (thymic) large B-cell lymphoma (C85.2-)
T-cell rich B-cell lymphoma (C83.3-)

C83.80 Other non-follicular lymphoma, unspecified site
Ex: See C83.00

C83.81 Other non-follicular lymphoma, lymph nodes of head, face, and neck
Ex: See C83.01

C83.82 Other non-follicular lymphoma, intrathoracic lymph nodes
Ex: See C83.02

C83.83 Other non-follicular lymphoma, intra-abdominal lymph nodes
Ex: See C83.03

C83.84 Other non-follicular lymphoma, lymph nodes of axilla and upper limb
Ex: See C83.04

C83.85 Other non-follicular lymphoma, lymph nodes of inguinal region and lower limb
Ex: See C83.05

C83.86 Other non-follicular lymphoma, intrapelvic lymph nodes
Ex: See C83.06

C83.87 Other non-follicular lymphoma, spleen
Ex: See C83.07

C83.88 Other non-follicular lymphoma, lymph nodes of multiple sites
Ex: See C83.00

C83.89 Other non-follicular lymphoma, extranodal and solid organ sites
Ex: See C83.00

● **C83.9 Non-follicular (diffuse) lymphoma, unspecified**

C83.90 Non-follicular (diffuse) lymphoma, unspecified, unspecified site
Ex: See C83.00

C83.91 Non-follicular (diffuse) lymphoma, unspecified, lymph nodes of head, face, and neck
Ex: See C83.01

C83.92 Non-follicular (diffuse) lymphoma, unspecified, intrathoracic lymph nodes
Ex: See C83.02

C83.93 Non-follicular (diffuse) lymphoma, unspecified, intra-abdominal lymph nodes
Ex: See C83.03

C83.94 Non-follicular (diffuse) lymphoma, unspecified, lymph nodes of axilla and upper limb
Ex: See C83.04

C83.95 Non-follicular (diffuse) lymphoma, unspecified, lymph nodes of inguinal region and lower limb
Ex: See C83.05

C83.96 Non-follicular (diffuse) lymphoma, unspecified, intrapelvic lymph nodes
Ex: See C83.06

C83.97 Non-follicular (diffuse) lymphoma, unspecified, spleen
Ex: See C83.07

C83.98 Non-follicular (diffuse) lymphoma, unspecified, lymph nodes of multiple sites
Ex: See C83.00

C83.99 Non-follicular (diffuse) lymphoma, unspecified, extranodal and solid organ sites
Ex: See C83.00

C84 Mature T/NK-cell lymphomas

Excludes1 personal history of non-Hodgkin lymphoma (Z85.72)

C84.0 Mycosis fungoides
Chronic or rapidly progressive form of cutaneous T-cell lymphoma; AKA granuloma fungoides

Excludes1 peripheral T-cell lymphoma, not classified (C84.4-)

C84.00 Mycosis fungoides, unspecified site
Ex: C82.50, C82.59, C83.10, C83.19, C84.00-C84.09, C84.40, C84.49, C84.60, C84.69-C84.70, C84.79, C84.90, C84.99, C84.A0, C84.A9-C84.Z0, C84.Z9, C85.10, C85.19-C85.20, C85.29-C85.80, C85.89-C85.90, C85.99, C86.4, C88.4, C96.4, C96.9, C96.Z, D49.81-D49.9

C84.01 Mycosis fungoides, lymph nodes of head, face, and neck
Ex: C82.51, C83.11, C84.00-C84.01, C84.08-C84.09, C84.41, C84.61, C84.71, C84.91, C84.A1, C84.Z1, C85.11, C85.21, C85.81, C85.91, C86.0, D49.81-D49.9

C84.02 Mycosis fungoides, intrathoracic lymph nodes
Ex: C82.52, C83.12, C84.00, C84.02, C84.08-C84.09, C84.42, C84.62, C84.72, C84.92, C84.A2, C84.Z2, C85.12, C85.22, C85.82, C85.92, D49.81-D49.9

C84.03 Mycosis fungoides, intra-abdominal lymph nodes
Ex: C82.53, C83.13, C84.00, C84.03, C84.08-C84.09, C84.43, C84.63, C84.73, C84.93, C84.A3, C84.Z3, C85.13, C85.23, C85.83, C85.93, C86.2-C86.3, D49.81-D49.9

C84.04 Mycosis fungoides, lymph nodes of axilla and upper limb
Ex: C82.54, C83.14, C84.00, C84.04, C84.08-C84.09, C84.44, C84.64, C84.74, C84.94, C84.A4, C84.Z4, C85.14, C85.24, C85.84, C85.94, D49.81-D49.9

C84.05 Mycosis fungoides, lymph nodes of inguinal region and lower limb
Ex: C82.55, C83.15, C84.00, C84.05, C84.08-C84.09, C84.45, C84.65, C84.75, C84.95, C84.A5, C84.Z5, C85.15, C85.25, C85.85, C85.95, D49.81-D49.9

C84.06 Mycosis fungoides, intrapelvic lymph nodes
Ex: C82.56, C83.16, C84.00, C84.06, C84.08-C84.09, C84.46, C84.66, C84.76, C84.96, C84.A6, C84.Z6, C85.16, C85.26, C85.86, C85.96, D49.81-D49.9

C84.07 Mycosis fungoides, spleen
Ex: C82.57, C83.17, C84.00, C84.07, C84.08-C84.09, C84.47, C84.67, C84.77, C84.97, C84.A7, C84.Z7, C85.17, C85.27, C85.87, C85.97, D49.81-D49.9

C84.08 Mycosis fungoides, lymph nodes of multiple sites
Ex: C82.58, C83.18, C84.00-C84.09, C84.48, C84.68, C84.78, C84.98, C84.A8, C84.Z8, C85.18, C85.28, C85.88, C85.98, D49.81-D49.9

C84.09 Mycosis fungoides, extranodal and solid organ sites
Ex: See C84.00

C84.1 Sézary disease
Type of cutaneous lymphoma affecting T-cells

C84.10 Sézary disease, unspecified site
Ex: C82.50, C82.59, C83.10, C83.19, C84.10-C84.19, C84.40, C84.49-C84.60, C84.69-C84.70, C84.79, C84.90, C84.99, C84.A0, C84.A9-C84.Z0, C84.Z9, C85.10, C85.19-C85.20, C85.29-C85.80, C85.89-C85.90, C85.99, C86.4, C88.4, C96.4, C96.9, C96.Z, D49.81-D49.9

C84.11 Sézary disease, lymph nodes of head, face, and neck
Ex: C82.51, C83.11, C84.10-C84.11, C84.18-C84.19, C84.41, C84.61, C84.71, C84.91, C84.A1, C84.Z1, C85.11, C85.21, C85.81, C85.91, C86.0, D49.81-D49.9

C84.12 Sézary disease, intrathoracic lymph nodes
Ex: C82.52, C83.12, C84.10, C84.12, C84.18-C84.19, C84.42, C84.62, C84.72, C84.92, C84.A2, C84.Z2, C85.12, C85.22, C85.82, C85.92, D49.81-D49.9

C84.13 Sézary disease, intra-abdominal lymph nodes
Ex: C82.53, C83.13, C84.10, C84.13, C84.18-C84.19, C84.43, C84.63, C84.73, C84.93, C84.A3, C84.Z3, C85.13, C85.23, C85.83, C85.93, C86.2-C86.3, D49.81-D49.9

C84.14 Sézary disease, lymph nodes of axilla and upper limb
Ex: C82.54, C83.14, C84.10, C84.14, C84.18-C84.19, C84.44, C84.64, C84.74, C84.94, C84.A4, C84.Z4, C85.14, C85.24, C85.84, C85.94, D49.81-D49.9

C84.15 Sézary disease, lymph nodes of inguinal region and lower limb
Ex: C82.55, C83.15, C84.10, C84.15, C84.18-C84.19, C84.45, C84.65, C84.75, C84.95, C84.A5, C84.Z5, C85.15, C85.25, C85.85, C85.95, D49.81-D49.9

C84.16 Sézary disease, intrapelvic lymph nodes
Ex: C82.56, C83.16, C84.10, C84.16, C84.18-C84.19, C84.46, C84.66, C84.76, C84.96, C84.A6, C84.Z6, C85.16, C85.26, C85.86, C85.96, D49.81-D49.9

C84.17 Sézary disease, spleen
Ex: C82.57, C83.17, C84.10, C84.17-C84.19, C84.47, C84.67, C84.77, C84.97, C84.A7, C84.Z7, C85.17, C85.27, C85.87, C85.97, C86.1, D49.81-D49.9

C84.18 Sézary disease, lymph nodes of multiple sites
Ex: C82.58, C83.18, C84.10-C84.19, C84.48, C84.68, C84.78, C84.98, C84.A8, C84.Z8, C85.18, C85.28, C85.88, C85.98, D49.81-D49.9

C84.19 Sézary disease, extranodal and solid organ sites
Ex: See C84.10

C84.4 Peripheral T-cell lymphoma, not classified
Diverse group of blood carcinomas originating from T-cells, requiring aggressive chemotherapy
Lennert's lymphoma
Lymphoepithelioid lymphoma
Mature T-cell lymphoma, not elsewhere classified

C84.40 Peripheral T-cell lymphoma, not classified, unspecified site
Ex: See C82.50

C84.41 Peripheral T-cell lymphoma, not classified, lymph nodes of head, face, and neck
Ex: See C82.51

C84.42 Peripheral T-cell lymphoma, not classified, intrathoracic lymph nodes
Ex: See C82.52

C84.43 Peripheral T-cell lymphoma, not classified, intra-abdominal lymph nodes
Ex: See C82.53

C84.44 Peripheral T-cell lymphoma, not classified, lymph nodes of axilla and upper limb
Ex: See C82.54

C84.45 Peripheral T-cell lymphoma, not classified, lymph nodes of inguinal region and lower limb
Ex: See C82.55

C84.46 Peripheral T-cell lymphoma, not classified, intrapelvic lymph nodes
Ex: See C82.56

C84.47 Peripheral T-cell lymphoma, not classified, spleen
Ex: See C82.57

C84.48 Peripheral T-cell lymphoma, not classified, lymph nodes of multiple sites
Ex: See C82.58

C84.49 Peripheral T-cell lymphoma, not classified, extranodal and solid organ sites
Ex: See C82.50

● **C84.6 Anaplastic large cell lymphoma, ALK-positive**
Anaplastic large cell lymphoma, CD30-positive

C84.60 Anaplastic large cell lymphoma, ALK-positive, unspecified site
Ex: See C82.50

C84.61 Anaplastic large cell lymphoma, ALK-positive, lymph nodes of head, face, and neck
Ex: See C82.51

C84.62 Anaplastic large cell lymphoma, ALK-positive, intrathoracic lymph nodes
Ex: See C82.52

C84.63 Anaplastic large cell lymphoma, ALK-positive, intra-abdominal lymph nodes
Ex: See C82.53

C84.64 Anaplastic large cell lymphoma, ALK-positive, lymph nodes of axilla and upper limb
Ex: See C82.54

C84.65 Anaplastic large cell lymphoma, ALK-positive, lymph nodes of inguinal region and lower limb
Ex: See C82.56

C84.66 Anaplastic large cell lymphoma, ALK-positive, intrapelvic lymph nodes
Ex: See C82.56

C84.67 Anaplastic large cell lymphoma, ALK-positive, spleen
Ex: See C82.57

C84.68 Anaplastic large cell lymphoma, ALK-positive, lymph nodes of multiple sites
Ex: See C82.58

C84.69 Anaplastic large cell lymphoma, ALK-positive, extranodal and solid organ sites
Ex: See C82.50

● **C84.7 Anaplastic large cell lymphoma, ALK-negative**

Excludes1 primary cutaneous CD30-positive T-cell proliferations (C86.6-)

C84.70 Anaplastic large cell lymphoma, ALK-negative, unspecified site
Ex: See C82.50

C84.71 Anaplastic large cell lymphoma, ALK-negative, lymph nodes of head, face, and neck
Ex: See C82.51

C84.72 Anaplastic large cell lymphoma, ALK-negative, intrathoracic lymph nodes
Ex: See C82.52

C84.73 Anaplastic large cell lymphoma, ALK-negative, intra-abdominal lymph nodes
Ex: See C82.53

C84.74 Anaplastic large cell lymphoma, ALK-negative, lymph nodes of axilla and upper limb
Ex: See C82.54

C84.75 Anaplastic large cell lymphoma, ALK-negative, lymph nodes of inguinal region and lower limb
Ex: See C82.55

Item 2–7 Lymphosarcoma, also known as malignant lymphoma, is a cancer of the lymph system exhibiting abnormal cells encompassing an entire lymph node creating a diffuse pattern without any definite organization. Diffuse pattern lymphoma has a more unfavorable survival outlook than those with a follicular or nodular pattern. Reticulosarcoma is the most common aggressive form of non-Hodgkin's lymphoma.

C84.76 Anaplastic large cell lymphoma, ALK-negative, intrapelvic lymph nodes
Ex: See C82.56

C84.77 Anaplastic large cell lymphoma, ALK-negative, spleen
Ex: See C82.57

C84.78 Anaplastic large cell lymphoma, ALK-negative, lymph nodes of multiple sites
Ex: See C82.58

C84.79 Anaplastic large cell lymphoma, ALK-negative, extranodal and solid organ sites
Ex: See C82.50

● **C84.A Cutaneous T-cell lymphoma, unspecified**

C84.A0 Cutaneous T-cell lymphoma, unspecified, unspecified site
Ex: See C82.50

C84.A1 Cutaneous T-cell lymphoma, unspecified lymph nodes of head, face, and neck
Ex: See C82.51

C84.A2 Cutaneous T-cell lymphoma, unspecified, intrathoracic lymph nodes
Ex: See C82.52

C84.A3 Cutaneous T-cell lymphoma, unspecified, intra-abdominal lymph nodes
Ex: See C82.53

C84.A4 Cutaneous T-cell lymphoma, unspecified, lymph nodes of axilla and upper limb
Ex: See C82.54

C84.A5 Cutaneous T-cell lymphoma, unspecified, lymph nodes of inguinal region and lower limb
Ex: See C82.55

C84.A6 Cutaneous T-cell lymphoma, unspecified, intrapelvic lymph nodes
Ex: See C82.56

C84.A7 Cutaneous T-cell lymphoma, unspecified, spleen
Ex: See C82.57

C84.A8 Cutaneous T-cell lymphoma, unspecified, lymph nodes of multiple sites
Ex: See C82.58

C84.A9 Cutaneous T-cell lymphoma, unspecified, extranodal and solid organ sites
Ex: See C82.50

● **C84.Z Other mature T/NK-cell lymphomas**

Note: If T-cell lineage or involvement is mentioned in conjunction with a specific lymphoma, code to the more specific description.

Excludes1 angioimmunoblastic T-cell lymphoma (C86.5)
blastic NK-cell lymphoma (C86.4)
enteropathy-type T-cell lymphoma (C86.2)
extranodal NK-cell lymphoma, nasal type (C86.0)
hepatosplenic T-cell lymphoma (C86.1)
primary cutaneous CD30-positive T-cell proliferations (C86.6)
subcutaneous panniculitis-like T-cell lymphoma (C86.3)
T-cell leukemia (C91.1-)

C84.Z0 Other mature T/NK-cell lymphomas, unspecified site
Ex: See C82.50

C84.Z1 Other mature T/NK-cell lymphomas, lymph nodes of head, face, and neck
Ex: See C82.51

C84.Z2 Other mature T/NK-cell lymphomas, intrathoracic lymph nodes
Ex: See C82.52

C84.Z3 Other mature T/NK-cell lymphomas, intra-abdominal lymph nodes
Ex: See C82.53

C84.Z4 Other mature T/NK-cell lymphomas, lymph nodes of axilla and upper limb
Ex: See C82.54

C84.Z5 Other mature T/NK-cell lymphomas, lymph nodes of inguinal region and lower limb
Ex: See C82.55

C84.Z6 Other mature T/NK-cell lymphomas, intrapelvic lymph nodes
Ex: See C82.56

C84.Z7 Other mature T/NK-cell lymphomas, spleen
Ex: See C82.57

C84.Z8 Other mature T/NK-cell lymphomas, lymph nodes of multiple sites
Ex: See C82.58

C84.Z9 Other mature T/NK-cell lymphomas, extranodal and solid organ sites
Ex: See C82.50

C84.9 Mature T/NK-cell lymphomas, unspecified
NK/T cell lymphoma NOS

Excludes1 mature T-cell lymphoma, not elsewhere classified (C84.4-)

C84.90 Mature T/NK-cell lymphomas, unspecified, unspecified site
Ex: See C82.50

C84.91 Mature T/NK-cell lymphomas, unspecified, lymph nodes of head, face, and neck
Ex: See C82.51

C84.92 Mature T/NK-cell lymphomas, unspecified, intrathoracic lymph nodes
Ex: See C82.52

C84.93 Mature T/NK-cell lymphomas, unspecified, intra-abdominal lymph nodes
Ex: See C82.53

C84.94 Mature T/NK-cell lymphomas, unspecified, lymph nodes of axilla and upper limb
Ex: See C82.54

C84.95 Mature T/NK-cell lymphomas, unspecified, lymph nodes of inguinal region and lower limb
Ex: See C82.55

C84.96 Mature T/NK-cell lymphomas, unspecified, intrapelvic lymph nodes
Ex: See C82.56

C84.97 Mature T/NK-cell lymphomas, unspecified, spleen
Ex: See C82.57

C84.98 Mature T/NK-cell lymphomas, unspecified, lymph nodes of multiple sites
Ex: See C82.58

C84.99 Mature T/NK-cell lymphomas, unspecified, extranodal and solid organ sites
Ex: See C82.50

C85 Other specified and unspecified types of non-Hodgkin lymphoma

Excludes1 other specified types of T/NK-cell lymphoma (C86.-)
personal history of non-Hodgkin lymphoma (Z85.72)

C85.1 Unspecified B-cell lymphoma

Note: If B-cell lineage or involvement is mentioned in conjunction with a specific lymphoma, code to the more specific description.

C85.10 Unspecified B-cell lymphoma, unspecified site
Ex: See C82.50

C85.11 Unspecified B-cell lymphoma, lymph nodes of head, face, and neck
Ex: See C82.51

C85.12 Unspecified B-cell lymphoma, intrathoracic lymph nodes
Ex: See C82.52

C85.13 Unspecified B-cell lymphoma, intra-abdominal lymph nodes
Ex: See C82.53

C85.14 Unspecified B-cell lymphoma, lymph nodes of axilla and upper limb
Ex: See C82.54

C85.15 Unspecified B-cell lymphoma, lymph nodes of inguinal region and lower limb
Ex: See C82.55

C85.16 Unspecified B-cell lymphoma, intrapelvic lymph nodes
Ex: See C82.56

C85.17 Unspecified B-cell lymphoma, spleen
Ex: See C82.57

C85.18 Unspecified B-cell lymphoma, lymph nodes of multiple sites
Ex: See C82.58

C85.19 Unspecified B-cell lymphoma, extranodal and solid organ sites
Ex: See C82.50

C85.2 Mediastinal (thymic) large B-cell lymphoma

C85.20 Mediastinal (thymic) large B-cell lymphoma, unspecified site
Ex: See C82.50

C85.21 Mediastinal (thymic) large B-cell lymphoma, lymph nodes of head, face, and neck
Ex: See C82.51

C85.22 Mediastinal (thymic) large B-cell lymphoma, intrathoracic lymph nodes
Ex: See C82.52

C85.23 Mediastinal (thymic) large B-cell lymphoma, intra-abdominal lymph nodes
Ex: See C82.53

C85.24 Mediastinal (thymic) large B-cell lymphoma, lymph nodes of axilla and upper limb
Ex: See C82.54

C85.25 Mediastinal (thymic) large B-cell lymphoma, lymph nodes of inguinal region and lower limb
Ex: See C82.55

C85.26 Mediastinal (thymic) large B-cell lymphoma, intrapelvic lymph nodes
Ex: See C82.56

C85.27 Mediastinal (thymic) large B-cell lymphoma, spleen
Ex: See C82.57

C85.28 Mediastinal (thymic) large B-cell lymphoma, lymph nodes of multiple sites
Ex: See C82.58

C85.29 Mediastinal (thymic) large B-cell lymphoma, extranodal and solid organ sites
Ex: See C82.50

C85.8 Other specified types of non-Hodgkin lymphoma

C85.80 Other specified types of non-Hodgkin lymphoma, unspecified site
Ex: See C82.50

C85.81 Other specified types of non-Hodgkin lymphoma, lymph nodes of head, face, and neck
Ex: See C82.51

C85.82 Other specified types of non-Hodgkin lymphoma, intrathoracic lymph nodes
Ex: See C82.52

C85.83 Other specified types of non-Hodgkin lymphoma, intra-abdominal lymph nodes
Ex: See C82.53

C85.84 Other specified types of non-Hodgkin lymphoma, lymph nodes of axilla and upper limb
Ex: See C82.54

C85.85 Other specified types of non-Hodgkin lymphoma, lymph nodes of inguinal region and lower limb
Ex: See C82.55

C85.86 Other specified types of non-Hodgkin lymphoma, intrapelvic lymph nodes
Ex: See C82.56

C85.87 Other specified types of non-Hodgkin lymphoma, spleen
Ex: See C82.57

C85.88 Other specified types of non-Hodgkin lymphoma, lymph nodes of multiple sites
Ex: See C82.58

C85.89 Other specified types of non-Hodgkin lymphoma, extranodal and solid organ sites
Ex: See C82.50

● **C85.9 Non-Hodgkin lymphoma, unspecified**
Lymphoma NOS
Malignant lymphoma NOS
Non-Hodgkin lymphoma NOS

C85.90 Non-Hodgkin lymphoma, unspecified, unspecified site
Ex: See C82.50

C85.91 Non-Hodgkin lymphoma, unspecified, lymph nodes of head, face, and neck
Ex: See C82.51

C85.92 Non-Hodgkin lymphoma, unspecified, intrathoracic lymph nodes
Ex: See C82.52

C85.93 Non-Hodgkin lymphoma, unspecified, intra-abdominal lymph nodes
Ex: See C82.53

C85.94 Non-Hodgkin lymphoma, unspecified, lymph nodes of axilla and upper limb
Ex: See C82.54

C85.95 Non-Hodgkin lymphoma, unspecified, lymph nodes of inguinal region and lower limb
Ex: See C82.55

C85.96 Non-Hodgkin lymphoma, unspecified, intrapelvic lymph nodes
Ex: See C82.56

C85.97 Non-Hodgkin lymphoma, unspecified, spleen
Ex: See C82.57

C85.98 Non-Hodgkin lymphoma, unspecified, lymph nodes of multiple sites
Ex: See C82.58

C85.99 Non-Hodgkin lymphoma, unspecified, extranodal and solid organ sites
Ex: See C82.50

● **C86 Other specified types of T/NK-cell lymphoma**
Excludes1 anaplastic large cell lymphoma, ALK negative (C84.7-)
anaplastic large cell lymphoma, ALK positive (C84.6-)
mature T/NK-cell lymphomas (C84.-)
other specified types of non-Hodgkin lymphoma (C85.8-)

C86.0 Extranodal NK/T-cell lymphoma, nasal type
Ex: See C82.51

C86.1 Hepatosplenic T-cell lymphoma
Alpha-beta and gamma delta types
Ex: See C82.57

C86.2 Enteropathy-type (intestinal) T-cell lymphoma
Enteropathy associated T-cell lymphoma
Ex: See C82.53

C86.3 Subcutaneous panniculitis-like T-cell lymphoma
Ex: See C82.53

C86.4 Blastic NK-cell lymphoma
Ex: See C82.50

C86.5 Angioimmunoblastic T-cell lymphoma
Angioimmunoblastic lymphadenopathy with dysproteinemia (AILD)
Ex: See C83.00

C86.6 Primary cutaneous CD30-positive T-cell proliferations
Lymphomatoid papulosis
Primary cutaneous anaplastic large cell lymphoma
Primary cutaneous CD30-positive large T-cell lymphoma
Ex: See C83.00

● **C88 Malignant immunoproliferative diseases and certain other B-cell lymphomas**
Diseases involving immune system
Excludes1 B-cell lymphoma, unspecified (C85.1-)
personal history of other malignant neoplasms of lymphoid, hematopoietic and related tissues (Z85.79)

C88.0 Waldenström's macroglobulinemia
Lymphoplasmacytic lymphoma with IgM-production
Macroglobulinemia (idiopathic) (primary)
Excludes1 small cell B-cell lymphoma (C83.0)

C88.2 Heavy chain disease
Franklin disease
Gamma heavy chain disease
Mu heavy chain disease
Ex: C88.2-C88.3, C88.8-C90.02, C90.10-C90.12, C90.20-C90.22, C90.30-C90.32, C91.00-C91.02, C91.10-C91.12, C91.30-C91.32, C91.50-C91.52, C91.60-C91.62, C91.90-C91.92, C91.A0-C91.A2, C91.Z0-C91.Z2, C92.00-C92.02, C92.10-C92.12, C92.20-C92.22, C92.30-C92.32, C92.40-C92.42, C92.50-C92.52, C92.60-C92.62, C92.90-C92.92, C92.A0-C92.A2, C92.Z0-C92.Z2, C93.00-C93.02, C93.10-C93.12, C93.30-C93.32, C93.90-C93.92, C93.Z0-C93.Z2, C94.00-C94.02, C94.20-C94.22, C94.30-C94.32, C94.80-C94.82, C95.00-C95.02, C95.10-C95.12, C95.90-C95.92, D49.81-D49.9

C88.3 Immunoproliferative small intestinal disease
Alpha heavy chain disease
Mediterranean lymphoma
Ex: See C88.2

C88.4 Extranodal marginal zone B-cell lymphoma of mucosa-associated lymphoid tissue [MALT-lymphoma]
Lymphoma of skin-associated lymphoid tissue [SALT-lymphoma]
Lymphoma of bronchial-associated lymphoid tissue [BALT-lymphoma]
Excludes1 high malignant (diffuse large B-cell) lymphoma (C83.3-)
Ex: See C82.50

C88.8 Other malignant immunoproliferative diseases
Ex: C88.2-C88.3, C88.8-C90.02, C90.10-C90.12, C90.20-C90.22, C90.30-C90.32, C91.00-C91.02, C91.10-C91.12, C91.30-C91.32, C91.40-C91.42, C91.50-C91.52, C91.60-C91.62, C91.90-C91.92, C91.A0-C91.A2, C91.Z0-C91.Z2, C92.00-C92.02, C92.10-C92.12, C92.20-C92.22, C92.30-C92.32, C92.40-C92.42, C92.50-C92.52, C92.60-C92.62, C92.90-C92.92, C92.A0-C92.A2, C92.Z0-C92.Z2, C93.00-C93.02, C93.10-C93.12, C93.30-C93.32, C93.90-C93.92, C93.Z0-C93.Z2, C94.00-C94.02, C94.20-C94.22, C94.30-C94.32, C94.40-C94.42, C94.6, C94.80-C94.82, C95.00-C95.02, C95.10-C95.12, C95.90-C95.92, D45-D46.22, D46.4, D46.9, D46.A-D46.Z, D47.0-D47.1, D47.3, D47.9, D47.Z2, D47.Z9, D48.7-D48.9, D49.81-D49.9

C88.9 Malignant immunoproliferative disease, unspecified
Immunoproliferative disease NOS
Ex: See C88.2

Item 2–8 **Multiple myeloma** is a cancer of a plasma cell (a type of white blood cell) and is an incurable but treatable disease. Immunoproliferative neoplasm is a term for diseases (mostly cancers), in which the immune system cells proliferate.

● **C90 Multiple myeloma and malignant plasma cell neoplasms**

Excludes1 personal history of other malignant neoplasms of lymphoid, hematopoietic and related tissues (Z85.79)

Ex **For category C90 CC codes:** C88.2-C88.3, C88.8-C90.02, C90.10-C90.12, C90.20-C90.22, C90.30-C90.32, C91.00-C91.02, C91.10-C91.12, C91.30-C91.32, C91.50-C91.52, C91.60-C91.62, C91.90-C91.92, C91.A0-C91.A2, C91.Z0-C91.Z2, C92.00-C92.02, C92.10-C92.12, C92.20-C92.22, C92.30-C92.32, C92.40-C92.42, C92.50-C92.52, C92.60-C92.62, C92.90-C92.92, C92.A0-C92.A2, C92.Z0-C92.Z2, C93.00-C93.02, C93.10-C93.12, C93.30-C93.32, C93.90-C93.92, C93.Z0-C93.Z2, C94.00-C94.02, C94.20-C94.22, C94.30-C94.32, C94.80-C94.82, C95.00-C95.02, C95.10-C95.12, C95.90-C95.92, D49.81-D49.9

● **C90.0 Multiple myeloma**
Kahler's disease
Medullary plasmacytoma
Myelomatosis
Plasma cell myeloma

Excludes1 solitary myeloma (C90.3-)
solitary plasmacytoma (C90.3-)

C90.00 Multiple myeloma not having achieved remission
Multiple myeloma with failed remission
Multiple myeloma NOS

C90.01 Multiple myeloma in remission

C90.02 Multiple myeloma in relapse

● **C90.1 Plasma cell leukemia**
Rare type of acute leukemia
Plasmacytic leukemia

C90.10 Plasma cell leukemia not having achieved remission
Plasma cell leukemia with failed remission
Plasma cell leukemia NOS

C90.11 Plasma cell leukemia in remission

C90.12 Plasma cell leukemia in relapse

● **C90.2 Extramedullary plasmacytoma**
Malignant monoclonal plasma cell tumor growing in soft tissue; AKA plasma cell dyscrasias

C90.20 Extramedullary plasmacytoma not having achieved remission
Extramedullary plasmacytoma with failed remission
Extramedullary plasmacytoma NOS

C90.21 Extramedullary plasmacytoma in remission

C90.22 Extramedullary plasmacytoma in relapse

● **C90.3 Solitary plasmacytoma**
Localized malignant plasma cell tumor NOS
Plasmacytoma NOS
Solitary myeloma

C90.30 Solitary plasmacytoma not having achieved remission
Solitary plasmacytoma with failed remission
Solitary plasmacytoma NOS

C90.31 Solitary plasmacytoma in remission

C90.32 Solitary plasmacytoma in relapse

Item 2–9 Leukemia is a cancer (acute or chronic) of the blood-forming tissues of the bone marrow. Blood cells all start out as stem cells. They mature and become red cells, white cells, or platelets. There are three main types of leukocytes (white cells that fight infection): monocytes, lymphocytes, and granulocytes. **Acute monocytic leukemia** (AML) affects monocytes. **Acute lymphoid leukemia** (ALL) affects lymphocytes, and **acute myeloid leukemia** (AML) affects cells that typically develop into white blood cells (not lymphocytes), though it may develop in other blood cells.

● **C91 Lymphoid leukemia**
Type of leukemia affecting circulating cells of lymphoid origin

Excludes1 personal history of leukemia (Z85.6)

Ex **For category C91 CC codes unless otherwise indicated:** C88.2-C88.3, C88.8-C90.02, C90.10-C90.12, C90.20-C90.22, C90.30-C90.32, C91.00-C91.02, C91.10-C91.12, C91.30-C91.32, C91.50-C91.52, C91.60-C91.62, C91.90-C91.92, C91.A0-C91.A2, C91.Z0-C91.Z2, C92.00-C92.02, C92.10-C92.12, C92.20-C92.22, C92.30-C92.32, C92.40-C92.42, C92.50-C92.52, C92.60-C92.62, C92.90-C92.92, C92.A0-C92.A2, C92.Z0-C92.Z2, C93.00-C93.02, C93.10-C93.12, C93.30-C93.32, C93.90-C93.92, C93.Z0-C93.Z2, C94.00-C94.02, C94.20-C94.22, C94.30-C94.32, C94.80-C94.82, C95.00-C95.02, C95.10-C95.12, C95.90-C95.92, D49.81-D49.9

● **C91.0 Acute lymphoblastic leukemia [ALL]**

Note: Code C91.0 should only be used for T-cell and B-cell precusor leukemia

C91.00 Acute lymphoblastic leukemia not having achieved remission
Acute lymphoblastic leukemia with failed remission
Acute lymphoblastic leukemia NOS

C91.01 Acute lymphoblastic leukemia, in remission

C91.02 Acute lymphoblastic leukemia, in relapse

● **C91.1 Chronic lymphocytic leukemia of B-cell type**
Lymphoplasmacytic leukemia
Richter syndrome

Excludes1 lymphoplasmacytic lymphoma (C83.0-)

C91.10 Chronic lymphocytic leukemia of B-cell type not having achieved remission
Chronic lymphocytic leukemia of B-cell type with failed remission
Chronic lymphocytic leukemia of B-cell type NOS

C91.11 Chronic lymphocytic leukemia of B-cell type in remission

C91.12 Chronic lymphocytic leukemia of B-cell type in relapse

● **C91.3 Prolymphocytic leukemia of B-cell type**
Chronic leukemia with symptoms of large number of circulating lymphocytes

C91.30 Prolymphocytic leukemia of B-cell type not having achieved remission
Prolymphocytic leukemia of B-cell type with failed remission
Prolymphocytic leukemia of B-cell type NOS

C91.31 Prolymphocytic leukemia of B-cell type, in remission

C91.32 Prolymphocytic leukemia of B-cell type, in relapse

● **C91.4 Hairy cell leukemia**
Chronic leukemia with splenomegaly and excessive number of abnormal large mononuclear cells covered by hairlike villi
Leukemic reticuloendotheliosis

Ex **For category C91.4 CC codes:** C82.50, C82.59, C83.10, C83.19, C84.40, C84.49-C84.60, C84.69-C84.70, C84.79, C84.90, C84.99, C84.A0, C84.A9-C84.Z0, C84.Z9, C85.10, C85.19-C85.20, C85.29-C85.80, C85.89-C85.90, C85.99, C86.4, C88.4, C91.40-C91.42, C96.4, C96.9, C96.Z, D49.81-D49.9

C91.40 Hairy cell leukemia not having achieved remission
Hairy cell leukemia with failed remission
Hairy cell leukemia NOS

C91.41 Hairy cell leukemia, in remission

C91.42 Hairy cell leukemia, in relapse

● **C91.5 Adult T-cell lymphoma/leukemia (HTLV-1-associated)**
Acute variant of adult T-cell lymphoma/leukemia (HTLV-1-associated)
Chronic variant of adult T-cell lymphoma/leukemia (HTLV-1-associated)
Lymphomatoid variant of adult T-cell lymphoma/leukemia (HTLV-1-associated)
Smouldering variant of adult T-cell lymphoma/leukemia (HTLV-1-associated)

C91.50 Adult T-cell lymphoma/leukemia (HTLV-1-associated) not having achieved remission A
Adult T-cell lymphoma/leukemia (HTLV-1-associated) with failed remission
Adult T-cell lymphoma/leukemia (HTLV-1-associated) NOS

C91.51 Adult T-cell lymphoma/leukemia (HTLV-1-associated), in remission A

C91.52 Adult T-cell lymphoma/leukemia (HTLV-1-associated), in relapse A

● **C91.6 Prolymphocytic leukemia of T-cell type**

C91.60 Prolymphocytic leukemia of T-cell type not having achieved remission
Prolymphocytic leukemia of T-cell type with failed remission
Prolymphocytic leukemia of T-cell type NOS

C91.61 Prolymphocytic leukemia of T-cell type, in remission

C91.62 Prolymphocytic leukemia of T-cell type, in relapse

● **C91.A Mature B-cell leukemia Burkitt-type**
Excludes1 Burkitt lymphoma (C83.7-)

C91.A0 Mature B-cell leukemia Burkitt-type not having achieved remission
Mature B-cell leukemia Burkitt-type with failed remission
Mature B-cell leukemia Burkitt-type NOS

C91.A1 Mature B-cell leukemia Burkitt-type, in remission

C91.A2 Mature B-cell leukemia Burkitt-type, in relapse

● **C91.Z Other lymphoid leukemia**
T-cell large granular lymphocytic leukemia (associated with rheumatoid arthritis)

C91.Z0 Other lymphoid leukemia not having achieved remission
Other lymphoid leukemia with failed remission
Other lymphoid leukemia NOS

C91.Z1 Other lymphoid leukemia, in remission

C91.Z2 Other lymphoid leukemia, in relapse

● **C91.9 Lymphoid leukemia, unspecified**

C91.90 Lymphoid leukemia, unspecified not having achieved remission
Lymphoid leukemia with failed remission
Lymphoid leukemia NOS

C91.91 Lymphoid leukemia, unspecified, in remission

C91.92 Lymphoid leukemia, unspecified, in relapse

● **C92 Myeloid leukemia**
Includes granulocytic leukemia
myelogenous leukemia
Excludes1 personal history of leukemia (Z85.6)
Ex For category C92 CC codes: C88.2-C88.3, C88.8-C90.02, C90.10-C90.12, C90.20-C90.22, C90.30-C90.32, C91.00-C91.02, C91.10-C91.12, C91.30-C91.32, C91.50-C91.52, C91.60-C91.62, C91.90-C91.92, C91.A0-C91.A2, C91.Z0-C91.Z2, C92.00-C92.02, C92.10-C92.12, C92.20-C92.22, C92.30-C92.32, C92.40-C92.42, C92.50-C92.52, C92.60-C92.62, C92.90-C92.92, C92.A0-C92.A2, C92.Z0-C92.Z2, C93.00-C93.02, C93.10-C93.12, C93.30-C93.32, C93.90-C93.92, C93.Z0-C93.Z2, C94.00-C94.02, C94.20-C94.22, C94.30-C94.32, C94.80-C94.82, C95.00-C95.02, C95.10-C95.12, C95.90-C95.92, D49.81-D49.9

● **C92.0 Acute myeloblastic leukemia**
Acute myeloblastic leukemia, minimal differentiation
Acute myeloblastic leukemia (with maturation)
Acute myeloblastic leukemia 1/ETO
Acute myeloblastic leukemia M0
Acute myeloblastic leukemia M1
Acute myeloblastic leukemia M2
Acute myeloblastic leukemia with t(8;21)
Acute myeloblastic leukemia (without a FAB classification) NOS
Refractory anemia with excess blasts in transformation [RAEB T]
Excludes1 acute exacerbation of chronic myeloid leukemia (C92.10)
refractory anemia with excess of blasts not in transformation (D46.2-)

C92.00 Acute myeloblastic leukemia, not having achieved remission
Acute myeloblastic leukemia with failed remission
Acute myeloblastic leukemia NOS

C92.01 Acute myeloblastic leukemia, in remission

C92.02 Acute myeloblastic leukemia, in relapse

● **C92.1 Chronic myeloid leukemia, BCR/ABL-positive**
Chronic myelogenous leukemia, Philadelphia chromosome (Ph1) positive
Chronic myelogenous leukemia, t(9;22) (q34;q11)
Chronic myelogenous leukemia with crisis of blast cells
Excludes1 atypical chronic myeloid leukemia BCR/ABL-negative (C92.2-)
chronic myelomonocytic leukemia (C93.1-)
chronic myeloproliferative disease (D47.1)

C92.10 Chronic myeloid leukemia, BCR/ABL-positive, not having achieved remission
Chronic myeloid leukemia, BCR/ABL-positive with failed remission
Chronic myeloid leukemia, BCR/ABL-positive NOS

C92.11 Chronic myeloid leukemia, BCR/ABL-positive, in remission

C92.12 Chronic myeloid leukemia, BCR/ABL-positive, in relapse

● **C92.2 Atypical chronic myeloid leukemia, BCR/ABL-negative**

C92.20 Atypical chronic myeloid leukemia, BCR/ABL-negative, not having achieved remission
Atypical chronic myeloid leukemia, BCR/ABL-negative with failed remission
Atypical chronic myeloid leukemia, BCR/ABL-negative NOS

C92.21 Atypical chronic myeloid leukemia, BCR/ABL-negative, in remission

C92.22 Atypical chronic myeloid leukemia, BCR/ABL-negative, in relapse

C92.3 Myeloid sarcoma
A malignant tumor of immature myeloid cells
Chloroma
Granulocytic sarcoma

C92.30 Myeloid sarcoma, not having achieved remission
Myeloid sarcoma with failed remission
Myeloid sarcoma NOS

C92.31 Myeloid sarcoma, in remission

C92.32 Myeloid sarcoma, in relapse

C92.4 Acute promyelocytic leukemia
AML M3
AML Me with t(15;17) and variants

C92.40 Acute promyelocytic leukemia, not having achieved remission
Acute promyelocytic leukemia with failed remission
Acute promyelocytic leukemia NOS

C92.41 Acute promyelocytic leukemia, in remission

C92.42 Acute promyelocytic leukemia, in relapse

C92.5 Acute myelomonocytic leukemia
AML M4
AML M4 Eo with inv(16) or t(16;16)

C92.50 Acute myelomonocytic leukemia, not having achieved remission
Acute myelomonocytic leukemia with failed remission
Acute myelomonocytic leukemia NOS

C92.51 Acute myelomonocytic leukemia, in remission

C92.52 Acute myelomonocytic leukemia, in relapse

C92.6 Acute myeloid leukemia with 11q23-abnormality
Acute myeloid leukemia with variation of MLL-gene

C92.60 Acute myeloid leukemia with 11q23-abnormality not having achieved remission
Acute myeloid leukemia with 11q23-abnormality with failed remission
Acute myeloid leukemia with 11q23-abnormality NOS

C92.61 Acute myeloid leukemia with 11q23-abnormality in remission

C92.62 Acute myeloid leukemia with 11q23-abnormality in relapse

C92.A Acute myeloid leukemia with multilineage dysplasia
Acute myeloid leukemia with dysplasia of remaining hematopoesis and/or myelodysplastic disease in its history

C92.A0 Acute myeloid leukemia with multilineage dysplasia, not having achieved remission
Acute myeloid leukemia with multilineage dysplasia with failed remission
Acute myeloid leukemia with multilineage dysplasia NOS

C92.A1 Acute myeloid leukemia with multilineage dysplasia, in remission

C92.A2 Acute myeloid leukemia with multilineage dysplasia, in relapse

C92.Z Other myeloid leukemia

C92.Z0 Other myeloid leukemia not having achieved remission
Myeloid leukemia NEC with failed remission
Myeloid leukemia NEC

C92.Z1 Other myeloid leukemia, in remission

C92.Z2 Other myeloid leukemia, in relapse

C92.9 Myeloid leukemia, unspecified

C92.90 Myeloid leukemia, unspecified, not having achieved remission
Myeloid leukemia, unspecified with failed remission
Myeloid leukemia, unspecified NOS

C92.91 Myeloid leukemia, unspecified in remission

C92.92 Myeloid leukemia, unspecified in relapse

C93 Monocytic leukemia

Includes monocytoid leukemia

Excludes1 personal history of leukemia (Z85.6)

Ex For category C93 CC codes: C88.2-C88.3, C88.8-C90.02, C90.10-C90.12, C90.20-C90.22, C90.30-C90.32, C91.00-C91.02, C91.10-C91.12, C91.30-C91.32, C91.50-C91.52, C91.60-C91.62, C91.90-C91.92, C91.A0-C91.A2, C91.Z0-C91.Z2, C92.00-C92.02, C92.10-C92.12, C92.20-C92.22, C92.30-C92.32, C92.40-C92.42, C92.50-C92.52, C92.60-C92.62, C92.90-C92.92, C92.A0-C92.A2, C92.Z0-C92.Z2, C93.00-C93.02, C93.10-C93.12, C93.30-C93.32, C93.90-C93.92, C93.Z0-C93.Z2, C94.00-C94.02, C94.20-C94.22, C94.30-C94.32, C94.80-C94.82, C95.00-C95.02, C95.10-C95.12, C95.90-C95.92, D49.81-D49.9

C93.0 Acute monoblastic/monocytic leukemia
AML M5
AML M5a
AML M5b

C93.00 Acute monoblastic/monocytic leukemia, not having achieved remission
Acute monoblastic/monocytic leukemia with failed remission
Acute monoblastic/monocytic leukemia NOS

C93.01 Acute monoblastic/monocytic leukemia, in remission

C93.02 Acute monoblastic/monocytic leukemia, in relapse

C93.1 Chronic myelomonocytic leukemia
Chronic monocytic leukemia
CMML-1
CMML-2
CMML with eosinophilia

C93.10 Chronic myelomonocytic leukemia not having achieved remission
Chronic myelomonocytic leukemia with failed remission
Chronic myelomonocytic leukemia NOS

C93.11 Chronic myelomonocytic leukemia, in remission

C93.12 Chronic myelomonocytic leukemia, in relapse

C93.3 Juvenile myelomonocytic leukemia

C93.30 Juvenile myelomonocytic leukemia, not having achieved remission P
Juvenile myelomonocytic leukemia with failed remission
Juvenile myelomonocytic leukemia NOS

C93.31 Juvenile myelomonocytic leukemia, in remission P

C93.32 Juvenile myelomonocytic leukemia, in relapse P

C93.Z Other monocytic leukemia

C93.Z0 Other monocytic leukemia, not having achieved remission
Other monocytic leukemia NOS

C93.Z1 Other monocytic leukemia, in remission

C93.Z2 Other monocytic leukemia, in relapse

C93.9 Monocytic leukemia, unspecified

C93.90 Monocytic leukemia, unspecified, not having achieved remission
Monocytic leukemia, unspecified with failed remission
Monocytic leukemia, unspecified NOS

C93.91 Monocytic leukemia, unspecified in remission

C93.92 Monocytic leukemia, unspecified in relapse

● **C94 Other leukemias of specified cell type**

Excludes1 leukemic reticuloendotheliosis (C91.4-)
myelodysplastic syndromes (D46.-)
personal history of leukemia (Z85.6)
plasma cell leukemia (C90.1-)

Ex: **For category C94 CC codes unless otherwise indicated:** C88.2-C88.3, C88.8-C90.02, C90.10-C90.12, C90.20-C90.22, C90.30-C90.32, C91.00-C91.02, C91.10-C91.12, C91.30-C91.32, C91.50-C91.52, C91.60-C91.62, C91.90-C91.92, C91.A0-C91.A2, C91.Z0-C91.Z2, C92.00-C92.02, C92.10-C92.12, C92.20-C92.22, C92.30-C92.32, C92.40-C92.42, C92.50-C92.52, C92.60-C92.62, C92.90-C92.92, C92.A0-C92.A2, C92.Z0-C92.Z2, C93.00-C93.02, C93.10-C93.12, C93.30-C93.32, C93.90-C93.92, C93.Z0-C93.Z2, C94.00-C94.02, C94.20-C94.22, C94.30-C94.32, C94.80-C94.82, C95.00-C95.02, C95.10-C95.12, C95.90-C95.92, D49.81-D49.9

● **C94.0 Acute erythroid leukemia**
Acute myeloid leukemia M6(a)(b)
Erythroleukemia

C94.00 Acute erythroid leukemia, not having achieved remission
Acute erythroid leukemia with failed remission
Acute erythroid leukemia NOS

C94.01 Acute erythroid leukemia, in remission

C94.02 Acute erythroid leukemia, in relapse

● **C94.2 Acute megakaryoblastic leukemia**
Acute myeloid leukemia M7
Acute megakaryocytic leukemia

C94.20 Acute megakaryoblastic leukemia not having achieved remission
Acute megakaryoblastic leukemia with failed remission
Acute megakaryoblastic leukemia NOS

C94.21 Acute megakaryoblastic leukemia, in remission

C94.22 Acute megakaryoblastic leukemia, in relapse

● **C94.3 Mast cell leukemia**

C94.30 Mast cell leukemia not having achieved remission
Mast cell leukemia with failed remission
Mast cell leukemia NOS

C94.31 Mast cell leukemia, in remission

C94.32 Mast cell leukemia, in relapse

● **C94.4 Acute panmyelosis with myelofibrosis**
Acute myelofibrosis

Excludes1 myelofibrosis NOS (D75.81)
secondary myelofibrosis NOS (D75.81)

Ex: **For category C94.4 CC codes:** C88.2-C88.3, C88.8-C88.9, C90.10-C90.11, C90.20-C90.21, C90.30-C90.31, C91.00-C91.02, C91.10-C91.12, C91.30-C91.32, C91.40-C91.42, C91.50-C91.52, C91.60-C91.62, C91.90-C91.92, C91.A0-C91.A2, C91.Z0-C91.Z2, C92.00-C92.02, C92.10-C92.12, C92.20-C92.22, C92.30-C92.32, C92.40-C92.42, C92.50-C92.52, C92.60-C92.62, C92.90-C92.92, C92.A0-C92.A2, C92.Z0-C92.Z2, C93.00-C93.02, C93.10-C93.12, C93.30-C93.32, C93.90-C93.92, C93.Z0-C93.Z2, C94.00-C94.02, C94.20-C94.22, C94.30-C94.32, C94.40-C94.42, C94.6, C94.80-C94.82, C95.00-C95.02, C95.10-C95.12, C95.90-C95.92, D45-D46.22, D46.4, D46.9, D46.A-D46.Z, D47.0-D47.1, D47.3, D47.9, D47.Z2, D47.Z9, D48.7-D48.9

C94.40 Acute panmyelosis with myelofibrosis not having achieved remission
Acute myelofibrosis NOS
Acute panmyelosis with myelofibrosis with failed remission
Acute panmyelosis NOS

C94.41 Acute panmyelosis with myelofibrosis, in remission

C94.42 Acute panmyelosis with myelofibrosis, in relapse

C94.6 Myelodysplastic disease, not classified
Myeloproliferative disease, not classified
Ex: See C94.4

● **C94.8 Other specified leukemias**
Aggressive NK-cell leukemia
Acute basophilic leukemia

C94.80 Other specified leukemias not having achieved remission
Other specified leukemia with failed remission
Other specified leukemias NOS

C94.81 Other specified leukemias, in remission

C94.82 Other specified leukemias, in relapse

● **C95 Leukemia of unspecified cell type**

Excludes1 personal history of leukemia (Z85.6)

Ex: **For category C95 CC codes:** C88.2-C88.3, C88.8-C90.02, C90.10-C90.12, C90.20-C90.22, C90.30-C90.32, C91.00-C91.02, C91.10-C91.12, C91.30-C91.32, C91.50-C91.52, C91.60-C91.62, C91.90-C91.92, C91.A0-C91.A2, C91.Z0-C91.Z2, C92.00-C92.02, C92.10-C92.12, C92.20-C92.22, C92.30-C92.32, C92.40-C92.42, C92.50-C92.52, C92.60-C92.62, C92.90-C92.92, C92.A0-C92.A2, C92.Z0-C92.Z2, C93.00-C93.02, C93.10-C93.12, C93.30-C93.32, C93.90-C93.92, C93.Z0-C93.Z2, C94.00-C94.02, C94.20-C94.22, C94.30-C94.32, C94.80-C94.82, C95.00-C95.02, C95.10-C95.12, C95.90-C95.92, D49.81-D49.9

● **C95.0 Acute leukemia of unspecified cell type**
Acute bilineal leukemia
Acute mixed lineage leukemia
Biphenotypic acute leukemia
Stem cell leukemia of unclear lineage

Excludes1 acute exacerbation of unspecified chronic leukemia (C95.10)

C95.00 Acute leukemia of unspecified cell type not having achieved remission
Acute leukemia of unspecified cell type with failed remission
Acute leukemia NOS

C95.01 Acute leukemia of unspecified cell type, in remission

C95.02 Acute leukemia of unspecified cell type, in relapse

● **C95.1 Chronic leukemia of unspecified cell type**

C95.10 Chronic leukemia of unspecified cell type not having achieved remission
Chronic leukemia of unspecified cell type with failed remission
Chronic leukemia NOS

C95.11 Chronic leukemia of unspecified cell type, in remission

C95.12 Chronic leukemia of unspecified cell type, in relapse

● **C95.9 Leukemia, unspecified**

C95.90 Leukemia, unspecified not having achieved remission
Leukemia, unspecified with failed remission
Leukemia NOS

C95.91 Leukemia, unspecified, in remission

C95.92 Leukemia, unspecified, in relapse

C96 Other and unspecified malignant neoplasms of lymphoid, hematopoietic and related tissue

Excludes1 personal history of other malignant neoplasms of lymphoid, hematopoietic and related tissues (Z85.79)

C96.0 Multifocal and multisystemic (disseminated) Langerhans-cell histiocytosis

Histiocytosis X, multisystemic
Letterer-Siwe disease

Excludes1 adult pulmonary Langerhans cell histiocytosis (J84.82)
multifocal and unisystemic Langerhans-cell histiocytosis (C96.5)
unifocal Langerhans-cell histiocytosis (C96.6)

Ex: C82.50, C82.59, C83.10, C83.19, C84.40, C84.49-C84.60, C84.69-C84.70, C84.79, C84.90, C84.99, C84.A0, C84.A9-C84.Z0, C84.Z9, C85.10, C85.19-C85.20, C85.29-C85.80, C85.89-C85.90, C85.99, C86.4, C88.4, C96.0, C96.4, C96.9, C96.Z, D49.81-D49.9

C96.2 Malignant mast cell tumor

Aggressive systemic mastocytosis
Mast cell sarcoma

Excludes1 indolent mastocytosis (D47.0)
mast cell leukemia (C94.30)
mastocytosis (congenital) (cutaneous) (Q82.2)

Ex: C82.50, C82.59, C83.10, C83.19, C84.40, C84.49-C84.60, C84.69-C84.70, C84.79, C84.90, C84.99, C84.A0, C84.A9-C84.Z0, C84.Z9, C85.10, C85.19-C85.20, C85.29-C85.80, C85.89-C85.90, C85.99, C86.4, C88.4, C96.2, C96.4, C96.9, C96.Z, D49.81-D49.9

C96.4 Sarcoma of dendritic cells (accessory cells)

Follicular dendritic cell sarcoma
Interdigitating dendritic cell sarcoma
Langerhans cell sarcoma

Ex: C96.4, C96.9, C96.Z, D49.81-D49.9

C96.5 Multifocal and unisystemic Langerhans-cell histiocytosis

Hand-Schüller-Christian disease
Histiocytosis X, multifocal

Excludes1 multifocal and multisystemic (disseminated) Langerhans-cell histiocytosis (C96.0)
unifocal Langerhans-cell histiocytosis (C96.6)

Ex: E71.310-E71.32, E71.40-E71.548, E80.4-E80.7, E88.40-E88.49, H49.811-H49.819

C96.6 Unifocal Langerhans-cell histiocytosis

Eosinophilic granuloma
Histiocytosis X, unifocal
Histiocytosis X NOS
Langerhans-cell histiocytosis NOS

Excludes1 multifocal and multisysemic (disseminated) Langerhans-cell histiocytosis (C96.0)
multifocal and unisystemic Langerhans-cell histiocytosis (C96.5)

Ex: See C96.5

C96.A Histiocytic sarcoma

Malignant histiocytosis

Ex: C82.50, C82.59, C83.10, C83.19, C84.40, C84.49-C84.60, C84.69-C84.70, C84.79, C84.90, C84.99, C84.A0, C84.A9-C84.Z0, C84.Z9, C85.10, C85.19-C85.20, C85.29-C85.80, C85.89-C85.90, C85.99, C86.4, C88.4, C96.4, C96.9, C96.A, C96.Z, D49.81-D49.9

C96.Z Other specified malignant neoplasms of lymphoid, hematopoietic and related tissue

Ex: See C96.4

C96.9 Malignant neoplasm of lymphoid, hematopoietic and related tissue, unspecified

Ex: See C96.4

In situ is carcinoma involving cells in localized tissues that has not spread to nearby tissues

IN SITU NEOPLASMS (D00-D09)

Includes Bowen's disease
erythroplasia
grade III intraepithelial neoplasia
Queyrat's erythroplasia

D00 Carcinoma in situ of oral cavity, esophagus and stomach

Excludes1 melanoma in situ (D03.-)

D00.0 Carcinoma in situ of lip, oral cavity and pharynx

Use additional code to identify:
exposure to environmental tobacco smoke (Z77.22)
exposure to tobacco smoke in the perinatal period (P96.81)
history of tobacco dependence (Z87.891)
occupational exposure to environmental tobacco smoke (Z57.31)
tobacco dependence (F17.-)
tobacco use (Z72.0)

Excludes1 carcinoma in situ of aryepiglottic fold or interarytenoid fold, laryngeal aspect (D02.0)
carcinoma in situ of epiglottis NOS (D02.0)
carcinoma in situ of epiglottis suprahyoid portion (D02.0)
carcinoma in situ of skin of lip (D03.0, D04.0)

D00.00 Carcinoma in situ of oral cavity, unspecified site

D00.01 Carcinoma in situ of labial mucosa and vermilion border

D00.02 Carcinoma in situ of buccal mucosa

D00.03 Carcinoma in situ of gingiva and edentulous alveolar ridge

D00.04 Carcinoma in situ of soft palate

D00.05 Carcinoma in situ of hard palate

D00.06 Carcinoma in situ of floor of mouth

D00.07 Carcinoma in situ of tongue

D00.08 Carcinoma in situ of pharynx

Carcinoma in situ of aryepiglottic fold NOS
Carcinoma in situ of hypopharyngeal aspect of aryepiglottic fold
Carcinoma in situ of marginal zone of aryepiglottic fold

D00.1 Carcinoma in situ of esophagus

D00.2 Carcinoma in situ of stomach

D01 Carcinoma in situ of other and unspecified digestive organs

Excludes1 melanoma in situ (D03.-)

D01.0 Carcinoma in situ of colon

Excludes1 carcinoma in situ of rectosigmoid junction (D01.1)

D01.1 Carcinoma in situ of rectosigmoid junction

D01.2 Carcinoma in situ of rectum

D01.3 Carcinoma in situ of anus and anal canal

Anal intraepithelial neoplasia III [AIN III] ◀
Severe dysplasia of anus ◀

Excludes1 anal intraepithelial neoplasia I and II [AIN I and AIN II] (K62.82) ◀
carcinoma in situ of anal margin (D04.5)
carcinoma in situ of anal skin (D04.5)
carcinoma in situ of perianal skin (D04.5)

D01.4 Carcinoma in situ of other and unspecified parts of intestine

Excludes1 carcinoma in situ of ampulla of Vater (D01.5)

D01.40 Carcinoma in situ of unspecified part of intestine

D01.49 Carcinoma in situ of other parts of intestine

D01.5 Carcinoma in situ of liver, gallbladder and bile ducts
Carcinoma in situ of ampulla of Vater

D01.7 Carcinoma in situ of other specified digestive organs
Carcinoma in situ of pancreas

D01.9 Carcinoma in situ of digestive organ, unspecified

● **D02 Carcinoma in situ of middle ear and respiratory system**
Use additional code to identify:
exposure to environmental tobacco smoke (Z77.22)
exposure to tobacco smoke in the perinatal period (P96.81)
history of tobacco dependence (Z87.891) ⟸
occupational exposure to environmental tobacco smoke (Z57.31)
tobacco dependence (F17.-)
tobacco use (Z72.0)
Excludes1 melanoma in situ (D03.-)

D02.0 Carcinoma in situ of larynx
Carcinoma in situ of aryepiglottic fold or interarytenoid fold, laryngeal aspect
Carcinoma in situ of epiglottis (suprahyoid portion)
Excludes1 carcinoma in situ of aryepiglottic fold or interarytenoid fold NOS (D00.08)
carcinoma in situ of hypopharyngeal aspect (D00.08)
carcinoma in situ of marginal zone (D00.08)

D02.1 Carcinoma in situ of trachea

● **D02.2 Carcinoma in situ of bronchus and lung**
D02.20 Carcinoma in situ of unspecified bronchus and lung
D02.21 Carcinoma in situ of right bronchus and lung
D02.22 Carcinoma in situ of left bronchus and lung

D02.3 Carcinoma in situ of other parts of respiratory system
Carcinoma in situ of accessory sinuses
Carcinoma in situ of middle ear
Carcinoma in situ of nasal cavities
Excludes1 carcinoma in situ of ear (external) (skin) (D04.2-)
carcinoma in situ of nose NOS (D09.8)
carcinoma in situ of skin of nose (D04.3)

D02.4 Carcinoma in situ of respiratory system, unspecified

● **D03 Melanoma in situ**
D03.0 Melanoma in situ of lip

● **D03.1 Melanoma in situ of eyelid, including canthus**
D03.10 Melanoma in situ of unspecified eyelid, including canthus
D03.11 Melanoma in situ of right eyelid, including canthus
D03.12 Melanoma in situ of left eyelid, including canthus

● **D03.2 Melanoma in situ of ear and external auricular canal**
D03.20 Melanoma in situ of unspecified ear and external auricular canal
D03.21 Melanoma in situ of right ear and external auricular canal
D03.22 Melanoma in situ of left ear and external auricular canal

● **D03.3 Melanoma in situ of other and unspecified parts of face**
D03.30 Melanoma in situ of unspecified part of face
D03.39 Melanoma in situ of other parts of face

D03.4 Melanoma in situ of scalp and neck

● **D03.5 Melanoma in situ of trunk**
D03.51 Melanoma in situ of anal skin
Melanoma in situ of anal margin
Melanoma in situ of perianal skin
D03.52 Melanoma in situ of breast (skin) (soft tissue)
D03.59 Melanoma in situ of other part of trunk

● **D03.6 Melanoma in situ of upper limb, including shoulder**
D03.60 Melanoma in situ of unspecified upper limb, including shoulder
D03.61 Melanoma in situ of right upper limb, including shoulder
D03.62 Melanoma in situ of left upper limb, including shoulder

● **D03.7 Melanoma in situ of lower limb, including hip**
D03.70 Melanoma in situ of unspecified lower limb, including hip
D03.71 Melanoma in situ of right lower limb, including hip
D03.72 Melanoma in situ of left lower limb, including hip

D03.8 Melanoma in situ of other sites
Melanoma in situ of scrotum
Excludes1 carcinoma in situ of scrotum (D07.61)

D03.9 Melanoma in situ, unspecified

● **D04 Carcinoma in situ of skin**
Excludes1 erythroplasia of Queyrat (penis) NOS (D07.4)
melanoma in situ (D03.-)

D04.0 Carcinoma in situ of skin of lip
Excludes1 carcinoma in situ of vermilion border of lip (D00.01)

● **D04.1 Carcinoma in situ of skin of eyelid, including canthus**
D04.10 Carcinoma in situ of skin of unspecified eyelid, including canthus
D04.11 Carcinoma in situ of skin of right eyelid, including canthus
D04.12 Carcinoma in situ of skin of left eyelid, including canthus

● **D04.2 Carcinoma in situ of skin of ear and external auricular canal**
D04.20 Carcinoma in situ of skin of unspecified ear and external auricular canal
D04.21 Carcinoma in situ of skin of right ear and external auricular canal
D04.22 Carcinoma in situ of skin of left ear and external auricular canal

● **D04.3 Carcinoma in situ of skin of other and unspecified parts of face**
D04.30 Carcinoma in situ of skin of unspecified part of face
D04.39 Carcinoma in situ of skin of other parts of face

D04.4 Carcinoma in situ of skin of scalp and neck

D04.5 Carcinoma in situ of skin of trunk
Carcinoma in situ of anal margin
Carcinoma in situ of anal skin
Carcinoma in situ of perianal skin
Carcinoma in situ of skin of breast
Excludes1 carcinoma in situ of anus NOS (D01.3)
carcinoma in situ of scrotum (D07.61)
carcinoma in situ of skin of genital organs (D07.-)

● **D04.6 Carcinoma in situ of skin of upper limb, including shoulder**
D04.60 Carcinoma in situ of skin of unspecified upper limb, including shoulder
D04.61 Carcinoma in situ of skin of right upper limb, including shoulder
D04.62 Carcinoma in situ of skin of left upper limb, including shoulder

● **D04.7 Carcinoma in situ of skin of lower limb, including hip**
D04.70 Carcinoma in situ of skin of unspecified lower limb, including hip
D04.71 Carcinoma in situ of skin of right lower limb, including hip
D04.72 Carcinoma in situ of skin of left lower limb, including hip

D04.8 Carcinoma in situ of skin of other sites
D04.9 Carcinoma in situ of skin, unspecified

D05 Carcinoma in situ of breast

Excludes1 carcinoma in situ of skin of breast (D04.5)
melanoma in situ of breast (skin) (D03.5)
Paget's disease of breast or nipple (C50.-)

D05.0 Lobular carcinoma in situ of breast

D05.00 Lobular carcinoma in situ of unspecified breast

D05.01 Lobular carcinoma in situ of right breast

D05.02 Lobular carcinoma in situ of left breast

D05.1 Intraductal carcinoma in situ of breast

D05.10 Intraductal carcinoma in situ of unspecified breast

D05.11 Intraductal carcinoma in situ of right breast

D05.12 Intraductal carcinoma in situ of left breast

D05.8 Other specified type of carcinoma in situ of breast

D05.80 Other specified type of carcinoma in situ of unspecified breast

D05.81 Other specified type of carcinoma in situ of right breast

D05.82 Other specified type of carcinoma in situ of left breast

D05.9 Unspecified type of carcinoma in situ of breast

D05.90 Unspecified type of carcinoma in situ of unspecified breast

D05.91 Unspecified type of carcinoma in situ of right breast

D05.92 Unspecified type of carcinoma in situ of left breast

D06 Carcinoma in situ of cervix uteri

Includes cervical adenocarcinoma in situ
cervical intraepithelial glandular neoplasia
cervical intraepithelial neoplasia III [CIN III]
severe dysplasia of cervix uteri

Excludes1 cervical intraepithelial neoplasia II [CIN II] (N87.1)
cytologic evidence of malignancy of cervix without histologic confirmation (R87.614)
high grade squamous intraepithelial lesion (HGSIL) of cervix (R87.613)
melanoma in situ of cervix (D03.5)
moderate cervical dysplasia (N87.1)

D06.0 Carcinoma in situ of endocervix ♀

D06.1 Carcinoma in situ of exocervix ♀

D06.7 Carcinoma in situ of other parts of cervix ♀

D06.9 Carcinoma in situ of cervix, unspecified ♀

D07 Carcinoma in situ of other and unspecified genital organs

Excludes1 melanoma in situ of trunk (D03.5)

D07.0 Carcinoma in situ of endometrium ♀

D07.1 Carcinoma in situ of vulva ♀
Severe dysplasia of vulva
Vulvar intraepithelial neoplasia III [VIN III]

Excludes1 moderate dysplasia of vulva (N90.1)
vulvar intraepithelial neoplasia II [VIN II] (N90.1)

D07.2 Carcinoma in situ of vagina ♀
Severe dysplasia of vagina
Vaginal intraepithelial neoplasia III [VIN III]

Excludes1 moderate dysplasia of vagina (N89.1)
vaginal intraepithelial neoplasia II [VIN II] (N89.1)

D07.3 Carcinoma in situ of other and unspecified female genital organs

D07.30 Carcinoma in situ of unspecified female genital organs ♀

D07.39 Carcinoma in situ of other female genital organs ♀

D07.4 Carcinoma in situ of penis ♂
Erythroplasia of Queyrat NOS

D07.5 Carcinoma in situ of prostate ♂
Prostatic intraepithelial neoplasia III (PIN III)
Severe dysplasia of prostate

Excludes1 dysplasia (mild) (moderate) of prostate (N42.3-)
prostatic intraepithelial neoplasia II [PIN II] (N42.3-)

D07.6 Carcinoma in situ of other and unspecified male genital organs

D07.60 Carcinoma in situ of unspecified male genital organs ♂

D07.61 Carcinoma in situ of scrotum ♂

D07.69 Carcinoma in situ of other male genital organs ♂

D09 Carcinoma in situ of other and unspecified sites

Excludes1 melanoma in situ (D03.-)

D09.0 Carcinoma in situ of bladder

D09.1 Carcinoma in situ of other and unspecified urinary organs

D09.10 Carcinoma in situ of unspecified urinary organ

D09.19 Carcinoma in situ of other urinary organs

D09.2 Carcinoma in situ of eye

Excludes1 carcinoma in situ of skin of eyelid (D04.1-)

D09.20 Carcinoma in situ of unspecified eye

D09.21 Carcinoma in situ of right eye

D09.22 Carcinoma in situ of left eye

D09.3 Carcinoma in situ of thyroid and other endocrine glands

Excludes1 carcinoma in situ of endocrine pancreas (D01.7)
carcinoma in situ of ovary (D07.39)
carcinoma in situ of testis (D07.69)

D09.8 Carcinoma in situ of other specified sites

D09.9 Carcinoma in situ, unspecified

BENIGN NEOPLASMS, EXCEPT BENIGN NEUROENDOCRINE TUMORS (D10-D36)

D10 Benign neoplasm of mouth and pharynx

D10.0 Benign neoplasm of lip
Benign neoplasm of lip (frenulum) (inner aspect) (mucosa) (vermilion border)

Excludes1 benign neoplasm of skin of lip (D22.0, D23.0)

D10.1 Benign neoplasm of tongue
Benign neoplasm of lingual tonsil

D10.2 Benign neoplasm of floor of mouth

D10.3 Benign neoplasm of other and unspecified parts of mouth

D10.30 Benign neoplasm of unspecified part of mouth

D10.39 Benign neoplasm of other parts of mouth
Benign neoplasm of minor salivary gland NOS

Excludes1 benign odontogenic neoplasms (D16.4-D16.5)
benign neoplasm of mucosa of lip (D10.0)
benign neoplasm of nasopharyngeal surface of soft palate (D10.6)

D10.4 Benign neoplasm of tonsil
Benign neoplasm of tonsil (faucial) (palatine)

Excludes1 benign neoplasm of lingual tonsil (D10.1)
benign neoplasm of pharyngeal tonsil (D10.6)
benign neoplasm of tonsillar fossa (D10.5)
benign neoplasm of tonsillar pillars (D10.5)

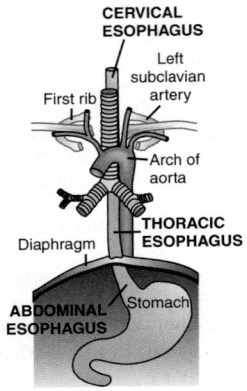

Figure 2-16 The esophagus is the muscular tube that connects the pharynx and the stomach. The 10 inch (25 cm) long esophagus is divided into three parts: **cervical, thoracic,** and **abdominal.**

D10.5 Benign neoplasm of other parts of oropharynx
Division of pharynx lying between soft palate and upper edge of epiglottis
Benign neoplasm of epiglottis, anterior aspect
Benign neoplasm of tonsillar fossa
Benign neoplasm of tonsillar pillars
Benign neoplasm of vallecula
Excludes1 benign neoplasm of epiglottis NOS (D14.1)
benign neoplasm of epiglottis, suprahyoid portion (D14.1)

D10.6 Benign neoplasm of nasopharynx
Segment of pharynx that lies above soft palate
Benign neoplasm of pharyngeal tonsil
Benign neoplasm of posterior margin of septum and choanae

D10.7 Benign neoplasm of hypopharynx
Segment of pharynx that lies below upper edge of epiglottis and opens into larynx and esophagus

D10.9 Benign neoplasm of pharynx, unspecified

● **D11 Benign neoplasm of major salivary glands**
Excludes1 benign neoplasms of specified minor salivary glands which are classified according to their anatomical location
benign neoplasms of minor salivary glands NOS (D10.39)

D11.0 Benign neoplasm of parotid gland

D11.7 Benign neoplasm of other major salivary glands
Benign neoplasm of sublingual salivary gland
Benign neoplasm of submandibular salivary gland

D11.9 Benign neoplasm of major salivary gland, unspecified

● **D12 Benign neoplasm of colon, rectum, anus and anal canal**
Excludes1 benign carcinoid tumors of the large intestine, and rectum (D3A.02-)
Coding Clinic: 2015, Q2, P14

D12.0 Benign neoplasm of cecum
Benign neoplasm of ileocecal valve

D12.1 Benign neoplasm of appendix
Excludes1 benign carcinoid tumor of the appendix (D3A.020)

D12.2 Benign neoplasm of ascending colon

D12.3 Benign neoplasm of transverse colon
Benign neoplasm of hepatic flexure
Benign neoplasm of splenic flexure
Flexure is a bending in a structure or organ. Note the three flexures illustrated in Figure 2–17. Hepatic = liver, sigmoid = colon, splenic = spleen.

D12.4 Benign neoplasm of descending colon
Coding Clinic: 2015, Q2, P14

D12.5 Benign neoplasm of sigmoid colon

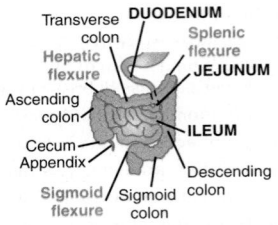

Figure 2-17 Small intestine and colon.

D12.6 Benign neoplasm of colon, unspecified
Adenomatosis of colon
Benign neoplasm of large intestine NOS
Polyposis (hereditary) of colon
Excludes1 inflammatory polyp of colon (K51.4-)
polyp of colon NOS (K63.5)

D12.7 Benign neoplasm of rectosigmoid junction
Angle where sigmoid colon becomes rectum

D12.8 Benign neoplasm of rectum
Excludes1 benign carcinoid tumor of the rectum (D3A.026)

D12.9 Benign neoplasm of anus and anal canal
Benign neoplasm of anus NOS
Excludes1 benign neoplasm of anal margin (D22.5, D23.5)
benign neoplasm of anal skin (D22.5, D23.5)
benign neoplasm of perianal skin (D22.5, D23.5)

● **D13 Benign neoplasm of other and ill-defined parts of digestive system**
Excludes1 benign stromal tumors of digestive system (D21.4)

D13.0 Benign neoplasm of esophagus

D13.1 Benign neoplasm of stomach
Excludes1 benign carcinoid tumor of the stomach (D3A.092)

D13.2 Benign neoplasm of duodenum
Excludes1 benign carcinoid tumor of the duodenum (D3A.010)

● **D13.3 Benign neoplasm of other and unspecified parts of small intestine**
Excludes1 benign carcinoid tumors of the small intestine (D3A.01-)
benign neoplasm of ileocecal valve (D12.0)

D13.30 Benign neoplasm of unspecified part of small intestine

D13.39 Benign neoplasm of other parts of small intestine

D13.4 Benign neoplasm of liver
Benign neoplasm of intrahepatic bile ducts

D13.5 Benign neoplasm of extrahepatic bile ducts
Extensions of common hepatic bile duct (tube that collects bile from liver)

D13.6 Benign neoplasm of pancreas
Excludes1 benign neoplasm of endocrine pancreas (D13.7)

D13.7 Benign neoplasm of endocrine pancreas
Pancreatic islets: Cells scattered throughout pancreas
Islet cell tumor
Benign neoplasm of islets of Langerhans
Use additional code to identify any functional activity.

D13.9 Benign neoplasm of ill-defined sites within the digestive system
Benign neoplasm of digestive system NOS
Benign neoplasm of intestine NOS
Benign neoplasm of spleen

D14 Benign neoplasm of middle ear and respiratory system

D14.0 Benign neoplasm of middle ear, nasal cavity and accessory sinuses

Benign neoplasm of cartilage of nose

Excludes1 benign neoplasm of auricular canal (external) (D22.2-, D23.2-)
benign neoplasm of bone of ear (D16.4)
benign neoplasm of bone of nose (D16.4)
benign neoplasm of cartilage of ear (D21.0)
benign neoplasm of ear (external) (skin) (D22.2-, D23.2-)
benign neoplasm of nose NOS (D36.7)
benign neoplasm of skin of nose (D22.39, D23.39)
benign neoplasm of olfactory bulb (D33.3)
benign neoplasm of posterior margin of septum and choanae (D10.6)
polyp of accessory sinus (J33.8)
polyp of ear (middle) (H74.4)
polyp of nasal (cavity) (J33.-)

D14.1 Benign neoplasm of larynx

Adenomatous polyp of larynx
Benign neoplasm of epiglottis (suprahyoid portion)
Horseshoe shaped bone in anterior midline of neck between chin and thyroid cartilage

Excludes1 benign neoplasm of epiglottis, anterior aspect (D10.5)
polyp (nonadenomatous) of vocal cord or larynx (J38.1)

D14.2 Benign neoplasm of trachea

D14.3 Benign neoplasm of bronchus and lung

Excludes1 benign carcinoid tumor of the bronchus and lung (D3A.090)

D14.30 Benign neoplasm of unspecified bronchus and lung

D14.31 Benign neoplasm of right bronchus and lung

D14.32 Benign neoplasm of left bronchus and lung

D14.4 Benign neoplasm of respiratory system, unspecified

D15 Benign neoplasm of other and unspecified intrathoracic organs

Excludes1 benign neoplasm of mesothelial tissue (D19.-)

D15.0 Benign neoplasm of thymus

Excludes1 benign carcinoid tumor of the thymus (D3A.091)

D15.1 Benign neoplasm of heart

Excludes1 benign neoplasm of great vessels (D21.3)

D15.2 Benign neoplasm of mediastinum

D15.7 Benign neoplasm of other specified intrathoracic organs

D15.9 Benign neoplasm of intrathoracic organ, unspecified

D16 Benign neoplasm of bone and articular cartilage

Excludes1 benign neoplasm of connective tissue of ear (D21.0)
benign neoplasm of connective tissue of eyelid (D21.0)
benign neoplasm of connective tissue of larynx (D14.1)
benign neoplasm of connective tissue of nose (D14.0)
benign neoplasm of synovia (D21.-)

D16.0 Benign neoplasm of scapula and long bones of upper limb

D16.00 Benign neoplasm of scapula and long bones of unspecified upper limb

D16.01 Benign neoplasm of scapula and long bones of right upper limb

D16.02 Benign neoplasm of scapula and long bones of left upper limb

D16.1 Benign neoplasm of short bones of upper limb

D16.10 Benign neoplasm of short bones of unspecified upper limb

D16.11 Benign neoplasm of short bones of right upper limb

D16.12 Benign neoplasm of short bones of left upper limb

D16.2 Benign neoplasm of long bones of lower limb

D16.20 Benign neoplasm of long bones of unspecified lower limb

D16.21 Benign neoplasm of long bones of right lower limb

D16.22 Benign neoplasm of long bones of left lower limb

D16.3 Benign neoplasm of short bones of lower limb

D16.30 Benign neoplasm of short bones of unspecified lower limb

D16.31 Benign neoplasm of short bones of right lower limb

D16.32 Benign neoplasm of short bones of left lower limb

D16.4 Benign neoplasm of bones of skull and face

Benign neoplasm of maxilla (superior)
Benign neoplasm of orbital bone
Cavity or socket of skull in which eye and its appendages are located
Keratocyst of maxilla
Keratocystic odontogenic tumor of maxilla

Excludes2 benign neoplasm of lower jaw bone (D16.5) ◀

D16.5 Benign neoplasm of lower jaw bone

Keratocyst of mandible
Keratocystic odontogenic tumor of mandible

D16.6 Benign neoplasm of vertebral column

Excludes1 benign neoplasm of sacrum and coccyx (D16.8)

D16.7 Benign neoplasm of ribs, sternum and clavicle

D16.8 Benign neoplasm of pelvic bones, sacrum and coccyx

D16.9 Benign neoplasm of bone and articular cartilage, unspecified

D17 Benign lipomatous neoplasm

Slow-growing benign tumors (rubbery masses) of mature fat cells enclosed in a thin fibrous capsule

D17.0 Benign lipomatous neoplasm of skin and subcutaneous tissue of head, face and neck

D17.1 Benign lipomatous neoplasm of skin and subcutaneous tissue of trunk

D17.2 Benign lipomatous neoplasm of skin and subcutaneous tissue of limb

D17.20 Benign lipomatous neoplasm of skin and subcutaneous tissue of unspecified limb

D17.21 Benign lipomatous neoplasm of skin and subcutaneous tissue of right arm

D17.22 Benign lipomatous neoplasm of skin and subcutaneous tissue of left arm

D17.23 Benign lipomatous neoplasm of skin and subcutaneous tissue of right leg

D17.24 Benign lipomatous neoplasm of skin and subcutaneous tissue of left leg

D17.3 Benign lipomatous neoplasm of skin and subcutaneous tissue of other and unspecified sites

D17.30 Benign lipomatous neoplasm of skin and subcutaneous tissue of unspecified sites

D17.39 Benign lipomatous neoplasm of skin and subcutaneous tissue of other sites

D17.4 Benign lipomatous neoplasm of intrathoracic organs

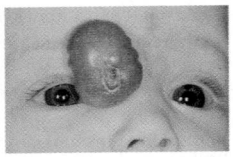

Figure 2-18 Hemangioma of skin and subcutaneous tissue. (From Yanoff: Ophthalmology, ed 3, Mosby, Inc., 2008)

Item 2–10 Hemangiomas are abnormally dense collections of dilated capillaries that occur on the skin or in internal organs. Hemangiomas are both deep and superficial and undergo a rapid growth phase when the size increases rapidly, followed by a rest phase, in which the tumor changes very little, followed by an involutional phase in which the tumor begins to and can disappear altogether. **Lymphangiomas** or cystic hygroma are benign collections of overgrown lymph vessels and, although rare, may occur anywhere but most commonly on the head and neck of children and infants. Visceral organs, lungs, and gastrointestinal tract may also be involved.

D17.5 Benign lipomatous neoplasm of intra-abdominal organs
Excludes1 benign lipomatous neoplasm of peritoneum and retroperitoneum (D17.79)

D17.6 Benign lipomatous neoplasm of spermatic cord ♂

● **D17.7 Benign lipomatous neoplasm of other sites**
- **D17.71 Benign lipomatous neoplasm of kidney**
- **D17.72 Benign lipomatous neoplasm of other genitourinary organ**
- **D17.79 Benign lipomatous neoplasm of other sites**
  Benign lipomatous neoplasm of peritoneum
  Benign lipomatous neoplasm of retroperitoneum

D17.9 Benign lipomatous neoplasm, unspecified
Lipoma NOS

● **D18 Hemangioma and lymphangioma, any site**
Excludes1 benign neoplasm of glomus jugulare (D35.6)
blue or pigmented nevus (D22.-)
nevus NOS (D22.-)
vascular nevus (Q82.5)

● **D18.0 Hemangioma**
Common type of vascular malformation
Angioma NOS
Cavernous nevus
- **D18.00 Hemangioma unspecified site**
- **D18.01 Hemangioma of skin and subcutaneous tissue**
- **D18.02 Hemangioma of intracranial structures**
- **D18.03 Hemangioma of intra-abdominal structures**
- **D18.09 Hemangioma of other sites**

D18.1 Lymphangioma, any site

● **D19 Benign neoplasm of mesothelial tissue**
Mesothelial tissue is the membrane lining several body cavities
- **D19.0 Benign neoplasm of mesothelial tissue of pleura**
- **D19.1 Benign neoplasm of mesothelial tissue of peritoneum**
- **D19.7 Benign neoplasm of mesothelial tissue of other sites**
- **D19.9 Benign neoplasm of mesothelial tissue, unspecified**
  Benign mesothelioma NOS

● **D20 Benign neoplasm of soft tissue of retroperitoneum and peritoneum**
Excludes1 benign lipomatous neoplasm of peritoneum and retroperitoneum (D17.79)
benign neoplasm of mesothelial tissue (D19.-)
- **D20.0 Benign neoplasm of soft tissue of retroperitoneum**
- **D20.1 Benign neoplasm of soft tissue of peritoneum**

● **D21 Other benign neoplasms of connective and other soft tissue**
Includes benign neoplasm of blood vessel
benign neoplasm of bursa
benign neoplasm of cartilage
benign neoplasm of fascia
benign neoplasm of fat
benign neoplasm of ligament, except uterine
benign neoplasm of lymphatic channel
benign neoplasm of muscle
benign neoplasm of synovia
benign neoplasm of tendon (sheath)
benign stromal tumors
Excludes1 benign neoplasm of articular cartilage (D16.-)
benign neoplasm of cartilage of larynx (D14.1)
benign neoplasm of cartilage of nose (D14.0)
benign neoplasm of connective tissue of breast (D24.-)
benign neoplasm of peripheral nerves and autonomic nervous system (D36.1-)
benign neoplasm of peritoneum (D20.1)
benign neoplasm of retroperitoneum (D20.0)
benign neoplasm of uterine ligament, any (D28.2)
benign neoplasm of vascular tissue (D18.-)
hemangioma (D18.0-)
lipomatous neoplasm (D17.-)
lymphangioma (D18.1)
uterine leiomyoma (D25.-)

D21.0 Benign neoplasm of connective and other soft tissue of head, face and neck
Benign neoplasm of connective tissue of ear
Benign neoplasm of connective tissue of eyelid
Excludes1 benign neoplasm of connective tissue of orbit (D31.6-)

● **D21.1 Benign neoplasm of connective and other soft tissue of upper limb, including shoulder**
- **D21.10 Benign neoplasm of connective and other soft tissue of unspecified upper limb, including shoulder**
- **D21.11 Benign neoplasm of connective and other soft tissue of right upper limb, including shoulder**
- **D21.12 Benign neoplasm of connective and other soft tissue of left upper limb, including shoulder**

● **D21.2 Benign neoplasm of connective and other soft tissue of lower limb, including hip**
- **D21.20 Benign neoplasm of connective and other soft tissue of unspecified lower limb, including hip**
- **D21.21 Benign neoplasm of connective and other soft tissue of right lower limb, including hip**
- **D21.22 Benign neoplasm of connective and other soft tissue of left lower limb, including hip**

D21.3 Benign neoplasm of connective and other soft tissue of thorax
Benign neoplasm of axilla
Benign neoplasm of diaphragm
Benign neoplasm of great vessels
Excludes1 benign neoplasm of heart (D15.1)
benign neoplasm of mediastinum (D15.2)
benign neoplasm of thymus (D15.0)

D21.4 Benign neoplasm of connective and other soft tissue of abdomen Benign stromal tumors of abdomen

D21.5 Benign neoplasm of connective and other soft tissue of pelvis
Excludes1 benign neoplasm of any uterine ligament (D28.2)
uterine leiomyoma (D25.-)

D21.6 Benign neoplasm of connective and other soft tissue of trunk, unspecified
Benign neoplasm of back NOS

D21.9 Benign neoplasm of connective and other soft tissue, unspecified

◀ New ◀ Revised ~~deleted~~ Deleted Excludes 1 Excludes 2 Includes Use additional Code first Code also Unspecified
OGCR Official Guidelines ● Unacceptable Principal Diagnosis X Assign placeholder X ● Use Additional Character(s) ▶ Manifestation Code Coding Clinic

D22 Melanocytic nevi

Includes atypical nevus
blue hairy pigmented nevus
nevus NOS

D22.0 Melanocytic nevi of lip
Skin lesions composed of nests of nevus cells with macules/papules

D22.1 Melanocytic nevi of eyelid, including canthus
- **D22.10 Melanocytic nevi of unspecified eyelid, including canthus**
- **D22.11 Melanocytic nevi of right eyelid, including canthus**
- **D22.12 Melanocytic nevi of left eyelid, including canthus**

D22.2 Melanocytic nevi of ear and external auricular canal
- **D22.20 Melanocytic nevi of unspecified ear and external auricular canal**
- **D22.21 Melanocytic nevi of right ear and external auricular canal**
- **D22.22 Melanocytic nevi of left ear and external auricular canal**

D22.3 Melanocytic nevi of other and unspecified parts of face
- **D22.30 Melanocytic nevi of unspecified part of face**
- **D22.39 Melanocytic nevi of other parts of face**

D22.4 Melanocytic nevi of scalp and neck

D22.5 Melanocytic nevi of trunk
Melanocytic nevi of anal margin
Melanocytic nevi of anal skin
Melanocytic nevi of perianal skin
Melanocytic nevi of skin of breast

D22.6 Melanocytic nevi of upper limb, including shoulder
- **D22.60 Melanocytic nevi of unspecified upper limb, including shoulder**
- **D22.61 Melanocytic nevi of right upper limb, including shoulder**
- **D22.62 Melanocytic nevi of left upper limb, including shoulder**

D22.7 Melanocytic nevi of lower limb, including hip
- **D22.70 Melanocytic nevi of unspecified lower limb, including hip**
- **D22.71 Melanocytic nevi of right lower limb, including hip**
- **D22.72 Melanocytic nevi of left lower limb, including hip**

D22.9 Melanocytic nevi, unspecified

D23 Other benign neoplasms of skin

Includes benign neoplasm of hair follicles
benign neoplasm of sebaceous glands
benign neoplasm of sweat glands

Excludes1 benign lipomatous neoplasms of skin (D17.0-D17.3)
melanocytic nevi (D22.-)

D23.0 Other benign neoplasm of skin of lip
Excludes1 benign neoplasm of vermilion border of lip (D10.0)

D23.1 Other benign neoplasm of skin of eyelid, including canthus
- **D23.10 Other benign neoplasm of skin unspecified of eyelid, including canthus**
- **D23.11 Other benign neoplasm of skin of right eyelid, including canthus**
- **D23.12 Other benign neoplasm of skin of left eyelid, including canthus**

D23.2 Other benign neoplasm of skin of ear and external auricular canal
- **D23.20 Other benign neoplasm of skin of unspecified ear and external auricular canal**
- **D23.21 Other benign neoplasm of skin of right ear and external auricular canal**
- **D23.22 Other benign neoplasm of skin of left ear and external auricular canal**

D23.3 Other benign neoplasm of skin of other and unspecified parts of face
- **D23.30 Other benign neoplasm of skin of unspecified part of face**
- **D23.39 Other benign neoplasm of skin of other parts of face**

D23.4 Other benign neoplasm of skin of scalp and neck

D23.5 Other benign neoplasm of skin of trunk
Other benign neoplasm of anal margin
Other benign neoplasm of anal skin
Other benign neoplasm of perianal skin
Other benign neoplasm of skin of breast
Excludes1 benign neoplasm of anus NOS (D12.9)

D23.6 Other benign neoplasm of skin of upper limb, including shoulder
- **D23.60 Other benign neoplasm of skin of unspecified upper limb, including shoulder**
- **D23.61 Other benign neoplasm of skin of right upper limb, including shoulder**
- **D23.62 Other benign neoplasm of skin of left upper limb, including shoulder**

D23.7 Other benign neoplasm of skin of lower limb, including hip
- **D23.70 Other benign neoplasm of skin of unspecified lower limb, including hip**
- **D23.71 Other benign neoplasm of skin of right lower limb, including hip**
- **D23.72 Other benign neoplasm of skin of left lower limb, including hip**

D23.9 Other benign neoplasm of skin, unspecified

D24 Benign neoplasm of breast

Includes benign neoplasm of connective tissue of breast
benign neoplasm of soft parts of breast
fibroadenoma of breast

Excludes2 adenofibrosis of breast (N60.2)
benign cyst of breast (N60.-)
benign mammary dysplasia (N60.-)
benign neoplasm of skin of breast (D22.5, D23.5)
fibrocystic disease of breast (N60.-)

D24.1 Benign neoplasm of right breast

D24.2 Benign neoplasm of left breast

D24.9 Benign neoplasm of unspecified breast

D25 Leiomyoma of uterus
Benign tumors or nodules of the uterine wall

Includes uterine fibroid
uterine fibromyoma
uterine myoma

D25.0 Submucous leiomyoma of uterus ♀

D25.1 Intramural leiomyoma of uterus ♀
Interstitial leiomyoma of uterus

D25.2 Subserosal leiomyoma of uterus ♀
Subperitoneal leiomyoma of uterus

D25.9 Leiomyoma of uterus, unspecified ♀

D26 Other benign neoplasms of uterus
- **D26.0 Other benign neoplasm of cervix uteri ♀**
- **D26.1 Other benign neoplasm of corpus uteri ♀**
- **D26.7 Other benign neoplasm of other parts of uterus ♀**
- **D26.9 Other benign neoplasm of uterus, unspecified ♀**

Item 2–11 Teratoma: terat = monster, oma = mass, tumor. Alternate terms: dermoid cyst of the ovary, ovarian teratoma. Teratomas are neoplasms and arise from germ cells (ovaries in female and testes in male) and can be benign or malignant. Teratomas have been known to contain hair, nails, and teeth, giving them a bizarre ("monster") appearance.

● **D27 Benign neoplasm of ovary**

Use additional code to identify any functional activity.

Excludes2 corpus albicans cyst (N83.2-)
corpus luteum cyst (N83.1-)
endometrial cyst (N80.1)
follicular (atretic) cyst (N83.0-)
graafian follicle cyst (N83.0-)
ovarian cyst NEC (N83.2-)
ovarian retention cyst (N83.2-)

D27.0 Benign neoplasm of right ovary ♀

D27.1 Benign neoplasm of left ovary ♀

D27.9 Benign neoplasm of unspecified ovary ♀

● **D28 Benign neoplasm of other and unspecified female genital organs**

Includes adenomatous polyp
benign neoplasm of skin of female genital organs
benign teratoma

Excludes1 epoophoron cyst (Q50.5)
fimbrial cyst (Q50.4)
Gartner's duct cyst (Q52.4)
parovarian cyst (Q50.5)

D28.0 Benign neoplasm of vulva ♀

D28.1 Benign neoplasm of vagina ♀

D28.2 Benign neoplasm of uterine tubes and ligaments ♀
Benign neoplasm of fallopian tube
Benign neoplasm of uterine ligament (broad) (round)

D28.7 Benign neoplasm of other specified female genital organs ♀

D28.9 Benign neoplasm of female genital organ, unspecified ♀

● **D29 Benign neoplasm of male genital organs**

Includes benign neoplasm of skin of male genital organs

D29.0 Benign neoplasm of penis ♂

D29.1 Benign neoplasm of prostate ♂

Excludes1 enlarged prostate (N40.-)

● **D29.2 Benign neoplasm of testis**

Use additional code to identify any functional activity.

D29.20 Benign neoplasm of unspecified testis ♂

D29.21 Benign neoplasm of right testis ♂

D29.22 Benign neoplasm of left testis ♂

● **D29.3 Benign neoplasm of epididymis**

D29.30 Benign neoplasm of unspecified epididymis ♂

D29.31 Benign neoplasm of right epididymis ♂

D29.32 Benign neoplasm of left epididymis ♂

D29.4 Benign neoplasm of scrotum ♂
Benign neoplasm of skin of scrotum

D29.8 Benign neoplasm of other specified male genital organs ♂
Benign neoplasm of seminal vesicle
Benign neoplasm of spermatic cord
Benign neoplasm of tunica vaginalis

D29.9 Benign neoplasm of male genital organ, unspecified ♂

● **D30 Benign neoplasm of urinary organs**

● **D30.0 Benign neoplasm of kidney**

Excludes1 benign carcinoid tumor of the kidney (D3A.093)
benign neoplasm of renal calyces (D30.1-)
benign neoplasm of renal pelvis (D30.1-)

D30.00 Benign neoplasm of unspecified kidney

D30.01 Benign neoplasm of right kidney

D30.02 Benign neoplasm of left kidney

● **D30.1 Benign neoplasm of renal pelvis**

D30.10 Benign neoplasm of unspecified renal pelvis

D30.11 Benign neoplasm of right renal pelvis

D30.12 Benign neoplasm of left renal pelvis

● **D30.2 Benign neoplasm of ureter**

Excludes1 benign neoplasm of ureteric orifice of bladder (D30.3)

D30.20 Benign neoplasm of unspecified ureter

D30.21 Benign neoplasm of right ureter

D30.22 Benign neoplasm of left ureter

D30.3 Benign neoplasm of bladder
Benign neoplasm of ureteric orifice of bladder
Benign neoplasm of urethral orifice of bladder

D30.4 Benign neoplasm of urethra

Excludes1 benign neoplasm of urethral orifice of bladder (D30.3)

D30.8 Benign neoplasm of other specified urinary organs
Benign neoplasm of paraurethral glands

D30.9 Benign neoplasm of urinary organ, unspecified
Benign neoplasm of urinary system NOS

● **D31 Benign neoplasm of eye and adnexa**

Excludes1 benign neoplasm of connective tissue of eyelid (D21.0)
benign neoplasm of optic nerve (D33.3)
benign neoplasm of skin of eyelid (D22.1-, D23.1-)

● **D31.0 Benign neoplasm of conjunctiva**

D31.00 Benign neoplasm of unspecified conjunctiva

D31.01 Benign neoplasm of right conjunctiva

D31.02 Benign neoplasm of left conjunctiva

● **D31.1 Benign neoplasm of cornea**

D31.10 Benign neoplasm of unspecified cornea

D31.11 Benign neoplasm of right cornea

D31.12 Benign neoplasm of left cornea

● **D31.2 Benign neoplasm of retina**

Excludes1 dark area on retina (D49.81)
hemangioma of retina (D49.81)
neoplasm of unspecified behavior of retina and choroid (D49.81)
retinal freckle (D49.81)

D31.20 Benign neoplasm of unspecified retina

D31.21 Benign neoplasm of right retina

D31.22 Benign neoplasm of left retina

● **D31.3 Benign neoplasm of choroid**

D31.30 Benign neoplasm of unspecified choroid

D31.31 Benign neoplasm of right choroid

D31.32 Benign neoplasm of left choroid

● **D31.4 Benign neoplasm of ciliary body**

D31.40 Benign neoplasm of unspecified ciliary body

D31.41 Benign neoplasm of right ciliary body

D31.42 Benign neoplasm of left ciliary body

● **D31.5 Benign neoplasm of lacrimal gland and duct**
Benign neoplasm of lacrimal sac
Benign neoplasm of nasolacrimal duct

D31.50 Benign neoplasm of unspecified lacrimal gland and duct

D31.51 Benign neoplasm of right lacrimal gland and duct

D31.52 Benign neoplasm of left lacrimal gland and duct

● **D31.6 Benign neoplasm of unspecified site of orbit**
Benign neoplasm of connective tissue of orbit
Benign neoplasm of extraocular muscle
Benign neoplasm of peripheral nerves of orbit
Benign neoplasm of retrobulbar tissue
Benign neoplasm of retro-ocular tissue

Excludes1 benign neoplasm of orbital bone (D16.4)

D31.60 Benign neoplasm of unspecified site of unspecified orbit

D31.61 Benign neoplasm of unspecified site of right orbit

D31.62 Benign neoplasm of unspecified site of left orbit

● **D31.9 Benign neoplasm of unspecified part of eye**
Benign neoplasm of eyeball

D31.90 Benign neoplasm of unspecified part of unspecified eye

D31.91 Benign neoplasm of unspecified part of right eye

D31.92 Benign neoplasm of unspecified part of left eye

● **D32 Benign neoplasm of meninges**

D32.0 Benign neoplasm of cerebral meninges

D32.1 Benign neoplasm of spinal meninges

D32.9 Benign neoplasm of meninges, unspecified
Meningioma NOS

● **D33 Benign neoplasm of brain and other parts of central nervous system**

Excludes1 angioma (D18.0-)
benign neoplasm of meninges (D32.-)
benign neoplasm of peripheral nerves and autonomic nervous system (D36.1-)
hemangioma (D18.0-)
neurofibromatosis (Q85.0-)
retro-ocular benign neoplasm (D31.6-)

D33.0 Benign neoplasm of brain, supratentorial
Benign neoplasm of cerebral ventricle
Benign neoplasm of cerebrum
Benign neoplasm of frontal lobe
Benign neoplasm of occipital lobe
Benign neoplasm of parietal lobe
Benign neoplasm of temporal lobe

Excludes1 benign neoplasm of fourth ventricle (D33.1)

D33.1 Benign neoplasm of brain, infratentorial
Benign neoplasm of brain stem
Benign neoplasm of cerebellum
Benign neoplasm of fourth ventricle

D33.2 Benign neoplasm of brain, unspecified

D33.3 Benign neoplasm of cranial nerves
Benign neoplasm of olfactory bulb

D33.4 Benign neoplasm of spinal cord

D33.7 Benign neoplasm of other specified parts of central nervous system

D33.9 Benign neoplasm of central nervous system, unspecified
Benign neoplasm of nervous system (central) NOS

D34 Benign neoplasm of thyroid gland
Use additional code to identify any functional activity.

● **D35 Benign neoplasm of other and unspecified endocrine glands**
Use additional code to identify any functional activity.

Excludes1 benign neoplasm of endocrine pancreas (D13.7)
benign neoplasm of ovary (D27.-)
benign neoplasm of testis (D29.2.-)
benign neoplasm of thymus (D15.0)

● **D35.0 Benign neoplasm of adrenal gland**

D35.00 Benign neoplasm of unspecified adrenal gland

D35.01 Benign neoplasm of right adrenal gland

D35.02 Benign neoplasm of left adrenal gland

D35.1 Benign neoplasm of parathyroid gland

D35.2 Benign neoplasm of pituitary gland

D35.3 Benign neoplasm of craniopharyngeal duct

D35.4 Benign neoplasm of pineal gland

D35.5 Benign neoplasm of carotid body

D35.6 Benign neoplasm of aortic body and other paraganglia
Benign tumor of glomus jugulare

D35.7 Benign neoplasm of other specified endocrine glands

D35.9 Benign neoplasm of endocrine gland, unspecified
Benign neoplasm of unspecified endocrine gland

● **D36 Benign neoplasm of other and unspecified sites**

D36.0 Benign neoplasm of lymph nodes

Excludes1 lymphangioma (D18.1)

● **D36.1 Benign neoplasm of peripheral nerves and autonomic nervous system**

Excludes1 benign neoplasm of peripheral nerves of orbit (D31.6-)
neurofibromatosis (Q85.0-)

D36.10 Benign neoplasm of peripheral nerves and autonomic nervous system, unspecified

D36.11 Benign neoplasm of peripheral nerves and autonomic nervous system of face, head, and neck

D36.12 Benign neoplasm of peripheral nerves and autonomic nervous system, upper limb, including shoulder

D36.13 Benign neoplasm of peripheral nerves and autonomic nervous system of lower limb, including hip

D36.14 Benign neoplasm of peripheral nerves and autonomic nervous system of thorax

D36.15 Benign neoplasm of peripheral nerves and autonomic nervous system of abdomen

D36.16 Benign neoplasm of peripheral nerves and autonomic nervous system of pelvis

D36.17 Benign neoplasm of peripheral nerves and autonomic nervous system of trunk, unspecified

D36.7 Benign neoplasm of other specified sites
Benign neoplasm of nose NOS

D36.9 Benign neoplasm, unspecified site

BENIGN NEUROENDOCRINE TUMORS (D3A)

● **D3A Benign neuroendocrine tumors**
Code also any associated multiple endocrine neoplasia [MEN] syndromes (E31.2-)
Use additional code to identify any associated endocrine syndrome, such as:
carcinoid syndrome (E34.0)

Excludes2 benign pancreatic islet cell tumors (D13.7)

● **D3A.0 Benign carcinoid tumors**

D3A.00 Benign carcinoid tumor of unspecified site
Carcinoid tumor NOS

● **D3A.01 Benign carcinoid tumors of the small intestine**

D3A.010 Benign carcinoid tumor of the duodenum

D3A.011 Benign carcinoid tumor of the jejunum

D3A.012 Benign carcinoid tumor of the ileum

D3A.019 Benign carcinoid tumor of the small intestine, unspecified portion

● **D3A.02 Benign carcinoid tumors of the appendix, large intestine, and rectum**

D3A.020 Benign carcinoid tumor of the appendix

D3A.021 Benign carcinoid tumor of the cecum

D3A.022 Benign carcinoid tumor of the ascending colon

D3A.023 Benign carcinoid tumor of the transverse colon

D3A.024 Benign carcinoid tumor of the descending colon

D3A.025 Benign carcinoid tumor of the sigmoid colon

D3A.026 Benign carcinoid tumor of the rectum

D3A.029 Benign carcinoid tumor of the large intestine, unspecified portion

Benign carcinoid tumor of the colon NOS

● **D3A.09 Benign carcinoid tumors of other sites**

D3A.090 Benign carcinoid tumor of the bronchus and lung

D3A.091 Benign carcinoid tumor of the thymus

D3A.092 Benign carcinoid tumor of the stomach

D3A.093 Benign carcinoid tumor of the kidney

D3A.094 Benign carcinoid tumor of the foregut unspecified ◄

D3A.095 Benign carcinoid tumor of the midgut unspecified ◄

D3A.096 Benign carcinoid tumor of the hindgut unspecified ◄

D3A.098 Benign carcinoid tumors of other sites

D3A.8 Other benign neuroendocrine tumors

Neuroendocrine tumor NOS

NEOPLASMS OF UNCERTAIN BEHAVIOR, POLYCYTHEMIA VERA AND MYELODYSPLASTIC SYNDROMES (D37-D48)

Note: Categories D37-D44, and D48 classify by site neoplasms of uncertain behavior, i.e., histologic confirmation whether the neoplasm is malignant or benign cannot be made.

Excludes1 neoplasms of unspecified behavior (D49.-)

● **D37 Neoplasm of uncertain behavior of oral cavity and digestive organs**

Excludes1 stromal tumors of uncertain behavior of digestive system (D48.1)

● **D37.0 Neoplasm of uncertain behavior of lip, oral cavity and pharynx**

Excludes1 neoplasm of uncertain behavior of aryepiglottic fold or interarytenoid fold, laryngeal aspect (D38.0)
neoplasm of uncertain behavior of epiglottis NOS (D38.0)
neoplasm of uncertain behavior of skin of lip (D48.5)
neoplasm of uncertain behavior of suprahyoid portion of epiglottis (D38.0)

D37.01 Neoplasm of uncertain behavior of lip

Neoplasm of uncertain behavior of vermilion border of lip

D37.02 Neoplasm of uncertain behavior of tongue

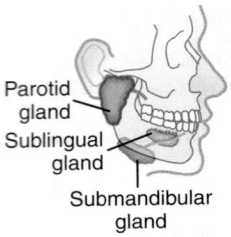

Figure 2-19 Major salivary glands.

● **D37.03 Neoplasm of uncertain behavior of the major salivary glands**

D37.030 Neoplasm of uncertain behavior of the parotid salivary glands

D37.031 Neoplasm of uncertain behavior of the sublingual salivary glands

D37.032 Neoplasm of uncertain behavior of the submandibular salivary glands

D37.039 Neoplasm of uncertain behavior of the major salivary glands, unspecified

D37.04 Neoplasm of uncertain behavior of the minor salivary glands

Neoplasm of uncertain behavior of submucosal salivary glands of lip
Neoplasm of uncertain behavior of submucosal salivary glands of cheek
Neoplasm of uncertain behavior of submucosal salivary glands of hard palate
Neoplasm of uncertain behavior of submucosal salivary glands of soft palate

D37.05 Neoplasm of uncertain behavior of pharynx

Neoplasm of uncertain behavior of aryepiglottic fold of pharynx NOS
Neoplasm of uncertain behavior of hypopharyngeal aspect of aryepiglottic fold of pharynx
Neoplasm of uncertain behavior of marginal zone of aryepiglottic fold of pharynx

D37.09 Neoplasm of uncertain behavior of other specified sites of the oral cavity

D37.1 Neoplasm of uncertain behavior of stomach

D37.2 Neoplasm of uncertain behavior of small intestine

D37.3 Neoplasm of uncertain behavior of appendix

D37.4 Neoplasm of uncertain behavior of colon

D37.5 Neoplasm of uncertain behavior of rectum

Neoplasm of uncertain behavior of rectosigmoid junction

Rectosigmoid junction: Angle where sigmoid colon becomes rectum

D37.6 Neoplasm of uncertain behavior of liver, gallbladder and bile ducts

Neoplasm of uncertain behavior of ampulla of Vater

Ampulla of Vater: Enlarged segment of ducts from liver and pancreas at entry point to small intestine

D37.8 Neoplasm of uncertain behavior of other specified digestive organs

Neoplasm of uncertain behavior of anal canal
Neoplasm of uncertain behavior of anal sphincter
Neoplasm of uncertain behavior of anus NOS
Neoplasm of uncertain behavior of esophagus
Neoplasm of uncertain behavior of intestine NOS
Neoplasm of uncertain behavior of pancreas

Excludes1 neoplasm of uncertain behavior of anal margin (D48.5)
neoplasm of uncertain behavior of anal skin (D48.5)
neoplasm of uncertain behavior of perianal skin (D48.5)

D37.9 Neoplasm of uncertain behavior of digestive organ, unspecified

D38 Neoplasm of uncertain behavior of middle ear and respiratory and intrathoracic organs

Excludes1 neoplasm of uncertain behavior of heart (D48.7)

D38.0 Neoplasm of uncertain behavior of larynx
Neoplasm of uncertain behavior of aryepiglottic fold or interarytenoid fold, laryngeal aspect
Neoplasm of uncertain behavior of epiglottis (suprahyoid portion)

Excludes1 neoplasm of uncertain behavior of aryepiglottic fold or interarytenoid fold NOS (D37.05)
neoplasm of uncertain behavior of hypopharyngeal aspect of aryepiglottic fold (D37.05)
neoplasm of uncertain behavior of marginal zone of aryepiglottic fold (D37.05)

D38.1 Neoplasm of uncertain behavior of trachea, bronchus and lung

D38.2 Neoplasm of uncertain behavior of pleura

D38.3 Neoplasm of uncertain behavior of mediastinum

D38.4 Neoplasm of uncertain behavior of thymus

D38.5 Neoplasm of uncertain behavior of other respiratory organs
Neoplasm of uncertain behavior of accessory sinuses
Neoplasm of uncertain behavior of cartilage of nose
Neoplasm of uncertain behavior of middle ear
Neoplasm of uncertain behavior of nasal cavities

Excludes1 neoplasm of uncertain behavior of ear (external) (skin) (D48.5)
neoplasm of uncertain behavior of nose NOS (D48.7)
neoplasm of uncertain behavior of skin of nose (D48.5)

D38.6 Neoplasm of uncertain behavior of respiratory organ, unspecified

D39 Neoplasm of uncertain behavior of female genital organs

D39.0 Neoplasm of uncertain behavior of uterus ♀

D39.1 Neoplasm of uncertain behavior of ovary
Use additional code to identify any functional activity.

D39.10 Neoplasm of uncertain behavior of unspecified ovary ♀

D39.11 Neoplasm of uncertain behavior of right ovary ♀

D39.12 Neoplasm of uncertain behavior of left ovary ♀

D39.2 Neoplasm of uncertain behavior of placenta ♀ M
Chorioadenoma destruens
Invasive hydatidiform mole
Malignant hydatidiform mole

Excludes1 hydatidiform mole NOS (O01.9)

D39.8 Neoplasm of uncertain behavior of other specified female genital organs ♀
Neoplasm of uncertain behavior of skin of female genital organs

D39.9 Neoplasm of uncertain behavior of female genital organ, unspecified ♀

D40 Neoplasm of uncertain behavior of male genital organs

D40.0 Neoplasm of uncertain behavior of prostate ♂

D40.1 Neoplasm of uncertain behavior of testis

D40.10 Neoplasm of uncertain behavior of unspecified testis ♂

D40.11 Neoplasm of uncertain behavior of right testis ♂

D40.12 Neoplasm of uncertain behavior of left testis ♂

D40.8 Neoplasm of uncertain behavior of other specified male genital organs ♂
Neoplasm of uncertain behavior of skin of male genital organs

D40.9 Neoplasm of uncertain behavior of male genital organ, unspecified ♂

D41 Neoplasm of uncertain behavior of urinary organs

D41.0 Neoplasm of uncertain behavior of kidney

Excludes1 neoplasm of uncertain behavior of renal pelvis (D41.1-)

D41.00 Neoplasm of uncertain behavior of unspecified kidney

D41.01 Neoplasm of uncertain behavior of right kidney

D41.02 Neoplasm of uncertain behavior of left kidney

D41.1 Neoplasm of uncertain behavior of renal pelvis

D41.10 Neoplasm of uncertain behavior of unspecified renal pelvis

D41.11 Neoplasm of uncertain behavior of right renal pelvis

D41.12 Neoplasm of uncertain behavior of left renal pelvis

D41.2 Neoplasm of uncertain behavior of ureter

D41.20 Neoplasm of uncertain behavior of unspecified ureter

D41.21 Neoplasm of uncertain behavior of right ureter

D41.22 Neoplasm of uncertain behavior of left ureter

D41.3 Neoplasm of uncertain behavior of urethra

D41.4 Neoplasm of uncertain behavior of bladder

D41.8 Neoplasm of uncertain behavior of other specified urinary organs

D41.9 Neoplasm of uncertain behavior of unspecified urinary organ

D42 Neoplasm of uncertain behavior of meninges

D42.0 Neoplasm of uncertain behavior of cerebral meninges

D42.1 Neoplasm of uncertain behavior of spinal meninges

D42.9 Neoplasm of uncertain behavior of meninges, unspecified

D43 Neoplasm of uncertain behavior of brain and central nervous system

Excludes1 neoplasm of uncertain behavior of peripheral nerves and autonomic nervous system (D48.2)

D43.0 Neoplasm of uncertain behavior of brain, supratentorial
Superior to tentorium of cerebellum
Neoplasm of uncertain behavior of cerebral ventricle
Neoplasm of uncertain behavior of cerebrum
Neoplasm of uncertain behavior of frontal lobe
Neoplasm of uncertain behavior of occipital lobe
Neoplasm of uncertain behavior of parietal lobe
Neoplasm of uncertain behavior of temporal lobe

Excludes1 neoplasm of uncertain behavior of fourth ventricle (D43.1)

D43.1 Neoplasm of uncertain behavior of brain, infratentorial
Beneath the tentorium of cerebellum
Neoplasm of uncertain behavior of brain stem
Neoplasm of uncertain behavior of cerebellum
Neoplasm of uncertain behavior of fourth ventricle

D43.2 Neoplasm of uncertain behavior of brain, unspecified

D43.3 Neoplasm of uncertain behavior of cranial nerves

D43.4 Neoplasm of uncertain behavior of spinal cord

D43.8 Neoplasm of uncertain behavior of other specified parts of central nervous system

D43.9 Neoplasm of uncertain behavior of central nervous system, unspecified
Neoplasm of uncertain behavior of nervous system (central) NOS

D44 Neoplasm of uncertain behavior of endocrine glands

Excludes1 multiple endocrine adenomatosis (E31.2-)
multiple endocrine neoplasia (E31.2-)
neoplasm of uncertain behavior of endocrine pancreas (D37.8)
neoplasm of uncertain behavior of ovary (D39.1-)
neoplasm of uncertain behavior of testis (D40.1-)
neoplasm of uncertain behavior of thymus (D38.4)

D44.0 Neoplasm of uncertain behavior of thyroid gland

D44.1 Neoplasm of uncertain behavior of adrenal gland

Use additional code to identify any functional activity.

D44.10 Neoplasm of uncertain behavior of unspecified adrenal gland

D44.11 Neoplasm of uncertain behavior of right adrenal gland

D44.12 Neoplasm of uncertain behavior of left adrenal gland

D44.2 Neoplasm of uncertain behavior of parathyroid gland

D44.3 Neoplasm of uncertain behavior of pituitary gland

Use additional code to identify any functional activity.

D44.4 Neoplasm of uncertain behavior of craniopharyngeal duct

D44.5 Neoplasm of uncertain behavior of pineal gland

D44.6 Neoplasm of uncertain behavior of carotid body

D44.7 Neoplasm of uncertain behavior of aortic body and other paraganglia

D44.9 Neoplasm of uncertain behavior of unspecified endocrine gland

D45 Polycythemia vera

Excludes1 familial polycythemia (D75.0)
secondary polycythemia (D75.1)

Primary polycythemia. Secondary polycythemia is D75.1. Check your documentation. Polycythemia is caused by too many red blood cells, which increase the thickness of blood (viscosity). This can cause engorgement of the spleen (splenomegaly) with extra RBCs and potential clot formation.

D46 Myelodysplastic syndromes

Use additional code for adverse effect, if applicable, to identify drug (T36-T50 with fifth or sixth character 5)

Excludes2 drug-induced aplastic anemia (D61.1)

D46.0 Refractory anemia without ring sideroblasts, so stated

Refractory anemia without sideroblasts, without excess of blasts

D46.1 Refractory anemia with ring sideroblasts RARS

D46.2 Refractory anemia with excess of blasts [RAEB]

Form of myelodysplasia with increased immature white blood cells (blasts) in bone marrow

D46.20 Refractory anemia with excess of blasts, unspecified RAEB NOS

D46.21 Refractory anemia with excess of blasts 1 RAEB 1

Bone marrow disease which results in insufficient RBCs (anemia) in which level of blasts is less than 10%

D46.22 Refractory anemia with excess of blasts 2 RAEB 2

Bone marrow disease manifested by insufficient numbers of RBCs (anemia) with level of blasts 10-20%

Ex: See C94.4

D46.A Refractory cytopenia with multilineage dysplasia

D46.B Refractory cytopenia with multilineage dysplasia and ring sideroblasts

RCMD RS

D46.C Myelodysplastic syndrome with isolated del(5q) chromosomal abnormality

Myelodysplastic syndrome with 5q deletion
5q minus syndrome NOS

Ex: See C94.4

D46.4 Refractory anemia, unspecified

D46.Z Other myelodysplastic syndromes

Excludes1 chronic myelomonocytic leukemia (C93.1-)

D46.9 Myelodysplastic syndrome, unspecified

Myelodysplasia NOS

D47 Other neoplasms of uncertain behavior of lymphoid, hematopoietic and related tissue

D47.0 Histiocytic and mast cell tumors of uncertain behavior

Indolent systemic mastocytosis
Mast cell tumor NOS
Mastocytoma NOS

Excludes1 malignant mast cell tumor (C96.2)
mastocytosis (congenital) (cutaneous) (Q82.2)

Ex: C88.8, C94.40-C94.42, C94.6, D45-D46.22, D46.4, D46.9, D46.A-D46.C, D46.Z, D47.0-D47.1, D47.3, D47.9, D47.Z2, D47.Z9, D75.81, Z51.0

D47.1 Chronic myeloproliferative disease

Chronic neutrophilic leukemia
Myeloproliferative disease, unspecified

Excludes1 atypical chronic myeloid leukemia BCR/ABL-negative (C92.2-)
chronic myeloid leukemia BCR/ABL-positive (C92.1-)
myelofibrosis NOS (D75.81)
myelophthisic anemia (D61.82)
myelophthisis (D61.82)
secondary myelofibrosis NOS (D75.81)

Ex: See C94.4

D47.2 Monoclonal gammopathy

Monoclonal gammopathy of undetermined significance [MGUS]

D47.3 Essential (hemorrhagic) thrombocythemia

Essential thrombocytosis
Idiopathic hemorrhagic thrombocythemia

D47.4 Osteomyelofibrosis

Chronic idiopathic myelofibrosis
Myelofibrosis (idiopathic) (with myeloid metaplasia)
Myelosclerosis (megakaryocytic) with myeloid metaplasia
Secondary myelofibrosis in myeloproliferative disease

Excludes1 acute myelofibrosis (C94.4-)

D47.Z Other specified neoplasms of uncertain behavior of lymphoid, hematopoietic and related tissue

D47.Z1 Post-transplant lymphoproliferative disorder (PTLD)

Code first complications of transplanted organs and tissue (T86.-)

Ex: D47.Z1, D78.81-D78.89, E89.810-E89.89, H59.011-H59.019, H59.031-H59.099, H59.811-H59.89, H95.811-H95.89, I97.3, M96.89, N98.1-N98.9, T86.850-T86.99

D47.Z2 Castleman disease

Code also if applicable human herpesvirus 8 infection (B10.89)

Excludes2 Kaposi's sarcoma (C46-)

Ex: See C94.4

D47.Z9 Other specified neoplasms of uncertain behavior of lymphoid, hematopoietic and related tissue

Histiocytic tumors of uncertain behavior

Ex: See C94.4

D47.9 Neoplasm of uncertain behavior of lymphoid, hematopoietic and related tissue, unspecified

Lymphoproliferative disease NOS

Ex: See C94.4

D48 Neoplasm of uncertain behavior of other and unspecified sites

Excludes1 neurofibromatosis (nonmalignant) (Q85.0-)

D48.0 Neoplasm of uncertain behavior of bone and articular cartilage

Excludes1 neoplasm of uncertain behavior of cartilage of ear (D48.1)
neoplasm of uncertain behavior of cartilage of larynx (D38.0)
neoplasm of uncertain behavior of cartilage of nose (D38.5)
neoplasm of uncertain behavior of connective tissue of eyelid (D48.1)
neoplasm of uncertain behavior of synovia (D48.1)

D48.1 Neoplasm of uncertain behavior of connective and other soft tissue

Neoplasm of uncertain behavior of connective tissue of ear
Neoplasm of uncertain behavior of connective tissue of eyelid
Stromal tumors of uncertain behavior of digestive system

Excludes1 neoplasm of uncertain behavior of articular cartilage (D48.0)
neoplasm of uncertain behavior of cartilage of larynx (D38.0)
neoplasm of uncertain behavior of cartilage of nose (D38.5)
neoplasm of uncertain behavior of connective tissue of breast (D48.6-)

D48.2 Neoplasm of uncertain behavior of peripheral nerves and autonomic nervous system

Excludes1 neoplasm of uncertain behavior of peripheral nerves of orbit (D48.7)

D48.3 Neoplasm of uncertain behavior of retroperitoneum

D48.4 Neoplasm of uncertain behavior of peritoneum

D48.5 Neoplasm of uncertain behavior of skin

Neoplasm of uncertain behavior of anal margin
Neoplasm of uncertain behavior of anal skin
Neoplasm of uncertain behavior of perianal skin
Neoplasm of uncertain behavior of skin of breast

Excludes1 neoplasm of uncertain behavior of anus NOS (D37.8)
neoplasm of uncertain behavior of skin of genital organs (D39.8, D40.8)
neoplasm of uncertain behavior of vermilion border of lip (D37.0)

D48.6 Neoplasm of uncertain behavior of breast

Neoplasm of uncertain behavior of connective tissue of breast
Cystosarcoma phyllodes

Excludes1 neoplasm of uncertain behavior of skin of breast (D48.5)

D48.60 Neoplasm of uncertain behavior of unspecified breast

D48.61 Neoplasm of uncertain behavior of right breast

D48.62 Neoplasm of uncertain behavior of left breast

D48.7 Neoplasm of uncertain behavior of other specified sites

Neoplasm of uncertain behavior of eye
Neoplasm of uncertain behavior of heart
Neoplasm of uncertain behavior of peripheral nerves of orbit

Excludes1 neoplasm of uncertain behavior of connective tissue (D48.1)
neoplasm of uncertain behavior of skin of eyelid (D48.5)

D48.9 Neoplasm of uncertain behavior, unspecified

D49 Neoplasms of unspecified behavior

Note: Category D49 classifies by site neoplasms of unspecified morphology and behavior. The term 'mass,' unless otherwise stated, is not to be regarded as a neoplastic growth.

Includes 'growth' NOS
neoplasm NOS
new growth NOS
tumor NOS

Excludes1 neoplasms of uncertain behavior (D37-D44, D48)

D49.0 Neoplasm of unspecified behavior of digestive system

Excludes1 neoplasm of unspecified behavior of margin of anus (D49.2)
neoplasm of unspecified behavior of perianal skin (D49.2)
neoplasm of unspecified behavior of skin of anus (D49.2)

D49.1 Neoplasm of unspecified behavior of respiratory system

D49.2 Neoplasm of unspecified behavior of bone, soft tissue, and skin

Excludes1 neoplasm of unspecified behavior of anal canal (D49.0)
neoplasm of unspecified behavior of anus NOS (D49.0)
neoplasm of unspecified behavior of bone marrow (D49.89)
neoplasm of unspecified behavior of cartilage of larynx (D49.1)
neoplasm of unspecified behavior of cartilage of nose (D49.1)
neoplasm of unspecified behavior of connective tissue of breast (D49.3)
neoplasm of unspecified behavior of skin of genital organs (D49.59) ◀
neoplasm of unspecified behavior of vermilion border of lip (D49.0)

D49.3 Neoplasm of unspecified behavior of breast

Excludes1 neoplasm of unspecified behavior of skin of breast (D49.2)

D49.4 Neoplasm of unspecified behavior of bladder

D49.5 Neoplasm of unspecified behavior of other genitourinary organs

D49.51 Neoplasm of unspecified behavior of kidney ◀

D49.511 Neoplasm of unspecified behavior of right kidney ◀

D49.512 Neoplasm of unspecified behavior of left kidney ◀

D49.519 Neoplasm of unspecified behavior of unspecified kidney ◀

D49.59 Neoplasm of unspecified behavior of other genitourinary organ ◀

D49.6 Neoplasm of unspecified behavior of brain

Excludes1 neoplasm of unspecified behavior of cerebral meninges (D49.7)
neoplasm of unspecified behavior of cranial nerves (D49.7)

D49.7 Neoplasm of unspecified behavior of endocrine glands and other parts of nervous system

Excludes1 neoplasm of unspecified behavior of peripheral, sympathetic, and parasympathetic nerves and ganglia (D49.2)

D49.8 Neoplasm of unspecified behavior of other specified sites

Excludes1 neoplasm of unspecified behavior of eyelid (skin) (D49.2)
neoplasm of unspecified behavior of eyelid cartilage (D49.2)
neoplasm of unspecified behavior of great vessels (D49.2)
neoplasm of unspecified behavior of optic nerve (D49.7)

D49.81 Neoplasm of unspecified behavior of retina and choroid

Dark area on retina
Retinal freckle

D49.89 Neoplasm of unspecified behavior of other specified sites

D49.9 Neoplasm of unspecified behavior of unspecified site

OGCR Chapter-Specific Coding Guidelines

3. **Chapter 3: Disease of the blood and blood-forming organs and certain disorders involving the immune mechanism (D50-D89)**
Reserved for future guideline expansion

CHAPTER 3

DISEASES OF THE BLOOD AND BLOOD-FORMING ORGANS AND CERTAIN DISORDERS INVOLVING THE IMMUNE MECHANISM (D50-D89)

Excludes2 autoimmune disease (systemic) NOS (M35.9)
certain conditions originating in the perinatal period (P00-P96)
complications of pregnancy, childbirth and the puerperium (O00-O9A)
congenital malformations, deformations and chromosomal abnormalities (Q00-Q99)
endocrine, nutritional and metabolic diseases (E00-E88)
human immunodeficiency virus [HIV] disease (B20)
injury, poisoning and certain other consequences of external causes (S00-T88)
neoplasms (C00-D49)
symptoms, signs and abnormal clinical and laboratory findings, not elsewhere classified (R00-R94)

This chapter contains the following blocks:

D50-D53	Nutritional anemias
D55-D59	Hemolytic anemias
D60-D64	Aplastic and other anemias and other bone marrow failure syndromes
D65-D69	Coagulation defects, purpura and other hemorrhagic conditions
D70-D77	Other disorders of blood and blood-forming organs
D78	Intraoperative and postprocedural complications of the spleen
D80-D89	Certain disorders involving the immune mechanism

NUTRITIONAL ANEMIAS (D50-D53)

D50 Iron deficiency anemia
A disease characterized by a decrease in the number of red cells (hemoglobin) in the blood.
Includes asiderotic anemia
hypochromic anemia

D50.0 Iron deficiency anemia secondary to blood loss (chronic)
Posthemorrhagic anemia (chronic)
Excludes1 acute posthemorrhagic anemia (D62)
congenital anemia from fetal blood loss (P61.3)

D50.1 Sideropenic dysphagia
Web-like growth of membranes in throat that makes swallowing difficult
Kelly-Paterson syndrome
Plummer-Vinson syndrome

D50.8 Other iron deficiency anemias
Iron deficiency anemia due to inadequate dietary iron intake

D50.9 Iron deficiency anemia, unspecified

D51 Vitamin B12 deficiency anemia
Excludes1 vitamin B12 deficiency (E53.8)

D51.0 Vitamin B12 deficiency anemia due to intrinsic factor deficiency
Addison anemia
Biermer anemia
Pernicious (congenital) anemia
Congenital intrinsic factor deficiency

D51.1 Vitamin B12 deficiency anemia due to selective vitamin B12 malabsorption with proteinuria
Imerslund (Gräsbeck) syndrome
Megaloblastic hereditary anemia

D51.2 Transcobalamin II deficiency

D51.3 Other dietary vitamin B12 deficiency anemia
Vegan anemia

D51.8 Other vitamin B12 deficiency anemias

D51.9 Vitamin B12 deficiency anemia, unspecified

D52 Folate deficiency anemia
Excludes1 folate deficiency without anemia (E53.8)

D52.0 Dietary folate deficiency anemia
Nutritional megaloblastic anemia

D52.1 Drug-induced folate deficiency anemia
Use additional code for adverse effect, if applicable, to identify drug (T36-T50 with fifth or sixth character 5)

D52.8 Other folate deficiency anemias

D52.9 Folate deficiency anemia, unspecified
Folic acid deficiency anemia NOS

D53 Other nutritional anemias
Includes megaloblastic anemia unresponsive to vitamin B12 or folate therapy

D53.0 Protein deficiency anemia
Amino-acid deficiency anemia
Orotaciduric anemia
Excludes1 Lesch-Nyhan syndrome (E79.1)

D53.1 Other megaloblastic anemias, not elsewhere classified
Megaloblastic anemia NOS
Excludes1 Di Guglielmo's disease (C94.0)

D53.2 Scorbutic anemia
Anemia resulting from deficiency of ascorbic acid (vitamin C)
Excludes1 scurvy (E54)

D53.8 Other specified nutritional anemias
Anemia associated with deficiency of copper
Anemia associated with deficiency of molybdenum
Anemia associated with deficiency of zinc
Excludes1 nutritional deficiencies without anemia, such as:
copper deficiency NOS (E61.0)
molybdenum deficiency NOS (E61.5)
zinc deficiency NOS (E60)

D53.9 Nutritional anemia, unspecified
Simple chronic anemia
Excludes1 anemia NOS (D64.9)

HEMOLYTIC ANEMIAS (D55-D59)

D55 Anemia due to enzyme disorders
Excludes1 drug-induced enzyme deficiency anemia (D59.2)

D55.0 Anemia due to glucose-6-phosphate dehydrogenase [G6PD] deficiency
Favism
G6PD deficiency anemia

D55.1 Anemia due to other disorders of glutathione metabolism
Anemia (due to) enzyme deficiencies, except G6PD, related to the hexose monophosphate [HMP] shunt pathway
Anemia (due to) hemolytic nonspherocytic (hereditary), type I

D55.2 Anemia due to disorders of glycolytic enzymes
Hemolytic nonspherocytic (hereditary) anemia, type II
Hexokinase deficiency anemia
Pyruvate kinase [PK] deficiency anemia
Triose-phosphate isomerase deficiency anemia
Excludes1 disorders of glycolysis not associated with anemia (E74.8)

D55.3 Anemia due to disorders of nucleotide metabolism

D55.8 Other anemias due to enzyme disorders

D55.9 Anemia due to enzyme disorder, unspecified

D56 Thalassemia
Hereditary disorders characterized by low production of hemoglobin or excessive destruction of red blood cells
Excludes1 sickle-cell thalassemia (D57.4-)

D56.0 Alpha thalassemia
Alpha thalassemia major
Hemoglobin H Constant Spring
Hemoglobin H disease
Hydrops fetalis due to alpha thalassemia
Severe alpha thalassemia
Triple gene defect alpha thalassemia
Use additional code, if applicable, for hydrops fetalis due to alpha thalassemia (P56.99)
Excludes1 alpha thalassemia trait or minor (D56.3)
asymptomatic alpha thalassemia (D56.3)
hydrops fetalis due to isoimmunization (P56.0)
hydrops fetalis not due to immune hemolysis (P83.2)

D56.1 Beta thalassemia
Beta thalassemia major
Cooley's anemia
Homozygous beta thalassemia
Severe beta thalassemia
Thalassemia intermedia
Thalassemia major
Excludes1 beta thalassemia minor (D56.3)
beta thalassemia trait (D56.3)
delta-beta thalassemia (D56.2)
hemoglobin E-beta thalassemia (D56.5)
sickle-cell beta thalassemia (D57.4-)

D56.2 Delta-beta thalassemia
Homozygous delta-beta thalassemia
Excludes1 delta-beta thalassemia minor (D56.3)
delta-beta thalassemia trait (D56.3)

D56.3 Thalassemia minor
Genetic disorders that have in common defective production of hemoglobin
Alpha thalassemia minor
Alpha thalassemia silent carrier
Alpha thalassemia trait
Beta thalassemia minor
Beta thalassemia trait
Delta-beta thalassemia minor
Delta-beta thalassemia trait
Thalassemia trait NOS
Excludes1 alpha thalassemia (D56.0)
beta thalassemia (D56.1)
delta-beta thalassemia (D56.2)
hemoglobin E-beta thalassemia (D56.5)
sickle-cell trait (D57.3)

D56.4 Hereditary persistence of fetal hemoglobin [HPFH]
Persistent production of hemoglobin

D56.5 Hemoglobin E-beta thalassemia
Excludes1 beta thalassemia (D56.1)
beta thalassemia minor (D56.3)
beta thalassemia trait (D56.3)
delta-beta thalassemia (D56.2)
delta-beta thalassemia trait (D56.3)
hemoglobin E disease (D58.2)
other hemoglobinopathies (D58.2)
sickle-cell beta thalassemia (D57.4-)

D56.8 Other thalassemias
Dominant thalassemia
Hemoglobin C thalassemia
Mixed thalassemia
Thalassemia with other hemoglobinopathy
Excludes1 hemoglobin C disease (D58.2)
hemoglobin E disease (D58.2)
other hemoglobinopathies (D58.2)
sickle cell anemia (D57.-)
sickle-cell thalassemia (D57.4)

D56.9 Thalassemia, unspecified
Mediterranean anemia (with other hemoglobinopathy)

D57 Sickle-cell disorders
Inherited disease in which red blood cells, normally disc-shaped, become crescent shaped
Use additional code for any associated fever (R50.81)
Excludes1 other hemoglobinopathies (D58.-)
For category D57 CC codes: D47.4, D50.0-D64.9, D68.312, D68.51-D68.69, D75.81, D75.89-D75.9, D77, D89.2

D57.0 Hb-SS disease with crisis
Sickle-cell disease NOS with crisis
Hb-SS disease with vasoocclusive pain

D57.00 Hb-SS disease with crisis, unspecified

D57.01 Hb-SS disease with acute chest syndrome

D57.02 Hb-SS disease with splenic sequestration

D57.1 Sickle-cell disease without crisis Hb-SS disease without crisis
Sickle-cell anemia NOS
Sickle-cell disease NOS
Sickle-cell disorder NOS

D57.2 Sickle-cell/Hb-C disease
Hb-SC disease
Hb-S/Hb-C disease

D57.20 Sickle-cell/Hb-C disease without crisis

D57.21 Sickle-cell/Hb-C disease with crisis

D57.211 Sickle-cell/Hb-C disease with acute chest syndrome
CC when PDX is its own CC

D57.212 Sickle-cell/Hb-C disease with splenic sequestration

D57.219 Sickle-cell/Hb-C disease with crisis, unspecified
Sickle-cell/Hb-C disease with crisis NOS

D57.3 Sickle-cell trait
Hb-S trait
Heterozygous hemoglobin S

D57.4 Sickle-cell thalassemia
Sickle-cell beta thalassemia
Thalassemia Hb-S disease

D57.40 Sickle-cell thalassemia without crisis
Microdrepanocytosis
Sickle-cell thalassemia NOS

D57.41 Sickle-cell thalassemia with crisis
Sickle-cell "crisis" is precipitated when abnormally crescent-shaped red blood cells form clots and interrupt blood flow to major organs, causing severe pain and organ damage.
Sickle-cell thalassemia with vasoocclusive pain

D57.411 Sickle-cell thalassemia with acute chest syndrome
CC when PDX is its own CC

D57.412 Sickle-cell thalassemia with splenic sequestration

D57.419 Sickle-cell thalassemia with crisis, unspecified
Sickle-cell thalassemia with crisis NOS

● **D57.8 Other sickle-cell disorders**
Hb-SD disease
Hb-SE disease

D57.80 Other sickle-cell disorders without crisis

● **D57.81 Other sickle-cell disorders with crisis**

D57.811 Other sickle-cell disorders with acute chest syndrome

D57.812 Other sickle-cell disorders with splenic sequestration

D57.819 Other sickle-cell disorders with crisis, unspecified
Other sickle-cell disorders with crisis NOS

● **D58 Other hereditary hemolytic anemias**
Genetic condition in which bone marrow is unable to compensate for premature destruction of red blood cells
Excludes1 hemolytic anemia of the newborn (P55.-)

D58.0 Hereditary spherocytosis
Presence of spherocytes (spherically shaped red blood cells)
Acholuric (familial) jaundice
Congenital (spherocytic) hemolytic icterus
Minkowski-Chauffard syndrome

D58.1 Hereditary elliptocytosis
Presence of large numbers of elliptocytes in blood
Elliptocytosis (congenital)
Ovalocytosis (congenital) (hereditary)

D58.2 Other hemoglobinopathies
Abnormal hemoglobin NOS
Congenital Heinz body anemia
Hb-C disease
Hb-D disease
Hb-E disease
Hemoglobinopathy NOS
Unstable hemoglobin hemolytic disease
Excludes1 familial polycythemia (D75.0)
Hb-M disease (D74.0)
hemoglobin E-beta thalassemia (D56.5)
hereditary persistence of fetal hemoglobin [HPFH] (D56.4)
high-altitude polycythemia (D75.1)
methemoglobinemia (D74.-)
other hemoglobinopathies with thalassemia (D56.8)

D58.8 Other specified hereditary hemolytic anemias
Stomatocytosis
Ex: D50.0-D64.9, D75.9, P61.2-P61.4

D58.9 Hereditary hemolytic anemia, unspecified
Ex: See D58.8

● **D59 Acquired hemolytic anemia**
Ex: **For category D59 CC codes:** D47.4, D50.0-D64.9, D68.312, D68.51-D68.69, D75.81, D75.89-D75.9, D77, D89.2

D59.0 Drug-induced autoimmune hemolytic anemia
Use additional code for adverse effect, if applicable, to identify drug (T36-T50 with fifth or sixth character 5)

D59.1 Other autoimmune hemolytic anemias
Autoimmune hemolytic disease (cold type) (warm type)
Chronic cold hemagglutinin disease
Cold agglutinin disease
Cold agglutinin hemoglobinuria
Cold type (secondary) (symptomatic) hemolytic anemia
Warm type (secondary) (symptomatic) hemolytic anemia
Excludes1 Evans syndrome (D69.41)
hemolytic disease of newborn (P55.-)
paroxysmal cold hemoglobinuria (D59.6)

D59.2 Drug-induced nonautoimmune hemolytic anemia
Drug-induced enzyme deficiency anemia
Use additional code for adverse effect, if applicable, to identify drug (T36-T50 with fifth or sixth character 5)

D59.3 Hemolytic-uremic syndrome
Use additional code to identify associated:
E. coli infection (B96.2-)
Pneumococcal pneumonia (J13)
Shigella dysenteriae (A03.9)

D59.4 Other nonautoimmune hemolytic anemias
Mechanical hemolytic anemia
Microangiopathic hemolytic anemia
Toxic hemolytic anemia

D59.5 Paroxysmal nocturnal hemoglobinuria [Marchiafava-Micheli]
Excludes1 hemoglobinuria NOS (R82.3)

D59.6 Hemoglobinuria due to hemolysis from other external causes
Hemoglobinuria from exertion
March hemoglobinuria
Paroxysmal cold hemoglobinuria
Use additional code (Chapter 20) to identify external cause
Excludes1 hemoglobinuria NOS (R82.3)

D59.8 Other acquired hemolytic anemias

D59.9 Acquired hemolytic anemia, unspecified
Idiopathic hemolytic anemia, chronic

APLASTIC AND OTHER ANEMIAS AND OTHER BONE MARROW FAILURE SYNDROMES (D60-D64)

● **D60 Acquired pure red cell aplasia [erythroblastopenia]**
Deficiency of erythroblasts
Includes red cell aplasia (acquired) (adult) (with thymoma)
Excludes1 congenital red cell aplasia (D61.01)
Ex: **For category D60 CC codes:** D47.4, D50.0-D64.9, D68.312, D68.51-D68.69, D75.81, D75.89-D75.9, D77, D89.2

D60.0 Chronic acquired pure red cell aplasia
Lack of development of blood cell

D60.1 Transient acquired pure red cell aplasia

D60.8 Other acquired pure red cell aplasias

D60.9 Acquired pure red cell aplasia, unspecified

● **D61 Other aplastic anemias and other bone marrow failure syndromes**
Excludes1 neutropenia (D70.-)

● **D61.0 Constitutional aplastic anemia**
Condition where bone marrow is unable to produce blood cells

D61.01 Constitutional (pure) red blood cell aplasia
Blackfan-Diamond syndrome
Congenital (pure) red cell aplasia
Familial hypoplastic anemia
Primary (pure) red cell aplasia
Red cell (pure) aplasia of infants
Excludes1 acquired red cell aplasia (D60.9)
Ex: D50.0-D64.9, D75.9, P61.2-P61.4

D61.09 Other constitutional aplastic anemia
Fanconi's anemia
Pancytopenia with malformations
Ex: D50.0-D64.9, D69.3-D69.49, D75.9, P61.2-P61.4

D61.1 Drug-induced aplastic anemia
Use additional code for adverse effect, if applicable, to identify drug (T36-T50 with fifth or sixth character 5)
Ex: See D60

D61.2 Aplastic anemia due to other external agents
Code first, if applicable, toxic effects of substances chiefly nonmedicinal as to source (T51-T65)
Ex: See D60

D61.3 Idiopathic aplastic anemia
Ex: See D60

D61.8 Other specified aplastic anemias and other bone marrow failure syndromes

Ex: For category D61.8 CC codes unless otherwise indicated: D60.0-D60.9, D61.1-D64.9, D70.0-D70.9, D72.810-D72.820, D72.823, D72.825-D72.829, D75.9-D76.3, P61.2

D61.81 Pancytopenia

Marked deficiency of all the blood elements: Red blood cells (erythrocytes), white blood cells (leukocytes), and platelets (thrombocytes). Check laboratory results.

Excludes1 pancytopenia (due to) (with) aplastic anemia (D61.9)
pancytopenia (due to) (with) bone marrow infiltration (D61.82)
pancytopenia (due to) (with) congenital (pure) red cell aplasia (D61.01)
pancytopenia (due to) (with) hairy cell leukemia (C91.4-)
pancytopenia (due to) (with) human immunodeficiency virus disease (B20.-)
pancytopenia (due to) (with) leukoerythroblastic anemia (D61.82)
pancytopenia (due to) (with) myeloproliferative disease (D47.1)

Excludes2 pancytopenia (due to) (with) myelodysplastic syndromes (D46.-)

D61.810 Antineoplastic chemotherapy induced pancytopenia

Excludes2 aplastic anemia due to antineoplastic chemotherapy (D61.1)

D61.811 Other drug-induced pancytopenia

Excludes2 aplastic anemia due to drugs (D61.1)

D61.818 Other pancytopenia

D61.82 Myelophthisis

Leukoerythroblastic anemia
Myelophthisic anemia
Panmyelophthisis

Code also the underlying disorder, such as:
malignant neoplasm of breast (C50.-)
tuberculosis (A15.-)

Excludes1 idiopathic myelofibrosis (D47.1)
myelofibrosis NOS (D75.81)
myelofibrosis with myeloid metaplasia (D47.4)
primary myelofibrosis (D47.1)
secondary myelofibrosis (D75.81)

D61.89 Other specified aplastic anemias and other bone marrow failure syndromes

Ex: See D60

D61.9 Aplastic anemia, unspecified

Hypoplastic anemia NOS
Medullary hypoplasia

Ex: See D60

D62 Acute posthemorrhagic anemia

Excludes1 anemia due to chronic blood loss (D50.0)
blood loss anemia NOS (D50.0)
congenital anemia from fetal blood loss (P61.3)

Ex: D47.4, D50.0-D64.9, D68.312, D68.51-D68.69, D75.81, D75.89-D75.9, D77, D89.2, T79.2XX[A]

D63 Anemia in chronic diseases classified elsewhere

D63.0 Anemia in neoplastic disease

Code first neoplasm (C00-D49)

Excludes1 anemia due to antineoplastic chemotherapy (D64.81)
aplastic anemia due to antineoplastic chemotherapy (D61.1)

OGCR Section I.C.2.e.2.

2) Anemia associated with chemotherapy, immunotherapy and radiation therapy

When the admission/encounter is for management of an anemia associated with an adverse effect of the administration of chemotherapy or immunotherapy and the only treatment is for the anemia, the anemia code is sequenced first followed by the appropriate codes for the neoplasm and the adverse effect (T45.1X5, Adverse effect of antineoplastic and immunosuppressive drugs).

D63.1 Anemia in chronic kidney disease

Erythropoietin resistant anemia (EPO resistant anemia)

Code first underlying chronic kidney disease (CKD) (N18.-)

D63.8 Anemia in other chronic diseases classified elsewhere

Code first underlying disease, such as:
diphyllobothriasis (B70.0)
hookworm disease (B76.0-B76.9)
hypothyroidism (E00.0-E03.9)
malaria (B50.0-B54)
symptomatic late syphilis (A52.79)
tuberculosis (A18.89)

D64 Other anemias

Excludes1 refractory anemia (D46.-)
refractory anemia with excess blasts in transformation [RAEB T] (C92.0-)

D64.0 Hereditary sideroblastic anemia

Abnormal production RBCs (erythrocytes)

Sex-linked hypochromic sideroblastic anemia

D64.1 Secondary sideroblastic anemia due to disease

Code first underlying disease

D64.2 Secondary sideroblastic anemia due to drugs and toxins

Code first poisoning due to drug or toxin, if applicable (T36-T65 with fifth or sixth character 1-4 or 6)

Use additional code for adverse effect, if applicable, to identify drug (T36-T50 with fifth or sixth character 5)

D64.3 Other sideroblastic anemias

Sideroblastic anemia NOS
Pyridoxine-responsive sideroblastic anemia NEC

D64.4 Congenital dyserythropoietic anemia

Any of several rare hereditary anemias, mostly types of macrocytic anemia

Dyshematopoietic anemia (congenital)

Excludes1 Blackfan-Diamond syndrome (D61.01)
Di Guglielmo's disease (C94.0)

D64.8 Other specified anemias

D64.81 Anemia due to antineoplastic chemotherapy

Antineoplastic chemotherapy induced anemia

Excludes1 aplastic anemia due to antineoplastic chemotherapy (D61.1)

Excludes2 anemia in neoplastic disease (D63.0)

D64.89 Other specified anemias

Infantile pseudoleukemia

D64.9 Anemia, unspecified

COAGULATION DEFECTS, PURPURA AND OTHER HEMORRHAGIC CONDITIONS (D65-D69)

D65 Disseminated intravascular coagulation [defibrination syndrome]
Blood clots form and consume all coagulation proteins and platelets and disrupt normal coagulation, resulting in abnormal bleeding
Afibrinogenemia, acquired
Consumption coagulopathy
Diffuse or disseminated intravascular coagulation [DIC]
Fibrinolytic hemorrhage, acquired
Fibrinolytic purpura
Purpura fulminans
Excludes1 disseminated intravascular coagulation (complicating):
abortion or ectopic or molar pregnancy (O00-O07, O08.1)
in newborn (P60)
pregnancy, childbirth and the puerperium (O45.0, O46.0, O67.0, O72.3)
Ex: D47.4, D65-D69.9, D75.81-D75.9, D77, D89.2

D66 Hereditary factor VIII deficiency
Inherited coagulation disorder carried by females but most often affecting males
Classical hemophilia
Deficiency factor VIII (with functional defect)
Hemophilia NOS
Hemophilia A
Excludes1 factor VIII deficiency with vascular defect (D68.0)
Ex: See D65

D67 Hereditary factor IX deficiency
Christmas disease
Factor IX deficiency (with functional defect)
Hemophilia B
Plasma thromboplastin component [PTC] deficiency
Ex: See D65

D68 Other coagulation defects
Excludes1 abnormal coagulation profile (R79.1)
coagulation defects complicating abortion or ectopic or molar pregnancy (O00-O07, O08.1)
coagulation defects complicating pregnancy, childbirth and the puerperium (O45.0, O46.0, O67.0, O72.3)
Coding Clinic: 2016, Q1, P14

D68.0 Von Willebrand's disease
Congenital bleeding disorder
Angiohemophilia
Factor VIII deficiency with vascular defect
Vascular hemophilia
Excludes1 capillary fragility (hereditary) (D69.8)
factor VIII deficiency NOS (D66)
factor VIII deficiency with functional defect (D66)

D68.1 Hereditary factor XI deficiency
Deficiency of blood coagulation resulting in systemic blood-clotting defect
Hemophilia C
Plasma thromboplastin antecedent [PTA] deficiency
Rosenthal's disease

D68.2 Hereditary deficiency of other clotting factors
Blood clotting disorders caused by hereditary deficiencies of one or more clotting factors
AC globulin deficiency
Congenital afibrinogenemia
Deficiency of factor I [fibrinogen]
Deficiency of factor II [prothrombin]
Deficiency of factor V [labile]
Deficiency of factor VII [stable]
Deficiency of factor X [Stuart-Prower]
Deficiency of factor XII [Hageman]
Deficiency of factor XIII [fibrin stabilizing]
Dysfibrinogenemia (congenital)
Hypoproconvertinemia
Owren's disease
Proaccelerin deficiency

D68.3 Hemorrhagic disorder due to circulating anticoagulants
Blood clotting disorders caused by anticoagulants (warfarin and heparin)

D68.31 Hemorrhagic disorder due to intrinsic circulating anticoagulants, antibodies, or inhibitors

D68.311 Acquired hemophilia
Autoimmune hemophilia
Autoimmune inhibitors to clotting factors
Secondary hemophilia
Ex: D47.4, D65-D69.9, D75.82-D75.9, D77, D89.2

D68.312 Antiphospholipid antibody with hemorrhagic disorder
Lupus anticoagulant (LAC) with hemorrhagic disorder
Systemic lupus erythematosus [SLE] inhibitor with hemorrhagic disorder
Excludes1 antiphospholipid antibody, finding without diagnosis (R76.0)
antiphospholipid antibody syndrome (D68.61)
antiphospholipid antibody with hypercoagulable state (D68.61)
lupus anticoagulant (LAC) finding without diagnosis (R76.0)
lupus anticoagulant (LAC) with hypercoagulable state (D68.62)
systemic lupus erythematosus [SLE] inhibitor finding without diagnosis (R76.0)
systemic lupus erythematosus [SLE] inhibitor with hypercoagulable state (D68.62)
Ex: D47.4, D68.311-D68.318, D68.51-D68.69, D70.0-D72.9, D73.81, D75.81, D75.89-D77, D89.2

D68.318 Other hemorrhagic disorder due to intrinsic circulating anticoagulants, antibodies, or inhibitors
Antithromboplastinemia
Antithromboplastinogenemia
Hemorrhagic disorder due to intrinsic increase in antithrombin
Hemorrhagic disorder due to intrinsic increase in anti-VIIIa
Hemorrhagic disorder due to intrinsic increase in anti-IXa
Hemorrhagic disorder due to intrinsic increase in anti-XIa
Ex: See 68.31

D68.32 Hemorrhagic disorder due to extrinsic circulating anticoagulants
Drug-induced hemorrhagic disorder
Hemorrhagic disorder due to increase in anti-IIa
Hemorrhagic disorder due to increase in anti-Xa
Hyperheparinemia
Use additional code for adverse effect, if applicable, to identify drug (T45.515, T45.525)
Ex: D47.4, D65-D69.9, D75.81-D75.9, D77, D89.2
Coding Clinic: 2016, Q1, P14-15

D68.4 Acquired coagulation factor deficiency
Deficiency of coagulation factor due to liver disease
Deficiency of coagulation factor due to vitamin K deficiency
Excludes1 vitamin K deficiency of newborn (P53)
Ex: See D68.32

D68.5 Primary thrombophilia
AKA idiopathic thrombocytopenia, may be acquired or congenital and is a common cause of coagulation disorders.
Primary hypercoagulable states
Excludes1 antiphospholipid syndrome (D68.61)
lupus anticoagulant (D68.62)
secondary activated protein C resistance (D68.69)
secondary antiphospholipid antibody syndrome (D68.69)
secondary lupus anticoagulant with hypercoagulable state (D68.69)
secondary systemic lupus erythematosus [SLE] inhibitor with hypercoagulable state (D68.69)
systemic lupus erythematosus [SLE] inhibitor finding without diagnosis (R76.0)
systemic lupus erythematosus [SLE] inhibitor with hemorrhagic disorder (D68.312)
thrombotic thrombocytopenic purpura (M31.1)
Ex: **For category D68.5 CC codes:** D47.4, D68.312, D68.51-D68.69, D70.0-D72.9, D73.81, D75.81, D75.89-D77, D89.2

D68.51 Activated protein C resistance
Factor V Leiden mutation

D68.52 Prothrombin gene mutation

D68.59 Other primary thrombophilia
Antithrombin III deficiency
Hypercoagulable state NOS
Primary hypercoagulable state NEC
Primary thrombophilia NEC
Protein C deficiency
Protein S deficiency
Thrombophilia NOS

D68.6 Other thrombophilia
Other hypercoagulable states
Excludes1 diffuse or disseminated intravascular coagulation [DIC] (D65)
heparin induced thrombocytopenia (HIT) (D75.82)
hyperhomocysteinemia (E72.11)
Ex: **For category D68.6 CC codes:** D47.4, D68.312, D68.51-D68.69, D70.0-D72.9, D73.81, D75.81, D75.89-D77, D89.2

D68.61 Antiphospholipid syndrome
Anticardiolipin syndrome
Antiphospholipid antibody syndrome
Excludes1 anti-phospholipid antibody, finding without diagnosis (R76.0)
anti-phospholipid antibody with hemorrhagic disorder (D68.312)
lupus anticoagulant syndrome (D68.62)

D68.62 Lupus anticoagulant syndrome
Lupus anticoagulant
Presence of systemic lupus erythematosus [SLE] inhibitor
Excludes1 anticardiolipin syndrome (D68.61)
antiphospholipid syndrome (D68.61)
lupus anticoagulant (LAC) finding without diagnosis (R76.0)
lupus anticoagulant (LAC) with hemorrhagic disorder (D68.312)

D68.69 Other thrombophilia
Hypercoagulable states NEC
Secondary hypercoagulable state NOS

D68.8 Other specified coagulation defects
Excludes1 hemorrhagic disease of newborn (P53)
Ex: See D68.32

D68.9 Coagulation defect, unspecified
Ex: See D68.32

D69 Purpura and other hemorrhagic conditions
Group of conditions characterized by small hemorrhages in skin, mucous membranes, or serosal surfaces
Excludes1 benign hypergammaglobulinemic purpura (D89.0)
cryoglobulinemic purpura (D89.1)
essential (hemorrhagic) thrombocythemia (D47.3)
hemorrhagic thrombocythemia (D47.3)
purpura fulminans (D65)
thrombotic thrombocytopenic purpura (M31.1)
Waldenström hypergammaglobulinemic purpura (D89.0)

D69.0 Allergic purpura
Allergic vasculitis
Nonthrombocytopenic hemorrhagic purpura
Nonthrombocytopenic idiopathic purpura
Purpura anaphylactoid
Purpura Henoch(-Schönlein)
Purpura rheumatica
Vascular purpura
Excludes1 thrombocytopenic hemorrhagic purpura (D69.3)
Ex: See D68.32

D69.1 Qualitative platelet defects
Bernard-Soulier [giant platelet] syndrome
Glanzmann's disease
Grey platelet syndrome
Thromboasthenia (hemorrhagic) (hereditary)
Thrombocytopathy
Excludes1 von Willebrand's disease (D68.0)

D69.2 Other nonthrombocytopenic purpura
Purpura NOS
Purpura simplex
Senile purpura

D69.3 Immune thrombocytopenic purpura
Hemorrhagic (thrombocytopenic) purpura
Idiopathic thrombocytopenic purpura
Tidal platelet dysgenesis
Ex: See D68.32

● **D69.4 Other primary thrombocytopenia**
Excludes1 transient neonatal thrombocytopenia (P61.0)
Wiskott-Aldrich syndrome (D82.0)

D69.41 Evans syndrome
Acquired hemolytic anemia and thrombocytopenia
Ex: See D68.32

D69.42 Congenital and hereditary thrombocytopenia purpura
Congenital thrombocytopenia
Hereditary thrombocytopenia
Code first congential or hereditary disorder, such as:
thrombocytopenia with absent radius (TAR syndrome) (Q87.2)
Ex: See D68.32

D69.49 Other primary thrombocytopenia
Megakaryocytic hypoplasia
Primary thrombocytopenia NOS

● **D69.5 Secondary thrombocytopenia**
Acquired reduction of number of platelets required for blood clotting
Excludes1 heparin induced thrombocytopenia (HIT) (D75.82)
transient thrombocytopenia of newborn (P61.0)

D69.51 Posttransfusion purpura
Posttransfusion purpura from whole blood (fresh) or blood products PTP

D69.59 Other secondary thrombocytopenia

D69.6 Thrombocytopenia, unspecified

D69.8 Other specified hemorrhagic conditions
Capillary fragility (hereditary)
Vascular pseudohemophilia

D69.9 Hemorrhagic condition, unspecified

OTHER DISORDERS OF BLOOD AND BLOOD-FORMING ORGANS (D70-D77)

● **D70 Neutropenia**
Decrease in number of neutrophils (type of white blood cell)
Includes agranulocytosis
decreased absolute neurophile count (ANC)
Use additional code for any associated:
fever (R50.81)
mucositis (J34.81, K12.3-, K92.81, N76.81)
Excludes1 neutropenic splenomegaly (D73.81)
transient neonatal neutropenia (P61.5)

D70.0 Congenital agranulocytosis
Reduced numbers of neutrophils (type of white blood cell)
Congenital neutropenia
Infantile genetic agranulocytosis
Kostmann's disease

D70.1 Agranulocytosis secondary to cancer chemotherapy
Decreased numbers of granulocytes (type of white blood cell)
Code also *underlying neoplasm*
Use additional code for adverse effect, if applicable, to identify drug (T45.1X5)

D70.2 Other drug-induced agranulocytosis
Use additional code for adverse effect, if applicable, to identify drug (T36-T50 with fifth or sixth character 5)

D70.3 Neutropenia due to infection

D70.4 Cyclic neutropenia
Chronic neutropenia (low number of type of white blood cell)
Cyclic hematopoiesis
Periodic neutropenia

D70.8 Other neutropenia

D70.9 Neutropenia, unspecified

D71 Functional disorders of polymorphonuclear neutrophils
Polymorphonuclear: varying shapes of nucleus; AKA PMNs
Cell membrane receptor complex [CR3] defect
Chronic (childhood) granulomatous disease
Congenital dysphagocytosis
Progressive septic granulomatosis

● **D72 Other disorders of white blood cells**
Excludes1 basophilia (D72.824)
immunity disorders (D80-D89)
neutropenia (D70)
preleukemia (syndrome) (D46.9)

D72.0 Genetic anomalies of leukocytes
Alder (granulation) (granulocyte) anomaly
Alder syndrome
Hereditary leukocytic hypersegmentation
Hereditary leukocytic hyposegmentation
Hereditary leukomelanopathy
May-Hegglin (granulation) (granulocyte) anomaly
May-Hegglin syndrome
Pelger-Huët (granulation) (granulocyte) anomaly
Pelger-Huët syndrome
Excludes1 Chédiak (-Steinbrinck)-Higashi syndrome (E70.330)

D72.1 Eosinophilia
Formation and accumulation of high number of white cells in blood/tissue
Allergic eosinophilia
Hereditary eosinophilia
Excludes1 Löffler's syndrome (J82)
pulmonary eosinophilia (J82)

● **D72.8 Other specified disorders of white blood cells**
Excludes1 leukemia (C91-C95)

● **D72.81 Decreased white blood cell count**
Excludes1 neutropenia (D70.-)

D72.810 Lymphocytopenia
Decreased lymphocytes
Reduction in number of lympho cytes in blood

D72.818 Other decreased white blood cell count
Basophilic leukopenia
Eosinophilic leukopenia
Monocytopenia
Other decreased leukocytes
Plasmacytopenia

D72.819 Decreased white blood cell count, unspecified
Decreased leukocytes, unspecified
Leukocytopenia, unspecified
Leukopenia
Excludes1 malignant leukopenia (D70.9)

D72.82 Elevated white blood cell count
Excludes1 eosinophilia (D72.1)

D72.820 Lymphocytosis (symptomatic)
Elevated lymphocytes
Excess of normal lymphocytes

D72.821 Monocytosis (symptomatic)
Excludes1 infectious mononucleosis (B27.-)

D72.822 Plasmacytosis
Presence of excess plasma cells

D72.823 Leukemoid reaction
Basophilic leukemoid reaction
Leukemoid reaction NOS
Lymphocytic leukemoid reaction
Monocytic leukemoid reaction
Myelocytic leukemoid reaction
Neutrophilic leukemoid reaction

D72.824 Basophilia
Increase of basophils in blood

D72.825 Bandemia
Bandemia without diagnosis of specific infection
Excess number of band cells (immature white blood cells) released by bone marrow
Excludes1 confirmed infection -code to infection
leukemia (C91.-, C92.-, C93.-, C94.-, C95.-)

D72.828 Other elevated white blood cell count

D72.829 Elevated white blood cell count, unspecified
Elevated leukocytes, unspecified
Leukocytosis, unspecified

D72.89 Other specified disorders of white blood cells
Abnormality of white blood cells NEC

D72.9 Disorder of white blood cells, unspecified
Abnormal leukocyte differential NOS

D73 Diseases of spleen

D73.0 Hyposplenism
Diminished functioning of spleen
Atrophy of spleen
Excludes1 asplenia (congenital) (Q89.01)
postsurgical absence of spleen (Z90.81)

D73.1 Hypersplenism
Accelerated function of spleen
Excludes1 neutropenic splenomegaly (D73.81)
primary splenic neutropenia (D73.81)
splenitis, splenomegaly in late syphilis (A52.79)
splenitis, splenomegaly in tuberculosis (A18.85)
splenomegaly NOS (R16.1)
splenomegaly congenital (Q89.0)

D73.2 Chronic congestive splenomegaly
Enlargement of spleen

D73.3 Abscess of spleen

D73.4 Cyst of spleen

D73.5 Infarction of spleen
Splenic rupture, nontraumatic
Torsion of spleen
Excludes1 rupture of spleen due to Plasmodium vivax malaria (B51.0)
traumatic rupture of spleen (S36.03-)

D73.8 Other diseases of spleen

D73.81 Neutropenic splenomegaly
Werner-Schultz disease
Enlarged spleen responding to inadequate number of neutrophils

D73.89 Other diseases of spleen
Fibrosis of spleen NOS
Perisplenitis
Splenitis NOS

D73.9 Disease of spleen, unspecified

D74 Methemoglobinemia
Excessive methemoglobin (form of hemoglobin)
Ex: **For category D74 CC codes:** D56.4, D58.2-D59.2, D59.4-D59.9, D64.4-D64.9, D74.0-D74.9, D75.9

D74.0 Congenital methemoglobinemia
Congenital NADH-methemoglobin reductase deficiency
Hemoglobin-M [Hb-M] disease
Methemoglobinemia, hereditary

D74.8 Other methemoglobinemias
Acquired methemoglobinemia (with sulfhemoglobinemia)
Toxic methemoglobinemia

D74.9 Methemoglobinemia, unspecified

D75 Other and unspecified diseases of blood and blood-forming organs
Excludes2 acute lymphadenitis (L04.-)
chronic lymphadenitis (I88.1)
enlarged lymph nodes (R59.-)
hypergammaglobulinemia NOS (D89.2)
lymphadenitis NOS (I88.9)
mesenteric lymphadenitis (acute) (chronic) (I88.0)

D75.0 Familial erythrocytosis
Genetic mutation of gene that results in increased circulating RBCs
Benign polycythemia
Familial polycythemia
Excludes1 hereditary ovalocytosis (D58.1)

D75.1 Secondary polycythemia
Increase in total red cell mass
Acquired polycythemia
Emotional polycythemia
Erythrocytosis NOS
Hypoxemic polycythemia
Nephrogenous polycythemia
Polycythemia due to erythropoietin
Polycythemia due to fall in plasma volume
Polycythemia due to high altitude
Polycythemia due to stress
Polycythemia NOS
Relative polycythemia
Excludes1 polycythemia neonatorum (P61.1)
polycythemia vera (D45)

● **D75.8 Other specified diseases of blood and blood-forming organs**

▶ *D75.81 Myelofibrosis*

Replacing bone marrow by fibrous tissue
Myelofibrosis NOS
Secondary myelofibrosis NOS

Code first the underlying disorder, such as:
malignant neoplasm of breast (C50.-)

Use additional code, if applicable, for associated therapy-related myelodysplastic syndrome (D46.-)

Use additional code for adverse effect, if applicable, to identify drug (T45.1X5)

Excludes1 acute myelofibrosis (C94.4-)
idiopathic myelofibrosis (D47.1)
leukoerythroblastic anemia (D61.82)
myelofibrosis with myeloid metaplasia (D47.4)
myelophthisic anemia (D61.82)
myelophthisis (D61.82)
primary myelofibrosis (D47.1)

Ex: C88.2-C88.3, C88.8-C88.9, C90.10-C90.11, C90.20-C90.21, C90.30-C90.31, C91.00-C91.02, C91.10-C91.12, C91.30-C91.32, C91.40-C91.42, C91.50-C91.52, C91.60-C91.62, C91.90-C91.92, C91.A0-C91.A2, C91.Z0-C91.Z2, C92.00-C92.02, C92.10-C92.12, C92.20-C92.22, C92.30-C92.32, C92.40-C92.42, C92.50-C92.52, C92.60-C92.62, C92.90-C92.92, C92.A0-C92.A2, C92.Z0-C92.Z2, C93.00-C93.02, C93.10-C93.12, C93.30-C93.32, C93.90-C93.92, C93.Z0-C93.Z2, C94.00-C94.02, C94.20-C94.22, C94.30-C94.32, C94.40-C94.42, C94.6, C94.80-C94.82, C95.00-C95.02, C95.10-C95.12, C95.90-C95.92, D45-D46.22, D46.4, D46.9, D46.A-D46.Z, D47.0-D47.1, D47.3, D47.9, D47.Z2, D47.Z9, D48.7-D48.9

D75.82 Heparin induced thrombocytopenia (HIT)

D75.89 Other specified diseases of blood and blood-forming organs

D75.9 Disease of blood and blood-forming organs, unspecified

● **D76 Other specified diseases with participation of lymphoreticular and reticulohistiocytic tissue**

Excludes1 (Abt-) Letterer-Siwe disease (C96.0)
eosinophilic granuloma (C96.6)
Hand-Schüller-Christian disease (C96.5)
histiocytic medullary reticulosis (C96.9) ◀
histiocytic sarcoma (C96.A)
histiocytosis X, multifocal (C96.5)
histiocytosis X, unifocal (C96.6)
Langerhans-cell histiocytosis, multifocal (C96.5)
Langerhans-cell histiocytosis NOS (C96.6)
Langerhans-cell histiocytosis, unifocal (C96.6)
leukemic reticuloendotheliosis (C91.4-) ◀
lipomelanotic reticulosis (I89.8) ◀
malignant histiocytosis (C96.A)
malignant reticulosis (C86.0) ◀
nonlipid reticuloendotheliosis (C96.0) ◀

Ex: **For category D76 CC codes:** D60.0-D60.9, D61.1-D61.9, D65, D69.3-D70.9, D72.818-D72.819, D75.82, D75.9

D76.1 Hemophagocytic lymphohistiocytosis
Familial hemophagocytic reticulosis
Histiocytoses of mononuclear phagocytes

D76.2 Hemophagocytic syndrome, infection-associated

Use additional code to identify infectious agent or disease.

D76.3 Other histiocytosis syndromes
Reticulohistiocytoma (giant-cell)
Sinus histiocytosis with massive lymphadenopathy
Xanthogranuloma

▶ *D77 Other disorders of blood and blood-forming organs in diseases classified elsewhere*

Code first underlying disease, such as:
amyloidosis (E85.-)
congenital early syphilis (A50.0)
echinococcosis (B67.0-B67.9)
malaria (B50.0-B54)
schistosomiasis [bilharziasis] (B65.0-B65.9)
vitamin C deficiency (E54)

Excludes1 rupture of spleen due to Plasmodium vivax malaria (B51.0)
splenitis, splenomegaly in late syphilis (A52.79)
splenitis, splenomegaly in tuberculosis (A18.85)

INTRAOPERATIVE AND POSTPROCEDURAL COMPLICATIONS OF THE SPLEEN (D78)

● **D78 Intraoperative and postprocedural complications of the spleen**

● **D78.0 Intraoperative hemorrhage and hematoma of the spleen complicating a procedure**

Excludes1 intraoperative hemorrhage and hematoma of the spleen due to accidental puncture or laceration during a procedure (D78.1-)

Ex: **For category D78.0 CC codes:** D78.01-D78.02, D78.21-D78.89, H95.811-H95.89, I85.01, I85.11, I97.3, K21.9, K22.8, K23-K25.0, K25.2, K25.4, K25.6, K26.0, K26.2, K26.4, K26.6, K27.0, K27.2, K27.4, K27.6, K28.0, K28.2, K28.4, K28.6, K29.01, K29.21, K29.31, K29.41, K29.51, K29.61, K29.71, K29.81, K29.91, K31.811, K55.21, K57.01, K57.11, K57.13, K57.21, K57.31, K57.33, K57.41, K57.51, K57.53, K57.81, K57.91, K57.93, K62.5, K92.0-K92.2, M96.89, N98.1-N98.9, P54.1-P54.3, T81.10X-T81.19X[A], T81.82X[A], T81.89X-T81.9XX[A]

D78.01 Intraoperative hemorrhage and hematoma of the spleen complicating a procedure on the spleen

D78.02 Intraoperative hemorrhage and hematoma of the spleen complicating other procedure

● **D78.1 Accidental puncture and laceration of the spleen during a procedure**

Ex: **For category D78.1 CC codes:** D78.11-D78.12, D78.81-D78.89, E36.11-E36.8, E89.810-E89.89, G96.11, G97.41-G97.49, H59.011-H59.019, H59.031-H59.099, H59.211-H59.229, H59.811-H59.89, H95.31-H95.32, H95.811-H95.89, I97.3, I97.51-I97.52, J95.71-J95.72, K91.71-K91.72, L76.11-L76.12, L76.81-L76.82, M96.820-M96.821, M96.89, N98.1-N98.9, N99.71-N99.72, T81.82X[A], T81.89X-T81.9XX[A]

D78.11 Accidental puncture and laceration of the spleen during a procedure on the spleen

D78.12 Accidental puncture and laceration of the spleen during other procedure

● **D78.2 Postprocedural hemorrhage of the spleen following a procedure** ⇐

Ex: **For category D78.2 CC codes:** See D78.0

D78.21 Postprocedural hemorrhage of the spleen following a procedure on the spleen ⇐

D78.22 Postprocedural hemorrhage of the spleen following other procedure ⇐

● **D78.3 Postprocedural hematoma and seroma of the spleen following a procedure** ◀

Ex: **For category D78.3 CC codes:** See D78.0

D78.31 Postprocedural hematoma of the spleen following a procedure on the spleen ◀

D78.32 Postprocedural hematoma of the spleen following other procedure ◀

D78.33 Postprocedural seroma of the spleen following a procedure on the spleen ◀

D78.34 Postprocedural seroma of the spleen following other procedure ◀

D78.8 Other intraoperative and postprocedural complications of the spleen
Use additional code, if applicable, to further specify disorder
Ex: For category D78.8 CC codes: D78.81-D78.89, H95.811-H95.89, I97.3, M96.89, N98.1-N98.9, T81.82X[A], T81.89X-T81.9XX[A]

D78.81 Other intraoperative complications of the spleen

D78.89 Other postprocedural complications of the spleen

CERTAIN DISORDERS INVOLVING THE IMMUNE MECHANISM (D80-D89)

Includes defects in the complement system
immunodeficiency disorders, except human immunodeficiency virus [HIV] disease
sarcoidosis

Excludes1 autoimmune disease (systemic) NOS (M35.9)
functional disorders of polymorphonuclear neutrophils (D71)
human immunodeficiency virus [HIV] disease (B20)

D80 Immunodeficiency with predominantly antibody defects
Ex: For category D80 CC codes unless otherwise indicated: D80.0, D80.3-D81.4, D81.6-D81.7, D81.89-D84.0, D84.8-D84.9, D89.3-D89.9

D80.0 Hereditary hypogammaglobulinemia
Autosomal recessive agammaglobulinemia (Swiss type)
X-linked agammaglobulinemia [Bruton] (with growth hormone deficiency)

D80.1 Nonfamilial hypogammaglobulinemia
Abnormally low levels of all classes of immunoglobulins
Agammaglobulinemia with immunoglobulin-bearing B-lymphocytes
Common variable agammaglobulinemia [CVAgamma]
Hypogammaglobulinemia NOS
Ex: D80.0-D81.2, D81.4, D81.6-D81.7, D81.89-D84.0, D84.8-D84.9, D89.3-D89.9

D80.2 Selective deficiency of immunoglobulin A [IgA]
Ex: See D80.1

D80.3 Selective deficiency of immunoglobulin G [IgG] subclasses

D80.4 Selective deficiency of immunoglobulin M [IgM]

D80.5 Immunodeficiency with increased immunoglobulin M [IgM]

D80.6 Antibody deficiency with near-normal immunoglobulins or with hyperimmunoglobulinemia
Abnormally high levels of immunoglobulins in serum

D80.7 Transient hypogammaglobulinemia of infancy

D80.8 Other immunodeficiencies with predominantly antibody defects
Kappa light chain deficiency

D80.9 Immunodeficiency with predominantly antibody defects, unspecified

D81 Combined immunodeficiencies
Excludes1 autosomal recessive agammaglobulinemia (Swiss type) (D80.0)
Ex: For category D81 CC codes unless otherwise indicated: See D80

D81.0 Severe combined immunodeficiency [SCID] with reticular dysgenesis

D81.1 Severe combined immunodeficiency [SCID] with low T- and B-cell numbers

D81.2 Severe combined immunodeficiency [SCID] with low or normal B-cell numbers

D81.3 Adenosine deaminase [ADA] deficiency
Ex: D81.3, D81.5, D81.810, D84.1, E76.01-E76.9, E79.1-E80.29, E80.4-E80.7, E88.81

D81.4 Nezelof's syndrome

D81.5 Purine nucleoside phosphorylase [PNP] deficiency
Ex: See D81.3

D81.6 Major histocompatibility complex class I deficiency
Bare lymphocyte syndrome

D81.7 Major histocompatibility complex class II deficiency

D81.8 Other combined immunodeficiencies

D81.81 Biotin-dependent carboxylase deficiency
Multiple carboxylase deficiency
Excludes1 biotin-dependent carboxylase deficiency due to dietary deficiency of biotin (E53.8)

D81.810 Biotinidase deficiency

D81.818 Other biotin-dependent carboxylase deficiency
Holocarboxylase synthetase deficiency
Other multiple carboxylase deficiency

D81.819 Biotin-dependent carboxylase deficiency, unspecified
Multiple carboxylase deficiency, unspecified

D81.89 Other combined immunodeficiencies

D81.9 Combined immunodeficiency, unspecified
Severe combined immunodeficiency disorder [SCID] NOS

D82 Immunodeficiency associated with other major defects
Excludes1 ataxia telangiectasia [Louis-Bar] (G11.3)

D82.0 Wiskott-Aldrich syndrome
X-linked immunodeficiency
Immunodeficiency with thrombocytopenia and eczema
Ex: See D80

D82.1 Di George's syndrome
Congenital disorder with defective development of third and fourth pharyngeal pouches
Pharyngeal pouch syndrome
Thymic alymphoplasia
Thymic aplasia or hypoplasia with immunodeficiency
Ex: See D80

D82.2 Immunodeficiency with short-limbed stature

D82.3 Immunodeficiency following hereditary defective response to Epstein-Barr virus
X-linked lymphoproliferative disease

D82.4 Hyperimmunoglobulin E [IgE] syndrome
Suspected genetic defect that produces high levels of antibody immunoglobulin (IgE) that causes skin and lung infections and eczema

D82.8 Immunodeficiency associated with other specified major defects

D82.9 Immunodeficiency associated with major defect, unspecified

D83 Common variable immunodeficiency
Ex: For category D83 CC codes: See D80

D83.0 Common variable immunodeficiency with predominant abnormalities of B-cell numbers and function

D83.1 Common variable immunodeficiency with predominant immunoregulatory T-cell disorders

D83.2 Common variable immunodeficiency with autoantibodies to B- or T-cells

D83.8 Other common variable immunodeficiencies

D83.9 Common variable immunodeficiency, unspecified

D84 Other immunodeficiencies

D84.0 Lymphocyte function antigen-1 [LFA-1] defect

D84.1 Defects in the complement system
C1 esterase inhibitor [C1-INH] deficiency

D84.8 Other specified immunodeficiencies
Ex: See D80

D84.9 Immunodeficiency, unspecified
Ex: See D80

Item 3-1 Sarcoidosis: A symptom of an inflammation producing tiny lumps of cells (granulomas) in various organs, most commonly the lungs and lymph nodes, that affect organ function. Cause is unknown occurring primarily in 20- to 40-year-olds, African-American, especially women, and those of Asian, German, Irish, Scandinavian, and Puerto Rican heritage.

D86 Sarcoidosis

D86.0 Sarcoidosis of lung

D86.1 Sarcoidosis of lymph nodes

D86.2 Sarcoidosis of lung with sarcoidosis of lymph nodes

D86.3 Sarcoidosis of skin

D86.8 Sarcoidosis of other sites

D86.81 Sarcoid meningitis

D86.82 Multiple cranial nerve palsies in sarcoidosis

D86.83 Sarcoid iridocyclitis
Rare large tumor with irregular surface of iris

D86.84 Sarcoid pyelonephritis
Systemic disease of unknown etiology characterized by chronic granulomatous inflammation with tissue destruction of pelvis kidney
Tubulo-interstitial nephropathy in sarcoidosis

D86.85 Sarcoid myocarditis

D86.86 Sarcoid arthropathy
Polyarthritis in sarcoidosis

D86.87 Sarcoid myositis
Granumloma of muscle

D86.89 Sarcoidosis of other sites
Hepatic granuloma
Uveoparotid fever [Heerfordt]

D86.9 Sarcoidosis, unspecified

D89 Other disorders involving the immune mechanism, not elsewhere classified

Excludes1 hyperglobulinemia NOS (R77.1)
monoclonal gammopathy (of undetermined significance) (D47.2)

Excludes2 transplant failure and rejection (T86.-)

D89.0 Polyclonal hypergammaglobulinemia
Benign hypergammaglobulinemic purpura
Polyclonal gammopathy NOS

D89.1 Cryoglobulinemia
Cryoglobulin (proteins) in blood that precipitate temperatures below 98.6° F; usually symptomatic of underlying disease
Cryoglobulinemic purpura
Cryoglobulinemic vasculitis
Essential cryoglobulinemia
Idiopathic cryoglobulinemia
Mixed cryoglobulinemia
Primary cryoglobulinemia
Secondary cryoglobulinemia

D89.2 Hypergammaglobulinemia, unspecified

D89.3 Immune reconstitution syndrome
Immune reconstitution inflammatory syndrome [IRIS]
Use additional code for adverse effect, if applicable, to identify drug (T36-T50 with fifth or sixth character 5)

D89.4 Mast cell activation syndrome and related disorders ◀

Excludes1 aggressive systemic mastocytosis (C96.2) ◀
cutaneous mastocytosis (Q82.2) ◀
indolent systemic mastocytosis (D47.0) ◀
malignant mastocytoma (C96.2) ◀
mast cell leukemia (C94.3-) ◀
mastocytoma (D47.0) ◀
systemic mastocytosis associated with a clonal hematologic non-mast cell lineage disease (SM-AHNMD) (D47.0) ◀

D89.40 Mast cell activation, unspecified ◀
Mast cell activation disorder, unspecified ◀
Mast cell activation syndrome, NOS ◀

D89.41 Monoclonal mast cell activation syndrome ◀

D89.42 Idiopathic mast cell activation syndrome ◀

D89.43 Secondary mast cell activation ◀
Secondary mast cell activation syndrome ◀
Code also underlying etiology, if known ◀

D89.49 Other mast cell activation disorder ◀
Other mast cell activation syndrome ◀

D89.8 Other specified disorders involving the immune mechanism, not elsewhere classified

D89.81 Graft-versus-host disease
Code first underlying cause, such as:
complications of transplanted organs and tissue (T86.-)
complications of blood transfusion (T80.89)
Use additional code to identify associated manifestations, such as:
desquamative dermatitis (L30.8)
diarrhea (R19.7)
elevated bilirubin (R17)
hair loss (L65.9)
Ex For category D89.81 CC codes: D78.81-D78.89, D89.810-D89.813, E89.810-E89.89, H59.011-H59.019, H59.031-H59.099, H59.811-H59.89, H95.811-H95.89, I97.3, M96.89, N98.1-N98.9, T86.00-T86.09

D89.810 Acute graft-versus-host disease CC

D89.811 Chronic graft-versus-host disease CC

D89.812 Acute on chronic graft-versus-host disease CC

D89.813 Graft-versus-host disease, unspecified CC

D89.82 Autoimmune lymphoproliferative syndrome [ALPS]

D89.89 Other specified disorders involving the immune mechanism, not elsewhere classified

Excludes1 human immunodeficiency virus disease (B20)

D89.9 Disorder involving the immune mechanism, unspecified
Immune disease NOS
Coding Clinic: 2015, Q3, P22

CHAPTER 4

ENDOCRINE, NUTRITIONAL AND METABOLIC DISEASES (E00-E89)

OGCR Chapter-Specific Coding Guidelines

4. Chapter 4: Endocrine, Nutritional, and Metabolic Diseases (E00-E89)

a. Diabetes mellitus

The diabetes mellitus codes are combination codes that include the type of diabetes mellitus, the body system affected, and the complications affecting that body system. As many codes within a particular category as are necessary to describe all of the complications of the disease may be used. They should be sequenced based on the reason for a particular encounter. Assign as many codes from categories E08 – E13 as needed to identify all of the associated conditions that the patient has.

1) Type of diabetes

The age of a patient is not the sole determining factor, though most type 1 diabetics develop the condition before reaching puberty. For this reason type 1 diabetes mellitus is also referred to as juvenile diabetes.

2) Type of diabetes mellitus not documented

If the type of diabetes mellitus is not documented in the medical record the default is E11.-, Type 2 diabetes mellitus.

3) Diabetes mellitus and the use of insulin oral hypoglycemics

If the documentation in a medical record does not indicate the type of diabetes but does indicate that the patient uses insulin, code E11, Type 2 diabetes mellitus, should be assigned. Code Z79.4, Long-term (current) use of insulin **or Z79.84, Long term (current) use of oral hypoglycemic drugs,** should also be assigned to indicate that the patient uses insulin **or hypoglycemic drugs**. Code Z79.4 should not be assigned if insulin is given temporarily to bring a type 2 patient's blood sugar under control during an encounter.

4) Diabetes mellitus in pregnancy and gestational diabetes

See Section I.C.15. Diabetes mellitus in pregnancy.
See Section I.C.15. Gestational (pregnancy induced) diabetes

5) Complications due to insulin pump malfunction

(a) Underdose of insulin due to insulin pump failure

An underdose of insulin due to an insulin pump failure should be assigned to a code from subcategory T85.6, Mechanical complication of other specified internal and external prosthetic devices, implants and grafts, that specifies the type of pump malfunction, as the principal or first-listed code, followed by code T38.3X6-, Underdosing of insulin and oral hypoglycemic [antidiabetic] drugs. Additional codes for the type of diabetes mellitus and any associated complications due to the underdosing should also be assigned.

(b) Overdose of insulin due to insulin pump failure

The principal or first-listed code for an encounter due to an insulin pump malfunction resulting in an overdose of insulin, should also be T85.6-, Mechanical complication of other specified internal and external prosthetic devices, implants and grafts, followed by code T38.3X1-, Poisoning by insulin and oral hypoglycemic [antidiabetic] drugs, accidental (unintentional).

6) Secondary diabetes mellitus

Codes under categories E08, Diabetes mellitus due to underlying condition, E09, Drug or chemical induced diabetes mellitus and E13, Other specified diabetes mellitus, identify complications/manifestations associated with secondary diabetes mellitus. Secondary diabetes is always caused by another condition or event (e.g., cystic fibrosis, malignant neoplasm of pancreas, pancreatectomy, adverse effect of drug, or poisoning).

(a) Secondary diabetes mellitus and the use of insulin or hypoglycemic drugs

For patients who routinely use insulin **or hypoglycemic drugs,** code Z79.4, Long-term (current) use of insulin **or Z79.84, Long term (current) use of oral hypoglycemic drugs,** should also be assigned. Code Z79.4 should not be assigned if insulin is given temporarily to bring a patient's blood sugar under control during an encounter.

(b) Assigning and sequencing secondary diabetes codes and its causes

The sequencing of the secondary diabetes codes in relationship to codes for the cause of the diabetes is based on the Tabular List instructions for categories E08, E09 and E13.

(i) Secondary diabetes mellitus due to pancreatectomy For postpancreatectomy diabetes mellitus (lack of insulin due to the surgical removal of all or part of the pancreas), assign code E89.1, Postprocedural hypoinsulinemia. Assign a code from category E13 and a code from subcategory Z90.41-, Acquired absence of pancreas, as additional codes.

(ii) Secondary diabetes due to drugs Secondary diabetes may be caused by an adverse effect of correctly administered medications, poisoning or sequela of poisoning.

See section I.C.19.e for coding of adverse effects and poisoning, and section I.C.20 for external cause code reporting.

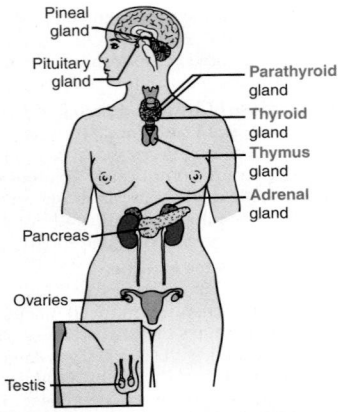

Figure 4-1 The endocrine system. (From Buck CJ: Step-by-Step Medical Coding, ed 2016, St. Louis, Elsevier, 2016)

CHAPTER 4

ENDOCRINE, NUTRITIONAL AND METABOLIC DISEASES (E00-E89)

All neoplasms, whether functionally active or not, are classified in Chapter 2. Appropriate codes in this chapter (i.e., E05.8, E07.0, E16-E31, E34.-) may be used as additional codes to indicate either functional activity by neoplasms and ectopic endocrine tissue or hyperfunction and hypofunction of endocrine glands associated with neoplasms and other conditions classified elsewhere.

Excludes1 transitory endocrine and metabolic disorders specific to newborn (P70-P74)

This chapter contains the following blocks:

E00-E07	Disorders of thyroid gland
E08-E13	Diabetes mellitus
E15-E16	Other disorders of glucose regulation and pancreatic internal secretion
E20-E35	Disorders of other endocrine glands
E36	Intraoperative complications of endocrine system
E40-E46	Malnutrition
E50-E64	Other nutritional deficiencies
E65-E68	Overweight, obesity and other hyperalimentation
E70-E88	Metabolic disorders
E89	Postprocedural endocrine and metabolic complications and disorders, not elsewhere classified

DISORDERS OF THYROID GLAND (E00-E07)

● **E00 Congenital iodine-deficiency syndrome**

Use additional code (F70-F79) to identify associated intellectual disabilities.

Excludes1 subclinical iodine-deficiency hypothyroidism (E02)

E00.0 Congenital iodine-deficiency syndrome, neurological type
Endemic cretinism, neurological type

E00.1 Congenital iodine-deficiency syndrome, myxedematous type
Dry, waxy type of swelling (nonpitting edema) with abnormal deposits of mucin in skin (mucinosis) and other tissues
Endemic hypothyroid cretinism
Endemic cretinism, myxedematous type

E00.2 Congenital iodine-deficiency syndrome, mixed type
Endemic cretinism, mixed type

E00.9 Congenital iodine-deficiency syndrome, unspecified
Congenital iodine-deficiency hypothyroidism NOS
Endemic cretinism NOS

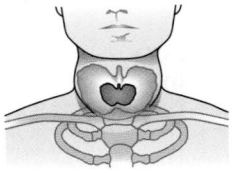

Figure 4-2 Goiter is an enlargement of the thyroid gland.

Item 4–1 Simple goiter indicates no nodules are present. The most common type of goiter is a **diffuse colloidal,** also called a **nontoxic** or **endemic** goiter.

● **E01 Iodine-deficiency related thyroid disorders and allied conditions**

Excludes1 congenital iodine-deficiency syndrome (E00.-)
subclinical iodine-deficiency hypothyroidism (E02)

E01.0 Iodine-deficiency related diffuse (endemic) goiter
Thyroid gland is enlarged

E01.1 Iodine-deficiency related multinodular (endemic) goiter
Iodine-deficiency related nodular goiter

E01.2 Iodine-deficiency related (endemic) goiter, unspecified
Endemic goiter NOS

E01.8 Other iodine-deficiency related thyroid disorders and allied conditions
Acquired iodine-deficiency hypothyroidism NOS

E02 Subclinical iodine-deficiency hypothyroidism

● **E03 Other hypothyroidism**

Excludes1 iodine-deficiency related hypothyroidism (E00-E02)
postprocedural hypothyroidism (E89.0)

E03.0 Congenital hypothyroidism with diffuse goiter
Congenital parenchymatous goiter (nontoxic)
Congenital goiter (nontoxic) NOS

Excludes1 transitory congenital goiter with normal function (P72.0)

E03.1 Congenital hypothyroidism without goiter
Aplasia of thyroid (with myxedema)
Congenital atrophy of thyroid
Congenital hypothyroidism NOS

E03.2 Hypothyroidism due to medicaments and other exogenous substances
Code first poisoning due to drug or toxin, if applicable (T36-T65 with fifth or sixth character 1-4 or 6)
Use additional code for adverse effect, if applicable, to identify drug (T36-T50 with fifth or sixth character 5)

E03.3 Postinfectious hypothyroidism

E03.4 Atrophy of thyroid (acquired)

Excludes1 congenital atrophy of thyroid (E03.1)

Item 4–2 Hypothyroidism is a condition in which there are insufficient levels of thyroxine. **Cretinism** is congenital hypothyroidism, which can result in mental and physical retardation.

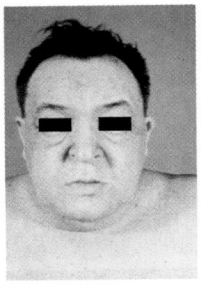

Figure 4-3 Typical appearance of patients with moderately severe primary hypothyroidism or myxedema. (From Larsen: Williams Textbook of Endocrinology, ed 10, Saunders, An Imprint of Elsevier, 2003)

E03.5 Myxedema coma
Often fatal complication of long-term hypothyroidism
Ex: B15.0-B19.9, E03.5, E08.00-E08.59, E08.618-E09.59, E09.618-E10.59, E10.618-E10.649, E10.69-E11.59, E11.618-E11.649, E11.69-E13.59, E13.618-E16.2, E89.1, G32.89, G89.0-G89.4, G93.81-G93.9, G96.8-G96.9, G98.0-G98.8, G99.8, I60.00-I62.9, K72.91, R29.700-R29.742, R40.0-R40.2124, R40.2210-R40.2224, R40.2310-R40.2324, R40.2340-R40.2344, R40.3-R41.3, R41.82, R41.9-R42, R44.8-R44.9, R45.83-R45.84, R46.0-R46.89, R52, R55, R68.0-R68.83, R68.89-R69, S02.0XX-S02.19X[A,B], S02.91X, S06.0X1[A], S06.0X9-S06.9X9[A]

E03.8 Other specified hypothyroidism

E03.9 Hypothyroidism, unspecified
Myxedema NOS

E04 Other nontoxic goiter
Excludes1 congenital goiter (NOS) (diffuse) (parenchymatous) (E03.0)
iodine-deficiency related goiter (E00-E02)

E04.0 Nontoxic diffuse goiter
Thyroid gland is enlarged
Diffuse (colloid) nontoxic goiter
Simple nontoxic goiter

E04.1 Nontoxic single thyroid nodule
Colloid nodule (cystic) (thyroid)
Nontoxic uninodular goiter
Thyroid (cystic) nodule NOS

E04.2 Nontoxic multinodular goiter
Enlarged thyroid gland with multiple nodules
Cystic goiter NOS
Multinodular (cystic) goiter NOS

E04.8 Other specified nontoxic goiter

E04.9 Nontoxic goiter, unspecified
Goiter NOS
Nodular goiter (nontoxic) NOS

E05 Thyrotoxicosis [hyperthyroidism]
Enlarged thyroid gland with multiple nodules
Excludes1 chronic thyroiditis with transient thyrotoxicosis (E06.2)
neonatal thyrotoxicosis (P72.1)
Ex: **For category E05 CC codes:** A17.9, A18.81-A18.82, A18.84, A18.89, E00.0-E03.4, E03.8-E07.1, E07.89-E07.9, E30.9, E34.1, E34.50-E35, E89.0

E05.0 Thyrotoxicosis with diffuse goiter
Exophthalmic or toxic goiter NOS
Graves' disease
Toxic diffuse goiter

E05.00 Thyrotoxicosis with diffuse goiter without thyrotoxic crisis or storm

E05.01 Thyrotoxicosis with diffuse goiter with thyrotoxic crisis or storm

E05.1 Thyrotoxicosis with toxic single thyroid nodule
Thyrotoxicosis with toxic uninodular goiter

E05.10 Thyrotoxicosis with toxic single thyroid nodule without thyrotoxic crisis or storm

E05.11 Thyrotoxicosis with toxic single thyroid nodule with thyrotoxic crisis or storm

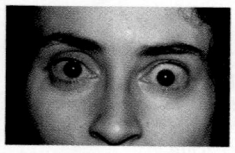

Figure 4-4 Graves' disease. In Graves' disease, exophthalmos often looks more pronounced than it actually is because of the extreme lid retraction that may occur. This patient, for instance, had minimal proptosis of the left eye but marked lid retraction. (Courtesy Dr. HG Scheie. From Yanoff M, Fine BS: Ocular Pathology, ed 6, St. Louis, Mosby, 2008)

Item 4–3 Thyrotoxicosis is a condition caused by excessive amounts of the thyroid hormone thyroxine production or hyperthyroidism. **Graves' disease is associated with hyperthyroidism** (known as **Basedow's disease** in Europe).

E05.2 Thyrotoxicosis with toxic multinodular goiter
Toxic nodular goiter NOS

E05.20 Thyrotoxicosis with toxic multinodular goiter without thyrotoxic crisis or storm

E05.21 Thyrotoxicosis with toxic multinodular goiter with thyrotoxic crisis or storm

E05.3 Thyrotoxicosis from ectopic thyroid tissue

E05.30 Thyrotoxicosis from ectopic thyroid tissue without thyrotoxic crisis or storm

E05.31 Thyrotoxicosis from ectopic thyroid tissue with thyrotoxic crisis or storm

E05.4 Thyrotoxicosis factitia

E05.40 Thyrotoxicosis factitia without thyrotoxic crisis or storm

E05.41 Thyrotoxicosis factitia with thyrotoxic crisis or storm

E05.8 Other thyrotoxicosis
Overproduction of thyroid-stimulating hormone

E05.80 Other thyrotoxicosis without thyrotoxic crisis or storm

E05.81 Other thyrotoxicosis with thyrotoxic crisis or storm

E05.9 Thyrotoxicosis, unspecified
Hyperthyroidism NOS

E05.90 Thyrotoxicosis, unspecified without thyrotoxic crisis or storm

E05.91 Thyrotoxicosis, unspecified with thyrotoxic crisis or storm

E06 Thyroiditis
An inflammation of the thyroid gland which results in an inability to convert iodine into thyroid hormone
Excludes1 postpartum thyroiditis (O90.5)

E06.0 Acute thyroiditis
Abscess of thyroid
Pyogenic thyroiditis
Suppurative thyroiditis
Use additional code (B95-B97) to identify infectious agent.
Ex: E06.0-E06.9

E06.1 Subacute thyroiditis
Inflammation of thyroid gland following viral upper respiratory infection
de Quervain thyroiditis
Giant-cell thyroiditis
Granulomatous thyroiditis
Nonsuppurative thyroiditis
Viral thyroiditis
Excludes1 autoimmune thyroiditis (E06.3)

E06.2 Chronic thyroiditis with transient thyrotoxicosis
Chronic inflammation of thyroid gland with intermittent overproduction of thyroid hormone
Excludes1 autoimmune thyroiditis (E06.3)

E06.3 Autoimmune thyroiditis
Hashimoto's thyroiditis
Hashitoxicosis (transient)
Lymphadenoid goiter
Lymphocytic thyroiditis
Struma lymphomatosa

E06.4 Drug-induced thyroiditis
Use additional code for adverse effect, if applicable, to identify drug (T36-T50 with fifth or sixth character 5)

E06.5 Other chronic thyroiditis
Chronic fibrous thyroiditis
Chronic thyroiditis NOS
Ligneous thyroiditis
Riedel thyroiditis

E06.9 Thyroiditis, unspecified

E07 Other disorders of thyroid

E07.0 Hypersecretion of calcitonin
C-cell hyperplasia of thyroid
Hypersecretion of thyrocalcitonin

E07.1 Dyshormogenetic goiter
Group of several types of goiter resulting from enzyme defects in hormone synthesis
Familial dyshormogenetic goiter
Pendred's syndrome
Excludes1 transitory congenital goiter with normal function (P72.0)

E07.8 Other specified disorders of thyroid

E07.81 Sick-euthyroid syndrome
Euthyroid sick-syndrome

E07.89 Other specified disorders of thyroid
Abnormality of thyroid-binding globulin
Hemorrhage of thyroid
Infarction of thyroid

E07.9 Disorder of thyroid, unspecified

OGCR Section I.C.4.a

Diabetes mellitus
The diabetes mellitus codes are combination codes that include the type of diabetes mellitus, body system affected, and the complications affecting that body system. As many codes within a particular category as are necessary to describe all of the complications of the disease may be used. They should be sequenced based on the reason for a particular visit. Assign as many codes from categories E08–E13 as needed to identify all of the associated conditions that the patient has.

DIABETES MELLITUS (E08-E13)

A metabolic disease that results in persistent hyperglycemia.

E08 Diabetes mellitus due to underlying condition

Code first the underlying condition, such as:
congenital rubella (P35.0)
Cushing's syndrome (E24.-)
cystic fibrosis (E84.-)
malignant neoplasm (C00-C96)
malnutrition (E40-E46)
pancreatitis and other diseases of the pancreas (K85-K86.-)

Use additional code to identify control using:
insulin (Z79.4)
oral antidiabetic drugs (Z79.84)
oral hypoglycemic drugs (Z79.84)

Excludes1 drug or chemical induced diabetes mellitus (E09.-)
gestational diabetes (O24.4-)
neonatal diabetes mellitus (P70.2)
postpancreatectomy diabetes mellitus (E13.-)
postprocedural diabetes mellitus (E13.-)
secondary diabetes mellitus NEC (E13.-)
type 1 diabetes mellitus (E10.-)
type 2 diabetes mellitus (E11.-)

E08.0 Diabetes mellitus due to underlying condition with hyperosmolarity
Ex: **For category E08.0 CC codes:** E08.00-E08.59, E08.618-E09.59, E09.618-E10.52, E10.59, E10.618-E10.649, E10.69-E11.59, E11.618-E11.649, E11.69-E13.59, E13.618-E16.2, E30.9, E34.1, E34.8-E35, E89.1

E08.00 *Diabetes mellitus due to underlying condition with hyperosmolarity without nonketotic hyperglycemic-hyperosmolar coma (NKHHC)*

E08.01 *Diabetes mellitus due to underlying condition with hyperosmolarity with coma*

E08.1 Diabetes mellitus due to underlying condition with ketoacidosis
Ex: **For category E08.1 CC codes:** See E08.0

E08.10 *Diabetes mellitus due to underlying condition with ketoacidosis without coma*

E08.11 *Diabetes mellitus due to underlying condition with ketoacidosis with coma*

E08.2 Diabetes mellitus due to underlying condition with kidney complications

E08.21 *Diabetes mellitus due to underlying condition with diabetic nephropathy*
Diabetes mellitus due to underlying condition with intercapillary glomerulosclerosis
Diabetes mellitus due to underlying condition with intracapillary glomerulonephrosis
Diabetes mellitus due to underlying condition with Kimmelstiel-Wilson disease

E08.22 *Diabetes mellitus due to underlying condition with diabetic chronic kidney disease*
Use additional code to identify stage of chronic kidney disease (N18.1-N18.6)

E08.29 *Diabetes mellitus due to underlying condition with other diabetic kidney complication*
Renal tubular degeneration in diabetes mellitus due to underlying condition

E08.3 Diabetes mellitus due to underlying condition with ophthalmic complications
Changes in blood vessels of retina in which blood vessels swell and leak fluid into retinal surface.

E08.31 Diabetes mellitus due to underlying condition with unspecified diabetic retinopathy

E08.311 *Diabetes mellitus due to underlying condition with unspecified diabetic retinopathy with macular edema*

E08.319 *Diabetes mellitus due to underlying condition with unspecified diabetic retinopathy without macular edema*

E08.32 Diabetes mellitus due to underlying condition with mild nonproliferative diabetic retinopathy
Diabetes mellitus due to underlying condition with nonproliferative diabetic retinopathy NOS
One of the following 7th characters is to be assigned to codes in subcategory E08.32 to designate laterality of the disease:

1	right eye
2	left eye
3	bilateral
9	unspecified eye

E08.321 *Diabetes mellitus due to underlying condition with mild nonproliferative diabetic retinopathy with macular edema*

E08.329 *Diabetes mellitus due to underlying condition with mild nonproliferative diabetic retinopathy without macular edema*

E08.33 Diabetes mellitus due to underlying condition with moderate nonproliferative diabetic retinopathy
One of the following 7th characters is to be assigned to codes in subcategory E08.33 to designate laterality of the disease:

1	right eye
2	left eye
3	bilateral
9	unspecified eye

E08.331 *Diabetes mellitus due to underlying condition with moderate nonproliferative diabetic retinopathy with macular edema*

E08.339 *Diabetes mellitus due to underlying condition with moderate nonproliferative diabetic retinopathy without macular edema*

E08.34 Diabetes mellitus due to underlying condition with severe nonproliferative diabetic retinopathy

One of the following 7th characters is to be assigned to codes in subcategory E08.34 to designate laterality of the disease: ◀

1	right eye ◀
2	left eye ◀
3	bilateral ◀
9	unspecified eye ◀

E08.341 Diabetes mellitus due to underlying condition with severe nonproliferative diabetic retinopathy with macular edema

E08.349 Diabetes mellitus due to underlying condition with severe nonproliferative diabetic retinopathy without macular edema

E08.35 Diabetes mellitus due to underlying condition with proliferative diabetic retinopathy

One of the following 7th characters is to be assigned to codes in subcategory E08.35 to designate laterality of the disease: ◀

1	right eye ◀
2	left eye ◀
3	bilateral ◀
9	unspecified eye ◀

E08.351 Diabetes mellitus due to underlying condition with proliferative diabetic retinopathy with macular edema

E08.352 Diabetes mellitus due to underlying condition with proliferative diabetic retinopathy with traction retinal detachment involving the macula ◀

Exc G89.0-G89.4, I70.261-I70.269, I96, R29.700-R29.742, R41.0-R41.3, R41.82, R41.9, R44.8, R44.9, R45.83, R45.84, R46.0-R46.89, R52, R68.0-R68.19, R68.81-R68.83, R68.89-R69

E08.353 Diabetes mellitus due to underlying condition with proliferative diabetic retinopathy with traction retinal detachment not involving the macula ◀

E08.354 Diabetes mellitus due to underlying condition with proliferative diabetic retinopathy with combined traction retinal detachment and rhegmatogenous retinal detachment ◀

E08.355 Diabetes mellitus due to underlying condition with stable proliferative diabetic retinopathy ◀

E08.359 Diabetes mellitus due to underlying condition with proliferative diabetic retinopathy without macular edema

E08.36 Diabetes mellitus due to underlying condition with diabetic cataract

X *E08.37 Diabetes mellitus due to underlying condition with diabetic macular edema, resolved following treatment* ◀

One of the following 7th characters is to be assigned to code E08.37 to designate laterality of the disease: ◀

1	right eye ◀
2	left eye ◀
3	bilateral ◀
9	unspecified eye ◀

E08.39 Diabetes mellitus due to underlying condition with other diabetic ophthalmic complication

Use additional code to identify manifestation, such as:
diabetic glaucoma (H40-H42)

E08.4 Diabetes mellitus due to underlying condition with neurological complications

E08.40 Diabetes mellitus due to underlying condition with diabetic neuropathy, unspecified

E08.41 Diabetes mellitus due to underlying condition with diabetic mononeuropathy

E08.42 Diabetes mellitus due to underlying condition with diabetic polyneuropathy

Diabetes mellitus due to underlying condition with diabetic neuralgia

E08.43 Diabetes mellitus due to underlying condition with diabetic autonomic (poly)neuropathy

Diabetes mellitus due to underlying condition with diabetic gastroparesis

E08.44 Diabetes mellitus due to underlying condition with diabetic amyotrophy

E08.49 Diabetes mellitus due to underlying condition with other diabetic neurological complication

E08.5 Diabetes mellitus due to underlying condition with circulatory complications

E08.51 Diabetes mellitus due to underlying condition with diabetic peripheral angiopathy without gangrene

E08.52 Diabetes mellitus due to underlying condition with diabetic peripheral angiopathy with gangrene

Diabetes mellitus due to underlying condition with diabetic gangrene

CC when PDx is its own CC

Exc G89.0-G89.4, I70.261-I70.269, I96, R41.0-R41.3, R41.82, R41.9, R44.8-R44.9, R45.83-R45.84, R46.0-R46.89, R52, R68.0-R68.19, R68.81-R68.83, R68.89-R69

E08.59 Diabetes mellitus due to underlying condition with other circulatory complications

E08.6 Diabetes mellitus due to underlying condition with other specified complications

E08.61 Diabetes mellitus due to underlying condition with diabetic arthropathy

E08.610 Diabetes mellitus due to underlying condition with diabetic neuropathic arthropathy

Diabetes mellitus due to underlying condition with Charcôt's joints

E08.618 Diabetes mellitus due to underlying condition with other diabetic arthropathy

E08.62 Diabetes mellitus due to underlying condition with skin complications

E08.620 Diabetes mellitus due to underlying condition with diabetic dermatitis

Diabetes mellitus due to underlying condition with diabetic necrobiosis lipoidica

E08.621 Diabetes mellitus due to underlying condition with foot ulcer

Use additional code to identify site of ulcer (L97.4-, L97.5-)

E08.622 Diabetes mellitus due to underlying condition with other skin ulcer

Use additional code to identify site of ulcer (L97.1-L97.9, L98.41-L98.49)

E08.628 Diabetes mellitus due to underlying condition with other skin complications

E08.63 Diabetes mellitus due to underlying condition with oral complications

E08.630 Diabetes mellitus due to underlying condition with periodontal disease

E08.638 Diabetes mellitus due to underlying condition with other oral complications

E08.64 Diabetes mellitus due to underlying condition with hypoglycemia

E08.641 Diabetes mellitus due to underlying condition with hypoglycemia with coma

Ex See E08.0

E08.649 Diabetes mellitus due to underlying condition with hypoglycemia without coma

E08.65 Diabetes mellitus due to underlying condition with hyperglycemia

E08.69 Diabetes mellitus due to underlying condition with other specified complication

Use additional code to identify complication

E08.8 Diabetes mellitus due to underlying condition with unspecified complications

E08.9 Diabetes mellitus due to underlying condition without complications

E09 Drug or chemical induced diabetes mellitus

Code first poisoning due to drug or toxin, if applicable (T36-T65 with fifth or sixth character 1-4 or 6)

Use additional code for adverse effect, if applicable, to identify drug (T36-T50 with fifth or sixth character 5)

Use additional code to identify control using:
insulin (Z79.4) ◀
oral antidiabetic drugs (Z79.84) ◀
oral hypoglycemic drugs (Z79.84) ◀

Excludes1 diabetes mellitus due to underlying condition (E08.-)
gestational diabetes (O24.4-)
neonatal diabetes mellitus (P70.2)
postpancreatectomy diabetes mellitus (E13.-)
postprocedural diabetes mellitus (E13.-)
secondary diabetes mellitus NEC (E13.-)
type 1 diabetes mellitus (E10.-)
type 2 diabetes mellitus (E11.-)

E09.0 Drug or chemical induced diabetes mellitus with hyperosmolarity

Ex For category E09.0 CC codes: See E08.0

E09.00 Drug or chemical induced diabetes mellitus with hyperosmolarity without nonketotic hyperglycemic-hyperosmolar coma (NKHHC)

E09.01 Drug or chemical induced diabetes mellitus with hyperosmolarity with coma

E09.1 Drug or chemical induced diabetes mellitus with ketoacidosis

Ex For category E09.1 CC codes: See E08.0

E09.10 Drug or chemical induced diabetes mellitus with ketoacidosis without coma

E09.11 Drug or chemical induced diabetes mellitus with ketoacidosis with coma

E09.2 Drug or chemical induced diabetes mellitus with kidney complications

E09.21 Drug or chemical induced diabetes mellitus with diabetic nephropathy
Drug or chemical induced diabetes mellitus with intercapillary glomerulosclerosis
Drug or chemical induced diabetes mellitus with intracapillary glomerulonephrosis
Drug or chemical induced diabetes mellitus with Kimmelstiel-Wilson disease

E09.22 Drug or chemical induced diabetes mellitus with diabetic chronic kidney disease

Use additional code to identify stage of chronic kidney disease (N18.1-N18.6)

E09.29 Drug or chemical induced diabetes mellitus with other diabetic kidney complication
Drug or chemical induced diabetes mellitus with renal tubular degeneration

E09.3 Drug or chemical induced diabetes mellitus with ophthalmic complications

E09.31 Drug or chemical induced diabetes mellitus with unspecified diabetic retinopathy

E09.311 Drug or chemical induced diabetes mellitus with unspecified diabetic retinopathy with macular edema

E09.319 Drug or chemical induced diabetes mellitus with unspecified diabetic retinopathy without macular edema

E09.32 Drug or chemical induced diabetes mellitus with mild nonproliferative diabetic retinopathy
Drug or chemical induced diabetes mellitus with nonproliferative diabetic retinopathy NOS

One of the following 7th characters is to be assigned to codes in subcategory E09.32 to designate laterality of the disease: ◀

1	right eye ◀
2	left eye ◀
3	bilateral ◀
9	unspecified eye ◀

E09.321 Drug or chemical induced diabetes mellitus with mild nonproliferative diabetic retinopathy with macular edema

E09.329 Drug or chemical induced diabetes mellitus with mild nonproliferative diabetic retinopathy without macular edema

E09.33 Drug or chemical induced diabetes mellitus with moderate nonproliferative diabetic retinopathy

One of the following 7th characters is to be assigned to codes in subcategory E09.33 to designate laterality of the disease: ◀

1	right eye ◀
2	left eye ◀
3	bilateral ◀
9	unspecified eye ◀

E09.331 Drug or chemical induced diabetes mellitus with moderate nonproliferative diabetic retinopathy with macular edema

E09.339 Drug or chemical induced diabetes mellitus with moderate nonproliferative diabetic retinopathy without macular edema

E09.34 Drug or chemical induced diabetes mellitus with severe nonproliferative diabetic retinopathy

One of the following 7th characters is to be assigned to codes in subcategory E09.34 to designate laterality of the disease: ◀

1	right eye ◀
2	left eye ◀
3	bilateral ◀
9	unspecified eye ◀

E09.341 Drug or chemical induced diabetes mellitus with severe nonproliferative diabetic retinopathy with macular edema

E09.349 Drug or chemical induced diabetes mellitus with severe nonproliferative diabetic retinopathy without macular edema

E09.35 Drug or chemical induced diabetes mellitus with proliferative diabetic retinopathy

One of the following 7th characters is to be assigned to codes in subcategory E09.35 to designate laterality of the disease: ◀

1	right eye ◀
2	left eye ◀
3	bilateral ◀
9	unspecified eye ◀

E09.351 Drug or chemical induced diabetes mellitus with proliferative diabetic retinopathy with macular edema

E09.352 Drug or chemical induced diabetes mellitus with proliferative diabetic retinopathy with traction retinal detachment involving the macula ◀

E09.353 Drug or chemical induced diabetes mellitus with proliferative diabetic retinopathy with traction retinal detachment not involving the macula ◀

E09.354 Drug or chemical induced diabetes mellitus with proliferative diabetic retinopathy with combined traction retinal detachment and rhegmatogenous retinal detachment ◀

E09.355 Drug or chemical induced diabetes mellitus with stable proliferative diabetic retinopathy ◀

E09.359 Drug or chemical induced diabetes mellitus with proliferative diabetic retinopathy without macular edema

E09.36 Drug or chemical induced diabetes mellitus with diabetic cataract

X **E09.37 Drug or chemical induced diabetes mellitus with diabetic macular edema, resolved following treatment ◀**

One of the following 7th characters is to be assigned to code E09.37 to designate laterality of the disease: ◀

1	right eye ◀
2	left eye ◀
3	bilateral ◀
9	unspecified eye ◀

E09.39 Drug or chemical induced diabetes mellitus with other diabetic ophthalmic complication

Use additional code to identify manifestation, such as:
diabetic glaucoma (H40-H42)

E09.4 Drug or chemical induced diabetes mellitus with neurological complications

E09.40 Drug or chemical induced diabetes mellitus with neurological complications with diabetic neuropathy, unspecified

E09.41 Drug or chemical induced diabetes mellitus with neurological complications with diabetic mononeuropathy

E09.42 Drug or chemical induced diabetes mellitus with neurological complications with diabetic polyneuropathy

Drug or chemical induced diabetes mellitus with diabetic neuralgia

E09.43 Drug or chemical induced diabetes mellitus with neurological complications with diabetic autonomic (poly)neuropathy

Drug or chemical induced diabetes mellitus with diabetic gastroparesis

E09.44 Drug or chemical induced diabetes mellitus with neurological complications with diabetic amyotrophy

E09.49 Drug or chemical induced diabetes mellitus with neurological complications with other diabetic neurological complication

E09.5 Drug or chemical induced diabetes mellitus with circulatory complications

E09.51 Drug or chemical induced diabetes mellitus with diabetic peripheral angiopathy without gangrene

E09.52 Drug or chemical induced diabetes mellitus with diabetic peripheral angiopathy with gangrene

Drug or chemical induced diabetes mellitus with diabetic gangrene
CC when PDx is its own CC
Ex: See E08.52

E09.59 Drug or chemical induced diabetes mellitus with other circulatory complications

E09.6 Drug or chemical induced diabetes mellitus with other specified complications

E09.61 Drug or chemical induced diabetes mellitus with diabetic arthropathy

E09.610 Drug or chemical induced diabetes mellitus with diabetic neuropathic arthropathy

Drug or chemical induced diabetes mellitus with Charcôt's joints
Progressive degeneration of weight-bearing joint

E09.618 Drug or chemical induced diabetes mellitus with other diabetic arthropathy

E09.62 Drug or chemical induced diabetes mellitus with skin complications

E09.620 Drug or chemical induced diabetes mellitus with diabetic dermatitis

Drug or chemical induced diabetes mellitus with diabetic necrobiosis lipoidica
Necrotizing skin condition

E09.621 Drug or chemical induced diabetes mellitus with foot ulcer

Use additional code to identify site of ulcer (L97.4-, L97.5-)

E09.622 Drug or chemical induced diabetes mellitus with other skin ulcer

Use additional code to identify site of ulcer (L97.1-L97.9, L98.41-L98.49)

E09.628 Drug or chemical induced diabetes mellitus with other skin complications

E09.63 Drug or chemical induced diabetes mellitus with oral complications

E09.630 Drug or chemical induced diabetes mellitus with periodontal disease

E09.638 Drug or chemical induced diabetes mellitus with other oral complications

E09.64 Drug or chemical induced diabetes mellitus with hypoglycemia

E09.641 Drug or chemical induced diabetes mellitus with hypoglycemia with coma

Ex: See E08.0

E09.649 Drug or chemical induced diabetes mellitus with hypoglycemia without coma

E09.65 Drug or chemical induced diabetes mellitus with hyperglycemia

E09.69 Drug or chemical induced diabetes mellitus with other specified complication

Use additional code to identify complication

E09.8 Drug or chemical induced diabetes mellitus with unspecified complications

E09.9 Drug or chemical induced diabetes mellitus without complications

● **E10 Type 1 diabetes mellitus**

Includes brittle diabetes (mellitus)
diabetes (mellitus) due to autoimmune process
diabetes (mellitus) due to immune mediated pancreatic islet beta-cell destruction
idiopathic diabetes (mellitus)
juvenile onset diabetes (mellitus)
ketosis-prone diabetes (mellitus)

Excludes1 diabetes mellitus due to underlying condition (E08.-)
drug or chemical induced diabetes mellitus (E09.-)
gestational diabetes (O24.4-)
hyperglycemia NOS (R73.9)
neonatal diabetes mellitus (P70.2)
postpancreatectomy diabetes mellitus (E13.-)
postprocedural diabetes mellitus (E13.-)
secondary diabetes mellitus NEC (E13.-)
type 2 diabetes mellitus (E11.-)

● **E10.1 Type 1 diabetes mellitus with ketoacidosis**
Acidosis accompanied by accumulation of ketone bodies (ketosis) in body tissues and fluids
Ex **For category E.10.1 CC codes:** E08.00-E08.59, E08.618-E09.59, E09.618-E10.59, E10.618-E10.649, E10.69-E11.59, E11.618-E11.649, E11.69-E13.59, E13.618-E16.2, E30.9, E34.1, E34.50-E35, E89.1

E10.10 Type 1 diabetes mellitus with ketoacidosis without coma
Coding Clinic: 2013, Q3, P20

E10.11 Type 1 diabetes mellitus with ketoacidosis with coma

● **E10.2 Type 1 diabetes mellitus with kidney complications**

E10.21 Type 1 diabetes mellitus with diabetic nephropathy
Type 1 diabetes mellitus with intercapillary glomerulosclerosis
Type 1 diabetes mellitus with intracapillary glomerulonephrosis
Type 1 diabetes mellitus with Kimmelstiel-Wilson disease

E10.22 Type 1 diabetes mellitus with diabetic chronic kidney disease
Use additional code to identify stage of chronic kidney disease (N18.1-N18.6)

E10.29 Type 1 diabetes mellitus with other diabetic kidney complication
Type 1 diabetes mellitus with renal tubular degeneration
Coding Clinic: 2016, Q1, P13

● **E10.3 Type 1 diabetes mellitus with ophthalmic complications**

● **E10.31 Type 1 diabetes mellitus with unspecified diabetic retinopathy**

E10.311 Type 1 diabetes mellitus with unspecified diabetic retinopathy with macular edema

E10.319 Type 1 diabetes mellitus with unspecified diabetic retinopathy without macular edema

● **E10.32 Type 1 diabetes mellitus with mild nonproliferative diabetic retinopathy**
Type 1 diabetes mellitus with nonproliferative diabetic retinopathy NOS
One of the following 7th characters is to be assigned to codes in subcategory E10.32 to designate laterality of the disease: ◀

1	right eye ◀
2	left eye ◀
3	bilateral ◀
9	unspecified eye ◀

● **E10.321 Type 1 diabetes mellitus with mild nonproliferative diabetic retinopathy with macular edema**

● **E10.329 Type 1 diabetes mellitus with mild nonproliferative diabetic retinopathy without macular edema**

● **E10.33 Type 1 diabetes mellitus with moderate nonproliferative diabetic retinopathy**
One of the following 7th characters is to be assigned to codes in subcategory E10.33 to designate laterality of the disease: ◀

1	right eye ◀
2	left eye ◀
3	bilateral ◀
9	unspecified eye ◀

● **E10.331 Type 1 diabetes mellitus with moderate nonproliferative diabetic retinopathy with macular edema**

● **E10.339 Type 1 diabetes mellitus with moderate nonproliferative diabetic retinopathy without macular edema**

● **E10.34 Type 1 diabetes mellitus with severe nonproliferative diabetic retinopathy**
One of the following 7th characters is to be assigned to codes in subcategory E10.34 to designate laterality of the disease: ◀

1	right eye ◀
2	left eye ◀
3	bilateral ◀
9	unspecified eye ◀

● **E10.341 Type 1 diabetes mellitus with severe nonproliferative diabetic retinopathy with macular edema**

● **E10.349 Type 1 diabetes mellitus with severe nonproliferative diabetic retinopathy without macular edema**

● **E10.35 Type 1 diabetes mellitus with proliferative diabetic retinopathy**
One of the following 7th characters is to be assigned to codes in subcategory E10.35 to designate laterality of the disease: ◀

1	right eye ◀
2	left eye ◀
3	bilateral ◀
9	unspecified eye ◀

● **E10.351 Type 1 diabetes mellitus with proliferative diabetic retinopathy with macular edema**

● **E10.352 Type 1 diabetes mellitus with proliferative diabetic retinopathy with traction retinal detachment involving the macula ◀**

● **E10.353 Type 1 diabetes mellitus with proliferative diabetic retinopathy with traction retinal detachment not involving the macula ◀**

● **E10.354 Type 1 diabetes mellitus with proliferative diabetic retinopathy with combined traction retinal detachment and rhegmatogenous retinal detachment ◀**

● **E10.355 Type 1 diabetes mellitus with stable proliferative diabetic retinopathy ◀**

● **E10.359 Type 1 diabetes mellitus with proliferative diabetic retinopathy without macular edema**

E10.36 Type 1 diabetes mellitus with diabetic cataract

X ● **E10.37 Type 1 diabetes mellitus with diabetic macular edema, resolved following treatment** ◀

One of the following 7th characters is to be assigned to code E10.37 to designate laterality of the disease: ◀

1	right eye ◀
2	left eye ◀
3	bilateral ◀
9	unspecified eye ◀

E10.39 Type 1 diabetes mellitus with other diabetic ophthalmic complication

Use additional code to identify manifestation, such as:
diabetic glaucoma (H40-H42)

● **E10.4 Type 1 diabetes mellitus with neurological complications**

E10.40 Type 1 diabetes mellitus with diabetic neuropathy, unspecified

E10.41 Type 1 diabetes mellitus with diabetic mononeuropathy

E10.42 Type 1 diabetes mellitus with diabetic polyneuropathy

Type 1 diabetes mellitus with diabetic neuralgia

E10.43 Type 1 diabetes mellitus with diabetic autonomic (poly)neuropathy

Type 1 diabetes mellitus with diabetic gastroparesis

E10.44 Type 1 diabetes mellitus with diabetic amyotrophy

E10.49 Type 1 diabetes mellitus with other diabetic neurological complication

● **E10.5 Type 1 diabetes mellitus with circulatory complications**

E10.51 Type 1 diabetes mellitus with diabetic peripheral angiopathy without gangrene

E10.52 Type 1 diabetes mellitus with diabetic peripheral angiopathy with gangrene

Type 1 diabetes mellitus with diabetic gangrene

CC when PDx is its own CC

Ex: See E08.52

E10.59 Type 1 diabetes mellitus with other circulatory complications

● **E10.6 Type 1 diabetes mellitus with other specified complications**

● **E10.61 Type 1 diabetes mellitus with diabetic arthropathy**

E10.610 Type 1 diabetes mellitus with diabetic neuropathic arthropathy

Type 1 diabetes mellitus with Charcôt's joints

E10.618 Type 1 diabetes mellitus with other diabetic arthropathy

● **E10.62 Type 1 diabetes mellitus with skin complications**

E10.620 Type 1 diabetes mellitus with diabetic dermatitis

Type 1 diabetes mellitus with diabetic necrobiosis lipoidica

E10.621 Type 1 diabetes mellitus with foot ulcer

Use additional code to identify site of ulcer (L97.4-, L97.5-)

E10.622 Type 1 diabetes mellitus with other skin ulcer

Use additional code to identify site of ulcer (L97.1-L97.9, L98.41-L98.49)

E10.628 Type 1 diabetes mellitus with other skin complications

● **E10.63 Type 1 diabetes mellitus with oral complications**

E10.630 Type 1 diabetes mellitus with periodontal disease

E10.638 Type 1 diabetes mellitus with other oral complications

● **E10.64 Type 1 diabetes mellitus with hypoglycemia**

E10.641 Type 1 diabetes mellitus with hypoglycemia with coma

Ex: See E10.1

E10.649 Type 1 diabetes mellitus with hypoglycemia without coma

Coding Clinic: 2016, Q1, P13

E10.65 Type 1 diabetes mellitus with hyperglycemia

Coding Clinic: 2013, Q3, P20

E10.69 Type 1 diabetes mellitus with other specified complication

Use additional code to identify complication

Use this code with E10.65 to report hyperosmolarity in a Type 1 patient

E10.8 Type 1 diabetes mellitus with unspecified complications

E10.9 Type 1 diabetes mellitus without complications

● **E11 Type 2 diabetes mellitus**

Includes diabetes (mellitus) due to insulin secretory defect
diabetes NOS
insulin resistant diabetes (mellitus)

Use additional code to identify control using: ◀
insulin (Z79.4) ◀
oral antidiabetic drugs (Z79.84) ◀
oral hypoglycemic drugs (Z79.84) ◀

Excludes1 diabetes mellitus due to underlying condition (E08.-)
drug or chemical induced diabetes mellitus (E09.-)
gestational diabetes (O24.4-)
neonatal diabetes mellitus (P70.2)
postpancreatectomy diabetes mellitus (E13.-)
postprocedural diabetes mellitus (E13.-)
secondary diabetes mellitus NEC (E13.-)
type 1 diabetes mellitus (E10.-)

Coding Clinic: 2016, Q2, P10

● **E11.0 Type 2 diabetes mellitus with hyperosmolarity**

Ex: For category E11.0 CC codes: See E08.0

E11.00 Type 2 diabetes mellitus with hyperosmolarity without nonketotic hyperglycemic-hyperosmolar coma (NKHHC)

E11.01 Type 2 diabetes mellitus with hyperosmolarity with coma

● **E11.2 Type 2 diabetes mellitus with kidney complications**

E11.21 Type 2 diabetes mellitus with diabetic nephropathy

Type 2 diabetes mellitus with intercapillary glomerulosclerosis
Type 2 diabetes mellitus with intracapillary glomerulonephrosis
Type 2 diabetes mellitus with Kimmelstiel-Wilson disease

E11.22 Type 2 diabetes mellitus with diabetic chronic kidney disease

Use additional code to identify stage of chronic kidney disease (N18.1-N18.6)

Coding Clinic: 2016, Q2, P36, Q1, P13

E11.29 Type 2 diabetes mellitus with other diabetic kidney complication

Type 2 diabetes mellitus with renal tubular degeneration

● **E11.3 Type 2 diabetes mellitus with ophthalmic complications**

● **E11.31 Type 2 diabetes mellitus with unspecified diabetic retinopathy**

E11.311 Type 2 diabetes mellitus with unspecified diabetic retinopathy with macular edema

E11.319 Type 2 diabetes mellitus with unspecified diabetic retinopathy without macular edema

Coding Clinic: 2013, Q3, P20

● **E11.32 Type 2 diabetes mellitus with mild nonproliferative diabetic retinopathy**

Type 2 diabetes mellitus with nonproliferative diabetic retinopathy NOS

One of the following 7th characters is to be assigned to codes in subcategory E11.32 to designate laterality of the disease: ◀

1	right eye ◀
2	left eye ◀
3	bilateral ◀
9	unspecified eye ◀

● **E11.321 Type 2 diabetes mellitus with mild nonproliferative diabetic retinopathy with macular edema**

● **E11.329 Type 2 diabetes mellitus with mild nonproliferative diabetic retinopathy without macular edema**

● **E11.33 Type 2 diabetes mellitus with moderate nonproliferative diabetic retinopathy**

One of the following 7th characters is to be assigned to codes in subcategory E11.33 to designate laterality of the disease: ◀

1	right eye ◀
2	left eye ◀
3	bilateral ◀
9	unspecified eye ◀

● **E11.331 Type 2 diabetes mellitus with moderate nonproliferative diabetic retinopathy with macular edema**

● **E11.339 Type 2 diabetes mellitus with moderate nonproliferative diabetic retinopathy without macular edema**

● **E11.34 Type 2 diabetes mellitus with severe nonproliferative diabetic retinopathy**

One of the following 7th characters is to be assigned to codes in subcategory E11.34 to designate laterality of the disease: ◀

1	right eye ◀
2	left eye ◀
3	bilateral ◀
9	unspecified eye ◀

● **E11.341 Type 2 diabetes mellitus with severe nonproliferative diabetic retinopathy with macular edema**

● **E11.349 Type 2 diabetes mellitus with severe nonproliferative diabetic retinopathy without macular edema**

● **E11.35 Type 2 diabetes mellitus with proliferative diabetic retinopathy**

One of the following 7th characters is to be assigned to codes in subcategory E11.35 to designate laterality of the disease: ◀

1	right eye ◀
2	left eye ◀
3	bilateral ◀
9	unspecified eye ◀

● **E11.351 Type 2 diabetes mellitus with proliferative diabetic retinopathy with macular edema**

● **E11.352 Type 2 diabetes mellitus with proliferative diabetic retinopathy with traction retinal detachment involving the macula ◀**

● **E11.353 Type 2 diabetes mellitus with proliferative diabetic retinopathy with traction retinal detachment not involving the macula ◀**

● **E11.354 Type 2 diabetes mellitus with proliferative diabetic retinopathy with combined traction retinal detachment and rhegmatogenous retinal detachment ◀**

● **E11.355 Type 2 diabetes mellitus with stable proliferative diabetic retinopathy ◀**

● **E11.359 Type 2 diabetes mellitus with proliferative diabetic retinopathy without macular edema**

E11.36 Type 2 diabetes mellitus with diabetic cataract

Coding Clinic: 2016, Q2, P36

X ● **E11.37 Type 2 diabetes mellitus with diabetic macular edema, resolved following treatment ◀**

One of the following 7th characters is to be assigned to code E11.37 to designate laterality of the disease: ◀

1	right eye ◀
2	left eye ◀
3	bilateral ◀
9	unspecified eye ◀

E11.39 Type 2 diabetes mellitus with other diabetic ophthalmic complication

Use additional code to identify manifestation, such as:
diabetic glaucoma (H40-H42)

● **E11.4 Type 2 diabetes mellitus with neurological complications**

E11.40 Type 2 diabetes mellitus with diabetic neuropathy, unspecified

E11.41 Type 2 diabetes mellitus with diabetic mononeuropathy

E11.42 Type 2 diabetes mellitus with diabetic polyneuropathy

Type 2 diabetes mellitus with diabetic neuralgia

Coding Clinic: 2016, Q1, P13

E11.43 Type 2 diabetes mellitus with diabetic autonomic (poly)neuropathy

Type 2 diabetes mellitus with diabetic gastroparesis

Coding Clinic: 2016, Q2, P36

E11.44 Type 2 diabetes mellitus with diabetic amyotrophy

Coding Clinic: 2016, Q2, P36

E11.49 Type 2 diabetes mellitus with other diabetic neurological complication

E11.5 Type 2 diabetes mellitus with circulatory complications

E11.51 Type 2 diabetes mellitus with diabetic peripheral angiopathy without gangrene

E11.52 Type 2 diabetes mellitus with diabetic peripheral angiopathy with gangrene

Type 2 diabetes mellitus with diabetic gangrene

CC when PDx is its own CC

Ex: See E08.52

E11.59 Type 2 diabetes mellitus with other circulatory complications

E11.6 Type 2 diabetes mellitus with other specified complications

E11.61 Type 2 diabetes mellitus with diabetic arthropathy

E11.610 Type 2 diabetes mellitus with diabetic neuropathic arthropathy

Type 2 diabetes mellitus with Charcôt's joints

Coding Clinic: 2016, Q2, P36

E11.618 Type 2 diabetes mellitus with other diabetic arthropathy

Coding Clinic: 2016, Q2, P36

E11.62 Type 2 diabetes mellitus with skin complications

E11.620 Type 2 diabetes mellitus with diabetic dermatitis

Type 2 diabetes mellitus with diabetic necrobiosis lipoidica

E11.621 Type 2 diabetes mellitus with foot ulcer

Use additional code to identify site of ulcer (L97.4-, L97.5-)

Coding Clinic: 2016, Q1, P12

E11.622 Type 2 diabetes mellitus with other skin ulcer

Use additional code to identify site of ulcer (L97.1-L97.9, L98.41-L98.49)

E11.628 Type 2 diabetes mellitus with other skin complications

E11.63 Type 2 diabetes mellitus with oral complications

E11.630 Type 2 diabetes mellitus with periodontal disease

E11.638 Type 2 diabetes mellitus with other oral complications

E11.64 Type 2 diabetes mellitus with hypoglycemia

E11.641 Type 2 diabetes mellitus with hypoglycemia with coma

Ex: See E08.0

E11.649 Type 2 diabetes mellitus with hypoglycemia without coma

Coding Clinic: 2015, Q3, P21

E11.65 Type 2 diabetes mellitus with hyperglycemia

Coding Clinic: 2013, Q3, P20

E11.69 Type 2 diabetes mellitus with other specified complication

Use additional code to identify complication

Use this code with E11.65 to report DKA in a Type 2 patient

E11.8 Type 2 diabetes mellitus with unspecified complications

E11.9 Type 2 diabetes mellitus without complications

MCE: Questionable admission when principal dx

Coding Clinic: 2016, Q2, P36

E13 Other specified diabetes mellitus

Includes diabetes mellitus due to genetic defects of beta-cell function
diabetes mellitus due to genetic defects in insulin action
postpancreatectomy diabetes mellitus
postprocedural diabetes mellitus
secondary diabetes mellitus NEC

Use additional code to identify control using:
insulin (Z79.4) ◀
oral antidiabetic drugs (Z79.84) ◀
oral hypoglycemic drugs (Z79.84) ◀

Excludes1 diabetes (mellitus) due to autoimmune process (E10.-)
diabetes (mellitus) due to immune mediated pancreatic islet beta-cell destruction (E10.-)
diabetes mellitus due to underlying condition (E08.-)
drug or chemical induced diabetes mellitus (E09.-)
gestational diabetes (O24.4-)
neonatal diabetes mellitus (P70.2)
type 1 diabetes mellitus (E10.-) ◀
type 2 diabetes mellitus (E11.-)

E13.0 Other specified diabetes mellitus with hyperosmolarity

Ex: For category E13.0 CC codes: See E08.0

E13.00 Other specified diabetes mellitus with hyperosmolarity without nonketotic hyperglycemic-hyperosmolar coma (NKHHC)

E13.01 Other specified diabetes mellitus with hyperosmolarity with coma

E13.1 Other specified diabetes mellitus with ketoacidosis

Ex: For category E13.1 CC codes: See E08.0

E13.10 Other specified diabetes mellitus with ketoacidosis without coma

Coding Clinic: 2016, Q2, P10; 2013, Q1, P26

E13.11 Other specified diabetes mellitus with ketoacidosis with coma

E13.2 Other specified diabetes mellitus with kidney complications

E13.21 Other specified diabetes mellitus with diabetic nephropathy

Other specified diabetes mellitus with intercapillary glomerulosclerosis
Other specified diabetes mellitus with intracapillary glomerulonephrosis
Other specified diabetes mellitus with Kimmelstiel-Wilson disease

E13.22 Other specified diabetes mellitus with diabetic chronic kidney disease

Use additional code to identify stage of chronic kidney disease (N18.1-N18.6)

E13.29 Other specified diabetes mellitus with other diabetic kidney complication

Other specified diabetes mellitus with renal tubular degeneration

E13.3 Other specified diabetes mellitus with ophthalmic complications

E13.31 Other specified diabetes mellitus with unspecified diabetic retinopathy

E13.311 Other specified diabetes mellitus with unspecified diabetic retinopathy with macular edema

E13.319 Other specified diabetes mellitus with unspecified diabetic retinopathy without macular edema

● **E13.32 Other specified diabetes mellitus with mild nonproliferative diabetic retinopathy**
Other specified diabetes mellitus with nonproliferative diabetic retinopathy NOS
One of the following 7th characters is to be assigned to codes in subcategory E13.32 to designate laterality of the disease: ◀

1	right eye ◀
2	left eye ◀
3	bilateral ◀
9	unspecified eye ◀

● **E13.321 Other specified diabetes mellitus with mild nonproliferative diabetic retinopathy with macular edema**

● **E13.329 Other specified diabetes mellitus with mild nonproliferative diabetic retinopathy without macular edema**

● **E13.33 Other specified diabetes mellitus with moderate nonproliferative diabetic retinopathy**
One of the following 7th characters is to be assigned to codes in subcategory E13.33 to designate laterality of the disease: ◀

1	right eye ◀
2	left eye ◀
3	bilateral ◀
9	unspecified eye ◀

● **E13.331 Other specified diabetes mellitus with moderate nonproliferative diabetic retinopathy with macular edema**

● **E13.339 Other specified diabetes mellitus with moderate nonproliferative diabetic retinopathy without macular edema**

● **E13.34 Other specified diabetes mellitus with severe nonproliferative diabetic retinopathy**
One of the following 7th characters is to be assigned to codes in subcategory E13.34 to designate laterality of the disease: ◀

1	right eye ◀
2	left eye ◀
3	bilateral ◀
9	unspecified eye ◀

● **E13.341 Other specified diabetes mellitus with severe nonproliferative diabetic retinopathy with macular edema**

● **E13.349 Other specified diabetes mellitus with severe nonproliferative diabetic retinopathy without macular edema**

● **E13.35 Other specified diabetes mellitus with proliferative diabetic retinopathy**
One of the following 7th characters is to be assigned to codes in subcategory E13.35 to designate laterality of the disease: ◀

1	right eye ◀
2	left eye ◀
3	bilateral ◀
9	unspecified eye ◀

● **E13.351 Other specified diabetes mellitus with proliferative diabetic retinopathy with macular edema**

● **E13.352 Other specified diabetes mellitus with proliferative diabetic retinopathy with traction retinal detachment involving the macula** ◀

● **E13.353 Other specified diabetes mellitus with proliferative diabetic retinopathy with traction retinal detachment not involving the macula** ◀

● **E13.354 Other specified diabetes mellitus with proliferative diabetic retinopathy with combined traction retinal detachment and rhegmatogenous retinal detachment** ◀

● **E13.355 Other specified diabetes mellitus with stable proliferative diabetic retinopathy** ◀

● **E13.359 Other specified diabetes mellitus with proliferative diabetic retinopathy without macular edema**

E13.36 Other specified diabetes mellitus with diabetic cataract

X ● **E13.37 Other specified diabetes mellitus with diabetic macular edema, resolved following treatment**
One of the following 7th characters is to be assigned to code E13.37 to designate laterality of the disease: ◀

1	right eye ◀
2	left eye ◀
3	bilateral ◀
9	unspecified eye ◀

E13.39 Other specified diabetes mellitus with other diabetic ophthalmic complication
Use additional code to identify manifestation, such as:
diabetic glaucoma (H40-H42)

● **E13.4 Other specified diabetes mellitus with neurological complications**

E13.40 Other specified diabetes mellitus with diabetic neuropathy, unspecified

E13.41 Other specified diabetes mellitus with diabetic mononeuropathy

E13.42 Other specified diabetes mellitus with diabetic polyneuropathy
Other specified diabetes mellitus with diabetic neuralgia

E13.43 Other specified diabetes mellitus with diabetic autonomic (poly)neuropathy
Other specified diabetes mellitus with diabetic gastroparesis

E13.44 Other specified diabetes mellitus with diabetic amyotrophy

E13.49 Other specified diabetes mellitus with other diabetic neurological complication

● **E13.5 Other specified diabetes mellitus with circulatory complications**

E13.51 Other specified diabetes mellitus with diabetic peripheral angiopathy without gangrene

E13.52 Other specified diabetes mellitus with diabetic peripheral angiopathy with gangrene
Other specified diabetes mellitus with diabetic gangrene
CC when PDx is its own CC
Ex See E08.52

E13.59 Other specified diabetes mellitus with other circulatory complications

● **E13.6 Other specified diabetes mellitus with other specified complications**

● **E13.61 Other specified diabetes mellitus with diabetic arthropathy**

E13.610 Other specified diabetes mellitus with diabetic neuropathic arthropathy
Other specified diabetes mellitus with Charcôt's joints

E13.618 Other specified diabetes mellitus with other diabetic arthropathy

● **E13.62 Other specified diabetes mellitus with skin complications**

E13.620 Other specified diabetes mellitus with diabetic dermatitis
Other specified diabetes mellitus with diabetic necrobiosis lipoidica

E13.621 Other specified diabetes mellitus with foot ulcer
Use additional code to identify site of ulcer (L97.4-, L97.5-)

E13.622 Other specified diabetes mellitus with other skin ulcer
Use additional code to identify site of ulcer (L97.1-L97.9, L98.41-L98.49)

E13.628 Other specified diabetes mellitus with other skin complications

● **E13.63 Other specified diabetes mellitus with oral complications**

E13.630 Other specified diabetes mellitus with periodontal disease

E13.638 Other specified diabetes mellitus with other oral complications

● **E13.64 Other specified diabetes mellitus with hypoglycemia**

E13.641 Other specified diabetes mellitus with hypoglycemia with coma CC MCC
Ex: See E08.0

E13.649 Other specified diabetes mellitus with hypoglycemia without coma

E13.65 Other specified diabetes mellitus with hyperglycemia

E13.69 Other specified diabetes mellitus with other specified complication
Use additional code to identify complication

E13.8 Other specified diabetes mellitus with unspecified complications

E13.9 Other specified diabetes mellitus without complications
MCE: Questionable admission when principal dx

OTHER DISORDERS OF GLUCOSE REGULATION AND PANCREATIC INTERNAL SECRETION (E15-E16)

E15 Nondiabetic hypoglycemic coma CC MCC

Includes drug-induced insulin coma in nondiabetic hyperinsulinism with hypoglycemic coma
hypoglycemic coma NOS

Ex: A74.81, A74.9, B33.3-B33.4, B34.1-B34.2, B34.4-B34.8, B97.10, B97.19-B97.29, B97.31-B97.39, B97.5-B97.6, B97.81-B97.89, E08.3211-E08.3299, E08.3311-E08.3499, E08.3511-E08.3599, E08.37X1-E08.37X9, E09.3211-E09.3319, E09.3391-E09.3399, E09.3411-E09.3419, E09.3491-E09.3499, E09.3511-E09.3599, E09.37X1-E09.37X9, E10.3211-E10.3599, E10.37X1-E10.37X9, E11.3211-E11.3599, E11.37X1-E11.37X9, E13.3211-E13.3599, E13.37X1-E13.37X9

● **E16 Other disorders of pancreatic internal secretion**

E16.0 Drug-induced hypoglycemia without coma

Excludes1 diabetes with hypoglycemia without coma (E09.692) ◀

Use additional code for adverse effect, if applicable, to identify drug (T36-T50 with fifth or sixth character 5)

E16.1 Other hypoglycemia
Functional hyperinsulinism
Functional nonhyperinsulinemic hypoglycemia
Hyperinsulinism NOS
Hyperplasia of pancreatic islet beta cells NOS

Excludes1 diabetes with hypoglycemia (E08.649, E10.649, E11.649, E13.649) ◀
hypoglycemia in infant of diabetic mother (P70.1)
neonatal hypoglycemia (P70.4)

E16.2 Hypoglycemia, unspecified

Excludes1 diabetes with hypoglycemia (E08.649, E10.649, E11.649, E13.649) ◀

E16.3 Increased secretion of glucagon
Hyperplasia of pancreatic endocrine cells with glucagon excess

E16.4 Increased secretion of gastrin
Hypergastrinemia
Hyperplasia of pancreatic endocrine cells with gastrin excess
Zollinger-Ellison syndrome

E16.8 Other specified disorders of pancreatic internal secretion
Increased secretion from endocrine pancreas of growth hormone-releasing hormone
Increased secretion from endocrine pancreas of pancreatic polypeptide
Increased secretion from endocrine pancreas of somatostatin
Increased secretion from endocrine pancreas of vasoactive-intestinal polypeptide

E16.9 Disorder of pancreatic internal secretion, unspecified
Islet-cell hyperplasia NOS
Pancreatic endocrine cell hyperplasia NOS

DISORDERS OF OTHER ENDOCRINE GLANDS (E20-E35)

Excludes1 galactorrhea (N64.3)
gynecomastia (N62)

● **E20 Hypoparathyroidism**
Greatly reduced function of parathyroid glands; AKA parathyroid insufficiency

Excludes1 Di George's syndrome (D82.1)
postprocedural hypoparathyroidism (E89.2)
tetany NOS (R29.0)
transitory neonatal hypoparathyroidism (P71.4)

E20.0 Idiopathic hypoparathyroidism
Rare condition, unknown cause; short dwarf-like with round face

E20.1 Pseudohypoparathyroidism
Hereditary condition resembling hypoparathyroidism, but caused by inability to respond to parathyroid hormone

E20.8 Other hypoparathyroidism

E20.9 Hypoparathyroidism, unspecified
Parathyroid tetany

● **E21 Hyperparathyroidism and other disorders of parathyroid gland**

Excludes1 adult osteomalacia (M83.-)
ectopic hyperparathyroidism (E34.2)
familial hypocalciuric hypercalcemia (E83.52)
hungry bone syndrome (E83.81)
infantile and juvenile osteomalacia (E55.0)

E21.0 Primary hyperparathyroidism
Hyperplasia of parathyroid
Osteitis fibrosa cystica generalisata [von Recklinghausen's disease of bone]

E21.1 Secondary hyperparathyroidism, not elsewhere classified

Excludes1 secondary hyperparathyroidism of renal origin (N25.81)

Item 4–4 Hyperparathyroidism is an overactive parathyroid gland that secretes excessive parathormone, causing increased levels of circulating calcium. This results in a loss of calcium in the bone (osteoporosis).

Hypoparathyroidism is an underactive parathyroid gland that results in decreased levels of circulating calcium. The primary manifestation is **tetany,** a continuous muscle spasm.

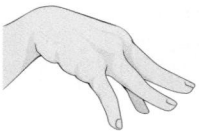

Figure 4-5 Tetany caused by hypoparathyroidism.

Item 4–5 Hyperadrenalism is overactivity of the adrenal cortex, which secretes corticosteroid hormones. Excessive glucocorticoid hormone results in hyperglycemia **(Cushing's syndrome),** and excessive aldosterone results in **Conn's syndrome. Adrenogenital syndrome** is the result of excessive secretion of androgens, male hormones, which stimulates premature sexual development. **Hypoadrenalism, Addison's disease,** is a condition in which the adrenal glands atrophy.

E21.2 Other hyperparathyroidism
Tertiary hyperparathyroidism
Excludes1 familial hypocalciuric hypercalcemia (E83.52)

E21.3 Hyperparathyroidism, unspecified

E21.4 Other specified disorders of parathyroid gland

E21.5 Disorder of parathyroid gland, unspecified

● **E22 Hyperfunction of pituitary gland**
Excludes1 Cushing's syndrome (E24.-)
Nelson's syndrome (E24.1)
overproduction of ACTH not associated with Cushing's disease (E27.0)
overproduction of pituitary ACTH (E24.0)
overproduction of thyroid-stimulating hormone (E05.8-)
Ex: For category E.22 CC codes unless otherwise indicated: E22.1-E22.9

E22.0 Acromegaly and pituitary gigantism
Chronic disease caused by hypersecretion of growth hormone
Overproduction of growth hormone
Excludes1 constitutional gigantism (E34.4)
constitutional tall stature (E34.4)
increased secretion from endocrine pancreas of growth hormone-releasing hormone (E16.8)

E22.1 Hyperprolactinemia
Increased levels of prolactin
Use additional code for adverse effect, if applicable, to identify drug (T36-T50 with fifth or sixth character 5)

E22.2 Syndrome of inappropriate secretion of antidiuretic hormone
Ex: E22.0-E23.7, E24.1, E30.9, E34.1, E34.4, E34.8-E35, E89.3

E22.8 Other hyperfunction of pituitary gland
Central precocious puberty

E22.9 Hyperfunction of pituitary gland, unspecified

● **E23 Hypofunction and other disorders of the pituitary gland**
Includes the listed conditions whether the disorder is in the pituitary or the hypothalamus
Excludes1 postprocedural hypopituitarism (E89.3)

E23.0 Hypopituitarism
Fertile eunuch syndrome
Hypogonadotropic hypogonadism
Idiopathic growth hormone deficiency
Isolated deficiency of gonadotropin
Isolated deficiency of growth hormone
Isolated deficiency of pituitary hormone
Kallmann's syndrome
Lorain-Levi short stature
Necrosis of pituitary gland (postpartum)
Panhypopituitarism
Pituitary cachexia
Pituitary insufficiency NOS
Pituitary short stature
Sheehan's syndrome
Simmonds' disease
Ex: E22.0-E23.7, E24.1, E30.9, E34.1, E34.4-E35, E89.3

E23.1 Drug-induced hypopituitarism
Use additional code for adverse effect, if applicable, to identify drug (T36-T50 with fifth or sixth character 5)

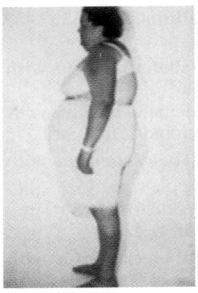

Figure 4-6 Centripetal and generalized obesity and dorsal kyphosis in a 30-year-old woman with Cushing's disease. (From Larsen: Williams Textbook of Endocrinology, ed 10, Saunders, An Imprint of Elsevier, 2003)

E23.2 Diabetes insipidus
Excludes1 nephrogenic diabetes insipidus (N25.1)
Ex: E22.1-E23.7, E24.1, E30.9, E34.1, E34.50-E35, E89.3

E23.3 Hypothalamic dysfunction, not elsewhere classified
Excludes1 Prader-Willi syndrome (Q87.1)
Russell-Silver syndrome (Q87.1)

E23.6 Other disorders of pituitary gland
Abscess of pituitary
Adiposogenital dystrophy

E23.7 Disorder of pituitary gland, unspecified

● **E24 Cushing's syndrome**
Excludes1 congenital adrenal hyperplasia (E25.0)
Ex: For category E24 CC codes: E24.0, E24.2-E26.9, E30.9, E34.1, E34.50-E35

E24.0 Pituitary-dependent Cushing's disease
Overproduction of pituitary ACTH
Pituitary-dependent hypercorticalism

E24.1 Nelson's syndrome

E24.2 Drug-induced Cushing's syndrome
Use additional code for adverse effect, if applicable, to identify drug (T36-T50 with fifth or sixth character 5)

E24.3 Ectopic ACTH syndrome

E24.4 Alcohol-induced pseudo-Cushing's syndrome

E24.8 Other Cushing's syndrome

E24.9 Cushing's syndrome, unspecified

● **E25 Adrenogenital disorders**
Disorder of production of steroid hormone in adrenal gland
Includes adrenogenital syndromes, virilizing or feminizing, whether acquired or due to adrenal hyperplasia consequent on inborn enzyme defects in hormone synthesis
female adrenal pseudohermaphroditism
female heterosexual precocious pseudopuberty
male isosexual precocious pseudopuberty
male macrogenitosomia praecox
male sexual precocity with adrenal hyperplasia
male virilization (female)
Excludes1 indeterminate sex and pseudohermaphroditism (Q56)
chromosomal abnormalities (Q90-Q99)

E25.0 Congenital adrenogenital disorders associated with enzyme deficiency
Congenital adrenal hyperplasia
21-Hydroxylase deficiency
Salt-losing congenital adrenal hyperplasia

E25.8 Other adrenogenital disorders
Idiopathic adrenogenital disorder
Use additional code for adverse effect, if applicable, to identify drug (T36-T50 with fifth or sixth character 5)

E25.9 Adrenogenital disorder, unspecified
Adrenogenital syndrome NOS

E26 Hyperaldosteronism
Abnormality of electrolyte metabolism caused by excessive secretion of aldosterone

E26.0 Primary hyperaldosteronism

E26.01 Conn's syndrome
Code also adrenal adenoma (D35.0-)

E26.02 Glucocorticoid-remediable aldosteronism
Familial aldosteronism type I

E26.09 Other primary hyperaldosteronism
Primary aldosteronism due to adrenal hyperplasia (bilateral)

E26.1 Secondary hyperaldosteronism

E26.8 Other hyperaldosteronism

E26.81 Bartter's syndrome

E26.89 Other hyperaldosteronism

E26.9 Hyperaldosteronism, unspecified
Aldosteronism NOS
Hyperaldosteronism NOS

E27 Other disorders of adrenal gland
Ex For category E27 CC codes: A17.9, A18.7, A18.82, A18.84, A18.89, E27.0-E27.9, E30.9, E34.1, E34.50-E35, E89.6

E27.0 Other adrenocortical overactivity
Overproduction of ACTH, not associated with Cushing's disease
Premature adrenarche
Excludes1 Cushing's syndrome (E24.-)

E27.1 Primary adrenocortical insufficiency
Addison's disease
Autoimmune adrenalitis
Excludes1 Addison only phenotype adrenoleukodystrophy (E71.528)
amyloidosis (E85.-)
tuberculous Addison's disease (A18.7)
Waterhouse-Friderichsen syndrome (A39.1)

E27.2 Addisonian crisis
Acute onset of adrenocortical insufficiency
Adrenal crisis
Adrenocortical crisis

E27.3 Drug-induced adrenocortical insufficiency
Use additional code for adverse effect, if applicable, to identify drug (T36-T50 with fifth or sixth character 5)

E27.4 Other and unspecified adrenocortical insufficiency
Excludes1 adrenoleukodystrophy [Addison-Schilder] (E71.528)
Waterhouse-Friderichsen syndrome (A39.1)

E27.40 Unspecified adrenocortical insufficiency
Adrenocortical insufficiency NOS
Hypoaldosteronism

E27.49 Other adrenocortical insufficiency
Adrenal hemorrhage
Adrenal infarction

E27.5 Adrenomedullary hyperfunction
Adrenomedullary hyperplasia
Catecholamine hypersecretion

E27.8 Other specified disorders of adrenal gland
Abnormality of cortisol-binding globulin

E27.9 Disorder of adrenal gland, unspecified

E28 Ovarian dysfunction
Excludes1 isolated gonadotropin deficiency (E23.0)
postprocedural ovarian failure (E89.4-)

E28.0 Estrogen excess ♀
Use additional code for adverse effect, if applicable, to identify drug (T36-T50 with fifth or sixth character 5)

E28.1 Androgen excess ♀
Hypersecretion of ovarian androgens
Use additional code for adverse effect, if applicable, to identify drug (T36-T50 with fifth or sixth character 5)

E28.2 Polycystic ovarian syndrome ♀
Sclerocystic ovary syndrome
Stein-Leventhal syndrome

E28.3 Primary ovarian failure
Excludes1 pure gonadal dysgenesis (Q99.1)
Turner's syndrome (Q96.-)

E28.31 Premature menopause

E28.310 Symptomatic premature menopause ♀ A
Symptoms such as flushing, sleeplessness, headache, lack of concentration, associated with premature menopause

E28.319 Asymptomatic premature menopause ♀ A
Premature menopause NOS

E28.39 Other primary ovarian failure ♀
Decreased estrogen
Resistant ovary syndrome

E28.8 Other ovarian dysfunction ♀
Ovarian hyperfunction NOS
Excludes1 postprocedural ovarian failure (E89.4-)

E28.9 Ovarian dysfunction, unspecified ♀

E29 Testicular dysfunction
Excludes1 androgen insensitivity syndrome (E34.5-)
azoospermia or oligospermia NOS (N46.0-N46.1)
isolated gonadotropin deficiency (E23.0)
Klinefelter's syndrome (Q98.0-Q98.1, Q98.4)

E29.0 Testicular hyperfunction ♂
Hypersecretion of testicular hormones

E29.1 Testicular hypofunction ♂
Defective biosynthesis of testicular androgen NOS
5-delta-Reductase deficiency (with male pseudohermaphroditism)
Testicular hypogonadism NOS
Use additional code for adverse effect, if applicable, to identify drug (T36-T50 with fifth or sixth character 5)
Excludes1 postprocedural testicular hypofunction (E89.5)

E29.8 Other testicular dysfunction ♂

E29.9 Testicular dysfunction, unspecified ♂

E30 Disorders of puberty, not elsewhere classified

E30.0 Delayed puberty
Constitutional delay of puberty
Delayed sexual development

E30.1 Precocious puberty P
Sexual maturation at earlier age than normal, or before age 8 in girls and 9 in boys, usually hormonal; AKA sexual precocity or pubertas praecox
Precocious menstruation
Excludes1 Albright (-McCune) (-Sternberg) syndrome (Q78.1)
central precocious puberty (E22.8)
congenital adrenal hyperplasia (E25.0)
female heterosexual precocious pseudopuberty (E25.-)
male isosexual precocious pseudopuberty (E25.-)

E30.8 Other disorders of puberty P
Premature thelarche

E30.9 Disorder of puberty, unspecified

● **E31 Polyglandular dysfunction**

Excludes1 ataxia telangiectasia [Louis-Bar] (G11.3)
dystrophia myotonica [Steinert] (G71.11)
pseudohypoparathyroidism (E20.1)

E31.0 Autoimmune polyglandular failure
Schmidt's syndrome

E31.1 Polyglandular hyperfunction

Excludes1 multiple endocrine adenomatosis (E31.2-)
multiple endocrine neoplasia (E31.2-)

● **E31.2 Multiple endocrine neoplasia [MEN] syndromes**
Adenomatous hyperplasia and malignant tumors in endocrine glands
Multiple endocrine adenomatosis

Code also any associated malignancies and other conditions associated with the syndromes

E31.20 Multiple endocrine neoplasia [MEN] syndrome, unspecified
Multiple endocrine adenomatosis NOS
Multiple endocrine neoplasia [MEN] syndrome NOS

E31.21 Multiple endocrine neoplasia [MEN] type I
Wermer's syndrome

E31.22 Multiple endocrine neoplasia [MEN] type IIA
Sipple's syndrome

E31.23 Multiple endocrine neoplasia [MEN] type IIB

E31.8 Other polyglandular dysfunction

E31.9 Polyglandular dysfunction, unspecified

● **E32 Diseases of thymus**

Excludes1 aplasia or hypoplasia of thymus with immunodeficiency (D82.1)
myasthenia gravis (G70.0)

E32.0 Persistent hyperplasia of thymus
Hypertrophy of thymus

E32.1 Abscess of thymus
Ex: E30.9, E32.0-E32.9, E34.1, E34.50-E35

E32.8 Other diseases of thymus

Excludes1 aplasia or hypoplasia with immunodeficiency (D82.1)
thymoma (D15.0)

E32.9 Disease of thymus, unspecified

● **E34 Other endocrine disorders**

Excludes1 pseudohypoparathyroidism (E20.1)

E34.0 Carcinoid syndrome

Note: May be used as an additional code to identify functional activity associated with a carcinoid tumor.
Ex: E30.9, E34.0-E34.2, E34.50-E35

E34.1 Other hypersecretion of intestinal hormones

E34.2 Ectopic hormone secretion, not elsewhere classified

Excludes1 ectopic ACTH syndrome (E24.3)

E34.3 Short stature due to endocrine disorder
Constitutional short stature
Laron-type short stature

Excludes1 achondroplastic short stature (Q77.4)
hypochondroplastic short stature (Q77.4)
nutritional short stature (E45)
pituitary short stature (E23.0)
progeria (E34.8)
renal short stature (N25.0)
Russell-Silver syndrome (Q87.1)
short-limbed stature with immunodeficiency (D82.2)
short stature in specific dysmorphic syndromes - code to syndrome - see Alphabetical Index
short stature NOS (R62.52)

E34.4 Constitutional tall stature
Constitutional gigantism

● **E34.5 Androgen insensitivity syndrome**

E34.50 Androgen insensitivity syndrome, unspecified
Androgen insensitivity NOS

E34.51 Complete androgen insensitivity syndrome
Complete androgen insensitivity
de Quervain syndrome
Goldberg-Maxwell syndrome

E34.52 Partial androgen insensitivity syndrome
Partial androgen insensitivity
Reifenstein syndrome

E34.8 Other specified endocrine disorders
Pineal gland dysfunction
Progeria

Excludes2 pseudohypoparathyroidism (E20.1)

E34.9 Endocrine disorder, unspecified
Endocrine disturbance NOS
Hormone disturbance NOS

▶ ***E35 Disorders of endocrine glands in diseases classified elsewhere***

Code first underlying disease, such as:
late congenital syphilis of thymus gland [Dubois disease] (A50.5)

Use additional code, if applicable, to identify:
sequelae of tuberculosis of other organs (B90.8)

Excludes1 Echinococcus granulosus infection of thyroid gland (B67.3)
meningococcal hemorrhagic adrenalitis (A39.1)
syphilis of endocrine gland (A52.79)
tuberculosis of adrenal gland, except calcification (A18.7)
tuberculosis of endocrine gland NEC (A18.82)
tuberculosis of thyroid gland (A18.81)
Waterhouse-Friderichsen syndrome (A39.1)

INTRAOPERATIVE COMPLICATIONS OF ENDOCRINE SYSTEM (E36)

● **E36 Intraoperative complications of endocrine system**

Excludes2 postprocedural endocrine and metabolic complications and disorders, not elsewhere classified (E89.-)

● **E36.0 Intraoperative hemorrhage and hematoma of an endocrine system organ or structure complicating a procedure**

Excludes1 intraoperative hemorrhage and hematoma of an endocrine system organ or structure due to accidental puncture or laceration during a procedure (E36.1-)

Ex: **For category E36.0 CC codes:** E36.01-E36.02, E36.8, E89.810-E89.89, H95.811-H95.89, I85.01, I85.11, I97.3, K21.9, K22.8, K23-K25.0, K25.2, K25.4, K25.6, K26.0, K26.2, K26.4, K26.6, K27.0, K27.2, K27.4, K27.6, K28.0, K28.2, K28.4, K28.6, K29.01, K29.21, K29.31, K29.41, K29.51, K29.61, K29.71, K29.81, K29.91, K31.811, K55.21, K57.01, K57.11, K57.13, K57.21, K57.31, K57.33, K57.41, K57.51, K57.53, K57.81, K57.91, K57.93, K62.5, K92.0-K92.2, M96.89, N98.1-N98.9, P54.1-P54.3, T81.10X-T81.19X[A], T81.82X[A], T81.89X-T81.9XX[A]

E36.01 Intraoperative hemorrhage and hematoma of an endocrine system organ or structure complicating an endocrine system procedure

E36.02 Intraoperative hemorrhage and hematoma of an endocrine system organ or structure complicating other procedure

● **E36.1 Accidental puncture and laceration of an endocrine system organ or structure during a procedure**

Ex: **For category E36.1 CC codes:** D78.11-D78.12, D78.81-D78.89, E36.11-E36.8, E89.810-E89.89, G96.11, G97.41-G97.49, H59.011-H59.019, H59.031-H59.099, H59.211-H59.229, H59.811-H59.89, H95.31-H95.32, H95.811-H95.89, I97.3, I97.51-I97.52, J95.71-J95.72, K91.71-K91.72, L76.11-L76.12, L76.81-L76.82, M96.820-M96.821, M96.89, N98.1-N98.9, N99.71-N99.72, T81.82X[A], T81.89X-T81.9XX[A]

E36.11 Accidental puncture and laceration of an endocrine system organ or structure during an endocrine system procedure

E36.12 Accidental puncture and laceration of an endocrine system organ or structure during other procedure

E36.8 Other intraoperative complications of endocrine system
Use additional code, if applicable, to further specify disorder

MALNUTRITION (E40-E46)

Excludes1 intestinal malabsorption (K90.-)
sequelae of protein-calorie malnutrition (E64.0)

Excludes2 nutritional anemias (D50-D53)
starvation (T73.0)

E40 Kwashiorkor
Malnutrition produced by severe protein deficiency
Severe malnutrition with nutritional edema with dyspigmentation of skin and hair
Excludes1 marasmic kwashiorkor (E42)
Ex: E40-E46, E64.0

E41 Nutritional marasmus
Severe malnutrition with marasmus
Excludes1 marasmic kwashiorkor (E42)
Ex: E40-E46, E64.0

E42 Marasmic kwashiorkor
Severe protein malnutrition
Intermediate form severe protein-calorie malnutrition
Severe protein-calorie malnutrition with signs of both kwashiorkor and marasmus
Ex: E40-E46, E64.0

E43 Unspecified severe protein-calorie malnutrition
Starvation edema
Ex: E40-E46, E64.0

E44 Protein-calorie malnutrition of moderate and mild degree
Ex: For category E44 CC codes: E40-E46, E64.0

E44.0 Moderate protein-calorie malnutrition

E44.1 Mild protein-calorie malnutrition

E45 Retarded development following protein-calorie malnutrition
Nutritional short stature
Nutritional stunting
Physical retardation due to malnutrition
Ex: E40-E46, E64.0

E46 Unspecified protein-calorie malnutrition
Malnutrition NOS
Protein-calorie imbalance NOS
Excludes1 nutritional deficiency NOS (E63.9)
Ex: E40-E46, E64.0

OTHER NUTRITIONAL DEFICIENCIES (E50-E64)

Excludes2 nutritional anemias (D50-D53)

E50 Vitamin A deficiency
Excludes1 sequelae of vitamin A deficiency (E64.1)

E50.0 Vitamin A deficiency with conjunctival xerosis

E50.1 Vitamin A deficiency with Bitot's spot and conjunctival xerosis
Bitot's spot in the young child

E50.2 Vitamin A deficiency with corneal xerosis

E50.3 Vitamin A deficiency with corneal ulceration and xerosis

E50.4 Vitamin A deficiency with keratomalacia
Eye disorder that results in dry cornea caused by vitamin A deficiency

E50.5 Vitamin A deficiency with night blindness

E50.6 Vitamin A deficiency with xerophthalmic scars of cornea
Abnormal dryness and thickening of conjunctiva and cornea due to vitamin A deficiency

E50.7 Other ocular manifestations of vitamin A deficiency
Xerophthalmia NOS

E50.8 Other manifestations of vitamin A deficiency
Follicular keratosis
Xeroderma

E50.9 Vitamin A deficiency, unspecified
Hypovitaminosis A NOS

E51 Thiamine deficiency
Excludes1 sequelae of thiamine deficiency (E64.8)

E51.1 Beriberi
Ex: For category E51.1 CC codes: D81.818-D81.819, E51.11-E53.9, E56.0, E56.8-E63.9, E64.8-E64.9

E51.11 Dry beriberi
Thiamine deficiency with nervous system manifestation most often caused by excessive alcohol consumption
Beriberi NOS
Beriberi with polyneuropathy

E51.12 Wet beriberi
Thiamine deficiency with cardiovascular manifestation most often caused by excessive alcohol consumption
Beriberi with cardiovascular manifestations
Cardiovascular beriberi
Shoshin disease

E51.2 Wernicke's encephalopathy
Acute disease of brain due to thiamine deficiency most often associated with excessive alcohol consumption
Ex: See E51.1

E51.8 Other manifestations of thiamine deficiency
Ex: See E51.1

E51.9 Thiamine deficiency, unspecified
Ex: See E51.1

Item 4–6 Bitot's spots are the result of a buildup of keratin debris found on the superficial surface the conjunctiva; oval, triangular, or irregular in shape; and a sign of vitamin A deficiency and associated with night blindness. The disease may progress to **keratomalacia,** which can result in eventual prolapse of the iris and loss of the lens.

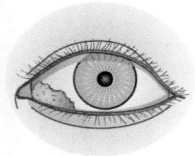

Figure 4-7 Bitot's spot on the conjunctiva.

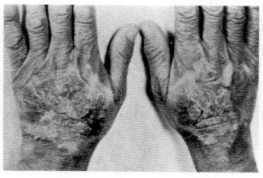

Figure 4-8 The sharply demarcated, characteristic scaling dermatitis of pellagra. (From Kumar: Robbins and Cotran: Pathologic Basis of Disease, ed 8, Saunders, An Imprint of Elsevier, 2009)

Item 4–7 Pellagra is associated with a deficiency of niacin and its precursor, **tryptophan.** Characteristics of the condition include diarrhea, dermatitis on exposed skin surfaces, dementia, and death. It is prevalent in developing countries where nutrition is inadequate. **Beriberi** is associated with thiamine deficiency.

E52 Niacin deficiency [pellagra]
Niacin (-tryptophan) deficiency
Nicotinamide deficiency
Pellagra (alcoholic)
Excludes1 sequelae of niacin deficiency (E64.8)

● **E53 Deficiency of other B group vitamins**
Excludes1 sequelae of vitamin B deficiency (E64.8)

E53.0 Riboflavin deficiency
Ariboflavinosis
Vitamin B2 deficiency
Ex: See E51.1

E53.1 Pyridoxine deficiency
Vitamin B6 deficiency
Excludes1 pyridoxine-responsive sideroblastic anemia (D64.3)

E53.8 Deficiency of other specified B group vitamins
Biotin deficiency
Cyanocobalamin deficiency
Folate deficiency
Folic acid deficiency
Pantothenic acid deficiency
Vitamin B12 deficiency
Excludes1 folate deficiency anemia (D52.-)
vitamin B12 deficiency anemia (D51.-)

E53.9 Vitamin B deficiency, unspecified

E54 Ascorbic acid deficiency
Deficiency of vitamin C
Scurvy
Excludes1 scorbutic anemia (D53.2)
sequelae of vitamin C deficiency (E64.2)

● **E55 Vitamin D deficiency**
Excludes1 adult osteomalacia (M83.-)
osteoporosis (M80.-)
sequelae of rickets (E64.3)

E55.0 Rickets, active
Infantile osteomalacia
Juvenile osteomalacia
Softening of bone
Excludes1 celiac rickets (K90.0)
Crohn's rickets (K50.-)
hereditary vitamin D-dependent rickets (E83.32)
inactive rickets (E64.3)
renal rickets (N25.0)
sequelae of rickets (E64.3)
vitamin D-resistant rickets (E83.31)
Ex: E55.0-E63.9, E64.3-E64.9, M83.0-M83.9

E55.9 Vitamin D deficiency, unspecified
Avitaminosis D

● **E56 Other vitamin deficiencies**
Excludes1 sequelae of other vitamin deficiencies (E64.8)

E56.0 Deficiency of vitamin E

E56.1 Deficiency of vitamin K
Excludes1 deficiency of coagulation factor due to vitamin K deficiency (D68.4)
vitamin K deficiency of newborn (P53)

E56.8 Deficiency of other vitamins

E56.9 Vitamin deficiency, unspecified

E58 Dietary calcium deficiency
Excludes1 disorders of calcium metabolism (E83.5-)
sequelae of calcium deficiency (E64.8)

E59 Dietary selenium deficiency
Keshan disease
Excludes1 sequelae of selenium deficiency (E64.8)

E60 Dietary zinc deficiency

● **E61 Deficiency of other nutrient elements**
Use additional code for adverse effect, if applicable, to identify drug (T36-T50 with fifth or sixth character 5)
Excludes1 disorders of mineral metabolism (E83.-)
iodine deficiency related thyroid disorders (E00-E02)
sequelae of malnutrition and other nutritional deficiencies (E64.-)

E61.0 Copper deficiency

E61.1 Iron deficiency
Excludes1 iron deficiency anemia (D50.-)

E61.2 Magnesium deficiency

E61.3 Manganese deficiency

E61.4 Chromium deficiency

E61.5 Molybdenum deficiency

E61.6 Vanadium deficiency

E61.7 Deficiency of multiple nutrient elements

E61.8 Deficiency of other specified nutrient elements

E61.9 Deficiency of nutrient element, unspecified

● **E63 Other nutritional deficiencies**
Excludes1 dehydration (E86.0)
failure to thrive, adult (R62.7)
failure to thrive, child (R62.51)
feeding problems in newborn (P92.-)
sequelae of malnutrition and other nutritional deficiencies (E64.-)

E63.0 Essential fatty acid [EFA] deficiency

E63.1 Imbalance of constituents of food intake

E63.8 Other specified nutritional deficiencies

E63.9 Nutritional deficiency, unspecified

● **E64 Sequelae of malnutrition and other nutritional deficiencies**
Pathological condition resulting from disease, injury, or other trauma
Note: This category is to be used to indicate conditions in categories E43, E44, E46, E50-E63 as the cause of sequelae, which are themselves classified elsewhere. The 'sequelae' include conditions specified as such; they also include the late effects of diseases classifiable to the above categories if the disease itself is no longer present
Code first condition resulting from (sequela) of malnutrition and other nutritional deficiencies

E64.0 Sequelae of protein-calorie malnutrition
Excludes2 retarded development following protein-calorie malnutrition (E45)
Ex: E40-E46, E64.0

E64.1 Sequelae of vitamin A deficiency

E64.2 Sequelae of vitamin C deficiency

E64.3 Sequelae of rickets

E64.8 Sequelae of other nutritional deficiencies

E64.9 Sequelae of unspecified nutritional deficiency

OVERWEIGHT, OBESITY AND OTHER HYPERALIMENTATION (E65-E68)

E65 Localized adiposity
Fat pad

● **E66 Overweight and obesity**
Code first obesity complicating pregnancy, childbirth and the puerperium, if applicable (O99.21-)
Use additional code to identify body mass index (BMI), if known (Z68.-)
Excludes1 adiposogenital dystrophy (E23.6)
lipomatosis NOS (E88.2)
lipomatosis dolorosa [Dercum] (E88.2)
Prader-Willi syndrome (Q87.1)

● **E66.0 Obesity due to excess calories**
E66.01 Morbid (severe) obesity due to excess calories
Excludes1 morbid (severe) obesity with alveolar hypoventilation (E66.2)
E66.09 Other obesity due to excess calories
MCE: Questionable admission when principal dx
E66.1 Drug-induced obesity
MCE: Questionable admission when principal dx
Use additional code for adverse effect, if applicable, to identify drug (T36-T50 with fifth or sixth character 5)
E66.2 Morbid (severe) obesity with alveolar hypoventilation
Uncommon condition of unknown cause leading to inadequate ventilation in lungs, even though lungs and airways are normal
Obesity hypoventilation syndrome (OHS) ◀
Pickwickian syndrome
Ex: E66.2, I27.0-I27.81, I27.89-I27.9
E66.3 Overweight
E66.8 Other obesity
MCE: Questionable admission when principal dx
E66.9 Obesity, unspecified
Obesity NOS
MCE: Questionable admission when principal dx

● **E67 Other hyperalimentation**
Ingestion of more than optimal amount of nutrients
Excludes1 hyperalimentation NOS (R63.2)
sequelae of hyperalimentation (E68)
E67.0 Hypervitaminosis A
E67.1 Hypercarotinemia
E67.2 Megavitamin-B6 syndrome
E67.3 Hypervitaminosis D
E67.8 Other specified hyperalimentation

E68 Sequelae of hyperalimentation
Code first condition resulting from (sequela) of hyperalimentation

METABOLIC DISORDERS (E70-E88)

Excludes1 androgen insensitivity syndrome (E34.5-)
congenital adrenal hyperplasia (E25.0)
Ehlers-Danlos syndrome (Q79.6)
hemolytic anemias attributable to enzyme disorders (D55.-)
Marfan's syndrome (Q87.4)
5-alpha-reductase deficiency (E29.1)

● **E70 Disorders of aromatic amino-acid metabolism**
Ex: **For category E70 CC codes:** C88.0, D47.2, D89.0-D89.1, E70.0-E71.30, E72.00-E72.02, E72.04-E74.9, E75.21-E75.249, E75.3, E75.5-E75.6, E77.0-E78.70, E78.79-E78.9, E88.09-E88.2, E88.89
E70.0 Classical phenylketonuria
Inherited disorder that increases to harmful levels amino acid phenylalanine
E70.1 Other hyperphenylalaninemias

● **E70.2 Disorders of tyrosine metabolism**
Excludes1 transitory tyrosinemia of newborn (P74.5)
E70.20 Disorder of tyrosine metabolism, unspecified
Tyrosine: Nonessential amino acid occurring in most proteins
E70.21 Tyrosinemia
Congenital amino acid metabolism
Hypertyrosinemia
E70.29 Other disorders of tyrosine metabolism
Alkaptonuria
Ochronosis

● **E70.3 Albinism**
Congenital condition of reduced or absent pigment in eyes, skin, and hair
E70.30 Albinism, unspecified
● **E70.31 Ocular albinism**
E70.310 X-linked ocular albinism
E70.311 Autosomal recessive ocular albinism
E70.318 Other ocular albinism
E70.319 Ocular albinism, unspecified
● **E70.32 Oculocutaneous albinism**
Partial or total lack of melanin pigment in eyes
Excludes1 Chediak-Higashi syndrome (E70.330)
Hermansky-Pudlak syndrome (E70.331)
E70.320 Tyrosinase negative oculocutaneous albinism
Albinism I
Oculocutaneous albinism ty-neg
E70.321 Tyrosinase positive oculocutaneous albinism
Albinism II
Oculocutaneous albinism ty-pos
E70.328 Other oculocutaneous albinism
Cross syndrome
E70.329 Oculocutaneous albinism, unspecified
● **E70.33 Albinism with hematologic abnormality**
E70.330 Chediak-Higashi syndrome
E70.331 Hermansky-Pudlak syndrome
E70.338 Other albinism with hematologic abnormality
E70.339 Albinism with hematologic abnormality, unspecified
E70.39 Other specified albinism
Piebaldism

● **E70.4 Disorders of histidine metabolism**
E70.40 Disorders of histidine metabolism, unspecified
E70.41 Histidinemia
E70.49 Other disorders of histidine metabolism
E70.5 Disorders of tryptophan metabolism
E70.8 Other disorders of aromatic amino-acid metabolism
E70.9 Disorder of aromatic amino-acid metabolism, unspecified

E71 Disorders of branched-chain amino-acid metabolism and fatty-acid metabolism

E71.0 Maple-syrup-urine disease
Due to defect in amino acid catabolism, causing severe ketoacidosis with smell of maple syrup in urine and on body
Ex: See E70

E71.1 Other disorders of branched-chain amino-acid metabolism
Ex: For category E71.1 CC codes: See E70

E71.11 Branched-chain organic acidurias

E71.110 Isovaleric acidemia

E71.111 3-methylglutaconic aciduria

E71.118 Other branched-chain organic acidurias

E71.12 Disorders of propionate metabolism

E71.120 Methylmalonic acidemia

E71.121 Propionic acidemia

E71.128 Other disorders of propionate metabolism

E71.19 Other disorders of branched-chain amino-acid metabolism
Hyperleucine-isoleucinemia
Hypervalinemia

E71.2 Disorder of branched-chain amino-acid metabolism, unspecified
Ex: See E70

E71.3 Disorders of fatty-acid metabolism
Excludes1 peroxisomal disorders (E71.5)
Refsum's disease (G60.1)
Schilder's disease (G37.0)
Excludes2 carnitine deficiency due to inborn error of metabolism (E71.42)

E71.30 Disorder of fatty-acid metabolism, unspecified

E71.31 Disorders of fatty-acid oxidation
Ex: For category E71.31 CC codes: C96.5-C96.6, E71.39-E71.548, E80.3, E88.40-E88.49, E88.89, H49.811-H49.819

E71.310 Long chain/very long chain acyl CoA dehydrogenase deficiency
LCAD
VLCAD

E71.311 Medium chain acyl CoA dehydrogenase deficiency
MCAD

E71.312 Short chain acyl CoA dehydrogenase deficiency
SCAD

E71.313 Glutaric aciduria type II
Glutaric aciduria type II A
Glutaric aciduria type II B
Glutaric aciduria type II C
Excludes1 glutaric aciduria (type 1) NOS (E72.3)

E71.314 Muscle carnitine palmitoyltransferase deficiency

E71.318 Other disorders of fatty-acid oxidation

E71.32 Disorders of ketone metabolism
Ex: See E71.31

E71.39 Other disorders of fatty-acid metabolism
Ex: E71.310-E71.32, E71.40-E71.548, E80.4-E80.7, E88.40-E88.49, H49.811-H49.819

E71.4 Disorders of carnitine metabolism
Excludes1 muscle carnitine palmitoyltransferase deficiency (E71.314)

E71.40 Disorder of carnitine metabolism, unspecified

E71.41 Primary carnitine deficiency

E71.42 Carnitine deficiency due to inborn errors of metabolism
Code also associated inborn error or metabolism

E71.43 Iatrogenic carnitine deficiency
Iatrogenic: Outcomes from activity of physicians
Carnitine deficiency due to hemodialysis
Carnitine deficiency due to Valproic acid therapy

E71.44 Other secondary carnitine deficiency

E71.440 Ruvalcaba-Myhre-Smith syndrome

E71.448 Other secondary carnitine deficiency

E71.5 Peroxisomal disorders
Class of conditions which lead to disorders of lipid metabolism
Excludes1 Schilder's disease (G37.0)
Ex: For category E71.5 CC codes: C96.5-C96.6, E71.310-E71.448, E80.3-E80.7, E88.40-E88.49, E88.89, H49.811-H49.819

E71.50 Peroxisomal disorder, unspecified

E71.51 Disorders of peroxisome biogenesis
Group 1 peroxisomal disorders
Excludes1 Refsum's disease (G60.1)

E71.510 Zellweger syndrome

E71.511 Neonatal adrenoleukodystrophy
Excludes1 X-linked adrenoleukodystrophy (E71.42-)

E71.518 Other disorders of peroxisome biogenesis

E71.52 X-linked adrenoleukodystrophy

E71.520 Childhood cerebral X-linked adrenoleukodystrophy

E71.521 Adolescent X-linked adrenoleukodystrophy

E71.522 Adrenomyeloneuropathy

E71.528 Other X-linked adrenoleukodystrophy
Addison only phenotype adrenoleukodystrophy
Addison-Schilder adrenoleukodystrophy

E71.529 X-linked adrenoleukodystrophy, unspecified type

E71.53 Other group 2 peroxisomal disorders

E71.54 Other peroxisomal disorders

E71.540 Rhizomelic chondrodysplasia punctata
Rare, severe, inherited disorder with limb shortening, bone and cartilage abnormalities, abnormal facial appearance, severe mental retardation, psychomotor retardation, and cataracts
Excludes1 chondrodysplasia punctata NOS (Q77.3)

E71.541 Zellweger-like syndrome

E71.542 Other group 3 peroxisomal disorders

E71.548 Other peroxisomal disorders

E72 Other disorders of amino-acid metabolism

Excludes1 disorders of:
aromatic amino-acid metabolism (E70.-)
branched-chain amino-acid metabolism (E71.0-E71.2)
fatty-acid metabolism (E71.3)
purine and pyrimidine metabolism (E79.-)
gout (M1A.-, M10.-)

Ex For category E72 CC codes unless otherwise noted: See E70

E72.0 Disorders of amino-acid transport

Excludes1 disorders of tryptophan metabolism (E70.5)

E72.00 Disorders of amino-acid transport, unspecified

E72.01 Cystinuria
Hereditary aminoaciduria due to impairment of renal transport with predominant symptom of urinary cystine calculi

E72.02 Hartnup's disease
Inborn error of metabolism

E72.03 Lowe's syndrome
X-linked disorder with rickets, hydrophthalmia, congenital glaucoma, cataracts, mental retardation, and renal tubule dysfunction

Use additional code for associated glaucoma (H42)

Ex No exclusion

E72.04 Cystinosis
Genetic disease with excessive depostits of amino acid cystine in cells
Fanconi (-de Toni) (-Debré) syndrome with cystinosis

Excludes1 Fanconi (-de Toni) (-Debré) syndrome without cystinosis (E72.09)

E72.09 Other disorders of amino-acid transport
Fanconi (-de Toni) (-Debré) syndrome, unspecified

E72.1 Disorders of sulfur-bearing amino-acid metabolism

Excludes1 cystinosis (E72.04)
cystinuria (E72.01)
transcobalamin II deficiency (D51.2)

E72.10 Disorders of sulfur-bearing amino-acid metabolism, unspecified

E72.11 Homocystinuria
Cystathionine synthase deficiency

E72.12 Methylenetetrahydrofolate reductase deficiency

E72.19 Other disorders of sulfur-bearing amino-acid metabolism
Cystathioninuria
Methioninemia
Sulfite oxidase deficiency

E72.2 Disorders of urea cycle metabolism

Excludes1 disorders of ornithine metabolism (E72.4)

E72.20 Disorder of urea cycle metabolism, unspecified
Hyperammonemia
Elevated levels of ammonia

Excludes1 hyperammonemia-hyperornithinemia-homocitrullinemia syndrome E72.4
transient hyperammonemia of newborn (P74.6)

E72.21 Argininemia
Disorder in which deficiency of enzyme arginase causes build up of arginine and ammonia in blood

E72.22 Arginosuccinic aciduria
Gene disorder of urea cycle resulting accumulation of ammonia

E72.23 Citrullinemia
Urea cycle disorder that causes ammonia and other toxic substances to accumulate in blood

E72.29 Other disorders of urea cycle metabolism

E72.3 Disorders of lysine and hydroxylysine metabolism
Glutaric aciduria NOS
Glutaric aciduria (type I)
Hydroxylysinemia
Hyperlysinemia

Excludes1 glutaric aciduria type II (E71.313)
Refsum's disease (G60.1)
Zellweger syndrome (E71.510)

E72.4 Disorders of ornithine metabolism
Hyperammonemia-Hyperornithinemia-Homocitrullinemia syndrome
Ornithinemia (types I, II)
Ornithine transcarbamylase deficiency

Excludes1 hereditary choroidal dystrophy (H31.2-)

E72.5 Disorders of glycine metabolism

E72.50 Disorder of glycine metabolism, unspecified

E72.51 Non-ketotic hyperglycinemia

E72.52 Trimethylaminuria

E72.53 Hyperoxaluria
Oxalosis
Oxaluria

E72.59 Other disorders of glycine metabolism
D-glycericacidemia
Hyperhydroxyprolinemia
Hyperprolinemia (types I, II)
Sarcosinemia

E72.8 Other specified disorders of amino-acid metabolism
Disorders of beta-amino-acid metabolism
Disorders of gamma-glutamyl cycle

E72.9 Disorder of amino-acid metabolism, unspecified

E73 Lactose intolerance
Intolerance for lactose, due to inherited deficiency of lactase activity in intestinal mucosa

E73.0 Congenital lactase deficiency

E73.1 Secondary lactase deficiency

E73.8 Other lactose intolerance

E73.9 Lactose intolerance, unspecified

E74 Other disorders of carbohydrate metabolism

Excludes1 diabetes mellitus (E08-E13)
hypoglycemia NOS (E16.2)
increased secretion of glucagon (E16.3)
mucopolysaccharidosis (E76.0-E76.3)

Ex For category E74 CC codes: See E70

E74.0 Glycogen storage disease

E74.00 Glycogen storage disease, unspecified

E74.01 von Gierke's disease
Type I glycogen storage disease

E74.02 Pompe disease
Cardiac glycogenosis
Type II glycogen storage disease

E74.03 Cori disease
Forbes' disease
Type III glycogen storage disease

E74.04 McArdle disease
Type V glycogen storage disease

E74.09 Other glycogen storage disease
Andersen disease
Hers disease
Tauri disease
Glycogen storage disease, types 0, IV, VI-XI
Liver phosphorylase deficiency
Muscle phosphofructokinase deficiency

E74.1 Disorders of fructose metabolism

Excludes1 muscle phosphofructokinase deficiency (E74.09)

E74.10 Disorder of fructose metabolism, unspecified

E74.11 Essential fructosuria
Fructokinase deficiency

E74.12 Hereditary fructose intolerance
Fructosemia

E74.19 Other disorders of fructose metabolism
Fructose-1, 6-diphosphatase deficiency

E74.2 Disorders of galactose metabolism

E74.20 Disorders of galactose metabolism, unspecified

E74.21 Galactosemia
Genetic disorders resulting from defective simple sugar (galactose) metabolism

E74.29 Other disorders of galactose metabolism
Galactokinase deficiency

E74.3 Other disorders of intestinal carbohydrate absorption

Excludes2 lactose intolerance (E73.-)

E74.31 Sucrase-isomaltase deficiency
Deficiency in metabolism in intestinal mucosa results in malabsorption of sucrose and starch

E74.39 Other disorders of intestinal carbohydrate absorption
Disorder of intestinal carbohydrate absorption NOS
Glucose-galactose malabsorption
Sucrase deficiency

E74.4 Disorders of pyruvate metabolism and gluconeogenesis
Deficiency of phosphoenolpyruvate carboxykinase
Deficiency of pyruvate carboxylase
Deficiency of pyruvate dehydrogenase

Excludes1 disorders of pyruvate metabolism and gluconeogenesis with anemia (D55.-)
Leigh's syndrome (G31.82)

E74.8 Other specified disorders of carbohydrate metabolism
Essential pentosuria
Renal glycosuria

E74.9 Disorder of carbohydrate metabolism, unspecified

E75 Disorders of sphingolipid metabolism and other lipid storage disorders

Excludes1 mucolipidosis, types I-III (E77.0-E77.1)
Refsum's disease (G60.1)

E75.0 GM2 gangliosidosis
Rare metabolic disorder that causes destruction of nerve cells of brain and spinal cord
Ex: **For category E75.0 CC codes:** E75.00-E75.19, E75.4, F84.2, G13.2-G13.8, G30.0-G31.82, G31.84-G31.9, G91.4, G94

E75.00 GM2 gangliosidosis, unspecified

E75.01 Sandhoff disease

E75.02 Tay-Sachs disease

E75.09 Other GM2 gangliosidosis
Adult GM2 gangliosidosis
Juvenile GM2 gangliosidosis

E75.1 Other and unspecified gangliosidosis
Ex: **For category E75.1 CC codes:** See E75.0

E75.10 Unspecified gangliosidosis
Gangliosidosis NOS

E75.11 Mucolipidosis IV
Disorder with symptoms of psychomotor retardation and severe visual impairment

E75.19 Other gangliosidosis
GM1 gangliosidosis
GM3 gangliosidosis

Item 4–8 Leukodystrophy is characterized by degeneration and/or failure of the myelin formation of the central nervous system and sometimes of the peripheral nervous system. The disease is inherited and progressive.

E75.2 Other sphingolipidosis
Lysosomal (a particle in a cytoplasm cell that contains digestive enzymes) storage diseases with symptoms of abnormal storage of amino acids

Excludes1 adrenoleukodystrophy [Addison-Schilder] (E71.528)

E75.21 Fabry (-Anderson) disease

E75.22 Gaucher disease

E75.23 Krabbe disease
Ex: E75.00-E75.19, E75.23, E75.25-E75.29, E75.4, F84.2, G13.2-G13.8, G31.2-G31.82, G32.89, G91.4, G93.81, G93.89-G94, G96.8-G96.9, G98.0-G98.8, G99.8

E75.24 Niemann-Pick disease

E75.240 Niemann-Pick disease type A

E75.241 Niemann-Pick disease type B

E75.242 Niemann-Pick disease type C

E75.243 Niemann-Pick disease type D

E75.248 Other Niemann-Pick disease

E75.249 Niemann-Pick disease, unspecified

E75.25 Metachromatic leukodystrophy
Ex: See E75.23

E75.29 Other sphingolipidosis
Farber's syndrome
Sulfatase deficiency
Sulfatide lipidosis
Ex: See E75.23

E75.3 Sphingolipidosis, unspecified

E75.4 Neuronal ceroid lipofuscinosis
Batten disease
Bielschowsky-Jansky disease
Kufs disease
Spielmeyer-Vogt disease
Ex: See E75.0

E75.5 Other lipid storage disorders
Cerebrotendinous cholesterosis [van Bogaert-Scherer-Epstein]
Wolman's disease

E75.6 Lipid storage disorder, unspecified

E76 Disorders of glycosaminoglycan metabolism
Ex: **For category E76 CC codes:** D81.3, D81.5, D81.810, D84.1, E76.01-E76.9, E79.1-E80.29, E80.4-E80.7, E85.0, E85.9, E88.81

E76.0 Mucopolysaccharidosis, type I
Inborn metabolic disorder of enzymes that break down carbohydrates

E76.01 Hurler's syndrome

E76.02 Hurler-Scheie syndrome

E76.03 Scheie's syndrome

E76.1 Mucopolysaccharidosis, type II
Inborn metabolic disorder of enzymes that break down carbohydrates occurs in 2-4 year old males
Hunter's syndrome

E76.2 Other mucopolysaccharidoses

E76.21 Morquio mucopolysaccharidoses

E76.210 Morquio A mucopolysaccharidoses
Classic Morquio syndrome
Morquio syndrome A
Mucopolysaccharidosis, type IVA

E76.211 Morquio B mucopolysaccharidoses
Morquio-like mucopolysaccharidoses
Morquio-like syndrome
Morquio syndrome B
Mucopolysaccharidosis, type IVB

E76.219 Morquio mucopolysaccharidoses, unspecified
Morquio syndrome
Mucopolysaccharidosis, type IV

E76.22 Sanfilippo mucopolysaccharidoses
Mucopolysaccharidosis, type III (A) (B) (C) (D)
Sanfilippo A syndrome
Sanfilippo B syndrome
Sanfilippo C syndrome
Sanfilippo D syndrome

E76.29 Other mucopolysaccharidoses
beta-Glucuronidase deficiency
Maroteaux-Lamy (mild) (severe) syndrome
Mucopolysaccharidosis, types VI, VII

E76.3 Mucopolysaccharidosis, unspecified

E76.8 Other disorders of glucosaminoglycan metabolism

E76.9 Glucosaminoglycan metabolism disorder, unspecified

E77 Disorders of glycoprotein metabolism

E77.0 Defects in post-translational modification of lysosomal enzymes
Mucolipidosis II [I-cell disease]
Mucolipidosis III [pseudo-Hurler polydystrophy]

E77.1 Defects in glycoprotein degradation
Aspartylglucosaminuria
Fucosidosis
Mannosidosis
Sialidosis [mucolipidosis I]

E77.8 Other disorders of glycoprotein metabolism

E77.9 Disorder of glycoprotein metabolism, unspecified

E78 Disorders of lipoprotein metabolism and other lipidemias
Excludes1 sphingolipidosis (E75.0-E75.3)

E78.0 Pure hypercholesterolemia
~~Familial hypercholesterolemia~~
~~Hyperlipidemia, Group A~~

E78.00 Pure hypercholesterolemia, unspecified ◀
Fredrickson's hyperlipoproteinemia, type IIa ◀
Hyperbetalipoproteinemia ◀
Low-density-lipoprotein-type [LDL] hyperlipoproteinemia ◀

E78.01 Familial hypercholesterolemia ◀

E78.1 Pure hyperglyceridemia
Elevated fasting triglycerides
Endogenous hyperglyceridemia
Fredrickson's hyperlipoproteinemia, type IV
Hyperlipidemia, group B
Hyperprebetalipoproteinemia
Very-low-density-lipoprotein-type [VLDL] hyperlipoproteinemia

E78.2 Mixed hyperlipidemia
Broad- or floating-betalipoproteinemia
Combined hyperlipidemia NOS
Elevated cholesterol with elevated triglycerides NEC
Fredrickson's hyperlipoproteinemia, type IIb or III
Hyperbetalipoproteinemia with prebetalipoproteinemia
Hypercholesteremia with endogenous hyperglyceridemia
Hyperlipidemia, group C
Tubo-eruptive xanthoma
Xanthoma tuberosum
Excludes1 cerebrotendinous cholesterosis [van Bogaert-Scherer-Epstein] (E75.5)
familial combined hyperlipidemia (E78.4)

E78.3 Hyperchylomicronemia
Chylomicron retention disease
Fredrickson's hyperlipoproteinemia, type I or V
Hyperlipidemia, group D
Mixed hyperglyceridemia

E78.4 Other hyperlipidemia
Familial combined hyperlipidemia

E78.5 Hyperlipidemia, unspecified

E78.6 Lipoprotein deficiency
Abetalipoproteinemia
Depressed HDL cholesterol
High-density lipoprotein deficiency
Hypoalphalipoproteinemia
Hypobetalipoproteinemia (familial)
Lecithin cholesterol acyltransferase deficiency
Tangier disease

E78.7 Disorders of bile acid and cholesterol metabolism
Excludes1 Niemann-Pick disease type C (E75.242)
For category E78.7 CC codes: E78.71-E78.72, Q87.1-Q87.89, Q89.8, Q99.2

E78.70 Disorder of bile acid and cholesterol metabolism, unspecified

E78.71 Barth syndrome

E78.72 Smith-Lemli-Opitz syndrome

E78.79 Other disorders of bile acid and cholesterol metabolism

E78.8 Other disorders of lipoprotein metabolism

E78.81 Lipoid dermatoarthritis

E78.89 Other lipoprotein metabolism disorders

E78.9 Disorder of lipoprotein metabolism, unspecified

E79 Disorders of purine and pyrimidine metabolism
Purines, along with pyrimidines, signal RNA and DNA production
Excludes1 Ataxia-telangiectasia (Q87.1)
Bloom's syndrome (Q82.8)
Cockayne's syndrome (Q87.1)
calculus of kidney (N20.0)
combined immunodeficiency disorders (D81.-)
Fanconi's anemia (D61.09)
gout (M1A.-, M10.-)
orotaciduric anemia (D53.0)
progeria (E34.8)
Werner's syndrome (E34.8)
xeroderma pigmentosum (Q82.1)
For category E79 CC codes: D81.3, D81.5, D81.810, D84.1, E76.01-E76.9, E79.1-E80.29, E80.4-E80.7, E88.81

E79.0 Hyperuricemia without signs of inflammatory arthritis and tophaceous disease
Asymptomatic hyperuricemia

E79.1 Lesch-Nyhan syndrome
HGPRT deficiency

E79.2 Myoadenylate deaminase deficiency

E79.8 Other disorders of purine and pyrimidine metabolism
Hereditary xanthinuria

E79.9 Disorder of purine and pyrimidine metabolism, unspecified

E80 Disorders of porphyrin and bilirubin metabolism
Group of chemical compounds in RBC's that combine with iron to form heme
Includes defects of catalase and peroxidase
For category E80 CC codes unless otherwise indicated: D81.3, D81.5, D81.810, D84.1, E76.01-E76.9, E79.1-E80.29, E80.4-E80.7, E88.81

E80.0 Hereditary erythropoietic porphyria
Congenital erythropoietic porphyria
Erythropoietic protoporphyria

E80.1 Porphyria cutanea tarda

E80.2 Other and unspecified porphyria

E80.20 Unspecified porphyria
Porphyria NOS

E80.21 Acute intermittent (hepatic) porphyria

E80.29 Other porphyria
Hereditary coproporphyria

E80.3 Defects of catalase and peroxidase
Acatalasia [Takahara]
E71.310-E71.32, E71.40-E71.548, E80.4-E80.7, E88.40-E88.49, H49.811-H49.819

E80.4 Gilbert syndrome

E80.5 Crigler-Najjar syndrome

E80.6 Other disorders of bilirubin metabolism
Dubin-Johnson syndrome
Rotor's syndrome

E80.7 Disorder of bilirubin metabolism, unspecified

E83 Disorders of mineral metabolism

Excludes1 dietary mineral deficiency (E58-E61)
parathyroid disorders (E20-E21)
vitamin D deficiency (E55.-)

E83.0 Disorders of copper metabolism

E83.00 Disorder of copper metabolism, unspecified

E83.01 Wilson's disease

Code also associated Kayser Fleischer ring (H18.04-)

E83.09 Other disorders of copper metabolism

Menkes' (kinky hair) (steely hair) disease

E83.1 Disorders of iron metabolism

Excludes1 iron deficiency anemia (D50.-)
sideroblastic anemia (D64.0-D64.3)

E83.10 Disorder of iron metabolism, unspecified

E83.11 Hemochromatosis

E83.110 Hereditary hemochromatosis

Bronzed diabetes
Pigmentary cirrhosis (of liver)
Primary (hereditary) hemochromatosis

E83.111 Hemochromatosis due to repeated red blood cell transfusions

Iron overload due to repeated red blood cell transfusions
Transfusion (red blood cell) associated hemochromatosis

E83.118 Other hemochromatosis

E83.119 Hemochromatosis, unspecified

E83.19 Other disorders of iron metabolism

Use additional code, if applicable, for idiopathic pulmonary hemosiderosis (J84.03)

E83.2 Disorders of zinc metabolism

Acrodermatitis enteropathica

E83.3 Disorders of phosphorus metabolism and phosphatases

Excludes1 adult osteomalacia (M83.-)
osteoporosis (M80.-)

E83.30 Disorder of phosphorus metabolism, unspecified

E83.31 Familial hypophosphatemia

Vitamin D-resistant osteomalacia
Vitamin D-resistant rickets

Excludes1 vitamin D-deficiency rickets (E55.0)

E83.32 Hereditary vitamin D-dependent rickets (type 1) (type 2)

25-hydroxyvitamin D 1-alpha-hydroxylase deficiency
Pseudovitamin D deficiency
Vitamin D receptor defect

E83.39 Other disorders of phosphorus metabolism

Acid phosphatase deficiency
Hypophosphatasia

E83.4 Disorders of magnesium metabolism

E83.40 Disorders of magnesium metabolism, unspecified

E83.41 Hypermagnesemia

E83.42 Hypomagnesemia

E83.49 Other disorders of magnesium metabolism

E83.5 Disorders of calcium metabolism

Excludes1 chondrocalcinosis (M11.1-M11.2)
hungry bone syndrome (E83.81)
hyperparathyroidism (E21.0-E21.3)

E83.50 Unspecified disorder of calcium metabolism

E83.51 Hypocalcemia

E83.52 Hypercalcemia

Familial hypocalciuric hypercalcemia

E83.59 Other disorders of calcium metabolism

Idiopathic hypercalciuria

E83.8 Other disorders of mineral metabolism

E83.81 Hungry bone syndrome

E83.89 Other disorders of mineral metabolism

E83.9 Disorder of mineral metabolism, unspecified

E84 Cystic fibrosis

Includes mucoviscidosis

Code also exocrine pancreatic insufficiency (K86.81) ◀

Ex For category E84 CC codes: E84.0-E84.9

E84.0 Cystic fibrosis with pulmonary manifestations

Use additional code to identify any infectious organism present, such as:
Pseudomonas (B96.5)

E84.1 Cystic fibrosis with intestinal manifestations

E84.11 Meconium ileus in cystic fibrosis N

Excludes1 meconium ileus not due to cystic fibrosis (P76.0)

E84.19 Cystic fibrosis with other intestinal manifestations

Distal intestinal obstruction syndrome

E84.8 Cystic fibrosis with other manifestations

E84.9 Cystic fibrosis, unspecified

E85 Amyloidosis

A disorder resulting from the abnormal deposition of a particular protein (amyloid) into tissues of the body

Excludes1 Alzheimer's disease (G30.0-)

Ex For category E85CC codes: E85.0-E85.9, E88.81

E85.0 Non-neuropathic heredofamilial amyloidosis

~~Familial Mediterranean fever~~
Hereditary amyloid nephropathy

E85.1 Neuropathic heredofamilial amyloidosis

Amyloid polyneuropathy (Portuguese)
Coding Clinic: 2012, Q4, P100

E85.2 Heredofamilial amyloidosis, unspecified

E85.3 Secondary systemic amyloidosis

Hemodialysis-associated amyloidosis

E85.4 Organ-limited amyloidosis

Localized amyloidosis

E85.8 Other amyloidosis

E85.9 Amyloidosis, unspecified

E86 Volume depletion

Excludes1 dehydration of newborn (P74.1)
hypovolemic shock NOS (R57.1)
postprocedural hypovolemic shock (T81.19)
traumatic hypovolemic shock (T79.4)

Use additional code(s) for any associated disorders of electrolyte and acid-base balance (E87.-) ◀

E86.0 Dehydration

Excessive loss of body water

E86.1 Hypovolemia

Diminished volume of circulating blood
Depletion of volume of plasma

E86.9 Volume depletion, unspecified

Item 4–9 Circulating fluid volume is regulated by the amount of water and sodium ingested, excreted by the kidneys into the urine, and lost through the gastrointestinal tract, lungs, and skin. To maintain blood volume within a normal range, the kidneys regulate the amount of water and sodium lost into the urine. Too much **(fluid overload)** or too little fluid volume **(volume depletion)** will affect blood pressure. Severe cases of vomiting, diarrhea, bleeding, and burns (fluid loss through exposed burn surface area) can contribute to fluid loss. Internal body environment must maintain a precise balance (homeostasis) between too much fluid and too little fluid. This complex balancing mechanism is critical to good health.

E87 Other disorders of fluid, electrolyte and acid-base balance

Excludes1 diabetes insipidus (E23.2)
electrolyte imbalance associated with hyperemesis gravidarum (O21.1)
electrolyte imbalance following ectopic or molar pregnancy (O08.5)
familial periodic paralysis (G72.3)

Ex: For category E87 CC codes: E86.0-E87.8

E87.0 Hyperosmolality and hypernatremia
Sodium [Na] excess
Sodium [Na] overload

E87.1 Hypo-osmolality and hyponatremia
Sodium [Na] deficiency

Excludes1 syndrome of inappropriate secretion of antidiuretic hormone (E22.2)

E87.2 Acidosis
Acidosis NOS
Lactic acidosis
Metabolic acidosis
Respiratory acidosis

Excludes1 diabetic acidosis - see categories E08-E10, E13 with ketoacidosis

E87.3 Alkalosis
Alkalosis NOS
Metabolic alkalosis
Respiratory alkalosis

E87.4 Mixed disorder of acid-base balance

E87.5 Hyperkalemia
Potassium [K] excess
Potassium [K] overload

E87.6 Hypokalemia
Potassium [K] deficiency

E87.7 Fluid overload

Excludes1 edema NOS (R60.9)
fluid retention (R60.9)

E87.70 Fluid overload, unspecified

E87.71 Transfusion associated circulatory overload
Fluid overload due to transfusion (blood) (blood components) TACO

E87.79 Other fluid overload

E87.8 Other disorders of electrolyte and fluid balance, not elsewhere classified
Electrolyte imbalance NOS
Hyperchloremia
Hypochloremia

E88 Other and unspecified metabolic disorders

Use additional codes for associated conditions

Excludes1 histiocytosis X (chronic) (C96.6)

E88.0 Disorders of plasma-protein metabolism, not elsewhere classified

Excludes1 disorder of lipoprotein metabolism (E78.-)
monoclonal gammopathy (of undetermined significance) (D47.2)
polyclonal hypergammaglobulinemia (D89.0)
Waldenström macroglobulinemia (C88.0)

E88.01 Alpha-1-antitrypsin deficiency AAT deficiency

E88.09 Other disorders of plasma-protein metabolism, not elsewhere classified
Bisalbuminemia

E88.1 Lipodystrophy, not elsewhere classified
Defective fat metabolism resulting in absence of subcutaneous fat
Lipodystrophy NOS

Excludes1 Whipple's disease (K90.81)

E88.2 Lipomatosis, not elsewhere classified
Abnormal tumorlike accumulations of fat in tissue
Lipomatosis NOS
Lipomatosis (Check) dolorosa [Dercum]

E88.3 Tumor lysis syndrome
Tumor lysis syndrome (spontaneous)
Tumor lysis syndrome following antineoplastic drug chemotherapy

Use additional code for adverse effect, if applicable, to identify drug (T45.1X5)

Ex: E08.21-E08.29, E09.21-E09.29, E88.3, N00.0-N01.9, N02.8-N02.9, N04.7-N05.1, N05.6-N06.1, N06.6-N07.1, N07.6-N08, N14.0-N15.0, N15.8-N17.9

E88.4 Mitochondrial metabolism disorders
Congenital disorder of metabolism

Excludes1 disorders of pyruvate metabolism (E74.4)
Kearns-Sayre syndrome (H49.81)
Leber's disease (H47.22)
Leigh's encephalopathy (G31.82)
Mitochondrial myopathy, NEC (G71.3)
Reye's syndrome (G93.7)

Ex: For category E88.4 CC codes: C96.5-C96.6, E71.310-E71.548, E80.3-E80.7, E88.89

E88.40 Mitochondrial metabolism disorder, unspecified

E88.41 MELAS syndrome
Mitochondrial myopathy, encephalopathy, lactic acidosis and stroke-like episodes

E88.42 MERRF syndrome
Myoclonic epilepsy associated with ragged-red fibers

Code also progressive myoclonic epilepsy (G40.3-)

E88.49 Other mitochondrial metabolism disorders

E88.8 Other specified metabolic disorders

E88.81 Metabolic syndrome
Dysmetabolic syndrome X

Use additional codes for associated manifestations, such as:
obesity (E66.-)

E88.89 Other specified metabolic disorders
Launois-Bensaude adenolipomatosis

Excludes1 adult pulmonary Langerhans cell histiocytosis (J84.82)

E88.9 Metabolic disorder, unspecified

POSTPROCEDURAL ENDOCRINE AND METABOLIC COMPLICATIONS AND DISORDERS, NOT ELSEWHERE CLASSIFIED (E89)

E89 Postprocedural endocrine and metabolic complications and disorders, not elsewhere classified

Excludes2 intraoperative complications of endocrine system organ or structure (E36.0-, E36.1-, E36.8)

E89.0 Postprocedural hypothyroidism
Postirradiation hypothyroidism
Postsurgical hypothyroidism

E89.1 Postprocedural hypoinsulinemia
Postpancreatectomy hyperglycemia
Postsurgical hypoinsulinemia

Use additional code, if applicable, to identify:
acquired absence of pancreas (Z90.41-)
diabetes mellitus (postpancreatectomy) (postprocedural) (E13.-)
insulin use (Z79.4)

Excludes1 transient postprocedural hyperglycemia (R73.9)
transient postprocedural hypoglycemia (E16.2)

Ex: E08.00-E08.59, E08.618-E09.59, E09.618-E10.59, E10.618-E10.649, E10.69-E11.59, E11.618-E11.649, E11.69-E13.59, E13.618-E16.2, E30.9, E34.1, E34.50-E35, E89.1

E89.2 Postprocedural hypoparathyroidism
Parathyroprival tetany

E89.3 Postprocedural hypopituitarism
Postirradiation hypopituitarism

● **E89.4 Postprocedural ovarian failure**

E89.40 Asymptomatic postprocedural ovarian failure ♀
Postprocedural ovarian failure NOS

E89.41 Symptomatic postprocedural ovarian failure ♀
Symptoms such as flushing, sleeplessness, headache, lack of concentration, associated with postprocedural menopause

E89.5 Postprocedural testicular hypofunction ♂

E89.6 Postprocedural adrenocortical (-medullary) hypofunction
Ex: A17.9, A18.7, A18.82, A18.84, A18.89, E27.0-E27.9, E30.9, E34.1, E34.50-E35, E89.6

● **E89.8 Other postprocedural endocrine and metabolic complications and disorders**
Ex: **For category E89.8 CC codes:** E36.8, E89.810-E89.89, H95.811-H95.89, I97.3, M96.89, N98.1-N98.9, T81.82X[A], T81.89X-T81.9XX[A]

● **E89.81 Postprocedural hemorrhage of an endocrine system organ or structure following a procedure**

E89.810 Postprocedural hemorrhage of an endocrine system organ or structure following an endocrine system procedure

E89.811 Postprocedural hemorrhage of an endocrine system organ or structure following other procedure

● **E89.82 Postprocedural hematoma and seroma of an endocrine system organ or structure** ◀

E89.820 Postprocedural hematoma of an endocrine system organ or structure following an endocrine system procedure ◀

E89.821 Postprocedural hematoma of an endocrine system organ or structure following other procedure ◀

E89.822 Postprocedural seroma of an endocrine system organ or structure following an endocrine system procedure ◀

E89.823 Postprocedural seroma of an endocrine system organ or structure following other procedure ◀

E89.89 Other postprocedural endocrine and metabolic complications and disorders
Use additional code, if applicable, to further specify disorder

CHAPTER 5

MENTAL, BEHAVIORAL AND NEURODEVELOPMENTAL DISORDERS (F01-F99)

OGCR Chapter-Specific Coding Guidelines

5. **Chapter 5: Mental, Behavioral and Neurodevelopmental disorders (F01 – F99)**

a. Pain disorders related to psychological factors

Assign code F45.41, for pain that is exclusively related to psychological disorders. As indicated by the Excludes 1 note under category G89, a code from category G89 should not be assigned with code F45.41

Code F45.42, Pain disorders with related psychological factors, should be used with a code from category G89, Pain, not elsewhere classified, if there is documentation of a psychological component for a patient with acute or chronic pain.

See Section I.C.6. Pain

c. Mental and behavioral disorders due to psychoactive substance use

1) In Remission

Selection of codes for "in remission" for categories F10-F19, Mental and behavioral disorders due to psychoactive substance use (categories F10-F19 with -.21) requires the provider's clinical judgment. The appropriate codes for "in remission" are assigned only on the basis of provider documentation (as defined in the Official Guidelines for Coding and Reporting).

2) Psychoactive Substance Use, Abuse And Dependence

When the provider documentation refers to use, abuse and dependence of the same substance (e.g. alcohol, opioid, cannabis, etc.), only one code should be assigned to identify the pattern of use based on the following hierarchy:

- If both use and abuse are documented, assign only the code for abuse
- If both abuse and dependence are documented, assign only the code for dependence
- If use, abuse and dependence are all documented, assign only the code for dependence
- If both use and dependence are documented, assign only the code for dependence.

3) Psychoactive Substance Use

As with all other diagnoses, the codes for psychoactive substance use (F10.9-, F11.9-, F12.9-, F13.9-, F14.9-, F15.9-, F16.9-) should only be assigned based on provider documentation and when they meet the definition of a reportable diagnosis (see Section III, Reporting Additional Diagnoses). The codes are to be used only when the psychoactive substance use is associated with a mental or behavioral disorder, and such a relationship is documented by the provider.

CHAPTER 5

MENTAL, BEHAVIORAL AND NEURODEVELOPMENTAL DISORDERS (F01-F99)

Includes disorders of psychological development

Excludes2 symptoms, signs and abnormal clinical laboratory findings, not elsewhere classified (R00-R99)

This chapter contains the following blocks:

F01-F09	Mental disorders due to known physiological conditions
F10-F19	Mental and behavioral disorders due to psychoactive substance use
F20-F29	Schizophrenia, schizotypal, delusional, and other non-mood psychotic disorders
F30-F39	Mood [affective] disorders
F40-F48	Anxiety, dissociative, stress-related, somatoform and other nonpsychotic mental disorders
F50-F59	Behavioral syndromes associated with physiological disturbances and physical factors
F60-F69	Disorders of adult personality and behavior
F70-F79	Intellectual disabilities
F80-F89	Pervasive and specific developmental disorders
F90-F98	Behavioral and emotional disorders with onset usually occurring in childhood and adolescence
F99	Unspecified mental disorder

MENTAL DISORDERS DUE TO KNOWN PHYSIOLOGICAL CONDITIONS (F01-F09)

This block comprises a range of mental disorders grouped together on the basis of their having in common a demonstrable etiology in cerebral disease, brain injury, or other insult leading to cerebral dysfunction. The dysfunction may be primary, as in diseases, injuries, and insults that affect the brain directly and selectively; or secondary, as in systemic diseases and disorders that attack the brain only as one of the multiple organs or systems of the body that are involved.

F01 Vascular dementia

Vascular dementia as a result of infarction of the brain due to vascular disease, including hypertensive cerebrovascular disease.

Includes arteriosclerotic dementia

Code first the underlying physiological condition or sequelae of cerebrovascular disease.

F01.5 Vascular dementia

F01.50 Vascular dementia without behavioral disturbance A

Major neurocognitive disorder without behavioral disturbance ◀

F01.51 Vascular dementia with behavioral disturbance A

Major neurocognitive disorder due to vascular disease, with behavioral disturbance ◀

Major neurocognitive disorder with aggressive behavior ◀

Major neurocognitive disorder with combative behavior ◀

Major neurocognitive disorder with violent behavior ◀

Vascular dementia with aggressive behavior

Vascular dementia with combative behavior

Vascular dementia with violent behavior

Use additional code, if applicable, to identify wandering in vascular dementia (Z91.83)

Ex: F01.51

F02 Dementia in other diseases classified elsewhere

Code first the underlying physiological condition, such as:
Alzheimer's (G30.-)
cerebral lipidosis (E75.4)
Creutzfeldt-Jakob disease (A81.0-)
dementia with Lewy bodies (G31.83)
dementia with Parkinsonism (G31.83) ◀
epilepsy and recurrent seizures (G40.-)
frontotemporal dementia (G31.09)
hepatolenticular degeneration (E83.0)
human immunodeficiency virus [HIV] disease (B20)
Huntington's disease (G10) ◀
hypercalcemia (E83.52)
hypothyroidism, acquired (E00-E03.-)
intoxications (T36-T65)
Jakob-Creutzfeldt disease (A81.0-)
multiple sclerosis (G35)
neurosyphilis (A52.17)
niacin deficiency [pellagra] (E52)
Parkinson's disease (G20)
Pick's disease (G31.01)
polyarteritis nodosa (M30.0)
prion disease (A81.9) ◀
systemic lupus erythematosus (M32.-)
traumatic brain injury (S06.-) ◀
trypanosomiasis (B56.-, B57.-)
vitamin B deficiency (E53.8)

Includes Major neurocognitive disorder in other diseases classified elsewhere ◀

Excludes2 dementia in alcohol and psychoactive substance disorders (F10-F19, with .17, .27, .97)
vascular dementia (F01.5-)

F02.8 Dementia in other diseases classified elsewhere

F02.80 Dementia in other diseases classified elsewhere without behavioral disturbance
Dementia in other diseases classified elsewhere NOS
Major neurocognitive disorder in other diseases classified elsewhere ◀
Coding Clinic: 2016, Q2, P6

F02.81 Dementia in other diseases classified elsewhere with behavioral disturbance
Dementia in other diseases classified elsewhere with aggressive behavior
Dementia in other diseases classified elsewhere with combative behavior
Dementia in other diseases classified elsewhere with violent behavior
Major neurocognitive disorder in other diseases classified elsewhere with aggressive behavior ◀
Major neurocognitive disorder in other diseases classified elsewhere with combative behavior ◀
Major neurocognitive disorder in other diseases classified elsewhere with violent behavior ◀
Use additional code, if applicable, to identify wandering in dementia in conditions classified elsewhere (Z91.83)
Ex: F02.81, F03.91

Item 5-1 Psychosis was a term formerly applied to any mental disorder but is now restricted to disturbances of a great magnitude in which there is a personality disintegration and loss of contact with reality.

F03 Unspecified dementia
Presenile dementia NOS
Presenile psychosis NOS
Primary degenerative dementia NOS
Senile dementia NOS
Senile dementia depressed or paranoid type
Senile psychosis NOS

Excludes1 senility NOS (R41.81)

Excludes2 mild memory disturbance due to known physiological condition (F06.8)
senile dementia with delirium or acute confusional state (F05)

F03.9 Unspecified dementia

F03.90 Unspecified dementia without behavioral disturbance A
Dementia NOS
Coding Clinic: 2012, Q4, P92

F03.91 Unspecified dementia with behavioral disturbance A
Unspecified dementia with aggressive behavior
Unspecified dementia with combative behavior
Unspecified dementia with violent behavior
Use additional code, if applicable, to identify wandering in unspecified dementia (Z91.83)
Ex: F02.81, F03.91

F04 Amnestic disorder due to known physiological condition
Korsakov's psychosis or syndrome, nonalcoholic
Code first the underlying physiological condition

Excludes1 amnesia NOS (R41.3)
anterograde amnesia (R41.1)
dissociative amnesia (F44.0)
retrograde amnesia (R41.2)

Excludes2 alcohol-induced or unspecified Korsakov's syndrome (F10.26, F10.96)
Korsakov's syndrome induced by other psychoactive substances (F13.26, F13.96, F19.16, F19.26, F19.96)

F05 Delirium due to known physiological condition
Acute or subacute brain syndrome
Acute or subacute confusional state (nonalcoholic)
Acute or subacute infective psychosis
Acute or subacute organic reaction
Acute or subacute psycho-organic syndrome
Delirium of mixed etiology
Delirium superimposed on dementia
Sundowning
Code first the underlying physiological condition

Excludes1 delirium NOS (R41.0)

Excludes2 delirium tremens alcohol-induced or unspecified (F10.231, F10.921)

Ex: F05, R45.851

F06 Other mental disorders due to known physiological condition

Includes mental disorders due to endocrine disorder
mental disorders due to exogenous hormone
mental disorders due to exogenous toxic substance
mental disorders due to primary cerebral disease
mental disorders due to somatic illness
mental disorders due to systemic disease affecting the brain

Code first the underlying physiological condition

Excludes1 unspecified dementia (F03)

Excludes2 delirium due to known physiological condition (F05)
dementia as classified in F01-F02
other mental disorders associated with alcohol and other psychoactive substances (F10-F19)

Ex **For category F06 CC codes:** F02.80-F02.81, F04-F06.8, F10.10-F11.19, F11.21-F13.19, F13.21-F14.19, F14.21-F15.19, F15.21-F16.19, F16.21-F17.209, F17.213-F17.219, F17.223-F17.229, F17.293-F18.19, F18.21-F19.19, F19.21-F19.99, F53-F55.8, R78

F06.0 Psychotic disorder with hallucinations due to known physiological condition

Organic hallucinatory state (nonalcoholic)

Excludes2 hallucinations and perceptual disturbance induced by alcohol and other psychoactive substances (F10-F19 with .151, .251, .951)
schizophrenia (F20.-)

F06.1 Catatonic disorder due to known physiological condition

Catatonia associated with another mental disorder ◀
Catatonia NOS ◀

Excludes1 catatonic stupor (R40.1)
stupor NOS (R40.1)

Excludes2 catatonic schizophrenia (F20.2)
dissociative stupor (F44.2)

F06.2 Psychotic disorder with delusions due to known physiological condition

Paranoid and paranoid-hallucinatory organic states
Schizophrenia-like psychosis in epilepsy

Excludes2 alcohol and drug-induced psychotic disorder (F10-F19 with .150, .250, .950)
brief psychotic disorder (F23)
delusional disorder (F22)
schizophrenia (F20.-)

F06.3 Mood disorder due to known physiological condition

Excludes2 mood disorders due to alcohol and other psychoactive substances (F10-F19 with .14, .24, .94)
mood disorders, not due to known physiological condition or unspecified (F30-F39)

F06.30 Mood disorder due to known physiological condition, unspecified

F06.31 Mood disorder due to known physiological condition with depressive features

F06.32 Mood disorder due to known physiological condition with major depressive-like episode

F06.33 Mood disorder due to known physiological condition with manic features

F06.34 Mood disorder due to known physiological condition with mixed features

F06.4 Anxiety disorder due to known physiological condition

Excludes2 anxiety disorders due to alcohol and other psychoactive substances (F10-F19 with .180, .280, .980)
anxiety disorders, not due to known physiological condition or unspecified (F40.-, F41.-)

F06.8 Other specified mental disorders due to known physiological condition

Epileptic psychosis NOS
Organic dissociative disorder
Organic emotionally labile [asthenic] disorder

F07 Personality and behavioral disorders due to known physiological condition

Code first the underlying physiological condition

F07.0 Personality change due to known physiological condition

Frontal lobe syndrome
Limbic epilepsy personality syndrome
Lobotomy syndrome
Organic personality disorder
Organic pseudopsychopathic personality
Organic pseudoretarded personality
Postleucotomy syndrome

Code first underlying physiological condition

Excludes1 mild cognitive impairment (G31.84)
postconcussional syndrome (F07.81)
postencephalitic syndrome (F07.89)
signs and symptoms involving emotional state (R45.-)

Excludes2 specific personality disorder (F60.-)

F07.8 Other personality and behavioral disorders due to known physiological condition

F07.81 Postconcussional syndrome

Postcontusional syndrome (encephalopathy)
Post-traumatic brain syndrome, nonpsychotic

Use additional code to identify associated post-traumatic headache, if applicable (G44.3-)

Excludes1 current concussion (brain) (S06.0-)
postencephalitic syndrome (F07.89)

F07.89 Other personality and behavioral disorders due to known physiological condition

Postencephalitic syndrome
Damage to temporal brain lobes with memory loss and abnormal behavior
Right hemispheric organic affective disorder

F07.9 Unspecified personality and behavioral disorder due to known physiological condition

Organic psychosyndrome
Due to exposure to organic solvents

F09 Unspecified mental disorder due to known physiological condition

Mental disorder NOS due to known physiological condition
Organic brain syndrome NOS
Organic mental disorder NOS
Organic psychosis NOS
Symptomatic psychosis NOS

Code first the underlying physiological condition

Excludes1 psychosis NOS (F29)

MENTAL AND BEHAVIORAL DISORDERS DUE TO PSYCHOACTIVE SUBSTANCE USE (F10-F19)

F10 Alcohol related disorders

Use additional code for blood alcohol level, if applicable (Y90.-)

Ex **For category F10 CC codes:** F02.80-F02.81, F04-F06.8, F10.10-F11.19, F11.21-F13.19, F13.21-F14.19, F14.21-F15.19, F15.21-F16.19, F16.21-F17.209, F17.213-F17.219, F17.223-F17.229, F17.293-F18.19, F18.21-F19.19, F19.21-F19.99, F53-F55.8, R78

F10.1 Alcohol abuse

Excludes1 alcohol dependence (F10.2-)
alcohol use, unspecified (F10.9-)

F10.10 Alcohol abuse, uncomplicated

Alcohol use disorder, mild ◀

F10.12 Alcohol abuse with intoxication

F10.120 Alcohol abuse with intoxication, uncomplicated

F10.121 Alcohol abuse with intoxication, delirium

F10.129 Alcohol abuse with intoxication, unspecified

F10.14 Alcohol abuse with alcohol-induced mood disorder
Alcohol use disorder, mild, with alcohol-induced bipolar or related disorder ◀
Alcohol use disorder, mild, with alcohol-induced depressive disorder ◀

● **F10.15 Alcohol abuse with alcohol-induced psychotic disorder**
F10.150 Alcohol abuse with alcohol-induced psychotic disorder with delusions
F10.151 Alcohol abuse with alcohol-induced psychotic disorder with hallucinations
F10.159 Alcohol abuse with alcohol-induced psychotic disorder, unspecified

● **F10.18 Alcohol abuse with other alcohol-induced disorders**
F10.180 Alcohol abuse with alcohol-induced anxiety disorder
F10.181 Alcohol abuse with alcohol-induced sexual dysfunction
F10.182 Alcohol abuse with alcohol-induced sleep disorder
F10.188 Alcohol abuse with other alcohol-induced disorder

F10.19 Alcohol abuse with unspecified alcohol-induced disorder

● **F10.2 Alcohol dependence**
Excludes1 alcohol abuse (F10.1-)
alcohol use, unspecified (F10.9-)
Excludes2 toxic effect of alcohol (T51.0-)

F10.20 Alcohol dependence, uncomplicated
Alcohol use disorder, moderate ◀
Alcohol use disorder, severe ◀

F10.21 Alcohol dependence, in remission

● **F10.22 Alcohol dependence with intoxication**
Acute drunkenness (in alcoholism)
Excludes2 alcohol dependence with withdrawal (F10.23-) ◀
F10.220 Alcohol dependence with intoxication, uncomplicated
F10.221 Alcohol dependence with intoxication delirium
F10.229 Alcohol dependence with intoxication, unspecified

● **F10.23 Alcohol dependence with withdrawal**
Excludes2 alcohol dependence with intoxication (F10.22-) ◀
F10.230 Alcohol dependence with withdrawal, uncomplicated
F10.231 Alcohol dependence with withdrawal delirium
F10.232 Alcohol dependence with withdrawal with perceptual disturbance
F10.239 Alcohol dependence with withdrawal, unspecified
Coding Clinic: 2015, Q2, P15

F10.24 Alcohol dependence with alcohol-induced mood disorder
Alcohol use disorder, moderate, with alcohol-induced bipolar or related disorder ◀
Alcohol use disorder, moderate, with alcohol-induced depressive disorder ◀
Alcohol use disorder, severe, with alcohol-induced bipolar or related disorder ◀
Alcohol use disorder, severe, with alcohol-induced depressive disorder ◀

● **F10.25 Alcohol dependence with alcohol-induced psychotic disorder**
F10.250 Alcohol dependence with alcohol-induced psychotic disorder with delusions
F10.251 Alcohol dependence with alcohol-induced psychotic disorder with hallucinations
F10.259 Alcohol dependence with alcohol-induced psychotic disorder, unspecified

F10.26 Alcohol dependence with alcohol-induced persisting amnestic disorder
Alcohol use disorder, moderate, with alcohol-induced major neurocognitive disorder, amnestic-confabulatory type ◀
Alcohol use disorder, severe, with alcohol-induced major neurocognitive disorder, amnestic-confabulatory type ◀

F10.27 Alcohol dependence with alcohol-induced persisting dementia
Alcohol use disorder, moderate, with alcohol-induced major neurocognitive disorder, nonamnestic-confabulatory type ◀
Alcohol use disorder, severe, with alcohol-induced major neurocognitive disorder, nonamnestic-confabulatory type ◀

● **F10.28 Alcohol dependence with other alcohol-induced disorders**
F10.280 Alcohol dependence with alcohol-induced anxiety disorder
F10.281 Alcohol dependence with alcohol-induced sexual dysfunction
F10.282 Alcohol dependence with alcohol-induced sleep disorder
F10.288 Alcohol dependence with other alcohol-induced disorder
Alcohol use disorder, moderate, with alcohol-induced mild neurocognitive disorder ◀
Alcohol use disorder, severe, with alcohol-induced mild neurocognitive disorder ◀

F10.29 Alcohol dependence with unspecified alcohol-induced disorder

● **F10.9 Alcohol use, unspecified**
Excludes1 alcohol abuse (F10.1-)
alcohol dependence (F10.2-)

● **F10.92 Alcohol use, unspecified with intoxication**
F10.920 Alcohol use, unspecified with intoxication, uncomplicated
F10.921 Alcohol use, unspecified with intoxication delirium
F10.929 Alcohol use, unspecified with intoxication, unspecified

F10.94 Alcohol use, unspecified with alcohol-induced mood disorder
Alcohol-induced bipolar or related disorder, without use disorder ◀
Alcohol-induced depressive disorder, without use disorder ◀

● **F10.95 Alcohol use, unspecified with alcohol-induced psychotic disorder**
F10.950 Alcohol use, unspecified with alcohol-induced psychotic disorder with delusions
F10.951 Alcohol use, unspecified with alcohol-induced psychotic disorder with hallucinations

F10.959 **Alcohol use, unspecified with alcohol-induced psychotic disorder, unspecified**
Alcohol-induced psychotic disorder without use disorder ◀

F10.96 **Alcohol use, unspecified with alcohol-induced persisting amnestic disorder**
Alcohol-induced major neurocognitive disorder, amnestic-confabulatory type, without use disorder ◀

F10.97 **Alcohol use, unspecified with alcohol-induced persisting dementia**
Alcohol-induced major neurocognitive disorder, nonamnestic-confabulatory type, without use disorder ◀

● **F10.98** **Alcohol use, unspecified with other alcohol-induced disorders**

F10.980 **Alcohol use, unspecified with alcohol-induced anxiety disorder**
Alcohol-induced anxiety disorder, without use disorder ◀

F10.981 **Alcohol use, unspecified with alcohol-induced sexual dysfunction**
Alcohol-induced sexual dysfunction, without use disorder ◀

F10.982 **Alcohol use, unspecified with alcohol-induced sleep disorder**
Alcohol-induced sleep disorder, without use disorder ◀

F10.988 **Alcohol use, unspecified with other alcohol-induced disorder**
Alcohol-induced mild neurocognitive disorder, without use disorder ◀

F10.99 **Alcohol use, unspecified with unspecified alcohol-induced disorder**

● **F11** **Opioid related disorders**
Ex: For category F11 CC codes unless otherwise indicated: F02.80-F02.81, F04-F06.8, F10.10-F11.19, F11.21-F13.19, F13.21-F14.19, F14.21-F15.19, F15.21-F16.19, F16.21-F17.209, F17.213-F17.219, F17.223-F17.229, F17.293-F18.19, F18.21-F19.19, F19.21-F19.99, F53-F55.8, R78

● **F11.1** **Opioid abuse**
Excludes1 opioid dependence (F11.2-)
opioid use, unspecified (F11.9-)

F11.10 **Opioid abuse, uncomplicated**
Opioid use disorder, mild ◀

● **F11.12** **Opioid abuse with intoxication**

F11.120 **Opioid abuse with intoxication, uncomplicated**

F11.121 **Opioid abuse with intoxication delirium**

F11.122 **Opioid abuse with intoxication with perceptual disturbance**

F11.129 **Opioid abuse with intoxication, unspecified**

F11.14 **Opioid abuse with opioid-induced mood disorder**
Opioid use disorder, mild, with opioid-induced depressive disorder ◀

● **F11.15** **Opioid abuse with opioid-induced psychotic disorder**

F11.150 **Opioid abuse with opioid-induced psychotic disorder with delusions**

F11.151 **Opioid abuse with opioid-induced psychotic disorder with hallucinations**

F11.159 **Opioid abuse with opioid-induced psychotic disorder, unspecified**

● **F11.18** **Opioid abuse with other opioid-induced disorder**

F11.181 **Opioid abuse with opioid-induced sexual dysfunction**

F11.182 **Opioid abuse with opioid-induced sleep disorder**

F11.188 **Opioid abuse with other opioid-induced disorder**

F11.19 **Opioid abuse with unspecified opioid-induced disorder**

● **F11.2** **Opioid dependence**
Excludes1 opioid abuse (F11.1-)
opioid use, unspecified (F11.9-)
Excludes2 opioid poisoning (T40.0--T40.2-)

F11.20 **Opioid dependence, uncomplicated**
Opioid use disorder, moderate ◀
Opioid use disorder, severe ◀
Ex: No exclusions

F11.21 **Opioid dependence, in remission**

● **F11.22** **Opioid dependence with intoxication**
Excludes1 opioid dependence with withdrawal (F11.23)

F11.220 **Opioid dependence with intoxication, uncomplicated**

F11.221 **Opioid dependence with intoxication delirium**

F11.222 **Opioid dependence with intoxication with perceptual disturbance**
Ex: No exclusions

F11.229 **Opioid dependence with intoxication, unspecified**

F11.23 **Opioid dependence with withdrawal**
Excludes1 opioid dependence with intoxication (F11.22-)

F11.24 **Opioid dependence with opioid-induced mood disorder**
Opioid use disorder, moderate, with opioid-induced depressive disorder ◀

● **F11.25** **Opioid dependence with opioid-induced psychotic disorder**

F11.250 **Opioid dependence with opioid-induced psychotic disorder with delusions**

F11.251 **Opioid dependence with opioid-induced psychotic disorder with hallucinations**

F11.259 **Opioid dependence with opioid-induced psychotic disorder, unspecified**
Ex: No exclusions

● **F11.28** **Opioid dependence with other opioid-induced disorder**
Ex: For category F11.28 CC codes: No exclusions

F11.281 **Opioid dependence with opioid-induced sexual dysfunction**

F11.282 **Opioid dependence with opioid-induced sleep disorder**

F11.288 **Opioid dependence with other opioid-induced disorder**

F11.29 **Opioid dependence with unspecified opioid-induced disorder**

● **F11.9** **Opioid use, unspecified**
Excludes1 opioid abuse (F11.1-)
opioid dependence (F11.2-)

F11.90 **Opioid use, unspecified, uncomplicated**

● **F11.92 Opioid use, unspecified with intoxication**

Excludes1 opioid use, unspecified with withdrawal (F11.93)

F11.920 Opioid use, unspecified with intoxication, uncomplicated

F11.921 Opioid use, unspecified with intoxication delirium

Opioid-induced delirium ◀

F11.922 Opioid use, unspecified with intoxication with perceptual disturbance

F11.929 Opioid use, unspecified with intoxication, unspecified

F11.93 Opioid use, unspecified with withdrawal

Excludes1 opioid use, unspecified with intoxication (F11.92-)

F11.94 Opioid use, unspecified with opioid-induced mood disorder

Opioid-induced depressive disorder, without use disorder ◀

● **F11.95 Opioid use, unspecified with opioid-induced psychotic disorder**

F11.950 Opioid use, unspecified with opioid-induced psychotic disorder with delusions

F11.951 Opioid use, unspecified with opioid-induced psychotic disorder with hallucinations

F11.959 Opioid use, unspecified with opioid-induced psychotic disorder, unspecified

● **F11.98 Opioid use, unspecified with other specified opioid-induced disorder**

F11.981 Opioid use, unspecified with opioid-induced sexual dysfunction

Opioid-induced sexual dysfunction, without use disorder ◀

F11.982 Opioid use, unspecified with opioid-induced sleep disorder

Opioid-induced sleep disorder, without use disorder ◀

F11.988 Opioid use, unspecified with other opioid-induced disorder

Opioid-induced anxiety disorder, without use disorder ◀

F11.99 Opioid use, unspecified with unspecified opioid-induced disorder

● **F12 Cannabis related disorders**

Includes marijuana

Ex: **For category F12 CC codes:** F02.80-F02.81, F04-F06.8, F10.10-F11.19, F11.21-F13.19, F13.21-F14.19, F14.21-F15.19, F15.21-F16.19, F16.21-F17.209, F17.213-F17.219, F17.223-F17.229, F17.293-F18.19, F18.21-F19.19, F19.21-F19.99, F53-F55.8, R78

● **F12.1 Cannabis abuse**

Excludes1 cannabis dependence (F12.2-)
cannabis use, unspecified (F12.9-)

F12.10 Cannabis abuse, uncomplicated

Cannabis use disorder, mild ◀

● **F12.12 Cannabis abuse with intoxication**

F12.120 Cannabis abuse with intoxication, uncomplicated

F12.121 Cannabis abuse with intoxication delirium

F12.122 Cannabis abuse with intoxication with perceptual disturbance

F12.129 Cannabis abuse with intoxication, unspecified

● **F12.15 Cannabis abuse with psychotic disorder**

F12.150 Cannabis abuse with psychotic disorder with delusions

F12.151 Cannabis abuse with psychotic disorder with hallucinations

F12.159 Cannabis abuse with psychotic disorder, unspecified

● **F12.18 Cannabis abuse with other cannabis-induced disorder**

F12.180 Cannabis abuse with cannabis-induced anxiety disorder

F12.188 Cannabis abuse with other cannabis-induced disorder

Cannabis use disorder, mild, with cannabis-induced sleep disorder ◀

F12.19 Cannabis abuse with unspecified cannabis-induced disorder

● **F12.2 Cannabis dependence**

Excludes1 cannabis abuse (F12.1-)
cannabis use, unspecified (F12.9-)

Excludes2 cannabis poisoning (T40.7-)

F12.20 Cannabis dependence, uncomplicated

Cannabis use disorder, moderate ◀
Cannabis use disorder, severe ◀

F12.21 Cannabis dependence, in remission

● **F12.22 Cannabis dependence with intoxication**

F12.220 Cannabis dependence with intoxication, uncomplicated

F12.221 Cannabis dependence with intoxication delirium

F12.222 Cannabis dependence with intoxication with perceptual disturbance

F12.229 Cannabis dependence with intoxication, unspecified

● **F12.25 Cannabis dependence with psychotic disorder**

F12.250 Cannabis dependence with psychotic disorder with delusions

F12.251 Cannabis dependence with psychotic disorder with hallucinations

F12.259 Cannabis dependence with psychotic disorder, unspecified

● **F12.28 Cannabis dependence with other cannabis-induced disorder**

F12.280 Cannabis dependence with cannabis-induced anxiety disorder

F12.288 Cannabis dependence with other cannabis-induced disorder

Cannabis use disorder, moderate, with cannabis-induced sleep disorder ◀
Cannabis use disorder, severe, with cannabis-induced sleep disorder ◀
Cannabis withdrawal ◀

F12.29 Cannabis dependence with unspecified cannabis-induced disorder

● **F12.9 Cannabis use, unspecified**

Excludes1 cannabis abuse (F12.1-)
cannabis dependence (F12.2-)

F12.90 Cannabis use, unspecified, uncomplicated

● **F12.92 Cannabis use, unspecified with intoxication**

F12.920 Cannabis use, unspecified with intoxication, uncomplicated

F12.921 Cannabis use, unspecified with intoxication delirium

F12.922 **Cannabis use, unspecified with intoxication with perceptual disturbance**

F12.929 **Cannabis use, unspecified with intoxication, unspecified**

● **F12.95** **Cannabis use, unspecified with psychotic disorder**

F12.950 **Cannabis use, unspecified with psychotic disorder with delusions**

F12.951 **Cannabis use, unspecified with psychotic disorder with hallucinations**

F12.959 **Cannabis use, unspecified with psychotic disorder, unspecified**

Cannabis-induced psychotic disorder, without use disorder ◀

● **F12.98** **Cannabis use, unspecified with other cannabis-induced disorder**

F12.980 **Cannabis use, unspecified with anxiety disorder**

Cannabis-induced anxiety disorder, without use disorder ◀

F12.988 **Cannabis use, unspecified with other cannabis-induced disorder**

Cannabis-induced sleep disorder, without use disorder ◀

F12.99 **Cannabis use, unspecified with unspecified cannabis-induced disorder**

● **F13** **Sedative, hypnotic, or anxiolytic related disorders**

Ex For category F13 CC codes unless otherwise indicated: F02.80-F02.81, F04-F06.8, F10.10-F11.19, F11.21-F13.19, F13.21-F14.19, F14.21-F15.19, F15.21-F16.19, F16.21-F17.209, F17.213-F17.219, F17.223-F17.229, F17.293-F18.19, F18.21-F19.19, F19.21-F19.99, F53-F55.8, R78

● **F13.1** **Sedative, hypnotic or anxiolytic-related abuse**

Excludes1 sedative, hypnotic or anxiolytic-related dependence (F13.2-)
sedative, hypnotic, or anxiolytic use, unspecified (F13.9-)

F13.10 **Sedative, hypnotic or anxiolytic abuse, uncomplicated**

Sedative, hypnotic, or anxiolytic use disorder, mild ◀

● **F13.12** **Sedative, hypnotic or anxiolytic abuse with intoxication**

F13.120 **Sedative, hypnotic or anxiolytic abuse with intoxication, uncomplicated**

F13.121 **Sedative, hypnotic or anxiolytic abuse with intoxication delirium**

F13.129 **Sedative, hypnotic or anxiolytic abuse with intoxication, unspecified**

F13.14 **Sedative, hypnotic or anxiolytic abuse with sedative, hypnotic or anxiolytic-induced mood disorder**

Sedative, hypnotic, or anxiolytic use disorder, mild, with sedative, hypnotic, or anxiolytic-induced bipolar or related disorder ◀

Sedative, hypnotic, or anxiolytic use disorder, mild, with sedative, hypnotic, or anxiolytic-induced depressive disorder ◀

● **F13.15** **Sedative, hypnotic or anxiolytic abuse with sedative, hypnotic or anxiolytic-induced psychotic disorder**

F13.150 **Sedative, hypnotic or anxiolytic abuse with sedative, hypnotic or anxiolytic-induced psychotic disorder with delusions**

F13.151 **Sedative, hypnotic or anxiolytic abuse with sedative, hypnotic or anxiolytic-induced psychotic disorder with hallucinations**

F13.159 **Sedative, hypnotic or anxiolytic abuse with sedative, hypnotic or anxiolytic-induced psychotic disorder, unspecified**

● **F13.18** **Sedative, hypnotic or anxiolytic abuse with other sedative, hypnotic or anxiolytic-induced disorders**

F13.180 **Sedative, hypnotic or anxiolytic abuse with sedative, hypnotic or anxiolytic-induced anxiety disorder**

F13.181 **Sedative, hypnotic or anxiolytic abuse with sedative, hypnotic or anxiolytic-induced sexual dysfunction**

F13.182 **Sedative, hypnotic or anxiolytic abuse with sedative, hypnotic or anxiolytic-induced sleep disorder**

F13.188 **Sedative, hypnotic or anxiolytic abuse with other sedative, hypnotic or anxiolytic-induced disorder**

F13.19 **Sedative, hypnotic or anxiolytic abuse with unspecified sedative, hypnotic or anxiolytic-induced disorder**

● **F13.2** **Sedative, hypnotic or anxiolytic-related dependence**

Excludes1 sedative, hypnotic or anxiolytic-related abuse (F13.1-)
sedative, hypnotic, or anxiolytic use, unspecified (F13.9-)

Excludes2 sedative, hypnotic, or anxiolytic poisoning (T42.-)

F13.20 **Sedative, hypnotic or anxiolytic dependence, uncomplicated**

Ex No exclusions

F13.21 **Sedative, hypnotic or anxiolytic dependence, in remission**

● **F13.22** **Sedative, hypnotic or anxiolytic dependence with intoxication**

Excludes1 sedative, hypnotic or anxiolytic dependence with withdrawal (F13.23-)

F13.220 **Sedative, hypnotic or anxiolytic dependence with intoxication, uncomplicated**

F13.221 **Sedative, hypnotic or anxiolytic dependence with intoxication delirium**

F13.229 **Sedative, hypnotic or anxiolytic dependence with intoxication, unspecified**

● **F13.23** **Sedative, hypnotic or anxiolytic dependence with withdrawal**

Sedative, hypnotic, or anxiolytic use disorder, moderate ◀

Sedative, hypnotic, or anxiolytic use disorder, severe ◀

Excludes1 sedative, hypnotic or anxiolytic dependence with intoxication (F13.22-)

F13.230 **Sedative, hypnotic or anxiolytic dependence with withdrawal, uncomplicated**

F13.231 **Sedative, hypnotic or anxiolytic dependence with withdrawal delirium**

F13.232 Sedative, hypnotic or anxiolytic dependence with withdrawal with perceptual disturbance
Sedative, hypnotic, or anxiolytic withdrawal with perceptual disturbances ◀

F13.239 Sedative, hypnotic or anxiolytic dependence with withdrawal, unspecified
Sedative, hypnotic, or anxiolytic withdrawal without perceptual disturbances ◀

F13.24 Sedative, hypnotic or anxiolytic dependence with sedative, hypnotic or anxiolytic-induced mood disorder
Sedative, hypnotic, or anxiolytic use disorder, moderate, with sedative, hypnotic, or anxiolytic-induced bipolar or related disorder ◀
Sedative, hypnotic, or anxiolytic use disorder, moderate, with sedative, hypnotic, or anxiolytic-induced depressive disorder ◀
Sedative, hypnotic, or anxiolytic use disorder, severe, with sedative, hypnotic, or anxiolytic-induced bipolar or related disorder ◀
Sedative, hypnotic, or anxiolytic use disorder, severe, with sedative, hypnotic, or anxiolytic-induced depressive disorder ◀

● **F13.25 Sedative, hypnotic or anxiolytic dependence with sedative, hypnotic or anxiolytic-induced psychotic disorder**

F13.250 Sedative, hypnotic or anxiolytic dependence with sedative, hypnotic or anxiolytic-induced psychotic disorder with delusions

F13.251 Sedative, hypnotic or anxiolytic dependence with sedative, hypnotic or anxiolytic-induced psychotic disorder with hallucinations

F13.259 Sedative, hypnotic or anxiolytic dependence with sedative, hypnotic or anxiolytic-induced psychotic disorder, unspecified
Ex No exclusions

F13.26 Sedative, hypnotic or anxiolytic dependence with sedative, hypnotic or anxiolytic-induced persisting amnestic disorder
Ex No exclusions

F13.27 Sedative, hypnotic or anxiolytic dependence with sedative, hypnotic or anxiolytic-induced persisting dementia
Sedative, hypnotic, or anxiolytic use disorder, moderate, with sedative, hypnotic, or anxiolytic-induced major neurocognitive disorder ◀
Sedative, hypnotic, or anxiolytic use disorder, severe, with sedative, hypnotic, or anxiolytic-induced major neurocognitive disorder ◀

● **F13.28 Sedative, hypnotic or anxiolytic dependence with other sedative, hypnotic or anxiolytic-induced disorders**
Ex For category F13.28 CC codes: No exclusions

F13.280 Sedative, hypnotic or anxiolytic dependence with sedative, hypnotic or anxiolytic-induced anxiety disorder

F13.281 Sedative, hypnotic or anxiolytic dependence with sedative, hypnotic or anxiolytic-induced sexual dysfunction

F13.282 Sedative, hypnotic or anxiolytic dependence with sedative, hypnotic or anxiolytic-induced sleep disorder

F13.288 Sedative, hypnotic or anxiolytic dependence with other sedative, hypnotic or anxiolytic-induced disorder
Sedative, hypnotic, or anxiolytic use disorder, moderate, with sedative, hypnotic, or anxiolytic-induced mild neurocognitive disorder ◀
Sedative, hypnotic, or anxiolytic use disorder, severe, with sedative, hypnotic, or anxiolytic-induced mild neurocognitive disorder ◀

F13.29 Sedative, hypnotic or anxiolytic dependence with unspecified sedative, hypnotic or anxiolytic-induced disorder

● **F13.9 Sedative, hypnotic or anxiolytic-related use, unspecified**
Excludes1 sedative, hypnotic or anxiolytic-related abuse (F13.1-)
sedative, hypnotic or anxiolytic-related dependence (F13.2-)

F13.90 Sedative, hypnotic, or anxiolytic use, unspecified, uncomplicated

● **F13.92 Sedative, hypnotic or anxiolytic use, unspecified with intoxication**
Excludes1 sedative, hypnotic or anxiolytic use, unspecified with withdrawal (F13.93-)

F13.920 Sedative, hypnotic or anxiolytic use, unspecified with intoxication, uncomplicated

F13.921 Sedative, hypnotic or anxiolytic use, unspecified with intoxication delirium
Sedative, hypnotic, or anxiolytic-induced delirium ◀

F13.929 Sedative, hypnotic or anxiolytic use, unspecified with intoxication, unspecified

● **F13.93 Sedative, hypnotic or anxiolytic use, unspecified with withdrawal**
Excludes1 sedative, hypnotic or anxiolytic use, unspecified with intoxication (F13.92-)

F13.930 Sedative, hypnotic or anxiolytic use, unspecified with withdrawal, uncomplicated

F13.931 Sedative, hypnotic or anxiolytic use, unspecified with withdrawal delirium

F13.932 Sedative, hypnotic or anxiolytic use, unspecified with withdrawal with perceptual disturbances

F13.939 Sedative, hypnotic or anxiolytic use, unspecified with withdrawal, unspecified

F13.94 Sedative, hypnotic or anxiolytic use, unspecified with sedative, hypnotic or anxiolytic-induced mood disorder
Sedative, hypnotic, or anxiolytic-induced bipolar or related disorder, without use disorder ◀
Sedative, hypnotic, or anxiolytic-induced depressive disorder, without use disorder ◀

F13.95 Sedative, hypnotic or anxiolytic use, unspecified with sedative, hypnotic or anxiolytic-induced psychotic disorder

F13.950 Sedative, hypnotic or anxiolytic use, unspecified with sedative, hypnotic or anxiolytic-induced psychotic disorder with delusions

F13.951 Sedative, hypnotic or anxiolytic use, unspecified with sedative, hypnotic or anxiolytic-induced psychotic disorder with hallucinations

F13.959 Sedative, hypnotic or anxiolytic use, unspecified with sedative, hypnotic or anxiolytic-induced psychotic disorder, unspecified

Sedative, hypnotic, or anxiolytic-induced psychotic disorder, without use disorder ◀

F13.96 Sedative, hypnotic or anxiolytic use, unspecified with sedative, hypnotic or anxiolytic-induced persisting amnestic disorder

F13.97 Sedative, hypnotic or anxiolytic use, unspecified with sedative, hypnotic or anxiolytic-induced persisting dementia

Sedative, hypnotic, or anxiolytic-induced major neurocognitive disorder, without use disorder ◀

F13.98 Sedative, hypnotic or anxiolytic use, unspecified with other sedative, hypnotic or anxiolytic-induced disorders

F13.980 Sedative, hypnotic or anxiolytic use, unspecified with sedative, hypnotic or anxiolytic-induced anxiety disorder

Sedative, hypnotic, or anxiolytic-induced anxiety disorder, without use disorder ◀

F13.981 Sedative, hypnotic or anxiolytic use, unspecified with sedative, hypnotic or anxiolytic-induced sexual dysfunction

Sedative, hypnotic, or anxiolytic-induced sexual dysfunction disorder, without use disorder ◀

F13.982 Sedative, hypnotic or anxiolytic use, unspecified with sedative, hypnotic or anxiolytic-induced sleep disorder

Sedative, hypnotic, or anxiolytic-induced sleep disorder, without use disorder ◀

F13.988 Sedative, hypnotic or anxiolytic use, unspecified with other sedative, hypnotic or anxiolytic-induced disorder

Sedative, hypnotic, or anxiolytic-induced mild neurocognitive disorder ◀

F13.99 Sedative, hypnotic or anxiolytic use, unspecified with unspecified sedative, hypnotic or anxiolytic-induced disorder

F14 Cocaine related disorders

Excludes2 other stimulant-related disorders (F15.-)

Ex: **For category F14 CC codes unless otherwise indicated:** F02.80-F02.81, F04-F06.8, F10.10-F11.19, F11.21-F13.19, F13.21-F14.19, F14.21-F15.19, F15.21-F16.19, F16.21-F17.209, F17.213-F17.219, F17.223-F17.229, F17.293-F18.19, F18.21-F19.19, F19.21-F19.99, F53-F55.8, R78

F14.1 Cocaine abuse

Excludes1 cocaine dependence (F14.2-)
cocaine use, unspecified (F14.9-)

F14.10 Cocaine abuse, uncomplicated

Cocaine use disorder, mild ◀

F14.12 Cocaine abuse with intoxication

F14.120 Cocaine abuse with intoxication, uncomplicated

F14.121 Cocaine abuse with intoxication with delirium

F14.122 Cocaine abuse with intoxication with perceptual disturbance

F14.129 Cocaine abuse with intoxication, unspecified

F14.14 Cocaine abuse with cocaine-induced mood disorder

Cocaine use disorder, mild, with cocaine-induced bipolar or related disorder ◀
Cocaine use disorder, mild, with cocaine-induced depressive disorder ◀

F14.15 Cocaine abuse with cocaine-induced psychotic disorder

F14.150 Cocaine abuse with cocaine-induced psychotic disorder with delusions

F14.151 Cocaine abuse with cocaine-induced psychotic disorder with hallucinations

F14.159 Cocaine abuse with cocaine-induced psychotic disorder, unspecified

F14.18 Cocaine abuse with other cocaine-induced disorder

F14.180 Cocaine abuse with cocaine-induced anxiety disorder

F14.181 Cocaine abuse with cocaine-induced sexual dysfunction

F14.182 Cocaine abuse with cocaine-induced sleep disorder

F14.188 Cocaine abuse with other cocaine-induced disorder

Cocaine use disorder, mild, with cocaine-induced obsessive-compulsive or related disorder ◀

F14.19 Cocaine abuse with unspecified cocaine-induced disorder

F14.2 Cocaine dependence

Excludes1 cocaine abuse (F14.1-)
cocaine use, unspecified (F14.9-)

Excludes2 cocaine poisoning (T40.5-)

F14.20 Cocaine dependence, uncomplicated

Cocaine use disorder, moderate ◀
Cocaine use disorder, severe ◀

Ex: No exclusions

F14.21 Cocaine dependence, in remission

F14.22 Cocaine dependence with intoxication

Excludes1 cocaine dependence with withdrawal (F14.23)

F14.220 Cocaine dependence with intoxication, uncomplicated

F14.221 Cocaine dependence with intoxication delirium

F14.222 Cocaine dependence with intoxication with perceptual disturbance

Ex: No exclusions

F14.229 Cocaine dependence with intoxication, unspecified

Ex: No exclusions

F14.23 Cocaine dependence with withdrawal

Excludes1 cocaine dependence with intoxication (F14.22-)

F14.24 Cocaine dependence with cocaine-induced mood disorder
Cocaine use disorder, moderate, with cocaine-induced bipolar or related disorder ◀
Cocaine use disorder, moderate, with cocaine-induced depressive disorder ◀
Cocaine use disorder, severe, with cocaine-induced bipolar or related disorder ◀
Cocaine use disorder, severe, with cocaine-induced depressive disorder ◀

● **F14.25 Cocaine dependence with cocaine-induced psychotic disorder**
F14.250 Cocaine dependence with cocaine-induced psychotic disorder with delusions
F14.251 Cocaine dependence with cocaine-induced psychotic disorder with hallucinations
F14.259 Cocaine dependence with cocaine-induced psychotic disorder, unspecified
Ex No exclusions

● **F14.28 Cocaine dependence with other cocaine-induced disorder**
Ex For category F14.28 CC codes: No exclusions
F14.280 Cocaine dependence with cocaine-induced anxiety disorder
F14.281 Cocaine dependence with cocaine-induced sexual dysfunction
F14.282 Cocaine dependence with cocaine-induced sleep disorder
F14.288 Cocaine dependence with other cocaine-induced disorder
Cocaine use disorder, moderate, with cocaine-induced obsessive-compulsive or related disorder ◀
Cocaine use disorder, severe, with cocaine-induced obsessive-compulsive or related disorder ◀
F14.29 Cocaine dependence with unspecified cocaine-induced disorder

● **F14.9 Cocaine use, unspecified**
Excludes1 cocaine abuse (F14.1-)
cocaine dependence (F14.2-)
F14.90 Cocaine use, unspecified, uncomplicated

● **F14.92 Cocaine use, unspecified with intoxication**
F14.920 Cocaine use, unspecified with intoxication, uncomplicated
F14.921 Cocaine use, unspecified with intoxication delirium
F14.922 Cocaine use, unspecified with intoxication with perceptual disturbance
F14.929 Cocaine use, unspecified with intoxication, unspecified
F14.94 Cocaine use, unspecified with cocaine-induced mood disorder
Cocaine-induced bipolar or related disorder, without use disorder ◀
Cocaine-induced depressive disorder, without use disorder ◀

● **F14.95 Cocaine use, unspecified with cocaine-induced psychotic disorder**
F14.950 Cocaine use, unspecified with cocaine-induced psychotic disorder with delusions
F14.951 Cocaine use, unspecified with cocaine-induced psychotic disorder with hallucinations
F14.959 Cocaine use, unspecified with cocaine-induced psychotic disorder, unspecified
Cocaine-induced psychotic disorder, without use disorder ◀

● **F14.98 Cocaine use, unspecified with other specified cocaine-induced disorder**
F14.980 Cocaine use, unspecified with cocaine-induced anxiety disorder
Cocaine-induced anxiety disorder, without use disorder ◀
F14.981 Cocaine use, unspecified with cocaine-induced sexual dysfunction
Cocaine-induced sexual dysfunction, without use disorder ◀
F14.982 Cocaine use, unspecified with cocaine-induced sleep disorder
Cocaine-induced sleep disorder, without use disorder ◀
F14.988 Cocaine use, unspecified with other cocaine-induced disorder
Cocaine-induced obsessive-compulsive or related disorder ◀
F14.99 Cocaine use, unspecified with unspecified cocaine-induced disorder

● **F15 Other stimulant related disorders**
Includes amphetamine-related disorders
caffeine
Excludes2 cocaine-related disorders (F14.-)
Ex For category F15 CC codes unless otherwise indicated: F02.80-F02.81, F04-F06.8, F10.10-F11.19, F11.21-F13.19, F13.21-F14.19, F14.21-F15.19, F15.21-F16.19, F16.21-F17.209, F17.213-F17.219, F17.223-F17.229, F17.293-F18.19, F18.21-F19.19, F19.21-F19.99, F53-F55.8, R78

● **F15.1 Other stimulant abuse**
Excludes1 other stimulant dependence (F15.2-)
other stimulant use, unspecified (F15.9-)
F15.10 Other stimulant abuse, uncomplicated
Amphetamine type substance use disorder, mild ◀
Other or unspecified stimulant use disorder, mild ◀

● **F15.12 Other stimulant abuse with intoxication**
F15.120 Other stimulant abuse with intoxication, uncomplicated
F15.121 Other stimulant abuse with intoxication delirium
F15.122 Other stimulant abuse with intoxication with perceptual disturbance
Amphetamine or other stimulant use disorder, mild, with amphetamine or other stimulant intoxication, with perceptual disturbances ◀
F15.129 Other stimulant abuse with intoxication, unspecified
Amphetamine or other stimulant use disorder, mild, with amphetamine or other stimulant intoxication, without perceptual disturbances ◀
F15.14 Other stimulant abuse with stimulant-induced mood disorder
Amphetamine or other stimulant use disorder, mild, with amphetamine or other stimulant-induced bipolar or related disorder ◀
Amphetamine or other stimulant use disorder, mild, with amphetamine or other stimulant-induced depressive disorder ◀

F15.15 Other stimulant abuse with stimulant-induced psychotic disorder

F15.150 Other stimulant abuse with stimulant-induced psychotic disorder with delusions CC

F15.151 Other stimulant abuse with stimulant-induced psychotic disorder with hallucinations CC

F15.159 Other stimulant abuse with stimulant-induced psychotic disorder, unspecified

F15.18 Other stimulant abuse with other stimulant-induced disorder

F15.180 Other stimulant abuse with stimulant-induced anxiety disorder

F15.181 Other stimulant abuse with stimulant-induced sexual dysfunction

F15.182 Other stimulant abuse with stimulant-induced sleep disorder

F15.188 Other stimulant abuse with other stimulant-induced disorder

Amphetamine or other stimulant use disorder, mild, with amphetamine or other stimulant-induced obsessive-compulsive or related disorder ◀

F15.19 Other stimulant abuse with unspecified stimulant-induced disorder

F15.2 Other stimulant dependence

Excludes1 other stimulant abuse (F15.1-)
other stimulant use, unspecified (F15.9-)

F15.20 Other stimulant dependence, uncomplicated CC

Amphetamine type substance use disorder, moderate ◀

Amphetamine type substance use disorder, severe ◀

Other or unspecified stimulant use disorder, moderate ◀

Other or unspecified stimulant use disorder, severe ◀

Ex: No exclusions

F15.21 Other stimulant dependence, in remission

F15.22 Other stimulant dependence with intoxication

Excludes1 other stimulant dependence with withdrawal (F15.23)

F15.220 Other stimulant dependence with intoxication, uncomplicated

F15.221 Other stimulant dependence with intoxication delirium CC

F15.222 Other stimulant dependence with intoxication with perceptual disturbance CC

Amphetamine or other stimulant use disorder, moderate, with amphetamine or other stimulant intoxication, with perceptual disturbances ◀

Amphetamine or other stimulant use disorder, severe, with amphetamine or other stimulant intoxication, with perceptual disturbances ◀

Ex: No exclusions

F15.229 Other stimulant dependence with intoxication, unspecified

Amphetamine or other stimulant use disorder, moderate, with amphetamine or other stimulant intoxication, without perceptual disturbances ◀

Amphetamine or other stimulant use disorder, severe, with amphetamine or other stimulant intoxication, without perceptual disturbances ◀

F15.23 Other stimulant dependence with withdrawal CC

Amphetamine or other stimulant withdrawal ◀

Excludes1 other stimulant dependence with intoxication (F15.22-)

F15.24 Other stimulant dependence with stimulant-induced mood disorder

Amphetamine or other stimulant use disorder, moderate, with amphetamine or other stimulant-induced bipolar or related disorder ◀

Amphetamine or other stimulant use disorder, moderate, with amphetamine or other stimulant-induced depressive disorder ◀

Amphetamine or other stimulant use disorder, severe, with amphetamine or other stimulant-induced bipolar or related disorder ◀

Amphetamine or other stimulant use disorder, severe, with amphetamine or other stimulant-induced depressive disorder ◀

F15.25 Other stimulant dependence with stimulant-induced psychotic disorder

F15.250 Other stimulant dependence with stimulant-induced psychotic disorder with delusions CC

F15.251 Other stimulant dependence with stimulant-induced psychotic disorder with hallucinations CC

F15.259 Other stimulant dependence with stimulant-induced psychotic disorder, unspecified CC

Ex: No exclusions

F15.28 Other stimulant dependence with other stimulant-induced disorder

Ex: For category F15.28 CC codes: No exclusions

F15.280 Other stimulant dependence with stimulant-induced anxiety disorder CC

F15.281 Other stimulant dependence with stimulant-induced sexual dysfunction CC

F15.282 Other stimulant dependence with stimulant-induced sleep disorder CC

F15.288 Other stimulant dependence with other stimulant-induced disorder CC

Amphetamine or other stimulant use disorder, moderate, with amphetamine or other stimulant-induced obsessive-compulsive or related disorder ◀

Amphetamine or other stimulant use disorder, severe, with amphetamine or other stimulant-induced obsessive-compulsive or related disorder ◀

F15.29 Other stimulant dependence with unspecified stimulant-induced disorder

F15.9 Other stimulant use, unspecified

Excludes1 other stimulant abuse (F15.1-)
other stimulant dependence (F15.2-)

F15.90 Other stimulant use, unspecified, uncomplicated

● **F15.92 Other stimulant use, unspecified with intoxication**

Excludes1 other stimulant use, unspecified with withdrawal (F15.93)

F15.920 Other stimulant use, unspecified with intoxication, uncomplicated

F15.921 Other stimulant use, unspecified with intoxication delirium

Amphetamine or other stimulant-induced delirium ◀

F15.922 Other stimulant use, unspecified with intoxication with perceptual disturbance

F15.929 Other stimulant use, unspecified with intoxication, unspecified

Caffeine intoxication ◀

F15.93 Other stimulant use, unspecified with withdrawal

Caffeine withdrawal ◀

Excludes1 other stimulant use, unspecified with intoxication (F15.92-)

F15.94 Other stimulant use, unspecified with stimulant-induced mood disorder

Amphetamine or other stimulant-induced bipolar or related disorder, without use disorder ◀

Amphetamine or other stimulant-induced depressive disorder, without use disorder ◀

● **F15.95 Other stimulant use, unspecified with stimulant-induced psychotic disorder**

F15.950 Other stimulant use, unspecified with stimulant-induced psychotic disorder with delusions

F15.951 Other stimulant use, unspecified with stimulant-induced psychotic disorder with hallucinations

F15.959 Other stimulant use, unspecified with stimulant-induced psychotic disorder, unspecified

Amphetamine or other stimulant-induced psychotic disorder, without use disorder ◀

● **F15.98 Other stimulant use, unspecified with other stimulant-induced disorder**

F15.980 Other stimulant use, unspecified with stimulant-induced anxiety disorder

Amphetamine or other stimulant-induced anxiety disorder, without use disorder ◀

Caffeine-induced anxiety disorder, without use disorder ◀

F15.981 Other stimulant use, unspecified with stimulant-induced sexual dysfunction

Amphetamine or other stimulant-induced sexual dysfunction, without use disorder ◀

F15.982 Other stimulant use, unspecified with stimulant-induced sleep disorder

Amphetamine or other stimulant-induced sleep disorder, without use disorder ◀

Caffeine-induced sleep disorder, without use disorder ◀

F15.988 Other stimulant use, unspecified with other stimulant-induced disorder

Amphetamine or other stimulant-induced obsessive-compulsive or related disorder, without use disorder ◀

F15.99 Other stimulant use, unspecified with unspecified stimulant-induced disorder

● **F16 Hallucinogen related disorders**

Includes ecstasy
PCP
phencyclidine

(Ex) **For category F16 CC codes unless otherwise indicated:** F02.80-F02.81, F04-F06.8, F10.10-F11.19, F11.21-F13.19, F13.21-F14.19, F14.21-F15.19, F15.21-F16.19, F16.21-F17.209, F17.213-F17.219, F17.223-F17.229, F17.293-F18.19, F18.21-F19.19, F19.21-F19.99, F53-F55.8, R78

● **F16.1 Hallucinogen abuse**

Excludes1 hallucinogen dependence (F16.2-)
hallucinogen use, unspecified (F16.9-)

F16.10 Hallucinogen abuse, uncomplicated

Other hallucinogen use disorder, mild ◀

Phencyclidine use disorder, mild ◀

● **F16.12 Hallucinogen abuse with intoxication**

F16.120 Hallucinogen abuse with intoxication, uncomplicated

F16.121 Hallucinogen abuse with intoxication with delirium

F16.122 Hallucinogen abuse with intoxication with perceptual disturbance

F16.129 Hallucinogen abuse with intoxication, unspecified

F16.14 Hallucinogen abuse with hallucinogen-induced mood disorder

Other hallucinogen use disorder, mild, with other hallucinogen-induced bipolar or related disorder ◀

Other hallucinogen use disorder, mild, with other hallucinogen-induced depressive disorder ◀

Phencyclidine use disorder, mild, with phencyclidine-induced bipolar or related disorder ◀

Phencyclidine use disorder, mild, with phencyclidine-induced depressive disorder ◀

● **F16.15 Hallucinogen abuse with hallucinogen-induced psychotic disorder**

F16.150 Hallucinogen abuse with hallucinogen-induced psychotic disorder with delusions

F16.151 Hallucinogen abuse with hallucinogen-induced psychotic disorder with hallucinations

F16.159 Hallucinogen abuse with hallucinogen-induced psychotic disorder, unspecified

● **F16.18 Hallucinogen abuse with other hallucinogen-induced disorder**

F16.180 Hallucinogen abuse with hallucinogen-induced anxiety disorder

F16.183 Hallucinogen abuse with hallucinogen persisting perception disorder (flashbacks)

F16.188 Hallucinogen abuse with other hallucinogen-induced disorder

F16.19 Hallucinogen abuse with unspecified hallucinogen-induced disorder

● **F16.2 Hallucinogen dependence**

Excludes1 hallucinogen abuse (F16.1-)
hallucinogen use, unspecified (F16.9-)

F16.20 Hallucinogen dependence, uncomplicated

Other hallucinogen use disorder, moderate ◀

Other hallucinogen use disorder, severe ◀

Phencyclidine use disorder, moderate ◀

Phencyclidine use disorder, severe ◀

(Ex) No exclusions

F16.21 Hallucinogen dependence, in remission

● **F16.22 Hallucinogen dependence with intoxication**
- **F16.220 Hallucinogen dependence with intoxication, uncomplicated**
- **F16.221 Hallucinogen dependence with intoxication with delirium** CC
- **F16.229 Hallucinogen dependence with intoxication, unspecified**

F16.24 Hallucinogen dependence with hallucinogen-induced mood disorder
- Other hallucinogen use disorder, moderate, with other hallucinogen-induced bipolar or related disorder ◀
- Other hallucinogen use disorder, moderate, with other hallucinogen-induced depressive disorder ◀
- Other hallucinogen use disorder, severe, with other hallucinogen-induced bipolar or related disorder ◀
- Other hallucinogen use disorder, severe, with other hallucinogen-induced depressive disorder ◀
- Phencyclidine use disorder, moderate, with phencyclidine-induced bipolar or related disorder ◀
- Phencyclidine use disorder, moderate, with phencyclidine-induced depressive disorder ◀
- Phencyclidine use disorder, severe, with phencyclidine-induced bipolar or related disorder ◀
- Phencyclidine use disorder, severe, with phencyclidine-induced depressive disorder ◀

● **F16.25 Hallucinogen dependence with hallucinogen-induced psychotic disorder**
- **F16.250 Hallucinogen dependence with hallucinogen-induced psychotic disorder with delusions** CC
- **F16.251 Hallucinogen dependence with hallucinogen-induced psychotic disorder with hallucinations** CC
- **F16.259 Hallucinogen dependence with hallucinogen-induced psychotic disorder, unspecified** CC
  - Ex: No exclusions

● **F16.28 Hallucinogen dependence with other hallucinogen-induced disorder**
  - Ex: For category F16.28 CC codes: No exclusions
- **F16.280 Hallucinogen dependence with hallucinogen-induced anxiety disorder** CC
- **F16.283 Hallucinogen dependence with hallucinogen persisting perception disorder (flashbacks)** CC
- **F16.288 Hallucinogen dependence with other hallucinogen-induced disorder** CC

F16.29 Hallucinogen dependence with unspecified hallucinogen-induced disorder

● **F16.9 Hallucinogen use, unspecified**
  - **Excludes1** hallucinogen abuse (F16.1-)
    hallucinogen dependence (F16.2-)
- **F16.90 Hallucinogen use, unspecified, uncomplicated**

● **F16.92 Hallucinogen use, unspecified with intoxication**
- **F16.920 Hallucinogen use, unspecified with intoxication, uncomplicated**
- **F16.921 Hallucinogen use, unspecified with intoxication with delirium** CC
  - Other hallucinogen intoxication delirium ◀
- **F16.929 Hallucinogen use, unspecified with intoxication, unspecified**

F16.94 Hallucinogen use, unspecified with hallucinogen-induced mood disorder
- Other hallucinogen-induced bipolar or related disorder, without use disorder ◀
- Other hallucinogen-induced depressive disorder, without use disorder ◀
- Phencyclidine-induced bipolar or related disorder, without use disorder ◀
- Phencyclidine-induced depressive disorder, without use disorder ◀

● **F16.95 Hallucinogen use, unspecified with hallucinogen-induced psychotic disorder**
- **F16.950 Hallucinogen use, unspecified with hallucinogen-induced psychotic disorder with delusions** CC
- **F16.951 Hallucinogen use, unspecified with hallucinogen-induced psychotic disorder with hallucinations** CC
- **F16.959 Hallucinogen use, unspecified with hallucinogen-induced psychotic disorder, unspecified**
  - Other hallucinogen-induced psychotic disorder, without use disorder ◀
  - Phencyclidine-induced psychotic disorder, without use disorder ◀

● **F16.98 Hallucinogen use, unspecified with other specified hallucinogen-induced disorder**
- **F16.980 Hallucinogen use, unspecified with hallucinogen-induced anxiety disorder**
  - Other hallucinogen-induced anxiety disorder, without use disorder ◀
  - Phencyclidine-induced anxiety disorder, without use disorder ◀
- **F16.983 Hallucinogen use, unspecified with hallucinogen persisting perception disorder (flashbacks)**
- **F16.988 Hallucinogen use, unspecified with other hallucinogen-induced disorder**

F16.99 Hallucinogen use, unspecified with unspecified hallucinogen-induced disorder

● **F17 Nicotine dependence**
  - **Excludes1** history of tobacco dependence (Z87.891)
    tobacco use NOS (Z72.0)
  - **Excludes2** tobacco use (smoking) during pregnancy, childbirth and the puerperium (O99.33-)
    toxic effect of nicotine (T65.2-)
  - Ex: For category F17 CC codes: F02.80-F02.81, F04-F06.8, F10.10-F11.19, F11.21-F13.19, F13.21-F14.19, F14.21-F15.19, F15.21-F16.19, F16.21-F17.209, F17.213-F17.219, F17.223-F17.229, F17.293-F18.19, F18.21-F19.19, F19.21-F19.99, F53-F55.8, R78

● **F17.2 Nicotine dependence**

● **F17.20 Nicotine dependence, unspecified**

● **F17.200 Nicotine dependence, unspecified, uncomplicated**
- Tobacco use disorder, mild ◀
- Tobacco use disorder, moderate ◀
- Tobacco use disorder, severe ◀
- **Coding Clinic: 2016, Q1, P37**

● **F17.201 Nicotine dependence, unspecified, in remission**
- **F17.203 Nicotine dependence unspecified, with withdrawal** CC
  - Tobacco withdrawal ◀
- **F17.208 Nicotine dependence, unspecified, with other nicotine-induced disorders**
- **F17.209 Nicotine dependence, unspecified, with unspecified nicotine-induced disorders**

● F17.21 Nicotine dependence, cigarettes
- ● F17.210 Nicotine dependence, cigarettes, uncomplicated
- ● F17.211 Nicotine dependence, cigarettes, in remission
- F17.213 Nicotine dependence, cigarettes, with withdrawal
- F17.218 Nicotine dependence, cigarettes, with other nicotine-induced disorders
- F17.219 Nicotine dependence, cigarettes, with unspecified nicotine-induced disorders

● F17.22 Nicotine dependence, chewing tobacco
- ● F17.220 Nicotine dependence, chewing tobacco, uncomplicated
- ● F17.221 Nicotine dependence, chewing tobacco, in remission
- F17.223 Nicotine dependence, chewing tobacco, with withdrawal
- F17.228 Nicotine dependence, chewing tobacco, with other nicotine-induced disorders
- F17.229 Nicotine dependence, chewing tobacco, with unspecified nicotine-induced disorders

● F17.29 Nicotine dependence, other tobacco product
- ● F17.290 Nicotine dependence, other tobacco product, uncomplicated
- ● F17.291 Nicotine dependence, other tobacco product, in remission
- F17.293 Nicotine dependence, other tobacco product, with withdrawal
- F17.298 Nicotine dependence, other tobacco product, with other nicotine-induced disorders
- F17.299 Nicotine dependence, other tobacco product, with unspecified nicotine-induced disorders

● F18 Inhalant related disorders

Includes volatile solvents

Ex: For category F18 CC codes unless otherwise indicated: F02.80-F02.81, F04-F06.8, F10.10-F11.19, F11.21-F13.19, F13.21-F14.19, F14.21-F15.19, F15.21-F16.19, F16.21-F17.209, F17.213-F17.219, F17.223-F17.229, F17.293-F18.19, F18.21-F19.19, F19.21-F19.99, F53-F55.8, R78

● F18.1 Inhalant abuse

Excludes1 inhalant dependence (F18.2-)
inhalant use, unspecified (F18.9-)

- F18.10 Inhalant abuse, uncomplicated
  - Inhalant use disorder, mild ◀
- ● F18.12 Inhalant abuse with intoxication
  - F18.120 Inhalant abuse with intoxication, uncomplicated
  - F18.121 Inhalant abuse with intoxication delirium
  - F18.129 Inhalant abuse with intoxication, unspecified
- F18.14 Inhalant abuse with inhalant-induced mood disorder
  - Inhalant use disorder, mild, with inhalant-induced depressive disorder ◀
- ● F18.15 Inhalant abuse with inhalant-induced psychotic disorder
  - F18.150 Inhalant abuse with inhalant-induced psychotic disorder with delusions
  - F18.151 Inhalant abuse with inhalant-induced psychotic disorder with hallucinations
  - F18.159 Inhalant abuse with inhalant-induced psychotic disorder, unspecified
- F18.17 Inhalant abuse with inhalant-induced dementia
  - Inhalant use disorder, mild, with inhalant-induced major neurocognitive disorder ◀
- ● F18.18 Inhalant abuse with other inhalant-induced disorders
  - F18.180 Inhalant abuse with inhalant-induced anxiety disorder
  - F18.188 Inhalant abuse with other inhalant-induced disorder
    - Inhalant use disorder, mild, with inhalant-induced mild neurocognitive disorder ◀
- F18.19 Inhalant abuse with unspecified inhalant-induced disorder

● F18.2 Inhalant dependence

Excludes1 inhalant abuse (F18.1-)
inhalant use, unspecified (F18.9-)

- F18.20 Inhalant dependence, uncomplicated
  - Inhalant use disorder, moderate ◀
  - Inhalant use disorder, severe ◀
  - Ex: No exclusions
- F18.21 Inhalant dependence, in remission
- ● F18.22 Inhalant dependence with intoxication
  - F18.220 Inhalant dependence with intoxication, uncomplicated
  - F18.221 Inhalant dependence with intoxication delirium
  - F18.229 Inhalant dependence with intoxication, unspecified
- F18.24 Inhalant dependence with inhalant-induced mood disorder
  - Inhalant use disorder, moderate, with inhalant-induced depressive disorder ◀
  - Inhalant use disorder, severe, with inhalant-induced depressive disorder ◀
- ● F18.25 Inhalant dependence with inhalant-induced psychotic disorder
  - F18.250 Inhalant dependence with inhalant-induced psychotic disorder with delusions
  - F18.251 Inhalant dependence with inhalant-induced psychotic disorder with hallucinations
  - F18.259 Inhalant dependence with inhalant-induced psychotic disorder, unspecified
    - Ex: No exclusions
- F18.27 Inhalant dependence with inhalant-induced dementia
  - Inhalant use disorder, moderate, with inhalant-induced major neurocognitive disorder ◀
  - Inhalant use disorder, severe, with inhalant-induced major neurocognitive disorder ◀
- ● F18.28 Inhalant dependence with other inhalant-induced disorders
  - Ex: For category F18.28 CC codes: No exclusions
  - F18.280 Inhalant dependence with inhalant-induced anxiety disorder
  - F18.288 Inhalant dependence with other inhalant-induced disorder
    - Inhalant use disorder, moderate, with inhalant-induced mild neurocognitive disorder ◀
    - Inhalant use disorder, severe, with inhalant-induced mild neurocognitive disorder ◀
- F18.29 Inhalant dependence with unspecified inhalant-induced disorder

● F18.9 Inhalant use, unspecified

Excludes1 inhalant abuse (F18.1-)
inhalant dependence (F18.2-)

- F18.90 Inhalant use, unspecified, uncomplicated

F18.92 Inhalant use, unspecified with intoxication
- **F18.920 Inhalant use, unspecified with intoxication, uncomplicated**
- **F18.921 Inhalant use, unspecified with intoxication with delirium**
- **F18.929 Inhalant use, unspecified with intoxication, unspecified**

F18.94 Inhalant use, unspecified with inhalant-induced mood disorder
Inhalant-induced depressive disorder ◀

F18.95 Inhalant use, unspecified with inhalant-induced psychotic disorder
- **F18.950 Inhalant use, unspecified with inhalant-induced psychotic disorder with delusions**
- **F18.951 Inhalant use, unspecified with inhalant-induced psychotic disorder with hallucinations**
- **F18.959 Inhalant use, unspecified with inhalant-induced psychotic disorder, unspecified**

F18.97 Inhalant use, unspecified with inhalant-induced persisting dementia
Inhalant-induced major neurocognitive disorder ◀

F18.98 Inhalant use, unspecified with other inhalant-induced disorders
- **F18.980 Inhalant use, unspecified with inhalant-induced anxiety disorder**
- **F18.988 Inhalant use, unspecified with other inhalant-induced disorder**
  Inhalant-induced mild neurocognitive disorder ◀

F18.99 Inhalant use, unspecified with unspecified inhalant-induced disorder

F19 Other psychoactive substance related disorders
Includes polysubstance drug use (indiscriminate drug use)
Ex For category F19 CC codes unless otherwise indicated: F02.80-F02.81, F04-F06.8, F10.10-F11.19, F11.21-F13.19, F13.21-F14.19, F14.21-F15.19, F15.21-F16.19, F16.21-F17.209, F17.213-F17.219, F17.223-F17.229, F17.293-F18.19, F18.21-F19.19, F19.21-F19.99, F53-F55.8, R78

F19.1 Other psychoactive substance abuse
Excludes1 other psychoactive substance dependence (F19.2-)
other psychoactive substance use, unspecified (F19.9-)

F19.10 Other psychoactive substance abuse, uncomplicated
Other (or unknown) substance use disorder, mild ◀

F19.12 Other psychoactive substance abuse with intoxication
- **F19.120 Other psychoactive substance abuse with intoxication, uncomplicated**
- **F19.121 Other psychoactive substance abuse with intoxication delirium**
- **F19.122 Other psychoactive substance abuse with intoxication with perceptual disturbances**
- **F19.129 Other psychoactive substance abuse with intoxication, unspecified**

F19.14 Other psychoactive substance abuse with psychoactive substance-induced mood disorder
Other (or unknown) substance use disorder, mild, with other (or unknown) substance-induced bipolar or related disorder ◀
Other (or unknown) substance use disorder, mild, with other (or unknown) substance-induced depressive disorder ◀

F19.15 Other psychoactive substance abuse with psychoactive substance-induced psychotic disorder
- **F19.150 Other psychoactive substance abuse with psychoactive substance-induced psychotic disorder with delusions**
- **F19.151 Other psychoactive substance abuse with psychoactive substance-induced psychotic disorder with hallucinations**
- **F19.159 Other psychoactive substance abuse with psychoactive substance-induced psychotic disorder, unspecified**

F19.16 Other psychoactive substance abuse with psychoactive substance-induced persisting amnestic disorder

F19.17 Other psychoactive substance abuse with psychoactive substance-induced persisting dementia
Other (or unknown) substance use disorder, mild, with other (or unknown) substance-induced major neurocognitive disorder ◀

F19.18 Other psychoactive substance abuse with other psychoactive substance-induced disorders
- **F19.180 Other psychoactive substance abuse with psychoactive substance-induced anxiety disorder**
- **F19.181 Other psychoactive substance abuse with psychoactive substance-induced sexual dysfunction**
- **F19.182 Other psychoactive substance abuse with psychoactive substance-induced sleep disorder**
- **F19.188 Other psychoactive substance abuse with other psychoactive substance-induced disorder**
  Other (or unknown) substance use disorder, mild, with other (or unknown) substance-induced mild neurocognitive disorder ◀
  Other (or unknown) substance use disorder, mild, with other (or unknown) substance-induced obsessive-compulsive or related disorder ◀

F19.19 Other psychoactive substance abuse with unspecified psychoactive substance-induced disorder

F19.2 Other psychoactive substance dependence
Excludes1 other psychoactive substance abuse (F19.1-)
other psychoactive substance use, unspecified (F19.9-)

F19.20 Other psychoactive substance dependence, uncomplicated
Other (or unknown) substance use disorder, moderate ◀
Other (or unknown) substance use disorder, severe ◀
Ex No exclusions

F19.21 Other psychoactive substance dependence, in remission

F19.22 Other psychoactive substance dependence with intoxication
Excludes1 other psychoactive substance dependence with withdrawal (F19.23-)
- **F19.220 Other psychoactive substance dependence with intoxication, uncomplicated**
- **F19.221 Other psychoactive substance dependence with intoxication delirium**

F19.222 **Other psychoactive substance dependence with intoxication with perceptual disturbance**
Ex: No exclusions

F19.229 **Other psychoactive substance dependence with intoxication, unspecified**

● F19.23 **Other psychoactive substance dependence with withdrawal**
Excludes1 other psychoactive substance dependence with intoxication (F19.22-)

F19.230 **Other psychoactive substance dependence with withdrawal, uncomplicated**

F19.231 **Other psychoactive substance dependence with withdrawal delirium**

F19.232 **Other psychoactive substance dependence with withdrawal with perceptual disturbance**

F19.239 **Other psychoactive substance dependence with withdrawal, unspecified**

F19.24 **Other psychoactive substance dependence with psychoactive substance-induced mood disorder**
Other (or unknown) substance use disorder, moderate, with other (or unknown) substance-induced bipolar or related disorder ◀
Other (or unknown) substance use disorder, moderate, with other (or unknown) substance-induced depressive disorder ◀
Other (or unknown) substance use disorder, severe, with other (or unknown) substance-induced bipolar or related disorder ◀
Other (or unknown) substance use disorder, severe, with other (or unknown) substance-induced depressive disorder ◀

● F19.25 **Other psychoactive substance dependence with psychoactive substance-induced psychotic disorder**

F19.250 **Other psychoactive substance dependence with psychoactive substance-induced psychotic disorder with delusions**

F19.251 **Other psychoactive substance dependence with psychoactive substance-induced psychotic disorder with hallucinations**

F19.259 **Other psychoactive substance dependence with psychoactive substance-induced psychotic disorder, unspecified**
Ex: No exclusions

F19.26 **Other psychoactive substance dependence with psychoactive substance-induced persisting amnestic disorder**
Ex: No exclusions

F19.27 **Other psychoactive substance dependence with psychoactive substance-induced persisting dementia**
Other (or unknown) substance use disorder, moderate, with other (or unknown) substance-induced major neurocognitive disorder ◀
Other (or unknown) substance use disorder, severe, with other (or unknown) substance-induced major neurocognitive disorder ◀

● F19.28 **Other psychoactive substance dependence with other psychoactive substance-induced disorders**
Ex: For category F19.28 CC codes: No exclusions

F19.280 **Other psychoactive substance dependence with psychoactive substance-induced anxiety disorder**

F19.281 **Other psychoactive substance dependence with psychoactive substance-induced sexual dysfunction**

F19.282 **Other psychoactive substance dependence with psychoactive substance-induced sleep disorder**

F19.288 **Other psychoactive substance dependence with other psychoactive substance-induced disorder**
Other (or unknown) substance use disorder, moderate, with other (or unknown) substance-induced mild neurocognitive disorder ◀
Other (or unknown) substance use disorder, severe, with other (or unknown) substance-induced mild neurocognitive disorder ◀
Other (or unknown) substance use disorder, moderate, with other (or unknown) substance-induced obsessive-compulsive or related disorder ◀
Other (or unknown) substance use disorder, severe, with other (or unknown) substance-induced obsessive-compulsive or related disorder ◀

F19.29 **Other psychoactive substance dependence with unspecified psychoactive substance-induced disorder**

● F19.9 **Other psychoactive substance use, unspecified**
Excludes1 other psychoactive substance abuse (F19.1-)
other psychoactive substance dependence (F19.2-)

F19.90 **Other psychoactive substance use, unspecified, uncomplicated**

● F19.92 **Other psychoactive substance use, unspecified with intoxication**
Excludes1 other psychoactive substance use, unspecified with withdrawal (F19.93)

F19.920 **Other psychoactive substance use, unspecified with intoxication, uncomplicated**

F19.921 **Other psychoactive substance use, unspecified with intoxication with delirium**
Other (or unknown) substance-induced delirium ◀

F19.922 **Other psychoactive substance use, unspecified with intoxication with perceptual disturbance**

F19.929 **Other psychoactive substance use, unspecified with intoxication, unspecified**

● F19.93 **Other psychoactive substance use, unspecified with withdrawal**
Excludes1 other psychoactive substance use, unspecified with intoxication (F19.92-)

F19.930 **Other psychoactive substance use, unspecified with withdrawal, uncomplicated**

F19.931 **Other psychoactive substance use, unspecified with withdrawal delirium**

F19.932 Other psychoactive substance use, unspecified with withdrawal with perceptual disturbance

F19.939 Other psychoactive substance use, unspecified with withdrawal, unspecified

F19.94 Other psychoactive substance use, unspecified with psychoactive substance-induced mood disorder
Other (or unknown) substance-induced bipolar or related disorder, without use disorder ◀
Other (or unknown) substance-induced depressive disorder, without use disorder ◀

● **F19.95 Other psychoactive substance use, unspecified with psychoactive substance-induced psychotic disorder**

F19.950 Other psychoactive substance use, unspecified with psychoactive substance-induced psychotic disorder with delusions

F19.951 Other psychoactive substance use, unspecified with psychoactive substance-induced psychotic disorder with hallucinations

F19.959 Other psychoactive substance use, unspecified with psychoactive substance-induced psychotic disorder, unspecified
Other or unknown substance-induced psychotic disorder, without use disorder ◀

F19.96 Other psychoactive substance use, unspecified with psychoactive substance-induced persisting amnestic disorder

F19.97 Other psychoactive substance use, unspecified with psychoactive substance-induced persisting dementia
Other (or unknown) substance-induced major neurocognitive disorder, without use disorder ◀

● **F19.98 Other psychoactive substance use, unspecified with other psychoactive substance-induced disorders**

F19.980 Other psychoactive substance use, unspecified with psychoactive substance-induced anxiety disorder
Other (or unknown) substance-induced anxiety disorder, without use disorder ◀

F19.981 Other psychoactive substance use, unspecified with psychoactive substance-induced sexual dysfunction
Other (or unknown) substance-induced sexual dysfunction, without use disorder ◀

F19.982 Other psychoactive substance use, unspecified with psychoactive substance-induced sleep disorder
Other (or unknown) substance-induced sleep disorder, without use disorder ◀

F19.988 Other psychoactive substance use, unspecified with other psychoactive substance-induced disorder
Other (or unknown) substance-induced mild neurocognitive disorder, without use disorder ◀
Other (or unknown) substance-induced obsessive-compulsive or related disorder, without use disorder ◀

F19.99 Other psychoactive substance use, unspecified with unspecified psychoactive substance-induced disorder

SCHIZOPHRENIA, SCHIZOTYPAL, DELUSIONAL, AND OTHER NON-MOOD PSYCHOTIC DISORDERS (F20-F29)

● **F20 Schizophrenia**
Personality disorders characterized by multiple mental and behavioral irregularities (may exhibit disorganized thinking, delusions, and auditory hallucinations)

Excludes1 brief psychotic disorder (F23)
cyclic schizophrenia (F25.0)
mood [affective] disorders with psychotic symptoms (F30.2, F31.2, F31.5, F31.64, F32.3, F33.3)
schizoaffective disorder (F25.-)
schizophrenic reaction NOS (F23)

Excludes2 schizophrenic reaction in:
alcoholism (F10.15-, F10.25-, F10.95-)
brain disease (F06.2)
epilepsy (F06.2)
psychoactive drug use (F11-F19 with .15, .25, .95)
schizotypal disorder (F21)

Ex: **For category F20 CC codes:** F07.0-F07.81, F07.9-F09, F20.0-F51.03, F51.12, F51.19, F51.3-F51.9, F52.5, F54, F59-F63.2, F63.81-F63.9, F68.10-F80.4, F80.82-F84.0, F84.3-F99, G44.201-G44.229, H93.25, R45.1-R45.2, R45.5-R45.82, R45.86-R45.87

F20.0 Paranoid schizophrenia
Paraphrenic schizophrenia

Excludes1 involutional paranoid state (F22)
paranoia (F22)

F20.1 Disorganized schizophrenia
Hebephrenic schizophrenia
Hebephrenia

F20.2 Catatonic schizophrenia
Schizophrenic catalepsy
Schizophrenic catatonia
Schizophrenic flexibilitas cerea

Excludes1 catatonic stupor (R40.1)

F20.3 Undifferentiated schizophrenia
Atypical schizophrenia

Excludes1 acute schizophrenia-like psychotic disorder (F23)

Excludes2 post-schizophrenic depression (F32.89) ◀

F20.5 Residual schizophrenia
Restzustand (schizophrenic)
Schizophrenic residual state

● **F20.8 Other schizophrenia**

F20.81 Schizophreniform disorder
Schizophreniform psychosis NOS

F20.89 Other schizophrenia
Cenesthopathic schizophrenia
Simple schizophrenia

F20.9 Schizophrenia, unspecified

F21 Schizotypal disorder
Personality disorder characterized by need for social isolation, odd behavior and thinking, and often unconventional beliefs
Borderline schizophrenia
Latent schizophrenia
Latent schizophrenic reaction
Prepsychotic schizophrenia
Prodromal schizophrenia
Pseudoneurotic schizophrenia
Pseudopsychopathic schizophrenia
Schizotypal personality disorder

Excludes2 Asperger's syndrome (F84.5)
schizoid personality disorder (F60.1)

F22 Delusional disorders
Delusional dysmorphophobia
Involutional paranoid state
Paranoia
Paranoia querulans
Paranoid psychosis
Paranoid state
Paraphrenia (late)
Sensitiver Beziehungswahn

Excludes1 mood [affective] disorders with psychotic symptoms (F30.2, F31.2, F31.5, F31.64, F32.3, F33.3)
paranoid schizophrenia (F20.0)

Excludes2 paranoid personality disorder (F60.0)
paranoid psychosis, psychogenic (F23)
paranoid reaction (F23)

F23 Brief psychotic disorder
Paranoid reaction
Psychogenic paranoid psychosis

Excludes2 mood [affective] disorders with psychotic symptoms (F30.2, F31.2, F31.5, F31.64, F32.3, F33.3)

Ex: No exclusions

F24 Shared psychotic disorder
Folie à deux
Induced paranoid disorder
Induced psychotic disorder

● **F25 Schizoaffective disorders**
Mental disorder exhibiting major depressive episode, manic episode, or mixed episode occurs with symptoms of schizophrenia, and mood disorder

Excludes1 mood [affective] disorders with psychotic symptoms (F30.2, F31.2, F31.5, F31.64, F32.3, F33.3)
schizophrenia (F20.-)

F25.0 Schizoaffective disorder, bipolar type
Cyclic schizophrenia
Schizoaffective disorder, manic type
Schizoaffective disorder, mixed type
Schizoaffective psychosis, bipolar type
Schizophreniform psychosis, manic type

F25.1 Schizoaffective disorder, depressive type
Schizoaffective psychosis, depressive type
Schizophreniform psychosis, depressive type

F25.8 Other schizoaffective disorders

F25.9 Schizoaffective disorder, unspecified
Schizoaffective psychosis NOS

F28 Other psychotic disorder not due to a substance or known physiological condition
Chronic hallucinatory psychosis

F29 Unspecified psychosis not due to a substance or known physiological condition
Psychosis NOS

Excludes1 mental disorder NOS (F99)
unspecified mental disorder due to known physiological condition (F09)

MOOD [AFFECTIVE] DISORDERS (F30-F39)

● **F30 Manic episode**
Elevated, expansive, or irritable mood

Includes bipolar disorder, single manic episode
mixed affective episode

Excludes1 bipolar disorder (F31.-)
major depressive disorder, single episode (F32.-)
major depressive disorder, recurrent (F33.-)

Ex: For category F30 CC codes unless otherwise indicated: See F20

● **F30.1 Manic episode without psychotic symptoms**

F30.10 Manic episode without psychotic symptoms, unspecified

F30.11 Manic episode without psychotic symptoms, mild

F30.12 Manic episode without psychotic symptoms, moderate

F30.13 Manic episode, severe, without psychotic symptoms
Ex: F30.13, F30.2, F31.13-F31.2, F31.4-F31.5, F31.63-F31.64

F30.2 Manic episode, severe with psychotic symptoms
Manic stupor
Mania with mood-congruent psychotic symptoms
Mania with mood-incongruent psychotic symptoms

F30.3 Manic episode in partial remission

F30.4 Manic episode in full remission

F30.8 Other manic episodes
Abnormality of mood resembling mania but less intense
Hypomania

F30.9 Manic episode, unspecified
Mania NOS

● **F31 Bipolar disorder**
Mood disorders with history of manic, mixed, or hypomanic episodes

Includes manic-depressive illness
manic-depressive psychosis
manic-depressive reaction

Excludes1 bipolar disorder, single manic episode (F30.-)
major depressive disorder, single episode (F32.-)
major depressive disorder, recurrent (F33.-)

Excludes2 cyclothymia (F34.0)

Ex: For category F31 CC codes unless otherwise indicated: See F20

F31.0 Bipolar disorder, current episode hypomanic

● **F31.1 Bipolar disorder, current episode manic without psychotic features**

F31.10 Bipolar disorder, current episode manic without psychotic features, unspecified

F31.11 Bipolar disorder, current episode manic without psychotic features, mild

F31.12 Bipolar disorder, current episode manic without psychotic features, moderate

F31.13 Bipolar disorder, current episode manic without psychotic features, severe
Ex: F31.13-F31.2, F31.63-F31.64

F31.2 Bipolar disorder, current episode manic severe with psychotic features
Bipolar disorder, current episode manic with mood-congruent psychotic symptoms
Bipolar disorder, current episode manic with mood-incongruent psychotic symptoms

● **F31.3 Bipolar disorder, current episode depressed, mild or moderate severity**

F31.30 Bipolar disorder, current episode depressed, mild or moderate severity, unspecified

F31.31 Bipolar disorder, current episode depressed, mild

F31.32 Bipolar disorder, current episode depressed, moderate

F31.4 Bipolar disorder, current episode depressed, severe, without psychotic features
Ex: F31.13-F31.2, F31.4-F31.5, F31.63-F31.64

F31.5 Bipolar disorder, current episode depressed, severe, with psychotic features
Bipolar disorder, current episode depressed with mood-incongruent psychotic symptoms
Bipolar disorder, current episode depressed with mood-congruent psychotic symptoms

● **F31.6 Bipolar disorder, current episode mixed**

F31.60 Bipolar disorder, current episode mixed, unspecified

F31.61 Bipolar disorder, current episode mixed, mild

F31.62 Bipolar disorder, current episode mixed, moderate

F31.63 Bipolar disorder, current episode mixed, severe, without psychotic features
Ex See F31.4

F31.64 Bipolar disorder, current episode mixed, severe, with psychotic features
Bipolar disorder, current episode mixed with mood-congruent psychotic symptoms
Bipolar disorder, current episode mixed with mood-incongruent psychotic symptoms

● **F31.7 Bipolar disorder, currently in remission**

F31.70 Bipolar disorder, currently in remission, most recent episode unspecified

F31.71 Bipolar disorder, in partial remission, most recent episode hypomanic

F31.72 Bipolar disorder, in full remission, most recent episode hypomanic

F31.73 Bipolar disorder, in partial remission, most recent episode manic

F31.74 Bipolar disorder, in full remission, most recent episode manic

F31.75 Bipolar disorder, in partial remission, most recent episode depressed

F31.76 Bipolar disorder, in full remission, most recent episode depressed

F31.77 Bipolar disorder, in partial remission, most recent episode mixed

F31.78 Bipolar disorder, in full remission, most recent episode mixed

● **F31.8 Other bipolar disorders**

F31.81 Bipolar II disorder

F31.89 Other bipolar disorder
Recurrent manic episodes NOS

F31.9 Bipolar disorder, unspecified

● **F32 Major depressive disorder, single episode**

Includes single episode of agitated depression
single episode of depressive reaction
single episode of major depression
single episode of psychogenic depression
single episode of reactive depression
single episode of vital depression

Excludes1 bipolar disorder (F31.-)
manic episode (F30.-)
recurrent depressive disorder (F33.-)

Excludes2 adjustment disorder (F43.2)

F32.0 Major depressive disorder, single episode, mild
Ex F32.0-F32.3, F33.0-F33.40, F33.9

F32.1 Major depressive disorder, single episode, moderate
Ex F32.0-F32.3, F33.0-F33.40, F33.9

F32.2 Major depressive disorder, single episode, severe without psychotic features
Ex F32.0-F32.3, F33.0-F33.40, F33.9

F32.3 Major depressive disorder, single episode, severe with psychotic features
Single episode of major depression with mood-congruent psychotic symptoms
Single episode of major depression with mood-incongruent psychotic symptoms
Single episode of major depression with psychotic symptoms
Single episode of psychogenic depressive psychosis
Single episode of psychotic depression
Single episode of reactive depressive psychosis
Ex F32.0-F32.3, F33.0-F33.40, F33.9

F32.4 Major depressive disorder, single episode, in partial remission

F32.5 Major depressive disorder, single episode, in full remission

● **F32.8 Other depressive episodes**

F32.81 Premenstrual dysphoric disorder ♀ ◀

Excludes1 premenstrual tension syndrome (N94.3) ◀

F32.89 Other specified depressive episodes ◀
Atypical depression ◀
Post-schizophrenic depression ◀
Single episode of 'masked' depression NOS ◀

F32.9 Major depressive disorder, single episode, unspecified
Depression NOS
Depressive disorder NOS
Major depression NOS

● **F33 Major depressive disorder, recurrent**

Includes recurrent episodes of depressive reaction
recurrent episodes of endogenous depression
recurrent episodes of major depression
recurrent episodes of psychogenic depression
recurrent episodes of reactive depression
recurrent episodes of seasonal depressive disorder
recurrent episodes of vital depression

Excludes1 bipolar disorder (F31.-)
manic episode (F30.-)

Ex **For category F33 CC codes unless otherwise indicated:** F32.0-F32.3, F33.0-F33.40, F33.9

F33.0 Major depressive disorder, recurrent, mild

F33.1 Major depressive disorder, recurrent, moderate

F33.2 Major depressive disorder, recurrent severe without psychotic features

F33.3 Major depressive disorder, recurrent, severe with psychotic symptoms
Endogenous depression with psychotic symptoms
Recurrent severe episodes of major depression with mood-congruent psychotic symptoms
Recurrent severe episodes of major depression with mood-incongruent psychotic symptoms
Recurrent severe episodes of major depression with psychotic symptoms
Recurrent severe episodes of psychogenic depressive psychosis
Recurrent severe episodes of psychotic depression
Recurrent severe episodes of reactive depressive psychosis
Ex See F20

● **F33.4 Major depressive disorder, recurrent, in remission**

F33.40 Major depressive disorder, recurrent, in remission, unspecified

F33.41 Major depressive disorder, recurrent, in partial remission

F33.42 Major depressive disorder, recurrent, in full remission

F33.8 Other recurrent depressive disorders
Recurrent brief depressive episodes
Ex See F20

F33.9 Major depressive disorder, recurrent, unspecified
Monopolar depression NOS

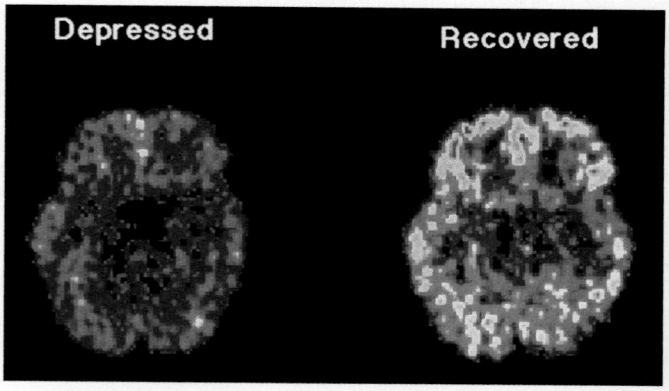

Figure 5-1 PET scan of depressed individual's brain before and after recovery. (From Fortinash KM: Psychiatric Mental Health Nursing, ed 4, St. Louis, Mosby, 2008)

● **F34 Persistent mood [affective] disorders**
Ex For category F34 CC codes: F07.0-F07.81, F07.9-F09, F20.0-F51.03, F51.12, F51.19, F51.3-F51.9, F52.5, F54, F59-F63.2, F63.81-F63.9, F68.10-F80.4, F80.82-F84.0, F84.3-F99, G44.201-G44.229, H93.25, R45.1-R45.2, R45.5-R45.82, R45.86-R45.87

F34.0 Cyclothymic disorder
Affective personality disorder
Cycloid personality
Cyclothymia
Cyclothymic personality

F34.1 Dysthymic disorder
Depressive neurosis
Depressive personality disorder
Dysthymia
Neurotic depression
Persistent anxiety depression
Persistent depressive disorder ◀
Excludes2 anxiety depression (mild or not persistent) (F41.8)

● **F34.8 Other persistent mood [affective] disorders**
Ex For category F34.8 CC codes: See F20

F34.81 Disruptive mood dysregulation disorder ◀
F34.89 Other specified persistent mood disorders ◀

F34.9 Persistent mood [affective] disorder, unspecified
Ex See F20

F39 Unspecified mood [affective] disorder
Affective psychosis NOS

ANXIETY, DISSOCIATIVE, STRESS-RELATED, SOMATOFORM AND OTHER NONPSYCHOTIC MENTAL DISORDERS (F40-F48)

● **F40 Phobic anxiety disorders**
Irrational fear with avoidance of the feared subject, activity, or situation even though the individual knows that the reaction is excessive

● **F40.0 Agoraphobia**
Intense, irrational fear of open spaces

F40.00 Agoraphobia, unspecified
F40.01 Agoraphobia with panic disorder
Panic disorder with agoraphobia
Excludes1 panic disorder without agoraphobia (F41.0)
F40.02 Agoraphobia without panic disorder

● **F40.1 Social phobias**
Anthropophobia
Social anxiety disorder of childhood
Social neurosis

F40.10 Social phobia, unspecified
F40.11 Social phobia, generalized

● **F40.2 Specific (isolated) phobias**
Excludes2 dysmorphophobia (nondelusional) (F45.22)
nosophobia (F45.22)

● **F40.21 Animal type phobia**
F40.210 Arachnophobia
Fear of spiders
F40.218 Other animal type phobia

● **F40.22 Natural environment type phobia**
F40.220 Fear of thunderstorms
F40.228 Other natural environment type phobia

● **F40.23 Blood, injection, injury type phobia**
F40.230 Fear of blood
F40.231 Fear of injections and transfusions
F40.232 Fear of other medical care
F40.233 Fear of injury

● **F40.24 Situational type phobia**
F40.240 Claustrophobia
Fear of closed spaces
F40.241 Acrophobia
Fear of heights
F40.242 Fear of bridges
F40.243 Fear of flying
F40.248 Other situational type phobia

● **F40.29 Other specified phobia**
F40.290 Androphobia
Fear of men
F40.291 Gynephobia
Fear of women
F40.298 Other specified phobia

F40.8 Other phobic anxiety disorders
Phobic anxiety disorder of childhood

F40.9 Phobic anxiety disorder, unspecified
Phobia NOS
Phobic state NOS

● **F41 Other anxiety disorders**
Excludes2 anxiety in:
acute stress reaction (F43.0)
transient adjustment reaction (F43.2)
neurasthenia (F48.8)
psychophysiologic disorders (F45.-)
separation anxiety (F93.0)

F41.0 Panic disorder [episodic paroxysmal anxiety] without agoraphobia
Panic attack
Panic state
Excludes1 panic disorder with agoraphobia (F40.01)

F41.1 Generalized anxiety disorder
Anxiety neurosis
Anxiety reaction
Anxiety state
Overanxious disorder
Excludes2 neurasthenia (F48.8)

F41.3 Other mixed anxiety disorders

F41.8 Other specified anxiety disorders
Anxiety depression (mild or not persistent)
Anxiety hysteria
Mixed anxiety and depressive disorder

F41.9 Anxiety disorder, unspecified
Anxiety NOS

● **F42 Obsessive-compulsive disorder**
Anxiety disorder with recurrent obsessions or compulsions
Excludes2 obsessive-compulsive personality (disorder) (F60.5)
obsessive-compulsive symptoms occurring in depression (F32-F33)
obsessive-compulsive symptoms occurring in schizophrenia (F20.-)

F42.2 Mixed obsessional thoughts and acts ◀
F42.3 Hoarding disorder ◀
F42.4 Excoriation (skin-picking) disorder ◀
Excludes1 factitial dermatitis (L98.1) ◀
other specified behavioral and emotional disorders with onset usually occurring in early childhood and adolescence (F98.8) ◀

F42.8 Other obsessive-compulsive disorder ◀
Anancastic neurosis ◀
Obsessive-compulsive neurosis ◀

F42.9 Obsessive-compulsive disorder, unspecified ◀

F43 Reaction to severe stress and adjustment disorders

F43.0 Acute stress reaction
Acute crisis reaction
Acute reaction to stress
Combat and operational stress reaction
Combat fatigue
Crisis state
Psychic shock

F43.1 Post-traumatic stress disorder (PTSD)
Traumatic neurosis

F43.10 Post-traumatic stress disorder, unspecified

F43.11 Post-traumatic stress disorder, acute

F43.12 Post-traumatic stress disorder, chronic

F43.2 Adjustment disorders
Culture shock
Grief reaction
Hospitalism in children

Excludes2 separation anxiety disorder of childhood (F93.0)

F43.20 Adjustment disorder, unspecified

F43.21 Adjustment disorder with depressed mood

F43.22 Adjustment disorder with anxiety

F43.23 Adjustment disorder with mixed anxiety and depressed mood

F43.24 Adjustment disorder with disturbance of conduct

F43.25 Adjustment disorder with mixed disturbance of emotions and conduct

F43.29 Adjustment disorder with other symptoms

F43.8 Other reactions to severe stress
Other specified trauma and stressor-related disorder ◀

F43.9 Reaction to severe stress, unspecified
Trauma and stressor-related disorder, NOS ◀

F44 Dissociative and conversion disorders

Includes conversion hysteria
conversion reaction
hysteria
hysterical psychosis

Excludes2 malingering [conscious simulation] (Z76.5)

F44.0 Dissociative amnesia
Sudden loss of memory for personal information

Excludes1 amnesia NOS (R41.3)
anterograde amnesia (R41.1)
dissociative amnesia with dissociative fugue (F44.1) ◀
retrograde amnesia (R41.2)

Excludes2 alcohol-or other psychoactive substance-induced amnestic disorder (F10, F13, F19 with .26, .96)
amnestic disorder due to known physiological condition (F04)
postictal amnesia in epilepsy (G40.-)

F44.1 Dissociative fugue
Characterized by episode of sudden, unexpected travel with amnesia for past and partial to total confusion about identity or assumption of new identity
Dissociative amnesia with dissociative fugue ◀

Excludes2 postictal fugue in epilepsy (G40.-)

F44.2 Dissociative stupor
Profound diminution or absence of voluntary movement and responsiveness to external stimuli

Excludes1 catatonic stupor (R40.1)
stupor NOS (R40.1)

Excludes2 catatonic disorder due to known physiological condition (F06.1)
depressive stupor (F32, F33)
manic stupor (F30, F31)

F44.4 Conversion disorder with motor symptom or deficit
Dissociative motor disorders
Psychogenic aphonia
Psychogenic dysphonia

F44.5 Conversion disorder with seizures or convulsions
Dissociative convulsions

F44.6 Conversion disorder with sensory symptom or deficit
Dissociative anesthesia and sensory loss
Psychogenic deafness

F44.7 Conversion disorder with mixed symptom presentation

F44.8 Other dissociative and conversion disorders

F44.81 Dissociative identity disorder
Multiple personality disorder

F44.89 Other dissociative and conversion disorders
Ganser's syndrome
Psychogenic confusion
Psychogenic twilight state
Trance and possession disorders

F44.9 Dissociative and conversion disorder, unspecified
Dissociative disorder NOS

OGCR Section I.C.5.a

Pain disorders related to psychological factors

Assign code F45.41, for pain that is exclusively psychological. Code F45.41, Pain disorder exclusively related to psychological factors, should be used following the appropriate code from category G89, Pain, not elsewhere classified, if there is documentation of a psychological component for a patient with acute or chronic pain.
See Section I.C.6. Pain

F45 Somatoform disorders
Mental disorders characterized by symptoms suggesting general medical condition

Excludes2 dissociative and conversion disorders (F44.-)
factitious disorders (F68.1-)
hair-plucking (F63.3)
lalling (F80.0)
lisping (F80.0)
malingering [conscious simulation] (Z76.5)
nail-biting (F98.8)
psychological or behavioral factors associated with disorders or diseases classified elsewhere (F54)
sexual dysfunction, not due to a substance or known physiological condition (F52.-)
thumb-sucking (F98.8)
tic disorders (in childhood and adolescence) (F95.-)
Tourette's syndrome (F95.2)
trichotillomania (F63.3)

F45.0 Somatization disorder
Briquet's disorder
Multiple psychosomatic disorder

F45.1 Undifferentiated somatoform disorder
Somatic symptom disorder ◀
Undifferentiated psychosomatic disorder

F45.2 Hypochondriacal disorders
Persistent, unrealistic preoccupation with possibility of having serious disease

Excludes2 delusional dysmorphophobia (F22)
fixed delusions about bodily functions or shape (F22)

F45.20 Hypochondriacal disorder, unspecified

F45.21 Hypochondriasis
Hypochondriacal neurosis
Illness anxiety disorder ◀

F45.22 Body dysmorphic disorder
Dysmorphophobia (nondelusional)
Nosophobia

F45.29 Other hypochondriacal disorders

F45.4 Pain disorders related to psychological factors

Excludes1 pain NOS (R52)

F45.41 Pain disorder exclusively related to psychological factors
Somatoform pain disorder (persistent)

F45.42 Pain disorder with related psychological factors
Code also associated acute or chronic pain (G89.-)

F45.8 Other somatoform disorders
Psychogenic dysmenorrhea
Psychogenic dysphagia, including 'globus hystericus'
Psychogenic pruritus
Psychogenic torticollis
Somatoform autonomic dysfunction
Teeth grinding
Excludes1 sleep related teeth grinding (G47.63)

F45.9 Somatoform disorder, unspecified
Psychosomatic disorder NOS

● **F48 Other nonpsychotic mental disorders**

F48.1 Depersonalization-derealization syndrome

F48.2 Pseudobulbar affect
Involuntary emotional expression disorder
Code first underlying cause, if known, such as:
amyotrophic lateral sclerosis (G12.21)
multiple sclerosis (G35)
sequelae of cerebrovascular disease (I69.-)
sequelae of traumatic intracranial injury (S06.-)

F48.8 Other specified nonpsychotic mental disorders
Dhat syndrome
Neurasthenia
Occupational neurosis, including writer's cramp
Psychasthenia
Psychasthenic neurosis
Psychogenic syncope

F48.9 Nonpsychotic mental disorder, unspecified
Neurosis NOS

BEHAVIORAL SYNDROMES ASSOCIATED WITH PHYSIOLOGICAL DISTURBANCES AND PHYSICAL FACTORS (F50-F59)

● **F50 Eating disorders**
Excludes1 anorexia NOS (R63.0)
feeding difficulties (R63.3)
polyphagia (R63.2)
Excludes2 feeding disorder in infancy or childhood (F98.2-)

● **F50.0 Anorexia nervosa**
Excludes1 loss of appetite (R63.0)
psychogenic loss of appetite (F50.89) ◀
Exc For category F50.0 CC codes: F45.9, F50.00-F50.9, F59, F98.21-F98.3

F50.00 Anorexia nervosa, unspecified

F50.01 Anorexia nervosa, restricting type

F50.02 Anorexia nervosa, binge eating/purging type
Excludes1 bulimia nervosa (F50.2)

F50.2 Bulimia nervosa
Bulimia NOS
Hyperorexia nervosa
Excludes1 anorexia nervosa, binge eating/purging type (F50.02)
Exc F50.00-F50.9, F98.21-F98.29

● **F50.8 Other eating disorders**
Excludes2 pica of infancy and childhood (F98.3)

F50.81 Binge eating disorder ◀

F50.89 Other specified eating disorder ◀
Pica in adults ◀
Psychogenic loss of appetite ◀

F50.9 Eating disorder, unspecified
Atypical anorexia nervosa
Atypical bulimia nervosa

● **F51 Sleep disorders not due to a substance or known physiological condition**
Excludes2 organic sleep disorders (G47.-)

● **F51.0 Insomnia not due to a substance or known physiological condition**
Excludes2 alcohol related insomnia (F10.182, F10.282, F10.982)
drug-related insomnia (F11.182, F11.282, F11.982, F13.182, F13.282, F13.982, F14.182, F14.282, F14.982, F15.182, F15.282, F15.982, F19.182, F19.282, F19.982)
insomnia NOS (G47.0-)
insomnia due to known physiological condition (G47.0-)
organic insomnia (G47.0-)
sleep deprivation (Z72.820)

F51.01 Primary insomnia
Idiopathic insomnia

F51.02 Adjustment insomnia

F51.03 Paradoxical insomnia

F51.04 Psychophysiologic insomnia

F51.05 Insomnia due to other mental disorder
Code also associated mental disorder

F51.09 Other insomnia not due to a substance or known physiological condition

● **F51.1 Hypersomnia not due to a substance or known physiological condition**
Hypersomnia: Excessive sleeping/sleepiness
Excludes2 alcohol related hypersomnia (F10.182, F10.282, F10.982)
drug-related hypersomnia (F11.182, F11.282, F11.982, F13.182, F13.282, F13.982, F14.182, F14.282, F14.982, F15.182, F15.282, F15.982, F19.182, F19.282, F19.982)
hypersomnia NOS (G47.10)
hypersomnia due to known physiological condition (G47.10)
idiopathic hypersomnia (G47.11, G47.12)
narcolepsy (G47.4-)

F51.11 Primary hypersomnia

F51.12 Insufficient sleep syndrome
Excludes1 sleep deprivation (Z72.820)

F51.13 Hypersomnia due to other mental disorder
Code also associated mental disorder

F51.19 Other hypersomnia not due to a substance or known physiological condition

F51.3 Sleepwalking [somnambulism]

F51.4 Sleep terrors [night terrors]

F51.5 Nightmare disorder
Dream anxiety disorder

F51.8 Other sleep disorders not due to a substance or known physiological condition

F51.9 Sleep disorder not due to a substance or known physiological condition, unspecified
Emotional sleep disorder NOS

● **F52 Sexual dysfunction not due to a substance or known physiological condition**
Excludes2 Dhat syndrome (F48.8)

F52.0 Hypoactive sexual desire disorder
Total loss of feeling of sexual pleasure
Lack or loss of sexual desire
Sexual anhedonia ◀
Excludes1 decreased libido (R68.82)

F52.1 Sexual aversion disorder
Sexual aversion and lack of sexual enjoyment

● **F52.2 Sexual arousal disorders**
Failure of genital response

F52.21 Male erectile disorder ♂
Psychogenic impotence
Excludes1 impotence of organic origin (N52.-)
impotence NOS (N52.-)

F52.22 Female sexual arousal disorder ♀
~~Frigidity~~

● **F52.3 Orgasmic disorder**
Inhibited orgasm
Psychogenic anorgasmy

F52.31 Female orgasmic disorder ♀

F52.32 Male orgasmic disorder ♂
Delayed ejaculation ◀

F52.4 Premature ejaculation ♂

F52.5 Vaginismus not due to a substance or known physiological condition ♀
Psychogenic vaginismus
Excludes2 vaginismus (due to a known physiological condition) (N94.2)

F52.6 Dyspareunia not due to a substance or known physiological condition ♀
Dyspareunia: Difficult or painful sexual intercourse
Genito-pelvic pain penetration disorder ◀
Psychogenic dyspareunia
Excludes2 dyspareunia (due to a known physiological condition) (N94.1-) ◀

F52.8 Other sexual dysfunction not due to a substance or known physiological condition
Excessive sexual drive
Nymphomania
Satyriasis

● **F52.9 Unspecified sexual dysfunction not due to a substance or known physiological condition**
Sexual dysfunction NOS

F53 Puerperal psychosis ♀ M
Postpartum depression
Acute mental illness with sudden onset following childbirth with symptoms of affective psychosis, disorientation, and confusion are prevalent
Excludes1 mood disorders with psychotic features (F30.2, F31.2, F31.5, F31.64, F32.3, F33.3)
postpartum dysphoria (O90.6)
psychosis in schizophrenia, schizotypal, delusional, and other psychotic disorders (F20-F29)

▶ ***F54 Psychological and behavioral factors associated with disorders or diseases classified elsewhere***
Psychological factors affecting physical conditions
Code first the associated physical disorder, such as:
asthma (J45.-)
dermatitis (L23-L25)
gastric ulcer (K25.-)
mucous colitis (K58.-)
ulcerative colitis (K51.-)
urticaria (L50.-)
Excludes2 tension-type headache (G44.2)

● **F55 Abuse of non-psychoactive substances**
Excludes2 abuse of psychoactive substances (F10-F19)

F55.0 Abuse of antacids

F55.1 Abuse of herbal or folk remedies

F55.2 Abuse of laxatives

F55.3 Abuse of steroids or hormones

F55.4 Abuse of vitamins

F55.8 Abuse of other non-psychoactive substances

F59 Unspecified behavioral syndromes associated with physiological disturbances and physical factors
Psychogenic physiological dysfunction NOS

DISORDERS OF ADULT PERSONALITY AND BEHAVIOR (F60-F69)

● **F60 Specific personality disorders**
Long-term patterns of thoughts and behaviors causing serious problems with relationships and work.

F60.0 Paranoid personality disorder
Hostile, devious, and combative response to disappointments
Expansive paranoid personality (disorder)
Fanatic personality (disorder)
Querulant personality (disorder)
Paranoid personality (disorder)
Sensitive paranoid personality (disorder)
Excludes2 paranoia (F22)
paranoia querulans (F22)
paranoid psychosis (F22)
paranoid schizophrenia (F20.0)
paranoid state (F22)

F60.1 Schizoid personality disorder
Detachment from social relationships with minimal emotional experiences and expressions
Excludes2 Asperger's syndrome (F84.5)
delusional disorder (F22)
schizoid disorder of childhood (F84.5)
schizophrenia (F20.-)
schizotypal disorder (F21)

F60.2 Antisocial personality disorder
Continuous and chronic antisocial behavior
Amoral personality (disorder)
Asocial personality (disorder)
Dissocial personality disorder
Psychopathic personality (disorder)
Sociopathic personality (disorder)
Excludes1 conduct disorders (F91.-)
Excludes2 borderline personality disorder (F60.3)

F60.3 Borderline personality disorder
Instability of mood, self-image or sense of self, and interpersonal relationships
Aggressive personality (disorder)
Emotionally unstable personality disorder
Explosive personality (disorder)
Excludes2 antisocial personality disorder (F60.2)

F60.4 Histrionic personality disorder
Personality disorder with excessive emotional and attention-seeking behavior
Hysterical personality (disorder)
Psychoinfantile personality (disorder)

F60.5 Obsessive-compulsive personality disorder
Anankastic personality (disorder)
Compulsive personality (disorder)
Obsessional personality (disorder)
Excludes2 obsessive-compulsive disorder (F42-) ◀

F60.6 Avoidant personality disorder
Anxious personality disorder

F60.7 Dependent personality disorder
Asthenic personality (disorder)
Inadequate personality (disorder)
Passive personality (disorder)

● **F60.8 Other specific personality disorders**

F60.81 Narcissistic personality disorder
Vanity, conceit, egotism or indifference to plight of others

F60.89 Other specific personality disorders
Eccentric personality disorder
'Haltlose' type personality disorder
Immature personality disorder
Passive-aggressive personality disorder
Psychoneurotic personality disorder
Self-defeating personality disorder

F60.9 Personality disorder, unspecified
Character disorder NOS
Character neurosis NOS
Pathological personality NOS

F63 Impulse disorders
Excludes2 habitual excessive use of alcohol or psychoactive substances (F10-F19)
impulse disorders involving sexual behavior (F65.-)

F63.0 Pathological gambling
Compulsive gambling
Excludes1 gambling and betting NOS (Z72.6)
Excludes2 excessive gambling by manic patients (F30, F31)
gambling in antisocial personality disorder (F60.2)

F63.1 Pyromania
Pathological fire-setting
Excludes2 fire-setting (by) (in):
adult with antisocial personality disorder (F60.2)
alcohol or psychoactive substance intoxication (F10-F19)
conduct disorders (F91.-)
mental disorders due to known physiological condition (F01-F09)
schizophrenia (F20.-)

F63.2 Kleptomania
Pathological stealing
Excludes1 shoplifting as the reason for observation for suspected mental disorder (Z03.8)
Excludes2 depressive disorder with stealing (F31-F33)
stealing due to underlying mental condition-code to mental condition
stealing in mental disorders due to known physiological condition (F01-F09)

F63.3 Trichotillomania
Hair plucking
Excludes2 other stereotyped movement disorder (F98.4)

F63.8 Other impulse disorders
F63.81 Intermittent explosive disorder
F63.89 Other impulse disorders

F63.9 Impulse disorder, unspecified
Impulse control disorder NOS

F64 Gender identity disorders

F64.0 Transsexualism ◀
Gender identity disorder in adolescence and adulthood ◀
Gender dysphoria in adolescents and adults ◀

F64.1 Dual role transvestism ⇐
Use additional code to identify sex reassignment status (Z87.890)
Excludes1 gender identity disorder in childhood (F64.2)
Excludes2 fetishistic transvestism (F65.1)

F64.2 Gender identity disorder of childhood P
Gender dysphoria in children ◀
Excludes1 gender identity disorder in adolescence and adulthood (F64.0) ⇐
Excludes2 sexual maturation disorder (F66)

F64.8 Other gender identity disorders

F64.9 Gender identity disorder, unspecified
Gender-role disorder NOS

F65 Paraphilias

F65.0 Fetishism
Intense sexual urges and arousing fantasies using inanimate objects

F65.1 Transvestic fetishism
Intense sexual urges, arousal, or orgasm associated with fantasized/actual cross-dressing
Fetishistic transvestism

F65.2 Exhibitionism

F65.3 Voyeurism
Sexual urges or arousal involving real or fantasized observation of unsuspecting people who are naked, disrobing, or engaging in sexual activity

F65.4 Pedophilia

F65.5 Sadomasochism
F65.50 Sadomasochism, unspecified
F65.51 Sexual masochism
F65.52 Sexual sadism

F65.8 Other paraphilias
F65.81 Frotteurism
Sexual arousal or orgasm is achieved by rubbing up against another person (or fantasies of), in crowded place with unsuspecting victim
F65.89 Other paraphilias
Necrophilia

F65.9 Paraphilia, unspecified
Sexual deviation NOS

F66 Other sexual disorders
Sexual maturation disorder
Sexual relationship disorder

F68 Other disorders of adult personality and behavior

F68.1 Factitious disorder
Compensation neurosis
Elaboration of physical symptoms for psychological reasons
Hospital hopper syndrome
Münchhausen's syndrome
Peregrinating patient
Excludes2 factitial dermatitis (L98.1)
person feigning illness (with obvious motivation) (Z76.5)
Ex: For category F68.1 CC codes: See F20
F68.10 Factitious disorder, unspecified
F68.11 Factitious disorder with predominantly psychological signs and symptoms
F68.12 Factitious disorder with predominantly physical signs and symptoms
F68.13 Factitious disorder with combined psychological and physical signs and symptoms

F68.8 Other specified disorders of adult personality and behavior

F69 Unspecified disorder of adult personality and behavior A

INTELLECTUAL DISABILITIES (F70-F79)

Code first any associated physical or developmental disorders
Excludes1 borderline intellectual functioning, IQ above 70 to 84 (R41.83)

F70 Mild intellectual disabilities
IQ level 50-55 to approximately 70
Mild mental subnormality

F71 Moderate intellectual disabilities
IQ level 35-40 to 50-55
Moderate mental subnormality

F72 Severe intellectual disabilities
IQ 20-25 to 35-40
Severe mental subnormality
Ex: F72-F73

F73 Profound intellectual disabilities
IQ level below 20-25
Profound mental subnormality
Ex: F72-F73

F78 Other intellectual disabilities

F79 Unspecified intellectual disabilities
Mental deficiency NOS
Mental subnormality NOS

PERVASIVE AND SPECIFIC DEVELOPMENTAL DISORDERS (F80-F89)

F80 Specific developmental disorders of speech and language

F80.0 Phonological disorder
Communication disorder of unknown cause, characterized by failure to use age-appropriate sounds
Dyslalia
Functional speech articulation disorder
Lalling
Lisping
Phonological developmental disorder
Speech articulation developmental disorder
Speech-sound disorder ◀
Excludes1 speech articulation impairment due to aphasia NOS (R47.01)
speech articulation impairment due to apraxia (R48.2)
Excludes2 speech articulation impairment due to hearing loss (F80.4)
speech articulation impairment due to intellectual disabilities (F70-F79)
speech articulation impairment with expressive language developmental disorder (F80.1)
speech articulation impairment with mixed receptive expressive language developmental disorder (F80.2)

F80.1 Expressive language disorder
Developmental dysphasia or aphasia, expressive type
Excludes1 mixed receptive-expressive language disorder (F80.2)
dysphasia and aphasia NOS (R47.-)
Excludes2 acquired aphasia with epilepsy [Landau-Kleffner] (G40.80-)
intellectual disabilities (F70-F79)
pervasive developmental disorders (F84.-)
selective mutism (F94.0)

F80.2 Mixed receptive-expressive language disorder
Developmental dysphasia or aphasia, receptive type
Developmental Wernicke's aphasia
Excludes1 central auditory processing disorder (H93.25)
dysphasia or aphasia NOS (R47.-)
expressive language disorder (F80.1)
expressive type dysphasia or aphasia (F80.1)
word deafness (H93.25)
Excludes2 acquired aphasia with epilepsy [Landau-Kleffner] (G40.80-)
intellectual disabilities (F70-F79)
pervasive developmental disorders (F84.-)
selective mutism (F94.0)

F80.4 Speech and language development delay due to hearing loss
Code also type of hearing loss (H90.-, H91.-)

F80.8 Other developmental disorders of speech or language

F80.81 Childhood onset fluency disorder
Cluttering NOS
Stuttering NOS
Excludes1 adult onset fluency disorder (F98.5)
fluency disorder in conditions classified elsewhere (R47.82)
fluency disorder (stuttering) following cerebrovascular disease (I69. with final characters -23)

F80.82 Social pragmatic communication disorder ◀
Excludes1 Asperger's syndrome (F84.5) ◀
autistic disorder (F84.0) ◀

F80.89 Other developmental disorders of speech and language

F80.9 Developmental disorder of speech and language, unspecified
Communication disorder NOS
Language disorder NOS

F81 Specific developmental disorders of scholastic skills

F81.0 Specific reading disorder
'Backward reading'
Developmental dyslexia
Specific reading retardation
Excludes1 alexia NOS (R48.0)
dyslexia NOS (R48.0)

F81.2 Mathematics disorder
Developmental acalculia
Developmental arithmetical disorder
Developmental Gerstmann's syndrome
Excludes1 acalculia NOS (R48.8)
Excludes2 arithmetical difficulties associated with a reading disorder (F81.0)
arithmetical difficulties associated with a spelling disorder (F81.81)
arithmetical difficulties due to inadequate teaching (Z55.8)

F81.8 Other developmental disorders of scholastic skills

F81.81 Disorder of written expression
Specific spelling disorder

F81.89 Other developmental disorders of scholastic skills

F81.9 Developmental disorder of scholastic skills, unspecified
Knowledge acquisition disability NOS
Learning disability NOS
Learning disorder NOS

F82 Specific developmental disorder of motor function
Clumsy child syndrome
Developmental coordination disorder
Developmental dyspraxia
Excludes1 abnormalities of gait and mobility (R26.-)
lack of coordination (R27.-)
Excludes2 lack of coordination secondary to intellectual disabilities (F70-F79)

F84 Pervasive developmental disorders
Use additional code to identify any associated medical condition and intellectual disabilities.
Ex: For category F84 CC codes unless otherwise indicated: See F20

F84.0 Autistic disorder
Autism spectrum disorder ◀
Infantile autism
Infantile psychosis
Kanner's syndrome
Excludes1 Asperger's syndrome (F84.5)

F84.2 Rett's syndrome
Neurodevelopmental disorder
Excludes1 Asperger's syndrome (F84.5)
Autistic disorder (F84.0)
other childhood disintegrative disorder (F84.3)
Ex: E75.00-E75.19, E75.4, F84.2, G13.2-G13.8, G30.0-G31.82, G31.84-G31.9, G91.4, G94

F84.3 Other childhood disintegrative disorder P
Dementia infantilis
At least two years of normal development followed by significant loss of language abilities, social skills, bowel/bladder control, motor skills
Disintegrative psychosis
Heller's syndrome
At least two years of normal development followed by significant loss of language abilities, social skills, bowel/bladder control, motor skills
Symbiotic psychosis
Abnormal relationship to mothering figure, characterized by intense separation anxiety, severe regression, giving up of useful speech, and autism
Use additional code to identify any associated neurological condition.
Excludes1 Asperger's syndrome (F84.5)
Autistic disorder (F84.0)
Rett's syndrome (F84.2)

F84.5 Asperger's syndrome
Developmental disorder
Asperger's disorder
Autistic psychopathy
Schizoid disorder of childhood

F84.8 Other pervasive developmental disorders
Overactive disorder associated with intellectual disabilities and stereotyped movements

F84.9 Pervasive developmental disorder, unspecified
Atypical autism

F88 Other disorders of psychological development
Developmental agnosia
Global developmental delay ◀
Other specified neurodevelopmental disorder ◀

F89 Unspecified disorder of psychological development
Developmental disorder NOS
Neurodevelopmental disorder NOS ◀

BEHAVIORAL AND EMOTIONAL DISORDERS WITH ONSET USUALLY OCCURRING IN CHILDHOOD AND ADOLESCENCE (F90-F98)

Note: Codes within categories F90-F98 may be used regardless of the age of a patient. These disorders generally have onset within the childhood or adolescent years, but may continue throughout life or not be diagnosed until adulthood.

● **F90 Attention-deficit hyperactivity disorders**
Attention deficit disorder with hyperactivity=ADHD
Includes attention deficit disorder with hyperactivity
attention deficit syndrome with hyperactivity
Excludes2 anxiety disorders (F40.-, F41.-)
mood [affective] disorders (F30-F39)
pervasive developmental disorders (F84.-)
schizophrenia (F20.-)

F90.0 Attention-deficit hyperactivity disorder, predominantly inattentive type

F90.1 Attention-deficit hyperactivity disorder, predominantly hyperactive type

F90.2 Attention-deficit hyperactivity disorder, combined type

F90.8 Attention-deficit hyperactivity disorder, other type

F90.9 Attention-deficit hyperactivity disorder, unspecified type
Attention-deficit hyperactivity disorder of childhood or adolescence NOS
Attention-deficit hyperactivity disorder NOS

● **F91 Conduct disorders**
Childhood/adolescence disruptive behavior disorder
Excludes1 antisocial behavior (Z72.81-)
antisocial personality disorder (F60.2)
Excludes2 conduct problems associated with attention-deficit hyperactivity disorder (F90.-)
mood [affective] disorders (F30-F39)
pervasive developmental disorders (F84.-)
schizophrenia (F20.-)

F91.0 Conduct disorder confined to family context

F91.1 Conduct disorder, childhood-onset type
Unsocialized conduct disorder
Conduct disorder, solitary aggressive type
Unsocialized aggressive disorder

F91.2 Conduct disorder, adolescent-onset type
Socialized conduct disorder
Conduct disorder, group type

F91.3 Oppositional defiant disorder

F91.8 Other conduct disorders
Other specified conduct disorder ◀
Other specified disruptive disorder ◀

F91.9 Conduct disorder, unspecified
Behavioral disorder NOS
Conduct disorder NOS
Disruptive behavior disorder NOS
Disruptive disorder NOS ◀

● **F93 Emotional disorders with onset specific to childhood**

F93.0 Separation anxiety disorder of childhood
Excludes2 mood [affective] disorders (F30-F39)
nonpsychotic mental disorders (F40-F48)
phobic anxiety disorder of childhood (F40.8)
social phobia (F40.1)

F93.8 Other childhood emotional disorders
Identity disorder
Excludes2 gender identity disorder of childhood (F64.2)

F93.9 Childhood emotional disorder, unspecified

● **F94 Disorders of social functioning with onset specific to childhood and adolescence**

F94.0 Selective mutism
Elective mutism
Excludes2 pervasive developmental disorders (F84.-)
schizophrenia (F20.-)
specific developmental disorders of speech and language (F80.-)
transient mutism as part of separation anxiety in young children (F93.0)

F94.1 Reactive attachment disorder of childhood
Use additional code to identify any associated failure to thrive or growth retardation
Excludes1 disinhibited attachment disorder of childhood (F94.2)
normal variation in pattern of selective attachment
Excludes2 Asperger's syndrome (F84.5)
maltreatment syndromes (T74.-)
sexual or physical abuse in childhood, resulting in psychosocial problems (Z62.81-)

F94.2 Disinhibited attachment disorder of childhood
Affectionless psychopathy
Institutional syndrome
Excludes1 reactive attachment disorder of childhood (F94.1)
Excludes2 Asperger's syndrome (F84.5)
attention-deficit hyperactivity disorders (F90.-)
hospitalism in children (F43.2-)

F94.8 Other childhood disorders of social functioning

F94.9 Childhood disorder of social functioning, unspecified

● F95 Tic disorder

Involuntary twitch

F95.0 Transient tic disorder

Provisional tic disorder ◀

F95.1 Chronic motor or vocal tic disorder

F95.2 Tourette's disorder

Combined vocal and multiple motor tic disorder [de la Tourette]

Tourette's syndrome

F95.8 Other tic disorders

F95.9 Tic disorder, unspecified

Tic NOS

● F98 Other behavioral and emotional disorders with onset usually occurring in childhood and adolescence

Excludes2 breath-holding spells (R06.89)
gender identity disorder of childhood (F64.2)
Kleine-Levin syndrome (G47.13)
obsessive-compulsive disorder (F42-) ◀
sleep disorders not due to a substance or known physiological condition (F51.-)

F98.0 Enuresis not due to a substance or known physiological condition

Enuresis: Urinary incontinence

Enuresis (primary) (secondary) of nonorganic origin
Functional enuresis
Psychogenic enuresis
Urinary incontinence of nonorganic origin

Excludes1 enuresis NOS (R32)

F98.1 Encopresis not due to a substance or known physiological condition

Encopresis: Fecal incontinence

Functional encopresis
Incontinence of feces of nonorganic origin
Psychogenic encopresis

Use additional code to identify the cause of any coexisting constipation.

Excludes1 encopresis NOS (R15.-)

● F98.2 Other feeding disorders of infancy and childhood

Excludes1 feeding difficulties (R63.3)

Excludes2 anorexia nervosa and other eating disorders (F50.-)
feeding problems of newborn (P92.-)
pica of infancy or childhood (F98.3)

F98.21 Rumination disorder of infancy

F98.29 Other feeding disorders of infancy and early childhood

F98.3 Pica of infancy and childhood

Craving and eating substances such as paint, clay, or dirt to replace a nutritional deficit in the body.

F98.4 Stereotyped movement disorders

Stereotype/habit disorder

Excludes1 abnormal involuntary movements (R25.-)

Excludes2 compulsions in obsessive-compulsive disorder (F42-) ◀
hair plucking (F63.3)
movement disorders of organic origin (G20-G25)
nail-biting (F98.8)
nose-picking (F98.8)
stereotypies that are part of a broader psychiatric condition (F01-F95)
thumb-sucking (F98.8)
tic disorders (F95.-)
trichotillomania (F63.3)

F98.5 Adult onset fluency disorder

Excludes1 childhood onset fluency disorder (F80.81)
dysphasia (R47.02)
fluency disorder in conditions classified elsewhere (R47.82)
fluency disorder (stuttering) following cerebrovascular disease (I69. with final characters -23)
tic disorders (F95.-)

F98.8 Other specified behavioral and emotional disorders with onset usually occurring in childhood and adolescence

Excessive masturbation
Nail-biting
Nose-picking
Thumb-sucking

F98.9 Unspecified behavioral and emotional disorders with onset usually occurring in childhood and adolescence

UNSPECIFIED MENTAL DISORDER (F99)

F99 Mental disorder, not otherwise specified

Mental illness NOS

Excludes1 unspecified mental disorder due to known physiological condition (F09)

Item 5–2 Enuresis: Bed wetting by children at night. Causes can be either psychological or medical (diabetes, urinary tract infections, or abnormalities). **Encopresis:** Overflow incontinence of bowels sometimes resulting from chronic constipation or fecal impaction. Check the documentation for additional diagnoses.

CHAPTER 6

DISEASES OF THE NERVOUS SYSTEM (G00-G99)

OGCR Chapter-Specific Coding Guidelines

6. Chapter 6: Diseases of the Nervous System (G00-G99)

a. Dominant/nondominant side

Codes from category G81, Hemiplegia and hemiparesis, and subcategories, G83.1, Monoplegia of lower limb, G83.2, Monoplegia of upper limb, and G83.3, Monoplegia, unspecified, identify whether the dominant or nondominant side is affected. Should the affected side be documented, but not specified as dominant or nondominant, and the classification system does not indicate a default, code selection is as follows:

- For ambidextrous patients, the default should be dominant.
- If the left side is affected, the default is non-dominant.
- If the right side is affected, the default is dominant.

b. Pain - Category G89

1) General coding information

Codes in category G89, Pain, not elsewhere classified, may be used in conjunction with codes from other categories and chapters to provide more detail about acute or chronic pain and neoplasm-related pain, unless otherwise indicated below.

If the pain is not specified as acute or chronic, post-thoracotomy, postprocedural, or neoplasm-related, do not assign codes from category G89.

A code from category G89 should not be assigned if the underlying (definitive) diagnosis is known, unless the reason for the encounter is pain control/management and not management of the underlying condition.

When an admission or encounter is for a procedure aimed at treating the underlying condition (e.g., spinal fusion, kyphoplasty), a code for the underlying condition (e.g., vertebral fracture, spinal stenosis) should be assigned as the principal diagnosis. No code from category G89 should be assigned.

(a) Category G89 Codes as Principal or First-Listed Diagnosis

Category G89 codes are acceptable as principal diagnosis or the first-listed code:

- When pain control or pain management is the reason for the admission/encounter (e.g., a patient with displaced intervertebral disc, nerve impingement and severe back pain presents for injection of steroid into the spinal canal). The underlying cause of the pain should be reported as an additional diagnosis, if known.
- When a patient is admitted for the insertion of a neurostimulator for pain control, assign the appropriate pain code as the principal or first-listed diagnosis. When an admission or encounter is for a procedure aimed at treating the underlying condition and a neurostimulator is inserted for pain control during the same admission/encounter, a code for the underlying condition should be assigned as the principal diagnosis and the appropriate pain code should be assigned as a secondary diagnosis.

(b) Use of Category G89 Codes in Conjunction with Site Specific Pain Codes

(i) Assigning Category G89 and Site-Specific Pain Codes

Codes from category G89 may be used in conjunction with codes that identify the site of pain (including codes from chapter 18) if the category G89 code provides additional information. For example, if the code describes the site of the pain, but does not fully describe whether the pain is acute or chronic, then both codes should be assigned.

(ii) Sequencing of Category G89 Codes with Site-Specific Pain Codes

The sequencing of category G89 codes with site-specific pain codes (including chapter 18 codes), is dependent on the circumstances of the encounter/admission as follows:

- If the encounter is for pain control or pain management, assign the code from category G89 followed by the code identifying the specific site of pain (e.g., encounter for pain management for acute neck pain from trauma is assigned code G89.11, Acute pain due to trauma, followed by code M54.2, Cervicalgia, to identify the site of pain).
- If the encounter is for any other reason except pain control or pain management, and a related definitive diagnosis has not been established (confirmed) by the provider, assign the code for the specific site of pain first, followed by the appropriate code from category G89.

2) Pain due to devices, implants and grafts

See Section I.C.19. Pain due to medical devices

3) Postoperative Pain

The provider's documentation should be used to guide the coding of postoperative pain, as well as *Section III. Reporting Additional Diagnoses* and *Section IV. Diagnostic Coding and Reporting in the Outpatient Setting.*

The default for post-thoracotomy and other postoperative pain not specified as acute or chronic is the code for the acute form.

Routine or expected postoperative pain immediately after surgery should not be coded.

(a) Postoperative pain not associated with specific postoperative complication

Postoperative pain not associated with a specific postoperative complication is assigned to the appropriate postoperative pain code in category G89.

(b) Postoperative pain associated with specific postoperative complication

Postoperative pain associated with a specific postoperative complication (such as painful wire sutures) is assigned to the appropriate code(s) found in Chapter 19, Injury, poisoning, and certain other consequences of external causes. If appropriate, use additional code(s) from category G89 to identify acute or chronic pain (G89.18 or G89.28).

4) Chronic pain

Chronic pain is classified to subcategory G89.2. There is no time frame defining when pain becomes chronic pain. The provider's documentation should be used to guide use of these codes.

5) Neoplasm Related Pain

Code G89.3 is assigned to pain documented as being related, associated or due to cancer, primary or secondary malignancy, or tumor. This code is assigned regardless of whether the pain is acute or chronic.

This code may be assigned as the principal or first-listed code when the stated reason for the admission/encounter is documented as pain control/pain management. The underlying neoplasm should be reported as an additional diagnosis.

When the reason for the admission/encounter is management of the neoplasm and the pain associated with the neoplasm is also documented, code G89.3 may be assigned as an additional diagnosis. It is not necessary to assign an additional code for the site of the pain.

See Section I.C.2 for instructions on the sequencing of neoplasms for all other stated reasons for the admission/encounter (except for pain control/pain management).

6) Chronic pain syndrome

Central pain syndrome (G89.0) and chronic pain syndrome (G89.4) are different than the term "chronic pain," and therefore codes should only be used when the provider has specifically documented this condition.

See Section I.C.5. Pain disorders related to psychological factors

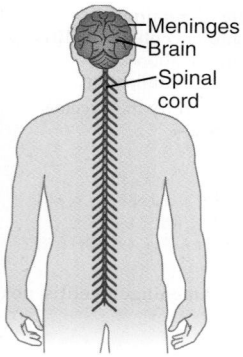

Figure 6-1 The brain and spinal cord make up the central nervous system.

Item 6–1 The two major classifications of the nervous system are the peripheral nervous system and the central nervous system (CNS). The central nervous system is comprised of the brain and the spinal cord. The peripheral nervous system is comprised of the parasympathetic and sympathetic systems. **Encephalitis** is the swelling of the brain. **Meningitis** is swelling of the covering of the brain, the meninges. Types and causes of brain infections are:

Type	Cause
purulent	bacterial
aseptic/abacterial	viral
chronic meningitis	mycobacterial and fungal

CHAPTER 6

DISEASES OF THE NERVOUS SYSTEM (G00-G99)

Excludes2 certain conditions originating in the perinatal period (P04-P96)
certain infectious and parasitic diseases (A00-B99)
complications of pregnancy, childbirth and the puerperium (O00-O9A)
congenital malformations, deformations, and chromosomal abnormalities (Q00-Q99)
endocrine, nutritional and metabolic diseases (E00-E88)
injury, poisoning and certain other consequences of external causes (S00-T88)
neoplasms (C00-D49)
symptoms, signs and abnormal clinical and laboratory findings, not elsewhere classified (R00-R94)

This chapter contains the following blocks:

G00-G09	Inflammatory diseases of the central nervous system
G10-G14	Systemic atrophies primarily affecting the central nervous system
G20-G26	Extrapyramidal and movement disorders
G30-G32	Other degenerative diseases of the nervous system
G35-G37	Demyelinating diseases of the central nervous system
G40-G47	Episodic and paroxysmal disorders
G50-G59	Nerve, nerve root and plexus disorders
G60-G65	Polyneuropathies and other disorders of the peripheral nervous system
G70-G73	Diseases of myoneural junction and muscle
G80-G83	Cerebral palsy and other paralytic syndromes
G89-G99	Other disorders of the nervous system

INFLAMMATORY DISEASES OF THE CENTRAL NERVOUS SYSTEM (G00-G09)

G00 Bacterial meningitis, not elsewhere classified
An infection of the cerebrospinal fluid surrounding the spinal cord and brain.

Includes bacterial arachnoiditis
bacterial leptomeningitis
bacterial meningitis
bacterial pachymeningitis

Excludes1 bacterial:
meningoencephalitis (G04.2)
meningomyelitis (G04.2)

Ex: **For category G00 CC codes:** 02.21, A17.0-A17.1, A27.81, A39.0, A50.41, A51.41, A52.13, A54.82, A54.84, A54.89-A54.9, A87.0-A87.9, B00.3, B02.1, B26.1, B37.5, B38.4, B45.1, B58.2, E08.40-E08.49, E08.618-E08.638, E08.649-E08.8, E09.40-E09.49, E09.618-E09.638, E09.649-E09.8, E10.40-E10.49, E10.618-E10.638, E10.649, E10.69, E10.8, E11.40-E11.49, E11.618-E11.638, E11.649, E11.69-E11.8, E13.40-E13.49, E13.618-E13.638, E13.649-E13.69, E13.8, G00.0-G03.9, G04.2, G32.89, G61.0, G96.8-G96.9, G98.0-G98.8, G99.8

G00.0 Hemophilus meningitis
Meningitis due to Hemophilus influenzae

G00.1 Pneumococcal meningitis
Meningitis due to Streptococcal pneumoniae ◀

G00.2 Streptococcal meningitis
Use additional code to further identify organism (B95.0-B95.5)

G00.3 Staphylococcal meningitis
Use additional code to further identify organism (B95.61-B95.8)

G00.8 Other bacterial meningitis
Meningitis due to Escherichia coli
Meningitis due to Friedländer bacillus
Meningitis due to Klebsiella
Use additional code to further identify organism (B96.-)

G00.9 Bacterial meningitis, unspecified
Meningitis due to gram-negative bacteria, unspecified
Purulent meningitis NOS
Pyogenic meningitis NOS
Suppurative meningitis NOS

G01 Meningitis in bacterial diseases classified elsewhere
Code first underlying disease

Excludes1 meningitis (in):
gonococcal (A54.81)
leptospirosis (A27.81)
listeriosis (A32.11)
Lyme disease (A69.21)
meningococcal (A39.0)
neurosyphilis (A52.13)
tuberculosis (A17.0)
meningoencephalitis and meningomyelitis in bacterial diseases classified elsewhere (G05)

Ex: See G00

G02 Meningitis in other infectious and parasitic diseases classified elsewhere
Code first underlying disease, such as:
African trypanosomiasis (B56.-)
poliovirus infection (A80.-)

Excludes1 candidal meningitis (B37.5)
coccidioidomycosis meningitis (B38.4)
cryptococcal meningitis (B45.1)
herpesviral [herpes simplex] meningitis (B00.3)
infectious mononucleosis complicated by meningitis (B27.- with fourth character 2)
measles complicated by meningitis (B05.1)
meningoencephalitis and meningomyelitis in other infectious and parasitic diseases classified elsewhere (G05)
mumps meningitis (B26.1)
rubella meningitis (B06.02)
varicella [chickenpox] meningitis (B01.0)
zoster meningitis (B02.1)

Ex: A02.21, A17.0-A17.1, A27.81, A39.0, A50.41, A51.41, A52.13, A54.82, A54.84, A54.89-A54.9, A87.0-A87.9, B00.3, B02.1, B26.1, B37.5, B38.4, B45.1, B58.2, G00.0-G03.9, G04.2, G32.89, G61.0, G96.8-G96.9, G98.0-G98.8, G99.8

● **G03 Meningitis due to other and unspecified causes**

Includes arachnoiditis NOS
leptomeningitis NOS
meningitis NOS
pachymeningitis NOS

Excludes1 meningoencephalitis (G04.-)
meningomyelitis (G04.-)

Ex: **For category G03 CC codes unless otherwise indicated:** See G00

G03.0 Nonpyogenic meningitis
Aseptic meningitis
Nonbacterial meningitis

G03.1 Chronic meningitis

G03.2 Benign recurrent meningitis [Mollaret]
Ex: A02.21, A17.0-A17.1, A27.81, A39.0, A50.41, A51.41, A52.13, A54.82-A54.84, A54.89-A54.9, A74.81-A74.9, A87.0-A87.9, A96.2, A98.3-A98.4, B26.1, B33.24, B33.4-B33.8, B34.1-B34.8, B37.5, B38.4, B45.1, B58.2, B92, B94.2-B94.9, B97.10, B97.19, B97.29, B97.5-B97.6, B97.81-B97.89, G00.0-G03.9, G04.2, G32.89, G61.0, G96.8-G96.9, G98.0-G98.8, G99.8

G03.8 Meningitis due to other specified causes

G03.9 Meningitis, unspecified
Arachnoiditis (spinal) NOS

● **G04 Encephalitis, myelitis and encephalomyelitis**

Includes acute ascending myelitis
meningoencephalitis
meningomyelitis

Excludes1 encephalopathy NOS (G93.40)
other noninfectious acute disseminated encephalomyelitis (noninfectious ADEM) (G04.81)

Excludes2 acute transverse myelitis (G37.3-)
alcoholic encephalopathy (G31.2)
benign myalgic encephalomyelitis (G93.3)
multiple sclerosis (G35)
subacute necrotizing myelitis (G37.4)
toxic encephalitis (G92)
toxic encephalopathy (G92)

● **G04.0 Acute disseminated encephalitis and encephalomyelitis (ADEM)**

Excludes1 acute necrotizing hemorrhagic encephalopathy (G04.3-)

Ex: **For category G04.0 CC codes unless otherwise indicated:** A02.21, A17.0-A17.1, A17.82, A27.81, A39.0, A50.41-A50.42, A51.41, A52.13-A52.14, A54.82, A54.84, A54.89-A54.9, A81.1, A81.82-A81.89, A83.0-A85.8, A87.0-A88.0, A88.8, A92.1-A92.8, A93.0, A96.2, A98.3-A98.4, B00.3-B00.4, B00.89-B01.11, B01.81-B02.23, B02.29, B02.7-B02.9, B04, B06.01, B08.04-B08.09, B08.20-B08.22, B08.60-B08.79, B09-B10.89, B26.1-B26.2, B27.00-B27.99, B33.1, B33.24, B33.4-B33.8, B34.1-B34.2, B34.4, B34.8, B37.5, B38.4, B45.1-B58.2, B92, B94.2, B94.8-B94.9, B97.10, B97.19-B97.29, B97.5-B97.6, B97.81-B97.89, G00.0-G04.01, G04.2, G04.31, G04.81-G05.4, G32.89, G37.0, G37.4-G37.5, G61.0, G96.8-G96.9, G98.0-G98.8, G99.8, J09.X3-J09.X9, J10.2-J10.89, J11.2-J11.89, L44.4, P35.2-P35.9, P37.0-P37.4, P37.8-P37.9

G04.00 Acute disseminated encephalitis and encephalomyelitis, unspecified

▶ ***G04.01 Postinfectious acute disseminated encephalitis and encephalomyelitis (postinfectious ADEM)***

Excludes1 post chickenpox encephalitis (B01.1)
post measles encephalitis (B05.0)
post measles myelitis (B05.1)

G04.02 Postimmunization acute disseminated encephalitis, myelitis and encephalomyelitis
Encephalitis, post immunization
Encephalomyelitis, post immunization
Use additional code to identify the vaccine (T50.A-, T50.B-, T50.Z-)
Ex: No exclusions

G04.1 Tropical spastic paraplegia
Ex: G04.1, G11.0-G12.9, G32.0-G37.3, G37.5-G37.9, G80.0-G80.2, G80.4-G80.9, G81.00-G83.9, G90.01-G90.09, G90.2, G90.4, G90.50-G90.9, G92, G93.40-G93.49, G93.81, G93.89-G95.9, G96.8-G96.9, G98.0-G99.8, I67.83, R53.2

G04.2 Bacterial meningoencephalitis and meningomyelitis, not elsewhere classified
Ex: See G00

● **G04.3 Acute necrotizing hemorrhagic encephalopathy**
Sudden and severe CNS disease with pathology of hemorrhages and necrosis of white matter

Excludes1 acute disseminated encephalitis and encephalomyelitis (G04.0-)

G04.30 Acute necrotizing hemorrhagic encephalopathy, unspecified
Ex: No exclusions

G04.31 Postinfectious acute necrotizing hemorrhagic encephalopathy
Ex: See G04.0

G04.32 Postimmunization acute necrotizing hemorrhagic encephalopathy
Use additional code to identify vaccine (T50.A-, T50.B-, T50.Z-)
Ex: No exclusions

G04.39 Other acute necrotizing hemorrhagic encephalopathy
Code also underlying etiology, if applicable
Ex: No exclusions

● **G04.8 Other encephalitis, myelitis and encephalomyelitis**
Code also any associated seizure (G40.-, R56.9)
Ex: **For category G04.8 CC codes:** See G04.0

G04.81 Other encephalitis and encephalomyelitis
Noninfectious acute disseminated encephalomyelitis (noninfectious ADEM)

G04.89 Other myelitis

● **G04.9 Encephalitis, myelitis and encephalomyelitis, unspecified**
Ex: **For category G04.9 CC codes:** A17.82, A28.1, A50.42, A52.14, A75.9, A79.9, A81.1, A81.82-A81.89, A83.0-A85.8, A87.2, A88.0, A88.8, A92.1-A92.8, A93.0, B00.4, B00.82, B01.11-B01.12, B04, B06.01, B08.09, B08.20-B08.22, B08.60-B08.79, B09, B10.01-B10.09, B26.2, B27.00-B27.99, B33.1, B45.0, B45.2-B45.9, B54, B58.2, B75, B97.10, B97.21, G04.00-G04.01, G04.31, G04.81-G05.4, G37.0, G37.4-G37.5, H66.40-H66.43, J09.X3-J09.X9, J10.2-J10.89, J11.2-J11.89, L44.4, M1A.10X0-M1A.19X1, M32.0-M32.9, P35.2-P35.9, P37.0-P37.9, T56.0X1-T56.0X4[A]

G04.90 Encephalitis and encephalomyelitis, unspecified
Ventriculitis (cerebral) NOS

G04.91 Myelitis, unspecified

G05 Encephalitis, myelitis and encephalomyelitis in diseases classified elsewhere

Code first underlying disease, such as:
human immunodeficiency virus [HIV] disease (B20)
poliovirus (A80.-)
suppurative otitis media (H66.01-H66.4)
trichinellosis (B75)

Excludes1 adenoviral encephalitis, myelitis and encephalomyelitis (A85.1)
congenital toxoplasmosis encephalitis, myelitis and encephalomyelitis (P37.1)
cytomegaloviral encephalitis, myelitis and encephalomyelitis (B25.8)
encephalitis, myelitis and encephalomyelitis (in) measles (B05.0)
encephalitis, myelitis and encephalomyelitis (in) systemic lupus erythematosus (M32.19)
enteroviral encephalitis, myelitis and encephalomyelitis (A85.0)
herpesviral [herpes simplex] encephalitis, myelitis and encephalomyelitis (B00.4)
listerial encephalitis, myelitis and encephalomyelitis (A32.12)
meningococcal encephalitis, myelitis and encephalomyelitis (A39.81)
mumps encephalitis, myelitis and encephalomyelitis (B26.2)
postchickenpox encephalitis, myelitis and encephalomyelitis (B01.1-)
rubella encephalitis, myelitis and encephalomyelitis (B06.01)
toxoplasmosis encephalitis, myelitis and encephalomyelitis (B58.2)
zoster encephalitis, myelitis and encephalomyelitis (B02.0)

Ex: **For category G05 CC codes:** See G04.0

G05.3 Encephalitis and encephalomyelitis in diseases classified elsewhere
Meningoencephalitis in diseases classified elsewhere

G05.4 Myelitis in diseases classified elsewhere
Meningomyelitis in diseases classified elsewhere

G06 Intracranial and intraspinal abscess and granuloma
An accumulation of pus in either the brain or spinal cord

Use additional code (B95-B97) to identify infectious agent.

G06.0 Intracranial abscess and granuloma
Brain [any part] abscess (embolic)
Cerebellar abscess (embolic)
Cerebral abscess (embolic)
Intracranial epidural abscess or granuloma
Intracranial extradural abscess or granuloma
Intracranial subdural abscess or granuloma
Otogenic abscess (embolic)

Excludes1 tuberculous intracranial abscess and granuloma (A17.81)

Ex: A06.6, A17.81, E08.40-E08.49, E08.618-E08.638, E08.649-E08.8, E09.40-E09.49, E09.618-E09.638, E09.649-E09.8, E10.40-E10.49, E10.618-E10.638, E10.649, E10.69-E10.8, E11.40-E11.49, E11.618-E11.638, E11.649, E11.69-E11.8, E13.40-E13.49, E13.618-E13.638, E13.649-E13.8, G06.0-G08, G93.81, G93.89-G93.9

G06.1 Intraspinal abscess and granuloma
Abscess (embolic) of spinal cord [any part]
Intraspinal epidural abscess or granuloma
Intraspinal extradural abscess or granuloma
Intraspinal subdural abscess or granuloma

Excludes1 tuberculous intraspinal abscess and granuloma (A17.81)

Ex: A06.6, A17.81, E08.40-A08.49, E08.618-E08.638, E08.649-E08.8, E09.40-E09.49, E09.618-E09.638, E09.649-E09.8, E10.40-E10.49, E10.618-E10.638, E10.649, E10.69-E10.8, E11.40-E11.49, E11.618-E11.638, E11.649, E11.69-E11.8, E13.40-E13.49, E13.618-E13.638, E13.649-E13.8, G06.1

G06.2 Extradural and subdural abscess, unspecified

Ex: A06.6, A17.81, E08.40-E08.49, E08.618-E08.638, E08.649-E08.8, E09.40-E09.49, E09.618-E09.638, E09.649-E09.8, E10.40-E10.49, E10.618-E10.638, E10.649, E10.69-E10.8, E11.40-E11.49, E11.618-E11.638, E11.649, E11.69-E11.8, E13.40-E13.49, E13.618-E13.638, E13.649-E13.8, G06.0-G06.2, G07-G08

G07 Intracranial and intraspinal abscess and granuloma in diseases classified elsewhere

Code first underlying disease, such as:
schistosomiasis granuloma of brain (B65.-)

Excludes1 abscess of brain:
amebic (A06.6)
chromomycotic (B43.1)
gonococcal (A54.82)
tuberculous (A17.81)
tuberculoma of meninges (A17.1)

Ex: See G06.2

G08 Intracranial and intraspinal phlebitis and thrombophlebitis
Septic embolism of intracranial or intraspinal venous sinuses and veins
Septic endophlebitis of intracranial or intraspinal venous sinuses and veins
Septic phlebitis of intracranial or intraspinal venous sinuses and veins
Septic thrombophlebitis of intracranial or intraspinal venous sinuses and veins
Septic thrombosis of intracranial or intraspinal venous sinuses and veins

Excludes1 intracranial phlebitis and thrombophlebitis complicating:
abortion, ectopic or molar pregnancy (O00-O07, O08.7)
pregnancy, childbirth and the puerperium (O22.5, O87.3)
nonpyogenic intracranial phlebitis and thrombophlebitis (I67.6)

Excludes2 intracranial phlebitis and thrombophlebitis complicating nonpyogenic intraspinal phlebitis and thrombophlebitis (G95.1)

Ex: See G06.2

G09 Sequelae of inflammatory diseases of central nervous system

Note: Category G09 is to be used to indicate conditions whose primary classification is to G00-G08 as the cause of sequelae, themselves classifiable elsewhere. The 'sequelae' include conditions specified as residuals.

Code first condition resulting from (sequela) of inflammatory diseases of central nervous system

SYSTEMIC ATROPHIES PRIMARILY AFFECTING THE CENTRAL NERVOUS SYSTEM (G10-G14)

G10 Huntington's disease
Genetic disease with degeneration of cells of the nervous system, including brain
Huntington's chorea
Huntington's dementia

Ex: G04.1, G20, G21.11-G21.9, G32.89-G37.9, G80.0-G80.2, G80.4-G80.9, G82.20-G83.0, G92, G93.1, G93.40-G93.6, G93.81, G93.89-G93.9, G96.8-G96.9, G98.0-G98.8, G99.8, I67.83, R53.2

Item 6–2 Huntington's chorea is an inherited degenerative disorder of the central nervous system and is characterized by ceaseless, jerky movements and progressive cognitive and behavioral deterioration.

G11 Hereditary ataxia
Genetic neurological disorder affecting coordination
Excludes2 cerebral palsy (G80.-)
hereditary and idiopathic neuropathy (G60.-)
metabolic disorders (E70-E88)
Ex: **For category G11 CC codes unless otherwise indicated:** G04.1, G10-G12.9, G21.0, G23.0-G25.79, G25.82-G26, G32.0-G37.9, G80.0-G83.9, G90.01-G90.09, G90.2-G90.9, G92-G93.1, G93.40-G93.49, G93.81, G93.89-G95.9, G96.8-G96.9, G98.0-G99.8, I67.83, R53.2

G11.0 Congenital nonprogressive ataxia

G11.1 Early-onset cerebellar ataxia
Early-onset cerebellar ataxia with essential tremor
Early-onset cerebellar ataxia with myoclonus [Hunt's ataxia]
Early-onset cerebellar ataxia with retained tendon reflexes
Friedreich's ataxia (autosomal recessive)
X-linked recessive spinocerebellar ataxia

G11.2 Late-onset cerebellar ataxia A

G11.3 Cerebellar ataxia with defective DNA repair
Ataxia telangiectasia [Louis-Bar]
Excludes2 Cockayne's syndrome (Q87.1)
other disorders of purine and pyrimidine metabolism (E79.-)
xeroderma pigmentosum (Q82.1)

G11.4 Hereditary spastic paraplegia
Ex: G04.1, G10-G12.9, G21.0, G23.0-G25.79, G25.82-G26, G32.0-G37.3, G37.5-G37.9, G80.0-G83.9, G90.01-G90.09, G90.2-G90.9, G92, G93.1, G93.40-G93.49, G93.81, G93.89-G93.9, G95.0-G95.9, G96.12-G96.9, G97.1, G98.0-G99.8, I67.83, R53.2

G11.8 Other hereditary ataxias

G11.9 Hereditary ataxia, unspecified
Hereditary cerebellar ataxia NOS
Hereditary cerebellar degeneration
Hereditary cerebellar disease
Hereditary cerebellar syndrome
Ex: G11.0-G11.9, G32.81

G12 Spinal muscular atrophy and related syndromes
Ex: **For category G12 CC codes:** E08.40-E08.49, E08.618-E08.638, E08.649-E08.8, E09.40-E09.49, E09.618-E09.638, E09.649-E09.8, E10.40-E10.49, E10.618-E10.638, E10.649, E10.69-E10.8, E11.40-E11.49, E11.618-E11.638, E11.649, E11.69-E11.8, E13.40-E13.49, E13.618-E13.638, E13.649-E13.8, G11.3, G11.8-G12.9, G32.0, G32.89, G90.01-G90.09, G90.2, G90.4, G90.50-G90.9, G95.0-G95.9, G96.8-G96.9, G98.0-G99.8

G12.0 Infantile spinal muscular atrophy, type I [Werdnig-Hoffman]

G12.1 Other inherited spinal muscular atrophy
Adult form spinal muscular atrophy
Childhood form, type II spinal muscular atrophy
Distal spinal muscular atrophy
Juvenile form, type III spinal muscular atrophy [Kugelberg-Welander]
Progressive bulbar palsy of childhood [Fazio-Londe]
Scapuloperoneal form spinal muscular atrophy

G12.2 Motor neuron disease
Progressive disease of motor neurons that carry impluses to muscles to move

G12.20 Motor neuron disease, unspecified

G12.21 Amyotrophic lateral sclerosis A
Lou Gehrig's disease (ALS)
Progressive spinal muscle atrophy

G12.22 Progressive bulbar palsy

G12.29 Other motor neuron disease
Familial motor neuron disease
Primary lateral sclerosis

G12.8 Other spinal muscular atrophies and related syndromes

G12.9 Spinal muscular atrophy, unspecified

G13 Systemic atrophies primarily affecting central nervous system in diseases classified elsewhere

G13.0 Paraneoplastic neuromyopathy and neuropathy
Carcinomatous neuromyopathy
Sensorial paraneoplastic neuropathy [Denny Brown]
Code first underlying neoplasm (C00-D49)

G13.1 Other systemic atrophy primarily affecting central nervous system in neoplastic disease
Paraneoplastic limbic encephalopathy
Code first underlying neoplasm (C00-D49)

G13.2 Systemic atrophy primarily affecting the central nervous system in myxedema
Code first underlying disease, such as:
hypothyroidism (E03.-)
myxedematous congenital iodine deficiency (E00.1)

G13.8 Systemic atrophy primarily affecting central nervous system in other diseases classified elsewhere
Code first underlying disease

G14 Postpolio syndrome
Includes Postpolio myelitic syndrome
Excludes1 sequelae of poliomyelitis (B91)

EXTRAPYRAMIDAL AND MOVEMENT DISORDERS (G20-G26)

G20 Parkinson's disease
Progressive disease of the nervous system that affects muscle coordination
Hemiparkinsonism
Idiopathic Parkinsonism or Parkinson's disease
Paralysis agitans
Parkinsonism or Parkinson's disease NOS
Primary Parkinsonism or Parkinson's disease
Excludes1 dementia with Parkinsonism (G31.83)
Coding Clinic: 2016, Q2, P7

G21 Secondary parkinsonism
Symptoms of Parkinson's caused by medicines, illness, or other nervous system disorder
Excludes1 dementia with Parkinsonism (G31.83)
Huntington's disease (G10)
Shy-Drager syndrome (G90.3)
syphilitic Parkinsonism (A52.19)

G21.0 Malignant neuroleptic syndrome
Use additional code for adverse effect, if applicable, to identify drug (T43.3X5, T43.4X5, T43.505, T43.595)
Excludes1 neuroleptic induced parkinsonism (G21.11)
Ex: G10, G21.0, G23.0-G25.79, G25.82-G26, G80.3, G81.00-G81.94, G90.3, G93.2, G93.40-G93.49, I67.83

G21.1 Other drug-induced secondary parkinsonism
Ex: **For category G21.1 CC codes:** G20, G21.11-G21.9

G21.11 Neuroleptic induced parkinsonism
Use additional code for adverse effect, if applicable, to identify drug (T43.3X5, T43.4X5, T43.505, T43.595)
Excludes1 malignant neuroleptic syndrome (G21.0)

G21.19 Other drug induced secondary parkinsonism
Use additional code for adverse effect, if applicable, to identify drug (T36-T50 with fifth or sixth character 5)

G21.2 Secondary parkinsonism due to other external agents
Code first (T51-T65) to identify external agent

G21.3 Postencephalitic parkinsonism

G21.4 Vascular parkinsonism

G21.8 Other secondary parkinsonism

G21.9 Secondary parkinsonism, unspecified

G23 Other degenerative diseases of basal ganglia

Excludes2 multi-system degeneration of the autonomic nervous system (G90.3)

Ex: For category G23 CC codes: G20, G21.11-G21.9, G90.01-G90.09, G93.40-G93.49, I67.83

G23.0 Hallervorden-Spatz disease
Pigmentary pallidal degeneration

G23.1 Progressive supranuclear ophthalmoplegia [Steele-Richardson-Olszewski]
Progressive supranuclear palsy

G23.2 Striatonigral degeneration

G23.8 Other specified degenerative diseases of basal ganglia
Calcification of basal ganglia

G23.9 Degenerative disease of basal ganglia, unspecified

G24 Dystonia
Involuntary movements

Includes dyskinesia

Excludes2 athetoid cerebral palsy (G80.3)

G24.0 Drug induced dystonia

Use additional code for adverse effect, if applicable, to identify drug (T36-T50 with fifth or sixth character 5)

G24.01 Drug induced subacute dyskinesia
Drug induced blepharospasm
Drug induced orofacial dyskinesia
Neuroleptic induced tardive dyskinesia
Tardive dyskinesia

G24.02 Drug induced acute dystonia
Acute dystonic reaction to drugs
Neuroleptic induced acute dystonia
Ex: G20, G21.11-G21.9, G25.70-G25.79, G25.89-G26, G80.3, G93.40, G93.41-G93.49, I67.83

G24.09 Other drug induced dystonia
Ex: See G24.02

G24.1 Genetic torsion dystonia
Dystonia deformans progressiva
Dystonia musculorum deformans
Familial torsion dystonia
Idiopathic familial dystonia
Idiopathic (torsion) dystonia NOS
(Schwalbe-) Ziehen-Oppenheim disease

G24.2 Idiopathic nonfamilial dystonia
Ex: See G24.02

G24.3 Spasmodic torticollis
Head tilts toward one side and chin is elevated and turned toward opposite side (wry neck)

Excludes1 congenital torticollis (Q68.0)
hysterical torticollis (F44.4)
ocular torticollis (R29.891)
psychogenic torticollis (F45.8)
torticollis NOS (M43.6)
traumatic recurrent torticollis (S13.4)

G24.4 Idiopathic orofacial dystonia
Orofacial dyskinesia

Excludes1 drug induced orofacial dyskinesia (G24.01)

G24.5 Blepharospasm
Tonic spasm of orbicularis oculi muscle, producing closure of eyelids

Excludes1 drug induced blepharospasm (G24.01)

G24.8 Other dystonia
Acquired torsion dystonia NOS
Ex: See G24.02

G24.9 Dystonia, unspecified
Dyskinesia NOS

G25 Other extrapyramidal and movement disorders
Extrapyramidal: Other than pyramidal tracts

Excludes2 sleep related movement disorders (G47.6-)

G25.0 Essential tremor
Familial tremor

Excludes1 tremor NOS (R25.1)

G25.1 Drug-induced tremor

Use additional code for adverse effect, if applicable, to identify drug (T36-T50 with fifth or sixth character 5)

G25.2 Other specified forms of tremor
Intention tremor

G25.3 Myoclonus
Shocklike contractions muscle(s)
Drug-induced myoclonus
Palatal myoclonus

Use additional code for adverse effect, if applicable, to identify drug (T36-T50 with fifth or sixth character 5)

Excludes1 facial myokymia (G51.4)
myoclonic epilepsy (G40.-)

G25.4 Drug-induced chorea

Use additional code for adverse effect, if applicable, to identify drug (T36-T50 with fifth or sixth character 5)

G25.5 Other chorea
Continual, involuntary, jerky, movements
Chorea NOS

Excludes1 chorea NOS with heart involvement (I02.0)
Huntington's chorea (G10)
rheumatic chorea (I02.-)
Sydenham's chorea (I02.-)

G25.6 Drug induced tics and other tics of organic origin

G25.61 Drug induced tics

Use additional code for adverse effect, if applicable, to identify drug (T36-T50 with fifth or sixth character 5)

G25.69 Other tics of organic origin

Excludes1 habit spasm (F95.9)
tic NOS (F95.9)
Tourette's syndrome (F95.2)

G25.7 Other and unspecified drug induced movement disorders

Use additional code for adverse effect, if applicable, to identify drug (T36-T50 with fifth or sixth character 5)

G25.70 Drug induced movement disorder, unspecified

G25.71 Drug induced akathisia
Drug induced acathisia
Neuroleptic induced acute akathisia

G25.79 Other drug induced movement disorders

G25.8 Other specified extrapyramidal and movement disorders

G25.81 Restless legs syndrome

G25.82 Stiff-man syndrome
Ex: G04.1, G10, G12.22, G20-G21.9, G24.01-G25.79, G25.82-G26, G32.89-G37.2, G37.5-G37.9, G80.0-G80.9, G82.20-G83.0, G92, G93.1, G93.40-G93.6, G93.81, G93.89-G93.9, G96.8-G96.9, G98.0-G98.8, G99.8, I67.83, R53.2

G25.83 Benign shuddering attacks

G25.89 Other specified extrapyramidal and movement disorders

G25.9 Extrapyramidal and movement disorder, unspecified
Ex: See G25.82

G26 Extrapyramidal and movement disorders in diseases classified elsewhere

Code first underlying disease

OTHER DEGENERATIVE DISEASES OF THE NERVOUS SYSTEM (G30-G32)

G30 Alzheimer's disease
Progressive central neurodegenerative disorder
Includes Alzheimer's dementia senile and presenile forms
Use additional code to identify:
delirium, if applicable (F05)
dementia with behavioral disturbance (F02.81)
dementia without behavioral disturbance (F02.80)
Excludes1 senile degeneration of brain NEC (G31.1)
senile dementia NOS (F03)
senility NOS (R41.81)

G30.0 Alzheimer's disease with early onset
G30.1 Alzheimer's disease with late onset A
G30.8 Other Alzheimer's disease
G30.9 Alzheimer's disease, unspecified
Coding Clinic: 2016, Q2, P6; 2012, Q4, P95

G31 Other degenerative diseases of nervous system, not elsewhere classified
Use additional code to identify:
dementia with behavioral disturbance (F02.81)
dementia without behavioral disturbance (F02.80)
Excludes2 Reye's syndrome (G93.7)

G31.0 Frontotemporal dementia
G31.01 Pick's disease
Primary progressive aphasia
Progressive isolated aphasia
G31.09 Other frontotemporal dementia
Frontal dementia

G31.1 Senile degeneration of brain, not elsewhere classified
Excludes1 Alzheimer's disease (G30.-)
senility NOS (R41.81)

G31.2 Degeneration of nervous system due to alcohol
Alcoholic cerebellar ataxia
Alcoholic cerebellar degeneration
Alcoholic cerebral degeneration
Alcoholic encephalopathy
Dysfunction of the autonomic nervous system due to alcohol
Code also associated alcoholism (F10.-)

G31.8 Other specified degenerative diseases of nervous system
G31.81 Alpers' disease
Rare neuronal degeneration of cerebral cortex disease of young children
Grey-matter degeneration
Ex: E75.00-E75.19, E75.4, F84.2, G13.2-G13.8, G30.0-G31.82, G31.84-G31.9, G91.4, G94
G31.82 Leigh's disease
Rare neurometabolic disorder that affects central nervous system
Subacute necrotizing encephalopathy
Ex: See G31.81
G31.83 Dementia with Lewy bodies
Closely allied to Parkinson's Disease
Dementia with Parkinsonism
Lewy body dementia
Lewy body disease
G31.84 Mild cognitive impairment, so stated
Excludes1 age related cognitive decline (R41.81)
altered mental status (R41.82)
cerebral degeneration (G31.9)
change in mental status (R41.82)
cognitive deficits following (sequelae of) cerebral hemorrhage or infarction (I69.01-, I69.11-, I69.21-, I69.31-, I69.81-, I69.91-)
cognitive impairment due to intracranial or head injury (S06.-)
dementia (F01.-, F02.-, F03)
mild memory disturbance (F06.8)
neurologic neglect syndrome (R41.4)
personality change, nonpsychotic (F68.8)
G31.85 Corticobasal degeneration
G31.89 Other specified degenerative diseases of nervous system
G31.9 Degenerative disease of nervous system, unspecified

G32 Other degenerative disorders of nervous system in diseases classified elsewhere
G32.0 Subacute combined degeneration of spinal cord in diseases classified elsewhere
Dana-Putnam syndrome
Sclerosis of spinal cord (combined) (dorsolateral) (posterolateral)
Code first underlying disease, such as:
anemia (D51.9)
dietary (D51.3)
pernicious (D51.0)
vitamin B12 deficiency (E53.8)
Excludes1 syphilitic combined degeneration of spinal cord (A52.11)
Ex: G04.1, G11.3, G11.8-G12.9, G32.0, G32.89-G37.3, G37.5-G37.9, G80.0-G83.9, G90.01-G90.09, G90.2, G90.4-G90.9, G93.1, G93.40-G93.49, G95.0-G96.9, G97.1, G98.0-G99.8, I67.83, R53.2

G32.8 Other specified degenerative disorders of nervous system in diseases classified elsewhere
Code first underlying disease, such as:
amyloidosis cerebral degeneration (E85.-)
cerebral degeneration (due to) hypothyroidism (E00.0-E03.9)
cerebral degeneration (due to) neoplasm (C00-D49)
cerebral degeneration (due to) vitamin B deficiency, except thiamine (E52-E53.-)
Excludes1 superior hemorrhagic polioencephalitis [Wernicke's encephalopathy] (E51.2)
G32.81 Cerebellar ataxia in diseases classified elsewhere
Code first underlying disease, such as:
celiac disease (with gluten ataxia) (K90.0)
cerebellar ataxia (in) neoplastic disease (paraneoplastic cerebellar degeneration) (C00-D49)
non-celiac gluten ataxia (M35.9)
Excludes1 systemic atrophy primarily affecting the central nervous system in alcoholic cerebellar ataxia (G31.2)
systemic atrophy primarily affecting the central nervous system in myxedema (G13.2)
Ex: G04.1, G10-G12.9, G21.0, G23.0-G25.79, G25.82-G26, G32.0-G37.9, G80.0-G83.9, G90.01-G90.09, G90.2-G90.9, G92-G93.1, G93.40-G93.49, G93.81, G93.89-G95.9, G96.8-G96.9, G98.0-G99.8, I67.83, R53.2
G32.89 Other specified degenerative disorders of nervous system in diseases classified elsewhere
Degenerative encephalopathy in diseases classified elsewhere

DEMYELINATING DISEASES OF THE CENTRAL NERVOUS SYSTEM (G35-G37)

G35 Multiple sclerosis
Destruction of central nervous system; four types: relapsing remitting, secondary progressive, primary progressive, and progressive relapsing
Disseminated multiple sclerosis
Generalized multiple sclerosis
Multiple sclerosis NOS
Multiple sclerosis of brain stem
Multiple sclerosis of cord

● **G36 Other acute disseminated demyelination**
Excludes1 postinfectious encephalitis and encephalomyelitis NOS (G04.01)
Ex: **For category G36 CC codes unless otherwise indicated:** G04.1, G10-G12.9, G21.0, G24.01-G25.79, G25.82-G26, G32.0-G37.3, G37.5, G37.8-G37.9, G80.0-G83.9, G90.01-G90.09, G90.2, G90.4-G90.9, G92, G93.40-G93.49, G93.81, G93.89-G95.9, G96.8-G96.9, G98.0-G99.8, I67.83, R53.2

G36.0 Neuromyelitis optica [Devic]
Inflammatory disorder in which immune system attacks optic nerves and spinal cord producing inflammation of optic nerve (optic neuritis) and spinal cord (myelitis)
Demyelination in optic neuritis
Excludes1 optic neuritis NOS (H46)
Ex: G36.0, G93.40-G93.49, I67.83

G36.1 Acute and subacute hemorrhagic leukoencephalitis [Hurst]

G36.8 Other specified acute disseminated demyelination

G36.9 Acute disseminated demyelination, unspecified

● **G37 Other demyelinating diseases of central nervous system**
Destruction of central nervous system

G37.0 Diffuse sclerosis of central nervous system
Periaxial encephalitis
Schilder's disease
Excludes1 X linked adrenoleukodystrophy (E71.52-)
Ex: A92.30-A92.39, B97.21, G93.40-G93.49, I67.83

G37.1 Central demyelination of corpus callosum
Ex: See G36

G37.2 Central pontine myelinolysis
Ex: See G36

G37.3 Acute transverse myelitis in demyelinating disease of central nervous system
Acute transverse myelitis NOS
Acute transverse myelopathy
Excludes1 multiple sclerosis (G35)
neuromyelitis optica [Devic] (G36.0)
Ex: A02.21, A17.0-A27.81, A39.0, A50.41, A51.41, A52.13, A54.82, A54.84, A54.89-A54.9, A87.0-A87.9, A96.2, A98.3-A98.4, B00.3, B00.89-B00.9, B02.0-B02.29, B02.7-B02.9, B10.81-B10.89, B26.1, B33.24-B33.8, B34.1-B34.2, B34.4-B34.8, B37.5, B38.4, B45.1, B58.2, B92, B94.2-B94.9, B97.10, B97.19, B97.29, B97.5-B97.6, B97.81-B97.89, E08.40-E08.49, E09.40-E09.49, E10.40-E10.49, E11.40-E11.49, E13.40-E13.49, G00.0-G03.9, G04.1-G04.2, G11.3, G11.8-G12.9, G32.0, G32.89-G37.2, G37.5-G37.9, G61.0, G80.0-G80.2, G80.4-G83.9, G90.01-G90.09, G90.2, G90.4-G90.9, G93.1, G93.40-G93.49, G95.0-G95.9, G96.12-G96.9, G97.1, G98.0-G99.8, I67.83, R53.2

G37.4 Subacute necrotizing myelitis of central nervous system
Ex: See G04.9

Item 6–3 Multiple sclerosis (MS) is a nervous system disease affecting the brain and spinal cord by damaging the myelin sheath surrounding and protecting nerve cells. The damage slows down/blocks messages between the brain and body. Symptoms are: visual disturbances, muscle weakness, coordination and balance issues, numbness, prickling, thinking and memory problems. The cause is unknown, though it is thought that it may be an autoimmune disease. It affects women more than men, between 20 and 40 years of age. MS can be mild, but it may cause the loss of ability to write, walk, and speak. There is no cure, but medication may slow or control symptoms.

G37.5 Concentric sclerosis [Baló] of central nervous system
Ex: See G37.0

G37.8 Other specified demyelinating diseases of central nervous system
Ex: See G36

G37.9 Demyelinating disease of central nervous system, unspecified
Ex: See G36

EPISODIC AND PAROXYSMAL DISORDERS (G40-G47)

● **G40 Epilepsy and recurrent seizures**
Note: The following terms are to be considered equivalent to intractable: pharmacoresistant (pharmacologically resistant), treatment resistant, refractory (medically) and poorly controlled
Excludes1 conversion disorder with seizures (F44.5)
convulsions NOS (R56.9)
post traumatic seizures (R56.1)
seizure (convulsive) NOS (R56.9)
seizure of newborn (P90)
Excludes2 hippocampal sclerosis (G93.81) ◀
mesial temporal sclerosis (G93.81) ◀
temporal sclerosis (G93.81) ◀
Todd's paralysis (G83.84) ◀

● **G40.0 Localization-related (focal) (partial) idiopathic epilepsy and epileptic syndromes with seizures of localized onset**
Benign childhood epilepsy with centrotemporal EEG spikes
Childhood epilepsy with occipital EEG paroxysms
Excludes1 adult onset localization-related epilepsy (G40.1-, G40.2-)

● **G40.00 Localization-related (focal) (partial) idiopathic epilepsy and epileptic syndromes with seizures of localized onset, not intractable**
Localization-related (focal) (partial) idiopathic epilepsy and epileptic syndromes with seizures of localized onset without intractability

G40.001 Localization-related (focal) (partial) idiopathic epilepsy and epileptic syndromes with seizures of localized onset, not intractable, with status epilepticus
Ex: G32.89, G40.001-G40.319, G40.401-G40.919, G40.A01-G40.B19, G93.40-G93.49, G93.9, G96.8-G96.9, G98.0-G98.8, G99.8. I67.83, R56.1

G40.009 Localization-related (focal) (partial) idiopathic epilepsy and epileptic syndromes with seizures of localized onset, not intractable, without status epilepticus
Localization-related (focal) (partial) idiopathic epilepsy and epileptic syndromes with seizures of localized onset NOS
Ex: See G40.001

G40.01 Localization-related (focal) (partial) idiopathic epilepsy and epileptic syndromes with seizures of localized onset, intractable

G40.011 Localization-related (focal) (partial) idiopathic epilepsy and epileptic syndromes with seizures of localized onset, intractable, with status epilepticus

Ex: E08.40-E08.49, E09.40-E09.49, E10.40-E10.49, E11.40-E11.49, E13.40-E13.49, G32.89, G40.001-G40.319, G40.401-G40.919, G40.A01-G40.A19, G40.B01-G40.B19, G93.81, G93.89-G93.9, G96.8-G96.9, G98.0-G98.8, G99.8, R56.1

G40.019 Localization-related (focal) (partial) idiopathic epilepsy and epileptic syndromes with seizures of localized onset, intractable, without status epilepticus

Ex: See G40.011

G40.1 Localization-related (focal) (partial) symptomatic epilepsy and epileptic syndromes with simple partial seizures

Attacks without alteration of consciousness
Epilepsia partialis continua [Kozhevnikof]
Simple partial seizures developing into secondarily generalized seizures

G40.10 Localization-related (focal) (partial) symptomatic epilepsy and epileptic syndromes with simple partial seizures, not intractable

Localization-related (focal) (partial) symptomatic epilepsy and epileptic syndromes with simple partial seizures without intractability

G40.101 Localization-related (focal) (partial) symptomatic epilepsy and epileptic syndromes with simple partial seizures, not intractable, with status epilepticus

Ex: See G40.001

G40.109 Localization-related (focal) (partial) symptomatic epilepsy and epileptic syndromes with simple partial seizures, not intractable, without status epilepticus

Localization-related (focal) (partial) symptomatic epilepsy and epileptic syndromes with simple partial seizures NOS

Ex: See G40.001

G40.11 Localization-related (focal) (partial) symptomatic epilepsy and epileptic syndromes with simple partial seizures, intractable

G40.111 Localization-related (focal) (partial) symptomatic epilepsy and epileptic syndromes with simple partial seizures, intractable, with status epilepticus

Ex: See G40.011

G40.119 Localization-related (focal) (partial) symptomatic epilepsy and epileptic syndromes with simple partial seizures, intractable, without status epilepticus

Ex: See G40.011

G40.2 Localization-related (focal) (partial) symptomatic epilepsy and epileptic syndromes with complex partial seizures

Attacks with alteration of consciousness, often with automatisms
Complex partial seizures developing into secondarily generalized seizures

G40.20 Localization-related (focal) (partial) symptomatic epilepsy and epileptic syndromes with complex partial seizures, not intractable

Localization-related (focal) (partial) symptomatic epilepsy and epileptic syndromes with complex partial seizures without intractability

G40.201 Localization-related (focal) (partial) symptomatic epilepsy and epileptic syndromes with complex partial seizures, not intractable, with status epilepticus

Ex: See G40.001

G40.209 Localization-related (focal) (partial) symptomatic epilepsy and epileptic syndromes with complex partial seizures, not intractable, without status epilepticus

Localization-related (focal) (partial) symptomatic epilepsy and epileptic syndromes with complex partial seizures NOS

Ex: See G40.001

G40.21 Localization-related (focal) (partial) symptomatic epilepsy and epileptic syndromes with complex partial seizures, intractable

G40.211 Localization-related (focal) (partial) symptomatic epilepsy and epileptic syndromes with complex partial seizures, intractable, with status epilepticus

Ex: See G40.011

G40.219 Localization-related (focal) (partial) symptomatic epilepsy and epileptic syndromes with complex partial seizures, intractable, without status epilepticus

Ex: See G40.011

G40.3 Generalized idiopathic epilepsy and epileptic syndromes

Code also MERRF syndrome, if applicable (E88.42)

G40.30 Generalized idiopathic epilepsy and epileptic syndromes, not intractable

Generalized idiopathic epilepsy and epileptic syndromes without intractability

G40.301 Generalized idiopathic epilepsy and epileptic syndromes, not intractable, with status epilepticus

Ex: E08.40-E08.49, E08.618-E08.638, E08.649-E08.8, E09.40-E09.49, E09.618-E09.638, E09.649-E09.8, E10.40-E10.49, E10.618-E10.638, E10.649, E10.69-E10.8, E11.40-E11.49, E11.618-E11.638, E11.649, E11.69-E11.8, E13.40-E13.49, E13.618-E13.638, E13.649-E13.8, G32.89, G40.001-G40.319, G40.401-G40.419, G40.501-G40.919, G40.A01-G40.B19, G93.81, G93.89-G93.9, G96.8-G96.9, G98.0-G98.8, G99.8, R56.1

G40.309 Generalized idiopathic epilepsy and epileptic syndromes, not intractable, without status epilepticus

Generalized idiopathic epilepsy and epileptic syndromes NOS

- **G40.31 Generalized idiopathic epilepsy and epileptic syndromes, intractable**
  - **G40.311 Generalized idiopathic epilepsy and epileptic syndromes, intractable, with status epilepticus**
    Ex: See G40.301
  - **G40.319 Generalized idiopathic epilepsy and epileptic syndromes, intractable, without status epilepticus**
    Ex: See G40.301
- **G40.A Absence epileptic syndrome**
  Childhood absence epilepsy [pyknolepsy]
  Juvenile absence epilepsy
  Absence epileptic syndrome, NOS
  - **G40.A0 Absence epileptic syndrome, not intractable**
    - **G40.A01 Absence epileptic syndrome, not intractable, with status epilepticus**
    - **G40.A09 Absence epileptic syndrome, not intractable, without status epilepticus**
  - **G40.A1 Absence epileptic syndrome, intractable**
    - **G40.A11 Absence epileptic syndrome, intractable, with status epilepticus**
      Ex: See G40.001
    - **G40.A19 Absence epileptic syndrome, intractable, without status epilepticus**
      Ex: See G40.001
- **G40.B Juvenile myoclonic epilepsy [impulsive petit mal]**
  Ex: For category G40.B CC codes: See G40.011
  - **G40.B0 Juvenile myoclonic epilepsy, not intractable**
    - **G40.B01 Juvenile myoclonic epilepsy, not intractable, with status epilepticus**
    - **G40.B09 Juvenile myoclonic epilepsy, not intractable, without status epilepticus**
  - **G40.B1 Juvenile myoclonic epilepsy, intractable**
    - **G40.B11 Juvenile myoclonic epilepsy, intractable, with status epilepticus**
    - **G40.B19 Juvenile myoclonic epilepsy, intractable, without status epilepticus**
- **G40.4 Other generalized epilepsy and epileptic syndromes**
  Epilepsy with grand mal seizures on awakening
  Epilepsy with myoclonic absences
  Epilepsy with myoclonic-astatic seizures
  Grand mal seizure NOS
  Nonspecific atonic epileptic seizures
  Nonspecific clonic epileptic seizures
  Nonspecific myoclonic epileptic seizures
  Nonspecific tonic epileptic seizures
  Nonspecific tonic-clonic epileptic seizures
  Symptomatic early myoclonic encephalopathy
  - **G40.40 Other generalized epilepsy and epileptic syndromes, not intractable**
    Other generalized epilepsy and epileptic syndromes without intractability
    Other generalized epilepsy and epileptic syndromes NOS
    - **G40.401 Other generalized epilepsy and epileptic syndromes, not intractable, with status epilepticus**
    - **G40.409 Other generalized epilepsy and epileptic syndromes, not intractable, without status epilepticus**
  - **G40.41 Other generalized epilepsy and epileptic syndromes, intractable**
    - **G40.411 Other generalized epilepsy and epileptic syndromes, intractable, with status epilepticus**
      Ex: See G40.011
    - **G40.419 Other generalized epilepsy and epileptic syndromes, intractable, without status epilepticus**
      Ex: See G40.011
- **G40.5 Epileptic seizures related to external causes**
  Epileptic seizures related to alcohol
  Epileptic seizures related to drugs
  Epileptic seizures related to hormonal changes
  Epileptic seizures related to sleep deprivation
  Epileptic seizures related to stress
  Code also, if applicable, associated epilepsy and recurrent seizures (G40.-)
  Use additional code for adverse effect, if applicable, to identify drug (T36-T50 with fifth or sixth character 5)
  Ex: For category G40.5 CC codes: See G40.011
  - **G40.50 Epileptic seizures related to external causes, not intractable**
    - **G40.501 Epileptic seizures related to external causes, not intractable, with status epilepticus**
    - **G40.509 Epileptic seizures related to external causes, not intractable, without status epilepticus**
      Epileptic seizures related to external causes, NOS
- **G40.8 Other epilepsy and recurrent seizures**
  Epilepsies and epileptic syndromes undetermined as to whether they are focal or generalized
  Landau-Kleffner syndrome
  Ex: For category G40.8 CC codes unless otherwise indicated: See G40.011
  - **G40.80 Other epilepsy**
    - **G40.801 Other epilepsy, not intractable, with status epilepticus**
      Other epilepsy without intractability with status epilepticus
    - **G40.802 Other epilepsy, not intractable, without status epilepticus**
      Other epilepsy NOS
      Other epilepsy without intractability without status epilepticus
    - **G40.803 Other epilepsy, intractable, with status epilepticus**
    - **G40.804 Other epilepsy, intractable, without status epilepticus**
  - **G40.81 Lennox-Gastaut syndrome**
    - **G40.811 Lennox-Gastaut syndrome, not intractable, with status epilepticus**
    - **G40.812 Lennox-Gastaut syndrome, not intractable, without status epilepticus**
    - **G40.813 Lennox-Gastaut syndrome, intractable, with status epilepticus**
    - **G40.814 Lennox-Gastaut syndrome, intractable, without status epilepticus**
  - **G40.82 Epileptic spasms**
    Infantile spasms
    Salaam attacks
    West's syndrome
    - **G40.821 Epileptic spasms, not intractable, with status epilepticus**
      Ex: See G40.001
    - **G40.822 Epileptic spasms, not intractable, without status epilepticus**
      Ex: See G40.001

G40.823 Epileptic spasms, intractable, with status epilepticus

G40.824 Epileptic spasms, intractable, without status epilepticus

G40.89 Other seizures

Excludes1 post traumatic seizures (R56.1)
recurrent seizures NOS (G40.909)
seizure NOS (R56.9)

G40.9 Epilepsy, unspecified

G40.90 Epilepsy, unspecified, not intractable
Epilepsy, unspecified, without intractability

G40.901 Epilepsy, unspecified, not intractable, with status epilepticus

G40.909 Epilepsy, unspecified, not intractable, without status epilepticus
Epilepsy NOS
Epileptic convulsions NOS
Epileptic fits NOS
Epileptic seizures NOS
Recurrent seizures NOS
Seizure disorder NOS

G40.91 Epilepsy, unspecified, intractable
Intractable seizure disorder NOS
Ex For category G40.91 CC codes: See G40.011

G40.911 Epilepsy, unspecified, intractable, with status epilepticus

G40.919 Epilepsy, unspecified, intractable, without status epilepticus

G43 Migraine

Note: The following terms are to be considered equivalent to intractable: pharmacoresistant (pharmacologically resistant), treatment resistant, refractory (medically) and poorly controlled

Use additional code for adverse effect, if applicable, to identify drug (T36-T50 with fifth or sixth character 5)

Excludes1 headache NOS (R51)
lower half migraine (G44.00)

Excludes2 headache syndromes (G44.-)

G43.0 Migraine without aura
Neurological disorder, generally recurring headaches without early symptom (aura)
Common migraine

Excludes1 chronic migraine without aura (G43.7-)

G43.00 Migraine without aura, not intractable
Neurological disorder, generally recurring headaches without early symptom (aura); resistant to cure, relief, or control
Migraine without aura without mention of refractory migraine

G43.001 Migraine without aura, not intractable, with status migrainosus

G43.009 Migraine without aura, not intractable, without status migrainosus
Migraine without aura NOS

G43.01 Migraine without aura, intractable
Intractable migraine: Not easily cured or managed; relentless pain from a migraine
Migraine without aura with refractory migraine

G43.011 Migraine without aura, intractable, with status migrainosus

G43.019 Migraine without aura, intractable, without status migrainosus

Item 6–4 Migraine headache is described as an intense pulsing or throbbing pain in one area of the head. It can be accompanied by extreme sensitivity to light (photophobic) and sound and is three times more common in women than in men. Symptoms include nausea and vomiting. Research indicates migraine headaches are caused by inherited abnormalities in genes that control the activities of certain cell populations in the brain.

G43.1 Migraine with aura
Basilar migraine
Classical migraine
Migraine equivalents
Migraine preceded or accompanied by transient focal neurological phenomena
Migraine triggered seizures
Migraine with acute-onset aura
Migraine with aura without headache (migraine equivalents)
Migraine with prolonged aura
Migraine with typical aura
Retinal migraine

Code also any associated seizure (G40.-, R56.9)

Excludes1 persistent migraine aura (G43.5-, G43.6-)

G43.10 Migraine with aura, not intractable
Migraine with aura without mention of refractory migraine

G43.101 Migraine with aura, not intractable, with status migrainosus

G43.109 Migraine with aura, not intractable, without status migrainosus
Migraine with aura NOS

G43.11 Migraine with aura, intractable
Migraine with aura with refractory migraine

G43.111 Migraine with aura, intractable, with status migrainosus

G43.119 Migraine with aura, intractable, without status migrainosus

G43.4 Hemiplegic migraine
Inherited migraine disorder causing temporary paralysis of one side of body followed by severe headache and nausea
Familial migraine
Sporadic migraine

G43.40 Hemiplegic migraine, not intractable
Hemiplegic migraine without refractory migraine

G43.401 Hemiplegic migraine, not intractable, with status migrainosus

G43.409 Hemiplegic migraine, not intractable, without status migrainosus
Hemiplegic migraine NOS

G43.41 Hemiplegic migraine, intractable
Hemiplegic migraine with refractory migraine

G43.411 Hemiplegic migraine, intractable, with status migrainosus

G43.419 Hemiplegic migraine, intractable, without status migrainosus

G43.5 Persistent migraine aura without cerebral infarction

G43.50 Persistent migraine aura without cerebral infarction, not intractable
Persistent migraine aura without cerebral infarction, without refractory migraine

G43.501 Persistent migraine aura without cerebral infarction, not intractable, with status migrainosus

G43.509 Persistent migraine aura without cerebral infarction, not intractable, without status migrainosus
Persistent migraine aura NOS

- **G43.51 Persistent migraine aura without cerebral infarction, intractable**
  Persistent migraine aura without cerebral infarction, with refractory migraine
  - **G43.511 Persistent migraine aura without cerebral infarction, intractable, with status migrainosus**
  - **G43.519 Persistent migraine aura without cerebral infarction, intractable, without status migrainosus**
- **G43.6 Persistent migraine aura with cerebral infarction**
  Visual, motor, or psychic disturbances, paresthesias, and related neurologic abnormalities accompanying migraine
  Code also the type of cerebral infarction (I63.-)
  - **G43.60 Persistent migraine aura with cerebral infarction, not intractable**
    Persistent migraine aura with cerebral infarction, without refractory migraine
    Ex: For category G43.6 CC codes: G43.601-G43.619, I63.00-I66.9
    - **G43.601 Persistent migraine aura with cerebral infarction, not intractable, with status migrainosus**
    - **G43.609 Persistent migraine aura with cerebral infarction, not intractable, without status migrainosus**
  - **G43.61 Persistent migraine aura with cerebral infarction, intractable**
    Persistent migraine aura with cerebral infarction, with refractory migraine
    - **G43.611 Persistent migraine aura with cerebral infarction, intractable, with status migrainosus**
    - **G43.619 Persistent migraine aura with cerebral infarction, intractable, without status migrainosus**
- **G43.7 Chronic migraine without aura**
  Transformed migraine
  Excludes1 migraine without aura (G43.0-)
  - **G43.70 Chronic migraine without aura, not intractable**
    Chronic migraine without aura, without refractory migraine
    - **G43.701 Chronic migraine without aura, not intractable, with status migrainosus**
    - **G43.709 Chronic migraine without aura, not intractable, without status migrainosus**
      Chronic migraine without aura NOS
  - **G43.71 Chronic migraine without aura, intractable**
    Chronic migraine without aura, with refractory migraine
    - **G43.711 Chronic migraine without aura, intractable, with status migrainosus**
    - **G43.719 Chronic migraine without aura, intractable, without status migrainosus**
- **G43.A Cyclical vomiting**
  - **G43.A0 Cyclical vomiting, not intractable**
    Cyclical vomiting, without refractory migraine
  - **G43.A1 Cyclical vomiting, intractable**
    Cyclical vomiting, with refractory migraine
- **G43.B Ophthalmoplegic migraine**
  - **G43.B0 Ophthalmoplegic migraine, not intractable**
    Ophthalmoplegic migraine, without refractory migraine
  - **G43.B1 Ophthalmoplegic migraine, intractable**
    Ophthalmoplegic migraine, with refractory migraine
- **G43.C Periodic headache syndromes in child or adult**
  - **G43.C0 Periodic headache syndromes in child or adult, not intractable**
    Periodic headache syndromes in child or adult, without refractory migraine
  - **G43.C1 Periodic headache syndromes in child or adult, intractable**
    Periodic headache syndromes in child or adult, with refractory migraine
- **G43.D Abdominal migraine**
  - **G43.D0 Abdominal migraine, not intractable**
    Abdominal migraine, without refractory migraine
  - **G43.D1 Abdominal migraine, intractable**
    Abdominal migraine, with refractory migraine
- **G43.8 Other migraine**
  - **G43.80 Other migraine, not intractable**
    Other migraine, without refractory migraine
    - **G43.801 Other migraine, not intractable, with status migrainosus**
    - **G43.809 Other migraine, not intractable, without status migrainosus**
  - **G43.81 Other migraine, intractable**
    Other migraine, with refractory migraine
    - **G43.811 Other migraine, intractable, with status migrainosus**
    - **G43.819 Other migraine, intractable, without status migrainosus**
  - **G43.82 Menstrual migraine, not intractable**
    Menstrual headache, not intractable
    Menstrual migraine, without refractory migraine
    Menstrually related migraine, not intractable
    Pre-menstrual headache, not intractable
    Pre-menstrual migraine, not intractable
    Pure menstrual migraine, not intractable
    Code also associated premenstrual tension syndrome (N94.3)
    - **G43.821 Menstrual migraine, not intractable, with status migrainosus ♀**
    - **G43.829 Menstrual migraine, not intractable, without status migrainosus ♀**
      Menstrual migraine NOS
  - **G43.83 Menstrual migraine, intractable**
    Menstrual headache, intractable
    Menstrual migraine, with refractory migraine
    Menstrually related migraine, intractable
    Pre-menstrual headache, intractable
    Pre-menstrual migraine, intractable
    Pure menstrual migraine, intractable
    Code also associated premenstrual tension syndrome (N94.3)
    - **G43.831 Menstrual migraine, intractable, with status migrainosus ♀**
    - **G43.839 Menstrual migraine, intractable, without status migrainosus ♀**
- **G43.9 Migraine, unspecified**
  - **G43.90 Migraine, unspecified, not intractable**
    Migraine, unspecified, without refractory migraine
    - **G43.901 Migraine, unspecified, not intractable, with status migrainosus**
      Status migrainosus NOS
    - **G43.909 Migraine, unspecified, not intractable, without status migrainosus**
      Migraine NOS

- **G43.91 Migraine, unspecified, intractable**
  Migraine, unspecified, with refractory migraine
  - **G43.911 Migraine, unspecified, intractable, with status migrainosus**
  - **G43.919 Migraine, unspecified, intractable, without status migrainosus**

- **G44 Other headache syndromes**
  Excludes1 headache NOS (R51)
  Excludes2 atypical facial pain (G50.1)
  headache due to lumbar puncture (G97.1)
  migraines (G43.-)
  trigeminal neuralgia (G50.0)
  - **G44.0 Cluster headaches and other trigeminal autonomic cephalgias (TAC)**
    - **G44.00 Cluster headache syndrome, unspecified**
      Ciliary neuralgia
      Cluster headache NOS
      Histamine cephalgia
      Lower half migraine
      Migrainous neuralgia
      - **G44.001 Cluster headache syndrome, unspecified, intractable**
      - **G44.009 Cluster headache syndrome, unspecified, not intractable**
        Cluster headache syndrome NOS
    - **G44.01 Episodic cluster headache**
      - **G44.011 Episodic cluster headache, intractable**
      - **G44.019 Episodic cluster headache, not intractable**
        Episodic cluster headache NOS
    - **G44.02 Chronic cluster headache**
      - **G44.021 Chronic cluster headache, intractable**
      - **G44.029 Chronic cluster headache, not intractable**
        Chronic cluster headache NOS
    - **G44.03 Episodic paroxysmal hemicrania**
      Paroxysmal hemicrania NOS
      - **G44.031 Episodic paroxysmal hemicrania, intractable**
      - **G44.039 Episodic paroxysmal hemicrania, not intractable**
        Episodic paroxysmal hemicrania NOS
    - **G44.04 Chronic paroxysmal hemicrania**
      Unilateral headache
      - **G44.041 Chronic paroxysmal hemicrania, intractable**
      - **G44.049 Chronic paroxysmal hemicrania, not intractable**
        Chronic paroxysmal hemicrania NOS
    - **G44.05 Short lasting unilateral neuralgiform headache with conjunctival injection and tearing (SUNCT)**
      - **G44.051 Short lasting unilateral neuralgiform headache with conjunctival injection and tearing (SUNCT), intractable**
      - **G44.059 Short lasting unilateral neuralgiform headache with conjunctival injection and tearing (SUNCT), not intractable**
        Short lasting unilateral neuralgiform headache with conjunctival injection and tearing (SUNCT) NOS
    - **G44.09 Other trigeminal autonomic cephalgias (TAC)**
      Cluster headaches
      - **G44.091 Other trigeminal autonomic cephalgias (TAC), intractable**
      - **G44.099 Other trigeminal autonomic cephalgias (TAC), not intractable**

G44.1 Vascular headache, not elsewhere classified
Excludes2 cluster headache (G44.0)
complicated headache syndromes (G44.5-)
drug-induced headache (G44.4-)
migraine (G43.-)
other specified headache syndromes (G44.8-)
post-traumatic headache (G44.3-)
tension-type headache (G44.2-)

- **G44.2 Tension-type headache**
  - **G44.20 Tension-type headache, unspecified**
    - **G44.201 Tension-type headache, unspecified, intractable**
    - **G44.209 Tension-type headache, unspecified, not intractable**
      Tension headache NOS
  - **G44.21 Episodic tension-type headache**
    - **G44.211 Episodic tension-type headache, intractable**
    - **G44.219 Episodic tension-type headache, not intractable**
      Episodic tension-type headache NOS
  - **G44.22 Chronic tension-type headache**
    - **G44.221 Chronic tension-type headache, intractable**
    - **G44.229 Chronic tension-type headache, not intractable**
      Chronic tension-type headache NOS
- **G44.3 Post-traumatic headache**
  - **G44.30 Post-traumatic headache, unspecified**
    - **G44.301 Post-traumatic headache, unspecified, intractable**
    - **G44.309 Post-traumatic headache, unspecified, not intractable**
      Post-traumatic headache NOS
  - **G44.31 Acute post-traumatic headache**
    - **G44.311 Acute post-traumatic headache, intractable**
    - **G44.319 Acute post-traumatic headache, not intractable**
      Acute post-traumatic headache NOS
  - **G44.32 Chronic post-traumatic headache**
    - **G44.321 Chronic post-traumatic headache, intractable**
    - **G44.329 Chronic post-traumatic headache, not intractable**
      Chronic post-traumatic headache NOS
- **G44.4 Drug-induced headache, not elsewhere classified**
  Medication overuse headache
  Use additional code for adverse effect, if applicable, to identify drug (T36-T50 with fifth or sixth character 5)
  - **G44.40 Drug-induced headache, not elsewhere classified, not intractable**
  - **G44.41 Drug-induced headache, not elsewhere classified, intractable**
- **G44.5 Complicated headache syndromes**
  - **G44.51 Hemicrania continua**
    Persistent unilateral headache
  - **G44.52 New daily persistent headache (NDPH)**
  - **G44.53 Primary thunderclap headache**
  - **G44.59 Other complicated headache syndrome**

◀ New ◀ Revised ~~deleted~~ Deleted Excludes 1 Excludes 2 Includes Use additional Code first Code also Unspecified
OGCR Official Guidelines ● Unacceptable Principal Diagnosis X Assign placeholder X ● Use Additional Character(s) ▶ Manifestation Code Coding Clinic

G44.8 Other specified headache syndromes

G44.81 Hypnic headache
Benign primary headaches

G44.82 Headache associated with sexual activity
Orgasmic headache
Preorgasmic headache

G44.83 Primary cough headache

G44.84 Primary exertional headache

G44.85 Primary stabbing headache

G44.89 Other headache syndrome

G45 Transient cerebral ischemic attacks and related syndromes

Excludes1 neonatal cerebral ischemia (P91.0)
transient retinal artery occlusion (H34.0-)

Ex: **For category G45 CC codes:** E08.51-E08.59, E08.618-E08.638, E08.649-E08.8, E09.51-E09.59, E09.618-E09.638, E09.649-E09.8, E10.51-E10.59, E10.618-E10.638, E10.649, E10.69-E10.8, E11.51-E11.59, E11.618-E11.638, E11.649, E11.69, E11.8, E13.51-E13.59, E13.618-E13.638, E13.649-E13.8, G45.0-G45.2, G45.8-G46.2, I63.00-I63.039, I63.09, I63.139, I63.19-I63.239, I63.29, I65.01-I65.9, I67.841-I67.848, I87.8-I87.9, I99.8-I99.9

G45.0 Vertebro-basilar artery syndrome

G45.1 Carotid artery syndrome (hemispheric)

G45.2 Multiple and bilateral precerebral artery syndromes

G45.3 Amaurosis fugax
Transient visual loss in one eye
Ex: G45.3, H34.00-H34.9

G45.4 Transient global amnesia
Episode of short-term memory loss, nonrecurrent, lasting few hours

Excludes1 amnesia NOS (R41.3)

G45.8 Other transient cerebral ischemic attacks and related syndromes

G45.9 Transient cerebral ischemic attack, unspecified
Spasm of cerebral artery
TIA
Transient cerebral ischemia NOS

G46 Vascular syndromes of brain in cerebrovascular diseases

Code first underlying cerebrovascular disease (I60-I69)

G46.0 Middle cerebral artery syndrome
Ex: See G45

G46.1 Anterior cerebral artery syndrome
Ex: See G45

G46.2 Posterior cerebral artery syndrome
Ex: See G45

G46.3 Brain stem stroke syndrome
Benedikt syndrome
Claude syndrome
Foville syndrome
Millard-Gubler syndrome
Wallenberg syndrome
Weber syndrome

G46.4 Cerebellar stroke syndrome

G46.5 Pure motor lacunar syndrome
Occlusion of single deep penetrating artery

G46.6 Pure sensory lacunar syndrome

G46.7 Other lacunar syndromes

G46.8 Other vascular syndromes of brain in cerebrovascular diseases

G47 Sleep disorders

Excludes2 nightmares (F51.5)
nonorganic sleep disorders (F51.-)
sleep terrors (F51.4)
sleepwalking (F51.3)

G47.0 Insomnia

Excludes2 alcohol related insomnia (F10.182, F10.282, F10.982)
drug-related insomnia (F11.182, F11.282, F11.982, F13.182, F13.282, F13.982, F14.182, F14.282, F14.982, F15.182, F15.282, F15.982, F19.182, F19.282, F19.982)
idiopathic insomnia (F51.01)
insomnia due to a mental disorder (F51.05)
insomnia not due to a substance or known physiological condition (F51.0-)
nonorganic insomnia (F51.0-)
primary insomnia (F51.01)
sleep apnea (G47.3-)

G47.00 Insomnia, unspecified
Insomnia NOS

G47.01 Insomnia due to medical condition
Code also associated medical condition

G47.09 Other insomnia

G47.1 Hypersomnia

Excludes2 alcohol-related hypersomnia (F10.182, F10.282, F10.982)
drug-related hypersomnia (F11.182, F11.282, F11.982, F13.182, F13.282, F13.982, F14.182, F14.282, F14.982, F15.182, F15.282, F15.982, F19.182, F19.282, F19.982)
hypersomnia due to a mental disorder (F51.13)
hypersomnia not due to a substance or known physiological condition (F51.1-)
primary hypersomnia (F51.11)
sleep apnea (G47.3-)

G47.10 Hypersomnia, unspecified
Hypersomnia NOS

G47.11 Idiopathic hypersomnia with long sleep time
Idiopathic hypersomnia NOS

G47.12 Idiopathic hypersomnia without long sleep time

G47.13 Recurrent hypersomnia
Kleine-Levin syndrome
Menstrual related hypersomnia

G47.14 Hypersomnia due to medical condition
Code also associated medical condition

G47.19 Other hypersomnia

G47.2 Circadian rhythm sleep disorders
Disorders of the sleep wake schedule
Inversion of nyctohemeral rhythm
Inversion of sleep rhythm

G47.20 Circadian rhythm sleep disorder, unspecified type
Sleep wake schedule disorder NOS

G47.21 Circadian rhythm sleep disorder, delayed sleep phase type
Delayed sleep phase syndrome

G47.22 Circadian rhythm sleep disorder, advanced sleep phase type

G47.23 Circadian rhythm sleep disorder, irregular sleep wake type
Irregular sleep-wake pattern

G47.24 **Circadian rhythm sleep disorder, free running type**
G47.25 **Circadian rhythm sleep disorder, jet lag type**
G47.26 **Circadian rhythm sleep disorder, shift work type**
▶ G47.27 ***Circadian rhythm sleep disorder in conditions classified elsewhere***
Code first underlying condition
G47.29 **Other circadian rhythm sleep disorder**

● G47.3 **Sleep apnea**
Characterized by episodes in which breathing stops during sleep
Code also any associated underlying condition
Excludes1 apnea NOS (R06.81)
Cheyne-Stokes breathing (R06.3)
pickwickian syndrome (E66.2)
sleep apnea of newborn (P28.3)
G47.30 **Sleep apnea, unspecified**
Sleep apnea NOS
G47.31 **Primary central sleep apnea**
G47.32 **High altitude periodic breathing**
G47.33 **Obstructive sleep apnea (adult) (pediatric)**
Excludes1 obstructive sleep apnea of newborn (P28.3)
G47.34 **Idiopathic sleep related nonobstructive alveolar hypoventilation**
Sleep related hypoxia
G47.35 **Congenital central alveolar hypoventilation syndrome**
▶ G47.36 ***Sleep related hypoventilation in conditions classified elsewhere***
Sleep related hypoxemia in conditions classified elsewhere
Code first underlying condition
▶ G47.37 ***Central sleep apnea in conditions classified elsewhere***
Code first underlying condition
G47.39 **Other sleep apnea**

● G47.4 **Narcolepsy and cataplexy**
Cataplexy *is a disorder evidenced by seizures including minor slacking of the facial muscles to complete collapse and often affects people who have* ***narcolepsy****, a disorder in which there is great difficulty remaining awake during the daytime.*
● G47.41 **Narcolepsy**
G47.411 **Narcolepsy with cataplexy**
G47.419 **Narcolepsy without cataplexy**
Narcolepsy NOS
● G47.42 **Narcolepsy in conditions classified elsewhere**
Code first underlying condition
▶ G47.421 ***Narcolepsy in conditions classified elsewhere with cataplexy***
▶ G47.429 ***Narcolepsy in conditions classified elsewhere without cataplexy***

● G47.5 **Parasomnia**
Excludes1 alcohol induced parasomnia (F10.182, F10.282, F10.982)
drug induced parasomnia (F11.182, F11.282, F11.982, F13.182, F13.282, F13.982, F14.182, F14.282, F14.982, F15.182, F15.282, F15.982, F19.182, F19.282, F19.982)
parasomnia not due to a substance or known physiological condition (F51.8)
G47.50 **Parasomnia, unspecified**
Parasomnia NOS
G47.51 **Confusional arousals**
G47.52 **REM sleep behavior disorder**
G47.53 **Recurrent isolated sleep paralysis**
▶ G47.54 ***Parasomnia in conditions classified elsewhere***
Code first underlying condition
G47.59 **Other parasomnia**

● G47.6 **Sleep related movement disorders**
Excludes2 restless legs syndrome (G25.81)
G47.61 **Periodic limb movement disorder**
Periodic limb movement disorder
G47.62 **Sleep related leg cramps**
G47.63 **Sleep related bruxism**
Excludes1 psychogenic bruxism (F45.8)
G47.69 **Other sleep related movement disorders**
G47.8 **Other sleep disorders**
G47.9 **Sleep disorder, unspecified**
Sleep disorder NOS

★ **(See Plate 118 on page 54.)**

NERVE, NERVE ROOT AND PLEXUS DISORDERS (G50-G59)

Excludes1 current traumatic nerve, nerve root and plexus disorders - see Injury, nerve by body region
neuralgia NOS (M79.2)
neuritis NOS (M79.2)
peripheral neuritis in pregnancy (O26.82-)
radiculitis NOS (M54.1-)

● G50 **Disorders of trigeminal nerve**
Includes disorders of 5th cranial nerve
G50.0 **Trigeminal neuralgia**
Syndrome of paroxysmal facial pain
Tic douloureux
G50.1 **Atypical facial pain**
G50.8 **Other disorders of trigeminal nerve**
G50.9 **Disorder of trigeminal nerve, unspecified**

● G51 **Facial nerve disorders**
Includes disorders of 7th cranial nerve
G51.0 **Bell's palsy**
Facial palsy
G51.1 **Geniculate ganglionitis**
Rare disorder with symptoms of severe pain deep in ear, spreading to ear canal, outer ear, mastoid or eye regions
Excludes1 postherpetic geniculate ganglionitis (B02.21)
G51.2 **Melkersson's syndrome**
Melkersson-Rosenthal syndrome
G51.3 **Clonic hemifacial spasm**
G51.4 **Facial myokymia**
Involuntary facial muscle movement
G51.8 **Other disorders of facial nerve**
G51.9 **Disorder of facial nerve, unspecified**

● G52 **Disorders of other cranial nerves**
Excludes2 disorders of acoustic [8th] nerve (H93.3)
disorders of optic [2nd] nerve (H46, H47.0)
paralytic strabismus due to nerve palsy (H49.0-H49.2)
G52.0 **Disorders of olfactory nerve**
Disorders of 1st cranial nerve
G52.1 **Disorders of glossopharyngeal nerve**
Disorder of 9th cranial nerve
Glossopharyngeal neuralgia
G52.2 **Disorders of vagus nerve**
Disorders of pneumogastric [10th] nerve

Item 6–5 Trigeminal neuralgia, tic douloureux, is a pain syndrome diagnosed from the patient's history alone. The condition is characterized by pain and a brief facial spasm or tic. Pain is unilateral and follows the sensory distribution of cranial nerve V, typically radiating to the maxillary (V2) or mandibular (V3) area.

Item 6–6 The most common facial nerve disorder is **Bell's Palsy,** which occurs suddenly and results in facial drooping unilaterally. This disorder is the result of a reaction to a virus that causes the facial nerve in the ear to swell resulting in pressure in the bony canal.

G52.3 Disorders of hypoglossal nerve
Disorders of 12th cranial nerve

G52.7 Disorders of multiple cranial nerves
Polyneuritis cranialis

G52.8 Disorders of other specified cranial nerves

G52.9 Cranial nerve disorder, unspecified

G53 Cranial nerve disorders in diseases classified elsewhere
Code first underlying disease, such as:
neoplasm (C00-D49)
Excludes1 multiple cranial nerve palsy in sarcoidosis (D86.82)
multiple cranial nerve palsy in syphilis (A52.15)
postherpetic geniculate ganglionitis (B02.21)
postherpetic trigeminal neuralgia (B02.22)

G54 Nerve root and plexus disorders
Raiculopathy (nerve root disorder) caused by pressure on nerve root, most common cause is herniation of intervertebral disk. Plexus disorders (plexopathies) are due to compression or injury.
Excludes1 current traumatic nerve root and plexus disorders - see nerve injury by body region
intervertebral disc disorders (M50-M51)
neuralgia or neuritis NOS (M79.2)
neuritis or radiculitis brachial NOS (M54.13)
neuritis or radiculitis lumbar NOS (M54.16)
neuritis or radiculitis lumbosacral NOS (M54.17)
neuritis or radiculitis thoracic NOS (M54.14)
radiculitis NOS (M54.10)
radiculopathy NOS (M54.10)
spondylosis (M47.-)

G54.0 Brachial plexus disorders
Thoracic outlet syndrome

G54.1 Lumbosacral plexus disorders

G54.2 Cervical root disorders, not elsewhere classified

G54.3 Thoracic root disorders, not elsewhere classified

G54.4 Lumbosacral root disorders, not elsewhere classified

G54.5 Neuralgic amyotrophy
Parsonage-Aldren-Turner syndrome
Shoulder-girdle neuritis
Excludes1 neuralgic amyotrophy in diabetes mellitus (E08-E13 with .44)

G54.6 Phantom limb syndrome with pain
Sensations (cramping, itching) in a limb that no longer exists

G54.7 Phantom limb syndrome without pain
Phantom limb syndrome NOS

G54.8 Other nerve root and plexus disorders

G54.9 Nerve root and plexus disorder, unspecified

G55 Nerve root and plexus compressions in diseases classified elsewhere
Code first underlying disease, such as:
neoplasm (C00-D49)
Excludes1 nerve root compression (due to) (in) ankylosing spondylitis (M45.-)
nerve root compression (due to) (in)dorsopathies (M53.-, M54.-)
nerve root compression (due to) (in)intervertebral disc disorders (M50.1.-, M51.1.-)
nerve root compression (due to) (in) spondylopathies (M46.-, M48.-)

★**(See Plates 472 and 473 on pages 56 and 57.)**

G56 Mononeuropathies of upper limb
Excludes1 current traumatic nerve disorder - see nerve injury by body region

G56.0 Carpal tunnel syndrome
G56.00 Carpal tunnel syndrome, unspecified upper limb
G56.01 Carpal tunnel syndrome, right upper limb
G56.02 Carpal tunnel syndrome, left upper limb
G56.03 Carpal tunnel syndrome, bilateral upper limbs ◀

G56.1 Other lesions of median nerve
G56.10 Other lesions of median nerve, unspecified side
G56.11 Other lesions of median nerve, right upper limb
G56.12 Other lesions of median nerve, left upper limb
G56.13 Other lesions of median nerve, bilateral upper limbs ◀

G56.2 Lesion of ulnar nerve
Tardy ulnar nerve palsy
G56.20 Lesion of ulnar nerve, unspecified upper limb
G56.21 Lesion of ulnar nerve, right upper limb
G56.22 Lesion of ulnar nerve, left upper limb
G56.23 Lesion of ulnar nerve, bilateral upper limbs ◀

G56.3 Lesion of radial nerve
G56.30 Lesion of radial nerve, unspecified upper limb
G56.31 Lesion of radial nerve, right upper limb
G56.32 Lesion of radial nerve, left upper limb
G56.33 Lesion of radial nerve, bilateral upper limbs ◀

G56.4 Causalgia of upper limb
Intense burning pain and sensitivity to slight touch
Complex regional pain syndrome II of upper limb
Excludes1 complex regional pain syndrome I of lower limb (G90.52-)
complex regional pain syndrome I of upper limb (G90.51-)
complex regional pain syndrome II of lower limb (G57.7-)
reflex sympathetic dystrophy of lower limb (G90.52-)
reflex sympathetic dystrophy (G90.51-)
G56.40 Causalgia of unspecified upper limb
G56.41 Causalgia of right upper limb
G56.42 Causalgia of left upper limb
G56.43 Causalgia of bilateral upper limbs ◀

G56.8 Other specified mononeuropathies of upper limb
Disease of a single nerve
Interdigital neuroma of upper limb
G56.80 Other specified mononeuropathies of unspecified upper limb
G56.81 Other specified mononeuropathies of right upper limb
G56.82 Other specified mononeuropathies of left upper limb
G56.83 Other specified mononeuropathies of bilateral upper limbs ◀

G56.9 Unspecified mononeuropathy of upper limb
Disease of a single nerve
G56.90 Unspecified mononeuropathy of unspecified upper limb
G56.91 Unspecified mononeuropathy of right upper limb
G56.92 Unspecified mononeuropathy of left upper limb
G56.93 Unspecified mononeuropathy of bilateral upper limbs ◀

● **G57 Mononeuropathies of lower limb**

Excludes1 current traumatic nerve disorder - see nerve injury by body region

★ **(See Plates 544 and 545 on pages 58 and 59.)**

● **G57.0 Lesion of sciatic nerve**

Excludes1 sciatica NOS (M54.3-)

Excludes2 sciatica attributed to intervertebral disc disorder (M51.1.-)

G57.00 Lesion of sciatic nerve, unspecified lower limb

G57.01 Lesion of sciatic nerve, right lower limb

G57.02 Lesion of sciatic nerve, left lower limb

G57.03 Lesion of sciatic nerve, bilateral lower limbs ◀

● **G57.1 Meralgia paresthetica**

Numbness or pain in outer thigh caused by injury to nerve

Lateral cutaneous nerve of thigh syndrome

G57.10 Meralgia paresthetica, unspecified lower limb

G57.11 Meralgia paresthetica, right lower limb

G57.12 Meralgia paresthetica, left lower limb

G57.13 Meralgia paresthetica, bilateral lower limbs ◀

● **G57.2 Lesion of femoral nerve**

G57.20 Lesion of femoral nerve, unspecified lower limb

G57.21 Lesion of femoral nerve, right lower limb

G57.22 Lesion of femoral nerve, left lower limb

G57.23 Lesion of femoral nerve, bilateral lower limbs ◀

● **G57.3 Lesion of lateral popliteal nerve**

Peroneal nerve palsy

G57.30 Lesion of lateral popliteal nerve, unspecified lower limb

G57.31 Lesion of lateral popliteal nerve, right lower limb

G57.32 Lesion of lateral popliteal nerve, left lower limb

G57.33 Lesion of lateral popliteal nerve, bilateral lower limbs ◀

● **G57.4 Lesion of medial popliteal nerve**

G57.40 Lesion of medial popliteal nerve, unspecified lower limb

G57.41 Lesion of medial popliteal nerve, right lower limb

G57.42 Lesion of medial popliteal nerve, left lower limb

G57.43 Lesion of medial popliteal nerve, bilateral lower limbs ◀

● **G57.5 Tarsal tunnel syndrome**

G57.50 Tarsal tunnel syndrome, unspecified lower limb

G57.51 Tarsal tunnel syndrome, right lower limb

G57.52 Tarsal tunnel syndrome, left lower limb

G57.53 Tarsal tunnel syndrome, bilateral lower limbs ◀

● **G57.6 Lesion of plantar nerve**

Morton's metatarsalgia

G57.60 Lesion of plantar nerve, unspecified lower limb

G57.61 Lesion of plantar nerve, right lower limb

G57.62 Lesion of plantar nerve, left lower limb

G57.63 Lesion of plantar nerve, bilateral lower limbs ◀

● **G57.7 Causalgia of lower limb**

Complex regional pain syndrome II of lower limb

Excludes1 complex regional pain syndrome I of lower limb (G90.52-)
complex regional pain syndrome I of upper limb (G90.51-)
complex regional pain syndrome II of upper limb (G56.4-)
reflex sympathetic dystrophy of lower limb (G90.52-)
reflex sympathetic dystrophy of upper limb (G90.51-)

G57.70 Causalgia of unspecified lower limb

G57.71 Causalgia of right lower limb

G57.72 Causalgia of left lower limb

G57.73 Causalgia of bilateral lower limbs ◀

● **G57.8 Other specified mononeuropathies of lower limb**

Interdigital neuroma of lower limb

G57.80 Other specified mononeuropathies of unspecified lower limb

G57.81 Other specified mononeuropathies of right lower limb

G57.82 Other specified mononeuropathies of left lower limb

G57.83 Other specified mononeuropathies of bilateral lower limbs ◀

● **G57.9 Unspecified mononeuropathy of lower limb**

G57.90 Unspecified mononeuropathy of unspecified lower limb

G57.91 Unspecified mononeuropathy of right lower limb

G57.92 Unspecified mononeuropathy of left lower limb

G57.93 Unspecified mononeuropathy of bilateral lower limbs ◀

● **G58 Other mononeuropathies**

G58.0 Intercostal neuropathy

G58.7 Mononeuritis multiplex

G58.8 Other specified mononeuropathies

G58.9 Mononeuropathy, unspecified

▶ ***G59 Mononeuropathy in diseases classified elsewhere***

Code first underlying disease

Excludes1 diabetic mononeuropathy (E08-E13 with .41)
syphilitic nerve paralysis (A52.19)
syphilitic neuritis (A52.15)
tuberculous mononeuropathy (A17.83)

POLYNEUROPATHIES AND OTHER DISORDERS OF THE PERIPHERAL NERVOUS SYSTEM (G60-G65)

Excludes1 neuralgia NOS (M79.2)
neuritis NOS (M79.2)
peripheral neuritis in pregnancy (O26.82-)
radiculitis NOS (M54.10)

● **G60 Hereditary and idiopathic neuropathy**

G60.0 Hereditary motor and sensory neuropathy

Charcot-Marie-Tooth disease
Déjerine-Sottas disease
Hereditary motor and sensory neuropathy, types I-IV
Hypertrophic neuropathy of infancy
Peroneal muscular atrophy (axonal type) (hypertrophic type)
Roussy-Lévy syndrome

G60.1 Refsum's disease

Genetic disorder affecting fatty acid metabolism

Infantile Refsum disease

Exc E11.42, G13.0, G13.1, G50.0-G65.2, M34.83

G60.2 Neuropathy in association with hereditary ataxia

G60.3 Idiopathic progressive neuropathy

G60.8 Other hereditary and idiopathic neuropathies

Dominantly inherited sensory neuropathy
Morvan's disease
Nelaton's syndrome
Recessively inherited sensory neuropathy

G60.9 Hereditary and idiopathic neuropathy, unspecified

● **G61 Inflammatory polyneuropathy**

G61.0 Guillain-Barré syndrome

Autoimmune disease affecting peripheral nervous system

Acute (post-)infective polyneuritis
Miller Fisher Syndrome

Exc A02.21, A17.0-A17.1, A27.81, A39.0, A39.89-A39.9, A49.3-A49.9, A50.41, A51.41, A52.13, A54.82, A54.84, A54.89-A54.9, A87.0-A87.9, B00.3, B02.1, B26.1, B37.5, B38.4, B45.1, B58.2, B92, B94.2-B94.9, B96.0, B96.6-B96.89, G00.0-G03.9, G04.2, G32.89, G61.0, G96.8-G96.9, G98.0-G98.8, G99.8

G61.1 Serum neuropathy

Use additional code for adverse effect, if applicable, to identify serum (T50.-)

Item 6-7 The **peripheral nervous system** consists of 31 pairs of spinal nerves, 12 pairs of cranial nerves, and the autonomic nerves, which are divided into the parasympathetic and sympathetic nerves. The cranial nerves are: olfactory (I), optic (II), oculomotor (III), trochlear (IV), trigeminal (V), abducens (VI), facial (VII), vestibulocochlear (VIII), glossopharyngeal (IX), vagus (X), accessory (XI), and hypoglossal (XII).

● **G61.8 Other inflammatory polyneuropathies**

G61.81 Chronic inflammatory demyelinating polyneuritis CC
Ex: G51.0-G54.5, G54.8-G60.9, G61.81-G61.89, G62.81-G62.89, G64

G61.82 Multifocal motor neuropathy ◀
MMN ◀

G61.89 Other inflammatory polyneuropathies

G61.9 Inflammatory polyneuropathy, unspecified

● **G62 Other and unspecified polyneuropathies**

G62.0 Drug-induced polyneuropathy
Use additional code for adverse effect, if applicable, to identify drug (T36-T50 with fifth or sixth character 5)

G62.1 Alcoholic polyneuropathy
Malfunction of many peripheral nerves throughout the body

G62.2 Polyneuropathy due to other toxic agents
Code first (T51-T65) to identify toxic agent

● **G62.8 Other specified polyneuropathies**

G62.81 Critical illness polyneuropathy CC
Acute motor neuropathy
Ex: G51.0-G54.5, G54.8-G60.9, G61.81-G61.9, G62.81, G62.89-G62.9, G64

G62.82 Radiation-induced polyneuropathy
Use additional external cause code (W88-W90, X39.0-) to identify cause

G62.89 Other specified polyneuropathies
Coding Clinic: 2016, Q2, P11

G62.9 Polyneuropathy, unspecified
Neuropathy NOS

▶ ***G63 Polyneuropathy in diseases classified elsewhere***
Code first underlying disease, such as:
amyloidosis (E85.-)
endocrine disease, except diabetes (E00-E07, E15-E16, E20-E34)
metabolic diseases (E70-E88)
neoplasm (C00-D49)
nutritional deficiency (E40-E64)

Excludes1 polyneuropathy (in):
diabetes mellitus (E08-E13 with .42)
diphtheria (A36.83)
infectious mononucleosis (B27.0-B27.9 with 1)
Lyme disease (A69.22)
mumps (B26.84)
postherpetic (B02.23)
rheumatoid arthritis (M05.33)
scleroderma (M34.83)
systemic lupus erythematosus (M32.19)

Coding Clinic: 2012, Q4, P100

G64 Other disorders of peripheral nervous system
Disorder of peripheral nervous system NOS

● **G65 Sequelae of inflammatory and toxic polyneuropathies**
Code first condition resulting from (sequela) of inflammatory and toxic polyneuropathies

G65.0 Sequelae of Guillain-Barré syndrome

G65.1 Sequelae of other inflammatory polyneuropathy

G65.2 Sequelae of toxic polyneuropathy

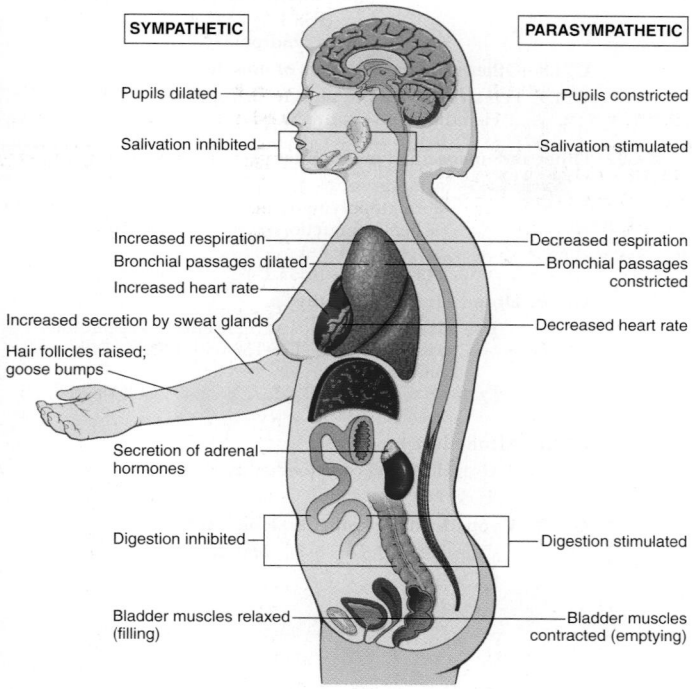

Figure 6-2 Actions of parasympathetic and sympathetic nerves. (From Chabner: The Language of Medicine, ed 9, St. Louis, Saunders, 2011)

DISEASES OF MYONEURAL JUNCTION AND MUSCLE (G70-G73)

G70 Myasthenia gravis and other myoneural disorders

Excludes1 botulism (A05.1, A48.51-A48.52)
transient neonatal myasthenia gravis (P94.0)

G70.0 Myasthenia gravis

Acquired and results in fatigable muscle weakness exacerbated by activity and improved with rest

G70.00 Myasthenia gravis without (acute) exacerbation
Myasthenia gravis NOS

G70.01 Myasthenia gravis with (acute) exacerbation
Myasthenia gravis in crisis
Ex: E08.40-E08.49, E08.618-E08.638, E08.649-E08.8, E09.40-E09.49, E09.618-E09.638, E09.649-E09.8, E10.40-E10.49, E10.618-E10.638, E10.649, E10.69-E10.8, E11.40-E11.49, E11.618-E11.638, E11.649, E11.69-E11.8, E13.40-E13.49, E13.618-E13.638, E13.649-E13.8, G32.89, G70.00-G70.01, G70.80-G70.81, G73.1-G73.3, G96.8-G96.9, G98.0-G98.8, G99.8

G70.1 Toxic myoneural disorders

Dysfunction at junction of muscle and motor nerve (myoneural junction)

Code first (T51-T65) to identify toxic agent

G70.2 Congenital and developmental myasthenia

G70.8 Other specified myoneural disorders

G70.80 Lambert-Eaton syndrome, unspecified
Lambert-Eaton syndrome NOS
Ex: See G70.01

G70.81 Lambert-Eaton syndrome in disease classified elsewhere

Code first underlying disease

Excludes1 Lambert-Eaton syndrome in neoplastic disease (G73.1)

Ex: See G70.01

G70.89 Other specified myoneural disorders

G70.9 Myoneural disorder, unspecified

G71 Primary disorders of muscles

Excludes2 arthrogryposis multiplex congenita (Q74.3)
metabolic disorders (E70-E88)
myositis (M60.-)

G71.0 Muscular dystrophy

Autosomal recessive, childhood type, muscular dystrophy resembling Duchenne or Becker muscular dystrophy
Benign [Becker] muscular dystrophy
Benign scapuloperoneal muscular dystrophy with early contractures [Emery-Dreifuss]
Congenital muscular dystrophy NOS
Congenital muscular dystrophy with specific morphological abnormalities of the muscle fiber
Distal muscular dystrophy
Facioscapulohumeral muscular dystrophy
Limb-girdle muscular dystrophy
Ocular muscular dystrophy
Oculopharyngeal muscular dystrophy
Scapuloperoneal muscular dystrophy
Severe [Duchenne] muscular dystrophy
Ex: E08.40-E08.49, E08.618-E08.638, E08.649-E08.8, E09.40-E09.49, E09.618-E09.638, E09.649-E09.8, E10.40-E10.49, E10.618-E10.638, E10.649, E10.69-E10.8, E11.40-E11.49, E11.618-E11.638, E11.649, E11.69-E11.8, E13.40-E13.49, E13.618-E13.638, E13.649-E13.8, G32.89, G71.0, G71.2, G96.8-G96.9, G98.0-G98.8, G99.8

Item 6–8 Muscular dystrophies (MD) are a group of rare inherited muscle diseases. Voluntary muscles become progressively weaker. In the late stages of MD, fat and connective tissue replace muscle fibers. In some types of muscular dystrophy, heart muscles, other involuntary muscles, and other organs are affected. **Myopathies** is a general term for neuromuscular diseases in which the muscle fibers dysfunction for any one of many reasons, resulting in muscular weakness.

G71.1 Myotonic disorders

Inherited disorder that affects muscles tone

G71.11 Myotonic muscular dystrophy
Dystrophia myotonica [Steinert]
Myotonia atrophica
Myotonic dystrophy
Proximal myotonic myopathy (PROMM)
Steinert disease

G71.12 Myotonia congenita
Acetazolamide responsive myotonia congenita
Dominant myotonia congenita [Thomsen disease]
Myotonia levior
Recessive myotonia congenita [Becker disease]

G71.13 Myotonic chondrodystrophy
Chondrodystrophic myotonia
Congenital myotonic chondrodystrophy
Schwartz-Jampel disease

G71.14 Drug induced myotonia

Use additional code for adverse effect, if applicable, to identify drug (T36-T50 with fifth or sixth character 5)

G71.19 Other specified myotonic disorders
Myotonia fluctuans
Myotonia permanens
Neuromyotonia [Isaacs]
Paramyotonia congenita (of von Eulenburg)
Pseudomyotonia
Symptomatic myotonia

G71.2 Congenital myopathies
Central core disease
Fiber-type disproportion
Minicore disease
Multicore disease
Myotubular (centronuclear) myopathy
Nemaline myopathy

Excludes1 arthrogryposis multiplex congenita (Q74.3)

Ex: See G71.0

G71.3 Mitochondrial myopathy, not elsewhere classified

Myopathies associated with increased number of enlarged, often abnormal, mitochondria in muscle fibers

Excludes1 Kearns-Sayre syndrome (H49.81)
Leber's disease (H47.21)
Leigh's encephalopathy (G31.82)
mitochondrial metabolism disorders (E88.4.-)
Reye's syndrome (G93.7)

G71.8 Other primary disorders of muscles

G71.9 Primary disorder of muscle, unspecified
Hereditary myopathy NOS

G72 Other and unspecified myopathies

Excludes1 arthrogryposis multiplex congenita (Q74.3)
dermatopolymyositis (M33.-)
ischemic infarction of muscle (M62.2-)
myositis (M60.-)
polymyositis (M33.2.-)

G72.0 Drug-induced myopathy

Use additional code for adverse effect, if applicable, to identify drug (T36-T50 with fifth or sixth character 5)

Ex: G32.89, G70.00-G71.0, G71.11-G72.3, G72.81-G73.7, G96.8-G96.9, G98.0-G98.8, G99.8

G72.1 Alcoholic myopathy

Use additional code to identify alcoholism (F10.-)

Ex: See G72.0

G72.2 Myopathy due to other toxic agents

Code first (T51-T65) to identify toxic agent

Ex: See G72.0

G72.3 Periodic paralysis
Familial periodic paralysis
Hyperkalemic periodic paralysis (familial)
Hypokalemic periodic paralysis (familial)
Myotonic periodic paralysis (familial)
Normokalemic paralysis (familial)
Potassium sensitive periodic paralysis
Excludes1 paramyotonia congenita (of von Eulenburg) (G71.19)

G72.4 Inflammatory and immune myopathies, not elsewhere classified
G72.41 Inclusion body myositis [IBM]
G72.49 Other inflammatory and immune myopathies, not elsewhere classified
Inflammatory myopathy NOS

G72.8 Other specified myopathies
G72.81 Critical illness myopathy
Acute necrotizing myopathy
Acute quadriplegic myopathy
Intensive care (ICU) myopathy
Myopathy of critical illness
Ex: G70.1-G72.3, G72.81-G73.7
G72.89 Other specified myopathies

G72.9 Myopathy, unspecified

G73 Disorders of myoneural junction and muscle in diseases classified elsewhere
Ex: For category G73 CC codes: See G70.01

G73.1 Lambert-Eaton syndrome in neoplastic disease
Rare autoimmune disorder affecting calcium channels of nerve-muscle (neuromuscular) junction
Code first underlying neoplasm (C00-D49)
Excludes1 Lambert-Eaton syndrome not associated with neoplasm (G70.80-G70.81)

G73.3 Myasthenic syndromes in other diseases classified elsewhere
Code first underlying disease, such as:
neoplasm (C00-D49)
thyrotoxicosis (E05.-)

G73.7 Myopathy in diseases classified elsewhere
Code first underlying disease, such as:
hyperparathyroidism (E21.0, E21.3)
hypoparathyroidism (E20.-)
glycogen storage disease (E74.0)
lipid storage disorders (E75.-)
Excludes1 myopathy in:
rheumatoid arthritis (M05.32)
sarcoidosis (D86.87)
scleroderma (M34.82)
sicca syndrome [Sjögren] (M35.03)
systemic lupus erythematosus (M32.19)

CEREBRAL PALSY AND OTHER PARALYTIC SYNDROMES (G80-G83)

G80 Cerebral palsy
Excludes1 hereditary spastic paraplegia (G11.4)

G80.0 Spastic quadriplegic cerebral palsy
Congenital spastic paralysis (cerebral)
Ex: E08.40-E08.49, E08.618-E08.638, E08.649-E08.8, E09.40-E09.49, E09.618-E09.638, E09.649-E09.8, E10.40-E10.49, E10.618-E10.638, E10.649, E10.69-E10.8, E11.40-E11.49, E11.618-E11.638, E11.649, E11.69-E11.8, E13.40-E13.49, E13.618-E13.638, E13.649-E13.8, G04.1, G32.89, G80.0-G80.2, G80.4-G83.9, G90.1, G93.81, G93.89-G93.9, G96.8-G96.9, G98.0-G98.8, G99.8, Q06.0-Q06.1, Q06.3, Q06.8-Q06.9, Q07.8-Q07.9, R53.2

G80.1 Spastic diplegic cerebral palsy
Spastic cerebral palsy NOS
Ex: G80.1, G93.40-G93.49, I67.83

G80.2 Spastic hemiplegic cerebral palsy
Ex: G80.2, G93.40-G93.49, I67.83

G80.3 Athetoid cerebral palsy
Result of damage to cerebellum or basal ganglia responsible for processing neuromuscular signals
Double athetosis (syndrome)
Dyskinetic cerebral palsy
Dystonic cerebral palsy
Vogt disease
Ex: G20, G21.11-G21.9, G25.70-G25.79, G25.89-G26, G80.0-G80.9, G93.40-G93.49, I67.83

G80.4 Ataxic cerebral palsy
Poor muscle tone and coordination

G80.8 Other cerebral palsy
Mixed cerebral palsy syndromes

G80.9 Cerebral palsy, unspecified
Cerebral palsy NOS

OGCR Section I.C.6.a.

Dominant/nondominant side
Codes from category G81, Hemiplegia and hemiparesis, and subcategories, G83.1, Monoplegia of lower limb, G83.2, Monoplegia of upper limb, and G83.3, Monoplegia, unspecified, identify whether the dominant and nondominant side is affected. Should the affected side be documented, but not specified as dominant or nondominant, and the classification system does not indicate a default, code selection is as follows:
- For ambidextrous patients, the default should be dominant.
- If the left side is affected, the default is non-dominant.
- If the right side is affected, the default is dominant.

G81 Hemiplegia and hemiparesis
Note: This category is to be used only when hemiplegia (complete)(incomplete) is reported without further specification, or is stated to be old or longstanding but of unspecified cause. The category is also for use in multiple coding to identify these types of hemiplegia resulting from any cause.
Excludes1 congenital cerebral palsy (G80.-)
hemiplegia and hemiparesis due to sequela of cerebrovascular disease (I69.05-, I69.15-, I69.25-, I69.35-, I69.85-, I69.95-)
Ex: For category G81 CC codes: G04.1, G11.0-G12.9, G32.0-G37.3, G37.5-G37.9, G80.0-G80.2, G80.4-G80.9, G81.00-G83.9, G90.01-G90.09, G90.2, G90.4, G90.50-G90.9, G92, G93.40-G93.49, G93.81, G93.89-G95.9, G96.8-G96.9, G98.0-G99.8, I67.83, R53.2
Coding Clinic: 2012, Q4, P106

G81.0 Flaccid hemiplegia
Paralysis of half of body with loss of tone of muscles of paralyzed part and absence of tendon reflexes
G81.00 Flaccid hemiplegia affecting unspecified side
G81.01 Flaccid hemiplegia affecting right dominant side
G81.02 Flaccid hemiplegia affecting left dominant side
G81.03 Flaccid hemiplegia affecting right nondominant side
G81.04 Flaccid hemiplegia affecting left nondominant side

Item 6–9 Hemiplegia is complete paralysis of one side of the body—arm, leg, and trunk. **Hemiparesis** is a generalized weakness or incomplete paralysis of one side of the body. If most activities (eating, writing) are performed with the right hand, the right is the dominant side, and the left is the nondominant side. **Quadriplegia,** also called tetraplegia, is the complete paralysis of all four limbs. **Quadriparesis** is the incomplete paralysis of all four limbs. Nerve damage in C1–C4 is associated with lower limb paralysis, and C5–C7 damage is associated with upper limb paralysis. **Diplegia** is the paralysis of the upper limbs. **Monoplegia** is the complete paralysis of one limb.

● **G81.1 Spastic hemiplegia**
Paralysis of half of body with spasticity of muscles of paralyzed part and increased tendon reflexes

G81.10 Spastic hemiplegia affecting unspecified side
G81.11 Spastic hemiplegia affecting right dominant side
G81.12 Spastic hemiplegia affecting left dominant side
G81.13 Spastic hemiplegia affecting right nondominant side
G81.14 Spastic hemiplegia affecting left nondominant side

● **G81.9 Hemiplegia, unspecified**

G81.90 Hemiplegia, unspecified affecting unspecified side
G81.91 Hemiplegia, unspecified affecting right dominant side
G81.92 Hemiplegia, unspecified affecting left dominant side
G81.93 Hemiplegia, unspecified affecting right nondominant side
G81.94 Hemiplegia, unspecified affecting left nondominant side
Coding Clinic: 2015, Q1, P26

● **G82 Paraplegia (paraparesis) and quadriplegia (quadriparesis)**

Note: This category is to be used only when the listed conditions are reported without further specification, or are stated to be old or longstanding but of unspecified cause. The category is also for use in multiple coding to identify these conditions resulting from any cause.

Excludes1 congenital cerebral palsy (G80.-)
functional quadriplegia (R53.2)
hysterical paralysis (F44.4)

● **G82.2 Paraplegia**
Paralysis of both lower limbs NOS
Paraparesis (lower) NOS
Paraplegia (lower) NOS
Ex: **For category G82.2 CC codes:** See G81

G82.20 Paraplegia, unspecified
G82.21 Paraplegia, complete
G82.22 Paraplegia, incomplete

● **G82.5 Quadriplegia**
Paralysis of all limbs; AKA tetraplegia
Ex: See G80.0

G82.50 Quadriplegia, unspecified
G82.51 Quadriplegia, C1-C4 complete
G82.52 Quadriplegia, C1-C4 incomplete
G82.53 Quadriplegia, C5-C7 complete
G82.54 Quadriplegia, C5-C7 incomplete

● **G83 Other paralytic syndromes**

Note: This category is to be used only when the listed conditions are reported without further specification, or are stated to be old or longstanding but of unspecified cause. The category is also for use in multiple coding to identify these conditions resulting from any cause.

Includes paralysis (complete) (incomplete), except as in G80-G82

G83.0 Diplegia of upper limbs
Paralysis affecting limbs on both sides; AKA bilateral paralysis
Diplegia (upper)
Paralysis of both upper limbs
Ex: G32.89, G82.50-G83.0, G83.5-G83.9, G96.8-G96.9, G98.0-G98.8, G99.8, R53.2

● **G83.1 Monoplegia of lower limb**
Paralysis of limb on one side
Paralysis of lower limb

Excludes1 monoplegia of lower limbs due to sequela of cerebrovascular disease (I69.04-, I69.14-, I69.24-, I69.34-, I69.84-, I69.94-)
Coding Clinic: 2012, Q4, P106

G83.10 Monoplegia of lower limb affecting unspecified side
G83.11 Monoplegia of lower limb affecting right dominant side
G83.12 Monoplegia of lower limb affecting left dominant side
G83.13 Monoplegia of lower limb affecting right nondominant side
G83.14 Monoplegia of lower limb affecting left nondominant side

● **G83.2 Monoplegia of upper limb**
Paralysis of upper limb

Excludes1 monoplegia of upper limbs due to sequela of cerebrovascular disease (I69.03-, I69.13-, I69.23-, I69.33-, I69.83-, I69.93-)
Coding Clinic: 2012, Q4, P106

G83.20 Monoplegia of upper limb affecting unspecified side
G83.21 Monoplegia of upper limb affecting right dominant side
G83.22 Monoplegia of upper limb affecting left dominant side
G83.23 Monoplegia of upper limb affecting right nondominant side
G83.24 Monoplegia of upper limb affecting left nondominant side

● **G83.3 Monoplegia, unspecified**
Coding Clinic: 2012, Q4, P106

G83.30 Monoplegia, unspecified affecting unspecified side
G83.31 Monoplegia, unspecified affecting right dominant side
G83.32 Monoplegia, unspecified affecting left dominant side
G83.33 Monoplegia, unspecified affecting right nondominant side
G83.34 Monoplegia, unspecified affecting left nondominant side

G83.4 Cauda equina syndrome
Aching pain due to compression of spinal nerve roots
Neurogenic bladder due to cauda equina syndrome

Excludes1 cord bladder NOS (G95.89)
neurogenic bladder NOS (N31.9)
Ex: G04.1, G32.89, G82.20-G82.54, G83.10-G83.14, G83.4-G83.9, G96.8-G96.9, G98.0-G98.8, G99.8, R53.2

G83.5 Locked-in state
Ex: G04.1, G32.89, G80.0-G83.9, G92, G93.40-G93.49, G93.81, G93.89-G93.9, G96.8-G96.9, G98.0-G98.8, G99.8, I67.83, R53.2

● **G83.8 Other specified paralytic syndromes**

Excludes1 paralytic syndromes due to current spinal cord injury-code to spinal cord injury (S14, S24, S34)

G83.81 Brown-Séquard syndrome
G83.82 Anterior cord syndrome
G83.83 Posterior cord syndrome
G83.84 Todd's paralysis (postepileptic)
G83.89 Other specified paralytic syndromes

G83.9 Paralytic syndrome, unspecified

OTHER DISORDERS OF THE NERVOUS SYSTEM (G89-G99)

G89 Pain, not elsewhere classified

Code also related psychological factors associated with pain (F45.42)

Excludes1 generalized pain NOS (R52)
pain disorders exclusively related to psychological factors (F45.41)
pain NOS (R52)

Excludes2 atypical face pain (G50.1)
headache syndromes (G44.-)
localized pain, unspecified type - code to pain by site, such as:
abdomen pain (R10.-)
back pain (M54.9)
breast pain (N64.4)
chest pain (R07.1-R07.9)
ear pain (H92.0-)
eye pain (H57.1)
headache (R51)
joint pain (M25.5-)
limb pain (M79.6-)
lumbar region pain (M54.5)
painful urination (R30.9)
pelvic and perineal pain (R10.2)
shoulder pain (M25.51-)
spine pain (M54.-)
throat pain (R07.0)
tongue pain (K14.6)
tooth pain (K08.8)
renal colic (N23)
migraines (G43.-)
myalgia (M79.1)
pain from prosthetic devices, implants, and grafts (T82.84, T83.84, T84.84, T85.84-)
phantom limb syndrome with pain (G54.6)
vulvar vestibulitis (N94.810)
vulvodynia (N94.81-)

G89.0 Central pain syndrome
Neurological condition causing intractable pain resulting from damage to CNS
Déjérine-Roussy syndrome
Myelopathic pain syndrome
Thalamic pain syndrome (hyperesthetic)

G89.1 Acute pain, not elsewhere classified

G89.11 Acute pain due to trauma

G89.12 Acute post-thoracotomy pain
Post-thoracotomy pain NOS

G89.18 Other acute postprocedural pain
Postoperative pain NOS
Postprocedural pain NOS

G89.2 Chronic pain, not elsewhere classified

Excludes1 causalgia, lower limb (G57.7-)
causalgia, upper limb (G56.4-)
central pain syndrome (G89.0)
chronic pain syndrome (G89.4)
complex regional pain syndrome II, lower limb (G57.7-)
complex regional pain syndrome II, upper limb (G56.4-)
neoplasm related chronic pain (G89.3)
reflex sympathetic dystrophy (G90.5-)

G89.21 Chronic pain due to trauma

G89.22 Chronic post-thoracotomy pain

G89.28 Other chronic postprocedural pain
Other chronic postoperative pain

G89.29 Other chronic pain

G89.3 Neoplasm related pain (acute) (chronic)
Cancer associated pain
Pain due to malignancy (primary) (secondary)
Tumor associated pain

G89.4 Chronic pain syndrome
Chronic pain associated with significant psychosocial dysfunction

G90 Disorders of autonomic nervous system

Excludes1 dysfunction of the autonomic nervous system due to alcohol (G31.2)

G90.0 Idiopathic peripheral autonomic neuropathy

G90.01 Carotid sinus syncope
Carotid sinus syndrome

G90.09 Other idiopathic peripheral autonomic neuropathy
Idiopathic peripheral autonomic neuropathy NOS

G90.1 Familial dysautonomia [Riley-Day]
Inherited disorder that affects nerve function

G90.2 Horner's syndrome
Due to damage of the sympathetic nervous system
Bernard(-Horner) syndrome
Cervical sympathetic dystrophy or paralysis

G90.3 Multi-system degeneration of the autonomic nervous system
Neurogenic orthostatic hypotension [Shy-Drager]

Excludes1 orthostatic hypotension NOS (I95.1)

Ex: G20, G21.11-G21.9, G90.01-G90.09, G93.40-G93.49, I67.83

G90.4 Autonomic dysreflexia
Syndrome resulting from lesions of spinal cord

Use additional code to identify the cause, such as:
fecal impaction (K56.41)
pressure ulcer (pressure area) (L89.-)
urinary tract infection (N39.0)

G90.5 Complex regional pain syndrome I (CRPS I)
Reflex sympathetic dystrophy

Excludes1 causalgia of lower limb (G57.7-)
causalgia of upper limb (G56.4-)
complex regional pain syndrome II of lower limb (G57.7-)
complex regional pain syndrome II of upper limb (G56.4-)

Ex: **For category G90.5 CC codes unless otherwise indicated:**
E08.40-E08.49, E09.40-E09.49, E10.40-E10.49, E11.40-E11.49, E13.40-E13.49, G04.1, G11.3, G11.8-G12.9, G32.0, G32.89-G37.3, G37.5-G37.9, G80.0-G80.2, G80.4-G83.9, G90.01-G90.09, G90.2, G90.4-G90.9, G93.1, G93.40-G93.49, G95.0-G95.9, G96.12-G96.9, G97.1, G98.0-G99.8, I67.83, R53.2

G90.50 Complex regional pain syndrome I, unspecified
Ex: G90.50-G90.59

G90.51 Complex regional pain syndrome I of upper limb

G90.511 Complex regional pain syndrome I of right upper limb

G90.512 Complex regional pain syndrome I of left upper limb

G90.513 Complex regional pain syndrome I of upper limb, bilateral

G90.519 Complex regional pain syndrome I of unspecified upper limb

G90.52 Complex regional pain syndrome I of lower limb

G90.521 Complex regional pain syndrome I of right lower limb

G90.522 Complex regional pain syndrome I of left lower limb

G90.523 Complex regional pain syndrome I of lower limb, bilateral

G90.529 Complex regional pain syndrome I of unspecified lower limb

G90.59 Complex regional pain syndrome I of other specified site

G90.8 Other disorders of autonomic nervous system

G90.9 Disorder of the autonomic nervous system, unspecified

G91 Hydrocephalus
Dilatation of cerebral ventricles, accompanied by accumulation of cerebrospinal fluid
Includes acquired hydrocephalus
Excludes1 Arnold-Chiari syndrome with hydrocephalus (Q07.-)
congenital hydrocephalus (Q03.-)
spina bifida with hydrocephalus (Q05.-)
Ex: **For category G91 CC codes unless otherwise indicated:** E08.40-E08.49, E08.618-E08.638, E08.649-E08.8, E09.40-E09.49, E09.618-E09.638, E09.649-E09.8, E10.40-E10.49, E10.618-E10.638, E10.649, E10.69-E10.8, E11.40-E11.49, E11.618-E11.638, E11.649, E11.69-E11.8, E13.40-E13.49, E13.618-E13.638, E13.649-E13.8, G13.2-G13.8, G31.2, G31.83-G31.9, G90.1, G91.0-G91.9, G93.81, G93.89-G94, Q03.0-Q03.9, Q04.4-Q04.8, Q05.0-Q05.4, Q05.9-Q06.1, Q06.3, Q06.8-Q06.9, Q07.02-Q07.9

G91.0 Communicating hydrocephalus
Secondary normal pressure hydrocephalus
Ex: G91.0-G91.3, G91.8-G91.9

G91.1 Obstructive hydrocephalus

G91.2 (Idiopathic) normal pressure hydrocephalus
Normal pressure hydrocephalus NOS
Ex: G91.0-G91.3, G91.8-G91.9

G91.3 Post-traumatic hydrocephalus, unspecified

G91.4 Hydrocephalus in diseases classified elsewhere
Code first underlying condition, such as:
congenital syphilis (A50.4-)
neoplasm (C00-D49)
Excludes1 hydrocephalus due to congenital toxoplasmosis (P37.1)

G91.8 Other hydrocephalus

G91.9 Hydrocephalus, unspecified

G92 Toxic encephalopathy
Disorder or disease of brain caused by chemicals
Toxic encephalitis
Toxic metabolic encephalopathy
Code first (T51-T65) to identify toxic agent
Ex: A17.82, A17,9, A18.82, A18.84, A18.89, A39.81, A50.42, A52.14, A83.0-A85.1, A85.8-A86, A88.8-A89, B00.4, B01.11, B10.01-B10.09, B26.2, B58.2, E08.40-E08.49, E08.618-E08.638, E08.649-E08.8, E09.40-E09.49, E09.618-E09.638, E09.649-E09.8, E10.40-E10.49, E10.618-E10.638, E10.649, E10.69-E10.8, E11.40-E11.49, E11.618-E11.638, E11.649, E11.69-E11.8, E13.40-E13.49, E13.618-E13.638, E13.649-E13.8, G04.00-G04.01, G04.31, G04.81-G05.4, G32.89, G37.3-G37.4, G92, G93.40-G93.49, G93.81, G93.89-G93.9, G96.8-G96.9, G98.0-G98.8, G99.8, I67.83

G93 Other disorders of brain

G93.0 Cerebral cysts
Arachnoid cyst
Porencephalic cyst, acquired
Excludes1 acquired periventricular cysts of newborn (P91.1)
congenital cerebral cysts (Q04.6)

G93.1 Anoxic brain damage, not elsewhere classified
Permanent brain damage by lack of oxygen perfusion through brain tissues.
Excludes1 cerebral anoxia due to anesthesia during labor and delivery (O74.3)
cerebral anoxia due to anesthesia during the puerperium (O89.2)
neonatal anoxia (P84)
Ex: E08.40-E08.49, E08.618-E08.638, E08.649-E08.8, E09.40-E09.49, E09.618-E09.638, E09.649-E09.8, E10.40-E10.49, E10.618-E10.638, E10.649, E10.69-E10.8, E11.40-E11.49, E11.618-E11.638, E11.649, E11.69-E11.8, E13.40-E13.49, E13.618-E13.638, E13.649-E13.8, G32.89, G93.1-G93.2, G96.8-G96.9, G98.0-G98.8, G99.8

G93.2 Benign intracranial hypertension
Excludes1 hypertensive encephalopathy (I67.4)

G93.3 Postviral fatigue syndrome
Benign myalgic encephalomyelitis
Excludes1 chronic fatigue syndrome NOS (R53.82)

G93.4 Other and unspecified encephalopathy
Excludes1 alcoholic encephalopathy (G31.2)
encephalopathy in diseases classified elsewhere (G94)
hypertensive encephalopathy (I67.4)
toxic (metabolic) encephalopathy (G92)

G93.40 Encephalopathy, unspecified
Ex: G21.0, G83.5, G93.41-G93.49, I67.83

G93.41 Metabolic encephalopathy
Septic encephalopathy
Ex: G21.0, G83.5, G93.40-G93.49, I67.83
Coding Clinic: 2015, Q3, P21

G93.49 Other encephalopathy
Encephalopathy NEC
Ex: G21.0, G83.5, G93.40-G93.41

G93.5 Compression of brain
Arnold-Chiari type 1 compression of brain
Compression of brain (stem)
Herniation of brain (stem)
Excludes1 diffuse traumatic compression of brain (S06.2-)
focal traumatic compression of brain (S06.3-)
Ex: G81.90, G93.82

G93.6 Cerebral edema
Excludes1 cerebral edema due to birth injury (P11.0)
traumatic cerebral edema (S06.1-)
Ex: G93.6, G93.82

G93.7 Reye's syndrome P
Life-threatening neurological condition, usually follows viral illness
Code first (T39.0-), if salicylates-induced
Ex: G93.7

G93.8 Other specified disorders of brain

G93.81 Temporal sclerosis
Hippocampal sclerosis
Mesial temporal sclerosis

G93.82 Brain death
Ex: B15.0-B19.9, E03.5, E08.00-E08.59, E08.618-E09.59, E09.618-E10.59, E10.618-E10.649, E10.69-E11.59, E11.618-E11.649, E11.69-E13.59, E13.618-E16.2, E89.1, G32.89, G89.0-G89.4, G93.81-G93.9, G96.8-G96.9, G98.0-G98.8, G99.8, I60.00-I62.9, K72.91, R29.700-R29.742, R40.0-R40.2124, R40.2210-R40.2224, R40.2310-R40.2324, R40.2340-R40.2344, R40.3-R41.3, R41.82, R41.9-R42, R44.8-R44.9, R45.83-R45.84, R46.0-R46.89, R52, R55, R68.0-R68.83, R68.89-R69, S02.0XX-S02.19X[A,B], S02.91X[A,B], S06.0X0-S06.0X1[A], S06.0X9-S06.9X9[A]

G93.89 Other specified disorders of brain
Postradiation encephalopathy

G93.9 Disorder of brain, unspecified

G94 Other disorders of brain in diseases classified elsewhere
Code first underlying disease
Excludes1 encephalopathy in congenital syphilis (A50.49)
encephalopathy in influenza (J09.X9, J10.81, J11.81)
encephalopathy in syphilis (A52.19)
hydrocephalus in diseases classified elsewhere (G91.4)

G95 Other and unspecified diseases of spinal cord

Excludes2 myelitis (G04.-)

G95.0 Syringomyelia and syringobulbia
(Ex) G04.1, G11.3, G11.8-G12.9, G32.0, G32.89-G37.3, G37.5-G37.9, G80.0-G80.2, G80.4-G83.9, G90.01-G90.09, G90.2, G90.4-G90.9, G93.40-G93.49, G93.81, G93.89-G93.9, G95.0-G95.9, G96.12-G96.9, G97.1, G98.0-G99.8, I67.83, R53.2

● **G95.1 Vascular myelopathies**
Excludes2 intraspinal phlebitis and thrombophlebitis, except non-pyogenic (G08)
(Ex) **For category G95.1 CC codes:** See G90.5

G95.11 Acute infarction of spinal cord (embolic) (nonembolic)
Anoxia of spinal cord
Arterial thrombosis of spinal cord

G95.19 Other vascular myelopathies
Edema of spinal cord
Hematomyelia
Nonpyogenic intraspinal phlebitis and thrombophlebitis
Subacute necrotic myelopathy

● **G95.2 Other and unspecified cord compression**
(Ex) **For category G95.2 CC codes:** E08.40-E08.49, E09.40-E09.49, E10.40-E10.49, E11.40-E11.49, E13.40-E13.49, G04.1, G11.3-G12.9, G32.0, G32.89-G37.9, G80.0-G80.2, G80.4-G83.9, G90.01-G90.09, G90.2, G90.4-G90.9, G93.1, G93.40-G93.49, G95.0-G95.9, G96.12-G96.9, G97.1, G98.0-G99.8, I67.83, R53.2

G95.20 Unspecified cord compression

G95.29 Other cord compression

● **G95.8 Other specified diseases of spinal cord**
Excludes1 neurogenic bladder NOS (N31.9)
neurogenic bladder due to cauda equina syndrome (G83.4)
neuromuscular dysfunction of bladder without spinal cord lesion (N31.-)
(Ex) **For category G95.8 CC codes:** See G90.5

G95.81 Conus medullaris syndrome
Damage to gray matter and/or nerve roots in lower end of spinal cord

G95.89 Other specified diseases of spinal cord
Cord bladder NOS
Drug-induced myelopathy
Radiation-induced myelopathy
Excludes1 myelopathy NOS (G95.9)

G95.9 Disease of spinal cord, unspecified
Myelopathy NOS
(Ex) See G95.2

● **G96 Other disorders of central nervous system**

G96.0 Cerebrospinal fluid leak
Excludes1 cerebrospinal fluid leak from spinal puncture (G97.0)
(Ex) E08.40-E08.49, E08.618-E08.638, E08.649-E08.8, E09.40-E09.49, E09.618-E09.638, E09.649-E09.8, E10.40-E10.49, E10.618-E10.638, E10.649, E10.69-E10.8, E11.40-E11.49, E11.618-E11.638, E11.649, E11.69-E11.8, E13.40-E13.49, E13.618-E13.638, E13.649-E13.8, G32.89, G96.0, G96.8-G96.9, G98.0-G98.8, G99.8

● **G96.1 Disorders of meninges, not elsewhere classified**

G96.11 Dural tear
Excludes1 accidental puncture or laceration of dura during a procedure (G97.41)
(Ex) D78.11-D78.12, D78.81-D78.89, E36.11-E36.8, E89.810-E89.89, G96.11, G97.41-G97.49, H59.011-H59.019, H59.031-H59.099, H59.211-H59.229, H59.811-H59.89, H95.31-H95.32, H95.811-H95.89, I97.3, I97.51-I97.52, J95.71-J95.72, K91.71-K91.72, L76.11-L76.12, L76.81-L76.82, M96.820-M96.821, M96.89, N98.1-N98.9, N99.71-N99.72, T81.82X[A], T81.89X-T81.9XX[A]

G96.12 Meningeal adhesions (cerebral) (spinal)

G96.19 Other disorders of meninges, not elsewhere classified

G96.8 Other specified disorders of central nervous system

G96.9 Disorder of central nervous system, unspecified

● **G97 Intraoperative and postprocedural complications and disorders of nervous system, not elsewhere classified**
Excludes2 intraoperative and postprocedural cerebrovascular infarction (I97.81-, I97.82-)

G97.0 Cerebrospinal fluid leak from spinal puncture
(Ex) D78.81-D78.89, E36.8, E89.810-E89.89, G97.0, G97.2-G97.32, G97.81-G97.82, H59.011-H59.019, H59.031-H59.099, H59.811-H59.89, H95.811-H95.89, I97.3, I97.810-I97.821, L76.81-L76.82, M96.89, N98.1-N98.9, T81.82X[A], T81.89X-T81.9XX[A]

G97.1 Other reaction to spinal and lumbar puncture
Headache due to lumbar puncture

G97.2 Intracranial hypotension following ventricular shunting
(Ex) See G97.0

● **G97.3 Intraoperative hemorrhage and hematoma of a nervous system organ or structure complicating a procedure**
Excludes1 intraoperative hemorrhage and hematoma of a nervous system organ or structure due to accidental puncture and laceration during a procedure (G97.4-)
(Ex) **For category G97.3 CC codes:** G97.0, G97.2-G97.32, G97.81-G97.82, H95.811-H95.89, I97.3, I97.810-I97.821, M96.89, N98.1-N98.9, T81.82X[A], T81.89X-T81.9XX[A]

G97.31 Intraoperative hemorrhage and hematoma of a nervous system organ or structure complicating a nervous system procedure

G97.32 Intraoperative hemorrhage and hematoma of a nervous system organ or structure complicating other procedure

● **G97.4 Accidental puncture and laceration of a nervous system organ or structure during a procedure**
(Ex) **For category G97.4 CC codes:** See G96.11

G97.41 Accidental puncture or laceration of dura during a procedure
Incidental (inadvertent) durotomy

G97.48 Accidental puncture and laceration of other nervous system organ or structure during a nervous system procedure

G97.49 Accidental puncture and laceration of other nervous system organ or structure during other procedure

● **G97.5 Postprocedural hemorrhage of a nervous system organ or structure following a procedure**
(Ex) **For category G97.5 CC codes:** G97.51-G97.52, G97.61-G97.64, H95.811-H95.89, I85.01, I85.11, I97.3, K21.9, K22.8, K23-K25.0, K25.2, K25.4, K25.6, K26.0, K26.2, K26.4, K26.6, K27.0, K27.2, K27.4, K27.6, K28.0, K28.2, K28.4, K28.6, K29.01, K29.21, K29.31, K29.41, K29.51, K29.61, K29.71, K29.81, K29.91, K31.811, K55.21, K57.01, K57.11, K57.13, K57.21, K57.31, K57.33, K57.41, K57.51, K57.53, K57.81, K57.91, K57.93, K62.5, K92.0-K92.2, M96.89, N98.1-N98.9, P54.1-P54.3, T81.10X-T81.19X[A], T81.82X-T81.9XX[A]

G97.51 Postprocedural hemorrhage of a nervous system organ or structure following a nervous system procedure

G97.52 Postprocedural hemorrhage of a nervous system organ or structure following other procedure

● **G97.6 Postprocedural hematoma and seroma of a nervous system organ or structure following a procedure**
(Ex) **For category G97.6 CC codes:** See G97.5

G97.61 Postprocedural hematoma of a nervous system organ or structure following a nervous system procedure

G97.62 Postprocedural hematoma of a nervous system organ or structure following other procedure

G97.63 Postprocedural seroma of a nervous system organ or structure following a nervous system procedure

G97.64 Postprocedural seroma of a nervous system organ or structure following other procedure

G97.8 Other intraoperative and postprocedural complications and disorders of nervous system

Use additional code to further specify disorder

Ex: For category G97.8 CC codes: See G97.0

G97.81 Other intraoperative complications of nervous system

G97.82 Other postprocedural complications and disorders of nervous system

G98 Other disorders of nervous system not elsewhere classified

Includes nervous system disorder NOS

G98.0 Neurogenic arthritis, not elsewhere classified

Nonsyphilitic neurogenic arthropathy NEC
Nonsyphilitic neurogenic spondylopathy NEC

Excludes1 spondylopathy (in):
syringomyelia and syringobulbia (G95.0)
tabes dorsalis (A52.11)

G98.8 Other disorders of nervous system

Nervous system disorder NOS

G99 Other disorders of nervous system in diseases classified elsewhere

G99.0 Autonomic neuropathy in diseases classified elsewhere

Code first underlying disease, such as:
amyloidosis (E85.-)
gout (M1A.-, M10.-)
hyperthyroidism (E05.-)

Excludes1 diabetic autonomic neuropathy (E08-E13 with .43)

Ex: G90.50-G90.59

G99.2 Myelopathy in diseases classified elsewhere

Code first underlying disease, such as:
neoplasm (C00-D49)

Excludes1 myelopathy in:
intervertebral disease (M50.0-, M51.0-)
spondylosis (M47.0-, M47.1-)

Ex: See G90.5

G99.8 Other specified disorders of nervous system in diseases classified elsewhere

Code first underlying disorder, such as:
amyloidosis (E85.-)
avitaminosis (E56.9)

Excludes1 nervous system involvement in:
cysticercosis (B69.0)
rubella (B06.0-)
syphilis (A52.1-)

CHAPTER 7

DISEASES OF THE EYE AND ADNEXA (H00-H59)

OGCR Chapter-Specific Coding Guidelines

7. **Chapter 7: Diseases of the Eye and Adnexa (H00-H59)**

a. **Glaucoma**

1) Assigning Glaucoma Codes

Assign as many codes from category H40, Glaucoma, as needed to identify the type of glaucoma, the affected eye, and the glaucoma stage.

2) Bilateral glaucoma with same type and stage

When a patient has bilateral glaucoma and both eyes are documented as being the same type and stage, and there is a code for bilateral glaucoma, report only the code for the type of glaucoma, bilateral, with the seventh character for the stage.

When a patient has bilateral glaucoma and both eyes are documented as being the same type and stage, and the classification does not provide a code for bilateral glaucoma (i.e. subcategories H40.10, H40.11 and H40.20) report only one code for the type of glaucoma with the appropriate seventh character for the stage.

3) Bilateral glaucoma stage with different types or stages

When a patient has bilateral glaucoma and each eye is documented as having a different type or stage, and the classification distinguishes laterality, assign the appropriate code for each eye rather than the code for bilateral glaucoma.

When a patient has bilateral glaucoma and each eye is documented as having a different type, and the classification does not distinguish laterality (i.e. subcategories H40.10, H40.11 and H40.20), assign one code for each type of glaucoma with the appropriate seventh character for the stage.

When a patient has bilateral glaucoma and each eye is documented as having the same type, but different stage, and the classification does not distinguish laterality (i.e. subcategories H40.10, H40.11 and H40.20), assign a code for the type of glaucoma for each eye with the seventh character for the specific glaucoma stage documented for each eye.

4) Patient admitted with glaucoma and stage evolves during the admission

If a patient is admitted with glaucoma and the stage progresses during the admission, assign the code for highest stage documented.

5) Indeterminate stage glaucoma

Assignment of the seventh character "4" for "indeterminate stage" should be based on the clinical documentation. The seventh character "4" is used for glaucomas whose stage cannot be clinically determined. This seventh character should not be confused with the seventh character "0", unspecified, which should be assigned when there is no documentation regarding the stage of the glaucoma.

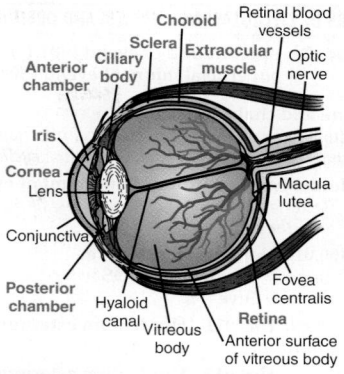

Figure 7–1 Eye and ocular adnexa. (From Buck CJ: Step-by-Step Medical Coding, ed 2016, St. Louis, Elsevier, 2016)

★ **(See Plate 87 on page 63.)**

CHAPTER 7

DISEASES OF THE EYE AND ADNEXA (H00-H59)

Note: Use an external cause code following the code for the eye condition, if applicable, to identify the cause of the eye condition

Excludes2
- certain conditions originating in the perinatal period (P04-P96)
- certain infectious and parasitic diseases (A00-B99)
- complications of pregnancy, childbirth and the puerperium (O00-O9A)
- congenital malformations, deformations, and chromosomal abnormalities (Q00-Q99)
- diabetes mellitus related eye conditions (E09.3-, E10.3-, E11.3-, E13.3-)
- endocrine, nutritional and metabolic diseases (E00-E88)
- injury (trauma) of eye and orbit (S05.-)
- injury, poisoning and certain other consequences of external causes (S00-T88)
- neoplasms (C00-D49)
- symptoms, signs and abnormal clinical and laboratory findings, not elsewhere classified (R00-R94)
- syphilis related eye disorders (A50.01, A50.3-, A51.43, A52.71)

This chapter contains the following blocks:

H00-H05	Disorders of eyelid, lacrimal system and orbit
H10-H11	Disorders of conjunctiva
H15-H22	Disorders of sclera, cornea, iris and ciliary body
H25-H28	Disorders of lens
H30-H36	Disorders of choroid and retina
H40-H42	Glaucoma
H43-H44	Disorders of vitreous body and globe
H46-H47	Disorders of optic nerve and visual pathways
H49-H52	Disorders of ocular muscles, binocular movement, accommodation and refraction
H53-H54	Visual disturbances and blindness
H55-H57	Other disorders of eye and adnexa
H59	Intraoperative and postprocedural complications and disorders of eye and adnexa, not elsewhere classified

DISORDERS OF EYELID, LACRIMAL SYSTEM AND ORBIT (H00-H05)

Excludes2 open wound of eyelid (S01.1-)
superficial injury of eyelid (S00.1-, S00.2-)

● **H00 Hordeolum and chalazion**
Hordeolum: inflammatory staphylococcal infection of sebaceous glands of eyelids; AKA stye. Chalazion: eyelid mass

● **H00.0 Hordeolum (externum) (internum) of eyelid**
Bacterial infection (staphylococcus) of the sebaceous gland of the eyelid (stye)

● **H00.01 Hordeolum externum**
Hordeolum NOS
Stye

H00.011 Hordeolum externum right upper eyelid
H00.012 Hordeolum externum right lower eyelid
H00.013 Hordeolum externum right eye, unspecified eyelid
H00.014 Hordeolum externum left upper eyelid
H00.015 Hordeolum externum left lower eyelid
H00.016 Hordeolum externum left eye, unspecified eyelid
H00.019 Hordeolum externum unspecified eye, unspecified eyelid

● **H00.02 Hordeolum internum**
Infection of meibomian gland

H00.021 Hordeolum internum right upper eyelid
H00.022 Hordeolum internum right lower eyelid
H00.023 Hordeolum internum right eye, unspecified eyelid
H00.024 Hordeolum internum left upper eyelid
H00.025 Hordeolum internum left lower eyelid
H00.026 Hordeolum internum left eye, unspecified eyelid
H00.029 Hordeolum internum unspecified eye, unspecified eyelid

● **H00.03 Abscess of eyelid**
Furuncle of eyelid

H00.031 Abscess of right upper eyelid
H00.032 Abscess of right lower eyelid
H00.033 Abscess of eyelid right eye, unspecified eyelid
H00.034 Abscess of left upper eyelid
H00.035 Abscess of left lower eyelid
H00.036 Abscess of eyelid left eye, unspecified eyelid
H00.039 Abscess of eyelid unspecified eye, unspecified eyelid

● **H00.1 Chalazion**
Often caused by accumulation of meibomian gland secretions resulting from a blockage of duct.
Meibomian (gland) cyst

Excludes2 infected meibomian gland (H00.02-)

H00.11 Chalazion right upper eyelid
H00.12 Chalazion right lower eyelid
H00.13 Chalazion right eye, unspecified eyelid
H00.14 Chalazion left upper eyelid
H00.15 Chalazion left lower eyelid
H00.16 Chalazion left eye, unspecified eyelid
H00.19 Chalazion unspecified eye, unspecified eyelid

● **H01 Other inflammation of eyelid**

● **H01.0 Blepharitis**
Inflammation of eyelids

Excludes1 blepharoconjunctivitis (H10.5-)

● **H01.00 Unspecified blepharitis**

H01.001 Unspecified blepharitis right upper eyelid
H01.002 Unspecified blepharitis right lower eyelid
H01.003 Unspecified blepharitis right eye, unspecified eyelid
H01.004 Unspecified blepharitis left upper eyelid
H01.005 Unspecified blepharitis left lower eyelid
H01.006 Unspecified blepharitis left eye, unspecified eyelid
H01.009 Unspecified blepharitis unspecified eye, unspecified eyelid

● **H01.01 Ulcerative blepharitis**

H01.011 Ulcerative blepharitis right upper eyelid
H01.012 Ulcerative blepharitis right lower eyelid
H01.013 Ulcerative blepharitis right eye, unspecified eyelid
H01.014 Ulcerative blepharitis left upper eyelid
H01.015 Ulcerative blepharitis left lower eyelid
H01.016 Ulcerative blepharitis left eye, unspecified eyelid
H01.019 Ulcerative blepharitis unspecified eye, unspecified eyelid

● **H01.02 Squamous blepharitis**

H01.021 Squamous blepharitis right upper eyelid
H01.022 Squamous blepharitis right lower eyelid
H01.023 Squamous blepharitis right eye, unspecified eyelid
H01.024 Squamous blepharitis left upper eyelid
H01.025 Squamous blepharitis left lower eyelid
H01.026 Squamous blepharitis left eye, unspecified eyelid
H01.029 Squamous blepharitis unspecified eye, unspecified eyelid

● **H01.1 Noninfectious dermatoses of eyelid**

● **H01.11 Allergic dermatitis of eyelid**
Contact dermatitis of eyelid

H01.111 Allergic dermatitis of right upper eyelid
H01.112 Allergic dermatitis of right lower eyelid
H01.113 Allergic dermatitis of right eye, unspecified eyelid
H01.114 Allergic dermatitis of left upper eyelid
H01.115 Allergic dermatitis of left lower eyelid
H01.116 Allergic dermatitis of left eye, unspecified eyelid
H01.119 Allergic dermatitis of unspecified eye, unspecified eyelid

- **H01.12** Discoid lupus erythematosus of eyelid
  - **H01.121** Discoid lupus erythematosus of right upper eyelid
  - **H01.122** Discoid lupus erythematosus of right lower eyelid
  - **H01.123** Discoid lupus erythematosus of right eye, unspecified eyelid
  - **H01.124** Discoid lupus erythematosus of left upper eyelid
  - **H01.125** Discoid lupus erythematosus of left lower eyelid
  - **H01.126** Discoid lupus erythematosus of left eye, unspecified eyelid
  - **H01.129** Discoid lupus erythematosus of unspecified eye, unspecified eyelid
- **H01.13** Eczematous dermatitis of eyelid
  - **H01.131** Eczematous dermatitis of right upper eyelid
  - **H01.132** Eczematous dermatitis of right lower eyelid
  - **H01.133** Eczematous dermatitis of right eye, unspecified eyelid
  - **H01.134** Eczematous dermatitis of left upper eyelid
  - **H01.135** Eczematous dermatitis of left lower eyelid
  - **H01.136** Eczematous dermatitis of left eye, unspecified eyelid
  - **H01.139** Eczematous dermatitis of unspecified eye, unspecified eyelid
- **H01.14** Xeroderma of eyelid
  Abnormally dry
  - **H01.141** Xeroderma of right upper eyelid
  - **H01.142** Xeroderma of right lower eyelid
  - **H01.143** Xeroderma of right eye, unspecified eyelid
  - **H01.144** Xeroderma of left upper eyelid
  - **H01.145** Xeroderma of left lower eyelid
  - **H01.146** Xeroderma of left eye, unspecified eyelid
  - **H01.149** Xeroderma of unspecified eye, unspecified eyelid
- **H01.8** Other specified inflammations of eyelid
- **H01.9** Unspecified inflammation of eyelid
  Inflammation of eyelid NOS

- **H02** Other disorders of eyelid
  Turning inward (inversion) of eyelid margin and ingrowing eyelashes
  Excludes1 congenital malformations of eyelid (Q10.0-Q10.3)
  - **H02.0** Entropion and trichiasis of eyelid
    - **H02.00** Unspecified entropion of eyelid
      - **H02.001** Unspecified entropion of right upper eyelid
      - **H02.002** Unspecified entropion of right lower eyelid
      - **H02.003** Unspecified entropion of right eye, unspecified eyelid
      - **H02.004** Unspecified entropion of left upper eyelid
      - **H02.005** Unspecified entropion of left lower eyelid
      - **H02.006** Unspecified entropion of left eye, unspecified eyelid
      - **H02.009** Unspecified entropion of unspecified eye, unspecified eyelid
    - **H02.01** Cicatricial entropion of eyelid
      Scar
      - **H02.011** Cicatricial entropion of right upper eyelid
      - **H02.012** Cicatricial entropion of right lower eyelid
      - **H02.013** Cicatricial entropion of right eye, unspecified eyelid
      - **H02.014** Cicatricial entropion of left upper eyelid
      - **H02.015** Cicatricial entropion of left lower eyelid
      - **H02.016** Cicatricial entropion of left eye, unspecified eyelid
      - **H02.019** Cicatricial entropion of unspecified eye, unspecified eyelid
    - **H02.02** Mechanical entropion of eyelid
      Turning inward (inversion) of eyelid margin due to lack of support
      - **H02.021** Mechanical entropion of right upper eyelid
      - **H02.022** Mechanical entropion of right lower eyelid
      - **H02.023** Mechanical entropion of right eye, unspecified eyelid
      - **H02.024** Mechanical entropion of left upper eyelid
      - **H02.025** Mechanical entropion of left lower eyelid
      - **H02.026** Mechanical entropion of left eye, unspecified eyelid
      - **H02.029** Mechanical entropion of unspecified eye, unspecified eyelid
    - **H02.03** Senile entropion of eyelid
      Turning inward (inversion) of eyelid margin due to aging
      - **H02.031** Senile entropion of right upper eyelid A
      - **H02.032** Senile entropion of right lower eyelid A
      - **H02.033** Senile entropion of right eye, unspecified eyelid A
      - **H02.034** Senile entropion of left upper eyelid A
      - **H02.035** Senile entropion of left lower eyelid A
      - **H02.036** Senile entropion of left eye, unspecified eyelid A
      - **H02.039** Senile entropion of unspecified eye, unspecified eyelid A
    - **H02.04** Spastic entropion of eyelid
      Turning inward (inversion) of eyelid margin caused by spasm of muscle
      - **H02.041** Spastic entropion of right upper eyelid
      - **H02.042** Spastic entropion of right lower eyelid
      - **H02.043** Spastic entropion of right eye, unspecified eyelid
      - **H02.044** Spastic entropion of left upper eyelid
      - **H02.045** Spastic entropion of left lower eyelid
      - **H02.046** Spastic entropion of left eye, unspecified eyelid
      - **H02.049** Spastic entropion of unspecified eye, unspecified eyelid

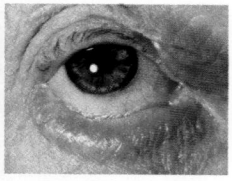

Figure 7-2 Right lower eyelid entropion. Note the inward rotation of the tarsal plate about the horizontal axis and the resultant contact between the mucocutaneous junction and ocular surface. (From Yanoff: Ophthalmology, ed 3, Mosby, Inc., 2008)

- **H02.05 Trichiasis without entropian**
  Ingrowing hairs of eyelashes
  - **H02.051 Trichiasis without entropian right upper eyelid**
  - **H02.052 Trichiasis without entropian right lower eyelid**
  - **H02.053 Trichiasis without entropian right eye, unspecified eyelid**
  - **H02.054 Trichiasis without entropian left upper eyelid**
  - **H02.055 Trichiasis without entropian left lower eyelid**
  - **H02.056 Trichiasis without entropian left eye, unspecified eyelid**
  - **H02.059 Trichiasis without entropian unspecified eye, unspecified eyelid**

- **H02.1 Ectropion of eyelid**
  Eversion (pulling away) of eyelid
  - **H02.10 Unspecified ectropion of eyelid**
    - **H02.101 Unspecified ectropion of right upper eyelid**
    - **H02.102 Unspecified ectropion of right lower eyelid**
    - **H02.103 Unspecified ectropion of right eye, unspecified eyelid**
    - **H02.104 Unspecified ectropion of left upper eyelid**
    - **H02.105 Unspecified ectropion of left lower eyelid**
    - **H02.106 Unspecified ectropion of left eye, unspecified eyelid**
    - **H02.109 Unspecified ectropion of unspecified eye, unspecified eyelid**
  - **H02.11 Cicatricial ectropion of eyelid**
    Pulling of eyelid down and away from eye due to scar or tightening
    - **H02.111 Cicatricial ectropion of right upper eyelid**
    - **H02.112 Cicatricial ectropion of right lower eyelid**
    - **H02.113 Cicatricial ectropion of right eye, unspecified eyelid**
    - **H02.114 Cicatricial ectropion of left upper eyelid**
    - **H02.115 Cicatricial ectropion of left lower eyelid**
    - **H02.116 Cicatricial ectropion of left eye, unspecified eyelid**
    - **H02.119 Cicatricial ectropion of unspecified eye, unspecified eyelid**
  - **H02.12 Mechanical ectropion of eyelid**
    Eversion (pulling away) of eyelid due to lack of support
    - **H02.121 Mechanical ectropion of right upper eyelid**
    - **H02.122 Mechanical ectropion of right lower eyelid**
    - **H02.123 Mechanical ectropion of right eye, unspecified eyelid**
    - **H02.124 Mechanical ectropion of left upper eyelid**
    - **H02.125 Mechanical ectropion of left lower eyelid**
    - **H02.126 Mechanical ectropion of left eye, unspecified eyelid**
    - **H02.129 Mechanical ectropion of unspecified eye, unspecified eyelid**
  - **H02.13 Senile ectropion of eyelid**
    Eversion (pulling away) of eyelid due to age
    - **H02.131 Senile ectropion of right upper eyelid** A
    - **H02.132 Senile ectropion of right lower eyelid** A
    - **H02.133 Senile ectropion of right eye, unspecified eyelid** A
    - **H02.134 Senile ectropion of left upper eyelid** A
    - **H02.135 Senile ectropion of left lower eyelid** A
    - **H02.136 Senile ectropion of left eye, unspecified eyelid** A
    - **H02.139 Senile ectropion of unspecified eye, unspecified eyelid** A
  - **H02.14 Spastic ectropion of eyelid**
    Eversion (pulling away) of eyelid due to tonic muscle spasm
    - **H02.141 Spastic ectropion of right upper eyelid**
    - **H02.142 Spastic ectropion of right lower eyelid**
    - **H02.143 Spastic ectropion of right eye, unspecified eyelid**
    - **H02.144 Spastic ectropion of left upper eyelid**
    - **H02.145 Spastic ectropion of left lower eyelid**
    - **H02.146 Spastic ectropion of left eye, unspecified eyelid**
    - **H02.149 Spastic ectropion of unspecified eye, unspecified eyelid**

- **H02.2 Lagophthalmos**
  Condition in which eye cannot completely close
  - **H02.20 Unspecified lagophthalmos**
    - **H02.201 Unspecified lagophthalmos right upper eyelid**
    - **H02.202 Unspecified lagophthalmos right lower eyelid**
    - **H02.203 Unspecified lagophthalmos right eye, unspecified eyelid**
    - **H02.204 Unspecified lagophthalmos left upper eyelid**
    - **H02.205 Unspecified lagophthalmos left lower eyelid**
    - **H02.206 Unspecified lagophthalmos left eye, unspecified eyelid**
    - **H02.209 Unspecified lagophthalmos unspecified eye, unspecified eyelid**
  - **H02.21 Cicatricial lagophthalmos**
    Upper or lower eyelid does not close due to scar or tightening
    - **H02.211 Cicatricial lagophthalmos right upper eyelid**
    - **H02.212 Cicatricial lagophthalmos right lower eyelid**
    - **H02.213 Cicatricial lagophthalmos right eye, unspecified eyelid**
    - **H02.214 Cicatricial lagophthalmos left upper eyelid**
    - **H02.215 Cicatricial lagophthalmos left lower eyelid**
    - **H02.216 Cicatricial lagophthalmos left eye, unspecified eyelid**
    - **H02.219 Cicatricial lagophthalmos unspecified eye, unspecified eyelid**

● **H02.22** Mechanical lagophthalmos
Inability to close lids due to structural disorder
- **H02.221** Mechanical lagophthalmos right upper eyelid
- **H02.222** Mechanical lagophthalmos right lower eyelid
- **H02.223** Mechanical lagophthalmos right eye, unspecified eyelid
- **H02.224** Mechanical lagophthalmos left upper eyelid
- **H02.225** Mechanical lagophthalmos left lower eyelid
- **H02.226** Mechanical lagophthalmos left eye, unspecified eyelid
- **H02.229** Mechanical lagophthalmos unspecified eye, unspecified eyelid

● **H02.23** Paralytic lagophthalmos
Eyelids do not close due to paralysis
- **H02.231** Paralytic lagophthalmos right upper eyelid
- **H02.232** Paralytic lagophthalmos right lower eyelid
- **H02.233** Paralytic lagophthalmos right eye, unspecified eyelid
- **H02.234** Paralytic lagophthalmos left upper eyelid
- **H02.235** Paralytic lagophthalmos left lower eyelid
- **H02.236** Paralytic lagophthalmos left eye, unspecified eyelid
- **H02.239** Paralytic lagophthalmos unspecified eye, unspecified eyelid

★ **(See Plate 81, middle, on page 65.)**

● **H02.3** Blepharochalasis
Relaxation of skin of eyelid, due to atrophy of intercellular tissue
Pseudoptosis
- **H02.30** Blepharochalasis unspecified eye, unspecified eyelid
- **H02.31** Blepharochalasis right upper eyelid
- **H02.32** Blepharochalasis right lower eyelid
- **H02.33** Blepharochalasis right eye, unspecified eyelid
- **H02.34** Blepharochalasis left upper eyelid
- **H02.35** Blepharochalasis left lower eyelid
- **H02.36** Blepharochalasis left eye, unspecified eyelid

● **H02.4** Ptosis of eyelid
Falling forward, drooping, sagging of eyelid

● **H02.40** Unspecified ptosis of eyelid
- **H02.401** Unspecified ptosis of right eyelid
- **H02.402** Unspecified ptosis of left eyelid
- **H02.403** Unspecified ptosis of bilateral eyelids
- **H02.409** Unspecified ptosis of unspecified eyelid

● **H02.41** Mechanical ptosis of eyelid
- **H02.411** Mechanical ptosis of right eyelid
- **H02.412** Mechanical ptosis of left eyelid
- **H02.413** Mechanical ptosis of bilateral eyelids
- **H02.419** Mechanical ptosis of unspecified eyelid

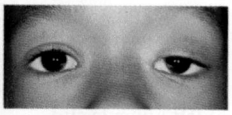

Figure 7-3 Ptosis of eyelid. (From Yanoff: Ophthalmology, ed 3, Mosby, Inc., 2008)

Item 7–1 Ptosis of eyelid is drooping of the upper eyelid over the pupil when the eyes are fully opened resulting from nerve or muscle damage, which may require surgical correction.

● **H02.42** Myogenic ptosis of eyelid
- **H02.421** Myogenic ptosis of right eyelid
- **H02.422** Myogenic ptosis of left eyelid
- **H02.423** Myogenic ptosis of bilateral eyelids
- **H02.429** Myogenic ptosis of unspecified eyelid

● **H02.43** Paralytic ptosis of eyelid
Neurogenic ptosis of eyelid
- **H02.431** Paralytic ptosis of right eyelid
- **H02.432** Paralytic ptosis of left eyelid
- **H02.433** Paralytic ptosis of bilateral eyelids
- **H02.439** Paralytic ptosis unspecified eyelid

● **H02.5** Other disorders affecting eyelid function
Excludes2 blepharospasm (G24.5)
organic tic (G25.69)
psychogenic tic (F95.-)

● **H02.51** Abnormal innervation syndrome
- **H02.511** Abnormal innervation syndrome right upper eyelid
- **H02.512** Abnormal innervation syndrome right lower eyelid
- **H02.513** Abnormal innervation syndrome right eye, unspecified eyelid
- **H02.514** Abnormal innervation syndrome left upper eyelid
- **H02.515** Abnormal innervation syndrome left lower eyelid
- **H02.516** Abnormal innervation syndrome left eye, unspecified eyelid
- **H02.519** Abnormal innervation syndrome unspecified eye, unspecified eyelid

● **H02.52** Blepharophimosis
Drooping of eyelid with reduced lid size
Ankyloblepharon
- **H02.521** Blepharophimosis right upper eyelid
- **H02.522** Blepharophimosis right lower eyelid
- **H02.523** Blepharophimosis right eye, unspecified eyelid
- **H02.524** Blepharophimosis left upper eyelid
- **H02.525** Blepharophimosis left lower eyelid
- **H02.526** Blepharophimosis left eye, unspecified eyelid
- **H02.529** Blepharophimosis unspecified eye, unspecified lid

● **H02.53** Eyelid retraction
Eyelid lag
- **H02.531** Eyelid retraction right upper eyelid
- **H02.532** Eyelid retraction right lower eyelid
- **H02.533** Eyelid retraction right eye, unspecified eyelid
- **H02.534** Eyelid retraction left upper eyelid
- **H02.535** Eyelid retraction left lower eyelid
- **H02.536** Eyelid retraction left eye, unspecified eyelid
- **H02.539** Eyelid retraction unspecified eye, unspecified lid

H02.59 Other disorders affecting eyelid function
Deficient blink reflex
Sensory disorders

- **H02.6 Xanthelasma of eyelid**
  Yellow-to-orange patches or pimples clustered together on eyelid
  - **H02.60 Xanthelasma of unspecified eye, unspecified eyelid**
  - **H02.61 Xanthelasma of right upper eyelid**
  - **H02.62 Xanthelasma of right lower eyelid**
  - **H02.63 Xanthelasma of right eye, unspecified eyelid**
  - **H02.64 Xanthelasma of left upper eyelid**
  - **H02.65 Xanthelasma of left lower eyelid**
  - **H02.66 Xanthelasma of left eye, unspecified eyelid**
- **H02.7 Other and unspecified degenerative disorders of eyelid and periocular area**
  - **H02.70 Unspecified degenerative disorders of eyelid and periocular area**
  - **H02.71 Chloasma of eyelid and periocular area**
    Dyspigmentation of eyelid
    Hyperpigmentation of eyelid
    - **H02.711 Chloasma of right upper eyelid and periocular area**
    - **H02.712 Chloasma of right lower eyelid and periocular area**
    - **H02.713 Chloasma of right eye, unspecified eyelid and periocular area**
    - **H02.714 Chloasma of left upper eyelid and periocular area**
    - **H02.715 Chloasma of left lower eyelid and periocular area**
    - **H02.716 Chloasma of left eye, unspecified eyelid and periocular area**
    - **H02.719 Chloasma of unspecified eye, unspecified eyelid and periocular area**
  - **H02.72 Madarosis of eyelid and periocular area**
    Loss of eyelashes and/or eyebrows
    Hypotrichosis of eyelid
    - **H02.721 Madarosis of right upper eyelid and periocular area**
    - **H02.722 Madarosis of right lower eyelid and periocular area**
    - **H02.723 Madarosis of right eye, unspecified eyelid and periocular area**
    - **H02.724 Madarosis of left upper eyelid and periocular area**
    - **H02.725 Madarosis of left lower eyelid and periocular area**
    - **H02.726 Madarosis of left eye, unspecified eyelid and periocular area**
    - **H02.729 Madarosis of unspecified eye, unspecified eyelid and periocular area**
  - **H02.73 Vitiligo of eyelid and periocular area**
    Skin pigmentation disease characterized by white patches
    Hypopigmentation of eyelid
    - **H02.731 Vitiligo of right upper eyelid and periocular area**
    - **H02.732 Vitiligo of right lower eyelid and periocular area**
    - **H02.733 Vitiligo of right eye, unspecified eyelid and periocular area**
    - **H02.734 Vitiligo of left upper eyelid and periocular area**
    - **H02.735 Vitiligo of left lower eyelid and periocular area**
    - **H02.736 Vitiligo of left eye, unspecified eyelid and periocular area**
    - **H02.739 Vitiligo of unspecified eye, unspecified eyelid and periocular area**
  - **H02.79 Other degenerative disorders of eyelid and periocular area**
- **H02.8 Other specified disorders of eyelid**
  - **H02.81 Retained foreign body in eyelid**
    Use additional code to identify the type of retained foreign body (Z18.-)
    Excludes1 laceration of eyelid with foreign body (S01.12-)
    retained intraocular foreign body (H44.6-, H44.7-)
    superficial foreign body of eyelid and periocular area (S00.25-)
    - **H02.811 Retained foreign body in right upper eyelid**
    - **H02.812 Retained foreign body in right lower eyelid**
    - **H02.813 Retained foreign body in right eye, unspecified eyelid**
    - **H02.814 Retained foreign body in left upper eyelid**
    - **H02.815 Retained foreign body in left lower eyelid**
    - **H02.816 Retained foreign body in left eye, unspecified eyelid**
    - **H02.819 Retained foreign body in unspecified eye, unspecified eyelid**
  - **H02.82 Cysts of eyelid**
    Sebaceous cyst of eyelid
    - **H02.821 Cysts of right upper eyelid**
    - **H02.822 Cysts of right lower eyelid**
    - **H02.823 Cysts of right eye, unspecified eyelid**
    - **H02.824 Cysts of left upper eyelid**
    - **H02.825 Cysts of left lower eyelid**
    - **H02.826 Cysts of left eye, unspecified eyelid**
    - **H02.829 Cysts of unspecified eye, unspecified eyelid**
  - **H02.83 Dermatochalasis of eyelid**
    Skin is inelastic and hangs loosely in folds
    - **H02.831 Dermatochalasis of right upper eyelid**
    - **H02.832 Dermatochalasis of right lower eyelid**
    - **H02.833 Dermatochalasis of right eye, unspecified eyelid**
    - **H02.834 Dermatochalasis of left upper eyelid**
    - **H02.835 Dermatochalasis of left lower eyelid**
    - **H02.836 Dermatochalasis of left eye, unspecified eyelid**
    - **H02.839 Dermatochalasis of unspecified eye, unspecified eyelid**
  - **H02.84 Edema of eyelid**
    Hyperemia of eyelid
    - **H02.841 Edema of right upper eyelid**
    - **H02.842 Edema of right lower eyelid**
    - **H02.843 Edema of right eye, unspecified eyelid**
    - **H02.844 Edema of left upper eyelid**
    - **H02.845 Edema of left lower eyelid**
    - **H02.846 Edema of left eye, unspecified eyelid**
    - **H02.849 Edema of unspecified eye, unspecified eyelid**
  - **H02.85 Elephantiasis of eyelid**
    Massive secondary lymphedema with hypertrophy of skin and subcutaneous tissues (pachyderma)
    - **H02.851 Elephantiasis of right upper eyelid**
    - **H02.852 Elephantiasis of right lower eyelid**
    - **H02.853 Elephantiasis of right eye, unspecified eyelid**
    - **H02.854 Elephantiasis of left upper eyelid**
    - **H02.855 Elephantiasis of left lower eyelid**

H02.856 Elephantiasis of left eye, unspecified eyelid
H02.859 Elephantiasis of unspecified eye, unspecified eyelid

● H02.86 Hypertrichosis of eyelid
Excessive growth of hair
H02.861 Hypertrichosis of right upper eyelid
H02.862 Hypertrichosis of right lower eyelid
H02.863 Hypertrichosis of right eye, unspecified eyelid
H02.864 Hypertrichosis of left upper eyelid
H02.865 Hypertrichosis of left lower eyelid
H02.866 Hypertrichosis of left eye, unspecified eyelid
H02.869 Hypertrichosis of unspecified eye, unspecified eyelid

● H02.87 Vascular anomalies of eyelid
H02.871 Vascular anomalies of right upper eyelid
H02.872 Vascular anomalies of right lower eyelid
H02.873 Vascular anomalies of right eye, unspecified eyelid
H02.874 Vascular anomalies of left upper eyelid
H02.875 Vascular anomalies of left lower eyelid
H02.876 Vascular anomalies of left eye, unspecified eyelid
H02.879 Vascular anomalies of unspecified eye, unspecified eyelid

H02.89 Other specified disorders of eyelid
Hemorrhage of eyelid

H02.9 Unspecified disorder of eyelid
Disorder of eyelid NOS

● H04 Disorders of lacrimal system
Excludes1 congenital malformations of lacrimal system (Q10.4-Q10.6)

● H04.0 Dacryoadenitis
Inflammation of lacrimal gland

● H04.00 Unspecified dacryoadenitis
H04.001 Unspecified dacryoadenitis, right lacrimal gland
H04.002 Unspecified dacryoadenitis, left lacrimal gland
H04.003 Unspecified dacryoadenitis, bilateral lacrimal glands
H04.009 Unspecified dacryoadenitis, unspecified lacrimal gland

● H04.01 Acute dacryoadenitis
H04.011 Acute dacryoadenitis, right lacrimal gland
H04.012 Acute dacryoadenitis, left lacrimal gland
H04.013 Acute dacryoadenitis, bilateral lacrimal glands
H04.019 Acute dacryoadenitis, unspecified lacrimal gland

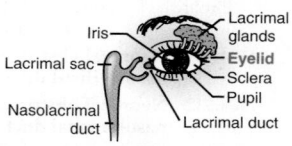

Figure 7-4 Lacrimal apparatus. (From Buck CJ: Step-by-Step Medical Coding, 2016, St. Louis, Elsevier, 2016)

★ **(See Plate 82 on page 67.)**

● H04.02 Chronic dacryoadenitis
H04.021 Chronic dacryoadenitis, right lacrimal gland
H04.022 Chronic dacryoadenitis, left lacrimal gland
H04.023 Chronic dacryoadenitis, bilateral lacrimal gland
H04.029 Chronic dacryoadenitis, unspecified lacrimal gland

● H04.03 Chronic enlargement of lacrimal gland
H04.031 Chronic enlargement of right lacrimal gland
H04.032 Chronic enlargement of left lacrimal gland
H04.033 Chronic enlargement of bilateral lacrimal glands
H04.039 Chronic enlargement of unspecified lacrimal gland

● H04.1 Other disorders of lacrimal gland

● H04.11 Dacryops
Watery eye or distention of lacrimal duct due to fluid
H04.111 Dacryops of right lacrimal gland
H04.112 Dacryops of left lacrimal gland
H04.113 Dacryops of bilateral lacrimal glands
H04.119 Dacryops of unspecified lacrimal gland

● H04.12 Dry eye syndrome
Tear film insufficiency, NOS
H04.121 Dry eye syndrome of right lacrimal gland
H04.122 Dry eye syndrome of left lacrimal gland
H04.123 Dry eye syndrome of bilateral lacrimal glands
H04.129 Dry eye syndrome of unspecified lacrimal gland

● H04.13 Lacrimal cyst
Lacrimal cystic degeneration
H04.131 Lacrimal cyst right lacrimal gland
H04.132 Lacrimal cyst left lacrimal gland
H04.133 Lacrimal cyst bilateral lacrimal glands
H04.139 Lacrimal cyst unspecified lacrimal gland

● H04.14 Primary lacrimal gland atrophy
H04.141 Primary lacrimal gland atrophy, right lacrimal gland
H04.142 Primary lacrimal gland atrophy, left lacrimal gland
H04.143 Primary lacrimal gland atrophy, bilateral lacrimal glands
H04.149 Primary lacrimal gland atrophy, unspecified lacrimal gland

● H04.15 Secondary lacrimal gland atrophy
H04.151 Secondary lacrimal gland atrophy, right lacrimal gland
H04.152 Secondary lacrimal gland atrophy, left lacrimal gland
H04.153 Secondary lacrimal gland atrophy, bilateral lacrimal glands
H04.159 Secondary lacrimal gland atrophy, unspecified lacrimal gland

● H04.16 Lacrimal gland dislocation
H04.161 Lacrimal gland dislocation, right lacrimal gland
H04.162 Lacrimal gland dislocation, left lacrimal gland

H04.163 Lacrimal gland dislocation, bilateral lacrimal glands
H04.169 Lacrimal gland dislocation, unspecified lacrimal gland
H04.19 Other specified disorders of lacrimal gland

● H04.2 Epiphora
Overflow of tears due to stricture of lacrimal passages; AKA lacrimation

● H04.20 Unspecified epiphora
H04.201 Unspecified epiphora, right lacrimal gland
H04.202 Unspecified epiphora, left lacrimal gland
H04.203 Unspecified epiphora, bilateral lacrimal glands
H04.209 Unspecified epiphora, unspecified lacrimal gland

● H04.21 Epiphora due to excess lacrimation
H04.211 Epiphora due to excess lacrimation, right lacrimal gland
H04.212 Epiphora due to excess lacrimation, left lacrimal gland
H04.213 Epiphora due to excess lacrimation, bilateral lacrimal glands
H04.219 Epiphora due to excess lacrimation, unspecified lacrimal gland

● H04.22 Epiphora due to insufficient drainage
H04.221 Epiphora due to insufficient drainage, right lacrimal gland
H04.222 Epiphora due to insufficient drainage, left lacrimal gland
H04.223 Epiphora due to insufficient drainage, bilateral lacrimal glands
H04.229 Epiphora due to insufficient drainage, unspecified lacrimal gland

● H04.3 Acute and unspecified inflammation of lacrimal passages
Excludes1 neonatal dacryocystitis (P39.1)

● H04.30 Unspecified dacryocystitis
H04.301 Unspecified dacryocystitis of right lacrimal passage
H04.302 Unspecified dacryocystitis of left lacrimal passage
H04.303 Unspecified dacryocystitis of bilateral lacrimal passages
H04.309 Unspecified dacryocystitis of unspecified lacrimal passage

● H04.31 Phlegmonous dacryocystitis
Cellulitis of lacrimal sac
H04.311 Phlegmonous dacryocystitis of right lacrimal passage
H04.312 Phlegmonous dacryocystitis of left lacrimal passage
H04.313 Phlegmonous dacryocystitis of bilateral lacrimal passages
H04.319 Phlegmonous dacryocystitis of unspecified lacrimal passage

● H04.32 Acute dacryocystitis
Acute dacryopericystitis
H04.321 Acute dacryocystitis of right lacrimal passage
H04.322 Acute dacryocystitis of left lacrimal passage
H04.323 Acute dacryocystitis of bilateral lacrimal passages
H04.329 Acute dacryocystitis of unspecified lacrimal passage

● H04.33 Acute lacrimal canaliculitis
H04.331 Acute lacrimal canaliculitis of right lacrimal passage
H04.332 Acute lacrimal canaliculitis of left lacrimal passage
H04.333 Acute lacrimal canaliculitis of bilateral lacrimal passages
H04.339 Acute lacrimal canaliculitis of unspecified lacrimal passage

● H04.4 Chronic inflammation of lacrimal passages

● H04.41 Chronic dacryocystitis
Inflammation of lacrimal sac
H04.411 Chronic dacryocystitis of right lacrimal passage
H04.412 Chronic dacryocystitis of left lacrimal passage
H04.413 Chronic dacryocystitis of bilateral lacrimal passages
H04.419 Chronic dacryocystitis of unspecified lacrimal passage

● H04.42 Chronic lacrimal canaliculitis
Inflammation of lacrimal ducts
H04.421 Chronic lacrimal canaliculitis of right lacrimal passage
H04.422 Chronic lacrimal canaliculitis of left lacrimal passage
H04.423 Chronic lacrimal canaliculitis of bilateral lacrimal passages
H04.429 Chronic lacrimal canaliculitis of unspecified lacrimal passage

● H04.43 Chronic lacrimal mucocele
Accumulation of mucous secretion
H04.431 Chronic lacrimal mucocele of right lacrimal passage
H04.432 Chronic lacrimal mucocele of left lacrimal passage
H04.433 Chronic lacrimal mucocele of bilateral lacrimal passages
H04.439 Chronic lacrimal mucocele of unspecified lacrimal passage

● H04.5 Stenosis and insufficiency of lacrimal passages

● H04.51 Dacryolith
Concretion in lacrimal sac/duct; AKA lacrimal calculus
H04.511 Dacryolith of right lacrimal passage
H04.512 Dacryolith of left lacrimal passage
H04.513 Dacryolith of bilateral lacrimal passages
H04.519 Dacryolith of unspecified lacrimal passage

● H04.52 Eversion of lacrimal punctum
Turning out of lacrimal drainage opening
H04.521 Eversion of right lacrimal punctum
H04.522 Eversion of left lacrimal punctum
H04.523 Eversion of bilateral lacrimal punctum
H04.529 Eversion of unspecified lacrimal punctum

● H04.53 Neonatal obstruction of nasolacrimal duct
Excludes1 congenital stenosis and stricture of lacrimal duct (Q10.5)
H04.531 Neonatal obstruction of right nasolacrimal duct N
H04.532 Neonatal obstruction of left nasolacrimal duct N
H04.533 Neonatal obstruction of bilateral nasolacrimal duct N
H04.539 Neonatal obstruction of unspecified nasolacrimal duct N

◀ New ◀ Revised ~~deleted~~ Deleted Excludes 1 Excludes 2 Includes Use additional Code first Code also Unspecified
OGCR Official Guidelines ● Unacceptable Principal Diagnosis X Assign placeholder X ● Use Additional Character(s) ▶ Manifestation Code Coding Clinic

- **H04.54** Stenosis of lacrimal canaliculi
  - **H04.541** Stenosis of right lacrimal canaliculi
  - **H04.542** Stenosis of left lacrimal canaliculi
  - **H04.543** Stenosis of bilateral lacrimal canaliculi
  - **H04.549** Stenosis of unspecified lacrimal canaliculi
- **H04.55** Acquired stenosis of nasolacrimal duct
  - **H04.551** Acquired stenosis of right nasolacrimal duct
  - **H04.552** Acquired stenosis of left nasolacrimal duct
  - **H04.553** Acquired stenosis of bilateral nasolacrimal duct
  - **H04.559** Acquired stenosis of unspecified nasolacrimal duct
- **H04.56** Stenosis of lacrimal punctum
  - **H04.561** Stenosis of right lacrimal punctum
  - **H04.562** Stenosis of left lacrimal punctum
  - **H04.563** Stenosis of bilateral lacrimal punctum
  - **H04.569** Stenosis of unspecified lacrimal punctum
- **H04.57** Stenosis of lacrimal sac
  - **H04.571** Stenosis of right lacrimal sac
  - **H04.572** Stenosis of left lacrimal sac
  - **H04.573** Stenosis of bilateral lacrimal sac
  - **H04.579** Stenosis of unspecified lacrimal sac
- **H04.6** Other changes of lacrimal passages
  - **H04.61** Lacrimal fistula
    - **H04.611** Lacrimal fistula right lacrimal passage
    - **H04.612** Lacrimal fistula left lacrimal passage
    - **H04.613** Lacrimal fistula bilateral lacrimal passages
    - **H04.619** Lacrimal fistula unspecified lacrimal passage
  - **H04.69** Other changes of lacrimal passages
- **H04.8** Other disorders of lacrimal system
  - **H04.81** Granuloma of lacrimal passages
    Inflammatory response due to infectious or noninfectious agents
    - **H04.811** Granuloma of right lacrimal passage
    - **H04.812** Granuloma of left lacrimal passage
    - **H04.813** Granuloma of bilateral lacrimal passages
    - **H04.819** Granuloma of unspecified lacrimal passage
  - **H04.89** Other disorders of lacrimal system
- **H04.9** Disorder of lacrimal system, unspecified

- **H05** Disorders of orbit

  Excludes1 congenital malformation of orbit (Q10.7)
  - **H05.0** Acute inflammation of orbit
    - **H05.00** Unspecified acute inflammation of orbit
    - **H05.01** Cellulitis of orbit
      Infection of soft tissue of orbit
      Abscess of orbit
      Ex: **For category H05.01 CC codes:** H05.00-H05.049
      - **H05.011** Cellulitis of right orbit
      - **H05.012** Cellulitis of left orbit
      - **H05.013** Cellulitis of bilateral orbits
      - **H05.019** Cellulitis of unspecified orbit
    - **H05.02** Osteomyelitis of orbit
      Infection of boney orbit of eye
      Ex: **For category H05.02 CC codes:** A02.24, A17.9, A18.03-A18.09, A18.82, A18.84, A18.89, H05.021-H05.029, M46.20-M46.39, M86.00-M86.9
      - **H05.021** Osteomyelitis of right orbit
      - **H05.022** Osteomyelitis of left orbit
      - **H05.023** Osteomyelitis of bilateral orbits
      - **H05.029** Osteomyelitis of unspecified orbit
    - **H05.03** Periostitis of orbit
      Inflammation of periosteum (membrane covering bone surface)
      Ex: **For category H05.03 CC codes:** A02.24, A17.9, A18.03-A18.09, A18.82, A18.84, A18.89, H05.031-H05.039, M46.20-M46.39, M86.00-M86.9
      - **H05.031** Periostitis of right orbit
      - **H05.032** Periostitis of left orbit
      - **H05.033** Periostitis of bilateral orbits
      - **H05.039** Periostitis of unspecified orbit
    - **H05.04** Tenonitis of orbit
      Inflammation of tenon capsule (space enclosing fascia of Tenon between eyeball and fat of orbit)
      - **H05.041** Tenonitis of right orbit
      - **H05.042** Tenonitis of left orbit
      - **H05.043** Tenonitis of bilateral orbits
      - **H05.049** Tenonitis of unspecified orbit
  - **H05.1** Chronic inflammatory disorders of orbit
    - **H05.10** Unspecified chronic inflammatory disorders of orbit
    - **H05.11** Granuloma of orbit
      Pseudotumor (inflammatory) of orbit
      - **H05.111** Granuloma of right orbit
      - **H05.112** Granuloma of left orbit
      - **H05.113** Granuloma of bilateral orbits
      - **H05.119** Granuloma of unspecified orbit
    - **H05.12** Orbital myositis
      Inflammation of extraocular muscles of orbit
      - **H05.121** Orbital myositis, right orbit
      - **H05.122** Orbital myositis, left orbit
      - **H05.123** Orbital myositis, bilateral
      - **H05.129** Orbital myositis, unspecified orbit
  - **H05.2** Exophthalmic conditions
    Bulging eyes
    - **H05.20** Unspecified exophthalmos
    - **H05.21** Displacement (lateral) of globe
      - **H05.211** Displacement (lateral) of globe, right eye
      - **H05.212** Displacement (lateral) of globe, left eye
      - **H05.213** Displacement (lateral) of globe, bilateral
      - **H05.219** Displacement (lateral) of globe, unspecified eye
    - **H05.22** Edema of orbit
      Orbital congestion
      - **H05.221** Edema of right orbit
      - **H05.222** Edema of left orbit
      - **H05.223** Edema of bilateral orbit
      - **H05.229** Edema of unspecified orbit
    - **H05.23** Hemorrhage of orbit
      - **H05.231** Hemorrhage of right orbit
      - **H05.232** Hemorrhage of left orbit
      - **H05.233** Hemorrhage of bilateral orbit
      - **H05.239** Hemorrhage of unspecified orbit

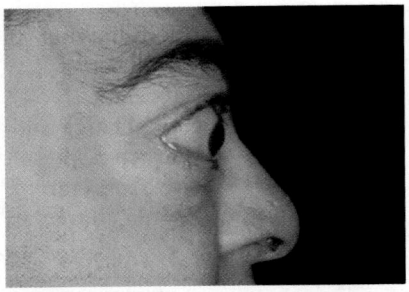

Figure 7-5 Exophthalmos. (From Stein: The Ophthalmic Assistant: Fundamentals and Clinical Practice, ed 6, London, Mosby, 1994)

- **H05.24 Constant exophthalmos**
  Constant bulging eyes, often symptom of Graves disease
  - H05.241 Constant exophthalmos, right eye
  - H05.242 Constant exophthalmos, left eye
  - H05.243 Constant exophthalmos, bilateral
  - H05.249 Constant exophthalmos, unspecified eye
- **H05.25 Intermittent exophthalmos**
  Intermittent bulging eye occurring with bending forward or sharp turning of head
  - H05.251 Intermittent exophthalmos, right eye
  - H05.252 Intermittent exophthalmos, left eye
  - H05.253 Intermittent exophthalmos, bilateral
  - H05.259 Intermittent exophthalmos, unspecified eye
- **H05.26 Pulsating exophthalmos**
  Bulging eyes with pulsation and bruit, often due to aneurysm pushing eye forward
  - H05.261 Pulsating exophthalmos, right eye
  - H05.262 Pulsating exophthalmos, left eye
  - H05.263 Pulsating exophthalmos, bilateral
  - H05.269 Pulsating exophthalmos, unspecified eye
- **H05.3 Deformity of orbit**
  - **Excludes1** congenital deformity of orbit (Q10.7)
    hypertelorism (Q75.2)
  - H05.30 Unspecified deformity of orbit
  - **H05.31 Atrophy of orbit**
    - H05.311 Atrophy of right orbit
    - H05.312 Atrophy of left orbit
    - H05.313 Atrophy of bilateral orbit
    - H05.319 Atrophy of unspecified orbit
  - **H05.32 Deformity of orbit due to bone disease**
    - Code also associated bone disease
    - H05.321 Deformity of right orbit due to bone disease
    - H05.322 Deformity of left orbit due to bone disease
    - H05.323 Deformity of bilateral orbits due to bone disease
    - H05.329 Deformity of unspecified orbit due to bone disease
  - **H05.33 Deformity of orbit due to trauma or surgery**
    - H05.331 Deformity of right orbit due to trauma or surgery
    - H05.332 Deformity of left orbit due to trauma or surgery
    - H05.333 Deformity of bilateral orbits due to trauma or surgery
    - H05.339 Deformity of unspecified orbit due to trauma or surgery
  - **H05.34 Enlargement of orbit**
    - H05.341 Enlargement of right orbit
    - H05.342 Enlargement of left orbit
    - H05.343 Enlargement of bilateral orbits
    - H05.349 Enlargement of unspecified orbit
  - **H05.35 Exostosis of orbit**
    - H05.351 Exostosis of right orbit
    - H05.352 Exostosis of left orbit
    - H05.353 Exostosis of bilateral orbits
    - H05.359 Exostosis of unspecified orbit
- **H05.4 Enophthalmos**
  Recessed eyeball into orbit
  - **H05.40 Unspecified enophthalmos**
    - H05.401 Unspecified enophthalmos, right eye
    - H05.402 Unspecified enophthalmos, left eye
    - H05.403 Unspecified enophthalmos, bilateral
    - H05.409 Unspecified enophthalmos, unspecified eye
  - **H05.41 Enophthalmos due to atrophy of orbital tissue**
    - H05.411 Enophthalmos due to atrophy of orbital tissue, right eye
    - H05.412 Enophthalmos due to atrophy of orbital tissue, left eye
    - H05.413 Enophthalmos due to atrophy of orbital tissue, bilateral
    - H05.419 Enophthalmos due to atrophy of orbital tissue, unspecified eye
  - **H05.42 Enophthalmos due to trauma or surgery**
    - H05.421 Enophthalmos due to trauma or surgery, right eye
    - H05.422 Enophthalmos due to trauma or surgery, left eye
    - H05.423 Enophthalmos due to trauma or surgery, bilateral
    - H05.429 Enophthalmos due to trauma or surgery, unspecified eye
- **H05.5 Retained (old) foreign body following penetrating wound of orbit**
  Retrobulbar foreign body
  - Use additional code to identify the type of retained foreign body (Z18.-)
  - **Excludes1** current penetrating wound of orbit (S05.4-)
  - **Excludes2** retained foreign body of eyelid (H02.81-)
    retained intraocular foreign body (H44.6-, H44.7-)
  - H05.50 Retained (old) foreign body following penetrating wound of unspecified orbit
  - H05.51 Retained (old) foreign body following penetrating wound of right orbit
  - H05.52 Retained (old) foreign body following penetrating wound of left orbit
  - H05.53 Retained (old) foreign body following penetrating wound of bilateral orbits
- **H05.8 Other disorders of orbit**
  - **H05.81 Cyst of orbit**
    Encephalocele of orbit
    - H05.811 Cyst of right orbit
    - H05.812 Cyst of left orbit
    - H05.813 Cyst of bilateral orbits
    - H05.819 Cyst of unspecified orbit

- H05.82 Myopathy of extraocular muscles
  Weakness of muscles of eye
  - H05.821 Myopathy of extraocular muscles, right orbit
  - H05.822 Myopathy of extraocular muscles, left orbit
  - H05.823 Myopathy of extraocular muscles, bilateral
  - H05.829 Myopathy of extraocular muscles, unspecified orbit
- H05.89 Other disorders of orbit
- H05.9 Unspecified disorder of orbit

DISORDERS OF CONJUNCTIVA (H10-H11)

★(See Plate 81, upper, on page 66.)

- H10 Conjunctivitis
  Inflammation of membrane of the inside of the eyelid or on surface of eye (conjunctiva)
  Excludes1 keratoconjunctivitis (H16.2-)
  - H10.0 Mucopurulent conjunctivitis
    - H10.01 Acute follicular conjunctivitis
      - H10.011 Acute follicular conjunctivitis, right eye
      - H10.012 Acute follicular conjunctivitis, left eye
      - H10.013 Acute follicular conjunctivitis, bilateral
      - H10.019 Acute follicular conjunctivitis, unspecified eye
    - H10.02 Other mucopurulent conjunctivitis
      - H10.021 Other mucopurulent conjunctivitis, right eye
      - H10.022 Other mucopurulent conjunctivitis, left eye
      - H10.023 Other mucopurulent conjunctivitis, bilateral
      - H10.029 Other mucopurulent conjunctivitis, unspecified eye
  - H10.1 Acute atopic conjunctivitis
    Acute papillary conjunctivitis
    - H10.10 Acute atopic conjunctivitis, unspecified eye
    - H10.11 Acute atopic conjunctivitis, right eye
    - H10.12 Acute atopic conjunctivitis, left eye
    - H10.13 Acute atopic conjunctivitis, bilateral
  - H10.2 Other acute conjunctivitis
    - H10.21 Acute toxic conjunctivitis
      Acute chemical conjunctivitis
      Code first (T51-T65) to identify chemical and intent
      Excludes1 burn and corrosion of eye and adnexa (T26.-)
      - H10.211 Acute toxic conjunctivitis, right eye
      - H10.212 Acute toxic conjunctivitis, left eye
      - H10.213 Acute toxic conjunctivitis, bilateral
      - H10.219 Acute toxic conjunctivitis, unspecified eye
    - H10.22 Pseudomembranous conjunctivitis
      - H10.221 Pseudomembranous conjunctivitis, right eye
      - H10.222 Pseudomembranous conjunctivitis, left eye
      - H10.223 Pseudomembranous conjunctivitis, bilateral
      - H10.229 Pseudomembranous conjunctivitis, unspecified eye
    - H10.23 Serous conjunctivitis, except viral
      Excludes1 viral conjunctivitis (B30.-)
      - H10.231 Serous conjunctivitis, except viral, right eye
      - H10.232 Serous conjunctivitis, except viral, left eye
      - H10.233 Serous conjunctivitis, except viral, bilateral
      - H10.239 Serous conjunctivitis, except viral, unspecified eye
  - H10.3 Unspecified acute conjunctivitis
    Excludes1 ophthalmia neonatorum NOS (P39.1)
    - H10.30 Unspecified acute conjunctivitis, unspecified eye
    - H10.31 Unspecified acute conjunctivitis, right eye
    - H10.32 Unspecified acute conjunctivitis, left eye
    - H10.33 Unspecified acute conjunctivitis, bilateral
  - H10.4 Chronic conjunctivitis
    - H10.40 Unspecified chronic conjunctivitis
      - H10.401 Unspecified chronic conjunctivitis, right eye
      - H10.402 Unspecified chronic conjunctivitis, left eye
      - H10.403 Unspecified chronic conjunctivitis, bilateral
      - H10.409 Unspecified chronic conjunctivitis, unspecified eye
    - H10.41 Chronic giant papillary conjunctivitis
      Inflammation of membrane of the inside of the eyelid or on surface of eye often associated with contact lens wear
      - H10.411 Chronic giant papillary conjunctivitis, right eye
      - H10.412 Chronic giant papillary conjunctivitis, left eye
      - H10.413 Chronic giant papillary conjunctivitis, bilateral
      - H10.419 Chronic giant papillary conjunctivitis, unspecified eye
    - H10.42 Simple chronic conjunctivitis
      - H10.421 Simple chronic conjunctivitis, right eye
      - H10.422 Simple chronic conjunctivitis, left eye
      - H10.423 Simple chronic conjunctivitis, bilateral
      - H10.429 Simple chronic conjunctivitis, unspecified eye
    - H10.43 Chronic follicular conjunctivitis
      Inflammation of membrane of the inside of the eyelid or on surface of eye due to topical medications or infection
      - H10.431 Chronic follicular conjunctivitis, right eye
      - H10.432 Chronic follicular conjunctivitis, left eye
      - H10.433 Chronic follicular conjunctivitis, bilateral
      - H10.439 Chronic follicular conjunctivitis, unspecified eye
    - H10.44 Vernal conjunctivitis
      Affecting children, especially boys in which there are flattened papules with thick, gelatinous exudate on conjunctivae on inside of upper lid
      Excludes1 vernal keratoconjunctivitis with limbar and corneal involvement (H16.26-)
    - H10.45 Other chronic allergic conjunctivitis

- **H10.5** Blepharoconjunctivitis
  Inflammation of eyelids and conjunctiva
  - **H10.50** Unspecified blepharoconjunctivitis
    - H10.501 Unspecified blepharoconjunctivitis, right eye
    - H10.502 Unspecified blepharoconjunctivitis, left eye
    - H10.503 Unspecified blepharoconjunctivitis, bilateral
    - H10.509 Unspecified blepharoconjunctivitis, unspecified eye
  - **H10.51** Ligneous conjunctivitis
    - H10.511 Ligneous conjunctivitis, right eye
    - H10.512 Ligneous conjunctivitis, left eye
    - H10.513 Ligneous conjunctivitis, bilateral
    - H10.519 Ligneous conjunctivitis, unspecified eye
  - **H10.52** Angular blepharoconjunctivitis
    - H10.521 Angular blepharoconjunctivitis, right eye
    - H10.522 Angular blepharoconjunctivitis, left eye
    - H10.523 Angular blepharoconjunctivitis, bilateral
    - H10.529 Angular blepharoconjunctivitis, unspecified eye
  - **H10.53** Contact blepharoconjunctivitis
    - H10.531 Contact blepharoconjunctivitis, right eye
    - H10.532 Contact blepharoconjunctivitis, left eye
    - H10.533 Contact blepharoconjunctivitis, bilateral
    - H10.539 Contact blepharoconjunctivitis, unspecified eye
- **H10.8** Other conjunctivitis
  - **H10.81** Pingueculitis
    Inflammation of a yellow, raised thickening on the white of the eye associated with chronic dry eyes
    Excludes1 pinguecula (H11.15-)
    - H10.811 Pingueculitis, right eye
    - H10.812 Pingueculitis, left eye
    - H10.813 Pingueculitis, bilateral
    - H10.819 Pingueculitis, unspecified eye
  - H10.89 Other conjunctivitis
- H10.9 Unspecified conjunctivitis

- **H11** Other disorders of conjunctiva
  Excludes1 keratoconjunctivitis (H16.2-)
  - **H11.0** Pterygium of eye
    Excludes1 pseudopterygium (H11.81-)
    - **H11.00** Unspecified pterygium of eye
      - H11.001 Unspecified pterygium of right eye
      - H11.002 Unspecified pterygium of left eye
      - H11.003 Unspecified pterygium of eye, bilateral
      - H11.009 Unspecified pterygium of unspecified eye
    - **H11.01** Amyloid pterygium
      - H11.011 Amyloid pterygium of right eye
      - H11.012 Amyloid pterygium of left eye
      - H11.013 Amyloid pterygium of eye, bilateral
      - H11.019 Amyloid pterygium of unspecified eye

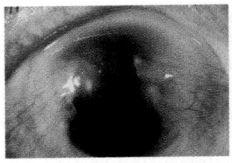

Figure 7-6 Double pterygium. Note both nasal and temporal pterygia in a 57-year-old farmer. (From Yanoff: Ophthalmology, ed 3, Mosby, Inc., 2008)

Item 7–2 Pterygium is Greek for batlike. The condition is characterized by a membrane that extends from the limbus to the center of the cornea and resembles a wing.

    - **H11.02** Central pterygium of eye
      - H11.021 Central pterygium of right eye
      - H11.022 Central pterygium of left eye
      - H11.023 Central pterygium of eye, bilateral
      - H11.029 Central pterygium of unspecified eye
    - **H11.03** Double pterygium of eye
      - H11.031 Double pterygium of right eye
      - H11.032 Double pterygium of left eye
      - H11.033 Double pterygium of eye, bilateral
      - H11.039 Double pterygium of unspecified eye
    - **H11.04** Peripheral pterygium of eye, stationary
      - H11.041 Peripheral pterygium, stationary, right eye
      - H11.042 Peripheral pterygium, stationary, left eye
      - H11.043 Peripheral pterygium, stationary, bilateral
      - H11.049 Peripheral pterygium, stationary, unspecified eye
    - **H11.05** Peripheral pterygium of eye, progressive
      - H11.051 Peripheral pterygium, progressive, right eye
      - H11.052 Peripheral pterygium, progressive, left eye
      - H11.053 Peripheral pterygium, progressive, bilateral
      - H11.059 Peripheral pterygium, progressive, unspecified eye
    - **H11.06** Recurrent pterygium of eye
      - H11.061 Recurrent pterygium of right eye
      - H11.062 Recurrent pterygium of left eye
      - H11.063 Recurrent pterygium of eye, bilateral
      - H11.069 Recurrent pterygium of unspecified eye
  - **H11.1** Conjunctival degenerations and deposits
    Excludes2 pseudopterygium (H11.81)
    - H11.10 Unspecified conjunctival degenerations
    - **H11.11** Conjunctival deposits
      - H11.111 Conjunctival deposits, right eye
      - H11.112 Conjunctival deposits, left eye
      - H11.113 Conjunctival deposits, bilateral
      - H11.119 Conjunctival deposits, unspecified eye
    - **H11.12** Conjunctival concretions
      White to yellow nodules within or beneath conjunctiva
      - H11.121 Conjunctival concretions, right eye
      - H11.122 Conjunctival concretions, left eye
      - H11.123 Conjunctival concretions, bilateral
      - H11.129 Conjunctival concretions, unspecified eye
    - **H11.13** Conjunctival pigmentations
      Conjunctival argyrosis [argyria]
      - H11.131 Conjunctival pigmentations, right eye
      - H11.132 Conjunctival pigmentations, left eye
      - H11.133 Conjunctival pigmentations, bilateral
      - H11.139 Conjunctival pigmentations, unspecified eye

- **H11.14 Conjunctival xerosis, unspecified**
  - **Excludes1** xerosis of conjunctiva due to vitamin A deficiency (E50.0, E50.1)
  - **H11.141 Conjunctival xerosis, unspecified, right eye**
  - **H11.142 Conjunctival xerosis, unspecified, left eye**
  - **H11.143 Conjunctival xerosis, unspecified, bilateral**
  - **H11.149 Conjunctival xerosis, unspecified, unspecified eye**
- **H11.15 Pinguecula**
  - *Yellowish spot near sclerocorneal junction, usually on nasal side; associated with aging*
  - **Excludes1** pingueculitis (H10.81-)
  - **H11.151 Pinguecula, right eye**
  - **H11.152 Pinguecula, left eye**
  - **H11.153 Pinguecula, bilateral**
  - **H11.159 Pinguecula, unspecified eye**
- **H11.2 Conjunctival scars**
  - **H11.21 Conjunctival adhesions and strands (localized)**
    - **H11.211 Conjunctival adhesions and strands (localized), right eye**
    - **H11.212 Conjunctival adhesions and strands (localized), left eye**
    - **H11.213 Conjunctival adhesions and strands (localized), bilateral**
    - **H11.219 Conjunctival adhesions and strands (localized), unspecified eye**
  - **H11.22 Conjunctival granuloma**
    - **H11.221 Conjunctival granuloma, right eye**
    - **H11.222 Conjunctival granuloma, left eye**
    - **H11.223 Conjunctival granuloma, bilateral**
    - **H11.229 Conjunctival granuloma, unspecified**
  - **H11.23 Symblepharon**
    - *Adhesion between tarsal conjunctiva and bulbar conjunctiva*
    - **H11.231 Symblepharon, right eye**
    - **H11.232 Symblepharon, left eye**
    - **H11.233 Symblepharon, bilateral**
    - **H11.239 Symblepharon, unspecified eye**
  - **H11.24 Scarring of conjunctiva**
    - **H11.241 Scarring of conjunctiva, right eye**
    - **H11.242 Scarring of conjunctiva, left eye**
    - **H11.243 Scarring of conjunctiva, bilateral**
    - **H11.249 Scarring of conjunctiva, unspecified eye**
- **H11.3 Conjunctival hemorrhage**
  - Subconjunctival hemorrhage
  - **H11.30 Conjunctival hemorrhage, unspecified eye**
  - **H11.31 Conjunctival hemorrhage, right eye**
  - **H11.32 Conjunctival hemorrhage, left eye**
  - **H11.33 Conjunctival hemorrhage, bilateral**
- **H11.4 Other conjunctival vascular disorders and cysts**
  - **H11.41 Vascular abnormalities of conjunctiva**
    - Conjunctival aneurysm
    - **H11.411 Vascular abnormalities of conjunctiva, right eye**
    - **H11.412 Vascular abnormalities of conjunctiva, left eye**
    - **H11.413 Vascular abnormalities of conjunctiva, bilateral**
    - **H11.419 Vascular abnormalities of conjunctiva, unspecified eye**
  - **H11.42 Conjunctival edema**
    - **H11.421 Conjunctival edema, right eye**
    - **H11.422 Conjunctival edema, left eye**
    - **H11.423 Conjunctival edema, bilateral**
    - **H11.429 Conjunctival edema, unspecified eye**
  - **H11.43 Conjunctival hyperemia**
    - **H11.431 Conjunctival hyperemia, right eye**
    - **H11.432 Conjunctival hyperemia, left eye**
    - **H11.433 Conjunctival hyperemia, bilateral**
    - **H11.439 Conjunctival hyperemia, unspecified eye**
  - **H11.44 Conjunctival cysts**
    - **H11.441 Conjunctival cysts, right eye**
    - **H11.442 Conjunctival cysts, left eye**
    - **H11.443 Conjunctival cysts, bilateral**
    - **H11.449 Conjunctival cysts, unspecified eye**
- **H11.8 Other specified disorders of conjunctiva**
  - **H11.81 Pseudopterygium of conjunctiva**
    - *Conjunctival scar attached to cornea*
    - **H11.811 Pseudopterygium of conjunctiva, right eye**
    - **H11.812 Pseudopterygium of conjunctiva, left eye**
    - **H11.813 Pseudopterygium of conjunctiva, bilateral**
    - **H11.819 Pseudopterygium of conjunctiva, unspecified eye**
  - **H11.82 Conjunctivochalasis**
    - *Conjunctiva bulges over eyelid margin or covers lower punctum*
    - **H11.821 Conjunctivochalasis, right eye**
    - **H11.822 Conjunctivochalasis, left eye**
    - **H11.823 Conjunctivochalasis, bilateral**
    - **H11.829 Conjunctivochalasis, unspecified eye**
  - **H11.89 Other specified disorders of conjunctiva**
- **H11.9 Unspecified disorder of conjunctiva**

DISORDERS OF SCLERA, CORNEA, IRIS AND CILIARY BODY (H15-H22)

- **H15 Disorders of sclera**
  - **H15.0 Scleritis**
    - *Inflammation of the white (sclera and episclera) of the eye.*
    - **H15.00 Unspecified scleritis**
      - **H15.001 Unspecified scleritis, right eye**
      - **H15.002 Unspecified scleritis, left eye**
      - **H15.003 Unspecified scleritis, bilateral**
      - **H15.009 Unspecified scleritis, unspecified eye**
    - **H15.01 Anterior scleritis**
      - **H15.011 Anterior scleritis, right eye**
      - **H15.012 Anterior scleritis, left eye**
      - **H15.013 Anterior scleritis, bilateral**
      - **H15.019 Anterior scleritis, unspecified eye**
    - **H15.02 Brawny scleritis**
      - *Swelling around the cornea that is gelantinous in appearance*
      - **H15.021 Brawny scleritis, right eye**
      - **H15.022 Brawny scleritis, left eye**
      - **H15.023 Brawny scleritis, bilateral**
      - **H15.029 Brawny scleritis, unspecified eye**
    - **H15.03 Posterior scleritis**
      - Sclerotenonitis
      - **H15.031 Posterior scleritis, right eye**
      - **H15.032 Posterior scleritis, left eye**
      - **H15.033 Posterior scleritis, bilateral**
      - **H15.039 Posterior scleritis, unspecified eye**

- H15.04 Scleritis with corneal involvement
  - H15.041 Scleritis with corneal involvement, right eye
  - H15.042 Scleritis with corneal involvement, left eye
  - H15.043 Scleritis with corneal involvement, bilateral
  - H15.049 Scleritis with corneal involvement, unspecified eye
- H15.05 Scleromalacia perforans
  Necrotic without inflammation; usually associated with rheumatoid arthritis
  - H15.051 Scleromalacia perforans, right eye
  - H15.052 Scleromalacia perforans, left eye
  - H15.053 Scleromalacia perforans, bilateral
  - H15.059 Scleromalacia perforans, unspecified eye
- H15.09 Other scleritis
  Scleral abscess
  - H15.091 Other scleritis, right eye
  - H15.092 Other scleritis, left eye
  - H15.093 Other scleritis, bilateral
  - H15.099 Other scleritis, unspecified eye
- H15.1 Episcleritis
  Inflammation of the white (sclera and episclera) of the eye.
  - H15.10 Unspecified episcleritis
    - H15.101 Unspecified episcleritis, right eye
    - H15.102 Unspecified episcleritis, left eye
    - H15.103 Unspecified episcleritis, bilateral
    - H15.109 Unspecified episcleritis, unspecified eye
  - H15.11 Episcleritis periodica fugax
    Transient, recurrent inflammation of portion of episclera (connective tissue on the surface of the sclera)
    - H15.111 Episcleritis periodica fugax, right eye
    - H15.112 Episcleritis periodica fugax, left eye
    - H15.113 Episcleritis periodica fugax, bilateral
    - H15.119 Episcleritis periodica fugax, unspecified eye
  - H15.12 Nodular episcleritis
    Characterized by tender, localized, moveable nodule within inflamed area
    - H15.121 Nodular episcleritis, right eye
    - H15.122 Nodular episcleritis, left eye
    - H15.123 Nodular episcleritis, bilateral
    - H15.129 Nodular episcleritis, unspecified eye
- H15.8 Other disorders of sclera
  Excludes2 blue sclera (Q13.5)
  degenerative myopia (H44.2-)
  - H15.81 Equatorial staphyloma
    - H15.811 Equatorial staphyloma, right eye
    - H15.812 Equatorial staphyloma, left eye
    - H15.813 Equatorial staphyloma, bilateral
    - H15.819 Equatorial staphyloma, unspecified eye
  - H15.82 Localized anterior staphyloma
    - H15.821 Localized anterior staphyloma, right eye
    - H15.822 Localized anterior staphyloma, left eye
    - H15.823 Localized anterior staphyloma, bilateral
    - H15.829 Localized anterior staphyloma, unspecified eye
  - H15.83 Staphyloma posticum
    - H15.831 Staphyloma posticum, right eye
    - H15.832 Staphyloma posticum, left eye
    - H15.833 Staphyloma posticum, bilateral
    - H15.839 Staphyloma posticum, unspecified eye
  - H15.84 Scleral ectasia
    - H15.841 Scleral ectasia, right eye
    - H15.842 Scleral ectasia, left eye
    - H15.843 Scleral ectasia, bilateral
    - H15.849 Scleral ectasia, unspecified eye
  - H15.85 Ring staphyloma
    - H15.851 Ring staphyloma, right eye
    - H15.852 Ring staphyloma, left eye
    - H15.853 Ring staphyloma, bilateral
    - H15.859 Ring staphyloma, unspecified eye
  - H15.89 Other disorders of sclera
- H15.9 Unspecified disorder of sclera

- H16 Keratitis
  - H16.0 Corneal ulcer
    - H16.00 Unspecified corneal ulcer
      - H16.001 Unspecified corneal ulcer, right eye
      - H16.002 Unspecified corneal ulcer, left eye
      - H16.003 Unspecified corneal ulcer, bilateral
      - H16.009 Unspecified corneal ulcer, unspecified eye
    - H16.01 Central corneal ulcer
      - H16.011 Central corneal ulcer, right eye
      - H16.012 Central corneal ulcer, left eye
      - H16.013 Central corneal ulcer, bilateral
      - H16.019 Central corneal ulcer, unspecified eye
    - H16.02 Ring corneal ulcer
      - H16.021 Ring corneal ulcer, right eye
      - H16.022 Ring corneal ulcer, left eye
      - H16.023 Ring corneal ulcer, bilateral
      - H16.029 Ring corneal ulcer, unspecified eye
    - H16.03 Corneal ulcer with hypopyon
      - H16.031 Corneal ulcer with hypopyon, right eye
      - H16.032 Corneal ulcer with hypopyon, left eye
      - H16.033 Corneal ulcer with hypopyon, bilateral
      - H16.039 Corneal ulcer with hypopyon, unspecified eye

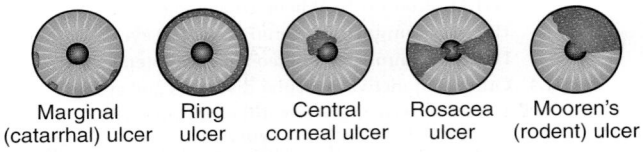

Figure 7-7 Corneal ulcers: marginal, ring, central corneal, rosacea, and Mooren's.

Item 7–3 An infected ulcer is usually called a **serpiginous** or **hypopyon** ulcer which is a pus sac in the anterior chamber of the eye. **Marginal** ulcers are usually asymptomatic, not primary, and are often superficial and simple. More severe marginal ulcers spread to form a ring ulcer. **Ring** ulcers can extend around the entire corneal periphery. **Central corneal** ulcers develop when there is an abrasion to the epithelium and an infection develops in the eroded area. The **pyocyaneal** ulcer is the most serious corneal infection, which, if left untreated, can lead to loss of the eye.

- **H16.04 Marginal corneal ulcer**
  - **H16.041 Marginal corneal ulcer, right eye**
  - **H16.042 Marginal corneal ulcer, left eye**
  - **H16.043 Marginal corneal ulcer, bilateral**
  - **H16.049 Marginal corneal ulcer, unspecified eye**
- **H16.05 Mooren's corneal ulcer**
  - **H16.051 Mooren's corneal ulcer, right eye**
  - **H16.052 Mooren's corneal ulcer, left eye**
  - **H16.053 Mooren's corneal ulcer, bilateral**
  - **H16.059 Mooren's corneal ulcer, unspecified eye**
- **H16.06 Mycotic corneal ulcer**
  - **H16.061 Mycotic corneal ulcer, right eye**
  - **H16.062 Mycotic corneal ulcer, left eye**
  - **H16.063 Mycotic corneal ulcer, bilateral**
  - **H16.069 Mycotic corneal ulcer, unspecified eye**
- **H16.07 Perforated corneal ulcer**
  - **H16.071 Perforated corneal ulcer, right eye**
  - **H16.072 Perforated corneal ulcer, left eye**
  - **H16.073 Perforated corneal ulcer, bilateral**
  - **H16.079 Perforated corneal ulcer, unspecified eye**

- **H16.1 Other and unspecified superficial keratitis without conjunctivitis**
  - **H16.10 Unspecified superficial keratitis**
    - **H16.101 Unspecified superficial keratitis, right eye**
    - **H16.102 Unspecified superficial keratitis, left eye**
    - **H16.103 Unspecified superficial keratitis, bilateral**
    - **H16.109 Unspecified superficial keratitis, unspecified eye**
  - **H16.11 Macular keratitis**
    - Areolar keratitis
    - Nummular keratitis
    - Stellate keratitis
    - Striate keratitis
    - **H16.111 Macular keratitis, right eye**
    - **H16.112 Macular keratitis, left eye**
    - **H16.113 Macular keratitis, bilateral**
    - **H16.119 Macular keratitis, unspecified eye**
  - **H16.12 Filamentary keratitis**
    - **H16.121 Filamentary keratitis, right eye**
    - **H16.122 Filamentary keratitis, left eye**
    - **H16.123 Filamentary keratitis, bilateral**
    - **H16.129 Filamentary keratitis, unspecified eye**
  - **H16.13 Photokeratitis**
    - Snow blindness
    - Welders' keratitis
    - **H16.131 Photokeratitis, right eye**
    - **H16.132 Photokeratitis, left eye**
    - **H16.133 Photokeratitis, bilateral**
    - **H16.139 Photokeratitis, unspecified eye**
  - **H16.14 Punctate keratitis**
    - **H16.141 Punctate keratitis, right eye**
    - **H16.142 Punctate keratitis, left eye**
    - **H16.143 Punctate keratitis, bilateral**
    - **H16.149 Punctate keratitis, unspecified eye**

- **H16.2 Keratoconjunctivitis**
  - **H16.20 Unspecified keratoconjunctivitis**
    - Superficial keratitis with conjunctivitis NOS
    - **H16.201 Unspecified keratoconjunctivitis, right eye**
    - **H16.202 Unspecified keratoconjunctivitis, left eye**
    - **H16.203 Unspecified keratoconjunctivitis, bilateral**
    - **H16.209 Unspecified keratoconjunctivitis, unspecified eye**
  - **H16.21 Exposure keratoconjunctivitis**
    - **H16.211 Exposure keratoconjunctivitis, right eye**
    - **H16.212 Exposure keratoconjunctivitis, left eye**
    - **H16.213 Exposure keratoconjunctivitis, bilateral**
    - **H16.219 Exposure keratoconjunctivitis, unspecified eye**
  - **H16.22 Keratoconjunctivitis sicca, not specified as Sjögren's**
    - **Excludes1** Sjogren's syndrome (M35.01)
    - **H16.221 Keratoconjunctivitis sicca, not specified as Sjögren's, right eye**
    - **H16.222 Keratoconjunctivitis sicca, not specified as Sjögren's, left eye**
    - **H16.223 Keratoconjunctivitis sicca, not specified as Sjögren's, bilateral**
    - **H16.229 Keratoconjunctivitis sicca, not specified as Sjögren's, unspecified eye**
  - **H16.23 Neurotrophic keratoconjunctivitis**
    - **H16.231 Neurotrophic keratoconjunctivitis, right eye**
    - **H16.232 Neurotrophic keratoconjunctivitis, left eye**
    - **H16.233 Neurotrophic keratoconjunctivitis, bilateral**
    - **H16.239 Neurotrophic keratoconjunctivitis, unspecified eye**
  - **H16.24 Ophthalmia nodosa**
    - **H16.241 Ophthalmia nodosa, right eye**
    - **H16.242 Ophthalmia nodosa, left eye**
    - **H16.243 Ophthalmia nodosa, bilateral**
    - **H16.249 Ophthalmia nodosa, unspecified eye**
  - **H16.25 Phlyctenular keratoconjunctivitis**
    - **H16.251 Phlyctenular keratoconjunctivitis, right eye**
    - **H16.252 Phlyctenular keratoconjunctivitis, left eye**
    - **H16.253 Phlyctenular keratoconjunctivitis, bilateral**
    - **H16.259 Phlyctenular keratoconjunctivitis, unspecified eye**
  - **H16.26 Vernal keratoconjunctivitis, with limbar and corneal involvement**
    - **Excludes1** vernal conjunctivitis without limbar and corneal involvement (H10.44)
    - **H16.261 Vernal keratoconjunctivitis, with limbar and corneal involvement, right eye**
    - **H16.262 Vernal keratoconjunctivitis, with limbar and corneal involvement, left eye**

H16.263 Vernal keratoconjunctivitis, with limbar and corneal involvement, bilateral
H16.269 Vernal keratoconjunctivitis, with limbar and corneal involvement, unspecified eye
● H16.29 Other keratoconjunctivitis
H16.291 Other keratoconjunctivitis, right eye
H16.292 Other keratoconjunctivitis, left eye
H16.293 Other keratoconjunctivitis, bilateral
H16.299 Other keratoconjunctivitis, unspecified eye
● H16.3 Interstitial and deep keratitis
● H16.30 Unspecified interstitial keratitis
H16.301 Unspecified interstitial keratitis, right eye
H16.302 Unspecified interstitial keratitis, left eye
H16.303 Unspecified interstitial keratitis, bilateral
H16.309 Unspecified interstitial keratitis, unspecified eye
● H16.31 Corneal abscess
H16.311 Corneal abscess, right eye
H16.312 Corneal abscess, left eye
H16.313 Corneal abscess, bilateral
H16.319 Corneal abscess, unspecified eye
● H16.32 Diffuse interstitial keratitis
Cogan's syndrome
H16.321 Diffuse interstitial keratitis, right eye
H16.322 Diffuse interstitial keratitis, left eye
H16.323 Diffuse interstitial keratitis, bilateral
H16.329 Diffuse interstitial keratitis, unspecified eye
● H16.33 Sclerosing keratitis
H16.331 Sclerosing keratitis, right eye
H16.332 Sclerosing keratitis, left eye
H16.333 Sclerosing keratitis, bilateral
H16.339 Sclerosing keratitis, unspecified eye
● H16.39 Other interstitial and deep keratitis
H16.391 Other interstitial and deep keratitis, right eye
H16.392 Other interstitial and deep keratitis, left eye
H16.393 Other interstitial and deep keratitis, bilateral
H16.399 Other interstitial and deep keratitis, unspecified eye
● H16.4 Corneal neovascularization
● H16.40 Unspecified corneal neovascularization
H16.401 Unspecified corneal neovascularization, right eye
H16.402 Unspecified corneal neovascularization, left eye
H16.403 Unspecified corneal neovascularization, bilateral
H16.409 Unspecified corneal neovascularization, unspecified eye
● H16.41 Ghost vessels (corneal)
H16.411 Ghost vessels (corneal), right eye
H16.412 Ghost vessels (corneal), left eye
H16.413 Ghost vessels (corneal), bilateral
H16.419 Ghost vessels (corneal), unspecified eye
● H16.42 Pannus (corneal)
H16.421 Pannus (corneal), right eye
H16.422 Pannus (corneal), left eye
H16.423 Pannus (corneal), bilateral
H16.429 Pannus (corneal), unspecified eye
● H16.43 Localized vascularization of cornea
H16.431 Localized vascularization of cornea, right eye
H16.432 Localized vascularization of cornea, left eye
H16.433 Localized vascularization of cornea, bilateral
H16.439 Localized vascularization of cornea, unspecified eye
● H16.44 Deep vascularization of cornea
H16.441 Deep vascularization of cornea, right eye
H16.442 Deep vascularization of cornea, left eye
H16.443 Deep vascularization of cornea, bilateral
H16.449 Deep vascularization of cornea, unspecified eye
● H16.8 Other keratitis
H16.9 Unspecified keratitis
● H17 Corneal scars and opacities
● H17.0 Adherent leukoma
H17.00 Adherent leukoma, unspecified eye
H17.01 Adherent leukoma, right eye
H17.02 Adherent leukoma, left eye
H17.03 Adherent leukoma, bilateral
● H17.1 Central corneal opacity
H17.10 Central corneal opacity, unspecified eye
H17.11 Central corneal opacity, right eye
H17.12 Central corneal opacity, left eye
H17.13 Central corneal opacity, bilateral
● H17.8 Other corneal scars and opacities
● H17.81 Minor opacity of cornea
Corneal nebula
H17.811 Minor opacity of cornea, right eye
H17.812 Minor opacity of cornea, left eye
H17.813 Minor opacity of cornea, bilateral
H17.819 Minor opacity of cornea, unspecified eye
● H17.82 Peripheral opacity of cornea
H17.821 Peripheral opacity of cornea, right eye
H17.822 Peripheral opacity of cornea, left eye
H17.823 Peripheral opacity of cornea, bilateral
H17.829 Peripheral opacity of cornea, unspecified eye
H17.89 Other corneal scars and opacities
H17.9 Unspecified corneal scar and opacity
● H18 Other disorders of cornea
● H18.0 Corneal pigmentations and deposits
● H18.00 Unspecified corneal deposit
H18.001 Unspecified corneal deposit, right eye
H18.002 Unspecified corneal deposit, left eye
H18.003 Unspecified corneal deposit, bilateral
H18.009 Unspecified corneal deposit, unspecified eye
● H18.01 Anterior corneal pigmentations
Staehli's line
H18.011 Anterior corneal pigmentations, right eye
H18.012 Anterior corneal pigmentations, left eye

H18.013 Anterior corneal pigmentations, bilateral
H18.019 Anterior corneal pigmentations, unspecified eye

● H18.02 Argentous corneal deposits
H18.021 Argentous corneal deposits, right eye
H18.022 Argentous corneal deposits, left eye
H18.023 Argentous corneal deposits, bilateral
H18.029 Argentous corneal deposits, unspecified eye

● H18.03 Corneal deposits in metabolic disorders
Code also associated metabolic disorder
H18.031 Corneal deposits in metabolic disorders, right eye
H18.032 Corneal deposits in metabolic disorders, left eye
H18.033 Corneal deposits in metabolic disorders, bilateral
H18.039 Corneal deposits in metabolic disorders, unspecified eye

● H18.04 Kayser-Fleischer ring
Code also associated Wilson's disease (E83.01)
H18.041 Kayser-Fleischer ring, right eye
H18.042 Kayser-Fleischer ring, left eye
H18.043 Kayser-Fleischer ring, bilateral
H18.049 Kayser-Fleischer ring, unspecified eye

● H18.05 Posterior corneal pigmentations
Krukenberg's spindle
H18.051 Posterior corneal pigmentations, right eye
H18.052 Posterior corneal pigmentations, left eye
H18.053 Posterior corneal pigmentations, bilateral
H18.059 Posterior corneal pigmentations, unspecified eye

● H18.06 Stromal corneal pigmentations
Hematocornea
H18.061 Stromal corneal pigmentations, right eye
H18.062 Stromal corneal pigmentations, left eye
H18.063 Stromal corneal pigmentations, bilateral
H18.069 Stromal corneal pigmentations, unspecified eye

● H18.1 Bullous keratopathy
H18.10 Bullous keratopathy, unspecified eye
H18.11 Bullous keratopathy, right eye
H18.12 Bullous keratopathy, left eye
H18.13 Bullous keratopathy, bilateral

● H18.2 Other and unspecified corneal edema
H18.20 Unspecified corneal edema

● H18.21 Corneal edema secondary to contact lens
Excludes2 other corneal disorders due to contact lens (H18.82-)
H18.211 Corneal edema secondary to contact lens, right eye
H18.212 Corneal edema secondary to contact lens, left eye
H18.213 Corneal edema secondary to contact lens, bilateral
H18.219 Corneal edema secondary to contact lens, unspecified eye

● H18.22 Idiopathic corneal edema
H18.221 Idiopathic corneal edema, right eye
H18.222 Idiopathic corneal edema, left eye
H18.223 Idiopathic corneal edema, bilateral
H18.229 Idiopathic corneal edema, unspecified eye

● H18.23 Secondary corneal edema
H18.231 Secondary corneal edema, right eye
H18.232 Secondary corneal edema, left eye
H18.233 Secondary corneal edema, bilateral
H18.239 Secondary corneal edema, unspecified eye

● H18.3 Changes of corneal membranes
H18.30 Unspecified corneal membrane change

● H18.31 Folds and rupture in Bowman's membrane
H18.311 Folds and rupture in Bowman's membrane, right eye
H18.312 Folds and rupture in Bowman's membrane, left eye
H18.313 Folds and rupture in Bowman's membrane, bilateral
H18.319 Folds and rupture in Bowman's membrane, unspecified eye

● H18.32 Folds in Descemet's membrane
H18.321 Folds in Descemet's membrane, right eye
H18.322 Folds in Descemet's membrane, left eye
H18.323 Folds in Descemet's membrane, bilateral
H18.329 Folds in Descemet's membrane, unspecified eye

● H18.33 Rupture in Descemet's membrane
H18.331 Rupture in Descemet's membrane, right eye
H18.332 Rupture in Descemet's membrane, left eye
H18.333 Rupture in Descemet's membrane, bilateral
H18.339 Rupture in Descemet's membrane, unspecified eye

● H18.4 Corneal degeneration
Excludes1 Mooren's ulcer (H16.0-)
recurrent erosion of cornea (H18.83-)
H18.40 Unspecified corneal degeneration

● H18.41 Arcus senilis
Senile corneal changes
H18.411 Arcus senilis, right eye
H18.412 Arcus senilis, left eye
H18.413 Arcus senilis, bilateral
H18.419 Arcus senilis, unspecified eye

● H18.42 Band keratopathy
H18.421 Band keratopathy, right eye
H18.422 Band keratopathy, left eye
H18.423 Band keratopathy, bilateral
H18.429 Band keratopathy, unspecified eye

H18.43 Other calcerous corneal degeneration

● H18.44 Keratomalacia
Excludes1 keratomalacia due to vitamin A deficiency (E50.4)
H18.441 Keratomalacia, right eye
H18.442 Keratomalacia, left eye
H18.443 Keratomalacia, bilateral
H18.449 Keratomalacia, unspecified eye

- H18.45 Nodular corneal degeneration
  - H18.451 Nodular corneal degeneration, right eye
  - H18.452 Nodular corneal degeneration, left eye
  - H18.453 Nodular corneal degeneration, bilateral
  - H18.459 Nodular corneal degeneration, unspecified eye
- H18.46 Peripheral corneal degeneration
  - H18.461 Peripheral corneal degeneration, right eye
  - H18.462 Peripheral corneal degeneration, left eye
  - H18.463 Peripheral corneal degeneration, bilateral
  - H18.469 Peripheral corneal degeneration, unspecified eye
  - H18.49 Other corneal degeneration
- H18.5 Hereditary corneal dystrophies
  - H18.50 Unspecified hereditary corneal dystrophies
  - H18.51 Endothelial corneal dystrophy
    Fuchs' dystrophy
  - H18.52 Epithelial (juvenile) corneal dystrophy
  - H18.53 Granular corneal dystrophy
  - H18.54 Lattice corneal dystrophy
  - H18.55 Macular corneal dystrophy
  - H18.59 Other hereditary corneal dystrophies
- H18.6 Keratoconus
  - H18.60 Keratoconus, unspecified
    - H18.601 Keratoconus, unspecified, right eye
    - H18.602 Keratoconus, unspecified, left eye
    - H18.603 Keratoconus, unspecified, bilateral
    - H18.609 Keratoconus, unspecified, unspecified eye
  - H18.61 Keratoconus, stable
    - H18.611 Keratoconus, stable, right eye
    - H18.612 Keratoconus, stable, left eye
    - H18.613 Keratoconus, stable, bilateral
    - H18.619 Keratoconus, stable, unspecified eye
  - H18.62 Keratoconus, unstable
    Acute hydrops
    - H18.621 Keratoconus, unstable, right eye
    - H18.622 Keratoconus, unstable, left eye
    - H18.623 Keratoconus, unstable, bilateral
    - H18.629 Keratoconus, unstable, unspecified eye

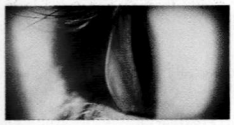

Figure 7-8 Lateral view of the displacement of the cone apex in keratoconus. (From Yanoff: Ophthalmology, ed 3, Mosby, Inc., 2008)

Item 7–4 Keratoconus results in corneal degeneration that begins in childhood, gradually changes the cornea from a round to cone shape, decreasing visual acuity. Treatment includes contact lenses. In severe cases the need for corneal transplant may be the treatment of choice; however, newer technologies may use high frequency radio energy to shrink the edges of the cornea, pulling the central area back to a more normal shape. It can help delay or avoid the need for a corneal transplantation.

- H18.7 Other and unspecified corneal deformities
  Excludes1 congenital malformations of cornea (Q13.3-Q13.4)
  - H18.70 Unspecified corneal deformity
  - H18.71 Corneal ectasia
    - H18.711 Corneal ectasia, right eye
    - H18.712 Corneal ectasia, left eye
    - H18.713 Corneal ectasia, bilateral
    - H18.719 Corneal ectasia, unspecified eye
  - H18.72 Corneal staphyloma
    - H18.721 Corneal staphyloma, right eye
    - H18.722 Corneal staphyloma, left eye
    - H18.723 Corneal staphyloma, bilateral
    - H18.729 Corneal staphyloma, unspecified eye
  - H18.73 Descemetocele
    - H18.731 Descemetocele, right eye
    - H18.732 Descemetocele, left eye
    - H18.733 Descemetocele, bilateral
    - H18.739 Descemetocele, unspecified eye
  - H18.79 Other corneal deformities
    - H18.791 Other corneal deformities, right eye
    - H18.792 Other corneal deformities, left eye
    - H18.793 Other corneal deformities, bilateral
    - H18.799 Other corneal deformities, unspecified eye
- H18.8 Other specified disorders of cornea
  - H18.81 Anesthesia and hypoesthesia of cornea
    - H18.811 Anesthesia and hypoesthesia of cornea, right eye
    - H18.812 Anesthesia and hypoesthesia of cornea, left eye
    - H18.813 Anesthesia and hypoesthesia of cornea, bilateral
    - H18.819 Anesthesia and hypoesthesia of cornea, unspecified eye
  - H18.82 Corneal disorder due to contact lens
    Excludes2 corneal edema due to contact lens (H18.21-)
    - H18.821 Corneal disorder due to contact lens, right eye
    - H18.822 Corneal disorder due to contact lens, left eye
    - H18.823 Corneal disorder due to contact lens, bilateral
    - H18.829 Corneal disorder due to contact lens, unspecified eye
  - H18.83 Recurrent erosion of cornea
    - H18.831 Recurrent erosion of cornea, right eye
    - H18.832 Recurrent erosion of cornea, left eye
    - H18.833 Recurrent erosion of cornea, bilateral
    - H18.839 Recurrent erosion of cornea, unspecified eye
  - H18.89 Other specified disorders of cornea
    - H18.891 Other specified disorders of cornea, right eye
    - H18.892 Other specified disorders of cornea, left eye
    - H18.893 Other specified disorders of cornea, bilateral
    - H18.899 Other specified disorders of cornea, unspecified eye
- H18.9 Unspecified disorder of cornea

- **H20 Iridocyclitis**
  - **H20.0 Acute and subacute iridocyclitis**
    Acute anterior uveitis
    Acute cyclitis
    Acute iritis
    Subacute anterior uveitis
    Subacute cyclitis
    Subacute iritis
    Excludes1 iridocyclitis, iritis, uveitis (due to) (in) diabetes mellitus (E08-E13 with .39)
    iridocyclitis, iritis, uveitis (due to) (in) diphtheria (A36.89)
    iridocyclitis, iritis, uveitis (due to) (in) gonococcal (A54.32)
    iridocyclitis, iritis, uveitis (due to) (in) herpes (simplex) (B00.51)
    iridocyclitis, iritis, uveitis (due to) (in) herpes zoster (B02.32)
    iridocyclitis, iritis, uveitis (due to) (in) late congenital syphilis (A50.39)
    iridocyclitis, iritis, uveitis (due to) (in) late syphilis (A52.71)
    iridocyclitis, iritis, uveitis (due to) (in) sarcoidosis (D86.83)
    iridocyclitis, iritis, uveitis (due to) (in) syphilis (A51.43)
    iridocyclitis, iritis, uveitis (due to) (in) toxoplasmosis (B58.09)
    iridocyclitis, iritis, uveitis (due to) (in) tuberculosis (A18.54)
    Ex: For category H20 CC codes: A18.54, H20.00-H20.9
    - **H20.00 Unspecified acute and subacute iridocyclitis**
    - **H20.01 Primary iridocyclitis**
      - **H20.011 Primary iridocyclitis, right eye**
      - **H20.012 Primary iridocyclitis, left eye**
      - **H20.013 Primary iridocyclitis, bilateral**
      - **H20.019 Primary iridocyclitis, unspecified eye**
    - **H20.02 Recurrent acute iridocyclitis**
      - **H20.021 Recurrent acute iridocyclitis, right eye**
      - **H20.022 Recurrent acute iridocyclitis, left eye**
      - **H20.023 Recurrent acute iridocyclitis, bilateral**
      - **H20.029 Recurrent acute iridocyclitis, unspecified eye**
    - **H20.03 Secondary infectious iridocyclitis**
      - **H20.031 Secondary infectious iridocyclitis, right eye**
      - **H20.032 Secondary infectious iridocyclitis, left eye**
      - **H20.033 Secondary infectious iridocyclitis, bilateral**
      - **H20.039 Secondary infectious iridocyclitis, unspecified eye**
    - **H20.04 Secondary noninfectious iridocyclitis**
      - **H20.041 Secondary noninfectious iridocyclitis, right eye**
      - **H20.042 Secondary noninfectious iridocyclitis, left eye**
      - **H20.043 Secondary noninfectious iridocyclitis, bilateral**
      - **H20.049 Secondary noninfectious iridocyclitis, unspecified eye**
    - **H20.05 Hypopyon**
      - **H20.051 Hypopyon, right eye**
      - **H20.052 Hypopyon, left eye**
      - **H20.053 Hypopyon, bilateral**
      - **H20.059 Hypopyon, unspecified eye**
  - **H20.1 Chronic iridocyclitis**
    Use additional code for any associated cataract (H26.21-)
    Excludes2 posterior cyclitis (H30.2-)
    - **H20.10 Chronic iridocyclitis, unspecified eye**
    - **H20.11 Chronic iridocyclitis, right eye**
    - **H20.12 Chronic iridocyclitis, left eye**
    - **H20.13 Chronic iridocyclitis, bilateral**
  - **H20.2 Lens-induced iridocyclitis**
    - **H20.20 Lens-induced iridocyclitis, unspecified eye**
    - **H20.21 Lens-induced iridocyclitis, right eye**
    - **H20.22 Lens-induced iridocyclitis, left eye**
    - **H20.23 Lens-induced iridocyclitis, bilateral**
  - **H20.8 Other iridocyclitis**
    Excludes2 glaucomatocyclitis crises (H40.4-)
    posterior cyclitis (H30.2-)
    sympathetic uveitis (H44.13-)
    - **H20.81 Fuchs' heterochromic cyclitis**
      - **H20.811 Fuchs' heterochromic cyclitis, right eye**
      - **H20.812 Fuchs' heterochromic cyclitis, left eye**
      - **H20.813 Fuchs' heterochromic cyclitis, bilateral**
      - **H20.819 Fuchs' heterochromic cyclitis, unspecified eye**
    - **H20.82 Vogt-Koyanagi syndrome**
      - **H20.821 Vogt-Koyanagi syndrome, right eye**
      - **H20.822 Vogt-Koyanagi syndrome, left eye**
      - **H20.823 Vogt-Koyanagi syndrome, bilateral**
      - **H20.829 Vogt-Koyanagi syndrome, unspecified eye**
  - **H20.9 Unspecified iridocyclitis**
    Uveitis NOS
- **H21 Other disorders of iris and ciliary body**
  Excludes2 sympathetic uveitis (H44.1-)
  - **H21.0 Hyphema**
    Excludes1 traumatic hyphema (S05.1-)
    - **H21.00 Hyphema, unspecified eye**
    - **H21.01 Hyphema, right eye**
    - **H21.02 Hyphema, left eye**
    - **H21.03 Hyphema, bilateral**
  - **H21.1 Other vascular disorders of iris and ciliary body**
    Neovascularization of iris or ciliary body
    Rubeosis iridis
    Rubeosis of iris
    - **H21.1X Other vascular disorders of iris and ciliary body**
      - **H21.1X1 Other vascular disorders of iris and ciliary body, right eye**
      - **H21.1X2 Other vascular disorders of iris and ciliary body, left eye**
      - **H21.1X3 Other vascular disorders of iris and ciliary body, bilateral**
      - **H21.1X9 Other vascular disorders of iris and ciliary body, unspecified eye**
  - **H21.2 Degeneration of iris and ciliary body**
    - **H21.21 Degeneration of chamber angle**
      - **H21.211 Degeneration of chamber angle, right eye**
      - **H21.212 Degeneration of chamber angle, left eye**
      - **H21.213 Degeneration of chamber angle, bilateral**
      - **H21.219 Degeneration of chamber angle, unspecified eye**

- H21.22 Degeneration of ciliary body
  - H21.221 Degeneration of ciliary body, right eye
  - H21.222 Degeneration of ciliary body, left eye
  - H21.223 Degeneration of ciliary body, bilateral
  - H21.229 Degeneration of ciliary body, unspecified eye
- H21.23 Degeneration of iris (pigmentary)
  Translucency of iris
  - H21.231 Degeneration of iris (pigmentary), right eye
  - H21.232 Degeneration of iris (pigmentary), left eye
  - H21.233 Degeneration of iris (pigmentary), bilateral
  - H21.239 Degeneration of iris (pigmentary), unspecified eye
- H21.24 Degeneration of pupillary margin
  - H21.241 Degeneration of pupillary margin, right eye
  - H21.242 Degeneration of pupillary margin, left eye
  - H21.243 Degeneration of pupillary margin, bilateral
  - H21.249 Degeneration of pupillary margin, unspecified eye
- H21.25 Iridoschisis
  - H21.251 Iridoschisis, right eye
  - H21.252 Iridoschisis, left eye
  - H21.253 Iridoschisis, bilateral
  - H21.259 Iridoschisis, unspecified eye
- H21.26 Iris atrophy (essential) (progressive)
  - H21.261 Iris atrophy (essential) (progressive), right eye
  - H21.262 Iris atrophy (essential) (progressive), left eye
  - H21.263 Iris atrophy (essential) (progressive), bilateral
  - H21.269 Iris atrophy (essential) (progressive), unspecified eye
- H21.27 Miotic pupillary cyst
  - H21.271 Miotic pupillary cyst, right eye
  - H21.272 Miotic pupillary cyst, left eye
  - H21.273 Miotic pupillary cyst, bilateral
  - H21.279 Miotic pupillary cyst, unspecified eye
- H21.29 Other iris atrophy
- H21.3 Cyst of iris, ciliary body and anterior chamber
  Excludes2 miotic pupillary cyst (H21.27-)
- H21.30 Idiopathic cysts of iris, ciliary body or anterior chamber
  Cyst of iris, ciliary body or anterior chamber NOS
  - H21.301 Idiopathic cysts of iris, ciliary body or anterior chamber, right eye
  - H21.302 Idiopathic cysts of iris, ciliary body or anterior chamber, left eye
  - H21.303 Idiopathic cysts of iris, ciliary body or anterior chamber, bilateral
  - H21.309 Idiopathic cysts of iris, ciliary body or anterior chamber, unspecified eye
- H21.31 Exudative cysts of iris or anterior chamber
  - H21.311 Exudative cysts of iris or anterior chamber, right eye
  - H21.312 Exudative cysts of iris or anterior chamber, left eye
  - H21.313 Exudative cysts of iris or anterior chamber, bilateral
  - H21.319 Exudative cysts of iris or anterior chamber, unspecified eye
- H21.32 Implantation cysts of iris, ciliary body or anterior chamber
  - H21.321 Implantation cysts of iris, ciliary body or anterior chamber, right eye
  - H21.322 Implantation cysts of iris, ciliary body or anterior chamber, left eye
  - H21.323 Implantation cysts of iris, ciliary body or anterior chamber, bilateral
  - H21.329 Implantation cysts of iris, ciliary body or anterior chamber, unspecified eye
- H21.33 Parasitic cyst of iris, ciliary body or anterior chamber
  Ex: For category H21.33 CC codes: H20.051-H20.059, H21.331-H21.339, H33.121-H33.129, H44.001-H44.029, H44.121-H44.129, H44.19
  - H21.331 Parasitic cyst of iris, ciliary body or anterior chamber, right eye
  - H21.332 Parasitic cyst of iris, ciliary body or anterior chamber, left eye
  - H21.333 Parasitic cyst of iris, ciliary body or anterior chamber, bilateral
  - H21.339 Parasitic cyst of iris, ciliary body or anterior chamber, unspecified eye
- H21.34 Primary cyst of pars plana
  - H21.341 Primary cyst of pars plana, right eye
  - H21.342 Primary cyst of pars plana, left eye
  - H21.343 Primary cyst of pars plana, bilateral
  - H21.349 Primary cyst of pars plana, unspecified eye
- H21.35 Exudative cyst of pars plana
  - H21.351 Exudative cyst of pars plana, right eye
  - H21.352 Exudative cyst of pars plana, left eye
  - H21.353 Exudative cyst of pars plana, bilateral
  - H21.359 Exudative cyst of pars plana, unspecified eye
- H21.4 Pupillary membranes
  Iris bombé
  Pupillary occlusion
  Pupillary seclusion
  Excludes1 congenital pupillary membranes (Q13.8)
  - H21.40 Pupillary membranes, unspecified eye
  - H21.41 Pupillary membranes, right eye
  - H21.42 Pupillary membranes, left eye
  - H21.43 Pupillary membranes, bilateral
- H21.5 Other and unspecified adhesions and disruptions of iris and ciliary body
  Excludes1 corectopia (Q13.2)
  - H21.50 Unspecified adhesions of iris
    Synechia (iris) NOS
    - H21.501 Unspecified adhesions of iris, right eye
    - H21.502 Unspecified adhesions of iris, left eye
    - H21.503 Unspecified adhesions of iris, bilateral
    - H21.509 Unspecified adhesions of iris and ciliary body, unspecified eye
  - H21.51 Anterior synechiae (iris)
    - H21.511 Anterior synechiae (iris), right eye
    - H21.512 Anterior synechiae (iris), left eye
    - H21.513 Anterior synechiae (iris), bilateral
    - H21.519 Anterior synechiae (iris), unspecified eye
  - H21.52 Goniosynechiae
    - H21.521 Goniosynechiae, right eye
    - H21.522 Goniosynechiae, left eye
    - H21.523 Goniosynechiae, bilateral
    - H21.529 Goniosynechiae, unspecified eye

- **H21.53** Iridodialysis
  - H21.531 Iridodialysis, right eye
  - H21.532 Iridodialysis, left eye
  - H21.533 Iridodialysis, bilateral
  - H21.539 Iridodialysis, unspecified eye
- **H21.54** Posterior synechiae (iris)
  - H21.541 Posterior synechiae (iris), right eye
  - H21.542 Posterior synechiae (iris), left eye
  - H21.543 Posterior synechiae (iris), bilateral
  - H21.549 Posterior synechiae (iris), unspecified eye
- **H21.55** Recession of chamber angle
  - H21.551 Recession of chamber angle, right eye
  - H21.552 Recession of chamber angle, left eye
  - H21.553 Recession of chamber angle, bilateral
  - H21.559 Recession of chamber angle, unspecified eye
- **H21.56** Pupillary abnormalities
  - Deformed pupil
  - Ectopic pupil
  - Rupture of sphincter, pupil
  - **Excludes1** congenital deformity of pupil (Q13.2-)
  - H21.561 Pupillary abnormality, right eye
  - H21.562 Pupillary abnormality, left eye
  - H21.563 Pupillary abnormality, bilateral
  - H21.569 Pupillary abnormality, unspecified eye
- **H21.8** Other specified disorders of iris and ciliary body
  - H21.81 Floppy iris syndrome
    - Intraoperative floppy iris syndrome (IFIS)
    - Use additional code for adverse effect, if applicable, to identify drug (T36-T50 with fifth or sixth character 5)
  - H21.82 Plateau iris syndrome (post-iridectomy) (postprocedural)
  - H21.89 Other specified disorders of iris and ciliary body
- H21.9 Unspecified disorder of iris and ciliary body

▶ *H22 Disorders of iris and ciliary body in diseases classified elsewhere*

Code first underlying disease, such as:
gout (M1A.-, M10.-)
leprosy (A30.-)
parasitic disease (B89)

DISORDERS OF LENS (H25-H28)

- **H25** Age-related cataract
  - Senile cataract
  - **Excludes2** capsular glaucoma with pseudoexfoliation of lens (H40.1-)
- **H25.0** Age-related incipient cataract
  - **H25.01** Cortical age-related cataract
    - H25.011 Cortical age-related cataract, right eye A
    - H25.012 Cortical age-related cataract, left eye A
    - H25.013 Cortical age-related cataract, bilateral A
    - H25.019 Cortical age-related cataract, unspecified eye A
  - **H25.03** Anterior subcapsular polar age-related cataract
    - H25.031 Anterior subcapsular polar age-related cataract, right eye A
    - H25.032 Anterior subcapsular polar age-related cataract, left eye A
    - H25.033 Anterior subcapsular polar age-related cataract, bilateral A
    - H25.039 Anterior subcapsular polar age-related cataract, unspecified eye A

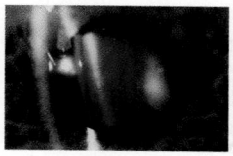

Figure 7-9 Age-related cataract. Nuclear sclerosis and cortical lens opacities are present. (From Yanoff: Ophthalmology, ed 3, Mosby, Inc., 2008)

Item 7–5 Senile cataracts are linked to the aging process. The most common area for the formation of a cataract is the cortical area of the lens. **Polar cataracts** can be either anterior or posterior. **Anterior polar cataracts** are more common and are small, white, capsular cataracts located on the anterior portion of the lens. **Total cataracts,** also called **complete** or **mature,** cause an opacity of all fibers of the lens. **Hypermature** describes a mature cataract with a swollen, milky cortex that covers the entire lens. **Immature**, also called **incipient,** cataracts have a clear cortex and are only slightly opaque. Treatment for all cataracts is the removal of the lens.

  - **H25.04** Posterior subcapsular polar age-related cataract
    - H25.041 Posterior subcapsular polar age-related cataract, right eye A
    - H25.042 Posterior subcapsular polar age-related cataract, left eye A
    - H25.043 Posterior subcapsular polar age-related cataract, bilateral A
    - H25.049 Posterior subcapsular polar age-related cataract, unspecified eye A
  - **H25.09** Other age-related incipient cataract
    - Coronary age-related cataract
    - Punctate age-related cataract
    - Water clefts
    - H25.091 Other age-related incipient cataract, right eye A
    - H25.092 Other age-related incipient cataract, left eye A
    - H25.093 Other age-related incipient cataract, bilateral A
    - H25.099 Other age-related incipient cataract, unspecified eye A
- **H25.1** Age-related nuclear cataract
  - Cataracta brunescens
  - Nuclear sclerosis cataract
  - H25.10 Age-related nuclear cataract, unspecified eye A
  - H25.11 Age-related nuclear cataract, right eye A
  - H25.12 Age-related nuclear cataract, left eye A
    - **Coding Clinic: 2016, Q1, P33**
  - H25.13 Age-related nuclear cataract, bilateral A
    - **Coding Clinic: 2016, Q1, P32**
- **H25.2** Age-related cataract, morgagnian type
  - Age-related hypermature cataract
  - H25.20 Age-related cataract, morgagnian type, unspecified eye A
  - H25.21 Age-related cataract, morgagnian type, right eye A
  - H25.22 Age-related cataract, morgagnian type, left eye A
  - H25.23 Age-related cataract, morgagnian type, bilateral A
- **H25.8** Other age-related cataract
  - **H25.81** Combined forms of age-related cataract
    - H25.811 Combined forms of age-related cataract, right eye A
    - H25.812 Combined forms of age-related cataract, left eye A
    - H25.813 Combined forms of age-related cataract, bilateral A
    - H25.819 Combined forms of age-related cataract, unspecified eye A
  - H25.89 Other age-related cataract A
- H25.9 Unspecified age-related cataract A

- H26 Other cataract
  - Excludes1 congenital cataract (Q12.0)
  - H26.0 Infantile and juvenile cataract
    - H26.00 Unspecified infantile and juvenile cataract
      - H26.001 Unspecified infantile and juvenile cataract, right eye P
      - H26.002 Unspecified infantile and juvenile cataract, left eye P
      - H26.003 Unspecified infantile and juvenile cataract, bilateral P
      - H26.009 Unspecified infantile and juvenile cataract, unspecified eye P
    - H26.01 Infantile and juvenile cortical, lamellar, or zonular cataract
      - H26.011 Infantile and juvenile cortical, lamellar, or zonular cataract, right eye P
      - H26.012 Infantile and juvenile cortical, lamellar, or zonular cataract, left eye P
      - H26.013 Infantile and juvenile cortical, lamellar, or zonular cataract, bilateral P
      - H26.019 Infantile and juvenile cortical, lamellar, or zonular cataract, unspecified eye P
    - H26.03 Infantile and juvenile nuclear cataract
      - H26.031 Infantile and juvenile nuclear cataract, right eye P
      - H26.032 Infantile and juvenile nuclear cataract, left eye P
      - H26.033 Infantile and juvenile nuclear cataract, bilateral P
      - H26.039 Infantile and juvenile nuclear cataract, unspecified eye P
    - H26.04 Anterior subcapsular polar infantile and juvenile cataract
      - H26.041 Anterior subcapsular polar infantile and juvenile cataract, right eye P
      - H26.042 Anterior subcapsular polar infantile and juvenile cataract, left eye P
      - H26.043 Anterior subcapsular polar infantile and juvenile cataract, bilateral P
      - H26.049 Anterior subcapsular polar infantile and juvenile cataract, unspecified eye P
    - H26.05 Posterior subcapsular polar infantile and juvenile cataract
      - H26.051 Posterior subcapsular polar infantile and juvenile cataract, right eye P
      - H26.052 Posterior subcapsular polar infantile and juvenile cataract, left eye P
      - H26.053 Posterior subcapsular polar infantile and juvenile cataract, bilateral P
      - H26.059 Posterior subcapsular polar infantile and juvenile cataract, unspecified eye P
    - H26.06 Combined forms of infantile and juvenile cataract
      - H26.061 Combined forms of infantile and juvenile cataract, right eye P
      - H26.062 Combined forms of infantile and juvenile cataract, left eye P
      - H26.063 Combined forms of infantile and juvenile cataract bilateral P
      - H26.069 Combined forms of infantile and juvenile cataract, unspecified eye P
    - H26.09 Other infantile and juvenile cataract P
- H26.1 Traumatic cataract
  - Use additional code (Chapter 20) to identify external cause
  - H26.10 Unspecified traumatic cataract
    - H26.101 Unspecified traumatic cataract, right eye
    - H26.102 Unspecified traumatic cataract, left eye
    - H26.103 Unspecified traumatic cataract, bilateral
    - H26.109 Unspecified traumatic cataract, unspecified eye
  - H26.11 Localized traumatic opacities
    - H26.111 Localized traumatic opacities, right eye
    - H26.112 Localized traumatic opacities, left eye
    - H26.113 Localized traumatic opacities, bilateral
    - H26.119 Localized traumatic opacities, unspecified eye
  - H26.12 Partially resolved traumatic cataract
    - H26.121 Partially resolved traumatic cataract, right eye
    - H26.122 Partially resolved traumatic cataract, left eye
    - H26.123 Partially resolved traumatic cataract, bilateral
    - H26.129 Partially resolved traumatic cataract, unspecified eye
  - H26.13 Total traumatic cataract
    - H26.131 Total traumatic cataract, right eye
    - H26.132 Total traumatic cataract, left eye
    - H26.133 Total traumatic cataract, bilateral
    - H26.139 Total traumatic cataract, unspecified eye
- H26.2 Complicated cataract
  - H26.20 Unspecified complicated cataract
    - Cataracta complicata NOS
  - H26.21 Cataract with neovascularization
    - Code also associated condition, such as: chronic iridocyclitis (H20.1-)
    - H26.211 Cataract with neovascularization, right eye
    - H26.212 Cataract with neovascularization, left eye
    - H26.213 Cataract with neovascularization, bilateral
    - H26.219 Cataract with neovascularization, unspecified eye
  - H26.22 Cataract secondary to ocular disorders (degenerative) (inflammatory)
    - Code also associated ocular disorder
    - H26.221 Cataract secondary to ocular disorders (degenerative) (inflammatory), right eye
    - H26.222 Cataract secondary to ocular disorders (degenerative) (inflammatory), left eye
    - H26.223 Cataract secondary to ocular disorders (degenerative) (inflammatory), bilateral
    - H26.229 Cataract secondary to ocular disorders (degenerative) (inflammatory), unspecified eye
  - H26.23 Glaucomatous flecks (subcapsular)
    - *Code first underlying glaucoma (H40-H42)*
    - H26.231 Glaucomatous flecks (subcapsular), right eye
    - H26.232 Glaucomatous flecks (subcapsular), left eye

H26.233 Glaucomatous flecks (subcapsular), bilateral
H26.239 Glaucomatous flecks (subcapsular), unspecified eye

● H26.3 Drug-induced cataract
Toxic cataract
Use additional code for adverse effect, if applicable, to identify drug (T36-T50 with fifth or sixth character 5)
H26.30 Drug-induced cataract, unspecified eye
H26.31 Drug-induced cataract, right eye
H26.32 Drug-induced cataract, left eye
H26.33 Drug-induced cataract, bilateral

● H26.4 Secondary cataract
H26.40 Unspecified secondary cataract
● H26.41 Soemmering's ring
H26.411 Soemmering's ring, right eye
H26.412 Soemmering's ring, left eye
H26.413 Soemmering's ring, bilateral
H26.419 Soemmering's ring, unspecified eye
● H26.49 Other secondary cataract
H26.491 Other secondary cataract, right eye
H26.492 Other secondary cataract, left eye
H26.493 Other secondary cataract, bilateral
H26.499 Other secondary cataract, unspecified eye
H26.8 Other specified cataract
H26.9 Unspecified cataract

● H27 Other disorders of lens
Excludes1 congenital lens malformations (Q12.-)
mechanical complications of intraocular lens implant (T85.2)
pseudophakia (Z96.1)

● H27.0 Aphakia
Acquired absence of lens
Acquired aphakia
Aphakia due to trauma
Excludes1 cataract extraction status (Z98.4-)
congenital absence of lens (Q12.3)
congenital aphakia (Q12.3)
H27.00 Aphakia, unspecified eye
H27.01 Aphakia, right eye
H27.02 Aphakia, left eye
H27.03 Aphakia, bilateral

● H27.1 Dislocation of lens
H27.10 Unspecified dislocation of lens
● H27.11 Subluxation of lens
H27.111 Subluxation of lens, right eye
H27.112 Subluxation of lens, left eye
H27.113 Subluxation of lens, bilateral
H27.119 Subluxation of lens, unspecified eye
● H27.12 Anterior dislocation of lens
H27.121 Anterior dislocation of lens, right eye
H27.122 Anterior dislocation of lens, left eye
H27.123 Anterior dislocation of lens, bilateral
H27.129 Anterior dislocation of lens, unspecified eye
● H27.13 Posterior dislocation of lens
H27.131 Posterior dislocation of lens, right eye
H27.132 Posterior dislocation of lens, left eye
H27.133 Posterior dislocation of lens, bilateral
H27.139 Posterior dislocation of lens, unspecified eye
H27.8 Other specified disorders of lens
H27.9 Unspecified disorder of lens

H28 Cataract in diseases classified elsewhere
Code first underlying disease, such as:
hypoparathyroidism (E20.-)
myotonia (G71.1-)
myxedema (E03.-)
protein-calorie malnutrition (E40-E46)
Excludes1 cataract in diabetes mellitus (E08.36, E09.36, E10.36, E11.36, E13.36)

DISORDERS OF CHOROID AND RETINA (H30-H36)

★ **(See Plate 90 on page 64.)**

● H30 Chorioretinal inflammation
● H30.0 Focal chorioretinal inflammation
Focal chorioretinitis
Focal choroiditis
Focal retinitis
Focal retinochoroiditis
● H30.00 Unspecified focal chorioretinal inflammation
Focal chorioretinitis NOS
Focal choroiditis NOS
Focal retinitis NOS
Focal retinochoroiditis NOS
H30.001 Unspecified focal chorioretinal inflammation, right eye
H30.002 Unspecified focal chorioretinal inflammation, left eye
H30.003 Unspecified focal chorioretinal inflammation, bilateral
H30.009 Unspecified focal chorioretinal inflammation, unspecified eye
● H30.01 Focal chorioretinal inflammation, juxtapapillary
H30.011 Focal chorioretinal inflammation, juxtapapillary, right eye
H30.012 Focal chorioretinal inflammation, juxtapapillary, left eye
H30.013 Focal chorioretinal inflammation, juxtapapillary, bilateral
H30.019 Focal chorioretinal inflammation, juxtapapillary, unspecified eye
● H30.02 Focal chorioretinal inflammation of posterior pole
H30.021 Focal chorioretinal inflammation of posterior pole, right eye
H30.022 Focal chorioretinal inflammation of posterior pole, left eye
H30.023 Focal chorioretinal inflammation of posterior pole, bilateral
H30.029 Focal chorioretinal inflammation of posterior pole, unspecified eye
● H30.03 Focal chorioretinal inflammation, peripheral
H30.031 Focal chorioretinal inflammation, peripheral, right eye
H30.032 Focal chorioretinal inflammation, peripheral, left eye
H30.033 Focal chorioretinal inflammation, peripheral, bilateral
H30.039 Focal chorioretinal inflammation, peripheral, unspecified eye
● H30.04 Focal chorioretinal inflammation, macular or paramacular
H30.041 Focal chorioretinal inflammation, macular or paramacular, right eye
H30.042 Focal chorioretinal inflammation, macular or paramacular, left eye
H30.043 Focal chorioretinal inflammation, macular or paramacular, bilateral
H30.049 Focal chorioretinal inflammation, macular or paramacular, unspecified eye

- **H30.1** Disseminated chorioretinal inflammation
  - Disseminated chorioretinitis
  - Disseminated choroiditis
  - Disseminated retinitis
  - Disseminated retinochoroiditis
  - **Excludes2** exudative retinopathy (H35.02-)
  - Ex For category H30.1 CC codes: H30.001-H30.93
  - **H30.10** Unspecified disseminated chorioretinal inflammation
    - Disseminated chorioretinitis NOS
    - Disseminated choroiditis NOS
    - Disseminated retinitis NOS
    - Disseminated retinochoroiditis NOS
    - H30.101 Unspecified disseminated chorioretinal inflammation, right eye
    - H30.102 Unspecified disseminated chorioretinal inflammation, left eye
    - H30.103 Unspecified disseminated chorioretinal inflammation, bilateral
    - H30.109 Unspecified disseminated chorioretinal inflammation, unspecified eye
  - **H30.11** Disseminated chorioretinal inflammation of posterior pole
    - H30.111 Disseminated chorioretinal inflammation of posterior pole, right eye
    - H30.112 Disseminated chorioretinal inflammation of posterior pole, left eye
    - H30.113 Disseminated chorioretinal inflammation of posterior pole, bilateral
    - H30.119 Disseminated chorioretinal inflammation of posterior pole, unspecified eye
  - **H30.12** Disseminated chorioretinal inflammation, peripheral
    - H30.121 Disseminated chorioretinal inflammation, peripheral right eye
    - H30.122 Disseminated chorioretinal inflammation, peripheral, left eye
    - H30.123 Disseminated chorioretinal inflammation, peripheral, bilateral
    - H30.129 Disseminated chorioretinal inflammation, peripheral, unspecified eye
  - **H30.13** Disseminated chorioretinal inflammation, generalized
    - H30.131 Disseminated chorioretinal inflammation, generalized, right eye
    - H30.132 Disseminated chorioretinal inflammation, generalized, left eye
    - H30.133 Disseminated chorioretinal inflammation, generalized, bilateral
    - H30.139 Disseminated chorioretinal inflammation, generalized, unspecified eye
  - **H30.14** Acute posterior multifocal placoid pigment epitheliopathy
    - H30.141 Acute posterior multifocal placoid pigment epitheliopathy, right eye
    - H30.142 Acute posterior multifocal placoid pigment epitheliopathy, left eye
    - H30.143 Acute posterior multifocal placoid pigment epitheliopathy, bilateral
    - H30.149 Acute posterior multifocal placoid pigment epitheliopathy, unspecified eye
- **H30.2** Posterior cyclitis
  - Pars planitis
  - H30.20 Posterior cyclitis, unspecified eye
  - H30.21 Posterior cyclitis, right eye
  - H30.22 Posterior cyclitis, left eye
  - H30.23 Posterior cyclitis, bilateral
- **H30.8** Other chorioretinal inflammations
  - **H30.81** Harada's disease
    - H30.811 Harada's disease, right eye
    - H30.812 Harada's disease, left eye
    - H30.813 Harada's disease, bilateral
    - H30.819 Harada's disease, unspecified eye
  - **H30.89** Other chorioretinal inflammations
    - Ex For category H30.89 CC codes: H30.001-H30.93
    - H30.891 Other chorioretinal inflammations, right eye
    - H30.892 Other chorioretinal inflammations, left eye
    - H30.893 Other chorioretinal inflammations, bilateral
    - H30.899 Other chorioretinal inflammations, unspecified eye
- **H30.9** Unspecified chorioretinal inflammation
  - Chorioretinitis NOS
  - Choroiditis NOS
  - Neuroretinitis NOS
  - Retinitis NOS
  - Retinochoroiditis NOS
  - Ex For category H30.9 CC codes: H30.001-H30.93
  - H30.90 Unspecified chorioretinal inflammation, unspecified eye
  - H30.91 Unspecified chorioretinal inflammation, right eye
  - H30.92 Unspecified chorioretinal inflammation, left eye
  - H30.93 Unspecified chorioretinal inflammation, bilateral

- **H31** Other disorders of choroid
  - **H31.0** Chorioretinal scars
    - **Excludes2** postsurgical chorioretinal scars (H59.81-)
    - **H31.00** Unspecified chorioretinal scars
      - H31.001 Unspecified chorioretinal scars, right eye
      - H31.002 Unspecified chorioretinal scars, left eye
      - H31.003 Unspecified chorioretinal scars, bilateral
      - H31.009 Unspecified chorioretinal scars, unspecified eye
    - **H31.01** Macula scars of posterior pole (postinflammatory) (post-traumatic)
      - **Excludes1** postprocedural chorioretinal scar (H59.81-)
      - H31.011 Macula scars of posterior pole (postinflammatory) (post-traumatic), right eye
      - H31.012 Macula scars of posterior pole (postinflammatory) (post-traumatic), left eye

H31.013 Macula scars of posterior pole (postinflammatory) (post-traumatic), bilateral
H31.019 Macula scars of posterior pole (postinflammatory) (post-traumatic), unspecified eye

● H31.02 Solar retinopathy
H31.021 Solar retinopathy, right eye
H31.022 Solar retinopathy, left eye
H31.023 Solar retinopathy, bilateral
H31.029 Solar retinopathy, unspecified eye

● H31.09 Other chorioretinal scars
H31.091 Other chorioretinal scars, right eye
H31.092 Other chorioretinal scars, left eye
H31.093 Other chorioretinal scars, bilateral
H31.099 Other chorioretinal scars, unspecified eye

● H31.1 Choroidal degeneration
Excludes2 angioid streaks of macula (H35.33)

● H31.10 Unspecified choroidal degeneration
Choroidal sclerosis NOS
H31.101 Choroidal degeneration, unspecified, right eye
H31.102 Choroidal degeneration, unspecified, left eye
H31.103 Choroidal degeneration, unspecified, bilateral
H31.109 Choroidal degeneration, unspecified, unspecified eye

● H31.11 Age-related choroidal atrophy
H31.111 Age-related choroidal atrophy, right eye A
H31.112 Age-related choroidal atrophy, left eye A
H31.113 Age-related choroidal atrophy, bilateral A
H31.119 Age-related choroidal atrophy, unspecified eye A

● H31.12 Diffuse secondary atrophy of choroid
H31.121 Diffuse secondary atrophy of choroid, right eye
H31.122 Diffuse secondary atrophy of choroid, left eye
H31.123 Diffuse secondary atrophy of choroid, bilateral
H31.129 Diffuse secondary atrophy of choroid, unspecified eye

● H31.2 Hereditary choroidal dystrophy
Excludes2 hyperornithinemia (E72.4)
ornithinemia (E72.4)
H31.20 Hereditary choroidal dystrophy, unspecified
H31.21 Choroideremia
H31.22 Choroidal dystrophy (central areolar) (generalized) (peripapillary)
H31.23 Gyrate atrophy, choroid
H31.29 Other hereditary choroidal dystrophy

● H31.3 Choroidal hemorrhage and rupture

● H31.30 Unspecified choroidal hemorrhage
H31.301 Unspecified choroidal hemorrhage, right eye
H31.302 Unspecified choroidal hemorrhage, left eye
H31.303 Unspecified choroidal hemorrhage, bilateral
H31.309 Unspecified choroidal hemorrhage, unspecified eye

● H31.31 Expulsive choroidal hemorrhage
H31.311 Expulsive choroidal hemorrhage, right eye
H31.312 Expulsive choroidal hemorrhage, left eye
H31.313 Expulsive choroidal hemorrhage, bilateral
H31.319 Expulsive choroidal hemorrhage, unspecified eye

● H31.32 Choroidal rupture
Ex For category H31.32 CC codes: H31.301-H32
H31.321 Choroidal rupture, right eye CC
H31.322 Choroidal rupture, left eye CC
H31.323 Choroidal rupture, bilateral CC
H31.329 Choroidal rupture, unspecified eye CC

● H31.4 Choroidal detachment
Ex For category H31.4 CC codes: H31.301-H32

● H31.40 Unspecified choroidal detachment
H31.401 Unspecified choroidal detachment, right eye CC
H31.402 Unspecified choroidal detachment, left eye CC
H31.403 Unspecified choroidal detachment, bilateral CC
H31.409 Unspecified choroidal detachment, unspecified eye CC

● H31.41 Hemorrhagic choroidal detachment
H31.411 Hemorrhagic choroidal detachment, right eye CC
H31.412 Hemorrhagic choroidal detachment, left eye CC
H31.413 Hemorrhagic choroidal detachment, bilateral CC
H31.419 Hemorrhagic choroidal detachment, unspecified eye CC

● H31.42 Serous choroidal detachment
H31.421 Serous choroidal detachment, right eye CC
H31.422 Serous choroidal detachment, left eye CC
H31.423 Serous choroidal detachment, bilateral CC
H31.429 Serous choroidal detachment, unspecified eye CC

H31.8 Other specified disorders of choroid
H31.9 Unspecified disorder of choroid

◗ *H32 Chorioretinal disorders in diseases classified elsewhere*
Code first underlying disease, such as:
congenital toxoplasmosis (P37.1)
histoplasmosis (B39.-)
leprosy (A30.-)
Excludes1 chorioretinitis (in):
toxoplasmosis (acquired) (B58.01)
tuberculosis (A18.53)

● H33 Retinal detachments and breaks
Excludes1 detachment of retinal pigment epithelium (H35.72-, H35.73-)

● H33.0 Retinal detachment with retinal break
Rhegmatogenous retinal detachment
Excludes1 serous retinal detachment (without retinal break) (H33.2-)

● H33.00 Unspecified retinal detachment with retinal break
H33.001 Unspecified retinal detachment with retinal break, right eye
H33.002 Unspecified retinal detachment with retinal break, left eye

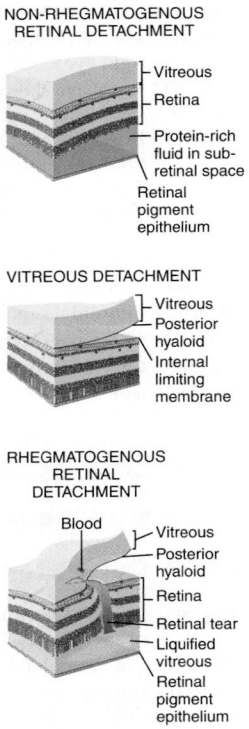

Figure 7-10 Retinal detachment. (From Kumar: Robbins and Cotran: Pathologic Basis of Disease, ed 7, Saunders, 2005)

Item 7–6 Retinal detachments and defects are conditions of the eye in which the retina separates from the underlying tissue. Initial detachment may be localized, requiring rapid treatment (medical emergency) to avoid the entire retina from detaching which leads to vision loss and blindness.

H33.003 **Unspecified retinal detachment with retinal break, bilateral**
H33.009 **Unspecified retinal detachment with retinal break, unspecified eye**

● **H33.01** **Retinal detachment with single break**
H33.011 **Retinal detachment with single break, right eye**
H33.012 **Retinal detachment with single break, left eye**
H33.013 **Retinal detachment with single break, bilateral**
H33.019 **Retinal detachment with single break, unspecified eye**

● **H33.02** **Retinal detachment with multiple breaks**
H33.021 **Retinal detachment with multiple breaks, right eye**
H33.022 **Retinal detachment with multiple breaks, left eye**
H33.023 **Retinal detachment with multiple breaks, bilateral**
H33.029 **Retinal detachment with multiple breaks, unspecified eye**

● **H33.03** **Retinal detachment with giant retinal tear**
H33.031 **Retinal detachment with giant retinal tear, right eye**
H33.032 **Retinal detachment with giant retinal tear, left eye**
H33.033 **Retinal detachment with giant retinal tear, bilateral**
H33.039 **Retinal detachment with giant retinal tear, unspecified eye**

● **H33.04** **Retinal detachment with retinal dialysis**
H33.041 **Retinal detachment with retinal dialysis, right eye**
H33.042 **Retinal detachment with retinal dialysis, left eye**
H33.043 **Retinal detachment with retinal dialysis, bilateral**
H33.049 **Retinal detachment with retinal dialysis, unspecified eye**

● **H33.05** **Total retinal detachment**
H33.051 **Total retinal detachment, right eye**
H33.052 **Total retinal detachment, left eye**
H33.053 **Total retinal detachment, bilateral**
H33.059 **Total retinal detachment, unspecified eye**

● **H33.1** **Retinoschisis and retinal cysts**
Excludes1 congenital retinoschisis (Q14.1)
microcystoid degeneration of retina (H35.42-)

● **H33.10** **Unspecified retinoschisis**
H33.101 **Unspecified retinoschisis, right eye**
H33.102 **Unspecified retinoschisis, left eye**
H33.103 **Unspecified retinoschisis, bilateral**
H33.109 **Unspecified retinoschisis, unspecified eye**

● **H33.11** **Cyst of ora serrata**
H33.111 **Cyst of ora serrata, right eye**
H33.112 **Cyst of ora serrata, left eye**
H33.113 **Cyst of ora serrata, bilateral**
H33.119 **Cyst of ora serrata, unspecified eye**

● **H33.12** **Parasitic cyst of retina**
Ex: **For category H33.12 CC codes:** H20.051-H20.059, H21.331-H21.339, H33.121-H33.129, H44.001-H44.029, H44.121-H44.129, H44.19
H33.121 **Parasitic cyst of retina, right eye**
H33.122 **Parasitic cyst of retina, left eye**
H33.123 **Parasitic cyst of retina, bilateral**
H33.129 **Parasitic cyst of retina, unspecified eye**

● **H33.19** **Other retinoschisis and retinal cysts**
Pseudocyst of retina
H33.191 **Other retinoschisis and retinal cysts, right eye**
H33.192 **Other retinoschisis and retinal cysts, left eye**
H33.193 **Other retinoschisis and retinal cysts, bilateral**
H33.199 **Other retinoschisis and retinal cysts, unspecified eye**

● **H33.2** **Serous retinal detachment**
Retinal detachment NOS
Retinal detachment without retinal break
Excludes1 central serous chorioretinopathy (H35.71-)
Ex: **For category H33.2 CC codes:** H33.001-H33.119, H33.191-H33.8, H35.70-H35.739
H33.20 **Serous retinal detachment, unspecified eye**
H33.21 **Serous retinal detachment, right eye**
H33.22 **Serous retinal detachment, left eye**
H33.23 **Serous retinal detachment, bilateral**

- **H33.3 Retinal breaks without detachment**
  - **Excludes1** chorioretinal scars after surgery for detachment (H59.81-)
    peripheral retinal degeneration without break (H35.4-)
  - **H33.30 Unspecified retinal break**
    - **H33.301 Unspecified retinal break, right eye**
    - **H33.302 Unspecified retinal break, left eye**
    - **H33.303 Unspecified retinal break, bilateral**
    - **H33.309 Unspecified retinal break, unspecified eye**
  - **H33.31 Horseshoe tear of retina without detachment**
    Operculum of retina without detachment
    - **H33.311 Horseshoe tear of retina without detachment, right eye**
    - **H33.312 Horseshoe tear of retina without detachment, left eye**
    - **H33.313 Horseshoe tear of retina without detachment, bilateral**
    - **H33.319 Horseshoe tear of retina without detachment, unspecified eye**
  - **H33.32 Round hole of retina without detachment**
    - **H33.321 Round hole, right eye**
    - **H33.322 Round hole, left eye**
    - **H33.323 Round hole, bilateral**
    - **H33.329 Round hole, unspecified eye**
  - **H33.33 Multiple defects of retina without detachment**
    - **H33.331 Multiple defects of retina without detachment, right eye**
    - **H33.332 Multiple defects of retina without detachment, left eye**
    - **H33.333 Multiple defects of retina without detachment, bilateral**
    - **H33.339 Multiple defects of retina without detachment, unspecified eye**
- **H33.4 Traction detachment of retina**
  Proliferative vitreo-retinopathy with retinal detachment
  - Ex: For category H33.4 CC codes: See H33.2
  - **H33.40 Traction detachment of retina, unspecified eye**
  - **H33.41 Traction detachment of retina, right eye**
  - **H33.42 Traction detachment of retina, left eye**
  - **H33.43 Traction detachment of retina, bilateral**
- **H33.8 Other retinal detachments**
  - Ex: See H33.2

- **H34 Retinal vascular occlusions**
  Blockage in vessel of the retina
  - **Excludes1** amaurosis fugax (G45.3)
  - Ex: For category H34 CC codes unless otherwise indicated: G45.3, H34.00-H34.9
  - **H34.0 Transient retinal artery occlusion**
    - **H34.00 Transient retinal artery occlusion, unspecified eye**
    - **H34.01 Transient retinal artery occlusion, right eye**
    - **H34.02 Transient retinal artery occlusion, left eye**
    - **H34.03 Transient retinal artery occlusion, bilateral**
  - **H34.1 Central retinal artery occlusion**
    - **H34.10 Central retinal artery occlusion, unspecified eye**
    - **H34.11 Central retinal artery occlusion, right eye**
    - **H34.12 Central retinal artery occlusion, left eye**
    - **H34.13 Central retinal artery occlusion, bilateral**
  - **H34.2 Other retinal artery occlusions**
    - **H34.21 Partial retinal artery occlusion**
      Hollenhorst's plaque
      Retinal microembolism
      - **H34.211 Partial retinal artery occlusion, right eye**
      - **H34.212 Partial retinal artery occlusion, left eye**
      - **H34.213 Partial retinal artery occlusion, bilateral**
      - **H34.219 Partial retinal artery occlusion, unspecified eye**
    - **H34.23 Retinal artery branch occlusion**
      - **H34.231 Retinal artery branch occlusion, right eye**
      - **H34.232 Retinal artery branch occlusion, left eye**
      - **H34.233 Retinal artery branch occlusion, bilateral**
      - **H34.239 Retinal artery branch occlusion, unspecified eye**
  - **H34.8 Other retinal vascular occlusions**
    - **H34.81 Central retinal vein occlusion**
      One of the following 7th characters is to be assigned to codes in subcategory H34.81 to designate the severity of the occlusion: ◀

0	with macular edema ◀
1	with retinal neovascularization ◀
2	stable ◀
	Old central retinal vein occlusion ◀

      - Ex: For category H34.81 CC codes: E08.3211-E08.3299, E08.3511-E08.3599, E08.37X1-E08.37X9, E09.3211-E09.3319, E09.3411-E09.3419, E09.3511-E09.3599, E09.37X1-E09.37X9, E10.3211-E10.3599, E10.37X1-E10.37X9, E11.3211-E11.3599, E11.37X1-E11.37X9, E13.3211-E13.3599, E13.37X1-E13.37X9, G45.3, H34.00-H34.239, H34.821-H34.9
      - **H34.811 Central retinal vein occlusion, right eye**
      - **H34.812 Central retinal vein occlusion, left eye**
      - **H34.813 Central retinal vein occlusion, bilateral**
      - **H34.819 Central retinal vein occlusion, unspecified eye**
    - **H34.82 Venous engorgement**
      Incipient retinal vein occlusion
      Partial retinal vein occlusion
      - **H34.821 Venous engorgement, right eye**
      - **H34.822 Venous engorgement, left eye**
      - **H34.823 Venous engorgement, bilateral**
      - **H34.829 Venous engorgement, unspecified eye**

● H34.83 Tributary (branch) retinal vein occlusion

One of the following 7th characters is to be assigned to codes in subcategory H34.83 to designate the severity of the occlusion: ◀

0	with macular edema ◀
1	with retinal neovascularization ◀
2	stable ◀
	Old tributary (branch) retinal vein occlusion ◀

● H34.831 Tributary (branch) retinal vein occlusion, right eye

● H34.832 Tributary (branch) retinal vein occlusion, left eye

● H34.833 Tributary (branch) retinal vein occlusion, bilateral

● H34.839 Tributary (branch) retinal vein occlusion, unspecified eye

H34.9 Unspecified retinal vascular occlusion

● H35 Other retinal disorders

Excludes2 diabetic retinal disorders (E08.311-E08.359, E09.311-E09.359, E10.311-E10.359, E11.311-E11.359, E13.311-E13.359)

● H35.0 Background retinopathy and retinal vascular changes

Code also any associated hypertension (I10.-)

OGCR Section I. C.9.a.5.

Hypertensive Retinopathy

Subcategory H35.0, Background retinopathy and retinal vascular changes, should be used with a code from category I10–I15, Hypertensive disease to include the systemic hypertension. The sequencing is based on the reason for the encounter.

H35.00 Unspecified background retinopathy

● H35.01 Changes in retinal vascular appearance

Retinal vascular sheathing

H35.011 Changes in retinal vascular appearance, right eye

H35.012 Changes in retinal vascular appearance, left eye

H35.013 Changes in retinal vascular appearance, bilateral

H35.019 Changes in retinal vascular appearance, unspecified eye

● H35.02 Exudative retinopathy

Coats retinopathy

H35.021 Exudative retinopathy, right eye

H35.022 Exudative retinopathy, left eye

H35.023 Exudative retinopathy, bilateral

H35.029 Exudative retinopathy, unspecified eye

● H35.03 Hypertensive retinopathy

H35.031 Hypertensive retinopathy, right eye

H35.032 Hypertensive retinopathy, left eye

H35.033 Hypertensive retinopathy, bilateral

H35.039 Hypertensive retinopathy, unspecified eye

● H35.04 Retinal micro-aneurysms, unspecified

H35.041 Retinal micro-aneurysms, unspecified, right eye

H35.042 Retinal micro-aneurysms, unspecified, left eye

H35.043 Retinal micro-aneurysms, unspecified, bilateral

H35.049 Retinal micro-aneurysms, unspecified, unspecified eye

● H35.05 Retinal neovascularization, unspecified

H35.051 Retinal neovascularization, unspecified, right eye

H35.052 Retinal neovascularization, unspecified, left eye

H35.053 Retinal neovascularization, unspecified, bilateral

H35.059 Retinal neovascularization, unspecified, unspecified eye

● H35.06 Retinal vasculitis

Eales disease

Retinal perivasculitis

H35.061 Retinal vasculitis, right eye

H35.062 Retinal vasculitis, left eye

H35.063 Retinal vasculitis, bilateral

H35.069 Retinal vasculitis, unspecified eye

● H35.07 Retinal telangiectasis

H35.071 Retinal telangiectasis, right eye

H35.072 Retinal telangiectasis, left eye

H35.073 Retinal telangiectasis, bilateral

H35.079 Retinal telangiectasis, unspecified eye

H35.09 Other intraretinal microvascular abnormalities

Retinal varices

H35.1 Retinopathy of prematurity

● H35.10 Retinopathy of prematurity, unspecified

Retinopathy of prematurity NOS

H35.101 Retinopathy of prematurity, unspecified, right eye

H35.102 Retinopathy of prematurity, unspecified, left eye

H35.103 Retinopathy of prematurity, unspecified, bilateral

H35.109 Retinopathy of prematurity, unspecified, unspecified eye

● H35.11 Retinopathy of prematurity, stage 0

H35.111 Retinopathy of prematurity, stage 0, right eye

H35.112 Retinopathy of prematurity, stage 0, left eye

H35.113 Retinopathy of prematurity, stage 0, bilateral

H35.119 Retinopathy of prematurity, stage 0, unspecified eye

● H35.12 Retinopathy of prematurity, stage 1

H35.121 Retinopathy of prematurity, stage 1, right eye

H35.122 Retinopathy of prematurity, stage 1, left eye

H35.123 Retinopathy of prematurity, stage 1, bilateral

H35.129 Retinopathy of prematurity, stage 1, unspecified eye

● H35.13 Retinopathy of prematurity, stage 2

H35.131 Retinopathy of prematurity, stage 2, right eye

H35.132 Retinopathy of prematurity, stage 2, left eye

H35.133 Retinopathy of prematurity, stage 2, bilateral

H35.139 Retinopathy of prematurity, stage 2, unspecified eye

● **H35.14 Retinopathy of prematurity, stage 3**
- **H35.141 Retinopathy of prematurity, stage 3, right eye**
- **H35.142 Retinopathy of prematurity, stage 3, left eye**
- **H35.143 Retinopathy of prematurity, stage 3, bilateral**
- **H35.149 Retinopathy of prematurity, stage 3, unspecified eye**

● **H35.15 Retinopathy of prematurity, stage 4**
- **H35.151 Retinopathy of prematurity, stage 4, right eye**
- **H35.152 Retinopathy of prematurity, stage 4, left eye**
- **H35.153 Retinopathy of prematurity, stage 4, bilateral**
- **H35.159 Retinopathy of prematurity, stage 4, unspecified eye**

● **H35.16 Retinopathy of prematurity, stage 5**
- **H35.161 Retinopathy of prematurity, stage 5, right eye**
- **H35.162 Retinopathy of prematurity, stage 5, left eye**
- **H35.163 Retinopathy of prematurity, stage 5, bilateral**
- **H35.169 Retinopathy of prematurity, stage 5, unspecified eye**

● **H35.17 Retrolental fibroplasia**
- **H35.171 Retrolental fibroplasia, right eye**
- **H35.172 Retrolental fibroplasia, left eye**
- **H35.173 Retrolental fibroplasia, bilateral**
- **H35.179 Retrolental fibroplasia, unspecified eye**

● **H35.2 Other non-diabetic proliferative retinopathy**
Proliferative vitreo-retinopathy

Excludes1 proliferative vitreo-retinopathy with retinal detachment (H33.4-)

- **H35.20 Other non-diabetic proliferative retinopathy, unspecified eye**
- **H35.21 Other non-diabetic proliferative retinopathy, right eye**
- **H35.22 Other non-diabetic proliferative retinopathy, left eye**
- **H35.23 Other non-diabetic proliferative retinopathy, bilateral**

● **H35.3 Degeneration of macula and posterior pole**
- **H35.30 Unspecified macular degeneration** A
  Age-related macular degeneration

● **H35.31 Nonexudative age-related macular degeneration**
Atrophic age-related macular degeneration
Dry age-related macular degeneration ◀
One of the following 7th characters is to be assigned to codes in subcategory H35.31 to designate the stage of the disease: ◀

0	stage unspecified ◀
1	early dry stage ◀
2	intermediate dry stage ◀
3	advanced atrophic without subfoveal involvement ◀ advanced dry stage ◀
4	advanced atrophic with subfoveal involvement ◀

- ● **H35.311 Nonexudative age-related macular degeneration, right eye** ◀ A
- ● **H35.312 Nonexudative age-related macular degeneration, left eye** ◀ A

Item 7–7 Macular degeneration is typically age-related, chronic, and is evidenced by deterioration of the macula (the part of the retina that provides for central field vision), resulting in blurred vision or a blind spot in the center of visual field while not affecting peripheral vision.

- ● **H35.313 Nonexudative age-related macular degeneration, bilateral** ◀ A
- ● **H35.319 Nonexudative age-related macular degeneration, unspecified eye** ◀ A

● **H35.32 Exudative age-related macular degeneration**
Wet age-related macular degeneration ◀
One of the following 7th characters is to be assigned to codes in subcategory H35.32 to designate the stage of the disease: ◀

0	stage unspecified ◀
1	with active choroidal neovascularization ◀
2	with inactive choroidal neovascularization ◀ with involuted or regressed neovascularization ◀
3	with inactive scar ◀

- ● **H35.321 Exudative age-related macular degeneration, right eye** ◀ A
- ● **H35.322 Exudative age-related macular degeneration, left eye** ◀ A
- ● **H35.323 Exudative age-related macular degeneration, bilateral** ◀ A
- ● **H35.329 Exudative age-related macular degeneration, unspecified eye** ◀ A

- **H35.33 Angioid streaks of macula**

● **H35.34 Macular cyst, hole, or pseudohole**
- **H35.341 Macular cyst, hole, or pseudohole, right eye**
- **H35.342 Macular cyst, hole, or pseudohole, left eye**
- **H35.343 Macular cyst, hole, or pseudohole, bilateral**
- **H35.349 Macular cyst, hole, or pseudohole, unspecified eye**

● **H35.35 Cystoid macular degeneration**

Excludes1 cystoid macular edema following cataract surgery (H59.03-)

- **H35.351 Cystoid macular degeneration, right eye**
- **H35.352 Cystoid macular degeneration, left eye**
- **H35.353 Cystoid macular degeneration, bilateral**
- **H35.359 Cystoid macular degeneration, unspecified eye**

● **H35.36 Drusen (degenerative) of macula**
- **H35.361 Drusen (degenerative) of macula, right eye**
- **H35.362 Drusen (degenerative) of macula, left eye**
- **H35.363 Drusen (degenerative) of macula, bilateral**
- **H35.369 Drusen (degenerative) of macula, unspecified eye**

- H35.37 Puckering of macula
  - H35.371 Puckering of macula, right eye
  - H35.372 Puckering of macula, left eye
  - H35.373 Puckering of macula, bilateral
  - H35.379 Puckering of macula, unspecified eye
- H35.38 Toxic maculopathy
  - *Code first poisoning due to drug or toxin, if applicable (T36-T65 with fifth or sixth character 1-4 or 6)*
  - Use additional code for adverse effect, if applicable, to identify drug (T36-T50 with fifth or sixth character 5)
  - H35.381 Toxic maculopathy, right eye
  - H35.382 Toxic maculopathy, left eye
  - H35.383 Toxic maculopathy, bilateral
  - H35.389 Toxic maculopathy, unspecified eye
- H35.4 Peripheral retinal degeneration
  - **Excludes1** hereditary retinal degeneration (dystrophy) (H35.5-)
    peripheral retinal degeneration with retinal break (H33.3-)
  - H35.40 Unspecified peripheral retinal degeneration
- H35.41 Lattice degeneration of retina
  - Palisade degeneration of retina
  - H35.411 Lattice degeneration of retina, right eye
  - H35.412 Lattice degeneration of retina, left eye
  - H35.413 Lattice degeneration of retina, bilateral
  - H35.419 Lattice degeneration of retina, unspecified eye
- H35.42 Microcystoid degeneration of retina
  - H35.421 Microcystoid degeneration of retina, right eye
  - H35.422 Microcystoid degeneration of retina, left eye
  - H35.423 Microcystoid degeneration of retina, bilateral
  - H35.429 Microcystoid degeneration of retina, unspecified eye
- H35.43 Paving stone degeneration of retina
  - H35.431 Paving stone degeneration of retina, right eye
  - H35.432 Paving stone degeneration of retina, left eye
  - H35.433 Paving stone degeneration of retina, bilateral
  - H35.439 Paving stone degeneration of retina, unspecified eye
- H35.44 Age-related reticular degeneration of retina
  - H35.441 Age-related reticular degeneration of retina, right eye A
  - H35.442 Age-related reticular degeneration of retina, left eye A
  - H35.443 Age-related reticular degeneration of retina, bilateral A
  - H35.449 Age-related reticular degeneration of retina, unspecified eye A
- H35.45 Secondary pigmentary degeneration
  - H35.451 Secondary pigmentary degeneration, right eye
  - H35.452 Secondary pigmentary degeneration, left eye
  - H35.453 Secondary pigmentary degeneration, bilateral
  - H35.459 Secondary pigmentary degeneration, unspecified eye
- H35.46 Secondary vitreoretinal degeneration
  - H35.461 Secondary vitreoretinal degeneration, right eye
  - H35.462 Secondary vitreoretinal degeneration, left eye
  - H35.463 Secondary vitreoretinal degeneration, bilateral
  - H35.469 Secondary vitreoretinal degeneration, unspecified eye
- H35.5 Hereditary retinal dystrophy
  - **Excludes1** dystrophies primarily involving Bruch's membrane (H31.1-)
  - H35.50 Unspecified hereditary retinal dystrophy
  - H35.51 Vitreoretinal dystrophy
  - H35.52 Pigmentary retinal dystrophy
    - Albipunctate retinal dystrophy
    - Retinitis pigmentosa
    - Tapetoretinal dystrophy
  - H35.53 Other dystrophies primarily involving the sensory retina
    - Stargardt's disease
  - H35.54 Dystrophies primarily involving the retinal pigment epithelium
    - Vitelliform retinal dystrophy
- H35.6 Retinal hemorrhage
  - H35.60 Retinal hemorrhage, unspecified eye
  - H35.61 Retinal hemorrhage, right eye
  - H35.62 Retinal hemorrhage, left eye
  - H35.63 Retinal hemorrhage, bilateral
- H35.7 Separation of retinal layers
  - **Excludes1** retinal detachment (serous) (H33.2-)
    rhegmatogenous retinal detachment (H33.0-)
  - Ex: **For category H35.7 CC codes:** H33.001-H33.119, H33.191-H33.8, H35.70-H35.739
  - H35.70 Unspecified separation of retinal layers
- H35.71 Central serous chorioretinopathy
  - H35.711 Central serous chorioretinopathy, right eye
  - H35.712 Central serous chorioretinopathy, left eye
  - H35.713 Central serous chorioretinopathy, bilateral
  - H35.719 Central serous chorioretinopathy, unspecified eye
- H35.72 Serous detachment of retinal pigment epithelium
  - H35.721 Serous detachment of retinal pigment epithelium, right eye
  - H35.722 Serous detachment of retinal pigment epithelium, left eye
  - H35.723 Serous detachment of retinal pigment epithelium, bilateral
  - H35.729 Serous detachment of retinal pigment epithelium, unspecified eye

- **H35.73 Hemorrhagic detachment of retinal pigment epithelium**
  - **H35.731 Hemorrhagic detachment of retinal pigment epithelium, right eye**
  - **H35.732 Hemorrhagic detachment of retinal pigment epithelium, left eye**
  - **H35.733 Hemorrhagic detachment of retinal pigment epithelium, bilateral**
  - **H35.739 Hemorrhagic detachment of retinal pigment epithelium, unspecified eye**
- **H35.8 Other specified retinal disorders**
  - **Excludes2** retinal hemorrhage (H35.6-)
  - **H35.81 Retinal edema**
    Retinal cotton wool spots
  - **H35.82 Retinal ischemia**
    Ex: H35.60-H35.63, H35.81-H35.89
  - **H35.89 Other specified retinal disorders**
- **H35.9 Unspecified retinal disorder**

H36 Retinal disorders in diseases classified elsewhere

Code first underlying disease, such as:
lipid storage disorders (E75.-)
sickle-cell disorders (D57.-)

Excludes1 arteriosclerotic retinopathy (H35.0-)
diabetic retinopathy (E08.3-, E09.3-, E10.3-, E11.3-, E13.3-)

GLAUCOMA (H40-H42)

- **H40 Glaucoma**
  Intraocular pressure (IOP) that is too high results from too much aqueous humor and because of excess production or inadequate drainage, optic nerve damage and vision loss may occur.
  - **Excludes1** absolute glaucoma (H44.51-)
    congenital glaucoma (Q15.0)
    traumatic glaucoma due to birth injury (P15.3)
  - **H40.0 Glaucoma suspect**
    - **H40.00 Preglaucoma, unspecified**
      - **H40.001 Preglaucoma, unspecified, right eye**
      - **H40.002 Preglaucoma, unspecified, left eye**
      - **H40.003 Preglaucoma, unspecified, bilateral**
      - **H40.009 Preglaucoma, unspecified, unspecified eye**
    - **H40.01 Open angle with borderline findings, low risk**
      Open angle, low risk
      - **H40.011 Open angle with borderline findings, low risk, right eye**
      - **H40.012 Open angle with borderline findings, low risk, left eye**
      - **H40.013 Open angle with borderline findings, low risk, bilateral**
      - **H40.019 Open angle with borderline findings, low risk, unspecified eye**
    - **H40.02 Open angle with borderline findings, high risk**
      Open angle, high risk
      - **H40.021 Open angle with borderline findings, high risk, right eye**
      - **H40.022 Open angle with borderline findings, high risk, left eye**
      - **H40.023 Open angle with borderline findings, high risk, bilateral**
      - **H40.029 Open angle with borderline findings, high risk, unspecified eye**
    - **H40.03 Anatomical narrow angle**
      Primary angle closure suspect
      - **H40.031 Anatomical narrow angle, right eye**
      - **H40.032 Anatomical narrow angle, left eye**
      - **H40.033 Anatomical narrow angle, bilateral**
      - **H40.039 Anatomical narrow angle, unspecified eye**
    - **H40.04 Steroid responder**
      - **H40.041 Steroid responder, right eye**
      - **H40.042 Steroid responder, left eye**
      - **H40.043 Steroid responder, bilateral**
      - **H40.049 Steroid responder, unspecified eye**
    - **H40.05 Ocular hypertension**
      - **H40.051 Ocular hypertension, right eye**
      - **H40.052 Ocular hypertension, left eye**
      - **H40.053 Ocular hypertension, bilateral**
      - **H40.059 Ocular hypertension, unspecified eye**
    - **H40.06 Primary angle closure without glaucoma damage**
      - **H40.061 Primary angle closure without glaucoma damage, right eye**
      - **H40.062 Primary angle closure without glaucoma damage, left eye**
      - **H40.063 Primary angle closure without glaucoma damage, bilateral**
      - **H40.069 Primary angle closure without glaucoma damage, unspecified eye**
  - **H40.1 Open-angle glaucoma**
    - X **H40.10 Unspecified open-angle glaucoma**
      One of the following 7th characters is to be assigned to code H40.10 to designate the stage of glaucoma

0	stage unspecified
1	mild stage
2	moderate stage
3	severe stage
4	indeterminate stage

    - **H40.11 Primary open-angle glaucoma**
      Chronic simple glaucoma
      One of the following 7th characters is to be assigned to each code in subcategory H40.11 to designate the stage of glaucoma ◀

0	stage unspecified
1	mild stage
2	moderate stage
3	severe stage
4	indeterminate stage

      - **H40.111 Primary open-angle glaucoma, right eye ◀**
      - **H40.112 Primary open-angle glaucoma, left eye ◀**
      - **H40.113 Primary open-angle glaucoma, bilateral ◀**
      - **H40.119 Primary open-angle glaucoma, unspecified eye ◀**
    - **H40.12 Low-tension glaucoma**
      One of the following 7th characters is to be assigned to each code in subcategory H40.12 to designate the stage of glaucoma

0	stage unspecified
1	mild stage
2	moderate stage
3	severe stage
4	indeterminate stage

      - **H40.121 Low-tension glaucoma, right eye**
      - **H40.122 Low-tension glaucoma, left eye**
      - **H40.123 Low-tension glaucoma, bilateral**
      - **H40.129 Low-tension glaucoma, unspecified eye**

● **H40.13 Pigmentary glaucoma**

One of the following 7th characters is to be assigned to each code in subcategory H40.13 to designate the stage of glaucoma

0	stage unspecified
1	mild stage
2	moderate stage
3	severe stage
4	indeterminate stage

●● **H40.131 Pigmentary glaucoma, right eye**

●● **H40.132 Pigmentary glaucoma, left eye**

●● **H40.133 Pigmentary glaucoma, bilateral**

●● **H40.139 Pigmentary glaucoma, unspecified eye**

● **H40.14 Capsular glaucoma with pseudoexfoliation of lens**

One of the following 7th characters is to be assigned to each code in subcategory H40.14 to designate the stage of glaucoma

0	stage unspecified
1	mild stage
2	moderate stage
3	severe stage
4	indeterminate stage

● **H40.141 Capsular glaucoma with pseudoexfoliation of lens, right eye**

● **H40.142 Capsular glaucoma with pseudoexfoliation of lens, left eye**

● **H40.143 Capsular glaucoma with pseudoexfoliation of lens, bilateral**

● **H40.149 Capsular glaucoma with pseudoexfoliation of lens, unspecified eye**

● **H40.15 Residual stage of open-angle glaucoma**

● **H40.151 Residual stage of open-angle glaucoma, right eye**

● **H40.152 Residual stage of open-angle glaucoma, left eye**

● **H40.153 Residual stage of open-angle glaucoma, bilateral**

● **H40.159 Residual stage of open-angle glaucoma, unspecified eye**

● **H40.2 Primary angle-closure glaucoma**

Excludes1 aqueous misdirection (H40.83-)
malignant glaucoma (H40.83-)

● **H40.20 Unspecified primary angle-closure glaucoma**

One of the following 7th characters is to be assigned to code H40.20 to designate the stage of glaucoma

0	stage unspecified
1	mild stage
2	moderate stage
3	severe stage
4	indeterminate stage

● **H40.21 Acute angle-closure glaucoma**

Acute angle-closure glaucoma attack
Acute angle-closure glaucoma crisis

Ex For category H40.21 CC codes: H40.211-H40.219

H40.211 Acute angle-closure glaucoma, right eye CC

H40.212 Acute angle-closure glaucoma, left eye CC

H40.213 Acute angle-closure glaucoma, bilateral CC

H40.219 Acute angle-closure glaucoma, unspecified eye CC

● **H40.22 Chronic angle-closure glaucoma**

Chronic primary angle closure glaucoma

One of the following 7th characters is to be assigned to each code in subcategory H40.22 to designate the stage of glaucoma

0	stage unspecified
1	mild stage
2	moderate stage
3	severe stage
4	indeterminate stage

● **H40.221 Chronic angle-closure glaucoma, right eye**

● **H40.222 Chronic angle-closure glaucoma, left eye**

● **H40.223 Chronic angle-closure glaucoma, bilateral**

● **H40.229 Chronic angle-closure glaucoma, unspecified eye**

● **H40.23 Intermittent angle-closure glaucoma**

H40.231 Intermittent angle-closure glaucoma, right eye

H40.232 Intermittent angle-closure glaucoma, left eye

H40.233 Intermittent angle-closure glaucoma, bilateral

H40.239 Intermittent angle-closure glaucoma, unspecified eye

● **H40.24 Residual stage of angle-closure glaucoma**

H40.241 Residual stage of angle-closure glaucoma, right eye

H40.242 Residual stage of angle-closure glaucoma, left eye

H40.243 Residual stage of angle-closure glaucoma, bilateral

H40.249 Residual stage of angle-closure glaucoma, unspecified eye

● **H40.3 Glaucoma secondary to eye trauma**

Code also underlying condition

One of the following 7th characters is to be assigned to each code in subcategory H40.3 to designate the stage of glaucoma

0	stage unspecified
1	mild stage
2	moderate stage
3	severe stage
4	indeterminate stage

X● **H40.30 Glaucoma secondary to eye trauma, unspecified eye**

X● **H40.31 Glaucoma secondary to eye trauma, right eye**

X● **H40.32 Glaucoma secondary to eye trauma, left eye**

X● **H40.33 Glaucoma secondary to eye trauma, bilateral**

● **H40.4 Glaucoma secondary to eye inflammation**

Code also underlying condition

One of the following 7th characters is to be assigned to each code in subcategory H40.4 to designate the stage of glaucoma

0	stage unspecified
1	mild stage
2	moderate stage
3	severe stage
4	indeterminate stage

X● **H40.40 Glaucoma secondary to eye inflammation, unspecified eye**

X● **H40.41 Glaucoma secondary to eye inflammation, right eye**

X● **H40.42 Glaucoma secondary to eye inflammation, left eye**

X● **H40.43 Glaucoma secondary to eye inflammation, bilateral**

● **H40.5 Glaucoma secondary to other eye disorders**

Code also underlying eye disorder

One of the following 7th characters is to be assigned to each code in subcategory H40.5 to designate the stage of glaucoma

0	stage unspecified
1	mild stage
2	moderate stage
3	severe stage
4	indeterminate stage

X● **H40.50 Glaucoma secondary to other eye disorders, unspecified eye**

X● **H40.51 Glaucoma secondary to other eye disorders, right eye**

X● **H40.52 Glaucoma secondary to other eye disorders, left eye**

X● **H40.53 Glaucoma secondary to other eye disorders, bilateral**

● **H40.6 Glaucoma secondary to drugs**

Use additional code for adverse effect, if applicable, to identify drug (T36-T50 with fifth or sixth character 5)

One of the following 7th characters is to be assigned to each code in subcategory H40.6 to designate the stage of glaucoma

0	stage unspecified
1	mild stage
2	moderate stage
3	severe stage
4	indeterminate stage

X● **H40.60 Glaucoma secondary to drugs, unspecified eye**

X● **H40.61 Glaucoma secondary to drugs, right eye**

X● **H40.62 Glaucoma secondary to drugs, left eye**

X● **H40.63 Glaucoma secondary to drugs, bilateral**

● **H40.8 Other glaucoma**

● **H40.81 Glaucoma with increased episcleral venous pressure**

H40.811 Glaucoma with increased episcleral venous pressure, right eye

H40.812 Glaucoma with increased episcleral venous pressure, left eye

H40.813 Glaucoma with increased episcleral venous pressure, bilateral

H40.819 Glaucoma with increased episcleral venous pressure, unspecified eye

● **H40.82 Hypersecretion glaucoma**

H40.821 Hypersecretion glaucoma, right eye

H40.822 Hypersecretion glaucoma, left eye

H40.823 Hypersecretion glaucoma, bilateral

H40.829 Hypersecretion glaucoma, unspecified eye

● **H40.83 Aqueous misdirection**

Malignant glaucoma

H40.831 Aqueous misdirection, right eye

H40.832 Aqueous misdirection, left eye

H40.833 Aqueous misdirection, bilateral

H40.839 Aqueous misdirection, unspecified eye

H40.89 Other specified glaucoma

H40.9 Unspecified glaucoma

▶ ***H42 Glaucoma in diseases classified elsewhere***

Code first underlying condition, such as:
amyloidosis (E85.-)
aniridia (Q13.1)
Lowe's syndrome (E72.03)
Reiger's anomaly (Q13.81)
specified metabolic disorder (E70-E88)

Excludes1 glaucoma (in) onchocerciasis (B73.02) ◀
glaucoma (in) syphilis (A52.71) ◀
glaucoma (in) tuberculous (A18.59) ◀

Excludes2 glaucoma (in) diabetes mellitus (E08.39, E09.39, E10.39, E11.39, E13.39) ◀

DISORDERS OF VITREOUS BODY AND GLOBE (H43-H44)

● **H43 Disorders of vitreous body**

● **H43.0 Vitreous prolapse**

Excludes1 vitreous syndrome following cataract surgery (H59.0-)
traumatic vitreous prolapse (S05.2-)

H43.00 Vitreous prolapse, unspecified eye

H43.01 Vitreous prolapse, right eye

H43.02 Vitreous prolapse, left eye

H43.03 Vitreous prolapse, bilateral

● **H43.1 Vitreous hemorrhage**

H43.10 Vitreous hemorrhage, unspecified eye

H43.11 Vitreous hemorrhage, right eye

H43.12 Vitreous hemorrhage, left eye

H43.13 Vitreous hemorrhage, bilateral

● **H43.2 Crystalline deposits in vitreous body**

H43.20 Crystalline deposits in vitreous body, unspecified eye

H43.21 Crystalline deposits in vitreous body, right eye

H43.22 Crystalline deposits in vitreous body, left eye

H43.23 Crystalline deposits in vitreous body, bilateral

- H43.3 Other vitreous opacities
  - H43.31 Vitreous membranes and strands
    - H43.311 Vitreous membranes and strands, right eye
    - H43.312 Vitreous membranes and strands, left eye
    - H43.313 Vitreous membranes and strands, bilateral
    - H43.319 Vitreous membranes and strands, unspecified eye
  - H43.39 Other vitreous opacities
    Vitreous floaters
    Small clumps of cells that float in the vitreous of the eye, appearing as black specks or dots in the field of vision and common in the aging eye.
    - H43.391 Other vitreous opacities, right eye
    - H43.392 Other vitreous opacities, left eye
    - H43.393 Other vitreous opacities, bilateral
    - H43.399 Other vitreous opacities, unspecified eye
- H43.8 Other disorders of vitreous body
  Excludes1 proliferative vitreo-retinopathy with retinal detachment (H33.4)
  Excludes2 vitreous abscess (H44.02-)
  - H43.81 Vitreous degeneration
    Vitreous detachment
    - H43.811 Vitreous degeneration, right eye
    - H43.812 Vitreous degeneration, left eye
    - H43.813 Vitreous degeneration, bilateral
    - H43.819 Vitreous degeneration, unspecified eye
  - H43.82 Vitreomacular adhesion
    Vitreomacular traction
    - H43.821 Vitreomacular adhesion, right eye A
    - H43.822 Vitreomacular adhesion, left eye A
    - H43.823 Vitreomacular adhesion, bilateral A
    - H43.829 Vitreomacular adhesion, unspecified eye A
  - H43.89 Other disorders of vitreous body
- H43.9 Unspecified disorder of vitreous body

- H44 Disorders of globe
  Includes disorders affecting multiple structures of eye
- H44.0 Purulent endophthalmitis
  Use additional code to identify organism
  Excludes1 bleb associated endophthalmitis (H59.4-)
  - H44.00 Unspecified purulent endophthalmitis
    Ex: For category H44.00 CC codes: H20.051-H20.059, H21.331-H21.339, H33.121-H33.129, H44.001-H44.029, H44.121-H44.129, H44.19
    - H44.001 Unspecified purulent endophthalmitis, right eye
    - H44.002 Unspecified purulent endophthalmitis, left eye
    - H44.003 Unspecified purulent endophthalmitis, bilateral
    - H44.009 Unspecified purulent endophthalmitis, unspecified eye
  - H44.01 Panophthalmitis (acute)
    Ex: For category H44.01 CC codes: See H44.00
    - H44.011 Panophthalmitis (acute), right eye
    - H44.012 Panophthalmitis (acute), left eye
    - H44.013 Panophthalmitis (acute), bilateral
    - H44.019 Panophthalmitis (acute), unspecified eye
  - H44.02 Vitreous abscess (chronic)
    Ex: For category H44.02 CC codes: H16.241-H16.249, H21.331-H21.339, H33.121-H33.129, H44.001-H44.19
    - H44.021 Vitreous abscess (chronic), right eye
    - H44.022 Vitreous abscess (chronic), left eye
    - H44.023 Vitreous abscess (chronic), bilateral
    - H44.029 Vitreous abscess (chronic), unspecified eye
- H44.1 Other endophthalmitis
  Excludes1 bleb associated endophthalmitis (H59.4-)
  Excludes2 ophthalmia nodosa (H16.2-)
  - H44.11 Panuveitis
    Ex: For category H44.11 CC codes: H44.111-H44.119, H44.131-H44.139
    - H44.111 Panuveitis, right eye
    - H44.112 Panuveitis, left eye
    - H44.113 Panuveitis, bilateral
    - H44.119 Panuveitis, unspecified eye
  - H44.12 Parasitic endophthalmitis, unspecified
    Ex: For category H44.12 CC codes: See H44.00
    - H44.121 Parasitic endophthalmitis, unspecified, right eye
    - H44.122 Parasitic endophthalmitis, unspecified, left eye
    - H44.123 Parasitic endophthalmitis, unspecified, bilateral
    - H44.129 Parasitic endophthalmitis, unspecified, unspecified eye
  - H44.13 Sympathetic uveitis
    Ex: For category H44.13 CC codes: See H44.11
    - H44.131 Sympathetic uveitis, right eye
    - H44.132 Sympathetic uveitis, left eye
    - H44.133 Sympathetic uveitis, bilateral
    - H44.139 Sympathetic uveitis, unspecified eye
  - H44.19 Other endophthalmitis
    Ex: See H44.00
- H44.2 Degenerative myopia
  Malignant myopia
  - H44.20 Degenerative myopia, unspecified eye
  - H44.21 Degenerative myopia, right eye
  - H44.22 Degenerative myopia, left eye
  - H44.23 Degenerative myopia, bilateral
- H44.3 Other and unspecified degenerative disorders of globe
  - H44.30 Unspecified degenerative disorder of globe
  - H44.31 Chalcosis
    - H44.311 Chalcosis, right eye
    - H44.312 Chalcosis, left eye
    - H44.313 Chalcosis, bilateral
    - H44.319 Chalcosis, unspecified eye
  - H44.32 Siderosis of eye
    - H44.321 Siderosis of eye, right eye
    - H44.322 Siderosis of eye, left eye
    - H44.323 Siderosis of eye, bilateral
    - H44.329 Siderosis of eye, unspecified eye
  - H44.39 Other degenerative disorders of globe
    - H44.391 Other degenerative disorders of globe, right eye
    - H44.392 Other degenerative disorders of globe, left eye
    - H44.393 Other degenerative disorders of globe, bilateral
    - H44.399 Other degenerative disorders of globe, unspecified eye

- **H44.4 Hypotony of eye**
  - H44.40 Unspecified hypotony of eye
  - **H44.41 Flat anterior chamber hypotony of eye**
    - H44.411 Flat anterior chamber hypotony of right eye
    - H44.412 Flat anterior chamber hypotony of left eye
    - H44.413 Flat anterior chamber hypotony of eye, bilateral
    - H44.419 Flat anterior chamber hypotony of unspecified eye
  - **H44.42 Hypotony of eye due to ocular fistula**
    - H44.421 Hypotony of right eye due to ocular fistula
    - H44.422 Hypotony of left eye due to ocular fistula
    - H44.423 Hypotony of eye due to ocular fistula, bilateral
    - H44.429 Hypotony of unspecified eye due to ocular fistula
  - **H44.43 Hypotony of eye due to other ocular disorders**
    - H44.431 Hypotony of eye due to other ocular disorders, right eye
    - H44.432 Hypotony of eye due to other ocular disorders, left eye
    - H44.433 Hypotony of eye due to other ocular disorders, bilateral
    - H44.439 Hypotony of eye due to other ocular disorders, unspecified eye
  - **H44.44 Primary hypotony of eye**
    - H44.441 Primary hypotony of right eye
    - H44.442 Primary hypotony of left eye
    - H44.443 Primary hypotony of eye, bilateral
    - H44.449 Primary hypotony of unspecified eye
- **H44.5 Degenerated conditions of globe**
  - H44.50 Unspecified degenerated conditions of globe
  - **H44.51 Absolute glaucoma**
    - H44.511 Absolute glaucoma, right eye
    - H44.512 Absolute glaucoma, left eye
    - H44.513 Absolute glaucoma, bilateral
    - H44.519 Absolute glaucoma, unspecified eye
  - **H44.52 Atrophy of globe**
    Phthisis bulbi
    - H44.521 Atrophy of globe, right eye
    - H44.522 Atrophy of globe, left eye
    - H44.523 Atrophy of globe, bilateral
    - H44.529 Atrophy of globe, unspecified eye
  - **H44.53 Leucocoria**
    - H44.531 Leucocoria, right eye
    - H44.532 Leucocoria, left eye
    - H44.533 Leucocoria, bilateral
    - H44.539 Leucocoria, unspecified eye
- **H44.6 Retained (old) intraocular foreign body, magnetic**
  Use additional code to identify magnetic foreign body (Z18.11)
  Excludes1 current intraocular foreign body (S05.-)
  Excludes2 retained foreign body in eyelid (H02.81-)
  retained (old) foreign body following penetrating wound of orbit (H05.5-)
  retained (old) intraocular foreign body, nonmagnetic (H44.7-)
  - **H44.60 Unspecified retained (old) intraocular foreign body, magnetic**
    - H44.601 Unspecified retained (old) intraocular foreign body, magnetic, right eye
    - H44.602 Unspecified retained (old) intraocular foreign body, magnetic, left eye
    - H44.603 Unspecified retained (old) intraocular foreign body, magnetic, bilateral
    - H44.609 Unspecified retained (old) intraocular foreign body, magnetic, unspecified eye
  - **H44.61 Retained (old) magnetic foreign body in anterior chamber**
    - H44.611 Retained (old) magnetic foreign body in anterior chamber, right eye
    - H44.612 Retained (old) magnetic foreign body in anterior chamber, left eye
    - H44.613 Retained (old) magnetic foreign body in anterior chamber, bilateral
    - H44.619 Retained (old) magnetic foreign body in anterior chamber, unspecified eye
  - **H44.62 Retained (old) magnetic foreign body in iris or ciliary body**
    - H44.621 Retained (old) magnetic foreign body in iris or ciliary body, right eye
    - H44.622 Retained (old) magnetic foreign body in iris or ciliary body, left eye
    - H44.623 Retained (old) magnetic foreign body in iris or ciliary body, bilateral
    - H44.629 Retained (old) magnetic foreign body in iris or ciliary body, unspecified eye
  - **H44.63 Retained (old) magnetic foreign body in lens**
    - H44.631 Retained (old) magnetic foreign body in lens, right eye
    - H44.632 Retained (old) magnetic foreign body in lens, left eye
    - H44.633 Retained (old) magnetic foreign body in lens, bilateral
    - H44.639 Retained (old) magnetic foreign body in lens, unspecified eye
  - **H44.64 Retained (old) magnetic foreign body in posterior wall of globe**
    - H44.641 Retained (old) magnetic foreign body in posterior wall of globe, right eye
    - H44.642 Retained (old) magnetic foreign body in posterior wall of globe, left eye
    - H44.643 Retained (old) magnetic foreign body in posterior wall of globe, bilateral
    - H44.649 Retained (old) magnetic foreign body in posterior wall of globe, unspecified eye
  - **H44.65 Retained (old) magnetic foreign body in vitreous body**
    - H44.651 Retained (old) magnetic foreign body in vitreous body, right eye
    - H44.652 Retained (old) magnetic foreign body in vitreous body, left eye
    - H44.653 Retained (old) magnetic foreign body in vitreous body, bilateral
    - H44.659 Retained (old) magnetic foreign body in vitreous body, unspecified eye

- H44.69 Retained (old) intraocular foreign body, magnetic, in other or multiple sites
  - H44.691 Retained (old) intraocular foreign body, magnetic, in other or multiple sites, right eye
  - H44.692 Retained (old) intraocular foreign body, magnetic, in other or multiple sites, left eye
  - H44.693 Retained (old) intraocular foreign body, magnetic, in other or multiple sites, bilateral
  - H44.699 Retained (old) intraocular foreign body, magnetic, in other or multiple sites, unspecified eye
- H44.7 Retained (old) intraocular foreign body, nonmagnetic

  Use additional code to identify nonmagnetic foreign body (Z18.01-Z18.10, Z18.12, Z18.2-Z18.9)

  Excludes1 current intraocular foreign body (S05.-)

  Excludes2 retained foreign body in eyelid (H02.81-)
  retained (old) foreign body following penetrating wound of orbit (H05.5-)
  retained (old) intraocular foreign body, magnetic (H44.6-)
  - H44.70 Unspecified retained (old) intraocular foreign body, nonmagnetic
    - H44.701 Unspecified retained (old) intraocular foreign body, nonmagnetic, right eye
    - H44.702 Unspecified retained (old) intraocular foreign body, nonmagnetic, left eye
    - H44.703 Unspecified retained (old) intraocular foreign body, nonmagnetic, bilateral
    - H44.709 Unspecified retained (old) intraocular foreign body, nonmagnetic, unspecified eye

      Retained (old) intraocular foreign body NOS
  - H44.71 Retained (nonmagnetic) (old) foreign body in anterior chamber
    - H44.711 Retained (nonmagnetic) (old) foreign body in anterior chamber, right eye
    - H44.712 Retained (nonmagnetic) (old) foreign body in anterior chamber, left eye
    - H44.713 Retained (nonmagnetic) (old) foreign body in anterior chamber, bilateral
    - H44.719 Retained (nonmagnetic) (old) foreign body in anterior chamber, unspecified eye
  - H44.72 Retained (nonmagnetic) (old) foreign body in iris or ciliary body
    - H44.721 Retained (nonmagnetic) (old) foreign body in iris or ciliary body, right eye
    - H44.722 Retained (nonmagnetic) (old) foreign body in iris or ciliary body, left eye
    - H44.723 Retained (nonmagnetic) (old) foreign body in iris or ciliary body, bilateral
    - H44.729 Retained (nonmagnetic) (old) foreign body in iris or ciliary body, unspecified eye
  - H44.73 Retained (nonmagnetic) (old) foreign body in lens
    - H44.731 Retained (nonmagnetic) (old) foreign body in lens, right eye
    - H44.732 Retained (nonmagnetic) (old) foreign body in lens, left eye
    - H44.733 Retained (nonmagnetic) (old) foreign body in lens, bilateral
    - H44.739 Retained (nonmagnetic) (old) foreign body in lens, unspecified eye
  - H44.74 Retained (nonmagnetic) (old) foreign body in posterior wall of globe
    - H44.741 Retained (nonmagnetic) (old) foreign body in posterior wall of globe, right eye
    - H44.742 Retained (nonmagnetic) (old) foreign body in posterior wall of globe, left eye
    - H44.743 Retained (nonmagnetic) (old) foreign body in posterior wall of globe, bilateral
    - H44.749 Retained (nonmagnetic) (old) foreign body in posterior wall of globe, unspecified eye
  - H44.75 Retained (nonmagnetic) (old) foreign body in vitreous body
    - H44.751 Retained (nonmagnetic) (old) foreign body in vitreous body, right eye
    - H44.752 Retained (nonmagnetic) (old) foreign body in vitreous body, left eye
    - H44.753 Retained (nonmagnetic) (old) foreign body in vitreous body, bilateral
    - H44.759 Retained (nonmagnetic) (old) foreign body in vitreous body, unspecified eye
  - H44.79 Retained (old) intraocular foreign body, nonmagnetic, in other or multiple sites
    - H44.791 Retained (old) intraocular foreign body, nonmagnetic, in other or multiple sites, right eye
    - H44.792 Retained (old) intraocular foreign body, nonmagnetic, in other or multiple sites, left eye
    - H44.793 Retained (old) intraocular foreign body, nonmagnetic, in other or multiple sites, bilateral
    - H44.799 Retained (old) intraocular foreign body, nonmagnetic, in other or multiple sites, unspecified eye
- H44.8 Other disorders of globe
  - H44.81 Hemophthalmos
    - H44.811 Hemophthalmos, right eye
    - H44.812 Hemophthalmos, left eye
    - H44.813 Hemophthalmos, bilateral
    - H44.819 Hemophthalmos, unspecified eye
  - H44.82 Luxation of globe
    - H44.821 Luxation of globe, right eye
    - H44.822 Luxation of globe, left eye
    - H44.823 Luxation of globe, bilateral
    - H44.829 Luxation of globe, unspecified eye
  - H44.89 Other disorders of globe
- H44.9 Unspecified disorder of globe

★ **(See Plate 86 on page 55.)**

DISORDERS OF OPTIC NERVE AND VISUAL PATHWAYS (H46-H47)

- H46 Optic neuritis

  Excludes2 ischemic optic neuropathy (H47.01-)
  neuromyelitis optica [Devic] (G36.0)

  Ex For category H46 CC codes: H46.00-H46.9
  - H46.0 Optic papillitis
    - H46.00 Optic papillitis, unspecified eye
    - H46.01 Optic papillitis, right eye
    - H46.02 Optic papillitis, left eye
    - H46.03 Optic papillitis, bilateral

◀ New ⟸ Revised ~~deleted~~ Deleted Excludes 1 Excludes 2 Includes Use additional Code first Code also Unspecified
OGCR Official Guidelines ● Unacceptable Principal Diagnosis X Assign placeholder X ● Use Additional Character(s) ▶ Manifestation Code Coding Clinic

- **H46.1 Retrobulbar neuritis**
  Retrobulbar neuritis NOS
  Excludes1 syphilitic retrobulbar neuritis (A52.15)
  - **H46.10 Retrobulbar neuritis, unspecified eye**
  - **H46.11 Retrobulbar neuritis, right eye**
  - **H46.12 Retrobulbar neuritis, left eye**
  - **H46.13 Retrobulbar neuritis, bilateral**
- **H46.2 Nutritional optic neuropathy**
- **H46.3 Toxic optic neuropathy**
  Code first (T51-T65) to identify cause
- **H46.8 Other optic neuritis**
- **H46.9 Unspecified optic neuritis**

- **H47 Other disorders of optic [2nd] nerve and visual pathways**
  - **H47.0 Disorders of optic nerve, not elsewhere classified**
    - **H47.01 Ischemic optic neuropathy**
      - **H47.011 Ischemic optic neuropathy, right eye**
      - **H47.012 Ischemic optic neuropathy, left eye**
      - **H47.013 Ischemic optic neuropathy, bilateral**
      - **H47.019 Ischemic optic neuropathy, unspecified eye**
    - **H47.02 Hemorrhage in optic nerve sheath**
      - **H47.021 Hemorrhage in optic nerve sheath, right eye**
      - **H47.022 Hemorrhage in optic nerve sheath, left eye**
      - **H47.023 Hemorrhage in optic nerve sheath, bilateral**
      - **H47.029 Hemorrhage in optic nerve sheath, unspecified eye**
    - **H47.03 Optic nerve hypoplasia**
      - **H47.031 Optic nerve hypoplasia, right eye**
      - **H47.032 Optic nerve hypoplasia, left eye**
      - **H47.033 Optic nerve hypoplasia, bilateral**
      - **H47.039 Optic nerve hypoplasia, unspecified eye**
    - **H47.09 Other disorders of optic nerve, not elsewhere classified**
      Compression of optic nerve
      - **H47.091 Other disorders of optic nerve, not elsewhere classified, right eye**
      - **H47.092 Other disorders of optic nerve, not elsewhere classified, left eye**
      - **H47.093 Other disorders of optic nerve, not elsewhere classified, bilateral**
      - **H47.099 Other disorders of optic nerve, not elsewhere classified, unspecified eye**
  - **H47.1 Papilledema**
    - **H47.10 Unspecified papilledema**
      Ex: A17.9, A18.50-A18.59, A18.82, A18.84, A18.89, A39.82, E08.311-E08.39, E08.618-E08.638, E08.649-E08.8, E09.311-E09.39, E09.618-E09.638, E09.649-E09.8, E10.311-E10.39, E10.618-E10.638, E10.649, E10.69-E10.8, E11.311-E11.39, E11.618-E11.638, E11.649, E11.69-E11.8, E13.311-E13.39, E13.618-E13.638, E13.649-E13.8, H47.10-H47.13, H47.231-H47.239, H47.331-H47.339, H57.8-H57.9, H59.40-H59.43, Q11.3, Q15.8-Q15.9
    - **H47.11 Papilledema associated with increased intracranial pressure**
      Ex: See H47.10
    - **H47.12 Papilledema associated with decreased ocular pressure**
    - **H47.13 Papilledema associated with retinal disorder**
    - **H47.14 Foster-Kennedy syndrome**
      - **H47.141 Foster-Kennedy syndrome, right eye**
      - **H47.142 Foster-Kennedy syndrome, left eye**
      - **H47.143 Foster-Kennedy syndrome, bilateral**
      - **H47.149 Foster-Kennedy syndrome, unspecified eye**

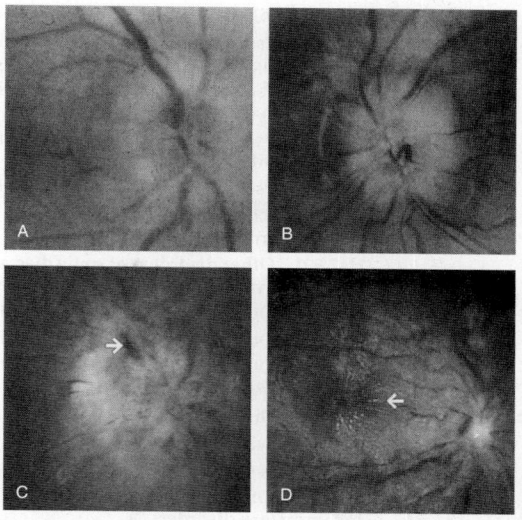

Figure 7-11 Papilledema. (From Behrma: Nelson Textbook of Pediatrics, ed 17, Saunders, 2004)

Item 7-8 Papilledema is swelling of the optic disc caused by increased intracranial pressure. It is most often bilateral and occurs quickly (hours) or over weeks of time. It is a common symptom of a brain tumor. The term should not be used to describe optic disc swelling with underlying infectious, infiltrative, or inflammatory etiologies.

- **H47.2 Optic atrophy**
  - **H47.20 Unspecified optic atrophy**
  - **H47.21 Primary optic atrophy**
    - **H47.211 Primary optic atrophy, right eye**
    - **H47.212 Primary optic atrophy, left eye**
    - **H47.213 Primary optic atrophy, bilateral**
    - **H47.219 Primary optic atrophy, unspecified eye**
  - **H47.22 Hereditary optic atrophy**
    Leber's optic atrophy
  - **H47.23 Glaucomatous optic atrophy**
    - **H47.231 Glaucomatous optic atrophy, right eye**
    - **H47.232 Glaucomatous optic atrophy, left eye**
    - **H47.233 Glaucomatous optic atrophy, bilateral**
    - **H47.239 Glaucomatous optic atrophy, unspecified eye**
  - **H47.29 Other optic atrophy**
    Temporal pallor of optic disc
    - **H47.291 Other optic atrophy, right eye**
    - **H47.292 Other optic atrophy, left eye**
    - **H47.293 Other optic atrophy, bilateral**
    - **H47.299 Other optic atrophy, unspecified eye**
- **H47.3 Other disorders of optic disc**
  - **H47.31 Coloboma of optic disc**
    - **H47.311 Coloboma of optic disc, right eye**
    - **H47.312 Coloboma of optic disc, left eye**
    - **H47.313 Coloboma of optic disc, bilateral**
    - **H47.319 Coloboma of optic disc, unspecified eye**
  - **H47.32 Drusen of optic disc**
    - **H47.321 Drusen of optic disc, right eye**
    - **H47.322 Drusen of optic disc, left eye**
    - **H47.323 Drusen of optic disc, bilateral**
    - **H47.329 Drusen of optic disc, unspecified eye**

- H47.33 Pseudopapilledema of optic disc
  - H47.331 Pseudopapilledema of optic disc, right eye
  - H47.332 Pseudopapilledema of optic disc, left eye
  - H47.333 Pseudopapilledema of optic disc, bilateral
  - H47.339 Pseudopapilledema of optic disc, unspecified eye
- H47.39 Other disorders of optic disc
  - H47.391 Other disorders of optic disc, right eye
  - H47.392 Other disorders of optic disc, left eye
  - H47.393 Other disorders of optic disc, bilateral
  - H47.399 Other disorders of optic disc, unspecified eye
- H47.4 Disorders of optic chiasm

  Code also underlying condition

  Ex: For category H47.4 CC codes: H47.41-H47.539
  - H47.41 Disorders of optic chiasm in (due to) inflammatory disorders
  - H47.42 Disorders of optic chiasm in (due to) neoplasm
  - H47.43 Disorders of optic chiasm in (due to) vascular disorders
  - H47.49 Disorders of optic chiasm in (due to) other disorders
- H47.5 Disorders of other visual pathways

  Disorders of optic tracts, geniculate nuclei and optic radiations

  Code also underlying condition

  Ex: For category H47.5 CC codes: H47.41-H47.539
  - H47.51 Disorders of visual pathways in (due to) inflammatory disorders
    - H47.511 Disorders of visual pathways in (due to) inflammatory disorders, right side
    - H47.512 Disorders of visual pathways in (due to) inflammatory disorders, left side
    - H47.519 Disorders of visual pathways in (due to) inflammatory disorders, unspecified side
  - H47.52 Disorders of visual pathways in (due to) neoplasm
    - H47.521 Disorders of visual pathways in (due to) neoplasm, right side
    - H47.522 Disorders of visual pathways in (due to) neoplasm, left side
    - H47.529 Disorders of visual pathways in (due to) neoplasm, unspecified side
  - H47.53 Disorders of visual pathways in (due to) vascular disorders
    - H47.531 Disorders of visual pathways in (due to) vascular disorders, right side
    - H47.532 Disorders of visual pathways in (due to) vascular disorders, left side
    - H47.539 Disorders of visual pathways in (due to) vascular disorders, unspecified side
- H47.6 Disorders of visual cortex

  Code also underlying condition

  Excludes1 injury to visual cortex S04.04

  Ex: For category H47.6 CC codes: H47.611-H47.9
  - H47.61 Cortical blindness
    - H47.611 Cortical blindness, right side of brain
    - H47.612 Cortical blindness, left side of brain
    - H47.619 Cortical blindness, unspecified side of brain
  - H47.62 Disorders of visual cortex in (due to) inflammatory disorders
    - H47.621 Disorders of visual cortex in (due to) inflammatory disorders, right side of brain
    - H47.622 Disorders of visual cortex in (due to) inflammatory disorders, left side of brain
    - H47.629 Disorders of visual cortex in (due to) inflammatory disorders, unspecified side of brain
  - H47.63 Disorders of visual cortex in (due to) neoplasm
    - H47.631 Disorders of visual cortex in (due to) neoplasm, right side of brain
    - H47.632 Disorders of visual cortex in (due to) neoplasm, left side of brain
    - H47.639 Disorders of visual cortex in (due to) neoplasm, unspecified side of brain
  - H47.64 Disorders of visual cortex in (due to) vascular disorders
    - H47.641 Disorders of visual cortex in (due to) vascular disorders, right side of brain
    - H47.642 Disorders of visual cortex in (due to) vascular disorders, left side of brain
    - H47.649 Disorders of visual cortex in (due to) vascular disorders, unspecified side of brain
- H47.9 Unspecified disorder of visual pathways

DISORDERS OF OCULAR MUSCLES, BINOCULAR MOVEMENT, ACCOMMODATION AND REFRACTION (H49-H52)

Excludes2 nystagmus and other irregular eye movements (H55)

- H49 Paralytic strabismus

  Excludes2 internal ophthalmoplegia (H52.51-)
  internuclear ophthalmoplegia (H51.2-)
  progressive supranuclear ophthalmoplegia (G23.1)
  - H49.0 Third [oculomotor] nerve palsy
    - H49.00 Third [oculomotor] nerve palsy, unspecified eye
    - H49.01 Third [oculomotor] nerve palsy, right eye
    - H49.02 Third [oculomotor] nerve palsy, left eye
    - H49.03 Third [oculomotor] nerve palsy, bilateral
  - H49.1 Fourth [trochlear] nerve palsy
    - H49.10 Fourth [trochlear] nerve palsy, unspecified eye
    - H49.11 Fourth [trochlear] nerve palsy, right eye
    - H49.12 Fourth [trochlear] nerve palsy, left eye
    - H49.13 Fourth [trochlear] nerve palsy, bilateral

Item 7–9 Strabismus or esotropia (crossed eyes) is a condition of the extraocular eye muscles, resulting in an inability of the eyes to focus and also affects depth perception.

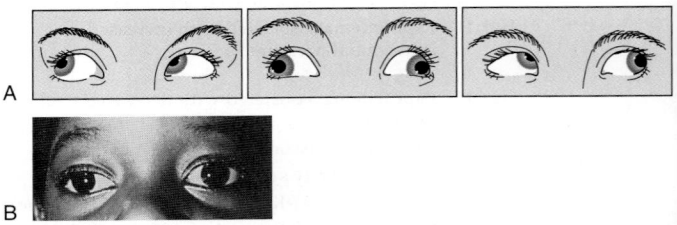

Figure 7-12 **A.** Image of strabismus. **B.** Exotropia. (**A** from Yanoff: Ophthalmology, ed 3, Mosby, Inc., 2008. **B** from Rakel: Textbook of Family Practice, ed 7, Saunders, 2007)

- **H49.2** Sixth [abducent] nerve palsy
  - **H49.20** Sixth [abducent] nerve palsy, unspecified eye
  - **H49.21** Sixth [abducent] nerve palsy, right eye
  - **H49.22** Sixth [abducent] nerve palsy, left eye
  - **H49.23** Sixth [abducent] nerve palsy, bilateral
- **H49.3** Total (external) ophthalmoplegia
  - **H49.30** Total (external) ophthalmoplegia, unspecified eye
  - **H49.31** Total (external) ophthalmoplegia, right eye
  - **H49.32** Total (external) ophthalmoplegia, left eye
  - **H49.33** Total (external) ophthalmoplegia, bilateral
- **H49.4** Progressive external ophthalmoplegia
  - **Excludes1** Kearns-Sayre syndrome (H49.81-)
  - **H49.40** Progressive external ophthalmoplegia, unspecified eye
  - **H49.41** Progressive external ophthalmoplegia, right eye
  - **H49.42** Progressive external ophthalmoplegia, left eye
  - **H49.43** Progressive external ophthalmoplegia, bilateral
- **H49.8** Other paralytic strabismus
  - **H49.81** Kearns-Sayre syndrome
    - Progressive external ophthalmoplegia with pigmentary retinopathy
    - Use additional code for other manifestation, such as:
      - heart block (I45.9)
    - Ex For category H49.81 CC codes: C96.5-C96.6, E71.310-E71.548, E80.3-E80.7, E88.89
    - **H49.811** Kearns-Sayre syndrome, right eye
    - **H49.812** Kearns-Sayre syndrome, left eye
    - **H49.813** Kearns-Sayre syndrome, bilateral
    - **H49.819** Kearns-Sayre syndrome, unspecified eye
  - **H49.88** Other paralytic strabismus
    - External ophthalmoplegia NOS
    - **H49.881** Other paralytic strabismus, right eye
    - **H49.882** Other paralytic strabismus, left eye
    - **H49.883** Other paralytic strabismus, bilateral
    - **H49.889** Other paralytic strabismus, unspecified eye
  - **H49.9** Unspecified paralytic strabismus
- **H50** Other strabismus
  - **H50.0** Esotropia
    - Convergent concomitant strabismus
    - **Excludes1** intermittent esotropia (H50.31-, H50.32)
    - **H50.00** Unspecified esotropia
    - **H50.01** Monocular esotropia
      - **H50.011** Monocular esotropia, right eye
      - **H50.012** Monocular esotropia, left eye
    - **H50.02** Monocular esotropia with A pattern
      - **H50.021** Monocular esotropia with A pattern, right eye
      - **H50.022** Monocular esotropia with A pattern, left eye
    - **H50.03** Monocular esotropia with V pattern
      - **H50.031** Monocular esotropia with V pattern, right eye
      - **H50.032** Monocular esotropia with V pattern, left eye
    - **H50.04** Monocular esotropia with other noncomitancies
      - **H50.041** Monocular esotropia with other noncomitancies, right eye
      - **H50.042** Monocular esotropia with other noncomitancies, left eye
    - **H50.05** Alternating esotropia
    - **H50.06** Alternating esotropia with A pattern
    - **H50.07** Alternating esotropia with V pattern
    - **H50.08** Alternating esotropia with other noncomitancies
  - **H50.1** Exotropia
    - *Misalignment in which one eye deviates outward (away from nose) while the other fixates normally*
    - Divergent concomitant strabismus
    - **Excludes1** intermittent exotropia (H50.33-, H50.34)
    - **H50.10** Unspecified exotropia
    - **H50.11** Monocular exotropia
      - **H50.111** Monocular exotropia, right eye
      - **H50.112** Monocular exotropia, left eye
    - **H50.12** Monocular exotropia with A pattern
      - **H50.121** Monocular exotropia with A pattern, right eye
      - **H50.122** Monocular exotropia with A pattern, left eye
    - **H50.13** Monocular exotropia with V pattern
      - **H50.131** Monocular exotropia with V pattern, right eye
      - **H50.132** Monocular exotropia with V pattern, left eye
    - **H50.14** Monocular exotropia with other noncomitancies
      - **H50.141** Monocular exotropia with other noncomitancies, right eye
      - **H50.142** Monocular exotropia with other noncomitancies, left eye
    - **H50.15** Alternating exotropia
    - **H50.16** Alternating exotropia with A pattern
    - **H50.17** Alternating exotropia with V pattern
    - **H50.18** Alternating exotropia with other noncomitancies
  - **H50.2** Vertical strabismus
    - Hypertropia
    - **H50.21** Vertical strabismus, right eye
    - **H50.22** Vertical strabismus, left eye
  - **H50.3** Intermittent heterotropia
    - *Displacement of an organ or part of an organ from its normal position*
    - **H50.30** Unspecified intermittent heterotropia
    - **H50.31** Intermittent monocular esotropia
      - **H50.311** Intermittent monocular esotropia, right eye
      - **H50.312** Intermittent monocular esotropia, left eye
    - **H50.32** Intermittent alternating esotropia
    - **H50.33** Intermittent monocular exotropia
      - **H50.331** Intermittent monocular exotropia, right eye
      - **H50.332** Intermittent monocular exotropia, left eye
    - **H50.34** Intermittent alternating exotropia
  - **H50.4** Other and unspecified heterotropia
    - **H50.40** Unspecified heterotropia
    - **H50.41** Cyclotropia
      - **H50.411** Cyclotropia, right eye
      - **H50.412** Cyclotropia, left eye
    - **H50.42** Monofixation syndrome
    - **H50.43** Accommodative component in esotropia

- H50.5 Heterophoria
  One or both eyes wander away from the position where both eyes are looking together in the same direction
  - H50.50 Unspecified heterophoria
  - H50.51 Esophoria
    Eye deviates inward (toward the nose)
  - H50.52 Exophoria
    Eye deviates outward (toward the ear)
  - H50.53 Vertical heterophoria
  - H50.54 Cyclophoria
  - H50.55 Alternating heterophoria
- H50.6 Mechanical strabismus
  - H50.60 Mechanical strabismus, unspecified
  - H50.61 Brown's sheath syndrome
    - H50.611 Brown's sheath syndrome, right eye
    - H50.612 Brown's sheath syndrome, left eye
  - H50.69 Other mechanical strabismus
    Strabismus due to adhesions
    Traumatic limitation of duction of eye muscle
- H50.8 Other specified strabismus
  - H50.81 Duane's syndrome
    - H50.811 Duane's syndrome, right eye
    - H50.812 Duane's syndrome, left eye
  - H50.89 Other specified strabismus
- H50.9 Unspecified strabismus

- H51 Other disorders of binocular movement
  - H51.0 Palsy (spasm) of conjugate gaze
  - H51.1 Convergence insufficiency and excess
    - H51.11 Convergence insufficiency
    - H51.12 Convergence excess
  - H51.2 Internuclear ophthalmoplegia
    - H51.20 Internuclear ophthalmoplegia, unspecified eye
    - H51.21 Internuclear ophthalmoplegia, right eye
    - H51.22 Internuclear ophthalmoplegia, left eye
    - H51.23 Internuclear ophthalmoplegia, bilateral
  - H51.8 Other specified disorders of binocular movement
  - H51.9 Unspecified disorder of binocular movement

- H52 Disorders of refraction and accommodation
  - H52.0 Hypermetropia
    - H52.00 Hypermetropia, unspecified eye
    - H52.01 Hypermetropia, right eye
    - H52.02 Hypermetropia, left eye
    - H52.03 Hypermetropia, bilateral
  - H52.1 Myopia
    Excludes1 degenerative myopia (H44.2-)
    - H52.10 Myopia, unspecified eye
    - H52.11 Myopia, right eye
    - H52.12 Myopia, left eye
    - H52.13 Myopia, bilateral
  - H52.2 Astigmatism
    - H52.20 Unspecified astigmatism
      - H52.201 Unspecified astigmatism, right eye
      - H52.202 Unspecified astigmatism, left eye
      - H52.203 Unspecified astigmatism, bilateral
      - H52.209 Unspecified astigmatism, unspecified eye
    - H52.21 Irregular astigmatism
      - H52.211 Irregular astigmatism, right eye
      - H52.212 Irregular astigmatism, left eye
      - H52.213 Irregular astigmatism, bilateral
      - H52.219 Irregular astigmatism, unspecified eye
    - H52.22 Regular astigmatism
      - H52.221 Regular astigmatism, right eye
      - H52.222 Regular astigmatism, left eye
      - H52.223 Regular astigmatism, bilateral
      - H52.229 Regular astigmatism, unspecified eye
  - H52.3 Anisometropia and aniseikonia
    - H52.31 Anisometropia
    - H52.32 Aniseikonia
  - H52.4 Presbyopia
  - H52.5 Disorders of accommodation
    - H52.51 Internal ophthalmoplegia (complete) (total)
      - H52.511 Internal ophthalmoplegia (complete) (total), right eye
      - H52.512 Internal ophthalmoplegia (complete) (total), left eye
      - H52.513 Internal ophthalmoplegia (complete) (total), bilateral
      - H52.519 Internal ophthalmoplegia (complete) (total), unspecified eye
    - H52.52 Paresis of accommodation
      - H52.521 Paresis of accommodation, right eye
      - H52.522 Paresis of accommodation, left eye
      - H52.523 Paresis of accommodation, bilateral
      - H52.529 Paresis of accommodation, unspecified eye
    - H52.53 Spasm of accommodation
      - H52.531 Spasm of accommodation, right eye
      - H52.532 Spasm of accommodation, left eye
      - H52.533 Spasm of accommodation, bilateral
      - H52.539 Spasm of accommodation, unspecified eye
  - H52.6 Other disorders of refraction
  - H52.7 Unspecified disorder of refraction

VISUAL DISTURBANCES AND BLINDNESS (H53-H54)

- H53 Visual disturbances
  - H53.0 Amblyopia ex anopsia
    Excludes1 amblyopia due to vitamin A deficiency (E50.5)
    - H53.00 Unspecified amblyopia
      - H53.001 Unspecified amblyopia, right eye
      - H53.002 Unspecified amblyopia, left eye
      - H53.003 Unspecified amblyopia, bilateral
      - H53.009 Unspecified amblyopia, unspecified eye
    - H53.01 Deprivation amblyopia
      - H53.011 Deprivation amblyopia, right eye
      - H53.012 Deprivation amblyopia, left eye
      - H53.013 Deprivation amblyopia, bilateral
      - H53.019 Deprivation amblyopia, unspecified eye

Item 7–10 Disorders of refraction: **Hypermetropia,** or farsightedness, means focus at a distance is adequate but not on close objects. **Myopia** is near-sightedness or short-sightedness and means the focus on nearby objects is clear but distant objects appear blurred. **Astigmatism** is warping of the curvature of the cornea so light rays entering do not meet a single focal point, resulting in a distorted image. **Anisometropia** is unequal refractive power in which one eye may be myopic (near-sighted) and the other hyperopic (far-sighted). **Presbyopia** is the loss of focus on near objects, which occurs with age because the lens loses elasticity.

- **H53.02 Refractive amblyopia**
  - **H53.021 Refractive amblyopia, right eye**
  - **H53.022 Refractive amblyopia, left eye**
  - **H53.023 Refractive amblyopia, bilateral**
  - **H53.029 Refractive amblyopia, unspecified eye**
- **H53.03 Strabismic amblyopia**
  - **Excludes1** strabismus (H50.-)
  - **H53.031 Strabismic amblyopia, right eye**
  - **H53.032 Strabismic amblyopia, left eye**
  - **H53.033 Strabismic amblyopia, bilateral**
  - **H53.039 Strabismic amblyopia, unspecified eye**
- **H53.04 Amblyopia suspect** ◀
  - **H53.041 Amblyopia suspect, right eye** ◀
  - **H53.042 Amblyopia suspect, left eye** ◀
  - **H53.043 Amblyopia suspect, bilateral** ◀
  - **H53.049 Amblyopia suspect, unspecified eye** ◀
- **H53.1 Subjective visual disturbances**
  - **Excludes1** subjective visual disturbances due to vitamin A deficiency (E50.5)
    visual hallucinations (R44.1)
  - **H53.10 Unspecified subjective visual disturbances**
  - **H53.11 Day blindness**
    Hemeralopia
  - **H53.12 Transient visual loss**
    Scintillating scotoma
    - **Excludes1** amaurosis fugax (G45.3-)
      transient retinal artery occlusion (H34.0-)
    - Ex **For category H53.12 CC codes:** H53.10-H53.139, H53.16, R44.1, R48.3
    - **H53.121 Transient visual loss, right eye** CC
    - **H53.122 Transient visual loss, left eye** CC
    - **H53.123 Transient visual loss, bilateral** CC
    - **H53.129 Transient visual loss, unspecified eye** CC
  - **H53.13 Sudden visual loss**
    - Ex **For category H53.13 CC codes:** See H53.12
    - **H53.131 Sudden visual loss, right eye** CC
    - **H53.132 Sudden visual loss, left eye** CC
    - **H53.133 Sudden visual loss, bilateral** CC
    - **H53.139 Sudden visual loss, unspecified eye** CC
  - **H53.14 Visual discomfort**
    Asthenopia
    Photophobia
    - **H53.141 Visual discomfort, right eye**
    - **H53.142 Visual discomfort, left eye**
    - **H53.143 Visual discomfort, bilateral**
    - **H53.149 Visual discomfort, unspecified**
  - **H53.15 Visual distortions of shape and size**
    Metamorphopsia
  - **H53.16 Psychophysical visual disturbances**
  - **H53.19 Other subjective visual disturbances**
    Visual halos
- **H53.2 Diplopia**
  Double vision
- **H53.3 Other and unspecified disorders of binocular vision**
  - **H53.30 Unspecified disorder of binocular vision**
  - **H53.31 Abnormal retinal correspondence**
  - **H53.32 Fusion with defective stereopsis**
  - **H53.33 Simultaneous visual perception without fusion**
  - **H53.34 Suppression of binocular vision**
- **H53.4 Visual field defects**
  - **H53.40 Unspecified visual field defects**
  - **H53.41 Scotoma involving central area**
    Central scotoma
    - **H53.411 Scotoma involving central area, right eye**
    - **H53.412 Scotoma involving central area, left eye**
    - **H53.413 Scotoma involving central area, bilateral**
    - **H53.419 Scotoma involving central area, unspecified eye**
  - **H53.42 Scotoma of blind spot area**
    Enlarged blind spot
    - **H53.421 Scotoma of blind spot area, right eye**
    - **H53.422 Scotoma of blind spot area, left eye**
    - **H53.423 Scotoma of blind spot area, bilateral**
    - **H53.429 Scotoma of blind spot area, unspecified eye**
  - **H53.43 Sector or arcuate defects**
    Arcuate scotoma
    Bjerrum scotoma
    - **H53.431 Sector or arcuate defects, right eye**
    - **H53.432 Sector or arcuate defects, left eye**
    - **H53.433 Sector or arcuate defects, bilateral**
    - **H53.439 Sector or arcuate defects, unspecified eye**
  - **H53.45 Other localized visual field defect**
    Peripheral visual field defect
    Ring scotoma NOS
    Scotoma NOS
    - **H53.451 Other localized visual field defect, right eye**
    - **H53.452 Other localized visual field defect, left eye**
    - **H53.453 Other localized visual field defect, bilateral**
    - **H53.459 Other localized visual field defect, unspecified eye**
  - **H53.46 Homonymous bilateral field defects**
    Homonymous hemianopia
    Homonymous hemianopsia
    Quadrant anopia
    Quadrant anopsia
    - **H53.461 Homonymous bilateral field defects, right side**
    - **H53.462 Homonymous bilateral field defects, left side**
    - **H53.469 Homonymous bilateral field defects, unspecified side**
      Homonymous bilateral field defects NOS
  - **H53.47 Heteronymous bilateral field defects**
    Heteronymous hemianop(s)ia
  - **H53.48 Generalized contraction of visual field**
    - **H53.481 Generalized contraction of visual field, right eye**
    - **H53.482 Generalized contraction of visual field, left eye**
    - **H53.483 Generalized contraction of visual field, bilateral**
    - **H53.489 Generalized contraction of visual field, unspecified eye**

● **H53.5 Color vision deficiencies**
Color blindness
Excludes2 day blindness (H53.11)
H53.50 Unspecified color vision deficiencies
Color blindness NOS
H53.51 Achromatopsia
H53.52 Acquired color vision deficiency
H53.53 Deuteranomaly
Deuteranopia
H53.54 Protanomaly
Protanopia
H53.55 Tritanomaly
Tritanopia
H53.59 Other color vision deficiencies

● **H53.6 Night blindness**
Excludes1 night blindness due to vitamin A deficiency (E50.5)
H53.60 Unspecified night blindness
H53.61 Abnormal dark adaptation curve
H53.62 Acquired night blindness
H53.63 Congenital night blindness
H53.69 Other night blindness

● **H53.7 Vision sensitivity deficiencies**
H53.71 Glare sensitivity
H53.72 Impaired contrast sensitivity

H53.8 Other visual disturbances
H53.9 Unspecified visual disturbance

● **H54 Blindness and low vision**
Note: For definition of visual impairment categories see table below.
Code first any associated underlying cause of the blindness
Excludes1 amaurosis fugax (G45.3)

H54.0 Blindness, both eyes
Visual impairment categories 3, 4, 5 in both eyes.

● **H54.1 Blindness, one eye, low vision other eye**
Visual impairment categories 3, 4, 5 in one eye, with categories 1 or 2 in the other eye.
H54.10 Blindness, one eye, low vision other eye, unspecified eyes
H54.11 Blindness, right eye, low vision left eye
H54.12 Blindness, left eye, low vision right eye

H54.2 Low vision, both eyes
Visual impairment categories 1 or 2 in both eyes.

H54.3 Unqualified visual loss, both eyes
Visual impairment category 9 in both eyes.

● **H54.4 Blindness, one eye**
Visual impairment categories 3, 4, 5 in one eye [normal vision in other eye]
H54.40 Blindness, one eye, unspecified eye
H54.41 Blindness, right eye, normal vision left eye
H54.42 Blindness, left eye, normal vision right eye

● **H54.5 Low vision, one eye**
Visual impairment categories 1 or 2 in one eye [normal vision in other eye].
H54.50 Low vision, one eye, unspecified eye
H54.51 Low vision, right eye, normal vision left eye
H54.52 Low vision, left eye, normal vision right eye

● **H54.6 Unqualified visual loss, one eye**
Visual impairment category 9 in one eye [normal vision in other eye].
H54.60 Unqualified visual loss, one eye, unspecified
H54.61 Unqualified visual loss, right eye, normal vision left eye
H54.62 Unqualified visual loss, left eye, normal vision right eye

● **H54.7 Unspecified visual loss**
Visual impairment category 9 NOS

H54.8 Legal blindness, as defined in USA
Blindness NOS according to USA definition
Excludes1 legal blindness with specification of impairment level (H54.0-H54.7)

Note: The table below gives a classification of severity of visual impairment recommended by a WHO Study Group on the Prevention of Blindness, Geneva, 6-10 November 1972.

The term 'low vision' in category H54 comprises categories 1 and 2 of the table, the term 'blindness' categories 3, 4 and 5, and the term 'unqualified visual loss' category 9.

If the extent of the visual field is taken into account, patients with a field no greater than 10 but greater than 5 around central fixation should be placed in category 3 and patients with a field no greater than 5 around central fixation should be placed in category 4, even if the central acuity is not impaired.

(Document 508 compliance requires all cells in the following table to be filled.)

Category of visual impairment	Visual acuity with best possible correction	
	Maximum less than:	Minimum equal to or better than:
—	6/18	6/60
3/10 (0.3)	1/10 (0.1)	—
20/70	20/200	—
—	6/60	3/60
1/10 (0.1)	1/20 (0.05)	—
20/200	20/400	—
—	3/60	1/60 (finger counting at one meter)
1/20 (0.05)	1/50 (0.02)	—
20/400	5/300 (20/1200)	—
—	1/60 (finger counting at one meter)	Light perception
1/50 (0.02)	—	—
5/300	—	—
—	No light perception	—
—	Undetermined or unspecified	—

OTHER DISORDERS OF EYE AND ADNEXA (H55-H57)

- **H55 Nystagmus and other irregular eye movements**
  - **H55.0 Nystagmus**
    Rapid, involuntary movements of the eyes in the horizontal or vertical direction
    - H55.00 Unspecified nystagmus
    - H55.01 Congenital nystagmus
    - H55.02 Latent nystagmus
    - H55.03 Visual deprivation nystagmus
    - H55.04 Dissociated nystagmus
    - H55.09 Other forms of nystagmus
  - **H55.8 Other irregular eye movements**
    - H55.81 Saccadic eye movements
    - H55.89 Other irregular eye movements
- **H57 Other disorders of eye and adnexa**
  - **H57.0 Anomalies of pupillary function**
    - H57.00 Unspecified anomaly of pupillary function
    - H57.01 Argyll Robertson pupil, atypical
      Excludes1 syphilitic Argyll Robertson pupil (A52.19)
    - H57.02 Anisocoria
    - H57.03 Miosis
    - H57.04 Mydriasis
    - **H57.05 Tonic pupil**
      - H57.051 Tonic pupil, right eye
      - H57.052 Tonic pupil, left eye
      - H57.053 Tonic pupil, bilateral
      - H57.059 Tonic pupil, unspecified eye
    - H57.09 Other anomalies of pupillary function
  - **H57.1 Ocular pain**
    - H57.10 Ocular pain, unspecified eye
    - H57.11 Ocular pain, right eye
    - H57.12 Ocular pain, left eye
    - H57.13 Ocular pain, bilateral
  - H57.8 Other specified disorders of eye and adnexa
  - **H57.9** Unspecified disorder of eye and adnexa

INTRAOPERATIVE AND POSTPROCEDURAL COMPLICATIONS AND DISORDERS OF EYE AND ADNEXA, NOT ELSEWHERE CLASSIFIED (H59)

- **H59 Intraoperative and postprocedural complications and disorders of eye and adnexa, not elsewhere classified**
  Excludes1 mechanical complication of intraocular lens (T85.2)
  mechanical complication of other ocular prosthetic devices, implants and grafts (T85.3)
  pseudophakia (Z96.1)
  secondary cataracts (H26.4-)
  - **H59.0 Disorders of the eye following cataract surgery**
    Ex: **For category H59.0 CC codes:** H59.011-H59.019, H59.031-H59.099, H59.811-H59.89, H95.811-H95.89, I97.3, M96.89, N98.1-N98.9, T81.82X[A], T81.89X-T81.9XX[A]
    - **H59.01 Keratopathy (bullous aphakic) following cataract surgery**
      Vitreal corneal syndrome
      Vitreous (touch) syndrome
      - H59.011 Keratopathy (bullous aphakic) following cataract surgery, right eye
      - H59.012 Keratopathy (bullous aphakic) following cataract surgery, left eye
      - H59.013 Keratopathy (bullous aphakic) following cataract surgery, bilateral
      - H59.019 Keratopathy (bullous aphakic) following cataract surgery, unspecified eye
    - **H59.02 Cataract (lens) fragments in eye following cataract surgery**
      - H59.021 Cataract (lens) fragments in eye following cataract surgery, right eye
      - H59.022 Cataract (lens) fragments in eye following cataract surgery, left eye
      - H59.023 Cataract (lens) fragments in eye following cataract surgery, bilateral
      - H59.029 Cataract (lens) fragments in eye following cataract surgery, unspecified eye
    - **H59.03 Cystoid macular edema following cataract surgery**
      - H59.031 Cystoid macular edema following cataract surgery, right eye
      - H59.032 Cystoid macular edema following cataract surgery, left eye
      - H59.033 Cystoid macular edema following cataract surgery, bilateral
      - H59.039 Cystoid macular edema following cataract surgery, unspecified eye
    - **H59.09 Other disorders of the eye following cataract surgery**
      - H59.091 Other disorders of the right eye following cataract surgery
      - H59.092 Other disorders of the left eye following cataract surgery
      - H59.093 Other disorders of the eye following cataract surgery, bilateral
      - H59.099 Other disorders of unspecified eye following cataract surgery
  - **H59.1 Intraoperative hemorrhage and hematoma of eye and adnexa complicating a procedure**
    Excludes1 intraoperative hemorrhage and hematoma of eye and adnexa due to accidental puncture or laceration during a procedure (H59.2-)
    Ex: **For category H59.1 CC codes:** H59.011-H59.019, H59.031-H59.129, H59.311-H59.329, H59.331-H59.369, H59.811-H59.89, H95.811-H95.89, I85.01, I85.11, I97.3, K21.9, K22.8, K23-K25.0, K25.2, K25.4, K25.6, K26.0, K26.2, K26.4, K26.6, K27.0, K27.2, K27.4, K27.6, K28.0, K28.2, K28.4, K28.6, K29.01, K29.21, K29.31, K29.41, K29.51, K29.61, K29.71, K29.81, K29.91, K31.811, K55.21, K57.01, K57.11, K57.13, K57.21, K57.31, K57.33, K57.41, K57.51, K57.53, K57.81, K57.91, K57.93, K62.5, K92.0-K92.2, M96.89, N98.1-N98.9, P54.1-P54.3, T81.10X-T81.19X[A], T81.82X[A], T81.89X-T81.9XX[A]
    - **H59.11 Intraoperative hemorrhage and hematoma of eye and adnexa complicating an ophthalmic procedure**
      - H59.111 Intraoperative hemorrhage and hematoma of right eye and adnexa complicating an ophthalmic procedure
      - H59.112 Intraoperative hemorrhage and hematoma of left eye and adnexa complicating an ophthalmic procedure
      - H59.113 Intraoperative hemorrhage and hematoma of eye and adnexa complicating an ophthalmic procedure, bilateral
      - H59.119 Intraoperative hemorrhage and hematoma of unspecified eye and adnexa complicating an ophthalmic procedure

- H59.12 Intraoperative hemorrhage and hematoma of eye and adnexa complicating other procedure
  - H59.121 Intraoperative hemorrhage and hematoma of right eye and adnexa complicating other procedure
  - H59.122 Intraoperative hemorrhage and hematoma of left eye and adnexa complicating other procedure
  - H59.123 Intraoperative hemorrhage and hematoma of eye and adnexa complicating other procedure, bilateral
  - H59.129 Intraoperative hemorrhage and hematoma of unspecified eye and adnexa complicating other procedure
- H59.2 Accidental puncture and laceration of eye and adnexa during a procedure

  Ex For category H59.2 CC codes: D78.11-D78.12, D78.81-D78.89, E36.11-E36.8, E89.810-E89.89, G96.11, G97.41-G97.49, H59.011-H59.019, H59.031-H59.099, H59.211-H59.229, H59.811-H59.89, H95.31-H95.32, H95.811-H95.89, I97.3, I97.51-I97.52, J95.71-J95.72, K91.71-K91.72, L76.11-L76.12, L76.81-L76.82, M96.820-M96.821, M96.89, N98.1-N98.9, N99.71-N99.72, T81.82X[A], T81.89X-T81.9XX[A]
  - H59.21 Accidental puncture and laceration of eye and adnexa during an ophthalmic procedure
    - H59.211 Accidental puncture and laceration of right eye and adnexa during an ophthalmic procedure
    - H59.212 Accidental puncture and laceration of left eye and adnexa during an ophthalmic procedure
    - H59.213 Accidental puncture and laceration of eye and adnexa during an ophthalmic procedure, bilateral
    - H59.219 Accidental puncture and laceration of unspecified eye and adnexa during an ophthalmic procedure
  - H59.22 Accidental puncture and laceration of eye and adnexa during other procedure
    - H59.221 Accidental puncture and laceration of right eye and adnexa during other procedure
    - H59.222 Accidental puncture and laceration of left eye and adnexa during other procedure
    - H59.223 Accidental puncture and laceration of eye and adnexa during other procedure, bilateral
    - H59.229 Accidental puncture and laceration of unspecified eye and adnexa during other procedure
- H59.3 Postprocedural hemorrhage, hematoma, and seroma of eye and adnexa following other procedure

  Ex For category H59.3 CC codes: See H59.1
  - H59.31 Postprocedural hemorrhage of eye and adnexa following an ophthalmic procedure
    - H59.311 Postprocedural hemorrhage of right eye and adnexa following an ophthalmic procedure
    - H59.312 Postprocedural hemorrhage of left eye and adnexa following an ophthalmic procedure
    - H59.313 Postprocedural hemorrhage of eye and adnexa following an ophthalmic procedure, bilateral
    - H59.319 Postprocedural hemorrhage of unspecified eye and adnexa following an ophthalmic procedure
  - H59.32 Postprocedural hemorrhage of eye and adnexa following other procedure
    - H59.321 Postprocedural hemorrhage of right eye and adnexa following other procedure
    - H59.322 Postprocedural hemorrhage of left eye and adnexa following other procedure
    - H59.323 Postprocedural hemorrhage of eye and adnexa following other procedure, bilateral
    - H59.329 Postprocedural hemorrhage of unspecified eye and adnexa following other procedure
  - H59.33 Postprocedural hematoma of eye and adnexa following an ophthalmic procedure
    - H59.331 Postprocedural hematoma of right eye and adnexa following an ophthalmic procedure
    - H59.332 Postprocedural hematoma of left eye and adnexa following an ophthalmic procedure
    - H59.333 Postprocedural hematoma of eye and adnexa following an ophthalmic procedure, bilateral
    - H59.339 Postprocedural hematoma of unspecified eye and adnexa following an ophthalmic procedure
  - H59.34 Postprocedural hematoma of eye and adnexa following other procedure
    - H59.341 Postprocedural hematoma of right eye and adnexa following other procedure
    - H59.342 Postprocedural hematoma of left eye and adnexa following other procedure
    - H59.343 Postprocedural hematoma of eye and adnexa following other procedure, bilateral
    - H59.349 Postprocedural hematoma of unspecified eye and adnexa following other procedure
  - H59.35 Postprocedural seroma of eye and adnexa following an ophthalmic procedure
    - H59.351 Postprocedural seroma of right eye and adnexa following an ophthalmic procedure
    - H59.352 Postprocedural seroma of left eye and adnexa following an ophthalmic procedure
    - H59.353 Postprocedural seroma of eye and adnexa following an ophthalmic procedure, bilateral
    - H59.359 Postprocedural seroma of unspecified eye and adnexa following an ophthalmic procedure
  - H59.36 Postprocedural seroma of eye and adnexa following other procedure
    - H59.361 Postprocedural seroma of right eye and adnexa following other procedure
    - H59.362 Postprocedural seroma of left eye and adnexa following other procedure
    - H59.363 Postprocedural seroma of eye and adnexa following other procedure, bilateral
    - H59.369 Postprocedural seroma of unspecified eye and adnexa following other procedure

◀ New ⇐ Revised ~~deleted~~ Deleted Excludes 1 Excludes 2 Includes Use additional Code first Code also Unspecified
OGCR Official Guidelines ● Unacceptable Principal Diagnosis X Assign placeholder X ● Use Additional Character(s) ◗ Manifestation Code Coding Clinic

H59.4 Inflammation (infection) of postprocedural bleb
Postprocedural blebitis

Excludes1 filtering (vitreous) bleb after glaucoma surgery status (Z98.83)

H59.40 Inflammation (infection) of postprocedural bleb, unspecified

H59.41 Inflammation (infection) of postprocedural bleb, stage 1

H59.42 Inflammation (infection) of postprocedural bleb, stage 2

H59.43 Inflammation (infection) of postprocedural bleb, stage 3
Bleb endophthalmitis

H59.8 Other intraoperative and postprocedural complications and disorders of eye and adnexa, not elsewhere classified
Ex: For category H59.8 CC codes: See H59.0

H59.81 Chorioretinal scars after surgery for detachment

H59.811 Chorioretinal scars after surgery for detachment, right eye

H59.812 Chorioretinal scars after surgery for detachment, left eye

H59.813 Chorioretinal scars after surgery for detachment, bilateral

H59.819 Chorioretinal scars after surgery for detachment, unspecified eye

H59.88 Other intraoperative complications of eye and adnexa, not elsewhere classified

H59.89 Other postprocedural complications and disorders of eye and adnexa, not elsewhere classified

CHAPTER 8

DISEASES OF THE EAR AND MASTOID PROCESS (H60-H95)

OGCR Chapter-Specific Coding Guidelines

8. Chapter 8: Diseases of the Ear and Mastoid Process (H60-H95)
Reserved for future guideline expansion

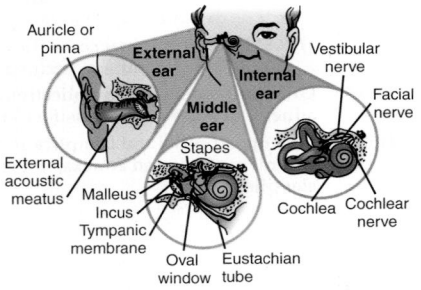

Figure 8-1 Auditory system. (From Buck CJ: Step-by-Step Medical Coding, ed 2016, St. Louis, Elsevier, 2016)

★**(See Plate 92 on page 68.)**

CHAPTER 8

DISEASES OF THE EAR AND MASTOID PROCESS (H60-H95)

Note: Use an external cause code following the code for the ear condition, if applicable, to identify the cause of the ear condition

Excludes2 certain conditions originating in the perinatal period (P04-P96)
certain infectious and parasitic diseases (A00-B99)
complications of pregnancy, childbirth and the puerperium (O00-O9A)
congenital malformations, deformations and chromosomal abnormalities (Q00-Q99)
endocrine, nutritional and metabolic diseases (E00-E88)
injury, poisoning and certain other consequences of external causes (S00-T88)
neoplasms (C00-D49)
symptoms, signs and abnormal clinical and laboratory findings, not elsewhere classified (R00-R94)

This chapter contains the following blocks:

H60-H62	Diseases of external ear
H65-H75	Diseases of middle ear and mastoid
H80-H83	Diseases of inner ear
H90-H94	Other disorders of ear
H95	Intraoperative and postprocedural complications and disorders of ear and mastoid process, not elsewhere classified

DISEASES OF EXTERNAL EAR (H60-H62)

● **H60 Otitis externa**

● **H60.0 Abscess of external ear**
Boil of external ear
Carbuncle of auricle or external auditory canal
Furuncle of external ear

H60.00 Abscess of external ear, unspecified ear
H60.01 Abscess of right external ear
H60.02 Abscess of left external ear
H60.03 Abscess of external ear, bilateral

● **H60.1 Cellulitis of external ear**
Cellulitis of auricle
Cellulitis of external auditory canal

H60.10 Cellulitis of external ear, unspecified ear
H60.11 Cellulitis of right external ear
H60.12 Cellulitis of left external ear
H60.13 Cellulitis of external ear, bilateral

● **H60.2 Malignant otitis externa**
Ex: For category H60.2 CC codes: H60.20-H60.23, H70.001-H70.13

H60.20 Malignant otitis externa, unspecified ear
H60.21 Malignant otitis externa, right ear
H60.22 Malignant otitis externa, left ear
H60.23 Malignant otitis externa, bilateral

● **H60.3 Other infective otitis externa**

● **H60.31 Diffuse otitis externa**

H60.311 Diffuse otitis externa, right ear
H60.312 Diffuse otitis externa, left ear
H60.313 Diffuse otitis externa, bilateral
H60.319 Diffuse otitis externa, unspecified ear

● **H60.32 Hemorrhagic otitis externa**

H60.321 Hemorrhagic otitis externa, right ear
H60.322 Hemorrhagic otitis externa, left ear
H60.323 Hemorrhagic otitis externa, bilateral
H60.329 Hemorrhagic otitis externa, unspecified ear

● **H60.33 Swimmer's ear**

H60.331 Swimmer's ear, right ear
H60.332 Swimmer's ear, left ear
H60.333 Swimmer's ear, bilateral
H60.339 Swimmer's ear, unspecified ear

● **H60.39 Other infective otitis externa**

H60.391 Other infective otitis externa, right ear
H60.392 Other infective otitis externa, left ear
H60.393 Other infective otitis externa, bilateral
H60.399 Other infective otitis externa, unspecified ear

● **H60.4 Cholesteatoma of external ear**
Keratosis obturans of external ear (canal)

Excludes2 cholesteatoma of middle ear (H71.-)
recurrent cholesteatoma of postmastoidectomy cavity (H95.0-)

H60.40 Cholesteatoma of external ear, unspecified ear
H60.41 Cholesteatoma of right external ear
H60.42 Cholesteatoma of left external ear
H60.43 Cholesteatoma of external ear, bilateral

● **H60.5 Acute noninfective otitis externa**

● **H60.50 Unspecified acute noninfective otitis externa**
Acute otitis externa NOS

H60.501 Unspecified acute noninfective otitis externa, right ear
H60.502 Unspecified acute noninfective otitis externa, left ear
H60.503 Unspecified acute noninfective otitis externa, bilateral
H60.509 Unspecified acute noninfective otitis externa, unspecified ear

● **H60.51 Acute actinic otitis externa**

H60.511 Acute actinic otitis externa, right ear
H60.512 Acute actinic otitis externa, left ear
H60.513 Acute actinic otitis externa, bilateral
H60.519 Acute actinic otitis externa, unspecified ear

- **H60.52** Acute chemical otitis externa
  - **H60.521** Acute chemical otitis externa, right ear
  - **H60.522** Acute chemical otitis externa, left ear
  - **H60.523** Acute chemical otitis externa, bilateral
  - **H60.529** Acute chemical otitis externa, unspecified ear
- **H60.53** Acute contact otitis externa
  - **H60.531** Acute contact otitis externa, right ear
  - **H60.532** Acute contact otitis externa, left ear
  - **H60.533** Acute contact otitis externa, bilateral
  - **H60.539** Acute contact otitis externa, unspecified ear
- **H60.54** Acute eczematoid otitis externa
  - **H60.541** Acute eczematoid otitis externa, right ear
  - **H60.542** Acute eczematoid otitis externa, left ear
  - **H60.543** Acute eczematoid otitis externa, bilateral
  - **H60.549** Acute eczematoid otitis externa, unspecified ear
- **H60.55** Acute reactive otitis externa
  - **H60.551** Acute reactive otitis externa, right ear
  - **H60.552** Acute reactive otitis externa, left ear
  - **H60.553** Acute reactive otitis externa, bilateral
  - **H60.559** Acute reactive otitis externa, unspecified ear
- **H60.59** Other noninfective acute otitis externa
  - **H60.591** Other noninfective acute otitis externa, right ear
  - **H60.592** Other noninfective acute otitis externa, left ear
  - **H60.593** Other noninfective acute otitis externa, bilateral
  - **H60.599** Other noninfective acute otitis externa, unspecified ear
- **H60.6** Unspecified chronic otitis externa
  - **H60.60** Unspecified chronic otitis externa, unspecified ear
  - **H60.61** Unspecified chronic otitis externa, right ear
  - **H60.62** Unspecified chronic otitis externa, left ear
  - **H60.63** Unspecified chronic otitis externa, bilateral
- **H60.8** Other otitis externa
  - **H60.8X** Other otitis externa
    - **H60.8X1** Other otitis externa, right ear
    - **H60.8X2** Other otitis externa, left ear
    - **H60.8X3** Other otitis externa, bilateral
    - **H60.8X9** Other otitis externa, unspecified ear
- **H60.9** Unspecified otitis externa
  - **H60.90** Unspecified otitis externa, unspecified ear
  - **H60.91** Unspecified otitis externa, right ear
  - **H60.92** Unspecified otitis externa, left ear
  - **H60.93** Unspecified otitis externa, bilateral

- **H61** Other disorders of external ear
  - **H61.0** Chondritis and perichondritis of external ear
    Chondrodermatitis nodularis chronica helicis
    Perichondritis of auricle
    Perichondritis of pinna
    - **H61.00** Unspecified perichondritis of external ear
      - **H61.001** Unspecified perichondritis of right external ear
      - **H61.002** Unspecified perichondritis of left external ear
      - **H61.003** Unspecified perichondritis of external ear, bilateral
      - **H61.009** Unspecified perichondritis of external ear, unspecified ear
    - **H61.01** Acute perichondritis of external ear
      - **H61.011** Acute perichondritis of right external ear
      - **H61.012** Acute perichondritis of left external ear
      - **H61.013** Acute perichondritis of external ear, bilateral
      - **H61.019** Acute perichondritis of external ear, unspecified ear
    - **H61.02** Chronic perichondritis of external ear
      - **H61.021** Chronic perichondritis of right external ear
      - **H61.022** Chronic perichondritis of left external ear
      - **H61.023** Chronic perichondritis of external ear, bilateral
      - **H61.029** Chronic perichondritis of external ear, unspecified ear
    - **H61.03** Chondritis of external ear
      Chondritis of auricle
      Chondritis of pinna
      - **H61.031** Chondritis of right external ear
      - **H61.032** Chondritis of left external ear
        Coding Clinic: 2015, Q1, P18
      - **H61.033** Chondritis of external ear, bilateral
      - **H61.039** Chondritis of external ear, unspecified ear
  - **H61.1** Noninfective disorders of pinna
    Excludes2 cauliflower ear (M95.1-)
    gouty tophi of ear (M1A.-)
    - **H61.10** Unspecified noninfective disorders of pinna
      Disorder of pinna NOS
      - **H61.101** Unspecified noninfective disorders of pinna, right ear
      - **H61.102** Unspecified noninfective disorders of pinna, left ear
      - **H61.103** Unspecified noninfective disorders of pinna, bilateral
      - **H61.109** Unspecified noninfective disorders of pinna, unspecified ear
    - **H61.11** Acquired deformity of pinna
      Acquired deformity of auricle
      Excludes2 cauliflower ear (M95.1-)
      - **H61.111** Acquired deformity of pinna, right ear
      - **H61.112** Acquired deformity of pinna, left ear
      - **H61.113** Acquired deformity of pinna, bilateral
      - **H61.119** Acquired deformity of pinna, unspecified ear
    - **H61.12** Hematoma of pinna
      Hematoma of auricle
      - **H61.121** Hematoma of pinna, right ear
      - **H61.122** Hematoma of pinna, left ear
      - **H61.123** Hematoma of pinna, bilateral
      - **H61.129** Hematoma of pinna, unspecified ear
    - **H61.19** Other noninfective disorders of pinna
      - **H61.191** Noninfective disorders of pinna, right ear
      - **H61.192** Noninfective disorders of pinna, left ear
      - **H61.193** Noninfective disorders of pinna, bilateral
      - **H61.199** Noninfective disorders of pinna, unspecified ear

● **H61.2 Impacted cerumen**
Wax in ear
H61.20 Impacted cerumen, unspecified ear
MCE: Questionable admission when principal dx
H61.21 Impacted cerumen, right ear
MCE: Questionable admission when principal dx
H61.22 Impacted cerumen, left ear
MCE: Questionable admission when principal dx
H61.23 Impacted cerumen, bilateral
MCE: Questionable admission when principal dx

● **H61.3 Acquired stenosis of external ear canal**
Collapse of external ear canal
Excludes1 postprocedural stenosis of external ear canal (H95.81-)

● **H61.30 Acquired stenosis of external ear canal, unspecified**
H61.301 Acquired stenosis of right external ear canal, unspecified
H61.302 Acquired stenosis of left external ear canal, unspecified
H61.303 Acquired stenosis of external ear canal, unspecified, bilateral
H61.309 Acquired stenosis of external ear canal, unspecified, unspecified ear

● **H61.31 Acquired stenosis of external ear canal secondary to trauma**
H61.311 Acquired stenosis of right external ear canal secondary to trauma
H61.312 Acquired stenosis of left external ear canal secondary to trauma
H61.313 Acquired stenosis of external ear canal secondary to trauma, bilateral
H61.319 Acquired stenosis of external ear canal secondary to trauma, unspecified ear

● **H61.32 Acquired stenosis of external ear canal secondary to inflammation and infection**
H61.321 Acquired stenosis of right external ear canal secondary to inflammation and infection
H61.322 Acquired stenosis of left external ear canal secondary to inflammation and infection
H61.323 Acquired stenosis of external ear canal secondary to inflammation and infection, bilateral
H61.329 Acquired stenosis of external ear canal secondary to inflammation and infection, unspecified ear

● **H61.39 Other acquired stenosis of external ear canal**
H61.391 Other acquired stenosis of right external ear canal
H61.392 Other acquired stenosis of left external ear canal
H61.393 Other acquired stenosis of external ear canal, bilateral
H61.399 Other acquired stenosis of external ear canal, unspecified ear

● **H61.8 Other specified disorders of external ear**

● **H61.81 Exostosis of external canal**
H61.811 Exostosis of right external canal
H61.812 Exostosis of left external canal
H61.813 Exostosis of external canal, bilateral
H61.819 Exostosis of external canal, unspecified ear

● **H61.89 Other specified disorders of external ear**
H61.891 Other specified disorders of right external ear
H61.892 Other specified disorders of left external ear
H61.893 Other specified disorders of external ear, bilateral
H61.899 Other specified disorders of external ear, unspecified ear

● **H61.9 Disorder of external ear, unspecified**
H61.90 Disorder of external ear, unspecified, unspecified ear
H61.91 Disorder of right external ear, unspecified
H61.92 Disorder of left external ear, unspecified
H61.93 Disorder of external ear, unspecified, bilateral

● **H62 Disorders of external ear in diseases classified elsewhere**

● **H62.4 Otitis externa in other diseases classified elsewhere**
Code first underlying disease, such as:
erysipelas (A46)
impetigo (L01.0)
Excludes1 otitis externa (in):
candidiasis (B37.84)
herpes viral [herpes simplex] (B00.1)
herpes zoster (B02.8)
▶ ***H62.40 Otitis externa in other diseases classified elsewhere, unspecified ear***
▶ ***H62.41 Otitis externa in other diseases classified elsewhere, right ear***
▶ ***H62.42 Otitis externa in other diseases classified elsewhere, left ear***
▶ ***H62.43 Otitis externa in other diseases classified elsewhere, bilateral***

● **H62.8 Other disorders of external ear in diseases classified elsewhere**
Code first underlying disease, such as:
gout (M1A.-, M10.-)

● **H62.8X Other disorders of external ear in diseases classified elsewhere**
▶ ***H62.8X1 Other disorders of right external ear in diseases classified elsewhere***
▶ ***H62.8X2 Other disorders of left external ear in diseases classified elsewhere***
▶ ***H62.8X3 Other disorders of external ear in diseases classified elsewhere, bilateral***
▶ ***H62.8X9 Other disorders of external ear in diseases classified elsewhere, unspecified ear***

DISEASES OF MIDDLE EAR AND MASTOID (H65-H75)

★ **(See Plate 94 on page 69.)**

● **H65 Nonsuppurative otitis media**
Bacterial or viral infection or inflammation of the middle ear; may result in fluid accumulation with pain and temporary hearing loss.
Includes nonsuppurative otitis media with myringitis
Use additional code for any associated perforated tympanic membrane (H72.-)
Use additional code to identify:
exposure to environmental tobacco smoke (Z77.22)
exposure to tobacco smoke in the perinatal period (P96.81)
history of tobacco dependence (Z87.891) ◀
occupational exposure to environmental tobacco smoke (Z57.31)
tobacco dependence (F17.-)
tobacco use (Z72.0)

● **H65.0 Acute serous otitis media**
Acute and subacute secretory otitis
H65.00 Acute serous otitis media, unspecified ear
H65.01 Acute serous otitis media, right ear
H65.02 Acute serous otitis media, left ear
H65.03 Acute serous otitis media, bilateral
H65.04 Acute serous otitis media, recurrent, right ear
H65.05 Acute serous otitis media, recurrent, left ear
H65.06 Acute serous otitis media, recurrent, bilateral
H65.07 Acute serous otitis media, recurrent, unspecified ear

H65.1 Other acute nonsuppurative otitis media

Excludes1 otitic barotrauma (T70.0)
otitis media (acute) NOS (H66.9)

H65.11 Acute and subacute allergic otitis media (mucoid) (sanguinous) (serous)

H65.111 Acute and subacute allergic otitis media (mucoid) (sanguinous) (serous), right ear

H65.112 Acute and subacute allergic otitis media (mucoid) (sanguinous) (serous), left ear

H65.113 Acute and subacute allergic otitis media (mucoid) (sanguinous) (serous), bilateral

H65.114 Acute and subacute allergic otitis media (mucoid) (sanguinous) (serous), recurrent, right ear

H65.115 Acute and subacute allergic otitis media (mucoid) (sanguinous) (serous), recurrent, left ear

H65.116 Acute and subacute allergic otitis media (mucoid) (sanguinous) (serous), recurrent, bilateral

H65.117 Acute and subacute allergic otitis media (mucoid) (sanguinous) (serous), recurrent, unspecified ear

H65.119 Acute and subacute allergic otitis media (mucoid) (sanguinous) (serous), unspecified ear

H65.19 Other acute nonsuppurative otitis media
Acute and subacute mucoid otitis media
Acute and subacute nonsuppurative otitis media NOS
Acute and subacute sanguinous otitis media
Acute and subacute seromucinous otitis media

H65.191 Other acute nonsuppurative otitis media, right ear

H65.192 Other acute nonsuppurative otitis media, left ear

H65.193 Other acute nonsuppurative otitis media, bilateral

H65.194 Other acute nonsuppurative otitis media, recurrent, right ear

H65.195 Other acute nonsuppurative otitis media, recurrent, left ear

H65.196 Other acute nonsuppurative otitis media, recurrent, bilateral

H65.197 Other acute nonsuppurative otitis media recurrent, unspecified ear

H65.199 Other acute nonsuppurative otitis media, unspecified ear

H65.2 Chronic serous otitis media
Chronic tubotympanal catarrh

H65.20 Chronic serous otitis media, unspecified ear

H65.21 Chronic serous otitis media, right ear

H65.22 Chronic serous otitis media, left ear

H65.23 Chronic serous otitis media, bilateral

H65.3 Chronic mucoid otitis media
Chronic mucinous otitis media
Chronic secretory otitis media
Chronic transudative otitis media
Glue ear

Excludes1 adhesive middle ear disease (H74.1)

H65.30 Chronic mucoid otitis media, unspecified ear

H65.31 Chronic mucoid otitis media, right ear

H65.32 Chronic mucoid otitis media, left ear

H65.33 Chronic mucoid otitis media, bilateral

H65.4 Other chronic nonsuppurative otitis media

H65.41 Chronic allergic otitis media

H65.411 Chronic allergic otitis media, right ear

H65.412 Chronic allergic otitis media, left ear

H65.413 Chronic allergic otitis media, bilateral

H65.419 Chronic allergic otitis media, unspecified ear

H65.49 Other chronic nonsuppurative otitis media
Chronic exudative otitis media
Chronic nonsuppurative otitis media NOS
Chronic otitis media with effusion (nonpurulent)
Chronic seromucinous otitis media

H65.491 Other chronic nonsuppurative otitis media, right ear

H65.492 Other chronic nonsuppurative otitis media, left ear

H65.493 Other chronic nonsuppurative otitis media, bilateral

H65.499 Other chronic nonsuppurative otitis media, unspecified ear

H65.9 Unspecified nonsuppurative otitis media
Allergic otitis media NOS
Catarrhal otitis media NOS
Exudative otitis media NOS
Mucoid otitis media NOS
Otitis media with effusion (nonpurulent) NOS
Secretory otitis media NOS
Seromucinous otitis media NOS
Serous otitis media NOS
Transudative otitis media NOS

H65.90 Unspecified nonsuppurative otitis media, unspecified ear

H65.91 Unspecified nonsuppurative otitis media, right ear

H65.92 Unspecified nonsuppurative otitis media, left ear

H65.93 Unspecified nonsuppurative otitis media, bilateral

H66 Suppurative and unspecified otitis media
Suppurative: Discharging pus

Includes suppurative and unspecified otitis media with myringitis

Use additional code to identify:
exposure to environmental tobacco smoke (Z77.22)
exposure to tobacco smoke in the perinatal period (P96.81)
history of tobacco dependence (Z87.891)
occupational exposure to environmental tobacco smoke (Z57.31)
tobacco dependence (F17.-)
tobacco use (Z72.0)

H66.0 Acute suppurative otitis media

H66.00 Acute suppurative otitis media without spontaneous rupture of ear drum

H66.001 Acute suppurative otitis media without spontaneous rupture of ear drum, right ear
Coding Clinic: 2016, Q1, P34

H66.002 Acute suppurative otitis media without spontaneous rupture of ear drum, left ear

H66.003 Acute suppurative otitis media without spontaneous rupture of ear drum, bilateral

H66.004 Acute suppurative otitis media without spontaneous rupture of ear drum, recurrent, right ear

H66.005 Acute suppurative otitis media without spontaneous rupture of ear drum, recurrent, left ear

H66.006 Acute suppurative otitis media without spontaneous rupture of ear drum, recurrent, bilateral

H66.007 Acute suppurative otitis media without spontaneous rupture of ear drum, recurrent, unspecified ear

H66.009 Acute suppurative otitis media without spontaneous rupture of ear drum, unspecified ear

H66.01 Acute suppurative otitis media with spontaneous rupture of ear drum

- **H66.011 Acute suppurative otitis media with spontaneous rupture of ear drum, right ear**
- **H66.012 Acute suppurative otitis media with spontaneous rupture of ear drum, left ear**
- **H66.013 Acute suppurative otitis media with spontaneous rupture of ear drum, bilateral**
- **H66.014 Acute suppurative otitis media with spontaneous rupture of ear drum, recurrent, right ear**
- **H66.015 Acute suppurative otitis media with spontaneous rupture of ear drum, recurrent, left ear**
- **H66.016 Acute suppurative otitis media with spontaneous rupture of ear drum, recurrent, bilateral**
- **H66.017 Acute suppurative otitis media with spontaneous rupture of ear drum, recurrent, unspecified ear**
- **H66.019 Acute suppurative otitis media with spontaneous rupture of ear drum, unspecified ear**

H66.1 Chronic tubotympanic suppurative otitis media
Benign chronic suppurative otitis media
Chronic tubotympanic disease
Use additional code for any associated perforated tympanic membrane (H72.-)

- **H66.10 Chronic tubotympanic suppurative otitis media, unspecified**
- **H66.11 Chronic tubotympanic suppurative otitis media, right ear**
- **H66.12 Chronic tubotympanic suppurative otitis media, left ear**
- **H66.13 Chronic tubotympanic suppurative otitis media, bilateral**

H66.2 Chronic atticoantral suppurative otitis media
Chronic atticoantral disease
Use additional code for any associated perforated tympanic membrane (H72.-)

- **H66.20 Chronic atticoantral suppurative otitis media, unspecified ear**
- **H66.21 Chronic atticoantral suppurative otitis media, right ear**
- **H66.22 Chronic atticoantral suppurative otitis media, left ear**
- **H66.23 Chronic atticoantral suppurative otitis media, bilateral**

H66.3 Other chronic suppurative otitis media
Chronic suppurative otitis media NOS
Use additional code for any associated perforated tympanic membrane (H72.-)
Excludes1 tuberculous otitis media (A18.6)

H66.3X Other chronic suppurative otitis media

- **H66.3X1 Other chronic suppurative otitis media, right ear**
- **H66.3X2 Other chronic suppurative otitis media, left ear**
- **H66.3X3 Other chronic suppurative otitis media, bilateral**
- **H66.3X9 Other chronic suppurative otitis media, unspecified ear**

H66.4 Suppurative otitis media, unspecified
Purulent otitis media NOS
Use additional code for any associated perforated tympanic membrane (H72.-)

- **H66.40 Suppurative otitis media, unspecified, unspecified ear**
- **H66.41 Suppurative otitis media, unspecified, right ear**
- **H66.42 Suppurative otitis media, unspecified, left ear**
- **H66.43 Suppurative otitis media, unspecified, bilateral**

H66.9 Otitis media, unspecified
Otitis media NOS
Acute otitis media NOS
Chronic otitis media NOS
Use additional code for any associated perforated tympanic membrane (H72.-)

- **H66.90 Otitis media, unspecified, unspecified ear**
- **H66.91 Otitis media, unspecified, right ear**
- **H66.92 Otitis media, unspecified, left ear**
- **H66.93 Otitis media, unspecified, bilateral**

H67 Otitis media in diseases classified elsewhere
Code first underlying disease, such as:
viral disease NEC (B00-B34)
Use additional code for any associated perforated tympanic membrane (H72.-)
Excludes1 otitis media in:
influenza (J09.X9, J10.83, J11.83)
measles (B05.3)
scarlet fever (A38.0)
tuberculosis (A18.6)

- *H67.1 Otitis media in diseases classified elsewhere, right ear*
- *H67.2 Otitis media in diseases classified elsewhere, left ear*
- *H67.3 Otitis media in diseases classified elsewhere, bilateral*
- *H67.9 Otitis media in diseases classified elsewhere, unspecified ear*

H68 Eustachian salpingitis and obstruction

H68.0 Eustachian salpingitis

H68.00 Unspecified Eustachian salpingitis

- **H68.001 Unspecified Eustachian salpingitis, right ear**
- **H68.002 Unspecified Eustachian salpingitis, left ear**
- **H68.003 Unspecified Eustachian salpingitis, bilateral**
- **H68.009 Unspecified Eustachian salpingitis, unspecified ear**

H68.01 Acute Eustachian salpingitis

- **H68.011 Acute Eustachian salpingitis, right ear**
- **H68.012 Acute Eustachian salpingitis, left ear**
- **H68.013 Acute Eustachian salpingitis, bilateral**
- **H68.019 Acute Eustachian salpingitis, unspecified ear**

H68.02 Chronic Eustachian salpingitis

- **H68.021 Chronic Eustachian salpingitis, right ear**
- **H68.022 Chronic Eustachian salpingitis, left ear**
- **H68.023 Chronic Eustachian salpingitis, bilateral**
- **H68.029 Chronic Eustachian salpingitis, unspecified ear**

- **H68.1 Obstruction of Eustachian tube**
  Stenosis of Eustachian tube
  Stricture of Eustachian tube
  - **H68.10 Unspecified obstruction of Eustachian tube**
    - H68.101 Unspecified obstruction of Eustachian tube, right ear
    - H68.102 Unspecified obstruction of Eustachian tube, left ear
    - H68.103 Unspecified obstruction of Eustachian tube, bilateral
    - H68.109 Unspecified obstruction of Eustachian tube, unspecified ear
  - **H68.11 Osseous obstruction of Eustachian tube**
    - H68.111 Osseous obstruction of Eustachian tube, right ear
    - H68.112 Osseous obstruction of Eustachian tube, left ear
    - H68.113 Osseous obstruction of Eustachian tube, bilateral
    - H68.119 Osseous obstruction of Eustachian tube, unspecified ear
  - **H68.12 Intrinsic cartilagenous obstruction of Eustachian tube**
    - H68.121 Intrinsic cartilagenous obstruction of Eustachian tube, right ear
    - H68.122 Intrinsic cartilagenous obstruction of Eustachian tube, left ear
    - H68.123 Intrinsic cartilagenous obstruction of Eustachian tube, bilateral
    - H68.129 Intrinsic cartilagenous obstruction of Eustachian tube, unspecified ear
  - **H68.13 Extrinsic cartilagenous obstruction of Eustachian tube**
    Compression of Eustachian tube
    - H68.131 Extrinsic cartilagenous obstruction of Eustachian tube, right ear
    - H68.132 Extrinsic cartilagenous obstruction of Eustachian tube, left ear
    - H68.133 Extrinsic cartilagenous obstruction of Eustachian tube, bilateral
    - H68.139 Extrinsic cartilagenous obstruction of Eustachian tube, unspecified ear
- **H69 Other and unspecified disorders of Eustachian tube**
  - **H69.0 Patulous Eustachian tube**
    - H69.00 Patulous Eustachian tube, unspecified ear
    - H69.01 Patulous Eustachian tube, right ear
    - H69.02 Patulous Eustachian tube, left ear
    - H69.03 Patulous Eustachian tube, bilateral
  - **H69.8 Other specified disorders of Eustachian tube**
    - H69.80 Other specified disorders of Eustachian tube, unspecified ear
    - H69.81 Other specified disorders of Eustachian tube, right ear
    - H69.82 Other specified disorders of Eustachian tube, left ear
    - H69.83 Other specified disorders of Eustachian tube, bilateral
  - **H69.9 Unspecified Eustachian tube disorder**
    - H69.90 Unspecified Eustachian tube disorder, unspecified ear
    - H69.91 Unspecified Eustachian tube disorder, right ear
    - H69.92 Unspecified Eustachian tube disorder, left ear
    - H69.93 Unspecified Eustachian tube disorder, bilateral
- **H70 Mastoiditis and related conditions**
  - **H70.0 Acute mastoiditis**
    Abscess of mastoid
    Empyema of mastoid
    Ex **For category H70.0 CC codes:** A17.9, A18.6, A18.82, A18.84, A18.89, H70.001-H70.213, H70.219-H70.93, H75.00-H75.83, H93.8X1-H93.93, H94.80-H95.199, Q16.1, Q16.9, Q17.3-Q17.9
    - **H70.00 Acute mastoiditis without complications**
      - H70.001 Acute mastoiditis without complications, right ear CC
      - H70.002 Acute mastoiditis without complications, left ear CC
      - H70.003 Acute mastoiditis without complications, bilateral CC
      - H70.009 Acute mastoiditis without complications, unspecified ear CC
    - **H70.01 Subperiosteal abscess of mastoid**
      - H70.011 Subperiosteal abscess of mastoid, right ear CC
      - H70.012 Subperiosteal abscess of mastoid, left ear CC
      - H70.013 Subperiosteal abscess of mastoid, bilateral CC
      - H70.019 Subperiosteal abscess of mastoid, unspecified ear CC
    - **H70.09 Acute mastoiditis with other complications**
      - H70.091 Acute mastoiditis with other complications, right ear CC
      - H70.092 Acute mastoiditis with other complications, left ear CC
      - H70.093 Acute mastoiditis with other complications, bilateral CC
      - H70.099 Acute mastoiditis with other complications, unspecified ear CC
  - **H70.1 Chronic mastoiditis**
    Caries of mastoid
    Fistula of mastoid
    Excludes1 tuberculous mastoiditis (A18.03)
    - H70.10 Chronic mastoiditis, unspecified ear
    - H70.11 Chronic mastoiditis, right ear
    - H70.12 Chronic mastoiditis, left ear
    - H70.13 Chronic mastoiditis, bilateral
  - **H70.2 Petrositis**
    Inflammation of petrous bone
    - **H70.20 Unspecified petrositis**
      - H70.201 Unspecified petrositis, right ear
      - H70.202 Unspecified petrositis, left ear
      - H70.203 Unspecified petrositis, bilateral
      - H70.209 Unspecified petrositis, unspecified ear
    - **H70.21 Acute petrositis**
      - H70.211 Acute petrositis, right ear
      - H70.212 Acute petrositis, left ear
      - H70.213 Acute petrositis, bilateral
      - H70.219 Acute petrositis, unspecified ear
    - **H70.22 Chronic petrositis**
      - H70.221 Chronic petrositis, right ear
      - H70.222 Chronic petrositis, left ear
      - H70.223 Chronic petrositis, bilateral
      - H70.229 Chronic petrositis, unspecified ear

Item 8–1 Mastoiditis is an infection of the portion of the temporal bone of the skull that is behind the ear (mastoid process) caused by an untreated otitis media, leading to an infection of the surrounding structures which may include the brain.

● H70.8 Other mastoiditis and related conditions

Excludes1 preauricular sinus and cyst (Q18.1)
sinus, fistula, and cyst of branchial cleft (Q18.0)

● H70.81 Postauricular fistula

H70.811 Postauricular fistula, right ear

H70.812 Postauricular fistula, left ear

H70.813 Postauricular fistula, bilateral

H70.819 Postauricular fistula, unspecified ear

● H70.89 Other mastoiditis and related conditions

H70.891 Other mastoiditis and related conditions, right ear

H70.892 Other mastoiditis and related conditions, left ear

H70.893 Other mastoiditis and related conditions, bilateral

H70.899 Other mastoiditis and related conditions, unspecified ear

● H70.9 Unspecified mastoiditis

H70.90 Unspecified mastoiditis, unspecified ear

H70.91 Unspecified mastoiditis, right ear

H70.92 Unspecified mastoiditis, left ear

H70.93 Unspecified mastoiditis, bilateral

● H71 Cholesteatoma of middle ear

Excludes2 cholesteatoma of external ear (H60.4-)
recurrent cholesteatoma of postmastoidectomy cavity (H95.0-)

● H71.0 Cholesteatoma of attic

H71.00 Cholesteatoma of attic, unspecified ear

H71.01 Cholesteatoma of attic, right ear

H71.02 Cholesteatoma of attic, left ear

H71.03 Cholesteatoma of attic, bilateral

● H71.1 Cholesteatoma of tympanum

H71.10 Cholesteatoma of tympanum, unspecified ear

H71.11 Cholesteatoma of tympanum, right ear

H71.12 Cholesteatoma of tympanum, left ear

H71.13 Cholesteatoma of tympanum, bilateral

● H71.2 Cholesteatoma of mastoid

H71.20 Cholesteatoma of mastoid, unspecified ear

H71.21 Cholesteatoma of mastoid, right ear

H71.22 Cholesteatoma of mastoid, left ear

H71.23 Cholesteatoma of mastoid, bilateral

● H71.3 Diffuse cholesteatosis

H71.30 Diffuse cholesteatosis, unspecified ear

H71.31 Diffuse cholesteatosis, right ear

H71.32 Diffuse cholesteatosis, left ear

H71.33 Diffuse cholesteatosis, bilateral

● H71.9 Unspecified cholesteatoma

H71.90 Unspecified cholesteatoma, unspecified ear

H71.91 Unspecified cholesteatoma, right ear

H71.92 Unspecified cholesteatoma, left ear

H71.93 Unspecified cholesteatoma, bilateral

★(See Plate 93 on page 69.)

● H72 Perforation of tympanic membrane

Hole or rupture in ear drum

Includes persistent post-traumatic perforation of ear drum
postinflammatory perforation of ear drum

Code first any associated otitis media (H65.-, H66.1-, H66.2-, H66.3-, H66.4-, H66.9-, H67.-)

Excludes1 acute suppurative otitis media with rupture of the tympanic membrane (H66.01-)
traumatic rupture of ear drum (S09.2-)

● H72.0 Central perforation of tympanic membrane

H72.00 Central perforation of tympanic membrane, unspecified ear

H72.01 Central perforation of tympanic membrane, right ear

H72.02 Central perforation of tympanic membrane, left ear

H72.03 Central perforation of tympanic membrane, bilateral

● H72.1 Attic perforation of tympanic membrane

Perforation of pars flaccida

H72.10 Attic perforation of tympanic membrane, unspecified ear

H72.11 Attic perforation of tympanic membrane, right ear

H72.12 Attic perforation of tympanic membrane, left ear

H72.13 Attic perforation of tympanic membrane, bilateral

● H72.2 Other marginal perforations of tympanic membrane

● H72.2X Other marginal perforations of tympanic membrane

H72.2X1 Other marginal perforations of tympanic membrane, right ear

H72.2X2 Other marginal perforations of tympanic membrane, left ear

H72.2X3 Other marginal perforations of tympanic membrane, bilateral

H72.2X9 Other marginal perforations of tympanic membrane, unspecified ear

● H72.8 Other perforations of tympanic membrane

● H72.81 Multiple perforations of tympanic membrane

H72.811 Multiple perforations of tympanic membrane, right ear

H72.812 Multiple perforations of tympanic membrane, left ear

H72.813 Multiple perforations of tympanic membrane, bilateral

H72.819 Multiple perforations of tympanic membrane, unspecified ear

● H72.82 Total perforations of tympanic membrane

H72.821 Total perforations of tympanic membrane, right ear

H72.822 Total perforations of tympanic membrane, left ear

H72.823 Total perforations of tympanic membrane, bilateral

H72.829 Total perforations of tympanic membrane, unspecified ear

● H72.9 Unspecified perforation of tympanic membrane

H72.90 Unspecified perforation of tympanic membrane, unspecified ear

H72.91 Unspecified perforation of tympanic membrane, right ear

H72.92 Unspecified perforation of tympanic membrane, left ear

H72.93 Unspecified perforation of tympanic membrane, bilateral

- **H73 Other disorders of tympanic membrane**
  - **H73.0 Acute myringitis**
    - **Excludes1** acute myringitis with otitis media (H65, H66)
    - **H73.00 Unspecified acute myringitis**
      Acute tympanitis NOS
      - **H73.001 Acute myringitis, right ear**
      - **H73.002 Acute myringitis, left ear**
      - **H73.003 Acute myringitis, bilateral**
      - **H73.009 Acute myringitis, unspecified ear**
    - **H73.01 Bullous myringitis**
      - **H73.011 Bullous myringitis, right ear**
      - **H73.012 Bullous myringitis, left ear**
      - **H73.013 Bullous myringitis, bilateral**
      - **H73.019 Bullous myringitis, unspecified ear**
    - **H73.09 Other acute myringitis**
      - **H73.091 Other acute myringitis, right ear**
      - **H73.092 Other acute myringitis, left ear**
      - **H73.093 Other acute myringitis, bilateral**
      - **H73.099 Other acute myringitis, unspecified ear**
  - **H73.1 Chronic myringitis**
    Chronic tympanitis
    - **Excludes1** chronic myringitis with otitis media (H65, H66)
    - **H73.10 Chronic myringitis, unspecified ear**
    - **H73.11 Chronic myringitis, right ear**
    - **H73.12 Chronic myringitis, left ear**
    - **H73.13 Chronic myringitis, bilateral**
  - **H73.2 Unspecified myringitis**
    - **H73.20 Unspecified myringitis, unspecified ear**
    - **H73.21 Unspecified myringitis, right ear**
    - **H73.22 Unspecified myringitis, left ear**
    - **H73.23 Unspecified myringitis, bilateral**
  - **H73.8 Other specified disorders of tympanic membrane**
    - **H73.81 Atrophic flaccid tympanic membrane**
      - **H73.811 Atrophic flaccid tympanic membrane, right ear**
      - **H73.812 Atrophic flaccid tympanic membrane, left ear**
      - **H73.813 Atrophic flaccid tympanic membrane, bilateral**
      - **H73.819 Atrophic flaccid tympanic membrane, unspecified ear**
    - **H73.82 Atrophic nonflaccid tympanic membrane**
      - **H73.821 Atrophic nonflaccid tympanic membrane, right ear**
      - **H73.822 Atrophic nonflaccid tympanic membrane, left ear**
      - **H73.823 Atrophic nonflaccid tympanic membrane, bilateral**
      - **H73.829 Atrophic nonflaccid tympanic membrane, unspecified ear**
    - **H73.89 Other specified disorders of tympanic membrane**
      - **H73.891 Other specified disorders of tympanic membrane, right ear**
      - **H73.892 Other specified disorders of tympanic membrane, left ear**
      - **H73.893 Other specified disorders of tympanic membrane, bilateral**
      - **H73.899 Other specified disorders of tympanic membrane, unspecified ear**
  - **H73.9 Unspecified disorder of tympanic membrane**
    - **H73.90 Unspecified disorder of tympanic membrane, unspecified ear**
    - **H73.91 Unspecified disorder of tympanic membrane, right ear**
    - **H73.92 Unspecified disorder of tympanic membrane, left ear**
    - **H73.93 Unspecified disorder of tympanic membrane, bilateral**
- **H74 Other disorders of middle ear mastoid**
  - **Excludes2** mastoiditis (H70.-)
  - **H74.0 Tympanosclerosis**
    - **H74.01 Tympanosclerosis, right ear**
    - **H74.02 Tympanosclerosis, left ear**
    - **H74.03 Tympanosclerosis, bilateral**
    - **H74.09 Tympanosclerosis, unspecified ear**
  - **H74.1 Adhesive middle ear disease**
    Adhesive otitis
    - **Excludes1** glue ear (H65.3-)
    - **H74.11 Adhesive right middle ear disease**
    - **H74.12 Adhesive left middle ear disease**
    - **H74.13 Adhesive middle ear disease, bilateral**
    - **H74.19 Adhesive middle ear disease, unspecified ear**
  - **H74.2 Discontinuity and dislocation of ear ossicles**
    - **H74.20 Discontinuity and dislocation of ear ossicles, unspecified ear**
    - **H74.21 Discontinuity and dislocation of right ear ossicles**
    - **H74.22 Discontinuity and dislocation of left ear ossicles**
    - **H74.23 Discontinuity and dislocation of ear ossicles, bilateral**
  - **H74.3 Other acquired abnormalities of ear ossicles**
    - **H74.31 Ankylosis of ear ossicles**
      - **H74.311 Ankylosis of ear ossicles, right ear**
      - **H74.312 Ankylosis of ear ossicles, left ear**
      - **H74.313 Ankylosis of ear ossicles, bilateral**
      - **H74.319 Ankylosis of ear ossicles, unspecified ear**
    - **H74.32 Partial loss of ear ossicles**
      - **H74.321 Partial loss of ear ossicles, right ear**
      - **H74.322 Partial loss of ear ossicles, left ear**
      - **H74.323 Partial loss of ear ossicles, bilateral**
      - **H74.329 Partial loss of ear ossicles, unspecified ear**
    - **H74.39 Other acquired abnormalities of ear ossicles**
      - **H74.391 Other acquired abnormalities of right ear ossicles**
      - **H74.392 Other acquired abnormalities of left ear ossicles**
      - **H74.393 Other acquired abnormalities of ear ossicles, bilateral**
      - **H74.399 Other acquired abnormalities of ear ossicles, unspecified ear**
  - **H74.4 Polyp of middle ear**
    - **H74.40 Polyp of middle ear, unspecified ear**
    - **H74.41 Polyp of right middle ear**
    - **H74.42 Polyp of left middle ear**
    - **H74.43 Polyp of middle ear, bilateral**

- H74.8 Other specified disorders of middle ear and mastoid
  - H74.8X Other specified disorders of middle ear and mastoid
    - H74.8X1 Other specified disorders of right middle ear and mastoid
    - H74.8X2 Other specified disorders of left middle ear and mastoid
    - H74.8X3 Other specified disorders of middle ear and mastoid, bilateral
    - H74.8X9 Other specified disorders of middle ear and mastoid, unspecified ear
- H74.9 Unspecified disorder of middle ear and mastoid
  - H74.90 Unspecified disorder of middle ear and mastoid, unspecified ear
  - H74.91 Unspecified disorder of right middle ear and mastoid
  - H74.92 Unspecified disorder of left middle ear and mastoid
  - H74.93 Unspecified disorder of middle ear and mastoid, bilateral

- H75 Other disorders of middle ear and mastoid in diseases classified elsewhere

  Code first underlying disease
  - H75.0 Mastoiditis in infectious and parasitic diseases classified elsewhere

    Excludes1 mastoiditis (in):
    syphilis (A52.77)
    tuberculosis (A18.03)
    - *H75.00 Mastoiditis in infectious and parasitic diseases classified elsewhere, unspecified ear*
    - *H75.01 Mastoiditis in infectious and parasitic diseases classified elsewhere, right ear*
    - *H75.02 Mastoiditis in infectious and parasitic diseases classified elsewhere, left ear*
    - *H75.03 Mastoiditis in infectious and parasitic diseases classified elsewhere, bilateral*
  - H75.8 Other specified disorders of middle ear and mastoid in diseases classified elsewhere
    - *H75.80 Other specified disorders of middle ear and mastoid in diseases classified elsewhere, unspecified ear*
    - *H75.81 Other specified disorders of right middle ear and mastoid in diseases classified elsewhere*
    - *H75.82 Other specified disorders of left middle ear and mastoid in diseases classified elsewhere*
    - *H75.83 Other specified disorders of middle ear and mastoid in diseases classified elsewhere, bilateral*

DISEASES OF INNER EAR (H80-H83)

★(See Plate 95 on page 69.)

- H80 Otosclerosis

  Inherited middle ear spongelike bone growth causing hearing loss

  Includes Otospongiosis
  - H80.0 Otosclerosis involving oval window, nonobliterative
    - H80.00 Otosclerosis involving oval window, nonobliterative, unspecified ear
    - H80.01 Otosclerosis involving oval window, nonobliterative, right ear
    - H80.02 Otosclerosis involving oval window, nonobliterative, left ear
    - H80.03 Otosclerosis involving oval window, nonobliterative, bilateral
  - H80.1 Otosclerosis involving oval window, obliterative
    - H80.10 Otosclerosis involving oval window, obliterative, unspecified ear
    - H80.11 Otosclerosis involving oval window, obliterative, right ear
    - H80.12 Otosclerosis involving oval window, obliterative, left ear
    - H80.13 Otosclerosis involving oval window, obliterative, bilateral
  - H80.2 Cochlear otosclerosis

    Otosclerosis involving otic capsule
    Otosclerosis involving round window
    - H80.20 Cochlear otosclerosis, unspecified ear
    - H80.21 Cochlear otosclerosis, right ear
    - H80.22 Cochlear otosclerosis, left ear
    - H80.23 Cochlear otosclerosis, bilateral
  - H80.8 Other otosclerosis
    - H80.80 Other otosclerosis, unspecified ear
    - H80.81 Other otosclerosis, right ear
    - H80.82 Other otosclerosis, left ear
    - H80.83 Other otosclerosis, bilateral
  - H80.9 Unspecified otosclerosis
    - H80.90 Unspecified otosclerosis, unspecified ear
    - H80.91 Unspecified otosclerosis, right ear
    - H80.92 Unspecified otosclerosis, left ear
    - H80.93 Unspecified otosclerosis, bilateral

- H81 Disorders of vestibular function

  Excludes1 epidemic vertigo (A88.1)
  vertigo NOS (R42)
  - H81.0 Ménière's disease

    Vestibular disorder that produces recurring symptoms including severe and intermittent hearing loss including the feeling of ear pressure or pain

    Labyrinthine hydrops
    Ménière's syndrome or vertigo
    - H81.01 Ménière's disease, right ear
    - H81.02 Ménière's disease, left ear
    - H81.03 Ménière's disease, bilateral
    - H81.09 Ménière's disease, unspecified ear
  - H81.1 Benign paroxysmal vertigo
    - H81.10 Benign paroxysmal vertigo, unspecified ear
    - H81.11 Benign paroxysmal vertigo, right ear
    - H81.12 Benign paroxysmal vertigo, left ear
    - H81.13 Benign paroxysmal vertigo, bilateral
  - H81.2 Vestibular neuronitis
    - H81.20 Vestibular neuronitis, unspecified ear
    - H81.21 Vestibular neuronitis, right ear
    - H81.22 Vestibular neuronitis, left ear
    - H81.23 Vestibular neuronitis, bilateral
  - H81.3 Other peripheral vertigo
    - H81.31 Aural vertigo
      - H81.311 Aural vertigo, right ear
      - H81.312 Aural vertigo, left ear
      - H81.313 Aural vertigo, bilateral
      - H81.319 Aural vertigo, unspecified ear
    - H81.39 Other peripheral vertigo

      Lermoyez' syndrome
      Otogenic vertigo
      Peripheral vertigo NOS
      - H81.391 Other peripheral vertigo, right ear
      - H81.392 Other peripheral vertigo, left ear
      - H81.393 Other peripheral vertigo, bilateral
      - H81.399 Other peripheral vertigo, unspecified ear
  - H81.4 Vertigo of central origin

    Central positional nystagmus
    - H81.41 Vertigo of central origin, right ear
    - H81.42 Vertigo of central origin, left ear
    - H81.43 Vertigo of central origin, bilateral
    - H81.49 Vertigo of central origin, unspecified ear

- **H81.8 Other disorders of vestibular function**
  - **H81.8X Other disorders of vestibular function**
    - **H81.8X1 Other disorders of vestibular function, right ear**
    - **H81.8X2 Other disorders of vestibular function, left ear**
    - **H81.8X3 Other disorders of vestibular function, bilateral**
    - **H81.8X9 Other disorders of vestibular function, unspecified ear**
- **H81.9 Unspecified disorder of vestibular function**
  Vertiginous syndrome NOS
  - **H81.90 Unspecified disorder of vestibular function, unspecified ear**
  - **H81.91 Unspecified disorder of vestibular function, right ear**
  - **H81.92 Unspecified disorder of vestibular function, left ear**
  - **H81.93 Unspecified disorder of vestibular function, bilateral**

- **H82 Vertiginous syndromes in diseases classified elsewhere**
  Code first underlying disease
  Excludes1 epidemic vertigo (A88.1)
  - *H82.1 Vertiginous syndromes in diseases classified elsewhere, right ear*
  - *H82.2 Vertiginous syndromes in diseases classified elsewhere, left ear*
  - *H82.3 Vertiginous syndromes in diseases classified elsewhere, bilateral*
  - *H82.9 Vertiginous syndromes in diseases classified elsewhere, unspecified ear*

- **H83 Other diseases of inner ear**
  - **H83.0 Labyrinthitis**
    Balance disorder that follows URI or head injury
    - **H83.01 Labyrinthitis, right ear**
    - **H83.02 Labyrinthitis, left ear**
    - **H83.03 Labyrinthitis, bilateral**
    - **H83.09 Labyrinthitis, unspecified ear**
  - **H83.1 Labyrinthine fistula**
    - **H83.11 Labyrinthine fistula, right ear**
    - **H83.12 Labyrinthine fistula, left ear**
    - **H83.13 Labyrinthine fistula, bilateral**
    - **H83.19 Labyrinthine fistula, unspecified ear**
  - **H83.2 Labyrinthine dysfunction**
    Labyrinthine hypersensitivity
    Labyrinthine hypofunction
    Labyrinthine loss of function
    - **H83.2X Labyrinthine dysfunction**
      - **H83.2X1 Labyrinthine dysfunction, right ear**
      - **H83.2X2 Labyrinthine dysfunction, left ear**
      - **H83.2X3 Labyrinthine dysfunction, bilateral**
      - **H83.2X9 Labyrinthine dysfunction, unspecified ear**
  - **H83.3 Noise effects on inner ear**
    Acoustic trauma of inner ear
    Noise-induced hearing loss of inner ear
    - **H83.3X Noise effects on inner ear**
      - **H83.3X1 Noise effects on right inner ear**
      - **H83.3X2 Noise effects on left inner ear**
      - **H83.3X3 Noise effects on inner ear, bilateral**
      - **H83.3X9 Noise effects on inner ear, unspecified ear**
  - **H83.8 Other specified diseases of inner ear**
    - **H83.8X Other specified diseases of inner ear**
      - **H83.8X1 Other specified diseases of right inner ear**
      - **H83.8X2 Other specified diseases of left inner ear**
      - **H83.8X3 Other specified diseases of inner ear, bilateral**
      - **H83.8X9 Other specified diseases of inner ear, unspecified ear**
  - **H83.9 Unspecified disease of inner ear**
    - **H83.90 Unspecified disease of inner ear, unspecified ear**
    - **H83.91 Unspecified disease of right inner ear**
    - **H83.92 Unspecified disease of left inner ear**
    - **H83.93 Unspecified disease of inner ear, bilateral**

OTHER DISORDERS OF EAR (H90-H94)

- **H90 Conductive and sensorineural hearing loss**
  Excludes1 deaf nonspeaking NEC (H91.3)
  deafness NOS (H91.9-)
  hearing loss NOS (H91.9-)
  noise-induced hearing loss (H83.3-)
  ototoxic hearing loss (H91.0-)
  sudden (idiopathic) hearing loss (H91.2-)
  - **H90.0 Conductive hearing loss, bilateral**
  - **H90.1 Conductive hearing loss, unilateral with unrestricted hearing on the contralateral side**
    - **H90.11 Conductive hearing loss, unilateral, right ear, with unrestricted hearing on the contralateral side**
    - **H90.12 Conductive hearing loss, unilateral, left ear, with unrestricted hearing on the contralateral side**
  - **H90.2 Conductive hearing loss, unspecified**
    Conductive deafness NOS
  - **H90.3 Sensorineural hearing loss, bilateral**
  - **H90.4 Sensorineural hearing loss, unilateral with unrestricted hearing on the contralateral side**
    - **H90.41 Sensorineural hearing loss, unilateral, right ear, with unrestricted hearing on the contralateral side**
    - **H90.42 Sensorineural hearing loss, unilateral, left ear, with unrestricted hearing on the contralateral side**
  - **H90.5 Unspecified sensorineural hearing loss**
    Central hearing loss NOS
    Congenital deafness NOS
    Neural hearing loss NOS
    Perceptive hearing loss NOS
    Sensorineural deafness NOS
    Sensory hearing loss NOS
    Excludes1 abnormal auditory perception (H93.2-)
    psychogenic deafness (F44.6)
  - **H90.6 Mixed conductive and sensorineural hearing loss, bilateral**
    Coding Clinic: 2015, Q2, P7
  - **H90.7 Mixed conductive and sensorineural hearing loss, unilateral with unrestricted hearing on the contralateral side**
    - **H90.71 Mixed conductive and sensorineural hearing loss, unilateral, right ear, with unrestricted hearing on the contralateral side**
    - **H90.72 Mixed conductive and sensorineural hearing loss, unilateral, left ear, with unrestricted hearing on the contralateral side**
  - **H90.8 Mixed conductive and sensorineural hearing loss, unspecified**

- **H90.A Conductive and sensorineural hearing loss with restricted hearing on the contralateral side ◀**
  - **H90.A1 Conductive hearing loss, unilateral, with restricted hearing on the contralateral side ◀**
    - **H90.A11 Conductive hearing loss, unilateral, right ear with restricted hearing on the contralateral side ◀**
    - **H90.A12 Conductive hearing loss, unilateral, left ear with restricted hearing on the contralateral side ◀**
  - **H90.A2 Sensorineural hearing loss, unilateral, with restricted hearing on the contralateral side ◀**
    - **H90.A21 Sensorineural hearing loss, unilateral, right ear, with restricted hearing on the contralateral side ◀**
    - **H90.A22 Sensorineural hearing loss, unilateral, left ear, with restricted hearing on the contralateral side ◀**
  - **H90.A3 Mixed conductive and sensorineural hearing loss, unilateral with restricted hearing on the contralateral side ◀**
    - **H90.A31 Mixed conductive and sensorineural hearing loss, unilateral, right ear with restricted hearing on the contralateral side ◀**
    - **H90.A32 Mixed conductive and sensorineural hearing loss, unilateral, left ear with restricted hearing on the contralateral side ◀**

- **H91 Other and unspecified hearing loss**

  Excludes1 abnormal auditory perception (H93.2-)
  hearing loss as classified in H90.-
  impacted cerumen (H61.2-)
  noise-induced hearing loss (H83.3-)
  psychogenic deafness (F44.6)
  transient ischemic deafness (H93.01-)

  - **H91.0 Ototoxic hearing loss**

    Code first poisoning due to drug or toxin, if applicable (T36-T65 with fifth or sixth character 1-4 or 6)

    Use additional code for adverse effect, if applicable, to identify drug (T36-T50 with fifth or sixth character 5)

    - **H91.01 Ototoxic hearing loss, right ear**
    - **H91.02 Ototoxic hearing loss, left ear**
    - **H91.03 Ototoxic hearing loss, bilateral**
    - **H91.09 Ototoxic hearing loss, unspecified ear**
  - **H91.1 Presbycusis**
    Presbyacusia
    - **H91.10 Presbycusis, unspecified ear**
    - **H91.11 Presbycusis, right ear**
    - **H91.12 Presbycusis, left ear**
    - **H91.13 Presbycusis, bilateral**
  - **H91.2 Sudden idiopathic hearing loss**
    Sudden hearing loss NOS
    - **H91.20 Sudden idiopathic hearing loss, unspecified ear**
    - **H91.21 Sudden idiopathic hearing loss, right ear**
    - **H91.22 Sudden idiopathic hearing loss, left ear**
    - **H91.23 Sudden idiopathic hearing loss, bilateral**
  - **H91.3 Deaf nonspeaking, not elsewhere classified**
  - **H91.8 Other specified hearing loss**
    - **H91.8X Other specified hearing loss**
      - **H91.8X1 Other specified hearing loss, right ear**
      - **H91.8X2 Other specified hearing loss, left ear**
      - **H91.8X3 Other specified hearing loss, bilateral**
      - **H91.8X9 Other specified hearing loss, unspecified ear**
  - **H91.9 Unspecified hearing loss**
    Deafness NOS
    High frequency deafness
    Low frequency deafness
    - **H91.90 Unspecified hearing loss, unspecified ear**
    - **H91.91 Unspecified hearing loss, right ear**
    - **H91.92 Unspecified hearing loss, left ear**
    - **H91.93 Unspecified hearing loss, bilateral**

- **H92 Otalgia and effusion of ear**
  - **H92.0 Otalgia**
    - **H92.01 Otalgia, right ear**
    - **H92.02 Otalgia, left ear**
    - **H92.03 Otalgia, bilateral**
    - **H92.09 Otalgia, unspecified ear**
  - **H92.1 Otorrhea**

    Excludes1 leakage of cerebrospinal fluid through ear (G96.0)

    - **H92.10 Otorrhea, unspecified ear**
    - **H92.11 Otorrhea, right ear**
    - **H92.12 Otorrhea, left ear**
    - **H92.13 Otorrhea, bilateral**
  - **H92.2 Otorrhagia**

    Excludes1 traumatic otorrhagia - code to injury

    - **H92.20 Otorrhagia, unspecified ear**
    - **H92.21 Otorrhagia, right ear**
    - **H92.22 Otorrhagia, left ear**
    - **H92.23 Otorrhagia, bilateral**

- **H93 Other disorders of ear, not elsewhere classified**
  - **H93.0 Degenerative and vascular disorders of ear**

    Excludes1 presbycusis (H91.1)

    - **H93.01 Transient ischemic deafness**
      - **H93.011 Transient ischemic deafness, right ear**
      - **H93.012 Transient ischemic deafness, left ear**
      - **H93.013 Transient ischemic deafness, bilateral**
      - **H93.019 Transient ischemic deafness, unspecified ear**
    - **H93.09 Unspecified degenerative and vascular disorders of ear**
      - **H93.091 Unspecified degenerative and vascular disorders of right ear**
      - **H93.092 Unspecified degenerative and vascular disorders of left ear**
      - **H93.093 Unspecified degenerative and vascular disorders of ear, bilateral**
      - **H93.099 Unspecified degenerative and vascular disorders of unspecified ear**
  - **H93.1 Tinnitus**

    Perception of sound (ringing, buzzing, humming, whistling tunes, or singing)

    - **H93.11 Tinnitus, right ear**
    - **H93.12 Tinnitus, left ear**
    - **H93.13 Tinnitus, bilateral**
    - **H93.19 Tinnitus, unspecified ear**
  - **H93.A Pulsatile tinnitus ◀**
    - **H93.A1 Pulsatile tinnitus, right ear ◀**
    - **H93.A2 Pulsatile tinnitus, left ear ◀**
    - **H93.A3 Pulsatile tinnitus, bilateral ◀**
    - **H93.A9 Pulsatile tinnitus, unspecified ear ◀**
  - **H93.2 Other abnormal auditory perceptions**

    Excludes2 auditory hallucinations (R44.0)

    - **H93.21 Auditory recruitment**
      - **H93.211 Auditory recruitment, right ear**
      - **H93.212 Auditory recruitment, left ear**
      - **H93.213 Auditory recruitment, bilateral**
      - **H93.219 Auditory recruitment, unspecified ear**

- **H93.22 Diplacusis**
  - **H93.221 Diplacusis, right ear**
  - **H93.222 Diplacusis, left ear**
  - **H93.223 Diplacusis, bilateral**
  - **H93.229 Diplacusis, unspecified ear**
- **H93.23 Hyperacusis**
  - **H93.231 Hyperacusis, right ear**
  - **H93.232 Hyperacusis, left ear**
  - **H93.233 Hyperacusis, bilateral**
  - **H93.239 Hyperacusis, unspecified ear**
- **H93.24 Temporary auditory threshold shift**
  - **H93.241 Temporary auditory threshold shift, right ear**
  - **H93.242 Temporary auditory threshold shift, left ear**
  - **H93.243 Temporary auditory threshold shift, bilateral**
  - **H93.249 Temporary auditory threshold shift, unspecified ear**
- **H93.25 Central auditory processing disorder**
  - Congenital auditory imperception
  - Word deafness
  - **Excludes1** mixed receptive-expressive language disorder (F80.2)
- **H93.29 Other abnormal auditory perceptions**
  - **H93.291 Other abnormal auditory perceptions, right ear**
  - **H93.292 Other abnormal auditory perceptions, left ear**
  - **H93.293 Other abnormal auditory perceptions, bilateral**
  - **H93.299 Other abnormal auditory perceptions, unspecified ear**
- **H93.3 Disorders of acoustic nerve**
  - Disorder of 8th cranial nerve
  - **Excludes1** acoustic neuroma (D33.3)
    syphilitic acoustic neuritis (A52.15)
  - **H93.3X Disorders of acoustic nerve**
    - **H93.3X1 Disorders of right acoustic nerve**
    - **H93.3X2 Disorders of left acoustic nerve**
    - **H93.3X3 Disorders of bilateral acoustic nerves**
    - **H93.3X9 Disorders of unspecified acoustic nerve**
- **H93.8 Other specified disorders of ear**
  - **H93.8X Other specified disorders of ear**
    - **H93.8X1 Other specified disorders of right ear**
    - **H93.8X2 Other specified disorders of left ear**
    - **H93.8X3 Other specified disorders of ear, bilateral**
    - **H93.8X9 Other specified disorders of ear, unspecified ear**
- **H93.9 Unspecified disorder of ear**
  - **H93.90 Unspecified disorder of ear, unspecified ear**
  - **H93.91 Unspecified disorder of right ear**
  - **H93.92 Unspecified disorder of left ear**
  - **H93.93 Unspecified disorder of ear, bilateral**

- **H94 Other disorders of ear in diseases classified elsewhere**
  - **H94.0 Acoustic neuritis in infectious and parasitic diseases classified elsewhere**
    - *Code first underlying disease, such as:*
      parasitic disease (B65-B89)
    - **Excludes1** acoustic neuritis (in):
      herpes zoster (B02.29)
      syphilis (A52.15)
    - ***H94.00 Acoustic neuritis in infectious and parasitic diseases classified elsewhere, unspecified ear***
    - ***H94.01 Acoustic neuritis in infectious and parasitic diseases classified elsewhere, right ear***
    - ***H94.02 Acoustic neuritis in infectious and parasitic diseases classified elsewhere, left ear***
    - ***H94.03 Acoustic neuritis in infectious and parasitic diseases classified elsewhere, bilateral***
  - **H94.8 Other specified disorders of ear in diseases classified elsewhere**
    - *Code first underlying disease, such as:*
      congenital syphilis (A50.0)
    - **Excludes1** aural myiasis (B87.4)
      syphilitic labyrinthitis (A52.79)
    - ***H94.80 Other specified disorders of ear in diseases classified elsewhere, unspecified ear***
    - ***H94.81 Other specified disorders of right ear in diseases classified elsewhere***
    - ***H94.82 Other specified disorders of left ear in diseases classified elsewhere***
    - ***H94.83 Other specified disorders of ear in diseases classified elsewhere, bilateral***

- **H95 Intraoperative and postprocedural complications and disorders of ear and mastoid process, not elsewhere classified**
  - **H95.0 Recurrent cholesteatoma of postmastoidectomy cavity**
    - **H95.00 Recurrent cholesteatoma of postmastoidectomy cavity, unspecified ear**
    - **H95.01 Recurrent cholesteatoma of postmastoidectomy cavity, right ear**
    - **H95.02 Recurrent cholesteatoma of postmastoidectomy cavity, left ear**
    - **H95.03 Recurrent cholesteatoma of postmastoidectomy cavity, bilateral ears**
  - **H95.1 Other disorders of ear and mastoid process following mastoidectomy**
    - **H95.11 Chronic inflammation of postmastoidectomy cavity**
      - **H95.111 Chronic inflammation of postmastoidectomy cavity, right ear**
      - **H95.112 Chronic inflammation of postmastoidectomy cavity, left ear**
      - **H95.113 Chronic inflammation of postmastoidectomy cavity, bilateral ears**
      - **H95.119 Chronic inflammation of postmastoidectomy cavity, unspecified ear**
    - **H95.12 Granulation of postmastoidectomy cavity**
      - **H95.121 Granulation of postmastoidectomy cavity, right ear**
      - **H95.122 Granulation of postmastoidectomy cavity, left ear**
      - **H95.123 Granulation of postmastoidectomy cavity, bilateral ears**
      - **H95.129 Granulation of postmastoidectomy cavity, unspecified ear**

● **H95.13 Mucosal cyst of postmastoidectomy cavity**

H95.131 Mucosal cyst of postmastoidectomy cavity, right ear

H95.132 Mucosal cyst of postmastoidectomy cavity, left ear

H95.133 Mucosal cyst of postmastoidectomy cavity, bilateral ears

H95.139 Mucosal cyst of postmastoidectomy cavity, unspecified ear

● **H95.19 Other disorders following mastoidectomy**

H95.191 Other disorders following mastoidectomy, right ear

H95.192 Other disorders following mastoidectomy, left ear

H95.193 Other disorders following mastoidectomy, bilateral ears

H95.199 Other disorders following mastoidectomy, unspecified ear

● **H95.2 Intraoperative hemorrhage and hematoma of ear and mastoid process complicating a procedure**

Excludes1 intraoperative hemorrhage and hematoma of ear and mastoid process due to accidental puncture or laceration during a procedure (H95.3-)

Ex. **For category H95.2 CC codes:** H95.21-H95.22, H95.41-H95.89, I85.01, I85.11, I97.3, K21.9, K22.8, K23-K25.2, K25.4, K25.6, K26.0, K26.2, K26.4, K26.6, K27.0, K27.2, K27.4, K27.6, K28.0, K28.2, K28.4, K28.6, K29.01, K29.21, K29.31, K29.41, K29.51, K29.61, K29.71, K29.81, K29.91, K31.811, K55.21, K57.01, K57.11, K57.13, K57.21, K57.31, K57.33, K57.41, K57.51, K57.53, K57.81, K57.91, K57.93, K62.5, K92.0-K92.2, M96.89, N98.1-N98.9, P54.1-P54.3, T81.10X-T81.19X[A], T81.82X[A], T81.89X-T81.9XX[A]

H95.21 Intraoperative hemorrhage and hematoma of ear and mastoid process complicating a procedure on the ear and mastoid process

H95.22 Intraoperative hemorrhage and hematoma of ear and mastoid process complicating other procedure

● **H95.3 Accidental puncture and laceration of ear and mastoid process during a procedure**

Ex. **For category H95.3 CC codes:** D78.11-D78.12, D78.81-D78.89, E36.11-E36.8, E89.810-E89.89, G96.11, G97.41-G97.49, H59.011-H59.019, H59.031-H59.099, H59.211-H59.229, H59.811-H59.89, H95.31-H95.32, H95.811-H95.89, I97.3, I97.51-I97.52, J95.71-J95.72, K91.71-K91.72, L76.11-L76.12, L76.81-L76.82, M96.820-M96.821, M96.89, N98.1-N98.9, N99.71-N99.72, T81.82X[A], T81.89X-T81.9XX[A]

H95.31 Accidental puncture and laceration of the ear and mastoid process during a procedure on the ear and mastoid process

H95.32 Accidental puncture and laceration of the ear and mastoid process during other procedure

● **H95.4 Postprocedural hemorrhage of ear and mastoid process following a procedure** ◀

Ex. **For category H95.4 CC codes:** See H95.2

H95.41 Postprocedural hemorrhage of ear and mastoid process following a procedure on the ear and mastoid process ◀

H95.42 Postprocedural hemorrhage of ear and mastoid process following other procedure ◀

● **H95.5 Postprocedural hematoma and seroma of ear and mastoid process following a procedure** ◀

Ex. **For category H95.5 CC codes:** See H95.2

H95.51 Postprocedural hematoma of ear and mastoid process following a procedure on the ear and mastoid process ◀

H95.52 Postprocedural hematoma of ear and mastoid process following other procedure ◀

H95.53 Postprocedural seroma of ear and mastoid process following a procedure on the ear and mastoid process ◀

H95.54 Postprocedural seroma of ear and mastoid process following other procedure ◀

● **H95.8 Other intraoperative and postprocedural complications and disorders of the ear and mastoid process, not elsewhere classified**

Excludes2 postprocedural complications and disorders following mastoidectomy (H95.0-, H95.1-)

Ex. **For category H95.8 CC codes:** D78.81-D78.89, E36.8, E89.810-E89.89, H59.011-H59.019, H59.031-H59.099, H59.811-H59.89, H95.811-H95.89, I97.3, L76.81-L76.82, M96.89, N98.1-N98.9, T81.82X[A], T81.89X-T81.9XX[A]

● **H95.81 Postprocedural stenosis of external ear canal**

H95.811 Postprocedural stenosis of right external ear canal

H95.812 Postprocedural stenosis of left external ear canal

H95.813 Postprocedural stenosis of external ear canal, bilateral

H95.819 Postprocedural stenosis of unspecified external ear canal

H95.88 Other intraoperative complications and disorders of the ear and mastoid process, not elsewhere classified

Use additional code, if applicable, to further specify disorder

H95.89 Other postprocedural complications and disorders of the ear and mastoid process, not elsewhere classified

Use additional code, if applicable, to further specify disorder

CHAPTER 9 DISEASES OF THE CIRCULATORY SYSTEM (I00-I99)

OGCR Chapter-Specific Coding Guidelines

9. Chapter 9: Diseases of the Circulatory System (I00-I99)

a. Hypertension

The classification presumes a causal relationship between hypertension and heart involvement and between hypertension and kidney involvement, as the two conditions are linked by the term "with" in the Alphabetic Index. These conditions should be coded as related even in the absence of provider documentation explicitly linking them, unless the documentation clearly states the conditions are unrelated.

For hypertension and conditions not specifically linked by relational terms such as "with," "associated with" or "due to" in the classification, provider documentation must link the conditions in order to code them as related.

1) Hypertension with Heart Disease

Hypertension with heart conditions classified to I50.- or I51.4-I51.9, are assigned to, a code from category I11, Hypertensive heart disease. Use an additional code from category I50, Heart failure, to identify the type of heart failure in those patients with heart failure.

The same heart conditions (I50.-, I51.4-I51.9) with hypertension, are coded separately **if the provider has specifically documented a different cause**. Sequence according to the circumstances of the admission/encounter.

2) Hypertensive Chronic Kidney Disease

Assign codes from category I12, Hypertensive chronic kidney disease, when both hypertension and a condition classifiable to category N18, Chronic kidney disease (CKD), are present. **CKD should not be coded as hypertensive if the physician has specifically documented a different cause.**

The appropriate code from category N18 should be used as a secondary code with a code from category I12 to identify the stage of chronic kidney disease.

See Section I.C.14. Chronic kidney disease.

If a patient has hypertensive chronic kidney disease and acute renal failure, an additional code for the acute renal failure is required.

3) Hypertensive Heart and Chronic Kidney Disease

Assign codes from combination category I13, Hypertensive heart and chronic kidney disease, when **there is hypertension with both heart and kidney involvement.** If heart failure is present, assign an additional code from category I50 to identify the type of heart failure.

The appropriate code from category N18, Chronic kidney disease, should be used as a secondary code with a code from category I13 to identify the stage of chronic kidney disease.

See Section I.C.14. Chronic kidney disease.

The codes in category I13, Hypertensive heart and chronic kidney disease, are combination codes that include hypertension, heart disease and chronic kidney disease. The Includes note at I13 specifies that the conditions included at I11 and I12 are included together in I13. If a patient has hypertension, heart disease and chronic kidney disease then a code from I13 should be used, not individual codes for hypertension, heart disease and chronic kidney disease, or codes from I11 or I12.

For patients with both acute renal failure and chronic kidney disease an additional code for acute renal failure is required.

4) Hypertensive Cerebrovascular Disease

For hypertensive cerebrovascular disease, first assign the appropriate code from categories I60-I69, followed by the appropriate hypertension code.

5) Hypertensive Retinopathy

Subcategory H35.0, Background retinopathy and retinal vascular changes, should be used with a code from category I10 – I15, Hypertensive disease to include the systemic hypertension. The sequencing is based on the reason for the encounter.

6) Hypertension, Secondary

Secondary hypertension is due to an underlying condition. Two codes are required: one to identify the underlying etiology and one from category I15 to identify the hypertension. Sequencing of codes is determined by the reason for admission/encounter.

7) Hypertension, Transient

Assign code R03.0, Elevated blood pressure reading without diagnosis of hypertension, unless patient has an established diagnosis of hypertension. Assign code O13.-, Gestational [pregnancy-induced] hypertension without significant proteinuria, or O14.-, Pre-eclampsia, for transient hypertension of pregnancy.

8) Hypertension, Controlled

This diagnostic statement usually refers to an existing state of hypertension under control by therapy. Assign the appropriate code from categories I10-I15, Hypertensive diseases.

9) Hypertension, Uncontrolled

Uncontrolled hypertension may refer to untreated hypertension or hypertension not responding to current therapeutic regimen. In either case, assign the appropriate code from categories I10-I15, Hypertensive diseases.

10) Hypertensive Crisis

Assign a code from category I16, Hypertensive crisis, for documented hypertensive urgency, hypertensive emergency or unspecified hypertensive crisis. Code also any identified hypertensive disease (I10-I15). The sequencing is based on the reason for the encounter.

b. Atherosclerotic Coronary Artery Disease and Angina

ICD-10-CM has combination codes for atherosclerotic heart disease with angina pectoris. The subcategories for these codes are I25.11, Atherosclerotic heart disease of native coronary artery with angina pectoris and I25.7, Atherosclerosis of coronary artery bypass graft(s) and coronary artery of transplanted heart with angina pectoris.

When using one of these combination codes it is not necessary to use an additional code for angina pectoris. A causal relationship can be assumed in a patient with both atherosclerosis and angina pectoris, unless the documentation indicates the angina is due to something other than the atherosclerosis.

If a patient with coronary artery disease is admitted due to an acute myocardial infarction (AMI), the AMI should be sequenced before the coronary artery disease.

See Section I.C.9. Acute myocardial infarction (AMI)

c. Intraoperative and Postprocedural Cerebrovascular Accident

Medical record documentation should clearly specify the cause-and-effect relationship between the medical intervention and the cerebrovascular accident in order to assign a code for intraoperative or postprocedural cerebrovascular accident.

Proper code assignment depends on whether it was an infarction or hemorrhage and whether it occurred intraoperatively or postoperatively. If it was a cerebral hemorrhage, code assignment depends on the type of procedure performed.

d. Sequelae of Cerebrovascular Disease

1) Category I69, Sequelae of Cerebrovascular disease

Category I69 is used to indicate conditions classifiable to categories I60-I67 as the causes of sequela (neurologic deficits), themselves classified elsewhere. These "late effects" include neurologic deficits that persist after initial onset of conditions classifiable to categories I60-I67. The neurologic deficits caused by cerebrovascular disease may be present from the onset or may arise at any time after the onset of the condition classifiable to categories I60-I67.

Codes from category I69, Sequelae of cerebrovascular disease, that specify hemiplegia, hemiparesis and monoplegia identify whether the dominant or nondominant side is affected. Should the affected side be documented, but not specified as dominant or nondominant, and the classification system does not indicate a default, code selection is as follows:

- For ambidextrous patients, the default should be dominant.
- If the left side is affected, the default is non-dominant.
- If the right side is affected, the default is dominant.

2) Codes from category I69 with codes from I60-I67

Codes from category I69 may be assigned on a health care record with codes from I60-I67, if the patient has a current cerebrovascular disease and deficits from an old cerebrovascular disease.

3) Codes from category I69 and Personal history of transient ischemic attack (TIA) and cerebral infarction (Z86.73)

Codes from category I69 should not be assigned if the patient does not have neurologic deficits.

See Section I.C.21. 4. History (of) for use of personal history codes

e. Acute myocardial infarction (AMI)

1) ST elevation myocardial infarction (STEMI) and non ST elevation myocardial infarction (NSTEMI)

The ICD-10-CM codes for acute myocardial infarction (AMI) identify the site, such as anterolateral wall or true posterior wall. Subcategories I21.0-I21.2 and code I21.3 are used for ST elevation myocardial infarction (STEMI). Code I21.4, Non-ST elevation (NSTEMI) myocardial infarction, is used for non ST elevation myocardial infarction (NSTEMI) and nontransmural MIs.

If NSTEMI evolves to STEMI, assign the STEMI code. If STEMI converts to NSTEMI due to thrombolytic therapy, it is still coded as STEMI.

For encounters occurring while the myocardial infarction is equal to, or less than, four weeks old, including transfers to another acute setting or a postacute setting, and the myocardial infarction **meets the definition for "other diagnoses" (see Section III, Reporting Additional Diagnoses)**, codes from category I21 may continue to be reported. For encounters after the 4 week time frame and the patient is still receiving care related to the myocardial infarction, the appropriate aftercare code should be assigned, rather than a code from category I21. For old or healed myocardial infarctions not requiring further care, code I25.2, Old myocardial infarction, may be assigned.

2) Acute myocardial infarction, unspecified

Code I21.3, ST elevation (STEMI) myocardial infarction of unspecified site, is the default for unspecified acute myocardial infarction. If only STEMI or transmural MI without the site is documented, assign code I21.3.

3) AMI documented as nontransmural or subendocardial but site provided

If an AMI is documented as nontransmural or subendocardial, but the site is provided, it is still coded as a subendocardial AMI.

See Section I.C.21.3 for information on coding status post administration of tPA in a different facility within the last 24 hours.

4) Subsequent acute myocardial infarction

A code from category I22, Subsequent ST elevation (STEMI) and non ST elevation (NSTEMI) myocardial infarction, is to be used when a patient who has suffered an AMI has a new AMI within the 4 week time frame of the initial AMI. A code from category I22 must be used in conjunction with a code from category I21. The sequencing of the I22 and I21 codes depends on the circumstances of the encounter.

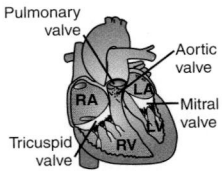

Figure 9-1 Cardiovascular valves.

Item 9–1 Rheumatic fever is the inflammation of the valve(s) of the heart, usually the mitral or aortic, which leads to valve damage. Rheumatic heart inflammations are usually **pericarditis** (sac surrounding heart), **endocarditis** (heart cavity), or **myocarditis** (heart muscle).

CHAPTER 9 DISEASES OF THE CIRCULATORY SYSTEM (I00-I99)

Excludes2 certain conditions originating in the perinatal period (P04-P96)
certain infectious and parasitic diseases (A00-B99)
complications of pregnancy, childbirth and the puerperium (O00-O9A)
congenital malformations, deformations, and chromosomal abnormalities (Q00-Q99)
endocrine, nutritional and metabolic diseases (E00-E88)
injury, poisoning and certain other consequences of external causes (S00-T88)
neoplasms (C00-D49)
symptoms, signs and abnormal clinical and laboratory findings, not elsewhere classified (R00-R94)
systemic connective tissue disorders (M30-M36)
transient cerebral ischemic attacks and related syndromes (G45.-)

This chapter contains the following blocks:

I00-I02	Acute rheumatic fever
I05-I09	Chronic rheumatic heart diseases
I10-I16	Hypertensive diseases ◀
I20-I25	Ischemic heart diseases
I26-I28	Pulmonary heart disease and diseases of pulmonary circulation
I30-I52	Other forms of heart disease
I60-I69	Cerebrovascular diseases
I70-I79	Diseases of arteries, arterioles and capillaries
I80-I89	Diseases of veins, lymphatic vessels and lymph nodes, not elsewhere classified
I95-I99	Other and unspecified disorders of the circulatory system

ACUTE RHEUMATIC FEVER (I00-I02)

I00 Rheumatic fever without heart involvement

Includes arthritis, rheumatic, acute or subacute

Excludes1 rheumatic fever with heart involvement (I01.0-I01.9)

● **I01 Rheumatic fever with heart involvement**

Excludes1 chronic diseases of rheumatic origin (I05-I09) unless rheumatic fever is also present or there is evidence of reactivation or activity of the rheumatic process.

I01.0 Acute rheumatic pericarditis

Any condition in I00 with pericarditis
Rheumatic pericarditis (acute)

Excludes1 acute pericarditis not specified as rheumatic (I30.-)

Ex: B33.23, I01.0, I09.2, I30.0-I30.9, I31.3-I32, I87.8, I99.8-I99.9

I01.1 Acute rheumatic endocarditis

Any condition in I00 with endocarditis or valvulitis
Acute rheumatic valvulitis

Ex: A01.00-A01.09, A39.51, A52.03, A78, B33.21, B37.6, I00, I01.1, I01.8-I02.0, I05.0-I07.9, I08.1-I08.3, I08.9, I09.1, I09.89-I09.9, I33.0-I39, I42.4, I87.8-I87.9, I99.8-I99.9, Q22.2, Q23.8-Q23.9, Q24.8, T82.6XX[A]

◀ New ◀ Revised ~~deleted~~ Deleted Excludes 1 Excludes 2 Includes Use additional Code first Code also Unspecified
OGCR Official Guidelines ● Unacceptable Principal Diagnosis X Assign placeholder X ● Use Additional Character(s) ▶ Manifestation Code Coding Clinic

Item 9–2 Rheumatic chorea, also called Sydenham's, juvenile, minor, simple, or St. Vitus' dance, is a major symptom of rheumatic fever and is characterized by ceaseless, involuntary, jerky, purposeless movements.

I01.2 Acute rheumatic myocarditis
Any condition in I00 with myocarditis
Ex: A52.06, B33.20-B33.22, I00, I01.2-I01.9, I09.0, I09.9, I23.0-I23.3, I23.6-I23.8, I40.0-I41, I51.0, I51.4, I87.8, I99.8-I99.9

I01.8 Other acute rheumatic heart disease
Any condition in I00 with other or multiple types of heart involvement
Acute rheumatic pancarditis
Ex: I01.0-I09.9, I50.20-I50.43

I01.9 Acute rheumatic heart disease, unspecified
Any condition in I00 with unspecified type of heart involvement
Rheumatic carditis, acute
Rheumatic heart disease, active or acute
Ex: I01.0-I09.9

I02 Rheumatic chorea
Includes Sydenham's chorea
Excludes1 chorea NOS (G25.5)
Huntington's chorea (G10)

I02.0 Rheumatic chorea with heart involvement
Chorea NOS with heart involvement
Rheumatic chorea with heart involvement of any type classifiable under I01.-
Ex: See I01.8

I02.9 Rheumatic chorea without heart involvement
Rheumatic chorea NOS
Ex: See I01.9

CHRONIC RHEUMATIC HEART DISEASES (I05-I09)

I05 Rheumatic mitral valve diseases
Includes conditions classifiable to both I05.0 and I05.2-I05.9, whether specified as rheumatic or not
Excludes1 mitral valve disease specified as nonrheumatic (I34.-)
mitral valve disease with aortic and/or tricuspid valve involvement (I08.-)

I05.0 Rheumatic mitral stenosis
Mitral (valve) obstruction (rheumatic)

I05.1 Rheumatic mitral insufficiency
Rheumatic mitral incompetence
Rheumatic mitral regurgitation
Excludes1 mitral insufficiency not specified as rheumatic (I34.0)

I05.2 Rheumatic mitral stenosis with insufficiency
Rheumatic mitral stenosis with incompetence or regurgitation

I05.8 Other rheumatic mitral valve diseases
Rheumatic mitral (valve) failure

I05.9 Rheumatic mitral valve disease, unspecified
Rheumatic mitral (valve) disorder (chronic) NOS

I06 Rheumatic aortic valve diseases
Excludes1 aortic valve disease not specified as rheumatic (I35.-)
aortic valve disease with mitral and/or tricuspid valve involvement (I08.-)

I06.0 Rheumatic aortic stenosis
Rheumatic aortic (valve) obstruction

I06.1 Rheumatic aortic insufficiency
Rheumatic aortic incompetence
Rheumatic aortic regurgitation

★ **(See Plate 244 on page 78.)**

Item 9–3 Mitral stenosis is the narrowing of the mitral valve separating the left atrium from the left ventricle. **Mitral insufficiency** is the improper closure of the mitral valve which may lead to enlargement (hypertrophy) of the left atrium.

Item 9–4 Aortic stenosis is the narrowing of the aortic valve located between the left ventricle and the aorta. **Aortic insufficiency** is the improper closure of the aortic valve which may lead to enlargement (hypertrophy) of the left ventricle.

I06.2 Rheumatic aortic stenosis with insufficiency
Rheumatic aortic stenosis with incompetence or regurgitation

I06.8 Other rheumatic aortic valve diseases

I06.9 Rheumatic aortic valve disease, unspecified
Rheumatic aortic (valve) disease NOS

I07 Rheumatic tricuspid valve diseases
Includes rheumatic tricuspid valve diseases specified as rheumatic or unspecified
Excludes1 tricuspid valve disease specified as nonrheumatic (I36.-)
tricuspid valve disease with aortic and/or mitral valve involvement (I08.-)

I07.0 Rheumatic tricuspid stenosis
Tricuspid (valve) stenosis (rheumatic)

I07.1 Rheumatic tricuspid insufficiency
Tricuspid (valve) insufficiency (rheumatic)

I07.2 Rheumatic tricuspid stenosis and insufficiency

I07.8 Other rheumatic tricuspid valve diseases

I07.9 Rheumatic tricuspid valve disease, unspecified
Rheumatic tricuspid valve disorder NOS

I08 Multiple valve diseases
Includes multiple valve diseases specified as rheumatic or unspecified
Excludes1 endocarditis, valve unspecified (I38)
multiple valve disease specified a nonrheumatic (I34.-, I35.-, I36.-, I37.-, I38.-, Q22.-, Q23.-, Q24.8-)
rheumatic valve disease NOS (I09.1)

I08.0 Rheumatic disorders of both mitral and aortic valves
Involvement of both mitral and aortic valves specified as rheumatic or unspecified

I08.1 Rheumatic disorders of both mitral and tricuspid valves

I08.2 Rheumatic disorders of both aortic and tricuspid valves

I08.3 Combined rheumatic disorders of mitral, aortic and tricuspid valves

I08.8 Other rheumatic multiple valve diseases

I08.9 Rheumatic multiple valve disease, unspecified

I09 Other rheumatic heart diseases

I09.0 Rheumatic myocarditis
Excludes1 myocarditis not specified as rheumatic (I51.4)
Ex: I00, I01.2-I01.9, I09.0, I09.9, I23.0-I23.3, I23.6-I23.8, I40.0-I41, I51.0, I51.4, I87.8-I87.9, I99.8-I99.9

I09.1 Rheumatic diseases of endocardium, valve unspecified
Rheumatic endocarditis (chronic)
Rheumatic valvulitis (chronic)
Excludes1 endocarditis, valve unspecified (I38)

I09.2 Chronic rheumatic pericarditis
Adherent pericardium, rheumatic
Chronic rheumatic mediastinopericarditis
Chronic rheumatic myopericarditis
Excludes1 chronic pericarditis not specified as rheumatic (I31.-)
Ex: See I01.0

I09.8 Other specified rheumatic heart diseases

I09.81 Rheumatic heart failure
Use additional code to identify type of heart failure (I50.-)
Ex: I09.81, I09.9, I11.0, I50.1-I50.9, I87.8-I87.9, I99.8-I99.9

I09.89 Other specified rheumatic heart diseases
Rheumatic disease of pulmonary valve

I09.9 Rheumatic heart disease, unspecified
Rheumatic carditis
Excludes1 rheumatoid carditis (M05.31)

Item 9–5 Hypertension is caused by high arterial blood pressure in the arteries. **Essential, primary,** or **idiopathic** hypertension occurs without identifiable organic cause. **Secondary** hypertension is that which has an organic cause. **Malignant** hypertension is severely elevated blood pressure. **Benign** hypertension is mildly elevated blood pressure.

HYPERTENSIVE DISEASES (I10-I16)

Use additional code to identify:
exposure to environmental tobacco smoke (Z77.22)
history of tobacco dependence (Z87.891)
occupational exposure to environmental tobacco smoke (Z57.31)
tobacco dependence (F17.-)
tobacco use (Z72.0)

Excludes1 neonatal hypertension (P29.2)
primary pulmonary hypertension (I27.0)

Excludes2 hypertensive disease complicating pregnancy, childbirth and the puerperium (O10-O11, O13-O16)

I10 Essential (primary) hypertension

Includes high blood pressure
hypertension (arterial) (benign) (essential) (malignant) (primary) (systemic)

Excludes1 hypertensive disease complicating pregnancy, childbirth and the puerperium (O10-O11, O13-O16)

Excludes2 essential (primary) hypertension involving vessels of brain (I60-I69)
essential (primary) hypertension involving vessels of eye (H35.0-)

MCE: Questionable admission when principal dx

I11 Hypertensive heart disease

Includes any condition in I51.4-I51.9 due to hypertension

I11.0 Hypertensive heart disease with heart failure
Hypertensive heart failure
Use additional code to identify type of heart failure (I50.-)

I11.9 Hypertensive heart disease without heart failure
Hypertensive heart disease NOS

OGCR Section I.C.9.a.2

Hypertensive Chronic Kidney Disease

Assign codes from category I12, Hypertensive chronic kidney disease, when both hypertension and a condition classifiable to category N18, Chronic kidney disease (CKD), are present. **CKD should not be coded as hypertensive if the physician has specifically documented a different cause.**

The appropriate code from category N18 should be used as a secondary code with a code from category I12 to identify the stage of chronic kidney disease.

See Section I.C.14. Chronic kidney disease.

If a patient has hypertensive chronic kidney disease and acute renal failure, an additional code for the acute renal failure is required.

I12 Hypertensive chronic kidney disease

Includes any condition in N18 and N26 - due to hypertension
arteriosclerosis of kidney
arteriosclerotic nephritis (chronic) (interstitial)
hypertensive nephropathy
nephrosclerosis

Excludes1 hypertension due to kidney disease (I15.0, I15.1)
renovascular hypertension (I15.0)
secondary hypertension (I15.-)

Excludes2 acute kidney failure (N17.-)

I12.0 Hypertensive chronic kidney disease with stage 5 chronic kidney disease or end stage renal disease
Use additional code to identify the stage of chronic kidney disease (N18.5, N18.6)
Ex: I10-I16.9, I87.8-I87.9, I99.8-I99.9, N18.6, N26.2

I12.9 Hypertensive chronic kidney disease with stage 1 through stage 4 chronic kidney disease, or unspecified chronic kidney disease
Hypertensive chronic kidney disease NOS
Hypertensive renal disease NOS
Use additional code to identify the stage of chronic kidney disease (N18.1-N18.4, N18.9)

OGCR Section I.c.9.a.3

Hypertensive Heart and Chronic Kidney Disease

Assign codes from combination category I13, Hypertensive heart and chronic kidney disease, when **there is hypertension with both heart and kidney involvement.** If heart failure is present, assign an additional code from category I50 to identify the type of heart failure.

The appropriate code from category N18, Chronic kidney disease, should be used as a secondary code with a code from category I13 to identify the stage of chronic kidney disease.

See Section I.C.14. Chronic kidney disease.

The codes in category I13, Hypertensive heart and chronic kidney disease, are combination codes that include hypertension, heart disease and chronic kidney disease. The Includes note at I13 specifies that the conditions included at I11 and I12 are included together in I13. If a patient has hypertension, heart disease and chronic kidney disease then a code from I13 should be used, not individual codes for hypertension, heart disease and chronic kidney disease, or codes from I11 or I12.

For patients with both acute renal failure and chronic kidney disease an additional code for acute renal failure is required.

I13 Hypertensive heart and chronic kidney disease

Includes any condition in I11.- with any condition in I12.-
cardiorenal disease
cardiovascular renal disease

Ex: **For category I13 CC codes:** I10-I16.9, I87.8-I87.9, I99.8-I99.9, N26.2

I13.0 Hypertensive heart and chronic kidney disease with heart failure and stage 1 through stage 4 chronic kidney disease, or unspecified chronic kidney disease
Use additional code to identify type of heart failure (I50.-)
Use additional code to identify stage of chronic kidney disease (N18.1-N18.4, N18.9)

I13.1 Hypertensive heart and chronic kidney disease without heart failure

I13.10 Hypertensive heart and chronic kidney disease without heart failure, with stage 1 through stage 4 chronic kidney disease, or unspecified chronic kidney disease
Hypertensive heart disease and hypertensive chronic kidney disease NOS
Use additional code to identify the stage of chronic kidney disease (N18.1-N18.4, N18.9)

I13.11 Hypertensive heart and chronic kidney disease without heart failure, with stage 5 chronic kidney disease, or end stage renal disease
Use additional code to identify the stage of chronic kidney disease (N18.5, N18.6)

I13.2 Hypertensive heart and chronic kidney disease with heart failure and with stage 5 chronic kidney disease, or end stage renal disease
Use additional code to identify type of heart failure (I50.-)
Use additional code to identify the stage of chronic kidney disease (N18.5, N18.6)

OGCR Section I.9.a.6

Hypertension, Secondary

Secondary hypertension is due to an underlying condition. Two codes are required: one to identify the underlying etiology and one from category I15 to identify the hypertension. Sequencing of codes is determined by the reason for admission/encounter.

I15 Secondary hypertension

Code also underlying condition

Excludes1 postprocedural hypertension (I97.3)

Excludes2 secondary hypertension involving vessels of brain (I60-I69)
secondary hypertension involving vessels of eye (H35.0-)

I15.0 Renovascular hypertension

I15.1 Hypertension secondary to other renal disorders

I15.2 Hypertension secondary to endocrine disorders

I15.8 Other secondary hypertension

I15.9 Secondary hypertension, unspecified

I16 Hypertensive crisis ◀

Code also any identified hypertensive disease (I10-I15) ◀

I16.0 Hypertensive urgency ◀

Ex: No exclusions

I16.1 Hypertensive emergency ◀

I16.9 Hypertensive crisis, unspecified ◀

Ex: No exclusions

ISCHEMIC HEART DISEASES (I20-I25)

Use additional code to identify presence of hypertension (I10-I16)

I20 Angina pectoris

Chest pain/discomfort due to lack of oxygen to the heart muscle. Principal symptom of myocardial infarction.

Use additional code to identify:
exposure to environmental tobacco smoke (Z77.22)
history of tobacco dependence (Z87.891)
occupational exposure to environmental tobacco smoke (Z57.31)
tobacco dependence (F17.-)
tobacco use (Z72.0)

Excludes1 angina pectoris with atherosclerotic heart disease of native coronary arteries (I25.1-)
atherosclerosis of coronary artery bypass graft(s) and coronary artery of transplanted heart with angina pectoris (I25.7-)
postinfarction angina (I23.7)

I20.0 Unstable angina

Accelerated angina
Crescendo angina
De novo effort angina
Intermediate coronary syndrome
Preinfarction syndrome
Worsening effort angina

Ex: I09.81, I11.0, I13.0, I13.2, I20.0-I22.9, I24.0, I24.8-I24.9, I25.5-I25.6, I25.82-I25.83, I25.89-I25.9, I50.1, I50.9, I87.8-I87.9, I99.8-I99.9, R57.0, R57.9

I20.1 Angina pectoris with documented spasm

Angiospastic angina
Prinzmetal angina
Spasm-induced angina
Variant angina

Ex: I20.0-I22.9, I24.0, I24.8-I24.9, I25.5-I25.6, I25.89-I25.9, I87.8-I87.9, I99.8-I99.9

I20.8 Other forms of angina pectoris

Angina equivalent
Angina of effort
Coronary slow flow syndrome
Stable angina ◀
Stenocardia

Use additional code(s) for symptoms associated with angina equivalent

I20.9 Angina pectoris, unspecified

Angina NOS
Anginal syndrome
Cardiac angina
Ischemic chest pain

I21 ST elevation (STEMI) and non-ST elevation (NSTEMI) myocardial infarction

Includes cardiac infarction
coronary (artery) embolism
coronary (artery) occlusion
coronary (artery) rupture
coronary (artery) thrombosis
infarction of heart, myocardium, or ventricle
myocardial infarction specified as acute or with a stated duration of 4 weeks (28 days) or less from onset

Use additional code, if applicable, to identify:
exposure to environmental tobacco smoke (Z77.22)
history of tobacco dependence (Z87.891)
occupational exposure to environmental tobacco smoke (Z57.31)
status post administration of tPA (rtPA) in a different facility within the last 24 hours prior to admission to current facility (Z92.82)
tobacco dependence (F17.-)
tobacco use (Z72.0)

Excludes2 old myocardial infarction (I25.2)
postmyocardial infarction syndrome (I24.1)
subsequent myocardial infarction (I22.-)

Ex: **For category I21 CC codes:** I21.01-I22.9, I87.8-I87.9, I99.8-I99.9

Coding Clinic: 2013, Q1, P25-26; 2012, Q4, P103

I21.0 ST elevation (STEMI) myocardial infarction of anterior wall

Coding Clinic: 2013, Q1, P26

I21.01 ST elevation (STEMI) myocardial infarction involving left main coronary artery

I21.02 ST elevation (STEMI) myocardial infarction involving left anterior descending coronary artery

ST elevation (STEMI) myocardial infarction involving diagonal coronary artery

Coding Clinic: 2013, Q1, P26

I21.09 ST elevation (STEMI) myocardial infarction involving other coronary artery of anterior wall

Acute transmural myocardial infarction of anterior wall
Anteroapical transmural (Q wave) infarction (acute)
Anterolateral transmural (Q wave) infarction (acute)
Anteroseptal transmural (Q wave) infarction (acute)
Transmural (Q wave) infarction (acute) (of) anterior (wall) NOS

Coding Clinic: 2012, Q4, P102, 104

● **I21.1 ST elevation (STEMI) myocardial infarction of inferior wall**
Coding Clinic: 2013, Q1, P26

I21.11 ST elevation (STEMI) myocardial infarction involving right coronary artery
Inferoposterior transmural (Q wave) infarction (acute)

I21.19 ST elevation (STEMI) myocardial infarction involving other coronary artery of inferior wall
Acute transmural myocardial infarction of inferior wall
Inferolateral transmural (Q wave) infarction (acute)
Transmural (Q wave) infarction (acute) (of) diaphragmatic wall
Transmural (Q wave) infarction (acute) (of) inferior (wall) NOS

Excludes2 ST elevation (STEMI) myocardial infarction involving left circumflex coronary artery (I21.21)

Coding Clinic: 2012, Q4, P97

● **I21.2 ST elevation (STEMI) myocardial infarction of other sites**
Ex: For category I21.2 CC codes: I21.01-I22.9, I87.8-I87.9, I99.8-I99.9
Coding Clinic: 2013, Q1, P26

I21.21 ST elevation (STEMI) myocardial infarction involving left circumflex coronary artery
ST elevation (STEMI) myocardial infarction involving oblique marginal coronary artery

I21.29 ST elevation (STEMI) myocardial infarction involving other sites
Acute transmural myocardial infarction of other sites
Apical-lateral transmural (Q wave) infarction (acute)
Basal-lateral transmural (Q wave) infarction (acute)
High lateral transmural (Q wave) infarction (acute)
Lateral (wall) NOS transmural (Q wave) infarction (acute)
Posterior (true) transmural (Q wave) infarction (acute)
Posterobasal transmural (Q wave) infarction (acute)
Posterolateral transmural (Q wave) infarction (acute)
Posteroseptal transmural (Q wave) infarction (acute)
Septal transmural (Q wave) infarction (acute) NOS

OGCR Section I.c.9.e.2

Acute myocardial infarction, unspecified
Code I21.3, ST elevation (STEMI) myocordial infarction of unspecified site, is the default for unspecified acute myocardial infarction. If only STEMI or transmural MI without the site is documented, assign I21.3.

I21.3 ST elevation (STEMI) myocardial infarction of unspecified site
Acute transmural myocardial infarction of unspecified site
Myocardial infarction (acute) NOS
Transmural (Q wave) myocardial infarction NOS
Ex: I21.01-I22.9, I87.8-I87.9, I99.8-I99.9
Coding Clinic: 2013, Q1, P26

I21.4 Non-ST elevation (NSTEMI) myocardial infarction
Acute subendocardial myocardial infarction
Non-Q wave myocardial infarction NOS
Nontransmural myocardial infarction NOS
Ex: I21.01-I22.9, I87.8-I87.9, I99.8-I99.9
Coding Clinic: 2015, Q2, P16; 2013, Q1, P26

● **I22 Subsequent ST elevation (STEMI) and non-ST elevation (NSTEMI) myocardial infarction**

Includes acute myocardial infarction occurring within four weeks (28 days) of a previous acute myocardial infarction, regardless of site
cardiac infarction
coronary (artery) embolism
coronary (artery) occlusion
coronary (artery) rupture
coronary (artery) thrombosis
infarction of heart, myocardium, or ventricle
recurrent myocardial infarction
reinfarction of myocardium
rupture of heart, myocardium, or ventricle

Use additional code, if applicable, to identify:
exposure to environmental tobacco smoke (Z77.22)
history of tobacco dependence (Z87.891)
occupational exposure to environmental tobacco smoke (Z57.31)
status post administration of tPA (rtPA) in a different facility within the last 24 hours prior to admission to current facility (Z92.82)
tobacco dependence (F17.-)
tobacco use (Z72.0)
Ex: For category I22 CC codes: I21.01-I22.9, I87.8-I87.9, I99.8-I99.9
Coding Clinic: 2013, Q1, P25; 2012, Q4, P103

I22.0 Subsequent ST elevation (STEMI) myocardial infarction of anterior wall
Subsequent acute transmural myocardial infarction of anterior wall
Subsequent transmural (Q wave) infarction (acute)(of) anterior (wall) NOS
Subsequent anteroapical transmural (Q wave) infarction (acute)
Subsequent anterolateral transmural (Q wave) infarction (acute)
Subsequent anteroseptal transmural (Q wave) infarction (acute)

I22.1 Subsequent ST elevation (STEMI) myocardial infarction of inferior wall
Subsequent acute transmural myocardial infarction of inferior wall
Subsequent transmural (Q wave) infarction (acute)(of) diaphragmatic wall
Subsequent transmural (Q wave) infarction (acute)(of) inferior (wall) NOS
Subsequent inferolateral transmural (Q wave) infarction (acute)
Subsequent inferoposterior transmural (Q wave) infarction (acute)
Coding Clinic: 2012, Q4, P97, 102, 104

I22.2 Subsequent non-ST elevation (NSTEMI) myocardial infarction
Subsequent acute subendocardial myocardial infarction
Subsequent non-Q wave myocardial infarction NOS
Subsequent nontransmural myocardial infarction NOS

I22.8 Subsequent ST elevation (STEMI) myocardial infarction of other sites
Subsequent acute transmural myocardial infarction of other sites
Subsequent apical-lateral transmural (Q wave) myocardial infarction (acute)
Subsequent basal-lateral transmural (Q wave) myocardial infarction (acute)
Subsequent high lateral transmural (Q wave) myocardial infarction (acute)
Subsequent transmural (Q wave) myocardial infarction (acute)(of) lateral (wall) NOS
Subsequent posterior (true) transmural (Q wave) myocardial infarction (acute)
Subsequent posterobasal transmural (Q wave) myocardial infarction (acute)
Subsequent posterolateral transmural (Q wave) myocardial infarction (acute)
Subsequent posteroseptal transmural (Q wave) myocardial infarction (acute)
Subsequent septal NOS transmural (Q wave) myocardial infarction (acute)

I22.9 Subsequent ST elevation (STEMI) myocardial infarction of unspecified site
Subsequent acute myocardial infarction of unspecified site
Subsequent myocardial infarction (acute) NOS

I23 Certain current complications following ST elevation (STEMI) and non-ST elevation (NSTEMI) myocardial infarction (within the 28 day period)
Ex For category I23 CC codes unless otherwise indicated: E78.71-E78.72, I23.0-I23.8, I40.0-I41, I51.0-I51.2, I51.4, I87.8-I87.9, I97.0-I97.191, I99.8-I99.9, P29.3, Q20.0-Q21.9, Q23.8-Q23.9, Q24.8-Q24.9, Q27.30, Q27.4, Q28.0-Q28.1, Q28.8-Q28.9, Q87.1-Q87.89, Q89.7-Q89.8, Q99.2

I23.0 Hemopericardium as current complication following acute myocardial infarction A
Excludes1 hemopericardium not specified as current complication following acute myocardial infarction (I31.2)

I23.1 Atrial septal defect as current complication following acute myocardial infarction A
Excludes1 acquired atrial septal defect not specified as current complication following acute myocardial infarction (I51.0)

I23.2 Ventricular septal defect as current complication following acute myocardial infarction A
Excludes1 acquired ventricular septal defect not specified as current complication following acute myocardial infarction (I51.0)

I23.3 Rupture of cardiac wall without hemopericardium as current complication following acute myocardial infarction A

I23.4 Rupture of chordae tendineae as current complication following acute myocardial infarction
Excludes1 rupture of chordae tendineae not specified as current complication following acute myocardial infarction (I51.1)
Ex I23.0-I23.4, I23.6-I23.8, I51.0-I51.1, I87.8-I87.9, I99.8-I99.9

I23.5 Rupture of papillary muscle as current complication following acute myocardial infarction
Excludes1 rupture of papillary muscle not specified as current complication following acute myocardial infarction (I51.2)
Ex I23.0-I23.3, I23.5-I23.8, I51.0, I51.2, I87.8-I87.9, I99.8-I99.9

I23.6 Thrombosis of atrium, auricular appendage, and ventricle as current complications following acute myocardial infarction A
Excludes1 thrombosis of atrium, auricular appendage, and ventricle not specified as current complication following acute myocardial infarction (I51.3)

I23.7 Postinfarction angina A
Coding Clinic: 2015, Q2, P16-17

I23.8 Other current complications following acute myocardial infarction A

I24 Other acute ischemic heart diseases
Excludes1 angina pectoris (I20.-)
transient myocardial ischemia in newborn (P29.4)
Ex For category I24 CC codes unless otherwise indicated: I20.0-I22.9, I24.0-I24.9, I25.5-I25.6, I25.89-I25.9, I87.8-I87.9, I99.8-I99.9

I24.0 Acute coronary thrombosis not resulting in myocardial infarction
Acute coronary (artery) (vein) embolism not resulting in myocardial infarction
Acute coronary (artery) (vein) occlusion not resulting in myocardial infarction
Acute coronary (artery) (vein) thromboembolism not resulting in myocardial infarction
Excludes1 atherosclerotic heart disease (I25.1-)
Coding Clinic: 2013, Q1, P24

I24.1 Dressler's syndrome
Postmyocardial infarction syndrome
Excludes1 postinfarction angina (I23.7)
Ex I24.0-I24.9, I87.8-I87.9, I99.8-I99.9

I24.8 Other forms of acute ischemic heart disease

I24.9 Acute ischemic heart disease, unspecified
Excludes1 ischemic heart disease (chronic) NOS (I25.9)

I25 Chronic ischemic heart disease
Use additional code to identify:
chronic total occlusion of coronary artery (I25.82)
exposure to environmental tobacco smoke (Z77.22)
history of tobacco dependence (Z87.891)
occupational exposure to environmental tobacco smoke (Z57.31)
tobacco dependence (F17.-)
tobacco use (Z72.0)

★ **(See Plates 218 and 219 on pages 74 and 75.)**

I25.1 Atherosclerotic heart disease of native coronary artery
Disease in which fatty deposits form on the walls of arteries
Atherosclerotic cardiovascular disease
Coronary (artery) atheroma
Coronary (artery) atherosclerosis
Coronary (artery) disease
Coronary (artery) sclerosis
Use additional code, if applicable, to identify:
coronary atherosclerosis due to calcified coronary lesion (I25.84)
coronary atherosclerosis due to lipid rich plaque (I25.83)
Excludes2 atheroembolism (I75.-)
atherosclerosis of coronary artery bypass graft(s) and transplanted heart (I25.7-)

I25.10 Atherosclerotic heart disease of native coronary artery without angina pectoris A
Atherosclerotic heart disease NOS
Coding Clinic: 2015, Q2, P17; 2012, Q4, P92

Item 9–6 Classification is based on the location of the atherosclerosis. **"Of native coronary artery"** indicates the atherosclerosis is within an original heart artery. **"Of autologous vein bypass graft"** indicates that the atherosclerosis is within a vein graft that was taken from within the patient. **"Of nonautologous biological bypass graft"** indicates the atherosclerosis is within a vessel grafted from other than the patient. **"Of artery bypass graft"** indicates the atherosclerosis is within an artery that was grafted from within the patient.

OGCR See Section I.9.b.

Atherosclerotic Coronary Artery Disease and Angina

ICD-10-CM has combination codes for atherosclerotic heart disease with angina pectoris. The subcategories for these codes are I25.11, Atherosclerotic heart disease of native coronary artery with angina pectoris and I25.7, Atherosclerosis of coronary artery bypass graft(s) and coronary artery of transplanted heart with angina pectoris.

When using one of these combination codes it is not necessary to use an additional code for angina pectoris. A causal relationship can be assumed in a patient with both atherosclerosis and angina pectoris, unless the documentation indicates the angina is due to something other than the atherosclerosis.

If a patient with coronary artery disease is admitted due to an acute myocardial infarction (AMI), the AMI should be sequenced before the coronary artery disease.

See Section I.C.9. Acute myocardial infarction (AMI)

I25.11 Atherosclerotic heart disease of native coronary artery with angina pectoris

I25.110 Atherosclerotic heart disease of native coronary artery with unstable angina pectoris A

Excludes1 unstable angina without atherosclerotic heart disease (I20.0)

CC when PDx is its own CC

Ex: See I20.0

I25.111 Atherosclerotic heart disease of native coronary artery with angina pectoris with documented spasm A

Excludes1 angina pectoris with documented spasm without atherosclerotic heart disease (I20.1)

I25.118 Atherosclerotic heart disease of native coronary artery with other forms of angina pectoris A

Excludes1 other forms of angina pectoris without atherosclerotic heart disease (I20.8)

Coding Clinic: 2015, Q2, P16-17

I25.119 Atherosclerotic heart disease of native coronary artery with unspecified angina pectoris A

Atherosclerotic heart disease with angina NOS

Atherosclerotic heart disease with ischemic chest pain

Excludes1 unspecified angina pectoris without atherosclerotic heart disease (I20.9)

I25.2 Old myocardial infarction

Healed myocardial infarction

Past myocardial infarction diagnosed by ECG or other investigation, but currently presenting no symptoms

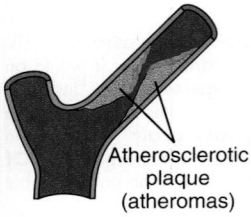

Figure 9-2 Atherosclerotic plaque.

I25.3 Aneurysm of heart

Mural aneurysm

Ventricular aneurysm

Ex: I25.3-I25.41

I25.4 Coronary artery aneurysm and dissection

I25.41 Coronary artery aneurysm

Coronary arteriovenous fistula, acquired

Excludes1 congenital coronary (artery) aneurysm (Q24.5)

I25.42 Coronary artery dissection

Ex: I25.42, I67.0, I77.2-I77.3, I77.5-I77.6, I77.70, I77.75-I77.79, I77.89-I77.9, M31.8-M31.9

I25.5 Ischemic cardiomyopathy

Excludes2 coronary atherosclerosis (I25.1-, I25.7-)

I25.6 Silent myocardial ischemia

I25.7 Atherosclerosis of coronary artery bypass graft(s) and coronary artery of transplanted heart with angina pectoris

Use additional code, if applicable, to identify:

coronary atherosclerosis due to calcified coronary lesion (I25.84)

coronary atherosclerosis due to lipid rich plaque (I25.83)

Excludes1 atherosclerosis of bypass graft(s) of transplanted heart without angina pectoris (I25.812)

atherosclerosis of coronary artery bypass graft(s) without angina pectoris (I25.810)

atherosclerosis of native coronary artery of transplanted heart without angina pectoris (I25.811)

embolism or thrombus of coronary artery bypass graft(s) (T82.8-)

I25.70 Atherosclerosis of coronary artery bypass graft(s), unspecified, with angina pectoris

I25.700 Atherosclerosis of coronary artery bypass graft(s), unspecified, with unstable angina pectoris A

Excludes1 unstable angina pectoris without atherosclerosis of coronary artery bypass graft (I20.0)

CC when PDx is its own CC

Ex: See I20.0

I25.701 Atherosclerosis of coronary artery bypass graft(s), unspecified, with angina pectoris with documented spasm A

Excludes1 angina pectoris with documented spasm without atherosclerosis of coronary artery bypass graft (I20.1)

I25.708 Atherosclerosis of coronary artery bypass graft(s), unspecified, with other forms of angina pectoris A

Excludes1 other forms of angina pectoris without atherosclerosis of coronary artery bypass graft (I20.8)

I25.709 Atherosclerosis of coronary artery bypass graft(s), unspecified, with unspecified angina pectoris A

Excludes1 unspecified angina pectoris without atherosclerosis of coronary artery bypass graft (I20.9)

● **I25.71 Atherosclerosis of autologous vein coronary artery bypass graft(s) with angina pectoris**

Ex For category I25.71 CC codes unless otherwise indicated: I25.10-I25.119, I25.700-I25.739, I25.760-I25.799, I25.812-I25.84

I25.710 Atherosclerosis of autologous vein coronary artery bypass graft(s) with unstable angina pectoris A

Excludes1 unstable angina without atherosclerosis of autologous vein coronary artery bypass graft(s) (I20.0)

CC when PDx is its own CC

Ex I09.81, I11.0, I13.0, I13.2, I20.0-I22.9, I24.0, I24.8-I25.119, I25.5-I25.739, I25.760-I25.799, I25.812-I25.9, I50.1, I50.9, I87.8-I87.9, I99.8-I99.9, R57.0, R57.9

I25.711 Atherosclerosis of autologous vein coronary artery bypass graft(s) with angina pectoris with documented spasm A

Excludes1 angina pectoris with documented spasm without atherosclerosis of autologous vein coronary artery bypass graft(s) (I20.1)

I25.718 Atherosclerosis of autologous vein coronary artery bypass graft(s) with other forms of angina pectoris A

Excludes1 other forms of angina pectoris without atherosclerosis of autologous vein coronary artery bypass graft(s) (I20.8)

I25.719 Atherosclerosis of autologous vein coronary artery bypass graft(s) with unspecified angina pectoris A

Excludes1 unspecified angina pectoris without atherosclerosis of autologous vein coronary artery bypass graft(s) (I20.9)

● **I25.72 Atherosclerosis of autologous artery coronary artery bypass graft(s) with angina pectoris**

Atherosclerosis of internal mammary artery graft with angina pectoris

Ex For category I25.72 CC codes unless otherwise indicated: See I25.71

I25.720 Atherosclerosis of autologous artery coronary artery bypass graft(s) with unstable angina pectoris A

Excludes1 unstable angina without atherosclerosis of autologous artery coronary artery bypass graft(s) (I20.0)

CC when PDx is its own CC

Ex See I25.710

I25.721 Atherosclerosis of autologous artery coronary artery bypass graft(s) with angina pectoris with documented spasm A

Excludes1 angina pectoris with documented spasm without atherosclerosis of autologous artery coronary artery bypass graft(s) (I20.1)

I25.728 Atherosclerosis of autologous artery coronary artery bypass graft(s) with other forms of angina pectoris A

Excludes1 other forms of angina pectoris without atherosclerosis of autologous artery coronary artery bypass graft(s) (I20.8)

I25.729 Atherosclerosis of autologous artery coronary artery bypass graft(s) with unspecified angina pectoris A

Excludes1 unspecified angina pectoris without atherosclerosis of autologous artery coronary artery bypass graft(s) (I20.9)

● **I25.73 Atherosclerosis of nonautologous biological coronary artery bypass graft(s) with angina pectoris**

Ex For category I25.73 CC codes unless otherwise indicated: See I25.71

I25.730 Atherosclerosis of nonautologous biological coronary artery bypass graft(s) with unstable angina pectoris A

Excludes1 unstable angina without atherosclerosis of nonautologous biological coronary artery bypass graft(s) (I20.0)

CC when PDx is its own CC

Ex See I25.710

I25.731 Atherosclerosis of nonautologous biological coronary artery bypass graft(s) with angina pectoris with documented spasm A

Excludes1 angina pectoris with documented spasm without atherosclerosis of nonautologous biological coronary artery bypass graft(s) (I20.1)

I25.738 Atherosclerosis of nonautologous biological coronary artery bypass graft(s) with other forms of angina pectoris A

Excludes1 other forms of angina pectoris without atherosclerosis of nonautologous biological coronary artery bypass graft(s) (I20.8)

I25.739 Atherosclerosis of nonautologous biological coronary artery bypass graft(s) with unspecified angina pectoris A

Excludes1 unspecified angina pectoris without atherosclerosis of nonautologous biological coronary artery bypass graft(s) (I20.9)

● **I25.75 Atherosclerosis of native coronary artery of transplanted heart with angina pectoris**

Excludes1 atherosclerosis of native coronary artery of transplanted heart without angina pectoris (I25.811)

Ex: For category I25.75 CC codes unless otherwise indicated: I25.10-I25.119, I25.700-I25.799, I25.811-I25.84

I25.750 Atherosclerosis of native coronary artery of transplanted heart with unstable angina

CC when PDx is its own CC

Ex: I09.81, I11.0, I13.0, I13.2, I20.0-I22.9, I24.0, I24.8-I25.119, I25.5-I25.799, I25.811-I25.9, I50.1, I50.9, I87.8-I87.9, I99.8-I99.9, R57.0, R57.9

I25.751 Atherosclerosis of native coronary artery of transplanted heart with angina pectoris with documented spasm

I25.758 Atherosclerosis of native coronary artery of transplanted heart with other forms of angina pectoris

I25.759 Atherosclerosis of native coronary artery of transplanted heart with unspecified angina pectoris

● **I25.76 Atherosclerosis of bypass graft of coronary artery of transplanted heart with angina pectoris**

Excludes1 atherosclerosis of bypass graft of coronary artery of transplanted heart without angina pectoris (I25.812)

Ex: For category I25.76 CC codes unless otherwise indicated: I25.10-I25.119, I25.700-I25.759, I25.790-I25.799, I25.811, I25.82-I25.84

I25.760 Atherosclerosis of bypass graft of coronary artery of transplanted heart with unstable angina A

CC when PDx is its own CC

Ex: I09.81, I11.0, I13.0, I13.2, I20.0-I22.9, I24.0, I24.8-I25.119, I25.5-I25.759, I25.790-I25.799, I25.811, I25.82-I25.9, I50.1, I50.9, I87.8-I87.9, I99.8-I99.9, R57.0, R57.9

I25.761 Atherosclerosis of bypass graft of coronary artery of transplanted heart with angina pectoris with documented spasm A

I25.768 Atherosclerosis of bypass graft of coronary artery of transplanted heart with other forms of angina pectoris A

I25.769 Atherosclerosis of bypass graft of coronary artery of transplanted heart with unspecified angina pectoris A

● **I25.79 Atherosclerosis of other coronary artery bypass graft(s) with angina pectoris** A

Ex: For category I25.79 CC codes unless otherwise indicated: No exclusions

I25.790 Atherosclerosis of other coronary artery bypass graft(s) with unstable angina pectoris

Excludes1 unstable angina without atherosclerosis of other coronary artery bypass graft(s) (I20.0)

CC when PDx is its own CC

Ex: See I20.0

I25.791 Atherosclerosis of other coronary artery bypass graft(s) with angina pectoris with documented spasm A

Excludes1 angina pectoris with documented spasm without atherosclerosis of other coronary artery bypass graft(s) (I20.1)

I25.798 Atherosclerosis of other coronary artery bypass graft(s) with other forms of angina pectoris A

Excludes1 other forms of angina pectoris without atherosclerosis of other coronary artery bypass graft(s) (I20.8)

I25.799 Atherosclerosis of other coronary artery bypass graft(s) with unspecified angina pectoris A

Excludes1 unspecified angina pectoris without atherosclerosis of other coronary artery bypass graft(s) (I20.9)

● **I25.8 Other forms of chronic ischemic heart disease**

● **I25.81 Atherosclerosis of other coronary vessels without angina pectoris**

Use additional code, if applicable, to identify:
coronary atherosclerosis due to calcified coronary lesion (I25.84)
coronary atherosclerosis due to lipid rich plaque (I25.83)

Excludes1 atherosclerotic heart disease of native coronary artery without angina pectoris (I25.10)

I25.810 Atherosclerosis of coronary artery bypass graft(s) without angina pectoris A

Atherosclerosis of coronary artery bypass graft NOS

Excludes1 atherosclerosis of coronary bypass graft(s) with angina pectoris (I25.70- -I25.73-, I25.79-)

Ex: No exclusions

I25.811 Atherosclerosis of native coronary artery of transplanted heart without angina pectoris

Atherosclerosis of native coronary artery of transplanted heart NOS

Excludes1 atherosclerosis of native coronary artery of transplanted heart with angina pectoris (I25.75-)

Ex: See I25.75

I25.812 Atherosclerosis of bypass graft of coronary artery of transplanted heart without angina pectoris A
Atherosclerosis of bypass graft of transplanted heart NOS
Excludes1 atherosclerosis of bypass graft of transplanted heart with angina pectoris (I25.76)

● **I25.82 Chronic total occlusion of coronary artery**
Complete occlusion of coronary artery
Total occlusion of coronary artery
Code first coronary atherosclerosis (I25.1-, I25.7-, I25.81-)
Excludes1 acute coronary occulsion with myocardial infarction (I21.-, I22.-)
acute coronary occulsion without myocardial infarction (I24.0)
Ex: See I25.76

● **I25.83 Coronary atherosclerosis due to lipid rich plaque** A
Code first coronary atherosclerosis (I25.1-, I25.7-, I25.81-)

● **I25.84 Coronary atherosclerosis due to calcified coronary lesion**
Coronary atherosclerosis due to severely calcified coronary lesion
Code first coronary atherosclerosis (I25.1-, I25.7-, I25.81-)

I25.89 Other forms of chronic ischemic heart disease

I25.9 Chronic ischemic heart disease, unspecified
Ischemic heart disease (chronic) NOS

PULMONARY HEART DISEASE AND DISEASES OF PULMONARY CIRCULATION (I26-I28)

● **I26 Pulmonary embolism**
Includes pulmonary (acute)(artery)(vein) infarction
pulmonary (acute)(artery)(vein) thromboembolism
pulmonary (acute)(artery)(vein) thrombosis
Excludes2 chronic pulmonary embolism (I27.82)
personal history of pulmonary embolism (Z86.711)
pulmonary embolism due to trauma (T79.0, T79.1)
pulmonary embolism due to complications of surgical and medical care (T80.0, T81.7-, T82.8-)
pulmonary embolism complicating abortion, ectopic or molar pregnancy (O00-O07, O08.2)
pulmonary embolism complicating pregnancy, childbirth and the puerperium (O88.-)
septic (non-pulmonary) arterial embolism (I76)

● **I26.0 Pulmonary embolism with acute cor pulmonale**
Ex: **For category I26.0 CC codes:** I26.01-I26.99, I27.2-I27.9, I74.01-I74.10, I74.19, I87.8-I87.9, I99.8-I99.9

● **I26.01 Septic pulmonary embolism with acute cor pulmonale**
Code first underlying infection
MCC when PDx is its own MCC

I26.02 Saddle embolus of pulmonary artery with acute cor pulmonale
MCC when PDx is its own MCC

I26.09 Other pulmonary embolism with acute cor pulmonale
Acute cor pulmonale NOS
MCC when PDx is its own MCC

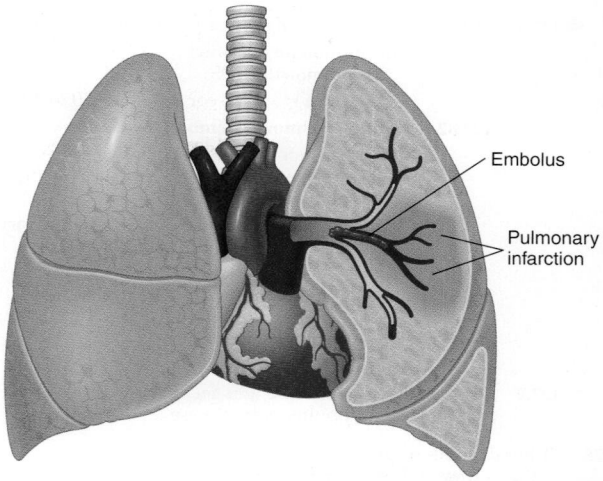

Figure 9-3 Pulmonary Embolism. (From Chabner: The Language of Medicine, ed 8, St. Louis, Saunders, 2007)

Item 9–7 Pulmonary heart disease or **cor pulmonale** is right ventricle hypertrophy or RVH as a result of a respiratory disorder increasing back flow pressure to the right ventricle. Left untreated, cor pulmonale leads to right-heart failure and death.

● **I26.9 Pulmonary embolism without acute cor pulmonale**

● **I26.90 Septic pulmonary embolism without acute cor pulmonale**
Code first underlying infection
Ex: I26.01-I26.99, I27.82, I74.01-I74.10, I74.19, I87.8-I87.9, I99.8-I99.9, T80.0XX[A], T81.718[A], T81.72X[A,] T82.817-T82.818[A]

I26.92 Saddle embolus of pulmonary artery without acute cor pulmonale
Ex: I26.01-I26.99, I27.82, I74.01-I74.10, I74.19, I87.8-I87.9, I99.8-I99.9

I26.99 Other pulmonary embolism without acute cor pulmonale
Acute pulmonary embolism NOS
Pulmonary embolism NOS
Ex: I26.01-I26.99, I27.82, I74.01-I74.10, I74.19, I87.8-I87.9, I99.8-I99.9, T80.0XX[A], T81.718[A], T81.72X[A], T82.817-T82.818[A]

● **I27 Other pulmonary heart diseases**

I27.0 Primary pulmonary hypertension
Excludes1 pulmonary hypertension NOS (I27.2)
secondary pulmonary hypertension (I27.2)
Ex: E66.2, I27.0, I27.2-I27.81, I27.89-I27.9, I28.8-I28.9, I87.8-I87.9, I99.8-I99.9

I27.1 Kyphoscoliotic heart disease
Ex: E66.2, I27.0-I27.81, I27.89-I27.9

I27.2 Other secondary pulmonary hypertension
Pulmonary hypertension NOS
Code also associated underlying condition
Coding Clinic: 2016, Q2, P8

● **I27.8 Other specified pulmonary heart diseases**

I27.81 Cor pulmonale (chronic)
Cor pulmonale NOS
Excludes1 acute cor pulmonale (I26.0-)

I27.82 Chronic pulmonary embolism
Use additional code, if applicable, for associated long-term (current) use of anticoagulants (Z79.01)
Excludes1 personal history of pulmonary embolism (Z86.711)
Ex: See I26.92

I27.89 Other specified pulmonary heart diseases
Eisenmenger's complex
Eisenmenger's syndrome
Excludes1 Eisenmenger's defect (Q21.8)

I27.9 Pulmonary heart disease, unspecified
Chronic cardiopulmonary disease

● **I28 Other diseases of pulmonary vessels**
Ex: For category I28 CC codes: I28.0-I28.9

I28.0 Arteriovenous fistula of pulmonary vessels
Excludes1 congenital arteriovenous fistula (Q25.72)

I28.1 Aneurysm of pulmonary artery
Excludes1 congenital aneurysm (Q25.79)
congenital arteriovenous aneurysm (Q25.72)

I28.8 Other diseases of pulmonary vessels
Pulmonary arteritis
Pulmonary endarteritis
Rupture of pulmonary vessels
Stenosis of pulmonary vessels
Stricture of pulmonary vessels

I28.9 Disease of pulmonary vessels, unspecified

OTHER FORMS OF HEART DISEASE (I30-I52)

● **I30 Acute pericarditis**
Inflammation of pericardium (sac surrounding the heart) caused by an infection
Includes acute mediastinopericarditis
acute myopericarditis
acute pericardial effusion
acute pleuropericarditis
acute pneumopericarditis
Excludes1 Dressler's syndrome (I24.1)
rheumatic pericarditis (acute) (I01.0)
Ex: For category I30 CC codes: I01.0, I09.2, I30.0-I30.9, I31.3-I32, I87.8-I87.9, I99.8-I99.9

I30.0 Acute nonspecific idiopathic pericarditis

I30.1 Infective pericarditis
Pneumococcal pericarditis
Pneumopyopericardium
Purulent pericarditis
Pyopericarditis
Pyopericardium
Pyopneumopericardium
Staphylococcal pericarditis
Streptococcal pericarditis
Suppurative pericarditis
Viral pericarditis
Use additional code (B95-B97) to identify infectious agent

I30.8 Other forms of acute pericarditis

I30.9 Acute pericarditis, unspecified

● **I31 Other diseases of pericardium**
Excludes1 diseases of pericardium specified as rheumatic (I09.2)
postcardiotomy syndrome (I97.0)
traumatic injury to pericardium (S26.-)
Ex: For category I31 CC codes unless otherwise indicated: B33.23, I01.0, I09.2, I30.0-I30.9, I31.3-I32, I87.8-I87.9, I99.8-I99.9

I31.0 Chronic adhesive pericarditis
Accretio cordis
Adherent pericardium
Adhesive mediastinopericarditis
Ex: I31.0-I31.9, I87.8, I99.8-I99.9

I31.1 Chronic constrictive pericarditis
Concretio cordis
Pericardial calcification
Ex: I31.0-I31.9, I87.8, I99.8-I99.9

I31.2 Hemopericardium, not elsewhere classified
Excludes1 hemopericardium as current complication following acute myocardial infarction (I23.0)
Ex: I31.0-I31.9, I87.8, I99.8-I99.9

I31.3 Pericardial effusion (noninflammatory)
Chylopericardium
Excludes1 acute pericardial effusion (I30.9)

● **I31.4 Cardiac tamponade**
Code first underlying cause

I31.8 Other specified diseases of pericardium
Epicardial plaques
Focal pericardial adhesions

I31.9 Disease of pericardium, unspecified
Pericarditis (chronic) NOS

▶ ***I32 Pericarditis in diseases classified elsewhere***
Code first underlying disease
Excludes1 pericarditis (in):
coxsackie (virus) (B33.23)
gonococcal (A54.83)
meningococcal (A39.53)
rheumatoid (arthritis) (M05.31)
syphilitic (A52.06)
systemic lupus erythematosus (M32.12)
tuberculosis (A18.84)
Ex: See I30

● **I33 Acute and subacute endocarditis**
Inflammation/infection of lining of heart, affecting heart valves including replacement valves and is usually caused by a bacterial infection
Excludes1 acute rheumatic endocarditis (I01.1)
endocarditis NOS (I38)
Ex: For category I33 CC codes: I01.1, I08.1-I08.3, I09.1, I33.0-I33.9, I38-I39, I87.8-I87.9, I99.8-I99.9

I33.0 Acute and subacute infective endocarditis
Bacterial endocarditis (acute) (subacute)
Infective endocarditis (acute) (subacute) NOS
Endocarditis lenta (acute) (subacute)
Malignant endocarditis (acute) (subacute)
Purulent endocarditis (acute) (subacute)
Septic endocarditis (acute) (subacute)
Ulcerative endocarditis (acute) (subacute)
Vegetative endocarditis (acute) (subacute)
Use additional code (B95-B97) to identify infectious agent

I33.9 Acute and subacute endocarditis, unspecified
Acute endocarditis NOS
Acute myoendocarditis NOS
Acute periendocarditis NOS
Subacute endocarditis NOS
Subacute myoendocarditis NOS
Subacute periendocarditis NOS

I34 Nonrheumatic mitral valve disorders

Excludes1 mitral valve disease (I05.9)
mitral valve failure (I05.8)
mitral valve stenosis (I05.0)
mitral valve disorder of unspecified cause with diseases of aortic and/or tricuspid valve(s) (I08.-)
mitral valve disorder of unspecified cause with mitral stenosis or obstruction (I05.0)
mitral valve disorder specified as congenital (Q23.2, Q23.3)
mitral valve disorder specified as rheumatic (I05.-)

I34.0 Nonrheumatic mitral (valve) insufficiency
Nonrheumatic mitral (valve) incompetence NOS
Nonrheumatic mitral (valve) regurgitation NOS

I34.1 Nonrheumatic mitral (valve) prolapse
Floppy nonrheumatic mitral valve syndrome
Excludes1 Marfan's syndrome (Q87.4-)

I34.2 Nonrheumatic mitral (valve) stenosis

I34.8 Other nonrheumatic mitral valve disorders

I34.9 Nonrheumatic mitral valve disorder, unspecified

I35 Nonrheumatic aortic valve disorders

Excludes1 aortic valve disorder of unspecified cause but with diseases of mitral and/or tricuspid valve(s) (I08.-)
aortic valve disorder specified as congenital (Q23.0, Q23.1)
aortic valve disorder specified as rheumatic (I06.-)
hypertrophic subaortic stenosis (I42.1)

I35.0 Nonrheumatic aortic (valve) stenosis

I35.1 Nonrheumatic aortic (valve) insufficiency
Nonrheumatic aortic (valve) incompetence NOS
Nonrheumatic aortic (valve) regurgitation NOS

I35.2 Nonrheumatic aortic (valve) stenosis with insufficiency

I35.8 Other nonrheumatic aortic valve disorders

I35.9 Nonrheumatic aortic valve disorder, unspecified

I36 Nonrheumatic tricuspid valve disorders

Excludes1 tricuspid valve disorders of unspecified cause (I07.-)
tricuspid valve disorders specified as congenital (Q22.4, Q22.8, Q22.9)
tricuspid valve disorders specified as rheumatic (I07.-)
tricuspid valve disorders with aortic and/or mitral valve involvement (I08.-)

I36.0 Nonrheumatic tricuspid (valve) stenosis

I36.1 Nonrheumatic tricuspid (valve) insufficiency
Nonrheumatic tricuspid (valve) incompetence
Nonrheumatic tricuspid (valve) regurgitation

I36.2 Nonrheumatic tricuspid (valve) stenosis with insufficiency

I36.8 Other nonrheumatic tricuspid valve disorders

I36.9 Nonrheumatic tricuspid valve disorder, unspecified

I37 Nonrheumatic pulmonary valve disorders

Excludes1 pulmonary valve disorder specified as congenital (Q22.1, Q22.2, Q22.3)
pulmonary valve disorder specified as rheumatic (I09.89)

I37.0 Nonrheumatic pulmonary valve stenosis

I37.1 Nonrheumatic pulmonary valve insufficiency
Nonrheumatic pulmonary valve incompetence
Nonrheumatic pulmonary valve regurgitation

I37.2 Nonrheumatic pulmonary valve stenosis with insufficiency

I37.8 Other nonrheumatic pulmonary valve disorders

I37.9 Nonrheumatic pulmonary valve disorder, unspecified

I38 Endocarditis, valve unspecified

Includes endocarditis (chronic) NOS
valvular incompetence NOS
valvular insufficiency NOS
valvular regurgitation NOS
valvular stenosis NOS
valvulitis (chronic) NOS

Excludes1 congenital insufficiency of cardiac valve NOS (Q24.8)
congenital stenosis of cardiac valve NOS (Q24.8)
endocardial fibroelastosis (I42.4)
endocarditis specified as rheumatic (I09.1)

Ex: I38-I39, I87.8-I87.9, I99.8-I99.9

I39 Endocarditis and heart valve disorders in diseases classified elsewhere

Code first underlying disease, such as:
Q fever (A78)

Excludes1 endocardial involvement in:
candidiasis (B37.6)
gonococcal infection (A54.83)
Libman-Sacks disease (M32.11)
listerosis (A32.82)
meningococcal infection (A39.51)
rheumatoid arthritis (M05.31)
syphilis (A52.03)
tuberculosis (A18.84)
typhoid fever (A01.02)

Ex: I38-I39, I87.8-I87.9, I99.8-I99.9

I40 Acute myocarditis

Inflammation of heart muscle due to infection (viral/bacterial)

Includes subacute myocarditis

Excludes1 acute rheumatic myocarditis (I01.2)

Ex: **For category I40 CC codes:** I01.2, I09.0, I23.0-I23.3, I23.6-I23.8, I40.0-I41, I51.0, I51.4, I87.8-I87.9, I99.8-I99.9

I40.0 Infective myocarditis
Septic myocarditis
Use additional code (B95-B97) to identify infectious agent

I40.1 Isolated myocarditis
Fiedler's myocarditis
Giant cell myocarditis
Idiopathic myocarditis

I40.8 Other acute myocarditis

I40.9 Acute myocarditis, unspecified

I41 Myocarditis in diseases classified elsewhere

Code first underlying disease, such as:
typhus (A75.0-A75.9)

Excludes1 myocarditis (in):
Chagas' disease (chronic) (B57.2)
acute (B57.0)
coxsackie (virus) infection (B33.22)
diphtheritic (A36.81)
gonococcal (A54.83)
influenzal (J09.X9, J10.82, J11.82)
meningococcal (A39.52)
mumps (B26.82)
rheumatoid arthritis (M05.31)
sarcoid (D86.85)
syphilis (A52.06)
toxoplasmosis (B58.81)
tuberculous (A18.84)

Ex: See I40

I42 Cardiomyopathy
Disease of the heart muscle resulting in an abnormally enlarged, weakened, thickened, and/or stiffened muscles
Includes myocardiopathy
Code first pre-existing cardiomyopathy complicating pregnancy and puerperium (O99.4)
Excludes2 ischemic cardiomyopathy (I25.5) ◀
peripartum cardiomyopathy (O90.3) ◀
ventricular hypertrophy (I51.7)
(Ex) **For category I42 CC codes:** I09.81, I11.0, I13.0, I13.2, I25.10-I25.119, I25.5-I25.799, I25.811-I25.9, I42.0-I44.1, I44.30-I44.39, I45.2-I45.4, I45.81-I45.89, I48.0-I49.1, I49.3-I49.8, I50.1, I50.9, I87.8-I87.9, I99.8-I99.9, Q24.6, R00.0-R00.2, R57.0, R57.9

I42.0 Dilated cardiomyopathy
Congestive cardiomyopathy

I42.1 Obstructive hypertrophic cardiomyopathy
Hypertrophic subaortic stenosis (idiopathic)

I42.2 Other hypertrophic cardiomyopathy
Nonobstructive hypertrophic cardiomyopathy

I42.3 Endomyocardial (eosinophilic) disease
Endomyocardial (tropical) fibrosis
Löffler's endocarditis

I42.4 Endocardial fibroelastosis
Congenital cardiomyopathy
Elastomyofibrosis

I42.5 Other restrictive cardiomyopathy
Constrictive cardiomyopathy NOS

I42.6 Alcoholic cardiomyopathy
Code also presence of alcoholism (F10.-)

I42.7 Cardiomyopathy due to drug and external agent
Code first poisoning due to drug or toxin, if applicable (T36-T65 with fifth or sixth character 1-4 or 6)
Use additional code for adverse effect, if applicable, to identify drug (T36-T50 with fifth or sixth character 5)

I42.8 Other cardiomyopathies

I42.9 Cardiomyopathy, unspecified
Cardiomyopathy (primary) (secondary) NOS

I43 *Cardiomyopathy in diseases classified elsewhere*
Code first underlying disease, such as:
amyloidosis (E85.-)
glycogen storage disease (E74.0)
gout (M10.0-)
thyrotoxicosis (E05.0-E05.9-)
Excludes1 cardiomyopathy (in):
coxsackie (virus) (B33.24)
diphtheria (A36.81)
sarcoidosis (D86.85)
tuberculosis (A18.84)
(Ex) See I42

I44 Atrioventricular and left bundle-branch block
Conduction problem resulting in arrhythmias/dysrhythmias due to a lack of electrical impulses being transmitted normally through the heart

I44.0 Atrioventricular block, first degree

I44.1 Atrioventricular block, second degree
Atrioventricular block, type I and II
Möbitz block, type I and II
Second degree block, type I and II
Wenckebach's block

I44.2 Atrioventricular block, complete
Complete heart block NOS
Third degree block
(Ex) I44.0-I49.02, I49.2, I49.8, I87.8-I87.9, I99.8-I99.9, R00.1

I44.3 Other and unspecified atrioventricular block
Atrioventricular block NOS

I44.30 Unspecified atrioventricular block

I44.39 Other atrioventricular block

I44.4 Left anterior fascicular block
MCE: Questionable admission when principal dx

I44.5 Left posterior fascicular block
MCE: Questionable admission when principal dx

I44.6 Other and unspecified fascicular block

I44.60 Unspecified fascicular block
Left bundle-branch hemiblock NOS
MCE: Questionable admission when principal dx

I44.69 Other fascicular block
MCE: Questionable admission when principal dx

I44.7 Left bundle-branch block, unspecified
MCE: Questionable admission when principal dx

I45 Other conduction disorders

I45.0 Right fascicular block
MCE: Questionable admission when principal dx

I45.1 Other and unspecified right bundle-branch block

I45.10 Unspecified right bundle-branch block
Right bundle-branch block NOS
MCE: Questionable admission when principal dx

I45.19 Other right bundle-branch block
MCE: Questionable admission when principal dx

I45.2 Bifascicular block
(Ex) See I44.2

I45.3 Trifascicular block
(Ex) See I44.2

I45.4 Nonspecific intraventricular block
Bundle-branch block NOS

I45.5 Other specified heart block
Sinoatrial block
Sinoauricular block
Excludes1 heart block NOS (I45.9)

I45.6 Pre-excitation syndrome
Accelerated atrioventricular conduction
Accessory atrioventricular conduction
Anomalous atrioventricular excitation
Lown-Ganong-Levine syndrome
Pre-excitation atrioventricular conduction
Wolff-Parkinson-White syndrome

I45.8 Other specified conduction disorders

I45.81 Long QT syndrome

I45.89 Other specified conduction disorders
Atrioventricular [AV] dissociation
Interference dissociation
Isorhythmic dissociation
Nonparoxysmal AV nodal tachycardia
(Ex) See I44.2
Coding Clinic: 2013, Q2, P32

I45.9 Conduction disorder, unspecified
Heart block NOS
Stokes-Adams syndrome

I46 Cardiac arrest
Excludes1 cardiogenic shock (R57.0)
(Ex) **For category I46 CC codes:** I46.2-I49.02, I49.2, I87.8-I87.9, I99.8-I99.9

I46.2 Cardiac arrest due to underlying cardiac condition
Code first underlying cardiac condition
MCC: If patient discharged alive

I46.8 Cardiac arrest due to other underlying condition
Code first underlying condition
MCC: If patient discharged alive

I46.9 Cardiac arrest, cause unspecified
MCC: If patient discharged alive

I47 Paroxysmal tachycardia
Code first tachycardia complicating:
abortion or ectopic or molar pregnancy (O00-O07, O08.8)
obstetric surgery and procedures (O75.4)
Excludes1 tachycardia NOS (R00.0)
sinoauricular tachycardia NOS (R00.0)
sinus [sinusal] tachycardia NOS (R00.0)
(Ex) **For category I47 CC codes:** See I44.2

I47.0 Re-entry ventricular arrhythmia

I47.1 Supraventricular tachycardia
Atrial (paroxysmal) tachycardia
Atrioventricular [AV] (paroxysmal) tachycardia
Atrioventricular re-entrant (nodal) tachycardia [AVNRT] [AVRT]
Junctional (paroxysmal) tachycardia
Nodal (paroxysmal) tachycardia

I47.2 Ventricular tachycardia
Coding Clinic: 2013, Q3, P23

I47.9 Paroxysmal tachycardia, unspecified
Bouveret (-Hoffman) syndrome

I48 Atrial fibrillation and flutter
Most common abnormal heart rhythm (arrhythmia) presenting as irregular, rapid beating (tachycardia) of the heart's upper chamber.
Ex: **For category I48 CC codes:** See I44.2

I48.0 Paroxysmal atrial fibrillation

I48.1 Persistent atrial fibrillation
Rapid contractions of the upper heart chamber

I48.2 Chronic atrial fibrillation
Permanent atrial fibrillation

I48.3 Typical atrial flutter
Type I atrial flutter

I48.4 Atypical atrial flutter
Type II atrial flutter

I48.9 Unspecified atrial fibrillation and atrial flutter

I48.91 Unspecified atrial fibrillation

I48.92 Unspecified atrial flutter

I49 Other cardiac arrhythmias
Code first cardiac arrhythmia complicating:
abortion or ectopic or molar pregnancy (O00-O07, O08.8)
obstetric surgery and procedures (O75.4)
Excludes1 bradycardia NOS (R00.1)
neonatal dysrhythmia (P29.1-)
sinoatrial bradycardia (R00.1)
sinus bradycardia (R00.1)
vagal bradycardia (R00.1)

I49.0 Ventricular fibrillation and flutter

I49.01 Ventricular fibrillation
MCC: If patient discharged alive
Ex: See I44.2

I49.02 Ventricular flutter
Ex: See I44.2

I49.1 Atrial premature depolarization
Atrial premature beats

I49.2 Junctional premature depolarization
Ex: See I44.2

I49.3 Ventricular premature depolarization

I49.4 Other and unspecified premature depolarization

I49.40 Unspecified premature depolarization
Premature beats NOS

I49.49 Other premature depolarization
Ectopic beats
Extrasystoles
Extrasystolic arrhythmias
Premature contractions

I49.5 Sick sinus syndrome
Tachycardia-bradycardia syndrome

I49.8 Other specified cardiac arrhythmias
Coronary sinus rhythm disorder
Ectopic rhythm disorder
Nodal rhythm disorder

I49.9 Cardiac arrhythmia, unspecified
Arrhythmia (cardiac) NOS

I50 Heart failure
Code first heart failure complicating abortion or ectopic or molar pregnancy (O00-O07, O08.8)
heart failure due to hypertension (I11.0)
heart failure due to hypertension with chronic kidney disease (I13.-)
heart failure following surgery (I97.13-)
obstetric surgery and procedures (O75.4)
rheumatic heart failure (I09.81)
Excludes1 neonatal cardiac failure (P29.0)
Excludes2 cardiac arrest (I46.-) ◀
Coding Clinic: 2016, Q1, P38; 2015, Q2, P15

I50.1 Left ventricular failure
Cardiac asthma
Edema of lung with heart disease NOS
Edema of lung with heart failure
Left heart failure
Pulmonary edema with heart disease NOS
Pulmonary edema with heart failure
Excludes1 edema of lung without heart disease or heart failure (J81.-)
pulmonary edema without heart disease or failure (J81.-)
Ex: I09.81, I11.0, I50.1-I50.9, I87.8-I87.9, I99.8-I99.9

I50.2 Systolic (congestive) heart failure
Excludes1 combined systolic (congestive) and diastolic (congestive) heart failure (I50.4-)
Ex: **For category I50.2 CC codes:** I09.81, I11.0, I50.1-I50.9, I87.8-I87.9, I99.8-I99.9, J81.0

I50.20 Unspecified systolic (congestive) heart failure

I50.21 Acute systolic (congestive) heart failure
Presenting a short and relatively severe episode

I50.22 Chronic systolic (congestive) heart failure
Long-lasting, presenting over time

I50.23 Acute on chronic systolic (congestive) heart failure
Combination code. What was a chronic condition now has an acute exacerbation (to make more severe).
Coding Clinic: 2013, Q2, P33

I50.3 Diastolic (congestive) heart failure
Excludes1 combined systolic (congestive) and diastolic (congestive) heart failure (I50.4-)
Ex: **For category I50.3 CC codes:** See I50.2

I50.30 Unspecified diastolic (congestive) heart failure

I50.31 Acute diastolic (congestive) heart failure

I50.32 Chronic diastolic (congestive) heart failure

I50.33 Acute on chronic diastolic (congestive) heart failure

I50.4 Combined systolic (congestive) and diastolic (congestive) heart failure
Ex: **For category I50.4 CC codes:** See I50.2

I50.40 Unspecified combined systolic (congestive) and diastolic (congestive) heart failure

I50.41 Acute combined systolic (congestive) and diastolic (congestive) heart failure

I50.42 Chronic combined systolic (congestive) and diastolic (congestive) heart failure

I50.43 Acute on chronic combined systolic (congestive) and diastolic (congestive) heart failure

Item 9–8 Congestive heart failure (CHF) is a condition in which the left ventricle of the heart cannot pump enough blood to the body. The blood flow from the heart slows or returns to the heart from the venous system back flow resulting in congestion (fluid accumulation) particularly in the abdomen. Most commonly, fluid collects in the lungs and results in shortness of breath, especially when in a reclining position.

I50.9 Heart failure, unspecified
Biventricular (heart) failure NOS
Cardiac, heart or myocardial failure NOS
Congestive heart disease
Congestive heart failure NOS
Right ventricular failure (secondary to left heart failure)
Excludes2 fluid overload (E87.70) ◀
Coding Clinic: 2015, Q2, P15; 2012, Q4, P92

● **I51 Complications and ill-defined descriptions of heart disease**
Excludes1 any condition in I51.4-I51.9 due to hypertension (I11.-)
any condition in I51.4-I51.9 due to hypertension and chronic kidney disease (I13.-)
heart disease specified as rheumatic (I00-I09)

I51.0 Cardiac septal defect, acquired A
Acquired septal atrial defect (old)
Acquired septal auricular defect (old)
Acquired septal ventricular defect (old)
Excludes1 cardiac septal defect as current complication following acute myocardial infarction (I23.1, I23.2)
(Ex) See I23

I51.1 Rupture of chordae tendineae, not elsewhere classified
Excludes1 rupture of chordae tendineae as current complication following acute myocardial infarction (I23.4)
(Ex) I23.0-I23.4, I23.6-I23.8, I51.0-I51.1, I87.8-I87.9, I99.8-I99.9

I51.2 Rupture of papillary muscle, not elsewhere classified
Excludes1 rupture of papillary muscle as current complication following acute myocardial infarction (I23.5)
(Ex) I23.0-I23.3, I23.5-I23.8, I51.0, I51.2, I87.8-I87.9, I99.8-I99.9

I51.3 Intracardiac thrombosis, not elsewhere classified
Apical thrombosis (old)
Atrial thrombosis (old)
Auricular thrombosis (old)
Mural thrombosis (old)
Ventricular thrombosis (old)
Excludes1 intracardiac thrombosis as current complication following acute myocardial infarction (I23.6)
Coding Clinic: 2013, Q1, P24

I51.4 Myocarditis, unspecified
Chronic (interstitial) myocarditis
Myocardial fibrosis
Myocarditis NOS
Excludes1 acute or subacute myocarditis (I40.-)

I51.5 Myocardial degeneration
Fatty degeneration of heart or myocardium
Myocardial disease
Senile degeneration of heart or myocardium

I51.7 Cardiomegaly
Cardiac dilatation
Cardiac hypertrophy
Ventricular dilatation

● **I51.8 Other ill-defined heart diseases**

I51.81 Takotsubo syndrome
Reversible left ventricular dysfunction following sudden emotional stress
Stress induced cardiomyopathy
Takotsubo cardiomyopathy
Transient left ventricular apical ballooning syndrome
(Ex) I09.81, I11.0, I50.1-I50.9, I51.81, I51.9-I52, I87.8-I87.9, I99.8-I99.9

I51.89 Other ill-defined heart diseases
Carditis (acute)(chronic)
Pancarditis (acute)(chronic)

I51.9 Heart disease, unspecified

▶ ***I52 Other heart disorders in diseases classified elsewhere***
Code first underlying disease, such as:
congenital syphilis (A50.5)
mucopolysaccharidosis (E76.3)
schistosomiasis (B65.0-B65.9)
Excludes1 heart disease (in):
gonococcal infection (A54.83)
meningococcal infection (A39.50)
rheumatoid arthritis (M05.31)
syphilis (A52.06)

CEREBROVASCULAR DISEASES (I60-I69)

Use additional code to identify presence of:
alcohol abuse and dependence (F10.-)
exposure to environmental tobacco smoke (Z77.22)
history of tobacco dependence (Z87.891) ⟸
hypertension (I10-I15)
occupational exposure to environmental tobacco smoke (Z57.31)
tobacco dependence (F17.-)
tobacco use (Z72.0)
Excludes1 transient cerebral ischemic attacks and related syndromes (G45.-)
traumatic intracranial hemorrhage (S06.-)
Coding Clinic: 2015, Q4, P40

● **I60 Nontraumatic subarachnoid hemorrhage**
Includes ruptured cerebral aneurysm
Excludes1 syphilitic ruptured cerebral aneurysm (A52.05)
Excludes2 sequelae of subarachnoid hemorrhage (I69.0-) ◀
(Ex) **For category I60 CC codes:** E03.5, G93.82, I60.00-I62.9, I87.8-I87.9, I99.8-I99.9, R40.0-R40.2224, R40.2310-R40.2324, R40.2340-R40.2344, R40.3-R40.4, S02.0XX[A,B], S02.101-S02.102[A,B], S02.109[A,B], S02.110-S02.19X[A,B], S02.91X[A,B], S06.0X0-S06.0X1[A], S06.0X9-S06.9X9[A]

● **I60.0 Nontraumatic subarachnoid hemorrhage from carotid siphon and bifurcation**
I60.00 Nontraumatic subarachnoid hemorrhage from unspecified carotid siphon and bifurcation
I60.01 Nontraumatic subarachnoid hemorrhage from right carotid siphon and bifurcation
I60.02 Nontraumatic subarachnoid hemorrhage from left carotid siphon and bifurcation

● **I60.1 Nontraumatic subarachnoid hemorrhage from middle cerebral artery**
I60.10 Nontraumatic subarachnoid hemorrhage from unspecified middle cerebral artery
I60.11 Nontraumatic subarachnoid hemorrhage from right middle cerebral artery
I60.12 Nontraumatic subarachnoid hemorrhage from left middle cerebral artery

I60.2 Nontraumatic subarachnoid hemorrhage from anterior communicating artery
~~I60.20 Nontraumatic subarachnoid hemorrhage from unspecified anterior communicating artery~~
~~I60.21 Nontraumatic subarachnoid hemorrhage from right anterior communicating artery~~
~~I60.22 Nontraumatic subarachnoid hemorrhage from left anterior communicating artery~~

● **I60.3 Nontraumatic subarachnoid hemorrhage from posterior communicating artery**
I60.30 Nontraumatic subarachnoid hemorrhage from unspecified posterior communicating artery
I60.31 Nontraumatic subarachnoid hemorrhage from right posterior communicating artery
I60.32 Nontraumatic subarachnoid hemorrhage from left posterior communicating artery

I60.4 Nontraumatic subarachnoid hemorrhage from basilar artery

● **I60.5 Nontraumatic subarachnoid hemorrhage from vertebral artery**

I60.50 Nontraumatic subarachnoid hemorrhage from unspecified vertebral artery

I60.51 Nontraumatic subarachnoid hemorrhage from right vertebral artery

I60.52 Nontraumatic subarachnoid hemorrhage from left vertebral artery

I60.6 Nontraumatic subarachnoid hemorrhage from other intracranial arteries

I60.7 Nontraumatic subarachnoid hemorrhage from unspecified intracranial artery

Ruptured (congenital) berry aneurysm
Ruptured (congenital) cerebral aneurysm
Subarachnoid hemorrhage (nontraumatic) from cerebral artery NOS
Subarachnoid hemorrhage (nontraumatic) from communicating artery NOS

Excludes1 berry aneurysm, nonruptured (I67.1)

I60.8 Other nontraumatic subarachnoid hemorrhage

Meningeal hemorrhage
Rupture of cerebral arteriovenous malformation

I60.9 Nontraumatic subarachnoid hemorrhage, unspecified

● **I61 Nontraumatic intracerebral hemorrhage**

Excludes2 sequelae of intracerebral hemorrhage (I69.1-) ◀

Ex: **For category I61 CC codes:** See I60

I61.0 Nontraumatic intracerebral hemorrhage in hemisphere, subcortical

Deep intracerebral hemorrhage (nontraumatic)

I61.1 Nontraumatic intracerebral hemorrhage in hemisphere, cortical

Cerebral lobe hemorrhage (nontraumatic)
Superficial intracerebral hemorrhage (nontraumatic)

I61.2 Nontraumatic intracerebral hemorrhage in hemisphere, unspecified

I61.3 Nontraumatic intracerebral hemorrhage in brain stem

I61.4 Nontraumatic intracerebral hemorrhage in cerebellum

I61.5 Nontraumatic intracerebral hemorrhage, intraventricular

I61.6 Nontraumatic intracerebral hemorrhage, multiple localized

I61.8 Other nontraumatic intracerebral hemorrhage

I61.9 Nontraumatic intracerebral hemorrhage, unspecified

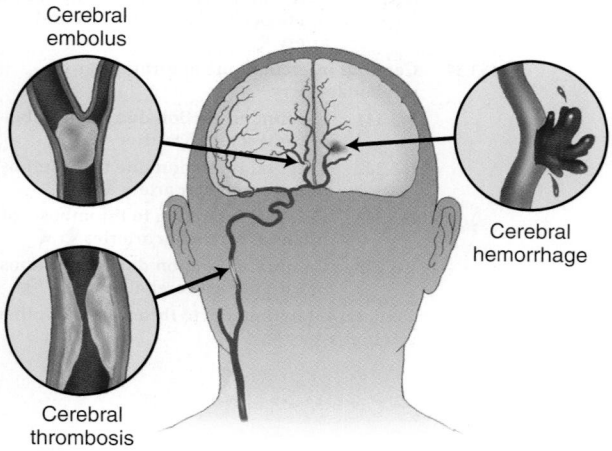

Figure 9-4 Events causing a stroke. (From Shiland: Mastering Healthcare Terminology, ed 1, St. Louis, Mosby, 2003)

● **I62 Other and unspecified nontraumatic intracranial hemorrhage**

Excludes2 sequelae of intracranial hemorrhage (I69.2) ◀

Ex: **For category I62 CC codes:** See I60

● **I62.0 Nontraumatic subdural hemorrhage**

I62.00 Nontraumatic subdural hemorrhage, unspecified

I62.01 Nontraumatic acute subdural hemorrhage

I62.02 Nontraumatic subacute subdural hemorrhage

I62.03 Nontraumatic chronic subdural hemorrhage

I62.1 Nontraumatic extradural hemorrhage

Nontraumatic epidural hemorrhage

I62.9 Nontraumatic intracranial hemorrhage, unspecified

★**(See Plate 141 on page 76.)**

● **I63 Cerebral infarction**

Includes occlusion and stenosis of cerebral and precerebral arteries, resulting in cerebral infarction

Use additional code, if applicable, to identify status post administration of tPA (rtPA) in a different facility within the last 24 hours prior to admission to current facility (Z92.82)

Use additional code, if known, to indicate National Institutes of Health Stroke Scale (NIHSS) score (R29.7-) ◀

Excludes2 sequelae of cerebral infarction (I69.3-) ◀

● **I63.0 Cerebral infarction due to thrombosis of precerebral arteries**

I63.00 Cerebral infarction due to thrombosis of unspecified precerebral artery

Ex: E08.51-E08.59, E08.618-E08.638, E08.649-E08.8, E09.51-E09.59, E09.618-E09.638, E09.649-E09.8, E10.51-E10.59, E10.618-E10.638, E10.649, E10.69-E10.8, E11.51-E11.59, E11.618-E11.638, E11.649, E11.69-E11.8, E13.51-E13.59, E13.618-E13.638, E13.649-E13.8, G43.601-G43.619, I63.00-I63.29, I65.01-I65.9, I87.8-I87.9, I99.8, I99.9

● **I63.01 Cerebral infarction due to thrombosis of vertebral artery**

Ex: **For category I63.01 CC codes unless otherwise indicated:** E08.51-E08.59, E08.618-E08.638, E08.649-E08.8, E09.51-E09.59, E09.618-E09.638, E09.649-E09.8, E10.51-E10.59, E10.618-E10.638, E10.649, E10.69-E10.8, E11.51-E11.59, E11.618-E11.638, E11.649, E11.69-E11.8, E13.51-E13.59, E13.618-E13.638, E13.649-E13.8, G43.601-G43.619, I63.00-I63.29, I65.01-I65.9, I87.8-I87.9, I99.8-I99.9

I63.011 Cerebral infarction due to thrombosis of right vertebral artery

I63.012 Cerebral infarction due to thrombosis of left vertebral artery

I63.013 Cerebral infarction due to thrombosis of bilateral vertebral arteries ◀

I63.019 Cerebral infarction due to thrombosis of unspecified vertebral artery

I63.02 Cerebral infarction due to thrombosis of basilar artery

Ex: See I63.00

● **I63.03 Cerebral infarction due to thrombosis of carotid artery**

Ex: **For category I63.03 CC codes:** E08.51-E08.59, E08.618-E08.638, E08.649-E08.8, E09.51-E09.59, E09.618-E09.638, E09.649-E09.8, E10.51-E10.59, E10.618-E10.638, E10.649, E10.69-E10.8, E11.51-E11.59, E11.618-E11.638, E11.649, E11.69-E11.8, E13.51-E13.59, E13.618-E13.638, E13.649-E13.8, G43.601-G43.619, I63.00-I63.29, I65.01-I65.9, I87.8-I87.9, I99.8-I99.9

I63.031 Cerebral infarction due to thrombosis of right carotid artery

I63.032 Cerebral infarction due to thrombosis of left carotid artery

I63.033 Cerebral infarction due to thrombosis of bilateral carotid arteries ◀

I63.039 Cerebral infarction due to thrombosis of unspecified carotid artery

I63.09 Cerebral infarction due to thrombosis of other precerebral artery

Ex: See I63.00

● I63.1 Cerebral infarction due to embolism of precerebral arteries

I63.10 Cerebral infarction due to embolism of unspecified precerebral artery

Ex: See I63.00

● I63.11 Cerebral infarction due to embolism of vertebral artery

Ex: For category I63.11 CC codes: See I63.01

I63.111 Cerebral infarction due to embolism of right vertebral artery

I63.112 Cerebral infarction due to embolism of left vertebral artery

I63.113 Cerebral infarction due to embolism of bilateral vertebral arteries ◀

I63.119 Cerebral infarction due to embolism of unspecified vertebral artery

I63.12 Cerebral infarction due to embolism of basilar artery

Ex: See I63.00

● I63.13 Cerebral infarction due to embolism of carotid artery

Ex: For category I63.13 CC codes: See I63.03

I63.131 Cerebral infarction due to embolism of right carotid artery

I63.132 Cerebral infarction due to embolism of left carotid artery

I63.133 Cerebral infarction due to embolism of bilateral carotid arteries ◀

I63.139 Cerebral infarction due to embolism of unspecified carotid artery

I63.19 Cerebral infarction due to embolism of other precerebral artery

Ex: See I63.00

● I63.2 Cerebral infarction due to unspecified occlusion or stenosis of precerebral arteries

I63.20 Cerebral infarction due to unspecified occlusion or stenosis of unspecified precerebral arteries

Ex: See I63.00

● I63.21 Cerebral infarction due to unspecified occlusion or stenosis of vertebral arteries

Ex: For category I63.21 CC codes: See I63.01

I63.211 Cerebral infarction due to unspecified occlusion or stenosis of right vertebral arteries

I63.212 Cerebral infarction due to unspecified occlusion or stenosis of left vertebral arteries

I63.213 Cerebral infarction due to unspecified occlusion or stenosis of bilateral vertebral arteries ◀

I63.219 Cerebral infarction due to unspecified occlusion or stenosis of unspecified vertebral arteries

I63.22 Cerebral infarction due to unspecified occlusion or stenosis of basilar arteries

Ex: See I63.00

● I63.23 Cerebral infarction due to unspecified occlusion or stenosis of carotid arteries

Ex: For category I63.23 CC codes: See I63.03

I63.231 Cerebral infarction due to unspecified occlusion or stenosis of right carotid arteries

I63.232 Cerebral infarction due to unspecified occlusion or stenosis of left carotid arteries

I63.233 Cerebral infarction due to unspecified occlusion or stenosis of bilateral carotid arteries ◀

I63.239 Cerebral infarction due to unspecified occlusion or stenosis of unspecified carotid arteries

I63.29 Cerebral infarction due to unspecified occlusion or stenosis of other precerebral arteries

Ex: See I63.00

● I63.3 Cerebral infarction due to thrombosis of cerebral arteries

Ex: For category I63.3 CC codes: E08.51-E08.59, E08.618-E08.638, E08.649-E08.8, E09.51-E09.59, E09.618-E09.638, E09.649-E09.8, E10.51-E10.59, E10.618-E10.638, E10.649, E10.69-E10.8, E11.51-E11.59, E11.618-E11.638, E11.649, E11.69-E11.8, E13.51-E13.59, E13.618-E13.638, E13.649-E13.8, G43.601-G43.619, I63.30-I63.9, I66.01-I66.9, I87.8-I87.9, I99.8-I99.9

I63.30 Cerebral infarction due to thrombosis of unspecified cerebral artery

● I63.31 Cerebral infarction due to thrombosis of middle cerebral artery

I63.311 Cerebral infarction due to thrombosis of right middle cerebral artery

I63.312 Cerebral infarction due to thrombosis of left middle cerebral artery

I63.313 Cerebral infarction due to thrombosis of bilateral middle cerebral arteries ◀

I63.319 Cerebral infarction due to thrombosis of unspecified middle cerebral artery

● I63.32 Cerebral infarction due to thrombosis of anterior cerebral artery

I63.321 Cerebral infarction due to thrombosis of right anterior cerebral artery

I63.322 Cerebral infarction due to thrombosis of left anterior cerebral artery

I63.323 Cerebral infarction due to thrombosis of bilateral anterior arteries ◀

I63.329 Cerebral infarction due to thrombosis of unspecified anterior cerebral artery

● I63.33 Cerebral infarction due to thrombosis of posterior cerebral artery

I63.331 Cerebral infarction due to thrombosis of right posterior cerebral artery

I63.332 Cerebral infarction due to thrombosis of left posterior cerebral artery

I63.333 Cerebral infarction to thrombosis of bilateral posterior arteries ◀

I63.339 Cerebral infarction due to thrombosis of unspecified posterior cerebral artery

● I63.34 Cerebral infarction due to thrombosis of cerebellar artery

I63.341 Cerebral infarction due to thrombosis of right cerebellar artery

I63.342 Cerebral infarction due to thrombosis of left cerebellar artery

I63.343 Cerebral infarction to thrombosis of bilateral cerebellar arteries ◀

I63.349 Cerebral infarction due to thrombosis of unspecified cerebellar artery

I63.39 Cerebral infarction due to thrombosis of other cerebral artery

- **I63.4** Cerebral infarction due to embolism of cerebral arteries
  Ex: For category I63.4 CC codes: See I63.3
  - **I63.40** Cerebral infarction due to embolism of unspecified cerebral artery
  - **I63.41** Cerebral infarction due to embolism of middle cerebral artery
    - **I63.411** Cerebral infarction due to embolism of right middle cerebral artery
    - **I63.412** Cerebral infarction due to embolism of left middle cerebral artery
    - **I63.413** Cerebral infarction due to embolism of bilateral middle cerebral arteries ◀
    - **I63.419** Cerebral infarction due to embolism of unspecified middle cerebral artery
  - **I63.42** Cerebral infarction due to embolism of anterior cerebral artery
    - **I63.421** Cerebral infarction due to embolism of right anterior cerebral artery
    - **I63.422** Cerebral infarction due to embolism of left anterior cerebral artery
    - **I63.423** Cerebral infarction due to embolism of bilateral anterior cerebral arteries ◀
    - **I63.429** Cerebral infarction due to embolism of unspecified anterior cerebral artery
  - **I63.43** Cerebral infarction due to embolism of posterior cerebral artery
    - **I63.431** Cerebral infarction due to embolism of right posterior cerebral artery
    - **I63.432** Cerebral infarction due to embolism of left posterior cerebral artery
    - **I63.433** Cerebral infarction due to embolism of bilateral posterior cerebral arteries ◀
    - **I63.439** Cerebral infarction due to embolism of unspecified posterior cerebral artery
  - **I63.44** Cerebral infarction due to embolism of cerebellar artery
    - **I63.441** Cerebral infarction due to embolism of right cerebellar artery
    - **I63.442** Cerebral infarction due to embolism of left cerebellar artery
    - **I63.443** Cerebral infarction due to embolism of bilateral cerebellar arteries ◀
    - **I63.449** Cerebral infarction due to embolism of unspecified cerebellar artery
  - **I63.49** Cerebral infarction due to embolism of other cerebral artery
- **I63.5** Cerebral infarction due to unspecified occlusion or stenosis of cerebral arteries
  Ex: For category I63.5 CC codes: See I63.3
  - **I63.50** Cerebral infarction due to unspecified occlusion or stenosis of unspecified cerebral artery
  - **I63.51** Cerebral infarction due to unspecified occlusion or stenosis of middle cerebral artery
    - **I63.511** Cerebral infarction due to unspecified occlusion or stenosis of right middle cerebral artery
    - **I63.512** Cerebral infarction due to unspecified occlusion or stenosis of left middle cerebral artery
    - **I63.513** Cerebral infarction due to unspecified occlusion or stenosis of bilateral middle arteries ◀
    - **I63.519** Cerebral infarction due to unspecified occlusion or stenosis of unspecified middle cerebral artery
  - **I63.52** Cerebral infarction due to unspecified occlusion or stenosis of anterior cerebral artery
    - **I63.521** Cerebral infarction due to unspecified occlusion or stenosis of right anterior cerebral artery
    - **I63.522** Cerebral infarction due to unspecified occlusion or stenosis of left anterior cerebral artery
    - **I63.523** Cerebral infarction due to unspecified occlusion or stenosis of bilateral anterior arteries ◀
    - **I63.529** Cerebral infarction due to unspecified occlusion or stenosis of unspecified anterior cerebral artery
  - **I63.53** Cerebral infarction due to unspecified occlusion or stenosis of posterior cerebral artery
    - **I63.531** Cerebral infarction due to unspecified occlusion or stenosis of right posterior cerebral artery
    - **I63.532** Cerebral infarction due to unspecified occlusion or stenosis of left posterior cerebral artery
    - **I63.533** Cerebral infarction due to unspecified occlusion or stenosis of bilateral posterior arteries ◀
    - **I63.539** Cerebral infarction due to unspecified occlusion or stenosis of unspecified posterior cerebral artery
  - **I63.54** Cerebral infarction due to unspecified occlusion or stenosis of cerebellar artery
    - **I63.541** Cerebral infarction due to unspecified occlusion or stenosis of right cerebellar artery
    - **I63.542** Cerebral infarction due to unspecified occlusion or stenosis of left cerebellar artery
    - **I63.543** Cerebral infarction due to unspecified occlusion or stenosis of bilateral cerebellar arteries ◀
    - **I63.549** Cerebral infarction due to unspecified occlusion or stenosis of unspecified cerebellar artery
  - **I63.59** Cerebral infarction due to unspecified occlusion or stenosis of other cerebral artery
- **I63.6** Cerebral infarction due to cerebral venous thrombosis, nonpyogenic
  Ex: See I63.3
- **I63.8** Other cerebral infarction
  Ex: See I63.3
- **I63.9** Cerebral infarction, unspecified
  Stroke NOS
  Ex: See I63.3
  Coding Clinic: 2015, Q1, P26

- **I65** Occlusion and stenosis of precerebral arteries, not resulting in cerebral infarction
  Includes embolism of precerebral artery
  narrowing of precerebral artery
  obstruction (complete) (partial) of precerebral artery
  thrombosis of precerebral artery
  Excludes1 insufficiency, NOS, of precerebral artery (G45.-)
  insufficiency of precerebral arteries causing cerebral infarction (I63.0-I63.2)
  - **I65.0** Occlusion and stenosis of vertebral artery
    - **I65.01** Occlusion and stenosis of right vertebral artery
    - **I65.02** Occlusion and stenosis of left vertebral artery
    - **I65.03** Occlusion and stenosis of bilateral vertebral arteries
    - **I65.09** Occlusion and stenosis of unspecified vertebral artery
  - **I65.1** Occlusion and stenosis of basilar artery

● **I65.2 Occlusion and stenosis of carotid artery**

I65.21 Occlusion and stenosis of right carotid artery

I65.22 Occlusion and stenosis of left carotid artery

I65.23 Occlusion and stenosis of bilateral carotid arteries

I65.29 Occlusion and stenosis of unspecified carotid artery

I65.8 Occlusion and stenosis of other precerebral arteries

I65.9 Occlusion and stenosis of unspecified precerebral artery
Occlusion and stenosis of precerebral artery NOS

● **I66 Occlusion and stenosis of cerebral arteries, not resulting in cerebral infarction**

Includes embolism of cerebral artery
narrowing of cerebral artery
obstruction (complete) (partial) of cerebral artery
thrombosis of cerebral artery

Excludes1 occlusion and stenosis of cerebral artery causing cerebral infarction (I63.3-I63.5)

● **I66.0 Occlusion and stenosis of middle cerebral artery**

I66.01 Occlusion and stenosis of right middle cerebral artery

I66.02 Occlusion and stenosis of left middle cerebral artery

I66.03 Occlusion and stenosis of bilateral middle cerebral arteries

I66.09 Occlusion and stenosis of unspecified middle cerebral artery

● **I66.1 Occlusion and stenosis of anterior cerebral artery**

I66.11 Occlusion and stenosis of right anterior cerebral artery

I66.12 Occlusion and stenosis of left anterior cerebral artery

I66.13 Occlusion and stenosis of bilateral anterior cerebral arteries

I66.19 Occlusion and stenosis of unspecified anterior cerebral artery

● **I66.2 Occlusion and stenosis of posterior cerebral artery**

I66.21 Occlusion and stenosis of right posterior cerebral artery

I66.22 Occlusion and stenosis of left posterior cerebral artery

I66.23 Occlusion and stenosis of bilateral posterior cerebral arteries

I66.29 Occlusion and stenosis of unspecified posterior cerebral artery

I66.3 Occlusion and stenosis of cerebellar arteries

I66.8 Occlusion and stenosis of other cerebral arteries
Occlusion and stenosis of perforating arteries

I66.9 Occlusion and stenosis of unspecified cerebral artery

● **I67 Other cerebrovascular diseases**

Excludes2 sequelae of the listed conditions (I69.8) ◀

I67.0 Dissection of cerebral arteries, nonruptured

Excludes1 ruptured cerebral arteries (I60.7)

Ex: I77.2-I77.3, I77.5-I77.6, I77.89-I77.9, M31.8-M31.9

I67.1 Cerebral aneurysm, nonruptured
Cerebral aneurysm NOS
Cerebral arteriovenous fistula, acquired
Internal carotid artery aneurysm, intracranial portion
Internal carotid artery aneurysm, NOS

Excludes1 congenital cerebral aneurysm, nonruptured (Q28.-)
ruptured cerebral aneurysm (I60.7)

I67.2 Cerebral atherosclerosis A
Atheroma of cerebral and precerebral arteries

I67.3 Progressive vascular leukoencephalopathy
Binswanger's disease

Ex: A17.82, A50.42, A52.14, A75.9, A79.9, A81.00-A81.9, A83.0-A85.8, A87.2, A88.0, A88.8, A92.1-A92.2, A92.4-A92.8, A93.0, B00.4, B00.82, B01.11-B01.12, B04, B06.01, B08.09, B08.20-B08.22, B08.60-B08.79, B09, B10.01-B10.09, B26.2, B27.00-B27.99, B33.1, B45.0, B45.2-B45.9, B58.2, B75, G04.00-G04.01, G04.31, G04.81-G05.4, G37.0, G37.4-G37.5, I67.3, J09.X3-J09.X9, J10.2-J10.89, J11.2-J11.89, L44.4, M1A.10X0-M1A.19X1, P35.2-P35.9, P37.0-P37.4, P37.8-P37.9, T56.0X1-T56.0X4[A]

I67.4 Hypertensive encephalopathy

Ex: E08.51-E08.59, E08.618-E08.638, E08.649-E08.8, E09.51-E09.59, E09.618-E09.638, E09.649-E09.8, E10.51-E10.59, E10.618-E10.638, E10.649, E10.69-E10.8, E11.51-E11.59, E11.618-E11.638, E11.649, E11.69-E11.8, E13.51-E13.59, E13.618-E13.638, E13.649-E13.8, I67.4, I87.8-I87.9, I99.8-I99.9

I67.5 Moyamoya disease

Ex: E08.51-E08.59, E08.618-E08.638, E08.649-E08.8, E09.51-E09.59, E09.618-E09.638, E09.649-E09.8, E10.51-E10.59, E10.618-E10.638, E10.649, E10.69-E10.8, E11.51-E11.59, E11.618-E11.638, E11.649, E11.69-E11.8, E13.51-E13.59, E13.618-E13.638, E13.649-E13.8, I67.5, I87.8-I87.9, I99.8-I99.9

I67.6 Nonpyogenic thrombosis of intracranial venous system
Nonpyogenic thrombosis of cerebral vein
Nonpyogenic thrombosis of intracranial venous sinus

Excludes1 nonpyogenic thrombosis of intracranial venous system causing infarction (I63.6)

Ex: E08.51-E08.59, E08.618-E08.638, E08.649-E08.8, E09.51-E09.59, E09.618-E09.638, E09.649-E09.8, E10.51-E10.59, E10.618-E10.638, E10.649, E10.69-E10.8, E11.51-E11.59, E11.618-E11.638, E11.649, E11.69-E11.8, E13.51-E13.59, E13.618-E13.638, E13.649-E13.8, I67.6, I87.8-I87.9, I99.8-I99.9

I67.7 Cerebral arteritis, not elsewhere classified
Granulomatous angiitis of the nervous system

Excludes1 allergic granulomatous angiitis (M30.1)

Ex: E08.51-E08.59, E08.618-E08.638, E08.649-E08.8, E09.51-E09.59, E09.618-E09.638, E09.649-E09.8, E10.51-E10.59, E10.618-E10.638, E10.649, E10.69-E10.8, E11.51-E11.59, E11.618-E11.638, E11.649, E11.69-E11.8, E13.51-E13.59, E13.618-E13.638, E13.649-E13.8, I67.7, I68.2, I87.8-I87.9, I99.8-I99.9

● **I67.8 Other specified cerebrovascular diseases**

I67.81 Acute cerebrovascular insufficiency
Acute cerebrovascular insufficiency unspecified as to location or reversibility

Ex: E08.51-E08.59, E08.618-E08.638, E08.649-E08.8, E09.51-E09.59, E09.618-E09.638, E09.649-E09.8, E10.51-E10.59, E10.618-E10.638, E10.649, E10.69-E10.8, E11.51-E11.59, E11.618-E11.638, E11.649, E11.69-E11.8, E13.51-E13.59, E13.618-E13.638, E13.649-E13.8, G45.0-G45.2, G45.8-G46.2, I60.00-I62.9, I63.30-I63.9, I66.01-I66.9, I67.81-I67.82, I67.841-I67.89, I87.8-I87.9, I99.8-I99.9

I67.82 Cerebral ischemia
Chronic cerebral ischemia

Ex: See I67.81

I67.83 Posterior reversible encephalopathy syndrome
PRES

Ex: G21.0, G83.5, G93.40-G93.41

● **I67.84 Cerebral vasospasm and vasoconstriction**

Ex: **For category I67.84 CC codes:** E08.51-E08.59, E08.618-E08.638, E08.649-E08.8, E09.51-E09.59, E09.618-E09.638, E09.649-E09.8, E10.51-E10.59, E10.618-E10.638, E10.649, E10.69-E10.8, E11.51-E11.59, E11.618-E11.638, E11.649, E11.69, E11.8, E13.51-E13.59, E13.618-E13.638, E13.649-E13.8, G45.0-G45.2, G45.8-G46.2, I63.00-I63.02, I63.033, I63.113, I63.133, I63.213, I63.233, I63.039, I63.09, I63.139, I63.19-I63.239, I63.29, I65.01-I65.9, I67.841-I67.848, I87.8-I87.9, I99.8-I99.9

I67.841 Reversible cerebrovascular vasoconstriction syndrome
Call-Fleming syndrome

Code first underlying condition, if applicable, such as eclampsia (O15.00-O15.9)

I67.848 Other cerebrovascular vasospasm and vasoconstriction

I67.89 Other cerebrovascular disease

Ex: See I67.81

I67.9 Cerebrovascular disease, unspecified

I68 Cerebrovascular disorders in diseases classified elsewhere

I68.0 Cerebral amyloid angiopathy

Code first underlying amyloidosis (E85.-)

I68.2 Cerebral arteritis in other diseases classified elsewhere

Code first underlying disease

Excludes1 cerebral arteritis (in):
listerosis (A32.89)
systemic lupus erythematosus (M32.19)
syphilis (A52.04)
tuberculosis (A18.89)

Ex: See I67.7

I68.8 Other cerebrovascular disorders in diseases classified elsewhere

Code first underlying disease

Excludes1 syphilitic cerebral aneurysm (A52.05)

OGCR Section I.c.9.d.

Sequelae of Cerebrovascular Disease

1) Category I69, Sequelae of Cerebrovascular disease

Category 169 is used to indicate conditions classifiable to categories I60-I67 as the causes of sequela (neurologic deficits), themselves classified elsewhere. These "late effects" include neurologic deficits that persist after initial onset of conditions classifiable to categories I60-I67. The neurologic deficits caused by cerebrovascular disease may be present from the onset of may arise at any time after the onset of the condition classifiable to categories I60-I67.

Codes from category I69, Sequelae of cerebrovascular disease, that specify hemiplegia, hemiparesis and monoplegia identify whether the dominant or nondominant side is affected. Should the affected side be documented, but not specified as dominant or nondominant, and the classification system does not indicate a default, code selection is as follows:

For ambidextrous patients, the default should be dominant.

If the left side is affected, the default is non-dominant.

If the right side is affected, the default is dominant.

2) Codes from category I69 with codes from I60-I67

Codes from category I69 may be assigned on a health care record with codes from I60-I67, if the patient has a current cerebrovascular disease and deficits from an old cerebrovascular disease.

I69 Sequelae of cerebrovascular disease

Note: Category I69 is to be used to indicate conditions in I60-I67 as the cause of sequelae. The 'sequelae' include conditions specified as such or as residuals which may occur at any time after the onset of the causal condition.

Excludes1 personal history of cerebral infarction without residual deficit (Z86.73)
personal history of prolonged reversible ischemic neurologic deficit (PRIND) (Z86.73)
personal history of reversible ischemic neurologcial deficit (RIND) (Z86.73)
sequelae of traumatic intracranial injury (S06.-)
transient ischemic attack (TIA) (G45.9)

Coding Clinic: 2015, Q4, P40; 2012, Q4, P107

I69.0 Sequelae of nontraumatic subarachnoid hemorrhage

I69.00 Unspecified sequelae of nontraumatic subarachnoid hemorrhage

I69.01 Cognitive deficits following nontraumatic subarachnoid hemorrhage

I69.010 Attention and concentration deficit following nontraumatic subarachnoid hemorrhage ◀

I69.011 Memory deficit following nontraumatic subarachnoid hemorrhage ◀

I69.012 Visuospatial deficit and spatial neglect following nontraumatic subarachnoid hemorrhage ◀

I69.013 Psychomotor deficit following nontraumatic subarachnoid hemorrhage ◀

I69.014 Frontal lobe and executive function deficit following nontraumatic subarachnoid hemorrhage ◀

I69.015 Cognitive social or emotional deficit following nontraumatic subarachnoid hemorrhage ◀

I69.018 Other symptoms and signs involving cognitive functions following nontraumatic subarachnoid hemorrhage ◀

I69.019 Unspecified symptoms and signs involving cognitive functions following nontraumatic subarachnoid hemorrhage ◀

I69.02 Speech and language deficits following nontraumatic subarachnoid hemorrhage

I69.020 Aphasia following nontraumatic subarachnoid hemorrhage

I69.021 Dysphasia following nontraumatic subarachnoid hemorrhage

I69.022 Dysarthria following nontraumatic subarachnoid hemorrhage

I69.023 Fluency disorder following nontraumatic subarachnoid hemorrhage

Stuttering following nontraumatic subarachnoid hemorrhage

I69.028 Other speech and language deficits following nontraumatic subarachnoid hemorrhage

I69.03 Monoplegia of upper limb following nontraumatic subarachnoid hemorrhage

I69.031 Monoplegia of upper limb following nontraumatic subarachnoid hemorrhage affecting right dominant side

I69.032 Monoplegia of upper limb following nontraumatic subarachnoid hemorrhage affecting left dominant side

I69.033 Monoplegia of upper limb following nontraumatic subarachnoid hemorrhage affecting right non-dominant side

I69.034 Monoplegia of upper limb following nontraumatic subarachnoid hemorrhage affecting left non-dominant side

I69.039 Monoplegia of upper limb following nontraumatic subarachnoid hemorrhage affecting unspecified side

I69.04 Monoplegia of lower limb following nontraumatic subarachnoid hemorrhage

I69.041 Monoplegia of lower limb following nontraumatic subarachnoid hemorrhage affecting right dominant side

I69.042 Monoplegia of lower limb following nontraumatic subarachnoid hemorrhage affecting left dominant side

I69.043 Monoplegia of lower limb following nontraumatic subarachnoid hemorrhage affecting right non-dominant side

I69.044 Monoplegia of lower limb following nontraumatic subarachnoid hemorrhage affecting left non-dominant side

I69.049 Monoplegia of lower limb following nontraumatic subarachnoid hemorrhage affecting unspecified side

I69.05 Hemiplegia and hemiparesis following nontraumatic subarachnoid hemorrhage

I69.051 Hemiplegia and hemiparesis following nontraumatic subarachnoid hemorrhage affecting right dominant side

Ex: I69.051-I69.052, I69.151-I69.152, I69.251-I69.252, I69.351-I69.352, I69.851-I69.852, I69.951-I69.952

I69.052 Hemiplegia and hemiparesis following nontraumatic subarachnoid hemorrhage affecting left dominant side

Ex: See I69.051

I69.053 Hemiplegia and hemiparesis following nontraumatic subarachnoid hemorrhage affecting right non-dominant side

Ex: I69.053-I69.054, I69.153-I69.154, I69.253-I69.254, I69.353-I69.354, I69.853-I69.854, I69.953-I69.954

I69.054 Hemiplegia and hemiparesis following nontraumatic subarachnoid hemorrhage affecting left non-dominant side

Ex: See I69.053

I69.059 Hemiplegia and hemiparesis following nontraumatic subarachnoid hemorrhage affecting unspecified side

Ex: I69.059, I69.159, I69.259, I69.359, I69.859, I69.959

I69.06 Other paralytic syndrome following nontraumatic subarachnoid hemorrhage

Use additional code to identify type of paralytic syndrome, such as:
locked-in state (G83.5)
quadriplegia (G82.5-)

Excludes1 hemiplegia/hemiparesis following nontraumatic subarachnoid hemorrhage (I69.05-)
monoplegia of lower limb following nontraumatic subarachnoid hemorrhage (I69.04-)
monoplegia of upper limb following nontraumatic subarachnoid hemorrhage (I69.03-)

I69.061 Other paralytic syndrome following nontraumatic subarachnoid hemorrhage affecting right dominant side

I69.062 Other paralytic syndrome following nontraumatic subarachnoid hemorrhage affecting left dominant side

I69.063 Other paralytic syndrome following nontraumatic subarachnoid hemorrhage affecting right non-dominant side

I69.064 Other paralytic syndrome following nontraumatic subarachnoid hemorrhage affecting left non-dominant side

I69.065 Other paralytic syndrome following nontraumatic subarachnoid hemorrhage, bilateral

I69.069 Other paralytic syndrome following nontraumatic subarachnoid hemorrhage affecting unspecified side

I69.09 Other sequelae of nontraumatic subarachnoid hemorrhage

I69.090 Apraxia following nontraumatic subarachnoid hemorrhage

I69.091 Dysphagia following nontraumatic subarachnoid hemorrhage

Use additional code to identify the type of dysphagia, if known (R13.1-)

I69.092 Facial weakness following nontraumatic subarachnoid hemorrhage

Facial droop following nontraumatic subarachnoid hemorrhage

I69.093 Ataxia following nontraumatic subarachnoid hemorrhage

I69.098 Other sequelae following nontraumatic subarachnoid hemorrhage

Alterations of sensation following nontraumatic subarachnoid hemorrhage
Disturbance of vision following nontraumatic subarachnoid hemorrhage

Use additional code to identify the sequelae

I69.1 Sequelae of nontraumatic intracerebral hemorrhage

I69.10 Unspecified sequelae of nontraumatic intracerebral hemorrhage

I69.11 Cognitive deficits following nontraumatic intracerebral hemorrhage

I69.110 Attention and concentration deficit following nontraumatic intracerebral hemorrhage ◀

I69.111 Memory deficit following nontraumatic intracerebral hemorrhage ◀

I69.112 Visuospatial deficit and spatial neglect following nontraumatic intracerebral hemorrhage ◀

I69.113 Psychomotor deficit following nontraumatic intracerebral hemorrhage ◀

I69.114 Frontal lobe and executive function deficit following nontraumatic intracerebral hemorrhage ◀

I69.115 Cognitive social or emotional deficit following nontraumatic intracerebral hemorrhage ◀

I69.118 Other symptoms and signs involving cognitive functions following nontraumatic intracerebral hemorrhage ◀

I69.119 Unspecified symptoms and signs involving cognitive functions following nontraumatic intracerebral hemorrhage ◀

I69.12 Speech and language deficits following nontraumatic intracerebral hemorrhage

I69.120 Aphasia following nontraumatic intracerebral hemorrhage

I69.121 Dysphasia following nontraumatic intracerebral hemorrhage

I69.122 Dysarthria following nontraumatic intracerebral hemorrhage

I69.123 Fluency disorder following nontraumatic intracerebral hemorrhage
Stuttering following nontraumatic intracerebral hemorrhage

I69.128 Other speech and language deficits following nontraumatic intracerebral hemorrhage

I69.13 Monoplegia of upper limb following nontraumatic intracerebral hemorrhage

I69.131 Monoplegia of upper limb following nontraumatic intracerebral hemorrhage affecting right dominant side

I69.132 Monoplegia of upper limb following nontraumatic intracerebral hemorrhage affecting left dominant side

I69.133 Monoplegia of upper limb following nontraumatic intracerebral hemorrhage affecting right non-dominant side

I69.134 Monoplegia of upper limb following nontraumatic intracerebral hemorrhage affecting left non-dominant side

I69.139 Monoplegia of upper limb following nontraumatic intracerebral hemorrhage affecting unspecified side

I69.14 Monoplegia of lower limb following nontraumatic intracerebral hemorrhage

I69.141 Monoplegia of lower limb following nontraumatic intracerebral hemorrhage affecting right dominant side

I69.142 Monoplegia of lower limb following nontraumatic intracerebral hemorrhage affecting left dominant side

I69.143 Monoplegia of lower limb following nontraumatic intracerebral hemorrhage affecting right non-dominant side

I69.144 Monoplegia of lower limb following nontraumatic intracerebral hemorrhage affecting left non-dominant side

I69.149 Monoplegia of lower limb following nontraumatic intracerebral hemorrhage affecting unspecified side

I69.15 Hemiplegia and hemiparesis following nontraumatic intracerebral hemorrhage

I69.151 Hemiplegia and hemiparesis following nontraumatic intracerebral hemorrhage affecting right dominant side
Ex See I69.051

I69.152 Hemiplegia and hemiparesis following nontraumatic intracerebral hemorrhage affecting left dominant side
Ex See I69.051

I69.153 Hemiplegia and hemiparesis following nontraumatic intracerebral hemorrhage affecting right non-dominant side
Ex See I69.053

I69.154 Hemiplegia and hemiparesis following nontraumatic intracerebral hemorrhage affecting left non-dominant side
Ex See I69.053

I69.159 Hemiplegia and hemiparesis following nontraumatic intracerebral hemorrhage affecting unspecified side
Ex See I69.059

I69.16 Other paralytic syndrome following nontraumatic intracerebral hemorrhage
Use additional code to identify type of paralytic syndrome, such as:
locked-in state (G83.5)
quadriplegia (G82.5-)
Excludes1 hemiplegia/hemiparesis following nontraumatic intracerebral hemorrhage (I69.15-)
monoplegia of lower limb following nontraumatic intracerebral hemorrhage (I69.14-)
monoplegia of upper limb following nontraumatic intracerebral hemorrhage (I69.13-)

I69.161 Other paralytic syndrome following nontraumatic intracerebral hemorrhage affecting right dominant side

I69.162 Other paralytic syndrome following nontraumatic intracerebral hemorrhage affecting left dominant side

I69.163 Other paralytic syndrome following nontraumatic intracerebral hemorrhage affecting right non-dominant side

I69.164 Other paralytic syndrome following nontraumatic intracerebral hemorrhage affecting left non-dominant side

I69.165 Other paralytic syndrome following nontraumatic intracerebral hemorrhage, bilateral

I69.169 Other paralytic syndrome following nontraumatic intracerebral hemorrhage affecting unspecified side

I69.19 Other sequelae of nontraumatic intracerebral hemorrhage

I69.190 Apraxia following nontraumatic intracerebral hemorrhage

I69.191 Dysphagia following nontraumatic intracerebral hemorrhage
Use additional code to identify the type of dysphagia, if known (R13.1-)

I69.192 Facial weakness following nontraumatic intracerebral hemorrhage
Facial droop following nontraumatic intracerebral hemorrhage

I69.193 Ataxia following nontraumatic intracerebral hemorrhage

I69.198 Other sequelae of nontraumatic intracerebral hemorrhage
Alteration of sensations following nontraumatic intracerebral hemorrhage
Disturbance of vision following nontraumatic intracerebral hemorrhage
Use additional code to identify the sequelae

● I69.2 **Sequelae of other nontraumatic intracranial hemorrhage**

I69.20 **Unspecified sequelae of other nontraumatic intracranial hemorrhage**

● I69.21 **Cognitive deficits following other nontraumatic intracranial hemorrhage**

I69.210 **Attention and concentration deficit following other nontraumatic intracranial hemorrhage** ◀

I69.211 **Memory deficit following other nontraumatic intracranial hemorrhage** ◀

I69.212 **Visuospatial deficit and spatial neglect following other nontraumatic intracranial hemorrhage** ◀

I69.213 **Psychomotor deficit following other nontraumatic intracranial hemorrhage** ◀

I69.214 **Frontal lobe and executive function deficit following other nontraumatic intracranial hemorrhage** ◀

I69.215 **Cognitive social or emotional deficit following other nontraumatic intracranial hemorrhage** ◀

I69.218 **Other symptoms and signs involving cognitive functions following other nontraumatic intracranial hemorrhage** ◀

I69.219 **Unspecified symptoms and signs involving cognitive functions following other nontraumatic intracranial hemorrhage** ◀

● I69.22 **Speech and language deficits following other nontraumatic intracranial hemorrhage**

I69.220 **Aphasia following other nontraumatic intracranial hemorrhage**

I69.221 **Dysphasia following other nontraumatic intracranial hemorrhage**

I69.222 **Dysarthria following other nontraumatic intracranial hemorrhage**

I69.223 **Fluency disorder following other nontraumatic intracranial hemorrhage**

Stuttering following other nontraumatic intracranial hemorrhage ⇐

I69.228 **Other speech and language deficits following other nontraumatic intracranial hemorrhage**

● I69.23 **Monoplegia of upper limb following other nontraumatic intracranial hemorrhage**

I69.231 **Monoplegia of upper limb following other nontraumatic intracranial hemorrhage affecting right dominant side**

I69.232 **Monoplegia of upper limb following other nontraumatic intracranial hemorrhage affecting left dominant side**

I69.233 **Monoplegia of upper limb following other nontraumatic intracranial hemorrhage affecting right non-dominant side**

I69.234 **Monoplegia of upper limb following other nontraumatic intracranial hemorrhage affecting left non-dominant side**

I69.239 **Monoplegia of upper limb following other nontraumatic intracranial hemorrhage affecting unspecified side**

● I69.24 **Monoplegia of lower limb following other nontraumatic intracranial hemorrhage**

I69.241 **Monoplegia of lower limb following other nontraumatic intracranial hemorrhage affecting right dominant side**

I69.242 **Monoplegia of lower limb following other nontraumatic intracranial hemorrhage affecting left dominant side**

I69.243 **Monoplegia of lower limb following other nontraumatic intracranial hemorrhage affecting right non-dominant side**

I69.244 **Monoplegia of lower limb following other nontraumatic intracranial hemorrhage affecting left non-dominant side**

I69.249 **Monoplegia of lower limb following other nontraumatic intracranial hemorrhage affecting unspecified side**

● I69.25 **Hemiplegia and hemiparesis following other nontraumatic intracranial hemorrhage**

I69.251 **Hemiplegia and hemiparesis following other nontraumatic intracranial hemorrhage affecting right dominant side**

Ex: See I69.051

I69.252 **Hemiplegia and hemiparesis following other nontraumatic intracranial hemorrhage affecting left dominant side**

Ex: See I69.051

I69.253 **Hemiplegia and hemiparesis following other nontraumatic intracranial hemorrhage affecting right non-dominant side**

Ex: See I69.053

I69.254 **Hemiplegia and hemiparesis following other nontraumatic intracranial hemorrhage affecting left non-dominant side**

Ex: See I69.053

I69.259 **Hemiplegia and hemiparesis following other nontraumatic intracranial hemorrhage affecting unspecified side**

Ex: See I69.059

● I69.26 **Other paralytic syndrome following other nontraumatic intracranial hemorrhage**

Use additional code to identify type of paralytic syndrome, such as:
locked-in state (G83.5)
quadriplegia (G82.5-)

Excludes1 hemiplegia/hemiparesis following other nontraumatic intracranial hemorrhage (I69.25-)
monoplegia of lower limb following other nontraumatic intracranial hemorrhage (I69.24-)
monoplegia of upper limb following other nontraumatic intracranial hemorrhage (I69.23-)

I69.261 **Other paralytic syndrome following other nontraumatic intracranial hemorrhage affecting right dominant side**

I69.262 **Other paralytic syndrome following other nontraumatic intracranial hemorrhage affecting left dominant side**

I69.263 **Other paralytic syndrome following other nontraumatic intracranial hemorrhage affecting right non-dominant side**

I69.264 **Other paralytic syndrome following other nontraumatic intracranial hemorrhage affecting left non-dominant side**

I69.265 **Other paralytic syndrome following other nontraumatic intracranial hemorrhage, bilateral**

I69.269 **Other paralytic syndrome following other nontraumatic intracranial hemorrhage affecting unspecified side**

● **I69.29** **Other sequelae of other nontraumatic intracranial hemorrhage**

I69.290 **Apraxia following other nontraumatic intracranial hemorrhage**

I69.291 **Dysphagia following other nontraumatic intracranial hemorrhage**

Use additional code to identify the type of dysphagia, if known (R13.1-)

I69.292 **Facial weakness following other nontraumatic intracranial hemorrhage**

Facial droop following other nontraumatic intracranial hemorrhage

I69.293 **Ataxia following other nontraumatic intracranial hemorrhage**

I69.298 **Other sequelae of other nontraumatic intracranial hemorrhage**

Alteration of sensation following other nontraumatic intracranial hemorrhage

Disturbance of vision following other nontraumatic intracranial hemorrhage

Use additional code to identify the sequelae

● **I69.3** **Sequelae of cerebral infarction**

Sequelae of stroke NOS

Coding Clinic: 2012, Q4, P92, 95

I69.30 **Unspecified sequelae of cerebral infarction**

● **I69.31** **Cognitive deficits following cerebral infarction**

I69.310 **Attention and concentration deficit following cerebral infarction** ◀

I69.311 **Memory deficit following cerebral infarction** ◀

I69.312 **Visuospatial deficit and spatial neglect following cerebral infarction** ◀

I69.313 **Psychomotor deficit following cerebral infarction** ◀

I69.314 **Frontal lobe and executive function deficit following cerebral infarction** ◀

I69.315 **Cognitive social or emotional deficit following cerebral infarction** ◀

I69.318 **Other symptoms and signs involving cognitive functions following cerebral infarction** ◀

I69.319 **Unspecified symptoms and signs involving cognitive functions following cerebral infarction** ◀

● **I69.32** **Speech and language deficits following cerebral infarction**

I69.320 **Aphasia following cerebral infarction**

I69.321 **Dysphasia following cerebral infarction**

Coding Clinic: 2012, Q4, P91

I69.322 **Dysarthria following cerebral infarction**

I69.323 **Fluency disorder following cerebral infarction**

Stuttering following cerebral infarction ◀

I69.328 **Other speech and language deficits following cerebral infarction**

● **I69.33** **Monoplegia of upper limb following cerebral infarction**

I69.331 **Monoplegia of upper limb following cerebral infarction affecting right dominant side**

I69.332 **Monoplegia of upper limb following cerebral infarction affecting left dominant side**

I69.333 **Monoplegia of upper limb following cerebral infarction affecting right non-dominant side**

I69.334 **Monoplegia of upper limb following cerebral infarction affecting left non-dominant side**

I69.339 **Monoplegia of upper limb following cerebral infarction affecting unspecified side**

● **I69.34** **Monoplegia of lower limb following cerebral infarction**

I69.341 **Monoplegia of lower limb following cerebral infarction affecting right dominant side**

I69.342 **Monoplegia of lower limb following cerebral infarction affecting left dominant side**

I69.343 **Monoplegia of lower limb following cerebral infarction affecting right non-dominant side**

I69.344 **Monoplegia of lower limb following cerebral infarction affecting left non-dominant side**

I69.349 **Monoplegia of lower limb following cerebral infarction affecting unspecified side**

● **I69.35** **Hemiplegia and hemiparesis following cerebral infarction**

I69.351 **Hemiplegia and hemiparesis following cerebral infarction affecting right dominant side**

Ex: See I69.051

Coding Clinic: 2015, Q1, P25

I69.352 **Hemiplegia and hemiparesis following cerebral infarction affecting left dominant side**

Ex: See I69.051

I69.353 **Hemiplegia and hemiparesis following cerebral infarction affecting right non-dominant side**

Ex: See I69.053

I69.354 **Hemiplegia and hemiparesis following cerebral infarction affecting left non-dominant side**

Ex: See I69.053

Coding Clinic: 2012, Q4, P91

I69.359 **Hemiplegia and hemiparesis following cerebral infarction affecting unspecified side**

Ex: See I69.059

● I69.36 Other paralytic syndrome following cerebral infarction

Use additional code to identify type of paralytic syndrome, such as:
locked-in state (G83.5)
quadriplegia (G82.5-)

Excludes1 hemiplegia/hemiparesis following cerebral infarction (I69.35-)
monoplegia of lower limb following cerebral infarction (I69.34-)
monoplegia of upper limb following cerebral infarction (I69.33-)

I69.361 Other paralytic syndrome following cerebral infarction affecting right dominant side

I69.362 Other paralytic syndrome following cerebral infarction affecting left dominant side

I69.363 Other paralytic syndrome following cerebral infarction affecting right non-dominant side

I69.364 Other paralytic syndrome following cerebral infarction affecting left non-dominant side

I69.365 Other paralytic syndrome following cerebral infarction, bilateral

I69.369 Other paralytic syndrome following cerebral infarction affecting unspecified side

● I69.39 Other sequelae of cerebral infarction

I69.390 Apraxia following cerebral infarction

I69.391 Dysphagia following cerebral infarction

Use additional code to identify the type of dysphagia, if known (R13.1-)

I69.392 Facial weakness following cerebral infarction

Facial droop following cerebral infarction

I69.393 Ataxia following cerebral infarction

I69.398 Other sequelae of cerebral infarction

Alteration of sensation following cerebral infarction
Disturbance of vision following cerebral infarction

Use additional code to identify the sequelae

● I69.8 Sequelae of other cerebrovascular diseases

Excludes1 sequelae of traumatic intracranial injury (S06.-)

I69.80 Unspecified sequelae of other cerebrovascular disease

● I69.81 Cognitive deficits following other cerebrovascular disease

I69.810 Attention and concentration deficit following other cerebrovascular disease ◀

I69.811 Memory deficit following other cerebrovascular disease ◀

I69.812 Visuospatial deficit and spatial neglect following other cerebrovascular disease ◀

I69.813 Psychomotor deficit following other cerebrovascular disease ◀

I69.814 Frontal lobe and executive function deficit following other cerebrovascular disease ◀

I69.815 Cognitive social or emotional deficit following other cerebrovascular disease ◀

I69.818 Other symptoms and signs involving cognitive functions following other cerebrovascular disease ◀

I69.819 Unspecified symptoms and signs involving cognitive functions following other cerebrovascular disease ◀

● I69.82 Speech and language deficits following other cerebrovascular disease

I69.820 Aphasia following other cerebrovascular disease

I69.821 Dysphasia following other cerebrovascular disease

I69.822 Dysarthria following other cerebrovascular disease

I69.823 Fluency disorder following other cerebrovascular disease

Stuttering following other cerebrovascular disease ⬅

I69.828 Other speech and language deficits following other cerebrovascular disease

● I69.83 Monoplegia of upper limb following other cerebrovascular disease

I69.831 Monoplegia of upper limb following other cerebrovascular disease affecting right dominant side

I69.832 Monoplegia of upper limb following other cerebrovascular disease affecting left dominant side

I69.833 Monoplegia of upper limb following other cerebrovascular disease affecting right non-dominant side

I69.834 Monoplegia of upper limb following other cerebrovascular disease affecting left non-dominant side

I69.839 Monoplegia of upper limb following other cerebrovascular disease affecting unspecified side

● I69.84 Monoplegia of lower limb following other cerebrovascular disease

I69.841 Monoplegia of lower limb following other cerebrovascular disease affecting right dominant side

I69.842 Monoplegia of lower limb following other cerebrovascular disease affecting left dominant side

I69.843 Monoplegia of lower limb following other cerebrovascular disease affecting right non-dominant side

I69.844 Monoplegia of lower limb following other cerebrovascular disease affecting left non-dominant side

I69.849 Monoplegia of lower limb following other cerebrovascular disease affecting unspecified side

● I69.85 Hemiplegia and hemiparesis following other cerebrovascular disease

I69.851 Hemiplegia and hemiparesis following other cerebrovascular disease affecting right dominant side

Ex: See I69.051

I69.852 Hemiplegia and hemiparesis following other cerebrovascular disease affecting left dominant side

Ex: See I69.051

◀ New ⬅ Revised ~~deleted~~ Deleted Excludes 1 Excludes 2 Includes Use additional Code first Code also Unspecified
OGCR Official Guidelines ● Unacceptable Principal Diagnosis X Assign placeholder X ● Use Additional Character(s) ▶ Manifestation Code Coding Clinic

I69.853 **Hemiplegia and hemiparesis following other cerebrovascular disease affecting right non-dominant side**
Ex: See I69.053

I69.854 **Hemiplegia and hemiparesis following other cerebrovascular disease affecting left non-dominant side**
Ex: See I69.053

I69.859 **Hemiplegia and hemiparesis following other cerebrovascular disease affecting unspecified side**
Ex: See I69.059

I69.86 **Other paralytic syndrome following other cerebrovascular disease**
Use additional code to identify type of paralytic syndrome, such as:
locked-in state (G83.5)
quadriplegia (G82.5-)
Excludes1 hemiplegia/hemiparesis following other cerebrovascular disease (I69.85-)
monoplegia of lower limb following other cerebrovascular disease (I69.84-)
monoplegia of upper limb following other cerebrovascular disease (I69.83-)

I69.861 **Other paralytic syndrome following other cerebrovascular disease affecting right dominant side**

I69.862 **Other paralytic syndrome following other cerebrovascular disease affecting left dominant side**

I69.863 **Other paralytic syndrome following other cerebrovascular disease affecting right non-dominant side**

I69.864 **Other paralytic syndrome following other cerebrovascular disease affecting left non-dominant side**

I69.865 **Other paralytic syndrome following other cerebrovascular disease, bilateral**

I69.869 **Other paralytic syndrome following other cerebrovascular disease affecting unspecified side**

I69.89 **Other sequelae of other cerebrovascular disease**

I69.890 **Apraxia following other cerebrovascular disease**

I69.891 **Dysphagia following other cerebrovascular disease**
Use additional code to identify the type of dysphagia, if known (R13.1-)

I69.892 **Facial weakness following other cerebrovascular disease**
Facial droop following other cerebrovascular disease

I69.893 **Ataxia following other cerebrovascular disease**

I69.898 **Other sequelae of other cerebrovascular disease**
Alteration of sensation following other cerebrovascular disease
Disturbance of vision following other cerebrovascular disease
Use additional code to identify the sequelae

I69.9 **Sequelae of unspecified cerebrovascular diseases**
Excludes1 sequelae of stroke (I69.3)
sequelae of traumatic intracranial injury (S06.-)

I69.90 **Unspecified sequelae of unspecified cerebrovascular disease**

I69.91 **Cognitive deficits following unspecified cerebrovascular disease**

I69.910 **Attention and concentration deficit following unspecified cerebrovascular disease**

I69.911 **Memory deficit following unspecified cerebrovascular disease**

I69.912 **Visuospatial deficit and spatial neglect following unspecified cerebrovascular disease**

I69.913 **Psychomotor deficit following unspecified cerebrovascular disease**

I69.914 **Frontal lobe and executive function deficit following unspecified cerebrovascular disease**

I69.915 **Cognitive social or emotional deficit following unspecified cerebrovascular disease**

I69.918 **Other symptoms and signs involving cognitive functions following unspecified cerebrovascular disease**

I69.919 **Unspecified symptoms and signs involving cognitive functions following unspecified cerebrovascular disease**

I69.92 **Speech and language deficits following unspecified cerebrovascular disease**

I69.920 **Aphasia following unspecified cerebrovascular disease**

I69.921 **Dysphasia following unspecified cerebrovascular disease**

I69.922 **Dysarthria following unspecified cerebrovascular disease**

I69.923 **Fluency disorder following unspecified cerebrovascular disease**
Stuttering following unspecified cerebrovascular disease

I69.928 **Other speech and language deficits following unspecified cerebrovascular disease**

I69.93 **Monoplegia of upper limb following unspecified cerebrovascular disease**

I69.931 **Monoplegia of upper limb following unspecified cerebrovascular disease affecting right dominant side**

I69.932 **Monoplegia of upper limb following unspecified cerebrovascular disease affecting left dominant side**

I69.933 **Monoplegia of upper limb following unspecified cerebrovascular disease affecting right non-dominant side**

I69.934 **Monoplegia of upper limb following unspecified cerebrovascular disease affecting left non-dominant side**

I69.939 **Monoplegia of upper limb following unspecified cerebrovascular disease affecting unspecified side**

● I69.94 **Monoplegia of lower limb following unspecified cerebrovascular disease**

I69.941 **Monoplegia of lower limb following unspecified cerebrovascular disease affecting right dominant side**

I69.942 **Monoplegia of lower limb following unspecified cerebrovascular disease affecting left dominant side**

I69.943 **Monoplegia of lower limb following unspecified cerebrovascular disease affecting right non-dominant side**

I69.944 **Monoplegia of lower limb following unspecified cerebrovascular disease affecting left non-dominant side**

I69.949 **Monoplegia of lower limb following unspecified cerebrovascular disease affecting unspecified side**

● I69.95 **Hemiplegia and hemiparesis following unspecified cerebrovascular disease**

I69.951 **Hemiplegia and hemiparesis following unspecified cerebrovascular disease affecting right dominant side**

Ex: See I69.051

I69.952 **Hemiplegia and hemiparesis following unspecified cerebrovascular disease affecting left dominant side**

Ex: See I69.051

I69.953 **Hemiplegia and hemiparesis following unspecified cerebrovascular disease affecting right non-dominant side**

Ex: See I69.053

I69.954 **Hemiplegia and hemiparesis following unspecified cerebrovascular disease affecting left non-dominant side**

Ex: See I69.053

I69.959 **Hemiplegia and hemiparesis following unspecified cerebrovascular disease affecting unspecified side**

Ex: See I69.059

● I69.96 **Other paralytic syndrome following unspecified cerebrovascular disease**

Use additional code to identify type of paralytic syndrome, such as:
locked-in state (G83.5)
quadriplegia (G82.5-)

Excludes1 hemiplegia/hemiparesis following unspecified cerebrovascular disease (I69.95-)
monoplegia of lower limb following unspecified cerebrovascular disease (I69.94-)
monoplegia of upper limb following unspecified cerebrovascular disease (I69.93-)

I69.961 **Other paralytic syndrome following unspecified cerebrovascular disease affecting right dominant side**

I69.962 **Other paralytic syndrome following unspecified cerebrovascular disease affecting left dominant side**

I69.963 **Other paralytic syndrome following unspecified cerebrovascular disease affecting right non-dominant side**

I69.964 **Other paralytic syndrome following unspecified cerebrovascular disease affecting left non-dominant side**

I69.965 **Other paralytic syndrome following unspecified cerebrovascular disease, bilateral**

I69.969 **Other paralytic syndrome following unspecified cerebrovascular disease affecting unspecified side**

● I69.99 **Other sequelae of unspecified cerebrovascular disease**

I69.990 **Apraxia following unspecified cerebrovascular disease**

I69.991 **Dysphagia following unspecified cerebrovascular disease**

Use additional code to identify the type of dysphagia, if known (R13.1-)

I69.992 **Facial weakness following unspecified cerebrovascular disease**

Facial droop following unspecified cerebrovascular disease

I69.993 **Ataxia following unspecified cerebrovascular disease**

I69.998 **Other sequelae following unspecified cerebrovascular disease**

Alteration in sensation following unspecified cerebrovascular disease
Disturbance of vision following unspecified cerebrovascular disease

Use additional code to identify the sequelae

DISEASES OF ARTERIES, ARTERIOLES AND CAPILLARIES (I70-I79)

● I70 **Atherosclerosis**

Includes arteriolosclerosis
arterial degeneration
arteriosclerosis
arteriosclerotic vascular disease
arteriovascular degeneration
atheroma
endarteritis deformans or obliterans
senile arteritis
senile endarteritis
vascular degeneration

Use additional code to identify:
exposure to environmental tobacco smoke (Z77.22)
history of tobacco dependence (Z87.891)
occupational exposure to environmental tobacco smoke (Z57.31)
tobacco dependence (F17.-)
tobacco use (Z72.0)

Excludes2 arteriosclerotic cardiovascular disease (I25.1-)
arteriosclerotic heart disease (I25.1-)
atheroembolism (I75.-)
cerebral atherosclerosis (I67.2)
coronary atherosclerosis (I25.1-)
mesenteric atherosclerosis (K55.1)
precerebral atherosclerosis (I67.2)
primary pulmonary atherosclerosis (I27.0)

I70.0 **Atherosclerosis of aorta** A

I70.1 **Atherosclerosis of renal artery** A

Goldblatt's kidney

Excludes2 atherosclerosis of renal arterioles (I12.-)

★ **(See Plates 500, 501, and 502 on pages 60 – 62.)**

● **I70.2 Atherosclerosis of native arteries of the extremities**
Mönckeberg's (medial) sclerosis
Use additional code, if applicable, to identify chronic total occlusion of artery of extremity (I70.92)
Excludes2 atherosclerosis of bypass graft of extremities (I70.30-I70.79)

● **I70.20 Unspecified atherosclerosis of native arteries of extremities**
I70.201 Unspecified atherosclerosis of native arteries of extremities, right leg A
I70.202 Unspecified atherosclerosis of native arteries of extremities, left leg A
I70.203 Unspecified atherosclerosis of native arteries of extremities, bilateral legs A
I70.208 Unspecified atherosclerosis of native arteries of extremities, other extremity A
I70.209 Unspecified atherosclerosis of native arteries of extremities, unspecified extremity A

● **I70.21 Atherosclerosis of native arteries of extremities with intermittent claudication**
I70.211 Atherosclerosis of native arteries of extremities with intermittent claudication, right leg A
I70.212 Atherosclerosis of native arteries of extremities with intermittent claudication, left leg A
I70.213 Atherosclerosis of native arteries of extremities with intermittent claudication, bilateral legs A
I70.218 Atherosclerosis of native arteries of extremities with intermittent claudication, other extremity A
I70.219 Atherosclerosis of native arteries of extremities with intermittent claudication, unspecified extremity A

● **I70.22 Atherosclerosis of native arteries of extremities with rest pain**
Includes any condition classifiable to I70.21-
I70.221 Atherosclerosis of native arteries of extremities with rest pain, right leg A
I70.222 Atherosclerosis of native arteries of extremities with rest pain, left leg A
I70.223 Atherosclerosis of native arteries of extremities with rest pain, bilateral legs A
I70.228 Atherosclerosis of native arteries of extremities with rest pain, other extremity A
I70.229 Atherosclerosis of native arteries of extremities with rest pain, unspecified extremity A

● **I70.23 Atherosclerosis of native arteries of right leg with ulceration**
Includes any condition classifiable to I70.211 and I70.221
Use additional code to identify severity of ulcer (L97.-)
I70.231 Atherosclerosis of native arteries of right leg with ulceration of thigh A
I70.232 Atherosclerosis of native arteries of right leg with ulceration of calf A
I70.233 Atherosclerosis of native arteries of right leg with ulceration of ankle A
I70.234 Atherosclerosis of native arteries of right leg with ulceration of heel and midfoot A
Atherosclerosis of native arteries of right leg with ulceration of plantar surface of midfoot
I70.235 Atherosclerosis of native arteries of right leg with ulceration of other part of foot A
Atherosclerosis of native arteries of right leg extremities with ulceration of toe
I70.238 Atherosclerosis of native arteries of right leg with ulceration of other part of lower right leg A
I70.239 Atherosclerosis of native arteries of right leg with ulceration of unspecified site A

● **I70.24 Atherosclerosis of native arteries of left leg with ulceration**
Includes any condition classifiable to I70.212 and I70.222
Use additional code to identify severity of ulcer (L97.-)
I70.241 Atherosclerosis of native arteries of left leg with ulceration of thigh A
I70.242 Atherosclerosis of native arteries of left leg with ulceration of calf A
I70.243 Atherosclerosis of native arteries of left leg with ulceration of ankle A
I70.244 Atherosclerosis of native arteries of left leg with ulceration of heel and midfoot A
Atherosclerosis of native arteries of left leg with ulceration of plantar surface of midfoot
I70.245 Atherosclerosis of native arteries of left leg with ulceration of other part of foot A
Atherosclerosis of native arteries of left leg extremities with ulceration of toe
I70.248 Atherosclerosis of native arteries of left leg with ulceration of other part of lower left leg A
I70.249 Atherosclerosis of native arteries of left leg with ulceration of unspecified site A

I70.25 Atherosclerosis of native arteries of other extremities with ulceration A
Includes any condition classifiable to I70.218 and I70.228
Use additional code to identify the severity of the ulcer (L98.49-)

● **I70.26 Atherosclerosis of native arteries of extremities with gangrene**
Includes any condition classifiable to I70.21-, I70.22-, I70.23-, I70.24-, and I70.25-
Use additional code to identify the severity of any ulcer (L97.-, L98.49-), if applicable
Exc **For category I70.26 CC codes:** G89.0-G89.4, I70.261-I70.269, I96, R29.700-R29.742, R41.0-R41.3, R41.82, R41.9, R44.8-R44.9, R45.83-R45.84, R46.0-R46.89, R52, R68.0-R68.19, R68.81-R68.83, R68.89-R69
I70.261 Atherosclerosis of native arteries of extremities with gangrene, right leg CC A
I70.262 Atherosclerosis of native arteries of extremities with gangrene, left leg CC A
I70.263 Atherosclerosis of native arteries of extremities with gangrene, bilateral legs CC A

I70.268 Atherosclerosis of native arteries of extremities with gangrene, other extremity A

I70.269 Atherosclerosis of native arteries of extremities with gangrene, unspecified extremity A

● I70.29 Other atherosclerosis of native arteries of extremities

I70.291 Other atherosclerosis of native arteries of extremities, right leg A

I70.292 Other atherosclerosis of native arteries of extremities, left leg A

I70.293 Other atherosclerosis of native arteries of extremities, bilateral legs A

I70.298 Other atherosclerosis of native arteries of extremities, other extremity A

I70.299 Other atherosclerosis of native arteries of extremities, unspecified extremity A

● I70.3 Atherosclerosis of unspecified type of bypass graft(s) of the extremities

Use additional code, if applicable, to identify chronic total occlusion of artery of extremity (I70.92)

Excludes1 embolism or thrombus of bypass graft(s) of extremities (T82.8-)

● I70.30 Unspecified atherosclerosis of unspecified type of bypass graft(s) of the extremities

70.301 Unspecified atherosclerosis of unspecified type of bypass graft(s) of the extremities, right leg A

I70.302 Unspecified atherosclerosis of unspecified type of bypass graft(s) of the extremities, left leg A

I70.303 Unspecified atherosclerosis of unspecified type of bypass graft(s) of the extremities, bilateral legs A

I70.308 Unspecified atherosclerosis of unspecified type of bypass graft(s) of the extremities, other extremity A

I70.309 Unspecified atherosclerosis of unspecified type of bypass graft(s) of the extremities, unspecified extremity A

● I70.31 Atherosclerosis of unspecified type of bypass graft(s) of the extremities with intermittent claudication

I70.311 Atherosclerosis of unspecified type of bypass graft(s) of the extremities with intermittent claudication, right leg A

I70.312 Atherosclerosis of unspecified type of bypass graft(s) of the extremities with intermittent claudication, left leg A

I70.313 Atherosclerosis of unspecified type of bypass graft(s) of the extremities with intermittent claudication, bilateral legs A

I70.318 Atherosclerosis of unspecified type of bypass graft(s) of the extremities with intermittent claudication, other extremity A

I70.319 Atherosclerosis of unspecified type of bypass graft(s) of the extremities with intermittent claudication, unspecified extremity A

● I70.32 Atherosclerosis of unspecified type of bypass graft(s) of the extremities with rest pain

Includes any condition classifiable to I70.31-

I70.321 Atherosclerosis of unspecified type of bypass graft(s) of the extremities with rest pain, right leg A

I70.322 Atherosclerosis of unspecified type of bypass graft(s) of the extremities with rest pain, left leg A

I70.323 Atherosclerosis of unspecified type of bypass graft(s) of the extremities with rest pain, bilateral legs A

I70.328 Atherosclerosis of unspecified type of bypass graft(s) of the extremities with rest pain, other extremity A

I70.329 Atherosclerosis of unspecified type of bypass graft(s) of the extremities with rest pain, unspecified extremity A

● I70.33 Atherosclerosis of unspecified type of bypass graft(s) of the right leg with ulceration

Includes any condition classifiable to I70.311 and I70.321

Use additional code to identify severity of ulcer (L97.-)

Ex: **For category I70.33 CC codes:** I70.231-I70.25, L44.8-L45, L94.2, L94.4, L97.101-L97.929, L98.411-L98.499, L98.7, L98.7-L99

I70.331 Atherosclerosis of unspecified type of bypass graft(s) of the right leg with ulceration of thigh A
CC when PDx is its own CC

I70.332 Atherosclerosis of unspecified type of bypass graft(s) of the right leg with ulceration of calf A
CC when PDx is its own CC

I70.333 Atherosclerosis of unspecified type of bypass graft(s) of the right leg with ulceration of ankle A
CC when PDx is its own CC

I70.334 Atherosclerosis of unspecified type of bypass graft(s) of the right leg with ulceration of heel and midfoot A
Atherosclerosis of unspecified type of bypass graft(s) of right leg with ulceration of plantar surface of midfoot
CC when PDx is its own CC

I70.335 Atherosclerosis of unspecified type of bypass graft(s) of the right leg with ulceration of other part of foot A
Atherosclerosis of unspecified type of bypass graft(s) of the right leg with ulceration of toe

I70.338 Atherosclerosis of unspecified type of bypass graft(s) of the right leg with ulceration of other part of lower leg A
CC when PDx is its own CC

I70.339 Atherosclerosis of unspecified type of bypass graft(s) of the right leg with ulceration of unspecified site A
CC when PDx is its own CC

● **I70.34 Atherosclerosis of unspecified type of bypass graft(s) of the left leg with ulceration**

Includes any condition classifiable to I70.312 and I70.322

Use additional code to identify severity of ulcer (L97.-)

Ex: **For category I70.34 CC codes:** See I70.33

I70.341 Atherosclerosis of unspecified type of bypass graft(s) of the left leg with ulceration of thigh A
CC when PDx is its own CC

I70.342 Atherosclerosis of unspecified type of bypass graft(s) of the left leg with ulceration of calf A
CC when PDx is its own CC

I70.343 Atherosclerosis of unspecified type of bypass graft(s) of the left leg with ulceration of ankle A
CC when PDx is its own CC

I70.344 Atherosclerosis of unspecified type of bypass graft(s) of the left leg with ulceration of heel and midfoot A
Atherosclerosis of unspecified type of bypass graft(s) of left leg with ulceration of plantar surface of midfoot
CC when PDx is its own CC

I70.345 Atherosclerosis of unspecified type of bypass graft(s) of the left leg with ulceration of other part of foot A
Atherosclerosis of unspecified type of bypass graft(s) of the left leg with ulceration of toe

I70.348 Atherosclerosis of unspecified type of bypass graft(s) of the left leg with ulceration of other part of lower leg A
CC when PDx is its own CC

I70.349 Atherosclerosis of unspecified type of bypass graft(s) of the left leg with ulceration of unspecified site A
CC when PDx is its own CC

I70.35 Atherosclerosis of unspecified type of bypass graft(s) of other extremity with ulceration A

Includes any condition classifiable to I70.318 and I70.328

Use additional code to identify severity of ulcer (L98.49-)

● **I70.36 Atherosclerosis of unspecified type of bypass graft(s) of the extremities with gangrene**

Includes any condition classifiable to I70.31-, I70.32-, I70.33-, I70.34-, I70.35

Use additional code to identify the severity of any ulcer (L97.-, L98.49-), if applicable

Ex: **For category I70.36 CC codes:** See I70.26

I70.361 Atherosclerosis of unspecified type of bypass graft(s) of the extremities with gangrene, right leg A
CC when PDx is its own CC

I70.362 Atherosclerosis of unspecified type of bypass graft(s) of the extremities with gangrene, left leg A
CC when PDx is its own CC

I70.363 Atherosclerosis of unspecified type of bypass graft(s) of the extremities with gangrene, bilateral legs A
CC when PDx is its own CC

I70.368 Atherosclerosis of unspecified type of bypass graft(s) of the extremities with gangrene, other extremity A
CC when PDx is its own CC

I70.369 Atherosclerosis of unspecified type of bypass graft(s) of the extremities with gangrene, unspecified extremity A
CC when PDx is its own CC

● **I70.39 Other atherosclerosis of unspecified type of bypass graft(s) of the extremities**

I70.391 Other atherosclerosis of unspecified type of bypass graft(s) of the extremities, right leg A

I70.392 Other atherosclerosis of unspecified type of bypass graft(s) of the extremities, left leg A

I70.393 Other atherosclerosis of unspecified type of bypass graft(s) of the extremities, bilateral legs A

I70.398 Other atherosclerosis of unspecified type of bypass graft(s) of the extremities, other extremity A

I70.399 Other atherosclerosis of unspecified type of bypass graft(s) of the extremities, unspecified extremity A

● **I70.4 Atherosclerosis of autologous vein bypass graft(s) of the extremities**

Use additional code, if applicable, to identify chronic total occlusion of artery of extremity (I70.92)

● **I70.40 Unspecified atherosclerosis of autologous vein bypass graft(s) of the extremities**

I70.401 Unspecified atherosclerosis of autologous vein bypass graft(s) of the extremities, right leg A

I70.402 Unspecified atherosclerosis of autologous vein bypass graft(s) of the extremities, left leg A

I70.403 Unspecified atherosclerosis of autologous vein bypass graft(s) of the extremities, bilateral legs A

I70.408 Unspecified atherosclerosis of autologous vein bypass graft(s) of the extremities, other extremity A

I70.409 Unspecified atherosclerosis of autologous vein bypass graft(s) of the extremities, unspecified extremity A

● **I70.41 Atherosclerosis of autologous vein bypass graft(s) of the extremities with intermittent claudication**

I70.411 Atherosclerosis of autologous vein bypass graft(s) of the extremities with intermittent claudication, right leg A

I70.412 Atherosclerosis of autologous vein bypass graft(s) of the extremities with intermittent claudication, left leg A

I70.413 Atherosclerosis of autologous vein bypass graft(s) of the extremities with intermittent claudication, bilateral legs A

I70.418 Atherosclerosis of autologous vein bypass graft(s) of the extremities with intermittent claudication, other extremity A

I70.419 Atherosclerosis of autologous vein bypass graft(s) of the extremities with intermittent claudication, unspecified extremity A

● **I70.42 Atherosclerosis of autologous vein bypass graft(s) of the extremities with rest pain**

Includes any condition classifiable to I70.41-

I70.421 Atherosclerosis of autologous vein bypass graft(s) of the extremities with rest pain, right leg A

I70.422 Atherosclerosis of autologous vein bypass graft(s) of the extremities with rest pain, left leg A

I70.423 **Atherosclerosis of autologous vein bypass graft(s) of the extremities with rest pain, bilateral legs** A

I70.428 **Atherosclerosis of autologous vein bypass graft(s) of the extremities with rest pain, other extremity** A

I70.429 **Atherosclerosis of autologous vein bypass graft(s) of the extremities with rest pain, unspecified extremity** A

● **I70.43** **Atherosclerosis of autologous vein bypass graft(s) of the right leg with ulceration**

Includes any condition classifiable to I70.411 and I70.421

Use additional code to identify severity of ulcer (L97.-)

Ex: **For category I70.43 CC codes:** See I70.33

I70.431 **Atherosclerosis of autologous vein bypass graft(s) of the right leg with ulceration of thigh** A
CC when PDx is its own CC

I70.432 **Atherosclerosis of autologous vein bypass graft(s) of the right leg with ulceration of calf** A
CC when PDx is its own CC

I70.433 **Atherosclerosis of autologous vein bypass graft(s) of the right leg with ulceration of ankle** A
CC when PDx is its own CC

I70.434 **Atherosclerosis of autologous vein bypass graft(s) of the right leg with ulceration of heel and midfoot** A
Atherosclerosis of autologous vein bypass graft(s) of right leg with ulceration of plantar surface of midfoot
CC when PDx is its own CC

I70.435 **Atherosclerosis of autologous vein bypass graft(s) of the right leg with ulceration of other part of foot** A
Atherosclerosis of autologous vein bypass graft(s) of right leg with ulceration of toe

I70.438 **Atherosclerosis of autologous vein bypass graft(s) of the right leg with ulceration of other part of lower leg** A
CC when PDx is its own CC

I70.439 **Atherosclerosis of autologous vein bypass graft(s) of the right leg with ulceration of unspecified site** A
CC when PDx is its own CC

● **I70.44** **Atherosclerosis of autologous vein bypass graft(s) of the left leg with ulceration**

Includes any condition classifiable to I70.412 and I70.422

Use additional code to identify severity of ulcer (L97.-)

Ex: **For category I70.44 CC codes:** See I70.33

I70.441 **Atherosclerosis of autologous vein bypass graft(s) of the left leg with ulceration of thigh** A
CC when PDx is its own CC

I70.442 **Atherosclerosis of autologous vein bypass graft(s) of the left leg with ulceration of calf** A
CC when PDx is its own CC

I70.443 **Atherosclerosis of autologous vein bypass graft(s) of the left leg with ulceration of ankle** A
CC when PDx is its own CC

I70.444 **Atherosclerosis of autologous vein bypass graft(s) of the left leg with ulceration of heel and midfoot** A
Atherosclerosis of autologous vein bypass graft(s) of left leg with ulceration of plantar surface of midfoot
CC when PDx is its own CC

I70.445 **Atherosclerosis of autologous vein bypass graft(s) of the left leg with ulceration of other part of foot** A
Atherosclerosis of autologous vein bypass graft(s) of left leg with ulceration of toe

I70.448 **Atherosclerosis of autologous vein bypass graft(s) of the left leg with ulceration of other part of lower leg** A
CC when PDx is its own CC

I70.449 **Atherosclerosis of autologous vein bypass graft(s) of the left leg with ulceration of unspecified site** A
CC when PDx is its own CC

I70.45 **Atherosclerosis of autologous vein bypass graft(s) of other extremity with ulceration** A

Includes any condition classifiable to I70.418, I70.428, and I70.438

Use additional code to identify severity of ulcer (L98.49-)

● **I70.46** **Atherosclerosis of autologous vein bypass graft(s) of the extremities with gangrene**

Includes any condition classifiable to I70.41-, I70.42-, and I70.43-, I70.44-, I70.45

Use additional code to identify the severity of any ulcer (L97.-, L98.49-), if applicable

Ex: **For category I70.46 CC codes:** See I70.26

I70.461 **Atherosclerosis of autologous vein bypass graft(s) of the extremities with gangrene, right leg** A
CC when PDx is its own CC

I70.462 **Atherosclerosis of autologous vein bypass graft(s) of the extremities with gangrene, left leg** A
CC when PDx is its own CC

I70.463 **Atherosclerosis of autologous vein bypass graft(s) of the extremities with gangrene, bilateral legs** A
CC when PDx is its own CC

I70.468 **Atherosclerosis of autologous vein bypass graft(s) of the extremities with gangrene, other extremity** A
CC when PDx is its own CC

I70.469 **Atherosclerosis of autologous vein bypass graft(s) of the extremities with gangrene, unspecified extremity** A
CC when PDx is its own CC

● **I70.49** **Other atherosclerosis of autologous vein bypass graft(s) of the extremities**

I70.491 **Other atherosclerosis of autologous vein bypass graft(s) of the extremities, right leg** A

I70.492 **Other atherosclerosis of autologous vein bypass graft(s) of the extremities, left leg** A

I70.493 **Other atherosclerosis of autologous vein bypass graft(s) of the extremities, bilateral legs** A

I70.498 **Other atherosclerosis of autologous vein bypass graft(s) of the extremities, other extremity** A

I70.499 **Other atherosclerosis of autologous vein bypass graft(s) of the extremities, unspecified extremity** A

I70.5 Atherosclerosis of nonautologous biological bypass graft(s) of the extremities

Use additional code, if applicable, to identify chronic total occlusion of artery of extremity (I70.92)

I70.50 Unspecified atherosclerosis of nonautologous biological bypass graft(s) of the extremities

- **I70.501 Unspecified atherosclerosis of nonautologous biological bypass graft(s) of the extremities, right leg** A
- **I70.502 Unspecified atherosclerosis of nonautologous biological bypass graft(s) of the extremities, left leg** A
- **I70.503 Unspecified atherosclerosis of nonautologous biological bypass graft(s) of the extremities, bilateral legs** A
- **I70.508 Unspecified atherosclerosis of nonautologous biological bypass graft(s) of the extremities, other extremity** A
- **I70.509 Unspecified atherosclerosis of nonautologous biological bypass graft(s) of the extremities, unspecified extremity** A

I70.51 Atherosclerosis of nonautologous biological bypass graft(s) of the extremities intermittent claudication

- **I70.511 Atherosclerosis of nonautologous biological bypass graft(s) of the extremities with intermittent claudication, right leg** A
- **I70.512 Atherosclerosis of nonautologous biological bypass graft(s) of the extremities with intermittent claudication, left leg** A
- **I70.513 Atherosclerosis of nonautologous biological bypass graft(s) of the extremities with intermittent claudication, bilateral legs** A
- **I70.518 Atherosclerosis of nonautologous biological bypass graft(s) of the extremities with intermittent claudication, other extremity** A
- **I70.519 Atherosclerosis of nonautologous biological bypass graft(s) of the extremities with intermittent claudication, unspecified extremity** A

I70.52 Atherosclerosis of nonautologous biological bypass graft(s) of the extremities with rest pain

Includes any condition classifiable to I70.51-

- **I70.521 Atherosclerosis of nonautologous biological bypass graft(s) of the extremities with rest pain, right leg** A
- **I70.522 Atherosclerosis of nonautologous biological bypass graft(s) of the extremities with rest pain, left leg** A
- **I70.523 Atherosclerosis of nonautologous biological bypass graft(s) of the extremities with rest pain, bilateral legs** A
- **I70.528 Atherosclerosis of nonautologous biological bypass graft(s) of the extremities with rest pain, other extremity** A
- **I70.529 Atherosclerosis of nonautologous biological bypass graft(s) of the extremities with rest pain, unspecified extremity** A

I70.53 Atherosclerosis of nonautologous biological bypass graft(s) of the right leg with ulceration

Includes any condition classifiable to I70.511 and I70.521

Use additional code to identify severity of ulcer (L97.-)

Ex: For category I70.53 CC codes: See I70.33

- **I70.531 Atherosclerosis of nonautologous biological bypass graft(s) of the right leg with ulceration of thigh** A
  CC when PDx is its own CC
- **I70.532 Atherosclerosis of nonautologous biological bypass graft(s) of the right leg with ulceration of calf** A
  CC when PDx is its own CC
- **I70.533 Atherosclerosis of nonautologous biological bypass graft(s) of the right leg with ulceration of ankle** A
  CC when PDx is its own CC
- **I70.534 Atherosclerosis of nonautologous biological bypass graft(s) of the right leg with ulceration of heel and midfoot** A
  Atherosclerosis of nonautologous biological bypass graft(s) of right leg with ulceration of plantar surface of midfoot
  CC when PDx is its own CC
- **I70.535 Atherosclerosis of nonautologous biological bypass graft(s) of the right leg with ulceration of other part of foot** A
  Atherosclerosis of nonautologous biological bypass graft(s) of the right leg with ulceration of toe
- **I70.538 Atherosclerosis of nonautologous biological bypass graft(s) of the right leg with ulceration of other part of lower leg** A
  CC when PDx is its own CC
- **I70.539 Atherosclerosis of nonautologous biological bypass graft(s) of the right leg with ulceration of unspecified site** A
  CC when PDx is its own CC

I70.54 Atherosclerosis of nonautologous biological bypass graft(s) of the left leg with ulceration

Includes any condition classifiable to I70.512 and I70.522

Use additional code to identify severity of ulcer (L97.-)

Ex: For category I70.54 CC codes: See I70.33

- **I70.541 Atherosclerosis of nonautologous biological bypass graft(s) of the left leg with ulceration of thigh** A
  CC when PDx is its own CC
- **I70.542 Atherosclerosis of nonautologous biological bypass graft(s) of the left leg with ulceration of calf** A
  CC when PDx is its own CC
- **I70.543 Atherosclerosis of nonautologous biological bypass graft(s) of the left leg with ulceration of ankle** A
  CC when PDx is its own CC
- **I70.544 Atherosclerosis of nonautologous biological bypass graft(s) of the left leg with ulceration of heel and midfoot** A
  Atherosclerosis of nonautologous biological bypass graft(s) of left leg with ulceration of plantar surface of midfoot
  CC when PDx is its own CC

I70.545 Atherosclerosis of nonautologous biological bypass graft(s) of the left leg with ulceration of other part of foot A

Atherosclerosis of nonautologous biological bypass graft(s) of the left leg with ulceration of toe

I70.548 Atherosclerosis of nonautologous biological bypass graft(s) of the left leg with ulceration of other part of lower leg A

CC when PDx is its own CC

I70.549 Atherosclerosis of nonautologous biological bypass graft(s) of the left leg with ulceration of unspecified site A

CC when PDx is its own CC

I70.55 Atherosclerosis of nonautologous biological bypass graft(s) of other extremity with ulceration A

Includes any condition classifiable to I70.518, I70.528, and I70.538

Use additional code to identify severity of ulcer (L98.49)

● **I70.56 Atherosclerosis of nonautologous biological bypass graft(s) of the extremities with gangrene**

Includes any condition classifiable to I70.51-, I70.52-, and I70.53-, I70.54-, I70.55

Use additional code to identify the severity of any ulcer (L97.-, L98.49-), if applicable

Ex: For category I70.56 CC codes: See I70.26

I70.561 Atherosclerosis of nonautologous biological bypass graft(s) of the extremities with gangrene, right leg A

CC when PDx is its own CC

I70.562 Atherosclerosis of nonautologous biological bypass graft(s) of the extremities with gangrene, left leg A

CC when PDx is its own CC

I70.563 Atherosclerosis of nonautologous biological bypass graft(s) of the extremities with gangrene, bilateral legs A

CC when PDx is its own CC

I70.568 Atherosclerosis of nonautologous biological bypass graft(s) of the extremities with gangrene, other extremity A

CC when PDx is its own CC

I70.569 Atherosclerosis of nonautologous biological bypass graft(s) of the extremities with gangrene, unspecified extremity A

CC when PDx is its own CC

● **I70.59 Other atherosclerosis of nonautologous biological bypass graft(s) of the extremities**

I70.591 Other atherosclerosis of nonautologous biological bypass graft(s) of the extremities, right leg A

I70.592 Other atherosclerosis of nonautologous biological bypass graft(s) of the extremities, left leg A

I70.593 Other atherosclerosis of nonautologous biological bypass graft(s) of the extremities, bilateral legs A

I70.598 Other atherosclerosis of nonautologous biological bypass graft(s) of the extremities, other extremity A

I70.599 Other atherosclerosis of nonautologous biological bypass graft(s) of the extremities, unspecified extremity A

● **I70.6 Atherosclerosis of nonbiological bypass graft(s) of the extremities**

Use additional code, if applicable, to identify chronic total occlusion of artery of extremity (I70.92)

● **I70.60 Unspecified atherosclerosis of nonbiological bypass graft(s) of the extremities**

I70.601 Unspecified atherosclerosis of nonbiological bypass graft(s) of the extremities, right leg A

I70.602 Unspecified atherosclerosis of nonbiological bypass graft(s) of the extremities, left leg A

I70.603 Unspecified atherosclerosis of nonbiological bypass graft(s) of the extremities, bilateral legs A

I70.608 Unspecified atherosclerosis of nonbiological bypass graft(s) of the extremities, other extremity A

I70.609 Unspecified atherosclerosis of nonbiological bypass graft(s) of the extremities, unspecified extremity A

● **I70.61 Atherosclerosis of nonbiological bypass graft(s) of the extremities with intermittent claudication**

I70.611 Atherosclerosis of nonbiological bypass graft(s) of the extremities with intermittent claudication, right leg A

I70.612 Atherosclerosis of nonbiological bypass graft(s) of the extremities with intermittent claudication, left leg A

I70.613 Atherosclerosis of nonbiological bypass graft(s) of the extremities with intermittent claudication, bilateral legs A

I70.618 Atherosclerosis of nonbiological bypass graft(s) of the extremities with intermittent claudication, other extremity A

I70.619 Atherosclerosis of nonbiological bypass graft(s) of the extremities with intermittent claudication, unspecified extremity A

● **I70.62 Atherosclerosis of nonbiological bypass graft(s) of the extremities with rest pain**

Includes any condition classifiable to I70.61-

I70.621 Atherosclerosis of nonbiological bypass graft(s) of the extremities with rest pain, right leg A

I70.622 Atherosclerosis of nonbiological bypass graft(s) of the extremities with rest pain, left leg A

I70.623 Atherosclerosis of nonbiological bypass graft(s) of the extremities with rest pain, bilateral legs A

I70.628 Atherosclerosis of nonbiological bypass graft(s) of the extremities with rest pain, other extremity A

I70.629 Atherosclerosis of nonbiological bypass graft(s) of the extremities with rest pain, unspecified extremity A

● **I70.63 Atherosclerosis of nonbiological bypass graft(s) of the right leg with ulceration**

Includes any condition classifiable to I70.611 and I70.621

Use additional code to identify severity of ulcer (L97.-)

Ex: For category I70.63 CC codes: See I70.33

I70.631 Atherosclerosis of nonbiological bypass graft(s) of the right leg with ulceration of thigh A
CC when PDx is its own CC

I70.632 Atherosclerosis of nonbiological bypass graft(s) of the right leg with ulceration of calf A
CC when PDx is its own CC

I70.633 Atherosclerosis of nonbiological bypass graft(s) of the right leg with ulceration of ankle A
CC when PDx is its own CC

I70.634 Atherosclerosis of nonbiological bypass graft(s) of the right leg with ulceration of heel and midfoot A
Atherosclerosis of nonbiological bypass graft(s) of right leg with ulceration of plantar surface of midfoot
CC when PDx is its own CC

I70.635 Atherosclerosis of nonbiological bypass graft(s) of the right leg with ulceration of other part of foot A
Atherosclerosis of nonbiological bypass graft(s) of the right leg with ulceration of toe

I70.638 Atherosclerosis of nonbiological bypass graft(s) of the right leg with ulceration of other part of lower leg A
CC when PDx is its own CC

I70.639 Atherosclerosis of nonbiological bypass graft(s) of the right leg with ulceration of unspecified site A
CC when PDx is its own CC

● **I70.64 Atherosclerosis of nonbiological bypass graft(s) of the left leg with ulceration**

Includes any condition classifiable to I70.612 and I70.622

Use additional code to identify severity of ulcer (L97.-)

Ex: For category I70.64 CC codes: See I70.33

I70.641 Atherosclerosis of nonbiological bypass graft(s) of the left leg with ulceration of thigh A
CC when PDx is its own CC

I70.642 Atherosclerosis of nonbiological bypass graft(s) of the left leg with ulceration of calf A
CC when PDx is its own CC

I70.643 Atherosclerosis of nonbiological bypass graft(s) of the left leg with ulceration of ankle A
CC when PDx is its own CC

I70.644 Atherosclerosis of nonbiological bypass graft(s) of the left leg with ulceration of heel and midfoot A
Atherosclerosis of nonbiological bypass graft(s) of left leg with ulceration of plantar surface of midfoot
CC when PDx is its own CC

I70.645 Atherosclerosis of nonbiological bypass graft(s) of the left leg with ulceration of other part of foot A
Atherosclerosis of nonbiological bypass graft(s) of the left leg with ulceration of toe

I70.648 Atherosclerosis of nonbiological bypass graft(s) of the left leg with ulceration of other part of lower leg A
CC when PDx is its own CC

I70.649 Atherosclerosis of nonbiological bypass graft(s) of the left leg with ulceration of unspecified site A
CC when PDx is its own CC

I70.65 Atherosclerosis of nonbiological bypass graft(s) of other extremity with ulceration A

Includes any condition classifiable to I70.618 and I70.628

Use additional code to identify severity of ulcer (L98.49-)

● **I70.66 Atherosclerosis of nonbiological bypass graft(s) of the extremities with gangrene**

Includes any condition classifiable to I70.61-, I70.62-, I70.63-, I70.64-, I70.65

Use additional code to identify the severity of any ulcer (L97.-, L98.49-), if applicable

Ex: For category I70.66 CC codes: See I70.26

I70.661 Atherosclerosis of nonbiological bypass graft(s) of the extremities with gangrene, right leg A
CC when PDx is its own CC

I70.662 Atherosclerosis of nonbiological bypass graft(s) of the extremities with gangrene, left leg A
CC when PDx is its own CC

I70.663 Atherosclerosis of nonbiological bypass graft(s) of the extremities with gangrene, bilateral legs A
CC when PDx is its own CC

I70.668 Atherosclerosis of nonbiological bypass graft(s) of the extremities with gangrene, other extremity A
CC when PDx is its own CC

I70.669 Atherosclerosis of nonbiological bypass graft(s) of the extremities with gangrene, unspecified extremity A
CC when PDx is its own CC

● **I70.69 Other atherosclerosis of nonbiological bypass graft(s) of the extremities**

I70.691 Other atherosclerosis of nonbiological bypass graft(s) of the extremities, right leg A

I70.692 Other atherosclerosis of nonbiological bypass graft(s) of the extremities, left leg A

I70.693 Other atherosclerosis of nonbiological bypass graft(s) of the extremities, bilateral legs A

I70.698 Other atherosclerosis of nonbiological bypass graft(s) of the extremities, other extremity A

I70.699 Other atherosclerosis of nonbiological bypass graft(s) of the extremities, unspecified extremity A

● **I70.7 Atherosclerosis of other type of bypass graft(s) of the extremities**

Use additional code, if applicable, to identify chronic total occlusion of artery of extremity (I70.92)

● **I70.70 Unspecified atherosclerosis of other type of bypass graft(s) of the extremities**

I70.701 Unspecified atherosclerosis of other type of bypass graft(s) of the extremities, right leg A

I70.702 Unspecified atherosclerosis of other type of bypass graft(s) of the extremities, left leg A

I70.703 **Unspecified atherosclerosis of other type of bypass graft(s) of the extremities, bilateral legs** A

I70.708 **Unspecified atherosclerosis of other type of bypass graft(s) of the extremities, other extremity** A

I70.709 **Unspecified atherosclerosis of other type of bypass graft(s) of the extremities, unspecified extremity** A

● I70.71 **Atherosclerosis of other type of bypass graft(s) of the extremities with intermittent claudication**

I70.711 **Atherosclerosis of other type of bypass graft(s) of the extremities with intermittent claudication, right leg** A

I70.712 **Atherosclerosis of other type of bypass graft(s) of the extremities with intermittent claudication, left leg** A

I70.713 **Atherosclerosis of other type of bypass graft(s) of the extremities with intermittent claudication, bilateral legs** A

I70.718 **Atherosclerosis of other type of bypass graft(s) of the extremities with intermittent claudication, other extremity** A

I70.719 **Atherosclerosis of other type of bypass graft(s) of the extremities with intermittent claudication, unspecified extremity** A

● I70.72 **Atherosclerosis of other type of bypass graft(s) of the extremities with rest pain**

Includes any condition classifiable to I70.71-

I70.721 **Atherosclerosis of other type of bypass graft(s) of the extremities with rest pain, right leg** A

I70.722 **Atherosclerosis of other type of bypass graft(s) of the extremities with rest pain, left leg** A

I70.723 **Atherosclerosis of other type of bypass graft(s) of the extremities with rest pain, bilateral legs** A

I70.728 **Atherosclerosis of other type of bypass graft(s) of the extremities with rest pain, other extremity** A

I70.729 **Atherosclerosis of other type of bypass graft(s) of the extremities with rest pain, unspecified extremity** A

● I70.73 **Atherosclerosis of other type of bypass graft(s) of the right leg with ulceration**

Includes any condition classifiable to I70.711 and I70.721

Use additional code to identify severity of ulcer (L97.-)

Ex **For category I70.73 CC codes:** See I70.33

I70.731 **Atherosclerosis of other type of bypass graft(s) of the right leg with ulceration of thigh** A
CC when PDx is its own CC

I70.732 **Atherosclerosis of other type of bypass graft(s) of the right leg with ulceration of calf** A
CC when PDx is its own CC

I70.733 **Atherosclerosis of other type of bypass graft(s) of the right leg with ulceration of ankle** A
CC when PDx is its own CC

I70.734 **Atherosclerosis of other type of bypass graft(s) of the right leg with ulceration of heel and midfoot** A
Atherosclerosis of other type of bypass graft(s) of right leg with ulceration of plantar surface of midfoot
CC when PDx is its own CC

I70.735 **Atherosclerosis of other type of bypass graft(s) of the right leg with ulceration of other part of foot** A
Atherosclerosis of other type of bypass graft(s) of right leg with ulceration of toe

I70.738 **Atherosclerosis of other type of bypass graft(s) of the right leg with ulceration of other part of lower leg** A
CC when PDx is its own CC

I70.739 **Atherosclerosis of other type of bypass graft(s) of the right leg with ulceration of unspecified site** A
CC when PDx is its own CC

● I70.74 **Atherosclerosis of other type of bypass graft(s) of the left leg with ulceration**

Includes any condition classifiable to I70.712 and I70.722

Use additional code to identify severity of ulcer (L97.-)

Ex **For category I70.74 CC codes:** See I70.33

I70.741 **Atherosclerosis of other type of bypass graft(s) of the left leg with ulceration of thigh** A
CC when PDx is its own CC

I70.742 **Atherosclerosis of other type of bypass graft(s) of the left leg with ulceration of calf** A
CC when PDx is its own CC

I70.743 **Atherosclerosis of other type of bypass graft(s) of the left leg with ulceration of ankle** A
CC when PDx is its own CC

I70.744 **Atherosclerosis of other type of bypass graft(s) of the left leg with ulceration of heel and midfoot** A
Atherosclerosis of other type of bypass graft(s) of left leg with ulceration of plantar surface of midfoot
CC when PDx is its own CC

I70.745 **Atherosclerosis of other type of bypass graft(s) of the left leg with ulceration of other part of foot** A
Atherosclerosis of other type of bypass graft(s) of left leg with ulceration of toe

I70.748 **Atherosclerosis of other type of bypass graft(s) of the left leg with ulceration of other part of lower leg** A
CC when PDx is its own CC

I70.749 **Atherosclerosis of other type of bypass graft(s) of the left leg with ulceration of unspecified site** A
CC when PDx is its own CC

I70.75 Atherosclerosis of other type of bypass graft(s) of other extremity with ulceration A

Includes any condition classifiable to I70.718 and I70.728

Use additional code to identify severity of ulcer (L98.49)

● **I70.76 Atherosclerosis of other type of bypass graft(s) of the extremities with gangrene**

Includes any condition classifiable to I70.71-, I70.72-, I70.73-, I70.74-, I70.75

Use additional code to identify the severity of any ulcer (L97.-, L98.49-), if applicable

Ex **For category I70.76 CC codes:** See I70.26

I70.761 Atherosclerosis of other type of bypass graft(s) of the extremities with gangrene, right leg A
CC when PDx is its own CC

I70.762 Atherosclerosis of other type of bypass graft(s) of the extremities with gangrene, left leg A
CC when PDx is its own CC

I70.763 Atherosclerosis of other type of bypass graft(s) of the extremities with gangrene, bilateral legs A
CC when PDx is its own CC

I70.768 Atherosclerosis of other type of bypass graft(s) of the extremities with gangrene, other extremity A
CC when PDx is its own CC

I70.769 Atherosclerosis of other type of bypass graft(s) of the extremities with gangrene, unspecified extremity A
CC when PDx is its own CC

● **I70.79 Other atherosclerosis of other type of bypass graft(s) of the extremities**

I70.791 Other atherosclerosis of other type of bypass graft(s) of the extremities, right leg A

I70.792 Other atherosclerosis of other type of bypass graft(s) of the extremities, left leg A

I70.793 Other atherosclerosis of other type of bypass graft(s) of the extremities, bilateral legs A

I70.798 Other atherosclerosis of other type of bypass graft(s) of the extremities, other extremity A

I70.799 Other atherosclerosis of other type of bypass graft(s) of the extremities, unspecified extremity A

I70.8 Atherosclerosis of other arteries A

● **I70.9 Other and unspecified atherosclerosis**

I70.90 Unspecified atherosclerosis A

I70.91 Generalized atherosclerosis A

● **I70.92 Chronic total occlusion of artery of the extremities** A
Complete occlusion of artery of the extremities
Total occlusion of artery of the extremities

Code first atherosclerosis of arteries of the extremities (I70.2-, I70.3-, I70.4-, I70.5-, I70.6-, I70.7-)

Ex I70.92, I73.81-I74.19, .I74.2-I77.2, I77.5-I77.6, I77.810-I77.819, I79.1-I79.8, M31.8-M31.9

● **I71 Aortic aneurysm and dissection**

Excludes1 aortic ectasia (I77.81-)
syphilitic aortic aneurysm (A52.01)
traumatic aortic aneurysm (S25.09, S35.09)

Ex **For category I71 CC codes:** E08.51-E08.59, E08.618-E08.638, E08.649-E08.8, E09.51-E09.59, E09.618-E09.638, E09.649, E09.65-E09.8, E10.51-E10.59, E10.618-E10.638, E10.649, E10.69-E10.8, E11.51-E11.59, E11.618-E11.638, E11.649, E11.69-E11.8, E13.51-E13.59, E13.618-E13.638, E13.649-E13.8, I71.00-I71.9, I77.810-I77.819, I79.0, I87.8-I87.9, I99.8-I99.9

● **I71.0 Dissection of aorta**

I71.00 Dissection of unspecified site of aorta

I71.01 Dissection of thoracic aorta

I71.02 Dissection of abdominal aorta

I71.03 Dissection of thoracoabdominal aorta

I71.1 Thoracic aortic aneurysm, ruptured

I71.2 Thoracic aortic aneurysm, without rupture

I71.3 Abdominal aortic aneurysm, ruptured

I71.4 Abdominal aortic aneurysm, without rupture

I71.5 Thoracoabdominal aortic aneurysm, ruptured

I71.6 Thoracoabdominal aortic aneurysm, without rupture

I71.8 Aortic aneurysm of unspecified site, ruptured
Rupture of aorta NOS

I71.9 Aortic aneurysm of unspecified site, without rupture
Aneurysm of aorta
Dilatation of aorta
Hyaline necrosis of aorta

● **I72 Other aneurysm**

Includes aneurysm (cirsoid) (false) (ruptured)

Excludes2 acquired aneurysm (I77.0)
aneurysm (of) aorta (I71.-)
aneurysm (of) arteriovenous NOS (Q27.3-)
carotid artery dissection (I77.71)
cerebral (nonruptured) aneurysm (I67.1)
coronary aneurysm (I25.4)
coronary artery dissection (I25.42)
dissection of artery NEC (I77.79)
dissection of precerebral artery, congenital (nonruptured) (Q28.1) ◀
heart aneurysm (I25.3)
iliac artery dissection (I77.72)
pulmonary artery aneurysm (I28.1)
renal artery dissection (I77.73)
retinal aneurysm (H35.0)
ruptured cerebral aneurysm (I60.7)
varicose aneurysm (I77.0)
vertebral artery dissection (I77.74)

I72.0 Aneurysm of carotid artery
Aneurysm of common carotid artery
Aneurysm of external carotid artery
Aneurysm of internal carotid artery, extracranial portion

Excludes1 aneurysm of internal carotid artery, intracranial portion (I67.1)
aneurysm of internal carotid artery NOS (I67.1)

I72.1 Aneurysm of artery of upper extremity

I72.2 Aneurysm of renal artery

I72.3 Aneurysm of iliac artery

I72.4 Aneurysm of artery of lower extremity

I72.5 Aneurysm of other precerebral arteries ◀
Aneurysm of basilar artery (trunk) ◀

Excludes2 aneurysm of carotid artery (I72.0) ◀
aneurysm of vertebral artery (I72.6) ◀
dissection of carotid artery (I77.71) ◀
dissection of other precerebral arteries (I77.75) ◀
dissection of vertebral artery (I77.74) ◀

I72.6 Aneurysm of vertebral artery ◀

Excludes2 dissection of vertebral artery (I77.74) ◀

I72.8 Aneurysm of other specified arteries

I72.9 Aneurysm of unspecified site

● **I73 Other peripheral vascular diseases**

Excludes2 chilblains (T69.1)
frostbite (T33-T34)
immersion hand or foot (T69.0-)
spasm of cerebral artery (G45.9)

● **I73.0 Raynaud's syndrome**

Diminishing oxygen supply to fingers, toes, nose, and ears when exposed to temperature changes or stress

Raynaud's disease
Raynaud's phenomenon (secondary)

I73.00 Raynaud's syndrome without gangrene

I73.01 Raynaud's syndrome with gangrene

CC when PDx is its own CC

Ex: See I70.26

I73.1 Thromboangiitis obliterans [Buerger's disease]

Inflammatory occlusive disease resulting in poor circulation to the legs, feet, and sometimes the hands due to progressive inflammatory narrowing and eventually obliteration of the small arteries

● **I73.8 Other specified peripheral vascular diseases**

Excludes1 diabetic (peripheral) angiopathy (E08-E13 with .51-.52)

I73.81 Erythromelalgia

I73.89 Other specified peripheral vascular diseases

Acrocyanosis
Erythrocyanosis
Simple acroparesthesia [Schultze's type]
Vasomotor acroparesthesia [Nothnagel's type]

I73.9 Peripheral vascular disease, unspecified

Intermittent claudication
Peripheral angiopathy NOS
Spasm of artery

Excludes1 atherosclerosis of the extremities (I70.2--I70.7-)

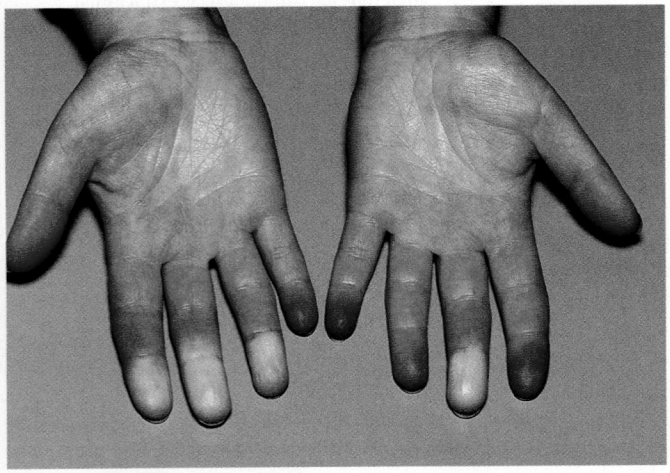

Figure 9-5 Raynaud's syndrome. (From Hallett: Comprehensive Vascular and Endovascular Surgery, ed 2, Philadelphia, Mosby Ltd., 2010)

● **I74 Arterial embolism and thrombosis**

Includes embolic infarction
embolic occlusion
thrombotic infarction
thrombotic occlusion

Code first embolism and thrombosis complicating abortion or ectopic or molar pregnancy (O00-O07, O08.2)
embolism and thrombosis complicating pregnancy, childbirth and the puerperium (O88.-)

Excludes2 atheroembolism (I75.-)
basilar embolism and thrombosis (I63.0-I63.2, I65.1)
carotid embolism and thrombosis (I63.0-I63.2, I65.2)
cerebral embolism and thrombosis (I63.3-I63.5, I66.-)
coronary embolism and thrombosis (I21-I25)
mesenteric embolism and thrombosis (K55.0-) ⇐
ophthalmic embolism and thrombosis (H34.-)
precerebral embolism and thrombosis NOS (I63.0-I63.2, I65.9)
pulmonary embolism and thrombosis (I26.-)
renal embolism and thrombosis (N28.0)
retinal embolism and thrombosis (H34.-)
septic embolism and thrombosis (I76)
vertebral embolism and thrombosis (I63.0-I63.2, I65.0)

● **I74.0 Embolism and thrombosis of abdominal aorta**

Ex: **For category I74.0 CC codes:** I26.01-I26.99, I27.82, I74.01-I74.10, I74.19, I87.8-I87.9, I99.8-I99.9

I74.01 Saddle embolus of abdominal aorta

I74.09 Other arterial embolism and thrombosis of abdominal aorta

Aortic bifurcation syndrome
Aortoiliac obstruction
Leriche's syndrome

● **I74.1 Embolism and thrombosis of other and unspecified parts of aorta**

Ex: **For category I74.1 CC codes unless otherwise indicated:** See I74.0

I74.10 Embolism and thrombosis of unspecified parts of aorta

I74.11 Embolism and thrombosis of thoracic aorta

Ex: E08.51-E08.59, E08.618-E08.638, E08.649-E08.8, E09.51-E09.59, E09.618-E09.638, E09.649, E09.65-E09.8, E10.51-E10.59, E10.618-E10.638, E10.649, E10.69-E10.8, E11.51-E11.59, E11.618-E11.638, E11.649, E11.69-E11.8, E13.51-E13.59, E13.618-E13.638, E13.649-E13.8, I74.11, I74.8-I74.9, I76, I87.8-I87.9, I99.8-I99.9

I74.19 Embolism and thrombosis of other parts of aorta

I74.2 Embolism and thrombosis of arteries of the upper extremities

Ex: E08.51-E08.59, E08.618-E08.638, E08.649-E08.8, E09.51-E09.59, E09.618-E09.638, E09.649, E09.65-E09.8, E10.51-E10.59, E10.618-E10.638, E10.649, E10.69-E10.8, E11.51-E11.59, E11.618-E11.638, E11.649, E11.69-E11.8, E13.51-E13.59, E13.618-E13.638, E13.649-E13.8, I74.2, I74.8-I74.9, I76, I87.8-I87.9, I99.8-I99.9

Item 9–9 An **embolus** is a mass of undissolved matter present in the blood that is transported by the blood current. A **thrombus** is a blood clot that occludes or shuts off a vessel. When a thrombus is dislodged, it becomes an embolus.

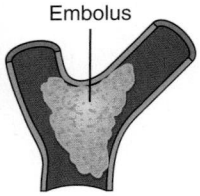

Figure 9-6 An arterial embolus.

I74.3 Embolism and thrombosis of arteries of the lower extremities
Ex: E08.51-E08.59, E08.618-E08.638, E08.649-E08.8, E09.51-E09.59, E09.618-E09.638, E09.649, E09.65-E09.8, E10.51-E10.59, E10.618-E10.638, E10.649, E10.69-E10.8, E11.51-E11.59, E11.618-E11.638, E11.649, E11.69-E11.8, E13.51-E13.59, E13.618-E13.638, E13.649-E13.8, I74.3-I74.4, I74.8-I74.9, I76, I87.8-I87.9, I99.8-I99.9

I74.4 Embolism and thrombosis of arteries of extremities, unspecified
Peripheral arterial embolism NOS
Ex: See I74.3

I74.5 Embolism and thrombosis of iliac artery
Ex: E08.51-E08.59, E08.618-E08.638, E08.649-E08.8, E09.51-E09.59, E09.618-E09.638, E09.649, E09.65-E09.8, E10.51-E10.59, E10.618-E10.638, E10.649, E10.69-E10.8, E11.51-E11.59, E11.618-E11.638, E11.649, E11.69-E11.8, E13.51-E13.59, E13.618-E13.638, E13.649-E13.8, I74.5-I74.9, I76, I87.8-I87.9, I99.8-I99.9

I74.8 Embolism and thrombosis of other arteries
Ex: E08.51-E08.59, E08.618-E08.638, E08.649-E08.8, E09.51-E09.59, E09.618-E09.638, E09.649, E09.65-E09.8, E10.51-E10.59, E10.618-E10.638, E10.649, E10.69-E10.8, E11.51-E11.59, E11.618-E11.638, E11.649, E11.69-E11.8, E13.51-E13.59, E13.618-E13.638, E13.649-E13.8, I74.8-I74.9, I76, I87.8-I87.9, I99.8-I99.9

I74.9 Embolism and thrombosis of unspecified artery
Ex: See I74.8

I75 Atheroembolism
Includes atherothrombotic microembolism
cholesterol embolism

I75.0 Atheroembolism of extremities

I75.01 Atheroembolism of upper extremity
Ex: **For category I75.01 CC codes:** E08.51-E08.59, E08.618-E08.638, E08.649-E08.8, E09.51-E09.59, E09.618-E09.638, E09.649, E09.65-E09.8, E10.51-E10.59, E10.618-E10.638, E10.649, E10.69-E10.8, E11.51-E11.59, E11.618-E11.638, E11.649, E11.69-E11.8, E13.51-E13.59, E13.618-E13.638, E13.649-E13.8, I74.8-I75.019, I76, I87.8-I87.9, I99.8-I99.9

I75.011 Atheroembolism of right upper extremity

I75.012 Atheroembolism of left upper extremity

I75.013 Atheroembolism of bilateral upper extremities

I75.019 Atheroembolism of unspecified upper extremity

I75.02 Atheroembolism of lower extremity
Ex: **For category I75.02 CC codes:** E08.51-E08.59, E08.618-E08.638, E08.649-E08.8, E09.51-E09.59, E09.618-E09.638, E09.649, E09.65-E09.8, E10.51-E10.59, E10.618-E10.638, E10.649, E10.69-E10.8, E11.51-E11.59, E11.618-E11.638, E11.649, E11.69-E11.8, E13.51-E13.59, E13.618-E13.638, E13.649-E13.8, I74.8-I74.9, I75.021-I75.029, I76, I87.8-I87.9, I99.8-I99.9

I75.021 Atheroembolism of right lower extremity

I75.022 Atheroembolism of left lower extremity

I75.023 Atheroembolism of bilateral lower extremities

I75.029 Atheroembolism of unspecified lower extremity

I75.8 Atheroembolism of other sites

I75.81 Atheroembolism of kidney
Use additional code for any associated acute kidney failure and chronic kidney disease (N17.-, N18.-)
Ex: E08.51-E08.59, E08.618-E08.638, E08.649-E08.8, E09.51-E09.59, E09.618-E09.638, E09.649, E09.65-E09.8, E10.51-E10.59, E10.618-E10.638, E10.649, E10.69-E10.8, E11.51-E11.59, E11.618-E11.638, E11.649, E11.69-E11.8, E13.51-E13.59, E13.618-E13.638, E13.649-E13.8, I74.8-I74.9, I75.81, I76, I87.8-I87.9, I99.8-I99.9

I75.89 Atheroembolism of other site
Ex: E08.51-E08.59, E08.618-E08.638, E08.649-E08.8, E09.51-E09.59, E09.618-E09.638, E09.649, E09.65-E09.8, E10.51-E10.59, E10.618-E10.638, E10.649, E10.69-E10.8, E11.51-E11.59, E11.618-E11.638, E11.649, E11.69-E11.8, E13.51-E13.59, E13.618-E13.638, E13.649-E13.8, I74.8-I74.9, I75.89, I76, I87.8-I87.9, I99.8-I99.9

I76 Septic arterial embolism
Code first underlying infection, such as:
infective endocarditis (I33.0)
lung abscess (J85.-)
Use additional code to identify the site of the embolism (I74.-)
Excludes2 septic pulmonary embolism (I26.01, I26.90)
Ex: See I74.8

I77 Other disorders of arteries and arterioles
Excludes2 collagen (vascular) diseases (M30-M36)
hypersensitivity angiitis (M31.0)
pulmonary artery (I28.-)

I77.0 Arteriovenous fistula, acquired
Aneurysmal varix
Arteriovenous aneurysm, acquired
Excludes1 arteriovenous aneurysm NOS (Q27.3-)
presence of arteriovenous shunt (fistula) for dialysis (Z99.2)
traumatic - see injury of blood vessel by body region
Excludes2 cerebral (I67.1)
coronary (I25.4)

I77.1 Stricture of artery
Narrowing of artery

I77.2 Rupture of artery
Erosion of artery
Fistula of artery
Ulcer of artery
Excludes1 traumatic rupture of artery - see injury of blood vessel by body region
Ex: I25.42, I67.0, I77.2, I77.70, I77.72-I77.79

I77.3 Arterial fibromuscular dysplasia
Fibromuscular hyperplasia (of) carotid artery
Fibromuscular hyperplasia (of) renal artery

I77.4 Celiac artery compression syndrome
Ex: I77.4

I77.5 Necrosis of artery
Ex: I77.5, M31.8-M31.9

I77.6 Arteritis, unspecified
Aortitis NOS
Endarteritis NOS
Excludes1 arteritis or endarteritis:
aortic arch (M31.4)
cerebral NEC (I67.7)
coronary (I25.89)
deformans (I70.-)
giant cell (M31.5., M31.6)
obliterans (I70.-)
senile (I70.-)

● **I77.7 Other arterial dissection**

Excludes2 dissection of aorta (I71.0-)
dissection of coronary artery (I25.42)

Ex: **For category I77.7 CC codes:** I77.2-I77.3, I77.5-I77.6, I77.89-I77.9, M31.8-M31.9

I77.70 Dissection of unspecified artery ◀

I77.71 Dissection of carotid artery

I77.72 Dissection of iliac artery

I77.73 Dissection of renal artery

I77.74 Dissection of vertebral artery

Excludes2 aneurysm of vertebral artery (I72.6) ◀

I77.75 Dissection of other precerebral arteries ◀

Dissection of basilar artery (trunk) ◀

Excludes2 aneurysm of carotid artery (I72.0) ◀
aneurysm of other precerebral arteries (I72.5) ◀
aneurysm of vertebral artery (I72.6) ◀
dissection of carotid artery (I77.71) ◀
dissection of vertebral artery (I77.74) ◀

I77.76 Dissection of artery of upper extremity ◀

I77.77 Dissection of artery of lower extremity ◀

I77.79 Dissection of other specified artery

● **I77.8 Other specified disorders of arteries and arterioles**

I77.81 Aortic ectasia

Ectasis aorta

Excludes1 aortic aneurysm and dissection (I71.0-)

I77.810 Thoracic aortic ectasia

I77.811 Abdominal aortic ectasia

I77.812 Thoracoabdominal aortic ectasia

I77.819 Aortic ectasia, unspecified site

I77.89 Other specified disorders of arteries and arterioles

I77.9 Disorder of arteries and arterioles, unspecified

● **I78 Diseases of capillaries**

I78.0 Hereditary hemorrhagic telangiectasia

Rendu-Osler-Weber disease

I78.1 Nevus, non-neoplastic

Araneus nevus
Senile nevus
Spider nevus
Stellar nevus

Excludes1 nevus NOS (D22.-)
vascular NOS (Q82.5)

Excludes2 blue nevus (D22.-)
flammeus nevus (Q82.5)
hairy nevus (D22.-)
melanocytic nevus (D22.-)
pigmented nevus (D22.-)
portwine nevus (Q82.5)
sanguineous nevus (Q82.5)
strawberry nevus (Q82.5)
verrucous nevus (Q82.5)

I78.8 Other diseases of capillaries

I78.9 Disease of capillaries, unspecified

● **I79 Disorders of arteries, arterioles and capillaries in diseases classified elsewhere**

▶ ***I79.0 Aneurysm of aorta in diseases classified elsewhere***

Code first underlying disease

Excludes1 syphilitic aneurysm (A52.01)

▶ ***I79.1 Aortitis in diseases classified elsewhere***

Code first underlying disease

Excludes1 syphilitic aortitis (A52.02)

▶ ***I79.8 Other disorders of arteries, arterioles and capillaries in diseases classified elsewhere***

Code first underlying disease, such as:
amyloidosis (E85.-)

Excludes1 diabetic (peripheral) angiopathy (E08-E13 with .51-.52)
syphilitic endarteritis (A52.09)
tuberculous endarteritis (A18.89)

DISEASES OF VEINS, LYMPHATIC VESSELS AND LYMPH NODES, NOT ELSEWHERE CLASSIFIED (I80-I89)

● **I80 Phlebitis and thrombophlebitis**

Inflammation of a vein with infiltration of walls (phlebitis).

Includes endophlebitis
inflammation, vein
periphlebitis
suppurative phlebitis

Code first phlebitis and thrombophlebitis complicating abortion, ectopic or molar pregnancy (O00-O07, O08.7)
phlebitis and thrombophlebitis complicating pregnancy, childbirth and the puerperium (O22.-, O87.-)

Excludes1 venous embolism and thrombosis of lower extremities (I82.4-, I82.5-, I82.81-)

● **I80.0 Phlebitis and thrombophlebitis of superficial vessels of lower extremities**

Phlebitis and thrombophlebitis of femoropopliteal vein

I80.00 Phlebitis and thrombophlebitis of superficial vessels of unspecified lower extremity

I80.01 Phlebitis and thrombophlebitis of superficial vessels of right lower extremity

I80.02 Phlebitis and thrombophlebitis of superficial vessels of left lower extremity

I80.03 Phlebitis and thrombophlebitis of superficial vessels of lower extremities, bilateral

● **I80.1 Phlebitis and thrombophlebitis of femoral vein**

Ex: **For category I80.1 CC codes:** E08.51-E08.59, E08.618-E08.638, E08.649-E08.8, E09.51-E09.59, E09.618-E09.638, E09.649, E09.65-E09.8, E10.51-E10.59, E10.618-E10.638, E10.649, E10.69-E10.8, E11.51-E11.59, E11.618-E11.638, E11.649, E11.69-E11.8, E13.51-E13.59, E13.618-E13.638, E13.649-E13.8, I80.00-I80.9, I87.8-I87.9, I99.8-I99.9

I80.10 Phlebitis and thrombophlebitis of unspecified femoral vein

I80.11 Phlebitis and thrombophlebitis of right femoral vein

I80.12 Phlebitis and thrombophlebitis of left femoral vein

I80.13 Phlebitis and thrombophlebitis of femoral vein, bilateral

● **I80.2 Phlebitis and thrombophlebitis of other and unspecified deep vessels of lower extremities**

Ex: **For category I80.2 CC codes:** See I80.1

● **I80.20 Phlebitis and thrombophlebitis of unspecified deep vessels of lower extremities**

I80.201 Phlebitis and thrombophlebitis of unspecified deep vessels of right lower extremity

I80.202 Phlebitis and thrombophlebitis of unspecified deep vessels of left lower extremity

I80.203 Phlebitis and thrombophlebitis of unspecified deep vessels of lower extremities, bilateral

I80.209 Phlebitis and thrombophlebitis of unspecified deep vessels of unspecified lower extremity

● **I80.21 Phlebitis and thrombophlebitis of iliac vein**

I80.211 Phlebitis and thrombophlebitis of right iliac vein

I80.212 Phlebitis and thrombophlebitis of left iliac vein

I80.213 **Phlebitis and thrombophlebitis of iliac vein, bilateral**

I80.219 **Phlebitis and thrombophlebitis of unspecified iliac vein**

● **I80.22** **Phlebitis and thrombophlebitis of popliteal vein**

I80.221 **Phlebitis and thrombophlebitis of right popliteal vein**

I80.222 **Phlebitis and thrombophlebitis of left popliteal vein**

I80.223 **Phlebitis and thrombophlebitis of popliteal vein, bilateral**

I80.229 **Phlebitis and thrombophlebitis of unspecified popliteal vein**

● **I80.23** **Phlebitis and thrombophlebitis of tibial vein**

I80.231 **Phlebitis and thrombophlebitis of right tibial vein**

I80.232 **Phlebitis and thrombophlebitis of left tibial vein**

I80.233 **Phlebitis and thrombophlebitis of tibial vein, bilateral**

I80.239 **Phlebitis and thrombophlebitis of unspecified tibial vein**

● **I80.29** **Phlebitis and thrombophlebitis of other deep vessels of lower extremities**

I80.291 **Phlebitis and thrombophlebitis of other deep vessels of right lower extremity**

I80.292 **Phlebitis and thrombophlebitis of other deep vessels of left lower extremity**

I80.293 **Phlebitis and thrombophlebitis of other deep vessels of lower extremity, bilateral**

I80.299 **Phlebitis and thrombophlebitis of other deep vessels of unspecified lower extremity**

I80.3 **Phlebitis and thrombophlebitis of lower extremities, unspecified**

I80.8 **Phlebitis and thrombophlebitis of other sites**

I80.9 **Phlebitis and thrombophlebitis of unspecified site**

I81 **Portal vein thrombosis**

Portal (vein) obstruction

Excludes2 hepatic vein thrombosis (I82.0)
phlebitis of portal vein (K75.1)

Ex: E08.51-E08.59, E08.618-E08.638, E08.649-E08.8, E09.51-E09.59, E09.618-E09.638, E09.649, E09.65-E09.8, E10.51-E10.59, E10.618-E10.638, E10.649, E10.69-E10.8, E11.51-E11.59, E11.618-E11.638, E11.649, E11.69-E11.8, E13.51-E13.59, E13.618-E13.638, E13.649-E13.8, I81, I82.210-I82.291, I82.401-I82.729, I82.811-I82.91, I82.A11-I82.C29, I87.8-I87.9, I99.8-I99.9

● **I82** **Other venous embolism and thrombosis**

Code first venous embolism and thrombosis complicating:
abortion, ectopic or molar pregnancy (O00-O07, O08.7)
pregnancy, childbirth and the puerperium (O22.-, O87.-)

Excludes2 venous embolism and thrombosis (of):
cerebral (I63.6, I67.6)
coronary (I21-I25)
intracranial and intraspinal, septic or NOS (G08)
intracranial, nonpyogenic (I67.6)
intraspinal, nonpyogenic (G95.1)
mesenteric (K55.0-)
portal (I81)
pulmonary (I26.-)

I82.0 **Budd-Chiari syndrome**

Hepatic vein thrombosis

Ex: E08.51-E08.59, E08.618-E08.638, E08.649-E08.8, E09.51-E09.59, E09.618-E09.638, E09.649, E09.65-E09.8, E10.51-E10.59, E10.618-E10.638, E10.649, E10.69-E10.8, E11.51-E11.59, E11.618-E11.638, E11.649, E11.69-E11.8, E13.51-E13.59, E13.618-E13.638, E13.649-E13.8, I82.0, I82.210-I82.291, I82.401-I82.729, I82.811-I82.91, I82.A11-I82.C29, I87.8-I87.9, I99.8-I99.9

I82.1 **Thrombophlebitis migrans**

"White leg" is the other term to describe a migrating thrombus.

Ex: E08.51-E08.59, E08.618-E08.638, E08.649-E08.8, E09.51-E09.59, E09.618-E09.638, E09.649, E09.65-E09.8, E10.51-E10.59, E10.618-E10.638, E10.649, E10.69-E10.8, E11.51-E11.59, E11.618-E11.638, E11.649, E11.69-E11.8, E13.51-E13.59, E13.618-E13.638, E13.649-E13.8, I82.1, I82.210-I82.291, I82.401-I82.729, I82.811-I82.91, I82.A11-I82.C29, I87.8-I87.9, I99.8-I99.9

● **I82.2** **Embolism and thrombosis of vena cava and other thoracic veins**

Ex: **For category I82.2 CC codes unless otherwise indicated:** E08.51-E08.59, E08.618-E08.638, E08.649-E08.8, E09.51-E09.59, E09.618-E09.638, E09.649, E09.65-E09.8, E10.51-E10.59, E10.618-E10.638, E10.649, E10.69-E10.8, E11.51-E11.59, E11.618-E11.638, E11.649, E11.69-E11.8, E13.51-E13.59, E13.618-E13.638, E13.649-E13.8, I82.210-I82.291, I82.401-I82.729, I82.811-I82.91, I82.A11-I82.C29, I87.8-I87.9, I99.8-I99.9

● **I82.21** **Embolism and thrombosis of superior vena cava**

I82.210 **Acute embolism and thrombosis of superior vena cava**

Embolism and thrombosis of superior vena cava NOS

I82.211 **Chronic embolism and thrombosis of superior vena cava**

● **I82.22** **Embolism and thrombosis of inferior vena cava**

Ex: **For category I82.22 CC codes:** E08.51-E08.59, E08.618-E08.638, E08.649-E08.8, E09.51-E09.59, E09.618-E09.638, E09.649, E09.65-E09.8, E10.51-E10.59, E10.618-E10.638, E10.649, E10.69-E10.8, E11.51-E11.59, E11.618-E11.638, E11.649, E11.69-E11.8, E13.51-E13.59, E13.618-E13.638, E13.649-E13.8, I82.210-I82.291, I82.401-I82.729, I82.811-I82.91, I82.A11-I82.C29, I87.8-I87.9, I99.8-I99.9

I82.220 **Acute embolism and thrombosis of inferior vena cava**

Embolism and thrombosis of inferior vena cava NOS

I82.221 **Chronic embolism and thrombosis of inferior vena cava**

● **I82.29** **Embolism and thrombosis of other thoracic veins**

Embolism and thrombosis of brachiocephalic (innominate) vein

I82.290 **Acute embolism and thrombosis of other thoracic veins**

I82.291 **Chronic embolism and thrombosis of other thoracic veins**

I82.3 **Embolism and thrombosis of renal vein**

Ex: E08.51-E08.59, E08.618-E08.638, E08.649-E08.8, E09.51-E09.59, E09.618-E09.638, E09.649, E09.65-E09.8, E10.51-E10.59, E10.618-E10.638, E10.649, E10.69-E10.8, E11.51-E11.59, E11.618-E11.638, E11.649, E11.69-E11.8, E13.51-E13.59, E13.618-E13.638, E13.649-E13.8, I82.210-I82.291, I82.3, I82.401-I82.729, I82.811-I82.91, I82.A11-I82.C29, I87.8-I87.9, I99.8-I99.9

I82.4 Acute embolism and thrombosis of deep veins of lower extremity

Ex For category I82.4 CC codes: See I82.2

I82.40 Acute embolism and thrombosis of unspecified deep veins of lower extremity

Deep vein thrombosis NOS
DVT NOS

Excludes1 acute embolism and thrombosis of unspecified deep veins of distal lower extremity (I82.4Z-)
acute embolism and thrombosis of unspecified deep veins of proximal lower extremity (I82.4Y-)

I82.401 Acute embolism and thrombosis of unspecified deep veins of right lower extremity

I82.402 Acute embolism and thrombosis of unspecified deep veins of left lower extremity

I82.403 Acute embolism and thrombosis of unspecified deep veins of lower extremity, bilateral

I82.409 Acute embolism and thrombosis of unspecified deep veins of unspecified lower extremity

I82.41 Acute embolism and thrombosis of femoral vein

I82.411 Acute embolism and thrombosis of right femoral vein

I82.412 Acute embolism and thrombosis of left femoral vein

I82.413 Acute embolism and thrombosis of femoral vein, bilateral

I82.419 Acute embolism and thrombosis of unspecified femoral vein

I82.42 Acute embolism and thrombosis of iliac vein

I82.421 Acute embolism and thrombosis of right iliac vein

I82.422 Acute embolism and thrombosis of left iliac vein

I82.423 Acute embolism and thrombosis of iliac vein, bilateral

I82.429 Acute embolism and thrombosis of unspecified iliac vein

I82.43 Acute embolism and thrombosis of popliteal vein

I82.431 Acute embolism and thrombosis of right popliteal vein

I82.432 Acute embolism and thrombosis of left popliteal vein

I82.433 Acute embolism and thrombosis of popliteal vein, bilateral

I82.439 Acute embolism and thrombosis of unspecified popliteal vein

I82.44 Acute embolism and thrombosis of tibial vein

I82.441 Acute embolism and thrombosis of right tibial vein

I82.442 Acute embolism and thrombosis of left tibial vein

I82.443 Acute embolism and thrombosis of tibial vein, bilateral

I82.449 Acute embolism and thrombosis of unspecified tibial vein

I82.49 Acute embolism and thrombosis of other specified deep vein of lower extremity

I82.491 Acute embolism and thrombosis of other specified deep vein of right lower extremity

I82.492 Acute embolism and thrombosis of other specified deep vein of left lower extremity

I82.493 Acute embolism and thrombosis of other specified deep vein of lower extremity, bilateral

I82.499 Acute embolism and thrombosis of other specified deep vein of unspecified lower extremity

I82.4Y Acute embolism and thrombosis of unspecified deep veins of proximal lower extremity

Acute embolism and thrombosis of deep vein of thigh NOS
Acute embolism and thrombosis of deep vein of upper leg NOS

I82.4Y1 Acute embolism and thrombosis of unspecified deep veins of right proximal lower extremity

I82.4Y2 Acute embolism and thrombosis of unspecified deep veins of left proximal lower extremity

I82.4Y3 Acute embolism and thrombosis of unspecified deep veins of proximal lower extremity, bilateral

I82.4Y9 Acute embolism and thrombosis of unspecified deep veins of unspecified proximal lower extremity

I82.4Z Acute embolism and thrombosis of unspecified deep veins of distal lower extremity

Acute embolism and thrombosis of deep vein of calf NOS
Acute embolism and thrombosis of deep vein of lower leg NOS

I82.4Z1 Acute embolism and thrombosis of unspecified deep veins of right distal lower extremity

I82.4Z2 Acute embolism and thrombosis of unspecified deep veins of left distal lower extremity

I82.4Z3 Acute embolism and thrombosis of unspecified deep veins of distal lower extremity, bilateral

I82.4Z9 Acute embolism and thrombosis of unspecified deep veins of unspecified distal lower extremity

I82.5 Chronic embolism and thrombosis of deep veins of lower extremity

Use additional code, if applicable, for associated long-term (current) use of anticoagulants (Z79.01)

Excludes1 personal history of venous embolism and thrombosis (Z86.718)

Ex For category I82.5 CC codes: See I82.2

I82.50 Chronic embolism and thrombosis of unspecified deep veins of lower extremity

Excludes1 chronic embolism and thrombosis of unspecified deep veins of distal lower extremity (I82.5Z-)
chronic embolism and thrombosis of unspecified deep veins of proximal lower extremity (I82.5Y-)

I82.501 Chronic embolism and thrombosis of unspecified deep veins of right lower extremity

I82.502 Chronic embolism and thrombosis of unspecified deep veins of left lower extremity

Item 9–10 Varicose/Varicosities (varix = singular, varices = plural): Enlarged, engorged, tortuous, twisted vascular vessels (veins, arteries, lymphatics). As such, the condition can present in various parts of the body, although the most familiar locations are the lower extremities. A common complication of varices is thrombophlebitis. Varicosities of the anus and rectum are called hemorrhoids.

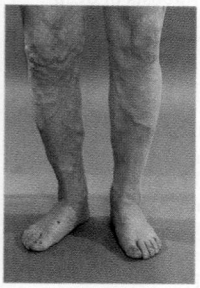

Figure 9-7 Varicose veins of the legs. (From Goldman: Cecil Medicine, ed 23, Saunders, 2008)

- I82.503 **Chronic embolism and thrombosis of unspecified deep veins of lower extremity, bilateral** CC
- I82.509 **Chronic embolism and thrombosis of unspecified deep veins of unspecified lower extremity** CC

● I82.51 **Chronic embolism and thrombosis of femoral vein**
- I82.511 **Chronic embolism and thrombosis of right femoral vein** CC
- I82.512 **Chronic embolism and thrombosis of left femoral vein** CC
- I82.513 **Chronic embolism and thrombosis of femoral vein, bilateral** CC
- I82.519 **Chronic embolism and thrombosis of unspecified femoral vein** CC

● I82.52 **Chronic embolism and thrombosis of iliac vein**
- I82.521 **Chronic embolism and thrombosis of right iliac vein** CC
- I82.522 **Chronic embolism and thrombosis of left iliac vein** CC
- I82.523 **Chronic embolism and thrombosis of iliac vein, bilateral** CC
- I82.529 **Chronic embolism and thrombosis of unspecified iliac vein** CC

● I82.53 **Chronic embolism and thrombosis of popliteal vein**
- I82.531 **Chronic embolism and thrombosis of right popliteal vein** CC
- I82.532 **Chronic embolism and thrombosis of left popliteal vein** CC
- I82.533 **Chronic embolism and thrombosis of popliteal vein, bilateral** CC
- I82.539 **Chronic embolism and thrombosis of unspecified popliteal vein** CC

● I82.54 **Chronic embolism and thrombosis of tibial vein**
- I82.541 **Chronic embolism and thrombosis of right tibial vein** CC
- I82.542 **Chronic embolism and thrombosis of left tibial vein** CC
- I82.543 **Chronic embolism and thrombosis of tibial vein, bilateral** CC
- I82.549 **Chronic embolism and thrombosis of unspecified tibial vein** CC

● I82.59 **Chronic embolism and thrombosis of other specified deep vein of lower extremity**
- I82.591 **Chronic embolism and thrombosis of other specified deep vein of right lower extremity** CC
- I82.592 **Chronic embolism and thrombosis of other specified deep vein of left lower extremity** CC
- I82.593 **Chronic embolism and thrombosis of other specified deep vein of lower extremity, bilateral** CC
- I82.599 **Chronic embolism and thrombosis of other specified deep vein of unspecified lower extremity** CC

● I82.5Y **Chronic embolism and thrombosis of unspecified deep veins of proximal lower extremity**
  - Chronic embolism and thrombosis of deep veins of thigh NOS
  - Chronic embolism and thrombosis of deep veins of upper leg NOS
- I82.5Y1 **Chronic embolism and thrombosis of unspecified deep veins of right proximal lower extremity** CC
- I82.5Y2 **Chronic embolism and thrombosis of unspecified deep veins of left proximal lower extremity** CC
- I82.5Y3 **Chronic embolism and thrombosis of unspecified deep veins of proximal lower extremity, bilateral** CC
- I82.5Y9 **Chronic embolism and thrombosis of unspecified deep veins of unspecified proximal lower extremity** CC

● I82.5Z **Chronic embolism and thrombosis of unspecified deep veins of distal lower extremity**
  - Chronic embolism and thrombosis of deep veins of calf NOS
  - Chronic embolism and thrombosis of deep veins of lower leg NOS
- I82.5Z1 **Chronic embolism and thrombosis of unspecified deep veins of right distal lower extremity** CC
- I82.5Z2 **Chronic embolism and thrombosis of unspecified deep veins of left distal lower extremity** CC
- I82.5Z3 **Chronic embolism and thrombosis of unspecified deep veins of distal lower extremity, bilateral** CC
- I82.5Z9 **Chronic embolism and thrombosis of unspecified deep veins of unspecified distal lower extremity** CC

● I82.6 **Acute embolism and thrombosis of veins of upper extremity**
  - Ex For category I82.6 CC codes: See I82.2

● I82.60 **Acute embolism and thrombosis of unspecified veins of upper extremity**
- I82.601 **Acute embolism and thrombosis of unspecified veins of right upper extremity** CC
- I82.602 **Acute embolism and thrombosis of unspecified veins of left upper extremity** CC
- I82.603 **Acute embolism and thrombosis of unspecified veins of upper extremity, bilateral** CC
- I82.609 **Acute embolism and thrombosis of unspecified veins of unspecified upper extremity** CC

- **I82.61 Acute embolism and thrombosis of superficial veins of upper extremity**
  - Acute embolism and thrombosis of antecubital vein
  - Acute embolism and thrombosis of basilic vein
  - Acute embolism and thrombosis of cephalic vein
  - **I82.611 Acute embolism and thrombosis of superficial veins of right upper extremity**
  - **I82.612 Acute embolism and thrombosis of superficial veins of left upper extremity**
  - **I82.613 Acute embolism and thrombosis of superficial veins of upper extremity, bilateral**
  - **I82.619 Acute embolism and thrombosis of superficial veins of unspecified upper extremity**
- **I82.62 Acute embolism and thrombosis of deep veins of upper extremity**
  - Acute embolism and thrombosis of brachial vein
  - Acute embolism and thrombosis of radial vein
  - Acute embolism and thrombosis of ulnar vein
  - **I82.621 Acute embolism and thrombosis of deep veins of right upper extremity**
  - **I82.622 Acute embolism and thrombosis of deep veins of left upper extremity**
  - **I82.623 Acute embolism and thrombosis of deep veins of upper extremity, bilateral**
  - **I82.629 Acute embolism and thrombosis of deep veins of unspecified upper extremity**
- **I82.7 Chronic embolism and thrombosis of veins of upper extremity**
  - Use additional code, if applicable, for associated long-term (current) use of anticoagulants (Z79.01)
  - **Excludes1** personal history of venous embolism and thrombosis (Z86.718)
  - Ex: **For category I82.7 CC codes:** See I82.2
- **I82.70 Chronic embolism and thrombosis of unspecified veins of upper extremity**
  - **I82.701 Chronic embolism and thrombosis of unspecified veins of right upper extremity**
  - **I82.702 Chronic embolism and thrombosis of unspecified veins of left upper extremity**
  - **I82.703 Chronic embolism and thrombosis of unspecified veins of upper extremity, bilateral**
  - **I82.709 Chronic embolism and thrombosis of unspecified veins of unspecified upper extremity**
- **I82.71 Chronic embolism and thrombosis of superficial veins of upper extremity**
  - Chronic embolism and thrombosis of antecubital vein
  - Chronic embolism and thrombosis of basilic vein
  - Chronic embolism and thrombosis of cephalic vein
  - **I82.711 Chronic embolism and thrombosis of superficial veins of right upper extremity**
  - **I82.712 Chronic embolism and thrombosis of superficial veins of left upper extremity**
  - **I82.713 Chronic embolism and thrombosis of superficial veins of upper extremity, bilateral**
  - **I82.719 Chronic embolism and thrombosis of superficial veins of unspecified upper extremity**
- **I82.72 Chronic embolism and thrombosis of deep veins of upper extremity**
  - Chronic embolism and thrombosis of brachial vein
  - Chronic embolism and thrombosis of radial vein
  - Chronic embolism and thrombosis of ulnar vein
  - **I82.721 Chronic embolism and thrombosis of deep veins of right upper extremity**
  - **I82.722 Chronic embolism and thrombosis of deep veins of left upper extremity**
  - **I82.723 Chronic embolism and thrombosis of deep veins of upper extremity, bilateral**
  - **I82.729 Chronic embolism and thrombosis of deep veins of unspecified upper extremity**
- **I82.A Embolism and thrombosis of axillary vein**
  - Ex: **For category I82.A CC codes:** See I82.2
  - **I82.A1 Acute embolism and thrombosis of axillary vein**
    - **I82.A11 Acute embolism and thrombosis of right axillary vein**
    - **I82.A12 Acute embolism and thrombosis of left axillary vein**
    - **I82.A13 Acute embolism and thrombosis of axillary vein, bilateral**
    - **I82.A19 Acute embolism and thrombosis of unspecified axillary vein**
  - **I82.A2 Chronic embolism and thrombosis of axillary vein**
    - **I82.A21 Chronic embolism and thrombosis of right axillary vein**
    - **I82.A22 Chronic embolism and thrombosis of left axillary vein**
    - **I82.A23 Chronic embolism and thrombosis of axillary vein, bilateral**
    - **I82.A29 Chronic embolism and thrombosis of unspecified axillary vein**
- **I82.B Embolism and thrombosis of subclavian vein**
  - Ex: **For category I82.B CC codes:** See I82.2
  - **I82.B1 Acute embolism and thrombosis of subclavian vein**
    - **I82.B11 Acute embolism and thrombosis of right subclavian vein**
    - **I82.B12 Acute embolism and thrombosis of left subclavian vein**
    - **I82.B13 Acute embolism and thrombosis of subclavian vein, bilateral**
    - **I82.B19 Acute embolism and thrombosis of unspecified subclavian vein**
  - **I82.B2 Chronic embolism and thrombosis of subclavian vein**
    - **I82.B21 Chronic embolism and thrombosis of right subclavian vein**
    - **I82.B22 Chronic embolism and thrombosis of left subclavian vein**
    - **I82.B23 Chronic embolism and thrombosis of subclavian vein, bilateral**
    - **I82.B29 Chronic embolism and thrombosis of unspecified subclavian vein**

I82.C Embolism and thrombosis of internal jugular vein
Ex: For category I82.C CC codes: See I82.2

I82.C1 Acute embolism and thrombosis of internal jugular vein

I82.C11 Acute embolism and thrombosis of right internal jugular vein

I82.C12 Acute embolism and thrombosis of left internal jugular vein

I82.C13 Acute embolism and thrombosis of internal jugular vein, bilateral

I82.C19 Acute embolism and thrombosis of unspecified internal jugular vein

I82.C2 Chronic embolism and thrombosis of internal jugular vein

I82.C21 Chronic embolism and thrombosis of right internal jugular vein

I82.C22 Chronic embolism and thrombosis of left internal jugular vein

I82.C23 Chronic embolism and thrombosis of internal jugular vein, bilateral

I82.C29 Chronic embolism and thrombosis of unspecified internal jugular vein

I82.8 Embolism and thrombosis of other specified veins
Use additional code, if applicable, for associated long-term (current) use of anticoagulants (Z79.01)
Ex: For category I82.8 CC codes: See I82.2

I82.81 Embolism and thrombosis of superficial veins of lower extremities
Embolism and thrombosis of saphenous vein (greater) (lesser)

I82.811 Embolism and thrombosis of superficial veins of right lower extremities

I82.812 Embolism and thrombosis of superficial veins of left lower extremities

I82.813 Embolism and thrombosis of superficial veins of lower extremities, bilateral

I82.819 Embolism and thrombosis of superficial veins of unspecified lower extremities

I82.89 Embolism and thrombosis of other specified veins

I82.890 Acute embolism and thrombosis of other specified veins

I82.891 Chronic embolism and thrombosis of other specified veins

I82.9 Embolism and thrombosis of unspecified vein
Ex: For category I82.9 CC codes: See I82.2

I82.90 Acute embolism and thrombosis of unspecified vein
Embolism of vein NOS
Thrombosis (vein) NOS

I82.91 Chronic embolism and thrombosis of unspecified vein

I83 Varicose veins of lower extremities
Excludes1 varicose veins complicating pregnancy (O22.0-)
varicose veins complicating the puerperium (O87.4)

I83.0 Varicose veins of lower extremities with ulcer
Use additional code to identify severity of ulcer (L97.-)

I83.00 Varicose veins of unspecified lower extremity with ulcer

I83.001 Varicose veins of unspecified lower extremity with ulcer of thigh A

I83.002 Varicose veins of unspecified lower extremity with ulcer of calf A

I83.003 Varicose veins of unspecified lower extremity with ulcer of ankle A

I83.004 Varicose veins of unspecified lower extremity with ulcer of heel and midfoot A
Varicose veins of unspecified lower extremity with ulcer of plantar surface of midfoot

I83.005 Varicose veins of unspecified lower extremity with ulcer other part of foot A
Varicose veins of unspecified lower extremity with ulcer of toe

I83.008 Varicose veins of unspecified lower extremity with ulcer other part of lower leg A

I83.009 Varicose veins of unspecified lower extremity with ulcer of unspecified site A

I83.01 Varicose veins of right lower extremity with ulcer

I83.011 Varicose veins of right lower extremity with ulcer of thigh A

I83.012 Varicose veins of right lower extremity with ulcer of calf A

I83.013 Varicose veins of right lower extremity with ulcer of ankle A

I83.014 Varicose veins of right lower extremity with ulcer of heel and midfoot A
Varicose veins of right lower extremity with ulcer of plantar surface of midfoot

I83.015 Varicose veins of right lower extremity with ulcer other part of foot A
Varicose veins of right lower extremity with ulcer of toe

I83.018 Varicose veins of right lower extremity with ulcer other part of lower leg A

I83.019 Varicose veins of right lower extremity with ulcer of unspecified site A

I83.02 Varicose veins of left lower extremity with ulcer

I83.021 Varicose veins of left lower extremity with ulcer of thigh A

I83.022 Varicose veins of left lower extremity with ulcer of calf A

I83.023 Varicose veins of left lower extremity with ulcer of ankle A

I83.024 Varicose veins of left lower extremity with ulcer of heel and midfoot A
Varicose veins of left lower extremity with ulcer of plantar surface of midfoot

I83.025 Varicose veins of left lower extremity with ulcer other part of foot A
Varicose veins of left lower extremity with ulcer of toe

I83.028 Varicose veins of left lower extremity with ulcer other part of lower leg A

I83.029 Varicose veins of left lower extremity with ulcer of unspecified site A

I83.1 Varicose veins of lower extremities with inflammation
~~Stasis dermatitis~~

I83.10 Varicose veins of unspecified lower extremity with inflammation A

I83.11 Varicose veins of right lower extremity with inflammation A

I83.12 Varicose veins of left lower extremity with inflammation A

● **I83.2 Varicose veins of lower extremities with both ulcer and inflammation**
Use additional code to identify severity of ulcer (L97.-)
Ex: For category I83.2 CC codes: I83.001-I83.229, I83.90-I83.93

● **I83.20 Varicose veins of unspecified lower extremity with both ulcer and inflammation**

I83.201 Varicose veins of unspecified lower extremity with both ulcer of thigh and inflammation A

I83.202 Varicose veins of unspecified lower extremity with both ulcer of calf and inflammation A

I83.203 Varicose veins of unspecified lower extremity with both ulcer of ankle and inflammation A

I83.204 Varicose veins of unspecified lower extremity with both ulcer of heel and midfoot and inflammation A
Varicose veins of unspecified lower extremity with both ulcer of plantar surface of midfoot and inflammation

I83.205 Varicose veins of unspecified lower extremity with both ulcer other part of foot and inflammation A
Varicose veins of unspecified lower extremity with both ulcer of toe and inflammation

I83.208 Varicose veins of unspecified lower extremity with both ulcer of other part of lower extremity and inflammation A

I83.209 Varicose veins of unspecified lower extremity with both ulcer of unspecified site and inflammation A

● **I83.21 Varicose veins of right lower extremity with both ulcer and inflammation**

I83.211 Varicose veins of right lower extremity with both ulcer of thigh and inflammation A

I83.212 Varicose veins of right lower extremity with both ulcer of calf and inflammation A

I83.213 Varicose veins of right lower extremity with both ulcer of ankle and inflammation A

I83.214 Varicose veins of right lower extremity with both ulcer of heel and midfoot and inflammation A
Varicose veins of right lower extremity with both ulcer of plantar surface of midfoot and inflammation

I83.215 Varicose veins of right lower extremity with both ulcer other part of foot and inflammation A
Varicose veins of right lower extremity with both ulcer of toe and inflammation

I83.218 Varicose veins of right lower extremity with both ulcer of other part of lower extremity and inflammation A

I83.219 Varicose veins of right lower extremity with both ulcer of unspecified site and inflammation A

● **I83.22 Varicose veins of left lower extremity with both ulcer and inflammation**

I83.221 Varicose veins of left lower extremity with both ulcer of thigh and inflammation A

I83.222 Varicose veins of left lower extremity with both ulcer of calf and inflammation A

I83.223 Varicose veins of left lower extremity with both ulcer of ankle and inflammation A

I83.224 Varicose veins of left lower extremity with both ulcer of heel and midfoot and inflammation A
Varicose veins of left lower extremity with both ulcer of plantar surface of midfoot and inflammation

I83.225 Varicose veins of left lower extremity with both ulcer other part of foot and inflammation A
Varicose veins of left lower extremity with both ulcer of toe and inflammation

I83.228 Varicose veins of left lower extremity with both ulcer of other part of lower extremity and inflammation A

I83.229 Varicose veins of left lower extremity with both ulcer of unspecified site and inflammation A

● **I83.8 Varicose veins of lower extremities with other complications**

● **I83.81 Varicose veins of lower extremities with pain**

I83.811 Varicose veins of right lower extremities with pain A

I83.812 Varicose veins of left lower extremities with pain A

I83.813 Varicose veins of bilateral lower extremities with pain A

I83.819 Varicose veins of unspecified lower extremities with pain A

● **I83.89 Varicose veins of lower extremities with other complications**
Varicose veins of lower extremities with edema
Varicose veins of lower extremities with swelling

I83.891 Varicose veins of right lower extremities with other complications A

I83.892 Varicose veins of left lower extremities with other complications A

I83.893 Varicose veins of bilateral lower extremities with other complications A

I83.899 Varicose veins of unspecified lower extremities with other complications A

● **I83.9 Asymptomatic varicose veins of lower extremities**
Phlebectasia of lower extremities
Varicose veins of lower extremities
Varix of lower extremities

I83.90 Asymptomatic varicose veins of unspecified lower extremity A
Varicose veins NOS

I83.91 Asymptomatic varicose veins of right lower extremity A

I83.92 Asymptomatic varicose veins of left lower extremity A

I83.93 Asymptomatic varicose veins of bilateral lower extremities A

I85 Esophageal varices
Use additional code to identify:
alcohol abuse and dependence (F10.-)

I85.0 Esophageal varices
Idiopathic esophageal varices
Primary esophageal varices

I85.00 Esophageal varices without bleeding
Esophageal varices NOS
Exc E16.4, I85.00-I85.01, I85.11, I87.8-I87.9, I99.8-I99.9, K22.6, K25.0-K28.9, K29.01, K29.21, K29.31, K29.41, K29.51, K29.61, K29.71, K29.81, K29.91, K31.811, K92.0-K92.2

I85.01 Esophageal varices with bleeding
Exc E16.4, I85.01, I85.11, I87.8-I87.9, I99.8-I99.9, K22.10-K22.11, K22.6-K22.70, K22.710-K22.719, K25.0-K28.9, K29.01, K29.21, K29.31, K29.41, K29.51, K29.61, K29.71, K29.81, K29.91, K31.811, K55.21, K57.01, K57.11, K57.13, K57.21, K57.31, K57.33, K57.41, K57.51, K57.53, K57.81, K57.91, K57.93, K62.5, K92.0-K92.2

I85.1 Secondary esophageal varices
Esophageal varices secondary to alcoholic liver disease
Esophageal varices secondary to cirrhosis of liver
Esophageal varices secondary to schistosomiasis
Esophageal varices secondary to toxic liver disease
Code first underlying disease

I85.10 Secondary esophageal varices without bleeding
Exc E16.4, I85.01, I85.10-I85.11, I87.8-I87.9, I99.8-I99.9, K22.6, K25.0-K28.9, K29.01, K29.21, K29.31, K29.41, K29.51, K29.61, K29.71, K29.81, K29.91, K31.811, K92.0-K92.2

I85.11 Secondary esophageal varices with bleeding
Exc I85.01, I85.11, I87.8-I87.9, I99.8-I99.9

I86 Varicose veins of other sites
Excludes1 varicose veins of unspecified site (I83.9-)
Excludes2 retinal varices (H35.0-)

I86.0 Sublingual varices

I86.1 Scrotal varices ♂
Varicocele

I86.2 Pelvic varices

I86.3 Vulval varices ♀
Excludes1 vulval varices complicating childbirth and the puerperium (O87.8)
vulval varices complicating pregnancy (O22.1-)

I86.4 Gastric varices

I86.8 Varicose veins of other specified sites A
Varicose ulcer of nasal septum

I87 Other disorders of veins

I87.0 Postthrombotic syndrome
Chronic venous hypertension due to deep vein thrombosis
Postphlebitic syndrome
Excludes1 chronic venous hypertension without deep vein thrombosis (I87.3-)

I87.00 Postthrombotic syndrome without complications
Asymptomatic Postthrombotic syndrome

I87.001 Postthrombotic syndrome without complications of right lower extremity

I87.002 Postthrombotic syndrome without complications of left lower extremity

I87.003 Postthrombotic syndrome without complications of bilateral lower extremity

I87.009 Postthrombotic syndrome without complications of unspecified extremity
Postthrombotic syndrome NOS

I87.01 Postthrombotic syndrome with ulcer
Use additional code to specify site and severity of ulcer (L97.-)
Exc For category I87.01 CC codes: I80.00-I80.9

I87.011 Postthrombotic syndrome with ulcer of right lower extremity

I87.012 Postthrombotic syndrome with ulcer of left lower extremity

I87.013 Postthrombotic syndrome with ulcer of bilateral lower extremity

I87.019 Postthrombotic syndrome with ulcer of unspecified lower extremity

I87.02 Postthrombotic syndrome with inflammation

I87.021 Postthrombotic syndrome with inflammation of right lower extremity

I87.022 Postthrombotic syndrome with inflammation of left lower extremity

I87.023 Postthrombotic syndrome with inflammation of bilateral lower extremity

I87.029 Postthrombotic syndrome with inflammation of unspecified lower extremity

I87.03 Postthrombotic syndrome with ulcer and inflammation
Use additional code to specify site and severity of ulcer (L97.-)
Exc For category I87.03 CC codes: I80.00-I80.9

I87.031 Postthrombotic syndrome with ulcer and inflammation of right lower extremity

I87.032 Postthrombotic syndrome with ulcer and inflammation of left lower extremity

I87.033 Postthrombotic syndrome with ulcer and inflammation of bilateral lower extremity

I87.039 Postthrombotic syndrome with ulcer and inflammation of unspecified lower extremity

I87.09 Postthrombotic syndrome with other complications

I87.091 Postthrombotic syndrome with other complications of right lower extremity

I87.092 Postthrombotic syndrome with other complications of left lower extremity

I87.093 Postthrombotic syndrome with other complications of bilateral lower extremity

I87.099 Postthrombotic syndrome with other complications of unspecified lower extremity

I87.1 Compression of vein
Stricture of vein
Vena cava syndrome (inferior) (superior)
Excludes2 compression of pulmonary vein (I28.8)
Exc I87.1

I87.2 Venous insufficiency (chronic) (peripheral)
Stasis dermatitis ◀
Excludes1 stasis dermatitis with varicose veins of lower extremities (I83.1-, I83.2-) ◀

● I87.3 **Chronic venous hypertension (idiopathic)**
Stasis edema
Excludes1 chronic venous hypertension due to deep vein thrombosis (I87.0-)
varicose veins of lower extremities (I83.-)

● I87.30 **Chronic venous hypertension (idiopathic) without complications**
Asymptomatic chronic venous hypertension (idiopathic)

I87.301 **Chronic venous hypertension (idiopathic) without complications of right lower extremity**

I87.302 **Chronic venous hypertension (idiopathic) without complications of left lower extremity**

I87.303 **Chronic venous hypertension (idiopathic) without complications of bilateral lower extremity**

I87.309 **Chronic venous hypertension (idiopathic) without complications of unspecified lower extremity**
Chronic venous hypertension NOS

● I87.31 **Chronic venous hypertension (idiopathic) with ulcer**
Use additional code to specify site and severity of ulcer (L97.-)
Ex: **For category I87.31 CC codes:** I83.001-I83.229, I83.90-I83.93, I87.2, I87.8-I87.9, I99.8-I99.9

I87.311 **Chronic venous hypertension (idiopathic) with ulcer of right lower extremity**

I87.312 **Chronic venous hypertension (idiopathic) with ulcer of left lower extremity**

I87.313 **Chronic venous hypertension (idiopathic) with ulcer of bilateral lower extremity**

I87.319 **Chronic venous hypertension (idiopathic) with ulcer of unspecified lower extremity**

● I87.32 **Chronic venous hypertension (idiopathic) with inflammation**

I87.321 **Chronic venous hypertension (idiopathic) with inflammation of right lower extremity**

I87.322 **Chronic venous hypertension (idiopathic) with inflammation of left lower extremity**

I87.323 **Chronic venous hypertension (idiopathic) with inflammation of bilateral lower extremity**

I87.329 **Chronic venous hypertension (idiopathic) with inflammation of unspecified lower extremity**

● I87.33 **Chronic venous hypertension (idiopathic) with ulcer and inflammation**
Use additional code to specify site and severity of ulcer (L97.-)
Ex: **For category I87.33 CC codes:** See I87.31

I87.331 **Chronic venous hypertension (idiopathic) with ulcer and inflammation of right lower extremity**

I87.332 **Chronic venous hypertension (idiopathic) with ulcer and inflammation of left lower extremity**

I87.333 **Chronic venous hypertension (idiopathic) with ulcer and inflammation of bilateral lower extremity**

I87.339 **Chronic venous hypertension (idiopathic) with ulcer and inflammation of unspecified lower extremity**

● I87.39 **Chronic venous hypertension (idiopathic) with other complications**

I87.391 **Chronic venous hypertension (idiopathic) with other complications of right lower extremity**

I87.392 **Chronic venous hypertension (idiopathic) with other complications of left lower extremity**

I87.393 **Chronic venous hypertension (idiopathic) with other complications of bilateral lower extremity**

I87.399 **Chronic venous hypertension (idiopathic) with other complications of unspecified lower extremity**

I87.8 **Other specified disorders of veins**
Phlebosclerosis
Venofibrosis

I87.9 **Disorder of vein, unspecified**

● I88 **Nonspecific lymphadenitis**
Excludes1 acute lymphadenitis, except mesenteric (L04.-)
enlarged lymph nodes NOS (R59.-)
human immunodeficiency virus [HIV] disease resulting in generalized lymphadenopathy (B20)

I88.0 **Nonspecific mesenteric lymphadenitis**
Mesenteric lymphadenitis (acute)(chronic)

I88.1 **Chronic lymphadenitis, except mesenteric**
Adenitis
Lymphadenitis

I88.8 **Other nonspecific lymphadenitis**

I88.9 **Nonspecific lymphadenitis, unspecified**
Lymphadenitis NOS

● I89 **Other noninfective disorders of lymphatic vessels and lymph nodes**
Excludes1 chylocele, tunica vaginalis (nonfilarial) NOS (N50.89)
enlarged lymph nodes NOS (R59.-)
filarial chylocele (B74.-)
hereditary lymphedema (Q82.0)

I89.0 **Lymphedema, not elsewhere classified**
Elephantiasis (nonfilarial) NOS
Lymphangiectasis
Obliteration, lymphatic vessel
Praecox lymphedema
Secondary lymphedema
Excludes1 postmastectomy lymphedema (I97.2)

I89.1 **Lymphangitis**
Chronic lymphangitis
Lymphangitis NOS
Subacute lymphangitis
Excludes1 acute lymphangitis (L03.-)

I89.8 **Other specified noninfective disorders of lymphatic vessels and lymph nodes**
Chylocele (nonfilarial)
Chylous ascites
Chylous cyst
Lipomelanotic reticulosis
Lymph node or vessel fistula
Lymph node or vessel infarction
Lymph node or vessel rupture

I89.9 **Noninfective disorder of lymphatic vessels and lymph nodes, unspecified**
Disease of lymphatic vessels NOS

OTHER AND UNSPECIFIED DISORDERS OF THE CIRCULATORY SYSTEM (I95-I99)

I95 Hypotension
Subnormal arterial blood pressure
Excludes1 cardiovascular collapse (R57.9)
maternal hypotension syndrome (O26.5-)
nonspecific low blood pressure reading NOS (R03.1)

I95.0 Idiopathic hypotension

I95.1 Orthostatic hypotension
Hypotension, postural
Moving from a sitting or reclining position to a standing position precipitates a sudden drop in blood pressure (hypotension).
Excludes1 neurogenic orthostatic hypotension [Shy-Drager] (G90.3)
orthostatic hypotension due to drugs (I95.2)

I95.2 Hypotension due to drugs
Orthostatic hypotension due to drugs
Use additional code for adverse effect, if applicable, to identify drug (T36-T50 with fifth or sixth character 5)

I95.3 Hypotension of hemodialysis
Intra-dialytic hypotension

I95.8 Other hypotension

I95.81 Postprocedural hypotension

I95.89 Other hypotension
Chronic hypotension

I95.9 Hypotension, unspecified

I96 Gangrene, not elsewhere classified
Gangrenous cellulitis
Excludes1 gangrene in atherosclerosis of native arteries of the extremities (I70.26)
gangrene of certain specified sites - *see* Alphabetical Index
gangrene in diabetes mellitus (E08-E13 with .52)
gangrene in hernia (K40.1, K40.4, K41.1, K41.4, K42.1, K43.1-, K44.1, K45.1, K46.1)
gangrene in other peripheral vascular diseases (I73.-)
gas gangrene (A48.0)
pyoderma gangrenosum (L88)
Ex: See I70.26
Coding Clinic: 2013, Q2, P35

I97 Intraoperative and postprocedural complications and disorders of circulatory system, not elsewhere classified
Excludes2 postprocedural shock (T81.1-)

I97.0 Postcardiotomy syndrome

I97.1 Other postprocedural cardiac functional disturbances
Excludes2 acute pulmonary insufficiency following thoracic surgery (J95.1)
intraoperative cardiac functional disturbances (I97.7-)
Ex: **For category I97.1 CC codes:** D78.81-D78.89, E36.8, E89.810-E89.89, H59.011-H59.019, H59.031-H59.099, H59.811-H59.89, H95.811-H95.89, I97.110-I97.191, I97.3, I97.710-I97.791, I97.88-I97.89, L76.81-L76.82, M96.89, N98.1-N98.9, T81.82X[A], T81.89X-T81.9XX[A]

I97.11 Postprocedural cardiac insufficiency

I97.110 Postprocedural cardiac insufficiency following cardiac surgery

I97.111 Postprocedural cardiac insufficiency following other surgery

I97.12 Postprocedural cardiac arrest

I97.120 Postprocedural cardiac arrest following cardiac surgery

I97.121 Postprocedural cardiac arrest following other surgery

I97.13 Postprocedural heart failure
Use additional code to identify the heart failure (I50.-)

I97.130 Postprocedural heart failure following cardiac surgery

I97.131 Postprocedural heart failure following other surgery

I97.19 Other postprocedural cardiac functional disturbances
Use additional code, if applicable, to further specify disorder

I97.190 Other postprocedural cardiac functional disturbances following cardiac surgery

I97.191 Other postprocedural cardiac functional disturbances following other surgery

I97.2 Postmastectomy lymphedema syndrome A
Elephantiasis due to mastectomy
Obliteration of lymphatic vessels

I97.3 Postprocedural hypertension

I97.4 Intraoperative hemorrhage and hematoma of a circulatory system organ or structure complicating a procedure
Excludes1 intraoperative hemorrhage and hematoma of a circulatory system organ or structure due to accidental puncture and laceration during a procedure (I97.5-)
Excludes2 intraoperative cerebrovascular hemorrhage complicating a procedure (G97.3-)
Ex: **For category I97.4 CC codes:** H95.811-H95.89, I85.01, I85.11, I97.3-I97.42, I97.610-I97.648, K21.9, K22.8, K23-K25.0, K25.2, K25.4, K25.6, K26.0, K26.2, K26.4, K26.6, K27.0, K27.2, K27.4, K27.6, K28.0, K28.2, K28.4, K28.6, K29.01, K29.21, K29.31, K29.41, K29.51, K29.61, K29.71, K29.81, K29.91, K31.811, K55.21, K57.01, K57.11, K57.13, K57.21, K57.31, K57.33, K57.41, K57.51, K57.53, K57.81, K57.91, K57.93, K62.5, K92.0-K92.2, M96.89, N98.1-N98.9, P54.1-P54.3, T81.10X-T81.19X[A], T81.82X[A], T81.89X-T81.9XX[A]

I97.41 Intraoperative hemorrhage and hematoma of a circulatory system organ or structure complicating a circulatory system procedure

I97.410 Intraoperative hemorrhage and hematoma of a circulatory system organ or structure complicating a cardiac catheterization

I97.411 Intraoperative hemorrhage and hematoma of a circulatory system organ or structure complicating a cardiac bypass

I97.418 Intraoperative hemorrhage and hematoma of a circulatory system organ or structure complicating other circulatory system procedure

I97.42 Intraoperative hemorrhage and hematoma of a circulatory system organ or structure complicating other procedure

I97.5 Accidental puncture and laceration of a circulatory system organ or structure during a procedure
Excludes2 accidental puncture and laceration of brain during a procedure (G97.4-)
Ex: **For category I97.5 CC codes:** D78.11-D78.12, D78.81-D78.89, E36.11-E36.8, E89.810-E89.89, G96.11, G97.41-G97.49, H59.011-H59.019, H59.031-H59.099, H59.211-H59.229, H59.811-H59.89, H95.31-H95.32, H95.811-H95.89, I97.3, I97.51-I97.52, J95.71-J95.72, K91.71-K91.72, L76.11-L76.12, L76.81-L76.82, M96.820-M96.821, M96.89, N98.1-N98.9, N99.71-N99.72, T81.82X[A], T81.89X-T81.9XX[A]

I97.51 Accidental puncture and laceration of a circulatory system organ or structure during a circulatory system procedure

I97.52 Accidental puncture and laceration of a circulatory system organ or structure during other procedure

● I97.6 **Postprocedural hemorrhage, hematoma and seroma of a circulatory system organ or structure following a procedure**

Excludes2 postprocedural cerebrovascular hemorrhage complicating a procedure (G97.5-)

Ex: **For category I97.6 CC codes:** See I97.4

● I97.61 **Postprocedural hemorrhage of a circulatory system organ or structure following a circulatory system procedure**

I97.610 **Postprocedural hemorrhage of a circulatory system organ or structure following a cardiac catheterization**

I97.611 **Postprocedural hemorrhage of a circulatory system organ or structure following cardiac bypass**

I97.618 **Postprocedural hemorrhage of a circulatory system organ or structure following other circulatory system procedure**

● I97.62 **Postprocedural hemorrhage, hematoma and seroma of a circulatory system organ or structure following other procedure**

I97.620 **Postprocedural hemorrhage of a circulatory system organ or structure following other procedure** ◀

I97.621 **Postprocedural hematoma of a circulatory system organ or structure following other procedure** ◀

I97.622 **Postprocedural seroma of a circulatory system organ or structure following other procedure** ◀

● I97.63 **Postprocedural hematoma of a circulatory system organ or structure following a circulatory system procedure** ◀

I97.630 **Postprocedural hematoma of a circulatory system organ or structure following a cardiac catheterization** ◀

I97.631 **Postprocedural hematoma of a circulatory system organ or structure following cardiac bypass** ◀

I97.638 **Postprocedural hematoma of a circulatory system organ or structure following other circulatory system procedure** ◀

● I97.64 **Postprocedural seroma of a circulatory system organ or structure following a circulatory system procedure** ◀

I97.640 **Postprocedural seroma of a circulatory system organ or structure following a cardiac catheterization** ◀

I97.641 **Postprocedural seroma of a circulatory system organ or structure following cardiac bypass** ◀

I97.648 **Postprocedural seroma of a circulatory system organ or structure following other circulatory system procedure** ◀

● I97.7 **Intraoperative cardiac functional disturbances**

Excludes2 acute pulmonary insufficiency following thoracic surgery (J95.1)
postprocedural cardiac functional disturbances (I97.1-)

Ex: **For category I97.7 CC codes:** See I97.1

● I97.71 **Intraoperative cardiac arrest**

I97.710 **Intraoperative cardiac arrest during cardiac surgery**

I97.711 **Intraoperative cardiac arrest during other surgery**

● I97.79 **Other intraoperative cardiac functional disturbances**

Use additional code, if applicable, to further specify disorder

I97.790 **Other intraoperative cardiac functional disturbances during cardiac surgery**

I97.791 **Other intraoperative cardiac functional disturbances during other surgery**

● I97.8 **Other intraoperative and postprocedural complications and disorders of the circulatory system, not elsewhere classified**

Use additional code, if applicable, to further specify disorder

Ex: **For category I97.8 CC codes unless otherwise indicated:** D78.81-D78.89, E36.8, E89.810-E89.89, G97.0, G97.2-G97.32, G97.81-G97.82, H59.011-H59.019, H59.031-H59.099, H59.811-H59.89, H95.811-H95.89, I97.3, I97.810-I97.821, L76.81-L76.82, M96.89, N98.1-N98.9, T81.82X[A], T81.89X-T81.9XX[A]

● I97.81 **Intraoperative cerebrovascular infarction**

I97.810 **Intraoperative cerebrovascular infarction during cardiac surgery**

I97.811 **Intraoperative cerebrovascular infarction during other surgery**

● I97.82 **Postprocedural cerebrovascular infarction**

I97.820 **Postprocedural cerebrovascular infarction following cardiac surgery**

I97.821 **Postprocedural cerebrovascular infarction following other surgery**

I97.88 **Other intraoperative complications of the circulatory system, not elsewhere classified**

Ex: See I97.1

I97.89 **Other postprocedural complications and disorders of the circulatory system, not elsewhere classified**

Ex: See I97.1

● I99 **Other and unspecified disorders of circulatory system**

I99.8 **Other disorder of circulatory system**

I99.9 **Unspecified disorder of circulatory system**

CHAPTER 10

DISEASES OF THE RESPIRATORY SYSTEM (J00-J99)

OGCR Chapter-Specific Coding Guidelines

10. Chapter 10: Diseases of the Respiratory System (J00-J99)

a. Chronic Obstructive Pulmonary Disease [COPD] and Asthma

1) Acute exacerbation of chronic obstructive bronchitis and asthma

The codes in categories J44 and J45 distinguish between uncomplicated cases and those in acute exacerbation. An acute exacerbation is a worsening or a decompensation of a chronic condition. An acute exacerbation is not equivalent to an infection superimposed on a chronic condition, though an exacerbation may be triggered by an infection.

b. Acute Respiratory Failure

1) Acute respiratory failure as principal diagnosis

A code from subcategory J96.0, Acute respiratory failure, or subcategory J96.2, Acute and chronic respiratory failure, may be assigned as a principal diagnosis when it is the condition established after study to be chiefly responsible for occasioning the admission to the hospital, and the selection is supported by the Alphabetic Index and Tabular List. However, chapter-specific coding guidelines (such as obstetrics, poisoning, HIV, newborn) that provide sequencing direction take precedence.

2) Acute respiratory failure as secondary diagnosis

Respiratory failure may be listed as a secondary diagnosis if it occurs after admission, or if it is present on admission, but does not meet the definition of principal diagnosis.

3) Sequencing of acute respiratory failure and another acute condition

When a patient is admitted with respiratory failure and another acute condition, (e.g., myocardial infarction, cerebrovascular accident, aspiration pneumonia), the principal diagnosis will not be the same in every situation. This applies whether the other acute condition is a respiratory or nonrespiratory condition. Selection of the principal diagnosis will be dependent on the circumstances of admission. If both the respiratory failure and the other acute condition are equally responsible for occasioning the admission to the hospital, and there are no chapter-specific sequencing rules, the guideline regarding two or more diagnoses that equally meet the definition for principal diagnosis *(Section II, C.)* may be applied in these situations.

If the documentation is not clear as to whether acute respiratory failure and another condition are equally responsible for occasioning the admission, query the provider for clarification.

c. Influenza due to certain identified influenza viruses

Code only confirmed cases of influenza due to certain identified influenza viruses (category J09), and due to other identified influenza virus (category J10). This is an exception to the hospital inpatient guideline Section II, H. (Uncertain Diagnosis).

In this context, "confirmation" does not require documentation of positive laboratory testing specific for avian or other novel influenza A or other identified influenza virus. However, coding should be based on the provider's diagnostic statement that the patient has avian influenza, or other novel influenza A, for category J09, or has another particular identified strain of influenza, such as H1N1 or H3N2, but not identified as novel or variant, for category J10.

If the provider records "suspected" or "possible" or "probable" avian influenza, or novel influenza, or other identified influenza, then the appropriate influenza code from category J11, Influenza due to unidentified influenza virus, should be assigned. A code from category J09, Influenza due to certain identified influenza viruses, should not be assigned nor should a code from category J10, Influenza due to other identified influenza virus.

d. Ventilator associated Pneumonia

1) Documentation of Ventilator associated Pneumonia

As with all procedural or postprocedural complications, code assignment is based on the provider's documentation of the relationship between the condition and the procedure.

Code J95.851, Ventilator associated pneumonia, should be assigned only when the provider has documented ventilator associated pneumonia (VAP). An additional code to identify the organism (e.g., Pseudomonas aeruginosa, code B96.5) should also be assigned. Do not assign an additional code from categories J12-J18 to identify the type of pneumonia.

Code J95.851 should not be assigned for cases where the patient has pneumonia and is on a mechanical ventilator and the provider has not specifically stated that the pneumonia is ventilator-associated pneumonia. If the documentation is unclear as to whether the patient has a pneumonia that is a complication attributable to the mechanical ventilator, query the provider.

2) Ventilator associated Pneumonia Develops after Admission

A patient may be admitted with one type of pneumonia (e.g., code J13, Pneumonia due to Streptococcus pneumonia) and subsequently develop VAP. In this instance, the principal diagnosis would be the appropriate code from categories J12-J18 for the pneumonia diagnosed at the time of admission. Code J95.851, Ventilator associated pneumonia, would be assigned as an additional diagnosis when the provider has also documented the presence of ventilator associated pneumonia.

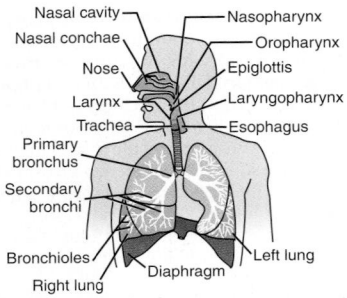

Figure 10-1 Respiratory system. (From Buck CJ: Step-by-Step Medical Coding, ed 2016, St. Louis, Elsevier, 2016)

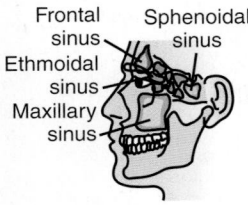

Figure 10-2 Paranasal sinuses. (From Buck CJ: Step-by-Step Medical Coding, ed 2016, St. Louis, Elsevier, 2016)

Item 10–1 Pharyngitis is painful inflammation of the pharynx (sore throat). Ninety percent of the infections are caused by a virus with the remaining being bacterial and rarely a fungus (candidiasis). Other irritants such as pollutants, chemicals, or smoke may cause similar symptoms.

CHAPTER 10

DISEASES OF THE RESPIRATORY SYSTEM (J00-J99)

Note: When a respiratory condition is described as occurring in more than one site and is not specifically indexed, it should be classified to the lower anatomic site (e.g., tracheobronchitis to bronchitis in J40).

Use additional code, where applicable, to identify:
exposure to environmental tobacco smoke (Z77.22)
exposure to tobacco smoke in the perinatal period (P96.81)
history of tobacco dependence (Z87.891) ◀
occupational exposure to environmental tobacco smoke (Z57.31)
tobacco dependence (F17.-)
tobacco use (Z72.0)

Excludes2 certain conditions originating in the perinatal period (P04-P96)
certain infectious and parasitic diseases (A00-B99)
complications of pregnancy, childbirth and the puerperium (O00-O99A)
congenital malformations, deformations and chromosomal abnormalities (Q00-Q99)
endocrine, nutritional and metabolic diseases (E00-E88)
injury, poisoning and certain other consequences of external causes (S00-T88)
neoplasms (C00-D49)
smoke inhalation (T59.81-)
symptoms, signs and abnormal clinical and laboratory findings, not elsewhere classified (R00-R94)

This chapter contains the following blocks:

J00-J06	Acute upper respiratory infections
J09-J18	Influenza and pneumonia
J20-J22	Other acute lower respiratory infections
J30-J39	Other diseases of upper respiratory tract
J40-J47	Chronic lower respiratory diseases
J60-J70	Lung diseases due to external agents
J80-J84	Other respiratory diseases principally affecting the interstitium
J85-J86	Suppurative and necrotic conditions of the lower respiratory tract
J90-J94	Other diseases of the pleura
J95	Intraoperative and postprocedural complications and disorders of respiratory system, not elsewhere classified
J96-J99	Other diseases of the respiratory system

ACUTE UPPER RESPIRATORY INFECTIONS (J00-J06)

Excludes1 chronic obstructive pulmonary disease with acute lower respiratory infection (J44.0)
influenza virus with other respiratory manifestations (J09.X2, J10.1, J11.1)

J00 Acute nasopharyngitis [common cold]
Acute rhinitis
Coryza (acute)
Infective nasopharyngitis NOS
Infective rhinitis
Nasal catarrh, acute
Nasopharyngitis NOS

Excludes1 acute pharyngitis (J02.-)
acute sore throat NOS (J02.9)
pharyngitis NOS (J02.9)
rhinitis NOS (J31.0)
sore throat NOS (J02.9)

Excludes2 allergic rhinitis (J30.1-J30.9)
chronic pharyngitis (J31.2)
chronic rhinitis (J31.0)
chronic sore throat (J31.2)
nasopharyngitis, chronic (J31.1)
vasomotor rhinitis (J30.0)

★ **(See Plate 49 on page 72.)**

● **J01 Acute sinusitis**

Includes acute abscess of sinus
acute empyema of sinus
acute infection of sinus
acute inflammation of sinus
acute suppuration of sinus

Use additional code (B95-B97) to identify infectious agent.

Excludes1 sinusitis NOS (J32.9)

Excludes2 chronic sinusitis (J32.0-J32.8)

● **J01.0 Acute maxillary sinusitis**
Acute antritis
J01.00 Acute maxillary sinusitis, unspecified
J01.01 Acute recurrent maxillary sinusitis

● **J01.1 Acute frontal sinusitis**
J01.10 Acute frontal sinusitis, unspecified
J01.11 Acute recurrent frontal sinusitis

● **J01.2 Acute ethmoidal sinusitis**
J01.20 Acute ethmoidal sinusitis, unspecified
J01.21 Acute recurrent ethmoidal sinusitis

● **J01.3 Acute sphenoidal sinusitis**
J01.30 Acute sphenoidal sinusitis, unspecified
J01.31 Acute recurrent sphenoidal sinusitis

● **J01.4 Acute pansinusitis**
J01.40 Acute pansinusitis, unspecified
J01.41 Acute recurrent pansinusitis

J01.8 Other acute sinusitis

J01.80 Other acute sinusitis
Acute sinusitis involving more than one sinus but not pansinusitis

J01.81 Other acute recurrent sinusitis
Acute recurrent sinusitis involving more than one sinus but not pansinusitis

J01.9 Acute sinusitis, unspecified

J01.90 Acute sinusitis, unspecified

J01.91 Acute recurrent sinusitis, unspecified

J02 Acute pharyngitis

Includes acute sore throat

Excludes1 acute laryngopharyngitis (J06.0)
peritonsillar abscess (J36)
pharyngeal abscess (J39.1)
retropharyngeal abscess (J39.0)

Excludes2 chronic pharyngitis (J31.2)

J02.0 Streptococcal pharyngitis
Septic pharyngitis
Streptococcal sore throat

Excludes2 scarlet fever (A38.-)

J02.8 Acute pharyngitis due to other specified organisms
Use additional code (B95-B97) to identify infectious agent

Excludes1 pharyngitis due to coxsackie virus (B08.5)
pharyngitis due to gonococcus (A54.5)
acute pharyngitis due to herpes [simplex] virus (B00.2)
acute pharyngitis due to infectious mononucleosis (B27.-)
enteroviral vesicular pharyngitis (B08.5)

J02.9 Acute pharyngitis, unspecified
Gangrenous pharyngitis (acute)
Infective pharyngitis (acute) NOS
Pharyngitis (acute) NOS
Sore throat (acute) NOS
Suppurative pharyngitis (acute)
Ulcerative pharyngitis (acute)

J03 Acute tonsillitis
Inflammation of pharyngeal tonsils caused by virus or bacteria

Excludes1 acute sore throat (J02.-)
hypertrophy of tonsils (J35.1)
peritonsillar abscess (J36)
sore throat NOS (J02.9)
streptococcal sore throat (J02.0)

Excludes2 chronic tonsillitis (J35.0)

J03.0 Streptococcal tonsillitis

J03.00 Acute streptococcal tonsillitis, unspecified

J03.01 Acute recurrent streptococcal tonsillitis

J03.8 Acute tonsillitis due to other specified organisms
Use additional code (B95-B97) to identify infectious agent.

Excludes1 diphtheritic tonsillitis (A36.0)
herpesviral pharyngotonsillitis (B00.2)
streptococcal tonsillitis (J03.0)
tuberculous tonsillitis (A15.8)
Vincent's tonsillitis (A69.1)

J03.80 Acute tonsillitis due to other specified organisms

J03.81 Acute recurrent tonsillitis due to other specified organisms

J03.9 Acute tonsillitis, unspecified
Follicular tonsillitis (acute)
Gangrenous tonsillitis (acute)
Infective tonsillitis (acute)
Tonsillitis (acute) NOS
Ulcerative tonsillitis (acute)

J03.90 Acute tonsillitis, unspecified

J03.91 Acute recurrent tonsillitis, unspecified

Item 10–2 Laryngitis is an inflammation of the larynx (voice box) resulting in hoarse voice or the complete loss of the voice. **Tracheitis** is an inflammation of the trachea (often following a URI) commonly caused by *staphylococcus aureus* resulting in inspiratory stridor (crowing sound on inspiration) and a croup like cough.

J04 Acute laryngitis and tracheitis
Use additional code (B95-B97) to identify infectious agent.

Excludes1 acute obstructive laryngitis [croup] and epiglottitis (J05.-)

Excludes2 laryngismus (stridulus) (J38.5)

J04.0 Acute laryngitis
Edematous laryngitis (acute)
Laryngitis (acute) NOS
Subglottic laryngitis (acute)
Suppurative laryngitis (acute)
Ulcerative laryngitis (acute)

Excludes1 acute obstructive laryngitis (J05.0)

Excludes2 chronic laryngitis (J37.0)

J04.1 Acute tracheitis
Acute viral tracheitis
Catarrhal tracheitis (acute)
Tracheitis (acute) NOS

Excludes2 chronic tracheitis (J42)

J04.10 Acute tracheitis without obstruction

J04.11 Acute tracheitis with obstruction
Ex: A15.8-A15.9, A17.9, A18.82, A18.84, A18.89, J04.10-J04.2, J05.10-J05.11, J22, J98.8-J98.9

J04.2 Acute laryngotracheitis
Laryngotracheitis NOS
Tracheitis (acute) with laryngitis (acute)

Excludes1 acute obstructive laryngotracheitis (J05.0)

Excludes2 chronic laryngotracheitis (J37.1)

J04.3 Supraglottitis, unspecified

J04.30 Supraglottitis, unspecified, without obstruction

J04.31 Supraglottitis, unspecified, with obstruction
Ex: A15.8-A15.9, A17.9, A18.82, A18.84, A18.89, J04.0-J04.2, J05.10-J05.11, J22, J98.8-J98.9

J05 Acute obstructive laryngitis [croup] and epiglottitis
Use additional code (B95-B97) to identify infectious agent.

J05.0 Acute obstructive laryngitis [croup]
Obstructive laryngitis (acute) NOS
Obstructive laryngotracheitis NOS

J05.1 Acute epiglottitis

Excludes2 epiglottitis, chronic (J37.0)

J05.10 Acute epiglottitis without obstruction
Epiglottitis NOS
Ex: J04.31, J05.10-J05.11

J05.11 Acute epiglottitis with obstruction
Ex: See J04.10

J06 Acute upper respiratory infections of multiple and unspecified sites

Excludes1 acute respiratory infection NOS (J22)
streptococcal pharyngitis (J02.0)

J06.0 Acute laryngopharyngitis

J06.9 Acute upper respiratory infection, unspecified
Upper respiratory disease, acute
Upper respiratory infection NOS

INFLUENZA AND PNEUMONIA (J09-J18)

Excludes2 allergic or eosinophilic pneumonia (J82)
aspiration pneumonia NOS (J69.0)
meconium pneumonia (P24.01)
neonatal aspiration pneumonia (P24.-)
pneumonia due to solids and liquids (J69.-)
congenital pneumonia (P23.9)
lipid pneumonia (J69.1)
rheumatic pneumonia (I00)
ventilator associated pneumonia (J95.851)

J09 Influenza due to certain identified influenza viruses

Excludes1 influenza due to other influenza viruses (J10.-)
influenza due to unidentified influenza virus (J11.-)
seasonal influenza due to other identified influenza virus (J10.-)
seasonal influenza due to unidentified influenza virus (J11.-)

J09.X Influenza due to identified novel influenza A virus
Avian influenza
Bird influenza
Influenza A/H5N1
Influenza of other animal origin, not bird or swine
Swine influenza virus (viruses that normally cause infections in pigs)

J09.X1 Influenza due to identified novel influenza A virus with pneumonia
Code also , if applicable, associated:
lung abscess (J85.1)
other specified type of pneumonia
Ex: A15.0-A15.9, A17.9, A18.82, A18.84, A18.89, A21.2, A22.1, A31.0, A37.01, A37.11, A37.81, A37.91, A42.0, A43.0, A48.1, B25.0, B39.0-B39.2, B44.0, B58.3, B59, B67.1, J09.X1-J09.X2, J10.00-J10.1, J11.00-J11.1, J12.0-J12.3, J12.89-J18.1, J18.8-J18.9, J22, J44.9, J47.0-J70.4, J70.8-J70.9, J98.4, J98.8-J98.9, Q33.4, R91.1

J09.X2 Influenza due to identified novel influenza A virus with other respiratory manifestations
Influenza due to identified novel influenza A virus NOS
Influenza due to identified novel influenza A virus with laryngitis
Influenza due to identified novel influenza A virus with pharyngitis
Influenza due to identified novel influenza A virus with upper respiratory symptoms
Use additional code, if applicable, for associated:
pleural effusion (J91.8)
sinusitis (J01.-)

J09.X3 Influenza due to identified novel influenza A virus with gastrointestinal manifestations
Influenza due to identified novel influenza A virus gastroenteritis
Excludes1 'intestinal flu' [viral gastroenteritis] (A08.-)

J09.X9 Influenza due to identified novel influenza A virus with other manifestations
Influenza due to identified novel influenza A virus with encephalopathy
Influenza due to identified novel influenza A virus with myocarditis
Influenza due to identified novel influenza A virus with otitis media
Use additional code to identify manifestation

J10 Influenza due to other identified influenza virus

Excludes1 influenza due to avian influenza virus (J09.X-)
influenza due to swine flu (J09.X-)
influenza due to unidentified influenza virus (J11.-)

J10.0 Influenza due to other identified influenza virus with pneumonia
Code also associated lung abscess, if applicable (J85.1)

J10.00 Influenza due to other identified influenza virus with unspecified type of pneumonia
Ex: See J09.X1

J10.01 Influenza due to other identified influenza virus with the same other identified influenza virus pneumonia
Ex: See J09.X1

J10.08 Influenza due to other identified influenza virus with other specified pneumonia
Code also other specified type of pneumonia
Ex: A15.0-A15.6, A15.8-A15.9, A17.9, A18.82, A18.84, A18.89, A21.2, A22.1, A31.0, A37.01, A37.11, A37.81, A37.91, A42.0, A43.0, A48.1, B25.0, B39.0-B39.2, B44.0, B58.3, B59, B67.1, J09.X1-J09.X2, J10.00-J10.1, J11.00-J11.1, J12.0-J12.3, J12.89-J18.1, J18.8-J18.9, J22, J44.0-J44.9, J45.21-J45.22, J45.31-J45.32, J45.41-J45.42, J45.51-J45.902, J47.0-J70.4, J70.8-J70.9, J98.4, J98.8-J99, Q33.4, R91.1

J10.1 Influenza due to other identified influenza virus with other respiratory manifestations
Influenza due to other identified influenza virus NOS
Influenza due to other identified influenza virus with laryngitis
Influenza due to other identified influenza virus with pharyngitis
Influenza due to other identified influenza virus with upper respiratory symptoms
Use additional code for associated pleural effusion, if applicable (J91.8)
Use additional code for associated sinusitis, if applicable (J01.-)

J10.2 Influenza due to other identified influenza virus with gastrointestinal manifestations
Influenza due to other identified influenza virus gastroenteritis
Excludes1 'intestinal flu' [viral gastroenteritis] (A08.-)

J10.8 Influenza due to other identified influenza virus with other manifestations

J10.81 Influenza due to other identified influenza virus with encephalopathy

J10.82 Influenza due to other identified influenza virus with myocarditis

J10.83 Influenza due to other identified influenza virus with otitis media
Use additional code for any associated perforated tympanic membrane (H72.-)

J10.89 Influenza due to other identified influenza virus with other manifestations
Use additional codes to identify the manifestations

J11 Influenza due to unidentified influenza virus

J11.0 Influenza due to unidentified influenza virus with pneumonia
Code also associated lung abscess, if applicable (J85.1)
Ex: For category J11.0 CC codes: See J09.X1

J11.00 Influenza due to unidentified influenza virus with unspecified type of pneumonia
Influenza with pneumonia NOS

J11.08 Influenza due to unidentified influenza virus with specified pneumonia
Code also other specified type of pneumonia

J11.1 Influenza due to unidentified influenza virus with other respiratory manifestations
Influenza NOS
Influenzal laryngitis NOS
Influenzal pharyngitis NOS
Influenza with upper respiratory symptoms NOS
Use additional code for associated pleural effusion, if applicable (J91.8)
Use additional code for associated sinusitis, if applicable (J01.-)

J11.2 Influenza due to unidentified influenza virus with gastrointestinal manifestations
Influenza gastroenteritis NOS
Excludes1 'intestinal flu' [viral gastroenteritis] (A08.-)

J11.8 Influenza due to unidentified influenza virus with other manifestations

J11.81 Influenza due to unidentified influenza virus with encephalopathy
Influenzal encephalopathy NOS

J11.82 Influenza due to unidentified influenza virus with myocarditis
Influenzal myocarditis NOS

J11.83 Influenza due to unidentified influenza virus with otitis media
Influenzal otitis media NOS
Use additional code for any associated perforated tympanic membrane (H72.-)

J11.89 Influenza due to unidentified influenza virus with other manifestations
Use additional codes to identify the manifestations

J12 Viral pneumonia, not elsewhere classified
Includes bronchopneumonia due to viruses other than influenza viruses
Code first associated influenza, if applicable (J09.X1, J10.0-, J11.0-)
Code also associated abscess, if applicable (J85.1)
Excludes1 aspiration pneumonia due to anesthesia during labor and delivery (O74.0)
aspiration pneumonia due to anesthesia during pregnancy (O29)
aspiration pneumonia due to anesthesia during puerperium (O89.0)
aspiration pneumonia due to solids and liquids (J69.-)
aspiration pneumonia NOS (J69.0)
congenital pneumonia (P23.0)
congenital rubella pneumonitis (P35.0)
interstitial pneumonia NOS (J84.9)
lipid pneumonia (J69.1)
neonatal aspiration pneumonia (P24.-)
Ex: **For category J12 CC codes unless otherwise indicated:** A15.0-A15.6, A15.8-A15.9, A17.9, A18.82, A18.84, A18.89, A20.2, A21.1, A22.1, A31.0, A37.01, A37.11, A37.81, A37.91, A42.0, A43.0, A48.1, B25.0, B39.0-B39.2, B44.0, B58.3, B59, B67.1, J09.X1-J09.X2, J10.00-J10.1, J11.00-J11.1, J12.0-J12.3, J12.81-J18.1, J18.8-J18.9, J22, J60-J70.4, J70.8-J70.9, J98.4, J98.8-J99, R91.1

J12.0 Adenoviral pneumonia

J12.1 Respiratory syncytial virus pneumonia

J12.2 Parainfluenza virus pneumonia

J12.3 Human metapneumovirus pneumonia

J12.8 Other viral pneumonia

J12.81 Pneumonia due to SARS-associated coronavirus
Severe acute respiratory syndrome NOS
Ex: A15.0-A15.6, A15.8-A15.9, A17.9, A18.82, A18.84, A18.89, A21.2, A22.1, A31.0, A37.01, A37.11, A37.81, A37.91, A42.0, A43.0, A48.1, B25.0, B39.0-B39.2, B44.0, B58.3, B59, B67.1, J09.X1-J09.X2, J10.00-J10.1, J11.00-J11.1, J12.0-J12.3, J12.81-J18.1, J18.8-J18.9, J22, J44.9, J47.0-J70.4, J70.8-J70.9, J98.4, J98.8-J99, Q33.4, R91.1

J12.89 Other viral pneumonia

J12.9 Viral pneumonia, unspecified

Item 10–3 Pneumonia is an infection of the lungs, caused by a variety of microorganisms, including viruses, most commonly the Streptococcus pneumoniae (pneumococcus) bacteria, fungi, and parasites. Pneumonia occurs when the immune system is weakened, often by a URI or influenza.

J13 Pneumonia due to Streptococcus pneumoniae
Bronchopneumonia due to S. pneumoniae
Code first associated influenza, if applicable (J09.X1, J10.0-, J11.0-)
Code also associated abscess, if applicable (J85.1)
Excludes1 congenital pneumonia due to S. pneumoniae (P23.6)
lobar pneumonia, unspecified organism (J18.1)
pneumonia due to other streptococci (J15.3-J15.4)
Ex: See J09.X1

J14 Pneumonia due to Hemophilus influenzae
Bronchopneumonia due to H. influenzae
Code first associated influenza, if applicable (J09.X1, J10.0-, J11.0-)
Code also associated abscess, if applicable (J85.1)
Excludes1 congenital pneumonia due to H. influenzae (P23.6)
Ex: See J09.X1

J15 Bacterial pneumonia, not elsewhere classified
Includes bronchopneumonia due to bacteria other than S. pneumoniae and H. influenzae
Code first associated influenza, if applicable (J09.X1, J10.0-, J11.0-)
Code also associated abscess, if applicable (J85.1)
Excludes1 chlamydial pneumonia (J16.0)
congenital pneumonia (P23.-)
Legionnaires' disease (A48.1)
spirochetal pneumonia (A69.8)
Ex: **For category J15 CC codes:** See J09.X1

J15.0 Pneumonia due to Klebsiella pneumoniae

J15.1 Pneumonia due to Pseudomonas

J15.2 Pneumonia due to staphylococcus

J15.20 Pneumonia due to staphylococcus, unspecified

J15.21 Pneumonia due to staphylococcus aureus

J15.211 Pneumonia due to Methicillin susceptible Staphylococcus aureus
MSSA pneumonia
Pneumonia due to Staphylococcus aureus NOS

J15.212 Pneumonia due to Methicillin resistant Staphylococcus aureus

J15.29 Pneumonia due to other staphylococcus

J15.3 Pneumonia due to streptococcus, group B

J15.4 Pneumonia due to other streptococci
Excludes1 pneumonia due to streptococcus, group B (J15.3)
pneumonia due to Streptococcus pneumoniae (J13)

J15.5 Pneumonia due to Escherichia coli

J15.6 Pneumonia due to other aerobic Gram-negative bacteria
Pneumonia due to Serratia marcescens

J15.7 Pneumonia due to Mycoplasma pneumoniae

J15.8 Pneumonia due to other specified bacteria

J15.9 Unspecified bacterial pneumonia
Pneumonia due to gram-positive bacteria

J16 Pneumonia due to other infectious organisms, not elsewhere classified

Code first associated influenza, if applicable (J09.X1, J10.0-, J11.0-)

Code also associated abscess, if applicable (J85.1)

Excludes1 congenital pneumonia (P23.-)
ornithosis (A70)
pneumocystosis (B59)
pneumonia NOS (J18.9)

Ex: For category J16 CC codes: See J09.X1

J16.0 Chlamydial pneumonia

J16.8 Pneumonia due to other specified infectious organisms

J17 Pneumonia in diseases classified elsewhere

Code first underlying disease, such as:
Q fever (A78)
rheumatic fever (I00)
schistosomiasis (B65.0-B65.9)

Excludes1 candidial pneumonia (B37.1)
chlamydial pneumonia (J16.0)
gonorrheal pneumonia (A54.84)
histoplasmosis pneumonia (B39.0-B39.2)
measles pneumonia (B05.2)
nocardiosis pneumonia (A43.0)
pneumocystosis (B59)
pneumonia due to Pneumocystis carinii (B59)
pneumonia due to Pneumocystis jiroveci (B59)
pneumonia in actinomycosis (A42.0)
pneumonia in anthrax (A22.1)
pneumonia in ascariasis (B77.81)
pneumonia in aspergillosis (B44.0-B44.1)
pneumonia in coccidioidomycosis (B38.0-B38.2)
pneumonia in cytomegalovirus disease (B25.0)
pneumonia in toxoplasmosis (B58.3)
rubella pneumonia (B06.81)
salmonella pneumonia (A02.22)
spirochetal infection NEC with pneumonia (A69.8)
tularemia pneumonia (A21.2)
typhoid fever with pneumonia (A01.03)
varicella pneumonia (B01.2)
whooping cough with pneumonia (A37 with fifth-character 1)

Ex: See J09.X1

J18 Pneumonia, unspecified organism

Code first associated influenza, if applicable (J09.X1, J10.0-, J11.0-)

Excludes1 abscess of lung with pneumonia (J85.1)
aspiration pneumonia due to anesthesia during labor and delivery (O74.0)
aspiration pneumonia due to anesthesia during pregnancy (O29)
aspiration pneumonia due to anesthesia during puerperium (O89.0)
aspiration pneumonia due to solids and liquids (J69.-)
aspiration pneumonia NOS (J69.0)
congenital pneumonia (P23.0)
drug-induced interstitial lung disorder (J70.2-J70.4)
interstitial pneumonia NOS (J84.9)
lipid pneumonia (J69.1)
neonatal aspiration pneumonia (P24.-)
pneumonitis due to external agents (J67-J70)
pneumonitis due to fumes and vapors (J68.0)
usual interstitial pneumonia (J84.17)

Ex: For category J18 CC code unless otherwise indicated: See J09.X1

J18.0 Bronchopneumonia, unspecified organism

Excludes1 hypostatic bronchopneumonia (J18.2)
lipid pneumonia (J69.1)

Excludes2 acute bronchiolitis (J21.-)
chronic bronchiolitis (J44.9)

J18.1 Lobar pneumonia, unspecified organism

J18.2 Hypostatic pneumonia, unspecified organism
Hypostatic bronchopneumonia
Passive pneumonia

Ex: J18.2, J22, J81.1, J98.4, J98.8-J99, R91.1

J18.8 Other pneumonia, unspecified organism

J18.9 Pneumonia, unspecified organism
Coding Clinic: 2012, Q4, P94

OTHER ACUTE LOWER RESPIRATORY INFECTIONS (J20-J22)

Excludes2 chronic obstructive pulmonary disease with acute lower respiratory infection (J44.0)

J20 Acute bronchitis

Inflammation/irritation of the bronchial tubes lasting 2-3 weeks, most commonly caused by a virus

Includes acute and subacute bronchitis (with) bronchospasm
acute and subacute bronchitis (with) tracheitis
acute and subacute bronchitis (with) tracheobronchitis, acute
acute and subacute fibrinous bronchitis
acute and subacute membranous bronchitis
acute and subacute purulent bronchitis
acute and subacute septic bronchitis

Excludes1 bronchitis NOS (J40)
tracheobronchitis NOS (J40)

Excludes2 acute bronchitis with bronchiectasis (J47.0)
acute bronchitis with chronic obstructive asthma (J44.0)
acute bronchitis with chronic obstructive pulmonary disease (J44.0)
allergic bronchitis NOS (J45.909-)
bronchitis due to chemicals, fumes and vapors (J68.0)
chronic bronchitis NOS (J42)
chronic mucopurulent bronchitis (J41.1)
chronic obstructive bronchitis (J44.-)
chronic obstructive tracheobronchitis (J44.-)
chronic simple bronchitis (J41.0)
chronic tracheobronchitis (J42)

J20.0 Acute bronchitis due to Mycoplasma pneumoniae

J20.1 Acute bronchitis due to Hemophilus influenzae

J20.2 Acute bronchitis due to streptococcus

J20.3 Acute bronchitis due to coxsackievirus

J20.4 Acute bronchitis due to parainfluenza virus

J20.5 Acute bronchitis due to respiratory syncytial virus

J20.6 Acute bronchitis due to rhinovirus

J20.7 Acute bronchitis due to echovirus

J20.8 Acute bronchitis due to other specified organisms

J20.9 Acute bronchitis, unspecified

J21 Acute bronchiolitis

Bronchiolitis obliterans with organizing pneumonia (BOOP) inflammation of bronchioles and surrounding tissue in lung

Includes acute bronchiolitis with bronchospasm

Excludes2 respiratory bronchiolitis interstitial lung disease (J84.115)

Ex: For category J21 CC codes unless otherwise indicated: J20.0-J21.9

J21.0 Acute bronchiolitis due to respiratory syncytial virus

Ex: J21.0

J21.1 Acute bronchiolitis due to human metapneumovirus

J21.8 Acute bronchiolitis due to other specified organisms

J21.9 Acute bronchiolitis, unspecified
Bronchiolitis (acute)

Excludes1 chronic bronchiolitis (J44.-)

J22 Unspecified acute lower respiratory infection
Acute (lower) respiratory (tract) infection NOS

Excludes1 upper respiratory infection (acute) (J06.9)

OTHER DISEASES OF UPPER RESPIRATORY TRACT (J30-J39)

J30 Vasomotor and allergic rhinitis

Includes spasmodic rhinorrhea

Excludes1 allergic rhinitis with asthma (bronchial) (J45.909)
rhinitis NOS (J31.0)

J30.0 Vasomotor rhinitis

J30.1 Allergic rhinitis due to pollen
Allergy NOS due to pollen
Hay fever
Pollinosis

J30.2 Other seasonal allergic rhinitis

J30.5 Allergic rhinitis due to food

J30.8 Other allergic rhinitis

J30.81 Allergic rhinitis due to animal (cat) (dog) hair and dander

J30.89 Other allergic rhinitis
Perennial allergic rhinitis

J30.9 Allergic rhinitis, unspecified

J31 Chronic rhinitis, nasopharyngitis and pharyngitis

Use additional code to identify:
exposure to environmental tobacco smoke (Z77.22)
exposure to tobacco smoke in the perinatal period (P96.81)
history of tobacco dependence (Z87.891)
occupational exposure to environmental tobacco smoke (Z57.31)
tobacco dependence (F17.-)
tobacco use (Z72.0)

J31.0 Chronic rhinitis
Atrophic rhinitis (chronic)
Granulomatous rhinitis (chronic)
Hypertrophic rhinitis (chronic)
Obstructive rhinitis (chronic)
Ozena
Purulent rhinitis (chronic)
Rhinitis (chronic) NOS
Ulcerative rhinitis (chronic)

Excludes1 allergic rhinitis (J30.1-J30.9)
vasomotor rhinitis (J30.0)

J31.1 Chronic nasopharyngitis

Excludes2 acute nasopharyngitis (J00)

J31.2 Chronic pharyngitis
Chronic sore throat
Atrophic pharyngitis (chronic)
Granular pharyngitis (chronic)
Hypertrophic pharyngitis (chronic)

Excludes2 acute pharyngitis (J02.9)

J32 Chronic sinusitis

Includes sinus abscess
sinus empyema
sinus infection
sinus suppuration

Use additional code to identify:
exposure to environmental tobacco smoke (Z77.22)
exposure to tobacco smoke in the perinatal period (P96.81)
history of tobacco dependence (Z87.891)
infectious agent (B95-B97)
occupational exposure to environmental tobacco smoke (Z57.31)
tobacco dependence (F17.-)
tobacco use (Z72.0)

Excludes2 acute sinusitis (J01.-)

J32.0 Chronic maxillary sinusitis
Antritis (chronic)
Maxillary sinusitis NOS

J32.1 Chronic frontal sinusitis
Frontal sinusitis NOS

Item 10–4 Nasal polyps are an abnormal growth of tissue (tumor) projecting from a mucous membrane and attached to the surface by a narrow elongated stalk (pedunculated). Nasal polyps usually originate in the ethmoid sinus but also may occur in the maxillary sinus. Symptoms are nasal block, sinusitis, anosmia, and secondary infections.

J32.2 Chronic ethmoidal sinusitis
Ethmoidal sinusitis NOS

Excludes1 Woakes' ethmoiditis (J33.1)

J32.3 Chronic sphenoidal sinusitis
Sphenoidal sinusitis NOS

J32.4 Chronic pansinusitis
Pansinusitis NOS

J32.8 Other chronic sinusitis
Sinusitis (chronic) involving more than one sinus but not pansinusitis

J32.9 Chronic sinusitis, unspecified
Sinusitis (chronic) NOS

J33 Nasal polyp

Use additional code to identify:
exposure to environmental tobacco smoke (Z77.22)
exposure to tobacco smoke in the perinatal period (P96.81)
history of tobacco dependence (Z87.891)
occupational exposure to environmental tobacco smoke (Z57.31)
tobacco dependence (F17.-)
tobacco use (Z72.0)

Excludes1 adenomatous polyps (D14.0)

J33.0 Polyp of nasal cavity
Choanal polyp
Nasopharyngeal polyp

J33.1 Polypoid sinus degeneration
Woakes' syndrome or ethmoiditis

J33.8 Other polyp of sinus
Accessory polyp of sinus
Ethmoidal polyp of sinus
Maxillary polyp of sinus
Sphenoidal polyp of sinus

J33.9 Nasal polyp, unspecified

J34 Other and unspecified disorders of nose and nasal sinuses

Excludes2 varicose ulcer of nasal septum (I86.8)

J34.0 Abscess, furuncle and carbuncle of nose
Cellulitis of nose
Necrosis of nose
Ulceration of nose

J34.1 Cyst and mucocele of nose and nasal sinus

J34.2 Deviated nasal septum
Deflection or deviation of septum (nasal) (acquired)

Excludes1 congenital deviated nasal septum (Q67.4)

J34.3 Hypertrophy of nasal turbinates

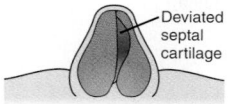

Figure 10-3 Deviated nasal septum.

Item 10–5 A **deviated nasal septum** is the displacement of the septal cartilage that separates the nares. This displacement causes obstructed air flow through the nasal passages. A child can be born with this displacement (congenital), or the condition may be acquired through trauma, such as a sports injury. Symptoms include nasal block, sinusitis, and related secondary infections. Septoplasty is surgical repair of this condition.

● **J34.8 Other specified disorders of nose and nasal sinuses**

J34.81 Nasal mucositis (ulcerative)

Code also type of associated therapy, such as:
antineoplastic and immunosuppressive drugs (T45.1X-)
radiological procedure and radiotherapy (Y84.2)

Excludes2 gastrointestinal mucositis (ulcerative) (K92.81)
mucositis (ulcerative) of vagina and vulva (N76.81)
oral mucositis (ulcerative) (K12.3-)

J34.89 Other specified disorders of nose and nasal sinuses

Perforation of nasal septum NOS
Rhinolith

J34.9 Unspecified disorder of nose and nasal sinuses

● **J35 Chronic diseases of tonsils and adenoids**

Use additional code to identify:
exposure to environmental tobacco smoke (Z77.22)
exposure to tobacco smoke in the perinatal period (P96.81)
history of tobacco dependence (Z87.891) ◀
occupational exposure to environmental tobacco smoke (Z57.31)
tobacco dependence (F17.-)
tobacco use (Z72.0)

● **J35.0 Chronic tonsillitis and adenoiditis**

Excludes2 acute tonsillitis (J03.-)

J35.01 Chronic tonsillitis

J35.02 Chronic adenoiditis

J35.03 Chronic tonsillitis and adenoiditis

J35.1 Hypertrophy of tonsils

Enlargement of tonsils

Excludes1 hypertrophy of tonsils with tonsillitis (J35.0-)

J35.2 Hypertrophy of adenoids

Enlargement of adenoids

Excludes1 hypertrophy of adenoids with adenoiditis (J35.0-)

J35.3 Hypertrophy of tonsils with hypertrophy of adenoids

Excludes1 hypertrophy of tonsils and adenoids with tonsillitis and adenoiditis (J35.03)

J35.8 Other chronic diseases of tonsils and adenoids

Adenoid vegetations
Amygdalolith
Calculus, tonsil
Cicatrix of tonsil (and adenoid)
Tonsillar tag
Ulcer of tonsil

J35.9 Chronic disease of tonsils and adenoids, unspecified

Disease (chronic) of tonsils and adenoids NOS

J36 Peritonsillar abscess

Includes abscess of tonsil
peritonsillar cellulitis
quinsy

Use additional code (B95-B97) to identify infectious agent.

Excludes1 acute tonsillitis (J03.-)
chronic tonsillitis (J35.0)
retropharyngeal abscess (J39.0)
tonsillitis NOS (J03.9-)

Ex: J22, J36, J98.8-J98.9

● **J37 Chronic laryngitis and laryngotracheitis**

Use additional code to identify:
exposure to environmental tobacco smoke (Z77.22)
exposure to tobacco smoke in the perinatal period (P96.81)
history of tobacco dependence (Z87.891) ◀
infectious agent (B95-B97)
occupational exposure to environmental tobacco smoke (Z57.31)
tobacco dependence (F17.-)
tobacco use (Z72.0)

J37.0 Chronic laryngitis

Catarrhal laryngitis
Hypertrophic laryngitis
Sicca laryngitis

Excludes2 acute laryngitis (J04.0)
obstructive (acute) laryngitis (J05.0)

J37.1 Chronic laryngotracheitis

Laryngitis, chronic, with tracheitis (chronic)
Tracheitis, chronic, with laryngitis

Excludes1 chronic tracheitis (J42)

Excludes2 acute laryngotracheitis (J04.2)
acute tracheitis (J04.1)

● **J38 Diseases of vocal cords and larynx, not elsewhere classified**

Use additional code to identify:
exposure to environmental tobacco smoke (Z77.22)
exposure to tobacco smoke in the perinatal period (P96.81)
history of tobacco dependence (Z87.891) ◀
occupational exposure to environmental tobacco smoke (Z57.31)
tobacco dependence (F17.-)
tobacco use (Z72.0)

Excludes1 congenital laryngeal stridor (P28.89)
obstructive laryngitis (acute) (J05.0)
postprocedural subglottic stenosis (J95.5)
stridor (R06.1)
ulcerative laryngitis (J04.0)

● **J38.0 Paralysis of vocal cords and larynx**

Laryngoplegia
Paralysis of glottis

J38.00 Paralysis of vocal cords and larynx, unspecified

J38.01 Paralysis of vocal cords and larynx, unilateral

J38.02 Paralysis of vocal cords and larynx, bilateral

J38.1 Polyp of vocal cord and larynx

Excludes1 adenomatous polyps (D14.1)

J38.2 Nodules of vocal cords

Chorditis (fibrinous)(nodosa)(tuberosa)
Singer's nodes
Teacher's nodes

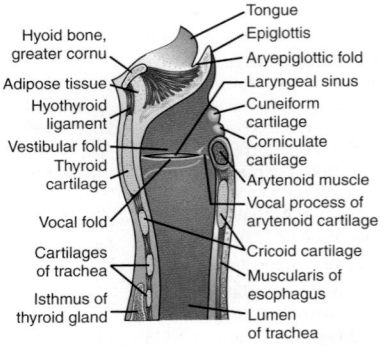

Figure 10-4 Coronal section of the larynx.

Item 10–6 The **larynx** extends from the tongue to the trachea and is divided into an upper and lower portion separated by folds. The framework of the larynx is cartilage composed of the single cricoid, thyroid, and epiglottic cartilages, and the paired arytenoid, cuneiform, and corniculate cartilages.

J38.3 Other diseases of vocal cords
Abscess of vocal cords
Cellulitis of vocal cords
Granuloma of vocal cords
Leukokeratosis of vocal cords
Leukoplakia of vocal cords

J38.4 Edema of larynx
Edema (of) glottis
Subglottic edema
Supraglottic edema
Excludes1 acute obstructive laryngitis [croup] (J05.0)
edematous laryngitis (J04.0)

J38.5 Laryngeal spasm
Laryngismus (stridulus)

J38.6 Stenosis of larynx

J38.7 Other diseases of larynx
Abscess of larynx
Cellulitis of larynx
Disease of larynx NOS
Necrosis of larynx
Pachyderma of larynx
Perichondritis of larynx
Ulcer of larynx

J39 Other diseases of upper respiratory tract
Excludes1 acute respiratory infection NOS (J22)
acute upper respiratory infection (J06.9)
upper respiratory inflammation due to chemicals, gases, fumes or vapors (J68.2)

J39.0 Retropharyngeal and parapharyngeal abscess
Peripharyngeal abscess
Excludes1 peritonsillar abscess (J36)
Ex: J22, J39.0-J39.1, J98.8-J98.9

J39.1 Other abscess of pharynx
Cellulitis of pharynx
Nasopharyngeal abscess
Ex: J22, J39.0-J39.1, J98.8-J98.9

J39.2 Other diseases of pharynx
Cyst of pharynx
Edema of pharynx
Excludes2 chronic pharyngitis (J31.2)
ulcerative pharyngitis (J02.9)

J39.3 Upper respiratory tract hypersensitivity reaction, site unspecified
Excludes1 hypersensitivity reaction of upper respiratory tract, such as:
extrinsic allergic alveolitis (J67.9)
pneumoconiosis (J60-J67.9)

J39.8 Other specified diseases of upper respiratory tract

J39.9 Disease of upper respiratory tract, unspecified

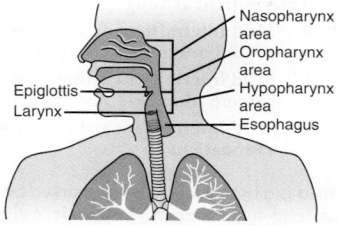

Figure 10-5 The pharynx.

Item 10–7 The **pharynx** is the passage for both food and air between the mouth and the esophagus and is divided into three areas: nasopharynx, oropharynx, and hypopharynx. The hypopharynx branches into the esophagus and the voice box.

Item 10–8 **Chronic bronchitis** is usually defined as being present in any patient who has persistent cough with sputum production for at least three months in at least two consecutive years. **Simple chronic bronchitis** is marked by a productive cough but no pathological airflow obstruction. **Chronic obstructive pulmonary disease (COPD)** is a group of conditions—bronchitis, emphysema, asthma, bronchiectasis, allergic alveolitis—marked by dyspnea. **Catarrhal** bronchitis is an acute form of bronchitis marked by profuse mucus and pus production (**mucopurulent** discharge). **Croupous** bronchitis, also known as pseudomembranous, fibrinous, plastic, exudative, or membranous, is marked by a violent cough and dyspnea.

CHRONIC LOWER RESPIRATORY DISEASES (J40-J47)

Excludes1 bronchitis due to chemicals, gases, fumes and vapors (J68.0)
Excludes2 cystic fibrosis (E84.-)

J40 Bronchitis, not specified as acute or chronic
Bronchitis NOS
Catarrhal bronchitis
Bronchitis with tracheitis NOS
Tracheobronchitis NOS
Use additional code to identify:
exposure to environmental tobacco smoke (Z77.22)
exposure to tobacco smoke in the perinatal period (P96.81)
history of tobacco dependence (Z87.891)
occupational exposure to environmental tobacco smoke (Z57.31)
tobacco dependence (F17.-)
tobacco use (Z72.0)
Excludes1 acute bronchitis (J20.-)
allergic bronchitis NOS (J45.909-)
asthmatic bronchitis NOS (J45.9-)
bronchitis due to chemicals, gases, fumes and vapors (J68.0)

J41 Simple and mucopurulent chronic bronchitis
Use additional code to identify:
exposure to environmental tobacco smoke (Z77.22)
exposure to tobacco smoke in the perinatal period (P96.81)
history of tobacco dependence (Z87.891)
occupational exposure to environmental tobacco smoke (Z57.31)
tobacco dependence (F17.-)
tobacco use (Z72.0)
Excludes1 chronic bronchitis NOS (J42)
chronic obstructive bronchitis (J44.-)

J41.0 Simple chronic bronchitis

J41.1 Mucopurulent chronic bronchitis

J41.8 Mixed simple and mucopurulent chronic bronchitis

J42 Unspecified chronic bronchitis
Chronic bronchitis NOS
Chronic tracheitis
Chronic tracheobronchitis
Use additional code to identify:
exposure to environmental tobacco smoke (Z77.22)
exposure to tobacco smoke in the perinatal period (P96.81)
history of tobacco dependence (Z87.891)
occupational exposure to environmental tobacco smoke (Z57.31)
tobacco dependence (F17.-)
tobacco use (Z72.0)
Excludes1 chronic asthmatic bronchitis (J44.-)
chronic bronchitis with airways obstruction (J44.-)
chronic emphysematous bronchitis (J44.-)
chronic obstructive pulmonary disease NOS (J44.9)
simple and mucopurulent chronic bronchitis (J41.-)

● **J43 Emphysema**

Use additional code to identify:
- exposure to environmental tobacco smoke (Z77.22)
- history of tobacco dependence (Z87.891) ⇐
- occupational exposure to environmental tobacco smoke (Z57.31)
- tobacco dependence (F17.-)
- tobacco use (Z72.0)

Excludes1 compensatory emphysema (J98.3)
- emphysema due to inhalation of chemicals, gases, fumes or vapors (J68.4)
- emphysema with chronic (obstructive) bronchitis (J44.-)
- emphysematous (obstructive) bronchitis (J44.-)
- interstitial emphysema (J98.2)
- mediastinal emphysema (J98.2)
- neonatal interstitial emphysema (P25.0)
- surgical (subcutaneous) emphysema (T81.82)
- traumatic subcutaneous emphysema (T79.7)

J43.0 Unilateral pulmonary emphysema [MacLeod's syndrome]
- Swyer-James syndrome
- Unilateral emphysema
- Unilateral hyperlucent lung
- Unilateral pulmonary artery functional hypoplasia
- Unilateral transparency of lung

J43.1 Panlobular emphysema
- Panacinar emphysema

J43.2 Centrilobular emphysema

J43.8 Other emphysema

J43.9 Emphysema, unspecified
- Bullous emphysema (lung)(pulmonary)
- Emphysema (lung)(pulmonary) NOS
- Emphysematous bleb
- Vesicular emphysema (lung)(pulmonary)

● **J44 Other chronic obstructive pulmonary disease**

Includes asthma with chronic obstructive pulmonary disease
- chronic asthmatic (obstructive) bronchitis
- chronic bronchitis with airways obstruction
- chronic bronchitis with emphysema
- chronic emphysematous bronchitis
- chronic obstructive asthma
- chronic obstructive bronchitis
- chronic obstructive tracheobronchitis

Code also type of asthma, if applicable (J45.-)

Use additional code to identify:
- exposure to environmental tobacco smoke (Z77.22)
- history of tobacco dependence (Z87.891) ⇐
- occupational exposure to environmental tobacco smoke (Z57.31)
- tobacco dependence (F17.-)
- tobacco use (Z72.0)

Excludes1 bronchiectasis (J47.-)
- chronic bronchitis NOS (J42)
- chronic simple and mucopurulent bronchitis (J41.-)
- chronic tracheitis (J42)
- chronic tracheobronchitis (J42)
- emphysema without chronic bronchitis (J43.-)

Excludes2 lung diseases due to external agents (J60-J70) ◀

J44.0 Chronic obstructive pulmonary disease with acute lower respiratory infection

Use additional code to identify the infection

Ex: J10.08, J41.1-J42, J44.0-J44.1

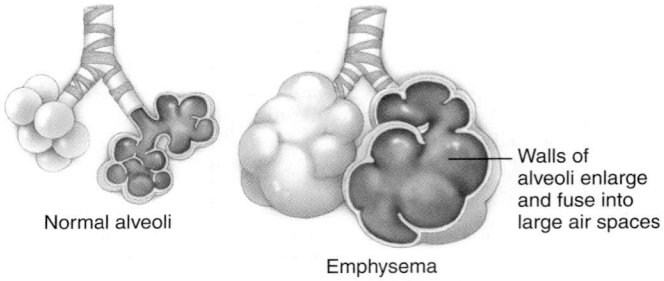

Figure 10-6 Emphysema. (From Shiland, BJ: Medical Terminology & Anatomy for ICD-10 Coding, ed 2, Mosby, 2015)

J44.1 Chronic obstructive pulmonary disease with (acute) exacerbation
- Decompensated COPD
- Decompensated COPD with (acute) exacerbation

Excludes2 chronic obstructive pulmonary disease [COPD] with acute bronchitis (J44.0)

Ex: J10.08, J41.1-J42, J44.0-J44.1

Coding Clinic: 2016, Q1, P36

J44.9 Chronic obstructive pulmonary disease, unspecified
- Chronic obstructive airway disease NOS
- Chronic obstructive lung disease NOS

Coding Clinic: 2016, Q1, P37

● **J45 Asthma**
- Allergic (predominantly) asthma
- Allergic bronchitis NOS
- Allergic rhinitis with asthma
- Atopic asthma
- Extrinsic allergic asthma
- Hay fever with asthma
- Idiosyncratic asthma
- Intrinsic nonallergic asthma
- Nonallergic asthma

Use additional code to identify:
- exposure to environmental tobacco smoke (Z77.22)
- exposure to tobacco smoke in the perinatal period (P96.81)
- history of tobacco dependence (Z87.891) ⇐
- occupational exposure to environmental tobacco smoke (Z57.31)
- tobacco dependence (F17.-)
- tobacco use (Z72.0)

Excludes1 detergent asthma (J69.8)
- eosinophilic asthma (J82)
- lung diseases due to external agents (J60-J70)
- miner's asthma (J60)
- wheezing NOS (R06.2)
- wood asthma (J67.8)

Excludes2 asthma with chronic obstructive pulmonary disease (J44.9)
- chronic asthmatic (obstructive) bronchitis (J44.9)
- chronic obstructive asthma (J44.9)

Ex: **For category J45 CC codes:** J10.08, J22, J45.20-J45.998, J98.4, J98.8-J99, R91.1

● **J45.2 Mild intermittent asthma**

J45.20 Mild intermittent asthma, uncomplicated
- Mild intermittent asthma NOS

J45.21 Mild intermittent asthma with (acute) exacerbation

J45.22 Mild intermittent asthma with status asthmaticus

Item 10–9 Asthma is a bronchial condition marked by airway obstruction, hyper-responsiveness, and inflammation. **Extrinsic** asthma, also known as allergic asthma, is characterized by the same symptoms that occur with exposure to allergens and is divided into the following types: **atopic, occupational, and allergic bronchopulmonary aspergillosis. Intrinsic** asthma occurs in patients who have no history of allergy or sensitivities to allergens and is divided into the following types: **nonreaginic and pharmacologic. Status asthmaticus** is the most severe form of asthma attack and can last for days or weeks.

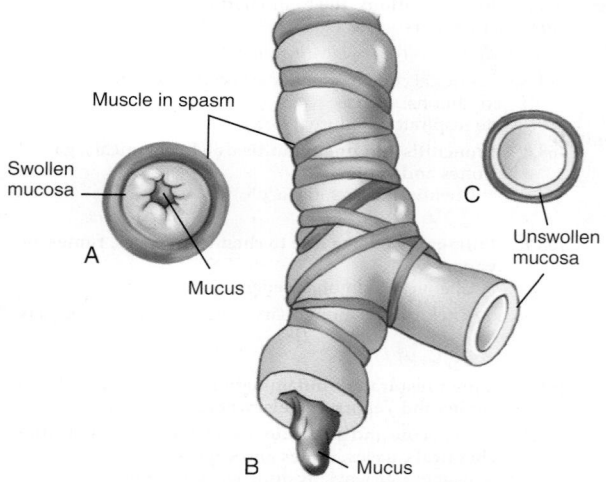

Figure 10-7 Factors causing expiratory obstruction in asthma. **A.** Cross section of a bronchiole occluded by muscle spasm, swollen mucosa, and mucus. **B.** Longitudinal section of an obstructed bronchiole. **C.** Cross-section of a clear bronchiole. (From Shiland: Mastering Healthcare Terminology, ed 1, St. Louis, Mosby, 2003)

● **J45.3 Mild persistent asthma**
- **J45.30 Mild persistent asthma, uncomplicated**
  Mild persistent asthma NOS
- **J45.31 Mild persistent asthma with (acute) exacerbation**
  Coding Clinic: 2016, Q1, P35
- **J45.32 Mild persistent asthma with status asthmaticus**

● **J45.4 Moderate persistent asthma**
- **J45.40 Moderate persistent asthma, uncomplicated**
  Moderate persistent asthma NOS
- **J45.41 Moderate persistent asthma with (acute) exacerbation**
- **J45.42 Moderate persistent asthma with status asthmaticus**

● **J45.5 Severe persistent asthma**
- **J45.50 Severe persistent asthma, uncomplicated**
  Severe persistent asthma NOS
- **J45.51 Severe persistent asthma with (acute) exacerbation**
- **J45.52 Severe persistent asthma with status asthmaticus**

● **J45.9 Other and unspecified asthma**
- ● **J45.90 Unspecified asthma**
  Asthmatic bronchitis NOS
  Childhood asthma NOS
  Late onset asthma
  - **J45.901 Unspecified asthma with (acute) exacerbation**
  - **J45.902 Unspecified asthma with status asthmaticus**
  - **J45.909 Unspecified asthma, uncomplicated**
    Asthma NOS
- ● **J45.99 Other asthma**
  - **J45.990 Exercise induced bronchospasm**
  - **J45.991 Cough variant asthma**
  - **J45.998 Other asthma**

● **J47 Bronchiectasis**
Includes bronchiolectasis
Use additional code to identify:
exposure to environmental tobacco smoke (Z77.22)
exposure to tobacco smoke in the perinatal period (P96.81)
history of tobacco dependence (Z87.891)
occupational exposure to environmental tobacco smoke (Z57.31)
tobacco dependence (F17.-)
tobacco use (Z72.0)
Excludes1 congenital bronchiectasis (Q33.4)
tuberculous bronchiectasis (current disease) (A15.0)
For category J47 CC codes: A17.9, A18.82, A18.84, A18.89, J09.X2, J10.08, J11.1, J44.9, J47.0-J47.1, J68.1, J68.4-J68.9, Q33.4
- **J47.0 Bronchiectasis with acute lower respiratory infection**
  Bronchiectasis with acute bronchitis
  Use additional code to identify the infection
- **J47.1 Bronchiectasis with (acute) exacerbation**
- **J47.9 Bronchiectasis, uncomplicated**
  Bronchiectasis NOS

LUNG DISEASES DUE TO EXTERNAL AGENTS (J60-J70)

Excludes2 asthma (J45.-)
malignant neoplasm of bronchus and lung (C34.-)

J60 Coalworker's pneumoconiosis A
Anthracosilicosis
Anthracosis
Black lung disease
Coalworker's lung
Excludes1 coalworker pneumoconiosis with tuberculosis, any type in A15 (J65)

J61 Pneumoconiosis due to asbestos and other mineral fibers A
Asbestosis
Excludes1 pleural plaque with asbestosis (J92.0)
pneumoconiosis with tuberculosis, any type in A15 (J65)

● **J62 Pneumoconiosis due to dust containing silica**
Includes silicotic fibrosis (massive) of lung
Excludes1 pneumoconiosis with tuberculosis, any type in A15 (J65)
- **J62.0 Pneumoconiosis due to talc dust**
- **J62.8 Pneumoconiosis due to other dust containing silica**
  Silicosis NOS

● **J63 Pneumoconiosis due to other inorganic dusts**
Excludes1 pneumoconiosis with tuberculosis, any type in A15 (J65)
- **J63.0 Aluminosis (of lung)**
- **J63.1 Bauxite fibrosis (of lung)**
- **J63.2 Berylliosis**
- **J63.3 Graphite fibrosis (of lung)**
- **J63.4 Siderosis**
- **J63.5 Stannosis**
- **J63.6 Pneumoconiosis due to other specified inorganic dusts**

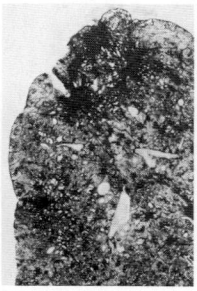

Figure 10-8 Progressive massive fibrosis superimposed on coal workers' pneumoconiosis. The large, blackened scars are located principally in the upper lobe. (From Cotran R, Kumar V, Collins T: Robbins Pathologic Basis of Disease, ed 8, Philadelphia, WB Saunders, 2009. Courtesy of Dr. Warner Laquer, Dr. Jerome Kleinerman, and the National Institute of Occupational Safety and Health, Morgantown, WV)

Item 10–10 Pneumoconiosis refers to a lung condition resulting from exposure to inorganic or organic airborne particles, such as coal dust or moldy hay, as well as chemical fumes and vapors, such as insecticides. In this condition, the lungs retain the airborne particles.

J64 Unspecified pneumoconiosis
Excludes1 pneumonoconiosis with tuberculosis, any type in A15 (J65)

J65 Pneumoconiosis associated with tuberculosis
Any condition in J60-J64 with tuberculosis, any type in A15
Silicotuberculosis

J66 Airway disease due to specific organic dust
Excludes2 allergic alveolitis (J67.-)
asbestosis (J61)
bagassosis (J67.1)
farmer's lung (J67.0)
hypersensitivity pneumonitis due to organic dust (J67.-)
reactive airways dysfunction syndrome (J68.3)

J66.0 Byssinosis
Airway disease due to cotton dust

J66.1 Flax-dressers' disease

J66.2 Cannabinosis

J66.8 Airway disease due to other specific organic dusts

J67 Hypersensitivity pneumonitis due to organic dust
Includes allergic alveolitis and pneumonitis due to inhaled organic dust and particles of fungal, actinomycetic or other origin
Excludes1 pneumonitis due to inhalation of chemicals, gases, fumes or vapors (J68.0)

J67.0 Farmer's lung
Harvester's lung
Haymaker's lung
Moldy hay disease

J67.1 Bagassosis
Bagasse disease
Bagasse pneumonitis

J67.2 Bird fancier's lung
Budgerigar fancier's disease or lung
Pigeon fancier's disease or lung

J67.3 Suberosis
Corkhandler's disease or lung
Corkworker's disease or lung

J67.4 Maltworker's lung
Alveolitis due to Aspergillus clavatus

J67.5 Mushroom-worker's lung

J67.6 Maple-bark-stripper's lung
Alveolitis due to Cryptostroma corticale
Cryptostromosis

J67.7 Air conditioner and humidifier lung
Allergic alveolitis due to fungal, thermophilic actinomycetes and other organisms growing in ventilation [air conditioning] systems
Ex: A15.0-A15.9, A17.9, A18.82, A18.84, A18.89, A21.2, A22.1, A31.0, A37.01, A37.11, A37.81, A37.91, A42.0, A43.0, A48.1, B25.0, B39.0-B39.2, B44.0, B58.3, B59, B67.1, J09.X1-J09.X2, J10.00-J10.1, J11.00-J11.1, J12.0-J12.3, J12.89-J18.1, J18.8-J18.9, J22, J44.9, J47.0-J70.4, J70.8-J70.9, J98.4, J98.8-J98.9, Q33.4, R91.1

J67.8 Hypersensitivity pneumonitis due to other organic dusts
Cheese-washer's lung
Coffee-worker's lung
Fish-meal worker's lung
Furrier's lung
Sequoiosis
Ex: See J67.7

J67.9 Hypersensitivity pneumonitis due to unspecified organic dust
Allergic alveolitis (extrinsic) NOS
Hypersensitivity pneumonitis NOS
Ex: See J67.7

J68 Respiratory conditions due to inhalation of chemicals, gases, fumes and vapors
Code first (T51-T65) to identify cause
Use additional code to identify associated respiratory conditions, such as:
acute respiratory failure (J96.0-)

J68.0 Bronchitis and pneumonitis due to chemicals, gases, fumes and vapors
Chemical bronchitis (acute)
Ex: See J67.7

J68.1 Pulmonary edema due to chemicals, gases, fumes and vapors
Chemical pulmonary edema (acute) (chronic)
Excludes1 pulmonary edema (acute) (chronic) NOS (J81.-)
Ex: See J67.7

J68.2 Upper respiratory inflammation due to chemicals, gases, fumes and vapors, not elsewhere classified

J68.3 Other acute and subacute respiratory conditions due to chemicals, gases, fumes and vapors
Reactive airways dysfunction syndrome

J68.4 Chronic respiratory conditions due to chemicals, gases, fumes and vapors
Emphysema (diffuse) (chronic) due to inhalation of chemicals, gases, fumes and vapors
Obliterative bronchiolitis (chronic) (subacute) due to inhalation of chemicals, gases, fumes and vapors
Pulmonary fibrosis (chronic) due to inhalation of chemicals, gases, fumes and vapors
Excludes1 chronic pulmonary edema due to chemicals, gases, fumes and vapors (J68.1)

J68.8 Other respiratory conditions due to chemicals, gases, fumes and vapors

J68.9 Unspecified respiratory condition due to chemicals, gases, fumes and vapors

J69 Pneumonitis due to solids and liquids
Excludes1 neonatal aspiration syndromes (P24.-)
postprocedural pneumonitis (J95.4)
Ex: For category J69 CC codes: See J67.7

J69.0 Pneumonitis due to inhalation of food and vomit
Aspiration pneumonia NOS
Aspiration pneumonia (due to) food (regurgitated)
Aspiration pneumonia (due to) gastric secretions
Aspiration pneumonia (due to) milk
Aspiration pneumonia (due to) vomit
Code also any associated foreign body in respiratory tract (T17.-)
Excludes1 chemical pneumonitis due to anesthesia (J95.4)
obstetric aspiration pneumonitis (O74.0)

J69.1 Pneumonitis due to inhalation of oils and essences
Exogenous lipoid pneumonia
Lipid pneumonia NOS
Code first (T51-T65) to identify substance
Excludes1 endogenous lipoid pneumonia (J84.89)

J69.8 Pneumonitis due to inhalation of other solids and liquids
Pneumonitis due to aspiration of blood
Pneumonitis due to aspiration of detergent
Code first (T51-T65) to identify substance

◀ New ◀ Revised ~~deleted~~ Deleted Excludes 1 Excludes 2 Includes Use additional Code first Code also Unspecified
OGCR Official Guidelines ● Unacceptable Principal Diagnosis X Assign placeholder X ● Use Additional Character(s) ▶ Manifestation Code Coding Clinic

J70 Respiratory conditions due to other external agents

J70.0 Acute pulmonary manifestations due to radiation
Radiation pneumonitis
Use additional code (W88-W90, X39.0-) to identify the external cause
Ex: See J67.7

J70.1 Chronic and other pulmonary manifestations due to radiation
Fibrosis of lung following radiation
Use additional code (W88-W90, X39.0-) to identify the external cause
Ex: See J67.7

J70.2 Acute drug-induced interstitial lung disorders
Use additional code for adverse effect, if applicable, to identify drug (T36-T50 with fifth or sixth character 5)
Excludes1 interstitial pneumonia NOS (J84.9)
lymphoid interstitial pneumonia (J84.2)

J70.3 Chronic drug-induced interstitial lung disorders
Use additional code for adverse effect, if applicable, to identify drug (T36-T50 with fifth or sixth character 5)
Excludes1 interstitial pneumonia NOS (J84.9)
lymphoid interstitial pneumonia (J84.2)

J70.4 Drug-induced interstitial lung disorders, unspecified
Use additional code for adverse effect, if applicable, to identify drug (T36-T50 with fifth or sixth character 5)
Excludes1 interstitial pneumonia NOS (J84.9)
lymphoid interstitial pneumonia (J84.2)

J70.5 Respiratory conditions due to smoke inhalation
Smoke inhalation NOS
Excludes1 smoke inhalation due to chemicals, gases, fumes and vapors (J68.9)

J70.8 Respiratory conditions due to other specified external agents
Code first (T51-T65) to identify the external agent

J70.9 Respiratory conditions due to unspecified external agent
Code first (T51-T65) to identify the external agent

OTHER RESPIRATORY DISEASES PRINCIPALLY AFFECTING THE INTERSTITIUM (J80-J84)

J80 Acute respiratory distress syndrome
Acute respiratory distress syndrome in adult or child
Adult hyaline membrane disease
Excludes1 respiratory distress syndrome in newborn (perinatal) (P22.0)
Ex: J22, J80, J96.00-J96.92, J98.8-J98.9, R09.2

J81 Pulmonary edema
Use additional code to identify:
exposure to environmental tobacco smoke (Z77.22)
history of tobacco dependence (Z87.891)
occupational exposure to environmental tobacco smoke (Z57.31)
tobacco dependence (F17.-)
tobacco use (Z72.0)
Excludes1 chemical (acute) pulmonary edema (J68.1)
hypostatic pneumonia (J18.2)
passive pneumonia (J18.2)
pulmonary edema due to external agents (J60-J70)
pulmonary edema with heart disease NOS (I50.1)
pulmonary edema with heart failure (I50.1)

J81.0 Acute pulmonary edema
Acute edema of lung
Ex: I09.81, I50.1-I50.9, J22, J81.0, J98.8-J98.9

J81.1 Chronic pulmonary edema
Pulmonary congestion (chronic) (passive)
Pulmonary edema NOS
Ex: J18.2, J22, J81.1, J98.4, J98.8-J99, R91.1

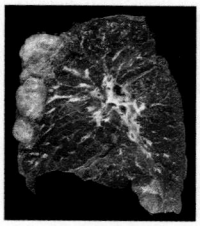

Figure 10-9 Bullous emphysema with large subpleural bullae *(upper left)*. (From Kumar: Robbins and Cotran: Pathologic Basis of Disease, ed 8, Saunders, An Imprint of Elsevier, 2009)

J82 Pulmonary eosinophilia, not elsewhere classified
Allergic pneumonia
Eosinophilic asthma
Eosinophilic pneumonia
Löffler's pneumonia
Tropical (pulmonary) eosinophilia NOS
Excludes1 pulmonary eosinophilia due to aspergillosis (B44.-)
pulmonary eosinophilia due to drugs (J70.2-J70.4)
pulmonary eosinophilia due to specified parasitic infection (B50-B83)
pulmonary eosinophilia due to systemic connective tissue disorders (M30-M36)
pulmonary infiltrate NOS (R91.8)
Ex: A15.0-A15.6, A15.8-A15.9, A17.9, A18.82, A18.84, A18.89, A20.2, A21.1, A22.1, A31.0, A37.01, A37.11, A37.81, A37.91, A42.0, A43.0, A48.1, B25.0, B39.0-B39.2, B44.0, B58.3, B59, B67.1, J09.X1-J09.X2, J10.00-J10.1, J11.00-J11.1, J12.0-J12.3, J12.89-J18.1, J18.8-J18.9, J22, J47.0-J70.4, J70.8-J70.9, J82, J98.4, J98.8-J99, Q33.4, R91.1

J84 Other interstitial pulmonary diseases
Excludes1 drug-induced interstitial lung disorders (J70.2-J70.4)
interstitial emphysema (J98.2)
lung diseases due to external agents (J60-J70)
Ex: **For category J84 CC codes unless otherwise indicated:** A15.0-A15.6, A15.8-A15.9, A17.9, A18.82, A18.84, A18.89, J22, J44.9, J47.0-J70.4, J70.8-J70.9, J84.01-J84.82, J84.89-J84.9, J98.4, J98.8-J99, Q33.4, R91.1

J84.0 Alveolar and parieto-alveolar conditions

J84.01 Alveolar proteinosis

J84.02 Pulmonary alveolar microlithiasis

J84.03 Idiopathic pulmonary hemosiderosis
Essential brown induration of lung
Code first underlying disease, such as:
disorders of iron metabolism (E83.1-)
Excludes1 acute idiopathic pulmonary hemorrhage in infants [AIPHI] (R04.81)

J84.09 Other alveolar and parieto-alveolar conditions

J84.1 Other interstitial pulmonary diseases with fibrosis
Excludes1 pulmonary fibrosis (chronic) due to inhalation of chemicals, gases, fumes or vapors (J68.4)
pulmonary fibrosis (chronic) following radiation (J70.1)

J84.10 Pulmonary fibrosis, unspecified
Capillary fibrosis of lung
Cirrhosis of lung (chronic) NOS
Fibrosis of lung (atrophic) (chronic) (confluent) (massive) (perialveolar) (peribronchial) NOS
Induration of lung (chronic) NOS
Postinflammatory pulmonary fibrosis

● **J84.11 Idiopathic interstitial pneumonia**
Excludes1 lymphoid interstitial pneumonia (J84.2)
pneumocystis pneumonia (B59)

J84.111 Idiopathic interstitial pneumonia, not otherwise specified

J84.112 Idiopathic pulmonary fibrosis
Cryptogenic fibrosing alveolitis
Idiopathic fibrosing alveolitis

J84.113 Idiopathic non-specific interstitial pneumonitis
Excludes1 non-specific interstitial pneumonia NOS, or due to known underlying cause (J84.89)

J84.114 Acute interstitial pneumonitis
Hamman-Rich syndrome
Excludes1 pneumocystis pneumonia (B59)

J84.115 Respiratory bronchiolitis interstitial lung disease

J84.116 Cryptogenic organizing pneumonia
Excludes1 organizing pneumonia NOS, or due to known underlying cause (J84.89)

J84.117 Desquamative interstitial pneumonia

▶ ***J84.17 Other interstitial pulmonary diseases with fibrosis in diseases classified elsewhere***
Interstitial pneumonia (nonspecific) (usual) due to collagen vascular disease
Interstitial pneumonia (nonspecific) (usual) in diseases classified elsewhere
Organizing pneumonia due to collagen vascular disease
Organizing pneumonia in diseases classified elsewhere
Code first underlying disease, such as:
progressive systemic sclerosis (M34.0)
rheumatoid arthritis (M05.00-M06.9)
systemic lupus erythematosis (M32.0-M32.9)

J84.2 Lymphoid interstitial pneumonia
Lymphoid interstitial pneumonitis

● **J84.8 Other specified interstitial pulmonary diseases**
Excludes1 exogenous lipoid pneumonia (J69.1)
unspecified lipoid pneumonia (J69.1)

J84.81 Lymphangioleiomyomatosis ♀
Lymphangiomyomatosis

J84.82 Adult pulmonary Langerhans cell histiocytosis A
Adult PLCH

J84.83 Surfactant mutations of the lung
Ex: J84.83-J84.848, P22.0-P28.5, P28.89-P29.2, P29.4, P29.89-P29.9, P84, P94.1-P96.0, P96.3-P96.5, P96.82-P96.89

● **J84.84 Other interstitial lung diseases of childhood**
Ex: **For category J84.84 CC codes:** See J84.83

J84.841 Neuroendocrine cell hyperplasia of infancy

J84.842 Pulmonary interstitial glycogenosis

J84.843 Alveolar capillary dysplasia with vein misalignment

J84.848 Other interstitial lung diseases of childhood

J84.89 Other specified interstitial pulmonary diseases
Endogenous lipoid pneumonia
Interstitial pneumonitis
Non-specific interstitial pneumonitis NOS
~~Organizing pneumonia due to known underlying cause~~
Organizing pneumonia NOS
Code first, if applicable:
poisoning due to drug or toxin (T51-T65 with fifth or sixth character to indicate intent), for toxic pneumonopathy
underlying cause of pneumonopathy, if known
Use additional code, for adverse effect, to identify drug (T36-T50 with fifth or sixth character 5), if drug-induced
Excludes1 cryptogenic organizing pneumonia (J84.116)
idiopathic non-specific interstitial pneumonitis (J84.113)
lipoid pneumonia, exogenous or unspecified (J69.1)
lymphoid interstitial pneumonia (J84.2)

J84.9 Interstitial pulmonary disease, unspecified
Interstitial pneumonia NOS

SUPPURATIVE AND NECROTIC CONDITIONS OF THE LOWER RESPIRATORY TRACT (J85-J86)

● **J85 Abscess of lung and mediastinum**
Use additional code (B95-B97) to identify infectious agent.
Ex: **For category J85 CC codes unless otherwise indicated:** A06.5, A15.0-A15.6, A15.8-A15.9, A17.9, A18.82, A18.84, A18.89, J22, J85.0-J85.2, J98.8-J98.9

J85.0 Gangrene and necrosis of lung

J85.1 Abscess of lung with pneumonia
Code also the type of pneumonia

J85.2 Abscess of lung without pneumonia
Abscess of lung NOS

J85.3 Abscess of mediastinum
Ex: J22, J85.3, J98.8-J98.9

Item 10–11 Empyema is a condition in which pus accumulates in a body cavity. Empyema **with fistula** occurs when the pus passes from one cavity to another organ or structure.

● **J86 Pyothorax**
Use additional code (B95-B97) to identify infectious agent.
Excludes1 abscess of lung (J85.-)
pyothorax due to tuberculosis (A15.6)
Ex: **For category J86 CC codes:** J22, J86.0-J86.9, J98.4, J98.8-J99, R91.1

J86.0 Pyothorax with fistula
Bronchocutaneous fistula
Bronchopleural fistula
Hepatopleural fistula
Mediastinal fistula
Pleural fistula
Thoracic fistula
Any condition classifiable to J86.9 with fistula

J86.9 Pyothorax without fistula
Abscess of pleura
Abscess of thorax
Empyema (chest) (lung) (pleura)
Fibrinopurulent pleurisy
Purulent pleurisy
Pyopneumothorax
Septic pleurisy
Seropurulent pleurisy
Suppurative pleurisy

OTHER DISEASES OF THE PLEURA (J90-J94)

J90 Pleural effusion, not elsewhere classified
Encysted pleurisy
Pleural effusion NOS
Pleurisy with effusion (exudative) (serous)
Excludes1 chylous (pleural) effusion (J94.0)
malignant pleural effusion (J91.0))
pleurisy NOS (R09.1)
tuberculous pleural effusion (A15.6)
Ex: A15.0-A15.6, A15.8-A15.9, A17.9, A18.82, A18.84, A18.89, J22, J90-J92.9, J94.0-J94.9, J98.4, J98.8-J99, R09.1, R91.1
Coding Clinic: 2015, Q2, P16

J91 Pleural effusion in conditions classified elsewhere
Excludes2 pleural effusion in heart failure (I50.-)
pleural effusion in systemic lupus erythematosus (M32.13)

J91.0 Malignant pleural effusion
Code first underlying neoplasm
Ex: C45.7-C45.9, C76.8, C78.2-C78.39, C79.89-C79.9, C7A.00, C7A.098, C7A.1-C7B.00, C7B.09-C7B.8, C80.0-C80.2, D49.81-D49.9, J90-J91.0, J94.0, J94.2

J91.8 Pleural effusion in other conditions classified elsewhere
Code first underlying disease, such as:
filariasis (B74.0-B74.9)
influenza (J09.X2, J10.1, J11.1)
Ex: See J90
Coding Clinic: 2015, Q2, P16

J92 Pleural plaque
Includes pleural thickening
J92.0 Pleural plaque with presence of asbestos
J92.9 Pleural plaque without asbestos
Pleural plaque NOS

J93 Pneumothorax and air leak
Collapsed lung
Excludes1 congenital or perinatal pneumothorax (P25.1)
postprocedural air leak (J95.812)
postprocedural pneumothorax (J95.811)
traumatic pneumothorax (S27.0)
tuberculous (current disease) pneumothorax (A15.-)
pyopneumothorax (J86.-)
Ex: For category J93 CC codes: J22, J93.0-J93.9, J95.811-J95.812, J98.4, J98.8-J99, R91.1

J93.0 Spontaneous tension pneumothorax
Tension pneumothorax (most serious type) occurs when air (positive pressure) collects in the pleural space

J93.1 Other spontaneous pneumothorax
J93.11 Primary spontaneous pneumothorax
J93.12 Secondary spontaneous pneumothorax
Code first underlying condition, such as:
catamenial pneumothorax due to endometriosis (N80.8)
cystic fibrosis (E84.-)
eosinophilic pneumonia (J82)
lymphangioleiomyomatosis (J84.81)
malignant neoplasm of bronchus and lung (C34.-)
Marfan's syndrome (Q87.4)
pneumonia due to Pneumocystis carinii (B59)
secondary malignant neoplasm of lung (C78.0-)
spontaneous rupture of the esophagus (K22.3)

J93.8 Other pneumothorax and air leak
J93.81 Chronic pneumothorax
J93.82 Other air leak
Persistent air leak
J93.83 Other pneumothorax
Acute pneumothorax
Spontaneous pneumothorax NOS

J93.9 Pneumothorax, unspecified
Pneumothorax NOS

J94 Other pleural conditions
Excludes1 pleurisy NOS (R09.1)
traumatic hemopneumothorax (S27.2)
traumatic hemothorax (S27.1)
tuberculous pleural conditions (current disease) (A15.-)
Ex: For category J94 CC codes unless otherwise indicated: See J90

J94.0 Chylous effusion
Chyliform effusion
J94.1 Fibrothorax
J94.2 Hemothorax
Hemopneumothorax
J94.8 Other specified pleural conditions
Hydropneumothorax
Hydrothorax
Ex: No exclusions
J94.9 Pleural condition, unspecified

INTRAOPERATIVE AND POSTPROCEDURAL COMPLICATIONS AND DISORDERS OF RESPIRATORY SYSTEM, NOT ELSEWHERE CLASSIFIED (J95)

J95 Intraoperative and postprocedural complications and disorders of respiratory system, not elsewhere classified
Excludes2 aspiration pneumonia (J69.-)
emphysema (subcutaneous) resulting from a procedure (T81.82)
hypostatic pneumonia (J18.2)
pulmonary manifestations due to radiation (J70.0- J70.1)

J95.0 Tracheostomy complications
Ex: For category J95.0 CC codes: J22, J39.8, J95.00-J95.09, J98.01-J98.09, J98.8-J98.9
J95.00 Unspecified tracheostomy complication
J95.01 Hemorrhage from tracheostomy stoma
J95.02 Infection of tracheostomy stoma
Use additional code to identify type of infection, such as:
cellulitis of neck (L03.8)
sepsis (A40, A41.-)
J95.03 Malfunction of tracheostomy stoma
Mechanical complication of tracheostomy stoma
Obstruction of tracheostomy airway
Tracheal stenosis due to tracheostomy
J95.04 Tracheo-esophageal fistula following tracheostomy
J95.09 Other tracheostomy complication

J95.1 Acute pulmonary insufficiency following thoracic surgery
Excludes2 functional disturbances following cardiac surgery (I97.0, I97.1-)
Ex: J22, J95.1-J95.3, J95.821-J95.822, J98.8-J98.9

J95.2 Acute pulmonary insufficiency following nonthoracic surgery
Excludes2 functional disturbances following cardiac surgery (I97.0, I97.1-)
Ex: See J95.1

J95.3 Chronic pulmonary insufficiency following surgery

Excludes2 functional disturbances following cardiac surgery (I97.0, I97.1-)

Ex: See J95.1

J95.4 Chemical pneumonitis due to anesthesia

Mendelson's syndrome
Postprocedural aspiration pneumonia

Use additional code for adverse effect, if applicable, to identify drug (T41.- with fifth or sixth character 5)

Excludes1 aspiration pneumonitis due to anesthesia complicating labor and delivery (O74.0)
aspiration pneumonitis due to anesthesia complicating pregnancy (O29)
aspiration pneumonitis due to anesthesia complicating the puerperium (O89.01)

Ex: D78.81-D78.89, E36.8, E89.810-E89.89, H59.011-H59.019, H59.031-H59.099, H59.811-H59.89, H95.811-H95.89, I97.3, J95.4-J95.5, J95.84, J95.851-J95.89, L76.81-L76.82, M96.89, N98.1-N98.9, T81.82X[A], T81.89X-T81.9XX[A]

J95.5 Postprocedural subglottic stenosis

Ex: See J95.4

● **J95.6 Intraoperative hemorrhage and hematoma of a respiratory system organ or structure complicating a procedure**

Excludes1 intraoperative hemorrhage and hematoma of a respiratory system organ or structure due to accidental puncture and laceration during procedure (J95.7-)

Ex: **For category J95.6 CC codes:** H95.811-H95.89, I85.01, I85.11, I97.3, J95.61-J95.62, J95.830-J95.831, J95.860-J95.863, K21.9, K22.8, K23-K25.0, K25.2, K25.4, K25.6, K26.0, K26.2, K26.4, K26.6, K27.0, K27.2, K27.4, K27.6, K28.0, K28.2, K28.4, K28.6, K29.01, K29.21, K29.31, K29.41, K29.51, K29.61, K29.71, K29.81, K29.91, K31.811, K55.21, K57.01, K57.11, K57.13, K57.21, K57.31, K57.33, K57.41, K57.51, K57.53, K57.81, K57.91, K57.93, K62.5, K92.0-K92.2, M96.89, N98.1-N98.9, P54.1-P54.3, T81.10X-T81.19X[A], T81.82X[A], T81.89X-T81.9XX[A]

J95.61 Intraoperative hemorrhage and hematoma of a respiratory system organ or structure complicating a respiratory system procedure

J95.62 Intraoperative hemorrhage and hematoma of a respiratory system organ or structure complicating other procedure

● **J95.7 Accidental puncture and laceration of a respiratory system organ or structure during a procedure**

Excludes2 postprocedural pneumothorax (J95.811)

Ex: **For category J95.7 CC codes:** D78.11-D78.12, D78.81-D78.89, E36.11-E36.8, E89.810-E89.89, G96.11, G97.41-G97.49, H59.011-H59.019, H59.031-H59.099, H59.211-H59.229, H59.811-H59.89, H95.31-H95.32, H95.811-H95.89, I97.3, I97.51-I97.52, J95.71-J95.72, K91.71-K91.72, L76.11-L76.12, L76.81-L76.82, M96.820-M96.821, M96.89, N98.1-N98.9, N99.71-N99.72, T81.82X[A], T81.89X-T81.9XX[A]

J95.71 Accidental puncture and laceration of a respiratory system organ or structure during a respiratory system procedure

J95.72 Accidental puncture and laceration of a respiratory system organ or structure during other procedure

● **J95.8 Other intraoperative and postprocedural complications and disorders of respiratory system, not elsewhere classified**

● **J95.81 Postprocedural pneumothorax and air leak**

Ex: **For category J95.81 CC codes:** J22, J93.0-J93.9, J95.811-J95.812, J98.4, J98.8-J99, R91.1

J95.811 Postprocedural pneumothorax

J95.812 Postprocedural air leak

● **J95.82 Postprocedural respiratory failure**

Excludes1 Respiratory failure in other conditions (J96.-)

Ex: **For category J95.82 CC codes:** See J95.1

J95.821 Acute postprocedural respiratory failure

Postprocedural respiratory failure NOS

J95.822 Acute and chronic postprocedural respiratory failure

● **J95.83 Postprocedural hemorrhage of a respiratory system organ or structure following a procedure**

Ex: **For category J95.83 CC codes:** See J95.6

J95.830 Postprocedural hemorrhage of a respiratory system organ or structure following a respiratory system procedure

J95.831 Postprocedural hemorrhage of a respiratory system organ or structure following other procedure

J95.84 Transfusion-related acute lung injury (TRALI)

Ex: See J95.4

● **J95.85 Complication of respirator [ventilator]**

J95.850 Mechanical complication of respirator

Excludes1 encounter for respirator [ventilator] dependence during power failure (Z99.12)

Ex: J95.850, Z99.0-Z99.12, Z99.81-Z99.89

J95.851 Ventilator associated pneumonia

Ventilator associated pneumonitis

Use additional code to identify the organism, if known (B95.-, B96.-, B97.-)

Excludes1 ventilator lung in newborn (P27.8)

Ex: See J95.4

J95.859 Other complication of respirator [ventilator]

Ex: See J95.4

● **J95.86 Postprocedural hematoma and seroma of a respiratory system organ or structure following a procedure** ◀

Ex: For Category J95.86 CC codes: See J95.6

J95.860 Postprocedural hematoma of a respiratory system organ or structure following a respiratory system procedure ◀

J95.861 Postprocedural hematoma of a respiratory system organ or structure following other procedure ◀

J95.862 Postprocedural seroma of a respiratory system organ or structure following a respiratory system procedure ◀

J95.863 Postprocedural seroma of a respiratory system organ or structure following other procedure ◀

J95.88 Other intraoperative complications of respiratory system, not elsewhere classified

Ex: See J95.4

J95.89 Other postprocedural complications and disorders of respiratory system, not elsewhere classified

Use additional code to identify disorder, such as:
aspiration pneumonia (J69.-)
bacterial or viral pneumonia (J12-J18)

Excludes2 acute pulmonary insufficiency following thoracic surgery (J95.1)
postprocedural subglottic stenosis (J95.5)

Ex: See J95.4

OTHER DISEASES OF THE RESPIRATORY SYSTEM (J96-J99)

● **J96 Respiratory failure, not elsewhere classified**

Excludes1 acute respiratory distress syndrome (J80)
cardiorespiratory failure (R09.2)
newborn respiratory distress syndrome (P22.0)
postprocedural respiratory failure (J95.82-)
respiratory arrest (R09.2)
respiratory arrest of newborn (P28.81)
respiratory failure of newborn (P28.5)

Ex: For category J96 CC codes: J22, J80, J96.00-J96.92, J98.8-J98.9, R09.2

● **J96.0 Acute respiratory failure**

J96.00 Acute respiratory failure, unspecified whether with hypoxia or hypercapnia

J96.01 Acute respiratory failure with hypoxia

J96.02 Acute respiratory failure with hypercapnia

● **J96.1 Chronic respiratory failure**

J96.10 Chronic respiratory failure, unspecified whether with hypoxia or hypercapnia

Coding Clinic: 2016, Q1, P38; 2015, Q1, P21

J96.11 Chronic respiratory failure with hypoxia

J96.12 Chronic respiratory failure with hypercapnia

● **J96.2 Acute and chronic respiratory failure**

Acute on chronic respiratory failure

J96.20 Acute and chronic respiratory failure, unspecified whether with hypoxia or hypercapnia

J96.21 Acute and chronic respiratory failure with hypoxia

J96.22 Acute and chronic respiratory failure with hypercapnia

● **J96.9 Respiratory failure, unspecified**

J96.90 Respiratory failure, unspecified, unspecified whether with hypoxia or hypercapnia

J96.91 Respiratory failure, unspecified with hypoxia

J96.92 Respiratory failure, unspecified with hypercapnia

● **J98 Other respiratory disorders**

Use additional code to identify:
exposure to environmental tobacco smoke (Z77.22)
exposure to tobacco smoke in the perinatal period (P96.81)
history of tobacco dependence (Z87.891)
occupational exposure to environmental tobacco smoke (Z57.31)
tobacco dependence (F17.-)
tobacco use (Z72.0)

Excludes1 newborn apnea (P28.4)
newborn sleep apnea (P28.3)

Excludes2 apnea NOS (R06.81)
sleep apnea (G47.3-)

● **J98.0 Diseases of bronchus, not elsewhere classified**

J98.01 Acute bronchospasm

Excludes1 acute bronchiolitis with bronchospasm (J21.-)
acute bronchitis with bronchospasm (J20.-)
asthma (J45.-)
exercise induced bronchospasm (J45.990)

J98.09 Other diseases of bronchus, not elsewhere classified

Broncholithiasis
Calcification of bronchus
Stenosis of bronchus
Tracheobronchial collapse
Tracheobronchial dyskinesia
Ulcer of bronchus

● **J98.1 Pulmonary collapse**

Excludes1 therapeutic collapse of lung status (Z98.3)

Ex: For category J98.1 CC codes: J22, J98.11-J98.19, J98.8-J98.9

J98.11 Atelectasis

Excludes1 newborn atelectasis
tuberculous atelectasis (current disease) (A15)

J98.19 Other pulmonary collapse

J98.2 Interstitial emphysema

Mediastinal emphysema

Excludes1 emphysema NOS (J43.9)
emphysema in newborn (P25.0)
surgical emphysema (subcutaneous) (T81.82)
traumatic subcutaneous emphysema (T79.7)

J98.3 Compensatory emphysema

J98.4 Other disorders of lung
Calcification of lung
Cystic lung disease (acquired)
Lung disease NOS
Pulmolithiasis
Excludes1 acute interstitial pneumonitis (J84.114)
pulmonary insufficiency following surgery (J95.1-J95.2)

● **J98.5 Diseases of mediastinum, not elsewhere classified**
Excludes2 abscess of mediastinum (J85.3)

J98.51 Mediastinitis ◀
Code first underlying condition, if applicable, such as postoperative mediastinitis (T81.-) ◀
Ex: No Exclusions ◀

J98.59 Other diseases of mediastinum, not elsewhere classified ◀
Fibrosis of mediastinum ◀
Hernia of mediastinum ◀
Retraction of mediastinum ◀
Ex: No Exclusions ◀

J98.6 Disorders of diaphragm
Diaphragmatitis
Paralysis of diaphragm
Relaxation of diaphragm
Excludes1 congenital malformation of diaphragm NEC (Q79.1)
congenital diaphragmatic hernia (Q79.0)
Excludes2 diaphragmatic hernia (K44.-)

J98.8 Other specified respiratory disorders

J98.9 Respiratory disorder, unspecified
Respiratory disease (chronic) NOS

◗ ***J99 Respiratory disorders in diseases classified elsewhere***
Code first underlying disease, such as:
amyloidosis (E85.-)
ankylosing spondylitis (M45)
congenital syphilis (A50.5)
cryoglobulinemia (D89.1)
early congenital syphilis (A50.0)
schistosomiasis (B65.0-B65.9)
Excludes1 respiratory disorders in:
amebiasis (A06.5)
blastomycosis (B40.0-B40.2)
candidiasis (B37.1)
coccidioidomycosis (B38.0-B38.2)
cystic fibrosis with pulmonary manifestations (E84.0)
dermatomyositis (M33.01, M33.11)
histoplasmosis (B39.0-B39.2)
late syphilis (A52.72, A52.73)
polymyositis (M33.21)
sicca syndrome (M35.02)
systemic lupus erythematosus (M32.13)
systemic sclerosis (M34.81)
Wegener's granulomatosis (M31.30-M31.31)

CHAPTER 11

DISEASES OF THE DIGESTIVE SYSTEM (KØØ-K95)

OGCR Chapter-Specific Coding Guidelines

11. Chapter 11: Diseases of the Digestive System (KØØ-K95)
Reserved for future guideline expansion

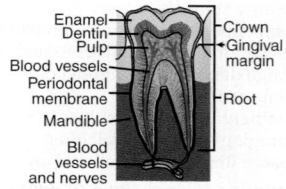

Figure 11-1 Anatomy of a tooth.

Item 11-1 **Anodontia** is the congenital absence of teeth. **Hypodontia** is partial anodontia. **Oligodontia** is the congenital absence of some teeth, whereas **supernumerary** is having more teeth than the normal number. **Mesiodens** are small extra teeth that often appear in pairs, although single small teeth are not uncommon.

CHAPTER 11

DISEASES OF THE DIGESTIVE SYSTEM (KØØ-K95)

Excludes2 certain conditions originating in the perinatal period (PØ4-P96)
certain infectious and parasitic diseases (AØØ-B99)
complications of pregnancy, childbirth and the puerperium (OØØ-O9A)
congenital malformations, deformations and chromosomal abnormalities (QØØ-Q99)
endocrine, nutritional and metabolic diseases (EØØ-E88)
injury, poisoning and certain other consequences of external causes (SØØ-T88)
neoplasms (CØØ-D49)
symptoms, signs and abnormal clinical and laboratory findings, not elsewhere classified (RØØ-R94)

This chapter contains the following blocks:

KØØ-K14	Diseases of oral cavity and salivary glands
K2Ø-K31	Diseases of esophagus, stomach and duodenum
K35-K38	Diseases of appendix
K4Ø-K46	Hernia
K5Ø-K52	Noninfective enteritis and colitis
K55-K64	Other diseases of intestines
K65-K68	Diseases of peritoneum and retroperitoneum
K7Ø-K77	Diseases of liver
K8Ø-K87	Disorders of gallbladder, biliary tract and pancreas
K9Ø-K95	Other diseases of the digestive system

DISEASES OF ORAL CAVITY AND SALIVARY GLANDS (KØØ-K14)

● **KØØ Disorders of tooth development and eruption**
Excludes2 embedded and impacted teeth (KØ1.-)

KØØ.Ø Anodontia
Hypodontia
Oligodontia
Excludes1 acquired absence of teeth (KØ8.1-)

KØØ.1 Supernumerary teeth
Distomolar
Fourth molar
Mesiodens
Paramolar
Supplementary teeth
Excludes2 supernumerary roots (KØØ.2)

KØØ.2 Abnormalities of size and form of teeth
Concrescence of teeth
Fusion of teeth
Gemination of teeth
Dens evaginatus
Dens in dente
Dens invaginatus
Enamel pearls
Macrodontia
Microdontia
Peg-shaped [conical] teeth
Supernumerary roots
Taurodontism
Tuberculum paramolare
Excludes1 abnormalities of teeth due to congenital syphilis (A5Ø.5)
tuberculum Carabelli, which is regarded as a normal variation and should not be coded

KØØ.3 Mottled teeth
Dental fluorosis
Mottling of enamel
Nonfluoride enamel opacities
Excludes2 deposits [accretions] on teeth (KØ3.6)

KØØ.4 Disturbances in tooth formation
Aplasia and hypoplasia of cementum
Dilaceration of tooth
Enamel hypoplasia (neonatal) (postnatal) (prenatal)
Regional odontodysplasia
Turner's tooth
Excludes1 Hutchinson's teeth and mulberry molars in congenital syphilis (A5Ø.5)
Excludes2 mottled teeth (KØØ.3)

KØØ.5 Hereditary disturbances in tooth structure, not elsewhere classified
Amelogenesis imperfecta
Dentinogenesis imperfecta
Odontogenesis imperfecta
Dentinal dysplasia
Shell teeth

KØØ.6 Disturbances in tooth eruption
Dentia praecox
Natal tooth
Neonatal tooth
Premature eruption of tooth
Premature shedding of primary [deciduous] tooth
Prenatal teeth
Retained [persistent] primary tooth
Excludes2 embedded and impacted teeth (KØ1.-)

KØØ.7 Teething syndrome

KØØ.8 Other disorders of tooth development
Color changes during tooth formation
Intrinsic staining of teeth NOS
Excludes2 posteruptive color changes (KØ3.7)

KØØ.9 Disorder of tooth development, unspecified
Disorder of odontogenesis NOS

● **KØ1 Embedded and impacted teeth**
Excludes1 abnormal position of fully erupted teeth (M26.3-)

KØ1.Ø Embedded teeth

KØ1.1 Impacted teeth

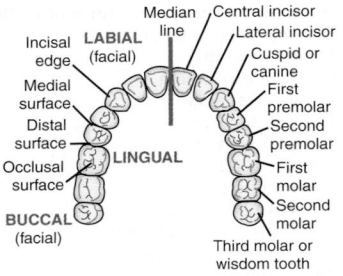

Figure 11-2 The permanent teeth within the dental arch.

Item 11-2 Each dental arch (jaw) normally contains 16 teeth. Tooth decay or **dental caries** is a disease of the enamel, dentin, and cementum of the tooth and can result in a cavity.

● **K02 Dental caries**
Includes caries of dentine ◀
dental cavities
early childhood caries ◀
pre-eruptive caries ◀
recurrent caries (dentino enamel junction) (enamel) (to the pulp) ◀
tooth decay

K02.3 Arrested dental caries
Arrested coronal and root caries

● **K02.5 Dental caries on pit and fissure surface**
Dental caries on chewing surface of tooth

K02.51 Dental caries on pit and fissure surface limited to enamel
White spot lesions [initial caries] on pit and fissure surface of tooth

K02.52 Dental caries on pit and fissure surface penetrating into dentin
Primary dental caries, cervical origin ◀

K02.53 Dental caries on pit and fissure surface penetrating into pulp

● **K02.6 Dental caries on smooth surface**

K02.61 Dental caries on smooth surface limited to enamel
White spot lesions [initial caries] on smooth surface of tooth

K02.62 Dental caries on smooth surface penetrating into dentin

K02.63 Dental caries on smooth surface penetrating into pulp

K02.7 Dental root caries

K02.9 Dental caries, unspecified

● **K03 Other diseases of hard tissues of teeth**
Excludes2 bruxism (F45.8)
dental caries (K02.-)
teeth-grinding NOS (F45.8)

K03.0 Excessive attrition of teeth
Approximal wear of teeth
Occlusal wear of teeth

K03.1 Abrasion of teeth
Dentifrice abrasion of teeth
Habitual abrasion of teeth
Occupational abrasion of teeth
Ritual abrasion of teeth
Traditional abrasion of teeth
Wedge defect NOS

K03.2 Erosion of teeth
Erosion of teeth due to diet
Erosion of teeth due to drugs and medicaments
Erosion of teeth due to persistent vomiting
Erosion of teeth NOS
Idiopathic erosion of teeth
Occupational erosion of teeth

K03.3 Pathological resorption of teeth
Internal granuloma of pulp
Resorption of teeth (external)

K03.4 Hypercementosis
Cementation hyperplasia

K03.5 Ankylosis of teeth

K03.6 Deposits [accretions] on teeth
Betel deposits [accretions] on teeth
Black deposits [accretions] on teeth
Extrinsic staining of teeth NOS
Green deposits [accretions] on teeth
Materia alba deposits [accretions] on teeth
Orange deposits [accretions] on teeth
Staining of teeth NOS
Subgingival dental calculus
Supragingival dental calculus
Tobacco deposits [accretions] on teeth

K03.7 Posteruptive color changes of dental hard tissues
Excludes2 deposits [accretions] on teeth (K03.6)

● **K03.8 Other specified diseases of hard tissues of teeth**

K03.81 Cracked tooth
Excludes1 asymptomatic craze lines in enamel - omit code
broken or fractured tooth due to trauma (S02.5)

K03.89 Other specified diseases of hard tissues of teeth

K03.9 Disease of hard tissues of teeth, unspecified

K04 Diseases of pulp and periapical tissues

● **K04.0 Pulpitis**
Acute pulpitis
Chronic (hyperplastic) (ulcerative) pulpitis
Ex for category K04.0 CC codes: K00.0-K08.9, M26.00-M26.9, M27.61-M27.69

K04.01 Reversible pulpitis ◀

K04.02 Irreversible pulpitis ◀

K04.1 Necrosis of pulp
Pulpal gangrene

K04.2 Pulp degeneration
Denticles
Pulpal calcifications
Pulpal stones

K04.3 Abnormal hard tissue formation in pulp
Secondary or irregular dentine

K04.4 Acute apical periodontitis of pulpal origin
Acute apical periodontitis NOS
Excludes1 acute periodontitis (K05.2-)
Ex See K04.0

K04.5 Chronic apical periodontitis
Apical or periapical granuloma
Apical periodontitis NOS
Excludes1 chronic periodontitis (K05.3-)

K04.6 Periapical abscess with sinus
Dental abscess with sinus
Dentoalveolar abscess with sinus

K04.7 Periapical abscess without sinus
Dental abscess without sinus
Dentoalveolar abscess without sinus
Periapical abscess without sinus

K04.8 Radicular cyst
Apical (periodontal) cyst
Periapical cyst
Residual radicular cyst
Excludes2 lateral periodontal cyst (K09.0)

● **K04.9 Other and unspecified diseases of pulp and periapical tissues**

K04.90 Unspecified diseases of pulp and periapical tissues

K04.99 Other diseases of pulp and periapical tissues

◀ New ◀ Revised ~~deleted~~ Deleted Excludes 1 Excludes 2 Includes Use additional Code first Code also Unspecified
OGCR Official Guidelines ● Unacceptable Principal Diagnosis X Assign placeholder X ● Use Additional Character(s) ▶ Manifestation Code Coding Clinic

Item 11-3 Acute gingivitis, also known as orilitis or ulitis, is the short-term, severe inflammation of the gums (gingiva) caused by bacteria. **Chronic gingivitis** is persistent inflammation of the gums. When the gingivitis moves into the periodontium it is called periodontitis, also known as paradentitis.

K05 Gingivitis and periodontal diseases
Use additional code to identify:
alcohol abuse and dependence (F10.-)
exposure to environmental tobacco smoke (Z77.22)
exposure to tobacco smoke in the perinatal period (P96.81)
history of tobacco dependence (Z87.891)
occupational exposure to environmental tobacco smoke (Z57.31)
tobacco dependence (F17.-)
tobacco use (Z72.0)

K05.0 Acute gingivitis
Excludes1 acute necrotizing ulcerative gingivitis (A69.1)
herpesviral [herpes simplex] gingivostomatitis (B00.2)

K05.00 Acute gingivitis, plaque induced
Acute gingivitis NOS
Plaque induced gingival disease ◀

K05.01 Acute gingivitis, non-plaque induced

K05.1 Chronic gingivitis
Desquamative gingivitis (chronic)
Gingivitis (chronic) NOS
Hyperplastic gingivitis (chronic)
Pregnancy associated gingivitis ◀
Simple marginal gingivitis (chronic)
Ulcerative gingivitis (chronic)
Code first, if applicable, diseases of the digestive system complicating pregnancy (O99.61-) ◀

K05.10 Chronic gingivitis, plaque induced
Chronic gingivitis NOS
Gingivitis NOS

K05.11 Chronic gingivitis, non-plaque induced

K05.2 Aggressive periodontitis
Acute pericoronitis
Excludes1 acute apical periodontitis (K04.4)
periapical abscess (K04.7)
periapical abscess with sinus (K04.6)

K05.20 Aggressive periodontitis, unspecified

K05.21 Aggressive periodontitis, localized
Periodontal abscess

K05.211 Aggressive periodontitis, localized, slight ◀

K05.212 Aggressive periodontitis, localized, moderate ◀

K05.213 Aggressive periodontitis, localized, severe ◀

K05.219 Aggressive periodontitis, localized, unspecified severity ◀

K05.22 Aggressive periodontitis, generalized

K05.221 Aggressive periodontitis, generalized, slight ◀

K05.222 Aggressive periodontitis, generalized, moderate ◀

K05.223 Aggressive periodontitis, generalized, severe ◀

K05.229 Aggressive periodontitis, generalized, unspecified severity ◀

K05.3 Chronic periodontitis
Chronic pericoronitis
Complex periodontitis
Periodontitis NOS
Simplex periodontitis
Excludes1 chronic apical periodontitis (K04.5)

K05.30 Chronic periodontitis, unspecified

K05.31 Chronic periodontitis, localized

K05.311 Chronic periodontitis, localized, slight ◀

K05.312 Chronic periodontitis, localized, moderate ◀

K05.313 Chronic periodontitis, localized, severe ◀

K05.319 Chronic periodontitis, localized, unspecified severity ◀

K05.32 Chronic periodontitis, generalized

K05.321 Chronic periodontitis, generalized, slight ◀

K05.322 Chronic periodontitis, generalized, moderate ◀

K05.323 Chronic periodontitis, generalized, severe ◀

K05.329 Chronic periodontitis, generalized, unspecified severity ◀

K05.4 Periodontosis
Juvenile periodontosis

K05.5 Other periodontal diseases
Combined periodontic-endodontic lesion ◀
Narrow gingival width (of periodontal soft tissue) ◀
Excludes2 leukoplakia of gingiva (K13.21)

K05.6 Periodontal disease, unspecified

K06 Other disorders of gingiva and edentulous alveolar ridge
Excludes2 acute gingivitis (K05.0)
atrophy of edentulous alveolar ridge (K08.2)
chronic gingivitis (K05.1)
gingivitis NOS (K05.1)

K06.0 Gingival recession
Gingival recession (generalized) (localized) (postinfective) (postprocedural)

K06.1 Gingival enlargement
Gingival fibromatosis

K06.2 Gingival and edentulous alveolar ridge lesions associated with trauma
Irritative hyperplasia of edentulous ridge [denture hyperplasia]
Use additional code (Chapter 20) to identify external cause or denture status (Z97.2)

K06.3 Horizontal alveolar bone loss ◀

K06.8 Other specified disorders of gingiva and edentulous alveolar ridge
Fibrous epulis
Flabby alveolar ridge
Giant cell epulis
Peripheral giant cell granuloma of gingiva
Pyogenic granuloma of gingiva
Vertical ridge deficiency ◀
Excludes2 gingival cyst (K09.0)

K06.9 Disorder of gingiva and edentulous alveolar ridge, unspecified

K08 Other disorders of teeth and supporting structures
Excludes2 dentofacial anomalies [including malocclusion] (M26.-)
disorders of jaw (M27.-)

K08.0 Exfoliation of teeth due to systemic causes
Code also underlying systemic condition

K08.1 Complete loss of teeth
Acquired loss of teeth, complete
Excludes1 congenital absence of teeth (K00.0)
exfoliation of teeth due to systemic causes (K08.0)
partial loss of teeth (K08.4-)

K08.10 Complete loss of teeth, unspecified cause
- **K08.101 Complete loss of teeth, unspecified cause, class I**
- **K08.102 Complete loss of teeth, unspecified cause, class II**
- **K08.103 Complete loss of teeth, unspecified cause, class III**
- **K08.104 Complete loss of teeth, unspecified cause, class IV**
- **K08.109 Complete loss of teeth, unspecified cause, unspecified class**
  Edentulism NOS

K08.11 Complete loss of teeth due to trauma
- **K08.111 Complete loss of teeth due to trauma, class I**
- **K08.112 Complete loss of teeth due to trauma, class II**
- **K08.113 Complete loss of teeth due to trauma, class III**
- **K08.114 Complete loss of teeth due to trauma, class IV**
- **K08.119 Complete loss of teeth due to trauma, unspecified class**

K08.12 Complete loss of teeth due to periodontal diseases
- **K08.121 Complete loss of teeth due to periodontal diseases, class I**
- **K08.122 Complete loss of teeth due to periodontal diseases, class II**
- **K08.123 Complete loss of teeth due to periodontal diseases, class III**
- **K08.124 Complete loss of teeth due to periodontal diseases, class IV**
- **K08.129 Complete loss of teeth due to periodontal diseases, unspecified class**

K08.13 Complete loss of teeth due to caries
- **K08.131 Complete loss of teeth due to caries, class I**
- **K08.132 Complete loss of teeth due to caries, class II**
- **K08.133 Complete loss of teeth due to caries, class III**
- **K08.134 Complete loss of teeth due to caries, class IV**
- **K08.139 Complete loss of teeth due to caries, unspecified class**

K08.19 Complete loss of teeth due to other specified cause
- **K08.191 Complete loss of teeth due to other specified cause, class I**
- **K08.192 Complete loss of teeth due to other specified cause, class II**
- **K08.193 Complete loss of teeth due to other specified cause, class III**
- **K08.194 Complete loss of teeth due to other specified cause, class IV**
- **K08.199 Complete loss of teeth due to other specified cause, unspecified class**

K08.2 Atrophy of edentulous alveolar ridge
- **K08.20 Unspecified atrophy of edentulous alveolar ridge**
  Atrophy of the mandible NOS
  Atrophy of the maxilla NOS
- **K08.21 Minimal atrophy of the mandible**
  Minimal atrophy of the edentulous mandible
- **K08.22 Moderate atrophy of the mandible**
  Moderate atrophy of the edentulous mandible
- **K08.23 Severe atrophy of the mandible**
  Severe atrophy of the edentulous mandible
- **K08.24 Minimal atrophy of maxilla**
  Minimal atrophy of the edentulous maxilla
- **K08.25 Moderate atrophy of the maxilla**
  Moderate atrophy of the edentulous maxilla
- **K08.26 Severe atrophy of the maxilla**
  Severe atrophy of the edentulous maxilla

K08.3 Retained dental root

K08.4 Partial loss of teeth
Acquired loss of teeth, partial
Excludes1 complete loss of teeth (K08.1-)
congenital absence of teeth (K00.0)
Excludes2 exfoliation of teeth due to systemic causes (K08.0)

K08.40 Partial loss of teeth, unspecified cause
- **K08.401 Partial loss of teeth, unspecified cause, class I**
- **K08.402 Partial loss of teeth, unspecified cause, class II**
- **K08.403 Partial loss of teeth, unspecified cause, class III**
- **K08.404 Partial loss of teeth, unspecified cause, class IV**
- **K08.409 Partial loss of teeth, unspecified cause, unspecified class**
  Tooth extraction status NOS

K08.41 Partial loss of teeth due to trauma
- **K08.411 Partial loss of teeth due to trauma, class I**
- **K08.412 Partial loss of teeth due to trauma, class II**
- **K08.413 Partial loss of teeth due to trauma, class III**
- **K08.414 Partial loss of teeth due to trauma, class IV**
- **K08.419 Partial loss of teeth due to trauma, unspecified class**

K08.42 Partial loss of teeth due to periodontal diseases
- **K08.421 Partial loss of teeth due to periodontal diseases, class I**
- **K08.422 Partial loss of teeth due to periodontal diseases, class II**
- **K08.423 Partial loss of teeth due to periodontal diseases, class III**
- **K08.424 Partial loss of teeth due to periodontal diseases, class IV**
- **K08.429 Partial loss of teeth due to periodontal diseases, unspecified class**

K08.43 Partial loss of teeth due to caries
- **K08.431 Partial loss of teeth due to caries, class I**
- **K08.432 Partial loss of teeth due to caries, class II**
- **K08.433 Partial loss of teeth due to caries, class III**
- **K08.434 Partial loss of teeth due to caries, class IV**
- **K08.439 Partial loss of teeth due to caries, unspecified class**

● **K08.49 Partial loss of teeth due to other specified cause**

K08.491 Partial loss of teeth due to other specified cause, class I

K08.492 Partial loss of teeth due to other specified cause, class II

K08.493 Partial loss of teeth due to other specified cause, class III

K08.494 Partial loss of teeth due to other specified cause, class IV

K08.499 Partial loss of teeth due to other specified cause, unspecified class

● **K08.5 Unsatisfactory restoration of tooth**
Defective bridge, crown, filling
Defective dental restoration

Excludes1 dental restoration status (Z98.811)

Excludes2 endosseous dental implant failure (M27.6-)
unsatisfactory endodontic treatment (M27.5-)

K08.50 Unsatisfactory restoration of tooth, unspecified
Defective dental restoration NOS

K08.51 Open restoration margins of tooth
Dental restoration failure of marginal integrity
Open margin on tooth restoration
Poor gingival margin to tooth restoration

K08.52 Unrepairable overhanging of dental restorative materials
Overhanging of tooth restoration

● **K08.53 Fractured dental restorative material**

Excludes1 cracked tooth (K03.81)
traumatic fracture of tooth (S02.5)

K08.530 Fractured dental restorative material without loss of material

K08.531 Fractured dental restorative material with loss of material

K08.539 Fractured dental restorative material, unspecified

K08.54 Contour of existing restoration of tooth biologically incompatible with oral health
Dental restoration failure of periodontal anatomical integrity
Unacceptable contours of existing restoration of tooth
Unacceptable morphology of existing restoration of tooth

K08.55 Allergy to existing dental restorative material
Use additional code to identify the specific type of allergy

K08.56 Poor aesthetic of existing restoration of tooth
Dental restoration aesthetically inadequate or displeasing

K08.59 Other unsatisfactory restoration of tooth
Other defective dental restoration

● **K08.8 Other specified disorders of teeth and supporting structures**

K08.81 Primary occlusal trauma ◀

K08.82 Secondary occlusal trauma ◀

K08.89 Other specified disorders of teeth and supporting structures ◀
Enlargement of alveolar ridge NOS ◀
Insufficient anatomic crown height ◀
Insufficient clinical crown length ◀
Irregular alveolar process ◀
Toothache NOS ◀

K08.9 Disorder of teeth and supporting structures, unspecified

● **K09 Cysts of oral region, not elsewhere classified**

Includes lesions showing histological features both of aneurysmal cyst and of another fibro-osseous lesion

Excludes2 cysts of jaw (M27.0-, M27.4-)
radicular cyst (K04.8)

K09.0 Developmental odontogenic cysts
Dentigerous cyst
Eruption cyst
Follicular cyst
Gingival cyst
Lateral periodontal cyst
Primordial cyst

Excludes2 keratocysts (D16.4, D16.5)
odontogenic keratocystic tumors (D16.4, D16.5)

K09.1 Developmental (nonodontogenic) cysts of oral region
Cyst (of) incisive canal
Cyst (of) palatine of papilla
Globulomaxillary cyst
Median palatal cyst
Nasoalveolar cyst
Nasolabial cyst
Nasopalatine duct cyst

K09.8 Other cysts of oral region, not elsewhere classified
Dermoid cyst
Epidermoid cyst
Lymphoepithelial cyst
Epstein's pearl

K09.9 Cyst of oral region, unspecified

★ **(See Plate 61 on page 73.)**

● **K11 Diseases of salivary glands**
Use additional code to identify:
alcohol abuse and dependence (F10.-)
exposure to environmental tobacco smoke (Z77.22)
exposure to tobacco smoke in the perinatal period (P96.81)
history of tobacco dependence (Z87.891) ◀
occupational exposure to environmental tobacco smoke (Z57.31)
tobacco dependence (F17.-)
tobacco use (Z72.0)

K11.0 Atrophy of salivary gland

K11.1 Hypertrophy of salivary gland

● **K11.2 Sialoadenitis**
Parotitis

Excludes1 epidemic parotitis (B26.-)
mumps (B26.-)
uveoparotid fever [Heerfordt] (D86.89)

K11.20 Sialoadenitis, unspecified

K11.21 Acute sialoadenitis

Excludes1 acute recurrent sialoadenitis (K11.22)

K11.22 Acute recurrent sialoadenitis

K11.23 Chronic sialoadenitis

Item 11–4 **Atrophy** is wasting away of a tissue or organ, whereas **hypertrophy** is overdevelopment or enlargement of a tissue or organ. **Sialoadenitis** is salivary gland inflammation. **Parotitis** is the inflammation of the parotid gland. In the epidemic form, parotitis is also known as mumps. **Sialolithiasis** is the formation of calculus within a salivary gland. **Mucocele** is a polyp composed of mucus.

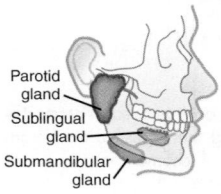

Figure 11-3 Major salivary glands.

K11.3 Abscess of salivary gland
(Ex) K11.0-K11.9, K31.89-K31.9, K92.81, R68.2

K11.4 Fistula of salivary gland
Excludes1 congenital fistula of salivary gland (Q38.4)
(Ex) See K11.3

K11.5 Sialolithiasis
Calculus of salivary gland or duct
Stone of salivary gland or duct

K11.6 Mucocele of salivary gland
Mucous extravasation cyst of salivary gland
Mucous retention cyst of salivary gland
Ranula

K11.7 Disturbances of salivary secretion
Hypoptyalism
Ptyalism
Xerostomia
Excludes2 dry mouth NOS (R68.2)

K11.8 Other diseases of salivary glands
Benign lymphoepithelial lesion of salivary gland
Mikulicz' disease
Necrotizing sialometaplasia
Sialectasia
Stenosis of salivary duct
Stricture of salivary duct
Excludes1 sicca syndrome [Sjögren] (M35.0-)

K11.9 Disease of salivary gland, unspecified
Sialoadenopathy NOS

● **K12 Stomatitis and related lesions**
Use additional code to identify:
alcohol abuse and dependence (F10.-)
exposure to environmental tobacco smoke (Z77.22)
exposure to tobacco smoke in the perinatal period (P96.81)
history of tobacco dependence (Z87.891) ⬅
occupational exposure to environmental tobacco smoke (Z57.31)
tobacco dependence (F17.-)
tobacco use (Z72.0)
Excludes1 cancrum oris (A69.0)
cheilitis (K13.0)
gangrenous stomatitis (A69.0)
herpesviral [herpes simplex] gingivostomatitis (B00.2)
noma (A69.0)

K12.0 Recurrent oral aphthae
Aphthous stomatitis (major) (minor)
Bednar's aphthae
Periadenitis mucosa necrotica recurrens
Recurrent aphthous ulcer
Stomatitis herpetiformis

K12.1 Other forms of stomatitis
Stomatitis NOS
Denture stomatitis
Ulcerative stomatitis
Vesicular stomatitis
Excludes1 acute necrotizing ulcerative stomatitis (A69.1)
Vincent's stomatitis (A69.1)

K12.2 Cellulitis and abscess of mouth
Cellulitis of mouth (floor)
Submandibular abscess
Excludes2 abscess of salivary gland (K11.3)
abscess of tongue (K14.0)
periapical abscess (K04.6-K04.7)
periodontal abscess (K05.21)
peritonsillar abscess (J36)
(Ex) K12.1-K12.39, K14.0, K14.2

● **K12.3 Oral mucositis (ulcerative)**
Mucositis (oral) (oropharyneal)
Excludes2 gastrointestinal mucositis (ulcerative) (K92.81)
mucositis (ulcerative) of vagina and vulva (N76.81)
nasal mucositis (ulcerative) (J34.81)

K12.30 Oral mucositis (ulcerative), unspecified

K12.31 Oral mucositis (ulcerative) due to antineoplastic therapy
Use additional code for adverse effect, if applicable, to identify antineoplastic and immunosuppressive drugs (T45.1X5)
Use additional code for other antineoplastic therapy, such as:
radiological procedure and radiotherapy (Y84.2)

K12.32 Oral mucositis (ulcerative) due to other drugs
Use additional code for adverse effect, if applicable, to identify drug (T36-T50 with fifth or sixth character 5)

K12.33 Oral mucositis (ulcerative) due to radiation
Use additional external cause code (W88-W90, X39.0-) to identify cause

K12.39 Other oral mucositis (ulcerative)
Viral oral mucositis (ulcerative)

● **K13 Other diseases of lip and oral mucosa**
Includes epithelial disturbances of tongue
Use additional code to identify:
alcohol abuse and dependence (F10.-)
exposure to environmental tobacco smoke (Z77.22)
exposure to tobacco smoke in the perinatal period (P96.81)
history of tobacco dependence (Z87.891) ⬅
occupational exposure to environmental tobacco smoke (Z57.31)
tobacco dependence (F17.-)
tobacco use (Z72.0)
Excludes2 certain disorders of gingiva and edentulous alveolar ridge (K05-K06)
cysts of oral region (K09.-)
diseases of tongue (K14.-)
stomatitis and related lesions (K12.-)

K13.0 Diseases of lips
Abscess of lips
Angular cheilitis
Cellulitis of lips
Cheilitis NOS
Cheilodynia
Cheilosis
Exfoliative cheilitis
Fistula of lips
Glandular cheilitis
Hypertrophy of lips
Perlèche NEC
Excludes1 ariboflavinosis (E53.0)
cheilitis due to radiation-related disorders (L55-L59)
congenital fistula of lips (Q38.0)
congenital hypertrophy of lips (Q18.6)
Perlèche due to candidiasis (B37.83)
Perlèche due to riboflavin deficiency (E53.0)

K13.1 Cheek and lip biting

Item 11-5 **Stomatitis** is the inflammation of the oral mucosa. **Mucositis** is the inflammation of the mucous membranes lining the digestive tract from the mouth to the anus. It is a common side effect of chemotherapy and of radiotherapy that involves any part of the digestive tract.

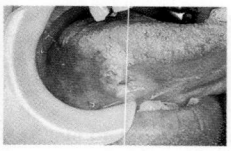

Figure 11-4 Oral leukoplakia and associated squamous carcinoma. (From Feldman: Sleisenger & Fordtran's Gastrointestinal and Liver Disease, ed 8, Saunders, An Imprint of Elsevier, 2006)

● **K13.2 Leukoplakia and other disturbances of oral epithelium, including tongue**

Excludes1 carcinoma in situ of oral epithelium (D00.0-)
hairy leukoplakia (K13.3)

K13.21 Leukoplakia of oral mucosa, including tongue
Considered precancerous and evidenced by thickened white patches of epithelium on mucous membranes
Leukokeratosis of oral mucosa
Leukoplakia of gingiva, lips, tongue

Excludes1 hairy leukoplakia (K13.3)
leukokeratosis nicotina palati (K13.24)

K13.22 Minimal keratinized residual ridge mucosa
Minimal keratinization of alveolar ridge mucosa

K13.23 Excessive keratinized residual ridge mucosa
Excessive keratinization of alveolar ridge mucosa

K13.24 Leukokeratosis nicotina palati
Smoker's palate

K13.29 Other disturbances of oral epithelium, including tongue
Erythroplakia of mouth or tongue
Focal epithelial hyperplasia of mouth or tongue
Leukoedema of mouth or tongue
Other oral epithelium disturbances

K13.3 Hairy leukoplakia

K13.4 Granuloma and granuloma-like lesions of oral mucosa
Eosinophilic granuloma
Granuloma pyogenicum
Verrucous xanthoma

K13.5 Oral submucous fibrosis
Submucous fibrosis of tongue

K13.6 Irritative hyperplasia of oral mucosa

Excludes2 irritative hyperplasia of edentulous ridge [denture hyperplasia] (K06.2)

● **K13.7 Other and unspecified lesions of oral mucosa**

K13.70 Unspecified lesions of oral mucosa

K13.79 Other lesions of oral mucosa
Focal oral mucinosis

★ **(See Plate 58 on page 71.)**

● **K14 Diseases of tongue**

Use additional code to identify:
alcohol abuse and dependence (F10.-)
exposure to environmental tobacco smoke (Z77.22)
history of tobacco dependence (Z87.891)
occupational exposure to environmental tobacco smoke (Z57.31)
tobacco dependence (F17.-)
tobacco use (Z72.0)

Excludes2 erythroplakia (K13.29)
focal epithelial hyperplasia (K13.29)
leukedema of tongue (K13.29)
leukoplakia of tongue (K13.21)
hairy leukoplakia (K13.3)
macroglossia (congenital) (Q38.2)
submucous fibrosis of tongue (K13.5)

K14.0 Glossitis
Abscess of tongue
Ulceration (traumatic) of tongue

Excludes1 atrophic glossitis (K14.4)

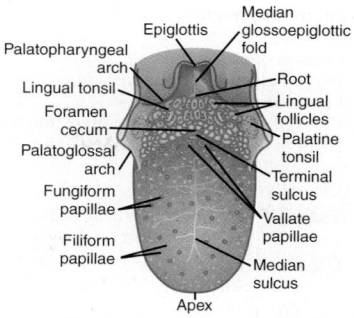

Figure 11-5 Structure of the tongue.

K14.1 Geographic tongue
Benign migratory glossitis
Glossitis areata exfoliativa

K14.2 Median rhomboid glossitis

K14.3 Hypertrophy of tongue papillae
Black hairy tongue
Coated tongue
Hypertrophy of foliate papillae
Lingua villosa nigra

K14.4 Atrophy of tongue papillae
Atrophic glossitis

K14.5 Plicated tongue
Fissured tongue
Furrowed tongue
Scrotal tongue

Excludes1 fissured tongue, congenital (Q38.3)

K14.6 Glossodynia
Glossopyrosis
Painful tongue

K14.8 Other diseases of tongue
Atrophy of tongue
Crenated tongue
Enlargement of tongue
Glossocele
Glossoptosis
Hypertrophy of tongue

K14.9 Disease of tongue, unspecified
Glossopathy NOS

DISEASES OF ESOPHAGUS, STOMACH AND DUODENUM (K20-K31)

Excludes2 hiatus hernia (K44.-)

● **K20 Esophagitis**

Use additional code to identify:
alcohol abuse and dependence (F10.-)

Excludes1 erosion of esophagus (K22.1-)
esophagitis with gastro-esophageal reflux disease (K21.0)
reflux esophagitis (K21.0)
ulcerative esophagitis (K22.1-)

Excludes2 eosinophilic gastritis or gastroenteritis (K52.81)

K20.0 Eosinophilic esophagitis

K20.8 Other esophagitis
Abscess of esophagus

K20.9 Esophagitis, unspecified
Esophagitis NOS

● **K21 Gastro-esophageal reflux disease**

Excludes1 newborn esophageal reflux (P78.83)

K21.0 Gastro-esophageal reflux disease with esophagitis
Reflux esophagitis

K21.9 Gastro-esophageal reflux disease without esophagitis
Esophageal reflux NOS
Coding Clinic: 2016, Q1, P18

● **K22 Other diseases of esophagus**

Excludes2 esophageal varices (I85.-)

K22.0 Achalasia of cardia
Achalasia NOS
Cardiospasm

Excludes1 congenital cardiospasm (Q39.5)

● **K22.1 Ulcer of esophagus**
Barrett's ulcer
Erosion of esophagus
Fungal ulcer of esophagus
Peptic ulcer of esophagus
Ulcer of esophagus due to ingestion of chemicals
Ulcer of esophagus due to ingestion of drugs and medicaments
Ulcerative esophagitis
Code first poisoning due to drug or toxin, if applicable (T36-T65 with fifth or sixth character 1-4 or 6)
Use additional code for adverse effect, if applicable, to identify drug (T36-T50 with fifth or sixth character 5)
Excludes1 Barrett's esophagus (K22.87-)

K22.10 Ulcer of esophagus without bleeding
Ulcer of esophagus NOS
Ex: K22.11, K22.8-K23, K31.82

K22.11 Ulcer of esophagus with bleeding
Excludes2 bleeding esophageal varices (I85.01, I85.11)
Ex: E16.4, I85.01, K22.10-K22.11, K22.6-K22.719, K25.0-K28.9, K29.01, K29.21, K29.31, K29.41, K29.51, K29.61, K29.71, K29.81, K29.91, K31.811, K31.89-K31.9, K55.21, K57.01, K57.11, K57.13, K57.21, K57.31, K57.33, K57.41, K57.51, K57.53, K57.81, K57.91, K57.93, K62.5, K92.0-K92.81

K22.2 Esophageal obstruction
Compression of esophagus
Constriction of esophagus
Stenosis of esophagus
Stricture of esophagus
Excludes1 congenital stenosis or stricture of esophagus (Q39.3)

K22.3 Perforation of esophagus
Rupture of esophagus
Excludes1 traumatic perforation of (thoracic) esophagus (S27.8-)
Ex: K21.9, K22.3, K22.6, K22.8-K23

K22.4 Dyskinesia of esophagus
Difficulty in moving
Corkscrew esophagus
Diffuse esophageal spasm
Spasm of esophagus
Excludes1 cardiospasm (K22.0)

K22.5 Diverticulum of esophagus, acquired
Esophageal pouch, acquired
Excludes1 diverticulum of esophagus (congenital) (Q39.6)

Item 11–6 Esophageal reflux is the return flow of the contents of the stomach to the esophagus and is referred to as GERD and/or "heartburn." **Gastroesophageal reflux** is the return flow of the contents of the stomach and duodenum to the esophagus. **Esophageal leukoplakia** are white areas on the mucous membrane of the esophagus for which no specific cause can be identified.

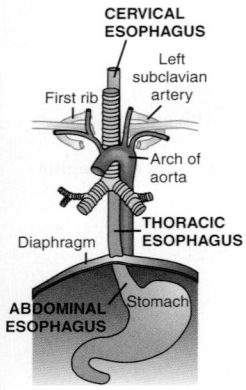

Figure 11-6 The esophagus is the muscular tube that connects the pharynx and the stomach. The 10 inch (25 cm) long esophagus is divided into three parts: **cervical, thoracic,** and **abdominal.**

Item 11–7 Achalasia is a condition in which the smooth muscle fibers of the esophagus do not relax. Most frequently, this condition occurs at the esophagogastric sphincter. **Cardiospasm,** also known as **megaesophagus,** is achalasia of the thoracic esophagus.

K22.6 Gastro-esophageal laceration-hemorrhage syndrome
Mallory-Weiss syndrome
Ex: E16.4, I85.01, K21.9, K22.10-K22.11, K22.3, K22.6-K28.9, K29.01, K29.21, K29.31, K29.41, K29.51, K29.61, K29.71, K29.81, K29.91, K31.811, K55.21, K57.01, K57.11, K57.13, K57.21, K57.31, K57.33, K57.41, K57.51, K57.53, K57.81, K57.91, K57.93, K62.5, K92.0-K92.2

● **K22.7 Barrett's esophagus**
Barrett's disease
Barrett's syndrome
Excludes1 Barrett's ulcer (K22.1)
malignant neoplasm of esophagus (C15.-)

K22.70 Barrett's esophagus without dysplasia
Barrett's esophagus NOS

● **K22.71 Barrett's esophagus with dysplasia**
K22.710 Barrett's esophagus with low grade dysplasia
K22.711 Barrett's esophagus with high grade dysplasia
K22.719 Barrett's esophagus with dysplasia, unspecified

K22.8 Other specified diseases of esophagus
Hemorrhage of esophagus NOS
Excludes2 esophageal varices (I85.-)
Paterson-Kelly syndrome (D50.1)

K22.9 Disease of esophagus, unspecified

▶ *K23 Disorders of esophagus in diseases classified elsewhere*
Code first underlying disease, such as:
congenital syphilis (A50.5)
Excludes1 late syphilis (A52.79)
megaesophagus due to Chagas' disease (B57.31)
tuberculosis (A18.83)

● **K25 Gastric ulcer**
Includes erosion (acute) of stomach
pylorus ulcer (peptic)
stomach ulcer (peptic)
Use additional code to identify:
alcohol abuse and dependence (F10.-)
Excludes1 acute gastritis (K29.0-)
peptic ulcer NOS (K27.-)
Ex: **For category K25 CC codes:** E16.4, I85.01, K22.10-K22.11, K22.6-K22.719, K25.0-K28.9, K29.01, K29.21, K29.31, K29.41, K29.51, K29.61, K29.71, K29.81, K29.91, K31.811, K31.89-K31.9, K55.21, K57.01, K57.11, K57.13, K57.21, K57.31, K57.33, K57.41, K57.51, K57.53, K57.81, K57.91, K57.93, K62.5, K92.0-K92.81

K25.0 Acute gastric ulcer with hemorrhage
K25.1 Acute gastric ulcer with perforation
K25.2 Acute gastric ulcer with both hemorrhage and perforation
K25.3 Acute gastric ulcer without hemorrhage or perforation
K25.4 Chronic or unspecified gastric ulcer with hemorrhage
K25.5 Chronic or unspecified gastric ulcer with perforation
K25.6 Chronic or unspecified gastric ulcer with both hemorrhage and perforation
K25.7 Chronic gastric ulcer without hemorrhage or perforation
K25.9 Gastric ulcer, unspecified as acute or chronic, without hemorrhage or perforation

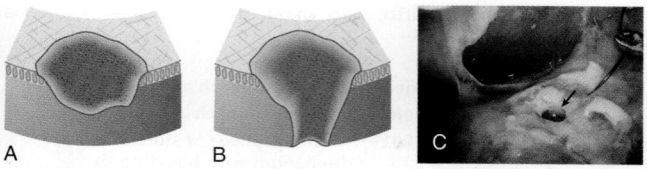

Figure 11-7 **A.** Ulcer. **B.** Perforated ulcer. **C.** Laparoscopic view of a perforated duodenal ulcer *(arrow)* with fibrinous exudate on the adjacent peritoneum. (**C** from Feldman: Sleisenger & Fordtran's Gastrointestinal and Liver Disease, ed 8, Saunders, An Imprint of Elsevier, 2006)

Item 11–8 **Gastric ulcers** are lesions of the stomach that result in the death of the tissue and a defect of the surface. **Perforated ulcers** are those in which the lesion penetrates the gastric wall, leaving a hole. **Peptic ulcers** are lesions of the stomach or the duodenum. **Peptic** refers to the gastric juice, pepsin.

● **K26 Duodenal ulcer**

Includes erosion (acute) of duodenum
duodenum ulcer (peptic)
postpyloric ulcer (peptic)

Use additional code to identify:
alcohol abuse and dependence (F10.-)

Excludes1 peptic ulcer NOS (K27.-)

Ex: **For category K26 CC codes unless otherwise indicated:** E16.4, I85.01, K22.10-K22.11, K22.6-K22.719, K25.0-K28.9, K29.01, K29.21, K29.31, K29.41, K29.51, K29.61, K29.71, K29.81, K29.91, K31.5, K31.811, K31.89-K31.9, K55.21, K57.01, K57.11, K57.13, K57.21, K57.31, K57.33, K57.41, K57.51, K57.53, K57.81, K57.91, K57.93, K62.5, K92.0-K92.81

K26.0 Acute duodenal ulcer with hemorrhage

K26.1 Acute duodenal ulcer with perforation

K26.2 Acute duodenal ulcer with both hemorrhage and perforation

K26.3 Acute duodenal ulcer without hemorrhage or perforation

Ex: E16.4, I85.01, K22.6, K25.0-K28.9, K29.01, K29.21, K29.31, K29.41, K29.51, K29.61, K29.71, K29.81, K29.91, K31.5, K31.811, K31.82, K31.89-K31.9, K55.21, K57.01, K57.11, K57.13, K57.21, K57.31, K57.33, K57.41, K57.51, K57.53, K57.81, K57.91, K57.93, K62.5, K92.0-K92.81

K26.4 Chronic or unspecified duodenal ulcer with hemorrhage

Coding Clinic: 2016, Q1, P14

K26.5 Chronic or unspecified duodenal ulcer with perforation

K26.6 Chronic or unspecified duodenal ulcer with both hemorrhage and perforation

K26.7 Chronic duodenal ulcer without hemorrhage or perforation

K26.9 Duodenal ulcer, unspecified as acute or chronic, without hemorrhage or perforation

● **K27 Peptic ulcer, site unspecified**

Includes gastroduodenal ulcer NOS
peptic ulcer NOS

Use additional code to identify:
alcohol abuse and dependence (F10.-)

Excludes1 peptic ulcer of newborn (P78.82)

Ex: **For category K27 CC codes:** See K26

K27.0 Acute peptic ulcer, site unspecified, with hemorrhage

K27.1 Acute peptic ulcer, site unspecified, with perforation

K27.2 Acute peptic ulcer, site unspecified, with both hemorrhage and perforation

K27.3 Acute peptic ulcer, site unspecified, without hemorrhage or perforation

K27.4 Chronic or unspecified peptic ulcer, site unspecified, with hemorrhage

K27.5 Chronic or unspecified peptic ulcer, site unspecified, with perforation

K27.6 Chronic or unspecified peptic ulcer, site unspecified, with both hemorrhage and perforation

K27.7 Chronic peptic ulcer, site unspecified, without hemorrhage or perforation

K27.9 Peptic ulcer, site unspecified, unspecified as acute or chronic, without hemorrhage or perforation

● **K28 Gastrojejunal ulcer**

Includes anastomotic ulcer (peptic) or erosion
gastrocolic ulcer (peptic) or erosion
gastrointestinal ulcer (peptic) or erosion
gastrojejunal ulcer (peptic) or erosion
jejunal ulcer (peptic) or erosion
marginal ulcer (peptic) or erosion
stomal ulcer (peptic) or erosion

Use additional code to identify:
alcohol abuse and dependence (F10.-)

Excludes1 primary ulcer of small intestine (K63.3)

Ex: **For category K28 CC codes:** See K25

K28.0 Acute gastrojejunal ulcer with hemorrhage

K28.1 Acute gastrojejunal ulcer with perforation

K28.2 Acute gastrojejunal ulcer with both hemorrhage and perforation

K28.3 Acute gastrojejunal ulcer without hemorrhage or perforation

K28.4 Chronic or unspecified gastrojejunal ulcer with hemorrhage

K28.5 Chronic or unspecified gastrojejunal ulcer with perforation

K28.6 Chronic or unspecified gastrojejunal ulcer with both hemorrhage and perforation

K28.7 Chronic gastrojejunal ulcer without hemorrhage or perforation

K28.9 Gastrojejunal ulcer, unspecified as acute or chronic, without hemorrhage or perforation

● **K29 Gastritis and duodenitis**

Excludes1 eosinophilic gastritis or gastroenteritis (K52.81)
Zollinger-Ellison syndrome (E16.4)

Ex: **For category K29 CC codes:** E16.4, I85.01, K22.10-K22.11, K22.6-K22.719, K25.0-K28.9, K29.01, K29.21, K29.31, K29.41, K29.51, K29.61, K29.71, K29.81, K29.91, K31.811, K55.21, K57.01, K57.11, K57.13, K57.21, K57.31, K57.33, K57.41, K57.51, K57.53, K57.81, K57.91, K57.93, K62.5, K92.0-K92.2

● **K29.0 Acute gastritis**

Use additional code to identify:
alcohol abuse and dependence (F10.-)

Excludes1 erosion (acute) of stomach (K25.-)

K29.00 Acute gastritis without bleeding

K29.01 Acute gastritis with bleeding

● **K29.2 Alcoholic gastritis**

Use additional code to identify:
alcohol abuse and dependence (F10.-)

K29.20 Alcoholic gastritis without bleeding

K29.21 Alcoholic gastritis with bleeding

● **K29.3 Chronic superficial gastritis**

K29.30 Chronic superficial gastritis without bleeding

K29.31 Chronic superficial gastritis with bleeding

● **K29.4 Chronic atrophic gastritis**

Gastric atrophy

K29.40 Chronic atrophic gastritis without bleeding

K29.41 Chronic atrophic gastritis with bleeding

● **K29.5 Unspecified chronic gastritis**

Chronic antral gastritis
Chronic fundal gastritis

K29.50 Unspecified chronic gastritis without bleeding

K29.51 Unspecified chronic gastritis with bleeding

Item 11–9 **Gastritis** is a severe inflammation of the stomach. **Atrophic gastritis** is a chronic inflammation of the stomach that results in destruction of the cells of the mucosa of the stomach. Duodenitis is an inflammation of the duodenum, the first section of the small intestine.

● **K29.6 Other gastritis**
Giant hypertrophic gastritis
Granulomatous gastritis
Ménétrier's disease

K29.60 Other gastritis without bleeding

K29.61 Other gastritis with bleeding

● **K29.7 Gastritis, unspecified**

K29.70 Gastritis, unspecified, without bleeding

K29.71 Gastritis, unspecified, with bleeding

● **K29.8 Duodenitis**

K29.80 Duodenitis without bleeding

K29.81 Duodenitis with bleeding

● **K29.9 Gastroduodenitis, unspecified**

K29.90 Gastroduodenitis, unspecified, without bleeding

K29.91 Gastroduodenitis, unspecified, with bleeding

K30 Functional dyspepsia
Indigestion
Excludes1 dyspepsia NOS (R10.13)
heartburn (R12)
nervous dyspepsia (F45.8)
neurotic dyspepsia (F45.8)
psychogenic dyspepsia (F45.8)

● **K31 Other diseases of stomach and duodenum**
Includes functional disorders of stomach
Excludes2 diabetic gastroparesis (E08.43, E09.43, E10.43, E11.43, E13.43)
diverticulum of duodenum (K57.00-K57.13)

K31.0 Acute dilatation of stomach
Acute distention of stomach
Exc K31.0

K31.1 Adult hypertrophic pyloric stenosis A
Pyloric stenosis NOS
Excludes1 congenital or infantile pyloric stenosis (Q40.0)
Exc K30-K31.1, K31.5, K31.84, Q38.5, Q40.0, Q40.8-Q41.9, Q43.4-Q43.9

K31.2 Hourglass stricture and stenosis of stomach
Excludes1 congenital hourglass stomach (Q40.2)
hourglass contraction of stomach (K31.89)

K31.3 Pylorospasm, not elsewhere classified
Excludes1 congenital or infantile pylorospasm (Q40.0)
neurotic pylorospasm (F45.8)
psychogenic pylorospasm (F45.8)

K31.4 Gastric diverticulum
Excludes1 congenital diverticulum of stomach (Q40.2)

K31.5 Obstruction of duodenum
Constriction of duodenum
Duodenal ileus (chronic)
Stenosis of duodenum
Narrowing
Stricture of duodenum
Narrowing
Volvulus of duodenum
Twisting/knotting
Excludes1 congenital stenosis of duodenum (Q41.0)
Exc K31.5, Q38.5, Q40.8-Q41.9, Q43.4-Q43.9

K31.6 Fistula of stomach and duodenum
Gastrocolic fistula
Gastrojejunocolic fistula
Exc K31.6, Q38.5, Q40.8-Q40.9, Q43.4-Q43.9

K31.7 Polyp of stomach and duodenum
Excludes1 adenomatous polyp of stomach (D13.1)

Item 11-10 Achlorhydria, also known as gastric anacidity, is the absence of gastric acid.

● **K31.8 Other specified diseases of stomach and duodenum**

● **K31.81 Angiodysplasia of stomach and duodenum**

K31.811 Angiodysplasia of stomach and duodenum with bleeding
Exc See K29

K31.819 Angiodysplasia of stomach and duodenum without bleeding
Angiodysplasia of stomach and duodenum NOS

K31.82 Dieulafoy lesion (hemorrhagic) of stomach and duodenum
Excludes2 Dieulafoy lesion of intestine (K63.81)
Exc E16.4, I85.01, K22.10-K22.11, K22.6-K22.719, K25.0-K28.9, K29.01, K29.21, K29.31, K29.41, K29.51, K29.61, K29.71, K29.81, K29.91, K31.811, K31.82, K55.21, K57.01, K57.11, K57.13, K57.21, K57.31, K57.33, K57.41, K57.51, K57.53, K57.81, K57.91, K57.93, K62.5, K92.0-K92.2

K31.83 Achlorhydria

K31.84 Gastroparesis
Gastroparalysis
Code first underlying disease, if known, such as:
anorexia nervosa (F50.0-)
diabetes mellitus (E08.43, E09.43, E10.43, E11.43, E13.43)
scleroderma (M34.-)

K31.89 Other diseases of stomach and duodenum

K31.9 Disease of stomach and duodenum, unspecified

DISEASES OF APPENDIX (K35-K38)

● **K35 Acute appendicitis**
Exc For category K35 CC codes: K31.89-K38.9, K92.81

K35.2 Acute appendicitis with generalized peritonitis
Appendicitis (acute) with generalized (diffuse) peritonitis following rupture or perforation of appendix
Perforated appendix NOS
Ruptured appendix NOS

K35.3 Acute appendicitis with localized peritonitis
Acute appendicitis with or without perforation or rupture with peritonitis NOS
Acute appendicitis with or without perforation or rupture with localized peritonitis
Acute appendicitis with peritoneal abscess

● **K35.8 Other and unspecified acute appendicitis**

K35.80 Unspecified acute appendicitis
Acute appendicitis NOS
Acute appendicitis without (localized) (generalized) peritonitis

K35.89 Other acute appendicitis

K36 Other appendicitis
Chronic appendicitis
Recurrent appendicitis

K37 Unspecified appendicitis
Excludes1 -unspecified appendicitis with peritonitis (K35.2-K35.3)

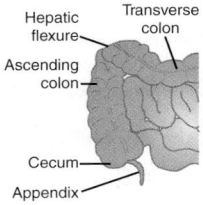

Figure 11-8 Acute appendicitis is the inflammation of the appendix, usually associated with obstruction. Most often this is a disease of adolescents and young adults.

● **K38 Other diseases of appendix**

K38.0 Hyperplasia of appendix

K38.1 Appendicular concretions
Fecalith of appendix
Stercolith of appendix

K38.2 Diverticulum of appendix

K38.3 Fistula of appendix

K38.8 Other specified diseases of appendix
Intussusception of appendix

K38.9 Disease of appendix, unspecified

HERNIA (K40-K46)

Note: Hernia with both gangrene and obstruction is classified to hernia with gangrene.

Includes acquired hernia
congenital [except diaphragmatic or hiatus] hernia
recurrent hernia

● **K40 Inguinal hernia**

Includes bubonocele
direct inguinal hernia
double inguinal hernia
indirect inguinal hernia
inguinal hernia NOS
oblique inguinal hernia
scrotal hernia

Ex: **For category K40 CC codes:** K31.89-K31.9, K40.00-K40.91, K45.0, K45.8-K46.0, K92.81

● **K40.0 Bilateral inguinal hernia, with obstruction, without gangrene**
Inguinal hernia (bilateral) causing obstruction without gangrene
Incarcerated inguinal hernia (bilateral) without gangrene
Irreducible inguinal hernia (bilateral) without gangrene
Strangulated inguinal hernia (bilateral) without gangrene

K40.00 Bilateral inguinal hernia, with obstruction, without gangrene, not specified as recurrent CC
Bilateral inguinal hernia, with obstruction, without gangrene NOS

K40.01 Bilateral inguinal hernia, with obstruction, without gangrene, recurrent CC

● **K40.1 Bilateral inguinal hernia, with gangrene**

K40.10 Bilateral inguinal hernia, with gangrene, not specified as recurrent CC
Bilateral inguinal hernia, with gangrene NOS

K40.11 Bilateral inguinal hernia, with gangrene, recurrent CC

Item 11-11 Hernias of the groin are the most common type, accounting for 80 percent of all hernias. There are two major types of inguinal hernias: indirect (oblique) affecting men only and direct. **Indirect inguinal hernias** result when the intestines emerge through the abdominal wall in an indirect fashion through the inguinal canal. **Direct inguinal hernias** penetrate through the abdominal wall in a direct fashion. **Femoral hernias** occur at the femoral ring where the femoral vessels enter the thigh and is most common in women. An abdominal wall hernia is also called a ventral or epigastric hernia and occurs in both sexes. Classification is based on location of the hernia and whether there is obstruction or gangrene.

Ventral, epigastric, or incisional hernia occurs on the abdominal surface caused by musculature weakness or a tear at a previous surgical site and is evidenced by a bulge that changes in size, becoming larger with exertion. An **incarcerated** hernia is one in which the intestines become trapped in the hernia. A **strangulated** hernia is one in which the blood supply to the intestines is lost. Hiatal hernia occurs when a loop of the stomach protrudes upward through the small opening in the diaphragm through which the esophagus passes, leaving the abdominal cavity and entering the chest. It occurs in both sexes.

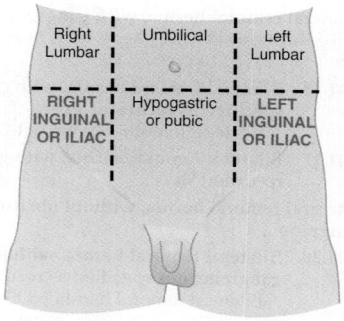

Figure 11-9 Inguinal hernias are those that are located in the inguinal or iliac areas of the abdomen.

● **K40.2 Bilateral inguinal hernia, without obstruction or gangrene**

K40.20 Bilateral inguinal hernia, without obstruction or gangrene, not specified as recurrent
Bilateral inguinal hernia NOS

K40.21 Bilateral inguinal hernia, without obstruction or gangrene, recurrent

● **K40.3 Unilateral inguinal hernia, with obstruction, without gangrene**
Inguinal hernia (unilateral) causing obstruction without gangrene
Incarcerated inguinal hernia (unilateral) without gangrene
Irreducible inguinal hernia (unilateral) without gangrene
Strangulated inguinal hernia (unilateral) without gangrene

K40.30 Unilateral inguinal hernia, with obstruction, without gangrene, not specified as recurrent CC
Inguinal hernia, with obstruction NOS
Unilateral inguinal hernia, with obstruction, without gangrene NOS

K40.31 Unilateral inguinal hernia, with obstruction, without gangrene, recurrent CC

● **K40.4 Unilateral inguinal hernia, with gangrene**

K40.40 Unilateral inguinal hernia, with gangrene, not specified as recurrent MC
Inguinal hernia with gangrene NOS
Unilateral inguinal hernia with gangrene NOS

K40.41 Unilateral inguinal hernia, with gangrene, recurrent MC

● **K40.9 Unilateral inguinal hernia, without obstruction or gangrene**

K40.90 Unilateral inguinal hernia, without obstruction or gangrene, not specified as recurrent
Inguinal hernia NOS
Unilateral inguinal hernia NOS

K40.91 Unilateral inguinal hernia, without obstruction or gangrene, recurrent

● **K41 Femoral hernia**

● **K41.0 Bilateral femoral hernia, with obstruction, without gangrene**
Femoral hernia (bilateral) causing obstruction, without gangrene
Incarcerated femoral hernia (bilateral), without gangrene
Irreducible femoral hernia (bilateral), without gangrene
Strangulated femoral hernia (bilateral), without gangrene

Ex: **For category K41.0 CC codes:** K31.89-K31.9, K41.00-K41.91, K45.0, K45.8-K46.0, K92.81

K41.00 Bilateral femoral hernia, with obstruction, without gangrene, not specified as recurrent CC
Bilateral femoral hernia, with obstruction, without gangrene NOS

K41.01 Bilateral femoral hernia, with obstruction, without gangrene, recurrent CC

● **K41.1 Bilateral femoral hernia, with gangrene**
Ex: For category K41.1 CC codes: K31.89-K31.9, K41.10-K41.21, K41.40-K41.91, K45.0, K45.8-K46.0, K92.81

K41.10 Bilateral femoral hernia, with gangrene, not specified as recurrent
Bilateral femoral hernia, with gangrene NOS

K41.11 Bilateral femoral hernia, with gangrene, recurrent

● **K41.2 Bilateral femoral hernia, without obstruction or gangrene**

K41.20 Bilateral femoral hernia, without obstruction or gangrene, not specified as recurrent
Bilateral femoral hernia NOS

K41.21 Bilateral femoral hernia, without obstruction or gangrene, recurrent

● **K41.3 Unilateral femoral hernia, with obstruction, without gangrene**
Femoral hernia (unilateral) causing obstruction, without gangrene
Incarcerated femoral hernia (unilateral), without gangrene
Irreducible femoral hernia (unilateral), without gangrene
Strangulated femoral hernia (unilateral), without gangrene
Ex: For category K41.3 CC codes: See K41.0

K41.30 Unilateral femoral hernia, with obstruction, without gangrene, not specified as recurrent
Femoral hernia, with obstruction NOS
Unilateral femoral hernia, with obstruction NOS

K41.31 Unilateral femoral hernia, with obstruction, without gangrene, recurrent

● **K41.4 Unilateral femoral hernia, with gangrene**
Ex: For category K41.4 CC codes: K41.1

K41.40 Unilateral femoral hernia, with gangrene, not specified as recurrent
Femoral hernia, with gangrene NOS
Unilateral femoral hernia, with gangrene NOS

K41.41 Unilateral femoral hernia, with gangrene, recurrent

● **K41.9 Unilateral femoral hernia, without obstruction or gangrene**

K41.90 Unilateral femoral hernia, without obstruction or gangrene, not specified as recurrent
Femoral hernia NOS
Unilateral femoral hernia NOS

K41.91 Unilateral femoral hernia, without obstruction or gangrene, recurrent

● **K42 Umbilical hernia**
Includes paraumbilical hernia
Excludes1 omphalocele (Q79.2)

K42.0 Umbilical hernia with obstruction, without gangrene
Umbilical hernia causing obstruction, without gangrene
Incarcerated umbilical hernia, without gangrene
Irreducible umbilical hernia, without gangrene
Strangulated umbilical hernia, without gangrene
Ex: K42.0-K42.1, K43.0-K43.1, K43.3-K43.4, K43.6-K43.7, K45.0, K45.8-K46.0

K42.1 Umbilical hernia with gangrene
Gangrenous umbilical hernia
Ex: K31.89-K31.9, K42.0-K43.9, K45.0, K45.8-K46.0, K46.9, K92.81

K42.9 Umbilical hernia without obstruction or gangrene
Umbilical hernia NOS

● **K43 Ventral hernia**

K43.0 Incisional hernia with obstruction, without gangrene
Incisional hernia causing obstruction, without gangrene
Incarcerated incisional hernia, without gangrene
Irreducible incisional hernia, without gangrene
Strangulated incisional hernia, without gangrene
Ex: See K42.0

K43.1 Incisional hernia with gangrene
Gangrenous incisional hernia
Ex: See K42.1

K43.2 Incisional hernia without obstruction or gangrene
Incisional hernia NOS

K43.3 Parastomal hernia with obstruction, without gangrene
Incarcerated parastomal hernia, without gangrene
Irreducible parastomal hernia, without gangrene
Parastomal hernia causing obstruction, without gangrene
Strangulated parastomal hernia, without gangrene
Ex: See K42.0

K43.4 Parastomal hernia with gangrene
Gangrenous parastomal hernia
Ex: See K42.1

K43.5 Parastomal hernia without obstruction or gangrene
Parastomal hernia NOS

K43.6 Other and unspecified ventral hernia with obstruction, without gangrene
Epigastric hernia causing obstruction, without gangrene
Hypogastric hernia causing obstruction, without gangrene
Incarcerated epigastric hernia without gangrene
Incarcerated hypogastric hernia without gangrene
Incarcerated midline hernia without gangrene
Incarcerated spigelian hernia without gangrene
Incarcerated subxiphoid hernia without gangrene
Irreducible epigastric hernia without gangrene
Irreducible hypogastric hernia without gangrene
Irreducible midline hernia without gangrene
Irreducible spigelian hernia without gangrene
Irreducible subxiphoid hernia without gangrene
Midline hernia causing obstruction, without gangrene
Spigelian hernia causing obstruction, without gangrene
Strangulated epigastric hernia without gangrene
Strangulated hypogastric hernia without gangrene
Strangulated midline hernia without gangrene
Strangulated spigelian hernia without gangrene
Strangulated subxiphoid hernia without gangrene
Subxiphoid hernia causing obstruction, without gangrene
Ex: See K42.0

K43.7 Other and unspecified ventral hernia with gangrene
Any condition listed under K43.6 specified as gangrenous
Ex: See K42.1

K43.9 Ventral hernia without obstruction or gangrene
Epigastric hernia
Ventral hernia NOS

● **K44 Diaphragmatic hernia**
Includes hiatus hernia (esophageal) (sliding)
paraesophageal hernia
Excludes1 congenital diaphragmatic hernia (Q79.0)
congenital hiatus hernia (Q40.1)
Ex: For category K44 CC codes: K44.0-K46.0

K44.0 Diaphragmatic hernia with obstruction, without gangrene
Diaphragmatic hernia causing obstruction
Incarcerated diaphragmatic hernia
Irreducible diaphragmatic hernia
Strangulated diaphragmatic hernia

K44.1 Diaphragmatic hernia with gangrene
Gangrenous diaphragmatic hernia

K44.9 Diaphragmatic hernia without obstruction or gangrene
Diaphragmatic hernia NOS

● **K45 Other abdominal hernia**

Includes abdominal hernia, specified site NEC
lumbar hernia
obturator hernia
pudendal hernia
retroperitoneal hernia
sciatic hernia

K45.0 Other specified abdominal hernia with obstruction, without gangrene
Other specified abdominal hernia causing obstruction
Other specified incarcerated abdominal hernia
Other specified irreducible abdominal hernia
Other specified strangulated abdominal hernia
Ex: K40.00-K46.9

K45.1 Other specified abdominal hernia with gangrene
Any condition listed under K45 specified as gangrenous
Ex: K31.89-K31.9, K40.00-K46.9, K92.81

K45.8 Other specified abdominal hernia without obstruction or gangrene

● **K46 Unspecified abdominal hernia**

Includes enterocele
epiplocele
hernia NOS
interstitial hernia
intestinal hernia
intra-abdominal hernia

Excludes1 vaginal enterocele (N81.5)

K46.0 Unspecified abdominal hernia with obstruction, without gangrene
Unspecified abdominal hernia causing obstruction
Unspecified incarcerated abdominal hernia
Unspecified irreducible abdominal hernia
Unspecified strangulated abdominal hernia
Ex: K40.00-K46.9

K46.1 Unspecified abdominal hernia with gangrene
Any condition listed under K46 specified as gangrenous
Ex: K31.89-K31.9, K40.00-K46.9, K92.81

K46.9 Unspecified abdominal hernia without obstruction or gangrene
Abdominal hernia NOS

★ **(See Plate 284 on page 77.)**

NONINFECTIVE ENTERITIS AND COLITIS (K50-K52)

Includes noninfective inflammatory bowel disease

Excludes1 irritable bowel syndrome (K58.-)
megacolon (K59.3-)

● **K50 Crohn's disease [regional enteritis]**

Includes granulomatous enteritis

Use additional code to identify manifestations, such as: pyoderma gangrenosum (L88)

Excludes1 ulcerative colitis (K51.-)

Ex: **For category K50 CC codes unless otherwise indicated:** K50.00-K51.919

● **K50.0 Crohn's disease of small intestine**
Crohn's disease [regional enteritis] of duodenum
Crohn's disease [regional enteritis] of ileum
Crohn's disease [regional enteritis] of jejunum
Regional ileitis
Terminal ileitis

Excludes1 Crohn's disease of both small and large intestine (K50.8-)

K50.00 Crohn's disease of small intestine without complications

● **K50.01 Crohn's disease of small intestine with complications**

K50.011 Crohn's disease of small intestine with rectal bleeding

K50.012 Crohn's disease of small intestine with intestinal obstruction
CC when PDx is its own CC

K50.013 Crohn's disease of small intestine with fistula
CC when PDx is its own CC

K50.014 Crohn's disease of small intestine with abscess
CC when PDx is its own CC
Coding Clinic: 2012, Q4, P104

K50.018 Crohn's disease of small intestine with other complication

K50.019 Crohn's disease of small intestine with unspecified complications

● **K50.1 Crohn's disease of large intestine**
Crohn's disease [regional enteritis] of colon
Crohn's disease [regional enteritis] of large bowel
Crohn's disease [regional enteritis] of rectum
Granulomatous colitis
Regional colitis

Excludes1 Crohn's disease of both small and large intestine (K50.8)

K50.10 Crohn's disease of large intestine without complications

● **K50.11 Crohn's disease of large intestine with complications**

K50.111 Crohn's disease of large intestine with rectal bleeding

K50.112 Crohn's disease of large intestine with intestinal obstruction
CC when PDx is its own CC

K50.113 Crohn's disease of large intestine with fistula
CC when PDx is its own CC

K50.114 Crohn's disease of large intestine with abscess
CC when PDx is its own CC
Coding Clinic: 2012, Q4, P104

K50.118 Crohn's disease of large intestine with other complication

K50.119 Crohn's disease of large intestine with unspecified complications

● **K50.8 Crohn's disease of both small and large intestine**

K50.80 Crohn's disease of both small and large intestine without complications

● **K50.81 Crohn's disease of both small and large intestine with complications**

K50.811 Crohn's disease of both small and large intestine with rectal bleeding

K50.812 Crohn's disease of both small and large intestine with intestinal obstruction
CC when PDx is its own CC

K50.813 Crohn's disease of both small and large intestine with fistula
CC when PDx is its own CC

K50.814 Crohn's disease of both small and large intestine with abscess
CC when PDx is its own CC
Coding Clinic: 2012, Q4, P104

K50.818 Crohn's disease of both small and large intestine with other complication

K50.819 Crohn's disease of both small and large intestine with unspecified complications

Item 11-12 Crohn's disease, also known as **regional enteritis,** is a chronic inflammatory disease of the intestines. Classification is based on location in the small (duodenum, ileum, jejunum) or large (cecum, colon, rectum, anal canal) intestine.

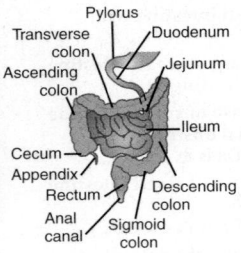

Figure 11-10 Small and large intestines.

● **K50.9 Crohn's disease, unspecified**
Ex: For category K50.9 CC codes: K50.00-K50.919

K50.90 Crohn's disease, unspecified, without complications
Crohn's disease NOS
Regional enteritis NOS

● **K50.91 Crohn's disease, unspecified, with complications**

K50.911 Crohn's disease, unspecified, with rectal bleeding

K50.912 Crohn's disease, unspecified, with intestinal obstruction
CC when PDx is its own CC

K50.913 Crohn's disease, unspecified, with fistula
CC when PDx is its own CC

K50.914 Crohn's disease, unspecified, with abscess
CC when PDx is its own CC
Coding Clinic: 2012, Q4, P104

K50.918 Crohn's disease, unspecified, with other complication

K50.919 Crohn's disease, unspecified, with unspecified complications

● **K51 Ulcerative colitis**
Use additional code to identify manifestations, such as: pyoderma gangrenosum (L88)
Excludes1 Crohn's disease [regional enteritis] (K50.-)
Ex: For category K51 CC codes unless otherwise indicated: K50.00-K51.919

● **K51.0 Ulcerative (chronic) pancolitis**
Backwash ileitis

K51.00 Ulcerative (chronic) pancolitis without complications
Ulcerative (chronic) pancolitis NOS

● **K51.01 Ulcerative (chronic) pancolitis with complications**

K51.011 Ulcerative (chronic) pancolitis with rectal bleeding

K51.012 Ulcerative (chronic) pancolitis with intestinal obstruction
CC when PDx is its own CC

K51.013 Ulcerative (chronic) pancolitis with fistula
CC when PDx is its own CC

K51.014 Ulcerative (chronic) pancolitis with abscess
CC when PDx is its own CC

K51.018 Ulcerative (chronic) pancolitis with other complication

K51.019 Ulcerative (chronic) pancolitis with unspecified complications

Item 11-13 Ulcerative colitis attacks the colonic mucosa and forms abscesses. The disease involves the intestines. Classification is based on the location:
- Enterocolitis: large and small intestine
- Ileocolitis: ileum and colon
- Proctitis: rectum
- Proctosigmoiditis: sigmoid colon and rectum

● **K51.2 Ulcerative (chronic) proctitis**

K51.20 Ulcerative (chronic) proctitis without complications
Ulcerative (chronic) proctitis NOS

● **K51.21 Ulcerative (chronic) proctitis with complications**

K51.211 Ulcerative (chronic) proctitis with rectal bleeding

K51.212 Ulcerative (chronic) proctitis with intestinal obstruction
CC when PDx is its own CC

K51.213 Ulcerative (chronic) proctitis with fistula
CC when PDx is its own CC

K51.214 Ulcerative (chronic) proctitis with abscess
CC when PDx is its own CC

K51.218 Ulcerative (chronic) proctitis with other complication

K51.219 Ulcerative (chronic) proctitis with unspecified complications

● **K51.3 Ulcerative (chronic) rectosigmoiditis**

K51.30 Ulcerative (chronic) rectosigmoiditis without complications
Ulcerative (chronic) rectosigmoiditis NOS

● **K51.31 Ulcerative (chronic) rectosigmoiditis with complications**

K51.311 Ulcerative (chronic) rectosigmoiditis with rectal bleeding

K51.312 Ulcerative (chronic) rectosigmoiditis with intestinal obstruction
CC when PDx is its own CC

K51.313 Ulcerative (chronic) rectosigmoiditis with fistula
CC when PDx is its own CC

K51.314 Ulcerative (chronic) rectosigmoiditis with abscess
CC when PDx is its own CC

K51.318 Ulcerative (chronic) rectosigmoiditis with other complication

K51.319 Ulcerative (chronic) rectosigmoiditis with unspecified complications

● **K51.4 Inflammatory polyps of colon**
Excludes1 adenomatous polyp of colon (D12.6)
polyposis of colon (D12.6)
polyps of colon NOS (K63.5)

K51.40 Inflammatory polyps of colon without complications
Inflammatory polyps of colon NOS

● **K51.41 Inflammatory polyps of colon with complications**

K51.411 Inflammatory polyps of colon with rectal bleeding

K51.412 Inflammatory polyps of colon with intestinal obstruction
CC when PDx is its own CC

K51.413 Inflammatory polyps of colon with fistula
CC when PDx is its own CC

K51.414 Inflammatory polyps of colon with abscess
CC when PDx is its own CC

K51.418 Inflammatory polyps of colon with other complication

K51.419 Inflammatory polyps of colon with unspecified complications

K51.5 Left sided colitis
Left hemicolitis

K51.50 Left sided colitis without complications
Left sided colitis NOS

K51.51 Left sided colitis with complications

K51.511 Left sided colitis with rectal bleeding

K51.512 Left sided colitis with intestinal obstruction
CC when PDx is its own CC

K51.513 Left sided colitis with fistula
CC when PDx is its own CC

K51.514 Left sided colitis with abscess
CC when PDx is its own CC

K51.518 Left sided colitis with other complication

K51.519 Left sided colitis with unspecified complications

K51.8 Other ulcerative colitis

K51.80 Other ulcerative colitis without complications

K51.81 Other ulcerative colitis with complications

K51.811 Other ulcerative colitis with rectal bleeding

K51.812 Other ulcerative colitis with intestinal obstruction
CC when PDx is its own CC

K51.813 Other ulcerative colitis with fistula
CC when PDx is its own CC

K51.814 Other ulcerative colitis with abscess
CC when PDx is its own CC

K51.818 Other ulcerative colitis with other complication

K51.819 Other ulcerative colitis with unspecified complications

K51.9 Ulcerative colitis, unspecified
Ex: For category K51.9 CC codes: K51.00-K51.919

K51.90 Ulcerative colitis, unspecified, without complications

K51.91 Ulcerative colitis, unspecified, with complications

K51.911 Ulcerative colitis, unspecified with rectal bleeding

K51.912 Ulcerative colitis, unspecified with intestinal obstruction
CC when PDx is its own CC

K51.913 Ulcerative colitis, unspecified with fistula
CC when PDx is its own CC

K51.914 Ulcerative colitis, unspecified with abscess
CC when PDx is its own CC

K51.918 Ulcerative colitis, unspecified with other complication

K51.919 Ulcerative colitis, unspecified with unspecified complications

K52 Other and unspecified noninfective gastroenteritis and colitis

K52.0 Gastroenteritis and colitis due to radiation
Ex: K52.0

K52.1 Toxic gastroenteritis and colitis
Drug-induced gastroenteritis and colitis
Code first (T51-T65) to identify toxic agent
Use additional code for adverse effect, if applicable, to identify drug (T36-T50 with fifth or sixth character 5)
Ex: K52.1

K52.2 Allergic and dietetic gastroenteritis and colitis
Food hypersensitivity gastroenteritis or colitis
Use additional code to identify type of food allergy (Z91.01-, Z91.02-)
Excludes2 allergic eosinophilic colitis (K52.82) ◀
allergic eosinophilic esophagitis (K20.0) ◀
allergic eosinophilic gastritis (K52.81) ◀
allergic eosinophilic gastroenteritis (K52.81) ◀
food protein-induced proctocolitis (K52.82) ◀

K52.21 Food protein-induced enterocolitis syndrome ◀
Use additional code for hypovolemic shock, if present (R57.1) ◀

K52.22 Food protein-induced enteropathy ◀

K52.29 Other allergic and dietetic gastroenteritis and colitis ◀
Food hypersensitivity gastroenteritis or colitis ◀
Immediate gastrointestinal hypersensitivity ◀

K52.3 Indeterminate colitis ◀
Colonic inflammatory bowel disease unclassified (IBDU) ◀
Excludes1 unspecified colitis (K52.9) ◀

K52.8 Other specified noninfective gastroenteritis and colitis

K52.81 Eosinophilic gastritis or gastroenteritis
Eosinophilic enteritis
Excludes2 eosinophilic esophagitis (K20.0) ◀

K52.82 Eosinophilic colitis
Allergic proctocolitis ◀
Food-induced eosinophilic proctocolitis ◀
Food protein-induced proctocolitis ◀
Milk protein-induced proctocolitis ◀

K52.83 Microscopic colitis ◀

K52.831 Collagenous colitis ◀

K52.832 Lymphocytic colitis ◀

K52.838 Other microscopic colitis ◀

K52.839 Microscopic colitis, unspecified ◀

K52.89 Other specified noninfective gastroenteritis and colitis

K52.9 Noninfective gastroenteritis and colitis, unspecified
Colitis NOS
Enteritis NOS
Gastroenteritis NOS
Ileitis NOS
Jejunitis NOS
Sigmoiditis NOS
Excludes1 diarrhea NOS (R19.7)
functional diarrhea (K59.1)
infectious gastroenteritis and colitis NOS (A09)
neonatal diarrhea (noninfective) (P78.3)
psychogenic diarrhea (F45.8)

OTHER DISEASES OF INTESTINES (K55-K64)

K55 Vascular disorders of intestine
Excludes1 necrotizing enterocolitis of newborn (P77.-)
Ex: For category K55 CC codes unless otherwise indicated: K55.021-K55.1, K55.30-K55.33

K55.0 Acute vascular disorders of intestine
Infarction of appendices epiploicae
Mesenteric (artery) (vein) embolism
Mesenteric (artery) (vein) infarction
Mesenteric (artery) (vein) thrombosis

K55.01 Acute (reversible) ischemia of small intestine ◀

K55.011 Focal (segmental) acute (reversible) ischemia of small intestine ◀

K55.012 Diffuse acute (reversible) ischemia of small intestine ◀

K55.019 Acute (reversible) ischemia of small intestine, extent unspecified ◀

● **K55.02 Acute infarction of small intestine** ◀
Gangrene of small intestine ◀
Necrosis of small intestine ◀

K55.021 Focal (segmental) acute infarction of small intestine ◀

K55.022 Diffuse acute infarction of small intestine ◀

K55.029 Acute infarction of small intestine, extent unspecified ◀

● **K55.03 Acute (reversible) ischemia of large intestine** ◀
Acute fulminant ischemic colitis ◀
Subacute ischemic colitis ◀

K55.031 Focal (segmental) acute (reversible) ischemia of large intestine ◀

K55.032 Diffuse acute (reversible) ischemia of large intestine ◀

K55.039 Acute (reversible) ischemia of large intestine, extent unspecified ◀

● **K55.04 Acute infarction of large intestine** ◀
Gangrene of large intestine ◀
Necrosis of large intestine ◀

K55.041 Focal (segmental) acute infarction of large intestine ◀

K55.042 Diffuse acute infarction of large intestine ◀

K55.049 Acute infarction of large intestine, extent unspecified ◀

● **K55.05 Acute (reversible) ischemia of intestine, part unspecified** ◀

K55.051 Focal (segmental) acute (reversible) ischemia of intestine, part unspecified ◀

K55.052 Diffuse acute (reversible) ischemia of intestine, part unspecified ◀

K55.059 Acute (reversible) ischemia of intestine, part and extent unspecified ◀

● **K55.06 Acute infarction of intestine, part unspecified** ◀
Acute intestinal infarction ◀
Gangrene of intestine ◀
Necrosis of intestine ◀

K55.061 Focal (segmental) acute infarction of intestine, part unspecified ◀

K55.062 Diffuse acute infarction of intestine, part unspecified ◀

K55.069 Acute infarction of intestine, part and extent unspecified ◀

K55.1 Chronic vascular disorders of intestine
Chronic ischemic colitis
Chronic ischemic enteritis
Chronic ischemic enterocolitis
Ischemic stricture of intestine
Mesenteric atherosclerosis
Mesenteric vascular insufficiency
Ex: K55.012-K55.069, K55.1, K55.30-K55.33, K55.8-K55.9

● **K55.2 Angiodysplasia of colon**

K55.20 Angiodysplasia of colon without hemorrhage

K55.21 Angiodysplasia of colon with hemorrhage
Ex: E16.4, I85.01, K22.10-K22.11, K22.6-K22.719, K25.0-K28.9, K29.01, K29.21, K29.31, K29.41, K29.51, K29.61, K29.71, K29.81, K29.91, K31.811, K55.21, K57.01, K57.11, K57.13, K57.21, K57.31, K57.33, K57.41, K57.51, K57.53, K57.81, K57.91, K57.93, K62.5, K92.0-K92.2

● **K55.3 Necrotizing enterocolitis** ◀

Excludes1 necrotizing enterocolitis of newborn (P77.-) ◀

Excludes2 necrotizing enterocolitis due to Clostridium difficile (A04.7) ◀

K55.30 Necrotizing enterocolitis, unspecified ◀
Necrotizing enterocolitis, NOS ◀

K55.31 Stage 1 necrotizing enterocolitis ◀
Necrotizing enterocolitis without pneumatosis, without perforation ◀

K55.32 Stage 2 necrotizing enterocolitis ◀
Necrotizing enterocolitis with pneumatosis, without perforation ◀

K55.33 Stage 3 necrotizing enterocolitis ◀
Necrotizing enterocolitis with perforation ◀
Necrotizing enterocolitis with pneumatosis and perforation ◀

K55.8 Other vascular disorders of intestine
Ex: See K55.1

K55.9 Vascular disorder of intestine, unspecified
Ischemic colitis
Ischemic enteritis
Ischemic enterocolitis
Ex: See K55.1

● **K56 Paralytic ileus and intestinal obstruction without hernia**

Excludes1 congenital stricture or stenosis of intestine (Q41-Q42)
cystic fibrosis with meconium ileus (E84.11)
ischemic stricture of intestine (K55.1)
meconium ileus NOS (P76.0)
neonatal intestinal obstructions classifiable to P76.-
obstruction of duodenum (K31.5)
postprocedural intestinal obstruction (K91.3)
stenosis of anus or rectum (K62.4)
intestinal obstruction with hernia (K40-K46)

Ex: **For category K56 CC codes:** K56.0-K56.3, K56.49-K56.7, K63.4, K63.89-K63.9, K92.89-K92.9, R11.13

K56.0 Paralytic ileus
Paralysis of bowel
Paralysis of colon
Paralysis of intestine

Excludes1 gallstone ileus (K56.3)
ileus NOS (K56.7)
obstructive ileus NOS (K56.69)

K56.1 Intussusception
Intussusception or invagination of bowel
Intussusception or invagination of colon
Intussusception or invagination of intestine
Intussusception or invagination of rectum

Excludes2 intussusception of appendix (K38.8)

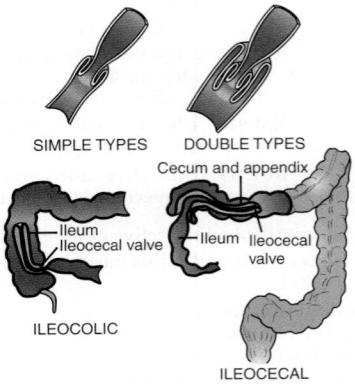

Figure 11-11 Types of intussusception.

Item 11-14 Intussusception is the prolapse (telescoping) of a part of the intestine into another adjacent part of the intestine. Intussusception may be enteric (ileoileal, jejunoileal, jejunojejunal), colic (colocolic), or intracolic (ileocecal, ileocolic).

Item 11-15 Volvulus is the twisting of a segment of the intestine, resulting in obstruction. Paralytic ileus is paralysis of the intestine. It need not be a complete paralysis, but it must prohibit the passage of food through the intestine and lead to intestinal blockage. It is a common aftermath of some types of surgery.

K56.2 Volvulus
Strangulation of colon or intestine
Torsion of colon or intestine
Twist of colon or intestine
Excludes2 volvulus of duodenum (K31.5)

K56.3 Gallstone ileus
Obstruction of intestine by gallstone

● **K56.4 Other impaction of intestine**

K56.41 Fecal impaction
Excludes1 constipation (K59.0-)
incomplete defecation (R15.0)

K56.49 Other impaction of intestine

K56.5 Intestinal adhesions [bands] with obstruction (postprocedural) (postinfection)
Abdominal hernia due to adhesions with obstruction
Peritoneal adhesions [bands] with intestinal obstruction (postprocedural) (postinfection)

● **K56.6 Other and unspecified intestinal obstruction**

K56.60 Unspecified intestinal obstruction Intestinal obstruction NOS
Excludes1 intestinal obstruction due to specified condition-code to condition

K56.69 Other intestinal obstruction
Enterostenosis NOS
Obstructive ileus NOS
Occlusion of colon or intestine NOS
Stenosis of colon or intestine NOS
Stricture of colon or intestine NOS
Excludes1 intestinal obstruction due to specified condition-code to condition

K56.7 Ileus, unspecified
Excludes1 obstructive ileus (K56.69)

● **K57 Diverticular disease of intestine**
Excludes1 congenital diverticulum of intestine (Q43.8)
Meckel's diverticulum (Q43.0)
Excludes2 diverticulum of appendix (K38.2)
For category K57 CC codes unless otherwise indicated: E16.4, I85.01, K22.10-K22.11, K22.6-K22.719, K25.0-K28.9, K29.01, K29.21, K29.31, K29.41, K29.51, K29.61, K29.71, K29.81, K29.91, K31.811, K55.21, K57.01, K57.11, K57.13, K57.21, K57.31, K57.33, K57.41, K57.51, K57.53, K57.81, K57.91, K57.93, K62.5, K92.0-K92.2

● **K57.0 Diverticulitis of small intestine with perforation and abscess**
Diverticulitis of small intestine with peritonitis
Excludes1 diverticulitis of both small and large intestine with perforation and abscess (K57.4-)

K57.00 Diverticulitis of small intestine with perforation and abscess without bleeding
CC when PDx is its own CC
K57.00-K57.13

K57.01 Diverticulitis of small intestine with perforation and abscess with bleeding
CC when PDx is its own CC

● **K57.1 Diverticular disease of small intestine without perforation or abscess**
Excludes1 diverticular disease of both small and large intestine without perforation or abscess (K57.5-)

K57.10 Diverticulosis of small intestine without perforation or abscess without bleeding
Diverticular disease of small intestine NOS

K57.11 Diverticulosis of small intestine without perforation or abscess with bleeding

K57.12 Diverticulitis of small intestine without perforation or abscess without bleeding
K57.00-K57.13

K57.13 Diverticulitis of small intestine without perforation or abscess with bleeding

● **K57.2 Diverticulitis of large intestine with perforation and abscess**
Diverticulitis of colon with peritonitis
Excludes1 diverticulitis of both small and large intestine with perforation and abscess (K57.4-)

K57.20 Diverticulitis of large intestine with perforation and abscess without bleeding
CC when PDx is its own CC
K57.20-K57.93

K57.21 Diverticulitis of large intestine with perforation and abscess with bleeding
CC when PDx is its own CC

● **K57.3 Diverticular disease of large intestine without perforation or abscess**
Excludes1 diverticular disease of both small and large intestine without perforation or abscess (K57.5-)

K57.30 Diverticulosis of large intestine without perforation or abscess without bleeding
Diverticular disease of colon NOS

K57.31 Diverticulosis of large intestine without perforation or abscess with bleeding

K57.32 Diverticulitis of large intestine without perforation or abscess without bleeding
K57.20-K57.93

K57.33 Diverticulitis of large intestine without perforation or abscess with bleeding

● **K57.4 Diverticulitis of both small and large intestine with perforation and abscess**
Diverticulitis of both small and large intestine with peritonitis

K57.40 Diverticulitis of both small and large intestine with perforation and abscess without bleeding
CC when PDx is its own CC
K57.20-K57.93

K57.41 Diverticulitis of both small and large intestine with perforation and abscess with bleeding
CC when PDx is its own CC

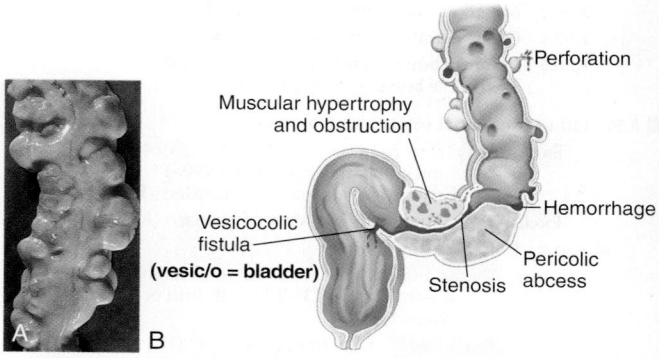

Figure 11-12 Diverticulosis. (From Shiland: Mastering Healthcare Terminology, ed 4, St. Louis, Mosby, 2012)

Item 11-16 Diverticula of the intestines are acquired herniations of the mucosa. Diverticulum (singular): Pocket or pouch that bulges outward through a weak spot (herniation) in the colon. Diverticula (plural). **Diverticulosis** is the condition of having diverticula. **Diverticulitis** is inflammation of these pouches or herniations. Classification is based on location (small intestine or colon) and whether it occurs with or without hemorrhage.

● **K57.5 Diverticular disease of both small and large intestine without perforation or abscess**

K57.50 Diverticulosis of both small and large intestine without perforation or abscess without bleeding
Diverticular disease of both small and large intestine NOS

K57.51 Diverticulosis of both small and large intestine without perforation or abscess with bleeding

K57.52 Diverticulitis of both small and large intestine without perforation or abscess without bleeding
CC when PDx is its own CC
Ex: K57.20-K57.93

K57.53 Diverticulitis of both small and large intestine without perforation or abscess with bleeding

● **K57.8 Diverticulitis of intestine, part unspecified, with perforation and abscess**
Diverticulitis of intestine NOS with peritonitis

K57.80 Diverticulitis of intestine, part unspecified, with perforation and abscess without bleeding
CC when PDx is its own CC
Ex: K57.20-K57.93

K57.81 Diverticulitis of intestine, part unspecified, with perforation and abscess with bleeding
CC when PDx is its own CC

● **K57.9 Diverticular disease of intestine, part unspecified, without perforation or abscess**

K57.90 Diverticulosis of intestine, part unspecified, without perforation or abscess without bleeding
Diverticular disease of intestine NOS

K57.91 Diverticulosis of intestine, part unspecified, without perforation or abscess with bleeding

K57.92 Diverticulitis of intestine, part unspecified, without perforation or abscess without bleeding
Ex: K57.20-K57.93

K57.93 Diverticulitis of intestine, part unspecified, without perforation or abscess with bleeding

● **K58 Irritable bowel syndrome**
Includes irritable colon
spastic colon

K58.0 Irritable bowel syndrome with diarrhea

K58.1 Irritable bowel syndrome with constipation ◀

K58.2 Mixed irritable bowel syndrome ◀

K58.8 Other irritable bowel syndrome ◀

K58.9 Irritable bowel syndrome without diarrhea
Irritable bowel syndrome NOS

● **K59 Other functional intestinal disorders**
Excludes1 change in bowel habit NOS (R19.4)
intestinal malabsorption (K90.-)
psychogenic intestinal disorders (F45.8)
Excludes2 functional disorders of stomach (K31.-)

● **K59.0 Constipation**
Use additional code for adverse effect, if applicable, to identify drug (T36-T50 with fifth or sixth character 5) ◀
Excludes1 fecal impaction (K56.41)
incomplete defecation (R15.0)

K59.00 Constipation, unspecified

K59.01 Slow transit constipation

K59.02 Outlet dysfunction constipation

K59.03 Drug induced constipation ◀
Use additional code for adverse effect, if applicable, to identify drug (T36-T50 with fifth or sixth character 5) ◀

K59.04 Chronic idiopathic constipation ◀
Functional constipation ◀

K59.09 Other constipation
Chronic constipation ◀

K59.1 Functional diarrhea
Excludes1 diarrhea NOS (R19.7)
irritable bowel syndrome with diarrhea (K58.0)

K59.2 Neurogenic bowel, not elsewhere classified
Ex: K58.0-K58.9, K59.1-K59.9, K91.0-K91.1

● **K59.3 Megacolon, not elsewhere classified**
Dilatation of colon
Code first, if applicable (T51-T65) to identify toxic agent ◀
Excludes1 congenital megacolon (aganglionic) (Q43.1)
megacolon (due to) (in) Chagas' disease (B57.32)
megacolon (due to) (in) Clostridium difficile (A04.7)
megacolon (due to) (in) Hirschsprung's disease (Q43.1)
Ex: For category K59.3 CC codes: See K59.2

K59.31 Toxic megacolon ◀

K59.39 Other megacolon ◀
Megacolon NOS ◀

K59.4 Anal spasm
Proctalgia fugax

K59.8 Other specified functional intestinal disorders
Atony of colon Pseudo-obstruction (acute) (chronic) of intestine

K59.9 Functional intestinal disorder, unspecified

● **K60 Fissure and fistula of anal and rectal regions**
Excludes1 fissure and fistula of anal and rectal regions with abscess or cellulitis (K61.-)
Excludes2 anal sphincter tear (healed) (nontraumatic) (old) (K62.81)

K60.0 Acute anal fissure

K60.1 Chronic anal fissure

K60.2 Anal fissure, unspecified

K60.3 Anal fistula

K60.4 Rectal fistula
Fistula of rectum to skin
Excludes1 rectovaginal fistula (N82.3)
vesicorectal fistula (N32.1)

K60.5 Anorectal fistula

● **K61 Abscess of anal and rectal regions**
Includes abscess of anal and rectal regions
cellulitis of anal and rectal regions
Ex: For category K61 CC codes: K61.0-K61.4

K61.0 Anal abscess
Perianal abscess
Excludes1 intrasphincteric abscess (K61.4)

K61.1 Rectal abscess
Perirectal abscess
Excludes1 ischiorectal abscess (K61.3)
Coding Clinic: 2012, Q4, P104

K61.2 Anorectal abscess

K61.3 Ischiorectal abscess
Abscess of ischiorectal fossa

K61.4 Intrasphincteric abscess

Item 11-17 A **fissure** is a groove in the surface, whereas a **fistula** is an abnormal passage. An **abscess** is an accumulation of pus in a tissue cavity resulting from a bacterial or parasitic infection.

K62 Other diseases of anus and rectum

Includes anal canal

Excludes2 colostomy and enterostomy malfunction (K94.0-, K91.4-)
fecal incontinence (R15.-)
hemorrhoids (K64.-)

K62.0 Anal polyp

K62.1 Rectal polyp

Excludes1 adenomatous polyp (D12.8)

K62.2 Anal prolapse
Prolapse of anal canal

K62.3 Rectal prolapse
Prolapse of rectal mucosa

K62.4 Stenosis of anus and rectum
Stricture of anus (sphincter)

K62.5 Hemorrhage of anus and rectum

Excludes1 gastrointestinal bleeding NOS (K92.2)
melena (K92.1)
neonatal rectal hemorrhage (P54.2)

Ex: See K57

K62.6 Ulcer of anus and rectum
Solitary ulcer of anus and rectum
Stercoral ulcer of anus and rectum

Excludes1 fissure and fistula of anus and rectum (K60.-)
ulcerative colitis (K51.-)

Ex: K62.6

K62.7 Radiation proctitis

Use additional code to identify the type of radiation (W90.-)

K62.8 Other specified diseases of anus and rectum

Excludes2 ulcerative proctitis (K51.2)

K62.81 Anal sphincter tear (healed) (nontraumatic) (old)
Tear of anus, nontraumatic

Use additional code for any associated fecal incontinence (R15.-)

Excludes2 anal fissure (K60.-)
anal sphincter tear (healed) (old) complicating delivery (O34.7-)
traumatic tear of anal sphincter (S31.831)

K62.82 Dysplasia of anus
Anal intraepithelial neoplasia I and II (AIN I and II) (histologically confirmed)
Dysplasia of anus NOS
Mild and moderate dysplasia of anus (histologically confirmed)

Excludes1 abnormal results from anal cytologic examination without histologic confirmation (R85.61-)
anal intraepithelial neoplasia III (D01.3)
carcinoma in situ of anus (D01.3)
HGSIL of anus (R85.613)
severe dysplasia of anus (D01.3)

K62.89 Other specified diseases of anus and rectum
Proctitis NOS

Use additional code for any associated fecal incontinence (R15.-)

K62.9 Disease of anus and rectum, unspecified

K63 Other diseases of intestine

K63.0 Abscess of intestine

Excludes1 abscess of intestine with Crohn's disease (K50.014, K50.114, K50.814, K50.914)
abscess of intestine with diverticular disease (K57.0, K57.2, K57.4, K57.8)
abscess of intestine with ulcerative colitis (K51.014, K51.214, K51.314, K51.414, K51.514, K51.814, K51.914)

Excludes2 abscess of anal and rectal regions (K61.-)
abscess of appendix (K35.3)

Ex: K63.0

K63.1 Perforation of intestine (nontraumatic)
Perforation (nontraumatic) of rectum

Excludes1 perforation (nontraumatic) of duodenum (K26.-)
perforation (nontraumatic) of intestine with diverticular disease (K57.0, K57.2, K57.4, K57.8)

Excludes2 perforation (nontraumatic) of appendix (K35.2, K35.3)

Ex: K63.1

K63.2 Fistula of intestine

Excludes1 fistula of duodenum (K31.6)
fistula of intestine with Crohn's disease (K50.013, K50.113, K50.813, K50.913)
fistula of intestine with ulcerative colitis (K51.013, K51.213, K51.313, K51.413, K51.513, K51.813, K51.913)

Excludes2 fistula of anal and rectal regions (K60.-)
fistula of appendix (K38.3)
intestinal-genital fistula, female (N82.2-N82.4)
vesicointestinal fistula (N32.1)

Ex: K63.2

K63.3 Ulcer of intestine
Primary ulcer of small intestine

Excludes1 duodenal ulcer (K26.-)
gastrointestinal ulcer (K28.-)
gastrojejunal ulcer (K28.-)
jejunal ulcer (K28.-)
peptic ulcer, site unspecified (K27.-)
ulcer of intestine with perforation (K63.1)
ulcer of anus or rectum (K62.6)
ulcerative colitis (K51.-)

Ex: K63.3

K63.4 Enteroptosis

K63.5 Polyp of colon

Excludes1 adenomatous polyp of colon (D12.6)
inflammatory polyp of colon (K51.4-)
polyposis of colon (D12.6)

Coding Clinic: 2015, Q2, P14

K63.8 Other specified diseases of intestine

K63.81 Dieulafoy lesion of intestine

Excludes2 Dieulafoy lesion of stomach and duodenum (K31.82)

Ex: E16.4, I85.01, K22.10-K22.11, K22.6-K22.719, K25.0-K28.9, K29.01, K29.21, K29.31, K29.41, K29.51, K29.61, K29.71, K29.81, K29.91, K31.811, K55.21, K57.01, K57.11, K57.13, K57.21, K57.31, K57.33, K57.41, K57.51, K57.53, K57.81, K57.91, K57.93, K62.5, K63.81, K92.0-K92.2

K63.89 Other specified diseases of intestine
Coding Clinic: 2013, Q2, P31

K63.9 Disease of intestine, unspecified

● **K64 Hemorrhoids and perianal venous thrombosis**

Includes piles

Excludes1 hemorrhoids complicating childbirth and the puerperium (O87.2)
hemorrhoids complicating pregnancy (O22.4)

K64.0 First degree hemorrhoids
Grade/stage I hemorrhoids
Hemorrhoids (bleeding) without prolapse outside of anal canal

K64.1 Second degree hemorrhoids
Grade/stage II hemorrhoids
Hemorrhoids (bleeding) that prolapse with straining, but retract spontaneously

K64.2 Third degree hemorrhoids
Grade/stage III hemorrhoids
Hemorrhoids (bleeding) that prolapse with straining and require manual replacement back inside anal canal

K64.3 Fourth degree hemorrhoids
Grade/stage IV hemorrhoids
Hemorrhoids (bleeding) with prolapsed tissue that cannot be manually replaced

K64.4 Residual hemorrhoidal skin tags
External hemorrhoids, NOS
Skin tags of anus

K64.5 Perianal venous thrombosis
External hemorrhoids with thrombosis
Perianal hematoma
Thrombosed hemorrhoids NOS

K64.8 Other hemorrhoids
Internal hemorrhoids, without mention of degree
Prolapsed hemorrhoids, degree not specified

K64.9 Unspecified hemorrhoids
Hemorrhoids (bleeding) NOS
Hemorrhoids (bleeding) without mention of degree

DISEASES OF PERITONEUM AND RETROPERITONEUM (K65-K68)

● **K65 Peritonitis**

Use additional code (B95-B97), to identify infectious agent

Excludes1 acute appendicitis with generalized peritonitis (K35.2)
aseptic peritonitis (T81.6)
benign paroxysmal peritonitis (E85.0)
chemical peritonitis (T81.6)
diverticulitis of both small and large intestine with peritonitis (K57.4-)
diverticulitis of colon with peritonitis (K57.2-)
diverticulitis of intestine, NOS, with peritonitis (K57.8-)
diverticulitis of small intestine with peritonitis (K57.0-)
gonococcal peritonitis (A54.85)
neonatal peritonitis (P78.0-P78.1)
pelvic peritonitis, female (N73.3-N73.5)
periodic familial peritonitis (E85.0)
peritonitis due to talc or other foreign substance (T81.6)
peritonitis in chlamydia (A74.81)
peritonitis in diphtheria (A36.89)
peritonitis in syphilis (late) (A52.74)
peritonitis in tuberculosis (A18.31)
peritonitis with or following abortion or ectopic or molar pregnancy (O00-O07, O08.0)
peritonitis with or following appendicitis (K35.-)
peritonitis with or following diverticular disease of intestine (K57.-)
puerperal peritonitis (O85)
retroperitoneal infections (K68.-)

Ex: **For category K65 CC codes:** K63.4, K63.89-K63.9, K65.0-K65.9, K67, K68.19-K68.9, K92.89-K92.9, R11.13

Item 11-18 Peritonitis is an inflammation of the lining (peritoneum) of the abdominal cavity and surface of the intestines.

Item 11-19 Retroperitoneal infections occur between the posterior parietal peritoneum and posterior abdominal wall where the kidneys, adrenal glands, ureters, duodenum, ascending colon, descending colon, pancreas, and the large vessels and nerves are located.

K65.0 Generalized (acute) peritonitis
Pelvic peritonitis (acute), male
Subphrenic peritonitis (acute)
Suppurative peritonitis (acute)

K65.1 Peritoneal abscess
Abdominopelvic abscess
Abscess (of) omentum
Abscess (of) peritoneum
Mesenteric abscess
Retrocecal abscess
Subdiaphragmatic abscess
Subhepatic abscess
Subphrenic abscess

K65.2 Spontaneous bacterial peritonitis

Excludes1 bacterial peritonitis NOS (K65.9)

K65.3 Choleperitonitis
Peritonitis due to bile

K65.4 Sclerosing mesenteritis
Fat necrosis of peritoneum
(Idiopathic) sclerosing mesenteric fibrosis
Mesenteric lipodystrophy
Mesenteric panniculitis
Retractile mesenteritis

K65.8 Other peritonitis
Chronic proliferative peritonitis
Peritonitis due to urine

K65.9 Peritonitis, unspecified
Bacterial peritonitis NOS
Coding Clinic: 2013, Q2, P31

● **K66 Other disorders of peritoneum**

Excludes2 ascites (R18.-)
peritoneal effusion (chronic) (R18.8)

K66.0 Peritoneal adhesions (postprocedural) (postinfection)
Adhesions (of) abdominal (wall)
Adhesions (of) diaphragm
Adhesions (of) intestine
Adhesions (of) male pelvis
Adhesions (of) omentum
Adhesions (of) stomach
Adhesive bands
Mesenteric adhesions

Excludes1 female pelvic adhesions [bands] (N73.6)
peritoneal adhesions with intestinal obstruction (K56.5)

K66.1 Hemoperitoneum

Excludes1 traumatic hemoperitoneum (S36.8-)

Ex: K66.1

K66.8 Other specified disorders of peritoneum

K66.9 Disorder of peritoneum, unspecified

▶ ***K67 Disorders of peritoneum in infectious diseases classified elsewhere***

Code first underlying disease, such as:
congenital syphilis (A50.0)
helminthiasis (B65.0-B83.9)

Excludes1 peritonitis in chlamydia (A74.81)
peritonitis in diphtheria (A36.89)
peritonitis in gonococcal (A54.85)
peritonitis in syphilis (late) (A52.74)
peritonitis in tuberculosis (A18.31)

Ex: See K65

● **K68 Disorders of retroperitoneum**

● **K68.1 Retroperitoneal abscess**

K68.11 Postprocedural retroperitoneal abscess
Ex: D78.81-D78.89, E36.8, E89.810-E89.89, H59.011-H59.019, H59.031-H59.099, H59.811-H59.89, H95.811-H95.89, I97.3, K68.11, L76.81-L76.82, M96.89, N98.1-N98.9, T81.4XX[A], T81.82X[A], T81.89X-T81.9XX[A]

K68.12 Psoas muscle abscess
Ex: K68.12, M60.00-M60.19, M61.00-M61.19, M61.30-M61.59, M62.3, M62.50-M62.59, M62.84, M62.89, M72.6

K68.19 Other retroperitoneal abscess
Ex: See K65

K68.9 Other disorders of retroperitoneum
Ex: See K65

DISEASES OF LIVER (K70-K77)

Excludes1 jaundice NOS (R17)
Excludes2 hemochromatosis (E83.11-)
Reye's syndrome (G93.7)
viral hepatitis (B15-B19)
Wilson's disease (E83.0)

● **K70 Alcoholic liver disease**
Use additional code to identify:
alcohol abuse and dependence (F10.-)

K70.0 Alcoholic fatty liver A

● **K70.1 Alcoholic hepatitis**

K70.10 Alcoholic hepatitis without ascites A

K70.11 Alcoholic hepatitis with ascites A

K70.2 Alcoholic fibrosis and sclerosis of liver A

● **K70.3 Alcoholic cirrhosis of liver**
Alcoholic cirrhosis NOS

K70.30 Alcoholic cirrhosis of liver without ascites A

K70.31 Alcoholic cirrhosis of liver with ascites A

● **K70.4 Alcoholic hepatic failure**
Acute alcoholic hepatic failure
Alcoholic hepatic failure NOS
Chronic alcoholic hepatic failure
Subacute alcoholic hepatic failure

K70.40 Alcoholic hepatic failure without coma A

K70.41 Alcoholic hepatic failure with coma A
MCC when PDx is its own MCC
Ex: K72.91, K76.5, K76.89-K76.9

K70.9 Alcoholic liver disease, unspecified A

● **K71 Toxic liver disease**
Includes drug-induced idiosyncratic (unpredictable) liver disease
drug-induced toxic (predictable) liver disease
Code first poisoning due to drug or toxin, if applicable (T36-T65 with fifth or sixth character 1-4 or 6)
Use additional code for adverse effect, if applicable, to identify drug (T36-T50 with fifth or sixth character 5)
Excludes2 alcoholic liver disease (K70.-)
Budd-Chiari syndrome (I82.0)

K71.0 Toxic liver disease with cholestasis
Cholestasis with hepatocyte injury
'Pure' cholestasis

● **K71.1 Toxic liver disease with hepatic necrosis**
Hepatic failure (acute) (chronic) due to drugs

K71.10 Toxic liver disease with hepatic necrosis, without coma

K71.11 Toxic liver disease with hepatic necrosis, with coma
MCC when PDx is its own MCC
Ex: K72.91, K76.5, K76.89-K76.9

Item 11-20 Cirrhosis is the progressive fibrosis of the liver resulting in loss of liver function. The main causes of cirrhosis of the liver are alcohol abuse, chronic hepatitis (inflammation of the liver), biliary disease, and excessive amounts of iron. **Alcoholic cirrhosis of the liver** is also called portal, Laënnec's, or fatty nutritional cirrhosis.

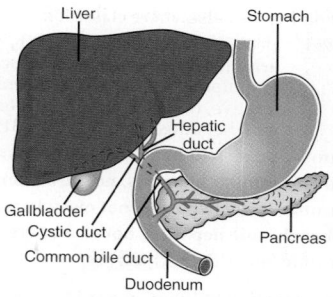

Figure 11-13 Liver and bile ducts.

K71.2 Toxic liver disease with acute hepatitis

K71.3 Toxic liver disease with chronic persistent hepatitis

K71.4 Toxic liver disease with chronic lobular hepatitis

● **K71.5 Toxic liver disease with chronic active hepatitis**
Toxic liver disease with lupoid hepatitis

K71.50 Toxic liver disease with chronic active hepatitis without ascites

K71.51 Toxic liver disease with chronic active hepatitis with ascites

K71.6 Toxic liver disease with hepatitis, not elsewhere classified

K71.7 Toxic liver disease with fibrosis and cirrhosis of liver

K71.8 Toxic liver disease with other disorders of liver
Toxic liver disease with focal nodular hyperplasia
Toxic liver disease with hepatic granulomas
Toxic liver disease with peliosis hepatis
Toxic liver disease with veno-occlusive disease of liver

K71.9 Toxic liver disease, unspecified

● **K72 Hepatic failure, not elsewhere classified**
Includes ~~acute hepatitis NEC, with hepatic failure~~
fulminant hepatitis NEC, with hepatic failure
hepatic encephalopathy NOS
liver (cell) necrosis with hepatic failure
malignant hepatitis NEC, with hepatic failure
yellow liver atrophy or dystrophy
Excludes1 alcoholic hepatic failure (K70.4)
hepatic failure with toxic liver disease (K71.1-)
icterus of newborn (P55-P59)
postprocedural hepatic failure (K91.82)
Excludes2 hepatic failure complicating abortion or ectopic or molar pregnancy (O00-O07, O08.8)
hepatic failure complicating pregnancy, childbirth and the puerperium (O26.6-)
viral hepatitis with hepatic coma (B15-B19) ◀

● **K72.0 Acute and subacute hepatic failure**
Acute non-viral hepatitis NOS ◀
Ex: For category K72.0 CC codes: K72.00-K72.01, K76.2-K76.3, K76.5, K76.89-K76.9
Coding Clinic: 2015, Q2, P17

K72.00 Acute and subacute hepatic failure without coma
Coding Clinic: 2015, Q2, P17

K72.01 Acute and subacute hepatic failure with coma
MCC when PDx is its own MCC

● **K72.1 Chronic hepatic failure**

K72.10 Chronic hepatic failure without coma

K72.11 Chronic hepatic failure with coma
MCC when PDx is its own MCC
Ex: K72.91, K76.5, K76.89-K76.9

● **K72.9 Hepatic failure, unspecified**

K72.90 Hepatic failure, unspecified without coma

K72.91 Hepatic failure, unspecified with coma
Hepatic coma NOS
Ex: K72.91, K76.5, K76.89-K76.9
Coding Clinic: 2016, Q2, P35

● **K73 Chronic hepatitis, not elsewhere classified**

Excludes1 alcoholic hepatitis (chronic) (K70.1-)
drug-induced hepatitis (chronic) (K71.-)
granulomatous hepatitis (chronic) NEC (K75.3)
reactive, nonspecific hepatitis (chronic) (K75.2)
viral hepatitis (chronic) (B15-B19)

K73.0 Chronic persistent hepatitis, not elsewhere classified
K73.1 Chronic lobular hepatitis, not elsewhere classified
K73.2 Chronic active hepatitis, not elsewhere classified
K73.8 Other chronic hepatitis, not elsewhere classified
K73.9 Chronic hepatitis, unspecified

● **K74 Fibrosis and cirrhosis of liver**

Code also, if applicable, viral hepatitis (acute) (chronic) (B15-B19)

Excludes1 alcoholic cirrhosis (of liver) (K70.3)
alcoholic fibrosis of liver (K70.2)
cardiac sclerosis of liver (K76.1)
cirrhosis (of liver) with toxic liver disease (K71.7)
congenital cirrhosis (of liver) (P78.81)
pigmentary cirrhosis (of liver) (E83.110)

K74.0 Hepatic fibrosis
K74.1 Hepatic sclerosis
K74.2 Hepatic fibrosis with hepatic sclerosis
K74.3 Primary biliary cirrhosis
Chronic nonsuppurative destructive cholangitis
K74.4 Secondary biliary cirrhosis
K74.5 Biliary cirrhosis, unspecified
● **K74.6 Other and unspecified cirrhosis of liver**
K74.60 Unspecified cirrhosis of liver
Cirrhosis (of liver) NOS
K74.69 Other cirrhosis of liver
Cryptogenic cirrhosis (of liver)
Macronodular cirrhosis (of liver)
Micronodular cirrhosis (of liver)
Mixed type cirrhosis (of liver)
Portal cirrhosis (of liver)
Postnecrotic cirrhosis (of liver)

● **K75 Other inflammatory liver diseases**

Excludes2 toxic liver disease (K71.-)

K75.0 Abscess of liver
Cholangitic hepatic abscess
Hematogenic hepatic abscess
Hepatic abscess NOS
Lymphogenic hepatic abscess
Pylephlebitic hepatic abscess

Excludes1 amebic liver abscess (A06.4)
cholangitis without liver abscess (K83.0)
pylephlebitis without liver abscess (K75.1)

Excludes2 acute or subacute hepatitis NOS (B17.9) ◀
acute or subacute non-viral hepatitis (K72.0) ◀
chronic hepatitis NEC (K73.8) ◀

Ex: A06.4, K75.0-K75.1, K76.5, K76.89-K76.9

K75.1 Phlebitis of portal vein
Pylephlebitis

Excludes1 pylephlebitic liver abscess (K75.0)

Ex: A06.4, K75.0-K75.1, K76.5, K76.89-K76.9

K75.2 Nonspecific reactive hepatitis

Excludes1 acute or subacute hepatitis (K72.0-)
chronic hepatitis NEC (K73.-)
viral hepatitis (B15-B19)

K75.3 Granulomatous hepatitis, not elsewhere classified

Excludes1 acute or subacute hepatitis (K72.0-)
chronic hepatitis NEC (K73.-)
viral hepatitis (B15-B19)

K75.4 Autoimmune hepatitis
Lupoid hepatitis NEC
● **K75.8 Other specified inflammatory liver diseases**
K75.81 Nonalcoholic steatohepatitis (NASH)
K75.89 Other specified inflammatory liver diseases
K75.9 Inflammatory liver disease, unspecified
Hepatitis NOS

Excludes1 acute or subacute hepatitis (K72.0-)
chronic hepatitis NEC (K73.-)
viral hepatitis (B15-B19)

Coding Clinic: 2015, Q2, P17

● **K76 Other diseases of liver**

Excludes2 alcoholic liver disease (K70.-)
amyloid degeneration of liver (E85.-)
cystic disease of liver (congenital) (Q44.6)
hepatic vein thrombosis (I82.0)
hepatomegaly NOS (R16.0)
pigmentary cirrhosis (of liver) (E83.110)
portal vein thrombosis (I81)
toxic liver disease (K71.-)

K76.0 Fatty (change of) liver, not elsewhere classified
Nonalcoholic fatty liver disease (NAFLD)

Excludes1 nonalcoholic steatohepatitis (NASH) (K75.81)

K76.1 Chronic passive congestion of liver
Cardiac cirrhosis
Cardiac sclerosis
K76.2 Central hemorrhagic necrosis of liver

Excludes1 liver necrosis with hepatic failure (K72.-)

Ex: K72.00-K72.01, K76.2-K76.3, K76.5, K76.89-K76.9

K76.3 Infarction of liver

Ex: See K76.2

K76.4 Peliosis hepatis
Hepatic angiomatosis
K76.5 Hepatic veno-occlusive disease

Excludes1 Budd-Chiari syndrome (I82.0)

K76.6 Portal hypertension

Use additional code for any associated complications, such as:
portal hypertensive gastropathy (K31.89)

Ex: K72.91, K76.5-K76.6, K76.89-K76.9

K76.7 Hepatorenal syndrome

Excludes1 hepatorenal syndrome following labor and delivery (O90.4)
postprocedural hepatorenal syndrome (K91.83) ◀

Ex: K76.5, K76.7, K76.89-K76.9

● **K76.8 Other specified diseases of liver**
● **K76.81 Hepatopulmonary syndrome**
Code first underlying liver disease, such as:
alcoholic cirrhosis of liver (K70.3-)
cirrhosis of liver without mention of alcohol (K74.6-)
K76.89 Other specified diseases of liver
Cyst (simple) of liver
Focal nodular hyperplasia of liver
Hepatoptosis
K76.9 Liver disease, unspecified

◗ ***K77 Liver disorders in diseases classified elsewhere***

Code first underlying disease, such as:
amyloidosis (E85.-)
congenital syphilis (A50.0, A50.5)
congenital toxoplasmosis (P37.1)
schistosomiasis (B65.0-B65.9)

Excludes1 alcoholic hepatitis (K70.1-)
alcoholic liver disease (K70.-)
cytomegaloviral hepatitis (B25.1)
herpesviral [herpes simplex] hepatitis (B00.81)
infectious mononucleosis with liver disease (B27.0-B27.9 with .9)
mumps hepatitis (B26.81)
sarcoidosis with liver disease (D86.89)
secondary syphilis with liver disease (A51.45)
syphilis (late) with liver disease (A52.74)
toxoplasmosis (acquired) hepatitis (B58.1)
tuberculosis with liver disease (A18.83)

Ex: No exclusions

DISORDERS OF GALLBLADDER, BILIARY TRACT AND PANCREAS (K80–K87)

K80 Cholelithiasis
Presence or formation of gallstones
Excludes1 retained cholelithiasis following cholecystectomy (K91.86)

K80.0 Calculus of gallbladder with acute cholecystitis
Any condition listed in K80.2 with acute cholecystitis
Check documentation for acute/chronic gallbladder/common bile duct either with or without obstruction.

K80.00 Calculus of gallbladder with acute cholecystitis without obstruction
Ex: K80.00-K80.21, K80.40, K80.44, K80.62-K80.63, K80.66-K80.67, K80.80, K81.0-K81.9, K82.9, K83.5-K83.9, K87

K80.01 Calculus of gallbladder with acute cholecystitis with obstruction
Ex: K80.00-K80.21, K80.62-K80.63, K80.66-K80.67, K80.80, K81.0-K81.9, K82.9, K83.5-K83.9, K87

K80.1 Calculus of gallbladder with other cholecystitis
Ex: For category K80.1 CC codes unless otherwise indicated: See K80.01

K80.10 Calculus of gallbladder with chronic cholecystitis without obstruction
Cholelithiasis with cholecystitis NOS

K80.11 Calculus of gallbladder with chronic cholecystitis with obstruction

K80.12 Calculus of gallbladder with acute and chronic cholecystitis without obstruction
Ex: See K80.00

K80.13 Calculus of gallbladder with acute and chronic cholecystitis with obstruction

K80.18 Calculus of gallbladder with other cholecystitis without obstruction

K80.19 Calculus of gallbladder with other cholecystitis with obstruction

K80.2 Calculus of gallbladder without cholecystitis
Cholecystolithiasis without cholecystitis
Cholelithiasis (without cholecystitis)
Colic (recurrent) of gallbladder (without cholecystitis)
Gallstone (impacted) of cystic duct (without cholecystitis)
Gallstone (impacted) of gallbladder (without cholecystitis)

K80.20 Calculus of gallbladder without cholecystitis without obstruction

K80.21 Calculus of gallbladder without cholecystitis with obstruction
Ex: See K80.01

K80.3 Calculus of bile duct with cholangitis
Any condition listed in K80.5 with cholangitis

K80.30 Calculus of bile duct with cholangitis, unspecified, without obstruction
CC when PDx is its own CC
Ex: K83.0, K83.5-K83.9, K87

K80.31 Calculus of bile duct with cholangitis, unspecified, with obstruction
CC when PDx is its own CC
Ex: K80.30-K80.71, K80.81-K81.9, K83.5-K83.9, K87

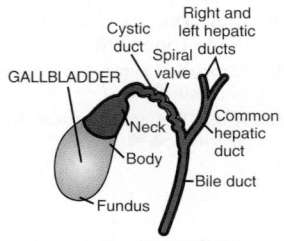

Figure 11-14 Gallbladder and bile ducts.

K80.32 Calculus of bile duct with acute cholangitis without obstruction
CC when PDx is its own CC
Ex: See K80.30

K80.33 Calculus of bile duct with acute cholangitis with obstruction
CC when PDx is its own CC
Ex: See K80.31

K80.34 Calculus of bile duct with chronic cholangitis without obstruction
CC when PDx is its own CC
Ex: See K80.30

K80.35 Calculus of bile duct with chronic cholangitis with obstruction
CC when PDx is its own CC
Ex: See K80.31

K80.36 Calculus of bile duct with acute and chronic cholangitis without obstruction
CC when PDx is its own CC
Ex: See K80.30

K80.37 Calculus of bile duct with acute and chronic cholangitis with obstruction
CC when PDx is its own CC
Ex: See K80.31

K80.4 Calculus of bile duct with cholecystitis
Any condition listed in K80.5 with cholecystitis (with cholangitis)
Ex: For category K80.4 CC codes: K80.30-K80.71, K80.81-K81.9, K83.5-K83.9, K87

K80.40 Calculus of bile duct with cholecystitis, unspecified, without obstruction

K80.41 Calculus of bile duct with cholecystitis, unspecified, with obstruction

K80.42 Calculus of bile duct with acute cholecystitis without obstruction

K80.43 Calculus of bile duct with acute cholecystitis with obstruction

K80.44 Calculus of bile duct with chronic cholecystitis without obstruction

K80.45 Calculus of bile duct with chronic cholecystitis with obstruction

K80.46 Calculus of bile duct with acute and chronic cholecystitis without obstruction

K80.47 Calculus of bile duct with acute and chronic cholecystitis with obstruction

K80.5 Calculus of bile duct without cholangitis or cholecystitis
Choledocholithiasis (without cholangitis or cholecystitis)
Gallstone (impacted) of bile duct NOS (without cholangitis or cholecystitis)
Gallstone (impacted) of common duct (without cholangitis or cholecystitis)
Gallstone (impacted) of hepatic duct (without cholangitis or cholecystitis)
Hepatic cholelithiasis (without cholangitis or cholecystitis)
Hepatic colic (recurrent) (without cholangitis or cholecystitis)

K80.50 Calculus of bile duct without cholangitis or cholecystitis without obstruction

K80.51 Calculus of bile duct without cholangitis or cholecystitis with obstruction
Ex: See K80.4

K80.6 Calculus of gallbladder and bile duct with cholecystitis

K80.60 Calculus of gallbladder and bile duct with cholecystitis, unspecified, without obstruction
Ex: See K80.4

K80.61 Calculus of gallbladder and bile duct with cholecystitis, unspecified, with obstruction
Ex: See K80.4

K80.62 Calculus of gallbladder and bile duct with acute cholecystitis without obstruction
Ex: K80.62-K80.63, K81.0-K81.9, K82.9, K83.5-K83.9, K87

K80.63 Calculus of gallbladder and bile duct with acute cholecystitis with obstruction
(Ex) See K80.62

K80.64 Calculus of gallbladder and bile duct with chronic cholecystitis without obstruction
(Ex) See K80.4

K80.65 Calculus of gallbladder and bile duct with chronic cholecystitis with obstruction
(Ex) See K80.4

K80.66 Calculus of gallbladder and bile duct with acute and chronic cholecystitis without obstruction
(Ex) K80.66-K80.67, K81.0-K81.9, K82.9, K83.5-K83.9, K87

K80.67 Calculus of gallbladder and bile duct with acute and chronic cholecystitis with obstruction
(Ex) See K80.66

● **K80.7 Calculus of gallbladder and bile duct without cholecystitis**

K80.70 Calculus of gallbladder and bile duct without cholecystitis without obstruction

K80.71 Calculus of gallbladder and bile duct without cholecystitis with obstruction
(Ex) See K80.4

● **K80.8 Other cholelithiasis**

K80.80 Other cholelithiasis without obstruction

K80.81 Other cholelithiasis with obstruction
(Ex) See K80.4

● **K81 Cholecystitis**
Chronic or acute inflammation of the gallbladder
Excludes1 cholecystitis with cholelithiasis (K80.-)

K81.0 Acute cholecystitis
Abscess of gallbladder
Angiocholecystitis
Emphysematous (acute) cholecystitis
Empyema of gallbladder
Gangrene of gallbladder
Gangrenous cholecystitis
Suppurative cholecystitis
(Ex) K80.00, K80.12, K80.62-K80.63, K80.66-K80.67, K81.0-K81.9, K82.9, K83.5-K83.9, K87

K81.1 Chronic cholecystitis

K81.2 Acute cholecystitis with chronic cholecystitis
(Ex) K81.0-K81.9, K82.9, K83.5-K83.9, K87

K81.9 Cholecystitis, unspecified

● **K82 Other diseases of gallbladder**
Excludes1 nonvisualization of gallbladder (R93.2)
postcholecystectomy syndrome (K91.5)
(Ex) **For category K82 CC codes:** K82.0-K82.9, K83.5-K83.9, K87

K82.0 Obstruction of gallbladder
Occlusion of cystic duct or gallbladder without cholelithiasis
Stenosis of cystic duct or gallbladder without cholelithiasis
Stricture of cystic duct or gallbladder without cholelithiasis
Excludes1 obstruction of gallbladder with cholelithiasis (K80.-)

K82.1 Hydrops of gallbladder
Mucocele of gallbladder

K82.2 Perforation of gallbladder
Rupture of cystic duct or gallbladder

K82.3 Fistula of gallbladder
Cholecystocolic fistula
Cholecystoduodenal fistula

K82.4 Cholesterolosis of gallbladder
Strawberry gallbladder
Excludes1 cholesterolosis of gallbladder with cholecystitis (K81.-)
cholesterolosis of gallbladder with cholelithiasis (K80.-)

K82.8 Other specified diseases of gallbladder
Adhesions of cystic duct or gallbladder
Atrophy of cystic duct or gallbladder
Cyst of cystic duct or gallbladder
Dyskinesia of cystic duct or gallbladder
Hypertrophy of cystic duct or gallbladder
Nonfunctioning of cystic duct or gallbladder
Ulcer of cystic duct or gallbladder

K82.9 Disease of gallbladder, unspecified

● **K83 Other diseases of biliary tract**
Excludes1 postcholecystectomy syndrome (K91.5)
Excludes2 conditions involving the gallbladder (K81-K82)
conditions involving the cystic duct (K81-K82)

K83.0 Cholangitis
Ascending cholangitis
Cholangitis NOS
Primary cholangitis
Recurrent cholangitis
Sclerosing cholangitis
Secondary cholangitis
Stenosing cholangitis
Suppurative cholangitis
Excludes1 cholangitic liver abscess (K75.0)
cholangitis with choledocholithiasis (K80.3-, K80.4-)
chronic nonsuppurative destructive cholangitis (K74.3)
(Ex) K83.0, K83.5-K83.9, K87

K83.1 Obstruction of bile duct
Occlusion of bile duct without cholelithiasis
Stenosis of bile duct without cholelithiasis
Stricture of bile duct without cholelithiasis
Excludes1 congenital obstruction of bile duct (Q44.3)
obstruction of bile duct with cholelithiasis (K80.-)
(Ex) K80.31, K80.33, K80.35, K80.37, K80.41, K80.43, K80.45, K80.47, K80.51, K80.81, K83.1, K83.5-K83.9, K87, Q44.2-Q44.3
Coding Clinic: 2016, Q1, P18

K83.2 Perforation of bile duct
Rupture of bile duct
(Ex) K83.2-K83.3, K83.5-K83.9, K87

K83.3 Fistula of bile duct
Choledochoduodenal fistula
(Ex) K83.2-K83.3, K83.5-K83.9, K87

K83.4 Spasm of sphincter of Oddi

K83.5 Biliary cyst

K83.8 Other specified diseases of biliary tract
Adhesions of biliary tract
Atrophy of biliary tract
Hypertrophy of biliary tract
Ulcer of biliary tract

K83.9 Disease of biliary tract, unspecified

● **K85 Acute pancreatitis**
Inflammatory process in which pancreatic enzymes autodigest the gland
Includes ~~abscess of pancreas~~
~~acute necrosis of pancreas~~
acute (recurrent) pancreatitis
~~gangrene of (gangrenous) pancreas~~
~~hemorrhagic pancreatitis~~
~~infective necrosis of pancreas~~
subacute pancreatitis
~~suppurative pancreatitis~~
(Ex) **For category K85 CC codes:** B25.2, K86.0-K86.1, K86.81-K86.9

● **K85.0 Idiopathic acute pancreatitis**

K85.00 Idiopathic acute pancreatitis without necrosis or infection ◀

K85.01 Idiopathic acute pancreatitis with uninfected necrosis ◀

K85.02 Idiopathic acute pancreatitis with infected necrosis ◀

● **K85.1 Biliary acute pancreatitis**
Gallstone pancreatitis

K85.10 Biliary acute pancreatitis without necrosis or infection ◀

K85.11 Biliary acute pancreatitis with uninfected necrosis ◀

K85.12 Biliary acute pancreatitis with infected necrosis ◀

● **K85.2 Alcohol induced acute pancreatitis**
Excludes2 alcohol induced chronic pancreatitis (K86.0)

K85.20 Alcohol induced acute pancreatitis without necrosis or infection ◀

K85.21 Alcohol induced acute pancreatitis with uninfected necrosis ◀

K85.22 Alcohol induced acute pancreatitis with infected necrosis ◀

● **K85.3 Drug induced acute pancreatitis**
Use additional code for adverse effect, if applicable, to identify drug (T36-T50 with fifth or sixth character 5)
Use additional code to identify drug abuse and dependence (F11.-F17.-)

K85.30 Drug induced acute pancreatitis without necrosis or infection ◀

K85.31 Drug induced acute pancreatitis with uninfected necrosis ◀

K85.32 Drug induced acute pancreatitis with infected necrosis ◀

● **K85.8 Other acute pancreatitis**

K85.80 Other acute pancreatitis without necrosis or infection ◀

K85.81 Other acute pancreatitis with uninfected necrosis ◀

K85.82 Other acute pancreatitis with infected necrosis ◀

● **K85.9 Acute pancreatitis, unspecified**
Pancreatitis NOS

K85.90 Acute pancreatitis without necrosis or infection, unspecified ◀

K85.91 Acute pancreatitis with uninfected necrosis, unspecified ◀

K85.92 Acute pancreatitis with infected necrosis, unspecified ◀

● **K86 Other diseases of pancreas**
Excludes2 fibrocystic disease of pancreas (E84.-)
islet cell tumor (of pancreas) (D13.7)
pancreatic steatorrhea (K90.3)

K86.0 Alcohol-induced chronic pancreatitis
Use additional code to identify:
alcohol abuse and dependence (F10.-)
Code also exocrine pancreatic insufficiency (K86.81) ◀
Excludes2 alcohol induced acute pancreatitis (K85.2-)
Ex: B25.2, E16.8, K85.00-K86.9

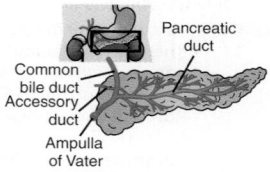

Figure 11-15 Pancreatic ductal system.

K86.1 Other chronic pancreatitis
Chronic pancreatitis NOS
Infectious chronic pancreatitis
Recurrent chronic pancreatitis
Relapsing chronic pancreatitis
Code also exocrine pancreatic insufficiency (K86.81) ◀
Ex: B25.2, E16.8, K85.00-K86.9

K86.2 Cyst of pancreas
Ex: K86.2-K86.9

K86.3 Pseudocyst of pancreas
Ex: K86.2-K86.9

● **K86.8 Other specified diseases of pancreas**

K86.81 Exocrine pancreatic insufficiency ◀

K86.89 Other specified diseases of pancreas ◀
Aseptic pancreatic necrosis, unrelated to acute pancreatitis ◀
Atrophy of pancreas ◀
Calculus of pancreas ◀
Cirrhosis of pancreas ◀
Fibrosis of pancreas ◀
Pancreatic fat necrosis, unrelated to acute pancreatitis ◀
Pancreatic infantilism ◀
Pancreatic necrosis NOS, unrelated to acute pancreatitis ◀

K86.9 Disease of pancreas, unspecified

▶ ***K87 Disorders of gallbladder, biliary tract and pancreas in diseases classified elsewhere***
Code first underlying disease
Excludes1 cytomegaloviral pancreatitis (B25.2)
mumps pancreatitis (B26.3)
syphilitic gallbladder (A52.74)
syphilitic pancreas (A52.74)
tuberculosis of gallbladder (A18.83)
tuberculosis of pancreas (A18.83)

OTHER DISEASES OF THE DIGESTIVE SYSTEM (K90-K95)

● **K90 Intestinal malabsorption**
Excludes1 intestinal malabsorption following gastrointestinal surgery (K91.2)
Ex: **For category K90 cc does unless otherwise indicated:** E84.19, K90.0-K90.49, K90.89-K90.9, K91.2

K90.0 Celiac disease
Celiac disease with steatorrhea ◀
Gluten-sensitive enteropathy
~~Idiopathic steatorrhea~~
Nontropical sprue
Use additional code for associated disorders including:
dermatitis herpetiformis (L13.0)
gluten ataxia (G32.81)
Code also exocrine pancreatic insufficiency (K86.81) ◀

K90.1 Tropical sprue
Sprue NOS
Tropical steatorrhea

K90.2 Blind loop syndrome, not elsewhere classified
Blind loop syndrome NOS
Excludes1 congenital blind loop syndrome (Q43.8)
postsurgical blind loop syndrome (K91.2)

K90.3 Pancreatic steatorrhea

● **K90.4 Other malabsorption due to intolerance**
Excludes2 gluten-sensitive enteropathy (K90.0)
lactose intolerance (E73.-)
Ex: **For category K90.4 CC codes:** E84.19, K90.0-K90.3, K90.41, K90.49, K90.89-K90.9, K91.2

K90.41 Non-celiac gluten sensitivity ◀
Gluten sensitivity NOS ◀
Non-celiac gluten sensitive enteropathy ◀

K90.49 Malabsorption due to intolerance, not elsewhere classified ◀
Malabsorption due to intolerance to carbohydrate ◀
Malabsorption due to intolerance to fat ◀
Malabsorption due to intolerance to protein ◀
Malabsorption due to intolerance to starch ◀

● **K90.8 Other intestinal malabsorption**

K90.81 Whipple's disease
Ex: K90.81

K90.89 Other intestinal malabsorption

K90.9 Intestinal malabsorption, unspecified

● **K91 Intraoperative and postprocedural complications and disorders of digestive system, not elsewhere classified**

Excludes2 complications of artificial opening of digestive system (K94.-)
complications of bariatric procedures (K95.-)
gastrojejunal ulcer (K28.-)
postprocedural (radiation) retroperitoneal abscess (K68.11)
radiation colitis (K52.0)
radiation gastroenteritis (K52.0)
radiation proctitis (K62.7)

K91.0 Vomiting following gastrointestinal surgery

K91.1 Postgastric surgery syndromes
Dumping syndrome
Postgastrectomy syndrome
Postvagotomy syndrome

K91.2 Postsurgical malabsorption, not elsewhere classified
Postsurgical blind loop syndrome

Excludes1 malabsorption osteomalacia in adults (M83.2)
malabsorption osteoporosis, postsurgical (M80.8-, M81.8)

Ex: K90.3-K90.49, K90.89-K90.9, K91.2

K91.3 Postprocedural intestinal obstruction
Ex: D78.81-D78.89, E36.8, E89.810-E89.89, H59.011-H59.019, H59.031-H59.099, H59.811-H59.89, H95.811-H95.89, I97.3, K91.3, K91.81-K91.83, K91.850-K91.89, K94.20-K95.89, L76.81-L76.82, M96.89, N98.1-N98.9, T81.710[A], T81.82X[A], T81.89X-T81.9XX[A]

K91.5 Postcholecystectomy syndrome

● **K91.6 Intraoperative hemorrhage and hematoma of a digestive system organ or structure complicating a procedure**

Excludes1 intraoperative hemorrhage and hematoma of a digestive system organ or structure due to accidental puncture and laceration during a procedure (K91.7-)

Ex: **For category K91.6 CC codes:** H95.811-H95.89, I85.01, I85.11, I97.3, K21.9, K22.8, K23-K25.0, K25.2, K25.4, K25.6, K26.0, K26.2, K26.4, K26.6, K27.0, K27.2, K27.4, K27.6, K28.0, K28.2, K28.4, K28.6, K29.01, K29.21, K29.31, K29.41, K29.51, K29.61, K29.71, K29.81, K29.91, K31.811, K55.21, K57.01, K57.11, K57.13, K57.21, K57.31, K57.33, K57.41, K57.51, K57.53, K57.81, K57.91, K57.93, K62.5, K91.61-K91.62, K91.840-K91.841, K91.870-K91.873, K92.0-K92.2, M96.89, N98.1-N98.9, P54.1-P54.3, T81.10X-T81.19X[A], T81.82X[A], T81.89X-T81.9XX[A]

K91.61 Intraoperative hemorrhage and hematoma of a digestive system organ or structure complicating a digestive system procedure

K91.62 Intraoperative hemorrhage and hematoma of a digestive system organ or structure complicating other procedure

● **K91.7 Accidental puncture and laceration of a digestive system organ or structure during a procedure**

Ex: **For category K91.7 CC codes:** D78.11-D78.12, D78.81-D78.89, E36.11-E36.8, E89.810-E89.89, G96.11, G97.41-G97.49, H59.011-H59.019, H59.031-H59.099, H59.211-H59.229, H59.811-H59.89, H95.31-H95.32, H95.811-H95.89, I97.3, I97.51-I97.52, J95.71-J95.72, K91.71-K91.72, L76.11-L76.12, L76.81-L76.82, M96.820-M96.821, M96.89, N98.1-N98.9, N99.71-N99.72, T81.82X[A], T81.89X-T81.9XX[A]

K91.71 Accidental puncture and laceration of a digestive system organ or structure during a digestive system procedure

K91.72 Accidental puncture and laceration of a digestive system organ or structure during other procedure

● **K91.8 Other intraoperative and postprocedural complications and disorders of digestive system**

Ex: **For category K91.8 CC codes unless otherwise indicated:** See K91.3

K91.81 Other intraoperative complications of digestive system

K91.82 Postprocedural hepatic failure

K91.83 Postprocedural hepatorenal syndrome

● **K91.84 Postprocedural hemorrhage of a digestive system organ or structure following a procedure**

Ex: **For category K91.84 CC codes:** K91.6

K91.840 Postprocedural hemorrhage of a digestive system organ or structure following a digestive system procedure
Coding Clinic: 2016, Q1, P15

K91.841 Postprocedural hemorrhage of a digestive system organ or structure following other procedure

● **K91.85 Complications of intestinal pouch**

K91.850 Pouchitis
Inflammation of internal ileoanal pouch

K91.858 Other complications of intestinal pouch

K91.86 Retained cholelithiasis following cholecystectomy

● **K91.87 Postprocedural hematoma and seroma of a digestive system organ or structure following a procedure**

Ex: **For category K97.87 CC codes:** See K91.6

K91.870 Postprocedural hematoma of a digestive system organ or structure following a digestive system procedure

K91.871 Postprocedural hematoma of a digestive system organ or structure following other procedure

K91.872 Postprocedural seroma of a digestive system organ or structure following a digestive system procedure

K91.873 Postprocedural seroma of a digestive system organ or structure following other procedure

K91.89 Other postprocedural complications and disorders of digestive system
Use additional code, if applicable, to further specify disorder

Excludes2 postprocedural retroperitoneal abscess (K68.11)

● **K92 Other diseases of digestive system**

Excludes1 neonatal gastrointestinal hemorrhage (P54.0-P54.3)

Ex: **For category K92 CC codes unless otherwise indicated:** E16.4, I85.01, K22.10-K22.11, K22.6-K22.719, K25.0-K28.9, K29.01, K29.21, K29.31, K29.41, K29.51, K29.61, K29.71, K29.81, K29.91, K31.811, K55.21, K57.01, K57.11, K57.13, K57.21, K57.31, K57.33, K57.41, K57.51, K57.53, K57.81, K57.91, K57.93, K62.5, K92.0-K92.2

K92.0 Hematemesis

K92.1 Melena

Excludes1 occult blood in feces (R19.5)

K92.2 Gastrointestinal hemorrhage, unspecified
Gastric hemorrhage NOS
Intestinal hemorrhage NOS

Excludes1 acute hemorrhagic gastritis (K29.01)
hemorrhage of anus and rectum (K62.5)
angiodysplasia of stomach with hemorrhage (K31.811)
diverticular disease with hemorrhage (K57.-)
gastritis and duodenitis with hemorrhage (K29.-)
peptic ulcer with hemorrhage (K25-K28)

K92.8 Other specified diseases of the digestive system

K92.81 Gastrointestinal mucositis (ulcerative)

Code also type of associated therapy, such as:
antineoplastic and immunosuppressive drugs (T45.1X-)
radiological procedure and radiotherapy (Y84.2)

Excludes2 mucositis (ulcerative) of vagina and vulva (N76.81)
nasal mucositis (ulcerative) (J34.81)
oral mucositis (ulcerative) (K12.3-)

Ex: E16.4, I85.01, K22.10-K22.11, K22.6-K22.719, K25.0-K28.9, K29.01, K29.21, K29.31, K29.41, K29.51, K29.61, K29.71, K29.81, K29.91, K31.811, K31.89-K31.9, K55.21, K57.01, K57.11, K57.13, K57.21, K57.31, K57.33, K57.41, K57.51, K57.53, K57.81, K57.91, K57.93, K62.5, K92.0-K92.81

K92.89 Other specified diseases of the digestive system

K92.9 Disease of digestive system, unspecified

K94 Complications of artificial openings of the digestive system

K94.0 Colostomy complications

Ex: For category K94.0 CC does unless otherwise indicated: K94.00-K94.19

K94.00 Colostomy complication, unspecified

K94.01 Colostomy hemorrhage

K94.02 Colostomy infection

Use additional code to specify type of infection, such as:
cellulitis of abdominal wall (L03.311)
sepsis (A40.-, A41.-)

K94.03 Colostomy malfunction

Mechanical complication of colostomy

Ex: D78.81-D78.89, E36.8, E89.810-E89.89, H59.011-H59.019, H59.031-H59.099, H59.811-H59.89, H95.811-H95.89, I97.3, K91.3, K91.81-K91.83, K91.850-K91.89, K94.00-K95.89, L76.81-L76.82, M96.89, N98.1-N98.9, T81.710[A], T81.82X[A], T81.89X-T81.9XX[A]

K94.09 Other complications of colostomy

K94.1 Enterostomy complications

Ex: For category K94.1 CC does unless otherwise indicated: K94.00-K94.19

K94.10 Enterostomy complication, unspecified

K94.11 Enterostomy hemorrhage

K94.12 Enterostomy infection

Use additional code to specify type of infection, such as:
cellulitis of abdominal wall (L03.311)
sepsis (A40.-, A41.-)

K94.13 Enterostomy malfunction

Mechanical complication of enterostomy

Ex: See K94.03

K94.19 Other complications of enterostomy

K94.2 Gastrostomy complications

K94.20 Gastrostomy complication, unspecified

K94.21 Gastrostomy hemorrhage

K94.22 Gastrostomy infection

Use additional code to specify type of infection, such as:
cellulitis of abdominal wall (L03.311)
sepsis (A40.-, A41.-)

Ex: See K91.3

K94.23 Gastrostomy malfunction

Mechanical complication of gastrostomy

Ex: See K91.3

K94.29 Other complications of gastrostomy

K94.3 Esophagostomy complications

Ex: For category K94.3 CC codes: See K91.3

K94.30 Esophagostomy complications, unspecified

K94.31 Esophagostomy hemorrhage

K94.32 Esophagostomy infection

Use additional code to identify the infection

K94.33 Esophagostomy malfunction

Mechanical complication of esophagostomy

K94.39 Other complications of esophagostomy

K95 Complications of bariatric procedures

Ex: For category K95 CC codes: See K91.3

K95.0 Complications of gastric band procedure

K95.01 Infection due to gastric band procedure

Use additional code to specify type of infection or organism, such as:
bacterial and viral infectious agents (B95.-, B96.-)
cellulitis of abdominal wall (L03.311)
sepsis (A40.-, A41.-)

K95.09 Other complications of gastric band procedure

Use additional code, if applicable, to further specify complication

K95.8 Complications of other bariatric procedure

Excludes1 complications of gastric band surgery (K95.0-)

K95.81 Infection due to other bariatric procedure

Use additional code to specify type of infection or organism, such as:
bacterial and viral infectious agents (B95.-, B96.-)
cellulitis of abdominal wall (L03.311)
sepsis (A40.-, A41.-)

K95.89 Other complications of other bariatric procedure

Use additional code, if applicable, to further specify complication

CHAPTER 12

DISEASES OF THE SKIN AND SUBCUTANEOUS TISSUE (L00-L99)

OGCR Chapter-Specific Coding Guidelines

12. Chapter 12: Diseases of the Skin and Subcutaneous Tissue (L00-L99)

a. Pressure ulcer stage codes

1) Pressure ulcer stages

Codes from category L89, Pressure ulcer, identify the site of the pressure ulcer as well as the stage of the ulcer.

The ICD-10-CM classifies pressure ulcer stages based on severity, which is designated by stages 1-4, unspecified stage and unstageable.

Assign as many codes from category L89 as needed to identify all the pressure ulcers the patient has, if applicable.

2) Unstageable pressure ulcers

Assignment of the code for unstageable pressure ulcer (L89.--0) should be based on the clinical documentation. These codes are used for pressure ulcers whose stage cannot be clinically determined (e.g., the ulcer is covered by eschar or has been treated with a skin or muscle graft) and pressure ulcers that are documented as deep tissue injury but not documented as due to trauma. This code should not be confused with the codes for unspecified stage (L89.--9). When there is no documentation regarding the stage of the pressure ulcer, assign the appropriate code for unspecified stage (L89.--9).

3) Documented pressure ulcer stage

Assignment of the pressure ulcer stage code should be guided by clinical documentation of the stage or documentation of the terms found in the Alphabetic Index. For clinical terms describing the stage that are not found in the Alphabetic Index, and there is no documentation of the stage, the provider should be queried.

4) Patients admitted with pressure ulcers documented as healed

No code is assigned if the documentation states that the pressure ulcer is completely healed.

5) Patients admitted with pressure ulcers documented as healing

Pressure ulcers described as healing should be assigned the appropriate pressure ulcer stage code based on the documentation in the medical record. If the documentation does not provide information about the stage of the healing pressure ulcer, assign the appropriate code for unspecified stage.

If the documentation is unclear as to whether the patient has a current (new) pressure ulcer or if the patient is being treated for a healing pressure ulcer, query the provider.

For ulcers that were present on admission but healed at the time of discharge, assign the code for the site and stage of the pressure ulcer at the time of admission.

6) Patient admitted with pressure ulcer evolving into another stage during the admission

If a patient is admitted with a pressure ulcer at one stage and it progresses to a higher stage, **two separate codes should be assigned: one code for the site and stage of the ulcer on admission and a second code for the same ulcer site and the highest stage reported during the stay.**

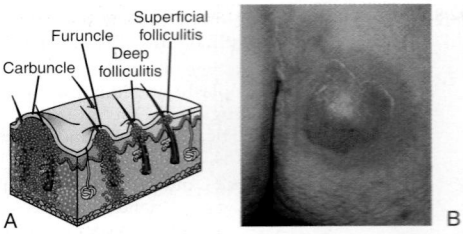

Figure 12-1 Furuncle, also known as a boil, is a staphylococcal infection. The organism enters the body through a hair follicle and so furuncles usually appear in hairy areas of the body. A cluster of furuncles is known as a carbuncle and involves infection into the deep subcutaneous fascia. These usually appear on the back and neck. (**B** from Habif: Clinical Dermatology, ed 5, Mosby, 2009)

CHAPTER 12

DISEASES OF THE SKIN AND SUBCUTANEOUS TISSUE (L00-L99)

Excludes2
- certain conditions originating in the perinatal period (P04-P96)
- certain infectious and parasitic diseases (A00-B99)
- complications of pregnancy, childbirth and the puerperium (O00-O9A)
- congenital malformations, deformations, and chromosomal abnormalities (Q00-Q99)
- endocrine, nutritional and metabolic diseases (E00-E88)
- lipomelanotic reticulosis (I89.8)
- neoplasms (C00-D49)
- symptoms, signs and abnormal clinical and laboratory findings, not elsewhere classified (R00-R94)
- systemic connective tissue disorders (M30-M36)
- viral warts (B07.-)

This chapter contains the following blocks:

L00-L08	Infections of the skin and subcutaneous tissue
L10-L14	Bullous disorders
L20-L30	Dermatitis and eczema
L40-L45	Papulosquamous disorders
L49-L54	Urticaria and erythema
L55-L59	Radiation-related disorders of the skin and subcutaneous tissue
L60-L75	Disorders of skin appendages
L76	Intraoperative and postprocedural complications of skin and subcutaneous tissue
L80-L99	Other disorders of the skin and subcutaneous tissue

INFECTIONS OF THE SKIN AND SUBCUTANEOUS TISSUE (L00-L08)

Use additional code (B95-B97) to identify infectious agent.

Excludes2 hordeolum (H00.0)
infective dermatitis (L30.3)
local infections of skin classified in Chapter 1
lupus panniculitis (L93.2)
panniculitis NOS (M79.3)
panniculitis of neck and back (M54.0-)
Perlèche NOS (K13.0)
Perlèche due to candidiasis (B37.0)
Perlèche due to riboflavin deficiency (E53.0)
pyogenic granuloma (L98.0)
relapsing panniculitis [Weber-Christian] (M35.6)
viral warts (B07.-)
zoster (B02.-)

L00 Staphylococcal scalded skin syndrome
Ritter's disease

Use additional code to identify percentage of skin exfoliation (L49.-)

Excludes1 bullous impetigo (L01.03)
pemphigus neonatorum (L01.03)
toxic epidermal necrolysis [Lyell] (L51.2)

L01 Impetigo
Contagious skin infection caused by a streptococcus or staphylococcus aureus, common skin infections among children

Excludes1 impetigo herpetiformis (L40.1)

L01.0 Impetigo
Impetigo contagiosa
Impetigo vulgaris

L01.00 Impetigo, unspecified
Impetigo NOS

L01.01 Non-bullous impetigo

L01.02 Bockhart's impetigo
Impetigo follicularis
Perifolliculitis NOS
Superficial pustular perifolliculitis

L01.03 Bullous impetigo
Impetigo neonatorum
Pemphigus neonatorum
Neonate = newborn

L01.09 Other impetigo
Ulcerative impetigo

L01.1 Impetiginization of other dermatoses

L02 Cutaneous abscess, furuncle and carbuncle

Use additional code to identify organism (B95-B96)

Excludes2 abscess of anus and rectal regions (K61.-)
abscess of female genital organs (external) (N76.4)
abscess of male genital organs (external) (N48.2, N49.-)

L02.0 Cutaneous abscess, furuncle and carbuncle of face

Excludes2 abscess of ear, external (H60.0)
abscess of eyelid (H00.0)
abscess of head [any part, except face] (L02.8)
abscess of lacrimal gland (H04.0)
abscess of lacrimal passages (H04.3)
abscess of mouth (K12.2)
abscess of nose (J34.0)
abscess of orbit (H05.0)
submandibular abscess (K12.2)

L02.01 Cutaneous abscess of face
Ex: No exclusions

L02.02 Furuncle of face
Boil of face
Folliculitis of face

L02.03 Carbuncle of face

L02.1 Cutaneous abscess, furuncle and carbuncle of neck

L02.11 Cutaneous abscess of neck
Ex: A17.9, A18.4, A18.82, A18.84, A18.89, A48.2-A48.4, A48.8-A49.9, B78.1, B95.0-B96.89, E83.2, L02.11, L02.811-L02.818, L02.91, L03.221-L03.222, L03.811-L03.91, L08.0-L08.9, L44.8-L45, L73.2, L88, L92.8, L94.2, L94.4, L98.0, L98.3, L98.7, L98.8, L99, Z16.10-Z16.39

L02.12 Furuncle of neck
Boil of neck
Folliculitis of neck

L02.13 Carbuncle of neck

L02.2 Cutaneous abscess, furuncle and carbuncle of trunk

Excludes1 non-newborn omphalitis (L08.82)
omphalitis of newborn (P38.-)

Excludes2 abscess of breast (N61.1)
abscess of buttocks (L02.3)
abscess of female external genital organs (N76.4)
abscess of male external genital organs (N48.2, N49.-)
abscess of hip (L02.4)

L02.21 Cutaneous abscess of trunk
Ex: **For category L02.21 CC codes:** A17.9, A18.4, A18.82, A18.84, A18.89, A48.2-A48.4, A48.8-A49.9, B78.1, B95.0-B96.89, E83.2, L02.211-L02.219, L02.811-L02.818, L02.91, L03.311-L03.316, L03.319-L03.326, L03.329-L03.91, L08.0, L08.81-L08.9, L44.8-L45, L73.2, L88, L92.8, L94.2, L94.4, L98.0, L98.3, L98.7, L98.8, L99, Z16.10-Z16.39

L02.211 Cutaneous abscess of abdominal wall

L02.212 Cutaneous abscess of back [any part, except buttock]

L02.213 Cutaneous abscess of chest wall

L02.214 Cutaneous abscess of groin

L02.215 Cutaneous abscess of perineum

L02.216 Cutaneous abscess of umbilicus

L02.219 Cutaneous abscess of trunk, unspecified

L02.22 Furuncle of trunk
Boil of trunk
Folliculitis of trunk

L02.221 Furuncle of abdominal wall

L02.222 Furuncle of back [any part, except buttock]

L02.223 Furuncle of chest wall

L02.224 Furuncle of groin

L02.225 Furuncle of perineum

L02.226 Furuncle of umbilicus

L02.229 Furuncle of trunk, unspecified

L02.23 Carbuncle of trunk

L02.231 Carbuncle of abdominal wall

L02.232 Carbuncle of back [any part, except buttock]

L02.233 Carbuncle of chest wall

L02.234 Carbuncle of groin

L02.235 Carbuncle of perineum

L02.236 Carbuncle of umbilicus

L02.239 Carbuncle of trunk, unspecified

L02.3 Cutaneous abscess, furuncle and carbuncle of buttock

Excludes1 pilonidal cyst with abscess (L05.01)

L02.31 Cutaneous abscess of buttock
Cutaneous abscess of gluteal region
Ex: A17.9, A18.4, A18.82, A18.84, A18.89, A48.2-A48.4, A48.8-A49.9, B78.1, B95.0-B96.89, E83.2, L02.31, L02.811-L02.818, L02.91, L03.317, L03.327, L03.811-L03.91, L08.0, L08.81-L08.9, L44.8-L45, L73.2, L88, L92.8, L94.2, L94.4, L98.0, L98.3, L98.7, L98.8, L99, Z16.10-Z16.39

L02.32 Furuncle of buttock
Boil of buttock
Folliculitis of buttock
Furuncle of gluteal region

L02.33 Carbuncle of buttock
Carbuncle of gluteal region

● **L02.4 Cutaneous abscess, furuncle and carbuncle of limb**
Excludes2 Cutaneous abscess, furuncle and carbuncle of groin (L02.214, L02.224, L02.234)
Cutaneous abscess, furuncle and carbuncle of hand (L02.5-)
Cutaneous abscess, furuncle and carbuncle of foot (L02.6-)

● **L02.41 Cutaneous abscess of limb**

L02.411 Cutaneous abscess of right axilla
Ex: A17.9, A18.4, A18.82, A18.84, A18.89, A48.2-A48.4, A48.8-A49.9, B78.1, B95.0-B96.89, E83.2, L02.411-L02.414, L02.811-L02.818, L02.91, L03.111-L03.114, L03.121-L03.124, L03.811-L03.91, L08.0, L08.81-L08.9, L44.8-L45, L73.2, L88, L92.8, L94.2, L94.4, L98.0, L98.3, L98.7, L98.8, L99, Z16.10-Z16.39

L02.412 Cutaneous abscess of left axilla
Ex: See L02.411

L02.413 Cutaneous abscess of right upper limb
Ex: See L02.411

L02.414 Cutaneous abscess of left upper limb
Ex: See L02.411

L02.415 Cutaneous abscess of right lower limb
Ex: A17.9, A18.4, A18.82, A18.84, A18.89, A48.2-A48.4, A48.8-A49.9, B78.1, B95.0-B96.89, E83.2, L02.415-L02.419, L02.811-L02.818, L02.91, L03.115-L03.119, L03.125-L03.129, L03.811-L03.91, L08.0, L08.81-L08.9, L44.8-L45, L73.2, L88, L92.8, L94.2, L94.4, L98.0, L98.3, L98.7, L98.8, L99, Z16.10-Z16.39

L02.416 Cutaneous abscess of left lower limb
Ex: See L02.415

L02.419 Cutaneous abscess of limb, unspecified
Ex: See L02.415

● **L02.42 Furuncle of limb**
Boil of limb
Folliculitis of limb

L02.421 Furuncle of right axilla
L02.422 Furuncle of left axilla
L02.423 Furuncle of right upper limb
L02.424 Furuncle of left upper limb
L02.425 Furuncle of right lower limb
L02.426 Furuncle of left lower limb
L02.429 Furuncle of limb, unspecified

● **L02.43 Carbuncle of limb**

L02.431 Carbuncle of right axilla
L02.432 Carbuncle of left axilla
L02.433 Carbuncle of right upper limb
L02.434 Carbuncle of left upper limb
L02.435 Carbuncle of right lower limb
L02.436 Carbuncle of left lower limb
L02.439 Carbuncle of limb, unspecified

● **L02.5 Cutaneous abscess, furuncle and carbuncle of hand**

● **L02.51 Cutaneous abscess of hand**
Ex: For category L02.51 CC codes: A17.9, A18.4, A18.82, A18.84, A18.89, A48.2-A48.4, A48.8-A49.9, B78.1, B95.0-B96.89, E83.2, L02.511-L02.519, L02.811-L02.818, L02.91, L03.811-L03.91, L08.0, L08.81-L08.9, L44.8-L45, L73.2, L88, L92.8, L94.2, L94.4, L98.0, L98.3, L98.7, L98.8, L99, Z16.10-Z16.39

L02.511 Cutaneous abscess of right hand
L02.512 Cutaneous abscess of left hand
L02.519 Cutaneous abscess of unspecified hand

● **L02.52 Furuncle hand**
Boil of hand
Folliculitis of hand

L02.521 Furuncle right hand
L02.522 Furuncle left hand
L02.529 Furuncle unspecified hand

● **L02.53 Carbuncle of hand**

L02.531 Carbuncle of right hand
L02.532 Carbuncle of left hand
L02.539 Carbuncle of unspecified hand

● **L02.6 Cutaneous abscess, furuncle and carbuncle of foot**

● **L02.61 Cutaneous abscess of foot**
Ex: For category L02.61 CC codes: A17.9, A18.4, A18.82, A18.84, A18.89, A48.2-A48.4, A48.8-A49.9, B78.1, B95.0-B96.89, E83.2, L02.611-L02.619, L02.811-L02.818, L02.91, L03.811-L03.91, L08.0, L08.81-L08.9, L44.8-L45, L73.2, L88, L92.8, L94.2, L94.4, L98.0, L98.3, L98.7, L98.8, L99, Z16.10-Z16.39

L02.611 Cutaneous abscess of right foot
L02.612 Cutaneous abscess of left foot
L02.619 Cutaneous abscess of unspecified foot

● **L02.62 Furuncle of foot**
Boil of foot
Folliculitis of foot

L02.621 Furuncle of right foot
L02.622 Furuncle of left foot
L02.629 Furuncle of unspecified foot

● **L02.63 Carbuncle of foot**

L02.631 Carbuncle of right foot
L02.632 Carbuncle of left foot
L02.639 Carbuncle of unspecified foot

● **L02.8 Cutaneous abscess, furuncle and carbuncle of other sites**

● **L02.81 Cutaneous abscess of other sites**
Ex: For category L02.81 CC codes: A17.9, A18.4, A18.82, A18.84, A18.89, A48.2-A48.4, A48.8-A49.9, B78.1, B95.0-B96.89, E83.2, L02.811-L02.818, L02.91, L03.811-L03.91, L08.0, L08.81-L08.9, L44.8-L45, L73.2, L88, L92.8, L94.2, L94.4, L98.0, L98.3, L98.7, L98.8, L99, Z16.10-Z16.39

L02.811 Cutaneous abscess of head [any part, except face]
L02.818 Cutaneous abscess of other sites

● **L02.82 Furuncle of other sites**
Boil of other sites
Folliculitis of other sites

L02.821 Furuncle of head [any part, except face]
L02.828 Furuncle of other sites

● **L02.83 Carbuncle of other sites**

L02.831 Carbuncle of head [any part, except face]
L02.838 Carbuncle of other sites

● **L02.9 Cutaneous abscess, furuncle and carbuncle, unspecified**

L02.91 Cutaneous abscess, unspecified
Ex: See L02.81

L02.92 Furuncle, unspecified
Boil NOS
Furunculosis NOS

L02.93 Carbuncle, unspecified

Item 12-1 **Onychia** is an inflammation of the tissue surrounding the nail with pus accumulation and loss of the nail, resulting from microscopic pathogens entering through small wounds. **Paronychia** is a nail disease also known as felon or whitlow and is a bacterial or fungal infection.

L03 Cellulitis and acute lymphangitis

Excludes2 cellulitis of anal and rectal region (K61.-)
cellulitis of external auditory canal (H60.1)
cellulitis of eyelid (H00.0)
cellulitis of female external genital organs (N76.4)
cellulitis of lacrimal apparatus (H04.3)
cellulitis of male external genital organs (N48.2, N49.-)
cellulitis of mouth (K12.2)
cellulitis of nose (J34.0)
eosinophilic cellulitis [Wells] (L98.3)
febrile neutrophilic dermatosis [Sweet] (L98.2)
lymphangitis (chronic) (subacute) (I89.1)

L03.0 Cellulitis and acute lymphangitis of finger and toe
Infection of nail
Onychia
Paronychia
Perionychia

L03.01 Cellulitis of finger
Felon
Whitlow

Excludes1 herpetic whitlow (B00.89)

L03.011 Cellulitis of right finger
L03.012 Cellulitis of left finger
L03.019 Cellulitis of unspecified finger

L03.02 Acute lymphangitis of finger
Hangnail with lymphangitis of finger

L03.021 Acute lymphangitis of right finger
L03.022 Acute lymphangitis of left finger
L03.029 Acute lymphangitis of unspecified finger

L03.03 Cellulitis of toe

L03.031 Cellulitis of right toe
L03.032 Cellulitis of left toe
L03.039 Cellulitis of unspecified toe

L03.04 Acute lymphangitis of toe
Hangnail with lymphangitis of toe

L03.041 Acute lymphangitis of right toe
L03.042 Acute lymphangitis of left toe
L03.049 Acute lymphangitis of unspecified toe

L03.1 Cellulitis and acute lymphangitis of other parts of limb

L03.11 Cellulitis of other parts of limb

Excludes2 cellulitis of fingers (L03.01-)
cellulitis of toes (L03.03-)
groin (L03.314)

L03.111 Cellulitis of right axilla
Ex: See L02.411

L03.112 Cellulitis of left axilla
Ex: See L02.411

L03.113 Cellulitis of right upper limb
Ex: See L02.411

L03.114 Cellulitis of left upper limb
Ex: See L02.411

L03.115 Cellulitis of right lower limb
Ex: See L02.415

L03.116 Cellulitis of left lower limb
Ex: See L02.415

L03.119 Cellulitis of unspecified part of limb
Ex: See L02.415

L03.12 Acute lymphangitis of other parts of limb

Excludes2 acute lymphangitis of fingers (L03.2-)
acute lymphangitis of toes (L03.04-)
acute lymphangitis of groin (L03.324)

L03.121 Acute lymphangitis of right axilla
Ex: See L02.411

L03.122 Acute lymphangitis of left axilla
Ex: See L02.411

L03.123 Acute lymphangitis of right upper limb
Ex: See L02.411

L03.124 Acute lymphangitis of left upper limb
Ex: See L02.411

L03.125 Acute lymphangitis of right lower limb
Ex: See L02.415

L03.126 Acute lymphangitis of left lower limb
Ex: See L02.415

L03.129 Acute lymphangitis of unspecified part of limb
Ex: See L02.415

L03.2 Cellulitis and acute lymphangitis of face and neck

L03.21 Cellulitis and acute lymphangitis of face

L03.211 Cellulitis of face

Excludes2 abscess of orbit (H05.01-) ◀
cellulitis of ear (H60.1-)
cellulitis of eyelid (H00.0-)
cellulitis of head (L03.81)
cellulitis of lacrimal apparatus (H04.3)
cellulitis of lip (K13.0)
cellulitis of mouth (K12.2)
cellulitis of nose (internal) (J34.0)
cellulitis of orbit (H05.01-) ◀
cellulitis of scalp (L03.81)

Ex: A17.9, A18.4, A18.82, A18.84, A18.89, A48.2-A48.4, A48.8-A49.9, B78.1, B95.0-B96.89, E83.2, L02.811-L02.818, L02.91, L03.211, L03.213, L03.811-L03.91, L08.0, L08.81-L08.9, L44.8-L45, L73.2, L88, L92.8, L94.2, L94.4, L98.0, L98.3, L98.7, L98.8, L99, Z16.10-Z16.39

L03.212 Acute lymphangitis of face
Ex: No exclusions

L03.213 Periorbital cellulitis ◀
Preseptal cellulitis ◀
Ex: See L03.211

L03.22 Cellulitis and acute lymphangitis of neck
Ex: For category L03.22 CC codes: See L02.11

L03.221 Cellulitis of neck
L03.222 Acute lymphangitis of neck

Item 12–2 Cellulitis is an acute spreading bacterial infection below the surface of the skin characterized by redness (erythema), warmth, swelling, pain, fever, chills, and enlarged lymph nodes ("swollen glands").

● **L03.3 Cellulitis and acute lymphangitis of trunk**

● **L03.31 Cellulitis of trunk**

Excludes2 cellulitis of anal and rectal regions (K61.-)
cellulitis of breast NOS (N61.0) ◀
cellulitis of female external genital organs (N76.4)
cellulitis of male external genital organs (N48.2, N49.-)
omphalitis of newborn (P38.-)
puerperal cellulitis of breast (O91.2)

Ex: **For category L03.31 CC codes unless otherwise indicated:** See L02.21

L03.311 Cellulitis of abdominal wall

Excludes2 cellulitis of umbilicus (L03.316)
cellulitis of groin (L03.314)

L03.312 Cellulitis of back [any part except buttock]

L03.313 Cellulitis of chest wall

L03.314 Cellulitis of groin

L03.315 Cellulitis of perineum

L03.316 Cellulitis of umbilicus

L03.317 Cellulitis of buttock

Ex: See L02.31

L03.319 Cellulitis of trunk, unspecified

● **L03.32 Acute lymphangitis of trunk**

Ex: **For category L03.32 CC codes unless otherwise indicated:** See L02.21

L03.321 Acute lymphangitis of abdominal wall

L03.322 Acute lymphangitis of back [any part except buttock]

L03.323 Acute lymphangitis of chest wall

L03.324 Acute lymphangitis of groin

L03.325 Acute lymphangitis of perineum

L03.326 Acute lymphangitis of umbilicus

L03.327 Acute lymphangitis of buttock

Ex: See L02.31

L03.329 Acute lymphangitis of trunk, unspecified

● **L03.8 Cellulitis and acute lymphangitis of other sites**

Ex: **For category L03.8 CC codes:** See L02.81

● **L03.81 Cellulitis of other sites**

L03.811 Cellulitis of head [any part, except face]
Cellulitis of scalp

Excludes2 cellulitis of face (L03.211)

L03.818 Cellulitis of other sites

● **L03.89 Acute lymphangitis of other sites**

L03.891 Acute lymphangitis of head [any part, except face]

L03.898 Acute lymphangitis of other sites

● **L03.9 Cellulitis and acute lymphangitis, unspecified**

Ex: **For category L03.9 CC codes:** See L02.81

L03.90 Cellulitis, unspecified

L03.91 Acute lymphangitis, unspecified

Excludes1 lymphangitis NOS (I89.1)

● **L04 Acute lymphadenitis**

Short-term inflammation of lymph nodes which can be regionalized to involve a given area of the lymph system or systemic involving much of the body

Includes abscess (acute) of lymph nodes, except mesenteric
acute lymphadenitis, except mesenteric

Excludes1 chronic or subacute lymphadenitis, except mesenteric (I88.1)
enlarged lymph nodes (R59.-)
human immunodeficiency virus [HIV] disease resulting in generalized lymphadenopathy (B20)
lymphadenitis NOS (I88.9)
nonspecific mesenteric lymphadenitis (I88.0)

L04.0 Acute lymphadenitis of face, head and neck

L04.1 Acute lymphadenitis of trunk

L04.2 Acute lymphadenitis of upper limb
Acute lymphadenitis of axilla
Acute lymphadenitis of shoulder

L04.3 Acute lymphadenitis of lower limb
Acute lymphadenitis of hip

Excludes2 acute lymphadenitis of groin (L04.1)

L04.8 Acute lymphadenitis of other sites

L04.9 Acute lymphadenitis, unspecified

● **L05 Pilonidal cyst and sinus**

● **L05.0 Pilonidal cyst and sinus with abscess**

Ex: **For category L05.0 CC codes:** L05.01-L05.92, L44.8-L45, L94.2, L94.4, L98.7, L98.8, L99

L05.01 Pilonidal cyst with abscess
Pilonidal abscess
Pilonidal dimple with abscess
Postanal dimple with abscess

Excludes2 congenital sacral dimple (Q82.6) ◀
parasacral dimple (Q82.6) ◀

L05.02 Pilonidal sinus with abscess
Coccygeal fistula with abscess
Coccygeal sinus with abscess
Pilonidal fistula with abscess

● **L05.9 Pilonidal cyst and sinus without abscess**

L05.91 Pilonidal cyst without abscess
Pilonidal dimple
Postanal dimple
Pilonidal cyst NOS

Excludes2 congenital sacral dimple (Q82.6) ◀
parasacral dimple (Q82.6) ◀

L05.92 Pilonidal sinus without abscess
Coccygeal fistula
Coccygeal sinus without abscess
Pilonidal fistula

● **L08 Other local infections of skin and subcutaneous tissue**

L08.0 Pyoderma
Dermatitis gangrenosa
Purulent dermatitis
Septic dermatitis
Suppurative dermatitis

Excludes1 pyoderma gangrenosum (L88)
pyoderma vegetans (L08.81)

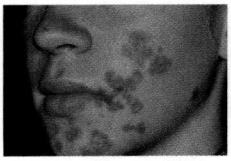

Figure 12-2 Impetigo. A thick, honey-yellow adherent crust covers the entire eroded surface. (From Habif: Clinical Dermatology, ed 4, Mosby, Inc., 2004)

Item 12–3 Abscess is a localized collection of pus in tissues or organs and is a sign of infection resulting in swelling and inflammation.

Item 12–4 Pilonidal cyst, also called a coccygeal cyst, is the result of a disorder called pilonidal disease. The cyst usually contains hair and pus.

L08.1 Erythrasma
Ex A42.81-A42.9, A43.1-A43.9, B47.1, L08.

L08.8 Other specified local infections of the skin and subcutaneous tissue
L08.81 Pyoderma vegetans
Excludes1 pyoderma gangrenosum (L88)
pyoderma NOS (L08.0)
L08.82 Omphalitis not of newborn
Excludes1 omphalitis of newborn (P38.-)
L08.89 Other specified local infections of the skin and subcutaneous tissue
L08.9 Local infection of the skin and subcutaneous tissue, unspecified

BULLOUS DISORDERS (L10-L14)

Excludes1 benign familial pemphigus [Hailey-Hailey] (Q82.8)
staphylococcal scalded skin syndrome (L00)
toxic epidermal necrolysis [Lyell] (L51.2)

L10 Pemphigus
Excludes1 pemphigus neonatorum (L01.03)
Ex For category L10 CC codes: L10.0-L10.9, L12.0-L12.1, L12.8-L12.9, L13.8-L14, L44.8-L45, L94.2, L94.4, L98.7, L98.8, L99
L10.0 Pemphigus vulgaris
L10.1 Pemphigus vegetans
L10.2 Pemphigus foliaceous
L10.3 Brazilian pemphigus [fogo selvagem]
L10.4 Pemphigus erythematosus
Senear-Usher syndrome
L10.5 Drug-induced pemphigus
Use additional code for adverse effect, if applicable, to identify drug (T36-T50 with fifth or sixth character 5)
L10.8 Other pemphigus
L10.81 Paraneoplastic pemphigus
L10.89 Other pemphigus
L10.9 Pemphigus, unspecified

L11 Other acantholytic disorders
L11.0 Acquired keratosis follicularis
Excludes1 keratosis follicularis (congenital) [Darier-White] (Q82.8)
L11.1 Transient acantholytic dermatosis [Grover]
L11.8 Other specified acantholytic disorders
L11.9 Acantholytic disorder, unspecified

L12 Pemphigoid
Excludes1 herpes gestationis (O26.4-)
impetigo herpetiformis (L40.1)
L12.0 Bullous pemphigoid
Ex See L10
L12.1 Cicatricial pemphigoid
Benign mucous membrane pemphigoid
L12.2 Chronic bullous disease of childhood P
Juvenile dermatitis herpetiformis
L12.3 Acquired epidermolysis bullosa
Excludes1 epidermolysis bullosa (congenital) (Q81.-)
Ex For category L12.3 CC codes: L00, L12.30-L12.35, L26, L30.4, L44.8-L45, L51.0-L54, L71.0-L71.9, L92.0, L93.0-L93.2, L94.2, L94.4, L95.1, L98.2, L98.7, L98.8, L99
L12.30 Acquired epidermolysis bullosa, unspecified
L12.31 Epidermolysis bullosa due to drug
Use additional code for adverse effect, if applicable, to identify drug (T36-T50 with fifth or sixth character 5)
L12.35 Other acquired epidermolysis bullosa
L12.8 Other pemphigoid
Ex See L10
L12.9 Pemphigoid, unspecified
Ex See L10

L13 Other bullous disorders
L13.0 Dermatitis herpetiformis
Duhring's disease
Hydroa herpetiformis
Excludes1 juvenile dermatitis herpetiformis (L12.2)
senile dermatitis herpetiformis (L12.0)
L13.1 Subcorneal pustular dermatitis
Sneddon-Wilkinson disease
L13.8 Other specified bullous disorders
L13.9 Bullous disorder, unspecified

L14 Bullous disorders in diseases classified elsewhere
Code first underlying disease

DERMATITIS AND ECZEMA (L20-L30)

Note: In this block the terms dermatitis and eczema are used synonymously and interchangeably.

Excludes2 chronic (childhood) granulomatous disease (D71)
dermatitis gangrenosa (L08.0)
dermatitis herpetiformis (L13.0)
dry skin dermatitis (L85.3)
factitial dermatitis (L98.1)
perioral dermatitis (L71.0)
radiation-related disorders of the skin and subcutaneous tissue (L55-L59)
stasis dermatitis (I87.2)

L20 Atopic dermatitis
L20.0 Besnier's prurigo
L20.8 Other atopic dermatitis
Excludes2 circumscribed neurodermatitis (L28.0)
L20.81 Atopic neurodermatitis
Diffuse neurodermatitis
L20.82 Flexural eczema
L20.83 Infantile (acute) (chronic) eczema P
L20.84 Intrinsic (allergic) eczema
L20.89 Other atopic dermatitis
L20.9 Atopic dermatitis, unspecified

L21 Seborrheic dermatitis
Excludes2 infective dermatitis (L30.3)
seborrheic keratosis (L82.-)
L21.0 Seborrhea capitis P
Cradle cap
L21.1 Seborrheic infantile dermatitis P
L21.8 Other seborrheic dermatitis
L21.9 Seborrheic dermatitis, unspecified
Seborrhea NOS

Item 12–5 Dermatitis herpetiformis, also known as Duhring's disease, is a systemic disease characterized by small blisters (3 to 5 mm) and occasionally large bullae (> 5 mm).

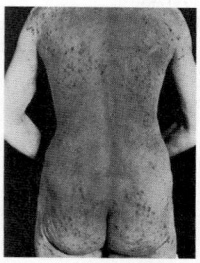

Figure 12-3 Dermatitis herpetiformis. (From Arnold HL, Odom RB, James WD: Andrews' Diseases of the Skin, Clinical Dermatology, ed 8, Philadelphia, WB Saunders, 1990)

Item 12–6 Seborrheic dermatitis is characterized by greasy, scaly, red patches and is associated with oily skin and scalp.

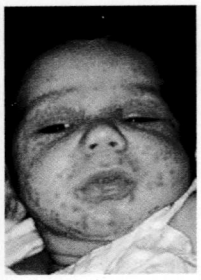

Figure 12-4 Seborrheic dermatitis. (From Cohen BA: Atlas of Pediatric Dermatology, St. Louis, Mosby, 1993)

Item 12–7 Atopic dermatitis, also known as atopic eczema, infantile eczema, disseminated neuro dermatitis, flexural eczema, and *prurigo diathesique* (Besnier), is characterized by intense itching and is often hereditary.

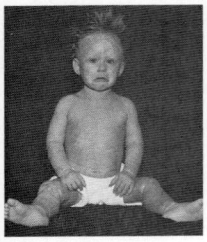

Figure 12-5 Atopic dermatitis. (From Moschella SL, Hurley HJ: Dermatology, ed 3, Philadelphia, WB Saunders, 1993)

L22 Diaper dermatitis
Diaper erythema
Diaper rash
Psoriasiform diaper rash

● **L23 Allergic contact dermatitis**
Excludes1 allergy NOS (T78.4Ø)
contact dermatitis NOS (L25.9)
dermatitis NOS (L3Ø.9)
Excludes2 dermatitis due to substances taken internally (L27.-)
dermatitis of eyelid (HØ1.1-)
diaper dermatitis (L22)
eczema of external ear (H6Ø.5-)
irritant contact dermatitis (L24.-)
perioral dermatitis (L71.Ø)
radiation-related disorders of the skin and subcutaneous tissue (L55-L59)

L23.Ø Allergic contact dermatitis due to metals
Allergic contact dermatitis due to chromium
Allergic contact dermatitis due to nickel

L23.1 Allergic contact dermatitis due to adhesives

L23.2 Allergic contact dermatitis due to cosmetics

L23.3 Allergic contact dermatitis due to drugs in contact with skin
Use additional code for adverse effect, if applicable, to identify drug (T36-T5Ø with fifth or sixth character 5)
Excludes2 dermatitis due to ingested drugs and medicaments (L27.Ø-L27.1)

L23.4 Allergic contact dermatitis due to dyes

L23.5 Allergic contact dermatitis due to other chemical products
Allergic contact dermatitis due to cement
Allergic contact dermatitis due to insecticide
Allergic contact dermatitis due to plastic
Allergic contact dermatitis due to rubber

L23.6 Allergic contact dermatitis due to food in contact with the skin
Excludes2 dermatitis due to ingested food (L27.2)

L23.7 Allergic contact dermatitis due to plants, except food
Excludes2 allergy NOS due to pollen (J3Ø.1)

● **L23.8 Allergic contact dermatitis due to other agents**

L23.81 Allergic contact dermatitis due to animal (cat) (dog) dander
Allergic contact dermatitis due to animal (cat) (dog) hair

L23.89 Allergic contact dermatitis due to other agents

L23.9 Allergic contact dermatitis, unspecified cause
Allergic contact eczema NOS

● **L24 Irritant contact dermatitis**
Excludes1 allergy NOS (T78.4Ø)
contact dermatitis NOS (L25.9)
dermatitis NOS (L3Ø.9)
Excludes2 allergic contact dermatitis (L23.-)
dermatitis due to substances taken internally (L27.-)
dermatitis of eyelid (HØ1.1-)
diaper dermatitis (L22)
eczema of external ear (H6Ø.5-)
perioral dermatitis (L71.Ø)
radiation-related disorders of the skin and subcutaneous tissue (L55-L59)

L24.Ø Irritant contact dermatitis due to detergents

L24.1 Irritant contact dermatitis due to oils and greases

L24.2 Irritant contact dermatitis due to solvents
Irritant contact dermatitis due to chlorocompound
Irritant contact dermatitis due to cyclohexane
Irritant contact dermatitis due to ester
Irritant contact dermatitis due to glycol
Irritant contact dermatitis due to hydrocarbon
Irritant contact dermatitis due to ketone

L24.3 Irritant contact dermatitis due to cosmetics

L24.4 Irritant contact dermatitis due to drugs in contact with skin
Use additional code for adverse effect, if applicable, to identify drug (T36-T5Ø with fifth or sixth character 5)

L24.5 Irritant contact dermatitis due to other chemical products
Irritant contact dermatitis due to cement
Irritant contact dermatitis due to insecticide
Irritant contact dermatitis due to plastic
Irritant contact dermatitis due to rubber

L24.6 Irritant contact dermatitis due to food in contact with skin
Excludes2 dermatitis due to ingested food (L27.2)

L24.7 Irritant contact dermatitis due to plants, except food
Excludes2 allergy NOS to pollen (J3Ø.1)

● **L24.8 Irritant contact dermatitis due to other agents**

L24.81 Irritant contact dermatitis due to metals
Irritant contact dermatitis due to chromium
Irritant contact dermatitis due to nickel

L24.89 Irritant contact dermatitis due to other agents
Irritant contact dermatitis due to dyes

L24.9 Irritant contact dermatitis, unspecified cause
Irritant contact eczema NOS

◀ New ⇐ Revised ~~deleted~~ Deleted Excludes 1 Excludes 2 Includes Use additional Code first Code also Unspecified
OGCR Official Guidelines ● Unacceptable Principal Diagnosis X Assign placeholder X ● Use Additional Character(s) ▶ Manifestation Code Coding Clinic

L25 Unspecified contact dermatitis

Excludes1 allergic contact dermatitis (L23.-)
allergy NOS (T78.40)
dermatitis NOS (L30.9)
irritant contact dermatitis (L24.-)

Excludes2 dermatitis due to ingested substances (L27.-)
dermatitis of eyelid (H01.1-)
eczema of external ear (H60.5-)
perioral dermatitis (L71.0)
radiation-related disorders of the skin and subcutaneous tissue (L55-L59)

L25.0 Unspecified contact dermatitis due to cosmetics

L25.1 Unspecified contact dermatitis due to drugs in contact with skin

Use additional code for adverse effect, if applicable, to identify drug (T36-T50 with fifth or sixth character 5)

Excludes2 dermatitis due to ingested drugs and medicaments (L27.0-L27.1)

L25.2 Unspecified contact dermatitis due to dyes

L25.3 Unspecified contact dermatitis due to other chemical products

Unspecified contact dermatitis due to cement
Unspecified contact dermatitis due to insecticide

L25.4 Unspecified contact dermatitis due to food in contact with skin

Excludes2 dermatitis due to ingested food (L27.2)

L25.5 Unspecified contact dermatitis due to plants, except food

Excludes1 nettle rash (L50.9)

Excludes2 allergy NOS due to pollen (J30.1)

L25.8 Unspecified contact dermatitis due to other agents

L25.9 Unspecified contact dermatitis, unspecified cause

Contact dermatitis (occupational) NOS
Contact eczema (occupational) NOS

L26 Exfoliative dermatitis

Hebra's pityriasis

Excludes1 Ritter's disease (L00)

L27 Dermatitis due to substances taken internally

Excludes1 allergy NOS (T78.40)

Excludes2 adverse food reaction, except dermatitis (T78.0-T78.1)
contact dermatitis (L23-L25)
drug photoallergic response (L56.1)
drug phototoxic response (L56.0)
urticaria (L50.-)

L27.0 Generalized skin eruption due to drugs and medicaments taken internally

Use additional code for adverse effect, if applicable, to identify drug (T36-T50 with fifth or sixth character 5)

L27.1 Localized skin eruption due to drugs and medicaments taken internally

Use additional code for adverse effect, if applicable, to identify drug (T36-T50 with fifth or sixth character 5)

L27.2 Dermatitis due to ingested food

Excludes2 dermatitis due to food in contact with skin (L23.6, L24.6, L25.4)

L27.8 Dermatitis due to other substances taken internally

L27.9 Dermatitis due to unspecified substance taken internally

L28 Lichen simplex chronicus and prurigo

L28.0 Lichen simplex chronicus

Circumscribed neurodermatitis
Lichen NOS

L28.1 Prurigo nodularis

L28.2 Other prurigo

Prurigo NOS
Prurigo Hebra
Prurigo mitis
Urticaria papulosa

L29 Pruritus

Excludes1 neurotic excoriation (L98.1)
psychogenic pruritus (F45.8)

L29.0 Pruritus ani

L29.1 Pruritus scroti ♂

L29.2 Pruritus vulvae ♀

L29.3 Anogenital pruritus, unspecified

L29.8 Other pruritus

L29.9 Pruritus, unspecified

Itch NOS

L30 Other and unspecified dermatitis

Excludes2 contact dermatitis (L23-L25)
dry skin dermatitis (L85.3)
small plaque parapsoriasis (L41.3)
stasis dermatitis (I87.2)

L30.0 Nummular dermatitis

L30.1 Dyshidrosis [pompholyx]

L30.2 Cutaneous autosensitization

Candidid [levurid]
Dermatophytid
Eczematid

L30.3 Infective dermatitis

Infectious eczematoid dermatitis

L30.4 Erythema intertrigo

L30.5 Pityriasis alba

L30.8 Other specified dermatitis

L30.9 Dermatitis, unspecified

Eczema NOS

PAPULOSQUAMOUS DISORDERS (L40-L45)

L40 Psoriasis

L40.0 Psoriasis vulgaris

Nummular psoriasis
Plaque psoriasis

L40.1 Generalized pustular psoriasis

Impetigo herpetiformis
Von Zumbusch's disease

L40.2 Acrodermatitis continua

L40.3 Pustulosis palmaris et plantaris

L40.4 Guttate psoriasis

L40.5 Arthropathic psoriasis

L40.50 Arthropathic psoriasis, unspecified

L40.51 Distal interphalangeal psoriatic arthropathy

L40.52 Psoriatic arthritis mutilans

L40.53 Psoriatic spondylitis

L40.54 Psoriatic juvenile arthropathy

L40.59 Other psoriatic arthropathy

L40.8 Other psoriasis

Flexural psoriasis

L40.9 Psoriasis, unspecified

Item 12–8 Psoriasis is a chronic, recurrent inflammatory skin disease characterized by small patches covered with thick silvery scales. **Parapsoriasis** is a treatment-resistant erythroderma. **Pityriasis rosea** is characterized by a herald patch that is a single large lesion and that usually appears on the trunk and is followed by scattered, smaller lesions.

● **L41 Parapsoriasis**
Excludes1 poikiloderma vasculare atrophicans (L94.5)
L41.0 Pityriasis lichenoides et varioliformis acuta
Mucha-Habermann disease
L41.1 Pityriasis lichenoides chronica
L41.3 Small plaque parapsoriasis
L41.4 Large plaque parapsoriasis
L41.5 Retiform parapsoriasis
L41.8 Other parapsoriasis
L41.9 Parapsoriasis, unspecified

L42 Pityriasis rosea

● **L43 Lichen planus**
Excludes1 lichen planopilaris (L66.1)
L43.0 Hypertrophic lichen planus
L43.1 Bullous lichen planus
L43.2 Lichenoid drug reaction
Use additional code for adverse effect, if applicable, to identify drug (T36-T50 with fifth or sixth character 5)
L43.3 Subacute (active) lichen planus
Lichen planus tropicus
L43.8 Other lichen planus
L43.9 Lichen planus, unspecified

● **L44 Other papulosquamous disorders**
L44.0 Pityriasis rubra pilaris
L44.1 Lichen nitidus
L44.2 Lichen striatus
L44.3 Lichen ruber moniliformis
L44.4 Infantile papular acrodermatitis [Gianotti-Crosti] P
L44.8 Other specified papulosquamous disorders
L44.9 Papulosquamous disorder, unspecified

▶ ***L45 Papulosquamous disorders in diseases classified elsewhere***
Code first underlying disease

URTICARIA AND ERYTHEMA (L49-L54)

Excludes1 Lyme disease (A69.2-)
rosacea (L71.-)

● **L49 Exfoliation due to erythematous conditions according to extent of body surface involved**
Code first erythematous condition causing exfoliation, such as:
Ritter's disease (L00)
(Staphylococcal) scalded skin syndrome (L00)
Stevens-Johnson syndrome (L51.1)
Stevens-Johnson syndrome-toxic epidermal necrolysis overlap syndrome (L51.3)
Toxic epidermal necrolysis (L51.2)
● **L49.0 Exfoliation due to erythematous condition involving less than 10 percent of body surface**
Exfoliation due to erythematous condition NOS
● **L49.1 Exfoliation due to erythematous condition involving 10-19 percent of body surface**
● **L49.2 Exfoliation due to erythematous condition involving 20-29 percent of body surface**
● **L49.3 Exfoliation due to erythematous condition involving 30-39 percent of body surface**
Ex L49.3
● **L49.4 Exfoliation due to erythematous condition involving 40-49 percent of body surface**
Ex L49.4
● **L49.5 Exfoliation due to erythematous condition involving 50-59 percent of body surface**
Ex L49.5

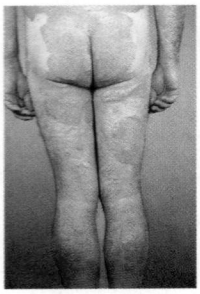

Figure 12-6 Erythematous plaques with silvery scales in a patient with psoriasis. (From Goldman: Cecil Textbook of Medicine, ed 22, Saunders, 2004)

● **L49.6 Exfoliation due to erythematous condition involving 60-69 percent of body surface**
Ex L49.6
● **L49.7 Exfoliation due to erythematous condition involving 70-79 percent of body surface**
Ex L49.7
● **L49.8 Exfoliation due to erythematous condition involving 80-89 percent of body surface**
Ex L49.8
● **L49.9 Exfoliation due to erythematous condition involving 90 or more percent of body surface**
Ex L49.9

● **L50 Urticaria**
Excludes1 allergic contact dermatitis (L23.-)
angioneurotic edema (T78.3)
giant urticaria (T78.3)
hereditary angio-edema (D84.1)
Quincke's edema (T78.3)
serum urticaria (T80.6-)
solar urticaria (L56.3)
urticaria neonatorum (P83.8)
urticaria papulosa (L28.2)
urticaria pigmentosa (Q82.2)
L50.0 Allergic urticaria
L50.1 Idiopathic urticaria
L50.2 Urticaria due to cold and heat
Excludes2 familial cold urticaria (M04.2) ◀
L50.3 Dermatographic urticaria
L50.4 Vibratory urticaria
L50.5 Cholinergic urticaria
L50.6 Contact urticaria
L50.8 Other urticaria
Chronic urticaria
Recurrent periodic urticaria
L50.9 Urticaria, unspecified

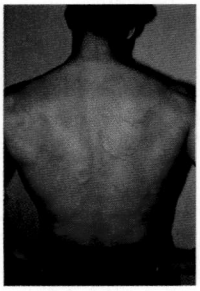

Figure 12-7 Urticaria (hives). *(Courtesy of David Effron, MD.)* (From Marx: Rosen's Emergency Medicine: Concepts and Clinical Practice, ed 6, Mosby, Inc., 2006)

Item 12–9 Urticaria is a vascular reaction in which wheals surrounded by a red halo appear and cause severe itching. The causes of urticaria or hives are extensive and varied (e.g., food, heat, cold, drugs, stress, infections).

L51 Erythema multiforme

Use additional code for adverse effect, if applicable, to identify drug (T36-T50 with fifth or sixth character 5)

Use additional code to identify associated manifestations, such as:
arthropathy associated with dermatological disorders (M14.8-)
conjunctival edema (H11.42)
conjunctivitis (H10.22-)
corneal scars and opacities (H17.-)
corneal ulcer (H16.0-)
edema of eyelid (H02.84)
inflammation of eyelid (H01.8)
keratoconjunctivitis sicca (H16.22-)
mechanical lagophthalmos (H02.22-)
stomatitis (K12.-)
symblepharon (H11.23-)

Use additional code to identify percentage of skin exfoliation (L49.-)

Excludes1 staphylococcal scalded skin syndrome (L00)
Ritter's disease (L00)

Ex: **For category L51 CC codes:** See L12.3

L51.0 Nonbullous erythema multiforme

L51.1 Stevens-Johnson syndrome

L51.2 Toxic epidermal necrolysis [Lyell]

L51.3 Stevens-Johnson syndrome-toxic epidermal necrolysis overlap syndrome
SJS-TEN overlap syndrome

L51.8 Other erythema multiforme

L51.9 Erythema multiforme, unspecified
Erythema iris
Erythema multiforme major NOS
Erythema multiforme minor NOS
Herpes iris

L52 Erythema nodosum

Excludes1 tuberculous erythema nodosum (A18.4)

L53 Other erythematous conditions

Excludes1 erythema ab igne (L59.0)
erythema due to external agents in contact with skin (L23-L25)
erythema intertrigo (L30.4)

Ex: **For category L53 CC codes:** L12.30-L12.35, L44.8-L45, L51.0-L53.3, L71.0-L71.9, L93.0-L93.2, L94.2, L94.4, L98.7, L98.8, L99

L53.0 Toxic erythema

Code first poisoning due to drug or toxin, if applicable (T36-T65 with fifth or sixth character 1-4 or 6)

Use additional code for adverse effect, if applicable, to identify drug (T36-T50 with fifth or sixth character 5)

Excludes1 neonatal erythema toxicum (P83.1)

L53.1 Erythema annulare centrifugum

L53.2 Erythema marginatum

L53.3 Other chronic figurate erythema

L53.8 Other specified erythematous conditions

L53.9 Erythematous condition, unspecified
Erythema NOS
Erythroderma NOS

L54 Erythema in diseases classified elsewhere

Code first underlying disease

RADIATION-RELATED DISORDERS OF THE SKIN AND SUBCUTANEOUS TISSUE (L55-L59)

L55 Sunburn

L55.0 Sunburn of first degree

L55.1 Sunburn of second degree

L55.2 Sunburn of third degree

L55.9 Sunburn, unspecified

L56 Other acute skin changes due to ultraviolet radiation

Use additional code to identify the source of the ultraviolet radiation (W89, X32)

L56.0 Drug phototoxic response

Use additional code for adverse effect, if applicable, to identify drug (T36-T50 with fifth or sixth character 5)

L56.1 Drug photoallergic response

Use additional code for adverse effect, if applicable, to identify drug (T36-T50 with fifth or sixth character 5)

L56.2 Photocontact dermatitis [berloque dermatitis]

L56.3 Solar urticaria

L56.4 Polymorphous light eruption

L56.5 Disseminated superficial actinic porokeratosis (DSAP)

L56.8 Other specified acute skin changes due to ultraviolet radiation

L56.9 Acute skin change due to ultraviolet radiation, unspecified

L57 Skin changes due to chronic exposure to nonionizing radiation

Use additional code to identify the source of the ultraviolet radiation (W89, X32)

L57.0 Actinic keratosis
Keratosis NOS
Senile keratosis
Solar keratosis

L57.1 Actinic reticuloid

L57.2 Cutis rhomboidalis nuchae

L57.3 Poikiloderma of Civatte

L57.4 Cutis laxa senilis
Elastosis senilis

L57.5 Actinic granuloma

L57.8 Other skin changes due to chronic exposure to nonionizing radiation
Farmer's skin
Sailor's skin
Solar dermatitis

L57.9 Skin changes due to chronic exposure to nonionizing radiation, unspecified

L58 Radiodermatitis

Use additional code to identify the source of the radiation (W88, W90)

L58.0 Acute radiodermatitis

L58.1 Chronic radiodermatitis

L58.9 Radiodermatitis, unspecified

L59 Other disorders of skin and subcutaneous tissue related to radiation

L59.0 Erythema ab igne [dermatitis ab igne]

L59.8 Other specified disorders of the skin and subcutaneous tissue related to radiation

L59.9 Disorder of the skin and subcutaneous tissue related to radiation, unspecified

DISORDERS OF SKIN APPENDAGES (L60-L75)

Excludes1 congenital malformations of integument (Q84.-)

L60 Nail disorders

Excludes2 clubbing of nails (R68.3)
onychia and paronychia (L03.0-)

L60.0 Ingrowing nail

L60.1 Onycholysis

L60.2 Onychogryphosis

L60.3 Nail dystrophy

L60.4 Beau's lines

L60.5 Yellow nail syndrome

L60.8 Other nail disorders

L60.9 Nail disorder, unspecified

Item 12-10 **Alopecia** is lack of hair and takes many forms. The most common is male pattern alopecia, also known as **androgenetic alopecia. Telogen effluvium** is early and excessive loss of hair resulting from a trauma to the hair follicle (fever, drugs, surgery, etc.).

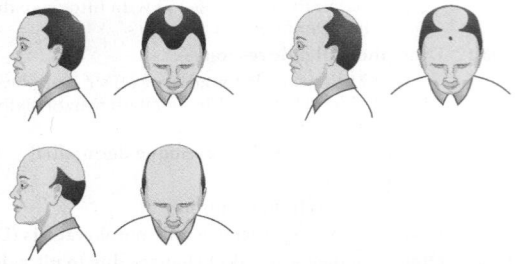

Figure 12-8 Male pattern alopecia.

L62 Nail disorders in diseases classified elsewhere
Code first underlying disease, such as:
pachydermoperiostosis (M89.4-)

L63 Alopecia areata
- **L63.0 Alopecia (capitis) totalis**
- **L63.1 Alopecia universalis**
- **L63.2 Ophiasis**
- **L63.8 Other alopecia areata**
- **L63.9 Alopecia areata, unspecified**

L64 Androgenic alopecia
Includes male-pattern baldness
- **L64.0 Drug-induced androgenic alopecia**
  Use additional code for adverse effect, if applicable, to identify drug (T36-T50 with fifth or sixth character 5)
- **L64.8 Other androgenic alopecia**
- **L64.9 Androgenic alopecia, unspecified**

L65 Other nonscarring hair loss
Use additional code for adverse effect, if applicable, to identify drug (T36-T50 with fifth or sixth character 5)
Excludes1 trichotillomania (F63.3)
- **L65.0 Telogen effluvium**
- **L65.1 Anagen effluvium**
- **L65.2 Alopecia mucinosa**
- **L65.8 Other specified nonscarring hair loss**
- **L65.9 Nonscarring hair loss, unspecified**
  Alopecia NOS

L66 Cicatricial alopecia [scarring hair loss]
- **L66.0 Pseudopelade**
- **L66.1 Lichen planopilaris**
  Follicular lichen planus
- **L66.2 Folliculitis decalvans**
- **L66.3 Perifolliculitis capitis abscedens**
- **L66.4 Folliculitis ulerythematosa reticulata**
- **L66.8 Other cicatricial alopecia**
  Coding Clinic: 2015, Q1, P19
- **L66.9 Cicatricial alopecia, unspecified**

L67 Hair color and hair shaft abnormalities
Excludes1 monilethrix (Q84.1)
pili annulati (Q84.1)
telogen effluvium (L65.0)
- **L67.0 Trichorrhexis nodosa**
- **L67.1 Variations in hair color**
  Canities
  Greyness, hair (premature)
  Heterochromia of hair
  Poliosis circumscripta, acquired
  Poliosis NOS
- **L67.8 Other hair color and hair shaft abnormalities**
  Fragilitas crinium
- **L67.9 Hair color and hair shaft abnormality, unspecified**

L68 Hypertrichosis
Includes excess hair
Excludes1 congenital hypertrichosis (Q84.2)
persistent lanugo (Q84.2)
- **L68.0 Hirsutism**
  Excessive growth of hair
- **L68.1 Acquired hypertrichosis lanuginosa**
- **L68.2 Localized hypertrichosis**
- **L68.3 Polytrichia**
- **L68.8 Other hypertrichosis**
- **L68.9 Hypertrichosis, unspecified**

L70 Acne
Excludes2 acne keloid (L73.0)
- **L70.0 Acne vulgaris**
- **L70.1 Acne conglobata**
- **L70.2 Acne varioliformis**
  Acne necrotica miliaris
- **L70.3 Acne tropica**
- **L70.4 Infantile acne** P
- **L70.5 Acné excoriée** ◀
  Acné excoriée des jeunes filles ◀
  Picker's acne
- **L70.8 Other acne**
- **L70.9 Acne, unspecified**

L71 Rosacea
Use additional code for adverse effect, if applicable, to identify drug (T36-T50 with fifth or sixth character 5)
- **L71.0 Perioral dermatitis**
- **L71.1 Rhinophyma**
- **L71.8 Other rosacea**
- **L71.9 Rosacea, unspecified**

L72 Follicular cysts of skin and subcutaneous tissue
- **L72.0 Epidermal cyst**
- **L72.1 Pilar and trichodermal cyst**
  - **L72.11 Pilar cyst**
  - **L72.12 Trichodermal cyst**
    Trichilemmal (proliferating) cyst
- **L72.3 Sebaceous cyst**
  Excludes2 pilar cyst (L72.11)
  trichilemmal (proliferating) cyst (L72.12)
- **L72.2 Steatocystoma multiplex**
- **L72.8 Other follicular cysts of the skin and subcutaneous tissue**
- **L72.9 Follicular cyst of the skin and subcutaneous tissue, unspecified**

L73 Other follicular disorders
- **L73.0 Acne keloid**
- **L73.1 Pseudofolliculitis barbae**
- **L73.2 Hidradenitis suppurativa**
- **L73.8 Other specified follicular disorders**
  Sycosis barbae
- **L73.9 Follicular disorder, unspecified**

L74 Eccrine sweat disorders
Excludes2 generalized hyperhidrosis (R61)
L74.0 Miliaria rubra
L74.1 Miliaria crystallina
L74.2 Miliaria profunda
Miliaria tropicalis
L74.3 Miliaria, unspecified
L74.4 Anhidrosis
Hypohidrosis
L74.5 Focal hyperhidrosis
L74.51 Primary focal hyperhidrosis
L74.510 Primary focal hyperhidrosis, axilla
L74.511 Primary focal hyperhidrosis, face
L74.512 Primary focal hyperhidrosis, palms
L74.513 Primary focal hyperhidrosis, soles
L74.519 Primary focal hyperhidrosis, unspecified
L74.52 Secondary focal hyperhidrosis
Frey's syndrome
L74.8 Other eccrine sweat disorders
L74.9 Eccrine sweat disorder, unspecified
Sweat gland disorder NOS

L75 Apocrine sweat disorders
Excludes1 dyshidrosis (L30.1)
hidradenitis suppurativa (L73.2)
L75.0 Bromhidrosis
L75.1 Chromhidrosis
L75.2 Apocrine miliaria
Fox-Fordyce disease
L75.8 Other apocrine sweat disorders
L75.9 Apocrine sweat disorder, unspecified
Intraoperative and postprocedural complications of skin and subcutaneous tissue (L76)

INTRAOPERATIVE AND POSTPROCEDURAL COMPLICATIONS OF SKIN AND SUBCUTANEOUS TISSUE (L76)

L76 Intraoperative and postprocedural complications of skin and subcutaneous tissue
Ex **For category L76 CC codes unless otherwise indicated:** H95.811-H95.89, I85.01, I85.11, I97.3, K21.9, K22.8, K23, K25.0, K25.2, K25.4, K25.6, K26.0, K26.2, K26.4, K26.6, K27.0, K27.2, K27.4, K27.6, K28.0, K28.2, K28.4, K28.6, K29.01, K29.21, K29.31, K29.41, K29.51, K29.61, K29.71, K29.81, K29.91, K31.811, K55.21, K57.01, K57.11, K57.13, K57.21, K57.31, K57.33, K57.41, K57.51, K57.53, K57.81, K57.91, K57.93, K62.5, K92.0-K92.2, L76.01-L76.02, L76.21-L76.82, M96.89, N98.1-N98.9, P54.1-P54.3, T81.10X-T81.19X[A], T81.82X[A], T81.89X-T81.9XX[A]
L76.0 Intraoperative hemorrhage and hematoma of skin and subcutaneous tissue complicating a procedure
Excludes1 intraoperative hemorrhage and hematoma of skin and subcutaneous tissue due to accidental puncture and laceration during a procedure (L76.1-)
L76.01 Intraoperative hemorrhage and hematoma of skin and subcutaneous tissue complicating a dermatologic procedure
L76.02 Intraoperative hemorrhage and hematoma of skin and subcutaneous tissue complicating other procedure
L76.1 Accidental puncture and laceration of skin and subcutaneous tissue during a procedure
Ex **For category L76.1 CC codes:** D78.11-D78.12, D78.81-D78.89, E36.11-E36.8, E89.810-E89.89, G96.11, G97.41-G97.49, H59.011-H59.019, H59.031-H59.099, H59.211-H59.229, H59.811-H59.89, H95.31-H95.32, H95.811-H95.89, I97.3, I97.51-I97.52, J95.71-J95.72, K91.71-K91.72, L76.11-L76.12, L76.81-L76.82, M96.820-M96.821, M96.89, N98.1-N98.9, N99.71-N99.72, T81.82X[A], T81.89X-T81.9XX[A]
L76.11 Accidental puncture and laceration of skin and subcutaneous tissue during a dermatologic procedure
L76.12 Accidental puncture and laceration of skin and subcutaneous tissue during other procedure
L76.2 Postprocedural hemorrhage of skin and subcutaneous tissue following a procedure
L76.21 Postprocedural hemorrhage of skin and subcutaneous tissue following a dermatologic procedure
L76.22 Postprocedural hemorrhage of skin and subcutaneous tissue following other procedure
L76.3 Postprocedural hematoma and seroma of skin and subcutaneous tissue following a procedure
L76.31 Postprocedural hematoma of skin and subcutaneous tissue following a dermatologic procedure
L76.32 Postprocedural hematoma of skin and subcutaneous tissue following other procedure
L76.33 Postprocedural seroma of skin and subcutaneous tissue following a dermatologic procedure
L76.34 Postprocedural seroma of skin and subcutaneous tissue following other procedure
L76.8 Other intraoperative and postprocedural complications of skin and subcutaneous tissue
Use additional code, if applicable, to further specify disorder
L76.81 Other intraoperative complications of skin and subcutaneous tissue
L76.82 Other postprocedural complications of skin and subcutaneous tissue

OTHER DISORDERS OF THE SKIN AND SUBCUTANEOUS TISSUE (L80-L99)

L80 Vitiligo
Excludes2 vitiligo of eyelids (H02.73-)
vitiligo of vulva (N90.89)

L81 Other disorders of pigmentation
Excludes1 birthmark NOS (Q82.5)
Peutz-Jeghers syndrome (Q85.8)
Excludes2 nevus - see Alphabetical Index
L81.0 Postinflammatory hyperpigmentation
L81.1 Chloasma
L81.2 Freckles
L81.3 Café au lait spots
L81.4 Other melanin hyperpigmentation
Lentigo
L81.5 Leukoderma, not elsewhere classified
L81.6 Other disorders of diminished melanin formation
L81.7 Pigmented purpuric dermatosis
Angioma serpiginosum
L81.8 Other specified disorders of pigmentation
Iron pigmentation
Tattoo pigmentation
L81.9 Disorder of pigmentation, unspecified

L82 Seborrheic keratosis
Includes basal cell papilloma
dermatosis papulosa nigra
Leser-Trélat disease
Excludes2 seborrheic dermatitis (L21.-)
L82.0 Inflamed seborrheic keratosis
L82.1 Other seborrheic keratosis
Seborrheic keratosis NOS

L83 Acanthosis nigricans
Confluent and reticulated papillomatosis

L84 Corns and callosities
Callus
Clavus

● **L85 Other epidermal thickening**

Excludes2 hypertrophic disorders of the skin (L91.-)

L85.0 Acquired ichthyosis

Excludes1 congenital ichthyosis (Q80.-)

L85.1 Acquired keratosis [keratoderma] palmaris et plantaris

Excludes1 inherited keratosis palmaris et plantaris (Q82.8)

L85.2 Keratosis punctata (palmaris et plantaris)

L85.3 Xerosis cutis

Dry skin dermatitis

L85.8 Other specified epidermal thickening

Cutaneous horn

L85.9 Epidermal thickening, unspecified

▶ *L86 Keratoderma in diseases classified elsewhere*

Firm horny papules that have a cobblestone appearance.

Code first underlying disease, such as:

Reiter's disease (M02.3-)

Excludes1 gonococcal keratoderma (A54.89)
gonococcal keratosis (A54.89)
keratoderma due to vitamin A deficiency (E50.8)
keratosis due to vitamin A deficiency (E50.8)
xeroderma due to vitamin A deficiency (E50.8)

● **L87 Transepidermal elimination disorders**

Excludes1 granuloma annulare (perforating) (L92.0)

L87.0 Keratosis follicularis et parafollicularis in cutem penetrans

Kyrle disease
Hyperkeratosis follicularis penetrans

L87.1 Reactive perforating collagenosis

L87.2 Elastosis perforans serpiginosa

L87.8 Other transepidermal elimination disorders

L87.9 Transepidermal elimination disorder, unspecified

L88 Pyoderma gangrenosum

Phagedenic pyoderma

Excludes1 dermatitis gangrenosa (L08.0)

Ex: L08.0, L08.81, L88

OGCR Section I.B.14.

General Coding Guidelines

Documentation for BMI, *Depth of* Non-pressure ulcers, Pressure Ulcer Stages, **Coma Scale, and** *NIH Stroke Scale*

For the Body Mass Index (BMI), depth of non-pressure chronic ulcers, pressure ulcer stage, **coma scale, and NIH stroke scale (NIHSS) codes,** code assignment may be based on medical record documentation from clinicians who are not the patient's provider (i.e., physician or other qualified healthcare practitioner legally accountable for establishing the patient's diagnosis), since this information is typically documented by other clinicians involved in the care of the patient (e.g., a dietitian often documents the BMI, a nurse often documents the pressure ulcer stages, **and an emergency medical technician often documents the coma scale**). However, the associated diagnosis (such as overweight, obesity, **acute stroke,** or pressure ulcer) must be documented by the patient's provider. If there is conflicting medical record documentation, either from the same clinician or different clinicians, the patient's attending provider should be queried for clarification.

The BMI, **coma scale, and NHSS** codes should only be reported as secondary diagnoses.

● **L89 Pressure ulcer**

Includes bed sore
decubitus ulcer
plaster ulcer
pressure area
pressure sore

Code first any associated gangrene (I96)

Excludes2 decubitus (trophic) ulcer of cervix (uteri) (N86)
diabetic ulcers (E08.621, E08.622, E09.621, E09.622, E10.621, E10.622, E11.621, E11.622, E13.621, E13.622)
non-pressure chronic ulcer of skin (L97.-)
skin infections (L00-L08)
varicose ulcer (I83.0, I83.2)

Ex: **For category L89 CC codes:** L89.000-L89.95, L97.101-L97.929, L98.411-L98.499

● **L89.0 Pressure ulcer of elbow**

● **L89.00 Pressure ulcer of unspecified elbow**

L89.000 Pressure ulcer of unspecified elbow, unstageable

L89.001 Pressure ulcer of unspecified elbow, stage 1

Healing pressure ulcer of unspecified elbow, stage 1
Pressure pre-ulcer skin changes limited to persistent focal edema, unspecified elbow

L89.002 Pressure ulcer of unspecified elbow, stage 2

Healing pressure ulcer of unspecified elbow, stage 2
Pressure ulcer with abrasion, blister, partial thickness skin loss involving epidermis and/or dermis, unspecified elbow

L89.003 Pressure ulcer of unspecified elbow, stage 3

Healing pressure ulcer of unspecified elbow, stage 3
Pressure ulcer with full thickness skin loss involving damage or necrosis of subcutaneous tissue, unspecified elbow
MCC when PDx is its own MCC

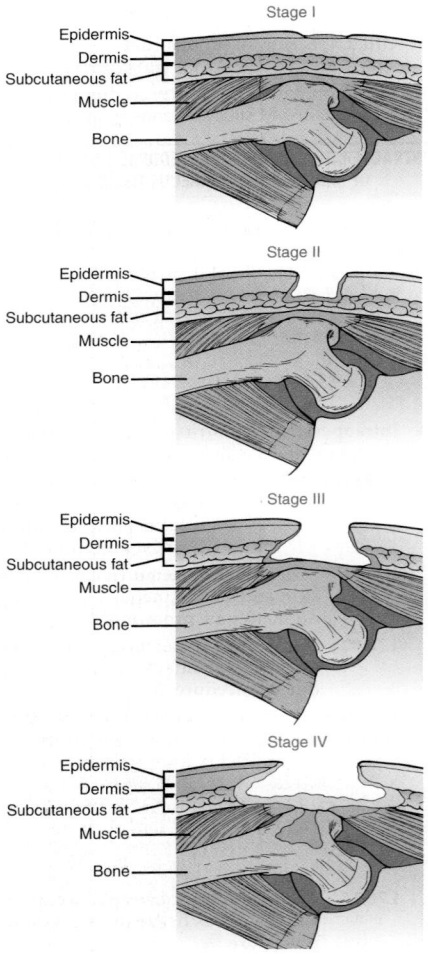

Figure 12-9 Stage I, II, III, and IV of pressure ulcers.

L89.004 Pressure ulcer of unspecified elbow, stage 4
Healing pressure ulcer of unspecified elbow, stage 4
Pressure ulcer with necrosis of soft tissues through to underlying muscle, tendon, or bone, unspecified elbow
MCC when PDx is its own MCC

L89.009 Pressure ulcer of unspecified elbow, unspecified stage
Healing pressure ulcer of elbow NOS
Healing pressure ulcer of unspecified elbow, unspecified stage

● **L89.01 Pressure ulcer of right elbow**

L89.010 Pressure ulcer of right elbow, unstageable

L89.011 Pressure ulcer of right elbow, stage 1
Healing pressure ulcer of right elbow, stage 1
Pressure pre-ulcer skin changes limited to persistent focal edema, right elbow

L89.012 Pressure ulcer of right elbow, stage 2
Healing pressure ulcer of right elbow, stage 2
Pressure ulcer with abrasion, blister, partial thickness skin loss involving epidermis and/or dermis, right elbow

L89.013 Pressure ulcer of right elbow, stage 3
Healing pressure ulcer of right elbow, stage 3
Pressure ulcer with full thickness skin loss involving damage or necrosis of subcutaneous tissue, right elbow
MCC when PDx is its own MCC

L89.014 Pressure ulcer of right elbow, stage 4
Healing pressure ulcer of right elbow, stage 4
Pressure ulcer with necrosis of soft tissues through to underlying muscle, tendon, or bone, right elbow
MCC when PDx is its own MCC

L89.019 Pressure ulcer of right elbow, unspecified stage
Healing pressure right of elbow NOS
Healing pressure ulcer of unspecified elbow, unspecified stage

● **L89.02 Pressure ulcer of left elbow**

L89.020 Pressure ulcer of left elbow, unstageable

L89.021 Pressure ulcer of left elbow, stage 1
Healing pressure ulcer of left elbow, stage 1
Pressure pre-ulcer skin changes limited to persistent focal edema, left elbow

L89.022 Pressure ulcer of left elbow, stage 2
Healing pressure ulcer of left elbow, stage 2
Pressure ulcer with abrasion, blister, partial thickness skin loss involving epidermis and/or dermis, left elbow

L89.023 Pressure ulcer of left elbow, stage 3
Healing pressure ulcer of left elbow, stage 3
Pressure ulcer with full thickness skin loss involving damage or necrosis of subcutaneous tissue, left elbow
MCC when PDx is its own MCC

L89.024 Pressure ulcer of left elbow, stage 4
Healing pressure ulcer of left elbow, stage 4
Pressure ulcer with necrosis of soft tissues through to underlying muscle, tendon, or bone, left elbow
MCC when PDx is its own MCC

L89.029 Pressure ulcer of left elbow, unspecified stage
Healing pressure ulcer of left of elbow NOS
Healing pressure ulcer of unspecified elbow, unspecified stage

● **L89.1 Pressure ulcer of back**

● **L89.10 Pressure ulcer of unspecified part of back**

L89.100 Pressure ulcer of unspecified part of back, unstageable

L89.101 Pressure ulcer of unspecified part of back, stage 1
Healing pressure ulcer of unspecified part of back, stage 1
Pressure pre-ulcer skin changes limited to persistent focal edema, unspecified part of back

L89.102 Pressure ulcer of unspecified part of back, stage 2
Healing pressure ulcer of unspecified part of back, stage 2
Pressure ulcer with abrasion, blister, partial thickness skin loss involving epidermis and/or dermis, unspecified part of back

L89.103 Pressure ulcer of unspecified part of back, stage 3
Healing pressure ulcer of unspecified part of back, stage 3
Pressure ulcer with full thickness skin loss involving damage or necrosis of subcutaneous tissue, unspecified part of back
MCC when PDx is its own MCC

L89.104 Pressure ulcer of unspecified part of back, stage 4
Healing pressure ulcer of unspecified part of back, stage 4
Pressure ulcer with necrosis of soft tissues through to underlying muscle, tendon, or bone, unspecified part of back
MCC when PDx is its own MCC

L89.109 Pressure ulcer of unspecified part of back, unspecified stage
Healing pressure ulcer of unspecified part of back NOS
Healing pressure ulcer of unspecified part of back, unspecified stage

● **L89.11 Pressure ulcer of right upper back**
Pressure ulcer of right shoulder blade

L89.110 Pressure ulcer of right upper back, unstageable

L89.111 Pressure ulcer of right upper back, stage 1
Healing pressure ulcer of right upper back, stage 1
Pressure pre-ulcer skin changes limited to persistent focal edema, right upper back

L89.112 Pressure ulcer of right upper back, stage 2
Healing pressure ulcer of right upper back, stage 2
Pressure ulcer with abrasion, blister, partial thickness skin loss involving epidermis and/or dermis, right upper back

L89.113 Pressure ulcer of right upper back, stage 3
Healing pressure ulcer of right upper back, stage 3
Pressure ulcer with full thickness skin loss involving damage or necrosis of subcutaneous tissue, right upper back
MCC when PDx is its own MCC

L89.114 Pressure ulcer of right upper back, stage 4
Healing pressure ulcer of right upper back, stage 4
Pressure ulcer with necrosis of soft tissues through to underlying muscle, tendon, or bone, right upper back
MCC when PDx is its own MCC

L89.119 Pressure ulcer of right upper back, unspecified stage
Healing pressure ulcer of right upper back NOS
Healing pressure ulcer of right upper back, unspecified stage

● **L89.12 Pressure ulcer of left upper back**
Pressure ulcer of left shoulder blade

L89.120 Pressure ulcer of left upper back, unstageable

L89.121 Pressure ulcer of left upper back, stage 1
Healing pressure ulcer of left upper back, stage 1
Pressure pre-ulcer skin changes limited to persistent focal edema, left upper back

L89.122 Pressure ulcer of left upper back, stage 2
Healing pressure ulcer of left upper back, stage 2
Pressure ulcer with abrasion, blister, partial thickness skin loss involving epidermis and/or dermis, left upper back

L89.123 Pressure ulcer of left upper back, stage 3
Healing pressure ulcer of left upper back, stage 3
Pressure ulcer with full thickness skin loss involving damage or necrosis of subcutaneous tissue, left upper back
MCC when PDx is its own MCC

L89.124 Pressure ulcer of left upper back, stage 4
Healing pressure ulcer of left upper back, stage 4
Pressure ulcer with necrosis of soft tissues through to underlying muscle, tendon, or bone, left upper back
MCC when PDx is its own MCC

L89.129 Pressure ulcer of left upper back, unspecified stage
Healing pressure ulcer of left upper back NOS
Healing pressure ulcer of left upper back, unspecified stage

● **L89.13 Pressure ulcer of right lower back**

L89.130 Pressure ulcer of right lower back, unstageable

L89.131 Pressure ulcer of right lower back, stage 1
Healing pressure ulcer of right lower back, stage 1
Pressure pre-ulcer skin changes limited to persistent focal edema, right lower back

L89.132 Pressure ulcer of right lower back, stage 2
Healing pressure ulcer of right lower back, stage 2
Pressure ulcer with abrasion, blister, partial thickness skin loss involving epidermis and/or dermis, right lower back

L89.133 Pressure ulcer of right lower back, stage 3
Healing pressure ulcer of right lower back, stage 3
Pressure ulcer with full thickness skin loss involving damage or necrosis of subcutaneous tissue, right lower back
MCC when PDx is its own MCC

L89.134 Pressure ulcer of right lower back, stage 4
Healing pressure ulcer of right lower back, stage 4
Pressure ulcer with necrosis of soft tissues through to underlying muscle, tendon, or bone, right lower back
MCC when PDx is its own MCC

L89.139 Pressure ulcer of right lower back, unspecified stage
Healing pressure ulcer of right lower back NOS
Healing pressure ulcer of right lower back, unspecified stage

● **L89.14 Pressure ulcer of left lower back**

L89.140 Pressure ulcer of left lower back, unstageable

L89.141 Pressure ulcer of left lower back, stage 1
Healing pressure ulcer of left lower back, stage 1
Pressure pre-ulcer skin changes limited to persistent focal edema, left lower back

L89.142 Pressure ulcer of left lower back, stage 2
Healing pressure ulcer of left lower back, stage 2
Pressure ulcer with abrasion, blister, partial thickness skin loss involving epidermis and/or dermis, left lower back

L89.143 Pressure ulcer of left lower back, stage 3
Healing pressure ulcer of left lower back, stage 3
Pressure ulcer with full thickness skin loss involving damage or necrosis of subcutaneous tissue, left lower back
MCC when PDx is its own MCC

L89.144 Pressure ulcer of left lower back, stage 4
Healing pressure ulcer of left lower back, stage 4
Pressure ulcer with necrosis of soft tissues through to underlying muscle, tendon, or bone, left lower back
MCC when PDx is its own MCC

L89.149 Pressure ulcer of left lower back, unspecified stage
Healing pressure ulcer of left lower back NOS
Healing pressure ulcer of left lower back, unspecified stage

L89.15 Pressure ulcer of sacral region
Pressure ulcer of coccyx
Pressure ulcer of tailbone

L89.150 Pressure ulcer of sacral region, unstageable

L89.151 Pressure ulcer of sacral region, stage 1
Healing pressure ulcer of sacral region, stage 1
Pressure pre-ulcer skin changes limited to persistent focal edema, sacral region

L89.152 Pressure ulcer of sacral region, stage 2
Healing pressure ulcer of sacral region, stage 2
Pressure ulcer with abrasion, blister, partial thickness skin loss involving epidermis and/or dermis, sacral region

L89.153 Pressure ulcer of sacral region, stage 3
Healing pressure ulcer of sacral region, stage 3
Pressure ulcer with full thickness skin loss involving damage or necrosis of subcutaneous tissue, sacral region
MCC when PDx is its own MCC

L89.154 Pressure ulcer of sacral region, stage 4
Healing pressure ulcer of sacral region, stage 4
Pressure ulcer with necrosis of soft tissues through to underlying muscle, tendon, or bone, sacral region
MCC when PDx is its own MCC

L89.159 Pressure ulcer of sacral region, unspecified stage
Healing pressure ulcer of sacral region NOS
Healing pressure ulcer of sacral region, unspecified stage

L89.2 Pressure ulcer of hip

L89.20 Pressure ulcer of unspecified hip

L89.200 Pressure ulcer of unspecified hip, unstageable

L89.201 Pressure ulcer of unspecified hip, stage 1
Healing pressure ulcer of unspecified hip back, stage 1
Pressure pre-ulcer skin changes limited to persistent focal edema, unspecified hip

L89.202 Pressure ulcer of unspecified hip, stage 2
Healing pressure ulcer of unspecified hip, stage 2
Pressure ulcer with abrasion, blister, partial thickness skin loss involving epidermis and/or dermis, unspecified hip

L89.203 Pressure ulcer of unspecified hip, stage 3
Healing pressure ulcer of unspecified hip, stage 3
Pressure ulcer with full thickness skin loss involving damage or necrosis of subcutaneous tissue, unspecified hip
MCC when PDx is its own MCC

L89.204 Pressure ulcer of unspecified hip, stage 4
Healing pressure ulcer of unspecified hip, stage 4
Pressure ulcer with necrosis of soft tissues through to underlying muscle, tendon, or bone, unspecified hip
MCC when PDx is its own MCC

L89.209 Pressure ulcer of unspecified hip, unspecified stage
Healing pressure ulcer of unspecified hip NOS
Healing pressure ulcer of unspecified hip, unspecified stage

L89.21 Pressure ulcer of right hip

L89.210 Pressure ulcer of right hip, unstageable

L89.211 Pressure ulcer of right hip, stage 1
Healing pressure ulcer of right hip back, stage 1
Pressure pre-ulcer skin changes limited to persistent focal edema, right hip

L89.212 Pressure ulcer of right hip, stage 2
Healing pressure ulcer of right hip, stage 2
Pressure ulcer with abrasion, blister, partial thickness skin loss involving epidermis and/or dermis, right hip

L89.213 Pressure ulcer of right hip, stage 3
Healing pressure ulcer of right hip, stage 3
Pressure ulcer with full thickness skin loss involving damage or necrosis of subcutaneous tissue, right hip
MCC when PDx is its own MCC

L89.214 Pressure ulcer of right hip, stage 4
Healing pressure ulcer of right hip, stage 4
Pressure ulcer with necrosis of soft tissues through to underlying muscle, tendon, or bone, right hip
MCC when PDx is its own MCC

L89.219 Pressure ulcer of right hip, unspecified stage
Healing pressure ulcer of right hip NOS
Healing pressure ulcer of right hip, unspecified stage

● **L89.22 Pressure ulcer of left hip**

L89.220 Pressure ulcer of left hip, unstageable

L89.221 Pressure ulcer of left hip, stage 1
- Healing pressure ulcer of left hip back, stage 1
- Pressure pre-ulcer skin changes limited to persistent focal edema, left hip

L89.222 Pressure ulcer of left hip, stage 2
- Healing pressure ulcer of left hip, stage 2
- Pressure ulcer with abrasion, blister, partial thickness skin loss involving epidermis and/or dermis, left hip

L89.223 Pressure ulcer of left hip, stage 3
- Healing pressure ulcer of left hip, stage 3
- Pressure ulcer with full thickness skin loss involving damage or necrosis of subcutaneous tissue, left hip
- MCC when PDx is its own MCC

L89.224 Pressure ulcer of left hip, stage 4
- Healing pressure ulcer of left hip, stage 4
- Pressure ulcer with necrosis of soft tissues through to underlying muscle, tendon, or bone, left hip
- MCC when PDx is its own MCC

L89.229 Pressure ulcer of left hip, unspecified stage
- Healing pressure ulcer of left hip NOS
- Healing pressure ulcer of left hip, unspecified stage

● **L89.3 Pressure ulcer of buttock**

● **L89.30 Pressure ulcer of unspecified buttock**

L89.300 Pressure ulcer of unspecified buttock, unstageable

L89.301 Pressure ulcer of unspecified buttock, stage 1
- Healing pressure ulcer of unspecified buttock, stage 1
- Pressure pre-ulcer skin changes limited to persistent focal edema, unspecified buttock

L89.302 Pressure ulcer of unspecified buttock, stage 2
- Healing pressure ulcer of unspecified buttock, stage 2
- Pressure ulcer with abrasion, blister, partial thickness skin loss involving epidermis and/or dermis, unspecified buttock

L89.303 Pressure ulcer of unspecified buttock, stage 3
- Healing pressure ulcer of unspecified buttock, stage 3
- Pressure ulcer with full thickness skin loss involving damage or necrosis of subcutaneous tissue, unspecified buttock
- MCC when PDx is its own MCC

L89.304 Pressure ulcer of unspecified buttock, stage 4
- Healing pressure ulcer of unspecified buttock, stage 4
- Pressure ulcer with necrosis of soft tissues through to underlying muscle, tendon, or bone, unspecified buttock
- MCC when PDx is its own MCC

L89.309 Pressure ulcer of unspecified buttock, unspecified stage
- Healing pressure ulcer of unspecified buttock NOS
- Healing pressure ulcer of unspecified buttock, unspecified stage

● **L89.31 Pressure ulcer of right buttock**

L89.310 Pressure ulcer of right buttock, unstageable

L89.311 Pressure ulcer of right buttock, stage 1
- Healing pressure ulcer of right buttock, stage 1
- Pressure pre-ulcer skin changes limited to persistent focal edema, right buttock

L89.312 Pressure ulcer of right buttock, stage 2
- Healing pressure ulcer of right buttock, stage 2
- Pressure ulcer with abrasion, blister, partial thickness skin loss involving epidermis and/or dermis, right buttock

L89.313 Pressure ulcer of right buttock, stage 3
- Healing pressure ulcer of right buttock, stage 3
- Pressure ulcer with full thickness skin loss involving damage or necrosis of subcutaneous tissue, right buttock
- MCC when PDx is its own MCC

L89.314 Pressure ulcer of right buttock, stage 4
- Healing pressure ulcer of right buttock, stage 4
- Pressure ulcer with necrosis of soft tissues through to underlying muscle, tendon, or bone, right buttock
- MCC when PDx is its own MCC

L89.319 Pressure ulcer of right buttock, unspecified stage
- Healing pressure ulcer of right buttock NOS
- Healing pressure ulcer of right buttock, unspecified stage

● **L89.32 Pressure ulcer of left buttock**

L89.320 Pressure ulcer of left buttock, unstageable

L89.321 Pressure ulcer of left buttock, stage 1
- Healing pressure ulcer of left buttock, stage 1
- Pressure pre-ulcer skin changes limited to persistent focal edema, left buttock

L89.322 Pressure ulcer of left buttock, stage 2
- Healing pressure ulcer of left buttock, stage 2
- Pressure ulcer with abrasion, blister, partial thickness skin loss involving epidermis and/or dermis, left buttock

L89.323 Pressure ulcer of left buttock, stage 3
Healing pressure ulcer of left buttock, stage 3
Pressure ulcer with full thickness skin loss involving damage or necrosis of subcutaneous tissue, left buttock
MCC when PDx is its own MCC

L89.324 Pressure ulcer of left buttock, stage 4
Healing pressure ulcer of left buttock, stage 4
Pressure ulcer with necrosis of soft tissues through to underlying muscle, tendon, or bone, left buttock
MCC when PDx is its own MCC

L89.329 Pressure ulcer of left buttock, unspecified stage
Healing pressure ulcer of left buttock NOS
Healing pressure ulcer of left buttock, unspecified stage

L89.4 Pressure ulcer of contiguous site of back, buttock and hip

L89.40 Pressure ulcer of contiguous site of back, buttock and hip, unspecified stage
Healing pressure ulcer of contiguous site of back, buttock and hip NOS
Healing pressure ulcer of contiguous site of back, buttock and hip, unspecified stage

L89.41 Pressure ulcer of contiguous site of back, buttock and hip, stage 1
Healing pressure ulcer of contiguous site of back, buttock and hip, stage 1
Pressure pre-ulcer skin changes limited to persistent focal edema, contiguous site of back, buttock and hip

L89.42 Pressure ulcer of contiguous site of back, buttock and hip, stage 2
Healing pressure ulcer of contiguous site of back, buttock and hip, stage 2
Pressure ulcer with abrasion, blister, partial thickness skin loss involving epidermis and/or dermis, contiguous site of back, buttock and hip

L89.43 Pressure ulcer of contiguous site of back, buttock and hip, stage 3
Healing pressure ulcer of contiguous site of back, buttock and hip, stage 3
Pressure ulcer with full thickness skin loss involving damage or necrosis of subcutaneous tissue, contiguous site of back, buttock and hip
MCC when PDx is its own MCC

L89.44 Pressure ulcer of contiguous site of back, buttock and hip, stage 4
Healing pressure ulcer of contiguous site of back, buttock and hip, stage 4
Pressure ulcer with necrosis of soft tissues through to underlying muscle, tendon, or bone, contiguous site of back, buttock and hip
MCC when PDx is its own MCC

L89.45 Pressure ulcer of contiguous site of back, buttock and hip, unstageable

L89.5 Pressure ulcer of ankle

L89.50 Pressure ulcer of unspecified ankle

L89.500 Pressure ulcer of unspecified ankle, unstageable

L89.501 Pressure ulcer of unspecified ankle, stage 1
Healing pressure ulcer of unspecified ankle, stage 1
Pressure pre-ulcer skin changes limited to persistent focal edema, unspecified ankle

L89.502 Pressure ulcer of unspecified ankle, stage 2
Healing pressure ulcer of unspecified ankle, stage 2
Pressure ulcer with abrasion, blister, partial thickness skin loss involving epidermis and/or dermis, unspecified ankle

L89.503 Pressure ulcer of unspecified ankle, stage 3
Healing pressure ulcer of unspecified ankle, stage 3
Pressure ulcer with full thickness skin loss involving damage or necrosis of subcutaneous tissue, unspecified ankle
MCC when PDx is its own MCC

L89.504 Pressure ulcer of unspecified ankle, stage 4
Healing pressure ulcer of unspecified ankle, stage 4
Pressure ulcer with necrosis of soft tissues through to underlying muscle, tendon, or bone, unspecified ankle
MCC when PDx is its own MCC

L89.509 Pressure ulcer of unspecified ankle, unspecified stage
Healing pressure ulcer of unspecified ankle NOS
Healing pressure ulcer of unspecified ankle, unspecified stage

L89.51 Pressure ulcer of right ankle

L89.510 Pressure ulcer of right ankle, unstageable

L89.511 Pressure ulcer of right ankle, stage 1
Healing pressure ulcer of right ankle, stage 1
Pressure pre-ulcer skin changes limited to persistent focal edema, right ankle

L89.512 Pressure ulcer of right ankle, stage 2
Healing pressure ulcer of right ankle, stage 2
Pressure ulcer with abrasion, blister, partial thickness skin loss involving epidermis and/or dermis, right ankle

L89.513 Pressure ulcer of right ankle, stage 3
Healing pressure ulcer of right ankle, stage 3
Pressure ulcer with full thickness skin loss involving damage or necrosis of subcutaneous tissue, right ankle
MCC when PDx is its own MCC

L89.514 Pressure ulcer of right ankle, stage 4
Healing pressure ulcer of right ankle, stage 4
Pressure ulcer with necrosis of soft tissues through to underlying muscle, tendon, or bone, right ankle
MCC when PDx is its own MCC

L89.519 Pressure ulcer of right ankle, unspecified stage
Healing pressure ulcer of right ankle NOS
Healing pressure ulcer of right ankle, unspecified stage

● **L89.52 Pressure ulcer of left ankle**

L89.520 Pressure ulcer of left ankle, unstageable

L89.521 Pressure ulcer of left ankle, stage 1
Healing pressure ulcer of left ankle, stage 1
Pressure pre-ulcer skin changes limited to persistent focal edema, left ankle ◀

L89.522 Pressure ulcer of left ankle, stage 2
Healing pressure ulcer of left ankle, stage 2
Pressure ulcer with abrasion, blister, partial thickness skin loss involving epidermis and/or dermis, left ankle

L89.523 Pressure ulcer of left ankle, stage 3
Healing pressure ulcer of left ankle, stage 3
Pressure ulcer with full thickness skin loss involving damage or necrosis of subcutaneous tissue, left ankle
MCC when PDx is its own MCC

L89.524 Pressure ulcer of left ankle, stage 4
Healing pressure ulcer of left ankle, stage 4
Pressure ulcer with necrosis of soft tissues through to underlying muscle, tendon, or bone, left ankle
MCC when PDx is its own MCC

L89.529 Pressure ulcer of left ankle, unspecified stage
Healing pressure ulcer of left ankle NOS
Healing pressure ulcer of left ankle, unspecified stage

● **L89.6 Pressure ulcer of heel**

● **L89.60 Pressure ulcer of unspecified heel**

L89.600 Pressure ulcer of unspecified heel, unstageable

L89.601 Pressure ulcer of unspecified heel, stage 1
Healing pressure ulcer of unspecified heel, stage 1
Pressure pre-ulcer skin changes limited to persistent focal edema, unspecified heel

L89.602 Pressure ulcer of unspecified heel, stage 2
Healing pressure ulcer of unspecified heel, stage 2
Pressure ulcer with abrasion, blister, partial thickness skin loss involving epidermis and/or dermis, unspecified heel

L89.603 Pressure ulcer of unspecified heel, stage 3
Healing pressure ulcer of unspecified heel, stage 3
Pressure ulcer with full thickness skin loss involving damage or necrosis of subcutaneous tissue, unspecified heel
MCC when PDx is its own MCC

L89.604 Pressure ulcer of unspecified heel, stage 4
Healing pressure ulcer of unspecified heel, stage 4
Pressure ulcer with necrosis of soft tissues through to underlying muscle, tendon, or bone, unspecified heel
MCC when PDx is its own MCC

L89.609 Pressure ulcer of unspecified heel, unspecified stage
Healing pressure ulcer of unspecified heel NOS
Healing pressure ulcer of unspecified heel, unspecified stage

● **L89.61 Pressure ulcer of right heel**

L89.610 Pressure ulcer of right heel, unstageable

L89.611 Pressure ulcer of right heel, stage 1
Healing pressure ulcer of right heel, stage 1
Pressure pre-ulcer skin changes limited to persistent focal edema, right heel

L89.612 Pressure ulcer of right heel, stage 2
Healing pressure ulcer of right heel, stage 2
Pressure ulcer with abrasion, blister, partial thickness skin loss involving epidermis and/or dermis, right heel

L89.613 Pressure ulcer of right heel, stage 3
Healing pressure ulcer of right heel, stage 3
Pressure ulcer with full thickness skin loss involving damage or necrosis of subcutaneous tissue, right heel
MCC when PDx is its own MCC

L89.614 Pressure ulcer of right heel, stage 4
Healing pressure ulcer of right heel, stage 4
Pressure ulcer with necrosis of soft tissues through to underlying muscle, tendon, or bone, right heel
MCC when PDx is its own MCC

L89.619 Pressure ulcer of right heel, unspecified stage
Healing pressure ulcer of right heel NOS
Healing pressure ulcer of unspecified heel, right stage

● **L89.62 Pressure ulcer of left heel**

L89.620 Pressure ulcer of left heel, unstageable

L89.621 Pressure ulcer of left heel, stage 1
Healing pressure ulcer of left heel, stage 1
Pressure pre-ulcer skin changes limited to persistent focal edema, left heel

L89.622 Pressure ulcer of left heel, stage 2
Healing pressure ulcer of left heel, stage 2
Pressure ulcer with abrasion, blister, partial thickness skin loss involving epidermis and/or dermis, left heel

L89.623 Pressure ulcer of left heel, stage 3
Healing pressure ulcer of left heel, stage 3
Pressure ulcer with full thickness skin loss involving damage or necrosis of subcutaneous tissue, left heel
MCC when PDx is its own MCC

L89.624 Pressure ulcer of left heel, stage 4
Healing pressure ulcer of left heel, stage 4
Pressure ulcer with necrosis of soft tissues through to underlying muscle, tendon, or bone, left heel
MCC when PDx is its own MCC

L89.629 Pressure ulcer of left heel, unspecified stage
Healing pressure ulcer of left heel NOS
Healing pressure ulcer of left heel, unspecified stage

L89.8 Pressure ulcer of other site

L89.81 Pressure ulcer of head
Pressure ulcer of face

L89.810 Pressure ulcer of head, unstageable

L89.811 Pressure ulcer of head, stage 1
Healing pressure ulcer of head, stage 1
Pressure pre-ulcer skin changes limited to persistent focal edema, head

L89.812 Pressure ulcer of head, stage 2
Healing pressure ulcer of head, stage 2
Pressure ulcer with abrasion, blister, partial thickness skin loss involving epidermis and/or dermis, head

L89.813 Pressure ulcer of head, stage 3
Healing pressure ulcer of head, stage 3
Pressure ulcer with full thickness skin loss involving damage or necrosis of subcutaneous tissue, head
MCC when PDx is its own MCC

L89.814 Pressure ulcer of head, stage 4
Healing pressure ulcer of head, stage 4
Pressure ulcer with necrosis of soft tissues through to underlying muscle, tendon, or bone, head
MCC when PDx is its own MCC

L89.819 Pressure ulcer of head, unspecified stage
Healing pressure ulcer of head NOS
Healing pressure ulcer of head, unspecified stage

L89.89 Pressure ulcer of other site

L89.890 Pressure ulcer of other site, unstageable

L89.891 Pressure ulcer of other site, stage 1
Healing pressure ulcer of other site, stage 1
Pressure pre-ulcer skin changes limited to persistent focal edema, other site

L89.892 Pressure ulcer of other site, stage 2
Healing pressure ulcer of other site, stage 2
Pressure ulcer with abrasion, blister, partial thickness skin loss involving epidermis and/or dermis, other site

L89.893 Pressure ulcer of other site, stage 3
Healing pressure ulcer of other site, stage 3
Pressure ulcer with full thickness skin loss involving damage or necrosis of subcutaneous tissue, other site
MCC when PDx is its own MCC

L89.894 Pressure ulcer of other site, stage 4
Healing pressure ulcer of other site, stage 4
Pressure ulcer with necrosis of soft tissues through to underlying muscle, tendon, or bone, other site
MCC when PDx is its own MCC

L89.899 Pressure ulcer of other site, unspecified stage
Healing pressure ulcer of other site NOS
Healing pressure ulcer of other site, unspecified stage

L89.9 Pressure ulcer of unspecified site

L89.90 Pressure ulcer of unspecified site, unspecified stage
Healing pressure ulcer of unspecified site NOS
Healing pressure ulcer of unspecified site, unspecified stage

L89.91 Pressure ulcer of unspecified site, stage 1
Healing pressure ulcer of unspecified site, stage 1
Pressure pre-ulcer skin changes limited to persistent focal edema, unspecified site

L89.92 Pressure ulcer of unspecified site, stage 2
Healing pressure ulcer of unspecified site, stage 2
Pressure ulcer with abrasion, blister, partial thickness skin loss involving epidermis and/or dermis, unspecified site

L89.93 Pressure ulcer of unspecified site, stage 3
Healing pressure ulcer of unspecified site, stage 3
Pressure ulcer with full thickness skin loss involving damage or necrosis of subcutaneous tissue, unspecified site
MCC when PDx is its own MCC

L89.94 Pressure ulcer of unspecified site, stage 4
Healing pressure ulcer of unspecified site, stage 4
Pressure ulcer with necrosis of soft tissues through to underlying muscle, tendon, or bone, unspecified site
MCC when PDx is its own MCC

L89.95 Pressure ulcer of unspecified site, unstageable

● **L90 Atrophic disorders of skin**

L90.0 Lichen sclerosus et atrophicus

Excludes2 lichen sclerosus of external female genital organs (N90.4)
lichen sclerosus of external male genital organs (N48.0)

L90.1 Anetoderma of Schweninger-Buzzi

L90.2 Anetoderma of Jadassohn-Pellizzari

L90.3 Atrophoderma of Pasini and Pierini

L90.4 Acrodermatitis chronica atrophicans

L90.5 Scar conditions and fibrosis of skin

Adherent scar (skin)
Cicatrix
Disfigurement of skin due to scar
Fibrosis of skin NOS
Scar NOS

Excludes2 hypertrophic scar (L91.0)
keloid scar (L91.0)

Coding Clinic: 2016, Q2, P5; 2015, Q1, P19

L90.6 Striae atrophicae

L90.8 Other atrophic disorders of skin

L90.9 Atrophic disorder of skin, unspecified

● **L91 Hypertrophic disorders of skin**

L91.0 Keloid scar

Hypertrophic scar
Keloid

Excludes2 acne keloid (L73.0)
scar NOS (L90.5)

L91.8 Other hypertrophic disorders of the skin

L91.9 Hypertrophic disorder of the skin, unspecified

● **L92 Granulomatous disorders of skin and subcutaneous tissue**

Excludes2 actinic granuloma (L57.5)

L92.0 Granuloma annulare

Perforating granuloma annulare

L92.1 Necrobiosis lipoidica, not elsewhere classified

Excludes1 necrobiosis lipoidica associated with diabetes mellitus (E08-E13 with .620)

L92.2 Granuloma faciale [eosinophilic granuloma of skin]

L92.3 Foreign body granuloma of the skin and subcutaneous tissue

Use additional code to identify the type of retained foreign body (Z18.-)

L92.8 Other granulomatous disorders of the skin and subcutaneous tissue

L92.9 Granulomatous disorder of the skin and subcutaneous tissue, unspecified

● **L93 Lupus erythematosus**

Use additional code for adverse effect, if applicable, to identify drug (T36-T50 with fifth or sixth character 5)

Excludes1 lupus exedens (A18.4)
lupus vulgaris (A18.4)
scleroderma (M34.-)
systemic lupus erythematosus (M32.-)

L93.0 Discoid lupus erythematosus

Lupus erythematosus NOS

L93.1 Subacute cutaneous lupus erythematosus

L93.2 Other local lupus erythematosus

Lupus erythematosus profundus
Lupus panniculitis

● **L94 Other localized connective tissue disorders**

Excludes1 systemic connective tissue disorders (M30-M36)

L94.0 Localized scleroderma [morphea]

Circumscribed scleroderma

L94.1 Linear scleroderma

En coup de sabre lesion

L94.2 Calcinosis cutis

L94.3 Sclerodactyly

L94.4 Gottron's papules

L94.5 Poikiloderma vasculare atrophicans

L94.6 Ainhum

L94.8 Other specified localized connective tissue disorders

L94.9 Localized connective tissue disorder, unspecified

● **L95 Vasculitis limited to skin, not elsewhere classified**

Excludes1 angioma serpiginosum (L81.7)
Henoch(-Schönlein) purpura (D69.0)
hypersensitivity angiitis (M31.0)
lupus panniculitis (L93.2)
panniculitis NOS (M79.3)
panniculitis of neck and back (M54.0-)
polyarteritis nodosa (M30.0)
relapsing panniculitis (M35.6)
rheumatoid vasculitis (M05.2)
serum sickness (T80.6-)
urticaria (L50.-)
Wegener's granulomatosis (M31.3-)

L95.0 Livedoid vasculitis

Atrophie blanche (en plaque)

L95.1 Erythema elevatum diutinum

L95.8 Other vasculitis limited to the skin

L95.9 Vasculitis limited to the skin, unspecified

● **L97 Non-pressure chronic ulcer of lower limb, not elsewhere classified**

Includes chronic ulcer of skin of lower limb NOS
non-healing ulcer of skin
non-infected sinus of skin
trophic ulcer NOS
tropical ulcer NOS
ulcer of skin of lower limb NOS

Code first any associated underlying condition, such as:
any associated gangrene (I96)
atherosclerosis of the lower extremities (I70.23-, I70.24-, I70.33-, I70.34-, I70.43-, I70.44-, I70.53-, I70.54-, I70.63-, I70.64-, I70.73-, I70.74-)
chronic venous hypertension (I87.31-, I87.33-)
diabetic ulcers (E08.621, E08.622, E09.621, E09.622, E10.621, E10.622, E11.621, E11.622, E13.621, E13.622)
postphlebitic syndrome (I87.01-, I87.03-)
postthrombotic syndrome (I87.01-, I87.03-)
varicose ulcer (I83.0-, I83.2-)

Excludes2 pressure ulcer (pressure area) (L89.-)
skin infections (L00-L08)
specific infections classified to A00-B99

Ex **For category L97 CC codes:** I70.231-I70.25, L44.8-L45, L94.2, L94.4, L97.101-L97.929, L98.411-L98.499, L98.7-L99

● **L97.1 Non-pressure chronic ulcer of thigh**

● **L97.10 Non-pressure chronic ulcer of unspecified thigh**

L97.101 Non-pressure chronic ulcer of unspecified thigh limited to breakdown of skin

L97.102 Non-pressure chronic ulcer of unspecified thigh with fat layer exposed

L97.103 Non-pressure chronic ulcer of unspecified thigh with necrosis of muscle

Item 12–11 Scleroderma means hard skin. It is a group of diseases that causes abnormal growth of connective tissues that support the skin and organs. There are two types: localized scleroderma affecting the skin and systemic scleroderma affecting blood vessels and internal organs and the skin.

L97.104 Non-pressure chronic ulcer of unspecified thigh with necrosis of bone

L97.109 Non-pressure chronic ulcer of unspecified thigh with unspecified severity

● L97.11 Non-pressure chronic ulcer of right thigh

L97.111 Non-pressure chronic ulcer of right thigh limited to breakdown of skin

L97.112 Non-pressure chronic ulcer of right thigh with fat layer exposed

L97.113 Non-pressure chronic ulcer of right thigh with necrosis of muscle

L97.114 Non-pressure chronic ulcer of right thigh with necrosis of bone

L97.119 Non-pressure chronic ulcer of right thigh with unspecified severity

● L97.12 Non-pressure chronic ulcer of left thigh

L97.121 Non-pressure chronic ulcer of left thigh limited to breakdown of skin

L97.122 Non-pressure chronic ulcer of left thigh with fat layer exposed

L97.123 Non-pressure chronic ulcer of left thigh with necrosis of muscle

L97.124 Non-pressure chronic ulcer of left thigh with necrosis of bone

L97.129 Non-pressure chronic ulcer of left thigh with unspecified severity

● L97.2 Non-pressure chronic ulcer of calf

● L97.20 Non-pressure chronic ulcer of unspecified calf

L97.201 Non-pressure chronic ulcer of unspecified calf limited to breakdown of skin

L97.202 Non-pressure chronic ulcer of unspecified calf with fat layer exposed

L97.203 Non-pressure chronic ulcer of unspecified calf with necrosis of muscle

L97.204 Non-pressure chronic ulcer of unspecified calf with necrosis of bone

L97.209 Non-pressure chronic ulcer of unspecified calf with unspecified severity

● L97.21 Non-pressure chronic ulcer of right calf

L97.211 Non-pressure chronic ulcer of right calf limited to breakdown of skin

L97.212 Non-pressure chronic ulcer of right calf with fat layer exposed

L97.213 Non-pressure chronic ulcer of right calf with necrosis of muscle

L97.214 Non-pressure chronic ulcer of right calf with necrosis of bone

L97.219 Non-pressure chronic ulcer of right calf with unspecified severity

● L97.22 Non-pressure chronic ulcer of left calf

L97.221 Non-pressure chronic ulcer of left calf limited to breakdown of skin

L97.222 Non-pressure chronic ulcer of left calf with fat layer exposed

L97.223 Non-pressure chronic ulcer of left calf with necrosis of muscle

L97.224 Non-pressure chronic ulcer of left calf with necrosis of bone

L97.229 Non-pressure chronic ulcer of left calf with unspecified severity

● L97.3 Non-pressure chronic ulcer of ankle

● L97.30 Non-pressure chronic ulcer of unspecified ankle

L97.301 Non-pressure chronic ulcer of unspecified ankle limited to breakdown of skin

L97.302 Non-pressure chronic ulcer of unspecified ankle with fat layer exposed

L97.303 Non-pressure chronic ulcer of unspecified ankle with necrosis of muscle

L97.304 Non-pressure chronic ulcer of unspecified ankle with necrosis of bone

L97.309 Non-pressure chronic ulcer of unspecified ankle with unspecified severity

● L97.31 Non-pressure chronic ulcer of right ankle

L97.311 Non-pressure chronic ulcer of right ankle limited to breakdown of skin

L97.312 Non-pressure chronic ulcer of right ankle with fat layer exposed

L97.313 Non-pressure chronic ulcer of right ankle with necrosis of muscle

L97.314 Non-pressure chronic ulcer of right ankle with necrosis of bone

L97.319 Non-pressure chronic ulcer of right ankle with unspecified severity

● L97.32 Non-pressure chronic ulcer of left ankle

L97.321 Non-pressure chronic ulcer of left ankle limited to breakdown of skin

L97.322 Non-pressure chronic ulcer of left ankle with fat layer exposed

L97.323 Non-pressure chronic ulcer of left ankle with necrosis of muscle

L97.324 Non-pressure chronic ulcer of left ankle with necrosis of bone

L97.329 Non-pressure chronic ulcer of left ankle with unspecified severity

● L97.4 Non-pressure chronic ulcer of heel and midfoot

Non-pressure chronic ulcer of plantar surface of midfoot

● L97.40 Non-pressure chronic ulcer of unspecified heel and midfoot

L97.401 Non-pressure chronic ulcer of unspecified heel and midfoot limited to breakdown of skin

L97.402 Non-pressure chronic ulcer of unspecified heel and midfoot with fat layer exposed

L97.403 Non-pressure chronic ulcer of unspecified heel and midfoot with necrosis of muscle

L97.404 Non-pressure chronic ulcer of unspecified heel and midfoot with necrosis of bone

L97.409 Non-pressure chronic ulcer of unspecified heel and midfoot with unspecified severity

● L97.41 Non-pressure chronic ulcer of right heel and midfoot

L97.411 Non-pressure chronic ulcer of right heel and midfoot limited to breakdown of skin

L97.412 Non-pressure chronic ulcer of right heel and midfoot with fat layer exposed

L97.413 Non-pressure chronic ulcer of right heel and midfoot with necrosis of muscle

L97.414 Non-pressure chronic ulcer of right heel and midfoot with necrosis of bone

L97.419 Non-pressure chronic ulcer of right heel and midfoot with unspecified severity

● L97.42 Non-pressure chronic ulcer of left heel and midfoot

L97.421 Non-pressure chronic ulcer of left heel and midfoot limited to breakdown of skin
Coding Clinic: 2016, Q1, P13

L97.422 Non-pressure chronic ulcer of left heel and midfoot with fat layer exposed

L97.423 Non-pressure chronic ulcer of left heel and midfoot with necrosis of muscle

L97.424 Non-pressure chronic ulcer of left heel and midfoot with necrosis of bone

L97.429 Non-pressure chronic ulcer of left heel and midfoot with unspecified severity

● L97.5 Non-pressure chronic ulcer of other part of foot
Non-pressure chronic ulcer of toe

● L97.50 Non-pressure chronic ulcer of other part of unspecified foot

L97.501 Non-pressure chronic ulcer of other part of unspecified foot limited to breakdown of skin

L97.502 Non-pressure chronic ulcer of other part of unspecified foot with fat layer exposed

L97.503 Non-pressure chronic ulcer of other part of unspecified foot with necrosis of muscle

L97.504 Non-pressure chronic ulcer of other part of unspecified foot with necrosis of bone

L97.509 Non-pressure chronic ulcer of other part of unspecified foot with unspecified severity

● L97.51 Non-pressure chronic ulcer of other part of right foot

L97.511 Non-pressure chronic ulcer of other part of right foot limited to breakdown of skin

L97.512 Non-pressure chronic ulcer of other part of right foot with fat layer exposed

L97.513 Non-pressure chronic ulcer of other part of right foot with necrosis of muscle

L97.514 Non-pressure chronic ulcer of other part of right foot with necrosis of bone

L97.519 Non-pressure chronic ulcer of other part of right foot with unspecified severity

● L97.52 Non-pressure chronic ulcer of other part of left foot

L97.521 Non-pressure chronic ulcer of other part of left foot limited to breakdown of skin

L97.522 Non-pressure chronic ulcer of other part of left foot with fat layer exposed

L97.523 Non-pressure chronic ulcer of other part of left foot with necrosis of muscle

L97.524 Non-pressure chronic ulcer of other part of left foot with necrosis of bone

L97.529 Non-pressure chronic ulcer of other part of left foot with unspecified severity

● L97.8 Non-pressure chronic ulcer of other part of lower leg

● L97.80 Non-pressure chronic ulcer of other part of unspecified lower leg

L97.801 Non-pressure chronic ulcer of other part of unspecified lower leg limited to breakdown of skin

L97.802 Non-pressure chronic ulcer of other part of unspecified lower leg with fat layer exposed

L97.803 Non-pressure chronic ulcer of other part of unspecified lower leg with necrosis of muscle

L97.804 Non-pressure chronic ulcer of other part of unspecified lower leg with necrosis of bone

L97.809 Non-pressure chronic ulcer of other part of unspecified lower leg with unspecified severity

● L97.81 Non-pressure chronic ulcer of other part of right lower leg

L97.811 Non-pressure chronic ulcer of other part of right lower leg limited to breakdown of skin

L97.812 Non-pressure chronic ulcer of other part of right lower leg with fat layer exposed

L97.813 Non-pressure chronic ulcer of other part of right lower leg with necrosis of muscle

L97.814 Non-pressure chronic ulcer of other part of right lower leg with necrosis of bone

L97.819 Non-pressure chronic ulcer of other part of right lower leg with unspecified severity

● L97.82 Non-pressure chronic ulcer of other part of left lower leg

L97.821 Non-pressure chronic ulcer of other part of left lower leg limited to breakdown of skin

L97.822 Non-pressure chronic ulcer of other part of left lower leg with fat layer exposed

L97.823 Non-pressure chronic ulcer of other part of left lower leg with necrosis of muscle

L97.824 Non-pressure chronic ulcer of other part of left lower leg with necrosis of bone

L97.829 Non-pressure chronic ulcer of other part of left lower leg with unspecified severity

● L97.9 Non-pressure chronic ulcer of unspecified part of lower leg

● L97.90 Non-pressure chronic ulcer of unspecified part of unspecified lower leg

L97.901 Non-pressure chronic ulcer of unspecified part of unspecified lower leg limited to breakdown of skin

L97.902 Non-pressure chronic ulcer of unspecified part of unspecified lower leg with fat layer exposed

◀ New ◀ Revised ~~deleted~~ Deleted Excludes 1 Excludes 2 Includes Use additional Code first Code also Unspecified
OGCR Official Guidelines ● Unacceptable Principal Diagnosis X Assign placeholder X ● Use Additional Character(s) ▶ Manifestation Code Coding Clinic

L97.903 Non-pressure chronic ulcer of unspecified part of unspecified lower leg with necrosis of muscle

L97.904 Non-pressure chronic ulcer of unspecified part of unspecified lower leg with necrosis of bone

L97.909 Non-pressure chronic ulcer of unspecified part of unspecified lower leg with unspecified severity

L97.91 Non-pressure chronic ulcer of unspecified part of right lower leg

L97.911 Non-pressure chronic ulcer of unspecified part of right lower leg limited to breakdown of skin

L97.912 Non-pressure chronic ulcer of unspecified part of right lower leg with fat layer exposed

L97.913 Non-pressure chronic ulcer of unspecified part of right lower leg with necrosis of muscle

L97.914 Non-pressure chronic ulcer of unspecified part of right lower leg with necrosis of bone

L97.919 Non-pressure chronic ulcer of unspecified part of right lower leg with unspecified severity

L97.92 Non-pressure chronic ulcer of unspecified part of left lower leg

L97.921 Non-pressure chronic ulcer of unspecified part of left lower leg limited to breakdown of skin

L97.922 Non-pressure chronic ulcer of unspecified part of left lower leg with fat layer exposed

L97.923 Non-pressure chronic ulcer of unspecified part of left lower leg with necrosis of muscle

L97.924 Non-pressure chronic ulcer of unspecified part of left lower leg with necrosis of bone

L97.929 Non-pressure chronic ulcer of unspecified part of left lower leg with unspecified severity

L98 Other disorders of skin and subcutaneous tissue, not elsewhere classified

L98.0 Pyogenic granuloma

Excludes2 pyogenic granuloma of gingiva (K06.8)
pyogenic granuloma of maxillary alveolar ridge (K04.5)
pyogenic granuloma of oral mucosa (K13.4)

L98.1 Factitial dermatitis
Neurotic excoriation

Excludes1 Excoriation (skin-picking) disorder (F42.4) ◀

L98.2 Febrile neutrophilic dermatosis [Sweet]

L98.3 Eosinophilic cellulitis [Wells]
Ex See L02.81

L98.4 Non-pressure chronic ulcer of skin, not elsewhere classified
Chronic ulcer of skin NOS
Tropical ulcer NOS
Ulcer of skin NOS

Excludes2 pressure ulcer (pressure area) (L89.-)
gangrene (I96)
skin infections (L00-L08)
specific infections classified to A00-B99
ulcer of lower limb NEC (L97.-)
varicose ulcer (I83.0-I82.2)

L98.41 Non-pressure chronic ulcer of buttock

L98.411 Non-pressure chronic ulcer of buttock limited to breakdown of skin

L98.412 Non-pressure chronic ulcer of buttock with fat layer exposed

L98.413 Non-pressure chronic ulcer of buttock with necrosis of muscle

L98.414 Non-pressure chronic ulcer of buttock with necrosis of bone

L98.419 Non-pressure chronic ulcer of buttock with unspecified severity

L98.42 Non-pressure chronic ulcer of back

L98.421 Non-pressure chronic ulcer of back limited to breakdown of skin

L98.422 Non-pressure chronic ulcer of back with fat layer exposed

L98.423 Non-pressure chronic ulcer of back with necrosis of muscle

L98.424 Non-pressure chronic ulcer of back with necrosis of bone

L98.429 Non-pressure chronic ulcer of back with unspecified severity

L98.49 Non-pressure chronic ulcer of skin of other sites
Non-pressure chronic ulcer of skin NOS

L98.491 Non-pressure chronic ulcer of skin of other sites limited to breakdown of skin

L98.492 Non-pressure chronic ulcer of skin of other sites with fat layer exposed

L98.493 Non-pressure chronic ulcer of skin of other sites with necrosis of muscle

L98.494 Non-pressure chronic ulcer of skin of other sites with necrosis of bone

L98.499 Non-pressure chronic ulcer of skin of other sites with unspecified severity

L98.5 Mucinosis of the skin
Focal mucinosis
Lichen myxedematosus
Reticular erythematous mucinosis

Excludes1 focal oral mucinosis (K13.79)
myxedema (E03.9)

L98.6 Other infiltrative disorders of the skin and subcutaneous tissue

Excludes1 hyalinosis cutis et mucosae (E78.89)

L98.7 Excessive and redundant skin and subcutaneous tissue ◀
Loose or sagging skin following bariatric surgery weight loss ◀
Loose or sagging skin following dietary weight loss ◀
Loose or sagging skin, NOS ◀

Excludes2 acquired excess or redundant skin of eyelid (H02.3-) ◀
congenital excess or redundant skin of eyelid (Q10.3) ◀
skin changes due to chronic exposure to nonionizing radiation (L57.-) ◀

L98.8 Other specified disorders of the skin and subcutaneous tissue
Coding Clinic: 2013, Q2, P32

L98.9 Disorder of the skin and subcutaneous tissue, unspecified

L99 *Other disorders of skin and subcutaneous tissue in diseases classified elsewhere*
Code first underlying disease, such as:
amyloidosis (E85.-)

Excludes1 skin disorders in diabetes (E08-E13 with .62)
skin disorders in gonorrhea (A54.89)
skin disorders in syphilis (A51.31, A52.79)

CHAPTER 13

DISEASES OF THE MUSCULOSKELETAL SYSTEM AND CONNECTIVE TISSUE (M00-M99)

OGCR Chapter-Specific Coding Guidelines

13. Chapter 13: Diseases of the Musculoskeletal System and Connective Tissue (M00-M99)

a. Site and laterality

Most of the codes within Chapter 13 have site and laterality designations. The site represents the bone, joint or the muscle involved. For some conditions where more than one bone, joint or muscle is usually involved, such as osteoarthritis, there is a "multiple sites" code available. For categories where no multiple site code is provided and more than one bone, joint or muscle is involved, multiple codes should be used to indicate the different sites involved.

1) Bone versus joint

For certain conditions, the bone may be affected at the upper or lower end, (e.g., avascular necrosis of bone, M87, Osteoporosis, M80, M81). Though the portion of the bone affected may be at the joint, the site designation will be the bone, not the joint.

b. Acute traumatic versus chronic or recurrent musculoskeletal conditions

Many musculoskeletal conditions are a result of previous injury or trauma to a site, or are recurrent conditions. Bone, joint or muscle conditions that are the result of a healed injury are usually found in chapter 13. Recurrent bone, joint or muscle conditions are also usually found in chapter 13. Any current, acute injury should be coded to the appropriate injury code from chapter 19. Chronic or recurrent conditions should generally be coded with a code from chapter 13. If it is difficult to determine from the documentation in the record which code is best to describe a condition, query the provider.

c. Coding of Pathologic Fractures

7th character A is for use as long as the patient is receiving active treatment for the fracture. While the patient may be seen by a new or different provider over the course of treatment for a pathological fracture, assignment of the 7th character is based on whether the patient is undergoing active treatment and not whether the provider is seeing the patient for the first time.

7th character, D is to be used for encounters after the patient has completed active treatment. The other 7th characters, listed under each subcategory in the Tabular List, are to be used for subsequent encounters for **routine care of fractures during the healing and recovery phase as well as** treatment of problems associated with the healing, such as malunions, nonunions, and sequelae.

Care for complications of surgical treatment for fracture repairs during the healing or recovery phase should be coded with the appropriate complication codes.

See Section I.C.19. Coding of traumatic fractures.

d. Osteoporosis

Osteoporosis is a systemic condition, meaning that all bones of the musculoskeletal system are affected. Therefore, site is not a component of the codes under category M81, Osteoporosis without current pathological fracture. The site codes under category M80, Osteoporosis with current pathological fracture, identify the site of the fracture, not the osteoporosis.

1) Osteoporosis without pathological fracture

Category M81, Osteoporosis without current pathological fracture, is for use for patients with osteoporosis who do not currently have a pathologic fracture due to the osteoporosis, even if they have had a fracture in the past. For patients with a history of osteoporosis fractures, status code Z87.310, Personal history of (healed) osteoporosis fracture, should follow the code from M81.

2) Osteoporosis with current pathological fracture

Category M80, Osteoporosis with current pathological fracture, is for patients who have a current pathologic fracture at the time of an encounter. The codes under M80 identify the site of the fracture. A code from category M80, not a traumatic fracture code, should be used for any patient with known osteoporosis who suffers a fracture, even if the patient had a minor fall or trauma, if that fall or trauma would not usually break a normal, healthy bone.

CHAPTER 13

DISEASES OF THE MUSCULOSKELETAL SYSTEM AND CONNECTIVE TISSUE (M00-M99)

Note: Use an external cause code following the code for the musculoskeletal condition, if applicable, to identify the cause of the musculoskeletal condition

Excludes2
- arthropathic psoriasis (L40.5-)
- certain conditions originating in the perinatal period (P04-P96)
- certain infectious and parasitic diseases (A00-B99)
- compartment syndrome (traumatic) (T79.A-)
- complications of pregnancy, childbirth and the puerperium (O00-O9A)
- congenital malformations, deformations, and chromosomal abnormalities (Q00-Q99)
- endocrine, nutritional and metabolic diseases (E00-E88)
- injury, poisoning and certain other consequences of external causes (S00-T88)
- neoplasms (C00-D49)
- symptoms, signs and abnormal clinical and laboratory findings, not elsewhere classified (R00-R94)

This chapter contains the following blocks:

M00-M02	Infectious arthropathies
M04	Autoinflammatory syndromes ◀
M05-M14	Inflammatory polyarthropathies
M15-M19	Osteoarthritis
M20-M25	Other joint disorders
M26-M27	Dentofacial anomalies [including malocclusion] and other disorders of jaw
M30-M36	Systemic connective tissue disorders
M40-M43	Deforming dorsopathies
M45-M49	Spondylopathies
M50-M54	Other dorsopathies
M60-M63	Disorders of muscles
M65-M67	Disorders of synovium and tendon
M70-M79	Other soft tissue disorders
M80-M85	Disorders of bone density and structure
M86-M90	Other osteopathies
M91-M94	Chondropathies
M95	Other disorders of the musculoskeletal system and connective tissue
M96	Intraoperative and postprocedural complications and disorders of musculoskeletal system, not elsewhere classified
M97	Periprosthetic fracture around internal prosthetic joint ◀
M99	Biomechanical lesions, not elsewhere classified

ARTHROPATHIES (M00-M25)

Includes Disorders affecting predominantly peripheral (limb) joints

INFECTIOUS ARTHROPATHIES (M00-M02)

Note: This block comprises arthropathies due to microbiological agents.

Distinction is made between the following types of etiological relationship:

a) direct infection of joint, where organisms invade synovial tissue and microbial antigen is present in the joint;

b) indirect infection, which may be of two types: a reactive arthropathy, where microbial infection of the body is established but neither organisms nor antigens can be identified in the joint, and a postinfective arthropathy, where microbial antigen is present but recovery of an organism is inconstant and evidence of local multiplication is lacking.

● **M00 Pyogenic arthritis**

● **M00.0 Staphylococcal arthritis and polyarthritis**

Use additional code (B95.61-B95.8) to identify bacterial agent

Excludes2 infection and inflammatory reaction due to internal joint prosthesis (T84.5-)

M00.00 Staphylococcal arthritis, unspecified joint CC

Ex: A17.9, A18.02, A18.09, A18.82, A18.84, A18.89, A39.83-A39.84, A54.40, A54.42-A54.43, A54.82, A54.84, A54.89-A54.9, B06.82, M00.00-M02.30, M02.319, M02.329, M02.339, M02.349, M02.359, M02.369, M02.379-M02.9, M05.40-M05.59, M05.70-M06.09, M06.20-M07.69, M11.00-M11.9, M12.10-M15.0, M15.3-M15.9, M16.2-M16.9, M17.2-M17.9, M18.2-M19.93, M24.10-M24.176, M25.00, M25.08-M25.18, M25.40-M25.676, M25.80-M25.9, M35.2, M36.1-M36.4, R26.2, R29.4

● **M00.01 Staphylococcal arthritis, shoulder**

Ex: **For category M00.01 CC codes:** A17.9, A18.02, A18.09, A18.82, A18.84, A18.89, A39.83-A39.84, A54.40, A54.42-A54.43, A54.82, A54.84, A54.89-A54.9, B06.82, M00.00-M02.30, M02.319, M02.38-M02.819, M02.88-M02.9, M05.40-M05.59, M05.70-M06.09, M06.20-M07.69, M11.00-M11.9, M11.20-M11.219, M11.28-M11.819, M11.88-M11.9, M12.10-M15.0, M15.3-M15.9, M19.011-M19.019, M19.111-M19.119, M19.211-M19.219, M19.90-M19.93, M24.10-M24.119, M25.00, M25.011-M25.019, M25.08-M25.119, M25.18, M25.40-M25.419, M25.48-M25.519, M25.541-M25.549, M25.60-M25.619, M25.80-M25.819, M25.9, M35.2, M36.1-M36.4, R26.2

M00.011 Staphylococcal arthritis, right shoulder CC

M00.012 Staphylococcal arthritis, left shoulder CC

M00.019 Staphylococcal arthritis, unspecified shoulder CC

● **M00.02 Staphylococcal arthritis, elbow**

Ex: **For category M00.02 CC codes:** A17.9, A18.02, A18.09, A18.82, A18.84, A18.89, A39.83-A39.84, A54.40, A54.42-A54.43, A54.82, A54.84, A54.89-A54.9, B06.82, M00.00-M02.30, M02.329, M02.38-M02.80, M02.821-M02.829, M02.88-M02.9, M05.40-M05.59, M05.70-M07.60, M07.621-M07.629, M07.68-M07.69, M11.00, M11.021-M11.029, M11.08-M11.10, M11.121-M11.129, M11.18-M11.20, M11.221-M11.229, M11.28-M11.80, M11.821-M11.829, M11.88-M11.9, M12.10, M12.121-M12.129, M12.18-M12.20, M12.221-M12.229, M12.28-M12.30, M12.321-M12.329, M12.38-M12.40, M12.421-M12.429, M12.48-M12.50, M12.521-M12.529, M12.58-M12.80, M12.821-M12.829, M12.88-M12.9, M13.0-M13.10, M13.121-M13.129, M13.80, M13.821-M13.829, M13.88-M13.89, M14.60-M15.9, M19.021-M19.029, M19.121-M19.129, M19.221-M19.229, M19.90-M19.93, M24.10, M24.121-M24.129, M25.00, M25.021-M25.029, M25.08-M25.10, M25.121-M25.129, M25.18, M25.40, M25.421-M25.429, M25.48-M25.50, M25.521-M25.529, M25.541-M25.549, M25.60, M25.621-M25.629, M25.80, M25.821-M25.829, M25.9, M35.2, M36.1-M36.4, R26.2

M00.021 Staphylococcal arthritis, right elbow CC

M00.022 Staphylococcal arthritis, left elbow CC

M00.029 Staphylococcal arthritis, unspecified elbow CC

● **M00.03 Staphylococcal arthritis, wrist**

Staphylococcal arthritis of carpal bones

Ex: **For category M00.03 CC codes:** A17.9, A18.02, A18.09, A18.82, A18.84, A18.89, A39.83-A39.84, A54.40, A54.42-A54.43, A54.82, A54.84, A54.89-A54.9, B06.82, M00.00-M02.30, M02.339, M02.38-M02.80, M02.831-M02.839, M02.88-M02.9, M05.40-M05.59, M05.70-M07.60, M07.631-M07.639, M07.68-M07.69, M11.00, M11.031-M11.039, M11.08-M11.10, M11.131-M11.139, M11.18-M11.20, M11.231-M11.239, M11.28-M11.80, M11.831-M11.839, M11.88-M11.9, M12.10, M12.131-M12.139, M12.18-M12.20, M12.231-M12.239, M12.28-M12.30, M12.331-M12.339, M12.38-M12.40, M12.431-M12.439, M12.48-M12.50, M12.531-M12.539, M12.58-M12.80, M12.831-M12.839, M12.88-M12.9, M13.0-M13.10, M13.131-M13.139, M13.80, M13.831-M13.839, M13.88-M15.9, M19.031-M19.039, M19.131-M19.139, M19.231-M19.239, M19.90-M19.93, M24.10, M24.131-M24.139, M25.00, M25.031-M25.039, M25.08-M25.10, M25.131-M25.139, M25.18, M25.40, M25.431-M25.439, M25.48-M25.50, M25.531-M25.539, M25.541-M25.549, M25.60, M25.631-M25.639, M25.80, M25.831-M25.839, M25.9, M35.2, M36.1-M36.4, R26.2

M00.031 Staphylococcal arthritis, right wrist CC

M00.032 Staphylococcal arthritis, left wrist CC

M00.039 Staphylococcal arthritis, unspecified wrist CC

● **M00.04 Staphylococcal arthritis, hand**

Staphylococcal arthritis of metacarpus and phalanges

Ex: **For category M00.04 CC codes:** A17.9, A18.02, A18.09, A18.82, A18.84, A18.89, A39.83-A39.84, A54.40, A54.42-A54.43, A54.82, A54.84, A54.89-A54.9, B06.82, M00.00, M00.041-M00.049, M00.08-M00.10, M00.141-M00.149, M00.18-M00.20, M00.241-M00.249, M00.28-M00.80, M00.841-M00.849, M00.88-M01.X0, M01.X41-M01.X49, M01.X8-M02.10, M02.141-M02.149, M02.18-M02.30, M02.349, M02.38-M02.80, M02.841-M02.849, M02.88-M02.9, M05.40-M05.59, M05.70-M06.09, M06.20-M07.60, M07.641-M07.649, M07.68-M07.69, M11.00, M11.041-M11.049, M11.08-M11.10, M11.141-M11.149, M11.18-M11.20, M11.241-M11.249, M11.28-M11.80, M11.841-M11.849, M11.88-M11.9, M12.10, M12.141-M12.149, M12.18-M12.20, M12.241-M12.249, M12.28-M12.30, M12.341-M12.349, M12.38-M12.40, M12.441-M12.449, M12.48-M12.50, M12.541-M12.549, M12.58-M12.80, M12.841-M12.849, M12.88-M13.10, M13.141-M13.149, M13.80, M13.841-M13.849, M13.88-M15.9, M18.0-M18.9, M19.041-M19.049, M19.141-M19.149, M19.241-M19.249, M19.90-M19.93, M24.10, M24.141-M24.149, M25.00, M25.041-M25.049, M25.08-M25.10, M25.141-M25.149, M25.18, M25.40, M25.441-M25.449, M25.48-M25.50, M25.541-M25.549, M25.60, M25.641-M25.649, M25.80, M25.841-M25.849, M25.9, M35.2, M36.1-M36.4, R26.2

M00.041 Staphylococcal arthritis, right hand CC

M00.042 Staphylococcal arthritis, left hand CC

M00.049 Staphylococcal arthritis, unspecified hand CC

● **M00.05 Staphylococcal arthritis, hip**

Ex: **For category M00.05 CC codes:** A17.9, A18.02, A18.09, A18.82, A18.84, A18.89, A39.83-A39.84, A54.40, A54.42-A54.43, A54.82, A54.84, A54.89-A54.9, B06.82, M00.00, M00.051-M00.059, M00.08-M00.10, M00.151-M00.159, M00.18-M00.20, M00.251-M00.259, M00.28-M00.29, M00.80, M00.851-M00.859, M00.88-M00.9, M01.X0, M01.X51-M01.X59 , M01.X8-M02.10, M02.151-M02.159, M02.18-M02.30, M02.359, M02.38-M02.80, M02.851-M02.9, M05.40-M05.59, M05.70-M06.09, M06.20-M06.39, M06.80-M07.60, M07.651-M07.659, M07.68-M07.69, M11.00, M11.051-M11.059, M11.08-M11.10, M11.151-M11.159, M11.18-M11.20, M11.251-M11.259, M11.28-M11.80, M11.851-M11.859, M11.88-M12.10, M12.151-M12.159, M12.18-M12.20, M12.251-M12.259, M12.28-M12.30, M12.351-M12.359, M12.38-M12.40, M12.451-M12.459, M12.48-M12.50, M12.551-M12.559, M12.58-M12.80, M12.851-M12.859, M12.88-M13.10, M13.151-M13.159, M13.80, M13.851-M13.859, M13.88-M15.0, M15.3-M16.9, M19.90-M19.93, M24.10, M24.151-M24.159, M25.00, M25.051-M25.059, M25.08-M25.10, M25.151-M25.159, M25.18, M25.40, M25.451-M25.459, M25.48-M25.559, M25.60, M25.651-M25.659, M25.80, M25.851-M25.859, M25.9, M35.2, M36.1-M36.4, R26.2, R29.4

M00.051 Staphylococcal arthritis, right hip CC

M00.052 Staphylococcal arthritis, left hip CC

M00.059 Staphylococcal arthritis, unspecified hip CC

● **M00.06 Staphylococcal arthritis, knee**

Ex: **For category M00.06 CC codes:** A17.9, A18.02, A18.09, A18.82, A18.84, A18.89, A39.83-A39.84, A54.40, A54.42-A54.43, A54.82, A54.84, A54.89-A54.9, B06.82, M00.00, M00.061-M00.069, M00.08-M00.10, M00.161-M00.169, M00.18-M00.20, M00.261-M00.269, M00.28-M00.29, M00.80, M00.861-M00.869, M00.88-M00.9, M01.X0, M01.X61-M01.X69 , M01.X8-M02.10, M02.161-M02.169, M02.18-M02.30, M02.369, M02.38-M02.80, M02.861-M02.869, M02.88-M02.9, M05.40-M05.59, M05.70-M06.09, M06.20-M06.39, M06.80-M07.60, M07.661-M07.669, M07.68-M07.69, M11.00, M11.061-M11.069, M11.08-M11.10, M11.161-M11.169, M11.18-M11.20, M11.261-M11.269, M11.28-M11.80, M11.861-M11.869, M11.88-M12.10, M12.161-M12.169, M12.18-M12.20, M12.261-M12.269, M12.28-M12.30, M12.361-M12.369, M12.38-M12.40, M12.461-M12.469, M12.48-M12.50, M12.561-M12.569, M12.58-M12.80, M12.861-M12.869, M12.88-M13.10, M13.161-M13.169, M13.80, M13.861-M13.869, M13.88-M15.0, M15.3-M15.9, M17.0-M17.9, M19.90-M19.93, M24.10, M25.00, M25.061-M25.069, M25.08-M25.10, M25.161-M25.169, M25.18, M25.40, M25.461-M25.469, M25.48-M25.50, M25.541-M25.549, M25.561-M25.569, M25.60, M25.661-M25.669, M25.80, M25.861-M25.869, M25.9, M35.2, M36.1-M36.4, R26.2

M00.061 Staphylococcal arthritis, right knee CC

M00.062 Staphylococcal arthritis, left knee CC

M00.069 Staphylococcal arthritis, unspecified knee CC

● **M00.07 Staphylococcal arthritis, ankle and foot**

Staphylococcal arthritis, tarsus, metatarsus and phalanges

Ex: **For category M00.07 CC codes:** A17.9, A18.02, A18.09, A18.82, A18.84, A18.89, A39.83-A39.84, A54.40, A54.42-A54.43, A54.82, A54.84, A54.89-A54.9, B06.82, M00.00, M00.071-M00.079, M00.08-M00.10, M00.171-M00.179, M00.18-M00.20, M00.271-M00.279, M00.28-M00.29, M00.80, M00.871-M00.879, M00.88-M00.9, M01.X0, M01.X71-M01.X79 , M01.X8-M02.10, M02.171-M02.179, M02.18-M02.9, M05.40-M05.59, M05.70-M06.09, M06.20-M06.39, M06.80-M07.60, M07.671-M07.679, M07.68-M07.69, M11.00, M11.071-M11.079, M11.08-M11.10, M11.171-M11.179, M11.18-M11.20, M11.271-M11.279, M11.28-M11.80, M11.871-M11.879, M11.88-M11.9, M12.10, M12.171-M12.179, M12.18-M12.20, M12.271-M12.279, M12.28-M12.30, M12.371-M12.379, M12.38-M12.40, M12.471-M12.479, M12.48-M12.50, M12.571-M12.579, M12.58-M12.80, M12.871-M12.879, M12.88-M13.10, M13.171-M13.179, M13.80, M13.871-M13.879, M13.88-M15.0, M15.3-M15.9, M19.071-M19.079, M19.171-M19.179, M19.271-M19.279, M19.90-M19.93, M24.10, M24.171-M24.176, M25.00, M25.071-M25.10, M25.171-M25.18, M25.40, M25.471-M25.50, M25.541-M25.549, M25.571-M25.60, M25.671-M25.676, M25.80, M25.871-M25.9, M35.2, M36.1-M36.4, R26.2

M00.071 Staphylococcal arthritis, right ankle and foot CC

M00.072 Staphylococcal arthritis, left ankle and foot CC

M00.079 Staphylococcal arthritis, unspecified ankle and foot CC

M00.08 Staphylococcal arthritis, vertebrae CC

Ex: See M00.00

M00.09 Staphylococcal polyarthritis CC

Ex: See M00.00

● **M00.1 Pneumococcal arthritis and polyarthritis**

M00.10 Pneumococcal arthritis, unspecified joint CC

Ex: See M00.00

● **M00.11 Pneumococcal arthritis, shoulder**

Ex: **For category M00.11 CC codes:** See M00.01

M00.111 Pneumococcal arthritis, right shoulder CC

M00.112 Pneumococcal arthritis, left shoulder CC

M00.119 Pneumococcal arthritis, unspecified shoulder CC

● **M00.12 Pneumococcal arthritis, elbow**

Ex: **For category M00.12 CC codes:** See M00.02

M00.121 Pneumococcal arthritis, right elbow CC

M00.122 Pneumococcal arthritis, left elbow CC

M00.129 Pneumococcal arthritis, unspecified elbow CC

● **M00.13 Pneumococcal arthritis, wrist**

Pneumococcal arthritis of carpal bones

Ex: **For category M00.13 CC codes:** See M00.03

M00.131 Pneumococcal arthritis, right wrist CC

M00.132 Pneumococcal arthritis, left wrist CC

M00.139 Pneumococcal arthritis, unspecified wrist CC

● **M00.14 Pneumococcal arthritis, hand**

Pneumococcal arthritis of metacarpus and phalanges

Ex: **For category M00.14 CC codes:** See M00.04

M00.141 Pneumococcal arthritis, right hand CC

M00.142 Pneumococcal arthritis, left hand CC

M00.149 Pneumococcal arthritis, unspecified hand CC

M00.15 Pneumococcal arthritis, hip
Ex: For category M00.15 CC codes: See M00.05
- **M00.151 Pneumococcal arthritis, right hip**
- **M00.152 Pneumococcal arthritis, left hip**
- **M00.159 Pneumococcal arthritis, unspecified hip**

M00.16 Pneumococcal arthritis, knee
Ex: For category M00.16 CC codes: See M00.06
- **M00.161 Pneumococcal arthritis, right knee**
- **M00.162 Pneumococcal arthritis, left knee**
- **M00.169 Pneumococcal arthritis, unspecified knee**

M00.17 Pneumococcal arthritis, ankle and foot
Pneumococcal arthritis, tarsus, metatarsus and phalanges
Ex: For category M00.17 CC codes: See M00.07
- **M00.171 Pneumococcal arthritis, right ankle and foot**
- **M00.172 Pneumococcal arthritis, left ankle and foot**
- **M00.179 Pneumococcal arthritis, unspecified ankle and foot**

M00.18 Pneumococcal arthritis, vertebrae
Ex: See M00.00

M00.19 Pneumococcal polyarthritis
Ex: See M00.00

M00.2 Other streptococcal arthritis and polyarthritis
Use additional code (B95.0-B95.2, B95.4-B95.5) to identify bacterial agent
- **M00.20 Other streptococcal arthritis, unspecified joint**
  Ex: See M00.00
- **M00.21 Other streptococcal arthritis, shoulder**
  Ex: For category M00.21 CC codes: See M00.01
  - **M00.211 Other streptococcal arthritis, right shoulder**
  - **M00.212 Other streptococcal arthritis, left shoulder**
  - **M00.219 Other streptococcal arthritis, unspecified shoulder**
- **M00.22 Other streptococcal arthritis, elbow**
  Ex: For category M00.22 CC codes: See M00.02
  - **M00.221 Other streptococcal arthritis, right elbow**
  - **M00.222 Other streptococcal arthritis, left elbow**
  - **M00.229 Other streptococcal arthritis, unspecified elbow**
- **M00.23 Other streptococcal arthritis, wrist**
  Other streptococcal arthritis of carpal bones
  Ex: For category M00.23 CC codes: See M00.03
  - **M00.231 Other streptococcal arthritis, right wrist**
  - **M00.232 Other streptococcal arthritis, left wrist**
  - **M00.239 Other streptococcal arthritis, unspecified wrist**
- **M00.24 Other streptococcal arthritis, hand**
  Other streptococcal arthritis metacarpus and phalanges
  Ex: For category M00.24 CC codes: See M00.04
  - **M00.241 Other streptococcal arthritis, right hand**
  - **M00.242 Other streptococcal arthritis, left hand**
  - **M00.249 Other streptococcal arthritis, unspecified hand**
- **M00.25 Other streptococcal arthritis, hip**
  Ex: For category M00.25 CC codes: See M00.05
  - **M00.251 Other streptococcal arthritis, right hip**
  - **M00.252 Other streptococcal arthritis, left hip**
  - **M00.259 Other streptococcal arthritis, unspecified hip**
- **M00.26 Other streptococcal arthritis, knee**
  Ex: For category M00.26 CC codes: See M00.06
  - **M00.261 Other streptococcal arthritis, right knee**
  - **M00.262 Other streptococcal arthritis, left knee**
  - **M00.269 Other streptococcal arthritis, unspecified knee**
- **M00.27 Other streptococcal arthritis, ankle and foot**
  Other streptococcal arthritis, tarsus, metatarsus and phalanges
  Ex: For category M00.27 CC codes: See M00.07
  - **M00.271 Other streptococcal arthritis, right ankle and foot**
  - **M00.272 Other streptococcal arthritis, left ankle and foot**
  - **M00.279 Other streptococcal arthritis, unspecified ankle and foot**
- **M00.28 Other streptococcal arthritis, vertebrae**
  Ex: See M00.00
- **M00.29 Other streptococcal polyarthritis**
  Ex: See M00.00

M00.8 Arthritis and polyarthritis due to other bacteria
Use additional code (B96) to identify bacteria
- **M00.80 Arthritis due to other bacteria, unspecified joint**
  Ex: See M00.00
- **M00.81 Arthritis due to other bacteria, shoulder**
  Ex: For category M00.81 CC codes: See M00.01
  - **M00.811 Arthritis due to other bacteria, right shoulder**
  - **M00.812 Arthritis due to other bacteria, left shoulder**
  - **M00.819 Arthritis due to other bacteria, unspecified shoulder**
- **M00.82 Arthritis due to other bacteria, elbow**
  Ex: For category M00.82 CC codes: See M00.02
  - **M00.821 Arthritis due to other bacteria, right elbow**
  - **M00.822 Arthritis due to other bacteria, left elbow**
  - **M00.829 Arthritis due to other bacteria, unspecified elbow**
- **M00.83 Arthritis due to other bacteria, wrist**
  Arthritis due to other bacteria, carpal bones
  Ex: For category M00.83 CC codes: See M00.03
  - **M00.831 Arthritis due to other bacteria, right wrist**
  - **M00.832 Arthritis due to other bacteria, left wrist**
  - **M00.839 Arthritis due to other bacteria, unspecified wrist**
- **M00.84 Arthritis due to other bacteria, hand**
  Arthritis due to other bacteria, metacarpus and phalanges
  Ex: For category M00.84 CC codes: See M00.04
  - **M00.841 Arthritis due to other bacteria, right hand**
  - **M00.842 Arthritis due to other bacteria, left hand**
  - **M00.849 Arthritis due to other bacteria, unspecified hand**

● **M00.85 Arthritis due to other bacteria, hip**
(Ex) **For category M00.85 CC codes:** See M00.05

M00.851 Arthritis due to other bacteria, right hip

M00.852 Arthritis due to other bacteria, left hip

M00.859 Arthritis due to other bacteria, unspecified hip

● **M00.86 Arthritis due to other bacteria, knee**
(Ex) **For category M00.86 CC codes:** See M00.06

M00.861 Arthritis due to other bacteria, right knee

M00.862 Arthritis due to other bacteria, left knee

M00.869 Arthritis due to other bacteria, unspecified knee

● **M00.87 Arthritis due to other bacteria, ankle and foot**
Arthritis due to other bacteria, tarsus, metatarsus, and phalanges
(Ex) **For category M00.87 CC codes:** See M00.07

M00.871 Arthritis due to other bacteria, right ankle and foot

M00.872 Arthritis due to other bacteria, left ankle and foot

M00.879 Arthritis due to other bacteria, unspecified ankle and foot

M00.88 Arthritis due to other bacteria, vertebrae
(Ex) See M00.00

M00.89 Polyarthritis due to other bacteria
(Ex) See M00.00

M00.9 Pyogenic arthritis, unspecified
Infective arthritis NOS
(Ex) See M00.00

● **M01 Direct infections of joint in infectious and parasitic diseases classified elsewhere**
Code first underlying disease, such as:
leprosy [Hansen's disease] (A30.-)
mycoses (B35-B49)
O'nyong-nyong fever (A92.1)
paratyphoid fever (A01.1-A01.4)

Excludes1
arthropathy in Lyme disease (A69.23)
gonococcal arthritis (A54.42)
meningococcal arthritis (A39.83)
mumps arthritis (B26.85)
postinfective arthropathy (M02.-)
postmeningococcal arthritis (A39.84)
reactive arthritis (M02.3)
rubella arthritis (B06.82)
sarcoidosis arthritis (D86.86)
typhoid fever arthritis (A01.04)
tuberculosis arthritis (A18.01-A18.02)

● **M01.X Direct infection of joint in infectious and parasitic diseases classified elsewhere**
(Ex) **For category M01.X CC codes unless otherwise indicated:** A02.23, A17.9, A18.02, A18.09, A18.82, A18.84, A18.89, A39.83-A39.84, A54.40, A54.42-A54.43, A54.82, A54.84, A54.89-A54.9, B06.82, M00.00, M00.011-M02.30, M02.319, M02.329, M02.339, M02.349, M02.359, M02.369, M02.379, M02.38-M02.9, M05.40-M05.59, M05.70-M07.69, M11.00-M15.0, M15.3-M15.9, M16.2-M16.9, M17.2-M17.9, M18.2-M18.9, M19.111-M19.93, M24.10-M24.176, M25.00, M25.08-M25.18, M25.40-M25.676, M25.80-M25.9, M35.2, M36.1-M36.4, R29.4

▶ *M01.X0 Direct infection of unspecified joint in infectious and parasitic diseases classified elsewhere*

● **M01.X1 Direct infection of shoulder joint in infectious and parasitic diseases classified elsewhere**
(Ex) **For category M01.X1 CC codes:** A02.23, A17.9, A18.02, A18.09, A18.82, A18.84, A18.89, A39.83-A39.84, A54.40, A54.42-A54.43, A54.82, A54.84, A54.89-A54.9, B06.82, M00.00, M00.011-M02.30, M02.319, M02.329, M02.339, M02.349, M02.359, M02.369, M02.379, M02.38-M02.9, M05.40-M05.59, M05.70-M07.69, M11.00-M15.0, M15.3-M15.9, M16.2-M16.9, M17.2-M17.9, M18.2-M18.9, M19.111-M19.93, M24.10-M24.176, M25.00, M25.08-M25.18, M25.40-M25.676, M25.80-M25.9, M35.2, M36.1-M36.4, R29.4

▶ *M01.X11 Direct infection of right shoulder in infectious and parasitic diseases classified elsewhere*

▶ *M01.X12 Direct infection of left shoulder in infectious and parasitic diseases classified elsewhere*

▶ *M01.X19 Direct infection of unspecified shoulder in infectious and parasitic diseases classified elsewhere*

● **M01.X2 Direct infection of elbow in infectious and parasitic diseases classified elsewhere**

▶ *M01.X21 Direct infection of right elbow in infectious and parasitic diseases classified elsewhere*

▶ *M01.X22 Direct infection of left elbow in infectious and parasitic diseases classified elsewhere*

▶ *M01.X29 Direct infection of unspecified elbow in infectious and parasitic diseases classified elsewhere*

● **M01.X3 Direct infection of wrist in infectious and parasitic diseases classified elsewhere**
Direct infection of carpal bones in infectious and parasitic diseases classified elsewhere

▶ *M01.X31 Direct infection of right wrist in infectious and parasitic diseases classified elsewhere*

▶ *M01.X32 Direct infection of left wrist in infectious and parasitic diseases classified elsewhere*

▶ *M01.X39 Direct infection of unspecified wrist in infectious and parasitic diseases classified elsewhere*

● **M01.X4 Direct infection of hand in infectious and parasitic diseases classified elsewhere**
Direct infection of metacarpus and phalanges in infectious and parasitic diseases classified elsewhere

▶ *M01.X41 Direct infection of right hand in infectious and parasitic diseases classified elsewhere*

▶ *M01.X42 Direct infection of left hand in infectious and parasitic diseases classified elsewhere*

▶ *M01.X49 Direct infection of unspecified hand in infectious and parasitic diseases classified elsewhere*

● **M01.X5 Direct infection of hip in infectious and parasitic diseases classified elsewhere**

▶ *M01.X51 Direct infection of right hip in infectious and parasitic diseases classified elsewhere*

▶ *M01.X52 Direct infection of left hip in infectious and parasitic diseases classified elsewhere*

▶ *M01.X59 Direct infection of unspecified hip in infectious and parasitic diseases classified elsewhere*

- **M01.X6 Direct infection of knee in infectious and parasitic diseases classified elsewhere**
  - *M01.X61 Direct infection of right knee in infectious and parasitic diseases classified elsewhere*
  - *M01.X62 Direct infection of left knee in infectious and parasitic diseases classified elsewhere*
  - *M01.X69 Direct infection of unspecified knee in infectious and parasitic diseases classified elsewhere*
- **M01.X7 Direct infection of ankle and foot in infectious and parasitic diseases classified elsewhere**
  Direct infection of tarsus, metatarsus and phalanges in infectious and parasitic diseases classified elsewhere
  - *M01.X71 Direct infection of right ankle and foot in infectious and parasitic diseases classified elsewhere*
  - *M01.X72 Direct infection of left ankle and foot in infectious and parasitic diseases classified elsewhere*
  - *M01.X79 Direct infection of unspecified ankle and foot in infectious and parasitic diseases classified elsewhere*
  - *M01.X8 Direct infection of vertebrae in infectious and parasitic diseases classified elsewhere*
  - *M01.X9 Direct infection of multiple joints in infectious and parasitic diseases classified elsewhere*

- **M02 Postinfective and reactive arthropathies**
  Code first underlying disease, such as:
  congenital syphilis [Clutton's joints] (A50.5)
  enteritis due to Yersinia enterocolitica (A04.6)
  infective endocarditis (I33.0)
  viral hepatitis (B15-B19)

  Excludes1 Behçet's disease (M35.2)
  direct infections of joint in infectious and parasitic diseases classified elsewhere (M01.-)
  postmeningococcal arthritis (A39.84)
  mumps arthritis (B26.85)
  rubella arthritis (B06.82)
  syphilis arthritis (late) (A52.77)
  rheumatic fever (I00)
  tabetic arthropathy [Charcôt's] (A52.16)

  For category M02 CC codes unless otherwise indicated: See M01.X

- **M02.0 Arthropathy following intestinal bypass**
  - **M02.00 Arthropathy following intestinal bypass, unspecified site**
  - **M02.01 Arthropathy following intestinal bypass, shoulder**
    - **M02.011 Arthropathy following intestinal bypass, right shoulder**
    - **M02.012 Arthropathy following intestinal bypass, left shoulder**
    - **M02.019 Arthropathy following intestinal bypass, unspecified shoulder**
  - **M02.02 Arthropathy following intestinal bypass, elbow**
    - **M02.021 Arthropathy following intestinal bypass, right elbow**
    - **M02.022 Arthropathy following intestinal bypass, left elbow**
    - **M02.029 Arthropathy following intestinal bypass, unspecified elbow**
  - **M02.03 Arthropathy following intestinal bypass, wrist**
    Arthropathy following intestinal bypass, carpal bones
    - **M02.031 Arthropathy following intestinal bypass, right wrist**
    - **M02.032 Arthropathy following intestinal bypass, left wrist**
    - **M02.039 Arthropathy following intestinal bypass, unspecified wrist**
  - **M02.04 Arthropathy following intestinal bypass, hand**
    Arthropathy following intestinal bypass, metacarpals and phalanges
    - **M02.041 Arthropathy following intestinal bypass, right hand**
    - **M02.042 Arthropathy following intestinal bypass, left hand**
    - **M02.049 Arthropathy following intestinal bypass, unspecified hand**
  - **M02.05 Arthropathy following intestinal bypass, hip**
    - **M02.051 Arthropathy following intestinal bypass, right hip**
    - **M02.052 Arthropathy following intestinal bypass, left hip**
    - **M02.059 Arthropathy following intestinal bypass, unspecified hip**
  - **M02.06 Arthropathy following intestinal bypass, knee**
    - **M02.061 Arthropathy following intestinal bypass, right knee**
    - **M02.062 Arthropathy following intestinal bypass, left knee**
    - **M02.069 Arthropathy following intestinal bypass, unspecified knee**
  - **M02.07 Arthropathy following intestinal bypass, ankle and foot**
    Arthropathy following intestinal bypass, tarsus, metatarsus and phalanges
    - **M02.071 Arthropathy following intestinal bypass, right ankle and foot**
    - **M02.072 Arthropathy following intestinal bypass, left ankle and foot**
    - **M02.079 Arthropathy following intestinal bypass, unspecified ankle and foot**
  - **M02.08 Arthropathy following intestinal bypass, vertebrae**
  - **M02.09 Arthropathy following intestinal bypass, multiple sites**
- **M02.1 Postdysenteric arthropathy**
  - **M02.10 Postdysenteric arthropathy, unspecified site**
  - **M02.11 Postdysenteric arthropathy, shoulder**
    - **M02.111 Postdysenteric arthropathy, right shoulder**
    - **M02.112 Postdysenteric arthropathy, left shoulder**
    - **M02.119 Postdysenteric arthropathy, unspecified shoulder**
  - **M02.12 Postdysenteric arthropathy, elbow**
    - **M02.121 Postdysenteric arthropathy, right elbow**
    - **M02.122 Postdysenteric arthropathy, left elbow**
    - **M02.129 Postdysenteric arthropathy, unspecified elbow**
  - **M02.13 Postdysenteric arthropathy, wrist**
    Postdysenteric arthropathy, carpal bones
    - **M02.131 Postdysenteric arthropathy, right wrist**
    - **M02.132 Postdysenteric arthropathy, left wrist**
    - **M02.139 Postdysenteric arthropathy, unspecified wrist**
  - **M02.14 Postdysenteric arthropathy, hand**
    Postdysenteric arthropathy, metacarpus and phalanges
    - **M02.141 Postdysenteric arthropathy, right hand**
    - **M02.142 Postdysenteric arthropathy, left hand**
    - **M02.149 Postdysenteric arthropathy, unspecified hand**

- **M02.15 Postdysenteric arthropathy, hip**
  - **M02.151 Postdysenteric arthropathy, right hip**
  - **M02.152 Postdysenteric arthropathy, left hip**
  - **M02.159 Postdysenteric arthropathy, unspecified hip**
- **M02.16 Postdysenteric arthropathy, knee**
  - Ex **For category M02.16 CC codes:** A02.23, A17.9, A18.02, A18.09, A18.82, A18.84, A18.89, A39.83-A39.84, A54.40, A54.42-A54.43, A54.82, A54.84, A54.89-A54.9, B06.82, M00.00, M00.011-M02.30, M02.319, M02.329, M02.339, M02.349, M02.359, M02.369, M02.379, M02.38-M02.9, M05.40-M05.59, M05.70-M07.69, M11.00-M15.0, M15.3-M15.9, M16.2-M16.9, M17.2-M17.9, M18.2-M18.9, M19.111-M19.93, M24.10-M24.176, M25.00, M25.08-M25.18, M25.40-M25.676, M25.80-M25.9, M35.2, M36.1-M36.4, R29.4
  - **M02.161 Postdysenteric arthropathy, right knee**
  - **M02.162 Postdysenteric arthropathy, left knee**
  - **M02.169 Postdysenteric arthropathy, unspecified knee**
- **M02.17 Postdysenteric arthropathy, ankle and foot**
  - Postdysenteric arthropathy, tarsus, metatarsus and phalanges
  - **M02.171 Postdysenteric arthropathy, right ankle and foot**
  - **M02.172 Postdysenteric arthropathy, left ankle and foot**
  - **M02.179 Postdysenteric arthropathy, unspecified ankle and foot**
- **M02.18 Postdysenteric arthropathy, vertebrae**
  - Ex A02.23, A17.9, A18.02, A18.09, A18.82, A18.84, A18.89, A39.83-A39.84, A54.40, A54.42-A54.43, A54.82, A54.84, A54.89-A54.9, B06.82, M00.00, M00.011-M02.30, M02.319, M02.329, M02.339, M02.349, M02.359, M02.369, M02.379, M02.38-M02.9, M05.40-M05.59, M05.70-M07.69, M11.00-M15.0, M15.3-M15.9, M16.2-M16.9, M17.2-M17.9, M18.2-M18.9, M19.111-M19.93, M24.10-M24.176, M25.00, M25.08-M25.18, M25.40-M25.676, M25.80-M25.9, M35.2, M36.1-M36.4, R29.4
- **M02.19 Postdysenteric arthropathy, multiple sites**
- **M02.2 Postimmunization arthropathy**
  - **M02.20 Postimmunization arthropathy, unspecified site**
  - **M02.21 Postimmunization arthropathy, shoulder**
    - **M02.211 Postimmunization arthropathy, right shoulder**
    - **M02.212 Postimmunization arthropathy, left shoulder**
    - **M02.219 Postimmunization arthropathy, unspecified shoulder**
  - **M02.22 Postimmunization arthropathy, elbow**
    - **M02.221 Postimmunization arthropathy, right elbow**
    - **M02.222 Postimmunization arthropathy, left elbow**
    - **M02.229 Postimmunization arthropathy, unspecified elbow**
  - **M02.23 Postimmunization arthropathy, wrist**
    - Postimmunization arthropathy, carpal bones
    - **M02.231 Postimmunization arthropathy, right wrist**
    - **M02.232 Postimmunization arthropathy, left wrist**
    - **M02.239 Postimmunization arthropathy, unspecified wrist**
  - **M02.24 Postimmunization arthropathy, hand**
    - Postimmunization arthropathy, metacarpus and phalanges
    - **M02.241 Postimmunization arthropathy, right hand**
    - **M02.242 Postimmunization arthropathy, left hand**
    - **M02.249 Postimmunization arthropathy, unspecified hand**
  - **M02.25 Postimmunization arthropathy, hip**
    - **M02.251 Postimmunization arthropathy, right hip**
    - **M02.252 Postimmunization arthropathy, left hip**
    - **M02.259 Postimmunization arthropathy, unspecified hip**
  - **M02.26 Postimmunization arthropathy, knee**
    - **M02.261 Postimmunization arthropathy, right knee**
    - **M02.262 Postimmunization arthropathy, left knee**
    - **M02.269 Postimmunization arthropathy, unspecified knee**
  - **M02.27 Postimmunization arthropathy, ankle and foot**
    - Postimmunization arthropathy, tarsus, metatarsus and phalanges
    - **M02.271 Postimmunization arthropathy, right ankle and foot**
    - **M02.272 Postimmunization arthropathy, left ankle and foot**
    - **M02.279 Postimmunization arthropathy, unspecified ankle and foot**
  - **M02.28 Postimmunization arthropathy, vertebrae**
  - **M02.29 Postimmunization arthropathy, multiple sites**
- **M02.3 Reiter's disease**
  - Reactive arthritis
  - **M02.30 Reiter's disease, unspecified site**
    - CC when PDx is its own CC
  - **M02.31 Reiter's disease, shoulder**
    - **M02.311 Reiter's disease, right shoulder**
      - CC when PDx is its own CC
    - **M02.312 Reiter's disease, left shoulder**
      - CC when PDx is its own CC
    - **M02.319 Reiter's disease, unspecified shoulder**
      - CC when PDx is its own CC
  - **M02.32 Reiter's disease, elbow**
    - **M02.321 Reiter's disease, right elbow**
      - CC when PDx is its own CC
    - **M02.322 Reiter's disease, left elbow**
      - CC when PDx is its own CC
    - **M02.329 Reiter's disease, unspecified elbow**
      - CC when PDx is its own CC
  - **M02.33 Reiter's disease, wrist**
    - Reiter's disease, carpal bones
    - **M02.331 Reiter's disease, right wrist**
      - CC when PDx is its own CC
    - **M02.332 Reiter's disease, left wrist**
      - CC when PDx is its own CC
    - **M02.339 Reiter's disease, unspecified wrist**
      - CC when PDx is its own CC
  - **M02.34 Reiter's disease, hand**
    - Reiter's disease, metacarpus and phalanges
    - **M02.341 Reiter's disease, right hand**
      - CC when PDx is its own CC
    - **M02.342 Reiter's disease, left hand**
      - CC when PDx is its own CC
    - **M02.349 Reiter's disease, unspecified hand**
      - CC when PDx is its own CC
  - **M02.35 Reiter's disease, hip**
    - **M02.351 Reiter's disease, right hip**
      - CC when PDx is its own CC
    - **M02.352 Reiter's disease, left hip**
      - CC when PDx is its own CC
    - **M02.359 Reiter's disease, unspecified hip**
      - CC when PDx is its own CC

- **M02.36 Reiter's disease, knee**
  - **M02.361 Reiter's disease, right knee**
    CC when PDx is its own CC
  - **M02.362 Reiter's disease, left knee**
    CC when PDx is its own CC
  - **M02.369 Reiter's disease, unspecified knee**
    CC when PDx is its own CC
- **M02.37 Reiter's disease, ankle and foot**
  Reiter's disease, tarsus, metatarsus and phalanges
  - **M02.371 Reiter's disease, right ankle and foot**
    CC when PDx is its own CC
  - **M02.372 Reiter's disease, left ankle and foot**
    CC when PDx is its own CC
  - **M02.379 Reiter's disease, unspecified ankle and foot**
    CC when PDx is its own CC
- **M02.38 Reiter's disease, vertebrae**
  CC when PDx is its own CC
- **M02.39 Reiter's disease, multiple sites**
  CC when PDx is its own CC
- **M02.8 Other reactive arthropathies**
  - *M02.80 Other reactive arthropathies, unspecified site*
  - **M02.81 Other reactive arthropathies, shoulder**
    Ex For category M02.81 CC codes: See M01.X1
    - *M02.811 Other reactive arthropathies, right shoulder*
    - *M02.812 Other reactive arthropathies, left shoulder*
    - *M02.819 Other reactive arthropathies, unspecified shoulder*
  - **M02.82 Other reactive arthropathies, elbow**
    - *M02.821 Other reactive arthropathies, right elbow*
    - *M02.822 Other reactive arthropathies, left elbow*
    - *M02.829 Other reactive arthropathies, unspecified elbow*
  - **M02.83 Other reactive arthropathies, wrist**
    Other reactive arthropathies, carpal bones
    - *M02.831 Other reactive arthropathies, right wrist*
    - *M02.832 Other reactive arthropathies, left wrist*
    - *M02.839 Other reactive arthropathies, unspecified wrist*
  - **M02.84 Other reactive arthropathies, hand**
    Other reactive arthropathies, metacarpus and phalanges
    - *M02.841 Other reactive arthropathies, right hand*
    - *M02.842 Other reactive arthropathies, left hand*
    - *M02.849 Other reactive arthropathies, unspecified hand*
  - **M02.85 Other reactive arthropathies, hip**
    - *M02.851 Other reactive arthropathies, right hip*
    - *M02.852 Other reactive arthropathies, left hip*
    - *M02.859 Other reactive arthropathies, unspecified hip*
  - **M02.86 Other reactive arthropathies, knee**
    - *M02.861 Other reactive arthropathies, right knee*
    - *M02.862 Other reactive arthropathies, left knee*
    - *M02.869 Other reactive arthropathies, unspecified knee*
  - **M02.87 Other reactive arthropathies, ankle and foot**
    Other reactive arthropathies, tarsus, metatarsus and phalanges
    - *M02.871 Other reactive arthropathies, right ankle and foot*
    - *M02.872 Other reactive arthropathies, left ankle and foot*
    - *M02.879 Other reactive arthropathies, unspecified ankle and foot*
  - *M02.88 Other reactive arthropathies, vertebrae*
  - *M02.89 Other reactive arthropathies, multiple sites*
- *M02.9 Reactive arthropathy, unspecified*

AUTOINFLAMMATORY SYNDROMES (M04)

- **M04 Autoinflammatory syndromes**
  Excludes2 Crohn's disease (K50.-)
  - **M04.1 Periodic fever syndromes**
    Familial Mediterranean fever
    Hyperimmunoglobin D syndrome
    Mevalonate kinase deficiency
    Tumor necrosis factor receptor associated periodic syndrome [TRAPS]
  - **M04.2 Cryopyrin-associated periodic syndromes**
    Chronic infantile neurological, cutaneous and articular syndrome [CINCA]
    Familial cold autoinflammatory syndrome
    Familial cold urticaria
    Muckle-Wells syndrome
    Neonatal onset multisystemic inflammatory disorder [NOMID]
  - **M04.8 Other autoinflammatory syndromes**
    Blau syndrome
    Deficiency of interleukin 1 receptor antagonist [DIRA]
    Majeed syndrome
    Periodic fever, aphthous stomatitis, pharyngitis, and adenopathy syndrome [PFAPA]
    Pyogenic arthritis, pyoderma gangrenosum, and acne syndrome [PAPA]
  - **M04.9 Autoinflammatory syndrome, unspecified**

INFLAMMATORY POLYARTHROPATHIES (M05-M14)

- **M05 Rheumatoid arthritis with rheumatoid factor**
  Excludes1 rheumatic fever (I00)
  juvenile rheumatoid arthritis (M08.-)
  rheumatoid arthritis of spine (M45.-)
  - **M05.0 Felty's syndrome**
    Rheumatoid arthritis with splenoadenomegaly and leukopenia
    - **M05.00 Felty's syndrome, unspecified site**
    - **M05.01 Felty's syndrome, shoulder**
      - **M05.011 Felty's syndrome, right shoulder**
      - **M05.012 Felty's syndrome, left shoulder**
      - **M05.019 Felty's syndrome, unspecified shoulder**
    - **M05.02 Felty's syndrome, elbow**
      - **M05.021 Felty's syndrome, right elbow**
      - **M05.022 Felty's syndrome, left elbow**
      - **M05.029 Felty's syndrome, unspecified elbow**
    - **M05.03 Felty's syndrome, wrist**
      Felty's syndrome, carpal bones
      - **M05.031 Felty's syndrome, right wrist**
      - **M05.032 Felty's syndrome, left wrist**
      - **M05.039 Felty's syndrome, unspecified wrist**

Item 13–1 Rheumatoid arthritis (RA) is a chronic systemic inflammatory autoimmune disease of undetermined etiology involving primarily the synovial membranes and articular structures of multiple joints. It can also affect other organs, including the eyes, blood vessels, heart, and lungs. The disease is often progressive. In late stages, deformity, ankylosis, and other **inflammatory polyarthropathies** develop.

- **M05.04 Felty's syndrome, hand**
  Felty's syndrome, metacarpus and phalanges
  - **M05.041 Felty's syndrome, right hand**
  - **M05.042 Felty's syndrome, left hand**
  - **M05.049 Felty's syndrome, unspecified hand**
- **M05.05 Felty's syndrome, hip**
  - **M05.051 Felty's syndrome, right hip**
  - **M05.052 Felty's syndrome, left hip**
  - **M05.059 Felty's syndrome, unspecified hip**
- **M05.06 Felty's syndrome, knee**
  - **M05.061 Felty's syndrome, right knee**
  - **M05.062 Felty's syndrome, left knee**
  - **M05.069 Felty's syndrome, unspecified knee**
- **M05.07 Felty's syndrome, ankle and foot**
  Felty's syndrome, tarsus, metatarsus and phalanges
  - **M05.071 Felty's syndrome, right ankle and foot**
  - **M05.072 Felty's syndrome, left ankle and foot**
  - **M05.079 Felty's syndrome, unspecified ankle and foot**
- **M05.09 Felty's syndrome, multiple sites**

- **M05.1 Rheumatoid lung disease with rheumatoid arthritis**
  - **M05.10 Rheumatoid lung disease with rheumatoid arthritis of unspecified site**
  - **M05.11 Rheumatoid lung disease with rheumatoid arthritis of shoulder**
    - **M05.111 Rheumatoid lung disease with rheumatoid arthritis of right shoulder**
    - **M05.112 Rheumatoid lung disease with rheumatoid arthritis of left shoulder**
    - **M05.119 Rheumatoid lung disease with rheumatoid arthritis of unspecified shoulder**
  - **M05.12 Rheumatoid lung disease with rheumatoid arthritis of elbow**
    - **M05.121 Rheumatoid lung disease with rheumatoid arthritis of right elbow**
    - **M05.122 Rheumatoid lung disease with rheumatoid arthritis of left elbow**
    - **M05.129 Rheumatoid lung disease with rheumatoid arthritis of unspecified elbow**
  - **M05.13 Rheumatoid lung disease with rheumatoid arthritis of wrist**
    Rheumatoid lung disease with rheumatoid arthritis, carpal bones
    - **M05.131 Rheumatoid lung disease with rheumatoid arthritis of right wrist**
    - **M05.132 Rheumatoid lung disease with rheumatoid arthritis of left wrist**
    - **M05.139 Rheumatoid lung disease with rheumatoid arthritis of unspecified wrist**
  - **M05.14 Rheumatoid lung disease with rheumatoid arthritis of hand**
    Rheumatoid lung disease with rheumatoid arthritis, metacarpus and phalanges
    - **M05.141 Rheumatoid lung disease with rheumatoid arthritis of right hand**
    - **M05.142 Rheumatoid lung disease with rheumatoid arthritis of left hand**
    - **M05.149 Rheumatoid lung disease with rheumatoid arthritis of unspecified hand**
  - **M05.15 Rheumatoid lung disease with rheumatoid arthritis of hip**
    - **M05.151 Rheumatoid lung disease with rheumatoid arthritis of right hip**
    - **M05.152 Rheumatoid lung disease with rheumatoid arthritis of left hip**
    - **M05.159 Rheumatoid lung disease with rheumatoid arthritis of unspecified hip**
  - **M05.16 Rheumatoid lung disease with rheumatoid arthritis of knee**
    - **M05.161 Rheumatoid lung disease with rheumatoid arthritis of right knee**
    - **M05.162 Rheumatoid lung disease with rheumatoid arthritis of left knee**
    - **M05.169 Rheumatoid lung disease with rheumatoid arthritis of unspecified knee**
  - **M05.17 Rheumatoid lung disease with rheumatoid arthritis of ankle and foot**
    Rheumatoid lung disease with rheumatoid arthritis, tarsus, metatarsus and phalanges
    - **M05.171 Rheumatoid lung disease with rheumatoid arthritis of right ankle and foot**
    - **M05.172 Rheumatoid lung disease with rheumatoid arthritis of left ankle and foot**
    - **M05.179 Rheumatoid lung disease with rheumatoid arthritis of unspecified ankle and foot**
  - **M05.19 Rheumatoid lung disease with rheumatoid arthritis of multiple sites**
- **M05.2 Rheumatoid vasculitis with rheumatoid arthritis**
  - **M05.20 Rheumatoid vasculitis with rheumatoid arthritis of unspecified site**
  - **M05.21 Rheumatoid vasculitis with rheumatoid arthritis of shoulder**
    - **M05.211 Rheumatoid vasculitis with rheumatoid arthritis of right shoulder**
    - **M05.212 Rheumatoid vasculitis with rheumatoid arthritis of left shoulder**
    - **M05.219 Rheumatoid vasculitis with rheumatoid arthritis of unspecified shoulder**
  - **M05.22 Rheumatoid vasculitis with rheumatoid arthritis of elbow**
    - **M05.221 Rheumatoid vasculitis with rheumatoid arthritis of right elbow**
    - **M05.222 Rheumatoid vasculitis with rheumatoid arthritis of left elbow**
    - **M05.229 Rheumatoid vasculitis with rheumatoid arthritis of unspecified elbow**
  - **M05.23 Rheumatoid vasculitis with rheumatoid arthritis of wrist**
    Rheumatoid vasculitis with rheumatoid arthritis, carpal bones
    - **M05.231 Rheumatoid vasculitis with rheumatoid arthritis of right wrist**
    - **M05.232 Rheumatoid vasculitis with rheumatoid arthritis of left wrist**
    - **M05.239 Rheumatoid vasculitis with rheumatoid arthritis of unspecified wrist**

◀ New ◀ Revised ~~deleted~~ Deleted Excludes 1 Excludes 2 Includes Use additional Code first Code also Unspecified
OGCR Official Guidelines ● Unacceptable Principal Diagnosis X Assign placeholder X ● Use Additional Character(s) ▶ Manifestation Code Coding Clinic

● **M05.24 Rheumatoid vasculitis with rheumatoid arthritis of hand**
Rheumatoid vasculitis with rheumatoid arthritis, metacarpus and phalanges
M05.241 Rheumatoid vasculitis with rheumatoid arthritis of right hand
M05.242 Rheumatoid vasculitis with rheumatoid arthritis of left hand
M05.249 Rheumatoid vasculitis with rheumatoid arthritis of unspecified hand

● **M05.25 Rheumatoid vasculitis with rheumatoid arthritis of hip**
M05.251 Rheumatoid vasculitis with rheumatoid arthritis of right hip
M05.252 Rheumatoid vasculitis with rheumatoid arthritis of left hip
M05.259 Rheumatoid vasculitis with rheumatoid arthritis of unspecified hip

● **M05.26 Rheumatoid vasculitis with rheumatoid arthritis of knee**
M05.261 Rheumatoid vasculitis with rheumatoid arthritis of right knee
M05.262 Rheumatoid vasculitis with rheumatoid arthritis of left knee
M05.269 Rheumatoid vasculitis with rheumatoid arthritis of unspecified knee

● **M05.27 Rheumatoid vasculitis with rheumatoid arthritis of ankle and foot**
Rheumatoid vasculitis with rheumatoid arthritis, tarsus, metatarsus and phalanges
M05.271 Rheumatoid vasculitis with rheumatoid arthritis of right ankle and foot
M05.272 Rheumatoid vasculitis with rheumatoid arthritis of left ankle and foot
M05.279 Rheumatoid vasculitis with rheumatoid arthritis of unspecified ankle and foot

M05.29 Rheumatoid vasculitis with rheumatoid arthritis of multiple sites

● **M05.3 Rheumatoid heart disease with rheumatoid arthritis**
Rheumatoid carditis
Rheumatoid endocarditis
Rheumatoid myocarditis
Rheumatoid pericarditis
M05.30 Rheumatoid heart disease with rheumatoid arthritis of unspecified site

● **M05.31 Rheumatoid heart disease with rheumatoid arthritis of shoulder**
M05.311 Rheumatoid heart disease with rheumatoid arthritis of right shoulder
M05.312 Rheumatoid heart disease with rheumatoid arthritis of left shoulder
M05.319 Rheumatoid heart disease with rheumatoid arthritis of unspecified shoulder

● **M05.32 Rheumatoid heart disease with rheumatoid arthritis of elbow**
M05.321 Rheumatoid heart disease with rheumatoid arthritis of right elbow
M05.322 Rheumatoid heart disease with rheumatoid arthritis of left elbow
M05.329 Rheumatoid heart disease with rheumatoid arthritis of unspecified elbow

● **M05.33 Rheumatoid heart disease with rheumatoid arthritis of wrist**
Rheumatoid heart disease with rheumatoid arthritis, carpal bones
M05.331 Rheumatoid heart disease with rheumatoid arthritis of right wrist
M05.332 Rheumatoid heart disease with rheumatoid arthritis of left wrist
M05.339 Rheumatoid heart disease with rheumatoid arthritis of unspecified wrist

● **M05.34 Rheumatoid heart disease with rheumatoid arthritis of hand**
Rheumatoid heart disease with rheumatoid arthritis, metacarpus and phalanges
M05.341 Rheumatoid heart disease with rheumatoid arthritis of right hand
M05.342 Rheumatoid heart disease with rheumatoid arthritis of left hand
M05.349 Rheumatoid heart disease with rheumatoid arthritis of unspecified hand

● **M05.35 Rheumatoid heart disease with rheumatoid arthritis of hip**
M05.351 Rheumatoid heart disease with rheumatoid arthritis of right hip
M05.352 Rheumatoid heart disease with rheumatoid arthritis of left hip
M05.359 Rheumatoid heart disease with rheumatoid arthritis of unspecified hip

● **M05.36 Rheumatoid heart disease with rheumatoid arthritis of knee**
M05.361 Rheumatoid heart disease with rheumatoid arthritis of right knee
M05.362 Rheumatoid heart disease with rheumatoid arthritis of left knee
M05.369 Rheumatoid heart disease with rheumatoid arthritis of unspecified knee

● **M05.37 Rheumatoid heart disease with rheumatoid arthritis of ankle and foot**
Rheumatoid heart disease with rheumatoid arthritis, tarsus, metatarsus and phalanges
M05.371 Rheumatoid heart disease with rheumatoid arthritis of right ankle and foot
M05.372 Rheumatoid heart disease with rheumatoid arthritis of left ankle and foot
M05.379 Rheumatoid heart disease with rheumatoid arthritis of unspecified ankle and foot

M05.39 Rheumatoid heart disease with rheumatoid arthritis of multiple sites

● **M05.4 Rheumatoid myopathy with rheumatoid arthritis**

Ex For category M05.4 CC codes: E08.40-E08.49, E08.618-E08.638, E08.649-E08.8, E09.40-E09.49, E09.618-E09.638, E09.649-E09.8, E10.40-E10.49, E10.618-E10.638, E10.649, E10.69-E10.8, E11.40-E11.49, E11.618-E11.638, E11.649, E11.69-E11.8, E13.40-E13.49, E13.618-E13.638, E13.649-E13.8, G32.89, G70.00-G72.3, G72.81-G73.7, G96.8-G96.9, G98.0-G98.8, G99.8

M05.40 Rheumatoid myopathy with rheumatoid arthritis of unspecified site
CC when PDx is its own CC

● **M05.41 Rheumatoid myopathy with rheumatoid arthritis of shoulder**

M05.411 Rheumatoid myopathy with rheumatoid arthritis of right shoulder
CC when PDx is its own CC

M05.412 Rheumatoid myopathy with rheumatoid arthritis of left shoulder
CC when PDx is its own CC

M05.419 Rheumatoid myopathy with rheumatoid arthritis of unspecified shoulder
CC when PDx is its own CC

● **M05.42 Rheumatoid myopathy with rheumatoid arthritis of elbow**

M05.421 Rheumatoid myopathy with rheumatoid arthritis of right elbow
CC when PDx is its own CC

M05.422 Rheumatoid myopathy with rheumatoid arthritis of left elbow
CC when PDx is its own CC

M05.429 Rheumatoid myopathy with rheumatoid arthritis of unspecified elbow
CC when PDx is its own CC

● **M05.43 Rheumatoid myopathy with rheumatoid arthritis of wrist**
Rheumatoid myopathy with rheumatoid arthritis, carpal bones

M05.431 Rheumatoid myopathy with rheumatoid arthritis of right wrist
CC when PDx is its own CC

M05.432 Rheumatoid myopathy with rheumatoid arthritis of left wrist
CC when PDx is its own CC

M05.439 Rheumatoid myopathy with rheumatoid arthritis of unspecified wrist
CC when PDx is its own CC

● **M05.44 Rheumatoid myopathy with rheumatoid arthritis of hand**
Rheumatoid myopathy with rheumatoid arthritis, metacarpus and phalanges

M05.441 Rheumatoid myopathy with rheumatoid arthritis of right hand
CC when PDx is its own CC

M05.442 Rheumatoid myopathy with rheumatoid arthritis of left hand
CC when PDx is its own CC

M05.449 Rheumatoid myopathy with rheumatoid arthritis of unspecified hand
CC when PDx is its own CC

● **M05.45 Rheumatoid myopathy with rheumatoid arthritis of hip**

M05.451 Rheumatoid myopathy with rheumatoid arthritis of right hip
CC when PDx is its own CC

M05.452 Rheumatoid myopathy with rheumatoid arthritis of left hip
CC when PDx is its own CC

M05.459 Rheumatoid myopathy with rheumatoid arthritis of unspecified hip
CC when PDx is its own CC

● **M05.46 Rheumatoid myopathy with rheumatoid arthritis of knee**

M05.461 Rheumatoid myopathy with rheumatoid arthritis of right knee
CC when PDx is its own CC

M05.462 Rheumatoid myopathy with rheumatoid arthritis of left knee
CC when PDx is its own CC

M05.469 Rheumatoid myopathy with rheumatoid arthritis of unspecified knee
CC when PDx is its own CC

● **M05.47 Rheumatoid myopathy with rheumatoid arthritis of ankle and foot**
Rheumatoid myopathy with rheumatoid arthritis, tarsus, metatarsus and phalanges

M05.471 Rheumatoid myopathy with rheumatoid arthritis of right ankle and foot
CC when PDx is its own CC

M05.472 Rheumatoid myopathy with rheumatoid arthritis of left ankle and foot
CC when PDx is its own CC

M05.479 Rheumatoid myopathy with rheumatoid arthritis of unspecified ankle and foot
CC when PDx is its own CC

M05.49 Rheumatoid myopathy with rheumatoid arthritis of multiple sites
CC when PDx is its own CC

● **M05.5 Rheumatoid polyneuropathy with rheumatoid arthritis**

M05.50 Rheumatoid polyneuropathy with rheumatoid arthritis of unspecified site

● **M05.51 Rheumatoid polyneuropathy with rheumatoid arthritis of shoulder**

M05.511 Rheumatoid polyneuropathy with rheumatoid arthritis of right shoulder

M05.512 Rheumatoid polyneuropathy with rheumatoid arthritis of left shoulder

M05.519 Rheumatoid polyneuropathy with rheumatoid arthritis of unspecified shoulder

● **M05.52 Rheumatoid polyneuropathy with rheumatoid arthritis of elbow**

M05.521 Rheumatoid polyneuropathy with rheumatoid arthritis of right elbow

M05.522 Rheumatoid polyneuropathy with rheumatoid arthritis of left elbow

M05.529 Rheumatoid polyneuropathy with rheumatoid arthritis of unspecified elbow

- **M05.53 Rheumatoid polyneuropathy with rheumatoid arthritis of wrist**
  Rheumatoid polyneuropathy with rheumatoid arthritis, carpal bones
  - **M05.531 Rheumatoid polyneuropathy with rheumatoid arthritis of right wrist**
  - **M05.532 Rheumatoid polyneuropathy with rheumatoid arthritis of left wrist**
  - **M05.539 Rheumatoid polyneuropathy with rheumatoid arthritis of unspecified wrist**
- **M05.54 Rheumatoid polyneuropathy with rheumatoid arthritis of hand**
  Rheumatoid polyneuropathy with rheumatoid arthritis, metacarpus and phalanges
  - **M05.541 Rheumatoid polyneuropathy with rheumatoid arthritis of right hand**
  - **M05.542 Rheumatoid polyneuropathy with rheumatoid arthritis of left hand**
  - **M05.549 Rheumatoid polyneuropathy with rheumatoid arthritis of unspecified hand**
- **M05.55 Rheumatoid polyneuropathy with rheumatoid arthritis of hip**
  - **M05.551 Rheumatoid polyneuropathy with rheumatoid arthritis of right hip**
  - **M05.552 Rheumatoid polyneuropathy with rheumatoid arthritis of left hip**
  - **M05.559 Rheumatoid polyneuropathy with rheumatoid arthritis of unspecified hip**
- **M05.56 Rheumatoid polyneuropathy with rheumatoid arthritis of knee**
  - **M05.561 Rheumatoid polyneuropathy with rheumatoid arthritis of right knee**
  - **M05.562 Rheumatoid polyneuropathy with rheumatoid arthritis of left knee**
  - **M05.569 Rheumatoid polyneuropathy with rheumatoid arthritis of unspecified knee**
- **M05.57 Rheumatoid polyneuropathy with rheumatoid arthritis of ankle and foot**
  Rheumatoid polyneuropathy with rheumatoid arthritis, tarsus, metatarsus and phalanges
  - **M05.571 Rheumatoid polyneuropathy with rheumatoid arthritis of right ankle and foot**
  - **M05.572 Rheumatoid polyneuropathy with rheumatoid arthritis of left ankle and foot**
  - **M05.579 Rheumatoid polyneuropathy with rheumatoid arthritis of unspecified ankle and foot**
- **M05.59 Rheumatoid polyneuropathy with rheumatoid arthritis of multiple sites**

- **M05.6 Rheumatoid arthritis with involvement of other organs and systems**
  - **M05.60 Rheumatoid arthritis of unspecified site with involvement of other organs and systems**
  - **M05.61 Rheumatoid arthritis of shoulder with involvement of other organs and systems**
    - **M05.611 Rheumatoid arthritis of right shoulder with involvement of other organs and systems**
    - **M05.612 Rheumatoid arthritis of left shoulder with involvement of other organs and systems**
    - **M05.619 Rheumatoid arthritis of unspecified shoulder with involvement of other organs and systems**
  - **M05.62 Rheumatoid arthritis of elbow with involvement of other organs and systems**
    - **M05.621 Rheumatoid arthritis of right elbow with involvement of other organs and systems**
    - **M05.622 Rheumatoid arthritis of left elbow with involvement of other organs and systems**
    - **M05.629 Rheumatoid arthritis of unspecified elbow with involvement of other organs and systems**
  - **M05.63 Rheumatoid arthritis of wrist with involvement of other organs and systems**
    Rheumatoid arthritis of carpal bones with involvement of other organs and systems
    - **M05.631 Rheumatoid arthritis of right wrist with involvement of other organs and systems**
    - **M05.632 Rheumatoid arthritis of left wrist with involvement of other organs and systems**
    - **M05.639 Rheumatoid arthritis of unspecified wrist with involvement of other organs and systems**
  - **M05.64 Rheumatoid arthritis of hand with involvement of other organs and systems**
    Rheumatoid arthritis of metacarpus and phalanges with involvement of other organs and systems
    - **M05.641 Rheumatoid arthritis of right hand with involvement of other organs and systems**
    - **M05.642 Rheumatoid arthritis of left hand with involvement of other organs and systems**
    - **M05.649 Rheumatoid arthritis of unspecified hand with involvement of other organs and systems**
  - **M05.65 Rheumatoid arthritis of hip with involvement of other organs and systems**
    - **M05.651 Rheumatoid arthritis of right hip with involvement of other organs and systems**
    - **M05.652 Rheumatoid arthritis of left hip with involvement of other organs and systems**
    - **M05.659 Rheumatoid arthritis of unspecified hip with involvement of other organs and systems**
  - **M05.66 Rheumatoid arthritis of knee with involvement of other organs and systems**
    - **M05.661 Rheumatoid arthritis of right knee with involvement of other organs and systems**
    - **M05.662 Rheumatoid arthritis of left knee with involvement of other organs and systems**
    - **M05.669 Rheumatoid arthritis of unspecified knee with involvement of other organs and systems**

● M05.67 Rheumatoid arthritis of ankle and foot with involvement of other organs and systems
Rheumatoid arthritis of tarsus, metatarsus and phalanges with involvement of other organs and systems
M05.671 Rheumatoid arthritis of right ankle and foot with involvement of other organs and systems
M05.672 Rheumatoid arthritis of left ankle and foot with involvement of other organs and systems
M05.679 Rheumatoid arthritis of unspecified ankle and foot with involvement of other organs and systems
M05.69 Rheumatoid arthritis of multiple sites with involvement of other organs and systems

● M05.7 Rheumatoid arthritis with rheumatoid factor without organ or systems involvement
M05.70 Rheumatoid arthritis with rheumatoid factor of unspecified site without organ or systems involvement

● M05.71 Rheumatoid arthritis with rheumatoid factor of shoulder without organ or systems involvement
M05.711 Rheumatoid arthritis with rheumatoid factor of right shoulder without organ or systems involvement
M05.712 Rheumatoid arthritis with rheumatoid factor of left shoulder without organ or systems involvement
M05.719 Rheumatoid arthritis with rheumatoid factor of unspecified shoulder without organ or systems involvement

● M05.72 Rheumatoid arthritis with rheumatoid factor of elbow without organ or systems involvement
M05.721 Rheumatoid arthritis with rheumatoid factor of right elbow without organ or systems involvement
M05.722 Rheumatoid arthritis with rheumatoid factor of left elbow without organ or systems involvement
M05.729 Rheumatoid arthritis with rheumatoid factor of unspecified elbow without organ or systems involvement

● M05.73 Rheumatoid arthritis with rheumatoid factor of wrist without organ or systems involvement
M05.731 Rheumatoid arthritis with rheumatoid factor of right wrist without organ or systems involvement
M05.732 Rheumatoid arthritis with rheumatoid factor of left wrist without organ or systems involvement
M05.739 Rheumatoid arthritis with rheumatoid factor of unspecified wrist without organ or systems involvement

● M05.74 Rheumatoid arthritis with rheumatoid factor of hand without organ or systems involvement
M05.741 Rheumatoid arthritis with rheumatoid factor of right hand without organ or systems involvement
M05.742 Rheumatoid arthritis with rheumatoid factor of left hand without organ or systems involvement
M05.749 Rheumatoid arthritis with rheumatoid factor of unspecified hand without organ or systems involvement

● M05.75 Rheumatoid arthritis with rheumatoid factor of hip without organ or systems involvement
M05.751 Rheumatoid arthritis with rheumatoid factor of right hip without organ or systems involvement
M05.752 Rheumatoid arthritis with rheumatoid factor of left hip without organ or systems involvement
M05.759 Rheumatoid arthritis with rheumatoid factor of unspecified hip without organ or systems involvement

● M05.76 Rheumatoid arthritis with rheumatoid factor of knee without organ or systems involvement
M05.761 Rheumatoid arthritis with rheumatoid factor of right knee without organ or systems involvement
M05.762 Rheumatoid arthritis with rheumatoid factor of left knee without organ or systems involvement
M05.769 Rheumatoid arthritis with rheumatoid factor of unspecified knee without organ or systems involvement

● M05.77 Rheumatoid arthritis with rheumatoid factor of ankle and foot without organ or systems involvement
M05.771 Rheumatoid arthritis with rheumatoid factor of right ankle and foot without organ or systems involvement
M05.772 Rheumatoid arthritis with rheumatoid factor of left ankle and foot without organ or systems involvement
M05.779 Rheumatoid arthritis with rheumatoid factor of unspecified ankle and foot without organ or systems involvement
M05.79 Rheumatoid arthritis with rheumatoid factor of multiple sites without organ or systems involvement

● M05.8 Other rheumatoid arthritis with rheumatoid factor
M05.80 Other rheumatoid arthritis with rheumatoid factor of unspecified site

● M05.81 Other rheumatoid arthritis with rheumatoid factor of shoulder
M05.811 Other rheumatoid arthritis with rheumatoid factor of right shoulder
M05.812 Other rheumatoid arthritis with rheumatoid factor of left shoulder
M05.819 Other rheumatoid arthritis with rheumatoid factor of unspecified shoulder

- M05.82 Other rheumatoid arthritis with rheumatoid factor of elbow
  - M05.821 Other rheumatoid arthritis with rheumatoid factor of right elbow
  - M05.822 Other rheumatoid arthritis with rheumatoid factor of left elbow
  - M05.829 Other rheumatoid arthritis with rheumatoid factor of unspecified elbow
- M05.83 Other rheumatoid arthritis with rheumatoid factor of wrist
  - M05.831 Other rheumatoid arthritis with rheumatoid factor of right wrist
  - M05.832 Other rheumatoid arthritis with rheumatoid factor of left wrist
  - M05.839 Other rheumatoid arthritis with rheumatoid factor of unspecified wrist
- M05.84 Other rheumatoid arthritis with rheumatoid factor of hand
  - M05.841 Other rheumatoid arthritis with rheumatoid factor of right hand
  - M05.842 Other rheumatoid arthritis with rheumatoid factor of left hand
  - M05.849 Other rheumatoid arthritis with rheumatoid factor of unspecified hand
- M05.85 Other rheumatoid arthritis with rheumatoid factor of hip
  - M05.851 Other rheumatoid arthritis with rheumatoid factor of right hip
  - M05.852 Other rheumatoid arthritis with rheumatoid factor of left hip
  - M05.859 Other rheumatoid arthritis with rheumatoid factor of unspecified hip
- M05.86 Other rheumatoid arthritis with rheumatoid factor of knee
  - M05.861 Other rheumatoid arthritis with rheumatoid factor of right knee
  - M05.862 Other rheumatoid arthritis with rheumatoid factor of left knee
  - M05.869 Other rheumatoid arthritis with rheumatoid factor of unspecified knee
- M05.87 Other rheumatoid arthritis with rheumatoid factor of ankle and foot
  - M05.871 Other rheumatoid arthritis with rheumatoid factor of right ankle and foot
  - M05.872 Other rheumatoid arthritis with rheumatoid factor of left ankle and foot
  - M05.879 Other rheumatoid arthritis with rheumatoid factor of unspecified ankle and foot
- M05.89 Other rheumatoid arthritis with rheumatoid factor of multiple sites
- M05.9 Rheumatoid arthritis with rheumatoid factor, unspecified

- M06 Other rheumatoid arthritis
  - M06.0 Rheumatoid arthritis without rheumatoid factor
    - M06.00 Rheumatoid arthritis without rheumatoid factor, unspecified site
    - M06.01 Rheumatoid arthritis without rheumatoid factor, shoulder
      - M06.011 Rheumatoid arthritis without rheumatoid factor, right shoulder
      - M06.012 Rheumatoid arthritis without rheumatoid factor, left shoulder
      - M06.019 Rheumatoid arthritis without rheumatoid factor, unspecified shoulder
    - M06.02 Rheumatoid arthritis without rheumatoid factor, elbow
      - M06.021 Rheumatoid arthritis without rheumatoid factor, right elbow
      - M06.022 Rheumatoid arthritis without rheumatoid factor, left elbow
      - M06.029 Rheumatoid arthritis without rheumatoid factor, unspecified elbow
    - M06.03 Rheumatoid arthritis without rheumatoid factor, wrist
      - M06.031 Rheumatoid arthritis without rheumatoid factor, right wrist
      - M06.032 Rheumatoid arthritis without rheumatoid factor, left wrist
      - M06.039 Rheumatoid arthritis without rheumatoid factor, unspecified wrist
    - M06.04 Rheumatoid arthritis without rheumatoid factor, hand
      - M06.041 Rheumatoid arthritis without rheumatoid factor, right hand
      - M06.042 Rheumatoid arthritis without rheumatoid factor, left hand
      - M06.049 Rheumatoid arthritis without rheumatoid factor, unspecified hand
    - M06.05 Rheumatoid arthritis without rheumatoid factor, hip
      - M06.051 Rheumatoid arthritis without rheumatoid factor, right hip
      - M06.052 Rheumatoid arthritis without rheumatoid factor, left hip
      - M06.059 Rheumatoid arthritis without rheumatoid factor, unspecified hip
    - M06.06 Rheumatoid arthritis without rheumatoid factor, knee
      - M06.061 Rheumatoid arthritis without rheumatoid factor, right knee
      - M06.062 Rheumatoid arthritis without rheumatoid factor, left knee
      - M06.069 Rheumatoid arthritis without rheumatoid factor, unspecified knee
    - M06.07 Rheumatoid arthritis without rheumatoid factor, ankle and foot
      - M06.071 Rheumatoid arthritis without rheumatoid factor, right ankle and foot
      - M06.072 Rheumatoid arthritis without rheumatoid factor, left ankle and foot
      - M06.079 Rheumatoid arthritis without rheumatoid factor, unspecified ankle and foot
    - M06.08 Rheumatoid arthritis without rheumatoid factor, vertebrae
    - M06.09 Rheumatoid arthritis without rheumatoid factor, multiple sites
  - M06.1 Adult-onset Still's disease A
    - **Excludes1** Still's disease NOS (M08.2-)
  - M06.2 Rheumatoid bursitis
    - M06.20 Rheumatoid bursitis, unspecified site
    - M06.21 Rheumatoid bursitis, shoulder
      - M06.211 Rheumatoid bursitis, right shoulder
      - M06.212 Rheumatoid bursitis, left shoulder
      - M06.219 Rheumatoid bursitis, unspecified shoulder
    - M06.22 Rheumatoid bursitis, elbow
      - M06.221 Rheumatoid bursitis, right elbow
      - M06.222 Rheumatoid bursitis, left elbow
      - M06.229 Rheumatoid bursitis, unspecified elbow

- M06.23 Rheumatoid bursitis, wrist
  - M06.231 Rheumatoid bursitis, right wrist
  - M06.232 Rheumatoid bursitis, left wrist
  - M06.239 Rheumatoid bursitis, unspecified wrist
- M06.24 Rheumatoid bursitis, hand
  - M06.241 Rheumatoid bursitis, right hand
  - M06.242 Rheumatoid bursitis, left hand
  - M06.249 Rheumatoid bursitis, unspecified hand
- M06.25 Rheumatoid bursitis, hip
  - M06.251 Rheumatoid bursitis, right hip
  - M06.252 Rheumatoid bursitis, left hip
  - M06.259 Rheumatoid bursitis, unspecified hip
- M06.26 Rheumatoid bursitis, knee
  - M06.261 Rheumatoid bursitis, right knee
  - M06.262 Rheumatoid bursitis, left knee
  - M06.269 Rheumatoid bursitis, unspecified knee
- M06.27 Rheumatoid bursitis, ankle and foot
  - M06.271 Rheumatoid bursitis, right ankle and foot
  - M06.272 Rheumatoid bursitis, left ankle and foot
  - M06.279 Rheumatoid bursitis, unspecified ankle and foot
- M06.28 Rheumatoid bursitis, vertebrae
- M06.29 Rheumatoid bursitis, multiple sites

- M06.3 Rheumatoid nodule
  - M06.30 Rheumatoid nodule, unspecified site
  - M06.31 Rheumatoid nodule, shoulder
    - M06.311 Rheumatoid nodule, right shoulder
    - M06.312 Rheumatoid nodule, left shoulder
    - M06.319 Rheumatoid nodule, unspecified shoulder
  - M06.32 Rheumatoid nodule, elbow
    - M06.321 Rheumatoid nodule, right elbow
    - M06.322 Rheumatoid nodule, left elbow
    - M06.329 Rheumatoid nodule, unspecified elbow
  - M06.33 Rheumatoid nodule, wrist
    - M06.331 Rheumatoid nodule, right wrist
    - M06.332 Rheumatoid nodule, left wrist
    - M06.339 Rheumatoid nodule, unspecified wrist
  - M06.34 Rheumatoid nodule, hand
    - M06.341 Rheumatoid nodule, right hand
    - M06.342 Rheumatoid nodule, left hand
    - M06.349 Rheumatoid nodule, unspecified hand
  - M06.35 Rheumatoid nodule, hip
    - M06.351 Rheumatoid nodule, right hip
    - M06.352 Rheumatoid nodule, left hip
    - M06.359 Rheumatoid nodule, unspecified hip
  - M06.36 Rheumatoid nodule, knee
    - M06.361 Rheumatoid nodule, right knee
    - M06.362 Rheumatoid nodule, left knee
    - M06.369 Rheumatoid nodule, unspecified knee
  - M06.37 Rheumatoid nodule, ankle and foot
    - M06.371 Rheumatoid nodule, right ankle and foot
    - M06.372 Rheumatoid nodule, left ankle and foot
    - M06.379 Rheumatoid nodule, unspecified ankle and foot
  - M06.38 Rheumatoid nodule, vertebrae
  - M06.39 Rheumatoid nodule, multiple sites
- M06.4 Inflammatory polyarthropathy
  - **Excludes1** polyarthritis NOS (M13.0)
- M06.8 Other specified rheumatoid arthritis
  - M06.80 Other specified rheumatoid arthritis, unspecified site
  - M06.81 Other specified rheumatoid arthritis, shoulder
    - M06.811 Other specified rheumatoid arthritis, right shoulder
    - M06.812 Other specified rheumatoid arthritis, left shoulder
    - M06.819 Other specified rheumatoid arthritis, unspecified shoulder
  - M06.82 Other specified rheumatoid arthritis, elbow
    - M06.821 Other specified rheumatoid arthritis, right elbow
    - M06.822 Other specified rheumatoid arthritis, left elbow
    - M06.829 Other specified rheumatoid arthritis, unspecified elbow
  - M06.83 Other specified rheumatoid arthritis, wrist
    - M06.831 Other specified rheumatoid arthritis, right wrist
    - M06.832 Other specified rheumatoid arthritis, left wrist
    - M06.839 Other specified rheumatoid arthritis, unspecified wrist
  - M06.84 Other specified rheumatoid arthritis, hand
    - M06.841 Other specified rheumatoid arthritis, right hand
    - M06.842 Other specified rheumatoid arthritis, left hand
    - M06.849 Other specified rheumatoid arthritis, unspecified hand
  - M06.85 Other specified rheumatoid arthritis, hip
    - M06.851 Other specified rheumatoid arthritis, right hip
    - M06.852 Other specified rheumatoid arthritis, left hip
    - M06.859 Other specified rheumatoid arthritis, unspecified hip
  - M06.86 Other specified rheumatoid arthritis, knee
    - M06.861 Other specified rheumatoid arthritis, right knee
    - M06.862 Other specified rheumatoid arthritis, left knee
    - M06.869 Other specified rheumatoid arthritis, unspecified knee
  - M06.87 Other specified rheumatoid arthritis, ankle and foot
    - M06.871 Other specified rheumatoid arthritis, right ankle and foot
    - M06.872 Other specified rheumatoid arthritis, left ankle and foot
    - M06.879 Other specified rheumatoid arthritis, unspecified ankle and foot
  - M06.88 Other specified rheumatoid arthritis, vertebrae
  - M06.89 Other specified rheumatoid arthritis, multiple sites
- M06.9 Rheumatoid arthritis, unspecified

◀ New ◀ Revised ~~deleted~~ Deleted Excludes 1 Excludes 2 Includes Use additional Code first Code also Unspecified
OGCR Official Guidelines ● Unacceptable Principal Diagnosis X Assign placeholder X ● Use Additional Character(s) ▶ Manifestation Code Coding Clinic

M07 Enteropathic arthropathies

Code also associated enteropathy, such as:
regional enteritis [Crohn's disease] (K50.-)
ulcerative colitis (K51.-)

Excludes1 psoriatic arthropathies (L40.5-)

M07.6 Enteropathic arthropathies

M07.60 Enteropathic arthropathies, unspecified site

M07.61 Enteropathic arthropathies, shoulder

M07.611 Enteropathic arthropathies, right shoulder

M07.612 Enteropathic arthropathies, left shoulder

M07.619 Enteropathic arthropathies, unspecified shoulder

M07.62 Enteropathic arthropathies, elbow

M07.621 Enteropathic arthropathies, right elbow

M07.622 Enteropathic arthropathies, left elbow

M07.629 Enteropathic arthropathies, unspecified elbow

M07.63 Enteropathic arthropathies, wrist

M07.631 Enteropathic arthropathies, right wrist

M07.632 Enteropathic arthropathies, left wrist

M07.639 Enteropathic arthropathies, unspecified wrist

M07.64 Enteropathic arthropathies, hand

M07.641 Enteropathic arthropathies, right hand

M07.642 Enteropathic arthropathies, left hand

M07.649 Enteropathic arthropathies, unspecified hand

M07.65 Enteropathic arthropathies, hip

M07.651 Enteropathic arthropathies, right hip

M07.652 Enteropathic arthropathies, left hip

M07.659 Enteropathic arthropathies, unspecified hip

M07.66 Enteropathic arthropathies, knee

M07.661 Enteropathic arthropathies, right knee

M07.662 Enteropathic arthropathies, left knee

M07.669 Enteropathic arthropathies, unspecified knee

M07.67 Enteropathic arthropathies, ankle and foot

M07.671 Enteropathic arthropathies, right ankle and foot

M07.672 Enteropathic arthropathies, left ankle and foot

M07.679 Enteropathic arthropathies, unspecified ankle and foot

M07.68 Enteropathic arthropathies, vertebrae

M07.69 Enteropathic arthropathies, multiple sites

M08 Juvenile arthritis

Code also any associated underlying condition, such as:
regional enteritis [Crohn's disease] (K50.-)
ulcerative colitis (K51.-)

Excludes1 arthropathy in Whipple's disease (M14.8)
Felty's syndrome (M05.0)
juvenile dermatomyositis (M33.0-)
psoriatic juvenile arthropathy (L40.54)

M08.0 Unspecified juvenile rheumatoid arthritis

Juvenile rheumatoid arthritis with or without rheumatoid factor

M08.00 Unspecified juvenile rheumatoid arthritis of unspecified site

M08.01 Unspecified juvenile rheumatoid arthritis, shoulder

M08.011 Unspecified juvenile rheumatoid arthritis, right shoulder

M08.012 Unspecified juvenile rheumatoid arthritis, left shoulder

M08.019 Unspecified juvenile rheumatoid arthritis, unspecified shoulder

M08.02 Unspecified juvenile rheumatoid arthritis of elbow

M08.021 Unspecified juvenile rheumatoid arthritis, right elbow

M08.022 Unspecified juvenile rheumatoid arthritis, left elbow

M08.029 Unspecified juvenile rheumatoid arthritis, unspecified elbow

M08.03 Unspecified juvenile rheumatoid arthritis, wrist

M08.031 Unspecified juvenile rheumatoid arthritis, right wrist

M08.032 Unspecified juvenile rheumatoid arthritis, left wrist

M08.039 Unspecified juvenile rheumatoid arthritis, unspecified wrist

M08.04 Unspecified juvenile rheumatoid arthritis, hand

M08.041 Unspecified juvenile rheumatoid arthritis, right hand

M08.042 Unspecified juvenile rheumatoid arthritis, left hand

M08.049 Unspecified juvenile rheumatoid arthritis, unspecified hand

M08.05 Unspecified juvenile rheumatoid arthritis, hip

M08.051 Unspecified juvenile rheumatoid arthritis, right hip

M08.052 Unspecified juvenile rheumatoid arthritis, left hip

M08.059 Unspecified juvenile rheumatoid arthritis, unspecified hip

M08.06 Unspecified juvenile rheumatoid arthritis, knee

M08.061 Unspecified juvenile rheumatoid arthritis, right knee

M08.062 Unspecified juvenile rheumatoid arthritis, left knee

M08.069 Unspecified juvenile rheumatoid arthritis, unspecified knee

M08.07 Unspecified juvenile rheumatoid arthritis, ankle and foot

M08.071 Unspecified juvenile rheumatoid arthritis, right ankle and foot

M08.072 Unspecified juvenile rheumatoid arthritis, left ankle and foot

M08.079 Unspecified juvenile rheumatoid arthritis, unspecified ankle and foot

M08.08 Unspecified juvenile rheumatoid arthritis, vertebrae

M08.09 Unspecified juvenile rheumatoid arthritis, multiple sites

M08.1 Juvenile ankylosing spondylitis

Excludes1 ankylosing spondylitis in adults (M45.0-)

M08.2 Juvenile rheumatoid arthritis with systemic onset

Still's disease NOS

Excludes1 adult-onset Still's disease (M06.1-)

M08.20 Juvenile rheumatoid arthritis with systemic onset, unspecified site

M08.21 Juvenile rheumatoid arthritis with systemic onset, shoulder

M08.211 Juvenile rheumatoid arthritis with systemic onset, right shoulder

M08.212 Juvenile rheumatoid arthritis with systemic onset, left shoulder

M08.219 Juvenile rheumatoid arthritis with systemic onset, unspecified shoulder

- M08.22 Juvenile rheumatoid arthritis with systemic onset, elbow
  - M08.221 Juvenile rheumatoid arthritis with systemic onset, right elbow
  - M08.222 Juvenile rheumatoid arthritis with systemic onset, left elbow
  - M08.229 Juvenile rheumatoid arthritis with systemic onset, unspecified elbow
- M08.23 Juvenile rheumatoid arthritis with systemic onset, wrist
  - M08.231 Juvenile rheumatoid arthritis with systemic onset, right wrist
  - M08.232 Juvenile rheumatoid arthritis with systemic onset, left wrist
  - M08.239 Juvenile rheumatoid arthritis with systemic onset, unspecified wrist
- M08.24 Juvenile rheumatoid arthritis with systemic onset, hand
  - M08.241 Juvenile rheumatoid arthritis with systemic onset, right hand
  - M08.242 Juvenile rheumatoid arthritis with systemic onset, left hand
  - M08.249 Juvenile rheumatoid arthritis with systemic onset, unspecified hand
- M08.25 Juvenile rheumatoid arthritis with systemic onset, hip
  - M08.251 Juvenile rheumatoid arthritis with systemic onset, right hip
  - M08.252 Juvenile rheumatoid arthritis with systemic onset, left hip
  - M08.259 Juvenile rheumatoid arthritis with systemic onset, unspecified hip
- M08.26 Juvenile rheumatoid arthritis with systemic onset, knee
  - M08.261 Juvenile rheumatoid arthritis with systemic onset, right knee
  - M08.262 Juvenile rheumatoid arthritis with systemic onset, left knee
  - M08.269 Juvenile rheumatoid arthritis with systemic onset, unspecified knee
- M08.27 Juvenile rheumatoid arthritis with systemic onset, ankle and foot
  - M08.271 Juvenile rheumatoid arthritis with systemic onset, right ankle and foot
  - M08.272 Juvenile rheumatoid arthritis with systemic onset, left ankle and foot
  - M08.279 Juvenile rheumatoid arthritis with systemic onset, unspecified ankle and foot
- M08.28 Juvenile rheumatoid arthritis with systemic onset, vertebrae
- M08.29 Juvenile rheumatoid arthritis with systemic onset, multiple sites

M08.3 Juvenile rheumatoid polyarthritis (seronegative)

- M08.4 Pauciarticular juvenile rheumatoid arthritis
  - M08.40 Pauciarticular juvenile rheumatoid arthritis, unspecified site
  - M08.41 Pauciarticular juvenile rheumatoid arthritis, shoulder
    - M08.411 Pauciarticular juvenile rheumatoid arthritis, right shoulder
    - M08.412 Pauciarticular juvenile rheumatoid arthritis, left shoulder
    - M08.419 Pauciarticular juvenile rheumatoid arthritis, unspecified shoulder
  - M08.42 Pauciarticular juvenile rheumatoid arthritis, elbow
    - M08.421 Pauciarticular juvenile rheumatoid arthritis, right elbow
    - M08.422 Pauciarticular juvenile rheumatoid arthritis, left elbow
    - M08.429 Pauciarticular juvenile rheumatoid arthritis, unspecified elbow
  - M08.43 Pauciarticular juvenile rheumatoid arthritis, wrist
    - M08.431 Pauciarticular juvenile rheumatoid arthritis, right wrist
    - M08.432 Pauciarticular juvenile rheumatoid arthritis, left wrist
    - M08.439 Pauciarticular juvenile rheumatoid arthritis, unspecified wrist
  - M08.44 Pauciarticular juvenile rheumatoid arthritis, hand
    - M08.441 Pauciarticular juvenile rheumatoid arthritis, right hand
    - M08.442 Pauciarticular juvenile rheumatoid arthritis, left hand
    - M08.449 Pauciarticular juvenile rheumatoid arthritis, unspecified hand
  - M08.45 Pauciarticular juvenile rheumatoid arthritis, hip
    - M08.451 Pauciarticular juvenile rheumatoid arthritis, right hip
    - M08.452 Pauciarticular juvenile rheumatoid arthritis, left hip
    - M08.459 Pauciarticular juvenile rheumatoid arthritis, unspecified hip
  - M08.46 Pauciarticular juvenile rheumatoid arthritis, knee
    - M08.461 Pauciarticular juvenile rheumatoid arthritis, right knee
    - M08.462 Pauciarticular juvenile rheumatoid arthritis, left knee
    - M08.469 Pauciarticular juvenile rheumatoid arthritis, unspecified knee
  - M08.47 Pauciarticular juvenile rheumatoid arthritis, ankle and foot
    - M08.471 Pauciarticular juvenile rheumatoid arthritis, right ankle and foot
    - M08.472 Pauciarticular juvenile rheumatoid arthritis, left ankle and foot
    - M08.479 Pauciarticular juvenile rheumatoid arthritis, unspecified ankle and foot
  - M08.48 Pauciarticular juvenile rheumatoid arthritis, vertebrae
- M08.8 Other juvenile arthritis
  - M08.80 Other juvenile arthritis, unspecified site
  - M08.81 Other juvenile arthritis, shoulder
    - M08.811 Other juvenile arthritis, right shoulder
    - M08.812 Other juvenile arthritis, left shoulder
    - M08.819 Other juvenile arthritis, unspecified shoulder
  - M08.82 Other juvenile arthritis, elbow
    - M08.821 Other juvenile arthritis, right elbow
    - M08.822 Other juvenile arthritis, left elbow
    - M08.829 Other juvenile arthritis, unspecified elbow
  - M08.83 Other juvenile arthritis, wrist
    - M08.831 Other juvenile arthritis, right wrist
    - M08.832 Other juvenile arthritis, left wrist
    - M08.839 Other juvenile arthritis, unspecified wrist

New Revised ~~deleted~~ Deleted Excludes 1 Excludes 2 Includes Use additional Code first Code also Unspecified
OGCR Official Guidelines Unacceptable Principal Diagnosis X Assign placeholder X Use Additional Character(s) Manifestation Code Coding Clinic

- **M08.84 Other juvenile arthritis, hand**
  - **M08.841 Other juvenile arthritis, right hand**
  - **M08.842 Other juvenile arthritis, left hand**
  - **M08.849 Other juvenile arthritis, unspecified hand**
- **M08.85 Other juvenile arthritis, hip**
  - **M08.851 Other juvenile arthritis, right hip**
  - **M08.852 Other juvenile arthritis, left hip**
  - **M08.859 Other juvenile arthritis, unspecified hip**
- **M08.86 Other juvenile arthritis, knee**
  - **M08.861 Other juvenile arthritis, right knee**
  - **M08.862 Other juvenile arthritis, left knee**
  - **M08.869 Other juvenile arthritis, unspecified knee**
- **M08.87 Other juvenile arthritis, ankle and foot**
  - **M08.871 Other juvenile arthritis, right ankle and foot**
  - **M08.872 Other juvenile arthritis, left ankle and foot**
  - **M08.879 Other juvenile arthritis, unspecified ankle and foot**
- **M08.88 Other juvenile arthritis, other specified site**
  Other juvenile arthritis, vertebrae
- **M08.89 Other juvenile arthritis, multiple sites**

- **M08.9 Juvenile arthritis, unspecified**
  Excludes1 juvenile rheumatoid arthritis, unspecified (M08.0-)
  - **M08.90 Juvenile arthritis, unspecified, unspecified site**
  - **M08.91 Juvenile arthritis, unspecified, shoulder**
    - **M08.911 Juvenile arthritis, unspecified, right shoulder**
    - **M08.912 Juvenile arthritis, unspecified, left shoulder**
    - **M08.919 Juvenile arthritis, unspecified, unspecified shoulder**
  - **M08.92 Juvenile arthritis, unspecified, elbow**
    - **M08.921 Juvenile arthritis, unspecified, right elbow**
    - **M08.922 Juvenile arthritis, unspecified, left elbow**
    - **M08.929 Juvenile arthritis, unspecified, unspecified elbow**
  - **M08.93 Juvenile arthritis, unspecified, wrist**
    - **M08.931 Juvenile arthritis, unspecified, right wrist**
    - **M08.932 Juvenile arthritis, unspecified, left wrist**
    - **M08.939 Juvenile arthritis, unspecified, unspecified wrist**
  - **M08.94 Juvenile arthritis, unspecified, hand**
    - **M08.941 Juvenile arthritis, unspecified, right hand**
    - **M08.942 Juvenile arthritis, unspecified, left hand**
    - **M08.949 Juvenile arthritis, unspecified, unspecified hand**
  - **M08.95 Juvenile arthritis, unspecified, hip**
    - **M08.951 Juvenile arthritis, unspecified, right hip**
    - **M08.952 Juvenile arthritis, unspecified, left hip**
    - **M08.959 Juvenile arthritis, unspecified, unspecified hip**
  - **M08.96 Juvenile arthritis, unspecified, knee**
    - **M08.961 Juvenile arthritis, unspecified, right knee**
    - **M08.962 Juvenile arthritis, unspecified, left knee**
    - **M08.969 Juvenile arthritis, unspecified, unspecified knee**
  - **M08.97 Juvenile arthritis, unspecified, ankle and foot**
    - **M08.971 Juvenile arthritis, unspecified, right ankle and foot**
    - **M08.972 Juvenile arthritis, unspecified, left ankle and foot**
    - **M08.979 Juvenile arthritis, unspecified, unspecified ankle and foot**
  - **M08.98 Juvenile arthritis, unspecified, vertebrae**
  - **M08.99 Juvenile arthritis, unspecified, multiple sites**

- **M1A Chronic gout**
  Use additional code to identify:
  Autonomic neuropathy in diseases classified elsewhere (G99.0)
  Calculus of urinary tract in diseases classified elsewhere (N22)
  Cardiomyopathy in diseases classified elsewhere (I43)
  Disorders of external ear in diseases classified elsewhere (H61.1-, H62.8-)
  Disorders of iris and ciliary body in diseases classified elsewhere (H22)
  Glomerular disorders in diseases classified elsewhere (N08)
  Excludes1 gout NOS (M10.-)
  Excludes2 acute gout (M10.-) ◀
  The appropriate 7th character is to be added to each code from category M1A

0	without tophus (tophi)
1	with tophus (tophi)

  - **M1A.0 Idiopathic chronic gout**
    Chronic gouty bursitis
    Primary chronic gout
    - X **M1A.00 Idiopathic chronic gout, unspecified site**
    - **M1A.01 Idiopathic chronic gout, shoulder**
      - **M1A.011 Idiopathic chronic gout, right shoulder**
      - **M1A.012 Idiopathic chronic gout, left shoulder**
      - **M1A.019 Idiopathic chronic gout, unspecified shoulder**
    - **M1A.02 Idiopathic chronic gout, elbow**
      - **M1A.021 Idiopathic chronic gout, right elbow**
      - **M1A.022 Idiopathic chronic gout, left elbow**
      - **M1A.029 Idiopathic chronic gout, unspecified elbow**
    - **M1A.03 Idiopathic chronic gout, wrist**
      - **M1A.031 Idiopathic chronic gout, right wrist**
      - **M1A.032 Idiopathic chronic gout, left wrist**
      - **M1A.039 Idiopathic chronic gout, unspecified wrist**
    - **M1A.04 Idiopathic chronic gout, hand**
      - **M1A.041 Idiopathic chronic gout, right hand**
      - **M1A.042 Idiopathic chronic gout, left hand**
      - **M1A.049 Idiopathic chronic gout, unspecified hand**
    - **M1A.05 Idiopathic chronic gout, hip**
      - **M1A.051 Idiopathic chronic gout, right hip**
      - **M1A.052 Idiopathic chronic gout, left hip**
      - **M1A.059 Idiopathic chronic gout, unspecified hip**
    - **M1A.06 Idiopathic chronic gout, knee**
      - **M1A.061 Idiopathic chronic gout, right knee**
      - **M1A.062 Idiopathic chronic gout, left knee**
      - **M1A.069 Idiopathic chronic gout, unspecified knee**

- M1A.07 Idiopathic chronic gout, ankle and foot
  - M1A.071 Idiopathic chronic gout, right ankle and foot
  - M1A.072 Idiopathic chronic gout, left ankle and foot
  - M1A.079 Idiopathic chronic gout, unspecified ankle and foot
- X M1A.08 Idiopathic chronic gout, vertebrae
- X M1A.09 Idiopathic chronic gout, multiple sites
- M1A.1 Lead-induced chronic gout

  Code first toxic effects of lead and its compounds (T56.0-)
- X M1A.10 Lead-induced chronic gout, unspecified site
- M1A.11 Lead-induced chronic gout, shoulder
  - M1A.111 Lead-induced chronic gout, right shoulder
  - M1A.112 Lead-induced chronic gout, left shoulder
  - M1A.119 Lead-induced chronic gout, unspecified shoulder
- M1A.12 Lead-induced chronic gout, elbow
  - M1A.121 Lead-induced chronic gout, right elbow
  - M1A.122 Lead-induced chronic gout, left elbow
  - M1A.129 Lead-induced chronic gout, unspecified elbow
- M1A.13 Lead-induced chronic gout, wrist
  - M1A.131 Lead-induced chronic gout, right wrist
  - M1A.132 Lead-induced chronic gout, left wrist
  - M1A.139 Lead-induced chronic gout, unspecified wrist
- M1A.14 Lead-induced chronic gout, hand
  - M1A.141 Lead-induced chronic gout, right hand
  - M1A.142 Lead-induced chronic gout, left hand
  - M1A.149 Lead-induced chronic gout, unspecified hand
- M1A.15 Lead-induced chronic gout, hip
  - M1A.151 Lead-induced chronic gout, right hip
  - M1A.152 Lead-induced chronic gout, left hip
  - M1A.159 Lead-induced chronic gout, unspecified hip
- M1A.16 Lead-induced chronic gout, knee
  - M1A.161 Lead-induced chronic gout, right knee
  - M1A.162 Lead-induced chronic gout, left knee
  - M1A.169 Lead-induced chronic gout, unspecified knee
- M1A.17 Lead-induced chronic gout, ankle and foot
  - M1A.171 Lead-induced chronic gout, right ankle and foot
  - M1A.172 Lead-induced chronic gout, left ankle and foot
  - M1A.179 Lead-induced chronic gout, unspecified ankle and foot
- X M1A.18 Lead-induced chronic gout, vertebrae
- X M1A.19 Lead-induced chronic gout, multiple sites
- M1A.2 Drug-induced chronic gout

  Use additional code for adverse effect, if applicable, to identify drug (T36-T50 with fifth or sixth character 5)
- X M1A.20 Drug-induced chronic gout, unspecified site
- M1A.21 Drug-induced chronic gout, shoulder
  - M1A.211 Drug-induced chronic gout, right shoulder
  - M1A.212 Drug-induced chronic gout, left shoulder
  - M1A.219 Drug-induced chronic gout, unspecified shoulder
- M1A.22 Drug-induced chronic gout, elbow
  - M1A.221 Drug-induced chronic gout, right elbow
  - M1A.222 Drug-induced chronic gout, left elbow
  - M1A.229 Drug-induced chronic gout, unspecified elbow
- M1A.23 Drug-induced chronic gout, wrist
  - M1A.231 Drug-induced chronic gout, right wrist
  - M1A.232 Drug-induced chronic gout, left wrist
  - M1A.239 Drug-induced chronic gout, unspecified wrist
- M1A.24 Drug-induced chronic gout, hand
  - M1A.241 Drug-induced chronic gout, right hand
  - M1A.242 Drug-induced chronic gout, left hand
  - M1A.249 Drug-induced chronic gout, unspecified hand
- M1A.25 Drug-induced chronic gout, hip
  - M1A.251 Drug-induced chronic gout, right hip
  - M1A.252 Drug-induced chronic gout, left hip
  - M1A.259 Drug-induced chronic gout, unspecified hip
- M1A.26 Drug-induced chronic gout, knee
  - M1A.261 Drug-induced chronic gout, right knee
  - M1A.262 Drug-induced chronic gout, left knee
  - M1A.269 Drug-induced chronic gout, unspecified knee
- M1A.27 Drug-induced chronic gout, ankle and foot
  - M1A.271 Drug-induced chronic gout, right ankle and foot
  - M1A.272 Drug-induced chronic gout, left ankle and foot
  - M1A.279 Drug-induced chronic gout, unspecified ankle and foot
- X M1A.28 Drug-induced chronic gout, vertebrae
- X M1A.29 Drug-induced chronic gout, multiple sites
- M1A.3 Chronic gout due to renal impairment

  Code first associated renal disease
- X M1A.30 Chronic gout due to renal impairment, unspecified site
- M1A.31 Chronic gout due to renal impairment, shoulder
  - M1A.311 Chronic gout due to renal impairment, right shoulder
  - M1A.312 Chronic gout due to renal impairment, left shoulder
  - M1A.319 Chronic gout due to renal impairment, unspecified shoulder
- M1A.32 Chronic gout due to renal impairment, elbow
  - M1A.321 Chronic gout due to renal impairment, right elbow
  - M1A.322 Chronic gout due to renal impairment, left elbow
  - M1A.329 Chronic gout due to renal impairment, unspecified elbow
- M1A.33 Chronic gout due to renal impairment, wrist
  - M1A.331 Chronic gout due to renal impairment, right wrist
  - M1A.332 Chronic gout due to renal impairment, left wrist
  - M1A.339 Chronic gout due to renal impairment, unspecified wrist

◀ New ◀ Revised ~~deleted~~ Deleted Excludes 1 Excludes 2 Includes Use additional Code first Code also Unspecified
OGCR Official Guidelines ● Unacceptable Principal Diagnosis X Assign placeholder X ● Use Additional Character(s) ▶ Manifestation Code Coding Clinic

- M1A.34 Chronic gout due to renal impairment, hand
  - M1A.341 Chronic gout due to renal impairment, right hand
  - M1A.342 Chronic gout due to renal impairment, left hand
  - M1A.349 Chronic gout due to renal impairment, unspecified hand
- M1A.35 Chronic gout due to renal impairment, hip
  - M1A.351 Chronic gout due to renal impairment, right hip
  - M1A.352 Chronic gout due to renal impairment, left hip
  - M1A.359 Chronic gout due to renal impairment, unspecified hip
- M1A.36 Chronic gout due to renal impairment, knee
  - M1A.361 Chronic gout due to renal impairment, right knee
  - M1A.362 Chronic gout due to renal impairment, left knee
  - M1A.369 Chronic gout due to renal impairment, unspecified knee
- M1A.37 Chronic gout due to renal impairment, ankle and foot
  - M1A.371 Chronic gout due to renal impairment, right ankle and foot
  - M1A.372 Chronic gout due to renal impairment, left ankle and foot
  - M1A.379 Chronic gout due to renal impairment, unspecified ankle and foot
- X M1A.38 Chronic gout due to renal impairment, vertebrae
- X M1A.39 Chronic gout due to renal impairment, multiple sites

M1A.4 Other secondary chronic gout

Code first associated condition

- X M1A.40 Other secondary chronic gout, unspecified site
- M1A.41 Other secondary chronic gout, shoulder
  - M1A.411 Other secondary chronic gout, right shoulder
  - M1A.412 Other secondary chronic gout, left shoulder
  - M1A.419 Other secondary chronic gout, unspecified shoulder
- M1A.42 Other secondary chronic gout, elbow
  - M1A.421 Other secondary chronic gout, right elbow
  - M1A.422 Other secondary chronic gout, left elbow
  - M1A.429 Other secondary chronic gout, unspecified elbow
- M1A.43 Other secondary chronic gout, wrist
  - M1A.431 Other secondary chronic gout, right wrist
  - M1A.432 Other secondary chronic gout, left wrist
  - M1A.439 Other secondary chronic gout, unspecified wrist
- M1A.44 Other secondary chronic gout, hand
  - M1A.441 Other secondary chronic gout, right hand
  - M1A.442 Other secondary chronic gout, left hand
  - M1A.449 Other secondary chronic gout, unspecified hand
- M1A.45 Other secondary chronic gout, hip
  - M1A.451 Other secondary chronic gout, right hip
  - M1A.452 Other secondary chronic gout, left hip
  - M1A.459 Other secondary chronic gout, unspecified hip
- M1A.46 Other secondary chronic gout, knee
  - M1A.461 Other secondary chronic gout, right knee
  - M1A.462 Other secondary chronic gout, left knee
  - M1A.469 Other secondary chronic gout, unspecified knee
- M1A.47 Other secondary chronic gout, ankle and foot
  - M1A.471 Other secondary chronic gout, right ankle and foot
  - M1A.472 Other secondary chronic gout, left ankle and foot
  - M1A.479 Other secondary chronic gout, unspecified ankle and foot
- X M1A.48 Other secondary chronic gout, vertebrae
- X M1A.49 Other secondary chronic gout, multiple sites

X M1A.9 Chronic gout, unspecified

M10 Gout

Accumulation of uric acid that results in swollen, red, hot, painful, stiff joints

Acute gout
Gout attack
Gout flare
Podagra

Use additional code to identify:
Autonomic neuropathy in diseases classified elsewhere (G99.0)
Calculus of urinary tract in diseases classified elsewhere (N22)
Cardiomyopathy in diseases classified elsewhere (I43)
Disorders of external ear in diseases classified elsewhere (H61.1-, H62.8-)
Disorders of iris and ciliary body in diseases classified elsewhere (H22)
Glomerular disorders in diseases classified elsewhere (N08)

Excludes2 chronic gout (M1A.-) ◀

- M10.0 Idiopathic gout
  - Gouty bursitis
  - Primary gout
  - M10.00 Idiopathic gout, unspecified site
  - M10.01 Idiopathic gout, shoulder
    - M10.011 Idiopathic gout, right shoulder
    - M10.012 Idiopathic gout, left shoulder
    - M10.019 Idiopathic gout, unspecified shoulder
  - M10.02 Idiopathic gout, elbow
    - M10.021 Idiopathic gout, right elbow
    - M10.022 Idiopathic gout, left elbow
    - M10.029 Idiopathic gout, unspecified elbow
  - M10.03 Idiopathic gout, wrist
    - M10.031 Idiopathic gout, right wrist
    - M10.032 Idiopathic gout, left wrist
    - M10.039 Idiopathic gout, unspecified wrist
  - M10.04 Idiopathic gout, hand
    - M10.041 Idiopathic gout, right hand
    - M10.042 Idiopathic gout, left hand
    - M10.049 Idiopathic gout, unspecified hand
  - M10.05 Idiopathic gout, hip
    - M10.051 Idiopathic gout, right hip
    - M10.052 Idiopathic gout, left hip
    - M10.059 Idiopathic gout, unspecified hip

- M10.06 Idiopathic gout, knee
  - M10.061 Idiopathic gout, right knee
  - M10.062 Idiopathic gout, left knee
  - M10.069 Idiopathic gout, unspecified knee
- M10.07 Idiopathic gout, ankle and foot
  - M10.071 Idiopathic gout, right ankle and foot
  - M10.072 Idiopathic gout, left ankle and foot
  - M10.079 Idiopathic gout, unspecified ankle and foot
- M10.08 Idiopathic gout, vertebrae
- M10.09 Idiopathic gout, multiple sites

- M10.1 Lead-induced gout
  - *Code first toxic effects of lead and its compounds (T56.0-)*
  - M10.10 Lead-induced gout, unspecified site
  - M10.11 Lead-induced gout, shoulder
    - M10.111 Lead-induced gout, right shoulder
    - M10.112 Lead-induced gout, left shoulder
    - M10.119 Lead-induced gout, unspecified shoulder
  - M10.12 Lead-induced gout, elbow
    - M10.121 Lead-induced gout, right elbow
    - M10.122 Lead-induced gout, left elbow
    - M10.129 Lead-induced gout, unspecified elbow
  - M10.13 Lead-induced gout, wrist
    - M10.131 Lead-induced gout, right wrist
    - M10.132 Lead-induced gout, left wrist
    - M10.139 Lead-induced gout, unspecified wrist
  - M10.14 Lead-induced gout, hand
    - M10.141 Lead-induced gout, right hand
    - M10.142 Lead-induced gout, left hand
    - M10.149 Lead-induced gout, unspecified hand
  - M10.15 Lead-induced gout, hip
    - M10.151 Lead-induced gout, right hip
    - M10.152 Lead-induced gout, left hip
    - M10.159 Lead-induced gout, unspecified hip
  - M10.16 Lead-induced gout, knee
    - M10.161 Lead-induced gout, right knee
    - M10.162 Lead-induced gout, left knee
    - M10.169 Lead-induced gout, unspecified knee
  - M10.17 Lead-induced gout, ankle and foot
    - M10.171 Lead-induced gout, right ankle and foot
    - M10.172 Lead-induced gout, left ankle and foot
    - M10.179 Lead-induced gout, unspecified ankle and foot
  - M10.18 Lead-induced gout, vertebrae
  - M10.19 Lead-induced gout, multiple sites

- M10.2 Drug-induced gout
  - Use additional code for adverse effect, if applicable, to identify drug (T36-T50 with fifth or sixth character 5)
  - M10.20 Drug-induced gout, unspecified site
  - M10.21 Drug-induced gout, shoulder
    - M10.211 Drug-induced gout, right shoulder
    - M10.212 Drug-induced gout, left shoulder
    - M10.219 Drug-induced gout, unspecified shoulder
  - M10.22 Drug-induced gout, elbow
    - M10.221 Drug-induced gout, right elbow
    - M10.222 Drug-induced gout, left elbow
    - M10.229 Drug-induced gout, unspecified elbow
  - M10.23 Drug-induced gout, wrist
    - M10.231 Drug-induced gout, right wrist
    - M10.232 Drug-induced gout, left wrist
    - M10.239 Drug-induced gout, unspecified wrist
  - M10.24 Drug-induced gout, hand
    - M10.241 Drug-induced gout, right hand
    - M10.242 Drug-induced gout, left hand
    - M10.249 Drug-induced gout, unspecified hand
  - M10.25 Drug-induced gout, hip
    - M10.251 Drug-induced gout, right hip
    - M10.252 Drug-induced gout, left hip
    - M10.259 Drug-induced gout, unspecified hip
  - M10.26 Drug-induced gout, knee
    - M10.261 Drug-induced gout, right knee
    - M10.262 Drug-induced gout, left knee
    - M10.269 Drug-induced gout, unspecified knee
  - M10.27 Drug-induced gout, ankle and foot
    - M10.271 Drug-induced gout, right ankle and foot
    - M10.272 Drug-induced gout, left ankle and foot
    - M10.279 Drug-induced gout, unspecified ankle and foot
  - M10.28 Drug-induced gout, vertebrae
  - M10.29 Drug-induced gout, multiple sites

- M10.3 Gout due to renal impairment
  - Code also associated renal disease
  - M10.30 Gout due to renal impairment, unspecified site
  - M10.31 Gout due to renal impairment, shoulder
    - M10.311 Gout due to renal impairment, right shoulder
    - M10.312 Gout due to renal impairment, left shoulder
    - M10.319 Gout due to renal impairment, unspecified shoulder
  - M10.32 Gout due to renal impairment, elbow
    - M10.321 Gout due to renal impairment, right elbow
    - M10.322 Gout due to renal impairment, left elbow
    - M10.329 Gout due to renal impairment, unspecified elbow
  - M10.33 Gout due to renal impairment, wrist
    - M10.331 Gout due to renal impairment, right wrist
    - M10.332 Gout due to renal impairment, left wrist
    - M10.339 Gout due to renal impairment, unspecified wrist
  - M10.34 Gout due to renal impairment, hand
    - M10.341 Gout due to renal impairment, right hand
    - M10.342 Gout due to renal impairment, left hand
    - M10.349 Gout due to renal impairment, unspecified hand
  - M10.35 Gout due to renal impairment, hip
    - M10.351 Gout due to renal impairment, right hip
    - M10.352 Gout due to renal impairment, left hip
    - M10.359 Gout due to renal impairment, unspecified hip
  - M10.36 Gout due to renal impairment, knee
    - M10.361 Gout due to renal impairment, right knee
    - M10.362 Gout due to renal impairment, left knee
    - M10.369 Gout due to renal impairment, unspecified knee

◀ New ◀ Revised ~~deleted~~ Deleted Excludes 1 Excludes 2 Includes Use additional Code first Code also Unspecified
OGCR Official Guidelines ● Unacceptable Principal Diagnosis X Assign placeholder X ● Use Additional Character(s) ▶ Manifestation Code Coding Clinic

- M10.37 Gout due to renal impairment, ankle and foot
  - M10.371 Gout due to renal impairment, right ankle and foot
  - M10.372 Gout due to renal impairment, left ankle and foot
  - M10.379 Gout due to renal impairment, unspecified ankle and foot
- M10.38 Gout due to renal impairment, vertebrae
- M10.39 Gout due to renal impairment, multiple sites
- M10.4 Other secondary gout
  - *Code first associated condition*
  - M10.40 Other secondary gout, unspecified site
  - M10.41 Other secondary gout, shoulder
    - M10.411 Other secondary gout, right shoulder
    - M10.412 Other secondary gout, left shoulder
    - M10.419 Other secondary gout, unspecified shoulder
  - M10.42 Other secondary gout, elbow
    - M10.421 Other secondary gout, right elbow
    - M10.422 Other secondary gout, left elbow
    - M10.429 Other secondary gout, unspecified elbow
  - M10.43 Other secondary gout, wrist
    - M10.431 Other secondary gout, right wrist
    - M10.432 Other secondary gout, left wrist
    - M10.439 Other secondary gout, unspecified wrist
  - M10.44 Other secondary gout, hand
    - M10.441 Other secondary gout, right hand
    - M10.442 Other secondary gout, left hand
    - M10.449 Other secondary gout, unspecified hand
  - M10.45 Other secondary gout, hip
    - M10.451 Other secondary gout, right hip
    - M10.452 Other secondary gout, left hip
    - M10.459 Other secondary gout, unspecified hip
  - M10.46 Other secondary gout, knee
    - M10.461 Other secondary gout, right knee
    - M10.462 Other secondary gout, left knee
    - M10.469 Other secondary gout, unspecified knee
  - M10.47 Other secondary gout, ankle and foot
    - M10.471 Other secondary gout, right ankle and foot
    - M10.472 Other secondary gout, left ankle and foot
    - M10.479 Other secondary gout, unspecified ankle and foot
  - M10.48 Other secondary gout, vertebrae
  - M10.49 Other secondary gout, multiple sites
- M10.9 Gout, unspecified
  - Gout NOS

- M11 Other crystal arthropathies
  - M11.0 Hydroxyapatite deposition disease
    - M11.00 Hydroxyapatite deposition disease, unspecified site
    - M11.01 Hydroxyapatite deposition disease, shoulder
      - M11.011 Hydroxyapatite deposition disease, right shoulder
      - M11.012 Hydroxyapatite deposition disease, left shoulder
      - M11.019 Hydroxyapatite deposition disease, unspecified shoulder
    - M11.02 Hydroxyapatite deposition disease, elbow
      - M11.021 Hydroxyapatite deposition disease, right elbow
      - M11.022 Hydroxyapatite deposition disease, left elbow
      - M11.029 Hydroxyapatite deposition disease, unspecified elbow
    - M11.03 Hydroxyapatite deposition disease, wrist
      - M11.031 Hydroxyapatite deposition disease, right wrist
      - M11.032 Hydroxyapatite deposition disease, left wrist
      - M11.039 Hydroxyapatite deposition disease, unspecified wrist
    - M11.04 Hydroxyapatite deposition disease, hand
      - M11.041 Hydroxyapatite deposition disease, right hand
      - M11.042 Hydroxyapatite deposition disease, left hand
      - M11.049 Hydroxyapatite deposition disease, unspecified hand
    - M11.05 Hydroxyapatite deposition disease, hip
      - M11.051 Hydroxyapatite deposition disease, right hip
      - M11.052 Hydroxyapatite deposition disease, left hip
      - M11.059 Hydroxyapatite deposition disease, unspecified hip
    - M11.06 Hydroxyapatite deposition disease, knee
      - M11.061 Hydroxyapatite deposition disease, right knee
      - M11.062 Hydroxyapatite deposition disease, left knee
      - M11.069 Hydroxyapatite deposition disease, unspecified knee
    - M11.07 Hydroxyapatite deposition disease, ankle and foot
      - M11.071 Hydroxyapatite deposition disease, right ankle and foot
      - M11.072 Hydroxyapatite deposition disease, left ankle and foot
      - M11.079 Hydroxyapatite deposition disease, unspecified ankle and foot
    - M11.08 Hydroxyapatite deposition disease, vertebrae
    - M11.09 Hydroxyapatite deposition disease, multiple sites
  - M11.1 Familial chondrocalcinosis
    - M11.10 Familial chondrocalcinosis, unspecified site
    - M11.11 Familial chondrocalcinosis, shoulder
      - M11.111 Familial chondrocalcinosis, right shoulder
      - M11.112 Familial chondrocalcinosis, left shoulder
      - M11.119 Familial chondrocalcinosis, unspecified shoulder
    - M11.12 Familial chondrocalcinosis, elbow
      - M11.121 Familial chondrocalcinosis, right elbow
      - M11.122 Familial chondrocalcinosis, left elbow
      - M11.129 Familial chondrocalcinosis, unspecified elbow
    - M11.13 Familial chondrocalcinosis, wrist
      - M11.131 Familial chondrocalcinosis, right wrist
      - M11.132 Familial chondrocalcinosis, left wrist
      - M11.139 Familial chondrocalcinosis, unspecified wrist

- M11.14 Familial chondrocalcinosis, hand
  - M11.141 Familial chondrocalcinosis, right hand
  - M11.142 Familial chondrocalcinosis, left hand
  - M11.149 Familial chondrocalcinosis, unspecified hand
- M11.15 Familial chondrocalcinosis, hip
  - M11.151 Familial chondrocalcinosis, right hip
  - M11.152 Familial chondrocalcinosis, left hip
  - M11.159 Familial chondrocalcinosis, unspecified hip
- M11.16 Familial chondrocalcinosis, knee
  - M11.161 Familial chondrocalcinosis, right knee
  - M11.162 Familial chondrocalcinosis, left knee
  - M11.169 Familial chondrocalcinosis, unspecified knee
- M11.17 Familial chondrocalcinosis, ankle and foot
  - M11.171 Familial chondrocalcinosis, right ankle and foot
  - M11.172 Familial chondrocalcinosis, left ankle and foot
  - M11.179 Familial chondrocalcinosis, unspecified ankle and foot
  - M11.18 Familial chondrocalcinosis, vertebrae
  - M11.19 Familial chondrocalcinosis, multiple sites
- M11.2 Other chondrocalcinosis
  Chondrocalcinosis NOS
  - M11.20 Other chondrocalcinosis, unspecified site
  - M11.21 Other chondrocalcinosis, shoulder
    - M11.211 Other chondrocalcinosis, right shoulder
    - M11.212 Other chondrocalcinosis, left shoulder
    - M11.219 Other chondrocalcinosis, unspecified shoulder
  - M11.22 Other chondrocalcinosis, elbow
    - M11.221 Other chondrocalcinosis, right elbow
    - M11.222 Other chondrocalcinosis, left elbow
    - M11.229 Other chondrocalcinosis, unspecified elbow
  - M11.23 Other chondrocalcinosis, wrist
    - M11.231 Other chondrocalcinosis, right wrist
    - M11.232 Other chondrocalcinosis, left wrist
    - M11.239 Other chondrocalcinosis, unspecified wrist
  - M11.24 Other chondrocalcinosis, hand
    - M11.241 Other chondrocalcinosis, right hand
    - M11.242 Other chondrocalcinosis, left hand
    - M11.249 Other chondrocalcinosis, unspecified hand
  - M11.25 Other chondrocalcinosis, hip
    - M11.251 Other chondrocalcinosis, right hip
    - M11.252 Other chondrocalcinosis, left hip
    - M11.259 Other chondrocalcinosis, unspecified hip
  - M11.26 Other chondrocalcinosis, knee
    - M11.261 Other chondrocalcinosis, right knee
    - M11.262 Other chondrocalcinosis, left knee
    - M11.269 Other chondrocalcinosis, unspecified knee
  - M11.27 Other chondrocalcinosis, ankle and foot
    - M11.271 Other chondrocalcinosis, right ankle and foot
    - M11.272 Other chondrocalcinosis, left ankle and foot
    - M11.279 Other chondrocalcinosis, unspecified ankle and foot
  - M11.28 Other chondrocalcinosis, vertebrae
  - M11.29 Other chondrocalcinosis, multiple sites
- M11.8 Other specified crystal arthropathies
  - M11.80 Other specified crystal arthropathies, unspecified site
  - M11.81 Other specified crystal arthropathies, shoulder
    - M11.811 Other specified crystal arthropathies, right shoulder
    - M11.812 Other specified crystal arthropathies, left shoulder
    - M11.819 Other specified crystal arthropathies, unspecified shoulder
  - M11.82 Other specified crystal arthropathies, elbow
    - M11.821 Other specified crystal arthropathies, right elbow
    - M11.822 Other specified crystal arthropathies, left elbow
    - M11.829 Other specified crystal arthropathies, unspecified elbow
  - M11.83 Other specified crystal arthropathies, wrist
    - M11.831 Other specified crystal arthropathies, right wrist
    - M11.832 Other specified crystal arthropathies, left wrist
    - M11.839 Other specified crystal arthropathies, unspecified wrist
  - M11.84 Other specified crystal arthropathies, hand
    - M11.841 Other specified crystal arthropathies, right hand
    - M11.842 Other specified crystal arthropathies, left hand
    - M11.849 Other specified crystal arthropathies, unspecified hand
  - M11.85 Other specified crystal arthropathies, hip
    - M11.851 Other specified crystal arthropathies, right hip
    - M11.852 Other specified crystal arthropathies, left hip
    - M11.859 Other specified crystal arthropathies, unspecified hip
  - M11.86 Other specified crystal arthropathies, knee
    - M11.861 Other specified crystal arthropathies, right knee
    - M11.862 Other specified crystal arthropathies, left knee
    - M11.869 Other specified crystal arthropathies, unspecified knee
  - M11.87 Other specified crystal arthropathies, ankle and foot
    - M11.871 Other specified crystal arthropathies, right ankle and foot
    - M11.872 Other specified crystal arthropathies, left ankle and foot
    - M11.879 Other specified crystal arthropathies, unspecified ankle and foot
  - M11.88 Other specified crystal arthropathies, vertebrae
  - M11.89 Other specified crystal arthropathies, multiple sites
- M11.9 Crystal arthropathy, unspecified

- M12 Other and unspecified arthropathy
  Excludes1 arthrosis (M15-M19)
  cricoarytenoid arthropathy (J38.7)
  - M12.0 Chronic postrheumatic arthropathy [Jaccoud]
    - M12.00 Chronic postrheumatic arthropathy [Jaccoud], unspecified site

- M12.01 Chronic postrheumatic arthropathy [Jaccoud], shoulder
  - M12.011 Chronic postrheumatic arthropathy [Jaccoud], right shoulder
  - M12.012 Chronic postrheumatic arthropathy [Jaccoud], left shoulder
  - M12.019 Chronic postrheumatic arthropathy [Jaccoud], unspecified shoulder
- M12.02 Chronic postrheumatic arthropathy [Jaccoud], elbow
  - M12.021 Chronic postrheumatic arthropathy [Jaccoud], right elbow
  - M12.022 Chronic postrheumatic arthropathy [Jaccoud], left elbow
  - M12.029 Chronic postrheumatic arthropathy [Jaccoud], unspecified elbow
- M12.03 Chronic postrheumatic arthropathy [Jaccoud], wrist
  - M12.031 Chronic postrheumatic arthropathy [Jaccoud], right wrist
  - M12.032 Chronic postrheumatic arthropathy [Jaccoud], left wrist
  - M12.039 Chronic postrheumatic arthropathy [Jaccoud], unspecified wrist
- M12.04 Chronic postrheumatic arthropathy [Jaccoud], hand
  - M12.041 Chronic postrheumatic arthropathy [Jaccoud], right hand
  - M12.042 Chronic postrheumatic arthropathy [Jaccoud], left hand
  - M12.049 Chronic postrheumatic arthropathy [Jaccoud], unspecified hand
- M12.05 Chronic postrheumatic arthropathy [Jaccoud], hip
  - M12.051 Chronic postrheumatic arthropathy [Jaccoud], right hip
  - M12.052 Chronic postrheumatic arthropathy [Jaccoud], left hip
  - M12.059 Chronic postrheumatic arthropathy [Jaccoud], unspecified hip
- M12.06 Chronic postrheumatic arthropathy [Jaccoud], knee
  - M12.061 Chronic postrheumatic arthropathy [Jaccoud], right knee
  - M12.062 Chronic postrheumatic arthropathy [Jaccoud], left knee
  - M12.069 Chronic postrheumatic arthropathy [Jaccoud], unspecified knee
- M12.07 Chronic postrheumatic arthropathy [Jaccoud], ankle and foot
  - M12.071 Chronic postrheumatic arthropathy [Jaccoud], right ankle and foot
  - M12.072 Chronic postrheumatic arthropathy [Jaccoud], left ankle and foot
  - M12.079 Chronic postrheumatic arthropathy [Jaccoud], unspecified ankle and foot
- M12.08 Chronic postrheumatic arthropathy [Jaccoud], other specified site
  - Chronic postrheumatic arthropathy [Jaccoud], vertebrae
- M12.09 Chronic postrheumatic arthropathy [Jaccoud], multiple sites
- M12.1 Kaschin-Beck disease
  - Osteochondroarthrosis deformans endemica
  - M12.10 Kaschin-Beck disease, unspecified site
  - M12.11 Kaschin-Beck disease, shoulder
    - M12.111 Kaschin-Beck disease, right shoulder
    - M12.112 Kaschin-Beck disease, left shoulder
    - M12.119 Kaschin-Beck disease, unspecified shoulder
  - M12.12 Kaschin-Beck disease, elbow
    - M12.121 Kaschin-Beck disease, right elbow
    - M12.122 Kaschin-Beck disease, left elbow
    - M12.129 Kaschin-Beck disease, unspecified elbow
  - M12.13 Kaschin-Beck disease, wrist
    - M12.131 Kaschin-Beck disease, right wrist
    - M12.132 Kaschin-Beck disease, left wrist
    - M12.139 Kaschin-Beck disease, unspecified wrist
  - M12.14 Kaschin-Beck disease, hand
    - M12.141 Kaschin-Beck disease, right hand
    - M12.142 Kaschin-Beck disease, left hand
    - M12.149 Kaschin-Beck disease, unspecified hand
  - M12.15 Kaschin-Beck disease, hip
    - M12.151 Kaschin-Beck disease, right hip
    - M12.152 Kaschin-Beck disease, left hip
    - M12.159 Kaschin-Beck disease, unspecified hip
  - M12.16 Kaschin-Beck disease, knee
    - M12.161 Kaschin-Beck disease, right knee
    - M12.162 Kaschin-Beck disease, left knee
    - M12.169 Kaschin-Beck disease, unspecified knee
  - M12.17 Kaschin-Beck disease, ankle and foot
    - M12.171 Kaschin-Beck disease, right ankle and foot
    - M12.172 Kaschin-Beck disease, left ankle and foot
    - M12.179 Kaschin-Beck disease, unspecified ankle and foot
  - M12.18 Kaschin-Beck disease, vertebrae
  - M12.19 Kaschin-Beck disease, multiple sites
- M12.2 Villonodular synovitis (pigmented)
  - M12.20 Villonodular synovitis (pigmented), unspecified site
  - M12.21 Villonodular synovitis (pigmented), shoulder
    - M12.211 Villonodular synovitis (pigmented), right shoulder
    - M12.212 Villonodular synovitis (pigmented), left shoulder
    - M12.219 Villonodular synovitis (pigmented), unspecified shoulder
  - M12.22 Villonodular synovitis (pigmented), elbow
    - M12.221 Villonodular synovitis (pigmented), right elbow
    - M12.222 Villonodular synovitis (pigmented), left elbow
    - M12.229 Villonodular synovitis (pigmented), unspecified elbow
  - M12.23 Villonodular synovitis (pigmented), wrist
    - M12.231 Villonodular synovitis (pigmented), right wrist
    - M12.232 Villonodular synovitis (pigmented), left wrist
    - M12.239 Villonodular synovitis (pigmented), unspecified wrist
  - M12.24 Villonodular synovitis (pigmented), hand
    - M12.241 Villonodular synovitis (pigmented), right hand
    - M12.242 Villonodular synovitis (pigmented), left hand
    - M12.249 Villonodular synovitis (pigmented), unspecified hand

- M12.25 Villonodular synovitis (pigmented), hip
  - M12.251 Villonodular synovitis (pigmented), right hip
  - M12.252 Villonodular synovitis (pigmented), left hip
  - M12.259 Villonodular synovitis (pigmented), unspecified hip
- M12.26 Villonodular synovitis (pigmented), knee
  - M12.261 Villonodular synovitis (pigmented), right knee
  - M12.262 Villonodular synovitis (pigmented), left knee
  - M12.269 Villonodular synovitis (pigmented), unspecified knee
- M12.27 Villonodular synovitis (pigmented), ankle and foot
  - M12.271 Villonodular synovitis (pigmented), right ankle and foot
  - M12.272 Villonodular synovitis (pigmented), left ankle and foot
  - M12.279 Villonodular synovitis (pigmented), unspecified ankle and foot
- M12.28 Villonodular synovitis (pigmented), other specified site
  - Villonodular synovitis (pigmented), vertebrae
- M12.29 Villonodular synovitis (pigmented), multiple sites

- M12.3 Palindromic rheumatism
  - M12.30 Palindromic rheumatism, unspecified site
  - M12.31 Palindromic rheumatism, shoulder
    - M12.311 Palindromic rheumatism, right shoulder
    - M12.312 Palindromic rheumatism, left shoulder
    - M12.319 Palindromic rheumatism, unspecified shoulder
  - M12.32 Palindromic rheumatism, elbow
    - M12.321 Palindromic rheumatism, right elbow
    - M12.322 Palindromic rheumatism, left elbow
    - M12.329 Palindromic rheumatism, unspecified elbow
  - M12.33 Palindromic rheumatism, wrist
    - M12.331 Palindromic rheumatism, right wrist
    - M12.332 Palindromic rheumatism, left wrist
    - M12.339 Palindromic rheumatism, unspecified wrist
  - M12.34 Palindromic rheumatism, hand
    - M12.341 Palindromic rheumatism, right hand
    - M12.342 Palindromic rheumatism, left hand
    - M12.349 Palindromic rheumatism, unspecified hand
  - M12.35 Palindromic rheumatism, hip
    - M12.351 Palindromic rheumatism, right hip
    - M12.352 Palindromic rheumatism, left hip
    - M12.359 Palindromic rheumatism, unspecified hip
  - M12.36 Palindromic rheumatism, knee
    - M12.361 Palindromic rheumatism, right knee
    - M12.362 Palindromic rheumatism, left knee
    - M12.369 Palindromic rheumatism, unspecified knee
  - M12.37 Palindromic rheumatism, ankle and foot
    - M12.371 Palindromic rheumatism, right ankle and foot
    - M12.372 Palindromic rheumatism, left ankle and foot
    - M12.379 Palindromic rheumatism, unspecified ankle and foot
  - M12.38 Palindromic rheumatism, other specified site
    - Palindromic rheumatism, vertebrae
  - M12.39 Palindromic rheumatism, multiple sites

- M12.4 Intermittent hydrarthrosis
  - M12.40 Intermittent hydrarthrosis, unspecified site
  - M12.41 Intermittent hydrarthrosis, shoulder
    - M12.411 Intermittent hydrarthrosis, right shoulder
    - M12.412 Intermittent hydrarthrosis, left shoulder
    - M12.419 Intermittent hydrarthrosis, unspecified shoulder
  - M12.42 Intermittent hydrarthrosis, elbow
    - M12.421 Intermittent hydrarthrosis, right elbow
    - M12.422 Intermittent hydrarthrosis, left elbow
    - M12.429 Intermittent hydrarthrosis, unspecified elbow
  - M12.43 Intermittent hydrarthrosis, wrist
    - M12.431 Intermittent hydrarthrosis, right wrist
    - M12.432 Intermittent hydrarthrosis, left wrist
    - M12.439 Intermittent hydrarthrosis, unspecified wrist
  - M12.44 Intermittent hydrarthrosis, hand
    - M12.441 Intermittent hydrarthrosis, right hand
    - M12.442 Intermittent hydrarthrosis, left hand
    - M12.449 Intermittent hydrarthrosis, unspecified hand
  - M12.45 Intermittent hydrarthrosis, hip
    - M12.451 Intermittent hydrarthrosis, right hip
    - M12.452 Intermittent hydrarthrosis, left hip
    - M12.459 Intermittent hydrarthrosis, unspecified hip
  - M12.46 Intermittent hydrarthrosis, knee
    - M12.461 Intermittent hydrarthrosis, right knee
    - M12.462 Intermittent hydrarthrosis, left knee
    - M12.469 Intermittent hydrarthrosis, unspecified knee
  - M12.47 Intermittent hydrarthrosis, ankle and foot
    - M12.471 Intermittent hydrarthrosis, right ankle and foot
    - M12.472 Intermittent hydrarthrosis, left ankle and foot
    - M12.479 Intermittent hydrarthrosis, unspecified ankle and foot
  - M12.48 Intermittent hydrarthrosis, other site
  - M12.49 Intermittent hydrarthrosis, multiple sites

- M12.5 Traumatic arthropathy
  - **Excludes1** current injury-see Alphabetic Index
    - post-traumatic osteoarthritis of first carpometacarpal joint (M18.2-M18.3)
    - post-traumatic osteoarthritis of hip (M16.4-M16.5)
    - post-traumatic osteoarthritis of knee (M17.2-M17.3)
    - post-traumatic osteoarthritis NOS (M19.1-)
    - post-traumatic osteoarthritis of other single joints (M19.1-)
  - M12.50 Traumatic arthropathy, unspecified site
  - M12.51 Traumatic arthropathy, shoulder
    - M12.511 Traumatic arthropathy, right shoulder
    - M12.512 Traumatic arthropathy, left shoulder
    - M12.519 Traumatic arthropathy, unspecified shoulder

- M12.52 Traumatic arthropathy, elbow
  - M12.521 Traumatic arthropathy, right elbow
  - M12.522 Traumatic arthropathy, left elbow
  - M12.529 Traumatic arthropathy, unspecified elbow
- M12.53 Traumatic arthropathy, wrist
  - M12.531 Traumatic arthropathy, right wrist
  - M12.532 Traumatic arthropathy, left wrist
  - M12.539 Traumatic arthropathy, unspecified wrist
- M12.54 Traumatic arthropathy, hand
  - M12.541 Traumatic arthropathy, right hand
  - M12.542 Traumatic arthropathy, left hand
  - M12.549 Traumatic arthropathy, unspecified hand
- M12.55 Traumatic arthropathy, hip
  - M12.551 Traumatic arthropathy, right hip
  - M12.552 Traumatic arthropathy, left hip
    - Coding Clinic: 2015, Q1, P17
  - M12.559 Traumatic arthropathy, unspecified hip
- M12.56 Traumatic arthropathy, knee
  - M12.561 Traumatic arthropathy, right knee
  - M12.562 Traumatic arthropathy, left knee
  - M12.569 Traumatic arthropathy, unspecified knee
- M12.57 Traumatic arthropathy, ankle and foot
  - M12.571 Traumatic arthropathy, right ankle and foot
  - M12.572 Traumatic arthropathy, left ankle and foot
  - M12.579 Traumatic arthropathy, unspecified ankle and foot
- M12.58 Traumatic arthropathy, other specified site
  - Traumatic arthropathy, vertebrae
- M12.59 Traumatic arthropathy, multiple sites
- M12.8 Other specific arthropathies, not elsewhere classified
  - Transient arthropathy
  - M12.80 Other specific arthropathies, not elsewhere classified, unspecified site
  - M12.81 Other specific arthropathies, not elsewhere classified, shoulder
    - M12.811 Other specific arthropathies, not elsewhere classified, right shoulder
    - M12.812 Other specific arthropathies, not elsewhere classified, left shoulder
    - M12.819 Other specific arthropathies, not elsewhere classified, unspecified shoulder
  - M12.82 Other specific arthropathies, not elsewhere classified, elbow
    - M12.821 Other specific arthropathies, not elsewhere classified, right elbow
    - M12.822 Other specific arthropathies, not elsewhere classified, left elbow
    - M12.829 Other specific arthropathies, not elsewhere classified, unspecified elbow
  - M12.83 Other specific arthropathies, not elsewhere classified, wrist
    - M12.831 Other specific arthropathies, not elsewhere classified, right wrist
    - M12.832 Other specific arthropathies, not elsewhere classified, left wrist
    - M12.839 Other specific arthropathies, not elsewhere classified, unspecified wrist
  - M12.84 Other specific arthropathies, not elsewhere classified, hand
    - M12.841 Other specific arthropathies, not elsewhere classified, right hand
    - M12.842 Other specific arthropathies, not elsewhere classified, left hand
    - M12.849 Other specific arthropathies, not elsewhere classified, unspecified hand
  - M12.85 Other specific arthropathies, not elsewhere classified, hip
    - M12.851 Other specific arthropathies, not elsewhere classified, right hip
    - M12.852 Other specific arthropathies, not elsewhere classified, left hip
    - M12.859 Other specific arthropathies, not elsewhere classified, unspecified hip
  - M12.86 Other specific arthropathies, not elsewhere classified, knee
    - M12.861 Other specific arthropathies, not elsewhere classified, right knee
    - M12.862 Other specific arthropathies, not elsewhere classified, left knee
    - M12.869 Other specific arthropathies, not elsewhere classified, unspecified knee
  - M12.87 Other specific arthropathies, not elsewhere classified, ankle and foot
    - M12.871 Other specific arthropathies, not elsewhere classified, right ankle and foot
    - M12.872 Other specific arthropathies, not elsewhere classified, left ankle and foot
    - M12.879 Other specific arthropathies, not elsewhere classified, unspecified ankle and foot
  - M12.88 Other specific arthropathies, not elsewhere classified, other specified site
    - Other specific arthropathies, not elsewhere classified, vertebrae
  - M12.89 Other specific arthropathies, not elsewhere classified, multiple sites
- M12.9 Arthropathy, unspecified

- M13 Other arthritis
  - **Excludes1** arthrosis (M15-M19)
    osteoarthritis (M15-M19)
  - M13.0 Polyarthritis, unspecified
  - M13.1 Monoarthritis, not elsewhere classified
    - M13.10 Monoarthritis, not elsewhere classified, unspecified site
    - M13.11 Monoarthritis, not elsewhere classified, shoulder
      - M13.111 Monoarthritis, not elsewhere classified, right shoulder
      - M13.112 Monoarthritis, not elsewhere classified, left shoulder
      - M13.119 Monoarthritis, not elsewhere classified, unspecified shoulder
    - M13.12 Monoarthritis, not elsewhere classified, elbow
      - M13.121 Monoarthritis, not elsewhere classified, right elbow
      - M13.122 Monoarthritis, not elsewhere classified, left elbow
      - M13.129 Monoarthritis, not elsewhere classified, unspecified elbow
    - M13.13 Monoarthritis, not elsewhere classified, wrist
      - M13.131 Monoarthritis, not elsewhere classified, right wrist
      - M13.132 Monoarthritis, not elsewhere classified, left wrist
      - M13.139 Monoarthritis, not elsewhere classified, unspecified wrist

- M13.14 Monoarthritis, not elsewhere classified, hand
  - M13.141 Monoarthritis, not elsewhere classified, right hand
  - M13.142 Monoarthritis, not elsewhere classified, left hand
  - M13.149 Monoarthritis, not elsewhere classified, unspecified hand
- M13.15 Monoarthritis, not elsewhere classified, hip
  - M13.151 Monoarthritis, not elsewhere classified, right hip
  - M13.152 Monoarthritis, not elsewhere classified, left hip
  - M13.159 Monoarthritis, not elsewhere classified, unspecified hip
- M13.16 Monoarthritis, not elsewhere classified, knee
  - M13.161 Monoarthritis, not elsewhere classified, right knee
  - M13.162 Monoarthritis, not elsewhere classified, left knee
  - M13.169 Monoarthritis, not elsewhere classified, unspecified knee
- M13.17 Monoarthritis, not elsewhere classified, ankle and foot
  - M13.171 Monoarthritis, not elsewhere classified, right ankle and foot
  - M13.172 Monoarthritis, not elsewhere classified, left ankle and foot
  - M13.179 Monoarthritis, not elsewhere classified, unspecified ankle and foot
- M13.8 Other specified arthritis
  - Allergic arthritis
  - **Excludes1** osteoarthritis (M15-M19)
  - M13.80 Other specified arthritis, unspecified site
- M13.81 Other specified arthritis, shoulder
  - M13.811 Other specified arthritis, right shoulder
  - M13.812 Other specified arthritis, left shoulder
  - M13.819 Other specified arthritis, unspecified shoulder
- M13.82 Other specified arthritis, elbow
  - M13.821 Other specified arthritis, right elbow
  - M13.822 Other specified arthritis, left elbow
  - M13.829 Other specified arthritis, unspecified elbow
- M13.83 Other specified arthritis, wrist
  - M13.831 Other specified arthritis, right wrist
  - M13.832 Other specified arthritis, left wrist
  - M13.839 Other specified arthritis, unspecified wrist
- M13.84 Other specified arthritis, hand
  - M13.841 Other specified arthritis, right hand
  - M13.842 Other specified arthritis, left hand
  - M13.849 Other specified arthritis, unspecified hand
- M13.85 Other specified arthritis, hip
  - M13.851 Other specified arthritis, right hip
  - M13.852 Other specified arthritis, left hip
  - M13.859 Other specified arthritis, unspecified hip
- M13.86 Other specified arthritis, knee
  - M13.861 Other specified arthritis, right knee
  - M13.862 Other specified arthritis, left knee
  - M13.869 Other specified arthritis, unspecified knee
- M13.87 Other specified arthritis, ankle and foot
  - M13.871 Other specified arthritis, right ankle and foot
  - M13.872 Other specified arthritis, left ankle and foot
  - M13.879 Other specified arthritis, unspecified ankle and foot
  - M13.88 Other specified arthritis, other site
  - M13.89 Other specified arthritis, multiple sites

- M14 Arthropathies in other diseases classified elsewhere
  - **Excludes1** arthropathy in:
    - diabetes mellitus (EØ8-E13 with .61-)
    - hematological disorders (M36.2-M36.3)
    - hypersensitivity reactions (M36.4)
    - neoplastic disease (M36.1)
    - neurosyphillis (A52.16)
    - sarcoidosis (D86.86)
  - enteropathic arthropathies (MØ7.Ø-)
  - juvenile psoriatic arthropathy (LØ.54)
  - lipoid dermatoarthritis (E78.81)
- M14.6 Charcôt's joint
  - Neuropathic arthropathy
  - **Excludes1** Charcôt's joint in diabetes mellitus (EØ8-E13 with .61Ø)
    - Charcôt's joint in tabes dorsalis (A52.16)
  - M14.6Ø Charcôt's joint, unspecified site
- M14.61 Charcôt's joint, shoulder
  - M14.611 Charcôt's joint, right shoulder
  - M14.612 Charcôt's joint, left shoulder
  - M14.619 Charcôt's joint, unspecified shoulder
- M14.62 Charcôt's joint, elbow
  - M14.621 Charcôt's joint, right elbow
  - M14.622 Charcôt's joint, left elbow
  - M14.629 Charcôt's joint, unspecified elbow
- M14.63 Charcôt's joint, wrist
  - M14.631 Charcôt's joint, right wrist
  - M14.632 Charcôt's joint, left wrist
  - M14.639 Charcôt's joint, unspecified wrist
- M14.64 Charcôt's joint, hand
  - M14.641 Charcôt's joint, right hand
  - M14.642 Charcôt's joint, left hand
  - M14.649 Charcôt's joint, unspecified hand
- M14.65 Charcôt's joint, hip
  - M14.651 Charcôt's joint, right hip
  - M14.652 Charcôt's joint, left hip
  - M14.659 Charcôt's joint, unspecified hip
- M14.66 Charcôt's joint, knee
  - M14.661 Charcôt's joint, right knee
  - M14.662 Charcôt's joint, left knee
  - M14.669 Charcôt's joint, unspecified knee
- M14.67 Charcôt's joint, ankle and foot
  - M14.671 Charcôt's joint, right ankle and foot
  - M14.672 Charcôt's joint, left ankle and foot
  - M14.679 Charcôt's joint, unspecified ankle and foot
  - M14.68 Charcôt's joint, vertebrae
  - M14.69 Charcôt's joint, multiple sites

M14.8 Arthropathies in other specified diseases classified elsewhere

Code first underlying disease, such as:
amyloidosis (E85.-)
erythema multiforme (L51.-)
erythema nodosum (L52)
hemochromatosis (E83.11-)
hyperparathyroidism (E21.-)
hypothyroidism (E00-E03)
sickle-cell disorders (D57.-)
thyrotoxicosis [hyperthyroidism] (E05.-)
Whipple's disease (K90.81)

M14.80 Arthropathies in other specified diseases classified elsewhere, unspecified site

M14.81 Arthropathies in other specified diseases classified elsewhere, shoulder

M14.811 Arthropathies in other specified diseases classified elsewhere, right shoulder

M14.812 Arthropathies in other specified diseases classified elsewhere, left shoulder

M14.819 Arthropathies in other specified diseases classified elsewhere, unspecified shoulder

M14.82 Arthropathies in other specified diseases classified elsewhere, elbow

M14.821 Arthropathies in other specified diseases classified elsewhere, right elbow

M14.822 Arthropathies in other specified diseases classified elsewhere, left elbow

M14.829 Arthropathies in other specified diseases classified elsewhere, unspecified elbow

M14.83 Arthropathies in other specified diseases classified elsewhere, wrist

M14.831 Arthropathies in other specified diseases classified elsewhere, right wrist

M14.832 Arthropathies in other specified diseases classified elsewhere, left wrist

M14.839 Arthropathies in other specified diseases classified elsewhere, unspecified wrist

M14.84 Arthropathies in other specified diseases classified elsewhere, hand

M14.841 Arthropathies in other specified diseases classified elsewhere, right hand

M14.842 Arthropathies in other specified diseases classified elsewhere, left hand

M14.849 Arthropathies in other specified diseases classified elsewhere, unspecified hand

M14.85 Arthropathies in other specified diseases classified elsewhere, hip

M14.851 Arthropathies in other specified diseases classified elsewhere, right hip

M14.852 Arthropathies in other specified diseases classified elsewhere, left hip

M14.859 Arthropathies in other specified diseases classified elsewhere, unspecified hip

M14.86 Arthropathies in other specified diseases classified elsewhere, knee

M14.861 Arthropathies in other specified diseases classified elsewhere, right knee

M14.862 Arthropathies in other specified diseases classified elsewhere, left knee

M14.869 Arthropathies in other specified diseases classified elsewhere, unspecified knee

M14.87 Arthropathies in other specified diseases classified elsewhere, ankle and foot

M14.871 Arthropathies in other specified diseases classified elsewhere, right ankle and foot

M14.872 Arthropathies in other specified diseases classified elsewhere, left ankle and foot

M14.879 Arthropathies in other specified diseases classified elsewhere, unspecified ankle and foot

M14.88 Arthropathies in other specified diseases classified elsewhere, vertebrae

M14.89 Arthropathies in other specified diseases classified elsewhere, multiple sites

OSTEOARTHRITIS (M15-M19)

Osteoarthritis is the most common degenerative joint disease and form of arthritis that breaks down the cartilage causing pain, swelling, and reduced motion in the joints.

Excludes2 osteoarthritis of spine (M47.-)

M15 Polyosteoarthritis

Includes arthritis of multiple sites
Excludes1 bilateral involvement of single joint (M16-M19)

M15.0 Primary generalized (osteo)arthritis

M15.1 Heberden's nodes (with arthropathy)
Interphalangeal distal osteoarthritis

M15.2 Bouchard's nodes (with arthropathy)
Juxtaphalangeal distal osteoarthritis

M15.3 Secondary multiple arthritis
Post-traumatic polyosteoarthritis

M15.4 Erosive (osteo)arthritis

M15.8 Other polyosteoarthritis

M15.9 Polyosteoarthritis, unspecified
Generalized osteoarthritis NOS

M16 Osteoarthritis of hip

M16.0 Bilateral primary osteoarthritis of hip

M16.1 Unilateral primary osteoarthritis of hip
Primary osteoarthritis of hip NOS

M16.10 Unilateral primary osteoarthritis, unspecified hip

M16.11 Unilateral primary osteoarthritis, right hip

M16.12 Unilateral primary osteoarthritis, left hip

M16.2 Bilateral osteoarthritis resulting from hip dysplasia

M16.3 Unilateral osteoarthritis resulting from hip dysplasia
Dysplastic osteoarthritis of hip NOS

M16.30 Unilateral osteoarthritis resulting from hip dysplasia, unspecified hip

M16.31 Unilateral osteoarthritis resulting from hip dysplasia, right hip

M16.32 Unilateral osteoarthritis resulting from hip dysplasia, left hip

M16.4 Bilateral post-traumatic osteoarthritis of hip

- M16.5 Unilateral post-traumatic osteoarthritis of hip
  Post-traumatic osteoarthritis of hip NOS
  - M16.50 Unilateral post-traumatic osteoarthritis, unspecified hip
  - M16.51 Unilateral post-traumatic osteoarthritis, right hip
  - M16.52 Unilateral post-traumatic osteoarthritis, left hip
- M16.6 Other bilateral secondary osteoarthritis of hip
- M16.7 Other unilateral secondary osteoarthritis of hip
  Secondary osteoarthritis of hip NOS
- M16.9 Osteoarthritis of hip, unspecified

- M17 Osteoarthritis of knee
  - M17.0 Bilateral primary osteoarthritis of knee
  - M17.1 Unilateral primary osteoarthritis of knee
    Primary osteoarthritis of knee NOS
    - M17.10 Unilateral primary osteoarthritis, unspecified knee
    - M17.11 Unilateral primary osteoarthritis, right knee
    - M17.12 Unilateral primary osteoarthritis, left knee
  - M17.2 Bilateral post-traumatic osteoarthritis of knee
  - M17.3 Unilateral post-traumatic osteoarthritis of knee
    Post-traumatic osteoarthritis of knee NOS
    - M17.30 Unilateral post-traumatic osteoarthritis, unspecified knee
    - M17.31 Unilateral post-traumatic osteoarthritis, right knee
    - M17.32 Unilateral post-traumatic osteoarthritis, left knee
  - M17.4 Other bilateral secondary osteoarthritis of knee
  - M17.5 Other unilateral secondary osteoarthritis of knee
    Secondary osteoarthritis of knee NOS
  - M17.9 Osteoarthritis of knee, unspecified

- M18 Osteoarthritis of first carpometacarpal joint
  - M18.0 Bilateral primary osteoarthritis of first carpometacarpal joints
  - M18.1 Unilateral primary osteoarthritis of first carpometacarpal joint
    Primary osteoarthritis of first carpometacarpal joint NOS
    - M18.10 Unilateral primary osteoarthritis of first carpometacarpal joint, unspecified hand
    - M18.11 Unilateral primary osteoarthritis of first carpometacarpal joint, right hand
    - M18.12 Unilateral primary osteoarthritis of first carpometacarpal joint, left hand
  - M18.2 Bilateral post-traumatic osteoarthritis of first carpometacarpal joints
  - M18.3 Unilateral post-traumatic osteoarthritis of first carpometacarpal joint
    Post-traumatic osteoarthritis of first carpometacarpal joint NOS
    - M18.30 Unilateral post-traumatic osteoarthritis of first carpometacarpal joint, unspecified hand
    - M18.31 Unilateral post-traumatic osteoarthritis of first carpometacarpal joint, right hand
    - M18.32 Unilateral post-traumatic osteoarthritis of first carpometacarpal joint, left hand
  - M18.4 Other bilateral secondary osteoarthritis of first carpometacarpal joints
  - M18.5 Other unilateral secondary osteoarthritis of first carpometacarpal joint
    Secondary osteoarthritis of first carpometacarpal joint NOS
    - M18.50 Other unilateral secondary osteoarthritis of first carpometacarpal joint, unspecified hand
    - M18.51 Other unilateral secondary osteoarthritis of first carpometacarpal joint, right hand
    - M18.52 Other unilateral secondary osteoarthritis of first carpometacarpal joint, left hand
  - M18.9 Osteoarthritis of first carpometacarpal joint, unspecified

- M19 Other and unspecified osteoarthritis
  Excludes1 polyarthritis (M15.-)
  Excludes2 arthrosis of spine (M47.-)
  hallux rigidus (M20.2)
  osteoarthritis of spine (M47.-)
  - M19.0 Primary osteoarthritis of other joints
    - M19.01 Primary osteoarthritis, shoulder
      - M19.011 Primary osteoarthritis, right shoulder
      - M19.012 Primary osteoarthritis, left shoulder
      - M19.019 Primary osteoarthritis, unspecified shoulder
    - M19.02 Primary osteoarthritis, elbow
      - M19.021 Primary osteoarthritis, right elbow
      - M19.022 Primary osteoarthritis, left elbow
      - M19.029 Primary osteoarthritis, unspecified elbow
    - M19.03 Primary osteoarthritis, wrist
      - M19.031 Primary osteoarthritis, right wrist
      - M19.032 Primary osteoarthritis, left wrist
      - M19.039 Primary osteoarthritis, unspecified wrist
    - M19.04 Primary osteoarthritis, hand
      Excludes2 primary osteoarthritis of first carpometacarpal joint (M18.0-, M18.1-)
      - M19.041 Primary osteoarthritis, right hand
      - M19.042 Primary osteoarthritis, left hand
      - M19.049 Primary osteoarthritis, unspecified hand
    - M19.07 Primary osteoarthritis ankle and foot
      - M19.071 Primary osteoarthritis, right ankle and foot
      - M19.072 Primary osteoarthritis, left ankle and foot
      - M19.079 Primary osteoarthritis, unspecified ankle and foot
  - M19.1 Post-traumatic osteoarthritis of other joints
    - M19.11 Post-traumatic osteoarthritis, shoulder
      - M19.111 Post-traumatic osteoarthritis, right shoulder
      - M19.112 Post-traumatic osteoarthritis, left shoulder
      - M19.119 Post-traumatic osteoarthritis, unspecified shoulder
    - M19.12 Post-traumatic osteoarthritis, elbow
      - M19.121 Post-traumatic osteoarthritis, right elbow
      - M19.122 Post-traumatic osteoarthritis, left elbow
      - M19.129 Post-traumatic osteoarthritis, unspecified elbow
    - M19.13 Post-traumatic osteoarthritis, wrist
      - M19.131 Post-traumatic osteoarthritis, right wrist
      - M19.132 Post-traumatic osteoarthritis, left wrist
      - M19.139 Post-traumatic osteoarthritis, unspecified wrist
    - M19.14 Post-traumatic osteoarthritis, hand
      Excludes2 post-traumatic osteoarthritis of first carpometacarpal joint (M18.2-, M18.3-)
      - M19.141 Post-traumatic osteoarthritis, right hand
      - M19.142 Post-traumatic osteoarthritis, left hand
      - M19.149 Post-traumatic osteoarthritis, unspecified hand

◀ New ⇐ Revised ~~deleted~~ Deleted Excludes 1 Excludes 2 Includes Use additional Code first Code also Unspecified
OGCR Official Guidelines ● Unacceptable Principal Diagnosis X Assign placeholder X ● Use Additional Character(s) ◗ Manifestation Code Coding Clinic

- **M19.17 Post-traumatic osteoarthritis, ankle and foot**
  - **M19.171 Post-traumatic osteoarthritis, right ankle and foot**
  - **M19.172 Post-traumatic osteoarthritis, left ankle and foot**
  - **M19.179 Post-traumatic osteoarthritis, unspecified ankle and foot**
- **M19.2 Secondary osteoarthritis of other joints**
  - **M19.21 Secondary osteoarthritis, shoulder**
    - **M19.211 Secondary osteoarthritis, right shoulder**
    - **M19.212 Secondary osteoarthritis, left shoulder**
    - **M19.219 Secondary osteoarthritis, unspecified shoulder**
  - **M19.22 Secondary osteoarthritis, elbow**
    - **M19.221 Secondary osteoarthritis, right elbow**
    - **M19.222 Secondary osteoarthritis, left elbow**
    - **M19.229 Secondary osteoarthritis, unspecified elbow**
  - **M19.23 Secondary osteoarthritis, wrist**
    - **M19.231 Secondary osteoarthritis, right wrist**
    - **M19.232 Secondary osteoarthritis, left wrist**
    - **M19.239 Secondary osteoarthritis, unspecified wrist**
  - **M19.24 Secondary osteoarthritis, hand**
    - **M19.241 Secondary osteoarthritis, right hand**
    - **M19.242 Secondary osteoarthritis, left hand**
    - **M19.249 Secondary osteoarthritis, unspecified hand**
  - **M19.27 Secondary osteoarthritis, ankle and foot**
    - **M19.271 Secondary osteoarthritis, right ankle and foot**
    - **M19.272 Secondary osteoarthritis, left ankle and foot**
    - **M19.279 Secondary osteoarthritis, unspecified ankle and foot**
- **M19.9 Osteoarthritis, unspecified site**
  - **M19.90 Unspecified osteoarthritis, unspecified site**
    - Arthrosis NOS
    - Arthritis NOS
    - Osteoarthritis NOS
  - **M19.91 Primary osteoarthritis, unspecified site**
    - Primary osteoarthritis NOS
  - **M19.92 Post-traumatic osteoarthritis, unspecified site**
    - Post-traumatic osteoarthritis NOS
  - **M19.93 Secondary osteoarthritis, unspecified site**
    - Secondary osteoarthritis NOS

OTHER JOINT DISORDERS (M20-M25)

Excludes2 joints of the spine (M40-M54)

- **M20 Acquired deformities of fingers and toes**

  Excludes1 acquired absence of fingers and toes (Z89.-)
  congenital absence of fingers and toes (Q71.3-, Q72.3-)
  congenital deformities and malformations of fingers and toes (Q66.-, Q68-Q70, Q74.-)
  - **M20.0 Deformity of finger(s)**

    Excludes1 clubbing of fingers (R68.3)
    palmar fascial fibromatosis [Dupuytren] (M72.0)
    trigger finger (M65.3)
    - **M20.00 Unspecified deformity of finger(s)**
      - **M20.001 Unspecified deformity of right finger(s)**
      - **M20.002 Unspecified deformity of left finger(s)**
      - **M20.009 Unspecified deformity of unspecified finger(s)**
    - **M20.01 Mallet finger**
      - **M20.011 Mallet finger of right finger(s)**
      - **M20.012 Mallet finger of left finger(s)**
      - **M20.019 Mallet finger of unspecified finger(s)**
    - **M20.02 Boutonnière deformity**
      - **M20.021 Boutonnière deformity of right finger(s)**
      - **M20.022 Boutonnière deformity of left finger(s)**
      - **M20.029 Boutonnière deformity of unspecified finger(s)**
    - **M20.03 Swan-neck deformity**
      - **M20.031 Swan-neck deformity of right finger(s)**
      - **M20.032 Swan-neck deformity of left finger(s)**
      - **M20.039 Swan-neck deformity of unspecified finger(s)**
    - **M20.09 Other deformity of finger(s)**
      - **M20.091 Other deformity of right finger(s)**
      - **M20.092 Other deformity of left finger(s)**
      - **M20.099 Other deformity of finger(s), unspecified finger(s)**
  - **M20.1 Hallux valgus (acquired)**

    Excludes2 bunion (M21.6-) ◀
    - **M20.10 Hallux valgus (acquired), unspecified foot**
    - **M20.11 Hallux valgus (acquired), right foot**
    - **M20.12 Hallux valgus (acquired), left foot**
  - **M20.2 Hallux rigidus**
    - **M20.20 Hallux rigidus, unspecified foot**
    - **M20.21 Hallux rigidus, right foot**
    - **M20.22 Hallux rigidus, left foot**
  - **M20.3 Hallux varus (acquired)**
    - **M20.30 Hallux varus (acquired), unspecified foot**
    - **M20.31 Hallux varus (acquired), right foot**
    - **M20.32 Hallux varus (acquired), left foot**
  - **M20.4 Other hammer toe(s) (acquired)**
    - **M20.40 Other hammer toe(s) (acquired), unspecified foot**
    - **M20.41 Other hammer toe(s) (acquired), right foot**
    - **M20.42 Other hammer toe(s) (acquired), left foot**

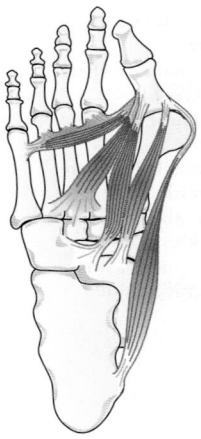

Figure 13-1 Hallux valgus or bunion.

Item 13–2 Hallux valgus or bunion is a sometimes painful structural deformity caused by an inflammation of the bursal sac at the base of the metatarsophalangeal joint (big toe). **Hallus varus** is a deviation of the great toe to the inner side of the foot or away from the next toe.

- M20.5 Other deformities of toe(s) (acquired)
  - M20.5X Other deformities of toe(s) (acquired)
    - M20.5X1 Other deformities of toe(s) (acquired), right foot
    - M20.5X2 Other deformities of toe(s) (acquired), left foot
    - M20.5X9 Other deformities of toe(s) (acquired), unspecified foot
- M20.6 Acquired deformities of toe(s), unspecified
  - M20.60 Acquired deformities of toe(s), unspecified, unspecified foot
  - M20.61 Acquired deformities of toe(s), unspecified, right foot
  - M20.62 Acquired deformities of toe(s), unspecified, left foot

- M21 Other acquired deformities of limbs

  Excludes1 acquired absence of limb (Z89.-)
  congenital absence of limbs (Q71-Q73)
  congenital deformities and malformations of limbs (Q65-Q66, Q68-Q74)

  Excludes2 acquired deformities of fingers or toes (M20.-)
  coxa plana (M91.2)

  - M21.0 Valgus deformity, not elsewhere classified

    Excludes1 metatarsus valgus (Q66.6)
    talipes calcaneovalgus (Q66.4)

    - M21.00 Valgus deformity, not elsewhere classified, unspecified site
    - M21.02 Valgus deformity, not elsewhere classified, elbow
      Cubitus valgus
      - M21.021 Valgus deformity, not elsewhere classified, right elbow
      - M21.022 Valgus deformity, not elsewhere classified, left elbow
      - M21.029 Valgus deformity, not elsewhere classified, unspecified elbow
    - M21.05 Valgus deformity, not elsewhere classified, hip
      - M21.051 Valgus deformity, not elsewhere classified, right hip
      - M21.052 Valgus deformity, not elsewhere classified, left hip
      - M21.059 Valgus deformity, not elsewhere classified, unspecified hip
    - M21.06 Valgus deformity, not elsewhere classified, knee
      Genu valgum
      Knock knee
      - M21.061 Valgus deformity, not elsewhere classified, right knee
      - M21.062 Valgus deformity, not elsewhere classified, left knee
      - M21.069 Valgus deformity, not elsewhere classified, unspecified knee
    - M21.07 Valgus deformity, not elsewhere classified, ankle
      - M21.071 Valgus deformity, not elsewhere classified, right ankle
      - M21.072 Valgus deformity, not elsewhere classified, left ankle
      - M21.079 Valgus deformity, not elsewhere classified, unspecified ankle

Item 13–3 Cubitus valgus is a deformity of the elbow resulting in an increased carrying angle in which the arm extends at the side and the palm faces forward, which results in the forearm and hand extended at a greater than 15 degrees.

Item 13–4 Cubitus varus is a deformity of the elbow resulting in the arm extended at the side and the palm facing forward so that the forearm and hand are held at less than 5 degrees, decreasing the carrying angle.

- M21.1 Varus deformity, not elsewhere classified

  Excludes1 metatarsus varus (Q66.22) ⇐
  tibia vara (M92.5)

  - M21.10 Varus deformity, not elsewhere classified, unspecified site
  - M21.12 Varus deformity, not elsewhere classified, elbow
    Cubitus varus, elbow
    - M21.121 Varus deformity, not elsewhere classified, right elbow
    - M21.122 Varus deformity, not elsewhere classified, left elbow
    - M21.129 Varus deformity, not elsewhere classified, unspecified elbow
  - M21.15 Varus deformity, not elsewhere classified, hip
    - M21.151 Varus deformity, not elsewhere classified, right hip
    - M21.152 Varus deformity, not elsewhere classified, left hip
    - M21.159 Varus deformity, not elsewhere classified, unspecified
  - M21.16 Varus deformity, not elsewhere classified, knee
    Bow leg
    Genu varum
    - M21.161 Varus deformity, not elsewhere classified, right knee
    - M21.162 Varus deformity, not elsewhere classified, left knee
    - M21.169 Varus deformity, not elsewhere classified, unspecified knee
  - M21.17 Varus deformity, not elsewhere classified, ankle
    - M21.171 Varus deformity, not elsewhere classified, right ankle
    - M21.172 Varus deformity, not elsewhere classified, left ankle
    - M21.179 Varus deformity, not elsewhere classified, unspecified ankle
- M21.2 Flexion deformity
  - M21.20 Flexion deformity, unspecified site
  - M21.21 Flexion deformity, shoulder
    - M21.211 Flexion deformity, right shoulder
    - M21.212 Flexion deformity, left shoulder
    - M21.219 Flexion deformity, unspecified shoulder
  - M21.22 Flexion deformity, elbow
    - M21.221 Flexion deformity, right elbow
    - M21.222 Flexion deformity, left elbow
    - M21.229 Flexion deformity, unspecified elbow
  - M21.23 Flexion deformity, wrist
    - M21.231 Flexion deformity, right wrist
    - M21.232 Flexion deformity, left wrist
    - M21.239 Flexion deformity, unspecified wrist
  - M21.24 Flexion deformity, finger joints
    - M21.241 Flexion deformity, right finger joints
    - M21.242 Flexion deformity, left finger joints
    - M21.249 Flexion deformity, unspecified finger joints
  - M21.25 Flexion deformity, hip
    - M21.251 Flexion deformity, right hip
    - M21.252 Flexion deformity, left hip
    - M21.259 Flexion deformity, unspecified hip
  - M21.26 Flexion deformity, knee
    - M21.261 Flexion deformity, right knee
    - M21.262 Flexion deformity, left knee
    - M21.269 Flexion deformity, unspecified knee

◀ New ⇐ Revised ~~deleted~~ Deleted Excludes 1 Excludes 2 Includes Use additional Code first Code also Unspecified
OGCR Official Guidelines ● Unacceptable Principal Diagnosis X Assign placeholder X ● Use Additional Character(s) ▶ Manifestation Code Coding Clinic

- M21.27 Flexion deformity, ankle and toes
  - M21.271 Flexion deformity, right ankle and toes
  - M21.272 Flexion deformity, left ankle and toes
  - M21.279 Flexion deformity, unspecified ankle and toes
- M21.3 Wrist or foot drop (acquired)
  - M21.33 Wrist drop (acquired)
    - M21.331 Wrist drop, right wrist
    - M21.332 Wrist drop, left wrist
    - M21.339 Wrist drop, unspecified wrist
  - M21.37 Foot drop (acquired)
    - M21.371 Foot drop, right foot
    - M21.372 Foot drop, left foot
    - M21.379 Foot drop, unspecified foot
- M21.4 Flat foot [pes planus] (acquired)
  - **Excludes1** congenital pes planus (Q66.5-)
  - M21.40 Flat foot [pes planus] (acquired), unspecified foot
  - M21.41 Flat foot [pes planus] (acquired), right foot
  - M21.42 Flat foot [pes planus] (acquired), left foot
- M21.5 Acquired clawhand, clubhand, clawfoot and clubfoot
  - **Excludes1** clubfoot, not specified as acquired (Q66.89)
  - M21.51 Acquired clawhand
    - M21.511 Acquired clawhand, right hand
    - M21.512 Acquired clawhand, left hand
    - M21.519 Acquired clawhand, unspecified hand
  - M21.52 Acquired clubhand
    - M21.521 Acquired clubhand, right hand
    - M21.522 Acquired clubhand, left hand
    - M21.529 Acquired clubhand, unspecified hand
  - M21.53 Acquired clawfoot
    - M21.531 Acquired clawfoot, right foot
    - M21.532 Acquired clawfoot, left foot
    - M21.539 Acquired clawfoot, unspecified foot
  - M21.54 Acquired clubfoot
    - M21.541 Acquired clubfoot, right foot
    - M21.542 Acquired clubfoot, left foot
    - M21.549 Acquired clubfoot, unspecified foot
- M21.6 Other acquired deformities of foot
  - **Excludes2** deformities of toe (acquired) (M20.1-M20.6-)
  - M21.61 Bunion ◀
    - M21.611 Bunion of right foot ◀
    - M21.612 Bunion of left foot ◀
    - M21.619 Bunion of unspecified foot ◀
  - M21.62 Bunionette ◀
    - M21.621 Bunionette of right foot ◀
    - M21.622 Bunionette of left foot ◀
    - M21.629 Bunionette of unspecified foot ◀
  - M21.6X Other acquired deformities of foot
    - M21.6X1 Other acquired deformities of right foot
    - M21.6X2 Other acquired deformities of left foot
    - M21.6X9 Other acquired deformities of unspecified foot
- M21.7 Unequal limb length (acquired)
  - **Note:** The site used should correspond to the shorter limb.
  - M21.70 Unequal limb length (acquired), unspecified site
  - M21.72 Unequal limb length (acquired), humerus
    - M21.721 Unequal limb length (acquired), right humerus
    - M21.722 Unequal limb length (acquired), left humerus
    - M21.729 Unequal limb length (acquired), unspecified humerus
  - M21.73 Unequal limb length (acquired), ulna and radius
    - M21.731 Unequal limb length (acquired), right ulna
    - M21.732 Unequal limb length (acquired), left ulna
    - M21.733 Unequal limb length (acquired), right radius
    - M21.734 Unequal limb length (acquired), left radius
    - M21.739 Unequal limb length (acquired), unspecified ulna and radius
  - M21.75 Unequal limb length (acquired), femur
    - M21.751 Unequal limb length (acquired), right femur
    - M21.752 Unequal limb length (acquired), left femur
    - M21.759 Unequal limb length (acquired), unspecified femur
  - M21.76 Unequal limb length (acquired), tibia and fibula
    - M21.761 Unequal limb length (acquired), right tibia
    - M21.762 Unequal limb length (acquired), left tibia
    - M21.763 Unequal limb length (acquired), right fibula
    - M21.764 Unequal limb length (acquired), left fibula
    - M21.769 Unequal limb length (acquired), unspecified tibia and fibula
- M21.8 Other specified acquired deformities of limbs
  - **Excludes2** coxa plana (M91.2)
  - M21.80 Other specified acquired deformities of unspecified limb
  - M21.82 Other specified acquired deformities of upper arm
    - M21.821 Other specified acquired deformities of right upper arm
    - M21.822 Other specified acquired deformities of left upper arm
    - M21.829 Other specified acquired deformities of unspecified upper arm
  - M21.83 Other specified acquired deformities of forearm
    - M21.831 Other specified acquired deformities of right forearm
    - M21.832 Other specified acquired deformities of left forearm
    - M21.839 Other specified acquired deformities of unspecified forearm
  - M21.85 Other specified acquired deformities of thigh
    - M21.851 Other specified acquired deformities of right thigh
    - M21.852 Other specified acquired deformities of left thigh
    - M21.859 Other specified acquired deformities of unspecified thigh

- M21.86 Other specified acquired deformities of lower leg
  - M21.861 Other specified acquired deformities of right lower leg
  - M21.862 Other specified acquired deformities of left lower leg
  - M21.869 Other specified acquired deformities of unspecified lower leg
- M21.9 Unspecified acquired deformity of limb and hand
  - M21.90 Unspecified acquired deformity of unspecified limb
  - M21.92 Unspecified acquired deformity of upper arm
    - M21.921 Unspecified acquired deformity of right upper arm
    - M21.922 Unspecified acquired deformity of left upper arm
    - M21.929 Unspecified acquired deformity of unspecified upper arm
  - M21.93 Unspecified acquired deformity of forearm
    - M21.931 Unspecified acquired deformity of right forearm
    - M21.932 Unspecified acquired deformity of left forearm
    - M21.939 Unspecified acquired deformity of unspecified forearm
  - M21.94 Unspecified acquired deformity of hand
    - M21.941 Unspecified acquired deformity of hand, right hand
    - M21.942 Unspecified acquired deformity of hand, left hand
    - M21.949 Unspecified acquired deformity of hand, unspecified hand
  - M21.95 Unspecified acquired deformity of thigh
    - M21.951 Unspecified acquired deformity of right thigh
    - M21.952 Unspecified acquired deformity of left thigh
    - M21.959 Unspecified acquired deformity of unspecified thigh
  - M21.96 Unspecified acquired deformity of lower leg
    - M21.961 Unspecified acquired deformity of right lower leg
    - M21.962 Unspecified acquired deformity of left lower leg
    - M21.969 Unspecified acquired deformity of unspecified lower leg

- M22 Disorder of patella

  Excludes1 traumatic dislocation of patella (S83.0-)
  - M22.0 Recurrent dislocation of patella
    - M22.00 Recurrent dislocation of patella, unspecified knee
    - M22.01 Recurrent dislocation of patella, right knee
    - M22.02 Recurrent dislocation of patella, left knee
  - M22.1 Recurrent subluxation of patella

    Incomplete dislocation of patella
    - M22.10 Recurrent subluxation of patella, unspecified knee
    - M22.11 Recurrent subluxation of patella, right knee
    - M22.12 Recurrent subluxation of patella, left knee
  - M22.2 Patellofemoral disorders
    - M22.2X Patellofemoral disorders
      - M22.2X1 Patellofemoral disorders, right knee
      - M22.2X2 Patellofemoral disorders, left knee
      - M22.2X9 Patellofemoral disorders, unspecified knee
  - M22.3 Other derangements of patella
    - M22.3X Other derangements of patella
      - M22.3X1 Other derangements of patella, right knee
      - M22.3X2 Other derangements of patella, left knee
      - M22.3X9 Other derangements of patella, unspecified knee
  - M22.4 Chondromalacia patellae
    - M22.40 Chondromalacia patellae, unspecified knee
    - M22.41 Chondromalacia patellae, right knee
    - M22.42 Chondromalacia patellae, left knee
  - M22.8 Other disorders of patella
    - M22.8X Other disorders of patella
      - M22.8X1 Other disorders of patella, right knee
      - M22.8X2 Other disorders of patella, left knee
      - M22.8X9 Other disorders of patella, unspecified knee
  - M22.9 Unspecified disorder of patella
    - M22.90 Unspecified disorder of patella, unspecified knee
    - M22.91 Unspecified disorder of patella, right knee
    - M22.92 Unspecified disorder of patella, left knee

- M23 Internal derangement of knee

  Excludes1 ankylosis (M24.66)
  current injury - see injury of knee and lower leg (S80-S89)
  deformity of knee (M21.-)
  osteochondritis dissecans (M93.2)
  recurrent dislocation or subluxation of joints (M24.4)
  recurrent dislocation or subluxation of patella (M22.0-M22.1)
  - M23.0 Cystic meniscus
    - M23.00 Cystic meniscus, unspecified meniscus

      Cystic meniscus, unspecified lateral meniscus
      Cystic meniscus, unspecified medial meniscus
      - M23.000 Cystic meniscus, unspecified lateral meniscus, right knee
      - M23.001 Cystic meniscus, unspecified lateral meniscus, left knee
      - M23.002 Cystic meniscus, unspecified lateral meniscus, unspecified knee
      - M23.003 Cystic meniscus, unspecified medial meniscus, right knee
      - M23.004 Cystic meniscus, unspecified medial meniscus, left knee
      - M23.005 Cystic meniscus, unspecified medial meniscus, unspecified knee
      - M23.006 Cystic meniscus, unspecified meniscus, right knee
      - M23.007 Cystic meniscus, unspecified meniscus, left knee
      - M23.009 Cystic meniscus, unspecified meniscus, unspecified knee
    - M23.01 Cystic meniscus, anterior horn of medial meniscus
      - M23.011 Cystic meniscus, anterior horn of medial meniscus, right knee
      - M23.012 Cystic meniscus, anterior horn of medial meniscus, left knee
      - M23.019 Cystic meniscus, anterior horn of medial meniscus, unspecified knee

- M23.02 Cystic meniscus, posterior horn of medial meniscus
  - M23.021 Cystic meniscus, posterior horn of medial meniscus, right knee
  - M23.022 Cystic meniscus, posterior horn of medial meniscus, left knee
  - M23.029 Cystic meniscus, posterior horn of medial meniscus, unspecified knee
- M23.03 Cystic meniscus, other medial meniscus
  - M23.031 Cystic meniscus, other medial meniscus, right knee
  - M23.032 Cystic meniscus, other medial meniscus, left knee
  - M23.039 Cystic meniscus, other medial meniscus, unspecified knee
- M23.04 Cystic meniscus, anterior horn of lateral meniscus
  - M23.041 Cystic meniscus, anterior horn of lateral meniscus, right knee
  - M23.042 Cystic meniscus, anterior horn of lateral meniscus, left knee
  - M23.049 Cystic meniscus, anterior horn of lateral meniscus, unspecified knee
- M23.05 Cystic meniscus, posterior horn of lateral meniscus
  - M23.051 Cystic meniscus, posterior horn of lateral meniscus, right knee
  - M23.052 Cystic meniscus, posterior horn of lateral meniscus, left knee
  - M23.059 Cystic meniscus, posterior horn of lateral meniscus, unspecified knee
- M23.06 Cystic meniscus, other lateral meniscus
  - M23.061 Cystic meniscus, other lateral meniscus, right knee
  - M23.062 Cystic meniscus, other lateral meniscus, left knee
  - M23.069 Cystic meniscus, other lateral meniscus, unspecified knee

★ **(See Plate 509 on page 79.)**

- M23.2 Derangement of meniscus due to old tear or injury
  Old bucket-handle tear
  - M23.20 Derangement of unspecified meniscus due to old tear or injury
    Derangement of unspecified lateral meniscus due to old tear or injury
    Derangement of unspecified medial meniscus due to old tear or injury
    - M23.200 Derangement of unspecified lateral meniscus due to old tear or injury, right knee
    - M23.201 Derangement of unspecified lateral meniscus due to old tear or injury, left knee
    - M23.202 Derangement of unspecified lateral meniscus due to old tear or injury, unspecified knee
    - M23.203 Derangement of unspecified medial meniscus due to old tear or injury, right knee
    - M23.204 Derangement of unspecified medial meniscus due to old tear or injury, left knee
    - M23.205 Derangement of unspecified medial meniscus due to old tear or injury, unspecified knee
    - M23.206 Derangement of unspecified meniscus due to old tear or injury, right knee
    - M23.207 Derangement of unspecified meniscus due to old tear or injury, left knee
    - M23.209 Derangement of unspecified meniscus due to old tear or injury, unspecified knee
  - M23.21 Derangement of anterior horn of medial meniscus due to old tear or injury
    - M23.211 Derangement of anterior horn of medial meniscus due to old tear or injury, right knee
    - M23.212 Derangement of anterior horn of medial meniscus due to old tear or injury, left knee
    - M23.219 Derangement of anterior horn of medial meniscus due to old tear or injury, unspecified knee
  - M23.22 Derangement of posterior horn of medial meniscus due to old tear or injury
    - M23.221 Derangement of posterior horn of medial meniscus due to old tear or injury, right knee
    - M23.222 Derangement of posterior horn of medial meniscus due to old tear or injury, left knee
    - M23.229 Derangement of posterior horn of medial meniscus due to old tear or injury, unspecified knee
  - M23.23 Derangement of other medial meniscus due to old tear or injury
    - M23.231 Derangement of other medial meniscus due to old tear or injury, right knee
    - M23.232 Derangement of other medial meniscus due to old tear or injury, left knee
    - M23.239 Derangement of other medial meniscus due to old tear or injury, unspecified knee
  - M23.24 Derangement of anterior horn of lateral meniscus due to old tear or injury
    - M23.241 Derangement of anterior horn of lateral meniscus due to old tear or injury, right knee
    - M23.242 Derangement of anterior horn of lateral meniscus due to old tear or injury, left knee
    - M23.249 Derangement of anterior horn of lateral meniscus due to old tear or injury, unspecified knee
  - M23.25 Derangement of posterior horn of lateral meniscus due to old tear or injury
    - M23.251 Derangement of posterior horn of lateral meniscus due to old tear or injury, right knee
    - M23.252 Derangement of posterior horn of lateral meniscus due to old tear or injury, left knee
    - M23.259 Derangement of posterior horn of lateral meniscus due to old tear or injury, unspecified knee
  - M23.26 Derangement of other lateral meniscus due to old tear or injury
    - M23.261 Derangement of other lateral meniscus due to old tear or injury, right knee
    - M23.262 Derangement of other lateral meniscus due to old tear or injury, left knee
    - M23.269 Derangement of other lateral meniscus due to old tear or injury, unspecified knee

- **M23.3 Other meniscus derangements**
  - Degenerate meniscus
  - Detached meniscus
  - Retained meniscus
  - **M23.30 Other meniscus derangements, unspecified meniscus**
    - Other meniscus derangements, unspecified lateral meniscus
    - Other meniscus derangements, unspecified medial meniscus
    - **M23.300 Other meniscus derangements, unspecified lateral meniscus, right knee**
    - **M23.301 Other meniscus derangements, unspecified lateral meniscus, left knee**
    - **M23.302 Other meniscus derangements, unspecified lateral meniscus, unspecified knee**
    - **M23.303 Other meniscus derangements, unspecified medial meniscus, right knee**
    - **M23.304 Other meniscus derangements, unspecified medial meniscus, left knee**
    - **M23.305 Other meniscus derangements, unspecified medial meniscus, unspecified knee**
    - **M23.306 Other meniscus derangements, unspecified meniscus, right knee**
    - **M23.307 Other meniscus derangements, unspecified meniscus, left knee**
    - **M23.309 Other meniscus derangements, unspecified meniscus, unspecified knee**
  - **M23.31 Other meniscus derangements, anterior horn of medial meniscus**
    - **M23.311 Other meniscus derangements, anterior horn of medial meniscus, right knee**
    - **M23.312 Other meniscus derangements, anterior horn of medial meniscus, left knee**
    - **M23.319 Other meniscus derangements, anterior horn of medial meniscus, unspecified knee**
  - **M23.32 Other meniscus derangements, posterior horn of medial meniscus**
    - **M23.321 Other meniscus derangements, posterior horn of medial meniscus, right knee**
    - **M23.322 Other meniscus derangements, posterior horn of medial meniscus, left knee**
    - **M23.329 Other meniscus derangements, posterior horn of medial meniscus, unspecified knee**
  - **M23.33 Other meniscus derangements, other medial meniscus**
    - **M23.331 Other meniscus derangements, other medial meniscus, right knee**
    - **M23.332 Other meniscus derangements, other medial meniscus, left knee**
    - **M23.339 Other meniscus derangements, other medial meniscus, unspecified knee**
  - **M23.34 Other meniscus derangements, anterior horn of lateral meniscus**
    - **M23.341 Other meniscus derangements, anterior horn of lateral meniscus, right knee**
    - **M23.342 Other meniscus derangements, anterior horn of lateral meniscus, left knee**
    - **M23.349 Other meniscus derangements, anterior horn of lateral meniscus, unspecified knee**
  - **M23.35 Other meniscus derangements, posterior horn of lateral meniscus**
    - **M23.351 Other meniscus derangements, posterior horn of lateral meniscus, right knee**
    - **M23.352 Other meniscus derangements, posterior horn of lateral meniscus, left knee**
    - **M23.359 Other meniscus derangements, posterior horn of lateral meniscus, unspecified knee**
  - **M23.36 Other meniscus derangements, other lateral meniscus**
    - **M23.361 Other meniscus derangements, other lateral meniscus, right knee**
    - **M23.362 Other meniscus derangements, other lateral meniscus, left knee**
    - **M23.369 Other meniscus derangements, other lateral meniscus, unspecified knee**
- **M23.4 Loose body in knee**
  - **M23.40 Loose body in knee, unspecified knee**
  - **M23.41 Loose body in knee, right knee**
  - **M23.42 Loose body in knee, left knee**
- **M23.5 Chronic instability of knee**
  - **M23.50 Chronic instability of knee, unspecified knee**
  - **M23.51 Chronic instability of knee, right knee**
  - **M23.52 Chronic instability of knee, left knee**
- **M23.6 Other spontaneous disruption of ligament(s) of knee**
  - **M23.60 Other spontaneous disruption of unspecified ligament of knee**
    - **M23.601 Other spontaneous disruption of unspecified ligament of right knee**
    - **M23.602 Other spontaneous disruption of unspecified ligament of left knee**
    - **M23.609 Other spontaneous disruption of unspecified ligament of unspecified knee**
  - **M23.61 Other spontaneous disruption of anterior cruciate ligament of knee**
    - **M23.611 Other spontaneous disruption of anterior cruciate ligament of right knee**
    - **M23.612 Other spontaneous disruption of anterior cruciate ligament of left knee**
    - **M23.619 Other spontaneous disruption of anterior cruciate ligament of unspecified knee**

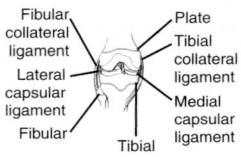

Figure 13-2 Collateral and cruciate ligament of knee. (From DeLee: DeLee and Drez's Orthopaedic Sports Medicine, ed 3, Saunders, 2009)

- **M23.62** Other spontaneous disruption of posterior cruciate ligament of knee
  - **M23.621** Other spontaneous disruption of posterior cruciate ligament of right knee
  - **M23.622** Other spontaneous disruption of posterior cruciate ligament of left knee
  - **M23.629** Other spontaneous disruption of posterior cruciate ligament of unspecified knee
- **M23.63** Other spontaneous disruption of medial collateral ligament of knee
  - **M23.631** Other spontaneous disruption of medial collateral ligament of right knee
  - **M23.632** Other spontaneous disruption of medial collateral ligament of left knee
  - **M23.639** Other spontaneous disruption of medial collateral ligament of unspecified knee
- **M23.64** Other spontaneous disruption of lateral collateral ligament of knee
  - **M23.641** Other spontaneous disruption of lateral collateral ligament of right knee
  - **M23.642** Other spontaneous disruption of lateral collateral ligament of left knee
  - **M23.649** Other spontaneous disruption of lateral collateral ligament of unspecified knee
- **M23.67** Other spontaneous disruption of capsular ligament of knee
  - **M23.671** Other spontaneous disruption of capsular ligament of right knee
  - **M23.672** Other spontaneous disruption of capsular ligament of left knee
  - **M23.679** Other spontaneous disruption of capsular ligament of unspecified knee
- **M23.8** Other internal derangements of knee
  - Laxity of ligament of knee
  - Snapping knee
  - **M23.8X** Other internal derangements of knee
    - **M23.8X1** Other internal derangements of right knee
    - **M23.8X2** Other internal derangements of left knee
    - **M23.8X9** Other internal derangements of unspecified knee
- **M23.9** Unspecified internal derangement of knee
  - **M23.90** Unspecified internal derangement of unspecified knee
  - **M23.91** Unspecified internal derangement of right knee
  - **M23.92** Unspecified internal derangement of left knee

- **M24** Other specific joint derangements
  - **Excludes1** current injury - see injury of joint by body region
  - **Excludes2** ganglion (M67.4)
    snapping knee (M23.8-)
    temporomandibular joint disorders (M26.6-)
- **M24.0** Loose body in joint
  - **Excludes2** loose body in knee (M23.4)
  - **M24.00** Loose body in unspecified joint
  - **M24.01** Loose body in shoulder
    - **M24.011** Loose body in right shoulder
    - **M24.012** Loose body in left shoulder
    - **M24.019** Loose body in unspecified shoulder
  - **M24.02** Loose body in elbow
    - **M24.021** Loose body in right elbow
    - **M24.022** Loose body in left elbow
    - **M24.029** Loose body in unspecified elbow
  - **M24.03** Loose body in wrist
    - **M24.031** Loose body in right wrist
    - **M24.032** Loose body in left wrist
    - **M24.039** Loose body in unspecified wrist
  - **M24.04** Loose body in finger joints
    - **M24.041** Loose body in right finger joint(s)
    - **M24.042** Loose body in left finger joint(s)
    - **M24.049** Loose body in unspecified finger joint(s)
  - **M24.05** Loose body in hip
    - **M24.051** Loose body in right hip
    - **M24.052** Loose body in left hip
    - **M24.059** Loose body in unspecified hip
  - **M24.07** Loose body in ankle and toe joints
    - **M24.071** Loose body in right ankle
    - **M24.072** Loose body in left ankle
    - **M24.073** Loose body in unspecified ankle
    - **M24.074** Loose body in right toe joint(s)
    - **M24.075** Loose body in left toe joint(s)
    - **M24.076** Loose body in unspecified toe joints
  - **M24.08** Loose body, other site
- **M24.1** Other articular cartilage disorders
  - **Excludes2** chondrocalcinosis (M11.1, M11.2-)
    internal derangement of knee (M23.-)
    metastatic calcification (E83.5)
    ochronosis (E70.2)
  - **M24.10** Other articular cartilage disorders, unspecified site
  - **M24.11** Other articular cartilage disorders, shoulder
    - **M24.111** Other articular cartilage disorders, right shoulder
    - **M24.112** Other articular cartilage disorders, left shoulder
    - **M24.119** Other articular cartilage disorders, unspecified shoulder
  - **M24.12** Other articular cartilage disorders, elbow
    - **M24.121** Other articular cartilage disorders, right elbow
    - **M24.122** Other articular cartilage disorders, left elbow
    - **M24.129** Other articular cartilage disorders, unspecified elbow
  - **M24.13** Other articular cartilage disorders, wrist
    - **M24.131** Other articular cartilage disorders, right wrist
    - **M24.132** Other articular cartilage disorders, left wrist
    - **M24.139** Other articular cartilage disorders, unspecified wrist
  - **M24.14** Other articular cartilage disorders, hand
    - **M24.141** Other articular cartilage disorders, right hand
    - **M24.142** Other articular cartilage disorders, left hand
    - **M24.149** Other articular cartilage disorders, unspecified hand

- M24.15 Other articular cartilage disorders, hip
  - M24.151 Other articular cartilage disorders, right hip
  - M24.152 Other articular cartilage disorders, left hip
  - M24.159 Other articular cartilage disorders, unspecified hip
- M24.17 Other articular cartilage disorders, ankle and foot
  - M24.171 Other articular cartilage disorders, right ankle
  - M24.172 Other articular cartilage disorders, left ankle
  - M24.173 Other articular cartilage disorders, unspecified ankle
  - M24.174 Other articular cartilage disorders, right foot
  - M24.175 Other articular cartilage disorders, left foot
  - M24.176 Other articular cartilage disorders, unspecified foot
- M24.2 Disorder of ligament
  - Instability secondary to old ligament injury
  - Ligamentous laxity NOS
  - **Excludes1** familial ligamentous laxity (M35.7)
  - **Excludes2** internal derangement of knee (M23.5-M23.89)
  - M24.20 Disorder of ligament, unspecified site
- M24.21 Disorder of ligament, shoulder
  - M24.211 Disorder of ligament, right shoulder
  - M24.212 Disorder of ligament, left shoulder
  - M24.219 Disorder of ligament, unspecified shoulder
- M24.22 Disorder of ligament, elbow
  - M24.221 Disorder of ligament, right elbow
  - M24.222 Disorder of ligament, left elbow
  - M24.229 Disorder of ligament, unspecified elbow
- M24.23 Disorder of ligament, wrist
  - M24.231 Disorder of ligament, right wrist
  - M24.232 Disorder of ligament, left wrist
  - M24.239 Disorder of ligament, unspecified wrist
- M24.24 Disorder of ligament, hand
  - M24.241 Disorder of ligament, right hand
  - M24.242 Disorder of ligament, left hand
  - M24.249 Disorder of ligament, unspecified hand
- M24.25 Disorder of ligament, hip
  - M24.251 Disorder of ligament, right hip
  - M24.252 Disorder of ligament, left hip
  - M24.259 Disorder of ligament, unspecified hip
- M24.27 Disorder of ligament, ankle and foot
  - M24.271 Disorder of ligament, right ankle
  - M24.272 Disorder of ligament, left ankle
  - M24.273 Disorder of ligament, unspecified ankle
  - M24.274 Disorder of ligament, right foot
  - M24.275 Disorder of ligament, left foot
  - M24.276 Disorder of ligament, unspecified foot
  - M24.28 Disorder of ligament, vertebrae

- M24.3 Pathological dislocation of joint, not elsewhere classified
  - **Excludes1** congenital dislocation or displacement of joint - see congenital malformations and deformations of the musculoskeletal system (Q65-Q79)
  - current injury - see injury of joints and ligaments by body region
  - recurrent dislocation of joint (M24.4-)
  - M24.30 Pathological dislocation of unspecified joint, not elsewhere classified
- M24.31 Pathological dislocation of shoulder, not elsewhere classified
  - M24.311 Pathological dislocation of right shoulder, not elsewhere classified
  - M24.312 Pathological dislocation of left shoulder, not elsewhere classified
  - M24.319 Pathological dislocation of unspecified shoulder, not elsewhere classified
- M24.32 Pathological dislocation of elbow, not elsewhere classified
  - M24.321 Pathological dislocation of right elbow, not elsewhere classified
  - M24.322 Pathological dislocation of left elbow, not elsewhere classified
  - M24.329 Pathological dislocation of unspecified elbow, not elsewhere classified
- M24.33 Pathological dislocation of wrist, not elsewhere classified
  - M24.331 Pathological dislocation of right wrist, not elsewhere classified
  - M24.332 Pathological dislocation of left wrist, not elsewhere classified
  - M24.339 Pathological dislocation of unspecified wrist, not elsewhere classified
- M24.34 Pathological dislocation of hand, not elsewhere classified
  - M24.341 Pathological dislocation of right hand, not elsewhere classified
  - M24.342 Pathological dislocation of left hand, not elsewhere classified
  - M24.349 Pathological dislocation of unspecified hand, not elsewhere classified
- M24.35 Pathological dislocation of hip, not elsewhere classified
  - M24.351 Pathological dislocation of right hip, not elsewhere classified
  - M24.352 Pathological dislocation of left hip, not elsewhere classified
  - M24.359 Pathological dislocation of unspecified hip, not elsewhere classified
- M24.36 Pathological dislocation of knee, not elsewhere classified
  - M24.361 Pathological dislocation of right knee, not elsewhere classified
  - M24.362 Pathological dislocation of left knee, not elsewhere classified
  - M24.369 Pathological dislocation of unspecified knee, not elsewhere classified
- M24.37 Pathological dislocation of ankle and foot, not elsewhere classified
  - M24.371 Pathological dislocation of right ankle, not elsewhere classified
  - M24.372 Pathological dislocation of left ankle, not elsewhere classified

◀ New ⇐ Revised ~~deleted~~ Deleted Excludes 1 Excludes 2 Includes Use additional Code first Code also Unspecified
OGCR Official Guidelines ● Unacceptable Principal Diagnosis X Assign placeholder X ● Use Additional Character(s) ▶ Manifestation Code Coding Clinic

M24.373 Pathological dislocation of unspecified ankle, not elsewhere classified
M24.374 Pathological dislocation of right foot, not elsewhere classified
M24.375 Pathological dislocation of left foot, not elsewhere classified
M24.376 Pathological dislocation of unspecified foot, not elsewhere classified

● M24.4 Recurrent dislocation of joint
Recurrent subluxation of joint
Excludes2 recurrent dislocation of patella (M22.0-M22.1)
recurrent vertebral dislocation (M43.3-, M43.4, M43.5-)
M24.40 Recurrent dislocation, unspecified joint
● M24.41 Recurrent dislocation, shoulder
M24.411 Recurrent dislocation, right shoulder
M24.412 Recurrent dislocation, left shoulder
M24.419 Recurrent dislocation, unspecified shoulder
● M24.42 Recurrent dislocation, elbow
M24.421 Recurrent dislocation, right elbow
M24.422 Recurrent dislocation, left elbow
M24.429 Recurrent dislocation, unspecified elbow
● M24.43 Recurrent dislocation, wrist
M24.431 Recurrent dislocation, right wrist
M24.432 Recurrent dislocation, left wrist
M24.439 Recurrent dislocation, unspecified wrist
● M24.44 Recurrent dislocation, hand and finger(s)
M24.441 Recurrent dislocation, right hand
M24.442 Recurrent dislocation, left hand
M24.443 Recurrent dislocation, unspecified hand
M24.444 Recurrent dislocation, right finger
M24.445 Recurrent dislocation, left finger
M24.446 Recurrent dislocation, unspecified finger
● M24.45 Recurrent dislocation, hip
M24.451 Recurrent dislocation, right hip
M24.452 Recurrent dislocation, left hip
M24.459 Recurrent dislocation, unspecified hip
● M24.46 Recurrent dislocation, knee
M24.461 Recurrent dislocation, right knee
M24.462 Recurrent dislocation, left knee
M24.469 Recurrent dislocation, unspecified knee
● M24.47 Recurrent dislocation, ankle, foot and toes
M24.471 Recurrent dislocation, right ankle
M24.472 Recurrent dislocation, left ankle
M24.473 Recurrent dislocation, unspecified ankle
M24.474 Recurrent dislocation, right foot
M24.475 Recurrent dislocation, left foot
M24.476 Recurrent dislocation, unspecified foot
M24.477 Recurrent dislocation, right toe(s)
M24.478 Recurrent dislocation, left toe(s)
M24.479 Recurrent dislocation, unspecified toe(s)

● M24.5 Contracture of joint
Excludes1 contracture of muscle without contracture of joint (M62.4-)
contracture of tendon (sheath) without contracture of joint (M62.4-)
Dupuytren's contracture (M72.0)
Excludes2 acquired deformities of limbs (M20-M21)
M24.50 Contracture, unspecified joint
● M24.51 Contracture, shoulder
M24.511 Contracture, right shoulder
M24.512 Contracture, left shoulder
M24.519 Contracture, unspecified shoulder
● M24.52 Contracture, elbow
M24.521 Contracture, right elbow
M24.522 Contracture, left elbow
M24.529 Contracture, unspecified elbow
● M24.53 Contracture, wrist
M24.531 Contracture, right wrist
M24.532 Contracture, left wrist
M24.539 Contracture, unspecified wrist
● M24.54 Contracture, hand
M24.541 Contracture, right hand
M24.542 Contracture, left hand
M24.549 Contracture, unspecified hand
● M24.55 Contracture, hip
M24.551 Contracture, right hip
Coding Clinic: 2016, Q2, P6
M24.552 Contracture, left hip
Coding Clinic: 2016, Q2, P6
M24.559 Contracture, unspecified hip
● M24.56 Contracture, knee
M24.561 Contracture, right knee
Coding Clinic: 2016, Q2, P6
M24.562 Contracture, left knee
Coding Clinic: 2016, Q2, P6
M24.569 Contracture, unspecified knee
● M24.57 Contracture, ankle and foot
M24.571 Contracture, right ankle
M24.572 Contracture, left ankle
M24.573 Contracture, unspecified ankle
M24.574 Contracture, right foot
M24.575 Contracture, left foot
M24.576 Contracture, unspecified foot

● M24.6 Ankylosis of joint
Excludes1 stiffness of joint without ankylosis (M25.6-)
Excludes2 spine (M43.2-)
M24.60 Ankylosis, unspecified joint
● M24.61 Ankylosis, shoulder
M24.611 Ankylosis, right shoulder
M24.612 Ankylosis, left shoulder
M24.619 Ankylosis, unspecified shoulder
● M24.62 Ankylosis, elbow
M24.621 Ankylosis, right elbow
M24.622 Ankylosis, left elbow
M24.629 Ankylosis, unspecified elbow
● M24.63 Ankylosis, wrist
M24.631 Ankylosis, right wrist
M24.632 Ankylosis, left wrist
M24.639 Ankylosis, unspecified wrist

Item 13–5 Ankylosis or arthrokleisis is a consolidation of a joint due to disease, injury, or surgical procedure. Spondylosis is the degeneration of the vertebral processes and formation of osteophytes and commonly occurs with age. **Spondylitis** or ankylosing spondylitis is a type of arthritis that affects the spine or backbone causing back pain and stiffness.

- M24.64 Ankylosis, hand
  - M24.641 Ankylosis, right hand
  - M24.642 Ankylosis, left hand
  - M24.649 Ankylosis, unspecified hand
- M24.65 Ankylosis, hip
  - M24.651 Ankylosis, right hip
  - M24.652 Ankylosis, left hip
  - M24.659 Ankylosis, unspecified hip
- M24.66 Ankylosis, knee
  - M24.661 Ankylosis, right knee
  - M24.662 Ankylosis, left knee
  - M24.669 Ankylosis, unspecified knee
- M24.67 Ankylosis, ankle and foot
  - M24.671 Ankylosis, right ankle
  - M24.672 Ankylosis, left ankle
  - M24.673 Ankylosis, unspecified ankle
  - M24.674 Ankylosis, right foot
  - M24.675 Ankylosis, left foot
  - M24.676 Ankylosis, unspecified foot

M24.7 Protrusio acetabuli

- M24.8 Other specific joint derangements, not elsewhere classified

  Excludes2 iliotibial band syndrome (M76.3)

  - M24.80 Other specific joint derangements of unspecified joint, not elsewhere classified
  - M24.81 Other specific joint derangements of shoulder, not elsewhere classified
    - M24.811 Other specific joint derangements of right shoulder, not elsewhere classified
    - M24.812 Other specific joint derangements of left shoulder, not elsewhere classified
    - M24.819 Other specific joint derangements of unspecified shoulder, not elsewhere classified
  - M24.82 Other specific joint derangements of elbow, not elsewhere classified
    - M24.821 Other specific joint derangements of right elbow, not elsewhere classified
    - M24.822 Other specific joint derangements of left elbow, not elsewhere classified
    - M24.829 Other specific joint derangements of unspecified elbow, not elsewhere classified
  - M24.83 Other specific joint derangements of wrist, not elsewhere classified
    - M24.831 Other specific joint derangements of right wrist, not elsewhere classified
    - M24.832 Other specific joint derangements of left wrist, not elsewhere classified
    - M24.839 Other specific joint derangements of unspecified wrist, not elsewhere classified
  - M24.84 Other specific joint derangements of hand, not elsewhere classified
    - M24.841 Other specific joint derangements of right hand, not elsewhere classified
    - M24.842 Other specific joint derangements of left hand, not elsewhere classified
    - M24.849 Other specific joint derangements of unspecified hand, not elsewhere classified
  - M24.85 Other specific joint derangements of hip, not elsewhere classified

    Irritable hip
    - M24.851 Other specific joint derangements of right hip, not elsewhere classified
    - M24.852 Other specific joint derangements of left hip, not elsewhere classified
    - M24.859 Other specific joint derangements of unspecified hip, not elsewhere classified
  - M24.87 Other specific joint derangements of ankle and foot, not elsewhere classified
    - M24.871 Other specific joint derangements of right ankle, not elsewhere classified
    - M24.872 Other specific joint derangements of left ankle, not elsewhere classified
    - M24.873 Other specific joint derangements of unspecified ankle, not elsewhere classified
    - M24.874 Other specific joint derangements of right foot, not elsewhere classified
    - M24.875 Other specific joint derangements left foot, not elsewhere classified
    - M24.876 Other specific joint derangements of unspecified foot, not elsewhere classified

M24.9 Joint derangement, unspecified

- M25 Other joint disorder, not elsewhere classified

  Excludes2 abnormality of gait and mobility (R26.-)
  acquired deformities of limb (M20-M21)
  calcification of bursa (M71.4-)
  calcification of shoulder (joint) (M75.3)
  calcification of tendon (M65.2-)
  difficulty in walking (R26.2)
  temporomandibular joint disorder (M26.6-)

  - M25.0 Hemarthrosis

    Excludes1 current injury - see injury of joint by body region
    hemophilic arthropathy (M36.2)

    - M25.00 Hemarthrosis, unspecified joint
      Ex: M25.00-M25.08, T79.A11A-T79.A29A
    - M25.01 Hemarthrosis, shoulder
      Ex: For category M25.01 CC codes: M25.00-M25.039, M25.08, T79.A11-T79.A19[A]
      - M25.011 Hemarthrosis, right shoulder
      - M25.012 Hemarthrosis, left shoulder
      - M25.019 Hemarthrosis, unspecified shoulder
    - M25.02 Hemarthrosis, elbow
      Ex: For category M25.02 CC codes: M25.00-M25.029, M25.08, T79.A11-T79.A19[A]
      - M25.021 Hemarthrosis, right elbow
      - M25.022 Hemarthrosis, left elbow
      - M25.029 Hemarthrosis, unspecified elbow
    - M25.03 Hemarthrosis, wrist
      Ex: For category M25.03 CC codes: M25.00-M25.049, M25.08, T79.A11-T79.A19[A]
      - M25.031 Hemarthrosis, right wrist
      - M25.032 Hemarthrosis, left wrist
      - M25.039 Hemarthrosis, unspecified wrist
    - M25.04 Hemarthrosis, hand
      Ex: For category M25.04 CC codes: M25.00, M25.031-M25.049, M25.08, T79.A11-T79.A19[A]
      - M25.041 Hemarthrosis, right hand
      - M25.042 Hemarthrosis, left hand
      - M25.049 Hemarthrosis, unspecified hand

New Revised ~~deleted~~ Deleted Excludes 1 Excludes 2 Includes Use additional Code first Code also Unspecified
OGCR Official Guidelines Unacceptable Principal Diagnosis X Assign placeholder X Use Additional Character(s) Manifestation Code Coding Clinic

- **M25.05 Hemarthrosis, hip**
  - Ex: For category M25.05 CC codes: See M25.00
  - M25.051 Hemarthrosis, right hip
  - M25.052 Hemarthrosis, left hip
  - M25.059 Hemarthrosis, unspecified hip
- **M25.06 Hemarthrosis, knee**
  - Ex: For category M25.06 CC codes: M25.00, M25.061-M25.08, T79.A21-T79.A29[A]
  - M25.061 Hemarthrosis, right knee
  - M25.062 Hemarthrosis, left knee
  - M25.069 Hemarthrosis, unspecified knee
- **M25.07 Hemarthrosis, ankle and foot**
  - Ex: For category M25.07 CC codes: See M25.06
  - M25.071 Hemarthrosis, right ankle
  - M25.072 Hemarthrosis, left ankle
  - M25.073 Hemarthrosis, unspecified ankle
  - M25.074 Hemarthrosis, right foot
  - M25.075 Hemarthrosis, left foot
  - M25.076 Hemarthrosis, unspecified foot
- M25.08 Hemarthrosis, other specified site
  - Hemarthrosis, vertebrae
  - Ex: See M25.00

- **M25.1 Fistula of joint**
  - M25.10 Fistula, unspecified joint
  - **M25.11 Fistula, shoulder**
    - M25.111 Fistula, right shoulder
    - M25.112 Fistula, left shoulder
    - M25.119 Fistula, unspecified shoulder
  - **M25.12 Fistula, elbow**
    - M25.121 Fistula, right elbow
    - M25.122 Fistula, left elbow
    - M25.129 Fistula, unspecified elbow
  - **M25.13 Fistula, wrist**
    - M25.131 Fistula, right wrist
    - M25.132 Fistula, left wrist
    - M25.139 Fistula, unspecified wrist
  - **M25.14 Fistula, hand**
    - M25.141 Fistula, right hand
    - M25.142 Fistula, left hand
    - M25.149 Fistula, unspecified hand
  - **M25.15 Fistula, hip**
    - M25.151 Fistula, right hip
    - M25.152 Fistula, left hip
    - M25.159 Fistula, unspecified hip
  - **M25.16 Fistula, knee**
    - M25.161 Fistula, right knee
    - M25.162 Fistula, left knee
    - M25.169 Fistula, unspecified knee
  - **M25.17 Fistula, ankle and foot**
    - M25.171 Fistula, right ankle
    - M25.172 Fistula, left ankle
    - M25.173 Fistula, unspecified ankle
    - M25.174 Fistula, right foot
    - M25.175 Fistula, left foot
    - M25.176 Fistula, unspecified foot
  - M25.18 Fistula, other specified site
    - Fistula, vertebrae
- **M25.2 Flail joint**
  - M25.20 Flail joint, unspecified joint
  - **M25.21 Flail joint, shoulder**
    - M25.211 Flail joint, right shoulder
    - M25.212 Flail joint, left shoulder
    - M25.219 Flail joint, unspecified shoulder
  - **M25.22 Flail joint, elbow**
    - M25.221 Flail joint, right elbow
    - M25.222 Flail joint, left elbow
    - M25.229 Flail joint, unspecified elbow
  - **M25.23 Flail joint, wrist**
    - M25.231 Flail joint, right wrist
    - M25.232 Flail joint, left wrist
    - M25.239 Flail joint, unspecified wrist
  - **M25.24 Flail joint, hand**
    - M25.241 Flail joint, right hand
    - M25.242 Flail joint, left hand
    - M25.249 Flail joint, unspecified hand
  - **M25.25 Flail joint, hip**
    - M25.251 Flail joint, right hip
    - M25.252 Flail joint, left hip
    - M25.259 Flail joint, unspecified hip
  - **M25.26 Flail joint, knee**
    - M25.261 Flail joint, right knee
    - M25.262 Flail joint, left knee
    - M25.269 Flail joint, unspecified knee
  - **M25.27 Flail joint, ankle and foot**
    - M25.271 Flail joint, right ankle and foot
    - M25.272 Flail joint, left ankle and foot
    - M25.279 Flail joint, unspecified ankle and foot
  - M25.28 Flail joint, other site
- **M25.3 Other instability of joint**
  - **Excludes1** instability of joint secondary to old ligament injury (M24.2-)
    - instability of joint secondary to removal of joint prosthesis (M96.8-)
  - **Excludes2** spinal instabilities (M53.2-)
  - M25.30 Other instability, unspecified joint
  - **M25.31 Other instability, shoulder**
    - M25.311 Other instability, right shoulder
    - M25.312 Other instability, left shoulder
    - M25.319 Other instability, unspecified shoulder
  - **M25.32 Other instability, elbow**
    - M25.321 Other instability, right elbow
    - M25.322 Other instability, left elbow
    - M25.329 Other instability, unspecified elbow
  - **M25.33 Other instability, wrist**
    - M25.331 Other instability, right wrist
    - M25.332 Other instability, left wrist
    - M25.339 Other instability, unspecified wrist
  - **M25.34 Other instability, hand**
    - M25.341 Other instability, right hand
    - M25.342 Other instability, left hand
    - M25.349 Other instability, unspecified hand
  - **M25.35 Other instability, hip**
    - M25.351 Other instability, right hip
    - M25.352 Other instability, left hip
    - M25.359 Other instability, unspecified hip
  - **M25.36 Other instability, knee**
    - M25.361 Other instability, right knee
    - M25.362 Other instability, left knee
    - M25.369 Other instability, unspecified knee
  - **M25.37 Other instability, ankle and foot**
    - M25.371 Other instability, right ankle
    - M25.372 Other instability, left ankle
    - M25.373 Other instability, unspecified ankle
    - M25.374 Other instability, right foot
    - M25.375 Other instability, left foot
    - M25.376 Other instability, unspecified foot

- M25.4 Effusion of joint
  - **Excludes1** hydrarthrosis in yaws (A66.6)
    intermittent hydrarthrosis (M12.4-)
    other infective (teno)synovitis (M65.1-)
  - M25.40 Effusion, unspecified joint
  - M25.41 Effusion, shoulder
    - M25.411 Effusion, right shoulder
    - M25.412 Effusion, left shoulder
    - M25.419 Effusion, unspecified shoulder
  - M25.42 Effusion, elbow
    - M25.421 Effusion, right elbow
    - M25.422 Effusion, left elbow
    - M25.429 Effusion, unspecified elbow
  - M25.43 Effusion, wrist
    - M25.431 Effusion, right wrist
    - M25.432 Effusion, left wrist
    - M25.439 Effusion, unspecified wrist
  - M25.44 Effusion, hand
    - M25.441 Effusion, right hand
    - M25.442 Effusion, left hand
    - M25.449 Effusion, unspecified hand
  - M25.45 Effusion, hip
    - M25.451 Effusion, right hip
    - M25.452 Effusion, left hip
    - M25.459 Effusion, unspecified hip
  - M25.46 Effusion, knee
    - M25.461 Effusion, right knee
    - M25.462 Effusion, left knee
    - M25.469 Effusion, unspecified knee
  - M25.47 Effusion, ankle and foot
    - M25.471 Effusion, right ankle
    - M25.472 Effusion, left ankle
    - M25.473 Effusion, unspecified ankle
    - M25.474 Effusion, right foot
    - M25.475 Effusion, left foot
    - M25.476 Effusion, unspecified foot
  - M25.48 Effusion, other site
- M25.5 Pain in joint
  - **Excludes2** pain in hand (M79.64-)
    pain in fingers (M79.64-)
    pain in foot (M79.67-)
    pain in limb (M79.6-)
    pain in toes (M79.67-)
  - M25.50 Pain in unspecified joint
  - M25.51 Pain in shoulder
    - M25.511 Pain in right shoulder
    - M25.512 Pain in left shoulder
    - M25.519 Pain in unspecified shoulder
  - M25.52 Pain in elbow
    - M25.521 Pain in right elbow
    - M25.522 Pain in left elbow
    - M25.529 Pain in unspecified elbow
  - M25.53 Pain in wrist
    - M25.531 Pain in right wrist
    - M25.532 Pain in left wrist
    - M25.539 Pain in unspecified wrist
  - M25.54 Pain in joints of hand ◀
    - M25.541 Pain in joints of right hand ◀
    - M25.542 Pain in joints of left hand ◀
    - M25.549 Pain in joints of unspecified hand ◀
      Pain in joints of hand NOS ◀
  - M25.55 Pain in hip
    - M25.551 Pain in right hip
    - M25.552 Pain in left hip
    - M25.559 Pain in unspecified hip
  - M25.56 Pain in knee
    - M25.561 Pain in right knee
    - M25.562 Pain in left knee
    - M25.569 Pain in unspecified knee
  - M25.57 Pain in ankle and joints of foot
    - M25.571 Pain in right ankle and joints of right foot
    - M25.572 Pain in left ankle and joints of left foot
    - M25.579 Pain in unspecified ankle and joints of unspecified foot
- M25.6 Stiffness of joint, not elsewhere classified
  - **Excludes1** ankylosis of joint (M24.6-)
    contracture of joint (M24.5-)
  - M25.60 Stiffness of unspecified joint, not elsewhere classified
  - M25.61 Stiffness of shoulder, not elsewhere classified
    - M25.611 Stiffness of right shoulder, not elsewhere classified
    - M25.612 Stiffness of left shoulder, not elsewhere classified
    - M25.619 Stiffness of unspecified shoulder, not elsewhere classified
  - M25.62 Stiffness of elbow, not elsewhere classified
    - M25.621 Stiffness of right elbow, not elsewhere classified
    - M25.622 Stiffness of left elbow, not elsewhere classified
    - M25.629 Stiffness of unspecified elbow, not elsewhere classified
  - M25.63 Stiffness of wrist, not elsewhere classified
    - M25.631 Stiffness of right wrist, not elsewhere classified
    - M25.632 Stiffness of left wrist, not elsewhere classified
    - M25.639 Stiffness of unspecified wrist, not elsewhere classified
  - M25.64 Stiffness of hand, not elsewhere classified
    - M25.641 Stiffness of right hand, not elsewhere classified
    - M25.642 Stiffness of left hand, not elsewhere classified
    - M25.649 Stiffness of unspecified hand, not elsewhere classified
  - M25.65 Stiffness of hip, not elsewhere classified
    - M25.651 Stiffness of right hip, not elsewhere classified
    - M25.652 Stiffness of left hip, not elsewhere classified
    - M25.659 Stiffness of unspecified hip, not elsewhere classified
  - M25.66 Stiffness of knee, not elsewhere classified
    - M25.661 Stiffness of right knee, not elsewhere classified
    - M25.662 Stiffness of left knee, not elsewhere classified
    - M25.669 Stiffness of unspecified knee, not elsewhere classified
  - M25.67 Stiffness of ankle and foot, not elsewhere classified
    - M25.671 Stiffness of right ankle, not elsewhere classified
    - M25.672 Stiffness of left ankle, not elsewhere classified
    - M25.673 Stiffness of unspecified ankle, not elsewhere classified
    - M25.674 Stiffness of right foot, not elsewhere classified

M25.675 Stiffness of left foot, not elsewhere classified
M25.676 Stiffness of unspecified foot, not elsewhere classified

● M25.7 Osteophyte
M25.70 Osteophyte, unspecified joint
● M25.71 Osteophyte, shoulder
M25.711 Osteophyte, right shoulder
M25.712 Osteophyte, left shoulder
M25.719 Osteophyte, unspecified shoulder
● M25.72 Osteophyte, elbow
M25.721 Osteophyte, right elbow
M25.722 Osteophyte, left elbow
M25.729 Osteophyte, unspecified elbow
● M25.73 Osteophyte, wrist
M25.731 Osteophyte, right wrist
M25.732 Osteophyte, left wrist
M25.739 Osteophyte, unspecified wrist
● M25.74 Osteophyte, hand
M25.741 Osteophyte, right hand
M25.742 Osteophyte, left hand
M25.749 Osteophyte, unspecified hand
● M25.75 Osteophyte, hip
M25.751 Osteophyte, right hip
M25.752 Osteophyte, left hip
M25.759 Osteophyte, unspecified hip
● M25.76 Osteophyte, knee
M25.761 Osteophyte, right knee
M25.762 Osteophyte, left knee
M25.769 Osteophyte, unspecified knee
● M25.77 Osteophyte, ankle and foot
M25.771 Osteophyte, right ankle
M25.772 Osteophyte, left ankle
M25.773 Osteophyte, unspecified ankle
M25.774 Osteophyte, right foot
M25.775 Osteophyte, left foot
M25.776 Osteophyte, unspecified foot
M25.78 Osteophyte, vertebrae
● M25.8 Other specified joint disorders
M25.80 Other specified joint disorders, unspecified joint
● M25.81 Other specified joint disorders, shoulder
M25.811 Other specified joint disorders, right shoulder
M25.812 Other specified joint disorders, left shoulder
M25.819 Other specified joint disorders, unspecified shoulder
● M25.82 Other specified joint disorders, elbow
M25.821 Other specified joint disorders, right elbow
M25.822 Other specified joint disorders, left elbow
M25.829 Other specified joint disorders, unspecified elbow
● M25.83 Other specified joint disorders, wrist
M25.831 Other specified joint disorders, right wrist
M25.832 Other specified joint disorders, left wrist
M25.839 Other specified joint disorders, unspecified wrist
● M25.84 Other specified joint disorders, hand
M25.841 Other specified joint disorders, right hand
M25.842 Other specified joint disorders, left hand
M25.849 Other specified joint disorders, unspecified hand
● M25.85 Other specified joint disorders, hip
M25.851 Other specified joint disorders, right hip
M25.852 Other specified joint disorders, left hip
M25.859 Other specified joint disorders, unspecified hip
● M25.86 Other specified joint disorders, knee
M25.861 Other specified joint disorders, right knee
M25.862 Other specified joint disorders, left knee
M25.869 Other specified joint disorders, unspecified knee
● M25.87 Other specified joint disorders, ankle and foot
M25.871 Other specified joint disorders, right ankle and foot
M25.872 Other specified joint disorders, left ankle and foot
M25.879 Other specified joint disorders, unspecified ankle and foot
M25.9 Joint disorder, unspecified

DENTOFACIAL ANOMALIES [INCLUDING MALOCCLUSION] AND OTHER DISORDERS OF JAW (M26-M27)

Excludes1 hemifacial atrophy or hypertrophy (Q67.4)
unilateral condylar hyperplasia or hypoplasia (M27.8)

● M26 Dentofacial anomalies [including malocclusion]
● M26.0 Major anomalies of jaw size
Excludes1 acromegaly (E22.0)
Robin's syndrome (Q87.0)
M26.00 Unspecified anomaly of jaw size
M26.01 Maxillary hyperplasia
M26.02 Maxillary hypoplasia
M26.03 Mandibular hyperplasia
M26.04 Mandibular hypoplasia
M26.05 Macrogenia
M26.06 Microgenia
M26.07 Excessive tuberosity of jaw
Entire maxillary tuberosity
M26.09 Other specified anomalies of jaw size
● M26.1 Anomalies of jaw-cranial base relationship
M26.10 Unspecified anomaly of jaw-cranial base relationship
M26.11 Maxillary asymmetry
M26.12 Other jaw asymmetry
M26.19 Other specified anomalies of jaw-cranial base relationship

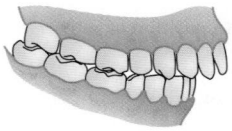

Figure 13-3 Dentofacial malocclusion.

Item 13–6 **Hyperplasia** is a condition of overdevelopment, whereas **hypoplasia** is a condition of underdevelopment. **Macrogenia** is overdevelopment of the chin, whereas **microgenia** is underdevelopment of the chin.

● **M26.2 Anomalies of dental arch relationship**

M26.20 Unspecified anomaly of dental arch relationship

● **M26.21 Malocclusion, Angle's class**

M26.211 Malocclusion, Angle's class I
Neutro-occlusion

M26.212 Malocclusion, Angle's class II
Disto-occlusion Division I
Disto-occlusion Division II

M26.213 Malocclusion, Angle's class III
Mesio-occlusion

M26.219 Malocclusion, Angle's class, unspecified

● **M26.22 Open occlusal relationship**

M26.220 Open anterior occlusal relationship
Anterior openbite

M26.221 Open posterior occlusal relationship
Posterior openbite

M26.23 Excessive horizontal overlap
Excessive horizontal overjet

M26.24 Reverse articulation
Crossbite (anterior) (posterior)

M26.25 Anomalies of interarch distance

M26.29 Other anomalies of dental arch relationship
Midline deviation of dental arch
Overbite (excessive) deep
Overbite (excessive) horizontal
Overbite (excessive) vertical
Posterior lingual occlusion of mandibular teeth

● **M26.3 Anomalies of tooth position of fully erupted tooth or teeth**

Excludes2 embedded and impacted teeth (KØ1.-)

M26.30 Unspecified anomaly of tooth position of fully erupted tooth or teeth
Abnormal spacing of fully erupted tooth or teeth NOS
Displacement of fully erupted tooth or teeth NOS
Transposition of fully erupted tooth or teeth NOS

M26.31 Crowding of fully erupted teeth

M26.32 Excessive spacing of fully erupted teeth
Diastema of fully erupted tooth or teeth NOS

M26.33 Horizontal displacement of fully erupted tooth or teeth
Tipped tooth or teeth
Tipping of fully erupted tooth

M26.34 Vertical displacement of fully erupted tooth or teeth
Extruded tooth
Infraeruption of tooth or teeth
Supraeruption of tooth or teeth

M26.35 Rotation of fully erupted tooth or teeth

M26.36 Insufficient interocclusal distance of fully erupted teeth (ridge)
Lack of adequate intermaxillary vertical dimension of fully erupted teeth

M26.37 Excessive interocclusal distance of fully erupted teeth
Excessive intermaxillary vertical dimension of fully erupted teeth
Loss of occlusal vertical dimension of fully erupted teeth

M26.39 Other anomalies of tooth position of fully erupted tooth or teeth

M26.4 Malocclusion, unspecified

● **M26.5 Dentofacial functional abnormalities**

Excludes1 bruxism (F45.8)
teeth-grinding NOS (F45.8)

M26.50 Dentofacial functional abnormalities, unspecified

M26.51 Abnormal jaw closure

M26.52 Limited mandibular range of motion

M26.53 Deviation in opening and closing of the mandible

M26.54 Insufficient anterior guidance
Insufficient anterior occlusal guidance

M26.55 Centric occlusion maximum intercuspation discrepancy

Excludes1 centric occlusion NOS (M26.59)

M26.56 Non-working side interference
Balancing side interference

M26.57 Lack of posterior occlusal support

M26.59 Other dentofacial functional abnormalities
Centric occlusion (of teeth) NOS
Malocclusion due to abnormal swallowing
Malocclusion due to mouth breathing
Malocclusion due to tongue, lip or finger habits

● **M26.6 Temporomandibular joint disorders**

Excludes2 current temporomandibular joint dislocation (SØ3.Ø)
current temporomandibular joint sprain (SØ3.4)

● **M26.60 Temporomandibular joint disorder, unspecified**

M26.601 Right temporomandibular joint disorder, unspecified ◀

M26.602 Left temporomandibular joint disorder, unspecified ◀

M26.603 Bilateral temporomandibular joint disorder, unspecified ◀

M26.609 Unspecified temporomandibular joint disorder, unspecified side ◀
Temporomandibular joint disorder NOS ◀

● **M26.61 Adhesions and ankylosis of temporomandibular joint**

M26.611 Adhesions and ankylosis of right temporomandibular joint ◀

M26.612 Adhesions and ankylosis of left temporomandibular joint ◀

M26.613 Adhesions and ankylosis of bilateral temporomandibular joint ◀

M26.619 Adhesions and ankylosis of temporomandibular joint, unspecified side ◀

● **M26.62 Arthralgia of temporomandibular joint**

M26.621 Arthralgia of right temporomandibular joint ◀

M26.622 Arthralgia of left temporomandibular joint ◀

M26.623 Arthralgia of bilateral temporomandibular joint ◀

M26.629 Arthralgia of temporomandibular joint, unspecified side ◀

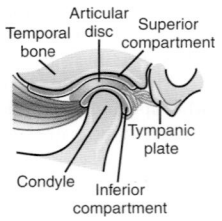

Figure 13-4 Temporomandibular joint.

Item 13–7 Dysfunction of the temporomandibular joint is termed **temporomandibular joint (TMJ) syndrome** and is characterized by pain and tenderness/spasm of the muscles of mastication, joint noise, and in the later stages, limited mandibular movement.

- **M26.63 Articular disc disorder of temporomandibular joint**
  - **M26.631 Articular disc disorder of right temporomandibular joint** ◀
  - **M26.632 Articular disc disorder of left temporomandibular joint** ◀
  - **M26.633 Articular disc disorder of bilateral temporomandibular joint** ◀
  - **M26.639 Articular disc disorder of temporomandibular joint, unspecified side** ◀
  - **M26.69 Other specified disorders of temporomandibular joint**
- **M26.7 Dental alveolar anomalies**
  - **M26.70 Unspecified alveolar anomaly**
  - **M26.71 Alveolar maxillary hyperplasia**
  - **M26.72 Alveolar mandibular hyperplasia**
  - **M26.73 Alveolar maxillary hypoplasia**
  - **M26.74 Alveolar mandibular hypoplasia**
  - **M26.79 Other specified alveolar anomalies**
- **M26.8 Other dentofacial anomalies**
  - **M26.81 Anterior soft tissue impingement**
    Anterior soft tissue impingement on teeth
  - **M26.82 Posterior soft tissue impingement**
    Posterior soft tissue impingement on teeth
  - **M26.89 Other dentofacial anomalies**
- **M26.9 Dentofacial anomaly, unspecified**

- **M27 Other diseases of jaws**
  - **M27.0 Developmental disorders of jaws**
    Latent bone cyst of jaw
    Stafne's cyst
    Torus mandibularis
    Torus palatinus
  - **M27.1 Giant cell granuloma, central**
    Giant cell granuloma NOS
    Excludes1 peripheral giant cell granuloma (K06.8)
  - **M27.2 Inflammatory conditions of jaws**
    Osteitis of jaw(s)
    Osteomyelitis (neonatal) jaw(s)
    Osteoradionecrosis jaw(s)
    Periostitis jaw(s)
    Sequestrum of jaw bone
    Use additional code (W88-W90, X39.0) to identify radiation, if radiation-induced
    Excludes2 osteonecrosis of jaw due to drug (M87.180)
  - **M27.3 Alveolitis of jaws**
    Alveolar osteitis
    Dry socket
  - **M27.4 Other and unspecified cysts of jaw**
    Excludes1 cysts of oral region (K09.-)
    latent bone cyst of jaw (M27.0)
    Stafne's cyst (M27.0)
    - **M27.40 Unspecified cyst of jaw**
      Cyst of jaw NOS
    - **M27.49 Other cysts of jaw**
      Aneurysmal cyst of jaw
      Hemorrhagic cyst of jaw
      Traumatic cyst of jaw
  - **M27.5 Periradicular pathology associated with previous endodontic treatment**
    - **M27.51 Perforation of root canal space due to endodontic treatment**
    - **M27.52 Endodontic overfill**
    - **M27.53 Endodontic underfill**
    - **M27.59 Other periradicular pathology associated with previous endodontic treatment**
  - **M27.6 Endosseous dental implant failure**
    - **M27.61 Osseointegration failure of dental implant**
      Hemorrhagic complications of dental implant placement
      Iatrogenic osseointegration failure of dental implant
      Osseointegration failure of dental implant due to complications of systemic disease
      Osseointegration failure of dental implant due to poor bone quality
      Pre-integration failure of dental implant NOS
      Pre-osseointegration failure of dental implant
    - **M27.62 Post-osseointegration biological failure of dental implant**
      Failure of dental implant due to lack of attached gingiva
      Failure of dental implant due to occlusal trauma (caused by poor prosthetic design)
      Failure of dental implant due to parafunctional habits
      Failure of dental implant due to periodontal infection (peri–implantitis)
      Failure of dental implant due to poor oral hygiene
      Iatrogenic post-osseointegration failure of dental implant
      Post-osseointegration failure of dental implant due to complications of systemic disease
    - **M27.63 Post-osseointegration mechanical failure of dental implant**
      Failure of dental prosthesis causing loss of dental implant
      Fracture of dental implant
      Excludes2 cracked tooth (K03.81)
      fractured dental restorative material with loss of material (K08.531)
      fractured dental restorative material without loss of material (K08.530)
      fractured tooth (S02.5)
    - **M27.69 Other endosseous dental implant failure**
      Dental implant failure NOS
  - **M27.8 Other specified diseases of jaws**
    Cherubism
    Exostosis
    Fibrous dysplasia
    Unilateral condylar hyperplasia
    Unilateral condylar hypoplasia
    Excludes1 jaw pain (R68.84)
  - **M27.9 Disease of jaws, unspecified**

SYSTEMIC CONNECTIVE TISSUE DISORDERS (M30-M36)

Includes autoimmune disease NOS
collagen (vascular) disease NOS
systemic autoimmune disease
systemic collagen (vascular) disease

Excludes1 autoimmune disease, single organ or single cell-type - code to relevant condition category

- **M30 Polyarteritis nodosa and related conditions**
  Excludes1 microscopic polyarteritis (M31.7)
  Ex: **For category M30 CC codes unless otherwise indicated:** E08.51-E08.59, E08.618-E08.638, E08.649-E08.8, E09.51-E09.59, E09.618-E09.638, E09.649-E09.8, E10.51-E10.59, E10.618-E10.638, E10.649, E10.69-E10.8, E11.51-E11.59, E11.618-E11.638, E11.649, E11.69-E11.8, E13.51-E13.59, E13.618-E13.638, E13.649-E13.8, I87.8-I87.9, I99.8-I99.9, M30.0-M31.7
  - **M30.0 Polyarteritis nodosa**
  - **M30.1 Polyarteritis with lung involvement [Churg-Strauss]**
    Allergic granulomatous angiitis
  - **M30.2 Juvenile polyarteritis**
  - **M30.3 Mucocutaneous lymph node syndrome [Kawasaki]**
    Ex: I87.8-I87.9, I99.8-I99.9, M30.0-M31.7
  - **M30.8 Other conditions related to polyarteritis nodosa**
    Polyangiitis overlap syndrome

M31 Other necrotizing vasculopathies
Ex: For category M31 CC codes unless otherwise indicated: See M30

M31.0 Hypersensitivity angiitis
Goodpasture's syndrome

M31.1 Thrombotic microangiopathy
Thrombotic thrombocytopenic purpura

M31.2 Lethal midline granuloma

M31.3 Wegener's granulomatosis
Necrotizing respiratory granulomatosis

M31.30 Wegener's granulomatosis without renal involvement
Wegener's granulomatosis NOS

M31.31 Wegener's granulomatosis with renal involvement

M31.4 Aortic arch syndrome [Takayasu]

M31.5 Giant cell arteritis with polymyalgia rheumatica

M31.6 Other giant cell arteritis

M31.7 Microscopic polyangiitis
Microscopic polyarteritis
Excludes1 polyarteritis nodosa (M30.0)

M31.8 Other specified necrotizing vasculopathies
Hypocomplementemic vasculitis
Septic vasculitis
Ex: I77.5, M31.8-M31.9

M31.9 Necrotizing vasculopathy, unspecified
Ex: I77.5, M31.8-M31.9

M32 Systemic lupus erythematosus (SLE)
Autoimmune inflammatory connective tissue disease of unknown cause that occurs most often in women
Excludes1 lupus erythematosus (discoid) (NOS) (L93.0)

M32.0 Drug-induced systemic lupus erythematosus
Use additional code for adverse effect, if applicable, to identify drug (T36-T50 with fifth or sixth character 5)

M32.1 Systemic lupus erythematosus with organ or system involvement

M32.10 Systemic lupus erythematosus, organ or system involvement unspecified

M32.11 Endocarditis in systemic lupus erythematosus
Libman-Sacks disease
CC when PDx is its own CC
Ex: I38-I39, I87.8-I87.9, I99.8-I99.9

M32.12 Pericarditis in systemic lupus erythematosus
Lupus pericarditis
CC when PDx is its own CC
Ex: I01.0, I09.2, I30.0-I30.9, I31.3-I32, I87.8-I87.9, I99.8-I99.9

M32.13 Lung involvement in systemic lupus erythematosus
Pleural effusion due to systemic lupus erythematosus

M32.14 Glomerular disease in systemic lupus erythematosus
Lupus renal disease NOS

M32.15 Tubulo-interstitial nephropathy in systemic lupus erythematosus

M32.19 Other organ or system involvement in systemic lupus erythematosus

M32.8 Other forms of systemic lupus erythematosus

M32.9 Systemic lupus erythematosus, unspecified
SLE NOS
Systemic lupus erythematosus NOS
Systemic lupus erythematosus without organ involvement

M33 Dermatopolymyositis
Ex: For category M33 CC codes unless otherwise indicated: M33.00-M33.19, M33.90-M33.99, M36.0

M33.0 Juvenile dermatopolymyositis

M33.00 Juvenile dermatopolymyositis, organ involvement unspecified

M33.01 Juvenile dermatopolymyositis with respiratory involvement

M33.02 Juvenile dermatopolymyositis with myopathy
CC when PDx is its own CC
Ex: E08.40-E08.49, E08.618-E08.638, E08.649-E08.8, E09.40-E09.49, E09.618-E09.638, E09.649-E09.8, E10.40-E10.49, E10.618-E10.638, E10.649, E10.69-E10.8, E11.40-E11.49, E11.618-E11.638, E11.649, E11.69-E11.8, E13.40-E13.49, E13.618-E13.638, E13.649-E13.8, G32.89, G70.00-G72.3, G72.81-G73.7, G96.8-G96.9, G98.0-G98.8, G99.8, M33.00-M33.19, M33.90-M33.99, M36.0

M33.09 Juvenile dermatopolymyositis with other organ involvement

M33.1 Other dermatopolymyositis

M33.10 Other dermatopolymyositis, organ involvement unspecified

M33.11 Other dermatopolymyositis with respiratory involvement

M33.12 Other dermatopolymyositis with myopathy
CC when PDx is its own CC
Ex: See M33.02

M33.19 Other dermatopolymyositis with other organ involvement

M33.2 Polymyositis

M33.20 Polymyositis, organ involvement unspecified
Ex: M33.20-M33.29

M33.21 Polymyositis with respiratory involvement
Ex: M33.20-M33.29

M33.22 Polymyositis with myopathy
CC when PDx is its own CC
Ex: E08.40-E08.49, E08.618-E08.638, E08.649-E08.8, E09.40-E09.49, E09.618-E09.638, E09.649-E09.8, E10.40-E10.49, E10.618-E10.638, E10.649, E10.69-E10.8, E11.40-E11.49, E11.618-E11.638, E11.649, E11.69-E11.8, E13.40-E13.49, E13.618-E13.638, E13.649-E13.8, G32.89, G70.00-G72.3, G72.81-G73.7, G96.8-G96.9, G98.0-G98.8, G99.8, M33.20-M33.29

M33.29 Polymyositis with other organ involvement
Ex: M33.20-M33.29

M33.9 Dermatopolymyositis, unspecified

M33.90 Dermatopolymyositis, unspecified, organ involvement unspecified

M33.91 Dermatopolymyositis, unspecified with respiratory involvement

M33.92 Dermatopolymyositis, unspecified with myopathy
CC when PDx is its own CC
Ex: See M33.02

M33.99 Dermatopolymyositis, unspecified with other organ involvement

M34 Systemic sclerosis [scleroderma]
Excludes1 circumscribed scleroderma (L94.0)
neonatal scleroderma (P83.8)

M34.0 Progressive systemic sclerosis

M34.1 CR(E)ST syndrome
Combination of calcinosis, Raynaud's phenomenon, esophageal dysfunction, sclerodactyly, telangiectasia

M34.2 Systemic sclerosis induced by drug and chemical
Code first poisoning due to drug or toxin, if applicable (T36-T65 with fifth or sixth character 1-4 or 6)
Use additional code for adverse effect, if applicable, to identify drug (T36-T50 with fifth or sixth character 5)

Item 13-8 Polymyalgia rheumatica is a syndrome characterized by aching and morning stiffness and is related to aging and hereditary predisposition.

M34.8 Other forms of systemic sclerosis

M34.81 Systemic sclerosis with lung involvement
CC when PDx is its own CC
Ex: No exclusions

M34.82 Systemic sclerosis with myopathy
CC when PDx is its own CC
Ex: E08.40-E08.49, E08.618-E08.638, E08.649-E08.8, E09.40-E09.49, E09.618-E09.638, E09.649-E09.8, E10.40-E10.49, E10.618-E10.638, E10.649, E10.69-E10.8, E11.40-E11.49, E11.618-E11.638, E11.649, E11.69-E11.8, E13.40-E13.49, E13.618-E13.638, E13.649-E13.8, G32.89, G70.00-G72.3, G72.81-G73.7, G96.8-G96.9, G98.0-G98.8, G99.8

M34.83 Systemic sclerosis with polyneuropathy

M34.89 Other systemic sclerosis

M34.9 Systemic sclerosis, unspecified

M35 Other systemic involvement of connective tissue
Excludes1 reactive perforating collagenosis (L87.1)

M35.0 Sicca syndrome [Sjögren]

M35.00 Sicca syndrome, unspecified

M35.01 Sicca syndrome with keratoconjunctivitis

M35.02 Sicca syndrome with lung involvement

M35.03 Sicca syndrome with myopathy
CC when PDx is its own CC
Ex: See M34.82

M35.04 Sicca syndrome with tubulo-interstitial nephropathy
Renal tubular acidosis in sicca syndrome

M35.09 Sicca syndrome with other organ involvement

M35.1 Other overlap syndromes
Mixed connective tissue disease
Excludes1 polyangiitis overlap syndrome (M30.8)
Ex: G72.41-G72.49, M35.1, M35.5, M35.8

M35.2 Behçet's disease
Ex: See M01.X

M35.3 Polymyalgia rheumatica
Excludes1 polymyalgia rheumatica with giant cell arteritis (M31.5)

M35.4 Diffuse (eosinophilic) fasciitis

M35.5 Multifocal fibrosclerosis
Ex: G72.41-G72.49, M35.1, M35.5, M35.8

M35.6 Relapsing panniculitis [Weber-Christian]
Excludes1 lupus panniculitis (L93.2)
panniculitis NOS (M79.3-)

M35.7 Hypermobility syndrome
Familial ligamentous laxity
Excludes1 Ehlers-Danlos syndrome (Q79.6)
ligamentous laxity, NOS (M24.2-)

M35.8 Other specified systemic involvement of connective tissue
Ex: G72.41-G72.49, M35.1, M35.5, M35.8

M35.9 Systemic involvement of connective tissue, unspecified
Autoimmune disease (systemic) NOS
Collagen (vascular) disease NOS

M36 Systemic disorders of connective tissue in diseases classified elsewhere
Excludes2 arthropathies in diseases classified elsewhere (M14.-)

M36.0 Dermato(poly)myositis in neoplastic disease
Code first underlying neoplasm (C00-D49)
Ex: M33.00-M33.19, M33.90-M33.99, M36.0

M36.1 Arthropathy in neoplastic disease
Code first underlying neoplasm, such as:
leukemia (C91-C95)
malignant histiocytosis (C96.A)
multiple myeloma (C90.0)

M36.2 Hemophilic arthropathy
Hemarthrosis in hemophilic arthropathy
Code first underlying disease, such as:
factor VIII deficiency (D66)
with vascular defect (D68.0)
factor IX deficiency (D67)
hemophilia (classical) (D66)
hemophilia B (D67)
hemophilia C (D68.1)

M36.3 Arthropathy in other blood disorders

M36.4 Arthropathy in hypersensitivity reactions classified elsewhere
Code first underlying disease, such as:
Henoch (-Schönlein) purpura (D69.0)
serum sickness (T80.6-)

M36.8 Systemic disorders of connective tissue in other diseases classified elsewhere
Code first underlying disease, such as:
alkaptonuria (E70.2)
hypogammaglobulinemia (D80.-)
ochronosis (E70.2)

DORSOPATHIES (M40-M54)

DEFORMING DORSOPATHIES (M40-M43)

M40 Kyphosis and lordosis
Excludes1 congenital kyphosis and lordosis (Q76.4)
kyphoscoliosis (M41.-)
postprocedural kyphosis and lordosis (M96.-)

M40.0 Postural kyphosis
Excludes1 osteochondrosis of spine (M42.-)

M40.00 Postural kyphosis, site unspecified

M40.03 Postural kyphosis, cervicothoracic region

M40.04 Postural kyphosis, thoracic region

M40.05 Postural kyphosis, thoracolumbar region

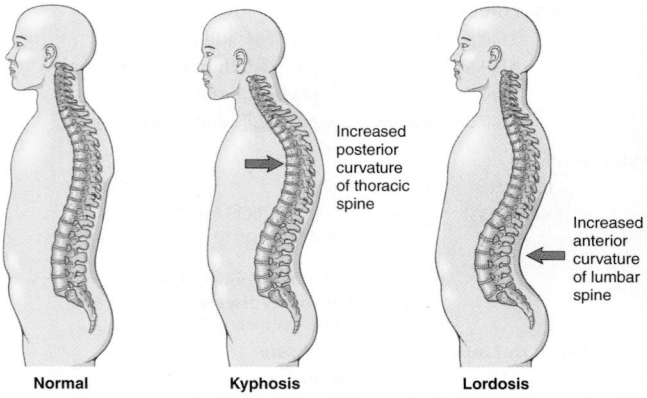

Figure 13-5 Kyphosis, Lordosis, Scoliosis. (From Chabner: The Language of Medicine, ed 8, St. Louis, Saunders, 2007)

Item 13–9 Kyphosis is an abnormal curvature of the spine. **Senile kyphosis** is a result of disc degeneration causing ossification (turning to bone). **Adolescent** or **juvenile** kyphosis is also known as **Scheuermann's disease,** a condition in which the discs of the lower thoracic spine herniate, causing the disc space to narrow and the spine to tilt forward. This condition is attributed to poor posture. Lordosis or swayback is an abnormal curvature of the spine resulting in an inward curve of the lumbar spine just above the buttocks. Scoliosis causes a sideways curve to the spine. The curves are S- or C-shaped, and it is most commonly acquired in late childhood and early teen years, when growth is fast.

- **M40.1 Other secondary kyphosis**
  - **M40.10 Other secondary kyphosis, site unspecified**
  - **M40.12 Other secondary kyphosis, cervical region**
  - **M40.13 Other secondary kyphosis, cervicothoracic region**
  - **M40.14 Other secondary kyphosis, thoracic region**
  - **M40.15 Other secondary kyphosis, thoracolumbar region**
- **M40.2 Other and unspecified kyphosis**
  - **M40.20 Unspecified kyphosis**
    - **M40.202 Unspecified kyphosis, cervical region**
    - **M40.203 Unspecified kyphosis, cervicothoracic region**
    - **M40.204 Unspecified kyphosis, thoracic region**
    - **M40.205 Unspecified kyphosis, thoracolumbar region**
    - **M40.209 Unspecified kyphosis, site unspecified**
  - **M40.29 Other kyphosis**
    - **M40.292 Other kyphosis, cervical region**
    - **M40.293 Other kyphosis, cervicothoracic region**
    - **M40.294 Other kyphosis, thoracic region**
    - **M40.295 Other kyphosis, thoracolumbar region**
    - **M40.299 Other kyphosis, site unspecified**
- **M40.3 Flatback syndrome**
  - **M40.30 Flatback syndrome, site unspecified**
  - **M40.35 Flatback syndrome, thoracolumbar region**
  - **M40.36 Flatback syndrome, lumbar region**
  - **M40.37 Flatback syndrome, lumbosacral region**
- **M40.4 Postural lordosis**
  - *Abnormal increase in the normal curvature of the lumbar spine (sway back)*
  - Acquired lordosis
  - **M40.40 Postural lordosis, site unspecified**
  - **M40.45 Postural lordosis, thoracolumbar region**
  - **M40.46 Postural lordosis, lumbar region**
  - **M40.47 Postural lordosis, lumbosacral region**
- **M40.5 Lordosis, unspecified**
  - **M40.50 Lordosis, unspecified, site unspecified**
  - **M40.55 Lordosis, unspecified, thoracolumbar region**
  - **M40.56 Lordosis, unspecified, lumbar region**
  - **M40.57 Lordosis, unspecified, lumbosacral region**

- **M41 Scoliosis**
  - **Includes** kyphoscoliosis
  - **Excludes1** congenital scoliosis NOS (Q67.5)
    congenital scoliosis due to bony malformation (Q76.3)
    postural congenital scoliosis (Q67.5)
    kyphoscoliotic heart disease (I27.1)
    postprocedural scoliosis (M96.-)
- **M41.0 Infantile idiopathic scoliosis**
  - **M41.00 Infantile idiopathic scoliosis, site unspecified**
  - **M41.02 Infantile idiopathic scoliosis, cervical region**
  - **M41.03 Infantile idiopathic scoliosis, cervicothoracic region**
  - **M41.04 Infantile idiopathic scoliosis, thoracic region**
  - **M41.05 Infantile idiopathic scoliosis, thoracolumbar region**
  - **M41.06 Infantile idiopathic scoliosis, lumbar region**
  - **M41.07 Infantile idiopathic scoliosis, lumbosacral region**
  - **M41.08 Infantile idiopathic scoliosis, sacral and sacrococcygeal region**
- **M41.1 Juvenile and adolescent idiopathic scoliosis**
  - **M41.11 Juvenile idiopathic scoliosis**
    - **M41.112 Juvenile idiopathic scoliosis, cervical region**
    - **M41.113 Juvenile idiopathic scoliosis, cervicothoracic region**
    - **M41.114 Juvenile idiopathic scoliosis, thoracic region**
    - **M41.115 Juvenile idiopathic scoliosis, thoracolumbar region**
    - **M41.116 Juvenile idiopathic scoliosis, lumbar region**
    - **M41.117 Juvenile idiopathic scoliosis, lumbosacral region**
    - **M41.119 Juvenile idiopathic scoliosis, site unspecified**
  - **M41.12 Adolescent scoliosis**
    - **M41.122 Adolescent idiopathic scoliosis, cervical region**
    - **M41.123 Adolescent idiopathic scoliosis, cervicothoracic region**
    - **M41.124 Adolescent idiopathic scoliosis, thoracic region**
    - **M41.125 Adolescent idiopathic scoliosis, thoracolumbar region**
    - **M41.126 Adolescent idiopathic scoliosis, lumbar region**
    - **M41.127 Adolescent idiopathic scoliosis, lumbosacral region**
    - **M41.129 Adolescent idiopathic scoliosis, site unspecified**
- **M41.2 Other idiopathic scoliosis**
  - **M41.20 Other idiopathic scoliosis, site unspecified**
  - **M41.22 Other idiopathic scoliosis, cervical region**
  - **M41.23 Other idiopathic scoliosis, cervicothoracic region**
  - **M41.24 Other idiopathic scoliosis, thoracic region**
  - **M41.25 Other idiopathic scoliosis, thoracolumbar region**
  - **M41.26 Other idiopathic scoliosis, lumbar region**
  - **M41.27 Other idiopathic scoliosis, lumbosacral region**
- **M41.3 Thoracogenic scoliosis**
  - **M41.30 Thoracogenic scoliosis, site unspecified**
  - **M41.34 Thoracogenic scoliosis, thoracic region**
  - **M41.35 Thoracogenic scoliosis, thoracolumbar region**
- **M41.4 Neuromuscular scoliosis**
  - Scoliosis secondary to cerebral palsy, Friedreich's ataxia, poliomyelitis and other neuromuscular disorders
  - Code also underlying condition
  - **M41.40 Neuromuscular scoliosis, site unspecified**
  - **M41.41 Neuromuscular scoliosis, occipito-atlanto-axial region**
  - **M41.42 Neuromuscular scoliosis, cervical region**
  - **M41.43 Neuromuscular scoliosis, cervicothoracic region**
  - **M41.44 Neuromuscular scoliosis, thoracic region**
  - **M41.45 Neuromuscular scoliosis, thoracolumbar region**
  - **M41.46 Neuromuscular scoliosis, lumbar region**
  - **M41.47 Neuromuscular scoliosis, lumbosacral region**

◀ New ◀ Revised ~~deleted~~ Deleted Excludes 1 Excludes 2 Includes Use additional Code first Code also Unspecified
OGCR Official Guidelines ● Unacceptable Principal Diagnosis X Assign placeholder X ● Use Additional Character(s) ▶ Manifestation Code Coding Clinic

- **M41.5 Other secondary scoliosis**
  - **M41.50 Other secondary scoliosis, site unspecified**
  - **M41.52 Other secondary scoliosis, cervical region**
  - **M41.53 Other secondary scoliosis, cervicothoracic region**
  - **M41.54 Other secondary scoliosis, thoracic region**
  - **M41.55 Other secondary scoliosis, thoracolumbar region**
  - **M41.56 Other secondary scoliosis, lumbar region**
  - **M41.57 Other secondary scoliosis, lumbosacral region**
- **M41.8 Other forms of scoliosis**
  - **M41.80 Other forms of scoliosis, site unspecified**
  - **M41.82 Other forms of scoliosis, cervical region**
  - **M41.83 Other forms of scoliosis, cervicothoracic region**
  - **M41.84 Other forms of scoliosis, thoracic region**
  - **M41.85 Other forms of scoliosis, thoracolumbar region**
  - **M41.86 Other forms of scoliosis, lumbar region**
  - **M41.87 Other forms of scoliosis, lumbosacral region**
- **M41.9 Scoliosis, unspecified**

- **M42 Spinal osteochondrosis**
  - **M42.0 Juvenile osteochondrosis of spine**
    Calvé's disease
    Scheuermann's disease
    Excludes1 postural kyphosis (M40.0)
    - **M42.00 Juvenile osteochondrosis of spine, site unspecified**
    - **M42.01 Juvenile osteochondrosis of spine, occipito-atlanto-axial region**
    - **M42.02 Juvenile osteochondrosis of spine, cervical region**
    - **M42.03 Juvenile osteochondrosis of spine, cervicothoracic region**
    - **M42.04 Juvenile osteochondrosis of spine, thoracic region**
    - **M42.05 Juvenile osteochondrosis of spine, thoracolumbar region**
    - **M42.06 Juvenile osteochondrosis of spine, lumbar region**
    - **M42.07 Juvenile osteochondrosis of spine, lumbosacral region**
    - **M42.08 Juvenile osteochondrosis of spine, sacral and sacrococcygeal region**
    - **M42.09 Juvenile osteochondrosis of spine, multiple sites in spine**
  - **M42.1 Adult osteochondrosis of spine**
    - **M42.10 Adult osteochondrosis of spine, site unspecified** A
    - **M42.11 Adult osteochondrosis of spine, occipitoatlanto-axial region** A
    - **M42.12 Adult osteochondrosis of spine, cervical region** A
    - **M42.13 Adult osteochondrosis of spine, cervicothoracic region** A
    - **M42.14 Adult osteochondrosis of spine, thoracic region** A
    - **M42.15 Adult osteochondrosis of spine, thoracolumbar region** A
    - **M42.16 Adult osteochondrosis of spine, lumbar region** A
    - **M42.17 Adult osteochondrosis of spine, lumbosacral region** A
    - **M42.18 Adult osteochondrosis of spine, sacral and sacrococcygeal region** A
    - **M42.19 Adult osteochondrosis of spine, multiple sites in spine** A
  - **M42.9 Spinal osteochondrosis, unspecified**

Item 13-10 Spondylolisthesis is a condition caused by the slipping forward of one disc over another.

- **M43 Other deforming dorsopathies**
  Excludes1 congenital spondylolysis and spondylolisthesis (Q76.2)
  hemivertebra (Q76.3-Q76.4)
  Klippel-Feil syndrome (Q76.1)
  lumbarization and sacralization (Q76.4)
  platyspondylisis (Q76.4)
  spina bifida occulta (Q76.0)
  spinal curvature in osteoporosis (M80.-)
  spinal curvature in Paget's disease of bone [osteitis deformans] (M88.-)
  - **M43.0 Spondylolysis**
    Excludes1 congenital spondylolysis (Q76.2)
    spondylolisthesis (M43.1)
    - **M43.00 Spondylolysis, site unspecified**
    - **M43.01 Spondylolysis, occipito-atlanto-axial region**
    - **M43.02 Spondylolysis, cervical region**
    - **M43.03 Spondylolysis, cervicothoracic region**
    - **M43.04 Spondylolysis, thoracic region**
    - **M43.05 Spondylolysis, thoracolumbar region**
    - **M43.06 Spondylolysis, lumbar region**
    - **M43.07 Spondylolysis, lumbosacral region**
    - **M43.08 Spondylolysis, sacral and sacrococcygeal region**
    - **M43.09 Spondylolysis, multiple sites in spine**
  - **M43.1 Spondylolisthesis**
    Excludes1 acute traumatic of lumbosacral region (S33.1)
    acute traumatic of sites other than lumbosacral - code to Fracture, vertebra, by region
    congenital spondylolisthesis (Q76.2)
    - **M43.10 Spondylolisthesis, site unspecified**
    - **M43.11 Spondylolisthesis, occipito-atlanto-axial region**
    - **M43.12 Spondylolisthesis, cervical region**
    - **M43.13 Spondylolisthesis, cervicothoracic region**
    - **M43.14 Spondylolisthesis, thoracic region**
    - **M43.15 Spondylolisthesis, thoracolumbar region**
    - **M43.16 Spondylolisthesis, lumbar region**
    - **M43.17 Spondylolisthesis, lumbosacral region**
    - **M43.18 Spondylolisthesis, sacral and sacrococcygeal region**
    - **M43.19 Spondylolisthesis, multiple sites in spine**
  - **M43.2 Fusion of spine**
    Ankylosis of spinal joint
    Excludes1 ankylosing spondylitis (M45.0-)
    congenital fusion of spine (Q76.4)
    Excludes2 arthrodesis status (Z98.1)
    pseudoarthrosis after fusion or arthrodesis (M96.0)
    - **M43.20 Fusion of spine, site unspecified**
    - **M43.21 Fusion of spine, occipito-atlanto-axial region**
    - **M43.22 Fusion of spine, cervical region**
    - **M43.23 Fusion of spine, cervicothoracic region**
    - **M43.24 Fusion of spine, thoracic region**
    - **M43.25 Fusion of spine, thoracolumbar region**
    - **M43.26 Fusion of spine, lumbar region**
    - **M43.27 Fusion of spine, lumbosacral region**
    - **M43.28 Fusion of spine, sacral and sacrococcygeal region**
  - **M43.3 Recurrent atlantoaxial dislocation with myelopathy**
  - **M43.4 Other recurrent atlantoaxial dislocation**

M43.5 Other recurrent vertebral dislocation

Excludes1 biomechanical lesions NEC (M99.-)

M43.5X Other recurrent vertebral dislocation

- **M43.5X2 Other recurrent vertebral dislocation, cervical region**
- **M43.5X3 Other recurrent vertebral dislocation, cervicothoracic region**
- **M43.5X4 Other recurrent vertebral dislocation, thoracic region**
- **M43.5X5 Other recurrent vertebral dislocation, thoracolumbar region**
- **M43.5X6 Other recurrent vertebral dislocation, lumbar region**
- **M43.5X7 Other recurrent vertebral dislocation, lumbosacral region**
- **M43.5X8 Other recurrent vertebral dislocation, sacral and sacrococcygeal region**
- **M43.5X9 Other recurrent vertebral dislocation, site unspecified**

M43.6 Torticollis

Excludes1 congenital (sternomastoid) torticollis (Q68.0)
current injury - see Injury, of spine, by body region ocular torticollis (R29.891)
psychogenic torticollis (F45.8)
spasmodic torticollis (G24.3)
torticollis due to birth injury (P15.2)

M43.8 Other specified deforming dorsopathies

Excludes2 kyphosis and lordosis (M40.-)
scoliosis (M41.-)

M43.8X Other specified deforming dorsopathies

- **M43.8X1 Other specified deforming dorsopathies, occipito-atlanto-axial region**
- **M43.8X2 Other specified deforming dorsopathies, cervical region**
- **M43.8X3 Other specified deforming dorsopathies, cervicothoracic region**
- **M43.8X4 Other specified deforming dorsopathies, thoracic region**
- **M43.8X5 Other specified deforming dorsopathies, thoracolumbar region**
- **M43.8X6 Other specified deforming dorsopathies, lumbar region**
- **M43.8X7 Other specified deforming dorsopathies, lumbosacral region**
- **M43.8X8 Other specified deforming dorsopathies, sacral and sacrococcygeal region**
- **M43.8X9 Other specified deforming dorsopathies, site unspecified**

M43.9 Deforming dorsopathy, unspecified
Curvature of spine NOS

SPONDYLOPATHIES (M45-M49)

M45 Ankylosing spondylitis
Rheumatoid arthritis of spine

Excludes1 arthropathy in Reiter's disease (M02.3-)
juvenile (ankylosing) spondylitis (M08.1)

Excludes2 Behçet's disease (M35.2)

- **M45.0 Ankylosing spondylitis of multiple sites in spine**
- **M45.1 Ankylosing spondylitis of occipito-atlanto-axial region**
- **M45.2 Ankylosing spondylitis of cervical region**
- **M45.3 Ankylosing spondylitis of cervicothoracic region**
- **M45.4 Ankylosing spondylitis of thoracic region**
- **M45.5 Ankylosing spondylitis of thoracolumbar region**
- **M45.6 Ankylosing spondylitis lumbar region**
- **M45.7 Ankylosing spondylitis of lumbosacral region**
- **M45.8 Ankylosing spondylitis sacral and sacrococcygeal region**
- **M45.9 Ankylosing spondylitis of unspecified sites in spine**

M46 Other inflammatory spondylopathies

M46.0 Spinal enthesopathy
Disorder of ligamentous or muscular attachments of spine

- **M46.00 Spinal enthesopathy, site unspecified**
- **M46.01 Spinal enthesopathy, occipito-atlanto-axial region**
- **M46.02 Spinal enthesopathy, cervical region**
- **M46.03 Spinal enthesopathy, cervicothoracic region**
- **M46.04 Spinal enthesopathy, thoracic region**
- **M46.05 Spinal enthesopathy, thoracolumbar region**
- **M46.06 Spinal enthesopathy, lumbar region**
- **M46.07 Spinal enthesopathy, lumbosacral region**
- **M46.08 Spinal enthesopathy, sacral and sacrococcygeal region**
- **M46.09 Spinal enthesopathy, multiple sites in spine**

M46.1 Sacroiliitis, not elsewhere classified

M46.2 Osteomyelitis of vertebra

Ex: **For category M46.2 CC codes:** A02.24, A17.9, A18.03, A18.09, A18.82, A18.84, A18.89, M46.20-M46.39, M86.00-M86.9

- **M46.20 Osteomyelitis of vertebra, site unspecified**
- **M46.21 Osteomyelitis of vertebra, occipito-atlanto-axial region**
- **M46.22 Osteomyelitis of vertebra, cervical region**
- **M46.23 Osteomyelitis of vertebra, cervicothoracic region**
- **M46.24 Osteomyelitis of vertebra, thoracic region**
- **M46.25 Osteomyelitis of vertebra, thoracolumbar region**
- **M46.26 Osteomyelitis of vertebra, lumbar region**
- **M46.27 Osteomyelitis of vertebra, lumbosacral region**
- **M46.28 Osteomyelitis of vertebra, sacral and sacrococcygeal region**

M46.3 Infection of intervertebral disc (pyogenic)

Use additional code (B95-B97) to identify infectious agent

Ex: **For category M46.3 CC codes:** A17.9, A18.01, A18.03, A18.09, A18.82, A18.84, A18.89, M46.20-M46.39, M86.00-M86.9

- **M46.30 Infection of intervertebral disc (pyogenic), site unspecified**
- **M46.31 Infection of intervertebral disc (pyogenic), occipito-atlanto-axial region**
- **M46.32 Infection of intervertebral disc (pyogenic), cervical region**
- **M46.33 Infection of intervertebral disc (pyogenic), cervicothoracic region**
- **M46.34 Infection of intervertebral disc (pyogenic), thoracic region**
- **M46.35 Infection of intervertebral disc (pyogenic), thoracolumbar region**
- **M46.36 Infection of intervertebral disc (pyogenic), lumbar region**
- **M46.37 Infection of intervertebral disc (pyogenic), lumbosacral region**
- **M46.38 Infection of intervertebral disc (pyogenic), sacral and sacrococcygeal region**
- **M46.39 Infection of intervertebral disc (pyogenic), multiple sites in spine**

M46.4 Discitis, unspecified

- **M46.40 Discitis, unspecified, site unspecified**
- **M46.41 Discitis, unspecified, occipito-atlanto-axial region**
- **M46.42 Discitis, unspecified, cervical region**
- **M46.43 Discitis, unspecified, cervicothoracic region**
- **M46.44 Discitis, unspecified, thoracic region**

M46.45 Discitis, unspecified, thoracolumbar region
M46.46 Discitis, unspecified, lumbar region
M46.47 Discitis, unspecified, lumbosacral region
M46.48 Discitis, unspecified, sacral and sacrococcygeal region
M46.49 Discitis, unspecified, multiple sites in spine

● M46.5 Other infective spondylopathies
M46.50 Other infective spondylopathies, site unspecified
M46.51 Other infective spondylopathies, occipitoatlanto-axial region
M46.52 Other infective spondylopathies, cervical region
M46.53 Other infective spondylopathies, cervicothoracic region
M46.54 Other infective spondylopathies, thoracic region
M46.55 Other infective spondylopathies, thoracolumbar region
M46.56 Other infective spondylopathies, lumbar region
M46.57 Other infective spondylopathies, lumbosacral region
M46.58 Other infective spondylopathies, sacral and sacrococcygeal region
M46.59 Other infective spondylopathies, multiple sites in spine

● M46.8 Other specified inflammatory spondylopathies
M46.80 Other specified inflammatory spondylopathies, site unspecified
M46.81 Other specified inflammatory spondylopathies, occipito-atlanto-axial region
M46.82 Other specified inflammatory spondylopathies, cervical region
M46.83 Other specified inflammatory spondylopathies, cervicothoracic region
M46.84 Other specified inflammatory spondylopathies, thoracic region
M46.85 Other specified inflammatory spondylopathies, thoracolumbar region
M46.86 Other specified inflammatory spondylopathies, lumbar region
M46.87 Other specified inflammatory spondylopathies, lumbosacral region
M46.88 Other specified inflammatory spondylopathies, sacral and sacrococcygeal region
M46.89 Other specified inflammatory spondylopathies, multiple sites in spine

● M46.9 Unspecified inflammatory spondylopathy
M46.90 Unspecified inflammatory spondylopathy, site unspecified
M46.91 Unspecified inflammatory spondylopathy, occipito-atlanto-axial region
M46.92 Unspecified inflammatory spondylopathy, cervical region
M46.93 Unspecified inflammatory spondylopathy, cervicothoracic region
M46.94 Unspecified inflammatory spondylopathy, thoracic region
M46.95 Unspecified inflammatory spondylopathy, thoracolumbar region
M46.96 Unspecified inflammatory spondylopathy, lumbar region
M46.97 Unspecified inflammatory spondylopathy, lumbosacral region
M46.98 Unspecified inflammatory spondylopathy, sacral and sacrococcygeal region
M46.99 Unspecified inflammatory spondylopathy, multiple sites in spine

● M47 Spondylosis
Includes arthrosis or osteoarthritis of spine
degeneration of facet joints

● M47.0 Anterior spinal and vertebral artery compression syndromes
Ex: For category M47.0 CC codes: M47.011-M47.029, M47.11-M47.13, M47.21-M47.23, M47.811-M47.813, M47.891-M47.893

● M47.01 Anterior spinal artery compression syndromes
M47.011 Anterior spinal artery compression syndromes, occipito-atlanto-axial region
M47.012 Anterior spinal artery compression syndromes, cervical region
M47.013 Anterior spinal artery compression syndromes, cervicothoracic region
M47.014 Anterior spinal artery compression syndromes, thoracic region
M47.015 Anterior spinal artery compression syndromes, thoracolumbar region
M47.016 Anterior spinal artery compression syndromes, lumbar region
M47.019 Anterior spinal artery compression syndromes, site unspecified

● M47.02 Vertebral artery compression syndromes
M47.021 Vertebral artery compression syndromes, occipito-atlanto-axial region
M47.022 Vertebral artery compression syndromes, cervical region
M47.029 Vertebral artery compression syndromes, site unspecified

● M47.1 Other spondylosis with myelopathy
Spondylogenic compression of spinal cord
Excludes1 vertebral subluxation (M43.3-M43.59)
M47.10 Other spondylosis with myelopathy, site unspecified
Ex: M25.78, M47.011-M47.16, M47.20-M47.9, M48.10-M48.38, M48.9
M47.11 Other spondylosis with myelopathy, occipito-atlanto-axial region
Ex: See M47.0
M47.12 Other spondylosis with myelopathy, cervical region
Ex: See M47.0
M47.13 Other spondylosis with myelopathy, cervicothoracic region
Ex: See M47.0
M47.14 Other spondylosis with myelopathy, thoracic region
Ex: M47.14-M47.15
M47.15 Other spondylosis with myelopathy, thoracolumbar region
Ex: M47.14-M47.15
M47.16 Other spondylosis with myelopathy, lumbar region
Ex: M46.40, M46.46-M46.49, M47.16, M47.26-M47.28, M47.816-M47.818, M47.896-M47.898, M51.06, M51.26-M51.27, M51.36-M51.37, M51.46-M51.47, M51.86-M51.9

● M47.2 Other spondylosis with radiculopathy
M47.20 Other spondylosis with radiculopathy, site unspecified
M47.21 Other spondylosis with radiculopathy, occipito-atlanto-axial region
M47.22 Other spondylosis with radiculopathy, cervical region
M47.23 Other spondylosis with radiculopathy, cervicothoracic region
M47.24 Other spondylosis with radiculopathy, thoracic region

M47.25 Other spondylosis with radiculopathy, thoracolumbar region
M47.26 Other spondylosis with radiculopathy, lumbar region
M47.27 Other spondylosis with radiculopathy, lumbosacral region
M47.28 Other spondylosis with radiculopathy, sacral and sacrococcygeal region

● M47.8 Other spondylosis
● M47.81 Spondylosis without myelopathy or radiculopathy
M47.811 Spondylosis without myelopathy or radiculopathy, occipito-atlanto-axial region
M47.812 Spondylosis without myelopathy or radiculopathy, cervical region
M47.813 Spondylosis without myelopathy or radiculopathy, cervicothoracic region
M47.814 Spondylosis without myelopathy or radiculopathy, thoracic region
M47.815 Spondylosis without myelopathy or radiculopathy, thoracolumbar region
M47.816 Spondylosis without myelopathy or radiculopathy, lumbar region
M47.817 Spondylosis without myelopathy or radiculopathy, lumbosacral region
M47.818 Spondylosis without myelopathy or radiculopathy, sacral and sacrococcygeal region
M47.819 Spondylosis without myelopathy or radiculopathy, site unspecified
● M47.89 Other spondylosis
M47.891 Other spondylosis, occipito-atlanto-axial region
M47.892 Other spondylosis, cervical region
M47.893 Other spondylosis, cervicothoracic region
M47.894 Other spondylosis, thoracic region
M47.895 Other spondylosis, thoracolumbar region
M47.896 Other spondylosis, lumbar region
M47.897 Other spondylosis, lumbosacral region
M47.898 Other spondylosis, sacral and sacrococcygeal region
M47.899 Other spondylosis, site unspecified
M47.9 Spondylosis, unspecified

● M48 Other spondylopathies
● M48.0 Spinal stenosis
Caudal stenosis
M48.00 Spinal stenosis, site unspecified
M48.01 Spinal stenosis, occipito-atlanto-axial region
M48.02 Spinal stenosis, cervical region
M48.03 Spinal stenosis, cervicothoracic region
M48.04 Spinal stenosis, thoracic region
M48.05 Spinal stenosis, thoracolumbar region
M48.06 Spinal stenosis, lumbar region
M48.07 Spinal stenosis, lumbosacral region
M48.08 Spinal stenosis, sacral and sacrococcygeal region
● M48.1 Ankylosing hyperostosis [Forestier]
Diffuse idiopathic skeletal hyperostosis [DISH]
M48.10 Ankylosing hyperostosis [Forestier], site unspecified
M48.11 Ankylosing hyperostosis [Forestier], occipito-atlanto-axial region
M48.12 Ankylosing hyperostosis [Forestier], cervical region
M48.13 Ankylosing hyperostosis [Forestier], cervicothoracic region
M48.14 Ankylosing hyperostosis [Forestier], thoracic region
M48.15 Ankylosing hyperostosis [Forestier], thoracolumbar region
M48.16 Ankylosing hyperostosis [Forestier], lumbar region
M48.17 Ankylosing hyperostosis [Forestier], lumbosacral region
M48.18 Ankylosing hyperostosis [Forestier], sacral and sacrococcygeal region
M48.19 Ankylosing hyperostosis [Forestier], multiple sites in spine
● M48.2 Kissing spine
M48.20 Kissing spine, site unspecified
M48.21 Kissing spine, occipito-atlanto-axial region
M48.22 Kissing spine, cervical region
M48.23 Kissing spine, cervicothoracic region
M48.24 Kissing spine, thoracic region
M48.25 Kissing spine, thoracolumbar region
M48.26 Kissing spine, lumbar region
M48.27 Kissing spine, lumbosacral region
● M48.3 Traumatic spondylopathy
Ex. For category M48.3 CC codes: M48.30-M48.38
M48.30 Traumatic spondylopathy, site unspecified
M48.31 Traumatic spondylopathy, occipito-atlanto-axial region
M48.32 Traumatic spondylopathy, cervical region
M48.33 Traumatic spondylopathy, cervicothoracic region
M48.34 Traumatic spondylopathy, thoracic region
M48.35 Traumatic spondylopathy, thoracolumbar region
M48.36 Traumatic spondylopathy, lumbar region
M48.37 Traumatic spondylopathy, lumbosacral region
M48.38 Traumatic spondylopathy, sacral and sacrococcygeal region
● M48.4 Fatigue fracture of vertebra
Stress fracture of vertebra
Excludes1 pathological fracture NOS (M84.4-)
pathological fracture of vertebra due to neoplasm (M84.58)
pathological fracture of vertebra due to other diagnosis (M84.68)
pathological fracture of vertebra due to osteoporosis (M80.-)
traumatic fracture of vertebrae (S12.0-S12.3-, S22.0-, S32.0-)

The appropriate 7th character is to be added to each code from subcategory M48.4:

A	initial encounter for fracture
D	subsequent encounter for fracture with routine healing
G	subsequent encounter for fracture with delayed healing
S	sequela of fracture

X● M48.40 Fatigue fracture of vertebra, site unspecified
X● M48.41 Fatigue fracture of vertebra, occipitoatlanto-axial region
X● M48.42 Fatigue fracture of vertebra, cervical region
X● M48.43 Fatigue fracture of vertebra, cervicothoracic region
X● M48.44 Fatigue fracture of vertebra, thoracic region
X● M48.45 Fatigue fracture of vertebra, thoracolumbar region

X● **M48.46 Fatigue fracture of vertebra, lumbar region**

X● **M48.47 Fatigue fracture of vertebra, lumbosacral region**

X● **M48.48 Fatigue fracture of vertebra, sacral and sacrococcygeal region**

● **M48.5 Collapsed vertebra, not elsewhere classified**

Collapsed vertebra NOS
Compression fracture of vertebra NOS ◀
Wedging of vertebra NOS

Excludes1 current injury - see Injury of spine, by body region
fatigue fracture of vertebra (M48.4)
pathological fracture of vertebra due to neoplasm (M84.58)
pathological fracture of vertebra due to other diagnosis (M84.68)
pathological fracture of vertebra due to osteoporosis (M80.-)
pathological fracture NOS (M84.4-)
stress fracture of vertebra (M48.4-)
traumatic fracture of vertebra (S12.-, S22.-, S32.-)

The appropriate 7th character is to be added to each code from subcategory M48.5:

A	initial encounter for fracture
D	subsequent encounter for fracture with routine healing
G	subsequent encounter for fracture with delayed healing
S	sequela of fracture

Ex: **For category M48.5 CC codes:** M48.40X-M48.58X[A], M80.00X-M80.88X[A], M84.30X-M84.68X[A], M84.750-M84.759[A]

X● **M48.50 Collapsed vertebra, not elsewhere classified, site unspecified** A

X● **M48.51 Collapsed vertebra, not elsewhere classified, occipito-atlanto-axial region** A

X● **M48.52 Collapsed vertebra, not elsewhere classified, cervical region** A

X● **M48.53 Collapsed vertebra, not elsewhere classified, cervicothoracic region** A

X● **M48.54 Collapsed vertebra, not elsewhere classified, thoracic region** A

X● **M48.55 Collapsed vertebra, not elsewhere classified, thoracolumbar region** A

X● **M48.56 Collapsed vertebra, not elsewhere classified, lumbar region** A

X● **M48.57 Collapsed vertebra, not elsewhere classified, lumbosacral region** A

X● **M48.58 Collapsed vertebra, not elsewhere classified, sacral and sacrococcygeal region** A

● **M48.8 Other specified spondylopathies**

Ossification of posterior longitudinal ligament

● **M48.8X Other specified spondylopathies**

M48.8X1 Other specified spondylopathies, occipito-atlanto-axial region

M48.8X2 Other specified spondylopathies, cervical region

M48.8X3 Other specified spondylopathies, cervicothoracic region

M48.8X4 Other specified spondylopathies, thoracic region

M48.8X5 Other specified spondylopathies, thoracolumbar region

M48.8X6 Other specified spondylopathies, lumbar region

M48.8X7 Other specified spondylopathies, lumbosacral region

M48.8X8 Other specified spondylopathies, sacral and sacrococcygeal region

M48.8X9 Other specified spondylopathies, site unspecified

M48.9 Spondylopathy, unspecified

● **M49 Spondylopathies in diseases classified elsewhere**

Includes curvature of spine in diseases classified elsewhere
deformity of spine in diseases classified elsewhere
kyphosis in diseases classified elsewhere
scoliosis in diseases classified elsewhere
spondylopathy in diseases classified elsewhere

Code first underlying disease, such as:
brucellosis (A23.-)
Charcot-Marie-Tooth disease (G60.0)
enterobacterial infections (A01-A04)
osteitis fibrosa cystica (E21.0)

Excludes1 curvature of spine in tuberculosis [Pott's] (A18.01)
enteropathic arthropathies (M07.-)
gonococcal spondylitis (A54.41)
neuropathic [tabes dorsalis] spondylitis (A52.11)
neuropathic spondylopathy in syringomyelia (G95.0)
neuropathic spondylopathy in tabes dorsalis (A52.11)
nonsyphilitic neuropathic spondylopathy NEC (G98.0)
spondylitis in syphilis (acquired) (A52.77)
tuberculous spondylitis (A18.01)
typhoid fever spondylitis (A01.05)

● **M49.8 Spondylopathy in diseases classified elsewhere**

◗ *M49.80 Spondylopathy in diseases classified elsewhere, site unspecified*

◗ *M49.81 Spondylopathy in diseases classified elsewhere, occipito-atlanto-axial region*

◗ *M49.82 Spondylopathy in diseases classified elsewhere, cervical region*

◗ *M49.83 Spondylopathy in diseases classified elsewhere, cervicothoracic region*

◗ *M49.84 Spondylopathy in diseases classified elsewhere, thoracic region*

◗ *M49.85 Spondylopathy in diseases classified elsewhere, thoracolumbar region*

◗ *M49.86 Spondylopathy in diseases classified elsewhere, lumbar region*

◗ *M49.87 Spondylopathy in diseases classified elsewhere, lumbosacral region*

◗ *M49.88 Spondylopathy in diseases classified elsewhere, sacral and sacrococcygeal region*

◗ *M49.89 Spondylopathy in diseases classified elsewhere, multiple sites in spine*

OTHER DORSOPATHIES (M50-M54)

Excludes1 current injury - see injury of spine by body region
discitis NOS (M46.4-)

● **M50 Cervical disc disorders**

Note: Code to the most superior level of disorder.

Includes cervicothoracic disc disorders with cervicalgia
cervicothoracic disc disorders

Coding Clinic: 2016, Q1, P17

● **M50.0 Cervical disc disorder with myelopathy**

Ex: **For category M50.0 CC codes:** M50.00-M50.03, M50.20-M50.23

M50.00 Cervical disc disorder with myelopathy, unspecified cervical region

M50.01 Cervical disc disorder with myelopathy, high cervical region

C2-C3 disc disorder with myelopathy
C3-C4 disc disorder with myelopathy
Coding Clinic: 2016, Q1, P17

● **M50.02 Cervical disc disorder with myelopathy, mid-cervical region**

M50.020 Cervical disc disorder with myelopathy, mid-cervical region, unspecified level ◀

M50.021 Cervical disc disorder at C4-C5 level with myelopathy ◀
C4-C5 disc disorder with myelopathy ◀

M50.022 Cervical disc disorder at C5-C6 level with myelopathy ◀
C5-C6 disc disorder with myelopathy ◀

M50.023 Cervical disc disorder at C6-C7 level with myelopathy ◀
C6-C7 disc disorder with myelopathy ◀

M50.03 Cervical disc disorder with myelopathy, cervicothoracic region
C7-T1 disc disorder with myelopathy

● **M50.1 Cervical disc disorder with radiculopathy**

Excludes2 brachial radiculitis NOS (M54.13)

M50.10 Cervical disc disorder with radiculopathy, unspecified cervical region

M50.11 Cervical disc disorder with radiculopathy, high cervical region
C2-C3 disc disorder with radiculopathy
C3 radiculopathy due to disc disorder
C3-C4 disc disorder with radiculopathy
C4 radiculopathy due to disc disorder

● **M50.12 Cervical disc disorder with radiculopathy, mid-cervical region**

M50.120 Mid-cervical disc disorder, unspecified ◀

M50.121 Cervical disc disorder at C4-C5 level with radiculopathy ◀
C4-C5 disc disorder with radiculopathy ◀
C5 radiculopathy due to disc disorder ◀

M50.122 Cervical disc disorder at C5-C6 level with radiculopathy ◀
C5-C6 disc disorder with radiculopathy ◀
C6 radiculopathy due to disc disorder ◀

M50.123 Cervical disc disorder at C6-C7 level with radiculopathy ◀
C6-C7 disc disorder with radiculopathy ◀
C7 radiculopathy due to disc disorder ◀

M50.13 Cervical disc disorder with radiculopathy, cervicothoracic region
C7-T1 disc disorder with radiculopathy
C8 radiculopathy due to disc disorder

● **M50.2 Other cervical disc displacement**

M50.20 Other cervical disc displacement, unspecified cervical region

M50.21 Other cervical disc displacement, high cervical region
Other C2-C3 cervical disc displacement
Other C3-C4 cervical disc displacement

● **M50.22 Other cervical disc displacement, mid-cervical region**

M50.220 Other cervical disc displacement, mid-cervical region, unspecified level ◀

M50.221 Other cervical disc displacement at C4-C5 level ◀
Other C4-C5 cervical disc displacement ◀

M50.222 Other cervical disc displacement at C5-C6 level ◀
Other C5-C6 cervical disc displacement ◀

M50.223 Other cervical disc displacement at C6-C7 level ◀
Other C6-C7 cervical disc displacement ◀

M50.23 Other cervical disc displacement, cervicothoracic region
Other C7-T1 cervical disc displacement

● **M50.3 Other cervical disc degeneration**

M50.30 Other cervical disc degeneration, unspecified cervical region

M50.31 Other cervical disc degeneration, high cervical region
Other C2-C3 cervical disc degeneration
Other C3-C4 cervical disc degeneration

● **M50.32 Other cervical disc degeneration, mid-cervical region**

M50.320 Other cervical disc degeneration, mid-cervical region, unspecified level ◀

M50.321 Other cervical disc degeneration at C4-C5 level ◀
Other C4-C5 cervical disc degeneration ◀

M50.322 Other cervical disc degeneration at C5-C6 level ◀
Other C5-C6 cervical disc degeneration ◀

M50.323 Other cervical disc degeneration at C6-C7 level ◀
Other C6-C7 cervical disc degeneration ◀

M50.33 Other cervical disc degeneration, cervicothoracic region
Other C7-T1 cervical disc degeneration

● **M50.8 Other cervical disc disorders**

M50.80 Other cervical disc disorders, unspecified cervical region

M50.81 Other cervical disc disorders, high cervical region
Other C2-C3 cervical disc disorders
Other C3-C4 cervical disc disorders

● **M50.82 Other cervical disc disorders, mid-cervical region**

M50.820 Other cervical disc disorders, mid-cervical region, unspecified level ◀

M50.821 Other cervical disc disorders at C4-C5 level ◀
Other C4-C5 cervical disc disorders ◀

M50.822 Other cervical disc disorders at C5-C6 level ◀
Other C5-C6 cervical disc disorders ◀

M50.823 Other cervical disc disorders at C6-C7 level ◀
Other C6-C7 cervical disc disorders ◀

M50.83 Other cervical disc disorders, cervicothoracic region
Other C7-T1 cervical disc disorders

- **M50.9 Cervical disc disorder, unspecified**
  - **M50.90 Cervical disc disorder, unspecified, unspecified cervical region**
  - **M50.91 Cervical disc disorder, unspecified, high cervical region**
    - C2-C3 cervical disc disorder, unspecified
    - C3-C4 cervical disc disorder, unspecified
  - **M50.92 Cervical disc disorder, unspecified, mid-cervical region**
    - **M50.920 Unspecified cervical disc disorder, mid-cervical region, unspecified level ◀**
    - **M50.921 Unspecified cervical disc disorder at C4-C5 level ◀**
      - Unspecified C4-C5 cervical disc disorder ◀
    - **M50.922 Unspecified cervical disc disorder at C5-C6 level ◀**
      - Unspecified C5-C6 cervical disc disorder ◀
    - **M50.923 Unspecified cervical disc disorder at C6-C7 level ◀**
      - Unspecified C6-C7 cervical disc disorder ◀
  - **M50.93 Cervical disc disorder, unspecified, cervicothoracic region**
    - C7-T1 cervical disc disorder, unspecified

- **M51 Thoracic, thoracolumbar, and lumbosacral intervertebral disc disorders**
  - **Excludes2** cervical and cervicothoracic disc disorders (M50.-)
    sacral and sacrococcygeal disorders (M53.3)
  - **M51.0 Thoracic, thoracolumbar and lumbosacral intervertebral disc disorders with myelopathy**
    - Ex For category M51.0 CC codes unless otherwise indicated: M51.04-M51.05, M51.24-M51.25
    - **M51.04 Intervertebral disc disorders with myelopathy, thoracic region** CC
    - **M51.05 Intervertebral disc disorders with myelopathy, thoracolumbar region** CC
    - **M51.06 Intervertebral disc disorders with myelopathy, lumbar region** CC
      - Ex M51.06, M51.24-M51.25
  - **M51.1 Thoracic, thoracolumbar and lumbosacral intervertebral disc disorders with radiculopathy**
    - Sciatica due to intervertebral disc disorder
    - **Excludes1** lumbar radiculitis NOS (M54.16)
      sciatica NOS (M54.3)
    - **M51.14 Intervertebral disc disorders with radiculopathy, thoracic region**
    - **M51.15 Intervertebral disc disorders with radiculopathy, thoracolumbar region**
    - **M51.16 Intervertebral disc disorders with radiculopathy, lumbar region**
    - **M51.17 Intervertebral disc disorders with radiculopathy, lumbosacral region**
  - **M51.2 Other thoracic, thoracolumbar and lumbosacral intervertebral disc displacement**
    - Lumbago due to displacement of intervertebral disc
    - **M51.24 Other intervertebral disc displacement, thoracic region**
    - **M51.25 Other intervertebral disc displacement, thoracolumbar region**
    - **M51.26 Other intervertebral disc displacement, lumbar region**
    - **M51.27 Other intervertebral disc displacement, lumbosacral region**
  - **M51.3 Other thoracic, thoracolumbar and lumbosacral intervertebral disc degeneration**
    - Coding Clinic: 2013, Q3, P22
    - **M51.34 Other intervertebral disc degeneration, thoracic region**
    - **M51.35 Other intervertebral disc degeneration, thoracolumbar region**
    - **M51.36 Other intervertebral disc degeneration, lumbar region**
    - **M51.37 Other intervertebral disc degeneration, lumbosacral region**
  - **M51.4 Schmorl's nodes**
    - **M51.44 Schmorl's nodes, thoracic region**
    - **M51.45 Schmorl's nodes, thoracolumbar region**
    - **M51.46 Schmorl's nodes, lumbar region**
    - **M51.47 Schmorl's nodes, lumbosacral region**
  - **M51.8 Other thoracic, thoracolumbar and lumbosacral intervertebral disc disorders**
    - **M51.84 Other intervertebral disc disorders, thoracic region**
    - **M51.85 Other intervertebral disc disorders, thoracolumbar region**
    - **M51.86 Other intervertebral disc disorders, lumbar region**
    - **M51.87 Other intervertebral disc disorders, lumbosacral region**
  - **M51.9 Unspecified thoracic, thoracolumbar and lumbosacral intervertebral disc disorder**

- **M53 Other and unspecified dorsopathies, not elsewhere classified**
  - **M53.0 Cervicocranial syndrome**
    - Posterior cervical sympathetic syndrome
  - **M53.1 Cervicobrachial syndrome**
    - **Excludes2** cervical disc disorder (M50.-)
      thoracic outlet syndrome (G54.0)
  - **M53.2 Spinal instabilities**
    - **M53.2X Spinal instabilities**
      - **M53.2X1 Spinal instabilities, occipito-atlanto-axial region**
      - **M53.2X2 Spinal instabilities, cervical region**
      - **M53.2X3 Spinal instabilities, cervicothoracic region**
      - **M53.2X4 Spinal instabilities, thoracic region**
      - **M53.2X5 Spinal instabilities, thoracolumbar region**
      - **M53.2X6 Spinal instabilities, lumbar region**
      - **M53.2X7 Spinal instabilities, lumbosacral region**
      - **M53.2X8 Spinal instabilities, sacral and sacrococcygeal region**
      - **M53.2X9 Spinal instabilities, site unspecified**
  - **M53.3 Sacrococcygeal disorders, not elsewhere classified**
    - Coccygodynia
  - **M53.8 Other specified dorsopathies**
    - **M53.80 Other specified dorsopathies, site unspecified**
    - **M53.81 Other specified dorsopathies, occipito-atlanto-axial region**
    - **M53.82 Other specified dorsopathies, cervical region**
    - **M53.83 Other specified dorsopathies, cervicothoracic region**
    - **M53.84 Other specified dorsopathies, thoracic region**
    - **M53.85 Other specified dorsopathies, thoracolumbar region**
    - **M53.86 Other specified dorsopathies, lumbar region**
    - **M53.87 Other specified dorsopathies, lumbosacral region**
    - **M53.88 Other specified dorsopathies, sacral and sacrococcygeal region**
  - **M53.9 Dorsopathy, unspecified**

M54 Dorsalgia

Excludes1 psychogenic dorsalgia (F45.41)

M54.0 Panniculitis affecting regions of neck and back

Excludes1 lupus panniculitis (L93.2)
panniculitis NOS (M79.3)
relapsing [Weber-Christian] panniculitis (M35.6)

M54.00 Panniculitis affecting regions of neck and back, site unspecified

M54.01 Panniculitis affecting regions of neck and back, occipito-atlanto-axial region

M54.02 Panniculitis affecting regions of neck and back, cervical region

M54.03 Panniculitis affecting regions of neck and back, cervicothoracic region

M54.04 Panniculitis affecting regions of neck and back, thoracic region

M54.05 Panniculitis affecting regions of neck and back, thoracolumbar region

M54.06 Panniculitis affecting regions of neck and back, lumbar region

M54.07 Panniculitis affecting regions of neck and back, lumbosacral region

M54.08 Panniculitis affecting regions of neck and back, sacral and sacrococcygeal region

M54.09 Panniculitis affecting regions, neck and back, multiple sites in spine

M54.1 Radiculopathy

Brachial neuritis or radiculitis NOS
Lumbar neuritis or radiculitis NOS
Lumbosacral neuritis or radiculitis NOS
Thoracic neuritis or radiculitis NOS
Radiculitis NOS

Excludes1 neuralgia and neuritis NOS (M79.2)
radiculopathy with cervical disc disorder (M50.1)
radiculopathy with lumbar and other intervertebral disc disorder (M51.1-)
radiculopathy with spondylosis (M47.2-)

M54.10 Radiculopathy, site unspecified

M54.11 Radiculopathy, occipito-atlanto-axial region

M54.12 Radiculopathy, cervical region

M54.13 Radiculopathy, cervicothoracic region

M54.14 Radiculopathy, thoracic region

M54.15 Radiculopathy, thoracolumbar region

M54.16 Radiculopathy, lumbar region

M54.17 Radiculopathy, lumbosacral region

M54.18 Radiculopathy, sacral and sacrococcygeal region

M54.2 Cervicalgia

Excludes1 cervicalgia due to intervertebral cervical disc disorder (M50.-)

M54.3 Sciatica

Excludes1 lesion of sciatic nerve (G57.0)
sciatica due to intervertebral disc disorder (M51.1-)
sciatica with lumbago (M54.4-)

M54.30 Sciatica, unspecified side

M54.31 Sciatica, right side

M54.32 Sciatica, left side

M54.4 Lumbago with sciatica

Excludes1 lumbago with sciatica due to intervertebral disc disorder (M51.1-)

M54.40 Lumbago with sciatica, unspecified side

M54.41 Lumbago with sciatica, right side

M54.42 Lumbago with sciatica, left side

Coding Clinic: 2016, Q2, P7

M54.5 Low back pain

Loin pain
Lumbago NOS

Excludes1 low back strain (S39.012)
lumbago due to intervertebral disc displacement (M51.2-)
lumbago with sciatica (M54.4-)

M54.6 Pain in thoracic spine

Excludes1 pain in thoracic spine due to intervertebral disc disorder (M51.)

M54.8 Other dorsalgia

Excludes1 dorsalgia in thoracic region (M54.6)
low back pain (M54.5)

M54.81 Occipital neuralgia

M54.89 Other dorsalgia

M54.9 Dorsalgia, unspecified

Backache NOS
Back pain NOS

SOFT TISSUE DISORDERS (M60-M79)

DISORDERS OF MUSCLES (M60-M63)

Excludes1 dermatopolymyositis (M33.-)
muscular dystrophies and myopathies (G71-G72)
myopathy in amyloidosis (E85.-)
myopathy in polyarteritis nodosa (M30.0)
myopathy in rheumatoid arthritis (M05.32)
myopathy in scleroderma (M34.-)
myopathy in Sjögren's syndrome (M35.03)
myopathy in systemic lupus erythematosus (M32.-)

M60 Myositis

Excludes2 inclusion body myositis [IBM] (G72.41)

M60.0 Infective myositis

Tropical pyomyositis

Use additional code (B95-B97) to identify infectious agent

Ex: **For category M60.0 CC codes:** K68.12, M60.000-M60.19, M61.00-M61.19, M61.30-M61.59, M62.3, M62.50-M62.59, M62.84, M62.89, M72.6

M60.00 Infective myositis, unspecified site

M60.000 Infective myositis, unspecified right arm

Infective myositis, right upper limb NOS

M60.001 Infective myositis, unspecified left arm

Infective myositis, left upper limb NOS

M60.002 Infective myositis, unspecified arm

Infective myositis, upper limb NOS

M60.003 Infective myositis, unspecified right leg

Infective myositis, right lower limb NOS

M60.004 Infective myositis, unspecified left leg

Infective myositis, left lower limb NOS

M60.005 Infective myositis, unspecified leg

Infective myositis, lower limb NOS

M60.009 Infective myositis, unspecified site

M60.01 Infective myositis, shoulder

M60.011 Infective myositis, right shoulder

M60.012 Infective myositis, left shoulder

M60.019 Infective myositis, unspecified shoulder

M60.02 Infective myositis, upper arm

M60.021 Infective myositis, right upper arm

M60.022 Infective myositis, left upper arm

M60.029 Infective myositis, unspecified upper arm

- M60.03 Infective myositis, forearm
  - M60.031 Infective myositis, right forearm
  - M60.032 Infective myositis, left forearm
  - M60.039 Infective myositis, unspecified forearm
- M60.04 Infective myositis, hand and fingers
  - M60.041 Infective myositis, right hand
  - M60.042 Infective myositis, left hand
  - M60.043 Infective myositis, unspecified hand
  - M60.044 Infective myositis, right finger(s)
  - M60.045 Infective myositis, left finger(s)
  - M60.046 Infective myositis, unspecified finger(s)
- M60.05 Infective myositis, thigh
  - M60.051 Infective myositis, right thigh
  - M60.052 Infective myositis, left thigh
  - M60.059 Infective myositis, unspecified thigh
- M60.06 Infective myositis, lower leg
  - M60.061 Infective myositis, right lower leg
  - M60.062 Infective myositis, left lower leg
  - M60.069 Infective myositis, unspecified lower leg
- M60.07 Infective myositis, ankle, foot and toes
  - M60.070 Infective myositis, right ankle
  - M60.071 Infective myositis, left ankle
  - M60.072 Infective myositis, unspecified ankle
  - M60.073 Infective myositis, right foot
  - M60.074 Infective myositis, left foot
  - M60.075 Infective myositis, unspecified foot
  - M60.076 Infective myositis, right toe(s)
  - M60.077 Infective myositis, left toe(s)
  - M60.078 Infective myositis, unspecified toe(s)
- M60.08 Infective myositis, other site
- M60.09 Infective myositis, multiple sites

- M60.1 Interstitial myositis
  - M60.10 Interstitial myositis of unspecified site
  - M60.11 Interstitial myositis, shoulder
    - M60.111 Interstitial myositis, right shoulder
    - M60.112 Interstitial myositis, left shoulder
    - M60.119 Interstitial myositis, unspecified shoulder
  - M60.12 Interstitial myositis, upper arm
    - M60.121 Interstitial myositis, right upper arm
    - M60.122 Interstitial myositis, left upper arm
    - M60.129 Interstitial myositis, unspecified upper arm
  - M60.13 Interstitial myositis, forearm
    - M60.131 Interstitial myositis, right forearm
    - M60.132 Interstitial myositis, left forearm
    - M60.139 Interstitial myositis, unspecified forearm
  - M60.14 Interstitial myositis, hand
    - M60.141 Interstitial myositis, right hand
    - M60.142 Interstitial myositis, left hand
    - M60.149 Interstitial myositis, unspecified hand
  - M60.15 Interstitial myositis, thigh
    - M60.151 Interstitial myositis, right thigh
    - M60.152 Interstitial myositis, left thigh
    - M60.159 Interstitial myositis, unspecified thigh
  - M60.16 Interstitial myositis, lower leg
    - M60.161 Interstitial myositis, right lower leg
    - M60.162 Interstitial myositis, left lower leg
    - M60.169 Interstitial myositis, unspecified lower leg
  - M60.17 Interstitial myositis, ankle and foot
    - M60.171 Interstitial myositis, right ankle and foot
    - M60.172 Interstitial myositis, left ankle and foot
    - M60.179 Interstitial myositis, unspecified ankle and foot
  - M60.18 Interstitial myositis, other site
  - M60.19 Interstitial myositis, multiple sites
- M60.2 Foreign body granuloma of soft tissue, not elsewhere classified

  Use additional code to identify the type of retained foreign body (Z18.-)

  Excludes1 foreign body granuloma of skin and subcutaneous tissue (L92.3)
  - M60.20 Foreign body granuloma of soft tissue, not elsewhere classified, unspecified site
  - M60.21 Foreign body granuloma of soft tissue, not elsewhere classified, shoulder
    - M60.211 Foreign body granuloma of soft tissue, not elsewhere classified, right shoulder
    - M60.212 Foreign body granuloma of soft tissue, not elsewhere classified, left shoulder
    - M60.219 Foreign body granuloma of soft tissue, not elsewhere classified, unspecified shoulder
  - M60.22 Foreign body granuloma of soft tissue, not elsewhere classified, upper arm
    - M60.221 Foreign body granuloma of soft tissue, not elsewhere classified, right upper arm
    - M60.222 Foreign body granuloma of soft tissue, not elsewhere classified, left upper arm
    - M60.229 Foreign body granuloma of soft tissue, not elsewhere classified, unspecified upper arm
  - M60.23 Foreign body granuloma of soft tissue, not elsewhere classified, forearm
    - M60.231 Foreign body granuloma of soft tissue, not elsewhere classified, right forearm
    - M60.232 Foreign body granuloma of soft tissue, not elsewhere classified, left forearm
    - M60.239 Foreign body granuloma of soft tissue, not elsewhere classified, unspecified forearm
  - M60.24 Foreign body granuloma of soft tissue, not elsewhere classified, hand
    - M60.241 Foreign body granuloma of soft tissue, not elsewhere classified, right hand
    - M60.242 Foreign body granuloma of soft tissue, not elsewhere classified, left hand
    - M60.249 Foreign body granuloma of soft tissue, not elsewhere classified, unspecified hand

- M60.25 Foreign body granuloma of soft tissue, not elsewhere classified, thigh
  - M60.251 Foreign body granuloma of soft tissue, not elsewhere classified, right thigh
  - M60.252 Foreign body granuloma of soft tissue, not elsewhere classified, left thigh
  - M60.259 Foreign body granuloma of soft tissue, not elsewhere classified, unspecified thigh
- M60.26 Foreign body granuloma of soft tissue, not elsewhere classified, lower leg
  - M60.261 Foreign body granuloma of soft tissue, not elsewhere classified, right lower leg
  - M60.262 Foreign body granuloma of soft tissue, not elsewhere classified, left lower leg
  - M60.269 Foreign body granuloma of soft tissue, not elsewhere classified, unspecified lower leg
- M60.27 Foreign body granuloma of soft tissue, not elsewhere classified, ankle and foot
  - M60.271 Foreign body granuloma of soft tissue, not elsewhere classified, right ankle and foot
  - M60.272 Foreign body granuloma of soft tissue, not elsewhere classified, left ankle and foot
  - M60.279 Foreign body granuloma of soft tissue, not elsewhere classified, unspecified ankle and foot
- M60.28 Foreign body granuloma of soft tissue, not elsewhere classified, other site

- M60.8 Other myositis
  - M60.80 Other myositis, unspecified site
  - M60.81 Other myositis shoulder
    - M60.811 Other myositis, right shoulder
    - M60.812 Other myositis, left shoulder
    - M60.819 Other myositis, unspecified shoulder
  - M60.82 Other myositis, upper arm
    - M60.821 Other myositis, right upper arm
    - M60.822 Other myositis, left upper arm
    - M60.829 Other myositis, unspecified upper arm
  - M60.83 Other myositis, forearm
    - M60.831 Other myositis, right forearm
    - M60.832 Other myositis, left forearm
    - M60.839 Other myositis, unspecified forearm
  - M60.84 Other myositis, hand
    - M60.841 Other myositis, right hand
    - M60.842 Other myositis, left hand
    - M60.849 Other myositis, unspecified hand
  - M60.85 Other myositis, thigh
    - M60.851 Other myositis, right thigh
    - M60.852 Other myositis, left thigh
    - M60.859 Other myositis, unspecified thigh
  - M60.86 Other myositis, lower leg
    - M60.861 Other myositis, right lower leg
    - M60.862 Other myositis, left lower leg
    - M60.869 Other myositis, unspecified lower leg
  - M60.87 Other myositis, ankle and foot
    - M60.871 Other myositis, right ankle and foot
    - M60.872 Other myositis, left ankle and foot
    - M60.879 Other myositis, unspecified ankle and foot
  - M60.88 Other myositis, other site
  - M60.89 Other myositis, multiple sites
- M60.9 Myositis, unspecified

- M61 Calcification and ossification of muscle
  - M61.0 Myositis ossificans traumatica
    - M61.00 Myositis ossificans traumatica, unspecified site
    - M61.01 Myositis ossificans traumatica, shoulder
      - M61.011 Myositis ossificans traumatica, right shoulder
      - M61.012 Myositis ossificans traumatica, left shoulder
      - M61.019 Myositis ossificans traumatica, unspecified shoulder
    - M61.02 Myositis ossificans traumatica, upper arm
      - M61.021 Myositis ossificans traumatica, right upper arm
      - M61.022 Myositis ossificans traumatica, left upper arm
      - M61.029 Myositis ossificans traumatica, unspecified upper arm
    - M61.03 Myositis ossificans traumatica, forearm
      - M61.031 Myositis ossificans traumatica, right forearm
      - M61.032 Myositis ossificans traumatica, left forearm
      - M61.039 Myositis ossificans traumatica, unspecified forearm
    - M61.04 Myositis ossificans traumatica, hand
      - M61.041 Myositis ossificans traumatica, right hand
      - M61.042 Myositis ossificans traumatica, left hand
      - M61.049 Myositis ossificans traumatica, unspecified hand
    - M61.05 Myositis ossificans traumatica, thigh
      - M61.051 Myositis ossificans traumatica, right thigh
      - M61.052 Myositis ossificans traumatica, left thigh
      - M61.059 Myositis ossificans traumatica, unspecified thigh
    - M61.06 Myositis ossificans traumatica, lower leg
      - M61.061 Myositis ossificans traumatica, right lower leg
      - M61.062 Myositis ossificans traumatica, left lower leg
      - M61.069 Myositis ossificans traumatica, unspecified lower leg
    - M61.07 Myositis ossificans traumatica, ankle and foot
      - M61.071 Myositis ossificans traumatica, right ankle and foot
      - M61.072 Myositis ossificans traumatica, left ankle and foot
      - M61.079 Myositis ossificans traumatica, unspecified ankle and foot
    - M61.08 Myositis ossificans traumatica, other site
    - M61.09 Myositis ossificans traumatica, multiple sites
  - M61.1 Myositis ossificans progressiva
    Fibrodysplasia ossificans progressiva
    - M61.10 Myositis ossificans progressiva, unspecified site
    - M61.11 Myositis ossificans progressiva, shoulder
      - M61.111 Myositis ossificans progressiva, right shoulder
      - M61.112 Myositis ossificans progressiva, left shoulder
      - M61.119 Myositis ossificans progressiva, unspecified shoulder

- **M61.12** Myositis ossificans progressiva, upper arm
  - M61.121 Myositis ossificans progressiva, right upper arm
  - M61.122 Myositis ossificans progressiva, left upper arm
  - M61.129 Myositis ossificans progressiva, unspecified arm
- **M61.13** Myositis ossificans progressiva, forearm
  - M61.131 Myositis ossificans progressiva, right forearm
  - M61.132 Myositis ossificans progressiva, left forearm
  - M61.139 Myositis ossificans progressiva, unspecified forearm
- **M61.14** Myositis ossificans progressiva, hand and finger(s)
  - M61.141 Myositis ossificans progressiva, right hand
  - M61.142 Myositis ossificans progressiva, left hand
  - M61.143 Myositis ossificans progressiva, unspecified hand
  - M61.144 Myositis ossificans progressiva, right finger(s)
  - M61.145 Myositis ossificans progressiva, left finger(s)
  - M61.146 Myositis ossificans progressiva, unspecified finger(s)
- **M61.15** Myositis ossificans progressiva, thigh
  - M61.151 Myositis ossificans progressiva, right thigh
  - M61.152 Myositis ossificans progressiva, left thigh
  - M61.159 Myositis ossificans progressiva, unspecified thigh
- **M61.16** Myositis ossificans progressiva, lower leg
  - M61.161 Myositis ossificans progressiva, right lower leg
  - M61.162 Myositis ossificans progressiva, left lower leg
  - M61.169 Myositis ossificans progressiva, unspecified lower leg
- **M61.17** Myositis ossificans progressiva, ankle, foot and toe(s)
  - M61.171 Myositis ossificans progressiva, right ankle
  - M61.172 Myositis ossificans progressiva, left ankle
  - M61.173 Myositis ossificans progressiva, unspecified ankle
  - M61.174 Myositis ossificans progressiva, right foot
  - M61.175 Myositis ossificans progressiva, left foot
  - M61.176 Myositis ossificans progressiva, unspecified foot
  - M61.177 Myositis ossificans progressiva, right toe(s)
  - M61.178 Myositis ossificans progressiva, left toe(s)
  - M61.179 Myositis ossificans progressiva, unspecified toe(s)
- M61.18 Myositis ossificans progressiva, other site
- M61.19 Myositis ossificans progressiva, multiple sites

- **M61.2** Paralytic calcification and ossification of muscle
  Myositis ossificans associated with quadriplegia or paraplegia
  - M61.20 Paralytic calcification and ossification of muscle, unspecified site
  - **M61.21** Paralytic calcification and ossification of muscle, shoulder
    - M61.211 Paralytic calcification and ossification of muscle, right shoulder
    - M61.212 Paralytic calcification and ossification of muscle, left shoulder
    - M61.219 Paralytic calcification and ossification of muscle, unspecified shoulder
  - **M61.22** Paralytic calcification and ossification of muscle, upper arm
    - M61.221 Paralytic calcification and ossification of muscle, right upper arm
    - M61.222 Paralytic calcification and ossification of muscle, left upper arm
    - M61.229 Paralytic calcification and ossification of muscle, unspecified upper arm
  - **M61.23** Paralytic calcification and ossification of muscle, forearm
    - M61.231 Paralytic calcification and ossification of muscle, right forearm
    - M61.232 Paralytic calcification and ossification of muscle, left forearm
    - M61.239 Paralytic calcification and ossification of muscle, unspecified forearm
  - **M61.24** Paralytic calcification and ossification of muscle, hand
    - M61.241 Paralytic calcification and ossification of muscle, right hand
    - M61.242 Paralytic calcification and ossification of muscle, left hand
    - M61.249 Paralytic calcification and ossification of muscle, unspecified hand
  - **M61.25** Paralytic calcification and ossification of muscle, thigh
    - M61.251 Paralytic calcification and ossification of muscle, right thigh
    - M61.252 Paralytic calcification and ossification of muscle, left thigh
    - M61.259 Paralytic calcification and ossification of muscle, unspecified thigh
  - **M61.26** Paralytic calcification and ossification of muscle, lower leg
    - M61.261 Paralytic calcification and ossification of muscle, right lower leg
    - M61.262 Paralytic calcification and ossification of muscle, left lower leg
    - M61.269 Paralytic calcification and ossification of muscle, unspecified lower leg
  - **M61.27** Paralytic calcification and ossification of muscle, ankle and foot
    - M61.271 Paralytic calcification and ossification of muscle, right ankle and foot
    - M61.272 Paralytic calcification and ossification of muscle, left ankle and foot
    - M61.279 Paralytic calcification and ossification of muscle, unspecified ankle and foot
  - M61.28 Paralytic calcification and ossification of muscle, other site
  - M61.29 Paralytic calcification and ossification of muscle, multiple sites

● M61.3 Calcification and ossification of muscles associated with burns
Myositis ossificans associated with burns
M61.30 Calcification and ossification of muscles associated with burns, unspecified site
● M61.31 Calcification and ossification of muscles associated with burns, shoulder
M61.311 Calcification and ossification of muscles associated with burns, right shoulder
M61.312 Calcification and ossification of muscles associated with burns, left shoulder
M61.319 Calcification and ossification of muscles associated with burns, unspecified shoulder
● M61.32 Calcification and ossification of muscles associated with burns, upper arm
M61.321 Calcification and ossification of muscles associated with burns, right upper arm
M61.322 Calcification and ossification of muscles associated with burns, left upper arm
M61.329 Calcification and ossification of muscles associated with burns, unspecified upper arm
● M61.33 Calcification and ossification of muscles associated with burns, forearm
M61.331 Calcification and ossification of muscles associated with burns, right forearm
M61.332 Calcification and ossification of muscles associated with burns, left forearm
M61.339 Calcification and ossification of muscles associated with burns, unspecified forearm
● M61.34 Calcification and ossification of muscles associated with burns, hand
M61.341 Calcification and ossification of muscles associated with burns, right hand
M61.342 Calcification and ossification of muscles associated with burns, left hand
M61.349 Calcification and ossification of muscles associated with burns, unspecified hand
● M61.35 Calcification and ossification of muscles associated with burns, thigh
M61.351 Calcification and ossification of muscles associated with burns, right thigh
M61.352 Calcification and ossification of muscles associated with burns, left thigh
M61.359 Calcification and ossification of muscles associated with burns, unspecified thigh
● M61.36 Calcification and ossification of muscles associated with burns, lower leg
M61.361 Calcification and ossification of muscles associated with burns, right lower leg
M61.362 Calcification and ossification of muscles associated with burns, left lower leg
M61.369 Calcification and ossification of muscles associated with burns, unspecified lower leg
● M61.37 Calcification and ossification of muscles associated with burns, ankle and foot
M61.371 Calcification and ossification of muscles associated with burns, right ankle and foot
M61.372 Calcification and ossification of muscles associated with burns, left ankle and foot
M61.379 Calcification and ossification of muscles associated with burns, unspecified ankle and foot
M61.38 Calcification and ossification of muscles associated with burns, other site
M61.39 Calcification and ossification of muscles associated with burns, multiple sites
● M61.4 Other calcification of muscle
Excludes1 calcific tendinitis NOS (M65.2-)
calcific tendinitis of shoulder (M75.3)
M61.40 Other calcification of muscle, unspecified site
● M61.41 Other calcification of muscle, shoulder
M61.411 Other calcification of muscle, right shoulder
M61.412 Other calcification of muscle, left shoulder
M61.419 Other calcification of muscle, unspecified shoulder
● M61.42 Other calcification of muscle, upper arm
M61.421 Other calcification of muscle, right upper arm
M61.422 Other calcification of muscle, left upper arm
M61.429 Other calcification of muscle, unspecified upper arm
● M61.43 Other calcification of muscle, forearm
M61.431 Other calcification of muscle, right forearm
M61.432 Other calcification of muscle, left forearm
M61.439 Other calcification of muscle, unspecified forearm
● M61.44 Other calcification of muscle, hand
M61.441 Other calcification of muscle, right hand
M61.442 Other calcification of muscle, left hand
M61.449 Other calcification of muscle, unspecified hand
● M61.45 Other calcification of muscle, thigh
M61.451 Other calcification of muscle, right thigh
M61.452 Other calcification of muscle, left thigh
M61.459 Other calcification of muscle, unspecified thigh
● M61.46 Other calcification of muscle, lower leg
M61.461 Other calcification of muscle, right lower leg
M61.462 Other calcification of muscle, left lower leg
M61.469 Other calcification of muscle, unspecified lower leg
● M61.47 Other calcification of muscle, ankle and foot
M61.471 Other calcification of muscle, right ankle and foot
M61.472 Other calcification of muscle, left ankle and foot
M61.479 Other calcification of muscle, unspecified ankle and foot
M61.48 Other calcification of muscle, other site
M61.49 Other calcification of muscle, multiple sites

- **M61.5 Other ossification of muscle**
  - **M61.50 Other ossification of muscle, unspecified site**
  - **M61.51 Other ossification of muscle, shoulder**
    - **M61.511 Other ossification of muscle, right shoulder**
    - **M61.512 Other ossification of muscle, left shoulder**
    - **M61.519 Other ossification of muscle, unspecified shoulder**
  - **M61.52 Other ossification of muscle, upper arm**
    - **M61.521 Other ossification of muscle, right upper arm**
    - **M61.522 Other ossification of muscle, left upper arm**
    - **M61.529 Other ossification of muscle, unspecified upper arm**
  - **M61.53 Other ossification of muscle, forearm**
    - **M61.531 Other ossification of muscle, right forearm**
    - **M61.532 Other ossification of muscle, left forearm**
    - **M61.539 Other ossification of muscle, unspecified forearm**
  - **M61.54 Other ossification of muscle, hand**
    - **M61.541 Other ossification of muscle, right hand**
    - **M61.542 Other ossification of muscle, left hand**
    - **M61.549 Other ossification of muscle, unspecified hand**
  - **M61.55 Other ossification of muscle, thigh**
    - **M61.551 Other ossification of muscle, right thigh**
    - **M61.552 Other ossification of muscle, left thigh**
    - **M61.559 Other ossification of muscle, unspecified thigh**
  - **M61.56 Other ossification of muscle, lower leg**
    - **M61.561 Other ossification of muscle, right lower leg**
    - **M61.562 Other ossification of muscle, left lower leg**
    - **M61.569 Other ossification of muscle, unspecified lower leg**
  - **M61.57 Other ossification of muscle, ankle and foot**
    - **M61.571 Other ossification of muscle, right ankle and foot**
    - **M61.572 Other ossification of muscle, left ankle and foot**
    - **M61.579 Other ossification of muscle, unspecified ankle and foot**
  - **M61.58 Other ossification of muscle, other site**
  - **M61.59 Other ossification of muscle, multiple sites**
- **M61.9 Calcification and ossification of muscle, unspecified**

- **M62 Other disorders of muscle**

  Excludes1 alcoholic myopathy (G72.1)
  cramp and spasm (R25.2)
  drug-induced myopathy (G72.0)
  myalgia (M79.1)
  stiff-man syndrome (G25.82)

  Excludes2 nontraumatic hematoma of muscle (M79.81)
  - **M62.0 Separation of muscle (nontraumatic)**
    Diastasis of muscle

    Excludes1 diastasis recti complicating pregnancy, labor and delivery (O71.8)
    traumatic separation of muscle - see strain of muscle by body region
    - **M62.00 Separation of muscle (nontraumatic), unspecified site**
    - **M62.01 Separation of muscle (nontraumatic), shoulder**
      - **M62.011 Separation of muscle (nontraumatic), right shoulder**
      - **M62.012 Separation of muscle (nontraumatic), left shoulder**
      - **M62.019 Separation of muscle (nontraumatic), unspecified shoulder**
    - **M62.02 Separation of muscle (nontraumatic), upper arm**
      - **M62.021 Separation of muscle (nontraumatic), right upper arm**
      - **M62.022 Separation of muscle (nontraumatic), left upper arm**
      - **M62.029 Separation of muscle (nontraumatic), unspecified upper arm**
    - **M62.03 Separation of muscle (nontraumatic), forearm**
      - **M62.031 Separation of muscle (nontraumatic), right forearm**
      - **M62.032 Separation of muscle (nontraumatic), left forearm**
      - **M62.039 Separation of muscle (nontraumatic), unspecified forearm**
    - **M62.04 Separation of muscle (nontraumatic), hand**
      - **M62.041 Separation of muscle (nontraumatic), right hand**
      - **M62.042 Separation of muscle (nontraumatic), left hand**
      - **M62.049 Separation of muscle (nontraumatic), unspecified hand**
    - **M62.05 Separation of muscle (nontraumatic), thigh**
      - **M62.051 Separation of muscle (nontraumatic), right thigh**
      - **M62.052 Separation of muscle (nontraumatic), left thigh**
      - **M62.059 Separation of muscle (nontraumatic), unspecified thigh**
    - **M62.06 Separation of muscle (nontraumatic), lower leg**
      - **M62.061 Separation of muscle (nontraumatic), right lower leg**
      - **M62.062 Separation of muscle (nontraumatic), left lower leg**
      - **M62.069 Separation of muscle (nontraumatic), unspecified lower leg**
    - **M62.07 Separation of muscle (nontraumatic), ankle and foot**
      - **M62.071 Separation of muscle (nontraumatic), right ankle and foot**
      - **M62.072 Separation of muscle (nontraumatic), left ankle and foot**
      - **M62.079 Separation of muscle (nontraumatic), unspecified ankle and foot**
    - **M62.08 Separation of muscle (nontraumatic), other site**
  - **M62.1 Other rupture of muscle (nontraumatic)**

    Excludes1 traumatic rupture of muscle - see strain of muscle by body region

    Excludes2 rupture of tendon (M66.-)
    - **M62.10 Other rupture of muscle (nontraumatic), unspecified site**
    - **M62.11 Other rupture of muscle (nontraumatic), shoulder**
      - **M62.111 Other rupture of muscle (nontraumatic), right shoulder**
      - **M62.112 Other rupture of muscle (nontraumatic), left shoulder**
      - **M62.119 Other rupture of muscle (nontraumatic), unspecified shoulder**

- M62.12 Other rupture of muscle (nontraumatic), upper arm
  - M62.121 Other rupture of muscle (nontraumatic), right upper arm
  - M62.122 Other rupture of muscle (nontraumatic), left upper arm
  - M62.129 Other rupture of muscle (nontraumatic), unspecified upper arm
- M62.13 Other rupture of muscle (nontraumatic), forearm
  - M62.131 Other rupture of muscle (nontraumatic), right forearm
  - M62.132 Other rupture of muscle (nontraumatic), left forearm
  - M62.139 Other rupture of muscle (nontraumatic), unspecified forearm
- M62.14 Other rupture of muscle (nontraumatic), hand
  - M62.141 Other rupture of muscle (nontraumatic), right hand
  - M62.142 Other rupture of muscle (nontraumatic), left hand
  - M62.149 Other rupture of muscle (nontraumatic), unspecified hand
- M62.15 Other rupture of muscle (nontraumatic), thigh
  - M62.151 Other rupture of muscle (nontraumatic), right thigh
  - M62.152 Other rupture of muscle (nontraumatic), left thigh
  - M62.159 Other rupture of muscle (nontraumatic), unspecified thigh
- M62.16 Other rupture of muscle (nontraumatic), lower leg
  - M62.161 Other rupture of muscle (nontraumatic), right lower leg
  - M62.162 Other rupture of muscle (nontraumatic), left lower leg
  - M62.169 Other rupture of muscle (nontraumatic), unspecified lower leg
- M62.17 Other rupture of muscle (nontraumatic), ankle and foot
  - M62.171 Other rupture of muscle (nontraumatic), right ankle and foot
  - M62.172 Other rupture of muscle (nontraumatic), left ankle and foot
  - M62.179 Other rupture of muscle (nontraumatic), unspecified ankle and foot
- M62.18 Other rupture of muscle (nontraumatic), other site
- M62.2 Nontraumatic ischemic infarction of muscle

  Excludes1 compartment syndrome (traumatic) (T79.A-)
  nontraumatic compartment syndrome (M79.A-)
  traumatic ischemia of muscle (T79.6)
  rhabdomyolysis (M62.82)
  Volkmann's ischemic contracture (T79.6)
  - M62.20 Nontraumatic ischemic infarction of muscle, unspecified site
  - M62.21 Nontraumatic ischemic infarction of muscle, shoulder
    - M62.211 Nontraumatic ischemic infarction of muscle, right shoulder
    - M62.212 Nontraumatic ischemic infarction of muscle, left shoulder
    - M62.219 Nontraumatic ischemic infarction of muscle, unspecified shoulder
  - M62.22 Nontraumatic ischemic infarction of muscle, upper arm
    - M62.221 Nontraumatic ischemic infarction of muscle, right upper arm
    - M62.222 Nontraumatic ischemic infarction of muscle, left upper arm
    - M62.229 Nontraumatic ischemic infarction of muscle, unspecified upper arm
  - M62.23 Nontraumatic ischemic infarction of muscle, forearm
    - M62.231 Nontraumatic ischemic infarction of muscle, right forearm
    - M62.232 Nontraumatic ischemic infarction of muscle, left forearm
    - M62.239 Nontraumatic ischemic infarction of muscle, unspecified forearm
  - M62.24 Nontraumatic ischemic infarction of muscle, hand
    - M62.241 Nontraumatic ischemic infarction of muscle, right hand
    - M62.242 Nontraumatic ischemic infarction of muscle, left hand
    - M62.249 Nontraumatic ischemic infarction of muscle, unspecified hand
  - M62.25 Nontraumatic ischemic infarction of muscle, thigh
    - M62.251 Nontraumatic ischemic infarction of muscle, right thigh
    - M62.252 Nontraumatic ischemic infarction of muscle, left thigh
    - M62.259 Nontraumatic ischemic infarction of muscle, unspecified thigh
  - M62.26 Nontraumatic ischemic infarction of muscle, lower leg
    - M62.261 Nontraumatic ischemic infarction of muscle, right lower leg
    - M62.262 Nontraumatic ischemic infarction of muscle, left lower leg
    - M62.269 Nontraumatic ischemic infarction of muscle, unspecified lower leg
  - M62.27 Nontraumatic ischemic infarction of muscle, ankle and foot
    - M62.271 Nontraumatic ischemic infarction of muscle, right ankle and foot
    - M62.272 Nontraumatic ischemic infarction of muscle, left ankle and foot
    - M62.279 Nontraumatic ischemic infarction of muscle, unspecified ankle and foot
  - M62.28 Nontraumatic ischemic infarction of muscle, other site
- M62.3 Immobility syndrome (paraplegic)
- M62.4 Contracture of muscle

CONTRACTURE OF TENDON (SHEATH)

Excludes1 contracture of joint (M24.5-)

- M62.40 Contracture of muscle, unspecified site
- M62.41 Contracture of muscle, shoulder
  - M62.411 Contracture of muscle, right shoulder
  - M62.412 Contracture of muscle, left shoulder
  - M62.419 Contracture of muscle, unspecified shoulder
- M62.42 Contracture of muscle, upper arm
  - M62.421 Contracture of muscle, right upper arm
  - M62.422 Contracture of muscle, left upper arm
  - M62.429 Contracture of muscle, unspecified upper arm

- M62.43 Contracture of muscle, forearm
  - M62.431 Contracture of muscle, right forearm
  - M62.432 Contracture of muscle, left forearm
  - M62.439 Contracture of muscle, unspecified forearm
- M62.44 Contracture of muscle, hand
  - M62.441 Contracture of muscle, right hand
  - M62.442 Contracture of muscle, left hand
  - M62.449 Contracture of muscle, unspecified hand
- M62.45 Contracture of muscle, thigh
  - M62.451 Contracture of muscle, right thigh
  - M62.452 Contracture of muscle, left thigh
  - M62.459 Contracture of muscle, unspecified thigh
- M62.46 Contracture of muscle, lower leg
  - M62.461 Contracture of muscle, right lower leg
  - M62.462 Contracture of muscle, left lower leg
  - M62.469 Contracture of muscle, unspecified lower leg
- M62.47 Contracture of muscle, ankle and foot
  - M62.471 Contracture of muscle, right ankle and foot
  - M62.472 Contracture of muscle, left ankle and foot
  - M62.479 Contracture of muscle, unspecified ankle and foot
- M62.48 Contracture of muscle, other site
- M62.49 Contracture of muscle, multiple sites

- M62.5 Muscle wasting and atrophy, not elsewhere classified
  Disuse atrophy NEC
  Excludes1 neuralgic amyotrophy (G54.5)
  progressive muscular atrophy (G12.29)
  sarcopenia (M62.84) ◀
  Excludes2 pelvic muscle wasting (N81.84)
  - M62.50 Muscle wasting and atrophy, not elsewhere classified, unspecified site
  - M62.51 Muscle wasting and atrophy, not elsewhere classified, shoulder
    - M62.511 Muscle wasting and atrophy, not elsewhere classified, right shoulder
    - M62.512 Muscle wasting and atrophy, not elsewhere classified, left shoulder
    - M62.519 Muscle wasting and atrophy, not elsewhere classified, unspecified shoulder
  - M62.52 Muscle wasting and atrophy, not elsewhere classified, upper arm
    - M62.521 Muscle wasting and atrophy, not elsewhere classified, right upper arm
    - M62.522 Muscle wasting and atrophy, not elsewhere classified, left upper arm
    - M62.529 Muscle wasting and atrophy, not elsewhere classified, unspecified upper arm
  - M62.53 Muscle wasting and atrophy, not elsewhere classified, forearm
    - M62.531 Muscle wasting and atrophy, not elsewhere classified, right forearm
    - M62.532 Muscle wasting and atrophy, not elsewhere classified, left forearm
    - M62.539 Muscle wasting and atrophy, not elsewhere classified, unspecified forearm
  - M62.54 Muscle wasting and atrophy, not elsewhere classified, hand
    - M62.541 Muscle wasting and atrophy, not elsewhere classified, right hand
    - M62.542 Muscle wasting and atrophy, not elsewhere classified, left hand
    - M62.549 Muscle wasting and atrophy, not elsewhere classified, unspecified hand
  - M62.55 Muscle wasting and atrophy, not elsewhere classified, thigh
    - M62.551 Muscle wasting and atrophy, not elsewhere classified, right thigh
    - M62.552 Muscle wasting and atrophy, not elsewhere classified, left thigh
    - M62.559 Muscle wasting and atrophy, not elsewhere classified, unspecified thigh
  - M62.56 Muscle wasting and atrophy, not elsewhere classified, lower leg
    - M62.561 Muscle wasting and atrophy, not elsewhere classified, right lower leg
    - M62.562 Muscle wasting and atrophy, not elsewhere classified, left lower leg
    - M62.569 Muscle wasting and atrophy, not elsewhere classified, unspecified lower leg
  - M62.57 Muscle wasting and atrophy, not elsewhere classified, ankle and foot
    - M62.571 Muscle wasting and atrophy, not elsewhere classified, right ankle and foot
    - M62.572 Muscle wasting and atrophy, not elsewhere classified, left ankle and foot
    - M62.579 Muscle wasting and atrophy, not elsewhere classified, unspecified ankle and foot
  - M62.58 Muscle wasting and atrophy, not elsewhere classified, other site
  - M62.59 Muscle wasting and atrophy, not elsewhere classified, multiple sites

- M62.8 Other specified disorders of muscle
  Excludes2 nontraumatic hematoma of muscle (M79.81)
  - M62.81 Muscle weakness (generalized)
    Excludes1 muscle weakness in sarcopenia (M62.84) ◀
  - M62.82 Rhabdomyolysis
    Excludes1 traumatic rhabdomyolysis (T79.6)
    Ex: K68.12, M60.000-M60.19, M61.00-M61.19, M61.30-M61.59, M62.3, M62.50-M62.59, M62.82, M62.84, M62.89, M72.6
  - M62.83 Muscle spasm
    - M62.830 Muscle spasm of back
    - M62.831 Muscle spasm of calf
      Charley-horse
    - M62.838 Other muscle spasm
  - M62.84 Sarcopenia ◀
    Age-related sarcopenia ◀
    Code first underlying disease, if applicable, such as:
    disorders of myoneural junction and muscle disease in diseases classified elsewhere (G73.-) ◀
    other and unspecified myopathies (G72.-) ◀
    primary disorders of muscles (G71.-) ◀
  - M62.89 Other specified disorders of muscle
    Muscle (sheath) hernia
- M62.9 Disorder of muscle, unspecified

● **M63 Disorders of muscle in diseases classified elsewhere**

Code first underlying disease, such as:
leprosy (A30.-)
neoplasm (C49.-, C79.89, D21.-, D48.1)
schistosomiasis (B65.-)
trichinellosis (B75)

Excludes1 myopathy in cysticercosis (B69.81)
myopathy in endocrine diseases (G73.7)
myopathy in metabolic diseases (G73.7)
myopathy in sarcoidosis (D86.87)
myopathy in secondary syphilis (A51.49)
myopathy in syphilis (late) (A52.78)
myopathy in toxoplasmosis (B58.82)
myopathy in tuberculosis (A18.09)

● **M63.8 Disorders of muscle in diseases classified elsewhere**

▶ *M63.80 Disorders of muscle in diseases classified elsewhere, unspecified site*

● **M63.81 Disorders of muscle in diseases classified elsewhere, shoulder**

▶ *M63.811 Disorders of muscle in diseases classified elsewhere, right shoulder*

▶ *M63.812 Disorders of muscle in diseases classified elsewhere, left shoulder*

▶ *M63.819 Disorders of muscle in diseases classified elsewhere, unspecified shoulder*

● **M63.82 Disorders of muscle in diseases classified elsewhere, upper arm**

▶ *M63.821 Disorders of muscle in diseases classified elsewhere, right upper arm*

▶ *M63.822 Disorders of muscle in diseases classified elsewhere, left upper arm*

▶ *M63.829 Disorders of muscle in diseases classified elsewhere, unspecified upper arm*

● **M63.83 Disorders of muscle in diseases classified elsewhere, forearm**

▶ *M63.831 Disorders of muscle in diseases classified elsewhere, right forearm*

▶ *M63.832 Disorders of muscle in diseases classified elsewhere, left forearm*

▶ *M63.839 Disorders of muscle in diseases classified elsewhere, unspecified forearm*

● **M63.84 Disorders of muscle in diseases classified elsewhere, hand**

▶ *M63.841 Disorders of muscle in diseases classified elsewhere, right hand*

▶ *M63.842 Disorders of muscle in diseases classified elsewhere, left hand*

▶ *M63.849 Disorders of muscle in diseases classified elsewhere, unspecified hand*

● **M63.85 Disorders of muscle in diseases classified elsewhere, thigh**

▶ *M63.851 Disorders of muscle in diseases classified elsewhere, right thigh*

▶ *M63.852 Disorders of muscle in diseases classified elsewhere, left thigh*

▶ *M63.859 Disorders of muscle in diseases classified elsewhere, unspecified thigh*

● **M63.86 Disorders of muscle in diseases classified elsewhere, lower leg**

▶ *M63.861 Disorders of muscle in diseases classified elsewhere, right lower leg*

▶ *M63.862 Disorders of muscle in diseases classified elsewhere, left lower leg*

▶ *M63.869 Disorders of muscle in diseases classified elsewhere, unspecified lower leg*

● **M63.87 Disorders of muscle in diseases classified elsewhere, ankle and foot**

▶ *M63.871 Disorders of muscle in diseases classified elsewhere, right ankle and foot*

▶ *M63.872 Disorders of muscle in diseases classified elsewhere, left ankle and foot*

▶ *M63.879 Disorders of muscle in diseases classified elsewhere, unspecified ankle and foot*

▶ *M63.88 Disorders of muscle in diseases classified elsewhere, other site*

▶ *M63.89 Disorders of muscle in diseases classified elsewhere, multiple sites*

DISORDERS OF SYNOVIUM AND TENDON (M65-M67)

● **M65 Synovitis and tenosynovitis**

Excludes1 chronic crepitant synovitis of hand and wrist (M70.0-)
current injury - see injury of ligament or tendon by body region
soft tissue disorders related to use, overuse and pressure (M70.-)

● **M65.0 Abscess of tendon sheath**

Use additional code (B95-B96) to identify bacterial agent

M65.00 Abscess of tendon sheath, unspecified site

● **M65.01 Abscess of tendon sheath, shoulder**

M65.011 Abscess of tendon sheath, right shoulder

M65.012 Abscess of tendon sheath, left shoulder

M65.019 Abscess of tendon sheath, unspecified shoulder

● **M65.02 Abscess of tendon sheath, upper arm**

M65.021 Abscess of tendon sheath, right upper arm

M65.022 Abscess of tendon sheath, left upper arm

M65.029 Abscess of tendon sheath, unspecified upper arm

● **M65.03 Abscess of tendon sheath, forearm**

M65.031 Abscess of tendon sheath, right forearm

M65.032 Abscess of tendon sheath, left forearm

M65.039 Abscess of tendon sheath, unspecified forearm

● **M65.04 Abscess of tendon sheath, hand**

M65.041 Abscess of tendon sheath, right hand

M65.042 Abscess of tendon sheath, left hand

M65.049 Abscess of tendon sheath, unspecified hand

● **M65.05 Abscess of tendon sheath, thigh**

M65.051 Abscess of tendon sheath, right thigh

M65.052 Abscess of tendon sheath, left thigh

M65.059 Abscess of tendon sheath, unspecified thigh

Item 13-11 Synovitis is an inflammation of a synovial membrane resulting in pain on motion and is characterized by fluctuating swelling due to effusion in a synovial sac. **Tenosynovitis** is an inflammation of a tendon sheath and occurs most commonly in the wrists, hands, and feet. Bursitis is inflammation of a bursa (fluid filled sac) caused by repetitive use, trauma, infection, or systemic inflammatory disease. Bursae act as protectors and facilitate movement between bones and overlapping muscles (deep bursae) or between bones and tendons/skin (superficial bursae).

- M65.06 Abscess of tendon sheath, lower leg
  - M65.061 Abscess of tendon sheath, right lower leg
  - M65.062 Abscess of tendon sheath, left lower leg
  - M65.069 Abscess of tendon sheath, unspecified lower leg
- M65.07 Abscess of tendon sheath, ankle and foot
  - M65.071 Abscess of tendon sheath, right ankle and foot
  - M65.072 Abscess of tendon sheath, left ankle and foot
  - M65.079 Abscess of tendon sheath, unspecified ankle and foot
- M65.08 Abscess of tendon sheath, other site
- M65.1 Other infective (teno)synovitis
  - M65.10 Other infective (teno)synovitis, unspecified site
  - M65.11 Other infective (teno)synovitis, shoulder
    - M65.111 Other infective (teno)synovitis, right shoulder
    - M65.112 Other infective (teno)synovitis, left shoulder
    - M65.119 Other infective (teno)synovitis, unspecified shoulder
  - M65.12 Other infective (teno)synovitis, elbow
    - M65.121 Other infective (teno)synovitis, right elbow
    - M65.122 Other infective (teno)synovitis, left elbow
    - M65.129 Other infective (teno)synovitis, unspecified elbow
  - M65.13 Other infective (teno)synovitis, wrist
    - M65.131 Other infective (teno)synovitis, right wrist
    - M65.132 Other infective (teno)synovitis, left wrist
    - M65.139 Other infective (teno)synovitis, unspecified wrist
  - M65.14 Other infective (teno)synovitis, hand
    - M65.141 Other infective (teno)synovitis, right hand
    - M65.142 Other infective (teno)synovitis, left hand
    - M65.149 Other infective (teno)synovitis, unspecified hand
  - M65.15 Other infective (teno)synovitis, hip
    - M65.151 Other infective (teno)synovitis, right hip
    - M65.152 Other infective (teno)synovitis, left hip
    - M65.159 Other infective (teno)synovitis, unspecified hip
  - M65.16 Other infective (teno)synovitis, knee
    - M65.161 Other infective (teno)synovitis, right knee
    - M65.162 Other infective (teno)synovitis, left knee
    - M65.169 Other infective (teno)synovitis, unspecified knee
  - M65.17 Other infective (teno)synovitis, ankle and foot
    - M65.171 Other infective (teno)synovitis, right ankle and foot
    - M65.172 Other infective (teno)synovitis, left ankle and foot
    - M65.179 Other infective (teno)synovitis, unspecified ankle and foot
  - M65.18 Other infective (teno)synovitis, other site
  - M65.19 Other infective (teno)synovitis, multiple sites
- M65.2 Calcific tendinitis

  Excludes1 tendinitis as classified in M75-M77
  calcified tendinitis of shoulder (M75.3)
  - M65.20 Calcific tendinitis, unspecified site
  - M65.22 Calcific tendinitis, upper arm
    - M65.221 Calcific tendinitis, right upper arm
    - M65.222 Calcific tendinitis, left upper arm
    - M65.229 Calcific tendinitis, unspecified upper arm
  - M65.23 Calcific tendinitis, forearm
    - M65.231 Calcific tendinitis, right forearm
    - M65.232 Calcific tendinitis, left forearm
    - M65.239 Calcific tendinitis, unspecified forearm
  - M65.24 Calcific tendinitis, hand
    - M65.241 Calcific tendinitis, right hand
    - M65.242 Calcific tendinitis, left hand
    - M65.249 Calcific tendinitis, unspecified hand
  - M65.25 Calcific tendinitis, thigh
    - M65.251 Calcific tendinitis, right thigh
    - M65.252 Calcific tendinitis, left thigh
    - M65.259 Calcific tendinitis, unspecified thigh
  - M65.26 Calcific tendinitis, lower leg
    - M65.261 Calcific tendinitis, right lower leg
    - M65.262 Calcific tendinitis, left lower leg
    - M65.269 Calcific tendinitis, unspecified lower leg
  - M65.27 Calcific tendinitis, ankle and foot
    - M65.271 Calcific tendinitis, right ankle and foot
    - M65.272 Calcific tendinitis, left ankle and foot
    - M65.279 Calcific tendinitis, unspecified ankle and foot
  - M65.28 Calcific tendinitis, other site
  - M65.29 Calcific tendinitis, multiple sites
- M65.3 Trigger finger

  Nodular tendinous disease
  - M65.30 Trigger finger, unspecified finger
  - M65.31 Trigger thumb
    - M65.311 Trigger thumb, right thumb
    - M65.312 Trigger thumb, left thumb
    - M65.319 Trigger thumb, unspecified thumb
  - M65.32 Trigger finger, index finger
    - M65.321 Trigger finger, right index finger
    - M65.322 Trigger finger, left index finger
    - M65.329 Trigger finger, unspecified index finger
  - M65.33 Trigger finger, middle finger
    - M65.331 Trigger finger, right middle finger
    - M65.332 Trigger finger, left middle finger
    - M65.339 Trigger finger, unspecified middle finger
  - M65.34 Trigger finger, ring finger
    - M65.341 Trigger finger, right ring finger
    - M65.342 Trigger finger, left ring finger
    - M65.349 Trigger finger, unspecified ring finger
  - M65.35 Trigger finger, little finger
    - M65.351 Trigger finger, right little finger
    - M65.352 Trigger finger, left little finger
    - M65.359 Trigger finger, unspecified little finger
- M65.4 Radial styloid tenosynovitis [de Quervain]

- M65.8 Other synovitis and tenosynovitis
  - M65.80 Other synovitis and tenosynovitis, unspecified site
  - M65.81 Other synovitis and tenosynovitis, shoulder
    - M65.811 Other synovitis and tenosynovitis, right shoulder
    - M65.812 Other synovitis and tenosynovitis, left shoulder
    - M65.819 Other synovitis and tenosynovitis, unspecified shoulder
  - M65.82 Other synovitis and tenosynovitis, upper arm
    - M65.821 Other synovitis and tenosynovitis, right upper arm
    - M65.822 Other synovitis and tenosynovitis, left upper arm
    - M65.829 Other synovitis and tenosynovitis, unspecified upper arm
  - M65.83 Other synovitis and tenosynovitis, forearm
    - M65.831 Other synovitis and tenosynovitis, right forearm
    - M65.832 Other synovitis and tenosynovitis, left forearm
    - M65.839 Other synovitis and tenosynovitis, unspecified forearm
  - M65.84 Other synovitis and tenosynovitis, hand
    - M65.841 Other synovitis and tenosynovitis, right hand
    - M65.842 Other synovitis and tenosynovitis, left hand
    - M65.849 Other synovitis and tenosynovitis, unspecified hand
  - M65.85 Other synovitis and tenosynovitis, thigh
    - M65.851 Other synovitis and tenosynovitis, right thigh
    - M65.852 Other synovitis and tenosynovitis, left thigh
    - M65.859 Other synovitis and tenosynovitis, unspecified thigh
  - M65.86 Other synovitis and tenosynovitis, lower leg
    - M65.861 Other synovitis and tenosynovitis, right lower leg
    - M65.862 Other synovitis and tenosynovitis, left lower leg
    - M65.869 Other synovitis and tenosynovitis, unspecified lower leg
  - M65.87 Other synovitis and tenosynovitis, ankle and foot
    - M65.871 Other synovitis and tenosynovitis, right ankle and foot
    - M65.872 Other synovitis and tenosynovitis, left ankle and foot
    - M65.879 Other synovitis and tenosynovitis, unspecified ankle and foot
  - M65.88 Other synovitis and tenosynovitis, other site
  - M65.89 Other synovitis and tenosynovitis, multiple sites
- M65.9 Synovitis and tenosynovitis, unspecified

- M66 Spontaneous rupture of synovium and tendon

  Includes rupture that occurs when a normal force is applied to tissues that are inferred to have less than normal strength

  Excludes2 rotator cuff syndrome (M75.1-)
  rupture where an abnormal force is applied to normal tissue - see injury of tendon by body region

  - M66.0 Rupture of popliteal cyst
  - M66.1 Rupture of synovium

    Rupture of synovial cyst

    Excludes2 rupture of popliteal cyst (M66.0)
    - M66.10 Rupture of synovium, unspecified joint
    - M66.11 Rupture of synovium, shoulder
      - M66.111 Rupture of synovium, right shoulder
      - M66.112 Rupture of synovium, left shoulder
      - M66.119 Rupture of synovium, unspecified shoulder
    - M66.12 Rupture of synovium, elbow
      - M66.121 Rupture of synovium, right elbow
      - M66.122 Rupture of synovium, left elbow
      - M66.129 Rupture of synovium, unspecified elbow
    - M66.13 Rupture of synovium, wrist
      - M66.131 Rupture of synovium, right wrist
      - M66.132 Rupture of synovium, left wrist
      - M66.139 Rupture of synovium, unspecified wrist
    - M66.14 Rupture of synovium, hand and fingers
      - M66.141 Rupture of synovium, right hand
      - M66.142 Rupture of synovium, left hand
      - M66.143 Rupture of synovium, unspecified hand
      - M66.144 Rupture of synovium, right finger(s)
      - M66.145 Rupture of synovium, left finger(s)
      - M66.146 Rupture of synovium, unspecified finger(s)
    - M66.15 Rupture of synovium, hip
      - M66.151 Rupture of synovium, right hip
      - M66.152 Rupture of synovium, left hip
      - M66.159 Rupture of synovium, unspecified hip
    - M66.17 Rupture of synovium, ankle, foot and toes
      - M66.171 Rupture of synovium, right ankle
      - M66.172 Rupture of synovium, left ankle
      - M66.173 Rupture of synovium, unspecified ankle
      - M66.174 Rupture of synovium, right foot
      - M66.175 Rupture of synovium, left foot
      - M66.176 Rupture of synovium, unspecified foot
      - M66.177 Rupture of synovium, right toe(s)
      - M66.178 Rupture of synovium, left toe(s)
      - M66.179 Rupture of synovium, unspecified toe(s)
    - M66.18 Rupture of synovium, other site
  - M66.2 Spontaneous rupture of extensor tendons
    - M66.20 Spontaneous rupture of extensor tendons, unspecified site
    - M66.21 Spontaneous rupture of extensor tendons, shoulder
      - M66.211 Spontaneous rupture of extensor tendons, right shoulder
      - M66.212 Spontaneous rupture of extensor tendons, left shoulder
      - M66.219 Spontaneous rupture of extensor tendons, unspecified shoulder

◀ New ◀ Revised ~~deleted~~ Deleted Excludes 1 Excludes 2 Includes Use additional Code first Code also Unspecified
OGCR Official Guidelines ● Unacceptable Principal Diagnosis X Assign placeholder X ● Use Additional Character(s) ▶ Manifestation Code Coding Clinic

- M66.22 Spontaneous rupture of extensor tendons, upper arm
  - M66.221 Spontaneous rupture of extensor tendons, right upper arm
  - M66.222 Spontaneous rupture of extensor tendons, left upper arm
  - M66.229 Spontaneous rupture of extensor tendons, unspecified upper arm
- M66.23 Spontaneous rupture of extensor tendons, forearm
  - M66.231 Spontaneous rupture of extensor tendons, right forearm
  - M66.232 Spontaneous rupture of extensor tendons, left forearm
  - M66.239 Spontaneous rupture of extensor tendons, unspecified forearm
- M66.24 Spontaneous rupture of extensor tendons, hand
  - M66.241 Spontaneous rupture of extensor tendons, right hand
  - M66.242 Spontaneous rupture of extensor tendons, left hand
  - M66.249 Spontaneous rupture of extensor tendons, unspecified hand
- M66.25 Spontaneous rupture of extensor tendons, thigh
  - M66.251 Spontaneous rupture of extensor tendons, right thigh
  - M66.252 Spontaneous rupture of extensor tendons, left thigh
  - M66.259 Spontaneous rupture of extensor tendons, unspecified thigh
- M66.26 Spontaneous rupture of extensor tendons, lower leg
  - M66.261 Spontaneous rupture of extensor tendons, right lower leg
  - M66.262 Spontaneous rupture of extensor tendons, left lower leg
  - M66.269 Spontaneous rupture of extensor tendons, unspecified lower leg
- M66.27 Spontaneous rupture of extensor tendons, ankle and foot
  - M66.271 Spontaneous rupture of extensor tendons, right ankle and foot
  - M66.272 Spontaneous rupture of extensor tendons, left ankle and foot
  - M66.279 Spontaneous rupture of extensor tendons, unspecified ankle and foot
- M66.28 Spontaneous rupture of extensor tendons, other site
- M66.29 Spontaneous rupture of extensor tendons, multiple sites

- M66.3 Spontaneous rupture of flexor tendons
  - M66.30 Spontaneous rupture of flexor tendons, unspecified site
  - M66.31 Spontaneous rupture of flexor tendons, shoulder
    - M66.311 Spontaneous rupture of flexor tendons, right shoulder
    - M66.312 Spontaneous rupture of flexor tendons, left shoulder
    - M66.319 Spontaneous rupture of flexor tendons, unspecified shoulder
  - M66.32 Spontaneous rupture of flexor tendons, upper arm
    - M66.321 Spontaneous rupture of flexor tendons, right upper arm
    - M66.322 Spontaneous rupture of flexor tendons, left upper arm
    - M66.329 Spontaneous rupture of flexor tendons, unspecified upper arm
  - M66.33 Spontaneous rupture of flexor tendons, forearm
    - M66.331 Spontaneous rupture of flexor tendons, right forearm
    - M66.332 Spontaneous rupture of flexor tendons, left forearm
    - M66.339 Spontaneous rupture of flexor tendons, unspecified forearm
  - M66.34 Spontaneous rupture of flexor tendons, hand
    - M66.341 Spontaneous rupture of flexor tendons, right hand
    - M66.342 Spontaneous rupture of flexor tendons, left hand
    - M66.349 Spontaneous rupture of flexor tendons, unspecified hand
  - M66.35 Spontaneous rupture of flexor tendons, thigh
    - M66.351 Spontaneous rupture of flexor tendons, right thigh
    - M66.352 Spontaneous rupture of flexor tendons, left thigh
    - M66.359 Spontaneous rupture of flexor tendons, unspecified thigh
  - M66.36 Spontaneous rupture of flexor tendons, lower leg
    - M66.361 Spontaneous rupture of flexor tendons, right lower leg
    - M66.362 Spontaneous rupture of flexor tendons, left lower leg
    - M66.369 Spontaneous rupture of flexor tendons, unspecified lower leg
  - M66.37 Spontaneous rupture of flexor tendons, ankle and foot
    - M66.371 Spontaneous rupture of flexor tendons, right ankle and foot
    - M66.372 Spontaneous rupture of flexor tendons, left ankle and foot
    - M66.379 Spontaneous rupture of flexor tendons, unspecified ankle and foot
  - M66.38 Spontaneous rupture of flexor tendons, other site
  - M66.39 Spontaneous rupture of flexor tendons, multiple sites
- M66.8 Spontaneous rupture of other tendons
  - M66.80 Spontaneous rupture of other tendons, unspecified site
  - M66.81 Spontaneous rupture of other tendons, shoulder
    - M66.811 Spontaneous rupture of other tendons, right shoulder
    - M66.812 Spontaneous rupture of other tendons, left shoulder
    - M66.819 Spontaneous rupture of other tendons, unspecified shoulder
  - M66.82 Spontaneous rupture of other tendons, upper arm
    - M66.821 Spontaneous rupture of other tendons, right upper arm
    - M66.822 Spontaneous rupture of other tendons, left upper arm
    - M66.829 Spontaneous rupture of other tendons, unspecified upper arm
  - M66.83 Spontaneous rupture of other tendons, forearm
    - M66.831 Spontaneous rupture of other tendons, right forearm
    - M66.832 Spontaneous rupture of other tendons, left forearm
    - M66.839 Spontaneous rupture of other tendons, unspecified forearm

- M66.84 Spontaneous rupture of other tendons, hand
  - M66.841 Spontaneous rupture of other tendons, right hand
  - M66.842 Spontaneous rupture of other tendons, left hand
  - M66.849 Spontaneous rupture of other tendons, unspecified hand
- M66.85 Spontaneous rupture of other tendons, thigh
  - M66.851 Spontaneous rupture of other tendons, right thigh
  - M66.852 Spontaneous rupture of other tendons, left thigh
  - M66.859 Spontaneous rupture of other tendons, unspecified thigh
- M66.86 Spontaneous rupture of other tendons, lower leg
  - M66.861 Spontaneous rupture of other tendons, right lower leg
  - M66.862 Spontaneous rupture of other tendons, left lower leg
  - M66.869 Spontaneous rupture of other tendons, unspecified lower leg
- M66.87 Spontaneous rupture of other tendons, ankle and foot
  - M66.871 Spontaneous rupture of other tendons, right ankle and foot
  - M66.872 Spontaneous rupture of other tendons, left ankle and foot
  - M66.879 Spontaneous rupture of other tendons, unspecified ankle and foot
- M66.88 Spontaneous rupture of other tendons, other
- M66.89 Spontaneous rupture of other tendons, multiple sites
- M66.9 Spontaneous rupture of unspecified tendon
  Rupture at musculotendinous junction, nontraumatic

- M67 Other disorders of synovium and tendon
  Excludes1 palmar fascial fibromatosis [Dupuytren] (M72.0)
  tendinitis NOS (M77.9-)
  xanthomatosis localized to tendons (E78.2)
- M67.0 Short Achilles tendon (acquired)
  - M67.00 Short Achilles tendon (acquired), unspecified ankle
  - M67.01 Short Achilles tendon (acquired), right ankle
  - M67.02 Short Achilles tendon (acquired), left ankle
- M67.2 Synovial hypertrophy, not elsewhere classified
  Excludes1 villonodular synovitis (pigmented) (M12.2-)
  - M67.20 Synovial hypertrophy, not elsewhere classified, unspecified site
  - M67.21 Synovial hypertrophy, not elsewhere classified, shoulder
    - M67.211 Synovial hypertrophy, not elsewhere classified, right shoulder
    - M67.212 Synovial hypertrophy, not elsewhere classified, left shoulder
    - M67.219 Synovial hypertrophy, not elsewhere classified, unspecified shoulder
  - M67.22 Synovial hypertrophy, not elsewhere classified, upper arm
    - M67.221 Synovial hypertrophy, not elsewhere classified, right upper arm
    - M67.222 Synovial hypertrophy, not elsewhere classified, left upper arm
    - M67.229 Synovial hypertrophy, not elsewhere classified, unspecified upper arm
  - M67.23 Synovial hypertrophy, not elsewhere classified, forearm
    - M67.231 Synovial hypertrophy, not elsewhere classified, right forearm
    - M67.232 Synovial hypertrophy, not elsewhere classified, left forearm
    - M67.239 Synovial hypertrophy, not elsewhere classified, unspecified forearm
  - M67.24 Synovial hypertrophy, not elsewhere classified, hand
    - M67.241 Synovial hypertrophy, not elsewhere classified, right hand
    - M67.242 Synovial hypertrophy, not elsewhere classified, left hand
    - M67.249 Synovial hypertrophy, not elsewhere classified, unspecified hand
  - M67.25 Synovial hypertrophy, not elsewhere classified, thigh
    - M67.251 Synovial hypertrophy, not elsewhere classified, right thigh
    - M67.252 Synovial hypertrophy, not elsewhere classified, left thigh
    - M67.259 Synovial hypertrophy, not elsewhere classified, unspecified thigh
  - M67.26 Synovial hypertrophy, not elsewhere classified, lower leg
    - M67.261 Synovial hypertrophy, not elsewhere classified, right lower leg
    - M67.262 Synovial hypertrophy, not elsewhere classified, left lower leg
    - M67.269 Synovial hypertrophy, not elsewhere classified, unspecified lower leg
  - M67.27 Synovial hypertrophy, not elsewhere classified, ankle and foot
    - M67.271 Synovial hypertrophy, not elsewhere classified, right ankle and foot
    - M67.272 Synovial hypertrophy, not elsewhere classified, left ankle and foot
    - M67.279 Synovial hypertrophy, not elsewhere classified, unspecified ankle and foot
  - M67.28 Synovial hypertrophy, not elsewhere classified, other site
  - M67.29 Synovial hypertrophy, not elsewhere classified, multiple sites
- M67.3 Transient synovitis
  Toxic synovitis
  Excludes1 palindromic rheumatism (M12.3-)
  - M67.30 Transient synovitis, unspecified site
  - M67.31 Transient synovitis, shoulder
    - M67.311 Transient synovitis, right shoulder
    - M67.312 Transient synovitis, left shoulder
    - M67.319 Transient synovitis, unspecified shoulder
  - M67.32 Transient synovitis, elbow
    - M67.321 Transient synovitis, right elbow
    - M67.322 Transient synovitis, left elbow
    - M67.329 Transient synovitis, unspecified elbow
  - M67.33 Transient synovitis, wrist
    - M67.331 Transient synovitis, right wrist
    - M67.332 Transient synovitis, left wrist
    - M67.339 Transient synovitis, unspecified wrist
  - M67.34 Transient synovitis, hand
    - M67.341 Transient synovitis, right hand
    - M67.342 Transient synovitis, left hand
    - M67.349 Transient synovitis, unspecified hand

- M67.35 Transient synovitis, hip
  - M67.351 Transient synovitis, right hip
  - M67.352 Transient synovitis, left hip
  - M67.359 Transient synovitis, unspecified hip
- M67.36 Transient synovitis, knee
  - M67.361 Transient synovitis, right knee
  - M67.362 Transient synovitis, left knee
  - M67.369 Transient synovitis, unspecified knee
- M67.37 Transient synovitis, ankle and foot
  - M67.371 Transient synovitis, right ankle and foot
  - M67.372 Transient synovitis, left ankle and foot
  - M67.379 Transient synovitis, unspecified ankle and foot
- M67.38 Transient synovitis, other site
- M67.39 Transient synovitis, multiple sites

- M67.4 Ganglion
  Ganglion of joint or tendon (sheath)
  Excludes1 ganglion in yaws (A66.6)
  Excludes2 cyst of bursa (M71.2-M71.3)
  cyst of synovium (M71.2-M71.3)
  - M67.40 Ganglion, unspecified site
  - M67.41 Ganglion, shoulder
    - M67.411 Ganglion, right shoulder
    - M67.412 Ganglion, left shoulder
    - M67.419 Ganglion, unspecified shoulder
  - M67.42 Ganglion, elbow
    - M67.421 Ganglion, right elbow
    - M67.422 Ganglion, left elbow
    - M67.429 Ganglion, unspecified elbow
  - M67.43 Ganglion, wrist
    - M67.431 Ganglion, right wrist
    - M67.432 Ganglion, left wrist
    - M67.439 Ganglion, unspecified wrist
  - M67.44 Ganglion, hand
    - M67.441 Ganglion, right hand
    - M67.442 Ganglion, left hand
    - M67.449 Ganglion, unspecified hand
  - M67.45 Ganglion, hip
    - M67.451 Ganglion, right hip
    - M67.452 Ganglion, left hip
    - M67.459 Ganglion, unspecified hip
  - M67.46 Ganglion, knee
    - M67.461 Ganglion, right knee
    - M67.462 Ganglion, left knee
    - M67.469 Ganglion, unspecified knee
  - M67.47 Ganglion, ankle and foot
    - M67.471 Ganglion, right ankle and foot
    - M67.472 Ganglion, left ankle and foot
    - M67.479 Ganglion, unspecified ankle and foot
  - M67.48 Ganglion, other site
  - M67.49 Ganglion, multiple sites

- M67.5 Plica syndrome
  Plica knee
  - M67.50 Plica syndrome, unspecified knee
  - M67.51 Plica syndrome, right knee
  - M67.52 Plica syndrome, left knee

- M67.8 Other specified disorders of synovium and tendon
  - M67.80 Other specified disorders of synovium and tendon, unspecified site
  - M67.81 Other specified disorders of synovium and tendon, shoulder
    - M67.811 Other specified disorders of synovium, right shoulder
    - M67.812 Other specified disorders of synovium, left shoulder
    - M67.813 Other specified disorders of tendon, right shoulder
    - M67.814 Other specified disorders of tendon, left shoulder
    - M67.819 Other specified disorders of synovium and tendon, unspecified shoulder
  - M67.82 Other specified disorders of synovium and tendon, elbow
    - M67.821 Other specified disorders of synovium, right elbow
    - M67.822 Other specified disorders of synovium, left elbow
    - M67.823 Other specified disorders of tendon, right elbow
    - M67.824 Other specified disorders of tendon, left elbow
    - M67.829 Other specified disorders of synovium and tendon, unspecified elbow
  - M67.83 Other specified disorders of synovium and tendon, wrist
    - M67.831 Other specified disorders of synovium, right wrist
    - M67.832 Other specified disorders of synovium, left wrist
    - M67.833 Other specified disorders of tendon, right wrist
    - M67.834 Other specified disorders of tendon, left wrist
    - M67.839 Other specified disorders of synovium and tendon, unspecified forearm
  - M67.84 Other specified disorders of synovium and tendon, hand
    - M67.841 Other specified disorders of synovium, right hand
    - M67.842 Other specified disorders of synovium, left hand
    - M67.843 Other specified disorders of tendon, right hand
    - M67.844 Other specified disorders of tendon, left hand
    - M67.849 Other specified disorders of synovium and tendon, unspecified hand
  - M67.85 Other specified disorders of synovium and tendon, hip
    - M67.851 Other specified disorders of synovium, right hip
    - M67.852 Other specified disorders of synovium, left hip
    - M67.853 Other specified disorders of tendon, right hip
    - M67.854 Other specified disorders of tendon, left hip
    - M67.859 Other specified disorders of synovium and tendon, unspecified hip
  - M67.86 Other specified disorders of synovium and tendon, knee
    - M67.861 Other specified disorders of synovium, right knee
    - M67.862 Other specified disorders of synovium, left knee
    - M67.863 Other specified disorders of tendon, right knee
    - M67.864 Other specified disorders of tendon, left knee
    - M67.869 Other specified disorders of synovium and tendon, unspecified knee

- M67.87 Other specified disorders of synovium and tendon, ankle and foot
  - M67.871 Other specified disorders of synovium, right ankle and foot
  - M67.872 Other specified disorders of synovium, left ankle and foot
  - M67.873 Other specified disorders of tendon, right ankle and foot
  - M67.874 Other specified disorders of tendon, left ankle and foot
  - M67.879 Other specified disorders of synovium and tendon, unspecified ankle and foot
- M67.88 Other specified disorders of synovium and tendon, other site
- M67.89 Other specified disorders of synovium and tendon, multiple sites
- M67.9 Unspecified disorder of synovium and tendon
  - M67.90 Unspecified disorder of synovium and tendon, unspecified site
  - M67.91 Unspecified disorder of synovium and tendon, shoulder
    - M67.911 Unspecified disorder of synovium and tendon, right shoulder
    - M67.912 Unspecified disorder of synovium and tendon, left shoulder
    - M67.919 Unspecified disorder of synovium and tendon, unspecified shoulder
  - M67.92 Unspecified disorder of synovium and tendon, upper arm
    - M67.921 Unspecified disorder of synovium and tendon, right upper arm
    - M67.922 Unspecified disorder of synovium and tendon, left upper arm
    - M67.929 Unspecified disorder of synovium and tendon, unspecified upper arm
  - M67.93 Unspecified disorder of synovium and tendon, forearm
    - M67.931 Unspecified disorder of synovium and tendon, right forearm
    - M67.932 Unspecified disorder of synovium and tendon, left forearm
    - M67.939 Unspecified disorder of synovium and tendon, unspecified forearm
  - M67.94 Unspecified disorder of synovium and tendon, hand
    - M67.941 Unspecified disorder of synovium and tendon, right hand
    - M67.942 Unspecified disorder of synovium and tendon, left hand
    - M67.949 Unspecified disorder of synovium and tendon, unspecified hand
  - M67.95 Unspecified disorder of synovium and tendon, thigh
    - M67.951 Unspecified disorder of synovium and tendon, right thigh
    - M67.952 Unspecified disorder of synovium and tendon, left thigh
    - M67.959 Unspecified disorder of synovium and tendon, unspecified thigh
  - M67.96 Unspecified disorder of synovium and tendon, lower leg
    - M67.961 Unspecified disorder of synovium and tendon, right lower leg
    - M67.962 Unspecified disorder of synovium and tendon, left lower leg
    - M67.969 Unspecified disorder of synovium and tendon, unspecified lower leg
  - M67.97 Unspecified disorder of synovium and tendon, ankle and foot
    - M67.971 Unspecified disorder of synovium and tendon, right ankle and foot
    - M67.972 Unspecified disorder of synovium and tendon, left ankle and foot
    - M67.979 Unspecified disorder of synovium and tendon, unspecified ankle and foot
  - M67.98 Unspecified disorder of synovium and tendon, other site
  - M67.99 Unspecified disorder of synovium and tendon, multiple sites

OTHER SOFT TISSUE DISORDERS (M70-M79)

- M70 Soft tissue disorders related to use, overuse and pressure

  Includes soft tissue disorders of occupational origin

  Use additional external cause code to identify activity causing disorder (Y93.-)

  Excludes1 bursitis NOS (M71.9-)

  Excludes2 bursitis of shoulder (M75.5)
  enthesopathies (M76-M77)
  pressure ulcer (pressure area) (L89.-)
  - M70.0 Crepitant synovitis (acute) (chronic) of hand and wrist
    - M70.03 Crepitant synovitis (acute) (chronic), wrist
      - M70.031 Crepitant synovitis (acute) (chronic), right wrist
      - M70.032 Crepitant synovitis (acute) (chronic), left wrist
      - M70.039 Crepitant synovitis (acute) (chronic), unspecified wrist
    - M70.04 Crepitant synovitis (acute) (chronic), hand
      - M70.041 Crepitant synovitis (acute) (chronic), right hand
      - M70.042 Crepitant synovitis (acute) (chronic), left hand
      - M70.049 Crepitant synovitis (acute) (chronic), unspecified hand
  - M70.1 Bursitis of hand
    - M70.10 Bursitis, unspecified hand
    - M70.11 Bursitis, right hand
    - M70.12 Bursitis, left hand
  - M70.2 Olecranon bursitis
    - M70.20 Olecranon bursitis, unspecified elbow
    - M70.21 Olecranon bursitis, right elbow
    - M70.22 Olecranon bursitis, left elbow
  - M70.3 Other bursitis of elbow
    - M70.30 Other bursitis of elbow, unspecified elbow
    - M70.31 Other bursitis of elbow, right elbow
    - M70.32 Other bursitis of elbow, left elbow
  - M70.4 Prepatellar bursitis
    - M70.40 Prepatellar bursitis, unspecified knee
    - M70.41 Prepatellar bursitis, right knee
    - M70.42 Prepatellar bursitis, left knee
  - M70.5 Other bursitis of knee
    - M70.50 Other bursitis of knee, unspecified knee
    - M70.51 Other bursitis of knee, right knee
    - M70.52 Other bursitis of knee, left knee
  - M70.6 Trochanteric bursitis

    Trochanteric tendinitis
    - M70.60 Trochanteric bursitis, unspecified hip
    - M70.61 Trochanteric bursitis, right hip
    - M70.62 Trochanteric bursitis, left hip

◀ New ◀ Revised ~~deleted~~ Deleted Excludes 1 Excludes 2 Includes Use additional Code first Code also Unspecified
OGCR Official Guidelines ● Unacceptable Principal Diagnosis X Assign placeholder X ● Use Additional Character(s) ▶ Manifestation Code Coding Clinic

- **M70.7** Other bursitis of hip
  Ischial bursitis
  - M70.70 Other bursitis of hip, unspecified hip
  - M70.71 Other bursitis of hip, right hip
  - M70.72 Other bursitis of hip, left hip
- **M70.8** Other soft tissue disorders related to use, overuse and pressure
  - M70.80 Other soft tissue disorders related to use, overuse and pressure of unspecified site
  - **M70.81** Other soft tissue disorders related to use, overuse and pressure of shoulder
    - M70.811 Other soft tissue disorders related to use, overuse and pressure, right shoulder
    - M70.812 Other soft tissue disorders related to use, overuse and pressure, left shoulder
    - M70.819 Other soft tissue disorders related to use, overuse and pressure, unspecified shoulder
  - **M70.82** Other soft tissue disorders related to use, overuse and pressure of upper arm
    - M70.821 Other soft tissue disorders related to use, overuse and pressure, right upper arm
    - M70.822 Other soft tissue disorders related to use, overuse and pressure, left upper arm
    - M70.829 Other soft tissue disorders related to use, overuse and pressure, unspecified upper arms
  - **M70.83** Other soft tissue disorders related to use, overuse and pressure of forearm
    - M70.831 Other soft tissue disorders related to use, overuse and pressure, right forearm
    - M70.832 Other soft tissue disorders related to use, overuse and pressure, left forearm
    - M70.839 Other soft tissue disorders related to use, overuse and pressure, unspecified forearm
  - **M70.84** Other soft tissue disorders related to use, overuse and pressure of hand
    - M70.841 Other soft tissue disorders related to use, overuse and pressure, right hand
    - M70.842 Other soft tissue disorders related to use, overuse and pressure, left hand
    - M70.849 Other soft tissue disorders related to use, overuse and pressure, unspecified hand
  - **M70.85** Other soft tissue disorders related to use, overuse and pressure of thigh
    - M70.851 Other soft tissue disorders related to use, overuse and pressure, right thigh
    - M70.852 Other soft tissue disorders related to use, overuse and pressure, left thigh
    - M70.859 Other soft tissue disorders related to use, overuse and pressure, unspecified thigh
  - **M70.86** Other soft tissue disorders related to use, overuse and pressure lower leg
    - M70.861 Other soft tissue disorders related to use, overuse and pressure, right lower leg
    - M70.862 Other soft tissue disorders related to use, overuse and pressure, left lower leg
    - M70.869 Other soft tissue disorders related to use, overuse and pressure, unspecified leg
  - **M70.87** Other soft tissue disorders related to use, overuse and pressure of ankle and foot
    - M70.871 Other soft tissue disorders related to use, overuse and pressure, right ankle and foot
    - M70.872 Other soft tissue disorders related to use, overuse and pressure, left ankle and foot
    - M70.879 Other soft tissue disorders related to use, overuse and pressure, unspecified ankle and foot
  - M70.88 Other soft tissue disorders related to use, overuse and pressure other site
  - M70.89 Other soft tissue disorders related to use, overuse and pressure multiple sites
- **M70.9** Unspecified soft tissue disorder related to use, overuse and pressure
  - M70.90 Unspecified soft tissue disorder related to use, overuse and pressure of unspecified site
  - **M70.91** Unspecified soft tissue disorder related to use, overuse and pressure of shoulder
    - M70.911 Unspecified soft tissue disorder related to use, overuse and pressure, right shoulder
    - M70.912 Unspecified soft tissue disorder related to use, overuse and pressure, left shoulder
    - M70.919 Unspecified soft tissue disorder related to use, overuse and pressure, unspecified shoulder
  - **M70.92** Unspecified soft tissue disorder related to use, overuse and pressure of upper arm
    - M70.921 Unspecified soft tissue disorder related to use, overuse and pressure, right upper arm
    - M70.922 Unspecified soft tissue disorder related to use, overuse and pressure, left upper arm
    - M70.929 Unspecified soft tissue disorder related to use, overuse and pressure, unspecified upper arm
  - **M70.93** Unspecified soft tissue disorder related to use, overuse and pressure of forearm
    - M70.931 Unspecified soft tissue disorder related to use, overuse and pressure, right forearm
    - M70.932 Unspecified soft tissue disorder related to use, overuse and pressure, left forearm
    - M70.939 Unspecified soft tissue disorder related to use, overuse and pressure, unspecified forearm
  - **M70.94** Unspecified soft tissue disorder related to use, overuse and pressure of hand
    - M70.941 Unspecified soft tissue disorder related to use, overuse and pressure, right hand
    - M70.942 Unspecified soft tissue disorder related to use, overuse and pressure, left hand
    - M70.949 Unspecified soft tissue disorder related to use, overuse and pressure, unspecified hand

- M70.95 Unspecified soft tissue disorder related to use, overuse and pressure of thigh
  - M70.951 Unspecified soft tissue disorder related to use, overuse and pressure, right thigh
  - M70.952 Unspecified soft tissue disorder related to use, overuse and pressure, left thigh
  - M70.959 Unspecified soft tissue disorder related to use, overuse and pressure, unspecified thigh
- M70.96 Unspecified soft tissue disorder related to use, overuse and pressure lower leg
  - M70.961 Unspecified soft tissue disorder related to use, overuse and pressure, right lower leg
  - M70.962 Unspecified soft tissue disorder related to use, overuse and pressure, left lower leg
  - M70.969 Unspecified soft tissue disorder related to use, overuse and pressure, unspecified lower leg
- M70.97 Unspecified soft tissue disorder related to use, overuse and pressure of ankle and foot
  - M70.971 Unspecified soft tissue disorder related to use, overuse and pressure, right ankle and foot
  - M70.972 Unspecified soft tissue disorder related to use, overuse and pressure, left ankle and foot
  - M70.979 Unspecified soft tissue disorder related to use, overuse and pressure, unspecified ankle and foot
- M70.98 Unspecified soft tissue disorder related to use, overuse and pressure other
- M70.99 Unspecified soft tissue disorder related to use, overuse and pressure multiple sites

- M71 Other bursopathies

  Excludes1 bunion (M20.1)
  bursitis related to use, overuse or pressure (M70.-)
  enthesopathies (M76-M77)

  - M71.0 Abscess of bursa

    Use additional code (B95.-, B96.-) to identify causative organism

    - M71.00 Abscess of bursa, unspecified site
    - M71.01 Abscess of bursa, shoulder
      - M71.011 Abscess of bursa, right shoulder
      - M71.012 Abscess of bursa, left shoulder
      - M71.019 Abscess of bursa, unspecified shoulder
    - M71.02 Abscess of bursa, elbow
      - M71.021 Abscess of bursa, right elbow
      - M71.022 Abscess of bursa, left elbow
      - M71.029 Abscess of bursa, unspecified elbow
    - M71.03 Abscess of bursa, wrist
      - M71.031 Abscess of bursa, right wrist
      - M71.032 Abscess of bursa, left wrist
      - M71.039 Abscess of bursa, unspecified wrist
    - M71.04 Abscess of bursa, hand
      - M71.041 Abscess of bursa, right hand
      - M71.042 Abscess of bursa, left hand
      - M71.049 Abscess of bursa, unspecified hand
    - M71.05 Abscess of bursa, hip
      - M71.051 Abscess of bursa, right hip
      - M71.052 Abscess of bursa, left hip
      - M71.059 Abscess of bursa, unspecified hip
    - M71.06 Abscess of bursa, knee
      - M71.061 Abscess of bursa, right knee
      - M71.062 Abscess of bursa, left knee
      - M71.069 Abscess of bursa, unspecified knee
    - M71.07 Abscess of bursa, ankle and foot
      - M71.071 Abscess of bursa, right ankle and foot
      - M71.072 Abscess of bursa, left ankle and foot
      - M71.079 Abscess of bursa, unspecified ankle and foot
    - M71.08 Abscess of bursa, other site
    - M71.09 Abscess of bursa, multiple sites
  - M71.1 Other infective bursitis

    Use additional code (B95.-, B96.-) to identify causative organism

    - M71.10 Other infective bursitis, unspecified site
    - M71.11 Other infective bursitis, shoulder
      - M71.111 Other infective bursitis, right shoulder
      - M71.112 Other infective bursitis, left shoulder
      - M71.119 Other infective bursitis, unspecified shoulder
    - M71.12 Other infective bursitis, elbow
      - M71.121 Other infective bursitis, right elbow
      - M71.122 Other infective bursitis, left elbow
      - M71.129 Other infective bursitis, unspecified elbow
    - M71.13 Other infective bursitis, wrist
      - M71.131 Other infective bursitis, right wrist
      - M71.132 Other infective bursitis, left wrist
      - M71.139 Other infective bursitis, unspecified wrist
    - M71.14 Other infective bursitis, hand
      - M71.141 Other infective bursitis, right hand
      - M71.142 Other infective bursitis, left hand
      - M71.149 Other infective bursitis, unspecified hand
    - M71.15 Other infective bursitis, hip
      - M71.151 Other infective bursitis, right hip
      - M71.152 Other infective bursitis, left hip
      - M71.159 Other infective bursitis, unspecified hip
    - M71.16 Other infective bursitis, knee
      - M71.161 Other infective bursitis, right knee
      - M71.162 Other infective bursitis, left knee
      - M71.169 Other infective bursitis, unspecified knee
    - M71.17 Other infective bursitis, ankle and foot
      - M71.171 Other infective bursitis, right ankle and foot
      - M71.172 Other infective bursitis, left ankle and foot
      - M71.179 Other infective bursitis, unspecified ankle and foot
    - M71.18 Other infective bursitis, other site
    - M71.19 Other infective bursitis, multiple sites
  - M71.2 Synovial cyst of popliteal space [Baker]

    Popliteal space = popliteal cavity, popliteal fossa. Depression in the posterior aspect of the knee (behind the knee).

    Excludes1 synovial cyst of popliteal space with rupture (M66.0)

    - M71.20 Synovial cyst of popliteal space [Baker], unspecified knee
    - M71.21 Synovial cyst of popliteal space [Baker], right knee
    - M71.22 Synovial cyst of popliteal space [Baker], left knee

- **M71.3 Other bursal cyst**
  Synovial cyst NOS
  Excludes1 synovial cyst with rupture (M66.1-)
  - **M71.30 Other bursal cyst, unspecified site**
  - **M71.31 Other bursal cyst, shoulder**
    - **M71.311 Other bursal cyst, right shoulder**
    - **M71.312 Other bursal cyst, left shoulder**
    - **M71.319 Other bursal cyst, unspecified shoulder**
  - **M71.32 Other bursal cyst, elbow**
    - **M71.321 Other bursal cyst, right elbow**
    - **M71.322 Other bursal cyst, left elbow**
    - **M71.329 Other bursal cyst, unspecified elbow**
  - **M71.33 Other bursal cyst, wrist**
    - **M71.331 Other bursal cyst, right wrist**
    - **M71.332 Other bursal cyst, left wrist**
    - **M71.339 Other bursal cyst, unspecified wrist**
  - **M71.34 Other bursal cyst, hand**
    - **M71.341 Other bursal cyst, right hand**
    - **M71.342 Other bursal cyst, left hand**
    - **M71.349 Other bursal cyst, unspecified hand**
  - **M71.35 Other bursal cyst, hip**
    - **M71.351 Other bursal cyst, right hip**
    - **M71.352 Other bursal cyst, left hip**
    - **M71.359 Other bursal cyst, unspecified hip**
  - **M71.37 Other bursal cyst, ankle and foot**
    - **M71.371 Other bursal cyst, right ankle and foot**
    - **M71.372 Other bursal cyst, left ankle and foot**
    - **M71.379 Other bursal cyst, unspecified ankle and foot**
  - **M71.38 Other bursal cyst, other site**
  - **M71.39 Other bursal cyst, multiple sites**
- **M71.4 Calcium deposit in bursa**
  Excludes2 calcium deposit in bursa of shoulder (M75.3)
  - **M71.40 Calcium deposit in bursa, unspecified site**
  - **M71.42 Calcium deposit in bursa, elbow**
    - **M71.421 Calcium deposit in bursa, right elbow**
    - **M71.422 Calcium deposit in bursa, left elbow**
    - **M71.429 Calcium deposit in bursa, unspecified elbow**
  - **M71.43 Calcium deposit in bursa, wrist**
    - **M71.431 Calcium deposit in bursa, right wrist**
    - **M71.432 Calcium deposit in bursa, left wrist**
    - **M71.439 Calcium deposit in bursa, unspecified wrist**
  - **M71.44 Calcium deposit in bursa, hand**
    - **M71.441 Calcium deposit in bursa, right hand**
    - **M71.442 Calcium deposit in bursa, left hand**
    - **M71.449 Calcium deposit in bursa, unspecified hand**
  - **M71.45 Calcium deposit in bursa, hip**
    - **M71.451 Calcium deposit in bursa, right hip**
    - **M71.452 Calcium deposit in bursa, left hip**
    - **M71.459 Calcium deposit in bursa, unspecified hip**
  - **M71.46 Calcium deposit in bursa, knee**
    - **M71.461 Calcium deposit in bursa, right knee**
    - **M71.462 Calcium deposit in bursa, left knee**
    - **M71.469 Calcium deposit in bursa, unspecified knee**
  - **M71.47 Calcium deposit in bursa, ankle and foot**
    - **M71.471 Calcium deposit in bursa, right ankle and foot**
    - **M71.472 Calcium deposit in bursa, left ankle and foot**
    - **M71.479 Calcium deposit in bursa, unspecified ankle and foot**
  - **M71.48 Calcium deposit in bursa, other site**
  - **M71.49 Calcium deposit in bursa, multiple sites**
- **M71.5 Other bursitis, not elsewhere classified**
  Excludes1 bursitis NOS (M71.9-)
  Excludes2 bursitis of shoulder (M75.5)
  bursitis of tibial collateral [Pellegrini-Stieda] (M76.4-)
  - **M71.50 Other bursitis, not elsewhere classified, unspecified site**
  - **M71.52 Other bursitis, not elsewhere classified, elbow**
    - **M71.521 Other bursitis, not elsewhere classified, right elbow**
    - **M71.522 Other bursitis, not elsewhere classified, left elbow**
    - **M71.529 Other bursitis, not elsewhere classified, unspecified elbow**
  - **M71.53 Other bursitis, not elsewhere classified, wrist**
    - **M71.531 Other bursitis, not elsewhere classified, right wrist**
    - **M71.532 Other bursitis, not elsewhere classified, left wrist**
    - **M71.539 Other bursitis, not elsewhere classified, unspecified wrist**
  - **M71.54 Other bursitis, not elsewhere classified, hand**
    - **M71.541 Other bursitis, not elsewhere classified, right hand**
    - **M71.542 Other bursitis, not elsewhere classified, left hand**
    - **M71.549 Other bursitis, not elsewhere classified, unspecified hand**
  - **M71.55 Other bursitis, not elsewhere classified, hip**
    - **M71.551 Other bursitis, not elsewhere classified, right hip**
    - **M71.552 Other bursitis, not elsewhere classified, left hip**
    - **M71.559 Other bursitis, not elsewhere classified, unspecified hip**
  - **M71.56 Other bursitis, not elsewhere classified, knee**
    - **M71.561 Other bursitis, not elsewhere classified, right knee**
    - **M71.562 Other bursitis, not elsewhere classified, left knee**
    - **M71.569 Other bursitis, not elsewhere classified, unspecified knee**
  - **M71.57 Other bursitis, not elsewhere classified, ankle and foot**
    - **M71.571 Other bursitis, not elsewhere classified, right ankle and foot**
    - **M71.572 Other bursitis, not elsewhere classified, left ankle and foot**
    - **M71.579 Other bursitis, not elsewhere classified, unspecified ankle and foot**
  - **M71.58 Other bursitis, not elsewhere classified, other site**

- **M71.8 Other specified bursopathies**
  - **M71.80 Other specified bursopathies, unspecified site**
  - **M71.81 Other specified bursopathies, shoulder**
    - **M71.811 Other specified bursopathies, right shoulder**
    - **M71.812 Other specified bursopathies, left shoulder**
    - **M71.819 Other specified bursopathies, unspecified shoulder**
  - **M71.82 Other specified bursopathies, elbow**
    - **M71.821 Other specified bursopathies, right elbow**
    - **M71.822 Other specified bursopathies, left elbow**
    - **M71.829 Other specified bursopathies, unspecified elbow**
  - **M71.83 Other specified bursopathies, wrist**
    - **M71.831 Other specified bursopathies, right wrist**
    - **M71.832 Other specified bursopathies, left wrist**
    - **M71.839 Other specified bursopathies, unspecified wrist**
  - **M71.84 Other specified bursopathies, hand**
    - **M71.841 Other specified bursopathies, right hand**
    - **M71.842 Other specified bursopathies, left hand**
    - **M71.849 Other specified bursopathies, unspecified hand**
  - **M71.85 Other specified bursopathies, hip**
    - **M71.851 Other specified bursopathies, right hip**
    - **M71.852 Other specified bursopathies, left hip**
    - **M71.859 Other specified bursopathies, unspecified hip**
  - **M71.86 Other specified bursopathies, knee**
    - **M71.861 Other specified bursopathies, right knee**
    - **M71.862 Other specified bursopathies, left knee**
    - **M71.869 Other specified bursopathies, unspecified knee**
  - **M71.87 Other specified bursopathies, ankle and foot**
    - **M71.871 Other specified bursopathies, right ankle and foot**
    - **M71.872 Other specified bursopathies, left ankle and foot**
    - **M71.879 Other specified bursopathies, unspecified ankle and foot**
  - **M71.88 Other specified bursopathies, other site**
  - **M71.89 Other specified bursopathies, multiple sites**
- **M71.9 Bursopathy, unspecified**
  Bursitis NOS

- **M72 Fibroblastic disorders**
  Excludes2 retroperitoneal fibromatosis (D48.3)
  - **M72.0 Palmar fascial fibromatosis [Dupuytren]** A
  - **M72.1 Knuckle pads**
  - **M72.2 Plantar fascial fibromatosis**
    Plantar fasciitis
  - **M72.4 Pseudosarcomatous fibromatosis**
    Nodular fasciitis
  - **M72.6 Necrotizing fasciitis**
    Use additional code (B95.-, B96.-) to identify causative organism
    Ex: See M60.0
  - **M72.8 Other fibroblastic disorders**
    Abscess of fascia
    Fasciitis NEC
    Other infective fasciitis
    Use additional code to (B95.-, B96.-) identify causative organism
    Excludes1 diffuse (eosinophilic) fasciitis (M35.4)
    necrotizing fasciitis (M72.6)
    nodular fasciitis (M72.4)
    perirenal fasciitis NOS (N13.5)
    perirenal fasciitis with infection (N13.6)
    plantar fasciitis (M72.2)
  - **M72.9 Fibroblastic disorder, unspecified**
    Fasciitis NOS
    Fibromatosis NOS

- **M75 Shoulder lesions**
  Excludes2 shoulder-hand syndrome (M89.0-)
  - **M75.0 Adhesive capsulitis of shoulder**
    Frozen shoulder
    Periarthritis of shoulder
    - **M75.00 Adhesive capsulitis of unspecified shoulder**
    - **M75.01 Adhesive capsulitis of right shoulder**
    - **M75.02 Adhesive capsulitis of left shoulder**
      Coding Clinic: 2015, Q2, P23
  - **M75.1 Rotator cuff tear or rupture, not specified as traumatic**
    Rotator cuff syndrome
    Supraspinatus syndrome
    Supraspinatus tear or rupture, not specified as traumatic
    Excludes1 tear of rotator cuff, traumatic (S46.01-)
    Gradual onset due to repetitive stress to rotator cuff
    - **M75.10 Unspecified rotator cuff tear or rupture, not specified as traumatic**
      - **M75.100 Unspecified rotator cuff tear or rupture of unspecified shoulder, not specified as traumatic**
      - **M75.101 Unspecified rotator cuff tear or rupture of right shoulder, not specified as traumatic**
      - **M75.102 Unspecified rotator cuff tear or rupture of left shoulder, not specified as traumatic**
    - **M75.11 Incomplete rotator cuff tear or rupture not specified as traumatic**
      - **M75.110 Incomplete rotator cuff tear or rupture of unspecified shoulder, not specified as traumatic**
      - **M75.111 Incomplete rotator cuff tear or rupture of right shoulder, not specified as traumatic**
      - **M75.112 Incomplete rotator cuff tear or rupture of left shoulder, not specified as traumatic**
    - **M75.12 Complete rotator cuff tear or rupture not specified as traumatic**
      - **M75.120 Complete rotator cuff tear or rupture of unspecified shoulder, not specified as traumatic**
      - **M75.121 Complete rotator cuff tear or rupture of right shoulder, not specified as traumatic**
      - **M75.122 Complete rotator cuff tear or rupture of left shoulder, not specified as traumatic**

- **M75.2 Bicipital tendinitis**
  - **M75.20 Bicipital tendinitis, unspecified shoulder**
  - **M75.21 Bicipital tendinitis, right shoulder**
  - **M75.22 Bicipital tendinitis, left shoulder**
- **M75.3 Calcific tendinitis of shoulder**
  Calcified bursa of shoulder
  - **M75.30 Calcific tendinitis of unspecified shoulder**
  - **M75.31 Calcific tendinitis of right shoulder**
  - **M75.32 Calcific tendinitis of left shoulder**
- **M75.4 Impingement syndrome of shoulder**
  - **M75.40 Impingement syndrome of unspecified shoulder**
  - **M75.41 Impingement syndrome of right shoulder**
  - **M75.42 Impingement syndrome of left shoulder**
- **M75.5 Bursitis of shoulder**
  - **M75.50 Bursitis of unspecified shoulder**
  - **M75.51 Bursitis of right shoulder**
  - **M75.52 Bursitis of left shoulder**
- **M75.8 Other shoulder lesions**
  - **M75.80 Other shoulder lesions, unspecified shoulder**
  - **M75.81 Other shoulder lesions, right shoulder**
  - **M75.82 Other shoulder lesions, left shoulder**
- **M75.9 Shoulder lesion, unspecified**
  - **M75.90 Shoulder lesion, unspecified, unspecified shoulder**
  - **M75.91 Shoulder lesion, unspecified, right shoulder**
  - **M75.92 Shoulder lesion, unspecified, left shoulder**

- **M76 Enthesopathies, lower limb, excluding foot**
  Excludes2 bursitis due to use, overuse and pressure (M70.-)
  enthesopathies of ankle and foot (M77.5-)
- **M76.0 Gluteal tendinitis**
  - **M76.00 Gluteal tendinitis, unspecified hip**
  - **M76.01 Gluteal tendinitis, right hip**
  - **M76.02 Gluteal tendinitis, left hip**
- **M76.1 Psoas tendinitis**
  - **M76.10 Psoas tendinitis, unspecified hip**
  - **M76.11 Psoas tendinitis, right hip**
  - **M76.12 Psoas tendinitis, left hip**
- **M76.2 Iliac crest spur**
  - **M76.20 Iliac crest spur, unspecified hip**
  - **M76.21 Iliac crest spur, right hip**
  - **M76.22 Iliac crest spur, left hip**
- **M76.3 Iliotibial band syndrome**
  - **M76.30 Iliotibial band syndrome, unspecified leg**
  - **M76.31 Iliotibial band syndrome, right leg**
  - **M76.32 Iliotibial band syndrome, left leg**
- **M76.4 Tibial collateral bursitis [Pellegrini-Stieda]**
  - **M76.40 Tibial collateral bursitis [Pellegrini-Stieda], unspecified leg**
  - **M76.41 Tibial collateral bursitis [Pellegrini-Stieda], right leg**
  - **M76.42 Tibial collateral bursitis [Pellegrini-Stieda], left leg**
- **M76.5 Patellar tendinitis**
  - **M76.50 Patellar tendinitis, unspecified knee**
  - **M76.51 Patellar tendinitis, right knee**
  - **M76.52 Patellar tendinitis, left knee**
- **M76.6 Achilles tendinitis**
  Achilles bursitis
  - **M76.60 Achilles tendinitis, unspecified leg**
  - **M76.61 Achilles tendinitis, right leg**
  - **M76.62 Achilles tendinitis, left leg**
- **M76.7 Peroneal tendinitis**
  - **M76.70 Peroneal tendinitis, unspecified leg**
  - **M76.71 Peroneal tendinitis, right leg**
  - **M76.72 Peroneal tendinitis, left leg**
- **M76.8 Other specified enthesopathies of lower limb, excluding foot**
  - **M76.81 Anterior tibial syndrome**
    - **M76.811 Anterior tibial syndrome, right leg**
    - **M76.812 Anterior tibial syndrome, left leg**
    - **M76.819 Anterior tibial syndrome, unspecified leg**
  - **M76.82 Posterior tibial tendinitis**
    - **M76.821 Posterior tibial tendinitis, right leg**
    - **M76.822 Posterior tibial tendinitis, left leg**
    - **M76.829 Posterior tibial tendinitis, unspecified leg**
  - **M76.89 Other specified enthesopathies of lower limb, excluding foot**
    - **M76.891 Other specified enthesopathies of right lower limb, excluding foot**
    - **M76.892 Other specified enthesopathies of left lower limb, excluding foot**
    - **M76.899 Other specified enthesopathies of unspecified lower limb, excluding foot**
- **M76.9 Unspecified enthesopathy, lower limb, excluding foot**

- **M77 Other enthesopathies**
  Excludes1 bursitis NOS (M71.9-)
  Excludes2 bursitis due to use, overuse and pressure (M70.-)
  osteophyte (M25.7)
  spinal enthesopathy (M46.0-)
- **M77.0 Medial epicondylitis**
  - **M77.00 Medial epicondylitis, unspecified elbow**
  - **M77.01 Medial epicondylitis, right elbow**
  - **M77.02 Medial epicondylitis, left elbow**
- **M77.1 Lateral epicondylitis**
  Tennis elbow
  - **M77.10 Lateral epicondylitis, unspecified elbow**
  - **M77.11 Lateral epicondylitis, right elbow**
  - **M77.12 Lateral epicondylitis, left elbow**
- **M77.2 Periarthritis of wrist**
  - **M77.20 Periarthritis, unspecified wrist**
  - **M77.21 Periarthritis, right wrist**
  - **M77.22 Periarthritis, left wrist**
- **M77.3 Calcaneal spur**
  - **M77.30 Calcaneal spur, unspecified foot**
  - **M77.31 Calcaneal spur, right foot**
  - **M77.32 Calcaneal spur, left foot**
- **M77.4 Metatarsalgia**
  Excludes1 Morton's metatarsalgia (G57.6)
  - **M77.40 Metatarsalgia, unspecified foot**
  - **M77.41 Metatarsalgia, right foot**
  - **M77.42 Metatarsalgia, left foot**
- **M77.5 Other enthesopathy of foot**
  - **M77.50 Other enthesopathy of unspecified foot**
  - **M77.51 Other enthesopathy of right foot**
  - **M77.52 Other enthesopathy of left foot**
- **M77.8 Other enthesopathies, not elsewhere classified**
- **M77.9 Enthesopathy, unspecified**
  Bone spur NOS
  Capsulitis NOS
  Periarthritis NOS
  Tendinitis NOS

● **M79 Other and unspecified soft tissue disorders, not elsewhere classified**

Excludes1 psychogenic rheumatism (F45.8)
soft tissue pain, psychogenic (F45.41)

M79.0 Rheumatism, unspecified

Excludes1 fibromyalgia (M79.7)
palindromic rheumatism (M12.3-)

M79.1 Myalgia

Myofascial pain syndrome

Excludes1 fibromyalgia (M79.7)
myositis (M60.-)

M79.2 Neuralgia and neuritis, unspecified

Excludes1 brachial radiculitis NOS (M54.1)
lumbosacral radiculitis NOS (M54.1)
mononeuropathies (G56-G58)
radiculitis NOS (M54.1)
sciatica (M54.3-M54.4)

M79.3 Panniculitis, unspecified

Excludes1 lupus panniculitis (L93.2)
neck and back panniculitis (M54.0-)
relapsing [Weber-Christian] panniculitis (M35.6)

M79.4 Hypertrophy of (infrapatellar) fat pad

M79.5 Residual foreign body in soft tissue

Excludes1 foreign body granuloma of skin and subcutaneous tissue (L92.3)
foreign body granuloma of soft tissue (M60.2-)

● **M79.6 Pain in limb, hand, foot, fingers and toes**

Excludes2 pain in joint (M25.5-)

● **M79.60 Pain in limb, unspecified**

M79.601 Pain in right arm
Pain in right upper limb NOS

M79.602 Pain in left arm
Pain in left upper limb NOS

M79.603 Pain in arm, unspecified
Pain in upper limb NOS

M79.604 Pain in right leg
Pain in right lower limb NOS

M79.605 Pain in left leg
Pain in left lower limb NOS

M79.606 Pain in leg, unspecified
Pain in lower limb NOS

M79.609 Pain in unspecified limb
Pain in limb NOS

● **M79.62 Pain in upper arm**

Pain in axillary region

M79.621 Pain in right upper arm

M79.622 Pain in left upper arm

M79.629 Pain in unspecified upper arm

● **M79.63 Pain in forearm**

M79.631 Pain in right forearm

M79.632 Pain in left forearm

M79.639 Pain in unspecified forearm

● **M79.64 Pain in hand and fingers**

M79.641 Pain in right hand

M79.642 Pain in left hand

M79.643 Pain in unspecified hand

M79.644 Pain in right finger(s)

M79.645 Pain in left finger(s)

M79.646 Pain in unspecified finger(s)

● **M79.65 Pain in thigh**

M79.651 Pain in right thigh

M79.652 Pain in left thigh

M79.659 Pain in unspecified thigh

● **M79.66 Pain in lower leg**

M79.661 Pain in right lower leg

M79.662 Pain in left lower leg

M79.669 Pain in unspecified lower leg

● **M79.67 Pain in foot and toes**

M79.671 Pain in right foot

M79.672 Pain in left foot

M79.673 Pain in unspecified foot

M79.674 Pain in right toe(s)

M79.675 Pain in left toe(s)

M79.676 Pain in unspecified toe(s)

M79.7 Fibromyalgia

Fibromyositis
Fibrositis
Myofibrositis

● **M79.A Nontraumatic compartment syndrome**

Code first, if applicable, associated postprocedural complication

Excludes1 compartment syndrome NOS (T79.A-)
fibromyalgia (M79.7) nontraumatic ischemic infarction of muscle (M62.2-)
traumatic compartment syndrome (T79.A-)

● **M79.A1 Nontraumatic compartment syndrome of upper extremity**

Nontraumatic compartment syndrome of shoulder, arm, forearm, wrist, hand, and fingers

Ex: **For category M79.A1 CC codes:** M70.80-M70.99, M79.81-M79.9, R29.898, S45.301-S45.899[A], S55.201-S55.899[A], S65.801-S65.899[A]

M79.A11 Nontraumatic compartment syndrome of right upper extremity

M79.A12 Nontraumatic compartment syndrome of left upper extremity

M79.A19 Nontraumatic compartment syndrome of unspecified upper extremity

● **M79.A2 Nontraumatic compartment syndrome of lower extremity**

Nontraumatic compartment syndrome of hip, buttock, thigh, leg, foot, and toes

Ex: **For category M79.A2 CC codes:** M70.80-M70.99, M79.81-M79.9, R29.898, S75.801-S75.899[A], S85.201-S85.899[A], S95.001-S95.099[A], S95.201-S95.899[A]

M79.A21 Nontraumatic compartment syndrome of right lower extremity

M79.A22 Nontraumatic compartment syndrome of left lower extremity

M79.A29 Nontraumatic compartment syndrome of unspecified lower extremity

M79.A3 Nontraumatic compartment syndrome of abdomen

Ex: S31.001[A], S31.011[A], S31.021[A], S31.031[A], S31.041[A], S31.051-S31.159[A], S31.600-S31.659[A], S31.831-S31.839[A], S36.00X-S37.599[A], S37.812-S37.99X[A], S38.3XX[A], S39.021-S39.023[A], T14.90-T14.91, T79.8XX-T79.9XX[A]

M79.A9 Nontraumatic compartment syndrome of other sites

Ex: S31.001[A], S31.011[A], S31.021[A], S31.031[A], S31.041[A], S31.051[A], S31.600-S31.659[A], S36.81X-S36.899[A]

● **M79.8 Other specified soft tissue disorders**

M79.81 Nontraumatic hematoma of soft tissue

Nontraumatic hematoma of muscle
Nontraumatic seroma of muscle and soft tissue

M79.89 Other specified soft tissue disorders

Polyalgia

M79.9 Soft tissue disorder, unspecified

OGCR See Section I.C., Chapter 13.d.

Osteoporosis

Osteoporosis is a systemic condition, meaning that all bones of the musculoskeletal system are affected. Therefore, site is not a component of the codes under category M81, Osteoporosis without current pathological fracture. The site codes under category M80, Osteoporosis with current pathological fracture, identify the site of the fracture, not the osteoporosis.

1) Osteoporosis without pathological fracture

Category M81, Osteoporosis without current pathological fracture, is for use for patients with osteoporosis who do not currently have a pathologic fracture due to the osteoporosis, even if they have had a fracture in the past. For patients with a history of osteoporosis fractures, status code Z87.310, Personal history of (healed) osteoporosis fracture, should follow the code from M81.

2) Osteoporosis with current pathological fracture

Category M80, Osteoporosis with current pathological fracture, is for patients who have a current pathologic fracture at the time of an encounter. The codes under M80 identify the site of the fracture. A code from category M80, not a traumatic fracture code, should be used for any patient with known osteoporosis who suffers a fracture, even if the patient had a minor fall or trauma, if that fall or trauma would not usually break a normal, healthy bone.

OSTEOPATHIES AND CHONDROPATHIES (M80-M94)

DISORDERS OF BONE DENSITY AND STRUCTURE (M80-M85)

M80 Osteoporosis with current pathological fracture

Excessive skeletal fragility (porous bone) resulting in bone fractures

Includes osteoporosis with current fragility fracture

Use additional code to identify major osseous defect, if applicable (M89.7-)

Excludes1 collapsed vertebra NOS (M48.5)
pathological fracture NOS (M84.4)
wedging of vertebra NOS (M48.5)

Excludes2 personal history of (healed) osteoporosis fracture (Z87.310)

The appropriate 7th character is to be added to each code from category M80:

A	initial encounter for fracture *All encounters involving diagnosis and treatment*
D	subsequent encounter for fracture with routine healing
G	subsequent encounter for fracture with delayed healing *Encounters for attention to casting or fixation devices, medication, and follow-up visits during the healing phase*
K	subsequent encounter for fracture with nonunion *Total failure of fracture healing*
P	subsequent encounter for fracture with malunion *Fracture ends do not heal together correctly.*
S	sequela

Ex: **For category M80[A] CC codes:** M48.40X-M48.58X[A], M80.00X-M80.88X[A], M84.30X-M84.68X[A], M84.750-M84.759[A] **For category M80[K,P] CC codes:** M80.00X-M80.88X[K,P], M84.30X-M84.68X[K,P], M84.750-M84.759[K,P], S02.0XX-S02.92X[K], S12.000-S12.691[K], S22.000-S22.9XX[K], S32.000-S32.9XX[K], S42.001-S42.92X[K,P], S49.001-S49.199[K,P], S52.001-S52.92X[K,M,N,P,Q,R], S59.001-S59.299[K,P], S62.001-S62.92X[K,P], S72.001-S72.92X[K,M,N,P,Q,R], S79.001-S79.199[K,P], S82.001-S82.92X[K,M,N,P,Q,R], S89.001-S89.399[K,P], S92.001-S92.919[K,P]

M80.0 Age-related osteoporosis with current pathological fracture

Involutional osteoporosis with current pathological fracture
Osteoporosis NOS with current pathological fracture
Postmenopausal osteoporosis with current pathological fracture
Senile osteoporosis with current pathological fracture

X **M80.00 Age-related osteoporosis with current pathological fracture, unspecified site**
A, K, P A

M80.01 Age-related osteoporosis with current pathological fracture, shoulder

M80.011 Age-related osteoporosis with current pathological fracture, right shoulder
A, K, P A

M80.012 Age-related osteoporosis with current pathological fracture, left shoulder
A, K, P A

M80.019 Age-related osteoporosis with current pathological fracture, unspecified shoulder A, K, P A

M80.02 Age-related osteoporosis with current pathological fracture, humerus

M80.021 Age-related osteoporosis with current pathological fracture, right humerus
A, K, P A

M80.022 Age-related osteoporosis with current pathological fracture, left humerus
A, K, P A

M80.029 Age-related osteoporosis with current pathological fracture, unspecified humerus A, K, P A

M80.03 Age-related osteoporosis with current pathological fracture, forearm

Age-related osteoporosis with current pathological fracture of wrist

M80.031 Age-related osteoporosis with current pathological fracture, right forearm
A, K, P A

M80.032 Age-related osteoporosis with current pathological fracture, left forearm
A, K, P A

M80.039 Age-related osteoporosis with current pathological fracture, unspecified forearm A, K, P A

M80.04 Age-related osteoporosis with current pathological fracture, hand

M80.041 Age-related osteoporosis with current pathological fracture, right hand
A, K, P A

M80.042 Age-related osteoporosis with current pathological fracture, left hand
A, K, P A

M80.049 Age-related osteoporosis with current pathological fracture, unspecified hand A, K, P A

M80.05 Age-related osteoporosis with current pathological fracture, femur

Age-related osteoporosis with current pathological fracture of hip

M80.051 Age-related osteoporosis with current pathological fracture, right femur
A, K, P A

M80.052 Age-related osteoporosis with current pathological fracture, left femur
A, K, P A

M80.059 Age-related osteoporosis with current pathological fracture, unspecified femur A, K, P A

M80.06 Age-related osteoporosis with current pathological fracture, lower leg

M80.061 Age-related osteoporosis with current pathological fracture, right lower leg
A, K, P A

M80.062 Age-related osteoporosis with current pathological fracture, left lower leg
A, K, P A

M80.069 Age-related osteoporosis with current pathological fracture, unspecified lower leg A, K, P A

- **M80.07 Age-related osteoporosis with current pathological fracture, ankle and foot**
  - **M80.071 Age-related osteoporosis with current pathological fracture, right ankle and foot** A, K, P A
  - **M80.072 Age-related osteoporosis with current pathological fracture, left ankle and foot** A, K, P A
  - **M80.079 Age-related osteoporosis with current pathological fracture, unspecified ankle and foot** A, K, P A
- X **M80.08 Age-related osteoporosis with current pathological fracture, vertebra(e)** A, K, P A
- **M80.8 Other osteoporosis with current pathological fracture**
  - Drug-induced osteoporosis with current pathological fracture
  - Idiopathic osteoporosis with current pathological fracture
  - Osteoporosis of disuse with current pathological fracture
  - Postoophorectomy osteoporosis with current pathological fracture
  - Postsurgical malabsorption osteoporosis with current pathological fracture
  - Post-traumatic osteoporosis with current pathological fracture
  - Use additional code for adverse effect, if applicable, to identify drug (T36-T50 with fifth or sixth character 5)
- X **M80.80 Other osteoporosis with current pathological fracture, unspecified site** A, K, P A
- **M80.81 Other osteoporosis with pathological fracture, shoulder**
  - **M80.811 Other osteoporosis with current pathological fracture, right shoulder** A, K, P
  - **M80.812 Other osteoporosis with current pathological fracture, left shoulder** A, K, P
  - **M80.819 Other osteoporosis with current pathological fracture, unspecified shoulder** A, K, P
- **M80.82 Other osteoporosis with current pathological fracture, humerus**
  - **M80.821 Other osteoporosis with current pathological fracture, right humerus** A, K, P
  - **M80.822 Other osteoporosis with current pathological fracture, left humerus** A, K, P
  - **M80.829 Other osteoporosis with current pathological fracture, unspecified humerus** A, K, P
- **M80.83 Other osteoporosis with current pathological fracture, forearm**
  - Other osteoporosis with current pathological fracture of wrist
  - **M80.831 Other osteoporosis with current pathological fracture, right forearm** A, K, P
  - **M80.832 Other osteoporosis with current pathological fracture, left forearm** A, K, P
  - **M80.839 Other osteoporosis with current pathological fracture, unspecified forearm** A, K, P
- **M80.84 Other osteoporosis with current pathological fracture, hand**
  - **M80.841 Other osteoporosis with current pathological fracture, right hand** A, K, P
  - **M80.842 Other osteoporosis with current pathological fracture, left hand** A, K, P
  - **M80.849 Other osteoporosis with current pathological fracture, unspecified hand** A, K, P
- **M80.85 Other osteoporosis with current pathological fracture, femur**
  - Other osteoporosis with current pathological fracture of hip
  - **M80.851 Other osteoporosis with current pathological fracture, right femur** A, K, P
  - **M80.852 Other osteoporosis with current pathological fracture, left femur** A, K, P
  - **M80.859 Other osteoporosis with current pathological fracture, unspecified femur** A, K, P
- **M80.86 Other osteoporosis with current pathological fracture, lower leg**
  - **M80.861 Other osteoporosis with current pathological fracture, right lower leg** A, K, P
  - **M80.862 Other osteoporosis with current pathological fracture, left lower leg** A, K, P
  - **M80.869 Other osteoporosis with current pathological fracture, unspecified lower leg** A, K, P
- **M80.87 Other osteoporosis with current pathological fracture, ankle and foot**
  - **M80.871 Other osteoporosis with current pathological fracture, right ankle and foot** A, K, P
  - **M80.872 Other osteoporosis with current pathological fracture, left ankle and foot** A, K, P
  - **M80.879 Other osteoporosis with current pathological fracture, unspecified ankle and foot** A, K, P
- X **M80.88 Other osteoporosis with current pathological fracture, vertebra(e)** A, K, P

- **M81 Osteoporosis without current pathological fracture**
  - Use additional code to identify:
    - major osseous defect, if applicable (M89.7-)
    - personal history of (healed) osteoporosis fracture, if applicable (Z87.310)
  - **Excludes1** osteoporosis with current pathological fracture (M80.-)
    - Sudeck's atrophy (M89.0)
  - **M81.0 Age-related osteoporosis without current pathological fracture** A
    - Involutional osteoporosis without current pathological fracture
    - Osteoporosis NOS
    - Postmenopausal osteoporosis without current pathological fracture
    - Senile osteoporosis without current pathological fracture
  - **M81.6 Localized osteoporosis [Lequesne]**
    - **Excludes1** Sudeck's atrophy (M89.0)

M81.8 Other osteoporosis without current pathological fracture
Drug-induced osteoporosis without current pathological fracture
Idiopathic osteoporosis without current pathological fracture
Osteoporosis of disuse without current pathological fracture
Postoophorectomy osteoporosis without current pathological fracture
Postsurgical malabsorption osteoporosis without current pathological fracture
Post-traumatic osteoporosis without current pathological fracture
Use additional code for adverse effect, if applicable, to identify drug (T36-T50 with fifth or sixth character 5)

● **M83 Adult osteomalacia**
Excludes1 infantile and juvenile osteomalacia (E55.0)
renal osteodystrophy (N25.0)
rickets (active) (E55.0)
rickets (active) sequelae (E64.3)
vitamin D-resistant osteomalacia (E83.3)
vitamin D-resistant rickets (active) (E83.3)

M83.0 Puerperal osteomalacia ♀ M
M83.1 Senile osteomalacia A
M83.2 Adult osteomalacia due to malabsorption A
Postsurgical malabsorption osteomalacia in adults
M83.3 Adult osteomalacia due to malnutrition A
M83.4 Aluminum bone disease
M83.5 Other drug-induced osteomalacia in adults A
Use additional code for adverse effect, if applicable, to identify drug (T36-T50 with fifth or sixth character 5)
M83.8 Other adult osteomalacia A
M83.9 Adult osteomalacia, unspecified A

● **M84 Disorder of continuity of bone**
Excludes2 traumatic fracture of bone-see fracture, by site
Ex: **For category M84[A] CC codes:** M48.40X-M48.58X[A], M80.00X-M80.88X[A], M84.30X-M84.68X[A], M84.750-M84.759[A] **For category M84[K,P] CC codes:** See M80[K,P]

● **M84.3 Stress fracture**
Fatigue fracture
March fracture
Stress fracture NOS
Stress reaction
Use additional external cause code(s) to identify the cause of the stress fracture
Excludes1 pathological fracture NOS (M84.4.-)
pathological fracture due to osteoporosis (M80.-)
traumatic fracture (S12.-, S22.-, S32.-, S42.-, S52.-, S62.-, S72.-, S82.-, S92.-)
Excludes2 personal history of (healed) stress (fatigue) fracture (Z87.312)
stress fracture of vertebra (M48.4-)
The appropriate 7th character is to be added to each code from subcategory M84.3:

A	initial encounter for fracture
D	subsequent encounter for fracture with routine healing
G	subsequent encounter for fracture with delayed healing
K	subsequent encounter for fracture with nonunion
P	subsequent encounter for fracture with malunion
S	sequela

Ex: See M84

X ● **M84.30 Stress fracture, unspecified site** K, P

● **M84.31 Stress fracture, shoulder**
● **M84.311 Stress fracture, right shoulder** K, P
● **M84.312 Stress fracture, left shoulder** K, P
● **M84.319 Stress fracture, unspecified shoulder** K, P

● **M84.32 Stress fracture, humerus**
● **M84.321 Stress fracture, right humerus** K, P
● **M84.322 Stress fracture, left humerus** K, P
● **M84.329 Stress fracture, unspecified humerus** K, P

● **M84.33 Stress fracture, ulna and radius**
● **M84.331 Stress fracture, right ulna** K, P
● **M84.332 Stress fracture, left ulna** K, P
● **M84.333 Stress fracture, right radius** K, P
● **M84.334 Stress fracture, left radius** K, P
● **M84.339 Stress fracture, unspecified ulna and radius** K, P

● **M84.34 Stress fracture, hand and fingers**
● **M84.341 Stress fracture, right hand** K, P
● **M84.342 Stress fracture, left hand** K, P
● **M84.343 Stress fracture, unspecified hand** K, P
● **M84.344 Stress fracture, right finger(s)** K, P
● **M84.345 Stress fracture, left finger(s)** K, P
● **M84.346 Stress fracture, unspecified finger(s)** K, P

● **M84.35 Stress fracture, pelvis and femur**
Stress fracture, hip
● **M84.350 Stress fracture, pelvis** K, P
● **M84.351 Stress fracture, right femur** K, P
● **M84.352 Stress fracture, left femur** K, P
● **M84.353 Stress fracture, unspecified femur** K, P
● **M84.359 Stress fracture, hip, unspecified** K, P

● **M84.36 Stress fracture, tibia and fibula**
● **M84.361 Stress fracture, right tibia** K, P
● **M84.362 Stress fracture, left tibia** K, P
● **M84.363 Stress fracture, right fibula** K, P
● **M84.364 Stress fracture, left fibula** K, P
● **M84.369 Stress fracture, unspecified tibia and fibula** K, P

● **M84.37 Stress fracture, ankle, foot and toes**
● **M84.371 Stress fracture, right ankle** K, P
● **M84.372 Stress fracture, left ankle** K, P
● **M84.373 Stress fracture, unspecified ankle** K, P
● **M84.374 Stress fracture, right foot** K, P
● **M84.375 Stress fracture, left foot** K, P
● **M84.376 Stress fracture, unspecified foot** K, P
● **M84.377 Stress fracture, right toe(s)** K, P
● **M84.378 Stress fracture, left toe(s)** K, P
● **M84.379 Stress fracture, unspecified toe(s)** K, P

X ● **M84.38 Stress fracture, other site** K, P
Excludes2 stress fracture of vertebra (M48.4-)

● **M84.4 Pathological fracture, not elsewhere classified**
Chronic fracture
Pathological fracture NOS

Excludes1 collapsed vertebra NEC (M48.5)
pathological fracture in neoplastic disease (M84.5-)
pathological fracture in osteoporosis (MØØ.-)
pathological fracture in other disease (M84.6-)
stress fracture (M84.3-)
traumatic fracture (S12.-, S22.-, S32.-, S42.-, S52.-, S62.-, S72.-, S82.-, S92.-)

Excludes2 personal history of (healed) pathological fracture (Z87.311)

The appropriate 7th character is to be added to each code from subcategory M84.4:

A	initial encounter for fracture
D	subsequent encounter for fracture with routine healing
G	subsequent encounter for fracture with delayed healing
K	subsequent encounter for fracture with nonunion
P	subsequent encounter for fracture with malunion
S	sequela

Ex See MØØ

X ● **M84.40 Pathological fracture, unspecified site** A, K, P

● **M84.41 Pathological fracture, shoulder**
- ● **M84.411 Pathological fracture, right shoulder** A, K, P
- ● **M84.412 Pathological fracture, left shoulder** A, K, P
- ● **M84.419 Pathological fracture, unspecified shoulder** A, K, P

● **M84.42 Pathological fracture, humerus**
- ● **M84.421 Pathological fracture, right humerus** A, K, P
- ● **M84.422 Pathological fracture, left humerus** A, K, P
- ● **M84.429 Pathological fracture, unspecified humerus** A, K, P

● **M84.43 Pathological fracture, ulna and radius**
- ● **M84.431 Pathological fracture, right ulna** A, K, P
- ● **M84.432 Pathological fracture, left ulna** A, K, P
- ● **M84.433 Pathological fracture, right radius** A, K, P
- ● **M84.434 Pathological fracture, left radius** A, K, P
- ● **M84.439 Pathological fracture, unspecified ulna and radius** A, K, P

● **M84.44 Pathological fracture, hand and fingers**
- ● **M84.441 Pathological fracture, right hand** A, K, P
- ● **M84.442 Pathological fracture, left hand** A, K, P
- ● **M84.443 Pathological fracture, unspecified hand** A, K, P
- ● **M84.444 Pathological fracture, right finger(s)** A, K, P
- ● **M84.445 Pathological fracture, left finger(s)** A, K, P
- ● **M84.446 Pathological fracture, unspecified finger(s)** A, K, P

● **M84.45 Pathological fracture, femur and pelvis**
- ● **M84.451 Pathological fracture, right femur** A, K, P
- ● **M84.452 Pathological fracture, left femur** A, K, P
- ● **M84.453 Pathological fracture, unspecified femur** A, K, P
- ● **M84.454 Pathological fracture, pelvis** A, K, P
- ● **M84.459 Pathological fracture, hip, unspecified** A, K, P

● **M84.46 Pathological fracture, tibia and fibula**
- ● **M84.461 Pathological fracture, right tibia** A, K, P
- ● **M84.462 Pathological fracture, left tibia** A, K, P
- ● **M84.463 Pathological fracture, right fibula** A, K, P
- ● **M84.464 Pathological fracture, left fibula** A, K, P
- ● **M84.469 Pathological fracture, unspecified tibia and fibula** A, K, P

● **M84.47 Pathological fracture, ankle, foot and toes**
- ● **M84.471 Pathological fracture, right ankle** A, K, P
- ● **M84.472 Pathological fracture, left ankle** A, K, P
- ● **M84.473 Pathological fracture, unspecified ankle** A, K, P
- ● **M84.474 Pathological fracture, right foot** A, K, P
- ● **M84.475 Pathological fracture, left foot** A, K, P
- ● **M84.476 Pathological fracture, unspecified foot** A, K, P
- ● **M84.477 Pathological fracture, right toe(s)** A, K, P
- ● **M84.478 Pathological fracture, left toe(s)** A, K, P
- ● **M84.479 Pathological fracture, unspecified toe(s)** A, K, P

X ● **M84.48 Pathological fracture, other site** A, K, P

OGCR Section I.a, Chapter 13.C.

Coding of Pathologic Fractures

7th character A is for use as long as the patient is receiving active treatment for the fracture. While the patient may be seen by a new or different provider over the course of treatment for a pathological fracture, assignment of the 7th character is based on whether the patient is undergoing active treatment and not whether the provider is seeing the patient for the first time.3. 7th character, D is to be used for encounters after the patient has completed active treatment. The other 7th characters, listed under each subcategory in the Tabular List, are to be used for subsequent encounters for **routine care of fractures during the healing and recovery phase as well as** treatment of problems associated with the healing, such as malunions, nonunions, and sequelae.

Care for complications of surgical treatment for fracture repairs during the healing or recovery phase should be coded with the appropriate complication codes.

See Section I.C.19. Coding of traumatic fractures.

M84.5 Pathological fracture in neoplastic disease

Code also underlying neoplasm

The appropriate 7th character is to be added to each code from subcategory M84.5:

A	initial encounter for fracture
D	subsequent encounter for fracture with routine healing
G	subsequent encounter for fracture with delayed healing
K	subsequent encounter for fracture with nonunion
P	subsequent encounter for fracture with malunion
S	sequela

Ex: See M80

X **M84.50 Pathological fracture in neoplastic disease, unspecified site** A, K, P CC

M84.51 Pathological fracture in neoplastic disease, shoulder

- **M84.511 Pathological fracture in neoplastic disease, right shoulder** A, K, P CC
- **M84.512 Pathological fracture in neoplastic disease, left shoulder** A, K, P CC
- **M84.519 Pathological fracture in neoplastic disease, unspecified shoulder** A, K, P CC

M84.52 Pathological fracture in neoplastic disease, humerus

- **M84.521 Pathological fracture in neoplastic disease, right humerus** A, K, P CC
- **M84.522 Pathological fracture in neoplastic disease, left humerus** A, K, P CC
- **M84.529 Pathological fracture in neoplastic disease, unspecified humerus** A, K, P CC

M84.53 Pathological fracture in neoplastic disease, ulna and radius

- **M84.531 Pathological fracture in neoplastic disease, right ulna** A, K, P CC
- **M84.532 Pathological fracture in neoplastic disease, left ulna** A, K, P CC
- **M84.533 Pathological fracture in neoplastic disease, right radius** A, K, P CC
- **M84.534 Pathological fracture in neoplastic disease, left radius** A, K, P CC
- **M84.539 Pathological fracture in neoplastic disease, unspecified ulna and radius** A, K, P CC

M84.54 Pathological fracture in neoplastic disease, hand

- **M84.541 Pathological fracture in neoplastic disease, right hand** A, K, P CC
- **M84.542 Pathological fracture in neoplastic disease, left hand** A, K, P CC
- **M84.549 Pathological fracture in neoplastic disease, unspecified hand** A, K, P CC

M84.55 Pathological fracture in neoplastic disease, pelvis and femur

- **M84.550 Pathological fracture in neoplastic disease, pelvis** A, K, P CC
- **M84.551 Pathological fracture in neoplastic disease, right femur** A, K, P CC
- **M84.552 Pathological fracture in neoplastic disease, left femur** A, K, P CC
- **M84.553 Pathological fracture in neoplastic disease, unspecified femur** A, K, P CC
- **M84.559 Pathological fracture in neoplastic disease, hip, unspecified** A, K, P CC

M84.56 Pathological fracture in neoplastic disease, tibia and fibula

- **M84.561 Pathological fracture in neoplastic disease, right tibia** A, K, P CC
- **M84.562 Pathological fracture in neoplastic disease, left tibia** A, K, P CC
- **M84.563 Pathological fracture in neoplastic disease, right fibula** A, K, P CC
- **M84.564 Pathological fracture in neoplastic disease, left fibula** A, K, P CC
- **M84.569 Pathological fracture in neoplastic disease, unspecified tibia and fibula** A, K, P CC

M84.57 Pathological fracture in neoplastic disease, ankle and foot

- **M84.571 Pathological fracture in neoplastic disease, right ankle** A, K, P CC
- **M84.572 Pathological fracture in neoplastic disease, left ankle** A, K, P CC
- **M84.573 Pathological fracture in neoplastic disease, unspecified ankle** A, K, P CC
- **M84.574 Pathological fracture in neoplastic disease, right foot** A, K, P CC
- **M84.575 Pathological fracture in neoplastic disease, left foot** A, K, P CC
- **M84.576 Pathological fracture in neoplastic disease, unspecified foot** A, K, P CC

X **M84.58 Pathological fracture in neoplastic disease, other specified site** A, K, P CC

Pathological fracture in neoplastic disease, vertebrae

M84.6 Pathological fracture in other disease

Code also underlying condition

Excludes1 pathological fracture in osteoporosis (M80.-)

The appropriate 7th character is to be added to each code from subcategory M84.6:

A	initial encounter for fracture
D	subsequent encounter for fracture with routine healing
G	subsequent encounter for fracture with delayed healing
K	subsequent encounter for fracture with nonunion
P	subsequent encounter for fracture with malunion
S	sequela

Ex: See M80

X **M84.60 Pathological fracture in other disease, unspecified site** A, K, P CC

- M84.61 Pathological fracture in other disease, shoulder
  - M84.611 Pathological fracture in other disease, right shoulder A, K, P
  - M84.612 Pathological fracture in other disease, left shoulder A, K, P
  - M84.619 Pathological fracture in other disease, unspecified shoulder A, K, P
- M84.62 Pathological fracture in other disease, humerus
  - M84.621 Pathological fracture in other disease, right humerus A, K, P
  - M84.622 Pathological fracture in other disease, left humerus A, K, P
  - M84.629 Pathological fracture in other disease, unspecified humerus A, K, P
- M84.63 Pathological fracture in other disease, ulna and radius
  - M84.631 Pathological fracture in other disease, right ulna A, K, P
  - M84.632 Pathological fracture in other disease, left ulna A, K, P
  - M84.633 Pathological fracture in other disease, right radius A, K, P
  - M84.634 Pathological fracture in other disease, left radius A, K, P
  - M84.639 Pathological fracture in other disease, unspecified ulna and radius A, K, P
- M84.64 Pathological fracture in other disease, hand
  - M84.641 Pathological fracture in other disease, right hand A, K, P
  - M84.642 Pathological fracture in other disease, left hand A, K, P
  - M84.649 Pathological fracture in other disease, unspecified hand A, K, P
- M84.65 Pathological fracture in other disease, pelvis and femur
  - M84.650 Pathological fracture in other disease, pelvis A, K, P
  - M84.651 Pathological fracture in other disease, right femur A, K, P
  - M84.652 Pathological fracture in other disease, left femur A, K, P
  - M84.653 Pathological fracture in other disease, unspecified femur A, K, P
  - M84.659 Pathological fracture in other disease, hip, unspecified A, K, P
- M84.66 Pathological fracture in other disease, tibia and fibula
  - M84.661 Pathological fracture in other disease, right tibia A, K, P
  - M84.662 Pathological fracture in other disease, left tibia A, K, P
  - M84.663 Pathological fracture in other disease, right fibula A, K, P
  - M84.664 Pathological fracture in other disease, left fibula A, K, P
  - M84.669 Pathological fracture in other disease, unspecified tibia and fibula A, K, P
- M84.67 Pathological fracture in other disease, ankle and foot
  - M84.671 Pathological fracture in other disease, right ankle A, K, P
  - M84.672 Pathological fracture in other disease, left ankle A, K, P
  - M84.673 Pathological fracture in other disease, unspecified ankle A, K, P
  - M84.674 Pathological fracture in other disease, right foot A, K, P
  - M84.675 Pathological fracture in other disease, left foot A, K, P
  - M84.676 Pathological fracture in other disease, unspecified foot A, K, P
- X M84.68 Pathological fracture in other disease, other site A, K, P
- M84.7 Nontraumatic fracture, not elsewhere classified ◀
  - M84.75 Atypical femoral fracture ◀

    The appropriate 7th character is to be added to each code from M84.75: ◀

A	initial encounter for fracture ◀
D	subsequent encounter for fracture with routine healing ◀
G	subsequent encounter for fracture with delayed healing ◀
K	subsequent encounter for fracture with nonunion ◀
P	subsequent encounter for fracture with malunion ◀
S	sequela ◀

    Ex. See M80 ◀
    - M84.750 Atypical femoral fracture, unspecified A, K, P ◀
    - M84.751 Incomplete atypical femoral fracture, right leg A, K, P ◀
    - M84.752 Incomplete atypical femoral fracture, left leg A, K, P ◀
    - M84.753 Incomplete atypical femoral fracture, unspecified leg A, K, P ◀
    - M84.754 Complete transverse atypical femoral fracture, right leg A, K, P ◀
    - M84.755 Complete transverse atypical femoral fracture, left leg A, K, P ◀
    - M84.756 Complete transverse atypical femoral fracture, unspecified leg A, K, P ◀
    - M84.757 Complete oblique atypical femoral fracture, right leg A, K, P ◀
    - M84.758 Complete oblique atypical femoral fracture, left leg A, K, P ◀
    - M84.759 Complete oblique atypical femoral fracture, unspecified leg A, K, P ◀
- M84.8 Other disorders of continuity of bone
  - M84.80 Other disorders of continuity of bone, unspecified site
  - M84.81 Other disorders of continuity of bone, shoulder
    - M84.811 Other disorders of continuity of bone, right shoulder
    - M84.812 Other disorders of continuity of bone, left shoulder
    - M84.819 Other disorders of continuity of bone, unspecified shoulder
  - M84.82 Other disorders of continuity of bone, humerus
    - M84.821 Other disorders of continuity of bone, right humerus
    - M84.822 Other disorders of continuity of bone, left humerus
    - M84.829 Other disorders of continuity of bone, unspecified humerus

- M84.83 Other disorders of continuity of bone, ulna and radius
  - M84.831 Other disorders of continuity of bone, right ulna
  - M84.832 Other disorders of continuity of bone, left ulna
  - M84.833 Other disorders of continuity of bone, right radius
  - M84.834 Other disorders of continuity of bone, left radius
  - M84.839 Other disorders of continuity of bone, unspecified ulna and radius
- M84.84 Other disorders of continuity of bone, hand
  - M84.841 Other disorders of continuity of bone, right hand
  - M84.842 Other disorders of continuity of bone, left hand
  - M84.849 Other disorders of continuity of bone, unspecified hand
- M84.85 Other disorders of continuity of bone, pelvic region and thigh
  - M84.851 Other disorders of continuity of bone, right pelvic region and thigh
  - M84.852 Other disorders of continuity of bone, left pelvic region and thigh
  - M84.859 Other disorders of continuity of bone, unspecified pelvic region and thigh
- M84.86 Other disorders of continuity of bone, tibia and fibula
  - M84.861 Other disorders of continuity of bone, right tibia
  - M84.862 Other disorders of continuity of bone, left tibia
  - M84.863 Other disorders of continuity of bone, right fibula
  - M84.864 Other disorders of continuity of bone, left fibula
  - M84.869 Other disorders of continuity of bone, unspecified tibia and fibula
- M84.87 Other disorders of continuity of bone, ankle and foot
  - M84.871 Other disorders of continuity of bone, right ankle and foot
  - M84.872 Other disorders of continuity of bone, left ankle and foot
  - M84.879 Other disorders of continuity of bone, unspecified ankle and foot
- M84.88 Other disorders of continuity of bone, other site
- M84.9 Disorder of continuity of bone, unspecified

- M85 Other disorders of bone density and structure

  Excludes1 osteogenesis imperfecta (Q78.0)
  osteopetrosis (Q78.2)
  osteopoikilosis (Q78.8)
  polyostotic fibrous dysplasia (Q78.1)

- M85.0 Fibrous dysplasia (monostotic)

  Excludes2 fibrous dysplasia of jaw (M27.8)

  - M85.00 Fibrous dysplasia (monostotic), unspecified site
- M85.01 Fibrous dysplasia (monostotic), shoulder
  - M85.011 Fibrous dysplasia (monostotic), right shoulder
  - M85.012 Fibrous dysplasia (monostotic), left shoulder
  - M85.019 Fibrous dysplasia (monostotic), unspecified shoulder
- M85.02 Fibrous dysplasia (monostotic), upper arm
  - M85.021 Fibrous dysplasia (monostotic), right upper arm
  - M85.022 Fibrous dysplasia (monostotic), left upper arm
  - M85.029 Fibrous dysplasia (monostotic), unspecified upper arm
- M85.03 Fibrous dysplasia (monostotic), forearm
  - M85.031 Fibrous dysplasia (monostotic), right forearm
  - M85.032 Fibrous dysplasia (monostotic), left forearm
  - M85.039 Fibrous dysplasia (monostotic), unspecified forearm
- M85.04 Fibrous dysplasia (monostotic), hand
  - M85.041 Fibrous dysplasia (monostotic), right hand
  - M85.042 Fibrous dysplasia (monostotic), left hand
  - M85.049 Fibrous dysplasia (monostotic), unspecified hand
- M85.05 Fibrous dysplasia (monostotic), thigh
  - M85.051 Fibrous dysplasia (monostotic), right thigh
  - M85.052 Fibrous dysplasia (monostotic), left thigh
  - M85.059 Fibrous dysplasia (monostotic), unspecified thigh
- M85.06 Fibrous dysplasia (monostotic), lower leg
  - M85.061 Fibrous dysplasia (monostotic), right lower leg
  - M85.062 Fibrous dysplasia (monostotic), left lower leg
  - M85.069 Fibrous dysplasia (monostotic), unspecified lower leg
- M85.07 Fibrous dysplasia (monostotic), ankle and foot
  - M85.071 Fibrous dysplasia (monostotic), right ankle and foot
  - M85.072 Fibrous dysplasia (monostotic), left ankle and foot
  - M85.079 Fibrous dysplasia (monostotic), unspecified ankle and foot
- M85.08 Fibrous dysplasia (monostotic), other site
- M85.09 Fibrous dysplasia (monostotic), multiple sites
- M85.1 Skeletal fluorosis
  - M85.10 Skeletal fluorosis, unspecified site
- M85.11 Skeletal fluorosis, shoulder
  - M85.111 Skeletal fluorosis, right shoulder
  - M85.112 Skeletal fluorosis, left shoulder
  - M85.119 Skeletal fluorosis, unspecified shoulder
- M85.12 Skeletal fluorosis, upper arm
  - M85.121 Skeletal fluorosis, right upper arm
  - M85.122 Skeletal fluorosis, left upper arm
  - M85.129 Skeletal fluorosis, unspecified upper arm
- M85.13 Skeletal fluorosis, forearm
  - M85.131 Skeletal fluorosis, right forearm
  - M85.132 Skeletal fluorosis, left forearm
  - M85.139 Skeletal fluorosis, unspecified forearm
- M85.14 Skeletal fluorosis, hand
  - M85.141 Skeletal fluorosis, right hand
  - M85.142 Skeletal fluorosis, left hand
  - M85.149 Skeletal fluorosis, unspecified hand

- M85.15 Skeletal fluorosis, thigh
  - M85.151 Skeletal fluorosis, right thigh
  - M85.152 Skeletal fluorosis, left thigh
  - M85.159 Skeletal fluorosis, unspecified thigh
- M85.16 Skeletal fluorosis, lower leg
  - M85.161 Skeletal fluorosis, right lower leg
  - M85.162 Skeletal fluorosis, left lower leg
  - M85.169 Skeletal fluorosis, unspecified lower leg
- M85.17 Skeletal fluorosis, ankle and foot
  - M85.171 Skeletal fluorosis, right ankle and foot
  - M85.172 Skeletal fluorosis, left ankle and foot
  - M85.179 Skeletal fluorosis, unspecified ankle and foot
- M85.18 Skeletal fluorosis, other site
- M85.19 Skeletal fluorosis, multiple sites

M85.2 Hyperostosis of skull

- M85.3 Osteitis condensans
  - M85.30 Osteitis condensans, unspecified site
  - M85.31 Osteitis condensans, shoulder
    - M85.311 Osteitis condensans, right shoulder
    - M85.312 Osteitis condensans, left shoulder
    - M85.319 Osteitis condensans, unspecified shoulder
  - M85.32 Osteitis condensans, upper arm
    - M85.321 Osteitis condensans, right upper arm
    - M85.322 Osteitis condensans, left upper arm
    - M85.329 Osteitis condensans, unspecified upper arm
  - M85.33 Osteitis condensans, forearm
    - M85.331 Osteitis condensans, right forearm
    - M85.332 Osteitis condensans, left forearm
    - M85.339 Osteitis condensans, unspecified forearm
  - M85.34 Osteitis condensans, hand
    - M85.341 Osteitis condensans, right hand
    - M85.342 Osteitis condensans, left hand
    - M85.349 Osteitis condensans, unspecified hand
  - M85.35 Osteitis condensans, thigh
    - M85.351 Osteitis condensans, right thigh
    - M85.352 Osteitis condensans, left thigh
    - M85.359 Osteitis condensans, unspecified thigh
  - M85.36 Osteitis condensans, lower leg
    - M85.361 Osteitis condensans, right lower leg
    - M85.362 Osteitis condensans, left lower leg
    - M85.369 Osteitis condensans, unspecified lower leg
  - M85.37 Osteitis condensans, ankle and foot
    - M85.371 Osteitis condensans, right ankle and foot
    - M85.372 Osteitis condensans, left ankle and foot
    - M85.379 Osteitis condensans, unspecified ankle and foot
  - M85.38 Osteitis condensans, other site
  - M85.39 Osteitis condensans, multiple sites
- M85.4 Solitary bone cyst

  Excludes2 solitary cyst of jaw (M27.4)
  - M85.40 Solitary bone cyst, unspecified site
  - M85.41 Solitary bone cyst, shoulder
    - M85.411 Solitary bone cyst, right shoulder
    - M85.412 Solitary bone cyst, left shoulder
    - M85.419 Solitary bone cyst, unspecified shoulder
  - M85.42 Solitary bone cyst, humerus
    - M85.421 Solitary bone cyst, right humerus
    - M85.422 Solitary bone cyst, left humerus
    - M85.429 Solitary bone cyst, unspecified humerus
  - M85.43 Solitary bone cyst, ulna and radius
    - M85.431 Solitary bone cyst, right ulna and radius
    - M85.432 Solitary bone cyst, left ulna and radius
    - M85.439 Solitary bone cyst, unspecified ulna and radius
  - M85.44 Solitary bone cyst, hand
    - M85.441 Solitary bone cyst, right hand
    - M85.442 Solitary bone cyst, left hand
    - M85.449 Solitary bone cyst, unspecified hand
  - M85.45 Solitary bone cyst, pelvis
    - M85.451 Solitary bone cyst, right pelvis
    - M85.452 Solitary bone cyst, left pelvis
    - M85.459 Solitary bone cyst, unspecified pelvis
  - M85.46 Solitary bone cyst, tibia and fibula
    - M85.461 Solitary bone cyst, right tibia and fibula
    - M85.462 Solitary bone cyst, left tibia and fibula
    - M85.469 Solitary bone cyst, unspecified tibia and fibula
  - M85.47 Solitary bone cyst, ankle and foot
    - M85.471 Solitary bone cyst, right ankle and foot
    - M85.472 Solitary bone cyst, left ankle and foot
    - M85.479 Solitary bone cyst, unspecified ankle and foot
  - M85.48 Solitary bone cyst, other site
- M85.5 Aneurysmal bone cyst

  Excludes2 aneurysmal cyst of jaw (M27.4)
  - M85.50 Aneurysmal bone cyst, unspecified site
  - M85.51 Aneurysmal bone cyst, shoulder
    - M85.511 Aneurysmal bone cyst, right shoulder
    - M85.512 Aneurysmal bone cyst, left shoulder
    - M85.519 Aneurysmal bone cyst, unspecified shoulder
  - M85.52 Aneurysmal bone cyst, upper arm
    - M85.521 Aneurysmal bone cyst, right upper arm
    - M85.522 Aneurysmal bone cyst, left upper arm
    - M85.529 Aneurysmal bone cyst, unspecified upper arm
  - M85.53 Aneurysmal bone cyst, forearm
    - M85.531 Aneurysmal bone cyst, right forearm
    - M85.532 Aneurysmal bone cyst, left forearm
    - M85.539 Aneurysmal bone cyst, unspecified forearm
  - M85.54 Aneurysmal bone cyst, hand
    - M85.541 Aneurysmal bone cyst, right hand
    - M85.542 Aneurysmal bone cyst, left hand
    - M85.549 Aneurysmal bone cyst, unspecified hand
  - M85.55 Aneurysmal bone cyst, thigh
    - M85.551 Aneurysmal bone cyst, right thigh
    - M85.552 Aneurysmal bone cyst, left thigh
    - M85.559 Aneurysmal bone cyst, unspecified thigh

- M85.56 Aneurysmal bone cyst, lower leg
  - M85.561 Aneurysmal bone cyst, right lower leg
  - M85.562 Aneurysmal bone cyst, left lower leg
  - M85.569 Aneurysmal bone cyst, unspecified lower leg
- M85.57 Aneurysmal bone cyst, ankle and foot
  - M85.571 Aneurysmal bone cyst, right ankle and foot
  - M85.572 Aneurysmal bone cyst, left ankle and foot
  - M85.579 Aneurysmal bone cyst, unspecified ankle and foot
- M85.58 Aneurysmal bone cyst, other site
- M85.59 Aneurysmal bone cyst, multiple sites

- M85.6 Other cyst of bone

  Excludes1 cyst of jaw NEC (M27.4)
  osteitis fibrosa cystica generalisata [von Recklinghausen's disease of bone] (E21.0)

- M85.60 Other cyst of bone, unspecified site
- M85.61 Other cyst of bone, shoulder
  - M85.611 Other cyst of bone, right shoulder
  - M85.612 Other cyst of bone, left shoulder
  - M85.619 Other cyst of bone, unspecified shoulder
- M85.62 Other cyst of bone, upper arm
  - M85.621 Other cyst of bone, right upper arm
  - M85.622 Other cyst of bone, left upper arm
  - M85.629 Other cyst of bone, unspecified upper arm
- M85.63 Other cyst of bone, forearm
  - M85.631 Other cyst of bone, right forearm
  - M85.632 Other cyst of bone, left forearm
  - M85.639 Other cyst of bone, unspecified forearm
- M85.64 Other cyst of bone, hand
  - M85.641 Other cyst of bone, right hand
  - M85.642 Other cyst of bone, left hand
  - M85.649 Other cyst of bone, unspecified hand
- M85.65 Other cyst of bone, thigh
  - M85.651 Other cyst of bone, right thigh
  - M85.652 Other cyst of bone, left thigh
  - M85.659 Other cyst of bone, unspecified thigh
- M85.66 Other cyst of bone, lower leg
  - M85.661 Other cyst of bone, right lower leg
  - M85.662 Other cyst of bone, left lower leg
  - M85.669 Other cyst of bone, unspecified lower leg
- M85.67 Other cyst of bone, ankle and foot
  - M85.671 Other cyst of bone, right ankle and foot
  - M85.672 Other cyst of bone, left ankle and foot
  - M85.679 Other cyst of bone, unspecified ankle and foot
- M85.68 Other cyst of bone, other site
- M85.69 Other cyst of bone, multiple sites

- M85.8 Other specified disorders of bone density and structure

  Hyperostosis of bones, except skull
  Osteosclerosis, acquired

  Excludes1 diffuse idiopathic skeletal hyperostosis [DISH] (M48.1)
  osteosclerosis congenita (Q77.4)
  osteosclerosis fragilitas (generalista) (Q78.2)
  osteosclerosis myelofibrosis (D75.81)

- M85.80 Other specified disorders of bone density and structure, unspecified site
- M85.81 Other specified disorders of bone density and structure, shoulder
  - M85.811 Other specified disorders of bone density and structure, right shoulder
  - M85.812 Other specified disorders of bone density and structure, left shoulder
  - M85.819 Other specified disorders of bone density and structure, unspecified shoulder
- M85.82 Other specified disorders of bone density and structure, upper arm
  - M85.821 Other specified disorders of bone density and structure, right upper arm
  - M85.822 Other specified disorders of bone density and structure, left upper arm
  - M85.829 Other specified disorders of bone density and structure, unspecified upper arm
- M85.83 Other specified disorders of bone density and structure, forearm
  - M85.831 Other specified disorders of bone density and structure, right forearm
  - M85.832 Other specified disorders of bone density and structure, left forearm
  - M85.839 Other specified disorders of bone density and structure, unspecified forearm
- M85.84 Other specified disorders of bone density and structure, hand
  - M85.841 Other specified disorders of bone density and structure, right hand
  - M85.842 Other specified disorders of bone density and structure, left hand
  - M85.849 Other specified disorders of bone density and structure, unspecified hand
- M85.85 Other specified disorders of bone density and structure, thigh
  - M85.851 Other specified disorders of bone density and structure, right thigh
  - M85.852 Other specified disorders of bone density and structure, left thigh
  - M85.859 Other specified disorders of bone density and structure, unspecified thigh
- M85.86 Other specified disorders of bone density and structure, lower leg
  - M85.861 Other specified disorders of bone density and structure, right lower leg
  - M85.862 Other specified disorders of bone density and structure, left lower leg
  - M85.869 Other specified disorders of bone density and structure, unspecified lower leg
- M85.87 Other specified disorders of bone density and structure, ankle and foot
  - M85.871 Other specified disorders of bone density and structure, right ankle and foot
  - M85.872 Other specified disorders of bone density and structure, left ankle and foot
  - M85.879 Other specified disorders of bone density and structure, unspecified ankle and foot
- M85.88 Other specified disorders of bone density and structure, other site
- M85.89 Other specified disorders of bone density and structure, multiple sites

M85.9 Disorder of bone density and structure, unspecified

OTHER OSTEOPATHIES (M86-M90)

Excludes1 postprocedural osteopathies (M96.-)

M86 Osteomyelitis

Use additional code (B95-B97) to identify infectious agent

Use additional code to identify major osseous defect, if applicable (M89.7-)

Excludes1 osteomyelitis due to:
echinococcus (B67.2)
gonococcus (A54.43)
salmonella (A02.24)

Excludes2 ostemyelitis of:
orbit (H05.0-)
petrous bone (H70.2-)
vertebra (M46.2-)

M86.0 Acute hematogenous osteomyelitis

M86.00 Acute hematogenous osteomyelitis, unspecified site

Ex: A17.9, A18.03-A18.09, A18.82, A18.84, A18.89, M46.20-M46.39, M86.00-M86.9

M86.01 Acute hematogenous osteomyelitis, shoulder

Ex: For category M86.01 CC codes: A17.9, A18.03-A18.09, A18.82, A18.84, A18.89, M46.20-M46.39, M86.00, M86.08-M86.10, M86.18-M86.20, M86.28-M86.319, M86.38-M86.419, M86.48-M86.519, M86.58-M86.619, M86.68-M86.8X1, M86.8X8-M86.9

M86.011 Acute hematogenous osteomyelitis, right shoulder

M86.012 Acute hematogenous osteomyelitis, left shoulder

M86.019 Acute hematogenous osteomyelitis, unspecified shoulder

M86.02 Acute hematogenous osteomyelitis, humerus

Ex: For category M86.02 CC codes: A17.9, A18.03-A18.09, A18.82, A18.84, A18.89, M46.20-M46.39, M86.00, M86.08-M86.10, M86.18-M86.20, M86.28-M86.30, M86.321-M86.329, M86.38-M86.40, M86.421-M86.429, M86.48-M86.50, M86.521-M86.529, M86.58-M86.60, M86.621-M86.629, M86.68-M86.69, M86.8X0, M86.8X2, M86.8X8-M86.9

M86.021 Acute hematogenous osteomyelitis, right humerus

M86.022 Acute hematogenous osteomyelitis, left humerus

M86.029 Acute hematogenous osteomyelitis, unspecified humerus

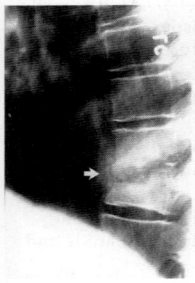

Figure 13-6 Osteomyelitis of the spine. A lateral view of the lower thoracic spine demonstrates destruction of the disk space *(arrow)* as well as destruction of the adjoining vertebral bodies. (From Mettler: Essentials of Radiology, ed 2, Saunders, An Imprint of Elsevier, 2005)

Item 13–12 Osteomyelitis is an inflammation of the bone. **Acute osteomyelitis** is a rapidly destructive, pus-producing infection capable of causing severe bone destruction. **Chronic osteomyelitis** can remain long after the initial acute episode has passed and may lead to a recurrence of the acute phase. **Brodie's abscess** is an encapsulated focal abscess that must be surgically drained. Periostitis is an inflammation of the periosteum, a dense membrane composed of fibrous connective tissue that closely wraps all bone, except those with articulating surfaces in joints, which are covered by synovial membranes.

M86.03 Acute hematogenous osteomyelitis, radius and ulna

Ex: For category M86.03 CC codes: A17.9, A18.03-A18.09, A18.82, A18.84, A18.89, M46.20-M46.39, M86.00, M86.08-M86.10, M86.18-M86.20, M86.28-M86.30, M86.331-M86.339, M86.38-M86.40, M86.431-M86.439, M86.48-M86.50, M86.531-M86.539, M86.58-M86.60, M86.631-M86.639, M86.68-M86.8X0, M86.8X3, M86.8X8-M86.9

M86.031 Acute hematogenous osteomyelitis, right radius and ulna

M86.032 Acute hematogenous osteomyelitis, left radius and ulna

M86.039 Acute hematogenous osteomyelitis, unspecified radius and ulna

M86.04 Acute hematogenous osteomyelitis, hand

Ex: For category M86.04 CC codes: A17.9, A18.03-A18.09, A18.82, A18.84, A18.89, M46.20-M46.39, M86.00, M86.08-M86.10, M86.18-M86.20, M86.28-M86.30, M86.341-M86.349, M86.38-M86.40, M86.441-M86.449, M86.48-M86.50, M86.541-M86.549, M86.58-M86.60, M86.41-M86.649, M86.68-M86.69, M86.8X0, M86.8X4, M86.8X8-M86.9

M86.041 Acute hematogenous osteomyelitis, right hand

M86.042 Acute hematogenous osteomyelitis, left hand

M86.049 Acute hematogenous osteomyelitis, unspecified hand

M86.05 Acute hematogenous osteomyelitis, femur

Ex: For category M86.05 CC codes: A17.9, A18.03-A18.09, A18.82, A18.84, A18.89, M46.20-M46.39, M86.00, M86.08-M86.10, M86.18-M86.20, M86.28-M86.30, M86.351-M86.359, M86.38-M86.40, M86.451-M86.459, M86.48-M86.50, M86.551-M86.559, M86.58-M86.60, M86.651-M86.659, M86.68-M86.8X0, M86.8X5, M86.8X8-M86.9

M86.051 Acute hematogenous osteomyelitis, right femur

M86.052 Acute hematogenous osteomyelitis, left femur

M86.059 Acute hematogenous osteomyelitis, unspecified femur

M86.06 Acute hematogenous osteomyelitis, tibia and fibula

Ex: For category M86.06 CC codes: A17.9, A18.03-A18.09, A18.82, A18.84, A18.89, M46.20-M46.39, M86.00, M86.08-M86.10, M86.18-M86.20, M86.28-M86.30, M86.361-M86.369, M86.38-M86.40, M86.461-M86.469, M86.48-M86.50, M86.561-M86.569, M86.58-M86.60, M86.661-M86.669, M86.68-M86.8X0, M86.8X6, M86.8X8-M86.9

M86.061 Acute hematogenous osteomyelitis, right tibia and fibula

M86.062 Acute hematogenous osteomyelitis, left tibia and fibula

M86.069 Acute hematogenous osteomyelitis, unspecified tibia and fibula

M86.07 Acute hematogenous osteomyelitis, ankle and foot

Ex: For category M86.07 CC codes: A17.9, A18.03-A18.09, A18.82, A18.84, A18.89, M46.20-M46.39, M86.00, M86.08-M86.10, M86.18-M86.20, M86.28-M86.30, M86.371-M86.379, M86.38-M86.40, M86.471-M86.479, M86.48-M86.50, M86.571-M86.579, M86.58-M86.60, M86.671-M86.679, M86.68-M86.8X0, M86.8X7-M86.9

M86.071 Acute hematogenous osteomyelitis, right ankle and foot

M86.072 Acute hematogenous osteomyelitis, left ankle and foot

M86.079 Acute hematogenous osteomyelitis, unspecified ankle and foot

M86.08 Acute hematogenous osteomyelitis, other sites
Ex: A17.9, A18.01, A18.03, A18.09, A18.82, A18.84, A18.89, M46.20-M46.39, M86.00-M86.9

M86.09 Acute hematogenous osteomyelitis, multiple sites
Ex: See M86.00

● M86.1 Other acute osteomyelitis

M86.10 Other acute osteomyelitis, unspecified site
Ex: See M86.00

● M86.11 Other acute osteomyelitis, shoulder
Ex: For category M86.11 CC codes: See M86.01

M86.111 Other acute osteomyelitis, right shoulder

M86.112 Other acute osteomyelitis, left shoulder

M86.119 Other acute osteomyelitis, unspecified shoulder

● M86.12 Other acute osteomyelitis, humerus
Ex: For category M86.12 CC codes: See M86.02

M86.121 Other acute osteomyelitis, right humerus

M86.122 Other acute osteomyelitis, left humerus

M86.129 Other acute osteomyelitis, unspecified humerus

● M86.13 Other acute osteomyelitis, radius and ulna
Ex: For category M86.13 CC codes: See M86.03

M86.131 Other acute osteomyelitis, right radius and ulna

M86.132 Other acute osteomyelitis, left radius and ulna

M86.139 Other acute osteomyelitis, unspecified radius and ulna

● M86.14 Other acute osteomyelitis, hand
Ex: For category M86.14 CC codes: See M86.04

M86.141 Other acute osteomyelitis, right hand

M86.142 Other acute osteomyelitis, left hand

M86.149 Other acute osteomyelitis, unspecified hand

● M86.15 Other acute osteomyelitis, femur
Ex: For category M86.15 CC codes: See M86.05

M86.151 Other acute osteomyelitis, right femur

M86.152 Other acute osteomyelitis, left femur

M86.159 Other acute osteomyelitis, unspecified femur

● M86.16 Other acute osteomyelitis, tibia and fibula
Ex: For category M86.16 CC codes: See M86.06

M86.161 Other acute osteomyelitis, right tibia and fibula

M86.162 Other acute osteomyelitis, left tibia and fibula

M86.169 Other acute osteomyelitis, unspecified tibia and fibula

● M86.17 Other acute osteomyelitis, ankle and foot
Ex: For category M86.17 CC codes: See M86.07

M86.171 Other acute osteomyelitis, right ankle and foot

M86.172 Other acute osteomyelitis, left ankle and foot

M86.179 Other acute osteomyelitis, unspecified ankle and foot

M86.18 Other acute osteomyelitis, other site
Ex: See M86.08

M86.19 Other acute osteomyelitis, multiple sites
Ex: See M86.00

● M86.2 Subacute osteomyelitis

M86.20 Subacute osteomyelitis, unspecified site
Ex: See M86.00

● M86.21 Subacute osteomyelitis, shoulder
Ex: For category M86.21 CC codes: See M86.01

M86.211 Subacute osteomyelitis, right shoulder

M86.212 Subacute osteomyelitis, left shoulder

M86.219 Subacute osteomyelitis, unspecified shoulder

● M86.22 Subacute osteomyelitis, humerus
Ex: For category M86.22 CC codes: See M86.02

M86.221 Subacute osteomyelitis, right humerus

M86.222 Subacute osteomyelitis, left humerus

M86.229 Subacute osteomyelitis, unspecified humerus

● M86.23 Subacute osteomyelitis, radius and ulna
Ex: For category M86.23 CC codes: See M86.03

M86.231 Subacute osteomyelitis, right radius and ulna

M86.232 Subacute osteomyelitis, left radius and ulna

M86.239 Subacute osteomyelitis, unspecified radius and ulna

● M86.24 Subacute osteomyelitis, hand
Ex: For category M86.24 CC codes: See M86.04

M86.241 Subacute osteomyelitis, right hand

M86.242 Subacute osteomyelitis, left hand

M86.249 Subacute osteomyelitis, unspecified hand

● M86.25 Subacute osteomyelitis, femur
Ex: For category M86.25 CC codes: See M86.05

M86.251 Subacute osteomyelitis, right femur

M86.252 Subacute osteomyelitis, left femur

M86.259 Subacute osteomyelitis, unspecified femur

● M86.26 Subacute osteomyelitis, tibia and fibula
Ex: For category M86.26 CC codes: See M86.06

M86.261 Subacute osteomyelitis, right tibia and fibula

M86.262 Subacute osteomyelitis, left tibia and fibula

M86.269 Subacute osteomyelitis, unspecified tibia and fibula

● M86.27 Subacute osteomyelitis, ankle and foot
Ex: For category M86.27 CC codes: See M86.07

M86.271 Subacute osteomyelitis, right ankle and foot

M86.272 Subacute osteomyelitis, left ankle and foot

M86.279 Subacute osteomyelitis, unspecified ankle and foot

M86.28 Subacute osteomyelitis, other site
Ex: See M86.08

M86.29 Subacute osteomyelitis, multiple sites
Ex: See M86.00

● M86.3 Chronic multifocal osteomyelitis
Ex: For category M86.3 CC codes unless otherwise indicated: A02.24, A17.9, A18.03, A18.09, A18.82, A18.84, A18.89, M46.20-M46.39, M86.00-M86.9

M86.30 Chronic multifocal osteomyelitis, unspecified site
Ex: M46.20-M46.39, M86.30-M86.9, M88.0-M88.9, M90.60-M90.69

- M86.31 Chronic multifocal osteomyelitis, shoulder
  - M86.311 Chronic multifocal osteomyelitis, right shoulder
  - M86.312 Chronic multifocal osteomyelitis, left shoulder
  - M86.319 Chronic multifocal osteomyelitis, unspecified shoulder
- M86.32 Chronic multifocal osteomyelitis, humerus
  - M86.321 Chronic multifocal osteomyelitis, right humerus
  - M86.322 Chronic multifocal osteomyelitis, left humerus
  - M86.329 Chronic multifocal osteomyelitis, unspecified humerus
- M86.33 Chronic multifocal osteomyelitis, radius and ulna
  - M86.331 Chronic multifocal osteomyelitis, right radius and ulna
  - M86.332 Chronic multifocal osteomyelitis, left radius and ulna
  - M86.339 Chronic multifocal osteomyelitis, unspecified radius and ulna
- M86.34 Chronic multifocal osteomyelitis, hand
  - M86.341 Chronic multifocal osteomyelitis, right hand
  - M86.342 Chronic multifocal osteomyelitis, left hand
  - M86.349 Chronic multifocal osteomyelitis, unspecified hand
- M86.35 Chronic multifocal osteomyelitis, femur
  - M86.351 Chronic multifocal osteomyelitis, right femur
  - M86.352 Chronic multifocal osteomyelitis, left femur
  - M86.359 Chronic multifocal osteomyelitis, unspecified femur
- M86.36 Chronic multifocal osteomyelitis, tibia and fibula
  - M86.361 Chronic multifocal osteomyelitis, right tibia and fibula
  - M86.362 Chronic multifocal osteomyelitis, left tibia and fibula
  - M86.369 Chronic multifocal osteomyelitis, unspecified tibia and fibula
- M86.37 Chronic multifocal osteomyelitis, ankle and foot
  - M86.371 Chronic multifocal osteomyelitis, right ankle and foot
  - M86.372 Chronic multifocal osteomyelitis, left ankle and foot
  - M86.379 Chronic multifocal osteomyelitis, unspecified ankle and foot
- M86.38 Chronic multifocal osteomyelitis, other site
- M86.39 Chronic multifocal osteomyelitis, multiple sites

- M86.4 Chronic osteomyelitis with draining sinus
  - Ex: For category M86.4 CC codes unless otherwise indicated: See M86.3
  - M86.40 Chronic osteomyelitis with draining sinus, unspecified site
    - Ex: See M86.30
  - M86.41 Chronic osteomyelitis with draining sinus, shoulder
    - M86.411 Chronic osteomyelitis with draining sinus, right shoulder
    - M86.412 Chronic osteomyelitis with draining sinus, left shoulder
    - M86.419 Chronic osteomyelitis with draining sinus, unspecified shoulder
  - M86.42 Chronic osteomyelitis with draining sinus, humerus
    - M86.421 Chronic osteomyelitis with draining sinus, right humerus
    - M86.422 Chronic osteomyelitis with draining sinus, left humerus
    - M86.429 Chronic osteomyelitis with draining sinus, unspecified humerus
  - M86.43 Chronic osteomyelitis with draining sinus, radius and ulna
    - M86.431 Chronic osteomyelitis with draining sinus, right radius and ulna
    - M86.432 Chronic osteomyelitis with draining sinus, left radius and ulna
    - M86.439 Chronic osteomyelitis with draining sinus, unspecified radius and ulna
  - M86.44 Chronic osteomyelitis with draining sinus, hand
    - M86.441 Chronic osteomyelitis with draining sinus, right hand
    - M86.442 Chronic osteomyelitis with draining sinus, left hand
    - M86.449 Chronic osteomyelitis with draining sinus, unspecified hand
  - M86.45 Chronic osteomyelitis with draining sinus, femur
    - M86.451 Chronic osteomyelitis with draining sinus, right femur
    - M86.452 Chronic osteomyelitis with draining sinus, left femur
    - M86.459 Chronic osteomyelitis with draining sinus, unspecified femur
  - M86.46 Chronic osteomyelitis with draining sinus, tibia and fibula
    - M86.461 Chronic osteomyelitis with draining sinus, right tibia and fibula
    - M86.462 Chronic osteomyelitis with draining sinus, left tibia and fibula
    - M86.469 Chronic osteomyelitis with draining sinus, unspecified tibia and fibula
  - M86.47 Chronic osteomyelitis with draining sinus, ankle and foot
    - M86.471 Chronic osteomyelitis with draining sinus, right ankle and foot
    - M86.472 Chronic osteomyelitis with draining sinus, left ankle and foot
    - M86.479 Chronic osteomyelitis with draining sinus, unspecified ankle and foot
  - M86.48 Chronic osteomyelitis with draining sinus, other site
  - M86.49 Chronic osteomyelitis with draining sinus, multiple sites
- M86.5 Other chronic hematogenous osteomyelitis
  - Ex: For category M86.5 CC codes unless otherwise indicated: See M86.3
  - M86.50 Other chronic hematogenous osteomyelitis, unspecified site
    - Ex: See M86.30
  - M86.51 Other chronic hematogenous osteomyelitis, shoulder
    - M86.511 Other chronic hematogenous osteomyelitis, right shoulder
    - M86.512 Other chronic hematogenous osteomyelitis, left shoulder
    - M86.519 Other chronic hematogenous osteomyelitis, unspecified shoulder

- M86.52 Other chronic hematogenous osteomyelitis, humerus
  - M86.521 Other chronic hematogenous osteomyelitis, right humerus
  - M86.522 Other chronic hematogenous osteomyelitis, left humerus
  - M86.529 Other chronic hematogenous osteomyelitis, unspecified humerus
- M86.53 Other chronic hematogenous osteomyelitis, radius and ulna
  - M86.531 Other chronic hematogenous osteomyelitis, right radius and ulna
  - M86.532 Other chronic hematogenous osteomyelitis, left radius and ulna
  - M86.539 Other chronic hematogenous osteomyelitis, unspecified radius and ulna
- M86.54 Other chronic hematogenous osteomyelitis, hand
  - M86.541 Other chronic hematogenous osteomyelitis, right hand
  - M86.542 Other chronic hematogenous osteomyelitis, left hand
  - M86.549 Other chronic hematogenous osteomyelitis, unspecified hand
- M86.55 Other chronic hematogenous osteomyelitis, femur
  - M86.551 Other chronic hematogenous osteomyelitis, right femur
  - M86.552 Other chronic hematogenous osteomyelitis, left femur
  - M86.559 Other chronic hematogenous osteomyelitis, unspecified femur
- M86.56 Other chronic hematogenous osteomyelitis, tibia and fibula
  - M86.561 Other chronic hematogenous osteomyelitis, right tibia and fibula
  - M86.562 Other chronic hematogenous osteomyelitis, left tibia and fibula
  - M86.569 Other chronic hematogenous osteomyelitis, unspecified tibia and fibula
- M86.57 Other chronic hematogenous osteomyelitis, ankle and foot
  - M86.571 Other chronic hematogenous osteomyelitis, right ankle and foot
  - M86.572 Other chronic hematogenous osteomyelitis, left ankle and foot
  - M86.579 Other chronic hematogenous osteomyelitis, unspecified ankle and foot
- M86.58 Other chronic hematogenous osteomyelitis, other site
- M86.59 Other chronic hematogenous osteomyelitis, multiple sites

- M86.6 Other chronic osteomyelitis
  - Ex: For category M86.6 CC codes unless otherwise indicated: See M86.3
  - M86.60 Other chronic osteomyelitis, unspecified site
    - Ex: See M86.30
  - M86.61 Other chronic osteomyelitis, shoulder
    - M86.611 Other chronic osteomyelitis, right shoulder
    - M86.612 Other chronic osteomyelitis, left shoulder
    - M86.619 Other chronic osteomyelitis, unspecified shoulder
  - M86.62 Other chronic osteomyelitis, humerus
    - M86.621 Other chronic osteomyelitis, right humerus
    - M86.622 Other chronic osteomyelitis, left humerus
    - M86.629 Other chronic osteomyelitis, unspecified humerus
  - M86.63 Other chronic osteomyelitis, radius and ulna
    - M86.631 Other chronic osteomyelitis, right radius and ulna
    - M86.632 Other chronic osteomyelitis, left radius and ulna
    - M86.639 Other chronic osteomyelitis, unspecified radius and ulna
  - M86.64 Other chronic osteomyelitis, hand
    - M86.641 Other chronic osteomyelitis, right hand
    - M86.642 Other chronic osteomyelitis, left hand
    - M86.649 Other chronic osteomyelitis, unspecified hand
  - M86.65 Other chronic osteomyelitis, thigh
    - M86.651 Other chronic osteomyelitis, right thigh
    - M86.652 Other chronic osteomyelitis, left thigh
    - M86.659 Other chronic osteomyelitis, unspecified thigh
  - M86.66 Other chronic osteomyelitis, tibia and fibula
    - M86.661 Other chronic osteomyelitis, right tibia and fibula
    - M86.662 Other chronic osteomyelitis, left tibia and fibula
    - M86.669 Other chronic osteomyelitis, unspecified tibia and fibula
  - M86.67 Other chronic osteomyelitis, ankle and foot
    - M86.671 Other chronic osteomyelitis, right ankle and foot
      - Coding Clinic: 2016, Q1, P13
    - M86.672 Other chronic osteomyelitis, left ankle and foot
    - M86.679 Other chronic osteomyelitis, unspecified ankle and foot
  - M86.68 Other chronic osteomyelitis, other site
  - M86.69 Other chronic osteomyelitis, multiple sites

- M86.8 Other osteomyelitis
  - Brodie's abscess
  - Ex: For category M86.8 CC codes unless otherwise indicated: See M86.3
  - M86.8X Other osteomyelitis
    - M86.8X0 Other osteomyelitis, multiple sites
    - M86.8X1 Other osteomyelitis, shoulder
    - M86.8X2 Other osteomyelitis, upper arm
    - M86.8X3 Other osteomyelitis, forearm
    - M86.8X4 Other osteomyelitis, hand
    - M86.8X5 Other osteomyelitis, thigh
    - M86.8X6 Other osteomyelitis, lower leg
    - M86.8X7 Other osteomyelitis, ankle and foot
    - M86.8X8 Other osteomyelitis, other site
    - M86.8X9 Other osteomyelitis, unspecified sites
      - Ex: See M86.30
- M86.9 Osteomyelitis, unspecified
  - Infection of bone NOS
  - Periostitis without osteomyelitis
  - Ex: See M86.30

M87 Osteonecrosis

Includes avascular necrosis of bone

Use additional code to identify major osseous defect, if applicable (M89.7-)

Excludes1 juvenile osteonecrosis (M91-M92)
osteochondropathies (M90-M93)

Ex: For category M87 CC codes unless otherwise indicated: M87.00-M87.9, M90.50-M90.59

M87.0 Idiopathic aseptic necrosis of bone

M87.00 Idiopathic aseptic necrosis of unspecified bone

M87.01 Idiopathic aseptic necrosis of shoulder

Idiopathic aseptic necrosis of clavicle and scapula

Ex: For category M87.01 CC codes: M87.00-M87.9, M90.50-M90.59

M87.011 Idiopathic aseptic necrosis of right shoulder

M87.012 Idiopathic aseptic necrosis of left shoulder

M87.019 Idiopathic aseptic necrosis of unspecified shoulder

M87.02 Idiopathic aseptic necrosis of humerus

Ex: For category M87.02 CC codes: See M87.01

M87.021 Idiopathic aseptic necrosis of right humerus

M87.022 Idiopathic aseptic necrosis of left humerus

M87.029 Idiopathic aseptic necrosis of unspecified humerus

M87.03 Idiopathic aseptic necrosis of radius, ulna and carpus

M87.031 Idiopathic aseptic necrosis of right radius

M87.032 Idiopathic aseptic necrosis of left radius

M87.033 Idiopathic aseptic necrosis of unspecified radius

M87.034 Idiopathic aseptic necrosis of right ulna

M87.035 Idiopathic aseptic necrosis of left ulna

M87.036 Idiopathic aseptic necrosis of unspecified ulna

M87.037 Idiopathic aseptic necrosis of right carpus

M87.038 Idiopathic aseptic necrosis of left carpus

M87.039 Idiopathic aseptic necrosis of unspecified carpus

M87.04 Idiopathic aseptic necrosis of hand and fingers

Idiopathic aseptic necrosis of metacarpals and phalanges of hands

M87.041 Idiopathic aseptic necrosis of right hand

M87.042 Idiopathic aseptic necrosis of left hand

M87.043 Idiopathic aseptic necrosis of unspecified hand

M87.044 Idiopathic aseptic necrosis of right finger(s)

M87.045 Idiopathic aseptic necrosis of left finger(s)

M87.046 Idiopathic aseptic necrosis of unspecified finger(s)

M87.05 Idiopathic aseptic necrosis of pelvis and femur

M87.050 Idiopathic aseptic necrosis of pelvis

M87.051 Idiopathic aseptic necrosis of right femur

Ex: M87.00-M87.9, M90.50-M90.59

M87.052 Idiopathic aseptic necrosis of left femur

Ex: See M87.501

M87.059 Idiopathic aseptic necrosis of unspecified femur

Idiopathic aseptic necrosis of hip NOS

Ex: See M87.501

M87.06 Idiopathic aseptic necrosis of tibia and fibula

M87.061 Idiopathic aseptic necrosis of right tibia

M87.062 Idiopathic aseptic necrosis of left tibia

M87.063 Idiopathic aseptic necrosis of unspecified tibia

M87.064 Idiopathic aseptic necrosis of right fibula

M87.065 Idiopathic aseptic necrosis of left fibula

M87.066 Idiopathic aseptic necrosis of unspecified fibula

M87.07 Idiopathic aseptic necrosis of ankle, foot and toes

Idiopathic aseptic necrosis of metatarsus, tarsus, and phalanges of toes

M87.071 Idiopathic aseptic necrosis of right ankle

M87.072 Idiopathic aseptic necrosis of left ankle

M87.073 Idiopathic aseptic necrosis of unspecified ankle

M87.074 Idiopathic aseptic necrosis of right foot

Ex: M87.00, M87.031-M87.819, M87.831-M87.849, M87.861-M87.9, M90.50, M90.521-M90.549, M90.561-M90.59

M87.075 Idiopathic aseptic necrosis of left foot

Ex: See M87.074

M87.076 Idiopathic aseptic necrosis of unspecified foot

Ex: See M87.074

M87.077 Idiopathic aseptic necrosis of right toe(s)

M87.078 Idiopathic aseptic necrosis of left toe(s)

M87.079 Idiopathic aseptic necrosis of unspecified toe(s)

M87.08 Idiopathic aseptic necrosis of bone, other site

M87.09 Idiopathic aseptic necrosis of bone, multiple sites

M87.1 Osteonecrosis due to drugs

Use additional code for adverse effect, if applicable, to identify drug (T36-T50 with fifth or sixth character 5)

Ex: See M87

M87.10 Osteonecrosis due to drugs, unspecified bone

M87.11 Osteonecrosis due to drugs, shoulder

M87.111 Osteonecrosis due to drugs, right shoulder

M87.112 Osteonecrosis due to drugs, left shoulder

M87.119 Osteonecrosis due to drugs, unspecified shoulder

- M87.12 Osteonecrosis due to drugs, humerus
  - Ex: For category M87.12 CC codes: See M87.01
  - M87.121 Osteonecrosis due to drugs, right humerus
  - M87.122 Osteonecrosis due to drugs, left humerus
  - M87.129 Osteonecrosis due to drugs, unspecified humerus
- M87.13 Osteonecrosis due to drugs of radius, ulna and carpus
  - M87.131 Osteonecrosis due to drugs of right radius
  - M87.132 Osteonecrosis due to drugs of left radius
  - M87.133 Osteonecrosis due to drugs of unspecified radius
  - M87.134 Osteonecrosis due to drugs of right ulna
  - M87.135 Osteonecrosis due to drugs of left ulna
  - M87.136 Osteonecrosis due to drugs of unspecified ulna
  - M87.137 Osteonecrosis due to drugs of right carpus
  - M87.138 Osteonecrosis due to drugs of left carpus
  - M87.139 Osteonecrosis due to drugs of unspecified carpus
- M87.14 Osteonecrosis due to drugs, hand and fingers
  - M87.141 Osteonecrosis due to drugs, right hand
  - M87.142 Osteonecrosis due to drugs, left hand
  - M87.143 Osteonecrosis due to drugs, unspecified hand
  - M87.144 Osteonecrosis due to drugs, right finger(s)
  - M87.145 Osteonecrosis due to drugs, left finger(s)
  - M87.146 Osteonecrosis due to drugs, unspecified finger(s)
- M87.15 Osteonecrosis due to drugs, pelvis and femur
  - Ex: For category M87.15 CC codes: See M87.051
  - M87.150 Osteonecrosis due to drugs, pelvis
  - M87.151 Osteonecrosis due to drugs, right femur
  - M87.152 Osteonecrosis due to drugs, left femur
  - M87.159 Osteonecrosis due to drugs, unspecified femur
- M87.16 Osteonecrosis due to drugs, tibia and fibula
  - M87.161 Osteonecrosis due to drugs, right tibia
  - M87.162 Osteonecrosis due to drugs, left tibia
  - M87.163 Osteonecrosis due to drugs, unspecified tibia
  - M87.164 Osteonecrosis due to drugs, right fibula
  - M87.165 Osteonecrosis due to drugs, left fibula
  - M87.166 Osteonecrosis due to drugs, unspecified fibula
- M87.17 Osteonecrosis due to drugs, ankle, foot and toes
  - M87.171 Osteonecrosis due to drugs, right ankle
  - M87.172 Osteonecrosis due to drugs, left ankle
  - M87.173 Osteonecrosis due to drugs, unspecified ankle
  - M87.174 Osteonecrosis due to drugs, right foot
    - Ex: See M87.074
  - M87.175 Osteonecrosis due to drugs, left foot
    - Ex: See M87.074
  - M87.176 Osteonecrosis due to drugs, unspecified foot
    - Ex: See M87.074
  - M87.177 Osteonecrosis due to drugs, right toe(s)
  - M87.178 Osteonecrosis due to drugs, left toe(s)
  - M87.179 Osteonecrosis due to drugs, unspecified toe(s)
- M87.18 Osteonecrosis due to drugs, other site
  - M87.180 Osteonecrosis due to drugs, jaw
  - M87.188 Osteonecrosis due to drugs, other site
- M87.19 Osteonecrosis due to drugs, multiple sites
- M87.2 Osteonecrosis due to previous trauma
  - Ex: See M87
  - M87.20 Osteonecrosis due to previous trauma, unspecified bone
- M87.21 Osteonecrosis due to previous trauma, shoulder
  - M87.211 Osteonecrosis due to previous trauma, right shoulder
  - M87.212 Osteonecrosis due to previous trauma, left shoulder
  - M87.219 Osteonecrosis due to previous trauma, unspecified shoulder
- M87.22 Osteonecrosis due to previous trauma, humerus
  - Ex: For category M87.22 CC codes: See M87.01
  - M87.221 Osteonecrosis due to previous trauma, right humerus
  - M87.222 Osteonecrosis due to previous trauma, left humerus
  - M87.229 Osteonecrosis due to previous trauma, unspecified humerus
- M87.23 Osteonecrosis due to previous trauma of radius, ulna and carpus
  - M87.231 Osteonecrosis due to previous trauma of right radius
  - M87.232 Osteonecrosis due to previous trauma of left radius
  - M87.233 Osteonecrosis due to previous trauma of unspecified radius
  - M87.234 Osteonecrosis due to previous trauma of right ulna
  - M87.235 Osteonecrosis due to previous trauma of left ulna
  - M87.236 Osteonecrosis due to previous trauma of unspecified ulna
  - M87.237 Osteonecrosis due to previous trauma of right carpus
  - M87.238 Osteonecrosis due to previous trauma of left carpus
  - M87.239 Osteonecrosis due to previous trauma of unspecified carpus

- M87.24 Osteonecrosis due to previous trauma, hand and fingers
  - M87.241 Osteonecrosis due to previous trauma, right hand
  - M87.242 Osteonecrosis due to previous trauma, left hand
  - M87.243 Osteonecrosis due to previous trauma, unspecified hand
  - M87.244 Osteonecrosis due to previous trauma, right finger(s)
  - M87.245 Osteonecrosis due to previous trauma, left finger(s)
  - M87.246 Osteonecrosis due to previous trauma, unspecified finger(s)
- M87.25 Osteonecrosis due to previous trauma, pelvis and femur
  - M87.250 Osteonecrosis due to previous trauma, pelvis
  - M87.251 Osteonecrosis due to previous trauma, right femur
    - Ex: See M87.051
  - M87.252 Osteonecrosis due to previous trauma, left femur
    - Ex: See M87.051
  - M87.256 Osteonecrosis due to previous trauma, unspecified femur
    - Ex: See M87.051
- M87.26 Osteonecrosis due to previous trauma, tibia and fibula
  - M87.261 Osteonecrosis due to previous trauma, right tibia
  - M87.262 Osteonecrosis due to previous trauma, left tibia
  - M87.263 Osteonecrosis due to previous trauma, unspecified tibia
  - M87.264 Osteonecrosis due to previous trauma, right fibula
  - M87.265 Osteonecrosis due to previous trauma, left fibula
  - M87.266 Osteonecrosis due to previous trauma, unspecified fibula
- M87.27 Osteonecrosis due to previous trauma, ankle, foot and toes
  - M87.271 Osteonecrosis due to previous trauma, right ankle
  - M87.272 Osteonecrosis due to previous trauma, left ankle
  - M87.273 Osteonecrosis due to previous trauma, unspecified ankle
  - M87.274 Osteonecrosis due to previous trauma, right foot
    - Ex: See M87.074
  - M87.275 Osteonecrosis due to previous trauma, left foot
    - Ex: See M87.074
  - M87.276 Osteonecrosis due to previous trauma, unspecified foot
    - Ex: See M87.074
  - M87.277 Osteonecrosis due to previous trauma, right toe(s)
  - M87.278 Osteonecrosis due to previous trauma, left toe(s)
  - M87.279 Osteonecrosis due to previous trauma, unspecified toe(s)
- M87.28 Osteonecrosis due to previous trauma, other site
- M87.29 Osteonecrosis due to previous trauma, multiple sites
- M87.3 Other secondary osteonecrosis
  - Ex: See M87
  - M87.30 Other secondary osteonecrosis, unspecified bone
- M87.31 Other secondary osteonecrosis, shoulder
  - M87.311 Other secondary osteonecrosis, right shoulder
  - M87.312 Other secondary osteonecrosis, left shoulder
  - M87.319 Other secondary osteonecrosis, unspecified shoulder
- M87.32 Other secondary osteonecrosis, humerus
  - Ex: For category M87.32 CC codes: See M87.01
  - M87.321 Other secondary osteonecrosis, right humerus
  - M87.322 Other secondary osteonecrosis, left humerus
  - M87.329 Other secondary osteonecrosis, unspecified humerus
- M87.33 Other secondary osteonecrosis of radius, ulna and carpus
  - M87.331 Other secondary osteonecrosis of right radius
  - M87.332 Other secondary osteonecrosis of left radius
  - M87.333 Other secondary osteonecrosis of unspecified radius
  - M87.334 Other secondary osteonecrosis of right ulna
  - M87.335 Other secondary osteonecrosis of left ulna
  - M87.336 Other secondary osteonecrosis of unspecified ulna
  - M87.337 Other secondary osteonecrosis of right carpus
  - M87.338 Other secondary osteonecrosis of left carpus
  - M87.339 Other secondary osteonecrosis of unspecified carpus
- M87.34 Other secondary osteonecrosis, hand and fingers
  - M87.341 Other secondary osteonecrosis, right hand
  - M87.342 Other secondary osteonecrosis, left hand
  - M87.343 Other secondary osteonecrosis, unspecified hand
  - M87.344 Other secondary osteonecrosis, right finger(s)
  - M87.345 Other secondary osteonecrosis, left finger(s)
  - M87.346 Other secondary osteonecrosis, unspecified finger(s)
- M87.35 Other secondary osteonecrosis, pelvis and femur
  - Ex: For category M87.35 CC codes: See M87.051
  - M87.350 Other secondary osteonecrosis, pelvis
  - M87.351 Other secondary osteonecrosis, right femur
  - M87.352 Other secondary osteonecrosis, left femur
  - M87.353 Other secondary osteonecrosis, unspecified femur

◀ New ⇐ Revised ~~deleted~~ Deleted Excludes 1 Excludes 2 Includes Use additional Code first Code also Unspecified
OGCR Official Guidelines ● Unacceptable Principal Diagnosis X Assign placeholder X ● Use Additional Character(s) ▶ Manifestation Code Coding Clinic

- M87.36 Other secondary osteonecrosis, tibia and fibula
  - M87.361 Other secondary osteonecrosis, right tibia
  - M87.362 Other secondary osteonecrosis, left tibia
  - M87.363 Other secondary osteonecrosis, unspecified tibia
  - M87.364 Other secondary osteonecrosis, right fibula
  - M87.365 Other secondary osteonecrosis, left fibula
  - M87.366 Other secondary osteonecrosis, unspecified fibula
- M87.37 Other secondary osteonecrosis, ankle and foot
  - M87.371 Other secondary osteonecrosis, right ankle
  - M87.372 Other secondary osteonecrosis, left ankle
  - M87.373 Other secondary osteonecrosis, unspecified ankle
  - M87.374 Other secondary osteonecrosis, right foot
    - Ex: See M87.074
  - M87.375 Other secondary osteonecrosis, left foot
    - Ex: See M87.074
  - M87.376 Other secondary osteonecrosis, unspecified foot
    - Ex: See M87.074
  - M87.377 Other secondary osteonecrosis, right toe(s)
  - M87.378 Other secondary osteonecrosis, left toe(s)
  - M87.379 Other secondary osteonecrosis, unspecified toe(s)
- M87.38 Other secondary osteonecrosis, other site
- M87.39 Other secondary osteonecrosis, multiple sites
- M87.8 Other osteonecrosis
  - Ex: See M87
  - M87.80 Other osteonecrosis, unspecified bone
  - M87.81 Other osteonecrosis, shoulder
    - M87.811 Other osteonecrosis, right shoulder
    - M87.812 Other osteonecrosis, left shoulder
    - M87.819 Other osteonecrosis, unspecified shoulder
  - M87.82 Other osteonecrosis, humerus
    - Ex: For category M87.82 CC codes: See M87.01
    - M87.821 Other osteonecrosis, right humerus
    - M87.822 Other osteonecrosis, left humerus
    - M87.829 Other osteonecrosis, unspecified humerus
  - M87.83 Other osteonecrosis of radius, ulna and carpus
    - M87.831 Other osteonecrosis of right radius
    - M87.832 Other osteonecrosis of left radius
    - M87.833 Other osteonecrosis of unspecified radius
    - M87.834 Other osteonecrosis of right ulna
    - M87.835 Other osteonecrosis of left ulna
    - M87.836 Other osteonecrosis of unspecified ulna
    - M87.837 Other osteonecrosis of right carpus
    - M87.838 Other osteonecrosis of left carpus
    - M87.839 Other osteonecrosis of unspecified carpus
  - M87.84 Other osteonecrosis, hand and fingers
    - M87.841 Other osteonecrosis, right hand
    - M87.842 Other osteonecrosis, left hand
    - M87.843 Other osteonecrosis, unspecified hand
    - M87.844 Other osteonecrosis, right finger(s)
    - M87.845 Other osteonecrosis, left finger(s)
    - M87.849 Other osteonecrosis, unspecified finger(s)
  - M87.85 Other osteonecrosis, pelvis and femur
    - Ex: For category M87.85 CC codes: See M87.051
    - M87.850 Other osteonecrosis, pelvis
    - M87.851 Other osteonecrosis, right femur
    - M87.852 Other osteonecrosis, left femur
    - M87.859 Other osteonecrosis, unspecified femur
  - M87.86 Other osteonecrosis, tibia and fibula
    - M87.861 Other osteonecrosis, right tibia
    - M87.862 Other osteonecrosis, left tibia
    - M87.863 Other osteonecrosis, unspecified tibia
    - M87.864 Other osteonecrosis, right fibula
    - M87.865 Other osteonecrosis, left fibula
    - M87.869 Other osteonecrosis, unspecified fibula
  - M87.87 Other osteonecrosis, ankle, foot and toes
    - M87.871 Other osteonecrosis, right ankle
    - M87.872 Other osteonecrosis, left ankle
    - M87.873 Other osteonecrosis, unspecified ankle
    - M87.874 Other osteonecrosis, right foot
      - Ex: See M87.074
    - M87.875 Other osteonecrosis, left foot
      - Ex: See M87.074
    - M87.876 Other osteonecrosis, unspecified foot
      - Ex: See M87.074
    - M87.877 Other osteonecrosis, right toe(s)
    - M87.878 Other osteonecrosis, left toe(s)
    - M87.879 Other osteonecrosis, unspecified toe(s)
  - M87.88 Other osteonecrosis, other site
  - M87.89 Other osteonecrosis, multiple sites
- M87.9 Osteonecrosis, unspecified
  - Necrosis of bone NOS
  - Ex: See M87

- M88 Osteitis deformans [Paget's disease of bone]
  - *Chronic disorder that results in enlarged and deformed bones. The excessive breakdown and formation of bone tissue causes bones to weaken and results in bone pain, arthritis, deformities, and fractures.*
  - **Excludes1** osteitis deformans in neoplastic disease (M90.6)
  - M88.0 Osteitis deformans of skull
  - M88.1 Osteitis deformans of vertebrae
  - M88.8 Osteitis deformans of other bones
    - M88.81 Osteitis deformans of shoulder
      - M88.811 Osteitis deformans of right shoulder
      - M88.812 Osteitis deformans of left shoulder
      - M88.819 Osteitis deformans of unspecified shoulder
    - M88.82 Osteitis deformans of upper arm
      - M88.821 Osteitis deformans of right upper arm
      - M88.822 Osteitis deformans of left upper arm
      - M88.829 Osteitis deformans of unspecified upper arm

- M88.83 Osteitis deformans of forearm
  - M88.831 Osteitis deformans of right forearm
  - M88.832 Osteitis deformans of left forearm
  - M88.839 Osteitis deformans of unspecified forearm
- M88.84 Osteitis deformans of hand
  - M88.841 Osteitis deformans of right hand
  - M88.842 Osteitis deformans of left hand
  - M88.849 Osteitis deformans of unspecified hand
- M88.85 Osteitis deformans of thigh
  - M88.851 Osteitis deformans of right thigh
  - M88.852 Osteitis deformans of left thigh
  - M88.859 Osteitis deformans of unspecified thigh
- M88.86 Osteitis deformans of lower leg
  - M88.861 Osteitis deformans of right lower leg
  - M88.862 Osteitis deformans of left lower leg
  - M88.869 Osteitis deformans of unspecified lower leg
- M88.87 Osteitis deformans of ankle and foot
  - M88.871 Osteitis deformans of right ankle and foot
  - M88.872 Osteitis deformans of left ankle and foot
  - M88.879 Osteitis deformans of unspecified ankle and foot
- M88.88 Osteitis deformans of other bones
  - **Excludes2** osteitis deformans of skull (M88.0)
    osteitis deformans of vertebrae (M88.1)
- M88.89 Osteitis deformans of multiple sites
- M88.9 Osteitis deformans of unspecified bone

- M89 Other disorders of bone
  - M89.0 Algoneurodystrophy
    Shoulder-hand syndrome
    Sudeck's atrophy
    - **Excludes1** causalgia, lower limb (G57.7-)
      causalgia, upper limb (G56.4-)
      complex regional pain syndrome II, lower limb (G57.7-)
      complex regional pain syndrome II, upper limb (G56.4-)
      reflex sympathetic dystrophy (G90.5-)
    - M89.00 Algoneurodystrophy, unspecified site
    - M89.01 Algoneurodystrophy, shoulder
      - M89.011 Algoneurodystrophy, right shoulder
      - M89.012 Algoneurodystrophy, left shoulder
      - M89.019 Algoneurodystrophy, unspecified shoulder
    - M89.02 Algoneurodystrophy, upper arm
      - M89.021 Algoneurodystrophy, right upper arm
      - M89.022 Algoneurodystrophy, left upper arm
      - M89.029 Algoneurodystrophy, unspecified upper arm
    - M89.03 Algoneurodystrophy, forearm
      - M89.031 Algoneurodystrophy, right forearm
      - M89.032 Algoneurodystrophy, left forearm
      - M89.039 Algoneurodystrophy, unspecified forearm
    - M89.04 Algoneurodystrophy, hand
      - M89.041 Algoneurodystrophy, right hand
      - M89.042 Algoneurodystrophy, left hand
      - M89.049 Algoneurodystrophy, unspecified hand
    - M89.05 Algoneurodystrophy, thigh
      - M89.051 Algoneurodystrophy, right thigh
      - M89.052 Algoneurodystrophy, left thigh
      - M89.059 Algoneurodystrophy, unspecified thigh
    - M89.06 Algoneurodystrophy, lower leg
      - M89.061 Algoneurodystrophy, right lower leg
      - M89.062 Algoneurodystrophy, left lower leg
      - M89.069 Algoneurodystrophy, unspecified lower leg
    - M89.07 Algoneurodystrophy, ankle and foot
      - M89.071 Algoneurodystrophy, right ankle and foot
      - M89.072 Algoneurodystrophy, left ankle and foot
      - M89.079 Algoneurodystrophy, unspecified ankle and foot
    - M89.08 Algoneurodystrophy, other site
    - M89.09 Algoneurodystrophy, multiple sites
  - M89.1 Physeal arrest
    Arrest of growth plate
    Epiphyseal arrest
    Growth plate arrest
    - M89.12 Physeal arrest, humerus
      - M89.121 Complete physeal arrest, right proximal humerus
      - M89.122 Complete physeal arrest, left proximal humerus
      - M89.123 Partial physeal arrest, right proximal humerus
      - M89.124 Partial physeal arrest, left proximal humerus
      - M89.125 Complete physeal arrest, right distal humerus
      - M89.126 Complete physeal arrest, left distal humerus
      - M89.127 Partial physeal arrest, right distal humerus
      - M89.128 Partial physeal arrest, left distal humerus
      - M89.129 Physeal arrest, humerus, unspecified
    - M89.13 Physeal arrest, forearm
      - M89.131 Complete physeal arrest, right distal radius
      - M89.132 Complete physeal arrest, left distal radius
      - M89.133 Partial physeal arrest, right distal radius
      - M89.134 Partial physeal arrest, left distal radius
      - M89.138 Other physeal arrest of forearm
      - M89.139 Physeal arrest, forearm, unspecified
    - M89.15 Physeal arrest, femur
      - M89.151 Complete physeal arrest, right proximal femur
      - M89.152 Complete physeal arrest, left proximal femur
      - M89.153 Partial physeal arrest, right proximal femur
      - M89.154 Partial physeal arrest, left proximal femur
      - M89.155 Complete physeal arrest, right distal femur
      - M89.156 Complete physeal arrest, left distal femur
      - M89.157 Partial physeal arrest, right distal femur
      - M89.158 Partial physeal arrest, left distal femur
      - M89.159 Physeal arrest, femur, unspecified

- M89.16 Physeal arrest, lower leg
  - M89.160 Complete physeal arrest, right proximal tibia
  - M89.161 Complete physeal arrest, left proximal tibia
  - M89.162 Partial physeal arrest, right proximal tibia
  - M89.163 Partial physeal arrest, left proximal tibia
  - M89.164 Complete physeal arrest, right distal tibia
  - M89.165 Complete physeal arrest, left distal tibia
  - M89.166 Partial physeal arrest, right distal tibia
  - M89.167 Partial physeal arrest, left distal tibia
  - M89.168 Other physeal arrest of lower leg
  - M89.169 Physeal arrest, lower leg, unspecified
- M89.18 Physeal arrest, other site
- M89.2 Other disorders of bone development and growth
  - M89.20 Other disorders of bone development and growth, unspecified site
  - M89.21 Other disorders of bone development and growth, shoulder
    - M89.211 Other disorders of bone development and growth, right shoulder
    - M89.212 Other disorders of bone development and growth, left shoulder
    - M89.219 Other disorders of bone development and growth, unspecified shoulder
  - M89.22 Other disorders of bone development and growth, humerus
    - M89.221 Other disorders of bone development and growth, right humerus
    - M89.222 Other disorders of bone development and growth, left humerus
    - M89.229 Other disorders of bone development and growth, unspecified humerus
  - M89.23 Other disorders of bone development and growth, ulna and radius
    - M89.231 Other disorders of bone development and growth, right ulna
    - M89.232 Other disorders of bone development and growth, left ulna
    - M89.233 Other disorders of bone development and growth, right radius
    - M89.234 Other disorders of bone development and growth, left radius
    - M89.239 Other disorders of bone development and growth, unspecified ulna and radius
  - M89.24 Other disorders of bone development and growth, hand
    - M89.241 Other disorders of bone development and growth, right hand
    - M89.242 Other disorders of bone development and growth, left hand
    - M89.249 Other disorders of bone development and growth, unspecified hand
  - M89.25 Other disorders of bone development and growth, femur
    - M89.251 Other disorders of bone development and growth, right femur
    - M89.252 Other disorders of bone development and growth, left femur
    - M89.259 Other disorders of bone development and growth, unspecified femur
  - M89.26 Other disorders of bone development and growth, tibia and fibula
    - M89.261 Other disorders of bone development and growth, right tibia
    - M89.262 Other disorders of bone development and growth, left tibia
    - M89.263 Other disorders of bone development and growth, right fibula
    - M89.264 Other disorders of bone development and growth, left fibula
    - M89.269 Other disorders of bone development and growth, unspecified lower leg
  - M89.27 Other disorders of bone development and growth, ankle and foot
    - M89.271 Other disorders of bone development and growth, right ankle and foot
    - M89.272 Other disorders of bone development and growth, left ankle and foot
    - M89.279 Other disorders of bone development and growth, unspecified ankle and foot
  - M89.28 Other disorders of bone development and growth, other site
  - M89.29 Other disorders of bone development and growth, multiple sites
- M89.3 Hypertrophy of bone
  - M89.30 Hypertrophy of bone, unspecified site
  - M89.31 Hypertrophy of bone, shoulder
    - M89.311 Hypertrophy of bone, right shoulder
    - M89.312 Hypertrophy of bone, left shoulder
    - M89.319 Hypertrophy of bone, unspecified shoulder
  - M89.32 Hypertrophy of bone, humerus
    - M89.321 Hypertrophy of bone, right humerus
    - M89.322 Hypertrophy of bone, left humerus
    - M89.329 Hypertrophy of bone, unspecified humerus
  - M89.33 Hypertrophy of bone, ulna and radius
    - M89.331 Hypertrophy of bone, right ulna
    - M89.332 Hypertrophy of bone, left ulna
    - M89.333 Hypertrophy of bone, right radius
    - M89.334 Hypertrophy of bone, left radius
    - M89.339 Hypertrophy of bone, unspecified ulna and radius
  - M89.34 Hypertrophy of bone, hand
    - M89.341 Hypertrophy of bone, right hand
    - M89.342 Hypertrophy of bone, left hand
    - M89.349 Hypertrophy of bone, unspecified hand
  - M89.35 Hypertrophy of bone, femur
    - M89.351 Hypertrophy of bone, right femur
    - M89.352 Hypertrophy of bone, left femur
    - M89.359 Hypertrophy of bone, unspecified femur
  - M89.36 Hypertrophy of bone, tibia and fibula
    - M89.361 Hypertrophy of bone, right tibia
    - M89.362 Hypertrophy of bone, left tibia
    - M89.363 Hypertrophy of bone, right fibula
    - M89.364 Hypertrophy of bone, left fibula
    - M89.369 Hypertrophy of bone, unspecified tibia and fibula

- M89.37 Hypertrophy of bone, ankle and foot
  - M89.371 Hypertrophy of bone, right ankle and foot
  - M89.372 Hypertrophy of bone, left ankle and foot
  - M89.379 Hypertrophy of bone, unspecified ankle and foot
- M89.38 Hypertrophy of bone, other site
- M89.39 Hypertrophy of bone, multiple sites

- M89.4 Other hypertrophic osteoarthropathy
  Marie-Bamberger disease
  Pachydermoperiostosis
  - M89.40 Other hypertrophic osteoarthropathy, unspecified site
  - M89.41 Other hypertrophic osteoarthropathy, shoulder
    - M89.411 Other hypertrophic osteoarthropathy, right shoulder
    - M89.412 Other hypertrophic osteoarthropathy, left shoulder
    - M89.419 Other hypertrophic osteoarthropathy, unspecified shoulder
  - M89.42 Other hypertrophic osteoarthropathy, upper arm
    - M89.421 Other hypertrophic osteoarthropathy, right upper arm
    - M89.422 Other hypertrophic osteoarthropathy, left upper arm
    - M89.429 Other hypertrophic osteoarthropathy, unspecified upper arm
  - M89.43 Other hypertrophic osteoarthropathy, forearm
    - M89.431 Other hypertrophic osteoarthropathy, right forearm
    - M89.432 Other hypertrophic osteoarthropathy, left forearm
    - M89.439 Other hypertrophic osteoarthropathy, unspecified forearm
  - M89.44 Other hypertrophic osteoarthropathy, hand
    - M89.441 Other hypertrophic osteoarthropathy, right hand
    - M89.442 Other hypertrophic osteoarthropathy, left hand
    - M89.449 Other hypertrophic osteoarthropathy, unspecified hand
  - M89.45 Other hypertrophic osteoarthropathy, thigh
    - M89.451 Other hypertrophic osteoarthropathy, right thigh
    - M89.452 Other hypertrophic osteoarthropathy, left thigh
    - M89.459 Other hypertrophic osteoarthropathy, unspecified thigh
  - M89.46 Other hypertrophic osteoarthropathy, lower leg
    - M89.461 Other hypertrophic osteoarthropathy, right lower leg
    - M89.462 Other hypertrophic osteoarthropathy, left lower leg
    - M89.469 Other hypertrophic osteoarthropathy, unspecified lower leg
  - M89.47 Other hypertrophic osteoarthropathy, ankle and foot
    - M89.471 Other hypertrophic osteoarthropathy, right ankle and foot
    - M89.472 Other hypertrophic osteoarthropathy, left ankle and foot
    - M89.479 Other hypertrophic osteoarthropathy, unspecified ankle and foot
  - M89.48 Other hypertrophic osteoarthropathy, other site
  - M89.49 Other hypertrophic osteoarthropathy, multiple sites

- M89.5 Osteolysis
  Use additional code to identify major osseous defect, if applicable (M89.7-)
  Excludes2 periprosthetic osteolysis of internal prosthetic joint (T84.05-)
  - M89.50 Osteolysis, unspecified site
  - M89.51 Osteolysis, shoulder
    - M89.511 Osteolysis, right shoulder
    - M89.512 Osteolysis, left shoulder
    - M89.519 Osteolysis, unspecified shoulder
  - M89.52 Osteolysis, upper arm
    - M89.521 Osteolysis, right upper arm
    - M89.522 Osteolysis, left upper arm
    - M89.529 Osteolysis, unspecified upper arm
  - M89.53 Osteolysis, forearm
    - M89.531 Osteolysis, right forearm
    - M89.532 Osteolysis, left forearm
    - M89.539 Osteolysis, unspecified forearm
  - M89.54 Osteolysis, hand
    - M89.541 Osteolysis, right hand
    - M89.542 Osteolysis, left hand
    - M89.549 Osteolysis, unspecified hand
  - M89.55 Osteolysis, thigh
    - M89.551 Osteolysis, right thigh
    - M89.552 Osteolysis, left thigh
    - M89.559 Osteolysis, unspecified thigh
  - M89.56 Osteolysis, lower leg
    - M89.561 Osteolysis, right lower leg
    - M89.562 Osteolysis, left lower leg
    - M89.569 Osteolysis, unspecified lower leg
  - M89.57 Osteolysis, ankle and foot
    - M89.571 Osteolysis, right ankle and foot
    - M89.572 Osteolysis, left ankle and foot
    - M89.579 Osteolysis, unspecified ankle and foot
  - M89.58 Osteolysis, other site
  - M89.59 Osteolysis, multiple sites

- M89.6 Osteopathy after poliomyelitis
  Use additional code (B91) to identify previous poliomyelitis
  Excludes1 postpolio syndrome (G14)
  - M89.60 Osteopathy after poliomyelitis, unspecified site
  - M89.61 Osteopathy after poliomyelitis, shoulder
    - M89.611 Osteopathy after poliomyelitis, right shoulder
    - M89.612 Osteopathy after poliomyelitis, left shoulder
    - M89.619 Osteopathy after poliomyelitis, unspecified shoulder
  - M89.62 Osteopathy after poliomyelitis, upper arm
    - M89.621 Osteopathy after poliomyelitis, right upper arm
    - M89.622 Osteopathy after poliomyelitis, left upper arm
    - M89.629 Osteopathy after poliomyelitis, unspecified upper arm
  - M89.63 Osteopathy after poliomyelitis, forearm
    - M89.631 Osteopathy after poliomyelitis, right forearm
    - M89.632 Osteopathy after poliomyelitis, left forearm
    - M89.639 Osteopathy after poliomyelitis, unspecified forearm

◀ New ◀ Revised ~~deleted~~ Deleted Excludes 1 Excludes 2 Includes Use additional Code first Code also Unspecified
OGCR Official Guidelines ● Unacceptable Principal Diagnosis X Assign placeholder X ● Use Additional Character(s) ▶ Manifestation Code Coding Clinic

- **M89.64 Osteopathy after poliomyelitis, hand**
  - **M89.641 Osteopathy after poliomyelitis, right hand**
  - **M89.642 Osteopathy after poliomyelitis, left hand**
  - **M89.649 Osteopathy after poliomyelitis, unspecified hand**
- **M89.65 Osteopathy after poliomyelitis, thigh**
  - **M89.651 Osteopathy after poliomyelitis, right thigh**
  - **M89.652 Osteopathy after poliomyelitis, left thigh**
  - **M89.659 Osteopathy after poliomyelitis, unspecified thigh**
- **M89.66 Osteopathy after poliomyelitis, lower leg**
  - **M89.661 Osteopathy after poliomyelitis, right lower leg**
  - **M89.662 Osteopathy after poliomyelitis, left lower leg**
  - **M89.669 Osteopathy after poliomyelitis, unspecified lower leg**
- **M89.67 Osteopathy after poliomyelitis, ankle and foot**
  - **M89.671 Osteopathy after poliomyelitis, right ankle and foot**
  - **M89.672 Osteopathy after poliomyelitis, left ankle and foot**
  - **M89.679 Osteopathy after poliomyelitis, unspecified ankle and foot**
- **M89.68 Osteopathy after poliomyelitis, other site**
- **M89.69 Osteopathy after poliomyelitis, multiple sites**

- **M89.7 Major osseous defect**

  Code first underlying disease, if known, such as:
  aseptic necrosis of bone (M87.-)
  malignant neoplasm of bone (C40.-)
  osteolysis (M89.5)
  osteomyelitis (M86.-)
  osteonecrosis (M87.-)
  osteoporosis (M80.-, M81.-)
  periprosthetic osteolysis (T84.05-)
  - **M89.70 Major osseous defect, unspecified site**
  - **M89.71 Major osseous defect, shoulder region**
    Major osseous defect clavicle or scapula
    - **M89.711 Major osseous defect, right shoulder region**
    - **M89.712 Major osseous defect, left shoulder region**
    - **M89.719 Major osseous defect, unspecified shoulder region**
  - **M89.72 Major osseous defect, humerus**
    - **M89.721 Major osseous defect, right humerus**
    - **M89.722 Major osseous defect, left humerus**
    - **M89.729 Major osseous defect, unspecified humerus**
  - **M89.73 Major osseous defect, forearm**
    Major osseous defect of radius and ulna
    - **M89.731 Major osseous defect, right forearm**
    - **M89.732 Major osseous defect, left forearm**
    - **M89.739 Major osseous defect, unspecified forearm**
  - **M89.74 Major osseous defect, hand**
    Major osseous defect of carpus, fingers, metacarpus
    - **M89.741 Major osseous defect, right hand**
    - **M89.742 Major osseous defect, left hand**
    - **M89.749 Major osseous defect, unspecified hand**
  - **M89.75 Major osseous defect, pelvic region and thigh**
    Major osseous defect of femur and pelvis
    - **M89.751 Major osseous defect, right pelvic region and thigh**
    - **M89.752 Major osseous defect, left pelvic region and thigh**
    - **M89.759 Major osseous defect, unspecified pelvic region and thigh**
  - **M89.76 Major osseous defect, lower leg**
    Major osseous defect of fibula and tibia
    - **M89.761 Major osseous defect, right lower leg**
    - **M89.762 Major osseous defect, left lower leg**
    - **M89.769 Major osseous defect, unspecified lower leg**
  - **M89.77 Major osseous defect, ankle and foot**
    Major osseous defect of metatarsus, tarsus, toes
    - **M89.771 Major osseous defect, right ankle and foot**
    - **M89.772 Major osseous defect, left ankle and foot**
    - **M89.779 Major osseous defect, unspecified ankle and foot**
  - **M89.78 Major osseous defect, other site**
  - **M89.79 Major osseous defect, multiple sites**
- **M89.8 Other specified disorders of bone**
  Infantile cortical hyperostoses
  Post-traumatic subperiosteal ossification
  - **M89.8X Other specified disorders of bone**
    - **M89.8X0 Other specified disorders of bone, multiple sites**
    - **M89.8X1 Other specified disorders of bone, shoulder**
    - **M89.8X2 Other specified disorders of bone, upper arm**
    - **M89.8X3 Other specified disorders of bone, forearm**
    - **M89.8X4 Other specified disorders of bone, hand**
    - **M89.8X5 Other specified disorders of bone, thigh**
    - **M89.8X6 Other specified disorders of bone, lower leg**
    - **M89.8X7 Other specified disorders of bone, ankle and foot**
    - **M89.8X8 Other specified disorders of bone, other site**
    - **M89.8X9 Other specified disorders of bone, unspecified site**
  - **M89.9 Disorder of bone, unspecified**

- **M90 Osteopathies in diseases classified elsewhere**

  Excludes1 osteochondritis, osteomyelitis, and osteopathy (in):
  cryptococcosis (B45.3)
  diabetes mellitus (E08-E13 with .69-)
  gonococcal (A54.43)
  neurogenic syphilis (A52.11)
  renal osteodystrophy (N25.0)
  salmonellosis (A02.24)
  secondary syphilis (A51.46)
  syphilis (late) (A52.77)
  - **M90.5 Osteonecrosis in diseases classified elsewhere**

    Code first underlying disease, such as:
    caisson disease (T70.3)
    hemoglobinopathy (D50-D64)
    Ex: **For category M90.5 CC codes unless otherwise indicated:**
    M87.00-M87.9, M90.50-M90.59
    - ***M90.50 Osteonecrosis in diseases classified elsewhere, unspecified site***
      CC when PDx is its own CC

M90.51 Osteonecrosis in diseases classified elsewhere, shoulder

Ex For category **M90.51** CC codes: M87.00-M87.9, M90.50-M90.59

M90.511 Osteonecrosis in diseases classified elsewhere, right shoulder
CC when PDx is its own CC

M90.512 Osteonecrosis in diseases classified elsewhere, left shoulder
CC when PDx is its own CC

M90.519 Osteonecrosis in diseases classified elsewhere, unspecified shoulder
CC when PDx is its own CC

M90.52 Osteonecrosis in diseases classified elsewhere, upper arm

M90.521 Osteonecrosis in diseases classified elsewhere, right upper arm
CC when PDx is its own CC

M90.522 Osteonecrosis in diseases classified elsewhere, left upper arm
CC when PDx is its own CC

M90.529 Osteonecrosis in diseases classified elsewhere, unspecified upper arm
CC when PDx is its own CC

M90.53 Osteonecrosis in diseases classified elsewhere, forearm

M90.531 Osteonecrosis in diseases classified elsewhere, right forearm
CC when PDx is its own CC

M90.532 Osteonecrosis in diseases classified elsewhere, left forearm
CC when PDx is its own CC

M90.539 Osteonecrosis in diseases classified elsewhere, unspecified forearm
CC when PDx is its own CC

M90.54 Osteonecrosis in diseases classified elsewhere, hand

M90.541 Osteonecrosis in diseases classified elsewhere, right hand
CC when PDx is its own CC

M90.542 Osteonecrosis in diseases classified elsewhere, left hand
CC when PDx is its own CC

M90.549 Osteonecrosis in diseases classified elsewhere, unspecified hand
CC when PDx is its own CC

M90.55 Osteonecrosis in diseases classified elsewhere, thigh

Ex For category **M90.55** CC codes: M87.00-M87.9, M90.50-M90.59, M87.9

M90.551 Osteonecrosis in diseases classified elsewhere, right thigh
CC when PDx is its own CC

M90.552 Osteonecrosis in diseases classified elsewhere, left thigh
CC when PDx is its own CC

M90.559 Osteonecrosis in diseases classified elsewhere, unspecified thigh
CC when PDx is its own CC

M90.56 Osteonecrosis in diseases classified elsewhere, lower leg

M90.561 Osteonecrosis in diseases classified elsewhere, right lower leg
CC when PDx is its own CC

M90.562 Osteonecrosis in diseases classified elsewhere, left lower leg
CC when PDx is its own CC

M90.569 Osteonecrosis in diseases classified elsewhere, unspecified lower leg
CC when PDx is its own CC

M90.57 Osteonecrosis in diseases classified elsewhere, ankle and foot

M90.571 Osteonecrosis in diseases classified elsewhere, right ankle and foot
CC when PDx is its own CC

M90.572 Osteonecrosis in diseases classified elsewhere, left ankle and foot
CC when PDx is its own CC

M90.579 Osteonecrosis in diseases classified elsewhere, unspecified ankle and foot
CC when PDx is its own CC

M90.58 Osteonecrosis in diseases classified elsewhere, other site
CC when PDx is its own CC

M90.59 Osteonecrosis in diseases classified elsewhere, multiple sites
CC when PDx is its own CC

M90.6 Osteitis deformans in neoplastic diseases

Osteitis deformans in malignant neoplasm of bone

Code first the neoplasm (C40.-, C41.-)

Excludes1 osteitis deformans [Paget's disease of bone] (M88.-)

M90.60 Osteitis deformans in neoplastic diseases, unspecified site

M90.61 Osteitis deformans in neoplastic diseases, shoulder

M90.611 Osteitis deformans in neoplastic diseases, right shoulder

M90.612 Osteitis deformans in neoplastic diseases, left shoulder

M90.619 Osteitis deformans in neoplastic diseases, unspecified shoulder

M90.62 Osteitis deformans in neoplastic diseases, upper arm

M90.621 Osteitis deformans in neoplastic diseases, right upper arm

M90.622 Osteitis deformans in neoplastic diseases, left upper arm

M90.629 Osteitis deformans in neoplastic diseases, unspecified upper arm

M90.63 Osteitis deformans in neoplastic diseases, forearm

M90.631 Osteitis deformans in neoplastic diseases, right forearm

M90.632 Osteitis deformans in neoplastic diseases, left forearm

M90.639 Osteitis deformans in neoplastic diseases, unspecified forearm

M90.64 Osteitis deformans in neoplastic diseases, hand

M90.641 Osteitis deformans in neoplastic diseases, right hand

M90.642 Osteitis deformans in neoplastic diseases, left hand

M90.649 Osteitis deformans in neoplastic diseases, unspecified hand

M90.65 Osteitis deformans in neoplastic diseases, thigh

M90.651 Osteitis deformans in neoplastic diseases, right thigh

M90.652 Osteitis deformans in neoplastic diseases, left thigh

M90.659 Osteitis deformans in neoplastic diseases, unspecified thigh

M90.66 Osteitis deformans in neoplastic diseases, lower leg

M90.661 Osteitis deformans in neoplastic diseases, right lower leg

M90.662 Osteitis deformans in neoplastic diseases, left lower leg

M90.669 Osteitis deformans in neoplastic diseases, unspecified lower leg

- **M90.67 Osteitis deformans in neoplastic diseases, ankle and foot**
  - *M90.671 Osteitis deformans in neoplastic diseases, right ankle and foot*
  - *M90.672 Osteitis deformans in neoplastic diseases, left ankle and foot*
  - *M90.679 Osteitis deformans in neoplastic diseases, unspecified ankle and foot*
- *M90.68 Osteitis deformans in neoplastic diseases, other site*
- *M90.69 Osteitis deformans in neoplastic diseases, multiple sites*

- **M90.8 Osteopathy in diseases classified elsewhere**
  Code first underlying disease, such as:
  rickets (E55.0)
  vitamin-D-resistant rickets (E83.3)
  - *M90.80 Osteopathy in diseases classified elsewhere, unspecified site*
  - **M90.81 Osteopathy in diseases classified elsewhere, shoulder**
    - *M90.811 Osteopathy in diseases classified elsewhere, right shoulder*
    - *M90.812 Osteopathy in diseases classified elsewhere, left shoulder*
    - *M90.819 Osteopathy in diseases classified elsewhere, unspecified shoulder*
  - **M90.82 Osteopathy in diseases classified elsewhere, upper arm**
    - *M90.821 Osteopathy in diseases classified elsewhere, right upper arm*
    - *M90.822 Osteopathy in diseases classified elsewhere, left upper arm*
    - *M90.829 Osteopathy in diseases classified elsewhere, unspecified upper arm*
  - **M90.83 Osteopathy in diseases classified elsewhere, forearm**
    - *M90.831 Osteopathy in diseases classified elsewhere, right forearm*
    - *M90.832 Osteopathy in diseases classified elsewhere, left forearm*
    - *M90.839 Osteopathy in diseases classified elsewhere, unspecified forearm*
  - **M90.84 Osteopathy in diseases classified elsewhere, hand**
    - *M90.841 Osteopathy in diseases classified elsewhere, right hand*
    - *M90.842 Osteopathy in diseases classified elsewhere, left hand*
    - *M90.849 Osteopathy in diseases classified elsewhere, unspecified hand*
  - **M90.85 Osteopathy in diseases classified elsewhere, thigh**
    - *M90.851 Osteopathy in diseases classified elsewhere, right thigh*
    - *M90.852 Osteopathy in diseases classified elsewhere, left thigh*
    - *M90.859 Osteopathy in diseases classified elsewhere, unspecified thigh*
  - **M90.86 Osteopathy in diseases classified elsewhere, lower leg**
    - *M90.861 Osteopathy in diseases classified elsewhere, right lower leg*
    - *M90.862 Osteopathy in diseases classified elsewhere, left lower leg*
    - *M90.869 Osteopathy in diseases classified elsewhere, unspecified lower leg*
  - **M90.87 Osteopathy in diseases classified elsewhere, ankle and foot**
    - *M90.871 Osteopathy in diseases classified elsewhere, right ankle and foot*
    - *M90.872 Osteopathy in diseases classified elsewhere, left ankle and foot*
    - *M90.879 Osteopathy in diseases classified elsewhere, unspecified ankle and foot*
  - *M90.88 Osteopathy in diseases classified elsewhere, other site*
  - *M90.89 Osteopathy in diseases classified elsewhere, multiple sites*

CHONDROPATHIES (M91-M94)

Excludes1 postprocedural chondropathies (M96.-)

- **M91 Juvenile osteochondrosis of hip and pelvis**
  Excludes1 slipped upper femoral epiphysis (nontraumatic) (M93.0)
  - **M91.0 Juvenile osteochondrosis of pelvis**
    Osteochondrosis (juvenile) of acetabulum
    Osteochondrosis (juvenile) of iliac crest [Buchanan]
    Osteochondrosis (juvenile) of ischiopubic synchondrosis [van Neck]
    Osteochondrosis (juvenile) of symphysis pubis [Pierson]
  - **M91.1 Juvenile osteochondrosis of head of femur [Legg-Calvé-Perthes]**
    - **M91.10 Juvenile osteochondrosis of head of femur [Legg-Calvé-Perthes], unspecified leg**
    - **M91.11 Juvenile osteochondrosis of head of femur [Legg-Calvé-Perthes], right leg**
    - **M91.12 Juvenile osteochondrosis of head of femur [Legg-Calvé-Perthes], left leg**
  - **M91.2 Coxa plana**
    Hip deformity due to previous juvenile osteochondrosis
    - **M91.20 Coxa plana, unspecified hip**
    - **M91.21 Coxa plana, right hip**
    - **M91.22 Coxa plana, left hip**
  - **M91.3 Pseudocoxalgia**
    - **M91.30 Pseudocoxalgia, unspecified hip**
    - **M91.31 Pseudocoxalgia, right hip**
    - **M91.32 Pseudocoxalgia, left hip**
  - **M91.4 Coxa magna**
    - **M91.40 Coxa magna, unspecified hip**
    - **M91.41 Coxa magna, right hip**
    - **M91.42 Coxa magna, left hip**
  - **M91.8 Other juvenile osteochondrosis of hip and pelvis**
    Juvenile osteochondrosis after reduction of congenital dislocation of hip
    - **M91.80 Other juvenile osteochondrosis of hip and pelvis, unspecified leg**
    - **M91.81 Other juvenile osteochondrosis of hip and pelvis, right leg**
    - **M91.82 Other juvenile osteochondrosis of hip and pelvis, left leg**
  - **M91.9 Juvenile osteochondrosis of hip and pelvis, unspecified**
    - **M91.90 Juvenile osteochondrosis of hip and pelvis, unspecified, unspecified leg**
    - **M91.91 Juvenile osteochondrosis of hip and pelvis, unspecified, right leg**
    - **M91.92 Juvenile osteochondrosis of hip and pelvis, unspecified, left leg**

M92 Other juvenile osteochondrosis

M92.0 Juvenile osteochondrosis of humerus
Osteochondrosis (juvenile) of capitulum of humerus [Panner]
Osteochondrosis (juvenile) of head of humerus [Haas]

M92.00 Juvenile osteochondrosis of humerus, unspecified arm

M92.01 Juvenile osteochondrosis of humerus, right arm

M92.02 Juvenile osteochondrosis of humerus, left arm

M92.1 Juvenile osteochondrosis of radius and ulna
Osteochondrosis (juvenile) of lower ulna [Burns]
Osteochondrosis (juvenile) of radial head [Brailsford]

M92.10 Juvenile osteochondrosis of radius and ulna, unspecified arm

M92.11 Juvenile osteochondrosis of radius and ulna, right arm

M92.12 Juvenile osteochondrosis of radius and ulna, left arm

M92.2 Juvenile osteochondrosis, hand

M92.20 Unspecified juvenile osteochondrosis, hand

M92.201 Unspecified juvenile osteochondrosis, right hand

M92.202 Unspecified juvenile osteochondrosis, left hand

M92.209 Unspecified juvenile osteochondrosis, unspecified hand

M92.21 Osteochondrosis (juvenile) of carpal lunate [Kienböck]

M92.211 Osteochondrosis (juvenile) of carpal lunate [Kienböck], right hand

M92.212 Osteochondrosis (juvenile) of carpal lunate [Kienböck], left hand

M92.219 Osteochondrosis (juvenile) of carpal lunate [Kienböck], unspecified hand

M92.22 Osteochondrosis (juvenile) of metacarpal heads [Mauclaire]

M92.221 Osteochondrosis (juvenile) of metacarpal heads [Mauclaire], right hand

M92.222 Osteochondrosis (juvenile) of metacarpal heads [Mauclaire], left hand

M92.229 Osteochondrosis (juvenile) of metacarpal heads [Mauclaire], unspecified hand

M92.29 Other juvenile osteochondrosis, hand

M92.291 Other juvenile osteochondrosis, right hand

M92.292 Other juvenile osteochondrosis, left hand

M92.299 Other juvenile osteochondrosis, unspecified hand

M92.3 Other juvenile osteochondrosis, upper limb

M92.30 Other juvenile osteochondrosis, unspecified upper limb

M92.31 Other juvenile osteochondrosis, right upper limb

M92.32 Other juvenile osteochondrosis, left upper limb

M92.4 Juvenile osteochondrosis of patella
Osteochondrosis (juvenile) of primary patellar center [Köhler]
Osteochondrosis (juvenile) of secondary patellar center [Sinding Larsen]

M92.40 Juvenile osteochondrosis of patella, unspecified knee

M92.41 Juvenile osteochondrosis of patella, right knee

M92.42 Juvenile osteochondrosis of patella, left knee

M92.5 Juvenile osteochondrosis of tibia and fibula
Osteochondrosis (juvenile) of proximal tibia [Blount]
Osteochondrosis (juvenile) of tibial tubercle [Osgood-Schlatter]
Tibia vara

M92.50 Juvenile osteochondrosis of tibia and fibula, unspecified leg

M92.51 Juvenile osteochondrosis of tibia and fibula, right leg

M92.52 Juvenile osteochondrosis of tibia and fibula, left leg

M92.6 Juvenile osteochondrosis of tarsus
Osteochondrosis (juvenile) of calcaneum [Sever]
Osteochondrosis (juvenile) of os tibiale externum [Haglund]
Osteochondrosis (juvenile) of talus [Diaz]
Osteochondrosis (juvenile) of tarsal navicular [Köhler]

M92.60 Juvenile osteochondrosis of tarsus, unspecified ankle

M92.61 Juvenile osteochondrosis of tarsus, right ankle

M92.62 Juvenile osteochondrosis of tarsus, left ankle

M92.7 Juvenile osteochondrosis of metatarsus
Osteochondrosis (juvenile) of fifth metatarsus [Iselin]
Osteochondrosis (juvenile) of second metatarsus [Freiberg]

M92.70 Juvenile osteochondrosis of metatarsus, unspecified foot

M92.71 Juvenile osteochondrosis of metatarsus, right foot

M92.72 Juvenile osteochondrosis of metatarsus, left foot

M92.8 Other specified juvenile osteochondrosis
Calcaneal apophysitis

M92.9 Juvenile osteochondrosis, unspecified
Juvenile apophysitis NOS
Juvenile epiphysitis NOS
Juvenile osteochondritis NOS
Juvenile osteochondrosis NOS

M93 Other osteochondropathies
Excludes2 osteochondrosis of spine (M42.-)

M93.0 Slipped upper femoral epiphysis (nontraumatic)
Use additional code for associated chondrolysis (M94.3)

M93.00 Unspecified slipped upper femoral epiphysis (nontraumatic)

M93.001 Unspecified slipped upper femoral epiphysis (nontraumatic), right hip

M93.002 Unspecified slipped upper femoral epiphysis (nontraumatic), left hip

M93.003 Unspecified slipped upper femoral epiphysis (nontraumatic), unspecified hip

M93.01 Acute slipped upper femoral epiphysis (nontraumatic)

M93.011 Acute slipped upper femoral epiphysis (nontraumatic), right hip

M93.012 Acute slipped upper femoral epiphysis (nontraumatic), left hip

M93.013 Acute slipped upper femoral epiphysis (nontraumatic), unspecified hip

M93.02 Chronic slipped upper femoral epiphysis (nontraumatic)

M93.021 Chronic slipped upper femoral epiphysis (nontraumatic), right hip

M93.022 Chronic slipped upper femoral epiphysis (nontraumatic), left hip

M93.023 Chronic slipped upper femoral epiphysis (nontraumatic), unspecified hip

- M93.03 Acute on chronic slipped upper femoral epiphysis (nontraumatic)
  - M93.031 Acute on chronic slipped upper femoral epiphysis (nontraumatic), right hip
  - M93.032 Acute on chronic slipped upper femoral epiphysis (nontraumatic), left hip
  - M93.033 Acute on chronic slipped upper femoral epiphysis (nontraumatic), unspecified hip
- M93.1 Kienböck's disease of adults A
  - Adult osteochondrosis of carpal lunates
- M93.2 Osteochondritis dissecans
  - M93.20 Osteochondritis dissecans of unspecified site
  - M93.21 Osteochondritis dissecans of shoulder
    - M93.211 Osteochondritis dissecans, right shoulder
    - M93.212 Osteochondritis dissecans, left shoulder
    - M93.219 Osteochondritis dissecans, unspecified shoulder
  - M93.22 Osteochondritis dissecans of elbow
    - M93.221 Osteochondritis dissecans, right elbow
    - M93.222 Osteochondritis dissecans, left elbow
    - M93.229 Osteochondritis dissecans, unspecified elbow
  - M93.23 Osteochondritis dissecans of wrist
    - M93.231 Osteochondritis dissecans, right wrist
    - M93.232 Osteochondritis dissecans, left wrist
    - M93.239 Osteochondritis dissecans, unspecified wrist
  - M93.24 Osteochondritis dissecans of joints of hand
    - M93.241 Osteochondritis dissecans, joints of right hand
    - M93.242 Osteochondritis dissecans, joints of left hand
    - M93.249 Osteochondritis dissecans, joints of unspecified hand
  - M93.25 Osteochondritis dissecans of hip
    - M93.251 Osteochondritis dissecans, right hip
    - M93.252 Osteochondritis dissecans, left hip
    - M93.259 Osteochondritis dissecans, unspecified hip
  - M93.26 Osteochondritis dissecans knee
    - M93.261 Osteochondritis dissecans, right knee
    - M93.262 Osteochondritis dissecans, left knee
    - M93.269 Osteochondritis dissecans, unspecified knee
  - M93.27 Osteochondritis dissecans of ankle and joints of foot
    - M93.271 Osteochondritis dissecans, right ankle and joints of right foot
    - M93.272 Osteochondritis dissecans, left ankle and joints of left foot
    - M93.279 Osteochondritis dissecans, unspecified ankle and joints of foot
  - M93.28 Osteochondritis dissecans other site
  - M93.29 Osteochondritis dissecans multiple sites
- M93.8 Other specified osteochondropathies
  - M93.80 Other specified osteochondropathies of unspecified site
  - M93.81 Other specified osteochondropathies of shoulder
    - M93.811 Other specified osteochondropathies, right shoulder
    - M93.812 Other specified osteochondropathies, left shoulder
    - M93.819 Other specified osteochondropathies, unspecified shoulder
  - M93.82 Other specified osteochondropathies of upper arm
    - M93.821 Other specified osteochondropathies, right upper arm
    - M93.822 Other specified osteochondropathies, left upper arm
    - M93.829 Other specified osteochondropathies, unspecified upper arm
  - M93.83 Other specified osteochondropathies of forearm
    - M93.831 Other specified osteochondropathies, right forearm
    - M93.832 Other specified osteochondropathies, left forearm
    - M93.839 Other specified osteochondropathies, unspecified forearm
  - M93.84 Other specified osteochondropathies of hand
    - M93.841 Other specified osteochondropathies, right hand
    - M93.842 Other specified osteochondropathies, left hand
    - M93.849 Other specified osteochondropathies, unspecified hand
  - M93.85 Other specified osteochondropathies of thigh
    - M93.851 Other specified osteochondropathies, right thigh
    - M93.852 Other specified osteochondropathies, left thigh
    - M93.859 Other specified osteochondropathies, unspecified thigh
  - M93.86 Other specified osteochondropathies lower leg
    - M93.861 Other specified osteochondropathies, right lower leg
    - M93.862 Other specified osteochondropathies, left lower leg
    - M93.869 Other specified osteochondropathies, unspecified lower leg
  - M93.87 Other specified osteochondropathies of ankle and foot
    - M93.871 Other specified osteochondropathies, right ankle and foot
    - M93.872 Other specified osteochondropathies, left ankle and foot
    - M93.879 Other specified osteochondropathies, unspecified ankle and foot
  - M93.88 Other specified osteochondropathies other
  - M93.89 Other specified osteochondropathies multiple sites

M93.9 Osteochondropathy, unspecified
Apophysitis NOS
Epiphysitis NOS
Osteochondritis NOS
Osteochondrosis NOS
M93.90 Osteochondropathy, unspecified of unspecified site
● M93.91 Osteochondropathy, unspecified of shoulder
M93.911 Osteochondropathy, unspecified, right shoulder
M93.912 Osteochondropathy, unspecified, left shoulder
M93.919 Osteochondropathy, unspecified, unspecified shoulder
● M93.92 Osteochondropathy, unspecified of upper arm
M93.921 Osteochondropathy, unspecified, right upper arm
M93.922 Osteochondropathy, unspecified, left upper arm
M93.929 Osteochondropathy, unspecified, unspecified upper arm
● M93.93 Osteochondropathy, unspecified of forearm
M93.931 Osteochondropathy, unspecified, right forearm
M93.932 Osteochondropathy, unspecified, left forearm
M93.939 Osteochondropathy, unspecified, unspecified forearm
● M93.94 Osteochondropathy, unspecified of hand
M93.941 Osteochondropathy, unspecified, right hand
M93.942 Osteochondropathy, unspecified, left hand
M93.949 Osteochondropathy, unspecified, unspecified hand
● M93.95 Osteochondropathy, unspecified of thigh
M93.951 Osteochondropathy, unspecified, right thigh
M93.952 Osteochondropathy, unspecified, left thigh
M93.959 Osteochondropathy, unspecified, unspecified thigh
● M93.96 Osteochondropathy, unspecified lower leg
M93.961 Osteochondropathy, unspecified, right lower leg
M93.962 Osteochondropathy, unspecified, left lower leg
M93.969 Osteochondropathy, unspecified, unspecified lower leg
● M93.97 Osteochondropathy, unspecified of ankle and foot
M93.971 Osteochondropathy, unspecified, right ankle and foot
M93.972 Osteochondropathy, unspecified, left ankle and foot
M93.979 Osteochondropathy, unspecified, unspecified ankle and foot
M93.98 Osteochondropathy, unspecified other
M93.99 Osteochondropathy, unspecified multiple sites

● M94 Other disorders of cartilage
M94.0 Chondrocostal junction syndrome [Tietze]
Costochondritis
M94.1 Relapsing polychondritis
● M94.2 Chondromalacia
Excludes1 chondromalacia patellae (M22.4)
M94.20 Chondromalacia, unspecified site
● M94.21 Chondromalacia, shoulder
M94.211 Chondromalacia, right shoulder
M94.212 Chondromalacia, left shoulder
M94.219 Chondromalacia, unspecified shoulder
● M94.22 Chondromalacia, elbow
M94.221 Chondromalacia, right elbow
M94.222 Chondromalacia, left elbow
M94.229 Chondromalacia, unspecified elbow
● M94.23 Chondromalacia, wrist
M94.231 Chondromalacia, right wrist
M94.232 Chondromalacia, left wrist
M94.239 Chondromalacia, unspecified wrist
● M94.24 Chondromalacia, joints of hand
M94.241 Chondromalacia, joints of right hand
M94.242 Chondromalacia, joints of left hand
M94.249 Chondromalacia, joints of unspecified hand
● M94.25 Chondromalacia, hip
M94.251 Chondromalacia, right hip
M94.252 Chondromalacia, left hip
M94.259 Chondromalacia, unspecified hip
● M94.26 Chondromalacia, knee
M94.261 Chondromalacia, right knee
M94.262 Chondromalacia, left knee
M94.269 Chondromalacia, unspecified knee
● M94.27 Chondromalacia, ankle and joints of foot
M94.271 Chondromalacia, right ankle and joints of right foot
M94.272 Chondromalacia, left ankle and joints of left foot
M94.279 Chondromalacia, unspecified ankle and joints of foot
M94.28 Chondromalacia, other site
M94.29 Chondromalacia, multiple sites
● M94.3 Chondrolysis
Code first any associated slipped upper femoral epiphysis (nontraumatic) (M93.0-)
● M94.35 Chondrolysis, hip
M94.351 Chondrolysis, right hip
M94.352 Chondrolysis, left hip
M94.359 Chondrolysis, unspecified hip
● M94.8 Other specified disorders of cartilage
● M94.8X Other specified disorders of cartilage
M94.8X0 Other specified disorders of cartilage, multiple sites
M94.8X1 Other specified disorders of cartilage, shoulder
M94.8X2 Other specified disorders of cartilage, upper arm
M94.8X3 Other specified disorders of cartilage, forearm
M94.8X4 Other specified disorders of cartilage, hand
M94.8X5 Other specified disorders of cartilage, thigh
M94.8X6 Other specified disorders of cartilage, lower leg
M94.8X7 Other specified disorders of cartilage, ankle and foot
M94.8X8 Other specified disorders of cartilage, other site
M94.8X9 Other specified disorders of cartilage, unspecified sites
M94.9 Disorder of cartilage, unspecified

◀ New ◀ Revised ~~deleted~~ Deleted Excludes 1 Excludes 2 Includes Use additional Code first Code also Unspecified
OGCR Official Guidelines ● Unacceptable Principal Diagnosis X Assign placeholder X ● Use Additional Character(s) ▶ Manifestation Code Coding Clinic

OTHER DISORDERS OF THE MUSCULOSKELETAL SYSTEM AND CONNECTIVE TISSUE (M95)

M95 Other acquired deformities of musculoskeletal system and connective tissue

Excludes2 acquired absence of limbs and organs (Z89-Z90)
acquired deformities of limbs (M20-M21)
congenital malformations and deformations of the musculoskeletal system (Q65-Q79)
deforming dorsopathies (M40-M43)
dentofacial anomalies [including malocclusion] (M26.-)
postprocedural musculoskeletal disorders (M96.-)

M95.0 Acquired deformity of nose

Excludes2 deviated nasal septum (J34.2)

M95.1 Cauliflower ear

Excludes2 other acquired deformities of ear (H61.1)

M95.10 Cauliflower ear, unspecified ear

M95.11 Cauliflower ear, right ear

M95.12 Cauliflower ear, left ear

M95.2 Other acquired deformity of head

M95.3 Acquired deformity of neck

M95.4 Acquired deformity of chest and rib

M95.5 Acquired deformity of pelvis

Excludes1 maternal care for known or suspected disproportion (O33.-)

M95.8 Other specified acquired deformities of musculoskeletal system

M95.9 Acquired deformity of musculoskeletal system, unspecified

INTRAOPERATIVE AND POSTPROCEDURAL COMPLICATIONS AND DISORDERS OF MUSCULOSKELETAL SYSTEM, NOT ELSEWHERE CLASSIFIED (M96)

M96 Intraoperative and postprocedural complications and disorders of musculoskeletal system, not elsewhere classified

Excludes2 arthropathy following intestinal bypass (M02.0-)
complications of internal orthopedic prosthetic devices, implants and grafts (T84.-)
disorders associated with osteoporosis (M80)
periprosthetic fracture around internal prosthetic joint (M97.-) ◀
presence of functional implants and other devices (Z96-Z97)

M96.0 Pseudarthrosis after fusion or arthrodesis

Ex: No exclusions

M96.1 Postlaminectomy syndrome, not elsewhere classified

M96.2 Postradiation kyphosis

M96.3 Postlaminectomy kyphosis

M96.4 Postsurgical lordosis

M96.5 Postradiation scoliosis

M96.6 Fracture of bone following insertion of orthopedic implant, joint prosthesis, or bone plate

Intraoperative fracture of bone during insertion of orthopedic implant, joint prosthesis, or bone plate

Excludes2 complication of internal orthopedic devices, implants or grafts (T84.-)

Ex: **For category M96.6 CC codes:** D78.81, D78.89, E36.8, E89.810-E89.89, H59.011-H59.019, H59.031-H59.819, H59.88-H59.89, H95.811-H95.89, I97.3, L76.81-L76.82, M96.621-M96.69, M96.89, M97.01X-M97.9XX[A], N98.1-N98.9, T81.82X[A], T81.89X-T81.9XX[A], T84.010-T84.039[A], T84.050-T84.9XX[A]

M96.62 Fracture of humerus following insertion of orthopedic implant, joint prosthesis, or bone plate

M96.621 Fracture of humerus following insertion of orthopedic implant, joint prosthesis, or bone plate, right arm

M96.622 Fracture of humerus following insertion of orthopedic implant, joint prosthesis, or bone plate, left arm

M96.629 Fracture of humerus following insertion of orthopedic implant, joint prosthesis, or bone plate, unspecified arm

M96.63 Fracture of radius or ulna following insertion of orthopedic implant, joint prosthesis, or bone plate

M96.631 Fracture of radius or ulna following insertion of orthopedic implant, joint prosthesis, or bone plate, right arm

M96.632 Fracture of radius or ulna following insertion of orthopedic implant, joint prosthesis, or bone plate, left arm

M96.639 Fracture of radius or ulna following insertion of orthopedic implant, joint prosthesis, or bone plate, unspecified arm

M96.65 Fracture of pelvis following insertion of orthopedic implant, joint prosthesis, or bone plate

M96.66 Fracture of femur following insertion of orthopedic implant, joint prosthesis, or bone plate

M96.661 Fracture of femur following insertion of orthopedic implant, joint prosthesis, or bone plate, right leg

M96.662 Fracture of femur following insertion of orthopedic implant, joint prosthesis, or bone plate, left leg

M96.669 Fracture of femur following insertion of orthopedic implant, joint prosthesis, or bone plate, unspecified leg

M96.67 Fracture of tibia or fibula following insertion of orthopedic implant, joint prosthesis, or bone plate

M96.671 Fracture of tibia or fibula following insertion of orthopedic implant, joint prosthesis, or bone plate, right leg

M96.672 Fracture of tibia or fibula following insertion of orthopedic implant, joint prosthesis, or bone plate, left leg

M96.679 Fracture of tibia or fibula following insertion of orthopedic implant, joint prosthesis, or bone plate, unspecified leg

M96.69 Fracture of other bone following insertion of orthopedic implant, joint prosthesis, or bone plate

● **M96.8 Other intraoperative and postprocedural complications and disorders of musculoskeletal system, not elsewhere classified**

● **M96.81 Intraoperative hemorrhage and hematoma of a musculoskeletal structure complicating a procedure**

Excludes1 intraoperative hemorrhage and hematoma of a musculoskeletal structure due to accidental puncture and laceration during a procedure (M96.82-)

Ex **For category M96.81 CC codes:** H95.811-H95.89, I85.01, I85.11, I97.3, K21.9, K22.8, K23-K25.2, K25.4, K25.6, K26.0, K26.2, K26.4, K26.6, K27.0, K27.2, K27.4, K27.6, K28.0, K28.2, K28.4, K28.6, K29.01, K29.21, K29.31, K29.41, K29.51, K29.61, K29.71, K29.81, K29.91, K31.811, K55.21, K57.01, K57.11, K57.13, K57.21, K57.31, K57.33, K57.41, K57.51, K57.53, K57.81, K57.91, K57.93, K62.5, K92.0-K92.2, M96.810-M96.811, M96.830-M96.89, N98.1-N98.9, P54.1-P54.3, T81.10X-T81.19X[A], T81.82X[A], T81.89X-T81.9XX[A]

M96.810 Intraoperative hemorrhage and hematoma of a musculoskeletal structure complicating a musculoskeletal system procedure

M96.811 Intraoperative hemorrhage and hematoma of a musculoskeletal structure complicating other procedure

● **M96.82 Accidental puncture and laceration of a musculoskeletal structure during a procedure**

Ex **For category M96.82 CC codes:** D78.11-D78.12, D78.81-D78.89, E36.11-E36.8, E89.810-E89.89, G96.11, G97.41-G97.49, H59.011-H59.019, H59.031-H59.099, H59.211-H59.229, H59.811-H59.89, H95.31-H95.32, H95.811-H95.89, I97.3, I97.51-I97.52, J95.71-J95.72, K91.71-K91.72, L76.11-L76.12, L76.81-L76.82, M96.820-M96.821, M96.89, N98.1-N98.9, N99.71-N99.72, T81.82X[A], T81.89X-T81.9XX[A]

M96.820 Accidental puncture and laceration of a musculoskeletal structure during a musculoskeletal system procedure

M96.821 Accidental puncture and laceration of a musculoskeletal structure during other procedure

● **M96.83 Postprocedural hemorrhage of a musculoskeletal structure following a procedure** ◀

Ex **For category M96.83 CC codes:** See M96.81

M96.830 Postprocedural hemorrhage of a musculoskeletal structure following a musculoskeletal system procedure ◀

M96.831 Postprocedural hemorrhage of a musculoskeletal structure following other procedure ◀

● **M96.84 Postprocedural hematoma and seroma of a musculoskeletal structure following a procedure** ◀

Ex **For category M96.84 CC codes:** See M96.81

M96.840 Postprocedural hematoma of a musculoskeletal structure following a musculoskeletal system procedure ◀

M96.841 Postprocedural hematoma of a musculoskeletal structure following other procedure ◀

M96.842 Postprocedural seroma of a musculoskeletal structure following a musculoskeletal system procedure ◀

M96.843 Postprocedural seroma of a musculoskeletal structure following other procedure ◀

M96.89 Other intraoperative and postprocedural complications and disorders of the musculoskeletal system

Instability of joint secondary to removal of joint prosthesis

Use additional code, if applicable, to further specify disorder

Ex D78.81-D78.89, E36.8, E89.810-E89.89, H59.011-H59.019, H59.031-H59.099, H59.811-H59.89, H95.811-H95.89, I97.3, L76.81-L76.82, M96.89, N98.1-N98.9, T81.82X[A], T81.89X-T81.9XX[A]

PERIPROSTHETIC FRACTURE AROUND INTERNAL PROSTHETIC JOINT (M97) ◀

● **M97 Periprosthetic fracture around internal prosthetic joint** ◀

Excludes2 fracture of bone following insertion of orthopedic implant, joint prosthesis or bone plate (M96.6-) ◀

breakage (fracture) of prosthetic joint (T84.01-) ◀

The appropriate 7th character is to be added to each code from category M97: ◀

A	initial encounter ◀
D	subsequent encounter ◀
S	sequela ◀

Ex **For category M97 CC codes:** See M96.6

● **M97.0 Periprosthetic fracture around internal prosthetic hip joint**

X ● **M97.01 Periprosthetic fracture around internal prosthetic right hip joint** A ◀

X ● **M97.02 Periprosthetic fracture around internal prosthetic left hip joint** A ◀

● **M97.1 Periprosthetic fracture around internal prosthetic knee joint** ◀

X ● **M97.11 Periprosthetic fracture around internal prosthetic right knee joint** A ◀

X ● **M97.12 Periprosthetic fracture around internal prosthetic left knee joint** A ◀

● **M97.2 Periprosthetic fracture around internal prosthetic ankle joint** ◀

X ● **M97.21 Periprosthetic fracture around internal prosthetic right ankle joint** A ◀

X ● **M97.22 Periprosthetic fracture around internal prosthetic left ankle joint** A ◀

● **M97.3 Periprosthetic fracture around internal prosthetic shoulder joint** ◀

X ● **M97.31 Periprosthetic fracture around internal prosthetic right shoulder joint** A ◀

X ● **M97.32 Periprosthetic fracture around internal prosthetic left shoulder joint** A ◀

● **M97.4 Periprosthetic fracture around internal prosthetic elbow joint** ◀

X ● **M97.41 Periprosthetic fracture around internal prosthetic right elbow joint** A ◀

X ● **M97.42 Periprosthetic fracture around internal prosthetic left elbow joint** A ◀

X ● **M97.8 Periprosthetic fracture around other internal prosthetic joint** A ◀
Periprosthetic fracture around internal prosthetic finger joint ◀
Periprosthetic fracture around internal prosthetic spinal joint ◀
Periprosthetic fracture around internal prosthetic toe joint ◀
Periprosthetic fracture around internal prosthetic wrist joint ◀
Use additional code to identify the joint (Z96.6-) ◀

X ● **M97.9 Periprosthetic fracture around unspecified internal prosthetic joint** A ◀

BIOMECHANICAL LESIONS, NOT ELSEWHERE CLASSIFIED (M99)

● **M99 Biomechanical lesions, not elsewhere classified**

Note: This category should not be used if the condition can be classified elsewhere.

● **M99.0 Segmental and somatic dysfunction**
- **M99.00 Segmental and somatic dysfunction of head region**
- **M99.01 Segmental and somatic dysfunction of cervical region**
- **M99.02 Segmental and somatic dysfunction of thoracic region**
- **M99.03 Segmental and somatic dysfunction of lumbar region**
- **M99.04 Segmental and somatic dysfunction of sacral region**
- **M99.05 Segmental and somatic dysfunction of pelvic region**
- **M99.06 Segmental and somatic dysfunction of lower extremity**
- **M99.07 Segmental and somatic dysfunction of upper extremity**
- **M99.08 Segmental and somatic dysfunction of rib cage**
- **M99.09 Segmental and somatic dysfunction of abdomen and other regions**

● **M99.1 Subluxation complex (vertebral)**
- **M99.10 Subluxation complex (vertebral) of head region**
  Ex: M99.10-M99.11, S03.8XX-S03.9XX[A], S12.000-S12.691[A,B], S12.9XX-S13.4XX[A], S13.8XX[A], S14.0XX-S14.108[A], S14.111-S14.118[A], S14.121-S14.128[A], S14.131-S14.138[A], S14.141-S14.148[A], S14.151-S14.158[A], S16.1XX[A], S29.011-S29.019[A], S38.3XX[A], S39.011-S39.013[A], T14.90-T14.91, T79.A0X-T79.9XX[A]
- **M99.11 Subluxation complex (vertebral) of cervical region**
  Ex: See M99.10
- **M99.12 Subluxation complex (vertebral) of thoracic region**
- **M99.13 Subluxation complex (vertebral) of lumbar region**
- **M99.14 Subluxation complex (vertebral) of sacral region**
- **M99.15 Subluxation complex (vertebral) of pelvic region**
- **M99.16 Subluxation complex (vertebral) of lower extremity**
- **M99.17 Subluxation complex (vertebral) of upper extremity**
- **M99.18 Subluxation complex (vertebral) of rib cage**
  Ex: M99.18, S43.201A-S43.226[A]
- **M99.19 Subluxation complex (vertebral) of abdomen and other regions**

● **M99.2 Subluxation stenosis of neural canal**
- **M99.20 Subluxation stenosis of neural canal of head region**
- **M99.21 Subluxation stenosis of neural canal of cervical region**
- **M99.22 Subluxation stenosis of neural canal of thoracic region**
- **M99.23 Subluxation stenosis of neural canal of lumbar region**
- **M99.24 Subluxation stenosis of neural canal of sacral region**
- **M99.25 Subluxation stenosis of neural canal of pelvic region**
- **M99.26 Subluxation stenosis of neural canal of lower extremity**
- **M99.27 Subluxation stenosis of neural canal of upper extremity**
- **M99.28 Subluxation stenosis of neural canal of rib cage**
- **M99.29 Subluxation stenosis of neural canal of abdomen and other regions**

● **M99.3 Osseous stenosis of neural canal**
- **M99.30 Osseous stenosis of neural canal of head region**
- **M99.31 Osseous stenosis of neural canal of cervical region**
- **M99.32 Osseous stenosis of neural canal of thoracic region**
- **M99.33 Osseous stenosis of neural canal of lumbar region**
- **M99.34 Osseous stenosis of neural canal of sacral region**
- **M99.35 Osseous stenosis of neural canal of pelvic region**
- **M99.36 Osseous stenosis of neural canal of lower extremity**
- **M99.37 Osseous stenosis of neural canal of upper extremity**
- **M99.38 Osseous stenosis of neural canal of rib cage**
- **M99.39 Osseous stenosis of neural canal of abdomen and other regions**

● **M99.4 Connective tissue stenosis of neural canal**
- **M99.40 Connective tissue stenosis of neural canal of head region**
- **M99.41 Connective tissue stenosis of neural canal of cervical region**
- **M99.42 Connective tissue stenosis of neural canal of thoracic region**
- **M99.43 Connective tissue stenosis of neural canal of lumbar region**
- **M99.44 Connective tissue stenosis of neural canal of sacral region**
- **M99.45 Connective tissue stenosis of neural canal of pelvic region**
- **M99.46 Connective tissue stenosis of neural canal of lower extremity**
- **M99.47 Connective tissue stenosis of neural canal of upper extremity**
- **M99.48 Connective tissue stenosis of neural canal of rib cage**
- **M99.49 Connective tissue stenosis of neural canal of abdomen and other regions**

- M99.5 Intervertebral disc stenosis of neural canal
  - M99.50 Intervertebral disc stenosis of neural canal of head region
  - M99.51 Intervertebral disc stenosis of neural canal of cervical region
  - M99.52 Intervertebral disc stenosis of neural canal of thoracic region
  - M99.53 Intervertebral disc stenosis of neural canal of lumbar region
  - M99.54 Intervertebral disc stenosis of neural canal of sacral region
  - M99.55 Intervertebral disc stenosis of neural canal of pelvic region
  - M99.56 Intervertebral disc stenosis of neural canal of lower extremity
  - M99.57 Intervertebral disc stenosis of neural canal of upper extremity
  - M99.58 Intervertebral disc stenosis of neural canal of rib cage
  - M99.59 Intervertebral disc stenosis of neural canal of abdomen and other regions
- M99.6 Osseous and subluxation stenosis of intervertebral foramina
  - M99.60 Osseous and subluxation stenosis of intervertebral foramina of head region
  - M99.61 Osseous and subluxation stenosis of intervertebral foramina of cervical region
  - M99.62 Osseous and subluxation stenosis of intervertebral foramina of thoracic region
  - M99.63 Osseous and subluxation stenosis of intervertebral foramina of lumbar region
  - M99.64 Osseous and subluxation stenosis of intervertebral foramina of sacral region
  - M99.65 Osseous and subluxation stenosis of intervertebral foramina of pelvic region
  - M99.66 Osseous and subluxation stenosis of intervertebral foramina of lower extremity
  - M99.67 Osseous and subluxation stenosis of intervertebral foramina of upper extremity
  - M99.68 Osseous and subluxation stenosis of intervertebral foramina of rib cage
  - M99.69 Osseous and subluxation stenosis of intervertebral foramina of abdomen and other regions
- M99.7 Connective tissue and disc stenosis of intervertebral foramina
  - M99.70 Connective tissue and disc stenosis of intervertebral foramina of head region
  - M99.71 Connective tissue and disc stenosis of intervertebral foramina of cervical region
  - M99.72 Connective tissue and disc stenosis of intervertebral foramina of thoracic region
  - M99.73 Connective tissue and disc stenosis of intervertebral foramina of lumbar region
  - M99.74 Connective tissue and disc stenosis of intervertebral foramina of sacral region
  - M99.75 Connective tissue and disc stenosis of intervertebral foramina of pelvic region
  - M99.76 Connective tissue and disc stenosis of intervertebral foramina of lower extremity
  - M99.77 Connective tissue and disc stenosis of intervertebral foramina of upper extremity
  - M99.78 Connective tissue and disc stenosis of intervertebral foramina of rib cage
  - M99.79 Connective tissue and disc stenosis of intervertebral foramina of abdomen and other regions
- M99.8 Other biomechanical lesions
  - M99.80 Other biomechanical lesions of head region
  - M99.81 Other biomechanical lesions of cervical region
  - M99.82 Other biomechanical lesions of thoracic region
  - M99.83 Other biomechanical lesions of lumbar region
  - M99.84 Other biomechanical lesions of sacral region
  - M99.85 Other biomechanical lesions of pelvic region
  - M99.86 Other biomechanical lesions of lower extremity
  - M99.87 Other biomechanical lesions of upper extremity
  - M99.88 Other biomechanical lesions of rib cage
  - M99.89 Other biomechanical lesions of abdomen and other regions
- M99.9 Biomechanical lesion, unspecified

CHAPTER 14

DISEASES OF THE GENITOURINARY SYSTEM (N00-N99)

OGCR Chapter-Specific Coding Guidelines

14. Chapter 14: Diseases of Genitourinary System (N00-N99)

a. Chronic kidney disease

1) Stages of chronic kidney disease (CKD)

The ICD-10-CM classifies CKD based on severity. The severity of CKD is designated by stages 1-5. Stage 2, code N18.2, equates to mild CKD; stage 3, code N18.3, equates to moderate CKD; and stage 4, code N18.4, equates to severe CKD. Code N18.6, End stage renal disease (ESRD), is assigned when the provider has documented end-stage-renal disease (ESRD).

If both a stage of CKD and ESRD are documented, assign code N18.6 only.

2) Chronic kidney disease and kidney transplant status

Patients who have undergone kidney transplant may still have some form of chronic kidney disease CKD because the kidney transplant may not fully restore kidney function. Therefore, the presence of CKD alone does not constitute a transplant complication. Assign the appropriate N18 code for the patient's stage of CKD and code Z94.0, Kidney transplant status. If a transplant complication such as failure or rejection or other transplant complication is documented, see section I.C.19.g for information on coding complications of a kidney transplant. If the documentation is unclear as to whether the patient has a complication of the transplant, query the provider.

3) Chronic kidney disease with other conditions

Patients with CKD may also suffer from other serious conditions, most commonly diabetes mellitus and hypertension. The sequencing of the CKD code in relationship to codes for other contributing conditions is based on the conventions in the Tabular List.

See I.C.9. Hypertensive chronic kidney disease.

See I.C.19. Chronic kidney disease and kidney transplant complications.

Item 14–1 Nephritis (inflammation) or **nephropathy** (disease) **with lesion of proliferative glomerulonephritis** results from a streptococcal infection.

Nephritis (inflammation) or **nephropathy** (disease) **with lesion of membranous glomerulonephritis** is characterized by deposits along the epithelial side of the basement membrane.

Nephritis (inflammation) or **nephropathy** (disease) **with lesion of membranoproliferative glomerulonephritis** is characterized by alterations in the basement membranes of the kidney and the glomerular cells.

Nephritis (inflammation) or **nephropathy** (disease) **with lesion of rapidly progressive glomerulonephritis** is characterized by rapid and progressive decline in renal function.

Nephritis (inflammation) or **nephropathy** (disease) **with lesion of renal cortical necrosis** is characterized by death of the cortical tissues.

Nephritis (inflammation) or **nephropathy** (disease) **with lesion of renal medullary necrosis** is characterized by death of the tissues that collect urine.

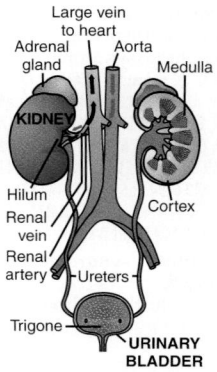

Figure 14-1 Kidneys within the urinary system.

Item 14–2 Glomerulonephritis is nephritis accompanied by inflammation of the glomeruli of the kidney, resulting in the degeneration of the glomeruli and the nephrons.

Acute glomerulonephritis primarily affects children and young adults and is usually a result of a streptococcal infection.

Proliferative glomerulonephritis is the acute form of the disease resulting from a streptococcal infection.

Rapidly progressive glomerulonephritis, also known as **crescentic** or **malignant glomerulonephritis**, is the acute form of the disease, which leads quickly to rapid and progressive decline in renal function.

CHAPTER 14

DISEASES OF THE GENITOURINARY SYSTEM (N00-N99)

Excludes2 certain conditions originating in the perinatal period (P04-P96)
certain infectious and parasitic diseases (A00-B99)
complications of pregnancy, childbirth and the puerperium (O00-O9A)
congenital malformations, deformations and chromosomal abnormalities (Q00-Q99)
endocrine, nutritional and metabolic diseases (E00-E88)
injury, poisoning and certain other consequences of external causes (S00-T88)
neoplasms (C00-D49)
symptoms, signs and abnormal clinical and laboratory findings, not elsewhere classified (R00-R94)

This chapter contains the following blocks:

N00-N08	Glomerular diseases
N10-N16	Renal tubulo-interstitial diseases
N17-N19	Acute kidney failure and chronic kidney disease
N20-N23	Urolithiasis
N25-N29	Other disorders of kidney and ureter
N30-N39	Other diseases of the urinary system
N40-N53	Diseases of male genital organs
N60-N65	Disorders of breast
N70-N77	Inflammatory diseases of female pelvic organs
N80-N98	Noninflammatory disorders of female genital tract
N99	Intraoperative and postprocedural complications and disorders of genitourinary system, not elsewhere classified

GLOMERULAR DISEASES (N00-N08)

Code also any associated kidney failure (N17-N19)

Excludes1 hypertensive chronic kidney disease (I12.-)

● **N00 Acute nephritic syndrome**

Includes acute glomerular disease
acute glomerulonephritis
acute nephritis

Excludes1 acute tubulo-interstitial nephritis (N10)
nephritic syndrome NOS (N05.-)

Ex **For category N00 CC codes unless otherwise indicated:** A17.9, A18.10-A18.11, A18.13, A18.82, A18.84, A18.89, A54.21, A54.29, A54.82, A54.84, A54.89-A54.9, A59.00, A59.8-A59.9, B37.41-B37.49, E08.21-E08.29, E08.618-E08.638, E08.649, E08.65-E08.8, E09.21-E09.29, E09.618-E09.638, E09.649-E09.8, E10.21-E10.29, E10.618-E10.638, E10.649, E10.69-E10.8, E11.21-E11.29, E11.618-E11.638, E11.649, E11.69-E11.8, E13.21-E13.29, E13.618-E13.638, E13.649-E13.69, E13.8, E88.3, M10.30-M10.39, N10, N11.10, N11.8, N11.9, N13.0-N13.39, N13.6, N14.0-N19, N25.0-N27.9, N28.1-N29, N36.41-N36.43, N36.8-N36.9, N39.8-N39.9, R31.0-R31.9

N00.0 Acute nephritic syndrome with minor glomerular abnormality CC
Acute nephritic syndrome with minimal change lesion

N00.1 Acute nephritic syndrome with focal and segmental glomerular lesions CC
Acute nephritic syndrome with focal and segmental hyalinosis
Acute nephritic syndrome with focal and segmental sclerosis
Acute nephritic syndrome with focal glomerulonephritis

N00.2 Acute nephritic syndrome with diffuse membranous glomerulonephritis

N00.3 Acute nephritic syndrome with diffuse mesangial proliferative glomerulonephritis

N00.4 Acute nephritic syndrome with diffuse endocapillary proliferative glomerulonephritis

N00.5 Acute nephritic syndrome with diffuse mesangiocapillary glomerulonephritis
Acute nephritic syndrome with membranoproliferative glomerulonephritis, types 1 and 3, or NOS

N00.6 Acute nephritic syndrome with dense deposit disease
Acute nephritic syndrome with membranoproliferative glomerulonephritis, type 2

N00.7 Acute nephritic syndrome with diffuse crescentic glomerulonephritis
Acute nephritic syndrome with extracapillary glomerulonephritis

N00.8 Acute nephritic syndrome with other morphologic changes
Acute nephritic syndrome with proliferative glomerulonephritis NOS
Ex: A17.9, A18.10-A18.11, A18.13, A18.82, A18.84, A18.89, A54.21, A54.29, A54.82, A54.84, A54.89-A54.9, A59.00, A59.8-A59.9, B37.41-B37.49, E08.21-E08.29, E09.21-E09.29, E88.3, M10.30-M10.39, N00.0-N13.39, N13.6, N14.0-N19, N25.0-N27.9, N28.1-N29, N36.41-N36.43, N36.8-N36.9, N39.8-N39.9, R31.0-R31.9

N00.9 Acute nephritic syndrome with unspecified morphologic changes

N01 Rapidly progressive nephritic syndrome

Includes rapidly progressive glomerular disease
rapidly progressive glomerulonephritis
rapidly progressive nephritis

Excludes1 nephritic syndrome NOS (N05.-)

Ex: For category N01 CC codes: See N00

N01.0 Rapidly progressive nephritic syndrome with minor glomerular abnormality
Rapidly progressive nephritic syndrome with minimal change lesion

N01.1 Rapidly progressive nephritic syndrome with focal and segmental glomerular lesions
Rapidly progressive nephritic syndrome with focal and segmental hyalinosis
Rapidly progressive nephritic syndrome with focal and segmental sclerosis
Rapidly progressive nephritic syndrome with focal glomerulonephritis

N01.2 Rapidly progressive nephritic syndrome with diffuse membranous glomerulonephritis

N01.3 Rapidly progressive nephritic syndrome with diffuse mesangial proliferative glomerulonephritis

N01.4 Rapidly progressive nephritic syndrome with diffuse endocapillary proliferative glomerulonephritis

N01.5 Rapidly progressive nephritic syndrome with diffuse mesangiocapillary glomerulonephritis
Rapidly progressive nephritic syndrome with membranoproliferative glomerulonephritis, types 1 and 3, or NOS

N01.6 Rapidly progressive nephritic syndrome with dense deposit disease
Rapidly progressive nephritic syndrome with membranoproliferative glomerulonephritis, type 2

N01.7 Rapidly progressive nephritic syndrome with diffuse crescentic glomerulonephritis
Rapidly progressive nephritic syndrome with extracapillary glomerulonephritis

N01.8 Rapidly progressive nephritic syndrome with other morphologic changes
Rapidly progressive nephritic syndrome with proliferative glomerulonephritis NOS

N01.9 Rapidly progressive nephritic syndrome with unspecified morphologic changes

N02 Recurrent and persistent hematuria

Excludes1 acute cystitis with hematuria (N30.01)
hematuria NOS (R31.9)
hematuria not associated with specified morphologic lesions (R31.-)

Ex: For category N02 CC codes unless otherwise indicated: A17.9, A18.10-A18.11, A18.13, A18.82, A18.84, A18.89, A54.21, A54.29, A54.82, A54.84, A54.89-A54.9, A59.00, A59.8-A59.9, B37.41-B37.49, E08.21-E08.29, E08.618-E08.638, E08.649, E08.65-E08.8, E09.21-E09.29, E09.618-E09.638, E09.649-E09.8, E10.21-E10.29, E10.618-E10.638, E10.649, E10.69-E10.8, E11.21-E11.29, E11.618-E11.638, E11.649, E11.69-E11.8, E13.21-E13.29, E13.618-E13.638, E13.649-E13.69, E13.8, M10.30-M10.39, N00.0-N13.39, N13.6, N14.0-N19, N25.0-N27.9, N28.1-N29, N36.41-N36.43, N36.8-N36.9, N39.8-N39.9, R31.0-R31.9

N02.0 Recurrent and persistent hematuria with minor glomerular abnormality
Recurrent and persistent hematuria with minimal change lesion

N02.1 Recurrent and persistent hematuria with focal and segmental glomerular lesions
Recurrent and persistent hematuria with focal and segmental hyalinosis
Recurrent and persistent hematuria with focal and segmental sclerosis
Recurrent and persistent hematuria with focal glomerulonephritis

N02.2 Recurrent and persistent hematuria with diffuse membranous glomerulonephritis

N02.3 Recurrent and persistent hematuria with diffuse mesangial proliferative glomerulonephritis

N02.4 Recurrent and persistent hematuria with diffuse endocapillary proliferative glomerulonephritis

N02.5 Recurrent and persistent hematuria with diffuse mesangiocapillary glomerulonephritis
Recurrent and persistent hematuria with membranoproliferative glomerulonephritis, types 1 and 3, or NOS

N02.6 Recurrent and persistent hematuria with dense deposit disease
Recurrent and persistent hematuria with membranoproliferative glomerulonephritis, type 2

N02.7 Recurrent and persistent hematuria with diffuse crescentic glomerulonephritis
Recurrent and persistent hematuria with extracapillary glomerulonephritis

N02.8 Recurrent and persistent hematuria with other morphologic changes
Recurrent and persistent hematuria with proliferative glomerulonephritis NOS
Ex: See N00

N02.9 Recurrent and persistent hematuria with unspecified morphologic changes
Ex: See N00

N03 Chronic nephritic syndrome

Includes chronic glomerular disease
chronic glomerulonephritis
chronic nephritis

Excludes1 chronic tubulo-interstitial nephritis (N11.-)
diffuse sclerosing glomerulonephritis (N05.8-)
nephritic syndrome NOS (N05.-)

Ex: For category N03 CC codes: A17.9, A18.10-A18.11, A18.13, A18.82, A18.84, A18.89, A54.21, A54.29, A54.82, A54.84, A54.89-A54.9, A59.00, A59.8-A59.9, A98.5, B37.41-B37.49, E08.21-E08.29, E08.618-E08.638, E08.649, E08.65-E08.8, E09.21-E09.29, E09.618-E09.638, E09.649-E09.8, E10.21-E10.29, E10.618-E10.638, E10.649, E10.69-E10.8, E11.21-E11.29, E11.618-E11.638, E11.649, E11.69-E11.8, E13.21-E13.29, E13.618-E13.638, E13.649-E13.69, E13.8, M10.30-M10.39, N00.0-N13.39, N13.6, N14.0-N19, N25.0-N27.9, N28.1-N29, N36.41-N36.43, N36.8-N36.9, N39.8-N39.9, R31.0-R31.9

N03.0 Chronic nephritic syndrome with minor glomerular abnormality
Chronic nephritic syndrome with minimal change lesion

Item 14–3 Chronic glomerulonephritis (GN) persists over a period of years, with remissions and exacerbation.

Chronic GN with lesion of proliferative glomerulonephritis results from a streptococcal infection.

Chronic GN with lesion of membranous glomerulonephritis, also known as membranous nephropathy, is characterized by deposits along the epithelial side of the basement membrane.

Chronic GN with lesion of membrano-proliferative glomerulonephritis (MPGN) is a group of disorders characterized by alterations in the basement membranes of the kidney and the glomerular cells.

Chronic GN with lesion of rapidly progressive glomerulonephritis is characterized by necrosis, endothelial proliferation, and mesangial proliferation. The condition is marked by rapid and progressive decline in renal function.

N03.1 Chronic nephritic syndrome with focal and segmental glomerular lesions CC
- Chronic nephritic syndrome with focal and segmental hyalinosis
- Chronic nephritic syndrome with focal and segmental sclerosis
- Chronic nephritic syndrome with focal glomerulonephritis

N03.2 Chronic nephritic syndrome with diffuse membranous glomerulonephritis CC

N03.3 Chronic nephritic syndrome with diffuse mesangial proliferative glomerulonephritis CC

N03.4 Chronic nephritic syndrome with diffuse endocapillary proliferative glomerulonephritis CC

N03.5 Chronic nephritic syndrome with diffuse mesangiocapillary glomerulonephritis CC
- Chronic nephritic syndrome with membranoproliferative glomerulonephritis, types 1 and 3, or NOS

N03.6 Chronic nephritic syndrome with dense deposit disease CC
- Chronic nephritic syndrome with membranoproliferative glomerulonephritis, type 2

N03.7 Chronic nephritic syndrome with diffuse crescentic glomerulonephritis CC
- Chronic nephritic syndrome with extracapillary glomerulonephritis

N03.8 Chronic nephritic syndrome with other morphologic changes CC
- Chronic nephritic syndrome with proliferative glomerulonephritis NOS

N03.9 Chronic nephritic syndrome with unspecified morphologic changes CC

● **N04 Nephrotic syndrome**

Includes congenital nephrotic syndrome
lipoid nephrosis

Ex: For category N04 CC codes unless otherwise indicated: See N02

N04.0 Nephrotic syndrome with minor glomerular abnormality CC
- Nephrotic syndrome with minimal change lesion

N04.1 Nephrotic syndrome with focal and segmental glomerular lesions CC
- Nephrotic syndrome with focal and segmental hyalinosis
- Nephrotic syndrome with focal and segmental sclerosis
- Nephrotic syndrome with focal glomerulonephritis

N04.2 Nephrotic syndrome with diffuse membranous glomerulonephritis CC

N04.3 Nephrotic syndrome with diffuse mesangial proliferative glomerulonephritis CC

N04.4 Nephrotic syndrome with diffuse endocapillary proliferative glomerulonephritis CC

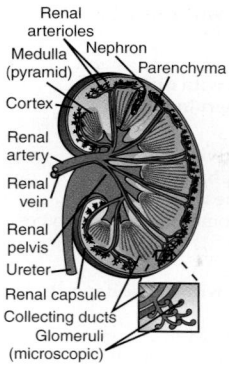

Figure 14-2 Kidney cross section.

Item 14–4 Nephrotic syndrome (NS) is marked by massive proteinuria (protein in the urine) and water retention. Patients with NS are particularly vulnerable to staphylococcal and pneumococcal infections. NS with lesion of proliferative glomerulonephritis results from a streptococcal infection. NS with lesion of membranous glomerulonephritis results in thickening of the capillary walls. NS with lesion of minimal change glomerulonephritis is usually a benign disorder that occurs mostly in children and requires electron microscopy (biopsy) to verify changes in the glomeruli.

N04.5 Nephrotic syndrome with diffuse mesangiocapillary glomerulonephritis CC
- Nephrotic syndrome with membranoproliferative glomerulonephritis, types 1 and 3, or NOS

N04.6 Nephrotic syndrome with dense deposit disease CC
- Nephrotic syndrome with membranoproliferative glomerulonephritis, type 2

N04.7 Nephrotic syndrome with diffuse crescentic glomerulonephritis CC
- Nephrotic syndrome with extracapillary glomerulonephritis

Ex: See N00

N04.8 Nephrotic syndrome with other morphologic changes CC
- Nephrotic syndrome with proliferative glomerulonephritis NOS

Ex: See N00

N04.9 Nephrotic syndrome with unspecified morphologic changes CC

Ex: See N00

● **N05 Unspecified nephritic syndrome**

Includes glomerular disease NOS
glomerulonephritis NOS
nephritis NOS
nephropathy NOS and renal disease NOS with morphological lesion specified in .0-.8

Excludes1 nephropathy NOS with no stated morphological lesion (N28.9)
renal disease NOS with no stated morphological lesion (N28.9)
tubulo-interstitial nephritis NOS (N12)

N05.0 Unspecified nephritic syndrome with minor glomerular abnormality
- Unspecified nephritic syndrome with minimal change lesion

N05.1 Unspecified nephritic syndrome with focal and segmental glomerular lesions
- Unspecified nephritic syndrome with focal and segmental hyalinosis
- Unspecified nephritic syndrome with focal and segmental sclerosis
- Unspecified nephritic syndrome with focal glomerulonephritis

N05.2 Unspecified nephritic syndrome with diffuse membranous glomerulonephritis CC

Ex: See N03

N05.3 Unspecified nephritic syndrome with diffuse mesangial proliferative glomerulonephritis
Ex See N03

N05.4 Unspecified nephritic syndrome with diffuse endocapillary proliferative glomerulonephritis
Ex See N03

N05.5 Unspecified nephritic syndrome with diffuse mesangiocapillary glomerulonephritis
Unspecified nephritic syndrome with membranoproliferative glomerulonephritis, types 1 and 3, or NOS
Ex See N03

N05.6 Unspecified nephritic syndrome with dense deposit disease
Unspecified nephritic syndrome with membranoproliferative glomerulonephritis, type 2

N05.7 Unspecified nephritic syndrome with diffuse crescentic glomerulonephritis
Unspecified nephritic syndrome with extracapillary glomerulonephritis

N05.8 Unspecified nephritic syndrome with other morphologic changes
Unspecified nephritic syndrome with proliferative glomerulonephritis NOS

N05.9 Unspecified nephritic syndrome with unspecified morphologic changes

● **N06 Isolated proteinuria with specified morphological lesion**
Excludes1 proteinuria not associated with specific morphologic lesions (R80.0)

N06.0 Isolated proteinuria with minor glomerular abnormality
Isolated proteinuria with minimal change lesion

N06.1 Isolated proteinuria with focal and segmental glomerular lesions
Isolated proteinuria with focal and segmental hyalinosis
Isolated proteinuria with focal and segmental sclerosis
Isolated proteinuria with focal glomerulonephritis

N06.2 Isolated proteinuria with diffuse membranous glomerulonephritis
Ex See N03

N06.3 Isolated proteinuria with diffuse mesangial proliferative glomerulonephritis
Ex See N03

N06.4 Isolated proteinuria with diffuse endocapillary proliferative glomerulonephritis
Ex See N03

N06.5 Isolated proteinuria with diffuse mesangiocapillary glomerulonephritis
Isolated proteinuria with membranoproliferative glomerulonephritis, types 1 and 3, or NOS
Ex See N03

N06.6 Isolated proteinuria with dense deposit disease
Isolated proteinuria with membranoproliferative glomerulonephritis, type 2

N06.7 Isolated proteinuria with diffuse crescentic glomerulonephritis
Isolated proteinuria with extracapillary glomerulonephritis

N06.8 Isolated proteinuria with other morphologic lesion
Isolated proteinuria with proliferative glomerulonephritis NOS

N06.9 Isolated proteinuria with unspecified morphologic lesion

● **N07 Hereditary nephropathy, not elsewhere classified**
Excludes2 Alport's syndrome (Q87.81-)
hereditary amyloid nephropathy (E85.-)
nail patella syndrome (Q87.2)
non-neuropathic heredofamilial amyloidosis (E85.-)

N07.0 Hereditary nephropathy, not elsewhere classified with minor glomerular abnormality
Hereditary nephropathy, not elsewhere classified with minimal change lesion

N07.1 Hereditary nephropathy, not elsewhere classified with focal and segmental glomerular lesions
Hereditary nephropathy, not elsewhere classified with focal and segmental hyalinosis
Hereditary nephropathy, not elsewhere classified with focal and segmental sclerosis
Hereditary nephropathy, not elsewhere classified with focal glomerulonephritis

N07.2 Hereditary nephropathy, not elsewhere classified with diffuse membranous glomerulonephritis
Ex See N03

N07.3 Hereditary nephropathy, not elsewhere classified with diffuse mesangial proliferative glomerulonephritis
Ex See N03

N07.4 Hereditary nephropathy, not elsewhere classified with diffuse endocapillary proliferative glomerulonephritis
Ex See N03

N07.5 Hereditary nephropathy, not elsewhere classified with diffuse mesangiocapillary glomerulonephritis
Hereditary nephropathy, not elsewhere classified with membranoproliferative glomerulonephritis, types 1 and 3, or NOS
Ex See N03

N07.6 Hereditary nephropathy, not elsewhere classified with dense deposit disease
Hereditary nephropathy, not elsewhere classified with membranoproliferative glomerulonephritis, type 2

N07.7 Hereditary nephropathy, not elsewhere classified with diffuse crescentic glomerulonephritis
Hereditary nephropathy, not elsewhere classified with extracapillary glomerulonephritis

N07.8 Hereditary nephropathy, not elsewhere classified with other morphologic lesions
Hereditary nephropathy, not elsewhere classified with proliferative glomerulonephritis NOS

N07.9 Hereditary nephropathy, not elsewhere classified with unspecified morphologic lesions

▶ ***N08 Glomerular disorders in diseases classified elsewhere***
Glomerulonephritis
Nephritis
Nephropathy
Code first underlying disease, such as:
amyloidosis (E85.-)
congenital syphilis (A50.5)
cryoglobulinemia (D89.1)
disseminated intravascular coagulation (D65)
gout (M1A.-, M10.-)
microscopic polyangiitis (M31.7)
multiple myeloma (C90.0-)
sepsis (A40.0-A41.9)
sickle-cell disease (D57.0-D57.8)
Excludes1 glomerulonephritis, nephritis and nephropathy (in):
antiglomerular basement membrane disease (M31.0)
diabetes (E08-E13 with .21)
gonococcal (A54.21)
Goodpasture's syndrome (M31.0)
hemolytic-uremic syndrome (D59.3)
lupus (M32.14)
mumps (B26.83)
syphilis (A52.75)
systemic lupus erythematosus (M32.14)
Wegener's granulomatosis (M31.31)
pyelonephritis in diseases classified elsewhere (N16)
renal tubulo-interstitial disorders classified elsewhere (N16)

◀ New ⇐ Revised ~~deleted~~ Deleted Excludes 1 Excludes 2 Includes Use additional Code first Code also Unspecified
OGCR Official Guidelines ● Unacceptable Principal Diagnosis X Assign placeholder X ● Use Additional Character(s) ▶ Manifestation Code Coding Clinic

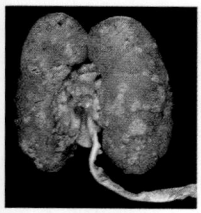

Figure 14-3 Acute pyelonephritis. Cortical surface exhibits grayish white areas of inflammation and abscess formation. (From Kumar: Robbins and Cotran: Pathologic Basis of Disease, ed 8, Saunders, An Imprint of Elsevier, 2009)

Item 14–5 Pyelonephritis is an infection of the kidneys and ureters and may be chronic or acute in one or both kidneys.

RENAL TUBULO-INTERSTITIAL DISEASES (N10-N16)

Includes pyelonephritis
Excludes1 pyeloureteritis cystica (N28.85)

N10 Acute pyelonephritis
Acute infectious interstitial nephritis
Acute pyelitis
Acute tubulo-interstitial nephritis
Hemoglobin nephrosis
Myoglobin nephrosis
Use additional code (B95-B97), to identify infectious agent
Ex: A17.9, A18.10-A18.11, A18.13, A18.82, A18.84, A18.89, A54.21, A54.29, A54.82, A54.84, A54.89-A54.9, A59.00, A59.8-A59.9, B37.41-B37.49, E08.21-E08.29, E08.618-E08.638, E08.649, E08.65-E08.8, E09.21-E09.29, E09.618-E09.638, E09.649-E09.8, E10.21-E10.29, E10.618-E10.638, E10.649, E10.69-E10.8, E11.21-E11.29, E11.618-E11.638, E11.649, E11.69-E11.8, E13.21-E13.29, E13.618-E13.638, E13.649-E13.69, E13.8, M10.30-M10.39, N00.0-N13.39, N13.6, N14.0-N19, N25.0-N27.9, N28.1-N29, N36.41-N36.43, N36.8-N36.9, N39.0, N39.8-N39.9, R31.0-R31.9, R82.71

N11 Chronic tubulo-interstitial nephritis
Includes chronic infectious interstitial nephritis
chronic pyelitis
chronic pyelonephritis
Use additional code (B95-B97), to identify infectious agent

N11.0 Nonobstructive reflux-associated chronic pyelonephritis
Pyelonephritis (chronic) associated with (vesicoureteral) reflux
Excludes1 vesicoureteral reflux NOS (N13.70)

N11.1 Chronic obstructive pyelonephritis
Pyelonephritis (chronic) associated with anomaly of pelviureteric junction
Pyelonephritis (chronic) associated with anomaly of pyeloureteric junction
Pyelonephritis (chronic) associated with crossing of vessel
Pyelonephritis (chronic) associated with kinking of ureter
Pyelonephritis (chronic) associated with obstruction of ureter
Pyelonephritis (chronic) associated with stricture of pelviureteric junction
Pyelonephritis (chronic) associated with stricture of ureter
Excludes1 calculous pyelonephritis (N20.9)
obstructive uropathy (N13.-)
CC when PDx is its own CC
Ex: N11.1, N13.4-N13.5, N13.8-N13.9, N28.82, N28.89-N30.91, N32.89-N33, N36.41-N36.43, N36.8-N36.9, N39.0, N39.8-N39.9, Q62.4-Q62.8, Q64.10-Q64.19, Q64.8-Q64.9, R31.0-R31.9, R82.71, Z90.6

N11.8 Other chronic tubulo-interstitial nephritis
Nonobstructive chronic pyelonephritis NOS
Ex: A17.9, A18.10-A18.11, A18.13, A18.82, A18.84, A18.89, A54.21, A54.29, A54.82, A54.84, A54.89-A54.9, A59.00, A59.8-A59.9, A98.5, B37.41-B37.49, E08.21-E08.29, E08.618-E08.638, E08.649, E08.65-E08.8, E09.21-E09.29, E09.618-E09.638, E09.649-E09.8, E10.21-E10.29, E10.618-E10.638, E10.649, E10.69-E10.8, E11.21-E11.29, E11.618-E11.638, E11.649, E11.69-E11.8, E13.21-E13.29, E13.618-E13.638, E13.649-E13.69, E13.8, M10.30-M10.39, N00.0-N13.39, N13.6, N14.0-N19, N25.0-N27.9, N28.1-N29, N36.41-N36.43, N36.8-N36.9, N39.8-N39.9, O23.01-O23.03, O23.11-O23.13, O23.21-O23.23, O23.31-O23.33, O23.41-O23.43, O23.511-O23.513, O23.521-O23.523, O23.591-O23.593, O23.91-O23.93, O86.11, O86.13-O86.29, R31.0-R31.9

N11.9 Chronic tubulo-interstitial nephritis, unspecified
Chronic interstitial nephritis NOS
Chronic pyelitis NOS
Chronic pyelonephritis NOS
Ex: A17.9, A18.10-A18.11, A18.13, A18.82, A18.84, A18.89, A54.21, A54.29, A54.82, A54.84, A54.89-A54.9, A59.00, A59.8-A59.9, B37.41-B37.49, E08.21-E08.29, E09.21-E09.29, M10.30-M10.39, N00.0-N13.39, N13.6, N14.0-N19, N25.0-N27.9, N28.1-N29, N36.41-N36.43, N36.8-N36.9, N39.0, N39.8-N39.9, R31.0-R31.9, R82.71

N12 Tubulo-interstitial nephritis, not specified as acute or chronic
Interstitial nephritis NOS
Pyelitis NOS
Pyelonephritis NOS
Excludes1 calculous pyelonephritis (N20.9)
Ex: See N11.9

N13 Obstructive and reflux uropathy
Excludes2 calculus of kidney and ureter without hydronephrosis (N20.-)
congenital obstructive defects of renal pelvis and ureter (Q62.0-Q62.3)
hydronephrosis with ureteropelvic junction obstruction (Q62.1)
obstructive pyelonephritis (N11.1)
Ex: For category N13 CC codes unless otherwise indicated: See N11.9

N13.0 Hydronephrosis with ureteropelvic junction obstruction
Hydronephrosis due to acquired occlusion of ureteropelvic junction
Excludes2 Hydronephrosis with ureteropelvic junction obstruction due to calculus (N13.2)
CC when PDx is its own CC

N13.1 Hydronephrosis with ureteral stricture, not elsewhere classified
Excludes1 hydronephrosis with ureteral stricture with infection (N13.6)
CC when PDx is its own CC

N13.2 Hydronephrosis with renal and ureteral calculous obstruction
Excludes1 hydronephrosis with renal and ureteral calculous obstruction with infection (N13.6)
CC when PDx is its own CC

N13.3 Other and unspecified hydronephrosis
Excludes1 hydronephrosis with infection (N13.6)
N13.30 Unspecified hydronephrosis
N13.39 Other hydronephrosis

N13.4 Hydroureter
Excludes1 congenital hydroureter (Q62.3-)
hydroureter with infection (N13.6)
vesicoureteral-reflux with hydroureter (N13.73-)
Ex: N11.1, N13.4-N13.5, N13.8-N13.9, N28.82, N28.89-N30.91, N32.89-N33, N36.41-N36.43, N36.8-N36.9, N39.0, N39.8-N39.9, Q62.4-Q62.8, Q64.10-Q64.19, Q64.8-Q64.9, R31.0-R31.9, R82.71

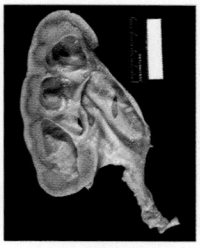

Figure 14-4 Hydronephrosis of the kidney, with marked dilatation of pelvis and calyces and thinning of renal parenchyma. (From Kumar: Robbins and Cotran: Pathologic Basis of Disease, ed 8, Saunders, An Imprint of Elsevier, 2009)

N13.5 Crossing vessel and stricture of ureter without hydronephrosis
Kinking and stricture of ureter without hydronephrosis
Excludes1 crossing vessel and stricture of ureter without hydronephrosis with infection (N13.6)

N13.6 Pyonephrosis
Conditions in N13.0-N13.5 with infection
Obstructive uropathy with infection
Use additional code (B95-B97), to identify infectious agent

● **N13.7 Vesicoureteral-reflux**
Excludes1 reflux-associated pyelonephritis (N11.0)

N13.70 Vesicoureteral-reflux, unspecified
Occurs when urine flows from bladder back into ureters
Vesicoureteral-reflux NOS

N13.71 Vesicoureteral-reflux without reflux nephropathy

● **N13.72 Vesicoureteral-reflux with reflux nephropathy without hydroureter**

N13.721 Vesicoureteral-reflux with reflux nephropathy without hydroureter, unilateral

N13.722 Vesicoureteral-reflux with reflux nephropathy without hydroureter, bilateral

N13.729 Vesicoureteral-reflux with reflux nephropathy without hydroureter, unspecified

● **N13.73 Vesicoureteral-reflux with reflux nephropathy with hydroureter**

N13.731 Vesicoureteral-reflux with reflux nephropathy with hydroureter, unilateral

N13.732 Vesicoureteral-reflux with reflux nephropathy with hydroureter, bilateral

N13.739 Vesicoureteral-reflux with reflux nephropathy with hydroureter, unspecified

N13.8 Other obstructive and reflux uropathy
Urinary tract obstruction due to specified cause
Code first, if applicable, any causal condition first, such as:
enlarged prostate (N40.1)
Ex: See N11.1

N13.9 Obstructive and reflux uropathy, unspecified
Urinary tract obstruction NOS

● **N14 Drug- and heavy-metal-induced tubulo-interstitial and tubular conditions**
Code first poisoning due to drug or toxin, if applicable (T36-T65 with fifth or sixth character 1-4 or 6)
Use additional code for adverse effect, if applicable, to identify drug (T36-T50 with fifth or sixth character 5)

N14.0 Analgesic nephropathy

N14.1 Nephropathy induced by other drugs, medicaments and biological substances

N14.2 Nephropathy induced by unspecified drug, medicament or biological substance

N14.3 Nephropathy induced by heavy metals

N14.4 Toxic nephropathy, not elsewhere classified

● **N15 Other renal tubulo-interstitial diseases**

N15.0 Balkan nephropathy
Balkan endemic nephropathy

N15.1 Renal and perinephric abscess
Ex: See N10

N15.8 Other specified renal tubulo-interstitial diseases

N15.9 Renal tubulo-interstitial disease, unspecified
Infection of kidney NOS
Excludes1 urinary tract infection NOS (N39.0)

N16 Renal tubulo-interstitial disorders in diseases classified elsewhere
Pyelonephritis
Tubulo-interstitial nephritis
Code first underlying disease, such as:
brucellosis (A23.0-A23.9)
cryoglobulinemia (D89.1)
glycogen storage disease (E74.0)
leukemia (C91-C95)
lymphoma (C81.0-C85.9, C96.0-C96.9)
multiple myeloma (C90.0-)
sepsis (A40.0-A41.9)
Wilson's disease (E83.0)
Excludes1 diphtheritic pyelonephritis and tubulo-interstitial nephritis (A36.84)
pyelonephritis and tubulo-interstitial nephritis in candidiasis (B37.49)
pyelonephritis and tubulo-interstitial nephritis in cystinosis (E72.04)
pyelonephritis and tubulo-interstitial nephritis in salmonella infection (A02.25)
pyelonephritis and tubulo-interstitial nephritis in sarcoidosis (D86.84)
pyelonephritis and tubulo-interstitial nephritis in sicca syndrome [Sjogren's] (M35.04)
pyelonephritis and tubulo-interstitial nephritis in systemic lupus erythematosus (M32.15)
pyelonephritis and tubulo-interstitial nephritis in toxoplasmosis (B58.83)
renal tubular degeneration in diabetes (E08-E13 with .29)
syphilitic pyelonephritis and tubulo-interstitial nephritis (A52.75)

ACUTE KIDNEY FAILURE AND CHRONIC KIDNEY DISEASE (N17-N19)

Excludes2 congenital renal failure (P96.0)
drug- and heavy-metal-induced tubulo-interstitial and tubular conditions (N14.-)
extrarenal uremia (R39.2)
hemolytic-uremic syndrome (D59.3)
hepatorenal syndrome (K76.7)
postpartum hepatorenal syndrome (O90.4)
posttraumatic renal failure (T79.5)
prerenal uremia (R39.2)
renal failure complicating abortion or ectopic or molar pregnancy (O00-O07, O08.4)
renal failure following labor and delivery (O90.4)
renal failure postprocedural (N99.0)

● **N17 Acute kidney failure**
Code also associated underlying condition
Excludes1 posttraumatic renal failure (T79.5)
Ex: **For category N17 CC codes unless otherwise indicated:** E08.21-E08.29, E08.618-E08.638, E08.649-E08.8, E09.21-E09.29, E09.618-E09.638, E09.649-E09.8, E10.21-E10.29, E10.618-E10.638, E10.649, E10.69-E10.8, E11.21-E11.29, E11.618-E11.638, E11.649, E11.69-E11.8, E13.21-E13.29, E13.618-E13.638, E13.649-E13.8, E88.3, M10.30-M10.39, N00.0-N13.39, N13.6, N14.0-N19, N25.0-N27.9, N28.1-N29, N36.41-N36.43, N36.8-N36.9, N39.8-N39.9, Q60.0-Q62.39, Q63.0-Q63.9, Q64.8-Q64.9, R31.0-R31.9

N17.0 Acute kidney failure with tubular necrosis
Acute tubular necrosis
Renal tubular necrosis
Tubular necrosis NOS

N17.1 Acute kidney failure with acute cortical necrosis
Acute cortical necrosis
Cortical necrosis NOS
Renal cortical necrosis

N17.2 Acute kidney failure with medullary necrosis
Medullary [papillary] necrosis NOS
Acute medullary [papillary] necrosis
Renal medullary [papillary] necrosis

◀ New ⇐ Revised ~~deleted~~ Deleted Excludes 1 Excludes 2 Includes Use additional Code first Code also Unspecified
OGCR Official Guidelines ● Unacceptable Principal Diagnosis X Assign placeholder X ● Use Additional Character(s) ◗ Manifestation Code Coding Clinic

Item 14–6 Decreased blood flow is the usual cause of **acute renal failure** that offers a good prognosis for recovery.

Chronic renal failure is usually the result of long-standing kidney disease and is a very serious condition that generally results in death.

N17.8 Other acute kidney failure
Ex: E08.21-E08.29, E08.618-E08.638, E08.649-E08.8, E09.21-E09.29, E09.618-E09.638, E09.649-E09.8, E10.21-E10.29, E10.618-E10.638, E10.649, E10.69-E10.8, E11.21-E11.29, E11.618-E11.638, E11.649, E11.69-E11.8, E13.21-E13.29, E13.618-E13.638, E13.649-E13.8, E88.3, M10.30-M10.39, N00.0-N13.39, N13.6, N14.0-N19, N25.0-N27.9, N28.1-N29, N36.41-N36.43, N36.8-N36.9, N39.8-N39.9, R31.0-R31.9

N17.9 Acute kidney failure, unspecified
Acute kidney injury (nontraumatic)
Excludes2 traumatic kidney injury (S37.0-)

N18 Chronic kidney disease (CKD)
Code first any associated:
diabetic chronic kidney disease (E08.22, E09.22, E10.22, E11.22, E13.22)
hypertensive chronic kidney disease (I12.-, I13.-)
Use additional code to identify kidney transplant status, if applicable, (Z94.0)

N18.1 Chronic kidney disease, stage 1

N18.2 Chronic kidney disease, stage 2 (mild)

N18.3 Chronic kidney disease, stage 3 (moderate)

N18.4 Chronic kidney disease, stage 4 (severe)
Ex: E08.21-E08.29, E08.618-E08.638, E08.649-E08.8, E09.21-E09.29, E09.618-E09.638, E09.649-E09.8, E10.21-E10.29, E10.618-E10.638, E10.649, E10.69-E10.8, E11.21-E11.29, E11.618-E11.638, E11.649, E11.69-E11.8, E13.21-E13.29, E13.618-E13.638, E13.649-E13.8, M10.30-M10.39, N00.0-N13.39, N13.6, N14.0-N19, N25.0-N27.9, N28.1-N29, N36.41-N36.43, N36.8-N36.9, N39.8-N39.9, Q60.0-Q62.39, Q63.0-Q63.9, Q64.8-Q64.9, R31.0-R31.9
Coding Clinic: 2013, Q1, P24

N18.5 Chronic kidney disease, stage 5
Excludes1 chronic kidney disease, stage 5 requiring chronic dialysis (N18.6)
Ex: See N18.4

N18.6 End stage renal disease
Chronic kidney disease requiring chronic dialysis
Use additional code to identify dialysis status (Z99.2)
Ex: E08.21-E08.29, E08.618-E08.638, E08.649-E08.8, E09.21-E09.29, E09.618-E09.638, E09.649-E09.8, E10.21-E10.29, E10.618-E10.638, E10.649, E10.69-E10.8, E11.21-E11.29, E11.618-E11.638, E11.649, E11.69-E11.8, E13.21-E13.29, E13.618-E13.638, E13.649-E13.8, I12.9, M10.30-M10.39, N00.0-N13.39, N13.6, N14.0-N19, N25.0-N27.9, N28.1-N29, N36.41-N36.43, N36.8-N36.9, N39.8-N39.9, Q60.0-Q62.39, Q63.0-Q63.9, Q64.8-Q64.9, R31.0-R31.9
Coding Clinic: 2016, Q1, P13

N18.9 Chronic kidney disease, unspecified
Chronic renal disease
Chronic renal failure NOS
Chronic renal insufficiency
Chronic uremia

N19 Unspecified kidney failure
Uremia NOS
Excludes1 acute kidney failure (N17.-)
chronic kidney disease (N18.-)
chronic uremia (N18.9)
extrarenal uremia (R39.2)
prerenal uremia (R39.2)
renal insufficiency (acute) (N28.9)
uremia of newborn (P96.0)

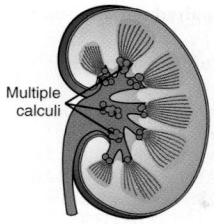

Figure 14-5 Multiple urinary calculi.

UROLITHIASIS (N20-N23)

N20 Calculus of kidney and ureter
Calculous pyelonephritis
Excludes1 nephrocalcinosis (E83.5)
that with hydronephrosis (N13.2)

N20.0 Calculus of kidney
Nephrolithiasis NOS
Renal calculus
Renal stone
Staghorn calculus
Stone in kidney

N20.1 Calculus of ureter
Ureteric stone
Ex: N11.1, N13.4-N13.5, N13.8-N13.9, N20.0-N22, N28.82, N28.89-N29, N36.41-N36.43, N36.8-N36.9, N39.8-N39.9, R31.0-R31.9

N20.2 Calculus of kidney with calculus of ureter
Ex: See N20.1

N20.9 Urinary calculus, unspecified

N21 Calculus of lower urinary tract
Includes calculus of lower urinary tract with cystitis and urethritis

N21.0 Calculus in bladder
Calculus in diverticulum of bladder
Urinary bladder stone
Excludes2 staghorn calculus (N20.0)
Coding Clinic: 2015, Q2, P9

N21.1 Calculus in urethra
Excludes2 calculus of prostate (N42.0)

N21.8 Other lower urinary tract calculus

N21.9 Calculus of lower urinary tract, unspecified
Excludes1 calculus of urinary tract NOS (N20.9)

N22 Calculus of urinary tract in diseases classified elsewhere
Code first underlying disease, such as:
gout (M1A.-, M10.-)
schistosomiasis (B65.0-B65.9)

N23 Unspecified renal colic

OTHER DISORDERS OF KIDNEY AND URETER (N25-N29)

Excludes2 disorders of kidney and ureter with urolithiasis (N20-N23)

N25 Disorders resulting from impaired renal tubular function
Excludes1 metabolic disorders classifiable to E70-E88

N25.0 Renal osteodystrophy
Azotemic osteodystrophy
Phosphate-losing tubular disorders
Renal rickets
Renal short stature

N25.1 Nephrogenic diabetes insipidus
Excludes1 diabetes insipidus NOS (E23.2)
Ex: A17.9, A18.10-A18.11, A18.13, A18.82, A18.84, A18.89, A54.21, A54.29, A54.82, A54.84, A54.89-A54.9, A59.00, A59.8-A59.9, A98.5, B37.41-B37.49, E08.21-E08.29, E08.618-E08.638, E08.649, E08.65-E08.8, E09.21-E09.29, E09.618-E09.638, E09.649-E09.8, E10.21-E10.29, E10.618-E10.638, E10.649, E10.69-E10.8, E11.21-E11.29, E11.618-E11.638, E11.649, E11.69-E11.8, E13.21-E13.29, E13.618-E13.638, E13.649-E13.69, E13.8, M10.30-M10.39, N00.0-N13.39, N13.6, N14.0-N19, N25.0-N27.9, N28.1-N29, N36.41-N36.43, N36.8-N36.9, N39.8-N39.9, R31.0-R31.9

● **N25.8 Other disorders resulting from impaired renal tubular function**

N25.81 Secondary hyperparathyroidism of renal origin

Excludes1 secondary hyperparathyroidism, non-renal (E21.1)

Ex: A17.9, A18.10-A18.11, A18.13, A18.82, A18.84, A18.89, A54.21, A54.29, A54.82, A54.84, A54.89-A54.9, A59.00, A59.8-A59.9, A98.5, B37.41-B37.49, E08.21-E08.29, E08.618-E08.638, E08.649, E08.65-E08.8, E09.21-E09.29, E09.618-E09.638, E09.649-E09.8, E10.21-E10.29, E10.618-E10.638, E10.649, E10.69-E10.8, E11.21-E11.29, E11.618-E11.638, E11.649, E11.69-E11.8, E13.21-E13.29, E13.618-E13.638, E13.649-E13.69, E13.8, M10.30-M10.39, N00.0-N13.39, N13.6, N14.0-N19, N25.0-N27.9, N28.1-N29, N36.41-N36.43, N36.8-N36.9, N39.8-N39.9, R31.0-R31.9

N25.89 Other disorders resulting from impaired renal tubular function

Hypokalemic nephropathy
Lightwood-Albright syndrome
Renal tubular acidosis NOS

N25.9 Disorder resulting from impaired renal tubular function, unspecified

● **N26 Unspecified contracted kidney**

Excludes1 contracted kidney due to hypertension (I12.-)
diffuse sclerosing glomerulonephritis (N05.8.-)
hypertensive nephrosclerosis (arteriolar) (arteriosclerotic) (I12.-)
small kidney of unknown cause (N27.-)

N26.1 Atrophy of kidney (terminal)

N26.2 Page kidney

N26.9 Renal sclerosis, unspecified

● **N27 Small kidney of unknown cause**

Includes oligonephronia

N27.0 Small kidney, unilateral

N27.1 Small kidney, bilateral

N27.9 Small kidney, unspecified

● **N28 Other disorders of kidney and ureter, not elsewhere classified**

N28.0 Ischemia and infarction of kidney

Renal artery embolism
Renal artery obstruction
Renal artery occlusion
Renal artery thrombosis
Renal infarct

Excludes1 atherosclerosis of renal artery (extrarenal part) (I70.1)
congenital stenosis of renal artery (Q27.1)
Goldblatt's kidney (I70.1)

Ex: N13.70-N13.739, N28.0, N28.9-N29

N28.1 Cyst of kidney, acquired

Cyst (multiple)(solitary) of kidney, acquired

Excludes1 cystic kidney disease (congenital) (Q61.-)

● **N28.8 Other specified disorders of kidney and ureter**

Excludes1 hydroureter (N13.4)
ureteric stricture with hydronephrosis (N13.1)
ureteric stricture without hydronephrosis (N13.5)

N28.81 Hypertrophy of kidney

N28.82 Megaloureter

N28.83 Nephroptosis

N28.84 Pyelitis cystica

Ex: See N11.9

N28.85 Pyeloureteritis cystica

Ex: See N11.9

N28.86 Ureteritis cystica

Ex: See N11.9

N28.89 Other specified disorders of kidney and ureter

N28.9 Disorder of kidney and ureter, unspecified

Nephropathy NOS
Renal disease (acute) NOS
Renal insufficiency (acute)

Excludes1 chronic renal insufficiency (N18.9)
unspecified nephritic syndrome (N05.-)

Coding Clinic: 2016, Q1, P13

▶ ***N29 Other disorders of kidney and ureter in diseases classified elsewhere***

Code first underlying disease, such as:
amyloidosis (E85.-)
nephrocalcinosis (E83.5)
schistosomiasis (B65.0-B65.9)

Excludes1 disorders of kidney and ureter in:
cystinosis (E72.0)
gonorrhea (A54.21)
syphilis (A52.75)
tuberculosis (A18.11)

OTHER DISEASES OF THE URINARY SYSTEM (N30-N39)

Excludes1 urinary infection (complicating):
abortion or ectopic or molar pregnancy (O00-O07, O08.8)
pregnancy, childbirth and the puerperium (O23.-, O75.3, O86.2-)

● **N30 Cystitis**

Infection of bladder and irritation in lower urinary tract

Use additional code to identify infectious agent (B95-B97)

Excludes1 prostatocystitis (N41.3)

● **N30.0 Acute cystitis**

Excludes1 irradiation cystitis (N30.4-)
trigonitis (N30.3-)

Ex: **For category N30.0 CC codes:** A17.9, A18.10, A18.12-A18.13, A18.82, A18.84, A18.89, A54.00-A54.02, A54.09-A54.1, A54.82, A54.84, A54.89-A54.9, A59.00, A59.8-A59.9, B37.41-B37.49, N11.1, N13.4-N13.5, N13.8-N13.9, N28.82, N28.89-N30.91, N32.89-N33, N36.41-N36.43, N36.8-N36.9, N39.0, N39.8-N39.9, R31.0-R31.9

N30.00 Acute cystitis without hematuria

N30.01 Acute cystitis with hematuria

● **N30.1 Interstitial cystitis (chronic)**

Ongoing infection of kidney glomeruli and tubules

N30.10 Interstitial cystitis (chronic) without hematuria

N30.11 Interstitial cystitis (chronic) with hematuria

● **N30.2 Other chronic cystitis**

N30.20 Other chronic cystitis without hematuria

N30.21 Other chronic cystitis with hematuria

● **N30.3 Trigonitis**

Inflammation of triangular area of bladder (where the ureters and urethra come together)

Urethrotrigonitis

N30.30 Trigonitis without hematuria

N30.31 Trigonitis with hematuria

● **N30.4 Irradiation cystitis**

Ex: **For category N30.4 CC codes:** See N30.0

N30.40 Irradiation cystitis without hematuria

N30.41 Irradiation cystitis with hematuria

● **N30.8 Other cystitis**

Abscess of bladder

N30.80 Other cystitis without hematuria

N30.81 Other cystitis with hematuria

● **N30.9 Cystitis, unspecified**

N30.90 Cystitis, unspecified without hematuria

N30.91 Cystitis, unspecified with hematuria

N31 Neuromuscular dysfunction of bladder, not elsewhere classified
Use additional code to identify any associated urinary incontinence (N39.3-N39.4-)
Excludes1 cord bladder NOS (G95.89)
neurogenic bladder due to cauda equina syndrome (G83.4)
neuromuscular dysfunction due to spinal cord lesion (G95.89)

N31.0 Uninhibited neuropathic bladder, not elsewhere classified

N31.1 Reflex neuropathic bladder, not elsewhere classified

N31.2 Flaccid neuropathic bladder, not elsewhere classified
Atonic (motor) (sensory) neuropathic bladder
Diminished tone of bladder muscle
Autonomous neuropathic bladder
Nonreflex neuropathic bladder

N31.8 Other neuromuscular dysfunction of bladder

N31.9 Neuromuscular dysfunction of bladder, unspecified
Neurogenic bladder dysfunction NOS

N32 Other disorders of bladder
Excludes2 calculus of bladder (N21.0)
cystocele (N81.1-)
hernia or prolapse of bladder, female (N81.1-)

N32.0 Bladder-neck obstruction
Bladder-neck stenosis (acquired)
Excludes1 congenital bladder-neck obstruction (Q64.3-)

N32.1 Vesicointestinal fistula
Vesicorectal fistula
Ex: A54.00-A54.02, A54.09-A54.1, A54.82, A54.84, A54.89-A54.9, N32.1-N32.2, N32.89-N33, N36.41-N36.43, N36.8-N36.9, N39.8-N39.9, R30.0, R30.9, R31.0-R31.9

N32.2 Vesical fistula, not elsewhere classified
Excludes1 fistula between bladder and female genital tract (N82.0-N82.1)
Ex: See N32.1

N32.3 Diverticulum of bladder
Formation of sac from a herniation of wall of bladder
Excludes1 congenital diverticulum of bladder (Q64.6)
diverticulitis of bladder (N30.8-)

N32.8 Other specified disorders of bladder

N32.81 Overactive bladder
Detrusor muscle hyperactivity
Excludes1 frequent urination due to specified bladder condition-code to condition

N32.89 Other specified disorders of bladder
Bladder hemorrhage
Bladder hypertrophy
Calcified bladder
Contracted bladder

N32.9 Bladder disorder, unspecified

N33 Bladder disorders in diseases classified elsewhere
Code first underlying disease, such as:
schistosomiasis (B65.0-B65.9)
Excludes1 bladder disorder in syphilis (A52.76)
bladder disorder in tuberculosis (A18.12)
candidal cystitis (B37.41)
chlamydial cystitis(A56.01)
cystitis in gonorrhea (A54.01)
cystitis in neurogenic bladder (N31.-)
diphtheritic cystitis (A36.85)
syphilitic cystitis (A52.76)
trichomonal cystitis (A59.03)

N34 Urethritis and urethral syndrome
Use additional code (B95-B97), to identify infectious agent
Excludes2 Reiter's disease (M02.3-)
urethritis in diseases with a predominantly sexual mode of transmission (A50-A64)
urethrotrigonitis (N30.3-)

N34.0 Urethral abscess
Abscess (of) Cowper's gland
Abscess (of) Littré's gland
Abscess (of) urethral (gland)
Periurethral abscess
Excludes1 urethral caruncle (N36.2)
Ex: A54.00-A54.02, A54.09-A54.1, A54.82, A54.84, A54.89-A54.9, A59.00, A59.03, A59.8-A59.9, B37.41-B37.49, N13.9, N34.0-N34.3, N35.111-N35.9, N36.41-N36.43, N36.8-N39.0, N39.8-N39.9, N44.1-N44.8, N47.6, N48.1-N48.9, N49.1-N49.9, N50.3-N50.89, N51, N53.11-N53.9, Q54.0-Q55.9, Q64.0, Q64.2-Q64.9, R30.0, R30.9-R31.9, R82.71

N34.1 Nonspecific urethritis
Nongonococcal urethritis
Nonvenereal urethritis

N34.2 Other urethritis
Inflammation of urethra
Meatitis, urethral
Postmenopausal urethritis
Ulcer of urethra (meatus)
Urethritis NOS

N34.3 Urethral syndrome, unspecified

N35 Urethral stricture
Narrowing of lumen of urethra caused by scarring due to infection or injury
Excludes1 congenital urethral stricture (Q64.3-)
postprocedural urethral stricture (N99.1-)

N35.0 Post-traumatic urethral stricture
Urethral stricture due to injury
Excludes1 postprocedural urethral stricture (N99.1-)

N35.01 Post-traumatic urethral stricture, male

N35.010 Post-traumatic urethral stricture, male, meatal ♂

N35.011 Post-traumatic bulbous urethral stricture

N35.012 Post-traumatic membranous urethral stricture

N35.013 Post-traumatic anterior urethral stricture

N35.014 Post-traumatic urethral stricture, male, unspecified ♂

N35.02 Post-traumatic urethral stricture, female

N35.021 Urethral stricture due to childbirth ♀

N35.028 Other post-traumatic urethral stricture, female ♀

N35.1 Postinfective urethral stricture, not elsewhere classified
Excludes1 urethral stricture associated with schistosomiasis (B65.-, N29)
gonococcal urethral stricture (A54.01)
syphilitic urethral stricture (A52.76)

N35.11 Postinfective urethral stricture, not elsewhere classified, male

N35.111 Postinfective urethral stricture, not elsewhere classified, male, meatal ♂

N35.112 Postinfective bulbous urethral stricture, not elsewhere classified

N35.113 Postinfective membranous urethral stricture, not elsewhere classified

N35.114 Postinfective anterior urethral stricture, not elsewhere classified

N35.119 Postinfective urethral stricture, not elsewhere classified, male, unspecified ♂

N35.12 Postinfective urethral stricture, not elsewhere classified, female ♀

N35.8 Other urethral stricture
Excludes1 postprocedural urethral stricture (N99.1-)

N35.9 Urethral stricture, unspecified

● N36 Other disorders of urethra

N36.0 Urethral fistula
Urethroperineal fistula
Urethrorectal fistula
Urinary fistula NOS
Excludes1 urethroscrotal fistula (N50.89)
urethrovaginal fistula (N82.1)
urethrovesicovaginal fistula (N82.1)
Ex: N13.9, N34.0, N34.2-N36.43, N36.5-N37, N39.8-N39.9, N44.1-N44.8, N47.6, N48.1-N48.9, N49.1-N49.9, N50.3-N50.89, N51, N53.11-N53.9, N99.110-N99.115, Q54.0-Q55.21, Q55.23-Q55.9, Q64.0, Q64.8-Q64.9, R30.0, R30.9-R31.9

N36.1 Urethral diverticulum

N36.2 Urethral caruncle

● N36.4 Urethral functional and muscular disorders
Use additional code to identify associated urinary stress incontinence (N39.3)

N36.41 Hypermobility of urethra

N36.42 Intrinsic sphincter deficiency (ISD)

N36.43 Combined hypermobility of urethra and intrinsic sphincter deficiency

N36.44 Muscular disorders of urethra
Bladder sphincter dyssynergy

N36.5 Urethral false passage

N36.8 Other specified disorders of urethra
Excludes1 congenital urethrocele (Q64.7) ◀
female urethrocele (N81.0) ◀

N36.9 Urethral disorder, unspecified

N37 Urethral disorders in diseases classified elsewhere
Code first underlying disease
Excludes1 urethritis (in):
candidal infection (B37.41)
chlamydial (A56.01)
gonorrhea (A54.01)
syphilis (A52.76)
trichomonal infection (A59.03)
tuberculosis (A18.13)

● N39 Other disorders of urinary system
Excludes2 hematuria NOS (R31.-)
recurrent or persistent hematuria (N02.-)
recurrent or persistent hematuria with specified morphological lesion (N02.-)
proteinuria NOS (R80.-)

N39.0 Urinary tract infection, site not specified
Use additional code (B95-B97), to identify infectious agent
Excludes1 candidiasis of urinary tract (B37.4-)
neonatal urinary tract infection (P39.3)
urinary tract infection of specified site, such as:
cystitis (N30.-)
urethritis (N34.-)
Ex: A54.82, A54.84, A54.89-A54.9, A59.00, A59.8-A59.9, B37.41-B37.49, N10, N11.9-N13.39, N13.6, N13.9, N15.1, N28.82, N28.84-N30.91, N34.1, N36.41-N36.43, N36.8-N36.9, N39.0, N39.8-N39.9, N99.511, R30.0, R30.9-R31.9, T83.511A
Coding Clinic: 2012, Q4, P94

N39.3 Stress incontinence (female) (male)
Code also any associated overactive bladder (N32.81)
Excludes1 mixed incontinence (N39.46)

● N39.4 Other specified urinary incontinence
Code also any associated overactive bladder (N32.81)
Excludes1 enuresis NOS (R32)
functional urinary incontinence (R39.81)
urinary incontinence associated with cognitive impairment (R39.81)
urinary incontinence NOS (R32)
urinary incontinence of nonorganic origin (F98.0)

N39.41 Urge incontinence
Excludes1 mixed incontinence (N39.46)

N39.42 Incontinence without sensory awareness
Insensible (urinary) incontinence ◀

N39.43 Post-void dribbling

N39.44 Nocturnal enuresis

N39.45 Continuous leakage

N39.46 Mixed incontinence
Urge and stress incontinence

● N39.49 Other specified urinary incontinence

N39.490 Overflow incontinence

N39.491 Coital incontinence ◀

N39.492 Postural (urinary) incontinence ◀

N39.498 Other specified urinary incontinence
Reflex incontinence
Total incontinence

N39.8 Other specified disorders of urinary system

N39.9 Disorder of urinary system, unspecified

DISEASES OF MALE GENITAL ORGANS (N40-N53)

★ **(See Plate 387 on page 53.)**

● N40 Benign prostatic hyperplasia
Includes adenofibromatous hypertrophy of prostate
benign hypertrophy of the prostate
Enlargement of prostate gland usually occurring with age and causing obstructed urine flow
benign prostatic hypertrophy
BPH
enlarged prostate ◀
nodular prostate
polyp of prostate
Excludes1 benign neoplasms of prostate (adenoma, benign) (fibroadenoma) (fibroma) (myoma) (D29.1)
malignant neoplasm of prostate (C61)

N40.0 Benign prostatic hyperplasia without lower urinary tract symptoms ♂ A
Enlarged prostate without LUTS
Enlarged prostate NOS

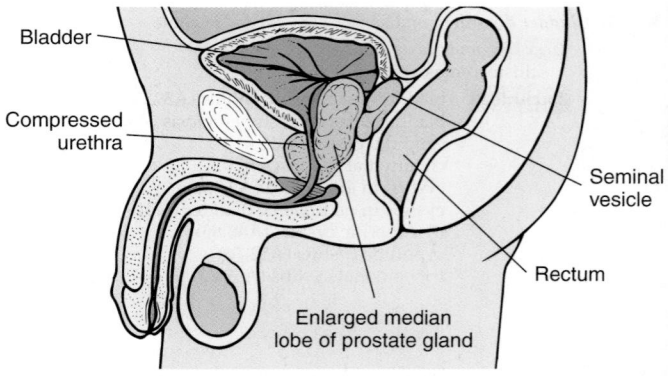

Figure 14-6 Benign prostatic hyperplasia. (From Shiland: Mastering Healthcare Terminology, ed 3, St. Louis, Mosby, 2010)

◀ New ◀ Revised ~~deleted~~ Deleted Excludes 1 Excludes 2 Includes Use additional Code first Code also Unspecified
OGCR Official Guidelines ● Unacceptable Principal Diagnosis X Assign placeholder X ● Use Additional Character(s) ▶ Manifestation Code Coding Clinic

N40.1 Benign prostatic hyperplasia with lower urinary tract symptoms ♂ A
Enlarged prostate with LUTS
Use additional code for associated symptoms, when specified:
incomplete bladder emptying (R39.14)
nocturia (R35.1)
straining on urination (R39.16)
urinary frequency (R35.0)
urinary hesitancy (R39.11)
urinary incontinence (N39.4-)
urinary obstruction (N13.8)
urinary retention (R33.8)
urinary urgency (R39.15)
weak urinary stream (R39.12)

N40.2 Nodular prostate without lower urinary tract symptoms ♂ A
Nodular prostate without LUTS

N40.3 Nodular prostate with lower urinary tract symptoms ♂ A
Use additional code for associated symptoms, when specified:
incomplete bladder emptying (R39.14)
nocturia (R35.1)
straining on urination (R39.16)
urinary frequency (R35.0)
urinary hesitancy (R39.11)
urinary incontinence (N39.4-)
urinary obstruction (N13.8)
urinary retention (R33.8)
urinary urgency (R39.15)
weak urinary stream (R39.12)

N41 Inflammatory diseases of prostate
Use additional code (B95-B97), to identify infectious agent

N41.0 Acute prostatitis ♂ A
Ex: A18.14, A54.22, A54.82, A54.84, A54.89-A54.9, A59.00, A59.02, A59.8-A59.9, B37.41-B37.49, N40.0-N42.9

N41.1 Chronic prostatitis ♂ A

N41.2 Abscess of prostate ♂ A
Ex: See N41.0

N41.3 Prostatocystitis ♂ A

N41.4 Granulomatous prostatitis ♂ A

N41.8 Other inflammatory diseases of prostate ♂ A

N41.9 Inflammatory disease of prostate, unspecified ♂ A
Prostatitis NOS

N42 Other and unspecified disorders of prostate

N42.0 Calculus of prostate ♂ A
Prostatic stone

N42.1 Congestion and hemorrhage of prostate ♂ A
Excludes1 enlarged prostate (N40.-)
hematuria (R31.-)
hyperplasia of prostate (N40.-)
inflammatory diseases of prostate (N41.-)

N42.3 Dysplasia of prostate

N42.30 Unspecified dysplasia of prostate ♂ ◀

N42.31 Prostatic intraepithelial neoplasia ♂ ◀
PIN ◀
Prostatic intraepithelial neoplasia I (PIN I) ◀
Prostatic intraepithelial neoplasia II (PIN II) ◀
Excludes1 prostatic intraepithelial neoplasia III (PIN III) (D07.5) ◀

N42.32 Atypical small acinar proliferation of prostate ♂ ◀

N42.39 Other dysplasia of prostate ♂ ◀

N42.8 Other specified disorders of prostate

N42.81 Prostatodynia syndrome ♂ A
Painful prostate syndrome

N42.82 Prostatosis syndrome ♂ A

N42.83 Cyst of prostate ♂ A

N42.89 Other specified disorders of prostate ♂ A

N42.9 Disorder of prostate, unspecified ♂ A

Item 14–7 Hydrocele is a sac of fluid accumulating in the testes membrane.

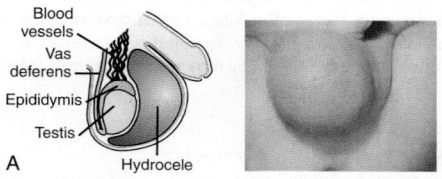

Figure 14-7 A. Hydrocele. **B.** Newborn with large right hydrocele. (**B** from Behrman: Nelson Textbook of Pediatrics, ed 18, Saunders, An Imprint of Elsevier, 2007)

N43 Hydrocele and spermatocele
Includes hydrocele of spermatic cord, testis or tunica vaginalis
Excludes1 congenital hydrocele (P83.5)

N43.0 Encysted hydrocele ♂

N43.1 Infected hydrocele ♂
Use additional code (B95-B97), to identify infectious agent
Ex: A59.00, A59.8-A59.9, B37.41-B37.49, N43.0-N43.3

N43.2 Other hydrocele ♂

N43.3 Hydrocele, unspecified ♂

N43.4 Spermatocele of epididymis
Spermatic cyst

N43.40 Spermatocele of epididymis, unspecified ♂

N43.41 Spermatocele of epididymis, single ♂

N43.42 Spermatocele of epididymis, multiple ♂

N44 Noninflammatory disorders of testis

N44.0 Torsion of testis
Ex: For category N44.0 CC codes: N44.00-N44.04

N44.00 Torsion of testis, unspecified ♂

N44.01 Extravaginal torsion of spermatic cord ♂

N44.02 Intravaginal torsion of spermatic cord ♂
Torsion of spermatic cord NOS

N44.03 Torsion of appendix testis ♂

N44.04 Torsion of appendix epididymis ♂

N44.1 Cyst of tunica albuginea testis ♂

N44.2 Benign cyst of testis ♂

N44.8 Other noninflammatory disorders of the testis ♂

N45 Orchitis and epididymitis
Orchitis is inflammation of one or both of the testes as a result of mumps or other infection, trauma, or metastasis. ***Epididymitis*** *is inflammation of the tubular structure that connects the testicle with the vas deferens.*
Use additional code (B95-B97), to identify infectious agent

N45.1 Epididymitis ♂

N45.2 Orchitis ♂

N45.3 Epididymo-orchitis ♂

N45.4 Abscess of epididymis or testis ♂
Ex: A54.23, A54.82, A54.84, A54.89-A54.9, A59.00, A59.8-A59.9, B26.0, B37.41-B37.49, N45.1-N45.4

Item 14-8 Male infertility is the inability of the female sex partner to conceive after one year of unprotected intercourse.

Azoospermia is no sperm ejaculated and **oligospermia** is few sperm ejaculated—both resulting in infertility. Extratesticular causes such as injury, infections, radiation, and chemotherapy may also cause male infertility.

N46 Male infertility
Excludes1 vasectomy status (Z98.52)

N46.0 Azoospermia
Absolute male infertility
Male infertility due to germinal (cell) aplasia
Male infertility due to spermatogenic arrest (complete)

N46.01 Organic azoospermia ♂ A
Azoospermia NOS

N46.02 Azoospermia due to extratesticular causes
Code also associated cause

N46.021 Azoospermia due to drug therapy ♂ A
N46.022 Azoospermia due to infection ♂ A
N46.023 Azoospermia due to obstruction of efferent ducts ♂ A
N46.024 Azoospermia due to radiation ♂ A
N46.025 Azoospermia due to systemic disease ♂ A
N46.029 Azoospermia due to other extratesticular causes ♂ A

N46.1 Oligospermia
Male infertility due to germinal cell desquamation
Male infertility due to hypospermatogenesis
Male infertility due to incomplete spermatogenic arrest

N46.11 Organic oligospermia ♂ A
Oligospermia NOS

N46.12 Oligospermia due to extratesticular causes
Code also associated cause

N46.121 Oligospermia due to drug therapy ♂ A
N46.122 Oligospermia due to infection ♂ A
N46.123 Oligospermia due to obstruction of efferent ducts ♂ A
N46.124 Oligospermia due to radiation ♂ A
N46.125 Oligospermia due to systemic disease ♂ A
N46.129 Oligospermia due to other extratesticular causes ♂ A

N46.8 Other male infertility ♂ A
N46.9 Male infertility, unspecified ♂ A

N47 Disorders of prepuce
N47.0 Adherent prepuce, newborn ♂ N
N47.1 Phimosis ♂
N47.2 Paraphimosis ♂
N47.3 Deficient foreskin ♂
N47.4 Benign cyst of prepuce ♂
N47.5 Adhesions of prepuce and glans penis ♂
N47.6 Balanoposthitis ♂
Use additional code (B95-B97), to identify infectious agent
Excludes1 balanitis (N48.1)
N47.7 Other inflammatory diseases of prepuce ♂
Use additional code (B95-B97), to identify infectious agent
N47.8 Other disorders of prepuce ♂

N48 Other disorders of penis

N48.0 Leukoplakia of penis ♂
Balanitis xerotica obliterans
Kraurosis of penis
Lichen sclerosus of external male genital organs
Excludes1 carcinoma in situ of penis (D07.4)

N48.1 Balanitis ♂
Use additional code (B95-B97), to identify infectious agent
Excludes1 amebic balanitis (A06.8)
balanitis xerotica obliterans (N48.0)
candidal balanitis (B37.42)
gonococcal balanitis (A54.23)
herpesviral [herpes simplex] balanitis (A60.01)

N48.2 Other inflammatory disorders of penis
Use additional code (B95-B97), to identify infectious agent
Excludes1 balanitis (N48.1)
balanitis xerotica obliterans (N48.0)
balanoposthitis (N47.6)
N48.21 Abscess of corpus cavernosum and penis ♂
N48.22 Cellulitis of corpus cavernosum and penis ♂
N48.29 Other inflammatory disorders of penis ♂

N48.3 Priapism
Painful erection
Code first underlying cause
Ex For category N48.3 CC codes: N47.6, N48.0-N48.9, N52.01-N52.9
N48.30 Priapism, unspecified ♂
N48.31 Priapism due to trauma ♂
N48.32 Priapism due to disease classified elsewhere ♂
N48.33 Priapism, drug-induced ♂
N48.39 Other priapism ♂

N48.5 Ulcer of penis ♂
N48.6 Induration penis plastica ♂
Peyronie's disease
Plastic induration of penis

N48.8 Other specified disorders of penis
N48.81 Thrombosis of superficial vein of penis ♂
N48.82 Acquired torsion of penis ♂
Acquired torsion of penis NOS
Excludes1 congenital torsion of penis (Q55.63)
N48.83 Acquired buried penis ♂
Excludes1 congenital hidden penis (Q55.64)
N48.89 Other specified disorders of penis ♂

N48.9 Disorder of penis, unspecified ♂

N49 Inflammatory disorders of male genital organs, not elsewhere classified
Use additional code (B95-B97), to identify infectious agent
Excludes1 inflammation of penis (N48.1, N48.2-)
orchitis and epididymitis (N45.-)
N49.0 Inflammatory disorders of seminal vesicle ♂
Vesiculitis NOS
N49.1 Inflammatory disorders of spermatic cord, tunica vaginalis and vas deferens ♂
Vasitis
N49.2 Inflammatory disorders of scrotum ♂
N49.3 Fournier gangrene ♂
N49.8 Inflammatory disorders of other specified male genital organs ♂
Inflammation of multiple sites in male genital organs
N49.9 Inflammatory disorder of unspecified male genital organ ♂
Abscess of unspecified male genital organ
Boil of unspecified male genital organ
Carbuncle of unspecified male genital organ
Cellulitis of unspecified male genital organ

New Revised ~~deleted~~ Deleted Excludes 1 Excludes 2 Includes Use additional Code first Code also Unspecified
OGCR Official Guidelines ● Unacceptable Principal Diagnosis X Assign placeholder X ● Use Additional Character(s) ▶ Manifestation Code Coding Clinic

Item 14–9 Seminal vesiculitis is an inflammation of the seminal vesicle. Spermatocele is a benign cystic accumulation of sperm arising from the head of the epididymis. Torsion of the testis is a medical emergency occurring most commonly in boys 7 to 12 years of age and results from a congenital abnormality of the covering of the testis allowing the testis to twist within its sac and cutting off the blood supply to the testis.

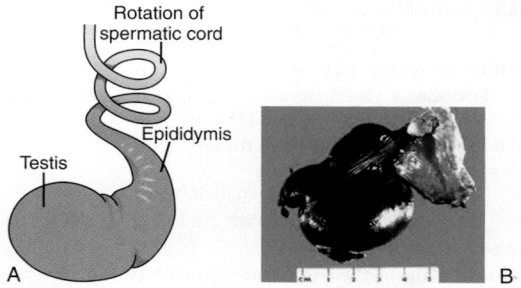

Figure 14-8 **A.** Torsion of testis. **B.** Torsion of the testis. (**B** from Kumar: Robbins and Cotran: Pathologic Basis of Disease, ed 8, Saunders, An Imprint of Elsevier, 2009)

● **N50 Other and unspecified disorders of male genital organs**
Excludes2 torsion of testis (N44.0-)
N50.0 Atrophy of testis ♂
N50.1 Vascular disorders of male genital organs ♂
Hematocele, NOS, of male genital organs
Hemorrhage of male genital organs
Thrombosis of male genital organs
N50.3 Cyst of epididymis ♂
● **N50.8 Other specified disorders of male genital organs**
● **N50.81 Testicular pain** ◀
N50.811 Right testicular pain ♂ ◀
N50.812 Left testicular pain ♂ ◀
N50.819 Testicular pain, unspecified ♂ ◀
N50.82 Scrotal pain ♂ ◀
N50.89 Other specified disorders of the male genital organs ♂ ◀
Atrophy of scrotum, seminal vesicle, spermatic cord, tunica vaginalis and vas deferens ◀
Chylocele, tunica vaginalis (nonfilarial) NOS ◀
Edema of scrotum, seminal vesicle, spermatic cord, tunica vaginalis and vas deferens ◀
Hypertrophy of scrotum, seminal vesicle, spermatic cord, tunica vaginalis and vas deferens ◀
Stricture of spermatic cord, tunica vaginalis, and vas deferens ◀
Ulcer of scrotum, seminal vesicle, spermatic cord, testis, tunica vaginalis and vas deferens ◀
Urethroscrotal fistula ◀
N50.9 Disorder of male genital organs, unspecified ♂

◗ *N51 Disorders of male genital organs in diseases classified elsewhere* ♂
Code first underlying disease, such as:
filariasis (B74.0-B74.9)
Excludes1 amebic balanitis (A06.8)
candidal balanitis (B37.42)
gonococcal balanitis (A54.23)
gonococcal prostatitis (A54.22)
herpesviral [herpes simplex] balanitis (A60.01)
trichomonal prostatitis (A59.02)
tuberculous prostatitis (A18.14)

● **N52 Male erectile dysfunction**
Excludes1 psychogenic impotence (F52.21)
● **N52.0 Vasculogenic erectile dysfunction**
N52.01 Erectile dysfunction due to arterial insufficiency ♂ A
N52.02 Corporo-venous occlusive erectile dysfunction ♂ A
N52.03 Combined arterial insufficiency and corporo-venous occlusive erectile dysfunction ♂ A
◗ *N52.1 Erectile dysfunction due to diseases classified elsewhere* ♂ A
Code first underlying disease
N52.2 Drug-induced erectile dysfunction ♂ A
● **N52.3 Postprocedural erectile dysfunction** ⇐
N52.31 Erectile dysfunction following radical prostatectomy ♂ A
N52.32 Erectile dysfunction following radical cystectomy ♂ A
N52.33 Erectile dysfunction following urethral surgery ♂ A
N52.34 Erectile dysfunction following simple prostatectomy ♂ A
N52.35 Erectile dysfunction following radiation therapy ♂ ◀ A
N52.36 Erectile dysfunction following interstitial seed therapy ♂ ◀ A
N52.37 Erectile dysfunction following prostate ablative therapy ♂ ◀ A
Erectile dysfunction following cryotherapy ◀
Erectile dysfunction following other prostate ablative therapies ◀
Erectile dysfunction following ultrasound ablative therapies ◀
N52.39 Other and unspecified postprocedural erectile dysfunction ♂ ⇐ A
N52.8 Other male erectile dysfunction ♂ A
N52.9 Male erectile dysfunction, unspecified ♂ A
Impotence NOS

● **N53 Other male sexual dysfunction**
Excludes1 psychogenic sexual dysfunction (F52.-)
● **N53.1 Ejaculatory dysfunction**
Excludes1 premature ejaculation (F52.4)
N53.11 Retarded ejaculation ♂
N53.12 Painful ejaculation ♂
N53.13 Anejaculatory orgasm ♂
N53.14 Retrograde ejaculation ♂
N53.19 Other ejaculatory dysfunction ♂
Ejaculatory dysfunction NOS
N53.8 Other male sexual dysfunction ♂
N53.9 Unspecified male sexual dysfunction ♂

DISORDERS OF BREAST (N60-N65)

Excludes1 disorders of breast associated with childbirth (O91-O92)

● **N60 Benign mammary dysplasia**
Benign lumpiness of breast
Includes fibrocystic mastopathy
● **N60.0 Solitary cyst of breast**
Cyst of breast
N60.01 Solitary cyst of right breast
N60.02 Solitary cyst of left breast
N60.09 Solitary cyst of unspecified breast

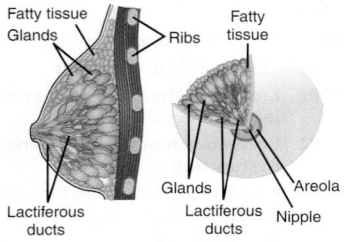

Figure 14-9 Breast.

● **N60.1 Diffuse cystic mastopathy**
Cystic breast
Fibrocystic disease of breast
Excludes1 diffuse cystic mastopathy with epithelial proliferation (N60.3-)
N60.11 Diffuse cystic mastopathy of right breast A
N60.12 Diffuse cystic mastopathy of left breast A
N60.19 Diffuse cystic mastopathy of unspecified breast A

● **N60.2 Fibroadenosis of breast**
Adenofibrosis of breast
Excludes2 fibroadenoma of breast (D24.-)
N60.21 Fibroadenosis of right breast
N60.22 Fibroadenosis of left breast
N60.29 Fibroadenosis of unspecified breast

● **N60.3 Fibrosclerosis of breast**
Cystic mastopathy with epithelial proliferation
N60.31 Fibrosclerosis of right breast
N60.32 Fibrosclerosis of left breast
N60.39 Fibrosclerosis of unspecified breast

● **N60.4 Mammary duct ectasia**
N60.41 Mammary duct ectasia of right breast
N60.42 Mammary duct ectasia of left breast
N60.49 Mammary duct ectasia of unspecified breast

● **N60.8 Other benign mammary dysplasias**
N60.81 Other benign mammary dysplasias of right breast
N60.82 Other benign mammary dysplasias of left breast
N60.89 Other benign mammary dysplasias of unspecified breast

● **N60.9 Unspecified benign mammary dysplasia**
N60.91 Unspecified benign mammary dysplasia of right breast
N60.92 Unspecified benign mammary dysplasia of left breast
N60.99 Unspecified benign mammary dysplasia of unspecified breast

● **N61 Inflammatory disorders of breast**
Excludes1 inflammatory carcinoma of breast (C50.9)
inflammatory disorder of breast associated with childbirth (O91.-)
neonatal infective mastitis (P39.0)
thrombophlebitis of breast [Mondor's disease] (I80.8)
N61.0 Mastitis without abscess ◀
Infective mastitis (acute) (nonpuerperal) (subacute) ◀
Mastitis (acute) (nonpuerperal) (subacute) NOS ◀
Cellulitis (acute) (nonpuerperal) (subacute) of breast NOS ◀
Cellulitis (acute) (nonpuerperal) (subacute) of nipple NOS ◀
N61.1 Abscess of the breast and nipple ◀
Abscess (acute) (chronic) (nonpuerperal) of areola ◀
Abscess (acute) (chronic) (nonpuerperal) of breast ◀
Carbuncle of breast ◀
Mastitis with abscess ◀

N62 Hypertrophy of breast
Gynecomastia
Hypertrophy of breast NOS
Massive pubertal hypertrophy of breast
Excludes1 breast engorgement of newborn (P83.4)
disproportion of reconstructed breast (N65.1)

N63 Unspecified lump in breast
Nodule(s) NOS in breast

● **N64 Other disorders of breast**
Excludes2 mechanical complication of breast prosthesis and implant (T85.4-)
N64.0 Fissure and fistula of nipple
● **N64.1 Fat necrosis of breast**
Fat necrosis (segmental) of breast
Code first breast necrosis due to breast graft (T85.898) ⇐
N64.2 Atrophy of breast
N64.3 Galactorrhea not associated with childbirth
Excessive or spontaneous flow of milk
N64.4 Mastodynia
● **N64.5 Other signs and symptoms in breast**
Excludes2 abnormal findings on diagnostic imaging of breast (R92.-)
N64.51 Induration of breast
N64.52 Nipple discharge
Excludes1 abnormal findings in nipple discharge (R89.-)
N64.53 Retraction of nipple
N64.59 Other signs and symptoms in breast
● **N64.8 Other specified disorders of breast**
N64.81 Ptosis of breast A
Excludes1 ptosis of native breast in relation to reconstructed breast (N65.1)
N64.82 Hypoplasia of breast A
Micromastia
Excludes1 congenital absence of breast (Q83.0)
hypoplasia of native breast in relation to reconstructed breast (N65.1)
N64.89 Other specified disorders of breast
Galactocele
Subinvolution of breast (postlactational)
N64.9 Disorder of breast, unspecified

● **N65 Deformity and disproportion of reconstructed breast**
N65.0 Deformity of reconstructed breast A
Contour irregularity in reconstructed breast
Excess tissue in reconstructed breast
Misshapen reconstructed breast
N65.1 Disproportion of reconstructed breast A
Breast asymmetry between native breast and reconstructed breast
Disproportion between native breast and reconstructed breast

◀ New ⇐ Revised ~~deleted~~ Deleted Excludes 1 Excludes 2 Includes Use additional Code first Code also Unspecified
OGCR Official Guidelines ● Unacceptable Principal Diagnosis X Assign placeholder X ● Use Additional Character(s) ◗ Manifestation Code Coding Clinic

INFLAMMATORY DISEASES OF FEMALE PELVIC ORGANS (N70-N77)

Excludes1 inflammatory diseases of female pelvic organs complicating:
abortion or ectopic or molar pregnancy (O00-O07, O08.0)
pregnancy, childbirth and the puerperium (O23.-, O75.3, O85, O86.-)

★**(See Plate 360 on page 80.)**

N70 Salpingitis and oophoritis
Oophoritis = inflammation of ovary
Salpingitis = inflammation of falloplan tube
Includes abscess (of) fallopian tube
abscess (of) ovary
pyosalpinx
salpingo-oophoritis
tubo-ovarian abscess
tubo-ovarian inflammatory disease
Use additional code (B95-B97), to identify infectious agent
Excludes1 gonococcal infection (A54.24)
tuberculous infection (A18.17)

N70.0 Acute salpingitis and oophoritis
Ex: **For category N70.0 CC codes:** A17.9, A18.10, A18.16-A18.18, A18.82, A18.84, A18.89, A54.03, A54.24, A54.82, A54.84, A54.89-A54.9, A59.00, A59.8-A59.9, B37.41-B37.49, N70.01-N71.9, N73.0-N74, N75.9, N76.5, N76.81-N76.89, N90.810-N90.818, N94.818-N94.9, N96, Q55.0-Q55.4, Q55.7-Q55.9

N70.01 Acute salpingitis ♀
N70.02 Acute oophoritis ♀
N70.03 Acute salpingitis and oophoritis ♀

N70.1 Chronic salpingitis and oophoritis
Hydrosalpinx

N70.11 Chronic salpingitis ♀
N70.12 Chronic oophoritis ♀
N70.13 Chronic salpingitis and oophoritis ♀

N70.9 Salpingitis and oophoritis, unspecified

N70.91 Salpingitis, unspecified ♀
N70.92 Oophoritis, unspecified ♀
N70.93 Salpingitis and oophoritis, unspecified ♀

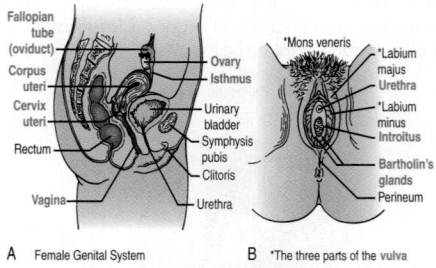

Figure 14-10 A. Female genital system. **B.** External female genital system. (From Buck CJ: Step-by-Step Medical Coding, ed 2016, St. Louis, Elsevier, 2016)

Item 14-10 Salpingitis is an infection of one or both fallopian tubes. **Oophoritis** is an infection of one or both ovaries.

N71 Inflammatory disease of uterus, except cervix
Includes endo (myo) metritis
metritis
myometritis
pyometra
uterine abscess
Use additional code (B95-B97), to identify infectious agent
Excludes1 hyperplastic endometritis (N85.0-)
infection of uterus following delivery (O85, O86.-)

N71.0 Acute inflammatory disease of uterus ♀
Ex: A17.9, A18.10, A18.16-A18.18, A18.82, A18.84, A18.89, A54.03, A54.24, A54.82, A54.84, A54.89-A54.9, A59.00, A59.8-A59.9, B37.41-B37.49, N70.01-N71.9, N72, N73.0-N74, N75.9, N76.5, N76.81-N76.89, N85.8-N85.9, N90.810-N90.818, N94.818-N94.9, N96, Q55.0-Q55.4, Q55.7-Q55.9

N71.1 Chronic inflammatory disease of uterus ♀
N71.9 Inflammatory disease of uterus, unspecified ♀

N72 Inflammatory disease of cervix uteri ♀
Includes cervicitis (with or without erosion or ectropion)
endocervicitis (with or without erosion or ectropion)
exocervicitis (with or without erosion or ectropion)
Use additional code (B95-B97), to identify infectious agent
Excludes1 erosion and ectropion of cervix without cervicitis (N86)

N73 Other female pelvic inflammatory diseases
Use additional code (B95-B97), to identify infectious agent

N73.0 Acute parametritis and pelvic cellulitis ♀
Abscess of broad ligament
Abscess of parametrium
Pelvic cellulitis, female
Ex: See N70.0

N73.1 Chronic parametritis and pelvic cellulitis ♀
Any condition in N73.0 specified as chronic
Excludes1 tuberculous parametritis and pelvic cellultis (A18.17)

N73.2 Unspecified parametritis and pelvic cellulitis ♀
Any condition in N73.0 unspecified whether acute or chronic

N73.3 Female acute pelvic peritonitis ♀
Ex: See N70.0

N73.4 Female chronic pelvic peritonitis ♀
Excludes1 tuberculous pelvic (female) peritonitis (A18.17)
Ex: See N70.0

N73.5 Female pelvic peritonitis, unspecified ♀
N73.6 Female pelvic peritoneal adhesions (postinfective) ♀
Excludes2 postprocedural pelvic peritoneal adhesions (N99.4)
N73.8 Other specified female pelvic inflammatory diseases ♀
N73.9 Female pelvic inflammatory disease, unspecified ♀
Female pelvic infection or inflammation NOS

N74 Female pelvic inflammatory disorders in diseases classified elsewhere ♀
Code first underlying disease
Excludes1 chlamydial cervicitis (A56.02)
chlamydial pelvic inflammatory disease (A56.11)
gonococcal cervicitis (A54.03)
gonococcal pelvic inflammatory disease (A54.24)
herpesviral [herpes simplex] cervicitis (A60.03)
herpesviral [herpes simplex] pelvic inflammatory disease (A60.09)
syphilitic cervicitis (A52.76)
syphilitic pelvic inflammatory disease (A52.76)
trichomonal cervicitis (A59.09)
tuberculous cervicitis (A18.16)
tuberculous pelvic inflammatory disease (A18.17)

● **N75 Diseases of Bartholin's gland**

N75.0 Cyst of Bartholin's gland ♀
Cysts filled with liquid or semisolid material

N75.1 Abscess of Bartholin's gland ♀
Localized collection of pus
Ex: A17.9, A18.10, A18.16-A18.18, A18.82, A18.84, A18.89, A59.00-A59.01, A59.8-A59.9, B37.3-B37.49, N75.0-N77.1, N84.3, N90.3, N90.60-N90.9, N94.810-N94.9, N96, Q55.0-Q55.4, Q55.7-Q55.9

N75.8 Other diseases of Bartholin's gland ♀
Bartholinitis

N75.9 Disease of Bartholin's gland, unspecified ♀

● **N76 Other inflammation of vagina and vulva**
Use additional code (B95-B97), to identify infectious agent
Excludes2 senile (atrophic) vaginitis (N95.2)
vulvar vestibulitis (N94.810)

N76.0 Acute vaginitis ♀
Acute vulvovaginitis
Vaginitis NOS
Vulvovaginitis NOS

N76.1 Subacute and chronic vaginitis ♀
Chronic vulvovaginitis
Subacute vulvovaginitis

N76.2 Acute vulvitis ♀
Vulvitis NOS

N76.3 Subacute and chronic vulvitis ♀

N76.4 Abscess of vulva ♀
Furuncle of vulva
Ex: See N75.1

N76.5 Ulceration of vagina ♀

N76.6 Ulceration of vulva ♀

● **N76.8 Other specified inflammation of vagina and vulva**

N76.81 Mucositis (ulcerative) of vagina and vulva ♀
Code also type of associated therapy, such as:
antineoplastic and immunosuppressive drugs (T45.1X-)
radiological procedure and radiotherapy (Y84.2)
Excludes2 gastrointestinal mucositis (ulcerative) (K92.81)
nasal mucositis (ulcerative) (J34.81)
oral mucositis (ulcerative) (K12.3-)
Ex: N72, N75.9, N76.5, N76.81-N76.89

N76.89 Other specified inflammation of vagina and vulva ♀

● **N77 Vulvovaginal ulceration and inflammation in diseases classified elsewhere**

▶ ***N77.0 Ulceration of vulva in diseases classified elsewhere ♀***
Code first underlying disease, such as:
Behçet's disease (M35.2)
Excludes1 ulceration of vulva in gonococcal infection (A54.02)
ulceration of vulva in herpesviral [herpes simplex] infection (A60.04)
ulceration of vulva in syphilis (A51.0)
ulceration of vulva in tuberculosis (A18.18)

▶ ***N77.1 Vaginitis, vulvitis and vulvovaginitis in diseases classified elsewhere ♀***
Code first underlying disease, such as:
pinworm (B80)
Excludes1 candidial vulvovaginitis (B37.3)
chlamydial vulvovaginitis (A56.02)
gonococcal vulvovaginitis (A54.02)
herpesviral [herpes simplex] vulvovaginitis (A60.04)
trichomonal vulvovaginitis (A59.01)
tuberculous vulvovaginitis (A18.18)
vulvovaginitis in early syphilis (A51.0)
vulvovaginitis in late syphilis (A52.76)

NONINFLAMMATORY DISORDERS OF FEMALE GENITAL TRACT (N80-N98)

● **N80 Endometriosis**

N80.0 Endometriosis of uterus ♀
Adenomyosis
Excludes1 stromal endometriosis (D39.0)

N80.1 Endometriosis of ovary ♀

N80.2 Endometriosis of fallopian tube ♀

N80.3 Endometriosis of pelvic peritoneum ♀

N80.4 Endometriosis of rectovaginal septum and vagina ♀

N80.5 Endometriosis of intestine ♀

N80.6 Endometriosis in cutaneous scar ♀

N80.8 Other endometriosis ♀

N80.9 Endometriosis, unspecified ♀

● **N81 Female genital prolapse**
Excludes1 genital prolapse complicating pregnancy, labor or delivery (O34.5-)
prolapse and hernia of ovary and fallopian tube (N83.4-) ◀
prolapse of vaginal vault after hysterectomy (N99.3)

N81.0 Urethrocele ♀
Excludes1 urethrocele with cystocele (N81.1-)
urethrocele with prolapse of uterus (N81.2-N81.4)

● **N81.1 Cystocele**
Cystocele with urethrocele
Cystourethrocele
Excludes1 cystocele with prolapse of uterus (N81.2-N81.4)

N81.10 Cystocele, unspecified ♀
Prolapse of (anterior) vaginal wall NOS

N81.11 Cystocele, midline ♀

N81.12 Cystocele, lateral ♀
Paravaginal cystocele

N81.2 Incomplete uterovaginal prolapse ♀
First degree uterine prolapse
Prolapse of cervix NOS
Second degree uterine prolapse
Excludes1 cervical stump prolaspe (N81.85)

N81.3 Complete uterovaginal prolapse ♀
Procidentia (uteri) NOS
Third degree uterine prolapse

N81.4 Uterovaginal prolapse, unspecified ♀
Prolapse of uterus NOS

Item 14–11 Endometriosis is a condition for which no clear cause has been identified. Endometrial tissue is expelled from the uterus into the abdominal cavity and can implant onto a variety of organs. Classification is based on the site of implant of the endometrial tissue.

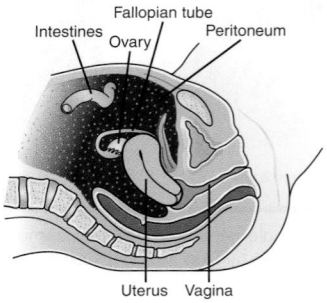

Figure 14-11 Sites of potential endometrial implants.

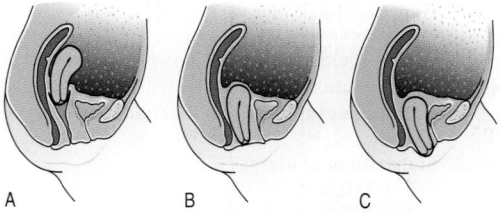

Figure 14-12 Three stages of uterine prolapse. **A.** Uterus is prolapsed. **B.** Vagina and uterus are prolapsed (incomplete uterovaginal prolapse). **C.** Vagina and uterus are completely prolapsed and are exposed through the external genitalia (complete uterovaginal prolapse).

N81.5 Vaginal enterocele ♀
Excludes1 enterocele with prolapse of uterus (N81.2-N81.4)

N81.6 Rectocele ♀
Prolapse of posterior vaginal wall
Use additional code for any associated fecal incontinence, if applicable (R15.-)
Excludes2 perineocele (N81.81)
rectal prolapse (K62.3)
rectocele with prolapse of uterus (N81.2-N81.4)

N81.8 Other female genital prolapse
N81.81 Perineocele ♀
N81.82 Incompetence or weakening of pubocervical tissue ♀
N81.83 Incompetence or weakening of rectovaginal tissue ♀
N81.84 Pelvic muscle wasting ♀
Disuse atrophy of pelvic muscles and anal sphincter
N81.85 Cervical stump prolapse ♀
N81.89 Other female genital prolapse ♀
Deficient perineum
Old laceration of muscles of pelvic floor

N81.9 Female genital prolapse, unspecified ♀

N82 Fistulae involving female genital tract
Excludes1 vesicointestinal fistulae (N32.1)
Ex For category N82 CC codes: N82.0-N82.9

N82.0 Vesicovaginal fistula ♀ CC
N82.1 Other female urinary-genital tract fistulae ♀ CC
Cervicovesical fistula
Ureterovaginal fistula
Urethrovaginal fistula
Uteroureteric fistula
Uterovesical fistula
N82.2 Fistula of vagina to small intestine ♀ CC
N82.3 Fistula of vagina to large intestine ♀ CC
Rectovaginal fistula
N82.4 Other female intestinal-genital tract fistulae ♀ CC
Intestinouterine fistula
N82.5 Female genital tract-skin fistulae ♀ CC
Uterus to abdominal wall fistula
Vaginoperineal fistula
N82.8 Other female genital tract fistulae ♀ CC
N82.9 Female genital tract fistula, unspecified ♀ CC

N83 Noninflammatory disorders of ovary, fallopian tube and broad ligament
Excludes2 hydrosalpinx (N70.1-)

N83.0 Follicular cyst of ovary
Cyst of graafian follicle
Hemorrhagic follicular cyst (of ovary)
N83.00 Follicular cyst of ovary, unspecified side ♀ ◀
N83.01 Follicular cyst of right ovary ♀ ◀
N83.02 Follicular cyst of left ovary ♀ ◀

N83.1 Corpus luteum cyst
Hemorrhagic corpus luteum cyst
N83.10 Corpus luteum cyst of ovary, unspecified side ♀ ◀
N83.11 Corpus luteum cyst of right ovary ♀ ◀
N83.12 Corpus luteum cyst of left ovary ♀ ◀

N83.2 Other and unspecified ovarian cysts
Excludes1 developmental ovarian cyst (Q50.1)
neoplastic ovarian cyst (D27.-)
polycystic ovarian syndrome (E28.2)
Stein-Leventhal syndrome (E28.2)

N83.20 Unspecified ovarian cysts
N83.201 Unspecified ovarian cyst, right side ♀ ◀
N83.202 Unspecified ovarian cyst, left side ♀ ◀
N83.209 Unspecified ovarian cyst, unspecified side ♀ ◀
Ovarian cyst, NOS ◀

N83.29 Other ovarian cysts
Retention cyst of ovary
Simple cyst of ovary
N83.291 Other ovarian cyst, right side ♀ ◀
N83.292 Other ovarian cyst, left side ♀ ◀
N83.299 Other ovarian cyst, unspecified side ♀ ◀

N83.3 Acquired atrophy of ovary and fallopian tube

N83.31 Acquired atrophy of ovary
N83.311 Acquired atrophy of right ovary ♀ ◀
N83.312 Acquired atrophy of left ovary ♀ ◀
N83.319 Acquired atrophy of ovary, unspecified side ♀ ◀
Acquired atrophy of ovary, NOS ◀

N83.32 Acquired atrophy of fallopian tube
N83.321 Acquired atrophy of right fallopian tube ♀ ◀
N83.322 Acquired atrophy of left fallopian tube ♀ ◀
N83.329 Acquired atrophy of fallopian tube, unspecified side ♀ ◀
Acquired atrophy of fallopian tube, NOS ◀

N83.33 Acquired atrophy of ovary and fallopian tube
N83.331 Acquired atrophy of right ovary and fallopian tube ♀ ◀
N83.332 Acquired atrophy of left ovary and fallopian tube ♀ ◀
N83.339 Acquired atrophy of ovary and fallopian tube, unspecified side ♀ ◀
Acquired atrophy of ovary and fallopian tube, NOS ◀

N83.4 Prolapse and hernia of ovary and fallopian tube
N83.40 Prolapse and hernia of ovary and fallopian tube, unspecified side ♀ ◀
Prolapse and hernia of ovary and fallopian tube, NOS ◀
N83.41 Prolapse and hernia of right ovary and fallopian tube ♀ ◀
N83.42 Prolapse and hernia of left ovary and fallopian tube ♀ ◀

● **N83.5 Torsion of ovary, ovarian pedicle and fallopian tube**
Torsion of accessory tube
Ex For category N83.5 CC codes: N83.00-N83.53, N83.6-N83.9, N99.83

● **N83.51 Torsion of ovary and ovarian pedicle**

N83.511 Torsion of right ovary and ovarian pedicle ♀ ◀

N83.512 Torsion of left ovary and ovarian pedicle ♀ ◀

N83.519 Torsion of ovary and ovarian pedicle, unspecified side ♀ ◀
Torsion of ovary and ovarian pedicle, NOS ◀

● **N83.52 Torsion of fallopian tube**
Torsion of hydatid of Morgagni

N83.521 Torsion of right fallopian tube ♀ ◀

N83.522 Torsion of left fallopian tube ♀ ◀

N83.529 Torsion of fallopian tube, unspecified side ♀ ◀
Torsion of fallopian tube, NOS ◀

N83.53 Torsion of ovary, ovarian pedicle and fallopian tube ♀

N83.6 Hematosalpinx ♀
Excludes1 hematosalpinx (with) (in):
hematocolpos (N89.7)
hematometra (N85.7)
tubal pregnancy (O00.1-) ◀

N83.7 Hematoma of broad ligament ♀

N83.8 Other noninflammatory disorders of ovary, fallopian tube and broad ligament ♀
Broad ligament laceration syndrome [Allen-Masters]

N83.9 Noninflammatory disorder of ovary, fallopian tube and broad ligament, unspecified ♀

● **N84 Polyp of female genital tract**
Excludes1 adenomatous polyp (D28.-)
placental polyp (O90.89)

N84.0 Polyp of corpus uteri ♀
Polyp of endometrium
Polyp of uterus NOS
Excludes1 polypoid endometrial hyperplasia (N85.0-)

N84.1 Polyp of cervix uteri ♀
Mucous polyp of cervix

N84.2 Polyp of vagina ♀

N84.3 Polyp of vulva ♀
Polyp of labia

N84.8 Polyp of other parts of female genital tract ♀

N84.9 Polyp of female genital tract, unspecified ♀

● **N85 Other noninflammatory disorders of uterus, except cervix**
Excludes1 endometriosis (N80.-)
inflammatory diseases of uterus (N71.-)
noninflammatory disorders of cervix, except malposition (N86-N88)
polyp of corpus uteri (N84.0)
uterine prolapse (N81.-)

● **N85.0 Endometrial hyperplasia**

N85.00 Endometrial hyperplasia, unspecified ♀
Hyperplasia (adenomatous) (cystic) (glandular) of endometrium
Hyperplastic endometritis

N85.01 Benign endometrial hyperplasia ♀
Endometrial hyperplasia (complex) (simple) without atypia

N85.02 Endometrial intraepithelial neoplasia [EIN] ♀
Endometrial hyperplasia with atypia
Excludes1 malignant neoplasm of endometrium (with endometrial intraepithelial neoplasia [EIN]) (C54.1)

N85.2 Hypertrophy of uterus ♀
Bulky or enlarged uterus
Excludes1 puerperal hypertrophy of uterus (O90.89)

N85.3 Subinvolution of uterus ♀
Excludes1 puerperal subinvolution of uterus (O90.89)

N85.4 Malposition of uterus ♀
Anteversion of uterus
Retroflexion of uterus
Retroversion of uterus
Excludes1 malposition of uterus complicating pregnancy, labor or delivery (O34.5-, O65.5)

N85.5 Inversion of uterus ♀
Excludes1 current obstetric trauma (O71.2)
postpartum inversion of uterus (O71.2)

N85.6 Intrauterine synechiae ♀

N85.7 Hematometra ♀
Hematosalpinx with hematometra
Excludes1 hematometra with hematocolpos (N89.7)

N85.8 Other specified noninflammatory disorders of uterus ♀
Atrophy of uterus, acquired
Fibrosis of uterus NOS

N85.9 Noninflammatory disorder of uterus, unspecified ♀
Disorder of uterus NOS

N86 Erosion and ectropion of cervix uteri ♀
Decubitus (trophic) ulcer of cervix
Eversion of cervix
Excludes1 erosion and ectropion of cervix with cervicitis (N72)

● **N87 Dysplasia of cervix uteri**
Excludes1 abnormal results from cervical cytologic examination without histologic confirmation (R87.61-)
carcinoma in situ of cervix uteri (D06.-)
cervical intraepithelial neoplasia III [CIN III] (D06.-)
HGSIL of cervix (R87.613)
severe dysplasia of cervix uteri (D06.-)

N87.0 Mild cervical dysplasia ♀
Cervical intraepithelial neoplasia I [CIN I]

N87.1 Moderate cervical dysplasia ♀
Cervical intraepithelial neoplasia II [CIN II]

N87.9 Dysplasia of cervix uteri, unspecified ♀
Anaplasia of cervix
Cervical atypism
Cervical dysplasia NOS

● **N88 Other noninflammatory disorders of cervix uteri**
Excludes2 inflammatory disease of cervix (N72)
polyp of cervix (N84.1)

N88.0 Leukoplakia of cervix uteri ♀

N88.1 Old laceration of cervix uteri ♀
Adhesions of cervix
Excludes1 current obstetric trauma (O71.3)

N88.2 Stricture and stenosis of cervix uteri ♀
Excludes1 stricture and stenosis of cervix uteri complicating labor (O65.5)

N88.3 Incompetence of cervix uteri ♀
Investigation and management of (suspected) cervical incompetence in a nonpregnant woman
Excludes1 cervical incompetence complicating pregnancy (O34.3-)

N88.4 Hypertrophic elongation of cervix uteri ♀

N88.8 Other specified noninflammatory disorders of cervix uteri ♀
Excludes1 current obstetric trauma (O71.3)

N88.9 Noninflammatory disorder of cervix uteri, unspecified ♀

N89 Other noninflammatory disorders of vagina

Excludes1 abnormal results from vaginal cytologic examination without histologic confirmation (R87.62-)
carcinoma in situ of vagina (D07.2)
HGSIL of vagina (R87.623)
inflammation of vagina (N76.-)
senile (atrophic) vaginitis (N95.2)
severe dysplasia of vagina (D07.2)
trichomonal leukorrhea (A59.00)
vaginal intraepithelial neoplasia [VAIN], grade III (D07.2)

N89.0 Mild vaginal dysplasia ♀
Vaginal intraepithelial neoplasia [VAIN], grade I

N89.1 Moderate vaginal dysplasia ♀
Vaginal intraepithelial neoplasia [VAIN], grade II

N89.3 Dysplasia of vagina, unspecified ♀

N89.4 Leukoplakia of vagina ♀

N89.5 Stricture and atresia of vagina ♀
Vaginal adhesions Vaginal stenosis

Excludes1 congenital atresia or stricture (Q52.4)
postprocedural adhesions of vagina (N99.2)

N89.6 Tight hymenal ring ♀
Rigid hymen Tight introitus

Excludes1 imperforate hymen (Q52.3)

N89.7 Hematocolpos ♀
Hematocolpos with hematometra or hematosalpinx

N89.8 Other specified noninflammatory disorders of vagina ♀
Leukorrhea NOS
Old vaginal laceration
Pessary ulcer of vagina

Excludes1 current obstetric trauma (O70.-, O71.4, O71.7-O71.8)
old laceration involving muscles of pelvic floor (N81.8)

N89.9 Noninflammatory disorder of vagina, unspecified ♀

N90 Other noninflammatory disorders of vulva and perineum

Excludes1 anogenital (venereal) warts (A63.0)
carcinoma in situ of vulva (D07.1)
condyloma acuminatum (A63.0)
current obstetric trauma (O70.-, O71.7-O71.8)
inflammation of vulva (N76.-)
severe dysplasia of vulva (D07.1)
vulvar intraepithelial neoplasm III [VIN III] (D07.1)

N90.0 Mild vulvar dysplasia ♀
Vulvar intraepithelial neoplasia [VIN], grade I

N90.1 Moderate vulvar dysplasia ♀
Vulvar intraepithelial neoplasia [VIN], grade II

N90.3 Dysplasia of vulva, unspecified ♀

N90.4 Leukoplakia of vulva ♀
Dystrophy of vulva
Kraurosis of vulva
Lichen sclerosus of external female genital organs

N90.5 Atrophy of vulva ♀
Stenosis of vulva

N90.6 Hypertrophy of vulva

N90.60 Unspecified hypertrophy of vulva ♀ ◀
Unspecified hypertrophy of labia ◀

N90.61 Childhood asymmetric labium majus enlargement ♀ ◀
CALME ◀

N90.69 Other specified hypertrophy of vulva ♀ ◀
Other specified hypertrophy of labia ◀

N90.7 Vulvar cyst ♀

N90.8 Other specified noninflammatory disorders of vulva and perineum

N90.81 Female genital mutilation status
Female genital cutting status

N90.810 Female genital mutilation status, unspecified ♀
Female genital cutting status, unspecified
Female genital mutilation status NOS

N90.811 Female genital mutilation Type I status ♀
Clitorectomy status
Female genital cutting Type I status

N90.812 Female genital mutilation Type II status ♀
Clitorectomy with excision of labia minora status
Female genital cutting Type II status

N90.813 Female genital mutilation Type III status ♀
Female genital cutting Type III status
Infibulation status

N90.818 Other female genital mutilation status ♀
Female genital cutting Type IV status
Female genital mutilation Type IV status
Other female genital cutting status

N90.89 Other specified noninflammatory disorders of vulva and perineum ♀
Adhesions of vulva
Hypertrophy of clitoris

N90.9 Noninflammatory disorder of vulva and perineum, unspecified ♀

N91 Absent, scanty and rare menstruation

Excludes1 ovarian dysfunction (E28.-)

N91.0 Primary amenorrhea ♀

N91.1 Secondary amenorrhea ♀

N91.2 Amenorrhea, unspecified ♀

N91.3 Primary oligomenorrhea ♀

N91.4 Secondary oligomenorrhea ♀

N91.5 Oligomenorrhea, unspecified ♀
Hypomenorrhea NOS

N92 Excessive, frequent and irregular menstruation

Excludes1 postmenopausal bleeding (N95.0)
precocious puberty (menstruation) (E30.1)

N92.0 Excessive and frequent menstruation with regular cycle ♀
Heavy periods NOS Polymenorrhea
Menorrhagia NOS

N92.1 Excessive and frequent menstruation with irregular cycle ♀
Irregular intermenstrual bleeding
Irregular, shortened intervals between menstrual bleeding
Menometrorrhagia
Metrorrhagia

N92.2 Excessive menstruation at puberty ♀ P
Excessive bleeding associated with onset of menstrual periods
Pubertal menorrhagia
Puberty bleeding

N92.3 Ovulation bleeding ♀
Regular intermenstrual bleeding

N92.4 Excessive bleeding in the premenopausal period ♀
Climacteric menorrhagia or metrorrhagia
Menopausal menorrhagia or metrorrhagia
Preclimacteric menorrhagia or metrorrhagia
Premenopausal menorrhagia or metrorrhagia

N92.5 Other specified irregular menstruation ♀

N92.6 Irregular menstruation, unspecified ♀
Irregular bleeding NOS
Irregular periods NOS

Excludes1 irregular menstruation with:
lengthened intervals or scanty bleeding (N91.3-N91.5)
shortened intervals or excessive bleeding (N92.1)

● **N93 Other abnormal uterine and vaginal bleeding**

Excludes1 neonatal vaginal hemorrhage (P54.6)
precocious puberty (menstruation) (E30.1)
pseudomenses (P54.6)

N93.0 Postcoital and contact bleeding ♀

N93.1 Pre-pubertal vaginal bleeding ♀ ◀

N93.8 Other specified abnormal uterine and vaginal bleeding ♀
Dysfunctional or functional uterine or vaginal bleeding NOS

N93.9 Abnormal uterine and vaginal bleeding, unspecified ♀

● **N94 Pain and other conditions associated with female genital organs and menstrual cycle**

N94.0 Mittelschmerz ♀
Ovulation pain

● **N94.1 Dyspareunia**
Painful intercourse/coitus

Excludes1 psychogenic dyspareunia (F52.6)

N94.10 Unspecified dyspareunia ♀ ◀

N94.11 Superficial (introital) dyspareunia ♀ ◀

N94.12 Deep dyspareunia ♀ ◀

N94.19 Other specified dyspareunia ♀ ◀

N94.2 Vaginismus ♀
Vagina tightness

Excludes1 psychogenic vaginismus (F52.5)

N94.3 Premenstrual tension syndrome ♀
AKA: PMS
Premenstrual dysphoric disorder

Code also associated menstrual migraine (G43.82-, G43.83-)

Excludes1 Premenstrual dysphoric disorder (F32.81) ◀

N94.4 Primary dysmenorrhea ♀
Lifelong painful menstruation

N94.5 Secondary dysmenorrhea ♀
Later onset of painful menstruation

N94.6 Dysmenorrhea, unspecified ♀

Excludes1 psychogenic dysmenorrhea (F45.8)

● **N94.8 Other specified conditions associated with female genital organs and menstrual cycle**

● **N94.81 Vulvodynia**

N94.810 Vulvar vestibulitis ♀

N94.818 Other vulvodynia ♀

N94.819 Vulvodynia, unspecified ♀
Vulvodynia NOS

N94.89 Other specified conditions associated with female genital organs and menstrual cycle ♀

N94.9 Unspecified condition associated with female genital organs and menstrual cycle ♀

● **N95 Menopausal and other perimenopausal disorders**
Menopausal and other perimenopausal disorders due to naturally occurring (age-related) menopause and perimenopause

Excludes1 excessive bleeding in the premenopausal period (N92.4)
menopausal and perimenopausal disorders due to artificial or premature menopause (E89.4-, E28.31-)
premature menopause (E28.31-)

Excludes2 postmenopausal osteoporosis (M81.0-)
postmenopausal osteoporosis with current pathological fracture (M80.0-)
postmenopausal urethritis (N34.2)

N95.0 Postmenopausal bleeding ♀

N95.1 Menopausal and female climacteric states ♀
Symptoms such as flushing, sleeplessness, headache, lack of concentration, associated with natural (age-related) menopause

Use additional code for associated symptoms

Excludes1 asymptomatic menopausal state (Z78.0)
symptoms associated with artificial menopause (E89.41)
symptoms associated with premature menopause (E28.310)

N95.2 Postmenopausal atrophic vaginitis ♀
Senile (atrophic) vaginitis

N95.8 Other specified menopausal and perimenopausal disorders ♀

N95.9 Unspecified menopausal and perimenopausal disorder ♀

N96 Recurrent pregnancy loss ♀
Investigation or care in a nonpregnant woman with history of recurrent pregnancy loss

Excludes1 recurrent pregnancy loss with current pregnancy (O26.2-)

● **N97 Female infertility**

Includes inability to achieve a pregnancy
sterility, female NOS

Excludes1 female infertility associated with:
hypopituitarism (E23.0)
Stein-Leventhal syndrome (E28.2)

Excludes2 incompetence of cervix uteri (N88.3)

N97.0 Female infertility associated with anovulation ♀

N97.1 Female infertility of tubal origin ♀
Female infertility associated with congenital anomaly of tube
Female infertility due to tubal block
Female infertility due to tubal occlusion
Female infertility due to tubal stenosis

N97.2 Female infertility of uterine origin ♀
Female infertility associated with congenital anomaly of uterus
Female infertility due to nonimplantation of ovum

N97.8 Female infertility of other origin ♀

N97.9 Female infertility, unspecified ♀

N98 Complications associated with artificial fertilization
Ex: For category N98 CC codes unless otherwise indicated: D78.81-D78.89, E36.8, E89.810-E89.89, H59.011-H59.019, H59.031-H59.099, H59.811-H59.89, H95.811-H95.89, I97.3, L76.81-L76.82, M96.89, N98.1-N98.9, T81.82X[A], T81.89X-T81.9XX[A]

N98.0 Infection associated with artificial insemination ♀
Ex: N98.0, T80.211-T80.29X[A], T82.7XX[A], T88.0XX[A]

N98.1 Hyperstimulation of ovaries ♀
Hyperstimulation of ovaries NOS
Hyperstimulation of ovaries associated with induced ovulation

N98.2 Complications of attempted introduction of fertilized ovum following in vitro fertilization ♀

N98.3 Complications of attempted introduction of embryo in embryo transfer ♀

N98.8 Other complications associated with artificial fertilization ♀

N98.9 Complication associated with artificial fertilization, unspecified ♀

INTRAOPERATIVE AND POSTPROCEDURAL COMPLICATIONS AND DISORDERS OF GENITOURINARY SYSTEM, NOT ELSEWHERE CLASSIFIED (N99)

N99 Intraoperative and postprocedural complications and disorders of genitourinary system, not elsewhere classified
Excludes2 irradiation cystitis (N30.4-)
postoophorectomy osteoporosis with current pathological fracture (M80.8-)
postoophorectomy osteoporosis without current pathological fracture (M81.8)

N99.0 Postprocedural (acute) (chronic) kidney failure
Use additional code to type of kidney disease

N99.1 Postprocedural urethral stricture
Postcatheterization urethral stricture

N99.11 Postprocedural urethral stricture, male

N99.110 Postprocedural urethral stricture, male, meatal ♂

N99.111 Postprocedural bulbous urethral stricture ♂

N99.112 Postprocedural membranous urethral stricture ♂

N99.113 Postprocedural anterior bulbous urethral stricture ♂

N99.114 Postprocedural urethral stricture, male, unspecified ♂

N99.115 Postprocedural fossa navicularis urethral stricture

N99.12 Postprocedural urethral stricture, female ♀

N99.2 Postprocedural adhesions of vagina ♀

N99.3 Prolapse of vaginal vault after hysterectomy ♀

N99.4 Postprocedural pelvic peritoneal adhesions
Excludes2 pelvic peritoneal adhesions NOS (N73.6)
postinfective pelvic peritoneal adhesions (N73.6)

N99.5 Complications of stoma of urinary tract
Excludes2 mechanical complication of urinary catheter (T83.0-)

N99.51 Complication of cystostomy

N99.510 Cystostomy hemorrhage
Ex: D78.81-D78.89, E36.8, E89.810-E89.89, H59.011-H59.019, H59.031-H59.099, H59.811-H59.89, H95.811-H95.89, I97.3, L76.81-L76.82, M96.89, N32.89, N33, N98.1-N98.9, N99.510-N99.518, T81.82X[A], T81.89X-T81.9XX[A], T83.010[A], T83.020[A], T83.030[A], T83.090[A], T83.110-T83.29X[A], T83.410-T83.69X[A], T83.712-T83.714[A], T83.718[A], T83.719A, T83.722-T83.724[A], T83.728-T83.9XX[A], T85.310-T85.311[A], T85.320-T85.321[A], T85.390-T85.391[A], T85.510-T85.9XX[A], T85.810D, T85.820D, T85.830D, T85.840D, T85.850D, T85.860D, T85.890D, T86.820-T86.829, T86.842-T86.849

N99.511 Cystostomy infection
Ex: D78.81-D78.89, E36.8, E89.810-E89.89, H59.011-H59.019, H59.031-H59.099, H59.811-H59.89, H95.811-H95.89, I97.3, L76.81-L76.82, M96.89, N32.89, N33, N39.0, N98.1-N98.9, N99.510-N99.518, R82.71, T81.82X[A], T81.89X-T81.9XX[A], T83.010[A], T83.020[A], T83.030[A], T83.090[A], T83.110-T83.29X[A], T83.410-T83.69X[A], T83.712-T83.714[A], T83.718[A], T83.719A, T83.722A-T83.724A, T83.728-T83.9XX[A], T85.310-T85.311[A], T85.320-T85.321[A], T85.390-T85.391[A], T85.510-T85.9XX[A], T85.810D, T85.820D, T85.830D, T85.840D, T85.850D, T85.860D, T85.890D, T86.842-T86.849

N99.512 Cystostomy malfunction
Ex: D78.81-D78.89, E36.8, E89.810-E89.89, H59.011-H59.019, H59.031-H59.099, H59.811-H59.89, H95.811-H95.89, I97.3, L76.81-L76.82, M96.89, N32.89, N33, N98.1-N98.9, N99.510-N99.518, T81.82XA, T81.89XA-T81.9XXA, T83.010[A], T83.020[A], T83.030[A], T83.090[A], T83.110-T83.29X[A], T83.410-T83.69X[A], T83.712-T83.714[A], T83.718[A], T83.719A, T83.722A-T83.724A, T83.728-T83.9XX[A]

N99.518 Other cystostomy complication
Ex: See N99.510

N99.52 Complication of incontinent external stoma of urinary tract

N99.520 Hemorrhage of incontinent external stoma of urinary tract

N99.521 Infection of incontinent external stoma of urinary tract

N99.522 Malfunction of incontinent external stoma of urinary tract

N99.523 Herniation of incontinent stoma of urinary tract

N99.524 Stenosis of incontinent stoma of urinary tract

N99.528 Other complication of incontinent external stoma of urinary tract

● N99.53 Complication of continent stoma of urinary tract

N99.530 Hemorrhage of continent stoma of urinary tract

N99.531 Infection of continent stoma of urinary tract

N99.532 Malfunction of continent stoma of urinary tract

N99.533 Herniation of continent stoma of urinary tract ◀

N99.534 Stenosis of continent stoma of urinary tract ◀

N99.538 Other complication of continent stoma of urinary tract

● N99.6 Intraoperative hemorrhage and hematoma of a genitourinary system organ or structure complicating a procedure

Excludes1 intraoperative hemorrhage and hematoma of a genitourinary system organ or structure due to accidental puncture or laceration during a procedure (N99.7-)

Ex: **For category N99.6 CC codes:** H95.811-H95.89, I85.01, I85.11, I97.3, K21.9, K22.8, K23-K25.0, K25.2, K25.4, K25.6, K26.0, K26.2, K26.4, K26.6, K27.0, K27.2, K27.4, K27.6, K28.0, K28.2, K28.4, K28.6, K29.01, K29.21, K29.31, K29.41, K29.51, K29.61, K29.71, K29.81, K29.91, K31.811, K55.21, K57.01, K57.11, K57.13, K57.21, K57.31, K57.33, K57.41, K57.51, K57.53, K57.81, K57.91, K57.93, K62.5, K92.0-K92.2, M96.89, N98.1-N98.9, N99.61-N99.62, N99.820-N99.821, N99.840-N99.843, P54.1-P54.3, T81.10X-T81.19X[A], T81.82X[A], T81.89X-T81.9XX[A]

N99.61 Intraoperative hemorrhage and hematoma of a genitourinary system organ or structure complicating a genitourinary system procedure

N99.62 Intraoperative hemorrhage and hematoma of a genitourinary system organ or structure complicating other procedure

● N99.7 Accidental puncture and laceration of a genitourinary system organ or structure during a procedure

Ex: **For category N99.7 CC codes:** D78.11-D78.12, D78.81-D78.89, E36.11-E36.8, E89.810-E89.89, G96.11, G97.41-G97.49, H59.011-H59.019, H59.031-H59.099, H59.211-H59.229, H59.811-H59.89, H95.31-H95.32, H95.811-H95.89, I97.3, I97.51-I97.52, J95.71-J95.72, K91.71-K91.72, L76.11-L76.12, L76.81-L76.82, M96.820-M96.821, M96.89, N98.1-N98.9, N99.71-N99.72, T81.82X[A], T81.89X-T81.9XX[A]

N99.71 Accidental puncture and laceration of a genitourinary system organ or structure during a genitourinary system procedure

N99.72 Accidental puncture and laceration of a genitourinary system organ or structure during other procedure

● N99.8 Other intraoperative and postprocedural complications and disorders of genitourinary system

N99.81 Other intraoperative complications of genitourinary system

● N99.82 Postprocedural hemorrhage of a genitourinary system organ or structure following a procedure

Ex: **For category N99.82 CC codes:** See N99.6

N99.820 Postprocedural hemorrhage of a genitourinary system organ or structure following a genitourinary system procedure

N99.821 Postprocedural hemorrhage of a genitourinary system organ or structure following other procedure

N99.83 Residual ovary syndrome ♀

● N99.84 Postprocedural hematoma and seroma of a genitourinary system organ or structure following a procedure ◀

Ex: **For category N99.84 CC codes:** See N99.6

N99.840 Postprocedural hematoma of a genitourinary system organ or structure following a genitourinary system procedure ◀

N99.841 Postprocedural hematoma of a genitourinary system organ or structure following other procedure ◀

N99.842 Postprocedural seroma of a genitourinary system organ or structure following a genitourinary system procedure ◀

N99.843 Postprocedural seroma of a genitourinary system organ or structure following other procedure ◀

N99.89 Other postprocedural complications and disorders of genitourinary system

CHAPTER 15

PREGNANCY, CHILDBIRTH AND THE PUERPERIUM (O00-O9A)

OGCR Chapter-Specific Coding Guidelines

15. Chapter 15: Pregnancy, Childbirth, and the Puerperium (O00-O9A)

a. General Rules for Obstetric Cases

1) Codes from chapter 15 and sequencing priority

Obstetric cases require codes from chapter 15, codes in the range O00-O9A, Pregnancy, Childbirth, and the Puerperium. Chapter 15 codes have sequencing priority over codes from other chapters. Additional codes from other chapters may be used in conjunction with chapter 15 codes to further specify conditions. Should the provider document that the pregnancy is incidental to the encounter, then code Z33.1, Pregnant state, incidental, should be used in place of any chapter 15 codes. It is the provider's responsibility to state that the condition being treated is not affecting the pregnancy.

2) Chapter 15 codes used only on the maternal record

Chapter 15 codes are to be used only on the maternal record, never on the record of the newborn.

3) Final character for trimester

The majority of codes in Chapter 15 have a final character indicating the trimester of pregnancy. The timeframes for the trimesters are indicated at the beginning of the chapter. If trimester is not a component of a code it is because the condition always occurs in a specific trimester, or the concept of trimester of pregnancy is not applicable. Certain codes have characters for only certain trimesters because the condition does not occur in all trimesters, but it may occur in more than just one.

Assignment of the final character for trimester should be based on the provider's documentation of the trimester (or number of weeks) for the current admission/encounter. This applies to the assignment of trimester for pre-existing conditions as well as those that develop during or are due to the pregnancy. The provider's documentation of the number of weeks may be used to assign the appropriate code identifying the trimester.

Whenever delivery occurs during the current admission, and there is an "in childbirth" option for the obstetric complication being coded, the "in childbirth" code should be assigned.

4) Selection of trimester for inpatient admissions that encompass more than one trimester

In instances when a patient is admitted to a hospital for complications of pregnancy during one trimester and remains in the hospital into a subsequent trimester, the trimester character for the antepartum complication code should be assigned on the basis of the trimester when the complication developed, not the trimester of the discharge. If the condition developed prior to the current admission/encounter or represents a pre-existing condition, the trimester character for the trimester at the time of the admission/encounter should be assigned.

5) Unspecified trimester

Each category that includes codes for trimester has a code for "unspecified trimester." The "unspecified trimester" code should rarely be used, such as when the documentation in the record is insufficient to determine the trimester and it is not possible to obtain clarification.

6) 7th character for Fetus Identification

Where applicable, a 7th character is to be assigned for certain categories (O31, O32, O33.3 - O33.6, O35, O36, O40, O41, O60.1, O60.2, O64, and O69) to identify the fetus for which the complication code applies.

Assign 7th character "0":

- For single gestations
- When the documentation in the record is insufficient to determine the fetus affected and it is not possible to obtain clarification.
- When it is not possible to clinically determine which fetus is affected.

b. Selection of OB Principal or First-listed Diagnosis

1) Routine outpatient prenatal visits

For routine outpatient prenatal visits when no complications are present, a code from category Z34, Encounter for supervision of normal pregnancy, should be used as the first-listed diagnosis. These codes should not be used in conjunction with chapter 15 codes.

2) ***Supervision of High-Risk Pregnancy***

Codes from category O09, Supervision of high-risk pregnancy, are intended for use only during the prenatal period. For complications during the labor or delivery episode as a result of a high-risk pregnancy, assign the applicable complication codes from Chapter 15. If there are no complications during the labor or delivery episode, assign code O80, Encounter for full-term uncomplicated delivery.

For routine prenatal outpatient visits for patients with high-risk pregnancies, a code from category O09, Supervision of high-risk pregnancy, should be used as the first-listed diagnosis. Secondary chapter 15 codes may be used in conjunction with these codes if appropriate.

3) Episodes when no delivery occurs

In episodes when no delivery occurs, the principal diagnosis should correspond to the principal complication of the pregnancy which necessitated the encounter. Should more than one complication exist, all of which are treated or monitored, any of the complications codes may be sequenced first.

4) When a delivery occurs

When an obstetric patient is admitted and delivers during that admission, the condition that prompted the admission should be sequenced as the principal diagnosis. If multiple conditions prompted the admission, sequence the one most related to the delivery as the principal diagnosis. A code for any complication of the delivery should be assigned as an additional diagnosis.

In cases of cesarean delivery, if the patient was admitted with a condition that resulted in the performance of a cesarean procedure, that condition should be selected as the principal diagnosis. If the reason for the admission was unrelated to the condition resulting in the cesarean delivery, the condition related to the reason for the admission should be selected as the principal diagnosis.

5) Outcome of delivery

A code from category Z37, Outcome of delivery, should be included on every maternal record when a delivery has occurred. These codes are not to be used on subsequent records or on the newborn record.

c. Pre-existing conditions versus conditions due to the pregnancy

Certain categories in Chapter 15 distinguish between conditions of the mother that existed prior to pregnancy (pre-existing) and those that are a direct result of pregnancy. When assigning codes from Chapter 15, it is important to assess if a condition was pre-existing prior to pregnancy or developed during or due to the pregnancy in order to assign the correct code.

Categories that do not distinguish between pre-existing and pregnancy-related conditions may be used for either. It is acceptable to use codes specifically for the puerperium with codes complicating pregnancy and childbirth if a condition arises postpartum during the delivery encounter.

d. Pre-existing hypertension in pregnancy

Category O10, Pre-existing hypertension complicating pregnancy, childbirth and the puerperium, includes codes for hypertensive heart and hypertensive chronic kidney disease. When assigning one of the O10 codes that includes hypertensive heart disease or hypertensive chronic kidney disease, it is necessary to add a secondary code from the appropriate hypertension category to specify the type of heart failure or chronic kidney disease.

See Section I.C.9. Hypertension.

e. Fetal Conditions Affecting the Management of the Mother

1) Codes from categories O35 and O36

Codes from categories O35, Maternal care for known or suspected fetal abnormality and damage, and O36, Maternal care for other fetal problems, are assigned only when the fetal condition is actually responsible for modifying the management of the mother, i.e., by requiring diagnostic studies, additional observation, special care, or termination of pregnancy. The fact that the fetal condition exists does not justify assigning a code from this series to the mother's record.

2) In utero surgery

In cases when surgery is performed on the fetus, a diagnosis code from category O35, Maternal care for known or suspected fetal abnormality and damage, should be assigned identifying the fetal condition. Assign the appropriate procedure code for the procedure performed.

No code from Chapter 16, the perinatal codes, should be used on the mother's record to identify fetal conditions. Surgery performed in utero on a fetus is still to be coded as an obstetric encounter.

f. HIV Infection in Pregnancy, Childbirth and the Puerperium

During pregnancy, childbirth or the puerperium, a patient admitted because of an HIV-related illness should receive a principal diagnosis from subcategory O98.7-, Human immunodeficiency [HIV] disease complicating pregnancy, childbirth and the puerperium, followed by the code(s) for the HIV-related illness(es).

Patients with asymptomatic HIV infection status admitted during pregnancy, childbirth, or the puerperium should receive codes of O98.7- and Z21, Asymptomatic human immunodeficiency virus [HIV] infection status.

g. Diabetes mellitus in pregnancy

Diabetes mellitus is a significant complicating factor in pregnancy. Pregnant women who are diabetic should be assigned a code from category O24, Diabetes mellitus in pregnancy, childbirth, and the puerperium, first, followed by the appropriate diabetes code(s) (E08-E13) from Chapter 4.

h. Long term use of insulin and oral hypoglycemics
Code Z79.4, Long-term (current) use of insulin **or code Z79.84, Long-term (current) use of oral hypoglycemic drugs,** should also be assigned if the diabetes mellitus is being treated with insulin **or oral medications. If the patient is treated with both oral medications and insulin, only the code for insulin-controlled should be assigned.**

i. Gestational (pregnancy induced) diabetes
Gestational (pregnancy induced) diabetes can occur during the second and third trimester of pregnancy in women who were not diabetic prior to pregnancy. Gestational diabetes can cause complications in the pregnancy similar to those of pre-existing diabetes mellitus. It also puts the woman at greater risk of developing diabetes after the pregnancy. Codes for gestational diabetes are in subcategory O24.4, Gestational diabetes mellitus. No other code from category O24, Diabetes mellitus in pregnancy, childbirth, and the puerperium, should be used with a code from O24.4.

The codes under subcategory O24.4 include diet controlled, insulin controlled**, and controlled by oral hypoglycemic drugs.** If a patient with gestational diabetes is treated with both diet and insulin, only the code for insulin-controlled is required. **If a patient with gestational diabetes is treated with both diet and oral hypoglycemic medications, only the code for "controlled by oral hypoglycemic drugs" is required.** Code Z79.4, Long-term (current) use of insulin **or code Z79.84, Long-term (current) use of oral hypoglycemic drugs,** should not be assigned with codes from subcategory O24.4.

An abnormal glucose tolerance in pregnancy is assigned a code from subcategory O99.81, Abnormal glucose complicating pregnancy, childbirth, and the puerperium.

j. Sepsis and septic shock complicating abortion, pregnancy, childbirth and the puerperium
When assigning a chapter 15 code for sepsis complicating abortion, pregnancy, childbirth, and the puerperium, a code for the specific type of infection should be assigned as an additional diagnosis. If severe sepsis is present, a code from subcategory R65.2, Severe sepsis, and code(s) for associated organ dysfunction(s) should also be assigned as additional diagnoses.

k. Puerperal sepsis
Code O85, Puerperal sepsis, should be assigned with a secondary code to identify the causal organism (e.g., for a bacterial infection, assign a code from category B95-B96, Bacterial infections in conditions classified elsewhere). A code from category A40, Streptococcal sepsis, or A41, Other sepsis, should not be used for puerperal sepsis. If applicable, use additional codes to identify severe sepsis (R65.2-) and any associated acute organ dysfunction.

l. Alcohol and tobacco use during pregnancy, childbirth and the puerperium

1) Alcohol use during pregnancy, childbirth and the puerperium
Codes under subcategory O99.31, Alcohol use complicating pregnancy, childbirth, and the puerperium, should be assigned for any pregnancy case when a mother uses alcohol during the pregnancy or postpartum. A secondary code from category F10, Alcohol related disorders, should also be assigned to identify manifestations of the alcohol use.

2) Tobacco use during pregnancy, childbirth and the puerperium
Codes under subcategory O99.33, Smoking (tobacco) complicating pregnancy, childbirth, and the puerperium, should be assigned for any pregnancy case when a mother uses any type of tobacco product during the pregnancy or postpartum. A secondary code from category F17, Nicotine dependence, should also be assigned to identify the type of nicotine dependence.

m. Poisoning, toxic effects, adverse effects and underdosing in a pregnant patient
A code from subcategory O9A.2, Injury, poisoning and certain other consequences of external causes complicating pregnancy, childbirth, and the puerperium, should be sequenced first, followed by the appropriate injury, poisoning, toxic effect, adverse effect or underdosing code, and then the additional code(s) that specifies the condition caused by the poisoning, toxic effect, adverse effect or underdosing.

See Section I.C.19. Adverse effects, poisoning, underdosing and toxic effects.

n. Normal Delivery, Code O80

1) Encounter for full term uncomplicated delivery
Code O80 should be assigned when a woman is admitted for a full-term normal delivery and delivers a single, healthy infant without any complications antepartum, during the delivery, or postpartum during the delivery episode. Code O80 is always a principal diagnosis. It is not to be used if any other code from chapter 15 is needed to describe a current complication of the antenatal, delivery, or perinatal period. Additional codes from other chapters may be used with code O80 if they are not related to or are in any way complicating the pregnancy.

2) Uncomplicated delivery with resolved antepartum complication
Code O80 may be used if the patient had a complication at some point during the pregnancy, but the complication is not present at the time of the admission for delivery.

3) Outcome of delivery for O80
Z37.0, Single live birth, is the only outcome of delivery code appropriate for use with O80.

o. The Peripartum and Postpartum Periods

1) Peripartum and postpartum periods
The postpartum period begins immediately after delivery and continues for six weeks following delivery. The peripartum period is defined as the last month of pregnancy to five months postpartum.

2) Peripartum and postpartum complication
A postpartum complication is any complication occurring within the six-week period.

3) Pregnancy-related complications after 6 week period
Chapter 15 codes may also be used to describe pregnancy-related complications after the peripartum or postpartum period if the provider documents that a condition is pregnancy related.

4) Admission for routine postpartum care following delivery outside hospital
When the mother delivers outside the hospital prior to admission and is admitted for routine postpartum care and no complications are noted, code Z39.0, Encounter for care and examination of mother immediately after delivery, should be assigned as the principal diagnosis.

5) Pregnancy associated cardiomyopathy
Pregnancy associated cardiomyopathy, code O90.3, is unique in that it may be diagnosed in the third trimester of pregnancy but may continue to progress months after delivery. For this reason, it is referred to as peripartum cardiomyopathy. Code O90.3 is only for use when the cardiomyopathy develops as a result of pregnancy in a woman who did not have pre-existing heart disease.

p. Code O94, Sequelae of complication of pregnancy, childbirth, and the puerperium

1) Code O94
Code O94, Sequelae of complication of pregnancy, childbirth, and the puerperium, is for use in those cases when an initial complication of a pregnancy develops a sequelae requiring care or treatment at a future date.

2) After the initial postpartum period
This code may be used at any time after the initial postpartum period.

3) Sequencing of Code O94
This code, like all sequela codes, is to be sequenced following the code describing the sequelae of the complication.

q. ***Termination of Pregnancy and Spontaneous abortions***

1) Abortion with Liveborn Fetus
When an attempted termination of pregnancy results in a liveborn fetus assign code Z33.2, Encounter for elective termination of pregnancy and a code from category Z37, Outcome of Delivery.

2) Retained Products of Conception following an abortion
Subsequent encounters for retained products of conception following a spontaneous abortion or elective termination of pregnancy are assigned the appropriate code from category O03, Spontaneous abortion, or codes O07.4, Failed attempted termination of pregnancy without complication and Z33.2, Encounter for elective termination of pregnancy. This advice is appropriate even when the patient was discharged previously with a discharge diagnosis of complete abortion.

3) Complications leading to abortion
Codes from Chapter 15 may be used as additional codes to identify any documented complications of the pregnancy in conjunction with codes in categories in O07 and O08.

r. Abuse in a pregnant patient
For suspected or confirmed cases of abuse of a pregnant patient, a code(s) from subcategories O9A.3, Physical abuse complicating pregnancy, childbirth, and the puerperium, O9A.4, Sexual abuse complicating pregnancy, childbirth, and the puerperium, and O9A.5, Psychological abuse complicating pregnancy, childbirth, and the puerperium, should be sequenced first, followed by the appropriate codes (if applicable) to identify any associated current injury due to physical abuse, sexual abuse, and the perpetrator of abuse.

See Section I.C.19. Adult and child abuse, neglect and other maltreatment.

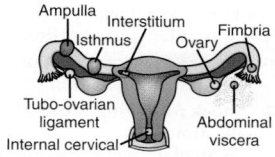

Figure 15-1 Implantation sites of ectopic pregnancy.

Item 15–1 **Ectopic** pregnancy most often occurs in the fallopian tube. Pregnancy outside the uterus may end in a lifethreatening rupture.

★**(See Plate 375 on page 52.)**

CHAPTER 15

PREGNANCY, CHILDBIRTH AND THE PUERPERIUM (O00-O9A)

Note: CODES FROM THIS CHAPTER ARE FOR USE ONLY ON MATERNAL RECORDS, NEVER ON NEWBORN RECORDS

Codes from this chapter are for use for conditions related to or aggravated by the pregnancy, childbirth, or by the puerperium (maternal causes or obstetric causes)

Trimesters are counted from the first day of the last menstrual period. They are defined as follows:

1st trimester - less than 14 weeks 0 days

2nd trimester - 14 weeks 0 days to less than 28 weeks 0 days

3rd trimester - 28 weeks 0 days until delivery

Use additional code from category Z3A, Weeks of gestation, to identify the specific week of the pregnancy, if known.

Excludes1 supervision of normal pregnancy (Z34.-)

Excludes2 mental and behavioral disorders associated with the puerperium (F53)
obstetrical tetanus (A34)
postpartum necrosis of pituitary gland (E23.0)
puerperal osteomalacia (M83.0)

This chapter contains the following blocks:

O00-O08	Pregnancy with abortive outcome
O09	Supervision of high risk pregnancy
O10-O16	Edema, proteinuria and hypertensive disorders in pregnancy, childbirth and the puerperium
O20-O29	Other maternal disorders predominantly related to pregnancy
O30-O48	Maternal care related to the fetus and amniotic cavity and possible delivery problems
O60-O77	Complications of labor and delivery
O80, O82	Encounter for delivery
O85-O92	Complications predominantly related to the puerperium
O94-O9A	Other obstetric conditions, not elsewhere classified

PREGNANCY WITH ABORTIVE OUTCOME (O00-O08)

Excludes1 continuing pregnancy in multiple gestation after abortion of one fetus or more (O31.1-, O31.3-)

O00 Ectopic pregnancy

Includes ruptured ectopic pregnancy

Use additional code from category O08 to identify any associated complication

Ex For category O00 CC codes: O00.00-O00.91

O00.0 Abdominal pregnancy

Excludes1 maternal care for viable fetus in abdominal pregnancy (O36.7-)

O00.00 Abdominal pregnancy without intrauterine pregnancy ♀ ◀ M
Abdominal pregnancy NOS ◀

O00.01 Abdominal pregnancy with intrauterine pregnancy ♀ ◀ M

Item 15–2 A **hydatidiform** mole is an overproduction of placental tissue. The tumor secretes a hormone, chorionic gonadotropic hormone (CGH), that indicates a positive pregnancy test. There is no viable fetus. More than 80% of hydatidiform moles are noncancerous.

O00.1 Tubal pregnancy
Fallopian pregnancy
Rupture of (fallopian) tube due to pregnancy
Tubal abortion

O00.10 Tubal pregnancy without intrauterine pregnancy ♀ ◀ M
Tubal pregnancy NOS ◀

O00.11 Tubal pregnancy with intrauterine pregnancy ♀ ◀ M

O00.2 Ovarian pregnancy

O00.20 Ovarian pregnancy without intrauterine pregnancy ♀ ◀ M
Ovarian pregnancy NOS ◀

O00.21 Ovarian pregnancy with intrauterine pregnancy ♀ ◀ M

O00.8 Other ectopic pregnancy
Cervical pregnancy
Cornual pregnancy
Intraligamentous pregnancy
Mural pregnancy

O00.80 Other ectopic pregnancy without intrauterine pregnancy ♀ ◀ M
Other ectopic pregnancy NOS ◀

O00.81 Other ectopic pregnancy with intrauterine pregnancy ♀ ◀ M

O00.9 Ectopic pregnancy, unspecified

O00.90 Unspecified ectopic pregnancy without intrauterine pregnancy ♀ ◀ M
Ectopic pregnancy NOS ◀

O00.91 Unspecified ectopic pregnancy with intrauterine pregnancy ♀ ◀ M

O01 Hydatidiform mole

Use additional code from category O08 to identify any associated complication

Excludes1 chorioadenoma (destruens) (D39.2)
malignant hydatidiform mole (D39.2)

O01.0 Classical hydatidiform mole ♀ M
Complete hydatidiform mole

O01.1 Incomplete and partial hydatidiform mole ♀ M

O01.9 Hydatidiform mole, unspecified ♀ M
Trophoblastic disease NOS
Vesicular mole NOS

O02 Other abnormal products of conception

Use additional code from category O08 to identify any associated complication

Excludes1 papyraceous fetus (O31.0-)

O02.0 Blighted ovum and nonhydatidiform mole ♀ M
Carneous mole
Fleshy mole
Intrauterine mole NOS
Molar pregnancy NEC
Pathological ovum

O02.1 Missed abortion ♀ M
Early fetal death, before completion of 20 weeks of gestation, with retention of dead fetus

Excludes1 failed induced abortion (O07.-)
fetal death (intrauterine) (late) (O36.4)
missed abortion with blighted ovum (O02.0)
missed abortion with hydatidiform mole (O01.-)
missed abortion with nonhydatidiform (O02.0)
missed abortion with other abnormal products of conception (O02.8-)
missed delivery (O36.4)
stillbirth (P95)

O02.8 Other specified abnormal products of conception

Excludes1 abnormal products of conception with blighted ovum (O02.0)
abnormal products of conception with hydatidiform mole (O01.-)
abnormal products of conception with nonhydatidiform mole (O02.0)

O02.81 Inappropriate change in quantitative human chorionic gonadotropin (hCG) in early pregnancy ♀ M
Biochemical pregnancy
Chemical pregnancy
Inappropriate level of quantitative human chorionic gonadotropin (hCG) for gestational age in early pregnancy

O02.89 Other abnormal products of conception ♀ M

O02.9 Abnormal product of conception, unspecified ♀ M

O03 Spontaneous abortion

Exc **For category O03 CC codes:** G70.1-G72.3, G72.81-G73.7, O11.4, O11.5, O12.04, O12.05, O12.14, O12.15, O12.24, O12.25, O13.4, O13.5, O14.04, O14.05, O14.14, O14.15, O14.24, O14.25, O14.94, O14.95, O16.4, O16.5, O20.0, O20.8, O20.9, O25.10-O25.3, O26.10-O26.93, O29.011-O26.63, O29.8X1-O29.93, O35.7XX0-O35.7XX9, O44.00, O44.53, O45.8X1-O45.93, O75.4, O75.81-O75.9, O80, O90.111-O99.355, O99.511-O99.73, O99.820, O99.824, O99.825, O99.840-O99.845, O99.89, O9A.111-O9A.53, Z33.2

Note: Incomplete abortion includes retained products of conception following spontaneous abortion.

Includes miscarriage

O03.0 Genital tract and pelvic infection following incomplete spontaneous abortion ♀ M
Endometritis following incomplete spontaneous abortion
Oophoritis following incomplete spontaneous abortion
Parametritis following incomplete spontaneous abortion
Pelvic peritonitis following incomplete spontaneous abortion
Salpingitis following incomplete spontaneous abortion
Salpingo-oophoritis following incomplete spontaneous abortion

Excludes1 sepsis following incomplete spontaneous abortion (O03.37)
urinary tract infection following incomplete spontaneous abortion (O03.38)

O03.1 Delayed or excessive hemorrhage following incomplete spontaneous abortion ♀ M
Afibrinogenemia following incomplete spontaneous abortion
Defibrination syndrome following incomplete spontaneous abortion
Hemolysis following incomplete spontaneous abortion
Intravascular coagulation following incomplete spontaneous abortion

O03.2 Embolism following incomplete spontaneous abortion ♀ M
Air embolism following incomplete spontaneous abortion
Amniotic fluid embolism following incomplete spontaneous abortion
Blood-clot embolism following incomplete spontaneous abortion
Embolism NOS following incomplete spontaneous abortion
Fat embolism following incomplete spontaneous abortion
Pulmonary embolism following incomplete spontaneous abortion
Pyemic embolism following incomplete spontaneous abortion
Septic or septicopyemic embolism following incomplete spontaneous abortion
Soap embolism following incomplete spontaneous abortion

O03.3 Other and unspecified complications following incomplete spontaneous abortion

O03.30 Unspecified complication following incomplete spontaneous abortion ♀ M

O03.31 Shock following incomplete spontaneous abortion ♀ M
Circulatory collapse following incomplete spontaneous abortion
Shock (postprocedural) following incomplete spontaneous abortion

Excludes1 shock due to infection following incomplete spontaneous abortion (O03.37)

O03.32 Renal failure following incomplete spontaneous abortion ♀ M
Kidney failure (acute) following incomplete spontaneous abortion
Oliguria following incomplete spontaneous abortion
Renal shutdown following incomplete spontaneous abortion
Renal tubular necrosis following incomplete spontaneous abortion
Uremia following incomplete spontaneous abortion

O03.33 Metabolic disorder following incomplete spontaneous abortion ♀ M

O03.34 Damage to pelvic organs following incomplete spontaneous abortion ♀ M
Laceration, perforation, tear or chemical damage of bladder following incomplete spontaneous abortion
Laceration, perforation, tear or chemical damage of bowel following incomplete spontaneous abortion
Laceration, perforation, tear or chemical damage of broad ligament following incomplete spontaneous abortion
Laceration, perforation, tear or chemical damage of cervix following incomplete spontaneous abortion
Laceration, perforation, tear or chemical damage of periurethral tissue following incomplete spontaneous abortion
Laceration, perforation, tear or chemical damage of uterus following incomplete spontaneous abortion
Laceration, perforation, tear or chemical damage of vagina following incomplete spontaneous abortion

O03.35 Other venous complications following incomplete spontaneous abortion ♀ M

O03.36 Cardiac arrest following incomplete spontaneous abortion ♀ M

O03.37 Sepsis following incomplete spontaneous abortion ♀ M
Use additional code to identify infectious agent (B95-B97)
Use additional code to identify severe sepsis, if applicable (R65.2-)

Excludes1 septic or septicopyemic embolism following incomplete spontaneous abortion (O03.2)

O03.38 Urinary tract infection following incomplete spontaneous abortion ♀ M
Cystitis following incomplete spontaneous abortion

O03.39 Incomplete spontaneous abortion with other complications ♀ M

O03.4 Incomplete spontaneous abortion without complication ♀ M

O03.5 Genital tract and pelvic infection following complete or unspecified spontaneous abortion ♀ M
- Endometritis following complete or unspecified spontaneous abortion
- Oophoritis following complete or unspecified spontaneous abortion
- Parametritis following complete or unspecified spontaneous abortion
- Pelvic peritonitis following complete or unspecified spontaneous abortion
- Salpingitis following complete or unspecified spontaneous abortion
- Salpingo-oophoritis following complete or unspecified spontaneous abortion

Excludes1 sepsis following complete or unspecified spontaneous abortion (O03.87)
urinary tract infection following complete or unspecified spontaneous abortion (O03.88)

O03.6 Delayed or excessive hemorrhage following complete or unspecified spontaneous abortion ♀ M
- Afibrinogenemia following complete or unspecified spontaneous abortion
- Defibrination syndrome following complete or unspecified spontaneous abortion
- Hemolysis following complete or unspecified spontaneous abortion
- Intravascular coagulation following complete or unspecified spontaneous abortion

O03.7 Embolism following complete or unspecified spontaneous abortion ♀ M
- Air embolism following complete or unspecified spontaneous abortion
- Amniotic fluid embolism following complete or unspecified spontaneous abortion
- Blood-clot embolism following complete or unspecified spontaneous abortion
- Embolism NOS following complete or unspecified spontaneous abortion
- Fat embolism following complete or unspecified spontaneous abortion
- Pulmonary embolism following complete or unspecified spontaneous abortion
- Pyemic embolism following complete or unspecified spontaneous abortion
- Septic or septicopyemic embolism following complete or unspecified spontaneous abortion
- Soap embolism following complete or unspecified spontaneous abortion

● **O03.8 Other and unspecified complications following complete or unspecified spontaneous abortion**

O03.80 Unspecified complication following complete or unspecified spontaneous abortion ♀ M

O03.81 Shock following complete or unspecified spontaneous abortion ♀ M
- Circulatory collapse following complete or unspecified spontaneous abortion
- Shock (postprocedural) following complete or unspecified spontaneous abortion

Excludes1 shock due to infection following complete or unspecified spontaneous abortion (O03.87)

O03.82 Renal failure following complete or unspecified spontaneous abortion ♀ M
- Kidney failure (acute) following complete or unspecified spontaneous abortion
- Oliguria following complete or unspecified spontaneous abortion
- Renal shutdown following complete or unspecified spontaneous abortion
- Renal tubular necrosis following complete or unspecified spontaneous abortion
- Uremia following complete or unspecified spontaneous abortion

O03.83 Metabolic disorder following complete or unspecified spontaneous abortion ♀ M

O03.84 Damage to pelvic organs following complete or unspecified spontaneous abortion ♀ M
- Laceration, perforation, tear or chemical damage of bladder following complete or unspecified spontaneous abortion
- Laceration, perforation, tear or chemical damage of bowel following complete or unspecified spontaneous abortion
- Laceration, perforation, tear or chemical damage of broad ligament following complete or unspecified spontaneous abortion
- Laceration, perforation, tear or chemical damage of cervix following complete or unspecified spontaneous abortion
- Laceration, perforation, tear or chemical damage of periurethral tissue following complete or unspecified spontaneous abortion
- Laceration, perforation, tear or chemical damage of uterus following complete or unspecified spontaneous abortion
- Laceration, perforation, tear or chemical damage of vagina following complete or unspecified spontaneous abortion

O03.85 Other venous complications following complete or unspecified spontaneous abortion ♀ M

O03.86 Cardiac arrest following complete or unspecified spontaneous abortion ♀ M

O03.87 Sepsis following complete or unspecified spontaneous abortion ♀ M

Use additional code to identify infectious agent (B95-B97)

Use additional code to identify severe sepsis, if applicable (R65.2-)

Excludes1 septic or septicopyemic embolism following complete or unspecified spontaneous abortion (O03.7)

O03.88 Urinary tract infection following complete or unspecified spontaneous abortion ♀ M
- Cystitis following complete or unspecified spontaneous abortion

O03.89 Complete or unspecified spontaneous abortion with other complications ♀ M

O03.9 Complete or unspecified spontaneous abortion without complication ♀ M
- Miscarriage NOS
- Spontaneous abortion NOS

● **O04 Complications following (induced) termination of pregnancy**

Includes complications following (induced) termination of pregnancy

Excludes1 encounter for elective termination of pregnancy, uncomplicated (Z33.2)
failed attempted termination of pregnancy (O07.-)

Ex: For category O04 CC codes unless otherwise indicated: See 003

O04.5 Genital tract and pelvic infection following (induced) termination of pregnancy ♀ M
- Endometritis following (induced) termination of pregnancy
- Oophoritis following (induced) termination of pregnancy
- Parametritis following (induced) termination of pregnancy
- Pelvic peritonitis following (induced) termination of pregnancy
- Salpingitis following (induced) termination of pregnancy
- Salpingo-oophoritis following (induced) termination of pregnancy

Excludes1 sepsis following (induced) termination of pregnancy (O04.87)
urinary tract infection following (induced) termination of pregnancy (O04.88)

O04.6 Delayed or excessive hemorrhage following (induced) termination of pregnancy ♀ M
- Afibrinogenemia following (induced) termination of pregnancy
- Defibrination syndrome following (induced) termination of pregnancy
- Hemolysis following (induced) termination of pregnancy
- Intravascular coagulation following (induced) termination of pregnancy

O04.7 Embolism following (induced) termination of pregnancy ♀ M
- Air embolism following (induced) termination of pregnancy
- Amniotic fluid embolism following (induced) termination of pregnancy
- Blood-clot embolism following (induced) termination of pregnancy
- Embolism NOS following (induced) termination of pregnancy
- Fat embolism following (induced) termination of pregnancy
- Pulmonary embolism following (induced) termination of pregnancy
- Pyemic embolism following (induced) termination of pregnancy
- Septic or septicopyemic embolism following (induced) termination of pregnancy
- Soap embolism following (induced) termination of pregnancy

● **O04.8 (Induced) termination of pregnancy with other and unspecified complications**

O04.80 (Induced) termination of pregnancy with unspecified complications ♀ M

O04.81 Shock following (induced) termination of pregnancy ♀ M
- Circulatory collapse following (induced) termination of pregnancy
- Shock (postprocedural) following (induced) termination of pregnancy

Excludes1 shock due to infection following (induced) termination of pregnancy (O04.87)

O04.82 Renal failure following (induced) termination of pregnancy ♀ M
- Kidney failure (acute) following (induced) termination of pregnancy
- Oliguria following (induced) termination of pregnancy
- Renal shutdown following (induced) termination of pregnancy
- Renal tubular necrosis following (induced) termination of pregnancy
- Uremia following (induced) termination of pregnancy

O04.83 Metabolic disorder following (induced) termination of pregnancy ♀ M

O04.84 Damage to pelvic organs following (induced) termination of pregnancy ♀ M
- Laceration, perforation, tear or chemical damage of bladder following (induced) termination of pregnancy
- Laceration, perforation, tear or chemical damage of bowel following (induced) termination of pregnancy
- Laceration, perforation, tear or chemical damage of broad ligament following (induced) termination of pregnancy
- Laceration, perforation, tear or chemical damage of cervix following (induced) termination of pregnancy
- Laceration, perforation, tear or chemical damage of periurethral tissue following (induced) termination of pregnancy
- Laceration, perforation, tear or chemical damage of uterus following (induced) termination of pregnancy
- Laceration, perforation, tear or chemical damage of vagina following (induced) termination of pregnancy

O04.85 Other venous complications following (induced) termination of pregnancy ♀ M

O04.86 Cardiac arrest following (induced) termination of pregnancy ♀ M

O04.87 Sepsis following (induced) termination of pregnancy ♀ M

Use additional code to identify infectious agent (B95-B97)

Use additional code to identify severe sepsis, if applicable (R65.2-)

Excludes1 septic or septicopyemic embolism following (induced) termination of pregnancy (O04.7)

Ex: 003.0-007.4, 011.4, 011.5, 012.04, 012.05, 012.14, 012.15, 012.24, 012.25, 013.4, 013.5, 014.04, 014.05, 014.14, 014.15, 014.24, 014.25, 014.94, 014.95, 016.4, 016.5, 020.0-020.9, 025.10-025.3, 026.10-026.13, 026.30-026.43, 026.63-026.819, 026.841-026.86, 026.891-026.93, 029.011-029.93, 035.7XX0-035.7XX9, 044.00-044.13, 044.20-044.53, 045.8X1-045.93, 075.4, 075.81, 075.89-075.9, 080, 090.89, 099.111-099.285, 099.330-099.335, 099.350-099.355, 099.511-099.73, 099.820-099.825, 099.840-09A.53, Z33.2

O04.88 Urinary tract infection following (induced) termination of pregnancy ♀ M
- Cystitis following (induced) termination of pregnancy

O04.89 (Induced) termination of pregnancy with other complications ♀ M

O07 Failed attempted termination of pregnancy

Includes failure of attempted induction of termination of pregnancy
incomplete elective abortion

Excludes1 incomplete spontaneous abortion (O03.0-)

O07.0 Genital tract and pelvic infection following failed attempted termination of pregnancy ♀ M

Endometritis following failed attempted termination of pregnancy
Oophoritis following failed attempted termination of pregnancy
Parametritis following failed attempted termination of pregnancy
Pelvic peritonitis following failed attempted termination of pregnancy
Salpingitis following failed attempted termination of pregnancy
Salpingo-oophoritis following failed attempted termination of pregnancy

Excludes1 sepsis following failed attempted termination of pregnancy (O07.37)
urinary tract infection following failed attempted termination of pregnancy (O07.38)

Ex: 003.0-007.4, 011.4, 011.5, 012.04, 012.05, 012.14, 012.15, 012.24, 012.25, 013.4, 013.5, 014.04, 014.05, 014.14, 014.15, 014.24, 014.25, 014.94, 014.95, 016.4, 016.5, 020.0-020.9, 025.10-025.3, 026.10-026.13, 026.30-026.43, 026.63-026.819, 026.841-026.86, 026.891-026.93, 029.011-029.93, 035.7XX0-035.7XX9, 044.00-044.13, 044.20-044.53, 045.8X1-045.93, 075.4, 075.81, 075.89-075.9, 080, 090.89, 099.111-099.285, 099.330-099.335, 099.350-099.355, 099.511-099.73, 099.820-099.825, 099.840-09A.53, Z33.2

O07.1 Delayed or excessive hemorrhage following failed attempted termination of pregnancy ♀ M

Afibrinogenemia following failed attempted termination of pregnancy
Defibrination syndrome following failed attempted termination of pregnancy
Hemolysis following failed attempted termination of pregnancy
Intravascular coagulation following failed attempted termination of pregnancy

Ex: 003.0-007.4, 011.4, 011.5, 012.04, 012.05, 012.14, 012.15, 012.24, 012.25, 013.4, 013.5, 014.04, 014.05, 014.14, 014.15, 014.24, 014.25, 014.94, 014.95, 016.4, 016.5, 020.0-020.9, 025.10-025.3, 026.10-026.13, 026.30-026.43, 026.63-026.819, 026.841-026.86, 026.891-026.93, 029.011-029.93, 035.7XX0-035.7XX9, 044.00-044.13, 044.20-044.53, 045.8X1-045.93, 075.4, 075.81, 075.89-075.9, 080, 090.89, 099.111-099.285, 099.330-099.335, 099.350-099.355, 099.511-099.73, 099.820-099.825, 099.840-09A.53, Z33.2

O07.2 Embolism following failed attempted termination of pregnancy ♀ M

Air embolism following failed attempted termination of pregnancy
Amniotic fluid embolism following failed attempted termination of pregnancy
Blood-clot embolism following failed attempted termination of pregnancy
Embolism NOS following failed attempted termination of pregnancy
Fat embolism following failed attempted termination of pregnancy
Pulmonary embolism following failed attempted termination of pregnancy
Pyemic embolism following failed attempted termination of pregnancy
Septic or septicopyemic embolism following failed attempted termination of pregnancy
Soap embolism following failed attempted termination of pregnancy

Ex: 003.0-007.4, 011.4, 011.5, 012.04, 012.05, 012.14, 012.15, 012.24, 012.25, 013.4, 013.5, 014.04, 014.05, 014.14, 014.15, 014.24, 014.25, 014.94, 014.95, 016.4, 016.5, 020.0-020.9, 025.10-025.3, 026.10-026.13, 026.30-026.43, 026.63-026.819, 026.841-026.86, 026.891-026.93, 029.011-029.93, 035.7XX0-035.7XX9, 044.00-044.13, 044.20-044.53, 045.8X1-045.93, 075.4, 075.81, 075.89-075.9, 080, 090.89, 099.111-099.285, 099.330-099.335, 099.350-099.355, 099.511-099.73, 099.820-099.825, 099.840-09A.53, Z33.2

O07.3 Failed attempted termination of pregnancy with other and unspecified complications

O07.30 Failed attempted termination of pregnancy with unspecified complications ♀ M

Ex: See 003

O07.31 Shock following failed attempted termination of pregnancy ♀ M

Circulatory collapse following failed attempted termination of pregnancy
Shock (postprocedural) following failed attempted termination of pregnancy

Excludes1 shock due to infection following failed attempted termination of pregnancy (O07.37)

Ex: 003.0-007.4, 011.4, 011.5, 012.04, 012.05, 012.14, 012.15, 012.24, 012.25, 013.4, 013.5, 014.04, 014.05, 014.14, 014.15, 014.24, 014.25, 014.94, 014.95, 016.4, 016.5, 020.0-020.9, 025.10-025.3, 026.10-026.13, 026.30-026.43, 026.63-026.819, 026.841-026.86, 026.891-026.93, 029.011-029.93, 035.7XX0-035.7XX9, 044.00-044.13, 044.20-044.53, 045.8X1-045.93, 075.4, 075.81, 075.89-075.9, 080, 090.89, 099.111-099.285, 099.330-099.335, 099.350-099.355, 099.511-099.73, 099.820-099.825, 099.840-09A.53, Z33.2

O07.32 Renal failure following failed attempted termination of pregnancy ♀ M

Kidney failure (acute) following failed attempted termination of pregnancy
Oliguria following failed attempted termination of pregnancy
Renal shutdown following failed attempted termination of pregnancy
Renal tubular necrosis following failed attempted termination of pregnancy
Uremia following failed attempted termination of pregnancy

Ex: 003.0-007.4, 011.4, 011.5, 012.04, 012.05, 012.14, 012.15, 012.24, 012.25, 013.4, 013.5, 014.04, 014.05, 014.14, 014.15, 014.24, 014.25, 014.94, 014.95, 016.4, 016.5, 020.0-020.9, 025.10-025.3, 026.10-026.13, 026.30-026.43, 026.63-026.819, 026.841-026.86, 026.891-026.93, 029.011-029.93, 035.7XX0-035.7XX9, 044.00-044.13, 044.20-044.53, 045.8X1-045.93, 075.4, 075.81, 075.89-075.9, 080, 090.89, 099.111-099.285, 099.330-099.335, 099.350-099.355, 099.511-099.73, 099.820-099.825, 099.840-09A.53, Z33.2

O07.33 Metabolic disorder following failed attempted termination of pregnancy ♀ M

Ex: See 003

O07.34 Damage to pelvic organs following failed attempted termination of pregnancy ♀ M

Laceration, perforation, tear or chemical damage of bladder following failed attempted termination of pregnancy
Laceration, perforation, tear or chemical damage of bowel following failed attempted termination of pregnancy
Laceration, perforation, tear or chemical damage of broad ligament following failed attempted termination of pregnancy
Laceration, perforation, tear or chemical damage of cervix following failed attempted termination of pregnancy
Laceration, perforation, tear or chemical damage of periurethral tissue following failed attempted termination of pregnancy
Laceration, perforation, tear or chemical damage of uterus following failed attempted termination of pregnancy
Laceration, perforation, tear or chemical damage of vagina following failed attempted termination of pregnancy

Ex: 003.0-007.4, 011.4, 011.5, 012.04, 012.05, 012.14, 012.15, 012.24, 012.25, 013.4, 013.5, 014.04, 014.05, 014.14, 014.15, 014.24, 014.25, 014.94, 014.95, 016.4, 016.5, 020.0-020.9, 025.10-025.3, 026.10-026.13, 026.30-026.43, 026.63-026.819, 026.841-026.86, 026.891-026.93, 029.011-029.93, 035.7XX0-035.7XX9, 044.00-044.13, 044.20-044.53, 045.8X1-045.93, 075.4, 075.81, 075.89-075.9, 080, 090.89, 099.111-099.285, 099.330-099.335, 099.350-099.355, 099.511-099.73, 099.820-099.825, 099.840-09A.53, Z33.2

O07.35 Other venous complications following failed attempted termination of pregnancy ♀ M
Ex: See O03

O07.36 Cardiac arrest following failed attempted termination of pregnancy ♀ M
Ex: See O03

O07.37 Sepsis following failed attempted termination of pregnancy ♀ M
Use additional code (B95-B97), to identify infectious agent
Use additional code (R65.2-) to identify severe sepsis, if applicable
Excludes1 septic or septicopyemic embolism following failed attempted termination of pregnancy (O07.2)
Ex: See O07.0

O07.38 Urinary tract infection following failed attempted termination of pregnancy ♀ M
Cystitis following failed attempted termination of pregnancy
Ex: See O03

O07.39 Failed attempted termination of pregnancy with other complications ♀ M
Ex: See O03

O07.4 Failed attempted termination of pregnancy without complication ♀ M

● O08 Complications following ectopic and molar pregnancy
This category is for use with categories O00-O02 to identify any associated complications.
Ex: **For category O08 CC codes unless otherwise indicated:** O08.2-O08.81, O08.83-O08.9, O11.4, O11.5, O12.04, O12.05, O12.14, O12.15, O12.24, O12.25, O13.4, O13.5, O14.04, O14.05, O14.14, O14.15, O14.24, O14.25, O14.94, O14.95, O16.4, O16.5, O20.0-O20.9, O25.10-O25.3, O26.10-O26.13, O26.30-O26.43, O26.63-O26.819, O26.841-O26.86, O26.891-O26.93, O29.011-O29.93, O35.7XX0-O35.7XX9, O44.00-O44.13, O44.20-O44.53, O45.8X1-O45.93, O75.4, O75.81, O75.89-O75.9, O80, O90.89, O99.111-O99.285, O99.330-O99.335, O99.350-O99.355, O99.511-O99.73, O99.820-O99.825, O99.840-O9A.53

O08.0 Genital tract and pelvic infection following ectopic and molar pregnancy ♀ M
Endometritis following ectopic and molar pregnancy
Oophoritis following ectopic and molar pregnancy
Parametritis following ectopic and molar pregnancy
Pelvic peritonitis following ectopic and molar pregnancy
Salpingitis following ectopic and molar pregnancy
Salpingo-oophoritis following ectopic and molar pregnancy
Excludes1 sepsis following ectopic and molar pregnancy (O08.82)
urinary tract infection (O08.83)
Ex: A34, O08.0, O08.2-O08.9, O11.4, O11.5, O12.04, O12.05, O12.14, O12.15, O12.24, O12.25, O13.4, O13.5, O14.04, O14.05, O14.14, O14.15, O14.24, O14.25, O14.94, O14.95, O16.4, O16.5, O20.0-O20.9, O25.10-O25.3, O26.10-O26.13, O26.30-O26.43, O26.63-O26.819, O26.841-O26.86, O26.891-O26.93, O29.011-O29.93, O35.7XX0-O35.7XX9, O44.00-O44.13, O44.20-O44.53, O45.8X1-O45.93, O75.4, O75.81, O75.89-O75.9, O80, O90.89, O99.111-O99.285, O99.330-O99.335, O99.350-O99.355, O99.511-O99.73, O99.820-O99.825, O99.840-O9A.53

O08.1 Delayed or excessive hemorrhage following ectopic and molar pregnancy ♀ M
Afibrinogenemia following ectopic and molar pregnancy
Defibrination syndrome following ectopic and molar pregnancy
Hemolysis following ectopic and molar pregnancy
Intravascular coagulation following ectopic and molar pregnancy
Excludes1 delayed or excessive hemorrhage due to incomplete abortion (O03.1)
Ex: O08.1-O08.81, O08.83-O08.9, O11.4, O11.5, O12.04, O12.05, O12.14, O12.15, O12.24, O12.25, O13.4, O13.5, O14.04, O14.05, O14.14, O14.15, O14.24, O14.25, O14.94, O14.95, O16.4, O16.5, O20.0-O20.9, O25.10-O25.3, O26.10-O26.13, O26.30-O26.43, O26.63-O26.819, O26.841-O26.86, O26.891-O26.93, O29.011-O29.93, O35.7XX0-O35.7XX9, O44.00-O44.13, O44.20-O44.53, O45.8X1-O45.93, O75.4, O75.81, O75.89-O75.9, O80, O90.89, O99.111-O99.285, O99.330-O99.335, O99.350-O99.355, O99.511-O99.73, O99.820-O99.825, O99.840-O9A.53

O08.2 Embolism following ectopic and molar pregnancy ♀ M
Air embolism following ectopic and molar pregnancy
Amniotic fluid embolism following ectopic and molar pregnancy
Blood-clot embolism following ectopic and molar pregnancy
Embolism NOS following ectopic and molar pregnancy
Fat embolism following ectopic and molar pregnancy
Pulmonary embolism following ectopic and molar pregnancy
Pyemic embolism following ectopic and molar pregnancy
Septic or septicopyemic embolism following ectopic and molar pregnancy
Soap embolism following ectopic and molar pregnancy

O08.3 Shock following ectopic and molar pregnancy ♀ M
Circulatory collapse following ectopic and molar pregnancy
Shock (postprocedural) following ectopic and molar pregnancy
Excludes1 shock due to infection following ectopic and molar pregnancy (O08.82)

O08.4 Renal failure following ectopic and molar pregnancy ♀ M
Kidney failure (acute) following ectopic and molar pregnancy
Oliguria following ectopic and molar pregnancy
Renal shutdown following ectopic and molar pregnancy
Renal tubular necrosis following ectopic and molar pregnancy
Uremia following ectopic and molar pregnancy

O08.5 Metabolic disorders following an ectopic and molar pregnancy ♀ M

O08.6 Damage to pelvic organs and tissues following an ectopic and molar pregnancy ♀ M
Laceration, perforation, tear or chemical damage of bladder following an ectopic and molar pregnancy
Laceration, perforation, tear or chemical damage of bowel following an ectopic and molar pregnancy
Laceration, perforation, tear or chemical damage of broad ligament following an ectopic and molar pregnancy
Laceration, perforation, tear or chemical damage of cervix following an ectopic and molar pregnancy
Laceration, perforation, tear or chemical damage of periurethral tissue following an ectopic and molar pregnancy
Laceration, perforation, tear or chemical damage of uterus following an ectopic and molar pregnancy
Laceration, perforation, tear or chemical damage of vagina following an ectopic and molar pregnancy

◀ New ⇐ Revised ~~deleted~~ Deleted Excludes 1 Excludes 2 Includes Use additional Code first Code also Unspecified
OGCR Official Guidelines ● Unacceptable Principal Diagnosis X Assign placeholder X ● Use Additional Character(s) ▶ Manifestation Code Coding Clinic

O08.7 Other venous complications following an ectopic and molar pregnancy ♀ M

O08.8 Other complications following an ectopic and molar pregnancy

O08.81 Cardiac arrest following an ectopic and molar pregnancy ♀ M

O08.82 Sepsis following ectopic and molar pregnancy ♀ M

Use additional code (B95-B97), to identify infectious agent

Use additional code (R65.2-) to identify severe sepsis, if applicable

Excludes1 septic or septicopyemic embolism following ectopic and molar pregnancy (O08.2)

Ex: See O08.0

O08.83 Urinary tract infection following an ectopic and molar pregnancy ♀ M

Cystitis following an ectopic and molar pregnancy

O08.89 Other complications following an ectopic and molar pregnancy ♀ M

O08.9 Unspecified complication following an ectopic and molar pregnancy ♀ M

SUPERVISION OF HIGH RISK PREGNANCY (O09)

O09 Supervision of high risk pregnancy

O09.0 Supervision of pregnancy with history of infertility

O09.00 Supervision of pregnancy with history of infertility, unspecified trimester ♀ M

O09.01 Supervision of pregnancy with history of infertility, first trimester ♀ M

O09.02 Supervision of pregnancy with history of infertility, second trimester ♀ M

O09.03 Supervision of pregnancy with history of infertility, third trimester ♀ M

O09.1 Supervision of pregnancy with history of ectopic pregnancy

O09.10 Supervision of pregnancy with history of ectopic pregnancy, unspecified trimester ♀ M

O09.11 Supervision of pregnancy with history of ectopic pregnancy, first trimester ♀ M

O09.12 Supervision of pregnancy with history of ectopic pregnancy, second trimester ♀ M

O09.13 Supervision of pregnancy with history of ectopic pregnancy, third trimester ♀ M

O09.A Supervision of pregnancy with history of molar pregnancy

O09.A0 Supervision of pregnancy with history of molar pregnancy, unspecified trimester ♀ M

O09.A1 Supervision of pregnancy with history of molar pregnancy, first trimester ♀ M

O09.A2 Supervision of pregnancy with history of molar pregnancy, second trimester ♀ M

O09.A3 Supervision of pregnancy with history of molar pregnancy, third trimester ♀ M

O09.2 Supervision of pregnancy with other poor reproductive or obstetric history

Excludes2 pregnancy care for patient with history of recurrent pregnancy loss (O26.2-)

O09.21 Supervision of pregnancy with history of pre-term labor

O09.211 Supervision of pregnancy with history of pre-term labor, first trimester ♀ M

O09.212 Supervision of pregnancy with history of pre-term labor, second trimester ♀ M

O09.213 Supervision of pregnancy with history of pre-term labor, third trimester ♀ M

O09.219 Supervision of pregnancy with history of pre-term labor, unspecified trimester ♀ M

O09.29 Supervision of pregnancy with other poor reproductive or obstetric history

Supervision of pregnancy with history of neonatal death

Supervision of pregnancy with history of stillbirth

O09.291 Supervision of pregnancy with other poor reproductive or obstetric history, first trimester ♀ M

O09.292 Supervision of pregnancy with other poor reproductive or obstetric history, second trimester ♀ M

O09.293 Supervision of pregnancy with other poor reproductive or obstetric history, third trimester ♀ M

O09.299 Supervision of pregnancy with other poor reproductive or obstetric history, unspecified trimester ♀ M

O09.3 Supervision of pregnancy with insufficient antenatal care

Supervision of concealed pregnancy

Supervision of hidden pregnancy

O09.30 Supervision of pregnancy with insufficient antenatal care, unspecified trimester ♀ M

O09.31 Supervision of pregnancy with insufficient antenatal care, first trimester ♀ M

O09.32 Supervision of pregnancy with insufficient antenatal care, second trimester ♀ M

O09.33 Supervision of pregnancy with insufficient antenatal care, third trimester ♀ M

O09.4 Supervision of pregnancy with grand multiparity

O09.40 Supervision of pregnancy with grand multiparity, unspecified trimester ♀ M

O09.41 Supervision of pregnancy with grand multiparity, first trimester ♀ M

O09.42 Supervision of pregnancy with grand multiparity, second trimester ♀ M

O09.43 Supervision of pregnancy with grand multiparity, third trimester ♀ M

O09.5 Supervision of elderly primigravida and multigravida

Pregnancy for a female 35 years and older at expected date of delivery

O09.51 Supervision of elderly primigravida

O09.511 Supervision of elderly primigravida, first trimester ♀ M

O09.512 Supervision of elderly primigravida, second trimester ♀ M

O09.513 Supervision of elderly primigravida, third trimester ♀ M

O09.519 Supervision of elderly primigravida, unspecified trimester ♀ M

- **O09.52 Supervision of elderly multigravida**
  - **O09.521 Supervision of elderly multigravida, first trimester ♀** M
  - **O09.522 Supervision of elderly multigravida, second trimester ♀** M
  - **O09.523 Supervision of elderly multigravida, third trimester ♀** M
  - **O09.529 Supervision of elderly multigravida, unspecified trimester ♀** M
- **O09.6 Supervision of young primigravida and multigravida**
  Supervision of pregnancy for a female less than 16 years old at expected date of delivery
  - **O09.61 Supervision of young primigravida**
    - **O09.611 Supervision of young primigravida, first trimester ♀** M
    - **O09.612 Supervision of young primigravida, second trimester ♀** M
    - **O09.613 Supervision of young primigravida, third trimester ♀** M
    - **O09.619 Supervision of young primigravida, unspecified trimester ♀** M
  - **O09.62 Supervision of young multigravida**
    - **O09.621 Supervision of young multigravida, first trimester ♀** M
    - **O09.622 Supervision of young multigravida, second trimester ♀** M
    - **O09.623 Supervision of young multigravida, third trimester ♀** M
    - **O09.629 Supervision of young multigravida, unspecified trimester ♀** M
- **O09.7 Supervision of high risk pregnancy due to social problems**
  - **O09.70 Supervision of high risk pregnancy due to social problems, unspecified trimester ♀** M
  - **O09.71 Supervision of high risk pregnancy due to social problems, first trimester ♀** M
  - **O09.72 Supervision of high risk pregnancy due to social problems, second trimester ♀** M
  - **O09.73 Supervision of high risk pregnancy due to social problems, third trimester ♀** M
- **O09.8 Supervision of other high risk pregnancies**
  - **O09.81 Supervision of pregnancy resulting from assisted reproductive technology**
    Supervision of pregnancy resulting from in-vitro fertilization
    Excludes2 gestational carrier status (Z33.3) ◀
    - **O09.811 Supervision of pregnancy resulting from assisted reproductive technology, first trimester ♀** M
    - **O09.812 Supervision of pregnancy resulting from assisted reproductive technology, second trimester ♀** M
    - **O09.813 Supervision of pregnancy resulting from assisted reproductive technology, third trimester ♀** M
    - **O09.819 Supervision of pregnancy resulting from assisted reproductive technology, unspecified trimester ♀** M
  - **O09.82 Supervision of pregnancy with history of in utero procedure during previous pregnancy**
    - **O09.821 Supervision of pregnancy with history of in utero procedure during previous pregnancy, first trimester ♀** M
    - **O09.822 Supervision of pregnancy with history of in utero procedure during previous pregnancy, second trimester ♀** M
    - **O09.823 Supervision of pregnancy with history of in utero procedure during previous pregnancy, third trimester ♀** M
    - **O09.829 Supervision of pregnancy with history of in utero procedure during previous pregnancy, unspecified trimester ♀** M
      Excludes1 supervision of pregnancy affected by in utero procedure during current pregnancy (O35.7)
  - **O09.89 Supervision of other high risk pregnancies**
    - **O09.891 Supervision of other high risk pregnancies, first trimester ♀** M
    - **O09.892 Supervision of other high risk pregnancies, second trimester ♀** M
    - **O09.893 Supervision of other high risk pregnancies, third trimester ♀** M
    - **O09.899 Supervision of other high risk pregnancies, unspecified trimester ♀** M
- **O09.9 Supervision of high risk pregnancy, unspecified**
  - **O09.90 Supervision of high risk pregnancy, unspecified, unspecified trimester ♀** M
  - **O09.91 Supervision of high risk pregnancy, unspecified, first trimester ♀** M
  - **O09.92 Supervision of high risk pregnancy, unspecified, second trimester ♀** M
  - **O09.93 Supervision of high risk pregnancy, unspecified, third trimester ♀** M

EDEMA, PROTEINURIA AND HYPERTENSIVE DISORDERS IN PREGNANCY, CHILDBIRTH AND THE PUERPERIUM (O10-O16)

- **O10 Pre-existing hypertension complicating pregnancy, childbirth and the puerperium**
  Includes pre-existing hypertension with pre-existing proteinuria complicating pregnancy, childbirth and the puerperium
  Excludes2 pre-existing hypertension with superimposed pre-eclampsia complicating pregnancy, childbirth and the puerperium (O11.-)
  Ex: **For category O10 CC codes:** 010.011-012.03, 012.04, 012.05, 012.14, 012.15, 012.20-016.9, 025.10-026.13, 026.30-026.43, 026.63-026.819, 026.841-026.86, 026.891-026.93, 029.011-029.93, 035.7XX0-035.7XX9, 075.4, 075.81, 075.89-075.9, 080, 090.89, 099.111-099.285, 099.330-099.335, 099.350-099.355, 099.511-099.73, 099.820-099.825, 099.840-09A.53
  - **O10.0 Pre-existing essential hypertension complicating pregnancy, childbirth and the puerperium**
    Any condition in I10 specified as a reason for obstetric care during pregnancy, childbirth or the puerperium
    - **O10.01 Pre-existing essential hypertension complicating pregnancy**
      - **O10.011 Pre-existing essential hypertension complicating pregnancy, first trimester ♀** M
      - **O10.012 Pre-existing essential hypertension complicating pregnancy, second trimester ♀** M
      - **O10.013 Pre-existing essential hypertension complicating pregnancy, third trimester ♀** M
      - **O10.019 Pre-existing essential hypertension complicating pregnancy, unspecified trimester ♀** M
    - **O10.02 Pre-existing essential hypertension complicating childbirth ♀** M
    - **O10.03 Pre-existing essential hypertension complicating the puerperium ♀** M

O10.1 Pre-existing hypertensive heart disease complicating pregnancy, childbirth and the puerperium
Any condition in I11 specified as a reason for obstetric care during pregnancy, childbirth or the puerperium
Use additional code from I11 to identify the type of hypertensive heart disease

O10.11 Pre-existing hypertensive heart disease complicating pregnancy

O10.111 Pre-existing hypertensive heart disease complicating pregnancy, first trimester ♀ M

O10.112 Pre-existing hypertensive heart disease complicating pregnancy, second trimester ♀ M

O10.113 Pre-existing hypertensive heart disease complicating pregnancy, third trimester ♀ M

O10.119 Pre-existing hypertensive heart disease complicating pregnancy, unspecified trimester ♀ M

O10.12 Pre-existing hypertensive heart disease complicating childbirth ♀ M

O10.13 Pre-existing hypertensive heart disease complicating the puerperium ♀ M

O10.2 Pre-existing hypertensive chronic kidney disease complicating pregnancy, childbirth and the puerperium
Any condition in I12 specified as a reason for obstetric care during pregnancy, childbirth or the puerperium
Use additional code from I12 to identify the type of hypertensive chronic kidney disease

O10.21 Pre-existing hypertensive chronic kidney disease complicating pregnancy

O10.211 Pre-existing hypertensive chronic kidney disease complicating pregnancy, first trimester ♀ M

O10.212 Pre-existing hypertensive chronic kidney disease complicating pregnancy, second trimester ♀ M

O10.213 Pre-existing hypertensive chronic kidney disease complicating pregnancy, third trimester ♀ M

O10.219 Pre-existing hypertensive chronic kidney disease complicating pregnancy, unspecified trimester ♀ M

O10.22 Pre-existing hypertensive chronic kidney disease complicating childbirth ♀ M

O10.23 Pre-existing hypertensive chronic kidney disease complicating the puerperium ♀ M

O10.3 Pre-existing hypertensive heart and chronic kidney disease complicating pregnancy, childbirth and the puerperium
Any condition in I13 specified as a reason for obstetric care during pregnancy, childbirth or the puerperium
Use additional code from I13 to identify the type of hypertensive heart and chronic kidney disease

O10.31 Pre-existing hypertensive heart and chronic kidney disease complicating pregnancy

O10.311 Pre-existing hypertensive heart and chronic kidney disease complicating pregnancy, first trimester ♀ M

O10.312 Pre-existing hypertensive heart and chronic kidney disease complicating pregnancy, second trimester ♀ M

O10.313 Pre-existing hypertensive heart and chronic kidney disease complicating pregnancy, third trimester ♀ M

O10.319 Pre-existing hypertensive heart and chronic kidney disease complicating pregnancy, unspecified trimester ♀ M

O10.32 Pre-existing hypertensive heart and chronic kidney disease complicating childbirth ♀ M

O10.33 Pre-existing hypertensive heart and chronic kidney disease complicating the puerperium ♀ M

O10.4 Pre-existing secondary hypertension complicating pregnancy, childbirth and the puerperium
Any condition in I15 specified as a reason for obstetric care during pregnancy, childbirth or the puerperium
Use additional code from I15 to identify the type of secondary hypertension

O10.41 Pre-existing secondary hypertension complicating pregnancy

O10.411 Pre-existing secondary hypertension complicating pregnancy, first trimester ♀ M

O10.412 Pre-existing secondary hypertension complicating pregnancy, second trimester ♀ M

O10.413 Pre-existing secondary hypertension complicating pregnancy, third trimester ♀ M

O10.419 Pre-existing secondary hypertension complicating pregnancy, unspecified trimester ♀ M

O10.42 Pre-existing secondary hypertension complicating childbirth ♀ M

O10.43 Pre-existing secondary hypertension complicating the puerperium ♀ M

O10.9 Unspecified pre-existing hypertension complicating pregnancy, childbirth and the puerperium

O10.91 Unspecified pre-existing hypertension complicating pregnancy

O10.911 Unspecified pre-existing hypertension complicating pregnancy, first trimester ♀ M

O10.912 Unspecified pre-existing hypertension complicating pregnancy, second trimester ♀ M

O10.913 Unspecified pre-existing hypertension complicating pregnancy, third trimester ♀ M

O10.919 Unspecified pre-existing hypertension complicating pregnancy, unspecified trimester ♀ M

O10.92 Unspecified pre-existing hypertension complicating childbirth ♀ M

O10.93 Unspecified pre-existing hypertension complicating the puerperium ♀ M

O11 Pre-existing hypertension with pre-eclampsia
Includes conditions in O10 complicated by pre-eclampsia
pre-eclampsia superimposed pre-existing hypertension
Use additional code from O10 to identify the type of hypertension
Ex For category O11 CC codes: See O10

O11.1 Pre-existing hypertension with pre-eclampsia, first trimester ♀ M

O11.2 Pre-existing hypertension with pre-eclampsia, second trimester ♀ M

O11.3 Pre-existing hypertension with pre-eclampsia, third trimester ♀ M

O11.4 Pre-existing hypertension with pre-eclampsia, complicating childbirth ♀ ◀ M

O11.5 Pre-existing hypertension with pre-eclampsia, complicating the puerperium ♀ ◀ M

O11.9 Pre-existing hypertension with pre-eclampsia, unspecified trimester ♀ M

● **O12 Gestational [pregnancy-induced] edema and proteinuria without hypertension**
Ex: For category O12 CC codes: 011.5, 012.05, 012.11-012.13, 012.15, 012.21-012.23, 012.25, 013.5, 014.05, 014.15, 014.25, 014.95, 016.5, 026.831-026.833, 090.89

● **O12.0 Gestational edema**
- **O12.00 Gestational edema, unspecified trimester ♀** M
- **O12.01 Gestational edema, first trimester ♀** M
- **O12.02 Gestational edema, second trimester ♀** M
- **O12.03 Gestational edema, third trimester ♀** M
- **O12.04 Gestational edema, complicating childbirth ♀ ◀** M
- **O12.05 Gestational edema, complicating the puerperium ♀ ◀** M

● **O12.1 Gestational proteinuria**
- **O12.10 Gestational proteinuria, unspecified trimester ♀** M
- **O12.11 Gestational proteinuria, first trimester ♀** M
- **O12.12 Gestational proteinuria, second trimester ♀** M
- **O12.13 Gestational proteinuria, third trimester ♀** M
- **O12.14 Gestational proteinuria, complicating childbirth ♀ ◀** M
- **O12.15 Gestational proteinuria, complicating the puerperium ♀ ◀** M

● **O12.2 Gestational edema with proteinuria**
- **O12.20 Gestational edema with proteinuria, unspecified trimester ♀** M
- **O12.21 Gestational edema with proteinuria, first trimester ♀** M
  CC when PDx is its own CC
- **O12.22 Gestational edema with proteinuria, second trimester ♀** M
  CC when PDx is its own CC
- **O12.23 Gestational edema with proteinuria, third trimester ♀** M
  CC when PDx is its own CC
- **O12.24 Gestational edema with proteinuria, complicating childbirth ♀ ◀** M
- **O12.25 Gestational edema with proteinuria, complicating the puerperium ♀ ◀** M

● **O13 Gestational [pregnancy-induced] hypertension without significant proteinuria**
Includes gestational hypertension NOS
transient hypertension of pregnancy ◀
- **O13.1 Gestational [pregnancy-induced] hypertension without significant proteinuria, first trimester ♀** M
- **O13.2 Gestational [pregnancy-induced] hypertension without significant proteinuria, second trimester ♀** M
- **O13.3 Gestational [pregnancy-induced] hypertension without significant proteinuria, third trimester ♀** M
- **O13.4 Gestational [pregnancy-induced] hypertension without significant proteinuria, complicating childbirth ♀ ◀** M
- **O13.5 Gestational [pregnancy-induced] hypertension without significant proteinuria, complicating the puerperium ♀ ◀** M
- **O13.9 Gestational [pregnancy-induced] hypertension without significant proteinuria, unspecified trimester ♀** M

● **O14 Pre-eclampsia**
Excludes1 pre-existing hypertension with pre-eclampsia (O11)
Ex: For category O14 CC codes: See O10

● **O14.0 Mild to moderate pre-eclampsia**
- **O14.00 Mild to moderate pre-eclampsia, unspecified trimester ♀** M
- **O14.02 Mild to moderate pre-eclampsia, second trimester ♀** M
- **O14.03 Mild to moderate pre-eclampsia, third trimester ♀** M
- **O14.04 Mild to moderate pre-eclampsia, complicating childbirth ♀ ◀** M
- **O14.05 Mild to moderate pre-eclampsia, complicating the puerperium ♀ ◀** M

● **O14.1 Severe pre-eclampsia**
Excludes1 HELLP syndrome (O14.2-)
H=hemolysis, EL=elevated liver enzymes, LP=low platelet count
- **O14.10 Severe pre-eclampsia, unspecified trimester ♀** M
- **O14.12 Severe pre-eclampsia, second trimester ♀** M
- **O14.13 Severe pre-eclampsia, third trimester ♀** M
- **O14.14 Severe pre-eclampsia complicating childbirth ♀ ◀** M
- **O14.15 Severe pre-eclampsia, complicating the puerperium ♀ ◀** M

● **O14.2 HELLP syndrome**
Severe pre-eclampsia with hemolysis, elevated liver enzymes and low platelet count (HELLP)
- **O14.20 HELLP syndrome (HELLP), unspecified trimester ♀** M
- **O14.22 HELLP syndrome (HELLP), second trimester ♀** M
- **O14.23 HELLP syndrome (HELLP), third trimester ♀** M
- **O14.24 HELLP syndrome, complicating childbirth ♀ ◀** M
- **O14.25 HELLP syndrome, complicating the puerperium ♀ ◀** M

● **O14.9 Unspecified pre-eclampsia**
- **O14.90 Unspecified pre-eclampsia, unspecified trimester ♀** M
- **O14.92 Unspecified pre-eclampsia, second trimester ♀** M
- **O14.93 Unspecified pre-eclampsia, third trimester ♀** M
- **O14.94 Unspecified pre-eclampsia, complicating childbirth ♀ ◀** M
- **O14.95 Unspecified pre-eclampsia, complicating the puerperium ♀ ◀** M

● **O15 Eclampsia**
Includes convulsions following conditions in O10-O14 and O16
Ex: For category O15 CC codes: See O10

● **O15.0 Eclampsia complicating pregnancy**
- **O15.00 Eclampsia complicating pregnancy, unspecified trimester ♀** M
- **O15.02 Eclampsia complicating pregnancy, second trimester ♀** M
- **O15.03 Eclampsia complicating pregnancy, third trimester ♀** M
- **O15.1 Eclampsia complicating labor ♀** M
- **O15.2 Eclampsia complicating the puerperium ♀** M
- **O15.9 Eclampsia, unspecified as to time period ♀** M
  Eclampsia NOS

● **O16 Unspecified maternal hypertension**
Ex: For category O16 CC codes: See O10
- **O16.1 Unspecified maternal hypertension, first trimester ♀** M
- **O16.2 Unspecified maternal hypertension, second trimester ♀** M
- **O16.3 Unspecified maternal hypertension, third trimester ♀** M
- **O16.4 Unspecified maternal hypertension, complicating childbirth ♀ ◀** M
- **O16.5 Unspecified maternal hypertension, complicating the puerperium ♀ ◀** M
- **O16.9 Unspecified maternal hypertension, unspecified trimester ♀** M

OTHER MATERNAL DISORDERS PREDOMINANTLY RELATED TO PREGNANCY (O20-O29)

Excludes2 maternal care related to the fetus and amniotic cavity and possible delivery problems (O30-O48)
maternal diseases classifiable elsewhere but complicating pregnancy, labor and delivery, and the puerperium (O98-O99)

O20 Hemorrhage in early pregnancy
Includes hemorrhage before completion of 20 weeks gestation
Excludes1 pregnancy with abortive outcome (O00-O08)
Ex: **For category O20 CC codes:** 011.4, 011.5, 012.04, 012.05, 012.14, 012.15, 012.24, 012.25, 013.4, 013.5, 014.04, 014.05, 014.14, 014.15, 014.24, 014.25, 014.94, 014.95, 016.4, 016.5, 020.0-020.9, 025.10-025.3, 026.10-026.13, 026.30-026.43, 026.63-026.819, 026.841-026.86, 026.891-026.93, 029.011-029.93, 035.7XX0-035.7XX9, 044.00-044.13, 044.20-044.53, 075.4, 075.81, 075.89-075.9, 080, 090.89, 099.111-099.119, 099.12-099.285, 099.330-099.335, 099.350-099.355, 099.511-099.73, 099.820-099.825, 099.840-09A.53

O20.0 Threatened abortion ♀ M
Hemorrhage specified as due to threatened abortion

O20.8 Other hemorrhage in early pregnancy ♀ M

O20.9 Hemorrhage in early pregnancy, unspecified ♀ M

O21 Excessive vomiting in pregnancy

O21.0 Mild hyperemesis gravidarum ♀ M
Hyperemesis gravidarum, mild or unspecified, starting before the end of the 20th week of gestation

O21.1 Hyperemesis gravidarum with metabolic disturbance ♀ M
Hyperemesis gravidarum, starting before the end of the 20th week of gestation, with metabolic disturbance such as carbohydrate depletion
Hyperemesis gravidarum, starting before the end of the 20th week of gestation, with metabolic disturbance such as dehydration
Hyperemesis gravidarum, starting before the end of the 20th week of gestation, with metabolic disturbance such as electrolyte imbalance

O21.2 Late vomiting of pregnancy ♀ M
Excessive vomiting starting after 20 completed weeks of gestation

O21.8 Other vomiting complicating pregnancy ♀ M
Vomiting due to diseases classified elsewhere, complicating pregnancy
Use additional code, to identify cause

O21.9 Vomiting of pregnancy, unspecified ♀ M

O22 Venous complications and hemorrhoids in pregnancy
Excludes1 venous complications of:
abortion NOS (O03.9)
ectopic or molar pregnancy (O08.7)
failed attempted abortion (O07.35)
induced abortion (O04.85)
spontaneous abortion (O03.89)
Excludes2 obstetric pulmonary embolism (O88.-)
venous complications and hemorrhoids of childbirth and the puerperium (O87.-)
Ex: **For category O22 CC codes unless otherwise indicated:** 022.20-022.93, 025.10-025.3, 026.10-026.13, 026.30-026.43, 026.63-026.819, 026.841-026.86, 026.891-026.93, 029.011-029.93, 035.7XX0-035.7XX9, 075.4, 075.81, 075.89-075.9, 080, 087.0-087.9, 090.89, 099.111-099.119, 099.12-099.285, 099.330-099.335, 099.350-099.355, 099.511-099.73, 099.820-099.825, 099.840-09A.53

O22.0 Varicose veins of lower extremity in pregnancy
Varicose veins NOS in pregnancy

O22.00 Varicose veins of lower extremity in pregnancy, unspecified trimester ♀ M

O22.01 Varicose veins of lower extremity in pregnancy, first trimester ♀ M

O22.02 Varicose veins of lower extremity in pregnancy, second trimester ♀ M

O22.03 Varicose veins of lower extremity in pregnancy, third trimester ♀ M

O22.1 Genital varices in pregnancy
Perineal varices in pregnancy
Vaginal varices in pregnancy
Vulval varices in pregnancy

O22.10 Genital varices in pregnancy, unspecified trimester ♀ M

O22.11 Genital varices in pregnancy, first trimester ♀ M

O22.12 Genital varices in pregnancy, second trimester ♀ M

O22.13 Genital varices in pregnancy, third trimester ♀ M

O22.2 Superficial thrombophlebitis in pregnancy
Phlebitis in pregnancy NOS
Thrombophlebitis of legs in pregnancy
Thrombosis in pregnancy NOS
Use additional code to identify the superficial thrombophlebitis (I80.0-)
Ex: **For category O22.2 CC codes:** 011.4, 011.5, 012.04, 012.05, 012.14, 012.15, 012.24, 012.25, 013.4, 013.5, 014.04, 014.05, 014.14, 014.15, 014.24, 014.25, 014.94, 014.95, 016.4, 016.5, 022.20-022.93, 025.10-025.3, 026.10-026.13, 026.30-026.43, 026.63-026.819, 026.841-026.86, 026.891-026.93, 029.011-029.93, 035.7XX0-035.7XX9, 075.4, 075.81, 075.89-075.9, 080, 087.0-087.9, 090.89, 099.111-099.119, 099.12-099.285, 099.330-099.335, 099.350-099.355, 099.511-099.73, 099.820-099.825, 099.840-09A.53

O22.20 Superficial thrombophlebitis in pregnancy, unspecified trimester ♀ M

O22.21 Superficial thrombophlebitis in pregnancy, first trimester ♀ M

O22.22 Superficial thrombophlebitis in pregnancy, second trimester ♀ M

O22.23 Superficial thrombophlebitis in pregnancy, third trimester ♀ M

O22.3 Deep phlebothrombosis in pregnancy
Deep vein thrombosis, antepartum
Use additional code to identify the deep vein thrombosis (I82.4-, I82.5-, I82.62-. I82.72-)
Use additional code, if applicable, for associated long-term (current) use of anticoagulants (Z79.01)
Ex: **For category O22.3 CC codes:** See O22.2

O22.30 Deep phlebothrombosis in pregnancy, unspecified trimester ♀ M

O22.31 Deep phlebothrombosis in pregnancy, first trimester ♀ M

O22.32 Deep phlebothrombosis in pregnancy, second trimester ♀ M

O22.33 Deep phlebothrombosis in pregnancy, third trimester ♀ M

O22.4 Hemorrhoids in pregnancy
Ex: **For category O22.4 CC codes:** See O22.2

O22.40 Hemorrhoids in pregnancy, unspecified trimester ♀ M

O22.41 Hemorrhoids in pregnancy, first trimester ♀ M

O22.42 Hemorrhoids in pregnancy, second trimester ♀ M

O22.43 Hemorrhoids in pregnancy, third trimester ♀ M

O22.5 Cerebral venous thrombosis in pregnancy
Cerebrovenous sinus thrombosis in pregnancy
Ex: **For category O22.5 CC codes:** See O22.2

O22.50 Cerebral venous thrombosis in pregnancy, unspecified trimester ♀ M

O22.51 Cerebral venous thrombosis in pregnancy, first trimester ♀ M

O22.52 Cerebral venous thrombosis in pregnancy, second trimester ♀ M

O22.53 Cerebral venous thrombosis in pregnancy, third trimester ♀ M

● O22.8 Other venous complications in pregnancy
Ex For category O22.8 CC codes: See O22.2
● O22.8X Other venous complications in pregnancy
O22.8X1 Other venous complications in pregnancy, first trimester ♀ M
O22.8X2 Other venous complications in pregnancy, second trimester ♀ M
O22.8X3 Other venous complications in pregnancy, third trimester ♀ M
O22.8X9 Other venous complications in pregnancy, unspecified trimester ♀ M

● O22.9 Venous complication in pregnancy, unspecified
Gestational phlebitis NOS
Gestational phlebopathy NOS
Gestational thrombosis NOS
Ex For category O22.9 CC codes: See O22.2
O22.90 Venous complication in pregnancy, unspecified, unspecified trimester ♀ M
O22.91 Venous complication in pregnancy, unspecified, first trimester ♀ M
O22.92 Venous complication in pregnancy, unspecified, second trimester ♀ M
O22.93 Venous complication in pregnancy, unspecified, third trimester ♀ M

● O23 Infections of genitourinary tract in pregnancy
Use additional code to identify organism (B95.-, B96.-)
Excludes2 gonococcal infections complicating pregnancy, childbirth and the puerperium (O98.2)
infections with a predominantly sexual mode of transmission NOS complicating pregnancy, childbirth and the puerperium (O98.3)
syphilis complicating pregnancy, childbirth and the puerperium (O98.1)
tuberculosis of genitourinary system complicating pregnancy, childbirth and the puerperium (O98.0)
venereal disease NOS complicating pregnancy, childbirth and the puerperium (O98.3)
Ex For category O23 CC codes: 011.4, 011.5, 012.04, 012.05, 012.14, 012.15, 012.24, 012.25, 013.4, 013.5, 014.04, 014.05, 014.14, 014.15, 014.24, 014.25, 014.94, 014.95, 016.4, 016.5, 023.00-023.93, 025.10-025.3, 026.10-026.13, 026.30-026.43, 026.63-026.819, 026.841-026.86, 026.891-026.93, 029.011-029.93, 035.7XX0-035.7XX9, 075.4, 075.81, 075.89-075.9, 080, 086.11, 086.13-086.29, 090.89, 099.111-099.285, 099.330-099.335, 099.350-099.355, 099.511-099.73, 099.820-099.825, 099.840-09A.53

● O23.0 Infections of kidney in pregnancy
Pyelonephritis in pregnancy
O23.00 Infections of kidney in pregnancy, unspecified trimester ♀ M
O23.01 Infections of kidney in pregnancy, first trimester ♀ M
O23.02 Infections of kidney in pregnancy, second trimester ♀ M
O23.03 Infections of kidney in pregnancy, third trimester ♀ M

● O23.1 Infections of bladder in pregnancy
O23.10 Infections of bladder in pregnancy, unspecified trimester ♀ M
O23.11 Infections of bladder in pregnancy, first trimester ♀ M
O23.12 Infections of bladder in pregnancy, second trimester ♀ M
O23.13 Infections of bladder in pregnancy, third trimester ♀ M

● O23.2 Infections of urethra in pregnancy
O23.20 Infections of urethra in pregnancy, unspecified trimester ♀ M
O23.21 Infections of urethra in pregnancy, first trimester ♀ M
O23.22 Infections of urethra in pregnancy, second trimester ♀ M
O23.23 Infections of urethra in pregnancy, third trimester ♀ M

● O23.3 Infections of other parts of urinary tract in pregnancy
O23.30 Infections of other parts of urinary tract in pregnancy, unspecified trimester ♀ M
O23.31 Infections of other parts of urinary tract in pregnancy, first trimester ♀ M
O23.32 Infections of other parts of urinary tract in pregnancy, second trimester ♀ M
O23.33 Infections of other parts of urinary tract in pregnancy, third trimester ♀ M

● O23.4 Unspecified infection of urinary tract in pregnancy
O23.40 Unspecified infection of urinary tract in pregnancy, unspecified trimester ♀ M
O23.41 Unspecified infection of urinary tract in pregnancy, first trimester ♀ M
O23.42 Unspecified infection of urinary tract in pregnancy, second trimester ♀ M
O23.43 Unspecified infection of urinary tract in pregnancy, third trimester ♀ M

● O23.5 Infections of the genital tract in pregnancy
● O23.51 Infection of cervix in pregnancy
O23.511 Infections of cervix in pregnancy, first trimester ♀ M
O23.512 Infections of cervix in pregnancy, second trimester ♀ M
O23.513 Infections of cervix in pregnancy, third trimester ♀ M
O23.519 Infections of cervix in pregnancy, unspecified trimester ♀ M
● O23.52 Salpingo-oophoritis in pregnancy
Oophoritis = inflammation of ovary
Salpingitis = inflammation of fallopian tube
Oophoritis in pregnancy
Salpingitis in pregnancy
O23.521 Salpingo-oophoritis in pregnancy, first trimester ♀ M
O23.522 Salpingo-oophoritis in pregnancy, second trimester ♀ M
O23.523 Salpingo-oophoritis in pregnancy, third trimester ♀ M
O23.529 Salpingo-oophoritis in pregnancy, unspecified trimester ♀ M
● O23.59 Infection of other part of genital tract in pregnancy
O23.591 Infection of other part of genital tract in pregnancy, first trimester ♀ M
O23.592 Infection of other part of genital tract in pregnancy, second trimester ♀ M
O23.593 Infection of other part of genital tract in pregnancy, third trimester ♀ M
O23.599 Infection of other part of genital tract in pregnancy, unspecified trimester ♀ M

● O23.9 Unspecified genitourinary tract infection in pregnancy
Genitourinary tract infection in pregnancy NOS
O23.90 Unspecified genitourinary tract infection in pregnancy, unspecified trimester ♀ M
O23.91 Unspecified genitourinary tract infection in pregnancy, first trimester ♀ M
O23.92 Unspecified genitourinary tract infection in pregnancy, second trimester ♀ M
O23.93 Unspecified genitourinary tract infection in pregnancy, third trimester ♀ M

◀ New ◀ Revised ~~deleted~~ Deleted Excludes 1 Excludes 2 Includes Use additional Code first Code also Unspecified
OGCR Official Guidelines ● Unacceptable Principal Diagnosis X Assign placeholder X ● Use Additional Character(s) ▶ Manifestation Code Coding Clinic

OGCR Section I.C.15.g.

Diabetes mellitus in pregnancy

Diabetes mellitus is a significant complicating factor in pregnancy. Pregnant women who are diabetic should be assigned a code from category O24, Diabetes mellitus in pregnancy, childbirth, and the puerperium, first, followed by the appropriate diabetes code(s) (E08-E13) from Chapter 4.

O24 Diabetes mellitus in pregnancy, childbirth, and the puerperium

Ex: For category O24 CC codes: 011.4, 011.5, 012.04, 012.05, 012.14, 012.15, 012.24, 012.25, 013.4, 013.5, 014.04, 014.05, 014.14, 014.15, 014.24, 014.25, 014.94, 014.95, 016.4, 016.5, 024.011-024.33, 024.811-025.3, 026.10-026.13, 026.30-026.43, 026.63-026.819, 026.841-026.86, 026.891-026.93, 029.011-029.93, 035.7XX0-035.7XX9, 075.4, 075.81, 075.89-075.9, 080, 090.89, 099.111-099.285, 099.330-099.335, 099.350-099.355, 099.511-099.73, 099.820-099.825, 099.840-09A.53

O24.0 Pre-existing type 1 diabetes mellitus, in pregnancy, childbirth and the puerperium

Juvenile onset diabetes mellitus, in pregnancy, childbirth and the puerperium

Ketosis-prone diabetes mellitus in pregnancy, childbirth and the puerperium

Use additional code from category E10 to further identify any manifestations

O24.01 Pre-existing type 1 diabetes mellitus, in pregnancy

O24.011 Pre-existing type 1 diabetes mellitus, in pregnancy, first trimester ♀ M

O24.012 Pre-existing type 1 diabetes mellitus, in pregnancy, second trimester ♀ M

O24.013 Pre-existing type 1 diabetes mellitus, in pregnancy, third trimester ♀ M

O24.019 Pre-existing type 1 diabetes mellitus, in pregnancy, unspecified trimester ♀ M

O24.02 Pre-existing type 1 diabetes mellitus, in childbirth ♀ M

O24.03 Pre-existing type 1 diabetes mellitus, in the puerperium ♀ M

O24.1 Pre-existing type 2 diabetes mellitus, in pregnancy, childbirth and the puerperium

Insulin-resistant diabetes mellitus in pregnancy, childbirth and the puerperium

Use additional code (for):
from category E11 to further identify any manifestations
long-term (current) use of insulin (Z79.4)

O24.11 Pre-existing type 2 diabetes mellitus, in pregnancy

O24.111 Pre-existing type 2 diabetes mellitus, in pregnancy, first trimester ♀ M

O24.112 Pre-existing type 2 diabetes mellitus, in pregnancy, second trimester ♀ M

O24.113 Pre-existing type 2 diabetes mellitus, in pregnancy, third trimester ♀ M

O24.119 Pre-existing type 2 diabetes mellitus, in pregnancy, unspecified trimester ♀ M

O24.12 Pre-existing type 2 diabetes mellitus, in childbirth ♀ M

O24.13 Pre-existing type 2 diabetes mellitus, in the puerperium ♀ M

O24.3 Unspecified pre-existing diabetes mellitus in pregnancy, childbirth and the puerperium

Use additional code (for):
from category E11 to further identify any manifestation
long-term (current) use of insulin (Z79.4)

O24.31 Unspecified pre-existing diabetes mellitus in pregnancy

O24.311 Unspecified pre-existing diabetes mellitus in pregnancy, first trimester ♀ M

O24.312 Unspecified pre-existing diabetes mellitus in pregnancy, second trimester ♀ M

O24.313 Unspecified pre-existing diabetes mellitus in pregnancy, third trimester ♀ M

O24.319 Unspecified pre-existing diabetes mellitus in pregnancy, unspecified trimester ♀ M

O24.32 Unspecified pre-existing diabetes mellitus in childbirth ♀ M

O24.33 Unspecified pre-existing diabetes mellitus in the puerperium ♀ M

O24.4 Gestational diabetes mellitus

Diabetes mellitus arising in pregnancy

Gestational diabetes mellitus NOS

O24.41 Gestational diabetes mellitus in pregnancy

O24.410 Gestational diabetes mellitus in pregnancy, diet controlled ♀ M

O24.414 Gestational diabetes mellitus in pregnancy, insulin controlled ♀ M

O24.415 Gestational diabetes mellitus in pregnancy, controlled by oral hypoglycemic drugs ♀ ◀ M

Gestational diabetes mellitus in pregnancy, controlled by oral antidiabetic drugs ◀

O24.419 Gestational diabetes mellitus in pregnancy, unspecified control ♀ M

Coding Clinic: 2015, Q4, P34

O24.42 Gestational diabetes mellitus in childbirth

O24.420 Gestational diabetes mellitus in childbirth, diet controlled ♀ M

O24.424 Gestational diabetes mellitus in childbirth, insulin controlled ♀ M

O24.425 Gestational diabetes mellitus in childbirth, controlled by oral hypoglycemic drugs ♀ ◀ M

Gestational diabetes mellitus in childbirth, controlled by oral antidiabetic drugs ◀

O24.429 Gestational diabetes mellitus in childbirth, unspecified control ♀ M

OGCR Section I.C.15.i.

Gestational (pregnancy induced) diabetes

Gestational (pregnancy induced) diabetes can occur during the second and third trimester of pregnancy in women who were not diabetic prior to pregnancy. Gestational diabetes can cause complications in the pregnancy similar to those of pre-existing diabetes mellitus. It also puts the woman at greater risk of developing diabetes after the pregnancy. Codes for gestational diabetes are in subcategory O24.4, Gestational diabetes mellitus. No other code from category O24, Diabetes mellitus in pregnancy, childbirth, and the puerperium, should be used with a code from O24.4

The codes under subcategory O24.4 include diet controlled, insulin controlled, **and controlled by oral hypoglycemic drugs.** If a patient with gestational diabetes is treated with both diet and insulin, only the code for insulin-controlled is required. **If a patient with gestational diabetes is treated with both diet and oral hypoglycemic medications, only the code for "controlled by oral hypoglycemic drugs" is required.** Code Z79.4, Long-term (current) use of insulin **or code Z79.84, Long-term (current) use of oral hypoglycemic drugs,** should not be assigned with codes from subcategory O24.4.

An abnormal glucose tolerance in pregnancy is assigned a code from subcategory O99.81, Abnormal glucose complicating pregnancy, childbirth, and the puerperium.

- **O24.43 Gestational diabetes mellitus in the puerperium**
  - **O24.430 Gestational diabetes mellitus in the puerperium, diet controlled ♀** M
  - **O24.434 Gestational diabetes mellitus in the puerperium, insulin controlled ♀** M
  - **O24.435 Gestational diabetes mellitus in puerperium, controlled by oral hypoglycemic drugs ♀ ◀** M
    - Gestational diabetes mellitus in puerperium, controlled by oral antidiabetic drugs ◀
  - **O24.439 Gestational diabetes mellitus in the puerperium, unspecified control ♀** M
- **O24.8 Other pre-existing diabetes mellitus in pregnancy, childbirth, and the puerperium**
  - Use additional code (for):
    - from categories E08, E09 and E13 to further identify any manifestation
    - long-term (current) use of insulin (Z79.4)
  - **O24.81 Other pre-existing diabetes mellitus in pregnancy**
    - **O24.811 Other pre-existing diabetes mellitus in pregnancy, first trimester ♀** M
    - **O24.812 Other pre-existing diabetes mellitus in pregnancy, second trimester ♀** M
    - **O24.813 Other pre-existing diabetes mellitus in pregnancy, third trimester ♀** M
    - **O24.819 Other pre-existing diabetes mellitus in pregnancy, unspecified trimester ♀** M
  - **O24.82 Other pre-existing diabetes mellitus in childbirth ♀** M
  - **O24.83 Other pre-existing diabetes mellitus in the puerperium ♀** M
- **O24.9 Unspecified diabetes mellitus in pregnancy, childbirth and the puerperium**
  - Use additional code for long-term (current) use of insulin (Z79.4)
  - *Unknown whether patient was diabetic before pregnancy occurred*
  - **O24.91 Unspecified diabetes mellitus in pregnancy**
    - **O24.911 Unspecified diabetes mellitus in pregnancy, first trimester ♀** M
    - **O24.912 Unspecified diabetes mellitus in pregnancy, second trimester ♀** M
    - **O24.913 Unspecified diabetes mellitus in pregnancy, third trimester ♀** M
    - **O24.919 Unspecified diabetes mellitus in pregnancy, unspecified trimester ♀** M
  - **O24.92 Unspecified diabetes mellitus in childbirth ♀** M
  - **O24.93 Unspecified diabetes mellitus in the puerperium ♀** M

- **O25 Malnutrition in pregnancy, childbirth and the puerperium**
  - **O25.1 Malnutrition in pregnancy**
    - **O25.10 Malnutrition in pregnancy, unspecified trimester ♀** M
    - **O25.11 Malnutrition in pregnancy, first trimester ♀** M
    - **O25.12 Malnutrition in pregnancy, second trimester ♀** M
    - **O25.13 Malnutrition in pregnancy, third trimester ♀** M
  - **O25.2 Malnutrition in childbirth ♀** M
  - **O25.3 Malnutrition in the puerperium ♀** M

- **O26 Maternal care for other conditions predominantly related to pregnancy**
  - **O26.0 Excessive weight gain in pregnancy**
    - **Excludes2** gestational edema (O12.0, O12.2)
    - **O26.00 Excessive weight gain in pregnancy, unspecified trimester ♀** M
    - **O26.01 Excessive weight gain in pregnancy, first trimester ♀** M
    - **O26.02 Excessive weight gain in pregnancy, second trimester ♀** M
    - **O26.03 Excessive weight gain in pregnancy, third trimester ♀** M
  - **O26.1 Low weight gain in pregnancy**
    - **O26.10 Low weight gain in pregnancy, unspecified trimester ♀** M
    - **O26.11 Low weight gain in pregnancy, first trimester ♀** M
    - **O26.12 Low weight gain in pregnancy, second trimester ♀** M
    - **O26.13 Low weight gain in pregnancy, third trimester ♀** M
  - **O26.2 Pregnancy care for patient with recurrent pregnancy loss**
    - **O26.20 Pregnancy care for patient with recurrent pregnancy loss, unspecified trimester ♀** M
    - **O26.21 Pregnancy care for patient with recurrent pregnancy loss, first trimester ♀** M
    - **O26.22 Pregnancy care for patient with recurrent pregnancy loss, second trimester ♀** M
    - **O26.23 Pregnancy care for patient with recurrent pregnancy loss, third trimester ♀** M
  - **O26.3 Retained intrauterine contraceptive device in pregnancy**
    - **O26.30 Retained intrauterine contraceptive device in pregnancy, unspecified trimester ♀** M
    - **O26.31 Retained intrauterine contraceptive device in pregnancy, first trimester ♀** M
    - **O26.32 Retained intrauterine contraceptive device in pregnancy, second trimester ♀** M
    - **O26.33 Retained intrauterine contraceptive device in pregnancy, third trimester ♀** M
  - **O26.4 Herpes gestationis**
    - **O26.40 Herpes gestationis, unspecified trimester ♀** M
    - **O26.41 Herpes gestationis, first trimester ♀** M
    - **O26.42 Herpes gestationis, second trimester ♀** M
    - **O26.43 Herpes gestationis, third trimester ♀** M
  - **O26.5 Maternal hypotension syndrome**
    - Supine hypotensive syndrome
    - **O26.50 Maternal hypotension syndrome, unspecified trimester ♀** M
    - **O26.51 Maternal hypotension syndrome, first trimester ♀** M
    - **O26.52 Maternal hypotension syndrome, second trimester ♀** M
    - **O26.53 Maternal hypotension syndrome, third trimester ♀** M

● **O26.6 Liver and biliary tract disorders in pregnancy, childbirth and the puerperium**

Use additional code to identify the specific disorder

Excludes2 hepatorenal syndrome following labor and delivery (O90.4)

● **O26.61 Liver and biliary tract disorders in pregnancy**

Ex For category O26.61 CC codes: 011.4, 011.5, 012.04, 012.05, 012.14, 012.15, 012.24, 012.25, 013.4, 013.5, 014.04, 014.05, 014.14, 014.15, 014.24, 014.25, 014.94, 014.95, 016.4, 016.5, 025.10-025.3, 026.10-026.13, 026.30-026.43, 026.611-026.819, 026.841-026.86, 026.891-026.93, 029.011-029.93, 035.7XX0-035.7XX9, 075.4, 075.81, 075.89-075.9, 080, 090.89, 099.111-099.285, 099.330-099.335, 099.350-099.355, 099.511-099.73, 099.820-099.825, 099.840-09A.53

O26.611 Liver and biliary tract disorders in pregnancy, first trimester ♀ M

O26.612 Liver and biliary tract disorders in pregnancy, second trimester ♀ M

O26.613 Liver and biliary tract disorders in pregnancy, third trimester ♀ M

O26.619 Liver and biliary tract disorders in pregnancy, unspecified trimester ♀ M

O26.62 Liver and biliary tract disorders in childbirth ♀ M

Ex See 026.61

O26.63 Liver and biliary tract disorders in the puerperium ♀ M

● **O26.7 Subluxation of symphysis (pubis) in pregnancy, childbirth and the puerperium**

Excludes1 traumatic separation of symphysis (pubis) during childbirth (O71.6)

● **O26.71 Subluxation of symphysis (pubis) in pregnancy**

O26.711 Subluxation of symphysis (pubis) in pregnancy, first trimester ♀ M

O26.712 Subluxation of symphysis (pubis) in pregnancy, second trimester ♀ M

O26.713 Subluxation of symphysis (pubis) in pregnancy, third trimester ♀ M

O26.719 Subluxation of symphysis (pubis) in pregnancy, unspecified trimester ♀ M

O26.72 Subluxation of symphysis (pubis) in childbirth ♀ M

O26.73 Subluxation of symphysis (pubis) in the puerperium ♀ M

● **O26.8 Other specified pregnancy related conditions**

● **O26.81 Pregnancy related exhaustion and fatigue**

O26.811 Pregnancy related exhaustion and fatigue, first trimester ♀ M

O26.812 Pregnancy related exhaustion and fatigue, second trimester ♀ M

O26.813 Pregnancy related exhaustion and fatigue, third trimester ♀ M

O26.819 Pregnancy related exhaustion and fatigue, unspecified trimester ♀ M

● **O26.82 Pregnancy related peripheral neuritis**

O26.821 Pregnancy related peripheral neuritis, first trimester ♀ M

O26.822 Pregnancy related peripheral neuritis, second trimester ♀ M

O26.823 Pregnancy related peripheral neuritis, third trimester ♀ M

O26.829 Pregnancy related peripheral neuritis, unspecified trimester ♀ M

● **O26.83 Pregnancy related renal disease**

Use additional code to identify the specific disorder

Ex For category O26.83 CC codes: 011.5, 012.05, 012.11-012.13, 012.15, 012.21-012.23, 012.25, 013.5, 014.05, 014.15, 014.25, 014.95, 016.5, 026.831-026.833, 090.89

O26.831 Pregnancy related renal disease, first trimester ♀ M

O26.832 Pregnancy related renal disease, second trimester ♀ M

O26.833 Pregnancy related renal disease, third trimester ♀ M

O26.839 Pregnancy related renal disease, unspecified trimester ♀ M

● **O26.84 Uterine size-date discrepancy complicating pregnancy**

Excludes1 encounter for suspected problem with fetal growth ruled out (Z03.74)

O26.841 Uterine size-date discrepancy, first trimester ♀ M

O26.842 Uterine size-date discrepancy, second trimester ♀ M

O26.843 Uterine size-date discrepancy, third trimester ♀ M

O26.849 Uterine size-date discrepancy, unspecified trimester ♀ M

● **O26.85 Spotting complicating pregnancy**

O26.851 Spotting complicating pregnancy, first trimester ♀ M

O26.852 Spotting complicating pregnancy, second trimester ♀ M

O26.853 Spotting complicating pregnancy, third trimester ♀ M

O26.859 Spotting complicating pregnancy, unspecified trimester ♀ M

O26.86 Pruritic urticarial papules and plaques of pregnancy (PUPPP) ♀ M

Polymorphic eruption of pregnancy

● **O26.87 Cervical shortening**

Excludes1 encounter for suspected cervical shortening ruled out (Z03.75)

Ex For category O26.87 CC codes: 026.872-026.879, 034.31-034.33

O26.872 Cervical shortening, second trimester ♀ M

O26.873 Cervical shortening, third trimester ♀ M

O26.879 Cervical shortening, unspecified trimester ♀ M

● **O26.89 Other specified pregnancy related conditions**

O26.891 Other specified pregnancy related conditions, first trimester ♀ M

O26.892 Other specified pregnancy related conditions, second trimester ♀ M

O26.893 Other specified pregnancy related conditions, third trimester ♀ M

Coding Clinic: 2015, Q3, P40

O26.899 Other specified pregnancy related conditions, unspecified trimester ♀ M

● **O26.9 Pregnancy related conditions, unspecified**

O26.90 Pregnancy related conditions, unspecified, unspecified trimester ♀ M

O26.91 Pregnancy related conditions, unspecified, first trimester ♀ M

O26.92 Pregnancy related conditions, unspecified, second trimester ♀ M

O26.93 Pregnancy related conditions, unspecified, third trimester ♀ M

- O28 Abnormal findings on antenatal screening of mother
  - **Excludes1** diagnostic findings classified elsewhere - see Alphabetical Index
  - O28.0 Abnormal hematological finding on antenatal screening of mother ♀ M
  - O28.1 Abnormal biochemical finding on antenatal screening of mother ♀ M
  - O28.2 Abnormal cytological finding on antenatal screening of mother ♀ M
  - O28.3 Abnormal ultrasonic finding on antenatal screening of mother ♀ M
  - O28.4 Abnormal radiological finding on antenatal screening of mother ♀ M
  - O28.5 Abnormal chromosomal and genetic finding on antenatal screening of mother ♀ M
  - O28.8 Other abnormal findings on antenatal screening of mother ♀ M
  - O28.9 Unspecified abnormal findings on antenatal screening of mother ♀ M

- O29 Complications of anesthesia during pregnancy
  - **Includes** maternal complications arising from the administration of a general, regional or local anesthetic, analgesic or other sedation during pregnancy
  - Use additional code, if necessary, to identify the complication
  - **Excludes2** complications of anesthesia during labor and delivery (O74.-)
    complications of anesthesia during the puerperium (O89.-)
  - O29.0 Pulmonary complications of anesthesia during pregnancy
    - O29.01 Aspiration pneumonitis due to anesthesia during pregnancy
      - Inhalation of stomach contents or secretions NOS due to anesthesia during pregnancy
      - Mendelson's syndrome due to anesthesia during pregnancy
      - O29.011 Aspiration pneumonitis due to anesthesia during pregnancy, first trimester ♀ M
      - O29.012 Aspiration pneumonitis due to anesthesia during pregnancy, second trimester ♀ M
      - O29.013 Aspiration pneumonitis due to anesthesia during pregnancy, third trimester ♀ M
      - O29.019 Aspiration pneumonitis due to anesthesia during pregnancy, unspecified trimester ♀ M
    - O29.02 Pressure collapse of lung due to anesthesia during pregnancy
      - O29.021 Pressure collapse of lung due to anesthesia during pregnancy, first trimester ♀ M
      - O29.022 Pressure collapse of lung due to anesthesia during pregnancy, second trimester ♀ M
      - O29.023 Pressure collapse of lung due to anesthesia during pregnancy, third trimester ♀ M
      - O29.029 Pressure collapse of lung due to anesthesia during pregnancy, unspecified trimester ♀ M
    - O29.09 Other pulmonary complications of anesthesia during pregnancy
      - O29.091 Other pulmonary complications of anesthesia during pregnancy, first trimester ♀ M
      - O29.092 Other pulmonary complications of anesthesia during pregnancy, second trimester ♀ M
      - O29.093 Other pulmonary complications of anesthesia during pregnancy, third trimester ♀ M
      - O29.099 Other pulmonary complications of anesthesia during pregnancy, unspecified trimester ♀ M
  - O29.1 Cardiac complications of anesthesia during pregnancy
    - O29.11 Cardiac arrest due to anesthesia during pregnancy
      - O29.111 Cardiac arrest due to anesthesia during pregnancy, first trimester ♀ M
      - O29.112 Cardiac arrest due to anesthesia during pregnancy, second trimester ♀ M
      - O29.113 Cardiac arrest due to anesthesia during pregnancy, third trimester ♀ M
      - O29.119 Cardiac arrest due to anesthesia during pregnancy, unspecified trimester ♀ M
    - O29.12 Cardiac failure due to anesthesia during pregnancy
      - O29.121 Cardiac failure due to anesthesia during pregnancy, first trimester ♀ M
      - O29.122 Cardiac failure due to anesthesia during pregnancy, second trimester ♀ M
      - O29.123 Cardiac failure due to anesthesia during pregnancy, third trimester ♀ M
      - O29.129 Cardiac failure due to anesthesia during pregnancy, unspecified trimester ♀ M
    - O29.19 Other cardiac complications of anesthesia during pregnancy
      - O29.191 Other cardiac complications of anesthesia during pregnancy, first trimester ♀ M
      - O29.192 Other cardiac complications of anesthesia during pregnancy, second trimester ♀ M
      - O29.193 Other cardiac complications of anesthesia during pregnancy, third trimester ♀ M
      - O29.199 Other cardiac complications of anesthesia during pregnancy, unspecified trimester ♀ M
  - O29.2 Central nervous system complications of anesthesia during pregnancy
    - O29.21 Cerebral anoxia due to anesthesia during pregnancy
      - O29.211 Cerebral anoxia due to anesthesia during pregnancy, first trimester ♀ M
      - O29.212 Cerebral anoxia due to anesthesia during pregnancy, second trimester ♀ M
      - O29.213 Cerebral anoxia due to anesthesia during pregnancy, third trimester ♀ M
      - O29.219 Cerebral anoxia due to anesthesia during pregnancy, unspecified trimester ♀ M
    - O29.29 Other central nervous system complications of anesthesia during pregnancy
      - O29.291 Other central nervous system complications of anesthesia during pregnancy, first trimester ♀ M
      - O29.292 Other central nervous system complications of anesthesia during pregnancy, second trimester ♀ M
      - O29.293 Other central nervous system complications of anesthesia during pregnancy, third trimester ♀ M
      - O29.299 Other central nervous system complications of anesthesia during pregnancy, unspecified trimester ♀ M

- **O29.3 Toxic reaction to local anesthesia during pregnancy**
  - **O29.3X Toxic reaction to local anesthesia during pregnancy**
    - **O29.3X1 Toxic reaction to local anesthesia during pregnancy, first trimester ♀** M
    - **O29.3X2 Toxic reaction to local anesthesia during pregnancy, second trimester ♀** M
    - **O29.3X3 Toxic reaction to local anesthesia during pregnancy, third trimester ♀** M
    - **O29.3X9 Toxic reaction to local anesthesia during pregnancy, unspecified trimester ♀** M
- **O29.4 Spinal and epidural anesthesia induced headache during pregnancy**
  - **O29.40 Spinal and epidural anesthesia induced headache during pregnancy, unspecified trimester ♀** M
  - **O29.41 Spinal and epidural anesthesia induced headache during pregnancy, first trimester ♀** M
  - **O29.42 Spinal and epidural anesthesia induced headache during pregnancy, second trimester ♀** M
  - **O29.43 Spinal and epidural anesthesia induced headache during pregnancy, third trimester ♀** M
- **O29.5 Other complications of spinal and epidural anesthesia during pregnancy**
  - **O29.5X Other complications of spinal and epidural anesthesia during pregnancy**
    - **O29.5X1 Other complications of spinal and epidural anesthesia during pregnancy, first trimester ♀** M
    - **O29.5X2 Other complications of spinal and epidural anesthesia during pregnancy, second trimester ♀** M
    - **O29.5X3 Other complications of spinal and epidural anesthesia during pregnancy, third trimester ♀** M
    - **O29.5X9 Other complications of spinal and epidural anesthesia during pregnancy, unspecified trimester ♀** M
- **O29.6 Failed or difficult intubation for anesthesia during pregnancy**
  - **O29.60 Failed or difficult intubation for anesthesia during pregnancy, unspecified trimester ♀** M
  - **O29.61 Failed or difficult intubation for anesthesia during pregnancy, first trimester ♀** M
  - **O29.62 Failed or difficult intubation for anesthesia during pregnancy, second trimester ♀** M
  - **O29.63 Failed or difficult intubation for anesthesia during pregnancy, third trimester ♀** M
- **O29.8 Other complications of anesthesia during pregnancy**
  - **O29.8X Other complications of anesthesia during pregnancy**
    - **O29.8X1 Other complications of anesthesia during pregnancy, first trimester ♀** M
    - **O29.8X2 Other complications of anesthesia during pregnancy, second trimester ♀** M
    - **O29.8X3 Other complications of anesthesia during pregnancy, third trimester ♀** M
    - **O29.8X9 Other complications of anesthesia during pregnancy, unspecified trimester ♀** M
- **O29.9 Unspecified complication of anesthesia during pregnancy**
  - **O29.90 Unspecified complication of anesthesia during pregnancy, unspecified trimester ♀** M
  - **O29.91 Unspecified complication of anesthesia during pregnancy, first trimester ♀** M
  - **O29.92 Unspecified complication of anesthesia during pregnancy, second trimester ♀** M
  - **O29.93 Unspecified complication of anesthesia during pregnancy, third trimester ♀** M

MATERNAL CARE RELATED TO THE FETUS AND AMNIOTIC CAVITY AND POSSIBLE DELIVERY PROBLEMS (O30-O48)

- **O30 Multiple gestation**
  Code also any complications specific to multiple gestation
  - **O30.0 Twin pregnancy**
    - **O30.00 Twin pregnancy, unspecified number of placenta and unspecified number of amniotic sacs**
      - **O30.001 Twin pregnancy, unspecified number of placenta and unspecified number of amniotic sacs, first trimester ♀** M
      - **O30.002 Twin pregnancy, unspecified number of placenta and unspecified number of amniotic sacs, second trimester ♀** M
      - **O30.003 Twin pregnancy, unspecified number of placenta and unspecified number of amniotic sacs, third trimester ♀** M
      - **O30.009 Twin pregnancy, unspecified number of placenta and unspecified number of amniotic sacs, unspecified trimester ♀** M
    - **O30.01 Twin pregnancy, monochorionic/monoamniotic**
      Twin pregnancy, one placenta, one amniotic sac
      Excludes1 conjoined twins (O30.02-)
      - **O30.011 Twin pregnancy, monochorionic/monoamniotic, first trimester ♀** M
      - **O30.012 Twin pregnancy, monochorionic/monoamniotic, second trimester ♀** M
      - **O30.013 Twin pregnancy, monochorionic/monoamniotic, third trimester ♀** M
      - **O30.019 Twin pregnancy, monochorionic/monoamniotic, unspecified trimester ♀** M
    - **O30.02 Conjoined twin pregnancy**
      - **O30.021 Conjoined twin pregnancy, first trimester ♀** M
      - **O30.022 Conjoined twin pregnancy, second trimester ♀** M
      - **O30.023 Conjoined twin pregnancy, third trimester ♀** M
      - **O30.029 Conjoined twin pregnancy, unspecified trimester ♀** M
    - **O30.03 Twin pregnancy, monochorionic/diamniotic**
      Twin pregnancy, one placenta, two amniotic sacs
      - **O30.031 Twin pregnancy, monochorionic/diamniotic, first trimester ♀** M
      - **O30.032 Twin pregnancy, monochorionic/diamniotic, second trimester ♀** M
      - **O30.033 Twin pregnancy, monochorionic/diamniotic, third trimester ♀** M
      - **O30.039 Twin pregnancy, monochorionic/diamniotic, unspecified trimester ♀** M

● O30.04 Twin pregnancy, dichorionic/diamniotic
Twin pregnancy, two placentae, two amniotic sacs
O30.041 Twin pregnancy, dichorionic/diamniotic, first trimester ♀ M
O30.042 Twin pregnancy, dichorionic/diamniotic, second trimester ♀ M
O30.043 Twin pregnancy, dichorionic/diamniotic, third trimester ♀ M
O30.049 Twin pregnancy, dichorionic/diamniotic, unspecified trimester ♀ M

● O30.09 Twin pregnancy, unable to determine number of placenta and number of amniotic sacs
O30.091 Twin pregnancy, unable to determine number of placenta and number of amniotic sacs, first trimester ♀ M
O30.092 Twin pregnancy, unable to determine number of placenta and number of amniotic sacs, second trimester ♀ M
O30.093 Twin pregnancy, unable to determine number of placenta and number of amniotic sacs, third trimester ♀ M
O30.099 Twin pregnancy, unable to determine number of placenta and number of amniotic sacs, unspecified trimester ♀ M

● O30.1 Triplet pregnancy
Ex For category O30.1 CC codes: O30.001-O30.019, O30.031-O31.23X9, O31.31X0-O32.9XX9, O80

● O30.10 Triplet pregnancy, unspecified number of placenta and unspecified number of amniotic sacs
O30.101 Triplet pregnancy, unspecified number of placenta and unspecified number of amniotic sacs, first trimester ♀ M
O30.102 Triplet pregnancy, unspecified number of placenta and unspecified number of amniotic sacs, second trimester ♀ M
O30.103 Triplet pregnancy, unspecified number of placenta and unspecified number of amniotic sacs, third trimester ♀ M
Coding Clinic: 2016, Q2, P8
O30.109 Triplet pregnancy, unspecified number of placenta and unspecified number of amniotic sacs, unspecified trimester ♀ M

● O30.11 Triplet pregnancy with two or more monochorionic fetuses
O30.111 Triplet pregnancy with two or more monochorionic fetuses, first trimester ♀ M
O30.112 Triplet pregnancy with two or more monochorionic fetuses, second trimester ♀ M
O30.113 Triplet pregnancy with two or more monochorionic fetuses, third trimester ♀ M
O30.119 Triplet pregnancy with two or more monochorionic fetuses, unspecified trimester ♀ M

● O30.12 Triplet pregnancy with two or more monoamniotic fetuses
O30.121 Triplet pregnancy with two or more monoamniotic fetuses, first trimester ♀ M
O30.122 Triplet pregnancy with two or more monoamniotic fetuses, second trimester ♀ M
O30.123 Triplet pregnancy with two or more monoamniotic fetuses, third trimester ♀ M
O30.129 Triplet pregnancy with two or more monoamniotic fetuses, unspecified trimester ♀ M

● O30.19 Triplet pregnancy, unable to determine number of placenta and number of amniotic sacs
O30.191 Triplet pregnancy, unable to determine number of placenta and number of amniotic sacs, first trimester ♀ M
O30.192 Triplet pregnancy, unable to determine number of placenta and number of amniotic sacs, second trimester ♀ M
O30.193 Triplet pregnancy, unable to determine number of placenta and number of amniotic sacs, third trimester ♀ M
O30.199 Triplet pregnancy, unable to determine number of placenta and number of amniotic sacs, unspecified trimester ♀ M

● O30.2 Quadruplet pregnancy
Ex For category O30.2 CC codes: See O30.1

● O30.20 Quadruplet pregnancy, unspecified number of placenta and unspecified number of amniotic sacs
O30.201 Quadruplet pregnancy, unspecified number of placenta and unspecified number of amniotic sacs, first trimester ♀ M
O30.202 Quadruplet pregnancy, unspecified number of placenta and unspecified number of amniotic sacs, second trimester ♀ M
O30.203 Quadruplet pregnancy, unspecified number of placenta and unspecified number of amniotic sacs, third trimester ♀ M
O30.209 Quadruplet pregnancy, unspecified number of placenta and unspecified number of amniotic sacs, unspecified trimester ♀ M

● O30.21 Quadruplet pregnancy with two or more monochorionic fetuses
O30.211 Quadruplet pregnancy with two or more monochorionic fetuses, first trimester ♀ M
O30.212 Quadruplet pregnancy with two or more monochorionic fetuses, second trimester ♀ M
O30.213 Quadruplet pregnancy with two or more monochorionic fetuses, third trimester ♀ M
O30.219 Quadruplet pregnancy with two or more monochorionic fetuses, unspecified trimester ♀ M

● O30.22 Quadruplet pregnancy with two or more monoamniotic fetuses
O30.221 Quadruplet pregnancy with two or more monoamniotic fetuses, first trimester ♀ M
O30.222 Quadruplet pregnancy with two or more monoamniotic fetuses, second trimester ♀ M
O30.223 Quadruplet pregnancy with two or more monoamniotic fetuses, third trimester ♀ M
O30.229 Quadruplet pregnancy with two or more monoamniotic fetuses, unspecified trimester ♀ M

O30.29 Quadruplet pregnancy, unable to determine number of placenta and number of amniotic sacs

- **O30.291 Quadruplet pregnancy, unable to determine number of placenta and number of amniotic sacs, first trimester ♀** M
- **O30.292 Quadruplet pregnancy, unable to determine number of placenta and number of amniotic sacs, second trimester ♀** M
- **O30.293 Quadruplet pregnancy, unable to determine number of placenta and number of amniotic sacs, third trimester ♀** M
- **O30.299 Quadruplet pregnancy, unable to determine number of placenta and number of amniotic sacs, unspecified trimester ♀** M

O30.8 Other specified multiple gestation

Multiple gestation pregnancy greater then quadruplets

Ex For category O30.8 CC codes: See O30.1

O30.80 Other specified multiple gestation, unspecified number of placenta and unspecified number of amniotic sacs

- **O30.801 Other specified multiple gestation, unspecified number of placenta and unspecified number of amniotic sacs, first trimester ♀** M
- **O30.802 Other specified multiple gestation, unspecified number of placenta and unspecified number of amniotic sacs, second trimester ♀** M
- **O30.803 Other specified multiple gestation, unspecified number of placenta and unspecified number of amniotic sacs, third trimester ♀** M
- **O30.809 Other specified multiple gestation, unspecified number of placenta and unspecified number of amniotic sacs, unspecified trimester ♀** M

O30.81 Other specified multiple gestation with two or more monochorionic fetuses

- **O30.811 Other specified multiple gestation with two or more monochorionic fetuses, first trimester ♀** M
- **O30.812 Other specified multiple gestation with two or more monochorionic fetuses, second trimester ♀** M
- **O30.813 Other specified multiple gestation with two or more monochorionic fetuses, third trimester ♀** M
- **O30.819 Other specified multiple gestation with two or more monochorionic fetuses, unspecified trimester ♀** M

O30.82 Other specified multiple gestation with two or more monoamniotic fetuses

- **O30.821 Other specified multiple gestation with two or more monoamniotic fetuses, first trimester ♀** M
- **O30.822 Other specified multiple gestation with two or more monoamniotic fetuses, second trimester ♀** M
- **O30.823 Other specified multiple gestation with two or more monoamniotic fetuses, third trimester ♀** M
- **O30.829 Other specified multiple gestation with two or more monoamniotic fetuses, unspecified trimester ♀** M

O30.89 Other specified multiple gestation, unable to determine number of placenta and number of amniotic sacs

- **O30.891 Other specified multiple gestation, unable to determine number of placenta and number of amniotic sacs, first trimester ♀** M
- **O30.892 Other specified multiple gestation, unable to determine number of placenta and number of amniotic sacs, second trimester ♀** M
- **O30.893 Other specified multiple gestation, unable to determine number of placenta and number of amniotic sacs, third trimester ♀** M
- **O30.899 Other specified multiple gestation, unable to determine number of placenta and number of amniotic sacs, unspecified trimester ♀** M

O30.9 Multiple gestation, unspecified

Multiple pregnancy NOS

- **O30.90 Multiple gestation, unspecified, unspecified trimester ♀** M
- **O30.91 Multiple gestation, unspecified, first trimester ♀** M
- **O30.92 Multiple gestation, unspecified, second trimester ♀** M
- **O30.93 Multiple gestation, unspecified, third trimester ♀** M

O31 Complications specific to multiple gestation

Excludes2 delayed delivery of second twin, triplet, etc. (O63.2)
malpresentation of one fetus or more (O32.9)
placental transfusion syndromes (O43.0-)

Coding Clinic: 2012, Q4, P107

One of the following 7th characters is to be assigned to each code under category O31. 7th character 0 is for single gestations and multiple gestations where the fetus is unspecified. 7th characters 1 through 9 are for cases of multiple gestations to identify the fetus for which the code applies. The appropriate code from category O30, Multiple gestation, must also be assigned when assigning a code from category O31 that has a 7th character of 1 through 9.

0	not applicable or unspecified
1	fetus 1
2	fetus 2
3	fetus 3
4	fetus 4
5	fetus 5
9	other fetus

O31.0 Papyraceous fetus

Fetus compressus

- X **O31.00 Papyraceous fetus, unspecified trimester ♀** M
- X **O31.01 Papyraceous fetus, first trimester ♀** M
- X **O31.02 Papyraceous fetus, second trimester ♀** M
- X **O31.03 Papyraceous fetus, third trimester ♀** M

O31.1 Continuing pregnancy after spontaneous abortion of one fetus or more

- X **O31.10 Continuing pregnancy after spontaneous abortion of one fetus or more, unspecified trimester ♀** M
- X **O31.11 Continuing pregnancy after spontaneous abortion of one fetus or more, first trimester ♀** M
- X **O31.12 Continuing pregnancy after spontaneous abortion of one fetus or more, second trimester ♀** M
- X **O31.13 Continuing pregnancy after spontaneous abortion of one fetus or more, third trimester ♀** M

● **O31.2 Continuing pregnancy after intrauterine death of one fetus or more**

X● **O31.20 Continuing pregnancy after intrauterine death of one fetus or more, unspecified trimester ♀** M

X● **O31.21 Continuing pregnancy after intrauterine death of one fetus or more, first trimester ♀** M

X● **O31.22 Continuing pregnancy after intrauterine death of one fetus or more, second trimester ♀** M

X● **O31.23 Continuing pregnancy after intrauterine death of one fetus or more, third trimester ♀** M

● **O31.3 Continuing pregnancy after elective fetal reduction of one fetus or more**

Continuing pregnancy after selective termination of one fetus or more

X● **O31.30 Continuing pregnancy after elective fetal reduction of one fetus or more, unspecified trimester ♀** M

X● **O31.31 Continuing pregnancy after elective fetal reduction of one fetus or more, first trimester ♀** M

X● **O31.32 Continuing pregnancy after elective fetal reduction of one fetus or more, second trimester ♀** M

X● **O31.33 Continuing pregnancy after elective fetal reduction of one fetus or more, third trimester ♀** M

● **O31.8 Other complications specific to multiple gestation**

Ex: For category O31.8 CC codes: See O30.1

● **O31.8X Other complications specific to multiple gestation**

● **O31.8X1 Other complications specific to multiple gestation, first trimester ♀** M

● **O31.8X2 Other complications specific to multiple gestation, second trimester ♀** M

● **O31.8X3 Other complications specific to multiple gestation, third trimester ♀** M

● **O31.8X9 Other complications specific to multiple gestation, unspecified trimester ♀** M

● **O32 Maternal care for malpresentation of fetus**

Includes the listed conditions as a reason for observation, hospitalization or other obstetric care of the mother, or for cesarean delivery before onset of labor

Excludes1 malpresentation of fetus with obstructed labor (O64.-)

Coding Clinic: 2012, Q4, P107

One of the following 7th characters is to be assigned to each code under category O32. 7th character 0 is for single gestations and multiple gestations where the fetus is unspecified. 7th characters 1 through 9 are for cases of multiple gestations to identify the fetus for which the code applies. The appropriate code from category O30, Multiple gestation, must also be assigned when assigning a code from category O32 that has a 7th character of 1 through 9.

0	not applicable or unspecified
1	fetus 1
2	fetus 2
3	fetus 3
4	fetus 4
5	fetus 5
9	other fetus

X● **O32.0 Maternal care for unstable lie ♀** M

X● **O32.1 Maternal care for breech presentation ♀** M

Maternal care for buttocks presentation
Maternal care for complete breech
Maternal care for frank breech

Excludes1 footling presentation (O32.8)
incomplete breech (O32.8)

X● **O32.2 Maternal care for transverse and oblique lie ♀** M

Maternal care for oblique presentation
Maternal care for transverse presentation

X● **O32.3 Maternal care for face, brow and chin presentation ♀** M

X● **O32.4 Maternal care for high head at term ♀** M

Maternal care for failure of head to enter pelvic brim

X● **O32.6 Maternal care for compound presentation ♀** M

X● **O32.8 Maternal care for other malpresentation of fetus ♀** M

Maternal care for footling presentation
Maternal care for incomplete breech

X● **O32.9 Maternal care for malpresentation of fetus, unspecified ♀** M

● **O33 Maternal care for disproportion**

Includes the listed conditions as a reason for observation, hospitalization or other obstetric care of the mother, or for cesarean delivery before onset of labor

Excludes1 disproportion with obstructed labor (O65-O66)

O33.0 Maternal care for disproportion due to deformity of maternal pelvic bones ♀ M

Maternal care for disproportion due to pelvic deformity causing disproportion NOS

Ex: O33.0

O33.1 Maternal care for disproportion due to generally contracted pelvis ♀ M

Maternal care for disproportion due to contracted pelvis NOS causing disproportion

O33.2 Maternal care for disproportion due to inlet contraction of pelvis ♀ M

Maternal care for disproportion due to inlet contraction (pelvis) causing disproportion

X● **O33.3 Maternal care for disproportion due to outlet contraction of pelvis ♀** M

Maternal care for disproportion due to mid-cavity contraction (pelvis)
Maternal care for disproportion due to outlet contraction (pelvis)

One of the following 7th characters is to be assigned to code O33.3. 7th character 0 is for single gestations and multiple gestations where the fetus is unspecified. 7th characters 1 through 9 are for cases of multiple gestations to identify the fetus for which the code applies. The appropriate code from category O30, Multiple gestation, must also be assigned when assigning code O33.3 with a 7th character of 1 through 9.

0	not applicable or unspecified
1	fetus 1
2	fetus 2
3	fetus 3
4	fetus 4
5	fetus 5
9	other fetus

X● **O33.4 Maternal care for disproportion of mixed maternal and fetal origin ♀** M

One of the following 7th characters is to be assigned to code O33.4. 7th character 0 is for single gestations and multiple gestations where the fetus is unspecified. 7th characters 1 through 9 are for cases of multiple gestations to identify the fetus for which the code applies. The appropriate code from category O30, Multiple gestation, must also be assigned when assigning code O33.4 with a 7th character of 1 through 9.

0	not applicable or unspecified
1	fetus 1
2	fetus 2
3	fetus 3
4	fetus 4
5	fetus 5
9	other fetus

X● **O33.5 Maternal care for disproportion due to unusually large fetus ♀** M

Maternal care for disproportion due to disproportion of fetal origin with normally formed fetus
Maternal care for disproportion due to fetal disproportion NOS

One of the following 7th characters is to be assigned to code O33.5. 7th character Ø is for single gestations and multiple gestations where the fetus is unspecified. 7th characters 1 through 9 are for cases of multiple gestations to identify the fetus for which the code applies. The appropriate code from category O3Ø, Multiple gestation, must also be assigned when assigning code O33.5 with a 7th character of 1 through 9.

Ø	not applicable or unspecified
1	fetus 1
2	fetus 2
3	fetus 3
4	fetus 4
5	fetus 5
9	other fetus

X● **O33.6 Maternal care for disproportion due to hydrocephalic fetus ♀** M

One of the following 7th characters is to be assigned to code O33.6. 7th character Ø is for single gestations and multiple gestations where the fetus is unspecified. 7th characters 1 through 9 are for cases of multiple gestations to identify the fetus for which the code applies. The appropriate code from category O3Ø, Multiple gestation, must also be assigned when assigning code O33.6 with a 7th character of 1 through 9.

Ø	not applicable or unspecified
1	fetus 1
2	fetus 2
3	fetus 3
4	fetus 4
5	fetus 5
9	other fetus

X● **O33.7 Maternal care for disproportion due to other fetal deformities ♀** M

Maternal care for disproportion due to fetal ascites
Maternal care for disproportion due to fetal hydrops
Maternal care for disproportion due to fetal meningomyelocele
Maternal care for disproportion due to fetal sacral teratoma
Maternal care for disproportion due to fetal tumor

Excludes1 obstructed labor due to other fetal deformities (O66.3)

One of the following 7th characters is to be assigned to code O33.7. 7th character Ø is for single gestations and multiple gestations where the fetus is unspecified. 7th characters 1 through 9 are for cases of multiple gestations to identify the fetus for which the code applies. The appropriate code from category O3Ø, Multiple gestation, must also be assigned when assigning code O33.7 with a 7th character of 1 through 9. ◀

Ø	not applicable or unspecified ◀
1	fetus 1 ◀
2	fetus 2 ◀
3	fetus 3 ◀
4	fetus 4 ◀
5	fetus 5 ◀
9	other fetus ◀

O33.8 Maternal care for disproportion of other origin ♀ M

O33.9 Maternal care for disproportion, unspecified ♀ M

Maternal care for disproportion due to cephalopelvic disproportion NOS
Maternal care for disproportion due to fetopelvic disproportion NOS

● **O34 Maternal care for abnormality of pelvic organs**

Includes the listed conditions as a reason for hospitalization or other obstetric care of the mother, or for cesarean delivery before onset of labor

Code first any associated obstructed labor (O65.5)

Use additional code for specific condition

● **O34.0 Maternal care for congenital malformation of uterus**

Maternal care for double uterus ◀
Maternal care for uterus bicornis ◀

O34.00 Maternal care for unspecified congenital malformation of uterus, unspecified trimester ♀ M

O34.01 Maternal care for unspecified congenital malformation of uterus, first trimester ♀ M

O34.02 Maternal care for unspecified congenital malformation of uterus, second trimester ♀ M

O34.03 Maternal care for unspecified congenital malformation of uterus, third trimester ♀ M

● **O34.1 Maternal care for benign tumor of corpus uteri**

Excludes2 maternal care for benign tumor of cervix (O34.4-)
maternal care for malignant neoplasm of uterus (O9A.1-)

O34.10 Maternal care for benign tumor of corpus uteri, unspecified trimester ♀ M

O34.11 Maternal care for benign tumor of corpus uteri, first trimester ♀ M

O34.12 Maternal care for benign tumor of corpus uteri, second trimester ♀ M

O34.13 Maternal care for benign tumor of corpus uteri, third trimester ♀ M

● **O34.2 Maternal care due to uterine scar from previous surgery**

● **O34.21 Maternal care for scar from previous cesarean delivery**

O34.211 Maternal care for low transverse scar from previous cesarean delivery ♀ ◀ M

O34.212 Maternal care for vertical scar from previous cesarean delivery ♀ ◀ M

Maternal care for classical scar from previous cesarean delivery ◀

O34.219 Maternal care for unspecified type scar from previous cesarean delivery ♀ ◀ M

O34.29 Maternal care due to uterine scar from other previous surgery ♀ M

Maternal care due to uterine scar from other transmural uterine incision ◀

● **O34.3 Maternal care for cervical incompetence**

Maternal care for cerclage with or without cervical incompetence
Maternal care for Shirodkar suture with or without cervical incompetence

Ex: **For category O34.3 CC codes:** 026.872-026.879, 034.31-034.33

O34.30 Maternal care for cervical incompetence, unspecified trimester ♀ M

O34.31 Maternal care for cervical incompetence, first trimester ♀ CC M

O34.32 Maternal care for cervical incompetence, second trimester ♀ CC M

O34.33 Maternal care for cervical incompetence, third trimester ♀ CC M

● **O34.4 Maternal care for other abnormalities of cervix**

O34.40 Maternal care for other abnormalities of cervix, unspecified trimester ♀ M

O34.41 Maternal care for other abnormalities of cervix, first trimester ♀ M

O34.42 Maternal care for other abnormalities of cervix, second trimester ♀ M

O34.43 Maternal care for other abnormalities of cervix, third trimester ♀ M

● O34.5 Maternal care for other abnormalities of gravid uterus

● O34.51 Maternal care for incarceration of gravid uterus

O34.511 Maternal care for incarceration of gravid uterus, first trimester ♀ M

O34.512 Maternal care for incarceration of gravid uterus, second trimester ♀ M

O34.513 Maternal care for incarceration of gravid uterus, third trimester ♀ M

O34.519 Maternal care for incarceration of gravid uterus, unspecified trimester ♀ M

● O34.52 Maternal care for prolapse of gravid uterus

O34.521 Maternal care for prolapse of gravid uterus, first trimester ♀ M

O34.522 Maternal care for prolapse of gravid uterus, second trimester ♀ M

O34.523 Maternal care for prolapse of gravid uterus, third trimester ♀ M

O34.529 Maternal care for prolapse of gravid uterus, unspecified trimester ♀ M

● O34.53 Maternal care for retroversion of gravid uterus

O34.531 Maternal care for retroversion of gravid uterus, first trimester ♀ M

O34.532 Maternal care for retroversion of gravid uterus, second trimester ♀ M

O34.533 Maternal care for retroversion of gravid uterus, third trimester ♀ M

O34.539 Maternal care for retroversion of gravid uterus, unspecified trimester ♀ M

● O34.59 Maternal care for other abnormalities of gravid uterus

O34.591 Maternal care for other abnormalities of gravid uterus, first trimester ♀ M

O34.592 Maternal care for other abnormalities of gravid uterus, second trimester ♀ M

O34.593 Maternal care for other abnormalities of gravid uterus, third trimester ♀ M

O34.599 Maternal care for other abnormalities of gravid uterus, unspecified trimester ♀ M

● O34.6 Maternal care for abnormality of vagina

Excludes2 maternal care for vaginal varices in pregnancy (O22.1-)

O34.60 Maternal care for abnormality of vagina, unspecified trimester ♀ M

O34.61 Maternal care for abnormality of vagina, first trimester ♀ M

O34.62 Maternal care for abnormality of vagina, second trimester ♀ M

O34.63 Maternal care for abnormality of vagina, third trimester ♀ M

● O34.7 Maternal care for abnormality of vulva and perineum

Excludes2 maternal care for perineal and vulval varices in pregnancy (O22.1-)

O34.70 Maternal care for abnormality of vulva and perineum, unspecified trimester ♀ M

O34.71 Maternal care for abnormality of vulva and perineum, first trimester ♀ M

O34.72 Maternal care for abnormality of vulva and perineum, second trimester ♀ M

O34.73 Maternal care for abnormality of vulva and perineum, third trimester ♀ M

● O34.8 Maternal care for other abnormalities of pelvic organs

O34.80 Maternal care for other abnormalities of pelvic organs, unspecified trimester ♀ M

O34.81 Maternal care for other abnormalities of pelvic organs, first trimester ♀ M

O34.82 Maternal care for other abnormalities of pelvic organs, second trimester ♀ M

O34.83 Maternal care for other abnormalities of pelvic organs, third trimester ♀ M

● O34.9 Maternal care for abnormality of pelvic organ, unspecified

O34.90 Maternal care for abnormality of pelvic organ, unspecified, unspecified trimester ♀ M

O34.91 Maternal care for abnormality of pelvic organ, unspecified, first trimester ♀ M

O34.92 Maternal care for abnormality of pelvic organ, unspecified, second trimester ♀ M

O34.93 Maternal care for abnormality of pelvic organ, unspecified, third trimester ♀ M

● O35 Maternal care for known or suspected fetal abnormality and damage

Includes the listed conditions in the fetus as a reason for hospitalization or other obstetric care to the mother, or for termination of pregnancy

Code also any associated maternal condition

Excludes1 encounter for suspected maternal and fetal conditions ruled out (Z03.7-)

One of the following 7th characters is to be assigned to each code under category O35. 7th character 0 is for single gestations and multiple gestations where the fetus is unspecified. 7th characters 1 through 9 are for cases of multiple gestations to identify the fetus for which the code applies. The appropriate code from category O30, Multiple gestation, must also be assigned when assigning a code from category O35 that has a 7th character of 1 through 9.

0	not applicable or unspecified
1	fetus 1
2	fetus 2
3	fetus 3
4	fetus 4
5	fetus 5
9	other fetus

X ● O35.0 Maternal care for (suspected) central nervous system malformation in fetus ♀ M

Maternal care for fetal anencephaly
Maternal care for fetal hydrocephalus
Maternal care for fetal spina bifida

Excludes2 chromosomal abnormality in fetus (O35.1)

X ● O35.1 Maternal care for (suspected) chromosomal abnormality in fetus ♀ M

X ● O35.2 Maternal care for (suspected) hereditary disease in fetus ♀ M

Excludes2 chromosomal abnormality in fetus (O35.1)

OGCR Section I.C.15.e.1.

Fetal Conditions Affecting the Management of the Mother

1) Code from categories O35 and O36

Codes from categories O35, Maternal care for known or suspected fetal abnormality and damage, and O36, Maternal care for other fetal problems, are assigned only when the fetal condition is actually responsible for modifying the management of the mother, i.e., by requiring diagnostic studies, additional observation, special care, or termination of pregnancy. The fact that the fetal condition exists does not justify assigning a code from this series to the mother's record.

2) In utero surgery

In cases when surgery is performed on the fetus, a diagnosis code from category O35, Maternal care for known or suspected fetal abnormality and damage, should be assigned identifying the fetal condition. Assign the appropriate procedure code for the procedure performed.

No code from Chapter 16, the perinatal codes, should be used on the mother's record to identify fetal conditions. Surgery performed in utero on a fetus is still to be coded as an obstetric encounter.

X● **O35.3 Maternal care for (suspected) damage to fetus from viral disease in mother ♀** M
Maternal care for damage to fetus from maternal cytomegalovirus infection
Maternal care for damage to fetus from maternal rubella

X● **O35.4 Maternal care for (suspected) damage to fetus from alcohol ♀** M

X● **O35.5 Maternal care for (suspected) damage to fetus by drugs ♀** M
Maternal care for damage to fetus from drug addiction

X● **O35.6 Maternal care for (suspected) damage to fetus by radiation ♀** M

X● **O35.7 Maternal care for (suspected) damage to fetus by other medical procedures ♀** M
Maternal care for damage to fetus by amniocentesis
Maternal care for damage to fetus by biopsy procedures
Maternal care for damage to fetus by hematological investigation
Maternal care for damage to fetus by intrauterine contraceptive device
Maternal care for damage to fetus by intrauterine surgery

X● **O35.8 Maternal care for other (suspected) fetal abnormality and damage ♀** M
Maternal care for damage to fetus from maternal listeriosis
Maternal care for damage to fetus from maternal toxoplasmosis

X● **O35.9 Maternal care for (suspected) fetal abnormality and damage, unspecified ♀** M

● **O36 Maternal care for other fetal problems**

Includes the listed conditions in the fetus as a reason for hospitalization or other obstetric care of the mother, or for termination of pregnancy

Excludes1 encounter for suspected maternal and fetal conditions ruled out (Z03.7-)
placental transfusion syndromes (O43.0-)

Excludes2 labor and delivery complicated by fetal stress (O77.-)

One of the following 7th characters is to be assigned to each code under category O36. 7th character 0 is for single gestations and multiple gestations where the fetus is unspecified. 7th characters 1 through 9 are for cases of multiple gestations to identify the fetus for which the code applies. The appropriate code from category O30, Multiple gestation, must also be assigned when assigning a code from category O36 that has a 7th character of 1 through 9.

0	not applicable or unspecified
1	fetus 1
2	fetus 2
3	fetus 3
4	fetus 4
5	fetus 5
9	other fetus

Coding Clinic: 2015, Q3, P40

● **O36.0 Maternal care for rhesus isoimmunization**
Maternal care for Rh incompatibility (with hydrops fetalis)
Ex: For category O36.0 CC codes: 036.0110-036.0139, 036.0910-036.0939

● **O36.01 Maternal care for anti-D [Rh] antibodies**

● **O36.011 Maternal care for anti-D [Rh] antibodies, first trimester ♀** M

● **O36.012 Maternal care for anti-D [Rh] antibodies, second trimester ♀** M

● **O36.013 Maternal care for anti-D [Rh] antibodies, third trimester ♀** M

● **O36.019 Maternal care for anti-D [Rh] antibodies, unspecified trimester ♀** M

● **O36.09 Maternal care for other rhesus isoimmunization**

● **O36.091 Maternal care for other rhesus isoimmunization, first trimester ♀** M

● **O36.092 Maternal care for other rhesus isoimmunization, second trimester ♀** M

● **O36.093 Maternal care for other rhesus isoimmunization, third trimester ♀** M
Coding Clinic: 2015, Q3, P40

● **O36.099 Maternal care for other rhesus isoimmunization, unspecified trimester ♀** M

● **O36.1 Maternal care for other isoimmunization**
Maternal care for ABO isoimmunization

● **O36.11 Maternal care for Anti-A sensitization**
Maternal care for isoimmunization NOS (with hydrops fetalis)

● **O36.111 Maternal care for Anti-A sensitization, first trimester ♀** M

● **O36.112 Maternal care for Anti-A sensitization, second trimester ♀** M

● **O36.113 Maternal care for Anti-A sensitization, third trimester ♀** M

● **O36.119 Maternal care for Anti-A sensitization, unspecified trimester ♀** M

● **O36.19 Maternal care for other isoimmunization**
Maternal care for Anti-B sensitization

● **O36.191 Maternal care for other isoimmunization, first trimester ♀** M

● **O36.192 Maternal care for other isoimmunization, second trimester ♀** M

● **O36.193 Maternal care for other isoimmunization, third trimester ♀** M

● **O36.199 Maternal care for other isoimmunization, unspecified trimester ♀** M

● **O36.2 Maternal care for hydrops fetalis**
Maternal care for hydrops fetalis NOS
Maternal care for hydrops fetalis not associated with isoimmunization

Excludes1 hydrops fetalis associated with ABO isoimmunization (O36.1-)
hydrops fetalis associated with rhesus isoimmunization (O36.0-)

● **O36.20 Maternal care for hydrops fetalis, unspecified trimester ♀** M

● **O36.21 Maternal care for hydrops fetalis, first trimester ♀** M

● **O36.22 Maternal care for hydrops fetalis, second trimester ♀** M

● **O36.23 Maternal care for hydrops fetalis, third trimester ♀** M

● **O36.4 Maternal care for intrauterine death ♀** M
Maternal care for intrauterine fetal death NOS
Maternal care for intrauterine fetal death after completion of 20 weeks of gestation
Maternal care for late fetal death
Maternal care for missed delivery

Excludes1 missed abortion (O02.1)
stillbirth (P95)

Ex: O36.4XX0-O36.4XX9

● O36.5 Maternal care for known or suspected poor fetal growth
● O36.51 Maternal care for known or suspected placental insufficiency
● O36.511 Maternal care for known or suspected placental insufficiency, first trimester ♀ M
● O36.512 Maternal care for known or suspected placental insufficiency, second trimester ♀ M
● O36.513 Maternal care for known or suspected placental insufficiency, third trimester ♀ M
● O36.519 Maternal care for known or suspected placental insufficiency, unspecified trimester ♀ M
● O36.59 Maternal care for other known or suspected poor fetal growth
Maternal care for known or suspected light-for-dates NOS
Maternal care for known or suspected small-for-dates NOS
● O36.591 Maternal care for other known or suspected poor fetal growth, first trimester ♀ M
● O36.592 Maternal care for other known or suspected poor fetal growth, second trimester ♀ M
● O36.593 Maternal care for other known or suspected poor fetal growth, third trimester ♀ M
● O36.599 Maternal care for other known or suspected poor fetal growth, unspecified trimester ♀ M
● O36.6 Maternal care for excessive fetal growth
Maternal care for known or suspected large-for-dates
X● O36.60 Maternal care for excessive fetal growth, unspecified trimester ♀ M
X● O36.61 Maternal care for excessive fetal growth, first trimester ♀ M
X● O36.62 Maternal care for excessive fetal growth, second trimester ♀ M
X● O36.63 Maternal care for excessive fetal growth, third trimester ♀ M
● O36.7 Maternal care for viable fetus in abdominal pregnancy
X● O36.70 Maternal care for viable fetus in abdominal pregnancy, unspecified trimester ♀ M
X● O36.71 Maternal care for viable fetus in abdominal pregnancy, first trimester ♀ M
X● O36.72 Maternal care for viable fetus in abdominal pregnancy, second trimester ♀ M
X● O36.73 Maternal care for viable fetus in abdominal pregnancy, third trimester ♀ M
● O36.8 Maternal care for other specified fetal problems
●X● O36.80 Pregnancy with inconclusive fetal viability ♀ M
Encounter to determine fetal viability of pregnancy
● O36.81 Decreased fetal movements
● O36.812 Decreased fetal movements, second trimester ♀ M
● O36.813 Decreased fetal movements, third trimester ♀ M
● O36.819 Decreased fetal movements, unspecified trimester ♀ M
● O36.82 Fetal anemia and thrombocytopenia
● O36.821 Fetal anemia and thrombocytopenia, first trimester ♀ M
● O36.822 Fetal anemia and thrombocytopenia, second trimester ♀ M
● O36.823 Fetal anemia and thrombocytopenia, third trimester ♀ M
● O36.829 Fetal anemia and thrombocytopenia, unspecified trimester ♀ M
● O36.89 Maternal care for other specified fetal problems
● O36.891 Maternal care for other specified fetal problems, first trimester ♀ M
● O36.892 Maternal care for other specified fetal problems, second trimester ♀ M
● O36.893 Maternal care for other specified fetal problems, third trimester ♀ M
● O36.899 Maternal care for other specified fetal problems, unspecified trimester ♀ M
● O36.9 Maternal care for fetal problem, unspecified
X● O36.90 Maternal care for fetal problem, unspecified, unspecified trimester ♀ M
X● O36.91 Maternal care for fetal problem, unspecified, first trimester ♀ M
X● O36.92 Maternal care for fetal problem, unspecified, second trimester ♀ M
X● O36.93 Maternal care for fetal problem, unspecified, third trimester ♀ M

● O40 Polyhydramnios
Overabundance of amniotic fluid
Includes hydramnios
Excludes1 encounter for suspected maternal and fetal conditions ruled out (Z03.7-)
One of the following 7th characters is to be assigned to each code under category O40. 7th character 0 is for single gestations and multiple gestations where the fetus is unspecified. 7th characters 1 through 9 are for cases of multiple gestations to identify the fetus for which the code applies. The appropriate code from category O30, Multiple gestation, must also be assigned when assigning a code from category O40 that has a 7th character of 1 through 9.

0	not applicable or unspecified
1	fetus 1
2	fetus 2
3	fetus 3
4	fetus 4
5	fetus 5
9	other fetus

X● O40.1 Polyhydramnios, first trimester ♀ M
X● O40.2 Polyhydramnios, second trimester ♀ M
X● O40.3 Polyhydramnios, third trimester ♀ M
X● O40.9 Polyhydramnios, unspecified trimester ♀ M

● O41 Other disorders of amniotic fluid and membranes
Excludes1 encounter for suspected maternal and fetal conditions ruled out (Z03.7-)
One of the following 7th characters is to be assigned to each code under category O41. 7th character 0 is for single gestations and multiple gestations where the fetus is unspecified. 7th characters 1 through 9 are for cases of multiple gestations to identify the fetus for which the code applies. The appropriate code from category O30, Multiple gestation, must also be assigned when assigning a code from category O41 that has a 7th character of 1 through 9.

0	not applicable or unspecified
1	fetus 1
2	fetus 2
3	fetus 3
4	fetus 4
5	fetus 5
9	other fetus

● O41.0 Oligohydramnios
Scant volume of amniotic fluid
Oligohydramnios without rupture of membranes
Ex For category O41.0 CC codes: O41.01X0-O41.03X9
X● O41.00 Oligohydramnios, unspecified trimester ♀ M
X● O41.01 Oligohydramnios, first trimester ♀ M
X● O41.02 Oligohydramnios, second trimester ♀ M
X● O41.03 Oligohydramnios, third trimester ♀ M

- **O41.1 Infection of amniotic sac and membranes**
  Ex For category O41.1 CC codes: 041.1010-041.1039, 041.1210-041.1239, 041.1410-041.1439
  - **O41.10 Infection of amniotic sac and membranes, unspecified**
    - **O41.101 Infection of amniotic sac and membranes, unspecified, first trimester ♀** M
    - **O41.102 Infection of amniotic sac and membranes, unspecified, second trimester ♀** M
    - **O41.103 Infection of amniotic sac and membranes, unspecified, third trimester ♀** M
    - **O41.109 Infection of amniotic sac and membranes, unspecified, unspecified trimester ♀** M
  - **O41.12 Chorioamnionitis**
    - **O41.121 Chorioamnionitis, first trimester ♀** M
    - **O41.122 Chorioamnionitis, second trimester ♀** M
    - **O41.123 Chorioamnionitis, third trimester ♀** M
    - **O41.129 Chorioamnionitis, unspecified trimester ♀** M
  - **O41.14 Placentitis**
    - **O41.141 Placentitis, first trimester ♀** M
    - **O41.142 Placentitis, second trimester ♀** M
    - **O41.143 Placentitis, third trimester ♀** M
    - **O41.149 Placentitis, unspecified trimester ♀** M
- **O41.8 Other specified disorders of amniotic fluid and membranes**
  - **O41.8X Other specified disorders of amniotic fluid and membranes**
    - **O41.8X1 Other specified disorders of amniotic fluid and membranes, first trimester ♀** M
    - **O41.8X2 Other specified disorders of amniotic fluid and membranes, second trimester ♀** M
    - **O41.8X3 Other specified disorders of amniotic fluid and membranes, third trimester ♀** M
    - **O41.8X9 Other specified disorders of amniotic fluid and membranes, unspecified trimester ♀** M
- **O41.9 Disorder of amniotic fluid and membranes, unspecified**
  - X **O41.90 Disorder of amniotic fluid and membranes, unspecified, unspecified trimester ♀** M
  - X **O41.91 Disorder of amniotic fluid and membranes, unspecified, first trimester ♀** M
  - X **O41.92 Disorder of amniotic fluid and membranes, unspecified, second trimester ♀** M
  - X **O41.93 Disorder of amniotic fluid and membranes, unspecified, third trimester ♀** M

- **O42 Premature rupture of membranes**
  - **O42.0 Premature rupture of membranes, onset of labor within 24 hours of rupture**
    - **O42.00 Premature rupture of membranes, onset of labor within 24 hours of rupture, unspecified weeks of gestation ♀** M
    - **O42.01 Preterm premature rupture of membranes, onset of labor within 24 hours of rupture**
      Premature rupture of membranes before 37 completed weeks of gestation
      - **O42.011 Preterm premature rupture of membranes, onset of labor within 24 hours of rupture, first trimester ♀** M
      - **O42.012 Preterm premature rupture of membranes, onset of labor within 24 hours of rupture, second trimester ♀** M
      - **O42.013 Preterm premature rupture of membranes, onset of labor within 24 hours of rupture, third trimester ♀** M
      - **O42.019 Preterm premature rupture of membranes, onset of labor within 24 hours of rupture, unspecified trimester ♀** M
    - **O42.02 Full-term premature rupture of membranes, onset of labor within 24 hours of rupture ♀** M
      Premature rupture of membranes at or after 37 completed weeks of gestation, onset of labor within 24 hours of rupture
  - **O42.1 Premature rupture of membranes, onset of labor more than 24 hours following rupture**
    - **O42.10 Premature rupture of membranes, onset of labor more than 24 hours following rupture, unspecified weeks of gestation ♀** M
    - **O42.11 Preterm premature rupture of membranes, onset of labor more than 24 hours following rupture**
      Premature rupture of membranes before 37 completed weeks of gestation
      - **O42.111 Preterm premature rupture of membranes, onset of labor more than 24 hours following rupture, first trimester ♀** M
      - **O42.112 Preterm premature rupture of membranes, onset of labor more than 24 hours following rupture, second trimester ♀** M
      - **O42.113 Preterm premature rupture of membranes, onset of labor more than 24 hours following rupture, third trimester ♀** M
      - **O42.119 Preterm premature rupture of membranes, onset of labor more than 24 hours following rupture, unspecified trimester ♀** M
    - **O42.12 Full-term premature rupture of membranes, onset of labor more than 24 hours following rupture ♀** M
      Premature rupture of membranes at or after 37 completed weeks of gestation, onset of labor more than 24 hours following rupture

- **O42.9 Premature rupture of membranes, unspecified as to length of time between rupture and onset of labor**
  - **O42.90 Premature rupture of membranes, unspecified as to length of time between rupture and onset of labor, unspecified weeks of gestation ♀** M
  - **O42.91 Preterm premature rupture of membranes, unspecified as to length of time between rupture and onset of labor**
    Premature rupture of membranes before 37 completed weeks of gestation
    - **O42.911 Preterm premature rupture of membranes, unspecified as to length of time between rupture and onset of labor, first trimester ♀** M
    - **O42.912 Preterm premature rupture of membranes, unspecified as to length of time between rupture and onset of labor, second trimester ♀** M
    - **O42.913 Preterm premature rupture of membranes, unspecified as to length of time between rupture and onset of labor, third trimester ♀** M
    - **O42.919 Preterm premature rupture of membranes, unspecified as to length of time between rupture and onset of labor, unspecified trimester ♀** M
  - **O42.92 Full-term premature rupture of membranes, unspecified as to length of time between rupture and onset of labor ♀** M
    Premature rupture of membranes at or after 37 completed weeks of gestation, unspecified as to length of time between rupture and onset of labor ◀

- **O43 Placental disorders**
  Excludes2 maternal care for poor fetal growth due to placental insufficiency (O36.5-)
  placenta previa (O44.-)
  placental polyp (O90.89)
  placentitis (O41.14-)
  premature separation of placenta [abruptio placentae] (O45.-)
  - **O43.0 Placental transfusion syndromes**
    - **O43.01 Fetomaternal placental transfusion syndrome**
      Maternofetal placental transfusion syndrome
      - **O43.011 Fetomaternal placental transfusion syndrome, first trimester ♀** M
      - **O43.012 Fetomaternal placental transfusion syndrome, second trimester ♀** M
      - **O43.013 Fetomaternal placental transfusion syndrome, third trimester ♀** M
      - **O43.019 Fetomaternal placental transfusion syndrome, unspecified trimester ♀** M
    - **O43.02 Fetus-to-fetus placental transfusion syndrome**
      - **O43.021 Fetus-to-fetus placental transfusion syndrome, first trimester ♀** M
      - **O43.022 Fetus-to-fetus placental transfusion syndrome, second trimester ♀** M
      - **O43.023 Fetus-to-fetus placental transfusion syndrome, third trimester ♀** M
      - **O43.029 Fetus-to-fetus placental transfusion syndrome, unspecified trimester ♀** M
  - **O43.1 Malformation of placenta**
    - **O43.10 Malformation of placenta, unspecified**
      Abnormal placenta NOS
      - **O43.101 Malformation of placenta, unspecified, first trimester ♀** M
      - **O43.102 Malformation of placenta, unspecified, second trimester ♀** M
      - **O43.103 Malformation of placenta, unspecified, third trimester ♀** M
      - **O43.109 Malformation of placenta, unspecified, unspecified trimester ♀** M
    - **O43.11 Circumvallate placenta**
      - **O43.111 Circumvallate placenta, first trimester ♀** M
      - **O43.112 Circumvallate placenta, second trimester ♀** M
      - **O43.113 Circumvallate placenta, third trimester ♀** M
      - **O43.119 Circumvallate placenta, unspecified trimester ♀** M
    - **O43.12 Velamentous insertion of umbilical cord**
      - **O43.121 Velamentous insertion of umbilical cord, first trimester ♀** M
      - **O43.122 Velamentous insertion of umbilical cord, second trimester ♀** M
      - **O43.123 Velamentous insertion of umbilical cord, third trimester ♀** M
      - **O43.129 Velamentous insertion of umbilical cord, unspecified trimester ♀** M
    - **O43.19 Other malformation of placenta**
      - **O43.191 Other malformation of placenta, first trimester ♀** M
      - **O43.192 Other malformation of placenta, second trimester ♀** M
      - **O43.193 Other malformation of placenta, third trimester ♀** M
      - **O43.199 Other malformation of placenta, unspecified trimester ♀** M
  - **O43.2 Morbidly adherent placenta**
    Code also associated third stage postpartum hemorrhage, if applicable (O72.0)
    Excludes1 retained placenta (O73.-)
    - **O43.21 Placenta accreta**
      - **O43.211 Placenta accreta, first trimester ♀** M
      - **O43.212 Placenta accreta, second trimester ♀** M
      - **O43.213 Placenta accreta, third trimester ♀** M
      - **O43.219 Placenta accreta, unspecified trimester ♀** M
    - **O43.22 Placenta increta**
      - **O43.221 Placenta increta, first trimester ♀** M
      - **O43.222 Placenta increta, second trimester ♀** M
      - **O43.223 Placenta increta, third trimester ♀** M
      - **O43.229 Placenta increta, unspecified trimester ♀** M
    - **O43.23 Placenta percreta**
      - **O43.231 Placenta percreta, first trimester ♀** M
      - **O43.232 Placenta percreta, second trimester ♀** M
      - **O43.233 Placenta percreta, third trimester ♀** M
      - **O43.239 Placenta percreta, unspecified trimester ♀** M
  - **O43.8 Other placental disorders**
    - **O43.81 Placental infarction**
      - **O43.811 Placental infarction, first trimester ♀** M
      - **O43.812 Placental infarction, second trimester ♀** M
      - **O43.813 Placental infarction, third trimester ♀** M
      - **O43.819 Placental infarction, unspecified trimester ♀** M
    - **O43.89 Other placental disorders**
      Placental dysfunction
      - **O43.891 Other placental disorders, first trimester ♀** M
      - **O43.892 Other placental disorders, second trimester ♀** M
      - **O43.893 Other placental disorders, third trimester ♀** M
      - **O43.899 Other placental disorders, unspecified trimester ♀** M

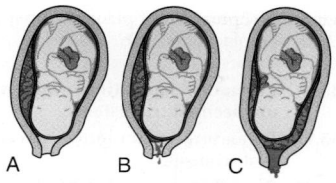

Figure 15-2 **A.** Marginal placento previa. **B.** Partial placenta previa. **C.** Total placento previa.

Item 15-3 **Placenta previa** is a condition in which the opening of the cervix is obstructed by the displaced placenta. The three types, marginal, partial, and total, are varying degrees of placenta displacement. Placenta abruption is the premature breaking away of the placenta from the site of the uterine implant before the delivery of the fetus.

- **O43.9 Unspecified placental disorder**
  - **O43.90 Unspecified placental disorder, unspecified trimester ♀** M
  - **O43.91 Unspecified placental disorder, first trimester ♀** M
  - **O43.92 Unspecified placental disorder, second trimester ♀** M
  - **O43.93 Unspecified placental disorder, third trimester ♀** M

- **O44 Placenta previa**
  - Ex: For category O44 CC codes: See O20
  - **O44.0 Complete placenta previa NOS or without hemorrhage**
    - Placenta previa NOS ◀
    - **O44.00 Complete placenta previa NOS or without hemorrhage, unspecified trimester ♀** M
    - **O44.01 Complete placenta previa NOS or without hemorrhage, first trimester ♀** M
    - **O44.02 Complete placenta previa NOS or without hemorrhage, second trimester ♀** M
    - **O44.03 Complete placenta previa NOS or without hemorrhage, third trimester ♀** M
  - **O44.1 Complete placenta previa with hemorrhage**
    - **Excludes1** labor and delivery complicated by hemorrhage from vasa previa (O69.4)
    - **O44.10 Complete placenta previa with hemorrhage, unspecified trimester ♀** M
    - **O44.11 Complete placenta previa with hemorrhage, first trimester ♀** M
    - **O44.12 Complete placenta previa with hemorrhage, second trimester ♀** M
    - **O44.13 Complete placenta previa with hemorrhage, third trimester ♀** M
  - **O44.2 Partial placenta previa without hemorrhage ◀**
    - Marginal placenta previa, NOS or without hemorrhage ◀
    - **O44.20 Partial placenta previa NOS or without hemorrhage, unspecified trimester ♀ ◀** M
    - **O44.21 Partial placenta previa NOS or without hemorrhage, first trimester ♀ ◀** M
    - **O44.22 Partial placenta previa NOS or without hemorrhage, second trimester ♀ ◀** M
    - **O44.23 Partial placenta previa NOS or without hemorrhage, third trimester ♀ ◀** M
  - **O44.3 Partial placenta previa with hemorrhage ◀**
    - Marginal placenta previa with hemorrhage ◀
    - **O44.30 Partial placenta previa with hemorrhage, unspecified trimester ♀ ◀** M
    - **O44.31 Partial placenta previa with hemorrhage, first trimester ♀ ◀** M
    - **O44.32 Partial placenta previa with hemorrhage, second trimester ♀ ◀** M
    - **O44.33 Partial placenta previa with hemorrhage, third trimester ♀ ◀** M
  - **O44.4 Low lying placenta NOS or without hemorrhage ◀**
    - Low implantation of placenta NOS or without hemorrhage ◀
    - **O44.40 Low lying placenta NOS or without hemorrhage, unspecified ♀ ◀** M
    - **O44.41 Low lying placenta NOS or without hemorrhage, first trimester ♀ ◀** M
    - **O44.42 Low lying placenta NOS or without hemorrhage, second trimester ♀ ◀** M
    - **O44.43 Low lying placenta NOS or without hemorrhage, third trimester ♀ ◀** M
  - **O44.5 Low lying placenta with hemorrhage ◀**
    - Low implantation of placenta with hemorrhage ◀
    - **O44.50 Low lying placenta with hemorrhage, unspecified trimester ♀ ◀** M
    - **O44.51 Low lying placenta with hemorrhage, first trimester ♀ ◀** M
    - **O44.52 Low lying placenta with hemorrhage, second trimester ♀ ◀** M
    - **O44.53 Low lying placenta with hemorrhage, third trimester ♀ ◀** M

- **O45 Premature separation of placenta [abruptio placentae]**
  - **O45.0 Premature separation of placenta with coagulation defect**
    - Ex: For category O45.0 CC codes: 011.4, 011.5, 012.04, 012.05, 012.14, 012.15, 012.24, 012.25, 013.4, 013.5, 014.04, 014.05, 014.14, 014.15, 014.24, 014.25, 014.94, 014.95, 016.4, 016.5, 025.10-025.3, 026.10-026.13, 026.30-026.43, 026.63-026.819, 026.841-026.86, 026.891-026.93, 029.011-029.93, 035.7XX0-035.7XX9, 045.001-045.099, 046.001-046.93, 067.0-067.9, 075.4, 075.81, 075.89-075.9, 080, 090.89, 099.111-099.285, 099.330-099.335, 099.350-099.355, 099.511-099.73, 099.820-099.825, 099.840-09A.53
    - **O45.00 Premature separation of placenta with coagulation defect, unspecified**
      - **O45.001 Premature separation of placenta with coagulation defect, unspecified, first trimester ♀** M
      - **O45.002 Premature separation of placenta with coagulation defect, unspecified, second trimester ♀** M

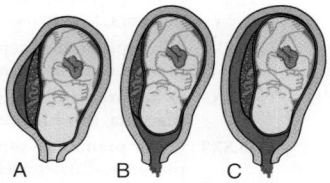

Figure 15-3 Abruptio placentae is classified according to the grade of separation of the placenta from the uterine wall. **A.** Mild separation in which hemorrhage is internal. **B.** Moderate separation in which there is external hemorrhage. **C.** Severe separation in which there is external hemorrhage and extreme separation.

O45.003 Premature separation of placenta with coagulation defect, unspecified, third trimester ♀ M

O45.009 Premature separation of placenta with coagulation defect, unspecified, unspecified trimester ♀ M

● O45.01 Premature separation of placenta with afibrinogenemia
Premature separation of placenta with hypofibrinogenemia

O45.011 Premature separation of placenta with afibrinogenemia, first trimester ♀ M

O45.012 Premature separation of placenta with afibrinogenemia, second trimester ♀ M

O45.013 Premature separation of placenta with afibrinogenemia, third trimester ♀ M

O45.019 Premature separation of placenta with afibrinogenemia, unspecified trimester ♀ M

● O45.02 Premature separation of placenta with disseminated intravascular coagulation

O45.021 Premature separation of placenta with disseminated intravascular coagulation, first trimester ♀ M

O45.022 Premature separation of placenta with disseminated intravascular coagulation, second trimester ♀ M

O45.023 Premature separation of placenta with disseminated intravascular coagulation, third trimester ♀ M

O45.029 Premature separation of placenta with disseminated intravascular coagulation, unspecified trimester ♀ M

● O45.09 Premature separation of placenta with other coagulation defect

O45.091 Premature separation of placenta with other coagulation defect, first trimester ♀ M

O45.092 Premature separation of placenta with other coagulation defect, second trimester ♀ M

O45.093 Premature separation of placenta with other coagulation defect, third trimester ♀ M

O45.099 Premature separation of placenta with other coagulation defect, unspecified trimester ♀ M

● O45.8 Other premature separation of placenta
Ex For category O45.8 CC codes: 011.4, 011.5, 012.04, 012.05, 012.14, 012.15, 012.24, 012.25, 013.4, 013.5, 014.04, 014.05, 014.14, 014.15, 014.24, 014.25, 014.94, 014.95, 016.4, 016.5, 020.0-020.9, 025.10-025.3, 026.10-026.13, 026.30-026.43, 026.63-026.819, 026.841-026.86, 026.891-026.93, 029.011-029.93, 035.7XX0-035.7XX9, 044.00-044.13, 044.20-044.53, 045.8X1-045.8X3, 045.91-045.93, 075.4, 075.81, 075.89-075.9, 080, 090.89, 099.111-099.285, 099.330-099.335, 099.350-099.355, 099.511-099.73, 099.820-099.825, 099.840-09A.53

● O45.8X Other premature separation of placenta

O45.8X1 Other premature separation of placenta, first trimester ♀ M

O45.8X2 Other premature separation of placenta, second trimester ♀ M

O45.8X3 Other premature separation of placenta, third trimester ♀ M

O45.8X9 Other premature separation of placenta, unspecified trimester ♀ M

● O45.9 Premature separation of placenta, unspecified
Abruptio placentae NOS
Ex For category O45.9 CC codes: See 045.8

O45.90 Premature separation of placenta, unspecified, unspecified trimester ♀ M

O45.91 Premature separation of placenta, unspecified, first trimester ♀ M

O45.92 Premature separation of placenta, unspecified, second trimester ♀ M

O45.93 Premature separation of placenta, unspecified, third trimester ♀ M

● O46 Antepartum hemorrhage, not elsewhere classified

Excludes 1 hemorrhage in early pregnancy (O20.-)
intrapartum hemorrhage NEC (O67.-)
placenta previa (O44.-)
premature separation of placenta [abruptio placentae] (O45.-)

● O46.0 Antepartum hemorrhage with coagulation defect
Ex For category O46.0 CC codes: See 045.0

● O46.00 Antepartum hemorrhage with coagulation defect, unspecified

O46.001 Antepartum hemorrhage with coagulation defect, unspecified, first trimester ♀ M

O46.002 Antepartum hemorrhage with coagulation defect, unspecified, second trimester ♀ M

O46.003 Antepartum hemorrhage with coagulation defect, unspecified, third trimester ♀ M

O46.009 Antepartum hemorrhage with coagulation defect, unspecified, unspecified trimester ♀ M

● O46.01 Antepartum hemorrhage with afibrinogenemia
Antepartum hemorrhage with hypofibrinogenemia

O46.011 Antepartum hemorrhage with afibrinogenemia, first trimester ♀ M

O46.012 Antepartum hemorrhage with afibrinogenemia, second trimester ♀ M

O46.013 Antepartum hemorrhage with afibrinogenemia, third trimester ♀ M

O46.019 Antepartum hemorrhage with afibrinogenemia, unspecified trimester ♀ M

● O46.02 Antepartum hemorrhage with disseminated intravascular coagulation

O46.021 Antepartum hemorrhage with disseminated intravascular coagulation, first trimester ♀ M

O46.022 Antepartum hemorrhage with disseminated intravascular coagulation, second trimester ♀ M

O46.023 Antepartum hemorrhage with disseminated intravascular coagulation, third trimester ♀ M

O46.029 Antepartum hemorrhage with disseminated intravascular coagulation, unspecified trimester ♀ M

- **O46.09 Antepartum hemorrhage with other coagulation defect**
  - **O46.091 Antepartum hemorrhage with other coagulation defect, first trimester ♀** M
  - **O46.092 Antepartum hemorrhage with other coagulation defect, second trimester ♀** M
  - **O46.093 Antepartum hemorrhage with other coagulation defect, third trimester ♀** M
  - **O46.099 Antepartum hemorrhage with other coagulation defect, unspecified trimester ♀** M
- **O46.8 Other antepartum hemorrhage**
  - **O46.8x Other antepartum hemorrhage**
    - **O46.8x1 Other antepartum hemorrhage, first trimester ♀** M
    - **O46.8x2 Other antepartum hemorrhage, second trimester ♀** M
    - **O46.8x3 Other antepartum hemorrhage, third trimester ♀** M
    - **O46.8x9 Other antepartum hemorrhage, unspecified trimester ♀** M
- **O46.9 Antepartum hemorrhage, unspecified**
  - **O46.90 Antepartum hemorrhage, unspecified, unspecified trimester ♀** M
  - **O46.91 Antepartum hemorrhage, unspecified, first trimester ♀** M
  - **O46.92 Antepartum hemorrhage, unspecified, second trimester ♀** M
  - **O46.93 Antepartum hemorrhage, unspecified, third trimester ♀** M

- **O47 False labor**

  Includes Braxton Hicks contractions
  threatened labor

  Excludes1 preterm labor (O60.-)

  Ex: **For category O47 CC codes:** 011.4, 011.5, 012.04, 012.05, 012.14, 012.15, 012.24, 012.25, 013.4, 013.5, 014.04, 014.05, 014.14, 014.15, 014.24, 014.25, 014.94, 014.95, 016.4, 016.5, 025.10-025.3, 026.10-026.13, 026.30-026.43, 026.63-026.819, 026.841-026.86, 026.891-026.93, 029.011-029.93, 035.7XX0-035.7XX9, 047.00-047.9, 060.00-060.23X9, 075.4, 075.81, 075.89-075.9, 080, 090.89, 099.111-099.285, 099.330-099.335, 099.350-099.355, 099.511-099.73, 099.820-099.825, 099.840-09A.53

- **O47.0 False labor before 37 completed weeks of gestation**
  - **O47.00 False labor before 37 completed weeks of gestation, unspecified trimester ♀** M
  - **O47.02 False labor before 37 completed weeks of gestation, second trimester ♀** M
  - **O47.03 False labor before 37 completed weeks of gestation, third trimester ♀** M
- **O47.1 False labor at or after 37 completed weeks of gestation ♀** M
- **O47.9 False labor, unspecified ♀** M

- **O48 Late pregnancy**
  - **O48.0 Post-term pregnancy ♀** M

    Pregnancy over 40 completed weeks to 42 completed weeks gestation
  - **O48.1 Prolonged pregnancy ♀** M

    Pregnancy which has advanced beyond 42 completed weeks gestation

COMPLICATIONS OF LABOR AND DELIVERY (O60-O77)

- **O60 Preterm labor**

  Includes onset (spontaneous) of labor before 37 completed weeks of gestation

  Excludes1 false labor (O47.0-)
  threatened labor NOS (O47.0-)

  Ex: **For category O60 CC codes:** See O47
  - **O60.0 Preterm labor without delivery**
    - **O60.00 Preterm labor without delivery, unspecified trimester ♀** M
    - **O60.02 Preterm labor without delivery, second trimester ♀** M
    - **O60.03 Preterm labor without delivery, third trimester ♀** M
  - **O60.1 Preterm labor with preterm delivery**

    One of the following 7th characters is to be assigned to each code under subcategory O60.1. 7th character 0 is for single gestations and multiple gestations where the fetus is unspecified. 7th characters 1 through 9 are for cases of multiple gestations to identify the fetus for which the code applies. The appropriate code from category O30, Multiple gestation, must also be assigned when assigning a code from subcategory O60.1 that has a 7th character of 1 through 9.

0	not applicable or unspecified
1	fetus 1
2	fetus 2
3	fetus 3
4	fetus 4
5	fetus 5
9	other fetus

    Coding Clinic: 2016, Q2, P11

    - X **O60.10 Preterm labor with preterm delivery, unspecified trimester ♀** M

      Preterm labor with delivery NOS
    - X **O60.12 Preterm labor second trimester with preterm delivery second trimester ♀** M
    - X **O60.13 Preterm labor second trimester with preterm delivery third trimester ♀** M
    - X **O60.14 Preterm labor third trimester with preterm delivery third trimester ♀** M

      Coding Clinic: 2016, Q2, P10

● **O60.2 Term delivery with preterm labor**

One of the following 7th characters is to be assigned to each code under subcategory O60.2. 7th character 0 is for single gestations and multiple gestations where the fetus is unspecified. 7th characters 1 through 9 are for cases of multiple gestations to identify the fetus for which the code applies. The appropriate code from category O30, Multiple gestation, must also be assigned when assigning a code from subcategory O60.2 that has a 7th character of 1 through 9.

0	not applicable or unspecified
1	fetus 1
2	fetus 2
3	fetus 3
4	fetus 4
5	fetus 5
9	other fetus

X● **O60.20 Term delivery with preterm labor, unspecified trimester ♀** M

X● **O60.22 Term delivery with preterm labor, second trimester ♀** M

X● **O60.23 Term delivery with preterm labor, third trimester ♀** M

● **O61 Failed induction of labor**

O61.0 Failed medical induction of labor ♀ M
- Failed induction (of labor) by oxytocin
- Failed induction (of labor) by prostaglandins

O61.1 Failed instrumental induction of labor ♀ M
- Failed mechanical induction (of labor)
- Failed surgical induction (of labor)

O61.8 Other failed induction of labor ♀ M

O61.9 Failed induction of labor, unspecified ♀ M

● **O62 Abnormalities of forces of labor**

O62.0 Primary inadequate contractions ♀ M
- Failure of cervical dilatation
- Primary hypotonic uterine dysfunction
- Uterine inertia during latent phase of labor

O62.1 Secondary uterine inertia ♀ M
- Arrested active phase of labor
- Secondary hypotonic uterine dysfunction

O62.2 Other uterine inertia ♀ M
- Atony of uterus without hemorrhage
- Atony of uterus NOS
- Desultory labor
- Hypotonic uterine dysfunction NOS
- Irregular labor
- Poor contractions
- Slow slope active phase of labor
- Uterine inertia NOS

Excludes1 atony of uterus with hemorrhage (postpartum) (O72.1)
postpartum atony of uterus without hemorrhage (O75.89)

O62.3 Precipitate labor ♀ M

O62.4 Hypertonic, incoordinate, and prolonged uterine contractions ♀ M
- Cervical spasm
- Contraction ring dystocia
- Dyscoordinate labor
- Hour-glass contraction of uterus
- Hypertonic uterine dysfunction
- Incoordinate uterine action
- Tetanic contractions
- Uterine dystocia NOS
- Uterine spasm

Excludes1 dystocia (fetal) (maternal) NOS (O66.9)

O62.8 Other abnormalities of forces of labor ♀ M

O62.9 Abnormality of forces of labor, unspecified ♀ M

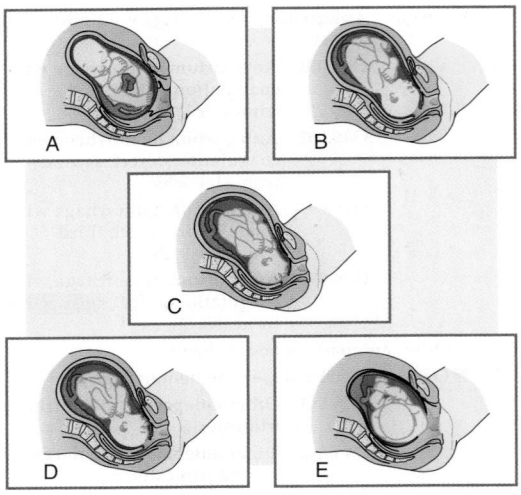

Figure 15-4 Five types of malposition and malpresentation of the fetus: **A.** Breech. **B.** Vertex. **C.** Face. **D.** Brow. **E.** Shoulder.

● **O63 Long labor**

O63.0 Prolonged first stage (of labor) ♀ M

O63.1 Prolonged second stage (of labor) ♀ M

O63.2 Delayed delivery of second twin, triplet, etc. ♀ M

O63.9 Long labor, unspecified ♀ M
- Prolonged labor NOS

Ex 011.4, 011.5, 012.04, 012.05, 012.14, 012.15, 012.24, 012.25, 013.4, 013.5, 014.04, 014.05, 014.14, 014.15, 014.24, 014.25, 014.94, 014.95, 016.4, 016.5, 025.10-025.3, 026.10-026.13, 026.30-026.43, 026.63-026.819, 026.841-026.86, 026.891-026.93, 029.011-029.93, 035.7XX0-035.7XX9, 036.8120-036.8199, 063.9, 071.00-071.1, 071.5, 071.81, 071.89-071.9, 075.4, 075.81, 075.89-075.9, 080, 090.89, 099.111-099.285, 099.330-099.335, 099.350-099.355, 099.511-099.73, 099.820-099.825, 099.840-09A.53

● **O64 Obstructed labor due to malposition and malpresentation of fetus**

One of the following 7th characters is to be assigned to each code under category O64. 7th character 0 is for single gestations and multiple gestations where the fetus is unspecified. 7th characters 1 through 9 are for cases of multiple gestations to identify the fetus for which the code applies. The appropriate code from category O30, Multiple gestation, must also be assigned when assigning a code from category O64 that has a 7th character of 1 through 9.

0	not applicable or unspecified
1	fetus 1
2	fetus 2
3	fetus 3
4	fetus 4
5	fetus 5
9	other fetus

X● **O64.0 Obstructed labor due to incomplete rotation of fetal head ♀** M
- Deep transverse arrest
- Obstructed labor due to persistent occipitoiliac (position)
- Obstructed labor due to persistent occipitoposterior (position)
- Obstructed labor due to persistent occipitosacral (position)
- Obstructed labor due to persistent occipitotransverse (position)

X● **O64.1 Obstructed labor due to breech presentation ♀** M
- Obstructed labor due to buttocks presentation
- Obstructed labor due to complete breech presentation
- Obstructed labor due to frank breech presentation

X● **O64.2 Obstructed labor due to face presentation ♀** M
Obstructed labor due to chin presentation

X● **O64.3 Obstructed labor due to brow presentation ♀** M

X● **O64.4 Obstructed labor due to shoulder presentation ♀** M
Prolapsed arm
Excludes1 impacted shoulders (O66.0)
shoulder dystocia (O66.0)

X● **O64.5 Obstructed labor due to compound presentation ♀** M

X● **O64.8 Obstructed labor due to other malposition and malpresentation ♀** M
Obstructed labor due to footling presentation
Obstructed labor due to incomplete breech presentation

X● **O64.9 Obstructed labor due to malposition and malpresentation, unspecified ♀** M

● **O65 Obstructed labor due to maternal pelvic abnormality**

O65.0 Obstructed labor due to deformed pelvis ♀ M

O65.1 Obstructed labor due to generally contracted pelvis ♀ M

O65.2 Obstructed labor due to pelvic inlet contraction ♀ M

O65.3 Obstructed labor due to pelvic outlet and mid-cavity contraction ♀ M

O65.4 Obstructed labor due to fetopelvic disproportion, unspecified ♀ M
Excludes1 dystocia due to abnormality of fetus (O66.2-O66.3)

O65.5 Obstructed labor due to abnormality of maternal pelvic organs ♀ M
Obstructed labor due to conditions listed in O34.-
Use additional code to identify abnormality of pelvic organs O34.-

O65.8 Obstructed labor due to other maternal pelvic abnormalities ♀ M

O65.9 Obstructed labor due to maternal pelvic abnormality, unspecified ♀ M

● **O66 Other obstructed labor**

O66.0 Obstructed labor due to shoulder dystocia ♀ M
Impacted shoulders

O66.1 Obstructed labor due to locked twins ♀ M

O66.2 Obstructed labor due to unusually large fetus ♀ M

O66.3 Obstructed labor due to other abnormalities of fetus ♀ M
Dystocia due to fetal ascites
Dystocia due to fetal hydrops
Dystocia due to fetal meningomyelocele
Dystocia due to fetal sacral teratoma
Dystocia due to fetal tumor
Dystocia due to hydrocephalic fetus
Use additional code to identify cause of obstruction

● **O66.4 Failed trial of labor**

O66.40 Failed trial of labor, unspecified ♀ M

O66.41 Failed attempted vaginal birth after previous cesarean delivery ♀ M
Code first rupture of uterus, if applicable (O71.0-, O71.1)

O66.5 Attempted application of vacuum extractor and forceps ♀ M
Attempted application of vacuum or forceps, with subsequent delivery by forceps or cesarean delivery

O66.6 Obstructed labor due to other multiple fetuses ♀ M

O66.8 Other specified obstructed labor ♀ M
Use additional code to identify cause of obstruction

O66.9 Obstructed labor, unspecified ♀ M
Dystocia NOS
Fetal dystocia NOS
Maternal dystocia NOS

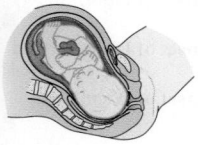

Figure 15-5 Hydrocephalic fetus causing disproportion.

● **O67 Labor and delivery complicated by intrapartum hemorrhage, not elsewhere classified**
Excludes1 antepartum hemorrhage NEC (O46.-)
placenta previa (O44.-)
premature separation of placenta [abruptio placentae] (O45.-)
Excludes2 postpartum hemorrhage (O72.-)

O67.0 Intrapartum hemorrhage with coagulation defect ♀ CC MCC M
Intrapartum hemorrhage (excessive) associated with afibrinogenemia
Intrapartum hemorrhage (excessive) associated with disseminated intravascular coagulation
Intrapartum hemorrhage (excessive) associated with hyperfibrinolysis
Intrapartum hemorrhage (excessive) associated with hypofibrinogenemia
Ex: See O45.0

O67.8 Other intrapartum hemorrhage ♀ M
Excessive intrapartum hemorrhage

O67.9 Intrapartum hemorrhage, unspecified ♀ M

O68 Labor and delivery complicated by abnormality of fetal acid-base balance ♀ CC M
Fetal acidemia complicating labor and delivery
Fetal acidosis complicating labor and delivery
Fetal alkalosis complicating labor and delivery
Fetal metabolic acidemia complicating labor and delivery
Excludes1 fetal stress NOS (O77.9)
labor and delivery complicated by electrocardiographic evidence of fetal stress (O77.8)
labor and delivery complicated by ultrasonic evidence of fetal stress (O77.8)
Excludes2 abnormality in fetal heart rate or rhythm (O76)
labor and delivery complicated by meconium in amniotic fluid (O77.0)
Ex: O68, O76, P03.811

● **O69 Labor and delivery complicated by umbilical cord complications**
One of the following 7th characters is to be assigned to each code under category O69. 7th character 0 is for single gestations and multiple gestations where the fetus is unspecified. 7th characters 1 through 9 are for cases of multiple gestations to identify the fetus for which the code applies. The appropriate code from category O30, Multiple gestation, must also be assigned when assigning a code from category O69 that has a 7th character of 1 through 9.

0	not applicable or unspecified
1	fetus 1
2	fetus 2
3	fetus 3
4	fetus 4
5	fetus 5
9	other fetus

X● **O69.0 Labor and delivery complicated by prolapse of cord ♀** M

X● **O69.1 Labor and delivery complicated by cord around neck, with compression ♀** M
Excludes1 labor and delivery complicated by cord around neck, without compression (O69.81)

X● **O69.2 Labor and delivery complicated by other cord entanglement, with compression ♀** M
Labor and delivery complicated by compression of cord NOS
Labor and delivery complicated by entanglement of cords of twins in monoamniotic sac
Labor and delivery complicated by knot in cord
Excludes1 labor and delivery complicated by other cord entanglement, without compression (O69.82)

X● **O69.3 Labor and delivery complicated by short cord ♀** M

X● **O69.4 Labor and delivery complicated by vasa previa ♀** M
Labor and delivery complicated by hemorrhage from vasa previa

X● **O69.5 Labor and delivery complicated by vascular lesion of cord ♀** M
Labor and delivery complicated by cord bruising
Labor and delivery complicated by cord hematoma
Labor and delivery complicated by thrombosis of umbilical vessels

● **O69.8 Labor and delivery complicated by other cord complications**

X● **O69.81 Labor and delivery complicated by cord around neck, without compression ♀** M

X● **O69.82 Labor and delivery complicated by other cord entanglement, without compression ♀** M

X● **O69.89 Labor and delivery complicated by other cord complications ♀** M

X● **O69.9 Labor and delivery complicated by cord complication, unspecified ♀** M

● **O70 Perineal laceration during delivery**
Includes episiotomy extended by laceration
Excludes1 obstetric high vaginal laceration alone (O71.4)

O70.0 First degree perineal laceration during delivery ♀ M
Perineal laceration, rupture or tear involving fourchette during delivery
Perineal laceration, rupture or tear involving labia during delivery
Perineal laceration, rupture or tear involving skin during delivery
Perineal laceration, rupture or tear involving vagina during delivery
Perineal laceration, rupture or tear involving vulva during delivery
Slight perineal laceration, rupture or tear during delivery

O70.1 Second degree perineal laceration during delivery ♀ M
Perineal laceration, rupture or tear during delivery as in O70.0, also involving pelvic floor
Perineal laceration, rupture or tear during delivery as in O70.0, also involving perineal muscles
Perineal laceration, rupture or tear during delivery as in O70.0, also involving vaginal muscles
Excludes1 perineal laceration involving anal sphincter (O70.2)
Coding Clinic: 2016, Q2, P34

● **O70.2 Third degree perineal laceration during delivery**
Perineal laceration, rupture or tear during delivery as in O70.1, also involving anal sphincter
Perineal laceration, rupture or tear during delivery as in O70.1, also involving rectovaginal septum
Perineal laceration, rupture or tear during delivery as in O70.1, also involving sphincter NOS
Excludes1 anal sphincter tear during delivery without third degree perineal laceration (O70.4)
perineal laceration involving anal or rectal mucosa (O70.3)
(Ex) **For category O70.2 CC codes:** 011.4, 011.5, 012.04, 012.05, 012.14, 012.15, 012.24, 012.25, 013.4, 013.5, 014.04, 014.05, 014.14, 014.15, 014.24, 014.25, 014.94, 014.95, 016.4, 016.5, 025.10-025.3, 026.10-026.13, 026.30-026.43, 026.63-026.819, 026.841-026.86, 026.891-026.93, 029.011-029.93, 035.7XX0-035.7XX9, 036.8120-036.8199, 070.4, 071.00-071.1, 071.5, 071.81, 071.89-071.9, 075.4, 075.81, 075.89-075.9, 080, 090.89, 099.111-099.285, 099.330-099.335, 099.350-099.355, 099.511-099.73, 099.820-099.825, 099.840-09A.53

O70.20 Third degree perineal laceration during delivery, unspecified ♀ ◀ M

O70.21 Third degree perineal laceration during delivery, IIIa ♀ ◀ M
Third degree perineal laceration during delivery with less than 50% of external anal sphincter (EAS) thickness torn ◀

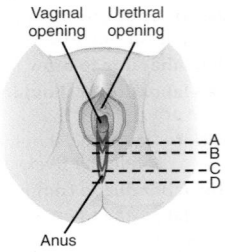

Figure 15-6 Perineal lacerations: **A.** First-degree is laceration of superficial tissues. **B.** Second-degree is limited to the pelvic floor and may involve the perineal or vaginal muscles. **C.** Third-degree involves the anal sphincter. **D.** Fourth-degree involves anal or rectal mucosa.

O70.22 Third degree perineal laceration during delivery, IIIb ♀ ◀ M
Third degree perineal laceration during delivery with more than 50% external anal sphincter (EAS) thickness torn ◀

O70.23 Third degree perineal laceration during delivery, IIIc ♀ ◀ M
Third degree perineal laceration during delivery with both external anal sphincter (EAS) and internal anal sphincter (IAS) torn ◀

O70.3 Fourth degree perineal laceration during delivery ♀ M
Perineal laceration, rupture or tear during delivery as in O70.2, also involving anal mucosa
Perineal laceration, rupture or tear during delivery as in O70.2, also involving rectal mucosa
(Ex) 011.4, 011.5, 012.04, 012.05, 012.14, 012.15, 012.24, 012.25, 013.4, 013.5, 014.04, 014.05, 014.14, 014.15, 014.24, 014.25, 014.94, 014.95, 016.4, 016.5, 025.10-025.3, 026.10-026.13, 026.30-026.43, 026.63-026.819, 026.841-026.86, 026.891-026.93, 029.011-029.93, 035.7XX0-035.7XX9, 036.8120-036.8199, 070.3, 071.00-071.1, 071.5, 071.81, 071.89-071.9, 075.4, 075.81, 075.89-075.9, 080, 090.89, 099.111-099.285, 099.330-099.335, 099.350-099.355, 099.511-099.73, 099.820-099.825, 099.840-09A.53

O70.4 Anal sphincter tear complicating delivery, not associated with third degree laceration ♀ M
Excludes1 anal sphincter tear with third degree perineal laceration (O70.2)
(Ex) 011.4, 011.5, 012.04, 012.05, 012.14, 012.15, 012.24, 012.25, 013.4, 013.5, 014.04, 014.05, 014.14, 014.15, 014.24, 014.25, 014.94, 014.95, 016.4, 016.5, 025.10-025.3, 026.10-026.13, 026.30-026.43, 026.63-026.819, 026.841-026.86, 026.891-026.93, 029.011-029.93, 035.7XX0-035.7XX9, 036.8120-036.8199, 070.20-070.23, 070.4, 071.00-071.1, 071.5, 071.81, 071.89-071.9, 075.4, 075.81, 075.89-075.9, 080, 090.89, 099.111-099.285, 099.330-099.335, 099.350-099.355, 099.511-099.73, 099.820-099.825, 099.840-09A.53

O70.9 Perineal laceration during delivery, unspecified ♀ M

● **O71 Other obstetric trauma**
Includes obstetric damage from instruments

● **O71.0 Rupture of uterus (spontaneous) before onset of labor**
Excludes1 disruption of (current) cesarean delivery wound (O90.0)
laceration of uterus, NEC (O71.81)
(Ex) **For category O71.0 CC codes:** 011.4, 011.5, 012.04, 012.05, 012.14, 012.15, 012.24, 012.25, 013.4, 013.5, 014.04, 014.05, 014.14, 014.15, 014.24, 014.25, 014.94, 014.95, 016.4, 016.5, 025.10-025.3, 026.10-026.13, 026.30-026.43, 026.63-026.819, 026.841-026.86, 026.891-026.93, 029.011-029.93, 035.7XX0-035.7XX9, 036.8120-036.8199, 071.00-071.1, 071.5, 071.81, 071.89-071.9, 075.4, 075.81, 075.89-075.9, 080, 090.89, 099.111-099.285, 099.330-099.335, 099.350-099.355, 099.511-099.73, 099.820-099.825, 099.840-09A.53

O71.00 Rupture of uterus before onset of labor, unspecified trimester ♀ M

O71.02 Rupture of uterus before onset of labor, second trimester ♀ M

O71.03 Rupture of uterus before onset of labor, third trimester ♀ M

O71.1 Rupture of uterus during labor ♀ M
Rupture of uterus not stated as occurring before onset of labor
Excludes1 disruption of cesarean delivery wound (O90.0)
laceration of uterus, NEC (O71.81)
Ex: See O71.0

O71.2 Postpartum inversion of uterus ♀ M
Ex: 011.4, 011.5, 012.04, 012.05, 012.14, 012.15, 012.24, 012.25, 013.4, 013.5, 014.04, 014.05, 014.14, 014.15, 014.24, 014.25, 014.94, 014.95, 016.4, 016.5, 025.10-025.3, 026.10-026.13, 026.30-026.43, 026.63-026.819, 026.841-026.86, 026.891-026.93, 029.011-029.93, 035.7XX0-035.7XX9, 036.8120-036.8199, 071.00-071.2, 071.5, 071.81, 071.89-071.9, 075.4, 075.81, 075.89-075.9, 080, 090.89, 099.111-099.285, 099.330-099.335, 099.350-099.355, 099.511-099.73, 099.820-099.825, 099.840-09A.53

O71.3 Obstetric laceration of cervix ♀ M
Annular detachment of cervix
Ex: 011.4, 011.5, 012.04, 012.05, 012.14, 012.15, 012.24, 012.25, 013.4, 013.5, 014.04, 014.05, 014.14, 014.15, 014.24, 014.25, 014.94, 014.95, 016.4, 016.5, 025.10-025.3, 026.10-026.13, 026.30-026.43, 026.63-026.819, 026.841-026.86, 026.891-026.93, 029.011-029.93, 035.7XX0-035.7XX9, 036.8120-036.8199, 071.00-071.1, 071.3, 071.5, 071.81, 071.89-071.9, 075.4, 075.81, 075.89-075.9, 080, 090.89, 099.111-099.285, 099.330-099.335, 099.350-099.355, 099.511-099.73, 099.820-099.825, 099.840-09A.53

O71.4 Obstetric high vaginal laceration alone ♀ M
Laceration of vaginal wall without perineal laceration
Excludes1 obstetric high vaginal laceration with perineal laceration (O70.-)
Ex: 011.4, 011.5, 012.04, 012.05, 012.14, 012.15, 012.24, 012.25, 013.4, 013.5, 014.04, 014.05, 014.14, 014.15, 014.24, 014.25, 014.94, 014.95, 016.4, 016.5, 025.10-025.3, 026.10-026.13, 026.30-026.43, 026.63-026.819, 026.841-026.86, 026.891-026.93, 029.011-029.93, 035.7XX0-035.7XX9, 036.8120-036.8199, 071.00-071.1, 071.4, 071.5, 071.81, 071.89-071.9, 075.4, 075.81, 075.89-075.9, 080, 090.89, 099.111-099.285, 099.330-099.335, 099.350-099.355, 099.511-099.73, 099.820-099.825, 099.840-09A.53

O71.5 Other obstetric injury to pelvic organs ♀ M
Obstetric injury to bladder
Obstetric injury to urethra
Excludes2 obstetric periurethral trauma (O71.82)
Ex: See O71.0

O71.6 Obstetric damage to pelvic joints and ligaments ♀ M
Obstetric avulsion of inner symphyseal cartilage
Obstetric damage to coccyx
Obstetric traumatic separation of symphysis (pubis)
Ex: 011.4, 011.5, 012.04, 012.05, 012.14, 012.15, 012.24, 012.25, 013.4, 013.5, 014.04, 014.05, 014.14, 014.15, 014.24, 014.25, 014.94, 014.95, 016.4, 016.5, 025.10-025.3, 026.10-026.13, 026.30-026.43, 026.63-026.819, 026.841-026.86, 026.891-026.93, 029.011-029.93, 035.7XX0-035.7XX9, 036.8120-036.8199, 071.00-071.1, 071.5-071.6, 071.81, 071.89-071.9, 075.4, 075.81, 075.89-075.9, 080, 090.89, 099.111-099.285, 099.330-099.335, 099.350-099.355, 099.511-099.73, 099.820-099.825, 099.840-09A.53

O71.7 Obstetric hematoma of pelvis ♀ M
Obstetric hematoma of perineum
Obstetric hematoma of vagina
Obstetric hematoma of vulva
Ex: 011.4, 011.5, 012.04, 012.05, 012.14, 012.15, 012.24, 012.25, 013.4, 013.5, 014.04, 014.05, 014.14, 014.15, 014.24, 014.25, 014.94, 014.95, 016.4, 016.5, 025.10-025.3, 026.10-026.13, 026.30-026.43, 026.63-026.819, 026.841-026.86, 026.891-026.93, 029.011-029.93, 035.7XX0-035.7XX9, 036.8120-036.8199, 071.00-071.1, 071.5, 071.7, 071.81, 071.89-071.9, 075.4, 075.81, 075.89-075.9, 080, 090.89, 099.111-099.285, 099.330-099.335, 099.350-099.355, 099.511-099.73, 099.820-099.825, 099.840-09A.53

O71.8 Other specified obstetric trauma
O71.81 Laceration of uterus, not elsewhere classified ♀ M
O71.82 Other specified trauma to perineum and vulva ♀ M
Obstetric periurethral trauma
O71.89 Other specified obstetric trauma ♀ M
O71.9 Obstetric trauma, unspecified ♀ M

O72 Postpartum hemorrhage
Includes hemorrhage after delivery of fetus or infant

O72.0 Third-stage hemorrhage ♀ M
Hemorrhage associated with retained, trapped or adherent placenta
Retained placenta NOS
Code also type of adherent placenta (O43.2-)
Ex: 011.4, 011.5, 012.04, 012.05, 012.14, 012.15, 012.24, 012.25, 013.4, 013.5, 014.04, 014.05, 014.14, 014.15, 014.24, 014.25, 014.94, 014.95, 016.4, 016.5, 025.10-025.3, 026.10-026.13, 026.30-026.43, 026.63-026.819, 026.841-026.86, 026.891-026.93, 029.011-029.93, 035.7XX0-035.7XX9, 036.8120-036.8199, 071.00-071.1, 071.5, 071.81, 071.89-071.9, 072.0, 075.4, 075.81, 075.89-075.9, 080, 090.89, 099.111-099.285, 099.330-099.335, 099.350-099.355, 099.511-099.73, 099.820-099.825, 099.840-09A.53

O72.1 Other immediate postpartum hemorrhage ♀ M
Hemorrhage following delivery of placenta
Postpartum hemorrhage (atonic) NOS
Uterine atony with hemorrhage
Excludes1 uterine atony NOS (O62.2)
uterine atony without hemorrhage (O62.2)
postpartum atony of uterus without hemorrhage (O75.89)
Ex: 011.4, 011.5, 012.04, 012.05, 012.14, 012.15, 012.24, 012.25, 013.4, 013.5, 014.04, 014.05, 014.14, 014.15, 014.24, 014.25, 014.94, 014.95, 016.4, 016.5, 025.10-025.3, 026.10-026.13, 026.30-026.43, 026.63-026.819, 026.841-026.86, 026.891-026.93, 029.011-029.93, 035.7XX0-035.7XX9, 036.8120-036.8199, 071.00-071.1, 071.5, 071.81, 071.89-071.9, 072.1, 075.4, 075.81, 075.89-075.9, 080, 090.89, 099.111-099.285, 099.330-099.335, 099.350-099.355, 099.511-099.73, 099.820-099.825, 099.840-09A.53

O72.2 Delayed and secondary postpartum hemorrhage ♀ M
Hemorrhage associated with retained portions of placenta or membranes after the first 24 hours following delivery of placenta
Retained products of conception NOS, following delivery
Ex: 011.4, 011.5, 012.04, 012.05, 012.14, 012.15, 012.24, 012.25, 013.4, 013.5, 014.04, 014.05, 014.14, 014.15, 014.24, 014.25, 014.94, 014.95, 016.4, 016.5, 025.10-025.3, 026.10-026.13, 026.30-026.43, 026.63-026.819, 026.841-026.86, 026.891-026.93, 029.011-029.93, 035.7XX0-035.7XX9, 036.8120-036.8199, 071.00-071.1, 071.5, 071.81, 071.89-071.9, 072.2, 075.4, 075.81, 075.89-075.9, 080, 090.89, 099.111-099.285, 099.330-099.335, 099.350-099.355, 099.511-099.73, 099.820-099.825, 099.840-09A.53

O72.3 Postpartum coagulation defects ♀ M
Postpartum afibrinogenemia
Postpartum fibrinolysis

O73 Retained placenta and membranes, without hemorrhage
Excludes1 placenta accreta (O43.21-)
placenta increta (O43.22-)
placenta percreta (O43.23-)

O73.0 Retained placenta without hemorrhage ♀ M
Adherent placenta, without hemorrhage
Trapped placenta without hemorrhage

O73.1 Retained portions of placenta and membranes, without hemorrhage ♀ M
Retained products of conception following delivery, without hemorrhage

O74 Complications of anesthesia during labor and delivery

Includes maternal complications arising from the administration of a general, regional or local anesthetic, analgesic or other sedation during labor and delivery

Use additional code, if applicable, to identify specific complication

O74.0 Aspiration pneumonitis due to anesthesia during labor and delivery ♀ M

Inhalation of stomach contents or secretions NOS due to anesthesia during labor and delivery

Mendelson's syndrome due to anesthesia during labor and delivery

O74.1 Other pulmonary complications of anesthesia during labor and delivery ♀ M

O74.2 Cardiac complications of anesthesia during labor and delivery ♀ M

O74.3 Central nervous system complications of anesthesia during labor and delivery ♀ M

O74.4 Toxic reaction to local anesthesia during labor and delivery ♀ M

O74.5 Spinal and epidural anesthesia-induced headache during labor and delivery ♀ M

O74.6 Other complications of spinal and epidural anesthesia during labor and delivery ♀ M

O74.7 Failed or difficult intubation for anesthesia during labor and delivery ♀ M

O74.8 Other complications of anesthesia during labor and delivery ♀ M

O74.9 Complication of anesthesia during labor and delivery, unspecified ♀ M

O75 Other complications of labor and delivery, not elsewhere classified

Excludes2 puerperal (postpartum) infection (O86.-)
puerperal (postpartum) sepsis (O85)

O75.0 Maternal distress during labor and delivery ♀ M

O75.1 Shock during or following labor and delivery ♀ M

Obstetric shock following labor and delivery

Ex: O11.4, O11.5, O12.04, O12.05, O12.14, O12.15, O12.24, O12.25, O13.4, O13.5, O14.04, O14.05, O14.14, O14.15, O14.24, O14.25, O14.94, O14.95, O16.4, O16.5, O25.10-O25.3, O26.10-O26.13, O26.30-O26.43, O26.63-O26.819, O26.841-O26.86, O26.891-O26.93, O29.011-O29.93, O35.7XX0-O35.7XX9, O75.1, O75.4, O75.81, O75.89-O75.9, O80, O90.89, O99.111-O99.285, O99.330-O99.335, O99.350-O99.355, O99.511-O99.73, O99.820-O99.825, O99.840-O9A.53

O75.2 Pyrexia during labor, not elsewhere classified ♀ M

Ex: O75.2

O75.3 Other infection during labor ♀ M

Sepsis during labor

Use additional code (B95-B97), to identify infectious agent

Ex: O11.4, O11.5, O12.04, O12.05, O12.14, O12.15, O12.24, O12.25, O13.4, O13.5, O14.04, O14.05, O14.14, O14.15, O14.24, O14.25, O14.94, O14.95, O16.4, O16.5, O25.10-O25.3, O26.10-O26.13, O26.30-O26.43, O26.63-O26.819, O26.841-O26.86, O26.891-O26.93, O29.011-O29.93, O35.7XX0-O35.7XX9, O75.3-O75.4, O75.81, O75.89-O75.9, O80, O90.89, O99.111-O99.285, O99.330-O99.335, O99.350-O99.355, O99.511-O99.73, O99.820-O99.825, O99.840-O9A.53

O75.4 Other complications of obstetric surgery and procedures ♀ M

Cardiac arrest following obstetric surgery or procedures

Cardiac failure following obstetric surgery or procedures

Cerebral anoxia following obstetric surgery or procedures

Pulmonary edema following obstetric surgery or procedures

Use additional code to identify specific complication

Excludes2 complications of anesthesia during labor and delivery (O74.-)
disruption of obstetrical (surgical) wound (O90.0-O90.1)
hematoma of obstetrical (surgical) wound (O90.2)
infection of obstetrical (surgical) wound (O86.0)

O75.5 Delayed delivery after artificial rupture of membranes ♀ M

O75.8 Other specified complications of labor and delivery

O75.81 Maternal exhaustion complicating labor and delivery ♀ M

O75.82 Onset (spontaneous) of labor after 37 completed weeks of gestation but before 39 completed weeks gestation, with delivery by (planned) cesarean section ♀ M

Delivery by (planned) cesarean section occurring after 37 completed weeks of gestation but before 39 completed weeks gestation due to (spontaneous) onset of labor

Code first to specify reason for planned cesarean section such as:
cephalopelvic disproportion (normally formed fetus) (O33.9)
previous cesarean delivery (O34.21)

O75.89 Other specified complications of labor and delivery ♀ M

O75.9 Complication of labor and delivery, unspecified ♀ M

O76 Abnormality in fetal heart rate and rhythm complicating labor and delivery ♀ M

Depressed fetal heart rate tones complicating labor and delivery

Fetal bradycardia complicating labor and delivery

Fetal heart rate decelerations complicating labor and delivery

Fetal heart rate irregularity complicating labor and delivery

Fetal heart rate abnormal variability complicating labor and delivery

Fetal tachycardia complicating labor and delivery

Non-reassuring fetal heart rate or rhythm complicating labor and delivery

Excludes1 fetal stress NOS (O77.9)
labor and delivery complicated by electrocardiographic evidence of fetal stress (O77.8)
labor and delivery complicated by ultrasonic evidence of fetal stress (O77.8)

Excludes2 fetal metabolic acidemia (O68)
other fetal stress (O77.0-O77.1)

O77 Other fetal stress complicating labor and delivery

O77.0 Labor and delivery complicated by meconium in amniotic fluid ♀ M

O77.1 Fetal stress in labor or delivery due to drug administration ♀ M

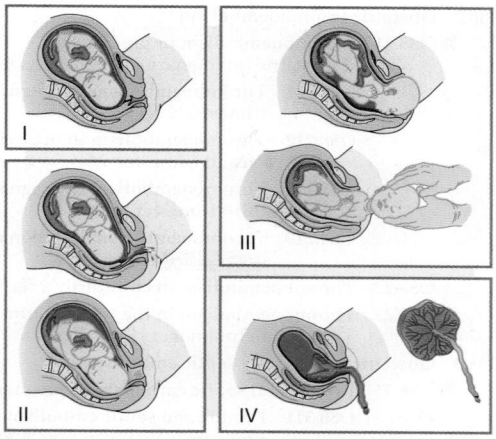

Figure 15-7 The four stages of normal delivery: **I.** Lightening, which occurs 2 to 4 weeks before birth, at which time the fetus turns with head toward the vagina. **II.** Regular contractions begin, the amniotic sac ruptures, and dilation is complete. **III.** Delivery of the head and rotation. **IV.** Expulsion of placenta.

O77.8 Labor and delivery complicated by other evidence of fetal stress ♀ M
Labor and delivery complicated by electrocardiographic evidence of fetal stress
Labor and delivery complicated by ultrasonic evidence of fetal stress
Excludes1 abnormality of fetal acid-base balance (O68)
abnormality in fetal heart rate or rhythm (O76)
fetal metabolic acidemia (O68)

O77.9 Labor and delivery complicated by fetal stress, unspecified ♀ M
Excludes1 abnormality of fetal acid-base balance (O68)
abnormality in fetal heart rate or rhythm (O76)
fetal metabolic acidemia (O68)

OGCR Section I.C., Chapter 15.n.

Normal Delivery, Code O80

1) Encounter for full term uncomplicated delivery

Code O80 should be assigned when a woman is admitted for a full-term normal delivery and delivers a single, healthy infant without any complications antepartum, during the delivery, or postpartum during the delivery episode. Code O80 is always a principal diagnosis. It is not to be used if any other code from chapter 15 is needed to describe a current complication of the antenatal, delivery, or perinatal period. Additional codes from other chapters may be used with code O80 if they are not related to or are in any way complicating the pregnancy.

2) Uncomplicated delivery with resolved antepartum complication

Code O80 may be used if the patient had a complication at some point during the pregnancy, but the complication is not present at the time of the admission for delivery.

3) Outcome of delivery for O80

Z37.0, Single live brith, is the only outcome of delivery code appropriate for use with O80.

ENCOUNTER FOR DELIVERY (O80-O82)

O80 Encounter for full-term uncomplicated delivery ♀ M
Delivery requiring minimal or no assistance, with or without episiotomy, without fetal manipulation [e.g., rotation version] or instrumentation [forceps] of a spontaneous, cephalic, vaginal, full-term, single, live-born infant. This code is for use as a single diagnosis code and is not to be used with any other code from chapter 15.
Use additional code to indicate outcome of delivery (Z37.0)

O82 Encounter for cesarean delivery without indication ♀ M
Use additional code to indicate outcome of delivery (Z37.0)

COMPLICATIONS PREDOMINANTLY RELATED TO THE PUERPERIUM (O85-O92)

Excludes2 mental and behavioral disorders associated with the puerperium (F53)
obstetrical tetanus (A34)
puerperal osteomalacia (M83.0)

O85 Puerperal sepsis ♀ M
Postpartum sepsis
Puerperal peritonitis
Puerperal pyemia
Use additional code (B95-B97), to identify infectious agent
Use additional code (R65.2-) to identify severe sepsis, if applicable
Excludes1 fever of unknown origin following delivery (O86.4)
genital tract infection following delivery (O86.1-)
obstetric pyemic and septic embolism (O88.3-)
puerperal septic thrombophlebitis (O86.81)
urinary tract infection following delivery (O86.2-)
Excludes2 sepsis during labor (O75.3)
Ex: 011.4, 011.5, 012.04, 012.05, 012.14, 012.15, 012.24, 012.25, 013.4, 013.5, 014.04, 014.05, 014.14, 014.15, 014.24, 014.25, 014.94, 014.95, 016.4, 016.5, 025.10-025.3, 026.10-026.13, 026.30-026.43, 026.63-026.819, 026.841-026.86, 026.891-026.93, 026.899-026.93, 029.011-029.93, 035.7XX0-035.7XX9, 075.4, 075.81, 075.89, 075.9, 080, 085, 086.12, 086.81-086.89, 090.89, 099.111-099.285, 099.330-099.335, 099.350-099.355, 099.511-099.73, 099.820-099.825, 099.840-09A.53

O86 Other puerperal infections
Use additional code (B95-B97), to identify infectious agent
Excludes2 infection during labor (O75.3)
obstetrical tetanus (A34)
Ex: For category O86 CC codes unless otherwise indicated: See O23

O86.0 Infection of obstetric surgical wound ♀ M
Infected cesarean delivery wound following delivery
Infected perineal repair following delivery

O86.1 Other infection of genital tract following delivery
O86.11 Cervicitis following delivery ♀ M
O86.12 Endometritis following delivery ♀ M
Ex: See O85
O86.13 Vaginitis following delivery ♀ M
O86.19 Other infection of genital tract following delivery ♀ M

O86.2 Urinary tract infection following delivery
O86.20 Urinary tract infection following delivery, unspecified ♀ M
Puerperal urinary tract infection NOS
O86.21 Infection of kidney following delivery ♀ M
O86.22 Infection of bladder following delivery ♀ M
Infection of urethra following delivery
O86.29 Other urinary tract infection following delivery ♀ M

O86.4 Pyrexia of unknown origin following delivery ♀ M
Puerperal infection NOS following delivery
Puerperal pyrexia NOS following delivery
Excludes2 pyrexia during labor (O75.2)
Ex: 011.4, 011.5, 012.04, 012.05, 012.14, 012.15, 012.24, 012.25, 013.4, 013.5, 014.04, 014.05, 014.14, 014.15, 014.24, 014.25, 014.94, 014.95, 016.4, 016.5, 022.20-022.93, 025.10-025.3, 026.10-026.13, 026.30-026.43, 026.63-026.819, 026.841-026.86, 026.891-026.93, 029.011-029.93, 035.7XX0-035.7XX9, 075.4, 075.81, 075.89-075.9, 080, 086.4-087.9, 090.89, 099.111-099.285, 099.330-099.335, 099.350-099.355, 099.511-099.73, 099.820-099.825, 099.840-09A.53

O86.8 Other specified puerperal infections
Ex: For category O86.8 CC codes: See O85
O86.81 Puerperal septic thrombophlebitis ♀ M
O86.89 Other specified puerperal infections ♀ M

O87 Venous complications and hemorrhoids in the puerperium

Includes venous complications in labor, delivery and the puerperium

Excludes2 obstetric embolism (O88.-)
puerperal septic thrombophlebitis (O86.81)
venous complications in pregnancy (O22.-)

Ex For category O87 CC codes: See O22.2

O87.0 Superficial thrombophlebitis in the puerperium ♀ M
Puerperal phlebitis NOS
Puerperal thrombosis NOS

O87.1 Deep phlebothrombosis in the puerperium ♀ M
Deep vein thrombosis, postpartum
Pelvic thrombophlebitis, postpartum

Use additional code to identify the deep vein thrombosis (I82.4-, I82.5-, I82.62-. I82.72-)

Use additional code, if applicable, for associated long-term (current) use of anticoagulants (Z79.01)

O87.2 Hemorrhoids in the puerperium ♀ M

O87.3 Cerebral venous thrombosis in the puerperium ♀ M
Cerebrovenous sinus thrombosis in the puerperium

O87.4 Varicose veins of lower extremity in the puerperium ♀ M

O87.8 Other venous complications in the puerperium ♀ M
Genital varices in the puerperium

O87.9 Venous complication in the puerperium, unspecified ♀ M
Puerperal phlebopathy NOS

O88 Obstetric embolism

Excludes1 embolism complicating abortion NOS (O03.2)
embolism complicating ectopic or molar pregnancy (O08.2)
embolism complicating failed attempted abortion (O07.2)
embolism complicating induced abortion (O04.7)
embolism complicating spontaneous abortion (O03.2, O03.7)

Ex For category O88 CC codes: 011.4, 011.5, 012.04, 012.05, 012.14, 012.15, 012.24, 012.25, 013.4, 013.5, 014.04, 014.05, 014.14, 014.15, 014.24, 014.25, 014.94, 014.95, 016.4, 016.5, 025.10-025.3, 026.10-026.93, 029.011-029.93, 035.7XX0-035.7XX9, 075.4, 075.81-080, 088.011-088.83, 090.89, 099.111-09A.53

O88.0 Obstetric air embolism

O88.01 Obstetric air embolism in pregnancy

O88.011 Air embolism in pregnancy, first trimester ♀ M

O88.012 Air embolism in pregnancy, second trimester ♀ M

O88.013 Air embolism in pregnancy, third trimester ♀ M

O88.019 Air embolism in pregnancy, unspecified trimester ♀ M

O88.02 Air embolism in childbirth ♀ M

O88.03 Air embolism in the puerperium ♀ M

O88.1 Amniotic fluid embolism
Anaphylactoid syndrome in pregnancy

O88.11 Amniotic fluid embolism in pregnancy

O88.111 Amniotic fluid embolism in pregnancy, first trimester ♀ M

O88.112 Amniotic fluid embolism in pregnancy, second trimester ♀ M

O88.113 Amniotic fluid embolism in pregnancy, third trimester ♀ M

O88.119 Amniotic fluid embolism in pregnancy, unspecified trimester ♀ M

O88.12 Amniotic fluid embolism in childbirth ♀ M

O88.13 Amniotic fluid embolism in the puerperium ♀ M

O88.2 Obstetric thromboembolism

O88.21 Thromboembolism in pregnancy
Obstetric (pulmonary) embolism NOS

O88.211 Thromboembolism in pregnancy, first trimester ♀ M

O88.212 Thromboembolism in pregnancy, second trimester ♀ M

O88.213 Thromboembolism in pregnancy, third trimester ♀ M

O88.219 Thromboembolism in pregnancy, unspecified trimester ♀ M

O88.22 Thromboembolism in childbirth ♀ M

O88.23 Thromboembolism in the puerperium ♀ M
Puerperal (pulmonary) embolism NOS

O88.3 Obstetric pyemic and septic embolism

O88.31 Pyemic and septic embolism in pregnancy

O88.311 Pyemic and septic embolism in pregnancy, first trimester ♀ M

O88.312 Pyemic and septic embolism in pregnancy, second trimester ♀ M

O88.313 Pyemic and septic embolism in pregnancy, third trimester ♀ M

O88.319 Pyemic and septic embolism in pregnancy, unspecified trimester ♀ M

O88.32 Pyemic and septic embolism in childbirth ♀ M

O88.33 Pyemic and septic embolism in the puerperium ♀ M

O88.8 Other obstetric embolism
Obstetric fat embolism

O88.81 Other embolism in pregnancy

O88.811 Other embolism in pregnancy, first trimester ♀ M

O88.812 Other embolism in pregnancy, second trimester ♀ M

O88.813 Other embolism in pregnancy, third trimester ♀ M

O88.819 Other embolism in pregnancy, unspecified trimester ♀ M

O88.82 Other embolism in childbirth ♀ M

O88.83 Other embolism in the puerperium ♀ M

O89 Complications of anesthesia during the puerperium

Includes maternal complications arising from the administration of a general, regional or local anesthetic, analgesic or other sedation during the puerperium

Use additional code, if applicable, to identify specific complication

O89.0 Pulmonary complications of anesthesia during the puerperium

O89.01 Aspiration pneumonitis due to anesthesia during the puerperium ♀ M
Inhalation of stomach contents or secretions NOS due to anesthesia during the puerperium
Mendelson's syndrome due to anesthesia during the puerperium

O89.09 Other pulmonary complications of anesthesia during the puerperium ♀ M

O89.1 Cardiac complications of anesthesia during the puerperium ♀ M

O89.2 Central nervous system complications of anesthesia during the puerperium ♀ M

O89.3 Toxic reaction to local anesthesia during the puerperium ♀ M

O89.4 Spinal and epidural anesthesia-induced headache during the puerperium ♀ M

O89.5 Other complications of spinal and epidural anesthesia during the puerperium ♀ M

O89.6 Failed or difficult intubation for anesthesia during the puerperium ♀ M

O89.8 Other complications of anesthesia during the puerperium ♀ M

O89.9 Complication of anesthesia during the puerperium, unspecified ♀ M

O90 Complications of the puerperium, not elsewhere classified

O90.0 Disruption of cesarean delivery wound ♀ M
Dehiscence of cesarean delivery wound
Excludes1 rupture of uterus (spontaneous) before onset of labor (O71.0-)
rupture of uterus during labor (O71.1)

O90.1 Disruption of perineal obstetric wound ♀ M
Disruption of wound of episiotomy
Disruption of wound of perineal laceration
Secondary perineal tear

O90.2 Hematoma of obstetric wound ♀ M

O90.3 Peripartum cardiomyopathy ♀ M
Conditions in I42.- arising during pregnancy and the puerperium
Excludes1 pre-existing heart disease complicating pregnancy and the puerperium (O99.4-)
Ex: 011.4, 011.5, 012.04, 012.05, 012.14, 012.15, 012.24, 012.25, 013.4, 013.5, 014.04, 014.05, 014.14, 014.15, 014.24, 014.25, 014.94, 014.95, 016.4, 016.5, 025.10-025.3, 026.10-026.13, 026.30-026.43, 026.63-026.819, 026.841-026.86, 026.891-026.93, 029.011-029.93, 035.7XX0-035.7XX9, 075.4, 075.81, 075.89-075.9, 080, 090.3, 090.89, 099.111-099.285, 099.330-099.335, 099.350-099.73, 099.820-099.825, 099.840-09A.53

O90.4 Postpartum acute kidney failure ♀ M
Hepatorenal syndrome following labor and delivery
Ex: 011.4, 011.5, 012.04, 012.05, 012.14, 012.15, 012.24, 012.25, 013.4, 013.5, 014.04, 014.05, 014.14, 014.15, 014.24, 014.25, 014.94, 014.95, 016.4, 016.5, 025.10-025.3, 026.10-026.13, 026.30-026.43, 026.63-026.819, 026.841-026.86, 026.891-026.93, 029.011-029.93, 035.7XX0-035.7XX9, 075.4, 075.81, 075.89-075.9, 080, 090.4, 090.89, 099.111-099.285, 099.330-099.335, 099.350-099.355, 099.511-099.73, 099.820-099.825, 099.840-09A.53

O90.5 Postpartum thyroiditis ♀ M

O90.6 Postpartum mood disturbance ♀ M
Postpartum blues Postpartum sadness
Postpartum dysphoria
Excludes1 postpartum depression (F53)
puerperal psychosis (F53)

O90.8 Other complications of the puerperium, not elsewhere classified

O90.81 Anemia of the puerperium ♀ M
Postpartum anemia NOS
Excludes1 pre-existing anemia complicating the puerperium (O99.03)

O90.89 Other complications of the puerperium, not elsewhere classified ♀ M
Placental polyp

O90.9 Complication of the puerperium, unspecified ♀ M

O91 Infections of breast associated with pregnancy, the puerperium and lactation
Use additional code to identify infection

O91.0 Infection of nipple associated with pregnancy, the puerperium and lactation

O91.01 Infection of nipple associated with pregnancy
Gestational abscess of nipple

O91.011 Infection of nipple associated with pregnancy, first trimester ♀ M

O91.012 Infection of nipple associated with pregnancy, second trimester ♀ M

O91.013 Infection of nipple associated with pregnancy, third trimester ♀ M

O91.019 Infection of nipple associated with pregnancy, unspecified trimester ♀ M

O91.02 Infection of nipple associated with the puerperium ♀ M
Puerperal abscess of nipple

O91.03 Infection of nipple associated with lactation ♀ M
Abscess of nipple associated with lactation

O91.1 Abscess of breast associated with pregnancy, the puerperium and lactation

O91.11 Abscess of breast associated with pregnancy
Gestational mammary abscess
Gestational purulent mastitis
Gestational subareolar abscess

O91.111 Abscess of breast associated with pregnancy, first trimester ♀ M

O91.112 Abscess of breast associated with pregnancy, second trimester ♀ M

O91.113 Abscess of breast associated with pregnancy, third trimester ♀ M

O91.119 Abscess of breast associated with pregnancy, unspecified trimester ♀ M

O91.12 Abscess of breast associated with the puerperium ♀ M
Puerperal mammary abscess
Puerperal purulent mastitis
Puerperal subareolar abscess

O91.13 Abscess of breast associated with lactation ♀ M
Mammary abscess associated with lactation
Purulent mastitis associated with lactation
Subareolar abscess associated with lactation

O91.2 Nonpurulent mastitis associated with pregnancy, the puerperium and lactation

O91.21 Nonpurulent mastitis associated with pregnancy
Gestational interstitial mastitis
Gestational lymphangitis of breast
Gestational mastitis NOS
Gestational parenchymatous mastitis

O91.211 Nonpurulent mastitis associated with pregnancy, first trimester ♀ M

O91.212 Nonpurulent mastitis associated with pregnancy, second trimester ♀ M

O91.213 Nonpurulent mastitis associated with pregnancy, third trimester ♀ M

O91.219 Nonpurulent mastitis associated with pregnancy, unspecified trimester ♀ M

O91.22 Nonpurulent mastitis associated with the puerperium ♀ M
Puerperal interstitial mastitis
Puerperal lymphangitis of breast
Puerperal mastitis NOS
Puerperal parenchymatous mastitis

O91.23 Nonpurulent mastitis associated with lactation ♀ M
Interstitial mastitis associated with lactation
Lymphangitis of breast associated with lactation
Mastitis NOS associated with lactation
Parenchymatous mastitis associated with lactation

● **O92 Other disorders of breast and disorders of lactation associated with pregnancy and the puerperium**

● **O92.0 Retracted nipple associated with pregnancy, the puerperium, and lactation**

● **O92.01 Retracted nipple associated with pregnancy**

O92.011 Retracted nipple associated with pregnancy, first trimester ♀ M

O92.012 Retracted nipple associated with pregnancy, second trimester ♀ M

O92.013 Retracted nipple associated with pregnancy, third trimester ♀ M

O92.019 Retracted nipple associated with pregnancy, unspecified trimester ♀ M

O92.02 Retracted nipple associated with the puerperium ♀ M

O92.03 Retracted nipple associated with lactation ♀ M

● **O92.1 Cracked nipple associated with pregnancy, the puerperium, and lactation**

Fissure of nipple, gestational or puerperal

● **O92.11 Cracked nipple associated with pregnancy**

O92.111 Cracked nipple associated with pregnancy, first trimester ♀ M

O92.112 Cracked nipple associated with pregnancy, second trimester ♀ M

O92.113 Cracked nipple associated with pregnancy, third trimester ♀ M

O92.119 Cracked nipple associated with pregnancy, unspecified trimester ♀ M

O92.12 Cracked nipple associated with the puerperium ♀ M

O92.13 Cracked nipple associated with lactation ♀ M

● **O92.2 Other and unspecified disorders of breast associated with pregnancy and the puerperium**

O92.20 Unspecified disorder of breast associated with pregnancy and the puerperium ♀ M

O92.29 Other disorders of breast associated with pregnancy and the puerperium ♀ M

O92.3 Agalactia ♀ M

Primary agalactia

Excludes1 elective agalactia (O92.5)
secondary agalactia (O92.5)
therapeutic agalactia (O92.5)

O92.4 Hypogalactia ♀ M

O92.5 Suppressed lactation ♀ M

Elective agalactia
Secondary agalactia
Therapeutic agalactia

Excludes1 primary agalactia (O92.3)

O92.6 Galactorrhea ♀ M

● **O92.7 Other and unspecified disorders of lactation**

O92.70 Unspecified disorders of lactation ♀ M

O92.79 Other disorders of lactation ♀ M

Puerperal galactocele

OTHER OBSTETRIC CONDITIONS, NOT ELSEWHERE CLASSIFIED (O94-O9A)

O94 Sequelae of complication of pregnancy, childbirth, and the puerperium ♀ M

Note: This category is to be used to indicate conditions in O00-O77.-, O85-O94 and O98-O9A.- as the cause of late effects. The 'sequelae' include conditions specified as such, or as late effects, which may occur at any time after the puerperium.

Code first condition resulting from (sequela) of complication of pregnancy, childbirth, and the puerperium

O98 Maternal infectious and parasitic diseases classifiable elsewhere but complicating pregnancy, childbirth and the puerperium

Includes the listed conditions when complicating the pregnant state, when aggravated by the pregnancy, or as a reason for obstetric care

Use additional code (Chapter 1), to identify specific infectious or parasitic disease

Excludes2 herpes gestationis (O26.4-)
infectious carrier state (O99.82-, O99.83-)
obstetrical tetanus (A34)
puerperal infection (O86.-)
puerperal sepsis (O85)
when the reason for maternal care is that the disease is known or suspected to have affected the fetus (O35-O36)

● **O98.0 Tuberculosis complicating pregnancy, childbirth and the puerperium**

Conditions in A15-A19

Ex **For category O98.0 CC codes:** 011.4, 011.5, 012.04, 012.05, 012.14, 012.15, 012.24, 012.25, 013.4, 013.5, 014.04, 014.05, 014.14, 014.15, 014.24, 014.25, 014.94, 014.95, 016.4, 016.5, 025.10-025.3, 026.10-026.13, 026.30-026.43, 026.63-026.819, 026.841-026.86, 026.891-026.93, 029.011-029.93, 035.7XX0-035.7XX9, 075.4, 075.81, 075.89-075.9, 080, 090.89, 098.011-098.03, 099.111-099.285, 099.330-099.335, 099.350-099.355, 099.511-099.73, 099.820-099.825, 099.840-09A.53

● **O98.01 Tuberculosis complicating pregnancy**

O98.011 Tuberculosis complicating pregnancy, first trimester ♀ M

O98.012 Tuberculosis complicating pregnancy, second trimester ♀ M

O98.013 Tuberculosis complicating pregnancy, third trimester ♀ M

O98.019 Tuberculosis complicating pregnancy, unspecified trimester ♀ M

O98.02 Tuberculosis complicating childbirth ♀ M

O98.03 Tuberculosis complicating the puerperium ♀ M

● **O98.1 Syphilis complicating pregnancy, childbirth and the puerperium**

Conditions in A50-A53

Ex **For category O98.1 CC codes:** 011.4, 012.04, 012.14, 012.24, 013.4, 014.04, 014.14, 014.24, 014.94, 016.4, 026.11-026.13, 026.31-026.33, 026.41-026.43, 026.63-026.713, 026.72-026.813, 026.86, 026.891-026.893, 026.90-026.93, 029.011-029.013, 029.021-029.023, 029.091-029.093, 029.111-029.113, 029.121-029.123, 029.191-029.193, 029.211-029.213, 029.291-029.293, 029.3X1-029.3X3, 029.41-029.5X3, 029.61-029.8X3, 029.91-029.93, 035.7XX0-035.7XX9, 098.111-098.33, 099.351-099.353, 099.355, 099.89

● **O98.11 Syphilis complicating pregnancy**

O98.111 Syphilis complicating pregnancy, first trimester ♀ M

O98.112 Syphilis complicating pregnancy, second trimester ♀ M

O98.113 Syphilis complicating pregnancy, third trimester ♀ M

O98.119 Syphilis complicating pregnancy, unspecified trimester ♀ M

O98.12 Syphilis complicating childbirth ♀ M

O98.13 Syphilis complicating the puerperium ♀ M

O98.2 Gonorrhea complicating pregnancy, childbirth and the puerperium
Conditions in A54.-
Ex: For category O98.2 CC codes: See O98.1

O98.21 Gonorrhea complicating pregnancy
- **O98.211 Gonorrhea complicating pregnancy, first trimester ♀** M
- **O98.212 Gonorrhea complicating pregnancy, second trimester ♀** M
- **O98.213 Gonorrhea complicating pregnancy, third trimester ♀** M
- **O98.219 Gonorrhea complicating pregnancy, unspecified trimester ♀** M

O98.22 Gonorrhea complicating childbirth ♀ M

O98.23 Gonorrhea complicating the puerperium ♀ M

O98.3 Other infections with a predominantly sexual mode of transmission complicating pregnancy, childbirth and the puerperium
Conditions in A55-A64
Ex: For category O98.3 CC codes: See O98.1

O98.31 Other infections with a predominantly sexual mode of transmission complicating pregnancy
- **O98.311 Other infections with a predominantly sexual mode of transmission complicating pregnancy, first trimester ♀** M
- **O98.312 Other infections with a predominantly sexual mode of transmission complicating pregnancy, second trimester ♀** M
- **O98.313 Other infections with a predominantly sexual mode of transmission complicating pregnancy, third trimester ♀** M
- **O98.319 Other infections with a predominantly sexual mode of transmission complicating pregnancy, unspecified trimester ♀** M

O98.32 Other infections with a predominantly sexual mode of transmission complicating childbirth ♀ M

O98.33 Other infections with a predominantly sexual mode of transmission complicating the puerperium ♀ M

O98.4 Viral hepatitis complicating pregnancy, childbirth and the puerperium
Conditions in B15-B19
Ex: For category O98.4 CC codes: 098.411-098.613, 098.711-098.93, 099.830-099.835

O98.41 Viral hepatitis complicating pregnancy
- **O98.411 Viral hepatitis complicating pregnancy, first trimester ♀** M
- **O98.412 Viral hepatitis complicating pregnancy, second trimester ♀** M
- **O98.413 Viral hepatitis complicating pregnancy, third trimester ♀** M
- **O98.419 Viral hepatitis complicating pregnancy, unspecified trimester ♀** M

O98.42 Viral hepatitis complicating childbirth ♀ M

O98.43 Viral hepatitis complicating the puerperium ♀ M

O98.5 Other viral diseases complicating pregnancy, childbirth and the puerperium
Conditions in A80-B09, B25-B34, R87.81-, R87.82-
Excludes:1 human immunodeficiency virus [HIV] disease complicating pregnancy, childbirth and the puerperium (O98.7-)
Ex: For category O98.5 CC codes: See O98.4

O98.51 Other viral diseases complicating pregnancy
- **O98.511 Other viral diseases complicating pregnancy, first trimester ♀** M
- **O98.512 Other viral diseases complicating pregnancy, second trimester ♀** M
- **O98.513 Other viral diseases complicating pregnancy, third trimester ♀** M
- **O98.519 Other viral diseases complicating pregnancy, unspecified trimester ♀** M

O98.52 Other viral diseases complicating childbirth ♀ M

O98.53 Other viral diseases complicating the puerperium ♀ M

O98.6 Protozoal diseases complicating pregnancy, childbirth and the puerperium
Conditions in B50-B64

O98.61 Protozoal diseases complicating pregnancy
Ex: For category O98.61 CC codes: 011.4, 011.5, 012.04, 012.05, 012.14, 012.15, 012.24, 012.25, 013.4, 013.5, 014.04, 014.05, 014.14, 014.15, 014.24, 014.25, 014.94, 014.95, 016.4, 016.5, 025.10-025.3, 026.10-026.13, 026.30-026.43, 026.63-026.819, 026.841-026.86, 026.891-026.93, 029.011-029.93, 035.7XX0-035.7XX9, 075.4, 075.81, 075.89-075.9, 080, 090.89, 098.411-098.93, 099.111-099.285, 099.330-099.335, 099.350-099.355, 099.511-099.73, 099.820-09A.53
- **O98.611 Protozoal diseases complicating pregnancy, first trimester ♀** M
- **O98.612 Protozoal diseases complicating pregnancy, second trimester ♀** M
- **O98.613 Protozoal diseases complicating pregnancy, third trimester ♀** M
- **O98.619 Protozoal diseases complicating pregnancy, unspecified trimester ♀** M

O98.62 Protozoal diseases complicating childbirth ♀ M
Ex: 011.4, 011.5, 012.04, 012.05, 012.14, 012.15, 012.24, 012.25, 013.4, 013.5, 014.04, 014.05, 014.14, 014.15, 014.24, 014.25, 014.94, 014.95, 016.4, 016.5, 025.10-025.3, 026.10-026.13, 026.30-026.43, 026.63-026.819, 026.841-026.86, 026.891-026.93, 029.011-029.93, 035.7XX0-035.7XX9, 075.4, 075.81, 075.89-075.9, 080, 090.89, 098.611-098.63, 099.111-099.285, 099.330-099.335, 099.350-099.355, 099.511-099.73, 099.820-09A.53

O98.63 Protozoal diseases complicating the puerperium ♀ M
Ex: See O98.62

● **O98.7 Human immunodeficiency virus [HIV] disease complicating pregnancy, childbirth and the puerperium**

Use additional code to identify the type of HIV disease:
Acquired immune deficiency syndrome (AIDS) (B20)
Asymptomatic HIV status (Z21)
HIV positive NOS (Z21)
Symptomatic HIV disease (B20)

OGCR Section I.C.15.f.

HIV Infection in Pregnancy, Childbirth and the Puerperium

During pregnancy, childbirth or the puerperium, a patient admitted because of an HIV-related illness should receive a principal diagnosis from subcategory O98.7-. Human immunodeficiency [HIV] disease complicating pregnancy, childbirth and the puerperium, followed by the code(s) for the HIV-related illness(es).

Patients with asymptomatic HIV infection status admitted during pregnancy, childbirth, or the puerperium should receive codes of O98.7- and Z21, Asymptomatic human immunodeficiency virus [HIV] infection status.

Ex **For category O98.7 CC codes:** See O98.4

● **O98.71 Human immunodeficiency virus [HIV] disease complicating pregnancy**

O98.711 Human immunodeficiency virus [HIV] disease complicating pregnancy, first trimester ♀ M

O98.712 Human immunodeficiency virus [HIV] disease complicating pregnancy, second trimester ♀ M

O98.713 Human immunodeficiency virus [HIV] disease complicating pregnancy, third trimester ♀ M

O98.719 Human immunodeficiency virus [HIV] disease complicating pregnancy, unspecified trimester ♀ M

O98.72 Human immunodeficiency virus [HIV] disease complicating childbirth ♀ M

O98.73 Human immunodeficiency virus [HIV] disease complicating the puerperium ♀ M

● **O98.8 Other maternal infectious and parasitic diseases complicating pregnancy, childbirth and the puerperium**

Ex **For category O98.8 CC codes:** See O98.4

● **O98.81 Other maternal infectious and parasitic diseases complicating pregnancy**

O98.811 Other maternal infectious and parasitic diseases complicating pregnancy, first trimester ♀ M

O98.812 Other maternal infectious and parasitic diseases complicating pregnancy, second trimester ♀ M

O98.813 Other maternal infectious and parasitic diseases complicating pregnancy, third trimester ♀ M

O98.819 Other maternal infectious and parasitic diseases complicating pregnancy, unspecified trimester ♀ M

O98.82 Other maternal infectious and parasitic diseases complicating childbirth ♀ M

O98.83 Other maternal infectious and parasitic diseases complicating the puerperium ♀ M

● **O98.9 Unspecified maternal infectious and parasitic disease complicating pregnancy, childbirth and the puerperium**

Ex **For category O98.9 CC codes:** See O98.4

● **O98.91 Unspecified maternal infectious and parasitic disease complicating pregnancy**

O98.911 Unspecified maternal infectious and parasitic disease complicating pregnancy, first trimester ♀ M

O98.912 Unspecified maternal infectious and parasitic disease complicating pregnancy, second trimester ♀ M

O98.913 Unspecified maternal infectious and parasitic disease complicating pregnancy, third trimester ♀ M

O98.919 Unspecified maternal infectious and parasitic disease complicating pregnancy, unspecified trimester ♀ M

O98.92 Unspecified maternal infectious and parasitic disease complicating childbirth ♀ M

O98.93 Unspecified maternal infectious and parasitic disease complicating the puerperium ♀ M

● **O99 Other maternal diseases classifiable elsewhere but complicating pregnancy, childbirth and the puerperium**

Includes: conditions which complicate the pregnant state, are aggravated by the pregnancy or are a main reason for obstetric care

Use additional code to identify specific condition

Excludes2 when the reason for maternal care is that the condition is known or suspected to have affected the fetus (O35-O36)

● **O99.0 Anemia complicating pregnancy, childbirth and the puerperium**

Conditions in D50-D64

Excludes1 anemia arising in the puerperium (O90.81)
postpartum anemia NOS (O90.81)

● **O99.01 Anemia complicating pregnancy**

O99.011 Anemia complicating pregnancy, first trimester ♀ M

O99.012 Anemia complicating pregnancy, second trimester ♀ M

O99.013 Anemia complicating pregnancy, third trimester ♀ M

O99.019 Anemia complicating pregnancy, unspecified trimester ♀ M

O99.02 Anemia complicating childbirth ♀ M

O99.03 Anemia complicating the puerperium ♀ M

Excludes1 postpartum anemia not pre-existing prior to delivery (O90.81)

● **O99.1 Other diseases of the blood and blood-forming organs and certain disorders involving the immune mechanism complicating pregnancy, childbirth and the puerperium**

Conditions in D65-D89

Excludes2 hemorrhage with coagulation defects (O45.-, O46.0-, O67.0, O72.3)

Ex **For category O99.1 CC codes unless otherwise indicated:** 025.11-025.3, 099.281-099.285, 099.511-099.513, 099.52-099.613, 099.62-099.713, 099.72-099.73, 099.820-099.825, 09A.111-09A.113, 09A.12-09A.213, 09A.22-09A.313, 09A.32-09A.413, 09A.42-09A.513, 09A.52-09A.53

● **O99.11 Other diseases of the blood and blood-forming organs and certain disorders involving the immune mechanism complicating pregnancy**

O99.111 Other diseases of the blood and blood-forming organs and certain disorders involving the immune mechanism complicating pregnancy, first trimester ♀ M

O99.112 Other diseases of the blood and blood-forming organs and certain disorders involving the immune mechanism complicating pregnancy, second trimester ♀ M

O99.113 Other diseases of the blood and blood-forming organs and certain disorders involving the immune mechanism complicating pregnancy, third trimester ♀ M

O99.119 Other diseases of the blood and blood-forming organs and certain disorders involving the immune mechanism complicating pregnancy, unspecified trimester ♀ M

Ex 025.10, 099.280, 099.519, 099.619, 099.719, 09A.119, 09A.219, 09A.319, 09A.419, 09A.519

O99.12 Other diseases of the blood and blood-forming organs and certain disorders involving the immune mechanism complicating childbirth ♀ M

O99.13 Other diseases of the blood and blood-forming organs and certain disorders involving the immune mechanism complicating the puerperium ♀ M

O99.2 Endocrine, nutritional and metabolic diseases complicating pregnancy, childbirth and the puerperium
Conditions in E00-E88

Excludes2 diabetes mellitus (O24.-)
malnutrition (O25.-)
postpartum thyroiditis (O90.5)

O99.21 Obesity complicating pregnancy, childbirth, and the puerperium
Use additional code to identify the type of obesity (E66.-)

O99.210 Obesity complicating pregnancy, unspecified trimester ♀ M

O99.211 Obesity complicating pregnancy, first trimester ♀ M

O99.212 Obesity complicating pregnancy, second trimester ♀ M

O99.213 Obesity complicating pregnancy, third trimester ♀ M

O99.214 Obesity complicating childbirth ♀ M

O99.215 Obesity complicating the puerperium ♀ M

O99.28 Other endocrine, nutritional and metabolic diseases complicating pregnancy, childbirth and the puerperium

O99.280 Endocrine, nutritional and metabolic diseases complicating pregnancy, unspecified trimester ♀ M

O99.281 Endocrine, nutritional and metabolic diseases complicating pregnancy, first trimester ♀ M

O99.282 Endocrine, nutritional and metabolic diseases complicating pregnancy, second trimester ♀ M

O99.283 Endocrine, nutritional and metabolic diseases complicating pregnancy, third trimester ♀ M

O99.284 Endocrine, nutritional and metabolic diseases complicating childbirth ♀ M

O99.285 Endocrine, nutritional and metabolic diseases complicating the puerperium ♀ M

O99.3 Mental disorders and diseases of the nervous system complicating pregnancy, childbirth and the puerperium

O99.31 Alcohol use complicating pregnancy, childbirth, and the puerperium
Use additional code(s) from F10 to identify manifestations of the alcohol use

O99.310 Alcohol use complicating pregnancy, unspecified trimester ♀ M

O99.311 Alcohol use complicating pregnancy, first trimester ♀ M

O99.312 Alcohol use complicating pregnancy, second trimester ♀ M

O99.313 Alcohol use complicating pregnancy, third trimester ♀ M

O99.314 Alcohol use complicating childbirth ♀ M

O99.315 Alcohol use complicating the puerperium ♀ M

O99.32 Drug use complicating pregnancy, childbirth, and the puerperium
Use additional code(s) from F11-F16 and F18-F19 to identify manifestations of the drug use
Ex **For category O99.32 CC codes:** 011.4, 011.5, 012.04, 012.05, 012.14, 012.15, 012.24, 012.25, 013.4, 013.5, 014.04, 014.05, 014.14, 014.15, 014.24, 014.25, 014.94, 014.95, 016.4, 016.5, 025.10-025.3, 026.10-026.13, 026.30-026.43, 026.63-026.819, 026.841-026.86, 026.891-026.93, 029.011-029.93, 035.7XX0-035.7XX9, 075.4, 075.81, 075.89-075.9, 080, 090.89, 099.111-099.285, 099.320-099.335, 099.350-099.355, 099.511-099.73, 099.820-099.825, 099.840-09A.53

O99.320 Drug use complicating pregnancy, unspecified trimester ♀ M

O99.321 Drug use complicating pregnancy, first trimester ♀ M

O99.322 Drug use complicating pregnancy, second trimester ♀ M

O99.323 Drug use complicating pregnancy, third trimester ♀ M

O99.324 Drug use complicating childbirth ♀ M

O99.325 Drug use complicating the puerperium ♀ M

O99.33 Tobacco use disorder complicating pregnancy, childbirth, and the puerperium
Smoking complicating pregnancy, childbirth, and the puerperium
Use additional code from category F17 to identify type of tobacco nicotine dependence

O99.330 Smoking (tobacco) complicating pregnancy, unspecified trimester ♀ M

O99.331 Smoking (tobacco) complicating pregnancy, first trimester ♀ M

O99.332 Smoking (tobacco) complicating pregnancy, second trimester ♀ M

O99.333 Smoking (tobacco) complicating pregnancy, third trimester ♀ M

O99.334 Smoking (tobacco) complicating childbirth ♀ M

O99.335 Smoking (tobacco) complicating the puerperium ♀ M

O99.34 Other mental disorders complicating pregnancy, childbirth, and the puerperium
Conditions in F01-F09 and F20-F99

Excludes2 postpartum mood disturbance (O90.6)
postnatal psychosis (F53)
puerperal psychosis (F53)

O99.340 Other mental disorders complicating pregnancy, unspecified trimester ♀ M

O99.341 Other mental disorders complicating pregnancy, first trimester ♀ M

O99.342 Other mental disorders complicating pregnancy, second trimester ♀ M

O99.343 Other mental disorders complicating pregnancy, third trimester ♀ M

O99.344 Other mental disorders complicating childbirth ♀ M

O99.345 Other mental disorders complicating the puerperium ♀ M

● **O99.35 Diseases of the nervous system complicating pregnancy, childbirth, and the puerperium**
Conditions in G00-G99

Excludes2 pregnancy related peripheral neuritis (O26.8-)

O99.350 Diseases of the nervous system complicating pregnancy, unspecified trimester ♀ M

O99.351 Diseases of the nervous system complicating pregnancy, first trimester ♀ M

O99.352 Diseases of the nervous system complicating pregnancy, second trimester ♀ M

O99.353 Diseases of the nervous system complicating pregnancy, third trimester ♀ M

O99.354 Diseases of the nervous system complicating childbirth ♀ M
Ex: See O99.1

O99.355 Diseases of the nervous system complicating the puerperium ♀ M
Ex: See O99.1

● **O99.4 Diseases of the circulatory system complicating pregnancy, childbirth and the puerperium**
Conditions in I00-I99

Excludes1 peripartum cardiomyopathy (O90.3)

Excludes2 hypertensive disorders (O10-O16)
obstetric embolism (O88.-)
venous complications and cerebrovenous sinus thrombosis in labor, childbirth and the puerperium (O87.-)
venous complications and cerebrovenous sinus thrombosis in pregnancy (O22.-)

Ex: **For category O99.4 CC codes unless otherwise indicated:** O11.4, O11.5, O12.04, O12.05, O12.14, O12.15, O12.24, O12.25, O13.4, O13.5, O14.04, O14.05, O14.14, O14.15, O14.24, O14.25, O14.94, O14.95, O16.4, O16.5, O25.10-O25.3, O26.10-O26.13, O26.30-O26.43, O26.63-O26.819, O26.841-O26.86, O26.891-O26.93, O29.011-O29.93, O35.7XX0-O35.7XX9, O75.4, O75.81, O75.89-O75.9, O80, O90.3, O90.89, O99.111-O99.285, O99.330-O99.335, O99.350-O99.73, O99.820-O99.825, O99.840-O9A.53

● **O99.41 Diseases of the circulatory system complicating pregnancy**
Coding Clinic: 2016, Q2, P8

O99.411 Diseases of the circulatory system complicating pregnancy, first trimester ♀ M

O99.412 Diseases of the circulatory system complicating pregnancy, second trimester ♀ M

O99.413 Diseases of the circulatory system complicating pregnancy, third trimester ♀ M

O99.419 Diseases of the circulatory system complicating pregnancy, unspecified trimester ♀ M

O99.42 Diseases of the circulatory system complicating childbirth ♀ M
Ex: O25.10-O25.3, O26.10-O26.13, O26.30-O26.43, O26.63-O26.819, O26.841-O26.86, O26.891-O26.93, O29.011-O29.93, O35.7XX0-O35.7XX9, O75.4, O75.81, O75.89-O75.9, O80, O90.3, O90.89, O99.111-O99.285, O99.330-O99.335, O99.350-O99.73, O99.820-O99.825, O99.840-O9A.53

O99.43 Diseases of the circulatory system complicating the puerperium ♀ M

● **O99.5 Diseases of the respiratory system complicating pregnancy, childbirth and the puerperium**
Conditions in J00-J99

● **O99.51 Diseases of the respiratory system complicating pregnancy**

O99.511 Diseases of the respiratory system complicating pregnancy, first trimester ♀ M

O99.512 Diseases of the respiratory system complicating pregnancy, second trimester ♀ M

O99.513 Diseases of the respiratory system complicating pregnancy, third trimester ♀ M

O99.519 Diseases of the respiratory system complicating pregnancy, unspecified trimester ♀ M

O99.52 Diseases of the respiratory system complicating childbirth ♀ M

O99.53 Diseases of the respiratory system complicating the puerperium ♀ M

● **O99.6 Diseases of the digestive system complicating pregnancy, childbirth and the puerperium**
Conditions in K00-K93

Excludes2 hemorrhoids in pregnancy (O22.4-) ◀
liver and biliary tract disorders in pregnancy, childbirth and the puerperium (O26.6-)

● **O99.61 Diseases of the digestive system complicating pregnancy**

O99.611 Diseases of the digestive system complicating pregnancy, first trimester ♀ M

O99.612 Diseases of the digestive system complicating pregnancy, second trimester ♀ M

O99.613 Diseases of the digestive system complicating pregnancy, third trimester ♀ M

O99.619 Diseases of the digestive system complicating pregnancy, unspecified trimester ♀ M

O99.62 Diseases of the digestive system complicating childbirth ♀ M

O99.63 Diseases of the digestive system complicating the puerperium ♀ M

● **O99.7 Diseases of the skin and subcutaneous tissue complicating pregnancy, childbirth and the puerperium**
Conditions in L00-L99

Excludes2 herpes gestationis (O26.4)
pruritic urticarial papules and plaques of pregnancy (PUPPP) (O26.86)

● **O99.71 Diseases of the skin and subcutaneous tissue complicating pregnancy**

O99.711 Diseases of the skin and subcutaneous tissue complicating pregnancy, first trimester ♀ M

O99.712 Diseases of the skin and subcutaneous tissue complicating pregnancy, second trimester ♀ M

O99.713 Diseases of the skin and subcutaneous tissue complicating pregnancy, third trimester ♀ M

O99.719 Diseases of the skin and subcutaneous tissue complicating pregnancy, unspecified trimester ♀ M

O99.72 Diseases of the skin and subcutaneous tissue complicating childbirth ♀ M

O99.73 Diseases of the skin and subcutaneous tissue complicating the puerperium ♀ M

O99.8 Other specified diseases and conditions complicating pregnancy, childbirth and the puerperium
Conditions in D00-D48, H00-H95, M00-N99, and Q00-Q99
Use additional code to identify condition
Excludes2 genitourinary infections in pregnancy (O23.-)
infection of genitourinary tract following delivery (O86.1-O86.3)
malignant neoplasm complicating pregnancy, childbirth and the puerperium (O9A.1-)
maternal care for known or suspected abnormality of maternal pelvic organs (O34.-)
postpartum acute kidney failure (O90.4)
traumatic injuries in pregnancy (O9A.2-)

O99.81 Abnormal glucose complicating pregnancy, childbirth and the puerperium
Excludes1 gestational diabetes (O24.4-)
O99.810 Abnormal glucose complicating pregnancy ♀ M
O99.814 Abnormal glucose complicating childbirth ♀ M
O99.815 Abnormal glucose complicating the puerperium ♀ M

O99.82 Streptococcus B carrier state complicating pregnancy, childbirth and the puerperium
Excludes1 Carrier of streptococcus group B (GBS) in a nonpregnant woman (Z22.330) ◀
O99.820 Streptococcus B carrier state complicating pregnancy ♀ M
O99.824 Streptococcus B carrier state complicating childbirth ♀ M
O99.825 Streptococcus B carrier state complicating the puerperium ♀ M

O99.83 Other infection carrier state complicating pregnancy, childbirth and the puerperium
Use additional code to identify the carrier state (Z22.-)
Ex **For category O99.83 CC codes:** 098.411-098.613, 098.711-098.93, 099.830-099.835
O99.830 Other infection carrier state complicating pregnancy ♀ CC M
O99.834 Other infection carrier state complicating childbirth ♀ CC M
O99.835 Other infection carrier state complicating the puerperium ♀ CC M

O99.84 Bariatric surgery status complicating pregnancy, childbirth and the puerperium
Gastric banding status complicating pregnancy, childbirth and the puerperium
Gastric bypass status for obesity complicating pregnancy, childbirth and the puerperium
Obesity surgery status complicating pregnancy, childbirth and the puerperium
O99.840 Bariatric surgery status complicating pregnancy, unspecified trimester ♀ M
O99.841 Bariatric surgery status complicating pregnancy, first trimester ♀ M
O99.842 Bariatric surgery status complicating pregnancy, second trimester ♀ M
O99.843 Bariatric surgery status complicating pregnancy, third trimester ♀ M
O99.844 Bariatric surgery status complicating childbirth ♀ M
O99.845 Bariatric surgery status complicating the puerperium ♀ M

O99.89 Other specified diseases and conditions complicating pregnancy, childbirth and the puerperium ♀ M

OGCR Section I.C.2.l.3.

Malignant neoplasm in a pregnant patient
When a pregnant woman has a malignant neoplasm, a code from subcategory O9A.1-, Malignant neoplasm complicating pregnancy, childbirth, and the puerperium, should be sequenced first, followed by the appropriate code from Chapter 2 to indicate the type of neoplasm.

O9A Maternal malignant neoplasms, traumatic injuries and abuse classifiable elsewhere but complicating pregnancy, childbirth and the puerperium

O9A.1 Malignant neoplasm complicating pregnancy, childbirth and the puerperium
Conditions in C00-C96
Use additional code to identify neoplasm
Excludes2 maternal care for benign tumor of corpus uteri (O34.1-)
maternal care for benign tumor of cervix (O34.4-)

O9A.11 Malignant neoplasm complicating pregnancy
O9A.111 Malignant neoplasm complicating pregnancy, first trimester ♀ M
O9A.112 Malignant neoplasm complicating pregnancy, second trimester ♀ M
O9A.113 Malignant neoplasm complicating pregnancy, third trimester ♀ M
O9A.119 Malignant neoplasm complicating pregnancy, unspecified trimester ♀ M

O9A.12 Malignant neoplasm complicating childbirth ♀ M

O9A.13 Malignant neoplasm complicating the puerperium ♀ M
Coding Clinic: 2015, Q3, P19

O9A.2 Injury, poisoning and certain other consequences of external causes complicating pregnancy, childbirth and the puerperium
Conditions in S00-T88, except T74 and T76
Use additional code(s) to identify the injury or poisoning
Excludes2 physical, sexual and psychological abuse complicating pregnancy, childbirth and the puerperium (O9A.3-, O9A.4-, O9A.5-)

O9A.21 Injury, poisoning and certain other consequences of external causes complicating pregnancy
O9A.211 Injury, poisoning and certain other consequences of external causes complicating pregnancy, first trimester ♀ M
O9A.212 Injury, poisoning and certain other consequences of external causes complicating pregnancy, second trimester ♀ M
O9A.213 Injury, poisoning and certain other consequences of external causes complicating pregnancy, third trimester ♀ M
O9A.219 Injury, poisoning and certain other consequences of external causes complicating pregnancy, unspecified trimester ♀ M

O9A.22 Injury, poisoning and certain other consequences of external causes complicating childbirth ♀ M

O9A.23 Injury, poisoning and certain other consequences of external causes complicating the puerperium ♀ M

● **O9A.3 Physical abuse complicating pregnancy, childbirth and the puerperium**
Conditions in T74.11 or T76.11
Use additional code (if applicable):
to identify any associated current injury due to physical abuse
to identify the perpetrator of abuse (Y07.-)
Excludes2 sexual abuse complicating pregnancy, childbirth and the puerperium (O9A.4)

● **O9A.31 Physical abuse complicating pregnancy**
O9A.311 Physical abuse complicating pregnancy, first trimester ♀ M
O9A.312 Physical abuse complicating pregnancy, second trimester ♀ M
O9A.313 Physical abuse complicating pregnancy, third trimester ♀ M
O9A.319 Physical abuse complicating pregnancy, unspecified trimester ♀ M
O9A.32 Physical abuse complicating childbirth ♀ M
O9A.33 Physical abuse complicating the puerperium ♀ M

● **O9A.4 Sexual abuse complicating pregnancy, childbirth and the puerperium**
Conditions in T74.21 or T76.21
Use additional code (if applicable):
to identify any associated current injury due to sexual abuse
to identify the perpetrator of abuse (Y07.-)

● **O9A.41 Sexual abuse complicating pregnancy**
O9A.411 Sexual abuse complicating pregnancy, first trimester ♀ M
O9A.412 Sexual abuse complicating pregnancy, second trimester ♀ M
O9A.413 Sexual abuse complicating pregnancy, third trimester ♀ M
O9A.419 Sexual abuse complicating pregnancy, unspecified trimester ♀ M
O9A.42 Sexual abuse complicating childbirth ♀ M
O9A.43 Sexual abuse complicating the puerperium ♀ M

● **O9A.5 Psychological abuse complicating pregnancy, childbirth and the puerperium**
Conditions in T74.31 or T76.31
Use additional code to identify the perpetrator of abuse (Y07.-)

● **O9A.51 Psychological abuse complicating pregnancy**
O9A.511 Psychological abuse complicating pregnancy, first trimester ♀ M
O9A.512 Psychological abuse complicating pregnancy, second trimester ♀ M
O9A.513 Psychological abuse complicating pregnancy, third trimester ♀ M
O9A.519 Psychological abuse complicating pregnancy, unspecified trimester ♀ M
O9A.52 Psychological abuse complicating childbirth ♀ M
O9A.53 Psychological abuse complicating the puerperium ♀ M

CHAPTER 16

CERTAIN CONDITIONS ORIGINATING IN THE PERINATAL PERIOD (P00-P96)

OGCR Chapter-Specific Coding Guidelines

16. Chapter 16: Certain Conditions Originating in the Perinatal Period (P00-P96)

For coding and reporting purposes the perinatal period is defined as before birth through the 28th day following birth. The following guidelines are provided for reporting purposes

a. General Perinatal Rules

1) Use of Chapter 16 Codes

Codes in this chapter are never for use on the maternal record. Codes from Chapter 15, the obstetric chapter, are never permitted on the newborn record. Chapter 16 codes may be used throughout the life of the patient if the condition is still present.

2) Principal Diagnosis for Birth Record

When coding the birth episode in a newborn record, assign a code from category Z38, Liveborn infants according to place of birth and type of delivery, as the principal diagnosis. A code from category Z38 is assigned only once, to a newborn at the time of birth. If a newborn is transferred to another institution, a code from category Z38 should not be used at the receiving hospital.

A code from category Z38 is used only on the newborn record, not on the mother's record.

3) Use of Codes from other Chapters with Codes from Chapter 16

Codes from other chapters may be used with codes from chapter 16 if the codes from the other chapters provide more specific detail. Codes for signs and symptoms may be assigned when a definitive diagnosis has not been established. If the reason for the encounter is a perinatal condition, the code from chapter 16 should be sequenced first.

4) Use of Chapter 16 Codes after the Perinatal Period

Should a condition originate in the perinatal period, and continue throughout the life of the patient, the perinatal code should continue to be used regardless of the patient's age.

5) Birth process or community acquired conditions

If a newborn has a condition that may be either due to the birth process or community acquired and the documentation does not indicate which it is, the default is due to the birth process and the code from Chapter 16 should be used. If the condition is community-acquired, a code from Chapter 16 should not be assigned.

6) Code all clinically significant conditions

All clinically significant conditions noted on routine newborn examination should be coded. A condition is clinically significant if it requires:

- clinical evaluation; or
- therapeutic treatment; or
- diagnostic procedures; or
- extended length of hospital stay; or
- increased nursing care and/or monitoring; or
- has implications for future health care needs

Note: The perinatal guidelines listed above are the same as the general coding guidelines for "additional diagnoses", except for the final point regarding implications for future health care needs. Codes should be assigned for conditions that have been specified by the provider as having implications for future health care needs.

b. Observation and Evaluation of Newborns for Suspected Conditions not Found

1) Assign a code from category Z05, Observation and evaluation of newborns and infants for suspected conditions ruled out, to identify those instances when a healthy newborn is evaluated for a suspected condition that is determined after study not to be present. Do not use a code from category Z05 when the patient has identified signs or symptoms of a suspected problem; in such cases code the sign or symptom.

2) A code from category Z05 may also be assigned as a principal or first-listed code for readmissions or encounters when the code from category Z38 code no longer applies. Codes from category Z05 are for use only for healthy newborns and infants for which no condition after study is found to be present.

3) Z05 on a birth record

A code from category Z05 is to be used as a secondary code after the code from category Z38, Liveborn infants according to place of birth and type of delivery.

c. Coding Additional Perinatal Diagnoses

1) Assigning codes for conditions that require treatment

Assign codes for conditions that require treatment or further investigation, prolong the length of stay, or require resource utilization.

2) Codes for conditions specified as having implications for future health care needs

Assign codes for conditions that have been specified by the provider as having implications for future health care needs.

Note: This guideline should not be used for adult patients.

d. Prematurity and Fetal Growth Retardation

Providers utilize different criteria in determining prematurity. A code for prematurity should not be assigned unless it is documented. Assignment of codes in categories P05, Disorders of newborn related to slow fetal growth and fetal malnutrition, and P07, Disorders of newborn related to short gestation and low birth weight, not elsewhere classified, should be based on the recorded birth weight and estimated gestational age. Codes from category P05 should not be assigned with codes from category P07.

When both birth weight and gestational age are available, two codes from category P07 should be assigned, with the code for birth weight sequenced before the code for gestational age.

e. Low birth weight and immaturity status

Codes from category P07, Disorders of newborn related to short gestation and low birth weight, not elsewhere classified, are for use for a child or adult who was premature or had a low birth weight as a newborn and this is affecting the patient's current health status.

See Section I.C.21. Factors influencing health status and contact with health services, Status.

f. Bacterial Sepsis of Newborn

Category P36, Bacterial sepsis of newborn, includes congenital sepsis. If a perinate is documented as having sepsis without documentation of congenital or community acquired, the default is congenital and a code from category P36 should be assigned. If the P36 code includes the causal organism, an additional code from category B95, Streptococcus, Staphylococcus, and Enterococcus as the cause of diseases classified elsewhere, or B96, Other bacterial agents as the cause of diseases classified elsewhere, should not be assigned. If the P36 code does not include the causal organism, assign an additional code from category B96. If applicable, use additional codes to identify severe sepsis (R65.2-) and any associated acute organ dysfunction.

g. Stillbirth

Code P95, Stillbirth, is only for use in institutions that maintain separate records for stillbirths. No other code should be used with P95. Code P95 should not be used on the mother's record.

CHAPTER 16

CERTAIN CONDITIONS ORIGINATING IN THE PERINATAL PERIOD (P00-P96)

Note: Codes from this chapter are for use on newborn records only, never on maternal records.

Includes conditions that have their origin in the fetal or perinatal period (before birth through the first 28 days after birth) even if morbidity occurs later

Excludes2 congenital malformations, deformations and chromosomal abnormalities (Q00-Q99)
endocrine, nutritional and metabolic diseases (E00-E88)
injury, poisoning and certain other consequences of external causes (S00-T88)
neoplasms (C00-D49)
tetanus neonatorum (A33)

This chapter contains the following blocks:

P00-P04	Newborn affected by maternal factors and by complications of pregnancy, labor, and delivery
P05-P08	Disorders of newborns related to length of gestation and fetal growth
P09	Abnormal findings on neonatal screening
P10-P15	Birth trauma
P19-P29	Respiratory and cardiovascular disorders specific to the perinatal period
P35-P39	Infections specific to the perinatal period
P50-P61	Hemorrhagic and hematological disorders of newborn
P70-P74	Transitory endocrine and metabolic disorders specific to newborn
P76-P78	Digestive system disorders of newborn
P80-P83	Conditions involving the integument and temperature regulation of newborn
P84	Other problems with newborn
P90-P96	Other disorders originating in the perinatal period

NEWBORN AFFECTED BY MATERNAL FACTORS AND BY COMPLICATIONS OF PREGNANCY, LABOR, AND DELIVERY (P00–P04)

Note: These codes are for use when the listed maternal conditions are specified as the cause of confirmed morbidity or potential morbidity which have their origin in the perinatal period (before birth through the first 28 days after birth).

● **P00 Newborn affected by maternal conditions that may be unrelated to present pregnancy**

Code first any current condition in newborn

Excludes2 encounter for observation of newborn for suspected diseases and conditions ruled out (Z05.-) ◀
newborn affected by maternal complications of pregnancy (P01.-) ◀
newborn affected by maternal endocrine and metabolic disorders (P70–P74)
newborn affected by noxious substances transmitted via placenta or breast milk (P04.-)

P00.0 Newborn affected by maternal hypertensive disorders
Newborn affected by maternal conditions classifiable to O10-O11, O13-O16

P00.1 Newborn affected by maternal renal and urinary tract diseases
Newborn affected by maternal conditions classifiable to N00-N39

P00.2 Newborn affected by maternal infectious and parasitic diseases
Newborn affected by maternal infectious disease classifiable to A00-B99, J09 and J10

Excludes1 infections specific to the perinatal period (P35-P39)
maternal genital tract or other localized infections (P00.8)

Coding Clinic: 2015, Q3, P21

P00.3 Newborn affected by other maternal circulatory and respiratory diseases
Newborn affected by maternal conditions classifiable to I00-I99, J00-J99, Q20-Q34 and not included in P00.0, P00.2

P00.4 Newborn affected by maternal nutritional disorders
Newborn affected by maternal disorders classifiable to E40-E64
Maternal malnutrition NOS

P00.5 Newborn affected by maternal injury
Newborn affected by maternal conditions classifiable to O9A.2-

P00.6 Newborn affected by surgical procedure on mother
Newborn affected by amniocentesis

Excludes1 Cesarean delivery for present delivery (P03.4)
damage to placenta from amniocentesis, cesarean delivery or surgical induction (P02.1)
previous surgery to uterus or pelvic organs (P03.89)

Excludes2 newborn affected by complication of (fetal) intrauterine procedure (P96.5)

P00.7 Newborn affected by other medical procedures on mother, not elsewhere classified
Newborn affected by radiation to mother

Excludes1 damage to placenta from amniocentesis, cesarean delivery or surgical induction (P02.1)
newborn affected by other complications of labor and delivery (P03.-)

● **P00.8 Newborn affected by other maternal conditions**

P00.81 Newborn affected by periodontal disease in mother

P00.89 Newborn affected by other maternal conditions
Newborn affected by conditions classifiable to T80-T88
Newborn affected by maternal genital tract or other localized infections
Newborn affected by maternal systemic lupus erythematosus

P00.9 Newborn affected by unspecified maternal condition

● **P01 Newborn affected by maternal complications of pregnancy**

Code first any current condition in newborn

Excludes2 encounter for observation of newborn for suspected diseases and conditions ruled out (Z05.-) ◀

P01.0 Newborn affected by incompetent cervix

P01.1 Newborn affected by premature rupture of membranes

P01.2 Newborn affected by oligohydramnios

Excludes1 oligohydramnios due to premature rupture of membranes (P01.1)

P01.3 Newborn affected by polyhydramnios
Excess of amniotic fluid, usually > 2000 mL
Newborn affected by hydramnios

P01.4 Newborn affected by ectopic pregnancy
Newborn affected by abdominal pregnancy

P01.5 Newborn affected by multiple pregnancy
Newborn affected by triplet (pregnancy)
Newborn affected by twin (pregnancy)

P01.6 Newborn affected by maternal death

P01.7 Newborn affected by malpresentation before labor
Newborn affected by breech presentation before labor
Newborn affected by external version before labor
Newborn affected by face presentation before labor
Newborn affected by transverse lie before labor
Newborn affected by unstable lie before labor

P01.8 Newborn affected by other maternal complications of pregnancy

P01.9 Newborn affected by maternal complication of pregnancy, unspecified

P02 Newborn affected by complications of placenta, cord and membranes

Code first any current condition in newborn

Excludes2 encounter for observation of newborn for suspected diseases and conditions ruled out (Z05.-)

P02.0 Newborn affected by placenta previa

P02.1 Newborn affected by other forms of placental separation and hemorrhage
- Newborn affected by abruptio placenta
- Newborn affected by accidental hemorrhage
- Newborn affected by antepartum hemorrhage
- Newborn affected by damage to placenta from amniocentesis, cesarean delivery or surgical induction
- Newborn affected by maternal blood loss
- Newborn affected by premature separation of placenta

P02.2 Newborn affected by other and unspecified morphological and functional abnormalities of placenta

P02.20 Newborn affected by unspecified morphological and functional abnormalities of placenta

P02.29 Newborn affected by other morphological and functional abnormalities of placenta
- Newborn affected by placental dysfunction
- Newborn affected by placental infarction
- Newborn affected by placental insufficiency

P02.3 Newborn affected by placental transfusion syndromes
- Newborn affected by placental and cord abnormalities resulting in twin-to-twin or other transplacental transfusion

P02.4 Newborn affected by prolapsed cord

P02.5 Newborn affected by other compression of umbilical cord
- Newborn affected by umbilical cord (tightly) around neck
- Newborn affected by entanglement of umbilical cord
- Newborn affected by knot in umbilical cord

P02.6 Newborn affected by other and unspecified conditions of umbilical cord

P02.60 Newborn affected by unspecified conditions of umbilical cord

P02.69 Newborn affected by other conditions of umbilical cord
- Newborn affected by short umbilical cord
- Newborn affected by vasa previa

Excludes1 newborn affected by single umbilical artery (Q27.0)

P02.7 Newborn affected by chorioamnionitis
- *Inflammation of chorion and amnion*
- Newborn affected by amnionitis
- Newborn affected by membranitis
- Newborn affected by placentitis

P02.8 Newborn affected by other abnormalities of membranes

P02.9 Newborn affected by abnormality of membranes, unspecified

P03 Newborn affected by other complications of labor and delivery

Code first any current condition in newborn

Excludes2 encounter for observation of newborn for suspected diseases and conditions ruled out (Z05.-)

P03.0 Newborn affected by breech delivery and extraction

P03.1 Newborn affected by other malpresentation, malposition and disproportion during labor and delivery
- Newborn affected by contracted pelvis
- Newborn affected by conditions classifiable to O64-O66
- Newborn affected by persistent occipitoposterior
- Newborn affected by transverse lie

P03.2 Newborn affected by forceps delivery

P03.3 Newborn affected by delivery by vacuum extractor [ventouse]

P03.4 Newborn affected by Cesarean delivery

P03.5 Newborn affected by precipitate delivery
- Newborn affected by rapid second stage

P03.6 Newborn affected by abnormal uterine contractions
- Newborn affected by conditions classifiable to O62.-, except O62.3
- Newborn affected by hypertonic labor
- Newborn affected by uterine inertia

P03.8 Newborn affected by other specified complications of labor and delivery

P03.81 Newborn affected by abnormality in fetal (intrauterine) heart rate or rhythm

Excludes1 neonatal cardiac dysrhythmia (P29.1-)

P03.810 Newborn affected by abnormality in fetal (intrauterine) heart rate or rhythm before the onset of labor

P03.811 Newborn affected by abnormality in fetal (intrauterine) heart rate or rhythm during labor

P03.819 Newborn affected by abnormality in fetal (intrauterine) heart rate or rhythm, unspecified as to time of onset

P03.82 Meconium passage during delivery

Excludes1 meconium aspiration (P24.00, P24.01)
meconium staining (P96.83)

P03.89 Newborn affected by other specified complications of labor and delivery
- Newborn affected by abnormality of maternal soft tissues
- Newborn affected by conditions classifiable to O60-O75 and by procedures used in labor and delivery not included in P02.- and P03.0-P03.6
- Newborn affected by induction of labor

P03.9 Newborn affected by complication of labor and delivery, unspecified

P04 Newborn affected by noxious substances transmitted via placenta or breast milk

Includes nonteratogenic effects of substances transmitted via placenta

Excludes2 congenital malformations (Q00-Q99)
encounter for observation of newborn for suspected diseases and conditions ruled out (Z05.-)
neonatal jaundice from excessive hemolysis due to drugs or toxins transmitted from mother (P58.4)
newborn in contact with and (suspected) exposures hazardous to health not transmitted via placenta or breast milk (Z77.-)

P04.0 Newborn affected by maternal anesthesia and analgesia in pregnancy, labor and delivery
- Newborn affected by reactions and intoxications from maternal opiates and tranquilizers administered during labor and delivery

P04.1 Newborn affected by other maternal medication
- Newborn affected by cancer chemotherapy
- Newborn affected by cytotoxic drugs

Excludes1 dysmorphism due to warfarin (Q86.2)
fetal hydantoin syndrome (Q86.1)
maternal use of drugs of addiction (P04.4-)

P04.2 Newborn affected by maternal use of tobacco
Newborn affected by exposure in utero to tobacco smoke
Excludes2 newborn exposure to environmental tobacco smoke (P96.81)

P04.3 Newborn affected by maternal use of alcohol
Excludes1 fetal alcohol syndrome (Q86.0)

● **P04.4 Newborn affected by maternal use of drugs of addiction**

P04.41 Newborn affected by maternal use of cocaine
'Crack baby'

P04.49 Newborn affected by maternal use of other drugs of addiction
Excludes2 newborn affected by maternal anesthesia and analgesia (P04.0)
withdrawal symptoms from maternal use of drugs of addiction (P96.1)

P04.5 Newborn affected by maternal use of nutritional chemical substances

P04.6 Newborn affected by maternal exposure to environmental chemical substances

P04.8 Newborn affected by other maternal noxious substances

P04.9 Newborn affected by maternal noxious substance, unspecified

OGCR Section I.C.16.d.

Prematurity and Fetal Growth Retardation

Providers utilize different criteria in determining prematurity. A code for prematurity should not be assigned unless it is documented. Assignment of codes in categories P05, Disorders of newborn related to slow fetal growth and fetal malnutrition, and P07, Disorders of newborn related to short gestation and low birth weight, not elsewhere classified, should be based on the recorded birth weight and estimated gestational age. Codes from category P05 should not be assigned with codes from category P07.

When both birth weight and gestational age are available, two codes from category P07 should be assigned, with the code for birth weight sequenced before the code for gestational age.

A code from P05 and codes from P07.2 and P07.3 may be used to specify weeks of gestation as documented by the provider in the record.

DISORDERS OF NEWBORN RELATED TO LENGTH OF GESTATION AND FETAL GROWTH (P05-P08)

● **P05 Disorders of newborn related to slow fetal growth and fetal malnutrition**

● **P05.0 Newborn light for gestational age**
Newborn light-for-dates
Weight below but length above 10th percentile for gestational age ◀

P05.00 Newborn light for gestational age, unspecified weight

P05.01 Newborn light for gestational age, less than 500 grams

P05.02 Newborn light for gestational age, 500-749 grams

P05.03 Newborn light for gestational age, 750-999 grams

P05.04 Newborn light for gestational age, 1000-1249 grams

P05.05 Newborn light for gestational age, 1250-1499 grams

P05.06 Newborn light for gestational age, 1500-1749 grams

P05.07 Newborn light for gestational age, 1750-1999 grams

P05.08 Newborn light for gestational age, 2000-2499 grams

P05.09 Newborn light for gestational age, 2500 grams and over ◀
Newborn light for gestational age, other ◀

● **P05.1 Newborn small for gestational age**
Newborn small-and-light-for-dates
Newborn small-for-dates
Weight and length below 10th percentile for gestational age ◀

P05.10 Newborn small for gestational age, unspecified weight

P05.11 Newborn small for gestational age, less than 500 grams

P05.12 Newborn small for gestational age, 500-749 grams

P05.13 Newborn small for gestational age, 750-999 grams

P05.14 Newborn small for gestational age, 1000-1249 grams

P05.15 Newborn small for gestational age, 1250-1499 grams

P05.16 Newborn small for gestational age, 1500-1749 grams

P05.17 Newborn small for gestational age, 1750-1999 grams

P05.18 Newborn small for gestational age, 2000-2499 grams

P05.19 Newborn small for gestational age, other ◀
Newborn small for gestational age, 2500 grams and over ◀

P05.2 Newborn affected by fetal (intrauterine) malnutrition not light or small for gestational age
Infant, not light or small for gestational age, showing signs of fetal malnutrition, such as dry, peeling skin and loss of subcutaneous tissue
Excludes1 newborn affected by fetal malnutrition with light for gestational age (P05.0-)
newborn affected by fetal malnutrition with small for gestational age (P05.1-)

P05.9 Newborn affected by slow intrauterine growth, unspecified
Newborn affected by fetal growth retardation NOS

● **P07 Disorders of newborn related to short gestation and low birth weight, not elsewhere classified**
Note: When both birth weight and gestational age of the newborn are available, both should be coded with birth weight sequenced before gestational age.
Includes the listed conditions, without further specification, as the cause of morbidity or additional care, in newborn

● **P07.0 Extremely low birth weight newborn**
Newborn birth weight 999 g. or less
Excludes1 low birth weight due to slow fetal growth and fetal malnutrition (P05.-) ◀

P07.00 Extremely low birth weight newborn, unspecified weight

P07.01 Extremely low birth weight newborn, less than 500 grams

P07.02 Extremely low birth weight newborn, 500-749 grams

P07.03 Extremely low birth weight newborn, 750-999 grams

P07.1 Other low birth weight newborn
Newborn birth weight 1000-2499 g.
Excludes1 low birth weight due to slow fetal growth and fetal malnutrition (P05.-) ◀

P07.10 Other low birth weight newborn, unspecified weight

P07.14 Other low birth weight newborn, 1000-1249 grams

P07.15 Other low birth weight newborn, 1250-1499 grams

P07.16 Other low birth weight newborn, 1500-1749 grams

P07.17 Other low birth weight newborn, 1750-1999 grams

P07.18 Other low birth weight newborn, 2000-2499 grams

P07.2 Extreme immaturity of newborn
Less than 28 completed weeks (less than 196 completed days) of gestation

P07.20 Extreme immaturity of newborn, unspecified weeks of gestation
Gestational age less than 28 completed weeks NOS

P07.21 Extreme immaturity of newborn, gestational age less than 23 completed weeks
Extreme immaturity of newborn, gestational age less than 23 weeks, 0 days

P07.22 Extreme immaturity of newborn, gestational age 23 completed weeks
Extreme immaturity of newborn, gestational age 23 weeks, 0 days through 23 weeks, 6 days

P07.23 Extreme immaturity of newborn, gestational age 24 completed weeks
Extreme immaturity of newborn, gestational age 24 weeks, 0 days through 24 weeks, 6 days

P07.24 Extreme immaturity of newborn, gestational age 25 completed weeks
Extreme immaturity of newborn, gestational age 25 weeks, 0 days through 25 weeks, 6 days

P07.25 Extreme immaturity of newborn, gestational age 26 completed weeks
Extreme immaturity of newborn, gestational age 26 weeks, 0 days through 26 weeks, 6 days

P07.26 Extreme immaturity of newborn, gestational age 27 completed weeks
Extreme immaturity of newborn, gestational age 27 weeks, 0 days through 27 weeks, 6 days

P07.3 Preterm [premature] newborn [other]
28 completed weeks or more but less than 37 completed weeks (196 completed days but less than 259 completed days) of gestation
Prematurity NOS

P07.30 Preterm newborn, unspecified weeks of gestation

P07.31 Preterm newborn, gestational age 28 completed weeks
Preterm newborn, gestational age 28 weeks, 0 days through 28 weeks, 6 days

P07.32 Preterm newborn, gestational age 29 completed weeks
Preterm newborn, gestational age 29 weeks, 0 days through 29 weeks, 6 days

P07.33 Preterm newborn, gestational age 30 completed weeks
Preterm newborn, gestational age 30 weeks, 0 days through 30 weeks, 6 days

P07.34 Preterm newborn, gestational age 31 completed weeks
Preterm newborn, gestational age 31 weeks, 0 days through 31 weeks, 6 days

P07.35 Preterm newborn, gestational age 32 completed weeks
Preterm newborn, gestational age 32 weeks, 0 days through 32 weeks, 6 days

P07.36 Preterm newborn, gestational age 33 completed weeks
Preterm newborn, gestational age 33 weeks, 0 days through 33 weeks, 6 days

P07.37 Preterm newborn, gestational age 34 completed weeks
Preterm newborn, gestational age 34 weeks, 0 days through 34 weeks, 6 days

P07.38 Preterm newborn, gestational age 35 completed weeks
Preterm newborn, gestational age 35 weeks, 0 days through 35 weeks, 6 days

P07.39 Preterm newborn, gestational age 36 completed weeks
Preterm newborn, gestational age 36 weeks, 0 days through 36 weeks, 6 days

P08 Disorders of newborn related to long gestation and high birth weight
Note: When both birth weight and gestational age of the newborn are available, priority of assignment should be given to birth weight.
Includes the listed conditions, without further specification, as causes of morbidity or additional care, in newborn

P08.0 Exceptionally large newborn baby
Usually implies a birth weight of 4500 g. or more
Excludes1 syndrome of infant of diabetic mother (P70.1)
syndrome of infant of mother with gestational diabetes (P70.0)

P08.1 Other heavy for gestational age newborn
Other newborn heavy- or large-for-dates regardless of period of gestation
Usually implies a birth weight of 4000 g. to 4499 g.
Excludes1 newborn with a birth weight of 4500 or more (P08.0)
syndrome of infant of diabetic mother (P70.1)
syndrome of infant of mother with gestational diabetes (P70.0)

P08.2 Late newborn, not heavy for gestational age

P08.21 Post-term newborn
Newborn with gestation period over 40 completed weeks to 42 completed weeks

P08.22 Prolonged gestation of newborn
Newborn with gestation period over 42 completed weeks (294 days or more), not heavy- or large-for-dates
Postmaturity NOS

ABNORMAL FINDINGS ON NEONATAL SCREENING (P09)

P09 Abnormal findings on neonatal screening
Use additional code to identify signs, symptoms and conditions associated with the screening
Excludes2 nonspecific serologic evidence of human immunodeficiency virus [HIV] (R75)

BIRTH TRAUMA (P10-P15)

● **P10 Intracranial laceration and hemorrhage due to birth injury**

Excludes1 intracranial hemorrhage of newborn NOS (P52.9)
intracranial hemorrhage of newborn due to anoxia or hypoxia (P52.-)
nontraumatic intracranial hemorrhage of newborn (P52.-)

Ex: **For category P10 CC codes unless otherwise indicated:** P10.0-P10.1, P10.4-P11.2, P11.9, P15.0-P15.9, P29.0-P29.2, P29.4, P29.89-P29.9, P52.4, P52.6-P52.9, P94.1-P94.9, P96.0, P96.3-P96.5, P96.82-P96.89

P10.0 Subdural hemorrhage due to birth injury
Subdural hematoma (localized) due to birth injury
Excludes1 subdural hemorrhage accompanying tentorial tear (P10.4)

P10.1 Cerebral hemorrhage due to birth injury

P10.2 Intraventricular hemorrhage due to birth injury
Ex: P10.2-P10.3, P29.0-P29.2, P29.4, P29.89-P29.9, P50.0-P50.9, P52.0-P52.3, P52.5, P53-P54.0, P54.6-P54.9, P60-P61.9, P94.1-P94.9, P96.0, P96.3-P96.5, P96.82-P96.89

P10.3 Subarachnoid hemorrhage due to birth injury
Ex: P10.2-P10.3, P29.0-P29.2, P29.4, P29.89-P29.9, P50.0-P50.9, P52.0-P52.3, P52.5, P53-P54.0, P54.6-P54.9, P60-P61.9, P91.2, P94.1-P94.9, P96.0, P96.3-P96.5, P96.82-P96.89

Item 16–1 The **peripheral nervous system** consists of 31 pairs of spinal nerves, 12 pairs of cranial nerves, and the autonomic nerves, which are divided into the parasympathetic and sympathetic nerves. The cranial nerves are: olfactory (I), optic (II), oculomotor (III), trochlear (IV), trigeminal (V), abducens (VI), facial (VII), vestibulocochlear (VIII), glossopharyngeal (IX), vagus (X), accessory (XI), and hypoglossal (XII).

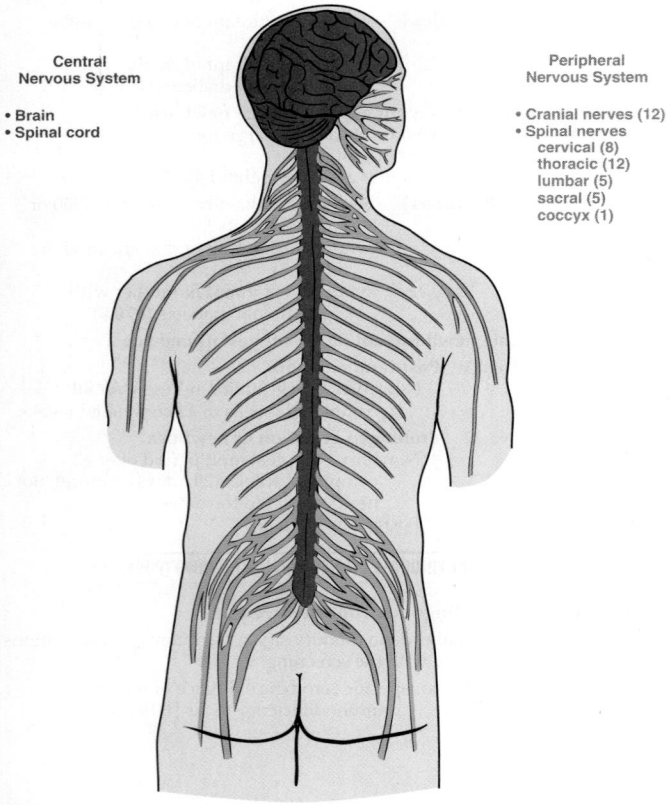

Figure 16-1 The central nervous system consists of the brain and spinal cord. The peripheral nervous system consists of nerves that lie outside the skull and spinal cord. (From Stoy: Mosby's EMT-Basic Textbook, ed 2, St. Louis, Mosby, 2007)

P10.4 Tentorial tear due to birth injury
Pertaining to tentorium of cerebellum (extension of dura mater that separates cerebellum from inferior portion of occipital lobes)

P10.8 Other intracranial lacerations and hemorrhages due to birth injury

P10.9 Unspecified intracranial laceration and hemorrhage due to birth injury

● **P11 Other birth injuries to central nervous system**

P11.0 Cerebral edema due to birth injury
Ex: See P10

P11.1 Other specified brain damage due to birth injury

P11.2 Unspecified brain damage due to birth injury
Ex: See P10

P11.3 Birth injury to facial nerve
Facial palsy due to birth injury

P11.4 Birth injury to other cranial nerves

P11.5 Birth injury to spine and spinal cord
Fracture of spine due to birth injury

P11.9 Birth injury to central nervous system, unspecified
Ex: See P10

● **P12 Birth injury to scalp**

P12.0 Cephalhematoma due to birth injury

P12.1 Chignon (from vacuum extraction) due to birth injury

P12.2 Epicranial subaponeurotic hemorrhage due to birth injury
Subgaleal hemorrhage
Ex: P10.0-P10.1, P10.4-P11.2, P11.9-P12.2, P15.0-P15.9, P29.0-P29.2, P29.4, P29.89-P29.9, P52.4, P52.6-P52.9, P94.1-P94.9, P96.0, P96.3-P96.5, P96.82-P96.89

P12.3 Bruising of scalp due to birth injury

P12.4 Injury of scalp of newborn due to monitoring equipment
Sampling incision of scalp of newborn
Scalp clip (electrode) injury of newborn

● **P12.8 Other birth injuries to scalp**

P12.81 Caput succedaneum

P12.89 Other birth injuries to scalp

P12.9 Birth injury to scalp, unspecified

● **P13 Birth injury to skeleton**

Excludes2 birth injury to spine (P11.5)

P13.0 Fracture of skull due to birth injury

P13.1 Other birth injuries to skull
Excludes1 cephalhematoma (P12.0)

P13.2 Birth injury to femur

P13.3 Birth injury to other long bones

P13.4 Fracture of clavicle due to birth injury

P13.8 Birth injuries to other parts of skeleton

P13.9 Birth injury to skeleton, unspecified

● **P14 Birth injury to peripheral nervous system**

P14.0 Erb's paralysis due to birth injury

P14.1 Klumpke's paralysis due to birth injury

P14.2 Phrenic nerve paralysis due to birth injury

P14.3 Other brachial plexus birth injuries

P14.8 Birth injuries to other parts of peripheral nervous system

P14.9 Birth injury to peripheral nervous system, unspecified

● **P15 Other birth injuries**

P15.0 Birth injury to liver
Rupture of liver due to birth injury

P15.1 Birth injury to spleen
Rupture of spleen due to birth injury

P15.2 Sternomastoid injury due to birth injury

P15.3 Birth injury to eye
Subconjunctival hemorrhage due to birth injury
Traumatic glaucoma due to birth injury

P15.4 Birth injury to face
Facial congestion due to birth injury

P15.5 Birth injury to external genitalia

P15.6 Subcutaneous fat necrosis due to birth injury

P15.8 Other specified birth injuries

P15.9 Birth injury, unspecified

RESPIRATORY AND CARDIOVASCULAR DISORDERS SPECIFIC TO THE PERINATAL PERIOD (P19-P29)

P19 Metabolic acidemia in newborn
Includes metabolic acidemia in newborn

P19.0 Metabolic acidemia in newborn first noted before onset of labor

P19.1 Metabolic acidemia in newborn first noted during labor

P19.2 Metabolic acidemia noted at birth

P19.9 Metabolic acidemia, unspecified

P22 Respiratory distress of newborn
Excludes1 respiratory arrest of newborn (P28.81)
respiratory failure of newborn NOS (P28.5)

P22.0 Respiratory distress syndrome of newborn
Cardiorespiratory distress syndrome of newborn
Hyaline membrane disease
Idiopathic respiratory distress syndrome [IRDS or RDS] of newborn
Pulmonary hypoperfusion syndrome
Respiratory distress syndrome, type I
Ex: J84.83-J84.848, P22.0-P28.5, P28.89-P29.2, P29.4, P29.89-P29.9, P84, P94.1-P96.0, P96.3-P96.5, P96.82-P96.89

P22.1 Transient tachypnea of newborn
Idiopathic tachypnea of newborn
Respiratory distress syndrome, type II
Wet lung syndrome

P22.8 Other respiratory distress of newborn

P22.9 Respiratory distress of newborn, unspecified

P23 Congenital pneumonia
Includes infective pneumonia acquired in utero or during birth
Excludes1 neonatal pneumonia resulting from aspiration (P24.-)
Ex: For category P23 CC codes: See P22.0

P23.0 Congenital pneumonia due to viral agent
Use additional code (B97) to identify organism
Excludes1 congenital rubella pneumonitis (P35.0)

P23.1 Congenital pneumonia due to Chlamydia

P23.2 Congenital pneumonia due to staphylococcus

P23.3 Congenital pneumonia due to streptococcus, group B

P23.4 Congenital pneumonia due to Escherichia coli

P23.5 Congenital pneumonia due to Pseudomonas

P23.6 Congenital pneumonia due to other bacterial agents
Congenital pneumonia due to Hemophilus influenzae
Congenital pneumonia due to Klebsiella pneumoniae
Congenital pneumonia due to Mycoplasma
Congenital pneumonia due to Streptococcus, except group B
Use additional code (B95-B96) to identify organism

P23.8 Congenital pneumonia due to other organisms

P23.9 Congenital pneumonia, unspecified

P24 Neonatal aspiration
Includes aspiration in utero and during delivery

P24.0 Meconium aspiration
Excludes1 meconium passage (without aspiration) during delivery (P03.82)
meconium staining (P96.83)

P24.00 Meconium aspiration without respiratory symptoms
Meconium aspiration NOS

P24.01 Meconium aspiration with respiratory symptoms
Meconium aspiration pneumonia
Meconium aspiration pneumonitis
Meconium aspiration syndrome NOS
Use additional code to identify any secondary pulmonary hypertension, if applicable (I27.2)
Ex: See P22.0

P24.1 Neonatal aspiration of (clear) amniotic fluid and mucus
Neonatal aspiration of liquor (amnii)

P24.10 Neonatal aspiration of (clear) amniotic fluid and mucus without respiratory symptoms
Neonatal aspiration of amniotic fluid and mucus NOS

P24.11 Neonatal aspiration of (clear) amniotic fluid and mucus with respiratory symptoms
Neonatal aspiration of amniotic fluid and mucus with pneumonia
Neonatal aspiration of amniotic fluid and mucus with pneumonitis
Use additional code to identify any secondary pulmonary hypertension, if applicable (I27.2)
Ex: See P22.0

P24.2 Neonatal aspiration of blood

P24.20 Neonatal aspiration of blood without respiratory symptoms
Neonatal aspiration of blood NOS

P24.21 Neonatal aspiration of blood with respiratory symptoms
Neonatal aspiration of blood with pneumonia
Neonatal aspiration of blood with pneumonitis
Use additional code to identify any secondary pulmonary hypertension, if applicable (I27.2)
Ex: See P22.0

P24.3 Neonatal aspiration of milk and regurgitated food
Neonatal aspiration of stomach contents

P24.30 Neonatal aspiration of milk and regurgitated food without respiratory symptoms
Neonatal aspiration of milk and regurgitated food NOS

P24.31 Neonatal aspiration of milk and regurgitated food with respiratory symptoms
Neonatal aspiration of milk and regurgitated food with pneumonia
Neonatal aspiration of milk and regurgitated food with pneumonitis
Use additional code to identify any secondary pulmonary hypertension, if applicable (I27.2)
Ex: See P22.0

● **P24.8 Other neonatal aspiration**

P24.80 Other neonatal aspiration without respiratory symptoms
Neonatal aspiration NEC

P24.81 Other neonatal aspiration with respiratory symptoms
Neonatal aspiration pneumonia NEC
Neonatal aspiration with pneumonitis NEC
Neonatal aspiration with pneumonia NOS
Neonatal aspiration with pneumonitis NOS
Use additional code to identify any secondary pulmonary hypertension, if applicable (I27.2)
Ex: See P22.0

P24.9 Neonatal aspiration, unspecified

● **P25 Interstitial emphysema and related conditions originating in the perinatal period**
Ex: For category P25 CC codes: See P22.0

P25.0 Interstitial emphysema originating in the perinatal period

P25.1 Pneumothorax originating in the perinatal period

P25.2 Pneumomediastinum originating in the perinatal period

P25.3 Pneumopericardium originating in the perinatal period

P25.8 Other conditions related to interstitial emphysema originating in the perinatal period

● **P26 Pulmonary hemorrhage originating in the perinatal period**
Excludes1 acute idiopathic hemorrhage in infants over 28 days old (R04.81)
Ex: For category P26 CC codes: See P22.0

P26.0 Tracheobronchial hemorrhage originating in the perinatal period

P26.1 Massive pulmonary hemorrhage originating in the perinatal period

P26.8 Other pulmonary hemorrhages originating in the perinatal period

P26.9 Unspecified pulmonary hemorrhage originating in the perinatal period

● **P27 Chronic respiratory disease originating in the perinatal period**
Excludes1 respiratory distress of newborn (P22.0-P22.9)
Ex: For category P27 CC codes: See P22.0

P27.0 Wilson-Mikity syndrome
Pulmonary dysmaturity

P27.1 Bronchopulmonary dysplasia originating in the perinatal period

P27.8 Other chronic respiratory diseases originating in the perinatal period
Congenital pulmonary fibrosis
Ventilator lung in newborn

P27.9 Unspecified chronic respiratory disease originating in the perinatal period

● **P28 Other respiratory conditions originating in the perinatal period**
Excludes1 congenital malformations of the respiratory system (Q30-Q34)

P28.0 Primary atelectasis of newborn
Failure of lungs to expand properly at birth
Primary failure to expand terminal respiratory units
Pulmonary hypoplasia associated with short gestation
Pulmonary immaturity NOS
Ex: See P22.0

● **P28.1 Other and unspecified atelectasis of newborn**
Ex: For category P28.1 CC codes: See P22.0

P28.10 Unspecified atelectasis of newborn
Atelectasis of newborn NOS

P28.11 Resorption atelectasis without respiratory distress syndrome
Excludes1 resorption atelectasis with respiratory distress syndrome (P22.0)

P28.19 Other atelectasis of newborn
Partial atelectasis of newborn
Secondary atelectasis of newborn

P28.2 Cyanotic attacks of newborn
Excludes1 apnea of newborn (P28.3-P28.4)
Ex: P22.8-P22.9, P28.2-P28.4, P28.81-P28.9, R06.81, R23.0

P28.3 Primary sleep apnea of newborn
Central sleep apnea of newborn
Obstructive sleep apnea of newborn
Sleep apnea of newborn NOS
Ex: P22.8-P22.9, P28.2, P28.4, P28.81-P28.9, R06.81

P28.4 Other apnea of newborn
Apnea of prematurity
Obstructive apnea of newborn
Excludes1 obstructive sleep apnea of newborn (P28.3)
Ex: P22.8-P22.9, P28.2-P28.4, P28.81-P28.9, R06.81

P28.5 Respiratory failure of newborn
Excludes1 respiratory arrest of newborn (P28.81)
respiratory distress of newborn (P22.0-)
Ex: See P22.0

● **P28.8 Other specified respiratory conditions of newborn**

P28.81 Respiratory arrest of newborn
Ex: P22.1-P22.9, P24.00, P24.10, P24.20, P24.30, P24.80, P28.2-P28.5, P28.89-P28.9, P29.81, R06.81, R09.2

P28.89 Other specified respiratory conditions of newborn
Congenital laryngeal stridor
Sniffles in newborn
Snuffles in newborn
Excludes1 early congenital syphilitic rhinitis (A50.05)

P28.9 Respiratory condition of newborn, unspecified
Respiratory depression in newborn

● **P29 Cardiovascular disorders originating in the perinatal period**
Excludes1 congenital malformations of the circulatory system (Q20-Q28)

P29.0 Neonatal cardiac failure

● **P29.1 Neonatal cardiac dysrhythmia**

P29.11 Neonatal tachycardia

P29.12 Neonatal bradycardia

P29.2 Neonatal hypertension

P29.3 Persistent fetal circulation
Delayed closure of ductus arteriosus
(Persistent) pulmonary hypertension of newborn
Ex: I27.0, I27.2-I27.81, I27.89-I27.9

P29.4 Transient myocardial ischemia in newborn

● **P29.8 Other cardiovascular disorders originating in the perinatal period**

P29.81 Cardiac arrest of newborn
Ex: P29.81

P29.89 Other cardiovascular disorders originating in the perinatal period

P29.9 Cardiovascular disorder originating in the perinatal period, unspecified

INFECTIONS SPECIFIC TO THE PERINATAL PERIOD (P35-P39)

Infections acquired in utero, during birth via the umbilicus, or during the first 28 days after birth

Excludes2 asymptomatic human immunodeficiency virus [HIV] infection status (Z21)
congenital gonococcal infection (A54.-)
congenital pneumonia (P23.-)
congenital syphilis (A50.-)
human immunodeficiency virus [HIV] disease (B20)
infant botulism (A48.51)
infectious diseases not specific to the perinatal period (A00-B99, J09, J10.-)
intestinal infectious disease (A00-A09)
laboratory evidence of human immunodeficiency virus [HIV] (R75)
tetanus neonatorum (A33)

P35 Congenital viral diseases

Includes infections acquired in utero or during birth

Ex: **For category P35 CC codes unless otherwise indicated:** A17.82, A28.1, A50.42, A52.14, A75.9, A79.9, A81.1, A81.82-A81.89, A83.0-A85.8, A87.2, A88.0, A88.8, A92.1-A92.8, A93.0, B00.4, B00.82, B01.11-B01.12, B04, B06.01, B08.09, B08.20-B08.22, B08.60-B08.79, B09, B10.01-B10.09, B26.2, B27.00-B27.99, B33.1, B45.0, B45.2-B45.9, B54, B58.2, B75, B97.10, B97.21, G04.00-G04.01, G04.31, G04.81-G05.4, G37.0, G37.4-G37.5, H66.40-H66.43, J09.X3-J09.X9, J10.2-J10.89, J11.2-J11.89, L44.4, M1A.10X0-M1A.19X1, M32.0-M32.9, P35.2-P35.9, P37.0-P37.9, T56.0X1-T56.0X4[A]

P35.0 Congenital rubella syndrome
Congenital rubella pneumonitis
Ex: P29.0-P29.2, P29.4, P29.89-P35.9, P37.0-P37.4, P37.8-P37.9, P94.1-P94.9, P96.0, P96.3-P96.5, P96.82-P96.89

P35.1 Congenital cytomegalovirus infection
Viruses transmitted by multiple routes that cause mild/subclinical infection
Ex: See P35.0

P35.2 Congenital herpesviral [herpes simplex] infection

P35.3 Congenital viral hepatitis

P35.8 Other congenital viral diseases
Congenital varicella [chickenpox]

P35.9 Congenital viral disease, unspecified

P36 Bacterial sepsis of newborn

Includes congenital sepsis

Use additional code(s), if applicable, to identify severe sepsis (R65.2-) and associated acute organ dysfunction(s)

Ex: **For category P36 CC codes:** P29.0-P29.2, P29.4, P29.89-P29.9, P36.0-P36.9, P37.5, P38.1-P39.9, P53, P60-P61.9, P94.1-P94.9, P96.0, P96.3-P96.5, P96.82-P96.89

P36.0 Sepsis of newborn due to streptococcus, group B

P36.1 Sepsis of newborn due to other and unspecified streptococci

P36.10 Sepsis of newborn due to unspecified streptococci

P36.19 Sepsis of newborn due to other streptococci

P36.2 Sepsis of newborn due to Staphylococcus aureus

P36.3 Sepsis of newborn due to other and unspecified staphylococci

P36.30 Sepsis of newborn due to unspecified staphylococci

P36.39 Sepsis of newborn due to other staphylococci

P36.4 Sepsis of newborn due to Escherichia coli

P36.5 Sepsis of newborn due to anaerobes

P36.8 Other bacterial sepsis of newborn
Use additional code from category B96 to identify organism

P36.9 Bacterial sepsis of newborn, unspecified

P37 Other congenital infectious and parasitic diseases

Excludes2 congenital syphilis (A50.-)
infectious neonatal diarrhea (A00-A09)
necrotizing enterocolitis in newborn (P77.-)
noninfectious neonatal diarrhea (P78.3)
ophthalmia neonatorum due to gonococcus (A54.31)
tetanus neonatorum (A33)

Ex: **For category P37 CC codes:** See P35

P37.0 Congenital tuberculosis

P37.1 Congenital toxoplasmosis
Parasitic infection, often causing mild flu-like illness
Hydrocephalus due to congenital toxoplasmosis

P37.2 Neonatal (disseminated) listeriosis
Acquired transplacentally or during/after parturition in which symptoms are those of sepsis

P37.3 Congenital falciparum malaria

P37.4 Other congenital malaria

P37.5 Neonatal candidiasis

P37.8 Other specified congenital infectious and parasitic diseases

P37.9 Congenital infectious or parasitic disease, unspecified

P38 Omphalitis of newborn
Inflammation of umbilicus

Excludes1 omphalitis not of newborn (L08.82)
tetanus omphalitis (A33)
umbilical hemorrhage of newborn (P51.-)

Ex: **For category P38 CC codes:** P39.2, P39.4-P39.9

P38.1 Omphalitis with mild hemorrhage

P38.9 Omphalitis without hemorrhage
Omphalitis of newborn NOS

P39 Other infections specific to the perinatal period

Use additional code to identify organism or specific infection

Ex: **For category P39 CC codes unless otherwise indicated:** A02.1, A20.7, A22.7, A39.2-A39.4, A40.9-A41.59, A41.81-A41.9, A42.7, A48.2, A48.4, A48.8-A49.9, B00.7, B92, B94.2-B96.89, P39.2-P39.9, P95, P96.9, R78.81

P39.0 Neonatal infective mastitis

Excludes1 breast engorgement of newborn (P83.4)
noninfective mastitis of newborn (P83.4)

Ex: See P38

P39.1 Neonatal conjunctivitis and dacryocystitis
Neonatal chlamydial conjunctivitis
Ophthalmia neonatorum NOS
Neonate = newborn

Excludes1 gonococcal conjunctivitis (A54.31)

P39.2 Intra-amniotic infection affecting newborn, not elsewhere classified

P39.3 Neonatal urinary tract infection

Ex: A49.9, N10-N11.0, N11.8-N12, N13.6, N15.1, N28.82, N28.84-N30.31, N30.80-N30.91, N36.9-N39.0, N39.9, N99.511, P39.2, P39.4-P39.9, R30.0, R30.9, T83.511A

P39.4 Neonatal skin infection
Neonatal pyoderma

Excludes1 pemphigus neonatorum (L00)
staphylococcal scalded skin syndrome (L00)

P39.8 Other specified infections specific to the perinatal period

P39.9 Infection specific to the perinatal period, unspecified

HEMORRHAGIC AND HEMATOLOGICAL DISORDERS OF NEWBORN (P50-P61)

Excludes1 congenital stenosis and stricture of bile ducts (Q44.3)
Crigler-Najjar syndrome (E80.5)
Dubin-Johnson syndrome (E80.6)
Gilbert syndrome (E80.4)
hereditary hemolytic anemias (D55-D58)

P50 Newborn affected by intrauterine (fetal) blood loss
Excludes1 congenital anemia from intrauterine (fetal) blood loss (P61.3)

P50.0 Newborn affected by intrauterine (fetal) blood loss from vasa previa
P50.1 Newborn affected by intrauterine (fetal) blood loss from ruptured cord
P50.2 Newborn affected by intrauterine (fetal) blood loss from placenta
P50.3 Newborn affected by hemorrhage into co-twin
P50.4 Newborn affected by hemorrhage into maternal circulation
P50.5 Newborn affected by intrauterine (fetal) blood loss from cut end of co-twin's cord
P50.8 Newborn affected by other intrauterine (fetal) blood loss
P50.9 Newborn affected by intrauterine (fetal) blood loss, unspecified
Newborn affected by fetal hemorrhage NOS

P51 Umbilical hemorrhage of newborn
Excludes1 omphalitis with mild hemorrhage (P38.1)
umbilical hemorrhage from cut end of co-twins cord (P50.5)

P51.0 Massive umbilical hemorrhage of newborn
P51.8 Other umbilical hemorrhages of newborn
Slipped umbilical ligature NOS
P51.9 Umbilical hemorrhage of newborn, unspecified

P52 Intracranial nontraumatic hemorrhage of newborn
Includes intracranial hemorrhage due to anoxia or hypoxia
Excludes1 intracranial hemorrhage due to birth injury (P10.-)
intracranial hemorrhage due to other injury (S06.-)

P52.0 Intraventricular (nontraumatic) hemorrhage, grade 1, of newborn
Subependymal hemorrhage (without intraventricular extension)
Bleeding into germinal matrix
Ex: P10.2-P10.3, P29.0-P29.2, P29.4, P29.89-P29.9, P50.0-P50.9, P52.0-P52.3, P52.5, P53-P54.0, P54.6-P54.9, P60-P61.9, P94.1-P94.9, P96.0, P96.3-P96.5, P96.82-P96.89

P52.1 Intraventricular (nontraumatic) hemorrhage, grade 2, of newborn
Subependymal hemorrhage with intraventricular extension
Bleeding into ventricle
Ex: See P52.0

P52.2 Intraventricular (nontraumatic) hemorrhage, grade 3 and grade 4, of newborn

P52.21 Intraventricular (nontraumatic) hemorrhage, grade 3, of newborn
Subependymal hemorrhage with intraventricular extension with enlargement of ventricle
Ex: See P52.0

P52.22 Intraventricular (nontraumatic) hemorrhage, grade 4, of newborn
Bleeding into cerebral cortex
Subependymal hemorrhage with intracerebral extension
Ex: See P52.0

P52.3 Unspecified intraventricular (nontraumatic) hemorrhage of newborn
Ex: See P52.0

P52.4 Intracerebral (nontraumatic) hemorrhage of newborn
Ex: P10.0-P10.1, P10.4-P11.2, P11.9, P15.0-P15.9, P29.0-P29.2, P29.4, P29.89-P29.9, P52.4, P52.6-P52.9, P94.1-P94.9, P96.0, P96.3-P96.5, P96.82-P96.89

P52.5 Subarachnoid (nontraumatic) hemorrhage of newborn
Ex: P10.2-P10.3, P29.0-P29.2, P29.4, P29.89-P29.9, P50.0-P50.9, P52.0-P52.3, P52.5, P53-P54.0, P54.6-P54.9, P60-P61.9, P91.2, P94.1-P94.9, P96.0, P96.3-P96.5, P96.82-P96.89

P52.6 Cerebellar (nontraumatic) and posterior fossa hemorrhage of newborn
Ex: See P52.4

P52.8 Other intracranial (nontraumatic) hemorrhages of newborn
Ex: See P52.4

P52.9 Intracranial (nontraumatic) hemorrhage of newborn, unspecified
Ex: See P52.4

P53 Hemorrhagic disease of newborn
Vitamin K deficiency of newborn
Ex: P29.0-P29.2, P29.4, P29.89-P29.9, P53, P60-P61.9, P94.1-P96.0, P96.3-P96.5, P96.82-P96.89

P54 Other neonatal hemorrhages
Excludes1 newborn affected by (intrauterine) blood loss (P50.-)
pulmonary hemorrhage originating in the perinatal period (P26.-)

P54.0 Neonatal hematemesis
Vomiting of blood
Excludes1 neonatal hematemesis due to swallowed maternal blood (P78.2)

P54.1 Neonatal melena
Dark-colored feces stained with blood pigments
Excludes1 neonatal melena due to swallowed maternal blood (P78.2)
Ex: P29.0-P29.2, P29.4, P29.89-P29.9, P50.0-P50.9, P53-P54.9, P60-P61.9, P94.1-P96.0, P96.3-P96.5, P96.82-P96.89

P54.2 Neonatal rectal hemorrhage
Ex: See P54.1

P54.3 Other neonatal gastrointestinal hemorrhage
Ex: See P54.1

P54.4 Neonatal adrenal hemorrhage
Ex: See P54.1

P54.5 Neonatal cutaneous hemorrhage
Neonatal bruising
Neonatal ecchymoses
Neonatal petechiae
Neonatal superficial hematomata
Excludes2 bruising of scalp due to birth injury (P12.3)
cephalhematoma due to birth injury (P12.0)

P54.6 Neonatal vaginal hemorrhage ♀
Neonatal pseudomenses
P54.8 Other specified neonatal hemorrhages
P54.9 Neonatal hemorrhage, unspecified

P55 Hemolytic disease of newborn
AKA erythroblastosis fetalis and is due to Rh isoimmunization, result of Rh blood factor incompatibilities between mother (Rh negative) and fetus (Rh positive)

P55.0 Rh isoimmunization of newborn
P55.1 ABO isoimmunization of newborn
Coding Clinic: 2015, Q3, P20
P55.8 Other hemolytic diseases of newborn
P55.9 Hemolytic disease of newborn, unspecified

P56 Hydrops fetalis due to hemolytic disease
Caused by maternal sensitization to fetal blood group antigen
Excludes1 hydrops fetalis NOS (P83.2)
Ex: **For category P56 CC codes:** P29.0-P29.2, P29.4, P29.89-P29.9, P55.0-P57.0, P94.1-P96.0, P96.3-P96.5, P96.82-P96.89

P56.0 Hydrops fetalis due to isoimmunization

P56.9 Hydrops fetalis due to other and unspecified hemolytic disease

P56.90 Hydrops fetalis due to unspecified hemolytic disease

P56.99 Hydrops fetalis due to other hemolytic disease

P57 Kernicterus
High levels of bilirubin in blood, with severe neural symptoms
Ex: **For category P57 CC codes unless otherwise indicated:** P29.0-P29.2, P29.4, P29.89-P29.9, P57.8-P59.9, P94.1-P96.0, P96.3-P96.5, P96.82-P96.89

P57.0 Kernicterus due to isoimmunization
Ex: See P56

P57.8 Other specified kernicterus
Excludes1 Crigler-Najjar syndrome (E80.5)

P57.9 Kernicterus, unspecified

P58 Neonatal jaundice due to other excessive hemolysis
Excludes1 jaundice due to isoimmunization (P55-P57)

P58.0 Neonatal jaundice due to bruising

P58.1 Neonatal jaundice due to bleeding

P58.2 Neonatal jaundice due to infection

P58.3 Neonatal jaundice due to polycythemia

P58.4 Neonatal jaundice due to drugs or toxins transmitted from mother or given to newborn
Code first poisoning due to drug or toxin, if applicable (T36-T65 with fifth or sixth character 1-4 or 6)
Use additional code for adverse effect, if applicable, to identify drug (T36-T50 with fifth or sixth character 5)

P58.41 Neonatal jaundice due to drugs or toxins transmitted from mother

P58.42 Neonatal jaundice due to drugs or toxins given to newborn

P58.5 Neonatal jaundice due to swallowed maternal blood

P58.8 Neonatal jaundice due to other specified excessive hemolysis

P58.9 Neonatal jaundice due to excessive hemolysis, unspecified

P59 Neonatal jaundice from other and unspecified causes
Excludes1 jaundice due to inborn errors of metabolism (E70-E88)
kernicterus (P57.-)

P59.0 Neonatal jaundice associated with preterm delivery
Hyperbilirubinemia of prematurity
Jaundice due to delayed conjugation associated with preterm delivery

P59.1 Inspissated bile syndrome
Ex: See P57

P59.2 Neonatal jaundice from other and unspecified hepatocellular damage
Excludes1 congenital viral hepatitis (P35.3)
Ex: **For category P59.2 CC codes unless otherwise indicated:** See P57

P59.20 Neonatal jaundice from unspecified hepatocellular damage

P59.29 Neonatal jaundice from other hepatocellular damage
Neonatal giant cell hepatitis
Neonatal (idiopathic) hepatitis

P59.3 Neonatal jaundice from breast milk inhibitor

P59.8 Neonatal jaundice from other specified causes

P59.9 Neonatal jaundice, unspecified
Neonatal physiological jaundice (intense)(prolonged) NOS
Coding Clinic: 2015, Q3, P20

P60 Disseminated intravascular coagulation of newborn
Defibrination syndrome of newborn
Ex: See P53

P61 Other perinatal hematological disorders
Excludes1 transient hypogammaglobulinemia of infancy (D80.7)

P61.0 Transient neonatal thrombocytopenia
Lack of sufficient numbers of circulating thrombocytes (platelets)
Neonatal thrombocytopenia due to exchange transfusion
Neonatal thrombocytopenia due to idiopathic maternal thrombocytopenia
Neonatal thrombocytopenia due to isoimmunization
Ex: See P53

P61.1 Polycythemia neonatorum
Neonate = newborn

P61.2 Anemia of prematurity
Ex: D50.0-D55.9, D56.4, D57.00-D57.3, D57.80-D64.9, D75.9, P61.2-P61.4

P61.3 Congenital anemia from fetal blood loss
Ex: See P61.2

P61.4 Other congenital anemias, not elsewhere classified
Congenital anemia NOS
Ex: See P61.2

P61.5 Transient neonatal neutropenia
Low levels of granulocytic neutrophilic white blood cells
Excludes1 congenital neutropenia (nontransient) (D70.0)
Ex: D50.1-D53.9, D56.4, D57.00-D57.20, D57.3, D57.811-D57.819, D58.2, D59.0-D59.1, D59.3, D60.0-D61.9, D63.0-D64.9, D75.9, P61.5, P61.8-P61.9

P61.6 Other transient neonatal disorders of coagulation
Ex: See P53

P61.8 Other specified perinatal hematological disorders

P61.9 Perinatal hematological disorder, unspecified

TRANSITORY ENDOCRINE AND METABOLIC DISORDERS SPECIFIC TO NEWBORN (P70-P74)

Includes transitory endocrine and metabolic disturbances caused by the infant's response to maternal endocrine and metabolic factors, or its adjustment to extrauterine environment

P70 Transitory disorders of carbohydrate metabolism specific to newborn

P70.0 Syndrome of infant of mother with gestational diabetes
Newborn (with hypoglycemia) affected by maternal gestational diabetes
Excludes1 newborn (with hypoglycemia) affected by maternal (pre-existing) diabetes mellitus (P70.1)
syndrome of infant of a diabetic mother (P70.1)

P70.1 Syndrome of infant of a diabetic mother
Newborn (with hypoglycemia) affected by maternal (pre-existing) diabetes mellitus
Excludes1 newborn (with hypoglycemia) affected by maternal gestational diabetes (P70.0)
syndrome of infant of mother with gestational diabetes (P70.0)

P70.2 Neonatal diabetes mellitus
Ex: P29.0-P29.2, P29.4, P29.89-P29.9, P70.0-P71.9, P72.1, P72.9-P74.4, P74.9, P94.0-P94.9, P96.0, P96.3-P96.5, P96.82-P96.89

P70.3 Iatrogenic neonatal hypoglycemia

P70.4 Other neonatal hypoglycemia
Transitory neonatal hypoglycemia

P70.8 Other transitory disorders of carbohydrate metabolism of newborn
Ex: P70.0-P70.4, P70.9-P71.9, P72.1, P72.9-P74.4, P74.9, P94.0

P70.9 Transitory disorder of carbohydrate metabolism of newborn, unspecified

P71 Transitory neonatal disorders of calcium and magnesium metabolism
Ex: For category P71 CC codes: See 70.2

P71.0 Cow's milk hypocalcemia in newborn

P71.1 Other neonatal hypocalcemia
Excludes1 neonatal hypoparathyroidism (P71.4)

P71.2 Neonatal hypomagnesemia

P71.3 Neonatal tetany without calcium or magnesium deficiency
Neonatal tetany NOS

P71.4 Transitory neonatal hypoparathyroidism

P71.8 Other transitory neonatal disorders of calcium and magnesium metabolism

P71.9 Transitory neonatal disorder of calcium and magnesium metabolism, unspecified

P72 Other transitory neonatal endocrine disorders
Excludes1 congenital hypothyroidism with or without goiter (E03.0-E03.1)
dyshormogenetic goiter (E07.1)
Pendred's syndrome (E07.1)
Ex: For category P72 CC codes unless otherwise noted: See P70.8

P72.0 Neonatal goiter, not elsewhere classified
Transitory congenital goiter with normal functioning

P72.1 Transitory neonatal hyperthyroidism
Neonatal thyrotoxicosis
Ex: See 70.2

P72.2 Other transitory neonatal disorders of thyroid function, not elsewhere classified
Transitory neonatal hypothyroidism

P72.8 Other specified transitory neonatal endocrine disorders

P72.9 Transitory neonatal endocrine disorder, unspecified

P74 Other transitory neonatal electrolyte and metabolic disturbances

P74.0 Late metabolic acidosis of newborn
Excludes1 (fetal) metabolic acidosis of newborn (P19)
Ex: See 70.2

P74.1 Dehydration of newborn

P74.2 Disturbances of sodium balance of newborn

P74.3 Disturbances of potassium balance of newborn

P74.4 Other transitory electrolyte disturbances of newborn

P74.5 Transitory tyrosinemia of newborn
Ex: See 70.8

P74.6 Transitory hyperammonemia of newborn
Ex: See 70.8

P74.8 Other transitory metabolic disturbances of newborn
Amino-acid metabolic disorders described as transitory
Ex: See 70.8

P74.9 Transitory metabolic disturbance of newborn, unspecified

DIGESTIVE SYSTEM DISORDERS OF NEWBORN (P76-P78)

P76 Other intestinal obstruction of newborn

P76.0 Meconium plug syndrome
Fetal stool obstruction in large intestine, present at birth; may be symptom of organic disease.
Meconium ileus NOS
Excludes1 meconium ileus in cystic fibrosis (E84.11)

P76.1 Transitory ileus of newborn
Temporary obstruction of ileus (small intestine)
Excludes1 Hirschsprung's disease (Q43.1)
Ex: P76.0-P78.9

P76.2 Intestinal obstruction due to inspissated milk
Being thickened, dried, or made less fluid

P76.8 Other specified intestinal obstruction of newborn
Excludes1 intestinal obstruction classifiable to K56.-

P76.9 Intestinal obstruction of newborn, unspecified

P77 Necrotizing enterocolitis of newborn
Ex: For category P77 CC codes: P29.0-P29.2, P29.4-P29.9, P76.0-P78.9, P94.1-P96.0, P96.3-P96.5, P96.82-P96.89

P77.1 Stage 1 necrotizing enterocolitis in newborn
Necrotizing enterocolitis without pneumatosis, without perforation

P77.2 Stage 2 necrotizing enterocolitis in newborn
Necrotizing enterocolitis with pneumatosis, without perforation

P77.3 Stage 3 necrotizing enterocolitis in newborn
Necrotizing enterocolitis with perforation
Necrotizing enterocolitis with pneumatosis and perforation

P77.9 Necrotizing enterocolitis in newborn, unspecified
Necrotizing enterocolitis in newborn, NOS

P78 Other perinatal digestive system disorders
Excludes1 cystic fibrosis (E84.0-E84.9)
neonatal gastrointestinal hemorrhages (P54.0-P54.3)

P78.0 Perinatal intestinal perforation
Meconium peritonitis
Ex: See P77

P78.1 Other neonatal peritonitis
Neonatal peritonitis NOS

P78.2 Neonatal hematemesis and melena due to swallowed maternal blood

P78.3 Noninfective neonatal diarrhea
Neonatal diarrhea NOS

P78.8 Other specified perinatal digestive system disorders

P78.81 Congenital cirrhosis (of liver)

P78.82 Peptic ulcer of newborn

P78.83 Newborn esophageal reflux
Neonatal esophageal reflux

P78.89 Other specified perinatal digestive system disorders

P78.9 Perinatal digestive system disorder, unspecified

CONDITIONS INVOLVING THE INTEGUMENT AND TEMPERATURE REGULATION OF NEWBORN (P80-P83)

P80 Hypothermia of newborn

P80.0 Cold injury syndrome
Severe and usually chronic hypothermia associated with a pink flushed appearance, edema and neurological and biochemical abnormalities.
Excludes1 mild hypothermia of newborn (P80.8)

P80.8 Other hypothermia of newborn
Mild hypothermia of newborn

P80.9 Hypothermia of newborn, unspecified

P81 Other disturbances of temperature regulation of newborn

P81.0 Environmental hyperthermia of newborn

P81.8 Other specified disturbances of temperature regulation of newborn

P81.9 Disturbance of temperature regulation of newborn, unspecified
Fever of newborn NOS

P83 Other conditions of integument specific to newborn

Excludes1 congenital malformations of skin and integument (Q80-Q84)
hydrops fetalis due to hemolytic disease (P56.-)
neonatal skin infection (P39.4)
staphylococcal scalded skin syndrome (L00)

Excludes2 cradle cap (L21.0)
diaper [napkin] dermatitis (L22)

P83.0 Sclerema neonatorum
Neonate = newborn
Ex: P83.0, P83.30-P83.39

P83.1 Neonatal erythema toxicum
Benign, generalized, transient pustules that become firm vesicles

P83.2 Hydrops fetalis not due to hemolytic disease
Severe, life-threatening problem of severe edema (swelling) as result of too much fluid leaving blood and entering tissue
Hydrops fetalis NOS
Ex: P29.0-P29.2, P29.4, P29.89-P29.9, P83.2, P94.1-P96.0, P96.3-P96.5, P96.82-P96.89

P83.3 Other and unspecified edema specific to newborn
Ex: For category P83.3 CC codes: P80.0-P83.0, P83.30-P83.39

P83.30 Unspecified edema specific to newborn

P83.39 Other edema specific to newborn

P83.4 Breast engorgement of newborn
Noninfective mastitis of newborn

P83.5 Congenital hydrocele ♂

P83.6 Umbilical polyp of newborn

P83.8 Other specified conditions of integument specific to newborn
Bronze baby syndrome
Neonatal scleroderma
Urticaria neonatorum

P83.9 Condition of the integument specific to newborn, unspecified

OTHER PROBLEMS WITH NEWBORN (P84)

P84 Other problems with newborn
Acidemia of newborn
Acidosis of newborn
Anoxia of newborn NOS
Asphyxia of newborn NOS
Hypercapnia of newborn
Hypoxemia of newborn
Hypoxia of newborn NOS
Mixed metabolic and respiratory acidosis of newborn

Excludes1 intracranial hemorrhage due to anoxia or hypoxia (P52.-)
hypoxic ischemic encephalopathy [HIE] (P91.6-)
late metabolic acidosis of newborn (P74.0)

OTHER DISORDERS ORIGINATING IN THE PERINATAL PERIOD (P90-P96)

P90 Convulsions of newborn

Excludes1 benign myoclonic epilepsy in infancy (G40.3-)
benign neonatal convulsions (familial) (G40.3-)
Ex: P29.0-P29.2, P29.4, P29.89-P29.9, P90, P91.8-P91.9, P94.1-P96.0, P96.3-P96.5, P96.82-P96.89

P91 Other disturbances of cerebral status of newborn

P91.0 Neonatal cerebral ischemia
Ex: P90-P91.1, P91.3-P91.5, P91.8-P91.9

P91.1 Acquired periventricular cysts of newborn
Ex: See P91.0

P91.2 Neonatal cerebral leukomalacia
Degeneration of white matter adjacent to cerebral ventricles following cerebral hypoxia or brain ischemia in neonates
Periventricular leukomalacia
Ex: P10.2-P10.3, P29.0-P29.2, P29.4, P29.89-P29.9, P50.0-P50.9, P52.0-P52.3, P52.5, P53-P54.0, P54.6-P54.9, P60-P61.9, P91.2, P94.1-P94.9, P96.0, P96.3-P96.5, P96.82-P96.89

P91.3 Neonatal cerebral irritability
Ex: See P91.0

P91.4 Neonatal cerebral depression
Ex: See P91.0

P91.5 Neonatal coma
Ex: See P91.0

P91.6 Hypoxic ischemic encephalopathy [HIE]
Ex: For category P91.6 CC codes: P84, P91.60-P91.63

P91.60 Hypoxic ischemic encephalopathy [HIE], unspecified

P91.61 Mild hypoxic ischemic encephalopathy [HIE]

P91.62 Moderate hypoxic ischemic encephalopathy [HIE]

P91.63 Severe hypoxic ischemic encephalopathy [HIE]

P91.8 Other specified disturbances of cerebral status of newborn

P91.9 Disturbance of cerebral status of newborn, unspecified

P92 Feeding problems of newborn

Excludes1 feeding problems in child over 28 days old (R63.3)

P92.0 Vomiting of newborn

Excludes1 vomiting of child over 28 days old (R11.-)

P92.01 Bilious vomiting of newborn

Excludes1 bilious vomiting in child over 28 days old (R11.14)
Ex: P92.01-P92.09

P92.09 Other vomiting of newborn

Excludes1 regurgitation of food in newborn (P92.1)

P92.1 Regurgitation and rumination of newborn

P92.2 Slow feeding of newborn

P92.3 Underfeeding of newborn

P92.4 Overfeeding of newborn

P92.5 Neonatal difficulty in feeding at breast

P92.6 Failure to thrive in newborn

Excludes1 failure to thrive in child over 28 days old (R62.51)

P92.8 Other feeding problems of newborn

P92.9 Feeding problem of newborn, unspecified

● **P93 Reactions and intoxications due to drugs administered to newborn**

Includes reactions and intoxications due to drugs administered to fetus affecting newborn

Excludes1 jaundice due to drugs or toxins transmitted from mother or given to newborn (P58.4-)
reactions and intoxications from maternal opiates, tranquilizers and other medication (P04.0-P04.1, P04.4)
withdrawal symptoms from maternal use of drugs of addiction (P96.1)
withdrawal symptoms from therapeutic use of drugs in newborn (P96.2)

Ex: **For category P93 CC codes:** P93.0-P93.8, P96.1-P96.2

P93.0 Grey baby syndrome
Grey syndrome from chloramphenicol administration in newborn

P93.8 Other reactions and intoxications due to drugs administered to newborn
Use additional code for adverse effect, if applicable, to identify drug (T36-T50 with fifth or sixth character 5)

● **P94 Disorders of muscle tone of newborn**

P94.0 Transient neonatal myasthenia gravis

Excludes1 myasthenia gravis (G70.0)

Ex: P29.0-P29.2, P29.4, P29.89-P29.9, P70.0-P71.9, P72.1, P72.9-P74.4, P74.9, P94.0-P94.9, P96.0, P96.3-P96.5, P96.82-P96.89

P94.1 Congenital hypertonia

P94.2 Congenital hypotonia
Floppy baby syndrome, unspecified

P94.8 Other disorders of muscle tone of newborn

P94.9 Disorder of muscle tone of newborn, unspecified

P95 Stillbirth
Deadborn fetus NOS
Fetal death of unspecified cause
Stillbirth NOS

Excludes1 maternal care for intrauterine death (O36.4)
missed abortion (O02.1)
outcome of delivery, stillbirth (Z37.1, Z37.3, Z37.4, Z37.7)

OGCR Section I.C.16.g.

Stillbirth
Code P95, Stillbirth, is only for use for institutions that maintain separate records for stillbirths. No other code should be used with P95. Code P95 should not be used on the mother's record.

● **P96 Other conditions originating in the perinatal period**

P96.0 Congenital renal failure
Uremia of newborn

P96.1 Neonatal withdrawal symptoms from maternal use of drugs of addiction
Drug withdrawal syndrome in infant of dependent mother
Neonatal abstinence syndrome

Excludes1 reactions and intoxications from maternal opiates and tranquilizers administered during labor and delivery (P04.0)

Ex: See P93

P96.2 Withdrawal symptoms from therapeutic use of drugs in newborn

Ex: See P93

P96.3 Wide cranial sutures of newborn
Neonatal craniotabes

P96.5 Complication to newborn due to (fetal) intrauterine procedure

Excludes2 newborn affected by amniocentesis (P00.6) ◄

● **P96.8 Other specified conditions originating in the perinatal period**

P96.81 Exposure to (parental) (environmental) tobacco smoke in the perinatal period

Excludes2 newborn affected by in utero exposure to tobacco (P04.2)
exposure to environmental tobacco smoke after the perinatal period (Z77.22)

P96.82 Delayed separation of umbilical cord

P96.83 Meconium staining

Excludes1 meconium aspiration (P24.00, P24.01)
meconium passage during delivery (P03.82)

P96.89 Other specified conditions originating in the perinatal period
Use additional code to specify condition

P96.9 Condition originating in the perinatal period, unspecified
Congenital debility NOS

CHAPTER 17

CONGENITAL MALFORMATIONS, DEFORMATIONS AND CHROMOSOMAL ABNORMALITIES (Q00-Q99)

OGCR Chapter-Specific Coding Guidelines

17. **Chapter 17: Congenital malformations, deformations, and chromosomal abnormalities (Q00-Q99)**
Assign an appropriate code(s) from categories Q00-Q99, Congenital malformations, deformations, and chromosomal abnormalities when a malformation/deformation or chromosomal abnormality is documented. A malformation/deformation/or chromosomal abnormality may be the principal/first-listed diagnosis on a record or a secondary diagnosis.

When a malformation/deformation/or chromosomal abnormality does not have a unique code assignment, assign additional code(s) for any manifestations that may be present.

When the code assignment specifically identifies the malformation/deformation/or chromosomal abnormality, manifestations that are an inherent component of the anomaly should not be coded separately. Additional codes should be assigned for manifestations that are not an inherent component.

Codes from Chapter 17 may be used throughout the life of the patient. If a congenital malformation or deformity has been corrected, a personal history code should be used to identify the history of the malformation or deformity. Although present at birth, malformation/deformation/or chromosomal abnormality may not be identified until later in life. Whenever the condition is diagnosed by the physician, it is appropriate to assign a code from codes Q00-Q99.

For the birth admission, the appropriate code from category Z38, Liveborn infants, according to place of birth and type of delivery, should be sequenced as the principal diagnosis, followed by any congenital anomaly codes, Q00-Q99.

CHAPTER 17

CONGENITAL MALFORMATIONS, DEFORMATIONS AND CHROMOSOMAL ABNORMALITIES (Q00-Q99)

Note: Codes from this chapter are not for use on maternal or fetal records

Excludes2 inborn errors of metabolism (E70-E88)

This chapter contains the following blocks:

Q00-Q07	Congenital malformations of the nervous system
Q10-Q18	Congenital malformations of eye, ear, face and neck
Q20-Q28	Congenital malformations of the circulatory system
Q30-Q34	Congenital malformations of the respiratory system
Q35-Q37	Cleft lip and cleft palate
Q38-Q45	Other congenital malformations of the digestive system
Q50-Q56	Congenital malformations of genital organs
Q60-Q64	Congenital malformations of the urinary system
Q65-Q79	Congenital malformations and deformations of the musculoskeletal system
Q80-Q89	Other congenital malformations
Q90-Q99	Chromosomal abnormalities, not elsewhere classified

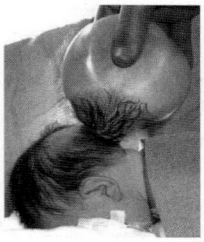

Figure 17-1 An infant with a large occipital encephalocele. The large skin-covered encephalocele is visible. (From Townsend: Sabiston Textbook of Surgery, ed 19, Saunders, An Imprint of Elsevier, 2012)

CONGENITAL MALFORMATIONS OF THE NERVOUS SYSTEM (Q00–Q07)

● **Q00 Anencephaly and similar malformations**
Ex For category Q00 CC codes: Q00.0-Q00.2

Q00.0 Anencephaly CC
Absence of skull with cerebral hemispheres missing or reduced to small masses attached to base of cranium
Acephaly
Acrania
Amyelencephaly
Hemianencephaly
Hemicephaly

Q00.1 Craniorachischisis CC
Developmental anomaly consisting of fissure of cranium and vertebral column

Q00.2 Iniencephaly CC
Developmental anomaly characterized by enlargement of foramen magnum and absence of laminae and spinous processes of cervical, dorsal

● **Q01 Encephalocele**
Sac-like protrusions of brain and membranes visible through an opening in skull
Includes Arnold-Chiari syndrome, type III
encephalocystocele
encephalomyelocele
hydroencephalocele
hydromeningocele, cranial
meningocele, cerebral
meningoencephalocele
Excludes1 Meckel-Gruber syndrome (Q61.9)
Ex For category Q01 CC codes: Q01.0-Q02, Q04.0-Q04.8

Q01.0 Frontal encephalocele CC
Q01.1 Nasofrontal encephalocele CC
Q01.2 Occipital encephalocele CC
Q01.8 Encephalocele of other sites CC
Q01.9 Encephalocele, unspecified CC

Q02 Microcephaly
Head size measures significantly below normal based on standardized charts
Includes hydromicrocephaly
micrencephalon
Excludes1 Meckel-Gruber syndrome (Q61.9)

● **Q03 Congenital hydrocephalus**
Accumulation of cerebrospinal fluid in ventricles resulting in swelling and enlargement
Includes hydrocephalus in newborn
Excludes1 Arnold-Chiari syndrome, type II (Q07.0-)
acquired hydrocephalus (G91.-)
hydrocephalus due to congenital toxoplasmosis (P37.1)
hydrocephalus with spina bifida (Q05.0-Q05.4)

Q03.0 Malformations of aqueduct of Sylvius
Anomaly of aqueduct of Sylvius
Obstruction of aqueduct of Sylvius, congenital
Stenosis of aqueduct of Sylvius

Q03.1 Atresia of foramina of Magendie and Luschka
Dandy-Walker syndrome

Q03.8 Other congenital hydrocephalus

Q03.9 Congenital hydrocephalus, unspecified

● **Q04 Other congenital malformations of brain**

Excludes1 cyclopia (Q87.0)
macrocephaly (Q75.3)

Ex For category Q04 CC codes Q04.0-Q04.3: Q01.0-Q02, Q04.0-Q04.8
For category Q04 CC codes Q04.4-Q04.8: Q04.4-Q04.8

Q04.0 Congenital malformations of corpus callosum
Agenesis of corpus callosum

Q04.1 Arhinencephaly
Congenital absence of olfactory bulbs, tract, or nerves

Q04.2 Holoprosencephaly
Failure of cleavage of forebrain (prosencephalon) resulting in incomplete or absent cortical separation and deficits in midline facial development

Q04.3 Other reduction deformities of brain
Absence of part of brain Agyria
Agenesis of part of brain
Cerebral cortex are not fully formed, brain surface is smooth
Aplasia of part of brain
Hydranencephaly
Hypoplasia of part of brain
Lissencephaly
Congenital malformation or absence of convolutions of cerebral cortex
Microgyria
Malformation of brain characterized by excessive number of small convolutions (gyri) on surface
Pachygyria
Reduction in number of sulci of cerebrum

Excludes1 congenital malformations of corpus callosum (Q04.0)

Q04.4 Septo-optic dysplasia of brain

Q04.5 Megalencephaly
Abnormally large brain

Q04.6 Congenital cerebral cysts
Porencephaly Schizencephaly

Excludes1 acquired porencephalic cyst (G93.0)

Q04.8 Other specified congenital malformations of brain
Arnold-Chiari syndrome, type IV
Macrogyria

Q04.9 Congenital malformation of brain, unspecified
Congenital anomaly NOS of brain
Congenital deformity NOS of brain
Congenital disease or lesion NOS of brain
Multiple anomalies NOS of brain, congenital

● **Q05 Spina bifida**
Developmental anomaly characterized by defective closure of vertebral arch, through which spinal cord and meninges may protrude

Includes hydromeningocele (spinal)
meningocele (spinal)
meningomyelocele
myelocele
myelomeningocele
rachischisis
spina bifida (aperta)(cystica)
syringomyelocele

Use additional code for any associated paraplegia (paraparesis) (G82.2-)

Excludes1 Arnold-Chiari syndrome, type II (Q07.0-)
spina bifida occulta (Q76.0)

Ex For category Q05 CC codes: E78.71-E78.72, G90.1, Q05.0-Q06.1, Q06.3, Q06.8-Q07.9, Q87.1-Q87.89, Q89.7-Q89.8, Q99.2

Q05.0 Cervical spina bifida with hydrocephalus

Q05.1 Thoracic spina bifida with hydrocephalus
Dorsal spina bifida with hydrocephalus
Thoracolumbar spina bifida with hydrocephalus

Q05.2 Lumbar spina bifida with hydrocephalus
Lumbosacral spina bifida with hydrocephalus

Q05.3 Sacral spina bifida with hydrocephalus

Q05.4 Unspecified spina bifida with hydrocephalus

Q05.5 Cervical spina bifida without hydrocephalus

Q05.6 Thoracic spina bifida without hydrocephalus
Dorsal spina bifida NOS
Thoracolumbar spina bifida NOS

Q05.7 Lumbar spina bifida without hydrocephalus
Lumbosacral spina bifida NOS

Q05.8 Sacral spina bifida without hydrocephalus

Q05.9 Spina bifida, unspecified

● **Q06 Other congenital malformations of spinal cord**

Q06.0 Amyelia
Congenital absence of spinal cord

Q06.1 Hypoplasia and dysplasia of spinal cord
Underdevelopment of spinal cord
Atelomyelia
Congenitally incomplete development of spinal cord
Myelatelia
Myelodysplasia of spinal cord
Defective development of spinal cord, especially lower segments

Q06.2 Diastematomyelia
Congenital anomaly, associated with spina bifida, in which spinal cord is split into halves and surrounded by dural sac

Q06.3 Other congenital cauda equina malformations

Q06.4 Hydromyelia
Dilation of central canal of spinal cord with increased fluid accumulation
Hydrorachis

Q06.8 Other specified congenital malformations of spinal cord

Q06.9 Congenital malformation of spinal cord, unspecified
Congenital anomaly NOS of spinal cord
Congenital deformity NOS of spinal cord
Congenital disease or lesion NOS of spinal cord

● **Q07 Other congenital malformations of nervous system**

Excludes2 congenital central alveolar hypoventilation syndrome (G47.35)
familial dysautonomia [Riley-Day] (G90.1)
neurofibromatosis (nonmalignant) (Q85.0-)

● **Q07.0 Arnold-Chiari syndrome**
Herniation of cerebellar tonsils and vermis through foramen magnum into spinal canal
Arnold-Chiari syndrome, type II

Excludes1 Arnold-Chiari syndrome, type III (Q01.-)
Arnold-Chiari syndrome, type IV (Q04.8)

Q07.00 Arnold-Chiari syndrome without spina bifida or hydrocephalus

Q07.01 Arnold-Chiari syndrome with spina bifida

Q07.02 Arnold-Chiari syndrome with hydrocephalus
Ex See Q05

Q07.03 Arnold-Chiari syndrome with spina bifida and hydrocephalus
Ex See Q05

Q07.8 Other specified congenital malformations of nervous system
Agenesis of nerve
Displacement of brachial plexus
Jaw-winking syndrome
Marcus Gunn's syndrome

Q07.9 Congenital malformation of nervous system, unspecified
Congenital anomaly NOS of nervous system
Congenital deformity NOS of nervous system
Congenital disease or lesion NOS of nervous system

CONGENITAL MALFORMATIONS OF EYE, EAR, FACE AND NECK (Q10-Q18)

Excludes2 cleft lip and cleft palate (Q35-Q37)
congenital malformation of cervical spine (Q05.0, Q05.5, Q67.5, Q76.0-Q76.4)
congenital malformation of larynx (Q31.-)
congenital malformation of lip NEC (Q38.0)
congenital malformation of nose (Q30.-)
congenital malformation of parathyroid gland (Q89.2)
congenital malformation of thyroid gland (Q89.2)

Q10 Congenital malformations of eyelid, lacrimal apparatus and orbit

Excludes1 cryptophthalmos NOS (Q11.2)
cryptophthalmos syndrome (Q87.0)

Q10.0 Congenital ptosis
Prolapse or drooping of upper eyelid from paralysis of third nerve or from sympathetic innervations

Q10.1 Congenital ectropion
Outward turning of eyelid

Q10.2 Congenital entropion
Inward turning of eyelid

Q10.3 Other congenital malformations of eyelid
Ablepharon
Blepharophimosis, congenital
Coloboma of eyelid
Congenital absence or agenesis of cilia
Congenital absence or agenesis of eyelid
Congenital accessory eyelid
Congenital accessory eye muscle
Congenital malformation of eyelid NOS

Q10.4 Absence and agenesis of lacrimal apparatus
Congenital absence of punctum lacrimale

Q10.5 Congenital stenosis and stricture of lacrimal duct

Q10.6 Other congenital malformations of lacrimal apparatus
Congenital malformation of lacrimal apparatus NOS

Q10.7 Congenital malformation of orbit

Q11 Anophthalmos, microphthalmos and macrophthalmos
Absence of eye and optic pit

Q11.0 Cystic eyeball

Q11.1 Other anophthalmos
Anophthalmos NOS
Agenesis of eye
Absence of eye
Aplasia of eye

Q11.2 Microphthalmos
Partial absence of eye and optic pit
Cryptophthalmos NOS
Dysplasia of eye
Hypoplasia of eye
Rudimentary eye

Excludes1 cryptophthalmos syndrome (Q87.0)

Q11.3 Macrophthalmos
Congenital enlargement of eyes

Excludes1 macrophthalmos in congenital glaucoma (Q15.0)

Q12 Congenital lens malformations

Q12.0 Congenital cataract

Q12.1 Congenital displaced lens

Q12.2 Coloboma of lens

Q12.3 Congenital aphakia

Q12.4 Spherophakia
Smaller, more spherical optic lens than normal

Q12.8 Other congenital lens malformations
Microphakia

Q12.9 Congenital lens malformation, unspecified

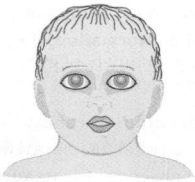

Figure 17-2 Bilateral congenital **hydrophthalmia,** in which the eyes are very large in comparison to the other facial features due to glaucoma.

Q13 Congenital malformations of anterior segment of eye

Q13.0 Coloboma of iris
Coloboma NOS

Q13.1 Absence of iris
Aniridia
Use additional code for associated glaucoma (H42)

Q13.2 Other congenital malformations of iris
Anisocoria, congenital
Atresia of pupil
Congenital malformation of iris NOS
Corectopia

Q13.3 Congenital corneal opacity

Q13.4 Other congenital corneal malformations
Congenital malformation of cornea NOS
Microcornea
Peter's anomaly

Q13.5 Blue sclera
Condition of unusual blueness of sclera; not harmful

Q13.8 Other congenital malformations of anterior segment of eye

Q13.81 Rieger's anomaly
Use additional code for associated glaucoma (H42)

Q13.89 Other congenital malformations of anterior segment of eye

Q13.9 Congenital malformation of anterior segment of eye, unspecified

Q14 Congenital malformations of posterior segment of eye

Excludes2 optic nerve hypoplasia (H47.03-)

Q14.0 Congenital malformation of vitreous humor
Congenital vitreous opacity

Q14.1 Congenital malformation of retina
Congenital retinal aneurysm

Q14.2 Congenital malformation of optic disc
Coloboma of optic disc

Q14.3 Congenital malformation of choroid

Q14.8 Other congenital malformations of posterior segment of eye
Coloboma of the fundus

Q14.9 Congenital malformation of posterior segment of eye, unspecified

Q15 Other congenital malformations of eye

Excludes1 congenital nystagmus (H55.01)
ocular albinism (E70.31-)
optic nerve hypoplasia (H47.03-)
retinitis pigmentosa (H35.52)

Q15.0 Congenital glaucoma
Axenfeld's anomaly
Buphthalmos
Congenital syndrome characterized by port-wine nevus covering portions of face and cranium
Glaucoma of childhood
Glaucoma of newborn
Hydrophthalmos
Keratoglobus, congenital, with glaucoma
Macrocornea with glaucoma
Macrophthalmos in congenital glaucoma
Megalocornea with glaucoma

Q15.8 Other specified congenital malformations of eye

Q15.9 Congenital malformation of eye, unspecified
Congenital anomaly of eye
Congenital deformity of eye

● **Q16 Congenital malformations of ear causing impairment of hearing**
Excludes1 congenital deafness (H90.-)

Q16.0 Congenital absence of (ear) auricle

Q16.1 Congenital absence, atresia and stricture of auditory canal (external)
Congenital atresia or stricture of osseous meatus

Q16.2 Absence of eustachian tube

Q16.3 Congenital malformation of ear ossicles
Congenital fusion of ear ossicles

Q16.4 Other congenital malformations of middle ear
Congenital malformation of middle ear NOS

Q16.5 Congenital malformation of inner ear
Congenital anomaly of membranous labyrinth
Congenital anomaly of organ of Corti

Q16.9 Congenital malformation of ear causing impairment of hearing, unspecified
Congenital absence of ear NOS

● **Q17 Other congenital malformations of ear**
Excludes1 congenital malformations of ear with impairment of hearing (Q16.0-Q16.9)
preauricular sinus (Q18.1)

Q17.0 Accessory auricle
Accessory tragus
Polyotia
Preauricular appendage or tag
Supernumerary ear
Supernumerary lobule

Q17.1 Macrotia
Enlarged ears

Q17.2 Microtia
An abnormally small or underdeveloped external ear

Q17.3 Other misshapen ear
Pointed ear

Q17.4 Misplaced ear
Low-set ears
Excludes1 cervical auricle (Q18.2)

Q17.5 Prominent ear
Bat ear

Q17.8 Other specified congenital malformations of ear
Congenital absence of lobe of ear

Q17.9 Congenital malformation of ear, unspecified
Congenital anomaly of ear NOS

● **Q18 Other congenital malformations of face and neck**
Excludes1 cleft lip and cleft palate (Q35-Q37)
conditions classified to Q67.0-Q67.4
congenital malformations of skull and face bones (Q75.-)
cyclopia (Q87.0)
dentofacial anomalies [including malocclusion] (M26.-)
malformation syndromes affecting facial appearance (Q87.0)
persistent thyroglossal duct (Q89.2)

Q18.0 Sinus, fistula and cyst of branchial cleft
Branchial vestige
Brachial remnants (cysts, fistula, skin tags) that are developmental anomalies

Q18.1 Preauricular sinus and cyst
Fistula of auricle, congenital
Cervicoaural fistula
Abnormal passage in neck originating from first branchial cleft

Q18.2 Other branchial cleft malformations
Branchial cleft malformation NOS
Cervical auricle
Otocephaly

Q18.3 Webbing of neck
Pterygium colli
Thick fold of skin on side of neck

Q18.4 Macrostomia
Results from failure of union of maxillary and mandibular processes, results in abnormally large mouth

Q18.5 Microstomia

Q18.6 Macrocheilia
Excessive size of lips
Hypertrophy of lip, congenital

Q18.7 Microcheilia
Abnormal smallness of lips

Q18.8 Other specified congenital malformations of face and neck
Medial cyst of face and neck
Medial fistula of face and neck
Medial sinus of face and neck

Q18.9 Congenital malformation of face and neck, unspecified
Congenital anomaly NOS of face and neck

CONGENITAL MALFORMATIONS OF THE CIRCULATORY SYSTEM (Q20-Q28)

● **Q20 Congenital malformations of cardiac chambers and connections**
Excludes1 dextrocardia with situs inversus (Q89.3)
mirror-image atrial arrangement with situs inversus (Q89.3)
Ex: **For category Q20 CC codes:** E78.71-E78.72, I23.0-I23.3, I23.6-I23.8, I51.0, P29.3, Q20.0-Q21.9, Q23.8-Q23.9, Q24.8-Q24.9, Q27.30, Q27.4, Q28.0-Q28.1, Q28.8-Q28.9, Q87.1-Q87.89, Q89.7-Q89.8, Q99.2

Q20.0 Common arterial trunk
Persistent truncus arteriosus
Excludes1 aortic septal defect (Q21.4)

Q20.1 Double outlet right ventricle
Taussig-Bing syndrome

Q20.2 Double outlet left ventricle

Q20.3 Discordant ventriculoarterial connection
Dextrotransposition of aorta
Transposition of great vessels (complete)

Q20.4 Double inlet ventricle
Common ventricle
Cor triloculare biatriatum
Single ventricle

Q20.5 Discordant atrioventricular connection
Corrected transposition
Levotransposition
Ventricular inversion

Q20.6 Isomerism of atrial appendages
Isomerism of atrial appendages with asplenia or polysplenia

Q20.8 Other congenital malformations of cardiac chambers and connections
Cor binoculare

Q20.9 Congenital malformation of cardiac chambers and connections, unspecified

● **Q21 Congenital malformations of cardiac septa**
Excludes1 acquired cardiac septal defect (I51.0)

Q21.0 Ventricular septal defect
Roger's disease
Ex: See Q20

Q21.1 Atrial septal defect
Coronary sinus defect
Patent or persistent foramen ovale
Patent or persistent ostium secundum defect (type II)
Patent or persistent sinus venosus defect
Ex: E78.71-E78.72, I23.0-I23.3, I23.6-I23.8, I51.0, Q20.0-Q20.9, Q21.1-Q21.9, Q23.8-Q23.9, Q24.8-Q24.9, Q27.30, Q27.4, Q28.0-Q28.1, Q28.8-Q28.9, Q87.2-Q87.3, Q87.5-Q87.89, Q89.7-Q89.8

Q21.2 Atrioventricular septal defect
Common atrioventricular canal
Endocardial cushion defect
Ostium primum atrial septal defect (type I)
Ex: See Q20

Q21.3 Tetralogy of Fallot
Ventricular septal defect with pulmonary stenosis or atresia, dextroposition of aorta and hypertrophy of right ventricle.
Ex: See Q20

Q21.4 Aortopulmonary septal defect
Aortic septal defect
Aortopulmonary window

Q21.8 Other congenital malformations of cardiac septa
Eisenmenger's defect
Pentalogy of Fallot
Excludes1 Eisenmenger's complex (I27.8)
Eisenmenger's syndrome (I27.8)

Q21.9 Congenital malformation of cardiac septum, unspecified
Septal (heart) defect NOS

Q22 Congenital malformations of pulmonary and tricuspid valves
Ex: **For category Q22 CC codes unless otherwise indicated:** E78.71-E78.72, P29.3, Q20.9, Q22.4-Q23.9, Q24.8-Q24.9, Q27.30, Q27.4, Q28.0-Q28.1, Q28.8-Q28.9, Q87.1-Q87.89, Q89.7-Q89.8, Q99.2

Q22.0 Pulmonary valve atresia
Ex: E78.71-E78.72, P29.3, Q20.9, Q22.0-Q22.3, Q23.8-Q23.9, Q24.8-Q24.9, Q27.30, Q27.4, Q28.0-Q28.1, Q28.8-Q28.9, Q87.1-Q87.89, Q89.7-Q89.8, Q99.2

Q22.1 Congenital pulmonary valve stenosis
Ex: See Q22.0

Q22.2 Congenital pulmonary valve insufficiency
Congenital pulmonary valve regurgitation
Ex: E78.71-E78.72, Q20.9, Q22.0-Q22.3, Q23.8-Q23.9, Q24.8-Q24.9, Q27.30, Q27.4, Q28.0-Q28.1, Q28.8-Q28.9, Q87.2-Q87.3, Q87.5-Q87.89, Q89.7-Q89.8

Q22.3 Other congenital malformations of pulmonary valve
Congenital malformation of pulmonary valve NOS
Supernumerary cusps of pulmonary valve
Ex: See Q22.2

Q22.4 Congenital tricuspid stenosis
Congenital tricuspid atresia

Q22.5 Ebstein's anomaly
Malformation of tricuspid valve

Q22.6 Hypoplastic right heart syndrome

Q22.8 Other congenital malformations of tricuspid valve

Q22.9 Congenital malformation of tricuspid valve, unspecified

Q23 Congenital malformations of aortic and mitral valves
Ex: **For category Q23 CC codes unless otherwise indicated:** See Q22

Q23.0 Congenital stenosis of aortic valve
Congenital aortic atresia
Congenital aortic stenosis NOS
Excludes1 congenital stenosis of aortic valve in hypoplastic left heart syndrome (Q23.4)
congenital subaortic stenosis (Q24.4)
supravalvular aortic stenosis (congenital) (Q25.3)

Q23.1 Congenital insufficiency of aortic valve
Bicuspid aortic valve
Congenital aortic insufficiency

Q23.2 Congenital mitral stenosis
Congenital mitral atresia

Q23.3 Congenital mitral insufficiency

Q23.4 Hypoplastic left heart syndrome

Q23.8 Other congenital malformations of aortic and mitral valves

Q23.9 Congenital malformation of aortic and mitral valves, unspecified

Q24 Other congenital malformations of heart
Excludes1 endocardial fibroelastosis (I42.4)

Q24.0 Dextrocardia
Heart is located in right hemithorax
Excludes1 dextrocardia with situs inversus (Q89.3)
isomerism of atrial appendages (with asplenia or polysplenia) (Q20.6)
mirror-image atrial arrangement with situs inversus (Q89.3)
Ex: E78.71-E78.72, Q20.9, Q23.8-Q24.4, Q24.8-Q24.9, Q27.30, Q27.4, Q28.0-Q28.1, Q28.8-Q28.9, Q87.2-Q87.3, Q87.5-Q87.89, Q89.7-Q89.8

Q24.1 Levocardia
Normal position of heart but related structures on wrong side
Ex: See Q24.0

Q24.2 Cor triatriatum
Congenital heart defect; left atrium is subdivided
Ex: E78.71-E78.72, P29.3, Q20.9, Q23.8-Q23.9, Q24.2-Q24.4, Q24.8-Q24.9, Q27.30, Q27.4, Q28.0-Q28.1, Q28.8-Q28.9, Q87.1-Q87.89, Q89.7-Q89.8, Q99.2

Q24.3 Pulmonary infundibular stenosis
Subvalvular pulmonic stenosis
Ex: See Q24.3

Q24.4 Congenital subaortic stenosis
Ex: See Q24.3

Q24.5 Malformation of coronary vessels
Congenital coronary (artery) aneurysm
Ex: Q20.9, Q23.8-Q23.9, Q24.5, Q24.8-Q24.9

Q24.6 Congenital heart block
Ex: E78.71-E78.72, P29.3, Q20.9, Q23.8-Q23.9, Q24.6-Q24.9, Q27.30, Q27.4, Q28.0-Q28.1, Q28.8-Q28.9, Q87.1-Q87.89, Q89.7-Q89.8, Q99.2

Q24.8 Other specified congenital malformations of heart
Congenital diverticulum of left ventricle
Congenital malformation of myocardium
Congenital malformation of pericardium
Malposition of heart
Uhl's disease

Q24.9 Congenital malformation of heart, unspecified
Congenital anomaly of heart
Congenital disease of heart

Q25 Congenital malformations of great arteries

Q25.0 Patent ductus arteriosus
Fetal blood vessel connecting left pulmonary artery directly to descending aorta
Patent ductus Botallo
Persistent ductus arteriosus
Ex: Q25.0, Q27.30, Q27.4, Q28.0-Q28.1, Q28.8

Q25.1 Coarctation of aorta
Coarctation of aorta (preductal) (postductal)
Stenosis of aorta ◀
Ex: E78.71-E78.72, Q25.1-Q25.3, Q27.30, Q27.4, Q28.0-Q28.1, Q28.8-Q28.9, Q87.2-Q87.3, Q87.5-Q87.89, Q89.7-Q89.8

Q25.2 Atresia of aorta
Ex: **For category Q25.2 CC codes:** E78.71-E78.72, P29.3, Q25.1-Q25.3, Q27.30, Q27.4, Q28.0-Q28.1, Q28.8-Q28.9, Q87.1-Q87.89, Q89.7-Q89.8, Q99.2

Q25.21 Interruption of aortic arch ◀
Atresia of aortic arch ◀

Q25.29 Other atresia of aorta ◀
Atresia of aorta ◀

Q25.3 Supravalvular aortic stenosis
Excludes1 congenital aortic stenosis NOS (Q23.0)
congenital stenosis of aortic valve (Q23.0)
Ex: See Q25.2

Q25.4 Other congenital malformations of aorta
Excludes1 hypoplasia of aorta in hypoplastic left heart syndrome (Q23.4)
Ex: **For category Q25.4 CC codes:** E78.71-E78.72, Q25.1-Q25.49, Q25.8-Q25.9, Q27.30, Q27.4, Q28.0-Q28.1, Q28.8-Q28.9, Q87.2-Q87.3, Q87.5-Q87.89, Q89.7-Q89.8

Q25.40 Congenital malformation of aorta unspecified ◀

Q25.41 Absence and aplasia of aorta ◀

Q25.42 Hypoplasia of aorta ◀

Q25.43 Congenital aneurysm of aorta ◀
Congenital aneurysm of aortic root ◀
Congenital aneurysm of aortic sinus ◀

Q25.44 Congenital dilation of aorta ◀

Q25.45 Double aortic arch ◀
Vascular ring of aorta ◀

Q25.46 Tortuous aortic arch ◀
Persistent convolutions of aortic arch ◀

Q25.47 Right aortic arch ◀
Persistent right aortic arch ◀

Q25.48 Anomalous origin of subclavian artery ◀

Q25.49 Other congenital malformations of aorta ◀

Q25.5 Atresia of pulmonary artery
Ex: Q25.5-Q25.79, Q27.30, Q27.4, Q28.0-Q28.1, Q28.8-Q28.9

Q25.6 Stenosis of pulmonary artery
Supravalvular pulmonary stenosis
Ex: See Q25.5

● **Q25.7 Other congenital malformations of pulmonary artery**
Ex: For category Q25.7 CC codes: See Q25.5

Q25.71 Coarctation of pulmonary artery

Q25.72 Congenital pulmonary arteriovenous malformation
Congenital pulmonary arteriovenous aneurysm

Q25.79 Other congenital malformations of pulmonary artery
Aberrant pulmonary artery
Agenesis of pulmonary artery
Congenital aneurysm of pulmonary artery
Congenital anomaly of pulmonary artery
Hypoplasia of pulmonary artery

Q25.8 Other congenital malformations of other great arteries
Ex: See Q25.4

Q25.9 Congenital malformation of great arteries, unspecified
Ex: See Q25.4

● **Q26 Congenital malformations of great veins**

Q26.0 Congenital stenosis of vena cava
Congenital stenosis of vena cava (inferior)(superior)
Ex: Q26.0-Q26.1, Q26.8, Q27.30, Q27.4, Q28.0-Q28.1, Q28.8-Q28.9

Q26.1 Persistent left superior vena cava
Ex: See Q26.0

Q26.2 Total anomalous pulmonary venous connection
Total anomalous pulmonary venous return [TAPVR], subdiaphragmatic
Total anomalous pulmonary venous return [TAPVR], supradiaphragmatic
Ex: Q26.2, Q27.30, Q27.4, Q28.0-Q28.1, Q28.8-Q28.9

Q26.3 Partial anomalous pulmonary venous connection
Partial anomalous pulmonary venous return
Ex: Q26.3-Q26.4, Q27.30, Q27.4, Q28.0-Q28.1, Q28.8-Q28.9

Q26.4 Anomalous pulmonary venous connection, unspecified
Ex: See Q26.3

Q26.5 Anomalous portal venous connection

Q26.6 Portal vein-hepatic artery fistula

Q26.8 Other congenital malformations of great veins
Absence of vena cava (inferior) (superior)
Azygos continuation of inferior vena cava
Persistent left posterior cardinal vein
Scimitar syndrome
Ex: See Q26.0

Q26.9 Congenital malformation of great vein, unspecified
Congenital anomaly of vena cava (inferior) (superior) NOS
Ex: Q26.9, Q27.30, Q27.4, Q28.0-Q28.1, Q28.8-Q28.9

● **Q27 Other congenital malformations of peripheral vascular system**
Excludes2 anomalies of cerebral and precerebral vessels (Q28.0-Q28.3)
anomalies of coronary vessels (Q24.5)
anomalies of pulmonary artery (Q25.5-Q25.7)
congenital retinal aneurysm (Q14.1)
hemangioma and lymphangioma (D18.-)

Q27.0 Congenital absence and hypoplasia of umbilical artery
Single umbilical artery

Q27.1 Congenital renal artery stenosis

Q27.2 Other congenital malformations of renal artery
Congenital malformation of renal artery NOS
Multiple renal arteries

● **Q27.3 Arteriovenous malformation (peripheral)**
Arteriovenous aneurysm
Excludes1 acquired arteriovenous aneurysm (I77.0)
Excludes2 arteriovenous malformation of cerebral vessels (Q28.2)
arteriovenous malformation of precerebral vessels (Q28.0)

Q27.30 Arteriovenous malformation, site unspecified
Ex: Q20.0-Q20.8, Q21.0-Q21.9, Q27.30, Q27.4, Q28.0-Q28.1, Q28.8

Q27.31 Arteriovenous malformation of vessel of upper limb

Q27.32 Arteriovenous malformation of vessel of lower limb

Q27.33 Arteriovenous malformation of digestive system vessel

Q27.34 Arteriovenous malformation of renal vessel

Q27.39 Arteriovenous malformation, other site

Q27.4 Congenital phlebectasia
Ex: See Q27.30

Q27.8 Other specified congenital malformations of peripheral vascular system
Absence of peripheral vascular system
Atresia of peripheral vascular system
Congenital aneurysm (peripheral)
Congenital stricture, artery
Congenital varix
Excludes1 arteriovenous malformation (Q27.3-)

Q27.9 Congenital malformation of peripheral vascular system, unspecified
Anomaly of artery or vein NOS

● **Q28 Other congenital malformations of circulatory system**
Excludes1 congenital aneurysm NOS (Q27.8)
congenital coronary aneurysm (Q24.5)
ruptured cerebral arteriovenous malformation (I60.8)
ruptured malformation of precerebral vessels (I72.0)
Excludes2 congenital peripheral aneurysm (Q27.8)
congenital pulmonary aneurysm (Q25.79)
congenital retinal aneurysm (Q14.1)

Q28.0 Arteriovenous malformation of precerebral vessels
Congenital arteriovenous precerebral aneurysm (nonruptured)
Ex: See Q27.30

Q28.1 Other malformations of precerebral vessels
Congenital malformation of precerebral vessels NOS
Congenital precerebral aneurysm (nonruptured)
Ex: See Q27.30

Q28.2 Arteriovenous malformation of cerebral vessels
Arteriovenous malformation of brain NOS
Congenital arteriovenous cerebral aneurysm (nonruptured)
Ex: Q27.30, Q27.4, Q28.0-Q28.9

Q28.3 Other malformations of cerebral vessels
Congenital cerebral aneurysm (nonruptured)
Congenital malformation of cerebral vessels NOS
Developmental venous anomaly
Ex: See Q28.2

Q28.8 Other specified congenital malformations of circulatory system
Congenital aneurysm, specified site NEC
Spinal vessel anomaly
Ex: See Q27.30

Q28.9 Congenital malformation of circulatory system, unspecified
Ex: Q20.0-Q28.9

CONGENITAL MALFORMATIONS OF THE RESPIRATORY SYSTEM (Q30-Q34)

Q30 Congenital malformations of nose
Excludes1 congenital deviation of nasal septum (Q67.4)

Q30.0 Choanal atresia
Atresia of nares (anterior) (posterior)
Congenital stenosis of nares (anterior) (posterior)

Q30.1 Agenesis and underdevelopment of nose
Congenital absent of nose

Q30.2 Fissured, notched and cleft nose

Q30.3 Congenital perforated nasal septum

Q30.8 Other congenital malformations of nose
Accessory nose
Congenital anomaly of nasal sinus wall

Q30.9 Congenital malformation of nose, unspecified

Q31 Congenital malformations of larynx
Excludes1 congenital laryngeal stridor NOS (P28.89)
Ex: For category Q31 CC codes: J39.8, J45.990, J98.09, Q31.1-Q32.4, Q34.0-Q34.9

Q31.0 Web of larynx
Glottic web of larynx
Subglottic web of larynx
Web of larynx NOS

Q31.1 Congenital subglottic stenosis

Q31.2 Laryngeal hypoplasia

Q31.3 Laryngocele

Q31.5 Congenital laryngomalacia

Q31.8 Other congenital malformations of larynx
Absence of larynx
Agenesis of larynx
Atresia of larynx
Congenital cleft thyroid cartilage
Congenital fissure of epiglottis
Congenital stenosis of larynx NEC
Posterior cleft of cricoid cartilage

Q31.9 Congenital malformation of larynx, unspecified

Q32 Congenital malformations of trachea and bronchus
Excludes1 congenital bronchiectasis (Q33.4)
Ex: For category Q32 CC codes: See Q31

Q32.0 Congenital tracheomalacia

Q32.1 Other congenital malformations of trachea
Atresia of trachea
Congenital anomaly of tracheal cartilage
Congenital dilatation of trachea
Congenital malformation of trachea
Congenital stenosis of trachea
Congenital tracheocele

Q32.2 Congenital bronchomalacia

Q32.3 Congenital stenosis of bronchus

Q32.4 Other congenital malformations of bronchus
Absence of bronchus
Agenesis of bronchus
Atresia of bronchus
Congenital diverticulum of bronchus
Congenital malformation of bronchus NOS

Q33 Congenital malformations of lung

Q33.0 Congenital cystic lung
Congenital cystic lung disease
Congenital honeycomb lung
Congenital polycystic lung disease
Excludes1 cystic fibrosis (E84.0)
cystic lung disease, acquired or unspecified (J98.4)
Ex: Q33.0-Q34.9

Q33.1 Accessory lobe of lung
Azygos lobe (fissured), lung

Q33.2 Sequestration of lung
Ex: Q33.0-Q34.9

Q33.3 Agenesis of lung
Congenital absence of lung (lobe)
Ex: Q33.0-Q34.9

Q33.4 Congenital bronchiectasis
Ex: J44.9, J47.0-J47.9, J68.1, J68.4-J68.9, Q33.4

Q33.5 Ectopic tissue in lung

Q33.6 Congenital hypoplasia and dysplasia of lung
Excludes1 pulmonary hypoplasia associated with short gestation (P28.0)
Ex: Q33.0-Q34.9

Q33.8 Other congenital malformations of lung

Q33.9 Congenital malformation of lung, unspecified

Q34 Other congenital malformations of respiratory system
Excludes2 congenital central alveolar hypoventilation syndrome (G47.35)

Q34.0 Anomaly of pleura

Q34.1 Congenital cyst of mediastinum

Q34.8 Other specified congenital malformations of respiratory system
Atresia of nasopharynx

Q34.9 Congenital malformation of respiratory system, unspecified
Congenital absence of respiratory system
Congenital anomaly of respiratory system NOS

CLEFT LIP AND CLEFT PALATE (Q35-Q37)

Use additional code to identify associated malformation of the nose (Q30.2)
Excludes1 Robin's syndrome (Q87.0)

Q35 Cleft palate
Includes fissure of palate
palatoschisis
Excludes1 cleft palate with cleft lip (Q37.-)

Q35.1 Cleft hard palate

Q35.3 Cleft soft palate

Q35.5 Cleft hard palate with cleft soft palate

Q35.7 Cleft uvula

Q35.9 Cleft palate, unspecified
Cleft palate NOS

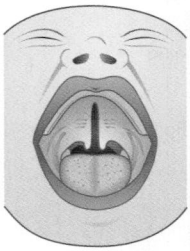

Figure 17-3 Cleft palate.

● **Q36 Cleft lip**

Includes cheiloschisis
congenital fissure of lip
harelip
labium leporinum

Excludes1 cleft lip with cleft palate (Q37.-)

Q36.0 Cleft lip, bilateral

Q36.1 Cleft lip, median

Q36.9 Cleft lip, unilateral
Cleft lip NOS

● **Q37 Cleft palate with cleft lip**

Includes cheilopalatoschisis

Q37.0 Cleft hard palate with bilateral cleft lip

Q37.1 Cleft hard palate with unilateral cleft lip
Cleft hard palate with cleft lip NOS

Q37.2 Cleft soft palate with bilateral cleft lip

Q37.3 Cleft soft palate with unilateral cleft lip
Cleft soft palate with cleft lip NOS

Q37.4 Cleft hard and soft palate with bilateral cleft lip

Q37.5 Cleft hard and soft palate with unilateral cleft lip
Cleft hard and soft palate with cleft lip NOS

Q37.8 Unspecified cleft palate with bilateral cleft lip

Q37.9 Unspecified cleft palate with unilateral cleft lip
Cleft palate with cleft lip NOS

OTHER CONGENITAL MALFORMATIONS OF THE DIGESTIVE SYSTEM (Q38-Q45)

● **Q38 Other congenital malformations of tongue, mouth and pharynx**

Excludes1 dentofacial anomalies (M26.-)
macrostomia (Q18.4)
microstomia (Q18.5)

Q38.0 Congenital malformations of lips, not elsewhere classified
Congenital fistula of lip
Congenital malformation of lip NOS
Van der Woude's syndrome

Excludes1 cleft lip (Q36.-)
cleft lip with cleft palate (Q37.-)
macrocheilia (Q18.6)
microcheilia (Q18.7)

Q38.1 Ankyloglossia
Restricted movement of tongue resulting in speech difficulty
Tongue tie

Q38.2 Macroglossia
Excessive size of tongue
Congenital hypertrophy of tongue

Q38.3 Other congenital malformations of tongue
Aglossia
Bifid tongue
Congenital adhesion of tongue
Congenital fissure of tongue
Congenital malformation of tongue NOS
Double tongue
Hypoglossia
Hypoplasia of tongue
Microglossia

Q38.4 Congenital malformations of salivary glands and ducts
Atresia of salivary glands and ducts
Congenital absence of salivary glands and ducts
Congenital accessory salivary glands and ducts
Congenital fistula of salivary gland

Q38.5 Congenital malformations of palate, not elsewhere classified
Congenital absence of uvula
Congenital malformation of palate NOS
Congenital high arched palate

Excludes1 cleft palate (Q35.-)
cleft palate with cleft lip (Q37.-)

Q38.6 Other congenital malformations of mouth
Congenital malformation of mouth NOS

Q38.7 Congenital pharyngeal pouch
Congenital diverticulum of pharynx

Excludes1 pharyngeal pouch syndrome (D82.1)

Q38.8 Other congenital malformations of pharynx
Congenital malformation of pharynx NOS
Imperforate pharynx

● **Q39 Congenital malformations of esophagus**

Ex: For category Q39 CC codes Q39.0-Q39.4: Q39.0-Q39.9, Q45.8-Q45.9
For category Q39 CC codes Q39.5-Q39.9: Q39.5-Q39.9, Q45.8-Q45.9

Q39.0 Atresia of esophagus without fistula
Atresia of esophagus NOS

Q39.1 Atresia of esophagus with tracheo-esophageal fistula
Atresia of esophagus with broncho-esophageal fistula

Q39.2 Congenital tracheo-esophageal fistula without atresia
Congenital tracheo-esophageal fistula NOS

Q39.3 Congenital stenosis and stricture of esophagus

Q39.4 Esophageal web

Q39.5 Congenital dilatation of esophagus
Congenital cardiospasm

Q39.6 Congenital diverticulum of esophagus
Congenital esophageal pouch

Q39.8 Other congenital malformations of esophagus
Congenital absence of esophagus
Congenital displacement of esophagus
Congenital duplication of esophagus

Q39.9 Congenital malformation of esophagus, unspecified

● **Q40 Other congenital malformations of upper alimentary tract**

Q40.0 Congenital hypertrophic pyloric stenosis
Congenital or infantile constriction
Congenital or infantile hypertrophy
Congenital or infantile spasm
Congenital or infantile stenosis
Congenital or infantile stricture

Q40.1 Congenital hiatus hernia
Congenital displacement of cardia through esophageal hiatus

Excludes1 congenital diaphragmatic hernia (Q79.0)

Q40.2 Other specified congenital malformations of stomach
Congenital displacement of stomach
Congenital diverticulum of stomach
Congenital hourglass stomach
Congenital duplication of stomach
Megalogastria
Microgastria

Q40.3 Congenital malformation of stomach, unspecified

Q40.8 Other specified congenital malformations of upper alimentary tract

Q40.9 Congenital malformation of upper alimentary tract, unspecified
Congenital anomaly of upper alimentary tract
Congenital deformity of upper alimentary tract

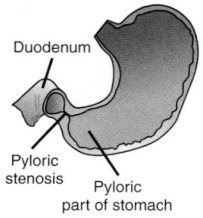

Figure 17-4 Pyloric stenosis.

Q41 Congenital absence, atresia and stenosis of small intestine

Includes congenital obstruction, occlusion or stricture of small intestine or intestine NOS

Excludes1 cystic fibrosis with intestinal manifestation (E84.11)
meconium ileus NOS (without cystic fibrosis) (P76.0)

Ex: For category Q41 CC codes: Q41.0-Q41.9, Q45.8-Q45.9

Q41.0 Congenital absence, atresia and stenosis of duodenum

Q41.1 Congenital absence, atresia and stenosis of jejunum
Apple peel syndrome
Imperforate jejunum

Q41.2 Congenital absence, atresia and stenosis of ileum

Q41.8 Congenital absence, atresia and stenosis of other specified parts of small intestine

Q41.9 Congenital absence, atresia and stenosis of small intestine, part unspecified
Congenital absence, atresia and stenosis of intestine NOS

Q42 Congenital absence, atresia and stenosis of large intestine

Includes congenital obstruction, occlusion and stricture of large intestine

Ex: For category Q42 CC codes: Q42.0-Q42.9, Q45.8-Q45.9

Q42.0 Congenital absence, atresia and stenosis of rectum with fistula

Q42.1 Congenital absence, atresia and stenosis of rectum without fistula
Imperforate rectum

Q42.2 Congenital absence, atresia and stenosis of anus with fistula

Q42.3 Congenital absence, atresia and stenosis of anus without fistula
Imperforate anus

Q42.8 Congenital absence, atresia and stenosis of other parts of large intestine

Q42.9 Congenital absence, atresia and stenosis of large intestine, part unspecified

Q43 Other congenital malformations of intestine

Ex: For category Q43 CC codes unless otherwise indicated: Q41.0-Q43.9

Q43.0 Meckel's diverticulum (displaced) (hypertrophic)
Congenital abnormality in which a pouch remains on the lower end of the small intestine
Persistent omphalomesenteric duct
Persistent vitelline duct

Q43.1 Hirschsprung's disease
Developmental disorder of enteric nervous system characterized by absence of ganglion cells in distal colon resulting in functional obstruction
Aganglionosis
Congenital (aganglionic) megacolon
Ex: Q43.1-Q43.2, Q45.8-Q45.9

Q43.2 Other congenital functional disorders of colon
Congenital dilatation of colon
Ex: Q43.1-Q43.2, Q45.8-Q45.9

Q43.3 Congenital malformations of intestinal fixation
Congenital omental, anomalous adhesions [bands]
Congenital peritoneal adhesions [bands]
Incomplete rotation of cecum and colon
Insufficient rotation of cecum and colon
Jackson's membrane
Malrotation of colon
Rotation failure of cecum and colon
Universal mesentery
Ex: Q43.3-Q43.9

Q43.4 Duplication of intestine

Q43.5 Ectopic anus
Anal opening in abnormal location

Q43.6 Congenital fistula of rectum and anus

Excludes1 congenital fistula of anus with absence, atresia and stenosis (Q42.2)
congenital fistula of rectum with absence, atresia and stenosis (Q42.0)
congenital rectovaginal fistula (Q52.2)
congenital urethrorectal fistula (Q64.73)
pilonidal fistula or sinus (L05.-)

Q43.7 Persistent cloaca
Malformation in which rectum, vagina, and urinary tract form one channel AKA congenital cloaca
Cloaca NOS

Q43.8 Other specified congenital malformations of intestine
Congenital blind loop syndrome
Congenital diverticulitis, colon
Congenital diverticulum, intestine
Dolichocolon
Megaloappendix
Megaloduodenum
Microcolon
Transposition of appendix
Transposition of colon
Transposition of intestine

Q43.9 Congenital malformation of intestine, unspecified

Q44 Congenital malformations of gallbladder, bile ducts and liver

Ex: For category Q44 CC codes unless otherwise indicated: Q44.0-Q44.7

Q44.0 Agenesis, aplasia and hypoplasia of gallbladder
Congenital absence of gallbladder

Q44.1 Other congenital malformations of gallbladder
Congenital malformation of gallbladder NOS
Intrahepatic gallbladder

Q44.2 Atresia of bile ducts
Ex: Q44.2-Q44.3, Q45.8-Q45.9

Q44.3 Congenital stenosis and stricture of bile ducts
Ex: Q44.2-Q44.3, Q45.8-Q45.9

Q44.4 Choledochal cyst

Q44.5 Other congenital malformations of bile ducts
Accessory hepatic duct
Biliary duct duplication
Congenital malformation of bile duct NOS
Cystic duct duplication

Q44.6 Cystic disease of liver
Fibrocystic disease of liver
Ex: Q44.0-Q44.1, Q44.4-Q44.7

Q44.7 Other congenital malformations of liver
Accessory liver
Alagille's syndrome
Congenital absence of liver
Congenital hepatomegaly
Congenital malformation of liver NOS

Q45 Other congenital malformations of digestive system

Excludes2 congenital diaphragmatic hernia (Q79.0)
congenital hiatus hernia (Q40.1)

Ex: For category Q45 CC codes: Q45.0-Q45.9

Q45.0 Agenesis, aplasia and hypoplasia of pancreas
Congenital absence of pancreas

Q45.1 Annular pancreas

Q45.2 Congenital pancreatic cyst

Q45.3 Other congenital malformations of pancreas and pancreatic duct
Accessory pancreas
Congenital malformation of pancreas or pancreatic duct NOS

Excludes1 congenital diabetes mellitus (E10.-)
cystic fibrosis (E84.0-E84.9)
fibrocystic disease of pancreas (E84.-)
neonatal diabetes mellitus (P70.2)

Q45.8 Other specified congenital malformations of digestive system
Absence (complete) (partial) of alimentary tract NOS
Duplication of digestive system
Malposition, congenital of digestive system

Q45.9 Congenital malformation of digestive system, unspecified
Congenital anomaly of digestive system
Congenital deformity of digestive system

CONGENITAL MALFORMATIONS OF GENITAL ORGANS (Q50-Q56)

Excludes1 androgen insensitivity syndrome (E34.5-)
syndromes associated with anomalies in the number and form of chromosomes (Q90-Q99)

● **Q50 Congenital malformations of ovaries, fallopian tubes and broad ligaments**

● **Q50.0 Congenital absence of ovary**
Excludes1 Turner's syndrome (Q96.-)
Q50.01 Congenital absence of ovary, unilateral ♀
Q50.02 Congenital absence of ovary, bilateral ♀

Q50.1 Developmental ovarian cyst ♀

Q50.2 Congenital torsion of ovary ♀

● **Q50.3 Other congenital malformations of ovary**
Q50.31 Accessory ovary ♀
Q50.32 Ovarian streak ♀
Inadequate ovaries with absent follicular and hormonal function
46, XX with streak gonads
Q50.39 Other congenital malformation of ovary ♀
Congenital malformation of ovary NOS

Q50.4 Embryonic cyst of fallopian tube ♀
Fimbrial cyst

Q50.5 Embryonic cyst of broad ligament ♀
Epoophoron cyst
Parovarian cyst

Q50.6 Other congenital malformations of fallopian tube and broad ligament ♀
Absence of fallopian tube and broad ligament
Accessory fallopian tube and broad ligament
Atresia of fallopian tube and broad ligament
Congenital malformation of fallopian tube or broad ligament NOS

● **Q51 Congenital malformations of uterus and cervix**

Q51.0 Agenesis and aplasia of uterus ♀
Congenital absence of uterus

● **Q51.1 Doubling of uterus with doubling of cervix and vagina**
Q51.10 Doubling of uterus with doubling of cervix and vagina without obstruction ♀
Doubling of uterus with doubling of cervix and vagina NOS
Q51.11 Doubling of uterus with doubling of cervix and vagina with obstruction ♀

Q51.2 Other doubling of uterus ♀
Doubling of uterus NOS
Septate uterus, complete or partial

Q51.3 Bicornate uterus ♀
Bicornate uterus, complete or partial
Birth defect in which uterus has two separate 'horns' that form top of uterus

Q51.4 Unicornate uterus ♀
Unicornate uterus with or without a separate uterine horn
Uterus with only one functioning horn
Uterus with half being undeveloped

Q51.5 Agenesis and aplasia of cervix ♀
Congenital absence of cervix

Q51.6 Embryonic cyst of cervix ♀

Q51.7 Congenital fistulae between uterus and digestive and urinary tracts ♀

● **Q51.8 Other congenital malformations of uterus and cervix**

● **Q51.81 Other congenital malformations of uterus**
Q51.810 Arcuate uterus ♀
Arcuatus uterus
Q51.811 Hypoplasia of uterus ♀
Q51.818 Other congenital malformations of uterus ♀
Müllerian anomaly of uterus NEC

● **Q51.82 Other congenital malformations of cervix**
Q51.820 Cervical duplication ♀
Q51.821 Hypoplasia of cervix ♀
Q51.828 Other congenital malformations of cervix ♀

Q51.9 Congenital malformation of uterus and cervix, unspecified ♀

● **Q52 Other congenital malformations of female genitalia**

Q52.0 Congenital absence of vagina ♀
Vaginal agenesis, total or partial

● **Q52.1 Doubling of vagina**
Excludes1 doubling of vagina with doubling of uterus and cervix (Q51.1-)
Q52.10 Doubling of vagina, unspecified ♀
Septate vagina NOS
Q52.11 Transverse vaginal septum ♀

● **Q52.12 Longitudinal vaginal septum**
~~Longitudinal vaginal septum with or without obstruction~~
Q52.120 Longitudinal vaginal septum, nonobstructing ♀ ◀
Q52.121 Longitudinal vaginal septum, obstructing, right side ♀ ◀
Q52.122 Longitudinal vaginal septum, obstructing, left side ♀ ◀
Q52.123 Longitudinal vaginal septum, microperforate, right side ♀ ◀
Q52.124 Longitudinal vaginal septum, microperforate, left side ♀ ◀
Q52.129 Other and unspecified longitudinal vaginal septum ♀ ◀

Q52.2 Congenital rectovaginal fistula ♀
Excludes1 cloaca (Q43.7)

Q52.3 Imperforate hymen ♀
Membrane (hymen) completely closes vaginal orifice

Q52.4 Other congenital malformations of vagina ♀
Canal of Nuck cyst, congenital
Congenital malformation of vagina NOS
Embryonic vaginal cyst
Gartner's duct cyst

Q52.5 Fusion of labia ♀

Q52.6 Congenital malformation of clitoris ♀

● **Q52.7 Other and unspecified congenital malformations of vulva**
Q52.70 Unspecified congenital malformations of vulva ♀
Congenital malformation of vulva NOS
Q52.71 Congenital absence of vulva ♀
Q52.79 Other congenital malformations of vulva ♀
Congenital cyst of vulva

Q52.8 Other specified congenital malformations of female genitalia ♀

Q52.9 Congenital malformation of female genitalia, unspecified ♀

● **Q53 Undescended and ectopic testicle**

● **Q53.0 Ectopic testis**
Q53.00 Ectopic testis, unspecified ♂
Q53.01 Ectopic testis, unilateral ♂
Q53.02 Ectopic testes, bilateral ♂

Item 17-1 Testes form in the abdomen of the male and only descend into the scrotum during normal embryonic development. "Ectopic" testes are out of their normal place or "retained" (left behind) in the abdomen. Crypto (hidden) orchism (testicle) is a major risk factor for testicular cancer.

ECTOPIC TESTES	CRYPTORCHID TESTES
Penile	Abdominal
Superficial inguinal (most common)	Inguinal
Femoral	Prepubic (most common)

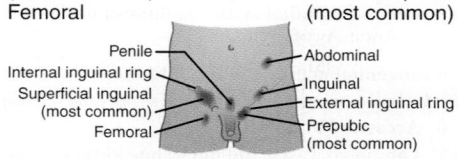

Figure 17-5 Undescended testes and the positions of the testes in various types of cryptorchidism or abnormal paths of descent.

- **Q53.1 Undescended testicle, unilateral**
  - **Q53.10 Unspecified undescended testicle, unilateral** ♂
  - **Q53.11 Abdominal testis, unilateral** ♂
  - **Q53.12 Ectopic perineal testis, unilateral** ♂
- **Q53.2 Undescended testicle, bilateral**
  - **Q53.20 Undescended testicle, unspecified, bilateral** ♂
  - **Q53.21 Abdominal testis, bilateral** ♂
  - **Q53.22 Ectopic perineal testis, bilateral** ♂
- **Q53.9 Undescended testicle, unspecified** ♂
  - Cryptorchism NOS

- **Q54 Hypospadias**
  - *Birth defect of male; urethra opens in abnormal location on shaft*
  - **Excludes1** epispadias (Q64.0)
  - **Q54.0 Hypospadias, balanic** ♂
    - Hypospadias, coronal
    - Hypospadias, glandular
  - **Q54.1 Hypospadias, penile** ♂
  - **Q54.2 Hypospadias, penoscrotal** ♂
  - **Q54.3 Hypospadias, perineal** ♂
  - **Q54.4 Congenital chordee** ♂
    - Chordee without hypospadias
  - **Q54.8 Other hypospadias** ♂
    - Hypospadias with intersex state
  - **Q54.9 Hypospadias, unspecified** ♂

- **Q55 Other congenital malformations of male genital organs**
  - **Excludes1** congenital hydrocele (P83.5)
    hypospadias (Q54.-)
  - **Q55.0 Absence and aplasia of testis** ♂
    - Monorchism
  - **Q55.1 Hypoplasia of testis and scrotum** ♂
    - Fusion of testes
  - **Q55.2 Other and unspecified congenital malformations of testis and scrotum**
    - **Q55.20 Unspecified congenital malformations of testis and scrotum** ♂
      - Congenital malformation of testis or scrotum NOS
    - **Q55.21 Polyorchism** ♂
      - *Developmental anomaly characterized by presence of more than two testes*
    - **Q55.22 Retractile testis** ♂
    - **Q55.23 Scrotal transposition** ♂
    - **Q55.29 Other congenital malformations of testis and scrotum** ♂
  - **Q55.3 Atresia of vas deferens** ♂
    - *Code first any associated cystic fibrosis (E84.-)*
  - **Q55.4 Other congenital malformations of vas deferens, epididymis, seminal vesicles and prostate** ♂
    - Absence or aplasia of prostate
    - Absence or aplasia of spermatic cord
    - Congenital malformation of vas deferens, epididymis, seminal vesicles or prostate NOS
  - **Q55.5 Congenital absence and aplasia of penis** ♂
  - **Q55.6 Other congenital malformations of penis**
    - **Q55.61 Curvature of penis (lateral)** ♂
    - **Q55.62 Hypoplasia of penis** ♂
      - *Underdevelopment penis*
      - Micropenis
    - **Q55.63 Congenital torsion of penis** ♂
      - **Excludes1** acquired torsion of penis (N48.82)
    - **Q55.64 Hidden penis** ♂
      - Buried penis
      - Concealed penis
      - **Excludes1** acquired buried penis (N48.83)
    - **Q55.69 Other congenital malformation of penis** ♂
      - Congenital malformation of penis NOS
  - **Q55.7 Congenital vasocutaneous fistula** ♂
    - *Abnormal opening between vas deferens and skin*
  - **Q55.8 Other specified congenital malformations of male genital organs** ♂
  - **Q55.9 Congenital malformation of male genital organ, unspecified** ♂
    - Congenital anomaly of male genital organ
    - Congenital deformity of male genital organ

- **Q56 Indeterminate sex and pseudohermaphroditism**
  - *Internal reproductive organs are opposite external physical characteristics.*
  - **Excludes1** 46,XX true hermaphrodite (Q99.1)
    androgen insensitivity syndrome (E34.5-)
    chimera 46,XX/46,XY true hermaphrodite (Q99.0)
    female pseudohermaphroditism with adrenocortical disorder (E25.-)
    pseudohermaphroditism with specified chromosomal anomaly (Q96-Q99)
    pure gonadal dysgenesis (Q99.1)
  - **Q56.0 Hermaphroditism, not elsewhere classified**
    - Ovotestis
  - **Q56.1 Male pseudohermaphroditism, not elsewhere classified** ♂
    - 46, XY with streak gonads
    - Male pseudohermaphroditism NOS
  - **Q56.2 Female pseudohermaphroditism, not elsewhere classified** ♀
    - Female pseudohermaphroditism NOS
  - **Q56.3 Pseudohermaphroditism, unspecified**
  - **Q56.4 Indeterminate sex, unspecified**
    - Ambiguous genitalia

CONGENITAL MALFORMATIONS OF THE URINARY SYSTEM (Q60-Q64)

- **Q60 Renal agenesis and other reduction defects of kidney**
  - **Includes** congenital absence of kidney
    congenital atrophy of kidney
    infantile atrophy of kidney
  - Ex For category Q60 CC codes: N13.9, Q60.0-Q60.6
  - **Q60.0 Renal agenesis, unilateral**
  - **Q60.1 Renal agenesis, bilateral**
  - **Q60.2 Renal agenesis, unspecified**
  - **Q60.3 Renal hypoplasia, unilateral**
  - **Q60.4 Renal hypoplasia, bilateral**
  - **Q60.5 Renal hypoplasia, unspecified**
  - **Q60.6 Potter's syndrome**

Q61 Cystic kidney disease
Cysts that develop in failing kidney due to end-stage renal disease
Excludes1 acquired cyst of kidney (N28.1)
Potter's syndrome (Q60.6)

Q61.0 Congenital renal cyst
Q61.00 Congenital renal cyst, unspecified
Cyst of kidney NOS (congenital)
Ex: N13.9, Q61.00, Q61.9
Q61.01 Congenital single renal cyst
Ex: N13.9, Q61.01
Q61.02 Congenital multiple renal cysts
Ex: N13.9, Q61.02, Q61.5-Q61.8

Q61.1 Polycystic kidney, infantile type
Polycystic kidney, autosomal recessive
Ex: For category Q61.1 CC codes: N13.9, Q61.11-Q61.3
Q61.11 Cystic dilatation of collecting ducts
Q61.19 Other polycystic kidney, infantile type

Q61.2 Polycystic kidney, adult type
Polycystic kidney, autosomal dominant
Ex: N13.9, Q61.11-Q61.3

Q61.3 Polycystic kidney, unspecified
Ex: N13.9, Q61.11-Q61.3

Q61.4 Renal dysplasia
Multicystic dysplastic kidney
Multicystic kidney (development)
Multicystic kidney disease
Multicystic renal dysplasia
Excludes1 polycystic kidney disease (Q61.11-Q61.3)
Ex: N13.9, Q61.4

Q61.5 Medullary cystic kidney
Nephronopthisis
Sponge kidney NOS
Ex: N13.9, Q61.02, Q61.5-Q61.8

Q61.8 Other cystic kidney diseases
Fibrocystic kidney
Fibrocystic renal degeneration or disease
Ex: N13.9, Q61.02, Q61.5-Q61.8

Q61.9 Cystic kidney disease, unspecified
Meckel-Gruber syndrome
Ex: N13.9, Q61.00, Q61.9

Q62 Congenital obstructive defects of renal pelvis and congenital malformations of ureter

Q62.0 Congenital hydronephrosis
Ex: N13.9, Q62.0-Q62.2, Q62.39

Q62.1 Congenital occlusion of ureter
Atresia and stenosis of ureter
Ex: For category Q62.1 CC codes: See Q62.0
Q62.10 Congenital occlusion of ureter, unspecified
Q62.11 Congenital occlusion of ureteropelvic junction
Q62.12 Congenital occlusion of ureterovesical orifice

Q62.2 Congenital megaureter
Congenital dilatation of ureter
Ex: See Q62.0

Q62.3 Other obstructive defects of renal pelvis and ureter
Ex: For category Q62.3 CC codes: See Q62.0
Q62.31 Congenital ureterocele, orthotopic
Q62.32 Cecoureterocele
Ectopic ureterocele
Q62.39 Other obstructive defects of renal pelvis and ureter
Ureteropelvic junction obstruction NOS

Q62.4 Agenesis of ureter
Congenital absence ureter

Q62.5 Duplication of ureter
Accessory ureter
Double ureter

Q62.6 Malposition of ureter
Q62.60 Malposition of ureter, unspecified
Q62.61 Deviation of ureter
Q62.62 Displacement of ureter
Q62.63 Anomalous implantation of ureter
Ectopia of ureter
Ectopic ureter
Q62.69 Other malposition of ureter

Q62.7 Congenital vesico-uretero-renal reflux

Q62.8 Other congenital malformations of ureter
Anomaly of ureter NOS

Q63 Other congenital malformations of kidney
Excludes1 congenital nephrotic syndrome (N04.-)

Q63.0 Accessory kidney

Q63.1 Lobulated, fused and horseshoe kidney

Q63.2 Ectopic kidney
Congenital displaced kidney
Malrotation of kidney

Q63.3 Hyperplastic and giant kidney
Compensatory hypertrophy of kidney

Q63.8 Other specified congenital malformations of kidney
Congenital renal calculi

Q63.9 Congenital malformation of kidney, unspecified

Q64 Other congenital malformations of urinary system

Q64.0 Epispadias ♂
Urethral opening somewhere on dorsum of penis
Excludes1 hypospadias (Q54.-)

Q64.1 Exstrophy of urinary bladder
Bladder is exposed, inside out, and protrudes through abdominal wall
Ex: For category Q64.1 CC codes: N13.9, Q64.10-Q64.19, Q64.8-Q64.9
Q64.10 Exstrophy of urinary bladder, unspecified
Ectopia vesicae
Q64.11 Supravesical fissure of urinary bladder
Q64.12 Cloacal extrophy of urinary bladder
Q64.19 Other exstrophy of urinary bladder
Extroversion of bladder

Q64.2 Congenital posterior urethral valves
Ex: N13.9, Q64.2-Q64.39, Q64.8-Q64.9

Q64.3 Other atresia and stenosis of urethra and bladder neck
Ex: For category Q64.3 CC codes: See Q64.2
Q64.31 Congenital bladder neck obstruction
Congenital obstruction of vesicourethral orifice
Q64.32 Congenital stricture of urethra
Q64.33 Congenital stricture of urinary meatus
Q64.39 Other atresia and stenosis of urethra and bladder neck
Atresia and stenosis of urethra and bladder neck NOS

Q64.4 Malformation of urachus
Cyst of urachus
Patent urachus
Prolapse of urachus

Q64.5 Congenital absence of bladder and urethra

Q64.6 Congenital diverticulum of bladder

Q64.7 Other and unspecified congenital malformations of bladder and urethra
Excludes1 congenital prolapse of bladder (mucosa) (Q79.4)
Q64.70 Unspecified congenital malformation of bladder and urethra
Malformation of bladder or urethra NOS
Q64.71 Congenital prolapse of urethra
Q64.72 Congenital prolapse of urinary meatus
Q64.73 Congenital urethrorectal fistula
Q64.74 Double urethra
Q64.75 Double urinary meatus
Q64.79 Other congenital malformations of bladder and urethra

Q64.8 Other specified congenital malformations of urinary system

Q64.9 Congenital malformation of urinary system, unspecified
Congenital anomaly NOS of urinary system
Congenital deformity NOS of urinary system

CONGENITAL MALFORMATIONS AND DEFORMATIONS OF THE MUSCULOSKELETAL SYSTEM (Q65-Q79)

Q65 Congenital deformities of hip
Excludes1 clicking hip (R29.4)

Q65.0 Congenital dislocation of hip, unilateral
Q65.00 Congenital dislocation of unspecified hip, unilateral
Q65.01 Congenital dislocation of right hip, unilateral
Q65.02 Congenital dislocation of left hip, unilateral
Q65.1 Congenital dislocation of hip, bilateral
Q65.2 Congenital dislocation of hip, unspecified
Q65.3 Congenital partial dislocation of hip, unilateral
Q65.30 Congenital partial dislocation of unspecified hip, unilateral
Q65.31 Congenital partial dislocation of right hip, unilateral
Q65.32 Congenital partial dislocation of left hip, unilateral
Q65.4 Congenital partial dislocation of hip, bilateral
Q65.5 Congenital partial dislocation of hip, unspecified
Q65.6 Congenital unstable hip
Congenital dislocatable hip
Q65.8 Other congenital deformities of hip
Q65.81 Congenital coxa valga
Q65.82 Congenital coxa vara
Q65.89 Other specified congenital deformities of hip
Anteversion of femoral neck
Congenital acetabular dysplasia
Q65.9 Congenital deformity of hip, unspecified

Q66 Congenital deformities of feet
Excludes1 reduction defects of feet (Q72.-)
valgus deformities (acquired) (M21.0-)
varus deformities (acquired) (M21.1-)
Q66.0 Congenital talipes equinovarus
Heel is turned inward from midline and foot is plantar flexed; AKA clubfoot
Q66.1 Congenital talipes calcaneovarus
Deformity of foot in which heel is turned toward midline of body and anterior of foot is elevated
Q66.2 Congenital metatarsus (primus) varus
Angulation of first metatarsal bone toward midline of body
Q66.21 Congenital metatarsus primus varus ◀
Q66.22 Congenital metatarsus adductus ◀
Congenital metatarsus varus ◀
Q66.3 Other congenital varus deformities of feet
Hallux varus, congenital
Q66.4 Congenital talipes calcaneovalgus
Q66.5 Congenital pes planus
Congenital flat foot
Congenital rigid flat foot
Congenital spastic (everted) flat foot
Excludes1 pes planus, acquired (M21.4)
Q66.50 Congenital pes planus, unspecified foot
Q66.51 Congenital pes planus, right foot
Q66.52 Congenital pes planus, left foot
Q66.6 Other congenital valgus deformities of feet
Inward angulation
Congenital metatarsus valgus
Q66.7 Congenital pes cavus

Item 17–2 Equinus foot is a term referring to the hoof of a horse. The deformity is usually congenital or spastic. Talipes equinovarus is referred to as clubfoot. The foot tends to be smaller than normal, with the heel pointing downward and the forefoot turning inward. The heel cord (Achilles tendon) is tight, causing the heel to be drawn up toward the leg.

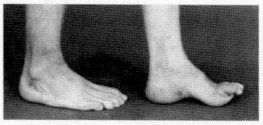

Figure 17-6 Supination and cavus deformity of forefoot. *(Courtesy Jay Cummings, MD.)* (From Canale: Campbell's Operative Orthopaedics, ed 11, Mosby, Inc., 2007)

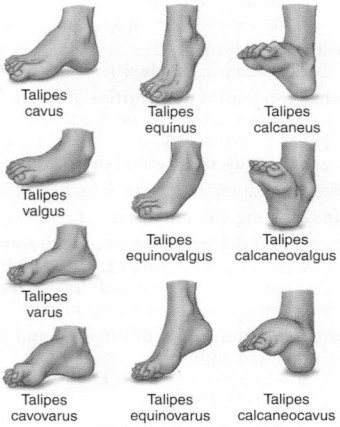

Figure 17-7 Talipes. (From Dorland: Dorland's Illustrated Medical Dictionary, ed 31, Saunders, 2007, p 1893)

Q66.8 Other congenital deformities of feet
Q66.80 Congenital vertical talus deformity, unspecified foot
Q66.81 Congenital vertical talus deformity, right foot
Q66.82 Congenital vertical talus deformity, left foot
Q66.89 Other specified congenital deformities of feet
Congenital asymmetric talipes
Congenital clubfoot NOS
Congenital talipes NOS
Congenital tarsal coalition
Hammer toe, congenital
Q66.9 Congenital deformity of feet, unspecified

Q67 Congenital musculoskeletal deformities of head, face, spine and chest
Excludes1 congenital malformation syndromes classified to Q87.-
Potter's syndrome (Q60.6)
Q67.0 Congenital facial asymmetry
Q67.1 Congenital compression facies
Q67.2 Dolichocephaly
Long head dimension
Q67.3 Plagiocephaly
Asymmetric shape of head resulting from irregular closure of cranial sutures
Q67.4 Other congenital deformities of skull, face and jaw
Congenital depressions in skull
Congenital hemifacial atrophy or hypertrophy
Deviation of nasal septum, congenital
Squashed or bent nose, congenital
Excludes1 dentofacial anomalies [including malocclusion] (M26.-)
syphilitic saddle nose (A50.5)

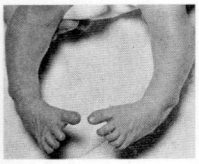

Figure 17-8 Mild to moderate inbowing of the lower leg. (From Jones KL: Smith's Recognizable Patterns of Human Malformation, ed 6, Philadelphia, Saunders, 2005)

Q67.5 Congenital deformity of spine
Congenital postural scoliosis
Congenital scoliosis NOS
Excludes1 infantile idiopathic scoliosis (M41.0)
scoliosis due to congenital bony malformation (Q76.3)
Ex: Q67.5, Q76.3, Q76.425-Q76.429

Q67.6 Pectus excavatum
Congenital funnel chest
Funnel-shaped chest depression

Q67.7 Pectus carinatum
Congenital pigeon chest

Q67.8 Other congenital deformities of chest
Congenital deformity of chest wall NOS
Ex: Q67.6-Q67.8, Q68.1, Q74.3

Q68 Other congenital musculoskeletal deformities
Excludes1 reduction defects of limb(s) (Q71-Q73)
Excludes2 congenital myotonic chondrodystrophy (G71.13)

Q68.0 Congenital deformity of sternocleidomastoid muscle
Congenital contracture of sternocleidomastoid (muscle)
Congenital (sternomastoid) torticollis
Sternomastoid tumor (congenital)

Q68.1 Congenital deformity of finger(s) and hand
Congenital clubfinger
Spade-like hand (congenital)
Ex: Q67.6-Q67.8, Q68.1, Q74.3

Q68.2 Congenital deformity of knee
Congenital dislocation of knee
Congenital genu recurvatum
Hyperextension of knee resulting from hypermobility

Q68.3 Congenital bowing of femur
Excludes1 anteversion of femur (neck) (Q65.89)

Q68.4 Congenital bowing of tibia and fibula

Q68.5 Congenital bowing of long bones of leg, unspecified

Q68.6 Discoid meniscus

Q68.8 Other specified congenital musculoskeletal deformities
Congenital deformity of clavicle
Congenital deformity of elbow
Congenital deformity of forearm
Congenital deformity of scapula
Congenital deformity of wrist
Congenital dislocation of elbow
Congenital dislocation of shoulder
Congenital dislocation of wrist

Q69 Polydactyly
AKA hyperdactyly, consists of supernumerary fingers or toes

Q69.0 Accessory finger(s)

Q69.1 Accessory thumb(s)

Q69.2 Accessory toe(s)
Accessory hallux

Q69.9 Polydactyly, unspecified
Supernumerary digit(s) NOS

Q70 Syndactyly
Webbing between distal phalanges of adjacent digits

Q70.0 Fused fingers
Complex syndactyly of fingers with synostosis

Q70.00 Fused fingers, unspecified hand

Q70.01 Fused fingers, right hand

Q70.02 Fused fingers, left hand

Q70.03 Fused fingers, bilateral

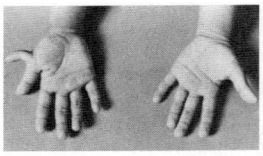

Figure 17-9 Polydactyly, congenital duplicated thumb. (From DeLee: DeLee and Drez's Orthopaedic Sports Medicine, ed 3, Saunders, An Imprint of Elsevier, 2009)

Q70.1 Webbed fingers
Simple syndactyly of fingers without synostosis

Q70.10 Webbed fingers, unspecified hand

Q70.11 Webbed fingers, right hand

Q70.12 Webbed fingers, left hand

Q70.13 Webbed fingers, bilateral

Q70.2 Fused toes
Complex syndactyly of toes with synostosis

Q70.20 Fused toes, unspecified foot

Q70.21 Fused toes, right foot

Q70.22 Fused toes, left foot

Q70.23 Fused toes, bilateral

Q70.3 Webbed toes
Simple syndactyly of toes without synostosis

Q70.30 Webbed toes, unspecified foot

Q70.31 Webbed toes, right foot

Q70.32 Webbed toes, left foot

Q70.33 Webbed toes, bilateral

Q70.4 Polysyndactyly, unspecified
Excludes1 specified syndactyly of hand and feet - code to specified conditions (Q70.0- -Q70.3-)
Extra and webbed digits

Q70.9 Syndactyly, unspecified
Symphalangy NOS

Q71 Reduction defects of upper limb

Q71.0 Congenital complete absence of upper limb

Q71.00 Congenital complete absence of unspecified upper limb

Q71.01 Congenital complete absence of right upper limb

Q71.02 Congenital complete absence of left upper limb

Q71.03 Congenital complete absence of upper limb, bilateral

Q71.1 Congenital absence of upper arm and forearm with hand present

Q71.10 Congenital absence of unspecified upper arm and forearm with hand present

Q71.11 Congenital absence of right upper arm and forearm with hand present

Q71.12 Congenital absence of left upper arm and forearm with hand present

Q71.13 Congenital absence of upper arm and forearm with hand present, bilateral

Q71.2 Congenital absence of both forearm and hand

Q71.20 Congenital absence of both forearm and hand, unspecified upper limb

Q71.21 Congenital absence of both forearm and hand, right upper limb

Q71.22 Congenital absence of both forearm and hand, left upper limb

Q71.23 Congenital absence of both forearm and hand, bilateral

Q71.3 Congenital absence of hand and finger

Q71.30 Congenital absence of unspecified hand and finger

Q71.31 Congenital absence of right hand and finger

Q71.32 Congenital absence of left hand and finger

Q71.33 Congenital absence of hand and finger, bilateral

◀ New ◀ Revised ~~deleted~~ Deleted Excludes 1 Excludes 2 Includes Use additional Code first Code also Unspecified
OGCR Official Guidelines ● Unacceptable Principal Diagnosis X Assign placeholder X ● Use Additional Character(s) ▶ Manifestation Code Coding Clinic

- **Q71.4 Longitudinal reduction defect of radius**
  Clubhand (congenital)
  Radial clubhand
  - **Q71.40 Longitudinal reduction defect of unspecified radius**
  - **Q71.41 Longitudinal reduction defect of right radius**
  - **Q71.42 Longitudinal reduction defect of left radius**
  - **Q71.43 Longitudinal reduction defect of radius, bilateral**
- **Q71.5 Longitudinal reduction defect of ulna**
  - **Q71.50 Longitudinal reduction defect of unspecified ulna**
  - **Q71.51 Longitudinal reduction defect of right ulna**
  - **Q71.52 Longitudinal reduction defect of left ulna**
  - **Q71.53 Longitudinal reduction defect of ulna, bilateral**
- **Q71.6 Lobster-claw hand**
  - **Q71.60 Lobster-claw hand, unspecified hand**
  - **Q71.61 Lobster-claw right hand**
  - **Q71.62 Lobster-claw left hand**
  - **Q71.63 Lobster-claw hand, bilateral**
- **Q71.8 Other reduction defects of upper limb**
  - **Q71.81 Congenital shortening of upper limb**
    - **Q71.811 Congenital shortening of right upper limb**
    - **Q71.812 Congenital shortening of left upper limb**
    - **Q71.813 Congenital shortening of upper limb, bilateral**
    - **Q71.819 Congenital shortening of unspecified upper limb**
  - **Q71.89 Other reduction defects of upper limb**
    - **Q71.891 Other reduction defects of right upper limb**
    - **Q71.892 Other reduction defects of left upper limb**
    - **Q71.893 Other reduction defects of upper limb, bilateral**
    - **Q71.899 Other reduction defects of unspecified upper limb**
- **Q71.9 Unspecified reduction defect of upper limb**
  - **Q71.90 Unspecified reduction defect of unspecified upper limb**
  - **Q71.91 Unspecified reduction defect of right upper limb**
  - **Q71.92 Unspecified reduction defect of left upper limb**
  - **Q71.93 Unspecified reduction defect of upper limb, bilateral**

- **Q72 Reduction defects of lower limb**
  - **Q72.0 Congenital complete absence of lower limb**
    - **Q72.00 Congenital complete absence of unspecified lower limb**
    - **Q72.01 Congenital complete absence of right lower limb**
    - **Q72.02 Congenital complete absence of left lower limb**
    - **Q72.03 Congenital complete absence of lower limb, bilateral**
  - **Q72.1 Congenital absence of thigh and lower leg with foot present**
    - **Q72.10 Congenital absence of unspecified thigh and lower leg with foot present**
    - **Q72.11 Congenital absence of right thigh and lower leg with foot present**
    - **Q72.12 Congenital absence of left thigh and lower leg with foot present**
    - **Q72.13 Congenital absence of thigh and lower leg with foot present, bilateral**
  - **Q72.2 Congenital absence of both lower leg and foot**
    - **Q72.20 Congenital absence of both lower leg and foot, unspecified lower limb**
    - **Q72.21 Congenital absence of both lower leg and foot, right lower limb**
    - **Q72.22 Congenital absence of both left lower leg and foot, left lower limb**
    - **Q72.23 Congenital absence of both lower leg and foot, bilateral**
  - **Q72.3 Congenital absence of foot and toe(s)**
    - **Q72.30 Congenital absence of unspecified foot and toe(s)**
    - **Q72.31 Congenital absence of right foot and toe(s)**
    - **Q72.32 Congenital absence of left foot and toe(s)**
    - **Q72.33 Congenital absence of foot and toe(s), bilateral**
  - **Q72.4 Longitudinal reduction defect of femur**
    Proximal femoral focal deficiency
    - **Q72.40 Longitudinal reduction defect of unspecified femur**
    - **Q72.41 Longitudinal reduction defect of right femur**
    - **Q72.42 Longitudinal reduction defect of left femur**
    - **Q72.43 Longitudinal reduction defect of femur, bilateral**
  - **Q72.5 Longitudinal reduction defect of tibia**
    - **Q72.50 Longitudinal reduction defect of unspecified tibia**
    - **Q72.51 Longitudinal reduction defect of right tibia**
    - **Q72.52 Longitudinal reduction defect of left tibia**
    - **Q72.53 Longitudinal reduction defect of tibia, bilateral**
  - **Q72.6 Longitudinal reduction defect of fibula**
    - **Q72.60 Longitudinal reduction defect of unspecified fibula**
    - **Q72.61 Longitudinal reduction defect of right fibula**
    - **Q72.62 Longitudinal reduction defect of left fibula**
    - **Q72.63 Longitudinal reduction defect of fibula, bilateral**
  - **Q72.7 Split foot**
    - **Q72.70 Split foot, unspecified lower limb**
    - **Q72.71 Split foot, right lower limb**
    - **Q72.72 Split foot, left lower limb**
    - **Q72.73 Split foot, bilateral**
  - **Q72.8 Other reduction defects of lower limb**
    - **Q72.81 Congenital shortening of lower limb**
      - **Q72.811 Congenital shortening of right lower limb**
      - **Q72.812 Congenital shortening of left lower limb**
      - **Q72.813 Congenital shortening of lower limb, bilateral**
      - **Q72.819 Congenital shortening of unspecified lower limb**
    - **Q72.89 Other reduction defects of lower limb**
      - **Q72.891 Other reduction defects of right lower limb**
      - **Q72.892 Other reduction defects of left lower limb**
      - **Q72.893 Other reduction defects of lower limb, bilateral**
      - **Q72.899 Other reduction defects of unspecified lower limb**
  - **Q72.9 Unspecified reduction defect of lower limb**
    - **Q72.90 Unspecified reduction defect of unspecified lower limb**
    - **Q72.91 Unspecified reduction defect of right lower limb**
    - **Q72.92 Unspecified reduction defect of left lower limb**
    - **Q72.93 Unspecified reduction defect of lower limb, bilateral**

● **Q73 Reduction defects of unspecified limb**

Q73.0 Congenital absence of unspecified limb(s)
Amelia NOS

Q73.1 Phocomelia, unspecified limb(s)
Phocomelia NOS
Absence/shortening of long bones primarily as a result of thalidomide

Q73.8 Other reduction defects of unspecified limb(s)
Longitudinal reduction deformity of unspecified limb(s)
Ectromelia of limb NOS
Gross hypoplasia or aplasia of one or more long bones of limb(s)
Hemimelia of limb NOS
Absence of one-half of long bone
Reduction defect of limb NOS

● **Q74 Other congenital malformations of limb(s)**

Excludes1 polydactyly (Q69.-)
reduction defect of limb (Q71-Q73)
syndactyly (Q70.-)

Q74.0 Other congenital malformations of upper limb(s), including shoulder girdle
Accessory carpal bones
Cleidocranial dysostosis
Congenital pseudarthrosis of clavicle
Macrodactylia (fingers)
Madelung's deformity
Radioulnar synostosis
Sprengel's deformity
Triphalangeal thumb

Q74.1 Congenital malformation of knee
Congenital absence of patella
Congenital dislocation of patella
Congenital genu valgum
Congenital genu varum
Rudimentary patella

Excludes1 congenital dislocation of knee (Q68.2)
congenital genu recurvatum (Q68.2)
nail patella syndrome (Q87.2)

Q74.2 Other congenital malformations of lower limb(s), including pelvic girdle
Congenital fusion of sacroiliac joint
Congenital malformation of ankle joint
Congenital malformation of sacroiliac joint

Excludes1 anteversion of femur (neck) (Q65.89)

Q74.3 Arthrogryposis multiplex congenita
Ex Q67.6-Q67.8, Q68.1, Q74.3

Q74.8 Other specified congenital malformations of limb(s)

Q74.9 Unspecified congenital malformation of limb(s)
Congenital anomaly of limb(s) NOS

● **Q75 Other congenital malformations of skull and face bones**

Excludes1 congenital malformation of face NOS (Q18.-)
congenital malformation syndromes classified to Q87.-
dentofacial anomalies [including malocclusion] (M26.-)
musculoskeletal deformities of head and face (Q67.0-Q67.4)
skull defects associated with congenital anomalies of brain such as:
anencephaly (Q00.0)
encephalocele (Q01.-)
hydrocephalus (Q03.-)
microcephaly (Q02)

Q75.0 Craniosynostosis
Premature closure of sutures of skull
Acrocephaly
Imperfect fusion of skull
Oxycephaly
Trigonocephaly

Q75.1 Craniofacial dysostosis
Congential deformity of head
Crouzon's disease

Item 17–3 Anencephalus is a congenital deformity of the cranial vault. **Craniosynostosis,** also known as craniostenosis and stenocephaly, signifies any form of congenital deformity of the skull that results from the premature closing of the sutures of the skull. **Inencephaly** is a deformity in which the head and neck are flexed backward to a great extent and the head is very large in comparison to the shortened body.

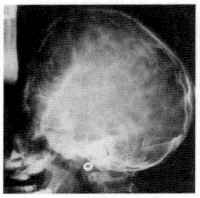

Figure 17-10 Generalized craniosynostosis in a 4-year-old girl without symptoms or signs of increased intracranial pressure. (From Bell WE, McCormick WF: Increased Intracranial Pressure in Children, ed 2, Philadelphia, WB Saunders, 1978, p 116)

Q75.2 Hypertelorism

Q75.3 Macrocephaly
Unusually large size of head; AKA megalocephaly

Q75.4 Mandibulofacial dysostosis
Franceschetti syndrome
Treacher Collins syndrome

Q75.5 Oculomandibular dysostosis
Ossification of occular and mandibular bones

Q75.8 Other specified congenital malformations of skull and face bones
Absence of skull bone, congenital
Congenital deformity of forehead
Platybasia

Q75.9 Congenital malformation of skull and face bones, unspecified
Congenital anomaly of face bones NOS
Congenital anomaly of skull NOS

● **Q76 Congenital malformations of spine and bony thorax**

Excludes1 congenital musculoskeletal deformities of spine and chest (Q67.5-Q67.8)

Q76.0 Spina bifida occulta

Excludes1 meningocele (spinal) (Q05.-)
spina bifida (aperta) (cystica) (Q05.-)

Q76.1 Klippel-Feil syndrome
Cervical fusion syndrome

Q76.2 Congenital spondylolisthesis
Congenital spondylolysis

Excludes1 spondylolisthesis (acquired) (M43.1-)
spondylolysis (acquired) (M43.0-)

Q76.3 Congenital scoliosis due to congenital bony malformation
Hemivertebra fusion or failure of segmentation with scoliosis
Ex Q67.5, Q76.3, Q76.425-Q76.429

● **Q76.4 Other congenital malformations of spine, not associated with scoliosis**

● **Q76.41 Congenital kyphosis**
Abnormal increase in convexity curvature of thoracic spinal column; AKA humpback

Q76.411 Congenital kyphosis, occipito-atlanto-axial region

Q76.412 Congenital kyphosis, cervical region

Q76.413 Congenital kyphosis, cervicothoracic region

Q76.414 Congenital kyphosis, thoracic region

Q76.415 Congenital kyphosis, thoracolumbar region

Q76.419 Congenital kyphosis, unspecified region

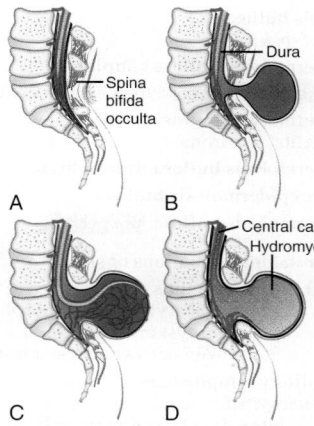

Figure 17-11 **A.** Spina bifida occulta. **B.** Meningocele. **C.** Myelomeningocele. **D.** Myelocystocele (syringomyelocele) or hydromyelia.

Item 17–4 **Spina bifida** is a midline spinal defect in which one or more vertebrae fail to fuse, leaving an opening in the vertebral canal. When the defect is not visible, it is called spina bifida occulta, and when it is visible, it is called spina bifida cystica.

● **Q76.42 Congenital lordosis**
An abnormal increase in curvature of lumbar spine (sway back)
Ex: **For category Q76.42 CC codes:** Q67.5, Q76.3, Q76.425-Q76.429

Q76.425 Congenital lordosis, thoracolumbar region CC
Q76.426 Congenital lordosis, lumbar region CC
Q76.427 Congenital lordosis, lumbosacral region CC
Q76.428 Congenital lordosis, sacral and sacrococcygeal region CC
Q76.429 Congenital lordosis, unspecified region CC

Q76.49 Other congenital malformations of spine, not associated with scoliosis
Congenital absence of vertebra NOS
Congenital fusion of spine NOS
Congenital malformation of lumbosacral (joint) (region) NOS
Congenital malformation of spine NOS
Hemivertebra NOS
Malformation of spine NOS
Platyspondylisis NOS
Supernumerary vertebra NOS

Q76.5 Cervical rib
Supernumerary rib in cervical region

Q76.6 Other congenital malformations of ribs CC
Accessory rib
Congenital absence of rib
Congenital fusion of ribs
Congenital malformation of ribs NOS
Excludes1 short rib syndrome (Q77.2)
Ex: Q76.5-Q76.9, Q77.2

Q76.7 Congenital malformation of sternum CC
Congenital absence of sternum
Sternum bifidum
Ex: Q76.5-Q76.9, Q77.2

Q76.8 Other congenital malformations of bony thorax CC
Ex: Q76.5-Q76.9, Q77.2

Q76.9 Congenital malformation of bony thorax, unspecified CC
Ex: Q76.5-Q76.9, Q77.2

● **Q77 Osteochondrodysplasia with defects of growth of tubular bones and spine**
Excludes1 mucopolysaccharidosis (E76.0-E76.3)
Excludes2 congenital myotonic chondrodystrophy (G71.13)

Q77.0 Achondrogenesis
Hypochondrogenesis

Q77.1 Thanatophoric short stature

Q77.2 Short rib syndrome CC
Asphyxiating thoracic dysplasia [Jeune]
Ex: Q76.5-Q76.9, Q77.2

Q77.3 Chondrodysplasia punctata
Benign cartilaginous neoplasms
Excludes1 rhizomelic chondrodysplasia punctata (E71.43)

Q77.4 Achondroplasia
Disturbance of epiphyseal chondroblastic growth and maturation, results in dwarfism
Hypochondroplasia
Osteosclerosis congenita

Q77.5 Diastrophic dysplasia

Q77.6 Chondroectodermal dysplasia
Defective development of skin, hair, teeth, with polydactyly and defect of cardiac septum
Ellis-van Creveld syndrome

Q77.7 Spondyloepiphyseal dysplasia

Q77.8 Other osteochondrodysplasia with defects of growth of tubular bones and spine

Q77.9 Osteochondrodysplasia with defects of growth of tubular bones and spine, unspecified

● **Q78 Other osteochondrodysplasias**
Disorder of development of bone and cartilage; common cause of dwarfism
Excludes2 congenital myotonic chondrodystrophy (G71.13)

Q78.0 Osteogenesis imperfecta CC
Fragilitas ossium
Osteopsathyrosis
Ex: Q77.3, Q77.6, Q78.0-Q78.3, Q78.5-Q78.9

Q78.1 Polyostotic fibrous dysplasia
Albright(-McCune)(-Sternberg) syndrome
Ex: See Q78.0

Q78.2 Osteopetrosis CC
Abnormally dense bone; AKA marble bones disease, ivory bones
Albers-Schönberg syndrome
Osteosclerosis NOS

Q78.3 Progressive diaphyseal dysplasia
Camurati-Engelmann syndrome

Q78.4 Enchondromatosis
Thinning of overlying cortex of bone and distorted length
Maffucci's syndrome
Ollier's disease

Q78.5 Metaphyseal dysplasia
Disturbance in enchondral bone growth, causing ends of shafts to remain larger than normal in circumference
Pyle's syndrome

Q78.6 Multiple congenital exostoses
Diaphyseal aclasis

Q78.8 Other specified osteochondrodysplasias
Osteopoikilosis

Q78.9 Osteochondrodysplasia, unspecified
Chondrodystrophy NOS
AKA skeletal dysplasia (dwarfism) caused by genetic mutations affecting hyaline cartilage capping long bones and vertebrae
Osteodystrophy NOS

● **Q79 Congenital malformations of musculoskeletal system, not elsewhere classified**

Excludes2 congenital (sternomastoid) torticollis (Q68.0)

Q79.0 Congenital diaphragmatic hernia

Excludes1 congenital hiatus hernia (Q40.1)

Ex Q40.1, Q79.0-Q79.1

Q79.1 Other congenital malformations of diaphragm

Absence of diaphragm
Congenital malformation of diaphragm NOS
Eventration of diaphragm

Ex Q40.1, Q79.0-Q79.1

Q79.2 Exomphalos

Abdominal hernia in which part of intestine protrudes at umbilicus; AKA exomphalos and exumbilication

Omphalocele

Excludes1 umbilical hernia (K42.-)

Ex Q79.2-Q79.59

Q79.3 Gastroschisis

Congenital fissure of anterior abdominal wall often with protrusion of small/large intestine

Ex Q79.2-Q79.59

Q79.4 Prune belly syndrome

Congenital prolapse of bladder mucosa
Eagle-Barrett syndrome

Ex Q79.2-Q79.59

● **Q79.5 Other congenital malformations of abdominal wall**

Excludes1 umbilical hernia (K42.-)

Ex For category Q79.5 CC codes: Q79.2-Q79.59

Q79.51 Congenital hernia of bladder

Q79.59 Other congenital malformations of abdominal wall

Q79.6 Ehlers-Danlos syndrome

Ex Q79.6

Group of inherited disorders of connective tissue; AKA cutis hyperelastica

Q79.8 Other congenital malformations of musculoskeletal system

Absence of muscle
Absence of tendon
Accessory muscle
Amyotrophia congenita
Congenital constricting bands
Congenital shortening of tendon
Poland syndrome

Q79.9 Congenital malformation of musculoskeletal system, unspecified

Congenital anomaly of musculoskeletal system NOS
Congenital deformity of musculoskeletal system NOS

OTHER CONGENITAL MALFORMATIONS (Q80-Q89)

● **Q80 Congenital ichthyosis**

Characterized by increased keratinization, resulting in noninflammatory scaling of skin

Excludes1 Refsum's disease (G60.1)

Q80.0 Ichthyosis vulgaris

Q80.1 X-linked ichthyosis

Q80.2 Lamellar ichthyosis

Collodion baby

Q80.3 Congenital bullous ichthyosiform erythroderma

Q80.4 Harlequin fetus

Q80.8 Other congenital ichthyosis

Q80.9 Congenital ichthyosis, unspecified

● **Q81 Epidermolysis bullosa**

Loosening of epidermis

Q81.0 Epidermolysis bullosa simplex

Excludes1 Cockayne's syndrome (Q87.1)

Q81.1 Epidermolysis bullosa letalis

Herlitz' syndrome

Q81.2 Epidermolysis bullosa dystrophica

Q81.8 Other epidermolysis bullosa

Q81.9 Epidermolysis bullosa, unspecified

● **Q82 Other congenital malformations of skin**

Excludes1 acrodermatitis enteropathica (E83.2)
congenital erythropoietic porphyria (E80.0)
pilonidal cyst or sinus (L05.-)
Sturge-Weber (-Dimitri) syndrome (Q85.8)

Q82.0 Hereditary lymphedema

Characterized by swelling of subcutaneous tissue caused by obstruction of lymphatic vessels and resulting edema of lymph fluid

Q82.1 Xeroderma pigmentosum

Dry, rough, discolored state of skin, and formation of scaly desquamation

Q82.2 Mastocytosis

Characterized by infiltrates of mast cells in tissues/organs

Urticaria pigmentosa

Excludes1 malignant mastocytosis (C96.2)

Q82.3 Incontinentia pigmenti

Characterized by hyperpigmented cutaneous

Q82.4 Ectodermal dysplasia (anhidrotic)

Absence/deficiency of tissues/structures, including teeth, hair, nails, and certain glands

Excludes1 Ellis-van Creveld syndrome (Q77.6)

Q82.5 Congenital non-neoplastic nevus

Birthmark NOS
Flammeus Nevus
Portwine Nevus
Sanguineous Nevus
Strawberry Nevus
Vascular Nevus NOS
Verrucous Nevus

Excludes2 Café au lait spots (L81.3)
lentigo (L81.4)
nevus NOS (D22.-)
araneus nevus (I78.1)
melanocytic nevus (D22.-)
pigmented nevus (D22.-)
spider nevus (I78.1)
stellar nevus (I78.1)

Q82.6 Congenital sacral dimple ◀

Parasacral dimple ◀

Excludes2 pilonidal cyst with abscess (L05.01) ◀
pilonidal cyst without abscess (L05.91) ◀

Q82.8 Other specified congenital malformations of skin

Abnormal palmar creases
Accessory skin tags
Benign familial pemphigus [Hailey-Hailey]
Congenital poikiloderma
Cutis laxa (hyperelastica)
Dermatoglyphic anomalies
Inherited keratosis palmaris et plantaris
Keratosis follicularis [Darier-White]

Excludes1 Ehlers-Danlos syndrome (Q79.6)

Coding Clinic: 2016, Q1, P17

Q82.9 Congenital malformation of skin, unspecified

Q83 Congenital malformations of breast

Excludes2 absence of pectoral muscle (Q79.8)
hypoplasia of breast (N64.82)
micromastia (N64.82)

Q83.0 Congenital absence of breast with absent nipple

Q83.1 Accessory breast
Supernumerary breast

Q83.2 Absent nipple

Q83.3 Accessory nipple
Supernumerary nipple

Q83.8 Other congenital malformations of breast

Q83.9 Congenital malformation of breast, unspecified

Q84 Other congenital malformations of integument

Q84.0 Congenital alopecia
Congenital atrichosis

Q84.1 Congenital morphological disturbances of hair, not elsewhere classified
Beaded hair
Monilethrix
Pili annulati

Excludes1 Menkes' kinky hair syndrome (E83.0)

Q84.2 Other congenital malformations of hair
Congenital hypertrichosis
Congenital malformation of hair NOS
Persistent lanugo

Q84.3 Anonychia
Absence of nail

Excludes1 nail patella syndrome (Q87.2)

Q84.4 Congenital leukonychia
Opaque, whitish discoloration of nails; AKA leukopathia unguium

Q84.5 Enlarged and hypertrophic nails
Congenital onychauxis
Pachyonychia

Q84.6 Other congenital malformations of nails
Congenital clubnail
Congenital koilonychia
Congenital malformation of nail NOS

Q84.8 Other specified congenital malformations of integument
Aplasia cutis congenita

Q84.9 Congenital malformation of integument, unspecified
Congenital anomaly of integument NOS
Congenital deformity of integument NOS

Q85 Phakomatoses, not elsewhere classified

Excludes1 ataxia telangiectasia [Louis-Bar] (G11.3)
familial dysautonomia [Riley-Day] (G90.1)

Q85.0 Neurofibromatosis (nonmalignant)
Developmental changes in nervous system and other structures, with formation of neurofibromas

Q85.00 Neurofibromatosis, unspecified

Q85.01 Neurofibromatosis, type 1
Von Recklinghausen disease

Q85.02 Neurofibromatosis, type 2
Acoustic neurofibromatosis

Q85.03 Schwannomatosis

Q85.09 Other neurofibromatosis

Q85.1 Tuberous sclerosis
Bourneville's disease
Epiloia
Ex: Q85.1-Q85.9, Q89.7, Q89.9

Q85.8 Other phakomatoses, not elsewhere classified
Peutz-Jeghers Syndrome
Sturge-Weber(-Dimitri) syndrome
von Hippel-Lindau syndrome

Excludes1 Meckel-Gruber syndrome (Q61.9)
Ex: Q85.8-Q85.9, Q89.9

Q85.9 Phakomatosis, unspecified
Hamartosis NOS
Ex: Q85.8-Q85.9, Q89.9

Q86 Congenital malformation syndromes due to known exogenous causes, not elsewhere classified

Excludes2 iodine-deficiency-related hypothyroidism (E00-E02)
nonteratogenic effects of substances transmitted via placenta or breast milk (P04.-)

Q86.0 Fetal alcohol syndrome (dysmorphic)

Q86.1 Fetal hydantoin syndrome
Meadow's syndrome

Q86.2 Dysmorphism due to warfarin

Q86.8 Other congenital malformation syndromes due to known exogenous causes

Q87 Other specified congenital malformation syndromes affecting multiple systems

Use additional code(s) to identify all associated manifestations

Q87.0 Congenital malformation syndromes predominantly affecting facial appearance
Acrocephalopolysyndactyly
Acrocephalosyndactyly [Apert]
Cryptophthalmos syndrome
Cyclopia
Goldenhar syndrome
Moebius syndrome
Oro-facial-digital syndrome
Robin syndrome
Whistling face

Q87.1 Congenital malformation syndromes predominantly associated with short stature
Aarskog syndrome
Cockayne syndrome
De Lange syndrome
Dubowitz syndrome
Noonan syndrome
Prader-Willi syndrome
Robinow-Silverman-Smith syndrome
Russell-Silver syndrome
Seckel syndrome

Excludes1 Ellis-van Creveld syndrome (Q77.6)
Smith-Lemli-Opitz syndrome (E78.72)
Ex: E78.71-E78.72, Q85.8-Q85.9, Q87.1-Q87.89, Q89.7-Q89.9, Q99.2

Q87.2 Congenital malformation syndromes predominantly involving limbs
Holt-Oram syndrome
Klippel-Trenaunay-Weber syndrome
Nail patella syndrome
Rubinstein-Taybi syndrome
Sirenomelia syndrome
Thrombocytopenia with absent radius [TAR] syndrome
VATER syndrome
Ex: E78.71-E78.72, Q87.1-Q87.89, Q89.8, Q99.2

Q87.3 Congenital malformation syndromes involving early overgrowth
Beckwith-Wiedemann syndrome
Sotos' syndrome
Weaver syndrome
Ex: See Q87.2

Q87.4 Marfan's syndrome
Ex: For category Q87.4 CC codes: See Q87.1

Q87.40 Marfan's syndrome, unspecified

Q87.41 Marfan's syndrome with cardiovascular manifestations

Q87.410 Marfan's syndrome with aortic dilation

Q87.418 Marfan's syndrome with other cardiovascular manifestations

Q87.42 Marfan's syndrome with ocular manifestations

Q87.43 Marfan's syndrome with skeletal manifestation

Q87.5 Other congenital malformation syndromes with other skeletal changes
Ex: See Q87.2

● **Q87.8 Other specified congenital malformation syndromes, not elsewhere classified**
Excludes1 Zellweger syndrome (E71.510)
Ex: For category Q87.8 CC codes: See Q87.2

Q87.81 Alport syndrome
Progressive sensorineural hearing loss, progressive pyelonephritis or glomerulonephritis, and ocular defects
Use additional code to identify stage of chronic kidney disease (N18.1-N18.6)

Q87.82 Arterial tortuosity syndrome ◀

Q87.89 Other specified congenital malformation syndromes, not elsewhere classified
Laurence-Moon (-Bardet)-Biedl syndrome

● **Q89 Other congenital malformations, not elsewhere classified**

● **Q89.0 Congenital absence and malformations of spleen**
Excludes1 isomerism of atrial appendages (with asplenia or polysplenia) (Q20.6)
Ex: For category Q87.8 CC codes: Q89.01-Q89.09, Q89.9

Q89.01 Asplenia (congenital)

Q89.09 Congenital malformations of spleen
Congenital splenomegaly

Q89.1 Congenital malformations of adrenal gland
Excludes1 adrenogenital disorders (E25.-)
congenital adrenal hyperplasia (E25.0)

Q89.2 Congenital malformations of other endocrine glands
Congenital malformation of parathyroid or thyroid gland
Persistent thyroglossal duct
Thyroglossal cyst
Excludes1 congenital goiter (E03.0)
congenital hypothyroidism (E03.1)

Q89.3 Situs inversus
Lateral transposition of viscera of thorax and abdomen
Dextrocardia with situs inversus
Mirror-image atrial arrangement with situs inversus
Situs inversus or transversus abdominalis
Situs inversus or transversus thoracis
Transposition of abdominal viscera
Transposition of thoracic viscera
Excludes1 dextrocardia NOS (Q24.0)
Ex: Q89.3, Q89.7, Q89.9

Q89.4 Conjoined twins
Craniopagus
Dicephaly
Pygopagus
Thoracopagus
Ex: Q89.4-Q89.7, Q89.9

Q89.7 Multiple congenital malformations, not elsewhere classified
Multiple congenital anomalies NOS
Multiple congenital deformities NOS
Excludes1 congenital malformation syndromes affecting multiple systems (Q87.-)
Ex: Q89.3, Q89.7, Q89.9

Q89.8 Other specified congenital malformations
Use additional code(s) to identify all associated manifestations
Ex: See Q87.2

Q89.9 Congenital malformation, unspecified
Congenital anomaly NOS
Congenital deformity NOS

CHROMOSOMAL ABNORMALITIES, NOT ELSEWHERE CLASSIFIED (Q90-Q99)

Excludes2 mitochondrial metabolic disorders (E88.4-)

● **Q90 Down syndrome**
Use additional code(s) to identify any associated physical conditions and degree of intellectual disabilities (F70-F79)

Q90.0 Trisomy 21, nonmosaicism (meiotic nondisjunction)
Trisomy 21, nondisjunction, accounts for 95% of Downs syndrome cases

Q90.1 Trisomy 21, mosaicism (mitotic nondisjunction)

Q90.2 Trisomy 21, translocation

Q90.9 Down syndrome, unspecified
Trisomy 21 NOS

● **Q91 Trisomy 18 and Trisomy 13**
Ex: For category Q91 CC codes: Q90.0-Q99.1, Q99.8-Q99.9

Q91.0 Trisomy 18, nonmosaicism (meiotic nondisjunction)

Q91.1 Trisomy 18, mosaicism (mitotic nondisjunction)

Q91.2 Trisomy 18, translocation

Q91.3 Trisomy 18, unspecified

Q91.4 Trisomy 13, nonmosaicism (meiotic nondisjunction)

Q91.5 Trisomy 13, mosaicism (mitotic nondisjunction)

Q91.6 Trisomy 13, translocation

Q91.7 Trisomy 13, unspecified

● **Q92 Other trisomies and partial trisomies of the autosomes, not elsewhere classified**
Includes unbalanced translocations and insertions
Excludes1 trisomies of chromosomes 13, 18, 21 (Q90-Q91)

Q92.0 Whole chromosome trisomy, nonmosaicism (meiotic nondisjunction)

Q92.1 Whole chromosome trisomy, mosaicism (mitotic nondisjunction)

Q92.2 Partial trisomy
Less than whole arm duplicated
Whole arm or more duplicated
Excludes1 partial trisomy due to unbalanced translocation (Q92.5)

Q92.5 Duplications with other complex rearrangements
Partial trisomy due to unbalanced translocations
Code also any associated deletions due to unbalanced translocations, inversions and insertions (Q93.7)

● **Q92.6 Marker chromosomes**
Trisomies due to dicentrics
Trisomies due to extra rings
Trisomies due to isochromosomes
Individual with marker heterochromatin

Q92.61 Marker chromosomes in normal individual

Q92.62 Marker chromosomes in abnormal individual

Q92.7 Triploidy and polyploidy

Q92.8 Other specified trisomies and partial trisomies of autosomes
Duplications identified by fluorescence in situ hybridization (FISH)
Duplications identified by in situ hybridization (ISH)
Duplications seen only at prometaphase

Q92.9 Trisomy and partial trisomy of autosomes, unspecified

● **Q93 Monosomies and deletions from the autosomes, not elsewhere classified**
Ex: For category Q93 CC codes unless otherwise indicated: Q90.0-Q99.1, Q99.8-Q99.9

Q93.0 Whole chromosome monosomy, nonmosaicism (meiotic nondisjunction)

Q93.1 Whole chromosome monosomy, mosaicism (mitotic nondisjunction)

Q93.2 Chromosome replaced with ring, dicentric or isochromosome

Q93.3 Deletion of short arm of chromosome 4
Wolff-Hirschorn syndrome

Q93.4 Deletion of short arm of chromosome 5
Cri-du-chat syndrome
Ex: Q90.0-Q99.1, Q99.8-Q99.9

Q93.5 Other deletions of part of a chromosome
Angelman syndrome

Q93.7 Deletions with other complex rearrangements
Deletions due to unbalanced translocations, inversions and insertions
Code also any associated duplications due to unbalanced translocations, inversions and insertions (Q92.5)

Q93.8 Other deletions from the autosomes

Q93.81 Velo-cardio-facial syndrome
Deletion 22q11.2
Ex: Q90.0-Q99.1, Q99.8-Q99.9

Q93.88 Other microdeletions Miller-Dieker syndrome
Smith-Magenis syndrome
Ex: Q90.0-Q99.1, Q99.8-Q99.9

Q93.89 Other deletions from the autosomes
Deletions identified by fluorescence in situ hybridization (FISH)
Deletions identified by in situ hybridization (ISH)
Deletions seen only at prometaphase

Q93.9 Deletion from autosomes, unspecified

Q95 Balanced rearrangements and structural markers, not elsewhere classified
Includes Robertsonian and balanced reciprocal translocations and insertions

Q95.0 Balanced translocation and insertion in normal individual

Q95.1 Chromosome inversion in normal individual

Q95.2 Balanced autosomal rearrangement in abnormal individual

Q95.3 Balanced sex/autosomal rearrangement in abnormal individual

Q95.5 Individual with autosomal fragile site

Q95.8 Other balanced rearrangements and structural markers

Q95.9 Balanced rearrangement and structural marker, unspecified

Q96 Turner's syndrome
Caused by missing or incomplete X chromosome affecting growth and sexual development
Excludes1 Noonan syndrome (Q87.1)

Q96.0 Karyotype 45, X ♀

Q96.1 Karyotype 46, X iso (Xq) ♀
Karyotype 46, isochromosome Xq

Q96.2 Karyotype 46, X with abnormal sex chromosome, except iso (Xq) ♀
Karyotype 46, X with abnormal sex chromosome, except isochromosome Xq

Q96.3 Mosaicism, 45, X/46, XX or XY ♀

Q96.4 Mosaicism, 45, X/other cell line(s) with abnormal sex chromosome ♀

Q96.8 Other variants of Turner's syndrome ♀

Q96.9 Turner's syndrome, unspecified ♀

Q97 Other sex chromosome abnormalities, female phenotype, not elsewhere classified
Excludes1 Turner's syndrome (Q96.-)

Q97.0 Karyotype 47, XXX ♀

Q97.1 Female with more than three X chromosomes ♀

Q97.2 Mosaicism, lines with various numbers of X chromosomes ♀

Q97.3 Female with 46, XY karyotype ♀

Q97.8 Other specified sex chromosome abnormalities, female phenotype ♀

Q97.9 Sex chromosome abnormality, female phenotype, unspecified ♀

Q98 Other sex chromosome abnormalities, male phenotype, not elsewhere classified

Q98.0 Klinefelter syndrome karyotype 47, XXY ♂

Q98.1 Klinefelter syndrome, male with more than two X chromosomes ♂

Q98.3 Other male with 46, XX karyotype ♂

Q98.4 Klinefelter syndrome, unspecified ♂

Q98.5 Karyotype 47, XYY

Q98.6 Male with structurally abnormal sex chromosome ♂

Q98.7 Male with sex chromosome mosaicism ♂

Q98.8 Other specified sex chromosome abnormalities, male phenotype ♂

Q98.9 Sex chromosome abnormality, male phenotype, unspecified ♂

Q99 Other chromosome abnormalities, not elsewhere classified

Q99.0 Chimera 46, XX/46, XY
Chimera 46, XX/46, XY true hermaphrodite

Q99.1 46, XX true hermaphrodite
46, XX with streak gonads
46, XY with streak gonads
Pure gonadal dysgenesis

Q99.2 Fragile X chromosome
Fragile X syndrome

Q99.8 Other specified chromosome abnormalities

Q99.9 Chromosomal abnormality, unspecified

CHAPTER 18

SYMPTOMS, SIGNS AND ABNORMAL CLINICAL AND LABORATORY FINDINGS, NOT ELSEWHERE CLASSIFIED (RØØ-R99)

OGCR Chapter-Specific Coding Guidelines

18. Chapter 18: Symptoms, signs, and abnormal clinical and laboratory findings, not elsewhere classified (RØØ-R99)

Chapter 18 includes symptoms, signs, abnormal results of clinical or other investigative procedures, and ill-defined conditions regarding which no diagnosis classifiable elsewhere is recorded. Signs and symptoms that point to a specific diagnosis have been assigned to a category in other chapters of the classification.

a. Use of symptom codes

Codes that describe symptoms and signs are acceptable for reporting purposes when a related definitive diagnosis has not been established (confirmed) by the provider.

b. Use of a symptom code with a definitive diagnosis code

Codes for signs and symptoms may be reported in addition to a related definitive diagnosis when the sign or symptom is not routinely associated with that diagnosis, such as the various signs and symptoms associated with complex syndromes. The definitive diagnosis code should be sequenced before the symptom code.

Signs or symptoms that are associated routinely with a disease process should not be assigned as additional codes, unless otherwise instructed by the classification.

c. Combination codes that include symptoms

ICD-10-CM contains a number of combination codes that identify both the definitive diagnosis and common symptoms of that diagnosis. When using one of these combination codes, an additional code should not be assigned for the symptom.

d. Repeated falls

Code R29.6, Repeated falls, is for use for encounters when a patient has recently fallen and the reason for the fall is being investigated.

Code Z91.81, History of falling, is for use when a patient has fallen in the past and is at risk for future falls. When appropriate, both codes R29.6 and Z91.81 may be assigned together.

e. Coma scale

The coma scale codes (R4Ø.2-) can be used in conjunction with traumatic brain injury codes, acute cerebrovascular disease or sequelae of cerebrovascular disease codes. These codes are primarily for use by trauma registries, but they may be used in any setting where this information is collected. **The coma scale may also be used to assess the status of the central nervous system for other non-trauma conditions, such as monitoring patients in the intensive care unit regardless of medical condition.** The coma scale codes should be sequenced after the diagnosis code(s).

These codes, one from each subcategory, are needed to complete the scale. The 7th character indicates when the scale was recorded. The 7th character should match for all three codes.

At a minimum, report the initial score documented on presentation at your facility. This may be a score from the emergency medicine technician (EMT) or in the emergency department. If desired, a facility may choose to capture multiple coma scale scores.

Assign code R4Ø.24, Glasgow coma scale, total score, when only the total score is documented in the medical record and not the individual score(s).

f. Functional quadriplegia

Functional quadriplegia (code R53.2) is the lack of ability to use one's limbs or to ambulate due to extreme debility. It is not associated with neurologic deficit or injury, and code R53.2 should not be used for cases of neurologic quadriplegia. It should only be assigned if functional quadriplegia is specifically documented in the medical record.

g. SIRS due to Non-Infectious Process

The systemic inflammatory response syndrome (SIRS) can develop as a result of certain non-infectious disease processes, such as trauma, malignant neoplasm, or pancreatitis. When SIRS is documented with a noninfectious condition, and no subsequent infection is documented, the code for the underlying condition, such as an injury, should be assigned, followed by code R65.1Ø, Systemic inflammatory response syndrome (SIRS) of non-infectious origin without acute organ dysfunction, or code R65.11, Systemic inflammatory response syndrome (SIRS) of non-infectious origin with acute organ dysfunction. If an associated acute organ dysfunction is documented, the appropriate code(s) for the specific type of organ dysfunction(s) should be assigned in addition to code R65.11. If acute organ dysfunction is documented, but it cannot be determined if the acute organ dysfunction is associated with SIRS or due to another condition (e.g., directly due to the trauma), the provider should be queried.

h. Death NOS

Code R99, Ill-defined and unknown cause of mortality, is only for use in the very limited circumstance when a patient who has already died is brought into an emergency department or other healthcare facility and is pronounced dead upon arrival. It does not represent the discharge disposition of death.

i. NIHSS Stroke Scale

The NIH stroke scale (NIHSS) codes (R29.7- -) can be used in conjunction with acute stroke codes (I63) to identify the patient's neurological status and the severity of the stroke. The stroke scale codes should be sequenced after the acute stroke diagnosis code(s).

At a minimum, report the initial score documented. If desired, a facility may choose to capture multiple stroke scale scores.

See Section I.B.14. for information concerning the medical record documentation that may be used for assignment of the NIHSS codes.

OGCR Section I.B.4.

Signs and symptoms

Codes that describe symptoms and signs, as opposed to diagnoses, are acceptable for reporting purposes when a related definitive diagnosis has not been established (confirmed) by the provider. Chapter 18 of ICD-10-CM, Symptoms, Signs, and Abnormal Clinical and Laboratory Findings, Not Elsewhere Classified (codes RØØ.Ø-R99) contains many, but not all codes for symptoms.

CHAPTER 18

SYMPTOMS, SIGNS AND ABNORMAL CLINICAL AND LABORATORY FINDINGS, NOT ELSEWHERE CLASSIFIED (RØØ-R99)

Note: This chapter includes symptoms, signs, abnormal results of clinical or other investigative procedures, and ill-defined conditions regarding which no diagnosis classifiable elsewhere is recorded.

Signs and symptoms that point rather definitely to a given diagnosis have been assigned to a category in other chapters of the classification. In general, categories in this chapter include the less well-defined conditions and symptoms that, without the necessary study of the case to establish a final diagnosis, point perhaps equally to two or more diseases or to two or more systems of the body. Practically all categories in the chapter could be designated 'not otherwise specified', 'unknown etiology' or 'transient'. The Alphabetical Index should be consulted to determine which symptoms and signs are to be allocated here and which to other chapters. The residual subcategories, numbered .8, are generally provided for other relevant symptoms that cannot be allocated elsewhere in the classification.

The conditions and signs or symptoms included in categories RØØ-R94 consist of:

(a) cases for which no more specific diagnosis can be made even after all the facts bearing on the case have been investigated;
(b) signs or symptoms existing at the time of initial encounter that proved to be transient and whose causes could not be determined;
(c) provisional diagnosis in a patient who failed to return for further investigation or care;
(d) cases referred elsewhere for investigation or treatment before the diagnosis was made;
(e) cases in which a more precise diagnosis was not available for any other reason;
(f) certain symptoms, for which supplementary information is provided, that represent important problems in medical care in their own right.

Excludes2 abnormal findings on antenatal screening of mother (O28.-)
certain conditions originating in the perinatal period (PØ4-P96)
signs and symptoms classified in the body system chapters
signs and symptoms of breast (N63, N64.5)

This chapter contains the following blocks:

RØØ-RØ9	Symptoms and signs involving the circulatory and respiratory systems
R1Ø-R19	Symptoms and signs involving the digestive system and abdomen
R2Ø-R23	Symptoms and signs involving the skin and subcutaneous tissue
R25-R29	Symptoms and signs involving the nervous and musculoskeletal systems
R3Ø-R39	Symptoms and signs involving the genitourinary system
R4Ø-R46	Symptoms and signs involving cognition, perception, emotional state and behavior
R47-R49	Symptoms and signs involving speech and voice
R5Ø-R69	General symptoms and signs
R7Ø-R79	Abnormal findings on examination of blood, without diagnosis
R8Ø-R82	Abnormal findings on examination of urine, without diagnosis
R83-R89	Abnormal findings on examination of other body fluids, substances and tissues, without diagnosis
R9Ø-R94	Abnormal findings on diagnostic imaging and in function studies, without diagnosis
R97	Abnormal tumor markers
R99	Ill-defined and unknown cause of mortality

SYMPTOMS AND SIGNS INVOLVING THE CIRCULATORY AND RESPIRATORY SYSTEMS (RØØ-RØ9)

RØØ Abnormalities of heart beat

Excludes1 abnormalities originating in the perinatal period (P29.1-)

Excludes2 specified arrhythmias (I47-I49) ◀

RØØ.Ø Tachycardia, unspecified
Rapid heart rate >1ØØ beats
Rapid heart beat
Sinoauricular tachycardia NOS
Sinus [sinusal] tachycardia NOS

Excludes1 neonatal tachycardia (P29.11)
paroxysmal tachycardia (I47.-)

RØØ.1 Bradycardia, unspecified
Slow heart rate, <6Ø
Sinoatrial bradycardia
Sinus bradycardia
Slow heart beat
Vagal bradycardia

Use additional code for adverse effect, if applicable, to identify drug (T36-T5Ø with fifth or sixth character 5)

Excludes1 neonatal bradycardia (P29.12)

RØØ.2 Palpitations
Awareness of heart beat

RØØ.8 Other abnormalities of heart beat

RØØ.9 Unspecified abnormalities of heart beat

● **R01 Cardiac murmurs and other cardiac sounds**
Excludes1 cardiac murmurs and sounds originating in the perinatal period (P29.8)

R01.0 Benign and innocent cardiac murmurs
Functional cardiac murmur

R01.1 Cardiac murmur, unspecified
Cardiac bruit NOS
Heart murmur NOS
Systolic murmur NOS ◀

R01.2 Other cardiac sounds
Cardiac dullness, increased or decreased
Precordial friction

OGCR Section I.C.9.a.7.

Hypertension, Transient
Assign code R03.0, Elevated blood pressure reading without diagnosis of hypertension, unless patient has an established diagnosis of hypertension. Assign code O13.-, Gestational [pregnancy-induced] hypertension with significant proteinuria, or O14.-, Pre-eclampsia, for transient hypertension of pregnancy.

● **R03 Abnormal blood-pressure reading, without diagnosis**

R03.0 Elevated blood-pressure reading, without diagnosis of hypertension
Note: This category is to be used to record an episode of elevated blood pressure in a patient in whom no formal diagnosis of hypertension has been made, or as an isolated incidental finding.
MCE: Questionable admission when principal dx

R03.1 Nonspecific low blood-pressure reading
Excludes1 hypotension (I95.-)
maternal hypotension syndrome (O26.5-)
neurogenic orthostatic hypotension (G90.3)

● **R04 Hemorrhage from respiratory passages**
Ex For category R04 CC codes: R04.2-R04.9, R09.3, R68.13

R04.0 Epistaxis
Hemorrhage from nose
Nosebleed

R04.1 Hemorrhage from throat
Excludes2 hemoptysis (R04.2)

R04.2 Hemoptysis
Blood-stained sputum
Cough with hemorrhage

● **R04.8 Hemorrhage from other sites in respiratory passages**

R04.81 Acute idiopathic pulmonary hemorrhage in infants P
AIPHI
Acute idiopathic hemorrhage in infants over 28 days old
Excludes1 perinatal pulmonary hemorrhage (P26.-)
von Willebrand's disease (D68.0)

R04.89 Hemorrhage from other sites in respiratory passages
Pulmonary hemorrhage NOS

R04.9 Hemorrhage from respiratory passages, unspecified

R05 Cough
Excludes1 cough with hemorrhage (R04.2)
smoker's cough (J41.0)

● **R06 Abnormalities of breathing**
Excludes1 acute respiratory distress syndrome (J80)
respiratory arrest (R09.2)
respiratory arrest of newborn (P28.81)
respiratory distress syndrome of newborn (P22.-)
respiratory failure (J96.-)
respiratory failure of newborn (P28.5)

● **R06.0 Dyspnea**
Excludes1 tachypnea NOS (R06.82)
transient tachypnea of newborn (P22.1)

R06.00 Dyspnea, unspecified

R06.01 Orthopnea

R06.02 Shortness of breath

R06.09 Other forms of dyspnea

R06.1 Stridor
Harsh, high-pitched breath sound
Excludes1 congenital laryngeal stridor (P28.89)
laryngismus (stridulus) (J38.5)

R06.2 Wheezing
Excludes1 Asthma (J45.-)
Coding Clinic: 2016, Q2, P34

R06.3 Periodic breathing
Cheyne-Stokes breathing
An abnormal pattern of breathing with gradually increasing and decreasing tidal volume with some periods of apnea
Ex J22, J80, J96.00-J96.92, J98.8-J98.9, R06.3, R06.81, R09.2

R06.4 Hyperventilation
Excludes1 psychogenic hyperventilation (F45.8)

R06.5 Mouth breathing
Excludes2 dry mouth NOS (R68.2)

R06.6 Hiccough
Excludes1 psychogenic hiccough (F45.8)

R06.7 Sneezing

● **R06.8 Other abnormalities of breathing**

R06.81 Apnea, not elsewhere classified
Apnea NOS
Excludes1 apnea (of) newborn (P28.4)
sleep apnea (G47.3-)
sleep apnea of newborn (primary) (P28.3)

R06.82 Tachypnea, not elsewhere classified
Tachypnea NOS
Excludes1 transitory tachypnea of newborn (P22.1)

R06.83 Snoring

R06.89 Other abnormalities of breathing
Breath-holding (spells)
Sighing

R06.9 Unspecified abnormalities of breathing

● **R07 Pain in throat and chest**
Excludes1 epidemic myalgia (B33.0)
Excludes2 jaw pain R68.84
pain in breast (N64.4)

R07.0 Pain in throat
Excludes1 chronic sore throat (J31.2)
sore throat (acute) NOS (J02.9)
Excludes2 dysphagia (R13.1-)
pain in neck (M54.2)

R07.1 Chest pain on breathing
Painful respiration

R07.2 Precordial pain

● **R07.8 Other chest pain**

R07.81 Pleurodynia
Pleurodynia NOS
Excludes1 epidemic pleurodynia (B33.0)

R07.82 Intercostal pain

R07.89 Other chest pain
Anterior chest-wall pain NOS

R07.9 Chest pain, unspecified

R09 Other symptoms and signs involving the circulatory and respiratory system

Excludes1 acute respiratory distress syndrome (J80)
respiratory arrest of newborn (P28.81)
respiratory distress syndrome of newborn (P22.0)
respiratory failure (J96.-)
respiratory failure of newborn (P28.5)

R09.0 Asphyxia and hypoxemia

Excludes1 asphyxia due to carbon monoxide (T58.-)
asphyxia due to foreign body in respiratory tract (T17.-)
birth (intrauterine) asphyxia (P84)
hypercapnia (R06.4)
hyperventilation (R06.4)
traumatic asphyxia (T71.-)

R09.01 Asphyxia

Ex G89.0-G89.4, J80, J96.00-J96.92, R09.01-R09.02, R09.2, R29.700-R29.742, R41.0-R41.3, R41.82, R41.9, R44.8-R44.9, R45.83-R45.84, R46.0-R46.89, R52, R68.0-R68.19, R68.81-R68.83, R68.89-R69

R09.02 Hypoxemia

R09.1 Pleurisy

Occurs when double membrane (pleura) lining chest cavity and lung surface becomes inflamed causing sharp pain on inspiration/expiration

Excludes1 pleurisy with effusion (J90)

R09.2 Respiratory arrest

Cardiorespiratory failure

Excludes1 cardiac arrest (I46.-)
respiratory arrest of newborn (P28.81)
respiratory distress of newborn (P22.0)
respiratory failure (J96.-)
respiratory failure of newborn (P28.5)
respiratory insufficiency (R06.89)
respiratory insufficiency of newborn (P28.5)

MCC: Only if patient discharged alive

Ex See R09.01

R09.3 Abnormal sputum

Abnormal amount of sputum
Abnormal color of sputum
Abnormal odor of sputum
Excessive sputum

Excludes1 blood-stained sputum (R04.2)

R09.8 Other specified symptoms and signs involving the circulatory and respiratory systems

R09.81 Nasal congestion

R09.82 Postnasal drip

R09.89 Other specified symptoms and signs involving the circulatory and respiratory systems

Bruit (arterial)
Abnormal chest percussion
Feeling of foreign body in throat
Friction sounds in chest
Chest tympany
Choking sensation
Rales
Wet rattling, clicking, crackling sounds on auscultation
Weak pulse

Excludes2 foreign body in throat (T17.2-)
wheezing (R06.2)

SYMPTOMS AND SIGNS INVOLVING THE DIGESTIVE SYSTEM AND ABDOMEN (R10-R19)

Excludes2 congenital or infantile pylorospasm (Q40.0) ◀
gastrointestinal hemorrhage (K92.0-K92.2) ◀
intestinal obstruction (K56.-) ◀
newborn gastrointestinal hemorrhage (P54.0-P54.3) ◀
newborn intestinal obstruction (P76.-) ◀
pylorospasm (K31.3) ◀
signs and symptoms involving the urinary system (R30-R39) ◀
symptoms referable to female genital organs (N94.-) ◀
symptoms referable to male genital organs (N48-N50) ◀

R10 Abdominal and pelvic pain

Excludes1 renal colic (N23)

Excludes2 dorsalgia (M54.-)
flatulence and related conditions (R14.-)

R10.0 Acute abdomen

Severe abdominal pain (generalized) (with abdominal rigidity)

Excludes1 abdominal rigidity NOS (R19.3)
generalized abdominal pain NOS (R10.84)
localized abdominal pain (R10.1-R10.3-)

R10.1 Pain localized to upper abdomen

R10.10 Upper abdominal pain, unspecified

R10.11 Right upper quadrant pain

R10.12 Left upper quadrant pain

R10.13 Epigastric pain

Dyspepsia

Excludes1 functional dyspepsia (K30)

R10.2 Pelvic and perineal pain

Excludes1 vulvodynia (N94.81)

R10.3 Pain localized to other parts of lower abdomen

R10.30 Lower abdominal pain, unspecified

R10.31 Right lower quadrant pain

R10.32 Left lower quadrant pain

R10.33 Periumbilical pain

R10.8 Other abdominal pain

R10.81 Abdominal tenderness

Abdominal tenderness NOS

R10.811 Right upper quadrant abdominal tenderness

R10.812 Left upper quadrant abdominal tenderness

R10.813 Right lower quadrant abdominal tenderness

R10.814 Left lower quadrant abdominal tenderness

R10.815 Periumbilic abdominal tenderness

R10.816 Epigastric abdominal tenderness

R10.817 Generalized abdominal tenderness

R10.819 Abdominal tenderness, unspecified site

R10.82 Rebound abdominal tenderness

R10.821 Right upper quadrant rebound abdominal tenderness

R10.822 Left upper quadrant rebound abdominal tenderness

R10.823 Right lower quadrant rebound abdominal tenderness

R10.824 **Left lower quadrant rebound abdominal tenderness**

R10.825 **Periumbilic rebound abdominal tenderness**

R10.826 **Epigastric rebound abdominal tenderness**

R10.827 **Generalized rebound abdominal tenderness**

R10.829 **Rebound abdominal tenderness, unspecified site**

R10.83 **Colic** P
Colic NOS
Infantile colic
Excludes1 colic in adult and child over 12 months old (R10.84)

R10.84 **Generalized abdominal pain**
Excludes1 generalized abdominal pain associated with acute abdomen (R10.0)

R10.9 **Unspecified abdominal pain**

● R11 **Nausea and vomiting**
Excludes1 cyclical vomiting associated with migraine (G43.A-)
excessive vomiting in pregnancy (O21.-)
hematemesis (K92.0)
neonatal hematemesis (P54.0)
newborn vomiting (P92.0-)
psychogenic vomiting (F50.89)
vomiting associated with bulimia nervosa (F50.2)
vomiting following gastrointestinal surgery (K91.0)

● R11.0 **Nausea**
Nausea NOS
Nausea without vomiting

● R11.1 **Vomiting**

R11.10 **Vomiting, unspecified**
Vomiting NOS

R11.11 **Vomiting without nausea**

R11.12 **Projectile vomiting**

R11.13 **Vomiting of fecal matter**

R11.14 **Bilious vomiting**
Bilious emesis

R11.2 **Nausea with vomiting, unspecified**
Persistent nausea with vomiting NOS

R12 **Heartburn**
Excludes1 dyspepsia NOS (R10.13)
functional dyspepsia (K30)

● R13 **Aphagia and dysphagia**

R13.0 **Aphagia**
Inability to swallow
Excludes1 psychogenic aphagia (F50.9)

● R13.1 **Dysphagia**
Difficulty swallowing
Code first, if applicable, dysphagia following cerebrovascular disease (I69. with final characters -91)
Excludes1 psychogenic dysphagia (F45.8)

R13.10 **Dysphagia, unspecified**
Difficulty in swallowing NOS

R13.11 **Dysphagia, oral phase**

R13.12 **Dysphagia, oropharyngeal phase**

R13.13 **Dysphagia, pharyngeal phase**

R13.14 **Dysphagia, pharyngoesophageal phase**

R13.19 **Other dysphagia**
Cervical dysphagia
Neurogenic dysphagia

● R14 **Flatulence and related conditions**
Excludes1 psychogenic aerophagy (F45.8)

R14.0 **Abdominal distension (gaseous)**
Bloating
Tympanites (abdominal) (intestinal)

R14.1 **Gas pain**

R14.2 **Eructation**
Belching air from stomach through mouth

R14.3 **Flatulence**

● R15 **Fecal incontinence**
Includes encopresis NOS
Excludes1 fecal incontinence of nonorganic origin (F98.1)

R15.0 **Incomplete defecation**
Excludes1 constipation (K59.0-)
fecal impaction (K56.41)

R15.1 **Fecal smearing**
Fecal soiling

R15.2 **Fecal urgency**

R15.9 **Full incontinence of feces**
Fecal incontinence NOS

● R16 **Hepatomegaly and splenomegaly, not elsewhere classified**
Enlargement of liver or spleen

R16.0 **Hepatomegaly, not elsewhere classified**
Hepatomegaly NOS

R16.1 **Splenomegaly, not elsewhere classified**
Splenomegaly NOS

R16.2 **Hepatomegaly with splenomegaly, not elsewhere classified**
Hepatosplenomegaly NOS

R17 **Unspecified jaundice**
Excludes1 neonatal jaundice (P55, P57-P59)
Ex: P57.8-P59.9, R17, R23.8-R23.9

● R18 **Ascites**
Includes fluid in peritoneal cavity
Excludes1 ascites in alcoholic cirrhosis (K70.31)
ascites in alcoholic hepatitis (K70.11)
ascites in toxic liver disease with chronic active hepatitis (K71.51)
Ex: **For category R18 CC codes:** G89.0-G89.4, R18.0-R19.09, R19.30-R19.37, R29.700-R29.742, R41.0-R41.3, R41.82, R41.9, R44.8-R44.9, R45.83-R45.84, R46.0-R46.89, R52, R68.0-R68.19, R68.81-R68.83, R68.89-R69

● R18.0 **Malignant ascites**
Code first malignancy, such as:
malignant neoplasm of ovary (C56.-)
secondary malignant neoplasm of retroperitoneum and peritoneum (C78.6)

R18.8 **Other ascites**
Ascites NOS
Peritoneal effusion (chronic)

● R19 **Other symptoms and signs involving the digestive system and abdomen**
Excludes1 acute abdomen (R10.0)

● R19.0 **Intra-abdominal and pelvic swelling, mass and lump**
Excludes1 abdominal distension (gaseous) (R14.-)
ascites (R18.-)

R19.00 **Intra-abdominal and pelvic swelling, mass and lump, unspecified site**

R19.01 **Right upper quadrant abdominal swelling, mass and lump**

R19.02 **Left upper quadrant abdominal swelling, mass and lump**

R19.03 **Right lower quadrant abdominal swelling, mass and lump**

R19.04 **Left lower quadrant abdominal swelling, mass and lump**

R19.05 Periumbilic swelling, mass or lump
Diffuse or generalized umbilical swelling or mass

R19.06 Epigastric swelling, mass or lump

R19.07 Generalized intra-abdominal and pelvic swelling, mass and lump
Diffuse or generalized intra-abdominal swelling or mass NOS
Diffuse or generalized pelvic swelling or mass NOS

R19.09 Other intra-abdominal and pelvic swelling, mass and lump

● **R19.1 Abnormal bowel sounds**

R19.11 Absent bowel sounds

R19.12 Hyperactive bowel sounds

R19.15 Other abnormal bowel sounds
Abnormal bowel sounds NOS

R19.2 Visible peristalsis
Hyperperistalsis

● **R19.3 Abdominal rigidity**
Excludes1 abdominal rigidity with severe abdominal pain (R10.0)

R19.30 Abdominal rigidity, unspecified site

R19.31 Right upper quadrant abdominal rigidity

R19.32 Left upper quadrant abdominal rigidity

R19.33 Right lower quadrant abdominal rigidity

R19.34 Left lower quadrant abdominal rigidity

R19.35 Periumbilic abdominal rigidity

R19.36 Epigastric abdominal rigidity

R19.37 Generalized abdominal rigidity

R19.4 Change in bowel habit
Excludes1 constipation (K59.0-)
functional diarrhea (K59.1)

R19.5 Other fecal abnormalities
Abnormal stool color
Bulky stools
Mucus in stools
Occult blood in feces
Occult blood in stools
Excludes1 melena (K92.1)
neonatal melena (P54.1)

R19.6 Halitosis

R19.7 Diarrhea, unspecified
Diarrhea NOS
Excludes1 functional diarrhea (K59.1)
neonatal diarrhea (P78.3)
psychogenic diarrhea (F45.8)

R19.8 Other specified symptoms and signs involving the digestive system and abdomen

SYMPTOMS AND SIGNS INVOLVING THE SKIN AND SUBCUTANEOUS TISSUE (R20-R23)

Excludes2 symptoms relating to breast (N64.4-N64.5)

● **R20 Disturbances of skin sensation**
Excludes1 dissociative anesthesia and sensory loss (F44.6)
psychogenic disturbances (F45.8)

R20.0 Anesthesia of skin
Loss of sensation

R20.1 Hypoesthesia of skin
Unpleasant abnormal sensation

R20.2 Paresthesia of skin
Abnormal touch sensation, including burning, prickling, often in absence of external stimulus
Formication Tingling skin
Pins and needles
Excludes1 acroparesthesia (I73.8)

R20.3 Hyperesthesia

R20.8 Other disturbances of skin sensation

R20.9 Unspecified disturbances of skin sensation

R21 Rash and other nonspecific skin eruption
Includes rash NOS
Excludes1 specified type of rash- code to condition
vesicular eruption (R23.8)

● **R22 Localized swelling, mass and lump of skin and subcutaneous tissue**
Includes subcutaneous nodules (localized) (superficial)
Excludes1 abnormal findings on diagnostic imaging (R90-R93)
edema (R60.-)
enlarged lymph nodes (R59.-)
localized adiposity (E65)
swelling of joint (M25.4-)

R22.0 Localized swelling, mass and lump, head

R22.1 Localized swelling, mass and lump, neck

R22.2 Localized swelling, mass and lump, trunk
Excludes1 intra-abdominal or pelvic mass and lump (R19.0-)
intra-abdominal or pelvic swelling (R19.0-)
Excludes2 breast mass and lump (N63)

● **R22.3 Localized swelling, mass and lump, upper limb**

R22.30 Localized swelling, mass and lump, unspecified upper limb

R22.31 Localized swelling, mass and lump, right upper limb

R22.32 Localized swelling, mass and lump, left upper limb

R22.33 Localized swelling, mass and lump, upper limb, bilateral

● **R22.4 Localized swelling, mass and lump, lower limb**

R22.40 Localized swelling, mass and lump, unspecified lower limb

R22.41 Localized swelling, mass and lump, right lower limb

R22.42 Localized swelling, mass and lump, left lower limb

R22.43 Localized swelling, mass and lump, lower limb, bilateral

R22.9 Localized swelling, mass and lump, unspecified

● **R23 Other skin changes**

R23.0 Cyanosis
Excludes1 acrocyanosis (I73.8)
cyanotic attacks of newborn (P28.2)

R23.1 Pallor
Clammy skin

R23.2 Flushing
Excessive blushing
Code first, if applicable, menopausal and female climacteric states (N95.1)

R23.3 Spontaneous ecchymoses
Small hemorrhagic spot of skin; AKA black and blue spot
Petechiae
Excludes1 ecchymoses of newborn (P54.5)
purpura (D69.-)

R23.4 Changes in skin texture
Desquamation of skin Scaling of skin
Induration of skin
Excludes1 epidermal thickening NOS (L85.9)

R23.8 Other skin changes

R23.9 Unspecified skin changes

SYMPTOMS AND SIGNS INVOLVING THE NERVOUS AND MUSCULOSKELETAL SYSTEMS (R25-R29)

● **R25 Abnormal involuntary movements**

Excludes1 specific movement disorders (G20-G26)
stereotyped movement disorders (F98.4)
tic disorders (F95.-)

R25.0 Abnormal head movements

R25.1 Tremor, unspecified

Excludes1 chorea NOS (G25.5)
essential tremor (G25.0)
hysterical tremor (F44.4)
intention tremor (G25.2)

R25.2 Cramp and spasm

Excludes2 carpopedal spasm (R29.0)
charley-horse (M62.831)
infantile spasms (G40.4-)
muscle spasm of back (M62.830)
muscle spasm of calf (M62.831)

R25.3 Fasciculation
Twitching NOS

R25.8 Other abnormal involuntary movements

R25.9 Unspecified abnormal involuntary movements

● **R26 Abnormalities of gait and mobility**

Excludes1 ataxia NOS (R27.0)
hereditary ataxia (G11.-)
locomotor (syphilitic) ataxia (A52.11)
immobility syndrome (paraplegic) (M62.3)

R26.0 Ataxic gait
Staggering gait

R26.1 Paralytic gait
Spastic gait

R26.2 Difficulty in walking, not elsewhere classified

Excludes1 falling (R29.6)
unsteadiness on feet (R26.81)

Coding Clinic: 2016, Q2, P7

● **R26.8 Other abnormalities of gait and mobility**

R26.81 Unsteadiness on feet

R26.89 Other abnormalities of gait and mobility

R26.9 Unspecified abnormalities of gait and mobility

● **R27 Other lack of coordination**

Excludes1 ataxic gait (R26.0)
hereditary ataxia (G11.-)
vertigo NOS (R42)

R27.0 Ataxia, unspecified

Excludes1 ataxia following cerebrovascular disease (I69. with final characters -93)

R27.8 Other lack of coordination

R27.9 Unspecified lack of coordination

● **R29 Other symptoms and signs involving the nervous and musculoskeletal systems**

R29.0 Tetany
Hyperexcitability of nerves and muscles characterized by spasm, twitching, and cramps
Carpopedal spasm

Excludes1 hysterical tetany (F44.5)
neonatal tetany (P71.3)
parathyroid tetany (E20.9)
post-thyroidectomy tetany (E89.2)

Exc A33, A35, G10-G11.2, G11.4, G20-G25.79, G25.82-G26, G32.81, G80.3, G81.10-G81.14, G89.0-G89.4, G90.3, R29.0, R29.700-R29.742, R41.0-R41.3, R41.82, R41.9, R44.8-R44.9, R45.83-R45.84, R46.0-R46.89, R52, R68.0-R68.19, R68.81-R68.83, R68.89-R69

R29.1 Meningismus
Exc R29.1, R29.810

R29.2 Abnormal reflex

Excludes2 abnormal pupillary reflex (H57.0)
hyperactive gag reflex (J39.2)
vasovagal reaction or syncope (R55)

R29.3 Abnormal posture

R29.4 Clicking hip

Excludes1 congenital deformities of hip (Q65.-)

R29.5 Transient paralysis
Code first any associated spinal cord injury (S14.0, S14.1-, S24.0, S24.1-, S34.0-, S34.1-)

Excludes1 transient ischemic attack (G45.9)

Exc R29.5, R29.810

R29.6 Repeated falls
Falling
Tendency to fall

Excludes2 at risk for falling (Z91.81)
history of falling (Z91.81)

OGCR Section I.C.18.d.

Repeated falls
Code R29.6, Repeated falls, is for use for encounters when a patient has recently fallen and the reason for the fall is being investigated.
Code Z91.81, History of falling, is for use when a patient has fallen in the past and is at risk for future falls.When appropriate, both codes R29.6 and Z91.81 may be assigned together.

Coding Clinic: 2016, Q2, P7

● **R29.7 National Institutes of Health Stroke Scale (NIHSS) score** ◀
Code first the type of cerebral infarction (I63-) ◀

● **R29.70 NIHSS score 0-9** ◀
- ● **R29.700 NIHSS score 0** ◀
- ● **R29.701 NIHSS score 1** ◀
- ● **R29.702 NIHSS score 2** ◀
- ● **R29.703 NIHSS score 3** ◀
- ● **R29.704 NIHSS score 4** ◀
- ● **R29.705 NIHSS score 5** ◀
- ● **R29.706 NIHSS score 6** ◀
- ● **R29.707 NIHSS score 7** ◀
- ● **R29.708 NIHSS score 8** ◀
- ● **R29.709 NIHSS score 9** ◀

● **R29.71 NIHSS score 10-19** ◀
- ● **R29.710 NIHSS score 10** ◀
- ● **R29.711 NIHSS score 11** ◀
- ● **R29.712 NIHSS score 12** ◀
- ● **R29.713 NIHSS score 13** ◀
- ● **R29.714 NIHSS score 14** ◀
- ● **R29.715 NIHSS score 15** ◀
- ● **R29.716 NIHSS score 16** ◀
- ● **R29.717 NIHSS score 17** ◀
- ● **R29.718 NIHSS score 18** ◀
- ● **R29.719 NIHSS score 19** ◀

● **R29.72 NIHSS score 20-29** ◀
- ● **R29.720 NIHSS score 20** ◀
- ● **R29.721 NIHSS score 21** ◀
- ● **R29.722 NIHSS score 22** ◀
- ● **R29.723 NIHSS score 23** ◀
- ● **R29.724 NIHSS score 24** ◀
- ● **R29.725 NIHSS score 25** ◀
- ● **R29.726 NIHSS score 26** ◀
- ● **R29.727 NIHSS score 27** ◀
- ● **R29.728 NIHSS score 28** ◀
- ● **R29.729 NIHSS score 29** ◀

OGCR Section I.C.18.i.

NIHSS Stroke Scale
The NIH stroke scale (NIHSS) codes (R29.7- -) can be used in conjunction with acute stroke codes (I63) to identify the patient's neurological status and the severity of the stroke. The stroke scale codes should be sequenced after the acute stroke diagnosis code(s).
At a minimum, report the initial score documented. If desired, a facility may choose to capture multiple stroke scale scores.

- **R29.73 NIHSS score 30-39** ◀
  - **R29.730 NIHSS score 30** ◀
  - **R29.731 NIHSS score 31** ◀
  - **R29.732 NIHSS score 32** ◀
  - **R29.733 NIHSS score 33** ◀
  - **R29.734 NIHSS score 34** ◀
  - **R29.735 NIHSS score 35** ◀
  - **R29.736 NIHSS score 36** ◀
  - **R29.737 NIHSS score 37** ◀
  - **R29.738 NIHSS score 38** ◀
  - **R29.739 NIHSS score 39** ◀
- **R29.74 NIHSS score 40-42** ◀
  - **R29.740 NIHSS score 40** ◀
  - **R29.741 NIHSS score 41** ◀
  - **R29.742 NIHSS score 42** ◀
- **R29.8 Other symptoms and signs involving the nervous and musculoskeletal systems**
  - **R29.81 Other symptoms and signs involving the nervous system**
    - **R29.810 Facial weakness**
      Facial droop
      Excludes1 Bell's palsy (G51.0)
      facial weakness following cerebrovascular disease (I69. with final characters -92)
    - **R29.818 Other symptoms and signs involving the nervous system**
  - **R29.89 Other symptoms and signs involving the musculoskeletal system**
    Excludes2 pain in limb (M79.6-)
    - **R29.890 Loss of height**
      Excludes1 osteoporosis (M80-M81)
    - **R29.891 Ocular torticollis**
      Excludes1 congenital (sterno-mastoid) torticollis Q68.0
      psychogenic torticollis (F45.8)
      spasmodic torticollis (G24.3)
      torticollis due to birth injury (P15.8)
      torticollis NOS M43.6
    - **R29.898 Other symptoms and signs involving the musculoskeletal system**
- **R29.9 Unspecified symptoms and signs involving the nervous and musculoskeletal systems**
  - **R29.90 Unspecified symptoms and signs involving the nervous system**
  - **R29.91 Unspecified symptoms and signs involving the musculoskeletal system**

SYMPTOMS AND SIGNS INVOLVING THE GENITOURINARY SYSTEM (R30-R39)

- **R30 Pain associated with micturition**
  Excludes1 psychogenic pain associated with micturition (F45.8)
  - **R30.0 Dysuria**
    Painful urination
    Strangury
  - **R30.1 Vesical tenesmus**
    Straining to urinate
  - **R30.9 Painful micturition, unspecified**
    Painful urination NOS
- **R31 Hematuria**
  Excludes1 hematuria included with underlying conditions, such as:
  acute cystitis with hematuria (N30.01)
  recurrent and persistent hematuria in glomerular diseases (N02.-)
  - **R31.0 Gross hematuria**
  - **R31.1 Benign essential microscopic hematuria**
  - **R31.2 Other microscopic hematuria**
    - **R31.21 Asymptomatic microscopic hematuria** ◀
      AMH ◀
    - **R31.29 Other microscopic hematuria** ◀
  - **R31.9 Hematuria, unspecified**
- **R32 Unspecified urinary incontinence**
  Enuresis NOS
  Excludes1 functional urinary incontinence (R39.81)
  nonorganic enuresis (F98.0)
  stress incontinence and other specified urinary incontinence (N39.3-N39.4-)
  urinary incontinence associated with cognitive impairment (R39.81)
- **R33 Retention of urine**
  Excludes1 psychogenic retention of urine (F45.8)
  - **R33.0 Drug induced retention of urine**
    Use additional code for adverse effect, if applicable, to identify drug (T36-T50 with fifth or sixth character 5)
  - **R33.8 Other retention of urine**
    Code first, if applicable, any causal condition, such as:
    enlarged prostate (N40.1)
  - **R33.9 Retention of urine, unspecified**
- **R34 Anuria and oliguria**
  Excludes1 anuria and oliguria complicating abortion or ectopic or molar pregnancy (O00-O07, O08.4)
  anuria and oliguria complicating pregnancy (O26.83-)
  anuria and oliguria complicating the puerperium (O90.4)
- **R35 Polyuria**
  Passage of excessive volume of urine
  Code first, if applicable, any causal condition, such as:
  enlarged prostate (N40.1)
  Excludes1 psychogenic polyuria (F45.8)
  - **R35.0 Frequency of micturition**
    Discharge or passage of urine; AKA uresis
  - **R35.1 Nocturia**
    Urinary frequency at night
  - **R35.8 Other polyuria**
    Polyuria NOS
- **R36 Urethral discharge**
  - **R36.0 Urethral discharge without blood**
  - **R36.1 Hematospermia** ♂
    Presence of blood in semen
  - **R36.9 Urethral discharge, unspecified**
    Penile discharge NOS
    Urethrorrhea
- **R37 Sexual dysfunction, unspecified**

● **R39 Other and unspecified symptoms and signs involving the genitourinary system**

R39.0 Extravasation of urine
Leakage, discharge
Ex: R30.1, R39.0, R39.2-R39.9

● **R39.1 Other difficulties with micturition**
Code first, if applicable, any causal condition, such as:
enlarged prostate (N40.1)

R39.11 Hesitancy of micturition

R39.12 Poor urinary stream
Weak urinary steam

R39.13 Splitting of urinary stream

R39.14 Feeling of incomplete bladder emptying

R39.15 Urgency of urination
Excludes1 urge incontinence (N39.41, N39.46)

R39.16 Straining to void

● **R39.19 Other difficulties with micturition**

R39.191 Need to immediately re-void ◀

R39.192 Position dependent micturition ◀

R39.198 Other difficulties with micturition ◀

R39.2 Extrarenal uremia
Prerenal uremia
Excludes1 uremia NOS (N19)

● **R39.8 Other symptoms and signs involving the genitourinary system**

R39.81 Functional urinary incontinence
Urinary incontinence due to cognitive impairment, or severe physical disability or immobility
Excludes1 stress incontinence and other specified urinary incontinence (N39.3-N39.4-)
urinary incontinence NOS (R32)

R39.82 Chronic bladder pain ◀

R39.89 Other symptoms and signs involving the genitourinary system

R39.9 Unspecified symptoms and signs involving the genitourinary system

SYMPTOMS AND SIGNS INVOLVING COGNITION, PERCEPTION, EMOTIONAL STATE AND BEHAVIOR (R40-R46)

Excludes2 symptoms and signs constituting part of a pattern of mental disorder (F01-F99) ◀
Coding Clinic: 2015, Q4, P40

● **R40 Somnolence, stupor and coma**
Excludes1 neonatal coma (P91.5)
somnolence, stupor and coma in diabetes (E08-E13)
somnolence, stupor and coma in hepatic failure (K72.-)
somnolence, stupor and coma in hypoglycemia (nondiabetic) (E15)

R40.0 Somnolence
Drowsiness
Excludes1 coma (R40.2-)

R40.1 Stupor
Lowered level of consciousness
Catatonic stupor
Semicoma
Excludes1 catatonic schizophrenia (F20.2)
coma (R40.2-)
depressive stupor (F31-F33)
dissociative stupor (F44.2)
manic stupor (F30.2)

OGCR Section I.C.18.e.

Coma scale

The coma scale codes (R40.2-) can be used in conjunction with traumatic brain injury codes, acute cerebrovascular disease or sequelae of cerebrovascular disease codes. These codes are primarily for use by trauma registries, but they may be used in any setting where this information is collected. **The coma scale may also be used to assess the status of the central nervous system for other non-trauma conditions, such as monitoring patients in the intensive care unit regardless of medical condition.** The coma scale codes should be sequenced after the diagnosis code(s).

These codes, one from each subcategory, are needed to complete the scale. The 7th character indicates when the scale was recorded. The 7th character should match for all three codes.

At a minimum, report the initial score documented on presentation at your facility. This may be a score from the emergency medicine technician (EMT) or in the emergency department. If desired, a facility may choose to capture multiple coma scale scores.

Assign code R40.24, Glasgow coma scale, total score, when only the total score is documented in the medical record and not the individual score(s).

● **R40.2 Coma**
Code first any associated:
fracture of skull (S02.-)
intracranial injury (S06.-)
Note: One code from each subcategory R40.21-R40-23 is required to complete the coma scale ⇐
Ex: **For category R40.2 CC codes:** B15.0-B19.9, E03.5, E08.00-E08.59, E08.618-E09.59, E09.618-E10.59, E10.618-E10.649, E10.69-E11.59, E11.618-E11.649, E11.69-E13.59, E13.618-E16.2, E89.1, G32.89, G89.0-G89.4, G93.81-G93.9, G96.8-G96.9, G98.0-G98.8, G99.8, I60.00-I62.9, K72.91, R29.700-R29.742, R40.0-R40.2124, R40.2210-R40.2224, R40.2310-R40.2324, R40.2340-R40.2344, R40.3-R41.3, R41.82, R41.9-R42, R44.8-R44.9, R45.83-R45.84, R46.0-R46.89, R52, R55, R68.0-R68.83, R68.89-R69, S02.0XX-S02.19X[A,B], S02.91X[A,B], S06.0X0-S06.0X1[A], S06.0X9-S06.9X9[A]

R40.20 Unspecified coma
Coma NOS
Unconsciousness NOS

● **R40.21 Coma scale, eyes open**
The following appropriate 7th character is to be added to subcategory R40.21-:

0	unspecified time
1	in the field [EMT or ambulance]
2	at arrival to emergency department
3	at hospital admission
4	24 hours or more after hospital admission

Coding Clinic: 2015, Q2, P18

● **R40.211 Coma scale, eyes open, never**

● **R40.212 Coma scale, eyes open, to pain**

● **R40.213 Coma scale, eyes open, to sound**

● **R40.214 Coma scale, eyes open, spontaneous**

● **R40.22 Coma scale, best verbal response**
The following appropriate 7th character is to be added to subcategory R40.22-:

0	unspecified time
1	in the field [EMT or ambulance]
2	at arrival to emergency department
3	at hospital admission
4	24 hours or more after hospital admission

Coding Clinic: 2015, Q2, P18

● **R40.221 Coma scale, best verbal response, none**

● **R40.222 Coma scale, best verbal response, incomprehensible words**

Glasgow Coma Scale

Eye Opening Response • Spontaneous--open with blinking at baseline	**4 points**
• To verbal stimuli, command, speech	**3 points**
• To pain only (not applied to face)	**2 points**
• No response	**1 point**
Verbal Response • Oriented	**5 points**
• Confused conversation, but able to answer questions	**4 points**
• Inappropriate words	**3 points**
• Incomprehensible speech	**2 points**
• No response	**1 point**
Motor Response • Obeys commands for movement	**6 points**
• Purposeful movement to painful stimulus	**5 points**
• Withdraws in response to pain	**4 points**
• Flexion in response to pain (decorticate posturing)	**3 points**
• Extension response in response to pain (decerebrate posturing)	**2 points**
• No response	**1 point**
Categorization: Coma: No eye opening, no ability to follow commands, no word verbalizations (3-8)	
Head Injury Classification: Severe Head Injury--GCS score of 8 or less Moderate Head Injury--GCS score of 9 to 12 Mild head injury--GCS score of 13 to 15	
(Adapted from: Advanced Trauma Life Support: Course for Physicians, American College of Surgeons, 1993). http://www.bt.cdc.gov/masscasulatires/gscale.asp	

Figure 18-1

R40.223 Coma scale, best verbal response, inappropriate words

R40.224 Coma scale, best verbal response, confused conversation

R40.225 Coma scale, best verbal response, oriented

R40.23 Coma scale, best motor response

The following appropriate 7th character is to be added to subcategory R40.23-:

0	unspecified time
1	in the field [EMT or ambulance]
2	at arrival to emergency department
3	at hospital admission
4	24 hours or more after hospital admission

Coding Clinic: 2015, Q2, P18

R40.231 Coma scale, best motor response, none MCC

R40.232 Coma scale, best motor response, extension MCC

R40.233 Coma scale, best motor response, abnormal

R40.234 Coma scale, best motor response, flexion withdrawal MCC

R40.235 Coma scale, best motor response, localizes pain

R40.236 Coma scale, best motor response, obeys commands

R40.24 Glasgow coma scale, total score

Note: Assign a code from subcategory R40.24, when only the total coma score is documented ◀

The following appropriate 7th character is to be added to subcategory R40.24-: ◀

0	unspecified time ◀
1	in the field [EMT or ambulance] ◀
2	at arrival to emergency department ◀
3	at hospital admission ◀
4	24 hours or more after hospital admission ◀

Coding Clinic: 2015, Q2, P18

R40.241 Glasgow coma scale score 13-15

R40.242 Glasgow coma scale score 9-12

R40.243 Glasgow coma scale score 3-8

R40.244 Other coma, without documented Glasgow coma scale score, or with partial score reported

R40.3 Persistent vegetative state CC

Exc See R40.2

R40.4 Transient alteration of awareness

R41 Other symptoms and signs involving cognitive functions and awareness

Excludes1 dissociative [conversion] disorders (F44.-)
mild cognitive impairment, so stated (G31.84)

R41.0 Disorientation, unspecified
Confusion NOS
Delirium NOS

R41.1 Anterograde amnesia

R41.2 Retrograde amnesia

R41.3 Other amnesia
Amnesia NOS
Memory loss NOS

Excludes1 amnestic disorder due to known physiologic condition (F04)
amnestic syndrome due to psychoactive substance use (F10-F19 with 5th character .6)
mild memory disturbance due to known physiological condition (F06.8)
transient global amnesia (G45.4)

R41.4 Neurologic neglect syndrome CC
Asomatognosia
Hemi-akinesia
Hemi-inattention
Hemispatial neglect
Left-sided neglect
Sensory neglect
Visuospatial neglect

Excludes1 visuospatial deficit (R41.842)

Exc R29.3, R29.6-R29.890, R29.90-R29.91, R41.4

R41.8 Other symptoms and signs involving cognitive functions and awareness

R41.81 Age-related cognitive decline A
Senility NOS

R41.82 Altered mental status, unspecified
Change in mental status NOS

Excludes1 altered level of consciousness (R40.-)
altered mental status due to known condition - code to condition
delirium NOS (R41.0)

Coding Clinic: 2012, Q4, P98

R41.83 Borderline intellectual functioning
IQ level 71 to 84

Excludes1 intellectual disabilities (F70-F79)

● R41.84 Other specified cognitive deficit
Excludes1 cognitive deficits as sequelae of cerebrovascular disease (I69.01-, I69.11-, I69.21-, I69.31-, I69.81-, I69.91-) ◀
R41.840 Attention and concentration deficit
Excludes1 attention-deficit hyperactivity disorders (F90.-)
R41.841 Cognitive communication deficit
R41.842 Visuospatial deficit
R41.843 Psychomotor deficit
R41.844 Frontal lobe and executive function deficit
R41.89 Other symptoms and signs involving cognitive functions and awareness
Anosognosia
R41.9 Unspecified symptoms and signs involving cognitive functions and awareness

R42 Dizziness and giddiness
Light-headedness
Vertigo NOS
Excludes1 vertiginous syndromes (H81.-)
vertigo from infrasound (T75.23)
Coding Clinic: 2015, Q4, P40

● R43 Disturbances of smell and taste
R43.0 Anosmia
Absence of sense of smell; AKA anosphresia and olfactory anesthesia
R43.1 Parosmia
R43.2 Parageusia
Perversion of sense of taste or bad taste in mouth; AKA dysgeusia
R43.8 Other disturbances of smell and taste
Mixed disturbance of smell and taste
R43.9 Unspecified disturbances of smell and taste

● R44 Other symptoms and signs involving general sensations and perceptions
Excludes1 alcoholic hallucinations (F1.5)
hallucinations in drug psychosis (F11-F19 with .5)
hallucinations in mood disorders with psychotic symptoms (F30.2, F31.5, F32.3, F33.3)
hallucinations in schizophrenia, schizotypal and delusional disorders (F20-F29)
Excludes2 disturbances of skin sensation (R20.-)
R44.0 Auditory hallucinations
Ex G89.0-G89.4, R29.700-R29.742, R41.0-R41.3, R41.82, R41.9-R42, R44.0, R44.2-R44.9, R45.83-R45.84, R46.0-R46.89, R52, R68.0-R68.19, R68.81-R68.83, R68.89-R69
R44.1 Visual hallucinations
R44.2 Other hallucinations
Ex See R44.0
R44.3 Hallucinations, unspecified
Ex See R44.0
R44.8 Other symptoms and signs involving general sensations and perceptions
R44.9 Unspecified symptoms and signs involving general sensations and perceptions

● R45 Symptoms and signs involving emotional state
R45.0 Nervousness
Nervous tension
R45.1 Restlessness and agitation
R45.2 Unhappiness
R45.3 Demoralization and apathy
Excludes1 anhedonia (R45.84)
R45.4 Irritability and anger
R45.5 Hostility
R45.6 Violent behavior
R45.7 State of emotional shock and stress, unspecified
● R45.8 Other symptoms and signs involving emotional state
R45.81 Low self-esteem
R45.82 Worries
R45.83 Excessive crying of child, adolescent or adult
Excludes1 excessive crying of infant (baby) R68.11
R45.84 Anhedonia
Total loss of feeling of pleasure in pleasurable acts
● R45.85 Homicidal and suicidal ideations
Excludes1 suicide attempt (T14.91)
● R45.850 Homicidal ideations
R45.851 Suicidal ideations
Ex F05
R45.86 Emotional lability
R45.87 Impulsiveness
R45.89 Other symptoms and signs involving emotional state

● R46 Symptoms and signs involving appearance and behavior
Excludes1 appearance and behavior in schizophrenia, schizotypal and delusional disorders (F20-F29)
mental and behavioral disorders (F01-F99)
R46.0 Very low level of personal hygiene
R46.1 Bizarre personal appearance
R46.2 Strange and inexplicable behavior
R46.3 Overactivity
R46.4 Slowness and poor responsiveness
Excludes1 stupor (R40.1)
R46.5 Suspiciousness and marked evasiveness
R46.6 Undue concern and preoccupation with stressful events
R46.7 Verbosity and circumstantial detail obscuring reason for contact
● R46.8 Other symptoms and signs involving appearance and behavior
● R46.81 Obsessive-compulsive behavior
Excludes1 obsessive-compulsive disorder (F42-) ⇐
● R46.89 Other symptoms and signs involving appearance and behavior

SYMPTOMS AND SIGNS INVOLVING SPEECH AND VOICE (R47-R49)

● R47 Speech disturbances, not elsewhere classified
Excludes1 autism (F84.0)
cluttering (F80.81)
specific developmental disorders of speech and language (F80.-)
stuttering (F80.81)
● R47.0 Dysphasia and aphasia
R47.01 Aphasia
Excludes1 aphasia following cerebrovascular disease (I69. with final characters -20)
progressive isolated aphasia (G31.01)
Ex F80.1, F80.81, I62.00-I66.9, R47.01-R47.9, R49.0-R49.9
R47.02 Dysphasia
Impairment in comprehension of speech, caused by left-sided brain damage
Excludes1 dysphasia following cerebrovascular disease (I69. with final characters -21)
R47.1 Dysarthria and anarthria
Motor speech disorder
Excludes1 dysarthria following cerebrovascular disease (I69. with final characters -22)

◀ New ⇐ Revised ~~deleted~~ Deleted Excludes 1 Excludes 2 Includes Use additional Code first Code also Unspecified
OGCR Official Guidelines ● Unacceptable Principal Diagnosis X Assign placeholder X ● Use Additional Character(s) ◗ Manifestation Code Coding Clinic

R47.8 Other speech disturbances

Excludes1 dysarthria following cerebrovascular disease (I69. with final characters -28)

R47.81 Slurred speech

R47.82 Fluency disorder in conditions classified elsewhere

Stuttering in conditions classified elsewhere

Code first underlying disease or condition, such as:
Parkinson's disease (G20)

Excludes1 adult onset fluency disorder (F98.5)
childhood onset fluency disorder (F80.81)
fluency disorder (stuttering) following cerebrovascular disease (I69. with final characters -23)

R47.89 Other speech disturbances

R47.9 Unspecified speech disturbances

R48 Dyslexia and other symbolic dysfunctions, not elsewhere classified

Excludes1 specific developmental disorders of scholastic skills (F81.-)

R48.0 Dyslexia and alexia

R48.1 Agnosia

Loss of ability to recognize objects, persons, sounds, shapes, or smells

Astereognosia (astereognosis)
Autotopagnosia

Excludes1 visual object agnosia (R48.3)

R48.2 Apraxia

Loss of ability to execute or carry out learned purposeful movements

Excludes1 apraxia following cerebrovascular disease (I69. with final characters -90)

R48.3 Visual agnosia

Prosopagnosia
Simultanagnosia (asimultagnosia)

R48.8 Other symbolic dysfunctions

Acalculia

Difficulty performing simple mathematical tasks resulting from neurological injury

Agraphia

R48.9 Unspecified symbolic dysfunctions

R49 Voice and resonance disorders

Excludes1 psychogenic voice and resonance disorders (F44.4)

R49.0 Dysphonia

Hoarseness

R49.1 Aphonia

Loss of voice

R49.2 Hypernasality and hyponasality

R49.21 Hypernasality

R49.22 Hyponasality

R49.8 Other voice and resonance disorders

R49.9 Unspecified voice and resonance disorder

Change in voice NOS
Resonance disorder NOS

GENERAL SYMPTOMS AND SIGNS (R50-R69)

R50 Fever of other and unknown origin

Excludes1 chills without fever (R68.83)
febrile convulsions (R56.0-)
fever of unknown origin during labor (O75.2)
fever of unknown origin in newborn (P81.9)
hypothermia due to illness (R68.0)
malignant hyperthermia due to anesthesia (T88.3)
puerperal pyrexia NOS (O86.4)

R50.2 Drug induced fever

Use additional code for adverse effect, if applicable, to identify drug (T36-T50 with fifth or sixth character 5)

Excludes1 postvaccination (postimmunization) fever (R50.83)

R50.8 Other specified fever

R50.81 Fever presenting with conditions classified elsewhere

Code first underlying condition when associated fever is present, such as with:
leukemia (C91-C95)
neutropenia (D70.-)
sickle-cell disease (D57.-)

R50.82 Postprocedural fever

Excludes1 postprocedural infection (T81.4-)
posttransfusion fever (R50.84)
postvaccination (postimmunization) fever (R50.83)

R50.83 Postvaccination fever

Postimmunization fever

R50.84 Febrile nonhemolytic transfusion reaction

FNHTR
Posttransfusion fever

R50.9 Fever, unspecified

Fever NOS
Fever of unknown origin [FUO]
Fever with chills
Fever with rigors
Hyperpyrexia NOS
Persistent fever
Pyrexia NOS

R51 Headache

Facial pain NOS

Excludes1 atypical face pain (G50.1)
migraine and other headache syndromes (G43-G44)
trigeminal neuralgia (G50.0)

R52 Pain, unspecified

Acute pain NOS
Generalized pain NOS
Pain NOS

Excludes1 acute and chronic pain, not elsewhere classified (G89.-)
localized pain, unspecified type - code to pain by site, such as:
abdomen pain (R10.-)
back pain (M54.9)
breast pain (N64.4)
chest pain (R07.1-R07.9)
ear pain (H92.0-)
eye pain (H57.1)
headache (R51)
joint pain (M25.5-)
limb pain (M79.6-)
lumbar region pain (M54.5)
pelvic and perineal pain (R10.2)
shoulder pain (M25.51-)
spine pain (M54.-)
throat pain (R07.0)
tongue pain (K14.6)
tooth pain (K08.8)
renal colic (N23)
pain disorders exclusively related to psychological factors (F45.41)

● **R53 Malaise and fatigue**

R53.0 Neoplastic (malignant) related fatigue
Code first associated neoplasm

R53.1 Weakness
Asthenia NOS
Excludes1 age-related weakness (R54)
muscle weakness (M62.8-)
sarcopenia (M62.84) ◀
senile asthenia (R54)

R53.2 Functional quadriplegia
Complete immobility due to severe physical disability or frailty
Excludes1 frailty NOS (R54)
hysterical paralysis (F44.4)
immobility syndrome (M62.3)
neurologic quadriplegia (G82.5-)
quadriplegia (G82.50)
Ex: E08.40-E08.49, E08.618-E08.638, E08.649-E08.8, E09.40-E09.49, E09.618-E09.638, E09.649-E09.8, E10.40-E10.49, E10.618-E10.638, E10.649, E10.69-E10.8, E11.40-E11.49, E11.618-E11.638, E11.649, E11.69-E11.8, E13.40-E13.49, E13.618-E13.638, E13.649-E13.8, G04.1, G32.89, G80.0-G80.2, G80.4-G83.9, G90.1, G93.81, G93.89-G93.9, G96.8-G96.9, G98.0-G98.8, G99.8, Q06.0-Q06.1, Q06.3, Q06.8-Q06.9, Q07.8-Q07.9, R53.2
Coding Clinic: 2016, Q2, P6

● **R53.8 Other malaise and fatigue**
Excludes1 combat exhaustion and fatigue (F43.0)
congenital debility (P96.9)
exhaustion and fatigue due to depressive episode (F32.-)
exhaustion and fatigue due to excessive exertion (T73.3)
exhaustion and fatigue due to exposure (T73.2)
exhaustion and fatigue due to heat (T67.-)
exhaustion and fatigue due to pregnancy (O26.8-)
exhaustion and fatigue due to recurrent depressive episode (F33)
exhaustion and fatigue due to senile debility (R54)

R53.81 Other malaise
Chronic debility
Debility NOS
General physical deterioration
Malaise NOS
Nervous debility
Excludes1 age-related physical debility (R54)

R53.82 Chronic fatigue, unspecified
Chronic fatigue syndrome NOS
Excludes1 postviral fatigue syndrome (G93.3)

R53.83 Other fatigue
Fatigue NOS
Lethargy
Lack of energy
Tiredness

R54 Age-related physical debility A
Frailty
Senile asthenia
Old age
Senile debility
Senescence
Excludes1 age-related cognitive decline (R41.81)
sarcopenia (M62.84) ◀
senile psychosis (F03)
senility NOS (R41.81)

R55 Syncope and collapse
Blackout
Fainting
Vasovagal attack
Excludes1 cardiogenic shock (R57.0)
carotid sinus syncope (G90.01)
heat syncope (T67.1)
neurocirculatory asthenia (F45.8)
neurogenic orthostatic hypotension (G90.3)
orthostatic hypotension (I95.1)
postprocedural shock (T81.1-)
psychogenic syncope (F48.8)
shock NOS (R57.9)
shock complicating or following abortion or ectopic or molar pregnancy (O00-O07, O08.3)
shock complicating or following labor and delivery (O75.1)
Stokes-Adams attack (I45.9)
unconsciousness NOS (R40.2-)

● **R56 Convulsions, not elsewhere classified**
Excludes1 dissociative convulsions and seizures (F44.5)
epileptic convulsions and seizures (G40.-)
newborn convulsions and seizures (P90)

● **R56.0 Febrile convulsions**
Ex: **For category R56.0 CC codes:** G32.89, G40.001-G40.319, G40.401-G40.919, G40.A01-G40.B19, G89.0-G89.4, G93.81, G93.89-G93.9, G96.8-G96.9, G98.0-G98.8, P90, P91.8-P91.9, R29.700-R29.742, R41.0-R41.3, R41.82, R41.9, R44.8-R44.9, R45.83-R45.84, R46.0-R46.89, R52, R56.00-R56.9, R68.0-R68.19, R68.81-R68.83, R68.89-R69

R56.00 Simple febrile convulsions
Febrile convulsion NOS
Febrile seizure NOS

R56.01 Complex febrile convulsions
Atypical febrile seizure
Complex febrile seizure
Complicated febrile seizure
Excludes1 status epilepticus (G40.901)

R56.1 Post traumatic seizures
Excludes1 post traumatic epilepsy (G40.-)
Ex: E08.40-E08.49, E09.40-E09.49, E10.40-E10.49, E11.40-E11.49, E13.40-E13.49, G32.89, G40.001-G40.319, G40.401-G40.919, G40.A01-G40.A19, G40.B01-G40.B19, G93.81, G93.89-G93.9, G96.8-G96.9, G98.0-G98.8, G99.8, R56.1

R56.9 Unspecified convulsions
Convulsion disorder
Recurrent convulsions
Fit NOS
Seizure(s) (convulsive) NOS

● **R57 Shock, not elsewhere classified**
Excludes1 anaphylactic shock NOS (T78.2)
anaphylactic reaction or shock due to adverse food reaction (T78.0-)
anaphylactic shock due to adverse effect of correct drug or medicament properly administered (T88.6)
anaphylactic shock due to serum (T80.5-)
anesthetic shock (T88.3)
electric shock (T75.4)
obstetric shock (O75.1)
postprocedural shock (T81.1-)
psychic shock (F43.0)
septic shock (R65.21)
shock complicating or following ectopic or molar pregnancy (O00-O07, O08.3)
shock due to lightning (T75.01)
traumatic shock (T79.4)
toxic shock syndrome (A48.3)
Ex: **For category R57 CC codes:** G89.0-G89.4, R09.89, R29.700-R29.742, R41.0-R41.3, R41.82, R41.9, R44.8-R44.9, R45.83-R45.84, R46.0-R46.89, R52, R57.0-R57.9, R65.21, R68.0-R68.19, R68.81-R68.83, R68.89-R69

R57.0 Cardiogenic shock
MCC: Only if patient discharged alive

R57.1 Hypovolemic shock
Decreased blood volume (loss)
MCC: Only if patient discharged alive

R57.8 Other shock
MCC: Only if patient discharged alive

R57.9 Shock, unspecified
Failure of peripheral circulation NOS
Resulting in significant blood pressure drop

R58 Hemorrhage, not elsewhere classified
Hemorrhage NOS
Excludes1 hemorrhage included with underlying conditions, such as:
acute duodenal ulcer with hemorrhage (K26.0)
acute gastritis with bleeding (K29.01)
ulcerative enterocolitis with rectal bleeding (K51.01)

R59 Enlarged lymph nodes
Includes swollen glands
Excludes1 lymphadenitis NOS (I88.9)
acute lymphadenitis (L04.-)
chronic lymphadenitis (I88.1)
mesenteric (acute) (chronic) lymphadenitis (I88.0)

R59.0 Localized enlarged lymph nodes

R59.1 Generalized enlarged lymph nodes
Lymphadenopathy NOS

R59.9 Enlarged lymph nodes, unspecified

R60 Edema, not elsewhere classified
Excludes1 angioneurotic edema (T78.3)
ascites (R18.-)
cerebral edema (G93.6)
cerebral edema due to birth injury (P11.0)
edema of larynx (J38.4)
edema of nasopharynx (J39.2)
edema of pharynx (J39.2)
gestational edema (O12.0-)
hereditary edema (Q82.0)
hydrops fetalis NOS (P83.2)
hydrothorax (J94.8)
nutritional edema (E40-E46)
hydrops fetalis NOS (P83.2)
newborn edema (P83.3)
pulmonary edema (J81.-)

R60.0 Localized edema

R60.1 Generalized edema

R60.9 Edema, unspecified
Fluid retention NOS

R61 Generalized hyperhidrosis
Excessive sweating
Night sweats
Secondary hyperhidrosis
Code first, if applicable, menopausal and female climacteric states (N95.1)
Excludes1 focal (primary) (secondary) hyperhidrosis (L74.5-)
Frey's syndrome (L74.52)
localized (primary) (secondary) hyperhidrosis (L74.5-)

R62 Lack of expected normal physiological development in childhood and adults
Excludes1 delayed puberty (E30.0)
gonadal dysgenesis (Q99.1)
hypopituitarism (E23.0)

R62.0 Delayed milestone in childhood P
Delayed attainment of expected physiological developmental stage
Late talker
Late walker

R62.5 Other and unspecified lack of expected normal physiological development in childhood
Excludes1 HIV disease resulting in failure to thrive (B20)
physical retardation due to malnutrition (E45)

R62.50 Unspecified lack of expected normal physiological development in childhood
Infantilism NOS

R62.51 Failure to thrive (child) P
Failure to gain weight
Excludes1 failure to thrive in child under 28 days old (P92.6)

R62.52 Short stature (child)
Lack of growth Short stature NOS
Physical retardation
Excludes1 short stature due to endocrine disorder (E34.3)

R62.59 Other lack of expected normal physiological development in childhood

R62.7 Adult failure to thrive A

R63 Symptoms and signs concerning food and fluid intake
Excludes1 bulimia NOS (F50.2)
eating disorders of nonorganic origin (F50.-)
malnutrition (E40-E46)

R63.0 Anorexia
Loss of appetite
Excludes1 anorexia nervosa (F50.0-)
loss of appetite of nonorganic origin (F50.89)

R63.1 Polydipsia
Excessive thirst

R63.2 Polyphagia
Excessive eating Hyperalimentation NOS

R63.3 Feeding difficulties
Feeding problem (elderly) (infant) NOS
Excludes1 feeding problems of newborn (P92.-)
infant feeding disorder of nonorganic origin (F98.2-)

R63.4 Abnormal weight loss

R63.5 Abnormal weight gain
Excludes1 excessive weight gain in pregnancy (O26.0-)
obesity (E66.-)

R63.6 Underweight
Use additional code to identify body mass index (BMI), if known (Z68.-)
Excludes1 abnormal weight loss (R63.4)
anorexia nervosa (F50.0-)
malnutrition (E40-E46)

R63.8 Other symptoms and signs concerning food and fluid intake

R64 Cachexia
Wasting syndrome
Code first underlying condition, if known
Excludes1 abnormal weight loss (R63.4)
nutritional marasmus (E41)
Ex G89.0-G89.4, R29.700-R29.742, R41.0-R41.3, R41.82, R41.9, R44.8-R44.9, R45.83-R45.84, R46.0-R46.89, R52, R64, R68.0-R68.19, R68.81-R68.83, R68.89-R69

OGCR Section I.C.18.g.

SIRS due to Non-Infectious Process

The systemic inflammatory response syndrome (SIRS) can develop as a result of certain non-infectious disease processes, such as trauma, malignant neoplasm, or pancreatitis. When SIRS is documented with a noninfectious condition, and no subsequent infection is documented, the code for the underlying condition, such as an injury, should be assigned, followed by code R65.10. Systemic inflammatory response syndrome (SIRS) of non-infectious origin without acute organ dysfunction, or code R65.11, Systemic inflammatory response syndrome (SIRS) of non-infectious origin with acute organ dysfunction. If an associated acute organ dysfunction is documented, the appropriate code(s) for the specific type of organ dysfunction(s) should be assigned in addition to code R65.11. If acute organ dysfunction is documented, but it cannot be determined if the acute organ dysfunction is associated with SIRS or due to another condition (e.g., directly due to the trauma), the provider should be queried.

R65 Symptoms and signs specifically associated with systemic inflammation and infection

Ex: **For category R65 CC codes unless otherwise indicated:** A02.1, A20.7, A22.7, A26.7, A32.7, A39.2-A39.4, A40.0-A40.1, A40.8-A41.9, A42.7, A48.2-A48.4, A48.8-A49.9, A54.86, B00.7, B3.77, B92, B94.2-B96.89, R65.10-R65.20, Z16.10-Z16.39

R65.1 Systemic inflammatory response syndrome (SIRS) of non-infectious origin

Code first underlying condition, such as:
heatstroke (T67.0)
injury and trauma (S00-T88)

Excludes1 sepsis - code to infection
severe sepsis (R65.2)

R65.10 Systemic inflammatory response syndrome (SIRS) of non-infectious origin without acute organ dysfunction
Systemic inflammatory response syndrome (SIRS) NOS

R65.11 Systemic inflammatory response syndrome (SIRS) of non-infectious origin with acute organ dysfunction
Use additional code to identify specific acute organ dysfunction, such as:
acute kidney failure (N17.-)
acute respiratory failure (J96.0-)
critical illness myopathy (G72.81)
critical illness polyneuropathy (G62.81)
disseminated intravascular coagulopathy [DIC] (D65)
encephalopathy (metabolic) (septic) (G93.41)
hepatic failure (K72.0-)

R65.2 Severe sepsis
Infection with associated acute organ dysfunction
Sepsis with acute organ dysfunction
Sepsis with multiple organ dysfunction
Systemic inflammatory response syndrome due to infectious process with acute organ dysfunction

Code first underlying infection, such as:
infection following a procedure (T81.4-)
infections following infusion, transfusion and therapeutic injection (T80.2-)
puerperal sepsis (O85)
sepsis following complete or unspecified spontaneous abortion (O03.87)
sepsis following ectopic and molar pregnancy (O08.82)
sepsis following incomplete spontaneous abortion (O03.37)
sepsis following (induced) termination of pregnancy (O04.87)
sepsis NOS (A41.9)

Use additional code to identify specific acute organ dysfunction, such as:
acute kidney failure (N17.-)
acute respiratory failure (J96.0-)
critical illness myopathy (G72.81)
critical illness polyneuropathy (G62.81)
disseminated intravascular coagulopathy [DIC] (D65)
encephalopathy (metabolic) (septic) (G93.41)
hepatic failure (K72.0-)

R65.20 Severe sepsis without septic shock
Severe sepsis NOS

R65.21 Severe sepsis with septic shock
MCC when PDx is its own MCC
Ex: See R57

R68 Other general symptoms and signs

R68.0 Hypothermia, not associated with low environmental temperature

Excludes1 hypothermia NOS (accidental) (T68)
hypothermia due to anesthesia (T88.51)
hypothermia due to low environmental temperature (T68)
newborn hypothermia (P80.-)

R68.1 Nonspecific symptoms peculiar to infancy

Excludes1 colic, infantile (R10.83)
neonatal cerebral irritability (P91.3)
teething syndrome (K00.7)

R68.11 Excessive crying of infant (baby) P

Excludes1 excessive crying of child, adolescent, or adult (R45.83)

R68.12 Fussy infant (baby) P
Irritable infant

R68.13 Apparent life threatening event in infant (ALTE) P
Apparent life threatening event in newborn
Code first confirmed diagnosis, if known
Use additional code(s) for associated signs and symptoms if no confirmed diagnosis established, or if signs and symptoms are not associated routinely with confirmed diagnosis, or provide additional information for cause of ALTE

R68.19 Other nonspecific symptoms peculiar to infancy P

R68.2 Dry mouth, unspecified

Excludes1 dry mouth due to dehydration (E86.0)
dry mouth due to sicca syndrome [Sjögren] (M35.0-)
salivary gland hyposecretion (K11.7)

R68.3 Clubbing of fingers
Clubbing of nails

Excludes1 congenital clubfinger (Q68.1)

R68.8 Other general symptoms and signs

R68.81 Early satiety

R68.82 Decreased libido A
Decreased sexual desire

R68.83 Chills (without fever)
Chills NOS

Excludes1 chills with fever (R50.9)

R68.84 Jaw pain
Mandibular pain
Maxilla pain

Excludes1 temporomandibular joint arthralgia (M26.62-)

R68.89 Other general symptoms and signs

R69 Illness, unspecified
Unknown and unspecified cases of morbidity

ABNORMAL FINDINGS ON EXAMINATION OF BLOOD, WITHOUT DIAGNOSIS (R70-R79)

Excludes2 abnormal findings on antenatal screening of mother (O28.-)
abnormalities of lipids (E78.-)
abnormalities of platelets and thrombocytes (D69.-)
abnormalities of white blood cells classified elsewhere (D70-D72)
coagulation hemorrhagic disorders (D65-D68)
diagnostic abnormal findings classified elsewhere —*see* Alphabetical Index
hemorrhagic and hematological disorders of newborn (P50-P61)

R70 Elevated erythrocyte sedimentation rate and abnormality of plasma viscosity

R70.0 Elevated erythrocyte sedimentation rate

R70.1 Abnormal plasma viscosity

R71 Abnormality of red blood cells

Excludes1 anemias (D50-D64)
anemia of premature infant (P61.2)
benign (familial) polycythemia (D75.0)
congenital anemias (P61.2-P61.4)
newborn anemia due to isoimmunization (P55.-)
polycythemia neonatorum (P61.1)
polycythemia NOS (D75.1)
polycythemia vera (D45)
secondary polycythemia (D75.1)

R71.0 Precipitous drop in hematocrit
Drop (precipitous) in hemoglobin
Drop in hematocrit
Blood volume that is red blood cells
Ex D62, D64.4-D64.9

R71.8 Other abnormality of red blood cells
Abnormal red-cell morphology NOS
Abnormal red-cell volume NOS
Anisocytosis
Red blood cells of unequal size
Poikilocytosis
Red blood cells of abnormal shape

R73 Elevated blood glucose level

Excludes1 diabetes mellitus (E08-E13)
diabetes mellitus in pregnancy, childbirth and the puerperium (O24.-)
neonatal disorders (P70.0-P70.2)
postsurgical hypoinsulinemia (E89.1)

R73.0 Abnormal glucose

Excludes1 abnormal glucose in pregnancy (O99.81-)
diabetes mellitus (E08-E13)
dysmetabolic syndrome X (E88.81)
gestational diabetes (O24.4-)
glycosuria (R81)
hypoglycemia (E16.2)

R73.01 Impaired fasting glucose
Elevated fasting glucose

R73.02 Impaired glucose tolerance (oral)
Elevated glucose tolerance

R73.03 Prediabetes ◀
Latent diabetes ◀

R73.09 Other abnormal glucose
Abnormal glucose NOS
Abnormal non-fasting glucose tolerance
~~Prediabetes~~

R73.9 Hyperglycemia, unspecified

R74 Abnormal serum enzyme levels

R74.0 Nonspecific elevation of levels of transaminase and lactic acid dehydrogenase [LDH]

R74.8 Abnormal levels of other serum enzymes
Abnormal level of acid phosphatase
Abnormal level of alkaline phosphatase
Abnormal level of amylase
Abnormal level of lipase [triacylglycerol lipase]

R74.9 Abnormal serum enzyme level, unspecified

OGCR Section I.C.1.2.e and f.

Patients with inconclusive HIV serology

e. Patients with inconclusive HIV serology, but no definitive diagnosis or manifestations of the illness, may be assigned code R75, Inconclusive laboratory evidence of human immunodeficiency virus [HIV].

f. Previously diagnosed HIV-related illness

Patients with any known prior diagnosis of an HIV-related illness should be coded to B20. Once a patient has developed an HIV-related illness, the patient should always be assigned code B20 on every subsequent admission/encounter. Patients previously diagnosed with any HIV illness (B20) should never be assigned to R75 or Z21, Asymptomatic human immunodeficiency virus [HIV] infection status.

R75 Inconclusive laboratory evidence of human immunodeficiency virus [HIV]
Nonconclusive HIV-test finding in infants

Excludes1 asymptomatic human immunodeficiency virus [HIV] infection status (Z21)
human immunodeficiency virus [HIV] disease (B20)

R76 Other abnormal immunological findings in serum

R76.0 Raised antibody titer

Excludes1 isoimmunization in pregnancy (O36.0-O36.1)
isoimmunization affecting newborn (P55.-)

R76.1 Nonspecific reaction to test for tuberculosis

R76.11 Nonspecific reaction to tuberculin skin test without active tuberculosis
Abnormal result of Mantoux test
PPD positive
Tuberculin (skin test) positive
Tuberculin (skin test) reactor

Excludes1 nonspecific reaction to cell mediated immunity measurement of gamma interferon antigen response without active tuberculosis (R76.12)

R76.12 Nonspecific reaction to cell mediated immunity measurement of gamma interferon antigen response without active tuberculosis
Nonspecific reaction to QuantiFERON-TB test (QFT) without active tuberculosis

Excludes1 nonspecific reaction to tuberculin skin test without active tuberculosis (R76.11)
positive tuberculin skin test (R76.11)

R76.8 Other specified abnormal immunological findings in serum
Raised level of immunoglobulins NOS

R76.9 Abnormal immunological finding in serum, unspecified

R77 Other abnormalities of plasma proteins

Excludes1 disorders of plasma-protein metabolism (E88.0)

R77.0 Abnormality of albumin

R77.1 Abnormality of globulin
Hyperglobulinemia NOS

R77.2 Abnormality of alphafetoprotein

R77.8 Other specified abnormalities of plasma proteins

R77.9 Abnormality of plasma protein, unspecified

R78 Findings of drugs and other substances, not normally found in blood

Use additional code to identify any retained foreign body, if applicable (Z18.-)

Excludes1 mental or behavioral disorders due to psychoactive substance use (F10-F19)

R78.0 Finding of alcohol in blood
Use additional external cause code (Y90.-), for detail regarding alcohol level.

R78.1 Finding of opiate drug in blood

R78.2 Finding of cocaine in blood

R78.3 Finding of hallucinogen in blood

R78.4 Finding of other drugs of addictive potential in blood

R78.5 Finding of other psychotropic drug in blood

R78.6 Finding of steroid agent in blood

R78.7 Finding of abnormal level of heavy metals in blood

R78.71 Abnormal lead level in blood

Excludes1 lead poisoning (T56.0-)

R78.79 Finding of abnormal level of heavy metals in blood

● **R78.8 Finding of other specified substances, not normally found in blood**

R78.81 Bacteremia
Blood poisoning/bacteremia
Excludes1 sepsis-code to specified infection
Ex B34.9, E07.81, G89.0-G89.4, R29.700-R29.742, R41.0-R41.3, R41.82, R41.9, R44.8-R44.9, R45.83-R45.84, R46.0-R46.89, R52, R68.0-R68.19, R68.81-R68.83, R68.89-R69, R70.1, R77.0-R77.9, R78.1-R78.6, R78.81, R78.9, R79.1-R79.89, R97.20, R97.21

R78.89 Finding of other specified substances, not normally found in blood
Finding of abnormal level of lithium in blood

R78.9 Finding of unspecified substance, not normally found in blood

● **R79 Other abnormal findings of blood chemistry**
Use additional code to identify any retained foreign body, if applicable (Z18.-)
Excludes1 abnormality of fluid, electrolyte or acid-base balance (E86-E87)
asymptomatic hyperuricemia (E79.0)
hyperglycemia NOS (R73.9)
hypoglycemia NOS (E16.2)
neonatal hypoglycemia (P70.3-P70.4)
specific findings indicating disorder of amino-acid metabolism (E70-E72)
specific findings indicating disorder of carbohydrate metabolism (E73-E74)
specific findings indicating disorder of lipid metabolism (E75.-)

R79.0 Abnormal level of blood mineral
Abnormal blood level of cobalt
Abnormal blood level of copper
Abnormal blood level of iron
Abnormal blood level of magnesium
Abnormal blood level of mineral NEC
Abnormal blood level of zinc
Excludes1 abnormal level of lithium (R78.89)
disorders of mineral metabolism (E83.-)
neonatal hypomagnesemia (P71.2)
nutritional mineral deficiency (E58-E61)

R79.1 Abnormal coagulation profile
Abnormal or prolonged bleeding time
Abnormal or prolonged coagulation time
Abnormal or prolonged partial thromboplastin time [PTT]
Abnormal or prolonged prothrombin time [PT]
Excludes1 coagulation defects (D68.-)

● **R79.8 Other specified abnormal findings of blood chemistry**

R79.81 Abnormal blood-gas level

R79.82 Elevated C-reactive protein (CRP)

R79.89 Other specified abnormal findings of blood chemistry

R79.9 Abnormal finding of blood chemistry, unspecified

ABNORMAL FINDINGS ON EXAMINATION OF URINE, WITHOUT DIAGNOSIS (R80-R82)

Excludes1 abnormal findings on antenatal screening of mother (O28.-)
diagnostic abnormal findings classified elsewhere - see Alphabetical Index
specific findings indicating disorder of amino-acid metabolism (E70-E72)
specific findings indicating disorder of carbohydrate metabolism (E73-E74)

● **R80 Proteinuria**
Excludes1 gestational proteinuria (O12.1-)

R80.0 Isolated proteinuria
Idiopathic proteinuria
Excludes1 isolated proteinuria with specific morphological lesion (N06.-)

R80.1 Persistent proteinuria, unspecified

R80.2 Orthostatic proteinuria, unspecified
Postural proteinuria

R80.3 Bence Jones proteinuria

R80.8 Other proteinuria

R80.9 Proteinuria, unspecified
Albuminuria NOS

R81 Glycosuria
Excludes1 renal glycosuria (E74.8)

● **R82 Other and unspecified abnormal findings in urine**
Includes chromoabnormalities in urine
Use additional code to identify any retained foreign body, if applicable (Z18.-)
Excludes2 hematuria (R31.-)

R82.0 Chyluria
White milky urine
Excludes1 filarial chyluria (B74.-)
Ex G89.0-G89.4, R29.700-R29.742, R41.0-R41.3, R41.82, R41.9, R44.8-R44.9, R45.83-R45.84, R46.0-R46.89, R52, R68.0-R68.19, R68.81-R68.83, R68.89-R69, R82.0, R82.5-R82.99

R82.1 Myoglobinuria
Presence of myoglobin (iron containing protein) in urine
Ex G89.0-G89.4, R29.700-R29.742, R41.0-R41.3, R41.82, R41.9, R44.8-R44.9, R45.83-R45.84, R46.0-R46.89, R52, R68.0-R68.19, R68.81-R68.83, R68.89-R69, R82.1, R82.3, R82.5-R82.99

R82.2 Biliuria
Presence of bile pigments/salts in urine

R82.3 Hemoglobinuria
Presence of hemoglobin in urine
Excludes1 hemoglobinuria due to hemolysis from external causes NEC (D59.6)
hemoglobinuria due to paroxysmal nocturnal [Marchiafava-Micheli] (D59.5)

R82.4 Acetonuria
Ketonuria

R82.5 Elevated urine levels of drugs, medicaments and biological substances
Elevated urine levels of catecholamines
Elevated urine levels of indoleacetic acid
Elevated urine levels of 17-ketosteroids
Elevated urine levels of steroids

R82.6 Abnormal urine levels of substances chiefly nonmedicinal as to source
Abnormal urine level of heavy metals

● **R82.7 Abnormal findings on microbiological examination of urine**
Excludes1 colonization status (Z22.-)

R82.71 Bacteriuria ◀

R82.79 Other abnormal findings on microbiological examination of urine ◀
Positive culture findings of urine ◀

R82.8 Abnormal findings on cytological and histological examination of urine

R82.9 Other and unspecified abnormal findings in urine

R82.90 Unspecified abnormal findings in urine

R82.91 Other chromoabnormalities of urine
Chromoconversion (dipstick)
Idiopathic dipstick converts positive for blood with no cellular forms in sediment

Excludes1 hemoglobinuria (R82.3)
myoglobinuria (R82.1)

R82.99 Other abnormal findings in urine
Cells and casts in urine
Crystalluria
Melanuria

ABNORMAL FINDINGS ON EXAMINATION OF OTHER BODY FLUIDS, SUBSTANCES AND TISSUES, WITHOUT DIAGNOSIS (R83-R89)

Excludes1 abnormal findings on antenatal screening of mother (O28.-)
diagnostic abnormal findings classified elsewhere - see Alphabetical Index

Excludes2 abnormal findings on examination of blood, without diagnosis (R70-R79)
abnormal findings on examination of urine, without diagnosis (R80-R82)
abnormal tumor markers (R97.-)

R83 Abnormal findings in cerebrospinal fluid

R83.0 Abnormal level of enzymes in cerebrospinal fluid

R83.1 Abnormal level of hormones in cerebrospinal fluid

R83.2 Abnormal level of other drugs, medicaments and biological substances in cerebrospinal fluid

R83.3 Abnormal level of substances chiefly nonmedicinal as to source in cerebrospinal fluid

R83.4 Abnormal immunological findings in cerebrospinal fluid

R83.5 Abnormal microbiological findings in cerebrospinal fluid
Positive culture findings in cerebrospinal fluid

Excludes1 colonization status (Z22.-)

R83.6 Abnormal cytological findings in cerebrospinal fluid

R83.8 Other abnormal findings in cerebrospinal fluid
Abnormal chromosomal findings in cerebrospinal fluid

R83.9 Unspecified abnormal finding in cerebrospinal fluid

R84 Abnormal findings in specimens from respiratory organs and thorax

Includes abnormal findings in bronchial washings
abnormal findings in nasal secretions
abnormal findings in pleural fluid
abnormal findings in sputum
abnormal findings in throat scrapings

Excludes1 blood-stained sputum (R04.2)

R84.0 Abnormal level of enzymes in specimens from respiratory organs and thorax

R84.1 Abnormal level of hormones in specimens from respiratory organs and thorax

R84.2 Abnormal level of other drugs, medicaments and biological substances in specimens from respiratory organs and thorax

R84.3 Abnormal level of substances chiefly nonmedicinal as to source in specimens from respiratory organs and thorax

R84.4 Abnormal immunological findings in specimens from respiratory organs and thorax

R84.5 Abnormal microbiological findings in specimens from respiratory organs and thorax
Positive culture findings in specimens from respiratory organs and thorax

Excludes1 colonization status (Z22.-)

R84.6 Abnormal cytological findings in specimens from respiratory organs and thorax

R84.7 Abnormal histological findings in specimens from respiratory organs and thorax

R84.8 Other abnormal findings in specimens from respiratory organs and thorax
Abnormal chromosomal findings in specimens from respiratory organs and thorax

R84.9 Unspecified abnormal finding in specimens from respiratory organs and thorax

R85 Abnormal findings in specimens from digestive organs and abdominal cavity

Includes abnormal findings in peritoneal fluid
abnormal findings in saliva

Excludes1 cloudy peritoneal dialysis effluent (R88.0)
fecal abnormalities (R19.5)

R85.0 Abnormal level of enzymes in specimens from digestive organs and abdominal cavity

R85.1 Abnormal level of hormones in specimens from digestive organs and abdominal cavity

R85.2 Abnormal level of other drugs, medicaments and biological substances in specimens from digestive organs and abdominal cavity

R85.3 Abnormal level of substances chiefly nonmedicinal as to source in specimens from digestive organs and abdominal cavity

R85.4 Abnormal immunological findings in specimens from digestive organs and abdominal cavity

R85.5 Abnormal microbiological findings in specimens from digestive organs and abdominal cavity
Positive culture findings in specimens from digestive organs and abdominal cavity

Excludes1 colonization status (Z22.-)

R85.6 Abnormal cytological findings in specimens from digestive organs and abdominal cavity

R85.61 Abnormal cytologic smear of anus

Excludes1 abnormal cytological findings in specimens from other digestive organs and abdominal cavity (R85.69)
carcinoma in situ of anus (histologically confirmed) (D01.3)
anal intraepithelial neoplasia I [AIN I] (K62.82)
anal intraepithelial neoplasia II [AIN II] (K62.82)
anal intraepithelial neoplasia III [AIN III] (D01.3)
dysplasia (mild) (moderate) of anus (histologically confirmed) (K62.82)
severe dysplasia of anus (histologically confirmed) (D01.3)

Excludes2 anal high risk human papillomavirus (HPV) DNA test positive (R85.81)
anal low risk human papillomavirus (HPV) DNA test positive (R85.82)

R85.610 Atypical squamous cells of undetermined significance on cytologic smear of anus (ASC-US)

R85.611 Atypical squamous cells cannot exclude high grade squamous intraepithelial lesion on cytologic smear of anus (ASC-H)

R85.612 Low grade squamous intraepithelial lesion on cytologic smear of anus (LGSIL)

R85.613 High grade squamous intraepithelial lesion on cytologic smear of anus (HGSIL)

R85.614 Cytologic evidence of malignancy on smear of anus

R85.615 Unsatisfactory cytologic smear of anus
Inadequate sample of cytologic smear of anus

R85.616 Satisfactory anal smear but lacking transformation zone

R85.618 Other abnormal cytological findings on specimens from anus

R85.619 Unspecified abnormal cytological findings in specimens from anus
Abnormal anal cytology NOS
Atypical glandular cells of anus NOS

R85.69 Abnormal cytological findings in specimens from other digestive organs and abdominal cavity

R85.7 Abnormal histological findings in specimens from digestive organs and abdominal cavity

● **R85.8 Other abnormal findings in specimens from digestive organs and abdominal cavity**

R85.81 Anal high risk human papillomavirus (HPV) DNA test positive
Excludes1 anogenital warts due to human papillomavirus (HPV) (A63.0)
condyloma acuminatum (A63.0)

R85.82 Anal low risk human papillomavirus (HPV) DNA test positive
Use additional code for associated human papillomavirus (B97.7)

R85.89 Other abnormal findings in specimens from digestive organs and abdominal cavity
Abnormal chromosomal findings in specimens from digestive organs and abdominal cavity

R85.9 Unspecified abnormal finding in specimens from digestive organs and abdominal cavity

● **R86 Abnormal findings in specimens from male genital organs**
Includes abnormal findings in prostatic secretions
abnormal findings in semen, seminal fluid
abnormal spermatozoa
Excludes1 azoospermia (N46.0-)
oligospermia (N46.1-)

R86.0 Abnormal level of enzymes in specimens from male genital organs ♂

R86.1 Abnormal level of hormones in specimens from male genital organs ♂

R86.2 Abnormal level of other drugs, medicaments and biological substances in specimens from male genital organs ♂

R86.3 Abnormal level of substances chiefly nonmedicinal as to source in specimens from male genital organs ♂

R86.4 Abnormal immunological findings in specimens from male genital organs ♂

R86.5 Abnormal microbiological findings in specimens from male genital organs ♂
Positive culture findings in specimens from male genital organs
Excludes1 colonization status (Z22.-)

R86.6 Abnormal cytological findings in specimens from male genital organs ♂

R86.7 Abnormal histological findings in specimens from male genital organs ♂

R86.8 Other abnormal findings in specimens from male genital organs ♂
Abnormal chromosomal findings in specimens from male genital organs

R86.9 Unspecified abnormal finding in specimens from male genital organs ♂

● **R87 Abnormal findings in specimens from female genital organs**
Includes abnormal findings in secretion and smears from cervix uteri
abnormal findings in secretion and smears from vagina
abnormal findings in secretion and smears from vulva

R87.0 Abnormal level of enzymes in specimens from female genital organs ♀

R87.1 Abnormal level of hormones in specimens from female genital organs ♀

R87.2 Abnormal level of other drugs, medicaments and biological substances in specimens from female genital organs ♀

R87.3 Abnormal level of substances chiefly nonmedicinal as to source in specimens from female genital organs ♀

R87.4 Abnormal immunological findings in specimens from female genital organs ♀

R87.5 Abnormal microbiological findings in specimens from female genital organs ♀
Positive culture findings in specimens from female genital organs
Excludes1 colonization status (Z22.-)

● **R87.6 Abnormal cytological findings in specimens from female genital organs**

● **R87.61 Abnormal cytological findings in specimens from cervix uteri**
Excludes1 abnormal cytological findings in specimens from other female genital organs (R87.69)
abnormal cytological findings in specimens from vagina (R87.62-)
carcinoma in situ of cervix uteri (histologically confirmed) (D06.-)
cervical intraepithelial neoplasia I [CIN I] (N87.0)
cervical intraepithelial neoplasia II [CIN II] (N87.1)
cervical intraepithelial neoplasia III [CIN III] (D06.-)
dysplasia (mild) (moderate) of cervix uteri (histologically confirmed) (N87.-)
severe dysplasia of cervix uteri (histologically confirmed) (D06.-)
Excludes2 cervical high risk human papillomavirus (HPV) DNA test positive (R87.810)
cervical low risk human papillomavirus (HPV) DNA test positive (R87.820)

R87.610 Atypical squamous cells of undetermined significance on cytologic smear of cervix (ASC-US) ♀

R87.611 Atypical squamous cells cannot exclude high grade squamous intraepithelial lesion on cytologic smear of cervix (ASC-H) ♀

R87.612 Low grade squamous intraepithelial lesion on cytologic smear of cervix (LGSIL) ♀

R87.613 High grade squamous intraepithelial lesion on cytologic smear of cervix (HGSIL) ♀

R87.614 Cytologic evidence of malignancy on smear of cervix ♀

R87.615 Unsatisfactory cytologic smear of cervix ♀
Inadequate sample of cytologic smear of cervix

R87.616 Satisfactory cervical smear but lacking transformation zone ♀

R87.618 Other abnormal cytological findings on specimens from cervix uteri ♀

R87.619 Unspecified abnormal cytological findings in specimens from cervix uteri ♀
- Abnormal cervical cytology NOS
- Abnormal Papanicolaou smear of cervix NOS
- Abnormal thin preparation smear of cervix NOS
- Atypical endocervial cells of cervix NOS
- Atypical endometrial cells of cervix NOS
- Atypical glandular cells of cervix NOS

R87.62 Abnormal cytological findings in specimens from vagina

Use additional code to identify acquired absence of uterus and cervix, if applicable (Z90.71-)

Excludes1 abnormal cytological findings in specimens from cervix uteri (R87.61-)
- abnormal cytological findings in specimens from other female genital organs (R87.69)
- carcinoma in situ of vagina (histologically confirmed) (D07.2)
- vaginal intraepithelial neoplasia I [VAIN I] (N89.0)
- vaginal intraepithelial neoplasia II [VAIN II] (N89.1)
- vaginal intraepithelial neoplasia III [VAIN III] (D07.2)
- dysplasia (mild) (moderate) of vagina (histologically confirmed) (N89.-)
- severe dysplasia of vagina (histologically confirmed) (D07.2)

Excludes2 vaginal high risk human papillomavirus (HPV) DNA test positive (R87.811)
- vaginal low risk human papillomavirus (HPV) DNA test positive (R87.821)

R87.620 Atypical squamous cells of undetermined significance on cytologic smear of vagina (ASC-US) ♀

R87.621 Atypical squamous cells cannot exclude high grade squamous intraepithelial lesion on cytologic smear of vagina (ASC-H) ♀

R87.622 Low grade squamous intraepithelial lesion on cytologic smear of vagina (LGSIL) ♀

R87.623 High grade squamous intraepithelial lesion on cytologic smear of vagina (HGSIL) ♀

R87.624 Cytologic evidence of malignancy on smear of vagina ♀

R87.625 Unsatisfactory cytologic smear of vagina ♀
- Inadequate sample of cytologic smear of vagina

R87.628 Other abnormal cytological findings on specimens from vagina ♀

R87.629 Unspecified abnormal cytological findings in specimens from vagina ♀
- Abnormal Papanicolaou smear of vagina NOS
- Abnormal thin preparation smear of vagina NOS
- Abnormal vaginal cytology NOS
- Atypical endocervical cells of vagina NOS
- Atypical endometrial cells of vagina NOS
- Atypical glandular cells of vagina NOS

R87.69 Abnormal cytological findings in specimens from other female genital organs ♀
- Abnormal cytological findings in specimens from female genital organs NOS

Excludes1 dysplasia of vulva (histologically confirmed) (N90.0-N90.3)

R87.7 Abnormal histological findings in specimens from female genital organs ♀

Excludes1 carcinoma in situ (histologically confirmed) of female genital organs (D06-D07.3)
- cervical intraepithelial neoplasia I [CIN I] (N87.0)
- cervical intraepithelial neoplasia II [CIN II] (N87.1)
- cervical intraepithelial neoplasia III [CIN III] (D06.-)
- dysplasia (mild) (moderate) of cervix uteri (histologically confirmed) (N87.-)
- dysplasia (mild) (moderate) of vagina (histologically confirmed) (N89.-)
- vaginal intraepithelial neoplasia I [VAIN I] (N89.0)
- vaginal intraepithelial neoplasia II [VAIN II] (N89.1)
- vaginal intraepithelial neoplasia III [VAIN III] (D07.2)
- severe dysplasia of cervix uteri (histologically confirmed) (D06.-)
- severe dysplasia of vagina (histologically confirmed) (D07.2)

R87.8 Other abnormal findings in specimens from female genital organs

R87.81 High risk human papillomavirus (HPV) DNA test positive from female genital organs

Excludes1 anogenital warts due to human papillomavirus (HPV) (A63.0)
- condyloma acuminatum (A63.0)

R87.810 Cervical high risk human papillomavirus (HPV) DNA test positive ♀

R87.811 Vaginal high risk human papillomavirus (HPV) DNA test positive ♀

R87.82 Low risk human papillomavirus (HPV) DNA test positive from female genital organs

Use additional code for associated human papillomavirus (B97.7)

R87.820 Cervical low risk human papillomavirus (HPV) DNA test positive ♀

R87.821 Vaginal low risk human papillomavirus (HPV) DNA test positive ♀

R87.89 Other abnormal findings in specimens from female genital organs ♀
- Abnormal chromosomal findings in specimens from female genital organs

R87.9 Unspecified abnormal finding in specimens from female genital organs ♀

● **R88 Abnormal findings in other body fluids and substances**

R88.0 Cloudy (hemodialysis) (peritoneal) dialysis effluent

R88.8 Abnormal findings in other body fluids and substances

● **R89 Abnormal findings in specimens from other organs, systems and tissues**

Includes abnormal findings in nipple discharge
abnormal findings in synovial fluid
abnormal findings in wound secretions

R89.0 Abnormal level of enzymes in specimens from other organs, systems and tissues

R89.1 Abnormal level of hormones in specimens from other organs, systems and tissues

R89.2 Abnormal level of other drugs, medicaments and biological substances in specimens from other organs, systems and tissues

R89.3 Abnormal level of substances chiefly nonmedicinal as to source in specimens from other organs, systems and tissues

R89.4 Abnormal immunological findings in specimens from other organs, systems and tissues

R89.5 Abnormal microbiological findings in specimens from other organs, systems and tissues
Positive culture findings in specimens from other organs, systems and tissues

Excludes1 colonization status (Z22.-)

R89.6 Abnormal cytological findings in specimens from other organs, systems and tissues

R89.7 Abnormal histological findings in specimens from other organs, systems and tissues

R89.8 Other abnormal findings in specimens from other organs, systems and tissues
Abnormal chromosomal findings in specimens from other organs, systems and tissues

R89.9 Unspecified abnormal finding in specimens from other organs, systems and tissues

ABNORMAL FINDINGS ON DIAGNOSTIC IMAGING AND IN FUNCTION STUDIES, WITHOUT DIAGNOSIS (R90-R94)

Includes nonspecific abnormal findings on diagnostic imaging by computerized axial tomography [CAT scan]
nonspecific abnormal findings on diagnostic imaging by magnetic resonance imaging [MRI][NMR]
nonspecific abnormal findings on diagnostic imaging by positron emission tomography [PET scan]
nonspecific abnormal findings on diagnostic imaging by thermography
nonspecific abnormal findings on diagnostic imaging by ultrasound [echogram]
nonspecific abnormal findings on diagnostic imaging by X-ray examination

Excludes1 abnormal findings on antenatal screening of mother (O28.-)
diagnostic abnormal findings classified elsewhere - see Alphabetical Index

● **R90 Abnormal findings on diagnostic imaging of central nervous system**

R90.0 Intracranial space-occupying lesion found on diagnostic imaging of central nervous system

● **R90.8 Other abnormal findings on diagnostic imaging of central nervous system**

R90.81 Abnormal echoencephalogram

R90.82 White matter disease, unspecified

R90.89 Other abnormal findings on diagnostic imaging of central nervous system
Other cerebrovascular abnormality found on diagnostic imaging of central nervous system

● **R91 Abnormal findings on diagnostic imaging of lung**

R91.1 Solitary pulmonary nodule
Coin lesion lung
Solitary pulmonary nodule, subsegmental branch of the bronchial tree

R91.8 Other nonspecific abnormal finding of lung field
Lung mass NOS found on diagnostic imaging of lung
Pulmonary infiltrate NOS
Shadow, lung

● **R92 Abnormal and inconclusive findings on diagnostic imaging of breast**

R92.0 Mammographic microcalcification found on diagnostic imaging of breast

Excludes2 mammographic calcification (calculus) found on diagnostic imaging of breast (R92.1)

R92.1 Mammographic calcification found on diagnostic imaging of breast
Mammographic calculus found on diagnostic imaging of breast

R92.2 Inconclusive mammogram
Dense breasts NOS
Inconclusive mammogram NEC
Inconclusive mammography due to dense breasts
Inconclusive mammography NEC
Coding Clinic: 2015, Q1, P24

R92.8 Other abnormal and inconclusive findings on diagnostic imaging of breast

● **R93 Abnormal findings on diagnostic imaging of other body structures**

R93.0 Abnormal findings on diagnostic imaging of skull and head, not elsewhere classified

Excludes1 intracranial space-occupying lesion found on diagnostic imaging (R90.0)

R93.1 Abnormal findings on diagnostic imaging of heart and coronary circulation
Abnormal echocardiogram NOS
Abnormal heart shadow

R93.2 Abnormal findings on diagnostic imaging of liver and biliary tract
Nonvisualization of gallbladder

R93.3 Abnormal findings on diagnostic imaging of other parts of digestive tract

● **R93.4 Abnormal findings on diagnostic imaging of urinary organs**

Excludes2 hypertrophy of kidney (N28.81) ◀

R93.41 Abnormal radiologic findings on diagnostic imaging of renal pelvis, ureter, or bladder ◀
Filling defect of bladder found on diagnostic imaging ◀
Filling defect of renal pelvis found on diagnostic imaging ◀
Filling defect of ureter found on diagnostic imaging ◀

● **R93.42 Abnormal radiologic findings on diagnostic imaging of kidney** ◀

R93.421 Abnormal radiologic findings on diagnostic imaging of right kidney ◀

R93.422 Abnormal radiologic findings on diagnostic imaging of left kidney ◀

R93.429 Abnormal radiologic findings on diagnostic imaging of unspecified kidney ◀

R93.49 Abnormal radiologic findings on diagnostic imaging of other urinary organs ◀

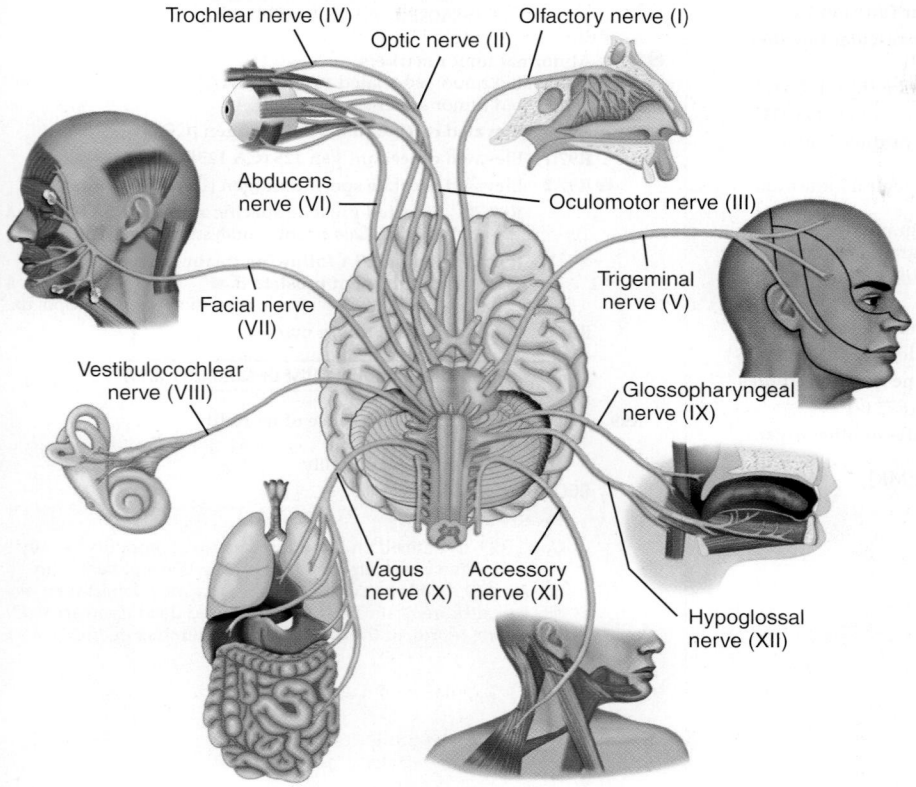

Figure 18-2 Cranial nerves. (From Patton and Thibodeau: Anatomy and physiology, ed 7, St. Louis, Mosby, 2009)

R93.5 Abnormal findings on diagnostic imaging of other abdominal regions, including retroperitoneum

R93.6 Abnormal findings on diagnostic imaging of limbs

Excludes2 abnormal finding in skin and subcutaneous tissue (R93.8)

R93.7 Abnormal findings on diagnostic imaging of other parts of musculoskeletal system

Excludes2 abnormal findings on diagnostic imaging of skull (R93.0)

R93.8 Abnormal findings on diagnostic imaging of other specified body structures

Abnormal finding by radioisotope localization of placenta
Abnormal radiological finding in skin and subcutaneous tissue
Mediastinal shift

R93.9 Diagnostic imaging inconclusive due to excess body fat of patient

● **R94 Abnormal results of function studies**

Includes abnormal results of radionuclide [radioisotope] uptake studies
abnormal results of scintigraphy

● **R94.0 Abnormal results of function studies of central nervous system**

R94.01 Abnormal electroencephalogram [EEG]

R94.02 Abnormal brain scan

R94.09 Abnormal results of other function studies of central nervous system

● **R94.1 Abnormal results of function studies of peripheral nervous system and special senses**

● **R94.11 Abnormal results of function studies of eye**

R94.110 Abnormal electro-oculogram [EOG]

R94.111 Abnormal electroretinogram [ERG]
Abnormal retinal function study

R94.112 Abnormal visually evoked potential [VEP]

R94.113 Abnormal oculomotor study

R94.118 Abnormal results of other function studies of eye

● **R94.12 Abnormal results of function studies of ear and other special senses**

R94.120 Abnormal auditory function study

R94.121 Abnormal vestibular function study

R94.128 Abnormal results of other function studies of ear and other special senses

● **R94.13 Abnormal results of function studies of peripheral nervous system**

R94.130 Abnormal response to nerve stimulation, unspecified

R94.131 Abnormal electromyogram [EMG]

Excludes1 electromyogram of eye (R94.113)

R94.138 Abnormal results of other function studies of peripheral nervous system

R94.2 Abnormal results of pulmonary function studies

Reduced ventilatory capacity
Reduced vital capacity

Item 18–1 The **peripheral nervous system** consists of 31 pairs of spinal nerves, 12 pairs of cranial nerves, and the autonomic nerves, which are divided into the parasympathetic and sympathetic nerves. The cranial nerves are: olfactory (I), optic (II), oculomotor (III), trochlear (IV), trigeminal (V), abducens (VI), facial (VII), vestibulocochlear (VIII), glossopharyngeal (IX), vagus (X), accessory (XI), and hypoglossal (XII).

● **R94.3 Abnormal results of cardiovascular function studies**

R94.30 Abnormal result of cardiovascular function study, unspecified

R94.31 Abnormal electrocardiogram [ECG] [EKG]

Excludes1 long QT syndrome (I45.81)

R94.39 Abnormal result of other cardiovascular function study

Abnormal electrophysiological intracardiac studies
Abnormal phonocardiogram
Abnormal vectorcardiogram

R94.4 Abnormal results of kidney function studies

Abnormal renal function test

R94.5 Abnormal results of liver function studies

R94.6 Abnormal results of thyroid function studies

R94.7 Abnormal results of other endocrine function studies

Excludes2 abnormal glucose (R73.0-)

R94.8 Abnormal results of function studies of other organs and systems

Abnormal basal metabolic rate [BMR]
Abnormal bladder function test
Abnormal splenic function test

ABNORMAL TUMOR MARKERS (R97)

● **R97 Abnormal tumor markers**

Elevated tumor associated antigens [TAA]
Elevated tumor specific antigens [TSA]

R97.0 Elevated carcinoembryonic antigen [CEA]

R97.1 Elevated cancer antigen 125 [CA 125] ♀

● **R97.2 Elevated prostate specific antigen [PSA]**

R97.20 Elevated prostate specific antigen [PSA] ♂ ◀ A

MCE: Questionable admission when principal dx

R97.21 Rising PSA following treatment for malignant neoplasm of prostate ♂ ◀ A

MCE: Questionable admission when principal dx

R97.8 Other abnormal tumor markers

ILL-DEFINED AND UNKNOWN CAUSE OF MORTALITY (R99)

R99 Ill-defined and unknown cause of mortality

Death (unexplained) NOS
Unspecified cause of mortality

OGCR Section I.C.18.h.

Death NOS

Code R99, Ill-defined and unknown cause of mortality, is only for use in the very limited circumstance when a patient who has already died is brought into the emergency department or other healthcare facility and is pronounced dead upon arrival. It does not represent the discharge disposition of death.

CHAPTER 19

INJURY, POISONING AND CERTAIN OTHER CONSEQUENCES OF EXTERNAL CAUSES (S00-T88)

OGCR Chapter-Specific Coding Guidelines

19. Chapter 19: Injury, poisoning, and certain other consequences of external causes (S00-T88)

a. Application of 7th Characters in Chapter 19

Most categories in chapter 19 have a 7th character requirement for each applicable code. Most categories in this chapter have three 7th character values (with the exception of fractures): A, initial encounter, D, subsequent encounter and S, sequela. Categories for traumatic fractures have additional 7th character values. **While the patient may be seen by a new or different provider over the course of treatment for an injury, assignment of the 7th character is based on whether the patient is undergoing active treatment and not whether the provider is seeing the patient for the first time.**

For complication codes, active treatment refers to treatment for the condition described by the code, even though it may be related to an earlier precipitating problem. For example, code T84.50XA, Infection and inflammatory reaction due to unspecified internal joint prosthesis, initial encounter, is used when active treatment is provided for the infection, even though the condition relates to the prosthetic device, implant or graft that was placed at a previous encounter.

7th character "A", initial encounter is used **for each encounter where** the patient is receiving active treatment for the condition.

7th character "D" subsequent encounter is used for encounters after the patient has **completed** active treatment of the condition and is receiving routine care for the condition during the healing or recovery phase.

The aftercare Z codes should not be used for aftercare for conditions such as injuries or poisonings, where 7th characters are provided to identify subsequent care. For example, for aftercare of an injury, assign the acute injury code with the 7th character "D" (subsequent encounter).

7th character "S", sequela, is for use for complications or conditions that arise as a direct result of a condition, such as scar formation after a burn. The scars are sequelae of the burn. When using 7th character "S", it is necessary to use both the injury code that precipitated the sequela and the code for the sequela itself. The "S" is added only to the injury code, not the sequela code. The 7th character "S" identifies the injury responsible for the sequela. The specific type of sequela (e.g. scar) is sequenced first, followed by the injury code.

See Section I.B.10. Sequelae, (Late Effects)

b. Coding of Injuries

When coding injuries, assign separate codes for each injury unless a combination code is provided, in which case the combination code is assigned. Code T07, Unspecified multiple injuries should not be assigned in the inpatient setting unless information for a more specific code is not available. Traumatic injury codes (S00-T14.9) are not to be used for normal, healing surgical wounds or to identify complications of surgical wounds.

The code for the most serious injury, as determined by the provider and the focus of treatment, is sequenced first.

1) Superficial injuries

Superficial injuries such as abrasions or contusions are not coded when associated with more severe injuries of the same site.

2) Primary injury with damage to nerves/blood vessels

When a primary injury results in minor damage to peripheral nerves or blood vessels, the primary injury is sequenced first with additional code(s) for injuries to nerves and spinal cord (such as category S04), and/or injury to blood vessels (such as category S15). When the primary injury is to the blood vessels or nerves, that injury should be sequenced first.

c. Coding of Traumatic Fractures

The principles of multiple coding of injuries should be followed in coding fractures. Fractures of specified sites are coded individually by site in accordance with both the provisions within categories S02, S12, S22, S32, S42, S49, S52, S59, S62, S72, S79, S82, S89, S92 and the level of detail furnished by medical record content.

A fracture not indicated as open or closed should be coded to closed. A fracture not indicated whether displaced or not displaced should be coded to displaced.

More specific guidelines are as follows:

1) Initial vs. Subsequent Encounter for Fractures

Traumatic fractures are coded using the appropriate 7th character for initial encounter (A, B, C) **for each encounter where** the patient is receiving active treatment for the fracture. The appropriate 7th character for initial encounter should also be assigned for a patient who delayed seeking treatment for the fracture or nonunion.

Fractures are coded using the appropriate 7th character for subsequent care for encounters after the patient has completed active treatment of the fracture and is receiving routine care for the fracture during the healing or recovery phase.

Care for complications of surgical treatment for fracture repairs during the healing or recovery phase should be coded with the appropriate complication codes.

Care of complications of fractures, such as malunion and nonunion, should be reported with the appropriate 7th character for subsequent care with nonunion (K, M, N,) or subsequent care with malunion (P, Q, R).

Malunion/nonunion: The appropriate 7th character for initial encounter should also be assigned for a patient who delayed seeking treatment for the fracture or nonunion.

The open fracture designations in the assignment of the 7th character for fractures of the forearm, femur and lower leg, including ankle are based on the Gustilo open fracture classification. When the Gustilo classification type is not specified for an open fracture, the 7th character for open fracture type I or II should be assigned (B, E, H, M, Q).

A code from category M80, not a traumatic fracture code, should be used for any patient with known osteoporosis who suffers a fracture, even if the patient had a minor fall or trauma, if that fall or trauma would not usually break a normal, healthy bone.

See Section I.C.13. Osteoporosis.

The aftercare Z codes should not be used for aftercare for traumatic fractures. For aftercare of a traumatic fracture, assign the acute fracture code with the appropriate 7th character.

2) Multiple fractures sequencing

Multiple fractures are sequenced in accordance with the severity of the fracture.

d. Coding of Burns and Corrosions

The ICD-10-CM makes a distinction between burns and corrosions. The burn codes are for thermal burns, except sunburns, that come from a heat source, such as a fire or hot appliance. The burn codes are also for burns resulting from electricity and radiation. Corrosions are burns due to chemicals. The guidelines are the same for burns and corrosions.

Current burns (T20-T25) are classified by depth, extent and by agent (X code). Burns are classified by depth as first degree (erythema), second degree (blistering), and third degree (full-thickness involvement). Burns of the eye and internal organs (T26-T28) are classified by site, but not by degree.

1) Sequencing of burn and related condition codes

Sequence first the code that reflects the highest degree of burn when more than one burn is present.

a. When the reason for the admission or encounter is for treatment of external multiple burns, sequence first the code that reflects the burn of the highest degree.
b. When a patient has both internal and external burns, the circumstances of admission govern the selection of the principal diagnosis or first-listed diagnosis.
c. When a patient is admitted for burn injuries and other related conditions such as smoke inhalation and/or respiratory failure, the circumstances of admission govern the selection of the principal or first-listed diagnosis.

2) Burns of the same local site
Classify burns of the same local site (three-character category level, T20-T28) but of different degrees to the subcategory identifying the highest degree recorded in the diagnosis.

3) Non-healing burns
Non-healing burns are coded as acute burns.

Necrosis of burned skin should be coded as a non-healed burn.

4) Infected Burn
For any documented infected burn site, use an additional code for the infection.

5) Assign separate codes for each burn site
When coding burns, assign separate codes for each burn site. Category T30, Burn and corrosion, body region unspecified is extremely vague and should rarely be used.

6) Burns and Corrosions Classified According to Extent of Body Surface Involved
Assign codes from category T31, Burns classified according to extent of body surface involved, or T32, Corrosions classified according to extent of body surface involved, when the site of the burn is not specified or when there is a need for additional data. It is advisable to use category T31 as additional coding when needed to provide data for evaluating burn mortality, such as that needed by burn units. It is also advisable to use category T31 as an additional code for reporting purposes when there is mention of a third-degree burn involving 20 percent or more of the body surface.

Categories T31 and T32 are based on the classic "rule of nines" in estimating body surface involved: head and neck are assigned nine percent, each arm nine percent, each leg 18 percent, the anterior trunk 18 percent, posterior trunk 18 percent, and genitalia one percent. Providers may change these percentage assignments where necessary to accommodate infants and children who have proportionately larger heads than adults, and patients who have large buttocks, thighs, or abdomen that involve burns.

7) Encounters for treatment of sequela of burns
Encounters for the treatment of the late effects of burns or corrosions (i.e., scars or joint contractures) should be coded with a burn or corrosion code with the 7th character "S" for sequela.

8) Sequelae with a late effect code and current burn
When appropriate, both a code for a current burn or corrosion with 7th character "A" or "D" and a burn or corrosion code with 7th character "S" may be assigned on the same record (when both a current burn and sequelae of an old burn exist). Burns and corrosions do not heal at the same rate and a current healing wound may still exist with sequela of a healed burn or corrosion.

See Section I.B.10. Sequela, (Late Effects)

9) Use of an external cause code with burns and corrosions
An external cause code should be used with burns and corrosions to identify the source and intent of the burn, as well as the place where it occurred.

e. Adverse Effects, Poisoning , Underdosing and Toxic Effects
Codes in categories T36-T65 are combination codes that include the substance that was taken as well as the intent. No additional external cause code is required for poisonings, toxic effects, adverse effects and underdosing codes.

1) Do not code directly from the Table of Drugs
Do not code directly from the Table of Drugs and Chemicals. Always refer back to the Tabular List.

2) Use as many codes as necessary to describe
Use as many codes as necessary to describe completely all drugs, medicinal or biological substances.

3) If the same code would describe the causative agent
If the same code would describe the causative agent for more than one adverse reaction, poisoning, toxic effect or underdosing, assign the code only once.

4) If two or more drugs, medicinal or biological substances
If two or more drugs, medicinal or biological substances are reported, code each individually unless a combination code is listed in the Table of Drugs and Chemicals.

5) The occurrence of drug toxicity is classified in ICD-10-CM as follows:

(a) Adverse Effect
When coding an adverse effect of a drug that has been correctly prescribed and properly administered, assign the appropriate code for the nature of the adverse effect followed by the appropriate code for the adverse effect of the drug (T36-T50). The code for the drug should have a 5th or 6th character "5" (for example T36.0X5-) Examples of the nature of an adverse effect are tachycardia, delirium, gastrointestinal hemorrhaging, vomiting, hypokalemia, hepatitis, renal failure, or respiratory failure.

(b) Poisoning
When coding a poisoning or reaction to the improper use of a medication (e.g., overdose, wrong substance given or taken in error, wrong route of administration), first assign the appropriate code from categories T36-T50. The poisoning codes have an associated intent as their 5th or 6th character (accidental, intentional self-harm, assault and undetermined). **If the intent of the poisoning is unknown or unspecified, code the intent as accidental intent. The undetermined intent is only for use if the documentation in the record specifies that the intent cannot be determined.** Use additional code(s) for all manifestations of poisonings.

If there is also a diagnosis of abuse or dependence of the substance, the abuse or dependence is assigned as an additional code.

Examples of poisoning include:

(i) Error was made in drug prescription
Errors made in drug prescription or in the administration of the drug by provider, nurse, patient, or other person.

(ii) Overdose of a drug intentionally taken If an overdose of a drug was intentionally taken or administered and resulted in drug toxicity, it would be coded as a poisoning.

(iii) Nonprescribed drug taken with correctly prescribed and properly administered drug.
If a nonprescribed drug or medicinal agent was taken in combination with a correctly prescribed and properly administered drug, any drug toxicity or other reaction resulting from the interaction of the two drugs would be classified as a poisoning.

(iv) Interaction of drug(s) and alcohol.
When a reaction results from the interaction of a drug(s) and alcohol, this would be classified as poisoning.

See Section I.C.4. if poisoning is the result of insulin pump malfunctions.

(c) Underdosing
Underdosing refers to taking less of a medication than is prescribed by a provider or a manufacturer's instruction. For

underdosing, assign the code from categories T36-T50 (fifth or sixth character "6").

Codes for underdosing should never be assigned as principal or first-listed codes. If a patient has a relapse or exacerbation of the medical condition for which the drug is prescribed because of the reduction in dose, then the medical condition itself should be coded.

Noncompliance (Z91.12-, Z91.13-) or complication of care (Y63.6-Y63.9) codes are to be used with an underdosing code to indicate intent, if known.

(d) Toxic Effects

When a harmful substance is ingested or comes in contact with a person, this is classified as a toxic effect. The toxic effect codes are in categories T51-T65.

Toxic effect codes have an associated intent: accidental, intentional self-harm, assault and undetermined.

f. Adult and child abuse, neglect and other maltreatment

Sequence first the appropriate code from categories T74.- (Adult and child abuse, neglect and other maltreatment, confirmed) or T76.- (Adult and child abuse, neglect and other maltreatment, suspected) for abuse, neglect and other maltreatment, followed by any accompanying mental health or injury code(s).

If the documentation in the medical record states abuse or neglect it is coded as confirmed (T74.-). It is coded as suspected if it is documented as suspected (T76.-).

For cases of confirmed abuse or neglect an external cause code from the assault section (X92-**Y09**) should be added to identify the cause of any physical injuries. A perpetrator code (Y07) should be added when the perpetrator of the abuse is known. For suspected cases of abuse or neglect, do not report external cause or perpetrator code.

If a suspected case of abuse, neglect or mistreatment is ruled out during an encounter code Z04.71, Encounter for examination and observation following alleged physical adult abuse, ruled out, or code Z04.72, Encounter for examination and observation following alleged child physical abuse, ruled out, should be used, not a code from T76.

If a suspected case of alleged rape or sexual abuse is ruled out during an encounter code Z04.41, Encounter for examination and observation following alleged **adult rape** or code Z04.42, Encounter for examination and observation following alleged **child** rape, should be used, not a code from T76.

See Section I.C.15. Abuse in a pregnant patient.

g. Complications of care

1) General guidelines for complications of care

(a) Documentation of complications of care

See Section I.B.16. for information on documentation of complications of care.

2) Pain due to medical devices

Pain associated with devices, implants or grafts left in a surgical site (for example painful hip prosthesis) is assigned to the appropriate code(s) found in Chapter 19, Injury, poisoning, and certain other consequences of external causes. Specific codes for pain due to medical devices are found in the T code section of the ICD-10-CM. Use additional code(s) from category G89 to identify acute or chronic pain due to presence of the device, implant or graft (G89.18 or G89.28).

3) Transplant complications

(a) Transplant complications other than kidney

Codes under category T86, Complications of transplanted organs and tissues, are for use for both complications and rejection of transplanted organs. A transplant complication code is only assigned if the complication affects the function of the transplanted organ. Two codes are required to fully describe a transplant complication: the appropriate code from category T86 and a secondary code that identifies the complication.

Pre-existing conditions or conditions that develop after the transplant are not coded as complications unless they affect the function of the transplanted organs.

See I.C.21. for transplant organ removal status

See I.C.2. for malignant neoplasm associated with transplanted organ.

(b) Kidney transplant complications

Patients who have undergone kidney transplant may still have some form of chronic kidney disease (CKD) because the kidney transplant may not fully restore kidney function. Code T86.1- should be assigned for documented complications of a kidney transplant, such as transplant failure or rejection or other transplant complication. Code T86.1- should not be assigned for post kidney transplant patients who have chronic kidney (CKD) unless a transplant complication such as transplant failure or rejection is documented. If the documentation is unclear as to whether the patient has a complication of the transplant, query the provider.

Conditions that affect the function of the transplanted kidney, other than CKD, should be assigned a code from subcategory T86.1, Complications of transplanted organ, Kidney, and a secondary code that identifies the complication.

For patients with CKD following a kidney transplant, but who do not have a complication such as failure or rejection, *see section I.C.14. Chronic kidney disease and kidney transplant status.*

4) Complication codes that include the external cause

As with certain other T codes, some of the complications of care codes have the external cause included in the code. The code includes the nature of the complication as well as the type of procedure that caused the complication. No external cause code indicating the type of procedure is necessary for these codes.

5) Complications of care codes within the body system chapters

Intraoperative and postprocedural complication codes are found within the body system chapters with codes specific to the organs and structures of that body system. These codes should be sequenced first, followed by a code(s) for the specific complication, if applicable.

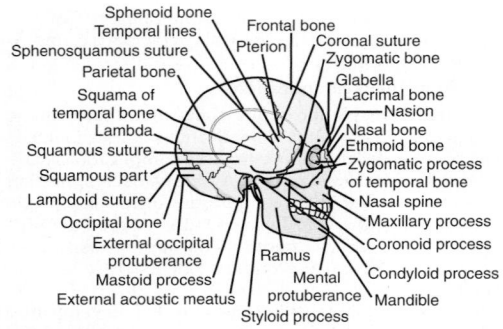

Figure 19-1 Lateral view of skull.

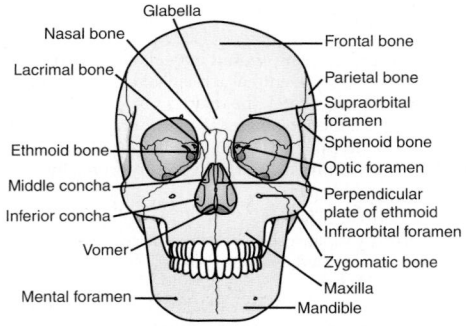

Figure 19-2 Frontal view of skull.

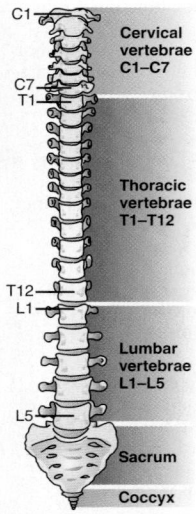

Figure 19-3 Anterior view of vertebral column.

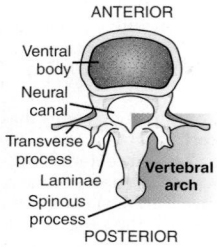

Figure 19-4 Vertebra viewed from above.

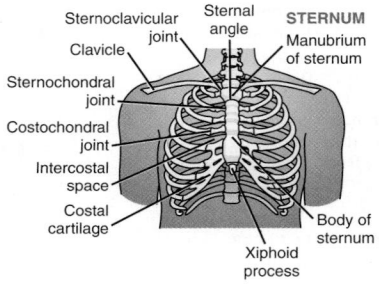

Figure 19-5 Anterior view of rib cage.

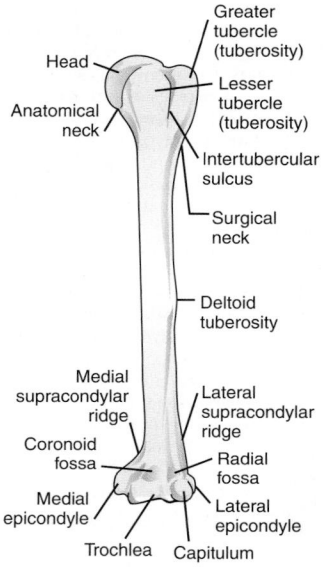

Figure 19-6 Anterior aspect of left humerus.

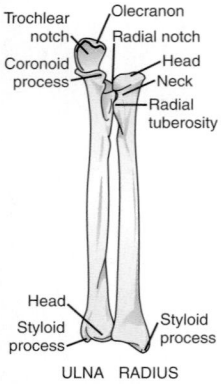

Figure 19-7 Anterior aspect of left radius and ulna.

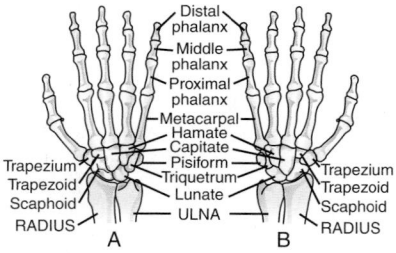

Figure 19-8 Right hand and wrist: **A.** Dorsal surface. **B.** Palmar surface.

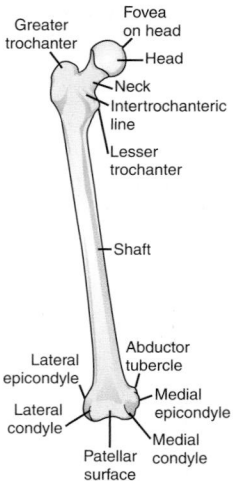

Figure 19-9 Anterior aspect of right femur.

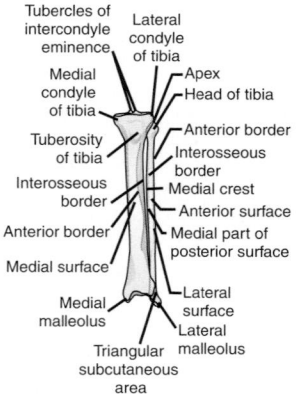

Figure 19-10 Anterior aspect of left tibia and fibula.

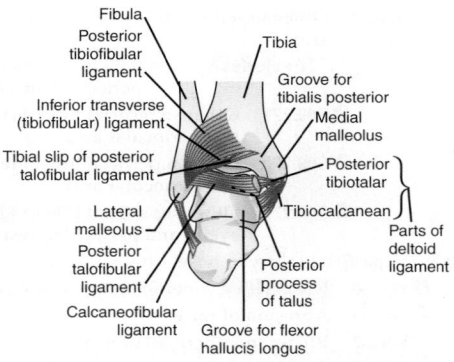

Figure 19-11 Posterior aspect of the left ankle joint.

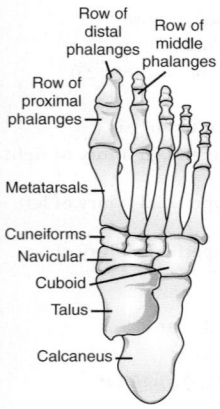

Figure 19-12 Right foot viewed from above.

CHAPTER 19

INJURY, POISONING AND CERTAIN OTHER CONSEQUENCES OF EXTERNAL CAUSES (S00-T88)

Note: Use secondary code(s) from Chapter 20, External causes of morbidity, to indicate cause of injury. Codes within the T section that include the external cause do not require an additional external cause code.

Use additional code to identify any retained foreign body, if applicable (Z18.-)

Excludes1 birth trauma (P10-P15)
obstetric trauma (O70-O71)

Note: The chapter uses the S-section for coding different types of injuries related to single body regions and the T-section to cover injuries to unspecified body regions as well as poisoning and certain other consequences of external causes.

This chapter contains the following blocks:

S00-S09	Injuries to the head
S10-S19	Injuries to the neck
S20-S29	Injuries to the thorax
S30-S39	Injuries to the abdomen, lower back, lumbar spine, pelvis and external genitals
S40-S49	Injuries to the shoulder and upper arm
S50-S59	Injuries to the elbow and forearm
S60-S69	Injuries to the wrist, hand, and fingers
S70-S79	Injuries to the hip and thigh
S80-S89	Injuries to the knee and lower leg
S90-S99	Injuries to the ankle and foot
T07	Injuries involving multiple body regions
T14	Injury of unspecified body region
T15-T19	Effects of foreign body entering through natural orifice
T20-T32	Burns and corrosions
T20-T25	Burns and corrosions of external body surface, specified by site
T26-T28	Burns and corrosions confined to eye and internal organs
T30-T32	Burns and corrosions of multiple and unspecified body regions
T33-T34	Frostbite
T36-T50	Poisoning by, adverse effect of and underdosing of drugs, medicaments and biological substances
T51-T65	Toxic effects of substances chiefly nonmedicinal as to source
T66-T78	Other and unspecified effects of external causes
T79	Certain early complications of trauma
T80-T88	Complications of surgical and medical care, not elsewhere classified

INJURIES TO THE HEAD (S00-S09)

Includes injuries of ear
injuries of eye
injuries of face [any part]
injuries of gum
injuries of jaw
injuries of oral cavity
injuries of palate
injuries of periocular area
injuries of scalp
injuries of temporomandibular joint area
injuries of tongue
injuries of tooth

Code also for any associated infection

Excludes2 burns and corrosions (T20-T32)
effects of foreign body in ear (T16)
effects of foreign body in larynx (T17.3)
effects of foreign body in mouth NOS (T18.0)
effects of foreign body in nose (T17.0-T17.1)
effects of foreign body in pharynx (T17.2)
effects of foreign body on external eye (T15.-)
frostbite (T33-T34)
insect bite or sting, venomous (T63.4)

● **S00 Superficial injury of head**

Excludes1 diffuse cerebral contusion (S06.2-)
focal cerebral contusion (S06.3-)
injury of eye and orbit (S05.-)
open wound of head (S01.-)

The appropriate 7th character is to be added to each code from category S00

A	initial encounter *All encounters involving diagnosis and treatment*
D	subsequent encounter *Encounters during the healing phase*
S	sequela

● **S00.0 Superficial injury of scalp**

X● **S00.00 Unspecified superficial injury of scalp**

X● **S00.01 Abrasion of scalp**

X● **S00.02 Blister (nonthermal) of scalp**

X● **S00.03 Contusion of scalp**
Bruise of scalp
Hematoma of scalp

X● **S00.04 External constriction of part of scalp**

X● **S00.05 Superficial foreign body of scalp**
Splinter in the scalp

X● **S00.06 Insect bite (nonvenomous) of scalp**

X● **S00.07 Other superficial bite of scalp**

Excludes1 open bite of scalp (S01.05)

- S00.1 Contusion of eyelid and periocular area
  Black eye
  Excludes2 contusion of eyeball and orbital tissues (S05.1)
  - X S00.10 Contusion of unspecified eyelid and periocular area
  - X S00.11 Contusion of right eyelid and periocular area
  - X S00.12 Contusion of left eyelid and periocular area
- S00.2 Other and unspecified superficial injuries of eyelid and periocular area
  Excludes2 superficial injury of conjunctiva and cornea (S05.0-)
  - S00.20 Unspecified superficial injury of eyelid and periocular area
    - S00.201 Unspecified superficial injury of right eyelid and periocular area
    - S00.202 Unspecified superficial injury of left eyelid and periocular area
    - S00.209 Unspecified superficial injury of unspecified eyelid and periocular area
  - S00.21 Abrasion of eyelid and periocular area
    - S00.211 Abrasion of right eyelid and periocular area
    - S00.212 Abrasion of left eyelid and periocular area
    - S00.219 Abrasion of unspecified eyelid and periocular area
  - S00.22 Blister (nonthermal) of eyelid and periocular area
    - S00.221 Blister (nonthermal) of right eyelid and periocular area
    - S00.222 Blister (nonthermal) of left eyelid and periocular area
    - S00.229 Blister (nonthermal) of unspecified eyelid and periocular area
  - S00.24 External constriction of eyelid and periocular area
    - S00.241 External constriction of right eyelid and periocular area
    - S00.242 External constriction of left eyelid and periocular area
    - S00.249 External constriction of unspecified eyelid and periocular area
  - S00.25 Superficial foreign body of eyelid and periocular area
    Splinter of eyelid and periocular area
    Excludes2 retained foreign body in eyelid (H02.81-)
    - S00.251 Superficial foreign body of right eyelid and periocular area
    - S00.252 Superficial foreign body of left eyelid and periocular area
    - S00.259 Superficial foreign body of unspecified eyelid and periocular area
  - S00.26 Insect bite (nonvenomous) of eyelid and periocular area
    - S00.261 Insect bite (nonvenomous) of right eyelid and periocular area
    - S00.262 Insect bite (nonvenomous) of left eyelid and periocular area
    - S00.269 Insect bite (nonvenomous) of unspecified eyelid and periocular area
  - S00.27 Other superficial bite of eyelid and periocular area
    Excludes1 open bite of eyelid and periocular area (S01.15)
    - S00.271 Other superficial bite of right eyelid and periocular area
    - S00.272 Other superficial bite of left eyelid and periocular area
    - S00.279 Other superficial bite of unspecified eyelid and periocular area
- S00.3 Superficial injury of nose
  - X S00.30 Unspecified superficial injury of nose
  - X S00.31 Abrasion of nose
  - X S00.32 Blister (nonthermal) of nose
  - X S00.33 Contusion of nose
    Bruise of nose
    Hematoma of nose
  - X S00.34 External constriction of nose
  - X S00.35 Superficial foreign body of nose
    Splinter in the nose
  - X S00.36 Insect bite (nonvenomous) of nose
  - X S00.37 Other superficial bite of nose
    Excludes1 open bite of nose (S01.25)
- S00.4 Superficial injury of ear
  - S00.40 Unspecified superficial injury of ear
    - S00.401 Unspecified superficial injury of right ear
    - S00.402 Unspecified superficial injury of left ear
    - S00.409 Unspecified superficial injury of unspecified ear
  - S00.41 Abrasion of ear
    - S00.411 Abrasion of right ear
    - S00.412 Abrasion of left ear
    - S00.419 Abrasion of unspecified ear
  - S00.42 Blister (nonthermal) of ear
    - S00.421 Blister (nonthermal) of right ear
    - S00.422 Blister (nonthermal) of left ear
    - S00.429 Blister (nonthermal) of unspecified ear
  - S00.43 Contusion of ear
    Bruise of ear
    Hematoma of ear
    - S00.431 Contusion of right ear
    - S00.432 Contusion of left ear
    - S00.439 Contusion of unspecified ear
  - S00.44 External constriction of ear
    - S00.441 External constriction of right ear
    - S00.442 External constriction of left ear
    - S00.449 External constriction of unspecified ear
  - S00.45 Superficial foreign body of ear
    Splinter in the ear
    - S00.451 Superficial foreign body of right ear
    - S00.452 Superficial foreign body of left ear
    - S00.459 Superficial foreign body of unspecified ear
  - S00.46 Insect bite (nonvenomous) of ear
    - S00.461 Insect bite (nonvenomous) of right ear
    - S00.462 Insect bite (nonvenomous) of left ear
    - S00.469 Insect bite (nonvenomous) of unspecified ear

- **S00.47 Other superficial bite of ear**
  - **Excludes1** open bite of ear (S01.35)
  - **S00.471 Other superficial bite of right ear**
  - **S00.472 Other superficial bite of left ear**
  - **S00.479 Other superficial bite of unspecified ear**
- **S00.5 Superficial injury of lip and oral cavity**
  - **S00.50 Unspecified superficial injury of lip and oral cavity**
    - **S00.501 Unspecified superficial injury of lip**
    - **S00.502 Unspecified superficial injury of oral cavity**
  - **S00.51 Abrasion of lip and oral cavity**
    - **S00.511 Abrasion of lip**
    - **S00.512 Abrasion of oral cavity**
  - **S00.52 Blister (nonthermal) of lip and oral cavity**
    - **S00.521 Blister (nonthermal) of lip**
    - **S00.522 Blister (nonthermal) of oral cavity**
  - **S00.53 Contusion of lip and oral cavity**
    - **S00.531 Contusion of lip**
      Bruise of lip
      Hematoma of oral cavity
    - **S00.532 Contusion of oral cavity**
      Bruise of lip
      Hematoma of oral cavity
  - **S00.54 External constriction of lip and oral cavity**
    - **S00.541 External constriction of lip**
    - **S00.542 External constriction of oral cavity**
  - **S00.55 Superficial foreign body of lip and oral cavity**
    - **S00.551 Superficial foreign body of lip**
      Splinter of lip and oral cavity
    - **S00.552 Superficial foreign body of oral cavity**
      Splinter of lip and oral cavity
  - **S00.56 Insect bite (nonvenomous) of lip and oral cavity**
    - **S00.561 Insect bite (nonvenomous) of lip**
    - **S00.562 Insect bite (nonvenomous) of oral cavity**
  - **S00.57 Other superficial bite of lip and oral cavity**
    - **S00.571 Other superficial bite of lip**
      - **Excludes1** open bite of lip (S01.551)
    - **S00.572 Other superficial bite of oral cavity**
      - **Excludes1** open bite of oral cavity (S01.552)
- **S00.8 Superficial injury of other parts of head**
  Superficial injuries of face [any part] ◀
  - X **S00.80 Unspecified superficial injury of other part of head**
  - X **S00.81 Abrasion of other part of head**
  - X **S00.82 Blister (nonthermal) of other part of head**
  - X **S00.83 Contusion of other part of head**
    Bruise of other part of head
    Hematoma of other part of head
  - X **S00.84 External constriction of other part of head**
  - X **S00.85 Superficial foreign body of other part of head**
    Splinter in other part of head
  - X **S00.86 Insect bite (nonvenomous) of other part of head**
  - X **S00.87 Other superficial bite of other part of head**
    - **Excludes1** open bite of other part of head (S01.85)
- **S00.9 Superficial injury of unspecified part of head**
  - X **S00.90 Unspecified superficial injury of unspecified part of head**
  - X **S00.91 Abrasion of unspecified part of head**
  - X **S00.92 Blister (nonthermal) of unspecified part of head**
  - X **S00.93 Contusion of unspecified part of head**
    Bruise of head
    Hematoma of head
  - X **S00.94 External constriction of unspecified part of head**
  - X **S00.95 Superficial foreign body of unspecified part of head**
    Splinter of head
  - X **S00.96 Insect bite (nonvenomous) of unspecified part of head**
  - X **S00.97 Other superficial bite of unspecified part of head**
    - **Excludes1** open bite of head (S01.95)
- **S01 Open wound of head**
  Code also any associated:
  injury of cranial nerve (S04.-)
  injury of muscle and tendon of head (S09.1-)
  intracranial injury (S06.-)
  wound infection
  - **Excludes1** open skull fracture (S02.- with 7th character B)
  - **Excludes2** injury of eye and orbit (S05.-)
    traumatic amputation of part of head (S08.-)

  The appropriate 7th character is to be added to each code from category S01

A	initial encounter
D	subsequent encounter
S	sequela

  - **S01.0 Open wound of scalp**
    - **Excludes1** avulsion of scalp (S08.0)
    - X **S01.00 Unspecified open wound of scalp**
    - X **S01.01 Laceration without foreign body of scalp**
    - X **S01.02 Laceration with foreign body of scalp**
      Coding Clinic: 2015, Q1, P5-7
    - X **S01.03 Puncture wound without foreign body of scalp**
    - X **S01.04 Puncture wound with foreign body of scalp**
    - X **S01.05 Open bite of scalp**
      Bite of scalp NOS
      - **Excludes1** superficial bite of scalp (S00.06, S00.07-)
  - **S01.1 Open wound of eyelid and periocular area**
    Open wound of eyelid and periocular area with or without involvement of lacrimal passages
    - **S01.10 Unspecified open wound of eyelid and periocular area**
      Ex **For category S01.10 CC codes:** S01.101-S01.159[A], S05.20X-S05.8X9[A], S05.91X-S05.92X[A], S38.3XX[A], T14.90-T14.91, T79.A0X-T79.9XX[A]
      - **S01.101 Unspecified open wound of right eyelid and periocular area** A
      - **S01.102 Unspecified open wound of left eyelid and periocular area** A
      - **S01.109 Unspecified open wound of unspecified eyelid and periocular area** A
    - **S01.11 Laceration without foreign body of eyelid and periocular area**
      - **S01.111 Laceration without foreign body of right eyelid and periocular area**
      - **S01.112 Laceration without foreign body of left eyelid and periocular area**
      - **S01.119 Laceration without foreign body of unspecified eyelid and periocular area**
    - **S01.12 Laceration with foreign body of eyelid and periocular area**
      - **S01.121 Laceration with foreign body of right eyelid and periocular area**
      - **S01.122 Laceration with foreign body of left eyelid and periocular area**
      - **S01.129 Laceration with foreign body of unspecified eyelid and periocular area**

- S01.13 Puncture wound without foreign body of eyelid and periocular area
  - S01.131 Puncture wound without foreign body of right eyelid and periocular area
  - S01.132 Puncture wound without foreign body of left eyelid and periocular area
  - S01.139 Puncture wound without foreign body of unspecified eyelid and periocular area
- S01.14 Puncture wound with foreign body of eyelid and periocular area
  - S01.141 Puncture wound with foreign body of right eyelid and periocular area
  - S01.142 Puncture wound with foreign body of left eyelid and periocular area
  - S01.149 Puncture wound with foreign body of unspecified eyelid and periocular area
- S01.15 Open bite of eyelid and periocular area
  Bite of eyelid and periocular area NOS
  Excludes1 superficial bite of eyelid and periocular area (S00.26, S00.27)
  - S01.151 Open bite of right eyelid and periocular area
  - S01.152 Open bite of left eyelid and periocular area
  - S01.159 Open bite of unspecified eyelid and periocular area

- S01.2 Open wound of nose
  - X S01.20 Unspecified open wound of nose
  - X S01.21 Laceration without foreign body of nose
    Coding Clinic: 2015, Q1, P5-6
  - X S01.22 Laceration with foreign body of nose
  - X S01.23 Puncture wound without foreign body of nose
  - X S01.24 Puncture wound with foreign body of nose
  - X S01.25 Open bite of nose
    Bite of nose NOS
    Excludes1 superficial bite of nose (S00.36, S00.37)

- S01.3 Open wound of ear
  - S01.30 Unspecified open wound of ear
    - S01.301 Unspecified open wound of right ear
    - S01.302 Unspecified open wound of left ear
    - S01.309 Unspecified open wound of unspecified ear
  - S01.31 Laceration without foreign body of ear
    - S01.311 Laceration without foreign body of right ear
    - S01.312 Laceration without foreign body of left ear
    - S01.319 Laceration without foreign body of unspecified ear
  - S01.32 Laceration with foreign body of ear
    - S01.321 Laceration with foreign body of right ear
    - S01.322 Laceration with foreign body of left ear
    - S01.329 Laceration with foreign body of unspecified ear
  - S01.33 Puncture wound without foreign body of ear
    - S01.331 Puncture wound without foreign body of right ear
    - S01.332 Puncture wound without foreign body of left ear
    - S01.339 Puncture wound without foreign body of unspecified ear
  - S01.34 Puncture wound with foreign body of ear
    - S01.341 Puncture wound with foreign body of right ear
    - S01.342 Puncture wound with foreign body of left ear
    - S01.349 Puncture wound with foreign body of unspecified ear
  - S01.35 Open bite of ear
    Bite of ear NOS
    Excludes1 superficial bite of ear (S00.46, S00.47)
    - S01.351 Open bite of right ear
    - S01.352 Open bite of left ear
    - S01.359 Open bite of unspecified ear

- S01.4 Open wound of cheek and temporomandibular area
  - S01.40 Unspecified open wound of cheek and temporomandibular area
    - S01.401 Unspecified open wound of right cheek and temporomandibular area
    - S01.402 Unspecified open wound of left cheek and temporomandibular area
    - S01.409 Unspecified open wound of unspecified cheek and temporomandibular area
  - S01.41 Laceration without foreign body of cheek and temporomandibular area
    - S01.411 Laceration without foreign body of right cheek and temporomandibular area
      Coding Clinic: 2015, Q1, P5-7
    - S01.412 Laceration without foreign body of left cheek and temporomandibular area
    - S01.419 Laceration without foreign body of unspecified cheek and temporomandibular area
  - S01.42 Laceration with foreign body of cheek and temporomandibular area
    - S01.421 Laceration with foreign body of right cheek and temporomandibular area
    - S01.422 Laceration with foreign body of left cheek and temporomandibular area
    - S01.429 Laceration with foreign body of unspecified cheek and temporomandibular area
  - S01.43 Puncture wound without foreign body of cheek and temporomandibular area
    - S01.431 Puncture wound without foreign body of right cheek and temporomandibular area
    - S01.432 Puncture wound without foreign body of left cheek and temporomandibular area
    - S01.439 Puncture wound without foreign body of unspecified cheek and temporomandibular area
  - S01.44 Puncture wound with foreign body of cheek and temporomandibular area
    - S01.441 Puncture wound with foreign body of right cheek and temporomandibular area
    - S01.442 Puncture wound with foreign body of left cheek and temporomandibular area
    - S01.449 Puncture wound with foreign body of unspecified cheek and temporomandibular area

- **S01.45 Open bite of cheek and temporomandibular area**
  Bite of cheek and temporomandibular area NOS
  Excludes2 superficial bite of cheek and temporomandibular area (S00.86, S00.87)
  - **S01.451 Open bite of right cheek and temporomandibular area**
  - **S01.452 Open bite of left cheek and temporomandibular area**
  - **S01.459 Open bite of unspecified cheek and temporomandibular area**
- **S01.5 Open wound of lip and oral cavity**
  Excludes2 tooth dislocation (S03.2)
  tooth fracture (S02.5)
  - **S01.50 Unspecified open wound of lip and oral cavity**
    - **S01.501 Unspecified open wound of lip**
    - **S01.502 Unspecified open wound of oral cavity**
  - **S01.51 Laceration of lip and oral cavity without foreign body**
    - **S01.511 Laceration without foreign body of lip**
    - **S01.512 Laceration without foreign body of oral cavity**
  - **S01.52 Laceration of lip and oral cavity with foreign body**
    - **S01.521 Laceration with foreign body of lip**
    - **S01.522 Laceration with foreign body of oral cavity**
  - **S01.53 Puncture wound of lip and oral cavity without foreign body**
    - **S01.531 Puncture wound without foreign body of lip**
    - **S01.532 Puncture wound without foreign body of oral cavity**
  - **S01.54 Puncture wound of lip and oral cavity with foreign body**
    - **S01.541 Puncture wound with foreign body of lip**
    - **S01.542 Puncture wound with foreign body of oral cavity**
  - **S01.55 Open bite of lip and oral cavity**
    - **S01.551 Open bite of lip**
      Bite of lip NOS
      Excludes1 superficial bite of lip (S00.571)
    - **S01.552 Open bite of oral cavity**
      Bite of oral cavity NOS
      Excludes1 superficial bite of oral cavity (S00.572)
- **S01.8 Open wound of other parts of head**
  - X **S01.80 Unspecified open wound of other part of head**
  - X **S01.81 Laceration without foreign body of other part of head**
  - X **S01.82 Laceration with foreign body of other part of head**
  - X **S01.83 Puncture wound without foreign body of other part of head**
  - X **S01.84 Puncture wound with foreign body of other part of head**
  - X **S01.85 Open bite of other part of head**
    Bite of other part of head NOS
    Excludes1 superficial bite of other part of head (S00.85)
- **S01.9 Open wound of unspecified part of head**
  - X **S01.90 Unspecified open wound of unspecified part of head**
  - X **S01.91 Laceration without foreign body of unspecified part of head**
  - X **S01.92 Laceration with foreign body of unspecified part of head**
  - X **S01.93 Puncture wound without foreign body of unspecified part of head**
  - X **S01.94 Puncture wound with foreign body of unspecified part of head**
  - X **S01.95 Open bite of unspecified part of head**
    Bite of head NOS
    Excludes1 superficial bite of head NOS (S00.97)

- **S02 Fracture of skull and facial bones**
  Note: A fracture not indicated as open or closed should be coded to closed
  The appropriate 7th character is to be added to each code from category S02

A	initial encounter for closed fracture
B	initial encounter for open fracture
D	subsequent encounter for fracture with routine healing
G	subsequent encounter for fracture with delayed healing
K	subsequent encounter for fracture with nonunion
S	sequela

  Code also any associated intracranial injury (S06.-)
  - X **S02.0 Fracture of vault of skull** A, K CC, B MCC, A, B UNC
    Fracture of frontal bone
    Fracture of parietal bone
    Ex **For category S02.0 CC codes S02.0[A,B]:** S01.90X-S01.95X[A], S02.0XX-S02.19X[A,B,S], S02.2XX-S02.82X[S], S02.91X[A,B,S], S02.92XS, S06.0X0-S07.9XX[A], S08.89X[A], S09.10X-S09.19X[A], S09.8XX-S09.90X[A], S09.92X-S09.93X[A], S16.8XX-S19.9XX[A], S38.3XX[A], T14.90-T14.91, T79.A0XA-T79.9XX[A] **For S02.0[K]:** M80.00X-M80.88X[K,P], M84.30X-M84.68X[K,P], M84.750-M84.759[K,P], S02.0XXK, S02.110-S02.2X[K], S02.400-S02.609[K], S02.63XK, S02.66XK, S02.69XK, S02.19X-S02.92X[K], S12.000-S12.691[K], S22.000-S22.9XX[K], S32.000-S32.9XX[K], S42.001-S42.92X[K,P], S49.001-S49.199[K,P], S52.001-S52.92X[K,M,N,P,Q,R], S59.001-S59.299[K,P], S62.001-S62.92X[K,P], S72.001-S72.92X[K,M,N,P,Q,R], S79.001-S79.199[K,P], S82.001-S82.92X[K,M,N,P,Q,R], S89.001-S89.399[K,P], S92.001-S92.919[K,P]
  - **S02.1 Fracture of base of skull**
    Excludes1 orbit NOS (S02.8)
    Excludes2 orbital floor (S02.3-)
    Ex **For category S02.1 CC codes S02.1[A,B]: For S02.1[A,B] CC codes:** See S02.0[A,B] **For S02.1[K] CC codes:** See S02.0[K]
    - **S02.10 Unspecified fracture of base of skull**
      - **S02.101 Fracture of base of skull, right side** A, K CC, B MCC, A, B UNC ◀
      - **S02.102 Fracture of base of skull, left side** A, K CC, B MCC, A, B UNC ◀
      - **S02.109 Fracture of base of skull, unspecified side** A, K CC, B MCC, A, B UNC ◀

- **S02.11 Fracture of occiput**
  - **S02.110 Type I occipital condyle fracture, unspecified side** A, K, B, A, B
  - **S02.111 Type II occipital condyle fracture, unspecified side** A, K, B, A, B
  - **S02.112 Type III occipital condyle fracture, unspecified side** A, K, B, A, B
  - **S02.113 Unspecified occipital condyle fracture** A, K, B, A, B
  - **S02.118 Other fracture of occiput, unspecified side** A, K, B, A, B
  - **S02.119 Unspecified fracture of occiput** A, K, B, A, B
  - **S02.11A Type I occipital condyle fracture, right side** A, K, B, A, B ◀
  - **S02.11B Type I occipital condyle fracture, left side** A, K, B, A, B ◀
  - **S02.11C Type II occipital condyle fracture, right side** A, K, B, A, B ◀
  - **S02.11D Type II occipital condyle fracture, left side** A, K, B, A, B ◀
  - **S02.11E Type III occipital condyle fracture, right side** A, K, B, A, B ◀
  - **S02.11F Type III occipital condyle fracture, left side** A, K, B, A, B ◀
  - **S02.11G Other fracture of occiput, right side** A, K, B, A, B ◀
  - **S02.11H Other fracture of occiput, left side** A, K, B, A, B ◀
- X **S02.19 Other fracture of base of skull** A, K, B, A, B
  - Fracture of anterior fossa of base of skull
  - Fracture of ethmoid sinus
  - Fracture of frontal sinus
  - Fracture of middle fossa of base of skull
  - Fracture of orbital roof
  - Fracture of posterior fossa of base of skull
  - Fracture of sphenoid
  - Fracture of temporal bone
- X **S02.2 Fracture of nasal bones** B, K, B
  - Ex: **For category S02.2 CC codes S02.2[B]:** S01.90X-S01.95X[A], S02.0XX-S02.2XX[A,B,S], S02.30X-S02.413[S], S02.42XS-S02.82X[S], S02.91X[A,B,S], S02.92X[S], S06.0X0-S07.9XX[A], S08.89X[A], S09.10X-S09.19X[A], S09.8XX-S09.90X[A], S09.92XA-S09.93X[A], S16.8XX-S19.9XX[A], S38.3XX[A], S92.811-S92.819[A,B], T14.90-T14.91, T79.A0X-T79.8XX[A] **For S02.2[K]:** See S02.0[K]
- **S02.3 Fracture of orbital floor**
  - **Excludes1** orbit NOS (S02.8)
  - **Excludes2** orbital roof (S02.1-)
  - Ex: **For category S02.3 CC codes S02.3[A,B]:** S01.90X-S01.95X[A], S02.0XX[A,B,S], S02.101-S02.2XX[A,B,S], S02.30X-S02.32X[A,B,S], S02.400-S02.413[S], S02.42X[A,B,S], S02.5XX-S02.69X[S], S02.80X-S02.92X[A,B,S], S06.0X0-S07.9XX[A], S08.89X[A], S09.10X-S09.19X[A], S09.8XX-S09.919X[A], S09.8XX-S09.90X[A]-S09.3X[A], S16.8XX-S19.9XX[A], S38.3XX[A], T14.90-T14.91, T79.8XX-T79.9XX[A], T79.A0X-T79.A9X[A] **For S02.3[K]:** See S02.0[K]
  - X **S02.30 Fracture of orbital floor, unspecified side** A, B, K, A, B ◀
  - X **S02.31 Fracture of orbital floor, right side** A, B, K, A, B ◀
  - X **S02.32 Fracture of orbital floor, left side** A, B, K, A, B ◀
- **S02.4 Fracture of malar, maxillary and zygoma bones**
  - Fracture of superior maxilla
  - Fracture of upper jaw (bone)
  - Fracture of zygomatic process of temporal bone
  - Ex: **For category S02.4 CC codes S02.4[A,B]:** N13.0, S01.90X- S01.95X[A], S02.0XX[A,B,S], S02.101-S02.413[A,B,S], S02.42XS, S02.5XXS, S02.600[A,B,S]-S02.69X[A,B,S], S02.91[A,B,S], S02.92XS, S06.0X0-S07.9XX[A], S08.89X[A], S09.10X-S09.19X[A], S09.8XX-S09.90X[A], S09.92X-S09.93X[A], S16.8XX-S19.9XX[A], S38.3XX[A], T14.90-T14.91, T79.8XX-T79.9XX[A], T79.A0X-T79.A9X[A] **For S02.4[K]:** See S02.0[K] **unless otherwise indicated**
  - **S02.40 Fracture of malar, maxillary and zygoma bones, unspecified**
    - **S02.400 Malar fracture unspecified side** A, B, K, A, B
    - **S02.401 Maxillary fracture, unspecified side** A, B, K, A, B
    - **S02.402 Zygomatic fracture, unspecified side** A, B, K, A, B
    - **S02.40A Malar fracture, right side** A, B, K, A, B ◀
    - **S02.40B Malar fracture, left side** A, B, K, A, B ◀
    - **S02.40C Maxillary fracture, right side** A, B, K, A, B ◀
    - **S02.40D Maxillary fracture, left side** A, B, K, A, B ◀
    - **S02.40E Zygomatic fracture, right side** A, B, K, A, B ◀
    - **S02.40F Zygomatic fracture, left side** A, B, K, A, B ◀
  - **S02.41 LeFort fracture**
    - **S02.411 LeFort I fracture** A, B, K, A, B
    - **S02.412 LeFort II fracture** A, B, K, A, B
    - **S02.413 LeFort III fracture** A, B, K, A, B
  - X **S02.42 Fracture of alveolus of maxilla** A, B, K, A, B
    - Ex: **For S02.42[A,B]:** See S02.3[A,B] **For S02.42[K]:** See S02.0[K]
- X **S02.5 Fracture of tooth (traumatic) Broken tooth** K
  - **Excludes1** cracked tooth (nontraumatic) (K03.81)
  - Ex: See S02.0[K]
- **S02.6 Fracture of mandible**
  - Fracture of lower jaw (bone)
  - Ex: **For category S02.6 CC codes S02.6[A,B]:** See S02.4[A,B] **For S02.6[K]:** See S02.0[K]
  - **S02.60 Fracture of mandible of unspecified site**
    - **S02.600 Fracture of unspecified part of body of mandible, unspecified side** A, B, K, A, B
    - **S02.601 Fracture of unspecified part of body of right mandible** A, B, K, A, B ◀
    - **S02.602 Fracture of unspecified part of body of left mandible** A, B, K, A, B ◀
    - **S02.609 Fracture of mandible, unspecified** A, B, K, A, B
  - **S02.61 Fracture of condylar process of mandible**
    - **S02.610 Fracture of condylar process of mandible, unspecified side** A, B, K, A, B ◀
    - **S02.611 Fracture of condylar process of right mandible** A, B, K, A, B ◀
    - **S02.612 Fracture of condylar process of left mandible** A, B, K, A, B ◀
  - **S02.62 Fracture of subcondylar process of mandible**
    - **S02.620 Fracture of subcondylar process of mandible, unspecified side** A, B, K, A, B ◀
    - **S02.621 Fracture of subcondylar process of right mandible** A, B, K, A, B ◀
    - **S02.622 Fracture of subcondylar process of left mandible** A, B, K, A, B ◀

- **S02.63 Fracture of coronoid process of mandible**
  - **S02.630 Fracture of coronoid process of mandible, unspecified side** A, B, K, A, B ◀
  - **S02.631 Fracture of coronoid process of right mandible** A, B, K, A, B ◀
  - **S02.632 Fracture of coronoid process of left mandible** A, B, K, A, B ◀
- **S02.64 Fracture of ramus of mandible**
  - **S02.640 Fracture of ramus of mandible, unspecified side** A, B, K, A, B ◀
  - **S02.641 Fracture of ramus of right mandible** A, B, K, A, B ◀
  - **S02.642 Fracture of ramus of left mandible** A, B, K, A, B ◀
- **S02.65 Fracture of angle of mandible**
  - **S02.650 Fracture of angle of mandible, unspecified side** A, B, K, A, B ◀
  - **S02.651 Fracture of angle of right mandible** A, B, K, A, B ◀
  - **S02.652 Fracture of angle of left mandible** A, B, K, A, B ◀
- X **S02.66 Fracture of symphysis of mandible** A, B, K, A, B
- **S02.67 Fracture of alveolus of mandible**
  - **S02.670 Fracture of alveolus of mandible, unspecified side** A, B, K, A, B ◀
  - **S02.671 Fracture of alveolus of right mandible** A, B, K, A, B ◀
  - **S02.672 Fracture of alveolus of left mandible** A, B, K, A, B ◀
- X **S02.69 Fracture of mandible of other specified site** A, B, K, A, B
- **S02.8 Fractures of other specified skull and facial bones**
  Fracture of orbit NOS
  Fracture of palate
  Excludes1 fracture of orbital floor (S02.3-)
  fracture of orbital roof (S02.1-)
  Ex **For category S02.8 CC codes S02.8[A,B]:** See S02.3[A,B] **For S02.8[K]:** See S02.0[K]
  - X **S02.80 Fracture of other specified skull and facial bones, unspecified side** A, B, K, A, B ◀
  - X **S02.81 Fracture of other specified skull and facial bones, right side** A, B, K, A, B ◀
  - X **S02.82 Fracture of other specified skull and facial bones, left side** A, B, K, A, B ◀
- **S02.9 Fracture of unspecified skull and facial bones**
  - X **S02.91 Unspecified fracture of skull** A, K, B, A, B
    Ex **For category S02.91 CC codes S02.91[A,B]:** See S02.0[A,B] **For S02.91[K]:** See S02.0[K]
  - X **S02.92 Unspecified fracture of facial bones** A, B, K, A, B
    Ex **For category S02.92 CC codes S02.92[A,B]:** See S02.3[A,B] **For S02.92[K]:** See S02.0[K]

- **S03 Dislocation and sprain of joints and ligaments of head**
  Includes avulsion of joint (capsule) or ligament of head
  laceration of cartilage, joint (capsule) or ligament of head
  sprain of cartilage, joint (capsule) or ligament of head
  traumatic hemarthrosis of joint or ligament of head
  traumatic rupture of joint or ligament of head
  traumatic subluxation of joint or ligament of head
  traumatic tear of joint or ligament of head
  Code also any associated open wound
  Excludes2 Strain of muscle or tendon of head (S09.1)
  The appropriate 7th character is to be added to each code from category S03

A	initial encounter
D	subsequent encounter
S	sequela

  - **S03.0 Dislocation of jaw**
    Dislocation of jaw (cartilage) (meniscus)
    Dislocation of mandible
    Dislocation of temporomandibular (joint)
    - X **S03.00 Dislocation of jaw, unspecified side** ◀
    - X **S03.01 Dislocation of jaw, right side** ◀
    - X **S03.02 Dislocation of jaw, left side** ◀
    - X **S03.03 Dislocation of jaw, bilateral side** ◀
  - X **S03.1 Dislocation of septal cartilage of nose**
  - X **S03.2 Dislocation of tooth**
  - **S03.4 Sprain of jaw**
    Sprain of temporomandibular (joint) (ligament)
    - X **S03.40 Sprain of jaw, unspecified side** ◀
    - X **S03.41 Sprain of jaw, right side** ◀
    - X **S03.42 Sprain of jaw, left side** ◀
    - X **S03.43 Sprain of jaw, bilateral side** ◀
  - X **S03.8 Sprain of joints and ligaments of other parts of head**
  - X **S03.9 Sprain of joints and ligaments of unspecified parts of head**

- **S04 Injury of cranial nerve**
  The selection of side should be based on the side of the body being affected
  Code first any associated intracranial injury (S06.-)
  Code also any associated:
  open wound of head (S01.-)
  skull fracture (S02.-)
  The appropriate 7th character is to be added to each code from category S04

A	initial encounter
D	subsequent encounter
S	sequela

  - **S04.0 Injury of optic nerve and pathways**
    Use additional code to identify any visual field defect or blindness (H53.4-, H54)
    Ex **For category S04.0 CC codes:** S04.011-S04.049[A], S04.811A-S04.9XX[A]
    - **S04.01 Injury of optic nerve**
      Injury of 2nd cranial nerve
      - **S04.011 Injury of optic nerve, right eye** A
      - **S04.012 Injury of optic nerve, left eye** A
      - **S04.019 Injury of optic nerve, unspecified eye** A
        Injury of optic nerve NOS

CHAPTER 19 (S00-T88)

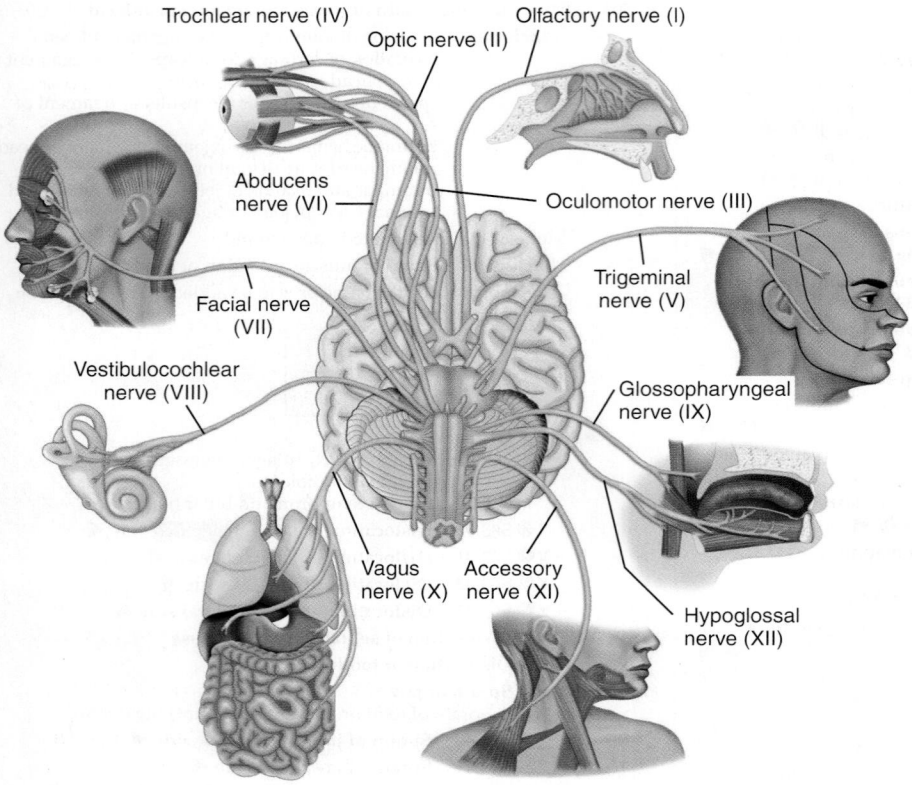

Figure 19-13 Cranial nerves. (From Patton and Thibodeau: Anatomy and physiology, ed 7, St. Louis, Mosby, 2009)

X ● **S04.02 Injury of optic chiasm** A

● **S04.03 Injury of optic tract and pathways**
Injury of optic radiation

● **S04.031 Injury of optic tract and pathways, right eye** A

● **S04.032 Injury of optic tract and pathways, left eye** A

● **S04.039 Injury of optic tract and pathways, unspecified eye** A
Injury of optic tract and pathways NOS

● **S04.04 Injury of visual cortex**

● **S04.041 Injury of visual cortex, right eye** A

● **S04.042 Injury of visual cortex, left eye** A

● **S04.049 Injury of visual cortex, unspecified eye** A
Injury of visual cortex NOS

● **S04.1 Injury of oculomotor nerve**
Injury of 3rd cranial nerve
Ex: For category S04.1 CC codes: S04.10X-S04.12X[A], S04.811-S04.9XX[A]

X ● **S04.10 Injury of oculomotor nerve, unspecified side** A

X ● **S04.11 Injury of oculomotor nerve, right side** A

X ● **S04.12 Injury of oculomotor nerve, left side** A

● **S04.2 Injury of trochlear nerve**
Injury of 4th cranial nerve
Ex: For category S04.2 CC codes: S04.20X-S04.22X[A], S04.811-S04.9XX[A]

X ● **S04.20 Injury of trochlear nerve, unspecified side** A

X ● **S04.21 Injury of trochlear nerve, right side** A

X ● **S04.22 Injury of trochlear nerve, left side** A

● **S04.3 Injury of trigeminal nerve**
Injury of 5th cranial nerve
Ex: For category S04.3 CC codes: S04.30XA-S04.32X[A], S04.811-S04.9XX[A]

X ● **S04.30 Injury of trigeminal nerve, unspecified side** A

X ● **S04.31 Injury of trigeminal nerve, right side** A

X ● **S04.32 Injury of trigeminal nerve, left side** A

● **S04.4 Injury of abducent nerve**
Injury of 6th cranial nerve
Ex: For category S04.4 CC codes: S04.40X-S04.42X[A], S04.811-S04.9XX[A]

X ● **S04.40 Injury of abducent nerve, unspecified side** A

X ● **S04.41 Injury of abducent nerve, right side** A

X ● **S04.42 Injury of abducent nerve, left side** A

● **S04.5 Injury of facial nerve**
Injury of 7th cranial nerve
Ex: For category S04.5 CC codes: S04.50X-S04.52X[A], S04.811-S04.9XX[A]

X ● **S04.50 Injury of facial nerve, unspecified side** A

X ● **S04.51 Injury of facial nerve, right side** A

X ● **S04.52 Injury of facial nerve, left side** A

● **S04.6 Injury of acoustic nerve**
Injury of auditory nerve
Injury of 8th cranial nerve
Ex: For category S04.6 CC codes: S04.60X-S04.62X[A], S04.811-S04.9XX[A]

X ● **S04.60 Injury of acoustic nerve, unspecified side** A

X ● **S04.61 Injury of acoustic nerve, right side** A

X ● **S04.62 Injury of acoustic nerve, left side** A

● **S04.7 Injury of accessory nerve**
Injury of 11th cranial nerve
Ex: For category S04.7 CC codes: S04.70X-S04.9XX[A]

X ● **S04.70 Injury of accessory nerve, unspecified side** A

X ● **S04.71 Injury of accessory nerve, right side** A

X ● **S04.72 Injury of accessory nerve, left side** A

- **S04.8 Injury of other cranial nerves**
  Ex: For category S04.8 CC codes: S04.811-S04.9XX[A]
  - **S04.81 Injury of olfactory [1st] nerve**
    - **S04.811 Injury of olfactory [1st] nerve, right side** A
    - **S04.812 Injury of olfactory [1st] nerve, left side** A
    - **S04.819 Injury of olfactory [1st] nerve, unspecified side** A
  - **S04.89 Injury of other cranial nerves**
    Injury of vagus [10th] nerve
    - **S04.891 Injury of other cranial nerves, right side** A
    - **S04.892 Injury of other cranial nerves, left side** A
    - **S04.899 Injury of other cranial nerves, unspecified side** A
  - X **S04.9 Injury of unspecified cranial nerve** A
    Ex: S04.811-S04.9XX[A]

- **S05 Injury of eye and orbit**
  Includes open wound of eye and orbit
  Excludes2 2nd cranial [optic] nerve injury (S04.0-)
  3rd cranial [oculomotor] nerve injury (S04.1-)
  open wound of eyelid and periocular area (S01.1-)
  orbital bone fracture (S02.1-, S02.3-, S02.8-)
  superficial injury of eyelid (S00.1-S00.2)

  The appropriate 7th character is to be added to each code from category S05

A	initial encounter
D	subsequent encounter
S	sequela

  - **S05.0 Injury of conjunctiva and corneal abrasion without foreign body**
    Excludes1 foreign body in conjunctival sac (T15.1)
    foreign body in cornea (T15.0)
    Ex: For category S05 CC codes unless otherwise indicated: S01.101-S01.159[A], S05.20X-S05.8X9[A], S05.91X-S05.92X[A], S38.3XX[A], T14.90-T14.91, T79.A0X-T79.9XX[A]
    - X **S05.00 Injury of conjunctiva and corneal abrasion without foreign body, unspecified eye**
    - X **S05.01 Injury of conjunctiva and corneal abrasion without foreign body, right eye**
    - X **S05.02 Injury of conjunctiva and corneal abrasion without foreign body, left eye**
  - **S05.1 Contusion of eyeball and orbital tissues**
    Traumatic hyphema
    Excludes2 black eye NOS (S00.1)
    contusion of eyelid and periocular area (S00.1)
    - X **S05.10 Contusion of eyeball and orbital tissues, unspecified eye**
    - X **S05.11 Contusion of eyeball and orbital tissues, right eye**
    - X **S05.12 Contusion of eyeball and orbital tissues, left eye**
  - **S05.2 Ocular laceration and rupture with prolapse or loss of intraocular tissue**
    - X **S05.20 Ocular laceration and rupture with prolapse or loss of intraocular tissue, unspecified eye** A
    - X **S05.21 Ocular laceration and rupture with prolapse or loss of intraocular tissue, right eye** A
    - X **S05.22 Ocular laceration and rupture with prolapse or loss of intraocular tissue, left eye** A
  - **S05.3 Ocular laceration without prolapse or loss of intraocular tissue**
    Laceration of eye NOS
    - X **S05.30 Ocular laceration without prolapse or loss of intraocular tissue, unspecified eye** A
    - X **S05.31 Ocular laceration without prolapse or loss of intraocular tissue, right eye** A
    - X **S05.32 Ocular laceration without prolapse or loss of intraocular tissue, left eye** A
  - **S05.4 Penetrating wound of orbit with or without foreign body**
    Excludes2 retained (old) foreign body following penetrating wound in orbit (H05.5-)
    - X **S05.40 Penetrating wound of orbit with or without foreign body, unspecified eye** A
    - X **S05.41 Penetrating wound of orbit with or without foreign body, right eye** A
    - X **S05.42 Penetrating wound of orbit with or without foreign body, left eye** A
  - **S05.5 Penetrating wound with foreign body of eyeball**
    Excludes2 retained (old) intraocular foreign body (H44.6-, H44.7)
    Ex: For category S05.5 CC codes: S01.101-S01.159[A], S05.20X-S05.8X9[A], S05.91X-S05.92X[A], S38.3XX[A], T14.90-T14.91, T79.8XX-T79.9XX[A]
    - X **S05.50 Penetrating wound with foreign body of unspecified eyeball** A
    - X **S05.51 Penetrating wound with foreign body of right eyeball** A
    - X **S05.52 Penetrating wound with foreign body of left eyeball** A
  - **S05.6 Penetrating wound without foreign body of eyeball**
    Ocular penetration NOS
    - X **S05.60 Penetrating wound without foreign body of unspecified eyeball**
    - X **S05.61 Penetrating wound without foreign body of right eyeball**
    - X **S05.62 Penetrating wound without foreign body of left eyeball**
  - **S05.7 Avulsion of eye**
    Traumatic enucleation
    - X **S05.70 Avulsion of unspecified eye** A
    - X **S05.71 Avulsion of right eye** A
    - X **S05.72 Avulsion of left eye** A
  - **S05.8 Other injuries of eye and orbit**
    Lacrimal duct injury
    - **S05.8X Other injuries of eye and orbit**
      - **S05.8X1 Other injuries of right eye and orbit** A
      - **S05.8X2 Other injuries of left eye and orbit** A
      - **S05.8X9 Other injuries of unspecified eye and orbit** A
  - **S05.9 Unspecified injury of eye and orbit**
    Injury of eye NOS
    - X **S05.90 Unspecified injury of unspecified eye and orbit**
    - X **S05.91 Unspecified injury of right eye and orbit** A
    - X **S05.92 Unspecified injury of left eye and orbit** A

● **S06 Intracranial injury**

Includes traumatic brain injury

Code also any associated:
open wound of head (S01.-)
skull fracture (S02.-)

Excludes1 head injury NOS (S09.90)

The appropriate 7th character is to be added to each code from category S06

A	initial encounter
D	subsequent encounter
S	sequela

Ex: **For category S06 CC codes unless otherwise indicated: For S06[A,B]:** See S02.4[A,B] **For S06[S]:** See S02.0[K]

Coding Clinic: 2015, Q4, P40

● **S06.0 Concussion**

Commotio cerebri

Excludes1 concussion with other intracranial injuries classified in subcategories S06.1- to S06.6- , S06.81- and S06.82- code to specified intracranial injury ◄

● **S06.0X Concussion**

● **S06.0X0 Concussion without loss of consciousness**

● **S06.0X1 Concussion with loss of consciousness of 30 minutes or less** A CC, A MCC

~~S06.0X2 Concussion with loss of consciousness of 31 minutes to 59 minutes~~

~~S06.0X3 Concussion with loss of consciousness of 1 hour to 5 hours 59 minutes~~

~~S06.0X4 Concussion with loss of consciousness of 6 hours to 24 hours~~

~~S06.0X5 Concussion with loss of consciousness greater than 24 hours with return to pre-existing conscious level~~

~~S06.0X6 Concussion with loss of consciousness greater than 24 hours without return to pre-existing conscious level with patient surviving~~

~~S06.0X7 Concussion with loss of consciousness of any duration with death due to brain injury prior to regaining consciousness~~

~~S06.0X8 Concussion with loss of consciousness of any duration with death due to other cause prior to regaining consciousness~~

● **S06.0X9 Concussion with loss of consciousness of unspecified duration** A CC, A MCC

Concussion NOS

● **S06.1 Traumatic cerebral edema**

Diffuse traumatic cerebral edema
Focal traumatic cerebral edema

● **S06.1X Traumatic cerebral edema**

● **S06.1X0 Traumatic cerebral edema without loss of consciousness** A MCC

MCC when PDx is its own MCC

Ex: G93.6, G93.82

Coding Clinic: 2015, Q1, P12

● **S06.1X1 Traumatic cerebral edema with loss of consciousness of 30 minutes or less** A CC, A MCC

MCC when PDx is its own MCC

Ex: G93.6, G93.82, S01.90X-S01.95X[A], S02.0XX-S02.19X[A,B,S], S02.2XXS-S02.82X[S], S02.91X[A,B,S], S02.92X[S], S06.0X0-S07.9XX[A], S08.89X-S09.19X[A], S09.8XX-S09.90X[A], S09.92X-S09.93X[A], S16.8XX-S19.9XX[A], S38.3XX[A], T14.90-T14.91, T79.8XX-T79.9XX[A], T79.A0X-T79.A9X[A]

● **S06.1X2 Traumatic cerebral edema with loss of consciousness of 31 minutes to 59 minutes** A CC, A MCC

MCC when PDx is its own MCC

Ex: See S06.1X1

● **S06.1X3 Traumatic cerebral edema with loss of consciousness of 1 hour to 5 hours 59 minutes** A CC, A MCC

MCC when PDx is its own MCC

Ex: See S06.1X1

● **S06.1X4 Traumatic cerebral edema with loss of consciousness of 6 hours to 24 hours** A CC, A MCC

MCC when PDx is its own MCC

Ex: See S06.1X1

● **S06.1X5 Traumatic cerebral edema with loss of consciousness greater than 24 hours with return to pre-existing conscious level** A CC, A MCC

MCC when PDx is its own MCC

Ex: See S06.1X1

● **S06.1X6 Traumatic cerebral edema with loss of consciousness greater than 24 hours without return to pre-existing conscious level with patient surviving** A CC, A MCC

MCC when PDx is its own MCC

● **S06.1X7 Traumatic cerebral edema with loss of consciousness of any duration with death due to brain injury prior to regaining consciousness** A CC, A MCC

MCC when PDx is its own MCC

● **S06.1X8 Traumatic cerebral edema with loss of consciousness of any duration with death due to other cause prior to regaining consciousness** A CC, A MCC

MCC when PDx is its own MCC

● **S06.1X9 Traumatic cerebral edema with loss of consciousness of unspecified duration** A CC, A MCC

Traumatic cerebral edema NOS

MCC when PDx is its own MCC

Ex: See S06.1X1

● **S06.2 Diffuse traumatic brain injury**

Diffuse axonal brain injury

Excludes1 traumatic diffuse cerebral edema (S06.1X-)

● **S06.2X Diffuse traumatic brain injury**

● **S06.2X0 Diffuse traumatic brain injury without loss of consciousness**

● **S06.2X1 Diffuse traumatic brain injury with loss of consciousness of 30 minutes or less** A CC, A MCC

● **S06.2X2 Diffuse traumatic brain injury with loss of consciousness of 31 minutes to 59 minutes** A CC, A MCC

● **S06.2X3 Diffuse traumatic brain injury with loss of consciousness of 1 hour to 5 hours 59 minutes** A CC, A MCC

● **S06.2X4 Diffuse traumatic brain injury with loss of consciousness of 6 hours to 24 hours** A CC, A MCC

- **S06.2X5** Diffuse traumatic brain injury with loss of consciousness greater than 24 hours with return to pre-existing conscious levels A, A
- **S06.2X6** Diffuse traumatic brain injury with loss of consciousness greater than 24 hours without return to pre-existing conscious level with patient surviving A, A
- **S06.2X7** Diffuse traumatic brain injury with loss of consciousness of any duration with death due to brain injury prior to regaining consciousness A, A
- **S06.2X8** Diffuse traumatic brain injury with loss of consciousness of any duration with death due to other cause prior to regaining consciousness A, A
- **S06.2X9** Diffuse traumatic brain injury with loss of consciousness of unspecified duration A, A
  Diffuse traumatic brain injury NOS

S06.3 Focal traumatic brain injury

Excludes1 any condition classifiable to S06.4-S06.6
focal cerebral edema (S06.1)

S06.30 Unspecified focal traumatic brain injury

- **S06.300** Unspecified focal traumatic brain injury without loss of consciousness
- **S06.301** Unspecified focal traumatic brain injury with loss of consciousness of 30 minutes or less A, A
- **S06.302** Unspecified focal traumatic brain injury with loss of consciousness of 31 minutes to 59 minutes A, A
- **S06.303** Unspecified focal traumatic brain injury with loss of consciousness of 1 hour to 5 hours 59 minutes A, A
- **S06.304** Unspecified focal traumatic brain injury with loss of consciousness of 6 hours to 24 hours A, A
- **S06.305** Unspecified focal traumatic brain injury with loss of consciousness greater than 24 hours with return to pre-existing conscious level A, A
- **S06.306** Unspecified focal traumatic brain injury with loss of consciousness greater than 24 hours without return to pre-existing conscious level with patient surviving A, A
- **S06.307** Unspecified focal traumatic brain injury with loss of consciousness of any duration with death due to brain injury prior to regaining consciousness A, A
- **S06.308** Unspecified focal traumatic brain injury with loss of consciousness of any duration with death due to other cause prior to regaining consciousness A, A
- **S06.309** Unspecified focal traumatic brain injury with loss of consciousness of unspecified duration A, A
  Unspecified focal traumatic brain injury NOS

S06.31 Contusion and laceration of right cerebrum

- **S06.310** Contusion and laceration of right cerebrum without loss of consciousness A, A
- **S06.311** Contusion and laceration of right cerebrum with loss of consciousness of 30 minutes or less A, A
- **S06.312** Contusion and laceration of right cerebrum with loss of consciousness of 31 minutes to 59 minutes A, A
- **S06.313** Contusion and laceration of right cerebrum with loss of consciousness of 1 hour to 5 hours 59 minutes A, A
- **S06.314** Contusion and laceration of right cerebrum with loss of consciousness of 6 hours to 24 hours A, A
- **S06.315** Contusion and laceration of right cerebrum with loss of consciousness greater than 24 hours with return to pre-existing conscious level A, A
- **S06.316** Contusion and laceration of right cerebrum with loss of consciousness greater than 24 hours without return to pre-existing conscious level with patient surviving A, A
- **S06.317** Contusion and laceration of right cerebrum with loss of consciousness of any duration with death due to brain injury prior to regaining consciousness A, A
- **S06.318** Contusion and laceration of right cerebrum with loss of consciousness of any duration with death due to other cause prior to regaining consciousness A, A
- **S06.319** Contusion and laceration of right cerebrum with loss of consciousness of unspecified duration A, A
  Contusion and laceration of right cerebrum NOS

S06.32 Contusion and laceration of left cerebrum

- **S06.320** Contusion and laceration of left cerebrum without loss of consciousness A, A
- **S06.321** Contusion and laceration of left cerebrum with loss of consciousness of 30 minutes or less A, A
- **S06.322** Contusion and laceration of left cerebrum with loss of consciousness of 31 minutes to 59 minutes A, A
- **S06.323** Contusion and laceration of left cerebrum with loss of consciousness of 1 hour to 5 hours 59 minutes A, A
- **S06.324** Contusion and laceration of left cerebrum with loss of consciousness of 6 hours to 24 hours A, A
- **S06.325** Contusion and laceration of left cerebrum with loss of consciousness greater than 24 hours with return to pre-existing conscious level A, A
- **S06.326** Contusion and laceration of left cerebrum with loss of consciousness greater than 24 hours without return to pre-existing conscious level with patient surviving A, A
- **S06.327** Contusion and laceration of left cerebrum with loss of consciousness of any duration with death due to brain injury prior to regaining consciousness A, A

- **S06.328** Contusion and laceration of left cerebrum with loss of consciousness of any duration with death due to other cause prior to regaining consciousness A, A
- **S06.329** Contusion and laceration of left cerebrum with loss of consciousness of unspecified duration A, A
  Contusion and laceration of left cerebrum NOS

S06.33 Contusion and laceration of cerebrum, unspecified

- **S06.330** Contusion and laceration of cerebrum, unspecified, without loss of consciousness A, A
- **S06.331** Contusion and laceration of cerebrum, unspecified, with loss of consciousness of 30 minutes or less A, A
- **S06.332** Contusion and laceration of cerebrum, unspecified, with loss of consciousness of 31 minutes to 59 minutes A, A
- **S06.333** Contusion and laceration of cerebrum, unspecified, with loss of consciousness of 1 hour to 5 hours 59 minutes A, A
- **S06.334** Contusion and laceration of cerebrum, unspecified, with loss of consciousness of 6 hours to 24 hours A, A
- **S06.335** Contusion and laceration of cerebrum, unspecified, with loss of consciousness greater than 24 hours with return to pre-existing conscious level A, A
- **S06.336** Contusion and laceration of cerebrum, unspecified, with loss of consciousness greater than 24 hours without return to pre-existing conscious level with patient surviving A, A
- **S06.337** Contusion and laceration of cerebrum, unspecified, with loss of consciousness of any duration with death due to brain injury prior to regaining consciousness A, A
- **S06.338** Contusion and laceration of cerebrum, unspecified, with loss of consciousness of any duration with death due to other cause prior to regaining consciousness A, A
- **S06.339** Contusion and laceration of cerebrum, unspecified, with loss of consciousness of unspecified duration A, A
  Contusion and laceration of cerebrum NOS

S06.34 Traumatic hemorrhage of right cerebrum
Traumatic intracerebral hemorrhage and hematoma of right cerebrum

- **S06.340** Traumatic hemorrhage of right cerebrum without loss of consciousness A, A
  Coding Clinic: 2015, Q1, P12
- **S06.341** Traumatic hemorrhage of right cerebrum with loss of consciousness of 30 minutes or less A, A
- **S06.342** Traumatic hemorrhage of right cerebrum with loss of consciousness of 31 minutes to 59 minutes A, A
- **S06.343** Traumatic hemorrhage of right cerebrum with loss of consciousness of 1 hours to 5 hours 59 minutes A, A
- **S06.344** Traumatic hemorrhage of right cerebrum with loss of consciousness of 6 hours to 24 hours A, A
- **S06.345** Traumatic hemorrhage of right cerebrum with loss of consciousness greater than 24 hours with return to pre-existing conscious level A, A
- **S06.346** Traumatic hemorrhage of right cerebrum with loss of consciousness greater than 24 hours without return to pre-existing conscious level with patient surviving A, A
- **S06.347** Traumatic hemorrhage of right cerebrum with loss of consciousness of any duration with death due to brain injury prior to regaining consciousness A, A
- **S06.348** Traumatic hemorrhage of right cerebrum with loss of consciousness of any duration with death due to other cause prior to regaining consciousness A, A
- **S06.349** Traumatic hemorrhage of right cerebrum with loss of consciousness of unspecified duration A, A
  Traumatic hemorrhage of right cerebrum NOS

S06.35 Traumatic hemorrhage of left cerebrum
Traumatic intracerebral hemorrhage and hematoma of left cerebrum

- **S06.350** Traumatic hemorrhage of left cerebrum without loss of consciousness A, A
- **S06.351** Traumatic hemorrhage of left cerebrum with loss of consciousness of 30 minutes or less A, A
- **S06.352** Traumatic hemorrhage of left cerebrum with loss of consciousness of 31 minutes to 59 minutes A, A
- **S06.353** Traumatic hemorrhage of left cerebrum with loss of consciousness of 1 hours to 5 hours 59 minutes A, A
- **S06.354** Traumatic hemorrhage of left cerebrum with loss of consciousness of 6 hours to 24 hours A, A
- **S06.355** Traumatic hemorrhage of left cerebrum with loss of consciousness greater than 24 hours with return to pre-existing conscious level A, A
- **S06.356** Traumatic hemorrhage of left cerebrum with loss of consciousness greater than 24 hours without return to pre-existing conscious level with patient surviving A, A
- **S06.357** Traumatic hemorrhage of left cerebrum with loss of consciousness of any duration with death due to brain injury prior to regaining consciousness A, A
- **S06.358** Traumatic hemorrhage of left cerebrum with loss of consciousness of any duration with death due to other cause prior to regaining consciousness A, A

- **S06.359** **Traumatic hemorrhage of left cerebrum with loss of consciousness of unspecified duration** A CC, A MCC
  Traumatic hemorrhage of left cerebrum NOS

- **S06.36** **Traumatic hemorrhage of cerebrum, unspecified**
  Traumatic intracerebral hemorrhage and hematoma, unspecified
  - **S06.360** **Traumatic hemorrhage of cerebrum, unspecified, without loss of consciousness** A CC, A MCC
  - **S06.361** **Traumatic hemorrhage of cerebrum, unspecified, with loss of consciousness of 30 minutes or less** A MCC, A MCC
  - **S06.362** **Traumatic hemorrhage of cerebrum, unspecified, with loss of consciousness of 31 minutes to 59 minutes** A CC, A MCC
  - **S06.363** **Traumatic hemorrhage of cerebrum, unspecified, with loss of consciousness of 1 hours to 5 hours 59 minutes** A CC, A MCC
  - **S06.364** **Traumatic hemorrhage of cerebrum, unspecified, with loss of consciousness of 6 hours to 24 hours** A MCC, A MCC
  - **S06.365** **Traumatic hemorrhage of cerebrum, unspecified, with loss of consciousness greater than 24 hours with return to pre-existing conscious level** A CC, A MCC
  - **S06.366** **Traumatic hemorrhage of cerebrum, unspecified, with loss of consciousness greater than 24 hours without return to pre-existing conscious level with patient surviving** A MCC, A MCC
  - **S06.367** **Traumatic hemorrhage of cerebrum, unspecified, with loss of consciousness of any duration with death due to brain injury prior to regaining consciousness** A MCC, A MCC
  - **S06.368** **Traumatic hemorrhage of cerebrum, unspecified, with loss of consciousness of any duration with death due to other cause prior to regaining consciousness** A MCC, A MCC
  - **S06.369** **Traumatic hemorrhage of cerebrum, unspecified, with loss of consciousness of unspecified duration** A MCC, A MCC
    Traumatic hemorrhage of cerebrum NOS

- **S06.37** **Contusion, laceration, and hemorrhage of cerebellum**
  - **S06.370** **Contusion, laceration, and hemorrhage of cerebellum without loss of consciousness** A CC, A MCC
    Ex: No exclusions
  - **S06.371** **Contusion, laceration, and hemorrhage of cerebellum with loss of consciousness of 30 minutes or less** A CC, A MCC
  - **S06.372** **Contusion, laceration, and hemorrhage of cerebellum with loss of consciousness of 31 minutes to 59 minutes** A CC, A MCC
  - **S06.373** **Contusion, laceration, and hemorrhage of cerebellum with loss of consciousness of 1 hour to 5 hours 59 minutes** A CC, A MCC
  - **S06.374** **Contusion, laceration, and hemorrhage of cerebellum with loss of consciousness of 6 hours to 24 hours** A CC, A MCC
  - **S06.375** **Contusion, laceration, and hemorrhage of cerebellum with loss of consciousness greater than 24 hours with return to pre-existing conscious level** A CC, A MCC
  - **S06.376** **Contusion, laceration, and hemorrhage of cerebellum with loss of consciousness greater than 24 hours without return to pre-existing conscious level with patient surviving** A MCC, A MCC
  - **S06.377** **Contusion, laceration, and hemorrhage of cerebellum with loss of consciousness of any duration with death due to brain injury prior to regaining consciousness** A MCC, A MCC
  - **S06.378** **Contusion, laceration, and hemorrhage of cerebellum with loss of consciousness of any duration with death due to other cause prior to regaining consciousness** A MCC, A MCC
  - **S06.379** **Contusion, laceration, and hemorrhage of cerebellum with loss of consciousness of unspecified duration** A CC, A MCC
    Contusion, laceration, and hemorrhage of cerebellum NOS

- **S06.38** **Contusion, laceration, and hemorrhage of brainstem**
  - **S06.380** **Contusion, laceration, and hemorrhage of brainstem without loss of consciousness** A MCC, A MCC
    Ex: No exclusions
  - **S06.381** **Contusion, laceration, and hemorrhage of brainstem with loss of consciousness of 30 minutes or less** A CC, A MCC
  - **S06.382** **Contusion, laceration, and hemorrhage of brainstem with loss of consciousness of 31 minutes to 59 minutes** A CC, A MCC
  - **S06.383** **Contusion, laceration, and hemorrhage of brainstem with loss of consciousness of 1 hour to 5 hours 59 minutes** A CC, A MCC
  - **S06.384** **Contusion, laceration, and hemorrhage of brainstem with loss of consciousness of 6 hours to 24 hours** A CC, A MCC
  - **S06.385** **Contusion, laceration, and hemorrhage of brainstem with loss of consciousness greater than 24 hours with return to pre-existing conscious level** A CC, A MCC
  - **S06.386** **Contusion, laceration, and hemorrhage of brainstem with loss of consciousness greater than 24 hours without return to pre-existing conscious level with patient surviving** A MCC, A MCC
  - **S06.387** **Contusion, laceration, and hemorrhage of brainstem with loss of consciousness of any duration with death due to brain injury prior to regaining consciousness** A MCC, A MCC

- **S06.388** **Contusion, laceration, and hemorrhage of brainstem with loss of consciousness of any duration with death due to other cause prior to regaining consciousness** A, A
- **S06.389** **Contusion, laceration, and hemorrhage of brainstem with loss of consciousness of unspecified duration** A, A
  Contusion, laceration, and hemorrhage of brainstem NOS

S06.4 Epidural hemorrhage
Situated outside dura mater
Extradural hemorrhage NOS
Intracranial hemorrhage due to trauma
Extradural hemorrhage (traumatic)

- **S06.4X Epidural hemorrhage**
  - **S06.4X0** **Epidural hemorrhage without loss of consciousness** A, A
  - **S06.4X1** **Epidural hemorrhage with loss of consciousness of 30 minutes or less** A, A
  - **S06.4X2** **Epidural hemorrhage with loss of consciousness of 31 minutes to 59 minutes** A, A
  - **S06.4X3** **Epidural hemorrhage with loss of consciousness of 1 hour to 5 hours 59 minutes** A, A
  - **S06.4X4** **Epidural hemorrhage with loss of consciousness of 6 hours to 24 hours** A, A
  - **S06.4X5** **Epidural hemorrhage with loss of consciousness greater than 24 hours with return to pre-existing conscious level** A, A
  - **S06.4X6** **Epidural hemorrhage with loss of consciousness greater than 24 hours without return to pre-existing conscious level with patient surviving** A, A
  - **S06.4X7** **Epidural hemorrhage with loss of consciousness of any duration with death due to brain injury prior to regaining consciousness** A, A
  - **S06.4X8** **Epidural hemorrhage with loss of consciousness of any duration with death due to other causes prior to regaining consciousness** A, A
  - **S06.4X9** **Epidural hemorrhage with loss of consciousness of unspecified duration** A, A
    Epidural hemorrhage NOS

S06.5 Traumatic subdural hemorrhage

- **S06.5X Traumatic subdural hemorrhage**
  - **S06.5X0** **Traumatic subdural hemorrhage without loss of consciousness** A, A
    Coding Clinic: 2015, Q3, P37
  - **S06.5X1** **Traumatic subdural hemorrhage with loss of consciousness of 30 minutes or less** A, A
  - **S06.5X2** **Traumatic subdural hemorrhage with loss of consciousness of 31 minutes to 59 minutes** A, A
  - **S06.5X3** **Traumatic subdural hemorrhage with loss of consciousness of 1 hour to 5 hours 59 minutes** A, A
  - **S06.5X4** **Traumatic subdural hemorrhage with loss of consciousness of 6 hours to 24 hours** A, A
  - **S06.5X5** **Traumatic subdural hemorrhage with loss of consciousness greater than 24 hours with return to pre-existing conscious level** A, A
  - **S06.5X6** **Traumatic subdural hemorrhage with loss of consciousness greater than 24 hours without return to pre-existing conscious level with patient surviving** A, A
  - **S06.5X7** **Traumatic subdural hemorrhage with loss of consciousness of any duration with death due to brain injury before regaining consciousness** A, A
  - **S06.5X8** **Traumatic subdural hemorrhage with loss of consciousness of any duration with death due to other cause before regaining consciousness** A, A
  - **S06.5X9** **Traumatic subdural hemorrhage with loss of consciousness of unspecified duration** A, A
    Traumatic subdural hemorrhage NOS

S06.6 Traumatic subarachnoid hemorrhage
Between arachnoid and pia mater

- **S06.6X Traumatic subarachnoid hemorrhage**
  - **S06.6X0** **Traumatic subarachnoid hemorrhage without loss of consciousness** A, A
    Coding Clinic: 2015, Q3, P37
  - **S06.6X1** **Traumatic subarachnoid hemorrhage with loss of consciousness of 30 minutes or less** A, A
  - **S06.6X2** **Traumatic subarachnoid hemorrhage with loss of consciousness of 31 minutes to 59 minutes** A, A
  - **S06.6X3** **Traumatic subarachnoid hemorrhage with loss of consciousness of 1 hour to 5 hours 59 minutes** A, A
  - **S06.6X4** **Traumatic subarachnoid hemorrhage with loss of consciousness of 6 hours to 24 hours** A, A
  - **S06.6X5** **Traumatic subarachnoid hemorrhage with loss of consciousness greater than 24 hours with return to pre-existing conscious level** A, A
  - **S06.6X6** **Traumatic subarachnoid hemorrhage with loss of consciousness greater than 24 hours without return to pre-existing conscious level with patient surviving** A, A
  - **S06.6X7** **Traumatic subarachnoid hemorrhage with loss of consciousness of any duration with death due to brain injury prior to regaining consciousness** A, A
  - **S06.6X8** **Traumatic subarachnoid hemorrhage with loss of consciousness of any duration with death due to other cause prior to regaining consciousness** A, A
  - **S06.6X9** **Traumatic subarachnoid hemorrhage with loss of consciousness of unspecified duration** A, A
    Traumatic subarachnoid hemorrhage NOS

S06.8 Other specified intracranial injuries

- **S06.81** **Injury of right internal carotid artery, intracranial portion, not elsewhere classified**
  - **S06.810** **Injury of right internal carotid artery, intracranial portion, not elsewhere classified without loss of consciousness**
  - **S06.811** **Injury of right internal carotid artery, intracranial portion, not elsewhere classified with loss of consciousness of 30 minutes or less** A, A

- **S06.812** Injury of right internal carotid artery, intracranial portion, not elsewhere classified with loss of consciousness of 31 minutes to 59 minutes A CC, A MCC
- **S06.813** Injury of right internal carotid artery, intracranial portion, not elsewhere classified with loss of consciousness of 1 hour to 5 hours 59 minutes A CC, A MCC
- **S06.814** Injury of right internal carotid artery, intracranial portion, not elsewhere classified with loss of consciousness of 6 hours to 24 hours A CC, A MCC
- **S06.815** Injury of right internal carotid artery, intracranial portion, not elsewhere classified with loss of consciousness greater than 24 hours with return to pre-existing conscious level A CC, A MCC
- **S06.816** Injury of right internal carotid artery, intracranial portion, not elsewhere classified with loss of consciousness greater than 24 hours without return to pre-existing conscious level with patient surviving A CC, A MCC
- **S06.817** Injury of right internal carotid artery, intracranial portion, not elsewhere classified with loss of consciousness of any duration with death due to brain injury prior to regaining consciousness A CC, A MCC
- **S06.818** Injury of right internal carotid artery, intracranial portion, not elsewhere classified with loss of consciousness of any duration with death due to other cause prior to regaining consciousness A CC, A MCC
- **S06.819** Injury of right internal carotid artery, intracranial portion, not elsewhere classified with loss of consciousness of unspecified duration A CC, A MCC
  - Injury of right internal carotid artery, intracranial portion, not elsewhere classified NOS

- **S06.82** Injury of left internal carotid artery, intracranial portion, not elsewhere classified
  - **S06.820** Injury of left internal carotid artery, intracranial portion, not elsewhere classified without loss of consciousness
  - **S06.821** Injury of left internal carotid artery, intracranial portion, not elsewhere classified with loss of consciousness of 30 minutes or less A CC, A MCC
  - **S06.822** Injury of left internal carotid artery, intracranial portion, not elsewhere classified with loss of consciousness of 31 minutes to 59 minutes A CC, A MCC
  - **S06.823** Injury of left internal carotid artery, intracranial portion, not elsewhere classified with loss of consciousness of 1 hour to 5 hours 59 minutes A CC, A MCC
  - **S06.824** Injury of left internal carotid artery, intracranial portion, not elsewhere classified with loss of consciousness of 6 hours to 24 hours A CC, A MCC
  - **S06.825** Injury of left internal carotid artery, intracranial portion, not elsewhere classified with loss of consciousness greater than 24 hours with return to pre-existing conscious level A CC, A MCC
  - **S06.826** Injury of left internal carotid artery, intracranial portion, not elsewhere classified with loss of consciousness greater than 24 hours without return to pre-existing conscious level with patient surviving A CC, A MCC
  - **S06.827** Injury of left internal carotid artery, intracranial portion, not elsewhere classified with loss of consciousness of any duration with death due to brain injury prior to regaining consciousness A CC, A MCC
  - **S06.828** Injury of left internal carotid artery, intracranial portion, not elsewhere classified with loss of consciousness of any duration with death due to other cause prior to regaining consciousness A CC, A MCC
  - **S06.829** Injury of left internal carotid artery, intracranial portion, not elsewhere classified with loss of consciousness of unspecified duration A CC, A MCC
    - Injury of left internal carotid artery, intracranial portion, not elsewhere classified NOS

- **S06.89** Other specified intracranial injury
  - **Excludes1** concussion (S06.0X-) ◀
  - **S06.890** Other specified intracranial injury without loss of consciousness
  - **S06.891** Other specified intracranial injury with loss of consciousness of 30 minutes or less A CC, A MCC
  - **S06.892** Other specified intracranial injury with loss of consciousness of 31 minutes to 59 minutes A CC, A MCC
  - **S06.893** Other specified intracranial injury with loss of consciousness of 1 hour to 5 hours 59 minutes A CC, A MCC
  - **S06.894** Other specified intracranial injury with loss of consciousness of 6 hours to 24 hours A CC, A MCC
  - **S06.895** Other specified intracranial injury with loss of consciousness greater than 24 hours with return to pre-existing conscious level A CC, A MCC
  - **S06.896** Other specified intracranial injury with loss of consciousness greater than 24 hours without return to pre-existing conscious level with patient surviving A CC, A MCC
  - **S06.897** Other specified intracranial injury with loss of consciousness of any duration with death due to brain injury prior to regaining consciousness A CC, A MCC
  - **S06.898** Other specified intracranial injury with loss of consciousness of any duration with death due to other cause prior to regaining consciousness A CC, A MCC
  - **S06.899** Other specified intracranial injury with loss of consciousness of unspecified duration A CC, A MCC

S06.9 Unspecified intracranial injury
Brain injury NOS
Head injury NOS with loss of consciousness
Traumatic brain injury NOS ◀

Excludes1 conditions classifiable to S06.0- to S06.8-code to specified intracranial injury ◀
head injury NOS (S09.90)

S06.9X Unspecified intracranial injury

S06.9X0 Unspecified intracranial injury without loss of consciousness

S06.9X1 Unspecified intracranial injury with loss of consciousness of 30 minutes or less A CC, A MCC

S06.9X2 Unspecified intracranial injury with loss of consciousness of 31 minutes to 59 minutes A CC, A MCC

S06.9X3 Unspecified intracranial injury with loss of consciousness of 1 hour to 5 hours 59 minutes A CC, A MCC

S06.9X4 Unspecified intracranial injury with loss of consciousness of 6 hours to 24 hours A CC, A MCC

S06.9X5 Unspecified intracranial injury with loss of consciousness greater than 24 hours with return to pre-existing conscious level A CC, A MCC

S06.9X6 Unspecified intracranial injury with loss of consciousness greater than 24 hours without return to pre-existing conscious level with patient surviving A MCC, A MCC

S06.9X7 Unspecified intracranial injury with loss of consciousness of any duration with death due to brain injury prior to regaining consciousness A MCC, A MCC

S06.9X8 Unspecified intracranial injury with loss of consciousness of any duration with death due to other cause prior to regaining consciousness A MCC, A MCC

S06.9X9 Unspecified intracranial injury with loss of consciousness of unspecified duration A CC, A MCC

S07 Crushing injury of head
Use additional code for all associated injuries, such as:
intracranial injuries (S06.-)
skull fractures (S02.-)

The appropriate 7th character is to be added to each code from category S07

A	initial encounter
D	subsequent encounter
S	sequela

Ex: **For category S07 CC codes:** S01.90X-S01.95X[A], S02.0XX-S02.92X[S], S07.0XX-S07.9XX[A], S08.89X-S09.19X[A], S09.8XXA-S09.90X[A], S09.92XA-S09.93X[A], S16.8XX-S19.9XX[A], T14.90-T14.91, T79.8XX-T79.9XX[A], T79.A0X-T79.A9X[A]

X **S07.0 Crushing injury of face** A CC, A MCC

X **S07.1 Crushing injury of skull** A CC, A MCC

X **S07.8 Crushing injury of other parts of head** A CC, A MCC

X **S07.9 Crushing injury of head, part unspecified** A CC, A MCC

S08 Avulsion and traumatic amputation of part of head
An amputation not identified as partial or complete should be coded to complete

The appropriate 7th character is to be added to each code from category S08

A	initial encounter
D	subsequent encounter
S	sequela

X **S08.0 Avulsion of scalp**

S08.1 Traumatic amputation of ear

S08.11 Complete traumatic amputation of ear

S08.111 Complete traumatic amputation of right ear

S08.112 Complete traumatic amputation of left ear

S08.119 Complete traumatic amputation of unspecified ear

S08.12 Partial traumatic amputation of ear

S08.121 Partial traumatic amputation of right ear

S08.122 Partial traumatic amputation of left ear

S08.129 Partial traumatic amputation of unspecified ear

S08.8 Traumatic amputation of other parts of head

S08.81 Traumatic amputation of nose

S08.811 Complete traumatic amputation of nose

S08.812 Partial traumatic amputation of nose

X **S08.89 Traumatic amputation of other parts of head**

S09 Other and unspecified injuries of head
The appropriate 7th character is to be added to each code from category S09

A	initial encounter
D	subsequent encounter
S	sequela

X **S09.0 Injury of blood vessels of head, not elsewhere classified** A CC

Excludes1 injury of cerebral blood vessels (S06.-)
injury of precerebral blood vessels (S15.-)

Ex: S09.0XX[A], S15.101-S15.199[A], S15.8XX-S15.9XX[A], T14.90-T14.91, T79.8XX-T79.9XX[A], T79.A0X-T79.A9X[A]

S09.1 Injury of muscle and tendon of head
Code also any associated open wound (S01.-)

Excludes2 sprain to joints and ligament of head (S03.9)

X **S09.10 Unspecified injury of muscle and tendon of head**
Injury of muscle and tendon of head NOS

X **S09.11 Strain of muscle and tendon of head**

X **S09.12 Laceration of muscle and tendon of head**

X **S09.19 Other specified injury of muscle and tendon of head**

S09.2 Traumatic rupture of ear drum

Excludes1 traumatic rupture of ear drum due to blast injury (S09.31-)

Ex: **For category S09.2 CC codes:** S01.301-S01.359[A], S08.111-S08.129[A], S09.20X-S09.399[A], S09.91X[A], S38.3XX[A],T14.90-T14.91, T79.8XX-T79.9XX[A]

X **S09.20 Traumatic rupture of unspecified ear drum** A CC

X **S09.21 Traumatic rupture of right ear drum** A CC

X **S09.22 Traumatic rupture of left ear drum** A CC

● **S09.3 Other specified and unspecified injury of middle and inner ear**

Excludes1 injury to ear NOS (S09.91-)

Excludes2 injury to external ear (S00.4-, S01.3-, S08.1-)

Ex For category S09.3 CC codes: See S09.2

● **S09.30 Unspecified injury of middle and inner ear**

● **S09.301 Unspecified injury of right middle and inner ear** A

● **S09.302 Unspecified injury of left middle and inner ear** A

● **S09.309 Unspecified injury of unspecified middle and inner ear** A

● **S09.31 Primary blast injury of ear**
Blast injury of ear NOS

● **S09.311 Primary blast injury of right ear** A

● **S09.312 Primary blast injury of left ear** A

● **S09.313 Primary blast injury of ear, bilateral** A

● **S09.319 Primary blast injury of unspecified ear** A

● **S09.39 Other specified injury of middle and inner ear**
Secondary blast injury to ear

● **S09.391 Other specified injury of right middle and inner ear** A

● **S09.392 Other specified injury of left middle and inner ear** A

● **S09.399 Other specified injury of unspecified middle and inner ear** A

X● **S09.8 Other specified injuries of head**

● **S09.9 Unspecified injury of face and head**

X● **S09.90 Unspecified injury of head**
Head injury NOS

Excludes1 brain injury NOS (S06.9-)
head injury NOS with loss of consciousness (S06.9-)
intracranial injury NOS (S06.9-)

X● **S09.91 Unspecified injury of ear**
Injury of ear NOS

X● **S09.92 Unspecified injury of nose**
Injury of nose NOS

X● **S09.93 Unspecified injury of face**
Injury of face NOS

INJURIES TO THE NECK (S10-S19)

Includes injuries of nape
injuries of supraclavicular region
injuries of throat

Excludes2 burns and corrosions (T20-T32)
effects of foreign body in esophagus (T18.1)
effects of foreign body in larynx (T17.3)
effects of foreign body in pharynx (T17.2)
effects of foreign body in trachea (T17.4)
frostbite (T33-T34)
insect bite or sting, venomous (T63.4)

● **S10 Superficial injury of neck**

The appropriate 7th character is to be added to each code from category S10

A	initial encounter
D	subsequent encounter
S	sequela

X● **S10.0 Contusion of throat**
Contusion of cervical esophagus
Contusion of larynx
Contusion of pharynx
Contusion of trachea

● **S10.1 Other and unspecified superficial injuries of throat**

X● **S10.10 Unspecified superficial injuries of throat**

X● **S10.11 Abrasion of throat**

X● **S10.12 Blister (nonthermal) of throat**

X● **S10.14 External constriction of part of throat**

X● **S10.15 Superficial foreign body of throat**
Splinter in the throat

X● **S10.16 Insect bite (nonvenomous) of throat**

X● **S10.17 Other superficial bite of throat**

Excludes1 open bite of throat (S11.85)

● **S10.8 Superficial injury of other specified parts of neck**

X● **S10.80 Unspecified superficial injury of other specified part of neck**

X● **S10.81 Abrasion of other specified part of neck**

X● **S10.82 Blister (nonthermal) of other specified part of neck**

X● **S10.83 Contusion of other specified part of neck**

X● **S10.84 External constriction of other specified part of neck**

X● **S10.85 Superficial foreign body of other specified part of neck**
Splinter in other part of neck

X● **S10.86 Insect bite of other specified part of neck**

X● **S10.87 Other superficial bite of other specified part of neck**

Excludes1 open bite of other specified parts of neck (S11.85)

● **S10.9 Superficial injury of unspecified part of neck**

X● **S10.90 Unspecified superficial injury of unspecified part of neck**

X● **S10.91 Abrasion of unspecified part of neck**

X● **S10.92 Blister (nonthermal) of unspecified part of neck**

X● **S10.93 Contusion of unspecified part of neck**

X● **S10.94 External constriction of unspecified part of neck**

X● **S10.95 Superficial foreign body of unspecified part of neck**

X● **S10.96 Insect bite of unspecified part of neck**

X● **S10.97 Other superficial bite of unspecified part of neck**

● **S11 Open wound of neck**

Code also any associated:
spinal cord injury (S14.0, S14.1-)
wound infection

Excludes2 open fracture of vertebra (S12.- with 7th character B)

The appropriate 7th character is to be added to each code from category S11

A	initial encounter
D	subsequent encounter
S	sequela

● **S11.0 Open wound of larynx and trachea**

Ex For category S11.0 CC codes: S11.011-S11.039[A], S11.80X-S11.95X[A], S13.4XX[A], S13.8XX[A], S16.1XX-S16.2XX[A], S38.3XX[A], T14.90-T14.91, T79.8XX-T79.9XX[A], T79.A0X-T79.A9X[A]

● **S11.01 Open wound of larynx**

Excludes2 open wound of vocal cord (S11.03)

● **S11.011 Laceration without foreign body of larynx** A

● **S11.012 Laceration with foreign body of larynx** A

● **S11.013 Puncture wound without foreign body of larynx** A

● **S11.014 Puncture wound with foreign body of larynx** A

● **S11.015 Open bite of larynx** A
Bite of larynx NOS

● **S11.019 Unspecified open wound of larynx** A

● **S11.02 Open wound of trachea**
Open wound of cervical trachea
Open wound of trachea NOS
Excludes2 open wound of thoracic trachea (S27.5-)

● **S11.021 Laceration without foreign body of trachea A**

● **S11.022 Laceration with foreign body of trachea A**

● **S11.023 Puncture wound without foreign body of trachea A**

● **S11.024 Puncture wound with foreign body of trachea A**

● **S11.025 Open bite of trachea A**
Bite of trachea NOS

● **S11.029 Unspecified open wound of trachea A**

● **S11.03 Open wound of vocal cord**

● **S11.031 Laceration without foreign body of vocal cord A**

● **S11.032 Laceration with foreign body of vocal cord A**

● **S11.033 Puncture wound without foreign body of vocal cord A**

● **S11.034 Puncture wound with foreign body of vocal cord A**

● **S11.035 Open bite of vocal cord A**
Bite of vocal cord NOS

● **S11.039 Unspecified open wound of vocal cord A**

● **S11.1 Open wound of thyroid gland**
Ex: For category S11.1 CC codes unless otherwise indicated: S11.10X-S11.15X[A], S11.80X-S11.95X[A], S13.4XX[A], S13.8XX[A], S16.1XX-S16.2XX[A], S38.3XX[A], T14.90-T14.91, T79.8XX-T79.9XX[A]

X● **S11.10 Unspecified open wound of thyroid gland A**

X● **S11.11 Laceration without foreign body of thyroid gland A**

X● **S11.12 Laceration with foreign body of thyroid gland A**
Ex: S11.10X-S11.15X[A], S11.80X-S11.95X[A], S13.4XX[A], S13.8XX[A], S16.1XX-S16.2XX[A], S38.3XX[A], T14.90-T14.91, T79.8XX-T79.9XX[A], T79.A0XA-T79.A9X[A]

X● **S11.13 Puncture wound without foreign body of thyroid gland A**

X● **S11.14 Puncture wound with foreign body of thyroid gland A**
Ex: See S11.12

X● **S11.15 Open bite of thyroid gland A**
Bite of thyroid gland NOS

● **S11.2 Open wound of pharynx and cervical esophagus**
Excludes1 open wound of esophagus NOS (S27.8-)
Ex: For category S11.2 CC codes unless otherwise indicated: S11.20X-S11.95X[A], S13.4XX[A], S13.8XX[A], S16.1XX-S16.2XX[A], S38.3XX[A], T14.90-T14.91, T79.8XX-T79.9XX[A]

X● **S11.20 Unspecified open wound of pharynx and cervical esophagus A**

X● **S11.21 Laceration without foreign body of pharynx and cervical esophagus A**

X● **S11.22 Laceration with foreign body of pharynx and cervical esophagus A**
Ex: S11.20X-S11.95X[A], S13.4XX[A], S13.8XX[A], S16.1XX-S16.2XX[A], S38.3XX[A], T14.90-T14.91, T79.8XX-T79.9XX[A], T79.A0X-T79.A9X[A]

X● **S11.23 Puncture wound without foreign body of pharynx and cervical esophagus A**

X● **S11.24 Puncture wound with foreign body of pharynx and cervical esophagus A**
Ex: See S11.22

X● **S11.25 Open bite of pharynx and cervical esophagus A**
Bite of pharynx and cervical esophagus NOS

● **S11.8 Open wound of other specified parts of neck**

X● **S11.80 Unspecified open specified wound of other part of neck**

X● **S11.81 Laceration without foreign body of other specified part of neck**

X● **S11.82 Laceration with foreign body of other specified part of neck**

X● **S11.83 Puncture wound without foreign body of other specified part of neck**

X● **S11.84 Puncture wound with foreign body of other specified part of neck**

X● **S11.85 Open bite of other specified part of neck**
Bite of other part of neck NOS
Excludes1 superficial bite of other specified part of neck (S10.87)

X● **S11.89 Other open wound of other part of neck**

● **S11.9 Open wound of unspecified part of neck**

X● **S11.90 Unspecified open wound of unspecified part of neck**

X● **S11.91 Laceration without foreign body of unspecified part of neck**

X● **S11.92 Laceration with foreign body of unspecified part of neck**

X● **S11.93 Puncture wound without foreign body of unspecified part of neck**

X● **S11.94 Puncture wound with foreign body of unspecified part of neck**

X● **S11.95 Open bite of unspecified part of neck**
Bite of neck NOS
Excludes1 superficial bite of neck (S10.97)

● **S12 Fracture of cervical vertebra and other parts of neck**
Note: A fracture not indicated as displaced or nondisplaced should be coded to displaced
A fracture not indicated as open or closed should be coded to closed
Includes fracture of cervical neural arch
fracture of cervical spine
fracture of cervical spinous process
fracture of cervical transverse process
fracture of cervical vertebral arch
fracture of neck
Code first any associated cervical spinal cord injury (S14.0, S14.1-)
The appropriate 7th character is to be added to all codes from subcategories S12.0-S12.6

A	initial encounter for closed fracture
B	initial encounter for open fracture
D	subsequent encounter for fracture with routine healing
G	subsequent encounter for fracture with delayed healing
K	subsequent encounter for fracture with nonunion
S	sequela

Ex: For category S12 CC codes S12[A,B]: M48.40X-M48.58X[S], M80.08X[S], M80.88X[S], M84.350[S], M84.454[S], M84.550[S], M84.58X[S], M84.650[S], M99.10-M99.11, M99.15-M99.17, M99.19, S03.1XX[A], S03.8XX-S03.9XX[A], S12.000-S12.691{A,B,S], S12.8XX[S], S12.9XX[A,S], S13.0XX-S13.4XX[A], S13.8XXA-S14.159[A], S16.1XX[A], S22.000-S22.9XX[S], S23.20X-S23.29X[A], S23.9XX[A], S24.109[A], S24.119[A], S24.139[A], S24.149[A], S24.159[A], S29.001-S29.019[A], S29.091-S29.9XX[A], S32.000-S32.9XX[S], S33.30X-S33.39X[A], S33.9XX[A], S38.1XX[A], S38.3XX-S39.013[A], S39.091-S39.94X[A], T14.90-T14.91, T79.8XX-T79.9XX[A], T79.A0X-T79.A9X[A] For S12[K]: See S02.0[K] unless otherwise indicated

● **S12.0 Fracture of first cervical vertebra**
Atlas

● **S12.00 Unspecified fracture of first cervical vertebra**

● **S12.000 Unspecified displaced fracture of first cervical vertebra A, K, B, A, B**

● **S12.001 Unspecified nondisplaced fracture of first cervical vertebra A, K, B, A, B**

X S12.01 Stable burst fracture of first cervical vertebra A, K CC, B MCC, A, B HAC

X S12.02 Unstable burst fracture of first cervical vertebra A, K CC, B MCC, A, B HAC

S12.03 Posterior arch fracture of first cervical vertebra

S12.030 Displaced posterior arch fracture of first cervical vertebra A, K CC, B MCC, A, B HAC

S12.031 Nondisplaced posterior arch fracture of first cervical vertebra A, K CC, B MCC, A, B HAC

S12.04 Lateral mass fracture of first cervical vertebra

S12.040 Displaced lateral mass fracture of first cervical vertebra A, K CC, B MCC, A, B HAC

S12.041 Nondisplaced lateral mass fracture of first cervical vertebra A, K CC, B MCC, A, B HAC

S12.09 Other fracture of first cervical vertebra

S12.090 Other displaced fracture of first cervical vertebra A, K CC, B MCC, A, B HAC

S12.091 Other nondisplaced fracture of first cervical vertebra A, K CC, B MCC, A, B HAC

S12.1 Fracture of second cervical vertebra
Axis

S12.10 Unspecified fracture of second cervical vertebra

S12.100 Unspecified displaced fracture of second cervical vertebra A, K CC, B MCC, A, B HAC

S12.101 Unspecified nondisplaced fracture of second cervical vertebra A, K CC, B MCC, A, B HAC

S12.11 Type II dens fracture

S12.110 Anterior displaced Type II dens fracture A, K CC, B MCC, A, B HAC

S12.111 Posterior displaced Type II dens fracture A, K CC, B MCC, A, B HAC

S12.112 Nondisplaced Type II dens fracture A, K CC, B MCC, A, B HAC

S12.12 Other dens fracture

S12.120 Other displaced dens fracture A, K CC, B MCC, A, B HAC

S12.121 Other nondisplaced dens fracture A, K CC, B MCC, A, B HAC

S12.13 Unspecified traumatic spondylolisthesis of second cervical vertebra

S12.130 Unspecified traumatic displaced spondylolisthesis of second cervical vertebra A, K CC, B MCC, A, B HAC

S12.131 Unspecified traumatic nondisplaced spondylolisthesis of second cervical vertebra A, K CC, B MCC, A, B HAC

X S12.14 Type III traumatic spondylolisthesis of second cervical vertebra A, K CC, B MCC, A, B HAC

S12.15 Other traumatic spondylolisthesis of second cervical vertebra

S12.150 Other traumatic displaced spondylolisthesis of second cervical vertebra A, K CC, B MCC, A, B HAC

S12.151 Other traumatic nondisplaced spondylolisthesis of second cervical vertebra A, K CC, B MCC, A, B HAC

S12.19 Other fracture of second cervical vertebra

S12.190 Other displaced fracture of second cervical vertebra A, K CC, B MCC, A, B HAC

S12.191 Other nondisplaced fracture of second cervical vertebra A, K CC, B MCC, A, B HAC

S12.2 Fracture of third cervical vertebra

S12.20 Unspecified fracture of third cervical vertebra

S12.200 Unspecified displaced fracture of third cervical vertebra A, K CC, B MCC, A, B HAC

S12.201 Unspecified nondisplaced fracture of third cervical vertebra A, K CC, B MCC, A, B HAC

S12.23 Unspecified traumatic spondylolisthesis of third cervical vertebra

S12.230 Unspecified traumatic displaced spondylolisthesis of third cervical vertebra A, K CC, B MCC, A, B HAC

S12.231 Unspecified traumatic nondisplaced spondylolisthesis of third cervical vertebra A, K CC, B MCC, A, B HAC

X S12.24 Type III traumatic spondylolisthesis of third cervical vertebra A, K CC, B MCC, A, B HAC

S12.25 Other traumatic spondylolisthesis of third cervical vertebra

S12.250 Other traumatic displaced spondylolisthesis of third cervical vertebra A, K CC, B MCC, A, B HAC

S12.251 Other traumatic nondisplaced spondylolisthesis of third cervical vertebra A, K CC, B MCC, A, B HAC

S12.29 Other fracture of third cervical vertebra

S12.290 Other displaced fracture of third cervical vertebra A, K CC, B MCC, A, B HAC

S12.291 Other nondisplaced fracture of third cervical vertebra A, K CC, B MCC, A, B HAC

S12.3 Fracture of fourth cervical vertebra

S12.30 Unspecified fracture of fourth cervical vertebra

S12.300 Unspecified displaced fracture of fourth cervical vertebra A, K CC, B MCC, A, B HAC

S12.301 Unspecified nondisplaced fracture of fourth cervical vertebra A, K CC, B MCC, A, B HAC

S12.33 Unspecified traumatic spondylolisthesis of fourth cervical vertebra

S12.330 Unspecified traumatic displaced spondylolisthesis of fourth cervical vertebra A, K CC, B MCC, A, B HAC

S12.331 Unspecified traumatic nondisplaced spondylolisthesis of fourth cervical vertebra A, K CC, B MCC, A, B HAC

X S12.34 Type III traumatic spondylolisthesis of fourth cervical vertebra A, K CC, B MCC, A, B HAC

S12.35 Other traumatic spondylolisthesis of fourth cervical vertebra

S12.350 Other traumatic displaced spondylolisthesis of fourth cervical vertebra A, K CC, B MCC, A, B HAC

S12.351 Other traumatic nondisplaced spondylolisthesis of fourth cervical vertebra A, K CC, B MCC, A, B HAC

S12.39 Other fracture of fourth cervical vertebra

S12.390 Other displaced fracture of fourth cervical vertebra A, K CC, B MCC, A, B HAC

S12.391 Other nondisplaced fracture of fourth cervical vertebra A, K CC, B MCC, A, B HAC

- S12.4 Fracture of fifth cervical vertebra
  - S12.40 Unspecified fracture of fifth cervical vertebra
    - S12.400 Unspecified displaced fracture of fifth cervical vertebra A, K, B, A, B
    - S12.401 Unspecified nondisplaced fracture of fifth cervical vertebra A, K, B, A, B
  - S12.43 Unspecified traumatic spondylolisthesis of fifth cervical vertebra
    - S12.430 Unspecified traumatic displaced spondylolisthesis of fifth cervical vertebra A, K, B, A, B
    - S12.431 Unspecified traumatic nondisplaced spondylolisthesis of fifth cervical vertebra A, K, B, A, B
  - X S12.44 Type III traumatic spondylolisthesis of fifth cervical vertebra A, K, B, A, B
  - S12.45 Other traumatic spondylolisthesis of fifth cervical vertebra
    - S12.450 Other traumatic displaced spondylolisthesis of fifth cervical vertebra A, K, B, A, B
    - S12.451 Other traumatic nondisplaced spondylolisthesis of fifth cervical vertebra A, K, B, A, B
  - S12.49 Other fracture of fifth cervical vertebra
    - S12.490 Other displaced fracture of fifth cervical vertebra A, K, B, A, B
    - S12.491 Other nondisplaced fracture of fifth cervical vertebra A, K, B, A, B
- S12.5 Fracture of sixth cervical vertebra
  - S12.50 Unspecified fracture of sixth cervical vertebra
    - S12.500 Unspecified displaced fracture of sixth cervical vertebra A, K, B, A, B
    - S12.501 Unspecified nondisplaced fracture of sixth cervical vertebra A, K, B, A, B
  - S12.53 Unspecified traumatic spondylolisthesis of sixth cervical vertebra
    - S12.530 Unspecified traumatic displaced spondylolisthesis of sixth cervical vertebra A, K, B, A, B
    - S12.531 Unspecified traumatic nondisplaced spondylolisthesis of sixth cervical vertebra A, K, B, A, B
  - X S12.54 Type III traumatic spondylolisthesis of sixth cervical vertebra A, K, B, A, B
  - S12.55 Other traumatic spondylolisthesis of sixth cervical vertebra
    - S12.550 Other traumatic displaced spondylolisthesis of sixth cervical vertebra A, K, B, A, B
    - S12.551 Other traumatic nondisplaced spondylolisthesis of sixth cervical vertebra A, K, B, A, B
  - S12.59 Other fracture of sixth cervical vertebra
    - S12.590 Other displaced fracture of sixth cervical vertebra A, K, B, A, B
    - S12.591 Other nondisplaced fracture of sixth cervical vertebra A, K, B, A, B
- S12.6 Fracture of seventh cervical vertebra
  - S12.60 Unspecified fracture of seventh cervical vertebra
    - S12.600 Unspecified displaced fracture of seventh cervical vertebra A, K, B, A, B
    - S12.601 Unspecified nondisplaced fracture of seventh cervical vertebra A, K, B, A, B
  - S12.63 Unspecified traumatic spondylolisthesis of seventh cervical vertebra
    - S12.630 Unspecified traumatic displaced spondylolisthesis of seventh cervical vertebra A, K, B, A, B
    - S12.631 Unspecified traumatic nondisplaced spondylolisthesis of seventh cervical vertebra A, K, B, A, B
  - X S12.64 Type III traumatic spondylolisthesis of seventh cervical vertebra A, K, B, A, B
  - S12.65 Other traumatic spondylolisthesis of seventh cervical vertebra
    - S12.650 Other traumatic displaced spondylolisthesis of seventh cervical vertebra A, K, B, A, B
    - S12.651 Other traumatic nondisplaced spondylolisthesis of seventh cervical vertebra A, K, B, A, B
  - S12.69 Other fracture of seventh cervical vertebra
    - S12.690 Other displaced fracture of seventh cervical vertebra A, K, B, A, B
    - S12.691 Other nondisplaced fracture of seventh cervical vertebra A, K, B, A, B
- X S12.8 Fracture of other parts of neck A, A

  Hyoid bone
  Larynx
  Thyroid cartilage
  Trachea

  The appropriate 7th character is to be added to code S12.8

A	initial encounter
D	subsequent encounter
S	sequela

  Ex S03.8XX-S03.9XX[A], S12.8XX[A], S29.011-S29.019[A], S38.3XX[A] S39.011-S39.013[A], T14.90-T14.91, T79.8XX-T79.9XX[A] T79.A0XA-T79.A9X[A]

- X S12.9 Fracture of neck, unspecified A, A

  Fracture of neck NOS
  Fracture of cervical spine NOS
  Fracture of cervical vertebra NOS

  The appropriate 7th character is to be added to code S12.9

A	initial encounter
D	subsequent encounter
S	sequela

S13 Dislocation and sprain of joints and ligaments at neck level

Includes avulsion of joint or ligament at neck level
laceration of cartilage, joint or ligament at neck level
sprain of cartilage, joint or ligament at neck level
traumatic hemarthrosis of joint or ligament at neck level
traumatic rupture of joint or ligament at neck level
traumatic subluxation of joint or ligament at neck level
traumatic tear of joint or ligament at neck level

Code also any associated open wound

Excludes2 strain of muscle or tendon at neck level (S16.1)

The appropriate 7th character is to be added to each code from category S13

A	initial encounter
D	subsequent encounter
S	sequela

Ex **For category S13 CC codes:** M99.10-M99.11, S03.8XX-S03.9XX[A], S12.000-S12.691[A,B], S12.9XX-S13.4XX[A], S13.8XX[A], S14.0XX-S14.108[A], S14.111-S14.118[A], S14.121-S14.128[A], S14.131-S14.138[A], S14.141-S14.148[A], S14.151-S14.158[A], S16.1XX[A], S29.011-S29.019[A], S38.3XX[A], S39.011-S39.013[A], T14.90-T14.91, T79.A0X-T79.9XX[A]

X **S13.0 Traumatic rupture of cervical intervertebral disc** A CC, A MCC

Excludes1 rupture or displacement (nontraumatic) of cervical intervertebral disc NOS (M50.-)

S13.1 Subluxation and dislocation of cervical vertebrae

Code also any associated:
open wound of neck (S11.-)
spinal cord injury (S14.1-)

Excludes2 fracture of cervical vertebrae (S12.0-S12.3-)

S13.10 Subluxation and dislocation of unspecified cervical vertebrae

S13.100 Subluxation of unspecified cervical vertebrae A CC, A MCC

S13.101 Dislocation of unspecified cervical vertebrae A CC, A MCC

S13.11 Subluxation and dislocation of C_0/C_1 cervical vertebrae

Subluxation and dislocation of atlantooccipital joint
Subluxation and dislocation of atloidooccipital joint
Subluxation and dislocation of occipitoatloid joint

S13.110 Subluxation of C_0/C_1 cervical vertebrae A CC, A MCC

S13.111 Dislocation of C_0/C_1 cervical vertebrae A CC, A MCC

S13.12 Subluxation and dislocation of C_1/C_2 cervical vertebrae

Subluxation and dislocation of atlantoaxial joint

S13.120 Subluxation of C_1/C_2 cervical vertebrae A CC, A MCC

S13.121 Dislocation of C_1/C_2 cervical vertebrae A CC, A MCC

S13.13 Subluxation and dislocation of C_2/C_3 cervical vertebrae

S13.130 Subluxation of C_2/C_3 cervical vertebrae A CC, A MCC

S13.131 Dislocation of C_2/C_3 cervical vertebrae A CC, A MCC

S13.14 Subluxation and dislocation of C_3/C_4 cervical vertebrae

S13.140 Subluxation of C_3/C_4 cervical vertebrae A CC, A MCC

S13.141 Dislocation of C_3/C_4 cervical vertebrae A CC, A MCC

S13.15 Subluxation and dislocation of C_4/C_5 cervical vertebrae

S13.150 Subluxation of C_4/C_5 cervical vertebrae A CC, A MCC

S13.151 Dislocation of C_4/C_5 cervical vertebrae A CC, A MCC

S13.16 Subluxation and dislocation of C_5/C_6 cervical vertebrae

S13.160 Subluxation of C_5/C_6 cervical vertebrae A CC, A MCC

S13.161 Dislocation of C_5/C_6 cervical vertebrae A CC, A MCC

S13.17 Subluxation and dislocation of C_6/C_7 cervical vertebrae

S13.170 Subluxation of C_6/C_7 cervical vertebrae A CC, A MCC

S13.171 Dislocation of C_6/C_7 cervical vertebrae A CC, A MCC

S13.18 Subluxation and dislocation of C_7/T_1 cervical vertebrae

S13.180 Subluxation of C_7/T_1 cervical vertebrae A CC, A MCC

S13.181 Dislocation of C_7/T_1 cervical vertebrae A CC, A MCC

S13.2 Dislocation of other and unspecified parts of neck

X **S13.20 Dislocation of unspecified parts of neck** A CC, A MCC

X **S13.29 Dislocation of other parts of neck** A CC, A MCC

X **S13.4 Sprain of ligaments of cervical spine**

Sprain of anterior longitudinal (ligament), cervical
Sprain of atlanto-axial (joints)
Sprain of atlanto-occipital (joints)
Whiplash injury of cervical spine

X **S13.5 Sprain of thyroid region**

Sprain of cricoarytenoid (joint) (ligament)
Sprain of cricothyroid (joint) (ligament)
Sprain of thyroid cartilage

X **S13.8 Sprain of joints and ligaments of other parts of neck**

X **S13.9 Sprain of joints and ligaments of unspecified parts of neck**

S14 Injury of nerves and spinal cord at neck level

Note: Code to highest level of cervical cord injury

Code also any associated:
fracture of cervical vertebra (S12.0--S12.6.-)
open wound of neck (S11.-)
transient paralysis (R29.5)

The appropriate 7th character is to be added to each code from category S14

A	initial encounter
D	subsequent encounter
S	sequela

Ex **For category S14 CC codes:** M48.40X-M48.58X[S], M80.08X[S], M80.88X[S], M84.350[S], M84.454[S], M84.550[S], M84.58X[S], M84.650[S], M99.10-M99.11, M99.15-M99.17, M99.19, S03.1XX[A], S12.000-S12.691[A,B,S], S12.8XX[S], S12.9XX[A,S], S13.0XX-S13.29X[A], S13.9XX-S14.159[A], S22.000-S22.9XX[S], S23.20X-S23.29X[A], S23.9XX[A], S24.109[A], S24.119[A], S24.139[A], S24.149[A], S24.159[A], S29.001-S29.009[A], S29.091-S29.9XX[A], S32.000-S32.9XX[S], S33.30X-S33.39X[A], S33.9XX[A], S38.1XX[A], S39.001-S39.003[A], S39.091-S39.94X[A], T14.90-T14.91, T79.8XX-T79.9XX[A], T79.A0X-T79.A9X[A]

X **S14.0 Concussion and edema of cervical spinal cord A**

S14.1 Other and unspecified injuries of cervical spinal cord

S14.10 Unspecified injury of cervical spinal cord

- **S14.101 Unspecified injury at C_1 level of cervical spinal cord A, A**
- **S14.102 Unspecified injury at C_2 level of cervical spinal cord A, A**
- **S14.103 Unspecified injury at C_3 level of cervical spinal cord A, A**
- **S14.104 Unspecified injury at C_4 level of cervical spinal cord A, A**
- **S14.105 Unspecified injury at C_5 level of cervical spinal cord A, A**
- **S14.106 Unspecified injury at C_6 level of cervical spinal cord A, A**
- **S14.107 Unspecified injury at C_7 level of cervical spinal cord A, A**
- **S14.108 Unspecified injury at C_8 level of cervical spinal cord A**
- **S14.109 Unspecified injury at unspecified level of cervical spinal cord A**
  Injury of cervical spinal cord NOS

S14.11 Complete lesion of cervical spinal cord

- **S14.111 Complete lesion at C_1 level of cervical spinal cord A, A**
- **S14.112 Complete lesion at C_2 level of cervical spinal cord A, A**
- **S14.113 Complete lesion at C_3 level of cervical spinal cord A, A**
- **S14.114 Complete lesion at C_4 level of cervical spinal cord A, A**
- **S14.115 Complete lesion at C_5 level of cervical spinal cord A, A**
- **S14.116 Complete lesion at C_6 level of cervical spinal cord A, A**
- **S14.117 Complete lesion at C_7 level of cervical spinal cord A, A**
- **S14.118 Complete lesion at C_8 level of cervical spinal cord A**
- **S14.119 Complete lesion at unspecified level of cervical spinal cord**

S14.12 Central cord syndrome of cervical spinal cord

- **S14.121 Central cord syndrome at C_1 level of cervical spinal cord A, A**
- **S14.122 Central cord syndrome at C_2 level of cervical spinal cord A, A**
- **S14.123 Central cord syndrome at C_3 level of cervical spinal cord A, A**
- **S14.124 Central cord syndrome at C_4 level of cervical spinal cord A, A**
- **S14.125 Central cord syndrome at C_5 level of cervical spinal cord A, A**
- **S14.126 Central cord syndrome at C_6 level of cervical spinal cord A, A**
- **S14.127 Central cord syndrome at C_7 level of cervical spinal cord A, A**
- **S14.128 Central cord syndrome at C_8 level of cervical spinal cord A**
- **S14.129 Central cord syndrome at unspecified level of cervical spinal cord**

S14.13 Anterior cord syndrome of cervical spinal cord

- **S14.131 Anterior cord syndrome at C_1 level of cervical spinal cord A, A**
- **S14.132 Anterior cord syndrome at C_2 level of cervical spinal cord A, A**
- **S14.133 Anterior cord syndrome at C_3 level of cervical spinal cord A, A**
- **S14.134 Anterior cord syndrome at C_4 level of cervical spinal cord A, A**
- **S14.135 Anterior cord syndrome at C_5 level of cervical spinal cord A, A**
- **S14.136 Anterior cord syndrome at C_6 level of cervical spinal cord A, A**
- **S14.137 Anterior cord syndrome at C_7 level of cervical spinal cord A, A**
- **S14.138 Anterior cord syndrome at C_8 level of cervical spinal cord A**
- **S14.139 Anterior cord syndrome at unspecified level of cervical spinal cord**

S14.14 Brown-Séquard syndrome of cervical spinal cord

- **S14.141 Brown-Séquard syndrome at C_1 level of cervical spinal cord A**
- **S14.142 Brown-Séquard syndrome at C_2 level of cervical spinal cord A**
- **S14.143 Brown-Séquard syndrome at C_3 level of cervical spinal cord A**
- **S14.144 Brown-Séquard syndrome at C_4 level of cervical spinal cord A**
- **S14.145 Brown-Séquard syndrome at C_5 level of cervical spinal cord A**
- **S14.146 Brown-Séquard syndrome at C_6 level of cervical spinal cord A**
- **S14.147 Brown-Séquard syndrome at C_7 level of cervical spinal cord A**
- **S14.148 Brown-Séquard syndrome at C_8 level of cervical spinal cord A**
- **S14.149 Brown-Séquard syndrome at unspecified level of cervical spinal cord**

S14.15 Other incomplete lesions of cervical spinal cord
Incomplete lesion of cervical spinal cord NOS
Posterior cord syndrome of cervical spinal cord

- **S14.151 Other incomplete lesion at C_1 level of cervical spinal cord A, A**
- **S14.152 Other incomplete lesion at C_2 level of cervical spinal cord A, A**
- **S14.153 Other incomplete lesion at C_3 level of cervical spinal cord A, A**
- **S14.154 Other incomplete lesion at C_4 level of cervical spinal cord A, A**
- **S14.155 Other incomplete lesion at C_5 level of cervical spinal cord A, A**
- **S14.156 Other incomplete lesion at C_6 level of cervical spinal cord A, A**
- **S14.157 Other incomplete lesion at C_7 level of cervical spinal cord A, A**
- **S14.158 Other incomplete lesion at C_8 level of cervical spinal cord A**
- **S14.159 Other incomplete lesion at unspecified level of cervical spinal cord**

X● **S14.2 Injury of nerve root of cervical spine**
X● **S14.3 Injury of brachial plexus**
X● **S14.4 Injury of peripheral nerves of neck**
X● **S14.5 Injury of cervical sympathetic nerves**
X● **S14.8 Injury of other specified nerves of neck**
X● **S14.9 Injury of unspecified nerves of neck**

● **S15 Injury of blood vessels at neck level**

Code also any associated open wound (S11.-)

The appropriate 7th character is to be added to each code from category S15

A	initial encounter
D	subsequent encounter
S	sequela

● **S15.0 Injury of carotid artery of neck**
Injury of carotid artery (common) (external) (internal, extracranial portion)
Injury of carotid artery NOS
Excludes1 injury of internal carotid artery, intracranial portion (S06.8)
Ex **For category S15.0 CC codes:** S09.0XX[A], S15.009[A], S15.029[A], S15.099-S15.199[A], S15.8XX-S15.9XX[A], T14.90-T14.91, T79.8XX-T79.9XX[A], T79.A0X-T79.A9X[A]

● **S15.00 Unspecified injury of carotid artery**
● **S15.001 Unspecified injury of right carotid artery** A
● **S15.002 Unspecified injury of left carotid artery** A
● **S15.009 Unspecified injury of unspecified carotid artery** A

● **S15.01 Minor laceration of carotid artery**
Incomplete transection of carotid artery
Laceration of carotid artery NOS
Superficial laceration of carotid artery
● **S15.011 Minor laceration of right carotid artery** A
● **S15.012 Minor laceration of left carotid artery** A
● **S15.019 Minor laceration of unspecified carotid artery** A

● **S15.02 Major laceration of carotid artery**
Complete transection of carotid artery
Traumatic rupture of carotid artery
● **S15.021 Major laceration of right carotid artery** A
● **S15.022 Major laceration of left carotid artery** A
● **S15.029 Major laceration of unspecified carotid artery** A

● **S15.09 Other specified injury of carotid artery**
● **S15.091 Other specified injury of right carotid artery** A
● **S15.092 Other specified injury of left carotid artery** A
● **S15.099 Other specified injury of unspecified carotid artery** A

● **S15.1 Injury of vertebral artery**
Ex **For category S15.1 CC codes:** S09.0XX[A], S15.101-S15.199[A] S15.8XX-S15.9XX[A], T14.90-T14.91, T79.8XX-T79.9XX[A] T79.A0X-T79.A9X[A]

● **S15.10 Unspecified injury of vertebral artery**
● **S15.101 Unspecified injury of right vertebral artery** A
● **S15.102 Unspecified injury of left vertebral artery** A
● **S15.109 Unspecified injury of unspecified vertebral artery** A

● **S15.11 Minor laceration of vertebral artery**
Incomplete transection of vertebral artery
Laceration of vertebral artery NOS
Superficial laceration of vertebral artery
● **S15.111 Minor laceration of right vertebral artery** A
● **S15.112 Minor laceration of left vertebral artery** A
● **S15.119 Minor laceration of unspecified vertebral artery** A

● **S15.12 Major laceration of vertebral artery**
Complete transection of vertebral artery
Traumatic rupture of vertebral artery
● **S15.121 Major laceration of right vertebral artery** A
● **S15.122 Major laceration of left vertebral artery** A
● **S15.129 Major laceration of unspecified vertebral artery** A

● **S15.19 Other specified injury of vertebral artery**
● **S15.191 Other specified injury of right vertebral artery** A
● **S15.192 Other specified injury of left vertebral artery** A
● **S15.199 Other specified injury of unspecified vertebral artery** A

● **S15.2 Injury of external jugular vein**
Ex **For category S15.2 CC codes:** See S15.1

● **S15.20 Unspecified injury of external jugular vein**
● **S15.201 Unspecified injury of right external jugular vein** A
● **S15.202 Unspecified injury of left external jugular vein** A
● **S15.209 Unspecified injury of unspecified external jugular vein** A

● **S15.21 Minor laceration of external jugular vein**
Incomplete transection of external jugular vein
Laceration of external jugular vein NOS
Superficial laceration of external jugular vein
● **S15.211 Minor laceration of right external jugular vein** A
● **S15.212 Minor laceration of left external jugular vein** A
● **S15.219 Minor laceration of unspecified external jugular vein** A

● **S15.22 Major laceration of external jugular vein**
Complete transection of external jugular vein
Traumatic rupture of external jugular vein
● **S15.221 Major laceration of right external jugular vein** A
● **S15.222 Major laceration of left external jugular vein** A
● **S15.229 Major laceration of unspecified external jugular vein** A

● **S15.29 Other specified injury of external jugular vein**
● **S15.291 Other specified injury of right external jugular vein** A
● **S15.292 Other specified injury of left external jugular vein** A
● **S15.299 Other specified injury of unspecified external jugular vein** A

● **S15.3 Injury of internal jugular vein**
Ex **For category S15.3 CC codes:** See S15.1

● **S15.30 Unspecified injury of internal jugular vein**
● **S15.301 Unspecified injury of right internal jugular vein** A
● **S15.302 Unspecified injury of left internal jugular vein** A
● **S15.309 Unspecified injury of unspecified internal jugular vein** A

S15.31 Minor laceration of internal jugular vein
Incomplete transection of internal jugular vein
Laceration of internal jugular vein NOS
Superficial laceration of internal jugular vein

S15.311 Minor laceration of right internal jugular vein A

S15.312 Minor laceration of left internal jugular vein A

S15.319 Minor laceration of unspecified internal jugular vein A

S15.32 Major laceration of internal jugular vein
Complete transection of internal jugular vein
Traumatic rupture of internal jugular vein

S15.321 Major laceration of right internal jugular vein A

S15.322 Major laceration of left internal jugular vein A

S15.329 Major laceration of unspecified internal jugular vein A

S15.39 Other specified injury of internal jugular vein

S15.391 Other specified injury of right internal jugular vein A

S15.392 Other specified injury of left internal jugular vein A

S15.399 Other specified injury of unspecified internal jugular vein A

X **S15.8 Injury of other specified blood vessels at neck level** A
Ex See S15.1

X **S15.9 Injury of unspecified blood vessel at neck level** A
Ex See S15.1

S16 Injury of muscle, fascia and tendon at neck level
Code also any associated open wound (S11.-)
Excludes2 sprain of joint or ligament at neck level (S13.9)
The appropriate 7th character is to be added to each code from category S16

A	initial encounter
D	subsequent encounter
S	sequela

X **S16.1 Strain of muscle, fascia and tendon at neck level**

X **S16.2 Laceration of muscle, fascia and tendon at neck level**

X **S16.8 Other specified injury of muscle, fascia and tendon at neck level**

X **S16.9 Unspecified injury of muscle, fascia and tendon at neck level**

S17 Crushing injury of neck
Use additional code for all associated injuries, such as:
injury of blood vessels (S15.-)
open wound of neck (S11.-)
spinal cord injury (S14.0, S14.1-)
vertebral fracture (S12.0--S12.3-)
The appropriate 7th character is to be added to each code from category S17

A	initial encounter
D	subsequent encounter
S	sequela

Ex For category S17 CC codes: See S07

X **S17.0 Crushing injury of larynx and trachea** A, A

X **S17.8 Crushing injury of other specified parts of neck** A, A

X **S17.9 Crushing injury of neck, part unspecified** A, A

S19 Other and unspecified injuries of neck
The appropriate 7th character is to be added to each code from category S19

A	initial encounter
D	subsequent encounter
S	sequela

S19.8 Other specified injuries of neck

X **S19.80 Other specified injuries of unspecified part of neck**

X **S19.81 Other specified injuries of larynx**

X **S19.82 Other specified injuries of cervical trachea**
Excludes2 other specified injury of thoracic trachea (S27.5-)

X **S19.83 Other specified injuries of vocal cord**

X **S19.84 Other specified injuries of thyroid gland**

X **S19.85 Other specified injuries of pharynx and cervical esophagus**

X **S19.89 Other specified injuries of other specified part of neck**

X **S19.9 Unspecified injury of neck**

INJURIES TO THE THORAX (S20-S29)

Includes injuries of breast
injuries of chest (wall)
injuries of interscapular area

Excludes2 burns and corrosions (T20-T32)
effects of foreign body in bronchus (T17.5)
effects of foreign body in esophagus (T18.1)
effects of foreign body in lung (T17.8)
effects of foreign body in trachea (T17.4)
frostbite (T33-T34)
injuries of axilla
injuries of clavicle
injuries of scapular region
injuries of shoulder
insect bite or sting, venomous (T63.4)

S20 Superficial injury of thorax
The appropriate 7th character is to be added to each code from category S20

A	initial encounter
D	subsequent encounter
S	sequela

S20.0 Contusion of breast

X **S20.00 Contusion of breast, unspecified breast**

X **S20.01 Contusion of right breast**

X **S20.02 Contusion of left breast**

S20.1 Other and unspecified superficial injuries of breast

S20.10 Unspecified superficial injuries of breast

S20.101 Unspecified superficial injuries of breast, right breast

S20.102 Unspecified superficial injuries of breast, left breast

S20.109 Unspecified superficial injuries of breast, unspecified breast

S20.11 Abrasion of breast

S20.111 Abrasion of breast, right breast

S20.112 Abrasion of breast, left breast

S20.119 Abrasion of breast, unspecified breast

S20.12 Blister (nonthermal) of breast

S20.121 Blister (nonthermal) of breast, right breast

S20.122 Blister (nonthermal) of breast, left breast

S20.129 Blister (nonthermal) of breast, unspecified breast

- S20.14 External constriction of part of breast
  - S20.141 External constriction of part of breast, right breast
  - S20.142 External constriction of part of breast, left breast
  - S20.149 External constriction of part of breast, unspecified breast
- S20.15 Superficial foreign body of breast
  Splinter in the breast
  - S20.151 Superficial foreign body of breast, right breast
  - S20.152 Superficial foreign body of breast, left breast
  - S20.159 Superficial foreign body of breast, unspecified breast
- S20.16 Insect bite (nonvenomous) of breast
  - S20.161 Insect bite (nonvenomous) of breast, right breast
  - S20.162 Insect bite (nonvenomous) of breast, left breast
  - S20.169 Insect bite (nonvenomous) of breast, unspecified breast
- S20.17 Other superficial bite of breast
  Excludes1 open bite of breast (S21.05-)
  - S20.171 Other superficial bite of breast, right breast
  - S20.172 Other superficial bite of breast, left breast
  - S20.179 Other superficial bite of breast, unspecified breast
- S20.2 Contusion of thorax
  - X S20.20 Contusion of thorax, unspecified
  - S20.21 Contusion of front wall of thorax
    - S20.211 Contusion of right front wall of thorax
    - S20.212 Contusion of left front wall of thorax
    - S20.219 Contusion of unspecified front wall of thorax
  - S20.22 Contusion of back wall of thorax
    - S20.221 Contusion of right back wall of thorax
    - S20.222 Contusion of left back wall of thorax
    - S20.229 Contusion of unspecified back wall of thorax
- S20.3 Other and unspecified superficial injuries of front wall of thorax
  - S20.30 Unspecified superficial injuries of front wall of thorax
    - S20.301 Unspecified superficial injuries of right front wall of thorax
    - S20.302 Unspecified superficial injuries of left front wall of thorax
    - S20.309 Unspecified superficial injuries of unspecified front wall of thorax
  - S20.31 Abrasion of front wall of thorax
    - S20.311 Abrasion of right front wall of thorax
    - S20.312 Abrasion of left front wall of thorax
    - S20.319 Abrasion of unspecified front wall of thorax
  - S20.32 Blister (nonthermal) of front wall of thorax
    - S20.321 Blister (nonthermal) of right front wall of thorax
    - S20.322 Blister (nonthermal) of left front wall of thorax
    - S20.329 Blister (nonthermal) of unspecified front wall of thorax
  - S20.34 External constriction of front wall of thorax
    - S20.341 External constriction of right front wall of thorax
    - S20.342 External constriction of left front wall of thorax
    - S20.349 External constriction of unspecified front wall of thorax
  - S20.35 Superficial foreign body of front wall of thorax
    Splinter in front wall of thorax
    - S20.351 Superficial foreign body of right front wall of thorax
    - S20.352 Superficial foreign body of left front wall of thorax
    - S20.359 Superficial foreign body of unspecified front wall of thorax
  - S20.36 Insect bite (nonvenomous) of front wall of thorax
    - S20.361 Insect bite (nonvenomous) of right front wall of thorax
    - S20.362 Insect bite (nonvenomous) of left front wall of thorax
    - S20.369 Insect bite (nonvenomous) of unspecified front wall of thorax
  - S20.37 Other superficial bite of front wall of thorax
    Excludes1 open bite of front wall of thorax (S21.14)
    - S20.371 Other superficial bite of right front wall of thorax
    - S20.372 Other superficial bite of left front wall of thorax
    - S20.379 Other superficial bite of unspecified front wall of thorax
- S20.4 Other and unspecified superficial injuries of back wall of thorax
  - S20.40 Unspecified superficial injuries of back wall of thorax
    - S20.401 Unspecified superficial injuries of right back wall of thorax
    - S20.402 Unspecified superficial injuries of left back wall of thorax
    - S20.409 Unspecified superficial injuries of unspecified back wall of thorax
  - S20.41 Abrasion of back wall of thorax
    - S20.411 Abrasion of right back wall of thorax
    - S20.412 Abrasion of left back wall of thorax
    - S20.419 Abrasion of unspecified back wall of thorax
  - S20.42 Blister (nonthermal) of back wall of thorax
    - S20.421 Blister (nonthermal) of right back wall of thorax
    - S20.422 Blister (nonthermal) of left back wall of thorax
    - S20.429 Blister (nonthermal) of unspecified back wall of thorax
  - S20.44 External constriction of back wall of thorax
    - S20.441 External constriction of right back wall of thorax
    - S20.442 External constriction of left back wall of thorax
    - S20.449 External constriction of unspecified back wall of thorax
  - S20.45 Superficial foreign body of back wall of thorax
    Splinter of back wall of thorax
    - S20.451 Superficial foreign body of right back wall of thorax
    - S20.452 Superficial foreign body of left back wall of thorax
    - S20.459 Superficial foreign body of unspecified back wall of thorax

- S20.46 Insect bite (nonvenomous) of back wall of thorax
  - S20.461 Insect bite (nonvenomous) of right back wall of thorax
  - S20.462 Insect bite (nonvenomous) of left back wall of thorax
  - S20.469 Insect bite (nonvenomous) of unspecified back wall of thorax
- S20.47 Other superficial bite of back wall of thorax
  - **Excludes1** open bite of back wall of thorax (S21.24)
  - S20.471 Other superficial bite of right back wall of thorax
  - S20.472 Other superficial bite of left back wall of thorax
  - S20.479 Other superficial bite of unspecified back wall of thorax
- S20.9 Superficial injury of unspecified parts of thorax
  - **Excludes1** contusion of thorax NOS (S20.20)
  - X S20.90 Unspecified superficial injury of unspecified parts of thorax
    - Superficial injury of thoracic wall NOS
  - X S20.91 Abrasion of unspecified parts of thorax
  - X S20.92 Blister (nonthermal) of unspecified parts of thorax
  - X S20.94 External constriction of unspecified parts of thorax
  - X S20.95 Superficial foreign body of unspecified parts of thorax
    - Splinter in thorax NOS
  - X S20.96 Insect bite (nonvenomous) of unspecified parts of thorax
  - X S20.97 Other superficial bite of unspecified parts of thorax
    - **Excludes1** open bite of thorax NOS (S21.95)

- S21 Open wound of thorax

  Code also any associated injury such as:
  - injury of heart (S26.-)
  - injury of intrathoracic organs (S27.-)
  - rib fracture (S22.3-, S22.4-)
  - spinal cord injury (S24.0-, S24.1-)
  - traumatic hemothorax (S27.1)
  - traumatic hemopneumothorax (S27.3)
  - traumatic pneumothorax (S27.0)
  - wound infection

  Excludes1 traumatic amputation (partial) of thorax (S28.1)

  The appropriate 7th character is to be added to each code from category S21

A	initial encounter
D	subsequent encounter
S	sequela

- S21.0 Open wound of breast
  - S21.00 Unspecified open wound of breast
    - S21.001 Unspecified open wound of right breast
    - S21.002 Unspecified open wound of left breast
    - S21.009 Unspecified open wound of unspecified breast

Item 19–1 **Pneumothorax** is a collection of gas (positive air pressure) in the pleural space resulting in the lung collapsing. A tension pneumothorax is life-threatening and is a result of air in the pleural space causing a displacement in the mediastinal structures and cardiopulmonary function compromise. A traumatic pneumothorax results from blunt or penetrating injury that disrupts the parietal/visceral pleura. **Hemothorax** is blood or bloody fluid in the pleural cavity as a result of traumatic blood vessel rupture or inflammation of the lungs from pneumonia.

- S21.01 Laceration without foreign body of breast
  - S21.011 Laceration without foreign body of right breast
  - S21.012 Laceration without foreign body of left breast
  - S21.019 Laceration without foreign body of unspecified breast
- S21.02 Laceration with foreign body of breast
  - S21.021 Laceration with foreign body of right breast
  - S21.022 Laceration with foreign body of left breast
  - S21.029 Laceration with foreign body of unspecified breast
- S21.03 Puncture wound without foreign body of breast
  - S21.031 Puncture wound without foreign body of right breast
  - S21.032 Puncture wound without foreign body of left breast
  - S21.039 Puncture wound without foreign body of unspecified breast
- S21.04 Puncture wound with foreign body of breast
  - S21.041 Puncture wound with foreign body of right breast
  - S21.042 Puncture wound with foreign body of left breast
  - S21.049 Puncture wound with foreign body of unspecified breast
- S21.05 Open bite of breast
  - Bite of breast NOS
  - **Excludes1** superficial bite of breast (S20.17)
  - S21.051 Open bite of right breast
  - S21.052 Open bite of left breast
  - S21.059 Open bite of unspecified breast
- S21.1 Open wound of front wall of thorax without penetration into thoracic cavity
  - Open wound of chest without penetration into thoracic cavity
  - Ex **For category S21.1 CC codes:** S21.101-S21.159[A], S21.301-S21.95X[A], S23.3XX[A], S23.8XX[A], S27.50X-S27.69X[A], S27.892A-S28.1XX[A], S29.021[A], S29.029[A], S38.3XX[A], T14.90-T14.91, T79.7XX[A] T79.8XX-T79.9XX[A], T79.A0X-T79.A9X[A]
  - S21.10 Unspecified open wound of front wall of thorax without penetration into thoracic cavity
    - S21.101 Unspecified open wound of right front wall of thorax without penetration into thoracic cavity A
    - S21.102 Unspecified open wound of left front wall of thorax without penetration into thoracic cavity A
    - S21.109 Unspecified open wound of unspecified front wall of thorax without penetration into thoracic cavity A
  - S21.11 Laceration without foreign body of front wall of thorax without penetration into thoracic cavity
    - S21.111 Laceration without foreign body of right front wall of thorax without penetration into thoracic cavity A
    - S21.112 Laceration without foreign body of left front wall of thorax without penetration into thoracic cavity A
    - S21.119 Laceration without foreign body of unspecified front wall of thorax without penetration into thoracic cavity A

- **S21.12** Laceration with foreign body of front wall of thorax without penetration into thoracic cavity
  - **S21.121** Laceration with foreign body of right front wall of thorax without penetration into thoracic cavity A
  - **S21.122** Laceration with foreign body of left front wall of thorax without penetration into thoracic cavity A
  - **S21.129** Laceration with foreign body of unspecified front wall of thorax without penetration into thoracic cavity A
- **S21.13** Puncture wound without foreign body of front wall of thorax without penetration into thoracic cavity
  - **S21.131** Puncture wound without foreign body of right front wall of thorax without penetration into thoracic cavity A
  - **S21.132** Puncture wound without foreign body of left front wall of thorax without penetration into thoracic cavity A
  - **S21.139** Puncture wound without foreign body of unspecified front wall of thorax without penetration into thoracic cavity A
- **S21.14** Puncture wound with foreign body of front wall of thorax without penetration into thoracic cavity
  - **S21.141** Puncture wound with foreign body of right front wall of thorax without penetration into thoracic cavity A
  - **S21.142** Puncture wound with foreign body of left front wall of thorax without penetration into thoracic cavity A
  - **S21.149** Puncture wound with foreign body of unspecified front wall of thorax without penetration into thoracic cavity A
- **S21.15** Open bite of front wall of thorax without penetration into thoracic cavity
  Bite of front wall of thorax NOS
  Excludes1 superficial bite of front wall of thorax (S20.37)
  - **S21.151** Open bite of right front wall of thorax without penetration into thoracic cavity A
  - **S21.152** Open bite of left front wall of thorax without penetration into thoracic cavity A
  - **S21.159** Open bite of unspecified front wall of thorax without penetration into thoracic cavity A
- **S21.2** Open wound of back wall of thorax without penetration into thoracic cavity
  - **S21.20** Unspecified open wound of back wall of thorax without penetration into thoracic cavity
    - **S21.201** Unspecified open wound of right back wall of thorax without penetration into thoracic cavity
    - **S21.202** Unspecified open wound of left back wall of thorax without penetration into thoracic cavity
    - **S21.209** Unspecified open wound of unspecified back wall of thorax without penetration into thoracic cavity
- **S21.21** Laceration without foreign body of back wall of thorax without penetration into thoracic cavity
  - **S21.211** Laceration without foreign body of right back wall of thorax without penetration into thoracic cavity
  - **S21.212** Laceration without foreign body of left back wall of thorax without penetration into thoracic cavity
  - **S21.219** Laceration without foreign body of unspecified back wall of thorax without penetration into thoracic cavity
- **S21.22** Laceration with foreign body of back wall of thorax without penetration into thoracic cavity
  - **S21.221** Laceration with foreign body of right back wall of thorax without penetration into thoracic cavity
  - **S21.222** Laceration with foreign body of left back wall of thorax without penetration into thoracic cavity
  - **S21.229** Laceration with foreign body of unspecified back wall of thorax without penetration into thoracic cavity
- **S21.23** Puncture wound without foreign body of back wall of thorax without penetration into thoracic cavity
  - **S21.231** Puncture wound without foreign body of right back wall of thorax without penetration into thoracic cavity
  - **S21.232** Puncture wound without foreign body of left back wall of thorax without penetration into thoracic cavity
  - **S21.239** Puncture wound without foreign body of unspecified back wall of thorax without penetration into thoracic cavity
- **S21.24** Puncture wound with foreign body of back wall of thorax without penetration into thoracic cavity
  - **S21.241** Puncture wound with foreign body of right back wall of thorax without penetration into thoracic cavity
  - **S21.242** Puncture wound with foreign body of left back wall of thorax without penetration into thoracic cavity
  - **S21.249** Puncture wound with foreign body of unspecified back wall of thorax without penetration into thoracic cavity
- **S21.25** Open bite of back wall of thorax without penetration into thoracic cavity
  Bite of back wall of thorax NOS
  Excludes1 superficial bite of back wall of thorax (S20.47)
  - **S21.251** Open bite of right back wall of thorax without penetration into thoracic cavity
  - **S21.252** Open bite of left back wall of thorax without penetration into thoracic cavity
  - **S21.259** Open bite of unspecified back wall of thorax without penetration into thoracic cavity

● S21.3 Open wound of front wall of thorax with penetration into thoracic cavity
Open wound of chest with penetration into thoracic cavity
Ex: For category S21.3 CC codes unless otherwise indicated: S21.101-S21.159[A], S21.301A-S21.95X[A], S27.50X-S27.69X[A] S27.892-S27.9XX[A], S28.1XX[A], S29.021[A], S29.029[A], S38.3XX[A], T14.90-T14.91, T79.7XX[A], T79.8XX-T79.9XX[A], T79.A0X-T79.A9X[A]

● S21.30 Unspecified open wound of front wall of thorax with penetration into thoracic cavity

● S21.301 Unspecified open wound of right front wall of thorax with penetration into thoracic cavity A

● S21.302 Unspecified open wound of left front wall of thorax with penetration into thoracic cavity A

● S21.309 Unspecified open wound of unspecified front wall of thorax with penetration into thoracic cavity A
Ex: S21.101A-S21.159[A], S21.301-S21.95X[A], S27.0XX-S27.2XX[A], S27.309[A], S27.329[A], S27.339[A], S27.409[A], S27.50X-S27.69X[A], S27.803[A], S27.892-S28.1XX[A], S29.021[A], S29.029[A], S38.3XX[A], T14.90-T14.91, T79.7XX[A], T79.8XX-T79.9XX[A] T79.A0X-T79.A9X[A]

● S21.31 Laceration without foreign body of front wall of thorax with penetration into thoracic cavity

● S21.311 Laceration without foreign body of right front wall of thorax with penetration into thoracic cavity A

● S21.312 Laceration without foreign body of left front wall of thorax with penetration into thoracic cavity A

● S21.319 Laceration without foreign body of unspecified front wall of thorax with penetration into thoracic cavity A

● S21.32 Laceration with foreign body of front wall of thorax with penetration into thoracic cavity

● S21.321 Laceration with foreign body of right front wall of thorax with penetration into thoracic cavity A

● S21.322 Laceration with foreign body of left front wall of thorax with penetration into thoracic cavity A

● S21.329 Laceration with foreign body of unspecified front wall of thorax with penetration into thoracic cavity A

● S21.33 Puncture wound without foreign body of front wall of thorax with penetration into thoracic cavity

● S21.331 Puncture wound without foreign body of right front wall of thorax with penetration into thoracic cavity A

● S21.332 Puncture wound without foreign body of left front wall of thorax with penetration into thoracic cavity A

● S21.339 Puncture wound without foreign body of unspecified front wall of thorax with penetration into thoracic cavity A

● S21.34 Puncture wound with foreign body of front wall of thorax with penetration into thoracic cavity

● S21.341 Puncture wound with foreign body of right front wall of thorax with penetration into thoracic cavity A

● S21.342 Puncture wound with foreign body of left front wall of thorax with penetration into thoracic cavity A

● S21.349 Puncture wound with foreign body of unspecified front wall of thorax with penetration into thoracic cavity A

● S21.35 Open bite of front wall of thorax with penetration into thoracic cavity
Excludes1 superficial bite of front wall of thorax (S20.37)

● S21.351 Open bite of right front wall of thorax with penetration into thoracic cavity A

● S21.352 Open bite of left front wall of thorax with penetration into thoracic cavity A

● S21.359 Open bite of unspecified front wall of thorax with penetration into thoracic cavity A

● S21.4 Open wound of back wall of thorax with penetration into thoracic cavity
Ex: For category S21.4 CC codes: See S21.3

● S21.40 Unspecified open wound of back wall of thorax with penetration into thoracic cavity

● S21.401 Unspecified open wound of right back wall of thorax with penetration into thoracic cavity A

● S21.402 Unspecified open wound of left back wall of thorax with penetration into thoracic cavity A

● S21.409 Unspecified open wound of unspecified back wall of thorax with penetration into thoracic cavity A

● S21.41 Laceration without foreign body of back wall of thorax with penetration into thoracic cavity

● S21.411 Laceration without foreign body of right back wall of thorax with penetration into thoracic cavity A

● S21.412 Laceration without foreign body of left back wall of thorax with penetration into thoracic cavity A

● S21.419 Laceration without foreign body of unspecified back wall of thorax with penetration into thoracic cavity A

● S21.42 Laceration with foreign body of back wall of thorax with penetration into thoracic cavity

● S21.421 Laceration with foreign body of right back wall of thorax with penetration into thoracic cavity A

● S21.422 Laceration with foreign body of left back wall of thorax with penetration into thoracic cavity A

● S21.429 Laceration with foreign body of unspecified back wall of thorax with penetration into thoracic cavity A

S21.43 Puncture wound without foreign body of back wall of thorax with penetration into thoracic cavity

S21.431 Puncture wound without foreign body of right back wall of thorax with penetration into thoracic cavity A

S21.432 Puncture wound without foreign body of left back wall of thorax with penetration into thoracic cavity A

S21.439 Puncture wound without foreign body of unspecified back wall of thorax with penetration into thoracic cavity A

S21.44 Puncture wound with foreign body of back wall of thorax with penetration into thoracic cavity

S21.441 Puncture wound with foreign body of right back wall of thorax with penetration into thoracic cavity A

S21.442 Puncture wound with foreign body of left back wall of thorax with penetration into thoracic cavity A

S21.449 Puncture wound with foreign body of unspecified back wall of thorax with penetration into thoracic cavity A

S21.45 Open bite of back wall of thorax with penetration into thoracic cavity

Bite of back wall of thorax NOS

Excludes1 superficial bite of back wall of thorax (S20.47)

S21.451 Open bite of right back wall of thorax with penetration into thoracic cavity A

S21.452 Open bite of left back wall of thorax with penetration into thoracic cavity A

S21.459 Open bite of unspecified back wall of thorax with penetration into thoracic cavity A

S21.9 Open wound of unspecified part of thorax

Open wound of thoracic wall NOS

Ex **For category S21.9 CC codes:** See S21.1

X **S21.90 Unspecified open wound of unspecified part of thorax** A

X **S21.91 Laceration without foreign body of unspecified part of thorax** A

X **S21.92 Laceration with foreign body of unspecified part of thorax** A

X **S21.93 Puncture wound without foreign body of unspecified part of thorax** A

X **S21.94 Puncture wound with foreign body of unspecified part of thorax** A

X **S21.95 Open bite of unspecified part of thorax** A

Excludes1 superficial bite of thorax (S20.97)

S22 Fracture of rib(s), sternum and thoracic spine

Note: A fracture not indicated as displaced or nondisplaced should be coded to displaced

A fracture not indicated as open or closed should be coded to closed

Includes fracture of thoracic neural arch
fracture of thoracic spinous process
fracture of thoracic transverse process
fracture of thoracic vertebra
fracture of thoracic vertebral arch

Code first any associated:
injury of intrathoracic organ (S27.-)
spinal cord injury (S24.0-, S24.1-)

Excludes1 transection of thorax (S28.1)

Excludes2 fracture of clavicle (S42.0-)
fracture of scapula (S42.1-)

The appropriate 7th character is to be added to each code from category S22

A	initial encounter for closed fracture
B	initial encounter for open fracture
D	subsequent encounter for fracture with routine healing
G	subsequent encounter for fracture with delayed healing
K	subsequent encounter for fracture with nonunion
S	sequela

S22.0 Fracture of thoracic vertebra

Ex **For category S22.0 CC codes S22.0[A,B]:** M48.40X-M48.58X[S], M80.08X[S], M80.88X[S], M83.50[S], M84.454[S], M84.550[S], M84.580X[S], M84.650[S], M99.12, M99.15-M99.17, M99.19, S03.1XX[A], S03.8XX-S03.9XX[A], S12.000-S12.9XX[S], S13.9XX[A], S14.109[A], S14.119[A], S14.129[A], S14.139[A], S14.149[A], S14.159[A], S22.000-S22.089[A,B,S], S22.20XS-S23.3XX[A], S23.8XX-S24.159[A], S29.001-S29.019[A], S29.091-S29.9XX[A], S32.000-S32.9XX[S], S32.9XX[S], S33.30X-S33.39X[A], S33.9XX[A], S38.1XX[A], S38.3XX[A], S39.001-S39.013[A], S39.091A-S39.94X[A], T14.90-T14.91, T79.8XX-T79.9XX[A], T79.A0X-T79.A9X[A] **For S22.0[K]:** See S02.0[K]

S22.00 Fracture of unspecified thoracic vertebra

S22.000 Wedge compression fracture of unspecified thoracic vertebra A, K, B, A, B

S22.001 Stable burst fracture of unspecified thoracic vertebra A, K, B, A, B

S22.002 Unstable burst fracture of unspecified thoracic vertebra A, K, B, A, B

S22.008 Other fracture of unspecified thoracic vertebra A, K, B, A, B

S22.009 Unspecified fracture of unspecified thoracic vertebra A, K, B, A, B

S22.01 Fracture of first thoracic vertebra

S22.010 Wedge compression fracture of first thoracic vertebra A, K, B, A, B

S22.011 Stable burst fracture of first thoracic vertebra A, K, B, A, B

S22.012 Unstable burst fracture of first thoracic vertebra A, K, B, A, B

S22.018 Other fracture of first thoracic vertebra A, K, B, A, B

S22.019 Unspecified fracture of first thoracic vertebra A, K, B, A, B

- S22.02 Fracture of second thoracic vertebra
  - S22.020 Wedge compression fracture of second thoracic vertebra A, K, B, A, B
  - S22.021 Stable burst fracture of second thoracic vertebra A, K, B, A, B
  - S22.022 Unstable burst fracture of second thoracic vertebra A, K, B, A, B
  - S22.028 Other fracture of second thoracic vertebra A, K, B, A, B
  - S22.029 Unspecified fracture of second thoracic vertebra A, K, B, A, B
- S22.03 Fracture of third thoracic vertebra
  - S22.030 Wedge compression fracture of third thoracic vertebra A, K, B, A, B
  - S22.031 Stable burst fracture of third thoracic vertebra A, K, B, A, B
  - S22.032 Unstable burst fracture of third thoracic vertebra A, K, B, A, B
  - S22.038 Other fracture of third thoracic vertebra A, K, B, A, B
  - S22.039 Unspecified fracture of third thoracic vertebra A, K, B, A, B
- S22.04 Fracture of fourth thoracic vertebra
  - S22.040 Wedge compression fracture of fourth thoracic vertebra A, K, B, A, B
  - S22.041 Stable burst fracture of fourth thoracic vertebra A, K, B, A, B
  - S22.042 Unstable burst fracture of fourth thoracic vertebra A, K, B, A, B
  - S22.048 Other fracture of fourth thoracic vertebra A, K, B, A, B
  - S22.049 Unspecified fracture of fourth thoracic vertebra A, K, B, A, B
- S22.05 Fracture of T_5-T_6 vertebra
  - S22.050 Wedge compression fracture of T_5-T_6 vertebra A, K, B, A, B
  - S22.051 Stable burst fracture of T_5-T_6 vertebra A, K, B, A, B
  - S22.052 Unstable burst fracture of T_5-T_6 vertebra A, K, B, A, B
  - S22.058 Other fracture of T_5-T_6 vertebra A, K, B, A, B
  - S22.059 Unspecified fracture of T_5-T_6 vertebra A, K, B, A, B
- S22.06 Fracture of T_7-T_8 vertebra
  - S22.060 Wedge compression fracture of T_7-T_8 vertebra A, K, B, A, B
  - S22.061 Stable burst fracture of T_7-T_8 vertebra A, K, B, A, B
  - S22.062 Unstable burst fracture of T_7-T_8 vertebra A, K, B, A, B
  - S22.068 Other fracture of T_7-T_8 thoracic vertebra A, K, B, A, B
  - S22.069 Unspecified fracture of T_7-T_8 vertebra A, K, B, A, B
- S22.07 Fracture of T_9-T_{10} vertebra
  - S22.070 Wedge compression fracture of T_9-T_{10} vertebra A, K, B, A, B
  - S22.071 Stable burst fracture of T_9-T_{10} vertebra A, K, B, A, B
  - S22.072 Unstable burst fracture of T_9-T_{10} vertebra A, K, B, A, B
  - S22.078 Other fracture of T_9-T_{10} vertebra A, K, B, A, B
  - S22.079 Unspecified fracture of T_9-T_{10} vertebra A, K, B, A, B
- S22.08 Fracture of T_{11}-T_{12} vertebra
  - S22.080 Wedge compression fracture of T_{11}-T_{12} vertebra A, K, B, A, B
  - S22.081 Stable burst fracture of T_{11}-T_{12} vertebra A, K, B, A, B
  - S22.082 Unstable burst fracture of T_{11}-T_{12} vertebra A, K, B, A, B
  - S22.088 Other fracture of T_{11}-T_{12} vertebra A, K, B, A, B
  - S22.089 Unspecified fracture of T_{11}-T_{12} vertebra A, K, B, A, B
- S22.2 Fracture of sternum

  Ex: **For category S22.2 CC codes S22.2[A,B]:** S03.8XX-S03.9XX[A], S22.20X-S22.24X[A,B], S22.5XX[A,B], S29.011-S29.019[A], S38.3XX[A], S39.011-S39.013[A], T14.90-T14.91, T79.8XX-T79.9XX[A], T79.A0X-T79.A9X[A] **For S22.2[K]:** See S02.0[K]
  - X S22.20 Unspecified fracture of sternum A, K, B, A, B
  - X S22.21 Fracture of manubrium A, K, B, A, B
  - X S22.22 Fracture of body of sternum A, K, B, A, B
  - X S22.23 Sternal manubrial dissociation A, K, B, A, B
  - X S22.24 Fracture of xiphoid process A, K, B, A, B
- S22.3 Fracture of one rib

  Ex: **For category S22.3 CC codes S22.3[A]:** S03.8XX-S03.9XX[A], S22.20X-S22.5XX[A,B], S29.011-S29.019[A], S38.3XX[A], S39.011-S39.013[A], T14.90-T14.91, T79.8XX-T79.9XX[A], T79.A0X-T79.A9X[A] **For S22.3[B]:** S03.8XX-S03.9XX[A], S22.31X-S22.5XX[A,B], S29.011-S29.019[A], S38.3XX[A], S39.011-S39.013[A], T14.90-T14.91, T79.8XX-T79.9XX[A], T79.A0X-T79.A9X[A] **For S22.3[K]:** See S02.0[K]
  - X S22.31 Fracture of one rib, right side A, K, B, A, B
  - X S22.32 Fracture of one rib, left side A, K, B, A, B
  - X S22.39 Fracture of one rib, unspecified side A, K, B, A, B
- S22.4 Multiple fractures of ribs

  Fractures of two or more ribs

  Excludes1 flail chest (S22.5-)

  Ex: **For category S22.4 CC codes S22.4[A,B]:** See S22.3[B] **For S22.49[B]:** No exclusions **For S22.4[K]:** See S02.0[K]
  - X S22.41 Multiple fractures of ribs, right side A, K, B, A, B
  - X S22.42 Multiple fractures of ribs, left side A, K, B, A, B
  - X S22.43 Multiple fractures of ribs, bilateral A, K, B, A, B
  - X S22.49 Multiple fractures of ribs, unspecified side A, K, B, A, B

X● **S22.5 Flail chest** K, A, B, A, B
Unstable chest due to sternum and/or rib fracture
Ex: **For category S22.5 CC codes S22.5[A,B]:** S03.8XX-S03.9XX[A], S22.20X-S22.5XX[A,B], S29.011-S29.019[A], S38.3XX[A], S39.011-S39.013[A], T14.90-T14.91, T79.8XX-T79.9XX[A], T79.A0X-T79.A9X[A] **For S22.5[K]:** See S02.0[K]

X● **S22.9 Fracture of bony thorax, part unspecified** A, K, B, A, B
Ex: **For category S22.9 CC codes S22.9[A,B]:** M80.00X-M80.019[A], M80.041A-M80.049[A], M80.80X-M80.819[A], M80.841-M80.849[A], M84.40X-M84.419[A], M84.441-M84.446[A], M84.454[A], M84.474-M84.519[A], M84.541-M84.550[A], M84.574-M84.576[A], M84.60X-M84.619[A], M84.641-M84.650[A], M84.674-M84.68X[A], S03.8XX-S03.9XX[A], S22.9XX-S22.9XX[A,B], S29.011A-S29.019[A], S32.301-S32.9XX[A,B], S33.4XX[A], S33.6XX-S33.8XX[A], S38.3XX[A], S39.011-S39.013[A], S73.001-S73.199[A], S76.001-S76.019[A], S76.091-S76.119[A], S76.191-S76.219[A], S76.291-S76.319[A], S76.391-S76.819[A], S76.891-S76.919[A], S76.991-S76.999[A], S79.811-S79.929[A], T14.90-T14.91, T79.8XX-T79.9XX[A], T79.A9X[A] **For S22.9[K]:** See S02.0[K]

● **S23 Dislocation and sprain of joints and ligaments of thorax**

Includes avulsion of joint or ligament of thorax
laceration of cartilage, joint or ligament of thorax
sprain of cartilage, joint or ligament of thorax
traumatic hemarthrosis of joint or ligament of thorax
traumatic rupture of joint or ligament of thorax
traumatic subluxation of joint or ligament of thorax
traumatic tear of joint or ligament of thorax

Code also any associated open wound

Excludes2 dislocation, sprain of sternoclavicular joint (S43.2, S43.6)
strain of muscle or tendon of thorax (S29.01-)

The appropriate 7th character is to be added to each code from category S23

A	initial encounter
D	subsequent encounter
S	sequela

X● **S23.0 Traumatic rupture of thoracic intervertebral disc**
Excludes1 rupture or displacement (nontraumatic) of thoracic intervertebral disc NOS (M51.- with fifth character 4)

● **S23.1 Subluxation and dislocation of thoracic vertebra**
Code also any associated
open wound of thorax (S21.-)
spinal cord injury (S24.0-, S24.1-)
Excludes2 fracture of thoracic vertebrae (S22.0-)

● **S23.10 Subluxation and dislocation of unspecified thoracic vertebra**
● **S23.100 Subluxation of unspecified thoracic vertebra**
● **S23.101 Dislocation of unspecified thoracic vertebra**

● **S23.11 Subluxation and dislocation of T_1/T_2 thoracic vertebra**
● **S23.110 Subluxation of T_1/T_2 thoracic vertebra**
● **S23.111 Dislocation of T_1/T_2 thoracic vertebra**

● **S23.12 Subluxation and dislocation of T_2/T_3-T_3/T_4 thoracic vertebra**
● **S23.120 Subluxation of T_2/T_3 thoracic vertebra**
● **S23.121 Dislocation of T_2/T_3 thoracic vertebra**
● **S23.122 Subluxation of T_3/T_4 thoracic vertebra**
● **S23.123 Dislocation of T_3/T_4 thoracic vertebra**

● **S23.13 Subluxation and dislocation of T_4/T_5-T_5/T_6 thoracic vertebra**
● **S23.130 Subluxation of T_4/T_5 thoracic vertebra**
● **S23.131 Dislocation of T_4/T_5 thoracic vertebra**
● **S23.132 Subluxation of T_5/T_6 thoracic vertebra**
● **S23.133 Dislocation of T_5/T_6 thoracic vertebra**

● **S23.14 Subluxation and dislocation of T_6/T_7-T_7/T_8 thoracic vertebra**
● **S23.140 Subluxation of T_6/T_7 thoracic vertebra**
● **S23.141 Dislocation of T_6/T_7 thoracic vertebra**
● **S23.142 Subluxation of T_7/T_8 thoracic vertebra**
● **S23.143 Dislocation of T_7/T_8 thoracic vertebra**

● **S23.15 Subluxation and dislocation of T_8/T_9-T_9/T_{10} thoracic vertebra**
● **S23.150 Subluxation of T_8/T_9 thoracic vertebra**
● **S23.151 Dislocation of T_8/T_9 thoracic vertebra**
● **S23.152 Subluxation of T_9/T_{10} thoracic vertebra**
● **S23.153 Dislocation of T_9/T_{10} thoracic vertebra**

● **S23.16 Subluxation and dislocation of T_{10}/T_{11}-T_{11}/T_{12} thoracic vertebra**
● **S23.160 Subluxation of T_{10}/T_{11} thoracic vertebra**
● **S23.161 Dislocation of T_{10}/T_{11} thoracic vertebra**
● **S23.162 Subluxation of T_{11}/T_{12} thoracic vertebra**
● **S23.163 Dislocation of T_{11}/T_{12} thoracic vertebra**

● **S23.17 Subluxation and dislocation of T_{12}/L_1 thoracic vertebra**
● **S23.170 Subluxation of T_{12}/L_1 thoracic vertebra**
● **S23.171 Dislocation of T_{12}/L_1 thoracic vertebra**

● **S23.2 Dislocation of other and unspecified parts of thorax**
X● **S23.20 Dislocation of unspecified part of thorax**
X● **S23.29 Dislocation of other parts of thorax**

X● **S23.3 Sprain of ligaments of thoracic spine**

● **S23.4 Sprain of ribs and sternum**
X● **S23.41 Sprain of ribs**
● **S23.42 Sprain of sternum**
● **S23.420 Sprain of sternoclavicular (joint) (ligament)**
● **S23.421 Sprain of chondrosternal joint**
● **S23.428 Other sprain of sternum**
● **S23.429 Unspecified sprain of sternum**

X● **S23.8 Sprain of other specified parts of thorax**
X● **S23.9 Sprain of unspecified parts of thorax**

● **S24 Injury of nerves and spinal cord at thorax level**

Note: Code to highest level of thoracic spinal cord injury.

Injuries to the spinal cord (S24.0 and S24.1) refer to the cord level and not bone level injury, and can affect nerve roots at and below the level given.

Code also any associated:
fracture of thoracic vertebra (S22.0-)
open wound of thorax (S21.-)
transient paralysis (R29.5)

Excludes2 injury of brachial plexus (S14.3)

The appropriate 7th character is to be added to each code from category S24

A	initial encounter
D	subsequent encounter
S	sequela

Ex: **For category S24 CC codes:** M48.40X-M48.58X[S], M80.08X[S], M80.88X[S], M84.350[S], M84.454[S], M84.550[S], M84.58[S], M84.650[S], M99.15-M99.17, M99.19, S03.1XX[A], S12.000-S12.9XX[S], S13.9XX[A], S14.109[A], S14.119[A], S14.129[A], S14.139[A], S14.149[A], S14.159[A], S22.000-S22.9XX[S], S23.20X-S23.29X[A], S23.9XX-S24.159[A], S29.001-S29.009[A], S29.091-S29.9XX[A], S32.000-S32.9XX[S], S33.30X-S33.39X[A], S33.9XX[A], S38.1XX[A], S39.001-S39.003[A], S39.091-S39.94X[A], T14.90-T14.91, T79.8XX-T79.9XX[A], T79.A0X-T79.A9X[A]

X● **S24.0 Concussion and edema of thoracic spinal cord A** OB

● **S24.1 Other and unspecified injuries of thoracic spinal cord**

● **S24.10 Unspecified injury of thoracic spinal cord**

● **S24.101 Unspecified injury at T_1 level of thoracic spinal cord A** OB, **A** OB

● **S24.102 Unspecified injury at T_2-T_6 level of thoracic spinal cord A** OB, **A** OB

● **S24.103 Unspecified injury at T_7-T_{10} level of thoracic spinal cord A** OB, **A** OB

● **S24.104 Unspecified injury at T_{11}-T_{12} level of thoracic spinal cord A** OB, **A** OB

● **S24.109 Unspecified injury at unspecified level of thoracic spinal cord A** OB
Injury of thoracic spinal cord NOS

● **S24.11 Complete lesion of thoracic spinal cord**

● **S24.111 Complete lesion at T_1 level of thoracic spinal cord A** OB, **A** OB

● **S24.112 Complete lesion at T_2-T_6 level of thoracic spinal cord A** OB, **A** OB

● **S24.113 Complete lesion at T_7-T_{10} level of thoracic spinal cord A** OB, **A** OB

● **S24.114 Complete lesion at T_{11}-T_{12} level of thoracic spinal cord A** OB, **A** OB

● **S24.119 Complete lesion at unspecified level of thoracic spinal cord**

● **S24.13 Anterior cord syndrome of thoracic spinal cord**

● **S24.131 Anterior cord syndrome at T_1 level of thoracic spinal cord A** OB, **A** OB

● **S24.132 Anterior cord syndrome at T_2-T_6 level of thoracic spinal cord A** OB, **A** OB

● **S24.133 Anterior cord syndrome at T_7-T_{10} level of thoracic spinal cord A** OB, **A** OB

● **S24.134 Anterior cord syndrome at T_{11}-T_{12} level of thoracic spinal cord A** OB, **A** OB

● **S24.139 Anterior cord syndrome at unspecified level of thoracic spinal cord**

● **S24.14 Brown-Séquard syndrome of thoracic spinal cord**

● **S24.141 Brown-Séquard syndrome at T_1 level of thoracic spinal cord A** OB

● **S24.142 Brown-Séquard syndrome at T_2-T_6 level of thoracic spinal cord A** OB

● **S24.143 Brown-Séquard syndrome at T_7-T_{10} level of thoracic spinal cord A** OB

● **S24.144 Brown-Séquard syndrome at T_{11}-T_{12} level of thoracic spinal cord A** OB

● **S24.149 Brown-Séquard syndrome at unspecified level of thoracic spinal cord**

● **S24.15 Other incomplete lesions of thoracic spinal cord**
Incomplete lesion of thoracic spinal cord NOS
Posterior cord syndrome of thoracic spinal cord

● **S24.151 Other incomplete lesion at T_1 level of thoracic spinal cord A** OB, **A** OB

● **S24.152 Other incomplete lesion at T_2-T_6 level of thoracic spinal cord A** OB, **A** OB

● **S24.153 Other incomplete lesion at T_7-T_{10} level of thoracic spinal cord A** OB, **A** OB

● **S24.154 Other incomplete lesion at T_{11}-T_{12} level of thoracic spinal cord A** OB, **A** OB

● **S24.159 Other incomplete lesion at unspecified level of thoracic spinal cord**

X● **S24.2 Injury of nerve root of thoracic spine**

X● **S24.3 Injury of peripheral nerves of thorax**

X● **S24.4 Injury of thoracic sympathetic nervous system**
Injury of cardiac plexus
Injury of esophageal plexus
Injury of pulmonary plexus
Injury of stellate ganglion
Injury of thoracic sympathetic ganglion

X● **S24.8 Injury of other specified nerves of thorax**

X● **S24.9 Injury of unspecified nerve of thorax**

● **S25 Injury of blood vessels of thorax**

The appropriate 7th character is to be added to each code from category S25

A	initial encounter
D	subsequent encounter
S	sequela

Code also any associated open wound (S21.-)

● **S25.0 Injury of thoracic aorta**
Injury of aorta NOS
Ex: **For category S25.0 CC codes:** S25.00XA-S25.09X[A], T14.90-T14.91, T79.8XX-T79.9XX[A], T79.A0X-T79.A9X[A]

X● **S25.00 Unspecified injury of thoracic aorta A** OB

X● **S25.01 Minor laceration of thoracic aorta A** OB
Incomplete transection of thoracic aorta
Laceration of thoracic aorta NOS
Superficial laceration of thoracic aorta

X● **S25.02 Major laceration of thoracic aorta A** OB
Complete transection of thoracic aorta
Traumatic rupture of thoracic aorta

X● **S25.09 Other specified injury of thoracic aorta A** OB

- **S25.1 Injury of innominate or subclavian artery**
  Ex: For category S25.1 CC codes: S25.101-S25.199[A], T14.90-T14.91, T79.8XX-T79.9XX[A], T79.A0X-T79.A9X[A]
  - **S25.10 Unspecified injury of innominate or subclavian artery**
    - **S25.101 Unspecified injury of right innominate or subclavian artery A**
    - **S25.102 Unspecified injury of left innominate or subclavian artery A**
    - **S25.109 Unspecified injury of unspecified innominate or subclavian artery A**
  - **S25.11 Minor laceration of innominate or subclavian artery**
    Incomplete transection of innominate or subclavian artery
    Laceration of innominate or subclavian artery NOS
    Superficial laceration of innominate or subclavian artery
    - **S25.111 Minor laceration of right innominate or subclavian artery A**
    - **S25.112 Minor laceration of left innominate or subclavian artery A**
    - **S25.119 Minor laceration of unspecified innominate or subclavian artery A**
  - **S25.12 Major laceration of innominate or subclavian artery**
    Complete transection of innominate or subclavian artery
    Traumatic rupture of innominate or subclavian artery
    - **S25.121 Major laceration of right innominate or subclavian artery A**
    - **S25.122 Major laceration of left innominate or subclavian artery A**
    - **S25.129 Major laceration of unspecified innominate or subclavian artery A**
  - **S25.19 Other specified injury of innominate or subclavian artery**
    - **S25.191 Other specified injury of right innominate or subclavian artery A**
    - **S25.192 Other specified injury of left innominate or subclavian artery A**
    - **S25.199 Other specified injury of unspecified innominate or subclavian artery A**
- **S25.2 Injury of superior vena cava**
  Injury of vena cava NOS
  Ex: For category S25.2 CC codes: S25.20X-S25.29X[A], T14.90-T14.91, T79.8XX-T79.9XX[A], T79.A0XA-T79.A9X[A]
  - X **S25.20 Unspecified injury of superior vena cava A**
  - X **S25.21 Minor laceration of superior vena cava A**
    Incomplete transection of superior vena cava
    Laceration of superior vena cava NOS
    Superficial laceration of superior vena cava
  - X **S25.22 Major laceration of superior vena cava A**
    Complete transection of superior vena cava
    Traumatic rupture of superior vena cava
  - X **S25.29 Other specified injury of superior vena cava A**
- **S25.3 Injury of innominate or subclavian vein**
  Ex: For category S25.3 CC codes: S25.301-S25.399[A], T14.90-T14.91, T79.8XX-T79.9XX[A], T79.A0X-T79.A9X[A]
  - **S25.30 Unspecified injury of innominate or subclavian vein**
    - **S25.301 Unspecified injury of right innominate or subclavian vein A**
    - **S25.302 Unspecified injury of left innominate or subclavian vein A**
    - **S25.309 Unspecified injury of unspecified innominate or subclavian vein A**
  - **S25.31 Minor laceration of innominate or subclavian vein**
    Incomplete transection of innominate or subclavian vein
    Laceration of innominate or subclavian vein NOS
    Superficial laceration of innominate or subclavian vein
    - **S25.311 Minor laceration of right innominate or subclavian vein A**
    - **S25.312 Minor laceration of left innominate or subclavian vein A**
    - **S25.319 Minor laceration of unspecified innominate or subclavian vein A**
  - **S25.32 Major laceration of innominate or subclavian vein**
    Complete transection of innominate or subclavian vein
    Traumatic rupture of innominate or subclavian vein
    - **S25.321 Major laceration of right innominate or subclavian vein A**
    - **S25.322 Major laceration of left innominate or subclavian vein A**
    - **S25.329 Major laceration of unspecified innominate or subclavian vein A**
  - **S25.39 Other specified injury of innominate or subclavian vein**
    - **S25.391 Other specified injury of right innominate or subclavian vein A**
    - **S25.392 Other specified injury of left innominate or subclavian vein A**
    - **S25.399 Other specified injury of unspecified innominate or subclavian vein A**
- **S25.4 Injury of pulmonary blood vessels**
  Ex: For category S25.4 CC codes unless otherwise indicated: S25.401-S25.499[A], T14.90-T14.91, T79.8XX-T79.9XX[A], T79.A0X-T79.A9X[A]
  - **S25.40 Unspecified injury of pulmonary blood vessels**
    - **S25.401 Unspecified injury of right pulmonary blood vessels A**
    - **S25.402 Unspecified injury of left pulmonary blood vessels A**
    - **S25.409 Unspecified injury of unspecified pulmonary blood vessels A**
  - **S25.41 Minor laceration of pulmonary blood vessels**
    Incomplete transection of pulmonary blood vessels
    Laceration of pulmonary blood vessels NOS
    Superficial laceration of pulmonary blood vessels
    - **S25.411 Minor laceration of right pulmonary blood vessels A**
    - **S25.412 Minor laceration of left pulmonary blood vessels A**
    - **S25.419 Minor laceration of unspecified pulmonary blood vessels A**
  - **S25.42 Major laceration of pulmonary blood vessels**
    Complete transection of pulmonary blood vessels
    Traumatic rupture of pulmonary blood vessels
    - **S25.421 Major laceration of right pulmonary blood vessels A**
      Ex: S25.401[A]-S25.499[A], T14.90-T14.91, T79.A0X[A]-T79.9XX[A]
    - **S25.422 Major laceration of left pulmonary blood vessels A**
    - **S25.429 Major laceration of unspecified pulmonary blood vessels A**

- **S25.49 Other specified injury of pulmonary blood vessels**
  - **S25.491 Other specified injury of right pulmonary blood vessels** A
  - **S25.492 Other specified injury of left pulmonary blood vessels** A
  - **S25.499 Other specified injury of unspecified pulmonary blood vessels** A

- **S25.5 Injury of intercostal blood vessels**
  Ex: For category S25.5 CC codes: S25.501-S25.899[A]
  - **S25.50 Unspecified injury of intercostal blood vessels**
    - **S25.501 Unspecified injury of intercostal blood vessels, right side** A
    - **S25.502 Unspecified injury of intercostal blood vessels, left side** A
    - **S25.509 Unspecified injury of intercostal blood vessels, unspecified side** A
  - **S25.51 Laceration of intercostal blood vessels**
    - **S25.511 Laceration of intercostal blood vessels, right side** A
    - **S25.512 Laceration of intercostal blood vessels, left side** A
    - **S25.519 Laceration of intercostal blood vessels, unspecified side** A
  - **S25.59 Other specified injury of intercostal blood vessels**
    - **S25.591 Other specified injury of intercostal blood vessels, right side** A
    - **S25.592 Other specified injury of intercostal blood vessels, left side** A
    - **S25.599 Other specified injury of intercostal blood vessels, unspecified side** A

- **S25.8 Injury of other blood vessels of thorax**
  Injury of azygos vein
  Injury of mammary artery or vein
  Ex: For category S25.8 CC codes: S25.00X-S25.99X[A]
  - **S25.80 Unspecified injury of other blood vessels of thorax**
    - **S25.801 Unspecified injury of other blood vessels of thorax, right side** A
    - **S25.802 Unspecified injury of other blood vessels of thorax, left side** A
    - **S25.809 Unspecified injury of other blood vessels of thorax, unspecified side** A
  - **S25.81 Laceration of other blood vessels of thorax**
    - **S25.811 Laceration of other blood vessels of thorax, right side** A
    - **S25.812 Laceration of other blood vessels of thorax, left side** A
    - **S25.819 Laceration of other blood vessels of thorax, unspecified side** A
  - **S25.89 Other specified injury of other blood vessels of thorax**
    - **S25.891 Other specified injury of other blood vessels of thorax, right side** A
    - **S25.892 Other specified injury of other blood vessels of thorax, left side** A
    - **S25.899 Other specified injury of other blood vessels of thorax, unspecified side** A

- **S25.9 Injury of unspecified blood vessel of thorax**
  Ex: For category S25.9 CC codes: S25.00X-S25.99X[A]
  - X **S25.90 Unspecified injury of unspecified blood vessel of thorax** A
  - X **S25.91 Laceration of unspecified blood vessel of thorax** A
  - X **S25.99 Other specified injury of unspecified blood vessel of thorax** A

- **S26 Injury of heart**
  The appropriate 7th character is to be added to each code from category S26

A	initial encounter
D	subsequent encounter
S	sequela

  Code also any associated:
  open wound of thorax (S21.-)
  traumatic hemopneumothorax (S27.2)
  traumatic hemothorax (S27.1)
  traumatic pneumothorax (S27.0)
  - **S26.0 Injury of heart with hemopericardium**
    Hemopericardium: effusion of blood within pericardium
    Ex: For category S26.0 CC codes unless otherwise indicated: S21.101-S21.159[A], S21.301-S21.95X[A], S26.00X-S26.99X[A] S27.50X-S27.69X[A], S27.892-S27.9XX[A], S28.1XX[A], S29.021[A], S29.029[A], S38.3XX[A], T14.90-T14.91, T79.7XX-T79.9XX[A], T79.A0X-T79.A9X[A]
    - X **S26.00 Unspecified injury of heart with hemopericardium** A
      Ex: S21.301-S21.459[A], S26.00X-S26.99X[A], S27.50X-S27.69X[A], S27.892-S27.9XX[A], T14.90-T14.91
    - X **S26.01 Contusion of heart with hemopericardium** A
    - **S26.02 Laceration of heart with hemopericardium**
      - **S26.020 Mild laceration of heart with hemopericardium** A
        Laceration of heart without penetration of heart chamber
      - **S26.021 Moderate laceration of heart with hemopericardium** A
        Laceration of heart with penetration of heart chamber
      - **S26.022 Major laceration of heart with hemopericardium** A
        Laceration of heart with penetration of multiple heart chambers
    - X **S26.09 Other injury of heart with hemopericardium** A
      Ex: See 26.00
  - **S26.1 Injury of heart without hemopericardium**
    Hemopericardium: effusion of blood within pericardium
    - X **S26.10 Unspecified injury of heart without hemopericardium** A
      Ex: See S26.00
    - X **S26.11 Contusion of heart without hemopericardium** A
    - X **S26.12 Laceration of heart without hemopericardium** A
    - X **S26.19 Other injury of heart without hemopericardium** A
      Ex: See S26.00

Item 19–2 Pneumothorax is a collection of gas (positive air pressure) in the pleural space resulting in the lung collapsing. A tension pneumothorax is life-threatening and is a result of air in the pleural space causing a displacement in the mediastinal structures and cardiopulmonary function compromise. A traumatic pneumothorax results from blunt or penetrating injury that disrupts the parietal/visceral pleura. **Hemothorax** is blood or bloody fluid in the pleural cavity as a result of traumatic blood vessel rupture or inflammation of the lungs from pneumonia.

◀ New ◀ Revised ~~deleted~~ Deleted Excludes 1 Excludes 2 Includes Use additional Code first Code also Unspecified
OGCR Official Guidelines ● Unacceptable Principal Diagnosis X Assign placeholder X ● Use Additional Character(s) ▶ Manifestation Code Coding Clinic

- **S26.9 Injury of heart, unspecified with or without hemopericardium**
  Hemopericardium: effusion of blood within pericardium
  - X **S26.90 Unspecified injury of heart, unspecified with or without hemopericardium** A
    Ex: See S26.00
  - X **S26.91 Contusion of heart, unspecified with or without hemopericardium** A
  - X **S26.92 Laceration of heart, unspecified with or without hemopericardium** A
    Laceration of heart NOS
  - X **S26.99 Other injury of heart, unspecified with or without hemopericardium** A
    Ex: See S26.00

- **S27 Injury of other and unspecified intrathoracic organs**
  Code also any associated open wound of thorax (S21.-)
  Excludes2 injury of cervical esophagus (S10-S19)
  injury of trachea (cervical) (S10-S19)
  The appropriate 7th character is to be added to each code from category S27

A	initial encounter
D	subsequent encounter
S	sequela

  - X **S27.0 Traumatic pneumothorax** A
    Excludes1 spontaneous pneumothorax (J93.-)
    Ex: S21.101-S21.159[A], S21.301-S21.95X[A], S27.0XX-S27.399[A] S27.50X-S27.69X[A], S27.892-S27.9XX[A], S28.1XX[A], S29.021[A], S29.029[A], S38.3XX[A], T14.90-T14.91, T79.7XX-T79.9XX[A], T79.A0X-T79.A9X[A]
  - X **S27.1 Traumatic hemothorax** A
    Ex: See S27.0
  - X **S27.2 Traumatic hemopneumothorax** A
    Ex: See S27.0
  - **S27.3 Other and unspecified injuries of lung**
    Ex: **For category S27.3 CC codes unless otherwise indicated:** S21.101-S21.159[A], S21.301-S21.95X[A], S27.301-S27.399[A] S27.50X-S27.69X[A], S27.892-S27.9XX[A], S28.1XX[A], S29.021[A], S29.029[A], S38.3XX[A], T14.90-T14.91, T79.7XX-T79.9XX[A], T79.A9X[A]
    - **S27.30 Unspecified injury of lung**
      - **S27.301 Unspecified injury of lung, unilateral** A
      - **S27.302 Unspecified injury of lung, bilateral** A
      - **S27.309 Unspecified injury of lung, unspecified** A
    - **S27.31 Primary blast injury of lung**
      Blast injury of lung NOS
      - **S27.311 Primary blast injury of lung, unilateral** A
      - **S27.312 Primary blast injury of lung, bilateral** A
      - **S27.319 Primary blast injury of lung, unspecified** A
    - **S27.32 Contusion of lung**
      - **S27.321 Contusion of lung, unilateral** A
      - **S27.322 Contusion of lung, bilateral** A
      - **S27.329 Contusion of lung, unspecified** A
    - **S27.33 Laceration of lung**
      Ex: **For category S27.33 CC codes:** S21.101-S21.159[A], S21.301-S21.95X[A], S27.301-S27.399[A], S27.50X-S27.69X[A], S27.892-S27.9XX[A], S28.1XX[A], S29.021[A], S29.029[A], S38.3XX[A], T14.90-T14.91, T79.7XX-T79.9XX[A], T79.A0X-T79.A9X[A]
      - **S27.331 Laceration of lung, unilateral** A
      - **S27.332 Laceration of lung, bilateral** A
      - **S27.339 Laceration of lung, unspecified** A
    - **S27.39 Other injuries of lung**
      Secondary blast injury of lung
      - **S27.391 Other injuries of lung, unilateral** A
      - **S27.392 Other injuries of lung, bilateral** A
      - **S27.399 Other injuries of lung, unspecified** A
  - **S27.4 Injury of bronchus**
    Ex: **For category S27.4 CC codes:** S21.101-S21.159[A], S21.301-S21.95X[A], S27.401-S27.69X[A], S27.892-S27.9XX[A], S28.1XX[A], S29.021[A], S29.029[A], S38.3XX[A], T14.90-T14.91, T79.7XX-T79.9XX[A], T79.A0X-T79.A9X[A]
    - **S27.40 Unspecified injury of bronchus**
      - **S27.401 Unspecified injury of bronchus, unilateral** A
      - **S27.402 Unspecified injury of bronchus, bilateral** A
      - **S27.409 Unspecified injury of bronchus, unspecified** A
    - **S27.41 Primary blast injury of bronchus**
      Blast injury of bronchus NOS
      - **S27.411 Primary blast injury of bronchus, unilateral** A
      - **S27.412 Primary blast injury of bronchus, bilateral** A
      - **S27.419 Primary blast injury of bronchus, unspecified** A
    - **S27.42 Contusion of bronchus**
      - **S27.421 Contusion of bronchus, unilateral** A
      - **S27.422 Contusion of bronchus, bilateral** A
      - **S27.429 Contusion of bronchus, unspecified** A
    - **S27.43 Laceration of bronchus**
      - **S27.431 Laceration of bronchus, unilateral** A
      - **S27.432 Laceration of bronchus, bilateral** A
      - **S27.439 Laceration of bronchus, unspecified** A
    - **S27.49 Other injury of bronchus**
      Secondary blast injury of bronchus
      - **S27.491 Other injury of bronchus, unilateral** A
      - **S27.492 Other injury of bronchus, bilateral** A
      - **S27.499 Other injury of bronchus, unspecified** A

- S27.5 Injury of thoracic trachea
  - Ex: For category S27.5 CC codes: See S21.3
  - X S27.50 Unspecified injury of thoracic trachea A
  - X S27.51 Primary blast injury of thoracic trachea A
    - Blast injury of thoracic trachea NOS
  - X S27.52 Contusion of thoracic trachea A
  - X S27.53 Laceration of thoracic trachea A
  - X S27.59 Other injury of thoracic trachea A
    - Secondary blast injury of thoracic trachea
- S27.6 Injury of pleura
  - Ex: For category S27.6 CC codes: See S21.3
  - X S27.60 Unspecified injury of pleura A
  - X S27.63 Laceration of pleura A
  - X S27.69 Other injury of pleura A
- S27.8 Injury of other specified intrathoracic organs
  - S27.80 Injury of diaphragm
    - Ex: For category S27.80 CC codes: S21.101-S21.159[A], S21.301-S21.95X[A], S27.50X-S27.809[A], S27.892-S27.9XX[A], S28.1XX[A], S29.021[A], S29.029[A], S38.3XX[A], T14.90-T14.91, T79.7XX-T79.9XX[A], T79.A9X[A]
    - S27.802 Contusion of diaphragm A
    - S27.803 Laceration of diaphragm A
    - S27.808 Other injury of diaphragm A
    - S27.809 Unspecified injury of diaphragm A
  - S27.81 Injury of esophagus (thoracic part)
    - Ex: For category S27.81 CC codes: S21.101-S21.159[A], S21.301-S21.95X[A], S27.50X-S27.69X[A], S27.812-S27.9XX[A], S28.1XX[A], S29.021[A], S29.029[A], S38.3XX[A], T14.90-T14.91, T79.7XX-T79.9XX[A], T79.A0X-T79.A9X[A]
    - S27.812 Contusion of esophagus (thoracic part) A
    - S27.813 Laceration of esophagus (thoracic part) A
    - S27.818 Other injury of esophagus (thoracic part) A
    - S27.819 Unspecified injury of esophagus (thoracic part) A
  - S27.89 Injury of other specified intrathoracic organs
    - Injury of lymphatic thoracic duct
    - Injury of thymus gland
    - Ex: For category S27.89 CC codes: See S21.3
    - S27.892 Contusion of other specified intrathoracic organs A
    - S27.893 Laceration of other specified intrathoracic organs A
    - S27.898 Other injury of other specified intrathoracic organs A
    - S27.899 Unspecified injury of other specified intrathoracic organs A
  - X S27.9 Injury of unspecified intrathoracic organ A
    - Ex: S21.101-S21.159[A], S21.301-S21.95X[A], S27.50X-S27.69X[A], S27.892-S27.9XX[A], S28.1XX[A], S29.021[A], S29.029[A], S38.3XX[A], T14.90-T14.91, T79.7XX-T79.9XX[A], T79.A3X-T79.A9X[A]
- S28 Crushing injury of thorax, and traumatic amputation of part of thorax
  - The appropriate 7th character is to be added to each code from category S28

A	initial encounter
D	subsequent encounter
S	sequela

  - X S28.0 Crushed chest
    - Use additional code for all associated injuries
    - **Excludes1** flail chest (S22.5)
  - X S28.1 Traumatic amputation (partial) of part of thorax, except breast A
    - Ex: For category S28.1 CC codes: See S21.1
- S28.2 Traumatic amputation of breast
  - S28.21 Complete traumatic amputation of breast
    - Traumatic amputation of breast NOS
    - S28.211 Complete traumatic amputation of right breast
    - S28.212 Complete traumatic amputation of left breast
    - S28.219 Complete traumatic amputation of unspecified breast
  - S28.22 Partial traumatic amputation of breast
    - S28.221 Partial traumatic amputation of right breast
    - S28.222 Partial traumatic amputation of left breast
    - S28.229 Partial traumatic amputation of unspecified breast
- S29 Other and unspecified injuries of thorax
  - Code also any associated open wound (S21.-)
  - The appropriate 7th character is to be added to each code from category S29

A	initial encounter
D	subsequent encounter
S	sequela

  - S29.0 Injury of muscle and tendon at thorax level
    - S29.00 Unspecified injury of muscle and tendon of thorax
      - S29.001 Unspecified injury of muscle and tendon of front wall of thorax
      - S29.002 Unspecified injury of muscle and tendon of back wall of thorax
      - S29.009 Unspecified injury of muscle and tendon of unspecified wall of thorax
    - S29.01 Strain of muscle and tendon of thorax
      - S29.011 Strain of muscle and tendon of front wall of thorax
      - S29.012 Strain of muscle and tendon of back wall of thorax
      - S29.019 Strain of muscle and tendon of unspecified wall of thorax
    - S29.02 Laceration of muscle and tendon of thorax
      - Ex: For category S29.02 CC codes: See S21.1
      - S29.021 Laceration of muscle and tendon of front wall of thorax A
      - S29.022 Laceration of muscle and tendon of back wall of thorax
      - S29.029 Laceration of muscle and tendon of unspecified wall of thorax A
    - S29.09 Other injury of muscle and tendon of thorax
      - S29.091 Other injury of muscle and tendon of front wall of thorax
      - S29.092 Other injury of muscle and tendon of back wall of thorax
      - S29.099 Other injury of muscle and tendon of unspecified wall of thorax
  - X S29.8 Other specified injuries of thorax
  - X S29.9 Unspecified injury of thorax

INJURIES TO THE ABDOMEN, LOWER BACK, LUMBAR SPINE PELVIS AND EXTERNAL GENITALS (S30-S39)

Includes injuries to the abdominal wall
injuries to the anus
injuries to the buttock
injuries to the external genitalia
injuries to the flank
injuries to the groin

Excludes2 burns and corrosions (T20-T32)
effects of foreign body in anus and rectum (T18.5)
effects of foreign body in genitourinary tract (T19.-)
effects of foreign body in stomach, small intestine and colon (T18.2-T18.4)
frostbite (T33-T34)
insect bite or sting, venomous (T63.4)

S30 Superficial injury of abdomen, lower back, pelvis and external genitals

Excludes2 superficial injury of hip (S70.-)

The appropriate 7th character is to be added to each code from category S30

A	initial encounter
D	subsequent encounter
S	sequela

X **S30.0 Contusion of lower back and pelvis**
Contusion of buttock

X **S30.1 Contusion of abdominal wall**
Contusion of flank
Contusion of groin

S30.2 Contusion of external genital organs

S30.20 Contusion of unspecified external genital organ

S30.201 Contusion of unspecified external genital organ, male ♂

S30.202 Contusion of unspecified external genital organ, female ♀

X **S30.21 Contusion of penis ♂**

X **S30.22 Contusion of scrotum and testes ♂**

X **S30.23 Contusion of vagina and vulva ♀**

X **S30.3 Contusion of anus**

S30.8 Other superficial injuries of abdomen, lower back, pelvis and external genitals

S30.81 Abrasion of abdomen, lower back, pelvis and external genitals

S30.810 Abrasion of lower back and pelvis

S30.811 Abrasion of abdominal wall

S30.812 Abrasion of penis ♂

S30.813 Abrasion of scrotum and testes ♂

S30.814 Abrasion of vagina and vulva ♀

S30.815 Abrasion of unspecified external genital organs, male ♂

S30.816 Abrasion of unspecified external genital organs, female ♀

S30.817 Abrasion of anus

S30.82 Blister (nonthermal) of abdomen, lower back, pelvis and external genitals

S30.820 Blister (nonthermal) of lower back and pelvis

S30.821 Blister (nonthermal) of abdominal wall

S30.822 Blister (nonthermal) of penis ♂

S30.823 Blister (nonthermal) of scrotum and testes ♂

S30.824 Blister (nonthermal) of vagina and vulva ♀

S30.825 Blister (nonthermal) of unspecified external genital organs, male ♂

S30.826 Blister (nonthermal) of unspecified external genital organs, female ♀

S30.827 Blister (nonthermal) of anus

S30.84 External constriction of abdomen, lower back, pelvis and external genitals

S30.840 External constriction of lower back and pelvis

S30.841 External constriction of abdominal wall

S30.842 External constriction of penis ♂
Hair tourniquet syndrome of penis
Use additional cause code to identify the constricting item (W49.0-)

S30.843 External constriction of scrotum and testes ♂

S30.844 External constriction of vagina and vulva ♀

S30.845 External constriction of unspecified external genital organs, male ♂

S30.846 External constriction of unspecified external genital organs, female ♀

S30.85 Superficial foreign body of abdomen, lower back, pelvis and external genitals
Splinter in the abdomen, lower back, pelvis and external genitals

S30.850 Superficial foreign body of lower back and pelvis

S30.851 Superficial foreign body of abdominal wall

S30.852 Superficial foreign body of penis ♂

S30.853 Superficial foreign body of scrotum and testes ♂

S30.854 Superficial foreign body of vagina and vulva ♀

S30.855 Superficial foreign body of unspecified external genital organs, male ♂

S30.856 Superficial foreign body of unspecified external genital organs, female ♀

S30.857 Superficial foreign body of anus

S30.86 Insect bite (nonvenomous) of abdomen, lower back, pelvis and external genitals

S30.860 Insect bite (nonvenomous) of lower back and pelvis

S30.861 Insect bite (nonvenomous) of abdominal wall

S30.862 Insect bite (nonvenomous) of penis ♂

S30.863 Insect bite (nonvenomous) of scrotum and testes ♂

S30.864 Insect bite (nonvenomous) of vagina and vulva ♀

S30.865 Insect bite (nonvenomous) of unspecified external genital organs, male ♂

S30.866 Insect bite (nonvenomous) of unspecified external genital organs, female ♀

S30.867 Insect bite (nonvenomous) of anus

- **S30.87 Other superficial bite of abdomen, lower back, pelvis and external genitals**
  - **Excludes1** open bite of abdomen, lower back, pelvis and external genitals (S31.05, S31.15, S31.25, S31.35, S31.45, S31.55)
  - **S30.870 Other superficial bite of lower back and pelvis**
  - **S30.871 Other superficial bite of abdominal wall**
  - **S30.872 Other superficial bite of penis ♂**
  - **S30.873 Other superficial bite of scrotum and testes ♂**
  - **S30.874 Other superficial bite of vagina and vulva ♀**
  - **S30.875 Other superficial bite of unspecified external genital organs, male ♂**
  - **S30.876 Other superficial bite of unspecified external genital organs, female ♀**
  - **S30.877 Other superficial bite of anus**
- **S30.9 Unspecified superficial injury of abdomen, lower back, pelvis and external genitals**
  - X **S30.91 Unspecified superficial injury of lower back and pelvis**
  - X **S30.92 Unspecified superficial injury of abdominal wall**
  - X **S30.93 Unspecified superficial injury of penis ♂**
  - X **S30.94 Unspecified superficial injury of scrotum and testes ♂**
  - X **S30.95 Unspecified superficial injury of vagina and vulva ♀**
  - X **S30.96 Unspecified superficial injury of unspecified external genital organs, male ♂**
  - X **S30.97 Unspecified superficial injury of unspecified external genital organs, female ♀**
  - X **S30.98 Unspecified superficial injury of anus**

- **S31 Open wound of abdomen, lower back, pelvis and external genitals**

  Code also any associated:
  spinal cord injury (S24.0, S24.1-, S34.0-, S34.1-)
  wound infection

  Excludes1 traumatic amputation of part of abdomen, lower back and pelvis (S38.2-, S38.3)

  Excludes2 open wound of hip (S71.00-S71.02)
  open fracture of pelvis (S32.1--S32.9 with 7th character B)

  The appropriate 7th character is to be added to each code from category S31

A	initial encounter
D	subsequent encounter
S	sequela

- **S31.0 Open wound of lower back and pelvis**

  Ex: **For category S31.0 CC codes:** S31.001[A], S31.011[A], S31.021[A], S31.031[A], S31.041[A], S31.051[A], S31.100-S31.159[A] S31.600-S31.659[A], S31.831-S31.839[A], S36.81X-S36.99X[A], S38.3XX[A], S39.021-S39.023[A], T14.90-T14.91, T79.8XX-T79.9XX[A] T79.A0X-T79.A9X[A]

  - **S31.00 Unspecified open wound of lower back and pelvis**
    - **S31.000 Unspecified open wound of lower back and pelvis without penetration into retroperitoneum**
      Unspecified open wound of lower back and pelvis NOS
    - **S31.001 Unspecified open wound of lower back and pelvis with penetration into retroperitoneum A**
  - **S31.01 Laceration without foreign body of lower back and pelvis**
    - **S31.010 Laceration without foreign body of lower back and pelvis without penetration into retroperitoneum**
      Laceration without foreign body of lower back and pelvis NOS
    - **S31.011 Laceration without foreign body of lower back and pelvis with penetration into retroperitoneum A**
  - **S31.02 Laceration with foreign body of lower back and pelvis**
    - **S31.020 Laceration with foreign body of lower back and pelvis without penetration into retroperitoneum**
      Laceration with foreign body of lower back and pelvis NOS
    - **S31.021 Laceration with foreign body of lower back and pelvis with penetration into retroperitoneum A**
  - **S31.03 Puncture wound without foreign body of lower back and pelvis**
    - **S31.030 Puncture wound without foreign body of lower back and pelvis without penetration into retroperitoneum**
      Puncture wound without foreign body of lower back and pelvis NOS
    - **S31.031 Puncture wound without foreign body of lower back and pelvis with penetration into retroperitoneum A**
  - **S31.04 Puncture wound with foreign body of lower back and pelvis**
    - **S31.040 Puncture wound with foreign body of lower back and pelvis without penetration into retroperitoneum**
      Puncture wound with foreign body of lower back and pelvis NOS
    - **S31.041 Puncture wound with foreign body of lower back and pelvis with penetration into retroperitoneum A**
  - **S31.05 Open bite of lower back and pelvis**
    Bite of lower back and pelvis NOS
    - **Excludes1** superficial bite of lower back and pelvis (S30.860, S30.870)
    - **S31.050 Open bite of lower back and pelvis without penetration into retroperitoneum**
      Open bite of lower back and pelvis NOS
    - **S31.051 Open bite of lower back and pelvis with penetration into retroperitoneum A**
- **S31.1 Open wound of abdominal wall without penetration into peritoneal cavity**
  Open wound of abdominal wall NOS
  - **Excludes2** open wound of abdominal wall with penetration into peritoneal cavity (S31.6-)
  - **S31.10 Unspecified open wound of abdominal wall without penetration into peritoneal cavity**
    - **S31.100 Unspecified open wound of abdominal wall, right upper quadrant without penetration into peritoneal cavity**
    - **S31.101 Unspecified open wound of abdominal wall, left upper quadrant without penetration into peritoneal cavity**

- S31.102 Unspecified open wound of abdominal wall, epigastric region without penetration into peritoneal cavity
- S31.103 Unspecified open wound of abdominal wall, right lower quadrant without penetration into peritoneal cavity
- S31.104 Unspecified open wound of abdominal wall, left lower quadrant without penetration into peritoneal cavity
- S31.105 Unspecified open wound of abdominal wall, periumbilic region without penetration into peritoneal cavity
- S31.109 Unspecified open wound of abdominal wall, unspecified quadrant without penetration into peritoneal cavity
  - Unspecified open wound of abdominal wall NOS
- S31.11 Laceration without foreign body of abdominal wall without penetration into peritoneal cavity
  - S31.110 Laceration without foreign body of abdominal wall, right upper quadrant without penetration into peritoneal cavity
  - S31.111 Laceration without foreign body of abdominal wall, left upper quadrant without penetration into peritoneal cavity
  - S31.112 Laceration without foreign body of abdominal wall, epigastric region without penetration into peritoneal cavity
  - S31.113 Laceration without foreign body of abdominal wall, right lower quadrant without penetration into peritoneal cavity
  - S31.114 Laceration without foreign body of abdominal wall, left lower quadrant without penetration into peritoneal cavity
  - S31.115 Laceration without foreign body of abdominal wall, periumbilic region without penetration into peritoneal cavity
  - S31.119 Laceration without foreign body of abdominal wall, unspecified quadrant without penetration into peritoneal cavity
- S31.12 Laceration with foreign body of abdominal wall without penetration into peritoneal cavity
  - S31.120 Laceration of abdominal wall with foreign body, right upper quadrant without penetration into peritoneal cavity
  - S31.121 Laceration of abdominal wall with foreign body, left upper quadrant without penetration into peritoneal cavity
  - S31.122 Laceration of abdominal wall with foreign body, epigastric region without penetration into peritoneal cavity
  - S31.123 Laceration of abdominal wall with foreign body, right lower quadrant without penetration into peritoneal cavity
  - S31.124 Laceration of abdominal wall with foreign body, left lower quadrant without penetration into peritoneal cavity
  - S31.125 Laceration of abdominal wall with foreign body, periumbilic region without penetration into peritoneal cavity
  - S31.129 Laceration of abdominal wall with foreign body, unspecified quadrant without penetration into peritoneal cavity
- S31.13 Puncture wound of abdominal wall without foreign body without penetration into peritoneal cavity
  - S31.130 Puncture wound of abdominal wall without foreign body, right upper quadrant without penetration into peritoneal cavity
  - S31.131 Puncture wound of abdominal wall without foreign body, left upper quadrant without penetration into peritoneal cavity
  - S31.132 Puncture wound of abdominal wall without foreign body, epigastric region without penetration into peritoneal cavity
  - S31.133 Puncture wound of abdominal wall without foreign body, right lower quadrant without penetration into peritoneal cavity
  - S31.134 Puncture wound of abdominal wall without foreign body, left lower quadrant without penetration into peritoneal cavity
  - S31.135 Puncture wound of abdominal wall without foreign body, periumbilic region without penetration into peritoneal cavity
  - S31.139 Puncture wound of abdominal wall without foreign body, unspecified quadrant without penetration into peritoneal cavity
- S31.14 Puncture wound of abdominal wall with foreign body without penetration into peritoneal cavity
  - S31.140 Puncture wound of abdominal wall with foreign body, right upper quadrant without penetration into peritoneal cavity
  - S31.141 Puncture wound of abdominal wall with foreign body, left upper quadrant without penetration into peritoneal cavity
  - S31.142 Puncture wound of abdominal wall with foreign body, epigastric region without penetration into peritoneal cavity
  - S31.143 Puncture wound of abdominal wall with foreign body, right lower quadrant without penetration into peritoneal cavity
  - S31.144 Puncture wound of abdominal wall with foreign body, left lower quadrant without penetration into peritoneal cavity
  - S31.145 Puncture wound of abdominal wall with foreign body, periumbilic region without penetration into peritoneal cavity
  - S31.149 Puncture wound of abdominal wall with foreign body, unspecified quadrant without penetration into peritoneal cavity

- S31.15 **Open bite of abdominal wall without penetration into peritoneal cavity**
  Bite of abdominal wall NOS
  Excludes1 superficial bite of abdominal wall (S30.871)
  - S31.150 **Open bite of abdominal wall, right upper quadrant without penetration into peritoneal cavity**
  - S31.151 **Open bite of abdominal wall, left upper quadrant without penetration into peritoneal cavity**
  - S31.152 **Open bite of abdominal wall, epigastric region without penetration into peritoneal cavity**
  - S31.153 **Open bite of abdominal wall, right lower quadrant without penetration into peritoneal cavity**
  - S31.154 **Open bite of abdominal wall, left lower quadrant without penetration into peritoneal cavity**
  - S31.155 **Open bite of abdominal wall, periumbilic region without penetration into peritoneal cavity**
  - S31.159 **Open bite of abdominal wall, unspecified quadrant without penetration into peritoneal cavity**
- S31.2 **Open wound of penis**
  - X S31.20 **Unspecified open wound of penis ♂**
  - X S31.21 **Laceration without foreign body of penis ♂**
  - X S31.22 **Laceration with foreign body of penis ♂**
  - X S31.23 **Puncture wound without foreign body of penis ♂**
  - X S31.24 **Puncture wound with foreign body of penis ♂**
  - X S31.25 **Open bite of penis ♂**
    Bite of penis NOS
    Excludes1 superficial bite of penis (S30.862, S30.872)
- S31.3 **Open wound of scrotum and testes**
  - X S31.30 **Unspecified open wound of scrotum and testes ♂**
  - X S31.31 **Laceration without foreign body of scrotum and testes ♂**
  - X S31.32 **Laceration with foreign body of scrotum and testes ♂**
  - X S31.33 **Puncture wound without foreign body of scrotum and testes ♂**
  - X S31.34 **Puncture wound with foreign body of scrotum and testes ♂**
  - X S31.35 **Open bite of scrotum and testes ♂**
    Bite of scrotum and testes NOS
    Excludes1 superficial bite of scrotum and testes (S30.863, S30.873)
- S31.4 **Open wound of vagina and vulva**
  Excludes1 injury to vagina and vulva during delivery (O70.-, O71.4)
  - X S31.40 **Unspecified open wound of vagina and vulva ♀**
  - X S31.41 **Laceration without foreign body of vagina and vulva ♀**
  - X S31.42 **Laceration with foreign body of vagina and vulva ♀**
  - X S31.43 **Puncture wound without foreign body of vagina and vulva ♀**
  - X S31.44 **Puncture wound with foreign body of vagina and vulva ♀**
  - X S31.45 **Open bite of vagina and vulva ♀**
    Bite of vagina and vulva NOS
    Excludes1 superficial bite of vagina and vulva (S30.864, S30.874)
- S31.5 **Open wound of unspecified external genital organs**
  Excludes1 traumatic amputation of external genital organs (S38.21, S38.22)
  - S31.50 **Unspecified open wound of unspecified external genital organs**
    - S31.501 **Unspecified open wound of unspecified external genital organs, male ♂**
    - S31.502 **Unspecified open wound of unspecified external genital organs, female ♀**
  - S31.51 **Laceration without foreign body of unspecified external genital organs**
    - S31.511 **Laceration without foreign body of unspecified external genital organs, male ♂**
    - S31.512 **Laceration without foreign body of unspecified external genital organs, female ♀**
  - S31.52 **Laceration with foreign body of unspecified external genital organs**
    - S31.521 **Laceration with foreign body of unspecified external genital organs, male ♂**
    - S31.522 **Laceration with foreign body of unspecified external genital organs, female ♀**
  - S31.53 **Puncture wound without foreign body of unspecified external genital organs**
    - S31.531 **Puncture wound without foreign body of unspecified external genital organs, male ♂**
    - S31.532 **Puncture wound without foreign body of unspecified external genital organs, female ♀**
  - S31.54 **Puncture wound with foreign body of unspecified external genital organs**
    - S31.541 **Puncture wound with foreign body of unspecified external genital organs, male ♂**
    - S31.542 **Puncture wound with foreign body of unspecified external genital organs, female ♀**
  - S31.55 **Open bite of unspecified external genital organs**
    Bite of unspecified external genital organs NOS
    Excludes1 superficial bite of unspecified external genital organs (S30.865, S30.866, S30.875, S30.876)
    - S31.551 **Open bite of unspecified external genital organs, male ♂**
    - S31.552 **Open bite of unspecified external genital organs, female ♀**
- S31.6 **Open wound of abdominal wall with penetration into peritoneal cavity**
  Ex For category S31.6 CC codes: See S31.0
  - S31.60 **Unspecified open wound of abdominal wall with penetration into peritoneal cavity**
    - S31.600 **Unspecified open wound of abdominal wall, right upper quadrant with penetration into peritoneal cavity A**
    - S31.601 **Unspecified open wound of abdominal wall, left upper quadrant with penetration into peritoneal cavity A**
    - S31.602 **Unspecified open wound of abdominal wall, epigastric region with penetration into peritoneal cavity A**

- S31.603 Unspecified open wound of abdominal wall, right lower quadrant with penetration into peritoneal cavity A
- S31.604 Unspecified open wound of abdominal wall, left lower quadrant with penetration into peritoneal cavity A
- S31.605 Unspecified open wound of abdominal wall, periumbilic region with penetration into peritoneal cavity A
- S31.609 Unspecified open wound of abdominal wall, unspecified quadrant with penetration into peritoneal cavity A

- S31.61 Laceration without foreign body of abdominal wall with penetration into peritoneal cavity
  - S31.610 Laceration without foreign body of abdominal wall, right upper quadrant with penetration into peritoneal cavity A
  - S31.611 Laceration without foreign body of abdominal wall, left upper quadrant with penetration into peritoneal cavity A
  - S31.612 Laceration without foreign body of abdominal wall, epigastric region with penetration into peritoneal cavity A
  - S31.613 Laceration without foreign body of abdominal wall, right lower quadrant with penetration into peritoneal cavity A,
    Coding Clinic: 2015, Q4, P37
  - S31.614 Laceration without foreign body of abdominal wall, left lower quadrant with penetration into peritoneal cavity A
  - S31.615 Laceration without foreign body of abdominal wall, periumbilic region with penetration into peritoneal cavity A
  - S31.619 Laceration without foreign body of abdominal wall, unspecified quadrant with penetration into peritoneal cavity A

- S31.62 Laceration with foreign body of abdominal wall with penetration into peritoneal cavity
  - S31.620 Laceration with foreign body of abdominal wall, right upper quadrant with penetration into peritoneal cavity A
  - S31.621 Laceration with foreign body of abdominal wall, left upper quadrant with penetration into peritoneal cavity A
  - S31.622 Laceration with foreign body of abdominal wall, epigastric region with penetration into peritoneal cavity A
  - S31.623 Laceration with foreign body of abdominal wall, right lower quadrant with penetration into peritoneal cavity A
  - S31.624 Laceration with foreign body of abdominal wall, left lower quadrant with penetration into peritoneal cavity A
  - S31.625 Laceration with foreign body of abdominal wall, periumbilic region with penetration into peritoneal cavity A
  - S31.629 Laceration with foreign body of abdominal wall, unspecified quadrant with penetration into peritoneal cavity A

- S31.63 Puncture wound without foreign body of abdominal wall with penetration into peritoneal cavity
  - S31.630 Puncture wound without foreign body of abdominal wall, right upper quadrant with penetration into peritoneal cavity A
  - S31.631 Puncture wound without foreign body of abdominal wall, left upper quadrant with penetration into peritoneal cavity A
  - S31.632 Puncture wound without foreign body of abdominal wall, epigastric region with penetration into peritoneal cavity A
  - S31.633 Puncture wound without foreign body of abdominal wall, right lower quadrant with penetration into peritoneal cavity A
  - S31.634 Puncture wound without foreign body of abdominal wall, left lower quadrant with penetration into peritoneal cavity A
  - S31.635 Puncture wound without foreign body of abdominal wall, periumbilic region with penetration into peritoneal cavity A
  - S31.639 Puncture wound without foreign body of abdominal wall, unspecified quadrant with penetration into peritoneal cavity A

- S31.64 Puncture wound with foreign body of abdominal wall with penetration into peritoneal cavity
  - S31.640 Puncture wound with foreign body of abdominal wall, right upper quadrant with penetration into peritoneal cavity A
  - S31.641 Puncture wound with foreign body of abdominal wall, left upper quadrant with penetration into peritoneal cavity A
  - S31.642 Puncture wound with foreign body of abdominal wall, epigastric region with penetration into peritoneal cavity A
  - S31.643 Puncture wound with foreign body of abdominal wall, right lower quadrant with penetration into peritoneal cavity A
  - S31.644 Puncture wound with foreign body of abdominal wall, left lower quadrant with penetration into peritoneal cavity A
  - S31.645 Puncture wound with foreign body of abdominal wall, periumbilic region with penetration into peritoneal cavity A
  - S31.649 Puncture wound with foreign body of abdominal wall, unspecified quadrant with penetration into peritoneal cavity A

- **S31.65 Open bite of abdominal wall with penetration into peritoneal cavity**
  - **Excludes1** superficial bite of abdominal wall (S30.861, S30.871)
  - **S31.650 Open bite of abdominal wall, right upper quadrant with penetration into peritoneal cavity** A
  - **S31.651 Open bite of abdominal wall, left upper quadrant with penetration into peritoneal cavity** A
  - **S31.652 Open bite of abdominal wall, epigastric region with penetration into peritoneal cavity** A
  - **S31.653 Open bite of abdominal wall, right lower quadrant with penetration into peritoneal cavity** A
  - **S31.654 Open bite of abdominal wall, left lower quadrant with penetration into peritoneal cavity** A
  - **S31.655 Open bite of abdominal wall, periumbilic region with penetration into peritoneal cavity** A
  - **S31.659 Open bite of abdominal wall, unspecified quadrant with penetration into peritoneal cavity** A
- **S31.8 Open wound of other parts of abdomen, lower back and pelvis**
  - **S31.80 Open wound of unspecified buttock**
    - **S31.801 Laceration without foreign body of unspecified buttock**
    - **S31.802 Laceration with foreign body of unspecified buttock**
    - **S31.803 Puncture wound without foreign body of unspecified buttock**
    - **S31.804 Puncture wound with foreign body of unspecified buttock**
    - **S31.805 Open bite of unspecified buttock**
      Bite of buttock NOS
      - **Excludes1** superficial bite of buttock (S30.870)
    - **S31.809 Unspecified open wound of unspecified buttock**
  - **S31.81 Open wound of right buttock**
    - **S31.811 Laceration without foreign body of right buttock**
    - **S31.812 Laceration with foreign body of right buttock**
    - **S31.813 Puncture wound without foreign body of right buttock**
    - **S31.814 Puncture wound with foreign body of right buttock**
    - **S31.815 Open bite of right buttock**
      Bite of right buttock NOS
      - **Excludes1** superficial bite of buttock (S30.870)
    - **S31.819 Unspecified open wound of right buttock**
  - **S31.82 Open wound of left buttock**
    - **S31.821 Laceration without foreign body of left buttock**
    - **S31.822 Laceration with foreign body of left buttock**
    - **S31.823 Puncture wound without foreign body of left buttock**
    - **S31.824 Puncture wound with foreign body of left buttock**
    - **S31.825 Open bite of left buttock**
      Bite of left buttock NOS
      - **Excludes1** superficial bite of buttock (S30.870)
    - **S31.829 Unspecified open wound of left buttock**
  - **S31.83 Open wound of anus**
    - **S31.831 Laceration without foreign body of anus**
    - **S31.832 Laceration with foreign body of anus**
    - **S31.833 Puncture wound without foreign body of anus**
    - **S31.834 Puncture wound with foreign body of anus**
    - **S31.835 Open bite of anus**
      Bite of anus NOS
      - **Excludes1** superficial bite of anus (S30.877)
    - **S31.839 Unspecified open wound of anus**
- **S32 Fracture of lumbar spine and pelvis**

  Note: A fracture not indicated as displaced or nondisplaced should be coded to displaced

  A fracture not indicated as opened or closed should be coded to closed

  Includes fracture of lumbosacral neural arch
  fracture of lumbosacral spinous process
  fracture of lumbosacral transverse process
  fracture of lumbosacral vertebra
  fracture of lumbosacral vertebral arch

  Code first any associated spinal cord and spinal nerve injury (S34.-)

  Excludes1 transection of abdomen (S38.3)

  Excludes2 fracture of hip NOS (S72.0-)

  The appropriate 7th character is to be added to each code from category S32

A	initial encounter for closed fracture
B	initial encounter for open fracture
D	subsequent encounter for fracture with routine healing
G	subsequent encounter for fracture with delayed healing
K	subsequent encounter for fracture with nonunion
S	sequela

  - **S32.0 Fracture of lumbar vertebra**
    Fracture of lumbar spine NOS
    Ex **For category S32.0 CC codes S32.0[A,B]:** M48.40X-M48.58X[S], M80.08X[S], M80.88X[S], M84.350[S], M84.454[S], M84.550[S], M84.58X[S], M84.650[S], M99.13, M99.15-M99.17, M99.19, S03.1XX[A], S03.8XX-S03.9XX[A], S12.000-S12.9XX[S], S13.9XX[A], S14.109[A], S14.119[A], S14.129[A], S14.139[A], S14.149[A], S14.159[A], S22.000-S22.9XX[S], S23.20X-S23.29X[A], S23.9XX[A], S24.109[A], S24.119[A], S24.139[A], S24.149[A], S24.159[A], S29.001-S29.019[A], S29.091-S29.9XX[A], S32.000-S32.059[A,B,S], S32.10X-S32.9XX[S], S33.0XX-S33.141[A], S33.30X-S33.39X[A], S33.5XX[A], S33.9XX[A], S34.01X[A], S34.101-S34.129[A], S38.1XX[A], S38.3XX-S39.013[A], S39.091-S39.94X[A], T14.90-T14.91, T79.8XX-T79.9XX[A], T79.A0X-T79.A9X[A] **For S32.0[K]:** See S02.0[K]
    - **S32.00 Fracture of unspecified lumbar vertebra**
      - **S32.000 Wedge compression fracture of unspecified lumbar vertebra** A, K, B, A, B
      - **S32.001 Stable burst fracture of unspecified lumbar vertebra** A, K, B, A, B
      - **S32.002 Unstable burst fracture of unspecified lumbar vertebra** A, K, B, A, B
      - **S32.008 Other fracture of unspecified lumbar vertebra** A, K, B, A, B
      - **S32.009 Unspecified fracture of unspecified lumbar vertebra** A, K, B, A, B

- **S32.01** Fracture of first lumbar vertebra
  - **S32.010** Wedge compression fracture of first lumbar vertebra A, K, B, A, B
  - **S32.011** Stable burst fracture of first lumbar vertebra A, K, B, A, B
  - **S32.012** Unstable burst fracture of first lumbar vertebra A, K, B, A, B
  - **S32.018** Other fracture of first lumbar vertebra A, K, B, A, B
  - **S32.019** Unspecified fracture of first lumbar vertebra A, K, B, A, B
- **S32.02** Fracture of second lumbar vertebra
  - **S32.020** Wedge compression fracture of second lumbar vertebra A, K, B, A, B
  - **S32.021** Stable burst fracture of second lumbar vertebra A, K, B, A, B
  - **S32.022** Unstable burst fracture of second lumbar vertebra A, K, B, A, B
  - **S32.028** Other fracture of second lumbar vertebra A, K, B, A, B
  - **S32.029** Unspecified fracture of second lumbar vertebra A, K, B, A, B
- **S32.03** Fracture of third lumbar vertebra
  - **S32.030** Wedge compression fracture of third lumbar vertebra A, K, B, A, B
  - **S32.031** Stable burst fracture of third lumbar vertebra A, K, B, A, B
  - **S32.032** Unstable burst fracture of third lumbar vertebra A, K, B, A, B
  - **S32.038** Other fracture of third lumbar vertebra A, K, B, A, B
  - **S32.039** Unspecified fracture of third lumbar vertebra A, K, B, A, B
- **S32.04** Fracture of fourth lumbar vertebra
  - **S32.040** Wedge compression fracture of fourth lumbar vertebra A, K, B, A, B
  - **S32.041** Stable burst fracture of fourth lumbar vertebra A, K, B, A, B
  - **S32.042** Unstable burst fracture of fourth lumbar vertebra A, K, B, A, B
  - **S32.048** Other fracture of fourth lumbar vertebra A, K, B, A, B
  - **S32.049** Unspecified fracture of fourth lumbar vertebra A, K, B, A, B
- **S32.05** Fracture of fifth lumbar vertebra
  - **S32.050** Wedge compression fracture of fifth lumbar vertebra A, K, B, A, B
  - **S32.051** Stable burst fracture of fifth lumbar vertebra A, K, B, A, B
  - **S32.052** Unstable burst fracture of fifth lumbar vertebra A, K, B, A, B
  - **S32.058** Other fracture of fifth lumbar vertebra A, K, B, A, B
  - **S32.059** Unspecified fracture of fifth lumbar vertebra A, K, B, A, B

- **S32.1** Fracture of sacrum

  For vertical fractures, code to most medial fracture extension

  Use two codes if both a vertical and transverse fracture are present

  Code also any associated fracture of pelvic ring (S32.8-)

  Ex: **For category S32.1 CC codes S32.1[A,B]:** M48.40X-M48.58X[S], M80.08X[S], M80.88X[S], M84.350[S], M84.454[S], M84.550[S], M84.58X[S], M84.650[S], M99.14-M99.17, M99.19, S03.1XX[A], S03.8XX-S03.9XX[A], S12.000-S12.9XX[S], S13.9XX[A], S14.109[A], S14.119[A], S14.129[A], S14.139[A], S14.149[A], S14.159[A], S22.000-S22.9XX[S], S23.20X[A], S23.29X[A], S23.9XX[A], S24.109[A], S24.119[A], S24.139[A], S24.149[A], S24.159[A], S29.001-S29.019[A], S29.091-S29.9XX[A], S32.000-S32.059[S], S32.10X-S32.2XX[A,B,S], S32.301-S32.9XX[S], S33.2XX-S33.4XX[A], S33.6XX-S33.9XX[A], S34.02X[A], S34.131-S34.3XX[A], S38.1XX[A], S38.3XX[A], S39.001-S39.013[A], S39.091-39.94X[A], T14.90-T14.91, T79.8XX-T79.9XX[A], T79.A0X-T79.A9X[A] **For S32.1[K]:** See S02.0[K]

  - X **S32.10** Unspecified fracture of sacrum A, K, B, A, B
  - **S32.11** Zone I fracture of sacrum

    Vertical sacral ala fracture of sacrum
    - **S32.110** Nondisplaced Zone I fracture of sacrum A, K, B, A, B
    - **S32.111** Minimally displaced Zone I fracture of sacrum A, K, B, A, B
    - **S32.112** Severely displaced Zone I fracture of sacrum A, K, B, A, B
    - **S32.119** Unspecified Zone I fracture of sacrum A, K, B, A, B
  - **S32.12** Zone II fracture of sacrum

    Vertical foraminal region fracture of sacrum
    - **S32.120** Nondisplaced Zone II fracture of sacrum A, K, B, A, B
    - **S32.121** Minimally displaced Zone II fracture of sacrum A, K, B, A, B
    - **S32.122** Severely displaced Zone II fracture of sacrum A, K, B, A, B
    - **S32.129** Unspecified Zone II fracture of sacrum A, K, B, A, B
  - **S32.13** Zone III fracture of sacrum

    Vertical fracture into spinal canal region of sacrum
    - **S32.130** Nondisplaced Zone III fracture of sacrum A, K, B, A, B
    - **S32.131** Minimally displaced Zone III fracture of sacrum A, K, B, A, B
    - **S32.132** Severely displaced Zone III fracture of sacrum A, K, B, A, B
    - **S32.139** Unspecified Zone III fracture of sacrum A, K, B, A, B
  - X **S32.14** Type 1 fracture of sacrum A, K, B, A, B

    Transverse flexion fracture of sacrum without displacement
  - X **S32.15** Type 2 fracture of sacrum A, K, B, A, B

    Transverse flexion fracture of sacrum with posterior displacement
  - X **S32.16** Type 3 fracture of sacrum A, K, B, A, B

    Transverse extension fracture of sacrum with anterior displacement
  - X **S32.17** Type 4 fracture of sacrum A, K, B, A, B

    Transverse segmental comminution of upper sacrum
  - X **S32.19** Other fracture of sacrum A, K, B, A, B
- X **S32.2** Fracture of coccyx A, K, B, A, B

  Ex: **For category S32.2 CC codes S32.2[A,B]:** See S32.1 [A,B]
  For S32.2[K]: See S02.0[K]

- **S32.3** Fracture of ilium

  Excludes1 fracture of ilium with associated disruption of pelvic ring (S32.8-)

  Ex: **For category S32.3 CC codes S32.3[A]:** See S22.9 **For S32.3[B]:** M48.40X-M48.58X[A], M80.00X-M80.88X[A], M84.30X-M84.68X[A], M84.750-M84.759[A], S03.8XX-S03.9XX[A], S22.9XX[A,B], S29.011-S29.019[A], S32.301-S32.399[A,B], S32.810-S32.9XX[A,B], S33.4XX[A], S33.6XX-S33.8XX[A], S38.3XX[A], S39.011-S39.013[A], S73.001-S73.199[A], S76.001-S76.019[A], S76.091-S76.119[A], S76.191-S76.219[A], S76.291-S76.319[A], S76.391-S76.819[A], S76.891-S76.919[A], S76.991-S76.999[A], S79.811-S79.929[A], T14.90-T14.91, T79.8XX-T79.9XX[A], T79.A0X-T79.A9X[A]
  For S32.3[K]: See S02.0[K]

  - **S32.30** Unspecified fracture of ilium
    - **S32.301** Unspecified fracture of right ilium A, K, B, A, B
    - **S32.302** Unspecified fracture of left ilium A, K, B, A, B
    - **S32.309** Unspecified fracture of unspecified ilium A, K, B, A, B
  - **S32.31** Avulsion fracture of ilium
    - **S32.311** Displaced avulsion fracture of right ilium A, K, B, A, B
    - **S32.312** Displaced avulsion fracture of left ilium A, K, B, A, B
    - **S32.313** Displaced avulsion fracture of unspecified ilium A, K, B, A, B
    - **S32.314** Nondisplaced avulsion fracture of right ilium A, K, B, A, B
    - **S32.315** Nondisplaced avulsion fracture of left ilium A, K, B, A, B
    - **S32.316** Nondisplaced avulsion fracture of unspecified ilium A, K, B, A, B
  - **S32.39** Other fracture of ilium
    - **S32.391** Other fracture of right ilium A, K, B, A, B
    - **S32.392** Other fracture of left ilium A, K, B, A, B
    - **S32.399** Other fracture of unspecified ilium A, K, B, A, B

- **S32.4** Fracture of acetabulum

  Code also any associated fracture of pelvic ring (S32.8-)

  Ex: **For category S32.4 CC codes S32.4[A]:** M48.40X-M48.58X[A], M80.00X-M80.88X[A], M84.30X-M84.68X[A], M84.750-M84.759[A], S03.8XX-S03.9XX[A], S22.9XX [A,B], S29.011-S29.019[A], S32.401-S32.499[A,B], S32.810-S32.811[A,B], S32.89X-S32.9XX[A,B], S33.4XX[A], S33.6XX-S33.8XX[A], S38.3XX[A], S39.011-S39.013[A], S73.001-S73.199[A], S76.001-S76.019[A], S76.091-S76.119[A], S76.191-S76.219[A], S76.291-S76.319[A], S76.391-S76.819[A], S76.891-S76.919[A], S76.991-S76.999[A], S79.811-S79.829[A], S79.911-S79.929[A], T14.90-T14.91, T79.8XX-T79.9XX[A], T79.A0X-T79.A9X[A] **For S32.4[B]:** S03.8XX-S03.9XX[A], S22.9XX [A,B], S29.011-S29.019[A], S32.401-S32.499[A,B], S32.810-S32.811[A,B], S32.89X-S32.9XX[A,B], S33.4XX[A], S33.6XX-S33.8XX[A], S38.3XX[A], S39.011-S39.013[A], S73.001-S73.199[A], S76.001-S76.019[A], S76.091-S76.119[A], S76.191-S76.219[A], S76.291-S76.319[A], S76.391-S76.819[A], S76.891-S76.919[A], S76.991-S76.999[A], S79.811-S79.929[A], T14.90-T14.91, T79.A0X-T79.A9X[A], T79.8XX-T79.9XX[A]
  For S32.4[K]: See S02.0[K]

  - **S32.40** Unspecified fracture of acetabulum
    - **S32.401** Unspecified fracture of right acetabulum K, A, B, A, B
    - **S32.402** Unspecified fracture of left acetabulum K, A, B, A, B
    - **S32.409** Unspecified fracture of unspecified acetabulum K, A, B, A, B
  - **S32.41** Fracture of anterior wall of acetabulum
    - **S32.411** Displaced fracture of anterior wall of right acetabulum K, A, B, A, B
    - **S32.412** Displaced fracture of anterior wall of left acetabulum K, A, B, A, B
    - **S32.413** Displaced fracture of anterior wall of unspecified acetabulum K, A, B, A, B
    - **S32.414** Nondisplaced fracture of anterior wall of right acetabulum K, A, B, A, B
    - **S32.415** Nondisplaced fracture of anterior wall of left acetabulum K, A, B, A, B
    - **S32.416** Nondisplaced fracture of anterior wall of unspecified acetabulum K, A, B, A, B
  - **S32.42** Fracture of posterior wall of acetabulum
    - **S32.421** Displaced fracture of posterior wall of right acetabulum K, A, B, A, B
    - **S32.422** Displaced fracture of posterior wall of left acetabulum K, A, B, A, B
    - **S32.423** Displaced fracture of posterior wall of unspecified acetabulum K, A, B, A, B
    - **S32.424** Nondisplaced fracture of posterior wall of right acetabulum K, A, B, A, B
    - **S32.425** Nondisplaced fracture of posterior wall of left acetabulum K, A, B, A, B
    - **S32.426** Nondisplaced fracture of posterior wall of unspecified acetabulum K, A, B, A, B
  - **S32.43** Fracture of anterior column [iliopubic] of acetabulum
    - **S32.431** Displaced fracture of anterior column [iliopubic] of right acetabulum K, A, B, A, B
    - **S32.432** Displaced fracture of anterior column [iliopubic] of left acetabulum K, A, B, A, B
    - **S32.433** Displaced fracture of anterior column [iliopubic] of unspecified acetabulum K, A, B, A, B
    - **S32.434** Nondisplaced fracture of anterior column [iliopubic] of right acetabulum K, A, B, A, B
    - **S32.435** Nondisplaced fracture of anterior column [iliopubic] of left acetabulum K, A, B, A, B
    - **S32.436** Nondisplaced fracture of anterior column [iliopubic] of unspecified acetabulum K, A, B, A, B
  - **S32.44** Fracture of posterior column [ilioischial] of acetabulum
    - **S32.441** Displaced fracture of posterior column [ilioischial] of right acetabulum K, A, B, A, B
    - **S32.442** Displaced fracture of posterior column [ilioischial] of left acetabulum K, A, B, A, B
    - **S32.443** Displaced fracture of posterior column [ilioischial] of unspecified acetabulum K, A, B, A, B
    - **S32.444** Nondisplaced fracture of posterior column [ilioischial] of right acetabulum K, A, B, A, B
    - **S32.445** Nondisplaced fracture of posterior column [ilioischial] of left acetabulum K, A, B, A, B
    - **S32.446** Nondisplaced fracture of posterior column [ilioischial] of unspecified acetabulum K, A, B, A, B

- **S32.45** Transverse fracture of acetabulum
  - **S32.451** Displaced transverse fracture of right acetabulum K, A, B, A, B
  - **S32.452** Displaced transverse fracture of left acetabulum K, A, B, A, B
  - **S32.453** Displaced transverse fracture of unspecified acetabulum K, A, B, A, B
  - **S32.454** Nondisplaced transverse fracture of right acetabulum K, A, B, A, B
  - **S32.455** Nondisplaced transverse fracture of left acetabulum K, A, B, A, B
  - **S32.456** Nondisplaced transverse fracture of unspecified acetabulum K, A, B, A, B
- **S32.46** Associated transverse-posterior fracture of acetabulum
  - **S32.461** Displaced associated transverse-posterior fracture of right acetabulum K, A, B, A, B
  - **S32.462** Displaced associated transverse-posterior fracture of left acetabulum K, A, B, A, B
  - **S32.463** Displaced associated transverse-posterior fracture of unspecified acetabulum K, A, B, A, B
  - **S32.464** Nondisplaced associated transverse-posterior fracture of right acetabulum K, A, B, A, B
  - **S32.465** Nondisplaced associated transverse-posterior fracture of left acetabulum K, A, B, A, B
  - **S32.466** Nondisplaced associated transverse-posterior fracture of unspecified acetabulum K, A, B, A, B
- **S32.47** Fracture of medial wall of acetabulum
  - **S32.471** Displaced fracture of medial wall of right acetabulum K, A, B, A, B
  - **S32.472** Displaced fracture of medial wall of left acetabulum K, A, B, A, B
  - **S32.473** Displaced fracture of medial wall of unspecified acetabulum K, A, B, A, B
  - **S32.474** Nondisplaced fracture of medial wall of right acetabulum K, A, B, A, B
  - **S32.475** Nondisplaced fracture of medial wall of left acetabulum K, A, B, A, B
  - **S32.476** Nondisplaced fracture of medial wall of unspecified acetabulum K, A, B, A, B
- **S32.48** Dome fracture of acetabulum
  - **S32.481** Displaced dome fracture of right acetabulum K, A, B, A, B
  - **S32.482** Displaced dome fracture of left acetabulum K, A, B, A, B
  - **S32.483** Displaced dome fracture of unspecified acetabulum K, A, B, A, B
  - **S32.484** Nondisplaced dome fracture of right acetabulum K, A, B, A, B
  - **S32.485** Nondisplaced dome fracture of left acetabulum K, A, B, A, B
  - **S32.486** Nondisplaced dome fracture of unspecified acetabulum K, A, B, A, B
- **S32.49** Other fracture of acetabulum
  - **S32.491** Other fracture of right acetabulum K, A, B, A, B
  - **S32.492** Other fracture of left acetabulum K, A, B, A, B
  - **S32.499** Other fracture of unspecified acetabulum K, A, B, A, B
- **S32.5** Fracture of pubis

  Excludes1 fracture of pubis with associated disruption of pelvic ring (S32.8-)

  Ex: **For category S32.5 CC codes S32.5[A,B]:** M48.40X-M48.58X[A], M80.00X-M80.88X[A], M84.30X-M84.68X[A], M84.750-M84.759[A], S03.8XX-S03.9XX[A], S22.9XX [A,B], S29.011-S29.019[A], S32.501A-S32.599[A,B], S32.810-S32.811[A,B], S32.89X-S32.9XX[A,B], S33.4XX[A], S33.6XX-S33.8XX[A], S38.3XX-S39.013[A], S73.001-S73.199[A], S76.001-S76.019[A], S76.091-S76.119[A], S76.191-S76.219[A], S76.291-S76.319[A], S76.391-S76.819[A], S76.891-S76.919[A], S76.991-S76.999[A], S79.811-S79.929[A], T14.90-T14.91,T79.A0X-T79.A9X[A], T79.8XX-T79.9XX[A] **For S32.5[K]:** See S02.0[K]
  - **S32.50** Unspecified fracture of pubis
    - **S32.501** Unspecified fracture of right pubis A, K, B, A, B
    - **S32.502** Unspecified fracture of left pubis A, K, B, A, B
    - **S32.509** Unspecified fracture of unspecified pubis A, K, B, A, B
  - **S32.51** Fracture of superior rim of pubis
    - **S32.511** Fracture of superior rim of right pubis A, K, B, A, B
    - **S32.512** Fracture of superior rim of left pubis A, K, B, A, B
    - **S32.519** Fracture of superior rim of unspecified pubis A, K, B, A, B
  - **S32.59** Other specified fracture of pubis
    - **S32.591** Other specified fracture of right pubis A, K, B, A, B
    - **S32.592** Other specified fracture of left pubis A, K, B, A, B
    - **S32.599** Other specified fracture of unspecified pubis A, K, B, A, B
- **S32.6** Fracture of ischium

  Excludes1 fracture of ischium with associated disruption of pelvic ring (S32.8-)

  Ex: **For category S32.6 CC codes S32.6[A]:** S32.601-S32.699[A] **For S32.6[B]:** M48.40X-M48.58X[A], M80.00X-M80.88X[A], M84.30X-M84.68X[A], M84.750-M84.759[A], S03.8XX-S03.9XX[A], S22.9XX[A,B], S29.011-S29.019[A], S32.601-S32.811[A,B], S32.89X-S32.9XX[A,B], S33.4XX[A], S33.6XX-S33.8XX[A], S38.3XX[A], S39.011-S39.013[A], S73.001-S73.199[A], S76.001-S76.019[A], S76.091-S76.119[A], S76.191-S76.219[A], S76.291-S76.319[A], S76.391-S76.819[A], S76.891-S76.919[A], S76.991-S76.999[A], S79.811-S79.929[A], T14.90-T14.91, T79.A0X-T79.A9X[A], T79.8XX-T79.9XX[A] **For S32.5[K]:** See S02.0[K]
  - **S32.60** Unspecified fracture of ischium
    - **S32.601** Unspecified fracture of right ischium A, K, B, A, B
    - **S32.602** Unspecified fracture of left ischium A, K, B, A, B
    - **S32.609** Unspecified fracture of unspecified ischium A, K, B, A, B

● **S32.61 Avulsion fracture of ischium**

● **S32.611 Displaced avulsion fracture of right ischium** A, K, B, A, B

● **S32.612 Displaced avulsion fracture of left ischium** A, K, B, A, B

● **S32.613 Displaced avulsion fracture of unspecified ischium** A, K, B, A, B

● **S32.614 Nondisplaced avulsion fracture of right ischium** A, K, B, A, B

● **S32.615 Nondisplaced avulsion fracture of left ischium** A, K, B, A, B

● **S32.616 Nondisplaced avulsion fracture of unspecified ischium** A, K, B, A, B

● **S32.69 Other specified fracture of ischium**

● **S32.691 Other specified fracture of right ischium** A, K, B, A, B

● **S32.692 Other specified fracture of left ischium** A, K, B, A, B

● **S32.699 Other specified fracture of unspecified ischium** A, K, B, A, B

● **S32.8 Fracture of other parts of pelvis**

Code also any associated:
fracture of acetabulum (S32.4-)
sacral fracture (S32.1-)

● **S32.81 Multiple fractures of pelvis with disruption of pelvic ring**

Multiple pelvic fractures with disruption of pelvic circle

Ex: **For category S32.81 CC codes S32.81[A,B]:** M48.40X-M48.58X[A], M80.00X-M80.88X[A], M84.30X-M84.68X[A], M84.750-M84.759[A], S03.8XX-S03.9XX[A], S22.9XX[A,B], S29.011-S29.019[A], S32.301-S32.811[A,B], S32.89X-S32.9XX[A,B], S33.4XX[A], S33.6XX-S33.8XX[A], S38.3XX[A], S39.011-S39.013[A], S73.001-S73.199[A], S76.001-S76.019[A], S76.091-S76.119[A], S76.191-S76.219[A], S76.291-S76.319[A], S76.391-S76.819[A], S76.891-S76.919[A], S76.991-S76.999[A], S79.811-S79.929[A], T14.90-T14.91, T79.A0X-T79.A9X[A], T79.8XX-T79.9XX[A] **For S32.81[K]:** See S02.0[K]

● **S32.810 Multiple fractures of pelvis with stable disruption of pelvic ring** A, K, B, A, B

● **S32.811 Multiple fractures of pelvis with unstable disruption of pelvic ring** A, K, B, A, B

X ● **S32.82 Multiple fractures of pelvis without disruption of pelvic ring** A, K, B, A, B

Multiple pelvic fractures without disruption of pelvic circle

Ex: **For category S32.82 CC codes S32.82[A,B]:** S32.89X[A] **For S32.81[K]:** See S32.0[K]

X ● **S32.89 Fracture of other parts of pelvis** A, K, B, A, B

Ex: **For category S32.89 CC codes S32.89[A,B]:** M48.40X-M48.58X[A], M80.00X-M80.88X[A], M84.30X-M84.68X[A], M84.750-M84.759[A], S03.8XX-S03.9XX[A], S22.9XX[A,B], S29.011-S29.019[A], S32.301-S32.9XX[A,B], S33.4XX[A], S33.6XX-S33.8XX[A], S38.3XX[A], S39.011-S39.013[A], S73.001-S73.199[A], S76.001-S76.019[A], S76.091-S76.119[A], S76.191-S76.219[A], 76.291-S76.319[A], S76.391-S76.819[A], S76.891-S76.919[A], S76.991-S76.999[A], S79.811-S79.929[A], T14.90-T14.91, T79.A0X-T79.A9X[A], T79.8XX-T79.9XX[A] **For S32.89[K]:** See S02.0[K]

X ● **S32.9 Fracture of unspecified parts of lumbosacral spine and pelvis** A, K, B, A, B

Fracture of lumbosacral spine NOS
Fracture of pelvis NOS

Ex: **For category S32.9 CC codes S32.9[A,B]:** See S32.81 **For S32.9[K]:** See S32.0[K]

Coding Clinic: 2012, Q4, P93

● **S33 Dislocation and sprain of joints and ligaments of lumbar spine and pelvis**

Includes avulsion of joint or ligament of lumbar spine and pelvis
laceration of cartilage, joint or ligament of lumbar spine and pelvis
sprain of cartilage, joint or ligament of lumbar spine and pelvis
traumatic hemarthrosis of joint or ligament of lumbar spine and pelvis
traumatic rupture of joint or ligament of lumbar spine and pelvis
traumatic subluxation of joint or ligament of lumbar spine and pelvis
traumatic tear of joint or ligament of lumbar spine and pelvis

Code also any associated open wound

Excludes1 nontraumatic rupture or displacement of lumbar intervertebral disc NOS (M51.-)
obstetric damage to pelvic joints and ligaments (O71.6)

Excludes2 dislocation and sprain of joints and ligaments of hip (S73.-)
strain of muscle of lower back and pelvis (S39.01-)

The appropriate 7th character is to be added to each code from category S33

A	initial encounter
D	subsequent encounter
S	sequela

X ● **S33.0 Traumatic rupture of lumbar intervertebral disc**

Excludes1 rupture or displacement (nontraumatic) of lumbar intervertebral disc NOS (M51.- with fifth character 6)

● **S33.1 Subluxation and dislocation of lumbar vertebra**

Code also any associated:
open wound of abdomen, lower back and pelvis (S31)
spinal cord injury (S24.0, S24.1-, S34.0-, S34.1-)

Excludes2 fracture of lumbar vertebrae (S32.0-)

● **S33.10 Subluxation and dislocation of unspecified lumbar vertebra**

● **S33.100 Subluxation of unspecified lumbar vertebra**

● **S33.101 Dislocation of unspecified lumbar vertebra**

● **S33.11 Subluxation and dislocation of L_1/L_2 lumbar vertebra**

● **S33.110 Subluxation of L_1/L_2 lumbar vertebra**

● **S33.111 Dislocation of L_1/L_2 lumbar vertebra**

● **S33.12 Subluxation and dislocation of L_2/L_3 lumbar vertebra**

● **S33.120 Subluxation of L_2/L_3 lumbar vertebra**

● **S33.121 Dislocation of L_2/L_3 lumbar vertebra**

● **S33.13 Subluxation and dislocation of L_3/L_4 lumbar vertebra**

● **S33.130 Subluxation of L_3/L_4 lumbar vertebra**

● **S33.131 Dislocation of L_3/L_4 lumbar vertebra**

● **S33.14 Subluxation and dislocation of L_4/L_5 lumbar vertebra**

● **S33.140 Subluxation of L_4/L_5 lumbar vertebra**

● **S33.141 Dislocation of L_4/L_5 lumbar vertebra**

X ● **S33.2 Dislocation of sacroiliac and sacrococcygeal joint**

● **S33.3 Dislocation of other and unspecified parts of lumbar spine and pelvis**

X ● **S33.30 Dislocation of unspecified parts of lumbar spine and pelvis**

X ● **S33.39 Dislocation of other parts of lumbar spine and pelvis**

X● **S33.4** **Traumatic rupture of symphysis pubis**
X● **S33.5** **Sprain of ligaments of lumbar spine**
X● **S33.6** **Sprain of sacroiliac joint**
X● **S33.8** **Sprain of other parts of lumbar spine and pelvis**
X● **S33.9** **Sprain of unspecified parts of lumbar spine and pelvis**

● **S34** **Injury of lumbar and sacral spinal cord and nerves at abdomen, lower back and pelvis level**

Note: Code to highest level of lumbar cord injury

Injuries to the spinal cord (S34.0 and S34.1) refer to the cord level and not bone level injury, and can affect nerve roots at and below the level given.

The appropriate 7th character is to be added to each code from category S34

A	initial encounter
D	subsequent encounter
S	sequela

Code also any associated:
fracture of vertebra (S22.0-, S32.0-)
open wound of abdomen, lower back and pelvis (S31.-)
transient paralysis (R29.5)

Ex **For category S34 CC codes unless otherwise indicated:** M48.40X-M48.58X[S], M80.08X[S], M80.88X[S], M84.350[S], M84.454[S], M84.550[S], M84.58X[S], M84.650[S], M99.15-M99.17, M99.19, S03.1XX[A], S12.000-S12.9XX[S], S13.9XX[A], S14.109[A], S14.119[A], S14.129[A], S14.139[A], S14.149[A], S14.159[A], S22.000-S22.9XX[S], S23.20X[A], S23.29X[A], S23.9XX[A], S24.109[A], S24.119[A], S24.139[A], S24.149[A]c, S24.159[A], S29.001-S29.009[A], S29.091-S29.9XX[A], S32.000-S32.9XX[S], S33.30X-S33.39X[A], S33.9XX-S34.01X[A], S34.101-S34.129[A], S38.1XX[A], S39.001-S39.003[A], S39.091-S39.94X[A], T14.90-T14.91, T79.A0X-T79.A9X[A], T79.8XX-T79.9XX[A]

● **S34.0** **Concussion and edema of lumbar and sacral spinal cord**

X● **S34.01** **Concussion and edema of lumbar spinal cord** A

X● **S34.02** **Concussion and edema of sacral spinal cord** A

Concussion and edema of conus medullaris

Ex M48.40X-M48.58X[S], M80.08X[S], M80.88X[S], M84.350[S], M84.454[S], M84.550[S], M84.58X[S], M84.650[S], M99.15-M99.17, M99.19, S03.1XX[A], S12.000-S12.9XX[S], S13.9XX[A], S14.109[A], S14.119[A], S14.129[A], S14.139[A], S14.149[A], S14.159[A], S22.000-S22.9XX[S], S23.20X-S23.29X[A], S23.9XX[A], S24.109[A], S24.119[A], S24.139[A], S24.149[A], S24.159[A], S29.001-S29.009[A], S29.091-S29.9XX[A], S32.000-S32.9XX[S], S33.30X-S33.39X[A], S33.9XX[A], S34.02X[A], S34.131-S34.139[A], S34.3XX[A], S38.1XX[A], S39.001-S39.003[A], S39.091-S39.94X[A], T14.90-T14.91, T79.A0X-T79.A9X[A], T79.8XX-T79.9XX[A]

● **S34.1** **Other and unspecified injury of lumbar and sacral spinal cord**

● **S34.10** **Unspecified injury to lumbar spinal cord**

● **S34.101** **Unspecified injury to L_1 level of lumbar spinal cord** A, A
Unspecified injury to lumbar spinal cord level 1 ◀

● **S34.102** **Unspecified injury to L_2 level of lumbar spinal cord** A, A
Unspecified injury to lumbar spinal cord level 2 ◀

● **S34.103** **Unspecified injury to L_3 level of lumbar spinal cord** A, A
Unspecified injury to lumbar spinal cord level 3 ◀

● **S34.104** **Unspecified injury to L_4 level of lumbar spinal cord** A, A
Unspecified injury to lumbar spinal cord level 4 ◀

● **S34.105** **Unspecified injury to L_5 level of lumbar spinal cord** A, A
Unspecified injury to lumbar spinal cord level 5 ◀

● **S34.109** **Unspecified injury to unspecified level of lumbar spinal cord** A, A

● **S34.11** **Complete lesion of lumbar spinal cord**

● **S34.111** **Complete lesion of L_1 level of lumbar spinal cord** A, A
Complete lesion of lumbar spinal cord level 1 ◀

● **S34.112** **Complete lesion of L_2 level of lumbar spinal cord** A, A
Complete lesion of lumbar spinal cord level 2 ◀

● **S34.113** **Complete lesion of L_3 level of lumbar spinal cord** A, A
Complete lesion of lumbar spinal cord level 3 ◀

● **S34.114** **Complete lesion of L_4 level of lumbar spinal cord** A, A
Complete lesion of lumbar spinal cord level 4 ◀

● **S34.115** **Complete lesion of L_5 level of lumbar spinal cord** A, A
Complete lesion of lumbar spinal cord level 5 ◀

● **S34.119** **Complete lesion of unspecified level of lumbar spinal cord** A, A

● **S34.12** **Incomplete lesion of lumbar spinal cord**

● **S34.121** **Incomplete lesion of L_1 level of lumbar spinal cord** A, A
Incomplete lesion of lumbar spinal cord level 1 ◀

● **S34.122** **Incomplete lesion of L_2 level of lumbar spinal cord** A, A
Incomplete lesion of lumbar spinal cord level 2 ◀

● **S34.123** **Incomplete lesion of L_3 level of lumbar spinal cord** A, A
Incomplete lesion of lumbar spinal cord level 3 ◀

● **S34.124** **Incomplete lesion of L_4 level of lumbar spinal cord** A, A
Incomplete lesion of lumbar spinal cord level 4 ◀

● **S34.125** **Incomplete lesion of L_5 level of lumbar spinal cord** A, A
Incomplete lesion of lumbar spinal cord level 5 ◀

● **S34.129** **Incomplete lesion of unspecified level of lumbar spinal cord** A, A

● **S34.13** **Other and unspecified injury to sacral spinal cord**

Other injury to conus medullaris

Ex **For category S34.13 CC codes:** See S32.04

● **S34.131** **Complete lesion of sacral spinal cord** A, A
Complete lesion of conus medullaris

● **S34.132** **Incomplete lesion of sacral spinal cord** A, A
Incomplete lesion of conus medullaris

● **S34.139** **Unspecified injury to sacral spinal cord** A, A
Unspecified injury of conus medullaris

- **S34.2 Injury of nerve root of lumbar and sacral spine**
  - X **S34.21 Injury of nerve root of lumbar spine**
  - X **S34.22 Injury of nerve root of sacral spine**
- X **S34.3 Injury of cauda equina A, A**
  - Ex See S32.04
- X **S34.4 Injury of lumbosacral plexus**
- X **S34.5 Injury of lumbar, sacral and pelvic sympathetic nerves**
  - Injury of celiac ganglion or plexus
  - Injury of hypogastric plexus
  - Injury of mesenteric plexus (inferior) (superior)
  - Injury of splanchnic nerve
- X **S34.6 Injury of peripheral nerve(s) at abdomen, lower back and pelvis level**
- X **S34.8 Injury of other nerves at abdomen, lower back and pelvis level**
- X **S34.9 Injury of unspecified nerves at abdomen, lower back and pelvis level**

- **S35 Injury of blood vessels at abdomen, lower back and pelvis level**

  The appropriate 7th character is to be added to each code from category S35

A	initial encounter
D	subsequent encounter
S	sequela

  Code also any associated open wound (S31.-)

- **S35.0 Injury of abdominal aorta**
  - **Excludes1** injury of aorta NOS (S25.0)
  - Ex **For category S35.0 CC codes:** S35.00X-S35.09X[A], S35.8X1-S35.99X[A], T14.90-T14.91, T79.A0X-T79.A9X[A], T79.8XX-T79.9XX[A]
  - X **S35.00 Unspecified injury of abdominal aorta A**
  - X **S35.01 Minor laceration of abdominal aorta A**
    - Incomplete transection of abdominal aorta
    - Laceration of abdominal aorta NOS
    - Superficial laceration of abdominal aorta
  - X **S35.02 Major laceration of abdominal aorta A**
    - Complete transection of abdominal aorta
    - Traumatic rupture of abdominal aorta
  - X **S35.09 Other injury of abdominal aorta A**
- **S35.1 Injury of inferior vena cava**
  - Injury of hepatic vein
  - **Excludes1** injury of vena cava NOS (S25.2)
  - Ex **For category S35.1 CC codes:** S35.10X-S35.19X[A], S35.8X1-S35.99X[A], T14.90-T14.91, T79.A0X-T79.A9X[A], T79.8XX-T79.9XX[A]
  - X **S35.10 Unspecified injury of inferior vena cava A**
  - X **S35.11 Minor laceration of inferior vena cava A**
    - Incomplete transection of inferior vena cava
    - Laceration of inferior vena cava NOS
    - Superficial laceration of inferior vena cava
  - X **S35.12 Major laceration of inferior vena cava A**
    - Complete transection of inferior vena cava
    - Traumatic rupture of inferior vena cava
  - X **S35.19 Other injury of inferior vena cava A**
- **S35.2 Injury of celiac or mesenteric artery and branches**
  - **S35.21 Injury of celiac artery**
    - Ex **For category S35.21 CC codes:** S35.211-S35.219[A], S35.8X1-S35.99X[A], T14.90-T14.91, T79.A0X-T79.A9X[A], T79.8XX-T79.9XX[A]
    - **S35.211 Minor laceration of celiac artery A**
      - Incomplete transection of celiac artery
      - Laceration of celiac artery NOS
      - Superficial laceration of celiac artery
    - **S35.212 Major laceration of celiac artery A**
      - Complete transection of celiac artery
      - Traumatic rupture of celiac artery
    - **S35.218 Other injury of celiac artery A**
    - **S35.219 Unspecified injury of celiac artery A**
  - **S35.22 Injury of superior mesenteric artery**
    - Ex **For category S35.22 CC codes:** S35.221-S35.229[A], S35.8X1-S35.99X[A], T14.90-T14.91, T79.A0X-T79.A9X[A], T79.8XX-T79.9XX[A]
    - **S35.221 Minor laceration of superior mesenteric artery A**
      - Incomplete transection of superior mesenteric artery
      - Laceration of superior mesenteric artery NOS
      - Superficial laceration of superior mesenteric artery
    - **S35.222 Major laceration of superior mesenteric artery A**
      - Complete transection of superior mesenteric artery
      - Traumatic rupture of superior mesenteric artery
    - **S35.228 Other injury of superior mesenteric artery A**
    - **S35.229 Unspecified injury of superior mesenteric artery A**
  - **S35.23 Injury of inferior mesenteric artery**
    - Ex **For category S35.23 CC codes:** S35.231-S35.239[A], S35.8X1-S35.99X[A], T14.90-T14.91, T79.A0X-T79.A9X[A], T79.8XX-T79.9XX[A]
    - **S35.231 Minor laceration of inferior mesenteric artery A**
      - Incomplete transection of inferior mesenteric artery
      - Laceration of inferior mesenteric artery NOS
      - Superficial laceration of inferior mesenteric artery
    - **S35.232 Major laceration of inferior mesenteric artery A**
      - Complete transection of inferior mesenteric artery
      - Traumatic rupture of inferior mesenteric artery
    - **S35.238 Other injury of inferior mesenteric artery A**
    - **S35.239 Unspecified injury of inferior mesenteric artery A**
  - **S35.29 Injury of branches of celiac and mesenteric artery**
    - Injury of gastric artery
    - Injury of gastroduodenal artery
    - Injury of hepatic artery
    - Injury of splenic artery
    - Ex **For category S35.29 CC codes unless otherwise indicated:** S35.292-S35.298[A], S35.8X1-S35.99X[A], T14.90-T14.91, T79.A0X-T79.A9X[A], T79.8XX-T79.9XX[A]
    - **S35.291 Minor laceration of branches of celiac and mesenteric artery A**
      - Incomplete transection of branches of celiac and mesenteric artery
      - Laceration of branches of celiac and mesenteric artery NOS
      - Superficial laceration of branches of celiac and mesenteric artery
      - Ex S35.291[A], S35.8X1-S35.99X[A], T14.90-T14.91, T79.8XX-T79.9XX[A], T79.A0X[A], T79.A3X-T79.A9X[A]
    - **S35.292 Major laceration of branches of celiac and mesenteric artery A**
      - Complete transection of branches of celiac and mesenteric artery
      - Traumatic rupture of branches of celiac and mesenteric artery

- S35.298 Other injury of branches of celiac and mesenteric artery A
- S35.299 Unspecified injury of branches of celiac and mesenteric artery A
  Ex: S35.299[A], S35.8X1-S35.99X[A], T14.90-T14.91, T79.A0X-T79.A9X[A], T79.8XX-T79.9XX[A]

- S35.3 Injury of portal or splenic vein and branches
  - S35.31 Injury of portal vein
    Ex: **For category S35.31 CC codes:** S35.311-S35.319[A], S35.8X1-S35.99X[A], T14.90-T14.91, T79.A0X-T79.A9X[A], T79.8XX-T79.9XX[A]
    - S35.311 Laceration of portal vein A
    - S35.318 Other specified injury of portal vein A
    - S35.319 Unspecified injury of portal vein A
  - S35.32 Injury of splenic vein
    Ex: **For category S35.32 CC codes:** S35.321-S35.329[A], S35.8X1-S35.99X[A], T14.90-T14.91, T79.A0X-T79.A9X[A], T79.8XX-T79.9XX[A]
    - S35.321 Laceration of splenic vein A
    - S35.328 Other specified injury of splenic vein A
    - S35.329 Unspecified injury of splenic vein A
  - S35.33 Injury of superior mesenteric vein
    Ex: **For category S35.33 CC codes:** S35.331-S35.339[A], S35.8X1-S35.99X[A], T14.90-T14.91, T79.A0X-T79.A9X[A], T79.8XX-T79.9XX[A]
    - S35.331 Laceration of superior mesenteric vein A
    - S35.338 Other specified injury of superior mesenteric vein A
    - S35.339 Unspecified injury of superior mesenteric vein A
  - S35.34 Injury of inferior mesenteric vein
    Ex: **For category S35.34 CC codes:** S35.341-S35.349[A], S35.8X1-S35.99X[A], T14.90-T14.91, T79.A0X-T79.A9X[A], T79.8XX-T79.9XX[A]
    - S35.341 Laceration of inferior mesenteric vein A
    - S35.348 Other specified injury of inferior mesenteric vein A
    - S35.349 Unspecified injury of inferior mesenteric vein A
- S35.4 Injury of renal blood vessels
  - S35.40 Unspecified injury of renal blood vessel
    Ex: **For category S35.40 CC codes S35.401-S35.403:** S35.401-S35.403[A], S35.411-S35.413[A], S35.491-S35.493[A], S35.8X1-S35.99X[A], T14.90-T14.91, T79.A0X-T79.A9X[A], T79.8XX-T79.9XX[A] **For category S35.40 CC codes S35.404-S35.406:** S35.404-S35.406[A], S35.414-S35.416[A], S35.494-S35.496[A], S35.8X1-S35.99X[A], T14.90-T14.91, T79.A0X-T79.A9X[A], T79.8XX-T79.9XX[A]
    - S35.401 Unspecified injury of right renal artery A
    - S35.402 Unspecified injury of left renal artery A
    - S35.403 Unspecified injury of unspecified renal artery A
    - S35.404 Unspecified injury of right renal vein A
    - S35.405 Unspecified injury of left renal vein A
    - S35.406 Unspecified injury of unspecified renal vein A
  - S35.41 Laceration of renal blood vessel
    Ex: **For category S35.41 CC codes S35.411-S35.413:** See S35.401-S35.403 **For category S35.41 CC codes S35.414-S35.416:** See 35.404-S35.406
    - S35.411 Laceration of right renal artery A
    - S35.412 Laceration of left renal artery A
    - S35.413 Laceration of unspecified renal artery A
    - S35.414 Laceration of right renal vein A
    - S35.415 Laceration of left renal vein A
    - S35.416 Laceration of unspecified renal vein A
  - S35.49 Other specified injury of renal blood vessel
    Ex: **For category S35.49 CC codes S35.491-S35.493:** See S35.401-S35.403 **For category S35.49 CC codes S35.494-S35.496:** See 35.404-S35.406
    - S35.491 Other specified injury of right renal artery A
    - S35.492 Other specified injury of left renal artery A
    - S35.493 Other specified injury of unspecified renal artery A
    - S35.494 Other specified injury of right renal vein A
    - S35.495 Other specified injury of left renal vein A
    - S35.496 Other specified injury of unspecified renal vein A
- S35.5 Injury of iliac blood vessels
  - X S35.50 Injury of unspecified iliac blood vessel(s) A
    Ex: S35.50X-S35.516[A], S35.59X-S35.99X[A], T14.90-T14.91, T79.A0X-T79.A9X[A], T79.8XX-T79.9XX[A]
  - S35.51 Injury of iliac artery or vein
    Injury of hypogastric artery or vein
    Ex: **For category S35.51 CC codes S35.511-S35.513:** S35.50X-S35.513[A], S35.59X-S35.99X[A], T14.90-T14.91, T79.A0X-T79.A9X[A], T79.8XX-T79.9XX[A] **For category S35.51 CC codes S35.514-S35.516:** S35.50X[A], S35.514-S35.516[A], S35.59X-S35.99X[A], T14.90-T14.91, T79.A0X-T79.A9X[A], T79.8XX-T79.9XX[A]
    - S35.511 Injury of right iliac artery A
    - S35.512 Injury of left iliac artery A
    - S35.513 Injury of unspecified iliac artery A
    - S35.514 Injury of right iliac vein A
    - S35.515 Injury of left iliac vein A
    - S35.516 Injury of unspecified iliac vein A
  - S35.53 Injury of uterine artery or vein
    Ex: **For category S35.53 CC codes S35.531-S35.533:** S35.50X[A], S35.531-S35.533[A], S35.59X-S35.99X[A], T14.90-T14.91, T79.8XX-T79.9XX[A], T79.A0X[A], T79.A3X-T79.A9X[A] **For category S35.53 CC codes S35.534-S35.536:** S35.50X[A], S35.534-S35.536[A], S35.59X-S35.99X[A], T14.90-T14.91, T79.8XX-T79.9XX[A], T79.A0X[A], T79.A3X-T79.A9X[A]
    - S35.531 Injury of right uterine artery ♀ A
    - S35.532 Injury of left uterine artery ♀ A
    - S35.533 Injury of unspecified uterine artery ♀ A
    - S35.534 Injury of right uterine vein ♀ A
    - S35.535 Injury of left uterine vein ♀ A
    - S35.536 Injury of unspecified uterine vein ♀ A
  - X S35.59 Injury of other iliac blood vessels A
    Ex: See S35.50

● **S35.8 Injury of other blood vessels at abdomen, lower back and pelvis level**
Injury of ovarian artery or vein
Ex: **For category S35.8 CC codes:** S35.8X1-S35.99X[A], T14.90-T14.91, T79.8XX-T79.9XX[A], T79.A0X[A], T79.A3X-T79.A9X[A]

● **S35.8X Injury of other blood vessels at abdomen, lower back and pelvis level**

● **S35.8X1 Laceration of other blood vessels at abdomen, lower back and pelvis level A**

● **S35.8X8 Other specified injury of other blood vessels at abdomen, lower back and pelvis level A**

● **S35.8X9 Unspecified injury of other blood vessels at abdomen, lower back and pelvis level A**

● **S35.9 Injury of unspecified blood vessel at abdomen, lower back and pelvis level**
Ex: **For category S35.9 CC codes:** S35.00X-S35.99X[A], T14.90-T14.91, T79.8XX-T79.9XX[A], T79.A0X[A], T79.A3X-T79.A9X[A]

X● **S35.90 Unspecified injury of unspecified blood vessel at abdomen, lower back and pelvis level A**

X● **S35.91 Laceration of unspecified blood vessel at abdomen, lower back and pelvis level A**

X● **S35.99 Other specified injury of unspecified blood vessel at abdomen, lower back and pelvis level A**

● **S36 Injury of intra-abdominal organs**
The appropriate 7th character is to be added to each code from category S36

A	initial encounter
D	subsequent encounter
S	sequela

Code also any associated open wound (S31.-)

● **S36.0 Injury of spleen**
Ex: **For category S36.0 CC codes:** S31.001[A], S31.011[A], S31.021[A], S31.031[A], S31.041[A], S31.051[A], S31.100-S31.159[A], S31.600-S31.659[A], S31.831-S31.839[A], S36.00X-S36.09X[A], S36.81X-S36.99X[A], S38.3XX[A], S39.021-S39.023[A], T14.90-T14.91, T79.8XX-T79.9XX[A], T79.A0X-T79.A9X[A]

X● **S36.00 Unspecified injury of spleen A**

● **S36.02 Contusion of spleen**

● **S36.020 Minor contusion of spleen A**
Contusion of spleen less than 2 cm

● **S36.021 Major contusion of spleen A**
Contusion of spleen greater than 2 cm

● **S36.029 Unspecified contusion of spleen A**
Coding Clinic: 2015, Q2, P36, Q1, P11

● **S36.03 Laceration of spleen**

● **S36.030 Superficial (capsular) laceration of spleen A**
Laceration of spleen less than 1 cm
Minor laceration of spleen

● **S36.031 Moderate laceration of spleen A**
Laceration of spleen 1 to 3 cm
Coding Clinic: 2015, Q2, P36, Q1, P11

● **S36.032 Major laceration of spleen A**
Avulsion of spleen
Laceration of spleen greater than 3 cm
Massive laceration of spleen
Multiple moderate lacerations of spleen
Stellate laceration of spleen

● **S36.039 Unspecified laceration of spleen A**

X● **S36.09 Other injury of spleen A**

● **S36.1 Injury of liver and gallbladder and bile duct**

● **S36.11 Injury of liver**
Ex: **For category S36.11 CC codes:** S31.001[A], S31.011[A], S31.021[A], S31.031[A], S31.041[A], S31.051[A], S31.100-S31.159[A], S31.600-S31.659[A], S31.831-S31.839[A], S36.112-S36.119[A], S36.81X-S36.99X[A], S38.3XX[A], S39.021-S39.023[A], T14.90-T14.91, T79.8XX-T79.9XX[A], T79.A0XA-T79.A9X[A]

● **S36.112 Contusion of liver A**

● **S36.113 Laceration of liver, unspecified degree A**

● **S36.114 Minor laceration of liver A**
Laceration involving capsule only, or, without significant involvement of hepatic parenchyma [i.e., less than 1 cm deep]

● **S36.115 Moderate laceration of liver A**
Laceration involving parenchyma but without major disruption of parenchyma [i.e., less than 10 cm long and less than 3 cm deep]

● **S36.116 Major laceration of liver A**
Laceration with significant disruption of hepatic parenchyma [i.e., greater than 10 cm long and 3 cm deep]
Multiple moderate lacerations, with or without hematoma
Stellate laceration of liver

● **S36.118 Other injury of liver A**

● **S36.119 Unspecified injury of liver A**
Coding Clinic: 2015, Q2, P17

● **S36.12 Injury of gallbladder**
Ex: **For category S36.12 CC codes:** S31.001[A], S31.011[A], S31.021[A], S31.031[A], S31.041[A], S31.051[A], S31.100-S31.159[A], S31.600-S31.659[A], S31.831-S31.839[A], S36.122-S36.13X[A], S36.81X-S36.99X[A], S38.3XX[A], S39.021-S39.023[A], T14.90-T14.91, T79.8XX-T79.9XX[A], T79.A0X-T79.A9X[A]

● **S36.122 Contusion of gallbladder A**

● **S36.123 Laceration of gallbladder A**

● **S36.128 Other injury of gallbladder A**

● **S36.129 Unspecified injury of gallbladder A**

X● **S36.13 Injury of bile duct A**
Ex: See S36.12

● **S36.2 Injury of pancreas**
Ex: **For category S36.2 CC codes:** M79.A3, S31.001[A], S31.011[A], S31.021[A], S31.031[A], S31.041[A], S31.051[A], S31.100-S31.159[A], S31.600-S31.659[A], S31.831-S31.839[A], S36.200-S36.299[A], S36.81X-S36.99X[A], S38.3XX[A], S39.021-S39.023[A], T14.90-T14.91, T79.8XX-T79.9XX[A], T79.A3X-T79.A9X[A]

● **S36.20 Unspecified injury of pancreas**

● **S36.200 Unspecified injury of head of pancreas A**

● **S36.201 Unspecified injury of body of pancreas A**

● **S36.202 Unspecified injury of tail of pancreas A**

● **S36.209 Unspecified injury of unspecified part of pancreas A**

● **S36.22 Contusion of pancreas**

● **S36.220 Contusion of head of pancreas A**

● **S36.221 Contusion of body of pancreas A**

● **S36.222 Contusion of tail of pancreas A**

● **S36.229 Contusion of unspecified part of pancreas A**

- **S36.23 Laceration of pancreas, unspecified degree**
  - **S36.230 Laceration of head of pancreas, unspecified degree** A
  - **S36.231 Laceration of body of pancreas, unspecified degree** A
  - **S36.232 Laceration of tail of pancreas, unspecified degree** A
  - **S36.239 Laceration of unspecified part of pancreas, unspecified degree** A
- **S36.24 Minor laceration of pancreas**
  - **S36.240 Minor laceration of head of pancreas** A
  - **S36.241 Minor laceration of body of pancreas** A
  - **S36.242 Minor laceration of tail of pancreas** A
  - **S36.249 Minor laceration of unspecified part of pancreas** A
- **S36.25 Moderate laceration of pancreas**
  - **S36.250 Moderate laceration of head of pancreas** A
  - **S36.251 Moderate laceration of body of pancreas** A
  - **S36.252 Moderate laceration of tail of pancreas** A
  - **S36.259 Moderate laceration of unspecified part of pancreas** A
- **S36.26 Major laceration of pancreas**
  - **S36.260 Major laceration of head of pancreas** A
  - **S36.261 Major laceration of body of pancreas** A
  - **S36.262 Major laceration of tail of pancreas** A
  - **S36.269 Major laceration of unspecified part of pancreas** A
- **S36.29 Other injury of pancreas**
  - **S36.290 Other injury of head of pancreas** A
  - **S36.291 Other injury of body of pancreas** A
  - **S36.292 Other injury of tail of pancreas** A
  - **S36.299 Other injury of unspecified part of pancreas** A
- **S36.3 Injury of stomach**

  Ex: **For category S36.3 CC codes:** M79.A3, S31.001[A], S31.011[A], S31.021[A], S31.031[A], S31.041[A], S31.051[A], S31.100-S31.159[A], S31.600-S31.659[A], S31.831-S31.839[A], S36.30X-S36.39X[A], S36.81X-S36.99X[A], S38.3XX[A], S39.021-S39.023[A], T14.90-T14.91, T79.8XX-T799.XX[A], T79.A3X-T79.A9X[A]

  - X **S36.30 Unspecified injury of stomach** A
  - X **S36.32 Contusion of stomach** A
  - X **S36.33 Laceration of stomach** A
  - X **S36.39 Other injury of stomach** A
- **S36.4 Injury of small intestine**

  Ex: **For category S36.4 CC codes:** M79.A3, S31.001[A], S31.011[A], S31.021[A], S31.031[A], S31.041[A], S31.051[A], S31.100-S31.159[A], S31.600-S31.659[A], S31.831-S31.839[A], S36.400-S36.499[A], S36.81X-S36.99X[A], S38.3XX[A], S39.021-S39.023[A], T14.90-T14.91, T79.8XX-T79.9XX[A], T79.A3X-T79.A9X[A]

  - **S36.40 Unspecified injury of small intestine**
    - **S36.400 Unspecified injury of duodenum** A
    - **S36.408 Unspecified injury of other part of small intestine** A
    - **S36.409 Unspecified injury of unspecified part of small intestine** A
  - **S36.41 Primary blast injury of small intestine**

    Blast injury of small intestine NOS
    - **S36.410 Primary blast injury of duodenum** A
    - **S36.418 Primary blast injury of other part of small intestine** A
    - **S36.419 Primary blast injury of unspecified part of small intestine** A
  - **S36.42 Contusion of small intestine**
    - **S36.420 Contusion of duodenum** A
    - **S36.428 Contusion of other part of small intestine** A
    - **S36.429 Contusion of unspecified part of small intestine** A
  - **S36.43 Laceration of small intestine**
    - **S36.430 Laceration of duodenum** A
    - **S36.438 Laceration of other part of small intestine** A
    - **S36.439 Laceration of unspecified part of small intestine** A
  - **S36.49 Other injury of small intestine**
    - **S36.490 Other injury of duodenum** A
    - **S36.498 Other injury of other part of small intestine** A
    - **S36.499 Other injury of unspecified part of small intestine** A
- **S36.5 Injury of colon**

  Excludes2 injury of rectum (S36.6-)

  Ex: **For category S36.5 CC codes:** M79.A3, S31.001[A], S31.011[A], S31.021[A], S31.031[A], S31.041[A], S31.051[A], S31.100-S31.159[A], S31.600-S31.659[A], S31.831-S31.839[A], S36.500-S36.99X[A], S38.3XX[A], S39.021-S39.023[A], T14.90-T14.91, T79.8XX-T79.9XX[A], T79.A3X-T79.A9X[A]

  - **S36.50 Unspecified injury of colon**
    - **S36.500 Unspecified injury of ascending [right] colon** A
    - **S36.501 Unspecified injury of transverse colon** A
    - **S36.502 Unspecified injury of descending [left] colon** A
    - **S36.503 Unspecified injury of sigmoid colon** A
    - **S36.508 Unspecified injury of other part of colon** A
    - **S36.509 Unspecified injury of unspecified part of colon** A
  - **S36.51 Primary blast injury of colon**

    Blast injury of colon NOS
    - **S36.510 Primary blast injury of ascending [right] colon** A
    - **S36.511 Primary blast injury of transverse colon** A
    - **S36.512 Primary blast injury of descending [left] colon** A
    - **S36.513 Primary blast injury of sigmoid colon** A
    - **S36.518 Primary blast injury of other part of colon** A
    - **S36.519 Primary blast injury of unspecified part of colon** A
  - **S36.52 Contusion of colon**
    - **S36.520 Contusion of ascending [right] colon** A
    - **S36.521 Contusion of transverse colon** A
    - **S36.522 Contusion of descending [left] colon** A
    - **S36.523 Contusion of sigmoid colon** A
    - **S36.528 Contusion of other part of colon** A
    - **S36.529 Contusion of unspecified part of colon** A

- S36.53 Laceration of colon
  - S36.530 Laceration of ascending [right] colon A
  - S36.531 Laceration of transverse colon A
  - S36.532 Laceration of descending [left] colon A
  - S36.533 Laceration of sigmoid colon A
  - S36.538 Laceration of other part of colon A
  - S36.539 Laceration of unspecified part of colon A
- S36.59 Other injury of colon
  Secondary blast injury of colon
  - S36.590 Other injury of ascending [right] colon A
  - S36.591 Other injury of transverse colon A
  - S36.592 Other injury of descending [left] colon A
  - S36.593 Other injury of sigmoid colon A
  - S36.598 Other injury of other part of colon A
  - S36.599 Other injury of unspecified part of colon A
- S36.6 Injury of rectum
  Ex: For category S36.6 CC codes: See S36.5
  - X S36.60 Unspecified injury of rectum A
  - X S36.61 Primary blast injury of rectum A
    Blast injury of rectum NOS
  - X S36.62 Contusion of rectum A
  - X S36.63 Laceration of rectum A
  - X S36.69 Other injury of rectum A
    Secondary blast injury of rectum
- S36.8 Injury of other intra-abdominal organs
  Ex: For category S36.8 CC codes: See S31.0
  - X S36.81 Injury of peritoneum A
  - S36.89 Injury of other intra-abdominal organs
    Injury of retroperitoneum
    - S36.892 Contusion of other intra-abdominal organs A
    - S36.893 Laceration of other intra-abdominal organs A
    - S36.898 Other injury of other intra-abdominal organs A
    - S36.899 Unspecified injury of other intra-abdominal organs A
- S36.9 Injury of unspecified intra-abdominal organ
  Ex: For category S36.9 CC codes: See S31.0
  - X S36.90 Unspecified injury of unspecified intra-abdominal organ A
  - X S36.92 Contusion of unspecified intra-abdominal organ A
  - X S36.93 Laceration of unspecified intra-abdominal organ A
  - X S36.99 Other injury of unspecified intra-abdominal organ A

- S37 Injury of urinary and pelvic organs
  Code also any associated open wound (S31.-)
  Excludes1 obstetric trauma to pelvic organs (O71.-)
  Excludes2 injury of peritoneum (S36.81)
  injury of retroperitoneum (S36.89-)
  The appropriate 7th character is to be added to each code from category S37

A	initial encounter
D	subsequent encounter
S	sequela

- S37.0 Injury of kidney
  Excludes2 acute kidney injury (nontraumatic) (N17.9)
  Ex: For category S37.0 CC codes: S31.001[A], S31.011[A], S31.021[A], S31.031[A], S31.041[A], S31.051[A], S31.100-S31.159[A], S31.600-S31.659[A], S31.831-S31.839[A], S36.81X-S37.099[A], S38.3XX[A], S39.021-S39.023[A], T14.90-T14.91, T79.8XX-T79.9XX[A], T79.A0X-T79.A9X[A]
  - S37.00 Unspecified injury of kidney
    - S37.001 Unspecified injury of right kidney A
    - S37.002 Unspecified injury of left kidney A
    - S37.009 Unspecified injury of unspecified kidney A
  - S37.01 Minor contusion of kidney
    Contusion of kidney less than 2 cm
    Contusion of kidney NOS
    - S37.011 Minor contusion of right kidney A
    - S37.012 Minor contusion of left kidney A
    - S37.019 Minor contusion of unspecified kidney A
  - S37.02 Major contusion of kidney
    Contusion of kidney greater than 2 cm
    - S37.021 Major contusion of right kidney A
    - S37.022 Major contusion of left kidney A
    - S37.029 Major contusion of unspecified kidney A
  - S37.03 Laceration of kidney, unspecified degree
    - S37.031 Laceration of right kidney, unspecified degree A
    - S37.032 Laceration of left kidney, unspecified degree A
    - S37.039 Laceration of unspecified kidney, unspecified degree A
  - S37.04 Minor laceration of kidney
    Laceration of kidney less than 1 cm
    - S37.041 Minor laceration of right kidney A
    - S37.042 Minor laceration of left kidney A
    - S37.049 Minor laceration of unspecified kidney A
  - S37.05 Moderate laceration of kidney
    Laceration of kidney 1 to 3 cm
    - S37.051 Moderate laceration of right kidney A
    - S37.052 Moderate laceration of left kidney A
    - S37.059 Moderate laceration of unspecified kidney A
  - S37.06 Major laceration of kidney
    Avulsion of kidney
    Laceration of kidney greater than 3 cm
    Massive laceration of kidney
    Multiple moderate lacerations of kidney
    Stellate laceration of kidney
    - S37.061 Major laceration of right kidney A
    - S37.062 Major laceration of left kidney A
    - S37.069 Major laceration of unspecified kidney A
  - S37.09 Other injury of kidney
    - S37.091 Other injury of right kidney A
    - S37.092 Other injury of left kidney A
    - S37.099 Other injury of unspecified kidney A

- S37.1 Injury of ureter
  - Ex: For category S37.1 CC codes: S31.001[A], S31.011[A], S31.021[A], S31.031[A], S31.041[A], S31.051[A], S31.100-S31.159[A], S31.600-S31.659[A], S31.831-S31.839[A], S36.81X-S36.99X[A], S37.10X-S37.19X[A], S37.401-S37.599[A], S37.822-S37.99X[A], S38.3XX[A], S39.021-S39.023[A], T14.90-T14.91, T79.8XX-T79.9XX[A], T79.A0X-T79.A9X[A]
  - X S37.10 Unspecified injury of ureter A
  - X S37.12 Contusion of ureter A
  - X S37.13 Laceration of ureter A
  - X S37.19 Other injury of ureter A
- S37.2 Injury of bladder
  - Ex: For category S37.2 CC codes: S31.001[A], S31.011[A], S31.021[A], S31.031[A], S31.041[A], S31.051[A], S31.100-S31.159[A], S31.600-S31.659[A], S31.831-S31.839[A], S36.81X-S36.99X[A], S37.20X-S37.599[A], S37.822-S37.99X[A], S38.3XX[A], S39.021-S39.023[A], T14.90-T14.91, T79.8XX-T79.9XX[A], T79.A0X-T79.A9X[A]
  - X S37.20 Unspecified injury of bladder A
  - X S37.22 Contusion of bladder A
  - X S37.23 Laceration of bladder A
  - X S37.29 Other injury of bladder A
- S37.3 Injury of urethra
  - Ex: For category S37.3 CC codes: See S37.2
  - X S37.30 Unspecified injury of urethra A
  - X S37.32 Contusion of urethra A
  - X S37.33 Laceration of urethra A
  - X S37.39 Other injury of urethra A
- S37.4 Injury of ovary
  - S37.40 Unspecified injury of ovary
    - S37.401 Unspecified injury of ovary, unilateral ♀
    - S37.402 Unspecified injury of ovary, bilateral ♀
    - S37.409 Unspecified injury of ovary, unspecified ♀
  - S37.42 Contusion of ovary
    - S37.421 Contusion of ovary, unilateral ♀
    - S37.422 Contusion of ovary, bilateral ♀
    - S37.429 Contusion of ovary, unspecified ♀
  - S37.43 Laceration of ovary
    - S37.431 Laceration of ovary, unilateral ♀
    - S37.432 Laceration of ovary, bilateral ♀
    - S37.439 Laceration of ovary, unspecified ♀
  - S37.49 Other injury of ovary
    - S37.491 Other injury of ovary, unilateral ♀
    - S37.492 Other injury of ovary, bilateral ♀
    - S37.499 Other injury of ovary, unspecified ♀
- S37.5 Injury of fallopian tube
  - S37.50 Unspecified injury of fallopian tube
    - S37.501 Unspecified injury of fallopian tube, unilateral ♀
    - S37.502 Unspecified injury of fallopian tube, bilateral ♀
    - S37.509 Unspecified injury of fallopian tube, unspecified ♀
  - S37.51 Primary blast injury of fallopian tube
    Blast injury of fallopian tube NOS
    - S37.511 Primary blast injury of fallopian tube, unilateral ♀
    - S37.512 Primary blast injury of fallopian tube, bilateral ♀
    - S37.519 Primary blast injury of fallopian tube, unspecified ♀
  - S37.52 Contusion of fallopian tube
    - S37.521 Contusion of fallopian tube, unilateral ♀
    - S37.522 Contusion of fallopian tube, bilateral ♀
    - S37.529 Contusion of fallopian tube, unspecified ♀
  - S37.53 Laceration of fallopian tube
    - S37.531 Laceration of fallopian tube, unilateral ♀
    - S37.532 Laceration of fallopian tube, bilateral ♀
    - S37.539 Laceration of fallopian tube, unspecified ♀
  - S37.59 Other injury of fallopian tube
    Secondary blast injury of fallopian tube
    - S37.591 Other injury of fallopian tube, unilateral ♀
    - S37.592 Other injury of fallopian tube, bilateral ♀
    - S37.599 Other injury of fallopian tube, unspecified ♀
- S37.6 Injury of uterus
  - **Excludes1** injury to gravid uterus (O9A.2-)
    injury to uterus during delivery (O71.-)
  - Ex: For category S37.6 CC codes: S31.001[A], S31.011[A], S31.021[A], S31.031[A], S31.041[A], S31.051[A], S31.100-S31.159[A], S31.600-S31.659[A], S31.831-S31.839[A], S36.81X-S36.99X[A], S37.401-S37.69X[A], S37.822-S37.99X[A], S38.3XX[A], S39.021-S39.023[A], T14.90-T14.91, T79.8XX-T79.9XX[A], T79.A0X-T79.A9X[A]
  - X S37.60 Unspecified injury of uterus ♀ A
  - X S37.62 Contusion of uterus ♀ A
  - X S37.63 Laceration of uterus ♀ A
  - X S37.69 Other injury of uterus ♀ A
- S37.8 Injury of other urinary and pelvic organs
  - S37.81 Injury of adrenal gland
    - Ex: For category S37.81 CC codes: S31.001[A], S31.011[A], S31.021[A], S31.031[A], S31.041[A], S31.051[A], S31.100-S31.159[A], S31.600-S31.659[A], S31.831-S31.839[A], S36.81X-S36.99X[A], S37.812-S37.819[A], S38.3XX[A], S39.021-S39.023[A], T14.90-T14.91, T79.8XX-T79.9XX[A], T79.A0X-T79.A9X[A]
    - S37.812 Contusion of adrenal gland A
    - S37.813 Laceration of adrenal gland A
    - S37.818 Other injury of adrenal gland A
    - S37.819 Unspecified injury of adrenal gland A
  - S37.82 Injury of prostate
    - S37.822 Contusion of prostate ♂
    - S37.823 Laceration of prostate ♂
    - S37.828 Other injury of prostate ♂
    - S37.829 Unspecified injury of prostate ♂
  - S37.89 Injury of other urinary and pelvic organ
    - Ex: For category S37.89 CC codes: S31.001[A], S31.011[A], S31.021[A], S31.031[A], S31.041[A], S31.051[A], S31.100-S31.159[A], S31.600-S31.659[A], S31.831-S31.839[A], S36.81X-S36.99X[A], S37.401-S37.599[A], S37.822-S37.99X[A], S38.3XX[A], S39.021-S39.023[A], T14.90-T14.91, T79.8XX-T79.9XX[A], T79.A0X-T79.A9X[A]
    - S37.892 Contusion of other urinary and pelvic organ A
    - S37.893 Laceration of other urinary and pelvic organ A
    - S37.898 Other injury of other urinary and pelvic organ A
    - S37.899 Unspecified injury of other urinary and pelvic organ A

● S37.9 Injury of unspecified urinary and pelvic organ
Ex For category S37.9 CC codes: See S37.89

X ● S37.90 Unspecified injury of unspecified urinary and pelvic organ A

X ● S37.92 Contusion of unspecified urinary and pelvic organ A

X ● S37.93 Laceration of unspecified urinary and pelvic organ A

X ● S37.99 Other injury of unspecified urinary and pelvic organ A

● S38 Crushing injury and traumatic amputation of abdomen, lower back, pelvis and external genitals

An amputation not identified as partial or complete should be coded to complete

The appropriate 7th character is to be added to each code from category S38

A	initial encounter
D	subsequent encounter
S	sequela

● S38.0 Crushing injury of external genital organs

Use additional code for any associated injuries

● S38.00 Crushing injury of unspecified external genital organs

● S38.001 Crushing injury of unspecified external genital organs, male ♂

● S38.002 Crushing injury of unspecified external genital organs, female ♀

X ● S38.01 Crushing injury of penis ♂

X ● S38.02 Crushing injury of scrotum and testis ♂

X ● S38.03 Crushing injury of vulva ♀

X ● S38.1 Crushing injury of abdomen, lower back, and pelvis

Use additional code for all associated injuries, such as:
fracture of thoracic or lumbar spine and pelvis (S22.0-, S32.-)
injury to intra-abdominal organs (S36.-)
injury to urinary and pelvic organs (S37.-)
open wound of abdominal wall (S31.-)
spinal cord injury (S34.0, S34.1-)

Excludes2 crushing injury of external genital organs (S38.0-)

● S38.2 Traumatic amputation of external genital organs

● S38.21 Traumatic amputation of female external genital organs

Traumatic amputation of clitoris
Traumatic amputation of labium (majus) (minus)
Traumatic amputation of vulva

● S38.211 Complete traumatic amputation of female external genital organs ♀

● S38.212 Partial traumatic amputation of female external genital organs ♀

● S38.22 Traumatic amputation of penis

● S38.221 Complete traumatic amputation of penis ♂

● S38.222 Partial traumatic amputation of penis ♂

● S38.23 Traumatic amputation of scrotum and testis

● S38.231 Complete traumatic amputation of scrotum and testis ♂

● S38.232 Partial traumatic amputation of scrotum and testis ♂

X ● S38.3 Transection (partial) of abdomen

● S39 Other and unspecified injuries of abdomen, lower back, pelvis and external genitals

Code also any associated open wound (S31.-)

Excludes2 sprain of joints and ligaments of lumbar spine and pelvis (S33.-)

The appropriate 7th character is to be added to each code from category S39

A	initial encounter
D	subsequent encounter
S	sequela

● S39.0 Injury of muscle, fascia and tendon of abdomen, lower back and pelvis

● S39.00 Unspecified injury of muscle, fascia and tendon of abdomen, lower back and pelvis

● S39.001 Unspecified injury of muscle, fascia and tendon of abdomen

● S39.002 Unspecified injury of muscle, fascia and tendon of lower back

● S39.003 Unspecified injury of muscle, fascia and tendon of pelvis

● S39.01 Strain of muscle, fascia and tendon of abdomen, lower back and pelvis

● S39.011 Strain of muscle, fascia and tendon of abdomen

● S39.012 Strain of muscle, fascia and tendon of lower back

● S39.013 Strain of muscle, fascia and tendon of pelvis

● S39.02 Laceration of muscle, fascia and tendon of abdomen, lower back and pelvis

● S39.021 Laceration of muscle, fascia and tendon of abdomen

● S39.022 Laceration of muscle, fascia and tendon of lower back

● S39.023 Laceration of muscle, fascia and tendon of pelvis

● S39.09 Other injury of muscle, fascia and tendon of abdomen, lower back and pelvis

● S39.091 Other injury of muscle, fascia and tendon of abdomen

● S39.092 Other injury of muscle, fascia and tendon of lower back

● S39.093 Other injury of muscle, fascia and tendon of pelvis

● S39.8 Other specified injuries of abdomen, lower back, pelvis and external genitals

X ● S39.81 Other specified injuries of abdomen

X ● S39.82 Other specified injuries of lower back

X ● S39.83 Other specified injuries of pelvis

● S39.84 Other specified injuries of external genitals

● S39.840 Fracture of corpus cavernosum penis ♂

● S39.848 Other specified injuries of external genitals

● S39.9 Unspecified injury of abdomen, lower back, pelvis and external genitals

X ● S39.91 Unspecified injury of abdomen

X ● S39.92 Unspecified injury of lower back

X ● S39.93 Unspecified injury of pelvis

X ● S39.94 Unspecified injury of external genitals

INJURIES TO THE SHOULDER AND UPPER ARM (S40-S49)

Includes injuries of axilla injuries of scapular region

Excludes2 burns and corrosions (T20-T32)
frostbite (T33-T34)
injuries of elbow (S50-S59)
insect bite or sting, venomous (T63.4)

S40 Superficial injury of shoulder and upper arm

The appropriate 7th character is to be added to each code from category S40

A	initial encounter
D	subsequent encounter
S	sequela

S40.0 Contusion of shoulder and upper arm
- **S40.01 Contusion of shoulder**
  - **S40.011 Contusion of right shoulder**
  - **S40.012 Contusion of left shoulder**
  - **S40.019 Contusion of unspecified shoulder**
- **S40.02 Contusion of upper arm**
  - **S40.021 Contusion of right upper arm**
  - **S40.022 Contusion of left upper arm**
  - **S40.029 Contusion of unspecified upper arm**

S40.2 Other superficial injuries of shoulder
- **S40.21 Abrasion of shoulder**
  - **S40.211 Abrasion of right shoulder**
  - **S40.212 Abrasion of left shoulder**
  - **S40.219 Abrasion of unspecified shoulder**
- **S40.22 Blister (nonthermal) of shoulder**
  - **S40.221 Blister (nonthermal) of right shoulder**
  - **S40.222 Blister (nonthermal) of left shoulder**
  - **S40.229 Blister (nonthermal) of unspecified shoulder**
- **S40.24 External constriction of shoulder**
  - **S40.241 External constriction of right shoulder**
  - **S40.242 External constriction of left shoulder**
  - **S40.249 External constriction of unspecified shoulder**
- **S40.25 Superficial foreign body of shoulder**
  Splinter in the shoulder
  - **S40.251 Superficial foreign body of right shoulder**
  - **S40.252 Superficial foreign body of left shoulder**
  - **S40.259 Superficial foreign body of unspecified shoulder**
- **S40.26 Insect bite (nonvenomous) of shoulder**
  - **S40.261 Insect bite (nonvenomous) of right shoulder**
  - **S40.262 Insect bite (nonvenomous) of left shoulder**
  - **S40.269 Insect bite (nonvenomous) of unspecified shoulder**
- **S40.27 Other superficial bite of shoulder**
  Excludes1 open bite of shoulder (S41.05)
  - **S40.271 Other superficial bite of right shoulder**
  - **S40.272 Other superficial bite of left shoulder**
  - **S40.279 Other superficial bite of unspecified shoulder**

S40.8 Other superficial injuries of upper arm
- **S40.81 Abrasion of upper arm**
  - **S40.811 Abrasion of right upper arm**
  - **S40.812 Abrasion of left upper arm**
  - **S40.819 Abrasion of unspecified upper arm**
- **S40.82 Blister (nonthermal) of upper arm**
  - **S40.821 Blister (nonthermal) of right upper arm**
  - **S40.822 Blister (nonthermal) of left upper arm**
  - **S40.829 Blister (nonthermal) of unspecified upper arm**
- **S40.84 External constriction of upper arm**
  - **S40.841 External constriction of right upper arm**
  - **S40.842 External constriction of left upper arm**
  - **S40.849 External constriction of unspecified upper arm**
- **S40.85 Superficial foreign body of upper arm**
  Splinter in the upper arm
  - **S40.851 Superficial foreign body of right upper arm**
  - **S40.852 Superficial foreign body of left upper arm**
  - **S40.859 Superficial foreign body of unspecified upper arm**
- **S40.86 Insect bite (nonvenomous) of upper arm**
  - **S40.861 Insect bite (nonvenomous) of right upper arm**
  - **S40.862 Insect bite (nonvenomous) of left upper arm**
  - **S40.869 Insect bite (nonvenomous) of unspecified upper arm**
- **S40.87 Other superficial bite of upper arm**
  Excludes1 open bite of upper arm (S41.14)
  Excludes2 other superficial bite of shoulder (S40.27-)
  - **S40.871 Other superficial bite of right upper arm**
  - **S40.872 Other superficial bite of left upper arm**
  - **S40.879 Other superficial bite of unspecified upper arm**

S40.9 Unspecified superficial injury of shoulder and upper arm
- **S40.91 Unspecified superficial injury of shoulder**
  - **S40.911 Unspecified superficial injury of right shoulder**
  - **S40.912 Unspecified superficial injury of left shoulder**
  - **S40.919 Unspecified superficial injury of unspecified shoulder**
- **S40.92 Unspecified superficial injury of upper arm**
  - **S40.921 Unspecified superficial injury of right upper arm**
  - **S40.922 Unspecified superficial injury of left upper arm**
  - **S40.929 Unspecified superficial injury of unspecified upper arm**

S41 Open wound of shoulder and upper arm

Code also any associated wound infection

Excludes1 traumatic amputation of shoulder and upper arm (S48.-)

Excludes2 open fracture of shoulder and upper arm (S42.- with 7th character B or C)

The appropriate 7th character is to be added to each code from category S41

A	initial encounter
D	subsequent encounter
S	sequela

S41.0 Open wound of shoulder

S41.00 Unspecified open wound of shoulder

S41.001 Unspecified open wound of right shoulder

S41.002 Unspecified open wound of left shoulder

S41.009 Unspecified open wound of unspecified shoulder

S41.01 Laceration without foreign body of shoulder

S41.011 Laceration without foreign body of right shoulder

S41.012 Laceration without foreign body of left shoulder

S41.019 Laceration without foreign body of unspecified shoulder

S41.02 Laceration with foreign body of shoulder

S41.021 Laceration with foreign body of right shoulder

S41.022 Laceration with foreign body of left shoulder

S41.029 Laceration with foreign body of unspecified shoulder

S41.03 Puncture wound without foreign body of shoulder

S41.031 Puncture wound without foreign body of right shoulder

S41.032 Puncture wound without foreign body of left shoulder

S41.039 Puncture wound without foreign body of unspecified shoulder

S41.04 Puncture wound with foreign body of shoulder

S41.041 Puncture wound with foreign body of right shoulder

S41.042 Puncture wound with foreign body of left shoulder

S41.049 Puncture wound with foreign body of unspecified shoulder

S41.05 Open bite of shoulder

Bite of shoulder NOS

Excludes1 superficial bite of shoulder (S40.27)

S41.051 Open bite of right shoulder

S41.052 Open bite of left shoulder

S41.059 Open bite of unspecified shoulder

S41.1 Open wound of upper arm

S41.10 Unspecified open wound of upper arm

S41.101 Unspecified open wound of right upper arm

S41.102 Unspecified open wound of left upper arm

S41.109 Unspecified open wound of unspecified upper arm

S41.11 Laceration without foreign body of upper arm

S41.111 Laceration without foreign body of right upper arm

S41.112 Laceration without foreign body of left upper arm

S41.119 Laceration without foreign body of unspecified upper arm

S41.12 Laceration with foreign body of upper arm

S41.121 Laceration with foreign body of right upper arm

S41.122 Laceration with foreign body of left upper arm

S41.129 Laceration with foreign body of unspecified upper arm

S41.13 Puncture wound without foreign body of upper arm

S41.131 Puncture wound without foreign body of right upper arm

S41.132 Puncture wound without foreign body of left upper arm

S41.139 Puncture wound without foreign body of unspecified upper arm

S41.14 Puncture wound with foreign body of upper arm

S41.141 Puncture wound with foreign body of right upper arm

S41.142 Puncture wound with foreign body of left upper arm

S41.149 Puncture wound with foreign body of unspecified upper arm

S41.15 Open bite of upper arm

Bite of upper arm NOS

Excludes1 superficial bite of upper arm (S40.87)

S41.151 Open bite of right upper arm

S41.152 Open bite of left upper arm

S41.159 Open bite of unspecified upper arm

S42 Fracture of shoulder and upper arm

Note: A fracture not indicated as displaced or nondisplaced should be coded to displaced

A fracture not indicated as open or closed should be coded to closed

Excludes1 traumatic amputation of shoulder and upper arm (S48.-)

The appropriate 7th character is to be added to all codes from category S42

A	initial encounter for closed fracture
B	initial encounter for open fracture
D	subsequent encounter for fracture with routine healing
G	subsequent encounter for fracture with delayed healing
K	subsequent encounter for fracture with nonunion
P	subsequent encounter for fracture with malunion
S	sequela

S42.0 Fracture of clavicle

Ex: **For S42.0[B]:** S42.001-S42.036[A,B], S62.90X[B] **For S42.0[K,P]:** See S02.0[K]

S42.00 Fracture of unspecified part of clavicle

S42.001 Fracture of unspecified part of right clavicle B, K, P, B

S42.002 Fracture of unspecified part of left clavicle B, K, P, B

S42.009 Fracture of unspecified part of unspecified clavicle B, K, P, B

Coding Clinic: 2012, Q4, P3

S42.01 Fracture of sternal end of clavicle

S42.011 Anterior displaced fracture of sternal end of right clavicle B, K, P, B

S42.012 Anterior displaced fracture of sternal end of left clavicle B, K, P, B

S42.013 Anterior displaced fracture of sternal end of unspecified clavicle B, K, P, B

Displaced fracture of sternal end of clavicle NOS

- S42.014 Posterior displaced fracture of sternal end of right clavicle B, K, P, B
- S42.015 Posterior displaced fracture of sternal end of left clavicle B, K, P, B
- S42.016 Posterior displaced fracture of sternal end of unspecified clavicle B, K, P, B
- S42.017 Nondisplaced fracture of sternal end of right clavicle B, K, P, B
- S42.018 Nondisplaced fracture of sternal end of left clavicle B, K, P, B
- S42.019 Nondisplaced fracture of sternal end of unspecified clavicle B, K, P, B

- S42.02 Fracture of shaft of clavicle
  - S42.021 Displaced fracture of shaft of right clavicle B, K, P, B
  - S42.022 Displaced fracture of shaft of left clavicle B, K, P, B
  - S42.023 Displaced fracture of shaft of unspecified clavicle B, K, P, B
  - S42.024 Nondisplaced fracture of shaft of right clavicle B, K, P, B
  - S42.025 Nondisplaced fracture of shaft of left clavicle B, K, P, B
  - S42.026 Nondisplaced fracture of shaft of unspecified clavicle B, K, P, B

- S42.03 Fracture of lateral end of clavicle
  Fracture of acromial end of clavicle
  - S42.031 Displaced fracture of lateral end of right clavicle B, K, P, B
  - S42.032 Displaced fracture of lateral end of left clavicle B, K, P, B
  - S42.033 Displaced fracture of lateral end of unspecified clavicle B, K, P, B
  - S42.034 Nondisplaced fracture of lateral end of right clavicle B, K, P, B
  - S42.035 Nondisplaced fracture of lateral end of left clavicle B, K, P, B
  - S42.036 Nondisplaced fracture of lateral end of unspecified clavicle B, K, P, B

- S42.1 Fracture of scapula
  Ex For S42.1[B]: S42.101-S42.199[A,B], S62.90X[B] For S42.1[K,P]: See S02.0[K]
  - S42.10 Fracture of unspecified part of scapula
    - S42.101 Fracture of unspecified part of scapula, right shoulder B, K, P, B
    - S42.102 Fracture of unspecified part of scapula, left shoulder B, K, P, B
    - S42.109 Fracture of unspecified part of scapula, unspecified shoulder B, K, P, B
  - S42.11 Fracture of body of scapula
    - S42.111 Displaced fracture of body of scapula, right shoulder B, K, P, B
    - S42.112 Displaced fracture of body of scapula, left shoulder B, K, P, B
    - S42.113 Displaced fracture of body of scapula, unspecified shoulder B, K, P, B
    - S42.114 Nondisplaced fracture of body of scapula, right shoulder B, K, P, B
    - S42.115 Nondisplaced fracture of body of scapula, left shoulder B, K, P, B
    - S42.116 Nondisplaced fracture of body of scapula, unspecified shoulder B, K, P, B
  - S42.12 Fracture of acromial process
    - S42.121 Displaced fracture of acromial process, right shoulder B, K, P, B
    - S42.122 Displaced fracture of acromial process, left shoulder B, K, P, B
    - S42.123 Displaced fracture of acromial process, unspecified shoulder B, K, P, B
    - S42.124 Nondisplaced fracture of acromial process, right shoulder B, K, P, B
    - S42.125 Nondisplaced fracture of acromial process, left shoulder B, K, P, B
    - S42.126 Nondisplaced fracture, of acromial process, unspecified shoulder B, K, P, B
  - S42.13 Fracture of coracoid process
    - S42.131 Displaced fracture of coracoid process, right shoulder B, K, P, B
    - S42.132 Displaced fracture of coracoid process, left shoulder B, K, P, B
    - S42.133 Displaced fracture of coracoid process, unspecified shoulder B, K, P, B
    - S42.134 Nondisplaced fracture of coracoid process, right shoulder B, K, P, B
    - S42.135 Nondisplaced fracture of coracoid process, left shoulder B, K, P, B
    - S42.136 Nondisplaced fracture of coracoid process, unspecified shoulder B, K, P, B
  - S42.14 Fracture of glenoid cavity of scapula
    - S42.141 Displaced fracture of glenoid cavity of scapula, right shoulder B, K, P, B
    - S42.142 Displaced fracture of glenoid cavity of scapula, left shoulder B, K, P, B
    - S42.143 Displaced fracture of glenoid cavity of scapula, unspecified shoulder B, K, P, B
    - S42.144 Nondisplaced fracture of glenoid cavity of scapula, right shoulder B, K, P, B
    - S42.145 Nondisplaced fracture of glenoid cavity of scapula, left shoulder B, K, P, B
    - S42.146 Nondisplaced fracture of glenoid cavity of scapula, unspecified shoulder B, K, P, B
  - S42.15 Fracture of neck of scapula
    - S42.151 Displaced fracture of neck of scapula, right shoulder B, K, P, B
    - S42.152 Displaced fracture of neck of scapula, left shoulder B, K, P, B
    - S42.153 Displaced fracture of neck of scapula, unspecified shoulder B, K, P, B
    - S42.154 Nondisplaced fracture of neck of scapula, right shoulder B, K, P, B
    - S42.155 Nondisplaced fracture of neck of scapula, left shoulder B, K, P, B
    - S42.156 Nondisplaced fracture of neck of scapula, unspecified shoulder B, K, P, B
  - S42.19 Fracture of other part of scapula
    - S42.191 Fracture of other part of scapula, right shoulder B, K, P, B
    - S42.192 Fracture of other part of scapula, left shoulder B, K, P, B
    - S42.199 Fracture of other part of scapula, unspecified shoulder B, K, P, B

S42.2 Fracture of upper end of humerus
Fracture of proximal end of humerus

Excludes2 fracture of shaft of humerus (S42.3-)
physeal fracture of upper end of humerus (S49.0-)

S42.20 Unspecified fracture of upper end of humerus

S42.201 Unspecified fracture of upper end of right humerus A, K, P, B, A, B

Ex: **For S42.201[A]:** S42.201[A,B], S42.202[B], S42.209-S42.211[A,B], S42.212[B], S42.213-S42.214[A,B], S42.215[B], S42.216-S42.221[A,B], S42.222[B], S42.223-S42.224[A,B], S42.225[B], S42.226-S42.231[A,B], S42.232[B], S42.239-S42.241[A,B], S42.242[B], S42.249-S42.251[A,B], S42.252[B], S42.253-S42.254[A,B], S42.255[B], S42.256-S42.261[A,B], S42.262[B], S42.263-S42.264[A,B], S42.265[B], S42.266[A,B], S42.271[A], S42.279[A], S42.291[A,B], S42.292[B], S42.293-S42.294[A,B], S42.295[B], S42.296-S42.301[A,B], S42.302[B], S42.309[A,B], S42.311[A], S42.319[A], S42.321[A,B], S42.322[B], S42.323-S42.324[A,B], S42.325[B], S42.326-S42.331[A,B], S42.332[B], S42.333-S42.334[A,B], S42.335[B], S42.336-S42.341[A,B], S42.342[B], S42.343-S42.344[A,B], S42.345[B], S42.346-S42.351[A,B], S42.352[B], S42.353-S42.354[A,B], S42.355[B], S42.356-S42.361[A,B], S42.362[B], S42.363-S42.364[A,B], S42.365[B], S42.366-S42.391[A,B], S42.392[B], S42.399-S42.401[A,B], S42.402[B], S42.409-S42.411[A,B], S42.412[B], S42.413-S42.414[A,B], S42.415[B], S42.416-S42.421[A,B], S42.422[B], S42.423-S42.424[A,B], S42.425[B], S42.426-S42.431[A,B], S42.432[B], S42.433-S42.434[A,B], S42.435[B], S42.436-S42.441[A,B], S42.442[B], S42.443-S42.444[A,B], S42.445[B], S42.446-S42.447[A,B], S42.448[B], S42.449-S42.451[A,B], S42.452[B], S42.453-S42.454[A,B], S42.455[B], S42.456-S42.461[A,B], S42.462[B], S42.463-S42.464[A,B], S42.465[B], S42.466-S42.471[A,B], S42.472[B], S42.473-S42.474[A,B], S42.475[B], S42.476 [A,B], S42.481[A], S42.489[A], S42.491[A,B], S42.492[B], S42.493-S42.494[A,B], S42.495[B], S42.496-S42.92X[A,B], S49.001[A], S49.009-S49.011[A], S49.019-S49.021[A], S49.029-S49.031[A], S49.039-S49.041[A], S49.049-S49.091[A], S49.099-S49.101[A], S49.109-S49.111[A], S49.119-S49.121[A], S49.129-S49.131[A], S49.139-S49.141[A], S49.149-S49.191[A], S49.199[A]
For S42.201[B]: S42.201-S42.266[B], S42.291-S42.296[B], S42.301-S42.309[A,B], S42.311-S42.319[A], S42.321-S42.476[A,B], S42.481-S42.489[A], S42.491-S42.92X[A,B], S49.101-S49.199[A], S62.90X[B]
For S42.201[K,P]: See S02.0[K]

S42.202 Unspecified fracture of upper end of left humerus A, K, P, B, A, B

Ex: **For category S42.202 CC codes**
S42.202[A]: S42.201[B], S42.202-S42.209[A,B], S42.211[B], S42.212-S42.213[A,B], S42.214[B], S42.215-S42.216[A,B], S42.221[B], S42.222-S42.223[A,B], S42.224[B], S42.225-S42.226[A,B], S42.231[B], S42.232-S42.239[A,B], S42.241[B], S42.242-S42.249[A,B], S42.251[B], S42.252-S42.253[A,B], S42.254[B], S42.255-S42.256[A,B], S42.261[B], S42.262-S42.263[A,B], S42.264[B], S42.265-S42.266[A,B], S42.272-S42.279[A], S42.291[B], S42.292-S42.293[A,B], S42.294[B], S42.295-S42.296[A,B], S42.301[B], S42.302-S42.309[A,B], S42.312-S42.319[A], S42.321[B], S42.322-S42.323[A,B], S42.324[B], S42.325-S42.326[A,B], S42.331[B], S42.332-S42.333[A,B], S42.334[B], S42.335-S42.336[A,B], S42.341[B], S42.342-S42.343[A,B], S42.344[B], S42.345-S42.346[A,B], S42.351[B], S42.352-S42.353[A,B], S42.354[B], S42.355-S42.356[A,B], S42.361[B], S42.362-S42.363[A,B], S42.364[B], S42.365-S42.366[A,B], S42.391[B], S42.392-S42.399[A,B], S42.401[B], S42.402-S42.409[A,B], S42.411[B], S42.412-S42.413[A,B], S42.414[B], S42.415-S42.416[A,B], S42.421[B], S42.422-S42.423[A,B], S42.424[B], S42.425-S42.426[A,B], S42.431[B], S42.432-S42.433[A,B], S42.434[B], S42.435-S42.436[A,B], S42.441[B], S42.442-S42.443[A,B], S42.444[B], S42.445-S42.446[A,B], S42.447[B], S42.448-S42.449[A,B], S42.451[B], S42.452-S42.453[A,B], S42.454[B], S42.455-S42.456[A,B], S42.461[B], S42.462-S42.463[A,B], S42.464[B], S42.465-S42.466[A,B], S42.471[B], S42.472-S42.473[A,B], S42.474[B], S42.475-S42.476[A,B], S42.482-S42.489[A], S42.491[B], S42.492-S42.493[A,B], S42.494[B], S42.495-S42.92X[A,B], S49.002-S49.009[A], S49.012-S49.019[A], S49.022-S49.029[A], S49.032-S49.039[A], S49.042-S49.049[A], S49.092-S49.099[A], S49.102-S49.109[A], S49.112-S49.119[A], S49.122-S49.129[A], S49.132-S49.139[A], S49.142-S49.149[A], S49.192-S49.199[A]
For S42.202[B]: See S42.201[B]
For S42.202[K,P]: See S02.0[K]

S42.209 Unspecified fracture of upper end of unspecified humerus A, K, P, B, A, B

Ex: **For S42.209[A]:** S42.201-S42.266[A,B], S42.271-S42.279[A], S42.291-S42.309[A,B], S42.311-S42.319[A], S42.321-S42.476[A,B], S42.481-S42.489[A], S42.491-S42.92X[A,B], S49.001-S49.199[A] **For S42.202[B]:** See S42.201[B] **For S42.202[K,P]:** See S02.0[K]

- **S42.21 Unspecified fracture of surgical neck of humerus**
  Fracture of neck of humerus NOS
  - **S42.211 Unspecified displaced fracture of surgical neck of right humerus** A, K, P CC, B MCC, A, B HAC
    Ex For S42.211[A]: See S42.201[A]
    For S42.211[B]: See S42.201[B]
    For S42.211[K,P]: See S02.0[K]
  - **S42.212 Unspecified displaced fracture of surgical neck of left humerus** A, K, P CC, B MCC, A, B HAC
    Ex For S42.212[A]: See S42.202[A]
    For S42.212[B]: See S42.201[B]
    For S42.212[K,P]: See S02.0[K]
  - **S42.213 Unspecified displaced fracture of surgical neck of unspecified humerus** A, K, P CC, B MCC, A, B HAC
    Ex For S42.213[A]: See S42.209[A]
    For S42.213[B]: See S42.201[B]
    For S42.213[K,P]: See S02.0[K]
  - **S42.214 Unspecified nondisplaced fracture of surgical neck of right humerus** A, K, P CC, B MCC, A, B HAC
    Ex For S42.214[A]: See S42.201[A]
    For S42.214[B]: See S42.201[B]
    For S42.214[K,P]: See S02.0[K]
  - **S42.215 Unspecified nondisplaced fracture of surgical neck of left humerus** A, K, P CC, B MCC, A, B HAC
    Ex For S42.215[A]: See S42.202[A]
    For S42.215[B]: See S42.201[B]
    For S42.215[K,P]: See S02.0[K]
  - **S42.216 Unspecified nondisplaced fracture of surgical neck of unspecified humerus** A, K, P CC, B MCC, A, B HAC
    Ex For S42.216[A]: See S42.209[A]
    For S42.216[B]: See S42.201[B]
    For S42.216[K,P]: See S02.0[K]
- **S42.22 2-part fracture of surgical neck of humerus**
  - **S42.221 2-part displaced fracture of surgical neck of right humerus** A, K, P CC, B MCC, A, B HAC
    Ex For S42.221[A]: See S42.201[A]
    For S42.221[B]: See S42.201[B]
    For S42.221[K,P]: See S02.0[K]
  - **S42.222 2-part displaced fracture of surgical neck of left humerus** A, K, P CC, B MCC, A, B HAC
    Ex For S42.222[A]: See S42.202[A]
    For S42.222[B]: See S42.201[B]
    For S42.222[K,P]: See S02.0[K]
  - **S42.223 2-part displaced fracture of surgical neck of unspecified humerus** A, K, P CC, B MCC, A, B HAC
    Ex For S42.223[A]: See S42.209[A]
    For S42.223[B]: See S42.201[B]
    For S42.223[K,P]: See S02.0[K]
  - **S42.224 2-part nondisplaced fracture of surgical neck of right humerus** A, K, P CC, B MCC, A, B HAC
    Ex For S42.224[A]: See S42.201[A]
    For S42.224[B]: See S42.201[B]
    For S42.224[K,P]: See S02.0[K]
  - **S42.225 2-part nondisplaced fracture of surgical neck of left humerus** A, K, P CC, B MCC, A, B HAC
    Ex For S42.225[A]: See S42.202[A]
    For S42.225[B]: See S42.201[B]
    For S42.225[K,P]: See S02.0[K]
  - **S42.226 2-part nondisplaced fracture of surgical neck of unspecified humerus** A, K, P CC, B MCC, A, B HAC
    Ex For S42.226[A]: See S42.209[A]
    For S42.226[B]: See S42.201[B]
    For S42.226[K,P]: See S02.0[K]
- **S42.23 3-part fracture of surgical neck of humerus**
  - **S42.231 3-part fracture of surgical neck of right humerus** A, K, P CC, B MCC, A, B HAC
    Ex For S42.231[A]: See S42.201[A]
    For S42.231[B]: See S42.201[B]
    For S42.231[K,P]: See S02.0[K]
  - **S42.232 3-part fracture of surgical neck of left humerus** A, K, P CC, B MCC, A, B HAC
    Ex For S42.232[A]: See S42.202[A]
    For S42.232[B]: See S42.201[B]
    For S42.232[K,P]: See S02.0[K]
  - **S42.239 3-part fracture of surgical neck of unspecified humerus** A, K, P CC, B MCC, A, B HAC
    Ex For S42.239[A]: See S42.209[A]
    For S42.239[B]: See S42.201[B]
    For S42.239[K,P]: See S02.0[K]
- **S42.24 4-part fracture of surgical neck of humerus**
  - **S42.241 4-part fracture of surgical neck of right humerus** A, K, P CC, B MCC, A, B HAC
    Ex For S42.241[A]: See S42.201[A]
    For S42.241[B]: See S42.201[B]
    For S42.241[K,P]: See S02.0[K]
  - **S42.242 4-part fracture of surgical neck of left humerus** A, K, P CC, B MCC, A, B HAC
    Ex For S42.242[A]: See S42.202[A]
    For S42.242[B]: See S42.201[B]
    For S42.242[K,P]: See S02.0[K]
  - **S42.249 4-part fracture of surgical neck of unspecified humerus** A, K, P CC, B MCC, A, B HAC
    Ex For S42.249[A]: See S42.209[A]
    For S42.249[B]: See S42.201[B]
    For S42.249[K,P]: See S02.0[K]
- **S42.25 Fracture of greater tuberosity of humerus**
  - **S42.251 Displaced fracture of greater tuberosity of right humerus** A, K, P CC, B MCC, A, B HAC
    Ex For S42.251[A]: See S42.201[A]
    For S42.251[B]: See S42.201[B]
    For S42.251[K,P]: See S02.0[K]
  - **S42.252 Displaced fracture of greater tuberosity of left humerus** A, K, P CC, B MCC, A, B HAC
    Ex For S42.252[A]: See S42.202[A]
    For S42.252[B]: See S42.201[B]
    For S42.252[K,P]: See S02.0[K]
  - **S42.253 Displaced fracture of greater tuberosity of unspecified humerus** A, K, P CC, B MCC, A, B HAC
    Ex For category S42.253 CC codes
    S42.253[A]: See S42.209[A]
    For S42.253[B]: See S42.201[B]
    For S42.253[K,P]: See S02.0[K]
  - **S42.254 Nondisplaced fracture of greater tuberosity of right humerus** A, K, P CC, B MCC, A, B HAC
    Ex For S42.254[A]: See S42.201[A]
    For S42.254[B]: See S42.201[B]
    For S42.254[K,P]: See S02.0[K]
  - **S42.255 Nondisplaced fracture of greater tuberosity of left humerus** A, K, P CC, B MCC, A, B HAC
    Ex For S42.255[A]: See S42.202[A]
    For S42.255[B]: See S42.201[B]
    For S42.255[K,P]: See S02.0[K]
  - **S42.256 Nondisplaced fracture of greater tuberosity of unspecified humerus** A, K, P CC, B MCC, A, B HAC
    Ex For S42.256[A]: See S42.209[A]
    For S42.256[B]: See S42.201[B]
    For S42.256[K,P]: See S02.0[K]

S42.26 Fracture of lesser tuberosity of humerus

S42.261 Displaced fracture of lesser tuberosity of right humerus A, K, P, B, A, B

Ex: **For S42.261[A]:** See S42.201[A]
For S42.261[B]: See S42.201[B]
For S42.261[K,P]: See S02.0[K]

S42.262 Displaced fracture of lesser tuberosity of left humerus A, K, P, B, A, B

Ex: **For S42.262[A]:** See S42.202[A]
For S42.262[B]: See S42.201[B]
For S42.262[K,P]: See S02.0[K]

S42.263 Displaced fracture of lesser tuberosity of unspecified humerus A, K, P, B, A, B

Ex: **For S42.263[A]:** See S42.209[A]
For S42.263[B]: See S42.201[B]
For S42.263[K,P]: See S02.0[K]

S42.264 Nondisplaced fracture of lesser tuberosity of right humerus A, K, P, B, A, B

Ex: **For S42.264[A]:** See S42.201[A]
For S42.264[B]: See S42.201[B]
For S42.264[K,P]: See S02.0[K]

S42.265 Nondisplaced fracture of lesser tuberosity of left humerus A, K, P, B, A, B

Ex: **For S42.265[A]:** See S42.202[A]
For S42.265[B]: See S42.201[B]
For S42.265[K,P]: See S02.0[K]

S42.266 Nondisplaced fracture of lesser tuberosity of unspecified humerus A, K, P, B, A, B

Ex: **For S42.266[A]:** See S42.209[A]
For S42.266[B]: See S42.201[B]
For S42.266[K,P]: See S02.0[K]

S42.27 Torus fracture of upper end of humerus

The appropriate 7th character is to be added to all codes in subcategory S42.27

A	initial encounter for closed fracture
D	subsequent encounter for fracture with routine healing
G	subsequent encounter for fracture with delayed healing
K	subsequent encounter for fracture with nonunion
P	subsequent encounter for fracture with malunion
S	sequela

S42.271 Torus fracture of upper end of right humerus A, K, P, A

Ex: **For S42.271[A]:** See S42.201[A]
For S42.271[K,P]: See S02.0[K]

S42.272 Torus fracture of upper end of left humerus A, K, P, A

Ex: **For S42.272[A]:** See S42.202[A]
For S42.272[K,P]: See S02.0[K]

S42.279 Torus fracture of upper end of unspecified humerus A, K, P, A

Ex: **For S42.279[A]:** See S42.209[A]
For S42.279[K,P]: See S02.0[K]

S42.29 Other fracture of upper end of humerus

Fracture of anatomical neck of humerus
Fracture of articular head of humerus

S42.291 Other displaced fracture of upper end of right humerus A, K, P, B, A, B

Ex: **For S42.291[A]:** See S42.201[A]
For S42.291[B]: See S42.201[B]
For S42.291[K,P]: See S02.0[K]

S42.292 Other displaced fracture of upper end of left humerus A, K, P, B, A, B

Ex: **For S42.292[A]:** See S42.202[A]
For S42.292[B]: See S42.201[B]
For S42.292[K,P]: See S02.0[K]

S42.293 Other displaced fracture of upper end of unspecified humerus A, K, P, B, A, B

Ex: **For S42.293[A]:** See S42.209[A]
For S42.293[B]: See S42.201[B]
For S42.293[K,P]: See S02.0[K]

S42.294 Other nondisplaced fracture of upper end of right humerus A, K, P, B, A, B

Ex: **For S42.294[A]:** See S42.201[A]
For S42.294[B]: See S42.201[B]
For S42.294[K,P]: See S02.0[K]

S42.295 Other nondisplaced fracture of upper end of left humerus A, K, P, B, A, B

Ex: **For S42.295[A]:** See S42.202[A]
For S42.295[B]: See S42.201[B]
For S42.295[K,P]: See S02.0[K]

S42.296 Other nondisplaced fracture of upper end of unspecified humerus A, K, P, B, A, B

Ex: **For S42.296[A]:** See S42.209[A]
For S42.296[B]: See S42.201[B]
For S42.296[K,P]: See S02.0[K]

S42.3 Fracture of shaft of humerus

Fracture of humerus NOS
Fracture of upper arm NOS

Excludes2 physeal fractures of upper end of humerus (S49.0-)
physeal fractures of lower end of humerus (S49.1-)

S42.30 Unspecified fracture of shaft of humerus

S42.301 Unspecified fracture of shaft of humerus, right arm A, K, P, B, A, B

Ex: **For S42.301[A]:** See S42.201[A]
For S42.301[B]: See S42.201[B]
For S42.301[K,P]: See S02.0[K]

S42.302 Unspecified fracture of shaft of humerus, left arm A, K, P, B, A, B

Ex: **For S42.302[A]:** See S42.202[A]
For S42.302[B]: See S42.201[B]
For S42.302[K,P]: See S02.0[K]

S42.309 Unspecified fracture of shaft of humerus, unspecified arm A, K, P, B, A, B

Ex: **For S42.309[A]:** See S42.209[A]
For S42.309[B]: See S42.201[B]
For S42.309[K,P]: See S02.0[K]

- S43.005 Unspecified dislocation of left shoulder joint
- S43.006 Unspecified dislocation of unspecified shoulder joint

- S43.01 Anterior subluxation and dislocation of humerus
  - S43.011 Anterior subluxation of right humerus
  - S43.012 Anterior subluxation of left humerus
  - S43.013 Anterior subluxation of unspecified humerus
  - S43.014 Anterior dislocation of right humerus
  - S43.015 Anterior dislocation of left humerus
  - S43.016 Anterior dislocation of unspecified humerus
- S43.02 Posterior subluxation and dislocation of humerus
  - S43.021 Posterior subluxation of right humerus
  - S43.022 Posterior subluxation of left humerus
  - S43.023 Posterior subluxation of unspecified humerus
  - S43.024 Posterior dislocation of right humerus
  - S43.025 Posterior dislocation of left humerus
  - S43.026 Posterior dislocation of unspecified humerus
- S43.03 Inferior subluxation and dislocation of humerus
  - S43.031 Inferior subluxation of right humerus
  - S43.032 Inferior subluxation of left humerus
  - S43.033 Inferior subluxation of unspecified humerus
  - S43.034 Inferior dislocation of right humerus
  - S43.035 Inferior dislocation of left humerus
  - S43.036 Inferior dislocation of unspecified humerus
- S43.08 Other subluxation and dislocation of shoulder joint
  - S43.081 Other subluxation of right shoulder joint
  - S43.082 Other subluxation of left shoulder joint
  - S43.083 Other subluxation of unspecified shoulder joint
  - S43.084 Other dislocation of right shoulder joint
  - S43.085 Other dislocation of left shoulder joint
  - S43.086 Other dislocation of unspecified shoulder joint

- S43.1 Subluxation and dislocation of acromioclavicular joint
  - S43.10 Unspecified dislocation of acromioclavicular joint
    - S43.101 Unspecified dislocation of right acromioclavicular joint
    - S43.102 Unspecified dislocation of left acromioclavicular joint
    - S43.109 Unspecified dislocation of unspecified acromioclavicular joint
  - S43.11 Subluxation of acromioclavicular joint
    - S43.111 Subluxation of right acromioclavicular joint
    - S43.112 Subluxation of left acromioclavicular joint
    - S43.119 Subluxation of unspecified acromioclavicular joint
  - S43.12 Dislocation of acromioclavicular joint, 100%-200% displacement
    - S43.121 Dislocation of right acromioclavicular joint, 100%-200% displacement
    - S43.122 Dislocation of left acromioclavicular joint, 100%-200% displacement
    - S43.129 Dislocation of unspecified acromioclavicular joint, 100%-200% displacement
  - S43.13 Dislocation of acromioclavicular joint, greater than 200% displacement
    - S43.131 Dislocation of right acromioclavicular joint, greater than 200% displacement
    - S43.132 Dislocation of left acromioclavicular joint, greater than 200% displacement
    - S43.139 Dislocation of unspecified acromioclavicular joint, greater than 200% displacement
  - S43.14 Inferior dislocation of acromioclavicular joint
    - S43.141 Inferior dislocation of right acromioclavicular joint
    - S43.142 Inferior dislocation of left acromioclavicular joint
    - S43.149 Inferior dislocation of unspecified acromioclavicular joint
  - S43.15 Posterior dislocation of acromioclavicular joint
    - S43.151 Posterior dislocation of right acromioclavicular joint
    - S43.152 Posterior dislocation of left acromioclavicular joint
    - S43.159 Posterior dislocation of unspecified acromioclavicular joint

- S43.2 Subluxation and dislocation of sternoclavicular joint
  - S43.20 Unspecified subluxation and dislocation of sternoclavicular joint
    - S43.201 Unspecified subluxation of right sternoclavicular joint A, A
      Ex: M99.18, S43.201[A], S43.203-S43.204[A], S43.206[A], S43.211[A], S43.213-S43.214[A], S43.216[A], S43.221[A], S43.223-S43.224[A], S43.226[A]
    - S43.202 Unspecified subluxation of left sternoclavicular joint A, A
      Ex: M99.18, S43.202-S43.203[A], S43.205-S43.206[A], S43.212-S43.213[A], S43.215-S43.216[A], S43.222-S43.223[A], S43.225-S43.226[A]
    - S43.203 Unspecified subluxation of unspecified sternoclavicular joint A, A
      Ex: M99.18, S43.201-S43.226[A]
    - S43.204 Unspecified dislocation of right sternoclavicular joint A, A
      Ex: See S43.201
    - S43.205 Unspecified dislocation of left sternoclavicular joint A, A
      Ex: See S43.202
    - S43.206 Unspecified dislocation of unspecified sternoclavicular joint A, A
      Ex: See S43.203
  - S43.21 Anterior subluxation and dislocation of sternoclavicular joint
    - S43.211 Anterior subluxation of right sternoclavicular joint A, A
      Ex: See S43.201
    - S43.212 Anterior subluxation of left sternoclavicular joint A, A
      Ex: See S43.202
    - S43.213 Anterior subluxation of unspecified sternoclavicular joint A, A
      Ex: See S43.203

◀ New ◀ Revised ~~deleted~~ Deleted Excludes 1 Excludes 2 Includes Use additional Code first Code also Unspecified
OGCR Official Guidelines ● Unacceptable Principal Diagnosis X Assign placeholder X ● Use Additional Character(s) ▶ Manifestation Code Coding Clinic

- **S52.04** Fracture of coronoid process of ulna
  Ex: For category S52.04 CC codes S52.04[B,C]: See S52.00[B,C] For S52.04[K,M,N,P,Q,R]: See S02.0[K]
  - **S52.041** Displaced fracture of coronoid process of right ulna K, M, N, P, Q, R CC, B, C MCC, B, C HAC
  - **S52.042** Displaced fracture of coronoid process of left ulna K, M, N, P, Q, R CC, B, C MCC, B, C HAC
  - **S52.043** Displaced fracture of coronoid process of unspecified ulna K, M, N, P, Q, R CC, B, C MCC, B, C HAC
  - **S52.044** Nondisplaced fracture of coronoid process of right ulna K, M, N, P, Q, R CC, B, C MCC, B, C HAC
  - **S52.045** Nondisplaced fracture of coronoid process of left ulna K, M, N, P, Q, R CC, B, C MCC, B, C HAC
  - **S52.046** Nondisplaced fracture of coronoid process of unspecified ulna K, M, N, P, Q, R CC, B, C MCC, B, C HAC
- **S52.09** Other fracture of upper end of ulna
  Ex: For category S52.09 CC codes S52.09[B,C]: See S52.00[B,C] For S52.09[K,M,N,P,Q,R]: See S02.0[K]
  - **S52.091** Other fracture of upper end of right ulna K, M, N, P, Q, R CC, B, C MCC, B, C HAC
  - **S52.092** Other fracture of upper end of left ulna K, M, N, P, Q, R CC, B, C MCC, B, C HAC
  - **S52.099** Other fracture of upper end of unspecified ulna K, M, N, P, Q, R CC, B, C MCC, B, C HAC
- **S52.1** Fracture of upper end of radius
  Fracture of proximal end of radius
  Excludes2 physeal fractures of upper end of radius (S59.2-)
  fracture of shaft of radius (S52.3-)
- **S52.10** Unspecified fracture of upper end of radius
  Ex: For category S52.10 CC codes S52.10[B,C]: See S52.00[B,C] For S52.10[K,M,N,P,Q,R]: See S02.0[K]
  - **S52.101** Unspecified fracture of upper end of right radius K, M, N, P, Q, R CC, B, C MCC, B, C HAC
  - **S52.102** Unspecified fracture of upper end of left radius K, M, N, P, Q, R CC, B, C MCC, B, C HAC
  - **S52.109** Unspecified fracture of upper end of unspecified radius K, M, N, P, Q, R CC, B, C MCC, B, C HAC
- **S52.11** Torus fracture of upper end of radius
  The appropriate 7th character is to be added to all codes in subcategory S52.11

A	initial encounter for closed fracture
D	subsequent encounter for fracture with routine healing
G	subsequent encounter for fracture with delayed healing
K	subsequent encounter for fracture with nonunion
P	subsequent encounter for fracture with malunion
S	sequela

  - **S52.111** Torus fracture of upper end of right radius A, K, P CC, A HAC
    Ex: For code S52.111[A]: See S52.011[A] For S52.111[K,P]: See S02.0[K]
  - **S52.112** Torus fracture of upper end of left radius A, K, P CC, A HAC
    Ex: For code S52.112[A]: See S52.012[A] For S52.112[K,P]: See S02.0[K]
  - **S52.119** Torus fracture of upper end of unspecified radius A, K, P CC, A HAC
    Ex: For code S52.119[A]: See S52.019[A] For S52.119[K,P]: See S02.0[K]
- **S52.12** Fracture of head of radius
  Ex: For category S52.12 CC codes S52.12[B,C]: See S52.00[B,C] For S52.12[K,M,N,P,Q,R]: See S02.0[K]
  - **S52.121** Displaced fracture of head of right radius K, M, N, P, Q, R CC, B, C MCC, B, C HAC
  - **S52.122** Displaced fracture of head of left radius K, M, N, P, Q, R CC, B, C MCC, B, C HAC
  - **S52.123** Displaced fracture of head of unspecified radius K, M, N, P, Q, R CC, B, C MCC, B, C HAC
  - **S52.124** Nondisplaced fracture of head of right radius K, M, N, P, Q, R CC, B, C MCC, B, C HAC
  - **S52.125** Nondisplaced fracture of head of left radius K, M, N, P, Q, R CC, B, C MCC, B, C HAC
  - **S52.126** Nondisplaced fracture of head of unspecified radius K, M, N, P, Q, R CC, B, C MCC, B, C HAC
- **S52.13** Fracture of neck of radius
  Ex: For category S52.13 CC codes S52.13[B,C]: See S52.00[B,C] For S52.13[K,M,N,P,Q,R]: See S02.0[K]
  - **S52.131** Displaced fracture of neck of right radius K, M, N, P, Q, R CC, B, C MCC, B, C HAC
  - **S52.132** Displaced fracture of neck of left radius K, M, N, P, Q, R CC, B, C MCC, B, C HAC
  - **S52.133** Displaced fracture of neck of unspecified radius K, M, N, P, Q, R CC, B, C MCC, B, C HAC
  - **S52.134** Nondisplaced fracture of neck of right radius K, M, N, P, Q, R CC, B, C MCC, B, C HAC
  - **S52.135** Nondisplaced fracture of neck of left radius K, M, N, P, Q, R CC, B, C MCC, B, C HAC
  - **S52.136** Nondisplaced fracture of neck of unspecified radius K, M, N, P, Q, R CC, B, C MCC, B, C HAC
- **S52.18** Other fracture of upper end of radius
  Ex: For category S52.18 CC codes S52.18[B,C]: See S52.00[B,C] For S52.18[K,M,N,P,Q,R]: See S02.0[K]
  - **S52.181** Other fracture of upper end of right radius K, M, N, P, Q, R CC, B, C MCC, B, C HAC
  - **S52.182** Other fracture of upper end of left radius K, M, N, P, Q, R CC, B, C MCC, B, C HAC
  - **S52.189** Other fracture of upper end of unspecified radius K, M, N, P, Q, R CC, B, C MCC, B, C HAC

● **S52.2 Fracture of shaft of ulna**

● **S52.20 Unspecified fracture of shaft of ulna**
Fracture of ulna NOS

● **S52.201 Unspecified fracture of shaft of right ulna** A, K, M, N, P, Q, R, B, C, A, B, C
Ex: For code S52.201[A]: See S52.011[A]
For S52.201[B,C]: See S52.00[B,C]
For S52.201[K,M,N,P,Q,R]: See S02.0[K]

● **S52.202 Unspecified fracture of shaft of left ulna** A, K, M, N, P, Q, R, B, C, A, B, C
Ex: For code S52.202[A]: See S52.012[A] For code S52.202[B,C]: See S52.00[B,C]
For S52.202[K,M,N,P,Q,R]: See S02.0[K]

● **S52.209 Unspecified fracture of shaft of unspecified ulna**
A, K, M, N, P, Q, R, B, C, A, B, C
Ex: For code S52.209[A]: See S52.019[A] For code S52.209[B,C]: See S52.00[B,C]
For S52.209[K,M,N,P,Q,R]: See S02.0[K]

● **S52.21 Greenstick fracture of shaft of ulna**
The appropriate 7th character is to be added to all codes in subcategory S52.21

A	initial encounter for closed fracture
D	subsequent encounter for fracture with routine healing
G	subsequent encounter for fracture with delayed healing
K	subsequent encounter for fracture with nonunion
P	subsequent encounter for fracture with malunion
S	sequela

● **S52.211 Greenstick fracture of shaft of right ulna** A, K, P, A
Ex: For code S52.211[A]: See S52.011[A]
For S52.211[K,P]: See S02.0[K]

● **S52.212 Greenstick fracture of shaft of left ulna** A, K, P, A
Ex: For code S52.212[A]: See S52.012[A]
For S52.202[K,P]: See S02.0[K]

● **S52.219 Greenstick fracture of shaft of unspecified ulna** A, K, P, A
Ex: For code S52.219[A]: See S52.019[A]
For S52.219[K,P]: See S02.0[K]

● **S52.22 Transverse fracture of shaft of ulna**

● **S52.221 Displaced transverse fracture of shaft of right ulna** A, K, M, N, P, Q, R, B, C, A, B, C
Ex: For code S52.221[A]: See S52.011[A]
For S52.221[B,C]: See S52.00[B,C]
For S52.221[K,M,N,P,Q,R]: See S02.0[K]

● **S52.222 Displaced transverse fracture of shaft of left ulna** A, K, M, N, P, Q, R, B, C, A, B, C
Ex: For code S52.222[A]: See S52.012[A] For code S52.222[B,C]: See S52.00[B,C]
For S52.222[K,M,N,P,Q,R]: See S02.0[K]

● **S52.223 Displaced transverse fracture of shaft of unspecified ulna**
A, K, M, N, P, Q, R, B, C, A, B, C
Ex: For code S52.223[A]: See S52.019[A] For code S52.223[B,C]: See S52.00[B,C]
For S52.223[K,M,N,P,Q,R]: See S02.0[K]

● **S52.224 Nondisplaced transverse fracture of shaft of right ulna**
A, K, M, N, P, Q, R, B, C, A, B, C
Ex: For code S52.224[A]: See S52.011[A]
For S52.224[B,C]: See S52.00[B,C]
For S52.224[K,M,N,P,Q,R]: See S02.0[K]

● **S52.225 Nondisplaced transverse fracture of shaft of left ulna**
A, K, M, N, P, Q, R, B, C, A, B, C
Ex: For code S52.225[A]: See S52.012[A] For code S52.225[B,C]: See S52.00[B,C]
For S52.225[K,M,N,P,Q,R]: See S02.0[K]

● **S52.226 Nondisplaced transverse fracture of shaft of unspecified ulna**
A, K, M, N, P, Q, R, B, C, A, B, C
Ex: For code S52.226[A]: See S52.019[A] For code S52.226[B,C]: See S52.00[B,C]
For S52.226[K,M,N,P,Q,R]: See S02.0[K]

● **S52.23 Oblique fracture of shaft of ulna**

● **S52.231 Displaced oblique fracture of shaft of right ulna** A, K, M, N, P, Q, R, B, C, A, B, C
Ex: For code S52.231[A]: See S52.011[A]
For S52.231[B,C]: See S52.00[B,C]
For S52.231[K,M,N,P,Q,R]: See S02.0[K]

● **S52.232 Displaced oblique fracture of shaft of left ulna** A, K, M, N, P, Q, R, B, C, A, B, C
Ex: For code S52.232[A]: See S52.012[A] For code S52.232[B,C]: See S52.00[B,C]
For S52.232[K,M,N,P,Q,R]: See S02.0[K]

● **S52.233 Displaced oblique fracture of shaft of unspecified ulna**
A, K, M, N, P, Q, R, B, C, A, B, C
Ex: For code S52.233[A]: See S52.019[A] For code S52.233[B,C]: See S52.00[B,C]
For S52.233[K,M,N,P,Q,R]: See S02.0[K]

● **S52.234 Nondisplaced oblique fracture of shaft of right ulna**
A, K, M, N, P, Q, R, B, C, A, B, C
Ex: For code S52.234[A]: See S52.011[A]
For S52.234[B,C]: See S52.00[B,C]
For S52.234[K,M,N,P,Q,R]: See S02.0[K]

● **S52.235 Nondisplaced oblique fracture of shaft of left ulna**
A, K, M, N, P, Q, R, B, C, A, B, C
Ex: For code S52.235[A]: See S52.012[A] For code S52.235[B,C]: See S52.00[B,C]
For S52.235[K,M,N,P,Q,R]: See S02.0[K]

● **S52.236 Nondisplaced oblique fracture of shaft of unspecified ulna**
A, K, M, N, P, Q, R, B, C, A, B, C
Ex: For code S52.236[A]: See S52.019[A] For code S52.236[B,C]: See S52.00[B,C]
For S52.236[K,M,N,P,Q,R]: See S02.0[K]

● S52.56 Barton's fracture

● S52.561 Barton's fracture of right radius
A, K, M, N, P, Q, R, B, C, A, B, C
Ex: For code S52.561[A]: See S52.011[A]
For S52.561[B,C]: See S52.00[B,C]
For S52.561[K,M,N,P,Q,R]: See S02.0[K]

● S52.562 Barton's fracture of left radius
A, K, M, N, P, Q, R, B, C, A, B, C
Ex: For code S52.562[A]: See S52.012[A] For code S52.562[B,C]: See S52.00[B,C]
For S52.562[K,M,N,P,Q,R]: See S02.0[K]

● S52.569 Barton's fracture of unspecified radius
A, K, M, N, P, Q, R, B, C, A, B, C
Ex: For code S52.569[A]: See S52.019[A] For code S52.569[B,C]: See S52.00[B,C]
For S52.569[K,M,N,P,Q,R]: See S02.0[K]

● S52.57 Other intraarticular fracture of lower end of radius

● S52.571 Other intraarticular fracture of lower end of right radius
A, K, M, N, P, Q, R, B, C, A, B, C
Ex: For code S52.571[A]: See S52.011[A]
For S52.571[B,C]: See S52.00[B,C]
For S52.571[K,M,N,P,Q,R]: See S02.0[K]

● S52.572 Other intraarticular fracture of lower end of left radius
A, K, M, N, P, Q, R, B, C, A, B, C
Ex: For code S52.572[A]: See S52.012[A] For code S52.572[B,C]: See S52.00[B,C]
For S52.572[K,M,N,P,Q,R]: See S02.0[K]

● S52.579 Other intraarticular fracture of lower end of unspecified radius
A, K, M, N, P, Q, R, B, C, A, B, C
Ex: For code S52.579[A]: See S52.019[A] For code S52.579[B,C]: See S52.00[B,C]
For S52.579[K,M,N,P,Q,R]: See S02.0[K]

● S52.59 Other fractures of lower end of radius

● S52.591 Other fractures of lower end of right radius A, K, M, N, P, Q, R, B, C, A, B, C
Ex: For code S52.591[A]: See S52.011[A]
For S52.591[B,C]: See S52.00[B,C]
For S52.591[K,M,N,P,Q,R]: See S02.0[K]

● S52.592 Other fractures of lower end of left radius A, K, M, N, P, Q, R, B, C, A, B, C
Ex: For code S52.592[A]: See S52.012[A] For code S52.592[B,C]: See S52.00[B,C]
For S52.592[K,M,N,P,Q,R]: See S02.0[K]

● S52.599 Other fractures of lower end of unspecified radius
A, K, M, N, P, Q, R, B, C, A, B, C
Ex: For code S52.599[A]: See S52.019[A] For code S52.599[B,C]: See S52.00[B,C]
For S52.599[K,M,N,P,Q,R]: See S02.0[K]

● S52.6 Fracture of lower end of ulna

● S52.60 Unspecified fracture of lower end of ulna

● S52.601 Unspecified fracture of lower end of right ulna A, K, M, N, P, Q, R, B, C, A, B, C
Ex: For code S52.601[A]: See S52.011[A]
For S52.601[B,C]: See S52.00[B,C]
For S52.601[K,M,N,P,Q,R]: See S02.0[K]

● S52.602 Unspecified fracture of lower end of left ulna A, K, M, N, P, Q, R, B, C, A, B, C
Ex: For code S52.602[A]: See S52.012[A] For code S52.602[B,C]: See S52.00[B,C]
For S52.602[K,M,N,P,Q,R]: See S02.0[K]

● S52.609 Unspecified fracture of lower end of unspecified ulna
A, K, M, N, P, Q, R, B, C, A, B, C
Ex: For code S52.609[A]: See S52.019[A] For code S52.609[B,C]: See S52.00[B,C]
For S52.609[K,M,N,P,Q,R]: See S02.0[K]

● S52.61 Fracture of ulna styloid process

● S52.611 Displaced fracture of right ulna styloid process A, K, M, N, P, Q, R, B, C, A, B, C
Ex: For code S52.611[A]: See S52.011[A]
For S52.611[B,C]: See S52.00[B,C]
For S52.611[K,M,N,P,Q,R]: See S02.0[K]

● S52.612 Displaced fracture of left ulna styloid process A, K, M, N, P, Q, R, B, C, A, B, C
Ex: For code S52.612[A]: See S52.012[A] For code S52.612[B,C]: See S52.00[B,C]
For S52.612[K,M,N,P,Q,R]: See S02.0[K]

● S52.613 Displaced fracture of unspecified ulna styloid process A, K, M, N, P, Q, R, B, C, A, B, C
Ex: For code S52.613[A]: See S52.019[A] For code S52.613[B,C]: See S52.00[B,C]
For S52.613[K,M,N,P,Q,R]: See S02.0[K]

● S52.614 Nondisplaced fracture of right ulna styloid process A, K, M, N, P, Q, R, B, C, A, B, C
Ex: For code S52.614[A]: See S52.011[A]
For S52.614[B,C]: See S52.00[B,C]
For S52.614[K,M,N,P,Q,R]: See S02.0[K]

● S52.615 Nondisplaced fracture of left ulna styloid process A, K, M, N, P, Q, R, B, C, A, B, C
Ex: For code S52.615[A]: See S52.012[A] For code S52.615[B,C]: See S52.00[B,C]
For S52.615[K,M,N,P,Q,R]: See S02.0[K]

● S52.616 Nondisplaced fracture of unspecified ulna styloid process
A, K, M, N, P, Q, R, B, C, A, B, C
Ex: For code S52.616[A]: See S52.019[A] For code S52.616[B,C]: See S52.00[B,C]
For S52.616[K,M,N,P,Q,R]: See S02.0[K]

S58.1 Traumatic amputation at level between elbow and wrist

S58.11 Complete traumatic amputation at level between elbow and wrist

S58.111 Complete traumatic amputation at level between elbow and wrist, right arm A CC
Ex: See S48.011

S58.112 Complete traumatic amputation at level between elbow and wrist, left arm A CC
Ex: See S48.012

S58.119 Complete traumatic amputation at level between elbow and wrist, unspecified arm A CC
Ex: See S48.019

S58.12 Partial traumatic amputation at level between elbow and wrist

S58.121 Partial traumatic amputation at level between elbow and wrist, right arm A CC
Ex: See S48.011

S58.122 Partial traumatic amputation at level between elbow and wrist, left arm A CC
Ex: See S48.012

S58.129 Partial traumatic amputation at level between elbow and wrist, unspecified arm A CC
Ex: See S48.019

S58.9 Traumatic amputation of forearm, level unspecified

Excludes1 traumatic amputation of wrist (S68.-)

S58.91 Complete traumatic amputation of forearm, level unspecified

S58.911 Complete traumatic amputation of right forearm, level unspecified A CC
Ex: See S48.011

S58.912 Complete traumatic amputation of left forearm, level unspecified A CC
Ex: See S48.012

S58.919 Complete traumatic amputation of unspecified forearm, level unspecified A CC
Ex: See S48.019

S58.92 Partial traumatic amputation of forearm, level unspecified

S58.921 Partial traumatic amputation of right forearm, level unspecified A CC
Ex: See S48.011

S58.922 Partial traumatic amputation of left forearm, level unspecified A CC
Ex: See S48.012

S58.929 Partial traumatic amputation of unspecified forearm, level unspecified A CC
Ex: See S48.019

S59 Other and unspecified injuries of elbow and forearm

Excludes2 other and unspecified injuries of wrist and hand (S69.-)

The appropriate 7th character is to be added to each code from subcategories S59.0, S59.1, and S59.2

A	initial encounter for closed fracture
D	subsequent encounter for fracture with routine healing
G	subsequent encounter for fracture with delayed healing
K	subsequent encounter for fracture with nonunion
P	subsequent encounter for fracture with malunion
S	sequela

S59.0 Physeal fracture of lower end of ulna

S59.00 Unspecified physeal fracture of lower end of ulna

S59.001 Unspecified physeal fracture of lower end of ulna, right arm A, K, P CC, A MCC
Ex: **For code S59.001[A]:** See S52.011[A]
For S59.001[K,P]: See S02.0[K]

S59.002 Unspecified physeal fracture of lower end of ulna, left arm A, K, P CC, A MCC
Ex: **For code S59.002[A]:** See S52.012[A]
For S59.002[K,P]: See S02.0[K]

S59.009 Unspecified physeal fracture of lower end of ulna, unspecified arm A, K, P CC, A MCC
Ex: **For code S59.009[A]:** See S52.019[A]
For S59.009[K,P]: See S02.0[K]

S59.01 Salter-Harris Type I physeal fracture of lower end of ulna

S59.011 Salter-Harris Type I physeal fracture of lower end of ulna, right arm A, K, P CC, A MCC
Ex: **For code S59.011[A]:** See S52.011[A]
For S59.011[K,P]: See S02.0[K]

S59.012 Salter-Harris Type I physeal fracture of lower end of ulna, left arm A, K, P CC, A MCC
Ex: **For code S59.012[A]:** See S52.012[A]
For S59.012[K,P]: See S02.0[K]

S59.019 Salter-Harris Type I physeal fracture of lower end of ulna, unspecified arm A, K, P CC, A MCC
Ex: **For code S59.019[A]:** See S52.019[A]
For S59.019[K,P]: See S02.0[K]

Item 19-4 SALTER-HARRIS TYPE 1: epiphysis is completely separated from end of bone, or metaphysic growth plate remains attached to epiphysis

SALTER-HARRIS TYPE 2: epiphysis and growth plate are partially separated from metaphysis, which is cracked—most common type

SALTER-HARRIS TYPE 3: fracture occurring through epiphysis and separates part of epiphysis and growth plate from metaphysis fracture, usually at distal end of tibia

SALTER-HARRIS TYPE 4: fracture runs through epiphysis, across growth plate, into metaphysic, surgery is required to restore joint surface to normal and align growth plate

INJURIES TO THE WRIST, HAND AND FINGERS (S60-S69)

Excludes2 burns and corrosions (T20-T32)
frostbite (T33-T34)
insect bite or sting, venomous (T63.4)

S60 Superficial injury of wrist, hand and fingers

The appropriate 7th character is to be added to each code from category S60

A	initial encounter
D	subsequent encounter
S	sequela

S60.0 Contusion of finger without damage to nail

Excludes1 contusion involving nail (matrix) (S60.1)

X **S60.00 Contusion of unspecified finger without damage to nail**
Contusion of finger(s) NOS

S60.01 Contusion of thumb without damage to nail
- **S60.011 Contusion of right thumb without damage to nail**
- **S60.012 Contusion of left thumb without damage to nail**
- **S60.019 Contusion of unspecified thumb without damage to nail**

S60.02 Contusion of index finger without damage to nail
- **S60.021 Contusion of right index finger without damage to nail**
- **S60.022 Contusion of left index finger without damage to nail**
- **S60.029 Contusion of unspecified index finger without damage to nail**

S60.03 Contusion of middle finger without damage to nail
- **S60.031 Contusion of right middle finger without damage to nail**
- **S60.032 Contusion of left middle finger without damage to nail**
- **S60.039 Contusion of unspecified middle finger without damage to nail**

S60.04 Contusion of ring finger without damage to nail
- **S60.041 Contusion of right ring finger without damage to nail**
- **S60.042 Contusion of left ring finger without damage to nail**
- **S60.049 Contusion of unspecified ring finger without damage to nail**

S60.05 Contusion of little finger without damage to nail
- **S60.051 Contusion of right little finger without damage to nail**
- **S60.052 Contusion of left little finger without damage to nail**
- **S60.059 Contusion of unspecified little finger without damage to nail**

S60.1 Contusion of finger with damage to nail

X **S60.10 Contusion of unspecified finger with damage to nail**

S60.11 Contusion of thumb with damage to nail
- **S60.111 Contusion of right thumb with damage to nail**
- **S60.112 Contusion of left thumb with damage to nail**
- **S60.119 Contusion of unspecified thumb with damage to nail**

S60.12 Contusion of index finger with damage to nail
- **S60.121 Contusion of right index finger with damage to nail**
- **S60.122 Contusion of left index finger with damage to nail**
- **S60.129 Contusion of unspecified index finger with damage to nail**

S60.13 Contusion of middle finger with damage to nail
- **S60.131 Contusion of right middle finger with damage to nail**
- **S60.132 Contusion of left middle finger with damage to nail**
- **S60.139 Contusion of unspecified middle finger with damage to nail**

S60.14 Contusion of ring finger with damage to nail
- **S60.141 Contusion of right ring finger with damage to nail**
- **S60.142 Contusion of left ring finger with damage to nail**
- **S60.149 Contusion of unspecified ring finger with damage to nail**

S60.15 Contusion of little finger with damage to nail
- **S60.151 Contusion of right little finger with damage to nail**
- **S60.152 Contusion of left little finger with damage to nail**
- **S60.159 Contusion of unspecified little finger with damage to nail**

S60.2 Contusion of wrist and hand

Excludes2 contusion of fingers (S60.0-, S60.1-)

S60.21 Contusion of wrist
- **S60.211 Contusion of right wrist**
- **S60.212 Contusion of left wrist**
- **S60.219 Contusion of unspecified wrist**

S60.22 Contusion of hand
- **S60.221 Contusion of right hand**
- **S60.222 Contusion of left hand**
- **S60.229 Contusion of unspecified hand**

S60.3 Other superficial injuries of thumb

S60.31 Abrasion of thumb
- **S60.311 Abrasion of right thumb**
- **S60.312 Abrasion of left thumb**
- **S60.319 Abrasion of unspecified thumb**

S60.32 Blister (nonthermal) of thumb
- **S60.321 Blister (nonthermal) of right thumb**
- **S60.322 Blister (nonthermal) of left thumb**
- **S60.329 Blister (nonthermal) of unspecified thumb**

S60.34 External constriction of thumb
Hair tourniquet syndrome of thumb
Use additional cause code to identify the constricting item (W49.0-)
- **S60.341 External constriction of right thumb**
- **S60.342 External constriction of left thumb**
- **S60.349 External constriction of unspecified thumb**

S60.35 Superficial foreign body of thumb
Splinter in the thumb
- **S60.351 Superficial foreign body of right thumb**
- **S60.352 Superficial foreign body of left thumb**
- **S60.359 Superficial foreign body of unspecified thumb**

New Revised ~~deleted~~ Deleted Excludes 1 Excludes 2 Includes Use additional Code first Code also Unspecified
OGCR Official Guidelines ● Unacceptable Principal Diagnosis X Assign placeholder X ● Use Additional Character(s) ▶ Manifestation Code Coding Clinic

- S61.33 Puncture wound without foreign body of finger with damage to nail
  - S61.330 Puncture wound without foreign body of right index finger with damage to nail
  - S61.331 Puncture wound without foreign body of left index finger with damage to nail
  - S61.332 Puncture wound without foreign body of right middle finger with damage to nail
  - S61.333 Puncture wound without foreign body of left middle finger with damage to nail
  - S61.334 Puncture wound without foreign body of right ring finger with damage to nail
  - S61.335 Puncture wound without foreign body of left ring finger with damage to nail
  - S61.336 Puncture wound without foreign body of right little finger with damage to nail
  - S61.337 Puncture wound without foreign body of left little finger with damage to nail
  - S61.338 Puncture wound without foreign body of other finger with damage to nail
    Puncture wound without foreign body of specified finger with unspecified laterality with damage to nail
  - S61.339 Puncture wound without foreign body of unspecified finger with damage to nail
- S61.34 Puncture wound with foreign body of finger with damage to nail
  - S61.340 Puncture wound with foreign body of right index finger with damage to nail
  - S61.341 Puncture wound with foreign body of left index finger with damage to nail
  - S61.342 Puncture wound with foreign body of right middle finger with damage to nail
  - S61.343 Puncture wound with foreign body of left middle finger with damage to nail
  - S61.344 Puncture wound with foreign body of right ring finger with damage to nail
  - S61.345 Puncture wound with foreign body of left ring finger with damage to nail
  - S61.346 Puncture wound with foreign body of right little finger with damage to nail
  - S61.347 Puncture wound with foreign body of left little finger with damage to nail
  - S61.348 Puncture wound with foreign body of other finger with damage to nail
    Puncture wound with foreign body of specified finger with unspecified laterality with damage to nail
  - S61.349 Puncture wound with foreign body of unspecified finger with damage to nail
- S61.35 Open bite of finger with damage to nail
  Bite of finger with damage to nail NOS
  Excludes1 superficial bite of finger (S60.46-, S60.47-)
  - S61.350 Open bite of right index finger with damage to nail
  - S61.351 Open bite of left index finger with damage to nail
  - S61.352 Open bite of right middle finger with damage to nail
  - S61.353 Open bite of left middle finger with damage to nail
  - S61.354 Open bite of right ring finger with damage to nail
  - S61.355 Open bite of left ring finger with damage to nail
  - S61.356 Open bite of right little finger with damage to nail
  - S61.357 Open bite of left little finger with damage to nail
  - S61.358 Open bite of other finger with damage to nail
    Open bite of specified finger with unspecified laterality with damage to nail
  - S61.359 Open bite of unspecified finger with damage to nail
- S61.4 Open wound of hand
  - S61.40 Unspecified open wound of hand
    - S61.401 Unspecified open wound of right hand
    - S61.402 Unspecified open wound of left hand
    - S61.409 Unspecified open wound of unspecified hand
  - S61.41 Laceration without foreign body of hand
    - S61.411 Laceration without foreign body of right hand
    - S61.412 Laceration without foreign body of left hand
    - S61.419 Laceration without foreign body of unspecified hand
  - S61.42 Laceration with foreign body of hand
    - S61.421 Laceration with foreign body of right hand
    - S61.422 Laceration with foreign body of left hand
    - S61.429 Laceration with foreign body of unspecified hand
  - S61.43 Puncture wound without foreign body of hand
    - S61.431 Puncture wound without foreign body of right hand
    - S61.432 Puncture wound without foreign body of left hand
    - S61.439 Puncture wound without foreign body of unspecified hand
  - S61.44 Puncture wound with foreign body of hand
    - S61.441 Puncture wound with foreign body of right hand
    - S61.442 Puncture wound with foreign body of left hand
    - S61.449 Puncture wound with foreign body of unspecified hand
  - S61.45 Open bite of hand
    Bite of hand NOS
    Excludes1 superficial bite of hand (S60.56-, S60.57-)
    - S61.451 Open bite of right hand
    - S61.452 Open bite of left hand
    - S61.459 Open bite of unspecified hand
- S61.5 Open wound of wrist
  - S61.50 Unspecified open wound of wrist
    - S61.501 Unspecified open wound of right wrist
    - S61.502 Unspecified open wound of left wrist
    - S61.509 Unspecified open wound of unspecified wrist

◀ New ◀ Revised ~~deleted~~ Deleted Excludes 1 Excludes 2 Includes Use additional Code first Code also Unspecified
OGCR Official Guidelines ● Unacceptable Principal Diagnosis X Assign placeholder X ● Use Additional Character(s) ▶ Manifestation Code Coding Clinic

S42.31 Greenstick fracture of shaft of humerus

The appropriate 7th character is to be added to all codes in subcategory S42.31

A	initial encounter for closed fracture
D	subsequent encounter for fracture with routine healing
G	subsequent encounter for fracture with delayed healing
K	subsequent encounter for fracture with nonunion
P	subsequent encounter for fracture with malunion
S	sequela

S42.311 Greenstick fracture of shaft of humerus, right arm A, K, P CC, A MCC
Ex: **For category S42.311 CC codes**
S42.311[A]: S42.311[A], S42.319-S42.321[A], S42.323-S42.324[A], S42.326-S42.331[A], S42.333-S42.334[A], S42.336-S42.341[A], S42.343-S42.344[A], S42.346-S42.351[A], S42.353-S42.354[A], S42.356-S42.361[A], S42.363-S42.364[A], S42.366-S42.391[A], S42.399[A]
For S42.311[K,P]: See S02.0[K]

S42.312 Greenstick fracture of shaft of humerus, left arm A, K, P CC, A MCC
Ex: **For category S42.312 CC codes**
S42.312[A]: S42.312-S42.319[A], S42.322-S42.323[A], S42.325-S42.326[A], S42.332-S42.333[A], S42.335-S42.336[A], S42.342-S42.343[A], S42.345-S42.346[A], S42.352-S42.353[A], S42.355-S42.356[A], S42.362-S42.363[A], S42.365-S42.366[A], S42.392-S42.399[A] **For S42.312[K,P]:** See S02.0[K]

S42.319 Greenstick fracture of shaft of humerus, unspecified arm A, K, P CC, A MCC
Ex: **For category S42.319 CC codes**
S42.319[A]: S42.311-S42.399[A]
For S42.319[K,P]: See S02.0[K]

S42.32 Transverse fracture of shaft of humerus

S42.321 Displaced transverse fracture of shaft of humerus, right arm A, K, P CC, B MCC, A, B MCC
Ex: **For category S42.321 CC codes**
S42.321[A]: See S42.311[A]
For S42.321[B]: See S42.201[B]
For S42.321[K,P]: See S02.0[K]

S42.322 Displaced transverse fracture of shaft of humerus, left arm A, K, P CC, B MCC, A, B MCC
Ex: **For category S42.322 CC codes**
S42.322[A]: See S42.312[A]
For S42.322[B]: See S42.201[B]
For S42.322[K,P]: See S02.0[K]

S42.323 Displaced transverse fracture of shaft of humerus, unspecified arm A, K, P CC, B MCC, A, B MCC
Ex: **For category S42.323 CC codes**
S42.323[A]: S42.311-S42.399[A]
For S42.323[B]: See S42.201[B]
For S42.313[K,P]: See S02.0[K]

S42.324 Nondisplaced transverse fracture of shaft of humerus, right arm A, K, P CC, B MCC, A, B MCC
Ex: **For category S42.324 CC codes**
S42.324[A]: See S42.311[A]
For S42.324[B]: See S42.201[B]
For S42.324[K,P]: See S02.0[K]

S42.325 Nondisplaced transverse fracture of shaft of humerus, left arm A, K, P CC, B MCC, A, B MCC
Ex: **For category S42.325 CC codes**
S42.325[A]: See S42.312[A]
For S42.325[B]: See S42.201[B]
For S42.325[K,P]: See S02.0[K]

S42.326 Nondisplaced transverse fracture of shaft of humerus, unspecified arm A, K, P CC, B MCC, A, B MCC
Ex: **For category S42.326 CC codes**
S42.326[A]: S42.311-S42.399[A]
For S42.326[B]: See S42.201[B]
For S42.316[K,P]: See S02.0[K]

S42.33 Oblique fracture of shaft of humerus

S42.331 Displaced oblique fracture of shaft of humerus, right arm A, K, P CC, B MCC, A, B MCC
Ex: **For category S42.331 CC codes**
S42.331[A]: See S42.311[A]
For S42.331[B]: See S42.201[B]
For S42.331[K,P]: See S02.0[K]

S42.332 Displaced oblique fracture of shaft of humerus, left arm A, K, P CC, B MCC, A, B MCC
Ex: **For category S42.332 CC codes**
S42.332[A]: See S42.312[A]
For S42.332[B]: See S42.201[B]
For S42.332[K,P]: See S02.0[K]

S42.333 Displaced oblique fracture of shaft of humerus, unspecified arm A, K, P CC, B MCC, A, B MCC
Ex: **For category S42.333 CC codes**
S42.333[A]: S42.311-S42.399[A]
For S42.333[B]: See S42.201[B]
For S42.333[K,P]: See S02.0[K]

S42.334 Nondisplaced oblique fracture of shaft of humerus, right arm A, K, P CC, B MCC, A, B MCC
Ex: **For category S42.334 CC codes**
S42.334[A]: See S42.311[A]
For S42.334[B]: See S42.201[B]
For S42.334[K,P]: See S02.0[K]

S42.335 Nondisplaced oblique fracture of shaft of humerus, left arm A, K, P CC, B MCC, A, B MCC
Ex: **For category S42.335 CC codes**
S42.335[A]: See S42.312[A]
For S42.335[B]: See S42.201[B]
For S42.335[K,P]: See S02.0[K]

S42.336 Nondisplaced oblique fracture of shaft of humerus, unspecified arm A, K, P CC, B MCC, A, B MCC
Ex: **For category S42.336 CC codes**
S42.336[A]: S42.311-S42.399[A]
For S42.336[B]: See S42.201[B]
For S42.336[K,P]: See S02.0[K]

S42.34 Spiral fracture of shaft of humerus

S42.341 Displaced spiral fracture of shaft of humerus, right arm A, K, P CC, B MCC, A, B MCC
Ex: **For category S42.341 CC codes**
S42.341[A]: See S42.311[A]
For S42.341[B]: See S42.201[B]
For S42.341[K,P]: See S02.0[K]

S42.342 Displaced spiral fracture of shaft of humerus, left arm A, K, P CC, B MCC, A, B MCC
Ex: **For category S42.342 CC codes**
S42.342[A]: See S42.312[A]
For S42.342[B]: See S42.201[B]
For S42.342[K,P]: See S02.0[K]

- **S42.343** Displaced spiral fracture of shaft of humerus, unspecified arm A, K, P, B, A, B
  - Ex: For category S42.343 CC codes
    - S42.343[A]: S42.311-S42.399[A]
    - For S42.343[B]: See S42.201[B]
    - For S42.343[K,P]: See S02.0[K]
- **S42.344** Nondisplaced spiral fracture of shaft of humerus, right arm A, K, P, B, A, B
  - Ex: For category S42.344 CC codes
    - S42.344[A]: See S42.311[A]
    - For S42.344[B]: See S42.201[B]
    - For S42.344[K,P]: See S02.0[K]
- **S42.345** Nondisplaced spiral fracture of shaft of humerus, left arm A, K, P, B, A, B
  - Ex: For category S42.345 CC codes
    - S42.345[A]: See S42.312[A]
    - For S42.345[B]: See S42.201[B]
    - For S42.345[K,P]: See S02.0[K]
- **S42.346** Nondisplaced spiral fracture of shaft of humerus, unspecified arm A, K, P, B, A, B
  - Ex: For category S42.346 CC codes
    - S42.346[A]: S42.311-S42.399[A]
    - For S42.346[B]: See S42.201[B]
    - For S42.346[K,P]: See S02.0[K]

- **S42.35** Comminuted fracture of shaft of humerus
  - **S42.351** Displaced comminuted fracture of shaft of humerus, right arm A, K, P, B, A, B
    - Ex: For category S42.351 CC codes
      - S42.351[A]: See S42.311[A]
      - For S42.351[B]: See S42.201[B]
      - For S42.351[K,P]: See S02.0[K]
  - **S42.352** Displaced comminuted fracture of shaft of humerus, left arm A, K, P, B, A, B
    - Ex: For category S42.352 CC codes
      - S42.352[A]: See S42.312[A]
      - For S42.352[B]: See S42.201[B]
      - For S42.352[K,P]: See S02.0[K]
  - **S42.353** Displaced comminuted fracture of shaft of humerus, unspecified arm A, K, P, B, A, B
    - Ex: For category S42.353 CC codes
      - S42.353[A]: S42.311-S42.399[A]
      - For S42.353[B]: See S42.201[B]
      - For S42.353[K,P]: See S02.0[K]
  - **S42.354** Nondisplaced comminuted fracture of shaft of humerus, right arm A, K, P, B, A, B
    - Ex: For category S42.354 CC codes
      - S42.354[A]: See S42.311[A]
      - For S42.354[B]: See S42.201[B]
      - For S42.354[K,P]: See S02.0[K]
  - **S42.355** Nondisplaced comminuted fracture of shaft of humerus, left arm A, K, P, B, A, B
    - Ex: For category S42.355 CC codes
      - S42.355[A]: See S42.312[A]
      - For S42.355[B]: See S42.201[B]
      - For S42.355[K,P]: See S02.0[K]
  - **S42.356** Nondisplaced comminuted fracture of shaft of humerus, unspecified arm A, K, P, B, A, B
    - Ex: For category S42.356 CC codes
      - S42.356[A]: S42.311-S42.399[A]
      - For S42.356[B]: See S42.201[B]
      - For S42.356[K,P]: See S02.0[K]

- **S42.36** Segmental fracture of shaft of humerus
  - **S42.361** Displaced segmental fracture of shaft of humerus, right arm A, K, P, B, A, B
    - Ex: For category S42.361 CC codes
      - S42.361[A]: See S42.311[A]
      - For S42.361[B]: See S42.201[B]
      - For S42.361[K,P]: See S02.0[K]
  - **S42.362** Displaced segmental fracture of shaft of humerus, left arm A, K, P, B, A, B
    - Ex: For category S42.362 CC codes
      - S42.362[A]: See S42.312[A]
      - For S42.362[B]: See S42.201[B]
      - For S42.362[K,P]: See S02.0[K]
  - **S42.363** Displaced segmental fracture of shaft of humerus, unspecified arm A, K, P, B, A, B
    - Ex: For category S42.363 CC codes
      - S42.363[A]: S42.311-S42.399[A]
      - For S42.363[B]: See S42.201[B]
      - For S42.363[K,P]: See S02.0[K]
  - **S42.364** Nondisplaced segmental fracture of shaft of humerus, right arm A, K, P, B, A, B
    - Ex: For category S42.364 CC codes
      - S42.364[A]: See S42.311[A]
      - For S42.364[B]: See S42.201[B]
      - For S42.364[K,P]: See S02.0[K]
  - **S42.365** Nondisplaced segmental fracture of shaft of humerus, left arm A, K, P, B, A, B
    - Ex: For category S42.365 CC codes
      - S42.365[A]: See S42.312[A]
      - For S42.365[B]: See S42.201[B]
      - For S42.365[K,P]: See S02.0[K]
  - **S42.366** Nondisplaced segmental fracture of shaft of humerus, unspecified arm A, K, P, B, A, B
    - Ex: For category S42.366 CC codes
      - S42.366[A]: S42.311-S42.399[A]
      - For S42.366[B]: See S42.201[B]
      - For S42.366[K,P]: See S02.0[K]

- **S42.39** Other fracture of shaft of humerus
  - **S42.391** Other fracture of shaft of right humerus A, K, P, B, A, B
    - Ex: For category S42.391 CC codes
      - S42.391[A]: See S42.311[A]
      - For S42.391[B]: See S42.201[B]
      - For S42.391[K,P]: See S02.0[K]
  - **S42.392** Other fracture of shaft of left humerus A, K, P, B, A, B
    - Ex: For category S42.392 CC codes
      - S42.392[A]: See S42.312[A]
      - For S42.392[B]: See S42.201[B]
      - For S42.392[K,P]: See S02.0[K]
  - **S42.399** Other fracture of shaft of unspecified humerus A, K, P, B, A, B
    - Ex: For category S42.399 CC codes
      - S42.399[A]: S42.311-S42.399[A]
      - For S42.399[B]: See S42.201[B]
      - For S42.399[K,P]: See S02.0[K]

◀ New ◀ Revised ~~deleted~~ Deleted Excludes 1 Excludes 2 Includes Use additional Code first Code also Unspecified
OGCR Official Guidelines ● Unacceptable Principal Diagnosis X Assign placeholder X ● Use Additional Character(s) ▶ Manifestation Code Coding Clinic

S42.4 Fracture of lower end of humerus
Fracture of distal end of humerus

Excludes2 fracture of shaft of humerus (S42.3-)
physeal fracture of lower end of humerus (S49.1-)

S42.40 Unspecified fracture of lower end of humerus
Fracture of elbow NOS

S42.401 Unspecified fracture of lower end of right humerus A, K, P CC, B MCC, A, B HAC
Ex: For S42.401[A]: See S42.201[A]
For S42.401[B]: See S42.201[B]
For S42.401[K,P]: See S02.0[K]

S42.402 Unspecified fracture of lower end of left humerus A, K, P CC, B MCC, A, B HAC
Ex: For S42.402[A]: See S42.202[A]
For S42.402[B]: See S42.201[B]
For S42.402[K,P]: See S02.0[K]

S42.409 Unspecified fracture of lower end of unspecified humerus A, K, P CC, B MCC, A, B HAC
Ex: For S42.409[A]: See S42.209[A]
For S42.409[B]: See S42.201[B]
For S42.409[K,P]: See S02.0[K]

S42.41 Simple supracondylar fracture without intercondylar fracture of humerus

S42.411 Displaced simple supracondylar fracture without intercondylar fracture of right humerus A, K, P CC, B MCC, A, B HAC
Ex: For S42.411[A]: See S42.201[A]
For S42.411[B]: See S42.201[B]
For S42.411[K,P]: See S02.0[K]

S42.412 Displaced simple supracondylar fracture without intercondylar fracture of left humerus A, K, P CC, B MCC, A, B HAC
Ex: For S42.412[A]: See S42.202[A]
For S42.412[B]: See S42.201[B]
For S42.412[K,P]: See S02.0[K]

S42.413 Displaced simple supracondylar fracture without intercondylar fracture of unspecified humerus A, K, P CC, B MCC, A, B HAC
Ex: For S42.413[A]: See S42.209[A]
For S42.413[B]: See S42.201[B]
For S42.413[K,P]: See S02.0[K]

S42.414 Nondisplaced simple supracondylar fracture without intercondylar fracture of right humerus A, K, P CC, B MCC, A, B HAC
Ex: For S42.414[A]: See S42.201[A]
For S42.414[B]: See S42.201[B]
For S42.414[K,P]: See S02.0[K]

S42.415 Nondisplaced simple supracondylar fracture without intercondylar fracture of left humerus A, K, P CC, B MCC, A, B HAC
Ex: For S42.415[A]: See S42.202[A]
For S42.415[B]: See S42.201[B]
For S42.415[K,P]: See S02.0[K]

S42.416 Nondisplaced simple supracondylar fracture without intercondylar fracture of unspecified humerus A, K, P CC, B MCC, A, B HAC
Ex: For S42.416[A]: See S42.209[A]
For S42.416[B]: See S42.201[B]
For S42.416[K,P]: See S02.0[K]

S42.42 Comminuted supracondylar fracture without intercondylar fracture of humerus

S42.421 Displaced comminuted supracondylar fracture without intercondylar fracture of right humerus A, K, P CC, B MCC, A, B HAC
Ex: For S42.421[A]: See S42.201[A]
For S42.421[B]: See S42.201[B]
For S42.421[K,P]: See S02.0[K]

S42.422 Displaced comminuted supracondylar fracture without intercondylar fracture of left humerus A, K, P CC, B MCC, A, B HAC
Ex: For S42.422[A]: See S42.202[A]
For S42.422[B]: See S42.201[B]
For S42.422[K,P]: See S02.0[K]

S42.423 Displaced comminuted supracondylar fracture without intercondylar fracture of unspecified humerus A, K, P CC, B MCC, A, B HAC
Ex: For S42.423[A]: See S42.209[A]
For S42.423[B]: See S42.201[B]
For S42.423[K,P]: See S02.0[K]

S42.424 Nondisplaced comminuted supracondylar fracture without intercondylar fracture of right humerus A, K, P CC, B MCC, A, B HAC
Ex: For S42.424[A]: See S42.201[A]
For S42.424[B]: See S42.201[B]
For S42.424[K,P]: See S02.0[K]

S42.425 Nondisplaced comminuted supracondylar fracture without intercondylar fracture of left humerus A, K, P CC, B MCC, A, B HAC
Ex: For S42.425[A]: See S42.202[A]
For S42.425[B]: See S42.201[B]
For S42.425[K,P]: See S02.0[K]

S42.426 Nondisplaced comminuted supracondylar fracture without intercondylar fracture of unspecified humerus A, K, P CC, B MCC, A, B HAC
Ex: For S42.426[A]: See S42.209[A]
For S42.426[B]: See S42.201[B]
For S42.426[K,P]: See S02.0[K]

S42.43 Fracture (avulsion) of lateral epicondyle of humerus

S42.431 Displaced fracture (avulsion) of lateral epicondyle of right humerus A, K, P CC, B MCC, A, B HAC
Ex: For S42.431[A]: See S42.201[A]
For S42.431[B]: See S42.201[B]
For S42.431[K,P]: See S02.0[K]

S42.432 Displaced fracture (avulsion) of lateral epicondyle of left humerus A, K, P CC, B MCC, A, B HAC
Ex: For S42.432[A]: See S42.202[A]
For S42.432[B]: See S42.201[B]
For S42.432[K,P]: See S02.0[K]

S42.433 Displaced fracture (avulsion) of lateral epicondyle of unspecified humerus A, K, P CC, B MCC, A, B HAC
Ex: For S42.433[A]: See S42.209[A]
For S42.433[B]: See S42.201[B]
For S42.433[K,P]: See S02.0[K]

S42.434 Nondisplaced fracture (avulsion) of lateral epicondyle of right humerus A, K, P CC, B MCC, A, B HAC
Ex: For S42.434[A]: See S42.201[A]
For S42.434[B]: See S42.201[B]
For S42.434[K,P]: See S02.0[K]

● **S42.435** **Nondisplaced fracture (avulsion) of lateral epicondyle of left humerus** A, K, P, B, A, B
Ex: **For S42.435[A]:** See S42.202[A]
For S42.435[B]: See S42.201[B]
For S42.435[K,P]: See S02.0[K]

● **S42.436** **Nondisplaced fracture (avulsion) of lateral epicondyle of unspecified humerus** A, K, P, B, A, B
Ex: **For S42.436[A]:** See S42.209[A]
For S42.436[B]: See S42.201[B]
For S42.436[K,P]: See S02.0[K]

● **S42.44** **Fracture (avulsion) of medial epicondyle of humerus**

● **S42.441** **Displaced fracture (avulsion) of medial epicondyle of right humerus** A, K, P, B, A, B
Ex: **For S42.441[A]:** See S42.201[A]
For S42.441[B]: See S42.201[B]
For S42.441[K,P]: See S02.0[K]

● **S42.442** **Displaced fracture (avulsion) of medial epicondyle of left humerus** A, K, P, B, A, B
Ex: **For S42.442[A]:** See S42.202[A]
For S42.442[B]: See S42.201[B]
For S42.442[K,P]: See S02.0[K]

● **S42.443** **Displaced fracture (avulsion) of medial epicondyle of unspecified humerus** A, K, P, B, A, B
Ex: **For S42.443[A]:** See S42.209[A]
For S42.443[B]: See S42.201[B]
For S42.443[K,P]: See S02.0[K]

● **S42.444** **Nondisplaced fracture (avulsion) of medial epicondyle of right humerus** A, K, P, B, A, B
Ex: **For S42.444[A]:** See S42.201[A]
For S42.444[B]: See S42.201[B]
For S42.444[K,P]: See S02.0[K]

● **S42.445** **Nondisplaced fracture (avulsion) of medial epicondyle of left humerus** A, K, P, B, A, B
Ex: **For S42.445[A]:** See S42.202[A]
For S42.445[B]: See S42.201[B]
For S42.445[K,P]: See S02.0[K]

● **S42.446** **Nondisplaced fracture (avulsion) of medial epicondyle of unspecified humerus** A, K, P, B, A, B
Ex: **For S42.446[A]:** See S42.209[A]
For S42.446[B]: See S42.201[B]
For S42.446[K,P]: See S02.0[K]

● **S42.447** **Incarcerated fracture (avulsion) of medial epicondyle of right humerus** A, K, P, B, A, B
Ex: **For S42.447[A]:** See S42.201[A]
For S42.447[B]: See S42.201[B]
For S42.447[K,P]: See S02.0[K]

● **S42.448** **Incarcerated fracture (avulsion) of medial epicondyle of left humerus** A, K, P, B, A, B
Ex: **For S42.448[A]:** See S42.202[A]
For S42.448[B]: See S42.201[B]
For S42.448[K,P]: See S02.0[K]

● **S42.449** **Incarcerated fracture (avulsion) of medial epicondyle of unspecified humerus** A, K, P, B, A, B
Ex: **For S42.449[A]:** See S42.209[A]
For S42.449[B]: See S42.201[B]
For S42.449[K,P]: See S02.0[K]

● **S42.45** **Fracture of lateral condyle of humerus**
Fracture of capitellum of humerus

● **S42.451** **Displaced fracture of lateral condyle of right humerus** A, K, P, B, A, B
Ex: **For S42.451[A]:** See S42.201[A]
For S42.451[B]: See S42.201[B]
For S42.451[K,P]: See S02.0[K]

● **S42.452** **Displaced fracture of lateral condyle of left humerus** A, K, P, B, A, B
Ex: **For S42.452[A]:** See S42.202[A]
For S42.452[B]: See S42.201[B]
For S42.452[K,P]: See S02.0[K]

● **S42.453** **Displaced fracture of lateral condyle of unspecified humerus** A, K, P, B, A, B
Ex: **For S42.453[A]:** See S42.209[A]
For S42.453[B]: See S42.201[B]
For S42.453[K,P]: See S02.0[K]

● **S42.454** **Nondisplaced fracture of lateral condyle of right humerus** A, K, P, B, A, B
Ex: **For S42.454[A]:** See S42.201[A]
For S42.454[B]: See S42.201[B]
For S42.454[K,P]: See S02.0[K]

● **S42.455** **Nondisplaced fracture of lateral condyle of left humerus** A, K, P, B, A, B
Ex: **For S42.455[A]:** See S42.202[A]
For S42.455[B]: See S42.201[B]
For S42.455[K,P]: See S02.0[K]

● **S42.456** **Nondisplaced fracture of lateral condyle of unspecified humerus** A, K, P, B, A, B
Ex: **For S42.456[A]:** See S42.209[A]
For S42.456[B]: See S42.201[B]
For S42.456[K,P]: See S02.0[K]

● **S42.46** **Fracture of medial condyle of humerus**
Trochlea fracture of humerus

● **S42.461** **Displaced fracture of medial condyle of right humerus** A, K, P, B, A, B
Ex: **For S42.461[A]:** See S42.201[A]
For S42.461[B]: See S42.201[B]
For S42.461[K,P]: See S02.0[K]

● **S42.462** **Displaced fracture of medial condyle of left humerus** A, K, P, B, A, B
Ex: **For S42.462[A]:** See S42.202[A]
For S42.462[B]: See S42.201[B]
For S42.462[K,P]: See S02.0[K]

● **S42.463** **Displaced fracture of medial condyle of unspecified humerus** A, K, P, B, A, B
Ex: **For S42.463[A]:** See S42.209[A]
For S42.463[B]: See S42.201[B]
For S42.463[K,P]: See S02.0[K]

● **S42.464** **Nondisplaced fracture of medial condyle of right humerus** A, K, P, B, A, B
Ex: **For S42.464[A]:** See S42.201[A]
For S42.464[B]: See S42.201[B]
For S42.464[K,P]: See S02.0[K]

● **S42.465** **Nondisplaced fracture of medial condyle of left humerus** A, K, P, B, A, B
Ex: **For S42.465[A]:** See S42.202[A]
For S42.465[B]: See S42.201[B]
For S42.465[K,P]: See S02.0[K]

● **S42.466** **Nondisplaced fracture of medial condyle of unspecified humerus** A, K, P, B, A, B
Ex: **For S42.466[A]:** See S42.209[A]
For S42.466[B]: See S42.201[B]
For S42.466[K,P]: See S02.0[K]

● **S42.47 Transcondylar fracture of humerus**

● **S42.471 Displaced transcondylar fracture of right humerus** A, K, P CC, B MCC, A, B HAC
Ex: **For S42.471[A]:** See S42.201[A]
For S42.471[B]: See S42.201[B]
For S42.471[K,P]: See S02.0[K]

● **S42.472 Displaced transcondylar fracture of left humerus** A, K, P CC, B MCC, A, B HAC
Ex: **For S42.472[A]:** See S42.202[A]
For S42.472[B]: See S42.201[B]
For S42.472[K,P]: See S02.0[K]

● **S42.473 Displaced transcondylar fracture of unspecified humerus** A, K, P CC, B MCC, A, B HAC
Ex: **For S42.473[A]:** See S42.209[A]
For S42.473[B]: See S42.201[B]
For S42.473[K,P]: See S02.0[K]

● **S42.474 Nondisplaced transcondylar fracture of right humerus** A, K, P CC, B MCC, A, B HAC
Ex: **For S42.474[A]:** See S42.201[A]
For S42.474[B]: See S42.201[B]
For S42.474[K,P]: See S02.0[K]

● **S42.475 Nondisplaced transcondylar fracture of left humerus** A, K, P CC, B MCC, A, B HAC
Ex: **For S42.475[A]:** See S42.202[A]
For S42.475[B]: See S42.201[B]
For S42.475[K,P]: See S02.0[K]

● **S42.476 Nondisplaced transcondylar fracture of unspecified humerus** A, K, P CC, B MCC, A, B HAC
Ex: **For S42.476[A]:** See S42.209[A]
For S42.476[B]: See S42.201[B]
For S42.476[K,P]: See S02.0[K]

● **S42.48 Torus fracture of lower end of humerus**
The appropriate 7th character is to be added to all codes in subcategory S42.48

A	initial encounter for closed fracture
D	subsequent encounter for fracture with routine healing
G	subsequent encounter for fracture with delayed healing
K	subsequent encounter for fracture with nonunion
P	subsequent encounter for fracture with malunion
S	sequela

● **S42.481 Torus fracture of lower end of right humerus** A, K, P CC, A HAC
Ex: **For S42.481[A]:** See S42.201[A]
For S42.481[K,P]: See S02.0[K]

● **S42.482 Torus fracture of lower end of left humerus** A, K, P CC, A HAC
Ex: **For S42.482[A]:** See S42.202[A]
For S42.482[K,P]: See S02.0[K]

● **S42.489 Torus fracture of lower end of unspecified humerus** A, K, P CC, A HAC
Ex: **For S42.489[A]:** See S42.209[A]
For S42.489[K,P]: See S02.0[K]

● **S42.49 Other fracture of lower end of humerus**

● **S42.491 Other displaced fracture of lower end of right humerus** A, K, P CC, B MCC, A, B HAC
Ex: **For S42.491[A]:** See S42.201[A]
For S42.491[B]: See S42.201[B]
For S42.491[K,P]: See S02.0[K]

● **S42.492 Other displaced fracture of lower end of left humerus** A, K, P CC, B MCC, A, B HAC
Ex: **For S42.492[A]:** See S42.202[A]
For S42.492[B]: See S42.201[B]
For S42.492[K,P]: See S02.0[K]

● **S42.493 Other displaced fracture of lower end of unspecified humerus** A, K, P CC, B MCC, A, B HAC
Ex: **For S42.493[A]:** See S42.209[A]
For S42.493[B]: See S42.201[B]
For S42.493[K,P]: See S02.0[K]

● **S42.494 Other nondisplaced fracture of lower end of right humerus** A, K, P CC, B MCC, A, B HAC
Ex: **For S42.494[A]:** See S42.201[A]
For S42.494[B]: See S42.201[B]
For S42.494[K,P]: See S02.0[K]

● **S42.495 Other nondisplaced fracture of lower end of left humerus** A, K, P CC, B MCC, A, B HAC
Ex: **For S42.495[A]:** See S42.202[A]
For S42.495[B]: See S42.201[B]
For S42.495[K,P]: See S02.0[K]

● **S42.496 Other nondisplaced fracture of lower end of unspecified humerus** A, K, P CC, B MCC, A, B HAC
Ex: **For S42.496[A]:** See S42.209[A]
For S42.496[B]: See S42.201[B]
For S42.496[K,P]: See S02.0[K]

● **S42.9 Fracture of shoulder girdle, part unspecified**
Fracture of shoulder NOS
Ex: **For category S42.9 CC codes S42.9[A]:** See S42.209[A] **For S42.9[B]:** See S42.201[B] **For S42.9[K,P]:** See S02.0[K]

X● **S42.90 Fracture of unspecified shoulder girdle, part unspecified** A, K, P CC, B MCC, A, B HAC

X● **S42.91 Fracture of right shoulder girdle, part unspecified** A, K, P CC, B MCC, A, B HAC

X● **S42.92 Fracture of left shoulder girdle, part unspecified** A, K, P CC, B MCC, A, B HAC

● **S43 Dislocation and sprain of joints and ligaments of shoulder girdle**

Includes avulsion of joint or ligament of shoulder girdle
laceration of cartilage, joint or ligament of shoulder girdle
sprain of cartilage, joint or ligament of shoulder girdle
traumatic hemarthrosis of joint or ligament of shoulder girdle
traumatic rupture of joint or ligament of shoulder girdle
traumatic subluxation of joint or ligament of shoulder girdle
traumatic tear of joint or ligament of shoulder girdle

Code also any associated open wound

Excludes2 strain of muscle, fascia and tendon of shoulder and upper arm (S46.-)

The appropriate 7th character is to be added to each code from category S43

A	initial encounter
D	subsequent encounter
S	sequela

● **S43.0 Subluxation and dislocation of shoulder joint**
Dislocation of glenohumeral joint
Subluxation of glenohumeral joint

● **S43.00 Unspecified subluxation and dislocation of shoulder joint**
Dislocation of humerus NOS
Subluxation of humerus NOS

● **S43.001 Unspecified subluxation of right shoulder joint**

● **S43.002 Unspecified subluxation of left shoulder joint**

● **S43.003 Unspecified subluxation of unspecified shoulder joint**

● **S43.004 Unspecified dislocation of right shoulder joint**

- S43.005 Unspecified dislocation of left shoulder joint
- S43.006 Unspecified dislocation of unspecified shoulder joint
- S43.01 Anterior subluxation and dislocation of humerus
  - S43.011 Anterior subluxation of right humerus
  - S43.012 Anterior subluxation of left humerus
  - S43.013 Anterior subluxation of unspecified humerus
  - S43.014 Anterior dislocation of right humerus
  - S43.015 Anterior dislocation of left humerus
  - S43.016 Anterior dislocation of unspecified humerus
- S43.02 Posterior subluxation and dislocation of humerus
  - S43.021 Posterior subluxation of right humerus
  - S43.022 Posterior subluxation of left humerus
  - S43.023 Posterior subluxation of unspecified humerus
  - S43.024 Posterior dislocation of right humerus
  - S43.025 Posterior dislocation of left humerus
  - S43.026 Posterior dislocation of unspecified humerus
- S43.03 Inferior subluxation and dislocation of humerus
  - S43.031 Inferior subluxation of right humerus
  - S43.032 Inferior subluxation of left humerus
  - S43.033 Inferior subluxation of unspecified humerus
  - S43.034 Inferior dislocation of right humerus
  - S43.035 Inferior dislocation of left humerus
  - S43.036 Inferior dislocation of unspecified humerus
- S43.08 Other subluxation and dislocation of shoulder joint
  - S43.081 Other subluxation of right shoulder joint
  - S43.082 Other subluxation of left shoulder joint
  - S43.083 Other subluxation of unspecified shoulder joint
  - S43.084 Other dislocation of right shoulder joint
  - S43.085 Other dislocation of left shoulder joint
  - S43.086 Other dislocation of unspecified shoulder joint
- S43.1 Subluxation and dislocation of acromioclavicular joint
  - S43.10 Unspecified dislocation of acromioclavicular joint
    - S43.101 Unspecified dislocation of right acromioclavicular joint
    - S43.102 Unspecified dislocation of left acromioclavicular joint
    - S43.109 Unspecified dislocation of unspecified acromioclavicular joint
  - S43.11 Subluxation of acromioclavicular joint
    - S43.111 Subluxation of right acromioclavicular joint
    - S43.112 Subluxation of left acromioclavicular joint
    - S43.119 Subluxation of unspecified acromioclavicular joint
  - S43.12 Dislocation of acromioclavicular joint, 100%-200% displacement
    - S43.121 Dislocation of right acromioclavicular joint, 100%-200% displacement
    - S43.122 Dislocation of left acromioclavicular joint, 100%-200% displacement
    - S43.129 Dislocation of unspecified acromioclavicular joint, 100%-200% displacement
  - S43.13 Dislocation of acromioclavicular joint, greater than 200% displacement
    - S43.131 Dislocation of right acromioclavicular joint, greater than 200% displacement
    - S43.132 Dislocation of left acromioclavicular joint, greater than 200% displacement
    - S43.139 Dislocation of unspecified acromioclavicular joint, greater than 200% displacement
  - S43.14 Inferior dislocation of acromioclavicular joint
    - S43.141 Inferior dislocation of right acromioclavicular joint
    - S43.142 Inferior dislocation of left acromioclavicular joint
    - S43.149 Inferior dislocation of unspecified acromioclavicular joint
  - S43.15 Posterior dislocation of acromioclavicular joint
    - S43.151 Posterior dislocation of right acromioclavicular joint
    - S43.152 Posterior dislocation of left acromioclavicular joint
    - S43.159 Posterior dislocation of unspecified acromioclavicular joint
- S43.2 Subluxation and dislocation of sternoclavicular joint
  - S43.20 Unspecified subluxation and dislocation of sternoclavicular joint
    - S43.201 Unspecified subluxation of right sternoclavicular joint A, A
      Ex: M99.18, S43.201[A], S43.203-S43.204[A], S43.206[A], S43.211[A], S43.213-S43.214[A], S43.216[A], S43.221[A], S43.223-S43.224[A], S43.226[A]
    - S43.202 Unspecified subluxation of left sternoclavicular joint A, A
      Ex: M99.18, S43.202-S43.203[A], S43.205-S43.206[A], S43.212-S43.213[A], S43.215-S43.216[A], S43.222-S43.223[A], S43.225-S43.226[A]
    - S43.203 Unspecified subluxation of unspecified sternoclavicular joint A, A
      Ex: M99.18, S43.201-S43.226[A]
    - S43.204 Unspecified dislocation of right sternoclavicular joint A, A
      Ex: See S43.201
    - S43.205 Unspecified dislocation of left sternoclavicular joint A, A
      Ex: See S43.202
    - S43.206 Unspecified dislocation of unspecified sternoclavicular joint A, A
      Ex: See S43.203
  - S43.21 Anterior subluxation and dislocation of sternoclavicular joint
    - S43.211 Anterior subluxation of right sternoclavicular joint A, A
      Ex: See S43.201
    - S43.212 Anterior subluxation of left sternoclavicular joint A, A
      Ex: See S43.202
    - S43.213 Anterior subluxation of unspecified sternoclavicular joint A, A
      Ex: See S43.203

- **S43.214** Anterior dislocation of right sternoclavicular joint A, A
  - Ex: See S43.201
- **S43.215** Anterior dislocation of left sternoclavicular joint A, A
  - Ex: See S43.202
- **S43.216** Anterior dislocation of unspecified sternoclavicular joint A, A
  - Ex: See S43.203
- **S43.22** Posterior subluxation and dislocation of sternoclavicular joint
  - **S43.221** Posterior subluxation of right sternoclavicular joint A, A
    - Ex: See S43.201
  - **S43.222** Posterior subluxation of left sternoclavicular joint A, A
    - Ex: See S43.202
  - **S43.223** Posterior subluxation of unspecified sternoclavicular joint A, A
    - Ex: See S43.203
  - **S43.224** Posterior dislocation of right sternoclavicular joint A, A
    - Ex: See S43.201
  - **S43.225** Posterior dislocation of left sternoclavicular joint A, A
    - Ex: See S43.202
  - **S43.226** Posterior dislocation of unspecified sternoclavicular joint A, A
    - Ex: See S43.203
- **S43.3** Subluxation and dislocation of other and unspecified parts of shoulder girdle
  - **S43.30** Subluxation and dislocation of unspecified parts of shoulder girdle
    - Dislocation of shoulder girdle NOS
    - Subluxation of shoulder girdle NOS
    - **S43.301** Subluxation of unspecified parts of right shoulder girdle
    - **S43.302** Subluxation of unspecified parts of left shoulder girdle
    - **S43.303** Subluxation of unspecified parts of unspecified shoulder girdle
    - **S43.304** Dislocation of unspecified parts of right shoulder girdle
    - **S43.305** Dislocation of unspecified parts of left shoulder girdle
    - **S43.306** Dislocation of unspecified parts of unspecified shoulder girdle
  - **S43.31** Subluxation and dislocation of scapula
    - **S43.311** Subluxation of right scapula
    - **S43.312** Subluxation of left scapula
    - **S43.313** Subluxation of unspecified scapula
    - **S43.314** Dislocation of right scapula
    - **S43.315** Dislocation of left scapula
    - **S43.316** Dislocation of unspecified scapula
  - **S43.39** Subluxation and dislocation of other parts of shoulder girdle
    - **S43.391** Subluxation of other parts of right shoulder girdle
    - **S43.392** Subluxation of other parts of left shoulder girdle
    - **S43.393** Subluxation of other parts of unspecified shoulder girdle
    - **S43.394** Dislocation of other parts of right shoulder girdle
    - **S43.395** Dislocation of other parts of left shoulder girdle
    - **S43.396** Dislocation of other parts of unspecified shoulder girdle
- **S43.4** Sprain of shoulder joint
  - **S43.40** Unspecified sprain of shoulder joint
    - **S43.401** Unspecified sprain of right shoulder joint
    - **S43.402** Unspecified sprain of left shoulder joint
    - **S43.409** Unspecified sprain of unspecified shoulder joint
  - **S43.41** Sprain of coracohumeral (ligament)
    - **S43.411** Sprain of right coracohumeral (ligament)
    - **S43.412** Sprain of left coracohumeral (ligament)
    - **S43.419** Sprain of unspecified coracohumeral (ligament)
  - **S43.42** Sprain of rotator cuff capsule
    - *Encounters during the healing phase*
    - **Excludes1** rotator cuff syndrome (complete) (incomplete), not specified as traumatic (M75.1-)
    - **Excludes2** injury of tendon of rotator cuff (S46.0-)
    - **S43.421** Sprain of right rotator cuff capsule
    - **S43.422** Sprain of left rotator cuff capsule
    - **S43.429** Sprain of unspecified rotator cuff capsule
  - **S43.43** Superior glenoid labrum lesion
    - SLAP lesion
    - **S43.431** Superior glenoid labrum lesion of right shoulder
    - **S43.432** Superior glenoid labrum lesion of left shoulder
    - **S43.439** Superior glenoid labrum lesion of unspecified shoulder
  - **S43.49** Other sprain of shoulder joint
    - **S43.491** Other sprain of right shoulder joint
    - **S43.492** Other sprain of left shoulder joint
    - **S43.499** Other sprain of unspecified shoulder joint
- **S43.5** Sprain of acromioclavicular joint
  - Sprain of acromioclavicular ligament
  - X **S43.50** Sprain of unspecified acromioclavicular joint
  - X **S43.51** Sprain of right acromioclavicular joint
  - X **S43.52** Sprain of left acromioclavicular joint
- **S43.6** Sprain of sternoclavicular joint
  - X **S43.60** Sprain of unspecified sternoclavicular joint
  - X **S43.61** Sprain of right sternoclavicular joint
  - X **S43.62** Sprain of left sternoclavicular joint
- **S43.8** Sprain of other specified parts of shoulder girdle
  - X **S43.80** Sprain of other specified parts of unspecified shoulder girdle
  - X **S43.81** Sprain of other specified parts of right shoulder girdle
  - X **S43.82** Sprain of other specified parts of left shoulder girdle
- **S43.9** Sprain of unspecified parts of shoulder girdle
  - X **S43.90** Sprain of unspecified parts of unspecified shoulder girdle
    - Sprain of shoulder girdle NOS
  - X **S43.91** Sprain of unspecified parts of right shoulder girdle
  - X **S43.92** Sprain of unspecified parts of left shoulder girdle

S44 Injury of nerves at shoulder and upper arm level

Code also any associated open wound (S41.-)

Excludes2 injury of brachial plexus (S14.3-)

The appropriate 7th character is to be added to each code from category S44

A	initial encounter
D	subsequent encounter
S	sequela

S44.0 Injury of ulnar nerve at upper arm level

Excludes1 ulnar nerve NOS (S54.0)

X **S44.00 Injury of ulnar nerve at upper arm level, unspecified arm**

X **S44.01 Injury of ulnar nerve at upper arm level, right arm**

X **S44.02 Injury of ulnar nerve at upper arm level, left arm**

S44.1 Injury of median nerve at upper arm level

Excludes1 median nerve NOS (S54.1)

X **S44.10 Injury of median nerve at upper arm level, unspecified arm**

X **S44.11 Injury of median nerve at upper arm level, right arm**

X **S44.12 Injury of median nerve at upper arm level, left arm**

S44.2 Injury of radial nerve at upper arm level

Excludes1 radial nerve NOS (S54.2)

X **S44.20 Injury of radial nerve at upper arm level, unspecified arm**

X **S44.21 Injury of radial nerve at upper arm level, right arm**

X **S44.22 Injury of radial nerve at upper arm level, left arm**

S44.3 Injury of axillary nerve

X **S44.30 Injury of axillary nerve, unspecified arm**

X **S44.31 Injury of axillary nerve, right arm**

X **S44.32 Injury of axillary nerve, left arm**

S44.4 Injury of musculocutaneous nerve

X **S44.40 Injury of musculocutaneous nerve, unspecified arm**

X **S44.41 Injury of musculocutaneous nerve, right arm**

X **S44.42 Injury of musculocutaneous nerve, left arm**

S44.5 Injury of cutaneous sensory nerve at shoulder and upper arm level

X **S44.50 Injury of cutaneous sensory nerve at shoulder and upper arm level, unspecified arm**

X **S44.51 Injury of cutaneous sensory nerve at shoulder and upper arm level, right arm**

X **S44.52 Injury of cutaneous sensory nerve at shoulder and upper arm level, left arm**

S44.8 Injury of other nerves at shoulder and upper arm level

S44.8X Injury of other nerves at shoulder and upper arm level

S44.8X1 Injury of other nerves at shoulder and upper arm level, right arm

S44.8X2 Injury of other nerves at shoulder and upper arm level, left arm

S44.8X9 Injury of other nerves at shoulder and upper arm level, unspecified arm

S44.9 Injury of unspecified nerve at shoulder and upper arm level

X **S44.90 Injury of unspecified nerve at shoulder and upper arm level, unspecified arm**

X **S44.91 Injury of unspecified nerve at shoulder and upper arm level, right arm**

X **S44.92 Injury of unspecified nerve at shoulder and upper arm level, left arm**

S45 Injury of blood vessels at shoulder and upper arm level

Code also any associated open wound (S41.-)

Excludes2 injury of subclavian artery (S25.1)
injury of subclavian vein (S25.3)

The appropriate 7th character is to be added to each code from category S45

A	initial encounter
D	subsequent encounter
S	sequela

S45.0 Injury of axillary artery

S45.00 Unspecified injury of axillary artery

S45.001 Unspecified injury of axillary artery, right side A

Ex: S45.001[A], S45.009-S45.011[A], S45.019-S45.091[A], S45.099[A], S45.301[A], S45.309-S45.311[A], S45.319-S45.391[A], S45.399-S45.801[A], S45.809-S45.811[A], S45.819-S45.891[A], S45.899-S45.901[A], S45.909-S45.911[A], S45.919-S45.991[A], S45.999[A], S55.201[A], S55.209-S55.211[A], S55.219-S55.291[A], S55.299-S55.801[A], S55.809-S55.811[A], S55.819-S55.891[A], S55.899-S55.901[A], S55.909-S55.911[A], S55.919-S55.991[A], S55.999[A], S65.801[A], S65.809-S65.811[A], S65.819-S65.891[A], S65.899-S65.901[A], S65.909-S65.911[A], S65.919-S65.991[A], S65.999[A]

S45.002 Unspecified injury of axillary artery, left side A

Ex: S45.002-S45.009[A], S45.012-S45.019[A], S45.092-S45.099[A], S45.302-S45.309[A], S45.312-S45.319[A], S45.392-S45.399[A], S45.802-S45.809[A], S45.812-S45.819[A], S45.892-S45.899[A], S45.902-S45.909[A], S45.912-S45.919[A], S45.992-S45.999[A], S55.202-S55.209[A], S55.212-S55.219[A], S55.292-S55.299[A], S55.802-S55.809[A], S55.812-S55.819[A], S55.892-S55.899[A], S55.902-S55.909[A], S55.912-S55.919[A], S55.992-S55.999[A], S65.802-S65.809[A], S65.812-S65.819[A], S65.892-S65.899[A], S65.902-S65.909[A], S65.912-S65.919[A], S65.992-S65.999[A]

S45.009 Unspecified injury of axillary artery, unspecified side A

Ex: S45.001-S45.099[A], S45.301-S45.399[A], S45.801-S45.999[A], S55.201-S55.999[A], S65.801-S65.999[A]

S45.01 Laceration of axillary artery

S45.011 Laceration of axillary artery, right side A

Ex: See S45.001

S45.012 Laceration of axillary artery, left side A

Ex: See S45.002

S45.019 Laceration of axillary artery, unspecified side A

Ex: See S45.009

S45.09 Other specified injury of axillary artery

S45.091 Other specified injury of axillary artery, right side A

Ex: See S45.001

S45.092 Other specified injury of axillary artery, left side A

Ex: See S45.002

S45.099 Other specified injury of axillary artery, unspecified side A

Ex: See S45.009

- **S45.1 Injury of brachial artery**
  - **S45.10 Unspecified injury of brachial artery**
    - **S45.101 Unspecified injury of brachial artery, right side A**
      Ex: S45.101[A], S45.109-S45.111[A], S45.119-S45.191[A], S45.199-S45.201[A], S45.209A-S45.211[A], S45.219-S45.291[A], S45.299-S45.301[A], S45.309-S45.311[A], S45.319-S45.391[A], S45.399-S45.801[A], S45.809-S45.811[A], S45.819-S45.891[A], S45.899-S45.901[A], S45.909-S45.911[A], S45.919-S45.991[A], S45.999[A], S55.201[A], S55.209-S55.211[A], S55.219-S55.291[A], S55.299-S55.801[A], S55.809-S55.811[A], S55.819-S55.891[A], S55.899-S55.901[A], S55.909-S55.911[A], S55.919-S55.991[A], S55.999[A], S65.801[A], S65.809-S65.811[A], S65.819-S65.891[A], S65.899-S65.901[A], S65.909-S65.911[A], S65.919-S65.991[A], S65.999[A]
    - **S45.102 Unspecified injury of brachial artery, left side A**
      Ex: S45.102-S45.109[A], S45.112-S45.119[A], S45.192-S45.199[A], S45.202-S45.209[A], S45.212-S45.219[A], S45.292-S45.299[A], S45.302-S45.309[A], S45.312-S45.319[A], S45.392-S45.399[A], S45.802-S45.809[A], S45.812-S45.819[A], S45.892-S45.899[A], S45.902-S45.909[A], S45.912-S45.919[A], S45.992-S45.999[A], S55.202-S55.209[A], S55.212-S55.219[A], S55.292-S55.299[A], S55.802-S55.809[A], S55.812-S55.819[A], S55.892-S55.899[A], S55.902-S55.909[A], S55.912-S55.919[A], S55.992-S55.999[A], S65.802-S65.809[A], S65.812-S65.819[A], S65.892-S65.899[A], S65.902-S65.909[A], S65.912-S65.919[A], S65.992-S65.999[A]
    - **S45.109 Unspecified injury of brachial artery, unspecified side A**
      Ex: S45.101-S45.999[A], S55.201-S55.999[A], S65.801-S65.999[A]
  - **S45.11 Laceration of brachial artery**
    - **S45.111 Laceration of brachial artery, right side A**
      Ex: See S45.101
    - **S45.112 Laceration of brachial artery, left side A**
      Ex: See S45.102
    - **S45.119 Laceration of brachial artery, unspecified side A**
      Ex: See S45.109
  - **S45.19 Other specified injury of brachial artery**
    - **S45.191 Other specified injury of brachial artery, right side A**
      Ex: See S45.101
    - **S45.192 Other specified injury of brachial artery, left side A**
      Ex: See S45.102
    - **S45.199 Other specified injury of brachial artery, unspecified side A**
      Ex: See S45.109
- **S45.2 Injury of axillary or brachial vein**
  - **S45.20 Unspecified injury of axillary or brachial vein**
    - **S45.201 Unspecified injury of axillary or brachial vein, right side A**
      Ex: See S45.101
    - **S45.202 Unspecified injury of axillary or brachial vein, left side A**
      Ex: See S45.102
    - **S45.209 Unspecified injury of axillary or brachial vein, unspecified side A**
      Ex: See S45.109
  - **S45.21 Laceration of axillary or brachial vein**
    - **S45.211 Laceration of axillary or brachial vein, right side A**
      Ex: See S45.101
    - **S45.212 Laceration of axillary or brachial vein, left side A**
      Ex: See S45.102
    - **S45.219 Laceration of axillary or brachial vein, unspecified side A**
      Ex: See S45.109
  - **S45.29 Other specified injury of axillary or brachial vein**
    - **S45.291 Other specified injury of axillary or brachial vein, right side A**
      Ex: See S45.101
    - **S45.292 Other specified injury of axillary or brachial vein, left side A**
      Ex: See S45.102
    - **S45.299 Other specified injury of axillary or brachial vein, unspecified side A**
      Ex: See S45.109
- **S45.3 Injury of superficial vein at shoulder and upper arm level**
  - **S45.30 Unspecified injury of superficial vein at shoulder and upper arm level**
    - **S45.301 Unspecified injury of superficial vein at shoulder and upper arm level, right arm A**
      Ex: S45.301[A], S45.309-S45.311[A], S45.319-S45.391[A], S45.399-S45.801[A], S45.809-S45.811[A], S45.819-S45.891[A], S45.899-S45.901[A], S45.909-S45.911[A], S45.919-S45.991[A], S45.999[A], S55.001[A], S55.009-S55.011[A], S55.019-S55.091[A], S55.099[A], S55.201[A], S55.209-S55.211[A], S55.219-S55.291[A], S55.299-S55.801[A], S55.809-S55.811[A], S55.819-S55.891[A], S55.899-S55.901[A], S55.909-S55.911[A], S55.919-S55.991[A], S55.999[A], S65.001[A], S65.009-S65.011[A], S65.019-S65.091[A], S65.099[A], S65.201[A], S65.209-S65.211[A], S65.219-S65.291[A], S65.299-S65.301[A], S65.309-S65.311[A], S65.319-S65.391[A], S65.399-S65.401[A], S65.409-S65.411[A], S65.419-S65.491[A], S65.499-S65.500[A], S65.502[A], S65.504[A], S65.506[A], S65.508-S65.510[A], S65.512[A], S65.514[A], S65.516[A], S65.518-S65.590[A], S65.592[A], S65.594[A], S65.596[A], S65.598-S65.801[A], S65.809-S65.811[A], S65.819-S65.891[A], S65.899-S65.901[A], S65.909-S65.911[A], S65.919-S65.991[A], S65.999[A]
    - **S45.302 Unspecified injury of superficial vein at shoulder and upper arm level, left arm A**
      Ex: S45.302-S45.309[A], S45.312-S45.319[A], S45.392-S45.399[A], S45.802-S45.809[A], S45.812-S45.819[A], S45.892-S45.899[A], S45.902-S45.909[A], S45.912-S45.919[A], S45.992-S45.999[A], S55.002-S55.009[A], S55.012-S55.019[A], S55.092-S55.099[A], S55.202-S55.209[A], S55.212-S55.219[A], S55.292-S55.299[A], S55.802-S55.809[A], S55.812-S55.819[A], S55.892-S55.899[A], S55.902-S55.909[A], S55.912-S55.919[A], S55.992-S55.999[A], S65.002-S65.009[A], S65.012-S65.019[A], S65.092-S65.099[A], S65.202-S65.209[A], S65.212-S65.219[A], S65.292-S65.299[A], S65.302-S65.309[A], S65.312-S65.319[A]. S65.392-S65.399[A], S65.402-S65.409[A], S65.412-S65.419[A], S65.492-S65.499[A], S65.501[A], S65.503[A], S65.505[A], S65.507-S65.509[A], S65.511[A], S65.513[A], S65.515[A], S65.517-S65.519[A], S65.591[A], S65.593[A], S65.595[A], S65.597-S65.599[A], S65.802-S65.809[A], S65.812-S65.819[A], S65.892-S65.899[A], S65.902-S65.909[A], S65.912-S65.919[A], S65.992-S65.999[A]

- S45.309 Unspecified injury of superficial vein at shoulder and upper arm level, unspecified arm A
  - Ex: S45.301-S45.999[A], S55.001-S55.099[A], S55.201-S55.999[A], S65.001-S65.099[A], S65.201-S65.999[A]
- S45.31 Laceration of superficial vein at shoulder and upper arm level
  - S45.311 Laceration of superficial vein at shoulder and upper arm level, right arm A
    - Ex: See S45.301
  - S45.312 Laceration of superficial vein at shoulder and upper arm level, left arm A
    - Ex: See S45.302
  - S45.319 Laceration of superficial vein at shoulder and upper arm level, unspecified arm A
    - Ex: See S45.309
- S45.39 Other specified injury of superficial vein at shoulder and upper arm level
  - S45.391 Other specified injury of superficial vein at shoulder and upper arm level, right arm A
    - Ex: See S45.301
  - S45.392 Other specified injury of superficial vein at shoulder and upper arm level, left arm A
    - Ex: See S45.302
  - S45.399 Other specified injury of superficial vein at shoulder and upper arm level, unspecified arm A
    - Ex: See S45.309
- S45.8 Injury of other specified blood vessels at shoulder and upper arm level
  - S45.80 Unspecified injury of other specified blood vessels at shoulder and upper arm level
    - S45.801 Unspecified injury of other specified blood vessels at shoulder and upper arm level, right arm A
      - Ex: See S45.301
    - S45.802 Unspecified injury of other specified blood vessels at shoulder and upper arm level, left arm A
      - Ex: See S45.302
    - S45.809 Unspecified injury of other specified blood vessels at shoulder and upper arm level, unspecified arm A
      - Ex: See S45.309
  - S45.81 Laceration of other specified blood vessels at shoulder and upper arm level
    - S45.811 Laceration of other specified blood vessels at shoulder and upper arm level, right arm A
      - Ex: See S45.301
    - S45.812 Laceration of other specified blood vessels at shoulder and upper arm level, left arm A
      - Ex: See S45.302
    - S45.819 Laceration of other specified blood vessels at shoulder and upper arm level, unspecified arm A
      - Ex: See S45.309
  - S45.89 Other specified injury of other specified blood vessels at shoulder and upper arm level
    - S45.891 Other specified injury of other specified blood vessels at shoulder and upper arm level, right arm A
      - Ex: See S45.301
    - S45.892 Other specified injury of other specified blood vessels at shoulder and upper arm level, left arm A
      - Ex: See S45.302
    - S45.899 Other specified injury of other specified blood vessels at shoulder and upper arm level, unspecified arm A
      - Ex: See S45.309
- S45.9 Injury of unspecified blood vessel at shoulder and upper arm level
  - S45.90 Unspecified injury of unspecified blood vessel at shoulder and upper arm level
    - S45.901 Unspecified injury of unspecified blood vessel at shoulder and upper arm level, right arm A
      - Ex: See S45.301
    - S45.902 Unspecified injury of unspecified blood vessel at shoulder and upper arm level, left arm A
      - Ex: See S45.302
    - S45.909 Unspecified injury of unspecified blood vessel at shoulder and upper arm level, unspecified arm A
      - Ex: See S45.309
  - S45.91 Laceration of unspecified blood vessel at shoulder and upper arm level
    - S45.911 Laceration of unspecified blood vessel at shoulder and upper arm level, right arm A
      - Ex: See S45.301
    - S45.912 Laceration of unspecified blood vessel at shoulder and upper arm level, left arm A
      - Ex: See S45.302
    - S45.919 Laceration of unspecified blood vessel at shoulder and upper arm level, unspecified arm A
      - Ex: See S45.309
  - S45.99 Other specified injury of unspecified blood vessel at shoulder and upper arm level
    - S45.991 Other specified injury of unspecified blood vessel at shoulder and upper arm level, right arm A
      - Ex: See S45.301
    - S45.992 Other specified injury of unspecified blood vessel at shoulder and upper arm level, left arm A
      - Ex: See S45.302
    - S45.999 Other specified injury of unspecified blood vessel at shoulder and upper arm level, unspecified arm A
      - Ex: See S45.309

S46 Injury of muscle, fascia and tendon at shoulder and upper arm level

Code also any associated open wound (S41.-)

Excludes2 injury of muscle, fascia and tendon at elbow (S56.-)
sprain of joints and ligaments of shoulder girdle (S43.9)

The appropriate 7th character is to be added to each code from category S46

A	initial encounter
D	subsequent encounter
S	sequela

S46.0 Injury of muscle(s) and tendon(s) of the rotator cuff of shoulder

S46.00 Unspecified injury of muscle(s) and tendon(s) of the rotator cuff of shoulder

S46.001 Unspecified injury of muscle(s) and tendon(s) of the rotator cuff of right shoulder

S46.002 Unspecified injury of muscle(s) and tendon(s) of the rotator cuff of left shoulder

S46.009 Unspecified injury of muscle(s) and tendon(s) of the rotator cuff of unspecified shoulder

S46.01 Strain of muscle(s) and tendon(s) of the rotator cuff of shoulder

Acute onset due to trauma to rotator cuff muscle/tendon

S46.011 Strain of muscle(s) and tendon(s) of the rotator cuff of right shoulder

S46.012 Strain of muscle(s) and tendon(s) of the rotator cuff of left shoulder

S46.019 Strain of muscle(s) and tendon(s) of the rotator cuff of unspecified shoulder

S46.02 Laceration of muscle(s) and tendon(s) of the rotator cuff of shoulder

S46.021 Laceration of muscle(s) and tendon(s) of the rotator cuff of right shoulder A

Ex: S41.001[A], S41.009-S41.011[A], S41.019-S41.021[A], S41.029-S41.031[A], S41.039-S41.041[A], S41.049-S41.051[A], S41.059-S41.101[A], S41.109-S41.111[A], S41.119-S41.121[A], S41.129-S41.131[A], S41.139-S41.141[A], S41.149-S41.151[A], S41.159[A], S46.021[A], S46.029[A], S46.121[A], S46.129[A], S46.221[A], S46.229[A], S46.321[A], S46.329[A], S46.821[A], S46.829[A], S46.921[A], S46.929[A]

S46.022 Laceration of muscle(s) and tendon(s) of the rotator cuff of left shoulder A

Ex: S41.002-S41.009[A], S41.012-S41.019[A], S41.022-S41.029[A], S41.032-S41.039[A], S41.042-S41.049[A], S41.052-S41.059[A], S41.102-S41.109[A], S41.112-S41.119[A], S41.122-S41.129[A], S41.132-S41.139[A], S41.142-S41.149[A], S41.152-S41.159[A], S46.022-S46.029[A], S46.122-S46.129[A], S46.222-S46.229[A], S46.322-S46.329[A], S46.822-S46.829[A], S46.922-S46.929[A]

S46.029 Laceration of muscle(s) and tendon(s) of the rotator cuff of unspecified shoulder A

Ex: S41.001-S41.159[A], S46.021-S46.029[A], S46.121-S46.129[A], S46.221-S46.229[A], S46.321-S46.329[A], S46.821-S46.829[A], S46.921-S46.929[A]

S46.09 Other injury of muscle(s) and tendon(s) of the rotator cuff of shoulder

S46.091 Other injury of muscle(s) and tendon(s) of the rotator cuff of right shoulder

S46.092 Other injury of muscle(s) and tendon(s) of the rotator cuff of left shoulder

S46.099 Other injury of muscle(s) and tendon(s) of the rotator cuff of unspecified shoulder

S46.1 Injury of muscle, fascia and tendon of long head of biceps

S46.10 Unspecified injury of muscle, fascia and tendon of long head of biceps

S46.101 Unspecified injury of muscle, fascia and tendon of long head of biceps, right arm

S46.102 Unspecified injury of muscle, fascia and tendon of long head of biceps, left arm

S46.109 Unspecified injury of muscle, fascia and tendon of long head of biceps, unspecified arm

S46.11 Strain of muscle, fascia and tendon of long head of biceps

S46.111 Strain of muscle, fascia and tendon of long head of biceps, right arm

S46.112 Strain of muscle, fascia and tendon of long head of biceps, left arm

S46.119 Strain of muscle, fascia and tendon of long head of biceps, unspecified arm

S46.12 Laceration of muscle, fascia and tendon of long head of biceps

S46.121 Laceration of muscle, fascia and tendon of long head of biceps, right arm A

Ex: See S46.021

S46.122 Laceration of muscle, fascia and tendon of long head of biceps, left arm A

Ex: See S46.022

S46.129 Laceration of muscle, fascia and tendon of long head of biceps, unspecified arm A

Ex: See S46.029

S46.19 Other injury of muscle, fascia and tendon of long head of biceps

S46.191 Other injury of muscle, fascia and tendon of long head of biceps, right arm

S46.192 Other injury of muscle, fascia and tendon of long head of biceps, left arm

S46.199 Other injury of muscle, fascia and tendon of long head of biceps, unspecified arm

S46.2 Injury of muscle, fascia and tendon of other parts of biceps

S46.20 Unspecified injury of muscle, fascia and tendon of other parts of biceps

S46.201 Unspecified injury of muscle, fascia and tendon of other parts of biceps, right arm

S46.202 Unspecified injury of muscle, fascia and tendon of other parts of biceps, left arm

S46.209 Unspecified injury of muscle, fascia and tendon of other parts of biceps, unspecified arm

- S46.21 Strain of muscle, fascia and tendon of other parts of biceps
  - S46.211 Strain of muscle, fascia and tendon of other parts of biceps, right arm
  - S46.212 Strain of muscle, fascia and tendon of other parts of biceps, left arm
  - S46.219 Strain of muscle, fascia and tendon of other parts of biceps, unspecified arm
- S46.22 Laceration of muscle, fascia and tendon of other parts of biceps
  - S46.221 Laceration of muscle, fascia and tendon of other parts of biceps, right arm A
    Ex: See S46.021
  - S46.222 Laceration of muscle, fascia and tendon of other parts of biceps, left arm A
    Ex: See S46.022
  - S46.229 Laceration of muscle, fascia and tendon of other parts of biceps, unspecified arm A
    Ex: See S46.029
- S46.29 Other injury of muscle, fascia and tendon of other parts of biceps
  - S46.291 Other injury of muscle, fascia and tendon of other parts of biceps, right arm
  - S46.292 Other injury of muscle, fascia and tendon of other parts of biceps, left arm
  - S46.299 Other injury of muscle, fascia and tendon of other parts of biceps, unspecified arm
- S46.3 Injury of muscle, fascia and tendon of triceps
  - S46.30 Unspecified injury of muscle, fascia and tendon of triceps
    - S46.301 Unspecified injury of muscle, fascia and tendon of triceps, right arm
    - S46.302 Unspecified injury of muscle, fascia and tendon of triceps, left arm
    - S46.309 Unspecified injury of muscle, fascia and tendon of triceps, unspecified arm
  - S46.31 Strain of muscle, fascia and tendon of triceps
    - S46.311 Strain of muscle, fascia and tendon of triceps, right arm
    - S46.312 Strain of muscle, fascia and tendon of triceps, left arm
    - S46.319 Strain of muscle, fascia and tendon of triceps, unspecified arm
  - S46.32 Laceration of muscle, fascia and tendon of triceps
    - S46.321 Laceration of muscle, fascia and tendon of triceps, right arm A
      Ex: See S46.021
    - S46.322 Laceration of muscle, fascia and tendon of triceps, left arm A
      Ex: See S46.022
    - S46.329 Laceration of muscle, fascia and tendon of triceps, unspecified arm A
      Ex: See S46.029
  - S46.39 Other injury of muscle, fascia and tendon of triceps
    - S46.391 Other injury of muscle, fascia and tendon of triceps, right arm
    - S46.392 Other injury of muscle, fascia and tendon of triceps, left arm
    - S46.399 Other injury of muscle, fascia and tendon of triceps, unspecified arm
- S46.8 Injury of other muscles, fascia and tendons at shoulder and upper arm level
  - S46.80 Unspecified injury of other muscles, fascia and tendons at shoulder and upper arm level
    - S46.801 Unspecified injury of other muscles, fascia and tendons at shoulder and upper arm level, right arm
    - S46.802 Unspecified injury of other muscles, fascia and tendons at shoulder and upper arm level, left arm
    - S46.809 Unspecified injury of other muscles, fascia and tendons at shoulder and upper arm level, unspecified arm
  - S46.81 Strain of other muscles, fascia and tendons at shoulder and upper arm level
    - S46.811 Strain of other muscles, fascia and tendons at shoulder and upper arm level, right arm
    - S46.812 Strain of other muscles, fascia and tendons at shoulder and upper arm level, left arm
    - S46.819 Strain of other muscles, fascia and tendons at shoulder and upper arm level, unspecified arm
  - S46.82 Laceration of other muscles, fascia and tendons at shoulder and upper arm level
    - S46.821 Laceration of other muscles, fascia and tendons at shoulder and upper arm level, right arm A
      Ex: See S46.021
    - S46.822 Laceration of other muscles, fascia and tendons at shoulder and upper arm level, left arm A
      Ex: See S46.022
    - S46.829 Laceration of other muscles, fascia and tendons at shoulder and upper arm level, unspecified arm A
      Ex: See S46.029
  - S46.89 Other injury of other muscles, fascia and tendons at shoulder and upper arm level
    - S46.891 Other injury of other muscles, fascia and tendons at shoulder and upper arm level, right arm
    - S46.892 Other injury of other muscles, fascia and tendons at shoulder and upper arm level, left arm
    - S46.899 Other injury of other muscles, fascia and tendons at shoulder and upper arm level, unspecified arm
- S46.9 Injury of unspecified muscle, fascia and tendon at shoulder and upper arm level
  - S46.90 Unspecified injury of unspecified muscle, fascia and tendon at shoulder and upper arm level
    - S46.901 Unspecified injury of unspecified muscle, fascia and tendon at shoulder and upper arm level, right arm
    - S46.902 Unspecified injury of unspecified muscle, fascia and tendon at shoulder and upper arm level, left arm
    - S46.909 Unspecified injury of unspecified muscle, fascia and tendon at shoulder and upper arm level, unspecified arm
  - S46.91 Strain of unspecified muscle, fascia and tendon at shoulder and upper arm level
    - S46.911 Strain of unspecified muscle, fascia and tendon at shoulder and upper arm level, right arm
    - S46.912 Strain of unspecified muscle, fascia and tendon at shoulder and upper arm level, left arm
    - S46.919 Strain of unspecified muscle, fascia and tendon at shoulder and upper arm level, unspecified arm

S46.92 Laceration of unspecified muscle, fascia and tendon at shoulder and upper arm level

S46.921 Laceration of unspecified muscle, fascia and tendon at shoulder and upper arm level, right arm A

Ex: See S46.021

S46.922 Laceration of unspecified muscle, fascia and tendon at shoulder and upper arm level, left arm A

Ex: See S46.022

S46.929 Laceration of unspecified muscle, fascia and tendon at shoulder and upper arm level, unspecified arm A

Ex: See S46.029

S46.99 Other injury of unspecified muscle, fascia and tendon at shoulder and upper arm level

S46.991 Other injury of unspecified muscle, fascia and tendon at shoulder and upper arm level, right arm

S46.992 Other injury of unspecified muscle, fascia and tendon at shoulder and upper arm level, left arm

S46.999 Other injury of unspecified muscle, fascia and tendon at shoulder and upper arm level, unspecified arm

S47 Crushing injury of shoulder and upper arm

Use additional code for all associated injuries

Excludes2 crushing injury of elbow (S57.0-)

The appropriate 7th character is to be added to each code from category S47

A	initial encounter
D	subsequent encounter
S	sequela

X **S47.1 Crushing injury of right shoulder and upper arm**

X **S47.2 Crushing injury of left shoulder and upper arm**

X **S47.9 Crushing injury of shoulder and upper arm, unspecified arm**

S48 Traumatic amputation of shoulder and upper arm

An amputation not identified as partial or complete should be coded to complete

Excludes1 traumatic amputation at elbow level (S58.0)

The appropriate 7th character is to be added to each code from category S48

A	initial encounter
D	subsequent encounter
S	sequela

S48.0 Traumatic amputation at shoulder joint

S48.01 Complete traumatic amputation at shoulder joint

S48.011 Complete traumatic amputation at right shoulder joint A

Ex: S41.001[A], S41.009-S41.011[A], S41.019-S41.021[A], S41.029-S41.031[A], S41.039-S41.041[A], S41.049-S41.051[A], S41.059-S41.101[A], S41.109-S41.111[A], S41.119-S41.121[A], S41.129-S41.131[A], S41.139-S41.141[A], S41.149-S41.151[A], S41.159[A], S46.021[A], S46.029[A], S46.121[A], S46.129[A], S46.221[A], S46.229[A], S46.321[A], S46.329[A], S46.821[A], S46.829[A], S46.921[A], S46.929[A], S48.011[A], S48.019-S48.021[A], S48.029-S48.111[A], S48.119-S48.121[A], S48.129-S48.911[A], S48.919-S48.921[A], S48.929[A], S51.001[A], S51.009-S51.011[A], S51.019-S51.021[A], S51.029-S51.031[A], S51.039-S51.041[A], S51.049-S51.051[A], S51.059-S51.801[A], S51.809-S51.811[A], S51.819-S51.821[A], S51.829-S51.831[A], S51.839-S51.841[A], S51.849-S51.851[A], S51.859[A], S56.021[A], S56.029[A], S56.121[A], S56.123[A], S56.125[A], S56.127[A], S56.129[A], S56.221[A], S56.229[A], S56.321[A], S56.329[A], S56.421[A], S56.423[A], S56.425[A], S56.427[A], S56.429[A], S56.521[A], S56.529[A], S56.821[A], S56.829[A], S56.921[A], S56.929[A], S58.011[A], S58.019-S58.021[A], S58.029-S58.111[A], S58.119-S58.121[A], S58.129-S58.911[A], S58.919-S58.921[A], S58.929[A], S61.001[A], S61.009-S61.011[A], S61.019-S61.021[A], S61.029-S61.031[A], S61.039-S61.041[A], S61.049-S61.051[A], S61.059-S61.101[A], S61.109-S61.111[A], S61.119-S61.121[A], S61.129-S61.131[A], S61.139-S61.141[A], S61.149-S61.151[A], S61.159-S61.200[A], S61.202[A], S61.204[A], S61.206[A], S61.208-S61.210[A], S61.212[A], S61.214[A], S61.216[A], S61.218-S61.220[A], S61.222[A], S61.224[A], S61.226[A], S61.228-S61.230[A], S61.232[A], S61.234[A], S61.236[A], S61.238-S61.240[A], S61.242[A], S61.244[A], S61.246[A], S61.248-S61.250[A], S61.252[A], S61.254[A], S61.256[A], S61.258-S61.300[A], S61.302[A], S61.304[A], S61.306[A], S61.308-S61.310[A], S61.312[A], S61.314[A], S61.316[A], S61.318-S61.320[A], S61.322[A], S61.324[A], S61.326[A], S61.328-S61.330[A], S61.332[A], S61.334[A], S61.336[A], S61.338-S61.340[A], S61.342[A], S61.344[A], S61.346[A], S61.348-S61.350[A], S61.352[A], S61.354[A], S61.356[A], S61.358-S61.401[A], S61.409-S61.411[A], S61.419-S61.421[A], S61.429-S61.431[A], S61.439-S61.441[A], S61.449-S61.451[A], S61.459-S61.501[A], S61.509-S61.511[A], S61.519-S61.521[A], S61.529-S61.531[A], S61.539-S61.541[A], S61.549-S61.551[A], S61.559[A], S66.021[A], S66.029[A], S66.120[A], S66.122[A], S66.124[A], S66.126[A], S66.128-S66.129[A], S66.221[A], S66.229[A], S66.320[A], S66.322[A], S66.324[A], S66.326[A], S66.328-S66.329[A], S66.421[A], S66.429[A], S66.520[A], S66.522[A], S66.524[A], S66.526[A], S66.528-S66.529[A], S66.821[A], S66.829[A], S66.921[A], S66.929[A], S68.011[A], S68.019-S68.021[A], S68.029-S68.110[A], S68.112[A], S68.114[A], S68.116[A], S68.118-S68.120[A], S68.122[A], S68.124[A], S68.126[A], S68.128-S68.411[A], S68.419-S68.421[A], S68.429-S68.511[A], S68.519-S68.521[A], S68.529-S68.610[A], S68.612[A], S68.614[A], S68.616[A], S68.618-S68.620[A], S68.622[A], S68.624[A], S68.626[A], S68.628-S68.711[A], S68.719-S68.721[A], S68.729[A], T14.90-T14.91, T79.A0X-T79.9XX[A]

● **S48.012** **Complete traumatic amputation at left shoulder joint** A

Ex: S41.002-S41.009[A], S41.012-S41.019[A], S41.022-S41.029[A], S41.032-S41.039[A], S41.042-S41.049[A], S41.052-S41.059[A], S41.102-S41.109[A], S41.112-S41.119[A], S41.122-S41.129[A], S41.132-S41.139[A], S41.142-S41.149[A], S41.152-S41.159[A], S46.022-S46.029[A], S46.122-S46.129[A], S46.222-S46.229[A], S46.322-S46.329[A], S46.822-S46.829[A], S46.922-S46.929[A], S48.012-S48.019[A], S48.022-S48.029[A], S48.112-S48.119[A], S48.122-S48.129[A], S48.912-S48.919[A], S48.922-S48.929[A], S51.002-S51.009[A], S51.012-S51.019[A], S51.022-S51.029[A], S51.032-S51.039[A], S51.042-S51.049[A], S51.052-S51.059[A], S51.802-S51.809[A], S51.812-S51.819[A], S51.822-S51.829[A], S51.832-S51.839[A], S51.842-S51.849[A], S51.852-S51.859[A], S56.022-S56.029[A], S56.122[A], S56.124[A], S56.126[A], S56.128-S56.129[A], S56.222-S56.229[A], S56.322-S56.329[A], S56.422[A], S56.424[A], S56.426[A], S56.428-S56.429[A], S56.522-S56.529[A], S56.822-S56.829[A], S56.922-S56.929[A], S58.012-S58.019[A], S58.022-S58.029[A], S58.112-S58.119[A], S58.122-S58.129[A], S58.912-S58.919[A], S58.922-S58.929[A], S61.002-S61.009[A], S61.012-S61.019[A], S61.022-S61.029[A], S61.032-S61.039[A], S61.042-S61.049[A], S61.052-S61.059[A], S61.102-S61.109[A], S61.112-S61.119[A], S61.122-S61.129[A]. S61.132-S61.139[A], S61.142-S61.149[A], S61.152-S61.159[A], S61.201[A], S61.203[A], S61.205[A], S61.207-S61.209[A], S61.211[A], S61.213[A], S61.215[A], S61.217-S61.219[A], S61.221[A], S61.223[A], S61.225[A], S61.227-S61.229[A], S61.231[A], S61.233[A], S61.235[A], S61.237-S61.239[A], S61.241[A], S61.243[A], S61.245[A], S61.247-S61.249[A], S61.251[A], S61.253[A], S61.255[A], S61.257-S61.259[A], S61.301[A], S61.303[A], S61.305[A], S61.307-S61.309[A], S61.311[A], S61.313[A], S61.315[A], S61.317-S61.319[A], S61.321[A], S61.323[A], S61.325[A], S61.327-S61.329[A], S61.331[A], S61.333[A], S61.335[A], S61.337-S61.339[A], S61.341[A], S61.343[A], S61.345[A], S61.347-S61.349[A], S61.351[A], S61.353[A], S61.355[A], S61.357-S61.359[A], S61.402-S61.409[A], S61.412-S61.419[A], S61.422-S61.429[A], S61.432-S61.439[A], S61.442-S61.449[A], S61.452-S61.459[A], S61.502-S61.509[A], S61.512-S61.519[A], S61.522-S61.529[A], S61.532-S61.539[A], S61.542-S61.549[A], S61.552-S61.559[A], S66.022-S66.029[A], S66.121[A], S66.123[A], S66.125[A], S66.127-S66.129[A], S66.222-S66.229[A], S66.321[A], S66.323[A], S66.325[A], S66.327-S66.329[A], S66.422-S66.429[A], S66.521[A], S66.523[A], S66.525[A], S66.527-S66.529[A], S66.822-S66.829[A], S66.922-S66.929[A], S68.012-S68.019[A], S68.022-S68.029[A], S68.111[A], S68.113[A], S68.115[A], S68.117-S68.119[A], S68.121[A], S68.123[A], S68.125[A], S68.127-S68.129[A], S68.412-S68.419[A], S68.422-S68.429[A], S68.512-S68.519[A], S68.522-S68.529[A], S68.611[A], S68.613[A], S68.615[A], S68.617-S68.619[A], S68.621[A], S68.623[A], S68.625[A], S68.627-S68.629[A], S68.712-S68.719[A], S68.722-S68.729[A], T14.90-T14.91, T79.A0X-T79.9XX[A]

● **S48.019** **Complete traumatic amputation at unspecified shoulder joint** A

Ex: S41.001-S41.159[A], S46.021-S46.029[A], S46.121-S46.129[A], S46.221-S46.229[A], S46.321-S46.329[A], S46.821-S46.829[A], S46.921-S46.929[A], S48.011-S48.929[A], S51.001-S51.859[A], S56.021-S56.029[A], S56.121-S56.129[A], S56.221-S56.229[A], S56.321-S56.329[A], S56.421-S56.429[A], S56.521-S56.529[A], S56.821-S56.829[A], S56.921-S56.929[A], S58.011-S58.929[A], S61.001-S61.559[A], S66.021-S66.029[A], S66.120-S66.129[A], S66.221-S66.229[A], S66.320-S66.329[A], S66.421-S66.429[A], S66.520-S66.529[A], S66.821-S66.829[A], S66.921-S66.929[A], S68.011-S68.729[A], T14.90-T14.91, T79.A0X-T79.9XX[A]

● **S48.02** **Partial traumatic amputation at shoulder joint**

● **S48.021** **Partial traumatic amputation at right shoulder joint** A

Ex: See S48.011

● **S48.022** **Partial traumatic amputation at left shoulder joint** A

Ex: See S48.012

● **S48.029** **Partial traumatic amputation at unspecified shoulder joint** A

Ex: See S48.019

● **S48.1** **Traumatic amputation at level between shoulder and elbow**

● **S48.11** **Complete traumatic amputation at level between shoulder and elbow**

● **S48.111** **Complete traumatic amputation at level between right shoulder and elbow** A

Ex: See S48.011

● **S48.112** **Complete traumatic amputation at level between left shoulder and elbow** A

Ex: See S48.012

● **S48.119** **Complete traumatic amputation at level between unspecified shoulder and elbow** A

Ex: See S48.019

● **S48.12** **Partial traumatic amputation at level between shoulder and elbow**

● **S48.121** **Partial traumatic amputation at level between right shoulder and elbow** A

Ex: See S48.011

● **S48.122** **Partial traumatic amputation at level between left shoulder and elbow** A

Ex: See S48.012

● **S48.129** **Partial traumatic amputation at level between unspecified shoulder and elbow** A

Ex: See S48.019

● **S48.9** **Traumatic amputation of shoulder and upper arm, level unspecified**

● **S48.91** **Complete traumatic amputation of shoulder and upper arm, level unspecified**

● **S48.911** **Complete traumatic amputation of right shoulder and upper arm, level unspecified** A

Ex: See S48.011

● **S48.912** **Complete traumatic amputation of left shoulder and upper arm, level unspecified** A

Ex: See S48.012

● **S48.919** **Complete traumatic amputation of unspecified shoulder and upper arm, level unspecified** A

Ex: See S48.019

- **S48.92** Partial traumatic amputation of shoulder and upper arm, level unspecified
  - **S48.921** Partial traumatic amputation of right shoulder and upper arm, level unspecified A
    Ex: See S48.011
  - **S48.922** Partial traumatic amputation of left shoulder and upper arm, level unspecified A
    Ex: See S48.012
  - **S48.929** Partial traumatic amputation of unspecified shoulder and upper arm, level unspecified A
    Ex: See S48.019

- **S49** Other and unspecified injuries of shoulder and upper arm

The appropriate 7th character is to be added to each code from subcategories S49.0 and S49.1

A	initial encounter for closed fracture
D	subsequent encounter for fracture with routine healing
G	subsequent encounter for fracture with delayed healing
K	subsequent encounter for fracture with nonunion
P	subsequent encounter for fracture with malunion
S	sequela

- **S49.0** Physeal fracture of upper end of humerus
  - **S49.00** Unspecified physeal fracture of upper end of humerus
    - **S49.001** Unspecified physeal fracture of upper end of humerus, right arm A, K, P, A
      Ex: For S49.001[A]: See S42.201[A]
      For S49.001[K,P]: See S02.0[K]
    - **S49.002** Unspecified physeal fracture of upper end of humerus, left arm A, K, P, A
      Ex: For S49.002[A]: See S42.202[A]
      For S49.002[K,P]: See S02.0[K]
    - **S49.009** Unspecified physeal fracture of upper end of humerus, unspecified arm A, K, P, A
      Ex: For S49.009[A]: See S42.209[A]
      For S49.009[K,P]: See S02.0[K]
  - **S49.01** Salter-Harris Type I physeal fracture of upper end of humerus
    - **S49.011** Salter-Harris Type I physeal fracture of upper end of humerus, right arm A, K, P, A
      Ex: For S49.011[A]: See S42.201[A]
      For S49.011[K,P]: See S02.0[K]
    - **S49.012** Salter-Harris Type I physeal fracture of upper end of humerus, left arm A, K, P, A
      Ex: For S49.012[A]: See S42.202[A]
      For S49.012[K,P]: See S02.0[K]
    - **S49.019** Salter-Harris Type I physeal fracture of upper end of humerus, unspecified arm A, K, P, A
      Ex: For S49.019[A]: See S42.209[A]
      For S49.019[K,P]: See S02.0[K]

Item 19-3 SALTER-HARRIS TYPE 1: epiphysis is completely separated from end of bone, or metaphysic growth plate remains attached to epiphysis

SALTER-HARRIS TYPE 2: epiphysis and growth plate are partially separated from metaphysis, which is cracked—most common type

SALTER-HARRIS TYPE 3: fracture occurring through epiphysis and separates part of epiphysis and growth plate from metaphysis fracture, usually at distal end of tibia

SALTER-HARRIS TYPE 4: fracture runs through epiphysis, across growth plate, into metaphysic, surgery is required to restore joint surface to normal and align growth plate

  - **S49.02** Salter-Harris Type II physeal fracture of upper end of humerus
    - **S49.021** Salter-Harris Type II physeal fracture of upper end of humerus, right arm A, K, P, A
      Ex: For S49.021[A]: See S42.201[A]
      For S49.021[K,P]: See S02.0[K]
    - **S49.022** Salter-Harris Type II physeal fracture of upper end of humerus, left arm A, K, P, A
      Ex: For S49.022[A]: See S42.202[A]
      For S49.022[K,P]: See S02.0[K]
    - **S49.029** Salter-Harris Type II physeal fracture of upper end of humerus, unspecified arm A, K, P, A
      Ex: For S49.029[A]: See S42.209[A]
      For S49.029[K,P]: See S02.0[K]
  - **S49.03** Salter-Harris Type III physeal fracture of upper end of humerus
    - **S49.031** Salter-Harris Type III physeal fracture of upper end of humerus, right arm A, K, P, A
      Ex: For S49.031[A]: See S42.201[A]
      For S49.031[K,P]: See S02.0[K]
    - **S49.032** Salter-Harris Type III physeal fracture of upper end of humerus, left arm A, K, P, A
      Ex: For S49.032[A]: See S42.202[A]
      For S49.032[K,P]: See S02.0[K]
    - **S49.039** Salter-Harris Type III physeal fracture of upper end of humerus, unspecified arm A, K, P, A
      Ex: For S49.039[A]: See S42.209[A]
      For S49.039[K,P]: See S02.0[K]
  - **S49.04** Salter-Harris Type IV physeal fracture of upper end of humerus
    - **S49.041** Salter-Harris Type IV physeal fracture of upper end of humerus, right arm A, K, P, A
      Ex: For S49.041[A]: See S42.201[A]
      For S49.041[K,P]: See S02.0[K]
    - **S49.042** Salter-Harris Type IV physeal fracture of upper end of humerus, left arm A, K, P, A
      Ex: For S49.042[A]: See S42.202[A]
      For S49.042[K,P]: See S02.0[K]
    - **S49.049** Salter-Harris Type IV physeal fracture of upper end of humerus, unspecified arm A, K, P, A
      Ex: For S49.049[A]: See S42.209[A]
      For S49.049[K,P]: See S02.0[K]
  - **S49.09** Other physeal fracture of upper end of humerus
    - **S49.091** Other physeal fracture of upper end of humerus, right arm A, K, P, A
      Ex: For S49.091[A]: See S42.201[A]
      For S49.091[K,P]: See S02.0[K]
    - **S49.092** Other physeal fracture of upper end of humerus, left arm A, K, P, A
      Ex: For S49.092[A]: See S42.202[A]
      For S49.092[K,P]: See S02.0[K]
    - **S49.099** Other physeal fracture of upper end of humerus, unspecified arm A, K, P, A
      Ex: For S49.099[A]: See S42.209[A]
      For S49.099[K,P]: See S02.0[K]

● **S49.1 Physeal fracture of lower end of humerus**

● **S49.10 Unspecified physeal fracture of lower end of humerus**

● **S49.101 Unspecified physeal fracture of lower end of humerus, right arm** A, K, P, A
Ex: **For S49.101[A]:** See S42.201[A]
For S49.101[K,P]: See S02.0[K]

● **S49.102 Unspecified physeal fracture of lower end of humerus, left arm** A, K, P, A
Ex: **For S49.102[A]:** See S42.202[A]
For S49.102[K,P]: See S02.0[K]

● **S49.109 Unspecified physeal fracture of lower end of humerus, unspecified arm** A, K, P, A
Ex: **For S49.109[A]:** See S42.209[A]
For S49.109[K,P]: See S02.0[K]

● **S49.11 Salter-Harris Type I physeal fracture of lower end of humerus**

● **S49.111 Salter-Harris Type I physeal fracture of lower end of humerus, right arm** A, K, P, A
Ex: **For S49.111[A]:** See S42.201[A]
For S49.111[K,P]: See S02.0[K]

● **S49.112 Salter-Harris Type I physeal fracture of lower end of humerus, left arm** A, K, P, A
Ex: **For S49.112[A]:** See S42.202[A]
For S49.112[K,P]: See S02.0[K]

● **S49.119 Salter-Harris Type I physeal fracture of lower end of humerus, unspecified arm** A, K, P, A
Ex: **For S49.119[A]:** See S42.209[A]
For S49.119[K,P]: See S02.0[K]

● **S49.12 Salter-Harris Type II physeal fracture of lower end of humerus**

● **S49.121 Salter-Harris Type II physeal fracture of lower end of humerus, right arm** A, K, P, A
Ex: **For S49.121[A]:** See S42.201[A]
For S49.121[K,P]: See S02.0[K]

● **S49.122 Salter-Harris Type II physeal fracture of lower end of humerus, left arm** A, K, P, A
Ex: **For S49.122[A]:** See S42.202[A]
For S49.122[K,P]: See S02.0[K]

● **S49.129 Salter-Harris Type II physeal fracture of lower end of humerus, unspecified arm** A, K, P, A
Ex: **For S49.129[A]:** See S42.209[A]
For S49.129[K,P]: See S02.0[K]

● **S49.13 Salter-Harris Type III physeal fracture of lower end of humerus**

● **S49.131 Salter-Harris Type III physeal fracture of lower end of humerus, right arm** A, K, P, A
Ex: **For S49.131[A]:** See S42.201[A]
For S49.131[K,P]: See S02.0[K]

● **S49.132 Salter-Harris Type III physeal fracture of lower end of humerus, left arm** A, K, P, A
Ex: **For S49.132[A]:** See S42.202[A]
For S49.132[K,P]: See S02.0[K]

● **S49.139 Salter-Harris Type III physeal fracture of lower end of humerus, unspecified arm** A, K, P, A
Ex: **For S49.139[A]:** See S42.209[A]
For S49.139[K,P]: See S02.0[K]

● **S49.14 Salter-Harris Type IV physeal fracture of lower end of humerus**

● **S49.141 Salter-Harris Type IV physeal fracture of lower end of humerus, right arm** A, K, P, A
Ex: **For S49.141[A]:** See S42.201[A]
For S49.141[K,P]: See S02.0[K]

● **S49.142 Salter-Harris Type IV physeal fracture of lower end of humerus, left arm** A, K, P, A
Ex: **For S49.142[A]:** See S42.202[A]
For S49.142[K,P]: See S02.0[K]

● **S49.149 Salter-Harris Type IV physeal fracture of lower end of humerus, unspecified arm** A, K, P, A
Ex: **For S49.149[A]:** See S42.209[A]
For S49.149[K,P]: See S02.0[K]

● **S49.19 Other physeal fracture of lower end of humerus**

● **S49.191 Other physeal fracture of lower end of humerus, right arm** A, K, P, A
Ex: **For S49.191[A]:** See S42.201[A]
For S49.191[K,P]: See S02.0[K]

● **S49.192 Other physeal fracture of lower end of humerus, left arm** A, K, P, A
Ex: **For S49.192[A]:** See S42.202[A]
For S49.192[K,P]: See S02.0[K]

● **S49.199 Other physeal fracture of lower end of humerus, unspecified arm** A, K, P, A
Ex: **For S49.199[A]:** See S42.209[A]
For S49.199[K,P]: See S02.0[K]

● **S49.8 Other specified injuries of shoulder and upper arm**

The appropriate 7th character is to be added to each code in subcategory S49.8

A	initial encounter
D	subsequent encounter
S	sequela

X● **S49.80 Other specified injuries of shoulder and upper arm, unspecified arm**

X● **S49.81 Other specified injuries of right shoulder and upper arm**

X● **S49.82 Other specified injuries of left shoulder and upper arm**

● **S49.9 Unspecified injury of shoulder and upper arm**

The appropriate 7th character is to be added to each code in subcategory S49.9

A	initial encounter
D	subsequent encounter
S	sequela

X● **S49.90 Unspecified injury of shoulder and upper arm, unspecified arm**

X● **S49.91 Unspecified injury of right shoulder and upper arm**

X● **S49.92 Unspecified injury of left shoulder and upper arm**

INJURIES TO THE ELBOW AND FOREARM (S50-S59)

Excludes2 burns and corrosions (T20-T32)
frostbite (T33-T34)
injuries of wrist and hand (S60-S69)
insect bite or sting, venomous (T63.4)

S50 Superficial injury of elbow and forearm

Excludes2 superficial injury of wrist and hand (S60.-)

The appropriate 7th character is to be added to each code from category S50

A	initial encounter
D	subsequent encounter
S	sequela

S50.0 Contusion of elbow
- X **S50.00 Contusion of unspecified elbow**
- X **S50.01 Contusion of right elbow**
- X **S50.02 Contusion of left elbow**

S50.1 Contusion of forearm
- X **S50.10 Contusion of unspecified forearm**
- X **S50.11 Contusion of right forearm**
- X **S50.12 Contusion of left forearm**

S50.3 Other superficial injuries of elbow
- **S50.31 Abrasion of elbow**
  - **S50.311 Abrasion of right elbow**
  - **S50.312 Abrasion of left elbow**
  - **S50.319 Abrasion of unspecified elbow**
- **S50.32 Blister (nonthermal) of elbow**
  - **S50.321 Blister (nonthermal) of right elbow**
  - **S50.322 Blister (nonthermal) of left elbow**
  - **S50.329 Blister (nonthermal) of unspecified elbow**
- **S50.34 External constriction of elbow**
  - **S50.341 External constriction of right elbow**
  - **S50.342 External constriction of left elbow**
  - **S50.349 External constriction of unspecified elbow**
- **S50.35 Superficial foreign body of elbow**
  Splinter in the elbow
  - **S50.351 Superficial foreign body of right elbow**
  - **S50.352 Superficial foreign body of left elbow**
  - **S50.359 Superficial foreign body of unspecified elbow**
- **S50.36 Insect bite (nonvenomous) of elbow**
  - **S50.361 Insect bite (nonvenomous) of right elbow**
  - **S50.362 Insect bite (nonvenomous) of left elbow**
  - **S50.369 Insect bite (nonvenomous) of unspecified elbow**
- **S50.37 Other superficial bite of elbow**
  Excludes1 open bite of elbow (S51.04)
  - **S50.371 Other superficial bite of right elbow**
  - **S50.372 Other superficial bite of left elbow**
  - **S50.379 Other superficial bite of unspecified elbow**

S50.8 Other superficial injuries of forearm
- **S50.81 Abrasion of forearm**
  - **S50.811 Abrasion of right forearm**
  - **S50.812 Abrasion of left forearm**
  - **S50.819 Abrasion of unspecified forearm**
- **S50.82 Blister (nonthermal) of forearm**
  - **S50.821 Blister (nonthermal) of right forearm**
  - **S50.822 Blister (nonthermal) of left forearm**
  - **S50.829 Blister (nonthermal) of unspecified forearm**
- **S50.84 External constriction of forearm**
  - **S50.841 External constriction of right forearm**
  - **S50.842 External constriction of left forearm**
  - **S50.849 External constriction of unspecified forearm**
- **S50.85 Superficial foreign body of forearm**
  Splinter in the forearm
  - **S50.851 Superficial foreign body of right forearm**
  - **S50.852 Superficial foreign body of left forearm**
  - **S50.859 Superficial foreign body of unspecified forearm**
- **S50.86 Insect bite (nonvenomous) of forearm**
  - **S50.861 Insect bite (nonvenomous) of right forearm**
  - **S50.862 Insect bite (nonvenomous) of left forearm**
  - **S50.869 Insect bite (nonvenomous) of unspecified forearm**
- **S50.87 Other superficial bite of forearm**
  Excludes1 open bite of forearm (S51.84)
  - **S50.871 Other superficial bite of right forearm**
  - **S50.872 Other superficial bite of left forearm**
  - **S50.879 Other superficial bite of unspecified forearm**

S50.9 Unspecified superficial injury of elbow and forearm
- **S50.90 Unspecified superficial injury of elbow**
  - **S50.901 Unspecified superficial injury of right elbow**
  - **S50.902 Unspecified superficial injury of left elbow**
  - **S50.909 Unspecified superficial injury of unspecified elbow**
- **S50.91 Unspecified superficial injury of forearm**
  - **S50.911 Unspecified superficial injury of right forearm**
  - **S50.912 Unspecified superficial injury of left forearm**
  - **S50.919 Unspecified superficial injury of unspecified forearm**

S51 Open wound of elbow and forearm

Code also any associated wound infection

Excludes1 open fracture of elbow and forearm (S52.- with open fracture 7th character)
traumatic amputation of elbow and forearm (S58.-)

Excludes2 open wound of wrist and hand (S61.-)

The appropriate 7th character is to be added to each code from category S51

A	initial encounter
D	subsequent encounter
S	sequela

S51.0 Open wound of elbow
- **S51.00 Unspecified open wound of elbow**
  - **S51.001 Unspecified open wound of right elbow**
    Coding Clinic: 2012, Q4, P108
  - **S51.002 Unspecified open wound of left elbow**
  - **S51.009 Unspecified open wound of unspecified elbow**
    Open wound of elbow NOS

- **S51.01 Laceration without foreign body of elbow**
  - **S51.011 Laceration without foreign body of right elbow**
  - **S51.012 Laceration without foreign body of left elbow**
  - **S51.019 Laceration without foreign body of unspecified elbow**
- **S51.02 Laceration with foreign body of elbow**
  - **S51.021 Laceration with foreign body of right elbow**
  - **S51.022 Laceration with foreign body of left elbow**
  - **S51.029 Laceration with foreign body of unspecified elbow**
- **S51.03 Puncture wound without foreign body of elbow**
  - **S51.031 Puncture wound without foreign body of right elbow**
  - **S51.032 Puncture wound without foreign body of left elbow**
  - **S51.039 Puncture wound without foreign body of unspecified elbow**
- **S51.04 Puncture wound with foreign body of elbow**
  - **S51.041 Puncture wound with foreign body of right elbow**
  - **S51.042 Puncture wound with foreign body of left elbow**
  - **S51.049 Puncture wound with foreign body of unspecified elbow**
- **S51.05 Open bite of elbow**
  Bite of elbow NOS
  Excludes1 superficial bite of elbow (S50.36, S50.37)
  - **S51.051 Open bite, right elbow**
  - **S51.052 Open bite, left elbow**
  - **S51.059 Open bite, unspecified elbow**

- **S51.8 Open wound of forearm**
  Excludes2 open wound of elbow (S51.0-)
  - **S51.80 Unspecified open wound of forearm**
    - **S51.801 Unspecified open wound of right forearm**
    - **S51.802 Unspecified open wound of left forearm**
    - **S51.809 Unspecified open wound of unspecified forearm**
      Open wound of forearm NOS
  - **S51.81 Laceration without foreign body of forearm**
    - **S51.811 Laceration without foreign body of right forearm**
    - **S51.812 Laceration without foreign body of left forearm**
    - **S51.819 Laceration without foreign body of unspecified forearm**
  - **S51.82 Laceration with foreign body of forearm**
    - **S51.821 Laceration with foreign body of right forearm**
    - **S51.822 Laceration with foreign body of left forearm**
    - **S51.829 Laceration with foreign body of unspecified forearm**
  - **S51.83 Puncture wound without foreign body of forearm**
    - **S51.831 Puncture wound without foreign body of right forearm**
    - **S51.832 Puncture wound without foreign body of left forearm**
    - **S51.839 Puncture wound without foreign body of unspecified forearm**
  - **S51.84 Puncture wound with foreign body of forearm**
    - **S51.841 Puncture wound with foreign body of right forearm**
    - **S51.842 Puncture wound with foreign body of left forearm**
    - **S51.849 Puncture wound with foreign body of unspecified forearm**
  - **S51.85 Open bite of forearm**
    Bite of forearm NOS
    Excludes1 superficial bite of forearm (S50.86, S50.87)
    - **S51.851 Open bite of right forearm**
    - **S51.852 Open bite of left forearm**
    - **S51.859 Open bite of unspecified forearm**

- **S52 Fracture of forearm**

Note: A fracture not identified as displaced or nondisplaced should be coded to displaced

A fracture not designated as open or closed should be coded to closed

The open fracture designations are based on the Gustilo open fracture classification

Excludes1 traumatic amputation of forearm (S58.-)

Excludes2 fracture at wrist and hand level (S62.-)

The appropriate 7th character is to be added to all codes from category S52

A	initial encounter for closed fracture
B	initial encounter for open fracture type I or II initial encounter for open fracture NOS
C	initial encounter for open fracture type IIIA, IIIB, or IIIC
D	subsequent encounter for closed fracture with routine healing
E	subsequent encounter for open fracture type I or II with routine healing
F	subsequent encounter for open fracture type IIIA, IIIB, or IIIC with routine healing
G	subsequent encounter for closed fracture with delayed healing
H	subsequent encounter for open fracture type I or II with delayed healing
J	subsequent encounter for open fracture type IIIA, IIIB, or IIIC with delayed healing
K	subsequent encounter for closed fracture with nonunion
M	subsequent encounter for open fracture type I or II with nonunion
N	subsequent encounter for open fracture type IIIA, IIIB, or IIIC with nonunion
P	subsequent encounter for closed fracture with malunion
Q	subsequent encounter for open fracture type I or II with malunion
R	subsequent encounter for open fracture type IIIA, IIIB, or IIIC with malunion
S	sequela

Coding Clinic: 2016, Q1, P33

S52.0 Fracture of upper end of ulna

Fracture of proximal end of ulna

Excludes2 fracture of elbow NOS (S42.40-)
fractures of shaft of ulna (S52.2-)

S52.00 Unspecified fracture of upper end of ulna

Ex **For category S52.00 CC codes S52.00[B,C]:** S52.001-S52.009[B,C], S52.021-S52.109[B,C], S52.121-S52.189[B,C], S52.201-S52.209[A,B,C], S52.211-S52.219[A], S52.221-S52.266[A,B,C], S52.271-S52.279[B,C], S52.281-S52.309[A,B,C], S52.311-S52.319[A], S52.321-S52.516[A,B,C], S52.531-S52.616[A,B,C], S52.691-S52.92X[A,B,C], S59.001-S59.099[A], S59.201-S59.299[A], S62.90X[B]

For S52.00[K,M,N,P,Q,R]: See S02.0[K]

S52.001 Unspecified fracture of upper end of right ulna K, M, N, P, Q, R CC, **B, C** MCC, B, C HA

S52.002 Unspecified fracture of upper end of left ulna K, M, N, P, Q, R CC, **B, C** MCC, B, C HA

S52.009 Unspecified fracture of upper end of unspecified ulna K, M, N, P, Q, R CC, **B, C** MCC, B, C HA

S52.01 Torus fracture of upper end of ulna

The appropriate 7th character is to be added to all codes in subcategory S52.01

A	initial encounter for closed fracture
D	subsequent encounter for fracture with routine healing
G	subsequent encounter for fracture with delayed healing
K	subsequent encounter for fracture with nonunion
P	subsequent encounter for fracture with malunion
S	sequela

S52.011 Torus fracture of upper end of right ulna A, K, P CC, A HA

Ex **For code S52.011[A]:** S52.001 [A,B,C], S52.002 [B,C], S52.009 [A,B,C], S52.011[A], S52.019[A], S52.021[A,B,C], S52.022[B,C], S52.023-S52.024[A,B,C], S52.025[B,C], S52.026-S52.031[A,B,C], S52.032[B,C], S52.033-S52.034[A,B,C], S52.035[B,C], S52.036-S52.041[A,B,C], S52.042[B,C], S52.043-S52.044[A,B,C], S52.045[B,C], S52.046-S52.091[A,B,C], S52.092[B,C], S52.099-S52.101[A,B,C], S52.102[B,C], S52.109[A,B,C], S52.111[A], S52.119[A], S52.121[A,B,C], S52.122[B,C], S52.123-S52.124[A,B,C], S52.125[B,C], S52.126-S52.131[A,B,C], S52.132[B,C], S52.133-S52.134[A,B,C], S52.135[B, C], S52.136-S52.181[A,B,C], S52.182[B,C], S52.189-S52.201[A,B,C], S52.202[B,C], S52.209[A,B,C], S52.211[A], S52.219[A], S52.221[A,B,C], S52.222[B,C], S52.223-S52.224[A,B,C], S52.225[B,C], S52.226-S52.231[C], S52.232[B,C], S52.233-S52.234[A,B,C], S52.235[B,C], S52.236-S52.241[C], S52.242[B,C], S52.243-S52.244[A,B,C], S52.245[B,C], S52.246-S52.251[A,B,C], S52.252[B,C], S52.253-S52.254[A,B,C], S52.255[B,C], S52.256-S52.261[A,B,C], S52.262[BC], S52.263-S52.264[A,B,C], S52.265[B,C], S52.266-S52.271[A,B,C], S52.272[B,C], S52.279-S52.281[A,B,C], S52.282[B,C], S52.283-S52.291[A,B,C], S52.292[B,C], S52.299-S52.301[A,B,C], S52.302[B,C], S52.309[A,B,C], S52.311[A], S52.319[A], S52.321[A,B,C], S52.322[B,C], S52.323-S52.324[A,B,C], S52.325[B,C], S52.326-S52.331[A,B,C], S52.332[B,C], S52.333-S52.334[A,B,C], S52.335[B,C], S52.336-S52.341[A,B,C], S52.342[B,C], S52.343-S52.344[A,B,C], S52.345[B,C], S52.346-S52.351[A,B,C], S52.352[B,C], S52.353-S52.354[A,B,C], S52.355[B,C], S52.356-S52.361[A,B,C], S52.362[B,C], S52.363-S52.364[A,B,C], S52.365[B,C], S52.366-S52.371[A,B,C], S52.372[B,C], S52.379-S52.381[A,B,C], S52.382[B,C], S52.389-S52.391[A,B,C], S52.392[B,C], S52.399-S52.501[A,B,C], S52.502[B,C], S52.509-S52.511[A,B,C], S52.512[B,C], S52.513-S52.514[A,B,C], S52.515[B,C], S52.16[A,B,C], S52.521[A], S52.529[A], S52.531[A,B,C], S52.532[B,C], S52.539-S52.541[A,B,C], S52.542[B,C], S52.549-S52.551[A,B,C], S52.552[B,C], S52.559-S52.561[A,B,C], S52.562[B,C], S52.569-S52.571[A,B,C], S52.572[B,C], S52.579-S52.591[A,B,C], S52.592[B,C], S52.599-S52.601[A,B,C], S52.602[B,C], S52.609-S52.611[A,B,C], S52.612[B,C], S52.613-S52.614[A,B,C], S52.615[B,C], S52.616[A,B,C], S52.621[A], S52.629[A], S52.691[A,B,C], S52.692[B,C], S52.699-S52.92X[A,B,C], S59.001[A], S59.009-S59.011[A], S59.019-S59.021[A], S59.029-S59.031[A], S59.039-S59.041[A], S59.049-S59.091[A], S59.099-S59.101[A], S59.109-S59.111[A], S59.119-S59.121[A], S59.129-S59.131[A], S59.139-S59.141[A], S59.149-S59.191[A], S59.199-S59.201[A], S59.209-S59.211[A], S59.219-S59.221[A], S59.229-S59.231[A], S59.239-S59.241[A], S59.249-S59.291[A], S59.299[A]

For S52.011[K,P]: See S02.0[K]

● **S52.012** **Torus fracture of upper end of left ulna** A, K, P, A

Ex: **For code S52.012[A]:** S52.001[B,C], S52.002-S52.009[A,B,C], S52.012-S52.019[A], S52.021[B,C], S52.022-S52.023[A,B,C], S52.024[B,C], S52.025-S52.026[A,B,C], S52.031[B,C], S52.032-S52.033[A,B,C], S52.034[B,C], S52.035-S52.036[A,B,C], S52.041[B,C], S52.042-S52.043[A,B,C], S52.044[B,C], S52.045-S52.046[A,B,C], S52.091[B,C], S52.092-S52.099[A,B,C], S52.101[B,C], S52.102-S52.109[A,B,C], S52.112-S52.119[A], S52.121[B,C], S52.122-S52.123[A,B,C], S52.124[B,C], S52.125-S52.126[A,B,C], S52.131[B,C], S52.132-S52.133[A,B,C], S52.134[B,C], S52.135-S52.136[A,B,C], S52.181[B,C], S52.182-S52.189[A,B,C], S52.201[B,C], S52.202-S52.209[A,B,C], S52.212-S52.219[A], S52.221[B,C], S52.222-S52.223[A,B,C], S52.224[B,C], S52.225-S52.226[A,B,C], S52.231[B,C], S52.232-S52.233[A,B,C], S52.234[B,C], S52.235-S52.236[A,B,C], S52.241[B,C], S52.242-S52.243[A,B,C], S52.244[B,C], S52.245-S52.246[A,B,C], S52.251[B,C], S52.252-S52.253[A,B,C], S52.254[B,C], S52.255-S52.256[A,B,C], S52.261[B,C], S52.262-S52.263[A,B,C], S52.264[B,C], S52.265-S52.266[A,B,C], S52.271[B,C], S52.272-S52.279[A,B,C], S52.281[B,C], S52.282-S52.283[A,B,C], S52.291[B,C], S52.292-S52.299[A,B,C], S52.301[B,C], S52.302-S52.309[A,B,C], S52.312-S52.319[A], S52.321[B,C], S52.322-S52.323[A,B,C], S52.324[B,C], S52.325-S52.326[A,B,C], S52.331[B,C], S52.332-S52.333[A,B,C], S52.334[B,C], S52.335-S52.336[A,B,C], S52.341[B,C], S52.342-S52.343[A,B,C], S52.344[B,C], S52.345-S52.346[A,B,C], S52.351[B,C], S52.352-S52.353[A,B,C], S52.354[B,C], S52.355-S52.356[A,B,C], S52.361[B,C], S52.362-S52.363[A,B,C], S52.364[B,C], S52.365-S52.366[A,B,C], S52.371[B,C], S52.372-S52.379[A,B,C], S52.381[B,C], S52.382-S52.389[A,B,C], S52.391[B,C], S52.392-S52.399[A,B,C], S52.501[B,C], S52.502-S52.509[A,B,C], S52.511[B,C], S52.512-S52.513[A,B,C], S52.514[B,C], S52.515-S52.516[A,B,C], S52.522-S52.529[A], S52.531[B,C], S52.532-S52.539[A,B,C], S52.541[B,C], S52.542-S52.549[A,B,C], S52.551[B,C], S52.552-S52.559[A,B,C], S52.561[B,C], S52.562-S52.569[A,B,C], S52.571[B,C], S52.572-S52.579[A,B,C], S52.591[B,C], S52.592-S52.599[A,B,C], S52.601[B,C], S52.602-S52.609[A,B,C], S52.611[B,C], S52.612-S52.613[A,B,C], S52.614[B,C], S52.615-S52.616[A,B,C], S52.622-S52.629[A], S52.691[B,C], S52.692-S52.92X[A,B,C], S59.002-S59.009[A], S59.012-S59.019[A], S59.022-S59.029[A], S59.032-S59.039[A], S59.042-S59.049[A], S59.092-S59.099[A], S59.102-S59.109[A], S59.112-S59.119[A], S59.122-S59.129[A], S59.132-S59.139[A], S59.142-S59.149[A], S59.192-S59.199[A], S59.202-S59.209[A], S59.212-S59.219[A], S59.222-S59.229[A], S59.232-S59.239[A], S59.242-S59.249[A], S59.292-S59.299[A] **For S52.012[K,P]:** See S02.0[K]

● **S52.019** **Torus fracture of upper end of unspecified ulna** A, K, P, A

Ex: **For code S52.019[A]:** S52.001-S52.009[A,B,C], S52.011-S52.019[A], S52.021-S52.109[A,B,C], S52.111-S52.119[A], S52.121-S52.209[A,B,C], S52.211-S52.219[A], S52.221-S52.309[A,B,C], S52.311-S52.319[A], S52.321-S52.516[A,B,C], S52.521-S52.529[A], S52.531-S52.616[A,B,C], S52.621-S52.629[A], S52.691-S52.92X[A,B,C], S59.001-S59.299[A] **For S52.019[K,P]:** See S02.0[K]

● **S52.02** **Fracture of olecranon process without intraarticular extension of ulna**

Ex: **For category S52.02 CC codes S52.02[B,C]:** S52.001-S52.009[B,C], S52.021-S52.109[B,C], S52.121-S52.189[B,C], S52.201-S52.209[A,B,C], S52.211-S52.219[A], S52.221-S52.266[A,B,C], S52.271-S52.279[B,C], S52.281-S52.309[A,B,C], S52.311-S52.319[A], S52.321-S52.516[A,B,C], S52.531-S52.549[B,C], S52.551-S52.616[A,B,C], S52.691-S52.92X[A,B,C], S59.001-S59.099[A], S59.201-S59.299[A], S62.90X[B] **For S52.02[K,M,N,P,Q,R]:** See S02.0[K]

● **S52.021** **Displaced fracture of olecranon process without intraarticular extension of right ulna** K, M, N, P, Q, R, B, C, B, C

● **S52.022** **Displaced fracture of olecranon process without intraarticular extension of left ulna** K, M, N, P, Q, R, B, C, B, C

● **S52.023** **Displaced fracture of olecranon process without intraarticular extension of unspecified ulna** K, M, N, P, Q, R, B, C, B, C

● **S52.024** **Nondisplaced fracture of olecranon process without intraarticular extension of right ulna** K, M, N, P, Q, R, B, C, B, C

● **S52.025** **Nondisplaced fracture of olecranon process without intraarticular extension of left ulna** K, M, N, P, Q, R, B, C, B, C

● **S52.026** **Nondisplaced fracture of olecranon process without intraarticular extension of unspecified ulna** K, M, N, P, Q, R, B, C, B, C

● **S52.03** **Fracture of olecranon process with intraarticular extension of ulna**

Ex: **For category S52.03 CC codes S52.03[B,C]:** See S52.02[B,C] **For S52.03[K,M,N,P,Q,R]:** See S02.0[K]

● **S52.031** **Displaced fracture of olecranon process with intraarticular extension of right ulna** K, M, N, P, Q, R, B, C, B, C

● **S52.032** **Displaced fracture of olecranon process with intraarticular extension of left ulna** K, M, N, P, Q, R, B, C, B, C

● **S52.033** **Displaced fracture of olecranon process with intraarticular extension of unspecified ulna** K, M, N, P, Q, R, B, C, B, C

● **S52.034** **Nondisplaced fracture of olecranon process with intraarticular extension of right ulna** K, M, N, P, Q, R, B, C, B, C

● **S52.035** **Nondisplaced fracture of olecranon process with intraarticular extension of left ulna** K, M, N, P, Q, R, B, C, B, C

● **S52.036** **Nondisplaced fracture of olecranon process with intraarticular extension of unspecified ulna** K, M, N, P, Q, R, B, C, B, C

- **S52.04 Fracture of coronoid process of ulna**
  Ex: For category S52.04 CC codes S52.04[B,C]: See S52.00[B,C] For S52.04[K,M,N,P,Q,R]: See S02.0[K]
  - **S52.041 Displaced fracture of coronoid process of right ulna** K, M, N, P, Q, R, B, C, B, C
  - **S52.042 Displaced fracture of coronoid process of left ulna** K, M, N, P, Q, R, B, C, B, C
  - **S52.043 Displaced fracture of coronoid process of unspecified ulna** K, M, N, P, Q, R, B, C, B, C
  - **S52.044 Nondisplaced fracture of coronoid process of right ulna** K, M, N, P, Q, R, B, C, B, C
  - **S52.045 Nondisplaced fracture of coronoid process of left ulna** K, M, N, P, Q, R, B, C, B, C
  - **S52.046 Nondisplaced fracture of coronoid process of unspecified ulna** K, M, N, P, Q, R, B, C, B, C
- **S52.09 Other fracture of upper end of ulna**
  Ex: For category S52.09 CC codes S52.09[B,C]: See S52.00[B,C] For S52.09[K,M,N,P,Q,R]: See S02.0[K]
  - **S52.091 Other fracture of upper end of right ulna** K, M, N, P, Q, R, B, C, B, C
  - **S52.092 Other fracture of upper end of left ulna** K, M, N, P, Q, R, B, C, B, C
  - **S52.099 Other fracture of upper end of unspecified ulna** K, M, N, P, Q, R, B, C, B, C
- **S52.1 Fracture of upper end of radius**
  Fracture of proximal end of radius
  Excludes2 physeal fractures of upper end of radius (S59.2-)
  fracture of shaft of radius (S52.3-)
- **S52.10 Unspecified fracture of upper end of radius**
  Ex: For category S52.10 CC codes S52.10[B,C]: See S52.00[B,C] For S52.10[K,M,N,P,Q,R]: See S02.0[K]
  - **S52.101 Unspecified fracture of upper end of right radius** K, M, N, P, Q, R, B, C, B, C
  - **S52.102 Unspecified fracture of upper end of left radius** K, M, N, P, Q, R, B, C, B, C
  - **S52.109 Unspecified fracture of upper end of unspecified radius** K, M, N, P, Q, R, B, C, B, C
- **S52.11 Torus fracture of upper end of radius**
  The appropriate 7th character is to be added to all codes in subcategory S52.11

A	initial encounter for closed fracture
D	subsequent encounter for fracture with routine healing
G	subsequent encounter for fracture with delayed healing
K	subsequent encounter for fracture with nonunion
P	subsequent encounter for fracture with malunion
S	sequela

  - **S52.111 Torus fracture of upper end of right radius** A, K, P, A
    Ex: For code S52.111[A]: See S52.011[A] For S52.111[K,P]: See S02.0[K]
  - **S52.112 Torus fracture of upper end of left radius** A, K, P, A
    Ex: For code S52.112[A]: See S52.012[A] For S52.112[K,P]: See S02.0[K]
  - **S52.119 Torus fracture of upper end of unspecified radius** A, K, P, A
    Ex: For code S52.119[A]: See S52.019[A] For S52.119[K,P]: See S02.0[K]
- **S52.12 Fracture of head of radius**
  Ex: For category S52.12 CC codes S52.12[B,C]: See S52.00[B,C] For S52.12[K,M,N,P,Q,R]: See S02.0[K]
  - **S52.121 Displaced fracture of head of right radius** K, M, N, P, Q, R, B, C, B, C
  - **S52.122 Displaced fracture of head of left radius** K, M, N, P, Q, R, B, C, B, C
  - **S52.123 Displaced fracture of head of unspecified radius** K, M, N, P, Q, R, B, C, B, C
  - **S52.124 Nondisplaced fracture of head of right radius** K, M, N, P, Q, R, B, C, B, C
  - **S52.125 Nondisplaced fracture of head of left radius** K, M, N, P, Q, R, B, C, B, C
  - **S52.126 Nondisplaced fracture of head of unspecified radius** K, M, N, P, Q, R, B, C, B, C
- **S52.13 Fracture of neck of radius**
  Ex: For category S52.13 CC codes S52.13[B,C]: See S52.00[B,C] For S52.13[K,M,N,P,Q,R]: See S02.0[K]
  - **S52.131 Displaced fracture of neck of right radius** K, M, N, P, Q, R, B, C, B, C
  - **S52.132 Displaced fracture of neck of left radius** K, M, N, P, Q, R, B, C, B, C
  - **S52.133 Displaced fracture of neck of unspecified radius** K, M, N, P, Q, R, B, C, B, C
  - **S52.134 Nondisplaced fracture of neck of right radius** K, M, N, P, Q, R, B, C, B, C
  - **S52.135 Nondisplaced fracture of neck of left radius** K, M, N, P, Q, R, B, C, B, C
  - **S52.136 Nondisplaced fracture of neck of unspecified radius** K, M, N, P, Q, R, B, C, B, C
- **S52.18 Other fracture of upper end of radius**
  Ex: For category S52.18 CC codes S52.18[B,C]: See S52.00[B,C] For S52.18[K,M,N,P,Q,R]: See S02.0[K]
  - **S52.181 Other fracture of upper end of right radius** K, M, N, P, Q, R, B, C, B, C
  - **S52.182 Other fracture of upper end of left radius** K, M, N, P, Q, R, B, C, B, C
  - **S52.189 Other fracture of upper end of unspecified radius** K, M, N, P, Q, R, B, C, B, C

S52.2 Fracture of shaft of ulna

S52.20 Unspecified fracture of shaft of ulna
Fracture of ulna NOS

S52.201 Unspecified fracture of shaft of right ulna A, K, M, N, P, Q, R, B, C, A, B, C
Ex: For code S52.201[A]: See S52.011[A]
For S52.201[B,C]: See S52.00[B,C]
For S52.201[K,M,N,P,Q,R]: See S02.0[K]

S52.202 Unspecified fracture of shaft of left ulna A, K, M, N, P, Q, R, B, C, A, B, C
Ex: For code S52.202[A]: See S52.012[A] For code S52.202[B,C]: See S52.00[B,C]
For S52.202[K,M,N,P,Q,R]: See S02.0[K]

S52.209 Unspecified fracture of shaft of unspecified ulna
A, K, M, N, P, Q, R, B, C, A, B, C
Ex: For code S52.209[A]: See S52.019[A] For code S52.209[B,C]: See S52.00[B,C]
For S52.209[K,M,N,P,Q,R]: See S02.0[K]

S52.21 Greenstick fracture of shaft of ulna

The appropriate 7th character is to be added to all codes in subcategory S52.21

A	initial encounter for closed fracture
D	subsequent encounter for fracture with routine healing
G	subsequent encounter for fracture with delayed healing
K	subsequent encounter for fracture with nonunion
P	subsequent encounter for fracture with malunion
S	sequela

S52.211 Greenstick fracture of shaft of right ulna A, K, P, A
Ex: For code S52.211[A]: See S52.011[A]
For S52.211[K,P]: See S02.0[K]

S52.212 Greenstick fracture of shaft of left ulna A, K, P, A
Ex: For code S52.212[A]: See S52.012[A]
For S52.202[K,P]: See S02.0[K]

S52.219 Greenstick fracture of shaft of unspecified ulna A, K, P, A
Ex: For code S52.219[A]: See S52.019[A]
For S52.219[K,P]: See S02.0[K]

S52.22 Transverse fracture of shaft of ulna

S52.221 Displaced transverse fracture of shaft of right ulna A, K, M, N, P, Q, R, B, C, A, B, C
Ex: For code S52.221[A]: See S52.011[A]
For S52.221[B,C]: See S52.00[B,C]
For S52.221[K,M,N,P,Q,R]: See S02.0[K]

S52.222 Displaced transverse fracture of shaft of left ulna A, K, M, N, P, Q, R, B, C, A, B, C
Ex: For code S52.222[A]: See S52.012[A] For code S52.222[B,C]: See S52.00[B,C]
For S52.222[K,M,N,P,Q,R]: See S02.0[K]

S52.223 Displaced transverse fracture of shaft of unspecified ulna
A, K, M, N, P, Q, R, B, C, A, B, C
Ex: For code S52.223[A]: See S52.019[A] For code S52.223[B,C]: See S52.00[B,C]
For S52.223[K,M,N,P,Q,R]: See S02.0[K]

S52.224 Nondisplaced transverse fracture of shaft of right ulna
A, K, M, N, P, Q, R, B, C, A, B, C
Ex: For code S52.224[A]: See S52.011[A]
For S52.224[B,C]: See S52.00[B,C]
For S52.224[K,M,N,P,Q,R]: See S02.0[K]

S52.225 Nondisplaced transverse fracture of shaft of left ulna
A, K, M, N, P, Q, R, B, C, A, B, C
Ex: For code S52.225[A]: See S52.012[A] For code S52.225[B,C]: See S52.00[B,C]
For S52.225[K,M,N,P,Q,R]: See S02.0[K]

S52.226 Nondisplaced transverse fracture of shaft of unspecified ulna
A, K, M, N, P, Q, R, B, C, A, B, C
Ex: For code S52.226[A]: See S52.019[A] For code S52.226[B,C]: See S52.00[B,C]
For S52.226[K,M,N,P,Q,R]: See S02.0[K]

S52.23 Oblique fracture of shaft of ulna

S52.231 Displaced oblique fracture of shaft of right ulna A, K, M, N, P, Q, R, B, C, A, B, C
Ex: For code S52.231[A]: See S52.011[A]
For S52.231[B,C]: See S52.00[B,C]
For S52.231[K,M,N,P,Q,R]: See S02.0[K]

S52.232 Displaced oblique fracture of shaft of left ulna A, K, M, N, P, Q, R, B, C, A, B, C
Ex: For code S52.232[A]: See S52.012[A] For code S52.232[B,C]: See S52.00[B,C]
For S52.232[K,M,N,P,Q,R]: See S02.0[K]

S52.233 Displaced oblique fracture of shaft of unspecified ulna
A, K, M, N, P, Q, R, B, C, A, B, C
Ex: For code S52.233[A]: See S52.019[A] For code S52.233[B,C]: See S52.00[B,C]
For S52.233[K,M,N,P,Q,R]: See S02.0[K]

S52.234 Nondisplaced oblique fracture of shaft of right ulna
A, K, M, N, P, Q, R, B, C, A, B, C
Ex: For code S52.234[A]: See S52.011[A]
For S52.234[B,C]: See S52.00[B,C]
For S52.234[K,M,N,P,Q,R]: See S02.0[K]

S52.235 Nondisplaced oblique fracture of shaft of left ulna
A, K, M, N, P, Q, R, B, C, A, B, C
Ex: For code S52.235[A]: See S52.012[A] For code S52.235[B,C]: See S52.00[B,C]
For S52.235[K,M,N,P,Q,R]: See S02.0[K]

S52.236 Nondisplaced oblique fracture of shaft of unspecified ulna
A, K, M, N, P, Q, R, B, C, A, B, C
Ex: For code S52.236[A]: See S52.019[A] For code S52.236[B,C]: See S52.00[B,C]
For S52.236[K,M,N,P,Q,R]: See S02.0[K]

● **S52.24 Spiral fracture of shaft of ulna**

● **S52.241 Displaced spiral fracture of shaft of ulna, right arm** A, K, M, N, P, Q, R, B, C, A, B, C
Ex: **For code S52.241[A]:** See S52.011[A] **For S52.241[B,C]:** See S52.00[B,C] **For S52.241[K,M,N,P,Q,R]:** See S02.0[K]

● **S52.242 Displaced spiral fracture of shaft of ulna, left arm** A, K, M, N, P, Q, R, B, C, A, B, C
Ex: **For code S52.242[A]:** See S52.012[A] **For code S52.242[B,C]:** See S52.00[B,C] **For S52.242[K,M,N,P,Q,R]:** See S02.0[K]

● **S52.243 Displaced spiral fracture of shaft of ulna, unspecified arm**
A, K, M, N, P, Q, R, B, C, A, B, C
Ex: **For code S52.243[A]:** See S52.019[A] **For code S52.243[B,C]:** See S52.00[B,C] **For S52.243[K,M,N,P,Q,R]:** See S02.0[K]

● **S52.244 Nondisplaced spiral fracture of shaft of ulna, right arm**
A, K, M, N, P, Q, R, B, C, A, B, C
Ex: **For code S52.244[A]:** See S52.011[A] **For S52.244[B,C]:** See S52.00[B,C] **For S52.244[K,M,N,P,Q,R]:** See S02.0[K]

● **S52.245 Nondisplaced spiral fracture of shaft of ulna, left arm** A, K, M, N, P, Q, R, B, C, A, B, C
Ex: **For code S52.245[A]:** See S52.012[A] **For code S52.245[B,C]:** See S52.00[B,C] **For S52.245[K,M,N,P,Q,R]:** See S02.0[K]

● **S52.246 Nondisplaced spiral fracture of shaft of ulna, unspecified arm**
A, K, M, N, P, Q, R, B, C, A, B, C
Ex: **For code S52.246[A]:** See S52.019[A] **For code S52.246[B,C]:** See S52.00[B,C] **For S52.246[K,M,N,P,Q,R]:** See S02.0[K]

● **S52.25 Comminuted fracture of shaft of ulna**

● **S52.251 Displaced comminuted fracture of shaft of ulna, right arm**
A, K, M, N, P, Q, R, B, C, A, B, C
Ex: **For code S52.251[A]:** See S52.011[A] **For S52.251[B,C]:** See S52.00[B,C] **For S52.251[K,M,N,P,Q,R]:** See S02.0[K]

● **S52.252 Displaced comminuted fracture of shaft of ulna, left arm**
A, K, M, N, P, Q, R, B, C, A, B, C
Ex: **For code S52.252[A]:** See S52.012[A] **For code S52.252[B,C]:** See S52.00[B,C] **For S52.252[K,M,N,P,Q,R]:** See S02.0[K]

● **S52.253 Displaced comminuted fracture of shaft of ulna, unspecified arm**
A, K, M, N, P, Q, R, B, C, A, B, C
Ex: **For code S52.253[A]:** See S52.019[A] **For code S52.253[B,C]:** See S52.00[B,C] **For S52.253[K,M,N,P,Q,R]:** See S02.0[K]

● **S52.254 Nondisplaced comminuted fracture of shaft of ulna, right arm**
A, K, M, N, P, Q, R, B, C, A, B, C
Ex: **For code S52.254[A]:** See S52.011[A] **For S52.254[B,C]:** See S52.00[B,C] **For S52.254[K,M,N,P,Q,R]:** See S02.0[K]

● **S52.255 Nondisplaced comminuted fracture of shaft of ulna, left arm**
A, K, M, N, P, Q, R, B, C, A, B, C
Ex: **For code S52.255[A]:** See S52.012[A] **For code S52.255[B,C]:** See S52.00[B,C] **For S52.255[K,M,N,P,Q,R]:** See S02.0[K]

● **S52.256 Nondisplaced comminuted fracture of shaft of ulna, unspecified arm**
A, K, M, N, P, Q, R, B, C, A, B, C
Ex: **For code S52.256[A]:** See S52.019[A] **For code S52.256[B,C]:** See S52.00[B,C] **For S52.256[K,M,N,P,Q,R]:** See S02.0[K]

● **S52.26 Segmental fracture of shaft of ulna**

● **S52.261 Displaced segmental fracture of shaft of ulna, right arm**
A, K, M, N, P, Q, R, B, C, A, B, C
Ex: **For code S52.261[A]:** See S52.011[A] **For S52.261[B,C]:** See S52.00[B,C] **For S52.261[K,M,N,P,Q,R]:** S02.0[K]

● **S52.262 Displaced segmental fracture of shaft of ulna, left arm** A, K, M, N, P, Q, R, B, C, A, B, C
Ex: **For code S52.262[A]:** See S52.012[A] **For code S52.262[B,C]:** See S52.00[B,C] **For S52.262[K,M,N,P,Q,R]:** See S02.0[K]

● **S52.263 Displaced segmental fracture of shaft of ulna, unspecified arm**
A, K, M, N, P, Q, R, B, C, A, B, C
Ex: **For code S52.263[A]:** See S52.019[A] **For code S52.263[B,C]:** See S52.00[B,C] **For S52.263[K,M,N,P,Q,R]:** See S02.0[K]

● **S52.264 Nondisplaced segmental fracture of shaft of ulna, right arm**
A, K, M, N, P, Q, R, B, C, A, B, C
Ex: **For code S52.264[A]:** See S52.011[A] **For S52.264[B,C]:** See S52.00[B,C] **For S52.264[K,M,N,P,Q,R]:** See S02.0[K]

● **S52.265 Nondisplaced segmental fracture of shaft of ulna, left arm**
A, K, M, N, P, Q, R, B, C, A, B, C
Ex: **For code S52.265[A]:** See S52.012[A] **For code S52.265[B,C]:** See S52.00[B,C] **For S52.265[K,M,N,P,Q,R]:** See S02.0[K]

● **S52.266 Nondisplaced segmental fracture of shaft of ulna, unspecified arm**
A, K, M, N, P, Q, R, B, C, A, B, C
Ex: **For code S52.266[A]:** See S52.019[A] **For code S52.266[B,C]:** See S52.00[B,C] **For S52.266[K,M,N,P,Q,R]:** See S02.0[K]

● **S52.27 Monteggia's fracture of ulna**
Fracture of upper shaft of ulna with dislocation of radial head
Ex: **For category S52.27 CC codes S52.27[B,C]:** See S52.00[B,C] **For S52.27[K,M,N,P,Q,R]:** See S02.0[K]

● **S52.271 Monteggia's fracture of right ulna**
K, M, N, P, Q, R, B, C, B, C

● **S52.272 Monteggia's fracture of left ulna**
K, M, N, P, Q, R, B, C, B, C

● **S52.279 Monteggia's fracture of unspecified ulna** K, M, N, P, Q, R, B, C, B, C

- **S52.28 Bent bone of ulna**
  - **S52.281 Bent bone of right ulna**
    A, K, M, N, P, Q, R, B, C, A, B, C
    Ex: For code S52.281[A]: See S52.011[A]
    For S52.281[B,C]: See S52.00[B,C]
    For S52.281[K,M,N,P,Q,R]: See S02.0[K]
  - **S52.282 Bent bone of left ulna**
    A, K, M, N, P, Q, R, B, C, A, B, C
    Ex: For code S52.282[A]: See S52.012[A] For code S52.282[B,C]: See S52.00[B,C]
    For S52.282[K,M,N,P,Q,R]: See S02.0[K]
  - **S52.283 Bent bone of unspecified ulna**
    A, K, M, N, P, Q, R, B, C, A, B, C
    Ex: For code S52.283[A]: See S52.019[A] For code S52.283[B,C]: See S52.00[B,C]
    For S52.283[K,M,N,P,Q,R]: See S02.0[K]
- **S52.29 Other fracture of shaft of ulna**
  - **S52.291 Other fracture of shaft of right ulna**
    A, K, M, N, P, Q, R, B, C, A, B, C
    Ex: For code S52.291[A]: See S52.011[A]
    For S52.291[B,C]: See S52.00[B,C]
    For S52.291[K,M,N,P,Q,R]: See S02.0[K]
  - **S52.292 Other fracture of shaft of left ulna**
    A, K, M, N, P, Q, R, B, C, A, B, C
    Ex: For code S52.292[A]: See S52.012[A] For code S52.292[B,C]: See S52.00[B,C]
    For S52.292[K,M,N,P,Q,R]: See S02.0[K]
  - **S52.299 Other fracture of shaft of unspecified ulna**
    A, K, M, N, P, Q, R, B, C, A, B, C
    Ex: For code S52.299[A]: See S52.019[A] For code S52.299[B,C]: See S52.00[B,C]
    For S52.299[K,M,N,P,Q,R]: See S02.0[K]
- **S52.3 Fracture of shaft of radius**
  - **S52.30 Unspecified fracture of shaft of radius**
    - **S52.301 Unspecified fracture of shaft of right radius**
      A, K, M, N, P, Q, R, B, C, A, B, C
      Ex: For code S52.301[A]: See S52.011[A]
      For S52.301[B,C]: See S52.00[B,C]
      For S52.301[K,M,N,P,Q,R]: See S02.0[K]
    - **S52.302 Unspecified fracture of shaft of left radius**
      A, K, M, N, P, Q, R, B, C, A, B, C
      Ex: For code S52.302[A]: See S52.012[A] For code S52.302[B,C]: See S52.00[B,C]
      For S52.302[K,M,N,P,Q,R]: See S02.0[K]
    - **S52.309 Unspecified fracture of shaft of unspecified radius**
      A, K, M, N, P, Q, R, B, C, A, B, C
      Ex: For code S52.309[A]: See S52.019[A] For code S52.309[B,C]: See S52.00[B,C]
      For S52.309[K,M,N,P,Q,R]: See S02.0[K]
- **S52.31 Greenstick fracture of shaft of radius**

  The appropriate 7th character is to be added to all codes in subcategory S52.31

A	initial encounter for closed fracture
D	subsequent encounter for fracture with routine healing
G	subsequent encounter for fracture with delayed healing
K	subsequent encounter for fracture with nonunion
P	subsequent encounter for fracture with malunion
S	sequela

  - **S52.311 Greenstick fracture of shaft of radius, right arm** A, K, P, A
    Ex: For code S52.311[A]: See S52.011[A]
    For S52.311[K,P]: See S02.0[K]
  - **S52.312 Greenstick fracture of shaft of radius, left arm** A, K, P, A
    Ex: For code S52.312[A]: See S52.012[A]
    For S52.312[K,P]: See S02.0[K]
  - **S52.319 Greenstick fracture of shaft of radius, unspecified arm** A, K, P, A
    Ex: For code S52.319[A]: See S52.019[A]
    For S52.319[K,P]: See S02.0[K]
- **S52.32 Transverse fracture of shaft of radius**
  - **S52.321 Displaced transverse fracture of shaft of right radius** A, K, M, N, P, Q, R, B, C, A, B, C
    Ex: For code S52.321[A]: See S52.011[A]
    For S52.321[B,C]: See S52.00[B,C]
    For S52.321[K,M,N,P,Q,R]: See S02.0[K]
  - **S52.322 Displaced transverse fracture of shaft of left radius** A, K, M, N, P, Q, R, B, C, A, B, C
    Ex: For code S52.322[A]: See S52.012[A] For code S52.322[B,C]: See S52.00[B,C]
    For S52.322[K,M,N,P,Q,R]: See S02.0[K]
  - **S52.323 Displaced transverse fracture of shaft of unspecified radius**
    A, K, M, N, P, Q, R, B, C, A, B, C
    Ex: For code S52.323[A]: See S52.019[A] For code S52.323[B,C]: See S52.00[B,C]
    For S52.323[K,M,N,P,Q,R]: See S02.0[K]
  - **S52.324 Nondisplaced transverse fracture of shaft of right radius**
    A, K, M, N, P, Q, R, B, C, A, B, C
    Ex: For code S52.324[A]: See S52.011[A]
    For S52.324[B,C]: See S52.00[B,C]
    For S52.324[K,M,N,P,Q,R]: See S02.0[K]
  - **S52.325 Nondisplaced transverse fracture of shaft of left radius**
    A, K, M, N, P, Q, R, B, C, A, B, C
    Ex: For code S52.325[A]: See S52.012[A] For code S52.325[B,C]: See S52.00[B,C]
    For S52.325[K,M,N,P,Q,R]: See S02.0[K]
  - **S52.326 Nondisplaced transverse fracture of shaft of unspecified radius**
    A, K, M, N, P, Q, R, B, C, A, B, C
    Ex: For code S52.326[A]: See S52.019[A] For code S52.326[B,C]: See S52.00[B,C]
    For S52.326[K,M,N,P,Q,R]: See S02.0[K]

- **S52.33 Oblique fracture of shaft of radius**
  - **S52.331 Displaced oblique fracture of shaft of right radius** A, K, M, N, P, Q, R CC, B, C MCC, A, B, C HAC
    Ex: **For code S52.331[A]:** See S52.011[A]
    For S52.331[B,C]: See S52.00[B,C]
    For S52.331[K,M,N,P,Q,R]: See S02.0[K]
  - **S52.332 Displaced oblique fracture of shaft of left radius** A, K, M, N, P, Q, R CC, B, C MCC, A, B, C HAC
    Ex: **For code S52.332[A]:** See S52.012[A] **For code S52.332[B,C]:** See S52.00[B,C]
    For S52.332[K,M,N,P,Q,R]: See S02.0[K]
  - **S52.333 Displaced oblique fracture of shaft of unspecified radius**
    A, K, M, N, P, Q, R CC, B, C MCC, A, B, C HAC
    Ex: **For code S52.333[A]:** See S52.019[A] **For code S52.333[B,C]:** See S52.00[B,C]
    For S52.333[K,M,N,P,Q,R]: See S02.0[K]
  - **S52.334 Nondisplaced oblique fracture of shaft of right radius**
    A, K, M, N, P, Q, R CC, B, C MCC, A, B, C HAC
    Ex: **For code S52.334[A]:** See S52.011[A]
    For S52.334[B,C]: See S52.00[B,C]
    For S52.334[K,M,N,P,Q,R]: See S02.0[K]
  - **S52.335 Nondisplaced oblique fracture of shaft of left radius**
    A, K, M, N, P, Q, R CC, B, C MCC, A, B, C HAC
    Ex: **For code S52.335[A]:** See S52.012[A] **For code S52.335[B,C]:** See S52.00[B,C]
    For S52.335[K,M,N,P,Q,R]: See S02.0[K]
  - **S52.336 Nondisplaced oblique fracture of shaft of unspecified radius**
    A, K, M, N, P, Q, R CC, B, C MCC, A, B, C HAC
    Ex: **For code S52.336[A]:** See S52.019[A] **For code S52.336[B,C]:** See S52.00[B,C]
    For S52.336[K,M,N,P,Q,R]: See S02.0[K]
- **S52.34 Spiral fracture of shaft of radius**
  - **S52.341 Displaced spiral fracture of shaft of radius, right arm**
    A, K, M, N, P, Q, R CC, B, C MCC, A, B, C HAC
    Ex: **For code S52.341[A]:** See S52.011[A]
    For S52.341[B,C]: See S52.00[B,C]
    For S52.341[K,M,N,P,Q,R]: See S02.0[K]
  - **S52.342 Displaced spiral fracture of shaft of radius, left arm** A, K, M, N, P, Q, R CC, B, C MCC, A, B, C HAC
    Ex: **For code S52.342[A]:** See S52.012[A] **For code S52.342[B,C]:** See S52.00[B,C]
    For S52.342[K,M,N,P,Q,R]: See S02.0[K]
  - **S52.343 Displaced spiral fracture of shaft of radius, unspecified arm**
    A, K, M, N, P, Q, R CC, B, C MCC, A, B, C HAC
    Ex: **For code S52.343[A]:** See S52.019[A] **For code S52.343[B,C]:** See S52.00[B,C]
    For S52.343[K,M,N,P,Q,R]: See S02.0[K]
  - **S52.344 Nondisplaced spiral fracture of shaft of radius, right arm**
    A, K, M, N, P, Q, R CC, B, C MCC, A, B, C HAC
    Ex: **For code S52.344[A]:** See S52.011[A]
    For S52.344[B,C]: See S52.00[B,C]
    For S52.344[K,M,N,P,Q,R]: See S02.0[K]
  - **S52.345 Nondisplaced spiral fracture of shaft of radius, left arm**
    A, K, M, N, P, Q, R CC, B, C MCC, A, B, C HAC
    Ex: **For code S52.345[A]:** See S52.012[A] **For code S52.345[B,C]:** See S52.00[B,C]
    For S52.345[K,M,N,P,Q,R]: See S02.0[K]
  - **S52.346 Nondisplaced spiral fracture of shaft of radius, unspecified arm**
    A, K, M, N, P, Q, R CC, B, C MCC, A, B, C HAC
    Ex: **For code S52.346[A]:** See S52.019[A] **For code S52.346[B,C]:** See S52.00[B,C]
    For S52.346[K,M,N,P,Q,R]: See S02.0[K]
- **S52.35 Comminuted fracture of shaft of radius**
  - **S52.351 Displaced comminuted fracture of shaft of radius, right arm**
    A, K, M, N, P, Q, R CC, B, C MCC, A, B, C HAC
    Ex: **For code S52.351[A]:** See S52.011[A]
    For S52.351[B,C]: See S52.00[B,C]
    For S52.351[K,M,N,P,Q,R]: See S02.0[K]
  - **S52.352 Displaced comminuted fracture of shaft of radius, left arm**
    A, K, M, N, P, Q, R CC, B, C MCC, A, B, C HAC
    Ex: **For code S52.352[A]:** See S52.012[A] **For code S52.352[B,C]:** See S52.00[B,C]
    For S52.352[K,M,N,P,Q,R]: See S02.0[K]
  - **S52.353 Displaced comminuted fracture of shaft of radius, unspecified arm**
    A, K, M, N, P, Q, R CC, B, C MCC, A, B, C HAC
    Ex: **For code S52.353[A]:** See S52.019[A] **For code S52.353[B,C]:** See S52.00[B,C]
    For S52.353[K,M,N,P,Q,R]: See S02.0[K]
  - **S52.354 Nondisplaced comminuted fracture of shaft of radius, right arm**
    A, K, M, N, P, Q, R CC, B, C MCC, A, B, C HAC
    Ex: **For code S52.354[A]:** See S52.011[A]
    For S52.354[B,C]: See S52.00[B,C]
    For S52.354[K,M,N,P,Q,R]: See S02.0[K]
  - **S52.355 Nondisplaced comminuted fracture of shaft of radius, left arm**
    A, K, M, N, P, Q, R CC, B, C MCC, A, B, C HAC
    Ex: **For code S52.355[A]:** See S52.012[A] **For code S52.355[B,C]:** See S52.00[B,C]
    For S52.355[K,M,N,P,Q,R]: See S02.0[K]
  - **S52.356 Nondisplaced comminuted fracture of shaft of radius, unspecified arm**
    A, K, M, N, P, Q, R CC, B, C MCC, A, B, C HAC
    Ex: **For code S52.356[A]:** See S52.019[A] **For code S52.356[B,C]:** See S52.00[B,C]
    For S52.356[K,M,N,P,Q,R]: See S02.0[K]

● **S52.36 Segmental fracture of shaft of radius**

● **S52.361 Displaced segmental fracture of shaft of radius, right arm**
A, K, M, N, P, Q, R, B, C, A, B, C
Ex: **For code S52.361[A]:** See S52.011[A]
For S52.361[B,C]: See S52.00[B,C]
For S52.361[K,M,N,P,Q,R]: See S02.0[K]

● **S52.362 Displaced segmental fracture of shaft of radius, left arm**
A, K, M, N, P, Q, R, B, C, A, B, C
Ex: **For code S52.362[A]:** See S52.012[A] **For code S52.362[B,C]:** See S52.00[B,C]
For S52.362[K,M,N,P,Q,R]: See S02.0[K]

● **S52.363 Displaced segmental fracture of shaft of radius, unspecified arm**
A, K, M, N, P, Q, R, B, C, A, B, C
Ex: **For code S52.363[A]:** See S52.019[A] **For code S52.363[B,C]:** See S52.00[B,C]
For S52.363[K,M,N,P,Q,R]: See S02.0[K]

● **S52.364 Nondisplaced segmental fracture of shaft of radius, right arm**
A, K, M, N, P, Q, R, B, C, A, B, C
Ex: **For code S52.364[A]:** See S52.011[A]
For S52.364[B,C]: See S52.00[B,C]
For S52.364[K,M,N,P,Q,R]: See S02.0[K]

● **S52.365 Nondisplaced segmental fracture of shaft of radius, left arm**
A, K, M, N, P, Q, R, B, C, A, B, C
Ex: **For code S52.365[A]:** See S52.012[A] **For code S52.365[B,C]:** See S52.00[B,C]
For S52.365[K,M,N,P,Q,R]: See S02.0[K]

● **S52.366 Nondisplaced segmental fracture of shaft of radius, unspecified arm**
A, K, M, N, P, Q, R, B, C, A, B, C
Ex: **For code S52.366[A]:** See S52.019[A] **For code S52.366[B,C]:** See S52.00[B,C]
For S52.366[K,M,N,P,Q,R]: See S02.0[K]

● **S52.37 Galeazzi's fracture**
Fracture of lower shaft of radius with radioulnar joint dislocation

● **S52.371 Galeazzi's fracture of right radius**
A, K, M, N, P, Q, R, B, C, A, B, C
Ex: **For code S52.371[A]:** See S52.011[A]
For S52.371[B,C]: See S52.00[B,C]
For S52.371[K,M,N,P,Q,R]: See S02.0[K]

● **S52.372 Galeazzi's fracture of left radius**
A, K, M, N, P, Q, R, B, C, A, B, C
Ex: **For code S52.372[A]:** See S52.012[A] **For code S52.372[B,C]:** See S52.00[B,C]
For S52.372[K,M,N,P,Q,R]: See S02.0[K]

● **S52.379 Galeazzi's fracture of unspecified radius** A, K, M, N, P, Q, R, B, C, A, B, C
Ex: **For code S52.379[A]:** See S52.019[A] **For code S52.379[B,C]:** See S52.00[B,C]
For S52.379[K,M,N,P,Q,R]: See S02.0[K]

● **S52.38 Bent bone of radius**

● **S52.381 Bent bone of right radius**
A, K, M, N, P, Q, R, B, C, A, B, C
Ex: **For code S52.381[A]:** See S52.011[A]
For S52.381[B,C]: See S52.00[B,C]
For S52.381[K,M,N,P,Q,R]: See S02.0[K]

● **S52.382 Bent bone of left radius**
A, K, M, N, P, Q, R, B, C, A, B, C
Ex: **For code S52.382[A]:** See S52.012[A] **For code S52.382[B,C]:** See S52.00[B,C]
For S52.382[K,M,N,P,Q,R]: See S02.0[K]

● **S52.389 Bent bone of unspecified radius**
A, K, M, N, P, Q, R, B, C, A, B, C
Ex: **For code S52.389[A]:** See S52.019[A] **For code S52.389[B,C]:** See S52.00[B,C]
For S52.389[K,M,N,P,Q,R]: See S02.0[K]

● **S52.39 Other fracture of shaft of radius**

● **S52.391 Other fracture of shaft of radius, right arm** A, K, M, N, P, Q, R, B, C, A, B, C
Ex: **For code S52.391[A]:** See S52.011[A]
For S52.391[B,C]: See S52.00[B,C]
For S52.391[K,M,N,P,Q,R]: See S02.0[K]

● **S52.392 Other fracture of shaft of radius, left arm** A, K, M, N, P, Q, R, B, C, A, B, C
Ex: **For code S52.392[A]:** See S52.012[A] **For code S52.392[B,C]:** See S52.00[B,C]
For S52.392[K,M,N,P,Q,R]: See S02.0[K]

● **S52.399 Other fracture of shaft of radius, unspecified arm** A, K, M, N, P, Q, R, B, C, A, B, C
Ex: **For code S52.399[A]:** See S52.019[A] **For code S52.399[B,C]:** See S52.00[B,C]
For S52.399[K,M,N,P,Q,R]: See S02.0[K]

● **S52.5 Fracture of lower end of radius**
Fracture of distal end of radius
Excludes2 physeal fractures of lower end of radius (S59.2-)

● **S52.50 Unspecified fracture of the lower end of radius**

● **S52.501 Unspecified fracture of the lower end of right radius** A, K, M, N, P, Q, R, B, C, A, B, C
Ex: **For code S52.501[A]:** See S52.011[A]
For S52.501[B,C]: See S52.00[B,C]
For S52.501[K,M,N,P,Q,R]: See S02.0[K]

● **S52.502 Unspecified fracture of the lower end of left radius** A, K, M, N, P, Q, R, B, C, A, B, C
Ex: **For code S52.502[A]:** See S52.012[A] **For code S52.502[B,C]:** See S52.00[B,C]
For S52.502[K,M,N,P,Q,R]: See S02.0[K]

● **S52.509 Unspecified fracture of the lower end of unspecified radius**
A, K, M, N, P, Q, R, B, C, A, B, C
Ex: **For code S52.509[A]:** See S52.019[A] **For code S52.509[B,C]:** See S52.00[B,C]
For S52.509[K,M,N,P,Q,R]: See S02.0[K]

● **S52.51 Fracture of radial styloid process**

● **S52.511 Displaced fracture of right radial styloid process** A, K, M, N, P, Q, R CC, B, C MCC, A, B, C HAC
Ex: **For code S52.511[A]:** See S52.011[A]
For S52.511[B,C]: See S52.00[B,C]
For S52.511[K,M,N,P,Q,R]: See S02.0[K]

● **S52.512 Displaced fracture of left radial styloid process** A, K, M, N, P, Q, R CC, B, C MCC, A, B, C HAC
Ex: **For code S52.512[A]:** See S52.012[A] **For code S52.512[B,C]:** See S52.00[B,C]
For S52.512[K,M,N,P,Q,R]: See S02.0[K]

● **S52.513 Displaced fracture of unspecified radial styloid process**
A, K, M, N, P, Q, R CC, B, C MCC, A, B, C HAC
Ex: **For code S52.513[A]:** See S52.019[A] **For code S52.513[B,C]:** See S52.00[B,C]
For S52.513[K,M,N,P,Q,R]: See S02.0[K]

● **S52.514 Nondisplaced fracture of right radial styloid process** A, K, M, N, P, Q, R CC, B, C MCC, A, B, C HAC
Ex: **For code S52.514[A]:** See S52.011[A]
For S52.514[B,C]: See S52.00[B,C]
For S52.514[K,M,N,P,Q,R]: See S02.0[K]

● **S52.515 Nondisplaced fracture of left radial styloid process** A, K, M, N, P, Q, R CC, B, C MCC, A, B, C HAC
Ex: **For code S52.515[A]:** See S52.012[A] **For code S52.515[B,C]:** See S52.00[B,C]
For S52.515[K,M,N,P,Q,R]: See S02.0[K]

● **S52.516 Nondisplaced fracture of unspecified radial styloid process**
A, K, M, N, P, Q, R CC, B, C MCC, A, B, C HAC
Ex: **For code S52.516[A]:** See S52.019[A] **For code S52.516[B,C]:** See S52.00[B,C]
For S52.516[K,M,N,P,Q,R]: See S02.0[K]

● **S52.52 Torus fracture of lower end of radius**

The appropriate 7th character is to be added to all codes in subcategory S52.52

A	initial encounter for closed fracture
D	subsequent encounter for fracture with routine healing
G	subsequent encounter for fracture with delayed healing
K	subsequent encounter for fracture with nonunion
P	subsequent encounter for fracture with malunion
S	sequela

● **S52.521 Torus fracture of lower end of right radius** A, K, P CC, A HAC
Ex: **For code S52.521[A]:** See S52.011[A]
For S52.521[K,P]: See S02.0[K]

● **S52.522 Torus fracture of lower end of left radius** A, K, P CC, A HAC
Ex: **For code S52.522[A]:** See S52.012[A]
For S52.522[K,P]: See S02.0[K]

● **S52.529 Torus fracture of lower end of unspecified radius** A, K, P CC, A HAC
Ex: **For code S52.529[A]:** See S52.019[A]
For S52.529[K,P]: See S02.0[K]

● **S52.53 Colles' fracture**

● **S52.531 Colles' fracture of right radius**
A, K, M, N, P, Q, R CC, B, C MCC, A, B, C HAC
Ex: **For code S52.531[A]:** See S52.011[A]
For S52.531[B,C]: See S52.00[B,C]
For S52.531[K,M,N,P,Q,R]: See S02.0[K]

● **S52.532 Colles' fracture of left radius**
A, K, M, N, P, Q, R CC, B, C MCC, A, B, C HAC
Ex: **For code S52.532[A]:** See S52.012[A] **For code S52.532[B,C]:** See S52.00[B,C]
For S52.532[K,M,N,P,Q,R]: See S02.0[K]
Coding Clinic: 2016, Q2, P5

● **S52.539 Colles' fracture of unspecified radius**
A, K, M, N, P, Q, R CC, B, C MCC, A, B, C HAC
Ex: **For code S52.539[A]:** See S52.019[A] **For code S52.539[B,C]:** See S52.00[B,C]
For S52.539[K,M,N,P,Q,R]: See S02.0[K]

● **S52.54 Smith's fracture**

● **S52.541 Smith's fracture of right radius**
A, K, M, N, P, Q, R CC, B, C MCC, A, B, C HAC
Ex: **For code S52.541[A]:** See S52.011[A]
For S52.541[B,C]: See S52.00[B,C]
For S52.541[K,M,N,P,Q,R]: See S02.0[K]

● **S52.542 Smith's fracture of left radius**
A, K, M, N, P, Q, R CC, B, C MCC, A, B, C HAC
Ex: **For code S52.542[A]:** See S52.012[A] **For code S52.542[B,C]:** See S52.00[B,C]
For S52.542[K,M,N,P,Q,R]: See S02.0[K]

● **S52.549 Smith's fracture of unspecified radius**
A, K, M, N, P, Q, R CC, B, C MCC, A, B, C HAC
Ex: **For code S52.549[A]:** See S52.019[A] **For code S52.549[B,C]:** See S52.00[B,C]
For S52.549[K,M,N,P,Q,R]: See S02.0[K]

● **S52.55 Other extraarticular fracture of lower end of radius**

● **S52.551 Other extraarticular fracture of lower end of right radius**
A, K, M, N, P, Q, R CC, B, C MCC, A, B, C HAC
Ex: **For code S52.551[A]:** See S52.011[A]
For S52.551[B,C]: See S52.00[B,C]
For S52.551[K,M,N,P,Q,R]: See S02.0[K]

● **S52.552 Other extraarticular fracture of lower end of left radius**
A, K, M, N, P, Q, R CC, B, C MCC, A, B, C HAC
Ex: **For code S52.552[A]:** See S52.012[A] **For code S52.552[B,C]:** See S52.00[B,C]
For S52.552[K,M,N,P,Q,R]: See S02.0[K]

● **S52.559 Other extraarticular fracture of lower end of unspecified radius**
A, K, M, N, P, Q, R CC, B, C MCC, A, B, C HAC
Ex: **For code S52.559[A]:** See S52.019[A] **For code S52.559[B,C]:** See S52.00[B,C]
For S52.559[K,M,N,P,Q,R]: See S02.0[K]

- **S52.56 Barton's fracture**
  - **S52.561 Barton's fracture of right radius** A, K, M, N, P, Q, R, B, C, A, B, C
    - Ex: For code S52.561[A]: See S52.011[A]
      For S52.561[B,C]: See S52.00[B,C]
      For S52.561[K,M,N,P,Q,R]: See S02.0[K]
  - **S52.562 Barton's fracture of left radius** A, K, M, N, P, Q, R, B, C, A, B, C
    - Ex: For code S52.562[A]: See S52.012[A] For code S52.562[B,C]: See S52.00[B,C]
      For S52.562[K,M,N,P,Q,R]: See S02.0[K]
  - **S52.569 Barton's fracture of unspecified radius** A, K, M, N, P, Q, R, B, C, A, B, C
    - Ex: For code S52.569[A]: See S52.019[A] For code S52.569[B,C]: See S52.00[B,C]
      For S52.569[K,M,N,P,Q,R]: See S02.0[K]
- **S52.57 Other intraarticular fracture of lower end of radius**
  - **S52.571 Other intraarticular fracture of lower end of right radius** A, K, M, N, P, Q, R, B, C, A, B, C
    - Ex: For code S52.571[A]: See S52.011[A]
      For S52.571[B,C]: See S52.00[B,C]
      For S52.571[K,M,N,P,Q,R]: See S02.0[K]
  - **S52.572 Other intraarticular fracture of lower end of left radius** A, K, M, N, P, Q, R, B, C, A, B, C
    - Ex: For code S52.572[A]: See S52.012[A] For code S52.572[B,C]: See S52.00[B,C]
      For S52.572[K,M,N,P,Q,R]: See S02.0[K]
  - **S52.579 Other intraarticular fracture of lower end of unspecified radius** A, K, M, N, P, Q, R, B, C, A, B, C
    - Ex: For code S52.579[A]: See S52.019[A] For code S52.579[B,C]: See S52.00[B,C]
      For S52.579[K,M,N,P,Q,R]: See S02.0[K]
- **S52.59 Other fractures of lower end of radius**
  - **S52.591 Other fractures of lower end of right radius** A, K, M, N, P, Q, R, B, C, A, B, C
    - Ex: For code S52.591[A]: See S52.011[A]
      For S52.591[B,C]: See S52.00[B,C]
      For S52.591[K,M,N,P,Q,R]: See S02.0[K]
  - **S52.592 Other fractures of lower end of left radius** A, K, M, N, P, Q, R, B, C, A, B, C
    - Ex: For code S52.592[A]: See S52.012[A] For code S52.592[B,C]: See S52.00[B,C]
      For S52.592[K,M,N,P,Q,R]: See S02.0[K]
  - **S52.599 Other fractures of lower end of unspecified radius** A, K, M, N, P, Q, R, B, C, A, B, C
    - Ex: For code S52.599[A]: See S52.019[A] For code S52.599[B,C]: See S52.00[B,C]
      For S52.599[K,M,N,P,Q,R]: See S02.0[K]
- **S52.6 Fracture of lower end of ulna**
  - **S52.60 Unspecified fracture of lower end of ulna**
    - **S52.601 Unspecified fracture of lower end of right ulna** A, K, M, N, P, Q, R, B, C, A, B, C
      - Ex: For code S52.601[A]: See S52.011[A]
        For S52.601[B,C]: See S52.00[B,C]
        For S52.601[K,M,N,P,Q,R]: See S02.0[K]
    - **S52.602 Unspecified fracture of lower end of left ulna** A, K, M, N, P, Q, R, B, C, A, B, C
      - Ex: For code S52.602[A]: See S52.012[A] For code S52.602[B,C]: See S52.00[B,C]
        For S52.602[K,M,N,P,Q,R]: See S02.0[K]
    - **S52.609 Unspecified fracture of lower end of unspecified ulna** A, K, M, N, P, Q, R, B, C, A, B, C
      - Ex: For code S52.609[A]: See S52.019[A] For code S52.609[B,C]: See S52.00[B,C]
        For S52.609[K,M,N,P,Q,R]: See S02.0[K]
  - **S52.61 Fracture of ulna styloid process**
    - **S52.611 Displaced fracture of right ulna styloid process** A, K, M, N, P, Q, R, B, C, A, B, C
      - Ex: For code S52.611[A]: See S52.011[A]
        For S52.611[B,C]: See S52.00[B,C]
        For S52.611[K,M,N,P,Q,R]: See S02.0[K]
    - **S52.612 Displaced fracture of left ulna styloid process** A, K, M, N, P, Q, R, B, C, A, B, C
      - Ex: For code S52.612[A]: See S52.012[A] For code S52.612[B,C]: See S52.00[B,C]
        For S52.612[K,M,N,P,Q,R]: See S02.0[K]
    - **S52.613 Displaced fracture of unspecified ulna styloid process** A, K, M, N, P, Q, R, B, C, A, B, C
      - Ex: For code S52.613[A]: See S52.019[A] For code S52.613[B,C]: See S52.00[B,C]
        For S52.613[K,M,N,P,Q,R]: See S02.0[K]
    - **S52.614 Nondisplaced fracture of right ulna styloid process** A, K, M, N, P, Q, R, B, C, A, B, C
      - Ex: For code S52.614[A]: See S52.011[A]
        For S52.614[B,C]: See S52.00[B,C]
        For S52.614[K,M,N,P,Q,R]: See S02.0[K]
    - **S52.615 Nondisplaced fracture of left ulna styloid process** A, K, M, N, P, Q, R, B, C, A, B, C
      - Ex: For code S52.615[A]: See S52.012[A] For code S52.615[B,C]: See S52.00[B,C]
        For S52.615[K,M,N,P,Q,R]: See S02.0[K]
    - **S52.616 Nondisplaced fracture of unspecified ulna styloid process** A, K, M, N, P, Q, R, B, C, A, B, C
      - Ex: For code S52.616[A]: See S52.019[A] For code S52.616[B,C]: See S52.00[B,C]
        For S52.616[K,M,N,P,Q,R]: See S02.0[K]

S52.62 Torus fracture of lower end of ulna

The appropriate 7th character is to be added to all codes in subcategory S52.62

A	initial encounter for closed fracture
D	subsequent encounter for fracture with routine healing
G	subsequent encounter for fracture with delayed healing
K	subsequent encounter for fracture with nonunion
P	subsequent encounter for fracture with malunion
S	sequela

S52.621 Torus fracture of lower end of right ulna A, K, P CC, A HAC

Ex: **For code S52.621[A]:** See S52.011[A] **For S52.621[K,P]:** See S02.0[K]

S52.622 Torus fracture of lower end of left ulna A, K, P CC, A HAC

Ex: **For code S52.622[A]:** See S52.012[A] **For S52.622[K,P]:** See S02.0[K]

S52.629 Torus fracture of lower end of unspecified ulna A, K, P CC, A HAC

Ex: **For code S52.629[A]:** See S52.019[A] **For S52.629[K,P]:** See S02.0[K]

S52.69 Other fracture of lower end of ulna

S52.691 Other fracture of lower end of right ulna A, K, M, N, P, Q, R CC, **B, C** MCC, A, B, C HAC

Ex: **For code S52.691[A]:** See S52.011[A] **For S52.691[B,C]:** See S52.00[B,C] **For S52.691[K,M,N,P,Q,R]:** See S02.0[K]

S52.692 Other fracture of lower end of left ulna A, K, M, N, P, Q, R CC, **B, C** MCC, A, B, C HAC

Ex: **For code S52.692[A]:** See S52.012[A] **For code S52.692[B,C]:** See S52.00[B,C] **For S52.692[K,M,N,P,Q,R]:** See S02.0[K]

S52.699 Other fracture of lower end of unspecified ulna A, K, M, N, P, Q, R CC, **B, C** MCC, A, B, C HAC

Ex: **For code S52.699[A]:** See S52.019[A] **For code S52.699[B,C]:** See S52.00[B,C] **For S52.699[K,M,N,P,Q,R]:** See S02.0[K]

S52.9 Unspecified fracture of forearm

Ex: **For category S52.9 CC codes S52.9[A]:** See S52.019[A] **For code S52.9[B,C]:** See S52.00[B,C] **For S52.9[K,M,N,P,Q,R]:** See S02.0[K]

X **S52.90 Unspecified fracture of unspecified forearm** A, K, M, N, P, Q, R CC, **B, C** MCC, A, B, C HAC

X **S52.91 Unspecified fracture of right forearm** A, K, M, N, P, Q, R CC, **B, C** MCC, A, B, C HAC

X **S52.92 Unspecified fracture of left forearm** A, K, M, N, P, Q, R CC, **B, C** MCC, A, B, C HAC

S53 Dislocation and sprain of joints and ligaments of elbow

Includes avulsion of joint or ligament of elbow
laceration of cartilage, joint or ligament of elbow
sprain of cartilage, joint or ligament of elbow
traumatic hemarthrosis of joint or ligament of elbow
traumatic rupture of joint or ligament of elbow
traumatic subluxation of joint or ligament of elbow
traumatic tear of joint or ligament of elbow

Code also any associated open wound

Excludes2 strain of muscle, fascia and tendon at forearm level (S56.-)

The appropriate 7th character is to be added to each code from category S53

A	initial encounter
D	subsequent encounter
S	sequela

S53.0 Subluxation and dislocation of radial head

Dislocation of radiohumeral joint
Subluxation of radiohumeral joint

Excludes1 Monteggia's fracture-dislocation (S52.27-)

S53.00 Unspecified subluxation and dislocation of radial head

S53.001 Unspecified subluxation of right radial head

S53.002 Unspecified subluxation of left radial head

S53.003 Unspecified subluxation of unspecified radial head

S53.004 Unspecified dislocation of right radial head

S53.005 Unspecified dislocation of left radial head

S53.006 Unspecified dislocation of unspecified radial head

S53.01 Anterior subluxation and dislocation of radial head

Anteriomedial subluxation and dislocation of radial head

S53.011 Anterior subluxation of right radial head

S53.012 Anterior subluxation of left radial head

S53.013 Anterior subluxation of unspecified radial head

S53.014 Anterior dislocation of right radial head

S53.015 Anterior dislocation of left radial head

S53.016 Anterior dislocation of unspecified radial head

- S53.02 Posterior subluxation and dislocation of radial head
  - Posteriolateral subluxation and dislocation of radial head
  - S53.021 Posterior subluxation of right radial head
  - S53.022 Posterior subluxation of left radial head
  - S53.023 Posterior subluxation of unspecified radial head
  - S53.024 Posterior dislocation of right radial head
  - S53.025 Posterior dislocation of left radial head
  - S53.026 Posterior dislocation of unspecified radial head
- S53.03 Nursemaid's elbow
  - S53.031 Nursemaid's elbow, right elbow
    - Coding Clinic: 2015, Q1, P7-8
  - S53.032 Nursemaid's elbow, left elbow
  - S53.033 Nursemaid's elbow, unspecified elbow
- S53.09 Other subluxation and dislocation of radial head
  - S53.091 Other subluxation of right radial head
  - S53.092 Other subluxation of left radial head
  - S53.093 Other subluxation of unspecified radial head
  - S53.094 Other dislocation of right radial head
  - S53.095 Other dislocation of left radial head
  - S53.096 Other dislocation of unspecified radial head
- S53.1 Subluxation and dislocation of ulnohumeral joint
  - Subluxation and dislocation of elbow NOS
  - **Excludes1** dislocation of radial head alone (S53.0-)
- S53.10 Unspecified subluxation and dislocation of ulnohumeral joint
  - S53.101 Unspecified subluxation of right ulnohumeral joint
  - S53.102 Unspecified subluxation of left ulnohumeral joint
  - S53.103 Unspecified subluxation of unspecified ulnohumeral joint
  - S53.104 Unspecified dislocation of right ulnohumeral joint
  - S53.105 Unspecified dislocation of left ulnohumeral joint
  - S53.106 Unspecified dislocation of unspecified ulnohumeral joint
- S53.11 Anterior subluxation and dislocation of ulnohumeral joint
  - S53.111 Anterior subluxation of right ulnohumeral joint
  - S53.112 Anterior subluxation of left ulnohumeral joint
  - S53.113 Anterior subluxation of unspecified ulnohumeral joint
  - S53.114 Anterior dislocation of right ulnohumeral joint
    - Coding Clinic: 2012, Q4, P108
  - S53.115 Anterior dislocation of left ulnohumeral joint
  - S53.116 Anterior dislocation of unspecified ulnohumeral joint
- S53.12 Posterior subluxation and dislocation of ulnohumeral joint
  - S53.121 Posterior subluxation of right ulnohumeral joint
  - S53.122 Posterior subluxation of left ulnohumeral joint
  - S53.123 Posterior subluxation of unspecified ulnohumeral joint
  - S53.124 Posterior dislocation of right ulnohumeral joint
  - S53.125 Posterior dislocation of left ulnohumeral joint
  - S53.126 Posterior dislocation of unspecified ulnohumeral joint
- S53.13 Medial subluxation and dislocation of ulnohumeral joint
  - S53.131 Medial subluxation of right ulnohumeral joint
  - S53.132 Medial subluxation of left ulnohumeral joint
  - S53.133 Medial subluxation of unspecified ulnohumeral joint
  - S53.134 Medial dislocation of right ulnohumeral joint
  - S53.135 Medial dislocation of left ulnohumeral joint
  - S53.136 Medial dislocation of unspecified ulnohumeral joint
- S53.14 Lateral subluxation and dislocation of ulnohumeral joint
  - S53.141 Lateral subluxation of right ulnohumeral joint
  - S53.142 Lateral subluxation of left ulnohumeral joint
  - S53.143 Lateral subluxation of unspecified ulnohumeral joint
  - S53.144 Lateral dislocation of right ulnohumeral joint
  - S53.145 Lateral dislocation of left ulnohumeral joint
  - S53.146 Lateral dislocation of unspecified ulnohumeral joint
- S53.19 Other subluxation and dislocation of ulnohumeral joint
  - S53.191 Other subluxation of right ulnohumeral joint
  - S53.192 Other subluxation of left ulnohumeral joint
  - S53.193 Other subluxation of unspecified ulnohumeral joint
  - S53.194 Other dislocation of right ulnohumeral joint
  - S53.195 Other dislocation of left ulnohumeral joint
  - S53.196 Other dislocation of unspecified ulnohumeral joint
- S53.2 Traumatic rupture of radial collateral ligament
  - **Excludes1** sprain of radial collateral ligament NOS (S53.43-)
  - X S53.20 Traumatic rupture of unspecified radial collateral ligament
  - X S53.21 Traumatic rupture of right radial collateral ligament
  - X S53.22 Traumatic rupture of left radial collateral ligament

- **S53.3 Traumatic rupture of ulnar collateral ligament**
  - **Excludes1** sprain of ulnar collateral ligament (S53.44-)
  - X **S53.30 Traumatic rupture of unspecified ulnar collateral ligament**
  - X **S53.31 Traumatic rupture of right ulnar collateral ligament**
  - X **S53.32 Traumatic rupture of left ulnar collateral ligament**
- **S53.4 Sprain of elbow**
  - **Excludes2** traumatic rupture of radial collateral ligament (S53.2-)
    traumatic rupture of ulnar collateral ligament (S53.3-)
  - **S53.40 Unspecified sprain of elbow**
    - **S53.401 Unspecified sprain of right elbow**
    - **S53.402 Unspecified sprain of left elbow**
    - **S53.409 Unspecified sprain of unspecified elbow**
      Sprain of elbow NOS
  - **S53.41 Radiohumeral (joint) sprain**
    - **S53.411 Radiohumeral (joint) sprain of right elbow**
    - **S53.412 Radiohumeral (joint) sprain of left elbow**
    - **S53.419 Radiohumeral (joint) sprain of unspecified elbow**
  - **S53.42 Ulnohumeral (joint) sprain**
    - **S53.421 Ulnohumeral (joint) sprain of right elbow**
    - **S53.422 Ulnohumeral (joint) sprain of left elbow**
    - **S53.429 Ulnohumeral (joint) sprain of unspecified elbow**
  - **S53.43 Radial collateral ligament sprain**
    - **S53.431 Radial collateral ligament sprain of right elbow**
    - **S53.432 Radial collateral ligament sprain of left elbow**
    - **S53.439 Radial collateral ligament sprain of unspecified elbow**
  - **S53.44 Ulnar collateral ligament sprain**
    - **S53.441 Ulnar collateral ligament sprain of right elbow**
    - **S53.442 Ulnar collateral ligament sprain of left elbow**
    - **S53.449 Ulnar collateral ligament sprain of unspecified elbow**
  - **S53.49 Other sprain of elbow**
    - **S53.491 Other sprain of right elbow**
    - **S53.492 Other sprain of left elbow**
    - **S53.499 Other sprain of unspecified elbow**

- **S54 Injury of nerves at forearm level**
  Code also any associated open wound (S51.-)
  - **Excludes2** injury of nerves at wrist and hand level (S64.-)
  The appropriate 7th character is to be added to each code from category S54

A	initial encounter
D	subsequent encounter
S	sequela

  - **S54.0 Injury of ulnar nerve at forearm level**
    Injury of ulnar nerve NOS
    - X **S54.00 Injury of ulnar nerve at forearm level, unspecified arm**
    - X **S54.01 Injury of ulnar nerve at forearm level, right arm**
    - X **S54.02 Injury of ulnar nerve at forearm level, left arm**
  - **S54.1 Injury of median nerve at forearm level**
    Injury of median nerve NOS
    - X **S54.10 Injury of median nerve at forearm level, unspecified arm**
    - X **S54.11 Injury of median nerve at forearm level, right arm**
    - X **S54.12 Injury of median nerve at forearm level, left arm**
  - **S54.2 Injury of radial nerve at forearm level**
    Injury of radial nerve NOS
    - X **S54.20 Injury of radial nerve at forearm level, unspecified arm**
    - X **S54.21 Injury of radial nerve at forearm level, right arm**
    - X **S54.22 Injury of radial nerve at forearm level, left arm**
  - **S54.3 Injury of cutaneous sensory nerve at forearm level**
    - X **S54.30 Injury of cutaneous sensory nerve at forearm level, unspecified arm**
    - X **S54.31 Injury of cutaneous sensory nerve at forearm level, right arm**
    - X **S54.32 Injury of cutaneous sensory nerve at forearm level, left arm**
  - **S54.8 Injury of other nerves at forearm level**
    - **S54.8X Injury of other nerves at forearm level**
      - **S54.8X1 Injury of other nerves at forearm level, right arm**
      - **S54.8X2 Injury of other nerves at forearm level, left arm**
      - **S54.8X9 Injury of other nerves at forearm level, unspecified arm**
  - **S54.9 Injury of unspecified nerve at forearm level**
    - X **S54.90 Injury of unspecified nerve at forearm level, unspecified arm**
    - X **S54.91 Injury of unspecified nerve at forearm level, right arm**
    - X **S54.92 Injury of unspecified nerve at forearm level, left arm**

S55 Injury of blood vessels at forearm level

Code also any associated open wound (S51.-)

Excludes2 injury of blood vessels at wrist and hand level (S65.-)
injury of brachial vessels (S45.1-S45.2)

The appropriate 7th character is to be added to each code from category S55

A	initial encounter
D	subsequent encounter
S	sequela

S55.0 Injury of ulnar artery at forearm level

S55.00 Unspecified injury of ulnar artery at forearm level

S55.001 Unspecified injury of ulnar artery at forearm level, right arm A

Ex: S45.301[A], S45.309-S45.311[A], S45.319-S45.391[A], S45.399-S45.801[A], S45.809-S45.811[A], S45.819-S45.891[A], S45.899-S45.901[A], S45.909-S45.911[A], S45.919-S45.991[A], S45.999[A], S55.001[A], S55.009-S55.011[A], S55.019-S55.091[A], S55.099[A], S55.201[A], S55.209-S55.211[A], S55.219-S55.291[A], S55.299-S55.801[A], S55.809-S55.811[A], S55.819-S55.891[A], S55.899-S55.901[A], S55.909-S55.911[A], S55.919-S55.991[A], S55.999[A], S65.001[A], S65.009-S65.011[A], S65.019-S65.091[A], S65.099[A], S65.801[A], S65.809-S65.811[A], S65.819-S65.891[A], S65.899-S65.901[A], S65.909-S65.911[A], S65.919-S65.991[A], S65.999[A]

S55.002 Unspecified injury of ulnar artery at forearm level, left arm A

Ex: S45.302-S45.309[A], S45.312-S45.319[A], S45.392-S45.399[A], S45.802-S45.809[A], S45.812-S45.819[A], S45.892-S45.899[A], S45.902-S45.909[A], S45.912-S45.919[A], S45.992-S45.999[A], S55.002-S55.009[A], S55.012-S55.019[A], S55.092-S55.099[A], S55.202-S55.209[A], S55.212-S55.219[A], S55.292-S55.299[A], S55.802-S55.809[A], S55.812-S55.819[A], S55.892-S55.899[A], S55.902-S55.909[A], S55.912-S55.919[A], S55.992-S55.999[A], S65.002-S65.009[A], S65.012-S65.019[A], S65.092-S65.099[A], S65.802-S65.809[A] S65.812-S65.819[A], S65.892-S65.899[A], S65.902-S65.909[A], S65.912-S65.919[A], S65.992-S65.999[A]

S55.009 Unspecified injury of ulnar artery at forearm level, unspecified arm A

Ex: S45.301-S45.999[A], S55.001-S55.099[A], S55.201-S55.999[A], S65.001-S65.099[A], S65.801-S65.999[A]

S55.01 Laceration of ulnar artery at forearm level

S55.011 Laceration of ulnar artery at forearm level, right arm A

Ex: See S55.001

S55.012 Laceration of ulnar artery at forearm level, left arm A

Ex: See S55.002

S55.019 Laceration of ulnar artery at forearm level, unspecified arm A

Ex: See S55.009

S55.09 Other specified injury of ulnar artery at forearm level

S55.091 Other specified injury of ulnar artery at forearm level, right arm A

Ex: See S55.001

S55.092 Other specified injury of ulnar artery at forearm level, left arm A

Ex: See S55.002

S55.099 Other specified injury of ulnar artery at forearm level, unspecified arm A

Ex: See S55.009

S55.1 Injury of radial artery at forearm level

S55.10 Unspecified injury of radial artery at forearm level

S55.101 Unspecified injury of radial artery at forearm level, right arm A

Ex: S45.301[A], S45.309-S45.311[A], S45.319-S45.391[A], S45.399-S45.801[A], S45.809-S45.811[A], S45.819-S45.891[A], S45.899-S45.901[A], S45.909-S45.911[A], S45.919-S45.991[A], S45.999[A], S55.101[A], S55.109-S55.111[A], S55.119-S55.191[A], S55.199-S55.201[A], S55.209-S55.211[A], S55.219-S55.291[A], S55.299-S55.801[A], S55.809-S55.811[A], S55.819-S55.891[A], S55.899-S55.901[A], S55.909-S55.911[A], S55.919-S55.991[A], S55.999[A], S65.101[A], S65.109-S65.111[A], S65.119-S65.191[A], S65.199[A], S65.801[A], S65.809-S65.811[A], S65.819-S65.891[A], S65.899-S65.901[A], S65.909-S65.911[A], S65.919-S65.991[A], S65.999[A]

S55.102 Unspecified injury of radial artery at forearm level, left arm A

Ex: S45.302-S45.309[A], S45.312-S45.319[A], S45.392-S45.399[A], S45.802-S45.809[A], S45.812-S45.819[A], S45.892-S45.899[A], S45.902-S45.909[A], S45.912-S45.919[A], S45.992-S45.999[A], S55.102-S55.109[A], S55.112-S55.119[A], S55.192-S55.199[A], S55.202-S55.209[A], S55.212-S55.219[A], S55.292-S55.299[A], S55.802A-S55.809[A], S55.812-S55.819[A], S55.892-S55.899[A], S55.902-S55.909[A], S55.912-S55.919[A], S55.992-S55.999[A], S65.102-S65.109[A], S65.112-S65.119[A], S65.192-S65.199[A], S65.802-S65.809[A], S65.812-S65.819[A], S65.892-S65.899[A], S65.902-S65.909[A], S65.912-S65.919[A], S65.992-S65.999[A]

S55.109 Unspecified injury of radial artery at forearm level, unspecified arm A

Ex: S45.301-S45.999[A], S55.101-S55.999[A], S65.101-S65.199[A], S65.801-S65.999[A]

S55.11 Laceration of radial artery at forearm level

S55.111 Laceration of radial artery at forearm level, right arm A

Ex: See S55.101

S55.112 Laceration of radial artery at forearm level, left arm A

Ex: See S55.102

S55.119 Laceration of radial artery at forearm level, unspecified arm A

Ex: See S55.109

- S55.19 Other specified injury of radial artery at forearm level
  - S55.191 Other specified injury of radial artery at forearm level, right arm A
    Ex: See S55.101
  - S55.192 Other specified injury of radial artery at forearm level, left arm A
    Ex: See S55.102
  - S55.199 Other specified injury of radial artery at forearm level, unspecified arm A
    Ex: See S55.109
- S55.2 Injury of vein at forearm level
  - S55.20 Unspecified injury of vein at forearm level
    - S55.201 Unspecified injury of vein at forearm level, right arm A
      Ex: See S45.301
    - S55.202 Unspecified injury of vein at forearm level, left arm A
      Ex: See S45.302
    - S55.209 Unspecified injury of vein at forearm level, unspecified arm A
      Ex: See S45.309
  - S55.21 Laceration of vein at forearm level
    - S55.211 Laceration of vein at forearm level, right arm A
      Ex: See S45.301
    - S55.212 Laceration of vein at forearm level, left arm A
      Ex: See S45.302
    - S55.219 Laceration of vein at forearm level, unspecified arm A
      Ex: See S45.309
  - S55.29 Other specified injury of vein at forearm level
    - S55.291 Other specified injury of vein at forearm level, right arm A
      Ex: See S45.301
    - S55.292 Other specified injury of vein at forearm level, left arm A
      Ex: See S45.302
    - S55.299 Other specified injury of vein at forearm level, unspecified arm A
      Ex: See S45.309
- S55.8 Injury of other blood vessels at forearm level
  - S55.80 Unspecified injury of other blood vessels at forearm level
    - S55.801 Unspecified injury of other blood vessels at forearm level, right arm A
      Ex: See S45.301
    - S55.802 Unspecified injury of other blood vessels at forearm level, left arm A
      Ex: See S45.302
    - S55.809 Unspecified injury of other blood vessels at forearm level, unspecified arm A
      Ex: See S45.309
  - S55.81 Laceration of other blood vessels at forearm level
    - S55.811 Laceration of other blood vessels at forearm level, right arm A
      Ex: See S45.301
    - S55.812 Laceration of other blood vessels at forearm level, left arm A
      Ex: See S45.302
    - S55.819 Laceration of other blood vessels at forearm level, unspecified arm A
      Ex: See S45.309
  - S55.89 Other specified injury of other blood vessels at forearm level
    - S55.891 Other specified injury of other blood vessels at forearm level, right arm A
      Ex: See S45.301
    - S55.892 Other specified injury of other blood vessels at forearm level, left arm A
      Ex: See S45.302
    - S55.899 Other specified injury of other blood vessels at forearm level, unspecified arm A
      Ex: See S45.309
- S55.9 Injury of unspecified blood vessel at forearm level
  - S55.90 Unspecified injury of unspecified blood vessel at forearm level
    - S55.901 Unspecified injury of unspecified blood vessel at forearm level, right arm A
      Ex: See S45.301
    - S55.902 Unspecified injury of unspecified blood vessel at forearm level, left arm A
      Ex: See S45.302
    - S55.909 Unspecified injury of unspecified blood vessel at forearm level, unspecified arm A
      Ex: See S45.309
  - S55.91 Laceration of unspecified blood vessel at forearm level
    - S55.911 Laceration of unspecified blood vessel at forearm level, right arm A
      Ex: See S45.301
    - S55.912 Laceration of unspecified blood vessel at forearm level, left arm A
      Ex: See S45.302
    - S55.919 Laceration of unspecified blood vessel at forearm level, unspecified arm A
      Ex: See S45.309
  - S55.99 Other specified injury of unspecified blood vessel at forearm level
    - S55.991 Other specified injury of unspecified blood vessel at forearm level, right arm A
      Ex: See S45.301
    - S55.992 Other specified injury of unspecified blood vessel at forearm level, left arm A
      Ex: See S45.302
    - S55.999 Other specified injury of unspecified blood vessel at forearm level, unspecified arm A
      Ex: See S45.309

S56 Injury of muscle, fascia and tendon at forearm level

Code also any associated open wound (S51.-)

Excludes2 injury of muscle, fascia and tendon at or below wrist (S66.-)
sprain of joints and ligaments of elbow (S53.4-)

The appropriate 7th character is to be added to each code from category S56

A	initial encounter
D	subsequent encounter
S	sequela

S56.0 Injury of flexor muscle, fascia and tendon of thumb at forearm level

S56.00 Unspecified injury of flexor muscle, fascia and tendon of thumb at forearm level

S56.001 Unspecified injury of flexor muscle, fascia and tendon of right thumb at forearm level

S56.002 Unspecified injury of flexor muscle, fascia and tendon of left thumb at forearm level

S56.009 Unspecified injury of flexor muscle, fascia and tendon of unspecified thumb at forearm level

S56.01 Strain of flexor muscle, fascia and tendon of thumb at forearm level

S56.011 Strain of flexor muscle, fascia and tendon of right thumb at forearm level

S56.012 Strain of flexor muscle, fascia and tendon of left thumb at forearm level

S56.019 Strain of flexor muscle, fascia and tendon of unspecified thumb at forearm level

S56.02 Laceration of flexor muscle, fascia and tendon of thumb at forearm level

S56.021 Laceration of flexor muscle, fascia and tendon of right thumb at forearm level A

Ex: S51.001[A], S51.009-S51.011[A], S51.019-S51.021[A], S51.029-S51.031[A], S51.039-S51.041[A], S51.049-S51.051[A], S51.059-S51.801[A], S51.809-S51.811[A], S51.819-S51.821[A]. S51.829-S51.831[A], S51.839-S51.841[A], S51.849-S51.851[A], S51.859[A], S56.021[A], S56.029[A], S56.121[A], S56.123[A], S56.125[A], S56.127[A], S56.129[A], S56.221[A], S56.229[A], S56.321[A], S56.329[A], S56.421[A], S56.423[A], S56.425[A], S56.427[A], S56.429[A], S56.521[A], S56.529[A], S56.821[A], S56.829[A], S56.921[A], S56.929[A], S61.501[A], S61.509-S61.511[A], S61.519-S61.521[A], S61.529-S61.531[A], S61.539-S61.541[A], S61.549-S61.551[A], S61.559[A]

S56.022 Laceration of flexor muscle, fascia and tendon of left thumb at forearm level A

Ex: S51.002-S51.009[A], S51.012-S51.019[A], S51.022-S51.029[A], S51.032-S51.039[A], S51.042-S51.049[A], S51.052-S51.059[A], S51.802-S51.809[A], S51.812-S51.819[A], S51.822-S51.829[A], S51.832-S51.839[A], S51.842-S51.849[A], S51.852-S51.859[A], S56.022-S56.029[A], S56.122[A], S56.124[A], S56.126[A], S56.128-S56.129[A], S56.222-S56.229[A], S56.322-S56.329[A], S56.422[A], S56.424[A], S56.426[A], S56.428-S56.429[A], S56.522-S56.529[A], S56.822-S56.829[A], S56.922-S56.929[A], S61.502-S61.509[A], S61.512-S61.519[A], S61.522-S61.529[A], S61.532-S61.539[A], S61.542-S61.549[A], S61.552-S61.559[A]

S56.029 Laceration of flexor muscle, fascia and tendon of unspecified thumb at forearm level A

Ex: S51.001-S51.859[A], S56.021-S56.029[A], S56.121-S56.129[A], S56.221-S56.229[A], S56.321-S56.329[A], S56.421-S56.429[A], S56.521-S56.529[A], S56.821-S56.829[A], S56.921-S56.929[A], S61.501-S61.559[A]

S56.09 Other injury of flexor muscle, fascia and tendon of thumb at forearm level

S56.091 Other injury of flexor muscle, fascia and tendon of right thumb at forearm level

S56.092 Other injury of flexor muscle, fascia and tendon of left thumb at forearm level

S56.099 Other injury of flexor muscle, fascia and tendon of unspecified thumb at forearm level

S56.1 Injury of flexor muscle, fascia and tendon of other and unspecified finger at forearm level

S56.10 Unspecified injury of flexor muscle, fascia and tendon of other and unspecified finger at forearm level

S56.101 Unspecified injury of flexor muscle, fascia and tendon of right index finger at forearm level

S56.102 Unspecified injury of flexor muscle, fascia and tendon of left index finger at forearm level

S56.103 Unspecified injury of flexor muscle, fascia and tendon of right middle finger at forearm level

S56.104 Unspecified injury of flexor muscle, fascia and tendon of left middle finger at forearm level

S56.105 Unspecified injury of flexor muscle, fascia and tendon of right ring finger at forearm level

S56.106 Unspecified injury of flexor muscle, fascia and tendon of left ring finger at forearm level

S56.107 Unspecified injury of flexor muscle, fascia and tendon of right little finger at forearm level

S56.108 Unspecified injury of flexor muscle, fascia and tendon of left little finger at forearm level

S56.109 Unspecified injury of flexor muscle, fascia and tendon of unspecified finger at forearm level

- S56.11 Strain of flexor muscle, fascia and tendon of other and unspecified finger at forearm level
  - S56.111 Strain of flexor muscle, fascia and tendon of right index finger at forearm level
  - S56.112 Strain of flexor muscle, fascia and tendon of left index finger at forearm level
  - S56.113 Strain of flexor muscle, fascia and tendon of right middle finger at forearm level
  - S56.114 Strain of flexor muscle, fascia and tendon of left middle finger at forearm level
  - S56.115 Strain of flexor muscle, fascia and tendon of right ring finger at forearm level
  - S56.116 Strain of flexor muscle, fascia and tendon of left ring finger at forearm level
  - S56.117 Strain of flexor muscle, fascia and tendon of right little finger at forearm level
  - S56.118 Strain of flexor muscle, fascia and tendon of left little finger at forearm level
  - S56.119 Strain of flexor muscle, fascia and tendon of finger of unspecified finger at forearm level
- S56.12 Laceration of flexor muscle, fascia and tendon of other and unspecified finger at forearm level
  - S56.121 Laceration of flexor muscle, fascia and tendon of right index finger at forearm level A
    - Ex: See S56.021
  - S56.122 Laceration of flexor muscle, fascia and tendon of left index finger at forearm level A
    - Ex: See S56.022
  - S56.123 Laceration of flexor muscle, fascia and tendon of right middle finger at forearm level A
    - Ex: See S56.021
  - S56.124 Laceration of flexor muscle, fascia and tendon of left middle finger at forearm level A
    - Ex: See S56.022
  - S56.125 Laceration of flexor muscle, fascia and tendon of right ring finger at forearm level A
    - Ex: See S56.021
  - S56.126 Laceration of flexor muscle, fascia and tendon of left ring finger at forearm level A
    - Ex: See S56.022
  - S56.127 Laceration of flexor muscle, fascia and tendon of right little finger at forearm level A
    - Ex: See S56.021
  - S56.128 Laceration of flexor muscle, fascia and tendon of left little finger at forearm level A
    - Ex: See S56.022
  - S56.129 Laceration of flexor muscle, fascia and tendon of unspecified finger at forearm level A
    - Ex: See S56.029
- S56.19 Other injury of flexor muscle, fascia and tendon of other and unspecified finger at forearm level
  - S56.191 Other injury of flexor muscle, fascia and tendon of right index finger at forearm level
  - S56.192 Other injury of flexor muscle, fascia and tendon of left index finger at forearm level
  - S56.193 Other injury of flexor muscle, fascia and tendon of right middle finger at forearm level
  - S56.194 Other injury of flexor muscle, fascia and tendon of left middle finger at forearm level
  - S56.195 Other injury of flexor muscle, fascia and tendon of right ring finger at forearm level
  - S56.196 Other injury of flexor muscle, fascia and tendon of left ring finger at forearm level
  - S56.197 Other injury of flexor muscle, fascia and tendon of right little finger at forearm level
  - S56.198 Other injury of flexor muscle, fascia and tendon of left little finger at forearm level
  - S56.199 Other injury of flexor muscle, fascia and tendon of unspecified finger at forearm level
- S56.2 Injury of other flexor muscle, fascia and tendon at forearm level
  - S56.20 Unspecified injury of other flexor muscle, fascia and tendon at forearm level
    - S56.201 Unspecified injury of other flexor muscle, fascia and tendon at forearm level, right arm
    - S56.202 Unspecified injury of other flexor muscle, fascia and tendon at forearm level, left arm
    - S56.209 Unspecified injury of other flexor muscle, fascia and tendon at forearm level, unspecified arm
  - S56.21 Strain of other flexor muscle, fascia and tendon at forearm level
    - S56.211 Strain of other flexor muscle, fascia and tendon at forearm level, right arm
    - S56.212 Strain of other flexor muscle, fascia and tendon at forearm level, left arm
    - S56.219 Strain of other flexor muscle, fascia and tendon at forearm level, unspecified arm
  - S56.22 Laceration of other flexor muscle, fascia and tendon at forearm level
    - S56.221 Laceration of other flexor muscle, fascia and tendon at forearm level, right arm A
      - Ex: See S56.021
    - S56.222 Laceration of other flexor muscle, fascia and tendon at forearm level, left arm A
      - Ex: See S56.022
    - S56.229 Laceration of other flexor muscle, fascia and tendon at forearm level, unspecified arm A
      - Ex: See S56.029

- S56.29 Other injury of other flexor muscle, fascia and tendon at forearm level
  - S56.291 Other injury of other flexor muscle, fascia and tendon at forearm level, right arm
  - S56.292 Other injury of other flexor muscle, fascia and tendon at forearm level, left arm
  - S56.299 Other injury of other flexor muscle, fascia and tendon at forearm level, unspecified arm
- S56.3 Injury of extensor or abductor muscles, fascia and tendons of thumb at forearm level
  - S56.30 Unspecified injury of extensor or abductor muscles, fascia and tendons of thumb at forearm level
    - S56.301 Unspecified injury of extensor or abductor muscles, fascia and tendons of right thumb at forearm level
    - S56.302 Unspecified injury of extensor or abductor muscles, fascia and tendons of left thumb at forearm level
    - S56.309 Unspecified injury of extensor or abductor muscles, fascia and tendons of unspecified thumb at forearm level
  - S56.31 Strain of extensor or abductor muscles, fascia and tendons of thumb at forearm level
    - S56.311 Strain of extensor or abductor muscles, fascia and tendons of right thumb at forearm level
    - S56.312 Strain of extensor or abductor muscles, fascia and tendons of left thumb at forearm level
    - S56.319 Strain of extensor or abductor muscles, fascia and tendons of unspecified thumb at forearm level
  - S56.32 Laceration of extensor or abductor muscles, fascia and tendons of thumb at forearm level
    - S56.321 Laceration of extensor or abductor muscles, fascia and tendons of right thumb at forearm level A
      Ex: See S56.021
    - S56.322 Laceration of extensor or abductor muscles, fascia and tendons of left thumb at forearm level A
      Ex: See S56.022
    - S56.329 Laceration of extensor or abductor muscles, fascia and tendons of unspecified thumb at forearm level A
      Ex: See S56.029
  - S56.39 Other injury of extensor or abductor muscles, fascia and tendons of thumb at forearm level
    - S56.391 Other injury of extensor or abductor muscles, fascia and tendons of right thumb at forearm level
    - S56.392 Other injury of extensor or abductor muscles, fascia and tendons of left thumb at forearm level
    - S56.399 Other injury of extensor or abductor muscles, fascia and tendons of unspecified thumb at forearm level
- S56.4 Injury of extensor muscle, fascia and tendon of other and unspecified finger at forearm level
  - S56.40 Unspecified injury of extensor muscle, fascia and tendon of other and unspecified finger at forearm level
    - S56.401 Unspecified injury of extensor muscle, fascia and tendon of right index finger at forearm level
    - S56.402 Unspecified injury of extensor muscle, fascia and tendon of left index finger at forearm level
    - S56.403 Unspecified injury of extensor muscle, fascia and tendon of right middle finger at forearm level
    - S56.404 Unspecified injury of extensor muscle, fascia and tendon of left middle finger at forearm level
    - S56.405 Unspecified injury of extensor muscle, fascia and tendon of right ring finger at forearm level
    - S56.406 Unspecified injury of extensor muscle, fascia and tendon of left ring finger at forearm level
    - S56.407 Unspecified injury of extensor muscle, fascia and tendon of right little finger at forearm level
    - S56.408 Unspecified injury of extensor muscle, fascia and tendon of left little finger at forearm level
    - S56.409 Unspecified injury of extensor muscle, fascia and tendon of unspecified finger at forearm level
  - S56.41 Strain of extensor muscle, fascia and tendon of other and unspecified finger at forearm level
    - S56.411 Strain of extensor muscle, fascia and tendon of right index finger at forearm level
    - S56.412 Strain of extensor muscle, fascia and tendon of left index finger at forearm level
    - S56.413 Strain of extensor muscle, fascia and tendon of right middle finger at forearm level
    - S56.414 Strain of extensor muscle, fascia and tendon of left middle finger at forearm level
    - S56.415 Strain of extensor muscle, fascia and tendon of right ring finger at forearm level
    - S56.416 Strain of extensor muscle, fascia and tendon of left ring finger at forearm level
    - S56.417 Strain of extensor muscle, fascia and tendon of right little finger at forearm level
    - S56.418 Strain of extensor muscle, fascia and tendon of left little finger at forearm level
    - S56.419 Strain of extensor muscle, fascia and tendon of finger, unspecified finger at forearm level

- **S56.42** Laceration of extensor muscle, fascia and tendon of other and unspecified finger at forearm level
  - **S56.421** Laceration of extensor muscle, fascia and tendon of right index finger at forearm level A
    Ex: See S56.021
  - **S56.422** Laceration of extensor muscle, fascia and tendon of left index finger at forearm level A
    Ex: See S56.022
  - **S56.423** Laceration of extensor muscle, fascia and tendon of right middle finger at forearm level A
    Ex: See S56.021
  - **S56.424** Laceration of extensor muscle, fascia and tendon of left middle finger at forearm level A
    Ex: See S56.022
  - **S56.425** Laceration of extensor muscle, fascia and tendon of right ring finger at forearm level A
    Ex: See S56.021
  - **S56.426** Laceration of extensor muscle, fascia and tendon of left ring finger at forearm level A
    Ex: See S56.022
  - **S56.427** Laceration of extensor muscle, fascia and tendon of right little finger at forearm level A
    Ex: See S56.021
  - **S56.428** Laceration of extensor muscle, fascia and tendon of left little finger at forearm level A
    Ex: See S56.022
  - **S56.429** Laceration of extensor muscle, fascia and tendon of unspecified finger at forearm level A
    Ex: See S56.029
- **S56.49** Other injury of extensor muscle, fascia and tendon of other and unspecified finger at forearm level
  - **S56.491** Other injury of extensor muscle, fascia and tendon of right index finger at forearm level
  - **S56.492** Other injury of extensor muscle, fascia and tendon of left index finger at forearm level
  - **S56.493** Other injury of extensor muscle, fascia and tendon of right middle finger at forearm level
  - **S56.494** Other injury of extensor muscle, fascia and tendon of left middle finger at forearm level
  - **S56.495** Other injury of extensor muscle, fascia and tendon of right ring finger at forearm level
  - **S56.496** Other injury of extensor muscle, fascia and tendon of left ring finger at forearm level
  - **S56.497** Other injury of extensor muscle, fascia and tendon of right little finger at forearm level
  - **S56.498** Other injury of extensor muscle, fascia and tendon of left little finger at forearm level
  - **S56.499** Other injury of extensor muscle, fascia and tendon of unspecified finger at forearm level
- **S56.5** Injury of other extensor muscle, fascia and tendon at forearm level
  - **S56.50** Unspecified injury of other extensor muscle, fascia and tendon at forearm level
    - **S56.501** Unspecified injury of other extensor muscle, fascia and tendon at forearm level, right arm
    - **S56.502** Unspecified injury of other extensor muscle, fascia and tendon at forearm level, left arm
    - **S56.509** Unspecified injury of other extensor muscle, fascia and tendon at forearm level, unspecified arm
  - **S56.51** Strain of other extensor muscle, fascia and tendon at forearm level
    - **S56.511** Strain of other extensor muscle, fascia and tendon at forearm level, right arm
    - **S56.512** Strain of other extensor muscle, fascia and tendon at forearm level, left arm
    - **S56.519** Strain of other extensor muscle, fascia and tendon at forearm level, unspecified arm
  - **S56.52** Laceration of other extensor muscle, fascia and tendon at forearm level
    - **S56.521** Laceration of other extensor muscle, fascia and tendon at forearm level, right arm A
      Ex: See S56.021
    - **S56.522** Laceration of other extensor muscle, fascia and tendon at forearm level, left arm A
      Ex: See S56.022
    - **S56.529** Laceration of other extensor muscle, fascia and tendon at forearm level, unspecified arm A
      Ex: See S56.029
  - **S56.59** Other injury of other extensor muscle, fascia and tendon at forearm level
    - **S56.591** Other injury of other extensor muscle, fascia and tendon at forearm level, right arm
    - **S56.592** Other injury of other extensor muscle, fascia and tendon at forearm level, left arm
    - **S56.599** Other injury of other extensor muscle, fascia and tendon at forearm level, unspecified arm
- **S56.8** Injury of other muscles, fascia and tendons at forearm level
  - **S56.80** Unspecified injury of other muscles, fascia and tendons at forearm level
    - **S56.801** Unspecified injury of other muscles, fascia and tendons at forearm level, right arm
    - **S56.802** Unspecified injury of other muscles, fascia and tendons at forearm level, left arm
    - **S56.809** Unspecified injury of other muscles, fascia and tendons at forearm level, unspecified arm
  - **S56.81** Strain of other muscles, fascia and tendons at forearm level
    - **S56.811** Strain of other muscles, fascia and tendons at forearm level, right arm
    - **S56.812** Strain of other muscles, fascia and tendons at forearm level, left arm
    - **S56.819** Strain of other muscles, fascia and tendons at forearm level, unspecified arm

- S56.82 Laceration of other muscles, fascia and tendons at forearm level
  - S56.821 Laceration of other muscles, fascia and tendons at forearm level, right arm A
    Ex: See S56.021
  - S56.822 Laceration of other muscles, fascia and tendons at forearm level, left arm A
    Ex: See S56.022
  - S56.829 Laceration of other muscles, fascia and tendons at forearm level, unspecified arm A
    Ex: See S56.029
- S56.89 Other injury of other muscles, fascia and tendons at forearm level
  - S56.891 Other injury of other muscles, fascia and tendons at forearm level, right arm
  - S56.892 Other injury of other muscles, fascia and tendons at forearm level, left arm
  - S56.899 Other injury of other muscles, fascia and tendons at forearm level, unspecified arm
- S56.9 Injury of unspecified muscles, fascia and tendons at forearm level
  - S56.90 Unspecified injury of unspecified muscles, fascia and tendons at forearm level
    - S56.901 Unspecified injury of unspecified muscles, fascia and tendons at forearm level, right arm
    - S56.902 Unspecified injury of unspecified muscles, fascia and tendons at forearm level, left arm
    - S56.909 Unspecified injury of unspecified muscles, fascia and tendons at forearm level, unspecified arm
  - S56.91 Strain of unspecified muscles, fascia and tendons at forearm level
    - S56.911 Strain of unspecified muscles, fascia and tendons at forearm level, right arm
    - S56.912 Strain of unspecified muscles, fascia and tendons at forearm level, left arm
    - S56.919 Strain of unspecified muscles, fascia and tendons at forearm level, unspecified arm
  - S56.92 Laceration of unspecified muscles, fascia and tendons at forearm level
    - S56.921 Laceration of unspecified muscles, fascia and tendons at forearm level, right arm A
      Ex: See S56.021
    - S56.922 Laceration of unspecified muscles, fascia and tendons at forearm level, left arm A
      Ex: See S56.022
    - S56.929 Laceration of unspecified muscles, fascia and tendons at forearm level, unspecified arm A
      Ex: See S56.029
  - S56.99 Other injury of unspecified muscles, fascia and tendons at forearm level
    - S56.991 Other injury of unspecified muscles, fascia and tendons at forearm level, right arm
    - S56.992 Other injury of unspecified muscles, fascia and tendons at forearm level, left arm
    - S56.999 Other injury of unspecified muscles, fascia and tendons at forearm level, unspecified arm

- S57 Crushing injury of elbow and forearm

  Use additional code(s) for all associated injuries

  Excludes2 crushing injury of wrist and hand (S67.-)

  The appropriate 7th character is to be added to each code from category S57

A	initial encounter
D	subsequent encounter
S	sequela

  - S57.0 Crushing injury of elbow
    - X S57.00 Crushing injury of unspecified elbow
    - X S57.01 Crushing injury of right elbow
    - X S57.02 Crushing injury of left elbow
  - S57.8 Crushing injury of forearm
    - X S57.80 Crushing injury of unspecified forearm
    - X S57.81 Crushing injury of right forearm
    - X S57.82 Crushing injury of left forearm

- S58 Traumatic amputation of elbow and forearm

  An amputation not identified as partial or complete should be coded to complete

  Excludes1 traumatic amputation of wrist and hand (S68.-)

  The appropriate 7th character is to be added to each code from category S58

A	initial encounter
D	subsequent encounter
S	sequela

  - S58.0 Traumatic amputation at elbow level
    - S58.01 Complete traumatic amputation at elbow level
      - S58.011 Complete traumatic amputation at elbow level, right arm A
        Ex: See S48.011
      - S58.012 Complete traumatic amputation at elbow level, left arm A
        Ex: See S48.012
      - S58.019 Complete traumatic amputation at elbow level, unspecified arm A
        Ex: See S48.019
    - S58.02 Partial traumatic amputation at elbow level
      - S58.021 Partial traumatic amputation at elbow level, right arm A
        Ex: See S48.011
      - S58.022 Partial traumatic amputation at elbow level, left arm A
        Ex: See S48.012
      - S58.029 Partial traumatic amputation at elbow level, unspecified arm A
        Ex: See S48.019

S58.1 Traumatic amputation at level between elbow and wrist

S58.11 Complete traumatic amputation at level between elbow and wrist

S58.111 Complete traumatic amputation at level between elbow and wrist, right arm A
Ex: See S48.011

S58.112 Complete traumatic amputation at level between elbow and wrist, left arm A
Ex: See S48.012

S58.119 Complete traumatic amputation at level between elbow and wrist, unspecified arm A
Ex: See S48.019

S58.12 Partial traumatic amputation at level between elbow and wrist

S58.121 Partial traumatic amputation at level between elbow and wrist, right arm A
Ex: See S48.011

S58.122 Partial traumatic amputation at level between elbow and wrist, left arm A
Ex: See S48.012

S58.129 Partial traumatic amputation at level between elbow and wrist, unspecified arm A
Ex: See S48.019

S58.9 Traumatic amputation of forearm, level unspecified

Excludes1 traumatic amputation of wrist (S68.-)

S58.91 Complete traumatic amputation of forearm, level unspecified

S58.911 Complete traumatic amputation of right forearm, level unspecified A
Ex: See S48.011

S58.912 Complete traumatic amputation of left forearm, level unspecified A
Ex: See S48.012

S58.919 Complete traumatic amputation of unspecified forearm, level unspecified A
Ex: See S48.019

S58.92 Partial traumatic amputation of forearm, level unspecified

S58.921 Partial traumatic amputation of right forearm, level unspecified A
Ex: See S48.011

S58.922 Partial traumatic amputation of left forearm, level unspecified A
Ex: See S48.012

S58.929 Partial traumatic amputation of unspecified forearm, level unspecified A
Ex: See S48.019

S59 Other and unspecified injuries of elbow and forearm

Excludes2 other and unspecified injuries of wrist and hand (S69.-)

The appropriate 7th character is to be added to each code from subcategories S59.0, S59.1, and S59.2

A	initial encounter for closed fracture
D	subsequent encounter for fracture with routine healing
G	subsequent encounter for fracture with delayed healing
K	subsequent encounter for fracture with nonunion
P	subsequent encounter for fracture with malunion
S	sequela

S59.0 Physeal fracture of lower end of ulna

S59.00 Unspecified physeal fracture of lower end of ulna

S59.001 Unspecified physeal fracture of lower end of ulna, right arm A, K, P, A
Ex: **For code S59.001[A]:** See S52.011[A]
For S59.001[K,P]: See S02.0[K]

S59.002 Unspecified physeal fracture of lower end of ulna, left arm A, K, P, A
Ex: **For code S59.002[A]:** See S52.012[A]
For S59.002[K,P]: See S02.0[K]

S59.009 Unspecified physeal fracture of lower end of ulna, unspecified arm A, K, P, A
Ex: **For code S59.009[A]:** See S52.019[A]
For S59.009[K,P]: See S02.0[K]

S59.01 Salter-Harris Type I physeal fracture of lower end of ulna

S59.011 Salter-Harris Type I physeal fracture of lower end of ulna, right arm A, K, P, A
Ex: **For code S59.011[A]:** See S52.011[A]
For S59.011[K,P]: See S02.0[K]

S59.012 Salter-Harris Type I physeal fracture of lower end of ulna, left arm A, K, P, A
Ex: **For code S59.012[A]:** See S52.012[A]
For S59.012[K,P]: See S02.0[K]

S59.019 Salter-Harris Type I physeal fracture of lower end of ulna, unspecified arm A, K, P, A
Ex: **For code S59.019[A]:** See S52.019[A]
For S59.019[K,P]: See S02.0[K]

Item 19-4 SALTER-HARRIS TYPE 1: epiphysis is completely separated from end of bone, or metaphysic growth plate remains attached to epiphysis

SALTER-HARRIS TYPE 2: epiphysis and growth plate are partially separated from metaphysis, which is cracked—most common type

SALTER-HARRIS TYPE 3: fracture occurring through epiphysis and separates part of epiphysis and growth plate from metaphysis fracture, usually at distal end of tibia

SALTER-HARRIS TYPE 4: fracture runs through epiphysis, across growth plate, into metaphysic, surgery is required to restore joint surface to normal and align growth plate

- **S59.02** Salter-Harris Type II physeal fracture of lower end of ulna
  - **S59.021** Salter-Harris Type II physeal fracture of lower end of ulna, right arm
    A, K, P, A
    Ex: For code S59.021[A]: See S52.011[A]
    For S59.021[K,P]: See S02.0[K]
  - **S59.022** Salter-Harris Type II physeal fracture of lower end of ulna, left arm
    A, K, P, A
    Ex: For code S59.022[A]: See S52.012[A]
    For S59.022[K,P]: See S02.0[K]
  - **S59.029** Salter-Harris Type II physeal fracture of lower end of ulna, unspecified arm
    A, K, P, A
    Ex: For code S59.029[A]: See S52.019[A]
    For S59.029[K,P]: See S02.0[K]
- **S59.03** Salter-Harris Type III physeal fracture of lower end of ulna
  - **S59.031** Salter-Harris Type III physeal fracture of lower end of ulna, right arm
    A, K, P, A
    Ex: For code S59.031[A]: See S52.011[A]
    For S59.031[K,P]: See S02.0[K]
  - **S59.032** Salter-Harris Type III physeal fracture of lower end of ulna, left arm
    A, K, P, A
    Ex: For code S59.032[A]: See S52.012[A]
    For S59.032[K,P]: See S02.0[K]
  - **S59.039** Salter-Harris Type III physeal fracture of lower end of ulna, unspecified arm
    A, K, P, A
    Ex: For code S59.039[A]: See S52.019[A]
    For S59.039[K,P]: See S02.0[K]
- **S59.04** Salter-Harris Type IV physeal fracture of lower end of ulna
  - **S59.041** Salter-Harris Type IV physeal fracture of lower end of ulna, right arm
    A, K, P, A
    Ex: For code S59.041[A]: See S52.011[A]
    For S59.041[K,P]: See S02.0[K]
  - **S59.042** Salter-Harris Type IV physeal fracture of lower end of ulna, left arm
    A, K, P, A
    Ex: For code S59.042[A]: See S52.012[A]
    For S59.042[K,P]: See S02.0[K]
  - **S59.049** Salter-Harris Type IV physeal fracture of lower end of ulna, unspecified arm
    A, K, P, A
    Ex: For code S59.049[A]: See S52.019[A]
    For S59.049[K,P]: See S02.0[K]
- **S59.09** Other physeal fracture of lower end of ulna
  - **S59.091** Other physeal fracture of lower end of ulna, right arm A, K, P, A
    Ex: For code S59.091[A]: See S52.011[A]
    For S59.091[K,P]: See S02.0[K]
  - **S59.092** Other physeal fracture of lower end of ulna, left arm A, K, P, A
    Ex: For code S59.092[A]: See S52.012[A]
    For S59.092[K,P]: See S02.0[K]
  - **S59.099** Other physeal fracture of lower end of ulna, unspecified arm A, K, P, A
    Ex: For code S59.099[A]: See S52.019[A]
    For S59.099[K,P]: See S02.0[K]
- **S59.1** Physeal fracture of upper end of radius
  Ex: For category S59.1 CC codes: See S02.0[K]
  - **S59.10** Unspecified physeal fracture of upper end of radius
    - **S59.101** Unspecified physeal fracture of upper end of radius, right arm K, P
    - **S59.102** Unspecified physeal fracture of upper end of radius, left arm K, P
    - **S59.109** Unspecified physeal fracture of upper end of radius, unspecified arm K, P
  - **S59.11** Salter-Harris Type I physeal fracture of upper end of radius
    - **S59.111** Salter-Harris Type I physeal fracture of upper end of radius, right arm K, P
    - **S59.112** Salter-Harris Type I physeal fracture of upper end of radius, left arm K, P
    - **S59.119** Salter-Harris Type I physeal fracture of upper end of radius, unspecified arm K, P
  - **S59.12** Salter-Harris Type II physeal fracture of upper end of radius
    - **S59.121** Salter-Harris Type II physeal fracture of upper end of radius, right arm K, P
    - **S59.122** Salter-Harris Type II physeal fracture of upper end of radius, left arm K, P
    - **S59.129** Salter-Harris Type II physeal fracture of upper end of radius, unspecified arm K, P
  - **S59.13** Salter-Harris Type III physeal fracture of upper end of radius
    - **S59.131** Salter-Harris Type III physeal fracture of upper end of radius, right arm K, P
    - **S59.132** Salter-Harris Type III physeal fracture of upper end of radius, left arm K, P
    - **S59.139** Salter-Harris Type III physeal fracture of upper end of radius, unspecified arm K, P
  - **S59.14** Salter-Harris Type IV physeal fracture of upper end of radius
    - **S59.141** Salter-Harris Type IV physeal fracture of upper end of radius, right arm K, P
    - **S59.142** Salter-Harris Type IV physeal fracture of upper end of radius, left arm K, P
    - **S59.149** Salter-Harris Type IV physeal fracture of upper end of radius, unspecified arm K, P
  - **S59.19** Other physeal fracture of upper end of radius
    - **S59.191** Other physeal fracture of upper end of radius, right arm K, P
    - **S59.192** Other physeal fracture of upper end of radius, left arm K, P
    - **S59.199** Other physeal fracture of upper end of radius, unspecified arm K, P

New Revised ~~deleted~~ Deleted Excludes 1 Excludes 2 Includes Use additional Code first Code also Unspecified
OGCR Official Guidelines Unacceptable Principal Diagnosis X Assign placeholder X Use Additional Character(s) Manifestation Code Coding Clinic

- **S59.2 Physeal fracture of lower end of radius**
  - **S59.20 Unspecified physeal fracture of lower end of radius**
    - **S59.201 Unspecified physeal fracture of lower end of radius, right arm** A, K, P, A
      - For code S59.201[A]: See S52.011[A]
      - For S59.201[K,P]: See S02.0[K]
    - **S59.202 Unspecified physeal fracture of lower end of radius, left arm** A, K, P, A
      - For code S59.202[A]: See S52.012[A]
      - For S59.202[K,P]: See S02.0[K]
    - **S59.209 Unspecified physeal fracture of lower end of radius, unspecified arm** A, K, P, A
      - For code S59.209[A]: See S52.019[A]
      - For S59.209[K,P]: See S02.0[K]
  - **S59.21 Salter-Harris Type I physeal fracture of lower end of radius**
    - **S59.211 Salter-Harris Type I physeal fracture of lower end of radius, right arm** A, K, P, A
      - For code S59.211[A]: See S52.011[A]
      - For S59.211[K,P]: See S02.0[K]
    - **S59.212 Salter-Harris Type I physeal fracture of lower end of radius, left arm** A, K, P, A
      - For code S59.212[A]: See S52.012[A]
      - For S59.212[K,P]: See S02.0[K]
    - **S59.219 Salter-Harris Type I physeal fracture of lower end of radius, unspecified arm** A, K, P, A
      - For code S59.219[A]: See S52.019[A]
      - For S59.219[K,P]: See S02.0[K]
  - **S59.22 Salter-Harris Type II physeal fracture of lower end of radius**
    - **S59.221 Salter-Harris Type II physeal fracture of lower end of radius, right arm** A, K, P, A
      - For code S59.221[A]: See S52.011[A]
      - For S59.221[K,P]: See S02.0[K]
    - **S59.222 Salter-Harris Type II physeal fracture of lower end of radius, left arm** A, K, P, A
      - For code S59.222[A]: See S52.012[A]
      - For S59.222[K,P]: See S02.0[K]
    - **S59.229 Salter-Harris Type II physeal fracture of lower end of radius, unspecified arm** A, K, P, A
      - For code S59.229[A]: See S52.019[A]
      - For S59.229[K,P]: See S02.0[K]
  - **S59.23 Salter-Harris Type III physeal fracture of lower end of radius**
    - **S59.231 Salter-Harris Type III physeal fracture of lower end of radius, right arm** A, K, P, A
      - For code S59.231[A]: See S52.011[A]
      - For S59.231[K,P]: See S02.0[K]
    - **S59.232 Salter-Harris Type III physeal fracture of lower end of radius, left arm** A, K, P, A
      - For code S59.232[A]: See S52.012[A]
      - For S59.232[K,P]: See S02.0[K]
    - **S59.239 Salter-Harris Type III physeal fracture of lower end of radius, unspecified arm** A, K, P, A
      - For code S59.239[A]: See S52.019[A]
      - For S59.239[K,P]: See S02.0[K]
  - **S59.24 Salter-Harris Type IV physeal fracture of lower end of radius**
    - **S59.241 Salter-Harris Type IV physeal fracture of lower end of radius, right arm** A, K, P, A
      - For code S59.241[A]: See S52.011[A]
      - For S59.241[K,P]: See S02.0[K]
    - **S59.242 Salter-Harris Type IV physeal fracture of lower end of radius, left arm** A, K, P, A
      - For code S59.242[A]: See S52.012[A]
      - For S59.242[K,P]: See S02.0[K]
    - **S59.249 Salter-Harris Type IV physeal fracture of lower end of radius, unspecified arm** A, K, P, A
      - For code S59.249[A]: See S52.019[A]
      - For S59.249[K,P]: See S02.0[K]
  - **S59.29 Other physeal fracture of lower end of radius**
    - **S59.291 Other physeal fracture of lower end of radius, right arm** A, K, P, A
      - For code S59.291[A]: See S52.011[A]
      - For S59.291[K,P]: See S02.0[K]
    - **S59.292 Other physeal fracture of lower end of radius, left arm** A, K, P, A
      - For code S59.292[A]: See S52.012[A]
      - For S59.292[K,P]: See S02.0[K]
    - **S59.299 Other physeal fracture of lower end of radius, unspecified arm** A, K, P, A
      - For code S59.299[A]: See S52.019[A]
      - For S59.299[K,P]: See S02.0[K]
- **S59.8 Other specified injuries of elbow and forearm**

  The appropriate 7th character is to be added to each code in subcategory S59.8

A	initial encounter
D	subsequent encounter
S	sequela

  - **S59.80 Other specified injuries of elbow**
    - **S59.801 Other specified injuries of right elbow**
    - **S59.802 Other specified injuries of left elbow**
    - **S59.809 Other specified injuries of unspecified elbow**
  - **S59.81 Other specified injuries of forearm**
    - **S59.811 Other specified injuries right forearm**
    - **S59.812 Other specified injuries left forearm**
    - **S59.819 Other specified injuries unspecified forearm**
- **S59.9 Unspecified injury of elbow and forearm**

  The appropriate 7th character is to be added to each code in subcategory S59.9

A	initial encounter
D	subsequent encounter
S	sequela

  - **S59.90 Unspecified injury of elbow**
    - **S59.901 Unspecified injury of right elbow**
    - **S59.902 Unspecified injury of left elbow**
    - **S59.909 Unspecified injury of unspecified elbow**
  - **S59.91 Unspecified injury of forearm**
    - **S59.911 Unspecified injury of right forearm**
    - **S59.912 Unspecified injury of left forearm**
    - **S59.919 Unspecified injury of unspecified forearm**

INJURIES TO THE WRIST, HAND AND FINGERS (S60-S69)

Excludes2 burns and corrosions (T20-T32)
frostbite (T33-T34)
insect bite or sting, venomous (T63.4)

S60 Superficial injury of wrist, hand and fingers

The appropriate 7th character is to be added to each code from category S60

A	initial encounter
D	subsequent encounter
S	sequela

S60.0 Contusion of finger without damage to nail

Excludes1 contusion involving nail (matrix) (S60.1)

X **S60.00 Contusion of unspecified finger without damage to nail**

Contusion of finger(s) NOS

S60.01 Contusion of thumb without damage to nail

S60.011 Contusion of right thumb without damage to nail

S60.012 Contusion of left thumb without damage to nail

S60.019 Contusion of unspecified thumb without damage to nail

S60.02 Contusion of index finger without damage to nail

S60.021 Contusion of right index finger without damage to nail

S60.022 Contusion of left index finger without damage to nail

S60.029 Contusion of unspecified index finger without damage to nail

S60.03 Contusion of middle finger without damage to nail

S60.031 Contusion of right middle finger without damage to nail

S60.032 Contusion of left middle finger without damage to nail

S60.039 Contusion of unspecified middle finger without damage to nail

S60.04 Contusion of ring finger without damage to nail

S60.041 Contusion of right ring finger without damage to nail

S60.042 Contusion of left ring finger without damage to nail

S60.049 Contusion of unspecified ring finger without damage to nail

S60.05 Contusion of little finger without damage to nail

S60.051 Contusion of right little finger without damage to nail

S60.052 Contusion of left little finger without damage to nail

S60.059 Contusion of unspecified little finger without damage to nail

S60.1 Contusion of finger with damage to nail

X **S60.10 Contusion of unspecified finger with damage to nail**

S60.11 Contusion of thumb with damage to nail

S60.111 Contusion of right thumb with damage to nail

S60.112 Contusion of left thumb with damage to nail

S60.119 Contusion of unspecified thumb with damage to nail

S60.12 Contusion of index finger with damage to nail

S60.121 Contusion of right index finger with damage to nail

S60.122 Contusion of left index finger with damage to nail

S60.129 Contusion of unspecified index finger with damage to nail

S60.13 Contusion of middle finger with damage to nail

S60.131 Contusion of right middle finger with damage to nail

S60.132 Contusion of left middle finger with damage to nail

S60.139 Contusion of unspecified middle finger with damage to nail

S60.14 Contusion of ring finger with damage to nail

S60.141 Contusion of right ring finger with damage to nail

S60.142 Contusion of left ring finger with damage to nail

S60.149 Contusion of unspecified ring finger with damage to nail

S60.15 Contusion of little finger with damage to nail

S60.151 Contusion of right little finger with damage to nail

S60.152 Contusion of left little finger with damage to nail

S60.159 Contusion of unspecified little finger with damage to nail

S60.2 Contusion of wrist and hand

Excludes2 contusion of fingers (S60.0-, S60.1-)

S60.21 Contusion of wrist

S60.211 Contusion of right wrist

S60.212 Contusion of left wrist

S60.219 Contusion of unspecified wrist

S60.22 Contusion of hand

S60.221 Contusion of right hand

S60.222 Contusion of left hand

S60.229 Contusion of unspecified hand

S60.3 Other superficial injuries of thumb

S60.31 Abrasion of thumb

S60.311 Abrasion of right thumb

S60.312 Abrasion of left thumb

S60.319 Abrasion of unspecified thumb

S60.32 Blister (nonthermal) of thumb

S60.321 Blister (nonthermal) of right thumb

S60.322 Blister (nonthermal) of left thumb

S60.329 Blister (nonthermal) of unspecified thumb

S60.34 External constriction of thumb

Hair tourniquet syndrome of thumb

Use additional cause code to identify the constricting item (W49.0-)

S60.341 External constriction of right thumb

S60.342 External constriction of left thumb

S60.349 External constriction of unspecified thumb

S60.35 Superficial foreign body of thumb

Splinter in the thumb

S60.351 Superficial foreign body of right thumb

S60.352 Superficial foreign body of left thumb

S60.359 Superficial foreign body of unspecified thumb

- **S60.36 Insect bite (nonvenomous) of thumb**
  - **S60.361 Insect bite (nonvenomous) of right thumb**
  - **S60.362 Insect bite (nonvenomous) of left thumb**
  - **S60.369 Insect bite (nonvenomous) of unspecified thumb**
- **S60.37 Other superficial bite of thumb**
  - **Excludes1** open bite of thumb (S61.05-, S61.15-)
  - **S60.371 Other superficial bite of right thumb**
  - **S60.372 Other superficial bite of left thumb**
  - **S60.379 Other superficial bite of unspecified thumb**
- **S60.39 Other superficial injuries of thumb**
  - **S60.391 Other superficial injuries of right thumb**
  - **S60.392 Other superficial injuries of left thumb**
  - **S60.399 Other superficial injuries of unspecified thumb**
- **S60.4 Other superficial injuries of other fingers**
  - **S60.41 Abrasion of fingers**
    - **S60.410 Abrasion of right index finger**
    - **S60.411 Abrasion of left index finger**
    - **S60.412 Abrasion of right middle finger**
    - **S60.413 Abrasion of left middle finger**
    - **S60.414 Abrasion of right ring finger**
    - **S60.415 Abrasion of left ring finger**
    - **S60.416 Abrasion of right little finger**
    - **S60.417 Abrasion of left little finger**
    - **S60.418 Abrasion of other finger**
      Abrasion of specified finger with unspecified laterality
    - **S60.419 Abrasion of unspecified finger**
  - **S60.42 Blister (nonthermal) of fingers**
    - **S60.420 Blister (nonthermal) of right index finger**
    - **S60.421 Blister (nonthermal) of left index finger**
    - **S60.422 Blister (nonthermal) of right middle finger**
    - **S60.423 Blister (nonthermal) of left middle finger**
    - **S60.424 Blister (nonthermal) of right ring finger**
    - **S60.425 Blister (nonthermal) of left ring finger**
    - **S60.426 Blister (nonthermal) of right little finger**
    - **S60.427 Blister (nonthermal) of left little finger**
    - **S60.428 Blister (nonthermal) of other finger**
      Blister (nonthermal) of specified finger with unspecified laterality
    - **S60.429 Blister (nonthermal) of unspecified finger**
  - **S60.44 External constriction of fingers**
    Hair tourniquet syndrome of finger
    Use additional cause code to identify the constricting item (W49.0-)
    - **S60.440 External constriction of right index finger**
    - **S60.441 External constriction of left index finger**
    - **S60.442 External constriction of right middle finger**
    - **S60.443 External constriction of left middle finger**
    - **S60.444 External constriction of right ring finger**
    - **S60.445 External constriction of left ring finger**
    - **S60.446 External constriction of right little finger**
    - **S60.447 External constriction of left little finger**
    - **S60.448 External constriction of other finger**
      External constriction of specified finger with unspecified laterality
    - **S60.449 External constriction of unspecified finger**
  - **S60.45 Superficial foreign body of fingers**
    Splinter in the finger(s)
    - **S60.450 Superficial foreign body of right index finger**
    - **S60.451 Superficial foreign body of left index finger**
    - **S60.452 Superficial foreign body of right middle finger**
    - **S60.453 Superficial foreign body of left middle finger**
    - **S60.454 Superficial foreign body of right ring finger**
    - **S60.455 Superficial foreign body of left ring finger**
    - **S60.456 Superficial foreign body of right little finger**
    - **S60.457 Superficial foreign body of left little finger**
    - **S60.458 Superficial foreign body of other finger**
      Superficial foreign body of specified finger with unspecified laterality
    - **S60.459 Superficial foreign body of unspecified finger**
  - **S60.46 Insect bite (nonvenomous) of fingers**
    - **S60.460 Insect bite (nonvenomous) of right index finger**
    - **S60.461 Insect bite (nonvenomous) of left index finger**
    - **S60.462 Insect bite (nonvenomous) of right middle finger**
    - **S60.463 Insect bite (nonvenomous) of left middle finger**
    - **S60.464 Insect bite (nonvenomous) of right ring finger**
    - **S60.465 Insect bite (nonvenomous) of left ring finger**
    - **S60.466 Insect bite (nonvenomous) of right little finger**
    - **S60.467 Insect bite (nonvenomous) of left little finger**
    - **S60.468 Insect bite (nonvenomous) of other finger**
      Insect bite (nonvenomous) of specified finger with unspecified laterality
    - **S60.469 Insect bite (nonvenomous) of unspecified finger**

- S60.47 Other superficial bite of fingers
  - **Excludes1** open bite of fingers (S61.25-, S61.35-)
  - S60.470 Other superficial bite of right index finger
  - S60.471 Other superficial bite of left index finger
  - S60.472 Other superficial bite of right middle finger
  - S60.473 Other superficial bite of left middle finger
  - S60.474 Other superficial bite of right ring finger
  - S60.475 Other superficial bite of left ring finger
  - S60.476 Other superficial bite of right little finger
  - S60.477 Other superficial bite of left little finger
  - S60.478 Other superficial bite of other finger
    Other superficial bite of specified finger with unspecified laterality
  - S60.479 Other superficial bite of unspecified finger
- S60.5 Other superficial injuries of hand
  - **Excludes2** superficial injuries of fingers (S60.3-, S60.4-)
  - S60.51 Abrasion of hand
    - S60.511 Abrasion of right hand
    - S60.512 Abrasion of left hand
    - S60.519 Abrasion of unspecified hand
  - S60.52 Blister (nonthermal) of hand
    - S60.521 Blister (nonthermal) of right hand
    - S60.522 Blister (nonthermal) of left hand
    - S60.529 Blister (nonthermal) of unspecified hand
  - S60.54 External constriction of hand
    - S60.541 External constriction of right hand
    - S60.542 External constriction of left hand
    - S60.549 External constriction of unspecified hand
  - S60.55 Superficial foreign body of hand
    Splinter in the hand
    - S60.551 Superficial foreign body of right hand
    - S60.552 Superficial foreign body of left hand
    - S60.559 Superficial foreign body of unspecified hand
  - S60.56 Insect bite (nonvenomous) of hand
    - S60.561 Insect bite (nonvenomous) of right hand
    - S60.562 Insect bite (nonvenomous) of left hand
    - S60.569 Insect bite (nonvenomous) of unspecified hand
  - S60.57 Other superficial bite of hand
    - **Excludes1** open bite of hand (S61.45-)
    - S60.571 Other superficial bite of hand of right hand
    - S60.572 Other superficial bite of hand of left hand
    - S60.579 Other superficial bite of hand of unspecified hand
- S60.8 Other superficial injuries of wrist
  - S60.81 Abrasion of wrist
    - S60.811 Abrasion of right wrist
    - S60.812 Abrasion of left wrist
    - S60.819 Abrasion of unspecified wrist
  - S60.82 Blister (nonthermal) of wrist
    - S60.821 Blister (nonthermal) of right wrist
    - S60.822 Blister (nonthermal) of left wrist
    - S60.829 Blister (nonthermal) of unspecified wrist
  - S60.84 External constriction of wrist
    - S60.841 External constriction of right wrist
    - S60.842 External constriction of left wrist
    - S60.849 External constriction of unspecified wrist
  - S60.85 Superficial foreign body of wrist
    Splinter in the wrist
    - S60.851 Superficial foreign body of right wrist
    - S60.852 Superficial foreign body of left wrist
    - S60.859 Superficial foreign body of unspecified wrist
  - S60.86 Insect bite (nonvenomous) of wrist
    - S60.861 Insect bite (nonvenomous) of right wrist
    - S60.862 Insect bite (nonvenomous) of left wrist
    - S60.869 Insect bite (nonvenomous) of unspecified wrist
  - S60.87 Other superficial bite of wrist
    - **Excludes1** open bite of wrist (S61.55)
    - S60.871 Other superficial bite of right wrist
    - S60.872 Other superficial bite of left wrist
    - S60.879 Other superficial bite of unspecified wrist
- S60.9 Unspecified superficial injury of wrist, hand and fingers
  - S60.91 Unspecified superficial injury of wrist
    - S60.911 Unspecified superficial injury of right wrist
    - S60.912 Unspecified superficial injury of left wrist
    - S60.919 Unspecified superficial injury of unspecified wrist
  - S60.92 Unspecified superficial injury of hand
    - S60.921 Unspecified superficial injury of right hand
    - S60.922 Unspecified superficial injury of left hand
    - S60.929 Unspecified superficial injury of unspecified hand
  - S60.93 Unspecified superficial injury of thumb
    - S60.931 Unspecified superficial injury of right thumb
    - S60.932 Unspecified superficial injury of left thumb
    - S60.939 Unspecified superficial injury of unspecified thumb
  - S60.94 Unspecified superficial injury of other fingers
    - S60.940 Unspecified superficial injury of right index finger
    - S60.941 Unspecified superficial injury of left index finger
    - S60.942 Unspecified superficial injury of right middle finger
    - S60.943 Unspecified superficial injury of left middle finger

◀ New ⇐ Revised ~~deleted~~ Deleted Excludes 1 Excludes 2 Includes Use additional Code first Code also Unspecified
OGCR Official Guidelines ● Unacceptable Principal Diagnosis X Assign placeholder X ● Use Additional Character(s) ▶ Manifestation Code Coding Clinic

- **S60.944** **Unspecified superficial injury of right ring finger**
- **S60.945** **Unspecified superficial injury of left ring finger**
- **S60.946** **Unspecified superficial injury of right little finger**
- **S60.947** **Unspecified superficial injury of left little finger**
- **S60.948** **Unspecified superficial injury of other finger**
  Unspecified superficial injury of specified finger with unspecified laterality
- **S60.949** **Unspecified superficial injury of unspecified finger**

S61 Open wound of wrist, hand and fingers

Code also any associated wound infection

Excludes1 open fracture of wrist, hand and finger (S62.- with 7th character B)
traumatic amputation of wrist and hand (S68.-)

The appropriate 7th character is to be added to each code from category S61

A	initial encounter
D	subsequent encounter
S	sequela

S61.0 Open wound of thumb without damage to nail

Excludes1 open wound of thumb with damage to nail (S61.1-)

- **S61.00 Unspecified open wound of thumb without damage to nail**
  - **S61.001** **Unspecified open wound of right thumb without damage to nail**
  - **S61.002** **Unspecified open wound of left thumb without damage to nail**
  - **S61.009** **Unspecified open wound of unspecified thumb without damage to nail**
- **S61.01 Laceration without foreign body of thumb without damage to nail**
  - **S61.011** **Laceration without foreign body of right thumb without damage to nail**
  - **S61.012** **Laceration without foreign body of left thumb without damage to nail**
  - **S61.019** **Laceration without foreign body of unspecified thumb without damage to nail**
- **S61.02 Laceration with foreign body of thumb without damage to nail**
  - **S61.021** **Laceration with foreign body of right thumb without damage to nail**
  - **S61.022** **Laceration with foreign body of left thumb without damage to nail**
  - **S61.029** **Laceration with foreign body of unspecified thumb without damage to nail**
- **S61.03 Puncture wound without foreign body of thumb without damage to nail**
  - **S61.031** **Puncture wound without foreign body of right thumb without damage to nail**
  - **S61.032** **Puncture wound without foreign body of left thumb without damage to nail**
  - **S61.039** **Puncture wound without foreign body of unspecified thumb without damage to nail**
- **S61.04 Puncture wound with foreign body of thumb without damage to nail**
  - **S61.041** **Puncture wound with foreign body of right thumb without damage to nail**
  - **S61.042** **Puncture wound with foreign body of left thumb without damage to nail**
  - **S61.049** **Puncture wound with foreign body of unspecified thumb without damage to nail**
- **S61.05 Open bite of thumb without damage to nail**
  Bite of thumb NOS

  Excludes1 superficial bite of thumb (S60.36-, S60.37-)
  - **S61.051** **Open bite of right thumb without damage to nail**
  - **S61.052** **Open bite of left thumb without damage to nail**
  - **S61.059** **Open bite of unspecified thumb without damage to nail**

S61.1 Open wound of thumb with damage to nail

- **S61.10 Unspecified open wound of thumb with damage to nail**
  - **S61.101** **Unspecified open wound of right thumb with damage to nail**
  - **S61.102** **Unspecified open wound of left thumb with damage to nail**
  - **S61.109** **Unspecified open wound of unspecified thumb with damage to nail**
- **S61.11 Laceration without foreign body of thumb with damage to nail**
  - **S61.111** **Laceration without foreign body of right thumb with damage to nail**
  - **S61.112** **Laceration without foreign body of left thumb with damage to nail**
  - **S61.119** **Laceration without foreign body of unspecified thumb with damage to nail**
- **S61.12 Laceration with foreign body of thumb with damage to nail**
  - **S61.121** **Laceration with foreign body of right thumb with damage to nail**
  - **S61.122** **Laceration with foreign body of left thumb with damage to nail**
  - **S61.129** **Laceration with foreign body of unspecified thumb with damage to nail**
- **S61.13 Puncture wound without foreign body of thumb with damage to nail**
  - **S61.131** **Puncture wound without foreign body of right thumb with damage to nail**
  - **S61.132** **Puncture wound without foreign body of left thumb with damage to nail**
  - **S61.139** **Puncture wound without foreign body of unspecified thumb with damage to nail**
- **S61.14 Puncture wound with foreign body of thumb with damage to nail**
  - **S61.141** **Puncture wound with foreign body of right thumb with damage to nail**
  - **S61.142** **Puncture wound with foreign body of left thumb with damage to nail**
  - **S61.149** **Puncture wound with foreign body of unspecified thumb with damage to nail**

- **S61.15 Open bite of thumb with damage to nail**
  Bite of thumb with damage to nail NOS
  Excludes1 superficial bite of thumb (S60.36-, S60.37-)
  - **S61.151 Open bite of right thumb with damage to nail**
  - **S61.152 Open bite of left thumb with damage to nail**
  - **S61.159 Open bite of unspecified thumb with damage to nail**
- **S61.2 Open wound of other finger without damage to nail**
  Excludes1 open wound of finger involving nail (matrix) (S61.3-)
  Excludes2 open wound of thumb without damage to nail (S61.0-)
  - **S61.20 Unspecified open wound of other finger without damage to nail**
    - **S61.200 Unspecified open wound of right index finger without damage to nail**
    - **S61.201 Unspecified open wound of left index finger without damage to nail**
    - **S61.202 Unspecified open wound of right middle finger without damage to nail**
    - **S61.203 Unspecified open wound of left middle finger without damage to nail**
    - **S61.204 Unspecified open wound of right ring finger without damage to nail**
    - **S61.205 Unspecified open wound of left ring finger without damage to nail**
    - **S61.206 Unspecified open wound of right little finger without damage to nail**
    - **S61.207 Unspecified open wound of left little finger without damage to nail**
    - **S61.208 Unspecified open wound of other finger without damage to nail**
      Unspecified open wound of specified finger with unspecified laterality without damage to nail
    - **S61.209 Unspecified open wound of unspecified finger without damage to nail**
  - **S61.21 Laceration without foreign body of finger without damage to nail**
    - **S61.210 Laceration without foreign body of right index finger without damage to nail**
    - **S61.211 Laceration without foreign body of left index finger without damage to nail**
    - **S61.212 Laceration without foreign body of right middle finger without damage to nail**
    - **S61.213 Laceration without foreign body of left middle finger without damage to nail**
    - **S61.214 Laceration without foreign body of right ring finger without damage to nail**
    - **S61.215 Laceration without foreign body of left ring finger without damage to nail**
    - **S61.216 Laceration without foreign body of right little finger without damage to nail**
    - **S61.217 Laceration without foreign body of left little finger without damage to nail**
    - **S61.218 Laceration without foreign body of other finger without damage to nail**
      Laceration without foreign body of specified finger with unspecified laterality without damage to nail
    - **S61.219 Laceration without foreign body of unspecified finger without damage to nail**
  - **S61.22 Laceration with foreign body of finger without damage to nail**
    - **S61.220 Laceration with foreign body of right index finger without damage to nail**
    - **S61.221 Laceration with foreign body of left index finger without damage to nail**
    - **S61.222 Laceration with foreign body of right middle finger without damage to nail**
    - **S61.223 Laceration with foreign body of left middle finger without damage to nail**
    - **S61.224 Laceration with foreign body of right ring finger without damage to nail**
    - **S61.225 Laceration with foreign body of left ring finger without damage to nail**
    - **S61.226 Laceration with foreign body of right little finger without damage to nail**
    - **S61.227 Laceration with foreign body of left little finger without damage to nail**
    - **S61.228 Laceration with foreign body of other finger without damage to nail**
      Laceration with foreign body of specified finger with unspecified laterality without damage to nail
    - **S61.229 Laceration with foreign body of unspecified finger without damage to nail**
  - **S61.23 Puncture wound without foreign body of finger without damage to nail**
    - **S61.230 Puncture wound without foreign body of right index finger without damage to nail**
    - **S61.231 Puncture wound without foreign body of left index finger without damage to nail**
    - **S61.232 Puncture wound without foreign body of right middle finger without damage to nail**
    - **S61.233 Puncture wound without foreign body of left middle finger without damage to nail**
    - **S61.234 Puncture wound without foreign body of right ring finger without damage to nail**
    - **S61.235 Puncture wound without foreign body of left ring finger without damage to nail**
    - **S61.236 Puncture wound without foreign body of right little finger without damage to nail**
    - **S61.237 Puncture wound without foreign body of left little finger without damage to nail**
    - **S61.238 Puncture wound without foreign body of other finger without damage to nail**
      Puncture wound without foreign body of specified finger with unspecified laterality without damage to nail
    - **S61.239 Puncture wound without foreign body of unspecified finger without damage to nail**

◀ New ⇐ Revised ~~deleted~~ Deleted Excludes 1 Excludes 2 Includes Use additional Code first Code also Unspecified
OGCR Official Guidelines ● Unacceptable Principal Diagnosis X Assign placeholder X ● Use Additional Character(s) ▶ Manifestation Code Coding Clinic

- **S61.24 Puncture wound with foreign body of finger without damage to nail**
  - **S61.240 Puncture wound with foreign body of right index finger without damage to nail**
  - **S61.241 Puncture wound with foreign body of left index finger without damage to nail**
  - **S61.242 Puncture wound with foreign body of right middle finger without damage to nail**
  - **S61.243 Puncture wound with foreign body of left middle finger without damage to nail**
  - **S61.244 Puncture wound with foreign body of right ring finger without damage to nail**
  - **S61.245 Puncture wound with foreign body of left ring finger without damage to nail**
  - **S61.246 Puncture wound with foreign body of right little finger without damage to nail**
  - **S61.247 Puncture wound with foreign body of left little finger without damage to nail**
  - **S61.248 Puncture wound with foreign body of other finger without damage to nail**
    Puncture wound with foreign body of specified finger with unspecified laterality without damage to nail
  - **S61.249 Puncture wound with foreign body of unspecified finger without damage to nail**
- **S61.25 Open bite of finger without damage to nail**
  Bite of finger without damage to nail NOS
  Excludes1 superficial bite of finger (S60.46-, S60.47-)
  - **S61.250 Open bite of right index finger without damage to nail**
  - **S61.251 Open bite of left index finger without damage to nail**
  - **S61.252 Open bite of right middle finger without damage to nail**
  - **S61.253 Open bite of left middle finger without damage to nail**
  - **S61.254 Open bite of right ring finger without damage to nail**
  - **S61.255 Open bite of left ring finger without damage to nail**
  - **S61.256 Open bite of right little finger without damage to nail**
  - **S61.257 Open bite of left little finger without damage to nail**
  - **S61.258 Open bite of other finger without damage to nail**
    Open bite of specified finger with unspecified laterality without damage to nail
  - **S61.259 Open bite of unspecified finger without damage to nail**
- **S61.3 Open wound of other finger with damage to nail**
  - **S61.30 Unspecified open wound of finger with damage to nail**
    - **S61.300 Unspecified open wound of right index finger with damage to nail**
    - **S61.301 Unspecified open wound of left index finger with damage to nail**
    - **S61.302 Unspecified open wound of right middle finger with damage to nail**
    - **S61.303 Unspecified open wound of left middle finger with damage to nail**
    - **S61.304 Unspecified open wound of right ring finger with damage to nail**
    - **S61.305 Unspecified open wound of left ring finger with damage to nail**
    - **S61.306 Unspecified open wound of right little finger with damage to nail**
    - **S61.307 Unspecified open wound of left little finger with damage to nail**
    - **S61.308 Unspecified open wound of other finger with damage to nail**
      Unspecified open wound of specified finger with unspecified laterality with damage to nail
    - **S61.309 Unspecified open wound of unspecified finger with damage to nail**
  - **S61.31 Laceration without foreign body of finger with damage to nail**
    - **S61.310 Laceration without foreign body of right index finger with damage to nail**
    - **S61.311 Laceration without foreign body of left index finger with damage to nail**
    - **S61.312 Laceration without foreign body of right middle finger with damage to nail**
    - **S61.313 Laceration without foreign body of left middle finger with damage to nail**
    - **S61.314 Laceration without foreign body of right ring finger with damage to nail**
    - **S61.315 Laceration without foreign body of left ring finger with damage to nail**
    - **S61.316 Laceration without foreign body of right little finger with damage to nail**
    - **S61.317 Laceration without foreign body of left little finger with damage to nail**
    - **S61.318 Laceration without foreign body of other finger with damage to nail**
      Laceration without foreign body of specified finger with unspecified laterality with damage to nail
    - **S61.319 Laceration without foreign body of unspecified finger with damage to nail**
  - **S61.32 Laceration with foreign body of finger with damage to nail**
    - **S61.320 Laceration with foreign body of right index finger with damage to nail**
    - **S61.321 Laceration with foreign body of left index finger with damage to nail**
    - **S61.322 Laceration with foreign body of right middle finger with damage to nail**
    - **S61.323 Laceration with foreign body of left middle finger with damage to nail**
    - **S61.324 Laceration with foreign body of right ring finger with damage to nail**
    - **S61.325 Laceration with foreign body of left ring finger with damage to nail**
    - **S61.326 Laceration with foreign body of right little finger with damage to nail**
    - **S61.327 Laceration with foreign body of left little finger with damage to nail**
    - **S61.328 Laceration with foreign body of other finger with damage to nail**
      Laceration with foreign body of specified finger with unspecified laterality with damage to nail
    - **S61.329 Laceration with foreign body of unspecified finger with damage to nail**

- S61.33 Puncture wound without foreign body of finger with damage to nail
  - S61.330 Puncture wound without foreign body of right index finger with damage to nail
  - S61.331 Puncture wound without foreign body of left index finger with damage to nail
  - S61.332 Puncture wound without foreign body of right middle finger with damage to nail
  - S61.333 Puncture wound without foreign body of left middle finger with damage to nail
  - S61.334 Puncture wound without foreign body of right ring finger with damage to nail
  - S61.335 Puncture wound without foreign body of left ring finger with damage to nail
  - S61.336 Puncture wound without foreign body of right little finger with damage to nail
  - S61.337 Puncture wound without foreign body of left little finger with damage to nail
  - S61.338 Puncture wound without foreign body of other finger with damage to nail
    Puncture wound without foreign body of specified finger with unspecified laterality with damage to nail
  - S61.339 Puncture wound without foreign body of unspecified finger with damage to nail
- S61.34 Puncture wound with foreign body of finger with damage to nail
  - S61.340 Puncture wound with foreign body of right index finger with damage to nail
  - S61.341 Puncture wound with foreign body of left index finger with damage to nail
  - S61.342 Puncture wound with foreign body of right middle finger with damage to nail
  - S61.343 Puncture wound with foreign body of left middle finger with damage to nail
  - S61.344 Puncture wound with foreign body of right ring finger with damage to nail
  - S61.345 Puncture wound with foreign body of left ring finger with damage to nail
  - S61.346 Puncture wound with foreign body of right little finger with damage to nail
  - S61.347 Puncture wound with foreign body of left little finger with damage to nail
  - S61.348 Puncture wound with foreign body of other finger with damage to nail
    Puncture wound with foreign body of specified finger with unspecified laterality with damage to nail
  - S61.349 Puncture wound with foreign body of unspecified finger with damage to nail
- S61.35 Open bite of finger with damage to nail
  Bite of finger with damage to nail NOS
  Excludes1 superficial bite of finger (S60.46-, S60.47-)
  - S61.350 Open bite of right index finger with damage to nail
  - S61.351 Open bite of left index finger with damage to nail
  - S61.352 Open bite of right middle finger with damage to nail
  - S61.353 Open bite of left middle finger with damage to nail
  - S61.354 Open bite of right ring finger with damage to nail
  - S61.355 Open bite of left ring finger with damage to nail
  - S61.356 Open bite of right little finger with damage to nail
  - S61.357 Open bite of left little finger with damage to nail
  - S61.358 Open bite of other finger with damage to nail
    Open bite of specified finger with unspecified laterality with damage to nail
  - S61.359 Open bite of unspecified finger with damage to nail
- S61.4 Open wound of hand
  - S61.40 Unspecified open wound of hand
    - S61.401 Unspecified open wound of right hand
    - S61.402 Unspecified open wound of left hand
    - S61.409 Unspecified open wound of unspecified hand
  - S61.41 Laceration without foreign body of hand
    - S61.411 Laceration without foreign body of right hand
    - S61.412 Laceration without foreign body of left hand
    - S61.419 Laceration without foreign body of unspecified hand
  - S61.42 Laceration with foreign body of hand
    - S61.421 Laceration with foreign body of right hand
    - S61.422 Laceration with foreign body of left hand
    - S61.429 Laceration with foreign body of unspecified hand
  - S61.43 Puncture wound without foreign body of hand
    - S61.431 Puncture wound without foreign body of right hand
    - S61.432 Puncture wound without foreign body of left hand
    - S61.439 Puncture wound without foreign body of unspecified hand
  - S61.44 Puncture wound with foreign body of hand
    - S61.441 Puncture wound with foreign body of right hand
    - S61.442 Puncture wound with foreign body of left hand
    - S61.449 Puncture wound with foreign body of unspecified hand
  - S61.45 Open bite of hand
    Bite of hand NOS
    Excludes1 superficial bite of hand (S60.56-, S60.57-)
    - S61.451 Open bite of right hand
    - S61.452 Open bite of left hand
    - S61.459 Open bite of unspecified hand
- S61.5 Open wound of wrist
  - S61.50 Unspecified open wound of wrist
    - S61.501 Unspecified open wound of right wrist
    - S61.502 Unspecified open wound of left wrist
    - S61.509 Unspecified open wound of unspecified wrist

- **S80.25 Superficial foreign body of knee**
  Splinter in the knee
  - **S80.251 Superficial foreign body, right knee**
  - **S80.252 Superficial foreign body, left knee**
  - **S80.259 Superficial foreign body, unspecified knee**
- **S80.26 Insect bite (nonvenomous) of knee**
  - **S80.261 Insect bite (nonvenomous), right knee**
  - **S80.262 Insect bite (nonvenomous), left knee**
  - **S80.269 Insect bite (nonvenomous), unspecified knee**
- **S80.27 Other superficial bite of knee**
  Excludes1 open bite of knee (S81.05-)
  - **S80.271 Other superficial bite of right knee**
  - **S80.272 Other superficial bite of left knee**
  - **S80.279 Other superficial bite of unspecified knee**

- **S80.8 Other superficial injuries of lower leg**
  - **S80.81 Abrasion of lower leg**
    - **S80.811 Abrasion, right lower leg**
    - **S80.812 Abrasion, left lower leg**
    - **S80.819 Abrasion, unspecified lower leg**
  - **S80.82 Blister (nonthermal) of lower leg**
    - **S80.821 Blister (nonthermal), right lower leg**
    - **S80.822 Blister (nonthermal), left lower leg**
    - **S80.829 Blister (nonthermal), unspecified lower leg**
  - **S80.84 External constriction of lower leg**
    - **S80.841 External constriction, right lower leg**
    - **S80.842 External constriction, left lower leg**
    - **S80.849 External constriction, unspecified lower leg**
  - **S80.85 Superficial foreign body of lower leg**
    Splinter in the lower leg
    - **S80.851 Superficial foreign body, right lower leg**
    - **S80.852 Superficial foreign body, left lower leg**
    - **S80.859 Superficial foreign body, unspecified lower leg**
  - **S80.86 Insect bite (nonvenomous) of lower leg**
    - **S80.861 Insect bite (nonvenomous), right lower leg**
    - **S80.862 Insect bite (nonvenomous), left lower leg**
    - **S80.869 Insect bite (nonvenomous), unspecified lower leg**
  - **S80.87 Other superficial bite of lower leg**
    Excludes1 open bite of lower leg (S81.85-)
    - **S80.871 Other superficial bite, right lower leg**
    - **S80.872 Other superficial bite, left lower leg**
    - **S80.879 Other superficial bite, unspecified lower leg**
- **S80.9 Unspecified superficial injury of knee and lower leg**
  - **S80.91 Unspecified superficial injury of knee**
    - **S80.911 Unspecified superficial injury of right knee**
    - **S80.912 Unspecified superficial injury of left knee**
    - **S80.919 Unspecified superficial injury of unspecified knee**
  - **S80.92 Unspecified superficial injury of lower leg**
    - **S80.921 Unspecified superficial injury of right lower leg**
    - **S80.922 Unspecified superficial injury of left lower leg**
    - **S80.929 Unspecified superficial injury of unspecified lower leg**

- **S81 Open wound of knee and lower leg**
  Code also any associated wound infection
  Excludes1 open fracture of knee and lower leg (S82.-)
  traumatic amputation of lower leg (S88.-)
  Excludes2 open wound of ankle and foot (S91.-)
  The appropriate 7th character is to be added to each code from category S81

A	initial encounter
D	subsequent encounter
S	sequela

  - **S81.0 Open wound of knee**
    - **S81.00 Unspecified open wound of knee**
      - **S81.001 Unspecified open wound, right knee**
      - **S81.002 Unspecified open wound, left knee**
      - **S81.009 Unspecified open wound, unspecified knee**
    - **S81.01 Laceration without foreign body of knee**
      - **S81.011 Laceration without foreign body, right knee**
      - **S81.012 Laceration without foreign body, left knee**
      - **S81.019 Laceration without foreign body, unspecified knee**
    - **S81.02 Laceration with foreign body of knee**
      - **S81.021 Laceration with foreign body, right knee**
      - **S81.022 Laceration with foreign body, left knee**
      - **S81.029 Laceration with foreign body, unspecified knee**
    - **S81.03 Puncture wound without foreign body of knee**
      - **S81.031 Puncture wound without foreign body, right knee**
      - **S81.032 Puncture wound without foreign body, left knee**
      - **S81.039 Puncture wound without foreign body, unspecified knee**
    - **S81.04 Puncture wound with foreign body of knee**
      - **S81.041 Puncture wound with foreign body, right knee**
      - **S81.042 Puncture wound with foreign body, left knee**
      - **S81.049 Puncture wound with foreign body, unspecified knee**
    - **S81.05 Open bite of knee**
      Bite of knee NOS
      Excludes1 superficial bite of knee (S80.27-)
      - **S81.051 Open bite, right knee**
      - **S81.052 Open bite, left knee**
      - **S81.059 Open bite, unspecified knee**

S81.8 Open wound of lower leg

S81.80 Unspecified open wound of lower leg

S81.801 Unspecified open wound, right lower leg

S81.802 Unspecified open wound, left lower leg

S81.809 Unspecified open wound, unspecified lower leg

S81.81 Laceration without foreign body of lower leg

S81.811 Laceration without foreign body, right lower leg

S81.812 Laceration without foreign body, left lower leg

S81.819 Laceration without foreign body, unspecified lower leg

S81.82 Laceration with foreign body of lower leg

S81.821 Laceration with foreign body, right lower leg

S81.822 Laceration with foreign body, left lower leg

S81.829 Laceration with foreign body, unspecified lower leg

S81.83 Puncture wound without foreign body of lower leg

S81.831 Puncture wound without foreign body, right lower leg

S81.832 Puncture wound without foreign body, left lower leg

S81.839 Puncture wound without foreign body, unspecified lower leg

S81.84 Puncture wound with foreign body of lower leg

S81.841 Puncture wound with foreign body, right lower leg

S81.842 Puncture wound with foreign body, left lower leg

S81.849 Puncture wound with foreign body, unspecified lower leg

S81.85 Open bite of lower leg

Bite of lower leg NOS

Excludes1 superficial bite of lower leg (S80.86-, S80.87-)

S81.851 Open bite, right lower leg

S81.852 Open bite, left lower leg

S81.859 Open bite, unspecified lower leg

S82 Fracture of lower leg, including ankle

Note: A fracture not indicated as displaced or nondisplaced should be coded to displaced

A fracture not indicated as open or closed should be coded to closed

The open fracture designations are based on the Gustilo open fracture classification

Includes fracture of malleolus

Excludes1 traumatic amputation of lower leg (S88.-)

Excludes2 fracture of foot, except ankle (S92.-)
periprosthetic fracture of prosthetic implant of knee (T84.042, T84.043)

The appropriate 7th character is to be added to all codes from category S82

A	initial encounter for closed fracture
B	initial encounter for open fracture type I or II initial encounter for open fracture NOS
C	initial encounter for open fracture type IIIA, IIIB, or IIIC
D	subsequent encounter for closed fracture with routine healing
E	subsequent encounter for open fracture type I or II with routine healing
F	subsequent encounter for open fracture type IIIA, IIIB, or IIIC with routine healing
G	subsequent encounter for closed fracture with delayed healing
H	subsequent encounter for open fracture type I or II with delayed healing
J	subsequent encounter for open fracture type IIIA, IIIB, or IIIC with delayed healing
K	subsequent encounter for closed fracture with nonunion
M	subsequent encounter for open fracture type I or II with nonunion
N	subsequent encounter for open fracture type IIIA, IIIB, or IIIC with nonunion
P	subsequent encounter for closed fracture with malunion
Q	subsequent encounter for open fracture type I or II with malunion
R	subsequent encounter for open fracture type IIIA, IIIB, or IIIC with malunion
S	sequela

S82.0 Fracture of patella

Knee cap

S82.00 Unspecified fracture of patella

S82.001 Unspecified fracture of right patella

A, B, C,K,M, N, P, Q, R, A, B, C

Ex **For S82.001[A]:** S82.001-S82.099[A,B,C]
For S82.001[B,C]: M80.00X-M80.019[A], M80.041-M80.049[A], M80.80X-M80.819[A], M80.841-M80.849[A], M84.40X-M84.419[A], M84.441-M84.446[A], M84.454[A], M84.474-M84.519[A], M84.541-M84.550[A], M84.574-M84.576[A], M84.60X-M84.619[A], M84.641-M84.650[A], M84.674-M84.68X[A], S03.8XX-S03.9XX[A], S29.011-S29.019[A], S38.3XX[A], S39.011-S39.013[A], S73.101-S73.199[A], S76.001-S76.019[A], S76.091-S76.119[A], S76.191-S76.219[A], S76.291-S76.319[A], S76.391-S76.819[A], S76.891-S76.919[A], S76.991-S76.999[A], S79.811-S79.929[A], S82.001-S82.099[B,C], S82.101-S82.156[A,B,C], S82.191-S82.299[A,B,C], S82.401-S82.499[A,B,C], S82.831-S82.839[A,B,C], S82.861-S82.866[A,B,C], S82.90X-S82.92X[A,B,C], S89.001-S89.099[A], S89.201-S89.299[A], T14.90-T14.91, T79.8XX-T79.9XX[A], T79.A9X[A]
For S82.001[K,M,N,P,Q,R]: See S02.0[K]

- **S82.002** Unspecified fracture of left patella
  A, B, C,K,M, N, P, Q, R, A, B, C
  Ex: **For S82.002[A]:** S82.001[B,C], S82.002-S82.009[A,B,C], S82.011[B,C], S82.012-S82.013[A,B,C], S82.014-S82.021[B,C], S82.022-S82.023[A,B,C], S82.024[B,C], S82.025-S82.026[A,B,C], S82.031-S82.033[A,B,C], S82.034[B,C], S82.035-S82.036[A,B,C], S82.041[B,C], S82.042-S82.043[A,B,C], S82.044[B,C], S82.045-S82.046[A,B,C], S82.091[B,C], S82.092-S82.099[A,B,C]
  For S82.002[B,C]: See S82.001[B,C]
  For S82.002[K,M,N,P,Q,R]: See S02.0[K]
- **S82.009** Unspecified fracture of unspecified patella A, B, C,K,M, N, P, Q, R, A, B, C
  Ex: **For S82.009[A]:** S82.001-S82.099[A,B,C]
  For S82.009[B,C]: See S82.001[B,C]
  For S82.009[K,M,N,P,Q,R]: See S02.0[K]
- **S82.01** Osteochondral fracture of patella
  - **S82.011** Displaced osteochondral fracture of right patella
    A, B, C,K,M, N, P, Q, R, A, B, C
    Ex: **For S82.011[A]:** See S82.001[A]
    For S82.011[B,C]: See S82.001[B,C]
    For S82.011[K,M,N,P,Q,R]: See S02.0[K]
  - **S82.012** Displaced osteochondral fracture of left patella A, B, C,K,M, N, P, Q, R, A, B, C
    Ex: **For S82.012[A]:** See S82.002[A]
    For S82.012[B,C]: See S82.001[B,C]
    For S82.012[K,M,N,P,Q,R]: See S02.0[K]
  - **S82.013** Displaced osteochondral fracture of unspecified patella
    A, B, C,K,M, N, P, Q, R, A, B, C
    Ex: **For S82.013[A]:** See S82.003
    For S82.013[B,C]: See S82.001[B,C]
    For S82.013[K,M,N,P,Q,R]: See S02.0[K]
  - **S82.014** Nondisplaced osteochondral fracture of right patella A, B, C,K,M, N, P, Q, R, A, B, C
    Ex: **For S82.014[A]:** See S82.001[A]
    For S82.014[B,C]: See S82.001[B,C]
    For S82.014[K,M,N,P,Q,R]: See S02.0[K]
  - **S82.015** Nondisplaced osteochondral fracture of left patella A, B, C,K,M, N, P, Q, R, A, B, C
    Ex: **For S82.015[A]:** See S82.002[A]
    For S82.015[B,C]: See S82.001[B,C]
    For S82.015[K,M,N,P,Q,R]: See S02.0[K]
  - **S82.016** Nondisplaced osteochondral fracture of unspecified patella A, B, C,K,M, N, P, Q, R, A, B, C
    Ex: **For S82.016[A]:** S82.001-S82.099[A,B,C]
    For S82.016[B,C]: See S82.001[B,C]
    For S82.016[K,M,N,P,Q,R]: See S02.0[K]
- **S82.02** Longitudinal fracture of patella
  - **S82.021** Displaced longitudinal fracture of right patella A, B, C,K,M, N, P, Q, R, A, B, C
    Ex: **For S82.021[A]:** See S82.001[A]
    For S82.021[B,C]: See S82.001[B,C]
    For S82.021[K,M,N,P,Q,R]: See S02.0[K]
  - **S82.022** Displaced longitudinal fracture of left patella A, B, C,K,M, N, P, Q, R, A, B, C
    Ex: **For S82.022[A]:** See S82.002[A]
    For S82.022[B,C]: See S82.001[B,C]
    For S82.022[K,M,N,P,Q,R]: See S02.0[K]
  - **S82.023** Displaced longitudinal fracture of unspecified patella A, B, C,K,M, N, P, Q, R, A, B, C
    Ex: **For S82.023[A]:** S82.001-S82.099[A,B,C]
    For S82.023[B,C]: See S82.001[B,C]
    For S82.023[K,M,N,P,Q,R]: See S02.0[K]
  - **S82.024** Nondisplaced longitudinal fracture of right patella A, B, C,K,M, N, P, Q, R, A, B, C
    Ex: **For S82.024[A]:** See S82.001[A]
    For S82.024[B,C]: See S82.001[B,C]
    For S82.024[K,M,N,P,Q,R]: See S02.0[K]
  - **S82.025** Nondisplaced longitudinal fracture of left patella A, B, C,K,M, N, P, Q, R, A, B, C
    Ex: **For S82.025[A]:** See S82.002[A]
    For S82.025[B,C]: See S82.001[B,C]
    For S82.025[K,M,N,P,Q,R]: See S02.0[K]
  - **S82.026** Nondisplaced longitudinal fracture of unspecified patella A, B, C,K,M, N, P, Q, R, A, B, C
    Ex: **For S82.026[A]:** S82.001-S82.099[A,B,C]
    For S82.026[B,C]: See S82.001[B,C]
    For S82.026[K,M,N,P,Q,R]: See S02.0[K]
- **S82.03** Transverse fracture of patella
  - **S82.031** Displaced transverse fracture of right patella A, B, C,K,M, N, P, Q, R, A, B, C
    Ex: **For S82.031[A]:** See S82.001[A]
    For S82.031[B,C]: See S82.001[B,C]
    For S82.031[K,M,N,P,Q,R]: See S02.0[K]
  - **S82.032** Displaced transverse fracture of left patella A, B, C,K,M, N, P, Q, R, A, B, C
    Ex: **For S82.032[A]:** See S82.002[A]
    For S82.032[B,C]: See S82.001[B,C]
    For S82.032[K,M,N,P,Q,R]: See S02.0[K]
  - **S82.033** Displaced transverse fracture of unspecified patella A, B, C,K,M, N, P, Q, R, A, B, C
    Ex: **For S82.033[A]:** S82.001-S82.099[A,B,C]
    For S82.033[B,C]: See S82.001[B,C]
    For S82.033[K,M,N,P,Q,R]: See S02.0[K]
  - **S82.034** Nondisplaced transverse fracture of right patella A, B, C,K,M, N, P, Q, R, A, B, C
    Ex: **For S82.034[A]:** See S82.001[A]
    For S82.034[B,C]: See S82.001[B,C]
    For S82.034[K,M,N,P,Q,R]: See S02.0[K]
  - **S82.035** Nondisplaced transverse fracture of left patella A, B, C,K,M, N, P, Q, R, A, B, C
    Ex: **For S82.035[A]:** See S82.002[A]
    For S82.035[B,C]: See S82.001[B,C]
    For S82.035[K,M,N,P,Q,R]: See S02.0[K]
  - **S82.036** Nondisplaced transverse fracture of unspecified patella A, B, C,K,M, N, P, Q, R, A, B, C
    Ex: **For S82.036[A]:** S82.001-S82.099[A,B,C]
    For S82.036[B,C]: See S82.001[B,C]
    For S82.036[K,M,N,P,Q,R]: See S02.0[K]

S82.04 Comminuted fracture of patella

S82.041 Displaced comminuted fracture of right patella A, B, C,K,M, N, P, Q, R, A, B, C

Ex: **For S82.041[A]:** See S82.001[A]
For S82.041[B,C]: See S82.001[B,C]
For S82.041[K,M,N,P,Q,R]: See S02.0[K]

S82.042 Displaced comminuted fracture of left patella A, B, C,K,M, N, P, Q, R, A, B, C

Ex: **For S82.042[A]:** See S82.002[A]
For S82.042[B,C]: See S82.001[B,C]
For S82.042[K,M,N,P,Q,R]: See S02.0[K]

S82.043 Displaced comminuted fracture of unspecified patella A, B, C,K,M, N, P, Q, R, A, B, C

Ex: **For S82.043[A]:** S82.001-S82.099[A,B,C]
For S82.043[B,C]: See S82.001[B,C]
For S82.043[K,M,N,P,Q,R]: See S02.0[K]

S82.044 Nondisplaced comminuted fracture of right patella A, B, C,K,M, N, P, Q, R, A, B, C

Ex: **For S82.044[A]:** See S82.001[A]
For S82.044[B,C]: See S82.001[B,C]
For S82.044[K,M,N,P,Q,R]: See S02.0[K]

S82.045 Nondisplaced comminuted fracture of left patella A, B, C,K,M, N, P, Q, R, A, B, C

Ex: **For S82.045[A]:** See S82.002[A]
For S82.045[B,C]: See S82.001[B,C]
For S82.045[K,M,N,P,Q,R]: See S02.0[K]

S82.046 Nondisplaced comminuted fracture of unspecified patella A, B, C,K,M, N, P, Q, R, A, B, C

Ex: **For S82.046[A]:** S82.001-S82.099[A,B,C]
For S82.046[B,C]: See S82.001[B,C]
For S82.046[K,M,N,P,Q,R]: See S02.0[K]

S82.09 Other fracture of patella

S82.091 Other fracture of right patella A, B, C,K,M, N, P, Q, R, A, B, C

Ex: **For S82.091[A]:** See S82.001[A]
For S82.091[B,C]: See S82.001[B,C]
For S82.091[K,M,N,P,Q,R]: See S02.0[K]

S82.092 Other fracture of left patella A, B, C,K,M, N, P, Q, R, A, B, C

Ex: **For S82.092[A]:** See S82.002[A]
For S82.092[B,C]: See S82.001[B,C]
For S82.092[K,M,N,P,Q,R]: See S02.0[K]

S82.099 Other fracture of unspecified patella A, B, C,K,M, N, P, Q, R, A, B, C

Ex: **For S82.099[A]:** S82.001-S82.099[A,B,C]
For S82.099[B,C]: See S82.001[B,C]
For S82.099[K,M,N,P,Q,R]: See S02.0[K]

S82.1 Fracture of upper end of tibia

Fracture of proximal end of tibia

Excludes2 fracture of shaft of tibia (S82.2-)
physeal fracture of upper end of tibia (S89.0-)

S82.10 Unspecified fracture of upper end of tibia

S82.101 Unspecified fracture of upper end of right tibia A, K, M, N, P, Q, R, B, C, A, B, C

Ex: **For S82.101[A]:** M80.00X-M80.019[A], M80.041-M80.049[A], M80.061-M80.819[A], M80.841-M80.849[A], M80.861-M80.879[A], M84.40X-M84.419[A], M84.441-M84.446[A], M84.454[A], M84.461-M84.519[A], M84.541-M84.550[A], M84.561-M84.619[A], M84.641-M84.650[A], M84.661-M84.68X[A], S03.8XX-S03.9XX[A], S29.011-S29.019[A], S38.3XX[A], S39.011-S39.013[A], S73.101[A], S73.109-S73.111[A], S73.119-S73.121[A], S73.129-S73.191[A], S73.199[A], S76.001[A], S76.009-S76.011[A], S76.019[A], S76.091[A], S76.099-S76.101[A], S76.109-S76.111[A], S76.119[A], S76.191[A], S76.199-S76.201[A], S76.209-S76.211[A], S76.219[A], S76.291[A], S76.299-S76.301[A], S76.309-S76.311[A], S76.319[A], S76.391[A], S76.399-S76.801[A], S76.809-S76.811[A], S76.819[A], S76.891[A], S76.899-S76.901[A], S76.909-S76.911[A], S76.919[A], S76.991[A], S76.999[A], S79.811[A], S79.819-S79.821[A], S79.829[A], S79.911[A], S79.919-S79.921[A], S79.929[A], S82.101[A,B,C], S82.102[B,C], S82.109-S82.111[A,B,C], S82.112[B,C], S82.113-S82.114[A,B,C], S82.115[B,C], S82.116-S82.121[A,B,C], S82.122[B,C], S82.123-S82.124[A,B,C], S82.125[B,C], S82.126-S82.131[A,B,C], S82.132[B,C], S82.133-S82.134[A,B,C], S82.135[B,C], S82.136-S82.141[A,B,C], S82.142[B,C], S82.143-S82.144[A,B,C], S82.145[B,C], S82.146-S82.151[A,B,C], S82.152[B,C], S82.153-S82.154[A,B,C], S82.155[B,C], S82.156[A,B,C], S82.191[A,B,C], S82.192[B,C], S82.199-S82.201[A,B,C], S82.202[B,C], S82.209-S82.221[A,B,C], S82.222[B,C], S82.223-S82.224[A,B,C], S82.225[B,C], S82.226-S82.231[A,B,C], S82.232[B,C], S82.233-S82.234[A,B,C], S82.235[B,C], S82.236-S82.241[A,B,C], S82.242[B,C], S82.243-S82.244[A,B,C], S82.245[B,C], S82.246-S82.251[A,B,C], S82.252[B,C], S82.253-S82.254[A,B,C], S82.255[B,C], S82.256-S82.261[A,B,C], S82.262[B,C], S82.263-S82.264[A,B,C], S82.265[B,C], S82.266-S82.291[A,B,C], S82.292[B,C], S82.299[A,B,C], S82.401[A,B,C], S82.402[B,C], S82.409-S82.421[A,B,C], S82.422[B,C], S82.423-S82.424[A,B,C], S82.425[B,C], S82.426-S82.431[A,B,C], S82.432[B,C], S82.433-S82.434[A,B,C], S82.435[B,C], S82.436-S82.441[A,B,C], S82.442[B,C], S82.443-S82.444[A,B,C], S82.445[B,C], S82.446-S82.451[A,B,C], S82.452[B,C], S82.453-S82.454[A,B,C], S82.455[B,C], S82.456-S82.461[A,B,C], S82.462[B,C], S82.463-S82.464[A,B,C], S82.465[B,C], S82.466-S82.491[A,B,C], S82.492[B,C], S82.499[A,B,C], S82.831[A,B,C], S82.831-S82.832[B,C], S82.839[A,B,C], S82.861[A,B,C], S82.862[B,C], S82.863-S82.864[A,B,C], S82.865[B,C], S82.866[A,B,C], S82.90X-S82.92X[A,B,C], S89.001[A], S89.009-S89.011[A], S89.019-S89.021[A], S89.029-S89.031[A], S89.039-S89.041[A], S89.049-S89.091[A], S89.099[A], S89.201[A], S89.209-S89.211[A], S89.219-S89.221[A], S89.229-S89.291[A], S89.299[A], T14.90-T14.91, T79.8XX-T79.9XX[A], T79.A9X[A] **For S82.101[B,C]:** M80.00X-M80.019[A], M80.041-M80.049[A], M80.061-M80.819[A], M80.841-M80.849[A], M80.861-M80.879[A], M84.40X-M84.419[A], M84.441-M84.446[A], M84.454[A], M84.461-M84.519[A], M84.541-M84.550[A], M84.561-M84.619[A], M84.641-M84.650[A], M84.661-M84.68X[A], S03.8XX-S03.9XX[A], S29.011-S29.019[A], S38.3XX[A], S39.011-S39.013[A], S73.101-S73.199[A], S76.001-S76.019[A], S76.091-S76.119[A], S76.191-S76.219[A], S76.291-S76.319[A], S76.391-S76.819[A], S76.891-S76.919[A], S76.991-S76.999[A], S79.811-S79.929[A], S82.101-S82.156[A,B,C], S82.191-S82.299[A,B,C], S82.401-S82.499[A,B,C], S82.831-S82.839[A,B,C], S82.861-S82.866[A,B,C], S82.90X-S82.92X[A,B,C], S89.001-S89.099[A], S89.201-S89.299[A], T14.90-T14.91, T79.8XX-T79.9XX[A], T79.A9X[A]
For S82.101[K,M,N,P,Q,R]: See S02.0[K]

● **S82.102** **Unspecified fracture of upper end of left tibia** A, K, M, N, P, Q, R CC, B, C MCC, A, B, C HAC

Ex: **For S82.102[A]:** M80.00X-M80.019[A], M80.041-M80.049[A], M80.061-M80.819[A], M80.841-M80.849[A], M80.861-M80.879[A], M84.40X-M84.419[A], M84.441-M84.446[A], M84.454[A], M84.461-M84.519[A], M84.541-M84.550[A], M84.561-M84.619[A], M84.641-M84.650[A], M84.661-M84.68X[A], S03.8XX-S03.9XX[A], S29.011-S29.019[A], S38.3XX[A], S39.011-S39.013[A], S73.102-S73.109[A], S73.112-S73.119[A], S73.122-S73.129[A], S73.192-S73.199[A], S76.002-S76.009[A], S76.012-S76.019[A], S76.092-S76.099[A], S76.102-S76.109[A], S76.112-S76.119[A], S76.192-S76.199[A], S76.202-S76.209[A], S76.212-S76.219[A], S76.292-S76.299[A], S76.302-S76.309[A], S76.312-S76.319[A], S76.392-S76.399[A], S76.802-S76.809[A], S76.812-S76.819[A], S76.892-S76.899[A], S76.902-S76.909[A], S76.912-S76.919[A], S76.992-S76.999[A], S79.812-S79.819[A], S79.822-S79.829[A], S79.912-S79.919[A], S79.922-S79.929[A], S82.101[B,C], S82.102-S82.109[A,B,C], S82.111[B,C], S82.112-S82.113[A,B,C], S82.114[B,C], S82.115-S82.116[A,B,C], S82.121[B,C], S82.122-S82.123[A,B,C], S82.124[B,C], S82.125-S82.126[A,B,C], S82.131[B,C], S82.132-S82.133[A,B,C], S82.134[B,C], S82.135-S82.136[A,B,C], S82.141[B,C], S82.142-S82.143[A,B,C], S82.144[B,C], S82.145-S82.146[A,B,C], S82.151[B,C], S82.152-S82.153[A,B,C], S82.154[B,C], S82.155-S82.156[A,B,C], S82.191[B,C], S82.192-S82.199[A,B,C], S82.201[B,C], S82.202-S82.209[A,B,C], S82.221[B,C], S82.222-S82.223[A,B,C], S82.224[B,C], S82.225-S82.226[A,B,C], S82.231[B,C], S82.232-S82.233[A,B,C], S82.234[B,C], S82.235-S82.236[A,B,C], S82.241[B,C], S82.242-S82.243[A,B,C], S82.244[B,C], S82.245-S82.246[A,B,C], S82.251[B,C], S82.252-S82.253[A,B,C], S82.254[B,C], S82.255-S82.256[A,B,C], S82.261[B,C], S82.262-S82.263[A,B,C], S82.264[B,C], S82.265-S82.266[A,B,C], S82.291[B,C], S82.292-S82.299[A,B,C], S82.401[B,C], S82.402-S82.409[A,B,C], S82.421[B,C], S82.422-S82.423[A,B,C], S82.424[B,C], S82.425-S82.426[A,B,C], S82.431[B,C], S82.432-S82.433[A,B,C], S82.434[B,C], S82.435-S82.436[A,B,C], S82.441[B,C], S82.442-S82.443[A,B,C], S82.444[B,C], S82.445-S82.446[A,B,C], S82.451[B,C], S82.452-S82.453[A,B,C], S82.454[B,C], S82.455-S82.456[A,B,C], S82.461[B,C], S82.462-S82.463[A,B,C], S82.464[B,C], S82.465-S82.466[A,B,C], S82.491[B,C], S82.492-S82.499[A,B,C], S82.831[B,C], S82.832-S82.839[A,B,C], S82.861[B,C], S82.862-S82.863[A,B,C], S82.864[B,C], S82.865-S82.866[A,B,C], S82.90X-S82.92X[A,B,C], S89.002-S89.009[A], S89.012-S89.019[A], S89.022-S89.029[A], S89.032-S89.039[A], S89.042-S89.049[A], S89.092-S89.099[A], S89.202-S89.209[A], S89.212-S89.219[A], S89.222-S89.229[A], S89.292-S89.299[A], T14.90-T14.91, T79.8XX-T79.9XX[A], T79.A9X[A]

For S82.102[B,C]: See S82.101[B,C]

For S82.102[K,M,N,P,Q,R]: See S02.0[K]

● **S82.109** **Unspecified fracture of upper end of unspecified tibia** A, K, M, N, P, Q, R CC, B, C MCC, A, B, C HAC

Ex: **For S82.109[A,B,C]:** See S82.101[B,C]

For S82.109[K,M,N,P,Q,R]: See S02.0[K]

● **S82.11** **Fracture of tibial spine**

● **S82.111** **Displaced fracture of right tibial spine** A, K, M, N, P, Q, R CC, B, C MCC, A, B, C HAC

Ex: **For S82.111[A]:** See S82.101[A]

For S82.111[B,C]: See S82.101[B,C]

For S82.111[K,M,N,P,Q,R]: See S02.0[K]

● **S82.112** **Displaced fracture of left tibial spine** A, K, M, N, P, Q, R CC, B, C MCC, A, B, C HAC

Ex: **For S82.112[A]:** See S82.102[A]

For S82.112[B,C]: See S82.101[B,C]

For S82.112[K,M,N,P,Q,R]: See S02.0[K]

● **S82.113** **Displaced fracture of unspecified tibial spine** A, K, M, N, P, Q, R CC, B, C MCC, A, B, C HAC

Ex: **For S82.113 [A,B,C]:** See S82.101[B,C]

For S82.113[K,M,N,P,Q,R]: See S02.0[K]

● **S82.114** **Nondisplaced fracture of right tibial spine** A, K, M, N, P, Q, R CC, B, C MCC, A, B, C HAC

Ex: **For S82.114[A]:** See S82.101[A]

For S82.114[B,C]: See S82.101[B,C]

For S82.114[K,M,N,P,Q,R]: See S02.0[K]

● **S82.115** **Nondisplaced fracture of left tibial spine** A, K, M, N, P, Q, R CC, B, C MCC, A, B, C HAC

Ex: **For S82.115[A]:** See S82.102[A]

For S82.115[B,C]: See S82.101[B,C]

For S82.115[K,M,N,P,Q,R]: See S02.0[K]

● **S82.116** **Nondisplaced fracture of unspecified tibial spine** A, K, M, N, P, Q, R CC, B, C MCC, A, B, C HAC

Ex: **For S82.116[A,B,C]:** See S82.101[B,C]

For S82.116[K,M,N,P,Q,R]: See S02.0[K]

● **S82.12** **Fracture of lateral condyle of tibia**

● **S82.121** **Displaced fracture of lateral condyle of right tibia** A, K, M, N, P, Q, R CC, B, C MCC, A, B, C HAC

Ex: **For S82.121[A]:** See S82.101[A]

For S82.121[B,C]: See S82.101[B,C]

For S82.121[K,M,N,P,Q,R]: See S02.0[K]

● **S82.122** **Displaced fracture of lateral condyle of left tibia** A, K, M, N, P, Q, R CC, B, C MCC, A, B, C HAC

Ex: **For S82.122[A]:** See S82.102[A]

For S82.122[B,C]: See S82.101[B,C]

For S82.122[K,M,N,P,Q,R]: See S02.0[K]

● **S82.123** **Displaced fracture of lateral condyle of unspecified tibia** A, K, M, N, P, Q, R CC, B, C MCC, A, B, C HAC

Ex: **For S82.123[A,B,C]:** See S82.101[B,C]

For S82.123[K,M,N,P,Q,R]: See S02.0[K]

● **S82.124** **Nondisplaced fracture of lateral condyle of right tibia** A, K, M, N, P, Q, R CC, B, C MCC, A, B, C HAC

Ex: **For S82.124[A]:** See S82.101[A]

For S82.124[B,C]: See S82.101[B,C]

For S82.124[K,M,N,P,Q,R]: See S02.0[K]

● **S82.125** **Nondisplaced fracture of lateral condyle of left tibia** A, K, M, N, P, Q, R CC, B, C MCC, A, B, C HAC

Ex: **For S82.125[A]:** See S82.102[A]

For S82.125[B,C]: See S82.101[B,C]

For S82.125[K,M,N,P,Q,R]: See S02.0[K]

● **S82.126** **Nondisplaced fracture of lateral condyle of unspecified tibia** A, K, M, N, P, Q, R CC, B, C MCC, A, B, C HAC

Ex: **For S82.126[A,B,C]:** See S82.101[B,C]

For S82.126[K,M,N,P,Q,R]: See S02.0[K]

- **S82.13 Fracture of medial condyle of tibia**
  - **S82.131 Displaced fracture of medial condyle of right tibia** A, K, M, N, P, Q, R, **B, C**, A, B, C
    - Ex: **For S82.131[A]:** See S82.101[A]
      For S82.131[B,C]: See S82.101[B,C]
      For S82.131[K,M,N,P,Q,R]: See S02.0[K]
  - **S82.132 Displaced fracture of medial condyle of left tibia** A, K, M, N, P, Q, R, **B, C**, A, B, C
    - Ex: **For S82.132[A]:** See S82.102[A]
      For S82.132[B,C]: See S82.101[B,C]
      For S82.132[K,M,N,P,Q,R]: See S02.0[K]
  - **S82.133 Displaced fracture of medial condyle of unspecified tibia** A, K, M, N, P, Q, R, **B, C**, A, B, C
    - Ex: **For S82.133[A,B,C]:** See S82.101[B,C]
      For S82.133[K,M,N,P,Q,R]: See S02.0[K]
  - **S82.134 Nondisplaced fracture of medial condyle of right tibia** A, K, M, N, P, Q, R, **B, C**, A, B, C
    - Ex: **For S82.134[A]:** See S82.101[A]
      For S82.134[B,C]: See S82.101[B,C]
      For S82.134[K,M,N,P,Q,R]: See S02.0[K]
  - **S82.135 Nondisplaced fracture of medial condyle of left tibia** A, K, M, N, P, Q, R, **B, C**, A, B, C
    - Ex: **For S82.135[A]:** See S82.102[A]
      For S82.135[B,C]: See S82.101[B,C]
      For S82.135[K,M,N,P,Q,R]: See S02.0[K]
  - **S82.136 Nondisplaced fracture of medial condyle of unspecified tibia** A, K, M, N, P, Q, R, **B, C**, A, B, C
    - Ex: **For S82.136[A,B,C]:** See S82.101[B,C]
      For S82.136[K,M,N,P,Q,R]: See S02.0[K]
- **S82.14 Bicondylar fracture of tibia**
  Fracture of tibial plateau NOS
  - **S82.141 Displaced bicondylar fracture of right tibia** A, K, M, N, P, Q, R, **B, C**, A, B, C
    - Ex: **For S82.141[A]:** See S82.101[A]
      For S82.141[B,C]: See S82.101[B,C]
      For S82.141[K,M,N,P,Q,R]: See S02.0[K]
  - **S82.142 Displaced bicondylar fracture of left tibia** A, K, M, N, P, Q, R, **B, C**, A, B, C
    - Ex: **For S82.142[A]:** See S82.102[A]
      For S82.142[B,C]: See S82.101[B,C]
      For S82.142[K,M,N,P,Q,R]: See S02.0[K]
  - **S82.143 Displaced bicondylar fracture of unspecified tibia** A, K, M, N, P, Q, R, **B, C**, A, B, C
    - Ex: **For S82.143[A,B,C]:** See S82.101[B,C]
      For S82.143[K,M,N,P,Q,R]: See S02.0[K]
  - **S82.144 Nondisplaced bicondylar fracture of right tibia** A, K, M, N, P, Q, R, **B, C**, A, B, C
    - Ex: **For S82.144[A]:** See S82.101[A]
      For S82.144[B,C]: See S82.101[B,C]
      For S82.144[K,M,N,P,Q,R]: See S02.0[K]
  - **S82.145 Nondisplaced bicondylar fracture of left tibia** A, K, M, N, P, Q, R, **B, C**, A, B, C
    - Ex: **For S82.145[A]:** See S82.102[A]
      For S82.145[B,C]: See S82.101[B,C]
      For S82.145[K,M,N,P,Q,R]: See S02.0[K]
  - **S82.146 Nondisplaced bicondylar fracture of unspecified tibia** A, K, M, N, P, Q, R, **B, C**, A, B, C
    - Ex: **For S82.146[A,B,C]:** See S82.101[B,C]
      For S82.146[K,M,N,P,Q,R]: See S02.0[K]
- **S82.15 Fracture of tibial tuberosity**
  - **S82.151 Displaced fracture of right tibial tuberosity** A, K, M, N, P, Q, R, **B, C**, A, B, C
    - Ex: **For S82.151[A]:** See S82.101[A]
      For S82.151[B,C]: See S82.101[B,C]
      For S82.151[K,M,N,P,Q,R]: See S02.0[K]
  - **S82.152 Displaced fracture of left tibial tuberosity** A, K, M, N, P, Q, R, **B, C**, A, B, C
    - Ex: **For S82.152[A]:** See S82.102[A]
      For S82.152[B,C]: See S82.101[B,C]
      For S82.152[K,M,N,P,Q,R]: See S02.0[K]
  - **S82.153 Displaced fracture of unspecified tibial tuberosity** A, K, M, N, P, Q, R, **B, C**, A, B, C
    - Ex: **For S82.153[A,B,C]:** See S82.101[B,C]
      For S82.153[K,M,N,P,Q,R]: See S02.0[K]
  - **S82.154 Nondisplaced fracture of right tibial tuberosity** A, K, M, N, P, Q, R, **B, C**, A, B, C
    - Ex: **For S82.154[A]:** See S82.101[A]
      For S82.154[B,C]: See S82.101[B,C]
      For S82.154[K,M,N,P,Q,R]: See S02.0[K]
  - **S82.155 Nondisplaced fracture of left tibial tuberosity** A, K, M, N, P, Q, R, **B, C**, A, B, C
    - Ex: **For S82.155[A]:** See S82.102[A]
      For S82.155[B,C]: See S82.101[B,C]
      For S82.155[K,M,N,P,Q,R]: See S02.0[K]
  - **S82.156 Nondisplaced fracture of unspecified tibial tuberosity** A, K, M, N, P, Q, R, **B, C**, A, B, C
    - Ex: **For S82.156[A,B,C]:** See S82.101[B,C]
      For S82.156[K,M,N,P,Q,R]: See S02.0[K]

S82.16 Torus fracture of upper end of tibia

The appropriate 7th character is to be added to all codes in subcategory S82.16

A	initial encounter for closed fracture
D	subsequent encounter for fracture with routine healing
G	subsequent encounter for fracture with delayed healing
K	subsequent encounter for fracture with nonunion
P	subsequent encounter for fracture with malunion
S	sequela

S82.161 Torus fracture of upper end of right tibia A, K, P CC, A MCC

Ex **For S82.161[A]:** S82.101[A,B,C], S82.102[B,C], S82.109-S82.111[A,B,C], S82.112[A,B], S82.113-S82.114[A,B,C], S82.115[B,C], S82.116-S82.121[A,B,C], S82.122[B,C], S82.123-S82.124[A,B,C], S82.125[B,C], S82.126-S82.131[A,B,C], S82.132[B,C], S82.133-S82.134[A,B,C], S82.135[B,C], S82.136-S82.141[A,B,C], S82.142[B,C], S82.143-S82.144[A,B,C], S82.145[B,C], S82.146-S82.151[A,B,C], S82.152[B,C], S82.153-S82.154[A,B,C], S82.155[B,C], S82.156[A,B,C], S82.161[A], S82.169[A], S82.191[A,B,C], S82.192[B,C], S82.199-S82.201[A,B,C], S82.202[B,C], S82.209-S82.221[A,B,C], S82.222[B,C], S82.223-S82.224[A,B,C], S82.225[B,C], S82.226-S82.231[A,B,C], S82.232[B,C], S82.233-S82.234[A,B,C], S82.235[B,C], S82.236-S82.241[A,B,C], S82.242[B,C], S82.243-S82.244[A,B,C], S82.245[B,C], S82.246-S82.251[A,B,C], S82.252[B,C], S82.253-S82.254[A,B,C], S82.255[B.C], S82.256-S82.261[A,B,C], S82.262[B,C], S82.263-S82.264[A,B,C], S82.265[B,C], S82.266-S82.291[A,B,C], S82.292[B,C], S82.299[A,B,C], S82.311[A], S82.319[A], S82.401[A,B,C], S82.402[B,C], S82.409-S82.421[A,B,C], S82.422[B,C], S82.423-S82.424[A,B,C], S82.425[B,C], S82.426-S82.431[A,B,C], S82.432[B,C], S82.433-S82.434[A,B,C], S82.435[B,C], S82.436-S82.441[A,B,C], S82.442[B,C], S82.443-S82.444[A,B,C], S82.445[B,C], S82.446-S82.451[A,B,C], S82.452[B,C], S82.453-S82.454[A,B,C], S82.455[B,C], S82.456-S82.461[A,B,C], S82.462[B,C], S82.463-S82.464[A,B,C], S82.465[B,C], S82.466-S82.491[A,B,C], S82.492[B,C], S82.499[A,B,C], S82.811[A], S82.819-S82.821[A], S82.829[A], S82.831[A,B,C], S82.832[B,C], S82.839[A,B,C], S82.861[A,B,C], S82.862[B,C], S82.863-S82.864[A,B,C], S82.865[B,C], S82.866[A,B,C], S89.001[A], S89.009-S89.011[A], S89.019-S89.021[A], S89.029-S89.031[A], S89.039-S89.041[A], S89.049-S89.091[A], S89.099[A], S89.201[A], S89.209-S89.211[A], S89.219-S89.221[A], S89.229-S89.291[A], S89.299[A] **For S82.161[K,P]:** See S02.0[K]

S82.162 Torus fracture of upper end of left tibia A, K, P CC, A MCC

Ex **For S82.162[A]:** S82.101[B,C], S82.102-S82.109[A,B,C], S82.111[B,C], S82.112-S82.113[A,B,C], S82.114[B,C], S82.115-S82.116[A,B,C], S82.121[B,C], S82.122-S82.123[A,B,C], S82.124[B,C], S82.125-S82.126[A,B,C], S82.131[B,C], S82.132-S82.133[A,B,C], S82.134[B,C], S82.135-S82.136[A,B,C], S82.141[B,C], S82.142-S82.143[A,B,C], S82.144[B,C], S82.145-S82.146[A,B,C], S82.151[B,C], S82.152-S82.153[A,B,C], S82.154[B,C], S82.155-S82.156[A,B,C], S82.162-S82.169[A], S82.191[B,C], S82.192-S82.199[A,B,C], S82.201[B,C], S82.202-S82.209[A,B,C], S82.221[B,C], S82.222-S82.223[A,B,C], S82.224[B,C], S82.225-S82.226[A,B,C], S82.231[B,C], S82.232-S82.233[A,B,C], S82.234[B,C], S82.235-S82.236[A,B,C], S82.241[B,C], S82.242-S82.243[A,B,C], S82.244[B,C], S82.245-S82.246[A,B,C], S82.251[B,C], S82.252-S82.253[A,B,C], S82.254[B,C], S82.255-S82.256[A,B,C], S82.261[B,C], S82.262-S82.263[A,B.C], S82.264[B,C], S82.265-S82.266[A,B.C], S82.291[B,C], S82.292-S82.299[A,B,C], S82.312-S82.319[A], S82.401[B,C], S82.402-S82.409[A,B,C], S82.421[B,C], S82.422-S82.423[A,B,C], S82.424[B,C], S82.425-S82.426[A,B,C], S82.431[B,C], S82.432-S82.433[A,B,C], S82.434[B,C], S82.435-S82.436[A,B,C], S82.441[B,C], S82.442-S82.443[A,B,C], S82.444[B,C], S82.445-S82.446[A,B,C], S82.451[B,C], S82.452-S82.453[A,B,C], S82.454[B,C], S82.455-S82.456[A,B,C], S82.461[B,C], S82.462-S82.463[A,B,C], S82.464[B,C], S82.465-S82.466[A,B,C], S82.491[B,C], S82.492-S82.499[A,B,C], S82.812-S82.819[A], S82.822-S82.829[A], S82.831[B,C], S82.832-S82.839[A,B,C], S82.861[B,C], S82.862-S82.863[A,B,C], S82.864[B,C], S82.865-S82.866[A,B,C], S89.002-S89.009[A], S89.012-S89.019[A], S89.022-S89.029[A], S89.032-S89.039[A], S89.042-S89.049[A], S89.092-S89.099[A], S89.202-S89.209[A], S89.212-S89.219[A], S89.222-S89.229[A], S89.292-S89.299[A] **For S82.162[K,P]:** See S02.0[K]

S82.169 Torus fracture of upper end of unspecified tibia A, K, P CC, A MCC

Ex **For S82.169[A]:** S82.101-S82.156[A,B,C], S82.161-S82.169[A], S82.191-S82.299[A,B,C], S82.311-S82.319[A], S82.401-S82.499[A,B,C], S82.811-S82.829[A], S82.831-S82.839[A,B,C], S82.861-S82.866[A,B,C], S89.001-S89.099[A], S89.201-S89.299[A] **S82.169[K,P]:** See S02.0[K]

- **S82.19 Other fracture of upper end of tibia**
  - **S82.191 Other fracture of upper end of right tibia** A, K, M, N, P, Q, R, **B, C**, A, B, C
    - Ex: **For S82.191[A]:** See S82.101[A]
      For S82.191[B,C]: See S82.101[B,C]
      For S82.191[K,M,N,P,Q,R]: See S02.0[K]
  - **S82.192 Other fracture of upper end of left tibia** A, K, M, N, P, Q, R, **B, C**, A, B, C
    - Ex: **For S82.192[A]:** See S82.102[A]
      For S82.192[B,C]: See S82.101[B,C]
      For S82.192[K,M,N,P,Q,R]: See S02.0[K]
  - **S82.199 Other fracture of upper end of unspecified tibia** A, K, M, N, P, Q, R, **B, C**, A, B, C
    - Ex: **For S82.199[A,B,C]:** See S82.101[B,C]
      For S82.199[K,M,N,P,Q,R]: See S02.0[K]
- **S82.2 Fracture of shaft of tibia**
  - **S82.20 Unspecified fracture of shaft of tibia**
    Fracture of tibia NOS
    - **S82.201 Unspecified fracture of shaft of right tibia** A, K, M, N, P, Q, R, **B, C**, A, B, C
      - Ex: **For S82.201[A]:** M80.00X-M80.019[A], M80.041-M80.049[A], M80.061-M80.819[A], M80.841-M80.849[A], M80.861-M80.879[A], M84.40X-M84.419[A], M84.441-M84.446[A], M84.454[A], M84.461-M84.519[A], M84.541-M84.550[A], M84.561-M84.576[A], M84.60X-M84.619[A], M84.641-M84.650[A], M84.661-M84.68X[A], S03.8XX-S03.9XX[A], S29.011-S29.019[A], S38.3XX[A], S39.011-S39.013[A], S73.101[A], S73.109-S73.111[A], S73.119-S73.121[A], S73.129-S73.191[A], S73.199[A], S76.001[A], S76.009-S76.011[A], S76.019[A], S76.091[A], S76.099-S76.101[A], S76.109-S76.111[A], S76.119[A], S76.191[A], S76.199-S76.201[A], S76.209-S76.211[A], S76.219[A], S76.291[A], S76.299-S76.301[A], S76.309-S76.311[A], S76.319[A], S76.391[A], S76.399-S76.801[A], S76.809-S76.811[A], S76.819[A], S76.891[A], S76.899-S76.901[A], S76.909-S76.911[A], S76.919[A], S76.991[A], S76.999[A], S79.811[A], S79.819-S79.821[A], S79.829-S79.911[A], S79.919-S79.921[A], S79.929[A], S82.101[A,B,C], S82.102[B,C], S82.109-S82.111[A,B,C], S82.112[B,C], S82.113-S82.114[A,B,C], S82.115[B,C], S82.116-S82.121[A,B,C], S82.122[B,C], S82.123-S82.124[A,B,C], S82.125[B,C], S82.126-S82.131[A,B,C], S82.132[B,C], S82.133-S82.134[A,B,C], S82.135[B,C], S82.136-S82.141[A,B,C], S82.142[B,C], S82.143-S82.144[A,B,C], S82.145[B,C], S82.146-S82.151[A,B,C], S82.152[B,C], S82.153-S82.154[A,B,C], S82.155[B,C], S82.156[A,B,C], S82.161[A], S82.169[A], S82.191[A,B,C], S82.192[B,C], S82.199-S82.201[A,B,C], S82.202[B,C], S82.209-S82.221[A,B,C], S82.222[B,C], S82.223-S82.224[A,B,C], S82.225[B,C], S82.226-S82.231[A,B,C], S82.232[B,C], S82.233-S82.234[A,B,C], S82.235[B,C], S82.236-S82.241[A,B,C], S82.242[B,C], S82.243-S82.244[A,B,C], S82.245[B,C], S82.246-S82.251[A,B,C], S82.252[B,C], S82.253-S82.254[A,B,C], S82.255[B,C], S82.256-S82.261[A,B,C], S82.262[B,C,], S82.263-S82.264[A,B,C], S82.265[B,C], S82.266-S82.291[A,B,C], S82.292[B,C], S82.299[A,B,C], S82.311[A], S82.319[A], S82.401[A,B,C], S82.402[B,C], S82.409-S82.421[A,B,C], S82.422[B,C], S82.423-S82.424[A,B,C], S82.425[B,C], S82.426-S82.431[A,B,C], S82.432[B,C], S82.433-S82.434[A,B,C], S82.435[B,C], S82.436-S82.441[A,B,C], S82.442[B,C], S82.443-S82.444[A,B,C], S82.445[B,C], S82.446-S82.451[A,B,C], S82.452[B,C,], S82.453-S82.454[A,B,C], S82.455[B,C], S82.456-S82.461[A,B,C], S82.462[B,C], S82.463-S82.464[A,B,C], S82.465[B,C], S82.466-S82.491[A,B,C], S82.492[B,C], S82.499[A,B,C], S82.811[A], S82.819-S82.821[A], S82.829[A], S82.831[A,B,C], S82.832[B,C], S82.839[A,B,C], S82.861[A,B,C], S82.862[B,C], S82.863-S82.864[A,B,C], S82.865[B,C], S82.866[A,B,C], S82.90X-S82.92X[A,B,C], S89.001[A], S89.009-S89.011[A], S89.019-S89.021[A], S89.029-S89.031[A], S89.039-S89.041[A], S89.049-S89.091[A], S89.099[A], S89.201[A], S89.209[A], S89.211-S89.219[A], S89.221-S89.229[A], S89.291-S89.299[A], T14.90-T14.91, T79.A9X-T79.9XX[A] **For S82.201[B,C]:** See S82.101[B,C] **For S82.201[K,M,N,P,Q,R]:** See S02.0[K]
    - **S82.202 Unspecified fracture of shaft of left tibia** A, K, M, N, P, Q, R, **B, C**, A, B, C
      - Ex: **For S82.202[A]:** See S82.102[A]
        For S82.202[B,C]: See S82.101[B,C]
        For S82.202[K,M,N,P,Q,R]: See S02.0[K]
    - **S82.209 Unspecified fracture of shaft of unspecified tibia** A, K, M, N, P, Q, R, **B, C**, A, B, C
      - Ex: **For S82.209[A,B,C]:** See S82.101[B,C]
        For S82.209[K,M,N,P,Q,R]: See S02.0[K]
- **S82.22 Transverse fracture of shaft of tibia**
  - **S82.221 Displaced transverse fracture of shaft of right tibia** A, K, M, N, P, Q, R, **B, C**, A, B, C
    - Ex: **For S82.221[A]:** See S82.101[A]
      For S82.221[B,C]: See S82.101[B,C]
      For S82.221[K,M,N,P,Q,R]: See S02.0[K]
  - **S82.222 Displaced transverse fracture of shaft of left tibia** A, K, M, N, P, Q, R, **B, C**, A, B, C
    - Ex: **For S82.222[A]:** See S82.102[A]
      For S82.222[B,C]: See S82.101[B,C]
      For S82.222[K,M,N,P,Q,R]: See S02.0[K]
  - **S82.223 Displaced transverse fracture of shaft of unspecified tibia** A, K, M, N, P, Q, R, **B, C**, A, B, C
    - Ex: **For S82.223[A,B,C]:** See S82.101[B,C]
      For S82.223[K,M,N,P,Q,R]: See S02.0[K]
  - **S82.224 Nondisplaced transverse fracture of shaft of right tibia** A, K, M, N, P, Q, R, **B, C**, A, B, C
    - Ex: **For S82.224[A]:** See S82.101[A]
      For S82.224[B,C]: See S82.101[B,C]
      For S82.224[K,M,N,P,Q,R]: See S02.0[K]
  - **S82.225 Nondisplaced transverse fracture of shaft of left tibia** A, K, M, N, P, Q, R, **B, C**, A, B, C
    - Ex: **For S82.225[A]:** See S82.102[A]
      For S82.225[B,C]: See S82.101[B,C]
      For S82.225[K,M,N,P,Q,R]: See S02.0[K]
  - **S82.226 Nondisplaced transverse fracture of shaft of unspecified tibia** A, K, M, N, P, Q, R, **B, C**, A, B, C
    - Ex: **For S82.226[A,B,C]:** See S82.101[B,C]
      For S82.226[K,M,N,P,Q,R]: See S02.0[K]

- **S82.23 Oblique fracture of shaft of tibia**
  - **S82.231 Displaced oblique fracture of shaft of right tibia** A, K, M, N, P, Q, R CC, B, C MCC, A, B, C UNC
    - Ex: **For S82.231[A]:** See S82.101[A]
    - **For S82.231[B,C]:** See S82.101[B,C]
    - **For S82.231[K,M,N,P,Q,R]:** See S02.0[K]
  - **S82.232 Displaced oblique fracture of shaft of left tibia** A, K, M, N, P, Q, R CC, B, C MCC, A, B, C UNC
    - Ex: **For S82.232[A]:** See S82.102[A]
    - **For S82.232[B,C]:** See S82.101[B,C]
    - **For S82.232[K,M,N,P,Q,R]:** See S02.0[K]
  - **S82.233 Displaced oblique fracture of shaft of unspecified tibia** A, K, M, N, P, Q, R CC, B, C MCC, A, B, C UNC
    - Ex: **For S82.233[A,B,C]:** See S82.101[B,C]
    - **For S82.233[K,M,N,P,Q,R]:** See S02.0[K]
  - **S82.234 Nondisplaced oblique fracture of shaft of right tibia** A, K, M, N, P, Q, R CC, B, C MCC, A, B, C UNC
    - Ex: **For S82.234[A]:** See S82.101[A]
    - **For S82.234[B,C]:** See S82.101[B,C]
    - **For S82.234[K,M,N,P,Q,R]:** See S02.0[K]
    - **Coding Clinic: 2015, Q1, P9-10**
  - **S82.235 Nondisplaced oblique fracture of shaft of left tibia** A, K, M, N, P, Q, R CC, B, C MCC, A, B, C UNC
    - Ex: **For S82.235[A]:** See S82.102[A]
    - **For S82.235[B,C]:** See S82.101[B,C]
    - **For S82.235[K,M,N,P,Q,R]:** See S02.0[K]
  - **S82.236 Nondisplaced oblique fracture of shaft of unspecified tibia** A, K, M, N, P, Q, R CC, B, C MCC, A, B, C UNC
    - Ex: **For S82.236[A,B,C]:** See S82.101[B,C]
    - **For S82.236[K,M,N,P,Q,R]:** See S02.0[K]
- **S82.24 Spiral fracture of shaft of tibia**
  Toddler fracture
  - **S82.241 Displaced spiral fracture of shaft of right tibia** A, K, M, N, P, Q, R CC, B, C MCC, A, B, C UNC
    - Ex: **For S82.241[A]:** See S82.101[A]
    - **For S82.241[B,C]:** See S82.101[B,C]
    - **For S82.241[K,M,N,P,Q,R]:** See S02.0[K]
  - **S82.242 Displaced spiral fracture of shaft of left tibia** A, K, M, N, P, Q, R CC, B, C MCC, A, B, C UNC
    - Ex: **For S82.242[A]:** See S82.102[A]
    - **For S82.242[B,C]:** See S82.101[B,C]
    - **For S82.242[K,M,N,P,Q,R]:** See S02.0[K]
  - **S82.243 Displaced spiral fracture of shaft of unspecified tibia** A, K, M, N, P, Q, R CC, B, C MCC, A, B, C UNC
    - Ex: **For S82.243[A,B,C]:** See S82.101[B,C]
    - **For S82.243[K,M,N,P,Q,R]:** See S02.0[K]
  - **S82.244 Nondisplaced spiral fracture of shaft of right tibia** A, K, M, N, P, Q, R CC, B, C MCC, A, B, C UNC
    - Ex: **For S82.244[A]:** See S82.101[A]
    - **For S82.244[B,C]:** See S82.101[B,C]
    - **For S82.244[K,M,N,P,Q,R]:** See S02.0[K]
  - **S82.245 Nondisplaced spiral fracture of shaft of left tibia** A, K, M, N, P, Q, R CC, B, C MCC, A, B, C UNC
    - Ex: **For S82.245[A]:** See S82.102[A]
    - **For S82.245[B,C]:** See S82.101[B,C]
    - **For S82.245[K,M,N,P,Q,R]:** See S02.0[K]
  - **S82.246 Nondisplaced spiral fracture of shaft of unspecified tibia** A, K, M, N, P, Q, R CC, B, C MCC, A, B, C UNC
    - Ex: **For S82.246[A,B,C]:** See S82.101[B,C]
    - **For S82.246[K,M,N,P,Q,R]:** See S02.0[K]
- **S82.25 Comminuted fracture of shaft of tibia**
  - **S82.251 Displaced comminuted fracture of shaft of right tibia** A, K, M, N, P, Q, R CC, B, C MCC, A, B, C UNC
    - Ex: **For S82.251[A]:** See S82.101[A]
    - **For S82.251[B,C]:** See S82.101[B,C]
    - **For S82.251[K,M,N,P,Q,R]:** See S02.0[K]
    - **Coding Clinic: 2015, Q2, P6**
  - **S82.252 Displaced comminuted fracture of shaft of left tibia** A, K, M, N, P, Q, R CC, B, C MCC, A, B, C UNC
    - Ex: **For S82.252[A]:** See S82.102[A]
    - **For S82.252[B,C]:** See S82.101[B,C]
    - **For S82.252[K,M,N,P,Q,R]:** See S02.0[K]
  - **S82.253 Displaced comminuted fracture of shaft of unspecified tibia** A, K, M, N, P, Q, R CC, B, C MCC, A, B, C UNC
    - Ex: **For S82.253[A,B,C]:** See S82.101[B,C]
    - **For S82.253[K,M,N,P,Q,R]:** See S02.0[K]
  - **S82.254 Nondisplaced comminuted fracture of shaft of right tibia** A, K, M, N, P, Q, R CC, B, C MCC, A, B, C UNC
    - Ex: **For S82.254[A]:** See S82.101[A]
    - **For S82.254[B,C]:** See S82.101[B,C]
    - **For S82.254[K,M,N,P,Q,R]:** See S02.0[K]
  - **S82.255 Nondisplaced comminuted fracture of shaft of left tibia** A, K, M, N, P, Q, R CC, B, C MCC, A, B, C UNC
    - Ex: **For S82.255[A]:** See S82.102[A]
    - **For S82.255[B,C]:** See S82.101[B,C]
    - **For S82.255[K,M,N,P,Q,R]:** See S02.0[K]
  - **S82.256 Nondisplaced comminuted fracture of shaft of unspecified tibia** A, K, M, N, P, Q, R CC, B, C MCC, A, B, C UNC
    - Ex: **For S82.256[A,B,C]:** See S82.101[B,C]
    - **For S82.256[K,M,N,P,Q,R]:** See S02.0[K]
- **S82.26 Segmental fracture of shaft of tibia**
  - **S82.261 Displaced segmental fracture of shaft of right tibia** A, K, M, N, P, Q, R CC, B, C MCC, A, B, C UNC
    - Ex: **For S82.261[A]:** See S82.101[A]
    - **For S82.261[B,C]:** See S82.101[B,C]
    - **For S82.261[K,M,N,P,Q,R]:** See S02.0[K]
  - **S82.262 Displaced segmental fracture of shaft of left tibia** A, K, M, N, P, Q, R CC, B, C MCC, A, B, C UNC
    - Ex: **For S82.262[A]:** See S82.102[A]
    - **For S82.262[B,C]:** See S82.101[B,C]
    - **For S82.262[K,M,N,P,Q,R]:** See S02.0[K]
  - **S82.263 Displaced segmental fracture of shaft of unspecified tibia** A, K, M, N, P, Q, R CC, B, C MCC, A, B, C UNC
    - Ex: **For S82.263[A,B,C]:** See S82.101[B,C]
    - **For S82.263[K,M,N,P,Q,R]:** See S02.0[K]
  - **S82.264 Nondisplaced segmental fracture of shaft of right tibia** A, K, M, N, P, Q, R CC, B, C MCC, A, B, C UNC
    - Ex: **For S82.264[A]:** See S82.101[A]
    - **For S82.264[B,C]:** See S82.101[B,C]
    - **For S82.264[K,M,N,P,Q,R]:** See S02.0[K]
  - **S82.265 Nondisplaced segmental fracture of shaft of left tibia** A, K, M, N, P, Q, R CC, B, C MCC, A, B, C UNC
    - Ex: **For S82.265[A]:** See S82.102[A]
    - **For S82.265[B,C]:** See S82.101[B,C]
    - **For S82.265[K,M,N,P,Q,R]:** See S02.0[K]
  - **S82.266 Nondisplaced segmental fracture of shaft of unspecified tibia** A, K, M, N, P, Q, R CC, B, C MCC, A, B, C UNC
    - Ex: **For S82.266[A,B,C]:** See S82.101[B,C]
    - **For S82.266[K,M,N,P,Q,R]:** See S02.0[K]

S82.29 Other fracture of shaft of tibia

S82.291 Other fracture of shaft of right tibia A, K, M, N, P, Q, R, B, C, A, B, C

Ex: **For S82.291[A]:** See S82.101[A]
For S82.291[B,C]: See S82.101[B,C]
For S82.291[K,M,N,P,Q,R]: See S02.0[K]

S82.292 Other fracture of shaft of left tibia A, K, M, N, P, Q, R, B, C, A, B, C

Ex: **For S82.292[A]:** See S82.102[A]
For S82.292[B,C]: See S82.101[B,C]
For S82.292[K,M,N,P,Q,R]: See S02.0[K]

S82.299 Other fracture of shaft of unspecified tibia A, K, M, N, P, Q, R, B, C, A, B, C

Ex: **For S82.299[A,B,C]:** See S82.101[B,C]
For S82.299[K,M,N,P,Q,R]: See S02.0[K]

S82.3 Fracture of lower end of tibia

Excludes1 bimalleolar fracture of lower leg (S82.84-)
fracture of medial malleolus alone (S82.5-)
Maisonneuve's fracture (S82.86-)
pilon fracture of distal tibia (S82.87-)
trimalleolar fractures of lower leg (S82.85-)

S82.30 Unspecified fracture of lower end of tibia

Ex: **For category S82.30 CC codes S82.30[B,C]:** M80.00X-M80.019[A], M80.041-M80.049[A], M80.061-M80.819[A], M80.841-M80.849[A], M80.861-M80.879[A], M84.40X-M84.419[A], M84.441-M84.446[A], M84.454[A], M84.461-M84.519[A], M84.541-M84.550[A], M84.561-M84.576[A], M84.60X-M84.619[A], M84.641-M84.650[A], M84.661-M84.68X[A], S03.8XX-S03.9XX[A], S29.011-S29.019[A], S38.3XX[A], S39.011-S39.013[A], S73.101-S73.199[A], S76.001-S76.019[A], S76.091-S76.119[A], S76.191-S76.219[A], S76.291-S76.319[A], S76.391-S76.819[A], S76.891-S76.919[A], S76.991-S76.999[A], S79.811-S79.929[A], S82.301-S82.309[A,B,C], S82.391-S82.399[A,B,C], S82.51X-S82.56X[B,C], S82.61X-S82.66X[A,B,C], S82.841-S82.856[A,B,C], S82.871-S82.876[B,C], S82.891-S82.92X[A,B,C], S89.101-S89.199[A], S89.301-S89.399[A], T14.90-T14.91, T79.A9X-T79.9XX[A] **For S82.30[K,M,N,P,Q,R]:** See S02.0[K]

S82.301 Unspecified fracture of lower end of right tibia B, C, K, M, N, P, Q, R, B, C

S82.302 Unspecified fracture of lower end of left tibia B, C, K, M, N, P, Q, R, B, C

S82.309 Unspecified fracture of lower end of unspecified tibia B, C, K, M, N, P, Q, R, B, C

S82.31 Torus fracture of lower end of tibia

The appropriate 7th character is to be added to all codes in subcategory S82.31

A	initial encounter for closed fracture
D	subsequent encounter for fracture with routine healing
G	subsequent encounter for fracture with delayed healing
K	subsequent encounter for fracture with nonunion
P	subsequent encounter for fracture with malunion
S	sequela

S82.311 Torus fracture of lower end of right tibia A, K, P, A

Ex: **For S82.311[A]:** See S82.161[A]
For S82.311[K,P]: See S02.0[K]

S82.312 Torus fracture of lower end of left tibia A, K, P, A

Ex: **For S82.312[A]:** See S82.162[A]
For S82.312[K,P]: See S02.0[K]

S82.319 Torus fracture of lower end of unspecified tibia A, K, P, A

Ex: **For S82.319[A]:** See S82.169[A]
S82.319[K,P]: See S02.0[K]

S82.39 Other fracture of lower end of tibia

Ex: **For category S82.39 CC codes S82.39[B,C]:** See S82.30[B,C] **For S82.39[K,M,N,P,Q,R]:** See S02.0[K]

S82.391 Other fracture of lower end of right tibia B, C, K, M, N, P, Q, R, B, C

S82.392 Other fracture of lower end of left tibia B, C, K, M, N, P, Q, R, B, C

Coding Clinic: 2015, Q1, P25

S82.399 Other fracture of lower end of unspecified tibia B, C, K, M, N, P, Q, R, B, C

S82.4 Fracture of shaft of fibula

Excludes2 fracture of lateral malleolus alone (S82.6-)

Ex: **For category S82.4 CC codes S82.4[B,C]:** See S82.101[B,C]
For S82.4[K,M,N,P,Q,R]: See S02.0[K]

S82.40 Unspecified fracture of shaft of fibula

S82.401 Unspecified fracture of shaft of right fibula K, M, N, P, Q, R, B, C, B, C

S82.402 Unspecified fracture of shaft of left fibula K, M, N, P, Q, R, B, C, B, C

S82.409 Unspecified fracture of shaft of unspecified fibula K, M, N, P, Q, R, B, C, B, C

S82.42 Transverse fracture of shaft of fibula

S82.421 Displaced transverse fracture of shaft of right fibula K, M, N, P, Q, R, B, C, B, C

S82.422 Displaced transverse fracture of shaft of left fibula K, M, N, P, Q, R, B, C, B, C

S82.423 Displaced transverse fracture of shaft of unspecified fibula K, M, N, P, Q, R, B, C, B, C

S82.424 Nondisplaced transverse fracture of shaft of right fibula K, M, N, P, Q, R, B, C, B, C

S82.425 Nondisplaced transverse fracture of shaft of left fibula K, M, N, P, Q, R, B, C, B, C

S82.426 Nondisplaced transverse fracture of shaft of unspecified fibula K, M, N, P, Q, R, B, C, B, C

S82.43 Oblique fracture of shaft of fibula

S82.431 Displaced oblique fracture of shaft of right fibula K, M, N, P, Q, R, B, C, B, C

S82.432 Displaced oblique fracture of shaft of left fibula K, M, N, P, Q, R, B, C, B, C

S82.433 Displaced oblique fracture of shaft of unspecified fibula K, M, N, P, Q, R, B, C, B, C

S82.434 Nondisplaced oblique fracture of shaft of right fibula K, M, N, P, Q, R, B, C, B, C

S82.435 Nondisplaced oblique fracture of shaft of left fibula K, M, N, P, Q, R, B, C, B, C

S82.436 Nondisplaced oblique fracture of shaft of unspecified fibula K, M, N, P, Q, R, B, C, B, C

- **S82.44 Spiral fracture of shaft of fibula**
  - **S82.441 Displaced spiral fracture of shaft of right fibula** K, M, N, P, Q, R CC, B, C MCC, B, C UNC
  - **S82.442 Displaced spiral fracture of shaft of left fibula** K, M, N, P, Q, R CC, B, C MCC, B, C UNC
  - **S82.443 Displaced spiral fracture of shaft of unspecified fibula** K, M, N, P, Q, R CC, B, C MCC, B, C UNC
  - **S82.444 Nondisplaced spiral fracture of shaft of right fibula** K, M, N, P, Q, R CC, B, C MCC, B, C UNC
  - **S82.445 Nondisplaced spiral fracture of shaft of left fibula** K, M, N, P, Q, R CC, B, C MCC, B, C UNC
  - **S82.446 Nondisplaced spiral fracture of shaft of unspecified fibula** K, M, N, P, Q, R CC, B, C MCC, B, C UNC
- **S82.45 Comminuted fracture of shaft of fibula**
  - **S82.451 Displaced comminuted fracture of shaft of right fibula** K, M, N, P, Q, R CC, B, C MCC, B, C UNC
  - **S82.452 Displaced comminuted fracture of shaft of left fibula** K, M, N, P, Q, R CC, B, C MCC, B, C UNC
  - **S82.453 Displaced comminuted fracture of shaft of unspecified fibula** K, M, N, P, Q, R CC, B, C MCC, B, C UNC
  - **S82.454 Nondisplaced comminuted fracture of shaft of right fibula** K, M, N, P, Q, R CC, B, C MCC, B, C UNC
  - **S82.455 Nondisplaced comminuted fracture of shaft of left fibula** K, M, N, P, Q, R CC, B, C MCC, B, C UNC
  - **S82.456 Nondisplaced comminuted fracture of shaft of unspecified fibula** K, M, N, P, Q, R CC, B, C MCC, B, C UNC
- **S82.46 Segmental fracture of shaft of fibula**
  - **S82.461 Displaced segmental fracture of shaft of right fibula** K, M, N, P, Q, R CC, B, C MCC, B, C UNC
  - **S82.462 Displaced segmental fracture of shaft of left fibula** K, M, N, P, Q, R CC, B, C MCC, B, C UNC
  - **S82.463 Displaced segmental fracture of shaft of unspecified fibula** K, M, N, P, Q, R CC, B, C MCC, B, C UNC
  - **S82.464 Nondisplaced segmental fracture of shaft of right fibula** K, M, N, P, Q, R CC, B, C MCC, B, C UNC
  - **S82.465 Nondisplaced segmental fracture of shaft of left fibula** K, M, N, P, Q, R CC, B, C MCC, B, C UNC
  - **S82.466 Nondisplaced segmental fracture of shaft of unspecified fibula** K, M, N, P, Q, R CC, B, C MCC, B, C UNC
- **S82.49 Other fracture of shaft of fibula**
  - **S82.491 Other fracture of shaft of right fibula** K, M, N, P, Q, R CC, B, C MCC, B, C UNC
  - **S82.492 Other fracture of shaft of left fibula** K, M, N, P, Q, R CC, B, C MCC, B, C UNC
  - **S82.499 Other fracture of shaft of unspecified fibula** K, M, N, P, Q, R CC, B, C MCC, B, C UNC
- **S82.5 Fracture of medial malleolus**

  Excludes1 pilon fracture of distal tibia (S82.87-)
  Salter-Harris type III of lower end of tibia (S89.13-)
  Salter-Harris type IV of lower end of tibia (S89.14-)

  Ex: **For category S82.5 CC codes S82.5[B,C]:** See S82.30[B,C]
  For S82.5[K,M,N,P,Q,R]: See S02.0[K]

  - X **S82.51 Displaced fracture of medial malleolus of right tibia** B, C, K, M, N, P, Q, R CC, B, C UNC
  - X **S82.52 Displaced fracture of medial malleolus of left tibia** B, C, K, M, N, P, Q, R CC, B, C UNC
  - X **S82.53 Displaced fracture of medial malleolus of unspecified tibia** B, C, K, M, N, P, Q, R CC, B, C UNC
  - X **S82.54 Nondisplaced fracture of medial malleolus of right tibia** B, C, K, M, N, P, Q, R CC, B, C UNC
  - X **S82.55 Nondisplaced fracture of medial malleolus of left tibia** B, C, K, M, N, P, Q, R CC, B, C UNC
  - X **S82.56 Nondisplaced fracture of medial malleolus of unspecified tibia** B, C, K, M, N, P, Q, R CC, B, C UNC
- **S82.6 Fracture of lateral malleolus**

  Excludes1 pilon fracture of distal tibia (S82.87-)

  Ex: **For category S82.6 CC codes S82.6[B,C]:** See S82.30[B,C]
  For S82.6[K,M,N,P,Q,R]: See S02.0[K]

  - X **S82.61 Displaced fracture of lateral malleolus of right fibula** B, C, K, M, N, P, Q, R CC, B, C UNC
  - X **S82.62 Displaced fracture of lateral malleolus of left fibula** B, C, K, M, N, P, Q, R CC, B, C UNC
  - X **S82.63 Displaced fracture of lateral malleolus of unspecified fibula** B, C, K, M, N, P, Q, R CC, B, C UNC
  - X **S82.64 Nondisplaced fracture of lateral malleolus of right fibula** B, C, K, M, N, P, Q, R CC, B, C UNC
  - X **S82.65 Nondisplaced fracture of lateral malleolus of left fibula** B, C, K, M, N, P, Q, R CC, B, C UNC
  - X **S82.66 Nondisplaced fracture of lateral malleolus of unspecified fibula** B, C, K, M, N, P, Q, R CC, B, C UNC
- **S82.8 Other fractures of lower leg**
  - **S82.81 Torus fracture of upper end of fibula**

    The appropriate 7th character is to be added to all codes in subcategory S82.81

A	initial encounter for closed fracture
D	subsequent encounter for fracture with routine healing
G	subsequent encounter for fracture with delayed healing
K	subsequent encounter for fracture with nonunion
P	subsequent encounter for fracture with malunion
S	sequela

    Ex: **For category S82.81 CC codes:** See S02.0[K]

    - **S82.811 Torus fracture of upper end of right fibula** K, P CC
    - **S82.812 Torus fracture of upper end of left fibula** K, P CC
    - **S82.819 Torus fracture of upper end of unspecified fibula** K, P CC

S82.82 Torus fracture of lower end of fibula

The appropriate 7th character is to be added to all codes in subcategory S82.82

A	initial encounter for closed fracture
D	subsequent encounter for fracture with routine healing
G	subsequent encounter for fracture with delayed healing
K	subsequent encounter for fracture with nonunion
P	subsequent encounter for fracture with malunion
S	sequela

Ex: **For category S82.82 CC codes:** See S02.0[K]

- **S82.821 Torus fracture of lower end of right fibula** K, P
- **S82.822 Torus fracture of lower end of left fibula** K, P
- **S82.829 Torus fracture of lower end of unspecified fibula** K, P

S82.83 Other fracture of upper and lower end of fibula

Ex: **For category S82.83 CC codes S82.83[B,C]:** See S82.101[B,C] **For S82.83[K,M,N,P,Q,R]:** See S02.0[K]

- **S82.831 Other fracture of upper and lower end of right fibula** K, M, N, P, Q, R, B, C, B, C
- **S82.832 Other fracture of upper and lower end of left fibula** K, M, N, P, Q, R, B, C, B, C
  Coding Clinic: 2015, Q1, P9-10
- **S82.839 Other fracture of upper and lower end of unspecified fibula** K, M, N, P, Q, R, B, C, B, C

S82.84 Bimalleolar fracture of lower leg

Ex: **For category S82.84 CC codes S82.84[B,C]:** See S82.30[B,C] **For S82.84[K,M,N,P,Q,R]:** See S02.0[K]

- **S82.841 Displaced bimalleolar fracture of right lower leg** B, C, K, M, N, P, Q, R, B, C
- **S82.842 Displaced bimalleolar fracture of left lower leg** B, C, K, M, N, P, Q, R, B, C
- **S82.843 Displaced bimalleolar fracture of unspecified lower leg** B, C, K, M, N, P, Q, R, B, C
- **S82.844 Nondisplaced bimalleolar fracture of right lower leg** B, C, K, M, N, P, Q, R, B, C
- **S82.845 Nondisplaced bimalleolar fracture of left lower leg** B, C, K, M, N, P, Q, R, B, C
- **S82.846 Nondisplaced bimalleolar fracture of unspecified lower leg** B, C, K, M, N, P, Q, R, B, C

S82.85 Trimalleolar fracture of lower leg

Ex: **For category S82.85 CC codes S82.85[B,C]:** See S82.30[B,C] **For S82.85[K,M,N,P,Q,R]:** See S02.0[K]

- **S82.851 Displaced trimalleolar fracture of right lower leg** B, C, K, M, N, P, Q, R, B, C
- **S82.852 Displaced trimalleolar fracture of left lower leg** B, C, K, M, N, P, Q, R, B, C
- **S82.853 Displaced trimalleolar fracture of unspecified lower leg** B, C, K, M, N, P, Q, R, B, C
- **S82.854 Nondisplaced trimalleolar fracture of right lower leg** B, C, K, M, N, P, Q, R, B, C
- **S82.855 Nondisplaced trimalleolar fracture of left lower leg** B, C, K, M, N, P, Q, R, B, C
- **S82.856 Nondisplaced trimalleolar fracture of unspecified lower leg** B, C, K, M, N, P, Q, R, B, C

S82.86 Maisonneuve's fracture

Ex: **For category S82.86 CC codes S82.86[B,C]:** See S82.101[B,C] **For S82.86[K,M,N,P,Q,R]:** See S02.0[K]

- **S82.861 Displaced Maisonneuve's fracture of right leg** K, M, N, P, Q, R, B, C, B, C
- **S82.862 Displaced Maisonneuve's fracture of left leg** K, M, N, P, Q, R, B, C, B, C
- **S82.863 Displaced Maisonneuve's fracture of unspecified leg** K, M, N, P, Q, R, B, C, B, C
- **S82.864 Nondisplaced Maisonneuve's fracture of right leg** K, M, N, P, Q, R, B, C, B, C
- **S82.865 Nondisplaced Maisonneuve's fracture of left leg** K, M, N, P, Q, R, B, C, B, C
- **S82.866 Nondisplaced Maisonneuve's fracture of unspecified leg** K, M, N, P, Q, R, B, C, B, C

S82.87 Pilon fracture of tibia

Ex: **For category S82.87 CC codes S82.87[B,C]:** See S82.30[B,C] **For S82.87[K,M,N,P,Q,R]:** See S02.0[K]

- **S82.871 Displaced pilon fracture of right tibia** B, C, K, M, N, P, Q, R, B, C
- **S82.872 Displaced pilon fracture of left tibia** B, C, K, M, N, P, Q, R, B, C
- **S82.873 Displaced pilon fracture of unspecified tibia** B, C, K, M, N, P, Q, R, B, C
- **S82.874 Nondisplaced pilon fracture of right tibia** B, C, K, M, N, P, Q, R, B, C
- **S82.875 Nondisplaced pilon fracture of left tibia** B, C, K, M, N, P, Q, R, B, C
- **S82.876 Nondisplaced pilon fracture of unspecified tibia** B, C, K, M, N, P, Q, R, B, C

S82.89 Other fractures of lower leg

Fracture of ankle NOS

Ex: **For category S82.89 CC codes S82.89[B,C]:** See S82.30[B,C] **For S82.89[K,M,N,P,Q,R]:** See S02.0[K]

- **S82.891 Other fracture of right lower leg** B, C, K, M, N, P, Q, R, B, C
- **S82.892 Other fracture of left lower leg** B, C, K, M, N, P, Q, R, B, C
- **S82.899 Other fracture of unspecified lower leg** B, C, K, M, N, P, Q, R, B, C

S82.9 Unspecified fracture of lower leg

Ex: **For category S82.9 CC codes S82.9[B,C]:** S72.001-S72.92X[A,B,C], S79.001-S79.199[A], S82.001-S82.156[A,B,C], S82.191-S82.309[A,B,C], S82.391-S82.66X[A,B,C], S82.831-S82.92X[A,B,C], S89.001-S89.399[A], S92.001-S92.599[A,B], S92.811-S92.919[A,B] **For S82.9[K,M,N,P,Q,R]:** See S02.0[K]

- X **S82.90 Unspecified fracture of unspecified lower leg** A, K, M, N, P, Q, R, B, C
- X **S82.91 Unspecified fracture of right lower leg** A, K, M, N, P, Q, R, B, C
- X **S82.92 Unspecified fracture of left lower leg** A, K, M, N, P, Q, R, B, C

S83 Dislocation and sprain of joints and ligaments of knee

Includes avulsion of joint or ligament of knee
laceration of cartilage, joint or ligament of knee
sprain of cartilage, joint or ligament of knee
traumatic hemarthrosis of joint or ligament of knee
traumatic rupture of joint or ligament of knee
traumatic subluxation of joint or ligament of knee
traumatic tear of joint or ligament of knee

Code also any associated open wound

Excludes1 derangement of patella (M22.0-M22.3)
injury of patellar ligament (tendon) (S76.1-)
internal derangement of knee (M23.-)
old dislocation of knee (M24.36)
pathological dislocation of knee (M24.36)
recurrent dislocation of knee (M22.0)

Excludes2 strain of muscle, fascia and tendon of lower leg (S86.-)

The appropriate 7th character is to be added to each code from category S83

A	initial encounter
D	subsequent encounter
S	sequela

S83.0 Subluxation and dislocation of patella

S83.00 Unspecified subluxation and dislocation of patella

S83.001 Unspecified subluxation of right patella
S83.002 Unspecified subluxation of left patella
S83.003 Unspecified subluxation of unspecified patella
S83.004 Unspecified dislocation of right patella
S83.005 Unspecified dislocation of left patella
S83.006 Unspecified dislocation of unspecified patella

S83.01 Lateral subluxation and dislocation of patella

S83.011 Lateral subluxation of right patella
S83.012 Lateral subluxation of left patella
S83.013 Lateral subluxation of unspecified patella
S83.014 Lateral dislocation of right patella
S83.015 Lateral dislocation of left patella
S83.016 Lateral dislocation of unspecified patella

S83.09 Other subluxation and dislocation of patella

S83.091 Other subluxation of right patella
S83.092 Other subluxation of left patella
S83.093 Other subluxation of unspecified patella
S83.094 Other dislocation of right patella
S83.095 Other dislocation of left patella
S83.096 Other dislocation of unspecified patella

S83.1 Subluxation and dislocation of knee

Excludes2 instability of knee prosthesis (T84.022, T84.023)

S83.10 Unspecified subluxation and dislocation of knee

S83.101 Unspecified subluxation of right knee
S83.102 Unspecified subluxation of left knee
S83.103 Unspecified subluxation of unspecified knee
S83.104 Unspecified dislocation of right knee
S83.105 Unspecified dislocation of left knee
S83.106 Unspecified dislocation of unspecified knee

S83.11 Anterior subluxation and dislocation of proximal end of tibia

Posterior subluxation and dislocation of distal end of femur

S83.111 Anterior subluxation of proximal end of tibia, right knee
S83.112 Anterior subluxation of proximal end of tibia, left knee
S83.113 Anterior subluxation of proximal end of tibia, unspecified knee
S83.114 Anterior dislocation of proximal end of tibia, right knee
S83.115 Anterior dislocation of proximal end of tibia, left knee
S83.116 Anterior dislocation of proximal end of tibia, unspecified knee

S83.12 Posterior subluxation and dislocation of proximal end of tibia

Anterior dislocation of distal end of femur

S83.121 Posterior subluxation of proximal end of tibia, right knee
S83.122 Posterior subluxation of proximal end of tibia, left knee
S83.123 Posterior subluxation of proximal end of tibia, unspecified knee
S83.124 Posterior dislocation of proximal end of tibia, right knee
S83.125 Posterior dislocation of proximal end of tibia, left knee
S83.126 Posterior dislocation of proximal end of tibia, unspecified knee

S83.13 Medial subluxation and dislocation of proximal end of tibia

S83.131 Medial subluxation of proximal end of tibia, right knee
S83.132 Medial subluxation of proximal end of tibia, left knee
S83.133 Medial subluxation of proximal end of tibia, unspecified knee
S83.134 Medial dislocation of proximal end of tibia, right knee
S83.135 Medial dislocation of proximal end of tibia, left knee
S83.136 Medial dislocation of proximal end of tibia, unspecified knee

S83.14 Lateral subluxation and dislocation of proximal end of tibia

S83.141 Lateral subluxation of proximal end of tibia, right knee
S83.142 Lateral subluxation of proximal end of tibia, left knee
S83.143 Lateral subluxation of proximal end of tibia, unspecified knee
S83.144 Lateral dislocation of proximal end of tibia, right knee
S83.145 Lateral dislocation of proximal end of tibia, left knee
S83.146 Lateral dislocation of proximal end of tibia, unspecified knee

S83.19 Other subluxation and dislocation of knee

S83.191 Other subluxation of right knee
S83.192 Other subluxation of left knee
S83.193 Other subluxation of unspecified knee
S83.194 Other dislocation of right knee
S83.195 Other dislocation of left knee
S83.196 Other dislocation of unspecified knee

- S83.2 Tear of meniscus, current injury
  - **Excludes1** old bucket-handle tear (M23.2)
  - S83.20 Tear of unspecified meniscus, current injury
    - Tear of meniscus of knee NOS
    - S83.200 Bucket-handle tear of unspecified meniscus, current injury, right knee
    - S83.201 Bucket-handle tear of unspecified meniscus, current injury, left knee
    - S83.202 Bucket-handle tear of unspecified meniscus, current injury, unspecified knee
    - S83.203 Other tear of unspecified meniscus, current injury, right knee
    - S83.204 Other tear of unspecified meniscus, current injury, left knee
    - S83.205 Other tear of unspecified meniscus, current injury, unspecified knee
    - S83.206 Unspecified tear of unspecified meniscus, current injury, right knee
    - S83.207 Unspecified tear of unspecified meniscus, current injury, left knee
    - S83.209 Unspecified tear of unspecified meniscus, current injury, unspecified knee
  - S83.21 Bucket-handle tear of medial meniscus, current injury
    - S83.211 Bucket-handle tear of medial meniscus, current injury, right knee
    - S83.212 Bucket-handle tear of medial meniscus, current injury, left knee
    - S83.219 Bucket-handle tear of medial meniscus, current injury, unspecified knee
  - S83.22 Peripheral tear of medial meniscus, current injury
    - S83.221 Peripheral tear of medial meniscus, current injury, right knee
    - S83.222 Peripheral tear of medial meniscus, current injury, left knee
    - S83.229 Peripheral tear of medial meniscus, current injury, unspecified knee
  - S83.23 Complex tear of medial meniscus, current injury
    - S83.231 Complex tear of medial meniscus, current injury, right knee
    - S83.232 Complex tear of medial meniscus, current injury, left knee
    - S83.239 Complex tear of medial meniscus, current injury, unspecified knee
  - S83.24 Other tear of medial meniscus, current injury
    - S83.241 Other tear of medial meniscus, current injury, right knee
    - S83.242 Other tear of medial meniscus, current injury, left knee
    - S83.249 Other tear of medial meniscus, current injury, unspecified knee
  - S83.25 Bucket-handle tear of lateral meniscus, current injury
    - S83.251 Bucket-handle tear of lateral meniscus, current injury, right knee
    - S83.252 Bucket-handle tear of lateral meniscus, current injury, left knee
    - S83.259 Bucket-handle tear of lateral meniscus, current injury, unspecified knee
  - S83.26 Peripheral tear of lateral meniscus, current injury
    - S83.261 Peripheral tear of lateral meniscus, current injury, right knee
    - S83.262 Peripheral tear of lateral meniscus, current injury, left knee
    - S83.269 Peripheral tear of lateral meniscus, current injury, unspecified knee
  - S83.27 Complex tear of lateral meniscus, current injury
    - S83.271 Complex tear of lateral meniscus, current injury, right knee
    - S83.272 Complex tear of lateral meniscus, current injury, left knee
    - S83.279 Complex tear of lateral meniscus, current injury, unspecified knee
  - S83.28 Other tear of lateral meniscus, current injury
    - S83.281 Other tear of lateral meniscus, current injury, right knee
    - S83.282 Other tear of lateral meniscus, current injury, left knee
    - S83.289 Other tear of lateral meniscus, current injury, unspecified knee
- S83.3 Tear of articular cartilage of knee, current
  - X S83.30 Tear of articular cartilage of unspecified knee, current
  - X S83.31 Tear of articular cartilage of right knee, current
  - X S83.32 Tear of articular cartilage of left knee, current
- S83.4 Sprain of collateral ligament of knee
  - S83.40 Sprain of unspecified collateral ligament of knee
    - S83.401 Sprain of unspecified collateral ligament of right knee
    - S83.402 Sprain of unspecified collateral ligament of left knee
    - S83.409 Sprain of unspecified collateral ligament of unspecified knee
  - S83.41 Sprain of medial collateral ligament of knee
    - Sprain of tibial collateral ligament
    - S83.411 Sprain of medial collateral ligament of right knee
    - S83.412 Sprain of medial collateral ligament of left knee
    - S83.419 Sprain of medial collateral ligament of unspecified knee
  - S83.42 Sprain of lateral collateral ligament of knee
    - Sprain of fibular collateral ligament
    - S83.421 Sprain of lateral collateral ligament of right knee
    - S83.422 Sprain of lateral collateral ligament of left knee
    - S83.429 Sprain of lateral collateral ligament of unspecified knee
- S83.5 Sprain of cruciate ligament of knee
  - S83.50 Sprain of unspecified cruciate ligament of knee
    - S83.501 Sprain of unspecified cruciate ligament of right knee
    - S83.502 Sprain of unspecified cruciate ligament of left knee
    - S83.509 Sprain of unspecified cruciate ligament of unspecified knee
  - S83.51 Sprain of anterior cruciate ligament of knee
    - S83.511 Sprain of anterior cruciate ligament of right knee
      - **Coding Clinic: 2016, Q2, P4**
    - S83.512 Sprain of anterior cruciate ligament of left knee
    - S83.519 Sprain of anterior cruciate ligament of unspecified knee

- **S83.52 Sprain of posterior cruciate ligament of knee**
  - **S83.521 Sprain of posterior cruciate ligament of right knee**
  - **S83.522 Sprain of posterior cruciate ligament of left knee**
  - **S83.529 Sprain of posterior cruciate ligament of unspecified knee**
- **S83.6 Sprain of the superior tibiofibular joint and ligament**
  - X **S83.60 Sprain of the superior tibiofibular joint and ligament, unspecified knee**
  - X **S83.61 Sprain of the superior tibiofibular joint and ligament, right knee**
  - X **S83.62 Sprain of the superior tibiofibular joint and ligament, left knee**
- **S83.8 Sprain of other specified parts of knee**
  - **S83.8X Sprain of other specified parts of knee**
    - **S83.8X1 Sprain of other specified parts of right knee**
    - **S83.8X2 Sprain of other specified parts of left knee**
    - **S83.8X9 Sprain of other specified parts of unspecified knee**
- **S83.9 Sprain of unspecified site of knee**
  - X **S83.90 Sprain of unspecified site of unspecified knee**
  - X **S83.91 Sprain of unspecified site of right knee**
  - X **S83.92 Sprain of unspecified site of left knee**

- **S84 Injury of nerves at lower leg level**

  Code also any associated open wound (S81.-)

  Excludes2 injury of nerves at ankle and foot level (S94.-)

  The appropriate 7th character is to be added to each code from category S84

A	initial encounter
D	subsequent encounter
S	sequela

- **S84.0 Injury of tibial nerve at lower leg level**
  - X **S84.00 Injury of tibial nerve at lower leg level, unspecified leg**
  - X **S84.01 Injury of tibial nerve at lower leg level, right leg**
  - X **S84.02 Injury of tibial nerve at lower leg level, left leg**
- **S84.1 Injury of peroneal nerve at lower leg level**
  - X **S84.10 Injury of peroneal nerve at lower leg level, unspecified leg**
  - X **S84.11 Injury of peroneal nerve at lower leg level, right leg**
  - X **S84.12 Injury of peroneal nerve at lower leg level, left leg**
- **S84.2 Injury of cutaneous sensory nerve at lower leg level**
  - X **S84.20 Injury of cutaneous sensory nerve at lower leg level, unspecified leg**
  - X **S84.21 Injury of cutaneous sensory nerve at lower leg level, right leg**
  - X **S84.22 Injury of cutaneous sensory nerve at lower leg level, left leg**
- **S84.8 Injury of other nerves at lower leg level**
  - **S84.80 Injury of other nerves at lower leg level**
    - **S84.801 Injury of other nerves at lower leg level, right leg**
    - **S84.802 Injury of other nerves at lower leg level, left leg**
    - **S84.809 Injury of other nerves at lower leg level, unspecified leg**
- **S84.9 Injury of unspecified nerve at lower leg level**
  - X **S84.90 Injury of unspecified nerve at lower leg level, unspecified leg**
  - X **S84.91 Injury of unspecified nerve at lower leg level, right leg**
  - X **S84.92 Injury of unspecified nerve at lower leg level, left leg**

- **S85 Injury of blood vessels at lower leg level**

  Code also any associated open wound (S81.-)

  Excludes2 injury of blood vessels at ankle and foot level (S95.-)

  The appropriate 7th character is to be added to each code from category S85

A	initial encounter
D	subsequent encounter
S	sequela

- **S85.0 Injury of popliteal artery**
  - **S85.00 Unspecified injury of popliteal artery**
    - **S85.001 Unspecified injury of popliteal artery, right leg A** MCC
      Ex: S75.801[A], S75.809-S75.811[A], S75.819-S75.891[A], S75.899-S75.901[A], S75.909-S75.911[A], S75.919-S75.991[A], S75.999[A], S85.001[A], S85.009-S85.011[A], S85.019-S85.091[A], S85.099[A], S85.201[A], S85.209-S85.211[A], S85.219-S85.291[A], S85.299[A], S85.801[A], S85.809-S85.811[A], S85.819-S85.891[A], S85.899-S85.901[A], S85.909-S85.911[A], S85.919-S85.991[A], S85.999[A], S95.001[A], S95.009-S95.011[A], S95.019-S95.091[A], S95.099-S95.201[A], S95.209-S95.211[A], S95.219-S95.291[A], S95.299-S95.801[A], S95.809-S95.811[A], S95.819-S95.891[A], S95.899-S95.901[A], S95.909-S95.911[A], S95.919-S95.991[A], S95.999[A]
    - **S85.002 Unspecified injury of popliteal artery, left leg A** MCC
      Ex: S75.802-S75.809[A], S75.812-S75.819[A], S75.892-S75.899[A], S75.902-S75.909[A], S75.912-S75.919[A], S75.992-S75.999[A], S85.002-S85.009[A], S85.012-S85.019[A], S85.092-S85.099[A], S85.202-S85.209[A], S85.212-S85.219[A], S85.292-S85.299[A], S85.802-S85.809[A], S85.812-S85.819[A], S85.892-S85.899[A], S85.902-S85.909[A], S85.912-S85.919[A], S85.992-S85.999[A], S95.002-S95.009[A], S95.012-S95.019[A], S95.092-S95.099[A], S95.202-S95.209[A], S95.212-S95.219[A], S95.292-S95.299[A], S95.802-S95.809[A], S95.812-S95.819[A], S95.892-S95.899[A], S95.902-S95.909[A], S95.912-S95.919[A], S95.992-S95.999[A]
    - **S85.009 Unspecified injury of popliteal artery, unspecified leg A** MCC
      Ex: S75.802-S75.809[A], S75.812-S75.819[A], S75.892-S75.899[A], S75.902-S75.909[A], S75.912-S75.919[A], S75.992-S75.999[A], S85.162-S85.169[A], S85.172-S85.179[A], S85.182-S85.189[A], S85.202-S85.209[A], S85.212-S85.219[A], S85.292-S85.299[A], S85.802-S85.809[A], S85.812-S85.819[A], S85.892-S85.899[A], S85.902-S85.909[A], S85.912-S85.919[A], S85.992-S85.999[A], S95.002-S95.009[A], S95.012-S95.019[A], S95.092-S95.099[A], S95.202-S95.209[A], S95.212-S95.219[A], S95.292-S95.299[A], S95.802-S95.809[A], S95.812-S95.819[A], S95.892-S95.899[A], S95.902-S95.909[A], S95.912-S95.919[A], S95.992-S95.999[A]

- **S85.01 Laceration of popliteal artery**
  - **S85.011 Laceration of popliteal artery, right leg A**
    Ex: See S85.001
  - **S85.012 Laceration of popliteal artery, left leg A**
    Ex: See S85.002
  - **S85.019 Laceration of popliteal artery, unspecified leg A**
    Ex: See S85.009
- **S85.09 Other specified injury of popliteal artery**
  - **S85.091 Other specified injury of popliteal artery, right leg A**
    Ex: See S85.001
  - **S85.092 Other specified injury of popliteal artery, left leg A**
    Ex: See S85.002
  - **S85.099 Other specified injury of popliteal artery, unspecified leg A**
    Ex: See S85.009
- **S85.1 Injury of tibial artery**
  - **S85.10 Unspecified injury of unspecified tibial artery**
    Injury of tibial artery NOS
    - **S85.101 Unspecified injury of unspecified tibial artery, right leg A**
      Ex: S75.801[A], S75.809-S75.811[A], S75.819-S75.891[A], S75.899-S75.901[A], S75.909-S75.911[A], S75.919-S75.991[A], S75.999[A], S85.101[A], S85.109-S85.111[A], S85.119-S85.121[A], S85.129[A], S85.201[A], S85.209-S85.211[A], S85.219-S85.291[A], S85.299[A], S85.801[A], S85.809-S85.811[A], S85.819-S85.891[A], S85.899-S85.901[A], S85.909-S85.911[A], S85.919-S85.991[A], S85.999[A], S95.001[A], S95.009-S95.011[A], S95.019-S95.091[A], S95.099-S95.201[A], S95.209-S95.211[A], S95.219-S95.291[A], S95.299-S95.801[A], S95.809-S95.811[A], S95.819-S95.891[A], S95.899-S95.901[A], S95.909-S95.911[A], S95.919-S95.991[A], S95.999[A]
    - **S85.102 Unspecified injury of unspecified tibial artery, left leg A**
      Ex: S75.802-S75.809[A], S75.812-S75.819[A], S75.892-S75.899[A], S75.902-S75.909[A], S75.912-S75.919[A], S75.992-S75.999[A], S85.102-S85.109[A], S85.112-S85.119[A], S85.122-S85.129[A], S85.202-S85.209[A], S85.212-S85.219[A], S85.292-S85.299[A], S85.802-S85.809[A], S85.812-S85.819[A], S85.892-S85.899[A], S85.902-S85.909[A], S85.912-S85.919[A], S85.992-S85.999[A], S95.002-S95.009[A], S95.012-S95.019[A], S95.092-S95.099[A], S95.202-S95.209[A], S95.212-S95.219[A], S95.292-S95.299[A], S95.802-S95.809[A], S95.812-S95.819[A], S95.892-S95.899[A], S95.902-S95.909[A], S95.912-S95.919[A], S95.992-S95.999[A]
    - **S85.109 Unspecified injury of unspecified tibial artery, unspecified leg A**
      Ex: S75.801-S75.999[A], S85.101-S85.129[A], S85.201-S85.299[A], S85.801-S85.999[A], S95.001-S95.099[A], S95.201-S95.999[A]
  - **S85.11 Laceration of unspecified tibial artery**
    - **S85.111 Laceration of unspecified tibial artery, right leg A**
      Ex: See S85.101
    - **S85.112 Laceration of unspecified tibial artery, left leg A**
      Ex: See S85.102
    - **S85.119 Laceration of unspecified tibial artery, unspecified leg A**
      Ex: See S85.109
  - **S85.12 Other specified injury of unspecified tibial artery**
    - **S85.121 Other specified injury of unspecified tibial artery, right leg A**
      Ex: See S85.101
    - **S85.122 Other specified injury of unspecified tibial artery, left leg A**
      Ex: See S85.102
    - **S85.129 Other specified injury of unspecified tibial artery, unspecified leg A**
      Ex: See S85.109
  - **S85.13 Unspecified injury of anterior tibial artery**
    - **S85.131 Unspecified injury of anterior tibial artery, right leg A**
      Ex: S75.801[A], S75.809-S75.811[A], S75.819-S75.891[A], S75.899-S75.901[A], S75.909-S75.911[A], S75.919-S75.991[A], S75.999[A], S85.131[A], S85.139-S85.141[A], S85.149-S85.151[A], S85.159[A], S85.201[A], S85.209-S85.211[A], S85.219-S85.291[A], S85.299[A], S85.801[A], S85.809-S85.811[A], S85.819-S85.891[A], S85.899-S85.901[A], S85.909-S85.911[A], S85.919-S85.991[A], S85.999[A], S95.001[A], S95.009-S95.011[A], S95.019-S95.091[A], S95.099-S95.201[A], S95.209-S95.211[A], S95.219-S95.291[A], S95.299-S95.801[A], S95.809-S95.811[A], S95.819-S95.891[A], S95.899-S95.901[A], S95.909-S95.911[A], S95.919-S95.991[A], S95.999[A]
    - **S85.132 Unspecified injury of anterior tibial artery, left leg A**
      Ex: S75.802-S75.809[A], S75.812-S75.819[A], S75.892-S75.899[A], S75.902-S75.909[A], S75.912-S75.919[A], S75.992-S75.999[A], S85.132-S85.139[A], S85.142-S85.149[A], S85.152-S85.159[A], S85.202-S85.209[A], S85.212-S85.219[A], S85.292-S85.299[A], S85.802-S85.809[A], S85.812-S85.819[A], S85.892-S85.899[A], S85.902-S85.909[A], S85.912-S85.919[A], S85.992-S85.999[A], S95.002-S95.009[A], S95.012-S95.019[A], S95.092-S95.099[A], S95.202-S95.209[A], S95.212-S95.219[A], S95.292-S95.299[A], S95.802-S95.809[A], S95.812-S95.819[A], S95.892-S95.899[A], S95.902-S95.909[A], S95.912-S95.919[A], S95.992-S95.999[A]
    - **S85.139 Unspecified injury of anterior tibial artery, unspecified leg A**
      Ex: S75.801-S75.999[A], S85.131-S85.159[A], S85.201-S85.299[A], S85.801-S85.999[A], S95.001-S95.099[A], S95.201-S95.999[A]

- **S85.14 Laceration of anterior tibial artery**
  - **S85.141 Laceration of anterior tibial artery, right leg A**
    Ex: See S85.131
  - **S85.142 Laceration of anterior tibial artery, left leg A**
    Ex: See S85.132
  - **S85.149 Laceration of anterior tibial artery, unspecified leg A**
    Ex: See S85.139
- **S85.15 Other specified injury of anterior tibial artery**
  - **S85.151 Other specified injury of anterior tibial artery, right leg A**
    Ex: See S85.131
  - **S85.152 Other specified injury of anterior tibial artery, left leg A**
    Ex: See S85.132
  - **S85.159 Other specified injury of anterior tibial artery, unspecified leg A**
    Ex: See S85.139
- **S85.16 Unspecified injury of posterior tibial artery**
  - **S85.161 Unspecified injury of posterior tibial artery, right leg A**
    Ex: S75.801[A], S75.809-S75.811[A], S75.819-S75.891[A], S75.899-S75.901[A], S75.909-S75.911[A], S75.919-S75.991[A], S75.999[A], S85.161[A], S85.169-S85.171[A], S85.179-S85.181[A], S85.189[A], S85.201[A], S85.209-S85.211[A], S85.219-S85.291[A], S85.299[A], S85.801[A], S85.809-S85.811[A], S85.819-S85.891[A], S85.899-S85.901[A], S85.909-S85.911[A], S85.919-S85.991[A], S85.999[A], S95.001[A], S95.009-S95.011[A], S95.019-S95.091[A], S95.099-S95.201[A], S95.209-S95.211[A], S95.219-S95.291[A], S95.299-S95.801[A], S95.809-S95.811[A], S95.819-S95.891[A], S95.899-S95.901[A], S95.909-S95.911[A], S95.919-S95.991[A], S95.999[A]
  - **S85.162 Unspecified injury of posterior tibial artery, left leg A**
    Ex: S75.802-S75.809[A], S75.812-S75.819[A], S75.892-S75.899[A], S75.902-S75.909[A], S75.912-S75.919[A], S75.992-S75.999[A], S85.162-S85.169[A], S85.172-S85.179[A], S85.182-S85.189[A], S85.202-S85.209[A], S85.212-S85.219[A], S85.292-S85.299[A], S85.802-S85.809[A], S85.812-S85.819[A], S85.892-S85.899[A], S85.902-S85.909[A], S85.912-S85.919[A], S85.992-S85.999[A], S95.002-S95.009[A], S95.012-S95.019[A], S95.092-S95.099[A], S95.202-S95.209[A], S95.212-S95.219[A], S95.292-S95.299[A], S95.802-S95.809[A], S95.812-S95.819[A], S95.892-S95.899[A], S95.902-S95.909[A], S95.912-S95.919[A], S95.992-S95.999[A]
  - **S85.169 Unspecified injury of posterior tibial artery, unspecified leg A**
    Ex: S75.801-S75.999[A], S85.161-S85.189[A], S85.201-S85.299[A], S85.801-S85.999[A], S95.001-S95.099[A], S95.201-S95.999[A]
- **S85.17 Laceration of posterior tibial artery**
  - **S85.171 Laceration of posterior tibial artery, right leg A**
    Ex: See S85.161
  - **S85.172 Laceration of posterior tibial artery, left leg A**
    Ex: See S85.162
  - **S85.179 Laceration of posterior tibial artery, unspecified leg A**
    Ex: See S85.169
- **S85.18 Other specified injury of posterior tibial artery**
  - **S85.181 Other specified injury of posterior tibial artery, right leg A**
    Ex: See S85.161
  - **S85.182 Other specified injury of posterior tibial artery, left leg A**
    Ex: See S85.162
  - **S85.189 Other specified injury of posterior tibial artery, unspecified leg A**
    Ex: See S85.169
- **S85.2 Injury of peroneal artery**
  - **S85.20 Unspecified injury of peroneal artery**
    - **S85.201 Unspecified injury of peroneal artery, right leg A**
      Ex: See S75.801
    - **S85.202 Unspecified injury of peroneal artery, left leg A**
      Ex: See S75.802
    - **S85.209 Unspecified injury of peroneal artery, unspecified leg A**
      Ex: See S75.809
  - **S85.21 Laceration of peroneal artery**
    - **S85.211 Laceration of peroneal artery, right leg A**
      Ex: See S75.801
    - **S85.212 Laceration of peroneal artery, left leg A**
      Ex: See S75.802
    - **S85.219 Laceration of peroneal artery, unspecified leg A**
      Ex: See S75.809
  - **S85.29 Other specified injury of peroneal artery**
    - **S85.291 Other specified injury of peroneal artery, right leg A**
      Ex: See S75.801
    - **S85.292 Other specified injury of peroneal artery, left leg A**
      Ex: See S75.802
    - **S85.299 Other specified injury of peroneal artery, unspecified leg A**
      Ex: See S75.809
- **S85.3 Injury of greater saphenous vein at lower leg level**
  Injury of greater saphenous vein NOS
  Injury of saphenous vein NOS
  - **S85.30 Unspecified injury of greater saphenous vein at lower leg level**
    - **S85.301 Unspecified injury of greater saphenous vein at lower leg level, right leg A**
      Ex: See S75.201
    - **S85.302 Unspecified injury of greater saphenous vein at lower leg level, left leg A**
      Ex: See S75.202
    - **S85.309 Unspecified injury of greater saphenous vein at lower leg level, unspecified leg A**
      Ex: See S75.209
  - **S85.31 Laceration of greater saphenous vein at lower leg level**
    - **S85.311 Laceration of greater saphenous vein at lower leg level, right leg A**
      Ex: See S75.201
    - **S85.312 Laceration of greater saphenous vein at lower leg level, left leg A**
      Ex: See S75.202
    - **S85.319 Laceration of greater saphenous vein at lower leg level, unspecified leg A**
      Ex: See S75.209

- S85.39 Other specified injury of greater saphenous vein at lower leg level
  - S85.391 Other specified injury of greater saphenous vein at lower leg level, right leg A
    - Ex: See S75.201
  - S85.392 Other specified injury of greater saphenous vein at lower leg level, left leg A
    - Ex: See S75.202
  - S85.399 Other specified injury of greater saphenous vein at lower leg level, unspecified leg A
    - Ex: See S75.209
- S85.4 Injury of lesser saphenous vein at lower leg level
  - S85.40 Unspecified injury of lesser saphenous vein at lower leg level
    - S85.401 Unspecified injury of lesser saphenous vein at lower leg level, right leg A
      - Ex: See S75.201
    - S85.402 Unspecified injury of lesser saphenous vein at lower leg level, left leg A
      - Ex: See S75.202
    - S85.409 Unspecified injury of lesser saphenous vein at lower leg level, unspecified leg A
      - Ex: See S75.209
  - S85.41 Laceration of lesser saphenous vein at lower leg level
    - S85.411 Laceration of lesser saphenous vein at lower leg level, right leg A
      - Ex: See S75.201
    - S85.412 Laceration of lesser saphenous vein at lower leg level, left leg A
      - Ex: See S75.202
    - S85.419 Laceration of lesser saphenous vein at lower leg level, unspecified leg A
      - Ex: See S75.209
  - S85.49 Other specified injury of lesser saphenous vein at lower leg level
    - S85.491 Other specified injury of lesser saphenous vein at lower leg level, right leg A
      - Ex: See S75.201
    - S85.492 Other specified injury of lesser saphenous vein at lower leg level, left leg A
      - Ex: See S75.202
    - S85.499 Other specified injury of lesser saphenous vein at lower leg level, unspecified leg A
      - Ex: See S75.209
- S85.5 Injury of popliteal vein
  - S85.50 Unspecified injury of popliteal vein
    - S85.501 Unspecified injury of popliteal vein, right leg A
      - Ex: S75.801[A], S75.809-S75.811[A], S75.819-S75.891[A], S75.899-S75.901[A], S75.909-S75.911[A], S75.919-S75.991[A], S75.999[A], S85.201[A], S85.209-S85.211[A], S85.219-S85.291[A], S85.299[A], S85.501[A], S85.509-S85.511[A], S85.519-S85.591[A], S85.599[A], S85.801[A], S85.809-S85.811[A], S85.819-S85.891[A], S85.899-S85.901[A], S85.909-S85.911[A], S85.919-S85.991[A], S85.999[A], S95.001[A], S95.009-S95.011[A], S95.019-S95.091[A], S95.099-S95.201[A], S95.209-S95.211[A], S95.219-S95.291[A], S95.299-S95.801[A], S95.809-S95.811[A], S95.819-S95.891[A], S95.899-S95.901[A], S95.909-S95.911[A], S95.919-S95.991[A], S95.999[A]
    - S85.502 Unspecified injury of popliteal vein, left leg A
      - Ex: S75.802-S75.809[A], S75.812-S75.819[A], S75.892-S75.899[A], S75.902-S75.909[A], S75.912-S75.919[A], S75.992-S75.999[A], S85.202-S85.209[A], S85.212-S85.219[A], S85.292-S85.299[A], S85.502-S85.509[A], S85.512-S85.519[A], S85.592-S85.599[A], S85.802-S85.809[A], S85.812-S85.819[A], S85.892-S85.899[A], S85.902-S85.909[A], S85.912-S85.919[A], S85.992-S85.999[A], S95.002-S95.009[A], S95.012-S95.019[A], S95.092-S95.099[A], S95.202-S95.209[A], S95.212-S95.219[A], S95.292-S95.299[A], S95.802-S95.809[A], S95.812-S95.819[A], S95.892-S95.899[A], S95.902-S95.909[A], S95.912-S95.919[A], S95.992-S95.999[A]
    - S85.509 Unspecified injury of popliteal vein, unspecified leg A
      - Ex: S75.801-S75.999[A], S85.201-S85.299[A], S85.501-S85.599[A], S85.801-S85.999[A], S95.001-S95.099[A], S95.201-S95.999[A]
  - S85.51 Laceration of popliteal vein
    - S85.511 Laceration of popliteal vein, right leg A
      - Ex: See S85.501
    - S85.512 Laceration of popliteal vein, left leg A
      - Ex: See S85.502
    - S85.519 Laceration of popliteal vein, unspecified leg A
      - Ex: See S85.509
  - S85.59 Other specified injury of popliteal vein
    - S85.591 Other specified injury of popliteal vein, right leg A
      - Ex: See S85.501
    - S85.592 Other specified injury of popliteal vein, left leg A
      - Ex: See S85.502
    - S85.599 Other specified injury of popliteal vein, unspecified leg A
      - Ex: See S85.509
- S85.8 Injury of other blood vessels at lower leg level
  - S85.80 Unspecified injury of other blood vessels at lower leg level
    - S85.801 Unspecified injury of other blood vessels at lower leg level, right leg A
      - Ex: See S75.801
    - S85.802 Unspecified injury of other blood vessels at lower leg level, left leg A
      - Ex: See S75.802
    - S85.809 Unspecified injury of other blood vessels at lower leg level, unspecified leg A
      - Ex: See S75.809
  - S85.81 Laceration of other blood vessels at lower leg level
    - S85.811 Laceration of other blood vessels at lower leg level, right leg A
      - Ex: See S75.801
    - S85.812 Laceration of other blood vessels at lower leg level, left leg A
      - Ex: See S75.802
    - S85.819 Laceration of other blood vessels at lower leg level, unspecified leg A
      - Ex: See S75.809

- **S85.89** Other specified injury of other blood vessels at lower leg level
  - **S85.891** Other specified injury of other blood vessels at lower leg level, right leg A
    Ex: See S75.801
  - **S85.892** Other specified injury of other blood vessels at lower leg level, left leg A
    Ex: See S75.802
  - **S85.899** Other specified injury of other blood vessels at lower leg level, unspecified leg A
    Ex: See S75.809
- **S85.9** Injury of unspecified blood vessel at lower leg level
  - **S85.90** Unspecified injury of unspecified blood vessel at lower leg level
    - **S85.901** Unspecified injury of unspecified blood vessel at lower leg level, right leg A
      Ex: See S75.801
    - **S85.902** Unspecified injury of unspecified blood vessel at lower leg level, left leg A
      Ex: See S75.802
    - **S85.909** Unspecified injury of unspecified blood vessel at lower leg level, unspecified leg A
      Ex: See S75.809
  - **S85.91** Laceration of unspecified blood vessel at lower leg level
    - **S85.911** Laceration of unspecified blood vessel at lower leg level, right leg A
      Ex: See S75.801
    - **S85.912** Laceration of unspecified blood vessel at lower leg level, left leg A
      Ex: See S75.802
    - **S85.919** Laceration of unspecified blood vessel at lower leg level, unspecified leg A
      Ex: See S75.809
  - **S85.99** Other specified injury of unspecified blood vessel at lower leg level
    - **S85.991** Other specified injury of unspecified blood vessel at lower leg level, right leg A
      Ex: See S75.801
    - **S85.992** Other specified injury of unspecified blood vessel at lower leg level, left leg A
      Ex: See S75.802
    - **S85.999** Other specified injury of unspecified blood vessel at lower leg level, unspecified leg A
      Ex: See S75.809

- **S86** Injury of muscle, fascia and tendon at lower leg level

  Code also any associated open wound (S81.-)

  Excludes2 injury of muscle, fascia and tendon at ankle (S96.-)
  injury of patellar ligament (tendon) (S76.1-)
  sprain of joints and ligaments of knee (S83.-)

  The appropriate 7th character is to be added to each code from category S86

A	initial encounter
D	subsequent encounter
S	sequela

- **S86.0** Injury of Achilles tendon
  - **S86.00** Unspecified injury of Achilles tendon
    - **S86.001** Unspecified injury of right Achilles tendon
    - **S86.002** Unspecified injury of left Achilles tendon
    - **S86.009** Unspecified injury of unspecified Achilles tendon
  - **S86.01** Strain of Achilles tendon
    - **S86.011** Strain of right Achilles tendon
    - **S86.012** Strain of left Achilles tendon
    - **S86.019** Strain of unspecified Achilles tendon
  - **S86.02** Laceration of Achilles tendon
    - **S86.021** Laceration of right Achilles tendon A
      Ex: S81.001[A], S81.009-S81.011[A], S81.019-S81.021[A], S81.029-S81.031[A], S81.039-S81.041[A], S81.049-S81.051[A], S81.059-S81.801[A], S81.809-S81.811[A], S81.819-S81.821[A], S81.829-S81.831[A], S81.839-S81.841[A], S81.849-S81.851[A], S81.859[A], S86.021[A], S86.029[A], S86.121[A], S86.129[A], S86.221[A], S86.229[A], S86.321[A], S86.329[A], S86.821[A], S86.829-S86.921[A], S86.929[A], S91.001[A], S91.009[A], S91.011[A], S91.019-S91.021[A], S91.029-S91.031[A], S91.039-S91.041[A], S91.049-S91.051[A], S91.059[A], S96.021[A], S96.029[A], S96.121[A], S96.129[A], S96.221[A], S96.229[A], S96.821[A], S96.829[A], S96.921[A], S96.929[A]
    - **S86.022** Laceration of left Achilles tendon A
      Ex: S81.002-S81.009[A], S81.012-S81.019[A], S81.022-S81.029[A], S81.032-S81.039[A], S81.042-S81.049[A], S81.052-S81.059[A], S81.802-S81.809[A], S81.812-S81.819[A], S81.822-S81.829[A], S81.832-S81.839[A], S81.842-S81.849[A], S81.852-S81.859[A], S86.022-S86.029[A], S86.122-S86.129[A], S86.222-S86.229[A], S86.322-S86.329[A], S86.822-S86.829[A], S86.922-S86.929[A], S91.002-S91.009[A], S91.012-S91.019[A], S91.022-S91.029[A], S91.032-S91.039[A], S91.042-S91.049[A], S91.052-S91.059[A], S96.022-S96.029[A], S96.122-S96.129[A], S96.222-S96.229[A], S96.822-S96.829[A], S96.922-S96.929[A]
    - **S86.029** Laceration of unspecified Achilles tendon A
      Ex: S81.001-S81.859[A], S86.021-S86.029[A], S86.121-S86.129[A], S86.221-S86.229[A], S86.321-S86.329[A], S86.821-S86.829[A], S86.921-S86.929[A], S91.001-S91.059[A], S96.021-S96.029[A], S96.121-S96.129[A], S96.221-S96.229[A], S96.821-S96.829[A], S96.921-S96.929[A]
  - **S86.09** Other specified injury of Achilles tendon
    - **S86.091** Other specified injury of right Achilles tendon
    - **S86.092** Other specified injury of left Achilles tendon
    - **S86.099** Other specified injury of unspecified Achilles tendon
- **S86.1** Injury of other muscle(s) and tendon(s) of posterior muscle group at lower leg level
  - **S86.10** Unspecified injury of other muscle(s) and tendon(s) of posterior muscle group at lower leg level
    - **S86.101** Unspecified injury of other muscle(s) and tendon(s) of posterior muscle group at lower leg level, right leg
    - **S86.102** Unspecified injury of other muscle(s) and tendon(s) of posterior muscle group at lower leg level, left leg
    - **S86.109** Unspecified injury of other muscle(s) and tendon(s) of posterior muscle group at lower leg level, unspecified leg

- S86.11 Strain of other muscle(s) and tendon(s) of posterior muscle group at lower leg level
  - S86.111 Strain of other muscle(s) and tendon(s) of posterior muscle group at lower leg level, right leg
  - S86.112 Strain of other muscle(s) and tendon(s) of posterior muscle group at lower leg level, left leg
  - S86.119 Strain of other muscle(s) and tendon(s) of posterior muscle group at lower leg level, unspecified leg
- S86.12 Laceration of other muscle(s) and tendon(s) of posterior muscle group at lower leg level
  - S86.121 Laceration of other muscle(s) and tendon(s) of posterior muscle group at lower leg level, right leg A
    Ex: See S86.021
  - S86.122 Laceration of other muscle(s) and tendon(s) of posterior muscle group at lower leg level, left leg A
    Ex: See S86.022
  - S86.129 Laceration of other muscle(s) and tendon(s) of posterior muscle group at lower leg level, unspecified leg A
    Ex: See S86.029
- S86.19 Other injury of other muscle(s) and tendon(s) of posterior muscle group at lower leg level
  - S86.191 Other injury of other muscle(s) and tendon(s) of posterior muscle group at lower leg level, right leg
  - S86.192 Other injury of other muscle(s) and tendon(s) of posterior muscle group at lower leg level, left leg
  - S86.199 Other injury of other muscle(s) and tendon(s) of posterior muscle group at lower leg level, unspecified leg
- S86.2 Injury of muscle(s) and tendon(s) of anterior muscle group at lower leg level
  - S86.20 Unspecified injury of muscle(s) and tendon(s) of anterior muscle group at lower leg level
    - S86.201 Unspecified injury of muscle(s) and tendon(s) of anterior muscle group at lower leg level, right leg
    - S86.202 Unspecified injury of muscle(s) and tendon(s) of anterior muscle group at lower leg level, left leg
    - S86.209 Unspecified injury of muscle(s) and tendon(s) of anterior muscle group at lower leg level, unspecified leg
  - S86.21 Strain of muscle(s) and tendon(s) of anterior muscle group at lower leg level
    - S86.211 Strain of muscle(s) and tendon(s) of anterior muscle group at lower leg level, right leg
    - S86.212 Strain of muscle(s) and tendon(s) of anterior muscle group at lower leg level, left leg
    - S86.219 Strain of muscle(s) and tendon(s) of anterior muscle group at lower leg level, unspecified leg
  - S86.22 Laceration of muscle(s) and tendon(s) of anterior muscle group at lower leg level
    - S86.221 Laceration of muscle(s) and tendon(s) of anterior muscle group at lower leg level, right leg A
      Ex: See S86.021
    - S86.222 Laceration of muscle(s) and tendon(s) of anterior muscle group at lower leg level, left leg A
      Ex: See S86.022
    - S86.229 Laceration of muscle(s) and tendon(s) of anterior muscle group at lower leg level, unspecified leg A
      Ex: See S86.029
  - S86.29 Other injury of muscle(s) and tendon(s) of anterior muscle group at lower leg level
    - S86.291 Other injury of muscle(s) and tendon(s) of anterior muscle group at lower leg level, right leg
    - S86.292 Other injury of muscle(s) and tendon(s) of anterior muscle group at lower leg level, left leg
    - S86.299 Other injury of muscle(s) and tendon(s) of anterior muscle group at lower leg level, unspecified leg
- S86.3 Injury of muscle(s) and tendon(s) of peroneal muscle group at lower leg level
  - S86.30 Unspecified injury of muscle(s) and tendon(s) of peroneal muscle group at lower leg level
    - S86.301 Unspecified injury of muscle(s) and tendon(s) of peroneal muscle group at lower leg level, right leg
    - S86.302 Unspecified injury of muscle(s) and tendon(s) of peroneal muscle group at lower leg level, left leg
    - S86.309 Unspecified injury of muscle(s) and tendon(s) of peroneal muscle group at lower leg level, unspecified leg
  - S86.31 Strain of muscle(s) and tendon(s) of peroneal muscle group at lower leg level
    - S86.311 Strain of muscle(s) and tendon(s) of peroneal muscle group at lower leg level, right leg
    - S86.312 Strain of muscle(s) and tendon(s) of peroneal muscle group at lower leg level, left leg
    - S86.319 Strain of muscle(s) and tendon(s) of peroneal muscle group at lower leg level, unspecified leg
  - S86.32 Laceration of muscle(s) and tendon(s) of peroneal muscle group at lower leg level
    - S86.321 Laceration of muscle(s) and tendon(s) of peroneal muscle group at lower leg level, right leg A
      Ex: See S86.021
    - S86.322 Laceration of muscle(s) and tendon(s) of peroneal muscle group at lower leg level, left leg A
      Ex: See S86.022
    - S86.329 Laceration of muscle(s) and tendon(s) of peroneal muscle group at lower leg level, unspecified leg A
      Ex: See S86.029

- **S86.39** Other injury of muscle(s) and tendon(s) of peroneal muscle group at lower leg level
  - **S86.391** Other injury of muscle(s) and tendon(s) of peroneal muscle group at lower leg level, right leg
  - **S86.392** Other injury of muscle(s) and tendon(s) of peroneal muscle group at lower leg level, left leg
  - **S86.399** Other injury of muscle(s) and tendon(s) of peroneal muscle group at lower leg level, unspecified leg
- **S86.8** Injury of other muscles and tendons at lower leg level
  - **S86.80** Unspecified injury of other muscles and tendons at lower leg level
    - **S86.801** Unspecified injury of other muscle(s) and tendon(s) at lower leg level, right leg
    - **S86.802** Unspecified injury of other muscle(s) and tendon(s) at lower leg level, left leg
    - **S86.809** Unspecified injury of other muscle(s) and tendon(s) at lower leg level, unspecified leg
  - **S86.81** Strain of other muscles and tendons at lower leg level
    - **S86.811** Strain of other muscle(s) and tendon(s) at lower leg level, right leg
    - **S86.812** Strain of other muscle(s) and tendon(s) at lower leg level, left leg
    - **S86.819** Strain of other muscle(s) and tendon(s) at lower leg level, unspecified leg
  - **S86.82** Laceration of other muscles and tendons at lower leg level
    - **S86.821** Laceration of other muscle(s) and tendon(s) at lower leg level, right leg A
      Ex: See S86.021
    - **S86.822** Laceration of other muscle(s) and tendon(s) at lower leg level, left leg A
      Ex: See S86.022
    - **S86.829** Laceration of other muscle(s) and tendon(s) at lower leg level, unspecified leg A
      Ex: See S86.029
  - **S86.89** Other injury of other muscles and tendons at lower leg level
    - **S86.891** Other injury of other muscle(s) and tendon(s) at lower leg level, right leg
    - **S86.892** Other injury of other muscle(s) and tendon(s) at lower leg level, left leg
    - **S86.899** Other injury of other muscle(s) and tendon(s) at lower leg level, unspecified leg
- **S86.9** Injury of unspecified muscle and tendon at lower leg level
  - **S86.90** Unspecified injury of unspecified muscle and tendon at lower leg level
    - **S86.901** Unspecified injury of unspecified muscle(s) and tendon(s) at lower leg level, right leg
    - **S86.902** Unspecified injury of unspecified muscle(s) and tendon(s) at lower leg level, left leg
    - **S86.909** Unspecified injury of unspecified muscle(s) and tendon(s) at lower leg level, unspecified leg
  - **S86.91** Strain of unspecified muscle and tendon at lower leg level
    - **S86.911** Strain of unspecified muscle(s) and tendon(s) at lower leg level, right leg
    - **S86.912** Strain of unspecified muscle(s) and tendon(s) at lower leg level, left leg
    - **S86.919** Strain of unspecified muscle(s) and tendon(s) at lower leg level, unspecified leg
  - **S86.92** Laceration of unspecified muscle and tendon at lower leg level
    - **S86.921** Laceration of unspecified muscle(s) and tendon(s) at lower leg level, right leg A
      Ex: See S86.021
    - **S86.922** Laceration of unspecified muscle(s) and tendon(s) at lower leg level, left leg A
      Ex: See S86.022
    - **S86.929** Laceration of unspecified muscle(s) and tendon(s) at lower leg level, unspecified leg A
      Ex: See S86.029
  - **S86.99** Other injury of unspecified muscle and tendon at lower leg level
    - **S86.991** Other injury of unspecified muscle(s) and tendon(s) at lower leg level, right leg
    - **S86.992** Other injury of unspecified muscle(s) and tendon(s) at lower leg level, left leg
    - **S86.999** Other injury of unspecified muscle(s) and tendon(s) at lower leg level, unspecified leg
- **S87** Crushing injury of lower leg

  Use additional code(s) for all associated injuries

  Excludes2 crushing injury of ankle and foot (S97.-)

  The appropriate 7th character is to be added to each code from category S87

A	initial encounter
D	subsequent encounter
S	sequela

  - **S87.0** Crushing injury of knee
    - X **S87.00** Crushing injury of unspecified knee
    - X **S87.01** Crushing injury of right knee
    - X **S87.02** Crushing injury of left knee
  - **S87.8** Crushing injury of lower leg
    - X **S87.80** Crushing injury of unspecified lower leg
    - X **S87.81** Crushing injury of right lower leg
    - X **S87.82** Crushing injury of left lower leg

S88 Traumatic amputation of lower leg

An amputation not identified as partial or complete should be coded to complete

Excludes1 traumatic amputation of ankle and foot (S98.-)

The appropriate 7th character is to be added to each code from category S88

A	initial encounter
D	subsequent encounter
S	sequela

S88.0 Traumatic amputation at knee level

S88.01 Complete traumatic amputation at knee level

S88.011 Complete traumatic amputation at knee level, right lower leg A
Ex: See S78.011

S88.012 Complete traumatic amputation at knee level, left lower leg A
Ex: See S78.012

S88.019 Complete traumatic amputation at knee level, unspecified lower leg A
Ex: See S78.019

S88.02 Partial traumatic amputation at knee level

S88.021 Partial traumatic amputation at knee level, right lower leg A
Ex: See S78.011

S88.022 Partial traumatic amputation at knee level, left lower leg A
Ex: See S78.012

S88.029 Partial traumatic amputation at knee level, unspecified lower leg A
Ex: See S78.019

S88.1 Traumatic amputation at level between knee and ankle

S88.11 Complete traumatic amputation at level between knee and ankle

S88.111 Complete traumatic amputation at level between knee and ankle, right lower leg A
Ex: See S78.011

S88.112 Complete traumatic amputation at level between knee and ankle, left lower leg A
Ex: See S78.012

S88.119 Complete traumatic amputation at level between knee and ankle, unspecified lower leg A
Ex: See S78.019

S88.12 Partial traumatic amputation at level between knee and ankle

S88.121 Partial traumatic amputation at level between knee and ankle, right lower leg A
Ex: See S78.011

S88.122 Partial traumatic amputation at level between knee and ankle, left lower leg A
Ex: See S78.012

S88.129 Partial traumatic amputation at level between knee and ankle, unspecified lower leg A
Ex: See S78.019

S88.9 Traumatic amputation of lower leg, level unspecified

S88.91 Complete traumatic amputation of lower leg, level unspecified

S88.911 Complete traumatic amputation of right lower leg, level unspecified A
Ex: See S78.011

S88.912 Complete traumatic amputation of left lower leg, level unspecified A
Ex: See S78.012

S88.919 Complete traumatic amputation of unspecified lower leg, level unspecified A
Ex: See S78.019

S88.92 Partial traumatic amputation of lower leg, level unspecified

S88.921 Partial traumatic amputation of right lower leg, level unspecified A
Ex: See S78.011

S88.922 Partial traumatic amputation of left lower leg, level unspecified A
Ex: See S78.012

S88.929 Partial traumatic amputation of unspecified lower leg, level unspecified A
Ex: See S78.019

S89 Other and unspecified injuries of lower leg

Note: A fracture not indicated as open or closed should be coded to closed

Excludes2 other and unspecified injuries of ankle and foot (S99.-)

The appropriate 7th character is to be added to each code from subcategories S89.0, S89.1, S89.2, and S89.3

A	initial encounter for closed fracture
D	subsequent encounter for fracture with routine healing
G	subsequent encounter for fracture with delayed healing
K	subsequent encounter for fracture with nonunion
P	subsequent encounter for fracture with malunion
S	sequela

S89.0 Physeal fracture of upper end of tibia

S89.00 Unspecified physeal fracture of upper end of tibia

S89.001 Unspecified physeal fracture of upper end of right tibia A, K, P, A
Ex: **For S89.001[A]:** See S82.101[A]
For S89.001[K,P]: See S02.0[K]

S89.002 Unspecified physeal fracture of upper end of left tibia A, K, P, A
Ex: **For S89.002[A]:** See S82.102[A]
For S89.002[K,P]: See S02.0[K]

S89.009 Unspecified physeal fracture of upper end of unspecified tibia A, K, P, A
Ex: **For S89.009[A]:** See S82.101[B,C]
For S89.009[K,P]: See S02.0[K]

S89.01 Salter-Harris Type I physeal fracture of upper end of tibia

S89.011 Salter-Harris Type I physeal fracture of upper end of right tibia A, K, P, A
Ex: **For S89.011[A]:** See S82.101[A]
For S89.011[K,P]: See S02.0[K]

S89.012 Salter-Harris Type I physeal fracture of upper end of left tibia A, K, P, A
Ex: **For S89.012[A]:** See S82.102[A]
For S89.012[K,P]: See S02.0[K]

S89.019 Salter-Harris Type I physeal fracture of upper end of unspecified tibia A, K, P, A
Ex: **For S89.019[A]:** See S82.101[B,C]
For S89.019[K,P]: See S02.0[K]

- **S89.02** Salter-Harris Type II physeal fracture of upper end of tibia
  - **S89.021** Salter-Harris Type II physeal fracture of upper end of right tibia A, K, P, A
    - Ex: For S89.021[A]: See S82.101[A]
    - For S89.021[K,P]: See S02.0[K]
  - **S89.022** Salter-Harris Type II physeal fracture of upper end of left tibia A, K, P, A
    - Ex: For S89.022[A]: See S82.102[A]
    - For S89.022[K,P]: See S02.0[K]
  - **S89.029** Salter-Harris Type II physeal fracture of upper end of unspecified tibia A, K, P, A
    - Ex: For S89.029[A]: See S82.101[B,C]
    - For S89.029[K,P]: See S02.0[K]
- **S89.03** Salter-Harris Type III physeal fracture of upper end of tibia
  - **S89.031** Salter-Harris Type III physeal fracture of upper end of right tibia A, K, P, A
    - Ex: For S89.031[A]: See S82.101[A]
    - For S89.031[K,P]: See S02.0[K]
  - **S89.032** Salter-Harris Type III physeal fracture of upper end of left tibia A, K, P, A
    - Ex: For S89.032[A]: See S82.102[A]
    - For S89.032[K,P]: See S02.0[K]
  - **S89.039** Salter-Harris Type III physeal fracture of upper end of unspecified tibia A, K, P, A
    - Ex: For S89.039[A]: See S82.101[B,C]
    - For S89.039[K,P]: See S02.0[K]
- **S89.04** Salter-Harris Type IV physeal fracture of upper end of tibia
  - **S89.041** Salter-Harris Type IV physeal fracture of upper end of right tibia A, K, P, A
    - Ex: For S89.041[A]: See S82.101[A]
    - For S89.041[K,P]: See S02.0[K]
  - **S89.042** Salter-Harris Type IV physeal fracture of upper end of left tibia A, K, P, A
    - Ex: For S89.042[A]: See S82.102[A]
    - For S89.042[K,P]: See S02.0[K]
  - **S89.049** Salter-Harris Type IV physeal fracture of upper end of unspecified tibia A, K, P, A
    - Ex: For S89.049[A]: See S82.101[B,C]
    - For S89.049[K,P]: See S02.0[K]
- **S89.09** Other physeal fracture of upper end of tibia
  - **S89.091** Other physeal fracture of upper end of right tibia A, K, P, A
    - Ex: For S89.091[A]: See S82.101[A]
    - For S89.091[K,P]: See S02.0[K]
  - **S89.092** Other physeal fracture of upper end of left tibia A, K, P, A
    - Ex: For S89.092[A]: See S82.102[A]
    - For S89.092[K,P]: See S02.0[K]
  - **S89.099** Other physeal fracture of upper end of unspecified tibia A, K, P, A
    - Ex: For S89.099[A]: See S82.101[B,C]
    - For S89.099[K,P]: See S02.0[K]
- **S89.1** Physeal fracture of lower end of tibia
  - Ex: For category S89.1 CC codes: See S02.0[K]
  - **S89.10** Unspecified physeal fracture of lower end of tibia
    - **S89.101** Unspecified physeal fracture of lower end of right tibia K, P
    - **S89.102** Unspecified physeal fracture of lower end of left tibia K, P
    - **S89.109** Unspecified physeal fracture of lower end of unspecified tibia K, P
  - **S89.11** Salter-Harris Type I physeal fracture of lower end of tibia
    - **S89.111** Salter-Harris Type I physeal fracture of lower end of right tibia K, P
    - **S89.112** Salter-Harris Type I physeal fracture of lower end of left tibia K, P
    - **S89.119** Salter-Harris Type I physeal fracture of lower end of unspecified tibia K, P
  - **S89.12** Salter-Harris Type II physeal fracture of lower end of tibia
    - **S89.121** Salter-Harris Type II physeal fracture of lower end of right tibia K, P
    - **S89.122** Salter-Harris Type II physeal fracture of lower end of left tibia K, P
    - **S89.129** Salter-Harris Type II physeal fracture of lower end of unspecified tibia K, P
  - **S89.13** Salter-Harris Type III physeal fracture of lower end of tibia
    - **Excludes1** fracture of medial malleolus (adult) (S82.5-)
    - **S89.131** Salter-Harris Type III physeal fracture of lower end of right tibia K, P
    - **S89.132** Salter-Harris Type III physeal fracture of lower end of left tibia K, P
    - **S89.139** Salter-Harris Type III physeal fracture of lower end of unspecified tibia K, P
  - **S89.14** Salter-Harris Type IV physeal fracture of lower end of tibia
    - **Excludes1** fracture of medial malleolus (adult) (S82.5-)
    - **S89.141** Salter-Harris Type IV physeal fracture of lower end of right tibia K, P
    - **S89.142** Salter-Harris Type IV physeal fracture of lower end of left tibia K, P
    - **S89.149** Salter-Harris Type IV physeal fracture of lower end of unspecified tibia K, P
  - **S89.19** Other physeal fracture of lower end of tibia
    - **S89.191** Other physeal fracture of lower end of right tibia K, P
    - **S89.192** Other physeal fracture of lower end of left tibia K, P
    - **S89.199** Other physeal fracture of lower end of unspecified tibia K, P
- **S89.2** Physeal fracture of upper end of fibula
  - Ex: For category S89.2 CC codes: See S02.0[K]
  - **S89.20** Unspecified physeal fracture of upper end of fibula
    - **S89.201** Unspecified physeal fracture of upper end of right fibula K, P
    - **S89.202** Unspecified physeal fracture of upper end of left fibula K, P
    - **S89.209** Unspecified physeal fracture of upper end of unspecified fibula K, P

- S89.21 Salter-Harris Type I physeal fracture of upper end of fibula
  - S89.211 Salter-Harris Type I physeal fracture of upper end of right fibula K, P
  - S89.212 Salter-Harris Type I physeal fracture of upper end of left fibula K, P
  - S89.219 Salter-Harris Type I physeal fracture of upper end of unspecified fibula K, P
- S89.22 Salter-Harris Type II physeal fracture of upper end of fibula
  - S89.221 Salter-Harris Type II physeal fracture of upper end of right fibula K, P
  - S89.222 Salter-Harris Type II physeal fracture of upper end of left fibula K, P
  - S89.229 Salter-Harris Type II physeal fracture of upper end of unspecified fibula K, P
- S89.29 Other physeal fracture of upper end of fibula
  - S89.291 Other physeal fracture of upper end of right fibula K, P
  - S89.292 Other physeal fracture of upper end of left fibula K, P
  - S89.299 Other physeal fracture of upper end of unspecified fibula K, P
- S89.3 Physeal fracture of lower end of fibula

  Ex For category S89.3 CC codes: See S02.0[K]
  - S89.30 Unspecified physeal fracture of lower end of fibula
    - S89.301 Unspecified physeal fracture of lower end of right fibula K, P
    - S89.302 Unspecified physeal fracture of lower end of left fibula K, P
    - S89.309 Unspecified physeal fracture of lower end of unspecified fibula K, P
  - S89.31 Salter-Harris Type I physeal fracture of lower end of fibula
    - S89.311 Salter-Harris Type I physeal fracture of lower end of right fibula K, P
    - S89.312 Salter-Harris Type I physeal fracture of lower end of left fibula K, P
    - S89.319 Salter-Harris Type I physeal fracture of lower end of unspecified fibula K, P
  - S89.32 Salter-Harris Type II physeal fracture of lower end of fibula
    - S89.321 Salter-Harris Type II physeal fracture of lower end of right fibula K, P
    - S89.322 Salter-Harris Type II physeal fracture of lower end of left fibula K, P
    - S89.329 Salter-Harris Type II physeal fracture of lower end of unspecified fibula K, P
  - S89.39 Other physeal fracture of lower end of fibula
    - S89.391 Other physeal fracture of lower end of right fibula K, P
    - S89.392 Other physeal fracture of lower end of left fibula K, P
    - S89.399 Other physeal fracture of lower end of unspecified fibula K, P
- S89.8 Other specified injuries of lower leg

  The appropriate 7th character is to be added to each code in subcategory S89.8

A	initial encounter
D	subsequent encounter
S	sequela

  - X S89.80 Other specified injuries of unspecified lower leg
  - X S89.81 Other specified injuries of right lower leg
  - X S89.82 Other specified injuries of left lower leg
- S89.9 Unspecified injury of lower leg

  The appropriate 7th character is to be added to each code in subcategory S89.9

A	initial encounter
D	subsequent encounter
S	sequela

  - X S89.90 Unspecified injury of unspecified lower leg
  - X S89.91 Unspecified injury of right lower leg
  - X S89.92 Unspecified injury of left lower leg

INJURIES TO THE ANKLE AND FOOT (S90-S99)

Excludes2 burns and corrosions (T20-T32)
fracture of ankle and malleolus (S82.-)
frostbite (T33-T34)
insect bite or sting, venomous (T63.4)

- S90 Superficial injury of ankle, foot and toes

  The appropriate 7th character is to be added to each code from category S90

A	initial encounter
D	subsequent encounter
S	sequela

  - S90.0 Contusion of ankle
    - X S90.00 Contusion of unspecified ankle
    - X S90.01 Contusion of right ankle
    - X S90.02 Contusion of left ankle
  - S90.1 Contusion of toe without damage to nail
    - S90.11 Contusion of great toe without damage to nail
      - S90.111 Contusion of right great toe without damage to nail
      - S90.112 Contusion of left great toe without damage to nail
      - S90.119 Contusion of unspecified great toe without damage to nail
    - S90.12 Contusion of lesser toe without damage to nail
      - S90.121 Contusion of right lesser toe(s) without damage to nail
      - S90.122 Contusion of left lesser toe(s) without damage to nail
      - S90.129 Contusion of unspecified lesser toe(s) without damage to nail

        Contusion of toe NOS
  - S90.2 Contusion of toe with damage to nail
    - S90.21 Contusion of great toe with damage to nail
      - S90.211 Contusion of right great toe with damage to nail
      - S90.212 Contusion of left great toe with damage to nail
      - S90.219 Contusion of unspecified great toe with damage to nail

- S90.22 Contusion of lesser toe with damage to nail
  - S90.221 Contusion of right lesser toe(s) with damage to nail
  - S90.222 Contusion of left lesser toe(s) with damage to nail
  - S90.229 Contusion of unspecified lesser toe(s) with damage to nail
- S90.3 Contusion of foot

  Excludes2 contusion of toes (S90.1-, S90.2-)
  - X S90.30 Contusion of unspecified foot

    Contusion of foot NOS
  - X S90.31 Contusion of right foot
  - X S90.32 Contusion of left foot
- S90.4 Other superficial injuries of toe
  - S90.41 Abrasion of toe
    - S90.411 Abrasion, right great toe
    - S90.412 Abrasion, left great toe
    - S90.413 Abrasion, unspecified great toe
    - S90.414 Abrasion, right lesser toe(s)
    - S90.415 Abrasion, left lesser toe(s)
    - S90.416 Abrasion, unspecified lesser toe(s)
  - S90.42 Blister (nonthermal) of toe
    - S90.421 Blister (nonthermal), right great toe
    - S90.422 Blister (nonthermal), left great toe
    - S90.423 Blister (nonthermal), unspecified great toe
    - S90.424 Blister (nonthermal), right lesser toe(s)
    - S90.425 Blister (nonthermal), left lesser toe(s)
    - S90.426 Blister (nonthermal), unspecified lesser toe(s)
  - S90.44 External constriction of toe

    Hair tourniquet syndrome of toe
    - S90.441 External constriction, right great toe
    - S90.442 External constriction, left great toe
    - S90.443 External constriction, unspecified great toe
    - S90.444 External constriction, right lesser toe(s)
    - S90.445 External constriction, left lesser toe(s)
    - S90.446 External constriction, unspecified lesser toe(s)
  - S90.45 Superficial foreign body of toe

    Splinter in the toe
    - S90.451 Superficial foreign body, right great toe
    - S90.452 Superficial foreign body, left great toe
    - S90.453 Superficial foreign body, unspecified great toe
    - S90.454 Superficial foreign body, right lesser toe(s)
    - S90.455 Superficial foreign body, left lesser toe(s)
    - S90.456 Superficial foreign body, unspecified lesser toe(s)
  - S90.46 Insect bite (nonvenomous) of toe
    - S90.461 Insect bite (nonvenomous), right great toe
    - S90.462 Insect bite (nonvenomous), left great toe
    - S90.463 Insect bite (nonvenomous), unspecified great toe
    - S90.464 Insect bite (nonvenomous), right lesser toe(s)
    - S90.465 Insect bite (nonvenomous), left lesser toe(s)
    - S90.466 Insect bite (nonvenomous), unspecified lesser toe(s)
  - S90.47 Other superficial bite of toe

    Excludes1 open bite of toe (S91.15-, S91.25-)
    - S90.471 Other superficial bite of right great toe
    - S90.472 Other superficial bite of left great toe
    - S90.473 Other superficial bite of unspecified great toe
    - S90.474 Other superficial bite of right lesser toe(s)
    - S90.475 Other superficial bite of left lesser toe(s)
    - S90.476 Other superficial bite of unspecified lesser toe(s)
- S90.5 Other superficial injuries of ankle
  - S90.51 Abrasion of ankle
    - S90.511 Abrasion, right ankle
    - S90.512 Abrasion, left ankle
    - S90.519 Abrasion, unspecified ankle
  - S90.52 Blister (nonthermal) of ankle
    - S90.521 Blister (nonthermal), right ankle
    - S90.522 Blister (nonthermal), left ankle
    - S90.529 Blister (nonthermal), unspecified ankle
  - S90.54 External constriction of ankle
    - S90.541 External constriction, right ankle
    - S90.542 External constriction, left ankle
    - S90.549 External constriction, unspecified ankle
  - S90.55 Superficial foreign body of ankle

    Splinter in the ankle
    - S90.551 Superficial foreign body, right ankle
    - S90.552 Superficial foreign body, left ankle
    - S90.559 Superficial foreign body, unspecified ankle
  - S90.56 Insect bite (nonvenomous) of ankle
    - S90.561 Insect bite (nonvenomous), right ankle
    - S90.562 Insect bite (nonvenomous), left ankle
    - S90.569 Insect bite (nonvenomous), unspecified ankle
  - S90.57 Other superficial bite of ankle

    Excludes1 open bite of ankle (S91.05-)
    - S90.571 Other superficial bite of ankle, right ankle
    - S90.572 Other superficial bite of ankle, left ankle
    - S90.579 Other superficial bite of ankle, unspecified ankle

- S90.8 Other superficial injuries of foot
  - S90.81 Abrasion of foot
    - S90.811 Abrasion, right foot
    - S90.812 Abrasion, left foot
    - S90.819 Abrasion, unspecified foot
  - S90.82 Blister (nonthermal) of foot
    - S90.821 Blister (nonthermal), right foot
    - S90.822 Blister (nonthermal), left foot
    - S90.829 Blister (nonthermal), unspecified foot
  - S90.84 External constriction of foot
    - S90.841 External constriction, right foot
    - S90.842 External constriction, left foot
    - S90.849 External constriction, unspecified foot
  - S90.85 Superficial foreign body of foot
    Splinter in the foot
    - S90.851 Superficial foreign body, right foot
    - S90.852 Superficial foreign body, left foot
    - S90.859 Superficial foreign body, unspecified foot
  - S90.86 Insect bite (nonvenomous) of foot
    - S90.861 Insect bite (nonvenomous), right foot
    - S90.862 Insect bite (nonvenomous), left foot
    - S90.869 Insect bite (nonvenomous), unspecified foot
  - S90.87 Other superficial bite of foot
    Excludes1 open bite of foot (S91.35-)
    - S90.871 Other superficial bite of right foot
    - S90.872 Other superficial bite of left foot
    - S90.879 Other superficial bite of unspecified foot
- S90.9 Unspecified superficial injury of ankle, foot and toe
  - S90.91 Unspecified superficial injury of ankle
    - S90.911 Unspecified superficial injury of right ankle
    - S90.912 Unspecified superficial injury of left ankle
    - S90.919 Unspecified superficial injury of unspecified ankle
  - S90.92 Unspecified superficial injury of foot
    - S90.921 Unspecified superficial injury of right foot
    - S90.922 Unspecified superficial injury of left foot
    - S90.929 Unspecified superficial injury of unspecified foot
  - S90.93 Unspecified superficial injury of toes
    - S90.931 Unspecified superficial injury of right great toe
    - S90.932 Unspecified superficial injury of left great toe
    - S90.933 Unspecified superficial injury of unspecified great toe
    - S90.934 Unspecified superficial injury of right lesser toe(s)
    - S90.935 Unspecified superficial injury of left lesser toe(s)
    - S90.936 Unspecified superficial injury of unspecified lesser toe(s)

- S91 Open wound of ankle, foot and toes
  Code also any associated wound infection
  Excludes1 open fracture of ankle, foot and toes (S92.-with 7th character B)
  traumatic amputation of ankle and foot (S98.-)
  The appropriate 7th character is to be added to each code from category S91

A	initial encounter
D	subsequent encounter
S	sequela

  - S91.0 Open wound of ankle
    - S91.00 Unspecified open wound of ankle
      - S91.001 Unspecified open wound, right ankle
      - S91.002 Unspecified open wound, left ankle
      - S91.009 Unspecified open wound, unspecified ankle
    - S91.01 Laceration without foreign body of ankle
      - S91.011 Laceration without foreign body, right ankle
      - S91.012 Laceration without foreign body, left ankle
      - S91.019 Laceration without foreign body, unspecified ankle
    - S91.02 Laceration with foreign body of ankle
      - S91.021 Laceration with foreign body, right ankle
      - S91.022 Laceration with foreign body, left ankle
      - S91.029 Laceration with foreign body, unspecified ankle
    - S91.03 Puncture wound without foreign body of ankle
      - S91.031 Puncture wound without foreign body, right ankle
      - S91.032 Puncture wound without foreign body, left ankle
      - S91.039 Puncture wound without foreign body, unspecified ankle
    - S91.04 Puncture wound with foreign body of ankle
      - S91.041 Puncture wound with foreign body, right ankle
      - S91.042 Puncture wound with foreign body, left ankle
      - S91.049 Puncture wound with foreign body, unspecified ankle
    - S91.05 Open bite of ankle
      Excludes1 superficial bite of ankle (S90.56-, S90.57-)
      - S91.051 Open bite, right ankle
      - S91.052 Open bite, left ankle
      - S91.059 Open bite, unspecified ankle
  - S91.1 Open wound of toe without damage to nail
    - S91.10 Unspecified open wound of toe without damage to nail
      - S91.101 Unspecified open wound of right great toe without damage to nail
      - S91.102 Unspecified open wound of left great toe without damage to nail
      - S91.103 Unspecified open wound of unspecified great toe without damage to nail

- S91.104 Unspecified open wound of right lesser toe(s) without damage to nail
- S91.105 Unspecified open wound of left lesser toe(s) without damage to nail
- S91.106 Unspecified open wound of unspecified lesser toe(s) without damage to nail
- S91.109 Unspecified open wound of unspecified toe(s) without damage to nail

- S91.11 Laceration without foreign body of toe without damage to nail
  - S91.111 Laceration without foreign body of right great toe without damage to nail
  - S91.112 Laceration without foreign body of left great toe without damage to nail
  - S91.113 Laceration without foreign body of unspecified great toe without damage to nail
  - S91.114 Laceration without foreign body of right lesser toe(s) without damage to nail
  - S91.115 Laceration without foreign body of left lesser toe(s) without damage to nail
  - S91.116 Laceration without foreign body of unspecified lesser toe(s) without damage to nail
  - S91.119 Laceration without foreign body of unspecified toe without damage to nail
- S91.12 Laceration with foreign body of toe without damage to nail
  - S91.121 Laceration with foreign body of right great toe without damage to nail
  - S91.122 Laceration with foreign body of left great toe without damage to nail
  - S91.123 Laceration with foreign body of unspecified great toe without damage to nail
  - S91.124 Laceration with foreign body of right lesser toe(s) without damage to nail
  - S91.125 Laceration with foreign body of left lesser toe(s) without damage to nail
  - S91.126 Laceration with foreign body of unspecified lesser toe(s) without damage to nail
  - S91.129 Laceration with foreign body of unspecified toe(s) without damage to nail
- S91.13 Puncture wound without foreign body of toe without damage to nail
  - S91.131 Puncture wound without foreign body of right great toe without damage to nail
  - S91.132 Puncture wound without foreign body of left great toe without damage to nail
  - S91.133 Puncture wound without foreign body of unspecified great toe without damage to nail
  - S91.134 Puncture wound without foreign body of right lesser toe(s) without damage to nail
  - S91.135 Puncture wound without foreign body of left lesser toe(s) without damage to nail
  - S91.136 Puncture wound without foreign body of unspecified lesser toe(s) without damage to nail
  - S91.139 Puncture wound without foreign body of unspecified toe(s) without damage to nail
- S91.14 Puncture wound with foreign body of toe without damage to nail
  - S91.141 Puncture wound with foreign body of right great toe without damage to nail
  - S91.142 Puncture wound with foreign body of left great toe without damage to nail
  - S91.143 Puncture wound with foreign body of unspecified great toe without damage to nail
  - S91.144 Puncture wound with foreign body of right lesser toe(s) without damage to nail
  - S91.145 Puncture wound with foreign body of left lesser toe(s) without damage to nail
  - S91.146 Puncture wound with foreign body of unspecified lesser toe(s) without damage to nail
  - S91.149 Puncture wound with foreign body of unspecified toe(s) without damage to nail
- S91.15 Open bite of toe without damage to nail
  Bite of toe NOS
  Excludes1 superficial bite of toe (S90.46-, S90.47-)
  - S91.151 Open bite of right great toe without damage to nail
  - S91.152 Open bite of left great toe without damage to nail
  - S91.153 Open bite of unspecified great toe without damage to nail
  - S91.154 Open bite of right lesser toe(s) without damage to nail
  - S91.155 Open bite of left lesser toe(s) without damage to nail
  - S91.156 Open bite of unspecified lesser toe(s) without damage to nail
  - S91.159 Open bite of unspecified toe(s) without damage to nail
- S91.2 Open wound of toe with damage to nail
  - S91.20 Unspecified open wound of toe with damage to nail
    - S91.201 Unspecified open wound of right great toe with damage to nail
    - S91.202 Unspecified open wound of left great toe with damage to nail
    - S91.203 Unspecified open wound of unspecified great toe with damage to nail
    - S91.204 Unspecified open wound of right lesser toe(s) with damage to nail
    - S91.205 Unspecified open wound of left lesser toe(s) with damage to nail
    - S91.206 Unspecified open wound of unspecified lesser toe(s) with damage to nail
    - S91.209 Unspecified open wound of unspecified toe(s) with damage to nail

- S91.21 Laceration without foreign body of toe with damage to nail
  - S91.211 Laceration without foreign body of right great toe with damage to nail
  - S91.212 Laceration without foreign body of left great toe with damage to nail
  - S91.213 Laceration without foreign body of unspecified great toe with damage to nail
  - S91.214 Laceration without foreign body of right lesser toe(s) with damage to nail
  - S91.215 Laceration without foreign body of left lesser toe(s) with damage to nail
  - S91.216 Laceration without foreign body of unspecified lesser toe(s) with damage to nail
  - S91.219 Laceration without foreign body of unspecified toe(s) with damage to nail
- S91.22 Laceration with foreign body of toe with damage to nail
  - S91.221 Laceration with foreign body of right great toe with damage to nail
  - S91.222 Laceration with foreign body of left great toe with damage to nail
  - S91.223 Laceration with foreign body of unspecified great toe with damage to nail
  - S91.224 Laceration with foreign body of right lesser toe(s) with damage to nail
  - S91.225 Laceration with foreign body of left lesser toe(s) with damage to nail
  - S91.226 Laceration with foreign body of unspecified lesser toe(s) with damage to nail
  - S91.229 Laceration with foreign body of unspecified toe(s) with damage to nail
- S91.23 Puncture wound without foreign body of toe with damage to nail
  - S91.231 Puncture wound without foreign body of right great toe with damage to nail
  - S91.232 Puncture wound without foreign body of left great toe with damage to nail
  - S91.233 Puncture wound without foreign body of unspecified great toe with damage to nail
  - S91.234 Puncture wound without foreign body of right lesser toe(s) with damage to nail
  - S91.235 Puncture wound without foreign body of left lesser toe(s) with damage to nail
  - S91.236 Puncture wound without foreign body of unspecified lesser toe(s) with damage to nail
  - S91.239 Puncture wound without foreign body of unspecified toe(s) with damage to nail
- S91.24 Puncture wound with foreign body of toe with damage to nail
  - S91.241 Puncture wound with foreign body of right great toe with damage to nail
  - S91.242 Puncture wound with foreign body of left great toe with damage to nail
  - S91.243 Puncture wound with foreign body of unspecified great toe with damage to nail
  - S91.244 Puncture wound with foreign body of right lesser toe(s) with damage to nail
  - S91.245 Puncture wound with foreign body of left lesser toe(s) with damage to nail
  - S91.246 Puncture wound with foreign body of unspecified lesser toe(s) with damage to nail
  - S91.249 Puncture wound with foreign body of unspecified toe(s) with damage to nail
- S91.25 Open bite of toe with damage to nail
  Bite of toe with damage to nail NOS
  Excludes1 superficial bite of toe (S90.46-, S90.47-)
  - S91.251 Open bite of right great toe with damage to nail
  - S91.252 Open bite of left great toe with damage to nail
  - S91.253 Open bite of unspecified great toe with damage to nail
  - S91.254 Open bite of right lesser toe(s) with damage to nail
  - S91.255 Open bite of left lesser toe(s) with damage to nail
  - S91.256 Open bite of unspecified lesser toe(s) with damage to nail
  - S91.259 Open bite of unspecified toe(s) with damage to nail
- S91.3 Open wound of foot
  - S91.30 Unspecified open wound of foot
    - S91.301 Unspecified open wound, right foot
    - S91.302 Unspecified open wound, left foot
    - S91.309 Unspecified open wound, unspecified foot
  - S91.31 Laceration without foreign body of foot
    - S91.311 Laceration without foreign body, right foot
    - S91.312 Laceration without foreign body, left foot
    - S91.319 Laceration without foreign body, unspecified foot
  - S91.32 Laceration with foreign body of foot
    - S91.321 Laceration with foreign body, right foot
    - S91.322 Laceration with foreign body, left foot
    - S91.329 Laceration with foreign body, unspecified foot
  - S91.33 Puncture wound without foreign body of foot
    - S91.331 Puncture wound without foreign body, right foot
    - S91.332 Puncture wound without foreign body, left foot
    - S91.339 Puncture wound without foreign body, unspecified foot
  - S91.34 Puncture wound with foreign body of foot
    - S91.341 Puncture wound with foreign body, right foot
    - S91.342 Puncture wound with foreign body, left foot
    - S91.349 Puncture wound with foreign body, unspecified foot
  - S91.35 Open bite of foot
    Excludes1 superficial bite of foot (S90.86-, S90.87-)
    - S91.351 Open bite, right foot
    - S91.352 Open bite, left foot
    - S91.359 Open bite, unspecified foot

S92 Fracture of foot and toe, except ankle

Note: A fracture not indicated as displaced or nondisplaced should be coded to displaced

A fracture not indicated as open or closed should be coded to closed

Excludes1 traumatic amputation of ankle and foot (S98.-)

Excludes2 fracture of ankle (S82.-)
fracture of malleolus (S82.-)

The appropriate 7th character is to be added to each code from category S92

A	initial encounter for closed fracture
B	initial encounter for open fracture
D	subsequent encounter for fracture with routine healing
G	subsequent encounter for fracture with delayed healing
K	subsequent encounter for fracture with nonunion
P	subsequent encounter for fracture with malunion
S	sequela

S92.0 Fracture of calcaneus

Heel bone Os calcis

Excludes2 Physeal fracture of calcaneus (S99.0-) ◀

Ex: **For category S92.0 CC codes S92.0[B]:** M80.00X-M80.019[A], M80.041-M80.049[A], M80.061-M80.819[A], M80.841-M80.849[A], M80.861-M80.879[A], M84.40X-M84.419[A], M84.441-M84.446[A], M84.454[A], M84.461-M84.519[A], M84.541-M84.550[A], M84.561-M84.576[A], M84.60X-M84.619[A], M84.641-M84.650[A], M84.661-M84.68X[A], S03.8XX-S03.9XX[A], S29.011-S29.019[A], S38.3XX[A], S39.011-S39.013[A], S73.101-S73.199[A], S76.001-S76.019[A], S76.091-S76.219[A], S76.291-S76.319[A], S76.391-S76.819[A], S76.891-S76.919[A], S76.991-S76.999[A], S79.811-S79.929[A], S82.90X-S82.92X[A,B,C], S92.001-S92.066[B], S92.101-S92.356[A,B], S92.811-S92.819[A,B], S92.901-S92.909[A,B], T14.90-T14.91, T79.A9X-T79.9XX[A] **For S92.0[K,P]:** See S02.0[K]

S92.00 Unspecified fracture of calcaneus

- **S92.001 Unspecified fracture of right calcaneus** B, K, P CC, B MCC
- **S92.002 Unspecified fracture of left calcaneus** B, K, P CC, B MCC
- **S92.009 Unspecified fracture of unspecified calcaneus** B, K, P CC, B MCC

S92.01 Fracture of body of calcaneus

- **S92.011 Displaced fracture of body of right calcaneus** B, K, P CC, B MCC
- **S92.012 Displaced fracture of body of left calcaneus** B, K, P CC, B MCC
- **S92.013 Displaced fracture of body of unspecified calcaneus** B, K, P CC, B MCC
- **S92.014 Nondisplaced fracture of body of right calcaneus** B, K, P CC, B MCC
- **S92.015 Nondisplaced fracture of body of left calcaneus** B, K, P CC, B MCC
- **S92.016 Nondisplaced fracture of body of unspecified calcaneus** B, K, P CC, B MCC

S92.02 Fracture of anterior process of calcaneus

- **S92.021 Displaced fracture of anterior process of right calcaneus** B, K, P CC, B MCC
- **S92.022 Displaced fracture of anterior process of left calcaneus** B, K, P CC, B MCC
- **S92.023 Displaced fracture of anterior process of unspecified calcaneus** B, K, P CC, B MCC
- **S92.024 Nondisplaced fracture of anterior process of right calcaneus** B, K, P CC, B MCC
- **S92.025 Nondisplaced fracture of anterior process of left calcaneus** B, K, P CC, B MCC
- **S92.026 Nondisplaced fracture of anterior process of unspecified calcaneus** B, K, P CC, B MCC

S92.03 Avulsion fracture of tuberosity of calcaneus

- **S92.031 Displaced avulsion fracture of tuberosity of right calcaneus** B, K, P CC, B MCC
- **S92.032 Displaced avulsion fracture of tuberosity of left calcaneus** B, K, P CC, B MCC
- **S92.033 Displaced avulsion fracture of tuberosity of unspecified calcaneus** B, K, P CC, B MCC
- **S92.034 Nondisplaced avulsion fracture of tuberosity of right calcaneus** B, K, P CC, B MCC
- **S92.035 Nondisplaced avulsion fracture of tuberosity of left calcaneus** B, K, P CC, B MCC
- **S92.036 Nondisplaced avulsion fracture of tuberosity of unspecified calcaneus** B, K, P CC, B MCC

S92.04 Other fracture of tuberosity of calcaneus

- **S92.041 Displaced other fracture of tuberosity of right calcaneus** B, K, P CC, B MCC
- **S92.042 Displaced other fracture of tuberosity of left calcaneus** B, K, P CC, B MCC
- **S92.043 Displaced other fracture of tuberosity of unspecified calcaneus** B, K, P CC, B MCC
- **S92.044 Nondisplaced other fracture of tuberosity of right calcaneus** B, K, P CC, B MCC
- **S92.045 Nondisplaced other fracture of tuberosity of left calcaneus** B, K, P CC, B MCC
- **S92.046 Nondisplaced other fracture of tuberosity of unspecified calcaneus** B, K, P CC, B MCC

S92.05 Other extraarticular fracture of calcaneus

- **S92.051 Displaced other extraarticular fracture of right calcaneus** B, K, P CC, B MCC
- **S92.052 Displaced other extraarticular fracture of left calcaneus** B, K, P CC, B MCC
- **S92.053 Displaced other extraarticular fracture of unspecified calcaneus** B, K, P CC, B MCC
- **S92.054 Nondisplaced other extraarticular fracture of right calcaneus** B, K, P CC, B MCC
- **S92.055 Nondisplaced other extraarticular fracture of left calcaneus** B, K, P CC, B MCC
- **S92.056 Nondisplaced other extraarticular fracture of unspecified calcaneus** B, K, P CC, B MCC

S92.06 Intraarticular fracture of calcaneus

- **S92.061 Displaced intraarticular fracture of right calcaneus** B, K, P CC, B MCC
- **S92.062 Displaced intraarticular fracture of left calcaneus** B, K, P CC, B MCC
- **S92.063 Displaced intraarticular fracture of unspecified calcaneus** B, K, P CC, B MCC
- **S92.064 Nondisplaced intraarticular fracture of right calcaneus** B, K, P CC, B MCC
- **S92.065 Nondisplaced intraarticular fracture of left calcaneus** B, K, P CC, B MCC
- **S92.066 Nondisplaced intraarticular fracture of unspecified calcaneus** B, K, P CC, B MCC

- **S92.1** Fracture of talus
  Astragalus
  Ex: For category S92.1 CC codes S92.1[B]: M80.00X-M80.019[A], M80.041-M80.049[A], M80.80X-M80.819[A], M80.841-M80.849[A], M84.40X-M84.419[A], M84.441-M84.446[A], M84.454[A], M84.474-M84.519[A], M84.541-M84.550[A], M84.574-M84.576[A], M84.60X-M84.619[A], M84.641-M84.650[A], M84.674-M84.68X[A], S03.8XX-S03.9XX[A], S29.011-S29.019[A], S38.3XX[A], S39.011-S39.013[A], S73.101-S73.199[A], S76.001-S76.019[A], S76.091-S76.219[A], S76.291-S76.319[A], S76.391-S76.819[A], S76.891-S76.919[A], S76.991-S76.999[A], S79.821-S79.929[A], S82.90X-S82.92X[A,B,C], S92.001-S92.066[B], S92.101-S92.356[A,B], S92.811-S92.819[A,B], S92.901-S92.909[A,B], T14.90-T14.91, T79.A9X-T79.9XX[A] For S92.1[K,P]: See S02.0[K]
  - **S92.10** Unspecified fracture of talus
    - **S92.101** Unspecified fracture of right talus B, K, P, B
    - **S92.102** Unspecified fracture of left talus B, K, P, B
    - **S92.109** Unspecified fracture of unspecified talus B, K, P, B
  - **S92.11** Fracture of neck of talus
    - **S92.111** Displaced fracture of neck of right talus B, K, P, B
    - **S92.112** Displaced fracture of neck of left talus B, K, P, B
    - **S92.113** Displaced fracture of neck of unspecified talus B, K, P, B
    - **S92.114** Nondisplaced fracture of neck of right talus B, K, P, B
    - **S92.115** Nondisplaced fracture of neck of left talus B, K, P, B
    - **S92.116** Nondisplaced fracture of neck of unspecified talus B, K, P, B
  - **S92.12** Fracture of body of talus
    - **S92.121** Displaced fracture of body of right talus B, K, P, B
    - **S92.122** Displaced fracture of body of left talus B, K, P, B
    - **S92.123** Displaced fracture of body of unspecified talus B, K, P, B
    - **S92.124** Nondisplaced fracture of body of right talus B, K, P, B
    - **S92.125** Nondisplaced fracture of body of left talus B, K, P, B
    - **S92.126** Nondisplaced fracture of body of unspecified talus B, K, P, B
  - **S92.13** Fracture of posterior process of talus
    - **S92.131** Displaced fracture of posterior process of right talus B, K, P, B
    - **S92.132** Displaced fracture of posterior process of left talus B, K, P, B
    - **S92.133** Displaced fracture of posterior process of unspecified talus B, K, P, B
    - **S92.134** Nondisplaced fracture of posterior process of right talus B, K, P, B
    - **S92.135** Nondisplaced fracture of posterior process of left talus B, K, P, B
    - **S92.136** Nondisplaced fracture of posterior process of unspecified talus B, K, P, B
  - **S92.14** Dome fracture of talus
    Excludes1 osteochondritis dissecans (M93.2)
    - **S92.141** Displaced dome fracture of right talus B, K, P, B
    - **S92.142** Displaced dome fracture of left talus B, K, P, B
    - **S92.143** Displaced dome fracture of unspecified talus B, K, P, B
    - **S92.144** Nondisplaced dome fracture of right talus B, K, P, B
    - **S92.145** Nondisplaced dome fracture of left talus B, K, P, B
    - **S92.146** Nondisplaced dome fracture of unspecified talus B, K, P, B
  - **S92.15** Avulsion fracture (chip fracture) of talus
    - **S92.151** Displaced avulsion fracture (chip fracture) of right talus B, K, P, B
    - **S92.152** Displaced avulsion fracture (chip fracture) of left talus B, K, P, B
    - **S92.153** Displaced avulsion fracture (chip fracture) of unspecified talus B, K, P, B
    - **S92.154** Nondisplaced avulsion fracture (chip fracture) of right talus B, K, P, B
    - **S92.155** Nondisplaced avulsion fracture (chip fracture) of left talus B, K, P, B
    - **S92.156** Nondisplaced avulsion fracture (chip fracture) of unspecified talus B, K, P, B
  - **S92.19** Other fracture of talus
    - **S92.191** Other fracture of right talus B, K, P, B
    - **S92.192** Other fracture of left talus B, K, P, B
    - **S92.199** Other fracture of unspecified talus B, K, P, B
- **S92.2** Fracture of other and unspecified tarsal bone(s)
  Ex: For category S92.2 CC codes S92.2[B]: See S92.1[B] For S92.2[K,P]: See S02.0[K] unless otherwise indicated
  - **S92.20** Fracture of unspecified tarsal bone(s)
    Ex: For category S92.20 CC codes S92.20[B]: S92.811-S92.819[A,B], S92.001-S92.919[A,B] For S92.20[K,P]: See S02.0[K]
    - **S92.201** Fracture of unspecified tarsal bone(s) of right foot B, K, P, B
    - **S92.202** Fracture of unspecified tarsal bone(s) of left foot B, K, P, B
    - **S92.209** Fracture of unspecified tarsal bone(s) of unspecified foot B, K, P, B
  - **S92.21** Fracture of cuboid bone
    - **S92.211** Displaced fracture of cuboid bone of right foot B, K, P, B
    - **S92.212** Displaced fracture of cuboid bone of left foot B, K, P, B
    - **S92.213** Displaced fracture of cuboid bone of unspecified foot B, K, P, B
    - **S92.214** Nondisplaced fracture of cuboid bone of right foot B, K, P, B
    - **S92.215** Nondisplaced fracture of cuboid bone of left foot B, K, P, B
    - **S92.216** Nondisplaced fracture of cuboid bone of unspecified foot B, K, P, B

- S92.22 Fracture of lateral cuneiform
  - S92.221 Displaced fracture of lateral cuneiform of right foot B, K, P, B
  - S92.222 Displaced fracture of lateral cuneiform of left foot B, K, P, B
  - S92.223 Displaced fracture of lateral cuneiform of unspecified foot B, K, P, B
  - S92.224 Nondisplaced fracture of lateral cuneiform of right foot B, K, P, B
  - S92.225 Nondisplaced fracture of lateral cuneiform of left foot B, K, P, B
  - S92.226 Nondisplaced fracture of lateral cuneiform of unspecified foot B, K, P, B
- S92.23 Fracture of intermediate cuneiform
  - S92.231 Displaced fracture of intermediate cuneiform of right foot B, K, P, B
  - S92.232 Displaced fracture of intermediate cuneiform of left foot B, K, P, B
  - S92.233 Displaced fracture of intermediate cuneiform of unspecified foot B, K, P, B
  - S92.234 Nondisplaced fracture of intermediate cuneiform of right foot B, K, P, B
  - S92.235 Nondisplaced fracture of intermediate cuneiform of left foot B, K, P, B
  - S92.236 Nondisplaced fracture of intermediate cuneiform of unspecified foot B, K, P, B
- S92.24 Fracture of medial cuneiform
  - S92.241 Displaced fracture of medial cuneiform of right foot B, K, P, B
  - S92.242 Displaced fracture of medial cuneiform of left foot B, K, P, B
  - S92.243 Displaced fracture of medial cuneiform of unspecified foot B, K, P, B
  - S92.244 Nondisplaced fracture of medial cuneiform of right foot B, K, P, B
  - S92.245 Nondisplaced fracture of medial cuneiform of left foot B, K, P, B
  - S92.246 Nondisplaced fracture of medial cuneiform of unspecified foot B, K, P, B
- S92.25 Fracture of navicular [scaphoid] of foot
  - S92.251 Displaced fracture of navicular [scaphoid] of right foot B, K, P, B
  - S92.252 Displaced fracture of navicular [scaphoid] of left foot B, K, P, B
  - S92.253 Displaced fracture of navicular [scaphoid] of unspecified foot B, K, P, B
  - S92.254 Nondisplaced fracture of navicular [scaphoid] of right foot B, K, P, B
  - S92.255 Nondisplaced fracture of navicular [scaphoid] of left foot B, K, P, B
  - S92.256 Nondisplaced fracture of navicular [scaphoid] of unspecified foot B, K, P, B
- S92.3 Fracture of metatarsal bone(s)

  Excludes2 Physeal fracture of metatarsal (S99.1-)

  Ex For category S92.3 CC codes S92.3[B]: See S92.1[B] For S92.3[K,P]: See S02.0[K]
  - S92.30 Fracture of unspecified metatarsal bone(s)
    - S92.301 Fracture of unspecified metatarsal bone(s), right foot B, K, P, B
    - S92.302 Fracture of unspecified metatarsal bone(s), left foot B, K, P, B
    - S92.309 Fracture of unspecified metatarsal bone(s), unspecified foot B, K, P, B
  - S92.31 Fracture of first metatarsal bone
    - S92.311 Displaced fracture of first metatarsal bone, right foot B, K, P, B
    - S92.312 Displaced fracture of first metatarsal bone, left foot B, K, P, B
    - S92.313 Displaced fracture of first metatarsal bone, unspecified foot B, K, P, B
    - S92.314 Nondisplaced fracture of first metatarsal bone, right foot B, K, P, B
    - S92.315 Nondisplaced fracture of first metatarsal bone, left foot B, K, P, B
    - S92.316 Nondisplaced fracture of first metatarsal bone, unspecified foot B, K, P, B
  - S92.32 Fracture of second metatarsal bone
    - S92.321 Displaced fracture of second metatarsal bone, right foot B, K, P, B
    - S92.322 Displaced fracture of second metatarsal bone, left foot B, K, P, B
    - S92.323 Displaced fracture of second metatarsal bone, unspecified foot B, K, P, B
    - S92.324 Nondisplaced fracture of second metatarsal bone, right foot B, K, P, B
    - S92.325 Nondisplaced fracture of second metatarsal bone, left foot B, K, P, B
    - S92.326 Nondisplaced fracture of second metatarsal bone, unspecified foot B, K, P, B
  - S92.33 Fracture of third metatarsal bone
    - S92.331 Displaced fracture of third metatarsal bone, right foot B, K, P, B
    - S92.332 Displaced fracture of third metatarsal bone, left foot B, K, P, B
    - S92.333 Displaced fracture of third metatarsal bone, unspecified foot B, K, P, B
    - S92.334 Nondisplaced fracture of third metatarsal bone, right foot B, K, P, B
    - S92.335 Nondisplaced fracture of third metatarsal bone, left foot B, K, P, B
    - S92.336 Nondisplaced fracture of third metatarsal bone, unspecified foot B, K, P, B

- S92.34 Fracture of fourth metatarsal bone
  - S92.341 Displaced fracture of fourth metatarsal bone, right foot B, K, P, B
  - S92.342 Displaced fracture of fourth metatarsal bone, left foot B, K, P, B
  - S92.343 Displaced fracture of fourth metatarsal bone, unspecified foot B, K, P, B
  - S92.344 Nondisplaced fracture of fourth metatarsal bone, right foot B, K, P, B
  - S92.345 Nondisplaced fracture of fourth metatarsal bone, left foot B, K, P, B
  - S92.346 Nondisplaced fracture of fourth metatarsal bone, unspecified foot B, K, P, B
- S92.35 Fracture of fifth metatarsal bone
  - S92.351 Displaced fracture of fifth metatarsal bone, right foot B, K, P, B
  - S92.352 Displaced fracture of fifth metatarsal bone, left foot B, K, P, B
  - S92.353 Displaced fracture of fifth metatarsal bone, unspecified foot B, K, P, B
  - S92.354 Nondisplaced fracture of fifth metatarsal bone, right foot B, K, P, B
  - S92.355 Nondisplaced fracture of fifth metatarsal bone, left foot B, K, P, B
  - S92.356 Nondisplaced fracture of fifth metatarsal bone, unspecified foot B, K, P, B
- S92.4 Fracture of great toe

  Excludes2 Physeal fracture of phalanx of toe (S99.2-) ◀

  Ex For category S92.4 CC codes: See S02.0[K]
  - S92.40 Unspecified fracture of great toe
    - S92.401 Displaced unspecified fracture of right great toe K, P
    - S92.402 Displaced unspecified fracture of left great toe K, P
    - S92.403 Displaced unspecified fracture of unspecified great toe K, P
    - S92.404 Nondisplaced unspecified fracture of right great toe K, P
    - S92.405 Nondisplaced unspecified fracture of left great toe K, P
    - S92.406 Nondisplaced unspecified fracture of unspecified great toe K, P
  - S92.41 Fracture of proximal phalanx of great toe
    - S92.411 Displaced fracture of proximal phalanx of right great toe K, P
    - S92.412 Displaced fracture of proximal phalanx of left great toe K, P
    - S92.413 Displaced fracture of proximal phalanx of unspecified great toe K, P
    - S92.414 Nondisplaced fracture of proximal phalanx of right great toe K, P
    - S92.415 Nondisplaced fracture of proximal phalanx of left great toe K, P
    - S92.416 Nondisplaced fracture of proximal phalanx of unspecified great toe K, P
  - S92.42 Fracture of distal phalanx of great toe
    - S92.421 Displaced fracture of distal phalanx of right great toe K, P
    - S92.422 Displaced fracture of distal phalanx of left great toe K, P
    - S92.423 Displaced fracture of distal phalanx of unspecified great toe K, P
    - S92.424 Nondisplaced fracture of distal phalanx of right great toe K, P
    - S92.425 Nondisplaced fracture of distal phalanx of left great toe K, P
    - S92.426 Nondisplaced fracture of distal phalanx of unspecified great toe K, P
  - S92.49 Other fracture of great toe
    - S92.491 Other fracture of right great toe K, P
    - S92.492 Other fracture of left great toe K, P
    - S92.499 Other fracture of unspecified great toe K, P
- S92.5 Fracture of lesser toe(s)

  Excludes2 Physeal fracture of phalanx of toe (S99.2-) ◀

  Ex For category S92.5 CC codes: See S02.0[K]
  - S92.50 Unspecified fracture of lesser toe(s)
    - S92.501 Displaced unspecified fracture of right lesser toe(s) K, P
    - S92.502 Displaced unspecified fracture of left lesser toe(s) K, P
    - S92.503 Displaced unspecified fracture of unspecified lesser toe(s) K, P
    - S92.504 Nondisplaced unspecified fracture of right lesser toe(s) K, P
    - S92.505 Nondisplaced unspecified fracture of left lesser toe(s) K, P
    - S92.506 Nondisplaced unspecified fracture of unspecified lesser toe(s) K, P
  - S92.51 Fracture of proximal phalanx of lesser toe(s)
    - S92.511 Displaced fracture of proximal phalanx of right lesser toe(s) K, P
    - S92.512 Displaced fracture of proximal phalanx of left lesser toe(s) K, P
    - S92.513 Displaced fracture of proximal phalanx of unspecified lesser toe(s) K, P
    - S92.514 Nondisplaced fracture of proximal phalanx of right lesser toe(s) K, P
    - S92.515 Nondisplaced fracture of proximal phalanx of left lesser toe(s) K, P
    - S92.516 Nondisplaced fracture of proximal phalanx of unspecified lesser toe(s) K, P
  - S92.52 Fracture of medial phalanx of lesser toe(s)
    - S92.521 Displaced fracture of medial phalanx of right lesser toe(s) K, P
    - S92.522 Displaced fracture of medial phalanx of left lesser toe(s) K, P
    - S92.523 Displaced fracture of medial phalanx of unspecified lesser toe(s) K, P
    - S92.524 Nondisplaced fracture of medial phalanx of right lesser toe(s) K, P
    - S92.525 Nondisplaced fracture of medial phalanx of left lesser toe(s) K, P
    - S92.526 Nondisplaced fracture of medial phalanx of unspecified lesser toe(s) K, P

- **S92.53 Fracture of distal phalanx of lesser toe(s)**
  - **S92.531 Displaced fracture of distal phalanx of right lesser toe(s)** K, P
  - **S92.532 Displaced fracture of distal phalanx of left lesser toe(s)** K, P
  - **S92.533 Displaced fracture of distal phalanx of unspecified lesser toe(s)** K, P
  - **S92.534 Nondisplaced fracture of distal phalanx of right lesser toe(s)** K, P
  - **S92.535 Nondisplaced fracture of distal phalanx of left lesser toe(s)** K, P
  - **S92.536 Nondisplaced fracture of distal phalanx of unspecified lesser toe(s)** K, P
- **S92.59 Other fracture of lesser toe(s)**
  - **S92.591 Other fracture of right lesser toe(s)** K, P
  - **S92.592 Other fracture of left lesser toe(s)** K, P
  - **S92.599 Other fracture of unspecified lesser toe(s)** K, P
- **S92.8 Other fracture of foot, except ankle** ◀

  Ex: **For category S92.8 CC codes S92.8[B]:** S92.001-S92.919[A,B]
  For S92.90[K,P]: See S02.0[K]
  - **S92.81 Other fracture of foot** ◀

    Sesamoid fracture of foot
    - **S92.811 Other fracture of right foot** B, K, P, B ◀
    - **S92.812 Other fracture of left foot** B, K, P, B ◀
    - **S92.819 Other fracture of unspecified foot** B, K, P, B ◀
- **S92.9 Unspecified fracture of foot and toe**
  - **S92.90 Unspecified fracture of foot**

    Ex: **For category S92.90 CC codes S92.90[B]:** S92.811-S92.819[A,B], S92.001-S92.919[A,B]
    For S92.90[K,P]: See S02.0[K]
    - **S92.901 Unspecified fracture of right foot** B, K, P, B
    - **S92.902 Unspecified fracture of left foot** B, K, P, B
    - **S92.909 Unspecified fracture of unspecified foot** B, K, P, B
  - **S92.91 Unspecified fracture of toe**

    Ex: **For category S92.91 CC codes:** See S02.0[K]
    - **S92.911 Unspecified fracture of right toe(s)** K, P
    - **S92.912 Unspecified fracture of left toe(s)** K, P
    - **S92.919 Unspecified fracture of unspecified toe(s)** K, P

- **S93 Dislocation and sprain of joints and ligaments at ankle, foot and toe level**

  Includes avulsion of joint or ligament of ankle, foot and toe
  laceration of cartilage, joint or ligament of ankle, foot and toe
  sprain of cartilage, joint or ligament of ankle, foot and toe
  traumatic hemarthrosis of joint or ligament of ankle, foot and toe
  traumatic rupture of joint or ligament of ankle, foot and toe
  traumatic subluxation of joint or ligament of ankle, foot and toe
  traumatic tear of joint or ligament of ankle, foot and toe

  Code also any associated open wound

  Excludes2 strain of muscle and tendon of ankle and foot (S96.-)

  The appropriate 7th character is to be added to each code from category S93

A	initial encounter
D	subsequent encounter
S	sequela

- **S93.0 Subluxation and dislocation of ankle joint**

  Subluxation and dislocation of astragalus
  Subluxation and dislocation of fibula, lower end
  Subluxation and dislocation of talus
  Subluxation and dislocation of tibia, lower end
  - X **S93.01 Subluxation of right ankle joint**
  - X **S93.02 Subluxation of left ankle joint**
  - X **S93.03 Subluxation of unspecified ankle joint**
  - X **S93.04 Dislocation of right ankle joint**
  - X **S93.05 Dislocation of left ankle joint**
  - X **S93.06 Dislocation of unspecified ankle joint**
- **S93.1 Subluxation and dislocation of toe**
  - **S93.10 Unspecified subluxation and dislocation of toe**

    Dislocation of toe NOS
    Subluxation of toe NOS
    - **S93.101 Unspecified subluxation of right toe(s)**
    - **S93.102 Unspecified subluxation of left toe(s)**
    - **S93.103 Unspecified subluxation of unspecified toe(s)**
    - **S93.104 Unspecified dislocation of right toe(s)**
    - **S93.105 Unspecified dislocation of left toe(s)**
    - **S93.106 Unspecified dislocation of unspecified toe(s)**
  - **S93.11 Dislocation of interphalangeal joint**
    - **S93.111 Dislocation of interphalangeal joint of right great toe**
    - **S93.112 Dislocation of interphalangeal joint of left great toe**
    - **S93.113 Dislocation of interphalangeal joint of unspecified great toe**
    - **S93.114 Dislocation of interphalangeal joint of right lesser toe(s)**
    - **S93.115 Dislocation of interphalangeal joint of left lesser toe(s)**
    - **S93.116 Dislocation of interphalangeal joint of unspecified lesser toe(s)**
    - **S93.119 Dislocation of interphalangeal joint of unspecified toe(s)**

- S93.12 Dislocation of metatarsophalangeal joint
  - S93.121 Dislocation of metatarsophalangeal joint of right great toe
  - S93.122 Dislocation of metatarsophalangeal joint of left great toe
  - S93.123 Dislocation of metatarsophalangeal joint of unspecified great toe
  - S93.124 Dislocation of metatarsophalangeal joint of right lesser toe(s)
  - S93.125 Dislocation of metatarsophalangeal joint of left lesser toe(s)
  - S93.126 Dislocation of metatarsophalangeal joint of unspecified lesser toe(s)
  - S93.129 Dislocation of metatarsophalangeal joint of unspecified toe(s)
- S93.13 Subluxation of interphalangeal joint
  - S93.131 Subluxation of interphalangeal joint of right great toe
  - S93.132 Subluxation of interphalangeal joint of left great toe
  - S93.133 Subluxation of interphalangeal joint of unspecified great toe
  - S93.134 Subluxation of interphalangeal joint of right lesser toe(s)
  - S93.135 Subluxation of interphalangeal joint of left lesser toe(s)
  - S93.136 Subluxation of interphalangeal joint of unspecified lesser toe(s)
  - S93.139 Subluxation of interphalangeal joint of unspecified toe(s)
- S93.14 Subluxation of metatarsophalangeal joint
  - S93.141 Subluxation of metatarsophalangeal joint of right great toe
  - S93.142 Subluxation of metatarsophalangeal joint of left great toe
  - S93.143 Subluxation of metatarsophalangeal joint of unspecified great toe
  - S93.144 Subluxation of metatarsophalangeal joint of right lesser toe(s)
  - S93.145 Subluxation of metatarsophalangeal joint of left lesser toe(s)
  - S93.146 Subluxation of metatarsophalangeal joint of unspecified lesser toe(s)
  - S93.149 Subluxation of metatarsophalangeal joint of unspecified toe(s)
- S93.3 Subluxation and dislocation of foot

  Excludes2 dislocation of toe (S93.1-)
  - S93.30 Unspecified subluxation and dislocation of foot

    Dislocation of foot NOS
    Subluxation of foot NOS
    - S93.301 Unspecified subluxation of right foot
    - S93.302 Unspecified subluxation of left foot
    - S93.303 Unspecified subluxation of unspecified foot
    - S93.304 Unspecified dislocation of right foot
    - S93.305 Unspecified dislocation of left foot
    - S93.306 Unspecified dislocation of unspecified foot
  - S93.31 Subluxation and dislocation of tarsal joint
    - S93.311 Subluxation of tarsal joint of right foot
    - S93.312 Subluxation of tarsal joint of left foot
    - S93.313 Subluxation of tarsal joint of unspecified foot
    - S93.314 Dislocation of tarsal joint of right foot
    - S93.315 Dislocation of tarsal joint of left foot
    - S93.316 Dislocation of tarsal joint of unspecified foot
  - S93.32 Subluxation and dislocation of tarsometatarsal joint
    - S93.321 Subluxation of tarsometatarsal joint of right foot
    - S93.322 Subluxation of tarsometatarsal joint of left foot
    - S93.323 Subluxation of tarsometatarsal joint of unspecified foot
    - S93.324 Dislocation of tarsometatarsal joint of right foot
    - S93.325 Dislocation of tarsometatarsal joint of left foot
    - S93.326 Dislocation of tarsometatarsal joint of unspecified foot
  - S93.33 Other subluxation and dislocation of foot
    - S93.331 Other subluxation of right foot
    - S93.332 Other subluxation of left foot
    - S93.333 Other subluxation of unspecified foot
    - S93.334 Other dislocation of right foot
    - S93.335 Other dislocation of left foot
    - S93.336 Other dislocation of unspecified foot
- S93.4 Sprain of ankle

  Injury to ligaments when one or more is stretched/torn

  Excludes2 injury of Achilles tendon (S86.0-)
  - S93.40 Sprain of unspecified ligament of ankle

    Sprain of ankle NOS
    Sprained ankle NOS
    - S93.401 Sprain of unspecified ligament of right ankle
    - S93.402 Sprain of unspecified ligament of left ankle
    - S93.409 Sprain of unspecified ligament of unspecified ankle
  - S93.41 Sprain of calcaneofibular ligament
    - S93.411 Sprain of calcaneofibular ligament of right ankle
    - S93.412 Sprain of calcaneofibular ligament of left ankle
    - S93.419 Sprain of calcaneofibular ligament of unspecified ankle
  - S93.42 Sprain of deltoid ligament
    - S93.421 Sprain of deltoid ligament of right ankle
    - S93.422 Sprain of deltoid ligament of left ankle
    - S93.429 Sprain of deltoid ligament of unspecified ankle
  - S93.43 Sprain of tibiofibular ligament
    - S93.431 Sprain of tibiofibular ligament of right ankle
    - S93.432 Sprain of tibiofibular ligament of left ankle
    - S93.439 Sprain of tibiofibular ligament of unspecified ankle

◀ New ◀ Revised ~~deleted~~ Deleted Excludes 1 Excludes 2 Includes Use additional Code first Code also Unspecified
OGCR Official Guidelines ● Unacceptable Principal Diagnosis X Assign placeholder X ● Use Additional Character(s) ▶ Manifestation Code Coding Clinic

- **S93.49 Sprain of other ligament of ankle**
  Sprain of internal collateral ligament
  Sprain of talofibular ligament
  - **S93.491 Sprain of other ligament of right ankle**
  - **S93.492 Sprain of other ligament of left ankle**
  - **S93.499 Sprain of other ligament of unspecified ankle**
- **S93.5 Sprain of toe**
  - **S93.50 Unspecified sprain of toe**
    - **S93.501 Unspecified sprain of right great toe**
    - **S93.502 Unspecified sprain of left great toe**
    - **S93.503 Unspecified sprain of unspecified great toe**
    - **S93.504 Unspecified sprain of right lesser toe(s)**
    - **S93.505 Unspecified sprain of left lesser toe(s)**
    - **S93.506 Unspecified sprain of unspecified lesser toe(s)**
    - **S93.509 Unspecified sprain of unspecified toe(s)**
  - **S93.51 Sprain of interphalangeal joint of toe**
    - **S93.511 Sprain of interphalangeal joint of right great toe**
    - **S93.512 Sprain of interphalangeal joint of left great toe**
    - **S93.513 Sprain of interphalangeal joint of unspecified great toe**
    - **S93.514 Sprain of interphalangeal joint of right lesser toe(s)**
    - **S93.515 Sprain of interphalangeal joint of left lesser toe(s)**
    - **S93.516 Sprain of interphalangeal joint of unspecified lesser toe(s)**
    - **S93.519 Sprain of interphalangeal joint of unspecified toe(s)**
  - **S93.52 Sprain of metatarsophalangeal joint of toe**
    - **S93.521 Sprain of metatarsophalangeal joint of right great toe**
    - **S93.522 Sprain of metatarsophalangeal joint of left great toe**
    - **S93.523 Sprain of metatarsophalangeal joint of unspecified great toe**
    - **S93.524 Sprain of metatarsophalangeal joint of right lesser toe(s)**
    - **S93.525 Sprain of metatarsophalangeal joint of left lesser toe(s)**
    - **S93.526 Sprain of metatarsophalangeal joint of unspecified lesser toe(s)**
    - **S93.529 Sprain of metatarsophalangeal joint of unspecified toe(s)**
- **S93.6 Sprain of foot**
  Excludes2 sprain of metatarsophalangeal joint of toe (S93.52-)
  sprain of toe (S93.5-)
  - **S93.60 Unspecified sprain of foot**
    - **S93.601 Unspecified sprain of right foot**
    - **S93.602 Unspecified sprain of left foot**
    - **S93.609 Unspecified sprain of unspecified foot**
  - **S93.61 Sprain of tarsal ligament of foot**
    - **S93.611 Sprain of tarsal ligament of right foot**
    - **S93.612 Sprain of tarsal ligament of left foot**
    - **S93.619 Sprain of tarsal ligament of unspecified foot**
  - **S93.62 Sprain of tarsometatarsal ligament of foot**
    - **S93.621 Sprain of tarsometatarsal ligament of right foot**
    - **S93.622 Sprain of tarsometatarsal ligament of left foot**
    - **S93.629 Sprain of tarsometatarsal ligament of unspecified foot**
  - **S93.69 Other sprain of foot**
    - **S93.691 Other sprain of right foot**
    - **S93.692 Other sprain of left foot**
    - **S93.699 Other sprain of unspecified foot**
- **S94 Injury of nerves at ankle and foot level**
  The appropriate 7th character is to be added to each code from category S94

A	initial encounter
D	subsequent encounter
S	sequela

  Code also any associated open wound (S91.-)
  - **S94.0 Injury of lateral plantar nerve**
    - X **S94.00 Injury of lateral plantar nerve, unspecified leg**
    - X **S94.01 Injury of lateral plantar nerve, right leg**
    - X **S94.02 Injury of lateral plantar nerve, left leg**
  - **S94.1 Injury of medial plantar nerve**
    - X **S94.10 Injury of medial plantar nerve, unspecified leg**
    - X **S94.11 Injury of medial plantar nerve, right leg**
    - X **S94.12 Injury of medial plantar nerve, left leg**
  - **S94.2 Injury of deep peroneal nerve at ankle and foot level**
    Injury of terminal, lateral branch of deep peroneal nerve
    - X **S94.20 Injury of deep peroneal nerve at ankle and foot level, unspecified leg**
    - X **S94.21 Injury of deep peroneal nerve at ankle and foot level, right leg**
    - X **S94.22 Injury of deep peroneal nerve at ankle and foot level, left leg**
  - **S94.3 Injury of cutaneous sensory nerve at ankle and foot level**
    - X **S94.30 Injury of cutaneous sensory nerve at ankle and foot level, unspecified leg**
    - X **S94.31 Injury of cutaneous sensory nerve at ankle and foot level, right leg**
    - X **S94.32 Injury of cutaneous sensory nerve at ankle and foot level, left leg**
  - **S94.8 Injury of other nerves at ankle and foot level**
    - **S94.8X Injury of other nerves at ankle and foot level**
      - **S94.8X1 Injury of other nerves at ankle and foot level, right leg**
      - **S94.8X2 Injury of other nerves at ankle and foot level, left leg**
      - **S94.8X9 Injury of other nerves at ankle and foot level, unspecified leg**
  - **S94.9 Injury of unspecified nerve at ankle and foot level**
    - X **S94.90 Injury of unspecified nerve at ankle and foot level, unspecified leg**
    - X **S94.91 Injury of unspecified nerve at ankle and foot level, right leg**
    - X **S94.92 Injury of unspecified nerve at ankle and foot level, left leg**

S95 Injury of blood vessels at ankle and foot level

Code also any associated open wound (S91.-)

Excludes2 injury of posterior tibial artery and vein (S85.1-, S85.8-)

The appropriate 7th character is to be added to each code from category S95

A	initial encounter
D	subsequent encounter
S	sequela

S95.0 Injury of dorsal artery of foot

S95.00 Unspecified injury of dorsal artery of foot

S95.001 Unspecified injury of dorsal artery of right foot A

Ex: See S75.801

S95.002 Unspecified injury of dorsal artery of left foot A

Ex: See S75.802

S95.009 Unspecified injury of dorsal artery of unspecified foot A

Ex: See S75.809

S95.01 Laceration of dorsal artery of foot

S95.011 Laceration of dorsal artery of right foot A

Ex: See S75.801

S95.012 Laceration of dorsal artery of left foot A

Ex: See S75.802

S95.019 Laceration of dorsal artery of unspecified foot A

Ex: See S75.809

S95.09 Other specified injury of dorsal artery of foot

S95.091 Other specified injury of dorsal artery of right foot A

Ex: See S75.801

S95.092 Other specified injury of dorsal artery of left foot A

Ex: See S75.802

S95.099 Other specified injury of dorsal artery of unspecified foot A

Ex: See S75.809

S95.1 Injury of plantar artery of foot

S95.10 Unspecified injury of plantar artery of foot

S95.101 Unspecified injury of plantar artery of right foot A

Ex: S75.801[A], S75.809-S75.811[A], S75.819-S75.891[A], S75.899-S75.901[A], S75.909-S75.911[A], S75.919-S75.991[A], S75.999[A], S85.201[A], S85.209-S85.211[A], S85.219-S85.291[A], S85.299[A], S85.801[A], S85.809-S85.811[A], S85.819-S85.891[A], S85.899-S85.901[A], S85.909-S85.911[A], S85.919-S85.991[A], S85.999[A], S95.001[A], S95.009-S95.011[A], S95.019-S95.091[A], S95.099-S95.201[A], S95.209-S95.211[A], S95.219-S95.291[A], S95.299-S95.801[A], S95.809-S95.811[A], S95.819-S95.891[A], S95.899-S95.901[A], S95.909-S95.911[A], S95.919-S95.991[A], S95.999[A]

S95.102 Unspecified injury of plantar artery of left foot A

Ex: S75.802-S75.809[A], S75.812-S75.819[A], S75.892-S75.899[A], S75.902-S75.909[A], S75.912-S75.919[A], S75.992-S75.999[A], S85.202-S85.209[A], S85.212-S85.219[A], S85.292-S85.299[A], S85.802-S85.809[A], S85.812-S85.819[A], S85.892-S85.899[A], S85.902-S85.909[A], S85.912-S85.919[A], S85.992-S85.999[A], S95.002-S95.009[A], S95.012-S95.019[A], S95.092-S95.099[A], S95.102-S95.109[A], S95.112-S95.119[A], S95.192-S95.199[A], S95.202-S95.209[A], S95.212-S95.219[A], S95.292-S95.299[A], S95.802-S95.809[A], S95.812-S95.819[A], S95.892-S95.899[A], S95.902-S95.909[A], S95.912-S95.919[A], S95.992-S95.999[A]

S95.109 Unspecified injury of plantar artery of unspecified foot A

Ex: S75.801-S75.999[A], S85.201-S85.299[A], S85.801-S85.999[A], S95.001-S95.099[A], S95.101-S95.999[A]

S95.11 Laceration of plantar artery of foot

S95.111 Laceration of plantar artery of right foot A

Ex: See S95.101

S95.112 Laceration of plantar artery of left foot A

Ex: See S95.102

S95.119 Laceration of plantar artery of unspecified foot A

Ex: See S95.109

S95.19 Other specified injury of plantar artery of foot

S95.191 Other specified injury of plantar artery of right foot A

Ex: See S95.101

S95.192 Other specified injury of plantar artery of left foot A

Ex: See S95.102

S95.199 Other specified injury of plantar artery of unspecified foot A

Ex: See S95.109

S95.2 Injury of dorsal vein of foot

S95.20 Unspecified injury of dorsal vein of foot

S95.201 Unspecified injury of dorsal vein of right foot A

Ex: See S75.801

S95.202 Unspecified injury of dorsal vein of left foot A

Ex: See S75.802

S95.209 Unspecified injury of dorsal vein of unspecified foot A

Ex: See S75.809

S95.21 Laceration of dorsal vein of foot

S95.211 Laceration of dorsal vein of right foot A

Ex: See S75.801

S95.212 Laceration of dorsal vein of left foot A

Ex: See S75.802

S95.219 Laceration of dorsal vein of unspecified foot A

Ex: See S75.809

S95.29 Other specified injury of dorsal vein of foot

S95.291 Other specified injury of dorsal vein of right foot A

Ex: See S75.801

S95.292 Other specified injury of dorsal vein of left foot A

Ex: See S75.802

S95.299 Other specified injury of dorsal vein of unspecified foot A

Ex: See S75.809

- **S95.8 Injury of other blood vessels at ankle and foot level**
  - **S95.80 Unspecified injury of other blood vessels at ankle and foot level**
    - **S95.801 Unspecified injury of other blood vessels at ankle and foot level, right leg A**
      Ex See S75.801
    - **S95.802 Unspecified injury of other blood vessels at ankle and foot level, left leg A**
      Ex See S75.802
    - **S95.809 Unspecified injury of other blood vessels at ankle and foot level, unspecified leg A**
      Ex See S75.809
  - **S95.81 Laceration of other blood vessels at ankle and foot level**
    - **S95.811 Laceration of other blood vessels at ankle and foot level, right leg A**
      Ex See S75.801
    - **S95.812 Laceration of other blood vessels at ankle and foot level, left leg A**
      Ex See S75.802
    - **S95.819 Laceration of other blood vessels at ankle and foot level, unspecified leg A**
      Ex See S75.809
  - **S95.89 Other specified injury of other blood vessels at ankle and foot level**
    - **S95.891 Other specified injury of other blood vessels at ankle and foot level, right leg A**
      Ex See S75.801
    - **S95.892 Other specified injury of other blood vessels at ankle and foot level, left leg A**
      Ex See S75.802
    - **S95.899 Other specified injury of other blood vessels at ankle and foot level, unspecified leg A**
      Ex See S75.809
- **S95.9 Injury of unspecified blood vessel at ankle and foot level**
  - **S95.90 Unspecified injury of unspecified blood vessel at ankle and foot level**
    - **S95.901 Unspecified injury of unspecified blood vessel at ankle and foot level, right leg A**
      Ex See S75.801
    - **S95.902 Unspecified injury of unspecified blood vessel at ankle and foot level, left leg A**
      Ex See S75.802
    - **S95.909 Unspecified injury of unspecified blood vessel at ankle and foot level, unspecified leg A**
      Ex See S75.809
  - **S95.91 Laceration of unspecified blood vessel at ankle and foot level**
    - **S95.911 Laceration of unspecified blood vessel at ankle and foot level, right leg A**
      Ex See S75.801
    - **S95.912 Laceration of unspecified blood vessel at ankle and foot level, left leg A**
      Ex See S75.802
    - **S95.919 Laceration of unspecified blood vessel at ankle and foot level, unspecified leg A**
      Ex See S75.809
  - **S95.99 Other specified injury of unspecified blood vessel at ankle and foot level**
    - **S95.991 Other specified injury of unspecified blood vessel at ankle and foot level, right leg A**
      Ex See S75.801
    - **S95.992 Other specified injury of unspecified blood vessel at ankle and foot level, left leg A**
      Ex See S75.802
    - **S95.999 Other specified injury of unspecified blood vessel at ankle and foot level, unspecified leg A**
      Ex See S75.809
- **S96 Injury of muscle and tendon at ankle and foot level**

  Code also any associated open wound (S91.-)

  Excludes2 injury of Achilles tendon (S86.0-)
  sprain of joints and ligaments of ankle and foot (S93.-)

  The appropriate 7th character is to be added to each code from category S96

A	initial encounter
D	subsequent encounter
S	sequela

  - **S96.0 Injury of muscle and tendon of long flexor muscle of toe at ankle and foot level**
    - **S96.00 Unspecified injury of muscle and tendon of long flexor muscle of toe at ankle and foot level**
      - **S96.001 Unspecified injury of muscle and tendon of long flexor muscle of toe at ankle and foot level, right foot**
      - **S96.002 Unspecified injury of muscle and tendon of long flexor muscle of toe at ankle and foot level, left foot**
      - **S96.009 Unspecified injury of muscle and tendon of long flexor muscle of toe at ankle and foot level, unspecified foot**
    - **S96.01 Strain of muscle and tendon of long flexor muscle of toe at ankle and foot level**
      - **S96.011 Strain of muscle and tendon of long flexor muscle of toe at ankle and foot level, right foot**
      - **S96.012 Strain of muscle and tendon of long flexor muscle of toe at ankle and foot level, left foot**
      - **S96.019 Strain of muscle and tendon of long flexor muscle of toe at ankle and foot level, unspecified foot**
    - **S96.02 Laceration of muscle and tendon of long flexor muscle of toe at ankle and foot level**
      - **S96.021 Laceration of muscle and tendon of long flexor muscle of toe at ankle and foot level, right foot A**
        Ex See S86.021
      - **S96.022 Laceration of muscle and tendon of long flexor muscle of toe at ankle and foot level, left foot A**
        Ex See S86.022
      - **S96.029 Laceration of muscle and tendon of long flexor muscle of toe at ankle and foot level, unspecified foot A**
        Ex See S86.029

- S96.09 Other injury of muscle and tendon of long flexor muscle of toe at ankle and foot level
  - S96.091 Other injury of muscle and tendon of long flexor muscle of toe at ankle and foot level, right foot
  - S96.092 Other injury of muscle and tendon of long flexor muscle of toe at ankle and foot level, left foot
  - S96.099 Other injury of muscle and tendon of long flexor muscle of toe at ankle and foot level, unspecified foot
- S96.1 Injury of muscle and tendon of long extensor muscle of toe at ankle and foot level
  - S96.10 Unspecified injury of muscle and tendon of long extensor muscle of toe at ankle and foot level
    - S96.101 Unspecified injury of muscle and tendon of long extensor muscle of toe at ankle and foot level, right foot
    - S96.102 Unspecified injury of muscle and tendon of long extensor muscle of toe at ankle and foot level, left foot
    - S96.109 Unspecified injury of muscle and tendon of long extensor muscle of toe at ankle and foot level, unspecified foot
  - S96.11 Strain of muscle and tendon of long extensor muscle of toe at ankle and foot level
    - S96.111 Strain of muscle and tendon of long extensor muscle of toe at ankle and foot level, right foot
    - S96.112 Strain of muscle and tendon of long extensor muscle of toe at ankle and foot level, left foot
    - S96.119 Strain of muscle and tendon of long extensor muscle of toe at ankle and foot level, unspecified foot
  - S96.12 Laceration of muscle and tendon of long extensor muscle of toe at ankle and foot level
    - S96.121 Laceration of muscle and tendon of long extensor muscle of toe at ankle and foot level, right foot A
      Ex: See S86.021
    - S96.122 Laceration of muscle and tendon of long extensor muscle of toe at ankle and foot level, left foot A
      Ex: See S86.022
    - S96.129 Laceration of muscle and tendon of long extensor muscle of toe at ankle and foot level, unspecified foot A
      Ex: See S86.029
  - S96.19 Other specified injury of muscle and tendon of long extensor muscle of toe at ankle and foot level
    - S96.191 Other specified injury of muscle and tendon of long extensor muscle of toe at ankle and foot level, right foot
    - S96.192 Other specified injury of muscle and tendon of long extensor muscle of toe at ankle and foot level, left foot
    - S96.199 Other specified injury of muscle and tendon of long extensor muscle of toe at ankle and foot level, unspecified foot
- S96.2 Injury of intrinsic muscle and tendon at ankle and foot level
  - S96.20 Unspecified injury of intrinsic muscle and tendon at ankle and foot level
    - S96.201 Unspecified injury of intrinsic muscle and tendon at ankle and foot level, right foot
    - S96.202 Unspecified injury of intrinsic muscle and tendon at ankle and foot level, left foot
    - S96.209 Unspecified injury of intrinsic muscle and tendon at ankle and foot level, unspecified foot
  - S96.21 Strain of intrinsic muscle and tendon at ankle and foot level
    - S96.211 Strain of intrinsic muscle and tendon at ankle and foot level, right foot
    - S96.212 Strain of intrinsic muscle and tendon at ankle and foot level, left foot
    - S96.219 Strain of intrinsic muscle and tendon at ankle and foot level, unspecified foot
  - S96.22 Laceration of intrinsic muscle and tendon at ankle and foot level
    - S96.221 Laceration of intrinsic muscle and tendon at ankle and foot level, right foot A
      Ex: See S86.021
    - S96.222 Laceration of intrinsic muscle and tendon at left ankle and foot level, left foot A
      Ex: See S86.022
    - S96.229 Laceration of intrinsic muscle and tendon at ankle and foot level, unspecified foot A
      Ex: See S86.029
  - S96.29 Other specified injury of intrinsic muscle and tendon at ankle and foot level
    - S96.291 Other specified injury of intrinsic muscle and tendon at ankle and foot level, right foot
    - S96.292 Other specified injury of intrinsic muscle and tendon at ankle and foot level, left foot
    - S96.299 Other specified injury of intrinsic muscle and tendon at ankle and foot level, unspecified foot
- S96.8 Injury of other specified muscles and tendons at ankle and foot level
  - S96.80 Unspecified injury of other specified muscles and tendons at ankle and foot level
    - S96.801 Unspecified injury of other specified muscles and tendons at ankle and foot level, right foot
    - S96.802 Unspecified injury of other specified muscles and tendons at ankle and foot level, left foot
    - S96.809 Unspecified injury of other specified muscles and tendons at ankle and foot level, unspecified foot
  - S96.81 Strain of other specified muscles and tendons at ankle and foot level
    - S96.811 Strain of other specified muscles and tendons at ankle and foot level, right foot
    - S96.812 Strain of other specified muscles and tendons at ankle and foot level, left foot
    - S96.819 Strain of other specified muscles and tendons at ankle and foot level, unspecified foot

- **S96.82 Laceration of other specified muscles and tendons at ankle and foot level**
  - **S96.821 Laceration of other specified muscles and tendons at ankle and foot level, right foot** A
    Ex: See S86.021
  - **S96.822 Laceration of other specified muscles and tendons at ankle and foot level, left foot** A
    Ex: See S86.022
  - **S96.829 Laceration of other specified muscles and tendons at ankle and foot level, unspecified foot** A
    Ex: See S86.029
- **S96.89 Other specified injury of other specified muscles and tendons at ankle and foot level**
  - **S96.891 Other specified injury of other specified muscles and tendons at ankle and foot level, right foot**
  - **S96.892 Other specified injury of other specified muscles and tendons at ankle and foot level, left foot**
  - **S96.899 Other specified injury of other specified muscles and tendons at ankle and foot level, unspecified foot**
- **S96.9 Injury of unspecified muscle and tendon at ankle and foot level**
  - **S96.90 Unspecified injury of unspecified muscle and tendon at ankle and foot level**
    - **S96.901 Unspecified injury of unspecified muscle and tendon at ankle and foot level, right foot**
    - **S96.902 Unspecified injury of unspecified muscle and tendon at ankle and foot level, left foot**
    - **S96.909 Unspecified injury of unspecified muscle and tendon at ankle and foot level, unspecified foot**
  - **S96.91 Strain of unspecified muscle and tendon at ankle and foot level**
    - **S96.911 Strain of unspecified muscle and tendon at ankle and foot level, right foot**
    - **S96.912 Strain of unspecified muscle and tendon at ankle and foot level, left foot**
    - **S96.919 Strain of unspecified muscle and tendon at ankle and foot level, unspecified foot**
  - **S96.92 Laceration of unspecified muscle and tendon at ankle and foot level**
    - **S96.921 Laceration of unspecified muscle and tendon at ankle and foot level, right foot** A
      Ex: See S86.021
    - **S96.922 Laceration of unspecified muscle and tendon at ankle and foot level, left foot** A
      Ex: See S86.022
    - **S96.929 Laceration of unspecified muscle and tendon at ankle and foot level, unspecified foot** A
      Ex: See S86.029
  - **S96.99 Other specified injury of unspecified muscle and tendon at ankle and foot level**
    - **S96.991 Other specified injury of unspecified muscle and tendon at ankle and foot level, right foot**
    - **S96.992 Other specified injury of unspecified muscle and tendon at ankle and foot level, left foot**
    - **S96.999 Other specified injury of unspecified muscle and tendon at ankle and foot level, unspecified foot**

- **S97 Crushing injury of ankle and foot**
  Use additional code(s) for all associated injuries
  The appropriate 7th character is to be added to each code from category S97

A	initial encounter
D	subsequent encounter
S	sequela

  - **S97.0 Crushing injury of ankle**
    - X **S97.00 Crushing injury of unspecified ankle**
    - X **S97.01 Crushing injury of right ankle**
    - X **S97.02 Crushing injury of left ankle**
  - **S97.1 Crushing injury of toe**
    - **S97.10 Crushing injury of unspecified toe(s)**
      - **S97.101 Crushing injury of unspecified right toe(s)**
      - **S97.102 Crushing injury of unspecified left toe(s)**
      - **S97.109 Crushing injury of unspecified toe(s)**
        Crushing injury of toe NOS
    - **S97.11 Crushing injury of great toe**
      - **S97.111 Crushing injury of right great toe**
      - **S97.112 Crushing injury of left great toe**
      - **S97.119 Crushing injury of unspecified great toe**
    - **S97.12 Crushing injury of lesser toe(s)**
      - **S97.121 Crushing injury of right lesser toe(s)**
      - **S97.122 Crushing injury of left lesser toe(s)**
      - **S97.129 Crushing injury of lesser toe(s), unspecified toe(s)**
  - **S97.8 Crushing injury of foot**
    - X **S97.80 Crushing injury of foot, unspecified side**
      Crushing injury of foot NOS
    - X **S97.81 Crushing injury of right foot**
    - X **S97.82 Crushing injury of left foot**

- **S98 Traumatic amputation of ankle and foot**
  An amputation not identified as partial or complete should be coded to complete
  The appropriate 7th character is to be added to each code from category S98

A	initial encounter
D	subsequent encounter
S	sequela

  - **S98.0 Traumatic amputation of foot at ankle level**
    - **S98.01 Complete traumatic amputation of foot at ankle level**
      - **S98.011 Complete traumatic amputation of right foot at ankle level** A
        Ex: See S78.011
      - **S98.012 Complete traumatic amputation of left foot at ankle level** A
        Ex: See S78.012
      - **S98.019 Complete traumatic amputation of unspecified foot at ankle level** A
        Ex: See S78.019
    - **S98.02 Partial traumatic amputation of foot at ankle level**
      - **S98.021 Partial traumatic amputation of right foot at ankle level** A
        Ex: See S78.011
      - **S98.022 Partial traumatic amputation of left foot at ankle level** A
        Ex: See S78.012
      - **S98.029 Partial traumatic amputation of unspecified foot at ankle level** A
        Ex: See S78.019

- S98.1 Traumatic amputation of one toe
  - S98.11 Complete traumatic amputation of great toe
    - S98.111 Complete traumatic amputation of right great toe
    - S98.112 Complete traumatic amputation of left great toe
    - S98.119 Complete traumatic amputation of unspecified great toe
  - S98.12 Partial traumatic amputation of great toe
    - S98.121 Partial traumatic amputation of right great toe
    - S98.122 Partial traumatic amputation of left great toe
    - S98.129 Partial traumatic amputation of unspecified great toe
  - S98.13 Complete traumatic amputation of one lesser toe
    Traumatic amputation of toe NOS
    - S98.131 Complete traumatic amputation of one right lesser toe
    - S98.132 Complete traumatic amputation of one left lesser toe
    - S98.139 Complete traumatic amputation of one unspecified lesser toe
  - S98.14 Partial traumatic amputation of one lesser toe
    - S98.141 Partial traumatic amputation of one right lesser toe
    - S98.142 Partial traumatic amputation of one left lesser toe
    - S98.149 Partial traumatic amputation of one unspecified lesser toe
- S98.2 Traumatic amputation of two or more lesser toes
  - S98.21 Complete traumatic amputation of two or more lesser toes
    - S98.211 Complete traumatic amputation of two or more right lesser toes
    - S98.212 Complete traumatic amputation of two or more left lesser toes
    - S98.219 Complete traumatic amputation of two or more unspecified lesser toes
  - S98.22 Partial traumatic amputation of two or more lesser toes
    - S98.221 Partial traumatic amputation of two or more right lesser toes
    - S98.222 Partial traumatic amputation of two or more left lesser toes
    - S98.229 Partial traumatic amputation of two or more unspecified lesser toes
- S98.3 Traumatic amputation of midfoot
  - S98.31 Complete traumatic amputation of midfoot
    - S98.311 Complete traumatic amputation of right midfoot A
      Ex: See S78.011
    - S98.312 Complete traumatic amputation of left midfoot A
      Ex: See S78.012
    - S98.319 Complete traumatic amputation of unspecified midfoot A
      Ex: See S78.019
  - S98.32 Partial traumatic amputation of midfoot
    - S98.321 Partial traumatic amputation of right midfoot A
      Ex: See S78.011
    - S98.322 Partial traumatic amputation of left midfoot A
      Ex: See S78.012
    - S98.329 Partial traumatic amputation of unspecified midfoot A
      Ex: See S78.019
- S98.9 Traumatic amputation of foot, level unspecified
  - S98.91 Complete traumatic amputation of foot, level unspecified
    - S98.911 Complete traumatic amputation of right foot, level unspecified A
      Ex: See S78.011
    - S98.912 Complete traumatic amputation of left foot, level unspecified A
      Ex: See S78.012
    - S98.919 Complete traumatic amputation of unspecified foot, level unspecified A
      Ex: See S78.019
  - S98.92 Partial traumatic amputation of foot, level unspecified
    - S98.921 Partial traumatic amputation of right foot, level unspecified A
      Ex: See S78.011
    - S98.922 Partial traumatic amputation of left foot, level unspecified A
      Ex: See S78.012
    - S98.929 Partial traumatic amputation of unspecified foot, level unspecified A
      Ex: See S78.019
- S99 Other and unspecified injuries of ankle and foot
  - S99.0 Physeal fracture of calcaneus ◀
    The appropriate 7th character is to be added to each code from subcategories S99.0 ◀

A	initial encounter for closed fracture ◀
B	initial encounter for open fracture ◀
D	subsequent encounter for fracture with routine healing ◀
G	subsequent encounter for fracture with delayed healing ◀
K	subsequent encounter for fracture with nonunion ◀
P	subsequent encounter for fracture with malunion ◀
S	sequela ◀

    - S99.00 Unspecified physeal fracture of calcaneus ◀
      - S99.001 Unspecified physeal fracture of right calcaneus ◀
      - S99.002 Unspecified physeal fracture of left calcaneus ◀
      - S99.009 Unspecified physeal fracture of unspecified calcaneus ◀
    - S99.01 Salter-Harris Type I physeal fracture of calcaneus ◀
      - S99.011 Salter-Harris Type I physeal fracture of right calcaneus ◀
      - S99.012 Salter-Harris Type I physeal fracture of left calcaneus ◀
      - S99.019 Salter-Harris Type I physeal fracture of unspecified calcaneus ◀
    - S99.02 Salter-Harris Type II physeal fracture of calcaneus ◀
      - S99.021 Salter-Harris Type II physeal fracture of right calcaneus ◀
      - S99.022 Salter-Harris Type II physeal fracture of left calcaneus ◀
      - S99.029 Salter-Harris Type II physeal fracture of unspecified calcaneus ◀

- **S99.03 Salter-Harris Type III physeal fracture of calcaneus**
  - **S99.031 Salter-Harris Type III physeal fracture of right calcaneus**
  - **S99.032 Salter-Harris Type III physeal fracture of left calcaneus**
  - **S99.039 Salter-Harris Type III physeal fracture of unspecified calcaneus**
- **S99.04 Salter-Harris Type IV physeal fracture of calcaneus**
  - **S99.041 Salter-Harris Type IV physeal fracture of right calcaneus**
  - **S99.042 Salter-Harris Type IV physeal fracture of left calcaneus**
  - **S99.049 Salter-Harris Type IV physeal fracture of unspecified calcaneus**
- **S99.09 Other physeal fracture of calcaneus**
  - **S99.091 Other physeal fracture of right calcaneus**
  - **S99.092 Other physeal fracture of left calcaneus**
  - **S99.099 Other physeal fracture of unspecified calcaneus**
- **S99.1 Physeal fracture of metatarsal**

  The appropriate 7th character is to be added to each code from subcategories S99.1

A	initial encounter for closed fracture
B	initial encounter for open fracture
D	subsequent encounter for fracture with routine healing
G	subsequent encounter for fracture with delayed healing
K	subsequent encounter for fracture with nonunion
P	subsequent encounter for fracture with malunion
S	sequela

- **S99.10 Unspecified physeal fracture of metatarsal**
  - **S99.101 Unspecified physeal fracture of right metatarsal**
  - **S99.102 Unspecified physeal fracture of left metatarsal**
  - **S99.109 Unspecified physeal fracture of unspecified metatarsal**
- **S99.11 Salter-Harris Type I physeal fracture of metatarsal**
  - **S99.111 Salter-Harris Type I physeal fracture of right metatarsal**
  - **S99.112 Salter-Harris Type I physeal fracture of left metatarsal**
  - **S99.119 Salter-Harris Type I physeal fracture of unspecified metatarsal**
- **S99.12 Salter-Harris Type II physeal fracture of metatarsal**
  - **S99.121 Salter-Harris Type II physeal fracture of right metatarsal**
  - **S99.122 Salter-Harris Type II physeal fracture of left metatarsal**
  - **S99.129 Salter-Harris Type II physeal fracture of unspecified metatarsal**
- **S99.13 Salter-Harris Type III physeal fracture of metatarsal**
  - **S99.131 Salter-Harris Type III physeal fracture of right metatarsal**
  - **S99.132 Salter-Harris Type III physeal fracture of left metatarsal**
  - **S99.139 Salter-Harris Type III physeal fracture of unspecified metatarsal**
- **S99.14 Salter-Harris Type IV physeal fracture of metatarsal**
  - **S99.141 Salter-Harris Type IV physeal fracture of right metatarsal**
  - **S99.142 Salter-Harris Type IV physeal fracture of left metatarsal**
  - **S99.149 Salter-Harris Type IV physeal fracture of unspecified metatarsal**
- **S99.19 Other physeal fracture of metatarsal**
  - **S99.191 Other physeal fracture of right metatarsal**
  - **S99.192 Other physeal fracture of left metatarsal**
  - **S99.199 Other physeal fracture of unspecified metatarsal**
- **S99.2 Physeal fracture of phalanx of toe**

  The appropriate 7th character is to be added to each code from subcategories S99.2

A	initial encounter for closed fracture
B	initial encounter for open fracture
D	subsequent encounter for fracture with routine healing
G	subsequent encounter for fracture with delayed healing
K	subsequent encounter for fracture with nonunion
P	subsequent encounter for fracture with malunion
S	sequela

- **S99.20 Unspecified physeal fracture of phalanx of toe**
  - **S99.201 Unspecified physeal fracture of phalanx of right toe**
  - **S99.202 Unspecified physeal fracture of phalanx of right toe**
  - **S99.209 Unspecified physeal fracture of phalanx of unspecified toe**
- **S99.21 Salter-Harris Type I physeal fracture of phalanx of toe**
  - **S99.211 Salter-Harris Type I physeal fracture of phalanx of right toe**
  - **S99.212 Salter-Harris Type I physeal fracture of phalanx of left toe**
  - **S99.219 Salter-Harris Type I physeal fracture of phalanx of unspecified toe**
- **S99.22 Salter-Harris Type II physeal fracture of phalanx of toe**
  - **S99.221 Salter-Harris Type II physeal fracture of phalanx of right toe**
  - **S99.222 Salter-Harris Type II physeal fracture of phalanx of left toe**
  - **S99.229 Salter-Harris Type II physeal fracture of phalanx of unspecified toe**

● S99.23 Salter-Harris Type III physeal fracture of phalanx of toe ◀
- ● S99.231 Salter-Harris Type III physeal fracture of phalanx of right toe ◀
- ● S99.232 Salter-Harris Type III physeal fracture of phalanx of left toe ◀
- ● S99.239 Salter-Harris Type III physeal fracture of phalanx of unspecified toe ◀

● S99.24 Salter-Harris Type IV physeal fracture of phalanx of toe ◀
- ● S99.241 Salter-Harris Type IV physeal fracture of phalanx of right toe ◀
- ● S99.242 Salter-Harris Type IV physeal fracture of phalanx of left toe ◀
- ● S99.249 Salter-Harris Type IV physeal fracture of phalanx of unspecified toe ◀

● S99.29 Other physeal fracture of phalanx of toe ◀
- ● S99.291 Other physeal fracture of phalanx of right toe ◀
- ● S99.292 Other physeal fracture of phalanx of left toe ◀
- ● S99.299 Other physeal fracture of phalanx of unspecified toe ◀

● S99.8 Other specified injuries of ankle and foot

The appropriate 7th character is to be added to each code from subcategory S99.8 ◀

A	initial encounter ◀
D	subsequent encounter ◀
S	sequela ◀

● S99.81 Other specified injuries of ankle
- ● S99.811 Other specified injuries of right ankle
- ● S99.812 Other specified injuries of left ankle
- ● S99.819 Other specified injuries of unspecified ankle

● S99.82 Other specified injuries of foot
- ● S99.821 Other specified injuries of right foot
- ● S99.822 Other specified injuries of left foot
- ● S99.829 Other specified injuries of unspecified foot

● S99.9 Unspecified injury of ankle and foot

The appropriate 7th character is to be added to each code from subcategory S99.9 ◀

A	initial encounter ◀
D	subsequent encounter ◀
S	sequela ◀

● S99.91 Unspecified injury of ankle
- ● S99.911 Unspecified injury of right ankle
- ● S99.912 Unspecified injury of left ankle
- ● S99.919 Unspecified injury of unspecified ankle

● S99.92 Unspecified injury of foot
- ● S99.921 Unspecified injury of right foot
- ● S99.922 Unspecified injury of left foot
- ● S99.929 Unspecified injury of unspecified foot

INJURY, POISONING AND CERTAIN OTHER CONSEQUENCES OF EXTERNAL CAUSES (T07-T88)

INJURIES INVOLVING MULTIPLE BODY REGIONS (T07)

Excludes1 burns and corrosions (T20-T32)
frostbite (T33-T34)
insect bite or sting, venomous (T63.4)
sunburn (L55.-)

T07 Unspecified multiple injuries

Excludes1 injury NOS (T14)

INJURY OF UNSPECIFIED BODY REGION (T14)

● T14 Injury of unspecified body region

Excludes1 multiple unspecified injuries (T07)

T14.8 Other injury of unspecified body region

Abrasion NOS	Fracture NOS
Contusion NOS	Skin injury NOS
Crush injury NOS	Vascular injury NOS

● T14.9 Unspecified injury

T14.90 Injury, unspecified
Injury NOS

T14.91 Suicide attempt
Attempted suicide NOS

EFFECTS OF FOREIGN BODY ENTERING THROUGH NATURAL ORIFICE (T15-T19)

Excludes2 foreign body accidentally left in operation wound (T81.5-)
foreign body in penetrating wound - see open wound by body region
residual foreign body in soft tissue (M79.5)
splinter, without open wound - see superficial injury by body region

● T15 Foreign body on external eye

Excludes2 foreign body in penetrating wound of orbit and eye ball (S05.4-, S05.5-)
open wound of eyelid and periocular area (S01.1-)
retained foreign body in eyelid (H02.8-)
retained (old) foreign body in penetrating wound of orbit and eye ball (H05.5-, H44.6-, H44.7-)
superficial foreign body of eyelid and periocular area (S00.25-)

The appropriate 7th character is to be added to each code from category T15

A	initial encounter
D	subsequent encounter
S	sequela

● T15.0 Foreign body in cornea
- X ● T15.00 Foreign body in cornea, unspecified eye
- X ● T15.01 Foreign body in cornea, right eye
- X ● T15.02 Foreign body in cornea, left eye

● T15.1 Foreign body in conjunctival sac
- X ● T15.10 Foreign body in conjunctival sac, unspecified eye
- X ● T15.11 Foreign body in conjunctival sac, right eye
- X ● T15.12 Foreign body in conjunctival sac, left eye

● T15.8 Foreign body in other and multiple parts of external eye
Foreign body in lacrimal punctum
- X ● T15.80 Foreign body in other and multiple parts of external eye, unspecified eye
- X ● T15.81 Foreign body in other and multiple parts of external eye, right eye
- X ● T15.82 Foreign body in other and multiple parts of external eye, left eye

- **T15.9 Foreign body on external eye, part unspecified**
  - X **T15.90 Foreign body on external eye, part unspecified, unspecified eye**
  - X **T15.91 Foreign body on external eye, part unspecified, right eye**
  - X **T15.92 Foreign body on external eye, part unspecified, left eye**

- **T16 Foreign body in ear**

  Includes foreign body in auditory canal

  The appropriate 7th character is to be added to each code from category T16

A	initial encounter
D	subsequent encounter
S	sequela

  - X **T16.1 Foreign body in right ear**
  - X **T16.2 Foreign body in left ear**
  - X **T16.9 Foreign body in ear, unspecified ear**

- **T17 Foreign body in respiratory tract**

  The appropriate 7th character is to be added to each code from category T17

A	initial encounter
D	subsequent encounter
S	sequela

  - X **T17.0 Foreign body in nasal sinus**
  - X **T17.1 Foreign body in nostril**
    Foreign body in nose NOS
  - **T17.2 Foreign body in pharynx**
    Foreign body in nasopharynx
    Foreign body in throat NOS
    - **T17.20 Unspecified foreign body in pharynx**
      - **T17.200 Unspecified foreign body in pharynx causing asphyxiation**
      - **T17.208 Unspecified foreign body in pharynx causing other injury**
    - **T17.21 Gastric contents in pharynx**
      Aspiration of gastric contents into pharynx
      Vomitus in pharynx
      - **T17.210 Gastric contents in pharynx causing asphyxiation**
      - **T17.218 Gastric contents in pharynx causing other injury**
    - **T17.22 Food in pharynx**
      Bones in pharynx
      Seeds in pharynx
      - **T17.220 Food in pharynx causing asphyxiation**
      - **T17.228 Food in pharynx causing other injury**
    - **T17.29 Other foreign object in pharynx**
      - **T17.290 Other foreign object in pharynx causing asphyxiation**
      - **T17.298 Other foreign object in pharynx causing other injury**
  - **T17.3 Foreign body in larynx**
    - **T17.30 Unspecified foreign body in larynx**
      - **T17.300 Unspecified foreign body in larynx causing asphyxiation**
      - **T17.308 Unspecified foreign body in larynx causing other injury**
    - **T17.31 Gastric contents in larynx**
      Aspiration of gastric contents into larynx
      Vomitus in larynx
      - **T17.310 Gastric contents in larynx causing asphyxiation**
      - **T17.318 Gastric contents in larynx causing other injury**
    - **T17.32 Food in larynx**
      Bones in larynx
      Seeds in larynx
      - **T17.320 Food in larynx causing asphyxiation**
      - **T17.328 Food in larynx causing other injury**
    - **T17.39 Other foreign object in larynx**
      - **T17.390 Other foreign object in larynx causing asphyxiation**
      - **T17.398 Other foreign object in larynx causing other injury**
  - **T17.4 Foreign body in trachea**
    Ex For category T17.4 CC codes: T17.400-T17.498[A]
    - **T17.40 Unspecified foreign body in trachea**
      - **T17.400 Unspecified foreign body in trachea causing asphyxiation** A
      - **T17.408 Unspecified foreign body in trachea causing other injury** A
    - **T17.41 Gastric contents in trachea**
      Aspiration of gastric contents into trachea
      Vomitus in trachea
      - **T17.410 Gastric contents in trachea causing asphyxiation** A
      - **T17.418 Gastric contents in trachea causing other injury** A
    - **T17.42 Food in trachea**
      Bones in trachea
      Seeds in trachea
      - **T17.420 Food in trachea causing asphyxiation** A
      - **T17.428 Food in trachea causing other injury** A
    - **T17.49 Other foreign object in trachea**
      - **T17.490 Other foreign object in trachea causing asphyxiation** A
      - **T17.498 Other foreign object in trachea causing other injury** A
  - **T17.5 Foreign body in bronchus**
    Ex For category T17.5 CC codes: T17.400-T17.998[A]
    - **T17.50 Unspecified foreign body in bronchus**
      - **T17.500 Unspecified foreign body in bronchus causing asphyxiation** A
      - **T17.508 Unspecified foreign body in bronchus causing other injury** A
    - **T17.51 Gastric contents in bronchus**
      Aspiration of gastric contents into bronchus
      Vomitus in bronchus
      - **T17.510 Gastric contents in bronchus causing asphyxiation** A
      - **T17.518 Gastric contents in bronchus causing other injury** A
    - **T17.52 Food in bronchus**
      Bones in bronchus
      Seeds in bronchus
      - **T17.520 Food in bronchus causing asphyxiation** A
      - **T17.528 Food in bronchus causing other injury** A
    - **T17.59 Other foreign object in bronchus**
      - **T17.590 Other foreign object in bronchus causing asphyxiation** A
      - **T17.598 Other foreign object in bronchus causing other injury** A

● **T17.8 Foreign body in other parts of respiratory tract**
Foreign body in bronchioles
Foreign body in lung
Ex: For category T17.8 CC codes: T17.400-T17.998[A]

● **T17.80 Unspecified foreign body in other parts of respiratory tract**

● **T17.800 Unspecified foreign body in other parts of respiratory tract causing asphyxiation** A

● **T17.808 Unspecified foreign body in other parts of respiratory tract causing other injury** A

● **T17.81 Gastric contents in other parts of respiratory tract**
Aspiration of gastric contents into other parts of respiratory tract
Vomitus in other parts of respiratory tract

● **T17.810 Gastric contents in other parts of respiratory tract causing asphyxiation** A

● **T17.818 Gastric contents in other parts of respiratory tract causing other injury** A

● **T17.82 Food in other parts of respiratory tract**
Bones in other parts of respiratory tract
Seeds in other parts of respiratory tract

● **T17.820 Food in other parts of respiratory tract causing asphyxiation** A

● **T17.828 Food in other parts of respiratory tract causing other injury** A

● **T17.89 Other foreign object in other parts of respiratory tract**

● **T17.890 Other foreign object in other parts of respiratory tract causing asphyxiation** A

● **T17.898 Other foreign object in other parts of respiratory tract causing other injury** A

● **T17.9 Foreign body in respiratory tract, part unspecified**

● **T17.90 Unspecified foreign body in respiratory tract, part unspecified**

● **T17.900 Unspecified foreign body in respiratory tract, part unspecified causing asphyxiation**

● **T17.908 Unspecified foreign body in respiratory tract, part unspecified causing other injury**

● **T17.91 Gastric contents in respiratory tract, part unspecified**
Aspiration of gastric contents into respiratory tract, part unspecified
Vomitus in trachea respiratory tract, part unspecified

● **T17.910 Gastric contents in respiratory tract, part unspecified causing asphyxiation**

● **T17.918 Gastric contents in respiratory tract, part unspecified causing other injury**

● **T17.92 Food in respiratory tract, part unspecified**
Bones in respiratory tract, part unspecified
Seeds in respiratory tract, part unspecified

● **T17.920 Food in respiratory tract, part unspecified causing asphyxiation**

● **T17.928 Food in respiratory tract, part unspecified causing other injury**

● **T17.99 Other foreign object in respiratory tract, part unspecified**

● **T17.990 Other foreign object in respiratory tract, part unspecified in causing asphyxiation**

● **T17.998 Other foreign object in respiratory tract, part unspecified causing other injury**

● **T18 Foreign body in alimentary tract**
Excludes2 foreign body in pharynx (T17.2-)
The appropriate 7th character is to be added to each code from category T18

A	initial encounter
D	subsequent encounter
S	sequela

X● **T18.0 Foreign body in mouth**

X● **T18.1 Foreign body in esophagus**
Excludes2 foreign body in respiratory tract (T17.-)

● **T18.10 Unspecified foreign body in esophagus**

● **T18.100 Unspecified foreign body in esophagus causing compression of trachea**
Unspecified foreign body in esophagus causing obstruction of respiration

● **T18.108 Unspecified foreign body in esophagus causing other injury**

● **T18.11 Gastric contents in esophagus**
Vomitus in esophagus

● **T18.110 Gastric contents in esophagus causing compression of trachea**
Gastric contents in esophagus causing obstruction of respiration

● **T18.118 Gastric contents in esophagus causing other injury**

● **T18.12 Food in esophagus**
Bones in esophagus
Seeds in esophagus

● **T18.120 Food in esophagus causing compression of trachea**
Food in esophagus causing obstruction of respiration

● **T18.128 Food in esophagus causing other injury**

● **T18.19 Other foreign object in esophagus**

● **T18.190 Other foreign object in esophagus causing compression of trachea**
Other foreign body in esophagus causing obstruction of respiration
Coding Clinic: 2015, Q1, P24

● **T18.198 Other foreign object in esophagus causing other injury**
Coding Clinic: 2015, Q1, P24

X● **T18.2 Foreign body in stomach**

X● **T18.3 Foreign body in small intestine**

X● **T18.4 Foreign body in colon**

X● **T18.5 Foreign body in anus and rectum**
Foreign body in rectosigmoid (junction)

X● **T18.8 Foreign body in other parts of alimentary tract**

X● **T18.9 Foreign body of alimentary tract, part unspecified**
Foreign body in digestive system NOS
Swallowed foreign body NOS

T19 Foreign body in genitourinary tract

Excludes2 complications due to implanted mesh (T83.7-)
mechanical complications of contraceptive device (intrauterine) (vaginal) (T83.3-)
presence of contraceptive device (intrauterine) (vaginal) (Z97.5)

The appropriate 7th character is to be added to each code from category T19

A	initial encounter
D	subsequent encounter
S	sequela

X **T19.0 Foreign body in urethra**
X **T19.1 Foreign body in bladder**
X **T19.2 Foreign body in vulva and vagina ♀**
X **T19.3 Foreign body in uterus ♀**
X **T19.4 Foreign body in penis ♂**
X **T19.8 Foreign body in other parts of genitourinary tract**
X **T19.9 Foreign body in genitourinary tract, part unspecified**

BURNS AND CORROSIONS (T20-T32)

Includes burns (thermal) from electrical heating appliances
burns (thermal) from electricity
burns (thermal) from flame
burns (thermal) from friction
burns (thermal) from hot air and hot gases
burns (thermal) from hot objects
burns (thermal) from lightning
burns (thermal) from radiation chemical
burn [corrosion] (external) (internal) scalds

Excludes2 erythema [dermatitis] ab igne (L59.0)
radiation-related disorders of the skin and subcutaneous tissue (L55-L59)
sunburn (L55.-)

OGCR Section I.C.19.d.

Burns and Corrosions

The ICD-10-CM makes a distinction between burn and corrosions. The burn codes are for thermal burns, except sunburns, that come from a heat source, such as a fire or hot appliance. The burn codes are also for burns resulting from electricity and radiation. Corrosions are burns due to chemicals. The guidelines for burns and corrosions are the same.

Current burns (T20-T25) are classified by depth, extent and by agent (X code). Burns are classified by depth as first degree (erythema), second degree (blistering), and third degree (full-thickness involvement). Burns of the eye and internal organs (T26-T28) are classified by site, but not by degree.

1) Sequencing of burn and related condition codes

Sequence first the code that reflects the highest degree of burn when more than one burn is present.

a. When the reason for the admission or encounter is for treatment of external multiple burns, sequence first the code that reflects the burn of the highest degree.

b. When a patient has both internal and external burns, the circumstances of admission govern the selection of the principal diagnosis or first-listed diagnosis.

c. When a patient is admitted for burn injuries and other related conditions such as smoke inhalation and/or respiratory failure, the circumstances of admission govern the selection of the principal or first-listed diagnosis.

2) Burns of the same local site

Classify burns of the same local site (three-character category level, T20-T28) but of different degrees to the subcategory identifying the highest degree recorded in the diagnosis.

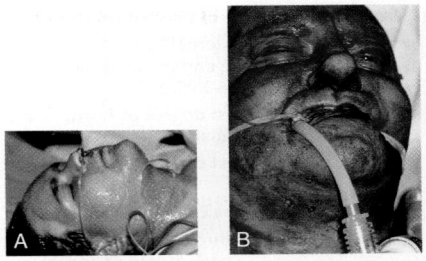

Figure 19-15 **A.** Second-degree burn. **B.** Third-degree burn. (From Cummings: Otolaryngology: Head & Neck Surgery, ed 4, Mosby, 2005)

BURNS AND CORROSIONS OF EXTERNAL BODY SURFACE, SPECIFIED BY SITE (T20-T25)

Includes burns and corrosions of first degree [erythema]
burns and corrosions of second degree [blisters] [epidermal loss]
burns and corrosions of third degree [deep necrosis of underlying tissue] [full-thickness skin loss]

Use additional code from category T31 or T32 to identify extent of body surface involved

T20 Burn and corrosion of head, face, and neck

Excludes2 burn and corrosion of ear drum (T28.41, T28.91)
burn and corrosion of eye and adnexa (T26.-)
burn and corrosion of mouth and pharynx (T28.0)

The appropriate 7th character is to be added to each code from category T20

A	initial encounter
D	subsequent encounter
S	sequela

T20.0 Burn of unspecified degree of head, face, and neck

Use additional external cause code to identify the source, place and intent of the burn (X00-X19, X75-X77, X96-X98, Y92)

X **T20.00 Burn of unspecified degree of head, face, and neck, unspecified site**

T20.01 Burn of unspecified degree of ear [any part, except ear drum]

Excludes2 burn of ear drum (T28.41-)

T20.011 Burn of unspecified degree of right ear [any part, except ear drum]

T20.012 Burn of unspecified degree of left ear [any part, except ear drum]

T20.019 Burn of unspecified degree of unspecified ear [any part, except ear drum]

X **T20.02 Burn of unspecified degree of lip(s)**
X **T20.03 Burn of unspecified degree of chin**
X **T20.04 Burn of unspecified degree of nose (septum)**
X **T20.05 Burn of unspecified degree of scalp [any part]**
X **T20.06 Burn of unspecified degree of forehead and cheek**
X **T20.07 Burn of unspecified degree of neck**
X **T20.09 Burn of unspecified degree of multiple sites of head, face, and neck**

CHAPTER 19 (S00-T88)

● **T20.1 Burn of first degree of head, face, and neck**

Use additional external cause code to identify the source, place and intent of the burn (X00-X19, X75-X77, X96-X98, Y92)

X● **T20.10 Burn of first degree of head, face, and neck, unspecified site**

● **T20.11 Burn of first degree of ear [any part, except ear drum]**

Excludes2 burn of ear drum (T28.41-)

● **T20.111 Burn of first degree of right ear [any part, except ear drum]**

● **T20.112 Burn of first degree of left ear [any part, except ear drum]**

● **T20.119 Burn of first degree of unspecified ear [any part, except ear drum]**

X● **T20.12 Burn of first degree of lip(s)**

X● **T20.13 Burn of first degree of chin**

X● **T20.14 Burn of first degree of nose (septum)**

X● **T20.15 Burn of first degree of scalp [any part]**

X● **T20.16 Burn of first degree of forehead and cheek**

X● **T20.17 Burn of first degree of neck**

X● **T20.19 Burn of first degree of multiple sites of head, face, and neck**

● **T20.2 Burn of second degree of head, face, and neck**

Use additional external cause code to identify the source, place and intent of the burn (X00-X19, X75-X77, X96-X98, Y92)

X● **T20.20 Burn of second degree of head, face, and neck, unspecified site**

● **T20.21 Burn of second degree of ear [any part, except ear drum]**

Excludes2 burn of ear drum (T28.41-)

● **T20.211 Burn of second degree of right ear [any part, except ear drum]**

● **T20.212 Burn of second degree of left ear [any part, except ear drum]**

● **T20.219 Burn of second degree of unspecified ear [any part, except ear drum]**

X● **T20.22 Burn of second degree of lip(s)**

X● **T20.23 Burn of second degree of chin**

X● **T20.24 Burn of second degree of nose (septum)**

X● **T20.25 Burn of second degree of scalp [any part]**

Coding Clinic: 2015, Q1, P19

X● **T20.26 Burn of second degree of forehead and cheek**

X● **T20.27 Burn of second degree of neck**

X● **T20.29 Burn of second degree of multiple sites of head, face, and neck**

● **T20.3 Burn of third degree of head, face, and neck**

Use additional external cause code to identify the source, place and intent of the burn (X00-X19, X75-X77, X96-X98, Y92)

X● **T20.30 Burn of third degree of head, face, and neck, unspecified site** A, A

Ex: T20.30X[A], T20.39X[A], T20.70X[A], T20.79X[A]

● **T20.31 Burn of third degree of ear [any part, except ear drum]**

Excludes2 burn of ear drum (T28.41-)

Ex: **For category T20.31 CC codes:** T20.311-T20.319[A], T20.39X[A], T20.711-T20.719[A], T20.79X[A]

● **T20.311 Burn of third degree of right ear [any part, except ear drum]** A, A

● **T20.312 Burn of third degree of left ear [any part, except ear drum]** A, A

Coding Clinic: 2015, Q1, P18

● **T20.319 Burn of third degree of unspecified ear [any part, except ear drum]** A, A

X● **T20.32 Burn of third degree of lip(s)** A, A

Ex: T20.32X[A], T20.39X[A], T20.72X[A], T20.79X[A]

X● **T20.33 Burn of third degree of chin** A, A

Ex: T20.33X[A], T20.39X[A], T20.73X[A], T20.79X[A]

X● **T20.34 Burn of third degree of nose (septum)** A, A

Ex: T20.34X[A], T20.39X[A], T20.74X[A], T20.79X[A]

X● **T20.35 Burn of third degree of scalp [any part]** A, A

Ex: T20.35X[A], T20.39X[A], T20.75X[A], T20.79X[A]

X● **T20.36 Burn of third degree of forehead and cheek** A, A

Ex: T20.36X[A], T20.39X[A], T20.76X[A], T20.79X[A]

X● **T20.37 Burn of third degree of neck** A, A

Ex: T20.37X-T20.39X[A], T20.77X-T20.79X[A]

X● **T20.39 Burn of third degree of multiple sites of head, face, and neck** A, A

Ex: T20.30X-T20.39X[A], T20.70X-T20.79X[A]

● **T20.4 Corrosion of unspecified degree of head, face, and neck**

Code first (T51-T65) to identify chemical and intent

Use additional external cause code to identify place (Y92)

X● **T20.40 Corrosion of unspecified degree of head, face, and neck, unspecified site**

● **T20.41 Corrosion of unspecified degree of ear [any part, except ear drum]**

Excludes2 corrosion of ear drum (T28.91-)

● **T20.411 Corrosion of unspecified degree of right ear [any part, except ear drum]**

● **T20.412 Corrosion of unspecified degree of left ear [any part, except ear drum]**

● **T20.419 Corrosion of unspecified degree of unspecified ear [any part, except ear drum]**

X● **T20.42 Corrosion of unspecified degree of lip(s)**

X● **T20.43 Corrosion of unspecified degree of chin**

X● **T20.44 Corrosion of unspecified degree of nose (septum)**

X● **T20.45 Corrosion of unspecified degree of scalp [any part]**

X● **T20.46 Corrosion of unspecified degree of forehead and cheek**

X● **T20.47 Corrosion of unspecified degree of neck**

X● **T20.49 Corrosion of unspecified degree of multiple sites of head, face, and neck**

● **T20.5 Corrosion of first degree of head, face, and neck**

Code first (T51-T65) to identify chemical and intent

Use additional external cause code to identify place (Y92)

X● **T20.50 Corrosion of first degree of head, face, and neck, unspecified site**

● **T20.51 Corrosion of first degree of ear [any part, except ear drum]**

Excludes2 corrosion of ear drum (T28.91-)

● **T20.511 Corrosion of first degree of right ear [any part, except ear drum]**

● **T20.512 Corrosion of first degree of left ear [any part, except ear drum]**

● **T20.519 Corrosion of first degree of unspecified ear [any part, except ear drum]**

X● **T20.52 Corrosion of first degree of lip(s)**

X● **T20.53 Corrosion of first degree of chin**

X● **T20.54 Corrosion of first degree of nose (septum)**

X● **T20.55 Corrosion of first degree of scalp [any part]**

X● **T20.56 Corrosion of first degree of forehead and cheek**

X● **T20.57 Corrosion of first degree of neck**

X● **T20.59 Corrosion of first degree of multiple sites of head, face, and neck**

T20.6 Corrosion of second degree of head, face, and neck
Code first (T51-T65) to identify chemical and intent
Use additional external cause code to identify place (Y92)

X **T20.60 Corrosion of second degree of head, face, and neck, unspecified site**

T20.61 Corrosion of second degree of ear [any part, except ear drum]
Excludes2 corrosion of ear drum (T28.91-)

T20.611 Corrosion of second degree of right ear [any part, except ear drum]

T20.612 Corrosion of second degree of left ear [any part, except ear drum]

T20.619 Corrosion of second degree of unspecified ear [any part, except ear drum]

X **T20.62 Corrosion of second degree of lip(s)**
X **T20.63 Corrosion of second degree of chin**
X **T20.64 Corrosion of second degree of nose (septum)**
X **T20.65 Corrosion of second degree of scalp [any part]**
X **T20.66 Corrosion of second degree of forehead and cheek**
X **T20.67 Corrosion of second degree of neck**
X **T20.69 Corrosion of second degree of multiple sites of head, face, and neck**

T20.7 Corrosion of third degree of head, face, and neck
Code first (T51-T65) to identify chemical and intent
Use additional external cause code to identify place (Y92)

X **T20.70 Corrosion of third degree of head, face, and neck, unspecified site** A CC, A MCC
Ex: See T20.30

T20.71 Corrosion of third degree of ear [any part, except ear drum]
Excludes2 corrosion of ear drum (T28.91-)
Ex: **For category T20.71 CC codes:** See T20.31

T20.711 Corrosion of third degree of right ear [any part, except ear drum] A CC, A MCC

T20.712 Corrosion of third degree of left ear [any part, except ear drum] A CC, A MCC

T20.719 Corrosion of third degree of unspecified ear [any part, except ear drum] A CC, A MCC

X **T20.72 Corrosion of third degree of lip(s)** A CC, A MCC
Ex: See T20.32

X **T20.73 Corrosion of third degree of chin** A CC, A MCC
Ex: See T20.33

X **T20.74 Corrosion of third degree of nose (septum)** A CC, A MCC
Ex: See T20.34

X **T20.75 Corrosion of third degree of scalp [any part]** A CC, A MCC
Ex: See T20.35

X **T20.76 Corrosion of third degree of forehead and cheek** A CC, A MCC
Ex: See T20.36

X **T20.77 Corrosion of third degree of neck** A CC, A MCC
Ex: See T20.37

X **T20.79 Corrosion of third degree of multiple sites of head, face, and neck** A CC, A MCC
Ex: See T20.39

T21 Burn and corrosion of trunk
Includes burns and corrosion of hip region
Excludes2 burns and corrosion of axilla (T22.- with fifth character 4)
burns and corrosion of scapular region (T22.- with fifth character 6)
burns and corrosion of shoulder (T22.- with fifth character 5)

The appropriate 7th character is to be added to each code from category T21

A	initial encounter
D	subsequent encounter
S	sequela

T21.0 Burn of unspecified degree of trunk
Use additional external cause code to identify the source, place and intent of the burn (X00-X19, X75-X77, X96-X98, Y92)

X **T21.00 Burn of unspecified degree of trunk, unspecified site**

X **T21.01 Burn of unspecified degree of chest wall**
Burn of of unspecified degree of breast

X **T21.02 Burn of unspecified degree of abdominal wall**
Burn of unspecified degree of flank
Burn of unspecified degree of groin

X **T21.03 Burn of unspecified degree of upper back**
Burn of unspecified degree of interscapular region

X **T21.04 Burn of unspecified degree of lower back**

X **T21.05 Burn of unspecified degree of buttock**
Burn of unspecified degree of anus

X **T21.06 Burn of unspecified degree of male genital region** ♂
Burn of unspecified degree of penis
Burn of unspecified degree of scrotum
Burn of unspecified degree of testis

X **T21.07 Burn of unspecified degree of female genital region** ♀
Burn of unspecified degree of labium (majus) (minus)
Burn of unspecified degree of perineum
Burn of unspecified degree of vulva
Excludes2 burn of vagina (T28.3)

X **T21.09 Burn of unspecified degree of other site of trunk**

T21.1 Burn of first degree of trunk
Use additional external cause code to identify the source, place and intent of the burn (X00-X19, X75-X77, X96-X98, Y92)

X **T21.10 Burn of first degree of trunk, unspecified site**

X **T21.11 Burn of first degree of chest wall**
Burn of first degree of breast

X **T21.12 Burn of first degree of abdominal wall**
Burn of first degree of flank
Burn of first degree of groin

X **T21.13 Burn of first degree of upper back**
Burn of first degree of interscapular region

X **T21.14 Burn of first degree of lower back**

X **T21.15 Burn of first degree of buttock**
Burn of first degree of anus

X **T21.16 Burn of first degree of male genital region** ♂
Burn of first degree of penis
Burn of first degree of scrotum
Burn of first degree of testis

X● **T21.17 Burn of first degree of female genital region ♀**
Burn of first degree of labium (majus) (minus)
Burn of first degree of perineum
Burn of first degree of vulva
Excludes2 burn of vagina (T28.3)

X● **T21.19 Burn of first degree of other site of trunk**

● **T21.2 Burn of second degree of trunk**
Use additional external cause code to identify the source, place and intent of the burn (X00-X19, X75-X77, X96-X98, Y92)

X● **T21.20 Burn of second degree of trunk, unspecified site**

X● **T21.21 Burn of second degree of chest wall**
Burn of second degree of breast

X● **T21.22 Burn of second degree of abdominal wall**
Burn of second degree of flank
Burn of second degree of groin

X● **T21.23 Burn of second degree of upper back**
Burn of second degree of interscapular region

X● **T21.24 Burn of second degree of lower back**

X● **T21.25 Burn of second degree of buttock**
Burn of second degree of anus

X● **T21.26 Burn of second degree of male genital region ♂**
Burn of second degree of penis
Burn of second degree of scrotum
Burn of second degree of testis

X● **T21.27 Burn of second degree of female genital region ♀**
Burn of second degree of labium (majus) (minus)
Burn of second degree of perineum
Burn of second degree of vulva
Excludes2 burn of vagina (T28.3)

X● **T21.29 Burn of second degree of other site of trunk**

● **T21.3 Burn of third degree of trunk**
Use additional external cause code to identify the source, place and intent of the burn (X00-X19, X75-X77, X96-X98, Y92)

X● **T21.30 Burn of third degree of trunk, unspecified site** A CC, A Unc
Ex: T21.30X[A], T21.39X[A], T21.70X[A], T21.79X[A]

X● **T21.31 Burn of third degree of chest wall** A CC, A Unc
Burn of third degree of breast
Ex: T21.30X-T21.31X[A], T21.39X[A], T21.70X-T21.71X[A], T21.79X[A]
Coding Clinic: 2016, Q2, P6

X● **T21.32 Burn of third degree of abdominal wall** A CC, A Unc
Burn of third degree of flank
Burn of third degree of groin
Ex: T21.30X[A], T21.32X[A], T21.39X[A], T21.70X[A], T21.72X[A], T21.79X[A]

X● **T21.33 Burn of third degree of upper back** A CC, A Unc
Burn of third degree of interscapular region
Ex: T21.30X[A], T21.33X-T21.35X[A], T21.39X[A], T21.70X[A], T21.73X-T21.75X[A], T21.79X[A]

X● **T21.34 Burn of third degree of lower back** A CC, A Unc
Ex: See T21.33

X● **T21.35 Burn of third degree of buttock** A CC, A Unc
Burn of third degree of anus
Ex: See T21.33

X● **T21.36 Burn of third degree of male genital region ♂** A CC, A Unc
Burn of third degree of penis
Burn of third degree of scrotum
Burn of third degree of testis
Ex: T21.30X[A], T21.36X-T21.39X[A], T21.70X[A], T21.76X-T21.79X[A]

X● **T21.37 Burn of third degree of female genital region ♀** A CC, A Unc
Burn of third degree of labium (majus) (minus)
Burn of third degree of perineum
Burn of third degree of vulva
Excludes2 burn of vagina (T28.3)
Ex: See T21.36

X● **T21.39 Burn of third degree of other site of trunk** A CC, A Unc
Ex: See T21.30

● **T21.4 Corrosion of unspecified degree of trunk**
Code first (T51-T65) to identify chemical and intent
Use additional external cause code to identify place (Y92)

X● **T21.40 Corrosion of unspecified degree of trunk, unspecified site**

X● **T21.41 Corrosion of unspecified degree of chest wall**
Corrosion of unspecified degree of breast

X● **T21.42 Corrosion of unspecified degree of abdominal wall**
Corrosion of unspecified degree of flank
Corrosion of unspecified degree of groin

X● **T21.43 Corrosion of unspecified degree of upper back**
Corrosion of unspecified degree of interscapular region

X● **T21.44 Corrosion of unspecified degree of lower back**

X● **T21.45 Corrosion of unspecified degree of buttock**
Corrosion of unspecified degree of anus

X● **T21.46 Corrosion of unspecified degree of male genital region ♂**
Corrosion of unspecified degree of penis
Corrosion of unspecified degree of scrotum
Corrosion of unspecified degree of testis

X● **T21.47 Corrosion of unspecified degree of female genital region ♀**
Corrosion of unspecified degree of labium (majus) (minus)
Corrosion of unspecified degree of perineum
Corrosion of unspecified degree of vulva
Excludes2 corrosion of vagina (T28.8)

X● **T21.49 Corrosion of unspecified degree of other site of trunk**

● **T21.5 Corrosion of first degree of trunk**
Code first (T51-T65) to identify chemical and intent
Use additional external cause code to identify place (Y92)

X● **T21.50 Corrosion of first degree of trunk, unspecified site**

X● **T21.51 Corrosion of first degree of chest wall**
Corrosion of first degree of breast

X● **T21.52 Corrosion of first degree of abdominal wall**
Corrosion of first degree of flank
Corrosion of first degree of groin

X● **T21.53 Corrosion of first degree of upper back**
Corrosion of first degree of interscapular region

X● **T21.54 Corrosion of first degree of lower back**

X● **T21.55 Corrosion of first degree of buttock**
Corrosion of first degree of anus

X● **T21.56 Corrosion of first degree of male genital region ♂**
Corrosion of first degree of penis
Corrosion of first degree of scrotum
Corrosion of first degree of testis

X● **T21.57 Corrosion of first degree of female genital region ♀**
Corrosion of first degree of labium (majus) (minus)
Corrosion of first degree of perineum
Corrosion of first degree of vulva
Excludes2 corrosion of vagina (T28.8)

X● **T21.59 Corrosion of first degree of other site of trunk**

● **T21.6 Corrosion of second degree of trunk**
Code first (T51-T65) to identify chemical and intent
Use additional external cause code to identify place (Y92)

X● **T21.60 Corrosion of second degree of trunk, unspecified site**

X● **T21.61 Corrosion of second degree of chest wall**
Corrosion of second degree of breast

X● **T21.62 Corrosion of second degree of abdominal wall**
Corrosion of second degree of flank
Corrosion of second degree of groin

X● **T21.63 Corrosion of second degree of upper back**
Corrosion of second degree of interscapular region

X● **T21.64 Corrosion of second degree of lower back**

X● **T21.65 Corrosion of second degree of buttock**
Corrosion of second degree of anus

X● **T21.66 Corrosion of second degree of male genital region ♂**
Corrosion of second degree of penis
Corrosion of second degree of scrotum
Corrosion of second degree of testis

X● **T21.67 Corrosion of second degree of female genital region ♀**
Corrosion of second degree of labium (majus) (minus)
Corrosion of second degree of perineum
Corrosion of second degree of vulva
Excludes2 corrosion of vagina (T28.8)

X● **T21.69 Corrosion of second degree of other site of trunk**

● **T21.7 Corrosion of third degree of trunk**
Code first (T51-T65) to identify chemical and intent
Use additional external cause code to identify place (Y92)

X● **T21.70 Corrosion of third degree of trunk, unspecified site** A CC, A MCC
Ex: See T21.30

X● **T21.71 Corrosion of third degree of chest wall** A CC, A MCC
Corrosion of third degree of breast
Ex: See T21.31

X● **T21.72 Corrosion of third degree of abdominal wall** A CC, A MCC
Corrosion of third degree of flank
Corrosion of third degree of groin
Ex: See T21.32

X● **T21.73 Corrosion of third degree of upper back** A CC, A MCC
Corrosion of third degree of interscapular region
Ex: See T21.33

X● **T21.74 Corrosion of third degree of lower back** A CC, A MCC
Ex: See T21.33

X● **T21.75 Corrosion of third degree of buttock** A CC, A MCC
Corrosion of third degree of anus
Ex: See T21.33

X● **T21.76 Corrosion of third degree of male genital region ♂** A CC, A MCC
Corrosion of third degree of penis
Corrosion of third degree of scrotum
Corrosion of third degree of testis
Ex: See T21.36

X● **T21.77 Corrosion of third degree of female genital region ♀** A CC, A MCC
Corrosion of third degree of labium (majus) (minus)
Corrosion of third degree of perineum
Corrosion of third degree of vulva
Excludes2 corrosion of vagina (T28.8)
Ex: See T21.36

X● **T21.79 Corrosion of third degree of other site of trunk** A CC, A MCC
Ex: See T21.30

● **T22 Burn and corrosion of shoulder and upper limb, except wrist and hand**
Excludes2 burn and corrosion of interscapular region (T21.-)
burn and corrosion of wrist and hand (T23.-)
The appropriate 7th character is to be added to each code from category T22

A	initial encounter
D	subsequent encounter
S	sequela

● **T22.0 Burn of unspecified degree of shoulder and upper limb, except wrist and hand**
Use additional external cause code to identify the source, place and intent of the burn (X00-X19, X75-X77, X96-X98, Y92)

X● **T22.00 Burn of unspecified degree of shoulder and upper limb, except wrist and hand, unspecified site**

● **T22.01 Burn of unspecified degree of forearm**
● **T22.011 Burn of unspecified degree of right forearm**
● **T22.012 Burn of unspecified degree of left forearm**
● **T22.019 Burn of unspecified degree of unspecified forearm**

● **T22.02 Burn of unspecified degree of elbow**
● **T22.021 Burn of unspecified degree of right elbow**
● **T22.022 Burn of unspecified degree of left elbow**
● **T22.029 Burn of unspecified degree of unspecified elbow**

● **T22.03 Burn of unspecified degree of upper arm**
● **T22.031 Burn of unspecified degree of right upper arm**
● **T22.032 Burn of unspecified degree of left upper arm**
● **T22.039 Burn of unspecified degree of unspecified upper arm**

● **T22.04 Burn of unspecified degree of axilla**
● **T22.041 Burn of unspecified degree of right axilla**
● **T22.042 Burn of unspecified degree of left axilla**
● **T22.049 Burn of unspecified degree of unspecified axilla**

- T22.05 Burn of unspecified degree of shoulder
  - T22.051 Burn of unspecified degree of right shoulder
  - T22.052 Burn of unspecified degree of left shoulder
  - T22.059 Burn of unspecified degree of unspecified shoulder
- T22.06 Burn of unspecified degree of scapular region
  - T22.061 Burn of unspecified degree of right scapular region
  - T22.062 Burn of unspecified degree of left scapular region
  - T22.069 Burn of unspecified degree of unspecified scapular region
- T22.09 Burn of unspecified degree of multiple sites of shoulder and upper limb, except wrist and hand
  - T22.091 Burn of unspecified degree of multiple sites of right shoulder and upper limb, except wrist and hand
  - T22.092 Burn of unspecified degree of multiple sites of left shoulder and upper limb, except wrist and hand
  - T22.099 Burn of unspecified degree of multiple sites of unspecified shoulder and upper limb, except wrist and hand

- T22.1 Burn of first degree of shoulder and upper limb, except wrist and hand

  Use additional external cause code to identify the source, place and intent of the burn (X00-X19, X75-X77, X96-X98, Y92)

  - X T22.10 Burn of first degree of shoulder and upper limb, except wrist and hand, unspecified site
  - T22.11 Burn of first degree of forearm
    - T22.111 Burn of first degree of right forearm
    - T22.112 Burn of first degree of left forearm
    - T22.119 Burn of first degree of unspecified forearm
  - T22.12 Burn of first degree of elbow
    - T22.121 Burn of first degree of right elbow
    - T22.122 Burn of first degree of left elbow
    - T22.129 Burn of first degree of unspecified elbow
  - T22.13 Burn of first degree of upper arm
    - T22.131 Burn of first degree of right upper arm
    - T22.132 Burn of first degree of left upper arm
    - T22.139 Burn of first degree of unspecified upper arm
  - T22.14 Burn of first degree of axilla
    - T22.141 Burn of first degree of right axilla
    - T22.142 Burn of first degree of left axilla
    - T22.149 Burn of first degree of unspecified axilla
  - T22.15 Burn of first degree of shoulder
    - T22.151 Burn of first degree of right shoulder
    - T22.152 Burn of first degree of left shoulder
    - T22.159 Burn of first degree of unspecified shoulder
  - T22.16 Burn of first degree of scapular region
    - T22.161 Burn of first degree of right scapular region
    - T22.162 Burn of first degree of left scapular region
    - T22.169 Burn of first degree of unspecified scapular region
  - T22.19 Burn of first degree of multiple sites of shoulder and upper limb, except wrist and hand
    - T22.191 Burn of first degree of multiple sites of right shoulder and upper limb, except wrist and hand
    - T22.192 Burn of first degree of multiple sites of left shoulder and upper limb, except wrist and hand
    - T22.199 Burn of first degree of multiple sites of unspecified shoulder and upper limb, except wrist and hand

- T22.2 Burn of second degree of shoulder and upper limb, except wrist and hand

  Use additional external cause code to identify the source, place and intent of the burn (X00-X19, X75-X77, X96-X98, Y92)

  - X T22.20 Burn of second degree of shoulder and upper limb, except wrist and hand, unspecified site
  - T22.21 Burn of second degree of forearm
    - T22.211 Burn of second degree of right forearm
    - T22.212 Burn of second degree of left forearm
    - T22.219 Burn of second degree of unspecified forearm
  - T22.22 Burn of second degree of elbow
    - T22.221 Burn of second degree of right elbow
    - T22.222 Burn of second degree of left elbow
    - T22.229 Burn of second degree of unspecified elbow
  - T22.23 Burn of second degree of upper arm
    - T22.231 Burn of second degree of right upper arm
    - T22.232 Burn of second degree of left upper arm
    - T22.239 Burn of second degree of unspecified upper arm
  - T22.24 Burn of second degree of axilla
    - T22.241 Burn of second degree of right axilla
    - T22.242 Burn of second degree of left axilla
    - T22.249 Burn of second degree of unspecified axilla
  - T22.25 Burn of second degree of shoulder
    - T22.251 Burn of second degree of right shoulder
    - T22.252 Burn of second degree of left shoulder
    - T22.259 Burn of second degree of unspecified shoulder
  - T22.26 Burn of second degree of scapular region
    - T22.261 Burn of second degree of right scapular region
    - T22.262 Burn of second degree of left scapular region
    - T22.269 Burn of second degree of unspecified scapular region
  - T22.29 Burn of second degree of multiple sites of shoulder and upper limb, except wrist and hand
    - T22.291 Burn of second degree of multiple sites of right shoulder and upper limb, except wrist and hand
    - T22.292 Burn of second degree of multiple sites of left shoulder and upper limb, except wrist and hand
    - T22.299 Burn of second degree of multiple sites of unspecified shoulder and upper limb, except wrist and hand

- **T22.3 Burn of third degree of shoulder and upper limb, except wrist and hand**
  Use additional external cause code to identify the source, place and intent of the burn (X00-X19, X75-X77, X96-X98, Y92)
  - X **T22.30 Burn of third degree of shoulder and upper limb, except wrist and hand, unspecified site** A CC, A MCC
    Ex: T22.30X[A], T22.391-T22.399[A], T22.70X[A], T22.791-T22.799[A]
  - **T22.31 Burn of third degree of forearm**
    Ex: **For category T22.31 CC codes:** T22.30X-T22.319[A], T22.391-T22.399[A], T22.70X-T22.719[A], T22.791-T22.799[A]
    - **T22.311 Burn of third degree of right forearm** A CC, A MCC
    - **T22.312 Burn of third degree of left forearm** A CC, A MCC
    - **T22.319 Burn of third degree of unspecified forearm** A CC, A MCC
  - **T22.32 Burn of third degree of elbow**
    Ex: **For category T22.32 CC codes:** T22.30X[A], T22.321-T22.329[A], T22.391-T22.399[A], T22.70X[A], T22.721-T22.729[A], T22.791-T22.799[A]
    - **T22.321 Burn of third degree of right elbow** A CC, A MCC
    - **T22.322 Burn of third degree of left elbow** A CC, A MCC
    - **T22.329 Burn of third degree of unspecified elbow** A CC, A MCC
  - **T22.33 Burn of third degree of upper arm**
    Ex: **For category T22.33 CC codes:** T22.30X[A], T22.331-T22.339[A], T22.391-T22.399[A], T22.70X[A], T22.731-T22.739[A], T22.791-T22.799[A]
    - **T22.331 Burn of third degree of right upper arm** A CC, A MCC
    - **T22.332 Burn of third degree of left upper arm** A CC, A MCC
    - **T22.339 Burn of third degree of unspecified upper arm** A CC, A MCC
  - **T22.34 Burn of third degree of axilla**
    Ex: **For category T22.34 CC codes:** T22.30X[A], T22.341-T22.349[A], T22.391-T22.399[A], T22.70X[A], T22.741-T22.749[A], T22.791-T22.799[A]
    - **T22.341 Burn of third degree of right axilla** A CC, A MCC
    - **T22.342 Burn of third degree of left axilla** A CC, A MCC
    - **T22.349 Burn of third degree of unspecified axilla** A CC, A MCC
  - **T22.35 Burn of third degree of shoulder**
    Ex: **For category T22.35 CC codes:** T22.30X[A], T22.351-T22.359[A], T22.391-T22.399[A], T22.70X[A], T22.751-T22.759[A], T22.791-T22.799[A]
    - **T22.351 Burn of third degree of right shoulder** A CC, A MCC
    - **T22.352 Burn of third degree of left shoulder** A CC, A MCC
    - **T22.359 Burn of third degree of unspecified shoulder** A CC, A MCC
  - **T22.36 Burn of third degree of scapular region**
    Ex: **For category T22.36 CC codes:** T22.30X[A], T22.361-T22.369[A], T22.391-T22.399[A], T22.70X[A], T22.761-T22.769[A], T22.791-T22.799[A]
    - **T22.361 Burn of third degree of right scapular region** A CC, A MCC
    - **T22.362 Burn of third degree of left scapular region** A CC, A MCC
    - **T22.369 Burn of third degree of unspecified scapular region** A CC, A MCC
  - **T22.39 Burn of third degree of multiple sites of shoulder and upper limb, except wrist and hand**
    Ex: **For category T22.39 CC codes:** See T22.30
    - **T22.391 Burn of third degree of multiple sites of right shoulder and upper limb, except wrist and hand** A CC, A MCC
    - **T22.392 Burn of third degree of multiple sites of left shoulder and upper limb, except wrist and hand** A CC, A MCC
    - **T22.399 Burn of third degree of multiple sites of unspecified shoulder and upper limb, except wrist and hand** A CC, A MCC
- **T22.4 Corrosion of unspecified degree of shoulder and upper limb, except wrist and hand**
  Code first (T51-T65) to identify chemical and intent
  Use additional external cause code to identify place (Y92)
  - X **T22.40 Corrosion of unspecified degree of shoulder and upper limb, except wrist and hand, unspecified site**
  - **T22.41 Corrosion of unspecified degree of forearm**
    - **T22.411 Corrosion of unspecified degree of right forearm**
    - **T22.412 Corrosion of unspecified degree of left forearm**
    - **T22.419 Corrosion of unspecified degree of unspecified forearm**
  - **T22.42 Corrosion of unspecified degree of elbow**
    - **T22.421 Corrosion of unspecified degree of right elbow**
    - **T22.422 Corrosion of unspecified degree of left elbow**
    - **T22.429 Corrosion of unspecified degree of unspecified elbow**
  - **T22.43 Corrosion of unspecified degree of upper arm**
    - **T22.431 Corrosion of unspecified degree of right upper arm**
    - **T22.432 Corrosion of unspecified degree of left upper arm**
    - **T22.439 Corrosion of unspecified degree of unspecified upper arm**
  - **T22.44 Corrosion of unspecified degree of axilla**
    - **T22.441 Corrosion of unspecified degree of right axilla**
    - **T22.442 Corrosion of unspecified degree of left axilla**
    - **T22.449 Corrosion of unspecified degree of unspecified axilla**
  - **T22.45 Corrosion of unspecified degree of shoulder**
    - **T22.451 Corrosion of unspecified degree of right shoulder**
    - **T22.452 Corrosion of unspecified degree of left shoulder**
    - **T22.459 Corrosion of unspecified degree of unspecified shoulder**
  - **T22.46 Corrosion of unspecified degree of scapular region**
    - **T22.461 Corrosion of unspecified degree of right scapular region**
    - **T22.462 Corrosion of unspecified degree of left scapular region**
    - **T22.469 Corrosion of unspecified degree of unspecified scapular region**

- T22.49 Corrosion of unspecified degree of multiple sites of shoulder and upper limb, except wrist and hand
  - T22.491 Corrosion of unspecified degree of multiple sites of right shoulder and upper limb, except wrist and hand
  - T22.492 Corrosion of unspecified degree of multiple sites of left shoulder and upper limb, except wrist and hand
  - T22.499 Corrosion of unspecified degree of multiple sites of unspecified shoulder and upper limb, except wrist and hand
- T22.5 Corrosion of first degree of shoulder and upper limb, except wrist and hand

  Code first (T51-T65) to identify chemical and intent

  Use additional external cause code to identify place (Y92)
  - X T22.50 Corrosion of first degree of shoulder and upper limb, except wrist and hand unspecified site
  - T22.51 Corrosion of first degree of forearm
    - T22.511 Corrosion of first degree of right forearm
    - T22.512 Corrosion of first degree of left forearm
    - T22.519 Corrosion of first degree of unspecified forearm
  - T22.52 Corrosion of first degree of elbow
    - T22.521 Corrosion of first degree of right elbow
    - T22.522 Corrosion of first degree of left elbow
    - T22.529 Corrosion of first degree of unspecified elbow
  - T22.53 Corrosion of first degree of upper arm
    - T22.531 Corrosion of first degree of right upper arm
    - T22.532 Corrosion of first degree of left upper arm
    - T22.539 Corrosion of first degree of unspecified upper arm
  - T22.54 Corrosion of first degree of axilla
    - T22.541 Corrosion of first degree of right axilla
    - T22.542 Corrosion of first degree of left axilla
    - T22.549 Corrosion of first degree of unspecified axilla
  - T22.55 Corrosion of first degree of shoulder
    - T22.551 Corrosion of first degree of right shoulder
    - T22.552 Corrosion of first degree of left shoulder
    - T22.559 Corrosion of first degree of unspecified shoulder
  - T22.56 Corrosion of first degree of scapular region
    - T22.561 Corrosion of first degree of right scapular region
    - T22.562 Corrosion of first degree of left scapular region
    - T22.569 Corrosion of first degree of unspecified scapular region
- T22.59 Corrosion of first degree of multiple sites of shoulder and upper limb, except wrist and hand
  - T22.591 Corrosion of first degree of multiple sites of right shoulder and upper limb, except wrist and hand
  - T22.592 Corrosion of first degree of multiple sites of left shoulder and upper limb, except wrist and hand
  - T22.599 Corrosion of first degree of multiple sites of unspecified shoulder and upper limb, except wrist and hand
- T22.6 Corrosion of second degree of shoulder and upper limb, except wrist and hand

  Code first (T51-T65) to identify chemical and intent

  Use additional external cause code to identify place (Y92)
  - X T22.60 Corrosion of second degree of shoulder and upper limb, except wrist and hand, unspecified site
  - T22.61 Corrosion of second degree of forearm
    - T22.611 Corrosion of second degree of right forearm
    - T22.612 Corrosion of second degree of left forearm
    - T22.619 Corrosion of second degree of unspecified forearm
  - T22.62 Corrosion of second degree of elbow
    - T22.621 Corrosion of second degree of right elbow
    - T22.622 Corrosion of second degree of left elbow
    - T22.629 Corrosion of second degree of unspecified elbow
  - T22.63 Corrosion of second degree of upper arm
    - T22.631 Corrosion of second degree of right upper arm
    - T22.632 Corrosion of second degree of left upper arm
    - T22.639 Corrosion of second degree of unspecified upper arm
  - T22.64 Corrosion of second degree of axilla
    - T22.641 Corrosion of second degree of right axilla
    - T22.642 Corrosion of second degree of left axilla
    - T22.649 Corrosion of second degree of unspecified axilla
  - T22.65 Corrosion of second degree of shoulder
    - T22.651 Corrosion of second degree of right shoulder
    - T22.652 Corrosion of second degree of left shoulder
    - T22.659 Corrosion of second degree of unspecified shoulder
  - T22.66 Corrosion of second degree of scapular region
    - T22.661 Corrosion of second degree of right scapular region
    - T22.662 Corrosion of second degree of left scapular region
    - T22.669 Corrosion of second degree of unspecified scapular region

- **T22.69** Corrosion of second degree of multiple sites of shoulder and upper limb, except wrist and hand
  - **T22.691** Corrosion of second degree of multiple sites of right shoulder and upper limb, except wrist and hand
  - **T22.692** Corrosion of second degree of multiple sites of left shoulder and upper limb, except wrist and hand
  - **T22.699** Corrosion of second degree of multiple sites of unspecified shoulder and upper limb, except wrist and hand
- **T22.7** Corrosion of third degree of shoulder and upper limb, except wrist and hand

  Code first (T51-T65) to identify chemical and intent

  Use additional external cause code to identify place (Y92)
  - X **T22.70** Corrosion of third degree of shoulder and upper limb, except wrist and hand, unspecified site A CC, A MCC

    Ex: See T22.30
- **T22.71** Corrosion of third degree of forearm

  Ex: For category T22.71 CC codes: See T22.31
  - **T22.711** Corrosion of third degree of right forearm A CC, A MCC
  - **T22.712** Corrosion of third degree of left forearm A CC, A MCC
  - **T22.719** Corrosion of third degree of unspecified forearm A CC, A MCC
- **T22.72** Corrosion of third degree of elbow

  Ex: For category T22.72 CC codes: See T22.32
  - **T22.721** Corrosion of third degree of right elbow A CC, A MCC
  - **T22.722** Corrosion of third degree of left elbow A CC, A MCC
  - **T22.729** Corrosion of third degree of unspecified elbow A CC, A MCC
- **T22.73** Corrosion of third degree of upper arm

  Ex: For category T22.73 CC codes: T22.33
  - **T22.731** Corrosion of third degree of right upper arm A CC, A MCC
  - **T22.732** Corrosion of third degree of left upper arm A CC, A MCC
  - **T22.739** Corrosion of third degree of unspecified upper arm A CC, A MCC
- **T22.74** Corrosion of third degree of axilla

  Ex: For category T22.74 CC codes: T22.34
  - **T22.741** Corrosion of third degree of right axilla A CC, A MCC
  - **T22.742** Corrosion of third degree of left axilla A CC, A MCC
  - **T22.749** Corrosion of third degree of unspecified axilla A CC, A MCC
- **T22.75** Corrosion of third degree of shoulder

  Ex: For category T22.75 CC codes: T22.35
  - **T22.751** Corrosion of third degree of right shoulder A CC, A MCC
  - **T22.752** Corrosion of third degree of left shoulder A CC, A MCC
  - **T22.759** Corrosion of third degree of unspecified shoulder A CC, A MCC
- **T22.76** Corrosion of third degree of scapular region

  Ex: For category T22.76 CC codes: T22.36
  - **T22.761** Corrosion of third degree of right scapular region A CC, A MCC
  - **T22.762** Corrosion of third degree of left scapular region A CC, A MCC
  - **T22.769** Corrosion of third degree of unspecified scapular region A CC, A MCC
- **T22.79** Corrosion of third degree of multiple sites of shoulder and upper limb, except wrist and hand

  Ex: For category T22.79 CC codes: See T22.30
  - **T22.791** Corrosion of third degree of multiple sites of right shoulder and upper limb, except wrist and hand A CC, A MCC
  - **T22.792** Corrosion of third degree of multiple sites of left shoulder and upper limb, except wrist and hand A CC, A MCC
  - **T22.799** Corrosion of third degree of multiple sites of unspecified shoulder and upper limb, except wrist and hand A CC, A MCC
- **T23** Burn and corrosion of wrist and hand

  The appropriate 7th character is to be added to each code from category T23

A	initial encounter
D	subsequent encounter
S	sequela

  - **T23.0** Burn of unspecified degree of wrist and hand

    Use additional external cause code to identify the source, place and intent of the burn (X00-X19, X75-X77, X96-X98, Y92)
    - **T23.00** Burn of unspecified degree of hand, unspecified site
      - **T23.001** Burn of unspecified degree of right hand, unspecified site
      - **T23.002** Burn of unspecified degree of left hand, unspecified site
      - **T23.009** Burn of unspecified degree of unspecified hand, unspecified site
    - **T23.01** Burn of unspecified degree of thumb (nail)
      - **T23.011** Burn of unspecified degree of right thumb (nail)
      - **T23.012** Burn of unspecified degree of left thumb (nail)
      - **T23.019** Burn of unspecified degree of unspecified thumb (nail)
    - **T23.02** Burn of unspecified degree of single finger (nail) except thumb
      - **T23.021** Burn of unspecified degree of single right finger (nail) except thumb
      - **T23.022** Burn of unspecified degree of single left finger (nail) except thumb
      - **T23.029** Burn of unspecified degree of unspecified single finger (nail) except thumb
    - **T23.03** Burn of unspecified degree of multiple fingers (nail), not including thumb
      - **T23.031** Burn of unspecified degree of multiple right fingers (nail), not including thumb
      - **T23.032** Burn of unspecified degree of multiple left fingers (nail), not including thumb
      - **T23.039** Burn of unspecified degree of unspecified multiple fingers (nail), not including thumb

- T23.04 Burn of unspecified degree of multiple fingers (nail), including thumb
  - T23.041 Burn of unspecified degree of multiple right fingers (nail), including thumb
  - T23.042 Burn of unspecified degree of multiple left fingers (nail), including thumb
  - T23.049 Burn of unspecified degree of unspecified multiple fingers (nail), including thumb
- T23.05 Burn of unspecified degree of palm
  - T23.051 Burn of unspecified degree of right palm
  - T23.052 Burn of unspecified degree of left palm
  - T23.059 Burn of unspecified degree of unspecified palm
- T23.06 Burn of unspecified degree of back of hand
  - T23.061 Burn of unspecified degree of back of right hand
  - T23.062 Burn of unspecified degree of back of left hand
  - T23.069 Burn of unspecified degree of back of unspecified hand
- T23.07 Burn of unspecified degree of wrist
  - T23.071 Burn of unspecified degree of right wrist
  - T23.072 Burn of unspecified degree of left wrist
  - T23.079 Burn of unspecified degree of unspecified wrist
- T23.09 Burn of unspecified degree of multiple sites of wrist and hand
  - T23.091 Burn of unspecified degree of multiple sites of right wrist and hand
  - T23.092 Burn of unspecified degree of multiple sites of left wrist and hand
  - T23.099 Burn of unspecified degree of multiple sites of unspecified wrist and hand

- T23.1 Burn of first degree of wrist and hand

  Use additional external cause code to identify the source, place and intent of the burn (X00-X19, X75-X77, X96-X98, Y92)
- T23.10 Burn of first degree of hand, unspecified site
  - T23.101 Burn of first degree of right hand, unspecified site
  - T23.102 Burn of first degree of left hand, unspecified site
  - T23.109 Burn of first degree of unspecified hand, unspecified site
- T23.11 Burn of first degree of thumb (nail)
  - T23.111 Burn of first degree of right thumb (nail)
  - T23.112 Burn of first degree of left thumb (nail)
  - T23.119 Burn of first degree of unspecified thumb (nail)
- T23.12 Burn of first degree of single finger (nail) except thumb
  - T23.121 Burn of first degree of single right finger (nail) except thumb
  - T23.122 Burn of first degree of single left finger (nail) except thumb
  - T23.129 Burn of first degree of unspecified single finger (nail) except thumb
- T23.13 Burn of first degree of multiple fingers (nail), not including thumb
  - T23.131 Burn of first degree of multiple right fingers (nail), not including thumb
  - T23.132 Burn of first degree of multiple left fingers (nail), not including thumb
  - T23.139 Burn of first degree of unspecified multiple fingers (nail), not including thumb
- T23.14 Burn of first degree of multiple fingers (nail), including thumb
  - T23.141 Burn of first degree of multiple right fingers (nail), including thumb
  - T23.142 Burn of first degree of multiple left fingers (nail), including thumb
  - T23.149 Burn of first degree of unspecified multiple fingers (nail), including thumb
- T23.15 Burn of first degree of palm
  - T23.151 Burn of first degree of right palm
  - T23.152 Burn of first degree of left palm
  - T23.159 Burn of first degree of unspecified palm
- T23.16 Burn of first degree of back of hand
  - T23.161 Burn of first degree of back of right hand
  - T23.162 Burn of first degree of back of left hand
  - T23.169 Burn of first degree of back of unspecified hand
- T23.17 Burn of first degree of wrist
  - T23.171 Burn of first degree of right wrist
  - T23.172 Burn of first degree of left wrist
  - T23.179 Burn of first degree of unspecified wrist
- T23.19 Burn of first degree of multiple sites of wrist and hand
  - T23.191 Burn of first degree of multiple sites of right wrist and hand
  - T23.192 Burn of first degree of multiple sites of left wrist and hand
  - T23.199 Burn of first degree of multiple sites of unspecified wrist and hand

- T23.2 Burn of second degree of wrist and hand

  Use additional external cause code to identify the source, place and intent of the burn (X00-X19, X75-X77, X96-X98, Y92)
- T23.20 Burn of second degree of hand, unspecified site
  - T23.201 Burn of second degree of right hand, unspecified site
  - T23.202 Burn of second degree of left hand, unspecified site
  - T23.209 Burn of second degree of unspecified hand, unspecified site
- T23.21 Burn of second degree of thumb (nail)
  - T23.211 Burn of second degree of right thumb (nail)
  - T23.212 Burn of second degree of left thumb (nail)
  - T23.219 Burn of second degree of unspecified thumb (nail)

◀ New ⇐ Revised ~~deleted~~ Deleted Excludes 1 Excludes 2 Includes Use additional Code first Code also Unspecified
OGCR Official Guidelines ● Unacceptable Principal Diagnosis X Assign placeholder X ● Use Additional Character(s) ▶ Manifestation Code Coding Clinic

- **T23.22** Burn of second degree of single finger (nail) except thumb
  - **T23.221** Burn of second degree of single right finger (nail) except thumb
  - **T23.222** Burn of second degree of single left finger (nail) except thumb
  - **T23.229** Burn of second degree of unspecified single finger (nail) except thumb
- **T23.23** Burn of second degree of multiple fingers (nail), not including thumb
  - **T23.231** Burn of second degree of multiple right fingers (nail), not including thumb
  - **T23.232** Burn of second degree of multiple left fingers (nail), not including thumb
  - **T23.239** Burn of second degree of unspecified multiple fingers (nail), not including thumb
- **T23.24** Burn of second degree of multiple fingers (nail), including thumb
  - **T23.241** Burn of second degree of multiple right fingers (nail), including thumb
  - **T23.242** Burn of second degree of multiple left fingers (nail), including thumb
  - **T23.249** Burn of second degree of unspecified multiple fingers (nail), including thumb
- **T23.25** Burn of second degree of palm
  - **T23.251** Burn of second degree of right palm
  - **T23.252** Burn of second degree of left palm
  - **T23.259** Burn of second degree of unspecified palm
- **T23.26** Burn of second degree of back of hand
  - **T23.261** Burn of second degree of back of right hand
  - **T23.262** Burn of second degree of back of left hand
  - **T23.269** Burn of second degree of back of unspecified hand
- **T23.27** Burn of second degree of wrist
  - **T23.271** Burn of second degree of right wrist
  - **T23.272** Burn of second degree of left wrist
  - **T23.279** Burn of second degree of unspecified wrist
- **T23.29** Burn of second degree of multiple sites of wrist and hand
  - **T23.291** Burn of second degree of multiple sites of right wrist and hand
  - **T23.292** Burn of second degree of multiple sites of left wrist and hand
  - **T23.299** Burn of second degree of multiple sites of unspecified wrist and hand
- **T23.3** Burn of third degree of wrist and hand

  Use additional external cause code to identify the source, place and intent of the burn (X00-X19, X75-X77, X96-X98, Y92)
  - **T23.30** Burn of third degree of hand, unspecified site

    Ex: **For category T23.30 CC codes:** T23.301-T23.309[A], T23.391-T23.399[A], T23.701-T23.709[A], T23.791-T23.799[A]
    - **T23.301** Burn of third degree of right hand, unspecified site A CC, A HAC

      Coding Clinic: 2015, Q1, P19
    - **T23.302** Burn of third degree of left hand, unspecified site A CC, A HAC

      Coding Clinic: 2016, Q2, P5
    - **T23.309** Burn of third degree of unspecified hand, unspecified site A CC, A HAC
  - **T23.31** Burn of third degree of thumb (nail)

    Ex: **For category T23.31 CC codes:** T23.301-T23.319[A], T23.391-T23.399[A], T23.701-T23.719[A], T23.791-T23.799[A]
    - **T23.311** Burn of third degree of right thumb (nail) A CC, A HAC
    - **T23.312** Burn of third degree of left thumb (nail) A CC, A HAC
    - **T23.319** Burn of third degree of unspecified thumb (nail) A CC, A HAC
  - **T23.32** Burn of third degree of single finger (nail) except thumb

    Ex: **For category T23.32 CC codes:** T23.301-T23.309[A], T23.321-T23.329[A], T23.391-T23.399[A], T23.701-T23.709[A], T23.721-T23.729[A], T23.791-T23.799[A]
    - **T23.321** Burn of third degree of single right finger (nail) except thumb A CC, A HAC
    - **T23.322** Burn of third degree of single left finger (nail) except thumb A CC, A HAC
    - **T23.329** Burn of third degree of unspecified single finger (nail) except thumb A CC, A HAC
  - **T23.33** Burn of third degree of multiple fingers (nail), not including thumb

    Ex: **For category T23.33 CC codes:** T23.301-T23.309[A], T23.331-T23.339[A], T23.391-T23.399[A], T23.701-709[A], T23.731-T23.739[A], T23.791-T23.799[A]
    - **T23.331** Burn of third degree of multiple right fingers (nail), not including thumb A CC, A HAC
    - **T23.332** Burn of third degree of multiple left fingers (nail), not including thumb A CC, A HAC
    - **T23.339** Burn of third degree of unspecified multiple fingers (nail), not including thumb A CC, A HAC
  - **T23.34** Burn of third degree of multiple fingers (nail), including thumb

    Ex: **For category T23.34 CC codes:** T23.301-T23.309[A], T23.341-T23.349[A], T23.391-T23.399[A], T23.701-T23.709[A], T23.741-T23.749[A], T23.791-T23.799[A]
    - **T23.341** Burn of third degree of multiple right fingers (nail), including thumb A CC, A HAC
    - **T23.342** Burn of third degree of multiple left fingers (nail), including thumb A CC, A HAC
    - **T23.349** Burn of third degree of unspecified multiple fingers (nail), including thumb A CC, A HAC
  - **T23.35** Burn of third degree of palm

    Ex: **For category T23.35 CC codes:** T23.301-T23.309[A], T23.351-T23.359[A], T23.391-T23.399[A], T23.701-T23.709[A], T23.751-T23.759[A], T23.791-T23.799[A]
    - **T23.351** Burn of third degree of right palm A CC, A HAC
    - **T23.352** Burn of third degree of left palm A CC, A HAC
    - **T23.359** Burn of third degree of unspecified palm A CC, A HAC
  - **T23.36** Burn of third degree of back of hand

    Ex: **For category T23.36 CC codes:** T23.301-T23.309[A], T23.361-T23.369[A], T23.391-T23.399[A], T23.701-T23.709[A], T23.761-T23.769[A], T23.791-T23.799[A]
    - **T23.361** Burn of third degree of back of right hand A CC, A HAC
    - **T23.362** Burn of third degree of back of left hand A CC, A HAC
    - **T23.369** Burn of third degree of back of unspecified hand A CC, A HAC

- T23.37 Burn of third degree of wrist
  - Ex For category T23.37 CC codes: T23.301-T23.309[A], T23.371-T23.379[A], T23.391-T23.399[A], T23.701-T23.709[A], T23.771-T23.779[A], T23.791-T23.799[A]
  - T23.371 Burn of third degree of right wrist A CC, A MCC
  - T23.372 Burn of third degree of left wrist A CC, A MCC
  - T23.379 Burn of third degree of unspecified wrist A CC, A MCC
- T23.39 Burn of third degree of multiple sites of wrist and hand
  - Ex For category T23.39 CC codes: T23.30
  - T23.391 Burn of third degree of multiple sites of right wrist and hand A CC, A MCC
  - T23.392 Burn of third degree of multiple sites of left wrist and hand A CC, A MCC
  - T23.399 Burn of third degree of multiple sites of unspecified wrist and hand A CC, A MCC
- T23.4 Corrosion of unspecified degree of wrist and hand
  - *Code first (T51-T65) to identify chemical and intent*
  - Use additional external cause code to identify place (Y92)
  - T23.40 Corrosion of unspecified degree of hand, unspecified site
    - T23.401 Corrosion of unspecified degree of right hand, unspecified site
    - T23.402 Corrosion of unspecified degree of left hand, unspecified site
    - T23.409 Corrosion of unspecified degree of unspecified hand, unspecified site
  - T23.41 Corrosion of unspecified degree of thumb (nail)
    - T23.411 Corrosion of unspecified degree of right thumb (nail)
    - T23.412 Corrosion of unspecified degree of left thumb (nail)
    - T23.419 Corrosion of unspecified degree of unspecified thumb (nail)
  - T23.42 Corrosion of unspecified degree of single finger (nail) except thumb
    - T23.421 Corrosion of unspecified degree of single right finger (nail) except thumb
    - T23.422 Corrosion of unspecified degree of single left finger (nail) except thumb
    - T23.429 Corrosion of unspecified degree of unspecified single finger (nail) except thumb
  - T23.43 Corrosion of unspecified degree of multiple fingers (nail), not including thumb
    - T23.431 Corrosion of unspecified degree of multiple right fingers (nail), not including thumb
    - T23.432 Corrosion of unspecified degree of multiple left fingers (nail), not including thumb
    - T23.439 Corrosion of unspecified degree of unspecified multiple fingers (nail), not including thumb
  - T23.44 Corrosion of unspecified degree of multiple fingers (nail), including thumb
    - T23.441 Corrosion of unspecified degree of multiple right fingers (nail), including thumb
    - T23.442 Corrosion of unspecified degree of multiple left fingers (nail), including thumb
    - T23.449 Corrosion of unspecified degree of unspecified multiple fingers (nail), including thumb
  - T23.45 Corrosion of unspecified degree of palm
    - T23.451 Corrosion of unspecified degree of right palm
    - T23.452 Corrosion of unspecified degree of left palm
    - T23.459 Corrosion of unspecified degree of unspecified palm
  - T23.46 Corrosion of unspecified degree of back of hand
    - T23.461 Corrosion of unspecified degree of back of right hand
    - T23.462 Corrosion of unspecified degree of back of left hand
    - T23.469 Corrosion of unspecified degree of back of unspecified hand
  - T23.47 Corrosion of unspecified degree of wrist
    - T23.471 Corrosion of unspecified degree of right wrist
    - T23.472 Corrosion of unspecified degree of left wrist
    - T23.479 Corrosion of unspecified degree of unspecified wrist
  - T23.49 Corrosion of unspecified degree of multiple sites of wrist and hand
    - T23.491 Corrosion of unspecified degree of multiple sites of right wrist and hand
    - T23.492 Corrosion of unspecified degree of multiple sites of left wrist and hand
    - T23.499 Corrosion of unspecified degree of multiple sites of unspecified wrist and hand
- T23.5 Corrosion of first degree of wrist and hand
  - *Code first (T51-T65) to identify chemical and intent*
  - Use additional external cause code to identify place (Y92)
  - T23.50 Corrosion of first degree of hand, unspecified site
    - T23.501 Corrosion of first degree of right hand, unspecified site
    - T23.502 Corrosion of first degree of left hand, unspecified site
    - T23.509 Corrosion of first degree of unspecified hand, unspecified site
  - T23.51 Corrosion of first degree of thumb (nail)
    - T23.511 Corrosion of first degree of right thumb (nail)
    - T23.512 Corrosion of first degree of left thumb (nail)
    - T23.519 Corrosion of first degree of unspecified thumb (nail)
  - T23.52 Corrosion of first degree of single finger (nail) except thumb
    - T23.521 Corrosion of first degree of single right finger (nail) except thumb
    - T23.522 Corrosion of first degree of single left finger (nail) except thumb
    - T23.529 Corrosion of first degree of unspecified single finger (nail) except thumb

- T23.53 Corrosion of first degree of multiple fingers (nail), not including thumb
  - T23.531 Corrosion of first degree of multiple right fingers (nail), not including thumb
  - T23.532 Corrosion of first degree of multiple left fingers (nail), not including thumb
  - T23.539 Corrosion of first degree of unspecified multiple fingers (nail), not including thumb
- T23.54 Corrosion of first degree of multiple fingers (nail), including thumb
  - T23.541 Corrosion of first degree of multiple right fingers (nail), including thumb
  - T23.542 Corrosion of first degree of multiple left fingers (nail), including thumb
  - T23.549 Corrosion of first degree of unspecified multiple fingers (nail), including thumb
- T23.55 Corrosion of first degree of palm
  - T23.551 Corrosion of first degree of right palm
  - T23.552 Corrosion of first degree of left palm
  - T23.559 Corrosion of first degree of unspecified palm
- T23.56 Corrosion of first degree of back of hand
  - T23.561 Corrosion of first degree of back of right hand
  - T23.562 Corrosion of first degree of back of left hand
  - T23.569 Corrosion of first degree of back of unspecified hand
- T23.57 Corrosion of first degree of wrist
  - T23.571 Corrosion of first degree of right wrist
  - T23.572 Corrosion of first degree of left wrist
  - T23.579 Corrosion of first degree of unspecified wrist
- T23.59 Corrosion of first degree of multiple sites of wrist and hand
  - T23.591 Corrosion of first degree of multiple sites of right wrist and hand
  - T23.592 Corrosion of first degree of multiple sites of left wrist and hand
  - T23.599 Corrosion of first degree of multiple sites of unspecified wrist and hand
- T23.6 Corrosion of second degree of wrist and hand

  Code first (T51-T65) to identify chemical and intent

  Use additional external cause code to identify place (Y92)
  - T23.60 Corrosion of second degree of hand, unspecified site
    - T23.601 Corrosion of second degree of right hand, unspecified site
    - T23.602 Corrosion of second degree of left hand, unspecified site
    - T23.609 Corrosion of second degree of unspecified hand, unspecified site
  - T23.61 Corrosion of second degree of thumb (nail)
    - T23.611 Corrosion of second degree of right thumb (nail)
    - T23.612 Corrosion of second degree of left thumb (nail)
    - T23.619 Corrosion of second degree of unspecified thumb (nail)
  - T23.62 Corrosion of second degree of single finger (nail) except thumb
    - T23.621 Corrosion of second degree of single right finger (nail) except thumb
    - T23.622 Corrosion of second degree of single left finger (nail) except thumb
    - T23.629 Corrosion of second degree of unspecified single finger (nail) except thumb
  - T23.63 Corrosion of second degree of multiple fingers (nail), not including thumb
    - T23.631 Corrosion of second degree of multiple right fingers (nail), not including thumb
    - T23.632 Corrosion of second degree of multiple left fingers (nail), not including thumb
    - T23.639 Corrosion of second degree of unspecified multiple fingers (nail), not including thumb
  - T23.64 Corrosion of second degree of multiple fingers (nail), including thumb
    - T23.641 Corrosion of second degree of multiple right fingers (nail), including thumb
    - T23.642 Corrosion of second degree of multiple left fingers (nail), including thumb
    - T23.649 Corrosion of second degree of unspecified multiple fingers (nail), including thumb
  - T23.65 Corrosion of second degree of palm
    - T23.651 Corrosion of second degree of right palm
    - T23.652 Corrosion of second degree of left palm
    - T23.659 Corrosion of second degree of unspecified palm
  - T23.66 Corrosion of second degree of back of hand
    - T23.661 Corrosion of second degree back of right hand
    - T23.662 Corrosion of second degree back of left hand
    - T23.669 Corrosion of second degree back of unspecified hand
  - T23.67 Corrosion of second degree of wrist
    - T23.671 Corrosion of second degree of right wrist
    - T23.672 Corrosion of second degree of left wrist
    - T23.679 Corrosion of second degree of unspecified wrist
  - T23.69 Corrosion of second degree of multiple sites of wrist and hand
    - T23.691 Corrosion of second degree of multiple sites of right wrist and hand
    - T23.692 Corrosion of second degree of multiple sites of left wrist and hand
    - T23.699 Corrosion of second degree of multiple sites of unspecified wrist and hand

- **T23.7 Corrosion of third degree of wrist and hand**
  Code first (T51-T65) to identify chemical and intent
  Use additional external cause code to identify place (Y92)
  - **T23.70 Corrosion of third degree of hand, unspecified site**
    Ex: For category T23.70 CC codes: See T23.30
    - **T23.701 Corrosion of third degree of right hand, unspecified site** A CC, A OB
    - **T23.702 Corrosion of third degree of left hand, unspecified site** A CC, A OB
    - **T23.709 Corrosion of third degree of unspecified hand, unspecified site** A CC, A OB
  - **T23.71 Corrosion of third degree of thumb (nail)**
    Ex: For category T23.71 CC codes: See T23.31
    - **T23.711 Corrosion of third degree of right thumb (nail)** A CC, A OB
    - **T23.712 Corrosion of third degree of left thumb (nail)** A CC, A OB
    - **T23.719 Corrosion of third degree of unspecified thumb (nail)** A CC, A OB
  - **T23.72 Corrosion of third degree of single finger (nail) except thumb**
    Ex: For category T23.72 CC codes: See T23.32
    - **T23.721 Corrosion of third degree of single right finger (nail) except thumb** A CC, A OB
    - **T23.722 Corrosion of third degree of single left finger (nail) except thumb** A CC, A OB
    - **T23.729 Corrosion of third degree of unspecified single finger (nail) except thumb** A CC, A OB
  - **T23.73 Corrosion of third degree of multiple fingers (nail), not including thumb**
    Ex: For category T23.73 CC codes: See T23.33
    - **T23.731 Corrosion of third degree of multiple right fingers (nail), not including thumb** A CC, A OB
    - **T23.732 Corrosion of third degree of multiple left fingers (nail), not including thumb** A CC, A OB
    - **T23.739 Corrosion of third degree of unspecified multiple fingers (nail), not including thumb** A CC, A OB
  - **T23.74 Corrosion of third degree of multiple fingers (nail), including thumb**
    Ex: For category T23.74 CC codes: See T23.34
    - **T23.741 Corrosion of third degree of multiple right fingers (nail), including thumb** A CC, A OB
    - **T23.742 Corrosion of third degree of multiple left fingers (nail), including thumb** A CC, A OB
    - **T23.749 Corrosion of third degree of unspecified multiple fingers (nail), including thumb** A CC, A OB
  - **T23.75 Corrosion of third degree of palm**
    Ex: For category T23.75 CC codes: See T23.35
    - **T23.751 Corrosion of third degree of right palm** A CC, A OB
    - **T23.752 Corrosion of third degree of left palm** A CC, A OB
    - **T23.759 Corrosion of third degree of unspecified palm** A CC, A OB
  - **T23.76 Corrosion of third degree of back of hand**
    Ex: For category T23.76 CC codes: See T23.36
    - **T23.761 Corrosion of third degree of back of right hand** A CC, A OB
    - **T23.762 Corrosion of third degree of back of left hand** A CC, A OB
    - **T23.769 Corrosion of third degree of back of unspecified hand** A CC, A OB
  - **T23.77 Corrosion of third degree of wrist**
    Ex: For category T23.77 CC codes: See T23.37
    - **T23.771 Corrosion of third degree of right wrist** A CC, A OB
    - **T23.772 Corrosion of third degree of left wrist** A CC, A OB
    - **T23.779 Corrosion of third degree of unspecified wrist** A CC, A OB
  - **T23.79 Corrosion of third degree of multiple sites of wrist and hand**
    Ex: For category T23.79 CC codes: T23.30
    - **T23.791 Corrosion of third degree of multiple sites of right wrist and hand** A CC, A OB
    - **T23.792 Corrosion of third degree of multiple sites of left wrist and hand** A CC, A OB
    - **T23.799 Corrosion of third degree of multiple sites of unspecified wrist and hand** A CC, A OB

- **T24 Burn and corrosion of lower limb, except ankle and foot**
  Excludes2 burn and corrosion of ankle and foot (T25.-)
  burn and corrosion of hip region (T21.-)
  The appropriate 7th character is to be added to each code from category T24

A	initial encounter
D	subsequent encounter
S	sequela

  - **T24.0 Burn of unspecified degree of lower limb, except ankle and foot**
    Use additional external cause code to identify the source, place and intent of the burn (X00-X19, X75-X77, X96-X98, Y92)
    - **T24.00 Burn of unspecified degree of unspecified site of lower limb, except ankle and foot**
      - **T24.001 Burn of unspecified degree of unspecified site of right lower limb, except ankle and foot**
      - **T24.002 Burn of unspecified degree of unspecified site of left lower limb, except ankle and foot**
      - **T24.009 Burn of unspecified degree of unspecified site of unspecified lower limb, except ankle and foot**
    - **T24.01 Burn of unspecified degree of thigh**
      - **T24.011 Burn of unspecified degree of right thigh**
      - **T24.012 Burn of unspecified degree of left thigh**
      - **T24.019 Burn of unspecified degree of unspecified thigh**
    - **T24.02 Burn of unspecified degree of knee**
      - **T24.021 Burn of unspecified degree of right knee**
      - **T24.022 Burn of unspecified degree of left knee**
      - **T24.029 Burn of unspecified degree of unspecified knee**

- **T24.03 Burn of unspecified degree of lower leg**
  - **T24.031 Burn of unspecified degree of right lower leg**
  - **T24.032 Burn of unspecified degree of left lower leg**
  - **T24.039 Burn of unspecified degree of unspecified lower leg**
- **T24.09 Burn of unspecified degree of multiple sites of lower limb, except ankle and foot**
  - **T24.091 Burn of unspecified degree of multiple sites of right lower limb, except ankle and foot**
  - **T24.092 Burn of unspecified degree of multiple sites of left lower limb, except ankle and foot**
  - **T24.099 Burn of unspecified degree of multiple sites of unspecified lower limb, except ankle and foot**
- **T24.1 Burn of first degree of lower limb, except ankle and foot**

  Use additional external cause code to identify the source, place and intent of the burn (X00-X19, X75-X77, X96-X98, Y92)
  - **T24.10 Burn of first degree of unspecified site of lower limb, except ankle and foot**
    - **T24.101 Burn of first degree of unspecified site of right lower limb, except ankle and foot**
    - **T24.102 Burn of first degree of unspecified site of left lower limb, except ankle and foot**
    - **T24.109 Burn of first degree of unspecified site of unspecified lower limb, except ankle and foot**
  - **T24.11 Burn of first degree of thigh**
    - **T24.111 Burn of first degree of right thigh**
    - **T24.112 Burn of first degree of left thigh**
    - **T24.119 Burn of first degree of unspecified thigh**
  - **T24.12 Burn of first degree of knee**
    - **T24.121 Burn of first degree of right knee**
    - **T24.122 Burn of first degree of left knee**
    - **T24.129 Burn of first degree of unspecified knee**
  - **T24.13 Burn of first degree of lower leg**
    - **T24.131 Burn of first degree of right lower leg**
    - **T24.132 Burn of first degree of left lower leg**
    - **T24.139 Burn of first degree of unspecified lower leg**
  - **T24.19 Burn of first degree of multiple sites of lower limb, except ankle and foot**
    - **T24.191 Burn of first degree of multiple sites of right lower limb, except ankle and foot**
    - **T24.192 Burn of first degree of multiple sites of left lower limb, except ankle and foot**
    - **T24.199 Burn of first degree of multiple sites of unspecified lower limb, except ankle and foot**
- **T24.2 Burn of second degree of lower limb, except ankle and foot**

  Use additional external cause code to identify the source, place and intent of the burn (X00-X19, X75-X77, X96-X98, Y92)
  - **T24.20 Burn of second degree of unspecified site of lower limb, except ankle and foot**
    - **T24.201 Burn of second degree of unspecified site of right lower limb, except ankle and foot**
    - **T24.202 Burn of second degree of unspecified site of left lower limb, except ankle and foot**
    - **T24.209 Burn of second degree of unspecified site of unspecified lower limb, except ankle and foot**
  - **T24.21 Burn of second degree of thigh**
    - **T24.211 Burn of second degree of right thigh**
    - **T24.212 Burn of second degree of left thigh**
    - **T24.219 Burn of second degree of unspecified thigh**
  - **T24.22 Burn of second degree of knee**
    - **T24.221 Burn of second degree of right knee**
    - **T24.222 Burn of second degree of left knee**
    - **T24.229 Burn of second degree of unspecified knee**
  - **T24.23 Burn of second degree of lower leg**
    - **T24.231 Burn of second degree of right lower leg**
    - **T24.232 Burn of second degree of left lower leg**
    - **T24.239 Burn of second degree of unspecified lower leg**
  - **T24.29 Burn of second degree of multiple sites of lower limb, except ankle and foot**
    - **T24.291 Burn of second degree of multiple sites of right lower limb, except ankle and foot**
    - **T24.292 Burn of second degree of multiple sites of left lower limb, except ankle and foot**
    - **T24.299 Burn of second degree of multiple sites of unspecified lower limb, except ankle and foot**
- **T24.3 Burn of third degree of lower limb, except ankle and foot**

  Use additional external cause code to identify the source, place and intent of the burn (X00-X19, X75-X77, X96-X98, Y92)
  - **T24.30 Burn of third degree of unspecified site of lower limb, except ankle and foot**

    Ex **For category T24.30 CC codes:** T24.301-T24.309[A], T24.391-T24.399[A], T24.701-T24.709[A], T24.791-T24.799[A], T25.391-T25.399[A], T25.791-T25.799[A]
    - **T24.301 Burn of third degree of unspecified site of right lower limb, except ankle and foot** A CC, A MCC
    - **T24.302 Burn of third degree of unspecified site of left lower limb, except ankle and foot** A CC, A MCC
    - **T24.309 Burn of third degree of unspecified site of unspecified lower limb, except ankle and foot** A CC, A MCC

- **T24.31 Burn of third degree of thigh**
  - Ex: For category T24.31 CC codes: T24.301-T24.309[A], T24.311-T24.319[A], T24.391-T24.399[A], T24.701-T24.709-T24.719[A], T24.791-T24.799[A], T25.391-T25.399[A], T25.791-T25.799[A]
  - **T24.311 Burn of third degree of right thigh** A CC, A UNC
  - **T24.312 Burn of third degree of left thigh** A CC, A UNC
  - **T24.319 Burn of third degree of unspecified thigh** A CC, A UNC
- **T24.32 Burn of third degree of knee**
  - Ex: For category T24.32 CC codes: T24.301-T24.309[A], T24.321-T24.329[A], T24.391-T24.399[A], T24.701-T24.709[A], T24.721-T24.729[A], T24.791-T24.799[A], T25.391-T25.399[A], T25.791-T25.799[A]
  - **T24.321 Burn of third degree of right knee** A CC, A UNC
  - **T24.322 Burn of third degree of left knee** A CC, A UNC
  - **T24.329 Burn of third degree of unspecified knee** A CC, A UNC
- **T24.33 Burn of third degree of lower leg**
  - Ex: For category T24.33 CC codes: T24.301-T24.309[A], T24.331-T24.339[A], T24.391-T24.399[A], T24.701-T24.709[A], T24.731-T24.739[A], T24.791-T24.799[A], T25.391-T25.399[A], T25.791-T25.799[A]
  - **T24.331 Burn of third degree of right lower leg** A CC, A UNC
  - **T24.332 Burn of third degree of left lower leg** A CC, A UNC
  - **T24.339 Burn of third degree of unspecified lower leg** A CC, A UNC
- **T24.39 Burn of third degree of multiple sites of lower limb, except ankle and foot**
  - Ex: For category T24.39 CC codes: See T24.30
  - **T24.391 Burn of third degree of multiple sites of right lower limb, except ankle and foot** A CC, A UNC
    - Coding Clinic: 2016, Q2, P5
  - **T24.392 Burn of third degree of multiple sites of left lower limb, except ankle and foot** A CC, A UNC
  - **T24.399 Burn of third degree of multiple sites of unspecified lower limb, except ankle and foot** A CC, A UNC
- **T24.4 Corrosion of unspecified degree of lower limb, except ankle and foot**
  - *Code first (T51-T65) to identify chemical and intent*
  - Use additional external cause code to identify place (Y92)
  - **T24.40 Corrosion of unspecified degree of unspecified site of lower limb, except ankle and foot**
    - **T24.401 Corrosion of unspecified degree of unspecified site of right lower limb, except ankle and foot**
    - **T24.402 Corrosion of unspecified degree of unspecified site of left lower limb, except ankle and foot**
    - **T24.409 Corrosion of unspecified degree of unspecified site of unspecified lower limb, except ankle and foot**
  - **T24.41 Corrosion of unspecified degree of thigh**
    - **T24.411 Corrosion of unspecified degree of right thigh**
    - **T24.412 Corrosion of unspecified degree of left thigh**
    - **T24.419 Corrosion of unspecified degree of unspecified thigh**
  - **T24.42 Corrosion of unspecified degree of knee**
    - **T24.421 Corrosion of unspecified degree of right knee**
    - **T24.422 Corrosion of unspecified degree of left knee**
    - **T24.429 Corrosion of unspecified degree of unspecified knee**
  - **T24.43 Corrosion of unspecified degree of lower leg**
    - **T24.431 Corrosion of unspecified degree of right lower leg**
    - **T24.432 Corrosion of unspecified degree of left lower leg**
    - **T24.439 Corrosion of unspecified degree of unspecified lower leg**
  - **T24.49 Corrosion of unspecified degree of multiple sites of lower limb, except ankle and foot**
    - **T24.491 Corrosion of unspecified degree of multiple sites of right lower limb, except ankle and foot**
    - **T24.492 Corrosion of unspecified degree of multiple sites of left lower limb, except ankle and foot**
    - **T24.499 Corrosion of unspecified degree of multiple sites of unspecified lower limb, except ankle and foot**
- **T24.5 Corrosion of first degree of lower limb, except ankle and foot**
  - *Code first (T51-T65) to identify chemical and intent*
  - Use additional external cause code to identify place (Y92)
  - **T24.50 Corrosion of first degree of unspecified site of lower limb, except ankle and foot**
    - **T24.501 Corrosion of first degree of unspecified site of right lower limb, except ankle and foot**
    - **T24.502 Corrosion of first degree of unspecified site of left lower limb, except ankle and foot**
    - **T24.509 Corrosion of first degree of unspecified site of unspecified lower limb, except ankle and foot**
  - **T24.51 Corrosion of first degree of thigh**
    - **T24.511 Corrosion of first degree of right thigh**
    - **T24.512 Corrosion of first degree of left thigh**
    - **T24.519 Corrosion of first degree of unspecified thigh**
  - **T24.52 Corrosion of first degree of knee**
    - **T24.521 Corrosion of first degree of right knee**
    - **T24.522 Corrosion of first degree of left knee**
    - **T24.529 Corrosion of first degree of unspecified knee**
  - **T24.53 Corrosion of first degree of lower leg**
    - **T24.531 Corrosion of first degree of right lower leg**
    - **T24.532 Corrosion of first degree of left lower leg**
    - **T24.539 Corrosion of first degree of unspecified lower leg**
  - **T24.59 Corrosion of first degree of multiple sites of lower limb, except ankle and foot**
    - **T24.591 Corrosion of first degree of multiple sites of right lower limb, except ankle and foot**
    - **T24.592 Corrosion of first degree of multiple sites of left lower limb, except ankle and foot**
    - **T24.599 Corrosion of first degree of multiple sites of unspecified lower limb, except ankle and foot**

- **T24.6 Corrosion of second degree of lower limb, except ankle and foot**
  Code first (T51-T65) to identify chemical and intent
  Use additional external cause code to identify place (Y92)
  - **T24.60 Corrosion of second degree of unspecified site of lower limb, except ankle and foot**
    - **T24.601 Corrosion of second degree of unspecified site of right lower limb, except ankle and foot**
    - **T24.602 Corrosion of second degree of unspecified site of left lower limb, except ankle and foot**
    - **T24.609 Corrosion of second degree of unspecified site of unspecified lower limb, except ankle and foot**
  - **T24.61 Corrosion of second degree of thigh**
    - **T24.611 Corrosion of second degree of right thigh**
    - **T24.612 Corrosion of second degree of left thigh**
    - **T24.619 Corrosion of second degree of unspecified thigh**
  - **T24.62 Corrosion of second degree of knee**
    - **T24.621 Corrosion of second degree of right knee**
    - **T24.622 Corrosion of second degree of left knee**
    - **T24.629 Corrosion of second degree of unspecified knee**
  - **T24.63 Corrosion of second degree of lower leg**
    - **T24.631 Corrosion of second degree of right lower leg**
    - **T24.632 Corrosion of second degree of left lower leg**
    - **T24.639 Corrosion of second degree of unspecified lower leg**
  - **T24.69 Corrosion of second degree of multiple sites of lower limb, except ankle and foot**
    - **T24.691 Corrosion of second degree of multiple sites of right lower limb, except ankle and foot**
    - **T24.692 Corrosion of second degree of multiple sites of left lower limb, except ankle and foot**
    - **T24.699 Corrosion of second degree of multiple sites of unspecified lower limb, except ankle and foot**
- **T24.7 Corrosion of third degree of lower limb, except ankle and foot**
  Code first (T51-T65) to identify chemical and intent
  Use additional external cause code to identify place (Y92)
  - **T24.70 Corrosion of third degree of unspecified site of lower limb, except ankle and foot**
    Ex For category T24.70 CC codes: See T24.30
    - **T24.701 Corrosion of third degree of unspecified site of right lower limb, except ankle and foot** A CC, A MCC
    - **T24.702 Corrosion of third degree of unspecified site of left lower limb, except ankle and foot** A CC, A MCC
    - **T24.709 Corrosion of third degree of unspecified site of unspecified lower limb, except ankle and foot** A CC, A MCC
  - **T24.71 Corrosion of third degree of thigh**
    Ex For category T24.71 CC codes: See T24.31
    - **T24.711 Corrosion of third degree of right thigh** A CC, A MCC
    - **T24.712 Corrosion of third degree of left thigh** A CC, A MCC
    - **T24.719 Corrosion of third degree of unspecified thigh** A CC, A MCC
  - **T24.72 Corrosion of third degree of knee**
    Ex For category T24.72 CC codes: See T24.32
    - **T24.721 Corrosion of third degree of right knee** A CC, A MCC
    - **T24.722 Corrosion of third degree of left knee** A CC, A MCC
    - **T24.729 Corrosion of third degree of unspecified knee** A CC, A MCC
  - **T24.73 Corrosion of third degree of lower leg**
    Ex For category T24.73 CC codes: See T24.33
    - **T24.731 Corrosion of third degree of right lower leg** A CC, A MCC
    - **T24.732 Corrosion of third degree of left lower leg** A CC, A MCC
    - **T24.739 Corrosion of third degree of unspecified lower leg** A CC, A MCC
  - **T24.79 Corrosion of third degree of multiple sites of lower limb, except ankle and foot**
    Ex For category T24.79 CC codes: See T24.30
    - **T24.791 Corrosion of third degree of multiple sites of right lower limb, except ankle and foot** A CC, A MCC
    - **T24.792 Corrosion of third degree of multiple sites of left lower limb, except ankle and foot** A CC, A MCC
    - **T24.799 Corrosion of third degree of multiple sites of unspecified lower limb, except ankle and foot** A CC, A MCC
- **T25 Burn and corrosion of ankle and foot**
  The appropriate 7th character is to be added to each code from category T25

A	initial encounter
D	subsequent encounter
S	sequela

  - **T25.0 Burn of unspecified degree of ankle and foot**
    Use additional external cause code to identify the source, place and intent of the burn (X00-X19, X75-X77, X96-X98, Y92)
    - **T25.01 Burn of unspecified degree of ankle**
      - **T25.011 Burn of unspecified degree of right ankle**
      - **T25.012 Burn of unspecified degree of left ankle**
      - **T25.019 Burn of unspecified degree of unspecified ankle**
    - **T25.02 Burn of unspecified degree of foot**
      Excludes2 burn of unspecified degree of toe(s) (nail) (T25.03-)
      - **T25.021 Burn of unspecified degree of right foot**
      - **T25.022 Burn of unspecified degree of left foot**
      - **T25.029 Burn of unspecified degree of unspecified foot**

- **T25.03 Burn of unspecified degree of toe(s) (nail)**
  - **T25.031 Burn of unspecified degree of right toe(s) (nail)**
  - **T25.032 Burn of unspecified degree of left toe(s) (nail)**
  - **T25.039 Burn of unspecified degree of unspecified toe(s) (nail)**
- **T25.09 Burn of unspecified degree of multiple sites of ankle and foot**
  - **T25.091 Burn of unspecified degree of multiple sites of right ankle and foot**
  - **T25.092 Burn of unspecified degree of multiple sites of left ankle and foot**
  - **T25.099 Burn of unspecified degree of multiple sites of unspecified ankle and foot**
- **T25.1 Burn of first degree of ankle and foot**

  Use additional external cause code to identify the source, place and intent of the burn (X00-X19, X75-X77, X96-X98, Y92)
  - **T25.11 Burn of first degree of ankle**
    - **T25.111 Burn of first degree of right ankle**
    - **T25.112 Burn of first degree of left ankle**
    - **T25.119 Burn of first degree of unspecified ankle**
  - **T25.12 Burn of first degree of foot**

    Excludes2 burn of first degree of toe(s) (nail) (T25.13-)
    - **T25.121 Burn of first degree of right foot**
    - **T25.122 Burn of first degree of left foot**
    - **T25.129 Burn of first degree of unspecified foot**
  - **T25.13 Burn of first degree of toe(s) (nail)**
    - **T25.131 Burn of first degree of right toe(s) (nail)**
    - **T25.132 Burn of first degree of left toe(s) (nail)**
    - **T25.139 Burn of first degree of unspecified toe(s) (nail)**
  - **T25.19 Burn of first degree of multiple sites of ankle and foot**
    - **T25.191 Burn of first degree of multiple sites of right ankle and foot**
    - **T25.192 Burn of first degree of multiple sites of left ankle and foot**
    - **T25.199 Burn of first degree of multiple sites of unspecified ankle and foot**
- **T25.2 Burn of second degree of ankle and foot**

  Use additional external cause code to identify the source, place and intent of the burn (X00-X19, X75-X77, X96-X98, Y92)
  - **T25.21 Burn of second degree of ankle**
    - **T25.211 Burn of second degree of right ankle**
    - **T25.212 Burn of second degree of left ankle**
    - **T25.219 Burn of second degree of unspecified ankle**
  - **T25.22 Burn of second degree of foot**

    Excludes2 burn of second degree of toe(s) (nail) (T25.23-)
    - **T25.221 Burn of second degree of right foot**
    - **T25.222 Burn of second degree of left foot**
    - **T25.229 Burn of second degree of unspecified foot**
  - **T25.23 Burn of second degree of toe(s) (nail)**
    - **T25.231 Burn of second degree of right toe(s) (nail)**
    - **T25.232 Burn of second degree of left toe(s) (nail)**
    - **T25.239 Burn of second degree of unspecified toe(s) (nail)**
  - **T25.29 Burn of second degree of multiple sites of ankle and foot**
    - **T25.291 Burn of second degree of multiple sites of right ankle and foot**
    - **T25.292 Burn of second degree of multiple sites of left ankle and foot**
    - **T25.299 Burn of second degree of multiple sites of unspecified ankle and foot**
- **T25.3 Burn of third degree of ankle and foot**

  Use additional external cause code to identify the source, place and intent of the burn (X00-X19, X75-X77, X96-X98, Y92)
  - **T25.31 Burn of third degree of ankle**

    Ex: **For category T25.31 CC codes:** T24.301-T24.309[A], T24.391-T24.399[A], T24.701-T24.709[A], T24.791-T24.799[A], T25.311-T25.319[A], T25.391-T25.399[A], T25.711-T25.719[A], T25.791-T25.799[A]
    - **T25.311 Burn of third degree of right ankle** A CC, A Unc
    - **T25.312 Burn of third degree of left ankle** A CC, A Unc
    - **T25.319 Burn of third degree of unspecified ankle** A CC, A Unc
  - **T25.32 Burn of third degree of foot**

    Excludes2 burn of third degree of toe(s) (nail) (T25.33-)

    Ex: **For category T25.32 CC codes:** T24.301-T24.309[A], T24.391-T24.399[A], T24.701-T24.709[A], T24.791-T24.799[A], T25.321-T25.329[A], T25.391-T25.399[A], T25.721-T25.729[A], T25.791-T25.799[A]
    - **T25.321 Burn of third degree of right foot** A CC, A Unc
    - **T25.322 Burn of third degree of left foot** A CC, A Unc
    - **T25.329 Burn of third degree of unspecified foot** A CC, A Unc
  - **T25.33 Burn of third degree of toe(s) (nail)**

    Ex: **For category T25.33 CC codes:** T24.301-T24.309[A], T24.391-T24.399[A], T24.701-T24.709[A], T24.791-T24.799[A], T25.331-T25.339[A], T25.391-T25.399[A] ,T25.731-T25.739[A], T25.791-T25.799[A]
    - **T25.331 Burn of third degree of right toe(s) (nail)** A CC, A Unc
    - **T25.332 Burn of third degree of left toe(s) (nail)** A CC, A Unc
    - **T25.339 Burn of third degree of unspecified toe(s) (nail)** A CC, A Unc
  - **T25.39 Burn of third degree of multiple sites of ankle and foot**

    Ex: **For category T25.39 CC codes:** See T24.30
    - **T25.391 Burn of third degree of multiple sites of right ankle and foot** A CC, A Unc
    - **T25.392 Burn of third degree of multiple sites of left ankle and foot** A CC, A Unc
    - **T25.399 Burn of third degree of multiple sites of unspecified ankle and foot** A CC, A Unc

- **T25.4 Corrosion of unspecified degree of ankle and foot**
  Code first (T51-T65) to identify chemical and intent
  Use additional external cause code to identify place (Y92)
  - **T25.41 Corrosion of unspecified degree of ankle**
    - **T25.411 Corrosion of unspecified degree of right ankle**
    - **T25.412 Corrosion of unspecified degree of left ankle**
    - **T25.419 Corrosion of unspecified degree of unspecified ankle**
  - **T25.42 Corrosion of unspecified degree of foot**
    Excludes2 corrosion of unspecified degree of toe(s) (nail) (T25.43-)
    - **T25.421 Corrosion of unspecified degree of right foot**
    - **T25.422 Corrosion of unspecified degree of left foot**
    - **T25.429 Corrosion of unspecified degree of unspecified foot**
  - **T25.43 Corrosion of unspecified degree of toe(s) (nail)**
    - **T25.431 Corrosion of unspecified degree of right toe(s) (nail)**
    - **T25.432 Corrosion of unspecified degree of left toe(s) (nail)**
    - **T25.439 Corrosion of unspecified degree of unspecified toe(s) (nail)**
  - **T25.49 Corrosion of unspecified degree of multiple sites of ankle and foot**
    - **T25.491 Corrosion of unspecified degree of multiple sites of right ankle and foot**
    - **T25.492 Corrosion of unspecified degree of multiple sites of left ankle and foot**
    - **T25.499 Corrosion of unspecified degree of multiple sites of unspecified ankle and foot**
- **T25.5 Corrosion of first degree of ankle and foot**
  Code first (T51-T65) to identify chemical and intent
  Use additional external cause code to identify place (Y92)
  - **T25.51 Corrosion of first degree of ankle**
    - **T25.511 Corrosion of first degree of right ankle**
    - **T25.512 Corrosion of first degree of left ankle**
    - **T25.519 Corrosion of first degree of unspecified ankle**
  - **T25.52 Corrosion of first degree of foot**
    Excludes2 corrosion of first degree of toe(s) (nail) (T25.53-)
    - **T25.521 Corrosion of first degree of right foot**
    - **T25.522 Corrosion of first degree of left foot**
    - **T25.529 Corrosion of first degree of unspecified foot**
  - **T25.53 Corrosion of first degree of toe(s) (nail)**
    - **T25.531 Corrosion of first degree of right toe(s) (nail)**
    - **T25.532 Corrosion of first degree of left toe(s) (nail)**
    - **T25.539 Corrosion of first degree of unspecified toe(s) (nail)**
  - **T25.59 Corrosion of first degree of multiple sites of ankle and foot**
    - **T25.591 Corrosion of first degree of multiple sites of right ankle and foot**
    - **T25.592 Corrosion of first degree of multiple sites of left ankle and foot**
    - **T25.599 Corrosion of first degree of multiple sites of unspecified ankle and foot**
- **T25.6 Corrosion of second degree of ankle and foot**
  Code first (T51-T65) to identify chemical and intent
  Use additional external cause code to identify place (Y92)
  - **T25.61 Corrosion of second degree of ankle**
    - **T25.611 Corrosion of second degree of right ankle**
    - **T25.612 Corrosion of second degree of left ankle**
    - **T25.619 Corrosion of second degree of unspecified ankle**
  - **T25.62 Corrosion of second degree of foot**
    Excludes2 corrosion of second degree of toe(s) (nail) (T25.63-)
    - **T25.621 Corrosion of second degree of right foot**
    - **T25.622 Corrosion of second degree of left foot**
    - **T25.629 Corrosion of second degree of unspecified foot**
  - **T25.63 Corrosion of second degree of toe(s) (nail)**
    - **T25.631 Corrosion of second degree of right toe(s) (nail)**
    - **T25.632 Corrosion of second degree of left toe(s) (nail)**
    - **T25.639 Corrosion of second degree of unspecified toe(s) (nail)**
  - **T25.69 Corrosion of second degree of multiple sites of ankle and foot**
    - **T25.691 Corrosion of second degree of right ankle and foot**
    - **T25.692 Corrosion of second degree of left ankle and foot**
    - **T25.699 Corrosion of second degree of unspecified ankle and foot**
- **T25.7 Corrosion of third degree of ankle and foot**
  Code first (T51-T65) to identify chemical and intent
  Use additional external cause code to identify place (Y92)
  - **T25.71 Corrosion of third degree of ankle**
    Ex: **For category T25.71 CC codes:** See T25.31
    - **T25.711 Corrosion of third degree of right ankle** A CC, A MCC
    - **T25.712 Corrosion of third degree of left ankle** A CC, A MCC
    - **T25.719 Corrosion of third degree of unspecified ankle** A CC, A MCC
  - **T25.72 Corrosion of third degree of foot**
    Excludes2 corrosion of third degree of toe(s) (nail) (T25.73-)
    Ex: **For category T25.72 CC codes:** See T25.32
    - **T25.721 Corrosion of third degree of right foot** A CC, A MCC
    - **T25.722 Corrosion of third degree of left foot** A CC, A MCC
    - **T25.729 Corrosion of third degree of unspecified foot** A CC, A MCC
  - **T25.73 Corrosion of third degree of toe(s) (nail)**
    Ex: **For category T25.73 CC codes:** See T25.33
    - **T25.731 Corrosion of third degree of right toe(s) (nail)** A CC, A MCC
    - **T25.732 Corrosion of third degree of left toe(s) (nail)** A CC, A MCC
    - **T25.739 Corrosion of third degree of unspecified toe(s) (nail)** A CC, A MCC

● **T25.79 Corrosion of third degree of multiple sites of ankle and foot**

Ex: **For category T25.79 CC codes:** See T24.30

● **T25.791 Corrosion of third degree of multiple sites of right ankle and foot** A CC, A Dx

● **T25.792 Corrosion of third degree of multiple sites of left ankle and foot** A CC, A Dx

● **T25.799 Corrosion of third degree of multiple sites of unspecified ankle and foot** A CC, A Dx

BURNS AND CORROSIONS CONFINED TO EYE AND INTERNAL ORGANS (T26-T28)

● **T26 Burn and corrosion confined to eye and adnexa**

The appropriate 7th character is to be added to each code from category T26

A	initial encounter
D	subsequent encounter
S	sequela

● **T26.0 Burn of eyelid and periocular area**

Use additional external cause code to identify the source, place and intent of the burn (X00-X19, X75-X77, X96-X98, Y92)

X● **T26.00 Burn of unspecified eyelid and periocular area**

X● **T26.01 Burn of right eyelid and periocular area**

X● **T26.02 Burn of left eyelid and periocular area**

● **T26.1 Burn of cornea and conjunctival sac**

Use additional external cause code to identify the source, place and intent of the burn (X00-X19, X75-X77, X96-X98, Y92)

X● **T26.10 Burn of cornea and conjunctival sac, unspecified eye**

X● **T26.11 Burn of cornea and conjunctival sac, right eye**

X● **T26.12 Burn of cornea and conjunctival sac, left eye**

● **T26.2 Burn with resulting rupture and destruction of eyeball**

Use additional external cause code to identify the source, place and intent of the burn (X00-X19, X75-X77, X96-X98, Y92)

Ex: **For category T26.2 CC codes:** No exclusions

X● **T26.20 Burn with resulting rupture and destruction of unspecified eyeball** A CC, A Dx

X● **T26.21 Burn with resulting rupture and destruction of right eyeball** A CC, A Dx

X● **T26.22 Burn with resulting rupture and destruction of left eyeball** A CC, A Dx

● **T26.3 Burns of other specified parts of eye and adnexa**

Use additional external cause code to identify the source, place and intent of the burn (X00-X19, X75-X77, X96-X98, Y92)

X● **T26.30 Burns of other specified parts of unspecified eye and adnexa**

X● **T26.31 Burns of other specified parts of right eye and adnexa**

X● **T26.32 Burns of other specified parts of left eye and adnexa**

● **T26.4 Burn of eye and adnexa, part unspecified**

Use additional external cause code to identify the source, place and intent of the burn (X00-X19, X75-X77, X96-X98, Y92)

X● **T26.40 Burn of unspecified eye and adnexa, part unspecified**

X● **T26.41 Burn of right eye and adnexa, part unspecified**

X● **T26.42 Burn of left eye and adnexa, part unspecified**

● **T26.5 Corrosion of eyelid and periocular area**

Code first (T51-T65) to identify chemical and intent

Use additional external cause code to identify place (Y92)

X● **T26.50 Corrosion of unspecified eyelid and periocular area**

X● **T26.51 Corrosion of right eyelid and periocular area**

X● **T26.52 Corrosion of left eyelid and periocular area**

● **T26.6 Corrosion of cornea and conjunctival sac**

Code first (T51-T65) to identify chemical and intent

Use additional external cause code to identify place (Y92)

X● **T26.60 Corrosion of cornea and conjunctival sac, unspecified eye**

X● **T26.61 Corrosion of cornea and conjunctival sac, right eye**

X● **T26.62 Corrosion of cornea and conjunctival sac, left eye**

● **T26.7 Corrosion with resulting rupture and destruction of eyeball**

Code first (T51-T65) to identify chemical and intent

Use additional external cause code to identify place (Y92)

Ex: **For category T26.7 CC codes:** No exclusions

X● **T26.70 Corrosion with resulting rupture and destruction of unspecified eyeball** A CC, A Dx

X● **T26.71 Corrosion with resulting rupture and destruction of right eyeball** A CC, A Dx

X● **T26.72 Corrosion with resulting rupture and destruction of left eyeball** A CC, A Dx

● **T26.8 Corrosions of other specified parts of eye and adnexa**

Code first (T51-T65) to identify chemical and intent

Use additional external cause code to identify place (Y92)

X● **T26.80 Corrosions of other specified parts of unspecified eye and adnexa**

X● **T26.81 Corrosions of other specified parts of right eye and adnexa**

X● **T26.82 Corrosions of other specified parts of left eye and adnexa**

● **T26.9 Corrosion of eye and adnexa, part unspecified**

Code first (T51-T65) to identify chemical and intent

Use additional external cause code to identify place (Y92)

X● **T26.90 Corrosion of unspecified eye and adnexa, part unspecified**

X● **T26.91 Corrosion of right eye and adnexa, part unspecified**

X● **T26.92 Corrosion of left eye and adnexa, part unspecified**

● **T27 Burn and corrosion of respiratory tract**

Use additional external cause code to identify the source and intent of the burn (X00-X19, X75-X77, X96-X98)

Use additional external cause code to identify place (Y92)

The appropriate 7th character is to be added to each code from category T27

A	initial encounter
D	subsequent encounter
S	sequela

Ex: **For category T27 CC codes:** T27.0XX-T27.7XX[A], T28.3XX-T28.49X[A], T28.8XX-T28.99X[A]

X● **T27.0 Burn of larynx and trachea** A CC, A Dx

X● **T27.1 Burn involving larynx and trachea with lung** A CC, A Dx

X● **T27.2 Burn of other parts of respiratory tract** A CC, A Dx

Burn of thoracic cavity

X● **T27.3** **Burn of respiratory tract, part unspecified** A, A
Code first (T51-T65) to identify chemical and intent for codes T27.4-T27.7

X● **T27.4** **Corrosion of larynx and trachea** A, A

X● **T27.5** **Corrosion involving larynx and trachea with lung** A, A

X● **T27.6** **Corrosion of other parts of respiratory tract** A, A

X● **T27.7** **Corrosion of respiratory tract, part unspecified** A, A

● **T28** **Burn and corrosion of other internal organs**

Use additional external cause code to identify the source and intent of the burn (X00-X19, X75-X77, X96-X98)

Use additional external cause code to identify place (Y92)

The appropriate 7th character is to be added to each code from category T28

A	initial encounter
D	subsequent encounter
S	sequela

X● **T28.0** **Burn of mouth and pharynx**

X● **T28.1** **Burn of esophagus** A, A
Ex: T28.1XX[A], T28.3XX-T28.49X[A], T28.6XX[A], T28.8XX-T28.99X[A]

X● **T28.2** **Burn of other parts of alimentary tract** A, A
Ex: T28.2XX-T28.49X[A], T28.7XX-T28.99X[A]

X● **T28.3** **Burn of internal genitourinary organs**

X● **T28.4** **Burns of other and unspecified internal organs**

X● **T28.40** **Burn of unspecified internal organ**

● **T28.41** **Burn of ear drum**

● **T28.411** **Burn of right ear drum**

● **T28.412** **Burn of left ear drum**

● **T28.419** **Burn of unspecified ear drum**

X● **T28.49** **Burn of other internal organ**
Code first (T51-T65) to identify chemical and intent for T28.5-T28.9-

X● **T28.5** **Corrosion of mouth and pharynx**

X● **T28.6** **Corrosion of esophagus** A, A
Ex: See T28.1

X● **T28.7** **Corrosion of other parts of alimentary tract** A, A
Ex: See T28.2

X● **T28.8** **Corrosion of internal genitourinary organs**

● **T28.9** **Corrosions of other and unspecified internal organs**

X● **T28.90** **Corrosions of unspecified internal organs**

● **T28.91** **Corrosions of ear drum**

● **T28.911** **Corrosions of right ear drum**

● **T28.912** **Corrosions of left ear drum**

● **T28.919** **Corrosions of unspecified ear drum**

X● **T28.99** **Corrosions of other internal organs**

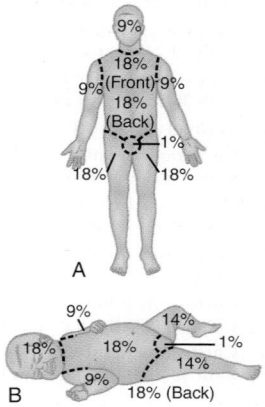

Figure 19-16 Rule of nines: percentages of total body area. (From Marx: Rosen's Emergency Medicine: Concepts and Clinical Practice, ed 6, Mosby, 2006)

OGCR Section I.C.19.d.5.

Assign separate code for each burn site

When coding burns, assign separate codes for each burn site. Category T30, Burn and corrosion, body region unspecified is extremely vague and should rarely be used.

BURNS AND CORROSIONS OF MULTIPLE AND UNSPECIFIED BODY REGIONS (T30-T32)

● **T30** **Burn and corrosion, body region unspecified**

T30.0 **Burn of unspecified body region, unspecified degree**
This code is not for inpatient use. Code to specified site and degree of burns
Burn NOS
Multiple burns NOS

T30.4 **Corrosion of unspecified body region, unspecified degree**
This code is not for inpatient use. Code to specified site and degree of corrosion
Corrosion NOS
Multiple corrosion NOS

● **T31** **Burns classified according to extent of body surface involved**

Note: This category is to be used as the primary code only when the site of the burn is unspecified. It should be used as a supplementary code with categories T20-T25 when the site is specified.
Ex: For category T31 CC codes: T31.0-T32.99

T31.0 **Burns involving less than 10% of body surface**

● **T31.1** **Burns involving 10-19% of body surface**

T31.10 **Burns involving 10-19% of body surface with 0% to 9% third degree burns**
Burns involving 10-19% of body surface NOS

T31.11 **Burns involving 10-19% of body surface with 10-19% third degree burns**

● **T31.2** **Burns involving 20-29% of body surface**

T31.20 **Burns involving 20-29% of body surface with 0% to 9% third degree burns**
Burns involving 20-29% of body surface NOS

T31.21 **Burns involving 20-29% of body surface with 10-19% third degree burns**

T31.22 **Burns involving 20-29% of body surface with 20-29% third degree burns**

● **T31.3** **Burns involving 30-39% of body surface**

T31.30 **Burns involving 30-39% of body surface with 0% to 9% third degree burns**
Burns involving 30-39% of body surface NOS

T31.31 **Burns involving 30-39% of body surface with 10-19% third degree burns**

T31.32 **Burns involving 30-39% of body surface with 20-29% third degree burns**

T31.33 **Burns involving 30-39% of body surface with 30-39% third degree burns**

● **T31.4** **Burns involving 40-49% of body surface**

T31.40 **Burns involving 40-49% of body surface with 0% to 9% third degree burns**
Burns involving 40-49% of body surface NOS

T31.41 **Burns involving 40-49% of body surface with 10-19% third degree burns**

T31.42 **Burns involving 40-49% of body surface with 20-29% third degree burns**

T31.43 **Burns involving 40-49% of body surface with 30-39% third degree burns**

T31.44 **Burns involving 40-49% of body surface with 40-49% third degree burns**

● **T31.5 Burns involving 50-59% of body surface**

T31.50 Burns involving 50-59% of body surface with 0% to 9% third degree burns
Burns involving 50-59% of body surface NOS

T31.51 Burns involving 50-59% of body surface with 10-19% third degree burns

T31.52 Burns involving 50-59% of body surface with 20-29% third degree burns

T31.53 Burns involving 50-59% of body surface with 30-39% third degree burns

T31.54 Burns involving 50-59% of body surface with 40-49% third degree burns

T31.55 Burns involving 50-59% of body surface with 50-59% third degree burns

● **T31.6 Burns involving 60-69% of body surface**

T31.60 Burns involving 60-69% of body surface with 0% to 9% third degree burns
Burns involving 60-69% of body surface NOS

T31.61 Burns involving 60-69% of body surface with 10-19% third degree burns

T31.62 Burns involving 60-69% of body surface with 20-29% third degree burns

T31.63 Burns involving 60-69% of body surface with 30-39% third degree burns

T31.64 Burns involving 60-69% of body surface with 40-49% third degree burns

T31.65 Burns involving 60-69% of body surface with 50-59% third degree burns

T31.66 Burns involving 60-69% of body surface with 60-69% third degree burns

● **T31.7 Burns involving 70-79% of body surface**

T31.70 Burns involving 70-79% of body surface with 0% to 9% third degree burns
Burns involving 70-79% of body surface NOS

T31.71 Burns involving 70-79% of body surface with 10-19% third degree burns

T31.72 Burns involving 70-79% of body surface with 20-29% third degree burns

T31.73 Burns involving 70-79% of body surface with 30-39% third degree burns

T31.74 Burns involving 70-79% of body surface with 40-49% third degree burns

T31.75 Burns involving 70-79% of body surface with 50-59% third degree burns

T31.76 Burns involving 70-79% of body surface with 60-69% third degree burns

T31.77 Burns involving 70-79% of body surface with 70-79% third degree burns

● **T31.8 Burns involving 80-89% of body surface**

T31.80 Burns involving 80-89% of body surface with 0% to 9% third degree burns
Burns involving 80-89% of body surface NOS

T31.81 Burns involving 80-89% of body surface with 10-19% third degree burns

T31.82 Burns involving 80-89% of body surface with 20-29% third degree burns

T31.83 Burns involving 80-89% of body surface with 30-39% third degree burns

T31.84 Burns involving 80-89% of body surface with 40-49% third degree burns

T31.85 Burns involving 80-89% of body surface with 50-59% third degree burns

T31.86 Burns involving 80-89% of body surface with 60-69% third degree burns

T31.87 Burns involving 80-89% of body surface with 70-79% third degree burns

T31.88 Burns involving 80-89% of body surface with 80-89% third degree burns

● **T31.9 Burns involving 90% or more of body surface**

T31.90 Burns involving 90% or more of body surface with 0% to 9% third degree burns
Burns involving 90% or more of body surface NOS

T31.91 Burns involving 90% or more of body surface with 10-19% third degree burns

T31.92 Burns involving 90% or more of body surface with 20-29% third degree burns

T31.93 Burns involving 90% or more of body surface with 30-39% third degree burns

T31.94 Burns involving 90% or more of body surface with 40-49% third degree burns

T31.95 Burns involving 90% or more of body surface with 50-59% third degree burns

T31.96 Burns involving 90% or more of body surface with 60-69% third degree burns

T31.97 Burns involving 90% or more of body surface with 70-79% third degree burns

T31.98 Burns involving 90% or more of body surface with 80-89% third degree burns

T31.99 Burns involving 90% or more of body surface with 90% or more third degree burns

● **T32 Corrosions classified according to extent of body surface involved**

Note: This category is to be used as the primary code only when the site of the corrosion is unspecified. It may be used as a supplementary code with categories T20-T25 when the site is specified.

Ex: For category T32 CC codes: T31.0-T32.99

T32.0 Corrosions involving less than 10% of body surface

● **T32.1 Corrosions involving 10-19% of body surface**

T32.10 Corrosions involving 10-19% of body surface with 0% to 9% third degree corrosion
Corrosions involving 10-19% of body surface NOS

T32.11 Corrosions involving 10-19% of body surface with 10-19% third degree corrosion

● **T32.2 Corrosions involving 20-29% of body surface**

T32.20 Corrosions involving 20-29% of body surface with 0% to 9% third degree corrosion

T32.21 Corrosions involving 20-29% of body surface with 10-19% third degree corrosion

T32.22 Corrosions involving 20-29% of body surface with 20-29% third degree corrosion

● **T32.3 Corrosions involving 30-39% of body surface**

T32.30 Corrosions involving 30-39% of body surface with 0% to 9% third degree corrosion

T32.31 Corrosions involving 30-39% of body surface with 10-19% third degree corrosion

T32.32 Corrosions involving 30-39% of body surface with 20-29% third degree corrosion

T32.33 Corrosions involving 30-39% of body surface with 30-39% third degree corrosion

● **T32.4 Corrosions involving 40-49% of body surface**

T32.40 Corrosions involving 40-49% of body surface with 0% to 9% third degree corrosion

T32.41 Corrosions involving 40-49% of body surface with 10-19% third degree corrosion

T32.42 Corrosions involving 40-49% of body surface with 20-29% third degree corrosion

T32.43 Corrosions involving 40-49% of body surface with 30-39% third degree corrosion

T32.44 Corrosions involving 40-49% of body surface with 40-49% third degree corrosion

● T32.5 Corrosions involving 50-59% of body surface
- T32.50 Corrosions involving 50-59% of body surface with 0% to 9% third degree corrosion
- T32.51 Corrosions involving 50-59% of body surface with 10-19% third degree corrosion
- T32.52 Corrosions involving 50-59% of body surface with 20-29% third degree corrosion
- T32.53 Corrosions involving 50-59% of body surface with 30-39% third degree corrosion
- T32.54 Corrosions involving 50-59% of body surface with 40-49% third degree corrosion
- T32.55 Corrosions involving 50-59% of body surface with 50-59% third degree corrosion

● T32.6 Corrosions involving 60-69% of body surface
- T32.60 Corrosions involving 60-69% of body surface with 0% to 9% third degree corrosion
- T32.61 Corrosions involving 60-69% of body surface with 10-19% third degree corrosion
- T32.62 Corrosions involving 60-69% of body surface with 20-29% third degree corrosion
- T32.63 Corrosions involving 60-69% of body surface with 30-39% third degree corrosion
- T32.64 Corrosions involving 60-69% of body surface with 40-49% third degree corrosion
- T32.65 Corrosions involving 60-69% of body surface with 50-59% third degree corrosion
- T32.66 Corrosions involving 60-69% of body surface with 60-69% third degree corrosion

● T32.7 Corrosions involving 70-79% of body surface
- T32.70 Corrosions involving 70-79% of body surface with 0% to 9% third degree corrosion
- T32.71 Corrosions involving 70-79% of body surface with 10-19% third degree corrosion
- T32.72 Corrosions involving 70-79% of body surface with 20-29% third degree corrosion
- T32.73 Corrosions involving 70-79% of body surface with 30-39% third degree corrosion
- T32.74 Corrosions involving 70-79% of body surface with 40-49% third degree corrosion
- T32.75 Corrosions involving 70-79% of body surface with 50-59% third degree corrosion
- T32.76 Corrosions involving 70-79% of body surface with 60-69% third degree corrosion
- T32.77 Corrosions involving 70-79% of body surface with 70-79% third degree corrosion

● T32.8 Corrosions involving 80-89% of body surface
- T32.80 Corrosions involving 80-89% of body surface with 0% to 9% third degree corrosion
- T32.81 Corrosions involving 80-89% of body surface with 10-19% third degree corrosion
- T32.82 Corrosions involving 80-89% of body surface with 20-29% third degree corrosion
- T32.83 Corrosions involving 80-89% of body surface with 30-39% third degree corrosion
- T32.84 Corrosions involving 80-89% of body surface with 40-49% third degree corrosion
- T32.85 Corrosions involving 80-89% of body surface with 50-59% third degree corrosion
- T32.86 Corrosions involving 80-89% of body surface with 60-69% third degree corrosion
- T32.87 Corrosions involving 80-89% of body surface with 70-79% third degree corrosion
- T32.88 Corrosions involving 80-89% of body surface with 80-89% third degree corrosion

● T32.9 Corrosions involving 90% or more of body surface
- T32.90 Corrosions involving 90% or more of body surface with 0% to 9% third degree corrosion
- T32.91 Corrosions involving 90% or more of body surface with 10-19% third degree corrosion
- T32.92 Corrosions involving 90% or more of body surface with 20-29% third degree corrosion
- T32.93 Corrosions involving 90% or more of body surface with 30-39% third degree corrosion
- T32.94 Corrosions involving 90% or more of body surface with 40-49% third degree corrosion
- T32.95 Corrosions involving 90% or more of body surface with 50-59% third degree corrosion
- T32.96 Corrosions involving 90% or more of body surface with 60-69% third degree corrosion
- T32.97 Corrosions involving 90% or more of body surface with 70-79% third degree corrosion
- T32.98 Corrosions involving 90% or more of body surface with 80-89% third degree corrosion
- T32.99 Corrosions involving 90% or more of body surface with 90% or more third degree corrosion

FROSTBITE (T33-T34)

Excludes2 hypothermia and other effects of reduced temperature (T68, T69.-)

● T33 Superficial frostbite

Includes frostbite with partial thickness skin loss

The appropriate 7th character is to be added to each code from category T33

A	initial encounter
D	subsequent encounter
S	sequela

● T33.0 Superficial frostbite of head

Ex: For category T33.0 CC codes: T33.011-T33.42X[A], T33.60X-T33.72X[A], T33.90X-T34.42X[A], T34.60X-T34.72X[A], T34.90X-T34.99X[A]

● T33.01 Superficial frostbite of ear

● T33.011 Superficial frostbite of right ear A, A

● T33.012 Superficial frostbite of left ear A, A

● T33.019 Superficial frostbite of unspecified ear A, A

X● T33.02 Superficial frostbite of nose A, A

X● T33.09 Superficial frostbite of other part of head A, A

X● T33.1 Superficial frostbite of neck A, A

Ex: See T33.0

X● T33.2 Superficial frostbite of thorax A, A

Ex: T33.011-T34.99X[A], T69.021-T69.029[A]

X● T33.3 Superficial frostbite of abdominal wall, lower back and pelvis A, A

Ex: See T33.2

CHAPTER 19 (S00-T88)

● T33.4 Superficial frostbite of arm
Excludes2 superficial frostbite of wrist and hand (T33.5-)
Ex: For category T33.4 CC codes: See T33.2
X● T33.40 Superficial frostbite of unspecified arm A CC, A Dx
X● T33.41 Superficial frostbite of right arm A CC, A Dx
X● T33.42 Superficial frostbite of left arm A CC, A Dx
● T33.5 Superficial frostbite of wrist, hand, and fingers
Ex: For category T33.5 CC codes: T33.2XX-T33.72X[A], T33.90X-T33.99X[A], T34.2XX-T34.72X[A], T34.90X-T34.99X[A]
● T33.51 Superficial frostbite of wrist
● T33.511 Superficial frostbite of right wrist A CC, A Dx
● T33.512 Superficial frostbite of left wrist A CC, A Dx
● T33.519 Superficial frostbite of unspecified wrist A CC, A Dx
● T33.52 Superficial frostbite of hand
Excludes2 superficial frostbite of fingers (T33.53-)
● T33.521 Superficial frostbite of right hand A CC, A Dx
● T33.522 Superficial frostbite of left hand A CC, A Dx
● T33.529 Superficial frostbite of unspecified hand A CC, A Dx
● T33.53 Superficial frostbite of finger(s)
● T33.531 Superficial frostbite of right finger(s) A CC, A Dx
● T33.532 Superficial frostbite of left finger(s) A CC, A Dx
● T33.539 Superficial frostbite of unspecified finger(s) A CC, A Dx
● T33.6 Superficial frostbite of hip and thigh
Ex: For category T33.6 CC codes: See T33.2
X● T33.60 Superficial frostbite of unspecified hip and thigh A CC, A Dx
X● T33.61 Superficial frostbite of right hip and thigh A CC, A Dx
X● T33.62 Superficial frostbite of left hip and thigh A CC, A Dx
● T33.7 Superficial frostbite of knee and lower leg
Excludes2 superficial frostbite of ankle and foot (T33.8-)
Ex: For category T33.7 CC codes: See T33.2
X● T33.70 Superficial frostbite of unspecified knee and lower leg A CC, A Dx
X● T33.71 Superficial frostbite of right knee and lower leg A CC, A Dx
X● T33.72 Superficial frostbite of left knee and lower leg A CC, A Dx
● T33.8 Superficial frostbite of ankle, foot, and toe(s)
Ex: For category T33.8 CC codes: T33.2XX-T33.42X[A], T33.60X-T33.99X[A], T34.2XX-T34.42X[A], T34.60X-T34.99X[A]
● T33.81 Superficial frostbite of ankle
● T33.811 Superficial frostbite of right ankle A CC, A Dx
● T33.812 Superficial frostbite of left ankle A CC, A Dx
● T33.819 Superficial frostbite of unspecified ankle A CC, A Dx
● T33.82 Superficial frostbite of foot
● T33.821 Superficial frostbite of right foot A CC, A Dx
● T33.822 Superficial frostbite of left foot A CC, A Dx
● T33.829 Superficial frostbite of unspecified foot A CC, A Dx
● T33.83 Superficial frostbite of toe(s)
● T33.831 Superficial frostbite of right toe(s) A CC, A Dx
● T33.832 Superficial frostbite of left toe(s) A CC, A Dx
● T33.839 Superficial frostbite of unspecified toe(s) A CC, A Dx
● T33.9 Superficial frostbite of other and unspecified sites
Ex: For category T33.9 CC codes: See T33.2
X● T33.90 Superficial frostbite of unspecified sites A CC, A Dx
Superficial frostbite NOS
X● T33.99 Superficial frostbite of other sites A CC, A Dx
Superficial frostbite of leg NOS
Superficial frostbite of trunk NOS

● T34 Frostbite with tissue necrosis
The appropriate 7th character is to be added to each code from category T34

A	initial encounter
D	subsequent encounter
S	sequela

● T34.0 Frostbite with tissue necrosis of head
Ex: For category T34.0 CC codes: See T33.0
● T34.01 Frostbite with tissue necrosis of ear
● T34.011 Frostbite with tissue necrosis of right ear A CC, A Dx
● T34.012 Frostbite with tissue necrosis of left ear A CC, A Dx
● T34.019 Frostbite with tissue necrosis of unspecified ear A CC, A Dx
X● T34.02 Frostbite with tissue necrosis of nose A CC, A Dx
X● T34.09 Frostbite with tissue necrosis of other part of head A CC, A Dx
X● T34.1 Frostbite with tissue necrosis of neck A CC, A Dx
Ex: See T33.0
X● T34.2 Frostbite with tissue necrosis of thorax A CC, A Dx
Ex: See T33.2
X● T34.3 Frostbite with tissue necrosis of abdominal wall, lower back and pelvis A CC, A Dx
Ex: See T33.2
● T34.4 Frostbite with tissue necrosis of arm
Excludes2 frostbite with tissue necrosis of wrist and hand (T34.5-)
Ex: For category T34.4 CC codes: See T33.2
X● T34.40 Frostbite with tissue necrosis of unspecified arm A CC, A Dx
X● T34.41 Frostbite with tissue necrosis of right arm A CC, A Dx
X● T34.42 Frostbite with tissue necrosis of left arm A CC, A Dx
● T34.5 Frostbite with tissue necrosis of wrist, hand, and finger(s)
Ex: For category T34.5 CC codes: See T33.5
● T34.51 Frostbite with tissue necrosis of wrist
● T34.511 Frostbite with tissue necrosis of right wrist A CC, A Dx
● T34.512 Frostbite with tissue necrosis of left wrist A CC, A Dx
● T34.519 Frostbite with tissue necrosis of unspecified wrist A CC, A Dx

- **T34.52 Frostbite with tissue necrosis of hand**
  - **Excludes2** frostbite with tissue necrosis of finger(s) (T34.53-)
  - **T34.521 Frostbite with tissue necrosis of right hand** A CC, A MCC
  - **T34.522 Frostbite with tissue necrosis of left hand** A CC, A MCC
  - **T34.529 Frostbite with tissue necrosis of unspecified hand** A CC, A MCC
- **T34.53 Frostbite with tissue necrosis of finger(s)**
  - **T34.531 Frostbite with tissue necrosis of right finger(s)** A CC, A MCC
  - **T34.532 Frostbite with tissue necrosis of left finger(s)** A CC, A MCC
  - **T34.539 Frostbite with tissue necrosis of unspecified finger(s)** A CC, A MCC
- **T34.6 Frostbite with tissue necrosis of hip and thigh**
  - Ex: For category T34.6 CC codes: See T33.2
  - X **T34.60 Frostbite with tissue necrosis of unspecified hip and thigh** A CC, A MCC
  - X **T34.61 Frostbite with tissue necrosis of right hip and thigh** A CC, A MCC
  - X **T34.62 Frostbite with tissue necrosis of left hip and thigh** A CC, A MCC
- **T34.7 Frostbite with tissue necrosis of knee and lower leg**
  - **Excludes2** frostbite with tissue necrosis of ankle and foot (T34.8-)
  - Ex: For category T34.7 CC codes: See T33.2
  - X **T34.70 Frostbite with tissue necrosis of unspecified knee and lower leg** A CC, A MCC
  - X **T34.71 Frostbite with tissue necrosis of right knee and lower leg** A CC, A MCC
  - X **T34.72 Frostbite with tissue necrosis of left knee and lower leg** A CC, A MCC
- **T34.8 Frostbite with tissue necrosis of ankle, foot, and toe(s)**
  - Ex: For category T34.8 CC codes: See T33.8
  - **T34.81 Frostbite with tissue necrosis of ankle**
    - **T34.811 Frostbite with tissue necrosis of right ankle** A CC, A MCC
    - **T34.812 Frostbite with tissue necrosis of left ankle** A CC, A MCC
    - **T34.819 Frostbite with tissue necrosis of unspecified ankle** A CC, A MCC
  - **T34.82 Frostbite with tissue necrosis of foot**
    - **T34.821 Frostbite with tissue necrosis of right foot** A CC, A MCC
    - **T34.822 Frostbite with tissue necrosis of left foot** A CC, A MCC
    - **T34.829 Frostbite with tissue necrosis of unspecified foot** A CC, A MCC
  - **T34.83 Frostbite with tissue necrosis of toe(s)**
    - **T34.831 Frostbite with tissue necrosis of right toe(s)** A CC, A MCC
    - **T34.832 Frostbite with tissue necrosis of left toe(s)** A CC, A MCC
    - **T34.839 Frostbite with tissue necrosis of unspecified toe(s)** A CC, A MCC
- **T34.9 Frostbite with tissue necrosis of other and unspecified sites**
  - Ex: For category T34.9 CC codes: See T33.2
  - X **T34.90 Frostbite with tissue necrosis of unspecified sites** A CC, A MCC
    - Frostbite with tissue necrosis NOS
  - X **T34.99 Frostbite with tissue necrosis of other sites** A CC, A MCC
    - Frostbite with tissue necrosis of leg NOS
    - Frostbite with tissue necrosis of trunk NOS

OGCR See Section I.C.19.e.

Adverse Effects, Poisoning , Underdosing and Toxic Effects

Codes in categories T36-T65 are combination codes that include the substance that was taken as well as the intent. No additional external cause code is required for poisonings, toxic effects, adverse effects and underdosing codes.

POISONING BY, ADVERSE EFFECTS OF AND UNDERDOSING OF DRUGS MEDICAMENTS AND BIOLOGICAL SUBSTANCES (T36-T50)

Includes adverse effect of correct substance properly administered
poisoning by overdose of substance
poisoning by wrong substance given or taken in error
underdosing by (inadvertently) (deliberately) taking less substance than prescribed or instructed

Code first, for adverse effects, the nature of the adverse effect, such as:
adverse effect NOS (T88.7)
aspirin gastritis (K29.-)
blood disorders (D56-D76)
contact dermatitis (L23-L25)
dermatitis due to substances taken internally (L27.-)
nephropathy (N14.0-N14.2)

Note: The drug giving rise to the adverse effect should be identified by use of codes from categories T36-T50 with fifth or sixth character 5.

Use additional code(s) to specify:
manifestations of poisoning
underdosing or failure in dosage during medical and surgical care (Y63.6, Y63.8-Y63.9)
underdosing of medication regimen (Z91.12-, Z91.13-)

Excludes1 toxic reaction to local anesthesia in pregnancy (O29.3-)

Excludes2 abuse and dependence of psychoactive substances (F10-F19)
abuse of non-dependence-producing substances (F55.-)
drug reaction and poisoning affecting newborn (P00-P96)
pathological drug intoxication (inebriation) (F10-F19)

- **T36 Poisoning by, adverse effect of and underdosing of systemic antibiotics**
  - **Excludes1** antineoplastic antibiotics (T45.1-)
    locally applied antibiotic NEC (T49.0)
    topically used antibiotic for ear, nose and throat (T49.6)
    topically used antibiotic for eye (T49.5)

  The appropriate 7th character is to be added to each code from category T36

A	initial encounter
D	subsequent encounter
S	sequela

  - **T36.0 Poisoning by, adverse effect of and underdosing of penicillins**
    - **T36.0X Poisoning by, adverse effect of and underdosing of penicillins**
      - **T36.0X1 Poisoning by penicillins, accidental (unintentional)**
        - Poisoning by penicillins NOS
      - **T36.0X2 Poisoning by penicillins, intentional self-harm**
      - **T36.0X3 Poisoning by penicillins, assault**
      - **T36.0X4 Poisoning by penicillins, undetermined**
      - **T36.0X5 Adverse effect of penicillins**
      - **T36.0X6 Underdosing of penicillins**

- **T36.1 Poisoning by, adverse effect of and underdosing of cephalosporins and other betalactam antibiotics**
  - **T36.1X Poisoning by, adverse effect of and underdosing of cephalosporins and other beta-lactam antibiotics**
    - **T36.1X1 Poisoning by cephalosporins and other beta-lactam antibiotics, accidental (unintentional)**
      Poisoning by cephalosporins and other beta-lactam antibiotics NOS
    - **T36.1X2 Poisoning by cephalosporins and other beta-lactam antibiotics, intentional self-harm**
    - **T36.1X3 Poisoning by cephalosporins and other beta-lactam antibiotics, assault**
    - **T36.1X4 Poisoning by cephalosporins and other beta-lactam antibiotics, undetermined**
    - **T36.1X5 Adverse effect of cephalosporins and other beta-lactam antibiotics**
    - **T36.1X6 Underdosing of cephalosporins and other beta-lactam antibiotics**
- **T36.2 Poisoning by, adverse effect of and underdosing of chloramphenicol group**
  - **T36.2X Poisoning by, adverse effect of and underdosing of chloramphenicol group**
    - **T36.2X1 Poisoning by chloramphenicol group, accidental (unintentional)**
      Poisoning by chloramphenicol group NOS
    - **T36.2X2 Poisoning by chloramphenicol group, intentional self-harm**
    - **T36.2X3 Poisoning by chloramphenicol group, assault**
    - **T36.2X4 Poisoning by chloramphenicol group, undetermined**
    - **T36.2X5 Adverse effect of chloramphenicol group**
    - **T36.2X6 Underdosing of chloramphenicol group**
- **T36.3 Poisoning by, adverse effect of and underdosing of macrolides**
  - **T36.3X Poisoning by, adverse effect of and underdosing of macrolides**
    - **T36.3X1 Poisoning by macrolides, accidental (unintentional)**
      Poisoning by macrolides NOS
    - **T36.3X2 Poisoning by macrolides, intentional self-harm**
    - **T36.3X3 Poisoning by macrolides, assault**
    - **T36.3X4 Poisoning by macrolides, undetermined**
    - **T36.3X5 Adverse effect of macrolides**
    - **T36.3X6 Underdosing of macrolides**
- **T36.4 Poisoning by, adverse effect of and underdosing of tetracyclines**
  - **T36.4X Poisoning by, adverse effect of and underdosing of tetracyclines**
    - **T36.4X1 Poisoning by tetracyclines, accidental (unintentional)**
      Poisoning by tetracyclines NOS
    - **T36.4X2 Poisoning by tetracyclines, intentional self-harm**
    - **T36.4X3 Poisoning by tetracyclines, assault**
    - **T36.4X4 Poisoning by tetracyclines, undetermined**
    - **T36.4X5 Adverse effect of tetracyclines**
    - **T36.4X6 Underdosing of tetracyclines**
- **T36.5 Poisoning by, adverse effect of and underdosing of aminoglycosides**
  Poisoning by, adverse effect of and underdosing of streptomycin
  - **T36.5X Poisoning by, adverse effect of and underdosing of aminoglycosides**
    - **T36.5X1 Poisoning by aminoglycosides, accidental (unintentional)**
      Poisoning by aminoglycosides NOS
    - **T36.5X2 Poisoning by aminoglycosides, intentional self-harm**
    - **T36.5X3 Poisoning by aminoglycosides, assault**
    - **T36.5X4 Poisoning by aminoglycosides, undetermined**
    - **T36.5X5 Adverse effect of aminoglycosides**
    - **T36.5X6 Underdosing of aminoglycosides**
- **T36.6 Poisoning by, adverse effect of and underdosing of rifampicins**
  - **T36.6X Poisoning by, adverse effect of and underdosing of rifampicins**
    - **T36.6X1 Poisoning by rifampicins, accidental (unintentional)**
      Poisoning by rifampicins NOS
    - **T36.6X2 Poisoning by rifampicins, intentional self-harm**
    - **T36.6X3 Poisoning by rifampicins, assault**
    - **T36.6X4 Poisoning by rifampicins, undetermined**
    - **T36.6X5 Adverse effect of rifampicins**
    - **T36.6X6 Underdosing of rifampicins**
- **T36.7 Poisoning by, adverse effect of and underdosing of antifungal antibiotics, systemically used**
  - **T36.7X Poisoning by, adverse effect of and underdosing of antifungal antibiotics, systemically used**
    - **T36.7X1 Poisoning by antifungal antibiotics, systemically used, accidental (unintentional)**
      Poisoning by antifungal antibiotics, systemically used NOS
    - **T36.7X2 Poisoning by antifungal antibiotics, systemically used, intentional self-harm**
    - **T36.7X3 Poisoning by antifungal antibiotics, systemically used, assault**
    - **T36.7X4 Poisoning by antifungal antibiotics, systemically used, undetermined**
    - **T36.7X5 Adverse effect of antifungal antibiotics, systemically used**
    - **T36.7X6 Underdosing of antifungal antibiotics, systemically used**
- **T36.8 Poisoning by, adverse effect of and underdosing of other systemic antibiotics**
  - **T36.8X Poisoning by, adverse effect of and underdosing of other systemic antibiotics**
    - **T36.8X1 Poisoning by other systemic antibiotics, accidental (unintentional)**
      Poisoning by other systemic antibiotics NOS
    - **T36.8X2 Poisoning by other systemic antibiotics, intentional self-harm**
    - **T36.8X3 Poisoning by other systemic antibiotics, assault**
    - **T36.8X4 Poisoning by other systemic antibiotics, undetermined**
    - **T36.8X5 Adverse effect of other systemic antibiotics**
    - **T36.8X6 Underdosing of other systemic antibiotics**

- **T36.9 Poisoning by, adverse effect of and underdosing of unspecified systemic antibiotic**
  - X **T36.91 Poisoning by unspecified systemic antibiotic, accidental (unintentional)**
    Poisoning by systemic antibiotic NOS
  - X **T36.92 Poisoning by unspecified systemic antibiotic, intentional self-harm**
  - X **T36.93 Poisoning by unspecified systemic antibiotic, assault**
  - X **T36.94 Poisoning by unspecified systemic antibiotic, undetermined**
  - X **T36.95 Adverse effect of unspecified systemic antibiotic**
  - X **T36.96 Underdosing of unspecified systemic antibiotic**

- **T37 Poisoning by, adverse effect of and underdosing of other systemic anti-infectives and antiparasitics**

  Excludes1 anti-infectives topically used for ear, nose and throat (T49.6-)
  anti-infectives topically used for eye (T49.5-)
  locally applied anti-infectives NEC (T49.0-)

  The appropriate 7th character is to be added to each code from category T37

A	initial encounter
D	subsequent encounter
S	sequela

- **T37.0 Poisoning by, adverse effect of and underdosing of sulfonamides**
  - **T37.0X Poisoning by, adverse effect of and underdosing of sulfonamides**
    - **T37.0X1 Poisoning by sulfonamides, accidental (unintentional)**
      Poisoning by sulfonamides NOS
    - **T37.0X2 Poisoning by sulfonamides, intentional self-harm**
    - **T37.0X3 Poisoning by sulfonamides, assault**
    - **T37.0X4 Poisoning by sulfonamides, undetermined**
    - **T37.0X5 Adverse effect of sulfonamides**
    - **T37.0X6 Underdosing of sulfonamides**
- **T37.1 Poisoning by, adverse effect of and underdosing of antimycobacterial drugs**

  Excludes1 rifampicins (T36.6-) streptomycin (T36.5-)
  - **T37.1X Poisoning by, adverse effect of and underdosing of antimycobacterial drugs**
    - **T37.1X1 Poisoning by antimycobacterial drugs, accidental (unintentional)**
      Poisoning by antimycobacterial drugs NOS
    - **T37.1X2 Poisoning by antimycobacterial drugs, intentional self-harm**
    - **T37.1X3 Poisoning by antimycobacterial drugs, assault**
    - **T37.1X4 Poisoning by antimycobacterial drugs, undetermined**
    - **T37.1X5 Adverse effect of antimycobacterial drugs**
    - **T37.1X6 Underdosing of antimycobacterial drugs**
- **T37.2 Poisoning by, adverse effect of and underdosing of antimalarials and drugs acting on other blood protozoa**

  Excludes1 hydroxyquinoline derivatives (T37.8-)
  - **T37.2X Poisoning by, adverse effect of and underdosing of antimalarials and drugs acting on other blood protozoa**
    - **T37.2X1 Poisoning by antimalarials and drugs acting on other blood protozoa, accidental (unintentional)**
      Poisoning by antimalarials and drugs acting on other blood protozoa NOS
    - **T37.2X2 Poisoning by antimalarials and drugs acting on other blood protozoa, intentional self-harm**
    - **T37.2X3 Poisoning by antimalarials and drugs acting on other blood protozoa, assault**
    - **T37.2X4 Poisoning by antimalarials and drugs acting on other blood protozoa, undetermined**
    - **T37.2X5 Adverse effect of antimalarials and drugs acting on other blood protozoa**
    - **T37.2X6 Underdosing of antimalarials and drugs acting on other blood protozoa**
- **T37.3 Poisoning by, adverse effect of and underdosing of other antiprotozoal drugs**
  - **T37.3X Poisoning by, adverse effect of and underdosing of other antiprotozoal drugs**
    - **T37.3X1 Poisoning by other antiprotozoal drugs, accidental (unintentional)**
      Poisoning by other antiprotozoal drugs NOS
    - **T37.3X2 Poisoning by other antiprotozoal drugs, intentional self-harm**
    - **T37.3X3 Poisoning by other antiprotozoal drugs, assault**
    - **T37.3X4 Poisoning by other antiprotozoal drugs, undetermined**
    - **T37.3X5 Adverse effect of other antiprotozoal drugs**
    - **T37.3X6 Underdosing of other antiprotozoal drugs**
- **T37.4 Poisoning by, adverse effect of and underdosing of anthelminthics**
  - **T37.4X Poisoning by, adverse effect of and underdosing of anthelminthics**
    - **T37.4X1 Poisoning by anthelminthics, accidental (unintentional)**
      Poisoning by anthelminthics NOS
    - **T37.4X2 Poisoning by anthelminthics, intentional self-harm**
    - **T37.4X3 Poisoning by anthelminthics, assault**
    - **T37.4X4 Poisoning by anthelminthics, undetermined**
    - **T37.4X5 Adverse effect of anthelminthics**
    - **T37.4X6 Underdosing of anthelminthics**

● **T37.5 Poisoning by, adverse effect of and underdosing of antiviral drugs**

Excludes1 amantadine (T42.8-)
cytarabine (T45.1-)

● **T37.5X Poisoning by, adverse effect of and underdosing of antiviral drugs**

● **T37.5X1 Poisoning by antiviral drugs, accidental (unintentional)**
Poisoning by antiviral drugs NOS

● **T37.5X2 Poisoning by antiviral drugs, intentional self-harm**

● **T37.5X3 Poisoning by antiviral drugs, assault**

● **T37.5X4 Poisoning by antiviral drugs, undetermined**

● **T37.5X5 Adverse effect of antiviral drugs**

● **T37.5X6 Underdosing of antiviral drugs**

● **T37.8 Poisoning by, adverse effect of and underdosing of other specified systemic anti-infectives and antiparasitics**
Poisoning by, adverse effect of and underdosing of hydroxyquinoline derivatives

Excludes1 antimalarial drugs (T37.2-)

● **T37.8X Poisoning by, adverse effect of and underdosing of other specified systemic anti-infectives and antiparasitics**

● **T37.8X1 Poisoning by other specified systemic anti-infectives and antiparasitics, accidental (unintentional)**
Poisoning by other specified systemic anti-infectives and antiparasitics NOS

● **T37.8X2 Poisoning by other specified systemic anti-infectives and antiparasitics, intentional self-harm**

● **T37.8X3 Poisoning by other specified systemic anti-infectives and antiparasitics, assault**

● **T37.8X4 Poisoning by other specified systemic anti-infectives and antiparasitics, undetermined**

● **T37.8X5 Adverse effect of other specified systemic anti-infectives and antiparasitics**

● **T37.8X6 Underdosing of other specified systemic anti-infectives and antiparasitics**

● **T37.9 Poisoning by, adverse effect of and underdosing of unspecified systemic anti-infective and antiparasitics**

X● **T37.91 Poisoning by unspecified systemic anti-infective and antiparasitics, accidental (unintentional)**
Poisoning by, adverse effect of and underdosing of systemic anti-infective and antiparasitics NOS

X● **T37.92 Poisoning by unspecified systemic anti-infective and antiparasitics, intentional self-harm**

X● **T37.93 Poisoning by unspecified systemic anti-infective and antiparasitics, assault**

X● **T37.94 Poisoning by unspecified systemic anti-infective and antiparasitics, undetermined**

X● **T37.95 Adverse effect of unspecified systemic anti-infective and antiparasitic**

X● **T37.96 Underdosing of unspecified systemic anti-infectives and antiparasitics**

● **T38 Poisoning by, adverse effect of and underdosing of hormones and their synthetic substitutes and antagonists, not elsewhere classified**

Excludes1 mineralocorticoids and their antagonists (T50.0-)
oxytocic hormones (T48.0-)
parathyroid hormones and derivatives (T50.9-)

The appropriate 7th character is to be added to each code from category T38

A	initial encounter
D	subsequent encounter
S	sequela

● **T38.0 Poisoning by, adverse effect of and underdosing of glucocorticoids and synthetic analogues**

Excludes1 glucocorticoids, topically used (T49.-)

● **T38.0X Poisoning by, adverse effect of and underdosing of glucocorticoids and synthetic analogues**

● **T38.0X1 Poisoning by glucocorticoids and synthetic analogues, accidental (unintentional)**
Poisoning by glucocorticoids and synthetic analogues NOS

● **T38.0X2 Poisoning by glucocorticoids and synthetic analogues, intentional self-harm**

● **T38.0X3 Poisoning by glucocorticoids and synthetic analogues, assault**

● **T38.0X4 Poisoning by glucocorticoids and synthetic analogues, undetermined**

● **T38.0X5 Adverse effect of glucocorticoids and synthetic analogues**

● **T38.0X6 Underdosing of glucocorticoids and synthetic analogues**

● **T38.1 Poisoning by, adverse effect of and underdosing of thyroid hormones and substitutes**

● **T38.1X Poisoning by, adverse effect of and underdosing of thyroid hormones and substitutes**

● **T38.1X1 Poisoning by thyroid hormones and substitutes, accidental (unintentional)**
Poisoning by thyroid hormones and substitutes NOS

● **T38.1X2 Poisoning by thyroid hormones and substitutes, intentional self-harm**

● **T38.1X3 Poisoning by thyroid hormones and substitutes, assault**

● **T38.1X4 Poisoning by thyroid hormones and substitutes, undetermined**

● **T38.1X5 Adverse effect of thyroid hormones and substitutes**

● **T38.1X6 Underdosing of thyroid hormones and substitutes**

● **T38.2 Poisoning by, adverse effect of and underdosing of antithyroid drugs**

● **T38.2X Poisoning by, adverse effect of and underdosing of antithyroid drugs**

● **T38.2X1 Poisoning by antithyroid drugs, accidental (unintentional)**
Poisoning by antithyroid drugs NOS

● **T38.2X2 Poisoning by antithyroid drugs, intentional self-harm**

● **T38.2X3 Poisoning by antithyroid drugs, assault**

● **T38.2X4 Poisoning by antithyroid drugs, undetermined**

● **T38.2X5 Adverse effect of antithyroid drugs**

● **T38.2X6 Underdosing of antithyroid drugs**

- **T38.3 Poisoning by, adverse effect of and underdosing of insulin and oral hypoglycemic [antidiabetic] drugs**
  - **T38.3X Poisoning by, adverse effect of and underdosing of insulin and oral hypoglycemic [antidiabetic] drugs**
    - **T38.3X1 Poisoning by insulin and oral hypoglycemic [antidiabetic] drugs, accidental (unintentional)**
      Poisoning by insulin and oral hypoglycemic [antidiabetic] drugs NOS
    - **T38.3X2 Poisoning by insulin and oral hypoglycemic [antidiabetic] drugs, intentional self-harm**
    - **T38.3X3 Poisoning by insulin and oral hypoglycemic [antidiabetic] drugs, assault**
    - **T38.3X4 Poisoning by insulin and oral hypoglycemic [antidiabetic] drugs, undetermined**
    - **T38.3X5 Adverse effect of insulin and oral hypoglycemic [antidiabetic] drugs**
    - **T38.3X6 Underdosing of insulin and oral hypoglycemic [antidiabetic] drugs**
- **T38.4 Poisoning by, adverse effect of and underdosing of oral contraceptives**
  Poisoning by, adverse effect of and underdosing of multiple- and single-ingredient oral contraceptive preparations
  - **T38.4X Poisoning by, adverse effect of and underdosing of oral contraceptives**
    - **T38.4X1 Poisoning by oral contraceptives, accidental (unintentional)**
      Poisoning by oral contraceptives NOS
    - **T38.4X2 Poisoning by oral contraceptives, intentional self-harm**
    - **T38.4X3 Poisoning by oral contraceptives, assault**
    - **T38.4X4 Poisoning by oral contraceptives, undetermined**
    - **T38.4X5 Adverse effect of oral contraceptives**
    - **T38.4X6 Underdosing of oral contraceptives**
- **T38.5 Poisoning by, adverse effect of and underdosing of other estrogens and progestogens**
  Poisoning by, adverse effect of and underdosing of estrogens and progestogens mixtures and substitutes
  - **T38.5X Poisoning by, adverse effect of and underdosing of other estrogens and progestogens**
    - **T38.5X1 Poisoning by other estrogens and progestogens, accidental (unintentional)**
      Poisoning by other estrogens and progestogens NOS
    - **T38.5X2 Poisoning by other estrogens and progestogens, intentional self-harm**
    - **T38.5X3 Poisoning by other estrogens and progestogens, assault**
    - **T38.5X4 Poisoning by other estrogens and progestogens, undetermined**
    - **T38.5X5 Adverse effect of other estrogens and progestogens**
    - **T38.5X6 Underdosing of other estrogens and progestogens**
- **T38.6 Poisoning by, adverse effect of and underdosing of antigonadotrophins, antiestrogens, antiandrogens, not elsewhere classified**
  Poisoning by, adverse effect of and underdosing of tamoxifen
  - **T38.6X Poisoning by, adverse effect of and underdosing of antigonadotrophins, antiestrogens, antiandrogens, not elsewhere classified**
    - **T38.6X1 Poisoning by antigonadotrophins, antiestrogens, antiandrogens, not elsewhere classified, accidental (unintentional)**
      Poisoning by antigonadotrophins, antiestrogens, antiandrogens, not elsewhere classified NOS
    - **T38.6X2 Poisoning by antigonadotrophins, antiestrogens, antiandrogens, not elsewhere classified, intentional self-harm**
    - **T38.6X3 Poisoning by antigonadotrophins, antiestrogens, antiandrogens, not elsewhere classified, assault**
    - **T38.6X4 Poisoning by antigonadotrophins, antiestrogens, antiandrogens, not elsewhere classified, undetermined**
    - **T38.6X5 Adverse effect of antigonadotrophins, antiestrogens, antiandrogens, not elsewhere classified**
    - **T38.6X6 Underdosing of antigonadotrophins, antiestrogens, antiandrogens, not elsewhere classified**
- **T38.7 Poisoning by, adverse effect of and underdosing of androgens and anabolic congeners**
  - **T38.7X Poisoning by, adverse effect of and underdosing of androgens and anabolic congeners**
    - **T38.7X1 Poisoning by androgens and anabolic congeners, accidental (unintentional)**
      Poisoning by androgens and anabolic congeners NOS
    - **T38.7X2 Poisoning by androgens and anabolic congeners, intentional self-harm**
    - **T38.7X3 Poisoning by androgens and anabolic congeners, assault**
    - **T38.7X4 Poisoning by androgens and anabolic congeners, undetermined**
    - **T38.7X5 Adverse effect of androgens and anabolic congeners**
    - **T38.7X6 Underdosing of androgens and anabolic congeners**
- **T38.8 Poisoning by, adverse effect of and underdosing of other and unspecified hormones and synthetic substitutes**
  - **T38.80 Poisoning by, adverse effect of and underdosing of unspecified hormones and synthetic substitutes**
    - **T38.801 Poisoning by unspecified hormones and synthetic substitutes, accidental (unintentional)**
      Poisoning by unspecified hormones and synthetic substitutes NOS
    - **T38.802 Poisoning by unspecified hormones and synthetic substitutes, intentional self-harm**
    - **T38.803 Poisoning by unspecified hormones and synthetic substitutes, assault**
    - **T38.804 Poisoning by unspecified hormones and synthetic substitutes, undetermined**
    - **T38.805 Adverse effect of unspecified hormones and synthetic substitutes**
    - **T38.806 Underdosing of unspecified hormones and synthetic substitutes**

- **T38.81 Poisoning by, adverse effect of and underdosing of anterior pituitary [adenohypophyseal] hormones**
  - **T38.811 Poisoning by anterior pituitary [adenohypophyseal] hormones, accidental (unintentional)**
    Poisoning by anterior pituitary [adenohypophyseal] hormones NOS
  - **T38.812 Poisoning by anterior pituitary [adenohypophyseal] hormones, intentional self-harm**
  - **T38.813 Poisoning by anterior pituitary [adenohypophyseal] hormones, assault**
  - **T38.814 Poisoning by anterior pituitary [adenohypophyseal] hormones, undetermined**
  - **T38.815 Adverse effect of anterior pituitary [adenohypophyseal] hormones**
  - **T38.816 Underdosing of anterior pituitary [adenohypophyseal] hormones**
- **T38.89 Poisoning by, adverse effect of and underdosing of other hormones and synthetic substitutes**
  - **T38.891 Poisoning by other hormones and synthetic substitutes, accidental (unintentional)**
    Poisoning by other hormones and synthetic substitutes NOS
  - **T38.892 Poisoning by other hormones and synthetic substitutes, intentional self-harm**
  - **T38.893 Poisoning by other hormones and synthetic substitutes, assault**
  - **T38.894 Poisoning by other hormones and synthetic substitutes, undetermined**
  - **T38.895 Adverse effect of other hormones and synthetic substitutes**
  - **T38.896 Underdosing of other hormones and synthetic substitutes**
- **T38.9 Poisoning by, adverse effect of and underdosing of other and unspecified hormone antagonists**
  - **T38.90 Poisoning by, adverse effect of and underdosing of unspecified hormone antagonists**
    - **T38.901 Poisoning by unspecified hormone antagonists, accidental (unintentional)**
      Poisoning by unspecified hormone antagonists NOS
    - **T38.902 Poisoning by unspecified hormone antagonists, intentional self-harm**
    - **T38.903 Poisoning by unspecified hormone antagonists, assault**
    - **T38.904 Poisoning by unspecified hormone antagonists, undetermined**
    - **T38.905 Adverse effect of unspecified hormone antagonists**
    - **T38.906 Underdosing of unspecified hormone antagonists**
  - **T38.99 Poisoning by, adverse effect of and underdosing of other hormone antagonists**
    - **T38.991 Poisoning by other hormone antagonists, accidental (unintentional)**
      Poisoning by other hormone antagonists NOS
    - **T38.992 Poisoning by other hormone antagonists, intentional self-harm**
    - **T38.993 Poisoning by other hormone antagonists, assault**
    - **T38.994 Poisoning by other hormone antagonists, undetermined**
    - **T38.995 Adverse effect of other hormone antagonists**
    - **T38.996 Underdosing of other hormone antagonists**

- **T39 Poisoning by, adverse effect of and underdosing of nonopioid analgesics, antipyretics and antirheumatics**
  The appropriate 7th character is to be added to each code from category T39

A	initial encounter
D	subsequent encounter
S	sequela

  - **T39.0 Poisoning by, adverse effect of and underdosing of salicylates**
    - **T39.01 Poisoning by, adverse effect of and underdosing of aspirin**
      Poisoning by, adverse effect of and underdosing of acetylsalicylic acid
      - **T39.011 Poisoning by aspirin, accidental (unintentional)**
      - **T39.012 Poisoning by aspirin, intentional self-harm**
      - **T39.013 Poisoning by aspirin, assault**
      - **T39.014 Poisoning by aspirin, undetermined**
      - **T39.015 Adverse effect of aspirin**
        Coding Clinic: 2016, Q1, P15
      - **T39.016 Underdosing of aspirin**
    - **T39.09 Poisoning by, adverse effect of and underdosing of other salicylates**
      - **T39.091 Poisoning by salicylates, accidental (unintentional)**
        Poisoning by salicylates NOS
      - **T39.092 Poisoning by salicylates, intentional self-harm**
      - **T39.093 Poisoning by salicylates, assault**
      - **T39.094 Poisoning by salicylates, undetermined**
      - **T39.095 Adverse effect of salicylates**
      - **T39.096 Underdosing of salicylates**
  - **T39.1 Poisoning by, adverse effect of and underdosing of 4-Aminophenol derivatives**
    - **T39.1X Poisoning by, adverse effect of and underdosing of 4-Aminophenol derivatives**
      - **T39.1X1 Poisoning by 4-Aminophenol derivatives, accidental (unintentional)**
        Poisoning by 4-Aminophenol derivatives NOS
      - **T39.1X2 Poisoning by 4-Aminophenol derivatives, intentional self-harm**
      - **T39.1X3 Poisoning by 4-Aminophenol derivatives, assault**
      - **T39.1X4 Poisoning by 4-Aminophenol derivatives, undetermined**
      - **T39.1X5 Adverse effect of 4-Aminophenol derivatives**
      - **T39.1X6 Underdosing of 4-Aminophenol derivatives**

- **T39.2 Poisoning by, adverse effect of and underdosing of pyrazolone derivatives**
  - **T39.2X Poisoning by, adverse effect of and underdosing of pyrazolone derivatives**
    - **T39.2X1 Poisoning by pyrazolone derivatives, accidental (unintentional)**
      Poisoning by pyrazolone derivatives NOS
    - **T39.2X2 Poisoning by pyrazolone derivatives, intentional self-harm**
    - **T39.2X3 Poisoning by pyrazolone derivatives, assault**
    - **T39.2X4 Poisoning by pyrazolone derivatives, undetermined**
    - **T39.2X5 Adverse effect of pyrazolone derivatives**
    - **T39.2X6 Underdosing of pyrazolone derivatives**
- **T39.3 Poisoning by, adverse effect of and underdosing of other nonsteroidal anti-inflammatory drugs [NSAID]**
  - **T39.31 Poisoning by, adverse effect of and underdosing of propionic acid derivatives**
    Poisoning by, adverse effect of and underdosing of fenoprofen
    Poisoning by, adverse effect of and underdosing of flurbiprofen
    Poisoning by, adverse effect of and underdosing of ibuprofen
    Poisoning by, adverse effect of and underdosing of ketoprofen
    Poisoning by, adverse effect of and underdosing of naproxen
    Poisoning by, adverse effect of and underdosing of oxaprozin
    - **T39.311 Poisoning by propionic acid derivatives, accidental (unintentional)**
    - **T39.312 Poisoning by propionic acid derivatives, intentional self-harm**
    - **T39.313 Poisoning by propionic acid derivatives, assault**
    - **T39.314 Poisoning by propionic acid derivatives, undetermined**
    - **T39.315 Adverse effect of propionic acid derivatives**
    - **T39.316 Underdosing of propionic acid derivatives**
  - **T39.39 Poisoning by, adverse effect of and underdosing of other nonsteroidal anti-inflammatory drugs [NSAID]**
    - **T39.391 Poisoning by other nonsteroidal anti-inflammatory drugs [NSAID], accidental (unintentional)**
      Poisoning by other nonsteroidal anti-inflammatory drugs NOS
    - **T39.392 Poisoning by other nonsteroidal anti-inflammatory drugs [NSAID], intentional self-harm**
    - **T39.393 Poisoning by other nonsteroidal anti-inflammatory drugs [NSAID], assault**
    - **T39.394 Poisoning by other nonsteroidal anti-inflammatory drugs [NSAID], undetermined**
    - **T39.395 Adverse effect of other nonsteroidal anti-inflammatory drugs [NSAID]**
    - **T39.396 Underdosing of other nonsteroidal anti-inflammatory drugs [NSAID]**
- **T39.4 Poisoning by, adverse effect of and underdosing of antirheumatics, not elsewhere classified**
  Excludes1 poisoning by, adverse effect of and underdosing of glucocorticoids (T38.0-)
  poisoning by, adverse effect of and underdosing of salicylates (T39.0-)
  - **T39.4X Poisoning by, adverse effect of and underdosing of antirheumatics, not elsewhere classified**
    - **T39.4X1 Poisoning by antirheumatics, not elsewhere classified, accidental (unintentional)**
      Poisoning by antirheumatics, not elsewhere classified NOS
    - **T39.4X2 Poisoning by antirheumatics, not elsewhere classified, intentional self-harm**
    - **T39.4X3 Poisoning by antirheumatics, not elsewhere classified, assault**
    - **T39.4X4 Poisoning by antirheumatics, not elsewhere classified, undetermined**
    - **T39.4X5 Adverse effect of antirheumatics, not elsewhere classified**
    - **T39.4X6 Underdosing of antirheumatics, not elsewhere classified**
- **T39.8 Poisoning by, adverse effect of and underdosing of other nonopioid analgesics and antipyretics, not elsewhere classified**
  - **T39.8X Poisoning by, adverse effect of and underdosing of other nonopioid analgesics and antipyretics, not elsewhere classified**
    - **T39.8X1 Poisoning by other nonopioid analgesics and antipyretics, not elsewhere classified, accidental (unintentional)**
      Poisoning by other nonopioid analgesics and antipyretics, not elsewhere classified NOS
    - **T39.8X2 Poisoning by other nonopioid analgesics and antipyretics, not elsewhere classified, intentional self-harm**
    - **T39.8X3 Poisoning by other nonopioid analgesics and antipyretics, not elsewhere classified, assault**
    - **T39.8X4 Poisoning by other nonopioid analgesics and antipyretics, not elsewhere classified, undetermined**
    - **T39.8X5 Adverse effect of other nonopioid analgesics and antipyretics, not elsewhere classified**
    - **T39.8X6 Underdosing of other nonopioid analgesics and antipyretics, not elsewhere classified**
- **T39.9 Poisoning by, adverse effect of and underdosing of unspecified nonopioid analgesic, antipyretic and antirheumatic**
  - X **T39.91 Poisoning by unspecified nonopioid analgesic, antipyretic and antirheumatic, accidental (unintentional)**
    Poisoning by nonopioid analgesic, antipyretic and antirheumatic NOS
  - X **T39.92 Poisoning by unspecified nonopioid analgesic, antipyretic and antirheumatic, intentional self-harm**
  - X **T39.93 Poisoning by unspecified nonopioid analgesic, antipyretic and antirheumatic, assault**
  - X **T39.94 Poisoning by unspecified nonopioid analgesic, antipyretic and antirheumatic, undetermined**
  - X **T39.95 Adverse effect of unspecified nonopioid analgesic, antipyretic and antirheumatic**
  - X **T39.96 Underdosing of unspecified nonopioid analgesic, antipyretic and antirheumatic**

T40 Poisoning by, adverse effect of and underdosing of narcotics and psychodysleptics [hallucinogens]

Excludes2 drug dependence and related mental and behavioral disorders due to psychoactive substance use (F10.-F19.-)

The appropriate 7th character is to be added to each code from category T40

A	initial encounter
D	subsequent encounter
S	sequela

T40.0 Poisoning by, adverse effect of and underdosing of opium

- **T40.0X Poisoning by, adverse effect of and underdosing of opium**
  - **T40.0X1 Poisoning by opium, accidental (unintentional)**
    Poisoning by opium NOS
  - **T40.0X2 Poisoning by opium, intentional self-harm**
  - **T40.0X3 Poisoning by opium, assault**
  - **T40.0X4 Poisoning by opium, undetermined**
  - **T40.0X5 Adverse effect of opium**
  - **T40.0X6 Underdosing of opium**

T40.1 Poisoning by and adverse effect of heroin

- **T40.1X Poisoning by and adverse effect of heroin**
  - **T40.1X1 Poisoning by heroin, accidental (unintentional)**
    Poisoning by heroin NOS
  - **T40.1X2 Poisoning by heroin, intentional self-harm**
  - **T40.1X3 Poisoning by heroin, assault**
  - **T40.1X4 Poisoning by heroin, undetermined**

T40.2 Poisoning by, adverse effect of and underdosing of other opioids

- **T40.2X Poisoning by, adverse effect of and underdosing of other opioids**
  - **T40.2X1 Poisoning by other opioids, accidental (unintentional)**
    Poisoning by other opioids NOS
  - **T40.2X2 Poisoning by other opioids, intentional self-harm**
  - **T40.2X3 Poisoning by other opioids, assault**
  - **T40.2X4 Poisoning by other opioids, undetermined**
  - **T40.2X5 Adverse effect of other opioids**
  - **T40.2X6 Underdosing of other opioids**

T40.3 Poisoning by, adverse effect of and underdosing of methadone

- **T40.3X Poisoning by, adverse effect of and underdosing of methadone**
  - **T40.3X1 Poisoning by methadone, accidental (unintentional)**
    Poisoning by methadone NOS
  - **T40.3X2 Poisoning by methadone, intentional self-harm**
  - **T40.3X3 Poisoning by methadone, assault**
  - **T40.3X4 Poisoning by methadone, undetermined**
  - **T40.3X5 Adverse effect of methadone**
  - **T40.3X6 Underdosing of methadone**

T40.4 Poisoning by, adverse effect of and underdosing of other synthetic narcotics

- **T40.4X Poisoning by, adverse effect of and underdosing of other synthetic narcotics**
  - **T40.4X1 Poisoning by other synthetic narcotics, accidental (unintentional)**
    Poisoning by other synthetic narcotics NOS
  - **T40.4X2 Poisoning by other synthetic narcotics, intentional self-harm**
  - **T40.4X3 Poisoning by other synthetic narcotics, assault**
  - **T40.4X4 Poisoning by other synthetic narcotics, undetermined**
  - **T40.4X5 Adverse effect of other synthetic narcotics**
  - **T40.4X6 Underdosing of other synthetic narcotics**

T40.5 Poisoning by, adverse effect of and underdosing of cocaine

- **T40.5X Poisoning by, adverse effect of and underdosing of cocaine**
  - **T40.5X1 Poisoning by cocaine, accidental (unintentional)**
    Poisoning by cocaine NOS
    Coding Clinic: 2016, Q2, P9
  - **T40.5X2 Poisoning by cocaine, intentional self-harm**
  - **T40.5X3 Poisoning by cocaine, assault**
  - **T40.5X4 Poisoning by cocaine, undetermined**
  - **T40.5X5 Adverse effect of cocaine**
  - **T40.5X6 Underdosing of cocaine**

T40.6 Poisoning by, adverse effect of and underdosing of other and unspecified narcotics

- **T40.60 Poisoning by, adverse effect of and underdosing of unspecified narcotics**
  - **T40.601 Poisoning by unspecified narcotics, accidental (unintentional)**
    Poisoning by narcotics NOS
  - **T40.602 Poisoning by unspecified narcotics, intentional self-harm**
  - **T40.603 Poisoning by unspecified narcotics, assault**
  - **T40.604 Poisoning by unspecified narcotics, undetermined**
  - **T40.605 Adverse effect of unspecified narcotics**
  - **T40.606 Underdosing of unspecified narcotics**
- **T40.69 Poisoning by, adverse effect of and underdosing of other narcotics**
  - **T40.691 Poisoning by other narcotics, accidental (unintentional)**
    Poisoning by other narcotics NOS
  - **T40.692 Poisoning by other narcotics, intentional self-harm**
  - **T40.693 Poisoning by other narcotics, assault**
  - **T40.694 Poisoning by other narcotics, undetermined**
  - **T40.695 Adverse effect of other narcotics**
  - **T40.696 Underdosing of other narcotics**

- **T40.7 Poisoning by, adverse effect of and underdosing of cannabis (derivatives)**
  - **T40.7X Poisoning by, adverse effect of and underdosing of cannabis (derivatives)**
    - **T40.7X1 Poisoning by cannabis (derivatives), accidental (unintentional)**
      Poisoning by cannabis NOS
    - **T40.7X2 Poisoning by cannabis (derivatives), intentional self-harm**
    - **T40.7X3 Poisoning by cannabis (derivatives), assault**
    - **T40.7X4 Poisoning by cannabis (derivatives), undetermined**
    - **T40.7X5 Adverse effect of cannabis (derivatives)**
    - **T40.7X6 Underdosing of cannabis (derivatives)**
- **T40.8 Poisoning by and adverse effect of lysergide [LSD]**
  - **T40.8X Poisoning by and adverse effect of lysergide [LSD]**
    - **T40.8X1 Poisoning by lysergide [LSD], accidental (unintentional)**
      Poisoning by lysergide [LSD] NOS
    - **T40.8X2 Poisoning by lysergide [LSD], intentional self-harm**
    - **T40.8X3 Poisoning by lysergide [LSD], assault**
    - **T40.8X4 Poisoning by lysergide [LSD], undetermined**
- **T40.9 Poisoning by, adverse effect of and underdosing of other and unspecified psychodysleptics [hallucinogens]**
  - **T40.90 Poisoning by, adverse effect of and underdosing of unspecified psychodysleptics [hallucinogens]**
    - **T40.901 Poisoning by unspecified psychodysleptics [hallucinogens], accidental (unintentional)**
    - **T40.902 Poisoning by unspecified psychodysleptics [hallucinogens], intentional self-harm**
    - **T40.903 Poisoning by unspecified psychodysleptics [hallucinogens], assault**
    - **T40.904 Poisoning by unspecified psychodysleptics [hallucinogens], undetermined**
    - **T40.905 Adverse effect of unspecified psychodysleptics [hallucinogens]**
    - **T40.906 Underdosing of unspecified psychodysleptics**
  - **T40.99 Poisoning by, adverse effect of and underdosing of other psychodysleptics [hallucinogens]**
    - **T40.991 Poisoning by other psychodysleptics [hallucinogens], accidental (unintentional)**
      Poisoning by other psychodysleptics [hallucinogens] NOS
    - **T40.992 Poisoning by other psychodysleptics [hallucinogens], intentional self-harm**
    - **T40.993 Poisoning by other psychodysleptics [hallucinogens], assault**
    - **T40.994 Poisoning by other psychodysleptics [hallucinogens], undetermined**
    - **T40.995 Adverse effect of other psychodysleptics [hallucinogens]**
    - **T40.996 Underdosing of other psychodysleptics**

- **T41 Poisoning by, adverse effect of and underdosing of anesthetics and therapeutic gases**

  Excludes1 benzodiazepines (T42.4-)
  cocaine (T40.5-)
  complications of anesthesia during pregnancy (O29.-)
  complications of anesthesia during labor and delivery (O74.-)
  complications of anesthesia during the puerperium (O89.-) opioids (T40.0-T40.2-)

  The appropriate 7th character is to be added to each code from category T41

A	initial encounter
D	subsequent encounter
S	sequela

- **T41.0 Poisoning by, adverse effect of and underdosing of inhaled anesthetics**

  Excludes1 oxygen (T41.5-)
  - **T41.0X Poisoning by, adverse effect of and underdosing of inhaled anesthetics**
    - **T41.0X1 Poisoning by inhaled anesthetics, accidental (unintentional)**
      Poisoning by inhaled anesthetics NOS
    - **T41.0X2 Poisoning by inhaled anesthetics, intentional self-harm**
    - **T41.0X3 Poisoning by inhaled anesthetics, assault**
    - **T41.0X4 Poisoning by inhaled anesthetics, undetermined**
    - **T41.0X5 Adverse effect of inhaled anesthetics**
    - **T41.0X6 Underdosing of inhaled anesthetics**
- **T41.1 Poisoning by, adverse effect of and underdosing of intravenous anesthetics**
  Poisoning by, adverse effect of and underdosing of thiobarbiturates
  - **T41.1X Poisoning by, adverse effect of and underdosing of intravenous anesthetics**
    - **T41.1X1 Poisoning by intravenous anesthetics, accidental (unintentional)**
      Poisoning by intravenous anesthetics NOS
    - **T41.1X2 Poisoning by intravenous anesthetics, intentional self-harm**
    - **T41.1X3 Poisoning by intravenous anesthetics, assault**
    - **T41.1X4 Poisoning by intravenous anesthetics, undetermined**
    - **T41.1X5 Adverse effect of intravenous anesthetics**
    - **T41.1X6 Underdosing of intravenous anesthetics**
- **T41.2 Poisoning by, adverse effect of and underdosing of other and unspecified general anesthetics**
  - **T41.20 Poisoning by, adverse effect of and underdosing of unspecified general anesthetics**
    - **T41.201 Poisoning by unspecified general anesthetics, accidental (unintentional)**
      Poisoning by general anesthetics NOS
    - **T41.202 Poisoning by unspecified general anesthetics, intentional self-harm**
    - **T41.203 Poisoning by unspecified general anesthetics, assault**
    - **T41.204 Poisoning by unspecified general anesthetics, undetermined**
    - **T41.205 Adverse effect of unspecified general anesthetics**
    - **T41.206 Underdosing of unspecified general anesthetics**

- **T41.29 Poisoning by, adverse effect of and underdosing of other general anesthetics**
  - **T41.291 Poisoning by other general anesthetics, accidental (unintentional)**
    Poisoning by other general anesthetics NOS
  - **T41.292 Poisoning by other general anesthetics, intentional self-harm**
  - **T41.293 Poisoning by other general anesthetics, assault**
  - **T41.294 Poisoning by other general anesthetics, undetermined**
  - **T41.295 Adverse effect of other general anesthetics**
  - **T41.296 Underdosing of other general anesthetics**
- **T41.3 Poisoning by, adverse effect of and underdosing of local anesthetics**
  Cocaine (topical)
  Excludes2 poisoning by cocaine used as a central nervous system stimulant (T40.5X1-T40.5X4)
  - **T41.3X Poisoning by, adverse effect of and underdosing of local anesthetics**
    - **T41.3X1 Poisoning by local anesthetics, accidental (unintentional)**
      Poisoning by local anesthetics NOS
    - **T41.3X2 Poisoning by local anesthetics, intentional self-harm**
    - **T41.3X3 Poisoning by local anesthetics, assault**
    - **T41.3X4 Poisoning by local anesthetics, undetermined**
    - **T41.3X5 Adverse effect of local anesthetics**
    - **T41.3X6 Underdosing of local anesthetics**
- **T41.4 Poisoning by, adverse effect of and underdosing of unspecified anesthetic**
  - X **T41.41 Poisoning by unspecified anesthetic, accidental (unintentional)**
    Poisoning by anesthetic NOS
  - X **T41.42 Poisoning by unspecified anesthetic, intentional self-harm**
  - X **T41.43 Poisoning by unspecified anesthetic, assault**
  - X **T41.44 Poisoning by unspecified anesthetic, undetermined**
  - X **T41.45 Adverse effect of unspecified anesthetic**
  - X **T41.46 Underdosing of unspecified anesthetics**
- **T41.5 Poisoning by, adverse effect of and underdosing of therapeutic gases**
  - **T41.5X Poisoning by, adverse effect of and underdosing of therapeutic gases**
    - **T41.5X1 Poisoning by therapeutic gases, accidental (unintentional)**
      Poisoning by therapeutic gases NOS
    - **T41.5X2 Poisoning by therapeutic gases, intentional self-harm**
    - **T41.5X3 Poisoning by therapeutic gases, assault**
    - **T41.5X4 Poisoning by therapeutic gases, undetermined**
    - **T41.5X5 Adverse effect of therapeutic gases**
    - **T41.5X6 Underdosing of therapeutic gases**
- **T42 Poisoning by, adverse effect of and underdosing of antiepileptic, sedative-hypnotic and antiparkinsonism drugs**
  Excludes2 drug dependence and related mental and behavioral disorders due to psychoactive substance use (F10.--F19.-)
  The appropriate 7th character is to be added to each code from category T42

A	initial encounter
D	subsequent encounter
S	sequela

- **T42.0 Poisoning by, adverse effect of and underdosing of hydantoin derivatives**
  - **T42.0X Poisoning by, adverse effect of and underdosing of hydantoin derivatives**
    - **T42.0X1 Poisoning by hydantoin derivatives, accidental (unintentional)**
      Poisoning by hydantoin derivatives NOS
    - **T42.0X2 Poisoning by hydantoin derivatives, intentional self-harm**
    - **T42.0X3 Poisoning by hydantoin derivatives, assault**
    - **T42.0X4 Poisoning by hydantoin derivatives, undetermined**
    - **T42.0X5 Adverse effect of hydantoin derivatives**
    - **T42.0X6 Underdosing of hydantoin derivatives**
- **T42.1 Poisoning by, adverse effect of and underdosing of iminostilbenes**
  Poisoning by, adverse effect of and underdosing of carbamazepine
  - **T42.1X Poisoning by, adverse effect of and underdosing of iminostilbenes**
    - **T42.1X1 Poisoning by iminostilbenes, accidental (unintentional)**
      Poisoning by iminostilbenes NOS
    - **T42.1X2 Poisoning by iminostilbenes, intentional self-harm**
    - **T42.1X3 Poisoning by iminostilbenes, assault**
    - **T42.1X4 Poisoning by iminostilbenes, undetermined**
    - **T42.1X5 Adverse effect of iminostilbenes**
    - **T42.1X6 Underdosing of iminostilbenes**
- **T42.2 Poisoning by, adverse effect of and underdosing of succinimides and oxazolidinediones**
  - **T42.2X Poisoning by, adverse effect of and underdosing of succinimides and oxazolidinediones**
    - **T42.2X1 Poisoning by succinimides and oxazolidinediones, accidental (unintentional)**
      Poisoning by succinimides and oxazolidinediones NOS
    - **T42.2X2 Poisoning by succinimides and oxazolidinediones, intentional self-harm**
    - **T42.2X3 Poisoning by succinimides and oxazolidinediones, assault**
    - **T42.2X4 Poisoning by succinimides and oxazolidinediones, undetermined**
    - **T42.2X5 Adverse effect of succinimides and oxazolidinediones**
    - **T42.2X6 Underdosing of succinimides and oxazolidinediones**

◀ New ◀ Revised ~~deleted~~ Deleted Excludes 1 Excludes 2 Includes Use additional Code first Code also Unspecified
OGCR Official Guidelines ● Unacceptable Principal Diagnosis X Assign placeholder X ● Use Additional Character(s) ▶ Manifestation Code Coding Clinic

- **T42.3 Poisoning by, adverse effect of and underdosing of barbiturates**
  - **Excludes1** poisoning by, adverse effect of and underdosing of thiobarbiturates (T41.1-)
  - **T42.3X Poisoning by, adverse effect of and underdosing of barbiturates**
    - **T42.3X1 Poisoning by barbiturates, accidental (unintentional)**
      - Poisoning by barbiturates NOS
    - **T42.3X2 Poisoning by barbiturates, intentional self-harm**
    - **T42.3X3 Poisoning by barbiturates, assault**
    - **T42.3X4 Poisoning by barbiturates, undetermined**
    - **T42.3X5 Adverse effect of barbiturates**
    - **T42.3X6 Underdosing of barbiturates**
- **T42.4 Poisoning by, adverse effect of and underdosing of benzodiazepines**
  - **T42.4X Poisoning by, adverse effect of and underdosing of benzodiazepines**
    - **T42.4X1 Poisoning by benzodiazepines, accidental (unintentional)**
      - Poisoning by benzodiazepines NOS
    - **T42.4X2 Poisoning by benzodiazepines, intentional self-harm**
    - **T42.4X3 Poisoning by benzodiazepines, assault**
    - **T42.4X4 Poisoning by benzodiazepines, undetermined**
    - **T42.4X5 Adverse effect of benzodiazepines**
    - **T42.4X6 Underdosing of benzodiazepines**
- **T42.5 Poisoning by, adverse effect of and underdosing of mixed antiepileptics**
  - **T42.5X Poisoning by, adverse effect of and underdosing of antiepileptics**
    - **T42.5X1 Poisoning by mixed antiepileptics, accidental (unintentional)**
      - Poisoning by mixed antiepileptics NOS
    - **T42.5X2 Poisoning by mixed antiepileptics, intentional self-harm**
    - **T42.5X3 Poisoning by mixed antiepileptics, assault**
    - **T42.5X4 Poisoning by mixed antiepileptics, undetermined**
    - **T42.5X5 Adverse effect of mixed antiepileptics**
    - **T42.5X6 Underdosing of mixed antiepileptics**
- **T42.6 Poisoning by, adverse effect of and underdosing of other antiepileptic and sedative-hypnotic drugs**
  - Poisoning by, adverse effect of and underdosing of methaqualone
  - Poisoning by, adverse effect of and underdosing of valproic acid
  - **Excludes1** poisoning by, adverse effect of and underdosing of carbamazepine (T42.1-)
  - **T42.6X Poisoning by, adverse effect of and underdosing of other antiepileptic and sedative-hypnotic drugs**
    - **T42.6X1 Poisoning by other antiepileptic and sedative-hypnotic drugs, accidental (unintentional)**
      - Poisoning by other antiepileptic and sedative-hypnotic drugs NOS
    - **T42.6X2 Poisoning by other antiepileptic and sedative-hypnotic drugs, intentional self-harm**
    - **T42.6X3 Poisoning by other antiepileptic and sedative-hypnotic drugs, assault**
    - **T42.6X4 Poisoning by other antiepileptic and sedative-hypnotic drugs, undetermined**
    - **T42.6X5 Adverse effect of other antiepileptic and sedative-hypnotic drugs**
    - **T42.6X6 Underdosing of other antiepileptic and sedative-hypnotic drugs**
- **T42.7 Poisoning by, adverse effect of and underdosing of unspecified antiepileptic and sedative-hypnotic drugs**
  - X **T42.71 Poisoning by unspecified antiepileptic and sedative-hypnotic drugs, accidental (unintentional)**
    - Poisoning by antiepileptic and sedative-hypnotic drugs NOS
  - X **T42.72 Poisoning by unspecified antiepileptic and sedative-hypnotic drugs, intentional self-harm**
  - X **T42.73 Poisoning by unspecified antiepileptic and sedative-hypnotic drugs, assault**
  - X **T42.74 Poisoning by unspecified antiepileptic and sedative-hypnotic drugs, undetermined**
  - X **T42.75 Adverse effect of unspecified antiepileptic and sedative-hypnotic drugs**
  - X **T42.76 Underdosing of unspecified antiepileptic and sedative-hypnotic drugs**
- **T42.8 Poisoning by, adverse effect of and underdosing of antiparkinsonism drugs and other central muscle-tone depressants**
  - Poisoning by, adverse effect of and underdosing of amantadine
  - **T42.8X Poisoning by, adverse effect of and underdosing of antiparkinsonism drugs and other central muscle-tone depressants**
    - **T42.8X1 Poisoning by antiparkinsonism drugs and other central muscle-tone depressants, accidental (unintentional)**
      - Poisoning by antiparkinsonism drugs and other central muscle-tone depressants NOS
    - **T42.8X2 Poisoning by antiparkinsonism drugs and other central muscle-tone depressants, intentional self-harm**
    - **T42.8X3 Poisoning by antiparkinsonism drugs and other central muscle-tone depressants, assault**
    - **T42.8X4 Poisoning by antiparkinsonism drugs and other central muscle-tone depressants, undetermined**
    - **T42.8X5 Adverse effect of antiparkinsonism drugs and other central muscle-tone depressants**
    - **T42.8X6 Underdosing of antiparkinsonism drugs and other central muscle-tone depressants**

T43 Poisoning by, adverse effect of and underdosing of psychotropic drugs, not elsewhere classified

Excludes1 appetite depressants (T50.5-)
barbiturates (T42.3-)
benzodiazepines (T42.4-)
methaqualone (T42.6-)
psychodysleptics [hallucinogens] (T40.7-T40.9-)

Excludes2 drug dependence and related mental and behavioral disorders due to psychoactive substance use (F10.--F19.-)

The appropriate 7th character is to be added to each code from category T43

A	initial encounter
D	subsequent encounter
S	sequela

T43.0 Poisoning by, adverse effect of and underdosing of tricyclic and tetracyclic antidepressants

T43.01 Poisoning by, adverse effect of and underdosing of tricyclic antidepressants

T43.011 Poisoning by tricyclic antidepressants, accidental (unintentional)
Poisoning by tricyclic antidepressants NOS

T43.012 Poisoning by tricyclic antidepressants, intentional self-harm

T43.013 Poisoning by tricyclic antidepressants, assault

T43.014 Poisoning by tricyclic antidepressants, undetermined

T43.015 Adverse effect of tricyclic antidepressants

T43.016 Underdosing of tricyclic antidepressants

T43.02 Poisoning by, adverse effect of and underdosing of tetracyclic antidepressants

T43.021 Poisoning by tetracyclic antidepressants, accidental (unintentional)
Poisoning by tetracyclic antidepressants NOS

T43.022 Poisoning by tetracyclic antidepressants, intentional self-harm

T43.023 Poisoning by tetracyclic antidepressants, assault

T43.024 Poisoning by tetracyclic antidepressants, undetermined

T43.025 Adverse effect of tetracyclic antidepressants

T43.026 Underdosing of tetracyclic antidepressants

T43.1 Poisoning by, adverse effect of and underdosing of monoamine-oxidase-inhibitor antidepressants

T43.1X Poisoning by, adverse effect of and underdosing of monoamine-oxidase-inhibitor antidepressants

T43.1X1 Poisoning by monoamine-oxidase-inhibitor antidepressants, accidental (unintentional)
Poisoning by monoamine-oxidase-inhibitor antidepressants NOS

T43.1X2 Poisoning by monoamine-oxidase-inhibitor antidepressants, intentional self-harm

T43.1X3 Poisoning by monoamine-oxidase-inhibitor antidepressants, assault

T43.1X4 Poisoning by monoamine-oxidase-inhibitor antidepressants, undetermined

T43.1X5 Adverse effect of monoamine-oxidase-inhibitor antidepressants

T43.1X6 Underdosing of monoamine-oxidase-inhibitor antidepressants

T43.2 Poisoning by, adverse effect of and underdosing of other and unspecified antidepressants

T43.20 Poisoning by, adverse effect of and underdosing of unspecified antidepressants

T43.201 Poisoning by unspecified antidepressants, accidental (unintentional)
Poisoning by antidepressants NOS

T43.202 Poisoning by unspecified antidepressants, intentional self-harm

T43.203 Poisoning by unspecified antidepressants, assault

T43.204 Poisoning by unspecified antidepressants, undetermined

T43.205 Adverse effect of unspecified antidepressants

T43.206 Underdosing of unspecified antidepressants

T43.21 Poisoning by, adverse effect of and underdosing of selective serotonin and norepinephrine reuptake inhibitors
Poisoning by, adverse effect of and underdosing of SSNRI antidepressants

T43.211 Poisoning by selective serotonin and norepinephrine reuptake inhibitors, accidental (unintentional)

T43.212 Poisoning by selective serotonin and norepinephrine reuptake inhibitors, intentional self-harm

T43.213 Poisoning by selective serotonin and norepinephrine reuptake inhibitors, assault

T43.214 Poisoning by selective serotonin and norepinephrine reuptake inhibitors, undetermined

T43.215 Adverse effect of selective serotonin and norepinephrine reuptake inhibitors

T43.216 Underdosing of selective serotonin and norepinephrine reuptake inhibitors

T43.22 Poisoning by, adverse effect of and underdosing of selective serotonin reuptake inhibitors
Poisoning by, adverse effect of and underdosing of SSRI antidepressants

T43.221 Poisoning by selective serotonin reuptake inhibitors, accidental (unintentional)

T43.222 Poisoning by selective serotonin reuptake inhibitors, intentional self-harm

T43.223 Poisoning by selective serotonin reuptake inhibitors, assault

T43.224 Poisoning by selective serotonin reuptake inhibitors, undetermined

T43.225 Adverse effect of selective serotonin reuptake inhibitors

T43.226 Underdosing of selective serotonin reuptake inhibitors

New Revised ~~deleted~~ Deleted Excludes 1 Excludes 2 Includes Use additional Code first Code also Unspecified
OGCR Official Guidelines Unacceptable Principal Diagnosis X Assign placeholder X Use Additional Character(s) Manifestation Code Coding Clinic

- **T43.29 Poisoning by, adverse effect of and underdosing of other antidepressants**
  - **T43.291 Poisoning by other antidepressants, accidental (unintentional)**
    Poisoning by other antidepressants NOS
  - **T43.292 Poisoning by other antidepressants, intentional self-harm**
  - **T43.293 Poisoning by other antidepressants, assault**
  - **T43.294 Poisoning by other antidepressants, undetermined**
  - **T43.295 Adverse effect of other antidepressants**
  - **T43.296 Underdosing of other antidepressants**
- **T43.3 Poisoning by, adverse effect of and underdosing of phenothiazine antipsychotics and neuroleptics**
  - **T43.3X Poisoning by, adverse effect of and underdosing of phenothiazine antipsychotics and neuroleptics**
    - **T43.3X1 Poisoning by phenothiazine antipsychotics and neuroleptics, accidental (unintentional)**
      Poisoning by phenothiazine antipsychotics and neuroleptics NOS
    - **T43.3X2 Poisoning by phenothiazine antipsychotics and neuroleptics, intentional self-harm**
    - **T43.3X3 Poisoning by phenothiazine antipsychotics and neuroleptics, assault**
    - **T43.3X4 Poisoning by phenothiazine antipsychotics and neuroleptics, undetermined**
    - **T43.3X5 Adverse effect of phenothiazine antipsychotics and neuroleptics**
    - **T43.3X6 Underdosing of phenothiazine antipsychotics and neuroleptics**
- **T43.4 Poisoning by, adverse effect of and underdosing of butyrophenone and thiothixene neuroleptics**
  - **T43.4X Poisoning by, adverse effect of and underdosing of butyrophenone and thiothixene neuroleptics**
    - **T43.4X1 Poisoning by butyrophenone and thiothixene neuroleptics, accidental (unintentional)**
      Poisoning by butyrophenone and thiothixene neuroleptics NOS
    - **T43.4X2 Poisoning by butyrophenone and thiothixene neuroleptics, intentional self-harm**
    - **T43.4X3 Poisoning by butyrophenone and thiothixene neuroleptics, assault**
    - **T43.4X4 Poisoning by butyrophenone and thiothixene neuroleptics, undetermined**
    - **T43.4X5 Adverse effect of butyrophenone and thiothixene neuroleptics**
    - **T43.4X6 Underdosing of butyrophenone and thiothixene neuroleptics**
- **T43.5 Poisoning by, adverse effect of and underdosing of other and unspecified antipsychotics and neuroleptics**
  Excludes1 poisoning by, adverse effect of and underdosing of rauwolfia (T46.5-)
  - **T43.50 Poisoning by, adverse effect of and underdosing of unspecified antipsychotics and neuroleptics**
    - **T43.501 Poisoning by unspecified antipsychotics and neuroleptics, accidental (unintentional)**
      Poisoning by antipsychotics and neuroleptics NOS
    - **T43.502 Poisoning by unspecified antipsychotics and neuroleptics, intentional self-harm**
    - **T43.503 Poisoning by unspecified antipsychotics and neuroleptics, assault**
    - **T43.504 Poisoning by unspecified antipsychotics and neuroleptics, undetermined**
    - **T43.505 Adverse effect of unspecified antipsychotics and neuroleptics**
    - **T43.506 Underdosing of unspecified antipsychotics and neuroleptics**
  - **T43.59 Poisoning by, adverse effect of and underdosing of other antipsychotics and neuroleptics**
    - **T43.591 Poisoning by other antipsychotics and neuroleptics, accidental (unintentional)**
      Poisoning by other antipsychotics and neuroleptics NOS
    - **T43.592 Poisoning by other antipsychotics and neuroleptics, intentional self-harm**
    - **T43.593 Poisoning by other antipsychotics and neuroleptics, assault**
    - **T43.594 Poisoning by other antipsychotics and neuroleptics, undetermined**
    - **T43.595 Adverse effect of other antipsychotics and neuroleptics**
    - **T43.596 Underdosing of other antipsychotics and neuroleptics**
- **T43.6 Poisoning by, adverse effect of and underdosing of psychostimulants**
  Excludes1 poisoning by, adverse effect of and underdosing of cocaine (T40.5-)
  - **T43.60 Poisoning by, adverse effect of and underdosing of unspecified psychostimulant**
    - **T43.601 Poisoning by unspecified psychostimulants, accidental (unintentional)**
      Poisoning by psychostimulants NOS
    - **T43.602 Poisoning by unspecified psychostimulants, intentional self-harm**
    - **T43.603 Poisoning by unspecified psychostimulants, assault**
    - **T43.604 Poisoning by unspecified psychostimulants, undetermined**
    - **T43.605 Adverse effect of unspecified psychostimulants**
    - **T43.606 Underdosing of unspecified psychostimulants**

- **T43.61 Poisoning by, adverse effect of and underdosing of caffeine**
  - **T43.611 Poisoning by caffeine, accidental (unintentional)**
    Poisoning by caffeine NOS
  - **T43.612 Poisoning by caffeine, intentional self-harm**
  - **T43.613 Poisoning by caffeine, assault**
  - **T43.614 Poisoning by caffeine, undetermined**
  - **T43.615 Adverse effect of caffeine**
  - **T43.616 Underdosing of caffeine**
- **T43.62 Poisoning by, adverse effect of and underdosing of amphetamines**
  Poisoning by, adverse effect of and underdosing of methamphetamines
  - **T43.621 Poisoning by amphetamines, accidental (unintentional)**
    Poisoning by amphetamines NOS
  - **T43.622 Poisoning by amphetamines, intentional self-harm**
  - **T43.623 Poisoning by amphetamines, assault**
  - **T43.624 Poisoning by amphetamines, undetermined**
  - **T43.625 Adverse effect of amphetamines**
  - **T43.626 Underdosing of amphetamines**
- **T43.63 Poisoning by, adverse effect of and underdosing of methylphenidate**
  - **T43.631 Poisoning by methylphenidate, accidental (unintentional)**
    Poisoning by methylphenidate NOS
  - **T43.632 Poisoning by methylphenidate, intentional self-harm**
  - **T43.633 Poisoning by methylphenidate, assault**
  - **T43.634 Poisoning by methylphenidate, undetermined**
  - **T43.635 Adverse effect of methylphenidate**
  - **T43.636 Underdosing of methylphenidate**
- **T43.69 Poisoning by, adverse effect of and underdosing of other psychostimulants**
  - **T43.691 Poisoning by other psychostimulants, accidental (unintentional)**
    Poisoning by other psychostimulants NOS
  - **T43.692 Poisoning by other psychostimulants, intentional self-harm**
  - **T43.693 Poisoning by other psychostimulants, assault**
  - **T43.694 Poisoning by other psychostimulants, undetermined**
  - **T43.695 Adverse effect of other psychostimulants**
  - **T43.696 Underdosing of other psychostimulants**
- **T43.8 Poisoning by, adverse effect of and underdosing of other psychotropic drugs**
  - **T43.8X Poisoning by, adverse effect of and underdosing of other psychotropic drugs**
    - **T43.8X1 Poisoning by other psychotropic drugs, accidental (unintentional)**
      Poisoning by other psychotropic drugs NOS
    - **T43.8X2 Poisoning by other psychotropic drugs, intentional self-harm**
    - **T43.8X3 Poisoning by other psychotropic drugs, assault**
    - **T43.8X4 Poisoning by other psychotropic drugs, undetermined**
    - **T43.8X5 Adverse effect of other psychotropic drugs**
    - **T43.8X6 Underdosing of other psychotropic drugs**
- **T43.9 Poisoning by, adverse effect of and underdosing of unspecified psychotropic drug**
  - X **T43.91 Poisoning by unspecified psychotropic drug, accidental (unintentional)**
    Poisoning by psychotropic drug NOS
  - X **T43.92 Poisoning by unspecified psychotropic drug, intentional self-harm**
  - X **T43.93 Poisoning by unspecified psychotropic drug, assault**
  - X **T43.94 Poisoning by unspecified psychotropic drug, undetermined**
  - X **T43.95 Adverse effect of unspecified psychotropic drug**
  - X **T43.96 Underdosing of unspecified psychotropic drug**

- **T44 Poisoning by, adverse effect of and underdosing of drugs primarily affecting the autonomic nervous system**
  The appropriate 7th character is to be added to each code from category T44

A	initial encounter
D	subsequent encounter
S	sequela

- **T44.0 Poisoning by, adverse effect of and underdosing of anticholinesterase agents**
  - **T44.0X Poisoning by, adverse effect of and underdosing of anticholinesterase agents**
    - **T44.0X1 Poisoning by anticholinesterase agents, accidental (unintentional)**
      Poisoning by anticholinesterase agents NOS
    - **T44.0X2 Poisoning by anticholinesterase agents, intentional self-harm**
    - **T44.0X3 Poisoning by anticholinesterase agents, assault**
    - **T44.0X4 Poisoning by anticholinesterase agents, undetermined**
    - **T44.0X5 Adverse effect of anticholinesterase agents**
    - **T44.0X6 Underdosing of anticholinesterase agents**
- **T44.1 Poisoning by, adverse effect of and underdosing of other parasympathomimetics [cholinergics]**
  - **T44.1X Poisoning by, adverse effect of and underdosing of other parasympathomimetics [cholinergics]**
    - **T44.1X1 Poisoning by other parasympathomimetics [cholinergics], accidental (unintentional)**
      Poisoning by other parasympathomimetics [cholinergics] NOS
    - **T44.1X2 Poisoning by other parasympathomimetics [cholinergics], intentional self-harm**
    - **T44.1X3 Poisoning by other parasympathomimetics [cholinergics], assault**
    - **T44.1X4 Poisoning by other parasympathomimetics [cholinergics], undetermined**
    - **T44.1X5 Adverse effect of other parasympathomimetics [cholinergics]**
    - **T44.1X6 Underdosing of other parasympathomimetics**

◀ New ◀ Revised ~~deleted~~ Deleted Excludes 1 Excludes 2 Includes Use additional Code first Code also Unspecified
OGCR Official Guidelines ● Unacceptable Principal Diagnosis X Assign placeholder X ● Use Additional Character(s) ▶ Manifestation Code Coding Clinic

- **T44.2 Poisoning by, adverse effect of and underdosing of ganglionic blocking drugs**
  - **T44.2X Poisoning by, adverse effect of and underdosing of ganglionic blocking drugs**
    - **T44.2X1 Poisoning by ganglionic blocking drugs, accidental (unintentional)**
      Poisoning by ganglionic blocking drugs NOS
    - **T44.2X2 Poisoning by ganglionic blocking drugs, intentional self-harm**
    - **T44.2X3 Poisoning by ganglionic blocking drugs, assault**
    - **T44.2X4 Poisoning by ganglionic blocking drugs, undetermined**
    - **T44.2X5 Adverse effect of ganglionic blocking drugs**
    - **T44.2X6 Underdosing of ganglionic blocking drugs**
- **T44.3 Poisoning by, adverse effect of and underdosing of other parasympatholytics [anticholinergics and antimuscarinics] and spasmolytics**
  Poisoning by, adverse effect of and underdosing of papaverine
  - **T44.3X Poisoning by, adverse effect of and underdosing of other parasympatholytics [anticholinergics and antimuscarinics] and spasmolytics**
    - **T44.3X1 Poisoning by other parasympatholytics [anticholinergics and antimuscarinics] and spasmolytics, accidental (unintentional)**
      Poisoning by other parasympatholytics [anticholinergics and antimuscarinics] and spasmolytics NOS
    - **T44.3X2 Poisoning by other parasympatholytics [anticholinergics and antimuscarinics] and spasmolytics, intentional self-harm**
    - **T44.3X3 Poisoning by other parasympatholytics [anticholinergics and antimuscarinics] and spasmolytics, assault**
    - **T44.3X4 Poisoning by other parasympatholytics [anticholinergics and antimuscarinics] and spasmolytics, undetermined**
    - **T44.3X5 Adverse effect of other parasympatholytics [anticholinergics and antimuscarinics] and spasmolytics**
    - **T44.3X6 Underdosing of other parasympatholytics [anticholinergics and antimuscarinics] and spasmolytics**
- **T44.4 Poisoning by, adverse effect of and underdosing of predominantly alpha-adrenoreceptor agonists**
  Poisoning by, adverse effect of and underdosing of metaraminol
  - **T44.4X Poisoning by, adverse effect of and underdosing of predominantly alpha-adrenoreceptor agonists**
    - **T44.4X1 Poisoning by predominantly alpha-adrenoreceptor agonists, accidental (unintentional)**
      Poisoning by predominantly alpha-adrenoreceptor agonists NOS
    - **T44.4X2 Poisoning by predominantly alpha-adrenoreceptor agonists, intentional self-harm**
    - **T44.4X3 Poisoning by predominantly alpha-adrenoreceptor agonists, assault**
    - **T44.4X4 Poisoning by predominantly alpha-adrenoreceptor agonists, undetermined**
    - **T44.4X5 Adverse effect of predominantly alpha-adrenoreceptor agonists**
    - **T44.4X6 Underdosing of predominantly alpha-adrenoreceptor agonists**
- **T44.5 Poisoning by, adverse effect of and underdosing of predominantly beta-adrenoreceptor agonists**
  Excludes1 poisoning by, adverse effect of and underdosing of beta-adrenoreceptor agonists used in asthma therapy (T48.6-)
  - **T44.5X Poisoning by, adverse effect of and underdosing of predominantly beta-adrenoreceptor agonists**
    - **T44.5X1 Poisoning by predominantly beta-adrenoreceptor agonists, accidental (unintentional)**
      Poisoning by predominantly beta-adrenoreceptor agonists NOS
    - **T44.5X2 Poisoning by predominantly beta-adrenoreceptor agonists, intentional self-harm**
    - **T44.5X3 Poisoning by predominantly beta-adrenoreceptor agonists, assault**
    - **T44.5X4 Poisoning by predominantly beta-adrenoreceptor agonists, undetermined**
    - **T44.5X5 Adverse effect of predominantly beta-adrenoreceptor agonists**
    - **T44.5X6 Underdosing of predominantly beta-adrenoreceptor agonists**
- **T44.6 Poisoning by, adverse effect of and underdosing of alpha-adrenoreceptor antagonists**
  Excludes1 poisoning by, adverse effect of and underdosing of ergot alkaloids (T48.0)
  - **T44.6X Poisoning by, adverse effect of and underdosing of alpha-adrenoreceptor antagonists**
    - **T44.6X1 Poisoning by alpha-adrenoreceptor antagonists, accidental (unintentional)**
      Poisoning by alpha-adrenoreceptor antagonists NOS
    - **T44.6X2 Poisoning by alpha-adrenoreceptor antagonists, intentional self-harm**
    - **T44.6X3 Poisoning by alpha-adrenoreceptor antagonists, assault**
    - **T44.6X4 Poisoning by alpha-adrenoreceptor antagonists, undetermined**
    - **T44.6X5 Adverse effect of alpha-adrenoreceptor antagonists**
    - **T44.6X6 Underdosing of alpha-adrenoreceptor antagonists**

- **T44.7 Poisoning by, adverse effect of and underdosing of beta-adrenoreceptor antagonists**
  - **T44.7X Poisoning by, adverse effect of and underdosing of beta-adrenoreceptor antagonists**
    - **T44.7X1 Poisoning by beta-adrenoreceptor antagonists, accidental (unintentional)**
      Poisoning by beta-adrenoreceptor antagonists NOS
    - **T44.7X2 Poisoning by beta-adrenoreceptor antagonists, intentional self-harm**
    - **T44.7X3 Poisoning by beta-adrenoreceptor antagonists, assault**
    - **T44.7X4 Poisoning by beta-adrenoreceptor antagonists, undetermined**
    - **T44.7X5 Adverse effect of beta-adrenoreceptor antagonists**
    - **T44.7X6 Underdosing of beta-adrenoreceptor antagonists**
- **T44.8 Poisoning by, adverse effect of and underdosing of centrally-acting and adrenergic-neuron-blocking agents**
  Excludes1 poisoning by, adverse effect of and underdosing of clonidine (T46.5)
  poisoning by, adverse effect of and underdosing of guanethidine (T46.5)
  - **T44.8X Poisoning by, adverse effect of and underdosing of centrally-acting and adrenergic-neuron-blocking agents**
    - **T44.8X1 Poisoning by centrally-acting and adrenergic-neuron-blocking agents, accidental (unintentional)**
      Poisoning by centrally-acting and adrenergic-neuron-blocking agents NOS
    - **T44.8X2 Poisoning by centrally-acting and adrenergic-neuron-blocking agents, intentional self-harm**
    - **T44.8X3 Poisoning by centrally-acting and adrenergic-neuron-blocking agents, assault**
    - **T44.8X4 Poisoning by centrally-acting and adrenergic-neuron-blocking agents, undetermined**
    - **T44.8X5 Adverse effect of centrally-acting and adrenergic-neuron-blocking agents**
    - **T44.8X6 Underdosing of centrally-acting and adrenergic-neuron-blocking agents**
- **T44.9 Poisoning by, adverse effect of and underdosing of other and unspecified drugs primarily affecting the autonomic nervous system**
  Poisoning by, adverse effect of and underdosing of drug stimulating both alpha and beta-adrenoreceptors
  - **T44.90 Poisoning by, adverse effect of and underdosing of unspecified drugs primarily affecting the autonomic nervous system**
    - **T44.901 Poisoning by unspecified drugs primarily affecting the autonomic nervous system, accidental (unintentional)**
      Poisoning by unspecified drugs primarily affecting the autonomic nervous system NOS
    - **T44.902 Poisoning by unspecified drugs primarily affecting the autonomic nervous system, intentional self-harm**
    - **T44.903 Poisoning by unspecified drugs primarily affecting the autonomic nervous system, assault**
    - **T44.904 Poisoning by unspecified drugs primarily affecting the autonomic nervous system, undetermined**
    - **T44.905 Adverse effect of unspecified drugs primarily affecting the autonomic nervous system**
    - **T44.906 Underdosing of unspecified drugs primarily affecting the autonomic nervous system**
  - **T44.99 Poisoning by, adverse effect of and underdosing of other drugs primarily affecting the autonomic nervous system**
    - **T44.991 Poisoning by other drug primarily affecting the autonomic nervous system, accidental (unintentional)**
      Poisoning by other drugs primarily affecting the autonomic nervous system NOS
    - **T44.992 Poisoning by other drug primarily affecting the autonomic nervous system, intentional self-harm**
    - **T44.993 Poisoning by other drug primarily affecting the autonomic nervous system, assault**
    - **T44.994 Poisoning by other drug primarily affecting the autonomic nervous system, undetermined**
    - **T44.995 Adverse effect of other drug primarily affecting the autonomic nervous system**
    - **T44.996 Underdosing of other drug primarily affecting the autonomic nervous system**

- **T45 Poisoning by, adverse effect of and underdosing of primarily systemic and hematological agents, not elsewhere classified**
  The appropriate 7th character is to be added to each code from category T45

A	initial encounter
D	subsequent encounter
S	sequela

  - **T45.0 Poisoning by, adverse effect of and underdosing of antiallergic and antiemetic drugs**
    Excludes1 poisoning by, adverse effect of and underdosing of phenothiazine-based neuroleptics (T43.3)
    - **T45.0X Poisoning by, adverse effect of and underdosing of antiallergic and antiemetic drugs**
      - **T45.0X1 Poisoning by antiallergic and antiemetic drugs, accidental (unintentional)**
        Poisoning by antiallergic and antiemetic drugs NOS
      - **T45.0X2 Poisoning by antiallergic and antiemetic drugs, intentional self-harm**
      - **T45.0X3 Poisoning by antiallergic and antiemetic drugs, assault**
      - **T45.0X4 Poisoning by antiallergic and antiemetic drugs, undetermined**
      - **T45.0X5 Adverse effect of antiallergic and antiemetic drugs**
      - **T45.0X6 Underdosing of antiallergic and antiemetic drugs**

- **T45.1 Poisoning by, adverse effect of and underdosing of antineoplastic and immunosuppressive drugs**
  - **Excludes1** poisoning by, adverse effect of and underdosing of tamoxifen (T38.6)
  - **T45.1X Poisoning by, adverse effect of and underdosing of antineoplastic and immunosuppressive drugs**
    - **T45.1X1 Poisoning by antineoplastic and immunosuppressive drugs, accidental (unintentional)**
      - Poisoning by antineoplastic and immunosuppressive drugs NOS
    - **T45.1X2 Poisoning by antineoplastic and immunosuppressive drugs, intentional self-harm**
    - **T45.1X3 Poisoning by antineoplastic and immunosuppressive drugs, assault**
    - **T45.1X4 Poisoning by antineoplastic and immunosuppressive drugs, undetermined**
    - **T45.1X5 Adverse effect of antineoplastic and immunosuppressive drugs**
    - **T45.1X6 Underdosing of antineoplastic and immunosuppressive drugs**
- **T45.2 Poisoning by, adverse effect of and underdosing of vitamins**
  - **Excludes2** poisoning by, adverse effect of and underdosing of nicotinic acid (derivatives) (T46.7)
    - poisoning by, adverse effect of and underdosing of iron (T45.4)
    - poisoning by, adverse effect of and underdosing of vitamin K (T45.7)
  - **T45.2X Poisoning by, adverse effect of and underdosing of vitamins**
    - **T45.2X1 Poisoning by vitamins, accidental (unintentional)**
      - Poisoning by vitamins NOS
    - **T45.2X2 Poisoning by vitamins, intentional self-harm**
    - **T45.2X3 Poisoning by vitamins, assault**
    - **T45.2X4 Poisoning by vitamins, undetermined**
    - **T45.2X5 Adverse effect of vitamins**
    - **T45.2X6 Underdosing of vitamins**
      - **Excludes1** vitamin deficiencies (E50-E56)
- **T45.3 Poisoning by, adverse effect of and underdosing of enzymes**
  - **T45.3X Poisoning by, adverse effect of and underdosing of enzymes**
    - **T45.3X1 Poisoning by enzymes, accidental (unintentional)**
      - Poisoning by enzymes NOS
    - **T45.3X2 Poisoning by enzymes, intentional self-harm**
    - **T45.3X3 Poisoning by enzymes, assault**
    - **T45.3X4 Poisoning by enzymes, undetermined**
    - **T45.3X5 Adverse effect of enzymes**
    - **T45.3X6 Underdosing of enzymes**
- **T45.4 Poisoning by, adverse effect of and underdosing of iron and its compounds**
  - **T45.4X Poisoning by, adverse effect of and underdosing of iron and its compounds**
    - **T45.4X1 Poisoning by iron and its compounds, accidental (unintentional)**
      - Poisoning by iron and its compounds NOS
    - **T45.4X2 Poisoning by iron and its compounds, intentional self-harm**
    - **T45.4X3 Poisoning by iron and its compounds, assault**
    - **T45.4X4 Poisoning by iron and its compounds, undetermined**
    - **T45.4X5 Adverse effect of iron and its compounds**
    - **T45.4X6 Underdosing of iron and its compounds**
      - **Excludes1** iron deficiency (E61.1)
- **T45.5 Poisoning by, adverse effect of and underdosing of anticoagulants and antithrombotic drugs**
  - **T45.51 Poisoning by, adverse effect of and underdosing of anticoagulants**
    - **T45.511 Poisoning by anticoagulants, accidental (unintentional)**
      - Poisoning by anticoagulants NOS
    - **T45.512 Poisoning by anticoagulants, intentional self-harm**
    - **T45.513 Poisoning by anticoagulants, assault**
    - **T45.514 Poisoning by anticoagulants, undetermined**
    - **T45.515 Adverse effect of anticoagulants**
      - **Coding Clinic: 2016, Q1, P14; 2013, Q2, P35**
    - **T45.516 Underdosing of anticoagulants**
  - **T45.52 Poisoning by, adverse effect of and underdosing of antithrombotic drugs**
    - Poisoning by, adverse effect of and underdosing of antiplatelet drugs
    - **Excludes2** poisoning by, adverse effect of and underdosing of aspirin (T39.01-)
      - poisoning by, adverse effect of and underdosing of acetylsalicylic acid (T39.01-)
    - **T45.521 Poisoning by antithrombotic drugs, accidental (unintentional)**
      - Poisoning by antithrombotic drug NOS
    - **T45.522 Poisoning by antithrombotic drugs, intentional self-harm**
    - **T45.523 Poisoning by antithrombotic drugs, assault**
    - **T45.524 Poisoning by antithrombotic drugs, undetermined**
    - **T45.525 Adverse effect of antithrombotic drugs**
      - **Coding Clinic: 2016, Q1, P15**
    - **T45.526 Underdosing of antithrombotic drugs**
- **T45.6 Poisoning by, adverse effect of and underdosing of fibrinolysis-affecting drugs**
  - **T45.60 Poisoning by, adverse effect of and underdosing of unspecified fibrinolysis-affecting drugs**
    - **T45.601 Poisoning by unspecified fibrinolysis-affecting drugs, accidental (unintentional)**
      - Poisoning by fibrinolysis-affecting drug NOS
    - **T45.602 Poisoning by unspecified fibrinolysis-affecting drugs, intentional self-harm**
    - **T45.603 Poisoning by unspecified fibrinolysis-affecting drugs, assault**
    - **T45.604 Poisoning by unspecified fibrinolysis-affecting drugs, undetermined**
    - **T45.605 Adverse effect of unspecified fibrinolysis-affecting drugs**
    - **T45.606 Underdosing of unspecified fibrinolysis-affecting drugs**

- **T45.61 Poisoning by, adverse effect of and underdosing of thrombolytic drugs**
  - **T45.611 Poisoning by thrombolytic drug, accidental (unintentional)**
    Poisoning by thrombolytic drug NOS
  - **T45.612 Poisoning by thrombolytic drug, intentional self-harm**
  - **T45.613 Poisoning by thrombolytic drug, assault**
  - **T45.614 Poisoning by thrombolytic drug, undetermined**
  - **T45.615 Adverse effect of thrombolytic drugs**
  - **T45.616 Underdosing of thrombolytic drugs**
- **T45.62 Poisoning by, adverse effect of and underdosing of hemostatic drugs**
  - **T45.621 Poisoning by hemostatic drug, accidental (unintentional)**
    Poisoning by hemostatic drug NOS
  - **T45.622 Poisoning by hemostatic drug, intentional self-harm**
  - **T45.623 Poisoning by hemostatic drug, assault**
  - **T45.624 Poisoning by hemostatic drug, undetermined**
  - **T45.625 Adverse effect of hemostatic drug**
  - **T45.626 Underdosing of hemostatic drugs**
- **T45.69 Poisoning by, adverse effect of and underdosing of other fibrinolysis-affecting drugs**
  - **T45.691 Poisoning by other fibrinolysis-affecting drugs, accidental (unintentional)**
    Poisoning by other fibrinolysis-affecting drug NOS
  - **T45.692 Poisoning by other fibrinolysis-affecting drugs, intentional self-harm**
  - **T45.693 Poisoning by other fibrinolysis-affecting drugs, assault**
  - **T45.694 Poisoning by other fibrinolysis-affecting drugs, undetermined**
  - **T45.695 Adverse effect of other fibrinolysis-affecting drugs**
  - **T45.696 Underdosing of other fibrinolysis-affecting drugs**
- **T45.7 Poisoning by, adverse effect of and underdosing of anticoagulant antagonists, vitamin K and other coagulants**
  - **T45.7X Poisoning by, adverse effect of and underdosing of anticoagulant antagonists, vitamin K and other coagulants**
    - **T45.7X1 Poisoning by anticoagulant antagonists, vitamin K and other coagulants, accidental (unintentional)**
      Poisoning by anticoagulant antagonists, vitamin K and other coagulants NOS
    - **T45.7X2 Poisoning by anticoagulant antagonists, vitamin K and other coagulants, intentional self-harm**
    - **T45.7X3 Poisoning by anticoagulant antagonists, vitamin K and other coagulants, assault**
    - **T45.7X4 Poisoning by anticoagulant antagonists, vitamin K and other coagulants, undetermined**
    - **T45.7X5 Adverse effect of anticoagulant antagonists, vitamin K and other coagulants**
    - **T45.7X6 Underdosing of anticoagulant antagonist, vitamin K and other coagulants**
      Excludes1 vitamin K deficiency (E56.1)
- **T45.8 Poisoning by, adverse effect of and underdosing of other primarily systemic and hematological agents**
  Poisoning by, adverse effect of and underdosing of liver preparations and other antianemic agents
  Poisoning by, adverse effect of and underdosing of natural blood and blood products
  Poisoning by, adverse effect of and underdosing of plasma substitute
  Excludes2 poisoning by, adverse effect of and underdosing of immunoglobulin (T50.Z1)
  poisoning by, adverse effect of and underdosing of iron (T45.4)
  transfusion reactions (T80.-)
  - **T45.8X Poisoning by, adverse effect of and underdosing of other primarily systemic and hematological agents**
    - **T45.8X1 Poisoning by other primarily systemic and hematological agents, accidental (unintentional)**
      Poisoning by other primarily systemic and hematological agents NOS
    - **T45.8X2 Poisoning by other primarily systemic and hematological agents, intentional self-harm**
    - **T45.8X3 Poisoning by other primarily systemic and hematological agents, assault**
    - **T45.8X4 Poisoning by other primarily systemic and hematological agents, undetermined**
    - **T45.8X5 Adverse effect of other primarily systemic and hematological agents**
    - **T45.8X6 Underdosing of other primarily systemic and hematological agents**
- **T45.9 Poisoning by, adverse effect of and underdosing of unspecified primarily systemic and hematological agent**
  - X **T45.91 Poisoning by unspecified primarily systemic and hematological agent, accidental (unintentional)**
    Poisoning by primarily systemic and hematological agent NOS
  - X **T45.92 Poisoning by unspecified primarily systemic and hematological agent, intentional self-harm**
  - X **T45.93 Poisoning by unspecified primarily systemic and hematological agent, assault**
  - X **T45.94 Poisoning by unspecified primarily systemic and hematological agent, undetermined**
  - X **T45.95 Adverse effect of unspecified primarily systemic and hematological agent**
  - X **T45.96 Underdosing of unspecified primarily systemic and hematological agent**

T46 Poisoning by, adverse effect of and underdosing of agents primarily affecting the cardiovascular system

Excludes1 poisoning by, adverse effect of and underdosing of metaraminol (T44.4)

The appropriate 7th character is to be added to each code from category T46

A	initial encounter
D	subsequent encounter
S	sequela

T46.0 Poisoning by, adverse effect of and underdosing of cardiac-stimulant glycosides and drugs of similar action

T46.0X Poisoning by, adverse effect of and underdosing of cardiac-stimulant glycosides and drugs of similar action

T46.0X1 Poisoning by cardiac-stimulant glycosides and drugs of similar action, accidental (unintentional)
Poisoning by cardiac-stimulant glycosides and drugs of similar action NOS

T46.0X2 Poisoning by cardiac-stimulant glycosides and drugs of similar action, intentional self-harm

T46.0X3 Poisoning by cardiac-stimulant glycosides and drugs of similar action, assault

T46.0X4 Poisoning by cardiac-stimulant glycosides and drugs of similar action, undetermined

T46.0X5 Adverse effect of cardiac-stimulant glycosides and drugs of similar action

T46.0X6 Underdosing of cardiac-stimulant glycosides and drugs of similar action

T46.1 Poisoning by, adverse effect of and underdosing of calcium-channel blockers

T46.1X Poisoning by, adverse effect of and underdosing of calcium-channel blockers

T46.1X1 Poisoning by calcium-channel blockers, accidental (unintentional)
Poisoning by calcium-channel blockers NOS

T46.1X2 Poisoning by calcium-channel blockers, intentional self-harm

T46.1X3 Poisoning by calcium-channel blockers, assault

T46.1X4 Poisoning by calcium-channel blockers, undetermined

T46.1X5 Adverse effect of calcium-channel blockers

T46.1X6 Underdosing of calcium-channel blockers

T46.2 Poisoning by, adverse effect of and underdosing of other antidysrhythmic drugs, not elsewhere classified

Excludes1 poisoning by, adverse effect of and underdosing of beta-adrenoreceptor antagonists (T44.7-)

T46.2X Poisoning by, adverse effect of and underdosing of other antidysrhythmic drugs

T46.2X1 Poisoning by other antidysrhythmic drugs, accidental (unintentional)
Poisoning by other antidysrhythmic drugs NOS

T46.2X2 Poisoning by other antidysrhythmic drugs, intentional self-harm

T46.2X3 Poisoning by other antidysrhythmic drugs, assault

T46.2X4 Poisoning by other antidysrhythmic drugs, undetermined

T46.2X5 Adverse effect of other antidysrhythmic drugs

T46.2X6 Underdosing of other antidysrhythmic drugs

T46.3 Poisoning by, adverse effect of and underdosing of coronary vasodilators
Poisoning by, adverse effect of and underdosing of dipyridamole

Excludes1 poisoning by, adverse effect of and underdosing of calcium-channel blockers (T46.1)

T46.3X Poisoning by, adverse effect of and underdosing of coronary vasodilators

T46.3X1 Poisoning by coronary vasodilators, accidental (unintentional)
Poisoning by coronary vasodilators NOS

T46.3X2 Poisoning by coronary vasodilators, intentional self-harm

T46.3X3 Poisoning by coronary vasodilators, assault

T46.3X4 Poisoning by coronary vasodilators, undetermined

T46.3X5 Adverse effect of coronary vasodilators

T46.3X6 Underdosing of coronary vasodilators

T46.4 Poisoning by, adverse effect of and underdosing of angiotensin-converting-enzyme inhibitors

T46.4X Poisoning by, adverse effect of and underdosing of angiotensin-converting-enzyme inhibitors

T46.4X1 Poisoning by angiotensin-converting-enzyme inhibitors, accidental (unintentional)
Poisoning by angiotensin-converting-enzyme inhibitors NOS

T46.4X2 Poisoning by angiotensin-converting-enzyme inhibitors, intentional self-harm

T46.4X3 Poisoning by angiotensin-converting-enzyme inhibitors, assault

T46.4X4 Poisoning by angiotensin-converting-enzyme inhibitors, undetermined

T46.4X5 Adverse effect of angiotensin-converting-enzyme inhibitors

T46.4X6 Underdosing of angiotensin-converting-enzyme inhibitors

- **T46.5 Poisoning by, adverse effect of and underdosing of other antihypertensive drugs**
  - **Excludes2** poisoning by, adverse effect of and underdosing of beta-adrenoreceptor antagonists (T44.7)
    poisoning by, adverse effect of and underdosing of calcium-channel blockers (T46.1)
    poisoning by, adverse effect of and underdosing of diuretics (T50.0-T50.2)
  - **T46.5X Poisoning by, adverse effect of and underdosing of other antihypertensive drugs**
    - **T46.5X1 Poisoning by other antihypertensive drugs, accidental (unintentional)**
      Poisoning by other antihypertensive drugs NOS
    - **T46.5X2 Poisoning by other antihypertensive drugs, intentional self-harm**
    - **T46.5X3 Poisoning by other antihypertensive drugs, assault**
    - **T46.5X4 Poisoning by other antihypertensive drugs, undetermined**
    - **T46.5X5 Adverse effect of other antihypertensive drugs**
    - **T46.5X6 Underdosing of other antihypertensive drugs**
- **T46.6 Poisoning by, adverse effect of and underdosing of antihyperlipidemic and antiarteriosclerotic drugs**
  - **T46.6X Poisoning by, adverse effect of and underdosing of antihyperlipidemic and antiarteriosclerotic drugs**
    - **T46.6X1 Poisoning by antihyperlipidemic and antiarteriosclerotic drugs, accidental (unintentional)**
      Poisoning by antihyperlipidemic and antiarteriosclerotic drugs NOS
    - **T46.6X2 Poisoning by antihyperlipidemic and antiarteriosclerotic drugs, intentional self-harm**
    - **T46.6X3 Poisoning by antihyperlipidemic and antiarteriosclerotic drugs, assault**
    - **T46.6X4 Poisoning by antihyperlipidemic and antiarteriosclerotic drugs, undetermined**
    - **T46.6X5 Adverse effect of antihyperlipidemic and antiarteriosclerotic drugs**
    - **T46.6X6 Underdosing of antihyperlipidemic and antiarteriosclerotic drugs**
- **T46.7 Poisoning by, adverse effect of and underdosing of peripheral vasodilators**
  Poisoning by, adverse effect of and underdosing of nicotinic acid (derivatives)
  - **Excludes1** poisoning by, adverse effect of and underdosing of papaverine (T44.3)
  - **T46.7X Poisoning by, adverse effect of and underdosing of peripheral vasodilators**
    - **T46.7X1 Poisoning by peripheral vasodilators, accidental (unintentional)**
      Poisoning by peripheral vasodilators NOS
    - **T46.7X2 Poisoning by peripheral vasodilators, intentional self-harm**
    - **T46.7X3 Poisoning by peripheral vasodilators, assault**
    - **T46.7X4 Poisoning by peripheral vasodilators, undetermined**
    - **T46.7X5 Adverse effect of peripheral vasodilators**
    - **T46.7X6 Underdosing of peripheral vasodilators**
- **T46.8 Poisoning by, adverse effect of and underdosing of antivaricose drugs, including sclerosing agents**
  - **T46.8X Poisoning by, adverse effect of and underdosing of antivaricose drugs, including sclerosing agents**
    - **T46.8X1 Poisoning by antivaricose drugs, including sclerosing agents, accidental (unintentional)**
      Poisoning by antivaricose drugs, including sclerosing agents NOS
    - **T46.8X2 Poisoning by antivaricose drugs, including sclerosing agents, intentional self-harm**
    - **T46.8X3 Poisoning by antivaricose drugs, including sclerosing agents, assault**
    - **T46.8X4 Poisoning by antivaricose drugs, including sclerosing agents, undetermined**
    - **T46.8X5 Adverse effect of antivaricose drugs, including sclerosing agents**
    - **T46.8X6 Underdosing of antivaricose drugs, including sclerosing agents**
- **T46.9 Poisoning by, adverse effect of and underdosing of other and unspecified agents primarily affecting the cardiovascular system**
  - **T46.90 Poisoning by, adverse effect of and underdosing of unspecified agents primarily affecting the cardiovascular system**
    - **T46.901 Poisoning by unspecified agents primarily affecting the cardiovascular system, accidental (unintentional)**
    - **T46.902 Poisoning by unspecified agents primarily affecting the cardiovascular system, intentional self-harm**
    - **T46.903 Poisoning by unspecified agents primarily affecting the cardiovascular system, assault**
    - **T46.904 Poisoning by unspecified agents primarily affecting the cardiovascular system, undetermined**
    - **T46.905 Adverse effect of unspecified agents primarily affecting the cardiovascular system**
    - **T46.906 Underdosing of unspecified agents primarily affecting the cardiovascular system**
  - **T46.99 Poisoning by, adverse effect of and underdosing of other agents primarily affecting the cardiovascular system**
    - **T46.991 Poisoning by other agents primarily affecting the cardiovascular system, accidental (unintentional)**
    - **T46.992 Poisoning by other agents primarily affecting the cardiovascular system, intentional self-harm**
    - **T46.993 Poisoning by other agents primarily affecting the cardiovascular system, assault**
    - **T46.994 Poisoning by other agents primarily affecting the cardiovascular system, undetermined**
    - **T46.995 Adverse effect of other agents primarily affecting the cardiovascular system**
    - **T46.996 Underdosing of other agents primarily affecting the cardiovascular system**

- **T47 Poisoning by, adverse effect of and underdosing of agents primarily affecting the gastrointestinal system**

  The appropriate 7th character is to be added to each code from category T47

A	initial encounter
D	subsequent encounter
S	sequela

  - **T47.0 Poisoning by, adverse effect of and underdosing of histamine H2-receptor blockers**
    - **T47.0X Poisoning by, adverse effect of and underdosing of histamine H2-receptor blockers**
      - **T47.0X1 Poisoning by histamine H2-receptor blockers, accidental (unintentional)**
        Poisoning by histamine H2-receptor blockers NOS
      - **T47.0X2 Poisoning by histamine H2-receptor blockers, intentional self-harm**
      - **T47.0X3 Poisoning by histamine H2-receptor blockers, assault**
      - **T47.0X4 Poisoning by histamine H2-receptor blockers, undetermined**
      - **T47.0X5 Adverse effect of histamine H2-receptor blockers**
      - **T47.0X6 Underdosing of histamine H2-receptor blockers**
  - **T47.1 Poisoning by, adverse effect of and underdosing of other antacids and anti-gastric-secretion drugs**
    - **T47.1X Poisoning by, adverse effect of and underdosing of other antacids and anti-gastric-secretion drugs**
      - **T47.1X1 Poisoning by other antacids and anti-gastric-secretion drugs, accidental (unintentional)**
        Poisoning by other antacids and anti-gastric-secretion drugs NOS
      - **T47.1X2 Poisoning by other antacids and anti-gastric-secretion drugs, intentional self-harm**
      - **T47.1X3 Poisoning by other antacids and anti-gastric-secretion drugs, assault**
      - **T47.1X4 Poisoning by other antacids and anti-gastric-secretion drugs, undetermined**
      - **T47.1X5 Adverse effect of other antacids and anti-gastric-secretion drugs**
      - **T47.1X6 Underdosing of other antacids and anti-gastric-secretion drugs**
  - **T47.2 Poisoning by, adverse effect of and underdosing of stimulant laxatives**
    - **T47.2X Poisoning by, adverse effect of and underdosing of stimulant laxatives**
      - **T47.2X1 Poisoning by stimulant laxatives, accidental (unintentional)**
        Poisoning by stimulant laxatives NOS
      - **T47.2X2 Poisoning by stimulant laxatives, intentional self-harm**
      - **T47.2X3 Poisoning by stimulant laxatives, assault**
      - **T47.2X4 Poisoning by stimulant laxatives, undetermined**
      - **T47.2X5 Adverse effect of stimulant laxatives**
      - **T47.2X6 Underdosing of stimulant laxatives**
  - **T47.3 Poisoning by, adverse effect of and underdosing of saline and osmotic laxatives**
    - **T47.3X Poisoning by and adverse effect of saline and osmotic laxatives**
      - **T47.3X1 Poisoning by saline and osmotic laxatives, accidental (unintentional)**
        Poisoning by saline and osmotic laxatives NOS
      - **T47.3X2 Poisoning by saline and osmotic laxatives, intentional self-harm**
      - **T47.3X3 Poisoning by saline and osmotic laxatives, assault**
      - **T47.3X4 Poisoning by saline and osmotic laxatives, undetermined**
      - **T47.3X5 Adverse effect of saline and osmotic laxatives**
      - **T47.3X6 Underdosing of saline and osmotic laxatives**
  - **T47.4 Poisoning by, adverse effect of and underdosing of other laxatives**
    - **T47.4X Poisoning by, adverse effect of and underdosing of other laxatives**
      - **T47.4X1 Poisoning by other laxatives, accidental (unintentional)**
        Poisoning by other laxatives NOS
      - **T47.4X2 Poisoning by other laxatives, intentional self-harm**
      - **T47.4X3 Poisoning by other laxatives, assault**
      - **T47.4X4 Poisoning by other laxatives, undetermined**
      - **T47.4X5 Adverse effect of other laxatives**
      - **T47.4X6 Underdosing of other laxatives**
  - **T47.5 Poisoning by, adverse effect of and underdosing of digestants**
    - **T47.5X Poisoning by, adverse effect of and underdosing of digestants**
      - **T47.5X1 Poisoning by digestants, accidental (unintentional)**
        Poisoning by digestants NOS
      - **T47.5X2 Poisoning by digestants, intentional self-harm**
      - **T47.5X3 Poisoning by digestants, assault**
      - **T47.5X4 Poisoning by digestants, undetermined**
      - **T47.5X5 Adverse effect of digestants**
      - **T47.5X6 Underdosing of digestants**
  - **T47.6 Poisoning by, adverse effect of and underdosing of antidiarrheal drugs**

    Excludes2 poisoning by, adverse effect of and underdosing of systemic antibiotics and other anti-infectives (T36-T37)
    - **T47.6X Poisoning by, adverse effect of and underdosing of antidiarrheal drugs**
      - **T47.6X1 Poisoning by antidiarrheal drugs, accidental (unintentional)**
        Poisoning by antidiarrheal drugs NOS
      - **T47.6X2 Poisoning by antidiarrheal drugs, intentional self-harm**
      - **T47.6X3 Poisoning by antidiarrheal drugs, assault**
      - **T47.6X4 Poisoning by antidiarrheal drugs, undetermined**
      - **T47.6X5 Adverse effect of antidiarrheal drugs**
      - **T47.6X6 Underdosing of antidiarrheal drugs**

- T47.7 Poisoning by, adverse effect of and underdosing of emetics
  - T47.7X Poisoning by, adverse effect of and underdosing of emetics
    - T47.7X1 Poisoning by emetics, accidental (unintentional)
      Poisoning by emetics NOS
    - T47.7X2 Poisoning by emetics, intentional self-harm
    - T47.7X3 Poisoning by emetics, assault
    - T47.7X4 Poisoning by emetics, undetermined
    - T47.7X5 Adverse effect of emetics
    - T47.7X6 Underdosing of emetics
- T47.8 Poisoning by, adverse effect of and underdosing of other agents primarily affecting gastrointestinal system
  - T47.8X Poisoning by, adverse effect of and underdosing of other agents primarily affecting gastrointestinal system
    - T47.8X1 Poisoning by other agents primarily affecting gastrointestinal system, accidental (unintentional)
      Poisoning by other agents primarily affecting gastrointestinal system NOS
    - T47.8X2 Poisoning by other agents primarily affecting gastrointestinal system, intentional self-harm
    - T47.8X3 Poisoning by other agents primarily affecting gastrointestinal system, assault
    - T47.8X4 Poisoning by other agents primarily affecting gastrointestinal system, undetermined
    - T47.8X5 Adverse effect of other agents primarily affecting gastrointestinal system
    - T47.8X6 Underdosing of other agents primarily affecting gastrointestinal system
- T47.9 Poisoning by, adverse effect of and underdosing of unspecified agents primarily affecting the gastrointestinal system
  - X T47.91 Poisoning by unspecified agents primarily affecting the gastrointestinal system, accidental (unintentional)
    Poisoning by agents primarily affecting the gastrointestinal system NOS
  - X T47.92 Poisoning by unspecified agents primarily affecting the gastrointestinal system, intentional self-harm
  - X T47.93 Poisoning by unspecified agents primarily affecting the gastrointestinal system, assault
  - X T47.94 Poisoning by unspecified agents primarily affecting the gastrointestinal system, undetermined
  - X T47.95 Adverse effect of unspecified agents primarily affecting the gastrointestinal system
  - X T47.96 Underdosing of unspecified agents primarily affecting the gastrointestinal system

- T48 Poisoning by, adverse effect of and underdosing of agents primarily acting on smooth and skeletal muscles and the respiratory system
  The appropriate 7th character is to be added to each code from category T48

A	initial encounter
D	subsequent encounter
S	sequela

- T48.0 Poisoning by, adverse effect of and underdosing of oxytocic drugs
  Excludes1 poisoning by, adverse effect of and underdosing of estrogens, progestogens and antagonists (T38.4-T38.6)
  - T48.0X Poisoning by, adverse effect of and underdosing of oxytocic drugs
    - T48.0X1 Poisoning by oxytocic drugs, accidental (unintentional)
      Poisoning by oxytocic drugs NOS
    - T48.0X2 Poisoning by oxytocic drugs, intentional self-harm
    - T48.0X3 Poisoning by oxytocic drugs, assault
    - T48.0X4 Poisoning by oxytocic drugs, undetermined
    - T48.0X5 Adverse effect of oxytocic drugs
    - T48.0X6 Underdosing of oxytocic drugs
- T48.1 Poisoning by, adverse effect of and underdosing of skeletal muscle relaxants [neuromuscular blocking agents]
  - T48.1X Poisoning by, adverse effect of and underdosing of skeletal muscle relaxants [neuromuscular blocking agents]
    - T48.1X1 Poisoning by skeletal muscle relaxants [neuromuscular blocking agents], accidental (unintentional)
      Poisoning by skeletal muscle relaxants [neuromuscular blocking agents] NOS
    - T48.1X2 Poisoning by skeletal muscle relaxants [neuromuscular blocking agents], intentional self-harm
    - T48.1X3 Poisoning by skeletal muscle relaxants [neuromuscular blocking agents], assault
    - T48.1X4 Poisoning by skeletal muscle relaxants [neuromuscular blocking agents], undetermined
    - T48.1X5 Adverse effect of skeletal muscle relaxants [neuromuscular blocking agents]
    - T48.1X6 Underdosing of skeletal muscle relaxants [neuromuscular blocking agents]
- T48.2 Poisoning by, adverse effect of and underdosing of other and unspecified drugs acting on muscles
  - T48.20 Poisoning by, adverse effect of and underdosing of unspecified drugs acting on muscles
    - T48.201 Poisoning by unspecified drugs acting on muscles, accidental (unintentional)
      Poisoning by unspecified drugs acting on muscles NOS
    - T48.202 Poisoning by unspecified drugs acting on muscles, intentional self-harm
    - T48.203 Poisoning by unspecified drugs acting on muscles, assault
    - T48.204 Poisoning by unspecified drugs acting on muscles, undetermined
    - T48.205 Adverse effect of unspecified drugs acting on muscles
    - T48.206 Underdosing of unspecified drugs acting on muscles

- **T48.29 Poisoning by, adverse effect of and underdosing of other drugs acting on muscles**
  - **T48.291 Poisoning by other drugs acting on muscles, accidental (unintentional)**
    Poisoning by other drugs acting on muscles NOS
  - **T48.292 Poisoning by other drugs acting on muscles, intentional self-harm**
  - **T48.293 Poisoning by other drugs acting on muscles, assault**
  - **T48.294 Poisoning by other drugs acting on muscles, undetermined**
  - **T48.295 Adverse effect of other drugs acting on muscles**
  - **T48.296 Underdosing of other drugs acting on muscles**
- **T48.3 Poisoning by, adverse effect of and underdosing of antitussives**
  - **T48.3X Poisoning by, adverse effect of and underdosing of antitussives**
    - **T48.3X1 Poisoning by antitussives, accidental (unintentional)**
      Poisoning by antitussives NOS
    - **T48.3X2 Poisoning by antitussives, intentional self-harm**
    - **T48.3X3 Poisoning by antitussives, assault**
    - **T48.3X4 Poisoning by antitussives, undetermined**
    - **T48.3X5 Adverse effect of antitussives**
    - **T48.3X6 Underdosing of antitussives**
- **T48.4 Poisoning by, adverse effect of and underdosing of expectorants**
  - **T48.4X Poisoning by, adverse effect of and underdosing of expectorants**
    - **T48.4X1 Poisoning by expectorants, accidental (unintentional)**
      Poisoning by expectorants NOS
    - **T48.4X2 Poisoning by expectorants, intentional self-harm**
    - **T48.4X3 Poisoning by expectorants, assault**
    - **T48.4X4 Poisoning by expectorants, undetermined**
    - **T48.4X5 Adverse effect of expectorants**
    - **T48.4X6 Underdosing of expectorants**
- **T48.5 Poisoning by, adverse effect of and underdosing of other anti-common-cold drugs**
  Poisoning by, adverse effect of and underdosing of decongestants

  Excludes2 poisoning by, adverse effect of and underdosing of antipyretics, NEC (T39.9-)
  poisoning by, adverse effect of and underdosing of non-steroidal antiinflammatory drugs (T39.3-)
  poisoning by, adverse effect of and underdosing of salicylates (T39.0-)
  - **T48.5X Poisoning by, adverse effect of and underdosing of other anti-common-cold drugs**
    - **T48.5X1 Poisoning by other anti-common-cold drugs, accidental (unintentional)**
      Poisoning by other anti-common-cold drugs NOS
    - **T48.5X2 Poisoning by other anti-common-cold drugs, intentional self-harm**
    - **T48.5X3 Poisoning by other anti-common-cold drugs, assault**
    - **T48.5X4 Poisoning by other anti-common-cold drugs, undetermined**
    - **T48.5X5 Adverse effect of other anti-common-cold drugs**
    - **T48.5X6 Underdosing of other anti-common-cold drugs**
- **T48.6 Poisoning by, adverse effect of and underdosing of antiasthmatics, not elsewhere classified**
  Poisoning by, adverse effect of and underdosing of beta-adrenoreceptor agonists used in asthma therapy

  Excludes1 poisoning by, adverse effect of and underdosing of beta-adrenoreceptor agonists not used in asthma therapy (T44.5)
  poisoning by, adverse effect of and underdosing of anterior pituitary [adenohypophyseal] hormones (T38.8)
  - **T48.6X Poisoning by, adverse effect of and underdosing of antiasthmatics**
    - **T48.6X1 Poisoning by antiasthmatics, accidental (unintentional)**
      Poisoning by antiasthmatics NOS
    - **T48.6X2 Poisoning by antiasthmatics, intentional self-harm**
    - **T48.6X3 Poisoning by antiasthmatics, assault**
    - **T48.6X4 Poisoning by antiasthmatics, undetermined**
    - **T48.6X5 Adverse effect of antiasthmatics**
    - **T48.6X6 Underdosing of antiasthmatics**
- **T48.9 Poisoning by, adverse effect of and underdosing of other and unspecified agents primarily acting on the respiratory system**
  - **T48.90 Poisoning by, adverse effect of and underdosing of unspecified agents primarily acting on the respiratory system**
    - **T48.901 Poisoning by unspecified agents primarily acting on the respiratory system, accidental (unintentional)**
    - **T48.902 Poisoning by unspecified agents primarily acting on the respiratory system, intentional self-harm**
    - **T48.903 Poisoning by unspecified agents primarily acting on the respiratory system, assault**
    - **T48.904 Poisoning by unspecified agents primarily acting on the respiratory system, undetermined**
    - **T48.905 Adverse effect of unspecified agents primarily acting on the respiratory system**
    - **T48.906 Underdosing of unspecified agents primarily acting on the respiratory system**
  - **T48.99 Poisoning by, adverse effect of and underdosing of other agents primarily acting on the respiratory system**
    - **T48.991 Poisoning by other agents primarily acting on the respiratory system, accidental (unintentional)**
    - **T48.992 Poisoning by other agents primarily acting on the respiratory system, intentional self-harm**
    - **T48.993 Poisoning by other agents primarily acting on the respiratory system, assault**
    - **T48.994 Poisoning by other agents primarily acting on the respiratory system, undetermined**
    - **T48.995 Adverse effect of other agents primarily acting on the respiratory system**
    - **T48.996 Underdosing of other agents primarily acting on the respiratory system**

● **T49 Poisoning by, adverse effect of and underdosing of topical agents primarily affecting skin and mucous membrane and by ophthalmological, otorhinorlaryngological and dental drugs**

Includes poisoning by, adverse effect of and underdosing of glucocorticoids, topically used

The appropriate 7th character is to be added to each code from category T49

A	initial encounter
D	subsequent encounter
S	sequela

● **T49.0 Poisoning by, adverse effect of and underdosing of local antifungal, anti-infective and anti-inflammatory drugs**

● **T49.0X Poisoning by, adverse effect of and underdosing of local antifungal, anti-infective and anti-inflammatory drugs**

● **T49.0X1 Poisoning by local antifungal, anti-infective and anti-inflammatory drugs, accidental (unintentional)**
Poisoning by local antifungal, anti-infective and anti-inflammatory drugs NOS

● **T49.0X2 Poisoning by local antifungal, anti-infective and anti-inflammatory drugs, intentional self-harm**

● **T49.0X3 Poisoning by local antifungal, anti-infective and anti-inflammatory drugs, assault**

● **T49.0X4 Poisoning by local antifungal, anti-infective and anti-inflammatory drugs, undetermined**

● **T49.0X5 Adverse effect of local antifungal, anti-infective and anti-inflammatory drugs**

● **T49.0X6 Underdosing of local antifungal, anti-infective and anti-inflammatory drugs**

● **T49.1 Poisoning by, adverse effect of and underdosing of antipruritics**

● **T49.1X Poisoning by, adverse effect of and underdosing of antipruritics**

● **T49.1X1 Poisoning by antipruritics, accidental (unintentional)**
Poisoning by antipruritics NOS

● **T49.1X2 Poisoning by antipruritics, intentional self-harm**

● **T49.1X3 Poisoning by antipruritics, assault**

● **T49.1X4 Poisoning by antipruritics, undetermined**

● **T49.1X5 Adverse effect of antipruritics**

● **T49.1X6 Underdosing of antipruritics**

● **T49.2 Poisoning by, adverse effect of and underdosing of local astringents and local detergents**

● **T49.2X Poisoning by, adverse effect of and underdosing of local astringents and local detergents**

● **T49.2X1 Poisoning by local astringents and local detergents, accidental (unintentional)**
Poisoning by local astringents and local detergents NOS

● **T49.2X2 Poisoning by local astringents and local detergents, intentional self-harm**

● **T49.2X3 Poisoning by local astringents and local detergents, assault**

● **T49.2X4 Poisoning by local astringents and local detergents, undetermined**

● **T49.2X5 Adverse effect of local astringents and local detergents**

● **T49.2X6 Underdosing of local astringents and local detergents**

● **T49.3 Poisoning by, adverse effect of and underdosing of emollients, demulcents and protectants**

● **T49.3X Poisoning by, adverse effect of and underdosing of emollients, demulcents and protectants**

● **T49.3X1 Poisoning by emollients, demulcents and protectants, accidental (unintentional)**
Poisoning by emollients, demulcents and protectants NOS

● **T49.3X2 Poisoning by emollients, demulcents and protectants, intentional self-harm**

● **T49.3X3 Poisoning by emollients, demulcents and protectants, assault**

● **T49.3X4 Poisoning by emollients, demulcents and protectants, undetermined**

● **T49.3X5 Adverse effect of emollients, demulcents and protectants**

● **T49.3X6 Underdosing of emollients, demulcents and protectants**

● **T49.4 Poisoning by, adverse effect of and underdosing of keratolytics, keratoplastics, and other hair treatment drugs and preparations**

● **T49.4X Poisoning by, adverse effect of and underdosing of keratolytics, keratoplastics, and other hair treatment drugs and preparations**

● **T49.4X1 Poisoning by keratolytics, keratoplastics, and other hair treatment drugs and preparations, accidental (unintentional)**
Poisoning by keratolytics, keratoplastics, and other hair treatment drugs and preparations NOS

● **T49.4X2 Poisoning by keratolytics, keratoplastics, and other hair treatment drugs and preparations, intentional self-harm**

● **T49.4X3 Poisoning by keratolytics, keratoplastics, and other hair treatment drugs and preparations, assault**

● **T49.4X4 Poisoning by keratolytics, keratoplastics, and other hair treatment drugs and preparations, undetermined**

● **T49.4X5 Adverse effect of keratolytics, keratoplastics, and other hair treatment drugs and preparations**

● **T49.4X6 Underdosing of keratolytics, keratoplastics, and other hair treatment drugs and preparations**

● **T49.5 Poisoning by, adverse effect of and underdosing of ophthalmological drugs and preparations**

● **T49.5X Poisoning by, adverse effect of and underdosing of ophthalmological drugs and preparations**

● **T49.5X1 Poisoning by ophthalmological drugs and preparations, accidental (unintentional)**
Poisoning by ophthalmological drugs and preparations NOS

● **T49.5X2 Poisoning by ophthalmological drugs and preparations, intentional self-harm**

● **T49.5X3 Poisoning by ophthalmological drugs and preparations, assault**

● **T49.5X4 Poisoning by ophthalmological drugs and preparations, undetermined**

● **T49.5X5 Adverse effect of ophthalmological drugs and preparations**

● **T49.5X6 Underdosing of ophthalmological drugs and preparations**

- **T49.6 Poisoning by, adverse effect of and underdosing of otorhinolaryngological drugs and preparations**
  - **T49.6X Poisoning by, adverse effect of and underdosing of otorhinolaryngological drugs and preparations**
    - **T49.6X1 Poisoning by otorhinolaryngological drugs and preparations, accidental (unintentional)**
      Poisoning by otorhinolaryngological drugs and preparations NOS
    - **T49.6X2 Poisoning by otorhinolaryngological drugs and preparations, intentional self-harm**
    - **T49.6X3 Poisoning by otorhinolaryngological drugs and preparations, assault**
    - **T49.6X4 Poisoning by otorhinolaryngological drugs and preparations, undetermined**
    - **T49.6X5 Adverse effect of otorhinolaryngological drugs and preparations**
    - **T49.6X6 Underdosing of otorhinolaryngological drugs and preparations**
- **T49.7 Poisoning by, adverse effect of and underdosing of dental drugs, topically applied**
  - **T49.7X Poisoning by, adverse effect of and underdosing of dental drugs, topically applied**
    - **T49.7X1 Poisoning by dental drugs, topically applied, accidental (unintentional)**
      Poisoning by dental drugs, topically applied NOS
    - **T49.7X2 Poisoning by dental drugs, topically applied, intentional self-harm**
    - **T49.7X3 Poisoning by dental drugs, topically applied, assault**
    - **T49.7X4 Poisoning by dental drugs, topically applied, undetermined**
    - **T49.7X5 Adverse effect of dental drugs, topically applied**
    - **T49.7X6 Underdosing of dental drugs, topically applied**
- **T49.8 Poisoning by, adverse effect of and underdosing of other topical agents**
  Poisoning by, adverse effect of and underdosing of spermicides
  - **T49.8X Poisoning by, adverse effect of and underdosing of other topical agents**
    - **T49.8X1 Poisoning by other topical agents, accidental (unintentional)**
      Poisoning by other topical agents NOS
    - **T49.8X2 Poisoning by other topical agents, intentional self-harm**
    - **T49.8X3 Poisoning by other topical agents, assault**
    - **T49.8X4 Poisoning by other topical agents, undetermined**
    - **T49.8X5 Adverse effect of other topical agents**
    - **T49.8X6 Underdosing of other topical agents**
- **T49.9 Poisoning by, adverse effect of and underdosing of unspecified topical agent**
  - X **T49.91 Poisoning by unspecified topical agent, accidental (unintentional)**
  - X **T49.92 Poisoning by unspecified topical agent, intentional self-harm**
  - X **T49.93 Poisoning by unspecified topical agent, assault**
  - X **T49.94 Poisoning by unspecified topical agent, undetermined**
  - X **T49.95 Adverse effect of unspecified topical agent**
  - X **T49.96 Underdosing of unspecified topical agent**
- **T50 Poisoning by, adverse effect of and underdosing of diuretics and other and unspecified drugs, medicaments and biological substances**
  The appropriate 7th character is to be added to each code from category T50

A	initial encounter
D	subsequent encounter
S	sequela

  - **T50.0 Poisoning by, adverse effect of and underdosing of mineralocorticoids and their antagonists**
    - **T50.0X Poisoning by, adverse effect of and underdosing of mineralocorticoids and their antagonists**
      - **T50.0X1 Poisoning by mineralocorticoids and their antagonists, accidental (unintentional)**
        Poisoning by mineralocorticoids and their antagonists NOS
      - **T50.0X2 Poisoning by mineralocorticoids and their antagonists, intentional self-harm**
      - **T50.0X3 Poisoning by mineralocorticoids and their antagonists, assault**
      - **T50.0X4 Poisoning by mineralocorticoids and their antagonists, undetermined**
      - **T50.0X5 Adverse effect of mineralocorticoids and their antagonists**
      - **T50.0X6 Underdosing of mineralocorticoids and their antagonists**
  - **T50.1 Poisoning by, adverse effect of and underdosing of loop [high-ceiling] diuretics**
    - **T50.1X Poisoning by, adverse effect of and underdosing of loop [high-ceiling] diuretics**
      - **T50.1X1 Poisoning by loop [high-ceiling] diuretics, accidental (unintentional)**
        Poisoning by loop [high-ceiling] diuretics NOS
      - **T50.1X2 Poisoning by loop [high-ceiling] diuretics, intentional self-harm**
      - **T50.1X3 Poisoning by loop [high-ceiling] diuretics, assault**
      - **T50.1X4 Poisoning by loop [high-ceiling] diuretics, undetermined**
      - **T50.1X5 Adverse effect of loop [high-ceiling] diuretics**
      - **T50.1X6 Underdosing of loop [high-ceiling] diuretics**

- **T50.2 Poisoning by, adverse effect of and underdosing of carbonic-anhydrase inhibitors, benzothiadiazides and other diuretics**
  Poisoning by, adverse effect of and underdosing of acetazolamide
  - **T50.2X Poisoning by, adverse effect of and underdosing of carbonic-anhydrase inhibitors, benzothiadiazides and other diuretics**
    - **T50.2X1 Poisoning by carbonic-anhydrase inhibitors, benzothiadiazides and other diuretics, accidental (unintentional)**
      Poisoning by carbonic-anhydrase inhibitors, benzothiadiazides and other diuretics NOS
    - **T50.2X2 Poisoning by carbonic-anhydrase inhibitors, benzothiadiazides and other diuretics, intentional self-harm**
    - **T50.2X3 Poisoning by carbonic-anhydrase inhibitors, benzothiadiazides and other diuretics, assault**
    - **T50.2X4 Poisoning by carbonic-anhydrase inhibitors, benzothiadiazides and other diuretics, undetermined**
    - **T50.2X5 Adverse effect of carbonic-anhydrase inhibitors, benzothiadiazides and other diuretics**
    - **T50.2X6 Underdosing of carbonic-anhydrase inhibitors, benzothiadiazides and other diuretics**
- **T50.3 Poisoning by, adverse effect of and underdosing of electrolytic, caloric and water-balance agents**
  Poisoning by, adverse effect of and underdosing of oral rehydration salts
  - **T50.3X Poisoning by, adverse effect of and underdosing of electrolytic, caloric and water-balance agents**
    - **T50.3X1 Poisoning by electrolytic, caloric and water-balance agents, accidental (unintentional)**
      Poisoning by electrolytic, caloric and water-balance agents NOS
    - **T50.3X2 Poisoning by electrolytic, caloric and water-balance agents, intentional self-harm**
    - **T50.3X3 Poisoning by electrolytic, caloric and water-balance agents, assault**
    - **T50.3X4 Poisoning by electrolytic, caloric and water-balance agents, undetermined**
    - **T50.3X5 Adverse effect of electrolytic, caloric and water-balance agents**
    - **T50.3X6 Underdosing of electrolytic, caloric and water-balance agents**
- **T50.4 Poisoning by, adverse effect of and underdosing of drugs affecting uric acid metabolism**
  - **T50.4X Poisoning by, adverse effect of and underdosing of drugs affecting uric acid metabolism**
    - **T50.4X1 Poisoning by drugs affecting uric acid metabolism, accidental (unintentional)**
      Poisoning by drugs affecting uric acid metabolism NOS
    - **T50.4X2 Poisoning by drugs affecting uric acid metabolism, intentional self-harm**
    - **T50.4X3 Poisoning by drugs affecting uric acid metabolism, assault**
    - **T50.4X4 Poisoning by drugs affecting uric acid metabolism, undetermined**
    - **T50.4X5 Adverse effect of drugs affecting uric acid metabolism**
    - **T50.4X6 Underdosing of drugs affecting uric acid metabolism**
- **T50.5 Poisoning by, adverse effect of and underdosing of appetite depressants**
  - **T50.5X Poisoning by, adverse effect of and underdosing of appetite depressants**
    - **T50.5X1 Poisoning by appetite depressants, accidental (unintentional)**
      Poisoning by appetite depressants NOS
    - **T50.5X2 Poisoning by appetite depressants, intentional self-harm**
    - **T50.5X3 Poisoning by appetite depressants, assault**
    - **T50.5X4 Poisoning by appetite depressants, undetermined**
    - **T50.5X5 Adverse effect of appetite depressants**
    - **T50.5X6 Underdosing of appetite depressants**
- **T50.6 Poisoning by, adverse effect of and underdosing of antidotes and chelating agents**
  Poisoning by, adverse effect of and underdosing of alcohol deterrents
  - **T50.6X Poisoning by, adverse effect of and underdosing of antidotes and chelating agents**
    - **T50.6X1 Poisoning by antidotes and chelating agents, accidental (unintentional)**
      Poisoning by antidotes and chelating agents NOS
    - **T50.6X2 Poisoning by antidotes and chelating agents, intentional self-harm**
    - **T50.6X3 Poisoning by antidotes and chelating agents, assault**
    - **T50.6X4 Poisoning by antidotes and chelating agents, undetermined**
    - **T50.6X5 Adverse effect of antidotes and chelating agents**
    - **T50.6X6 Underdosing of antidotes and chelating agents**
- **T50.7 Poisoning by, adverse effect of and underdosing of analeptics and opioid receptor antagonists**
  - **T50.7X Poisoning by, adverse effect of and underdosing of analeptics and opioid receptor antagonists**
    - **T50.7X1 Poisoning by analeptics and opioid receptor antagonists, accidental (unintentional)**
      Poisoning by analeptics and opioid receptor antagonists NOS
    - **T50.7X2 Poisoning by analeptics and opioid receptor antagonists, intentional self-harm**
    - **T50.7X3 Poisoning by analeptics and opioid receptor antagonists, assault**
    - **T50.7X4 Poisoning by analeptics and opioid receptor antagonists, undetermined**
    - **T50.7X5 Adverse effect of analeptics and opioid receptor antagonists**
    - **T50.7X6 Underdosing of analeptics and opioid receptor antagonists**

◀ New ⇐ Revised ~~deleted~~ Deleted Excludes 1 Excludes 2 Includes Use additional Code first Code also Unspecified
OGCR Official Guidelines ● Unacceptable Principal Diagnosis X Assign placeholder X ● Use Additional Character(s) ▶ Manifestation Code Coding Clinic

- **T50.8** Poisoning by, adverse effect of and underdosing of diagnostic agents
  - **T50.8X** Poisoning by, adverse effect of and underdosing of diagnostic agents
    - **T50.8X1** Poisoning by diagnostic agents, accidental (unintentional)
      Poisoning by diagnostic agents NOS
    - **T50.8X2** Poisoning by diagnostic agents, intentional self-harm
    - **T50.8X3** Poisoning by diagnostic agents, assault
    - **T50.8X4** Poisoning by diagnostic agents, undetermined
    - **T50.8X5** Adverse effect of diagnostic agents
    - **T50.8X6** Underdosing of diagnostic agents
- **T50.A** Poisoning by, adverse effect of and underdosing of bacterial vaccines
  - **T50.A1** Poisoning by, adverse effect of and underdosing of pertussis vaccine, including combinations with a pertussis component
    - **T50.A11** Poisoning by pertussis vaccine, including combinations with a pertussis component, accidental (unintentional)
    - **T50.A12** Poisoning by pertussis vaccine, including combinations with a pertussis component, intentional self-harm
    - **T50.A13** Poisoning by pertussis vaccine, including combinations with a pertussis component, assault
    - **T50.A14** Poisoning by pertussis vaccine, including combinations with a pertussis component, undetermined
    - **T50.A15** Adverse effect of pertussis vaccine, including combinations with a pertussis component
    - **T50.A16** Underdosing of pertussis vaccine, including combinations with a pertussis component
  - **T50.A2** Poisoning by, adverse effect of and underdosing of mixed bacterial vaccines without a pertussis component
    - **T50.A21** Poisoning by mixed bacterial vaccines without a pertussis component, accidental (unintentional)
    - **T50.A22** Poisoning by mixed bacterial vaccines without a pertussis component, intentional self-harm
    - **T50.A23** Poisoning by mixed bacterial vaccines without a pertussis component, assault
    - **T50.A24** Poisoning by mixed bacterial vaccines without a pertussis component, undetermined
    - **T50.A25** Adverse effect of mixed bacterial vaccines without a pertussis component
    - **T50.A26** Underdosing of mixed bacterial vaccines without a pertussis component
  - **T50.A9** Poisoning by, adverse effect of and underdosing of other bacterial vaccines
    - **T50.A91** Poisoning by other bacterial vaccines, accidental (unintentional)
    - **T50.A92** Poisoning by other bacterial vaccines, intentional self-harm
    - **T50.A93** Poisoning by other bacterial vaccines, assault
    - **T50.A94** Poisoning by other bacterial vaccines, undetermined
    - **T50.A95** Adverse effect of other bacterial vaccines
    - **T50.A96** Underdosing of other bacterial vaccines
- **T50.B** Poisoning by, adverse effect of and underdosing of viral vaccines
  - **T50.B1** Poisoning by, adverse effect of and underdosing of smallpox vaccines
    - **T50.B11** Poisoning by smallpox vaccines, accidental (unintentional)
    - **T50.B12** Poisoning by smallpox vaccines, intentional self-harm
    - **T50.B13** Poisoning by smallpox vaccines, assault
    - **T50.B14** Poisoning by smallpox vaccines, undetermined
    - **T50.B15** Adverse effect of smallpox vaccines
    - **T50.B16** Underdosing of smallpox vaccines
  - **T50.B9** Poisoning by, adverse effect of and underdosing of other viral vaccines
    - **T50.B91** Poisoning by other viral vaccines, accidental (unintentional)
    - **T50.B92** Poisoning by other viral vaccines, intentional self-harm
    - **T50.B93** Poisoning by other viral vaccines, assault
    - **T50.B94** Poisoning by other viral vaccines, undetermined
    - **T50.B95** Adverse effect of other viral vaccines
    - **T50.B96** Underdosing of other viral vaccines
- **T50.Z** Poisoning by, adverse effect of and underdosing of other vaccines and biological substances
  - **T50.Z1** Poisoning by, adverse effect of and underdosing of immunoglobulin
    - **T50.Z11** Poisoning by immunoglobulin, accidental (unintentional)
    - **T50.Z12** Poisoning by immunoglobulin, intentional self-harm
    - **T50.Z13** Poisoning by immunoglobulin, assault
    - **T50.Z14** Poisoning by immunoglobulin, undetermined
    - **T50.Z15** Adverse effect of immunoglobulin
    - **T50.Z16** Underdosing of immunoglobulin

- **T50.Z9** Poisoning by, adverse effect of and underdosing of other vaccines and biological substances
  - **T50.Z91** Poisoning by other vaccines and biological substances, accidental (unintentional)
  - **T50.Z92** Poisoning by other vaccines and biological substances, intentional self-harm
  - **T50.Z93** Poisoning by other vaccines and biological substances, assault
  - **T50.Z94** Poisoning by other vaccines and biological substances, undetermined
  - **T50.Z95** Adverse effect of other vaccines and biological substances
  - **T50.Z96** Underdosing of other vaccines and biological substances
- **T50.9** Poisoning by, adverse effect of and underdosing of other and unspecified drugs, medicaments and biological substances
  - **T50.90** Poisoning by, adverse effect of and underdosing of unspecified drugs, medicaments and biological substances
    - **T50.901** Poisoning by unspecified drugs, medicaments and biological substances, accidental (unintentional)
      Coding Clinic: 2015, Q1, P21
    - **T50.902** Poisoning by unspecified drugs, medicaments and biological substances, intentional self-harm
    - **T50.903** Poisoning by unspecified drugs, medicaments and biological substances, assault
    - **T50.904** Poisoning by unspecified drugs, medicaments and biological substances, undetermined
    - **T50.905** Adverse effect of unspecified drugs, medicaments and biological substances
    - **T50.906** Underdosing of unspecified drugs, medicaments and biological substances
  - **T50.99** Poisoning by, adverse effect of and underdosing of other drugs, medicaments and biological substances
    - **T50.991** Poisoning by other drugs, medicaments and biological substances, accidental (unintentional)
    - **T50.992** Poisoning by other drugs, medicaments and biological substances, intentional self-harm
    - **T50.993** Poisoning by other drugs, medicaments and biological substances, assault
    - **T50.994** Poisoning by other drugs, medicaments and biological substances, undetermined
    - **T50.995** Adverse effect of other drugs, medicaments and biological substances
    - **T50.996** Underdosing of other drugs, medicaments and biological substances

TOXIC EFFECTS OF SUBSTANCES CHIEFLY NONMEDICINAL AS TO SOURCE (T51-T65)

Note: When no intent is indicated code to accidental. Undetermined intent is only for use when there is specific documentation in the record that the intent of the toxic effect cannot be determined.

Use additional code(s): for all associated manifestations of toxic effect, such as:
respiratory conditions due to external agents (J60-J70)
personal history of foreign body fully removed (Z87.821)
to identify any retained foreign body, if applicable (Z18.-)

Excludes1 contact with and (suspected) exposure to toxic substances (Z77.-)

- **T51** Toxic effect of alcohol

  The appropriate 7th character is to be added to each code from category T51

A	initial encounter
D	subsequent encounter
S	sequela

  - **T51.0** Toxic effect of ethanol
    Toxic effect of ethyl alcohol
    Excludes2 acute alcohol intoxication or 'hangover' effects (F10.129, F10.229, F10.929)
    drunkenness (F10.129, F10.229, F10.929)
    pathological alcohol intoxication (F10.129, F10.229, F10.929)
    - **T51.0X** Toxic effect of ethanol
      - **T51.0X1** Toxic effect of ethanol, accidental (unintentional)
        Toxic effect of ethanol NOS
      - **T51.0X2** Toxic effect of ethanol, intentional self-harm
      - **T51.0X3** Toxic effect of ethanol, assault
      - **T51.0X4** Toxic effect of ethanol, undetermined
  - **T51.1** Toxic effect of methanol
    Toxic effect of methyl alcohol
    - **T51.1X** Toxic effect of methanol
      - **T51.1X1** Toxic effect of methanol, accidental (unintentional)
        Toxic effect of methanol NOS
      - **T51.1X2** Toxic effect of methanol, intentional self-harm
      - **T51.1X3** Toxic effect of methanol, assault
      - **T51.1X4** Toxic effect of methanol, undetermined
  - **T51.2** Toxic effect of 2-Propanol
    Toxic effect of isopropyl alcohol
    - **T51.2X** Toxic effect of 2-Propanol
      - **T51.2X1** Toxic effect of 2-Propanol, accidental (unintentional)
        Toxic effect of 2-Propanol NOS
      - **T51.2X2** Toxic effect of 2-Propanol, intentional self-harm
      - **T51.2X3** Toxic effect of 2-Propanol, assault
      - **T51.2X4** Toxic effect of 2-Propanol, undetermined
  - **T51.3** Toxic effect of fusel oil
    Toxic effect of amyl alcohol
    Toxic effect of butyl [1-butanol] alcohol
    Toxic effect of propyl [1-propanol] alcohol
    - **T51.3X** Toxic effect of fusel oil
      - **T51.3X1** Toxic effect of fusel oil, accidental (unintentional)
        Toxic effect of fusel oil NOS
      - **T51.3X2** Toxic effect of fusel oil, intentional self-harm
      - **T51.3X3** Toxic effect of fusel oil, assault
      - **T51.3X4** Toxic effect of fusel oil, undetermined

- **T51.8 Toxic effect of other alcohols**
  - **T51.8X Toxic effect of other alcohols**
    - **T51.8X1 Toxic effect of other alcohols, accidental (unintentional)**
      Toxic effect of other alcohols NOS
    - **T51.8X2 Toxic effect of other alcohols, intentional self-harm**
    - **T51.8X3 Toxic effect of other alcohols, assault**
    - **T51.8X4 Toxic effect of other alcohols, undetermined**
- **T51.9 Toxic effect of unspecified alcohol**
  - X **T51.91 Toxic effect of unspecified alcohol, accidental (unintentional)**
  - X **T51.92 Toxic effect of unspecified alcohol, intentional self-harm**
  - X **T51.93 Toxic effect of unspecified alcohol, assault**
  - X **T51.94 Toxic effect of unspecified alcohol, undetermined**

- **T52 Toxic effect of organic solvents**

  Excludes1 halogen derivatives of aliphatic and aromatic hydrocarbons (T53.-)

  The appropriate 7th character is to be added to each code from category T52

A	initial encounter
D	subsequent encounter
S	sequela

- **T52.0 Toxic effects of petroleum products**
  Toxic effects of gasoline [petrol]
  Toxic effects of kerosene [paraffin oil]
  Toxic effects of paraffin wax
  Toxic effects of ether petroleum
  Toxic effects of naphtha petroleum
  Toxic effects of spirit petroleum
  - **T52.0X Toxic effects of petroleum products**
    - **T52.0X1 Toxic effect of petroleum products, accidental (unintentional)**
      Toxic effects of petroleum products NOS
    - **T52.0X2 Toxic effect of petroleum products, intentional self-harm**
    - **T52.0X3 Toxic effect of petroleum products, assault**
    - **T52.0X4 Toxic effect of petroleum products, undetermined**
- **T52.1 Toxic effects of benzene**

  Excludes1 homologues of benzene (T52.2)
  nitroderivatives and aminoderivatives of benzene and its homologues (T65.3)
  - **T52.1X Toxic effects of benzene**
    - **T52.1X1 Toxic effect of benzene, accidental (unintentional)**
      Toxic effects of benzene NOS
    - **T52.1X2 Toxic effect of benzene, intentional self-harm**
    - **T52.1X3 Toxic effect of benzene, assault**
    - **T52.1X4 Toxic effect of benzene, undetermined**
- **T52.2 Toxic effects of homologues of benzene**
  Toxic effects of toluene [methylbenzene]
  Toxic effects of xylene [dimethylbenzene]
  - **T52.2X Toxic effects of homologues of benzene**
    - **T52.2X1 Toxic effect of homologues of benzene, accidental (unintentional)**
      Toxic effects of homologues of benzene NOS
    - **T52.2X2 Toxic effect of homologues of benzene, intentional self-harm**
    - **T52.2X3 Toxic effect of homologues of benzene, assault**
    - **T52.2X4 Toxic effect of homologues of benzene, undetermined**
- **T52.3 Toxic effects of glycols**
  - **T52.3X Toxic effects of glycols**
    - **T52.3X1 Toxic effect of glycols, accidental (unintentional)**
      Toxic effects of glycols NOS
    - **T52.3X2 Toxic effect of glycols, intentional self-harm**
    - **T52.3X3 Toxic effect of glycols, assault**
    - **T52.3X4 Toxic effect of glycols, undetermined**
- **T52.4 Toxic effects of ketones**
  - **T52.4X Toxic effects of ketones**
    - **T52.4X1 Toxic effect of ketones, accidental (unintentional)**
      Toxic effects of ketones NOS
    - **T52.4X2 Toxic effect of ketones, intentional self-harm**
    - **T52.4X3 Toxic effect of ketones, assault**
    - **T52.4X4 Toxic effect of ketones, undetermined**
- **T52.8 Toxic effects of other organic solvents**
  - **T52.8X Toxic effects of other organic solvents**
    - **T52.8X1 Toxic effect of other organic solvents, accidental (unintentional)**
      Toxic effects of other organic solvents NOS
    - **T52.8X2 Toxic effect of other organic solvents, intentional self-harm**
    - **T52.8X3 Toxic effect of other organic solvents, assault**
    - **T52.8X4 Toxic effect of other organic solvents, undetermined**
- **T52.9 Toxic effects of unspecified organic solvent**
  - X **T52.91 Toxic effect of unspecified organic solvent, accidental (unintentional)**
  - X **T52.92 Toxic effect of unspecified organic solvent, intentional self-harm**
  - X **T52.93 Toxic effect of unspecified organic solvent, assault**
  - X **T52.94 Toxic effect of unspecified organic solvent, undetermined**

- **T53 Toxic effect of halogen derivatives of aliphatic and aromatic hydrocarbons**

  The appropriate 7th character is to be added to each code from category T53

A	initial encounter
D	subsequent encounter
S	sequela

- **T53.0 Toxic effects of carbon tetrachloride**
  Toxic effects of tetrachloromethane
  - **T53.0X Toxic effects of carbon tetrachloride**
    - **T53.0X1 Toxic effect of carbon tetrachloride, accidental (unintentional)**
      Toxic effects of carbon tetrachloride NOS
    - **T53.0X2 Toxic effect of carbon tetrachloride, intentional self-harm**
    - **T53.0X3 Toxic effect of carbon tetrachloride, assault**
    - **T53.0X4 Toxic effect of carbon tetrachloride, undetermined**

- **T53.1 Toxic effects of chloroform**
  Toxic effects of trichloromethane
  - **T53.1X Toxic effects of chloroform**
    - **T53.1X1 Toxic effect of chloroform, accidental (unintentional)**
      Toxic effects of chloroform NOS
    - **T53.1X2 Toxic effect of chloroform, intentional self-harm**
    - **T53.1X3 Toxic effect of chloroform, assault**
    - **T53.1X4 Toxic effect of chloroform, undetermined**
- **T53.2 Toxic effects of trichloroethylene**
  Toxic effects of trichloroethene
  - **T53.2X Toxic effects of trichloroethylene**
    - **T53.2X1 Toxic effect of trichloroethylene, accidental (unintentional)**
      Toxic effects of trichloroethylene NOS
    - **T53.2X2 Toxic effect of trichloroethylene, intentional self-harm**
    - **T53.2X3 Toxic effect of trichloroethylene, assault**
    - **T53.2X4 Toxic effect of trichloroethylene, undetermined**
- **T53.3 Toxic effects of tetrachloroethylene**
  Toxic effects of perchloroethylene
  Toxic effect of tetrachloroethene
  - **T53.3X Toxic effects of tetrachloroethylene**
    - **T53.3X1 Toxic effect of tetrachloroethylene, accidental (unintentional)**
      Toxic effects of tetrachloroethylene NOS
    - **T53.3X2 Toxic effect of tetrachloroethylene, intentional self-harm**
    - **T53.3X3 Toxic effect of tetrachloroethylene, assault**
    - **T53.3X4 Toxic effect of tetrachloroethylene, undetermined**
- **T53.4 Toxic effects of dichloromethane**
  Toxic effects of methylene chloride
  - **T53.4X Toxic effects of dichloromethane**
    - **T53.4X1 Toxic effect of dichloromethane, accidental (unintentional)**
      Toxic effects of dichloromethane NOS
    - **T53.4X2 Toxic effect of dichloromethane, intentional self-harm**
    - **T53.4X3 Toxic effect of dichloromethane, assault**
    - **T53.4X4 Toxic effect of dichloromethane, undetermined**
- **T53.5 Toxic effects of chlorofluorocarbons**
  - **T53.5X Toxic effects of chlorofluorocarbons**
    - **T53.5X1 Toxic effect of chlorofluorocarbons, accidental (unintentional)**
      Toxic effects of chlorofluorocarbons NOS
    - **T53.5X2 Toxic effect of chlorofluorocarbons, intentional self-harm**
    - **T53.5X3 Toxic effect of chlorofluorocarbons, assault**
    - **T53.5X4 Toxic effect of chlorofluorocarbons, undetermined**
- **T53.6 Toxic effects of other halogen derivatives of aliphatic hydrocarbons**
  - **T53.6X Toxic effects of other halogen derivatives of aliphatic hydrocarbons**
    - **T53.6X1 Toxic effect of other halogen derivatives of aliphatic hydrocarbons, accidental (unintentional)**
      Toxic effects of other halogen derivatives of aliphatic hydrocarbons NOS
    - **T53.6X2 Toxic effect of other halogen derivatives of aliphatic hydrocarbons, intentional self-harm**
    - **T53.6X3 Toxic effect of other halogen derivatives of aliphatic hydrocarbons, assault**
    - **T53.6X4 Toxic effect of other halogen derivatives of aliphatic hydrocarbons, undetermined**
- **T53.7 Toxic effects of other halogen derivatives of aromatic hydrocarbons**
  - **T53.7X Toxic effects of other halogen derivatives of aromatic hydrocarbons**
    - **T53.7X1 Toxic effect of other halogen derivatives of aromatic hydrocarbons, accidental (unintentional)**
      Toxic effects of other halogen derivatives of aromatic hydrocarbons NOS
    - **T53.7X2 Toxic effect of other halogen derivatives of aromatic hydrocarbons, intentional self-harm**
    - **T53.7X3 Toxic effect of other halogen derivatives of aromatic hydrocarbons, assault**
    - **T53.7X4 Toxic effect of other halogen derivatives of aromatic hydrocarbons, undetermined**
- **T53.9 Toxic effects of unspecified halogen derivatives of aliphatic and aromatic hydrocarbons**
  - X **T53.91 Toxic effect of unspecified halogen derivatives of aliphatic and aromatic hydrocarbons, accidental (unintentional)**
  - X **T53.92 Toxic effect of unspecified halogen derivatives of aliphatic and aromatic hydrocarbons, intentional self-harm**
  - X **T53.93 Toxic effect of unspecified halogen derivatives of aliphatic and aromatic hydrocarbons, assault**
  - X **T53.94 Toxic effect of unspecified halogen derivatives of aliphatic and aromatic hydrocarbons, undetermined**

- **T54 Toxic effect of corrosive substances**
  The appropriate 7th character is to be added to each code from category T54

A	initial encounter
D	subsequent encounter
S	sequela

- **T54.0 Toxic effects of phenol and phenol homologues**
  - **T54.0X Toxic effects of phenol and phenol homologues**
    - **T54.0X1 Toxic effect of phenol and phenol homologues, accidental (unintentional)**
      Toxic effects of phenol and phenol homologues NOS
    - **T54.0X2 Toxic effect of phenol and phenol homologues, intentional self-harm**
    - **T54.0X3 Toxic effect of phenol and phenol homologues, assault**
    - **T54.0X4 Toxic effect of phenol and phenol homologues, undetermined**

- **T54.1 Toxic effects of other corrosive organic compounds**
  - **T54.1X Toxic effects of other corrosive organic compounds**
    - **T54.1X1 Toxic effect of other corrosive organic compounds, accidental (unintentional)**
      Toxic effects of other corrosive organic compounds NOS
    - **T54.1X2 Toxic effect of other corrosive organic compounds, intentional self-harm**
    - **T54.1X3 Toxic effect of other corrosive organic compounds, assault**
    - **T54.1X4 Toxic effect of other corrosive organic compounds, undetermined**
- **T54.2 Toxic effects of corrosive acids and acid-like substances**
  Toxic effects of hydrochloric acid
  Toxic effects of sulfuric acid
  - **T54.2X Toxic effects of corrosive acids and acid-like substances**
    - **T54.2X1 Toxic effect of corrosive acids and acid-like substances, accidental (unintentional)**
      Toxic effects of corrosive acids and acid-like substances NOS
    - **T54.2X2 Toxic effect of corrosive acids and acid-like substances, intentional self-harm**
    - **T54.2X3 Toxic effect of corrosive acids and acid-like substances, assault**
    - **T54.2X4 Toxic effect of corrosive acids and acid-like substances, undetermined**
- **T54.3 Toxic effects of corrosive alkalis and alkali-like substances**
  Toxic effects of potassium hydroxide
  Toxic effects of sodium hydroxide
  - **T54.3X Toxic effects of corrosive alkalis and alkali-like substances**
    - **T54.3X1 Toxic effect of corrosive alkalis and alkali-like substances, accidental (unintentional)**
      Toxic effects of corrosive alkalis and alkali-like substances NOS
    - **T54.3X2 Toxic effect of corrosive alkalis and alkali-like substances, intentional self-harm**
    - **T54.3X3 Toxic effect of corrosive alkalis and alkali-like substances, assault**
    - **T54.3X4 Toxic effect of corrosive alkalis and alkali-like substances, undetermined**
- **T54.9 Toxic effects of unspecified corrosive substance**
  - X **T54.91 Toxic effect of unspecified corrosive substance, accidental (unintentional)**
  - X **T54.92 Toxic effect of unspecified corrosive substance, intentional self-harm**
  - X **T54.93 Toxic effect of unspecified corrosive substance, assault**
  - X **T54.94 Toxic effect of unspecified corrosive substance, undetermined**

- **T55 Toxic effect of soaps and detergents**
  The appropriate 7th character is to be added to each code from category T55

A	initial encounter
D	subsequent encounter
S	sequela

  - **T55.0 Toxic effect of soaps**
    - **T55.0X Toxic effect of soaps**
      - **T55.0X1 Toxic effect of soaps, accidental (unintentional)**
        Toxic effect of soaps NOS
      - **T55.0X2 Toxic effect of soaps, intentional self-harm**
      - **T55.0X3 Toxic effect of soaps, assault**
      - **T55.0X4 Toxic effect of soaps, undetermined**
  - **T55.1 Toxic effect of detergents**
    - **T55.1X Toxic effect of detergents**
      - **T55.1X1 Toxic effect of detergents, accidental (unintentional)**
        Toxic effect of detergents NOS
      - **T55.1X2 Toxic effect of detergents, intentional self-harm**
      - **T55.1X3 Toxic effect of detergents, assault**
      - **T55.1X4 Toxic effect of detergents, undetermined**

- **T56 Toxic effect of metals**
  Includes toxic effects of fumes and vapors of metals
  toxic effects of metals from all sources, except medicinal substances
  Use additional code to identify any retained metal foreign body, if applicable (Z18.0-, T18.1-)
  Excludes1 arsenic and its compounds (T57.0)
  manganese and its compounds (T57.2)
  The appropriate 7th character is to be added to each code from category T56

A	initial encounter
D	subsequent encounter
S	sequela

  - **T56.0 Toxic effects of lead and its compounds**
    - **T56.0X Toxic effects of lead and its compounds**
      - **T56.0X1 Toxic effect of lead and its compounds, accidental (unintentional)**
        Toxic effects of lead and its compounds NOS
      - **T56.0X2 Toxic effect of lead and its compounds, intentional self-harm**
      - **T56.0X3 Toxic effect of lead and its compounds, assault**
      - **T56.0X4 Toxic effect of lead and its compounds, undetermined**
  - **T56.1 Toxic effects of mercury and its compounds**
    - **T56.1X Toxic effects of mercury and its compounds**
      - **T56.1X1 Toxic effect of mercury and its compounds, accidental (unintentional)**
        Toxic effects of mercury and its compounds NOS
      - **T56.1X2 Toxic effect of mercury and its compounds, intentional self-harm**
      - **T56.1X3 Toxic effect of mercury and its compounds, assault**
      - **T56.1X4 Toxic effect of mercury and its compounds, undetermined**

- **T56.2 Toxic effects of chromium and its compounds**
  - **T56.2X Toxic effects of chromium and its compounds**
    - **T56.2X1 Toxic effect of chromium and its compounds, accidental (unintentional)**
      Toxic effects of chromium and its compounds NOS
    - **T56.2X2 Toxic effect of chromium and its compounds, intentional self-harm**
    - **T56.2X3 Toxic effect of chromium and its compounds, assault**
    - **T56.2X4 Toxic effect of chromium and its compounds, undetermined**
- **T56.3 Toxic effects of cadmium and its compounds**
  - **T56.3X Toxic effects of cadmium and its compounds**
    - **T56.3X1 Toxic effect of cadmium and its compounds, accidental (unintentional)**
      Toxic effects of cadmium and its compounds NOS
    - **T56.3X2 Toxic effect of cadmium and its compounds, intentional self-harm**
    - **T56.3X3 Toxic effect of cadmium and its compounds, assault**
    - **T56.3X4 Toxic effect of cadmium and its compounds, undetermined**
- **T56.4 Toxic effects of copper and its compounds**
  - **T56.4X Toxic effects of copper and its compounds**
    - **T56.4X1 Toxic effect of copper and its compounds, accidental (unintentional)**
      Toxic effects of copper and its compounds NOS
    - **T56.4X2 Toxic effect of copper and its compounds, intentional self-harm**
    - **T56.4X3 Toxic effect of copper and its compounds, assault**
    - **T56.4X4 Toxic effect of copper and its compounds, undetermined**
- **T56.5 Toxic effects of zinc and its compounds**
  - **T56.5X Toxic effects of zinc and its compounds**
    - **T56.5X1 Toxic effect of zinc and its compounds, accidental (unintentional)**
      Toxic effects of zinc and its compounds NOS
    - **T56.5X2 Toxic effect of zinc and its compounds, intentional self-harm**
    - **T56.5X3 Toxic effect of zinc and its compounds, assault**
    - **T56.5X4 Toxic effect of zinc and its compounds, undetermined**
- **T56.6 Toxic effects of tin and its compounds**
  - **T56.6X Toxic effects of tin and its compounds**
    - **T56.6X1 Toxic effect of tin and its compounds, accidental (unintentional)**
      Toxic effects of tin and its compounds NOS
    - **T56.6X2 Toxic effect of tin and its compounds, intentional self-harm**
    - **T56.6X3 Toxic effect of tin and its compounds, assault**
    - **T56.6X4 Toxic effect of tin and its compounds, undetermined**
- **T56.7 Toxic effects of beryllium and its compounds**
  - **T56.7X Toxic effects of beryllium and its compounds**
    - **T56.7X1 Toxic effect of beryllium and its compounds, accidental (unintentional)**
      Toxic effects of beryllium and its compounds NOS
    - **T56.7X2 Toxic effect of beryllium and its compounds, intentional self-harm**
    - **T56.7X3 Toxic effect of beryllium and its compounds, assault**
    - **T56.7X4 Toxic effect of beryllium and its compounds, undetermined**
- **T56.8 Toxic effects of other metals**
  - **T56.81 Toxic effect of thallium**
    - **T56.811 Toxic effect of thallium, accidental (unintentional)**
      Toxic effect of thallium NOS
    - **T56.812 Toxic effect of thallium, intentional self-harm**
    - **T56.813 Toxic effect of thallium, assault**
    - **T56.814 Toxic effect of thallium, undetermined**
  - **T56.89 Toxic effects of other metals**
    - **T56.891 Toxic effect of other metals, accidental (unintentional)**
      Toxic effects of other metals NOS
    - **T56.892 Toxic effect of other metals, intentional self-harm**
    - **T56.893 Toxic effect of other metals, assault**
    - **T56.894 Toxic effect of other metals, undetermined**
- **T56.9 Toxic effects of unspecified metal**
  - X **T56.91 Toxic effect of unspecified metal, accidental (unintentional)**
  - X **T56.92 Toxic effect of unspecified metal, intentional self-harm**
  - X **T56.93 Toxic effect of unspecified metal, assault**
  - X **T56.94 Toxic effect of unspecified metal, undetermined**

- **T57 Toxic effect of other inorganic substances**

  The appropriate 7th character is to be added to each code from category T57

A	initial encounter
D	subsequent encounter
S	sequela

- **T57.0 Toxic effect of arsenic and its compounds**
  - **T57.0X Toxic effect of arsenic and its compounds**
    - **T57.0X1 Toxic effect of arsenic and its compounds, accidental (unintentional)**
      Toxic effect of arsenic and its compounds NOS
    - **T57.0X2 Toxic effect of arsenic and its compounds, intentional self-harm**
    - **T57.0X3 Toxic effect of arsenic and its compounds, assault**
    - **T57.0X4 Toxic effect of arsenic and its compounds, undetermined**

T57.1 Toxic effect of phosphorus and its compounds

Excludes1 organophosphate insecticides (T60.0)

T57.1X Toxic effect of phosphorus and its compounds

T57.1X1 Toxic effect of phosphorus and its compounds, accidental (unintentional)

Toxic effect of phosphorus and its compounds NOS

T57.1X2 Toxic effect of phosphorus and its compounds, intentional self-harm

T57.1X3 Toxic effect of phosphorus and its compounds, assault

T57.1X4 Toxic effect of phosphorus and its compounds, undetermined

T57.2 Toxic effect of manganese and its compounds

T57.2X Toxic effect of manganese and its compounds

T57.2X1 Toxic effect of manganese and its compounds, accidental (unintentional)

Toxic effect of manganese and its compounds NOS

T57.2X2 Toxic effect of manganese and its compounds, intentional self-harm

T57.2X3 Toxic effect of manganese and its compounds, assault

T57.2X4 Toxic effect of manganese and its compounds, undetermined

T57.3 Toxic effect of hydrogen cyanide

T57.3X Toxic effect of hydrogen cyanide

T57.3X1 Toxic effect of hydrogen cyanide, accidental (unintentional)

Toxic effect of hydrogen cyanide NOS

T57.3X2 Toxic effect of hydrogen cyanide, intentional self-harm

T57.3X3 Toxic effect of hydrogen cyanide, assault

T57.3X4 Toxic effect of hydrogen cyanide, undetermined

T57.8 Toxic effect of other specified inorganic substances

T57.8X Toxic effect of other specified inorganic substances

T57.8X1 Toxic effect of other specified inorganic substances, accidental (unintentional)

Toxic effect of other specified inorganic substances NOS

T57.8X2 Toxic effect of other specified inorganic substances, intentional self-harm

T57.8X3 Toxic effect of other specified inorganic substances, assault

T57.8X4 Toxic effect of other specified inorganic substances, undetermined

T57.9 Toxic effect of unspecified inorganic substance

X **T57.91 Toxic effect of unspecified inorganic substance, accidental (unintentional)**

X **T57.92 Toxic effect of unspecified inorganic substance, intentional self-harm**

X **T57.93 Toxic effect of unspecified inorganic substance, assault**

X **T57.94 Toxic effect of unspecified inorganic substance, undetermined**

T58 Toxic effect of carbon monoxide

Includes asphyxiation from carbon monoxide
toxic effect of carbon monoxide from all sources

The appropriate 7th character is to be added to each code from category T58

A	initial encounter
D	subsequent encounter
S	sequela

T58.0 Toxic effect of carbon monoxide from motor vehicle exhaust

Toxic effect of exhaust gas from gas engine
Toxic effect of exhaust gas from motor pump

X **T58.01 Toxic effect of carbon monoxide from motor vehicle exhaust, accidental (unintentional)**

X **T58.02 Toxic effect of carbon monoxide from motor vehicle exhaust, intentional self-harm**

X **T58.03 Toxic effect of carbon monoxide from motor vehicle exhaust, assault**

X **T58.04 Toxic effect of carbon monoxide from motor vehicle exhaust, undetermined**

T58.1 Toxic effect of carbon monoxide from utility gas

Toxic effect of acetylene
Toxic effect of gas NOS used for lighting, heating, cooking
Toxic effect of water gas

X **T58.11 Toxic effect of carbon monoxide from utility gas, accidental (unintentional)**

X **T58.12 Toxic effect of carbon monoxide from utility gas, intentional self-harm**

X **T58.13 Toxic effect of carbon monoxide from utility gas, assault**

X **T58.14 Toxic effect of carbon monoxide from utility gas, undetermined**

T58.2 Toxic effect of carbon monoxide from incomplete combustion of other domestic fuels

Toxic effect of carbon monoxide from incomplete combustion of coal, coke, kerosene, wood

T58.2X Toxic effect of carbon monoxide from incomplete combustion of other domestic fuels

T58.2X1 Toxic effect of carbon monoxide from incomplete combustion of other domestic fuels, accidental (unintentional)

T58.2X2 Toxic effect of carbon monoxide from incomplete combustion of other domestic fuels, intentional self-harm

T58.2X3 Toxic effect of carbon monoxide from incomplete combustion of other domestic fuels, assault

T58.2X4 Toxic effect of carbon monoxide from incomplete combustion of other domestic fuels, undetermined

T58.8 Toxic effect of carbon monoxide from other source

Toxic effect of carbon monoxide from blast furnace gas
Toxic effect of carbon monoxide from fuels in industrial use
Toxic effect of carbon monoxide from kiln vapor

T58.8X Toxic effect of carbon monoxide from other source

T58.8X1 Toxic effect of carbon monoxide from other source, accidental (unintentional)

T58.8X2 Toxic effect of carbon monoxide from other source, intentional self-harm

T58.8X3 Toxic effect of carbon monoxide from other source, assault

T58.8X4 Toxic effect of carbon monoxide from other source, undetermined

- T58.9 Toxic effect of carbon monoxide from unspecified source
  - X T58.91 Toxic effect of carbon monoxide from unspecified source, accidental (unintentional)
  - X T58.92 Toxic effect of carbon monoxide from unspecified source, intentional self-harm
  - X T58.93 Toxic effect of carbon monoxide from unspecified source, assault
  - X T58.94 Toxic effect of carbon monoxide from unspecified source, undetermined

- T59 Toxic effect of other gases, fumes and vapors

  Includes aerosol propellants

  Excludes1 chlorofluorocarbons (T53.5)

  The appropriate 7th character is to be added to each code from category T59

A	initial encounter
D	subsequent encounter
S	sequela

- T59.0 Toxic effect of nitrogen oxides
  - T59.0X Toxic effect of nitrogen oxides
    - T59.0X1 Toxic effect of nitrogen oxides, accidental (unintentional)
      Toxic effect of nitrogen oxides NOS
    - T59.0X2 Toxic effect of nitrogen oxides, intentional self-harm
    - T59.0X3 Toxic effect of nitrogen oxides, assault
    - T59.0X4 Toxic effect of nitrogen oxides, undetermined
- T59.1 Toxic effect of sulfur dioxide
  - T59.1X Toxic effect of sulfur dioxide
    - T59.1X1 Toxic effect of sulfur dioxide, accidental (unintentional)
      Toxic effect of sulfur dioxide NOS
    - T59.1X2 Toxic effect of sulfur dioxide, intentional self-harm
    - T59.1X3 Toxic effect of sulfur dioxide, assault
    - T59.1X4 Toxic effect of sulfur dioxide, undetermined
- T59.2 Toxic effect of formaldehyde
  - T59.2X Toxic effect of formaldehyde
    - T59.2X1 Toxic effect of formaldehyde, accidental (unintentional)
      Toxic effect of formaldehyde NOS
    - T59.2X2 Toxic effect of formaldehyde, intentional self-harm
    - T59.2X3 Toxic effect of formaldehyde, assault
    - T59.2X4 Toxic effect of formaldehyde, undetermined
- T59.3 Toxic effect of lacrimogenic gas
  Toxic effect of tear gas
  - T59.3X Toxic effect of lacrimogenic gas
    - T59.3X1 Toxic effect of lacrimogenic gas, accidental (unintentional)
      Toxic effect of lacrimogenic gas NOS
    - T59.3X2 Toxic effect of lacrimogenic gas, intentional self-harm
    - T59.3X3 Toxic effect of lacrimogenic gas, assault
    - T59.3X4 Toxic effect of lacrimogenic gas, undetermined
- T59.4 Toxic effect of chlorine gas
  - T59.4X Toxic effect of chlorine gas
    - T59.4X1 Toxic effect of chlorine gas, accidental (unintentional)
      Toxic effect of chlorine gas NOS
    - T59.4X2 Toxic effect of chlorine gas, intentional self-harm
    - T59.4X3 Toxic effect of chlorine gas, assault
    - T59.4X4 Toxic effect of chlorine gas, undetermined
- T59.5 Toxic effect of fluorine gas and hydrogen fluoride
  - T59.5X Toxic effect of fluorine gas and hydrogen fluoride
    - T59.5X1 Toxic effect of fluorine gas and hydrogen fluoride, accidental (unintentional)
      Toxic effect of fluorine gas and hydrogen fluoride NOS
    - T59.5X2 Toxic effect of fluorine gas and hydrogen fluoride, intentional self-harm
    - T59.5X3 Toxic effect of fluorine gas and hydrogen fluoride, assault
    - T59.5X4 Toxic effect of fluorine gas and hydrogen fluoride, undetermined
- T59.6 Toxic effect of hydrogen sulfide
  - T59.6X Toxic effect of hydrogen sulfide
    - T59.6X1 Toxic effect of hydrogen sulfide, accidental (unintentional)
      Toxic effect of hydrogen sulfide NOS
    - T59.6X2 Toxic effect of hydrogen sulfide, intentional self-harm
    - T59.6X3 Toxic effect of hydrogen sulfide, assault
    - T59.6X4 Toxic effect of hydrogen sulfide, undetermined
- T59.7 Toxic effect of carbon dioxide
  - T59.7X Toxic effect of carbon dioxide
    - T59.7X1 Toxic effect of carbon dioxide, accidental (unintentional)
      Toxic effect of carbon dioxide NOS
    - T59.7X2 Toxic effect of carbon dioxide, intentional self-harm
    - T59.7X3 Toxic effect of carbon dioxide, assault
    - T59.7X4 Toxic effect of carbon dioxide, undetermined
- T59.8 Toxic effect of other specified gases, fumes and vapors
  - T59.81 Toxic effect of smoke
    Smoke inhalation

    Excludes2 toxic effect of cigarette (tobacco) smoke (T65.22-)
    - T59.811 Toxic effect of smoke, accidental (unintentional)
      Toxic effect of smoke NOS
    - T59.812 Toxic effect of smoke, intentional self-harm
    - T59.813 Toxic effect of smoke, assault
    - T59.814 Toxic effect of smoke, undetermined
  - T59.89 Toxic effect of other specified gases, fumes and vapors
    - T59.891 Toxic effect of other specified gases, fumes and vapors, accidental (unintentional)
    - T59.892 Toxic effect of other specified gases, fumes and vapors, intentional self-harm
    - T59.893 Toxic effect of other specified gases, fumes and vapors, assault
    - T59.894 Toxic effect of other specified gases, fumes and vapors, undetermined

- **T59.9 Toxic effect of unspecified gases, fumes and vapors**
  - X **T59.91 Toxic effect of unspecified gases, fumes and vapors, accidental (unintentional)**
  - X **T59.92 Toxic effect of unspecified gases, fumes and vapors, intentional self-harm**
  - X **T59.93 Toxic effect of unspecified gases, fumes and vapors, assault**
  - X **T59.94 Toxic effect of unspecified gases, fumes and vapors, undetermined**

- **T60 Toxic effect of pesticides**

  Includes toxic effect of wood preservatives

  The appropriate 7th character is to be added to each code from category T60

A	initial encounter
D	subsequent encounter
S	sequela

- **T60.0 Toxic effect of organophosphate and carbamate insecticides**
  - **T60.0X Toxic effect of organophosphate and carbamate insecticides**
    - **T60.0X1 Toxic effect of organophosphate and carbamate insecticides, accidental (unintentional)**
      Toxic effect of organophosphate and carbamate insecticides NOS
    - **T60.0X2 Toxic effect of organophosphate and carbamate insecticides, intentional self-harm**
    - **T60.0X3 Toxic effect of organophosphate and carbamate insecticides, assault**
    - **T60.0X4 Toxic effect of organophosphate and carbamate insecticides, undetermined**
- **T60.1 Toxic effect of halogenated insecticides**

  Excludes1 chlorinated hydrocarbon (T53.-)
  - **T60.1X Toxic effect of halogenated insecticides**
    - **T60.1X1 Toxic effect of halogenated insecticides, accidental (unintentional)**
      Toxic effect of halogenated insecticides NOS
    - **T60.1X2 Toxic effect of halogenated insecticides, intentional self-harm**
    - **T60.1X3 Toxic effect of halogenated insecticides, assault**
    - **T60.1X4 Toxic effect of halogenated insecticides, undetermined**
- **T60.2 Toxic effect of other insecticides**
  - **T60.2X Toxic effect of other insecticides**
    - **T60.2X1 Toxic effect of other insecticides, accidental (unintentional)**
      Toxic effect of other insecticides NOS
    - **T60.2X2 Toxic effect of other insecticides, intentional self-harm**
    - **T60.2X3 Toxic effect of other insecticides, assault**
    - **T60.2X4 Toxic effect of other insecticides, undetermined**
- **T60.3 Toxic effect of herbicides and fungicides**
  - **T60.3X Toxic effect of herbicides and fungicides**
    - **T60.3X1 Toxic effect of herbicides and fungicides, accidental (unintentional)**
      Toxic effect of herbicides and fungicides NOS
    - **T60.3X2 Toxic effect of herbicides and fungicides, intentional self-harm**
    - **T60.3X3 Toxic effect of herbicides and fungicides, assault**
    - **T60.3X4 Toxic effect of herbicides and fungicides, undetermined**
- **T60.4 Toxic effect of rodenticides**

  Excludes1 strychnine and its salts (T65.1)
  thallium (T56.81-)
  - **T60.4X Toxic effect of rodenticides**
    - **T60.4X1 Toxic effect of rodenticides, accidental (unintentional)**
      Toxic effect of rodenticides NOS
    - **T60.4X2 Toxic effect of rodenticides, intentional self-harm**
    - **T60.4X3 Toxic effect of rodenticides, assault**
    - **T60.4X4 Toxic effect of rodenticides, undetermined**
- **T60.8 Toxic effect of other pesticides**
  - **T60.8X Toxic effect of other pesticides**
    - **T60.8X1 Toxic effect of other pesticides, accidental (unintentional)**
      Toxic effect of other pesticides NOS
    - **T60.8X2 Toxic effect of other pesticides, intentional self-harm**
    - **T60.8X3 Toxic effect of other pesticides, assault**
    - **T60.8X4 Toxic effect of other pesticides, undetermined**
- **T60.9 Toxic effect of unspecified pesticide**
  - X **T60.91 Toxic effect of unspecified pesticide, accidental (unintentional)**
  - X **T60.92 Toxic effect of unspecified pesticide, intentional self-harm**
  - X **T60.93 Toxic effect of unspecified pesticide, assault**
  - X **T60.94 Toxic effect of unspecified pesticide, undetermined**

- **T61 Toxic effect of noxious substances eaten as seafood**

  Excludes1 allergic reaction to food, such as:
  anaphylactic reaction or shock due to adverse food reaction (T78.0-)
  bacterial foodborne intoxications (A05.-)
  dermatitis (L23.6, L25.4, L27.2)
  food protein-induced enterocolitis syndrome (K52.21) ◀
  food protein-induced enteropathy (K52.22) ◀
  gastroenteritis (noninfective) (K52.29) ◀
  toxic effect of aflatoxin and other mycotoxins (T64)
  toxic effect of cyanides (T65.0-)
  toxic effect of harmful algae bloom (T65.82-)
  toxic effect of hydrogen cyanide (T57.3-)
  toxic effect of mercury (T56.1-)
  toxic effect of red tide (T65.82-)

  The appropriate 7th character is to be added to each code from category T61

A	initial encounter
D	subsequent encounter
S	sequela

- **T61.0 Ciguatera fish poisoning**
  - X **T61.01 Ciguatera fish poisoning, accidental (unintentional)**
  - X **T61.02 Ciguatera fish poisoning, intentional self-harm**
  - X **T61.03 Ciguatera fish poisoning, assault**
  - X **T61.04 Ciguatera fish poisoning, undetermined**
- **T61.1 Scombroid fish poisoning**
  Histamine-like syndrome
  - X **T61.11 Scombroid fish poisoning, accidental (unintentional)**
  - X **T61.12 Scombroid fish poisoning, intentional self-harm**
  - X **T61.13 Scombroid fish poisoning, assault**
  - X **T61.14 Scombroid fish poisoning, undetermined**

- **T61.7 Other fish and shellfish poisoning**
  - **T61.77 Other fish poisoning**
    - **T61.771 Other fish poisoning, accidental (unintentional)**
    - **T61.772 Other fish poisoning, intentional self-harm**
    - **T61.773 Other fish poisoning, assault**
    - **T61.774 Other fish poisoning, undetermined**
  - **T61.78 Other shellfish poisoning**
    - **T61.781 Other shellfish poisoning, accidental (unintentional)**
    - **T61.782 Other shellfish poisoning, intentional self-harm**
    - **T61.783 Other shellfish poisoning, assault**
    - **T61.784 Other shellfish poisoning, undetermined**
- **T61.8 Toxic effect of other seafood**
  - **T61.8X Toxic effect of other seafood**
    - **T61.8X1 Toxic effect of other seafood, accidental (unintentional)**
    - **T61.8X2 Toxic effect of other seafood, intentional self-harm**
    - **T61.8X3 Toxic effect of other seafood, assault**
    - **T61.8X4 Toxic effect of other seafood, undetermined**
- **T61.9 Toxic effect of unspecified seafood**
  - X **T61.91 Toxic effect of unspecified seafood, accidental (unintentional)**
  - X **T61.92 Toxic effect of unspecified seafood, intentional self-harm**
  - X **T61.93 Toxic effect of unspecified seafood, assault**
  - X **T61.94 Toxic effect of unspecified seafood, undetermined**

- **T62 Toxic effect of other noxious substances eaten as food**

  Excludes1 allergic reaction to food, such as:
  - anaphylactic shock (reaction) due to adverse food reaction (T78.0-)
  - dermatitis (L23.6, L25.4, L27.2)
  - food protein-induced enterocolitis syndrome (K52.21) ◀
  - food protein-induced enteropathy (K52.22) ◀
  - gastroenteritis (noninfective) (K52.29) ◀
  - bacterial food borne intoxications (A05.-)
  - toxic effect of aflatoxin and other mycotoxins (T64)
  - toxic effect of cyanides (T65.0-)
  - toxic effect of hydrogen cyanide (T57.3-)
  - toxic effect of mercury (T56.1-)

  The appropriate 7th character is to be added to each code from category T62

A	initial encounter
D	subsequent encounter
S	sequela

- **T62.0 Toxic effect of ingested mushrooms**
  - **T62.0X Toxic effect of ingested mushrooms**
    - **T62.0X1 Toxic effect of ingested mushrooms, accidental (unintentional)**
      Toxic effect of ingested mushrooms NOS
    - **T62.0X2 Toxic effect of ingested mushrooms, intentional self-harm**
    - **T62.0X3 Toxic effect of ingested mushrooms, assault**
    - **T62.0X4 Toxic effect of ingested mushrooms, undetermined**
- **T62.1 Toxic effect of ingested berries**
  - **T62.1X Toxic effect of ingested berries**
    - **T62.1X1 Toxic effect of ingested berries, accidental (unintentional)**
      Toxic effect of ingested berries NOS
    - **T62.1X2 Toxic effect of ingested berries, intentional self-harm**
    - **T62.1X3 Toxic effect of ingested berries, assault**
    - **T62.1X4 Toxic effect of ingested berries, undetermined**
- **T62.2 Toxic effect of other ingested (parts of) plant(s)**
  - **T62.2X Toxic effect of other ingested (parts of) plant(s)**
    - **T62.2X1 Toxic effect of other ingested (parts of) plant(s), accidental (unintentional)**
      Toxic effect of other ingested (parts of) plant(s) NOS
    - **T62.2X2 Toxic effect of other ingested (parts of) plant(s), intentional self-harm**
    - **T62.2X3 Toxic effect of other ingested (parts of) plant(s), assault**
    - **T62.2X4 Toxic effect of other ingested (parts of) plant(s), undetermined**
- **T62.8 Toxic effect of other specified noxious substances eaten as food**
  - **T62.8X Toxic effect of other specified noxious substances eaten as food**
    - **T62.8X1 Toxic effect of other specified noxious substances eaten as food, accidental (unintentional)**
      Toxic effect of other specified noxious substances eaten as food NOS
    - **T62.8X2 Toxic effect of other specified noxious substances eaten as food, intentional self-harm**
    - **T62.8X3 Toxic effect of other specified noxious substances eaten as food, assault**
    - **T62.8X4 Toxic effect of other specified noxious substances eaten as food, undetermined**
- **T62.9 Toxic effect of unspecified noxious substance eaten as food**
  - X **T62.91 Toxic effect of unspecified noxious substance eaten as food, accidental (unintentional)**
    Toxic effect of unspecified noxious substance eaten as food NOS
  - X **T62.92 Toxic effect of unspecified noxious substance eaten as food, intentional self-harm**
  - X **T62.93 Toxic effect of unspecified noxious substance eaten as food, assault**
  - X **T62.94 Toxic effect of unspecified noxious substance eaten as food, undetermined**

- **T63 Toxic effect of contact with venomous animals and plants**

  Includes bite or touch of venomous animal
  pricked or stuck by thorn or leaf

  Excludes2 ingestion of toxic animal or plant (T61.-, T62.-)

  The appropriate 7th character is to be added to each code from category T63

A	initial encounter
D	subsequent encounter
S	sequela

- **T63.0 Toxic effect of snake venom**
  - **T63.00 Toxic effect of unspecified snake venom**
    - **T63.001 Toxic effect of unspecified snake venom, accidental (unintentional)**
      Toxic effect of unspecified snake venom NOS
    - **T63.002 Toxic effect of unspecified snake venom, intentional self-harm**

- **T63.003 Toxic effect of unspecified snake venom, assault**
- **T63.004 Toxic effect of unspecified snake venom, undetermined**

- **T63.01 Toxic effect of rattlesnake venom**
  - **T63.011 Toxic effect of rattlesnake venom, accidental (unintentional)**
    Toxic effect of rattlesnake venom NOS
  - **T63.012 Toxic effect of rattlesnake venom, intentional self-harm**
  - **T63.013 Toxic effect of rattlesnake venom, assault**
  - **T63.014 Toxic effect of rattlesnake venom, undetermined**
- **T63.02 Toxic effect of coral snake venom**
  - **T63.021 Toxic effect of coral snake venom, accidental (unintentional)**
    Toxic effect of coral snake venom NOS
  - **T63.022 Toxic effect of coral snake venom, intentional self-harm**
  - **T63.023 Toxic effect of coral snake venom, assault**
  - **T63.024 Toxic effect of coral snake venom, undetermined**
- **T63.03 Toxic effect of taipan venom**
  - **T63.031 Toxic effect of taipan venom, accidental (unintentional)**
    Toxic effect of taipan venom NOS
  - **T63.032 Toxic effect of taipan venom, intentional self-harm**
  - **T63.033 Toxic effect of taipan venom, assault**
  - **T63.034 Toxic effect of taipan venom, undetermined**
- **T63.04 Toxic effect of cobra venom**
  - **T63.041 Toxic effect of cobra venom, accidental (unintentional)**
    Toxic effect of cobra venom NOS
  - **T63.042 Toxic effect of cobra venom, intentional self-harm**
  - **T63.043 Toxic effect of cobra venom, assault**
  - **T63.044 Toxic effect of cobra venom, undetermined**
- **T63.06 Toxic effect of venom of other North and South American snake**
  - **T63.061 Toxic effect of venom of other North and South American snake, accidental (unintentional)**
    Toxic effect of venom of other North and South American snake NOS
  - **T63.062 Toxic effect of venom of other North and South American snake, intentional self-harm**
  - **T63.063 Toxic effect of venom of other North and South American snake, assault**
  - **T63.064 Toxic effect of venom of other North and South American snake, undetermined**
- **T63.07 Toxic effect of venom of other Australian snake**
  - **T63.071 Toxic effect of venom of other Australian snake, accidental (unintentional)**
    Toxic effect of venom of other Australian snake NOS
  - **T63.072 Toxic effect of venom of other Australian snake, intentional self-harm**
  - **T63.073 Toxic effect of venom of other Australian snake, assault**
  - **T63.074 Toxic effect of venom of other Australian snake, undetermined**
- **T63.08 Toxic effect of venom of other African and Asian snake**
  - **T63.081 Toxic effect of venom of other African and Asian snake, accidental (unintentional)**
    Toxic effect of venom of other African and Asian snake NOS
  - **T63.082 Toxic effect of venom of other African and Asian snake, intentional self-harm**
  - **T63.083 Toxic effect of venom of other African and Asian snake, assault**
  - **T63.084 Toxic effect of venom of other African and Asian snake, undetermined**
- **T63.09 Toxic effect of venom of other snake**
  - **T63.091 Toxic effect of venom of other snake, accidental (unintentional)**
    Toxic effect of venom of other snake NOS
  - **T63.092 Toxic effect of venom of other snake, intentional self-harm**
  - **T63.093 Toxic effect of venom of other snake, assault**
  - **T63.094 Toxic effect of venom of other snake, undetermined**
- **T63.1 Toxic effect of venom of other reptiles**
  - **T63.11 Toxic effect of venom of gila monster**
    - **T63.111 Toxic effect of venom of gila monster, accidental (unintentional)**
      Toxic effect of venom of gila monster NOS
    - **T63.112 Toxic effect of venom of gila monster, intentional self-harm**
    - **T63.113 Toxic effect of venom of gila monster, assault**
    - **T63.114 Toxic effect of venom of gila monster, undetermined**
  - **T63.12 Toxic effect of venom of other venomous lizard**
    - **T63.121 Toxic effect of venom of other venomous lizard, accidental (unintentional)**
      Toxic effect of venom of other venomous lizard NOS
    - **T63.122 Toxic effect of venom of other venomous lizard, intentional self-harm**
    - **T63.123 Toxic effect of venom of other venomous lizard, assault**
    - **T63.124 Toxic effect of venom of other venomous lizard, undetermined**

- T63.19 Toxic effect of venom of other reptiles
  - T63.191 Toxic effect of venom of other reptiles, accidental (unintentional)
    Toxic effect of venom of other reptiles NOS
  - T63.192 Toxic effect of venom of other reptiles, intentional self-harm
  - T63.193 Toxic effect of venom of other reptiles, assault
  - T63.194 Toxic effect of venom of other reptiles, undetermined
- T63.2 Toxic effect of venom of scorpion
  - T63.2X Toxic effect of venom of scorpion
    - T63.2X1 Toxic effect of venom of scorpion, accidental (unintentional)
      Toxic effect of venom of scorpion NOS
    - T63.2X2 Toxic effect of venom of scorpion, intentional self-harm
    - T63.2X3 Toxic effect of venom of scorpion, assault
    - T63.2X4 Toxic effect of venom of scorpion, undetermined
- T63.3 Toxic effect of venom of spider
  - T63.30 Toxic effect of unspecified spider venom
    - T63.301 Toxic effect of unspecified spider venom, accidental (unintentional)
    - T63.302 Toxic effect of unspecified spider venom, intentional self-harm
    - T63.303 Toxic effect of unspecified spider venom, assault
    - T63.304 Toxic effect of unspecified spider venom, undetermined
  - T63.31 Toxic effect of venom of black widow spider
    - T63.311 Toxic effect of venom of black widow spider, accidental (unintentional)
    - T63.312 Toxic effect of venom of black widow spider, intentional self-harm
    - T63.313 Toxic effect of venom of black widow spider, assault
    - T63.314 Toxic effect of venom of black widow spider, undetermined
  - T63.32 Toxic effect of venom of tarantula
    - T63.321 Toxic effect of venom of tarantula, accidental (unintentional)
    - T63.322 Toxic effect of venom of tarantula, intentional self-harm
    - T63.323 Toxic effect of venom of tarantula, assault
    - T63.324 Toxic effect of venom of tarantula, undetermined
  - T63.33 Toxic effect of venom of brown recluse spider
    - T63.331 Toxic effect of venom of brown recluse spider, accidental (unintentional)
    - T63.332 Toxic effect of venom of brown recluse spider, intentional self-harm
    - T63.333 Toxic effect of venom of brown recluse spider, assault
    - T63.334 Toxic effect of venom of brown recluse spider, undetermined
  - T63.39 Toxic effect of venom of other spider
    - T63.391 Toxic effect of venom of other spider, accidental (unintentional)
    - T63.392 Toxic effect of venom of other spider, intentional self-harm
    - T63.393 Toxic effect of venom of other spider, assault
    - T63.394 Toxic effect of venom of other spider, undetermined
- T63.4 Toxic effect of venom of other arthropods
  - T63.41 Toxic effect of venom of centipedes and venomous millipedes
    - T63.411 Toxic effect of venom of centipedes and venomous millipedes, accidental (unintentional)
    - T63.412 Toxic effect of venom of centipedes and venomous millipedes, intentional self-harm
    - T63.413 Toxic effect of venom of centipedes and venomous millipedes, assault
    - T63.414 Toxic effect of venom of centipedes and venomous millipedes, undetermined
  - T63.42 Toxic effect of venom of ants
    - T63.421 Toxic effect of venom of ants, accidental (unintentional)
    - T63.422 Toxic effect of venom of ants, intentional self-harm
    - T63.423 Toxic effect of venom of ants, assault
    - T63.424 Toxic effect of venom of ants, undetermined
  - T63.43 Toxic effect of venom of caterpillars
    - T63.431 Toxic effect of venom of caterpillars, accidental (unintentional)
    - T63.432 Toxic effect of venom of caterpillars, intentional self-harm
    - T63.433 Toxic effect of venom of caterpillars, assault
    - T63.434 Toxic effect of venom of caterpillars, undetermined
  - T63.44 Toxic effect of venom of bees
    - T63.441 Toxic effect of venom of bees, accidental (unintentional)
    - T63.442 Toxic effect of venom of bees, intentional self-harm
    - T63.443 Toxic effect of venom of bees, assault
    - T63.444 Toxic effect of venom of bees, undetermined
  - T63.45 Toxic effect of venom of hornets
    - T63.451 Toxic effect of venom of hornets, accidental (unintentional)
    - T63.452 Toxic effect of venom of hornets, intentional self-harm
    - T63.453 Toxic effect of venom of hornets, assault
    - T63.454 Toxic effect of venom of hornets, undetermined
  - T63.46 Toxic effect of venom of wasps
    Toxic effect of yellow jacket
    - T63.461 Toxic effect of venom of wasps, accidental (unintentional)
    - T63.462 Toxic effect of venom of wasps, intentional self-harm
    - T63.463 Toxic effect of venom of wasps, assault
    - T63.464 Toxic effect of venom of wasps, undetermined

◀ New ◀ Revised ~~deleted~~ Deleted Excludes 1 Excludes 2 Includes Use additional Code first Code also Unspecified
OGCR Official Guidelines ● Unacceptable Principal Diagnosis X Assign placeholder X ● Use Additional Character(s) ▶ Manifestation Code Coding Clinic

- **T63.48 Toxic effect of venom of other arthropod**
  - **T63.481 Toxic effect of venom of other arthropod, accidental (unintentional)**
  - **T63.482 Toxic effect of venom of other arthropod, intentional self-harm**
  - **T63.483 Toxic effect of venom of other arthropod, assault**
  - **T63.484 Toxic effect of venom of other arthropod, undetermined**
- **T63.5 Toxic effect of contact with venomous fish**

  Excludes2 poisoning by ingestion of fish (T61.-)
  - **T63.51 Toxic effect of contact with stingray**
    - **T63.511 Toxic effect of contact with stingray, accidental (unintentional)**
    - **T63.512 Toxic effect of contact with stingray, intentional self-harm**
    - **T63.513 Toxic effect of contact with stingray, assault**
    - **T63.514 Toxic effect of contact with stingray, undetermined**
  - **T63.59 Toxic effect of contact with other venomous fish**
    - **T63.591 Toxic effect of contact with other venomous fish, accidental (unintentional)**
    - **T63.592 Toxic effect of contact with other venomous fish, intentional self-harm**
    - **T63.593 Toxic effect of contact with other venomous fish, assault**
    - **T63.594 Toxic effect of contact with other venomous fish, undetermined**
- **T63.6 Toxic effect of contact with other venomous marine animals**

  Excludes1 sea-snake venom (T63.Ø9)

  Excludes2 poisoning by ingestion of shellfish (T61.78-)
  - **T63.61 Toxic effect of contact with Portugese Man-o-war**

    Toxic effect of contact with bluebottle
    - **T63.611 Toxic effect of contact with Portugese Man-o-war, accidental (unintentional)**
    - **T63.612 Toxic effect of contact with Portugese Man-o-war, intentional self-harm**
    - **T63.613 Toxic effect of contact with Portugese Man-o-war, assault**
    - **T63.614 Toxic effect of contact with Portugese Man-o-war, undetermined**
  - **T63.62 Toxic effect of contact with other jellyfish**
    - **T63.621 Toxic effect of contact with other jellyfish, accidental (unintentional)**
    - **T63.622 Toxic effect of contact with other jellyfish, intentional self-harm**
    - **T63.623 Toxic effect of contact with other jellyfish, assault**
    - **T63.624 Toxic effect of contact with other jellyfish, undetermined**
  - **T63.63 Toxic effect of contact with sea anemone**
    - **T63.631 Toxic effect of contact with sea anemone, accidental (unintentional)**
    - **T63.632 Toxic effect of contact with sea anemone, intentional self-harm**
    - **T63.633 Toxic effect of contact with sea anemone, assault**
    - **T63.634 Toxic effect of contact with sea anemone, undetermined**
  - **T63.69 Toxic effect of contact with other venomous marine animals**
    - **T63.691 Toxic effect of contact with other venomous marine animals, accidental (unintentional)**
    - **T63.692 Toxic effect of contact with other venomous marine animals, intentional self-harm**
    - **T63.693 Toxic effect of contact with other venomous marine animals, assault**
    - **T63.694 Toxic effect of contact with other venomous marine animals, undetermined**
- **T63.7 Toxic effect of contact with venomous plant**
  - **T63.71 Toxic effect of contact with venomous marine plant**
    - **T63.711 Toxic effect of contact with venomous marine plant, accidental (unintentional)**
    - **T63.712 Toxic effect of contact with venomous marine plant, intentional self-harm**
    - **T63.713 Toxic effect of contact with venomous marine plant, assault**
    - **T63.714 Toxic effect of contact with venomous marine plant, undetermined**
  - **T63.79 Toxic effect of contact with other venomous plant**
    - **T63.791 Toxic effect of contact with other venomous plant, accidental (unintentional)**
    - **T63.792 Toxic effect of contact with other venomous plant, intentional self-harm**
    - **T63.793 Toxic effect of contact with other venomous plant, assault**
    - **T63.794 Toxic effect of contact with other venomous plant, undetermined**
- **T63.8 Toxic effect of contact with other venomous animals**
  - **T63.81 Toxic effect of contact with venomous frog**

    Excludes1 contact with nonvenomous frog (W62.Ø)
    - **T63.811 Toxic effect of contact with venomous frog, accidental (unintentional)**
    - **T63.812 Toxic effect of contact with venomous frog, intentional self-harm**
    - **T63.813 Toxic effect of contact with venomous frog, assault**
    - **T63.814 Toxic effect of contact with venomous frog, undetermined**
  - **T63.82 Toxic effect of contact with venomous toad**

    Excludes1 contact with nonvenomous toad (W62.1)
    - **T63.821 Toxic effect of contact with venomous toad, accidental (unintentional)**
    - **T63.822 Toxic effect of contact with venomous toad, intentional self-harm**
    - **T63.823 Toxic effect of contact with venomous toad, assault**
    - **T63.824 Toxic effect of contact with venomous toad, undetermined**

- **T63.83 Toxic effect of contact with other venomous amphibian**
  - **Excludes1** contact with nonvenomous amphibian (W62.9)
  - **T63.831 Toxic effect of contact with other venomous amphibian, accidental (unintentional)**
  - **T63.832 Toxic effect of contact with other venomous amphibian, intentional self-harm**
  - **T63.833 Toxic effect of contact with other venomous amphibian, assault**
  - **T63.834 Toxic effect of contact with other venomous amphibian, undetermined**
- **T63.89 Toxic effect of contact with other venomous animals**
  - **T63.891 Toxic effect of contact with other venomous animals, accidental (unintentional)**
  - **T63.892 Toxic effect of contact with other venomous animals, intentional self-harm**
  - **T63.893 Toxic effect of contact with other venomous animals, assault**
  - **T63.894 Toxic effect of contact with other venomous animals, undetermined**
- **T63.9 Toxic effect of contact with unspecified venomous animal**
  - X **T63.91 Toxic effect of contact with unspecified venomous animal, accidental (unintentional)**
  - X **T63.92 Toxic effect of contact with unspecified venomous animal, intentional self-harm**
  - X **T63.93 Toxic effect of contact with unspecified venomous animal, assault**
  - X **T63.94 Toxic effect of contact with unspecified venomous animal, undetermined**

- **T64 Toxic effect of aflatoxin and other mycotoxin food contaminants**

  The appropriate 7th character is to be added to each code from category T64

A	initial encounter
D	subsequent encounter
S	sequela

- **T64.0 Toxic effect of aflatoxin**
  - X **T64.01 Toxic effect of aflatoxin, accidental (unintentional)**
  - X **T64.02 Toxic effect of aflatoxin, intentional self-harm**
  - X **T64.03 Toxic effect of aflatoxin, assault**
  - X **T64.04 Toxic effect of aflatoxin, undetermined**
- **T64.8 Toxic effect of other mycotoxin food contaminants**
  - X **T64.81 Toxic effect of other mycotoxin food contaminants, accidental (unintentional)**
  - X **T64.82 Toxic effect of other mycotoxin food contaminants, intentional self-harm**
  - X **T64.83 Toxic effect of other mycotoxin food contaminants, assault**
  - X **T64.84 Toxic effect of other mycotoxin food contaminants, undetermined**

- **T65 Toxic effect of other and unspecified substances**

  The appropriate 7th character is to be added to each code from category T65

A	initial encounter
D	subsequent encounter
S	sequela

- **T65.0 Toxic effect of cyanides**
  - **Excludes1** hydrogen cyanide (T57.3-)
  - **T65.0X Toxic effect of cyanides**
    - **T65.0X1 Toxic effect of cyanides, accidental (unintentional)**
      - Toxic effect of cyanides NOS
    - **T65.0X2 Toxic effect of cyanides, intentional self-harm**
    - **T65.0X3 Toxic effect of cyanides, assault**
    - **T65.0X4 Toxic effect of cyanides, undetermined**
- **T65.1 Toxic effect of strychnine and its salts**
  - **T65.1X Toxic effect of strychnine and its salts**
    - **T65.1X1 Toxic effect of strychnine and its salts, accidental (unintentional)**
      - Toxic effect of strychnine and its salts NOS
    - **T65.1X2 Toxic effect of strychnine and its salts, intentional self-harm**
    - **T65.1X3 Toxic effect of strychnine and its salts, assault**
    - **T65.1X4 Toxic effect of strychnine and its salts, undetermined**
- **T65.2 Toxic effect of tobacco and nicotine**
  - **Excludes2** nicotine dependence (F17.-)
  - **T65.21 Toxic effect of chewing tobacco**
    - **T65.211 Toxic effect of chewing tobacco, accidental (unintentional)**
      - Toxic effect of chewing tobacco NOS
    - **T65.212 Toxic effect of chewing tobacco, intentional self-harm**
    - **T65.213 Toxic effect of chewing tobacco, assault**
    - **T65.214 Toxic effect of chewing tobacco, undetermined**
  - **T65.22 Toxic effect of tobacco cigarettes**
    - Toxic effect of tobacco smoke
    - Use additional code for exposure to second hand tobacco smoke (Z57.31, Z77.22)
    - **T65.221 Toxic effect of tobacco cigarettes, accidental (unintentional)**
      - Toxic effect of tobacco cigarettes NOS
    - **T65.222 Toxic effect of tobacco cigarettes, intentional self-harm**
    - **T65.223 Toxic effect of tobacco cigarettes, assault**
    - **T65.224 Toxic effect of tobacco cigarettes, undetermined**
  - **T65.29 Toxic effect of other tobacco and nicotine**
    - **T65.291 Toxic effect of other tobacco and nicotine, accidental (unintentional)**
      - Toxic effect of other tobacco and nicotine NOS
    - **T65.292 Toxic effect of other tobacco and nicotine, intentional self-harm**
    - **T65.293 Toxic effect of other tobacco and nicotine, assault**
    - **T65.294 Toxic effect of other tobacco and nicotine, undetermined**

- **T65.3 Toxic effect of nitroderivatives and aminoderivatives of benzene and its homologues**
  - Toxic effect of anilin [benzenamine]
  - Toxic effect of nitrobenzene
  - Toxic effect of trinitrotoluene
  - **T65.3X Toxic effect of nitroderivatives and aminoderivatives of benzene and its homologues**
    - **T65.3X1 Toxic effect of nitroderivatives and aminoderivatives of benzene and its homologues, accidental (unintentional)**
      - Toxic effect of nitroderivatives and aminoderivatives of benzene and its homologues NOS
    - **T65.3X2 Toxic effect of nitroderivatives and aminoderivatives of benzene and its homologues, intentional self-harm**
    - **T65.3X3 Toxic effect of nitroderivatives and aminoderivatives of benzene and its homologues, assault**
    - **T65.3X4 Toxic effect of nitroderivatives and aminoderivatives of benzene and its homologues, undetermined**
- **T65.4 Toxic effect of carbon disulfide**
  - **T65.4X Toxic effect of carbon disulfide**
    - **T65.4X1 Toxic effect of carbon disulfide, accidental (unintentional)**
      - Toxic effect of carbon disulfide NOS
    - **T65.4X2 Toxic effect of carbon disulfide, intentional self-harm**
    - **T65.4X3 Toxic effect of carbon disulfide, assault**
    - **T65.4X4 Toxic effect of carbon disulfide, undetermined**
- **T65.5 Toxic effect of nitroglycerin and other nitric acids and esters**
  - Toxic effect of 1,2,3-Propanetriol trinitrate
  - **T65.5X Toxic effect of nitroglycerin and other nitric acids and esters**
    - **T65.5X1 Toxic effect of nitroglycerin and other nitric acids and esters, accidental (unintentional)**
      - Toxic effect of nitroglycerin and other nitric acids and esters NOS
    - **T65.5X2 Toxic effect of nitroglycerin and other nitric acids and esters, intentional self-harm**
    - **T65.5X3 Toxic effect of nitroglycerin and other nitric acids and esters, assault**
    - **T65.5X4 Toxic effect of nitroglycerin and other nitric acids and esters, undetermined**
- **T65.6 Toxic effect of paints and dyes, not elsewhere classified**
  - **T65.6X Toxic effect of paints and dyes, not elsewhere classified**
    - **T65.6X1 Toxic effect of paints and dyes, not elsewhere classified, accidental (unintentional)**
      - Toxic effect of paints and dyes NOS
    - **T65.6X2 Toxic effect of paints and dyes, not elsewhere classified, intentional self-harm**
    - **T65.6X3 Toxic effect of paints and dyes, not elsewhere classified, assault**
    - **T65.6X4 Toxic effect of paints and dyes, not elsewhere classified, undetermined**
- **T65.8 Toxic effect of other specified substances**
  - **T65.81 Toxic effect of latex**
    - **T65.811 Toxic effect of latex, accidental (unintentional)**
      - Toxic effect of latex NOS
    - **T65.812 Toxic effect of latex, intentional self-harm**
    - **T65.813 Toxic effect of latex, assault**
    - **T65.814 Toxic effect of latex, undetermined**
  - **T65.82 Toxic effect of harmful algae and algae toxins**
    - Toxic effect of (harmful) algae bloom NOS
    - Toxic effect of blue-green algae bloom
    - Toxic effect of brown tide
    - Toxic effect of cyanobacteria bloom
    - Toxic effect of Florida red tide
    - Toxic effect of pfiesteria piscicida
    - Toxic effect of red tide
    - **T65.821 Toxic effect of harmful algae and algae toxins, accidental (unintentional)**
      - Toxic effect of harmful algae and algae toxins NOS
    - **T65.822 Toxic effect of harmful algae and algae toxins, intentional self-harm**
    - **T65.823 Toxic effect of harmful algae and algae toxins, assault**
    - **T65.824 Toxic effect of harmful algae and algae toxins, undetermined**
  - **T65.83 Toxic effect of fiberglass**
    - **T65.831 Toxic effect of fiberglass, accidental (unintentional)**
      - Toxic effect of fiberglass NOS
    - **T65.832 Toxic effect of fiberglass, intentional self-harm**
    - **T65.833 Toxic effect of fiberglass, assault**
    - **T65.834 Toxic effect of fiberglass, undetermined**
  - **T65.89 Toxic effect of other specified substances**
    - **T65.891 Toxic effect of other specified substances, accidental (unintentional)**
      - Toxic effect of other specified substances NOS
    - **T65.892 Toxic effect of other specified substances, intentional self-harm**
    - **T65.893 Toxic effect of other specified substances, assault**
    - **T65.894 Toxic effect of other specified substances, undetermined**
- **T65.9 Toxic effect of unspecified substance**
  - X **T65.91 Toxic effect of unspecified substance, accidental (unintentional)**
    - Poisoning NOS
  - X **T65.92 Toxic effect of unspecified substance, intentional self-harm**
  - X **T65.93 Toxic effect of unspecified substance, assault**
  - X **T65.94 Toxic effect of unspecified substance, undetermined**

OTHER AND UNSPECIFIED EFFECTS OF EXTERNAL CAUSES (T66-T78)

T66 Radiation sickness, unspecified

Excludes1 specified adverse effects of radiation, such as:
burns (T20-T31)
leukemia (C91-C95)
radiation gastroenteritis and colitis (K52.0)
radiation pneumonitis (J70.0)
radiation related disorders of the skin and subcutaneous tissue (L55-L59)
sunburn (L55.-)

The appropriate 7th character is to be added to code T66

A	initial encounter
D	subsequent encounter
S	sequela

T67 Effects of heat and light

Excludes1 erythema [dermatitis] ab igne (L59.0)
malignant hyperpyrexia due to anesthesia (T88.3)
radiation-related disorders of the skin and subcutaneous tissue (L55-L59)

Excludes2 burns (T20-T31)
sunburn (L55.-)
sweat disorder due to heat (L74-L75)

The appropriate 7th character is to be added to each code from category T67

A	initial encounter
D	subsequent encounter
S	sequela

X **T67.0 Heatstroke and sunstroke** A CC, A MCC
Heat apoplexy
Heat pyrexia
Siriasis
Thermoplegia
Use additional code(s) to identify any associated complications of heatstroke, such as:
coma and stupor (R40.-)
systemic inflammatory response syndrome (R65.1-)
Ex: T67.0XX-T67.9XX[A]

X **T67.1 Heat syncope**
Heat collapse

X **T67.2 Heat cramp**

X **T67.3 Heat exhaustion, anhydrotic**
Heat prostration due to water depletion
Excludes1 heat exhaustion due to salt depletion (T67.4)

X **T67.4 Heat exhaustion due to salt depletion**
Heat prostration due to salt (and water) depletion

X **T67.5 Heat exhaustion, unspecified**
Heat prostration NOS

X **T67.6 Heat fatigue, transient**

X **T67.7 Heat edema**

X **T67.8 Other effects of heat and light**

X **T67.9 Effect of heat and light, unspecified**

X **T68 Hypothermia**
Accidental hypothermia
Hypothermia NOS
Use additional code to identify source of exposure:
Exposure to excessive cold of man-made origin (W93)
Exposure to excessive cold of natural origin (X31)

Excludes1 hypothermia following anesthesia (T88.51)
hypothermia not associated with low environmental temperature (R68.0)
hypothermia of newborn (P80.-)

Excludes2 frostbite (T33-T34)

The appropriate 7th character is to be added to code T68

A	initial encounter
D	subsequent encounter
S	sequela

T69 Other effects of reduced temperature
Use additional code to identify source of exposure:
Exposure to excessive cold of man-made origin (W93)
Exposure to excessive cold of natural origin (X31)

Excludes2 frostbite (T33-T34)

The appropriate 7th character is to be added to each code from category T69

A	initial encounter
D	subsequent encounter
S	sequela

T69.0 Immersion hand and foot

T69.01 Immersion hand

T69.011 Immersion hand, right hand

T69.012 Immersion hand, left hand

T69.019 Immersion hand, unspecified hand

T69.02 Immersion foot
Trench foot
Ex: For category T69.02 CC codes: T33.2XX-T33.42X[A], T33.60X-T33.72X[A], T33.90X-T33.99X[A], T34.2XX-T34.42X[A], T34.60X-T34.72X[A], T34.90X-T34.99X[A], T69.021-T69.029[A]

T69.021 Immersion foot, right foot A CC, A MCC

T69.022 Immersion foot, left foot A CC, A MCC

T69.029 Immersion foot, unspecified foot A CC, A MCC

X **T69.1 Chilblains**

X **T69.8 Other specified effects of reduced temperature**

X **T69.9 Effect of reduced temperature, unspecified**

T70 Effects of air pressure and water pressure
The appropriate 7th character is to be added to each code from category T70

A	initial encounter
D	subsequent encounter
S	sequela

X **T70.0 Otitic barotrauma**
Aero-otitis media
Effects of change in ambient atmospheric pressure or water pressure on ears

X **T70.1 Sinus barotrauma**
Aerosinusitis
Effects of change in ambient atmospheric pressure on sinuses

T70.2 Other and unspecified effects of high altitude
Excludes2 polycythemia due to high altitude (D75.1)

X **T70.20 Unspecified effects of high altitude**

X **T70.29 Other effects of high altitude**
Alpine sickness
Anoxia due to high altitude
Barotrauma NOS
Hypobaropathy
Mountain sickness

X **T70.3 Caisson disease [decompression sickness]** A CC, A MCC
Compressed-air disease
Diver's palsy or paralysis
Ex: T70.3XX-T70.9XX[A]

X **T70.4 Effects of high-pressure fluids**
Hydraulic jet injection (industrial)
Pneumatic jet injection (industrial)
Traumatic jet injection (industrial)

X **T70.8 Other effects of air pressure and water pressure**

X **T70.9 Effect of air pressure and water pressure, unspecified**

T71 Asphyxiation
Mechanical suffocation
Traumatic suffocation

Excludes1 acute respiratory distress (syndrome) (J80)
anoxia due to high altitude (T70.2)
asphyxia NOS (R09.01)
asphyxia from carbon monoxide (T58.-)
asphyxia from inhalation of food or foreign body (T17.-)
asphyxia from other gases, fumes and vapors (T59.-)
respiratory distress (syndrome) in newborn (P22.-)

The appropriate 7th character is to be added to each code from category T71

A	initial encounter
D	subsequent encounter
S	sequela

Ex: For category T71 CC codes: T71.111-T71.9XX[A]

T71.1 Asphyxiation due to mechanical threat to breathing
Suffocation due to mechanical threat to breathing

T71.11 Asphyxiation due to smothering under pillow

T71.111 Asphyxiation due to smothering under pillow, accidental A CC, A MCC
Asphyxiation due to smothering under pillow NOS

T71.112 Asphyxiation due to smothering under pillow, intentional self-harm A CC, A MCC

T71.113 Asphyxiation due to smothering under pillow, assault A CC, A MCC

T71.114 Asphyxiation due to smothering under pillow, undetermined A CC, A MCC

T71.12 Asphyxiation due to plastic bag

T71.121 Asphyxiation due to plastic bag, accidental A CC, A MCC
Asphyxiation due to plastic bag NOS

T71.122 Asphyxiation due to plastic bag, intentional self-harm A CC, A MCC

T71.123 Asphyxiation due to plastic bag, assault A CC, A MCC

T71.124 Asphyxiation due to plastic bag, undetermined A CC, A MCC

T71.13 Asphyxiation due to being trapped in bed linens

T71.131 Asphyxiation due to being trapped in bed linens, accidental A CC, A MCC
Asphyxiation due to being trapped in bed linens NOS

T71.132 Asphyxiation due to being trapped in bed linens, intentional self-harm A CC, A MCC

T71.133 Asphyxiation due to being trapped in bed linens, assault A CC, A MCC

T71.134 Asphyxiation due to being trapped in bed linens, undetermined A CC, A MCC

T71.14 Asphyxiation due to smothering under another person's body (in bed)

T71.141 Asphyxiation due to smothering under another person's body (in bed), accidental A CC, A MCC
Asphyxiation due to smothering under another person's body (in bed) NOS

T71.143 Asphyxiation due to smothering under another person's body (in bed), assault A CC, A MCC

T71.144 Asphyxiation due to smothering under another person's body (in bed), undetermined A CC, A MCC

T71.15 Asphyxiation due to smothering in furniture

T71.151 Asphyxiation due to smothering in furniture, accidental A CC, A MCC
Asphyxiation due to smothering in furniture NOS

T71.152 Asphyxiation due to smothering in furniture, intentional self-harm A CC, A MCC

T71.153 Asphyxiation due to smothering in furniture, assault A CC, A MCC

T71.154 Asphyxiation due to smothering in furniture, undetermined A CC, A MCC

T71.16 Asphyxiation due to hanging
Hanging by window shade cord
Use additional code for any associated injuries, such as:
crushing injury of neck (S17.-)
fracture of cervical vertebrae (S12.0-S12.2-)
open wound of neck (S11.-)

T71.161 Asphyxiation due to hanging, accidental A CC, A MCC
Asphyxiation due to hanging NOS
Hanging NOS

T71.162 Asphyxiation due to hanging, intentional self-harm A CC, A MCC

T71.163 Asphyxiation due to hanging, assault A CC, A MCC

T71.164 Asphyxiation due to hanging, undetermined A CC, A MCC

T71.19 Asphyxiation due to mechanical
Threat to breathing due to other causes causes

T71.191 Asphyxiation due to mechanical threat to breathing due to other causes, accidental A CC, A MCC
Asphyxiation due to other causes NOS

T71.192 Asphyxiation due to mechanical threat to breathing due to other causes, intentional self-harm A CC, A MCC

T71.193 Asphyxiation due to mechanical threat to breathing due to other causes, assault A CC, A MCC

T71.194 Asphyxiation due to mechanical threat to breathing due to other causes, undetermined A CC, A MCC

● **T71.2 Asphyxiation due to systemic oxygen deficiency due to low oxygen content in ambient air**
Suffocation due to systemic oxygen deficiency due to low oxygen content in ambient air

X● **T71.20 Asphyxiation due to systemic oxygen deficiency due to low oxygen content in ambient air due to unspecified cause** A, A

X● **T71.21 Asphyxiation due to cave-in or falling earth** A, A
Use additional code for any associated cataclysm (X34-X38)

● **T71.22 Asphyxiation due to being trapped in a car trunk**

● **T71.221 Asphyxiation due to being trapped in a car trunk, accidental** A

● **T71.222 Asphyxiation due to being trapped in a car trunk, intentional self-harm** A

● **T71.223 Asphyxiation due to being trapped in a car trunk, assault** A

● **T71.224 Asphyxiation due to being trapped in a car trunk, undetermined** A

● **T71.23 Asphyxiation due to being trapped in a (discarded) refrigerator**

● **T71.231 Asphyxiation due to being trapped in a (discarded) refrigerator, accidental** A

● **T71.232 Asphyxiation due to being trapped in a (discarded) refrigerator, intentional self-harm** A

● **T71.233 Asphyxiation due to being trapped in a (discarded) refrigerator, assault** A

● **T71.234 Asphyxiation due to being trapped in a (discarded) refrigerator, undetermined** A

X● **T71.29 Asphyxiation due to being trapped in other low oxygen environment** A, A

X● **T71.9 Asphyxiation due to unspecified cause** A, A
Suffocation (by strangulation) due to unspecified cause
Suffocation NOS
Systemic oxygen deficiency due to low oxygen content in ambient air due to unspecified cause
Systemic oxygen deficiency due to mechanical threat to breathing due to unspecified cause
Traumatic asphyxia NOS

● **T73 Effects of other deprivation**
The appropriate 7th character is to be added to each code from category T73

A	initial encounter
D	subsequent encounter
S	sequela

X● **T73.0 Starvation**
Deprivation of food

X● **T73.1 Deprivation of water**

X● **T73.2 Exhaustion due to exposure**

X● **T73.3 Exhaustion due to excessive exertion**
Exhaustion due to overexertion

X● **T73.8 Other effects of deprivation**

X● **T73.9 Effect of deprivation, unspecified**

● **T74 Adult and child abuse, neglect and other maltreatment, confirmed**
Use additional code, if applicable, to identify any associated current injury
Use additional external cause code to identify perpetrator, if known (Y07.-)
Excludes1 abuse and maltreatment in pregnancy (O9A.3-, O9A.4-, O9A.5-)
adult and child maltreatment, suspected (T76.-)
The appropriate 7th character is to be added to each code from category T74

A	initial encounter
D	subsequent encounter
S	sequela

Ex **For category T74 CC codes unless otherwise indicated:** T74.01X-T74.92X[A], T76.01X-T76.92X[A]

● **T74.0 Neglect or abandonment, confirmed**

X● **T74.01 Adult neglect or abandonment, confirmed** A — A

X● **T74.02 Child neglect or abandonment, confirmed** A — P

● **T74.1 Physical abuse, confirmed**
Excludes2 sexual abuse (T74.2-)

X● **T74.11 Adult physical abuse, confirmed** A — A

X● **T74.12 Child physical abuse, confirmed** A — P
Excludes2 shaken infant syndrome (T74.4)

● **T74.2 Sexual abuse, confirmed**
Rape, confirmed
Sexual assault, confirmed

X● **T74.21 Adult sexual abuse, confirmed** A — A

X● **T74.22 Child sexual abuse, confirmed** A — P

● **T74.3 Psychological abuse, confirmed**

X● **T74.31 Adult psychological abuse, confirmed** — A

X● **T74.32 Child psychological abuse, confirmed** A — P

X● **T74.4 Shaken infant syndrome** A — P

● **T74.9 Unspecified maltreatment, confirmed**

X● **T74.91 Unspecified adult maltreatment, confirmed** A — A
Ex T74.91X[A], T76.91X[A]

X● **T74.92 Unspecified child maltreatment, confirmed** A — P

● **T75 Other and unspecified effects of other external causes**
Excludes1 adverse effects NEC (T78.-)
Excludes2 burns (electric) (T20-T31)
The appropriate 7th character is to be added to each code from category T75

A	initial encounter
D	subsequent encounter
S	sequela

● **T75.0 Effects of lightning**
Struck by lightning

X● **T75.00 Unspecified effects of lightning**
Struck by lightning NOS

X● **T75.01 Shock due to being struck by lightning**

X● **T75.09 Other effects of lightning**
Use additional code for other effects of lightning

X● **T75.1 Unspecified effects of drowning and nonfatal submersion** A, A
Immersion
Excludes1 specified effects of drowning code to effects
Ex T75.1XX[A]

T75.2 Effects of vibration

X **T75.20 Unspecified effects of vibration**

X **T75.21 Pneumatic hammer syndrome**

X **T75.22 Traumatic vasospastic syndrome**

X **T75.23 Vertigo from infrasound**

Excludes1 vertigo NOS (R42)

X **T75.29 Other effects of vibration**

X **T75.3 Motion sickness**

Airsickness
Seasickness
Travel sickness

Use additional external cause code to identify vehicle or type of motion (Y92.81-, Y93.5-)

X **T75.4 Electrocution**

Shock from electric current
Shock from electroshock gun (taser)

T75.8 Other specified effects of external causes

X **T75.81 Effects of abnormal gravitation [G] forces**

X **T75.82 Effects of weightlessness**

X **T75.89 Other specified effects of external causes**

T76 Adult and child abuse, neglect and other maltreatment, suspected

Use additional code, if applicable, to identify any associated current injury

Excludes1 adult and child maltreatment, confirmed (T74.-)
suspected abuse and maltreatment in pregnancy (O9A.3-, O9A.4-, O9A.5-)
suspected adult physical abuse, ruled out (Z04.71)
suspected adult sexual abuse, ruled out (Z04.41)
suspected child physical abuse, ruled out (Z04.72)
suspected child sexual abuse, ruled out (Z04.42)

The appropriate 7th character is to be added to each code from category T76

A	initial encounter
D	subsequent encounter
S	sequela

Ex **For category T76 CC codes unless otherwise indicated:** T74.01X-T74.92X[A], T76.01X-T76.92X[A]

T76.0 Neglect or abandonment, suspected

X **T76.01 Adult neglect or abandonment, suspected** A — A

X **T76.02 Child neglect or abandonment, suspected** A — P

T76.1 Physical abuse, suspected

X **T76.11 Adult physical abuse, suspected** A — A

X **T76.12 Child physical abuse, suspected** A — P

T76.2 Sexual abuse, suspected

Rape, suspected
Sexual abuse, suspected

Excludes1 alleged abuse, ruled out (Z04.7)

X **T76.21 Adult sexual abuse, suspected** A — A

X **T76.22 Child sexual abuse, suspected** A — P

T76.3 Psychological abuse, suspected

X **T76.31 Adult psychological abuse, suspected** — A

X **T76.32 Child psychological abuse, suspected** A — P

T76.9 Unspecified maltreatment, suspected

X **T76.91 Unspecified adult maltreatment, suspected** A — A

Ex T74.91X[A], T76.91X[A]

X **T76.92 Unspecified child maltreatment, suspected** A — P

T78 Adverse effects, not elsewhere classified

Excludes2 complications of surgical and medical care NEC (T80-T88)

The appropriate 7th character is to be added to each code from category T78

A	initial encounter
D	subsequent encounter
S	sequela

Ex **For category T78 CC codes:** T78.00X-T78.09X[A]

T78.0 Anaphylactic reaction due to food

Anaphylactic reaction due to adverse food reaction
Anaphylactic shock or reaction due to nonpoisonous foods
Anaphylactoid reaction due to food

X **T78.00 Anaphylactic reaction due to unspecified food** A

X **T78.01 Anaphylactic reaction due to peanuts** A

X **T78.02 Anaphylactic reaction due to shellfish (crustaceans)** A

X **T78.03 Anaphylactic reaction due to other fish** A

X **T78.04 Anaphylactic reaction due to fruits and vegetables** A

X **T78.05 Anaphylactic reaction due to tree nuts and seeds** A

Excludes2 anaphylactic reaction due to peanuts (T78.01) ◀

X **T78.06 Anaphylactic reaction due to food additives** A

X **T78.07 Anaphylactic reaction due to milk and dairy products** A

X **T78.08 Anaphylactic reaction due to eggs** A

X **T78.09 Anaphylactic reaction due to other food products** A

X **T78.1 Other adverse food reactions, not elsewhere classified**

Use additional code to identify the type of reaction, if applicable ◀

Excludes1 anaphylactic reaction or shock due to adverse food reaction (T78.0-)
anaphylactic reaction due to food (T78.0-)
bacterial food borne intoxications (A05.-)

Excludes2 allergic and dietetic gastroenteritis and colitis (K52.29) ◀
allergic rhinitis due to food (J30.5)
dermatitis due to food in contact with skin (L23.6, L24.6, L25.4)
dermatitis due to ingested food (L27.2)
food protein-induced enterocolitis syndrome (K52.21) ◀
food protein-induced enteropathy (K52.22) ◀

X **T78.2 Anaphylactic shock, unspecified** A

Occurs when allergic response triggers large quantities of histamines, prostaglandins, leukotrienes resulting in systemic vasodilation

Allergic shock
Anaphylactic reaction
Anaphylaxis

Excludes1 anaphylactic reaction or shock due to adverse effect of correct medicinal substance properly administered (T88.6)
anaphylactic reaction or shock due to adverse food reaction (T78.0-)
anaphylactic reaction or shock due to serum (T80.5-)

X **T78.3 Angioneurotic edema**

Allergic angioedema
Giant urticaria
Vascular disorder resulting from abnormalities of autonomic nervous system fibers supplying blood vessels
Quincke's edema

Excludes1 serum urticaria (T80.6-)
urticaria (L50.-)

● **T78.4 Other and unspecified allergy**

Excludes1 specified types of allergic reaction such as:
allergic diarrhea (K52.29) ⟸
allergic gastroenteritis and colitis (K52.29 ⟸)
dermatitis (L23-L25, L27.-)
food protein-induced enterocolitis syndrome (K52.21) ◀
food protein-induced enteropathy (K52.22) ◀
hay fever (J30.1)

X● **T78.40 Allergy, unspecified**
Allergic reaction NOS
Hypersensitivity NOS

X● **T78.41 Arthus phenomenon**
Arthus reaction

X● **T78.49 Other allergy**

X● **T78.8 Other adverse effects, not elsewhere classified**

CERTAIN EARLY COMPLICATIONS OF TRAUMA (T79)

● **T79 Certain early complications of trauma, not elsewhere classified**

Excludes2 acute respiratory distress syndrome (J80)
complications occurring during or following medical procedures (T80-T88)
complications of surgical and medical care NEC (T80-T88)
newborn respiratory distress syndrome (P22.0)

The appropriate 7th character is to be added to each code from category T79

A	initial encounter
D	subsequent encounter
S	sequela

X● **T79.0 Air embolism (traumatic) A**

Excludes1 air embolism complicating abortion or ectopic or molar pregnancy (O00-O07, O08.2)
air embolism complicating pregnancy, childbirth and the puerperium (O88.0)
air embolism following infusion, transfusion, and therapeutic injection (T80.0)
air embolism following procedure NEC (T81.7-)

Ex: D78.81-D78.89, E36.8, E89.810-E89.89, H59.011-H59.019, H59.031-H59.039, H59.091-H59.099, H59.811-H59.89, H95.811-H95.89, I97.3, L76.81-L76.82, M96.89, N98.1-N98.9, T14.90-T14.91, T79.0XX[A], T79.A0X- T79.9XX[A], T80.0XX[A], T81.82X[A], T81.89X-T81.9XX[A]

X● **T79.1 Fat embolism (traumatic) A**

Excludes1 fat embolism complicating:
abortion or ectopic or molar pregnancy (O00-O07, O08.2)
pregnancy, childbirth and the puerperium (O88.8)

Ex: D78.81-D78.89, E36.8, E89.810-E89.89, H59.011-H59.019, H59.031-H59.039, H59.091-H59.099, H59.811-H59.89, H95.811-H95.89, I97.3, L76.81-L76.82, M96.89, N98.1-N98.9, T14.90-T14.91, T79.0XX[A], T79.A0X- T79.9XX[A], T81.82X[A], T81.89X-T81.9XX[A]

X● **T79.2 Traumatic secondary and recurrent hemorrhage and seroma A**

Ex: D78.81-D78.89, E36.8, E89.810-E89.89, H59.011-H59.019, H59.031-H59.039, H59.091-H59.099, H59.811-H59.89, H95.811-H95.89, I97.3, L76.81-L76.82, M96.89, N98.1-N98.9, T14.90-T14.91, 79.2XX[A], T79.A0X-T79.9XX[A], T81.82X-T81.9XX[A]

X● **T79.4 Traumatic shock A**

Shock (immediate) (delayed) following injury

Excludes1 anaphylactic shock due to adverse food reaction (T78.0-)
anaphylactic shock due to correct medicinal substance properly administered (T88.6)
anaphylactic shock due to serum (T80.5-)
anaphylactic shock NOS (T78.2)
anesthetic shock (T88.2)
electric shock (T75.4)
nontraumatic shock NEC (R57.-)
obstetric shock (O75.1)
postprocedural shock (T81.1-)
septic shock (R65.21)
shock complicating abortion or ectopic or molar pregnancy (O00-O07, O08.3)
shock due to lightning (T75.01)
shock NOS (R57.9)

Ex: D78.81-D78.89, E36.8, E89.810-E89.89, H59.011-H59.019, H59.031-H59.039, H59.091-H59.099, H59.811-H59.89, H95.811-H95.89, I97.3, L76.81-L76.82, M96.89, N98.1-N98.9, T14.90-T14.91, T79.4XX[A], T79.A0X-T79.9XX[A], T81.82X-T81.9XX[A]

X● **T79.5 Traumatic anuria A**

Crush syndrome
Renal failure following crushing

Ex: D78.01-D78.02, D78.21-D78.22, D78.31-D78.34, D78.81-D78.89, E36.01-E36.02, E36.8, E89.810-E89.89, G97.51-G97.52, G97.61-G97.64, H59.011-H59.019, H59.031-H59.039, H59.091-H59.099, H59.111-H59.129, H59.311-H59.329, H59.331-H59.369, H59.811-H59.819, H59.88-H59.89, H95.21-H95.22, H95.41-H95.42, H95.51-H92.52, H95.551-H95.554, H95.811-H95.819, H95.88-H95.89, I97.3-I97.42, I97.610-I97.648, J95.61-J95.62, J95.830-J95.831, J95.860-J95.863, K91.61-K91.62, K91.840-K91.841, K91.870-K91.873, L76.01-L76.02, L76.21-L76.22, L76.31-L76.34, L76.81-L76.82, M96.810-M96.811, M96.830-M96.89, N98.1-N98.9, N99.61-N99.62, N99.820-N99.821, N99.840-N99.843, T14.90-T14.91, T79.5XX[A], T79. A0X-T79.9XX[A], T81.10X-T81.19X[A], T81.82X-T81.9XX[A], T88.2XX[A]

X● **T79.6 Traumatic ischemia of muscle**

Traumatic rhabdomyolysis
Volkmann's ischemic contracture

Excludes2 anterior tibial syndrome (M76.8)
compartment syndrome (traumatic) (T79.A-)
nontraumatic ischemia of muscle (M62.2-)

X● **T79.7 Traumatic subcutaneous emphysema A**

Excludes1 emphysema NOS (J43)
emphysema (subcutaneous) resulting from a procedure (T81.82)

Ex: D78.81-D78.89, E36.8, E89.810-E89.89, H59.011-H59.019, H59.031-H59.039, H59.091-H59.099, H59.811-H59.89, H95.811-H95.89, I97.3, L76.81-L76.82, M96.89, N98.1-N98.9, S21.101-S21.159[A], S21.301-S21.459[A], S21.90X-S21.95X[A], S27.0XX-S27.399[A], S27.50X-S27.809[A], S27.892—S27.9XX[A], S28.1XX[A], S29.021-S29.029[A], T14.90-T14.91, T79.7XX-T79.9XX[A], T81.82X-T81.9XX[A]

● **T79.A Traumatic compartment syndrome**

Excludes1 fibromyalgia (M79.7)
nontraumatic compartment syndrome (M79.A-)
traumatic ischemic infarction of muscle (T79.6)

Ex: **For category T79.A CC codes unless otherwise indicated:** M70.80-M70.99, M79.81-M79.9, R29.898

X● **T79.A0 Compartment syndrome, unspecified A**

Compartment syndrome NOS

Ex: S31.001[A], S31.011[A], S31.021[A], S31.031[A], S31.041[A], S31.051[A], S31.600-S31.659[A], S36.81X-S36.899[A]

● **T79.A1 Traumatic compartment syndrome of upper extremity**

Traumatic compartment syndrome of shoulder, arm, forearm, wrist, hand, and fingers

● **T79.A11 Traumatic compartment syndrome of right upper extremity A**

● **T79.A12 Traumatic compartment syndrome of left upper extremity A**

● **T79.A19 Traumatic compartment syndrome of unspecified upper extremity A**

● **T79.A2 Traumatic compartment syndrome of lower extremity**
Traumatic compartment syndrome of hip, buttock, thigh, leg, foot, and toes

● **T79.A21 Traumatic compartment syndrome of right lower extremity** A

● **T79.A22 Traumatic compartment syndrome of left lower extremity** A

● **T79.A29 Traumatic compartment syndrome of unspecified lower extremity** A

X● **T79.A3 Traumatic compartment syndrome of abdomen** A
Ex: S31.001[A], S31.011[A], S31.021[A], S31.031[A], S31.041[A], S31.051[A], S31.100-S31.159[A], S31.600-S31.659[A], S31.831-S31.839[A], S36.00X-S37.599[A], S37.812-S37.99X[A], S38.3XX[A], S39.021-S39.023[A], T14.90-T14.91, T79.8XX-T79.9XX[A]

X● **T79.A9 Traumatic compartment syndrome of other sites** A
Ex: See T79.A0

X● **T79.8 Other early complications of trauma**

X● **T79.9 Unspecified early complication of trauma**

COMPLICATIONS OF SURGICAL AND MEDICAL CARE NOT ELSEWHERE CLASSIFIED (T8Ø-T88)

Use additional code for adverse effect, if applicable, to identify drug (T36-T5Ø with fifth or sixth character 5)

Use additional code(s) to identify the specified condition resulting from the complication.

Use additional code to identify devices involved and details of circumstances (Y62-Y82)

Excludes2 any encounters with medical care for postprocedural conditions in which no complications are present, such as:
- artificial opening status (Z93.-)
- closure of external stoma (Z43.-)
- fitting and adjustment of external prosthetic device (Z44.-)

burns and corrosions from local applications and irradiation (T2Ø-T32)
complications of surgical procedures during pregnancy, childbirth and the puerperium (OØØ-O9A)
mechanical complication of respirator [ventilator] (J95.85Ø)
poisoning and toxic effects of drugs and chemicals (T36-T65 with fifth or sixth character 1-4 or 6)
postprocedural fever (R5Ø.82)
specified complications classified elsewhere, such as:
- cerebrospinal fluid leak from spinal puncture (G97.Ø)
- colostomy malfunction (K94.Ø-)
- disorders of fluid and electrolyte imbalance (E86-E87)
- functional disturbances following cardiac surgery (I97.Ø-I97.1)
- intraoperative and postprocedural complications of specified body systems (D78.-, E36.-, E89.-, G97.3-, G97.4, H59.3-, H59.-, H95.2-, H95.3, I97.4-, I97.5, J95.6-, J95.7, K91.6-, L76.-, M96.-, N99.-)
- ostomy complications (J95.Ø-, K94.-, N99.5-)
- postgastric surgery syndromes (K91.1)
- postlaminectomy syndrome NEC (M96.1)
- postmastectomy lymphedema syndrome (I97.2)
- postsurgical blind-loop syndrome (K91.2)
- ventilator associated pneumonia (J95.851)

● **T8Ø Complications following infusion, transfusion and therapeutic injection**

Includes complications following perfusion

Excludes2 bone marrow transplant rejection (T86.Ø1)
febrile nonhemolytic transfusion reaction (R5Ø.84)
fluid overload due to transfusion (E87.71)
posttransfusion purpura (D69.51)
transfusion associated circulatory overload (TACO) (E87.71)
transfusion (red blood cell) associated hemochromatosis (E83.111)
transfusion related acute lung injury (TRALI) (J95.84)

The appropriate 7th character is to be added to each code from category T8Ø

A	initial encounter
D	subsequent encounter
S	sequela

X● **T8Ø.Ø Air embolism following infusion, transfusion and therapeutic injection** A, A
Ex: T79.ØXX[A], T8Ø.ØXX[A]

X● **T8Ø.1 Vascular complications following infusion, transfusion and therapeutic injection** A

Use additional code to identify the vascular complication

Excludes2 extravasation of vesicant agent (T8Ø.81-)
infiltration of vesicant agent (T8Ø.81-)
vascular complications specified as due to prosthetic devices, implants and grafts (T82.8- T83.8-, T84.8-, T85.8-) ◀
postprocedural vascular complications (T81.7-)

Ex: T8Ø.1XX[A], T8Ø.81Ø-T8Ø.818[A], T8Ø.9ØX[A]

● **T8Ø.2 Infections following infusion, transfusion and therapeutic injection**

Use additional code to identify the specific infection, such as:
sepsis (A41.9)

Use additional code (R65.2-) to identify severe sepsis, if applicable

Excludes2 infections specified as due to prosthetic devices, implants and grafts (T82.6-T82.7, T83.5-T83.6, T84.5-T84.7, T85.7)
postprocedural infections (T81.4-) ◀

Ex: **For category T8Ø.2 CC codes:** Ex: N98.Ø, T8Ø.211-T8Ø.29X[A], T82.7XX[A], T88.ØXX[A]

● **T8Ø.21 Infection due to central venous catheter**
Infection due to pulmonary artery catheter (Swan-Ganz catheter) ◀

● **T8Ø.211 Bloodstream infection due to central venous catheter** A, A
- Catheter-related bloodstream infection (CRBSI) NOS
- Central line-associated bloodstream infection (CLABSI)
- Bloodstream infection due to Hickman catheter
- Bloodstream infection due to peripherally inserted central catheter (PICC)
- Bloodstream infection due to portacath (port-a-cath)
- Bloodstream infection due to pulmonary artery catheter ◀
- Bloodstream infection due to triple lumen catheter
- Bloodstream infection due to umbilical venous catheter

● **T80.212 Local infection due to central venous catheter** A, A
Exit or insertion site infection
Local infection due to Hickman catheter
Local infection due to peripherally inserted central catheter (PICC)
Local infection due to portacath (port-a-cath)
Local infection due to pulmonary artery catheter ◀
Local infection due to triple lumen catheter
Local infection due to umbilical venous catheter
Port or reservoir infection
Tunnel infection

● **T80.218 Other infection due to central venous catheter** A, A
Other central line-associated infection
Other infection due to Hickman catheter
Other infection due to peripherally inserted central catheter (PICC)
Other infection due to portacath (port-a-cath)
Other infection due to pulmonary artery catheter ◀
Other infection due to triple lumen catheter
Other infection due to umbilical venous catheter

● **T80.219 Unspecified infection due to central venous catheter** A, A
Central line-associated infection NOS
Unspecified infection due to Hickman catheter
Unspecified infection due to peripherally inserted central catheter (PICC)
Unspecified infection due to portacath (port-a-cath)
Unspecified infection due to pulmonary artery catheter ◀
Unspecified infection due to triple lumen catheter
Unspecified infection due to umbilical venous catheter

X● **T80.22 Acute infection following transfusion, infusion, or injection of blood and blood products** A

X● **T80.29 Infection following other infusion, transfusion and therapeutic injection** A

● **T80.3 ABO incompatibility reaction due to transfusion of blood or blood products**
Excludes1 minor blood group antigens reactions (Duffy) (E) (K(ell)) (Kidd) (Lewis) (M) (N) (P) (S) (T80.A)
Ex: **For category T80.3 CC codes unless otherwise indicated:** T80.30X-T80.A9X[A], T80.910-T80.92X[A]

X● **T80.30 ABO incompatibility reaction due to transfusion of blood or blood products, unspecified** A, A
ABO incompatibility blood transfusion NOS
Reaction to ABO incompatibility from transfusion NOS

● **T80.31 ABO incompatibility with hemolytic transfusion reaction**

● **T80.310 ABO incompatibility with acute hemolytic transfusion reaction** A, A
ABO incompatibility with hemolytic transfusion reaction less than 24 hours after transfusion
Acute hemolytic transfusion reaction (AHTR) due to ABO incompatibility

● **T80.311 ABO incompatibility with delayed hemolytic transfusion reaction** A, A
ABO incompatibility with hemolytic transfusion reaction 24 hours or more after transfusion
Delayed hemolytic transfusion reaction (DHTR) due to ABO incompatibility

● **T80.319 ABO incompatibility with hemolytic transfusion reaction, unspecified** A, A
ABO incompatibility with hemolytic transfusion reaction at unspecified time after transfusion
Hemolytic transfusion reaction (HTR) due to ABO incompatibility NOS

X● **T80.39 Other ABO incompatibility reaction due to transfusion of blood or blood products** A, A
Delayed serologic transfusion reaction (DSTR) from ABO incompatibility
Other ABO incompatible blood transfusion
Other reaction to ABO incompatible blood transfusion

● **T80.4 Rh incompatibility reaction due to transfusion of blood or blood products**
Reaction due to incompatibility of Rh antigens (C) (c) (D) (E) (e)
Ex: **For category T80.4 CC codes unless otherwise indicated:** See T80.3

X● **T80.40 Rh incompatibility reaction due to transfusion of blood or blood products, unspecified** A
Reaction due to Rh factor in transfusion NOS
Rh incompatible blood transfusion NOS

● **T80.41 Rh incompatibility with hemolytic transfusion reaction**

● **T80.410 Rh incompatibility with acute hemolytic transfusion reaction** A
Acute hemolytic transfusion reaction (AHTR) due to Rh incompatibility
Rh incompatibility with hemolytic transfusion reaction less than 24 hours after transfusion

● **T80.411 Rh incompatibility with delayed hemolytic transfusion reaction** A
Delayed hemolytic transfusion reaction (DHTR) due to Rh incompatibility
Rh incompatibility with hemolytic transfusion reaction 24 hours or more after transfusion

● **T80.419 Rh incompatibility with hemolytic transfusion reaction, unspecified** A
Rh incompatibility with hemolytic transfusion reaction at unspecified time after transfusion
Hemolytic transfusion reaction (HTR) due to Rh incompatibility NOS

X● **T80.49 Other Rh incompatibility reaction due to transfusion of blood or blood products** A
Delayed serologic transfusion reaction (DSTR) from Rh incompatibility
Other reaction to Rh incompatible blood transfusion
Ex: T80.30X-T80.419[A], T80.910-T80.92X[A], T80.A9X[A]

T80.A Non-ABO incompatibility reaction due to transfusion of blood or blood products
Reaction due to incompatibility of minor antigens (Duffy) (Kell) (Kidd) (Lewis) (M) (N) (P) (S)
Ex: For category T80.A CC codes unless otherwise indicated: See T80.49

X **T80.A0 Non-ABO incompatibility reaction due to transfusion of blood or blood products, unspecified** A
Non-ABO antigen incompatibility reaction from transfusion NOS

T80.A1 Non-ABO incompatibility with hemolytic transfusion reaction

T80.A10 Non-ABO incompatibility with acute hemolytic transfusion reaction A
Acute hemolytic transfusion reaction (AHTR) due to non-ABO incompatibility
Non-ABO incompatibility with hemolytic transfusion reaction less than 24 hours after transfusion

T80.A11 Non-ABO incompatibility with delayed hemolytic transfusion reaction A
Delayed hemolytic transfusion reaction (DHTR) due to non-ABO incompatibility
Non-ABO incompatibility with hemolytic transfusion reaction 24 or more hours after transfusion

T80.A19 Non-ABO incompatibility with hemolytic transfusion reaction, unspecified A
Hemolytic transfusion reaction (HTR) due to non-ABO incompatibility NOS
Non-ABO incompatibility with hemolytic transfusion reaction at unspecified time after transfusion

X **T80.A9 Other non-ABO incompatibility reaction due to transfusion of blood or blood products** A
Delayed serologic transfusion reaction (DSTR) from non-ABO incompatibility
Other reaction to non-ABO incompatible blood transfusion
Ex: See T80.3

T80.5 Anaphylactic reaction due to serum
Allergic reaction due to serum
Anaphylactic shock due to serum
Anaphylactoid reaction due to serum
Anaphylaxis due to serum

Excludes1 ABO incompatibility reaction due to transfusion of blood or blood products (T80.3-)
allergic reaction or shock NOS (T78.2)
anaphylactic reaction or shock NOS (T78.2)
anaphylactic reaction or shock due to adverse effect of correct medicinal substance properly administered (T88.6)
other serum reaction (T80.6-)

Ex: For category T80.5 CC codes: T80.51X-T80.69X[A]

X **T80.51 Anaphylactic reaction due to administration of blood and blood products** A

X **T80.52 Anaphylactic reaction due to vaccination** A

X **T80.59 Anaphylactic reaction due to other serum** A

T80.6 Other serum reactions
Intoxication by serum
Protein sickness
Serum rash
Serum sickness
Serum urticaria

Excludes2 serum hepatitis (B16-B19)

Ex: For category T80.6 CC codes unless otherwise indicated: T80.51X-T80.69X[A]

X **T80.61 Other serum reaction due to administration of blood and blood products** A

X **T80.62 Other serum reaction due to vaccination** A

X **T80.69 Other serum reaction due to other serum** A
Ex: T80.61X-T80.69X[A]

T80.8 Other complications following infusion, transfusion and therapeutic injection

T80.81 Extravasation of vesicant agent
Infiltration of vesicant agent
Ex: For category T80.81 CC codes: T80.1XX[A], T80.810-T80.818[A], T80.90X[A]

T80.810 Extravasation of vesicant antineoplastic chemotherapy A
Infiltration of vesicant antineoplastic chemotherapy

T80.818 Extravasation of other vesicant agent A
Infiltration of other vesicant agent

X **T80.89 Other complications following infusion, transfusion and therapeutic injection**
Delayed serologic transfusion reaction (DSTR), unspecified incompatibility
Use additional code to identify graft-versus-host reaction, if applicable, (D89.81-)

T80.9 Unspecified complication following infusion, transfusion and therapeutic injection

X **T80.90 Unspecified complication following infusion and therapeutic injection**

T80.91 Hemolytic transfusion reaction, unspecified incompatibility

Excludes1 ABO incompatibility with hemolytic transfusion reaction (T80.31-)
Non-ABO incompatibility with hemolytic transfusion reaction (T80.A1-)
Rh incompatibility with hemolytic transfusion reaction (T80.41-)

Ex: For category T80.91 CC codes unless otherwise indicated: See T80.3

T80.910 Acute hemolytic transfusion reaction, unspecified incompatibility A

T80.911 Delayed hemolytic transfusion reaction, unspecified incompatibility A

T80.919 Hemolytic transfusion reaction, unspecified incompatibility, unspecified as acute or delayed A
Hemolytic transfusion reaction NOS

X **T80.92 Unspecified transfusion reaction**
Transfusion reaction NOS

● **T81 Complications of procedures, not elsewhere classified**

Use additional code for adverse effect, if applicable, to identify drug (T36-T50 with fifth or sixth character 5)

Excludes2 complications following immunization (T88.0-T88.1)
complications following infusion, transfusion and therapeutic injection (T80.-)
complications of transplanted organs and tissue (T86.-)
poisoning and toxic effects of drugs and chemicals (T36-T65 with fifth or sixth character 1-4 or 6)
specified complications classified elsewhere, such as:
complication of prosthetic devices, implants and grafts (T82-T85)
dermatitis due to drugs and medicaments (L23.3, L24.4, L25.1, L27.0-L27.1)
endosseous dental implant failure (M27.6-)
floppy iris syndrome (IFIS) (intraoperative) H21.81
intraoperative and postprocedural complications of specific body system (D78.-, E36.-, E89.-, G97.3-, G97.4, H59.3-, H59.-, H95.2-, H95.3, I97.4-, I97.5, J95, K91.-, L76.-, M96.-, N99.-)
ostomy complications (J95.0-, K94.-, N99.5-)
plateau iris syndrome (post-iridectomy) (postprocedural) H21.82

The appropriate 7th character is to be added to each code from category T81

A	initial encounter
D	subsequent encounter
S	sequela

● **T81.1 Postprocedural shock**

Shock during or resulting from a procedure, not elsewhere classified

Excludes1 anaphylactic shock NOS (T78.2)
anaphylactic shock due to correct substance properly administered (T88.6)
anaphylactic shock due to serum (T80.5-)
anesthetic shock (T88.2)
electric shock (T75.4)
obstetric shock (O75.1)
septic shock (R65.21)
shock following abortion or ectopic or molar pregnancy (O00-O07, O08.3)
traumatic shock (T79.4)

Ex: **For category T81.1 CC codes:** D78.01-D78.02, D78.21-D78.22, D78.31-D78.34, D78.81-D78.89, E36.01-E36.02, E36.8, E89.810-E89.89, G97.51-G97.52, G97.61-G97.64, H59.011-H59.019, H59.031-H59.039, H59.091-H59.099, H59.111-H59.129, H59.311-H59.369, H59.331-H59.349, H59.811-H59.819, H59.88-H59.89, H95.21-H95.22, H95.41-H95.42, H59.51-H59.54, H95.811-H95.819, H95.88-H95.89, I97.3-I97.42, I97.610-I97.648, J95.61-J95.62, J95.830-J95.831, J95.860-J95.863, K91.61-K91.62, K91.840-K91.841, K91.870-K91.873, L76.01-L76.02, L76.21-L76.22, L76.31-L76.34, L76.81-L76.82, M96.810-M96.811, M96.830-M96.89, N98.1-N98.9, N99.61-N99.62, N99.820-N99.821, N99.840-N99.843, T79.4XX[A], T81.10X-T81.19X[A], T81.82X-T81.9XX[A], T88.2XX[A]

X● **T81.10 Postprocedural shock unspecified** A

Collapse NOS during or resulting from a procedure, not elsewhere classified
Postprocedural failure of peripheral circulation
Postprocedural shock NOS

X● **T81.11 Postprocedural cardiogenic shock** A

A●X● **T81.12 Postprocedural septic shock** A

Postprocedural endotoxic shock resulting from a procedure, not elsewhere classified
Postprocedural gram-negative shock resulting from a procedure, not elsewhere classified

Code first underlying infection

Use additional code, to identify any associated acute organ dysfunction, if applicable

X● **T81.19 Other postprocedural shock** A

Postprocedural hypovolemic shock

● **T81.3 Disruption of wound, not elsewhere classified**

Disruption of any suture materials or other closure methods

Excludes1 breakdown (mechanical) of permanent sutures (T85.612)
displacement of permanent sutures (T85.622)
disruption of cesarean delivery wound (O90.0)
disruption of perineal obstetric wound (O90.1)
mechanical complication of permanent sutures NEC (T85.692)

Ex: **For category T81.3 CC codes:** D78.81-D78.89, E36.8, E89.810-E89.89, H59.011-H59.019, H59.031-H59.039, H59.091-H59.099, H59.811-H59.89, H95.811-H95.89, I97.3, L76.81-L76.82, M96.89, N98.1-N98.9, T81.30X-T81.33X[A], T81.82X-T81.9XX[A]

X● **T81.30 Disruption of wound, unspecified** A

Disruption of wound NOS

X● **T81.31 Disruption of external operation (surgical) wound, not elsewhere classified** A

Excludes1 dehiscence of amputation stump (T87.81)

Dehiscence of operation wound NOS
Disruption of operation wound NOS
Disruption or dehiscence of closure of cornea
Disruption or dehiscence of closure of mucosa
Disruption or dehiscence of closure of skin and subcutaneous tissue
Full-thickness skin disruption or dehiscence
Superficial disruption or dehiscence of operation wound

Coding Clinic: 2015, Q1, P20

X● **T81.32 Disruption of internal operation (surgical) wound, not elsewhere classified** A

Deep disruption or dehiscence of operation wound NOS
Disruption or dehiscence of closure of internal organ or other internal tissue
Disruption or dehiscence of closure of muscle or muscle flap
Disruption or dehiscence of closure of ribs or rib cage
Disruption or dehiscence of closure of skull or craniotomy
Disruption or dehiscence of closure of sternum or sternotomy
Disruption or dehiscence of closure of tendon or ligament
Disruption or dehiscence of closure of superficial or muscular fascia

X● **T81.33 Disruption of traumatic injury wound repair** A

Disruption or dehiscence of closure of traumatic laceration (external) (internal)

X ● **T81.4 Infection following a procedure** A CC, A MCC
Intra-abdominal abscess following a procedure
Postprocedural infection, not elsewhere classified
Sepsis following a procedure
Stitch abscess following a procedure
Subphrenic abscess following a procedure
Wound abscess following a procedure
Use additional code to identify infection
Use additional code (R65.2-) to identify severe sepsis, if applicable
Excludes1 obstetric surgical wound infection (O86.0)
postprocedural fever NOS (R50.82)
postprocedural retroperitoneal abscess (K68.11)
Excludes2 bleb associated endophthalmitis (H59.4-)
infection due to infusion, transfusion and therapeutic injection (T80.2-)
infection due to prosthetic devices, implants and grafts (T82.6-T82.7, T83.5-T83.6, T84.5-T84.7, T85.7)
Ex: D78.81-D78.89, E36.8, E89.810-E89.89, H59.011-H59.019, H59.031-H59.099, H59.811-H59.89, H95.811-H95.89, I97.3, K68.11, L76.81-L76.82, M96.89, N98.1-N98.9, T81.4XX[A], T81.82X[A], T81.89X-T81.9XX[A]
Coding Clinic: 2015, Q4, P37

● **T81.5 Complications of foreign body accidentally left in body following procedure**
Ex: **For category T81.5 CC codes:** D78.81-D78.89, E36.8, E89.810-E89.89, H59.011-H59.019, H59.031-H59.039, H59.091-H59.099, H59.811-H59.89, H95.811-H95.89, I97.3, L76.81-L76.82, M96.89, N98.1-N98.9, T81.500-T81.599[A], T81.82X-T81.9XX[A]

● **T81.50 Unspecified complication of foreign body accidentally left in body following procedure**
● **T81.500 Unspecified complication of foreign body accidentally left in body following surgical operation** A CC, A MCC
● **T81.501 Unspecified complication of foreign body accidentally left in body following infusion or transfusion** A CC, A MCC
● **T81.502 Unspecified complication of foreign body accidentally left in body following kidney dialysis** A CC, A MCC
● **T81.503 Unspecified complication of foreign body accidentally left in body following injection or immunization** A CC, A MCC
● **T81.504 Unspecified complication of foreign body accidentally left in body following endoscopic examination** A CC, A MCC
● **T81.505 Unspecified complication of foreign body accidentally left in body following heart catheterization** A CC, A MCC
● **T81.506 Unspecified complication of foreign body accidentally left in body following aspiration, puncture or other catheterization** A CC, A MCC
● **T81.507 Unspecified complication of foreign body accidentally left in body following removal of catheter or packing** A CC, A MCC
● **T81.508 Unspecified complication of foreign body accidentally left in body following other procedure** A CC, A MCC
● **T81.509 Unspecified complication of foreign body accidentally left in body following unspecified procedure** A CC, A MCC

● **T81.51 Adhesions due to foreign body accidentally left in body following procedure**
● **T81.510 Adhesions due to foreign body accidentally left in body following surgical operation** A CC, A MCC
● **T81.511 Adhesions due to foreign body accidentally left in body following infusion or transfusion** A CC, A MCC
● **T81.512 Adhesions due to foreign body accidentally left in body following kidney dialysis** A CC, A MCC
● **T81.513 Adhesions due to foreign body accidentally left in body following injection or immunization** A CC, A MCC
● **T81.514 Adhesions due to foreign body accidentally left in body following endoscopic examination** A CC, A MCC
● **T81.515 Adhesions due to foreign body accidentally left in body following heart catheterization** A CC, A MCC
● **T81.516 Adhesions due to foreign body accidentally left in body following aspiration, puncture or other catheterization** A CC, A MCC
● **T81.517 Adhesions due to foreign body accidentally left in body following removal of catheter or packing** A CC, A MCC
● **T81.518 Adhesions due to foreign body accidentally left in body following other procedure** A CC, A MCC
● **T81.519 Adhesions due to foreign body accidentally left in body following unspecified procedure** A CC, A MCC

● **T81.52 Obstruction due to foreign body accidentally left in body following procedure**
● **T81.520 Obstruction due to foreign body accidentally left in body following surgical operation** A CC, A MCC
● **T81.521 Obstruction due to foreign body accidentally left in body following infusion or transfusion** A CC, A MCC
● **T81.522 Obstruction due to foreign body accidentally left in body following kidney dialysis** A CC, A MCC
● **T81.523 Obstruction due to foreign body accidentally left in body following injection or immunization** A CC, A MCC
● **T81.524 Obstruction due to foreign body accidentally left in body following endoscopic examination** A CC, A MCC
● **T81.525 Obstruction due to foreign body accidentally left in body following heart catheterization** A CC, A MCC
● **T81.526 Obstruction due to foreign body accidentally left in body following aspiration, puncture or other catheterization** A CC, A MCC
● **T81.527 Obstruction due to foreign body accidentally left in body following removal of catheter or packing** A CC, A MCC
● **T81.528 Obstruction due to foreign body accidentally left in body following other procedure** A CC, A MCC
● **T81.529 Obstruction due to foreign body accidentally left in body following unspecified procedure** A CC, A MCC

● T81.53 Perforation due to foreign body accidentally left in body following procedure

● T81.530 Perforation due to foreign body accidentally left in body following surgical operation A CC, A MCC

● T81.531 Perforation due to foreign body accidentally left in body following infusion or transfusion A CC, A MCC

● T81.532 Perforation due to foreign body accidentally left in body following kidney dialysis A CC, A MCC

● T81.533 Perforation due to foreign body accidentally left in body following injection or immunization A CC, A MCC

● T81.534 Perforation due to foreign body accidentally left in body following endoscopic examination A CC, A MCC

● T81.535 Perforation due to foreign body accidentally left in body following heart catheterization A CC, A MCC

● T81.536 Perforation due to foreign body accidentally left in body following aspiration, puncture or other catheterization A CC, A MCC

● T81.537 Perforation due to foreign body accidentally left in body following removal of catheter or packing A CC, A MCC

● T81.538 Perforation due to foreign body accidentally left in body following other procedure A CC, A MCC

● T81.539 Perforation due to foreign body accidentally left in body following unspecified procedure A CC, A MCC

● T81.59 Other complications of foreign body accidentally left in body following procedure

Excludes2 obstruction or perforation due to prosthetic devices and implants intentionally left in body (T82.0-T82.5, T83.0-T83.4, T83.7, T84.0-T84.4, T85.0-T85.6)

● T81.590 Other complications of foreign body accidentally left in body following surgical operation A CC, A MCC

● T81.591 Other complications of foreign body accidentally left in body following infusion or transfusion A CC, A MCC

● T81.592 Other complications of foreign body accidentally left in body following kidney dialysis A CC, A MCC

● T81.593 Other complications of foreign body accidentally left in body following injection or immunization A CC, A MCC

● T81.594 Other complications of foreign body accidentally left in body following endoscopic examination A CC, A MCC

● T81.595 Other complications of foreign body accidentally left in body following heart catheterization A CC, A MCC

● T81.596 Other complications of foreign body accidentally left in body following aspiration, puncture or other catheterization A CC, A MCC

● T81.597 Other complications of foreign body accidentally left in body following removal of catheter or packing A CC, A MCC

● T81.598 Other complications of foreign body accidentally left in body following other procedure A CC, A MCC

● T81.599 Other complications of foreign body accidentally left in body following unspecified procedure A CC, A MCC

● T81.6 Acute reaction to foreign substance accidentally left during a procedure

Excludes2 complications of foreign body accidentally left in body cavity or operation wound following procedure (T81.5-)

Ex: **For category T81.6 CC codes:** D78.81-D78.89, E36.8, E89.810-E89.89, H59.011-H59.019, H59.031-H59.039, H59.091-H59.099, H59.811-H59.89, H95.811-H95.89, I97.3, L76.81-L76.82, M96.89, N98.1-N98.9, T81.60X-T81.69X[A], T81.82X-T81.9XX[A]

X● T81.60 Unspecified acute reaction to foreign substance accidentally left during a procedure A CC, A MCC

X● T81.61 Aseptic peritonitis due to foreign substance accidentally left during a procedure A CC, A MCC

Chemical peritonitis

X● T81.69 Other acute reaction to foreign substance accidentally left during a procedure A CC, A MCC

● T81.7 Vascular complications following a procedure, not elsewhere classified

Air embolism following procedure NEC

Phlebitis or thrombophlebitis resulting from a procedure

Excludes1 embolism complicating abortion or ectopic or molar pregnancy (O00-O07, O08.2)

embolism complicating pregnancy, childbirth and the puerperium (O88.-)

traumatic embolism (T79.0)

Excludes2 embolism due to prosthetic devices, implants and grafts (T82.8, T83.81, T84.8-, T85.1-) ◄

embolism following infusion, transfusion and therapeutic injection (T80.0)

● T81.71 Complication of artery following a procedure, not elsewhere classified

Ex: **For category T81.71 CC codes T81.710-T81.711:** D78.81-D78.89, E36.8, E89.810-E89.89, H59.011-H59.019, H59.031-H59.039, H59.091-H59.099, H59.811-H59.89, H95.811-H95.89, I97.3, L76.81-L76.82, M96.89, N98.1-N98.9, T81.710-T81.72X[A], T81.82X-T81.9XX[A]

For T81.718-T81.719: D78.81-D78.89, E36.8, E89.810-E89.89, H59.011-H59.019, H59.031-H59.039, H59.091-H59.099, H59.811-H59.89, H95.811-H95.89, I97.3, L76.81-L76.82, M96.89, N98.1-N98.9, T81.718-T81.72X[A], T81.82X-T81.9XX[A]

● T81.710 Complication of mesenteric artery following a procedure, not elsewhere classified A CC

● T81.711 Complication of renal artery following a procedure, not elsewhere classified A CC

● T81.718 Complication of other artery following a procedure, not elsewhere classified A CC

● T81.719 Complication of unspecified artery following a procedure, not elsewhere classified A CC

X● T81.72 Complication of vein following a procedure, not elsewhere classified A CC

Ex: See T81.718-T81.719

- **T81.8 Other complications of procedures, not elsewhere classified**
  - **Excludes2** hypothermia following anesthesia (T88.51)
    malignant hyperpyrexia due to anesthesia (T88.3)
  - X **T81.81 Complication of inhalation therapy**
  - X **T81.82 Emphysema (subcutaneous) resulting from a procedure**
  - X **T81.83 Persistent postprocedural fistula** A
    - Ex: D78.81-D78.89, E36.8, E89.810-E89.89, H59.011-H59.019, H59.031-H59.039, H59.091-H59.099, H59.811-H59.89, H95.811-H95.89, I97.3, L76.81-L76.82, M96.89, N98.1-N98.9, T81.82X-T81.9XX[A]
  - X **T81.89 Other complications of procedures, not elsewhere classified**
    - Use additional code to specify complication, such as:
      postprocedural delirium (F05)
  - X **T81.9 Unspecified complication of procedure**

- **T82 Complications of cardiac and vascular prosthetic devices, implants and grafts**
  - **Excludes2** failure and rejection of transplanted organs and tissue (T86.-)
  - The appropriate 7th character is to be added to each code from category T82

A	initial encounter
D	subsequent encounter
S	sequela

  - **T82.0 Mechanical complication of heart valve prosthesis**
    - Mechanical complication of artificial heart valve
    - **Excludes1** mechanical complication of biological heart valve graft (T82.22-)
    - Ex: **For category T82.0 CC codes:** D78.81-D78.89, E36.8, E89.810-E89.89, H59.011-H59.019, H59.031-H59.039, H59.091-H59.099, H59.811-H59.89, H95.811-H95.89, I97.3, L76.81-L76.82, M96.89, N98.1-N98.9, T81.82X-T81.9XX[A], T82.01X-T82.09X[A]
    - X **T82.01 Breakdown (mechanical) of heart valve prosthesis** A
    - X **T82.02 Displacement of heart valve prosthesis** A
      - Malposition of heart valve prosthesis
    - X **T82.03 Leakage of heart valve prosthesis** A
    - X **T82.09 Other mechanical complication of heart valve prosthesis** A
      - Obstruction (mechanical) of heart valve prosthesis
      - Perforation of heart valve prosthesis
      - Protrusion of heart valve prosthesis
  - **T82.1 Mechanical complication of cardiac electronic device**
    - Ex: **For category T82.1 CC codes:** D78.81-D78.89, E36.8, E89.810-E89.89, H59.011-H59.019, H59.031-H59.039, H59.091-H59.099, H59.811-H59.89, H95.811-H95.89, I97.3, L76.81-L76.82, M96.89, N98.1-N98.9, T81.82X-T81.9XX[A], T82.110-T82.111[A], T82.120-T82.121[A], T82.190-T82.191[A]
    - **T82.11 Breakdown (mechanical) of cardiac electronic device**
      - **T82.110 Breakdown (mechanical) of cardiac electrode** A
      - **T82.111 Breakdown (mechanical) of cardiac pulse generator (battery)** A
      - **T82.118 Breakdown (mechanical) of other cardiac electronic device** A
        - Ex: D78.81-D78.89, E36.8, E89.810-E89.89, H59.011-H59.019, H59.031-H59.039, H59.091-H59.099, H59.811-H59.89, H95.811-H95.89, I97.3, L76.81-L76.82, M96.89, N98.1-N98.9, T81.82X-T81.9XX[A], T82.118[A], T82.128[A], T82.198[A], T82.221-T82.228[A], T82.512[A], T82.522[A], T82.532[A], T82.592[A], T82.594[A], T82.598[A]
      - **T82.119 Breakdown (mechanical) of unspecified cardiac electronic device** A
        - Ex: No Exclusions
    - **T82.12 Displacement of cardiac electronic device**
      - Malposition of cardiac electronic device
      - **T82.120 Displacement of cardiac electrode** A
      - **T82.121 Displacement of cardiac pulse generator (battery)** A
      - **T82.128 Displacement of other cardiac electronic device** A
        - Ex: See T82.118A
      - **T82.129 Displacement of unspecified cardiac electronic device** A
        - Ex: No Exclusions
    - **T82.19 Other mechanical complication of cardiac electronic device**
      - Leakage of cardiac electronic device
      - Obstruction of cardiac electronic device
      - Perforation of cardiac electronic device
      - Protrusion of cardiac electronic device
      - **T82.190 Other mechanical complication of cardiac electrode** A
      - **T82.191 Other mechanical complication of cardiac pulse generator (battery)** A
      - **T82.198 Other mechanical complication of other cardiac electronic device** A
        - Ex: See T82.118A
      - **T82.199 Other mechanical complication of unspecified cardiac device** A
        - Ex: No Exclusions
  - **T82.2 Mechanical complication of coronary artery bypass graft and biological heart valve graft**
    - **Excludes1** mechanical complication of artificial heart valve prosthesis (T82.0-)
    - **T82.21 Mechanical complication of coronary artery bypass graft**
      - Ex: **For category T82.21 CC codes:** D78.81-D78.89, E36.8, E89.810-E89.89, H59.011-H59.019, H59.031-H59.039, H59.091-H59.099, H59.811-H59.89, H95.811-H95.89, I97.3, L76.81-L76.82, M96.89, N98.1-N98.9, T81.82X-T81.9XX[A], T82.211-T82.218[A]
      - **T82.211 Breakdown (mechanical) of coronary artery bypass graft** A
      - **T82.212 Displacement of coronary artery bypass graft** A
        - Malposition of coronary artery bypass graft
      - **T82.213 Leakage of coronary artery bypass graft** A
      - **T82.218 Other mechanical complication of coronary artery bypass graft** A
        - Obstruction, mechanical of coronary artery bypass graft
        - Perforation of coronary artery bypass graft
        - Protrusion of coronary artery bypass graft
    - **T82.22 Mechanical complication of biological heart valve graft**
      - Ex: **For category T82.22 CC codes:** See T82.118A
      - **T82.221 Breakdown (mechanical) of biological heart valve graft** A
      - **T82.222 Displacement of biological heart valve graft** A
        - Malposition of biological heart valve graft

- T82.223 Leakage of biological heart valve graft A
- T82.228 Other mechanical complication of biological heart valve graft A
  - Obstruction of biological heart valve graft
  - Perforation of biological heart valve graft
  - Protrusion of biological heart valve graft

- T82.3 Mechanical complication of other vascular grafts
  - Ex: For category T82.3 CC codes: D78.81-D78.89, E36.8, E89.810-E89.89, H59.011-H59.019, H59.031-H59.039, H59.091-H59.099, H59.811-H59.89, H95.811-H95.89, I97.3, L76.81-L76.82, M96.89, N98.1-N98.9, T81.82X-T81.9XX[A], T82.310-T82.538[A], T82.590-T82.595[A]
  - T82.31 Breakdown (mechanical) of other vascular grafts
    - T82.310 Breakdown (mechanical) of aortic (bifurcation) graft (replacement) A
    - T82.311 Breakdown (mechanical) of carotid arterial graft (bypass) A
    - T82.312 Breakdown (mechanical) of femoral arterial graft (bypass) A
    - T82.318 Breakdown (mechanical) of other vascular grafts A
    - T82.319 Breakdown (mechanical) of unspecified vascular grafts A
  - T82.32 Displacement of other vascular grafts
    - Malposition of other vascular grafts
    - T82.320 Displacement of aortic (bifurcation) graft (replacement) A
    - T82.321 Displacement of carotid arterial graft (bypass) A
    - T82.322 Displacement of femoral arterial graft (bypass) A
    - T82.328 Displacement of other vascular grafts A
    - T82.329 Displacement of unspecified vascular grafts A
  - T82.33 Leakage of other vascular grafts
    - T82.330 Leakage of aortic (bifurcation) graft (replacement) A
    - T82.331 Leakage of carotid arterial graft (bypass) A
    - T82.332 Leakage of femoral arterial graft (bypass) A
    - T82.338 Leakage of other vascular grafts A
    - T82.339 Leakage of unspecified vascular graft A
  - T82.39 Other mechanical complication of other vascular grafts
    - Obstruction (mechanical) of other vascular grafts
    - Perforation of other vascular grafts
    - Protrusion of other vascular grafts
    - T82.390 Other mechanical complication of aortic (bifurcation) graft (replacement) A
    - T82.391 Other mechanical complication of carotid arterial graft (bypass) A
    - T82.392 Other mechanical complication of femoral arterial graft (bypass) A
    - T82.398 Other mechanical complication of other vascular grafts A
    - T82.399 Other mechanical complication of unspecified vascular grafts A

- T82.4 Mechanical complication of vascular dialysis catheter
  - Mechanical complication of hemodialysis catheter
  - Excludes1 mechanical complication of intraperitoneal dialysis catheter (T85.62)
  - Ex: For category T82.4 CC codes: See T82.3
  - X T82.41 Breakdown (mechanical) of vascular dialysis catheter A
  - X T82.42 Displacement of vascular dialysis catheter A
    - Malposition of vascular dialysis catheter
  - X T82.43 Leakage of vascular dialysis catheter A
  - X T82.49 Other complication of vascular dialysis catheter A
    - Obstruction (mechanical) of vascular dialysis catheter
    - Perforation of vascular dialysis catheter
    - Protrusion of vascular dialysis catheter

- T82.5 Mechanical complication of other cardiac and vascular devices and implants
  - Excludes2 mechanical complication of epidural and subdural infusion catheter (T85.61)
  - Ex: For category T82.5 CC codes unless otherwise indicated: See T82.3
  - T82.51 Breakdown (mechanical) of other cardiac and vascular devices and implants
    - T82.510 Breakdown (mechanical) of surgically created arteriovenous fistula A
    - T82.511 Breakdown (mechanical) of surgically created arteriovenous shunt A
    - T82.512 Breakdown (mechanical) of artificial heart A
      - Ex: See T82.118A
    - T82.513 Breakdown (mechanical) of balloon (counterpulsation) device A
    - T82.514 Breakdown (mechanical) of infusion catheter A
    - T82.515 Breakdown (mechanical) of umbrella device A
    - T82.518 Breakdown (mechanical) of other cardiac and vascular devices and implants A
    - T82.519 Breakdown (mechanical) of unspecified cardiac and vascular devices and implants A
      - Ex: D78.81-D78.89, E36.8, E89.810-E89.89, H59.011-H59.019, H59.031-H59.039, H59.091-H59.099, H59.811-H59.89, H95.811-H95.89, I97.3, L76.81-L76.82, M96.89, N98.1-N98.9, T81.82X-T81.9XX[A], T82.519[A], T82.539[A], T82.599-T82.9XX[A], T85.9XX[A]
  - T82.52 Displacement of other cardiac and vascular devices and implants
    - Malposition of other cardiac and vascular devices and implants
    - T82.520 Displacement of surgically created arteriovenous fistula A
    - T82.521 Displacement of surgically created arteriovenous shunt A
    - T82.522 Displacement of artificial heart A
      - Ex: See T82.118A
    - T82.523 Displacement of balloon (counterpulsation) device A
    - T82.524 Displacement of infusion catheter A
    - T82.525 Displacement of umbrella device A
    - T82.528 Displacement of other cardiac and vascular devices and implants A
    - T82.529 Displacement of unspecified cardiac and vascular devices and implants A

◀ New ⇐ Revised ~~deleted~~ Deleted Excludes 1 Excludes 2 Includes Use additional Code first Code also Unspecified
OGCR Official Guidelines ● Unacceptable Principal Diagnosis X Assign placeholder X ● Use Additional Character(s) ▶ Manifestation Code Coding Clinic

- **T82.53 Leakage of other cardiac and vascular devices and implants**
  - **T82.530 Leakage of surgically created arteriovenous fistula** A
  - **T82.531 Leakage of surgically created arteriovenous shunt** A
  - **T82.532 Leakage of artificial heart** A
    Ex: See T82.118A
  - **T82.533 Leakage of balloon (counterpulsation) device** A
  - **T82.534 Leakage of infusion catheter** A
  - **T82.535 Leakage of umbrella device** A
  - **T82.538 Leakage of other cardiac and vascular devices and implants** A
  - **T82.539 Leakage of unspecified cardiac and vascular devices and implants** A
    Ex: See T82.519
- **T82.59 Other mechanical complication of other cardiac and vascular devices and implants**
  Obstruction (mechanical) of other cardiac and vascular devices and implants
  Perforation of other cardiac and vascular devices and implants
  Protrusion of other cardiac and vascular devices and implants
  - **T82.590 Other mechanical complication of surgically created arteriovenous fistula** A
  - **T82.591 Other mechanical complication of surgically created arteriovenous shunt** A
  - **T82.592 Other mechanical complication of artificial heart** A
    Ex: See T82.118A
  - **T82.593 Other mechanical complication of balloon (counterpulsation) device** A
  - **T82.594 Other mechanical complication of infusion catheter** A
    Ex: See T82.118A
  - **T82.595 Other mechanical complication of umbrella device** A
  - **T82.598 Other mechanical complication of other cardiac and vascular devices and implants** A
    Ex: See T82.118A
  - **T82.599 Other mechanical complication of unspecified cardiac and vascular devices and implants** A
    Ex: See T82.519
- X **T82.6 Infection and inflammatory reaction due to cardiac valve prosthesis** A, A
  Use additional code to identify infection
  Ex: D78.81-D78.89, E36.8, E89.810-E89.89, H59.011-H59.019, H59.031-H59.039, H59.091-H59.099, H59.811-H59.89, H95.811-H95.89, I97.3, L76.81-L76.82, M96.89, N98.1-N98.9, T81.82X-T81.9XX[A], T82.01X-T82.118[A], T82.120-T82.128[A], T82.190-T82.198[A], T82.211-T82.9XX[A], T85.310-T85.311[A], T85.320-T85.321[A], T85.390-T85.391[A], T85.510-T85.738[A], T85.7XX[A], T85.810[A,D], T85.820[A,D], T85.830[A,D], T85.840[A,D], T85.850[A,D], T85.860[A,D], T85.890[A,D], T86.820-T86.829, T86.842-T86.849
- X **T82.7 Infection and inflammatory reaction due to other cardiac and vascular devices, implants and grafts** A, A
  Use additional code to identify infection
  Ex: See T82.6
- **T82.8 Other specified complications of cardiac and vascular prosthetic devices, implants and grafts**
  - **T82.81 Embolism due to cardiac and vascular prosthetic devices, implants and grafts**
    - **T82.817 Embolism due to cardiac prosthetic devices, implants and grafts** A
      Ex: D78.81-D78.89, E36.8, E89.810-E89.89, H59.011-H59.019, H59.031-H59.039, H59.091-H59.099, H59.811-H59.89, H95.811-H95.89, I97.3, L76.81-L76.82, M96.89, N98.1-N98.9, T81.82X-T81.9XX[A], T82.01X-T82.118[A], T82.120-T82.128[A], T82.190-T82.198[A], T82.221-T82.9XX[A], T85.310-T85.311[A], T85.320-T85.321[A], T85.390-T85.391[A], T85.510-T85.738[A], T85.79XA, 85.810[A,D], T85.820[A,D], T85.830[A,D], T85.840[A,D], T85.850[A,D], T85.860[A,D], T85.890[A,D], T85.9XX[A], T86.820-T86.829, T86.842-T86.849
      Coding Clinic: 2015, Q1, P20
    - **T82.818 Embolism due to vascular prosthetic devices, implants and grafts** A
      Ex: See T82.6
  - **T82.82 Fibrosis due to cardiac and vascular prosthetic devices, implants and grafts**
    - **T82.827 Fibrosis due to cardiac prosthetic devices, implants and grafts** A
      Ex: See T82.817
    - **T82.828 Fibrosis due to vascular prosthetic devices, implants and grafts** A
      Ex: See T82.6
  - **T82.83 Hemorrhage due to cardiac and vascular prosthetic devices, implants and grafts**
    - **T82.837 Hemorrhage due to cardiac prosthetic devices, implants and grafts** A
      Ex: See T82.817
    - **T82.838 Hemorrhage due to vascular prosthetic devices, implants and grafts** A
      Ex: See T82.6
  - **T82.84 Pain due to cardiac and vascular prosthetic devices, implants and grafts**
    - **T82.847 Pain due to cardiac prosthetic devices, implants and grafts** A
      Ex: See T82.817
    - **T82.848 Pain due to vascular prosthetic devices, implants and grafts** A
      Ex: See T82.6
  - **T82.85 Stenosis due to cardiac and vascular prosthetic devices, implants and grafts**
    - **T82.855 Stenosis of coronary artery stent** A ◀
      In-stent stenosis (restenosis) of coronary artery stent ◀
      Restenosis of coronary artery stent ◀
      Ex: D78.81-D78.89, E36.8, E89.810-E89.89, H59.011-H59.019, H59.031-H59.039, H59.091-H59.099, H59.811-H59.89, H95.811-H95.89, I60.2, I97.3, L76.81-L76.82, M96.89, N98.1-N98.9, S02.101-S02.82X[A,B], T81.82X-T81.9XX[A], T82.01X-T82.118[A], T82.120-T82.128[A], T82.190-T82.198[A], T82.221-T82.9XX[A], T85.310-T85.311[A], T85.320-T85.321[A], T85.390-T85.391[A], T85.510-T85.79X[A], T85.9XX[A], T86.820-T86.829, T86.842-T86.849

● **T82.856 Stenosis of peripheral vascular stent** A ◀
In-stent stenosis (restenosis) of peripheral vascular stent ◀
Restenosis of peripheral vascular stent ◀
Ex: D78.81-D78.89, E36.8, E89.810-E89.89, H59.011-H59.019, H59.031-H59.039, H59.091-H59.099, H59.811-H59.89, H95.811-H95.89, I60.2, I97.3, L76.81-L76.82, M96.89, N98.1-N98.9, S02.101-S02.82X[A,B], T81.82X-T81.9XX[A], T82.01X-T82.118[A], T82.120-T82.128[A], T82.190-T82.198[A], T82.221-T82.9XX[A], T85.310-T85.311[A], T85.320-T85.321[A], T85.390-T85.391[A], T85.510-T85.79X[A], T85.9XX[A], T86.820-T86.829, T86.842-T86.849

● **T82.857 Stenosis of other cardiac prosthetic devices, implants and grafts** A ⇐
Ex: See T82.817

● **T82.858 Stenosis of other vascular prosthetic devices, implants and grafts** A ⇐
Ex: See T82.6

● **T82.86 Thrombosis of cardiac and vascular prosthetic devices, implants and grafts**

● **T82.867 Thrombosis due to cardiac prosthetic devices, implants and grafts** A ⇐
Ex: See T82.817

● **T82.868 Thrombosis due to vascular prosthetic devices, implants and grafts** A ⇐
Ex: See T82.6

● **T82.89 Other specified complication of cardiac and vascular prosthetic devices, implants and grafts**

● **T82.897 Other specified complication of cardiac prosthetic devices, implants and grafts** A
Ex: See T82.817

● **T82.898 Other specified complication of vascular prosthetic devices, implants and grafts** A
Ex: See T82.6

X ● **T82.9 Unspecified complication of cardiac and vascular prosthetic device, implant and graft** A
Ex: See T82.817

● **T83 Complications of genitourinary prosthetic devices, implants and grafts**
Excludes2 failure and rejection of transplanted organs and tissue (T86.-)
The appropriate 7th character is to be added to each code from category T83

A	initial encounter
D	subsequent encounter
S	sequela

Ex: **For category T83 CC codes unless otherwise indicated:** D78.81-D78.89, E36.8, E89.810-E89.89, H59.011-H59.019, H59.031-H59.039, H59.091-H59.099, H59.811-H59.89, H95.811-H95.89, I97.3, L76.81-L76.82, M96.89, N98.1-N98.9, N99.510-N99.518, T81.82[A], T81.89-T81.9[A], T83.010[A], T83.020[A], T83.030[A], T83.090[A], T83.110-T83.29X[A], T83.410-T83.69[A], T83.712-T83.714[A], T83.718[A], T83.719A, T83.722-T83.724[A], T83.728-T83.9XX[A]

● **T83.0 Mechanical complication of urinary catheter** ⇐
Excludes2 complications of stoma of urinary tract (N99.5-)

● **T83.01 Breakdown (mechanical) of urinary catheter** ⇐

● **T83.010 Breakdown (mechanical) of cystostomy catheter** A

● **T83.011 Breakdown (mechanical) of indwelling urethral catheter** ◀

● **T83.012 Breakdown (mechanical) of nephrostomy catheter** ◀

● **T83.018 Breakdown (mechanical) of other urinary catheter** ⇐
Breakdown (mechanical) of Hopkins catheter ◀
Breakdown (mechanical) of ileostomy catheter ◀
Breakdown (mechanical) urostomy catheter ◀

● **T83.02 Displacement of urinary catheter** ⇐
Malposition of urinary catheter ⇐

● **T83.020 Displacement of cystostomy catheter** A

● **T83.021 Displacement of indwelling urethral catheter** ◀

● **T83.022 Displacement of nephrostomy catheter** ◀

● **T83.028 Displacement of other urinary catheter** ⇐
Displacement of Hopkins catheter ◀
Displacement of ileostomy catheter ◀
Displacement of urostomy catheter ◀

● **T83.03 Leakage of urinary catheter** ⇐

● **T83.030 Leakage of cystostomy catheter** A

● **T83.031 Leakage of indwelling urethral catheter** ◀

● **T83.032 Leakage of nephrostomy catheter** ◀

● **T83.038 Leakage of other urinary catheter** ⇐
Leakage of Hopkins catheter ◀
Leakage of ileostomy catheter ◀
Leakage of urostomy catheter ◀

● **T83.09 Other mechanical complication of urinary catheter** ⇐
Obstruction (mechanical) of urinary catheter ⇐
Perforation of urinary catheter ⇐
Protrusion of urinary catheter ⇐

● **T83.090 Other mechanical complication of cystostomy catheter** A

● **T83.091 Other mechanical complication of indwelling urethral catheter** ◀

● **T83.092 Other mechanical complication of nephrostomy catheter** ◀

● **T83.098 Other mechanical complication of other urinary catheter** ⇐
Other mechanical complication of Hopkins catheter ◀
Other mechanical complication of ileostomy catheter ◀
Other mechanical complication of urostomy catheter ◀

● **T83.1 Mechanical complication of other urinary devices and implants**

● **T83.11 Breakdown (mechanical) of other urinary devices and implants**

● **T83.110 Breakdown (mechanical) of urinary electronic stimulator device** A
Excludes2 Breakdown (mechanical) of electrode (lead) for sacral nerve neurostimulator (T85.111) ◀
Breakdown (mechanical) of implanted electronic sacral neurostimulator, pulse generator or receiver (T85.113) ◀

● **T83.111 Breakdown (mechanical) of implanted urinary sphincter** A ⇐

- **T83.112 Breakdown (mechanical) of indwelling ureteral stent** A
- **T83.113 Breakdown (mechanical) of other urinary stents** A ◀
  - Breakdown (mechanical) of ileal conduit stent ◀
  - Breakdown (mechanical) of nephroureteral stent ◀
  - Ex: D78.81-D78.89, E36.8, E89.810-E89.89, H59.011-H59.019, H59.031-H59.039, H59.091-H59.099, H59.811-H59.89, H95.811-H95.89, I60.2, I97.3, K55.011-K55.069, K55.30-K55.33, L76.81-76.82, M96.89, N98.1-N98.9, N99.510-N99.518, S02.101-S02.82X[A,B], T81.82[A], T81.89-T81.9[A], T83.010[A], T83.020[A], T83.030[A], T83.090[A], T83.110-T83.29X[A], T83.410-T83.498[A], T83.718[A], T83.728-T83.9XX[A]
- **T83.118 Breakdown (mechanical) of other urinary devices and implants** A

T83.12 Displacement of other urinary devices and implants
- Malposition of other urinary devices and implants
- **T83.120 Displacement of urinary electronic stimulator device** A
  - **Excludes2** Displacement of electrode (lead) for sacral nerve neurostimulator (T85.121) ◀
  - Displacement of implanted electronic sacral neurostimulator, pulse generator or receiver (T85.123) ◀
- **T83.121 Displacement of implanted urinary sphincter** A
- **T83.122 Displacement of indwelling ureteral stent** A
- **T83.123 Displacement of other urinary stents** A ◀
  - Displacement of ileal conduit stent ◀
  - Displacement of nephroureteral stent ◀
  - Ex: See T83.113A
- **T83.128 Displacement of other urinary devices and implants** A

T83.19 Other mechanical complication of other urinary devices and implants
- Leakage of other urinary devices and implants
- Obstruction (mechanical) of other urinary devices and implants
- Perforation of other urinary devices and implants
- Protrusion of other urinary devices and implants
- **T83.190 Other mechanical complication of urinary electronic stimulator device** A
  - **Excludes2** Other mechanical complication of electrode (lead) for sacral nerve neurostimulator (T85.191) ◀
  - Other mechanical complication of implanted electronic sacral neurostimulator, pulse generator or receiver (T85.193) ◀
- **T83.191 Other mechanical complication of implanted urinary sphincter** A
- **T83.192 Other mechanical complication of indwelling ureteral stent** A
- **T83.193 Other mechanical complication of other urinary stent** A ◀
  - Other mechanical complication of ileal conduit stent ◀
  - Other mechanical complication of nephroureteral stent ◀
  - Ex: See T83.113A
- **T83.198 Other mechanical complication of other urinary devices and implants** A

T83.2 Mechanical complication of graft of urinary organ
- X **T83.21 Breakdown (mechanical) of graft of urinary organ** A
- X **T83.22 Displacement of graft of urinary organ** A
  - Malposition of graft of urinary organ
- X **T83.23 Leakage of graft of urinary organ** A
- X **T83.24 Erosion of graft of urinary organ** A ◀
  - Ex: See T83.113A
- X **T83.25 Exposure of graft of urinary organ** A ◀
  - Ex: See T83.113A
- X **T83.29 Other mechanical complication of graft of urinary organ** A
  - Obstruction (mechanical) of graft of urinary organ
  - Perforation of graft of urinary organ
  - Protrusion of graft of urinary organ

T83.3 Mechanical complication of intrauterine contraceptive device
- X **T83.31 Breakdown (mechanical) of intrauterine contraceptive device** ♀
- X **T83.32 Displacement of intrauterine contraceptive device** ♀
  - Malposition of intrauterine contraceptive device
  - Missing string of intrauterine contraceptive device ◀
- X **T83.39 Other mechanical complication of intrauterine contraceptive device** ♀
  - Leakage of intrauterine contraceptive device
  - Obstruction (mechanical) of intrauterine contraceptive device
  - Perforation of intrauterine contraceptive device
  - Protrusion of intrauterine contraceptive device

T83.4 Mechanical complication of other prosthetic devices, implants and grafts of genital tract
- **T83.41 Breakdown (mechanical) of other prosthetic devices, implants and grafts of genital tract**
  - **T83.410 Breakdown (mechanical) of implanted penile prosthesis** ♂ A
    - Breakdown (mechanical) of penile prosthesis cylinder ◀
    - Breakdown (mechanical) of penile prosthesis pump ◀
    - Breakdown (mechanical) of penile prosthesis reservoir ◀
  - **T83.411 Breakdown (mechanical) of implanted testicular prosthesis** A ◀
    - Ex: See T83.113A
  - **T83.418 Breakdown (mechanical) of other prosthetic devices, implants and grafts of genital tract** A

● **T83.42 Displacement of other prosthetic devices, implants and grafts of genital tract**
Malposition of other prosthetic devices, implants and grafts of genital tract

● **T83.420 Displacement of implanted penile prosthesis** ♂ A
Displacement of penile prosthesis cylinder ◀
Displacement of penile prosthesis pump ◀
Displacement of penile prosthesis reservoir ◀

● **T83.421 Displacement of implanted testicular prosthesis** A ◀
Ex See T83.113A

● **T83.428 Displacement of other prosthetic devices, implants and grafts of genital tract** A

● **T83.49 Other mechanical complication of other prosthetic devices, implants and grafts of genital tract**
Leakage of other prosthetic devices, implants and grafts of genital tract
Obstruction, mechanical of other prosthetic devices, implants and grafts of genital tract
Perforation of other prosthetic devices, implants and grafts of genital tract
Protrusion of other prosthetic devices, implants and grafts of genital tract

● **T83.490 Other mechanical complication of implanted penile prosthesis** ♂ A
Other mechanical complication of penile prosthesis cylinder ◀
Other mechanical complication of penile prosthesis pump ◀
Other mechanical complication of penile prosthesis reservoir ◀

● **T83.491 Other mechanical complication of implanted testicular prosthesis** A ◀

● **T83.498 Other mechanical complication of other prosthetic devices, implants and grafts of genital tract** A

● **T83.5 Infection and inflammatory reaction due to prosthetic device, implant and graft in urinary system**
Use additional code to identify infection
Ex **For category T83.5 CC codes unless otherwise indicated:**
D78.81-D78.89, E36.8, E89.810-E89.89, H59.011-H59.019, H59.031-H59.039, H59.091-H59.099, H59.811-H59.89, H95.811-H95.89, I97.3, L76.81-L76.82, M96.89, N39.0, N98.1-N98.9, N99.510-N99.518, T81.82X-T81.9XX[A], T83.010[A], T83.020[A], T83.030[A], T83.090[A], T83.110-T83.29X[A], T83.410-T83.498[A], T83.510-T83.518[A], T83.590-T83.598[A], T83.61X-T83.69X[A], T83.712-T83.719[A], T83.722-T83.729[A], T83.79XA, T83.81X-T83.9XX[A], T85.310-T85.738[A], T85.79XA, T85.810[A,D], T85.820[A,D], T85.830[A,D], T85.840[A,D], T85.850[A,D], T85.860[A,D], T850.890[A,D], T85.9XX[A], T86.820-T86.849

● **T83.51 Infection and inflammatory reaction due to urinary catheter**
Excludes2 complications of stoma of urinary tract (N99.5-)

● **T83.510 Infection and inflammatory reaction due to cystostomy catheter** A ◀

● **T83.511 Infection and inflammatory reaction due to indwelling urethral catheter** A, Pr ◀
Ex D78.81-D78.89, E36.8, E89.810-E89.89, H59.011-H59.019, H59.031-H59.039, H59.091-H59.099, H59.811-H59.89, H95.811-H95.89, I97.3, L76.81-L76.82, M96.89, N98.1-N98.9, N99.510-N99.518, R82.71, T81.82X-T81.9XX[A], T83.010[A], T83.020[A], T83.030[A], T83.090[A], T83.110-T83.29X[A], T83.410-T83.498[A], T83.510-T83.518[A], T83.590-T83.598[A], T83.61X-T83.69X[A], T83.712-T83.719[A], T83.722-T83.729[A], T83.79XA, T83.81X-T83.9XX[A], T85.310-T85.311[A], T85.320-T85.321[A], T85.390-T85.391[A], T85.510-T85.79X[A], T85.810[A,D], T85.820[A,D], T85.830[A,D], T85.840[A,D], T85.850[A,D], T85.860[A,D], T850.890[A,D], T85.9XXA, T86.842-T86.849

● **T83.512 Infection and inflammatory reaction due to nephrostomy catheter** A ◀

● **T83.518 Infection and inflammatory reaction due to other urinary catheter** A, Pr ◀
Infection and inflammatory reaction due to Hopkins catheter ◀
Infection and inflammatory reaction due to ileostomy catheter ◀
Infection and inflammatory reaction due to urostomy catheter ◀

● **T83.59 Infection and inflammatory reaction due to prosthetic device, implant and graft in urinary system**

● **T83.590 Infection and inflammatory reaction due to implanted urinary neurostimulation device** A ◀
Excludes2 Infection and inflammatory reaction due to electrode lead of sacral nerve neurostimulator (T85.732) ◀
Infection and inflammatory reaction due to pulse generator or receiver of sacral nerve neurostimulator (T85.734) ◀

● **T83.591 Infection and inflammatory reaction due to implanted urinary sphincter** A ◀

● **T83.592 Infection and inflammatory reaction due to indwelling ureteral stent** A ◀

● **T83.593 Infection and inflammatory reaction due to other urinary stents** A ◀
Infection and inflammatory reaction due to ileal conduit stents ◀
Infection and inflammatory reaction due to nephroureteral stent ◀

● **T83.598 Infection and inflammatory reaction due to other prosthetic device, implant and graft in urinary system** A ◀

● **T83.6 Infection and inflammatory reaction due to prosthetic device, implant and graft in genital tract**
Use additional code to identify infection
Ex: For category T83.6: See T83.5

● **T83.61 Infection and inflammatory reaction due to implanted penile prosthesis** A ◀
Infection and inflammatory reaction due to penile prosthesis cylinder ◀
Infection and inflammatory reaction due to penile prosthesis pump ◀
Infection and inflammatory reaction due to penile prosthesis reservoir ◀

● **T83.62 Infection and inflammatory reaction due to implanted testicular prosthesis** A ◀

● **T83.69 Infection and inflammatory reaction due to other prosthetic device, implant and graft in genital tract** A ◀

● **T83.7 Complications due to implanted mesh and other prosthetic materials**
Ex: For Category T83.7 CC codes unless otherwise indicated: See T83.510A

● **T83.71 Erosion of implanted mesh and other prosthetic materials to surrounding organ or tissue**

● **T83.711 Erosion of implanted vaginal mesh to surrounding organ or tissue** ♀
Erosion of implanted vaginal mesh into pelvic floor muscles

● **T83.712 Erosion of implanted urethral mesh to surrounding organ or tissue** A ◀
Erosion of implanted female urethral sling ◀
Erosion of implanted male urethral sling ◀
Erosion of implanted urethral mesh into pelvic floor muscles ◀

● **T83.713 Erosion of implanted urethral bulking agent to surrounding organ or tissue** A ◀

● **T83.714 Erosion of implanted ureteral bulking agent to surrounding organ or tissue** A ◀

● **T83.718 Erosion of other implanted mesh to organ or tissue** A

● **T83.719 Erosion of other prosthetic materials to surrounding organ or tissue** A ◀

● **T83.72 Exposure of implanted mesh and other prosthetic materials into surrounding organ or tissue**
Extrusion of implanted mesh ◀

● **T83.721 Exposure of implanted vaginal mesh into vagina** ♀
Exposure of implanted vaginal mesh through vaginal wall

● **T83.722 Exposure of implanted urethral mesh into urethra** A ◀
Exposure of implanted female urethral sling ◀
Exposure of implanted male urethral sling ◀
Exposure of implanted urethral mesh through urethral wall ◀

● **T83.723 Exposure of implanted urethral bulking agent into urethra** A ◀

● **T83.724 Exposure of implanted ureteral bulking agent into ureter** A ◀

● **T83.728 Exposure of other implanted mesh into organ or tissue** A

● **T83.729 Exposure of other prosthetic materials into organ or tissue** A ◀

X● **T83.79 Other specified complications due to other genitourinary prosthetic materials** A ◀
Ex: See T83.5

● **T83.8 Other specified complications of genitourinary prosthetic devices, implants and grafts**
Ex: For category T83.8 CC codes: See T83.5

X● **T83.81 Embolism due to genitourinary prosthetic devices, implants and grafts** A

X● **T83.82 Fibrosis due to genitourinary prosthetic devices, implants and grafts** A

X● **T83.83 Hemorrhage due to genitourinary prosthetic devices, implants and grafts** A

X● **T83.84 Pain due to genitourinary prosthetic devices, implants and grafts** A

X● **T83.85 Stenosis due to genitourinary prosthetic devices, implants and grafts** A

X● **T83.86 Thrombosis due to genitourinary prosthetic devices, implants and grafts** A

X● **T83.89 Other specified complication of genitourinary prosthetic devices, implants and grafts** A

X● **T83.9 Unspecified complication of genitourinary prosthetic device, implant and graft** A
Ex: See T83.5

● **T84 Complications of internal orthopedic prosthetic devices, implants and grafts**
Excludes2 failure and rejection of transplanted organs and tissues (T86.-)
fracture of bone following insertion of orthopedic implant, joint prosthesis or bone plate (M96.6)
The appropriate 7th character is to be added to each code from category T84

A	initial encounter
D	subsequent encounter
S	sequela

Ex: D78.81, D78.89, E36.8, E89.810-E89.89, H59.011-H59.019, H59.031-H59.819, H59.88-H59.89, H95.811-H95.89, I97.3, L76.81-L76.82, M96.621-M96.69, M96.89, M97.01X-M97.9XX[A], N98.1-N98.9, T81.82X[A], T81.89X-T81.9XX[A], T84.010-T84.9XX[A]

● **T84.0 Mechanical complication of internal joint prosthesis**

● **T84.01 Broken internal joint prosthesis**
Breakage (fracture) of prosthetic joint
Broken prosthetic joint implant
Excludes1 periprosthetic joint implant fracture (T84.04)

● **T84.010 Broken internal right hip prosthesis** A

● **T84.011 Broken internal left hip prosthesis** A

● **T84.012 Broken internal right knee prosthesis** A

● **T84.013 Broken internal left knee prosthesis** A

● **T84.018 Broken internal joint prosthesis, other site** A
Use additional code to identify the joint (Z96.6-)

● **T84.019 Broken internal joint prosthesis, unspecified site** A

● **T84.02 Dislocation of internal joint prosthesis**
Instability of internal joint prosthesis
Subluxation of internal joint prosthesis

● **T84.020 Dislocation of internal right hip prosthesis** A

● **T84.021 Dislocation of internal left hip prosthesis** A

● **T84.022 Instability of internal right knee prosthesis** A

● **T84.023 Instability of internal left knee prosthesis** A

● **T84.028 Dislocation of other internal joint prosthesis** A
Use additional code to identify the joint (Z96.6-)

● **T84.029 Dislocation of unspecified internal joint prosthesis** A

T84.03 Mechanical loosening of internal prosthetic joint
Aseptic loosening of prosthetic joint

T84.030 Mechanical loosening of internal right hip prosthetic joint A

T84.031 Mechanical loosening of internal left hip prosthetic joint A

T84.032 Mechanical loosening of internal right knee prosthetic joint A

T84.033 Mechanical loosening of internal left knee prosthetic joint A

T84.038 Mechanical loosening of other internal prosthetic joint A
Use additional code to identify the joint (Z96.6-)

T84.039 Mechanical loosening of unspecified internal prosthetic joint A

~~T84.04 Periprosthetic fracture around internal prosthetic joint~~

~~T84.040 Periprosthetic fracture around internal prosthetic right hip joint~~

~~T84.041 Periprosthetic fracture around internal prosthetic left hip joint~~

~~T84.042 Periprosthetic fracture around internal prosthetic right knee joint~~

~~T84.043 Periprosthetic fracture around internal prosthetic left knee joint~~

~~T84.048 Periprosthetic fracture around other internal prosthetic joint~~

~~T84.049 Periprosthetic fracture around unspecified internal prosthetic joint~~

T84.05 Periprosthetic osteolysis of internal prosthetic joint
Use additional code to identify major osseous defect, if applicable (M89.7-)

T84.050 Periprosthetic osteolysis of internal prosthetic right hip joint A

T84.051 Periprosthetic osteolysis of internal prosthetic left hip joint A

T84.052 Periprosthetic osteolysis of internal prosthetic right knee joint A

T84.053 Periprosthetic osteolysis of internal prosthetic left knee joint A

T84.058 Periprosthetic osteolysis of other internal prosthetic joint A
Use additional code to identify the joint (Z96.6-)

T84.059 Periprosthetic osteolysis of unspecified internal prosthetic joint A

T84.06 Wear of articular bearing surface of internal prosthetic joint

T84.060 Wear of articular bearing surface of internal prosthetic right hip joint A

T84.061 Wear of articular bearing surface of internal prosthetic left hip joint A

T84.062 Wear of articular bearing surface of internal prosthetic right knee joint A

T84.063 Wear of articular bearing surface of internal prosthetic left knee joint A

T84.068 Wear of articular bearing surface of other internal prosthetic joint A
Use additional code to identify the joint (Z96.6-)

T84.069 Wear of articular bearing surface of unspecified internal prosthetic joint A

T84.09 Other mechanical complication of internal joint prosthesis
Prosthetic joint implant failure NOS

T84.090 Other mechanical complication of internal right hip prosthesis A

T84.091 Other mechanical complication of internal left hip prosthesis A

T84.092 Other mechanical complication of internal right knee prosthesis A

T84.093 Other mechanical complication of internal left knee prosthesis A

T84.098 Other mechanical complication of other internal joint prosthesis A
Use additional code to identify the joint (Z96.6-)

T84.099 Other mechanical complication of unspecified internal joint prosthesis A

T84.1 Mechanical complication of internal fixation device of bones of limb

Excludes2 mechanical complication of internal fixation device of bones of feet (T84.2-)
mechanical complication of internal fixation device of bones of fingers (T84.2-)
mechanical complication of internal fixation device of bones of hands (T84.2-)
mechanical complication of internal fixation device of bones of toes (T84.2-)

T84.11 Breakdown (mechanical) of internal fixation device of bones of limb

T84.110 Breakdown (mechanical) of internal fixation device of right humerus A

T84.111 Breakdown (mechanical) of internal fixation device of left humerus A

T84.112 Breakdown (mechanical) of internal fixation device of bone of right forearm A

T84.113 Breakdown (mechanical) of internal fixation device of bone of left forearm A

T84.114 Breakdown (mechanical) of internal fixation device of right femur A

T84.115 Breakdown (mechanical) of internal fixation device of left femur A

T84.116 Breakdown (mechanical) of internal fixation device of bone of right lower leg A

T84.117 Breakdown (mechanical) of internal fixation device of bone of left lower leg A

T84.119 Breakdown (mechanical) of internal fixation device of unspecified bone of limb A

T84.12 Displacement of internal fixation device of bones of limb
Malposition of internal fixation device of bones of limb

T84.120 Displacement of internal fixation device of right humerus A

T84.121 Displacement of internal fixation device of left humerus A

T84.122 Displacement of internal fixation device of bone of right forearm A

T84.123 Displacement of internal fixation device of bone of left forearm A

T84.124 Displacement of internal fixation device of right femur A

- **T84.125 Displacement of internal fixation device of left femur** A
- **T84.126 Displacement of internal fixation device of bone of right lower leg** A
- **T84.127 Displacement of internal fixation device of bone of left lower leg** A
- **T84.129 Displacement of internal fixation device of unspecified bone of limb** A

- **T84.19 Other mechanical complication of internal fixation device of bones of limb**
  - Obstruction (mechanical) of internal fixation device of bones of limb
  - Perforation of internal fixation device of bones of limb
  - Protrusion of internal fixation device of bones of limb
  - **T84.190 Other mechanical complication of internal fixation device of right humerus** A
  - **T84.191 Other mechanical complication of internal fixation device of left humerus** A
  - **T84.192 Other mechanical complication of internal fixation device of bone of right forearm** A
  - **T84.193 Other mechanical complication of internal fixation device of bone of left forearm** A
  - **T84.194 Other mechanical complication of internal fixation device of right femur** A
  - **T84.195 Other mechanical complication of internal fixation device of left femur** A
  - **T84.196 Other mechanical complication of internal fixation device of bone of right lower leg** A
  - **T84.197 Other mechanical complication of internal fixation device of bone of left lower leg** A
  - **T84.199 Other mechanical complication of internal fixation device of unspecified bone of limb** A

- **T84.2 Mechanical complication of internal fixation device of other bones**
  - **T84.21 Breakdown (mechanical) of internal fixation device of other bones**
    - **T84.210 Breakdown (mechanical) of internal fixation device of bones of hand and fingers** A
    - **T84.213 Breakdown (mechanical) of internal fixation device of bones of foot and toes** A
    - **T84.216 Breakdown (mechanical) of internal fixation device of vertebrae** A
    - **T84.218 Breakdown (mechanical) of internal fixation device of other bones** A
  - **T84.22 Displacement of internal fixation device of other bones**
    - Malposition of internal fixation device of other bones
    - **T84.220 Displacement of internal fixation device of bones of hand and fingers** A
    - **T84.223 Displacement of internal fixation device of bones of foot and toes** A
    - **T84.226 Displacement of internal fixation device of vertebrae** A
    - **T84.228 Displacement of internal fixation device of other bones** A
  - **T84.29 Other mechanical complication of internal fixation device of other bones**
    - Obstruction (mechanical) of internal fixation device of other bones
    - Perforation of internal fixation device of other bones
    - Protrusion of internal fixation device of other bones
    - **T84.290 Other mechanical complication of internal fixation device of bones of hand and fingers** A
    - **T84.293 Other mechanical complication of internal fixation device of bones of foot and toes** A
    - **T84.296 Other mechanical complication of internal fixation device of vertebrae** A
    - **T84.298 Other mechanical complication of internal fixation device of other bones** A

- **T84.3 Mechanical complication of other bone devices, implants and grafts**
  - **Excludes2** other complications of bone graft (T86.83-)
  - **T84.31 Breakdown (mechanical) of other bone devices, implants and grafts**
    - **T84.310 Breakdown (mechanical) of electronic bone stimulator** A
    - **T84.318 Breakdown (mechanical) of other bone devices, implants and grafts** A
  - **T84.32 Displacement of other bone devices, implants and grafts**
    - Malposition of other bone devices, implants and grafts
    - **T84.320 Displacement of electronic bone stimulator** A
    - **T84.328 Displacement of other bone devices, implants and grafts** A
  - **T84.39 Other mechanical complication of other bone devices, implants and grafts**
    - Obstruction (mechanical) of other bone devices, implants and grafts
    - Perforation of other bone devices, implants and grafts
    - Protrusion of other bone devices, implants and grafts
    - **T84.390 Other mechanical complication of electronic bone stimulator** A
    - **T84.398 Other mechanical complication of other bone devices, implants and grafts** A

- **T84.4 Mechanical complication of other internal orthopedic devices, implants and grafts**
  - **T84.41 Breakdown (mechanical) of other internal orthopedic devices, implants and grafts**
    - **T84.410 Breakdown (mechanical) of muscle and tendon graft** A
    - **T84.418 Breakdown (mechanical) of other internal orthopedic devices, implants and grafts** A
  - **T84.42 Displacement of other internal orthopedic devices, implants and grafts**
    - Malposition of other internal orthopedic devices, implants and grafts
    - **T84.420 Displacement of muscle and tendon graft** A
    - **T84.428 Displacement of other internal orthopedic devices, implants and grafts** A

● T84.49 **Other mechanical complication of other internal orthopedic devices, implants and grafts**
Mechanical complication of other internal orthopedic devices, implants and grafts NOS
Obstruction (mechanical) of other internal orthopedic devices, implants and grafts
Perforation of other internal orthopedic devices, implants and grafts
Protrusion of other internal orthopedic devices, implants and grafts

● T84.490 **Other mechanical complication of muscle and tendon graft** A

● T84.498 **Other mechanical complication of other internal orthopedic devices, implants and grafts** A

● T84.5 **Infection and inflammatory reaction due to internal joint prosthesis**
Use additional code to identify infection
Ex. **For category T84.5 CC codes:** D78.81-D78.89, E36.8, E89.810-E89.89, H59.011-H59.019, H59.031-H59.039, H59.091-H59.099, H59.811-H59.89, H95.811-H95.89, I97.3, L76.81-L76.82, M96.621-M96.69, M96.89, M97.01X-M97.02X[A], M97.11X-M97.12X[A], M97.21X-M97.22X[A], M97.31X-M97.32X[A], M97.41X-M97.42X[A], M97.8XXA, M97.9XXA, N98.1-N98.9, T81.82X-T81.9XX[A], T84.010-T84.039[A], T84.050-T84.9XX[A], T85.310-T85.311[A], T85.320-T85.321[A], T85.390-T85.391[A], T85.510-T85.738[A], T85.79XA, T85.810[A,D], T85.820[A,D], T85.830[A,D], T85.840[A,D], T85.850[A,D], T85.860[A,D], T85.890[A,D],T85.9XX[A], T86.820-T86.829, T86.842-T86.849
Coding Clinic: 2015, Q1, P16

X● T84.50 **Infection and inflammatory reaction due to unspecified internal joint prosthesis** A
Coding Clinic: 2015, Q1, P3

X● T84.51 **Infection and inflammatory reaction due to internal right hip prosthesis** A
Coding Clinic: 2015, Q4, P36

X● T84.52 **Infection and inflammatory reaction due to internal left hip prosthesis** A
Coding Clinic: 2015, Q1, P16-17

X● T84.53 **Infection and inflammatory reaction due to internal right knee prosthesis** A

X● T84.54 **Infection and inflammatory reaction due to internal left knee prosthesis** A

X● T84.59 **Infection and inflammatory reaction due to other internal joint prosthesis** A

● T84.6 **Infection and inflammatory reaction due to internal fixation device**
Use additional code to identify infection
Ex. **For category T84.6 CC codes:** See T84.5

X● T84.60 **Infection and inflammatory reaction due to internal fixation device of unspecified site** A, A

● T84.61 **Infection and inflammatory reaction due to internal fixation device of arm**

● T84.610 **Infection and inflammatory reaction due to internal fixation device of right humerus** A, A

● T84.611 **Infection and inflammatory reaction due to internal fixation device of left humerus** A, A

● T84.612 **Infection and inflammatory reaction due to internal fixation device of right radius** A, A

● T84.613 **Infection and inflammatory reaction due to internal fixation device of left radius** A, A

● T84.614 **Infection and inflammatory reaction due to internal fixation device of right ulna** A, A

● T84.615 **Infection and inflammatory reaction due to internal fixation device of left ulna** A, A

● T84.619 **Infection and inflammatory reaction due to internal fixation device of unspecified bone of arm** A, A

● T84.62 **Infection and inflammatory reaction due to internal fixation device of leg**

● T84.620 **Infection and inflammatory reaction due to internal fixation device of right femur** A

● T84.621 **Infection and inflammatory reaction due to internal fixation device of left femur** A

● T84.622 **Infection and inflammatory reaction due to internal fixation device of right tibia** A

● T84.623 **Infection and inflammatory reaction due to internal fixation device of left tibia** A

● T84.624 **Infection and inflammatory reaction due to internal fixation device of right fibula** A

● T84.625 **Infection and inflammatory reaction due to internal fixation device of left fibula** A

● T84.629 **Infection and inflammatory reaction due to internal fixation device of unspecified bone of leg** A

X● T84.63 **Infection and inflammatory reaction due to internal fixation device of spine** A, A

X● T84.69 **Infection and inflammatory reaction due to internal fixation device of other site** A, A

● T84.7 **Infection and inflammatory reaction due to other internal orthopedic prosthetic devices, implants and grafts** A, A
Use additional code to identify infection
Ex. See T84.5

● T84.8 **Other specified complications of internal orthopedic prosthetic devices, implants and grafts**
Ex. **For category T84.8 CC codes:** See T84.5

X● T84.81 **Embolism due to internal orthopedic prosthetic devices, implants and grafts** A

X● T84.82 **Fibrosis due to internal orthopedic prosthetic devices, implants and grafts** A

X● T84.83 **Hemorrhage due to internal orthopedic prosthetic devices, implants and grafts** A

X● T84.84 **Pain due to internal orthopedic prosthetic devices, implants and grafts** A

X● T84.85 **Stenosis due to internal orthopedic prosthetic devices, implants and grafts** A

X● T84.86 **Thrombosis due to internal orthopedic prosthetic devices, implants and grafts** A

X● T84.89 **Other specified complication of internal orthopedic prosthetic devices, implants and grafts** A

X● T84.9 **Unspecified complication of internal orthopedic prosthetic device, implant and graft** A
Ex. See T84.5

T85 Complications of other internal prosthetic devices, implants and grafts

Excludes2 failure and rejection of transplanted organs and tissue (T86.-)

The appropriate 7th character is to be added to each code from category T85

A	initial encounter
D	subsequent encounter
S	sequela

T85.0 Mechanical complication of ventricular intracranial (communicating) shunt

Ex **For category T85.0 CC codes:** D78.81-D78.89, E36.8, E89.810-E89.89, H59.011-H59.019, H59.031-H59.039, H59.091-H59.099, H59.811-H59.89, H95.811-H95.89, I97.3, L76.81-L76.82, M96.89, N98.1-N98.9, T81.82X-T81.9XX[A], T85.01X-T85.199[A]

X **T85.01 Breakdown (mechanical) of ventricular intracranial (communicating) shunt** A

X **T85.02 Displacement of ventricular intracranial (communicating) shunt** A

Malposition of ventricular intracranial (communicating) shunt

X **T85.03 Leakage of ventricular intracranial (communicating) shunt** A

X **T85.09 Other mechanical complication of ventricular intracranial (communicating) shunt** A

Obstruction (mechanical) of ventricular intracranial (communicating) shunt

Perforation of ventricular intracranial (communicating) shunt

Protrusion of ventricular intracranial (communicating) shunt

T85.1 Mechanical complication of implanted electronic stimulator of nervous system

Ex **For category T85.1 CC codes:** See T85.0

T85.11 Breakdown (mechanical) of implanted electronic stimulator of nervous system

T85.110 Breakdown (mechanical) of implanted electronic neurostimulator of brain electrode (lead) A

T85.111 Breakdown (mechanical) of implanted electronic neurostimulator of peripheral nerve electrode (lead) A

Breakdown of electrode (lead) for cranial nerve neurostimulators ◀

Breakdown of electrode (lead) for gastric neurostimulator ◀

Breakdown of electrode (lead) for sacral nerve neurostimulator ◀

Breakdown of electrode (lead) for vagal nerve neurostimulators ◀

T85.112 Breakdown (mechanical) of implanted electronic neurostimulator of spinal cord electrode (lead) A

T85.113 Breakdown (mechanical) of implanted electronic neurostimulator, generator A ◀

Breakdown (mechanical) of implanted electronic neurostimuator generator, brain, peripheral, gastric, spinal ◀

Breakdown (mechanical) of implanted electronic sacral neurostimulator, pulse generator or receiver ◀

T85.118 Breakdown (mechanical) of other implanted electronic stimulator of nervous system A

T85.12 Displacement of implanted electronic stimulator of nervous system

Malposition of implanted electronic stimulator of nervous system

T85.120 Displacement of implanted electronic neurostimulator of brain electrode (lead) A

T85.121 Displacement of implanted electronic neurostimulator of peripheral nerve electrode (lead) A

Displacement of electrode (lead) for cranial nerve neurostimulators ◀

Displacement of electrode (lead) for gastric neurostimulator ◀

Displacement of electrode (lead) for sacral nerve neurostimulator ◀

Displacement of electrode (lead) for vagal nerve neurostimulators ◀

T85.122 Displacement of implanted electronic neurostimulator of spinal cord electrode (lead) A

T85.123 Displacement of implanted electronic neurostimulator, generator A ◀

Displacement of implanted electronic neurostimulator generator, brain, peripheral, gastric, spinal ◀

Displacement of implanted electronic sacral neurostimulator, pulse generator or receiver ◀

T85.128 Displacement of other implanted electronic stimulator of nervous system A

● **T85.19 Other mechanical complication of implanted electronic stimulator of nervous system**
Leakage of implanted electronic stimulator of nervous system
Obstruction (mechanical) of implanted electronic stimulator of nervous system
Perforation of implanted electronic stimulator of nervous system
Protrusion of implanted electronic stimulator of nervous system

● **T85.190 Other mechanical complication of implanted electronic neurostimulator of brain electrode (lead)** A

● **T85.191 Other mechanical complication of implanted electronic neurostimulator of peripheral nerve electrode (lead)** A
Other mechanical complication of electrode (lead) for cranial nerve neurostimulators ◀
Other mechanical complication of electrode (lead) for gastric neurostimulator ◀
Other mechanical complication of electrode (lead) for sacral nerve neurostimulator ◀
Other mechanical complication of electrode (lead) for vagal nerve neurostimulators ◀

● **T85.192 Other mechanical complication of implanted electronic neurostimulator of spinal cord electrode (lead)** A

● **T85.193 Other mechanical complication of implanted electronic neurostimulator, generator** A ◀
Other mechanical complication of implanted electronic neurostimulator generator, brain, peripheral, gastric, spinal ◀
Other mechanical complication of implanted electronic sacral neurostimulator, pulse generator or receiver ◀
Ex: See T85.113A

● **T85.199 Other mechanical complication of other implanted electronic stimulator of nervous system** A

● **T85.2 Mechanical complication of intraocular lens**
Ex: **For category T85.2 CC codes:** D78.81-D78.89, E89.810-E89.89, H59.011-H59.019, H59.031-H59.039, H59.091-H59.099, H59.811-H59.89, H95.811-H95.89, I97.3, M96.89, N98.1-N98.9, T85.21X-T85.29X[A]

X● **T85.21 Breakdown (mechanical) of intraocular lens** A

X● **T85.22 Displacement of intraocular lens** A
Malposition of intraocular lens

X● **T85.29 Other mechanical complication of intraocular lens** A
Obstruction (mechanical) of intraocular lens
Perforation of intraocular lens
Protrusion of intraocular lens

● **T85.3 Mechanical complication of other ocular prosthetic devices, implants and grafts**
Excludes2 other complications of corneal graft (T86.84-)
Ex: **For category T85.3 CC codes:** H59.011-H59.019, H59.031-H59.819, H59.88-H59.89, H95.811-H95.89, I97.3, M96.89, N98.1-N98.9, T85.310-T85.311[A], T85.320-T85.321[A], T85.390-T85.391[A], T85.612A, T85.615A, T85.618A, T85.622A, T85.625A, T85.628A, T85.635A, T85.638A, T85.692A, T85.695A, T85.698-T85.738[A], T85.79XA, T85.810[A,D], T85.820[A,D], T85.830[A,D], T85.840[A,D], T85.850[A,D], T85.860[A,D], T85.890[A,D], T85.9XX[A], T86.842-T86.849

● **T85.31 Breakdown (mechanical) of other ocular prosthetic devices, implants and grafts**

● **T85.310 Breakdown (mechanical) of prosthetic orbit of right eye** A

● **T85.311 Breakdown (mechanical) of prosthetic orbit of left eye** A

● **T85.318 Breakdown (mechanical) of other ocular prosthetic devices, implants and grafts**

● **T85.32 Displacement of other ocular prosthetic devices, implants and grafts**
Malposition of other ocular prosthetic devices, implants and grafts

● **T85.320 Displacement of prosthetic orbit of right eye** A

● **T85.321 Displacement of prosthetic orbit of left eye** A

● **T85.328 Displacement of other ocular prosthetic devices, implants and grafts**

● **T85.39 Other mechanical complication of other ocular prosthetic devices, implants and grafts**
Obstruction (mechanical) of other ocular prosthetic devices, implants and grafts
Perforation of other ocular prosthetic devices, implants and grafts
Protrusion of other ocular prosthetic devices, implants and grafts

● **T85.390 Other mechanical complication of prosthetic orbit of right eye** A

● **T85.391 Other mechanical complication of prosthetic orbit of left eye** A

● **T85.398 Other mechanical complication of other ocular prosthetic devices, implants and grafts**

● **T85.4 Mechanical complication of breast prosthesis and implant**
Ex: **For category T85.4 CC codes:** D78.81-D78.89, E89.810-E89.89, H59.011-H59.019, H59.031-H59.039, H59.091-H59.099, H59.811-H59.89, H95.811-H95.89, I97.3, M96.89, N98.1-N98.9, T85.41X-T85.49X[A]

X● **T85.41 Breakdown (mechanical) of breast prosthesis and implant** A

X● **T85.42 Displacement of breast prosthesis and implant** A
Malposition of breast prosthesis and implant

X● **T85.43 Leakage of breast prosthesis and implant** A

X● **T85.44 Capsular contracture of breast implant** A

X● **T85.49 Other mechanical complication of breast prosthesis and implant** A
Obstruction (mechanical) of breast prosthesis and implant
Perforation of breast prosthesis and implant
Protrusion of breast prosthesis and implant

T85.5 Mechanical complication of gastrointestinal prosthetic devices, implants and grafts

Ex: **For category T85.5 CC codes:** H95.811-H95.89, I97.3, M96.89, N98.1-N98.9, T85.510-T85.598[A], T85.612A, T85.615A, T85.618A, T85.622A, T85.625A,T85.628A, T85.635A, T85.638A, T85.692A, T85.695A, T85.698-T85.738[A], T85.79XA, T85.810[A,D], T85.820[A,D], T85.830[A,D], T85.840[A,D], T85.850[A,D], T85.860[A,D], T85.890[A,D], T85.9XXA

T85.51 Breakdown (mechanical) of gastrointestinal prosthetic devices, implants and grafts

T85.510 Breakdown (mechanical) of bile duct prosthesis A

T85.511 Breakdown (mechanical) of esophageal anti-reflux device A

T85.518 Breakdown (mechanical) of other gastrointestinal prosthetic devices, implants and grafts A

T85.52 Displacement of gastrointestinal prosthetic devices, implants and grafts

Malposition of gastrointestinal prosthetic devices, implants and grafts

T85.520 Displacement of bile duct prosthesis A

T85.521 Displacement of esophageal anti-reflux device A

T85.528 Displacement of other gastrointestinal prosthetic devices, implants and grafts A

T85.59 Other mechanical complication of gastrointestinal prosthetic devices, implants and

Obstruction, mechanical of gastrointestinal prosthetic devices, implants and grafts

Perforation of gastrointestinal prosthetic devices, implants and grafts

Protrusion of gastrointestinal prosthetic devices, implants and grafts

T85.590 Other mechanical complication of bile duct prosthesis A

T85.591 Other mechanical complication of esophageal anti-reflux device A

T85.598 Other mechanical complication of other gastrointestinal prosthetic devices, implants and grafts A

T85.6 Mechanical complication of other specified internal and external prosthetic devices, implants and grafts

T85.61 Breakdown (mechanical) of other specified internal prosthetic devices, implants and grafts

T85.610 Breakdown (mechanical) of cranial or spinal infusion catheter A ◀

Breakdown (mechanical) of epidural infusion catheter ◀

Breakdown (mechanical) of intrathecal infusion catheter ◀

Breakdown (mechanical) of subarachnoid infusion catheter ◀

Breakdown (mechanical) of subdural infusion catheter ◀

Ex: H95.811-H95.89, I97.3, M96.89, N98.1-N98.9, T85.610A, T85.612A, T85.615A, T85.618-T85.620A, T85.622A, T85.625A, T85.628-T85.630A, T85.635A, T85.638-T85.690[A], T85.692A, T85.695A, T85.698-T85.738[A], T85.79XA, T85.810[A,D], T85.820[A,D], T85.830[A,D], T85.840[A,D], T85.850[A,D], T85.860[A,D], T85.890[A,D], T85.9XXA

T85.611 Breakdown (mechanical) of intraperitoneal dialysis catheter A

Excludes1 mechanical complication of vascular dialysis catheter (T82.4-)

Ex: H95.811-H95.89, I97.3, M96.89, N98.1-N98.9, T85.611-T85.612[A], T85.614-T85.618[A], T85.621-T85.622[A], T85.624-T85.628[A], T85.631-T85.638[A], T85.691-T85.692[A], T85.694-T85.738[A], T85.79XA, T85.810[A,D], T85.820[A,D], T85.830[A,D], T85.840[A,D], T85.850[A,D], T85.860[A,D], T85.890[A,D], T85.9XXA

T85.612 Breakdown (mechanical) of permanent sutures A

Excludes1 mechanical complication of permanent (wire) suture used in bone repair (T84.1-T84.2)

Ex: D78.81-D78.89, E89.810-E89.89, H59.011-H59.019, H59.031-H59.039, H59.091-H59.099, H59.811-H59.89, H95.811-H95.89, I97.3, M96.89, N98.1-N98.9, T85.310-T85.311[A], T85.320-T85.321[A], T85.390-T85.391[A], T85.510-T85.738A, T85.79XA, T85.810[A,D], T85.820[A,D], T85.830[A,D], T85.840[A,D], T85.850[A,D], T85.860[A,D], T85.890[A,D], T85.9XXA, T86.842-T86.849

T85.613 Breakdown (mechanical) of artificial skin graft and decellularized allodermis A

Failure of artificial skin graft and decellularized allodermis

Non-adherence of artificial skin graft and decellularized allodermis

Poor incorporation of artificial skin graft and decellularized allodermis

Shearing of artificial skin graft and decellularized allodermis

Ex: H95.811-H95.89, I97.3, M96.89, N98.1-N98.9, T85.612-T85.613[A], T85.615A, T85.618[A], T85.622-T85.623[A], T85.625A, T85.628[A], T85.635A, T85.638[A], T85.692-T85.693[A], T85.695A, T85.698-T85.738[A], T85.79XA, T85.810[A,D], T85.820[A,D], T85.830[A,D], T85.840[A,D], T85.850[A,D], T85.860[A,D], T85.890[A,D], T85.9XXA, T86.820-T86.829

T85.614 Breakdown (mechanical) of insulin pump A

Ex: H95.811-H95.89, I97.3, M96.621-M96.89, M97.01X-M97.9XX[A], N98.1-N98.9, N99.510-N99.518, T81.82X-T81.9XX[A], T82.01X-T82.118[A], T82.120-T82.128[A], T82.192-T82.198[A], T82.211-T83.010[A], T83.020[A], T83.030[A], T83.090[A], T83.110-T83.29X[A], T83.410-T83.69X[A], T83.712A-T83.714[A], T83.718[A], T83.719A, T83.722-T83.724[A], T83.728-T83.9XX[A], T84.010-T84.039[A], T84.050-T85.29X[A], T85.41X-T85.49X[A], T85.611-T85.618[A], T85.621-T85.622[A], T85.624-T85.628[A], T85.631-T85.638[A], T85.691-T85.692[A], T85.694-T85.738[A], T85.79XA, T85.810[A,D], T85.820[A,D], T85.830[A,D], T85.840[A,D], T85.850[A,D], T85.860[A,D], T85.890[A,D], T85.9XXA, T86.820-T86.829

● **T85.615 Breakdown (mechanical) of other nervous system device, implant or graft** A ◀
Breakdown (mechanical) of intrathecal infusion pump ◀
Ex: See T85.612

● **T85.618 Breakdown (mechanical) of other specified internal prosthetic devices, implants and grafts** A
Ex: See T85.612

● **T85.62 Displacement of other specified internal prosthetic devices, implants and grafts**
Malposition of other specified internal prosthetic devices, implants and grafts

● **T85.620 Displacement of cranial or spinal infusion catheter** A
Displacement of epidural infusion catheter ◀
Displacement of intrathecal infusion catheter ◀
Displacement of subarachnoid infusion catheter ◀
Displacement of subdural infusion catheter ◀
Ex: See T85.610

● **T85.621 Displacement of intraperitoneal dialysis catheter** A
Excludes1 mechanical complication of vascular dialysis catheter (T82.4-)
Ex: See T85.611

● **T85.622 Displacement of permanent sutures** A
Excludes1 mechanical complication of permanent (wire) suture used in bone repair (T84.1-T84.2)
Ex: See T85.612

● **T85.623 Displacement of artificial skin graft and decellularized allodermis** A
Dislodgement of artificial skin graft and decellularized allodermis
Displacement of artificial skin graft and decellularized allodermis
Ex: See T85.613

● **T85.624 Displacement of insulin pump** A
Ex: See T85.614

● **T85.625 Displacement of other nervous system device, implant or graft** A ◀
Displacement of intrathecal infusion pump ◀
Ex: See T85.612

● **T85.628 Displacement of other specified internal prosthetic devices, implants and grafts** A
Ex: See T85.612
Coding Clinic: 2015, Q1, P15

● **T85.63 Leakage of other specified internal prosthetic devices, implants and grafts**

● **T85.630 Leakage of cranial or spinal infusion catheter** A
Leakage of epidural infusion catheter ◀
Leakage of intrathecal infusion catheter ◀
Leakage of subdural infusion catheter ◀
Leakage of subarachnoid infusion catheter ◀
Ex: See T85.610

● **T85.631 Leakage of intraperitoneal dialysis catheter** A
Excludes1 mechanical complication of vascular dialysis catheter (T82.4)
Ex: See T85.611

● **T85.633 Leakage of insulin pump** A
Ex: See T85.614

● **T85.635 Leakage of other nervous system device, implant or graft** A ◀
Leakage of intrathecal infusion pump ◀
Ex: See T85.612

● **T85.638 Leakage of other specified internal prosthetic devices, implants and grafts** A
Ex: See T85.612

● **T85.69 Other mechanical complication of other specified internal prosthetic devices, implants and grafts**
Obstruction, mechanical of other specified internal prosthetic devices, implants and grafts
Perforation of other specified internal prosthetic devices, implants and grafts
Protrusion of other specified internal prosthetic devices, implants and grafts

● **T85.690 Other mechanical complication of cranial or spinal infusion catheter** A
Other mechanical complication of epidural infusion catheter ◀
Other mechanical complication of intrathecal infusion catheter ◀
Other mechanical complication of subarachnoid infusion catheter ◀
Other mechanical complication of subdural infusion catheter ◀
Ex: See T85.610

● **T85.691 Other mechanical complication of intraperitoneal dialysis catheter** A
Excludes1 mechanical complication of vascular dialysis catheter (T82.4)
Ex: See T85.611

● **T85.692 Other mechanical complication of permanent sutures** A
Excludes1 mechanical complication of permanent (wire) suture used in bone repair (T84.1-T84.2)
Ex: See T85.612

- **T85.693 Other mechanical complication of artificial skin graft and decellularized allodermis** A
  - Ex: See T85.613
- **T85.694 Other mechanical complication of insulin pump** A
  - Ex: See T85.614
- **T85.695 Other mechanical complication of other nervous system device, implant or graft** A ◀
  - Other mechanical complication of intrathecal infusion pump ◀
  - Ex: See T85.612
- **T85.698 Other mechanical complication of other specified internal prosthetic devices, implants and grafts** A
  - Mechanical complication of nonabsorbable surgical material NOS
  - Ex: See T85.612

- **T85.7 Infection and inflammatory reaction due to other internal prosthetic devices, implants and grafts**
  - Use additional code to identify infection
  - Ex: For category T85.7 CC codes unless otherwise indicated: D78.81-D78.89, E36.8, E89.810-E89.89, H59.011-H59.019, H59.031-H59.039, H59.091-H59.099, H59.811-H59.89, H95.811-H95.89, I97.3, L76.81-L76.82, M96.621-M96.89, M97.01X-M97.9XX[A], N98.1-N98.9, N99.510-N99.518, T81.82X-T81.9XX[A], T82.01X-T82.118[A], T82.120-T82.128[A], T82.192-T82.198[A], T82.211-T83.29X[A], T83.410-T83.69X[A], T83.712-T83.714[A], T83.718A, T83.719A, T83.722-T83.724[A], T83.728-T83.9XX[A], T84.010-T84.039[A], T84.050-T85.738[A], T85.79XA, T85.810[A,D], T85.820[A,D], T85.830[A,D], T85.840[A,D], T85.850[A,D], T85.860[A,D], T85.890[A,D], T85.9XX[A], T86.820-T86.849
  - X **T85.71 Infection and inflammatory reaction due to peritoneal dialysis catheter** A
    - Ex: See T85.612
  - X **T85.72 Infection and inflammatory reaction due to insulin pump** A
  - **T85.73 Infection and inflammatory reaction due to nervous system devices, implants and graft** ◀
    - **T85.730 Infection and inflammatory reaction due to ventricular intracranial (communicating) shunt** A ◀
    - **T85.731 Infection and inflammatory reaction due to implanted electronic neurostimulator of brain, electrode (lead)** A ◀
    - **T85.732 Infection and inflammatory reaction due to implanted electronic neurostimulator of peripheral nerve, electrode (lead)** A ◀
      - Infection and inflammatory reaction due to electrode (lead) for cranial nerve neurostimulators
      - Infection and inflammatory reaction due to electrode (lead) for gastric neurostimulator ◀
      - Infection and inflammatory reaction due to electrode (lead) for sacral nerve neurostimulator ◀
      - Infection and inflammatory reaction due to electrode (lead) for vagal nerve neurostimulators ◀
    - **T85.733 Infection and inflammatory reaction due to implanted electronic neurostimulator of spinal cord, electrode (lead)** A ◀
    - **T85.734 Infection and inflammatory reaction due to implanted electronic neurostimulator, generator** A ◀
      - Generator pocket infection ◀
    - **T85.735 Infection and inflammatory reaction due to cranial or spinal infusion catheter** A ◀
      - Infection and inflammatory reaction due to epidural catheter ◀
      - Infection and inflammatory reaction due to intrathecal infusion catheter ◀
      - Infection and inflammatory reaction due to subarachnoid catheter ◀
      - Infection and inflammatory reaction due to subdural catheter ◀
    - **T85.738 Infection and inflammatory reaction due to other nervous system device, implant or graft** A ◀
      - Infection and inflammatory reaction due to intrathecal infusion pump ◀
  - X **T85.79 Infection and inflammatory reaction due to other internal prosthetic devices, implants and grafts** A

- **T85.8 Other specified complications of internal prosthetic devices, implants and grafts, not elsewhere classified**
  - Ex: For category T85.8 CC codes: See T85.7
  - **T85.81 Embolism due to internal prosthetic devices, implants and grafts, not elsewhere classified**
    - **T85.810 Embolism due to nervous system prosthetic devices, implants and grafts** A, D ◀
    - **T85.818 Embolism due to other internal prosthetic devices, implants and grafts** ◀
  - **T85.82 Fibrosis due to internal prosthetic devices, implants and grafts, not elsewhere classified**
    - **T85.820 Fibrosis due to nervous system prosthetic devices, implants and grafts** A, D ◀
    - **T85.828 Fibrosis due to other internal prosthetic devices, implants and grafts** ◀
  - **T85.83 Hemorrhage due to internal prosthetic devices, implants and grafts, not elsewhere classified**
    - **T85.830 Hemorrhage due to nervous system prosthetic devices, implants and grafts** A, D ◀
    - **T85.838 Hemorrhage due to other internal prosthetic devices, implants and grafts** ◀
  - **T85.84 Pain due to internal prosthetic devices, implants and grafts, not elsewhere classified**
    - **T85.840 Pain due to nervous system prosthetic devices, implants and grafts** A, D ◀
    - **T85.848 Pain due to other internal prosthetic devices, implants and grafts** ◀
  - **T85.85 Stenosis due to internal prosthetic devices, implants and grafts, not elsewhere classified**
    - **T85.850 Stenosis due to nervous system prosthetic devices, implants and grafts** A, D ◀
    - **T85.858 Stenosis due to other internal prosthetic devices, implants and grafts** ◀

● T85.86 **Thrombosis due to internal prosthetic devices, implants and grafts, not elsewhere classified**

● T85.860 **Thrombosis due to nervous system prosthetic devices, implants and grafts** A, D ◀

● T85.868 **Thrombosis due to other internal prosthetic devices, implants and grafts** ◀

● T85.89 **Other specified complication of internal prosthetic devices, implants and grafts, not elsewhere classified**

● T85.890 **Other specified complication of nervous system prosthetic devices, implants and grafts** A, D ◀

● T85.898 **Other specified complication of other internal prosthetic devices, implants and grafts** ◀

X ● T85.9 **Unspecified complication of internal prosthetic device, implant and graft**

Complication of internal prosthetic device, implant and graft NOS

● T86 **Complications of transplanted organs and tissue**

Use additional code to identify other transplant complications, such as:
graft-versus-host disease (D89.81-)
malignancy associated with organ transplant (C80.2)
post-transplant lymphoproliferative disorders (PTLD) (D47.Z1)

● T86.0 **Complications of bone marrow transplant**

Ex: **For category T86.0 CC codes:** D78.81-D78.89, D89.810-D89.813, E89.810-E89.89, H59.011-H59.019, H59.031-H59.099, H59.811-H59.89, H95.811-H95.89, I97.3, M96.89, N98.1-N98.9, T86.00-T86.09

T86.00 **Unspecified complication of bone marrow transplant**

T86.01 **Bone marrow transplant rejection**

T86.02 **Bone marrow transplant failure**

T86.03 **Bone marrow transplant infection**

T86.09 **Other complications of bone marrow transplant**

● T86.1 **Complications of kidney transplant**

Ex: **For category T86.1 CC codes:** D78.81-D78.89, E89.810-E89.89, H59.011-H59.019, H59.031-H59.039, H59.091-H59.099, H59.811-H59.89, H95.811-H95.89, I97.3, M96.89, N98.1-N98.9, T86.10-T86.19

T86.10 **Unspecified complication of kidney transplant**

T86.11 **Kidney transplant rejection**

T86.12 **Kidney transplant failure**

Coding Clinic: 2013, Q1, P24

T86.13 **Kidney transplant infection**

Use additional code to specify infection

T86.19 **Other complication of kidney transplant**

OGCR Section I.C.19.g.3.

Organ Transplant Complications

Transplant Complications

(a) Transplant complications other than kidney

Codes under category T86, Complications of transplanted organs and tissues, are for use for both complications and rejection of transplanted organs. A transplant complication code is only assigned if the complication affects the function of the transplanted organ. Two codes are required to fully describe a transplant complication: the appropriate code from category T86 and a secondary code that identifies the complication.

Pre-existing conditions or conditions that develop after the transplant are not coded as complications unless they affect the function of the transplanted organs.

See I.C.21 for transplant organ removal status

See I.C.2 for malignant neoplasm associated with transplanted organ.

● T86.2 **Complications of heart transplant**

Excludes1 complication of:
artificial heart device (T82.5)
heart-lung transplant (T86.3)

Ex: **For category T86.2 CC codes:** D78.81-D78.89, E89.810-E89.89, H59.011-H59.019, H59.031-H59.039, H59.091-H59.099, H59.811-H59.89, H95.811-H95.89, I97.3, M96.89, N98.1-N98.9, T86.20-T86.39

T86.20 **Unspecified complication of heart transplant**

T86.21 **Heart transplant rejection**

T86.22 **Heart transplant failure**

T86.23 **Heart transplant infection**

Use additional code to specify infection

● T86.29 **Other complications of heart transplant**

T86.290 **Cardiac allograft vasculopathy**

Excludes1 atherosclerosis of coronary arteries (I25.75-, I25.76-, I25.81-)

T86.298 **Other complications of heart transplant**

● T86.3 **Complications of heart-lung transplant**

Ex: **For category T86.3 CC codes:** See T86.2

T86.30 **Unspecified complication of heart-lung transplant**

CC when PDx is its own CC

T86.31 **Heart-lung transplant rejection**

CC when PDx is its own CC

T86.32 **Heart-lung transplant failure**

CC when PDx is its own CC

T86.33 **Heart-lung transplant infection**

Use additional code to specify infection
CC when PDx is its own CC

T86.39 **Other complications of heart-lung transplant**

CC when PDx is its own CC

● T86.4 **Complications of liver transplant**

Ex: **For category T86.4 CC codes:** D78.81-D78.89, E89.810-E89.89, H59.011-H59.019, H59.031-H59.039, H59.091-H59.099, H59.811-H59.89, H95.811-H95.89, I97.3, M96.89, N98.1-N98.9, T86.40-T86.49

T86.40 **Unspecified complication of liver transplant**

T86.41 **Liver transplant rejection**

T86.42 **Liver transplant failure**

T86.43 **Liver transplant infection**

Use additional code to identify infection, such as:
Cytomegalovirus (CMV) infection (B25.-)

T86.49 **Other complications of liver transplant**

● T86.5 **Complications of stem cell transplant**

Complications from stem cells from peripheral blood
Complications from stem cells from umbilical cord

Ex: D78.81-D78.89, E89.810-E89.89, H59.011-H59.019, H59.031-H59.039, H59.091-H59.099, H59.811-H59.89, H95.811-H95.89, I97.3, M96.89, N98.1-N98.9, T86.5, T86.830-T86.839

● T86.8 **Complications of other transplanted organs and tissues**

● T86.81 **Complications of lung transplant**

Excludes1 complication of heart-lung transplant (T86.3-)

Ex: **For category T86.81 CC codes:** D78.81-D78.89, E89.810-E89.89, H59.011-H59.019, H59.031-H59.039, H59.091-H59.099, H59.811-H59.89, H95.811-H95.89, I97.3, M96.89, N98.1-N98.9, T86.810-T86.819

T86.810 **Lung transplant rejection**

T86.811 **Lung transplant failure**

T86.812 **Lung transplant infection**

Use additional code to specify infection

T86.818 **Other complications of lung transplant**

T86.819 **Unspecified complication of lung transplant**

● **T86.82 Complications of skin graft (allograft) (autograft)**

Excludes2 complication of artificial skin graft (T85.693)

Ex: **For category T86.82 CC codes:** D78.81-D78.89, E89.810-E89.89, H59.011-H59.019, H59.031-H59.039, H59.091-H59.099, H59.811-H59.89, H95.811-H95.89, I97.3, M96.89, N98.1-N98.9, T85.613[A], T85.623[A], T85.693[A], T86.820-T86.829

T86.820 Skin graft (allograft) rejection

T86.821 Skin graft (allograft) (autograft) failure

T86.822 Skin graft (allograft) (autograft) infection

Use additional code to specify infection

T86.828 Other complications of skin graft (allograft) (autograft)

T86.829 Unspecified complication of skin graft (allograft) (autograft)

● **T86.83 Complications of bone graft**

Excludes2 mechanical complications of bone graft (T84.3-)

Ex: **For category T86.83 CC codes:** H95.811-H95.89, I97.3, M96.89, N98.1-N98.9, T86.5, T86.830-T86.839

T86.830 Bone graft rejection

T86.831 Bone graft failure

T86.832 Bone graft infection

Use additional code to specify infection

T86.838 Other complications of bone graft

T86.839 Unspecified complication of bone graft

● **T86.84 Complications of corneal transplant**

Excludes2 mechanical complications of corneal graft (T85.3-)

Ex: **For category T86.84 CC codes unless otherwise indicated:** H59.011-H59.019, H59.031-H59.039, H59.091-H59.099, H59.811-H59.89, H95.811-H95.89, I97.3, M96.621-M96.89, M97.01X-M97.9XX[A], N98.1-N98.9, N99.510-N99.518, T81.82X[A], T81.89X-T81.9XX[A], T82.01X-T82.118[A], T82.120-T82.128[A], T82.192-T82.198[A], T82.211-T83.010[A], T83.020[A], T83.030[A], T83.090[A], T83.110-T83.29X[A], T83.410-T83.69X[A], T83.712A-T83.714A, T83.718A, T83.719[A], T83.722-T83.724[A], T83.728-T84.039[A], T84.050-T85.49X[A], T85.612[A], T85.615[A], T85.618[A], T85.622[A], T85.625[A], T85.628[A], T85.635A, T85.638[A], T85.692[A], T85.695A, T85.698, T85.738[A], T85.79XA, T85.810[A,D], T85.820[A,D], T85.830[A,D], T85.840[A,D], T85.850[A,D], T85.860[A,D], T85.890[A,D], T85.9XX[A], T86.820-T86.829, T86.840-T86.849

T86.840 Corneal transplant rejection

Ex: H59.031-H59.039, H59.091-H59.099, H59.811-H59.89, H95.811-H95.89, I97.3, M96.89, N98.1-N98.9, T85.318[A], T85.328[A], T85.398[A], T85.810[A,D], T85.820[A,D], T85.830[A,D], T85.840[A,D], T85.850[A,D], T85.860[A,D], T85.890[A,D], T86.840-T86.841

T86.841 Corneal transplant failure

Ex: See T86.840

T86.842 Corneal transplant infection

Use additional code to specify infection

T86.848 Other complications of corneal transplant

T86.849 Unspecified complication of corneal transplant

● **T86.85 Complication of intestine transplant**

Ex: **For category T86.85 CC codes:** D47.Z1, D78.81-D78.89, E89.810-E89.89, H59.011-H59.019, H59.031-H59.099, H59.811-H59.89, H95.811-H95.89, I97.3, M96.89, N98.1-N98.9, T86.850-T86.99

T86.850 Intestine transplant rejection

T86.851 Intestine transplant failure

T86.852 Intestine transplant infection

Use additional code to specify infection

T86.858 Other complications of intestine transplant

T86.859 Unspecified complication of intestine transplant

● **T86.89 Complications of other transplanted tissue**

Transplant failure or rejection of pancreas

Ex: **For category T86.89 CC codes:** D78.81-D78.89, E89.810-E89.89, H59.011-H59.019, H59.031-H59.039, H59.091-H59.099, H59.811-H59.89, H95.811-H95.89, I97.3, M96.89, N98.1-N98.9, T86.890-T86.899

T86.890 Other transplanted tissue rejection

T86.891 Other transplanted tissue failure

T86.892 Other transplanted tissue infection

Use additional code to specify infection

T86.898 Other complications of other transplanted tissue

T86.899 Unspecified complication of other transplanted tissue

● **T86.9 Complication of unspecified transplanted organ and tissue**

Ex: **For category T86.9 CC codes:** See T86.85

T86.90 Unspecified complication of unspecified transplanted organ and tissue

T86.91 Unspecified transplanted organ and tissue rejection

T86.92 Unspecified transplanted organ and tissue failure

T86.93 Unspecified transplanted organ and tissue infection

Use additional code to specify infection

T86.99 Other complications of unspecified transplanted organ and tissue

● **T87 Complications peculiar to reattachment and amputation**

● **T87.0 Complications of reattached (part of) upper extremity**

Ex: **For category T87.0 CC codes:** D78.81-D78.89, E36.8, E89.810-E89.89, H59.011-H59.019, H59.031-H59.039, H59.091-H59.099, H59.811-H59.89, H95.811-H95.89, I97.3, L76.81-L76.82, M96.89, N98.1-N98.9, T81.82X-T81.9XX[A], T87.0X1-T87.0X9

● **T87.0X Complications of reattached (part of) upper extremity**

T87.0X1 Complications of reattached (part of) right upper extremity

T87.0X2 Complications of reattached (part of) left upper extremity

T87.0X9 Complications of reattached (part of) unspecified upper extremity

● **T87.1 Complications of reattached (part of) lower extremity**

Ex: **For category T87.1 CC codes:** D78.81-D78.89, E36.8, E89.810-E89.89, H59.011-H59.019, H59.031-H59.039, H59.091-H59.099, H59.811-H59.89, H95.811-H95.89, I97.3, L76.81-L76.82, M96.89, N98.1-N98.9, T81.82X-T81.9XX[A], T87.1X1-T87.1X9

● **T87.1X Complications of reattached (part of) lower extremity**

T87.1X1 Complications of reattached (part of) right lower extremity

T87.1X2 Complications of reattached (part of) left lower extremity

T87.1X9 Complications of reattached (part of) unspecified lower extremity

T87.2 **Complications of other reattached body part**
Ex: D78.81-D78.89, E36.8, E89.810-E89.89, H59.011-H59.019, H59.031-H59.039, H59.091-H59.099, H59.811-H59.89, H95.811-H95.89, I97.3, L76.81-L76.82, M96.89, N98.1-N98.9, T81.82X-T81.9XX[A], T87.2

● T87.3 **Neuroma of amputation stump**
- T87.30 **Neuroma of amputation stump, unspecified extremity**
- T87.31 **Neuroma of amputation stump, right upper extremity**
- T87.32 **Neuroma of amputation stump, left upper extremity**
- T87.33 **Neuroma of amputation stump, right lower extremity**
- T87.34 **Neuroma of amputation stump, left lower extremity**

● T87.4 **Infection of amputation stump**
Ex: **For category T87.4 CC codes:** D78.81-D78.89, E36.8, E89.810-E89.89, H59.011-H59.019, H59.031-H59.039, H59.091-H59.099, H59.811-H59.89, H95.811-H95.89, I97.3, L76.81-L76.82, M96.89, N98.1-N98.9, T81.82X-T81.9XX[A], T87.40-T87.9
- T87.40 **Infection of amputation stump, unspecified extremity**
- T87.41 **Infection of amputation stump, right upper extremity**
- T87.42 **Infection of amputation stump, left upper extremity**
- T87.43 **Infection of amputation stump, right lower extremity**
- T87.44 **Infection of amputation stump, left lower extremity**

● T87.5 **Necrosis of amputation stump**
- T87.50 **Necrosis of amputation stump, unspecified extremity**
- T87.51 **Necrosis of amputation stump, right upper extremity**
- T87.52 **Necrosis of amputation stump, left upper extremity**
- T87.53 **Necrosis of amputation stump, right lower extremity**
- T87.54 **Necrosis of amputation stump, left lower extremity**

● T87.8 **Other complications of amputation stump**
- T87.81 **Dehiscence of amputation stump**
- T87.89 **Other complications of amputation stump**
  - Amputation stump contracture
  - Amputation stump contracture of next proximal joint
  - Amputation stump flexion
  - Amputation stump edema
  - Amputation stump hematoma
  - **Excludes2** phantom limb syndrome (G54.6-G54.7)

T87.9 **Unspecified complications of amputation stump**

● T88 **Other complications of surgical and medical care, not elsewhere classified**
Excludes2 complication following infusion, transfusion and therapeutic injection (T80.-)
complication following procedure NEC (T81.-)
complications of anesthesia in labor and delivery (O74.-)
complications of anesthesia in pregnancy (O29.-)
complications of anesthesia in puerperium (O89.-)
complications of devices, implants and grafts (T82-T85)
complications of obstetric surgery and procedure (O75.4)
dermatitis due to drugs and medicaments (L23.3, L24.4, L25.1, L27.0-L27.1)
poisoning and toxic effects of drugs and chemicals (T36-T65 with fifth or sixth character 1-4 or 6)
specified complications classified elsewhere

The appropriate 7th character is to be added to each code from category T88

A	initial encounter
D	subsequent encounter
S	sequela

X ● T88.0 **Infection following immunization** A
Sepsis following immunization
Ex: N98.0, T80.211-T80.29X[A], T82.7XX[A], T88.0XX[A]

X ● T88.1 **Other complications following immunization, not elsewhere classified** A
Generalized vaccinia
Rash following immunization
Excludes1 vaccinia not from vaccine (B08.011)
Excludes2 anaphylactic shock due to serum (T80.5-)
other serum reactions (T80.6-)
postimmunization arthropathy (M02.2)
postimmunization encephalitis (G04.02)
postimmunization fever (R50.83)
Ex: T88.1XX[A]

X ● T88.2 **Shock due to anesthesia** A
Use additional code for adverse effect, if applicable, to identify drug (T41.- with fifth or sixth character 5)
Excludes1 complications of anesthesia (in):
labor and delivery (O74.-)
pregnancy (O29.-)
puerperium (O89.-)
postprocedural shock NOS (T81.1-)
Ex: See T81.1

X ● T88.3 **Malignant hyperthermia due to anesthesia** A
Use additional code for adverse effect, if applicable, to identify drug (T41.- with fifth or sixth character 5)
Ex: D78.01-D78.02, D78.21-D78.89, E36.01-E36.02, E36.8, E89.810-E89.89, G97.51-G97.52, G97.61-G97.64, H59.011-H59.019, H59.031-H59.039, H59.091-H59.099, H59.111-H59.129, H59.311-H59.329, H59.331-H59.369, H59.811-H59.89, H95.21-H95.22, H95.41-H95.42, H95.51-H95.54, H95.811-H95.89, I97.3-I97.42, I97.610-I97.648, J95.61-J95.62, J95.830-J95.831, J95.860-J95.863, K91.61-K91.62, K91.840-K91.841, K91.870-K91.873, L76.01-L76.02, L76.21-L76.22, L76.31-L76.34, L76.81-L76.82, M96.810-M96.811, M96.830-M96.89, N98.1-N98.9, N99.61-N99.62, N99.820-N99.821, T79.4XX[A], T81.10X-T81.19X[A], T81.82X[A], T81.89X-T81.9XX[A], T88.2XX-T88.3XX[A]

X● **T88.4 Failed or difficult intubation**

X● **T88.5 Other complications of anesthesia**

Use additional code for adverse effect, if applicable, to identify drug (T41.- with fifth or sixth character 5)

X● **T88.51 Hypothermia following anesthesia**

X● **T88.52 Failed moderate sedation during procedure**

Failed conscious sedation during procedure

Excludes2 personal history of failed moderate sedation (Z92.83)

X● **T88.53 Unintended awareness under general anesthesia during procedure** ◀

Excludes2 personal history of unintended awareness under general anesthesia (Z92.84) ◀

X● **T88.59 Other complications of anesthesia**

X● **T88.6 Anaphylactic reaction due to adverse effect of correct drug or medicament properly administered** A

Anaphylactic shock due to adverse effect of correct drug or medicament properly administered

Anaphylactoid reaction NOS

Use additional code for adverse effect, if applicable, to identify drug (T36-T50 with fifth or sixth character 5)

Excludes1 anaphylactic reaction due to serum (T80.5-)

anaphylactic shock or reaction due to adverse food reaction (T78.0-)

Ex T78.00X-T78.09X[A]

X● **T88.7 Unspecified adverse effect of drug or medicament**

Drug hypersensitivity NOS

Drug reaction NOS

Use additional code for adverse effect, if applicable, to identify drug (T36-T50 with fifth or sixth character 5)

Excludes1 specified adverse effects of drugs and medicaments (A00-R94 and T80-T88.6, T88.8)

X● **T88.8 Other specified complications of surgical and medical care, not elsewhere classified**

Use additional code to identify the complication

X● **T88.9 Complication of surgical and medical care, unspecified**

CHAPTER 20

EXTERNAL CAUSES OF MORBIDITY (V00-Y99)

OGCR Chapter-Specific Coding Guidelines

20. Chapter 20: External Causes of Morbidity (V00-Y99)
The external causes of morbidity codes should never be sequenced as the first-listed or principal diagnosis.

External cause codes are intended to provide data for injury research and evaluation of injury prevention strategies. These codes capture how the injury or health condition happened (cause), the intent (unintentional or accidental; or intentional, such as suicide or assault), the place where the event occurred the activity of the patient at the time of the event, and the person's status (e.g., civilian, military).

There is no national requirement for mandatory ICD-10-CM external cause code reporting. Unless a provider is subject to a state-based external cause code reporting mandate or these codes are required by a particular payer, reporting of ICD-10-CM codes in Chapter 20, External Causes of Morbidity, is not required. In the absence of a mandatory reporting requirement, providers are encouraged to voluntarily report external cause codes, as they provide valuable data for injury research and evaluation of injury prevention strategies.

a. General External Cause Coding Guidelines

1) Used with any code in the range of A00.0-T88.9, Z00-Z99
An external cause code may be used with any code in the range of A00.0-T88.9, Z00-Z99, classification that is a health condition due to an external cause. Though they are most applicable to injuries, they are also valid for use with such things as infections or diseases due to an external source, and other health conditions, such as a heart attack that occurs during strenuous physical activity.

2) External cause code used for length of treatment
Assign the external cause code, with the appropriate 7th character (initial encounter, subsequent encounter or sequela) for each encounter for which the injury or condition is being treated.

Most categories in chapter 20 have a 7th character requirement for each applicable code. Most categories in this chapter have three 7th character values: A, initial encounter, D, subsequent encounter and S, sequela. While the patient may be seen by a new or different provider over the course of treatment for an injury or condition, assignment of the 7th character for external cause should match the 7th character of the code assigned for the associated injury or condition for the encounter.

3) Use the full range of external cause codes
Use the full range of external cause codes to completely describe the cause, the intent, the place of occurrence and if applicable, the activity of the patient at the time of the event, and the patient's status, for all injuries, and other health conditions due to an external cause.

4) Assign as many external cause codes as necessary
Assign as many external cause codes as necessary to fully explain each cause. If only one external code can be recorded, assign the code most related to the principal diagnosis.

5) The selection of the appropriate external cause code
The selection of the appropriate external cause code is guided by the Alphabetic Index of External Causes and by Inclusion and Exclusion notes in the Tabular List.

6) External cause code can never be a principal diagnosis
An external cause code can never be a principal (first-listed) diagnosis.

7) Combination external cause codes
Certain of the external cause codes are combination codes that identify sequential events that result in an injury, such as a fall which results in striking against an object. The injury may be due to either event or both. The combination external cause code used should correspond to the sequence of events regardless of which caused the most serious injury.

8) No external cause code needed in certain circumstances
No external cause code from Chapter 20 is needed if the external cause and intent are included in a code from another chapter (e.g. T36.0X1- Poisoning by penicillins, accidental (unintentional)).

b. Place of Occurrence Guideline
Codes from category Y92, Place of occurrence of the external cause, are secondary codes for use after other external cause codes to identify the location of the patient at the time of injury or other condition.

Generally, a place of occurrence code is **assigned** only once, at the initial encounter for treatment. **However, in the rare instance that a new injury occurs during hospitalization, an additional place of occurrence code may be assigned.** No 7th characters are used for Y92. Only one code from Y92 should be recorded on a medical record.

Do not use place of occurrence code Y92.9 if the place is not stated or is not applicable.

c. Activity Code
Assign a code from category Y93, Activity code, to describe the activity of the patient at the time the injury or other health condition occurred.

An activity code is used only once, at the initial encounter for treatment. Only one code from Y93 should be recorded on a medical record.

The activity codes are not applicable to poisonings, adverse effects, misadventures or sequela.

Do not assign Y93.9, Unspecified activity, if the activity is not stated.

A code from category Y93 is appropriate for use with external cause and intent codes if identifying the activity provides additional information about the event.

d. Place of Occurrence, Activity, and Status Codes Used with other External Cause Code
When applicable, place of occurrence, activity, and external cause status codes are sequenced after the main external cause code(s). Regardless of the number of external cause codes assigned, there should be only one place of occurrence code, one activity code, and one external cause status code assigned to an encounter.

e. If the Reporting Format Limits the Number of External Cause Codes

If the reporting format limits the number of external cause codes that can be used in reporting clinical data, report the code for the cause/intent most related to the principal diagnosis. If the format permits capture of additional external cause codes, the cause/intent, including medical misadventures, of the additional events should be reported rather than the codes for place, activity, or external status.

f. Multiple External Cause Coding Guidelines

More than one external cause code is required to fully describe the external cause of an illness or injury. The assignment of external cause codes should be sequenced in the following priority:

If two or more events cause separate injuries, an external cause code should be assigned for each cause. The first-listed external cause code will be selected in the following order:

External codes for child and adult abuse take priority over all other external cause codes.

See Section I.C.19., Child and Adult abuse guidelines.

External codes for terrorism events take priority over all other external cause codes except child and adult abuse.

External cause codes for cataclysmic events take priority over all other external cause codes except child and adult abuse and terrorism.

External cause codes for transport accidents take priority over all other external cause codes except cataclysmic events, child and adult abuse and terrorism.

Activity and external cause status codes are assigned following all causal (intent) external cause codes.

The first-listed external cause code should correspond to the cause of the most serious diagnosis due to an assault, accident, or self-harm, following the order of hierarchy listed above.

g. Child and Adult Abuse Guideline

Adult and child abuse, neglect and maltreatment are classified as assault. Any of the assault codes may be used to indicate the external cause of any injury resulting from the confirmed abuse.

For confirmed cases of abuse, neglect and maltreatment, when the perpetrator is known, a code from Y07, Perpetrator of maltreatment and neglect, should accompany any other assault codes.

See Section I.C.19. Adult and child abuse, neglect and other maltreatment

h. Unknown or Undetermined Intent Guideline

If the intent (accident, self-harm, assault) of the cause of an injury or other condition is unknown or unspecified, code the intent as accidental intent. All transport accident categories assume accidental intent.

1) Use of undetermined intent

External cause codes for events of undetermined intent are only for use if the documentation in the record specifies that the intent cannot be determined.

i. Sequelae (Late Effects) of External Cause Guidelines

1) Sequelae external cause codes

Sequela are reported using the external cause code with the 7th character "S" for sequela. These codes should be used with any report of a late effect or sequela resulting from a previous injury.

See Section I.B.10. Sequela, (Late Effects)

2) Sequela external cause code with a related current injury

A sequela external cause code should never be used with a related current nature of injury code.

3) Use of sequela external cause codes for subsequent visits

Use a late effect external cause code for subsequent visits when a late effect of the initial injury is being treated. Do not use a late effect external cause code for subsequent visits for follow-up care (e.g., to assess healing, to receive rehabilitative therapy) of the injury when no late effect of the injury has been documented.

j. Terrorism Guidelines

1) Cause of injury identified by the Federal Government (FBI) as terrorism

When the cause of an injury is identified by the Federal Government (FBI) as terrorism, the first-listed external cause code should be a code from category Y38, Terrorism. The definition of terrorism employed by the FBI is found at the inclusion note at the beginning of category Y38. Use additional code for place of occurrence (Y92.-). More than one Y38 code may be assigned if the injury is the result of more than one mechanism of terrorism.

2) Cause of an injury is suspected to be the result of terrorism

When the cause of an injury is suspected to be the result of terrorism a code from category Y38 should not be assigned. Suspected cases should be classified as assault.

3) Code Y38.9, Terrorism, secondary effects

Assign code Y38.9, Terrorism, secondary effects, for conditions occurring subsequent to the terrorist event. This code should not be assigned for conditions that are due to the initial terrorist act.

It is acceptable to assign code Y38.9 with another code from Y38 if there is an injury due to the initial terrorist event and an injury that is a subsequent result of the terrorist event.

k. External cause status

A code from category Y99, External cause status, should be assigned whenever any other external cause code is assigned for an encounter, including an Activity code, except for the events noted below. Assign a code from category Y99, External cause status, to indicate the work status of the person at the time the event occurred. The status code indicates whether the event occurred during military activity, whether a non-military person was at work, whether an individual including a student or volunteer was involved in a non-work activity at the time of the causal event.

A code from Y99, External cause status, should be assigned, when applicable, with other external cause codes, such as transport accidents and falls. The external cause status codes are not applicable to poisonings, adverse effects, misadventures or late effects.

Do not assign a code from category Y99 if no other external cause codes (cause, activity) are applicable for the encounter.

An external cause status code is used only once, at the initial encounter for treatment. Only one code from Y99 should be recorded on a medical record.

Do not assign code Y99.9, Unspecified external cause status, if the status is not stated.

CHAPTER 20

EXTERNAL CAUSES OF MORBIDITY (V00-Y99)

Note: This chapter permits the classification of environmental events and circumstances as the cause of injury, and other adverse effects. Where a code from this section is applicable, it is intended that it shall be used secondary to a code from another chapter of the Classification indicating the nature of the condition. Most often, the condition will be classifiable to Chapter 19, Injury, poisoning and certain other consequences of external causes (S00-T88). Other conditions that may be stated to be due to external causes are classified in Chapters I to XVIII. For these conditions, codes from Chapter 20 should be used to provide additional information as to the cause of the condition.

This chapter contains the following blocks:

V00-X58	Accidents
V00-V99	Transport accidents
V00-V09	Pedestrian injured in transport accident
V10-V19	Pedal cycle rider injured in transport accident
V20-V29	Motorcycle rider injured in transport accident
V30-V39	Occupant of three-wheeled motor vehicle injured in transport accident
V40-V49	Car occupant injured in transport accident
V50-V59	Occupant of pick-up truck or van injured in transport accident
V60-V69	Occupant of heavy transport vehicle injured in transport accident
V70-V79	Bus occupant injured in transport accident
V80-V89	Other land transport accidents
V90-V94	Water transport accidents
V95-V97	Air and space transport accidents
V98-V99	Other and unspecified transport accidents
W00-X58	Other external causes of accidental injury
W00-W19	Slipping, tripping, stumbling and falls
W20-W49	Exposure to inanimate mechanical forces
W50-W64	Exposure to animate mechanical forces
W65-W74	Accidental non-transport drowning and submersion
W85-W99	Exposure to electric current, radiation and extreme ambient air temperature and pressure
X00-X08	Exposure to smoke, fire and flames
X10-X19	Contact with heat and hot substances
X30-X39	Exposure to forces of nature
X50	Overexertion and strenuous or repetitive movements ◀
X52, X58	Accidental exposure to other specified factors
X71-X83	Intentional self-harm
X92-Y09 ⇐	Assault
Y21-Y33	Event of undetermined intent
Y35-Y38	Legal intervention, operations of war, military operations, and terrorism
Y62-Y84	Complications of medical and surgical care
Y62-Y69	Misadventures to patients during surgical and medical care
Y70-Y82	Medical devices associated with adverse incidents in diagnostic and therapeutic use
Y83-Y84	Surgical and other medical procedures as the cause of abnormal reaction of the patient, or of later complication, without mention of misadventure at the time of the procedure
Y90-Y99	Supplementary factors related to causes of morbidity classified elsewhere

ACCIDENTS (V00-X58)

TRANSPORT ACCIDENTS (V00-V99)

Note: This section is structured in 12 groups. Those relating to land transport accidents (V00-V89) reflect the victim's mode of transport and are subdivided to identify the victim's 'counterpart' or the type of event. The vehicle of which the injured person is an occupant is identified in the first two characters since it is seen as the most important factor to identify for prevention purposes. A transport accident is one in which the vehicle involved must be moving or running or in use for transport purposes at the time of the accident. ◀

Use additional code to identify:
- Airbag injury (W22.1)
- Type of street or road (Y92.4-)
- Use of cellular telephone and other electronic equipment at the time of the transport accident (Y93.C-)

Excludes1
- agricultural vehicles in stationary use or maintenance (W31.-)
- assault by crashing of motor vehicle (Y03.-)
- automobile or motor cycle in stationary use or maintenance - code to type of accident
- crashing of motor vehicle, undetermined intent (Y32)
- intentional self-harm by crashing of motor vehicle (X82)

Excludes2
- transport accidents due to cataclysm (X34-X38)

Note: Definitions related to transport accidents: ⇐

(a) A transport accident (V00-V99) is any accident involving a device designed primarily for, or used at the time primarily for, conveying persons or good from one place to another. ⇐

(b) A public highway [trafficway] or street is the entire width between property lines (or other boundary lines) of land open to the public as a matter of right or custom for purposes of moving persons or property from one place to another. A roadway is that part of the public highway designed, improved and customarily used for vehicular traffic.

(c) A traffic accident is any vehicle accident occurring on the public highway [i.e., originating on, terminating on, or involving a vehicle partially on the highway]. A vehicle accident is assumed to have occurred on the public highway unless another place is specified, except in the case of accidents involving only off-road motor vehicles, which are classified as nontraffic accidents unless the contrary is stated.

(d) A nontraffic accident is any vehicle accident that occurs entirely in any place other than a public highway.

(e) A pedestrian is any person involved in an accident who was not at the time of the accident riding in or on a motor vehicle, railway train, streetcar or animal-drawn or other vehicle, or on a pedal cycle or animal. This includes, a person changing a tire, working on a parked car, or a person on foot. It also includes the user of a pedestrian conveyance such as a baby-stroller, ice-skates, skis, sled, roller skates, a skateboard, nonmotorized or motorized wheelchair, motorized mobility scooter, or nonmotorized scooter. ⇐

(f) A driver is an occupant of a transport vehicle who is operating or intending to operate it.

(g) A passenger is any occupant of a transport vehicle other than the driver, except a person traveling on the outside of the vehicle.

(h) A person on the outside of a vehicle is any person being transported by a vehicle but not occupying the space normally reserved for the driver or passengers, or the space intended for the transport of property. This includes a person travelling on the bodywork, bumper, fender, roof, running board or step of a vehicle, as well as, hanging on the outside of the vehicle. ⇐

(i) A pedal cycle is any land transport vehicle operated solely by nonmotorized pedals including a bicycle or tricycle.

(j) A pedal cyclist is any person riding a pedal cycle or in a sidecar or trailer attached to a pedal cycle.

(k) A motorcycle is a two-wheeled motor vehicle with one or two riding saddles and sometimes with a third wheel for the support of a sidecar. The sidecar is considered part of the motorcycle. This includes a moped, motor scooter, or motorized bicycle.

(l) A motorcycle rider is any person riding a motorcycle or in a sidecar or trailer attached to the motorcycle.

(m) A three-wheeled motor vehicle is a motorized tricycle designed primarily for on-road use. This includes a motor-driven tricycle, a motorized rickshaw, or a three-wheeled motor car.

(n) A car [automobile] is a four-wheeled motor vehicle designed primarily for carrying up to 7 persons. A trailer being towed by the car is considered part of the car. It does not include a van or minivan—see definition (o)

(o) A pick-up truck or van is a four or six-wheeled motor vehicle designed for carrying passengers as well as property or cargo weighing less than the local limit for classification as a heavy goods vehicle, and not requiring a special driver's license. This includes a minivan and a sport-utility vehicle (SUV).

(p) A heavy transport vehicle is a motor vehicle designed primarily for carrying property, meeting local criteria for classification as a heavy goods vehicle in terms of weight and requiring a special driver's license.

(q) A bus (coach) is a motor vehicle designed or adapted primarily for carrying more than 10 passengers, and requiring a special driver's license.

(r) A railway train or railway vehicle is any device, with or without freight or passenger cars coupled to it, designed for traffic on a railway track. This includes subterranean (subways) or elevated trains.

(s) A streetcar is a device designed and used primarily for transporting passengers within a municipality, running on rails, usually subject to normal traffic control signals, and operated principally on a right-of-way that forms part of the roadway. This includes a tram or trolley that runs on rails. A trailer being towed by a streetcar is considered part of the streetcar.

(t) A special vehicle mainly used on industrial premises is a motor vehicle designed primarily for use within the buildings and premises of industrial or commercial establishments. This includes battery-powered airport passenger vehicles or baggage/mail trucks, forklifts, coal-cars in a coal mine, logging cars and trucks used in mines or quarries.

(u) A special vehicle mainly used in agriculture is a motor vehicle designed specifically for use in farming and agriculture (horticulture), to work the land, tend and harvest crops and transport materials on the farm. This includes harvesters, farm machinery and tractor and trailers.

(v) A special construction vehicle is a motor vehicle designed specifically for use on construction and demolition sites. This includes bulldozers, diggers, earth levellers, dump trucks, backhoes, front-end loaders, pavers, and mechanical shovels.

(w) A special all-terrain vehicle is a motor vehicle of special design to enable it to negotiate over rough or soft terrain, snow or sand. Examples of special design are high construction, special wheels and tires, tracks, and support on a cushion of air. This includes snow mobiles, all-terrain vehicles (ATV), and dune buggies. It does not include passenger vehicle designated as sport utility vehicles (SUV).

(x) A watercraft is any device designed for transporting passengers or goods on water. This includes motor or sail boats, ships, and hovercraft.

(y) An aircraft is any device for transporting passengers or goods in the air. This includes hot-air balloons, gliders, helicopters and airplanes.

(z) A military vehicle is any motorized vehicle operating on a public roadway owned by the military and being operated by a member of the military.

PEDESTRIAN INJURED IN TRANSPORT ACCIDENT (V00-V09)

Includes person changing tire on transport vehicle
person examining engine of vehicle broken down in (on side of) road

Excludes1 fall due to non-transport collision with other person (W03)
pedestrian on foot falling (slipping) on ice and snow (W00.-)
struck or bumped by another person (W51)

V00 Pedestrian conveyance accident

Use additional place of occurrence and activity external cause codes, if known (Y92.-, Y93.-)

Excludes1 collision with another person without fall (W51)
fall due to person on foot colliding with another person on foot (W03)
fall from non-moving wheelchair, nonmotorized scooter and motorized mobility scooter without collision (W05.-)
pedestrian (conveyance) collision with other land transport vehicle (V01-V09)
pedestrian on foot falling (slipping) on ice and snow (W00.-)

The appropriate 7th character is to be added to each code from category V00

A	initial encounter
D	subsequent encounter
S	sequela

V00.0 Pedestrian on foot injured in collision with pedestrian conveyance

X **V00.01 Pedestrian on foot injured in collision with roller-skater**

X **V00.02 Pedestrian on foot injured in collision with skateboarder**

X **V00.09 Pedestrian on foot injured in collision with other pedestrian conveyance**

V00.1 Rolling-type pedestrian conveyance accident

Excludes1 accident with babystroller (V00.82-)
accident with wheelchair (powered) (V00.81-)
accident with motorized mobility scooter (V00.83-)

V00.11 In-line roller-skate accident

V00.111 Fall from in-line roller-skates

V00.112 In-line roller-skater colliding with stationary object

V00.118 Other in-line roller-skate accident

Excludes1 roller-skater collision with other land transport vehicle (V01-V09 with 5th character 1)

V00.12 Non-in-line roller-skate accident

V00.121 Fall from non-in-line roller-skates

V00.122 Non-in-line roller-skater colliding with stationary object

V00.128 Other non-in-line roller-skating accident

Excludes1 roller-skater collision with other land transport vehicle (V01-V09 with 5th character 1)

- **V00.13 Skateboard accident**
  - **V00.131 Fall from skateboard**
  - **V00.132 Skateboarder colliding with stationary object**
  - **V00.138 Other skateboard accident**
    - **Excludes1** skateboarder collision with other land transport vehicle (V01-V09 with 5th character 2)
- **V00.14 Scooter (nonmotorized) accident**
  - **Excludes1** motorscooter accident (V20-V29)
  - **V00.141 Fall from scooter (nonmotorized)**
  - **V00.142 Scooter (nonmotorized) colliding with stationary object**
  - **V00.148 Other scooter (nonmotorized) accident**
    - **Excludes1** scooter (non-motorized) collision with other land transport vehicle (V01-V09 with fifth character 9)
- **V00.15 Heelies accident**
  - Rolling shoe
  - Wheeled shoe
  - Wheelies accident
  - **V00.151 Fall from heelies**
  - **V00.152 Heelies colliding with stationary object**
  - **V00.158 Other heelies accident**
- **V00.18 Accident on other rolling-type pedestrian conveyance**
  - **V00.181 Fall from other rolling-type pedestrian conveyance**
  - **V00.182 Pedestrian on other rolling-type pedestrian conveyance colliding with stationary object**
  - **V00.188 Other accident on other rolling-type pedestrian conveyance**
- **V00.2 Gliding-type pedestrian conveyance accident**
  - **V00.21 Ice-skates accident**
    - **V00.211 Fall from ice-skates**
    - **V00.212 Ice-skater colliding with stationary object**
    - **V00.218 Other ice-skates accident**
      - **Excludes1** ice-skater collision with other land transport vehicle (V01-V09 with 5th digit 9)
  - **V00.22 Sled accident**
    - **V00.221 Fall from sled**
    - **V00.222 Sledder colliding with stationary object**
    - **V00.228 Other sled accident**
      - **Excludes1** sled collision with other land transport vehicle (V01-V09 with 5th digit 9)
  - **V00.28 Other gliding-type pedestrian conveyance accident**
    - **V00.281 Fall from other gliding-type pedestrian conveyance**
    - **V00.282 Pedestrian on other gliding-type pedestrian conveyance colliding with stationary object**
    - **V00.288 Other accident on other gliding-type pedestrian conveyance**
      - **Excludes1** gliding-type pedestrian conveyance collision with other land transport vehicle (V01-V09 with 5th digit 9)
- **V00.3 Flat-bottomed pedestrian conveyance accident**
  - **V00.31 Snowboard accident**
    - **V00.311 Fall from snowboard**
    - **V00.312 Snowboarder colliding with stationary object**
    - **V00.318 Other snowboard accident**
      - **Excludes1** snowboarder collision with other land transport vehicle (V01-V09 with 5th digit 9)
  - **V00.32 Snow-ski accident**
    - **V00.321 Fall from snow-skis**
      - **Coding Clinic: 2015, Q1, P12**
    - **V00.322 Snow-skier colliding with stationary object**
    - **V00.328 Other snow-ski accident**
      - **Excludes1** snow-skier collision with other land transport vehicle (V01-V09 with 5th digit 9)
  - **V00.38 Other flat-bottomed pedestrian conveyance accident**
    - **V00.381 Fall from other flat-bottomed pedestrian conveyance**
    - **V00.382 Pedestrian on other flat-bottomed pedestrian conveyance colliding with stationary object**
    - **V00.388 Other accident on other flat-bottomed pedestrian conveyance**
- **V00.8 Accident on other pedestrian conveyance**
  - **V00.81 Accident with wheelchair (powered)**
    - **V00.811 Fall from moving wheelchair (powered)**
      - **Excludes1** fall from non-moving wheelchair (W05.0)
    - **V00.812 Wheelchair (powered) colliding with stationary object**
    - **V00.818 Other accident with wheelchair (powered)**
  - **V00.82 Accident with babystroller**
    - **V00.821 Fall from babystroller**
    - **V00.822 Babystroller colliding with stationary object**
    - **V00.828 Other accident with babystroller**

● **V00.83 Accident with motorized mobility scooter**

● **V00.831 Fall from motorized mobility scooter**

Excludes1 fall from non-moving motorized mobility scooter (W05.2)

● **V00.832 Motorized mobility scooter colliding with stationary object**

● **V00.838 Other accident with motorized mobility scooter**

● **V00.89 Accident on other pedestrian conveyance**

● **V00.891 Fall from other pedestrian conveyance**

● **V00.892 Pedestrian on other pedestrian conveyance colliding with stationary object**

● **V00.898 Other accident on other pedestrian conveyance**

Excludes1 other pedestrian (conveyance) collision with other land transport vehicle (V01-V09 with 5th digit 9)

● **V01 Pedestrian injured in collision with pedal cycle**

The appropriate 7th character is to be added to each code from category V01

A	initial encounter
D	subsequent encounter
S	sequela

● **V01.0 Pedestrian injured in collision with pedal cycle in nontraffic accident**

X● **V01.00 Pedestrian on foot injured in collision with pedal cycle in nontraffic accident**

Pedestrian NOS injured in collision with pedal cycle in nontraffic accident

X● **V01.01 Pedestrian on roller-skates injured in collision with pedal cycle in nontraffic accident**

X● **V01.02 Pedestrian on skateboard injured in collision with pedal cycle in nontraffic accident**

X● **V01.09 Pedestrian with other conveyance injured in collision with pedal cycle in nontraffic accident**

Pedestrian with babystroller injured in collision with pedal cycle in nontraffic accident
Pedestrian in wheelchair (powered) injured in collision with pedal cycle in nontraffic accident
Pedestrian in motorized mobility scooter injured in collision with pedal cycle in nontraffic accident
Pedestrian on ice-skates injured in collision with pedal cycle in nontraffic accident
Pedestrian on nonmotorized scooter injured in collision with pedal cycle in nontraffic accident
Pedestrian on sled injured in collision with pedal cycle in nontraffic accident
Pedestrian on snowboard injured in collision with pedal cycle in nontraffic accident
Pedestrian on snow-skis injured in collision with pedal cycle in nontraffic accident

● **V01.1 Pedestrian injured in collision with pedal cycle in traffic accident**

X● **V01.10 Pedestrian on foot injured in collision with pedal cycle in traffic accident**

Pedestrian NOS injured in collision with pedal cycle in traffic accident

X● **V01.11 Pedestrian on roller-skates injured in collision with pedal cycle in traffic accident**

X● **V01.12 Pedestrian on skateboard injured in collision with pedal cycle in traffic accident**

X● **V01.19 Pedestrian with other conveyance injured in collision with pedal cycle in traffic accident**

Pedestrian with babystroller injured in collision with pedal cycle in traffic accident
Pedestrian in wheelchair (powered) injured in collision with pedal cycle in traffic accident
Pedestrian in motorized mobility scooter injured in collision with pedal cycle in traffic accident
Pedestrian on ice-skates injured in collision with pedal cycle in traffic accident
Pedestrian on nonmotorized scooter injured in collision with pedal cycle in traffic accident
Pedestrian on sled injured in collision with pedal cycle in traffic accident
Pedestrian on snowboard injured in collision with pedal cycle in traffic accident
Pedestrian on snow-skis injured in collision with pedal cycle in traffic accident

● **V01.9 Pedestrian injured in collision with pedal cycle, unspecified whether traffic or nontraffic accident**

X● **V01.90 Pedestrian on foot injured in collision with pedal cycle, unspecified whether traffic or nontraffic accident**

Pedestrian NOS injured in collision with pedal cycle, unspecified whether traffic or nontraffic accident

X● **V01.91 Pedestrian on roller-skates injured in collision with pedal cycle, unspecified whether traffic or nontraffic accident**

X● **V01.92 Pedestrian on skateboard injured in collision with pedal cycle, unspecified whether traffic or nontraffic accident**

X● **V01.99 Pedestrian with other conveyance injured in collision with pedal cycle, unspecified whether traffic or nontraffic accident**

Pedestrian with babystroller injured in collision with pedal cycle, unspecified whether traffic or nontraffic accident
Pedestrian in wheelchair (powered) injured in collision with pedal cycle, unspecified whether traffic or nontraffic accident
Pedestrian in motorized mobility scooter injured in collision with pedal cycle, unspecified whether traffic or nontraffic accident
Pedestrian on ice-skates injured in collision with pedal cycle unspecified, whether traffic or nontraffic accident
Pedestrian on nonmotorized scooter injured in collision with pedal cycle, unspecified whether traffic or nontraffic accident
Pedestrian on sled injured in collision with pedal cycle unspecified, whether traffic or nontraffic accident
Pedestrian on snowboard injured in collision with pedal cycle, unspecified whether traffic or nontraffic accident
Pedestrian on snow-skis injured in collision with pedal cycle, unspecified whether traffic or nontraffic accident

● V02 Pedestrian injured in collision with two- or three-wheeled motor vehicle

The appropriate 7th character is to be added to each code from category V02

A	initial encounter
D	subsequent encounter
S	sequela

● V02.0 Pedestrian injured in collision with two- or three-wheeled motor vehicle in nontraffic accident

X● V02.00 Pedestrian on foot injured in collision with two- or three-wheeled motor vehicle in nontraffic accident

Pedestrian NOS injured in collision with two- or three-wheeled motor vehicle in nontraffic accident

X● V02.01 Pedestrian on roller-skates injured in collision with two- or three-wheeled motor vehicle in nontraffic accident

X● V02.02 Pedestrian on skateboard injured in collision with two- or three-wheeled motor vehicle in nontraffic accident

X● V02.09 Pedestrian with other conveyance injured in collision with two- or three-wheeled motor vehicle in nontraffic accident

Pedestrian with babystroller injured in collision with two- or three-wheeled motor vehicle in nontraffic accident
Pedestrian on ice-skates injured in collision with two- or three-wheeled motor vehicle in nontraffic accident
Pedestrian in wheelchair (powered) injured in collision with two- or three-wheeled motor vehicle in nontraffic accident
Pedestrian in motorized mobility scooter injured in collision with two- or three-wheeled motor vehicle in nontraffic accident
Pedestrian on nonmotorized scooter injured in collision with two- or three-wheeled motor vehicle in nontraffic accident
Pedestrian on sled injured in collision with two- or three-wheeled motor vehicle in nontraffic accident
Pedestrian on snowboard injured in collision with two- or three-wheeled motor vehicle in nontraffic accident
Pedestrian on snow-skis injured in collision with two- or three-wheeled motor vehicle in nontraffic accident

● V02.1 Pedestrian injured in collision with two- or three-wheeled motor vehicle in traffic accident

X● V02.10 Pedestrian on foot injured in collision with two- or three-wheeled motor vehicle in traffic accident

Pedestrian NOS injured in collision with two- or three-wheeled motor vehicle in traffic accident

X● V02.11 Pedestrian on roller-skates injured in collision with two- or three-wheeled motor vehicle in traffic accident

X● V02.12 Pedestrian on skateboard injured in collision with two- or three-wheeled motor vehicle in traffic accident

X● V02.19 Pedestrian with other conveyance injured in collision with two- or three-wheeled motor vehicle in traffic accident

Pedestrian with babystroller injured in collision with two- or three-wheeled motor vehicle in traffic accident
Pedestrian in wheelchair (powered) injured in collision with two- or three-wheeled motor vehicle in traffic accident
Pedestrian in motorized mobility scooter injured in collision with two- or three-wheeled motor vehicle in traffic accident
Pedestrian on ice-skates injured in collision with two- or three-wheeled motor vehicle in traffic accident
Pedestrian on nonmotorized scooter injured in collision with two- or three-wheeled motor vehicle in traffic accident
Pedestrian on sled injured in collision with two- or three-wheeled motor vehicle in traffic accident
Pedestrian on snowboard injured in collision with two- or three-wheeled motor vehicle in traffic accident
Pedestrian on snow-skis injured in collision with two- or three-wheeled motor vehicle in traffic accident

● V02.9 Pedestrian injured in collision with two- or three-wheeled motor vehicle, unspecified whether traffic or nontraffic accident

X● V02.90 Pedestrian on foot injured in collision with two- or three-wheeled motor vehicle, unspecified whether traffic or nontraffic accident

Pedestrian NOS injured in collision with two- or three-wheeled motor vehicle, unspecified whether traffic or nontraffic accident

X● V02.91 Pedestrian on roller-skates injured in collision with two- or three-wheeled motor vehicle, unspecified whether traffic or nontraffic accident

X● V02.92 Pedestrian on skateboard injured in collision with two- or three-wheeled motor vehicle, unspecified whether traffic or nontraffic accident

X● **V02.99 Pedestrian with other conveyance injured in collision with two- or three-wheeled motor vehicle, unspecified whether traffic or nontraffic accident**
- Pedestrian with babystroller injured in collision with two- or three-wheeled motor vehicle, unspecified whether traffic or nontraffic accident
- Pedestrian in wheelchair (powered) injured in collision with two- or three-wheeled motor vehicle, unspecified whether traffic or nontraffic accident
- Pedestrian in motorized mobility scooter injured in collision with two- or three-wheeled motor vehicle, unspecified whether traffic or nontraffic accident
- Pedestrian on ice-skates injured in collision with two- or three-wheeled motor vehicle, unspecified whether traffic or nontraffic accident
- Pedestrian on nonmotorized scooter injured in collision with two- or three-wheeled motor vehicle, unspecified whether traffic or nontraffic accident
- Pedestrian on sled injured in collision with two- or three-wheeled motor vehicle, unspecified whether traffic or nontraffic accident
- Pedestrian on snowboard injured in collision with two- or three-wheeled motor vehicle, unspecified whether traffic or nontraffic accident
- Pedestrian on snow-skis injured in collision with two- or three-wheeled motor vehicle, unspecified whether traffic or nontraffic accident

● **V03 Pedestrian injured in collision with car, pick-up truck or van**

The appropriate 7th character is to be added to each code from category V03

A	initial encounter
D	subsequent encounter
S	sequela

● **V03.0 Pedestrian injured in collision with car, pick-up truck or van in nontraffic accident**

X● **V03.00 Pedestrian on foot injured in collision with car, pick-up truck or van in nontraffic accident**
- Pedestrian NOS injured in collision with car, pick-up truck or van in nontraffic accident

X● **V03.01 Pedestrian on roller-skates injured in collision with car, pick-up truck or van in nontraffic accident**

X● **V03.02 Pedestrian on skateboard injured in collision with car, pick-up truck or van in nontraffic accident**

X● **V03.09 Pedestrian with other conveyance injured in collision with car, pick-up truck or van in nontraffic accident**
- Pedestrian with babystroller injured in collision with car, pick-up truck or van in nontraffic accident
- Pedestrian in wheelchair (powered) injured in collision with car, pick-up truck or van in nontraffic accident
- Pedestrian in motorized mobility scooter injured in collision with car, pick-up truck or van in nontraffic accident
- Pedestrian on ice-skates injured in collision with car, pick-up truck or van in nontraffic accident
- Pedestrian on nonmotorized scooter injured in collision with car, pick-up truck or van in nontraffic accident
- Pedestrian on sled injured in collision with car, pick-up truck or van in nontraffic accident
- Pedestrian on snowboard injured in collision with car, pick-up truck or van in nontraffic accident
- Pedestrian on snow-skis injured in collision with car, pick-up truck or van in nontraffic accident

● **V03.1 Pedestrian injured in collision with car, pick-up truck or van in traffic accident**

X● **V03.10 Pedestrian on foot injured in collision with car, pick-up truck or van in traffic accident**
- Pedestrian NOS injured in collision with car, pick-up truck or van in traffic accident

X● **V03.11 Pedestrian on roller-skates injured in collision with car, pick-up truck or van in traffic accident**

X● **V03.12 Pedestrian on skateboard injured in collision with car, pick-up truck or van in traffic accident**

X● **V03.19 Pedestrian with other conveyance injured in collision with car, pick-up truck or van in traffic accident**
- Pedestrian with babystroller injured in collision with car, pick-up truck or van in traffic accident
- Pedestrian in wheelchair (powered) injured in collision with car, pick-up truck or van in traffic accident
- Pedestrian in motorized mobility scooter injured in collision with car, pick-up truck or van in traffic accident
- Pedestrian on ice-skates injured in collision with car, pick-up truck or van in traffic accident
- Pedestrian on nonmotorized scooter injured in collision with car, pick-up truck or van in traffic accident
- Pedestrian on sled injured in collision with car, pick-up truck or van in traffic accident
- Pedestrian on snowboard injured in collision with car, pick-up truck or van in traffic accident
- Pedestrian on snow-skis injured in collision with car, pick-up truck or van in traffic accident

● **V03.9 Pedestrian injured in collision with car, pick-up truck or van, unspecified whether traffic or nontraffic accident**

X● **V03.90 Pedestrian on foot injured in collision with car, pick-up truck or van, unspecified whether traffic or nontraffic accident**
Pedestrian NOS injured in collision with car, pick-up truck or van, unspecified whether traffic or nontraffic accident

X● **V03.91 Pedestrian on roller-skates injured in collision with car, pick-up truck or van, unspecified whether traffic or nontraffic accident**

X● **V03.92 Pedestrian on skateboard injured in collision with car, pick-up truck or van, unspecified whether traffic or nontraffic accident**

X● **V03.99 Pedestrian with other conveyance injured in collision with car, pick-up truck or van, unspecified whether traffic or nontraffic accident**
Pedestrian with babystroller injured in collision with car, pick-up truck or van, unspecified whether traffic or nontraffic accident
Pedestrian in wheelchair (powered) injured in collision with car, pick-up truck or van, unspecified whether traffic or nontraffic accident
Pedestrian in motorized mobility scooter injured in collision with car, pick-up truck or van, unspecified whether traffic or nontraffic accident
Pedestrian on ice-skates injured in collision with car, pick-up truck or van, unspecified whether traffic or nontraffic accident
Pedestrian on nonmotorized scooter injured in collision with car, pick-up truck or van, unspecified whether traffic or nontraffic accident
Pedestrian on sled injured in collision with car, pick-up truck or van in nontraffic accident
Pedestrian on snowboard injured in collision with car, pick-up truck or van, unspecified whether traffic or nontraffic accident
Pedestrian on snow-skis injured in collision with car, pick-up truck or van, unspecified whether traffic or nontraffic accident

● **V04 Pedestrian injured in collision with heavy transport vehicle or bus**

Excludes1 pedestrian injured in collision with military vehicle (V09.01, V09.21)

The appropriate 7th character is to be added to each code from category V04

A	initial encounter
D	subsequent encounter
S	sequela

● **V04.0 Pedestrian injured in collision with heavy transport vehicle or bus in nontraffic accident**

X● **V04.00 Pedestrian on foot injured in collision with heavy transport vehicle or bus in nontraffic accident**
Pedestrian NOS injured in collision with heavy transport vehicle or bus in nontraffic accident

X● **V04.01 Pedestrian on roller-skates injured in collision with heavy transport vehicle or bus in nontraffic accident**

X● **V04.02 Pedestrian on skateboard injured in collision with heavy transport vehicle or bus in nontraffic accident**

X● **V04.09 Pedestrian with other conveyance injured in collision with heavy transport vehicle or bus in nontraffic accident**
Pedestrian with babystroller injured in collision with heavy transport vehicle or bus in nontraffic accident
Pedestrian in wheelchair (powered) injured in collision with heavy transport vehicle or bus in nontraffic accident
Pedestrian in motorized mobility scooter injured in collision with heavy transport vehicle or bus in nontraffic accident
Pedestrian on ice-skates injured in collision with heavy transport vehicle or bus in nontraffic accident
Pedestrian on nonmotorized scooter injured in collision with heavy transport vehicle or bus in nontraffic accident
Pedestrian on sled injured in collision with heavy transport vehicle or bus in nontraffic accident
Pedestrian on snowboard injured in collision with heavy transport vehicle or bus in nontraffic accident
Pedestrian on snow-skis injured in collision with heavy transport vehicle or bus in nontraffic accident

● **V04.1 Pedestrian injured in collision with heavy transport vehicle or bus in traffic accident**

X● **V04.10 Pedestrian on foot injured in collision with heavy transport vehicle or bus in traffic accident**
Pedestrian NOS injured in collision with heavy transport vehicle or bus in traffic accident

X● **V04.11 Pedestrian on roller-skates injured in collision with heavy transport vehicle or bus in traffic accident**

X● **V04.12 Pedestrian on skateboard injured in collision with heavy transport vehicle or bus in traffic accident**

X● **V04.19 Pedestrian with other conveyance injured in collision with heavy transport vehicle or bus in traffic accident**
Pedestrian with babystroller injured in collision with heavy transport vehicle or bus in traffic accident
Pedestrian in wheelchair (powered) injured in collision with heavy transport vehicle or bus in traffic accident
Pedestrian in motorized mobility scooter injured in collision with heavy transport vehicle or bus in traffic accident
Pedestrian on ice-skates injured in collision with heavy transport vehicle or bus in traffic accident
Pedestrian on nonmotorized scooter injured in collision with heavy transport vehicle or bus in traffic accident
Pedestrian on sled injured in collision with heavy transport vehicle or bus in traffic accident
Pedestrian on snowboard injured in collision with heavy transport vehicle or bus in traffic accident
Pedestrian on snow-skis injured in collision with heavy transport vehicle or bus in traffic accident

● **V04.9 Pedestrian injured in collision with heavy transport vehicle or bus, unspecified whether traffic or nontraffic accident**

X● **V04.90 Pedestrian on foot injured in collision with heavy transport vehicle or bus, unspecified whether traffic or nontraffic accident**

Pedestrian NOS injured in collision with heavy transport vehicle or bus, unspecified whether traffic or nontraffic accident

X● **V04.91 Pedestrian on roller-skates injured in collision with heavy transport vehicle or bus, unspecified whether traffic or nontraffic accident**

X● **V04.92 Pedestrian on skateboard injured in collision with heavy transport vehicle or bus, unspecified whether traffic or nontraffic accident**

X● **V04.99 Pedestrian with other conveyance injured in collision with heavy transport vehicle or bus, unspecified whether traffic or nontraffic accident**

Pedestrian with babystroller injured in collision with heavy transport vehicle or bus, unspecified whether traffic or nontraffic accident

Pedestrian in wheelchair (powered) injured in collision with heavy transport vehicle or bus, unspecified whether traffic or nontraffic accident

Pedestrian in motorized mobility scooter injured in collision with heavy transport vehicle or bus, unspecified whether traffic or nontraffic accident

Pedestrian on ice-skates injured in collision with heavy transport vehicle or bus, unspecified whether traffic or nontraffic accident

Pedestrian on nonmotorized scooter injured in collision with heavy transport vehicle or bus, unspecified whether traffic or nontraffic accident

Pedestrian on sled injured in collision with heavy transport vehicle or bus, unspecified whether traffic or nontraffic accident

Pedestrian on snowboard injured in collision with heavy transport vehicle or bus, unspecified whether traffic or nontraffic accident

Pedestrian on snow-skis injured in collision with heavy transport vehicle or bus, unspecified whether traffic or nontraffic accident

● **V05 Pedestrian injured in collision with railway train or railway vehicle**

The appropriate 7th character is to be added to each code from category V05

A	initial encounter
D	subsequent encounter
S	sequela

● **V05.0 Pedestrian injured in collision with railway train or railway vehicle in nontraffic accident**

X● **V05.00 Pedestrian on foot injured in collision with railway train or railway vehicle in nontraffic accident**

Pedestrian NOS injured in collision with railway train or railway vehicle in nontraffic accident

X● **V05.01 Pedestrian on roller-skates injured in collision with railway train or railway vehicle in nontraffic accident**

X● **V05.02 Pedestrian on skateboard injured in collision with railway train or railway vehicle in nontraffic accident**

X● **V05.09 Pedestrian with other conveyance injured in collision with railway train or railway vehicle in nontraffic accident**

Pedestrian with babystroller injured in collision with railway train or railway vehicle in nontraffic accident

Pedestrian in wheelchair (powered) injured in collision with railway train or railway vehicle in nontraffic accident

Pedestrian in motorized mobility scooter injured in collision with railway train or railway vehicle in nontraffic accident

Pedestrian on ice-skates injured in collision with railway train or railway vehicle in nontraffic accident

Pedestrian on nonmotorized scooter injured in collision with railway train or railway vehicle in nontraffic accident

Pedestrian on sled injured in collision with railway train or railway vehicle in nontraffic accident

Pedestrian on snowboard injured in collision with railway train or railway vehicle in nontraffic accident

Pedestrian on snow-skis injured in collision with railway train or railway vehicle in nontraffic accident

● **V05.1 Pedestrian injured in collision with railway train or railway vehicle in traffic accident**

X● **V05.10 Pedestrian on foot injured in collision with railway train or railway vehicle in traffic accident**

Pedestrian NOS injured in collision with railway train or railway vehicle in traffic accident

X● **V05.11 Pedestrian on roller-skates injured in collision with railway train or railway vehicle in traffic accident**

X● **V05.12 Pedestrian on skateboard injured in collision with railway train or railway vehicle in traffic accident**

X● **V05.19 Pedestrian with other conveyance injured in collision with railway train or railway vehicle in traffic accident**

Pedestrian with babystroller injured in collision with railway train or railway vehicle in traffic accident

Pedestrian in wheelchair (powered) injured in collision with railway train or railway vehicle in traffic accident

Pedestrian in motorized mobility scooter injured in collision with railway train or railway vehicle in traffic accident

Pedestrian on ice-skates injured in collision with railway train or railway vehicle in traffic accident

Pedestrian on nonmotorized scooter injured in collision with railway train or railway vehicle in traffic accident

Pedestrian on sled injured in collision with railway train or railway vehicle in traffic accident

Pedestrian on snowboard injured in collision with railway train or railway vehicle in traffic accident

Pedestrian on snow-skis injured in collision with railway train or railway vehicle in traffic accident

● **V05.9 Pedestrian injured in collision with railway train or railway vehicle, unspecified whether traffic or nontraffic accident**

X● **V05.90 Pedestrian on foot injured in collision with railway train or railway vehicle, unspecified whether traffic or nontraffic accident**
Pedestrian NOS injured in collision with railway train or railway vehicle, unspecified whether traffic or nontraffic accident

X● **V05.91 Pedestrian on roller-skates injured in collision with railway train or railway vehicle, unspecified whether traffic or nontraffic accident**

X● **V05.92 Pedestrian on skateboard injured in collision with railway train or railway vehicle, unspecified whether traffic or nontraffic accident**

X● **V05.99 Pedestrian with other conveyance injured in collision with railway train or railway vehicle, unspecified whether traffic or nontraffic accident**
Pedestrian with babystroller injured in collision with railway train or railway vehicle, unspecified whether traffic or nontraffic
Pedestrian in wheelchair (powered) injured in collision with railway train or railway vehicle, unspecified whether traffic or nontraffic
Pedestrian in motorized mobility scooter injured in collision with railway train or railway vehicle, unspecified whether traffic or nontraffic
Pedestrian on ice-skates injured in collision with railway train or railway vehicle, unspecified whether traffic or nontraffic
Pedestrian on nonmotorized scooter injured in collision with railway train or railway vehicle, unspecified whether traffic or nontraffic
Pedestrian on sled injured in collision with railway train or railway vehicle, unspecified whether traffic or nontraffic
Pedestrian on snowboard injured in collision with railway train or railway vehicle, unspecified whether traffic or nontraffic
Pedestrian on snow-skis injured in collision with railway train or railway vehicle, unspecified whether traffic or nontraffic

● **V06 Pedestrian injured in collision with other nonmotor vehicle**

Includes collision with animal-drawn vehicle, animal being ridden, nonpowered streetcar

Excludes1 pedestrian injured in collision with pedestrian conveyance (V00.0-)

The appropriate 7th character is to be added to each code from category V06

A	initial encounter
D	subsequent encounter
S	sequela

● **V06.0 Pedestrian injured in collision with other nonmotor vehicle in nontraffic accident**

X● **V06.00 Pedestrian on foot injured in collision with other nonmotor vehicle in nontraffic accident**
Pedestrian NOS injured in collision with other nonmotor vehicle in nontraffic accident

X● **V06.01 Pedestrian on roller-skates injured in collision with other nonmotor vehicle in nontraffic accident**

X● **V06.02 Pedestrian on skateboard injured in collision with other nonmotor vehicle in nontraffic accident**

X● **V06.09 Pedestrian with other conveyance injured in collision with other nonmotor vehicle in nontraffic accident**
Pedestrian with babystroller injured in collision with other nonmotor vehicle in nontraffic accident
Pedestrian in wheelchair (powered) injured in collision with other nonmotor vehicle in nontraffic accident
Pedestrian in motorized mobility scooter injured in collision with other nonmotor vehicle in nontraffic accident
Pedestrian on ice-skates injured in collision with other nonmotor vehicle in nontraffic accident
Pedestrian on nonmotorized scooter injured in collision with other nonmotor vehicle in nontraffic accident
Pedestrian on sled injured in collision with other nonmotor vehicle in nontraffic accident
Pedestrian on snowboard injured in collision with other nonmotor vehicle in nontraffic accident
Pedestrian on snow-skis injured in collision with other nonmotor vehicle in nontraffic accident

● **V06.1 Pedestrian injured in collision with other nonmotor vehicle in traffic accident**

X● **V06.10 Pedestrian on foot injured in collision with other nonmotor vehicle in traffic accident**
Pedestrian NOS injured in collision with other nonmotor vehicle in traffic accident

X● **V06.11 Pedestrian on roller-skates injured in collision with other nonmotor vehicle in traffic accident**

X● **V06.12 Pedestrian on skateboard injured in collision with other nonmotor vehicle in traffic accident**

X● **V06.19 Pedestrian with other conveyance injured in collision with other nonmotor vehicle in traffic accident**
Pedestrian with babystroller injured in collision with other nonmotor vehicle in nontraffic accident
Pedestrian in wheelchair (powered) injured in collision with other nonmotor vehicle in traffic accident
Pedestrian in motorized mobility scooter injured in collision with other nonmotor vehicle in traffic accident
Pedestrian on ice-skates injured in collision with other nonmotor vehicle in traffic accident
Pedestrian on nonmotorized scooter injured in collision with other nonmotor vehicle in traffic accident
Pedestrian on sled injured in collision with other nonmotor vehicle in traffic accident
Pedestrian on snowboard injured in collision with other nonmotor vehicle in traffic accident
Pedestrian on snow-skis injured in collision with other nonmotor vehicle in traffic accident

● **V06.9 Pedestrian injured in collision with other nonmotor vehicle, unspecified whether traffic or nontraffic accident**

X● **V06.90 Pedestrian on foot injured in collision with other nonmotor vehicle, unspecified whether traffic or nontraffic accident**
Pedestrian NOS injured in collision with other nonmotor vehicle, unspecified whether traffic or nontraffic accident

X● **V06.91 Pedestrian on roller-skates injured in collision with other nonmotor vehicle, unspecified whether traffic or nontraffic accident**

X● **V06.92 Pedestrian on skateboard injured in collision with other nonmotor vehicle, unspecified whether traffic or nontraffic accident**

X● **V06.99 Pedestrian with other conveyance injured in collision with other nonmotor vehicle, unspecified whether traffic or nontraffic accident**

Pedestrian with babystroller injured in collision with other nonmotor vehicle, unspecified whether traffic or nontraffic accident

Pedestrian in wheelchair (powered) injured in collision with other nonmotor vehicle, unspecified whether traffic or nontraffic accident

Pedestrian in motorized mobility scooter injured in collision with other nonmotor vehicle, unspecified whether traffic or nontraffic accident

Pedestrian on ice-skates injured in collision with other nonmotor vehicle, unspecified whether traffic or nontraffic accident

Pedestrian on nonmotorized scooter injured in collision with other nonmotor vehicle, unspecified whether traffic or nontraffic accident

Pedestrian on sled injured in collision with other nonmotor vehicle, unspecified whether traffic or nontraffic accident

Pedestrian on snowboard injured in collision with other nonmotor vehicle, unspecified whether traffic or nontraffic accident

Pedestrian on snow-skis injured in collision with other nonmotor vehicle, unspecified whether traffic or nontraffic accident

● **V09 Pedestrian injured in other and unspecified transport accidents**

The appropriate 7th character is to be added to each code from category V09

A	initial encounter
D	subsequent encounter
S	sequela

● **V09.0 Pedestrian injured in nontraffic accident involving other and unspecified motor vehicles**

X● **V09.00 Pedestrian injured in nontraffic accident involving unspecified motor vehicles**

X● **V09.01 Pedestrian injured in nontraffic accident involving military vehicle**

X● **V09.09 Pedestrian injured in nontraffic accident involving other motor vehicles**

Pedestrian injured in nontraffic accident by special vehicle

X● **V09.1 Pedestrian injured in unspecified nontraffic accident**

● **V09.2 Pedestrian injured in traffic accident involving other and unspecified motor vehicles**

X● **V09.20 Pedestrian injured in traffic accident involving unspecified motor vehicles**

X● **V09.21 Pedestrian injured in traffic accident involving military vehicle**

X● **V09.29 Pedestrian injured in traffic accident involving other motor vehicles**

X● **V09.3 Pedestrian injured in unspecified traffic accident**

X● **V09.9 Pedestrian injured in unspecified transport accident**

PEDAL CYCLE RIDER INJURED IN TRANSPORT ACCIDENT (V10-V19)

Includes any non-motorized vehicle, excluding an animal-drawn vehicle, or a sidecar or trailer attached to the pedal cycle

Excludes2 rupture of pedal cycle tire (W37.0)

● **V10 Pedal cycle rider injured in collision with pedestrian or animal**

Excludes1 pedal cycle rider collision with animal-drawn vehicle or animal being ridden (V16.-)

The appropriate 7th character is to be added to each code from category V10

A	initial encounter
D	subsequent encounter
S	sequela

X● **V10.0 Pedal cycle driver injured in collision with pedestrian or animal in nontraffic accident**

X● **V10.1 Pedal cycle passenger injured in collision with pedestrian or animal in nontraffic accident**

X● **V10.2 Unspecified pedal cyclist injured in collision with pedestrian or animal in nontraffic accident**

X● **V10.3 Person boarding or alighting a pedal cycle injured in collision with pedestrian or animal**

X● **V10.4 Pedal cycle driver injured in collision with pedestrian or animal in traffic accident**

X● **V10.5 Pedal cycle passenger injured in collision with pedestrian or animal in traffic accident**

X● **V10.9 Unspecified pedal cyclist injured in collision with pedestrian or animal in traffic accident**

● **V11 Pedal cycle rider injured in collision with other pedal cycle**

The appropriate 7th character is to be added to each code from category V11

A	initial encounter
D	subsequent encounter
S	sequela

X● **V11.0 Pedal cycle driver injured in collision with other pedal cycle in nontraffic accident**

X● **V11.1 Pedal cycle passenger injured in collision with other pedal cycle in nontraffic accident**

X● **V11.2 Unspecified pedal cyclist injured in collision with other pedal cycle in nontraffic accident**

X● **V11.3 Person boarding or alighting a pedal cycle injured in collision with other pedal cycle**

X● **V11.4 Pedal cycle driver injured in collision with other pedal cycle in traffic accident**

X● **V11.5 Pedal cycle passenger injured in collision with other pedal cycle in traffic accident**

X● **V11.9 Unspecified pedal cyclist injured in collision with other pedal cycle in traffic accident**

● **V12 Pedal cycle rider injured in collision with two- or three-wheeled motor vehicle**

The appropriate 7th character is to be added to each code from category V12

A	initial encounter
D	subsequent encounter
S	sequela

X● **V12.0 Pedal cycle driver injured in collision with two- or three-wheeled motor vehicle in nontraffic accident**

X● **V12.1 Pedal cycle passenger injured in collision with two- or three-wheeled motor vehicle in nontraffic accident**

X● **V12.2 Unspecified pedal cyclist injured in collision with two- or three-wheeled motor vehicle in nontraffic accident**

X● **V12.3 Person boarding or alighting a pedal cycle injured in collision with two- or three-wheeled motor vehicle**

X● **V12.4 Pedal cycle driver injured in collision with two- or three-wheeled motor vehicle in traffic accident**

X● **V12.5 Pedal cycle passenger injured in collision with two- or three-wheeled motor vehicle in traffic accident**

X● **V12.9 Unspecified pedal cyclist injured in collision with two- or three-wheeled motor vehicle in traffic accident**

● **V13 Pedal cycle rider injured in collision with car, pick-up truck or van**

The appropriate 7th character is to be added to each code from category V13

A	initial encounter
D	subsequent encounter
S	sequela

X● **V13.0 Pedal cycle driver injured in collision with car, pick-up truck or van in nontraffic accident**

X● **V13.1 Pedal cycle passenger injured in collision with car, pick-up truck or van in nontraffic accident**

X● **V13.2 Unspecified pedal cyclist injured in collision with car, pick-up truck or van in nontraffic accident**

X● **V13.3 Person boarding or alighting a pedal cycle injured in collision with car, pick-up truck or van**

X● **V13.4 Pedal cycle driver injured in collision with car, pick-up truck or van in traffic accident**

X● **V13.5 Pedal cycle passenger injured in collision with car, pick-up truck or van in traffic accident**

X● **V13.9 Unspecified pedal cyclist injured in collision with car, pick-up truck or van in traffic accident**

● **V14 Pedal cycle rider injured in collision with heavy transport vehicle or bus**

Excludes1 pedal cycle rider injured in collision with military vehicle (V19.81)

The appropriate 7th character is to be added to each code from category V14

A	initial encounter
D	subsequent encounter
S	sequela

X● **V14.0 Pedal cycle driver injured in collision with heavy transport vehicle or bus in nontraffic accident**

X● **V14.1 Pedal cycle passenger injured in collision with heavy transport vehicle or bus in nontraffic accident**

X● **V14.2 Unspecified pedal cyclist injured in collision with heavy transport vehicle or bus in nontraffic accident**

X● **V14.3 Person boarding or alighting a pedal cycle injured in collision with heavy transport vehicle or bus**

X● **V14.4 Pedal cycle driver injured in collision with heavy transport vehicle or bus in traffic accident**

X● **V14.5 Pedal cycle passenger injured in collision with heavy transport vehicle or bus in traffic accident**

X● **V14.9 Unspecified pedal cyclist injured in collision with heavy transport vehicle or bus in traffic accident**

● **V15 Pedal cycle rider injured in collision with railway train or railway vehicle**

The appropriate 7th character is to be added to each code from category V15

A	initial encounter
D	subsequent encounter
S	sequela

X● **V15.0 Pedal cycle driver injured in collision with railway train or railway vehicle in nontraffic accident**

X● **V15.1 Pedal cycle passenger injured in collision with railway train or railway vehicle in nontraffic accident**

X● **V15.2 Unspecified pedal cyclist injured in collision with railway train or railway vehicle in nontraffic accident**

X● **V15.3 Person boarding or alighting a pedal cycle injured in collision with railway train or railway vehicle**

X● **V15.4 Pedal cycle driver injured in collision with railway train or railway vehicle in traffic accident**

X● **V15.5 Pedal cycle passenger injured in collision with railway train or railway vehicle in traffic accident**

X● **V15.9 Unspecified pedal cyclist injured in collision with railway train or railway vehicle in traffic accident**

● **V16 Pedal cycle rider injured in collision with other nonmotor vehicle**

Includes collision with animal-drawn vehicle, animal being ridden, streetcar

The appropriate 7th character is to be added to each code from category V16

A	initial encounter
D	subsequent encounter
S	sequela

X● **V16.0 Pedal cycle driver injured in collision with other nonmotor vehicle in nontraffic accident**

X● **V16.1 Pedal cycle passenger injured in collision with other nonmotor vehicle in nontraffic accident**

X● **V16.2 Unspecified pedal cyclist injured in collision with other nonmotor vehicle in nontraffic accident**

X● **V16.3 Person boarding or alighting a pedal cycle injured in collision with other nonmotor vehicle in nontraffic accident**

X● **V16.4 Pedal cycle driver injured in collision with other nonmotor vehicle in traffic accident**

X● **V16.5 Pedal cycle passenger injured in collision with other nonmotor vehicle in traffic accident**

X● **V16.9 Unspecified pedal cyclist injured in collision with other nonmotor vehicle in traffic accident**

● **V17 Pedal cycle rider injured in collision with fixed or stationary object**

The appropriate 7th character is to be added to each code from category V17

A	initial encounter
D	subsequent encounter
S	sequela

X● **V17.0 Pedal cycle driver injured in collision with fixed or stationary object in nontraffic accident**

X● **V17.1 Pedal cycle passenger injured in collision with fixed or stationary object in nontraffic accident**

X● **V17.2 Unspecified pedal cyclist injured in collision with fixed or stationary object in nontraffic accident**

X● **V17.3 Person boarding or alighting a pedal cycle injured in collision with fixed or stationary object**

X● **V17.4 Pedal cycle driver injured in collision with fixed or stationary object in traffic accident**

X● **V17.5 Pedal cycle passenger injured in collision with fixed or stationary object in traffic accident**

X● **V17.9 Unspecified pedal cyclist injured in collision with fixed or stationary object in traffic accident**

● **V18 Pedal cycle rider injured in noncollision transport accident**

Includes fall or thrown from pedal cycle (without antecedent collision)
overturning pedal cycle NOS
overturning pedal cycle without collision

The appropriate 7th character is to be added to each code from category V18

A	initial encounter
D	subsequent encounter
S	sequela

X● **V18.0 Pedal cycle driver injured in noncollision transport accident in nontraffic accident**

X● **V18.1 Pedal cycle passenger injured in noncollision transport accident in nontraffic accident**

X● **V18.2 Unspecified pedal cyclist injured in noncollision transport accident in nontraffic accident**

X● **V18.3 Person boarding or alighting a pedal cycle injured in noncollision transport accident**

X● **V18.4 Pedal cycle driver injured in noncollision transport accident in traffic accident**

X● **V18.5 Pedal cycle passenger injured in noncollision transport accident in traffic accident**

X● **V18.9 Unspecified pedal cyclist injured in noncollision transport accident in traffic accident**

● **V19 Pedal cycle rider injured in other and unspecified transport accidents**

The appropriate 7th character is to be added to each code from category V19

A	initial encounter
D	subsequent encounter
S	sequela

● **V19.0 Pedal cycle driver injured in collision with other and unspecified motor vehicles in nontraffic accident**

X● **V19.00 Pedal cycle driver injured in collision with unspecified motor vehicles in nontraffic accident**

X● **V19.09 Pedal cycle driver injured in collision with other motor vehicles in nontraffic accident**

● **V19.1 Pedal cycle passenger injured in collision with other and unspecified motor vehicles in nontraffic accident**

X● **V19.10 Pedal cycle passenger injured in collision with unspecified motor vehicles in nontraffic accident**

X● **V19.19 Pedal cycle passenger injured in collision with other motor vehicles in nontraffic accident**

● **V19.2 Unspecified pedal cyclist injured in collision with other and unspecified motor vehicles in nontraffic accident**

X● **V19.20 Unspecified pedal cyclist injured in collision with unspecified motor vehicles in nontraffic accident**
Pedal cycle collision NOS, nontraffic

X● **V19.29 Unspecified pedal cyclist injured in collision with other motor vehicles in nontraffic accident**

X● **V19.3 Pedal cyclist (driver) (passenger) injured in unspecified nontraffic accident**
Pedal cycle accident NOS, nontraffic
Pedal cyclist injured in nontraffic accident NOS

● **V19.4 Pedal cycle driver injured in collision with other and unspecified motor vehicles in traffic accident**

X● **V19.40 Pedal cycle driver injured in collision with unspecified motor vehicles in traffic accident**

X● **V19.49 Pedal cycle driver injured in collision with other motor vehicles in traffic accident**

● **V19.5 Pedal cycle passenger injured in collision with other and unspecified motor vehicles in traffic accident**

X● **V19.50 Pedal cycle passenger injured in collision with unspecified motor vehicles in traffic accident**

X● **V19.59 Pedal cycle passenger injured in collision with other motor vehicles in traffic accident**

● **V19.6 Unspecified pedal cyclist injured in collision with other and unspecified motor vehicles in traffic accident**

X● **V19.60 Unspecified pedal cyclist injured in collision with unspecified motor vehicles in traffic accident**
Pedal cycle collision NOS (traffic)

X● **V19.69 Unspecified pedal cyclist injured in collision with other motor vehicles in traffic accident**

● **V19.8 Pedal cyclist (driver) (passenger) injured in other specified transport accidents**

X● **V19.81 Pedal cyclist (driver) (passenger) injured in transport accident with military vehicle**

X● **V19.88 Pedal cyclist (driver) (passenger) injured in other specified transport accidents**

X● **V19.9 Pedal cyclist (driver) (passenger) injured in unspecified traffic accident**
Pedal cycle accident NOS

MOTORCYCLE RIDER INJURED IN TRANSPORT ACCIDENT (V20-V29)

Includes moped motorcycle with sidecar motorized bicycle motor scooter

Excludes1 three-wheeled motor vehicle (V30-V39)

● **V20 Motorcycle rider injured in collision with pedestrian or animal**

Excludes1 motorcycle rider collision with animal-drawn vehicle or animal being ridden (V26.-)

The appropriate 7th character is to be added to each code from category V20

A	initial encounter
D	subsequent encounter
S	sequela

X● **V20.0 Motorcycle driver injured in collision with pedestrian or animal in nontraffic accident**

X● **V20.1 Motorcycle passenger injured in collision with pedestrian or animal in nontraffic accident**

X● **V20.2 Unspecified motorcycle rider injured in collision with pedestrian or animal in nontraffic accident**

X● **V20.3 Person boarding or alighting a motorcycle injured in collision with pedestrian or animal**

X● **V20.4 Motorcycle driver injured in collision with pedestrian or animal in traffic accident**

X● **V20.5 Motorcycle passenger injured in collision with pedestrian or animal in traffic accident**

X● **V20.9 Unspecified motorcycle rider injured in collision with pedestrian or animal in traffic accident**

● **V21 Motorcycle rider injured in collision with pedal cycle**

The appropriate 7th character is to be added to each code from category V21

A	initial encounter
D	subsequent encounter
S	sequela

X● **V21.0 Motorcycle driver injured in collision with pedal cycle in nontraffic accident**

X● **V21.1 Motorcycle passenger injured in collision with pedal cycle in nontraffic accident**

X● **V21.2 Unspecified motorcycle rider injured in collision with pedal cycle in nontraffic accident**

X● **V21.3 Person boarding or alighting a motorcycle injured in collision with pedal cycle**

X● **V21.4 Motorcycle driver injured in collision with pedal cycle in traffic accident**

X● **V21.5 Motorcycle passenger injured in collision with pedal cycle in traffic accident**

X● **V21.9 Unspecified motorcycle rider injured in collision with pedal cycle in traffic accident**

V22 Motorcycle rider injured in collision with two- or three-wheeled motor vehicle

The appropriate 7th character is to be added to each code from category V22

A	initial encounter
D	subsequent encounter
S	sequela

X **V22.0 Motorcycle driver injured in collision with two- or three-wheeled motor vehicle in nontraffic accident**

X **V22.1 Motorcycle passenger injured in collision with two- or three-wheeled motor vehicle in nontraffic accident**

X **V22.2 Unspecified motorcycle rider injured in collision with two- or three-wheeled motor vehicle in nontraffic accident**

X **V22.3 Person boarding or alighting a motorcycle injured in collision with two- or three-wheeled motor vehicle**

X **V22.4 Motorcycle driver injured in collision with two- or three-wheeled motor vehicle in traffic accident**

X **V22.5 Motorcycle passenger injured in collision with two- or three-wheeled motor vehicle in traffic accident**

X **V22.9 Unspecified motorcycle rider injured in collision with two- or three-wheeled motor vehicle in traffic accident**

V23 Motorcycle rider injured in collision with car, pick-up truck or van

The appropriate 7th character is to be added to each code from category V23

A	initial encounter
D	subsequent encounter
S	sequela

X **V23.0 Motorcycle driver injured in collision with car, pick-up truck or van in nontraffic accident**

X **V23.1 Motorcycle passenger injured in collision with car, pick-up truck or van in nontraffic accident**

X **V23.2 Unspecified motorcycle rider injured in collision with car, pick-up truck or van in nontraffic accident**

X **V23.3 Person boarding or alighting a motorcycle injured in collision with car, pick-up truck or van**

X **V23.4 Motorcycle driver injured in collision with car, pick-up truck or van in traffic accident**

X **V23.5 Motorcycle passenger injured in collision with car, pick-up truck or van in traffic accident**

X **V23.9 Unspecified motorcycle rider injured in collision with car, pick-up truck or van in traffic accident**

V24 Motorcycle rider injured in collision with heavy transport vehicle or bus

Excludes1 motorcycle rider injured in collision with military vehicle (V29.81)

The appropriate 7th character is to be added to each code from category V24

A	initial encounter
D	subsequent encounter
S	sequela

X **V24.0 Motorcycle driver injured in collision with heavy transport vehicle or bus in nontraffic accident**

X **V24.1 Motorcycle passenger injured in collision with heavy transport vehicle or bus in nontraffic accident**

X **V24.2 Unspecified motorcycle rider injured in collision with heavy transport vehicle or bus in nontraffic accident**

X **V24.3 Person boarding or alighting a motorcycle injured in collision with heavy transport vehicle or bus**

X **V24.4 Motorcycle driver injured in collision with heavy transport vehicle or bus in traffic accident**

X **V24.5 Motorcycle passenger injured in collision with heavy transport vehicle or bus in traffic accident**

X **V24.9 Unspecified motorcycle rider injured in collision with heavy transport vehicle or bus in traffic accident**

V25 Motorcycle rider injured in collision with railway train or railway vehicle

The appropriate 7th character is to be added to each code from category V25

A	initial encounter
D	subsequent encounter
S	sequela

X **V25.0 Motorcycle driver injured in collision with railway train or railway vehicle in nontraffic accident**

X **V25.1 Motorcycle passenger injured in collision with railway train or railway vehicle in nontraffic accident**

X **V25.2 Unspecified motorcycle rider injured in collision with railway train or railway vehicle in nontraffic accident**

X **V25.3 Person boarding or alighting a motorcycle injured in collision with railway train or railway vehicle**

X **V25.4 Motorcycle driver injured in collision with railway train or railway vehicle in traffic accident**

X **V25.5 Motorcycle passenger injured in collision with railway train or railway vehicle in traffic accident**

X **V25.9 Unspecified motorcycle rider injured in collision with railway train or railway vehicle in traffic accident**

V26 Motorcycle rider injured in collision with other nonmotor vehicle

Includes collision with animal-drawn vehicle, animal being ridden, streetcar

The appropriate 7th character is to be added to each code from category V26

A	initial encounter
D	subsequent encounter
S	sequela

X **V26.0 Motorcycle driver injured in collision with other nonmotor vehicle in nontraffic accident**

X **V26.1 Motorcycle passenger injured in collision with other nonmotor vehicle in nontraffic accident**

X **V26.2 Unspecified motorcycle rider injured in collision with other nonmotor vehicle in nontraffic accident**

X **V26.3 Person boarding or alighting a motorcycle injured in collision with other nonmotor vehicle**

X **V26.4 Motorcycle driver injured in collision with other nonmotor vehicle in traffic accident**

X **V26.5 Motorcycle passenger injured in collision with other nonmotor vehicle in traffic accident**

X **V26.9 Unspecified motorcycle rider injured in collision with other nonmotor vehicle in traffic accident**

V27 Motorcycle rider injured in collision with fixed or stationary object

The appropriate 7th character is to be added to each code from category V27

A	initial encounter
D	subsequent encounter
S	sequela

X **V27.0 Motorcycle driver injured in collision with fixed or stationary object in nontraffic accident**

X **V27.1 Motorcycle passenger injured in collision with fixed or stationary object in nontraffic accident**

X **V27.2 Unspecified motorcycle rider injured in collision with fixed or stationary object in nontraffic accident**

X **V27.3 Person boarding or alighting a motorcycle injured in collision with fixed or stationary object**

X **V27.4 Motorcycle driver injured in collision with fixed or stationary object in traffic accident**

X **V27.5 Motorcycle passenger injured in collision with fixed or stationary object in traffic accident**

X **V27.9 Unspecified motorcycle rider injured in collision with fixed or stationary object in traffic accident**

● **V28 Motorcycle rider injured in noncollision transport accident**

Includes fall or thrown from motorcycle (without antecedent collision)
overturning motorcycle NOS
overturning motorcycle without collision

The appropriate 7th character is to be added to each code from category V28

A	initial encounter
D	subsequent encounter
S	sequela

X● **V28.0 Motorcycle driver injured in noncollision transport accident in nontraffic accident**

X● **V28.1 Motorcycle passenger injured in noncollision transport accident in nontraffic accident**

X● **V28.2 Unspecified motorcycle rider injured in noncollision transport accident in nontraffic accident**

X● **V28.3 Person boarding or alighting a motorcycle injured in noncollision transport accident**

X● **V28.4 Motorcycle driver injured in noncollision transport accident in traffic accident**

X● **V28.5 Motorcycle passenger injured in noncollision transport accident in traffic accident**

X● **V28.9 Unspecified motorcycle rider injured in noncollision transport accident in traffic accident**

● **V29 Motorcycle rider injured in other and unspecified transport accidents**

The appropriate 7th character is to be added to each code from category V29

A	initial encounter
D	subsequent encounter
S	sequela

Coding Clinic: 2015, Q3, P20

● **V29.0 Motorcycle driver injured in collision with other and unspecified motor vehicles in nontraffic accident**

X● **V29.00 Motorcycle driver injured in collision with unspecified motor vehicles in nontraffic accident**

X● **V29.09 Motorcycle driver injured in collision with other motor vehicles in nontraffic accident**

● **V29.1 Motorcycle passenger injured in collision with other and unspecified motor vehicles in nontraffic accident**

X● **V29.10 Motorcycle passenger injured in collision with unspecified motor vehicles in nontraffic accident**

X● **V29.19 Motorcycle passenger injured in collision with other motor vehicles in nontraffic accident**

● **V29.2 Unspecified motorcycle rider injured in collision with other and unspecified motor vehicles in nontraffic accident**

X● **V29.20 Unspecified motorcycle rider injured in collision with unspecified motor vehicles in nontraffic accident**
Motorcycle collision NOS, nontraffic

X● **V29.29 Unspecified motorcycle rider injured in collision with other motor vehicles in nontraffic accident**

X● **V29.3 Motorcycle rider (driver) (passenger) injured in unspecified nontraffic accident**
Motorcycle accident NOS, nontraffic
Motorcycle rider injured in nontraffic accident NOS

● **V29.4 Motorcycle driver injured in collision with other and unspecified motor vehicles in traffic accident**

X● **V29.40 Motorcycle driver injured in collision with unspecified motor vehicles in traffic accident**

X● **V29.49 Motorcycle driver injured in collision with other motor vehicles in traffic accident**

● **V29.5 Motorcycle passenger injured in collision with other and unspecified motor vehicles in traffic accident**

X● **V29.50 Motorcycle passenger injured in collision with unspecified motor vehicles in traffic accident**

X● **V29.59 Motorcycle passenger injured in collision with other motor vehicles in traffic accident**

● **V29.6 Unspecified motorcycle rider injured in collision with other and unspecified motor vehicles in traffic accident**

X● **V29.60 Unspecified motorcycle rider injured in collision with unspecified motor vehicles in traffic accident**
Motorcycle collision NOS (traffic)

X● **V29.69 Unspecified motorcycle rider injured in collision with other motor vehicles in traffic accident**

● **V29.8 Motorcycle rider (driver) (passenger) injured in other specified transport accidents**

X● **V29.81 Motorcycle rider (driver) (passenger) injured in transport accident with military vehicle**

X● **V29.88 Motorcycle rider (driver) (passenger) injured in other specified transport accidents**

X● **V29.9 Motorcycle rider (driver) (passenger) injured in unspecified traffic accident**
Motorcycle accident NOS

OCCUPANT OF THREE-WHEELED MOTOR VEHICLE INJURED IN TRANSPORT ACCIDENT (V30-V39)

Includes motorized tricycle
motorized rickshaw
three-wheeled motor car

Excludes1 all-terrain vehicles (V86.-)
motorcycle with sidecar (V20-V29)
vehicle designed primarily for off-road use (V86.-)

● **V30 Occupant of three-wheeled motor vehicle injured in collision with pedestrian or animal**

Excludes1 three-wheeled motor vehicle collision with animal-drawn vehicle or animal being ridden (V36.-)

The appropriate 7th character is to be added to each code from category V30

A	initial encounter
D	subsequent encounter
S	sequela

X● **V30.0 Driver of three-wheeled motor vehicle injured in collision with pedestrian or animal in nontraffic accident**

X● **V30.1 Passenger in three-wheeled motor vehicle injured in collision with pedestrian or animal in nontraffic accident**

X● **V30.2 Person on outside of three-wheeled motor vehicle injured in collision with pedestrian or animal in nontraffic accident**

X● **V30.3 Unspecified occupant of three-wheeled motor vehicle injured in collision with pedestrian or animal in nontraffic accident**

X● **V30.4 Person boarding or alighting a three-wheeled motor vehicle injured in collision with pedestrian or animal**

X● **V30.5 Driver of three-wheeled motor vehicle injured in collision with pedestrian or animal in traffic accident**

X● **V30.6 Passenger in three-wheeled motor vehicle injured in collision with pedestrian or animal in traffic accident**

X● **V30.7 Person on outside of three-wheeled motor vehicle injured in collision with pedestrian or animal in traffic accident**

X● **V30.9 Unspecified occupant of three-wheeled motor vehicle injured in collision with pedestrian or animal in traffic accident**

V31 Occupant of three-wheeled motor vehicle injured in collision with pedal cycle

The appropriate 7th character is to be added to each code from category V31

A	initial encounter
D	subsequent encounter
S	sequela

X **V31.0 Driver of three-wheeled motor vehicle injured in collision with pedal cycle in nontraffic accident**

X **V31.1 Passenger in three-wheeled motor vehicle injured in collision with pedal cycle in nontraffic accident**

X **V31.2 Person on outside of three-wheeled motor vehicle injured in collision with pedal cycle in nontraffic accident**

X **V31.3 Unspecified occupant of three-wheeled motor vehicle injured in collision with pedal cycle in nontraffic accident**

X **V31.4 Person boarding or alighting a three-wheeled motor vehicle injured in collision with pedal cycle**

X **V31.5 Driver of three-wheeled motor vehicle injured in collision with pedal cycle in traffic accident**

X **V31.6 Passenger in three-wheeled motor vehicle injured in collision with pedal cycle in traffic accident**

X **V31.7 Person on outside of three-wheeled motor vehicle injured in collision with pedal cycle in traffic accident**

X **V31.9 Unspecified occupant of three-wheeled motor vehicle injured in collision with pedal cycle in traffic accident**

V32 Occupant of three-wheeled motor vehicle injured in collision with two- or three-wheeled motor vehicle

The appropriate 7th character is to be added to each code from category V32

A	initial encounter
D	subsequent encounter
S	sequela

X **V32.0 Driver of three-wheeled motor vehicle injured in collision with two- or three-wheeled motor vehicle in nontraffic accident**

X **V32.1 Passenger in three-wheeled motor vehicle injured in collision with two- or three-wheeled motor vehicle in nontraffic accident**

X **V32.2 Person on outside of three-wheeled motor vehicle injured in collision with two- or three-wheeled motor vehicle in nontraffic accident**

X **V32.3 Unspecified occupant of three-wheeled motor vehicle injured in collision with two- or three-wheeled motor vehicle in nontraffic accident**

X **V32.4 Person boarding or alighting a three-wheeled motor vehicle injured in collision with two- or three-wheeled motor vehicle**

X **V32.5 Driver of three-wheeled motor vehicle injured in collision with two- or three-wheeled motor vehicle in traffic accident**

X **V32.6 Passenger in three-wheeled motor vehicle injured in collision with two- or three-wheeled motor vehicle in traffic accident**

X **V32.7 Person on outside of three-wheeled motor vehicle injured in collision with two- or three-wheeled motor vehicle in traffic accident**

X **V32.9 Unspecified occupant of three-wheeled motor vehicle injured in collision with two- or three-wheeled motor vehicle in traffic accident**

V33 Occupant of three-wheeled motor vehicle injured in collision with car, pick-up truck or van

The appropriate 7th character is to be added to each code from category V33

A	initial encounter
D	subsequent encounter
S	sequela

X **V33.0 Driver of three-wheeled motor vehicle injured in collision with car, pick-up truck or van in nontraffic accident**

X **V33.1 Passenger in three-wheeled motor vehicle injured in collision with car, pick-up truck or van in nontraffic accident**

X **V33.2 Person on outside of three-wheeled motor vehicle injured in collision with car, pick-up truck or van in nontraffic accident**

X **V33.3 Unspecified occupant of three-wheeled motor vehicle injured in collision with car, pick-up truck or van in nontraffic accident**

X **V33.4 Person boarding or alighting a three-wheeled motor vehicle injured in collision with car, pick-up truck or van**

X **V33.5 Driver of three-wheeled motor vehicle injured in collision with car, pick-up truck or van in traffic accident**

X **V33.6 Passenger in three-wheeled motor vehicle injured in collision with car, pick-up truck or van in traffic accident**

X **V33.7 Person on outside of three-wheeled motor vehicle injured in collision with car, pick-up truck or van in traffic accident**

X **V33.9 Unspecified occupant of three-wheeled motor vehicle injured in collision with car, pick-up truck or van in traffic accident**

V34 Occupant of three-wheeled motor vehicle injured in collision with heavy transport vehicle or bus

Excludes1 occupant of three-wheeled motor vehicle injured in collision with military vehicle (V39.81)

The appropriate 7th character is to be added to each code from category V34

A	initial encounter
D	subsequent encounter
S	sequela

X **V34.0 Driver of three-wheeled motor vehicle injured in collision with heavy transport vehicle or bus in nontraffic accident**

X **V34.1 Passenger in three-wheeled motor vehicle injured in collision with heavy transport vehicle or bus in nontraffic accident**

X **V34.2 Person on outside of three-wheeled motor vehicle injured in collision with heavy transport vehicle or bus in nontraffic accident**

X **V34.3 Unspecified occupant of three-wheeled motor vehicle injured in collision with heavy transport vehicle or bus in nontraffic accident**

X **V34.4 Person boarding or alighting a three-wheeled motor vehicle injured in collision with heavy transport vehicle or bus**

X **V34.5 Driver of three-wheeled motor vehicle injured in collision with heavy transport vehicle or bus in traffic accident**

X **V34.6 Passenger in three-wheeled motor vehicle injured in collision with heavy transport vehicle or bus in traffic accident**

X **V34.7 Person on outside of three-wheeled motor vehicle injured in collision with heavy transport vehicle or bus in traffic accident**

X **V34.9 Unspecified occupant of three-wheeled motor vehicle injured in collision with heavy transport vehicle or bus in traffic accident**

● **V35 Occupant of three-wheeled motor vehicle injured in collision with railway train or railway vehicle**

The appropriate 7th character is to be added to each code from category V35

A	initial encounter
D	subsequent encounter
S	sequela

X● **V35.0 Driver of three-wheeled motor vehicle injured in collision with railway train or railway vehicle in nontraffic accident**

X● **V35.1 Passenger in three-wheeled motor vehicle injured in collision with railway train or railway vehicle in nontraffic accident**

X● **V35.2 Person on outside of three-wheeled motor vehicle injured in collision with railway train or railway vehicle in nontraffic accident**

X● **V35.3 Unspecified occupant of three-wheeled motor vehicle injured in collision with railway train or railway vehicle in nontraffic accident**

X● **V35.4 Person boarding or alighting a three-wheeled motor vehicle injured in collision with railway train or railway vehicle**

X● **V35.5 Driver of three-wheeled motor vehicle injured in collision with railway train or railway vehicle in traffic accident**

X● **V35.6 Passenger in three-wheeled motor vehicle injured in collision with railway train or railway vehicle in traffic accident**

X● **V35.7 Person on outside of three-wheeled motor vehicle injured in collision with railway train or railway vehicle in traffic accident**

X● **V35.9 Unspecified occupant of three-wheeled motor vehicle injured in collision with railway train or railway vehicle in traffic accident**

● **V36 Occupant of three-wheeled motor vehicle injured in collision with other nonmotor vehicle**

Includes collision with animal-drawn vehicle, animal being ridden, streetcar

The appropriate 7th character is to be added to each code from category V36

A	initial encounter
D	subsequent encounter
S	sequela

X● **V36.0 Driver of three-wheeled motor vehicle injured in collision with other nonmotor vehicle in nontraffic accident**

X● **V36.1 Passenger in three-wheeled motor vehicle injured in collision with other nonmotor vehicle in nontraffic accident**

X● **V36.2 Person on outside of three-wheeled motor vehicle injured in collision with other nonmotor vehicle in nontraffic accident**

X● **V36.3 Unspecified occupant of three-wheeled motor vehicle injured in collision with other nonmotor vehicle in nontraffic accident**

X● **V36.4 Person boarding or alighting a three-wheeled motor vehicle injured in collision with other nonmotor vehicle**

X● **V36.5 Driver of three-wheeled motor vehicle injured in collision with other nonmotor vehicle in traffic accident**

X● **V36.6 Passenger in three-wheeled motor vehicle injured in collision with other nonmotor vehicle in traffic accident**

X● **V36.7 Person on outside of three-wheeled motor vehicle injured in collision with other nonmotor vehicle in traffic accident**

X● **V36.9 Unspecified occupant of three-wheeled motor vehicle injured in collision with other nonmotor vehicle in traffic accident**

● **V37 Occupant of three-wheeled motor vehicle injured in collision with fixed or stationary object**

The appropriate 7th character is to be added to each code from category V37

A	initial encounter
D	subsequent encounter
S	sequela

X● **V37.0 Driver of three-wheeled motor vehicle injured in collision with fixed or stationary object in nontraffic accident**

X● **V37.1 Passenger in three-wheeled motor vehicle injured in collision with fixed or stationary object in nontraffic accident**

X● **V37.2 Person on outside of three-wheeled motor vehicle injured in collision with fixed or stationary object in nontraffic accident**

X● **V37.3 Unspecified occupant of three-wheeled motor vehicle injured in collision with fixed or stationary object in nontraffic accident**

X● **V37.4 Person boarding or alighting a three-wheeled motor vehicle injured in collision with fixed or stationary object**

X● **V37.5 Driver of three-wheeled motor vehicle injured in collision with fixed or stationary object in traffic accident**

X● **V37.6 Passenger in three-wheeled motor vehicle injured in collision with fixed or stationary object in traffic accident**

X● **V37.7 Person on outside of three-wheeled motor vehicle injured in collision with fixed or stationary object in traffic accident**

X● **V37.9 Unspecified occupant of three-wheeled motor vehicle injured in collision with fixed or stationary object in traffic accident**

● **V38 Occupant of three-wheeled motor vehicle injured in noncollision transport accident**

Includes fall or thrown from three-wheeled motor vehicle
overturning of three-wheeled motor vehicle NOS
overturning of three-wheeled motor vehicle without collision

The appropriate 7th character is to be added to each code from category V38

A	initial encounter
D	subsequent encounter
S	sequela

X● **V38.0 Driver of three-wheeled motor vehicle injured in noncollision transport accident in nontraffic accident**

X● **V38.1 Passenger in three-wheeled motor vehicle injured in noncollision transport accident in nontraffic accident**

X● **V38.2 Person on outside of three-wheeled motor vehicle injured in noncollision transport accident in nontraffic accident**

X● **V38.3 Unspecified occupant of three-wheeled motor vehicle injured in noncollision transport accident in nontraffic accident**

X● **V38.4 Person boarding or alighting a three-wheeled motor vehicle injured in noncollision transport accident**

X● **V38.5 Driver of three-wheeled motor vehicle injured in noncollision transport accident in traffic accident**

X● **V38.6 Passenger in three-wheeled motor vehicle injured in noncollision transport accident in traffic accident**

X● **V38.7 Person on outside of three-wheeled motor vehicle injured in noncollision transport accident in traffic accident**

X● **V38.9 Unspecified occupant of three-wheeled motor vehicle injured in noncollision transport accident in traffic accident**

V39 Occupant of three-wheeled motor vehicle injured in other and unspecified transport accidents

The appropriate 7th character is to be added to each code from category V39

A	initial encounter
D	subsequent encounter
S	sequela

V39.0 Driver of three-wheeled motor vehicle injured in collision with other and unspecified motor vehicles in nontraffic accident

X **V39.00 Driver of three-wheeled motor vehicle injured in collision with unspecified motor vehicles in nontraffic accident**

X **V39.09 Driver of three-wheeled motor vehicle injured in collision with other motor vehicles in nontraffic accident**

V39.1 Passenger in three-wheeled motor vehicle injured in collision with other and unspecified motor vehicles in nontraffic accident

X **V39.10 Passenger in three-wheeled motor vehicle injured in collision with unspecified motor vehicles in nontraffic accident**

X **V39.19 Passenger in three-wheeled motor vehicle injured in collision with other motor vehicles in nontraffic accident**

V39.2 Unspecified occupant of three-wheeled motor vehicle injured in collision with other and unspecified motor vehicles in nontraffic accident

X **V39.20 Unspecified occupant of three-wheeled motor vehicle injured in collision with unspecified motor vehicles in nontraffic accident**

Collision NOS involving three-wheeled motor vehicle, nontraffic

X **V39.29 Unspecified occupant of three-wheeled motor vehicle injured in collision with other motor vehicles in nontraffic accident**

X **V39.3 Occupant (driver) (passenger) of three-wheeled motor vehicle injured in unspecified nontraffic accident**

Accident NOS involving three-wheeled motor vehicle, nontraffic

Occupant of three-wheeled motor vehicle injured in nontraffic accident NOS

V39.4 Driver of three-wheeled motor vehicle injured in collision with other and unspecified motor vehicles in traffic accident

X **V39.40 Driver of three-wheeled motor vehicle injured in collision with unspecified motor vehicles in traffic accident**

X **V39.49 Driver of three-wheeled motor vehicle injured in collision with other motor vehicles in traffic accident**

V39.5 Passenger in three-wheeled motor vehicle injured in collision with other and unspecified motor vehicles in traffic accident

X **V39.50 Passenger in three-wheeled motor vehicle injured in collision with unspecified motor vehicles in traffic accident**

X **V39.59 Passenger in three-wheeled motor vehicle injured in collision with other motor vehicles in traffic accident**

V39.6 Unspecified occupant of three-wheeled motor vehicle injured in collision with other and unspecified motor vehicles in traffic accident

X **V39.60 Unspecified occupant of three-wheeled motor vehicle injured in collision with unspecified motor vehicles in traffic accident**

Collision NOS involving three-wheeled motor vehicle (traffic)

X **V39.69 Unspecified occupant of three-wheeled motor vehicle injured in collision with other motor vehicles in traffic accident**

V39.8 Occupant (driver) (passenger) of three-wheeled motor vehicle injured in other specified transport accidents

X **V39.81 Occupant (driver) (passenger) of three-wheeled motor vehicle injured in transport accident with military vehicle**

X **V39.89 Occupant (driver) (passenger) of three-wheeled motor vehicle injured in other specified transport accidents**

X **V39.9 Occupant (driver) (passenger) of three-wheeled motor vehicle injured in unspecified traffic accident**

Accident NOS involving three-wheeled motor vehicle

CAR OCCUPANT INJURED IN TRANSPORT ACCIDENT (V40-V49)

Includes a four-wheeled motor vehicle designed primarily for carrying passengers
automobile (pulling a trailer or camper)

Excludes1 bus (V50-V59)
minibus (V50-V59)
minivan (V50-V59)
motorcoach (V70-V79)
pick-up truck (V50-V59)
sport utility vehicle (SUV) (V50-V59)

V40 Car occupant injured in collision with pedestrian or animal

Excludes1 car collision with animal-drawn vehicle or animal being ridden (V46.-)

The appropriate 7th character is to be added to each code from category V40

A	initial encounter
D	subsequent encounter
S	sequela

X **V40.0 Car driver injured in collision with pedestrian or animal in nontraffic accident**

X **V40.1 Car passenger injured in collision with pedestrian or animal in nontraffic accident**

X **V40.2 Person on outside of car injured in collision with pedestrian or animal in nontraffic accident**

X **V40.3 Unspecified car occupant injured in collision with pedestrian or animal in nontraffic accident**

X **V40.4 Person boarding or alighting a car injured in collision with pedestrian or animal**

X **V40.5 Car driver injured in collision with pedestrian or animal in traffic accident**

X **V40.6 Car passenger injured in collision with pedestrian or animal in traffic accident**

X **V40.7 Person on outside of car injured in collision with pedestrian or animal in traffic accident**

X **V40.9 Unspecified car occupant injured in collision with pedestrian or animal in traffic accident**

V41 Car occupant injured in collision with pedal cycle

The appropriate 7th character is to be added to each code from category V41

A	initial encounter
D	subsequent encounter
S	sequela

X **V41.0 Car driver injured in collision with pedal cycle in nontraffic accident**

X **V41.1 Car passenger injured in collision with pedal cycle in nontraffic accident**

X **V41.2 Person on outside of car injured in collision with pedal cycle in nontraffic accident**

X **V41.3 Unspecified car occupant injured in collision with pedal cycle in nontraffic accident**

X **V41.4 Person boarding or alighting a car injured in collision with pedal cycle**

X **V41.5 Car driver injured in collision with pedal cycle in traffic accident**

X **V41.6 Car passenger injured in collision with pedal cycle in traffic accident**

X● V41.7 Person on outside of car injured in collision with pedal cycle in traffic accident

X● V41.9 Unspecified car occupant injured in collision with pedal cycle in traffic accident

● V42 Car occupant injured in collision with two- or three-wheeled motor vehicle

The appropriate 7th character is to be added to each code from category V42

A	initial encounter
D	subsequent encounter
S	sequela

X● V42.0 Car driver injured in collision with two- or three-wheeled motor vehicle in nontraffic accident

X● V42.1 Car passenger injured in collision with two- or three-wheeled motor vehicle in nontraffic accident

X● V42.2 Person on outside of car injured in collision with two- or three-wheeled motor vehicle in nontraffic accident

X● V42.3 Unspecified car occupant injured in collision with two- or three-wheeled motor vehicle in nontraffic accident

X● V42.4 Person boarding or alighting a car injured in collision with two- or three-wheeled motor vehicle

X● V42.5 Car driver injured in collision with two- or three-wheeled motor vehicle in traffic accident

X● V42.6 Car passenger injured in collision with two- or three-wheeled motor vehicle in traffic accident

X● V42.7 Person on outside of car injured in collision with two- or three-wheeled motor vehicle in traffic accident

X● V42.9 Unspecified car occupant injured in collision with two- or three-wheeled motor vehicle in traffic accident

● V43 Car occupant injured in collision with car, pick-up truck or van

The appropriate 7th character is to be added to each code from category V43

A	initial encounter
D	subsequent encounter
S	sequela

● V43.0 Car driver injured in collision with car, pick-up truck or van in nontraffic accident

X● V43.01 Car driver injured in collision with sport utility vehicle in nontraffic accident

X● V43.02 Car driver injured in collision with other type car in nontraffic accident

X● V43.03 Car driver injured in collision with pick-up truck in nontraffic accident

X● V43.04 Car driver injured in collision with van in nontraffic accident

● V43.1 Car passenger injured in collision with car, pick-up truck or van in nontraffic accident

X● V43.11 Car passenger injured in collision with sport utility vehicle in nontraffic accident

X● V43.12 Car passenger injured in collision with other type car in nontraffic accident

X● V43.13 Car passenger injured in collision with pick-up in nontraffic accident

X● V43.14 Car passenger injured in collision with van in nontraffic accident

● V43.2 Person on outside of car injured in collision with car, pick-up truck or van in nontraffic accident

X● V43.21 Person on outside of car injured in collision with sport utility vehicle in nontraffic accident

X● V43.22 Person on outside of car injured in collision with other type car in nontraffic accident

X● V43.23 Person on outside of car injured in collision with pick-up truck in nontraffic accident

X● V43.24 Person on outside of car injured in collision with van in nontraffic accident

● V43.3 Unspecified car occupant injured in collision with car, pick-up truck or van in nontraffic accident

X● V43.31 Unspecified car occupant injured in collision with sport utility vehicle in nontraffic accident

X● V43.32 Unspecified car occupant injured in collision with other type car in nontraffic accident

X● V43.33 Unspecified car occupant injured in collision with pick-up truck in nontraffic accident

X● V43.34 Unspecified car occupant injured in collision with van in nontraffic accident

● V43.4 Person boarding or alighting a car injured in collision with car, pick-up truck or van

X● V43.41 Person boarding or alighting a car injured in collision with sport utility vehicle

X● V43.42 Person boarding or alighting a car injured in collision with other type car

X● V43.43 Person boarding or alighting a car injured in collision with pick-up truck

X● V43.44 Person boarding or alighting a car injured in collision with van

● V43.5 Car driver injured in collision with car, pick-up truck or van in traffic accident

X● V43.51 Car driver injured in collision with sport utility vehicle in traffic accident

X● V43.52 Car driver injured in collision with other type car in traffic accident

X● V43.53 Car driver injured in collision with pick-up truck in traffic accident

X● V43.54 Car driver injured in collision with van in traffic accident

● V43.6 Car passenger injured in collision with car, pick-up truck or van in traffic accident

X● V43.61 Car passenger injured in collision with sport utility vehicle in traffic accident

Coding Clinic: 2015, Q1, P5-7

X● V43.62 Car passenger injured in collision with other type car in traffic accident

X● V43.63 Car passenger injured in collision with pick-up truck in traffic accident

X● V43.64 Car passenger injured in collision with van in traffic accident

● V43.7 Person on outside of car injured in collision with car, pick-up truck or van in traffic accident

X● V43.71 Person on outside of car injured in collision with sport utility vehicle in traffic accident

X● V43.72 Person on outside of car injured in collision with other type car in traffic accident

X● V43.73 Person on outside of car injured in collision with pick-up truck in traffic accident

X● V43.74 Person on outside of car injured in collision with van in traffic accident

● V43.9 Unspecified car occupant injured in collision with car, pick-up truck or van in traffic accident

X● V43.91 Unspecified car occupant injured in collision with sport utility vehicle in traffic accident

X● V43.92 Unspecified car occupant injured in collision with other type car in traffic accident

X● V43.93 Unspecified car occupant injured in collision with pick-up truck in traffic accident

X● V43.94 Unspecified car occupant injured in collision with van in traffic accident

● **V44 Car occupant injured in collision with heavy transport vehicle or bus**

Excludes1 car occupant injured in collision with military vehicle (V49.81)

The appropriate 7th character is to be added to each code from category V44

A	initial encounter
D	subsequent encounter
S	sequela

X● **V44.0 Car driver injured in collision with heavy transport vehicle or bus in nontraffic accident**

X● **V44.1 Car passenger injured in collision with heavy transport vehicle or bus in nontraffic accident**

X● **V44.2 Person on outside of car injured in collision with heavy transport vehicle or bus in nontraffic accident**

X● **V44.3 Unspecified car occupant injured in collision with heavy transport vehicle or bus in nontraffic accident**

X● **V44.4 Person boarding or alighting a car injured in collision with heavy transport vehicle or bus**

X● **V44.5 Car driver injured in collision with heavy transport vehicle or bus in traffic accident**

X● **V44.6 Car passenger injured in collision with heavy transport vehicle or bus in traffic accident**

X● **V44.7 Person on outside of car injured in collision with heavy transport vehicle or bus in traffic accident**

X● **V44.9 Unspecified car occupant injured in collision with heavy transport vehicle or bus in traffic accident**

● **V45 Car occupant injured in collision with railway train or railway vehicle**

The appropriate 7th character is to be added to each code from category V45

A	initial encounter
D	subsequent encounter
S	sequela

X● **V45.0 Car driver injured in collision with railway train or railway vehicle in nontraffic accident**

X● **V45.1 Car passenger injured in collision with railway train or railway vehicle in nontraffic accident**

X● **V45.2 Person on outside of car injured in collision with railway train or railway vehicle in nontraffic accident**

X● **V45.3 Unspecified car occupant injured in collision with railway train or railway vehicle in nontraffic accident**

X● **V45.4 Person boarding or alighting a car injured in collision with railway train or railway vehicle**

X● **V45.5 Car driver injured in collision with railway train or railway vehicle in traffic accident**

X● **V45.6 Car passenger injured in collision with railway train or railway vehicle in traffic accident**

X● **V45.7 Person on outside of car injured in collision with railway train or railway vehicle in traffic accident**

X● **V45.9 Unspecified car occupant injured in collision with railway train or railway vehicle in traffic accident**

● **V46 Car occupant injured in collision with other nonmotor vehicle**

Includes collision with animal-drawn vehicle, animal being ridden, streetcar

The appropriate 7th character is to be added to each code from category V46

A	initial encounter
D	subsequent encounter
S	sequela

X● **V46.0 Car driver injured in collision with other nonmotor vehicle in nontraffic accident**

X● **V46.1 Car passenger injured in collision with other nonmotor vehicle in nontraffic accident**

X● **V46.2 Person on outside of car injured in collision with other nonmotor vehicle in nontraffic accident**

X● **V46.3 Unspecified car occupant injured in collision with other nonmotor vehicle in nontraffic accident**

X● **V46.4 Person boarding or alighting a car injured in collision with other nonmotor vehicle**

X● **V46.5 Car driver injured in collision with other nonmotor vehicle in traffic accident**

X● **V46.6 Car passenger injured in collision with other nonmotor vehicle in traffic accident**

X● **V46.7 Person on outside of car injured in collision with other nonmotor vehicle in traffic accident**

X● **V46.9 Unspecified car occupant injured in collision with other nonmotor vehicle in traffic accident**

● **V47 Car occupant injured in collision with fixed or stationary object**

The appropriate 7th character is to be added to each code from category V47

A	initial encounter
D	subsequent encounter
S	sequela

X● **V47.0 Car driver injured in collision with fixed or stationary object in nontraffic accident**

~~V47.01 Driver of sport utility vehicle injured in collision with fixed or stationary object in nontraffic accident~~

~~V47.02 Driver of other type car injured in collision with fixed or stationary object in nontraffic accident~~

X● **V47.1 Car passenger injured in collision with fixed or stationary object in nontraffic accident**

~~V47.11 Passenger of sport utility vehicle injured in collision with fixed or stationary object in nontraffic accident~~

~~V47.12 Passenger of other type car injured in collision with fixed or stationary object in nontraffic accident~~

X● **V47.2 Person on outside of car injured in collision with fixed or stationary object in nontraffic accident**

X● **V47.3 Unspecified car occupant injured in collision with fixed or stationary object in nontraffic accident**

~~V47.31 Unspecified occupant of sport utility vehicle injured in collision with fixed or stationary object in nontraffic accident~~

~~V47.32 Unspecified occupant of other type car injured in collision with fixed or stationary object in nontraffic accident~~

X● **V47.4 Person boarding or alighting a car injured in collision with fixed or stationary object**

X● **V47.5 Car driver injured in collision with fixed or stationary object in traffic accident**

~~V47.51 Driver of sport utility vehicle injured in collision with fixed or stationary object in traffic accident~~

~~V47.52 Driver of other type car injured in collision with fixed or stationary object in traffic accident~~

X● **V47.6 Car passenger injured in collision with fixed or stationary object in traffic accident**

~~V47.61 Passenger of sport utility vehicle injured in collision with fixed or stationary object in traffic accident~~

~~V47.62 Passenger of other type car injured in collision with fixed or stationary object in traffic accident~~

X● **V47.7 Person on outside of car injured in collision with fixed or stationary object in traffic accident**

X● **V47.9 Unspecified car occupant injured in collision with fixed or stationary object in traffic accident**

~~V47.91 Unspecified occupant of sport utility vehicle injured in collision with fixed or stationary object in traffic accident~~

~~V47.92 Unspecified occupant of other type car injured in collision with fixed or stationary object in traffic accident~~

V48 Car occupant injured in noncollision transport accident

Includes overturning car NOS
overturning car without collision

The appropriate 7th character is to be added to each code from category V48

A	initial encounter
D	subsequent encounter
S	sequela

X **V48.0 Car driver injured in noncollision transport accident in nontraffic accident**

X **V48.1 Car passenger injured in noncollision transport accident in nontraffic accident**

X **V48.2 Person on outside of car injured in noncollision transport accident in nontraffic accident**

X **V48.3 Unspecified car occupant injured in noncollision transport accident in nontraffic accident**

X **V48.4 Person boarding or alighting a car injured in noncollision transport accident**

X **V48.5 Car driver injured in noncollision transport accident in traffic accident**

X **V48.6 Car passenger injured in noncollision transport accident in traffic accident**

X **V48.7 Person on outside of car injured in noncollision transport accident in traffic accident**

X **V48.9 Unspecified car occupant injured in noncollision transport accident in traffic accident**

V49 Car occupant injured in other and unspecified transport accidents

The appropriate 7th character is to be added to each code from category V49

A	initial encounter
D	subsequent encounter
S	sequela

V49.0 Driver injured in collision with other and unspecified motor vehicles in nontraffic accident

X **V49.00 Driver injured in collision with unspecified motor vehicles in nontraffic accident**

X **V49.09 Driver injured in collision with other motor vehicles in nontraffic accident**

V49.1 Passenger injured in collision with other and unspecified motor vehicles in nontraffic accident

X **V49.10 Passenger injured in collision with unspecified motor vehicles in nontraffic accident**

X **V49.19 Passenger injured in collision with other motor vehicles in nontraffic accident**

V49.2 Unspecified car occupant injured in collision with other and unspecified motor vehicles in nontraffic accident

X **V49.20 Unspecified car occupant injured in collision with unspecified motor vehicles in nontraffic accident**
Car collision NOS, nontraffic

X **V49.29 Unspecified car occupant injured in collision with other motor vehicles in nontraffic accident**

X **V49.3 Car occupant (driver) (passenger) injured in unspecified nontraffic accident**
Car accident NOS, nontraffic
Car occupant injured in nontraffic accident NOS

V49.4 Driver injured in collision with other and unspecified motor vehicles in traffic accident

X **V49.40 Driver injured in collision with unspecified motor vehicles in traffic accident**

X **V49.49 Driver injured in collision with other motor vehicles in traffic accident**

V49.5 Passenger injured in collision with other and unspecified motor vehicles in traffic accident

X **V49.50 Passenger injured in collision with unspecified motor vehicles in traffic accident**

X **V49.59 Passenger injured in collision with other motor vehicles in traffic accident**

V49.6 Unspecified car occupant injured in collision with other and unspecified motor vehicles in traffic accident

X **V49.60 Unspecified car occupant injured in collision with unspecified motor vehicles in traffic accident**
Car collision NOS (traffic)

X **V49.69 Unspecified car occupant injured in collision with other motor vehicles in traffic accident**

V49.8 Car occupant (driver) (passenger) injured in other specified transport accidents

X **V49.81 Car occupant (driver) (passenger) injured in transport accident with military vehicle**

X **V49.88 Car occupant (driver) (passenger) injured in other specified transport accidents**

X **V49.9 Car occupant (driver) (passenger) injured in unspecified traffic accident**
Car accident NOS
Coding Clinic: 2015, Q1, P11

OCCUPANT OF PICK-UP TRUCK OR VAN INJURED IN TRANSPORT ACCIDENT (V50-V59)

Includes a four- or six-wheel motor vehicle designed primarily for carrying passengers and property but weighing less than the local limit for classification as a heavy goods vehicle
minibus
minivan
sport utility vehicle (SUV)
truck
van

Excludes1 heavy transport vehicle (V60-V69)

V50 Occupant of pick-up truck or van injured in collision with pedestrian or animal

Excludes1 pick-up truck or van collision with animal-drawn vehicle or animal being ridden (V56.-)

The appropriate 7th character is to be added to each code from category V50

A	initial encounter
D	subsequent encounter
S	sequela

X **V50.0 Driver of pick-up truck or van injured in collision with pedestrian or animal in nontraffic accident**

X **V50.1 Passenger in pick-up truck or van injured in collision with pedestrian or animal in nontraffic accident**

X **V50.2 Person on outside of pick-up truck or van injured in collision with pedestrian or animal in nontraffic accident**

X **V50.3 Unspecified occupant of pick-up truck or van injured in collision with pedestrian or animal in nontraffic accident**

X **V50.4 Person boarding or alighting a pick-up truck or van injured in collision with pedestrian or animal**

X **V50.5 Driver of pick-up truck or van injured in collision with pedestrian or animal in traffic accident**

X **V50.6 Passenger in pick-up truck or van injured in collision with pedestrian or animal in traffic accident**

X **V50.7 Person on outside of pick-up truck or van injured in collision with pedestrian or animal in traffic accident**

X **V50.9 Unspecified occupant of pick-up truck or van injured in collision with pedestrian or animal in traffic accident**

● **V51 Occupant of pick-up truck or van injured in collision with pedal cycle**

The appropriate 7th character is to be added to each code from category V51

A	initial encounter
D	subsequent encounter
S	sequela

X● **V51.0 Driver of pick-up truck or van injured in collision with pedal cycle in nontraffic accident**

X● **V51.1 Passenger in pick-up truck or van injured in collision with pedal cycle in nontraffic accident**

X● **V51.2 Person on outside of pick-up truck or van injured in collision with pedal cycle in nontraffic accident**

X● **V51.3 Unspecified occupant of pick-up truck or van injured in collision with pedal cycle in nontraffic accident**

X● **V51.4 Person boarding or alighting a pick-up truck or van injured in collision with pedal cycle**

X● **V51.5 Driver of pick-up truck or van injured in collision with pedal cycle in traffic accident**

X● **V51.6 Passenger in pick-up truck or van injured in collision with pedal cycle in traffic accident**

X● **V51.7 Person on outside of pick-up truck or van injured in collision with pedal cycle in traffic accident**

X● **V51.9 Unspecified occupant of pick-up truck or van injured in collision with pedal cycle in traffic accident**

● **V52 Occupant of pick-up truck or van injured in collision with two- or three-wheeled motor vehicle**

The appropriate 7th character is to be added to each code from category V52

A	initial encounter
D	subsequent encounter
S	sequela

X● **V52.0 Driver of pick-up truck or van injured in collision with two- or three-wheeled motor vehicle in nontraffic accident**

X● **V52.1 Passenger in pick-up truck or van injured in collision with two- or three-wheeled motor vehicle in nontraffic accident**

X● **V52.2 Person on outside of pick-up truck or van injured in collision with two- or three-wheeled motor vehicle in nontraffic accident**

X● **V52.3 Unspecified occupant of pick-up truck or van injured in collision with two- or three-wheeled motor vehicle in nontraffic accident**

X● **V52.4 Person boarding or alighting a pick-up truck or van injured in collision with two- or three-wheeled motor vehicle**

X● **V52.5 Driver of pick-up truck or van injured in collision with two- or three-wheeled motor vehicle in traffic accident**

X● **V52.6 Passenger in pick-up truck or van injured in collision with two- or three-wheeled motor vehicle in traffic accident**

X● **V52.7 Person on outside of pick-up truck or van injured in collision with two- or three-wheeled motor vehicle in traffic accident**

X● **V52.9 Unspecified occupant of pick-up truck or van injured in collision with two- or three-wheeled motor vehicle in traffic accident**

● **V53 Occupant of pick-up truck or van injured in collision with car, pick-up truck or van**

The appropriate 7th character is to be added to each code from category V53

A	initial encounter
D	subsequent encounter
S	sequela

X● **V53.0 Driver of pick-up truck or van injured in collision with car, pick-up truck or van in nontraffic accident**

X● **V53.1 Passenger in pick-up truck or van injured in collision with car, pick-up truck or van in nontraffic accident**

X● **V53.2 Person on outside of pick-up truck or van injured in collision with car, pick-up truck or van in nontraffic accident**

X● **V53.3 Unspecified occupant of pick-up truck or van injured in collision with car, pick-up truck or van in nontraffic accident**

X● **V53.4 Person boarding or alighting a pick-up truck or van injured in collision with car, pick-up truck or van**

X● **V53.5 Driver of pick-up truck or van injured in collision with car, pick-up truck or van in traffic accident**

X● **V53.6 Passenger in pick-up truck or van injured in collision with car, pick-up truck or van in traffic accident**

X● **V53.7 Person on outside of pick-up truck or van injured in collision with car, pick-up truck or van in traffic accident**

X● **V53.9 Unspecified occupant of pick-up truck or van injured in collision with car, pick-up truck or van in traffic accident**

● **V54 Occupant of pick-up truck or van injured in collision with heavy transport vehicle or bus**

Excludes 1 occupant of pick-up truck or van injured in collision with military vehicle (V59.81)

The appropriate 7th character is to be added to each code from category V54

A	initial encounter
D	subsequent encounter
S	sequela

X● **V54.0 Driver of pick-up truck or van injured in collision with heavy transport vehicle or bus in nontraffic accident**

X● **V54.1 Passenger in pick-up truck or van injured in collision with heavy transport vehicle or bus in nontraffic accident**

X● **V54.2 Person on outside of pick-up truck or van injured in collision with heavy transport vehicle or bus in nontraffic accident**

X● **V54.3 Unspecified occupant of pick-up truck or van injured in collision with heavy transport vehicle or bus in nontraffic accident**

X● **V54.4 Person boarding or alighting a pick-up truck or van injured in collision with heavy transport vehicle or bus**

X● **V54.5 Driver of pick-up truck or van injured in collision with heavy transport vehicle or bus in traffic accident**

X● **V54.6 Passenger in pick-up truck or van injured in collision with heavy transport vehicle or bus in traffic accident**

X● **V54.7 Person on outside of pick-up truck or van injured in collision with heavy transport vehicle or bus in traffic accident**

X● **V54.9 Unspecified occupant of pick-up truck or van injured in collision with heavy transport vehicle or bus in traffic accident**

V55 Occupant of pick-up truck or van injured in collision with railway train or railway vehicle

The appropriate 7th character is to be added to each code from category V55

A	initial encounter
D	subsequent encounter
S	sequela

X **V55.0 Driver of pick-up truck or van injured in collision with railway train or railway vehicle in nontraffic accident**

X **V55.1 Passenger in pick-up truck or van injured in collision with railway train or railway vehicle in nontraffic accident**

X **V55.2 Person on outside of pick-up truck or van injured in collision with railway train or railway vehicle in nontraffic accident**

X **V55.3 Unspecified occupant of pick-up truck or van injured in collision with railway train or railway vehicle in nontraffic accident**

X **V55.4 Person boarding or alighting a pick-up truck or van injured in collision with railway train or railway vehicle**

X **V55.5 Driver of pick-up truck or van injured in collision with railway train or railway vehicle in traffic accident**

X **V55.6 Passenger in pick-up truck or van injured in collision with railway train or railway vehicle in traffic accident**

X **V55.7 Person on outside of pick-up truck or van injured in collision with railway train or railway vehicle in traffic accident**

X **V55.9 Unspecified occupant of pick-up truck or van injured in collision with railway train or railway vehicle in traffic accident**

V56 Occupant of pick-up truck or van injured in collision with other nonmotor vehicle

Includes collision with animal-drawn vehicle, animal being ridden, streetcar

The appropriate 7th character is to be added to each code from category V56

A	initial encounter
D	subsequent encounter
S	sequela

X **V56.0 Driver of pick-up truck or van injured in collision with other nonmotor vehicle in nontraffic accident**

X **V56.1 Passenger in pick-up truck or van injured in collision with other nonmotor vehicle in nontraffic accident**

X **V56.2 Person on outside of pick-up truck or van injured in collision with other nonmotor vehicle in nontraffic accident**

X **V56.3 Unspecified occupant of pick-up truck or van injured in collision with other nonmotor vehicle in nontraffic accident**

X **V56.4 Person boarding or alighting a pick-up truck or van injured in collision with other nonmotor vehicle**

X **V56.5 Driver of pick-up truck or van injured in collision with other nonmotor vehicle in traffic accident**

X **V56.6 Passenger in pick-up truck or van injured in collision with other nonmotor vehicle in traffic accident**

X **V56.7 Person on outside of pick-up truck or van injured in collision with other nonmotor vehicle in traffic accident**

X **V56.9 Unspecified occupant of pick-up truck or van injured in collision with other nonmotor vehicle in traffic accident**

V57 Occupant of pick-up truck or van injured in collision with fixed or stationary object

The appropriate 7th character is to be added to each code from category V57

A	initial encounter
D	subsequent encounter
S	sequela

X **V57.0 Driver of pick-up truck or van injured in collision with fixed or stationary object in nontraffic accident**

X **V57.1 Passenger in pick-up truck or van injured in collision with fixed or stationary object in nontraffic accident**

X **V57.2 Person on outside of pick-up truck or van injured in collision with fixed or stationary object in nontraffic accident**

X **V57.3 Unspecified occupant of pick-up truck or van injured in collision with fixed or stationary object in nontraffic accident**

X **V57.4 Person boarding or alighting a pick-up truck or van injured in collision with fixed or stationary object**

X **V57.5 Driver of pick-up truck or van injured in collision with fixed or stationary object in traffic accident**

X **V57.6 Passenger in pick-up truck or van injured in collision with fixed or stationary object in traffic accident**

X **V57.7 Person on outside of pick-up truck or van injured in collision with fixed or stationary object in traffic accident**

X **V57.9 Unspecified occupant of pick-up truck or van injured in collision with fixed or stationary object in traffic accident**

V58 Occupant of pick-up truck or van injured in noncollision transport accident

Includes overturning pick-up truck or van NOS
overturning pick-up truck or van without collision

The appropriate 7th character is to be added to each code from category V58

A	initial encounter
D	subsequent encounter
S	sequela

X **V58.0 Driver of pick-up truck or van injured in noncollision transport accident in nontraffic accident**

X **V58.1 Passenger in pick-up truck or van injured in noncollision transport accident in nontraffic accident**

X **V58.2 Person on outside of pick-up truck or van injured in noncollision transport accident in nontraffic accident**

X **V58.3 Unspecified occupant of pick-up truck or van injured in noncollision transport accident in nontraffic accident**

X **V58.4 Person boarding or alighting a pick-up truck or van injured in noncollision transport accident**

X **V58.5 Driver of pick-up truck or van injured in noncollision transport accident in traffic accident**

X **V58.6 Passenger in pick-up truck or van injured in noncollision transport accident in traffic accident**

X **V58.7 Person on outside of pick-up truck or van injured in noncollision transport accident in traffic accident**

X **V58.9 Unspecified occupant of pick-up truck or van injured in noncollision transport accident in traffic accident**

● **V59 Occupant of pick-up truck or van injured in other and unspecified transport accidents**

The appropriate 7th character is to be added to each code from category V59

A	initial encounter
D	subsequent encounter
S	sequela

● **V59.0 Driver of pick-up truck or van injured in collision with other and unspecified motor vehicles in nontraffic accident**

X● **V59.00 Driver of pick-up truck or van injured in collision with unspecified motor vehicles in nontraffic accident**

X● **V59.09 Driver of pick-up truck or van injured in collision with other motor vehicles in nontraffic accident**

● **V59.1 Passenger in pick-up truck or van injured in collision with other and unspecified motor vehicles in nontraffic accident**

X● **V59.10 Passenger in pick-up truck or van injured in collision with unspecified motor vehicles in nontraffic accident**

X● **V59.19 Passenger in pick-up truck or van injured in collision with other motor vehicles in nontraffic accident**

● **V59.2 Unspecified occupant of pick-up truck or van injured in collision with other and unspecified motor vehicles in nontraffic accident**

X● **V59.20 Unspecified occupant of pick-up truck or van injured in collision with unspecified motor vehicles in nontraffic accident**

Collision NOS involving pick-up truck or van, nontraffic

X● **V59.29 Unspecified occupant of pick-up truck or van injured in collision with other motor vehicles in nontraffic accident**

X● **V59.3 Occupant (driver) (passenger) of pick-up truck or van injured in unspecified nontraffic accident**

Accident NOS involving pick-up truck or van, nontraffic

Occupant of pick-up truck or van injured in nontraffic accident NOS

● **V59.4 Driver of pick-up truck or van injured in collision with other and unspecified motor vehicles in traffic accident**

X● **V59.40 Driver of pick-up truck or van injured in collision with unspecified motor vehicles in traffic accident**

X● **V59.49 Driver of pick-up truck or van injured in collision with other motor vehicles in traffic accident**

● **V59.5 Passenger in pick-up truck or van injured in collision with other and unspecified motor vehicles in traffic accident**

X● **V59.50 Passenger in pick-up truck or van injured in collision with unspecified motor vehicles in traffic accident**

X● **V59.59 Passenger in pick-up truck or van injured in collision with other motor vehicles in traffic accident**

● **V59.6 Unspecified occupant of pick-up truck or van injured in collision with other and unspecified motor vehicles in traffic accident**

X● **V59.60 Unspecified occupant of pick-up truck or van injured in collision with unspecified motor vehicles in traffic accident**

Collision NOS involving pick-up truck or van (traffic)

X● **V59.69 Unspecified occupant of pick-up truck or van injured in collision with other motor vehicles in traffic accident**

● **V59.8 Occupant (driver) (passenger) of pick-up truck or van injured in other specified transport accidents**

X● **V59.81 Occupant (driver) (passenger) of pick-up truck or van injured in transport accident with military vehicle**

X● **V59.88 Occupant (driver) (passenger) of pick-up truck or van injured in other specified transport accidents**

X● **V59.9 Occupant (driver) (passenger) of pick-up truck or van injured in unspecified traffic accident**

Accident NOS involving pick-up truck or van

OCCUPANT OF HEAVY TRANSPORT VEHICLE INJURED IN TRANSPORT ACCIDENT (V60-V69)

Includes 18 wheeler
armored car
panel truck

Excludes1 bus
motorcoach

● **V60 Occupant of heavy transport vehicle injured in collision with pedestrian or animal**

Excludes1 heavy transport vehicle collision with animal-drawn vehicle or animal being ridden (V66.-)

The appropriate 7th character is to be added to each code from category V60

A	initial encounter
D	subsequent encounter
S	sequela

X● **V60.0 Driver of heavy transport vehicle injured in collision with pedestrian or animal in nontraffic accident**

X● **V60.1 Passenger in heavy transport vehicle injured in collision with pedestrian or animal in nontraffic accident**

X● **V60.2 Person on outside of heavy transport vehicle injured in collision with pedestrian or animal in nontraffic accident**

X● **V60.3 Unspecified occupant of heavy transport vehicle injured in collision with pedestrian or animal in nontraffic accident**

X● **V60.4 Person boarding or alighting a heavy transport vehicle injured in collision with pedestrian or animal**

X● **V60.5 Driver of heavy transport vehicle injured in collision with pedestrian or animal in traffic accident**

X● **V60.6 Passenger in heavy transport vehicle injured in collision with pedestrian or animal in traffic accident**

X● **V60.7 Person on outside of heavy transport vehicle injured in collision with pedestrian or animal in traffic accident**

X● **V60.9 Unspecified occupant of heavy transport vehicle injured in collision with pedestrian or animal in traffic accident**

● **V61 Occupant of heavy transport vehicle injured in collision with pedal cycle**

The appropriate 7th character is to be added to each code from category V61

A	initial encounter
D	subsequent encounter
S	sequela

X● **V61.0 Driver of heavy transport vehicle injured in collision with pedal cycle in nontraffic accident**

X● **V61.1 Passenger in heavy transport vehicle injured in collision with pedal cycle in nontraffic accident**

X● **V61.2 Person on outside of heavy transport vehicle injured in collision with pedal cycle in nontraffic accident**

X● **V61.3 Unspecified occupant of heavy transport vehicle injured in collision with pedal cycle in nontraffic accident**

X● **V61.4 Person boarding or alighting a heavy transport vehicle injured in collision with pedal cycle while boarding or alighting**

X● **V61.5 Driver of heavy transport vehicle injured in collision with pedal cycle in traffic accident**

X● **V61.6** **Passenger in heavy transport vehicle injured in collision with pedal cycle in traffic accident**

X● **V61.7** **Person on outside of heavy transport vehicle injured in collision with pedal cycle in traffic accident**

X● **V61.9** **Unspecified occupant of heavy transport vehicle injured in collision with pedal cycle in traffic accident**

● **V62** **Occupant of heavy transport vehicle injured in collision with two- or three-wheeled motor vehicle**

The appropriate 7th character is to be added to each code from category V62

A	initial encounter
D	subsequent encounter
S	sequela

X● **V62.0** **Driver of heavy transport vehicle injured in collision with two- or three-wheeled motor vehicle in nontraffic accident**

X● **V62.1** **Passenger in heavy transport vehicle injured in collision with two- or three-wheeled motor vehicle in nontraffic accident**

X● **V62.2** **Person on outside of heavy transport vehicle injured in collision with two- or three-wheeled motor vehicle in nontraffic accident**

X● **V62.3** **Unspecified occupant of heavy transport vehicle injured in collision with two- or three-wheeled motor vehicle in nontraffic accident**

X● **V62.4** **Person boarding or alighting a heavy transport vehicle injured in collision with two- or three-wheeled motor vehicle**

X● **V62.5** **Driver of heavy transport vehicle injured in collision with two- or three-wheeled motor vehicle in traffic accident**

X● **V62.6** **Passenger in heavy transport vehicle injured in collision with two- or three-wheeled motor vehicle in traffic accident**

X● **V62.7** **Person on outside of heavy transport vehicle injured in collision with two- or three-wheeled motor vehicle in traffic accident**

X● **V62.9** **Unspecified occupant of heavy transport vehicle injured in collision with two- or three-wheeled motor vehicle in traffic accident**

● **V63** **Occupant of heavy transport vehicle injured in collision with car, pick-up truck or van**

The appropriate 7th character is to be added to each code from category V63

A	initial encounter
D	subsequent encounter
S	sequela

X● **V63.0** **Driver of heavy transport vehicle injured in collision with car, pick-up truck or van in nontraffic accident**

X● **V63.1** **Passenger in heavy transport vehicle injured in collision with car, pick-up truck or van in nontraffic accident**

X● **V63.2** **Person on outside of heavy transport vehicle injured in collision with car, pick-up truck or van in nontraffic accident**

X● **V63.3** **Unspecified occupant of heavy transport vehicle injured in collision with car, pick-up truck or van in nontraffic accident**

X● **V63.4** **Person boarding or alighting a heavy transport vehicle injured in collision with car, pick-up truck or van**

X● **V63.5** **Driver of heavy transport vehicle injured in collision with car, pick-up truck or van in traffic accident**

X● **V63.6** **Passenger in heavy transport vehicle injured in collision with car, pick-up truck or van in traffic accident**

X● **V63.7** **Person on outside of heavy transport vehicle injured in collision with car, pick-up truck or van in traffic accident**

X● **V63.9** **Unspecified occupant of heavy transport vehicle injured in collision with car, pick-up truck or van in traffic accident**

● **V64** **Occupant of heavy transport vehicle injured in collision with heavy transport vehicle or bus**

Excludes1 occupant of heavy transport vehicle injured in collision with military vehicle (V69.81)

The appropriate 7th character is to be added to each code from category V64

A	initial encounter
D	subsequent encounter
S	sequela

X● **V64.0** **Driver of heavy transport vehicle injured in collision with heavy transport vehicle or bus in nontraffic accident**

X● **V64.1** **Passenger in heavy transport vehicle injured in collision with heavy transport vehicle or bus in nontraffic accident**

X● **V64.2** **Person on outside of heavy transport vehicle injured in collision with heavy transport vehicle or bus in nontraffic accident**

X● **V64.3** **Unspecified occupant of heavy transport vehicle injured in collision with heavy transport vehicle or bus in nontraffic accident**

X● **V64.4** **Person boarding or alighting a heavy transport vehicle injured in collision with heavy transport vehicle or bus while boarding or alighting**

X● **V64.5** **Driver of heavy transport vehicle injured in collision with heavy transport vehicle or bus in traffic accident**

X● **V64.6** **Passenger in heavy transport vehicle injured in collision with heavy transport vehicle or bus in traffic accident**

X● **V64.7** **Person on outside of heavy transport vehicle injured in collision with heavy transport vehicle or bus in traffic accident**

X● **V64.9** **Unspecified occupant of heavy transport vehicle injured in collision with heavy transport vehicle or bus in traffic accident**

● **V65** **Occupant of heavy transport vehicle injured in collision with railway train or railway vehicle**

The appropriate 7th character is to be added to each code from category V65

A	initial encounter
D	subsequent encounter
S	sequela

X● **V65.0** **Driver of heavy transport vehicle injured in collision with railway train or railway vehicle in nontraffic accident**

X● **V65.1** **Passenger in heavy transport vehicle injured in collision with railway train or railway vehicle in nontraffic accident**

X● **V65.2** **Person on outside of heavy transport vehicle injured in collision with railway train or railway vehicle in nontraffic accident**

X● **V65.3** **Unspecified occupant of heavy transport vehicle injured in collision with railway train or railway vehicle in nontraffic accident**

X● **V65.4** **Person boarding or alighting a heavy transport vehicle injured in collision with railway train or railway vehicle**

X● **V65.5** **Driver of heavy transport vehicle injured in collision with railway train or railway vehicle in traffic accident**

X● **V65.6** **Passenger in heavy transport vehicle injured in collision with railway train or railway vehicle in traffic accident**

X● **V65.7** **Person on outside of heavy transport vehicle injured in collision with railway train or railway vehicle in traffic accident**

X● **V65.9** **Unspecified occupant of heavy transport vehicle injured in collision with railway train or railway vehicle in traffic accident**

● **V66 Occupant of heavy transport vehicle injured in collision with other nonmotor vehicle**

Includes collision with animal-drawn vehicle, animal being ridden, streetcar

The appropriate 7th character is to be added to each code from category V66

A	initial encounter
D	subsequent encounter
S	sequela

X● **V66.0 Driver of heavy transport vehicle injured in collision with other nonmotor vehicle in nontraffic accident**

X● **V66.1 Passenger in heavy transport vehicle injured in collision with other nonmotor vehicle in nontraffic accident**

X● **V66.2 Person on outside of heavy transport vehicle injured in collision with other nonmotor vehicle in nontraffic accident**

X● **V66.3 Unspecified occupant of heavy transport vehicle injured in collision with other nonmotor vehicle in nontraffic accident**

X● **V66.4 Person boarding or alighting a heavy transport vehicle injured in collision with other nonmotor vehicle**

X● **V66.5 Driver of heavy transport vehicle injured in collision with other nonmotor vehicle in traffic accident**

X● **V66.6 Passenger in heavy transport vehicle injured in collision with other nonmotor vehicle in traffic accident**

X● **V66.7 Person on outside of heavy transport vehicle injured in collision with other nonmotor vehicle in traffic accident**

X● **V66.9 Unspecified occupant of heavy transport vehicle injured in collision with other nonmotor vehicle in traffic accident**

● **V67 Occupant of heavy transport vehicle injured in collision with fixed or stationary object**

The appropriate 7th character is to be added to each code from category V67

A	initial encounter
D	subsequent encounter
S	sequela

X● **V67.0 Driver of heavy transport vehicle injured in collision with fixed or stationary object in nontraffic accident**

X● **V67.1 Passenger in heavy transport vehicle injured in collision with fixed or stationary object in nontraffic accident**

X● **V67.2 Person on outside of heavy transport vehicle injured in collision with fixed or stationary object in nontraffic accident**

X● **V67.3 Unspecified occupant of heavy transport vehicle injured in collision with fixed or stationary object in nontraffic accident**

X● **V67.4 Person boarding or alighting a heavy transport vehicle injured in collision with fixed or stationary object**

X● **V67.5 Driver of heavy transport vehicle injured in collision with fixed or stationary object in traffic accident**

X● **V67.6 Passenger in heavy transport vehicle injured in collision with fixed or stationary object in traffic accident**

X● **V67.7 Person on outside of heavy transport vehicle injured in collision with fixed or stationary object in traffic accident**

X● **V67.9 Unspecified occupant of heavy transport vehicle injured in collision with fixed or stationary object in traffic accident**

● **V68 Occupant of heavy transport vehicle injured in noncollision transport accident**

Includes overturning heavy transport vehicle NOS
overturning heavy transport vehicle without collision

The appropriate 7th character is to be added to each code from category V68

A	initial encounter
D	subsequent encounter
S	sequela

X● **V68.0 Driver of heavy transport vehicle injured in noncollision transport accident in nontraffic accident**

X● **V68.1 Passenger in heavy transport vehicle injured in noncollision transport accident in nontraffic accident**

X● **V68.2 Person on outside of heavy transport vehicle injured in noncollision transport accident in nontraffic accident**

X● **V68.3 Unspecified occupant of heavy transport vehicle injured in noncollision transport accident in nontraffic accident**

X● **V68.4 Person boarding or alighting a heavy transport vehicle injured in noncollision transport accident**

X● **V68.5 Driver of heavy transport vehicle injured in noncollision transport accident in traffic accident**

X● **V68.6 Passenger in heavy transport vehicle injured in noncollision transport accident in traffic accident**

X● **V68.7 Person on outside of heavy transport vehicle injured in noncollision transport accident in traffic accident**

X● **V68.9 Unspecified occupant of heavy transport vehicle injured in noncollision transport accident in traffic accident**

● **V69 Occupant of heavy transport vehicle injured in other and unspecified transport accidents**

The appropriate 7th character is to be added to each code from category V69

A	initial encounter
D	subsequent encounter
S	sequela

● **V69.0 Driver of heavy transport vehicle injured in collision with other and unspecified motor vehicles in nontraffic accident**

X● **V69.00 Driver of heavy transport vehicle injured in collision with unspecified motor vehicles in nontraffic accident**

X● **V69.09 Driver of heavy transport vehicle injured in collision with other motor vehicles in nontraffic accident**

● **V69.1 Passenger in heavy transport vehicle injured in collision with other and unspecified motor vehicles in nontraffic accident**

X● **V69.10 Passenger in heavy transport vehicle injured in collision with unspecified motor vehicles in nontraffic accident**

X● **V69.19 Passenger in heavy transport vehicle injured in collision with other motor vehicles in nontraffic accident**

● **V69.2 Unspecified occupant of heavy transport vehicle injured in collision with other and unspecified motor vehicles in nontraffic accident**

X● **V69.20 Unspecified occupant of heavy transport vehicle injured in collision with unspecified motor vehicles in nontraffic accident**

Collision NOS involving heavy transport vehicle, nontraffic

X● **V69.29 Unspecified occupant of heavy transport vehicle injured in collision with other motor vehicles in nontraffic accident**

X● **V69.3 Occupant (driver) (passenger) of heavy transport vehicle injured in unspecified nontraffic accident**
Accident NOS involving heavy transport vehicle, nontraffic
Occupant of heavy transport vehicle injured in nontraffic accident NOS

● **V69.4 Driver of heavy transport vehicle injured in collision with other and unspecified motor vehicles in traffic accident**

X● **V69.40 Driver of heavy transport vehicle injured in collision with unspecified motor vehicles in traffic accident**

X● **V69.49 Driver of heavy transport vehicle injured in collision with other motor vehicles in traffic accident**

● **V69.5 Passenger in heavy transport vehicle injured in collision with other and unspecified motor vehicles in traffic accident**

X● **V69.50 Passenger in heavy transport vehicle injured in collision with unspecified motor vehicles in traffic accident**

X● **V69.59 Passenger in heavy transport vehicle injured in collision with other motor vehicles in traffic accident**

● **V69.6 Unspecified occupant of heavy transport vehicle injured in collision with other and unspecified motor vehicles in traffic accident**

X● **V69.60 Unspecified occupant of heavy transport vehicle injured in collision with unspecified motor vehicles in traffic accident**
Collision NOS involving heavy transport vehicle (traffic)

X● **V69.69 Unspecified occupant of heavy transport vehicle injured in collision with other motor vehicles in traffic accident**

● **V69.8 Occupant (driver) (passenger) of heavy transport vehicle injured in other specified transport accidents**

X● **V69.81 Occupant (driver) (passenger) of heavy transport vehicle injured in transport accidents with military vehicle**

X● **V69.88 Occupant (driver) (passenger) of heavy transport vehicle injured in other specified transport accidents**

X● **V69.9 Occupant (driver) (passenger) of heavy transport vehicle injured in unspecified traffic accident**
Accident NOS involving heavy transport vehicle

BUS OCCUPANT INJURED IN TRANSPORT ACCIDENT (V70-V79)

Includes motorcoach
Excludes1 minibus (V50-V59)

● **V70 Bus occupant injured in collision with pedestrian or animal**
Excludes1 bus collision with animal-drawn vehicle or animal being ridden (V76.-)
The appropriate 7th character is to be added to each code from category V70

A	initial encounter
D	subsequent encounter
S	sequela

X● **V70.0 Driver of bus injured in collision with pedestrian or animal in nontraffic accident**

X● **V70.1 Passenger on bus injured in collision with pedestrian or animal in nontraffic accident**

X● **V70.2 Person on outside of bus injured in collision with pedestrian or animal in nontraffic accident**

X● **V70.3 Unspecified occupant of bus injured in collision with pedestrian or animal in nontraffic accident**

X● **V70.4 Person boarding or alighting from bus injured in collision with pedestrian or animal**

X● **V70.5 Driver of bus injured in collision with pedestrian or animal in traffic accident**

X● **V70.6 Passenger on bus injured in collision with pedestrian or animal in traffic accident**

X● **V70.7 Person on outside of bus injured in collision with pedestrian or animal in traffic accident**

X● **V70.9 Unspecified occupant of bus injured in collision with pedestrian or animal in traffic accident**

● **V71 Bus occupant injured in collision with pedal cycle**
The appropriate 7th character is to be added to each code from category V71

A	initial encounter
D	subsequent encounter
S	sequela

X● **V71.0 Driver of bus injured in collision with pedal cycle in nontraffic accident**

X● **V71.1 Passenger on bus injured in collision with pedal cycle in nontraffic accident**

X● **V71.2 Person on outside of bus injured in collision with pedal cycle in nontraffic accident**

X● **V71.3 Unspecified occupant of bus injured in collision with pedal cycle in nontraffic accident**

X● **V71.4 Person boarding or alighting from bus injured in collision with pedal cycle**

X● **V71.5 Driver of bus injured in collision with pedal cycle in traffic accident**

X● **V71.6 Passenger on bus injured in collision with pedal cycle in traffic accident**

X● **V71.7 Person on outside of bus injured in collision with pedal cycle in traffic accident**

X● **V71.9 Unspecified occupant of bus injured in collision with pedal cycle in traffic accident**

● **V72 Bus occupant injured in collision with two- or three-wheeled motor vehicle**
The appropriate 7th character is to be added to each code from category V72

A	initial encounter
D	subsequent encounter
S	sequela

X● **V72.0 Driver of bus injured in collision with two- or three-wheeled motor vehicle in nontraffic accident**

X● **V72.1 Passenger on bus injured in collision with two- or three-wheeled motor vehicle in nontraffic accident**

X● **V72.2 Person on outside of bus injured in collision with two- or three-wheeled motor vehicle in nontraffic accident**

X● **V72.3 Unspecified occupant of bus injured in collision with two- or three-wheeled motor vehicle in nontraffic accident**

X● **V72.4 Person boarding or alighting from bus injured in collision with two- or three-wheeled motor vehicle**

X● **V72.5 Driver of bus injured in collision with two- or three-wheeled motor vehicle in traffic accident**

X● **V72.6 Passenger on bus injured in collision with two- or three-wheeled motor vehicle in traffic accident**

X● **V72.7 Person on outside of bus injured in collision with two- or three-wheeled motor vehicle in traffic accident**

X● **V72.9 Unspecified occupant of bus injured in collision with two- or three-wheeled motor vehicle in traffic accident**

● **V73 Bus occupant injured in collision with car, pick-up truck or van**

The appropriate 7th character is to be added to each code from category V73

A	initial encounter
D	subsequent encounter
S	sequela

X● **V73.0 Driver of bus injured in collision with car, pick-up truck or van in nontraffic accident**

X● **V73.1 Passenger on bus injured in collision with car, pick-up truck or van in nontraffic accident**

X● **V73.2 Person on outside of bus injured in collision with car, pick-up truck or van in nontraffic accident**

X● **V73.3 Unspecified occupant of bus injured in collision with car, pick-up truck or van in nontraffic accident**

X● **V73.4 Person boarding or alighting from bus injured in collision with car, pick-up truck or van**

X● **V73.5 Driver of bus injured in collision with car, pick-up truck or van in traffic accident**

X● **V73.6 Passenger on bus injured in collision with car, pick-up truck or van in traffic accident**

X● **V73.7 Person on outside of bus injured in collision with car, pick-up truck or van in traffic accident**

X● **V73.9 Unspecified occupant of bus injured in collision with car, pick-up truck or van in traffic accident**

● **V74 Bus occupant injured in collision with heavy transport vehicle or bus**

Excludes1 bus occupant injured in collision with military vehicle (V79.81)

The appropriate 7th character is to be added to each code from category V74

A	initial encounter
D	subsequent encounter
S	sequela

X● **V74.0 Driver of bus injured in collision with heavy transport vehicle or bus in nontraffic accident**

X● **V74.1 Passenger on bus injured in collision with heavy transport vehicle or bus in nontraffic accident**

X● **V74.2 Person on outside of bus injured in collision with heavy transport vehicle or bus in nontraffic accident**

X● **V74.3 Unspecified occupant of bus injured in collision with heavy transport vehicle or bus in nontraffic accident**

X● **V74.4 Person boarding or alighting from bus injured in collision with heavy transport vehicle or bus**

X● **V74.5 Driver of bus injured in collision with heavy transport vehicle or bus in traffic accident**

X● **V74.6 Passenger on bus injured in collision with heavy transport vehicle or bus in traffic accident**

X● **V74.7 Person on outside of bus injured in collision with heavy transport vehicle or bus in traffic accident**

X● **V74.9 Unspecified occupant of bus injured in collision with heavy transport vehicle or bus in traffic accident**

● **V75 Bus occupant injured in collision with railway train or railway vehicle**

The appropriate 7th character is to be added to each code from category V75

A	initial encounter
D	subsequent encounter
S	sequela

X● **V75.0 Driver of bus injured in collision with railway train or railway vehicle in nontraffic accident**

X● **V75.1 Passenger on bus injured in collision with railway train or railway vehicle in nontraffic accident**

X● **V75.2 Person on outside of bus injured in collision with railway train or railway vehicle in nontraffic accident**

X● **V75.3 Unspecified occupant of bus injured in collision with railway train or railway vehicle in nontraffic accident**

X● **V75.4 Person boarding or alighting from bus injured in collision with railway train or railway vehicle**

X● **V75.5 Driver of bus injured in collision with railway train or railway vehicle in traffic accident**

X● **V75.6 Passenger on bus injured in collision with railway train or railway vehicle in traffic accident**

X● **V75.7 Person on outside of bus injured in collision with railway train or railway vehicle in traffic accident**

X● **V75.9 Unspecified occupant of bus injured in collision with railway train or railway vehicle in traffic accident**

● **V76 Bus occupant injured in collision with other nonmotor vehicle**

Includes collision with animal-drawn vehicle, animal being ridden, streetcar

The appropriate 7th character is to be added to each code from category V76

A	initial encounter
D	subsequent encounter
S	sequela

X● **V76.0 Driver of bus injured in collision with other nonmotor vehicle in nontraffic accident**

X● **V76.1 Passenger on bus injured in collision with other nonmotor vehicle in nontraffic accident**

X● **V76.2 Person on outside of bus injured in collision with other nonmotor vehicle in nontraffic accident**

X● **V76.3 Unspecified occupant of bus injured in collision with other nonmotor vehicle in nontraffic accident**

X● **V76.4 Person boarding or alighting from bus injured in collision with other nonmotor vehicle**

X● **V76.5 Driver of bus injured in collision with other nonmotor vehicle in traffic accident**

X● **V76.6 Passenger on bus injured in collision with other nonmotor vehicle in traffic accident**

X● **V76.7 Person on outside of bus injured in collision with other nonmotor vehicle in traffic accident**

X● **V76.9 Unspecified occupant of bus injured in collision with other nonmotor vehicle in traffic accident**

● **V77 Bus occupant injured in collision with fixed or stationary object**

The appropriate 7th character is to be added to each code from category V77

A	initial encounter
D	subsequent encounter
S	sequela

X● **V77.0 Driver of bus injured in collision with fixed or stationary object in nontraffic accident**

X● **V77.1 Passenger on bus injured in collision with fixed or stationary object in nontraffic accident**

X● **V77.2 Person on outside of bus injured in collision with fixed or stationary object in nontraffic accident**

X● **V77.3 Unspecified occupant of bus injured in collision with fixed or stationary object in nontraffic accident**

X● **V77.4 Person boarding or alighting from bus injured in collision with fixed or stationary object**

X● **V77.5 Driver of bus injured in collision with fixed or stationary object in traffic accident**

X● **V77.6 Passenger on bus injured in collision with fixed or stationary object in traffic accident**

X● **V77.7 Person on outside of bus injured in collision with fixed or stationary object in traffic accident**

X● **V77.9 Unspecified occupant of bus injured in collision with fixed or stationary object in traffic accident**

V78 Bus occupant injured in noncollision transport accident

Includes overturning bus NOS
overturning bus without collision

The appropriate 7th character is to be added to each code from category V78

A	initial encounter
D	subsequent encounter
S	sequela

X **V78.0 Driver of bus injured in noncollision transport accident in nontraffic accident**

X **V78.1 Passenger on bus injured in noncollision transport accident in nontraffic accident**

X **V78.2 Person on outside of bus injured in noncollision transport accident in nontraffic accident**

X **V78.3 Unspecified occupant of bus injured in noncollision transport accident in nontraffic accident**

X **V78.4 Person boarding or alighting from bus injured in noncollision transport accident**

X **V78.5 Driver of bus injured in noncollision transport accident in traffic accident**

X **V78.6 Passenger on bus injured in noncollision transport accident in traffic accident**

X **V78.7 Person on outside of bus injured in noncollision transport accident in traffic accident**

X **V78.9 Unspecified occupant of bus injured in noncollision transport accident in traffic accident**

V79 Bus occupant injured in other and unspecified transport accidents

The appropriate 7th character is to be added to each code from category V79

A	initial encounter
D	subsequent encounter
S	sequela

V79.0 Driver of bus injured in collision with other and unspecified motor vehicles in nontraffic accident

X **V79.00 Driver of bus injured in collision with unspecified motor vehicles in nontraffic accident**

X **V79.09 Driver of bus injured in collision with other motor vehicles in nontraffic accident**

V79.1 Passenger on bus injured in collision with other and unspecified motor vehicles in nontraffic accident

X **V79.10 Passenger on bus injured in collision with unspecified motor vehicles in nontraffic accident**

X **V79.19 Passenger on bus injured in collision with other motor vehicles in nontraffic accident**

V79.2 Unspecified bus occupant injured in collision with other and unspecified motor vehicles in nontraffic accident

X **V79.20 Unspecified bus occupant injured in collision with unspecified motor vehicles in nontraffic accident**
Bus collision NOS, nontraffic

X **V79.29 Unspecified bus occupant injured in collision with other motor vehicles in nontraffic accident**

X **V79.3 Bus occupant (driver) (passenger) injured in unspecified nontraffic accident**
Bus accident NOS, nontraffic
Bus occupant injured in nontraffic accident NOS

V79.4 Driver of bus injured in collision with other and unspecified motor vehicles in traffic accident

X **V79.40 Driver of bus injured in collision with unspecified motor vehicles in traffic accident**

X **V79.49 Driver of bus injured in collision with other motor vehicles in traffic accident**

V79.5 Passenger on bus injured in collision with other and unspecified motor vehicles in traffic accident

X **V79.50 Passenger on bus injured in collision with unspecified motor vehicles in traffic accident**

X **V79.59 Passenger on bus injured in collision with other motor vehicles in traffic accident**

V79.6 Unspecified bus occupant injured in collision with other and unspecified motor vehicles in traffic accident

X **V79.60 Unspecified bus occupant injured in collision with unspecified motor vehicles in traffic accident**
Bus collision NOS (traffic)

X **V79.69 Unspecified bus occupant injured in collision with other motor vehicles in traffic accident**

V79.8 Bus occupant (driver) (passenger) injured in other specified transport accidents

X **V79.81 Bus occupant (driver) (passenger) injured in transport accidents with military vehicle**

X **V79.88 Bus occupant (driver) (passenger) injured in other specified transport accidents**

X **V79.9 Bus occupant (driver) (passenger) injured in unspecified traffic accident**
Bus accident NOS

OTHER LAND TRANSPORT ACCIDENTS (V80-V89)

V80 Animal-rider or occupant of animal-drawn vehicle injured in transport accident

The appropriate 7th character is to be added to each code from category V80

A	initial encounter
D	subsequent encounter
S	sequela

V80.0 Animal-rider or occupant of animal drawn vehicle injured by fall from or being thrown from animal or animal-drawn vehicle in noncollision accident

V80.01 Animal-rider injured by fall from or being thrown from animal in noncollision accident

V80.010 Animal-rider injured by fall from or being thrown from horse in noncollision accident

V80.018 Animal-rider injured by fall from or being thrown from other animal in noncollision accident

X **V80.02 Occupant of animal-drawn vehicle injured by fall from or being thrown from animal-drawn vehicle in noncollision accident**
Overturning animal-drawn vehicle NOS
Overturning animal-drawn vehicle without collision

V80.1 Animal-rider or occupant of animal-drawn vehicle injured in collision with pedestrian or animal

Excludes1 animal-rider or animal-drawn vehicle collision with animal-drawn vehicle or animal being ridden (V80.7)

X **V80.11 Animal-rider injured in collision with pedestrian or animal**

X **V80.12 Occupant of animal-drawn vehicle injured in collision with pedestrian or animal**

V80.2 Animal-rider or occupant of animal-drawn vehicle injured in collision with pedal cycle

X **V80.21 Animal-rider injured in collision with pedal cycle**

X **V80.22 Occupant of animal-drawn vehicle injured in collision with pedal cycle**

● **V80.3 Animal-rider or occupant of animal-drawn vehicle injured in collision with two- or three-wheeled motor vehicle**

X● **V80.31 Animal-rider injured in collision with two- or three-wheeled motor vehicle**

X● **V80.32 Occupant of animal-drawn vehicle injured in collision with two- or three-wheeled motor vehicle**

● **V80.4 Animal-rider or occupant of animal-drawn vehicle injured in collision with car, pick-up truck, van, heavy transport vehicle or bus**

Excludes1 animal-rider injured in collision with military vehicle (V80.910)
occupant of animal-drawn vehicle injured in collision with military vehicle (V80.920)

X● **V80.41 Animal-rider injured in collision with car, pick-up truck, van, heavy transport vehicle or bus**

X● **V80.42 Occupant of animal-drawn vehicle injured in collision with car, pick-up truck, van, heavy transport vehicle or bus**

● **V80.5 Animal-rider or occupant of animal-drawn vehicle injured in collision with other specified motor vehicle**

X● **V80.51 Animal-rider injured in collision with other specified motor vehicle**

X● **V80.52 Occupant of animal-drawn vehicle injured in collision with other specified motor vehicle**

● **V80.6 Animal-rider or occupant of animal-drawn vehicle injured in collision with railway train or railway vehicle**

X● **V80.61 Animal-rider injured in collision with railway train or railway vehicle**

X● **V80.62 Occupant of animal-drawn vehicle injured in collision with railway train or railway vehicle**

● **V80.7 Animal-rider or occupant of animal-drawn vehicle injured in collision with other nonmotor vehicles**

● **V80.71 Animal-rider or occupant of animal-drawn vehicle injured in collision with animal being ridden**

● **V80.710 Animal-rider injured in collision with other animal being ridden**

● **V80.711 Occupant of animal-drawn vehicle injured in collision with animal being ridden**

● **V80.72 Animal-rider or occupant of animal-drawn vehicle injured in collision with other animal-drawn vehicle**

● **V80.720 Animal-rider injured in collision with animal-drawn vehicle**

● **V80.721 Occupant of animal-drawn vehicle injured in collision with other animal-drawn vehicle**

● **V80.73 Animal-rider or occupant of animal-drawn vehicle injured in collision with streetcar**

● **V80.730 Animal-rider injured in collision with streetcar**

● **V80.731 Occupant of animal-drawn vehicle injured in collision with streetcar**

● **V80.79 Animal-rider or occupant of animal-drawn vehicle injured in collision with other nonmotor vehicles**

● **V80.790 Animal-rider injured in collision with other nonmotor vehicles**

● **V80.791 Occupant of animal-drawn vehicle injured in collision with other nonmotor vehicles**

● **V80.8 Animal-rider or occupant of animal-drawn vehicle injured in collision with fixed or stationary object**

X● **V80.81 Animal-rider injured in collision with fixed or stationary object**

X● **V80.82 Occupant of animal-drawn vehicle injured in collision with fixed or stationary object**

● **V80.9 Animal-rider or occupant of animal-drawn vehicle injured in other and unspecified transport accidents**

● **V80.91 Animal-rider injured in other and unspecified transport accidents**

● **V80.910 Animal-rider injured in transport accident with military vehicle**

● **V80.918 Animal-rider injured in other transport accident**

● **V80.919 Animal-rider injured in unspecified transport accident**
Animal rider accident NOS

● **V80.92 Occupant of animal-drawn vehicle injured in other and unspecified transport accidents**

● **V80.920 Occupant of animal-drawn vehicle injured in transport accident with military vehicle**

● **V80.928 Occupant of animal-drawn vehicle injured in other transport accident**

● **V80.929 Occupant of animal-drawn vehicle injured in unspecified transport accident**
Animal-drawn vehicle accident NOS

● **V81 Occupant of railway train or railway vehicle injured in transport accident**

Includes derailment of railway train or railway vehicle
person on outside of train

Excludes1 streetcar (V82.-)

The appropriate 7th character is to be added to each code from category V81

A	initial encounter
D	subsequent encounter
S	sequela

X● **V81.0 Occupant of railway train or railway vehicle injured in collision with motor vehicle in nontraffic accident**

Excludes1 occupant of railway train or railway vehicle injured due to collision with military vehicle (V81.83)

X● **V81.1 Occupant of railway train or railway vehicle injured in collision with motor vehicle in traffic accident**

Excludes1 occupant of railway train or railway vehicle injured due to collision with military vehicle (V81.83)

X● **V81.2 Occupant of railway train or railway vehicle injured in collision with or hit by rolling stock**

X● **V81.3 Occupant of railway train or railway vehicle injured in collision with other object**
Railway collision NOS

X● **V81.4 Person injured while boarding or alighting from railway train or railway vehicle**

X● **V81.5 Occupant of railway train or railway vehicle injured by fall in railway train or railway vehicle**

X● **V81.6 Occupant of railway train or railway vehicle injured by fall from railway train or railway vehicle**

X● **V81.7 Occupant of railway train or railway vehicle injured in derailment without antecedent collision**

● **V81.8 Occupant of railway train or railway vehicle injured in other specified railway accidents**

X● **V81.81 Occupant of railway train or railway vehicle injured due to explosion or fire on train**

X● **V81.82 Occupant of railway train or railway vehicle injured due to object falling onto train**

Occupant of railway train or railway vehicle injured due to falling earth onto train
Occupant of railway train or railway vehicle injured due to falling rocks onto train
Occupant of railway train or railway vehicle injured due to falling snow onto train
Occupant of railway train or railway vehicle injured due to falling trees onto train

X● **V81.83 Occupant of railway train or railway vehicle injured due to collision with military vehicle**

X● **V81.89 Occupant of railway train or railway vehicle injured due to other specified railway accident**

X● **V81.9 Occupant of railway train or railway vehicle injured in unspecified railway accident**

Railway accident NOS

● **V82 Occupant of powered streetcar injured in transport accident**

Includes interurban electric car
person on outside of streetcar
tram (car)
trolley (car)

Excludes1 bus (V70-V79)
motorcoach (V70-V79)
nonpowered streetcar (V76.-)
train (V81.-)

The appropriate 7th character is to be added to each code from category V82

A	initial encounter
D	subsequent encounter
S	sequela

X● **V82.0 Occupant of streetcar injured in collision with motor vehicle in nontraffic accident**

X● **V82.1 Occupant of streetcar injured in collision with motor vehicle in traffic accident**

X● **V82.2 Occupant of streetcar injured in collision with or hit by rolling stock**

X● **V82.3 Occupant of streetcar injured in collision with other object**

Excludes1 collision with animal-drawn vehicle or animal being ridden (V82.8)

X● **V82.4 Person injured while boarding or alighting from streetcar**

X● **V82.5 Occupant of streetcar injured by fall in streetcar**

Excludes1 fall in streetcar:
while boarding or alighting (V82.4)
with antecedent collision (V82.0-V82.3)

X● **V82.6 Occupant of streetcar injured by fall from streetcar**

Excludes1 fall from streetcar:
while boarding or alighting (V82.4)
with antecedent collision (V82.0-V82.3)

X● **V82.7 Occupant of streetcar injured in derailment without antecedent collision**

Excludes1 occupant of streetcar injured in derailment with antecedent collision (V82.0-V82.3)

X● **V82.8 Occupant of streetcar injured in other specified transport accidents**

Streetcar collision with military vehicle
Streetcar collision with train or nonmotor vehicles

X● **V82.9 Occupant of streetcar injured in unspecified traffic accident**

Streetcar accident NOS

● **V83 Occupant of special vehicle mainly used on industrial premises injured in transport accident**

Includes battery-powered airport passenger vehicle
battery-powered truck (baggage) (mail)
coal-car in mine
forklift (truck)
logging car
self-propelled industrial truck
station baggage truck (powered)
tram, truck, or tub (powered) in mine or quarry

Excludes1 special construction vehicles (V85.-)
special industrial vehicle in stationary use or maintenance (W31.-)

The appropriate 7th character is to be added to each code from category V83

A	initial encounter
D	subsequent encounter
S	sequela

X● **V83.0 Driver of special industrial vehicle injured in traffic accident**

X● **V83.1 Passenger of special industrial vehicle injured in traffic accident**

X● **V83.2 Person on outside of special industrial vehicle injured in traffic accident**

X● **V83.3 Unspecified occupant of special industrial vehicle injured in traffic accident**

X● **V83.4 Person injured while boarding or alighting from special industrial vehicle**

X● **V83.5 Driver of special industrial vehicle injured in nontraffic accident**

X● **V83.6 Passenger of special industrial vehicle injured in nontraffic accident**

X● **V83.7 Person on outside of special industrial vehicle injured in nontraffic accident**

X● **V83.9 Unspecified occupant of special industrial vehicle injured in nontraffic accident**

Special-industrial-vehicle accident NOS

● **V84 Occupant of special vehicle mainly used in agriculture injured in transport accident**

Includes self-propelled farm machinery
tractor (and trailer)

Excludes1 animal-powered farm machinery accident (W30.8-)
contact with combine harvester (W30.0)
special agricultural vehicle in stationary use or maintenance (W30.-)

The appropriate 7th character is to be added to each code from category V84

A	initial encounter
D	subsequent encounter
S	sequela

X● **V84.0 Driver of special agricultural vehicle injured in traffic accident**

X● **V84.1 Passenger of special agricultural vehicle injured in traffic accident**

X● **V84.2 Person on outside of special agricultural vehicle injured in traffic accident**

X● **V84.3 Unspecified occupant of special agricultural vehicle injured in traffic accident**

X● **V84.4 Person injured while boarding or alighting from special agricultural vehicle**

X● **V84.5 Driver of special agricultural vehicle injured in nontraffic accident**

X● **V84.6 Passenger of special agricultural vehicle injured in nontraffic accident**

X● **V84.7 Person on outside of special agricultural vehicle injured in nontraffic accident**

X● **V84.9 Unspecified occupant of special agricultural vehicle injured in nontraffic accident**

Special-agricultural vehicle accident NOS

● **V85 Occupant of special construction vehicle injured in transport accident**

Includes bulldozer
digger
dump truck
earth-leveller
mechanical shovel
road-roller

Excludes1 special industrial vehicle (V83.-)
special construction vehicle in stationary use or maintenance (W31.-)

The appropriate 7th character is to be added to each code from category V85

A	initial encounter
D	subsequent encounter
S	sequela

X● **V85.0 Driver of special construction vehicle injured in traffic accident**

X● **V85.1 Passenger of special construction vehicle injured in traffic accident**

X● **V85.2 Person on outside of special construction vehicle injured in traffic accident**

X● **V85.3 Unspecified occupant of special construction vehicle injured in traffic accident**

X● **V85.4 Person injured while boarding or alighting from special construction vehicle**

X● **V85.5 Driver of special construction vehicle injured in nontraffic accident**

X● **V85.6 Passenger of special construction vehicle injured in nontraffic accident**

X● **V85.7 Person on outside of special construction vehicle injured in nontraffic accident**

X● **V85.9 Unspecified occupant of special construction vehicle injured in nontraffic accident**
Special-construction-vehicle accident NOS

● **V86 Occupant of special all-terrain or other off-road motor vehicle, injured in transport accident**

Excludes1 special all-terrain vehicle in stationary use or maintenance (W31.-)
sport-utility vehicle (V50-V59)
three-wheeled motor vehicle designed for on-road use (V30-V39)

The appropriate 7th character is to be added to each code from category V86

A	initial encounter
D	subsequent encounter
S	sequela

● **V86.0 Driver of special all-terrain or other off-road motor vehicle injured in traffic accident**

X● **V86.01 Driver of ambulance or fire engine injured in traffic accident**

X● **V86.02 Driver of snowmobile injured in traffic accident**

X● **V86.03 Driver of dune buggy injured in traffic accident**

X● **V86.04 Driver of military vehicle injured in traffic accident**

X● **V86.09 Driver of other off-road special all-terrain or other off-road vehicle injured in traffic accident**
Driver of dirt bike injured in traffic accident
Driver of go cart injured in traffic accident
Driver of golf cart injured in traffic accident

● **V86.1 Passenger of special all-terrain or other off-road motor vehicle injured in traffic accident**

X● **V86.11 Passenger of ambulance or fire engine injured in traffic accident**

X● **V86.12 Passenger of snowmobile injured in traffic accident**

X● **V86.13 Passenger of dune buggy injured in traffic accident**

X● **V86.14 Passenger of military vehicle injured in traffic accident**

X● **V86.19 Passenger of other off-road special all-terrain or other off-road off-road motor vehicle injured in traffic accident**
Passenger of dirt bike injured in traffic accident
Passenger of go cart injured in traffic accident
Passenger of golf cart injured in traffic accident

● **V86.2 Person on outside of special all-terrain or other off-road motor vehicle injured in traffic accident**

X● **V86.21 Person on outside of ambulance or fire engine injured in traffic accident**

X● **V86.22 Person on outside of snowmobile injured in traffic accident**

X● **V86.23 Person on outside of dune buggy injured in traffic accident**

X● **V86.24 Person on outside of military vehicle injured in traffic accident**

X● **V86.29 Person on outside of other special all-terrain or other off-road motor vehicle injured in traffic accident**
Person on outside of dirt bike injured in traffic accident
Person on outside of go cart in traffic accident
Person on outside of golf cart injured in traffic accident

● **V86.3 Unspecified occupant of special all-terrain or other off-road motor vehicle injured in traffic accident**

X● **V86.31 Unspecified occupant of ambulance or fire engine injured in traffic accident**

X● **V86.32 Unspecified occupant of snowmobile injured in traffic accident**

X● **V86.33 Unspecified occupant of dune buggy injured in traffic accident**

X● **V86.34 Unspecified occupant of military vehicle injured in traffic accident**

X● **V86.39 Unspecified occupant of other special all-terrain or other off-road motor vehicle injured in traffic accident**
Unspecified occupant of dirt bike injured in traffic accident
Unspecified occupant of go cart injured in traffic accident
Unspecified occupant of golf cart injured in traffic accident

● **V86.4 Person injured while boarding or alighting from special all-terrain or other off-road motor vehicle**

X● **V86.41 Person injured while boarding or alighting from ambulance or fire engine**

X● **V86.42 Person injured while boarding or alighting from snowmobile**

X● **V86.43 Person injured while boarding or alighting from dune buggy**

X● **V86.44 Person injured while boarding or alighting from military vehicle**

X● **V86.49 Person injured while boarding or alighting from other special all-terrain or other off-road motor vehicle**
Person injured while boarding or alighting from dirt bike
Person injured while boarding or alighting from go cart
Person injured while boarding or alighting from golf cart

● **V86.5 Driver of special all-terrain or other off-road motor vehicle injured in nontraffic accident**

X● **V86.51 Driver of ambulance or fire engine injured in nontraffic accident**

X● **V86.52 Driver of snowmobile injured in nontraffic accident**

X● **V86.53 Driver of dune buggy injured in nontraffic accident**

X● **V86.54 Driver of military vehicle injured in nontraffic accident**

X● **V86.59 Driver of other off-road special all-terrain or other off-road motor vehicle injured in nontraffic accident**
- Driver of dirt bike injured in nontraffic accident
- Driver of go cart injured in nontraffic accident
- Driver of golf cart injured in nontraffic accident

● **V86.6 Passenger of special all-terrain or other off-road motor vehicle injured in nontraffic accident**

X● **V86.61 Passenger of ambulance or fire engine injured in nontraffic accident**

X● **V86.62 Passenger of snowmobile injured in nontraffic accident**

X● **V86.63 Passenger of dune buggy injured in nontraffic accident**

X● **V86.64 Passenger of military vehicle injured in nontraffic accident**

X● **V86.69 Passenger of other special all-terrain or other off-road vehicle injured in nontraffic accident**
- Passenger of dirt bike injured in nontraffic accident
- Passenger of go cart injured in nontraffic accident
- Passenger of golf cart injured in nontraffic accident

● **V86.7 Person on outside of special all-terrain or other off-road motor vehicle injured in nontraffic accident**

X● **V86.71 Person on outside of ambulance or fire engine injured in nontraffic accident**

X● **V86.72 Person on outside of snowmobile injured in nontraffic accident**

X● **V86.73 Person on outside of dune buggy injured in nontraffic accident**

X● **V86.74 Person on outside of military vehicle injured in nontraffic accident**

X● **V86.79 Person on outside of other special all-terrain or other off-road motor vehicles injured in nontraffic accident**
- Person on outside of dirt bike injured in nontraffic accident
- Person on outside of go cart injured in nontraffic accident
- Person on outside of golf cart injured in nontraffic accident

● **V86.9 Unspecified occupant of special all-terrain or other off-road motor vehicle injured in nontraffic accident**

X● **V86.91 Unspecified occupant of ambulance or fire engine injured in nontraffic accident**

X● **V86.92 Unspecified occupant of snowmobile injured in nontraffic accident**

X● **V86.93 Unspecified occupant of dune buggy injured in nontraffic accident**

X● **V86.94 Unspecified occupant of military vehicle injured in nontraffic accident**

X● **V86.99 Unspecified occupant of other off-road special all-terrain or other off-road motor vehicle injured in nontraffic accident**
- All-terrain motor-vehicle accident NOS
- Off-road motor-vehicle accident NOS
- Other motor-vehicle accident NOS
- Unspecified occupant of dirt bike injured in nontraffic accident
- Unspecified occupant of go cart injured in nontraffic accident
- Unspecified occupant of golf cart injured in nontraffic accident
- Unspecified occupant of race car injured in nontraffic accident

● **V87 Traffic accident of specified type but victim's mode of transport unknown**

Excludes1 collision involving:
- pedal cycle (V10-V19)
- pedestrian (V01-V09)

The appropriate 7th character is to be added to each code from category V87

A	initial encounter
D	subsequent encounter
S	sequela

X● **V87.0 Person injured in collision between car and two- or three-wheeled powered vehicle (traffic)**

X● **V87.1 Person injured in collision between other motor vehicle and two- or three-wheeled motor vehicle (traffic)**

X● **V87.2 Person injured in collision between car and pick-up truck or van (traffic)**

X● **V87.3 Person injured in collision between car and bus (traffic)**

X● **V87.4 Person injured in collision between car and heavy transport vehicle (traffic)**

X● **V87.5 Person injured in collision between heavy transport vehicle and bus (traffic)**

X● **V87.6 Person injured in collision between railway train or railway vehicle and car (traffic)**

X● **V87.7 Person injured in collision between other specified motor vehicles (traffic)**

X● **V87.8 Person injured in other specified noncollision transport accidents involving motor vehicle (traffic)**

X● **V87.9 Person injured in other specified (collision) (noncollision) transport accidents involving nonmotor vehicle (traffic)**

● **V88 Nontraffic accident of specified type but victim's mode of transport unknown**

Excludes1 collision involving:
- pedal cycle (V10-V19)
- pedestrian (V01-V09)

The appropriate 7th character is to be added to each code from category V88

A	initial encounter
D	subsequent encounter
S	sequela

X● **V88.0 Person injured in collision between car and two- or three-wheeled motor vehicle, nontraffic**

X● **V88.1 Person injured in collision between other motor vehicle and two- or three-wheeled motor vehicle, nontraffic**

X● **V88.2 Person injured in collision between car and pick-up truck or van, nontraffic**

X● **V88.3 Person injured in collision between car and bus, nontraffic**

X● **V88.4 Person injured in collision between car and heavy transport vehicle, nontraffic**

X● **V88.5 Person injured in collision between heavy transport vehicle and bus, nontraffic**

X● **V88.6 Person injured in collision between railway train or railway vehicle and car, nontraffic**

X● **V88.7 Person injured in collision between other specified motor vehicle, nontraffic**

X● **V88.8 Person injured in other specified noncollision transport accidents involving motor vehicle, nontraffic**

X● **V88.9 Person injured in other specified (collision) (noncollision) transport accidents involving nonmotor vehicle, nontraffic**

● **V89 Motor- or nonmotor-vehicle accident, type of vehicle unspecified**

The appropriate 7th character is to be added to each code from category V89

A	initial encounter
D	subsequent encounter
S	sequela

X● **V89.0 Person injured in unspecified motor-vehicle accident, nontraffic**
Motor-vehicle accident NOS, nontraffic

X● **V89.1 Person injured in unspecified nonmotor-vehicle accident, nontraffic**
Nonmotor-vehicle accident NOS (nontraffic)

X● **V89.2 Person injured in unspecified motor-vehicle accident, traffic**
Motor-vehicle accident [MVA] NOS
Road (traffic) accident [RTA] NOS

X● **V89.3 Person injured in unspecified nonmotor-vehicle accident, traffic**
Nonmotor-vehicle traffic accident NOS

X● **V89.9 Person injured in unspecified vehicle accident**
Collision NOS

WATER TRANSPORT ACCIDENTS (V90-V94)

● **V90 Drowning and submersion due to accident to watercraft**

Excludes1 civilian water transport accident involving military watercraft (V94.81-)
fall into water not from watercraft (W16.-)
military watercraft accident in military or war operations (Y36.0-, Y37.0-)
water-transport–related drowning or submersion without accident to watercraft (V92.-)

The appropriate 7th character is to be added to each code from category V90

A	initial encounter
D	subsequent encounter
S	sequela

● **V90.0 Drowning and submersion due to watercraft overturning**

X● **V90.00 Drowning and submersion due to merchant ship overturning**

X● **V90.01 Drowning and submersion due to passenger ship overturning**
Drowning and submersion due to ferry-boat overturning
Drowning and submersion due to liner overturning

X● **V90.02 Drowning and submersion due to fishing boat overturning**

X● **V90.03 Drowning and submersion due to other powered watercraft overturning**
Drowning and submersion due to hovercraft (on open water) overturning
Drowning and submersion due to jet ski overturning

X● **V90.04 Drowning and submersion due to sailboat overturning**

X● **V90.05 Drowning and submersion due to canoe or kayak overturning**

X● **V90.06 Drowning and submersion due to (nonpowered) inflatable craft overturning**

X● **V90.08 Drowning and submersion due to other unpowered watercraft overturning**
Drowning and submersion due to windsurfer overturning

X● **V90.09 Drowning and submersion due to unspecified watercraft overturning**
Drowning and submersion due to boat NOS overturning
Drowning and submersion due to ship NOS overturning
Drowning and submersion due to watercraft NOS overturning

● **V90.1 Drowning and submersion due to watercraft sinking**

X● **V90.10 Drowning and submersion due to merchant ship sinking**

X● **V90.11 Drowning and submersion due to passenger ship sinking**
Drowning and submersion due to ferry-boat sinking
Drowning and submersion due to liner sinking

X● **V90.12 Drowning and submersion due to fishing boat sinking**

X● **V90.13 Drowning and submersion due to other powered watercraft sinking**
Drowning and submersion due to hovercraft (on open water) sinking
Drowning and submersion due to jet ski sinking

X● **V90.14 Drowning and submersion due to sailboat sinking**

X● **V90.15 Drowning and submersion due to canoe or kayak sinking**

X● **V90.16 Drowning and submersion due to (nonpowered) inflatable craft sinking**

X● **V90.18 Drowning and submersion due to other unpowered watercraft sinking**

X● **V90.19 Drowning and submersion due to unspecified watercraft sinking**
Drowning and submersion due to boat NOS sinking
Drowning and submersion due to ship NOS sinking
Drowning and submersion due to watercraft NOS sinking

● **V90.2 Drowning and submersion due to falling or jumping from burning watercraft**

X● **V90.20 Drowning and submersion due to falling or jumping from burning merchant ship**

X● **V90.21 Drowning and submersion due to falling or jumping from burning passenger ship**
Drowning and submersion due to falling or jumping from burning ferry-boat
Drowning and submersion due to falling or jumping from burning liner

X● **V90.22 Drowning and submersion due to falling or jumping from burning fishing boat**

X● **V90.23 Drowning and submersion due to falling or jumping from other burning powered watercraft**
Drowning and submersion due to falling and jumping from burning hovercraft (on open water)
Drowning and submersion due to falling and jumping from burning jet ski

X● **V90.24 Drowning and submersion due to falling or jumping from burning sailboat**

X● **V90.25 Drowning and submersion due to falling or jumping from burning canoe or kayak**

◀ New ⇐ Revised ~~deleted~~ Deleted Excludes 1 Excludes 2 Includes Use additional Code first Code also Unspecified
OGCR Official Guidelines ● Unacceptable Principal Diagnosis X Assign placeholder X ● Use Additional Character(s) ▶ Manifestation Code Coding Clinic

X● **V90.26 Drowning and submersion due to falling or jumping from burning (nonpowered) inflatable craft**

X● **V90.27 Drowning and submersion due to falling or jumping from burning water-skis**

X● **V90.28 Drowning and submersion due to falling or jumping from other burning unpowered watercraft**
- Drowning and submersion due to falling and jumping from burning surf-board
- Drowning and submersion due to falling and jumping from burning windsurfer

X● **V90.29 Drowning and submersion due to falling or jumping from unspecified burning watercraft**
- Drowning and submersion due to falling or jumping from burning boat NOS
- Drowning and submersion due to falling or jumping from burning ship NOS
- Drowning and submersion due to falling or jumping from burning watercraft NOS

● **V90.3 Drowning and submersion due to falling or jumping from crushed watercraft**

X● **V90.30 Drowning and submersion due to falling or jumping from crushed merchant ship**

X● **V90.31 Drowning and submersion due to falling or jumping from crushed passenger ship**
- Drowning and submersion due to falling and jumping from crushed ferry-boat
- Drowning and submersion due to falling and jumping from crushed liner

X● **V90.32 Drowning and submersion due to falling or jumping from crushed fishing boat**

X● **V90.33 Drowning and submersion due to falling or jumping from other crushed powered watercraft**
- Drowning and submersion due to falling and jumping from crushed hovercraft
- Drowning and submersion due to falling and jumping from crushed jet ski

X● **V90.34 Drowning and submersion due to falling or jumping from crushed sailboat**

X● **V90.35 Drowning and submersion due to falling or jumping from crushed canoe or kayak**

X● **V90.36 Drowning and submersion due to falling or jumping from crushed (nonpowered) inflatable craft**

X● **V90.37 Drowning and submersion due to falling or jumping from crushed water-skis**

X● **V90.38 Drowning and submersion due to falling or jumping from other crushed unpowered watercraft**
- Drowning and submersion due to falling and jumping from crushed surf-board
- Drowning and submersion due to falling and jumping from crushed windsurfer

X● **V90.39 Drowning and submersion due to falling or jumping from crushed unspecified watercraft**
- Drowning and submersion due to falling and jumping from crushed boat NOS
- Drowning and submersion due to falling and jumping from crushed ship NOS
- Drowning and submersion due to falling and jumping from crushed watercraft NOS

● **V90.8 Drowning and submersion due to other accident to watercraft**

X● **V90.80 Drowning and submersion due to other accident to merchant ship**

X● **V90.81 Drowning and submersion due to other accident to passenger ship**
- Drowning and submersion due to other accident to ferry-boat
- Drowning and submersion due to other accident to liner

X● **V90.82 Drowning and submersion due to other accident to fishing boat**

X● **V90.83 Drowning and submersion due to other accident to other powered watercraft**
- Drowning and submersion due to other accident to hovercraft (on open water)
- Drowning and submersion due to other accident to jet ski

X● **V90.84 Drowning and submersion due to other accident to sailboat**

X● **V90.85 Drowning and submersion due to other accident to canoe or kayak**

X● **V90.86 Drowning and submersion due to other accident to (nonpowered) inflatable craft**

X● **V90.87 Drowning and submersion due to other accident to water-skis**

X● **V90.88 Drowning and submersion due to other accident to other unpowered watercraft**
- Drowning and submersion due to other accident to surf-board
- Drowning and submersion due to other accident to windsurfer

X● **V90.89 Drowning and submersion due to other accident to unspecified watercraft**
- Drowning and submersion due to other accident to boat NOS
- Drowning and submersion due to other accident to ship NOS
- Drowning and submersion due to other accident to watercraft NOS

● **V91 Other injury due to accident to watercraft**

Includes any injury except drowning and submersion as a result of an accident to watercraft

Excludes1 civilian water transport accident involving military watercraft (V94.81-)
military watercraft accident in military or war operations (Y36, Y37.-)

Excludes2 drowning and submersion due to accident to watercraft (V90.-)

The appropriate 7th character is to be added to each code from category V91

A	initial encounter
D	subsequent encounter
S	sequela

● **V91.0 Burn due to watercraft on fire**

Excludes1 burn from localized fire or explosion on board ship without accident to watercraft (V93.-)

X● **V91.00 Burn due to merchant ship on fire**

X● **V91.01 Burn due to passenger ship on fire**
- Burn due to ferry-boat on fire
- Burn due to liner on fire

X● **V91.02 Burn due to fishing boat on fire**

X● **V91.03 Burn due to other powered watercraft on fire**
- Burn due to hovercraft (on open water) on fire
- Burn due to jet ski on fire

X● **V91.04 Burn due to sailboat on fire**

X● **V91.05 Burn due to canoe or kayak on fire**

X● **V91.06 Burn due to (nonpowered) inflatable craft on fire**

X● **V91.07 Burn due to water-skis on fire**

X● **V91.08 Burn due to other unpowered watercraft on fire**

X● **V91.09 Burn due to unspecified watercraft on fire**
- Burn due to boat NOS on fire
- Burn due to ship NOS on fire
- Burn due to watercraft NOS on fire

● **V91.1 Crushed between watercraft and other watercraft or other object due to collision**
Crushed by lifeboat after abandoning ship in a collision
Note: Select the specified type of watercraft that the victim was on at the time of the collision.

X● **V91.10 Crushed between merchant ship and other watercraft or other object due to collision**

X● **V91.11 Crushed between passenger ship and other watercraft or other object due to collision**
Crushed between ferry-boat and other watercraft or other object due to collision
Crushed between liner and other watercraft or other object due to collision

X● **V91.12 Crushed between fishing boat and other watercraft or other object due to collision**

X● **V91.13 Crushed between other powered watercraft and other watercraft or other object due to collision**
Crushed between hovercraft (on open water) and other watercraft or other object due to collision
Crushed between jet ski and other watercraft or other object due to collision

X● **V91.14 Crushed between sailboat and other watercraft or other object due to collision**

X● **V91.15 Crushed between canoe or kayak and other watercraft or other object due to collision**

X● **V91.16 Crushed between (nonpowered) inflatable craft and other watercraft or other object due to collision**

X● **V91.18 Crushed between other unpowered watercraft and other watercraft or other object due to collision**
Crushed between surfboard and other watercraft or other object due to collision
Crushed between windsurfer and other watercraft or other object due to collision

X● **V91.19 Crushed between unspecified watercraft and other watercraft or other object due to collision**
Crushed between boat NOS and other watercraft or other object due to collision
Crushed between ship NOS and other watercraft or other object due to collision
Crushed between watercraft NOS and other watercraft or other object due to collision

● **V91.2 Fall due to collision between watercraft and other watercraft or other object**
Fall while remaining on watercraft after collision
Note: Select the specified type of watercraft that the victim was on at the time of the collision.

Excludes1 crushed between watercraft and other watercraft and other object due to collision (V91.1-)
drowning and submersion due to falling from crushed watercraft (V90.3-)

X● **V91.20 Fall due to collision between merchant ship and other watercraft or other object**

X● **V91.21 Fall due to collision between passenger ship and other watercraft or other object**
Fall due to collision between ferry-boat and other watercraft or other object
Fall due to collision between liner and other watercraft or other object

X● **V91.22 Fall due to collision between fishing boat and other watercraft or other object**

X● **V91.23 Fall due to collision between other powered watercraft and other watercraft or other object**
Fall due to collision between hovercraft (on open water) and other watercraft or other object
Fall due to collision between jet ski and other watercraft or other object

X● **V91.24 Fall due to collision between sailboat and other watercraft or other object**

X● **V91.25 Fall due to collision between canoe or kayak and other watercraft or other object**

X● **V91.26 Fall due to collision between (nonpowered) inflatable craft and other watercraft or other object**

X● **V91.29 Fall due to collision between unspecified watercraft and other watercraft or other object**
Fall due to collision between boat NOS and other watercraft or other object
Fall due to collision between ship NOS and other watercraft or other object
Fall due to collision between watercraft NOS and other watercraft or other object

● **V91.3 Hit or struck by falling object due to accident to watercraft**
Hit or struck by falling object (part of damaged watercraft or other object) after falling or jumping from damaged watercraft

Excludes2 drowning or submersion due to fall or jumping from damaged watercraft (V90.2-, V90.3-)

X● **V91.30 Hit or struck by falling object due to accident to merchant ship**

X● **V91.31 Hit or struck by falling object due to accident to passenger ship**
Hit or struck by falling object due to accident to ferry-boat
Hit or struck by falling object due to accident to liner

X● **V91.32 Hit or struck by falling object due to accident to fishing boat**

X● **V91.33 Hit or struck by falling object due to accident to other powered watercraft**
Hit or struck by falling object due to accident to hovercraft (on open water)
Hit or struck by falling object due to accident to jet ski

X● **V91.34 Hit or struck by falling object due to accident to sailboat**

X● **V91.35 Hit or struck by falling object due to accident to canoe or kayak**

X● **V91.36 Hit or struck by falling object due to accident to (nonpowered) inflatable craft**

X● **V91.37 Hit or struck by falling object due to accident to water-skis**
Hit by water-skis after jumping off of waterskis

X● **V91.38 Hit or struck by falling object due to accident to other unpowered watercraft**
Hit or struck by surf-board after falling off damaged surf-board
Hit or struck by object after falling off damaged windsurfer

X● **V91.39 Hit or struck by falling object due to accident to unspecified watercraft**
Hit or struck by falling object due to accident to boat NOS
Hit or struck by falling object due to accident to ship NOS
Hit or struck by falling object due to accident to watercraft NOS

● **V91.8 Other injury due to other accident to watercraft**

X● **V91.80 Other injury due to other accident to merchant ship**

X● **V91.81 Other injury due to other accident to passenger ship**
- Other injury due to other accident to ferry-boat
- Other injury due to other accident to liner

X● **V91.82 Other injury due to other accident to fishing boat**

X● **V91.83 Other injury due to other accident to other powered watercraft**
- Other injury due to other accident to hovercraft (on open water)
- Other injury due to other accident to jet ski

X● **V91.84 Other injury due to other accident to sailboat**

X● **V91.85 Other injury due to other accident to canoe or kayak**

X● **V91.86 Other injury due to other accident to (nonpowered) inflatable craft**

X● **V91.87 Other injury due to other accident to water-skis**

X● **V91.88 Other injury due to other accident to other unpowered watercraft**
- Other injury due to other accident to surf-board
- Other injury due to other accident to windsurfer

X● **V91.89 Other injury due to other accident to unspecified watercraft**
- Other injury due to other accident to boat NOS
- Other injury due to other accident to ship NOS
- Other injury due to other accident to watercraft NOS

● **V92 Drowning and submersion due to accident on board watercraft, without accident to watercraft**

Excludes1 civilian water transport accident involving military watercraft (V94.81-)
drowning or submersion due to accident to watercraft (V90-V91)
drowning or submersion of diver who voluntarily jumps from boat not involved in an accident (W16.711, W16.721)
fall into water without watercraft (W16.-)
military watercraft accident in military or war operations (Y36, Y37)

The appropriate 7th character is to be added to each code from category V92

A	initial encounter
D	subsequent encounter
S	sequela

● **V92.0 Drowning and submersion due to fall off watercraft**
- Drowning and submersion due to fall from gangplank of watercraft
- Drowning and submersion due to fall overboard watercraft

Excludes2 hitting head on object or bottom of body of water due to fall from watercraft (V94.0-)

X● **V92.00 Drowning and submersion due to fall off merchant ship**

X● **V92.01 Drowning and submersion due to fall off passenger ship**
- Drowning and submersion due to fall off ferry-boat
- Drowning and submersion due to fall off liner

X● **V92.02 Drowning and submersion due to fall off fishing boat**

X● **V92.03 Drowning and submersion due to fall off other powered watercraft**
- Drowning and submersion due to fall off hovercraft (on open water)
- Drowning and submersion due to fall off jet ski

X● **V92.04 Drowning and submersion due to fall off sailboat**

X● **V92.05 Drowning and submersion due to fall off canoe or kayak**

X● **V92.06 Drowning and submersion due to fall off (nonpowered) inflatable craft**

X● **V92.07 Drowning and submersion due to fall off water-skis**

Excludes1 drowning and submersion due to falling off burning water-skis (V90.27)
drowning and submersion due to falling off crushed water-skis (V90.37)
hit by boat while water-skiing NOS (V94.X)

X● **V92.08 Drowning and submersion due to fall off other unpowered watercraft**
- Drowning and submersion due to fall off surf-board
- Drowning and submersion due to fall off windsurfer

Excludes1 drowning and submersion due to fall off burning unpowered watercraft (V90.28)
drowning and submersion due to fall off crushed unpowered watercraft (V90.38)
drowning and submersion due to fall off damaged unpowered watercraft (V90.88)
drowning and submersion due to rider of nonpowered watercraft being hit by other watercraft (V94.-)
other injury due to rider of nonpowered watercraft being hit by other watercraft (V94.-)

X● **V92.09 Drowning and submersion due to fall off unspecified watercraft**
- Drowning and submersion due to fall off boat NOS
- Drowning and submersion due to fall off ship
- Drowning and submersion due to fall off watercraft NOS

● **V92.1 Drowning and submersion due to being thrown overboard by motion of watercraft**

Excludes1 drowning and submersion due to fall off surf-board (V92.08)
drowning and submersion due to fall off water-skis (V92.07)
drowning and submersion due to fall off windsurfer (V92.08)

X● **V92.10 Drowning and submersion due to being thrown overboard by motion of merchant ship**

X● **V92.11 Drowning and submersion due to being thrown overboard by motion of passenger ship**
- Drowning and submersion due to being thrown overboard by motion of ferry-boat
- Drowning and submersion due to being thrown overboard by motion of liner

X● **V92.12 Drowning and submersion due to being thrown overboard by motion of fishing boat**

X● **V92.13 Drowning and submersion due to being thrown overboard by motion of other powered watercraft**
Drowning and submersion due to being thrown overboard by motion of hovercraft

X● **V92.14 Drowning and submersion due to being thrown overboard by motion of sailboat**

X● **V92.15 Drowning and submersion due to being thrown overboard by motion of canoe or kayak**

X● **V92.16 Drowning and submersion due to being thrown overboard by motion of (nonpowered) inflatable craft**

X● **V92.19 Drowning and submersion due to being thrown overboard by motion of unspecified watercraft**
Drowning and submersion due to being thrown overboard by motion of boat NOS
Drowning and submersion due to being thrown overboard by motion of ship NOS
Drowning and submersion due to being thrown overboard by motion of watercraft NOS

● **V92.2 Drowning and submersion due to being washed overboard from watercraft**
Code first any associated cataclysm (X37.0-)

X● **V92.20 Drowning and submersion due to being washed overboard from merchant ship**

X● **V92.21 Drowning and submersion due to being washed overboard from passenger ship**
Drowning and submersion due to being washed overboard from ferry-boat
Drowning and submersion due to being washed overboard from liner

X● **V92.22 Drowning and submersion due to being washed overboard from fishing boat**

X● **V92.23 Drowning and submersion due to being washed overboard from other powered watercraft**
Drowning and submersion due to being washed overboard from hovercraft (on open water)
Drowning and submersion due to being washed overboard from jet ski

X● **V92.24 Drowning and submersion due to being washed overboard from sailboat**

X● **V92.25 Drowning and submersion due to being washed overboard from canoe or kayak**

X● **V92.26 Drowning and submersion due to being washed overboard from (nonpowered) inflatable craft**

X● **V92.27 Drowning and submersion due to being washed overboard from water-skis**
Excludes1 drowning and submersion due to fall off water-skis (V92.07)

X● **V92.28 Drowning and submersion due to being washed overboard from other unpowered watercraft**
Drowning and submersion due to being washed overboard from surf-board
Drowning and submersion due to being washed overboard from windsurfer

X● **V92.29 Drowning and submersion due to being washed overboard from unspecified watercraft**
Drowning and submersion due to being washed overboard from boat NOS
Drowning and submersion due to being washed overboard from ship NOS
Drowning and submersion due to being washed overboard from watercraft NOS

● **V93 Other injury due to accident on board watercraft, without accident to watercraft**
Excludes1 civilian water transport accident involving military watercraft (V94.81-)
other injury due to accident to watercraft (V91.-)
military watercraft accident in military or war operations (Y36, Y37.-)
Excludes2 drowning and submersion due to accident on board watercraft, without accident to watercraft (V92.-)
The appropriate 7th character is to be added to each code from category V93

A	initial encounter
D	subsequent encounter
S	sequela

● **V93.0 Burn due to localized fire on board watercraft**
Excludes1 burn due to watercraft on fire (V91.0-)

X● **V93.00 Burn due to localized fire on board merchant vessel**

X● **V93.01 Burn due to localized fire on board passenger vessel**
Burn due to localized fire on board ferry-boat
Burn due to localized fire on board liner

X● **V93.02 Burn due to localized fire on board fishing boat**

X● **V93.03 Burn due to localized fire on board other powered watercraft**
Burn due to localized fire on board hovercraft
Burn due to localized fire on board jet ski

X● **V93.04 Burn due to localized fire on board sailboat**

X● **V93.09 Burn due to localized fire on board unspecified watercraft**
Burn due to localized fire on board boat NOS
Burn due to localized fire on board ship NOS
Burn due to localized fire on board watercraft NOS

● **V93.1 Other burn on board watercraft**
Burn due to source other than fire on board watercraft
Excludes1 burn due to watercraft on fire (V91.0-)

X● **V93.10 Other burn on board merchant vessel**

X● **V93.11 Other burn on board passenger vessel**
Other burn on board ferry-boat
Other burn on board liner

X● **V93.12 Other burn on board fishing boat**

X● **V93.13 Other burn on board other powered watercraft**
Other burn on board hovercraft
Other burn on board jet ski

X● **V93.14 Other burn on board sailboat**

X● **V93.19 Other burn on board unspecified watercraft**
Other burn on board boat NOS
Other burn on board ship NOS
Other burn on board watercraft NOS

● **V93.2 Heat exposure on board watercraft**
Excludes1 exposure to man-made heat not aboard watercraft (W92)
exposure to natural heat while on board watercraft (X30)
exposure to sunlight while on board watercraft (X32)
Excludes2 burn due to fire on board watercraft (V93.0-)

X● **V93.20 Heat exposure on board merchant ship**

X● **V93.21 Heat exposure on board passenger ship**
Heat exposure on board ferry-boat
Heat exposure on board liner

X● **V93.22 Heat exposure on board fishing boat**

X● **V93.23 Heat exposure on board other powered watercraft**
Heat exposure on board hovercraft

X● **V93.24 Heat exposure on board sailboat**

X● **V93.29 Heat exposure on board unspecified watercraft**
Heat exposure on board boat NOS
Heat exposure on board ship NOS
Heat exposure on board watercraft NOS

● **V93.3 Fall on board watercraft**
Excludes1 fall due to collision of watercraft (V91.2-)

X● **V93.30 Fall on board merchant ship**

X● **V93.31 Fall on board passenger ship**
Fall on board ferry-boat
Fall on board liner

X● **V93.32 Fall on board fishing boat**

X● **V93.33 Fall on board other powered watercraft**
Fall on board hovercraft (on open water)
Fall on board jet ski

X● **V93.34 Fall on board sailboat**

X● **V93.35 Fall on board canoe or kayak**

X● **V93.36 Fall on board (nonpowered) inflatable craft**

X● **V93.38 Fall on board other unpowered watercraft**

X● **V93.39 Fall on board unspecified watercraft**
Fall on board boat NOS
Fall on board ship NOS
Fall on board watercraft NOS

● **V93.4 Struck by falling object on board watercraft**
Hit by falling object on board watercraft
Excludes1 struck by falling object due to accident to watercraft (V91.3)

X● **V93.40 Struck by falling object on merchant ship**

X● **V93.41 Struck by falling object on passenger ship**
Struck by falling object on ferry-boat
Struck by falling object on liner

X● **V93.42 Struck by falling object on fishing boat**

X● **V93.43 Struck by falling object on other powered watercraft**
Struck by falling object on hovercraft

X● **V93.44 Struck by falling object on sailboat**

X● **V93.48 Struck by falling object on other unpowered watercraft**

X● **V93.49 Struck by falling object on unspecified watercraft**

● **V93.5 Explosion on board watercraft**
Boiler explosion on steamship
Excludes2 fire on board watercraft (V93.0-)

X● **V93.50 Explosion on board merchant ship**

X● **V93.51 Explosion on board passenger ship**
Explosion on board ferry-boat
Explosion on board liner

X● **V93.52 Explosion on board fishing boat**

X● **V93.53 Explosion on board other powered watercraft**
Explosion on board hovercraft
Explosion on board jet ski

X● **V93.54 Explosion on board sailboat**

X● **V93.59 Explosion on board unspecified watercraft**
Explosion on board boat NOS
Explosion on board ship NOS
Explosion on board watercraft NOS

● **V93.6 Machinery accident on board watercraft**
Excludes1 machinery explosion on board watercraft (V93.4-)
machinery fire on board watercraft (V93.0-)

X● **V93.60 Machinery accident on board merchant ship**

X● **V93.61 Machinery accident on board passenger ship**
Machinery accident on board ferry-boat
Machinery accident on board liner

X● **V93.62 Machinery accident on board fishing boat**

X● **V93.63 Machinery accident on board other powered watercraft**
Machinery accident on board hovercraft

X● **V93.64 Machinery accident on board sailboat**

X● **V93.69 Machinery accident on board unspecified watercraft**
Machinery accident on board boat NOS
Machinery accident on board ship NOS
Machinery accident on board watercraft NOS

● **V93.8 Other injury due to other accident on board watercraft**
Accidental poisoning by gases or fumes on watercraft

X● **V93.80 Other injury due to other accident on board merchant ship**

X● **V93.81 Other injury due to other accident on board passenger ship**
Other injury due to other accident on board ferry-boat
Other injury due to other accident on board liner

X● **V93.82 Other injury due to other accident on board fishing boat**

X● **V93.83 Other injury due to other accident on board other powered watercraft**
Other injury due to other accident on board hovercraft
Other injury due to other accident on board jet ski

X● **V93.84 Other injury due to other accident on board sailboat**

X● **V93.85 Other injury due to other accident on board canoe or kayak**

X● **V93.86 Other injury due to other accident on board (nonpowered) inflatable craft**

X● **V93.87 Other injury due to other accident on board water-skis**
Hit or struck by object while waterskiing

X● **V93.88 Other injury due to other accident on board other unpowered watercraft**
Hit or struck by object while surfing
Hit or struck by object while on board windsurfer

X● **V93.89 Other injury due to other accident on board unspecified watercraft**
Other injury due to other accident on board boat NOS
Other injury due to other accident on board ship NOS
Other injury due to other accident on board watercraft NOS

● **V94 Other and unspecified water transport accidents**
Excludes1 military watercraft accidents in military or war operations (Y36, Y37)

The appropriate 7th character is to be added to each code from category V94

A	initial encounter
D	subsequent encounter
S	sequela

X● **V94.0 Hitting object or bottom of body of water due to fall from watercraft**
Excludes2 drowning and submersion due to fall from watercraft (V92.0-)

● **V94.1 Bather struck by watercraft**
Swimmer hit by watercraft

X● **V94.11 Bather struck by powered watercraft**

X● **V94.12 Bather struck by nonpowered watercraft**

● **V94.2 Rider of nonpowered watercraft struck by other watercraft**

X● **V94.21 Rider of nonpowered watercraft struck by other nonpowered watercraft**
Canoer hit by other nonpowered watercraft
Surfer hit by other nonpowered watercraft
Windsurfer hit by other nonpowered watercraft

X● **V94.22 Rider of nonpowered watercraft struck by powered watercraft**
Canoer hit by motorboat
Surfer hit by motorboat
Windsurfer hit by motorboat

● **V94.3 Injury to rider of (inflatable) watercraft being pulled behind other watercraft**

X● **V94.31 Injury to rider of (inflatable) recreational watercraft being pulled behind other watercraft**
Injury to rider of inner-tube pulled behind motor boat

X● **V94.32 Injury to rider of non-recreational watercraft being pulled behind other watercraft**
Injury to occupant of dingy being pulled behind boat or ship
Injury to occupant of life-raft being pulled behind boat or ship

X● **V94.4 Injury to barefoot water-skier**
Injury to person being pulled behind boat or ship

● **V94.8 Other water transport accident**

● **V94.81 Water transport accident involving military watercraft**

● **V94.810 Civilian watercraft involved in water transport accident with military watercraft**
Passenger on civilian watercraft injured due to accident with military watercraft

● **V94.811 Civilian in water injured by military watercraft**

● **V94.818 Other water transport accident involving military watercraft**

X● **V94.89 Other water transport accident**

X● **V94.9 Unspecified water transport accident**
Water transport accident NOS

AIR AND SPACE TRANSPORT ACCIDENTS (V95-V97)

Excludes1 military aircraft accidents in military or war operations (Y36, Y37)

● **V95 Accident to powered aircraft causing injury to occupant**
The appropriate 7th character is to be added to each code from category V95

A	initial encounter
D	subsequent encounter
S	sequela

● **V95.0 Helicopter accident injuring occupant**

X● **V95.00 Unspecified helicopter accident injuring occupant**

X● **V95.01 Helicopter crash injuring occupant**

X● **V95.02 Forced landing of helicopter injuring occupant**

X● **V95.03 Helicopter collision injuring occupant**
Helicopter collision with any object, fixed, movable or moving

X● **V95.04 Helicopter fire injuring occupant**

X● **V95.05 Helicopter explosion injuring occupant**

X● **V95.09 Other helicopter accident injuring occupant**

● **V95.1 Ultralight, microlight or powered-glider accident injuring occupant**

X● **V95.10 Unspecified ultralight, microlight or powered-glider accident injuring occupant**

X● **V95.11 Ultralight, microlight or powered-glider crash injuring occupant**

X● **V95.12 Forced landing of ultralight, microlight or powered-glider injuring occupant**

X● **V95.13 Ultralight, microlight or powered-glider collision injuring occupant**
Ultralight, microlight or powered-glider collision with any object, fixed, movable or moving

X● **V95.14 Ultralight, microlight or powered-glider fire injuring occupant**

X● **V95.15 Ultralight, microlight or powered-glider explosion injuring occupant**

X● **V95.19 Other ultralight, microlight or powered-glider accident injuring occupant**

● **V95.2 Other private fixed-wing aircraft accident injuring occupant**

X● **V95.20 Unspecified accident to other private fixed-wing aircraft, injuring occupant**

X● **V95.21 Other private fixed-wing aircraft crash injuring occupant**

X● **V95.22 Forced landing of other private fixed-wing aircraft injuring occupant**

X● **V95.23 Other private fixed-wing aircraft collision injuring occupant**
Other private fixed-wing aircraft collision with any object, fixed, movable or moving

X● **V95.24 Other private fixed-wing aircraft fire injuring occupant**

X● **V95.25 Other private fixed-wing aircraft explosion injuring occupant**

X● **V95.29 Other accident to other private fixed-wing aircraft injuring occupant**

● **V95.3 Commercial fixed-wing aircraft accident injuring occupant**

X● **V95.30 Unspecified accident to commercial fixed-wing aircraft injuring occupant**

X● **V95.31 Commercial fixed-wing aircraft crash injuring occupant**

X● **V95.32 Forced landing of commercial fixed-wing aircraft injuring occupant**

X● **V95.33 Commercial fixed-wing aircraft collision injuring occupant**
Commercial fixed-wing aircraft collision with any object, fixed, movable or moving

X● **V95.34 Commercial fixed-wing aircraft fire injuring occupant**

X● **V95.35 Commercial fixed-wing aircraft explosion injuring occupant**

X● **V95.39 Other accident to commercial fixed-wing aircraft injuring occupant**

● **V95.4 Spacecraft accident injuring occupant**

X● **V95.40 Unspecified spacecraft accident injuring occupant**

X● **V95.41 Spacecraft crash injuring occupant**

X● **V95.42 Forced landing of spacecraft injuring occupant**

X● **V95.43 Spacecraft collision injuring occupant**
Spacecraft collision with any object, fixed, moveable or moving

X● **V95.44 Spacecraft fire injuring occupant**

X● **V95.45 Spacecraft explosion injuring occupant**

X● **V95.49 Other spacecraft accident injuring occupant**

X● **V95.8 Other powered aircraft accidents injuring occupant**

X● **V95.9 Unspecified aircraft accident injuring occupant**
Aircraft accident NOS
Air transport accident NOS

V96 Accident to nonpowered aircraft causing injury to occupant

The appropriate 7th character is to be added to each code from category V96

A	initial encounter
D	subsequent encounter
S	sequela

V96.0 Balloon accident injuring occupant

X **V96.00** **Unspecified balloon accident injuring occupant**

X **V96.01** **Balloon crash injuring occupant**

X **V96.02** **Forced landing of balloon injuring occupant**

X **V96.03** **Balloon collision injuring occupant**

Balloon collision with any object, fixed, moveable or moving

X **V96.04** **Balloon fire injuring occupant**

X **V96.05** **Balloon explosion injuring occupant**

X **V96.09** **Other balloon accident injuring occupant**

V96.1 Hang-glider accident injuring occupant

X **V96.10** **Unspecified hang-glider accident injuring occupant**

X **V96.11** **Hang-glider crash injuring occupant**

X **V96.12** **Forced landing of hang-glider injuring occupant**

X **V96.13** **Hang-glider collision injuring occupant**

Hang-glider collision with any object, fixed, moveable or moving

X **V96.14** **Hang-glider fire injuring occupant**

X **V96.15** **Hang-glider explosion injuring occupant**

X **V96.19** **Other hang-glider accident injuring occupant**

V96.2 Glider (nonpowered) accident injuring occupant

X **V96.20** **Unspecified glider (nonpowered) accident injuring occupant**

X **V96.21** **Glider (nonpowered) crash injuring occupant**

X **V96.22** **Forced landing of glider (nonpowered) injuring occupant**

X **V96.23** **Glider (nonpowered) collision injuring occupant**

Glider (nonpowered) collision with any object, fixed, moveable or moving

X **V96.24** **Glider (nonpowered) fire injuring occupant**

X **V96.25** **Glider (nonpowered) explosion injuring occupant**

X **V96.29** **Other glider (nonpowered) accident injuring occupant**

X **V96.8** **Other nonpowered-aircraft accidents injuring occupant**

Kite carrying a person accident injuring occupant

X **V96.9** **Unspecified nonpowered-aircraft accident injuring occupant**

Nonpowered-aircraft accident NOS

V97 Other specified air transport accidents

The appropriate 7th character is to be added to each code from category V97

A	initial encounter
D	subsequent encounter
S	sequela

X **V97.0** **Occupant of aircraft injured in other specified air transport accidents**

Fall in, on or from aircraft in air transport accident

Excludes1 accident while boarding or alighting aircraft (V97.1)

X **V97.1** **Person injured while boarding or alighting from aircraft**

V97.2 Parachutist accident

X **V97.21** **Parachutist entangled in object**

Parachutist landing in tree

X **V97.22** **Parachutist injured on landing**

X **V97.29** **Other parachutist accident**

V97.3 Person on ground injured in air transport accident

X **V97.31** **Hit by object falling from aircraft**

Hit by crashing aircraft
Injured by aircraft hitting house
Injured by aircraft hitting car

X **V97.32** **Injured by rotating propeller**

X **V97.33** **Sucked into jet engine**

X **V97.39** **Other injury to person on ground due to air transport accident**

V97.8 Other air transport accidents, not elsewhere classified

Excludes1 aircraft accident NOS (V95.9)
exposure to changes in air pressure during ascent or descent (W94.-)

V97.81 Air transport accident involving military aircraft

V97.810 Civilian aircraft involved in air transport accident with military aircraft

Passenger in civilian aircraft injured due to accident with military aircraft

V97.811 Civilian injured by military aircraft

V97.818 Other air transport accident involving military aircraft

X **V97.89** **Other air transport accidents, not elsewhere classified**

Injury from machinery on aircraft

OTHER AND UNSPECIFIED TRANSPORT ACCIDENTS (V98-V99)

Excludes1 vehicle accident, type of vehicle unspecified (V89.-)

V98 Other specified transport accidents

The appropriate 7th character is to be added to each code from category V98

A	initial encounter
D	subsequent encounter
S	sequela

X **V98.0** **Accident to, on or involving cable-car, not on rails**

Caught or dragged by cable-car, not on rails
Fall or jump from cable-car, not on rails
Object thrown from or in cable-car, not on rails

X **V98.1** **Accident to, on or involving land-yacht**

X **V98.2** **Accident to, on or involving ice yacht**

X **V98.3** **Accident to, on or involving ski lift**

Accident to, on or involving ski chair-lift
Accident to, on or involving ski-lift with gondola

X **V98.8** **Other specified transport accidents**

X **V99** **Unspecified transport accident**

The appropriate 7th character is to be added to code V99

A	initial encounter
D	subsequent encounter
S	sequela

OTHER EXTERNAL CAUSES OF ACCIDENTAL INJURY (W00-X58)

SLIPPING, TRIPPING, STUMBLING AND FALLS (W00-W19)

Excludes1 assault involving a fall (Y01-Y02)
fall from animal (V80.-)
fall (in) (from) machinery (in operation) (W28-W31)
fall (in) (from) transport vehicle (V01-V99)
intentional self-harm involving a fall (X80-X81)

Excludes2 at risk for fall (history of fall) Z91.81
fall (in) (from) burning building (X00.-)
fall into fire (X00-X04, X08-X09)

● **W00 Fall due to ice and snow**

Includes pedestrian on foot falling (slipping) on ice and snow

Excludes1 fall on (from) ice and snow involving pedestrian conveyance (V00.-)
fall from stairs and steps not due to ice and snow (W10.-)

The appropriate 7th character is to be added to each code from category W00

A	initial encounter
D	subsequent encounter
S	sequela

X● **W00.0 Fall on same level due to ice and snow**
Coding Clinic: 2016, Q2, P5

X● **W00.1 Fall from stairs and steps due to ice and snow**

X● **W00.2 Other fall from one level to another due to ice and snow**

X● **W00.9 Unspecified fall due to ice and snow**

● **W01 Fall on same level from slipping, tripping and stumbling**

Includes fall on moving sidewalk

Excludes1 fall due to bumping (striking) against object (W18.0-)
fall in shower or bathtub (W18.2-)
fall on same level NOS (W18.30)
fall on same level from slipping, tripping and stumbling due to ice or snow (W00.0)
fall off or from toilet (W18.1-)
slipping, tripping and stumbling NOS (W18.40)
slipping, tripping and stumbling without falling (W18.4-)

The appropriate 7th character is to be added to each code from category W01

A	initial encounter
D	subsequent encounter
S	sequela

X● **W01.0 Fall on same level from slipping, tripping and stumbling without subsequent striking against object**
Falling over animal

● **W01.1 Fall on same level from slipping, tripping and stumbling with subsequent striking against object**

X● **W01.10 Fall on same level from slipping, tripping and stumbling with subsequent striking against unspecified object**

● **W01.11 Fall on same level from slipping, tripping and stumbling with subsequent striking against sharp object**

● **W01.110 Fall on same level from slipping, tripping and stumbling with subsequent striking against sharp glass**

● **W01.111 Fall on same level from slipping, tripping and stumbling with subsequent striking against power tool or machine**

● **W01.118 Fall on same level from slipping, tripping and stumbling with subsequent striking against other sharp object**

● **W01.119 Fall on same level from slipping, tripping and stumbling with subsequent striking against unspecified sharp object**

● **W01.19 Fall on same level from slipping, tripping and stumbling with subsequent striking against other object**

● **W01.190 Fall on same level from slipping, tripping and stumbling with subsequent striking against furniture**

● **W01.198 Fall on same level from slipping, tripping and stumbling with subsequent striking against other object**

X● **W03 Other fall on same level due to collision with another person**
Fall due to non-transport collision with other person

Excludes1 collision with another person without fall (W51)
crushed or pushed by a crowd or human stampede (W52)
fall involving pedestrian conveyance (V00-V09)
fall due to ice or snow (W00)
fall on same level NOS (W18.30)

The appropriate 7th character is to be added to code W03

A	initial encounter
D	subsequent encounter
S	sequela

Coding Clinic: 2015, Q1, P9-10; 2012, Q4, P108

X● **W04 Fall while being carried or supported by other persons**
Accidentally dropped while being carried
The appropriate 7th character is to be added to code W04

A	initial encounter
D	subsequent encounter
S	sequel

● **W05 Fall from non-moving wheelchair, nonmotorized scooter and motorized mobility scooter**

Excludes1 fall from moving wheelchair (powered) (V00.811)
fall from moving motorized mobility scooter (V00.831)
fall from nonmotorized scooter (V00.141)

The appropriate 7th character is to be added to each code from category W05

A	initial encounter
D	subsequent encounter
S	sequela

X● **W05.0 Fall from non-moving wheelchair**

X● **W05.1 Fall from non-moving nonmotorized scooter**

X● **W05.2 Fall from non-moving motorized mobility scooter**

X● **W06 Fall from bed**

The appropriate 7th character is to be added to code W06

A	initial encounter
D	subsequent encounter
S	sequela

X● **W07 Fall from chair**

The appropriate 7th character is to be added to code W07

A	initial encounter
D	subsequent encounter
S	sequela

X● **W08 Fall from other furniture**

The appropriate 7th character is to be added to code W08

A	initial encounter
D	subsequent encounter
S	sequela

● **W09 Fall on and from playground equipment**

Excludes1 fall involving recreational machinery (W31)

The appropriate 7th character is to be added to each code from category W09

A	initial encounter
D	subsequent encounter
S	sequela

X● **W09.0 Fall on or from playground slide**

X● **W09.1 Fall from playground swing**

X● **W09.2 Fall on or from jungle gym**

X● **W09.8 Fall on or from other playground equipment**

● **W10 Fall on and from stairs and steps**

Excludes1 fall from stairs and steps due to ice and snow (W00.1)

The appropriate 7th character is to be added to each code from category W10

A	initial encounter
D	subsequent encounter
S	sequela

X● **W10.0 Fall (on) (from) escalator**

X● **W10.1 Fall (on) (from) sidewalk curb**

X● **W10.2 Fall (on) (from) incline**

Fall (on) (from) ramp

X● **W10.8 Fall (on) (from) other stairs and steps**

X● **W10.9 Fall (on) (from) unspecified stairs and steps**

X● **W11 Fall on and from ladder**

The appropriate 7th character is to be added to code W11

A	initial encounter
D	subsequent encounter
S	sequela

X● **W12 Fall on and from scaffolding**

The appropriate 7th character is to be added to code W12

A	initial encounter
D	subsequent encounter
S	sequela

● **W13 Fall from, out of or through building or structure**

The appropriate 7th character is to be added to each code from category W13

A	initial encounter
D	subsequent encounter
S	sequela

X● **W13.0 Fall from, out of or through balcony**

Fall from, out of or through railing

X● **W13.1 Fall from, out of or through bridge**

X● **W13.2 Fall from, out of or through roof**

X● **W13.3 Fall through floor**

X● **W13.4 Fall from, out of or through window**

Excludes2 fall with subsequent striking against sharp glass (W01.110)

X● **W13.8 Fall from, out of or through other building or structure**

Fall from, out of or through viaduct
Fall from, out of or through wall
Fall from, out of or through flag-pole

X● **W13.9 Fall from, out of or through building, not otherwise specified**

Excludes1 collapse of a building or structure (W20.-)
fall or jump from burning building or structure (X00.-)

X● **W14 Fall from tree**

The appropriate 7th character is to be added to code W14

A	initial encounter
D	subsequent encounter
S	sequela

X● **W15 Fall from cliff**

The appropriate 7th character is to be added to code W15

A	initial encounter
D	subsequent encounter
S	sequela

● **W16 Fall, jump or diving into water**

Excludes1 accidental non-watercraft drowning and submersion not involving fall (W65-W74)
effects of air pressure from diving (W94.-)
fall into water from watercraft (V90-V94)
hitting an object or against bottom when falling from watercraft (V94.0)

Excludes2 striking or hitting diving board (W21.4)

The appropriate 7th character is to be added to each code from category W16

A	initial encounter
D	subsequent encounter
S	sequela

● **W16.0 Fall into swimming pool**

Fall into swimming pool NOS

Excludes1 fall into empty swimming pool (W17.3)

● **W16.01 Fall into swimming pool striking water surface**

● **W16.011 Fall into swimming pool striking water surface causing drowning and submersion**

Excludes1 drowning and submersion while in swimming pool without fall (W67)

● **W16.012 Fall into swimming pool striking water surface causing other injury**

- **W16.02 Fall into swimming pool striking bottom**
  - **W16.021 Fall into swimming pool striking bottom causing drowning and submersion**
    - **Excludes1** drowning and submersion while in swimming pool without fall (W67)
  - **W16.022 Fall into swimming pool striking bottom causing other injury**
- **W16.03 Fall into swimming pool striking wall**
  - **W16.031 Fall into swimming pool striking wall causing drowning and submersion**
    - **Excludes1** drowning and submersion while in swimming pool without fall (W67)
  - **W16.032 Fall into swimming pool striking wall causing other injury**
- **W16.1 Fall into natural body of water**
  - Fall into lake
  - Fall into open sea
  - Fall into river
  - Fall into stream
- **W16.11 Fall into natural body of water striking water surface**
  - **W16.111 Fall into natural body of water striking water surface causing drowning and submersion**
    - **Excludes1** drowning and submersion while in natural body of water without fall (W69)
  - **W16.112 Fall into natural body of water striking water surface causing other injury**
- **W16.12 Fall into natural body of water striking bottom**
  - **W16.121 Fall into natural body of water striking bottom causing drowning and submersion**
    - **Excludes1** drowning and submersion while in natural body of water without fall (W69)
  - **W16.122 Fall into natural body of water striking bottom causing other injury**
- **W16.13 Fall into natural body of water striking side**
  - **W16.131 Fall into natural body of water striking side causing drowning and submersion**
    - **Excludes1** drowning and submersion while in natural body of water without fall (W69)
  - **W16.132 Fall into natural body of water striking side causing other injury**
- **W16.2 Fall in (into) filled bathtub or bucket of water**
  - **W16.21 Fall in (into) filled bathtub**
    - **Excludes1** fall into empty bathtub (W18.2)
  - **W16.211 Fall in (into) filled bathtub causing drowning and submersion**
    - **Excludes1** drowning and submersion while in filled bathtub without fall (W65)
  - **W16.212 Fall in (into) filled bathtub causing other injury**
- **W16.22 Fall in (into) bucket of water**
  - **W16.221 Fall in (into) bucket of water causing drowning and submersion**
  - **W16.222 Fall in (into) bucket of water causing other injury**
- **W16.3 Fall into other water**
  - Fall into fountain
  - Fall into reservoir
  - **W16.31 Fall into other water striking water surface**
    - **W16.311 Fall into other water striking water surface causing drowning and submersion**
      - **Excludes1** drowning and submersion while in other water without fall (W73)
    - **W16.312 Fall into other water striking water surface causing other injury**
  - **W16.32 Fall into other water striking bottom**
    - **W16.321 Fall into other water striking bottom causing drowning and submersion**
      - **Excludes1** drowning and submersion while in other water without fall (W73)
    - **W16.322 Fall into other water striking bottom causing other injury**
  - **W16.33 Fall into other water striking wall**
    - **W16.331 Fall into other water striking wall causing drowning and submersion**
      - **Excludes1** drowning and submersion while in other water without fall (W73)
    - **W16.332 Fall into other water striking wall causing other injury**
- **W16.4 Fall into unspecified water**
  - X **W16.41 Fall into unspecified water causing drowning and submersion**
  - X **W16.42 Fall into unspecified water causing other injury**
- **W16.5 Jumping or diving into swimming pool**
  - **W16.51 Jumping or diving into swimming pool striking water surface**
    - **W16.511 Jumping or diving into swimming pool striking water surface causing drowning and submersion**
      - **Excludes1** drowning and submersion while in swimming pool without jumping or diving (W67)
    - **W16.512 Jumping or diving into swimming pool striking water surface causing other injury**
  - **W16.52 Jumping or diving into swimming pool striking bottom**
    - **W16.521 Jumping or diving into swimming pool striking bottom causing drowning and submersion**
      - **Excludes1** drowning and submersion while in swimming pool without jumping or diving (W67)
    - **W16.522 Jumping or diving into swimming pool striking bottom causing other injury**

New Revised ~~deleted~~ Deleted Excludes 1 Excludes 2 Includes Use additional Code first Code also Unspecified
OGCR Official Guidelines ● Unacceptable Principal Diagnosis X Assign placeholder X ● Use Additional Character(s) ▶ Manifestation Code Coding Clinic

- **W16.53 Jumping or diving into swimming pool striking wall**
  - **W16.531 Jumping or diving into swimming pool striking wall causing drowning and submersion**
    - **Excludes1** drowning and submersion while in swimming pool without jumping or diving (W67)
  - **W16.532 Jumping or diving into swimming pool striking wall causing other injury**
- **W16.6 Jumping or diving into natural body of water**
  - Jumping or diving into lake
  - Jumping or diving into open sea
  - Jumping or diving into river
  - Jumping or diving into stream
  - **W16.61 Jumping or diving into natural body of water striking water surface**
    - **W16.611 Jumping or diving into natural body of water striking water surface causing drowning and submersion**
      - **Excludes1** drowning and submersion while in natural body of water without jumping or diving (W69)
    - **W16.612 Jumping or diving into natural body of water striking water surface causing other injury**
  - **W16.62 Jumping or diving into natural body of water striking bottom**
    - **W16.621 Jumping or diving into natural body of water striking bottom causing drowning and submersion**
      - **Excludes1** drowning and submersion while in natural body of water without jumping or diving (W69)
    - **W16.622 Jumping or diving into natural body of water striking bottom causing other injury**
- **W16.7 Jumping or diving from boat**
  - **Excludes1** fall from boat into water - see watercraft accident (V90-V94)
  - **W16.71 Jumping or diving from boat striking water surface**
    - **W16.711 Jumping or diving from boat striking water surface causing drowning and submersion**
    - **W16.712 Jumping or diving from boat striking water surface causing other injury**
  - **W16.72 Jumping or diving from boat striking bottom**
    - **W16.721 Jumping or diving from boat striking bottom causing drowning and submersion**
    - **W16.722 Jumping or diving from boat striking bottom causing other injury**
- **W16.8 Jumping or diving into other water**
  - Jumping or diving into fountain
  - Jumping or diving into reservoir
  - **W16.81 Jumping or diving into other water striking water surface**
    - **W16.811 Jumping or diving into other water striking water surface causing drowning and submersion**
      - **Excludes1** drowning and submersion while in other water without jumping or diving (W73)
    - **W16.812 Jumping or diving into other water striking water surface causing other injury**
  - **W16.82 Jumping or diving into other water striking bottom**
    - **W16.821 Jumping or diving into other water striking bottom causing drowning and submersion**
      - **Excludes1** drowning and submersion while in other water without jumping or diving (W73)
    - **W16.822 Jumping or diving into other water striking bottom causing other injury**
  - **W16.83 Jumping or diving into other water striking wall**
    - **W16.831 Jumping or diving into other water striking wall causing drowning and submersion**
      - **Excludes1** drowning and submersion while in other water without jumping or diving (W73)
    - **W16.832 Jumping or diving into other water striking wall causing other injury**
  - **W16.9 Jumping or diving into unspecified water**
    - X **W16.91 Jumping or diving into unspecified water causing drowning and submersion**
    - X **W16.92 Jumping or diving into unspecified water causing other injury**
- **W17 Other fall from one level to another**

  The appropriate 7th character is to be added to each code from category W17

A	initial encounter
D	subsequent encounter
S	sequela

- X **W17.0 Fall into well**
- X **W17.1 Fall into storm drain or manhole**
- X **W17.2 Fall into hole**
  - Fall into pit
- X **W17.3 Fall into empty swimming pool**
  - **Excludes1** fall into filled swimming pool (W16.0-)
- X **W17.4 Fall from dock**
- **W17.8 Other fall from one level to another**
  - X **W17.81 Fall down embankment (hill)**
  - X **W17.82 Fall from (out of) grocery cart**
    - Fall due to grocery cart tipping over
  - X **W17.89 Other fall from one level to another**
    - Fall from cherry picker
    - Fall from lifting device
    - Fall from mobile elevated work platform [MEWP]
    - Fall from sky lift
    - **Coding Clinic: 2015, Q2, P6**

W18 Other slipping, tripping and stumbling and falls

The appropriate 7th character is to be added to each code from category W18

A	initial encounter
D	subsequent encounter
S	sequela

W18.0 Fall due to bumping against object

Striking against object with subsequent fall

Excludes1 fall on same level due to slipping, tripping, or stumbling with subsequent striking against object (W01.1-)

X **W18.00 Striking against unspecified object with subsequent fall**

X **W18.01 Striking against sports equipment with subsequent fall**

X **W18.02 Striking against glass with subsequent fall**

X **W18.09 Striking against other object with subsequent fall**

W18.1 Fall from or off toilet

X **W18.11 Fall from or off toilet without subsequent striking against object**

Fall from (off) toilet NOS

X **W18.12 Fall from or off toilet with subsequent striking against object**

X **W18.2 Fall in (into) shower or empty bathtub**

Excludes1 fall in full bathtub causing drowning or submersion (W16.21-)

W18.3 Other and unspecified fall on same level

X **W18.30 Fall on same level, unspecified**

X **W18.31 Fall on same level due to stepping on an object**

Fall on same level due to stepping on an animal

Excludes1 slipping, tripping and stumbling without fall due to stepping on animal (W18.41)

X **W18.39 Other fall on same level**

W18.4 Slipping, tripping and stumbling without falling

Excludes1 collision with another person without fall (W51)

X **W18.40 Slipping, tripping and stumbling without falling, unspecified**

X **W18.41 Slipping, tripping and stumbling without falling due to stepping on object**

Slipping, tripping and stumbling without falling due to stepping on animal

Excludes1 slipping, tripping and stumbling with fall due to stepping on animal (W18.31)

X **W18.42 Slipping, tripping and stumbling without falling due to stepping into hole or opening**

X **W18.43 Slipping, tripping and stumbling without falling due to stepping from one level to another**

X **W18.49 Other slipping, tripping and stumbling without falling**

X **W19 Unspecified fall**

Accidental fall NOS

The appropriate 7th character is to be added to code W19

A	initial encounter
D	subsequent encounter
S	sequela

Coding Clinic: 2012, Q4, P95

EXPOSURE TO INANIMATE MECHANICAL FORCES (W20-W49)

Excludes1 assault (X92-Y09)
contact or collision with animals or persons (W50-W64)
exposure to inanimate mechanical forces involving military or war operations (Y36.-, Y37.-)
intentional self-harm (X71-X83)

W20 Struck by thrown, projected or falling object

Code first any associated:
cataclysm (X34-X39)
lightning strike (T75.00)

Excludes1 falling object in machinery accident (W24, W28-W31)
falling object in transport accident (V01-V99)
object set in motion by explosion (W35-W40)
object set in motion by firearm (W32-W34)
struck by thrown sports equipment (W21.-)

The appropriate 7th character is to be added to each code from category W20

A	initial encounter
D	subsequent encounter
S	sequela

X **W20.0 Struck by falling object in cave-in**

Excludes2 asphyxiation due to cave-in (T71.21)

X **W20.1 Struck by object due to collapse of building**

Excludes1 struck by object due to collapse of burning building (X00.2, X02.2)

X **W20.8 Other cause of strike by thrown, projected or falling object**

Excludes1 struck by thrown sports equipment (W21.-)

W21 Striking against or struck by sports equipment

Excludes1 assault with sports equipment (Y08.0-)
striking against or struck by sports equipment with subsequent fall (W18.01)

The appropriate 7th character is to be added to each code from category W21

A	initial encounter
D	subsequent encounter
S	sequela

W21.0 Struck by hit or thrown ball

X **W21.00 Struck by hit or thrown ball, unspecified type**

X **W21.01 Struck by football**

X **W21.02 Struck by soccer ball**

X **W21.03 Struck by baseball**

X **W21.04 Struck by golf ball**

X **W21.05 Struck by basketball**

X **W21.06 Struck by volleyball**

X **W21.07 Struck by softball**

X **W21.09 Struck by other hit or thrown ball**

W21.1 Struck by bat, racquet or club

X **W21.11 Struck by baseball bat**

X **W21.12 Struck by tennis racquet**

X **W21.13 Struck by golf club**

X **W21.19 Struck by other bat, racquet or club**

- **W21.2 Struck by hockey stick or puck**
  - **W21.21 Struck by hockey stick**
    - **W21.210 Struck by ice hockey stick**
    - **W21.211 Struck by field hockey stick**
  - **W21.22 Struck by hockey puck**
    - **W21.220 Struck by ice hockey puck**
    - **W21.221 Struck by field hockey puck**
- **W21.3 Struck by sports foot wear**
  - X **W21.31 Struck by shoe cleats**
    Stepped on by shoe cleats
  - X **W21.32 Struck by skate blades**
    Skated over by skate blades
  - X **W21.39 Struck by other sports foot wear**
- X **W21.4 Striking against diving board**
  Use additional code for subsequent falling into water, if applicable (W16.-)
- **W21.8 Striking against or struck by other sports equipment**
  - X **W21.81 Striking against or struck by football helmet**
  - X **W21.89 Striking against or struck by other sports equipment**
- X **W21.9 Striking against or struck by unspecified sports equipment**

- **W22 Striking against or struck by other objects**
  Excludes1 striking against or struck by object with subsequent fall (W18.09)
  The appropriate 7th character is to be added to each code from category W22

A	initial encounter
D	subsequent encounter
S	sequela

- **W22.0 Striking against stationary object**
  Excludes1 striking against stationary sports equipment (W21.8)
  - X **W22.01 Walked into wall**
  - X **W22.02 Walked into lamppost**
  - X **W22.03 Walked into furniture**
  - **W22.04 Striking against wall of swimming pool**
    - **W22.041 Striking against wall of swimming pool causing drowning and submersion**
      Excludes1 drowning and submersion while swimming without striking against wall (W67)
    - **W22.042 Striking against wall of swimming pool causing other injury**
  - X **W22.09 Striking against other stationary object**
- **W22.1 Striking against or struck by automobile airbag**
  - X **W22.10 Striking against or struck by unspecified automobile airbag**
  - X **W22.11 Striking against or struck by driver side automobile airbag**
  - X **W22.12 Striking against or struck by front passenger side automobile airbag**
  - X **W22.19 Striking against or struck by other automobile airbag**
- X **W22.8 Striking against or struck by other objects**
  Striking against or struck by object NOS
  Excludes1 struck by thrown, projected or falling object (W20.-)

- **W23 Caught, crushed, jammed or pinched in or between objects**
  Excludes1 injury caused by cutting or piercing instruments (W25-W27)
  injury caused by firearms malfunction (W32.1, W33.1-, W34.1-)
  injury caused by lifting and transmission devices (W24.-)
  injury caused by machinery (W28-W31)
  injury caused by nonpowered hand tools (W27.-)
  injury caused by transport vehicle being used as a means of transportation (V01-V99)
  injury caused by struck by thrown, projected or falling object (W20.-)
  The appropriate 7th character is to be added to each code from category W23

A	initial encounter
D	subsequent encounter
S	sequela

  - X **W23.0 Caught, crushed, jammed, or pinched between moving objects**
  - X **W23.1 Caught, crushed, jammed, or pinched between stationary objects**

- **W24 Contact with lifting and transmission devices, not elsewhere classified**
  Excludes1 transport accidents (V01-V99)
  The appropriate 7th character is to be added to each code from category W24

A	initial encounter
D	subsequent encounter
S	sequela

  - X **W24.0 Contact with lifting devices, not elsewhere classified**
    Contact with chain hoist
    Contact with drive belt
    Contact with pulley (block)
  - X **W24.1 Contact with transmission devices, not elsewhere classified**
    Contact with transmission belt or cable
- X **W25 Contact with sharp glass**
  Code first any associated:
  injury due to flying glass from explosion or firearm discharge (W32-W40)
  transport accident (V00-V99)
  Excludes1 fall on same level due to slipping, tripping and stumbling with subsequent striking against sharp glass (W01.10)
  striking against sharp glass with subsequent fall (W18.02)
  Excludes2 glass embedded in skin (W45) ◀
  The appropriate 7th character is to be added to code W25

A	initial encounter
D	subsequent encounter
S	sequela

- **W26 Contact with other sharp objects**
  Excludes2 sharp object(s) embedded in skin (W45) ◀
  The appropriate 7th character is to be added to each code from category W26

A	initial encounter
D	subsequent encounter
S	sequela

  - X **W26.0 Contact with knife**
    Excludes1 contact with electric knife (W29.1)
  - X **W26.1 Contact with sword or dagger**
  - X **W26.2 Contact with edge of stiff paper** ◀
    Paper cut ◀
  - X **W26.8 Contact with other sharp object(s), not elsewhere classified** ◀
    Contact with tin can lid ◀
  - X **W26.9 Contact with unspecified sharp object(s)** ◀

● **W27 Contact with nonpowered hand tool**

The appropriate 7th character is to be added to each code from category W27

A	initial encounter
D	subsequent encounter
S	sequela

X● **W27.0 Contact with workbench tool**
Contact with auger
Contact with axe
Contact with chisel
Contact with handsaw
Contact with screwdriver

X● **W27.1 Contact with garden tool**
Contact with hoe
Contact with nonpowered lawn mower
Contact with pitchfork
Contact with rake

X● **W27.2 Contact with scissors**

X● **W27.3 Contact with needle (sewing)**
Excludes1 contact with hypodermic needle (W46.-)

X● **W27.4 Contact with kitchen utensil**
Contact with fork
Contact with ice-pick
Contact with can-opener NOS

X● **W27.5 Contact with paper-cutter**

X● **W27.8 Contact with other nonpowered hand tool**
Contact with nonpowered sewing machine
Contact with shovel

X● **W28 Contact with powered lawn mower**
Powered lawn mower (commercial) (residential)
Excludes1 contact with nonpowered lawn mower (W27.1)
Excludes2 exposure to electric current (W86.-)
The appropriate 7th character is to be added to code W28

A	initial encounter
D	subsequent encounter
S	sequela

● **W29 Contact with other powered hand tools and household machinery**
Excludes1 contact with commercial machinery (W31.82)
contact with hot household appliance (X15)
contact with nonpowered hand tool (W27.-)
exposure to electric current (W86)
The appropriate 7th character is to be added to each code from category W29

A	initial encounter
D	subsequent encounter
S	sequela

X● **W29.0 Contact with powered kitchen appliance**
Contact with blender
Contact with can-opener
Contact with garbage disposal
Contact with mixer

X● **W29.1 Contact with electric knife**

X● **W29.2 Contact with other powered household machinery**
Contact with electric fan
Contact with powered dryer (clothes) (powered) (spin)
Contact with washing-machine
Contact with sewing machine

X● **W29.3 Contact with powered garden and outdoor hand tools and machinery**
Contact with chainsaw
Contact with edger
Contact with garden cultivator (tiller)
Contact with hedge trimmer
Contact with other powered garden tool
Excludes1 contact with powered lawn mower (W28)

X● **W29.4 Contact with nail gun**

X● **W29.8 Contact with other powered powered hand tools and household machinery**
Contact with do-it-yourself tool NOS

● **W30 Contact with agricultural machinery**
Includes animal-powered farm machine
Excludes1 agricultural transport vehicle accident (V01-V99)
explosion of grain store (W40.8)
exposure to electric current (W86.-)
The appropriate 7th character is to be added to each code from category W30

A	initial encounter
D	subsequent encounter
S	sequela

X● **W30.0 Contact with combine harvester**
Contact with reaper
Contact with thresher

X● **W30.1 Contact with power take-off devices (PTO)**

X● **W30.2 Contact with hay derrick**

X● **W30.3 Contact with grain storage elevator**
Excludes1 explosion of grain store (W40.8)

● **W30.8 Contact with other specified agricultural machinery**

X● **W30.81 Contact with agricultural transport vehicle in stationary use**
Contact with agricultural transport vehicle under repair, not on public roadway
Excludes1 agricultural transport vehicle accident (V01-V99)

X● **W30.89 Contact with other specified agricultural machinery**

X● **W30.9 Contact with unspecified agricultural machinery**
Contact with farm machinery NOS

● **W31 Contact with other and unspecified machinery**
Excludes1 contact with agricultural machinery (W30.-)
contact with machinery in transport under own power or being towed by a vehicle (V01-V99)
exposure to electric current (W86)
The appropriate 7th character is to be added to each code from category W31

A	initial encounter
D	subsequent encounter
S	sequela

X● **W31.0 Contact with mining and earth-drilling machinery**
Contact with bore or drill (land) (seabed)
Contact with shaft hoist
Contact with shaft lift
Contact with undercutter

X● **W31.1 Contact with metalworking machines**
Contact with abrasive wheel
Contact with forging machine
Contact with lathe
Contact with mechanical shears
Contact with metal drilling machine
Contact with milling machine
Contact with power press
Contact with rolling-mill
Contact with metal sawing machine

X● **W31.2 Contact with powered woodworking and forming machines**
Contact with band saw
Contact with bench saw
Contact with circular saw
Contact with molding machine
Contact with overhead plane
Contact with powered saw
Contact with radial saw
Contact with sander
Excludes1 nonpowered woodworking tools (W27.0)

X● **W31.3 Contact with prime movers**
Contact with gas turbine
Contact with internal combustion engine
Contact with steam engine
Contact with water driven turbine

● **W31.8 Contact with other specified machinery**

X● **W31.81 Contact with recreational machinery**
Contact with roller-coaster

X● **W31.82 Contact with other commercial machinery**
Contact with commercial electric fan
Contact with commercial kitchen appliances
Contact with commercial powered dryer (clothes) (powered) (spin)
Contact with commercial washing-machine
Contact with commercial sewing machine

Excludes1 contact with household machinery (W29.-)
contact with powered lawn mower (W28)

X● **W31.83 Contact with special construction vehicle in stationary use**
Contact with special construction vehicle under repair, not on public roadway

Excludes1 special construction vehicle accident (V01-V99)

X● **W31.89 Contact with other specified machinery**

X● **W31.9 Contact with unspecified machinery**
Contact with machinery NOS

● **W32 Accidental handgun discharge and malfunction**

Includes accidental discharge and malfunction of gun for single hand use
accidental discharge and malfunction of pistol
accidental discharge and malfunction of revolver
handgun discharge and malfunction NOS

Excludes1 accidental airgun discharge and malfunction (W34.010, W34.110)
accidental BB gun discharge and malfunction (W34.010, W34.110)
accidental pellet gun discharge and malfunction (W34.010, W34.110)
accidental shotgun discharge and malfunction (W33.01, W33.11)
assault by handgun discharge (X93)
handgun discharge involving legal intervention (Y35.0-)
handgun discharge involving military or war operations (Y36.4-)
intentional self-harm by handgun discharge (X72)
Very pistol discharge and malfunction (W34.09, W34.19)

The appropriate 7th character is to be added to each code from category W32

A	initial encounter
D	subsequent encounter
S	sequela

X● **W32.0 Accidental handgun discharge**

X● **W32.1 Accidental handgun malfunction**
Injury due to explosion of handgun (parts)
Injury due to malfunction of mechanism or component of handgun
Injury due to recoil of handgun
Powder burn from handgun

● **W33 Accidental rifle, shotgun and larger firearm discharge and malfunction**

Includes rifle, shotgun and larger firearm discharge and malfunction NOS

Excludes1 accidental airgun discharge and malfunction (W34.010, W34.110)
accidental BB gun discharge and malfunction (W34.010, W34.110)
accidental handgun discharge and malfunction (W32.-)
accidental pellet gun discharge and malfunction (W34.010, W34.110)
assault by rifle, shotgun and larger firearm discharge (X94)
firearm discharge involving legal intervention (Y35.0-)
firearm discharge involving military or war operations (Y36.4-)
intentional self-harm by rifle, shotgun and larger firearm discharge (X73)

The appropriate 7th character is to be added to each code from category W33

A	initial encounter
D	subsequent encounter
S	sequela

● **W33.0 Accidental rifle, shotgun and larger firearm discharge**

X● **W33.00 Accidental discharge of unspecified larger firearm**
Discharge of unspecified larger firearm NOS

X● **W33.01 Accidental discharge of shotgun**
Discharge of shotgun NOS

X● **W33.02 Accidental discharge of hunting rifle**
Discharge of hunting rifle NOS

X● **W33.03 Accidental discharge of machine gun**
Discharge of machine gun NOS

X● **W33.09 Accidental discharge of other larger firearm**
Discharge of other larger firearm NOS

● **W33.1 Accidental rifle, shotgun and larger firearm malfunction**
Injury due to explosion of rifle, shotgun and larger firearm (parts)
Injury due to malfunction of mechanism or component of rifle, shotgun and larger firearm
Injury due to piercing, cutting, crushing or pinching due to (by) slide trigger mechanism, scope or other gun part
Injury due to recoil of rifle, shotgun and larger firearm
Powder burn from rifle, shotgun and larger firearm

X● **W33.10 Accidental malfunction of unspecified larger firearm**
Malfunction of unspecified larger firearm NOS

X● **W33.11 Accidental malfunction of shotgun**
Malfunction of shotgun NOS

X● **W33.12 Accidental malfunction of hunting rifle**
Malfunction of hunting rifle NOS

X● **W33.13 Accidental malfunction of machine gun**
Malfunction of machine gun NOS

X● **W33.19 Accidental malfunction of other larger firearm**
Malfunction of other larger firearm NOS

W34 Accidental discharge and malfunction from other and unspecified firearms and guns

The appropriate 7th character is to be added to each code from category W34

A	initial encounter
D	subsequent encounter
S	sequela

W34.0 Accidental discharge from other and unspecified firearms and guns

X **W34.00 Accidental discharge from unspecified firearms or gun**
Discharge from firearm NOS
Gunshot wound NOS
Shot NOS
Coding Clinic: 2015, Q1, P17

W34.01 Accidental discharge of gas, air or spring-operated guns

W34.010 Accidental discharge of airgun
Accidental discharge of BB gun
Accidental discharge of pellet gun

W34.011 Accidental discharge of paintball gun
Accidental injury due to paintball discharge

W34.018 Accidental discharge of other gas, air or spring-operated gun

X **W34.09 Accidental discharge from other specified firearms**
Accidental discharge from Very pistol [flare]

W34.1 Accidental malfunction from other and unspecified firearms and guns

X **W34.10 Accidental malfunction from unspecified firearms or gun**
Firearm malfunction NOS

W34.11 Accidental malfunction of gas, air or spring-operated guns

W34.110 Accidental malfunction of airgun
Accidental malfunction of BB gun
Accidental malfunction of pellet gun

W34.111 Accidental malfunction of paintball gun
Accidental injury due to paintball gun malfunction

W34.118 Accidental malfunction of other gas, air or spring-operated gun

X **W34.19 Accidental malfunction from other specified firearms**
Accidental malfunction from Very pistol [flare]

X **W35 Explosion and rupture of boiler**

Excludes1 explosion and rupture of boiler on watercraft (V93.4)

The appropriate 7th character is to be added to code W35

A	initial encounter
D	subsequent encounter
S	sequela

W36 Explosion and rupture of gas cylinder

The appropriate 7th character is to be added to each code from category W36

A	initial encounter
D	subsequent encounter
S	sequela

X **W36.1 Explosion and rupture of aerosol can**

X **W36.2 Explosion and rupture of air tank**

X **W36.3 Explosion and rupture of pressurized-gas tank**

X **W36.8 Explosion and rupture of other gas cylinder**

X **W36.9 Explosion and rupture of unspecified gas cylinder**

W37 Explosion and rupture of pressurized tire, pipe or hose

The appropriate 7th character is to be added to each code from category W37

A	initial encounter
D	subsequent encounter
S	sequela

X **W37.0 Explosion of bicycle tire**

X **W37.8 Explosion and rupture of other pressurized tire, pipe or hose**

X **W38 Explosion and rupture of other specified pressurized devices**

The appropriate 7th character is to be added to code W38

A	initial encounter
D	subsequent encounter
S	sequela

X **W39 Discharge of firework**

The appropriate 7th character is to be added to code W39

A	initial encounter
D	subsequent encounter
S	sequela

W40 Explosion of other materials

Excludes1 assault by explosive material (X96)
explosion involving legal intervention (Y35.1-)
explosion involving military or war operations (Y36.0-, Y36.2-)
intentional self-harm by explosive material (X75)

The appropriate 7th character is to be added to each code from category W40

A	initial encounter
D	subsequent encounter
S	sequela

X **W40.0 Explosion of blasting material**
Explosion of blasting cap
Explosion of detonator
Explosion of dynamite
Explosion of explosive (any) used in blasting operations

X **W40.1 Explosion of explosive gases**
Explosion of acetylene
Explosion of butane
Explosion of coal gas
Explosion in mine NOS
Explosion of explosive gas
Explosion of fire damp
Explosion of gasoline fumes
Explosion of methane
Explosion of propane

X **W40.8 Explosion of other specified explosive materials**
Explosion in dump NOS
Explosion in factory NOS
Explosion in grain store
Explosion in munitions

Excludes1 explosion involving legal intervention (Y35.1-)
explosion involving military or war operations (Y36.0-, Y36.2-)

X **W40.9 Explosion of unspecified explosive materials**
Explosion NOS

W42 Exposure to noise

The appropriate 7th character is to be added to each code from category W42

A	initial encounter
D	subsequent encounter
S	sequela

X **W42.0 Exposure to supersonic waves**

X **W42.9 Exposure to other noise**
Exposure to sound waves NOS

● **W45 Foreign body or object entering through skin**

Includes foreign body or object embedded in skin ◀
nail embedded in skin ◀

Excludes2 contact with hand tools (nonpowered) (powered) (W27-W29)
contact with other sharp object(s) (W26.-) ◀
contact with sharp glass (W25.-)
struck by objects (W20-W22)

The appropriate 7th character is to be added to each code from category W45

A	initial encounter
D	subsequent encounter
S	sequela

X● **W45.0 Nail entering through skin**

~~W45.1 Paper entering through skin~~
~~Paper cut~~

~~W45.2 Lid of can entering through skin~~

X● **W45.8 Other foreign body or object entering through skin**
Splinter in skin NOS

● **W46 Contact with hypodermic needle**

The appropriate 7th character is to be added to each code from category W46

A	initial encounter
D	subsequent encounter
S	sequela

X● **W46.0 Contact with hypodermic needle**
Hypodermic needle stick NOS

X● **W46.1 Contact with contaminated hypodermic needle**

● **W49 Exposure to other inanimate mechanical forces**

Includes exposure to abnormal gravitational [G] forces
exposure to inanimate mechanical forces NEC

Excludes1 exposure to inanimate mechanical forces involving military or war operations (Y36.-, Y37.-)

The appropriate 7th character is to be added to each code from category W49

A	initial encounter
D	subsequent encounter
S	sequela

● **W49.0 Item causing external constriction**

X● **W49.01 Hair causing external constriction**

X● **W49.02 String or thread causing external constriction**

X● **W49.03 Rubber band causing external constriction**

X● **W49.04 Ring or other jewelry causing external constriction**

X● **W49.09 Other item causing external constriction**

X● **W49.9 Exposure to other inanimate mechanical forces**

EXPOSURE TO ANIMATE MECHANICAL FORCES (W50-W64)

Excludes1 toxic effect of contact with venomous animals and plants (T63.-)

● **W50 Accidental hit, strike, kick, twist, bite or scratch by another person**

Includes hit, strike, kick, twist, bite, or scratch by another person NOS

Excludes1 assault by bodily force (Y04)
struck by objects (W20-W22)

The appropriate 7th character is to be added to each code from category W50

A	initial encounter
D	subsequent encounter
S	sequela

X● **W50.0 Accidental hit or strike by another person**
Hit or strike by another person NOS

X● **W50.1 Accidental kick by another person**
Kick by another person NOS

X● **W50.2 Accidental twist by another person**
Twist by another person NOS
Coding Clinic: 2015, Q1, P8

X● **W50.3 Accidental bite by another person**
Human bite
Bite by another person NOS

X● **W50.4 Accidental scratch by another person**
Scratch by another person NOS

X● **W51 Accidental striking against or bumped into by another person**

Excludes1 assault by striking against or bumping into by another person (Y04.2)
fall due to collision with another person (W03)

The appropriate 7th character is to be added to code W51

A	initial encounter
D	subsequent encounter
S	sequela

X● **W52 Crushed, pushed or stepped on by crowd or human stampede**
Crushed, pushed or stepped on by crowd or human stampede with or without fall

The appropriate 7th character is to be added to code W52

A	initial encounter
D	subsequent encounter
S	sequela

● **W53 Contact with rodent**

Includes contact with saliva, feces or urine of rodent

The appropriate 7th character is to be added to each code from category W53

A	initial encounter
D	subsequent encounter
S	sequela

● **W53.0 Contact with mouse**

X● **W53.01 Bitten by mouse**

X● **W53.09 Other contact with mouse**

● **W53.1 Contact with rat**

X● **W53.11 Bitten by rat**

X● **W53.19 Other contact with rat**

● **W53.2 Contact with squirrel**

X● **W53.21 Bitten by squirrel**

X● **W53.29 Other contact with squirrel**

● **W53.8 Contact with other rodent**

X● **W53.81 Bitten by other rodent**

X● **W53.89 Other contact with other rodent**

● **W54 Contact with dog**

Includes contact with saliva, feces or urine of dog

The appropriate 7th character is to be added to each code from category W54

A	initial encounter
D	subsequent encounter
S	sequela

X● **W54.0 Bitten by dog**

X● **W54.1 Struck by dog**
Knocked over by dog

X● **W54.8 Other contact with dog**

W55 Contact with other mammals

Includes contact with saliva, feces or urine of mammal

Excludes1 animal being ridden - see transport accidents
bitten or struck by dog (W54)
bitten or struck by rodent (W53.-)
contact with marine mammals (W56.X-)

The appropriate 7th character is to be added to each code from category W55

A	initial encounter
D	subsequent encounter
S	sequela

W55.0 Contact with cat
- X **W55.01 Bitten by cat**
- X **W55.03 Scratched by cat**
- X **W55.09 Other contact with cat**

W55.1 Contact with horse
- X **W55.11 Bitten by horse**
- X **W55.12 Struck by horse**
- X **W55.19 Other contact with horse**

W55.2 Contact with cow
Contact with bull
- X **W55.21 Bitten by cow**
- X **W55.22 Struck by cow**
  Gored by bull
- X **W55.29 Other contact with cow**

W55.3 Contact with other hoof stock
Contact with goats
Contact with sheep
- X **W55.31 Bitten by other hoof stock**
- X **W55.32 Struck by other hoof stock**
  Gored by goat
  Gored by ram
- X **W55.39 Other contact with other hoof stock**

W55.4 Contact with pig
- X **W55.41 Bitten by pig**
- X **W55.42 Struck by pig**
- X **W55.49 Other contact with pig**

W55.5 Contact with raccoon
- X **W55.51 Bitten by raccoon**
- X **W55.52 Struck by raccoon**
- X **W55.59 Other contact with raccoon**

W55.8 Contact with other mammals
- X **W55.81 Bitten by other mammals**
- X **W55.82 Struck by other mammals**
- X **W55.89 Other contact with other mammals**

W56 Contact with nonvenomous marine animal

Excludes1 contact with venomous marine animal (T63.-)

The appropriate 7th character is to be added to each code from category W56

A	initial encounter
D	subsequent encounter
S	sequela

W56.0 Contact with dolphin
- X **W56.01 Bitten by dolphin**
- X **W56.02 Struck by dolphin**
- X **W56.09 Other contact with dolphin**

W56.1 Contact with sea lion
- X **W56.11 Bitten by sea lion**
- X **W56.12 Struck by sea lion**
- X **W56.19 Other contact with sea lion**

W56.2 Contact with orca
Contact with killer whale
- X **W56.21 Bitten by orca**
- X **W56.22 Struck by orca**
- X **W56.29 Other contact with orca**

W56.3 Contact with other marine mammals
- X **W56.31 Bitten by other marine mammals**
- X **W56.32 Struck by other marine mammals**
- X **W56.39 Other contact with other marine mammals**

W56.4 Contact with shark
- X **W56.41 Bitten by shark**
- X **W56.42 Struck by shark**
- X **W56.49 Other contact with shark**

W56.5 Contact with other fish
- X **W56.51 Bitten by other fish**
- X **W56.52 Struck by other fish**
- X **W56.59 Other contact with other fish**

W56.8 Contact with other nonvenomous marine animals
- X **W56.81 Bitten by other nonvenomous marine animals**
- X **W56.82 Struck by other nonvenomous marine animals**
- X **W56.89 Other contact with other nonvenomous marine animals**

X **W57 Bitten or stung by nonvenomous insect and other nonvenomous arthropods**

Excludes1 contact with venomous insects and arthropods (T63.2-, T63.3-, T63.4-)

The appropriate 7th character is to be added to code W57

A	initial encounter
D	subsequent encounter
S	sequela

W58 Contact with crocodile or alligator

The appropriate 7th character is to be added to each code from category W58

A	initial encounter
D	subsequent encounter
S	sequela

W58.0 Contact with alligator
- X **W58.01 Bitten by alligator**
- X **W58.02 Struck by alligator**
- X **W58.03 Crushed by alligator**
- X **W58.09 Other contact with alligator**

W58.1 Contact with crocodile
- X **W58.11 Bitten by crocodile**
- X **W58.12 Struck by crocodile**
- X **W58.13 Crushed by crocodile**
- X **W58.19 Other contact with crocodile**

W59 Contact with other nonvenomous reptiles

Excludes1 contact with venomous reptile (T63.0-, T63.1-)

The appropriate 7th character is to be added to each code from category W59

A	initial encounter
D	subsequent encounter
S	sequela

W59.0 Contact with nonvenomous lizards
- X **W59.01 Bitten by nonvenomous lizards**
- X **W59.02 Struck by nonvenomous lizards**
- X **W59.09 Other contact with nonvenomous lizards**
  Exposure to nonvenomous lizards

W59.1 Contact with nonvenomous snakes
- **X W59.11 Bitten by nonvenomous snake**
- **X W59.12 Struck by nonvenomous snake**
- **X W59.13 Crushed by nonvenomous snake**
- **X W59.19 Other contact with nonvenomous snake**

W59.2 Contact with turtles

Excludes1 contact with tortoises (W59.8-)
- **X W59.21 Bitten by turtle**
- **X W59.22 Struck by turtle**
- **X W59.29 Other contact with turtle**
  Exposure to turtles

W59.8 Contact with other nonvenomous reptiles
- **X W59.81 Bitten by other nonvenomous reptiles**
- **X W59.82 Struck by other nonvenomous reptiles**
- **X W59.83 Crushed by other nonvenomous reptiles**
- **X W59.89 Other contact with other nonvenomous reptiles**

X W60 Contact with nonvenomous plant thorns and spines and sharp leaves

Excludes1 contact with venomous plants (T63.X7-)

The appropriate 7th character is to be added to code W60

A	initial encounter
D	subsequent encounter
S	sequela

W61 Contact with birds (domestic) (wild)

Includes contact with excreta of birds

The appropriate 7th character is to be added to each code from category W61

A	initial encounter
D	subsequent encounter
S	sequela

W61.0 Contact with parrot
- **X W61.01 Bitten by parrot**
- **X W61.02 Struck by parrot**
- **X W61.09 Other contact with parrot**
  Exposure to parrots

W61.1 Contact with macaw
- **X W61.11 Bitten by macaw**
- **X W61.12 Struck by macaw**
- **X W61.19 Other contact with macaw**
  Exposure to macaws

W61.2 Contact with other psittacines
- **X W61.21 Bitten by other psittacines**
- **X W61.22 Struck by other psittacines**
- **X W61.29 Other contact with other psittacines**
  Exposure to other psittacines

W61.3 Contact with chicken
- **X W61.32 Struck by chicken**
- **X W61.33 Pecked by chicken**
- **X W61.39 Other contact with chicken**
  Exposure to chickens

W61.4 Contact with turkey
- **X W61.42 Struck by turkey**
- **X W61.43 Pecked by turkey**
- **X W61.49 Other contact with turkey**

W61.5 Contact with goose
- **X W61.51 Bitten by goose**
- **X W61.52 Struck by goose**
- **X W61.59 Other contact with goose**

W61.6 Contact with duck
- **X W61.61 Bitten by duck**
- **X W61.62 Struck by duck**
- **X W61.69 Other contact with duck**

W61.9 Contact with other birds
- **X W61.91 Bitten by other birds**
- **X W61.92 Struck by other birds**
- **X W61.99 Other contact with other birds**
  Contact with bird NOS

W62 Contact with nonvenomous amphibians

Excludes1 contact with venomous amphibians (T63.81-R63.83)

The appropriate 7th character is to be added to each code from category W62

A	initial encounter
D	subsequent encounter
S	sequela

- **X W62.0 Contact with nonvenomous frogs**
- **X W62.1 Contact with nonvenomous toads**
- **X W62.9 Contact with other nonvenomous amphibians**

X W64 Exposure to other animate mechanical forces

Includes exposure to nonvenomous animal NOS

Excludes1 contact with venomous animal (T63.-)

The appropriate 7th character is to be added to code W64

A	initial encounter
D	subsequent encounter
S	sequela

ACCIDENTAL NON-TRANSPORT DROWNING AND SUBMERSION (W65-W74)

Excludes1 accidental drowning and submersion due to fall into water (W16.-)
accidental drowning and submersion due to water transport accident (V90.-, V92.-)

Excludes2 accidental drowning and submersion due to cataclysm (X34-X39)

X W65 Accidental drowning and submersion while in bathtub

Excludes1 accidental drowning and submersion due to fall in (into) bathtub (W16.211)

The appropriate 7th character is to be added to code W65

A	initial encounter
D	subsequent encounter
S	sequela

X W67 Accidental drowning and submersion while in swimming pool

Excludes1 accidental drowning and submersion due to fall into swimming pool (W16.011, W16.021, W16.031)
accidental drowning and submersion due to striking into wall of swimming pool (W22.041)

The appropriate 7th character is to be added to code W67

A	initial encounter
D	subsequent encounter
S	sequela

X W69 Accidental drowning and submersion while in natural water

Accidental drowning and submersion while in lake
Accidental drowning and submersion while in open sea
Accidental drowning and submersion while in river
Accidental drowning and submersion while in stream

Excludes1 accidental drowning and submersion due to fall into natural body of water (W16.111, W16.121, W16.131)

The appropriate 7th character is to be added to code W69

A	initial encounter
D	subsequent encounter
S	sequela

X● **W73 Other specified cause of accidental non-transport drowning and submersion**
Accidental drowning and submersion while in quenching tank
Accidental drowning and submersion while in reservoir
Excludes1 accidental drowning and submersion due to fall into other water (W16.311, W16.321, W16.331)
The appropriate 7th character is to be added to code W73

A	initial encounter
D	subsequent encounter
S	sequela

X● **W74 Unspecified cause of accidental drowning and submersion**
Drowning NOS
The appropriate 7th character is to be added to code W74

A	initial encounter
D	subsequent encounter
S	sequela

EXPOSURE TO ELECTRIC CURRENT, RADIATION AND EXTREME AMBIENT AIR TEMPERATURE AND PRESSURE (W85-W99)

Excludes1 exposure to:
failure in dosage of radiation or temperature during surgical and medical care (Y63.2-Y63.5)
lightning (T75.0-)
natural cold (X31)
natural heat (X30)
natural radiation NOS (X39)
radiological procedure and radiotherapy (Y84.2)
sunlight (X32)

X● **W85 Exposure to electric transmission lines**
Broken power line
The appropriate 7th character is to be added to code W85

A	initial encounter
D	subsequent encounter
S	sequela

● **W86 Exposure to other specified electric current**
The appropriate 7th character is to be added to each code from category W86

A	initial encounter
D	subsequent encounter
S	sequela

X● **W86.0 Exposure to domestic wiring and appliances**
X● **W86.1 Exposure to industrial wiring, appliances and electrical machinery**
Exposure to conductors
Exposure to control apparatus
Exposure to electrical equipment and machinery
Exposure to transformers
X● **W86.8 Exposure to other electric current**
Exposure to wiring and appliances in or on farm (not farmhouse)
Exposure to wiring and appliances outdoors
Exposure to wiring and appliances in or on public building
Exposure to wiring and appliances in or on residential institutions
Exposure to wiring and appliances in or on schools

● **W88 Exposure to ionizing radiation**
Excludes1 exposure to sunlight (X32)
The appropriate 7th character is to be added to each code from category W88

A	initial encounter
D	subsequent encounter
S	sequela

X● **W88.0 Exposure to X-rays**
X● **W88.1 Exposure to radioactive isotopes**
X● **W88.8 Exposure to other ionizing radiation**

● **W89 Exposure to man-made visible and ultraviolet light**
Includes exposure to welding light (arc)
Excludes1 exposure to sunlight (X32) ◀
The appropriate 7th character is to be added to each code from category W89

A	initial encounter
D	subsequent encounter
S	sequela

X● **W89.0 Exposure to welding light (arc)**
X● **W89.1 Exposure to tanning bed**
X● **W89.8 Exposure to other man-made visible and ultraviolet light**
X● **W89.9 Exposure to unspecified man-made visible and ultraviolet light**

● **W90 Exposure to other nonionizing radiation**
Excludes1 exposure to sunlight (X32)
The appropriate 7th character is to be added to each code from category W90

A	initial encounter
D	subsequent encounter
S	sequela

X● **W90.0 Exposure to radiofrequency**
X● **W90.1 Exposure to infrared radiation**
X● **W90.2 Exposure to laser radiation**
X● **W90.8 Exposure to other nonionizing radiation**

X● **W92 Exposure to excessive heat of man-made origin**
The appropriate 7th character is to be added to code W92

A	initial encounter
D	subsequent encounter
S	sequela

● **W93 Exposure to excessive cold of man-made origin**
The appropriate 7th character is to be added to each code from category W93

A	initial encounter
D	subsequent encounter
S	sequela

● **W93.0 Contact with or inhalation of dry ice**
X● **W93.01 Contact with dry ice**
X● **W93.02 Inhalation of dry ice**
● **W93.1 Contact with or inhalation of liquid air**
X● **W93.11 Contact with liquid air**
Contact with liquid hydrogen
Contact with liquid nitrogen
X● **W93.12 Inhalation of liquid air**
Inhalation of liquid hydrogen
Inhalation of liquid nitrogen
X● **W93.2 Prolonged exposure in deep freeze unit or refrigerator**
X● **W93.8 Exposure to other excessive cold of man-made origin**

◀ New ⇐ Revised ~~deleted~~ Deleted Excludes 1 Excludes 2 Includes Use additional Code first Code also Unspecified
OGCR Official Guidelines ● Unacceptable Principal Diagnosis X Assign placeholder X ● Use Additional Character(s) ◗ Manifestation Code Coding Clinic

● **W94 Exposure to high and low air pressure and changes in air pressure**

The appropriate 7th character is to be added to each code from category W94

A	initial encounter
D	subsequent encounter
S	sequela

X● **W94.0 Exposure to prolonged high air pressure**

● **W94.1 Exposure to prolonged low air pressure**

X● **W94.11 Exposure to residence or prolonged visit at high altitude**

X● **W94.12 Exposure to other prolonged low air pressure**

● **W94.2 Exposure to rapid changes in air pressure during ascent**

X● **W94.21 Exposure to reduction in atmospheric pressure while surfacing from deep-water diving**

X● **W94.22 Exposure to reduction in atmospheric pressure while surfacing from underground**

X● **W94.23 Exposure to sudden change in air pressure in aircraft during ascent**

X● **W94.29 Exposure to other rapid changes in air pressure during ascent**

● **W94.3 Exposure to rapid changes in air pressure during descent**

X● **W94.31 Exposure to sudden change in air pressure in aircraft during descent**

X● **W94.32 Exposure to high air pressure from rapid descent in water**

X● **W94.39 Exposure to other rapid changes in air pressure during descent**

X● **W99 Exposure to other man-made environmental factors**

The appropriate 7th character is to be added to code W99

A	initial encounter
D	subsequent encounter
S	sequela

EXPOSURE TO SMOKE, FIRE AND FLAMES (X00-X08)

Excludes1 arson (X97)

Excludes2 explosions (W35-W40)
lightning (T75.0-)
transport accident (V01-V99)

● **X00 Exposure to uncontrolled fire in building or structure**

Includes conflagration in building or structure

Code first any associated cataclysm

Excludes2 exposure to ignition or melting of nightwear (X05)
exposure to ignition or melting of other clothing and apparel (X06.-)
exposure to other specified smoke, fire and flames (X08.-)

The appropriate 7th character is to be added to each code from category X00

A	initial encounter
D	subsequent encounter
S	sequela

X● **X00.0 Exposure to flames in uncontrolled fire in building or structure**

Coding Clinic: 2016, Q2, P5-6; 2015, Q1, P19

X● **X00.1 Exposure to smoke in uncontrolled fire in building or structure**

X● **X00.2 Injury due to collapse of burning building or structure in uncontrolled fire**

Excludes1 injury due to collapse of building not on fire (W20.1)

X● **X00.3 Fall from burning building or structure in uncontrolled fire**

X● **X00.4 Hit by object from burning building or structure in uncontrolled fire**

X● **X00.5 Jump from burning building or structure in uncontrolled fire**

X● **X00.8 Other exposure to uncontrolled fire in building or structure**

● **X01 Exposure to uncontrolled fire, not in building or structure**

Includes exposure to forest fire

The appropriate 7th character is to be added to each code from category X01

A	initial encounter
D	subsequent encounter
S	sequela

X● **X01.0 Exposure to flames in uncontrolled fire, not in building or structure**

X● **X01.1 Exposure to smoke in uncontrolled fire, not in building or structure**

X● **X01.3 Fall due to uncontrolled fire, not in building or structure**

X● **X01.4 Hit by object due to uncontrolled fire, not in building or structure**

X● **X01.8 Other exposure to uncontrolled fire, not in building or structure**

● **X02 Exposure to controlled fire in building or structure**

Includes exposure to fire in fireplace exposure to fire in stove

The appropriate 7th character is to be added to each code from category X02

A	initial encounter
D	subsequent encounter
S	sequela

X● **X02.0 Exposure to flames in controlled fire in building or structure**

X● **X02.1 Exposure to smoke in controlled fire in building or structure**

X● **X02.2 Injury due to collapse of burning building or structure in controlled fire**

Excludes1 injury due to collapse of building not on fire (W20.1)

X● **X02.3 Fall from burning building or structure in controlled fire**

X● **X02.4 Hit by object from burning building or structure in controlled fire**

X● **X02.5 Jump from burning building or structure in controlled fire**

X● **X02.8 Other exposure to controlled fire in building or structure**

● **X03 Exposure to controlled fire, not in building or structure**

Includes exposure to bon fire exposure to camp fire exposure to trash fire

The appropriate 7th character is to be added to each code from category X03

A	initial encounter
D	subsequent encounter
S	sequela

X● **X03.0 Exposure to flames in controlled fire, not in building or structure**

Coding Clinic: 2015, Q1, P19

X● **X03.1 Exposure to smoke in controlled fire, not in building or structure**

X● **X03.3 Fall due to controlled fire, not in building or structure**

X● **X03.4 Hit by object due to controlled fire, not in building or structure**

X● **X03.8 Other exposure to controlled fire, not in building or structure**

X●X04 Exposure to ignition of highly flammable material
Exposure to ignition of gasoline
Exposure to ignition of kerosene
Exposure to ignition of petrol

Excludes2 exposure to ignition or melting of nightwear (X05)
exposure to ignition or melting of other clothing and apparel (X06)

The appropriate 7th character is to be added to code X04

A	initial encounter
D	subsequent encounter
S	sequela

Coding Clinic: 2016, Q2, P4

X●X05 Exposure to ignition or melting of nightwear

Excludes2 exposure to uncontrolled fire in building or structure (X00.-)
exposure to uncontrolled fire, not in building or structure (X01.-)
exposure to controlled fire in building or structure (X02.-)
exposure to controlled fire, not in building or structure (X03.-)
exposure to ignition of highly flammable materials (X04.-)

The appropriate 7th character is to be added to code X05

A	initial encounter
D	subsequent encounter
S	sequela

●X06 Exposure to ignition or melting of other clothing and apparel

Excludes2 exposure to uncontrolled fire in building or structure (X00.-)
exposure to uncontrolled fire, not in building or structure (X01.-)
exposure to controlled fire in building or structure (X02.-)
exposure to controlled fire, not in building or structure (X03.-)
exposure to ignition of highly flammable materials (X04.-)

The appropriate 7th character is to be added to each code from category X06

A	initial encounter
D	subsequent encounter
S	sequela

X●X06.0 Exposure to ignition of plastic jewelry
X●X06.1 Exposure to melting of plastic jewelry
X●X06.2 Exposure to ignition of other clothing and apparel
X●X06.3 Exposure to melting of other clothing and apparel

●X08 Exposure to other specified smoke, fire and flames

The appropriate 7th character is to be added to each code from category X08

A	initial encounter
D	subsequent encounter
S	sequela

●X08.0 Exposure to bed fire
Exposure to mattress fire

X●X08.00 Exposure to bed fire due to unspecified burning material
X●X08.01 Exposure to bed fire due to burning cigarette
Coding Clinic: 2015, Q1, P19
X●X08.09 Exposure to bed fire due to other burning material

●X08.1 Exposure to sofa fire

X●X08.10 Exposure to sofa fire due to unspecified burning material
X●X08.11 Exposure to sofa fire due to burning cigarette
X●X08.19 Exposure to sofa fire due to other burning material

●X08.2 Exposure to other furniture fire

X●X08.20 Exposure to other furniture fire due to unspecified burning material
X●X08.21 Exposure to other furniture fire due to burning cigarette
X●X08.29 Exposure to other furniture fire due to other burning material

X●X08.8 Exposure to other specified smoke, fire and flames

CONTACT WITH HEAT AND HOT SUBSTANCES (X10-X19)

Excludes1 exposure to excessive natural heat (X30)
exposure to fire and flames (X00-X09)

●X10 Contact with hot drinks, food, fats and cooking oils

The appropriate 7th character is to be added to each code from category X10

A	initial encounter
D	subsequent encounter
S	sequela

X●X10.0 Contact with hot drinks
X●X10.1 Contact with hot food
X●X10.2 Contact with fats and cooking oils

●X11 Contact with hot tap-water

Includes contact with boiling tap-water
contact with boiling water NOS

Excludes1 contact with water heated on stove (X12)

The appropriate 7th character is to be added to each code from category X11

A	initial encounter
D	subsequent encounter
S	sequela

X●X11.0 Contact with hot water in bath or tub

Excludes1 contact with running hot water in bath or tub (X11.1)

X●X11.1 Contact with running hot water
Contact with hot water running out of hose
Contact with hot water running out of tap

X●X11.8 Contact with other hot tap-water
Contact with hot water in bucket
Contact with hot tap-water NOS

X●X12 Contact with other hot fluids
Contact with water heated on stove

Excludes1 hot (liquid) metals (X18)

The appropriate 7th character is to be added to code X12

A	initial encounter
D	subsequent encounter
S	sequela

●X13 Contact with steam and other hot vapors

The appropriate 7th character is to be added to each code from category X13

A	initial encounter
D	subsequent encounter
S	sequela

X●X13.0 Inhalation of steam and other hot vapors
X●X13.1 Other contact with steam and other hot vapors

● X14 Contact with hot air and other hot gases

The appropriate 7th character is to be added to each code from category X14

A	initial encounter
D	subsequent encounter
S	sequela

X● X14.0 Inhalation of hot air and gases

X● X14.1 Other contact with hot air and other hot gases

● X15 Contact with hot household appliances

Excludes1 contact with heating appliances (X16)
contact with powered household appliances (W29.-)
exposure to controlled fire in building or structure due to household appliance (X02.8)
exposure to household appliances electrical current (W86.0)

The appropriate 7th character is to be added to each code from category X15

A	initial encounter
D	subsequent encounter
S	sequela

X● X15.0 Contact with hot stove (kitchen)

X● X15.1 Contact with hot toaster

X● X15.2 Contact with hotplate

X● X15.3 Contact with hot saucepan or skillet

X● X15.8 Contact with other hot household appliances

Contact with cooker
Contact with kettle
Contact with light bulbs

X● X16 Contact with hot heating appliances, radiators and pipes

Excludes1 contact with powered appliances (W29.-)
exposure to controlled fire in building or structure due to appliance (X02.8)
exposure to industrial appliances electrical current (W86.1)

The appropriate 7th character is to be added to code X16

A	initial encounter
D	subsequent encounter
S	sequela

X● X17 Contact with hot engines, machinery and tools

Excludes1 contact with hot heating appliances, radiators and pipes (X16)
contact with hot household appliances (X15)

The appropriate 7th character is to be added to code X17

A	initial encounter
D	subsequent encounter
S	sequela

X● X18 Contact with other hot metals

Contact with liquid metal

The appropriate 7th character is to be added to code X18

A	initial encounter
D	subsequent encounter
S	sequela

X● X19 Contact with other heat and hot substances

Excludes1 objects that are not normally hot, e.g., an object made hot by a house fire (X00-X09)

The appropriate 7th character is to be added to code X19

A	initial encounter
D	subsequent encounter
S	sequela

EXPOSURE TO FORCES OF NATURE (X30-X39)

X● X30 Exposure to excessive natural heat

Exposure to excessive heat as the cause of sunstroke
Exposure to heat NOS

Excludes1 excessive heat of man-made origin (W92)
exposure to man-made radiation (W89)
exposure to sunlight (X32)
exposure to tanning bed (W89)

The appropriate 7th character is to be added to code X30

A	initial encounter
D	subsequent encounter
S	sequela

X● X31 Exposure to excessive natural cold

Excessive cold as the cause of chilblains NOS
Excessive cold as the cause of immersion foot or hand
Exposure to cold NOS
Exposure to weather conditions

Excludes1 cold of man-made origin (W93.-)
contact with or inhalation of dry ice (W93.-)
contact with or inhalation of liquefied gas (W93.-)

The appropriate 7th character is to be added to code X31

A	initial encounter
D	subsequent encounter
S	sequela

X● X32 Exposure to sunlight

Excludes1 ~~radiation-related disorders of the skin and subcutaneous tissue (L55-L59)~~
man-made radiation (tanning bed) (W89)

The appropriate 7th character is to be added to code X32

A	initial encounter
D	subsequent encounter
S	sequela

X● X34 Earthquake

Excludes2 tidal wave (tsunami) due to earthquake (X37.41)

The appropriate 7th character is to be added to code X34

A	initial encounter
D	subsequent encounter
S	sequela

X● X35 Volcanic eruption

Excludes2 tidal wave (tsunami) due to volcanic eruption (X37.41)

The appropriate 7th character is to be added to code X35

A	initial encounter
D	subsequent encounter
S	sequela

● X36 Avalanche, landslide and other earth movements

Includes victim of mudslide of cataclysmic nature

Excludes1 earthquake (X34)

Excludes2 transport accident involving collision with avalanche or landslide not in motion (V01-V99)

The appropriate 7th character is to be added to each code from category X36

A	initial encounter
D	subsequent encounter
S	sequela

X● X36.0 Collapse of dam or man-made structure causing earth movement

X● X36.1 Avalanche, landslide, or mudslide

● X37 Cataclysmic storm

The appropriate 7th character is to be added to each code from category X37

A	initial encounter
D	subsequent encounter
S	sequela

X● X37.0 Hurricane
Storm surge
Typhoon

X● X37.1 Tornado
Cyclone
Twister

X● X37.2 Blizzard (snow) (ice)

X● X37.3 Dust storm

● X37.4 Tidalwave

X● X37.41 Tidal wave due to earthquake or volcanic eruption
Tidal wave NOS
Tsunami

X● X37.42 Tidal wave due to storm

X● X37.43 Tidal wave due to landslide

X● X37.8 Other cataclysmic storms
Cloudburst
Torrential rain
Excludes2 flood (X38)

X● X37.9 Unspecified cataclysmic storm
Storm NOS
Excludes1 collapse of dam or man-made structure causing earth movement (X39.0)

X● X38 Flood
Flood arising from remote storm
Flood of cataclysmic nature arising from melting snow
Flood resulting directly from storm
Excludes1 collapse of dam or man-made structure causing earth movement (X39.0)
tidal wave NOS (X37.41)
tidal wave caused by storm (X37.2)

The appropriate 7th character is to be added to code X38

A	initial encounter
D	subsequent encounter
S	sequela

● X39 Exposure to other forces of nature

The appropriate 7th character is to be added to each code from category X39

A	initial encounter
D	subsequent encounter
S	sequela

● X39.0 Exposure to natural radiation
Excludes1 contact with and (suspected) exposure to radon and other naturally occuring radiation (Z77.123) ⇐
exposure to man-made radiation (W88-W90)
exposure to sunlight (X32)

X● X39.01 Exposure to radon

X● X39.08 Exposure to other natural radiation

X● X39.8 Other exposure to forces of nature

OVEREXERTION AND STRENUOUS OR REPETITIVE MOVEMENTS (X50) ◀

● X50 Overexertion and strenuous or repetitive movements ◀

The appropriate 7th character is to be added to each code from category X50 ◀

A	initial encounter ◀
D	subsequent encounter ◀
S	sequela ◀

X● X50.0 Overexertion from strenuous movement or load ◀
Lifting heavy objects ◀
Lifting weights ◀

X● X50.1 Overexertion from prolonged static or awkward postures ◀
Prolonged bending ◀
Prolonged kneeling ◀
Prolonged reaching ◀
Prolonged sitting ◀
Prolonged standing ◀
Prolonged twisting ◀
Static bending ◀
Static kneeling ◀
Static reaching ◀
Static sitting ◀
Static standing ◀
Static twisting ◀

X● X50.3 Overexertion from repetitive movements ◀
Use of hand as hammer ◀
Excludes2 Overuse from prolonged static or awkward postures (X50.1) ◀

X● X50.9 Other and unspecified overexertion or strenuous movements or postures ◀
Contact pressure ◀
Contact stress ◀

ACCIDENTAL EXPOSURE TO OTHER SPECIFIED FACTORS (X52, X58)

X● X52 Prolonged stay in weightless environment
Weightlessness in spacecraft (simulator)

The appropriate 7th character is to be added to code X52

A	initial encounter
D	subsequent encounter
S	sequela

X● X58 Exposure to other specified factors
Accident NOS
Exposure NOS

The appropriate 7th character is to be added to code X58

A	initial encounter
D	subsequent encounter
S	sequela

INTENTIONAL SELF-HARM (X71-X83)

Purposely self-inflicted injury
Suicide (attempted)

● X71 Intentional self-harm by drowning and submersion

The appropriate 7th character is to be added to each code from category X71

A	initial encounter
D	subsequent encounter
S	sequela

X● X71.0 Intentional self-harm by drowning and submersion while in bathtub

X● X71.1 Intentional self-harm by drowning and submersion while in swimming pool

X● X71.2 Intentional self-harm by drowning and submersion after jump into swimming pool

X●X71.3 Intentional self-harm by drowning and submersion in natural water

X●X71.8 Other intentional self-harm by drowning and submersion

X●X71.9 Intentional self-harm by drowning and submersion, unspecified

X●X72 Intentional self-harm by handgun discharge

Intentional self-harm by gun for single hand use
Intentional self-harm by pistol
Intentional self-harm by revolver

Excludes1 Very pistol (X74.8)

The appropriate 7th character is to be added to code X72

A	initial encounter
D	subsequent encounter
S	sequela

●X73 Intentional self-harm by rifle, shotgun and larger firearm discharge

Excludes1 airgun (X74.01)

The appropriate 7th character is to be added to each code from category X73

A	initial encounter
D	subsequent encounter
S	sequela

X●X73.0 Intentional self-harm by shotgun discharge

X●X73.1 Intentional self-harm by hunting rifle discharge

X●X73.2 Intentional self-harm by machine gun discharge

X●X73.8 Intentional self-harm by other larger firearm discharge

X●X73.9 Intentional self-harm by unspecified larger firearm discharge

●X74 Intentional self-harm by other and unspecified firearm and gun discharge

The appropriate 7th character is to be added to each code from category X74

A	initial encounter
D	subsequent encounter
S	sequela

●X74.0 Intentional self-harm by gas, air or spring-operated guns

X●X74.01 Intentional self-harm by airgun

Intentional self-harm by BB gun discharge
Intentional self-harm by pellet gun discharge

X●X74.02 Intentional self-harm by paintball gun

X●X74.09 Intentional self-harm by other gas, air or spring-operated gun

X●X74.8 Intentional self-harm by other firearm discharge

Intentional self-harm by Very pistol [flare] discharge

X●X74.9 Intentional self-harm by unspecified firearm discharge

X●X75 Intentional self-harm by explosive material

The appropriate 7th character is to be added to code X75

A	initial encounter
D	subsequent encounter
S	sequela

X●X76 Intentional self-harm by smoke, fire and flames

The appropriate 7th character is to be added to code X76

A	initial encounter
D	subsequent encounter
S	sequela

●X77 Intentional self-harm by steam, hot vapors and hot objects

The appropriate 7th character is to be added to each code from category X77

A	initial encounter
D	subsequent encounter
S	sequela

X●X77.0 Intentional self-harm by steam or hot vapors

X●X77.1 Intentional self-harm by hot tap water

X●X77.2 Intentional self-harm by other hot fluids

X●X77.3 Intentional self-harm by hot household appliances

X●X77.8 Intentional self-harm by other hot objects

X●X77.9 Intentional self-harm by unspecified hot objects

●X78 Intentional self-harm by sharp object

The appropriate 7th character is to be added to each code from category X78

A	initial encounter
D	subsequent encounter
S	sequela

X●X78.0 Intentional self-harm by sharp glass

X●X78.1 Intentional self-harm by knife

X●X78.2 Intentional self-harm by sword or dagger

X●X78.8 Intentional self-harm by other sharp object

X●X78.9 Intentional self-harm by unspecified sharp object

X●X79 Intentional self-harm by blunt object

The appropriate 7th character is to be added to code X79

A	initial encounter
D	subsequent encounter
S	sequela

X●X80 Intentional self-harm by jumping from a high place

Intentional fall from one level to another

The appropriate 7th character is to be added to code X80

A	initial encounter
D	subsequent encounter
S	sequela

●X81 Intentional self-harm by jumping or lying in front of moving object

The appropriate 7th character is to be added to each code from category X81

A	initial encounter
D	subsequent encounter
S	sequela

X●X81.0 Intentional self-harm by jumping or lying in front of motor vehicle

X●X81.1 Intentional self-harm by jumping or lying in front of (subway) train

X●X81.8 Intentional self-harm by jumping or lying in front of other moving object

●X82 Intentional self-harm by crashing of motor vehicle

The appropriate 7th character is to be added to each code from category X82

A	initial encounter
D	subsequent encounter
S	sequela

X●X82.0 Intentional collision of motor vehicle with other motor vehicle

X●X82.1 Intentional collision of motor vehicle with train

X●X82.2 Intentional collision of motor vehicle with tree

X●X82.8 Other intentional self-harm by crashing of motor vehicle

● X83 Intentional self-harm by other specified means

Excludes1 intentional self-harm by poisoning or contact with toxic substance - see Table of Drugs and Chemicals

The appropriate 7th character is to be added to each code from category X83

A	initial encounter
D	subsequent encounter
S	sequela

X● X83.0 Intentional self-harm by crashing of aircraft
X● X83.1 Intentional self-harm by electrocution
X● X83.2 Intentional self-harm by exposure to extremes of cold
X● X83.8 Intentional self-harm by other specified means

ASSAULT (X92-Y09)

Includes homicide injuries inflicted by another person with intent to injure or kill, by any means

Excludes1 injuries due to legal intervention (Y35.-)
injuries due to operations of war (Y36.-)
injuries due to terrorism (Y38.-)

● X92 Assault by drowning and submersion

The appropriate 7th character is to be added to each code from category X92

A	initial encounter
D	subsequent encounter
S	sequela

X● X92.0 Assault by drowning and submersion while in bathtub
X● X92.1 Assault by drowning and submersion while in swimming pool
X● X92.2 Assault by drowning and submersion after push into swimming pool
X● X92.3 Assault by drowning and submersion in natural water
X● X92.8 Other assault by drowning and submersion
X● X92.9 Assault by drowning and submersion, unspecified

X● X93 Assault by handgun discharge

Assault by discharge of gun for single hand use
Assault by discharge of pistol
Assault by discharge of revolver

Excludes1 Very pistol (X95.8)

The appropriate 7th character is to be added to code X93

A	initial encounter
D	subsequent encounter
S	sequela

● X94 Assault by rifle, shotgun and larger firearm discharge

Excludes1 airgun (X95.01)

The appropriate 7th character is to be added to each code from category X94

A	initial encounter
D	subsequent encounter
S	sequela

X● X94.0 Assault by shotgun
X● X94.1 Assault by hunting rifle
X● X94.2 Assault by machine gun
X● X94.8 Assault by other larger firearm discharge
X● X94.9 Assault by unspecified larger firearm discharge

● X95 Assault by other and unspecified firearm and gun discharge

The appropriate 7th character is to be added to each code from category X95

A	initial encounter
D	subsequent encounter
S	sequela

● X95.0 Assault by gas, air or spring-operated guns

X● X95.01 Assault by airgun discharge
Assault by BB gun discharge
Assault by pellet gun discharge

X● X95.02 Assault by paintball gun discharge
X● X95.09 Assault by other gas, air or spring-operated gun

X● X95.8 Assault by other firearm discharge
Assault by very pistol [flare] discharge

X● X95.9 Assault by unspecified firearm discharge

● X96 Assault by explosive material

Excludes1 incendiary device (X97)
terrorism involving explosive material (Y38.2-)

The appropriate 7th character is to be added to each code from category X96

A	initial encounter
D	subsequent encounter
S	sequela

X● X96.0 Assault by antipersonnel bomb

Excludes1 antipersonnel bomb use in military or war (Y36.2-)

X● X96.1 Assault by gasoline bomb
X● X96.2 Assault by letter bomb
X● X96.3 Assault by fertilizer bomb
X● X96.4 Assault by pipe bomb
X● X96.8 Assault by other specified explosive
X● X96.9 Assault by unspecified explosive

X● X97 Assault by smoke, fire and flames

Assault by arson
Assault by cigarettes
Assault by incendiary device

The appropriate 7th character is to be added to code X97

A	initial encounter
D	subsequent encounter
S	sequela

● X98 Assault by steam, hot vapors and hot objects

The appropriate 7th character is to be added to each code from category X98

A	initial encounter
D	subsequent encounter
S	sequela

X● X98.0 Assault by steam or hot vapors
X● X98.1 Assault by hot tap water
X● X98.2 Assault by hot fluids
X● X98.3 Assault by hot household appliances
X● X98.8 Assault by other hot objects
X● X98.9 Assault by unspecified hot objects

● **X99 Assault by sharp object**

Excludes1 assault by strike by sports equipment (Y08.0-)

The appropriate 7th character is to be added to each code from category X99

A	initial encounter
D	subsequent encounter
S	sequela

X● **X99.0 Assault by sharp glass**

X● **X99.1 Assault by knife**

X● **X99.2 Assault by sword or dagger**

X● **X99.8 Assault by other sharp object**

X● **X99.9 Assault by unspecified sharp object**

Assault by stabbing NOS

X● **Y00 Assault by blunt object**

Excludes1 assault by strike by sports equipment (Y08.0)

The appropriate 7th character is to be added to code Y00

A	initial encounter
D	subsequent encounter
S	sequela

X● **Y01 Assault by pushing from high place**

The appropriate 7th character is to be added to code Y01

A	initial encounter
D	subsequent encounter
S	sequela

● **Y02 Assault by pushing or placing victim in front of moving object**

The appropriate 7th character is to be added to each code from category Y02

A	initial encounter
D	subsequent encounter
S	sequela

X● **Y02.0 Assault by pushing or placing victim in front of motor vehicle**

X● **Y02.1 Assault by pushing or placing victim in front of (subway) train**

X● **Y02.8 Assault by pushing or placing victim in front of other moving object**

● **Y03 Assault by crashing of motor vehicle**

The appropriate 7th character is to be added to each code from category Y03

A	initial encounter
D	subsequent encounter
S	sequela

X● **Y03.0 Assault by being hit or run over by motor vehicle**

X● **Y03.8 Other assault by crashing of motor vehicle**

● **Y04 Assault by bodily force**

Excludes1 assault by:
submersion (X92.-)
use of weapon (X93-X95, X99, Y00)

The appropriate 7th character is to be added to each code from category Y04

A	initial encounter
D	subsequent encounter
S	sequela

X● **Y04.0 Assault by unarmed brawl or fight**

X● **Y04.1 Assault by human bite**

X● **Y04.2 Assault by strike against or bumped into by another person**

X● **Y04.8 Assault by other bodily force**

Assault by bodily force NOS

OGCR Section I.C.19.f.

Adult and child abuse, neglect and other maltreatment

Sequence first the appropriate code from categories T74.- or T76.- for abuse, neglect and other maltreatment, followed by any accompanying mental health or injury code(s).

If the documentation in the medical record states abuse or neglect it is coded as confirmed. It is coded as suspected if it is documented as suspected.

For cases of confirmed abuse or neglect an external cause code from the assault section (X92-Y08) should be added to identify the cause of any physical injuries. A perpetrator code (Y07) should be added when the perpetrator of the abuse is known. For suspected cases of abuse or neglect, do not report external cause or perpetrator code.

If a suspected case of abuse, neglect or mistreatment is ruled out during an encounter code Z04.71, Encounter for examination and observation following alleged physical adult abuse, ruled out, or code Z04.72, Encounter for examination and observation following alleged child physical abuse, ruled out, should be used, not a code from T76.

If a suspected case of alleged rape or sexual abuse is ruled out during an encounter code Z04.41, Encounter for examination and observation following alleged physical adult abuse, ruled out, or code Z04.42, Encounter for examination and observation following alleged rape or sexual abuse, ruled out, should be used, not a code from T76.

● **Y07 Perpetrator of assault, maltreatment and neglect**

Note: Codes from this category are for use only in cases of confirmed abuse (T74.-)

Selection of the correct perpetrator code is based on the relationship between the perpetrator and the victim

Includes perpetrator of abandonment
perpetrator of emotional neglect
perpetrator of mental cruelty
perpetrator of physical abuse
perpetrator of physical neglect
perpetrator of sexual abuse
perpetrator of torture

● **Y07.0 Spouse or partner, perpetrator of maltreatment and neglect**

Spouse or partner, perpetrator of maltreatment and neglect against spouse or partner

Y07.01 Husband, perpetrator of maltreatment and neglect

Y07.02 Wife, perpetrator of maltreatment and neglect

Y07.03 Male partner, perpetrator of maltreatment and neglect

Y07.04 Female partner, perpetrator of maltreatment and neglect

● **Y07.1 Parent (adoptive) (biological), perpetrator of maltreatment and neglect**

Y07.11 Biological father, perpetrator of maltreatment and neglect

Y07.12 Biological mother, perpetrator of maltreatment and neglect

Y07.13 Adoptive father, perpetrator of maltreatment and neglect

Y07.14 Adoptive mother, perpetrator of maltreatment and neglect

● **Y07.4 Other family member, perpetrator of maltreatment and neglect**

● **Y07.41 Sibling, perpetrator of maltreatment and neglect**

Excludes1 stepsibling, perpetrator of maltreatment and neglect (Y07.435, Y07.436)

Y07.410 Brother, perpetrator of maltreatment and neglect

Y07.411 Sister, perpetrator of maltreatment and neglect

● **Y07.42 Foster parent, perpetrator of maltreatment and neglect**

Y07.420 Foster father, perpetrator of maltreatment and neglect

Y07.421 Foster mother, perpetrator of maltreatment and neglect

● **Y07.43 Stepparent or stepsibling, perpetrator of maltreatment and neglect**

Y07.430 Stepfather, perpetrator of maltreatment and neglect

Y07.432 Male friend of parent (co-residing in household), perpetrator of maltreatment and neglect

Y07.433 Stepmother, perpetrator of maltreatment and neglect

Y07.434 Female friend of parent (co-residing in household), perpetrator of maltreatment and neglect

Y07.435 Stepbrother, perpetrator or maltreatment and neglect

Y07.436 Stepsister, perpetrator of maltreatment and neglect

● **Y07.49 Other family member, perpetrator of maltreatment and neglect**

Y07.490 Male cousin, perpetrator of maltreatment and neglect

Y07.491 Female cousin, perpetrator of maltreatment and neglect

Y07.499 Other family member, perpetrator of maltreatment and neglect

● **Y07.5 Non-family member, perpetrator of maltreatment and neglect**

Y07.50 Unspecified non-family member, perpetrator of maltreatment and neglect

● **Y07.51 Daycare provider, perpetrator of maltreatment and neglect**

Y07.510 At-home childcare provider, perpetrator of maltreatment and neglect

Y07.511 Daycare center childcare provider, perpetrator of maltreatment and neglect

Y07.512 At-home adultcare provider, perpetrator of maltreatment and neglect

Y07.513 Adultcare center provider, perpetrator of maltreatment and neglect

Y07.519 Unspecified daycare provider, perpetrator of maltreatment and neglect

● **Y07.52 Healthcare provider, perpetrator of maltreatment and neglect**

Y07.521 Mental health provider, perpetrator of maltreatment and neglect

Y07.528 Other therapist or healthcare provider, perpetrator of maltreatment and neglect

Nurse perpetrator of maltreatment and neglect
Occupational therapist perpetrator of maltreatment and neglect
Physical therapist perpetrator of maltreatment and neglect
Speech therapist perpetrator of maltreatment and neglect

Y07.529 Unspecified healthcare provider, perpetrator of maltreatment and neglect

Y07.53 Teacher or instructor, perpetrator of maltreatment and neglect

Coach, perpetrator of maltreatment and neglect

Y07.59 Other non-family member, perpetrator of maltreatment and neglect

Y07.9 Unspecified perpetrator of maltreatment and neglect

● **Y08 Assault by other specified means**

The appropriate 7th character is to be added to each code from category Y08

A	initial encounter
D	subsequent encounter
S	sequela

● **Y08.0 Assault by strike by sport equipment**

X● **Y08.01 Assault by strike by hockey stick**

X● **Y08.02 Assault by strike by baseball bat**

X● **Y08.09 Assault by strike by other specified type of sport equipment**

● **Y08.8 Assault by other specified means**

X● **Y08.81 Assault by crashing of aircraft**

X● **Y08.89 Assault by other specified means**

● **Y09 Assault by unspecified means**

Assassination (attempted) NOS
Homicide (attempted) NOS
Manslaughter (attempted) NOS
Murder (attempted) NOS

EVENT OF UNDETERMINED INTENT (Y21-Y33)

Undetermined intent is only for use when there is specific documentation in the record that the intent of the injury cannot be determined. If no such documentation is present, code to accidental (unintentional)

● **Y21 Drowning and submersion, undetermined intent**

The appropriate 7th character is to be added to each code from category Y21

A	initial encounter
D	subsequent encounter
S	sequela

X● **Y21.0 Drowning and submersion while in bathtub, undetermined intent**

X● **Y21.1 Drowning and submersion after fall into bathtub, undetermined intent**

X● **Y21.2 Drowning and submersion while in swimming pool, undetermined intent**

X● **Y21.3 Drowning and submersion after fall into swimming pool, undetermined intent**

X● **Y21.4 Drowning and submersion in natural water, undetermined intent**

X● **Y21.8 Other drowning and submersion, undetermined intent**

X● **Y21.9 Unspecified drowning and submersion, undetermined intent**

X● **Y22 Handgun discharge, undetermined intent**

Discharge of gun for single hand use, undetermined intent
Discharge of pistol, undetermined intent
Discharge of revolver, undetermined intent

Excludes2 very pistol (Y24.8)

The appropriate 7th character is to be added to code Y22

A	initial encounter
D	subsequent encounter
S	sequela

Y23 Rifle, shotgun and larger firearm discharge, undetermined intent

Excludes2 airgun (Y24.0)

The appropriate 7th character is to be added to each code from category Y23

A	initial encounter
D	subsequent encounter
S	sequela

X **Y23.0 Shotgun discharge, undetermined intent**
X **Y23.1 Hunting rifle discharge, undetermined intent**
X **Y23.2 Military firearm discharge, undetermined intent**
X **Y23.3 Machine gun discharge, undetermined intent**
X **Y23.8 Other larger firearm discharge, undetermined intent**
X **Y23.9 Unspecified larger firearm discharge, undetermined intent**

Y24 Other and unspecified firearm discharge, undetermined intent

The appropriate 7th character is to be added to each code from category Y24

A	initial encounter
D	subsequent encounter
S	sequela

X **Y24.0 Airgun discharge, undetermined intent**
BB gun discharge, undetermined intent
Pellet gun discharge, undetermined intent

X **Y24.8 Other firearm discharge, undetermined intent**
Paintball gun discharge, undetermined intent
Very pistol [flare] discharge, undetermined intent

X **Y24.9 Unspecified firearm discharge, undetermined intent**

X **Y25 Contact with explosive material, undetermined intent**

The appropriate 7th character is to be added to code Y25

A	initial encounter
D	subsequent encounter
S	sequela

X **Y26 Exposure to smoke, fire and flames, undetermined intent**

The appropriate 7th character is to be added to code Y26

A	initial encounter
D	subsequent encounter
S	sequela

Y27 Contact with steam, hot vapors and hot objects, undetermined intent

The appropriate 7th character is to be added to each code from category Y27

A	initial encounter
D	subsequent encounter
S	sequela

X **Y27.0 Contact with steam and hot vapors, undetermined intent**
X **Y27.1 Contact with hot tap water, undetermined intent**
X **Y27.2 Contact with hot fluids, undetermined intent**
X **Y27.3 Contact with hot household appliance, undetermined intent**
X **Y27.8 Contact with other hot objects, undetermined intent**
X **Y27.9 Contact with unspecified hot objects, undetermined intent**

Y28 Contact with sharp object, undetermined intent

The appropriate 7th character is to be added to each code from category Y28

A	initial encounter
D	subsequent encounter
S	sequela

X **Y28.0 Contact with sharp glass, undetermined intent**
X **Y28.1 Contact with knife, undetermined intent**
X **Y28.2 Contact with sword or dagger, undetermined intent**
X **Y28.8 Contact with other sharp object, undetermined intent**
X **Y28.9 Contact with unspecified sharp object, undetermined intent**

X **Y29 Contact with blunt object, undetermined intent**

The appropriate 7th character is to be added to code Y29

A	initial encounter
D	subsequent encounter
S	sequela

X **Y30 Falling, jumping or pushed from a high place, undetermined intent**

Victim falling from one level to another, undetermined intent

The appropriate 7th character is to be added to code Y30

A	initial encounter
D	subsequent encounter
S	sequela

X **Y31 Falling, lying or running before or into moving object, undetermined intent**

The appropriate 7th character is to be added to code Y31

A	initial encounter
D	subsequent encounter
S	sequela

X **Y32 Crashing of motor vehicle, undetermined intent**

The appropriate 7th character is to be added to code Y32

A	initial encounter
D	subsequent encounter
S	sequela

X **Y33 Other specified events, undetermined intent**

The appropriate 7th character is to be added to code Y33

A	initial encounter
D	subsequent encounter
S	sequela

LEGAL INTERVENTION, OPERATIONS OF WAR, MILITARY OPERATIONS, AND TERRORISM (Y35-Y38)

● **Y35 Legal intervention**

Includes any injury sustained as a result of an encounter with any law enforcement official, serving in any capacity at the time of the encounter, whether on-duty or off-duty. Includes: injury to law enforcement official, suspect and bystander

The appropriate 7th character is to be added to each code from category Y35

A	initial encounter
D	subsequent encounter
S	sequela

● **Y35.0 Legal intervention involving firearm discharge**

● **Y35.00 Legal intervention involving unspecified firearm discharge**
Legal intervention involving gunshot wound
Legal intervention involving shot NOS

● **Y35.001 Legal intervention involving unspecified firearm discharge, law enforcement official injured**

● **Y35.002 Legal intervention involving unspecified firearm discharge, bystander injured**

● **Y35.003 Legal intervention involving unspecified firearm discharge, suspect injured**

● **Y35.01 Legal intervention involving injury by machine gun**

● **Y35.011 Legal intervention involving injury by machine gun, law enforcement official injured**

● **Y35.012 Legal intervention involving injury by machine gun, bystander injured**

● **Y35.013 Legal intervention involving injury by machine gun, suspect injured**

● **Y35.02 Legal intervention involving injury by handgun**

● **Y35.021 Legal intervention involving injury by handgun, law enforcement official injured**

● **Y35.022 Legal intervention involving injury by handgun, bystander injured**

● **Y35.023 Legal intervention involving injury by handgun, suspect injured**

● **Y35.03 Legal intervention involving injury by rifle pellet**

● **Y35.031 Legal intervention involving injury by rifle pellet, law enforcement official injured**

● **Y35.032 Legal intervention involving injury by rifle pellet, bystander injured**

● **Y35.033 Legal intervention involving injury by rifle pellet, suspect injured**

● **Y35.04 Legal intervention involving injury by rubber bullet**

● **Y35.041 Legal intervention involving injury by rubber bullet, law enforcement official injured**

● **Y35.042 Legal intervention involving injury by rubber bullet, bystander injured**

● **Y35.043 Legal intervention involving injury by rubber bullet, suspect injured**

● **Y35.09 Legal intervention involving other firearm discharge**

● **Y35.091 Legal intervention involving other firearm discharge, law enforcement official injured**

● **Y35.092 Legal intervention involving other firearm discharge, bystander injured**

● **Y35.093 Legal intervention involving other firearm discharge, suspect injured**

● **Y35.1 Legal intervention involving explosives**

● **Y35.10 Legal intervention involving unspecified explosives**

● **Y35.101 Legal intervention involving unspecified explosives, law enforcement official injured**

● **Y35.102 Legal intervention involving unspecified explosives, bystander injured**

● **Y35.103 Legal intervention involving unspecified explosives, suspect injured**

● **Y35.11 Legal intervention involving injury by dynamite**

● **Y35.111 Legal intervention involving injury by dynamite, law enforcement official injured**

● **Y35.112 Legal intervention involving injury by dynamite, bystander injured**

● **Y35.113 Legal intervention involving injury by dynamite, suspect injured**

● **Y35.12 Legal intervention involving injury by explosive shell**

● **Y35.121 Legal intervention involving injury by explosive shell, law enforcement official injured**

● **Y35.122 Legal intervention involving injury by explosive shell, bystander injured**

● **Y35.123 Legal intervention involving injury by explosive shell, suspect injured**

● **Y35.19 Legal intervention involving other explosives**
Legal intervention involving injury by grenade
Legal intervention involving injury by mortar bomb

● **Y35.191 Legal intervention involving other explosives, law enforcement official injured**

● **Y35.192 Legal intervention involving other explosives, bystander injured**

● **Y35.193 Legal intervention involving other explosives, suspect injured**

● **Y35.2 Legal intervention involving gas**
Legal intervention involving asphyxiation by gas
Legal intervention involving poisoning by gas

● **Y35.20 Legal intervention involving unspecified gas**

● **Y35.201 Legal intervention involving unspecified gas, law enforcement official injured**

● **Y35.202 Legal intervention involving unspecified gas, bystander injured**

● **Y35.203 Legal intervention involving unspecified gas, suspect injured**

◀ New ◀ Revised ~~deleted~~ Deleted Excludes 1 Excludes 2 Includes Use additional Code first Code also Unspecified
OGCR Official Guidelines ● Unacceptable Principal Diagnosis X Assign placeholder X ● Use Additional Character(s) ▶ Manifestation Code Coding Clinic

- **Y35.21 Legal intervention involving injury by tear gas**
  - **Y35.211 Legal intervention involving injury by tear gas, law enforcement official injured**
  - **Y35.212 Legal intervention involving injury by tear gas, bystander injured**
  - **Y35.213 Legal intervention involving injury by tear gas, suspect injured**
- **Y35.29 Legal intervention involving other gas**
  - **Y35.291 Legal intervention involving other gas, law enforcement official injured**
  - **Y35.292 Legal intervention involving other gas, bystander injured**
  - **Y35.293 Legal intervention involving other gas, suspect injured**
- **Y35.3 Legal intervention involving blunt objects**
  Legal intervention involving being hit or struck by blunt object
  - **Y35.30 Legal intervention involving unspecified blunt objects**
    - **Y35.301 Legal intervention involving unspecified blunt objects, law enforcement official injured**
    - **Y35.302 Legal intervention involving unspecified blunt objects, bystander injured**
    - **Y35.303 Legal intervention involving unspecified blunt objects, suspect injured**
  - **Y35.31 Legal intervention involving baton**
    - **Y35.311 Legal intervention involving baton, law enforcement official injured**
    - **Y35.312 Legal intervention involving baton, bystander injured**
    - **Y35.313 Legal intervention involving baton, suspect injured**
  - **Y35.39 Legal intervention involving other blunt objects**
    - **Y35.391 Legal intervention involving other blunt objects, law enforcement official injured**
    - **Y35.392 Legal intervention involving other blunt objects, bystander injured**
    - **Y35.393 Legal intervention involving other blunt objects, suspect injured**
- **Y35.4 Legal intervention involving sharp objects**
  Legal intervention involving being cut by sharp objects
  Legal intervention involving being stabbed by sharp objects
  - **Y35.40 Legal intervention involving unspecified sharp objects**
    - **Y35.401 Legal intervention involving unspecified sharp objects, law enforcement official injured**
    - **Y35.402 Legal intervention involving unspecified sharp objects, bystander injured**
    - **Y35.403 Legal intervention involving unspecified sharp objects, suspect injured**
  - **Y35.41 Legal intervention involving bayonet**
    - **Y35.411 Legal intervention involving bayonet, law enforcement official injured**
    - **Y35.412 Legal intervention involving bayonet, bystander injured**
    - **Y35.413 Legal intervention involving bayonet, suspect injured**
  - **Y35.49 Legal intervention involving other sharp objects**
    - **Y35.491 Legal intervention involving other sharp objects, law enforcement official injured**
    - **Y35.492 Legal intervention involving other sharp objects, bystander injured**
    - **Y35.493 Legal intervention involving other sharp objects, suspect injured**
- **Y35.8 Legal intervention involving other specified means**
  - **Y35.81 Legal intervention involving manhandling**
    - **Y35.811 Legal intervention involving manhandling, law enforcement official injured**
    - **Y35.812 Legal intervention involving manhandling, bystander injured**
    - **Y35.813 Legal intervention involving manhandling, suspect injured**
  - **Y35.89 Legal intervention involving other specified means**
    - **Y35.891 Legal intervention involving other specified means, law enforcement official injured**
    - **Y35.892 Legal intervention involving other specified means, bystander injured**
    - **Y35.893 Legal intervention involving other specified means, suspect injured**
- **Y35.9 Legal intervention, means unspecified**
  - X **Y35.91 Legal intervention, means unspecified, law enforcement official injured**
  - X **Y35.92 Legal intervention, means unspecified, bystander injured**
  - X **Y35.93 Legal intervention, means unspecified, suspect injured**

- **Y36 Operations of war**

  Includes injuries to military personnel and civilians caused by war, civil insurrection, and peacekeeping missions

  Excludes1 injury to military personnel occurring during peacetime military operations (Y37.-)
  military vehicles involved in transport accidents with non-military vehicle during peacetime (V09.01, V09.21, V19.81, V29.81, V39.81, V49.81, V59.81, V69.81, V79.81)

  The appropriate 7th character is to be added to each code from category Y36

A	initial encounter
D	subsequent encounter
S	sequela

- **Y36.0 War operations involving explosion of marine weapons**
  Weapons and military watercraft
  - **Y36.00 War operations involving explosion of unspecified marine weapon**
    War operations involving underwater blast NOS
    - **Y36.000 War operations involving explosion of unspecified marine weapon, military personnel**
    - **Y36.001 War operations involving explosion of unspecified marine weapon, civilian**
  - **Y36.01 War operations involving explosion of depth-charge**
    - **Y36.010 War operations involving explosion of depth-charge, military personnel**
    - **Y36.011 War operations involving explosion of depth-charge, civilian**

- **Y36.02 War operations involving explosion of marine mine**
  - War operations involving explosion of marine mine, at sea or in harbor
  - **Y36.020 War operations involving explosion of marine mine, military personnel**
  - **Y36.021 War operations involving explosion of marine mine, civilian**
- **Y36.03 War operations involving explosion of sea-based artillery shell**
  - **Y36.030 War operations involving explosion of sea-based artillery shell, military personnel**
  - **Y36.031 War operations involving explosion of sea-based artillery shell, civilian**
- **Y36.04 War operations involving explosion of torpedo**
  - **Y36.040 War operations involving explosion of torpedo, military personnel**
  - **Y36.041 War operations involving explosion of torpedo, civilian**
- **Y36.05 War operations involving accidental detonation of onboard marine weapons**
  - **Y36.050 War operations involving accidental detonation of onboard marine weapons, military personnel**
  - **Y36.051 War operations involving accidental detonation of onboard marine weapons, civilian**
- **Y36.09 War operations involving explosion of other marine weapons**
  - **Y36.090 War operations involving explosion of other marine weapons, military personnel**
  - **Y36.091 War operations involving explosion of other marine weapons, civilian**
- **Y36.1 War operations involving destruction of aircraft**
  - **Y36.10 War operations involving unspecified destruction of aircraft**
    - **Y36.100 War operations involving unspecified destruction of aircraft, military personnel**
    - **Y36.101 War operations involving unspecified destruction of aircraft, civilian**
  - **Y36.11 War operations involving destruction of aircraft due to enemy fire or explosives**
    - War operations involving destruction of aircraft due to air to air missile
    - War operations involving destruction of aircraft due to explosive placed on aircraft
    - War operations involving destruction of aircraft due to rocket propelled grenade [RPG]
    - War operations involving destruction of aircraft due to small arms fire
    - War operations involving destruction of aircraft due to surface to air missile
    - **Y36.110 War operations involving destruction of aircraft due to enemy fire or explosives, military personnel**
    - **Y36.111 War operations involving destruction of aircraft due to enemy fire or explosives, civilian**
  - **Y36.12 War operations involving destruction of aircraft due to collision with other aircraft**
    - **Y36.120 War operations involving destruction of aircraft due to collision with other aircraft, military personnel**
    - **Y36.121 War operations involving destruction of aircraft due to collision with other aircraft, civilian**
  - **Y36.13 War operations involving destruction of aircraft due to onboard fire**
    - **Y36.130 War operations involving destruction of aircraft due to onboard fire, military personnel**
    - **Y36.131 War operations involving destruction of aircraft due to onboard fire, civilian**
  - **Y36.14 War operations involving destruction of aircraft due to accidental detonation of onboard munitions and explosives**
    - **Y36.140 War operations involving destruction of aircraft due to accidental detonation of onboard munitions and explosives, military personnel**
    - **Y36.141 War operations involving destruction of aircraft due to accidental detonation of onboard munitions and explosives, civilian**
  - **Y36.19 War operations involving other destruction of aircraft**
    - **Y36.190 War operations involving other destruction of aircraft, military personnel**
    - **Y36.191 War operations involving other destruction of aircraft, civilian**
- **Y36.2 War operations involving other explosions and fragments**

  Excludes1 war operations involving explosion of aircraft (Y36.1-)
  war operations involving explosion of marine weapons (Y36.0-)
  war operations involving explosion of nuclear weapons (Y36.5-)
  war operations involving explosion occurring after cessation of hostilities (Y36.8-)
  - **Y36.20 War operations involving unspecified explosion and fragments**
    - War operations involving air blast NOS
    - War operations involving blast NOS
    - War operations involving blast fragments NOS
    - War operations involving blast wave NOS
    - War operations involving blast wind NOS
    - War operations involving explosion NOS
    - War operations involving explosion of bomb NOS
    - **Y36.200 War operations involving unspecified explosion and fragments, military personnel**
    - **Y36.201 War operations involving unspecified explosion and fragments, civilian**
  - **Y36.21 War operations involving explosion of aerial bomb**
    - **Y36.210 War operations involving explosion of aerial bomb, military personnel**
    - **Y36.211 War operations involving explosion of aerial bomb, civilian**
  - **Y36.22 War operations involving explosion of guided missile**
    - **Y36.220 War operations involving explosion of guided missile, military personnel**
    - **Y36.221 War operations involving explosion of guided missile, civilian**

- **Y36.23 War operations involving explosion of improvised explosive device [IED]**
  - War operations involving explosion of person-borne improvised explosive device [IED]
  - War operations involving explosion of vehicle-borne improvised explosive device [IED]
  - War operations involving explosion of roadside improvised explosive device [IED]
  - **Y36.230 War operations involving explosion of improvised explosive device [IED], military personnel**
  - **Y36.231 War operations involving explosion of improvised explosive device [IED], civilian**
- **Y36.24 War operations involving explosion due to accidental detonation and discharge of own munitions or munitions launch device**
  - **Y36.240 War operations involving explosion due to accidental detonation and discharge of own munitions or munitions launch device, military personnel**
  - **Y36.241 War operations involving explosion due to accidental detonation and discharge of own munitions or munitions launch device, civilian**
- **Y36.25 War operations involving fragments from munitions**
  - **Y36.250 War operations involving fragments from munitions, military personnel**
  - **Y36.251 War operations involving fragments from munitions, civilian**
- **Y36.26 War operations involving fragments of improvised explosive device [IED]**
  - War operations involving fragments of person-borne improvised explosive device [IED]
  - War operations involving fragments of vehicle-borne improvised explosive device [IED]
  - War operations involving fragments of roadside improvised explosive device [IED]
  - **Y36.260 War operations involving fragments of improvised explosive device [IED], military personnel**
  - **Y36.261 War operations involving fragments of improvised explosive device [IED], civilian**
- **Y36.27 War operations involving fragments from weapons**
  - **Y36.270 War operations involving fragments from weapons, military personnel**
  - **Y36.271 War operations involving fragments from weapons, civilian**
- **Y36.29 War operations involving other explosions and fragments**
  - War operations involving explosion of grenade
  - War operations involving explosions of land mine
  - War operations involving shrapnel NOS
  - **Y36.290 War operations involving other explosions and fragments, military personnel**
  - **Y36.291 War operations involving other explosions and fragments, civilian**
- **Y36.3 War operations involving fires, conflagrations and hot substances**
  - War operations involving smoke, fumes, and heat from fires, conflagrations and hot substances

  Excludes1 war operations involving fires and conflagrations aboard military aircraft (Y36.1-)
  war operations involving fires and conflagrations aboard military watercraft (Y36.0-)
  war operations involving fires and conflagrations caused indirectly by conventional weapons (Y36.2-)
  war operations involving fires and thermal effects of nuclear weapons (Y36.53-)
  - **Y36.30 War operations involving unspecified fire, conflagration and hot substance**
    - **Y36.300 War operations involving unspecified fire, conflagration and hot substance, military personnel**
    - **Y36.301 War operations involving unspecified fire, conflagration and hot substance, civilian**
  - **Y36.31 War operations involving gasoline bomb**
    - War operations involving incendiary bomb
    - War operations involving petrol bomb
    - **Y36.310 War operations involving gasoline bomb, military personnel**
    - **Y36.311 War operations involving gasoline bomb, civilian**
  - **Y36.32 War operations involving incendiary bullet**
    - **Y36.320 War operations involving incendiary bullet, military personnel**
    - **Y36.321 War operations involving incendiary bullet, civilian**
  - **Y36.33 War operations involving flamethrower**
    - **Y36.330 War operations involving flamethrower, military personnel**
    - **Y36.331 War operations involving flamethrower, civilian**
  - **Y36.39 War operations involving other fires, conflagrations and hot substances**
    - **Y36.390 War operations involving other fires, conflagrations and hot substances, military personnel**
    - **Y36.391 War operations involving other fires, conflagrations and hot substances, civilian**
- **Y36.4 War operations involving firearm discharge and other forms of conventional warfare**
  - **Y36.41 War operations involving rubber bullets**
    - **Y36.410 War operations involving rubber bullets, military personnel**
    - **Y36.411 War operations involving rubber bullets, civilian**
  - **Y36.42 War operations involving firearms pellets**
    - **Y36.420 War operations involving firearms pellets, military personnel**
    - **Y36.421 War operations involving firearms pellets, civilian**

Y36.43 War operations involving other firearms discharge
War operations involving bullets NOS
Excludes1 war operations involving munitions fragments (Y36.25-)
war operations involving incendiary bullets (Y36.32-)
Y36.430 War operations involving other firearms discharge, military personnel
Y36.431 War operations involving other firearms discharge, civilian

Y36.44 War operations involving unarmed hand to hand combat
Excludes1 war operations involving combat using blunt or piercing object (Y36.45-)
war operations involving intentional restriction of air and airway (Y36.46-)
war operations involving unintentional restriction of air and airway (Y36.47-)
Y36.440 War operations involving unarmed hand to hand combat, military personnel
Y36.441 War operations involving unarmed hand to hand combat, civilian

Y36.45 War operations involving combat using blunt or piercing object
Y36.450 War operations involving combat using blunt or piercing object, military personnel
Y36.451 War operations involving combat using blunt or piercing object, civilian

Y36.46 War operations involving intentional restriction of air and airway
Y36.460 War operations involving intentional restriction of air and airway, military personnel
Y36.461 War operations involving intentional restriction of air and airway, civilian

Y36.47 War operations involving unintentional restriction of air and airway
Y36.470 War operations involving unintentional restriction of air and airway, military personnel
Y36.471 War operations involving unintentional restriction of air and airway, civilian

Y36.49 War operations involving other forms of conventional warfare
Y36.490 War operations involving other forms of conventional warfare, military personnel
Y36.491 War operations involving other forms of conventional warfare, civilian

Y36.5 War operations involving nuclear weapons
War operations involving dirty bomb NOS
Y36.50 War operations involving unspecified effect of nuclear weapon
Y36.500 War operations involving unspecified effect of nuclear weapon, military personnel
Y36.501 War operations involving unspecified effect of nuclear weapon, civilian

Y36.51 War operations involving direct blast effect of nuclear weapon
War operations involving blast pressure of nuclear weapon
Y36.510 War operations involving direct blast effect of nuclear weapon, military personnel
Y36.511 War operations involving direct blast effect of nuclear weapon, civilian

Y36.52 War operations involving indirect blast effect of nuclear weapon
War operations involving being thrown by blast of nuclear weapon
War operations involving being struck or crushed by blast debris of nuclear weapon
Y36.520 War operations involving indirect blast effect of nuclear weapon, military personnel
Y36.521 War operations involving indirect blast effect of nuclear weapon, civilian

Y36.53 War operations involving thermal radiation effect of nuclear weapon
War operations involving direct heat from nuclear weapon
War operation involving fireball effects from nuclear weapon
Y36.530 War operations involving thermal radiation effect of nuclear weapon, military personnel
Y36.531 War operations involving thermal radiation effect of nuclear weapon, civilian

Y36.54 War operation involving nuclear radiation effects of nuclear weapon
War operation involving acute radiation exposure from nuclear weapon
War operation involving exposure to immediate ionizing radiation from nuclear weapon
War operation involving fallout exposure from nuclear weapon
War operation involving secondary effects of nuclear weapons
Y36.540 War operation involving nuclear radiation effects of nuclear weapon, military personnel
Y36.541 War operation involving nuclear radiation effects of nuclear weapon, civilian

Y36.59 War operation involving other effects of nuclear weapons
Y36.590 War operation involving other effects of nuclear weapons, military personnel
Y36.591 War operation involving other effects of nuclear weapons, civilian

Y36.6 War operations involving biological weapons
Y36.6X War operations involving biological weapons
Y36.6X0 War operations involving biological weapons, military personnel
Y36.6X1 War operations involving biological weapons, civilian

- **Y36.7 War operations involving chemical weapons and other forms of unconventional warfare**

  Excludes1 war operations involving incendiary devices (Y36.3-, Y36.5-)

  - **Y36.7X War operations involving chemical weapons and other forms of unconventional warfare**
    - **Y36.7X0 War operations involving chemical weapons and other forms of unconventional warfare, military personnel**
    - **Y36.7X1 War operations involving chemical weapons and other forms of unconventional warfare, civilian**
- **Y36.8 War operations occurring after cessation of hostilities**

  War operations classifiable to categories Y36.0-Y36.8 but occurring after cessation of hostilities

  - **Y36.81 Explosion of mine placed during war operations but exploding after cessation of hostilities**
    - **Y36.810 Explosion of mine placed during war operations but exploding after cessation of hostilities, military personnel**
    - **Y36.811 Explosion of mine placed during war operations but exploding after cessation of hostilities, civilian**
  - **Y36.82 Explosion of bomb placed during war operations but exploding after cessation of hostilities**
    - **Y36.820 Explosion of bomb placed during war operations but exploding after cessation of hostilities, military personnel**
    - **Y36.821 Explosion of bomb placed during war operations but exploding after cessation of hostilities, civilian**
  - **Y36.88 Other war operations occurring after cessation of hostilities**
    - **Y36.880 Other war operations occurring after cessation of hostilities, military personnel**
    - **Y36.881 Other war operations occurring after cessation of hostilities, civilian**
  - **Y36.89 Unspecified war operations occurring after cessation of hostilities**
    - **Y36.890 Unspecified war operations occurring after cessation of hostilities, military personnel**
    - **Y36.891 Unspecified war operations occurring after cessation of hostilities, civilian**
- **Y36.9 Other and unspecified war operations**
  - X **Y36.90 War operations, unspecified**
  - X **Y36.91 War operations involving unspecified weapon of mass destruction [WMD]**
  - X **Y36.92 War operations involving friendly fire**

- **Y37 Military operations**

  Includes Injuries to military personnel and civilians occurring during peacetime on military property and during routine military exercises and operations

  Excludes1 military aircraft involved in aircraft accident with civilian aircraft (V97.81-)
  military vehicles involved in transport accident with civilian vehicle (V09.01, V09.21, V19.81, V29.81, V39.81, V49.81, V59.81, V69.81, V79.81)
  military watercraft involved in water transport accident with civilian watercraft (V94.81-)
  war operations (Y36.-)

  The appropriate 7th character is to be added to each code from category Y37

A	initial encounter
D	subsequent encounter
S	sequela

  - **Y37.0 Military operations involving explosion of marine weapons**
    - **Y37.00 Military operations involving explosion of unspecified marine weapon**

      Military operations involving underwater blast NOS
      - **Y37.000 Military operations involving explosion of unspecified marine weapon, military personnel**
      - **Y37.001 Military operations involving explosion of unspecified marine weapon, civilian**
    - **Y37.01 Military operations involving explosion of depth-charge**
      - **Y37.010 Military operations involving explosion of depth-charge, military personnel**
      - **Y37.011 Military operations involving explosion of depth-charge, civilian**
    - **Y37.02 Military operations involving explosion of marine mine**

      Military operations involving explosion of marine mine, at sea or in harbor
      - **Y37.020 Military operations involving explosion of marine mine, military personnel**
      - **Y37.021 Military operations involving explosion of marine mine, civilian**
    - **Y37.03 Military operations involving explosion of sea-based artillery shell**
      - **Y37.030 Military operations involving explosion of sea-based artillery shell, military personnel**
      - **Y37.031 Military operations involving explosion of sea-based artillery shell, civilian**
    - **Y37.04 Military operations involving explosion of torpedo**
      - **Y37.040 Military operations involving explosion of torpedo, military personnel**
      - **Y37.041 Military operations involving explosion of torpedo, civilian**
    - **Y37.05 Military operations involving accidental detonation of onboard marine weapons**
      - **Y37.050 Military operations involving accidental detonation of onboard marine weapons, military personnel**
      - **Y37.051 Military operations involving accidental detonation of onboard marine weapons, civilian**

- **Y37.09 Military operations involving explosion of other marine weapons**
  - **Y37.090 Military operations involving explosion of other marine weapons, military personnel**
  - **Y37.091 Military operations involving explosion of other marine weapons, civilian**
- **Y37.1 Military operations involving destruction of aircraft**
  - **Y37.10 Military operations involving unspecified destruction of aircraft**
    - **Y37.100 Military operations involving unspecified destruction of aircraft, military personnel**
    - **Y37.101 Military operations involving unspecified destruction of aircraft, civilian**
  - **Y37.11 Military operations involving destruction of aircraft due to enemy fire or explosives**
    - Military operations involving destruction of aircraft due to air to air missile
    - Military operations involving destruction of aircraft due to explosive placed on aircraft
    - Military operations involving destruction of aircraft due to rocket propelled grenade [RPG]
    - Military operations involving destruction of aircraft due to small arms fire
    - Military operations involving destruction of aircraft due to surface to air missile
    - **Y37.110 Military operations involving destruction of aircraft due to enemy fire or explosives, military personnel**
    - **Y37.111 Military operations involving destruction of aircraft due to enemy fire or explosives, civilian**
  - **Y37.12 Military operations involving destruction of aircraft due to collision with other aircraft**
    - **Y37.120 Military operations involving destruction of aircraft due to collision with other aircraft, military personnel**
    - **Y37.121 Military operations involving destruction of aircraft due to collision with other aircraft, civilian**
  - **Y37.13 Military operations involving destruction of aircraft due to onboard fire**
    - **Y37.130 Military operations involving destruction of aircraft due to onboard fire, military personnel**
    - **Y37.131 Military operations involving destruction of aircraft due to onboard fire, civilian**
  - **Y37.14 Military operations involving destruction of aircraft due to accidental detonation of onboard munitions and explosives**
    - **Y37.140 Military operations involving destruction of aircraft due to accidental detonation of onboard munitions and explosives, military personnel**
    - **Y37.141 Military operations involving destruction of aircraft due to accidental detonation of onboard munitions and explosives, civilian**
  - **Y37.19 Military operations involving other destruction of aircraft**
    - **Y37.190 Military operations involving other destruction of aircraft, military personnel**
    - **Y37.191 Military operations involving other destruction of aircraft, civilian**
- **Y37.2 Military operations involving other explosions and fragments**

  Excludes1 military operations involving explosion of aircraft (Y37.1-)
  military operations involving explosion of marine weapons (Y37.0-)
  military operations involving explosion of nuclear weapons (Y37.5-)
  - **Y37.20 Military operations involving unspecified explosion and fragments**
    - Military operations involving air blast NOS
    - Military operations involving blast NOS
    - Military operations involving blast fragments NOS
    - Military operations involving blast wave NOS
    - Military operations involving blast wind NOS
    - Military operations involving explosion NOS
    - Military operations involving explosion of bomb NOS
    - **Y37.200 Military operations involving unspecified explosion and fragments, military personnel**
    - **Y37.201 Military operations involving unspecified explosion and fragments, civilian**
  - **Y37.21 Military operations involving explosion of aerial bomb**
    - **Y37.210 Military operations involving explosion of aerial bomb, military personnel**
    - **Y37.211 Military operations involving explosion of aerial bomb, civilian**
  - **Y37.22 Military operations involving explosion of guided missile**
    - **Y37.220 Military operations involving explosion of guided missile, military personnel**
    - **Y37.221 Military operations involving explosion of guided missile, civilian**
  - **Y37.23 Military operations involving explosion of improvised explosive device [IED]**
    - Military operations involving explosion of person-borne improvised explosive device [IED]
    - Military operations involving explosion of vehicle-borne improvised explosive device [IED]
    - Military operations involving explosion of roadside improvised explosive device [IED]
    - **Y37.230 Military operations involving explosion of improvised explosive device [IED], military personnel**
    - **Y37.231 Military operations involving explosion of improvised explosive device [IED], civilian**
  - **Y37.24 Military operations involving explosion due to accidental detonation and discharge of own munitions or munitions launch device**
    - **Y37.240 Military operations involving explosion due to accidental detonation and discharge of own munitions or munitions launch device, military personnel**
    - **Y37.241 Military operations involving explosion due to accidental detonation and discharge of own munitions or munitions launch device, civilian**

◀ New ⇐ Revised ~~deleted~~ Deleted Excludes 1 Excludes 2 Includes Use additional Code first Code also Unspecified
OGCR Official Guidelines ● Unacceptable Principal Diagnosis X Assign placeholder X ● Use Additional Character(s) ▶ Manifestation Code Coding Clinic

- **Y37.25 Military operations involving fragments from munitions**
  - **Y37.250 Military operations involving fragments from munitions, military personnel**
  - **Y37.251 Military operations involving fragments from munitions, civilian**
- **Y37.26 Military operations involving fragments of improvised explosive device [IED]**
  - Military operations involving fragments of person-borne improvised explosive device [IED]
  - Military operations involving fragments of vehicle-borne improvised explosive device [IED]
  - Military operations involving fragments of roadside improvised explosive device [IED]
  - **Y37.260 Military operations involving fragments of improvised explosive device [IED], military personnel**
  - **Y37.261 Military operations involving fragments of improvised explosive device [IED], civilian**
- **Y37.27 Military operations involving fragments from weapons**
  - **Y37.270 Military operations involving fragments from weapons, military personnel**
  - **Y37.271 Military operations involving fragments from weapons, civilian**
- **Y37.29 Military operations involving other explosions and fragments**
  - Military operations involving explosion of grenade
  - Military operations involving explosions of land mine
  - Military operations involving shrapnel NOS
  - **Y37.290 Military operations involving other explosions and fragments, military personnel**
  - **Y37.291 Military operations involving other explosions and fragments, civilian**
- **Y37.3 Military operations involving fires, conflagrations and hot substances**
  - Military operations involving smoke, fumes, and heat from fires, conflagrations and hot substances
  - **Excludes1** military operations involving fires and conflagrations aboard military aircraft (Y37.1-)
    - military operations involving fires and conflagrations aboard military watercraft (Y37.0-)
    - military operations involving fires and conflagrations caused indirectly by conventional weapons (Y37.2-)
    - military operations involving fires and thermal effects of nuclear weapons (Y36.53-)
  - **Y37.30 Military operations involving unspecified fire, conflagration and hot substance**
    - **Y37.300 Military operations involving unspecified fire, conflagration and hot substance, military personnel**
    - **Y37.301 Military operations involving unspecified fire, conflagration and hot substance, civilian**
  - **Y37.31 Military operations involving gasoline bomb**
    - Military operations involving incendiary bomb
    - Military operations involving petrol bomb
    - **Y37.310 Military operations involving gasoline bomb, military personnel**
    - **Y37.311 Military operations involving gasoline bomb, civilian**
  - **Y37.32 Military operations involving incendiary bullet**
    - **Y37.320 Military operations involving incendiary bullet, military personnel**
    - **Y37.321 Military operations involving incendiary bullet, civilian**
  - **Y37.33 Military operations involving flamethrower**
    - **Y37.330 Military operations involving flamethrower, military personnel**
    - **Y37.331 Military operations involving flamethrower, civilian**
  - **Y37.39 Military operations involving other fires, conflagrations and hot substances**
    - **Y37.390 Military operations involving other fires, conflagrations and hot substances, military personnel**
    - **Y37.391 Military operations involving other fires, conflagrations and hot substances, civilian**
- **Y37.4 Military operations involving firearm discharge and other forms of conventional warfare**
  - **Y37.41 Military operations involving rubber bullets**
    - **Y37.410 Military operations involving rubber bullets, military personnel**
    - **Y37.411 Military operations involving rubber bullets, civilian**
  - **Y37.42 Military operations involving firearms pellets**
    - **Y37.420 Military operations involving firearms pellets, military personnel**
    - **Y37.421 Military operations involving firearms pellets, civilian**
  - **Y37.43 Military operations involving other firearms discharge**
    - Military operations involving bullets NOS
    - **Excludes1** military operations involving munitions fragments (Y37.25-)
      - military operations involving incendiary bullets (Y37.32-)
    - **Y37.430 Military operations involving other firearms discharge, military personnel**
    - **Y37.431 Military operations involving other firearms discharge, civilian**
  - **Y37.44 Military operations involving unarmed hand to hand combat**
    - **Excludes1** military operations involving combat using blunt or piercing object (Y37.45-)
      - military operations involving intentional restriction of air and airway (Y37.46-)
      - military operations involving unintentional restriction of air and airway (Y37.47-)
    - **Y37.440 Military operations involving unarmed hand to hand combat, military personnel**
    - **Y37.441 Military operations involving unarmed hand to hand combat, civilian**
  - **Y37.45 Military operations involving combat using blunt or piercing object**
    - **Y37.450 Military operations involving combat using blunt or piercing object, military personnel**
    - **Y37.451 Military operations involving combat using blunt or piercing object, civilian**

- **Y37.46 Military operations involving intentional restriction of air and airway**
  - **Y37.460 Military operations involving intentional restriction of air and airway, military personnel**
  - **Y37.461 Military operations involving intentional restriction of air and airway, civilian**
- **Y37.47 Military operations involving unintentional restriction of air and airway**
  - **Y37.470 Military operations involving unintentional restriction of air and airway, military personnel**
  - **Y37.471 Military operations involving unintentional restriction of air and airway, civilian**
- **Y37.49 Military operations involving other forms of conventional warfare**
  - **Y37.490 Military operations involving other forms of conventional warfare, military personnel**
  - **Y37.491 Military operations involving other forms of conventional warfare, civilian**
- **Y37.5 Military operations involving nuclear weapons**
  Military operation involving dirty bomb NOS
  - **Y37.50 Military operations involving unspecified effect of nuclear weapon**
    - **Y37.500 Military operations involving unspecified effect of nuclear weapon, military personnel**
    - **Y37.501 Military operations involving unspecified effect of nuclear weapon, civilian**
  - **Y37.51 Military operations involving direct blast effect of nuclear weapon**
    Military operations involving blast pressure of nuclear weapon
    - **Y37.510 Military operations involving direct blast effect of nuclear weapon, military personnel**
    - **Y37.511 Military operations involving direct blast effect of nuclear weapon, civilian**
  - **Y37.52 Military operations involving indirect blast effect of nuclear weapon**
    Military operations involving being thrown by blast of nuclear weapon
    Military operations involving being struck or crushed by blast debris of nuclear weapon
    - **Y37.520 Military operations involving indirect blast effect of nuclear weapon, military personnel**
    - **Y37.521 Military operations involving indirect blast effect of nuclear weapon, civilian**
  - **Y37.53 Military operations involving thermal radiation effect of nuclear weapon**
    Military operations involving direct heat from nuclear weapon
    Military operation involving fireball effects from nuclear weapon
    - **Y37.530 Military operations involving thermal radiation effect of nuclear weapon, military personnel**
    - **Y37.531 Military operations involving thermal radiation effect of nuclear weapon, civilian**
  - **Y37.54 Military operation involving nuclear radiation effects of nuclear weapon**
    Military operation involving acute radiation exposure from nuclear weapon
    Military operation involving exposure to immediate ionizing radiation from nuclear weapon
    Military operation involving fallout exposure from nuclear weapon
    Military operation involving secondary effects of nuclear weapons
    - **Y37.540 Military operation involving nuclear radiation effects of nuclear weapon, military personnel**
    - **Y37.541 Military operation involving nuclear radiation effects of nuclear weapon, civilian**
  - **Y37.59 Military operation involving other effects of nuclear weapons**
    - **Y37.590 Military operation involving other effects of nuclear weapons, military personnel**
    - **Y37.591 Military operation involving other effects of nuclear weapons, civilian**
- **Y37.6 Military operations involving biological weapons**
  - **Y37.6X Military operations involving biological weapons**
    - **Y37.6X0 Military operations involving biological weapons, military personnel**
    - **Y37.6X1 Military operations involving biological weapons, civilian**
- **Y37.7 Military operations involving chemical weapons and other forms of unconventional warfare**
  Excludes1 military operations involving incendiary devices (Y36.3-, Y36.5-)
  - **Y37.7X Military operations involving chemical weapons and other forms of unconventional warfare**
    - **Y37.7X0 Military operations involving chemical weapons and other forms of unconventional warfare, military personnel**
    - **Y37.7X1 Military operations involving chemical weapons and other forms of unconventional warfare, civilian**
- **Y37.9 Other and unspecified military operations**
  - X **Y37.90 Military operations, unspecified**
  - X **Y37.91 Military operations involving unspecified weapon of mass destruction [WMD]**
  - X **Y37.92 Military operations involving friendly fire**

Y38 Terrorism

These codes are for use to identify injuries resulting from the unlawful use of force or violence against persons or property to intimidate or coerce a government, the civilian population, or any segment thereof, in furtherance of political or social objective

Use additional code for place of occurrence (Y92.-)

The appropriate 7th character is to be added to each code from category Y38

A	initial encounter
D	subsequent encounter
S	sequela

Y38.0 Terrorism involving explosion of marine weapons
- Terrorism involving depth-charge
- Terrorism involving marine mine
- Terrorism involving mine NOS, at sea or in harbor
- Terrorism involving sea-based artillery shell
- Terrorism involving torpedo
- Terrorism involving underwater blast

Y38.0X Terrorism involving explosion of marine weapons

Y38.0X1 Terrorism involving explosion of marine weapons, public safety official injured

Y38.0X2 Terrorism involving explosion of marine weapons, civilian injured

Y38.0X3 Terrorism involving explosion of marine weapons, terrorist injured

Y38.1 Terrorism involving destruction of aircraft
- Terrorism involving aircraft burned
- Terrorism involving aircraft exploded
- Terrorism involving aircraft being shot down
- Terrorism involving aircraft used as a weapon

Y38.1X Terrorism involving destruction of aircraft

Y38.1X1 Terrorism involving destruction of aircraft, public safety official injured

Y38.1X2 Terrorism involving destruction of aircraft, civilian injured

Y38.1X3 Terrorism involving destruction of aircraft, terrorist injured

Y38.2 Terrorism involving other explosions and fragments
- Terrorism involving antipersonnel (fragments) bomb
- Terrorism involving blast NOS
- Terrorism involving explosion NOS
- Terrorism involving explosion of breech block
- Terrorism involving explosion of cannon block
- Terrorism involving explosion (fragments) of artillery shell
- Terrorism involving explosion (fragments) of bomb
- Terrorism involving explosion (fragments) of grenade
- Terrorism involving explosion (fragments) of guided missile
- Terrorism involving explosion (fragments) of land mine
- Terrorism involving explosion of mortar bomb
- Terrorism involving explosion of munitions
- Terrorism involving explosion (fragments) of rocket
- Terrorism involving explosion (fragments) of shell
- Terrorism involving shrapnel
- Terrorism involving mine NOS, on land

Excludes1 terrorism involving explosion of nuclear weapon (Y38.5)
terrorism involving suicide bomber (Y38.81)

Y38.2X Terrorism involving other explosions and fragments

Y38.2X1 Terrorism involving other explosions and fragments, public safety official injured

Y38.2X2 Terrorism involving other explosions and fragments, civilian injured

Y38.2X3 Terrorism involving other explosions and fragments, terrorist injured

Y38.3 Terrorism involving fires, conflagration and hot substances
- Terrorism involving conflagration NOS
- Terrorism involving fire NOS
- Terrorism involving petrol bomb

Excludes1 terrorism involving fire or heat of nuclear weapon (Y38.5)

Y38.3X Terrorism involving fires, conflagration and hot substances

Y38.3X1 Terrorism involving fires, conflagration and hot substances, public safety official injured

Y38.3X2 Terrorism involving fires, conflagration and hot substances, civilian injured

Y38.3X3 Terrorism involving fires, conflagration and hot substances, terrorist injured

Y38.4 Terrorism involving firearms
- Terrorism involving carbine bullet
- Terrorism involving machine gun bullet
- Terrorism involving pellets (shotgun)
- Terrorism involving pistol bullet
- Terrorism involving rifle bullet
- Terrorism involving rubber (rifle) bullet

Y38.4X Terrorism involving firearms

Y38.4X1 Terrorism involving firearms, public safety official injured

Y38.4X2 Terrorism involving firearms, civilian injured

Y38.4X3 Terrorism involving firearms, terrorist injured

Y38.5 Terrorism involving nuclear weapons
- Terrorism involving blast effects of nuclear weapon
- Terrorism involving exposure to ionizing radiation from nuclear weapon
- Terrorism involving fireball effect of nuclear weapon
- Terrorism involving heat from nuclear weapon

Y38.5X Terrorism involving nuclear weapons

Y38.5X1 Terrorism involving nuclear weapons, public safety official injured

Y38.5X2 Terrorism involving nuclear weapons, civilian injured

Y38.5X3 Terrorism involving nuclear weapons, terrorist injured

Y38.6 Terrorism involving biological weapons
- Terrorism involving anthrax
- Terrorism involving cholera
  - *A serious, often deadly, infectious disease of small intestine*
- Terrorism involving smallpox

Y38.6X Terrorism involving biological weapons

Y38.6X1 Terrorism involving biological weapons, public safety official injured

Y38.6X2 Terrorism involving biological weapons, civilian injured

Y38.6X3 Terrorism involving biological weapons, terrorist injured

Y38.7 Terrorism involving chemical weapons
- Terrorism involving gases, fumes, chemicals
- Terrorism involving hydrogen cyanide
- Terrorism involving phosgene
- Terrorism involving sarin

Y38.7X Terrorism involving chemical weapons

Y38.7X1 Terrorism involving chemical weapons, public safety official injured

Y38.7X2 Terrorism involving chemical weapons, civilian injured

Y38.7X3 Terrorism involving chemical weapons, terrorist injured

● **Y38.8 Terrorism involving other and unspecified means**

● **Y38.80 Terrorism involving unspecified means**
Terrorism NOS

● **Y38.81 Terrorism involving suicide bomber**

● **Y38.811 Terrorism involving suicide bomber, public safety official injured**

● **Y38.812 Terrorism involving suicide bomber, civilian injured**

● **Y38.89 Terrorism involving other means**
Terrorism involving drowning and submersion
Terrorism involving lasers
Terrorism involving piercing or stabbing instruments

● **Y38.891 Terrorism involving other means, public safety official injured**

● **Y38.892 Terrorism involving other means, civilian injured**

● **Y38.893 Terrorism involving other means, terrorist injured**

● **Y38.9 Terrorism, secondary effects**
Note: This code is for use to identify conditions occurring subsequent to a terrorist attack not those that are due to the initial terrorist attack.

● **Y38.9X Terrorism, secondary effects**

● **Y38.9X1 Terrorism, secondary effects, public safety official injured**

● **Y38.9X2 Terrorism, secondary effects, civilian injured categories**

COMPLICATIONS OF MEDICAL AND SURGICAL CARE (Y62-Y84)

Includes complications of medical devices surgical and medical procedures as the cause of abnormal reaction of the patient, or of later complication, without mention of misadventure at the time of the procedure

MISADVENTURES TO PATIENTS DURING SURGICAL AND MEDICAL CARE (Y62-Y69)

Excludes1 surgical and medical procedures as the cause of abnormal reaction of the patient, without mention of misadventure at the time of the procedure (Y83-Y84) ◀

Excludes2 breakdown or malfunctioning of medical device (during procedure) (after implantation) (ongoing use) (Y70-Y82)

● **Y62 Failure of sterile precautions during surgical and medical care**

Y62.0 Failure of sterile precautions during surgical operation

Y62.1 Failure of sterile precautions during infusion or transfusion

Y62.2 Failure of sterile precautions during kidney dialysis and other perfusion

Y62.3 Failure of sterile precautions during injection or immunization

Y62.4 Failure of sterile precautions during endoscopic examination

Y62.5 Failure of sterile precautions during heart catheterization

Y62.6 Failure of sterile precautions during aspiration, puncture and other catheterization

Y62.8 Failure of sterile precautions during other surgical and medical care

Y62.9 Failure of sterile precautions during unspecified surgical and medical care

● **Y63 Failure in dosage during surgical and medical care**

Excludes2 accidental overdose of drug or wrong drug given in error (T36-T50)

Y63.0 Excessive amount of blood or other fluid given during transfusion or infusion

Y63.1 Incorrect dilution of fluid used during infusion

Y63.2 Overdose of radiation given during therapy

Y63.3 Inadvertent exposure of patient to radiation during medical care

Y63.4 Failure in dosage in electroshock or insulin-shock therapy

Y63.5 Inappropriate temperature in local application and packing

Y63.6 Underdosing and nonadministration of necessary drug, medicament or biological substance

Y63.8 Failure in dosage during other surgical and medical care

Y63.9 Failure in dosage during unspecified surgical and medical care

● **Y64 Contaminated medical or biological substances**

Y64.0 Contaminated medical or biological substance, transfused or infused

Y64.1 Contaminated medical or biological substance, injected or used for immunization

Y64.8 Contaminated medical or biological substance administered by other means

Y64.9 Contaminated medical or biological substance administered by unspecified means
Administered contaminated medical or biological substance NOS

● **Y65 Other misadventures during surgical and medical care**

Y65.0 Mismatched blood in transfusion

Y65.1 Wrong fluid used in infusion

Y65.2 Failure in suture or ligature during surgical operation

Y65.3 Endotracheal tube wrongly placed during anesthetic procedure

Y65.4 Failure to introduce or to remove other tube or instrument

● **Y65.5 Performance of wrong procedure (operation)**

● **Y65.51 Performance of wrong procedure (operation) on correct patient**
Wrong device implanted into correct surgical site

Excludes1 performance of correct procedure (operation) on wrong side or body part (Y65.53)

MCE: Wrong procedure performed

● **Y65.52 Performance of procedure (operation) on patient not scheduled for surgery**
Performance of procedure (operation) intended for another patient
Performance of procedure (operation) on wrong patient
MCE: Wrong procedure performed

● **Y65.53 Performance of correct procedure (operation) on wrong side or body part**
Performance of correct procedure (operation) on wrong side
Performance of correct procedure (operation) on wrong site
MCE: Wrong procedure performed

Y65.8 Other specified misadventures during surgical and medical care

Y66 Nonadministration of surgical and medical care
Premature cessation of surgical and medical care

Excludes1 DNR status (Z66)
palliative care (Z51.5)

Y69 Unspecified misadventure during surgical and medical care

MEDICAL DEVICES ASSOCIATED WITH ADVERSE INCIDENTS IN DIAGNOSTIC AND THERAPEUTIC USE (Y70-Y82)

Includes breakdown or malfunction of medical devices (during use) (after implantation) (ongoing use)

Excludes2 breakdown or malfunctioning of medical device (after implantation) (during procedure) (ongoing use) (Y70-Y82) ◀
later complications following use of medical devices without breakdown or malfunctioning of device (Y83-Y84) ◀
misadventure to patients during surgical and medical care, classifiable to (Y62-Y69) ◀
surgical and other medical procedures as the cause of abnormal reaction of the patient, or of later complication, without mention of misadventure at the time of the procedure (Y83-Y84) ◀

● **Y70 Anesthesiology devices associated with adverse incidents**
- **Y70.0 Diagnostic and monitoring anesthesiology devices associated with adverse incidents**
- **Y70.1 Therapeutic (nonsurgical) and rehabilitative anesthesiology devices associated with adverse incidents**
- **Y70.2 Prosthetic and other implants, materials and accessory anesthesiology devices associated with adverse incidents**
- **Y70.3 Surgical instruments, materials and anesthesiology devices (including sutures) associated with adverse incidents**
- **Y70.8 Miscellaneous anesthesiology devices associated with adverse incidents, not elsewhere classified**

● **Y71 Cardiovascular devices associated with adverse incidents**
- **Y71.0 Diagnostic and monitoring cardiovascular devices associated with adverse incidents**
- **Y71.1 Therapeutic (nonsurgical) and rehabilitative cardiovascular devices associated with adverse incidents**
- **Y71.2 Prosthetic and other implants, materials and accessory cardiovascular devices associated with adverse incidents**
- **Y71.3 Surgical instruments, materials and cardiovascular devices (including sutures) associated with adverse incidents**
- **Y71.8 Miscellaneous cardiovascular devices associated with adverse incidents, not elsewhere classified**

● **Y72 Otorhinolaryngological devices associated with adverse incidents**
- **Y72.0 Diagnostic and monitoring otorhinolaryngological devices associated with adverse incidents**
- **Y72.1 Therapeutic (nonsurgical) and rehabilitative otorhinolaryngological devices associated with adverse incidents**
- **Y72.2 Prosthetic and other implants, materials and accessory otorhinolaryngological devices associated with adverse incidents**
- **Y72.3 Surgical instruments, materials and otorhinolaryngological devices (including sutures) associated with adverse incidents**
- **Y72.8 Miscellaneous otorhinolaryngological devices associated with adverse incidents, not elsewhere classified**

● **Y73 Gastroenterology and urology devices associated with adverse incidents**
- **Y73.0 Diagnostic and monitoring gastroenterology and urology devices associated with adverse incidents**
- **Y73.1 Therapeutic (nonsurgical) and rehabilitative gastroenterology and urology devices associated with adverse incidents**
- **Y73.2 Prosthetic and other implants, materials and accessory gastroenterology and urology devices associated with adverse incidents**
- **Y73.3 Surgical instruments, materials and gastroenterology and urology devices (including sutures) associated with adverse incidents**
- **Y73.8 Miscellaneous gastroenterology and urology devices associated with adverse incidents, not elsewhere classified**

● **Y74 General hospital and personal-use devices associated with adverse incidents**
- **Y74.0 Diagnostic and monitoring general hospital and personal-use devices associated with adverse incidents**
- **Y74.1 Therapeutic (nonsurgical) and rehabilitative general hospital and personal-use devices associated with adverse incidents**
- **Y74.2 Prosthetic and other implants, materials and accessory general hospital and personal-use devices associated with adverse incidents**
- **Y74.3 Surgical instruments, materials and general hospital and personal-use devices (including sutures) associated with adverse incidents**
- **Y74.8 Miscellaneous general hospital and personal-use devices associated with adverse incidents, not elsewhere classified**

● **Y75 Neurological devices associated with adverse incidents**
- **Y75.0 Diagnostic and monitoring neurological devices associated with adverse incidents**
- **Y75.1 Therapeutic (nonsurgical) and rehabilitative neurological devices associated with adverse incidents**
- **Y75.2 Prosthetic and other implants, materials and neurological devices associated with adverse incidents**
- **Y75.3 Surgical instruments, materials and neurological devices (including sutures) associated with adverse incidents**
- **Y75.8 Miscellaneous neurological devices associated with adverse incidents, not elsewhere classified**

● **Y76 Obstetric and gynecological devices associated with adverse incidents**
- **Y76.0 Diagnostic and monitoring obstetric and gynecological devices associated with adverse incidents ♀**
- **Y76.1 Therapeutic (nonsurgical) and rehabilitative obstetric and gynecological devices associated with adverse incidents ♀**
- **Y76.2 Prosthetic and other implants, materials and accessory obstetric and gynecological devices associated with adverse incidents ♀**
- **Y76.3 Surgical instruments, materials and obstetric and gynecological devices (including sutures) associated with adverse incidents ♀**
- **Y76.8 Miscellaneous obstetric and gynecological devices associated with adverse incidents, not elsewhere classified ♀**

● Y77 Ophthalmic devices associated with adverse incidents
- Y77.0 Diagnostic and monitoring ophthalmic devices associated with adverse incidents
- Y77.1 Therapeutic (nonsurgical) and rehabilitative ophthalmic devices associated with adverse incidents
- Y77.2 Prosthetic and other implants, materials and accessory ophthalmic devices associated with adverse incidents
- Y77.3 Surgical instruments, materials and ophthalmic devices (including sutures) associated with adverse incidents
- Y77.8 Miscellaneous ophthalmic devices associated with adverse incidents, not elsewhere classified

● Y78 Radiological devices associated with adverse incidents
- Y78.0 Diagnostic and monitoring radiological devices associated with adverse incidents
- Y78.1 Therapeutic (nonsurgical) and rehabilitative radiological devices associated with adverse incidents
- Y78.2 Prosthetic and other implants, materials and accessory radiological devices associated with adverse incidents
- Y78.3 Surgical instruments, materials and radiological devices (including sutures) associated with adverse incidents
- Y78.8 Miscellaneous radiological devices associated with adverse incidents, not elsewhere classified

● Y79 Orthopedic devices associated with adverse incidents
- Y79.0 Diagnostic and monitoring orthopedic devices associated with adverse incidents
- Y79.1 Therapeutic (nonsurgical) and rehabilitative orthopedic devices associated with adverse incidents
- Y79.2 Prosthetic and other implants, materials and accessory orthopedic devices associated with adverse incidents
- Y79.3 Surgical instruments, materials and orthopedic devices (including sutures) associated with adverse incidents
- Y79.8 Miscellaneous orthopedic devices associated with adverse incidents, not elsewhere classified

● Y80 Physical medicine devices associated with adverse incidents
- Y80.0 Diagnostic and monitoring physical medicine devices associated with adverse incidents
- Y80.1 Therapeutic (nonsurgical) and rehabilitative physical medicine devices associated with adverse incidents
- Y80.2 Prosthetic and other implants, materials and accessory physical medicine devices associated with adverse incidents
- Y80.3 Surgical instruments, materials and physical medicine devices (including sutures) associated with adverse incidents
- Y80.8 Miscellaneous physical medicine devices associated with adverse incidents, not elsewhere classified

● Y81 General- and plastic-surgery devices associated with adverse incidents
- Y81.0 Diagnostic and monitoring general- and plastic-surgery devices associated with adverse incidents
- Y81.1 Therapeutic (nonsurgical) and rehabilitative general- and plastic-surgery devices associated with adverse incidents
- Y81.2 Prosthetic and other implants, materials and accessory general- and plastic-surgery devices associated with adverse incidents
- Y81.3 Surgical instruments, materials and general- and plastic-surgery devices (including sutures) associated with adverse incidents
- Y81.8 Miscellaneous general- and plastic-surgery devices associated with adverse incidents, not elsewhere classified

● Y82 Other and unspecified medical devices associated with adverse incidents
- Y82.8 Other medical devices associated with adverse incidents
- Y82.9 Unspecified medical devices associated with adverse incidents

SURGICAL AND OTHER MEDICAL PROCEDURES AS THE CAUSE OF ABNORMAL REACTION OF THE PATIENT, OR OF LATER COMPLICATION, WITHOUT MENTION OF MISADVENTURE AT THE TIME OF THE PROCEDURE (Y83-Y84)

Excludes1 misadventures to patients during surgical and medical care, classifiable to (Y62-Y69)

Excludes2 breakdown or malfunctioning of medical device (after implantation) (during procedure) (ongoing use) (Y70-Y82) ◀

● Y83 Surgical operation and other surgical procedures as the cause of abnormal reaction of the patient, or of later complication, without mention of misadventure at the time of the procedure
- Y83.0 Surgical operation with transplant of whole organ as the cause of abnormal reaction of the patient, or of later complication, without mention of misadventure at the time of the procedure
- Y83.1 Surgical operation with implant of artificial internal device as the cause of abnormal reaction of the patient, or of later complication, without mention of misadventure at the time of the procedure
- Y83.2 Surgical operation with anastomosis, bypass or graft as the cause of abnormal reaction of the patient, or of later complication, without mention of misadventure at the time of the procedure
- Y83.3 Surgical operation with formation of external stoma as the cause of abnormal reaction of the patient, or of later complication, without mention of misadventure at the time of the procedure
- Y83.4 Other reconstructive surgery as the cause of abnormal reaction of the patient, or of later complication, without mention of misadventure at the time of the procedure
- Y83.5 Amputation of limb(s) as the cause of abnormal reaction of the patient, or of later complication, without mention of misadventure at the time of the procedure
- Y83.6 Removal of other organ (partial) (total) as the cause of abnormal reaction of the patient, or of later complication, without mention of misadventure at the time of the procedure
- Y83.8 Other surgical procedures as the cause of abnormal reaction of the patient, or of later complication, without mention of misadventure at the time of the procedure
- Y83.9 Surgical procedure, unspecified as the cause of abnormal reaction of the patient, or of later complication, without mention of misadventure at the time of the procedure

● Y84 Other medical procedures as the cause of abnormal reaction of the patient, or of later complication, without mention of misadventure at the time of the procedure
- Y84.0 Cardiac catheterization as the cause of abnormal reaction of the patient, or of later complication, without mention of misadventure at the time of the procedure
- Y84.1 Kidney dialysis as the cause of abnormal reaction of the patient, or of later complication, without mention of misadventure at the time of the procedure
- Y84.2 Radiological procedure and radiotherapy as the cause of abnormal reaction of the patient, or of later complication, without mention of misadventure at the time of the procedure
- Y84.3 Shock therapy as the cause of abnormal reaction of the patient, or of later complication, without mention of misadventure at the time of the procedure
- Y84.4 Aspiration of fluid as the cause of abnormal reaction of the patient, or of later complication, without mention of misadventure at the time of the procedure
- Y84.5 Insertion of gastric or duodenal sound as the cause of abnormal reaction of the patient, or of later complication, without mention of misadventure at the time of the procedure
- Y84.6 Urinary catheterization as the cause of abnormal reaction of the patient, or of later complication, without mention of misadventure at the time of the procedure
- Y84.7 Blood-sampling as the cause of abnormal reaction of the patient, or of later complication, without mention of misadventure at the time of the procedure

Y84.8 **Other medical procedures as the cause of abnormal reaction of the patient, or of later complication, without mention of misadventure at the time of the procedure**

Y84.9 **Medical procedure, unspecified as the cause of abnormal reaction of the patient, or of later complication, without mention of misadventure at the time of the procedure**

SUPPLEMENTARY FACTORS RELATED TO CAUSES OF MORBIDITY CLASSIFIED ELSEWHERE (Y90-Y99)

Note: These categories may be used to provide supplementary information concerning causes of morbidity. They are not to be used for single-condition coding.

● **Y90** **Evidence of alcohol involvement determined by blood alcohol level**

Code first any associated alcohol related disorders (F10)

Y90.0 **Blood alcohol level of less than 20 mg/100 ml**

Y90.1 **Blood alcohol level of 20-39 mg/100 ml**

Y90.2 **Blood alcohol level of 40-59 mg/100 ml**

Y90.3 **Blood alcohol level of 60-79 mg/100 ml**

Y90.4 **Blood alcohol level of 80-99 mg/100 ml**

Y90.5 **Blood alcohol level of 100-119 mg/100 ml**

Y90.6 **Blood alcohol level of 120-199 mg/100 ml**

Y90.7 **Blood alcohol level of 200-239 mg/100 ml**

Y90.8 **Blood alcohol level of 240 mg/100 ml or more**

Y90.9 **Presence of alcohol in blood, level not specified**

OGCR Section I.C.20.b.

Place of Occurrence Guideline

Codes from category Y92, Place of occurrence of the external cause, are secondary codes for use after other external cause codes to identify the location of the patient at the time of injury or other condition.

Generally, a place of occurrence code is assigned only once, at the initial encounter for treatment. However, in the rare instance that a new injury occurs during hospitalization, an additional place of occurrence code may be assigned. No 7th characters are used for Y92. Only one code from Y92 should be recorded on a medical record. A place of occurrence code should be used in conjunction with an activity code, Y93.

Do not use place of occurrence code Y92.9 if the place is not stated or is not applicable.

● **Y92** **Place of occurrence of the external cause**

The following category is for use, when relevant, to identify the place of occurrence of the external cause. Use in conjunction with an activity code.

Place of occurrence should be recorded only at the initial encounter for treatment

● **Y92.0** **Non-institutional (private) residence as the place of occurrence of the external cause**

Excludes1 abandoned or derelict house (Y92.89)
home under construction but not yet occupied (Y92.6-)
institutional place of residence (Y92.1-)

● **Y92.00** **Unspecified non-institutional (private) residence as the place of occurrence of the external cause**

Y92.000 **Kitchen of unspecified non-institutional (private) residence as the place of occurrence of the external cause**

Y92.001 **Dining room of unspecified non-institutional (private) residence as the place of occurrence of the external cause**

Y92.002 **Bathroom of unspecified non-institutional (private) residence single-family (private) house as the place of occurrence of the external cause**

Y92.003 **Bedroom of unspecified non-institutional (private) residence as the place of occurrence of the external cause**

Y92.007 **Garden or yard of unspecified non-institutional (private) residence as the place of occurrence of the external cause**

Y92.008 **Other place in unspecified non-institutional (private) residence as the place of occurrence of the external cause**

Y92.009 **Unspecified place in unspecified non-institutional (private) residence as the place of occurrence of the external cause**

Home (NOS) as the place of occurrence of the external cause

● **Y92.01** **Single-family non-institutional (private) house as the place of occurrence of the external cause**

Farmhouse as the place of occurrence of the external cause

Excludes1 barn (Y92.71)
chicken coop or hen house (Y92.72)
farm field (Y92.73)
orchard (Y92.74)
single family mobile home or trailer (Y92.02-)
slaughter house (Y92.86)

Y92.010 **Kitchen of single-family (private) house as the place of occurrence of the external cause**

Y92.011 **Dining room of single-family (private) house as the place of occurrence of the external cause**

Y92.012 **Bathroom of single-family (private) house as the place of occurrence of the external cause**

Y92.013 **Bedroom of single-family (private) house as the place of occurrence of the external cause**

Y92.014 **Private driveway to single-family (private) house as the place of occurrence of the external cause**

Y92.015 **Private garage of single-family (private) house as the place of occurrence of the external cause**

Y92.016 **Swimming pool in single-family (private) house or garden as the place of occurrence of the external cause**

Y92.017 **Garden or yard in single-family (private) house as the place of occurrence of the external cause**

Y92.018 **Other place in single-family (private) house as the place of occurrence of the external cause**

Y92.019 **Unspecified place in single-family (private) house as the place of occurrence of the external cause**

● Y92.02 Mobile home as the place of occurrence of the external cause

Y92.020 Kitchen in mobile home as the place of occurrence of the external cause

Y92.021 Dining room in mobile home as the place of occurrence of the external cause

Y92.022 Bathroom in mobile home as the place of occurrence of the external cause

Y92.023 Bedroom in mobile home as the place of occurrence of the external cause

Y92.024 Driveway of mobile home as the place of occurrence of the external cause

Y92.025 Garage of mobile home as the place of occurrence of the external cause

Y92.026 Swimming pool of mobile home as the place of occurrence of the external cause

Y92.027 Garden or yard of mobile home as the place of occurrence of the external cause

Y92.028 Other place in mobile home as the place of occurrence of the external cause

Y92.029 Unspecified place in mobile home as the place of occurrence of the external cause

● Y92.03 Apartment as the place of occurrence of the external cause

Condominium as the place of occurrence of the external cause

Co-op apartment as the place of occurrence of the external cause

Y92.030 Kitchen in apartment as the place of occurrence of the external cause

Y92.031 Bathroom in apartment as the place of occurrence of the external cause

Y92.032 Bedroom in apartment as the place of occurrence of the external cause

Y92.038 Other place in apartment as the place of occurrence of the external cause

Y92.039 Unspecified place in apartment as the place of occurrence of the external cause

● Y92.04 Boarding-house as the place of occurrence of the external cause

Y92.040 Kitchen in boarding-house as the place of occurrence of the external cause

Y92.041 Bathroom in boarding-house as the place of occurrence of the external cause

Y92.042 Bedroom in boarding-house as the place of occurrence of the external cause

Y92.043 Driveway of boarding-house as the place of occurrence of the external cause

Y92.044 Garage of boarding-house as the place of occurrence of the external cause

Y92.045 Swimming pool of boarding-house as the place of occurrence of the external cause

Y92.046 Garden or yard of boarding-house as the place of occurrence of the external cause

Y92.048 Other place in boarding-house as the place of occurrence of the external cause

Y92.049 Unspecified place in boarding-house as the place of occurrence of the external cause

● Y92.09 Other non-institutional residence as the place of occurrence of the external cause

Y92.090 Kitchen in other non-institutional residence as the place of occurrence of the external cause

Y92.091 Bathroom in other non-institutional residence as the place of occurrence of the external cause

Y92.092 Bedroom in other non-institutional residence as the place of occurrence of the external cause

Y92.093 Driveway of other non-institutional residence as the place of occurrence of the external cause

Y92.094 Garage of other non-institutional residence as the place of occurrence of the external cause

Y92.095 Swimming pool of other non-institutional residence as the place of occurrence of the external cause

Y92.096 Garden or yard of other non-institutional residence as the place of occurrence of the external cause

Y92.098 Other place in other non-institutional residence as the place of occurrence of the external cause

Y92.099 Unspecified place in other non-institutional residence as the place of occurrence of the external cause

● Y92.1 Institutional (nonprivate) residence as the place of occurrence of the external cause

Y92.10 Unspecified residential institution as the place of occurrence of the external cause

● Y92.11 Children's home and orphanage as the place of occurrence of the external cause

Y92.110 Kitchen in children's home and orphanage as the place of occurrence of the external cause

Y92.111 Bathroom in children's home and orphanage as the place of occurrence of the external cause

Y92.112 Bedroom in children's home and orphanage as the place of occurrence of the external cause

Y92.113 Driveway of children's home and orphanage as the place of occurrence of the external cause

Y92.114 Garage of children's home and orphanage as the place of occurrence of the external cause

Y92.115 Swimming pool of children's home and orphanage as the place of occurrence of the external cause

Y92.116 Garden or yard of children's home and orphanage as the place of occurrence of the external cause

Y92.118 Other place in children's home and orphanage as the place of occurrence of the external cause

Y92.119 Unspecified place in children's home and orphanage as the place of occurrence of the external cause

● **Y92.12 Nursing home as the place of occurrence of the external cause**
Home for the sick as the place of occurrence of the external cause
Hospice as the place of occurrence of the external cause
Y92.120 Kitchen in nursing home as the place of occurrence of the external cause
Y92.121 Bathroom in nursing home as the place of occurrence of the external cause
Y92.122 Bedroom in nursing home as the place of occurrence of the external cause
Y92.123 Driveway of nursing home as the place of occurrence of the external cause
Y92.124 Garage of nursing home as the place of occurrence of the external cause
Y92.125 Swimming pool of nursing home as the place of occurrence of the external cause
Y92.126 Garden or yard of nursing home as the place of occurrence of the external cause
Y92.128 Other place in nursing home as the place of occurrence of the external cause
Y92.129 Unspecified place in nursing home as the place of occurrence of the external cause

● **Y92.13 Military base as the place of occurrence of the external cause**
Excludes1 military training grounds (Y92.83)
Y92.130 Kitchen on military base as the place of occurrence of the external cause
Y92.131 Mess hall on military base as the place of occurrence of the external cause
Y92.133 Barracks on military base as the place of occurrence of the external cause
Y92.135 Garage on military base as the place of occurrence of the external cause
Y92.136 Swimming pool on military base as the place of occurrence of the external cause
Y92.137 Garden or yard on military base as the place of occurrence of the external cause
Y92.138 Other place on military base as the place of occurrence of the external cause
Y92.139 Unspecified place military base as the place of occurrence of the external cause

● **Y92.14 Prison as the place of occurrence of the external cause**
Y92.140 Kitchen in prison as the place of occurrence of the external cause
Y92.141 Dining room in prison as the place of occurrence of the external cause
Y92.142 Bathroom in prison as the place of occurrence of the external cause
Y92.143 Cell of prison as the place of occurrence of the external cause
Y92.146 Swimming pool of prison as the place of occurrence of the external cause
Y92.147 Courtyard of prison as the place of occurrence of the external cause
Y92.148 Other place in prison as the place of occurrence of the external cause
Y92.149 Unspecified place in prison as the place of occurrence of the external cause

● **Y92.15 Reform school as the place of occurrence of the external cause**
Y92.150 Kitchen in reform school as the place of occurrence of the external cause
Y92.151 Dining room in reform school as the place of occurrence of the external cause
Y92.152 Bathroom in reform school as the place of occurrence of the external cause
Y92.153 Bedroom in reform school as the place of occurrence of the external cause
Y92.154 Driveway of reform school as the place of occurrence of the external cause
Y92.155 Garage of reform school as the place of occurrence of the external cause
Y92.156 Swimming pool of reform school as the place of occurrence of the external cause
Y92.157 Garden or yard of reform school as the place of occurrence of the external cause
Y92.158 Other place in reform school as the place of occurrence of the external cause
Y92.159 Unspecified place in reform school as the place of occurrence of the external cause

● **Y92.16 School dormitory as the place of occurrence of the external cause**
Excludes1 reform school as the place of occurrence of the external cause (Y92.15-)
school buildings and grounds as the place of occurrence of the external cause (Y92.2-)
school sports and athletic areas as the place of occurrence of the external cause (Y92.3-)
Y92.160 Kitchen in school dormitory as the place of occurrence of the external cause
Y92.161 Dining room in school dormitory as the place of occurrence of the external cause
Y92.162 Bathroom in school dormitory as the place of occurrence of the external cause
Y92.163 Bedroom in school dormitory as the place of occurrence of the external cause
Y92.168 Other place in school dormitory as the place of occurrence of the external cause
Y92.169 Unspecified place in school dormitory as the place of occurrence of the external cause

● **Y92.19 Other specified residential institution as the place of occurrence of the external cause**

Y92.190 Kitchen in other specified residential institution as the place of occurrence of the external cause

Y92.191 Dining room in other specified residential institution as the place of occurrence of the external cause

Y92.192 Bathroom in other specified residential institution as the place of occurrence of the external cause

Y92.193 Bedroom in other specified residential institution as the place of occurrence of the external cause

Y92.194 Driveway of other specified residential institution as the place of occurrence of the external cause

Y92.195 Garage of other specified residential institution as the place of occurrence of the external cause

Y92.196 Pool of other specified residential institution as the place of occurrence of the external cause

Y92.197 Garden or yard of other specified residential institution as the place of occurrence of the external cause

Y92.198 Other place in other specified residential institution as the place of occurrence of the external cause

Y92.199 Unspecified place in other specified residential institution as the place of occurrence of the external cause

● **Y92.2 School, other institution and public administrative area as the place of occurrence of the external cause**

Building and adjacent grounds used by the general public or by a particular group of the public

Excludes1 building under construction as the place of occurrence of the external cause (Y92.6)
residential institution as the place of occurrence of the external cause (Y92.1)
school dormitory as the place of occurrence of the external cause (Y92.16-)
sports and athletics area of schools as the place of occurrence of the external cause (Y92.3-)

● **Y92.21 School (private) (public) (state) as the place of occurrence of the external cause**

Y92.210 Daycare center as the place of occurrence of the external cause

Y92.211 Elementary school as the place of occurrence of the external cause

Kindergarten as the place of occurrence of the external cause

Y92.212 Middle school as the place of occurrence of the external cause

Y92.213 High school as the place of occurrence of the external cause

Coding Clinic: 2012, Q4, P108

Y92.214 College as the place of occurrence of the external cause

University as the place of occurrence of the external cause

Y92.215 Trade school as the place of occurrence of the external cause

Y92.218 Other school as the place of occurrence of the external cause

Y92.219 Unspecified school as the place of occurrence of the external cause

Y92.22 Religious institution as the place of occurrence of the external cause

Church as the place of occurrence of the external cause
Mosque as the place of occurrence of the external cause
Synagogue as the place of occurrence of the external cause

● **Y92.23 Hospital as the place of occurrence of the external cause**

Excludes1 ambulatory (outpatient) health services establishments (Y92.53-)
home for the sick as the place of occurrence of the external cause (Y92.12-)
hospice as the place of occurrence of the external cause (Y92.12-)
nursing home as the place of occurrence of the external cause (Y92.12-)

Y92.230 Patient room in hospital as the place of occurrence of the external cause

Y92.231 Patient bathroom in hospital as the place of occurrence of the external cause

Y92.232 Corridor of hospital as the place of occurrence of the external cause

Y92.233 Cafeteria of hospital as the place of occurrence of the external cause

Y92.234 Operating room of hospital as the place of occurrence of the external cause

Y92.238 Other place in hospital as the place of occurrence of the external cause

Y92.239 Unspecified place in hospital as the place of occurrence of the external cause

● **Y92.24 Public administrative building as the place of occurrence of the external cause**

Y92.240 Courthouse as the place of occurrence of the external cause

Y92.241 Library as the place of occurrence of the external cause

Y92.242 Post office as the place of occurrence of the external cause

Y92.243 City hall as the place of occurrence of the external cause

Y92.248 Other public administrative building as the place of occurrence of the external cause

● **Y92.25 Cultural building as the place of occurrence of the external cause**

Y92.250 Art gallery as the place of occurrence of the external cause

Y92.251 Museum as the place of occurrence of the external cause

Y92.252 Music hall as the place of occurrence of the external cause

Y92.253 Opera house as the place of occurrence of the external cause

Y92.254 Theater (live) as the place of occurrence of the external cause

Y92.258 Other cultural public building as the place of occurrence of the external cause

Y92.26 Movie house or cinema as the place of occurrence of the external cause

Y92.29 Other specified public building as the place of occurrence of the external cause

Assembly hall as the place of occurrence of the external cause
Clubhouse as the place of occurrence of the external cause

Y92.3 Sports and athletics area as the place of occurrence of the external cause

Y92.31 Athletic court as the place of occurrence of the external cause

Excludes1 tennis court in private home or garden (Y92.09)

Y92.310 Basketball court as the place of occurrence of the external cause

Y92.311 Squash court as the place of occurrence of the external cause

Y92.312 Tennis court as the place of occurrence of the external cause

Y92.318 Other athletic court as the place of occurrence of the external cause

Y92.32 Athletic field as the place of occurrence of the external cause

Y92.320 Baseball field as the place of occurrence of the external cause

Y92.321 Football field as the place of occurrence of the external cause

Y92.322 Soccer field as the place of occurrence of the external cause

Y92.328 Other athletic field as the place of occurrence of the external cause

Cricket field as the place of occurrence of the external cause

Hockey field as the place of occurrence of the external cause

Y92.33 Skating rink as the place of occurrence of the external cause

Y92.330 Ice skating rink (indoor) (outdoor) as the place of occurrence of the external cause

Y92.331 Roller skating rink as the place of occurrence of the external cause

Y92.34 Swimming pool (public) as the place of occurrence of the external cause

Excludes1 swimming pool in private home or garden (Y92.016)

Y92.39 Other specified sports and athletic area as the place of occurrence of the external cause

Golf-course as the place of occurrence of the external cause

Gymnasium as the place of occurrence of the external cause

Riding-school as the place of occurrence of the external cause

Stadium as the place of occurrence of the external cause

Y92.4 Street, highway and other paved roadways as the place of occurrence of the external cause

Excludes1 private driveway of residence (Y92.014, Y92.024, Y92.043, Y92.093, Y92.113, Y92.123, Y92.154, Y92.194)

Y92.41 Street and highway as the place of occurrence of the external cause

Y92.410 Unspecified street and highway as the place of occurrence of the external cause

Road NOS as the place of occurrence of the external cause

Y92.411 Interstate highway as the place of occurrence of the external cause

Freeway as the place of occurrence of the external cause

Motorway as the place of occurrence of the external cause

Y92.412 Parkway as the place of occurrence of the external cause

Y92.413 State road as the place of occurrence of the external cause

Y92.414 Local residential or business street as the place of occurrence of the external cause

Y92.415 Exit ramp or entrance ramp of street or highway as the place of occurrence of the external cause

Y92.48 Other paved roadways as the place of occurrence of the external cause

Y92.480 Sidewalk as the place of occurrence of the external cause

Y92.481 Parking lot as the place of occurrence of the external cause

Y92.482 Bike path as the place of occurrence of the external cause

Y92.488 Other paved roadways as the place of occurrence of the external cause

Y92.5 Trade and service area as the place of occurrence of the external cause

Excludes1 garage in private home (Y92.015)
schools and other public administration buildings (Y92.2-)

Y92.51 Private commercial establishments as the place of occurrence of the external cause

Y92.510 Bank as the place of occurrence of the external cause

Y92.511 Restaurant or café as the place of occurrence of the external cause

Y92.512 Supermarket, store or market as the place of occurrence of the external cause

Y92.513 Shop (commercial) as the place of occurrence of the external cause

Y92.52 Service areas as the place of occurrence of the external cause

Y92.520 Airport as the place of occurrence of the external cause

Y92.521 Bus station as the place of occurrence of the external cause

Y92.522 Railway station as the place of occurrence of the external cause

Y92.523 Highway rest stop as the place of occurrence of the external cause

Y92.524 Gas station as the place of occurrence of the external cause

Petroleum station as the place of occurrence of the external cause

Service station as the place of occurrence of the external cause

Y92.53 Ambulatory health services establishments as the place of occurrence of the external cause

Y92.530 Ambulatory surgery center as the place of occurrence of the external cause

Outpatient surgery center, including that connected with a hospital as the place of occurrence of the external cause

Same day surgery center, including that connected with a hospital as the place of occurrence of the external cause

Y92.531 Health care provider office as the place of occurrence of the external cause

Physician office as the place of occurrence of the external cause

Y92.532 Urgent care center as the place of occurrence of the external cause

Y92.538 Other ambulatory health services establishments as the place of occurrence of the external cause

Y92.59 Other trade areas as the place of occurrence of the external cause
- Office building as the place of occurrence of the external cause
- Casino as the place of occurrence of the external cause
- Garage (commercial) as the place of occurrence of the external cause
- Hotel as the place of occurrence of the external cause
- Radio or television station as the place of occurrence of the external cause
- Shopping mall as the place of occurrence of the external cause
- Warehouse as the place of occurrence of the external cause

● **Y92.6 Industrial and construction area as the place of occurrence of the external cause**

Y92.61 Building [any] under construction as the place of occurrence of the external cause

Y92.62 Dock or shipyard as the place of occurrence of the external cause
- Dockyard as the place of occurrence of the external cause
- Dry dock as the place of occurrence of the external cause
- Shipyard as the place of occurrence of the external cause

Y92.63 Factory as the place of occurrence of the external cause
- Factory building as the place of occurrence of the external cause
- Factory premises as the place of occurrence of the external cause
- Industrial yard as the place of occurrence of the external cause

Y92.64 Mine or pit as the place of occurrence of the external cause
- Mine as the place of occurrence of the external cause

Y92.65 Oil rig as the place of occurrence of the external cause
- Pit (coal) (gravel) (sand) as the place of occurrence of the external cause

Y92.69 Other specified industrial and construction area as the place of occurrence of the external cause
- Gasworks as the place of occurrence of the external cause
- Power-station (coal) (nuclear) (oil) as the place of occurrence of the external cause
- Tunnel under construction as the place of occurrence of the external cause
- Workshop as the place of occurrence of the external cause

● **Y92.7 Farm as the place of occurrence of the external cause**
- Ranch as the place of occurrence of the external cause

Excludes1 farmhouse and home premises of farm (Y92.01-)

Y92.71 Barn as the place of occurrence of the external cause

Y92.72 Chicken coop as the place of occurrence of the external cause
- Hen house as the place of occurrence of the external cause

Y92.73 Farm field as the place of occurrence of the external cause

Y92.74 Orchard as the place of occurrence of the external cause

Y92.79 Other farm location as the place of occurrence of the external cause

● **Y92.8 Other places as the place of occurrence of the external cause**

● **Y92.81 Transport vehicle as the place of occurrence of the external cause**

Excludes1 transport accidents (V00-V99)

Y92.810 Car as the place of occurrence of the external cause

Y92.811 Bus as the place of occurrence of the external cause

Y92.812 Truck as the place of occurrence of the external cause

Y92.813 Airplane as the place of occurrence of the external cause

Y92.814 Boat as the place of occurrence of the external cause

Y92.815 Train as the place of occurrence of the external cause

Y92.816 Subway car as the place of occurrence of the external cause

Y92.818 Other transport vehicle as the place of occurrence of the external cause

● **Y92.82 Wilderness area**

Y92.820 Desert as the place of occurrence of the external cause

Y92.821 Forest as the place of occurrence of the external cause

Y92.828 Other wilderness area as the place of occurrence of the external cause
- Swamp as the place of occurrence of the external cause
- Mountain as the place of occurrence of the external cause
- Marsh as the place of occurrence of the external cause
- Prairie as the place of occurrence of the external cause

● **Y92.83 Recreation area as the place of occurrence of the external cause**

Y92.830 Public park as the place of occurrence of the external cause

Y92.831 Amusement park as the place of occurrence of the external cause

Y92.832 Beach as the place of occurrence of the external cause
- Seashore as the place of occurrence of the external cause

Y92.833 Campsite as the place of occurrence of the external cause

Y92.834 Zoological garden (zoo) as the place of occurrence of the external cause

Y92.838 Other recreation area as the place of occurrence of the external cause

Y92.84 Military training ground as the place of occurrence of the external cause

Y92.85 Railroad track as the place of occurrence of the external cause

Y92.86 Slaughter house as the place of occurrence of the external cause

Y92.89 Other specified places as the place of occurrence of the external cause
- Derelict house as the place of occurrence of the external cause

OGCR Section I.C.20.b.

Do not use place of occurrence code Y92.9 if the place is not stated or is not applicable.

Y92.9 Unspecified place or not applicable

◀ New ⇐ Revised ~~deleted~~ Deleted Excludes 1 Excludes 2 Includes Use additional Code first Code also Unspecified
OGCR Official Guidelines ● Unacceptable Principal Diagnosis X Assign placeholder X ● Use Additional Character(s) ▶ Manifestation Code Coding Clinic

OGCR See Section I.C.20.c.

Activity Code

Assign a code from category Y93, Activity code, to describe the activity of the patient at the time the injury or other health condition occurred.

An activity code is used only once, at the initial encounter for treatment. Only one code from Y93 should be recorded on a medical record.

The activity codes are not applicable to poisonings, adverse effects, misadventures or sequela.

Do not assign Y93.9, Unspecified activity, if the activity is not stated.

A code from category Y93 is appropriate for use with external cause and intent codes if identifying the activity provides additional information about the event.

● **Y93 Activity codes**

Note: Category Y93 is provided for use to indicate the activity of the person seeking healthcare for an injury or health condition, such as a heart attack while shoveling snow, which resulted from, or was contributed to, by the activity. These codes are appropriate for use for both acute injuries, such as those from chapter 19, and conditions that are due to the long-term, cumulative effects of an activity, such as those from chapter 13. They are also appropriate for use with external cause codes for cause and intent if identifying the activity provides additional information on the event. These codes should be used in conjunction with codes for external cause status (Y99) and place of occurrence (Y92).

This section contains the following broad activity categories:

- Y93.0 Activities involving walking and running
- Y93.1 Activities involving water and water craft
- Y93.2 Activities involving ice and snow
- Y93.3 Activities involving climbing, rappelling, and jumping off
- Y93.4 Activities involving dancing and other rhythmic movement
- Y93.5 Activities involving other sports and athletics played individually
- Y93.6 Activities involving other sports and athletics played as a team or group
- Y93.7 Activities involving other specified sports and athletics
- Y93.A Activities involving other cardiorespiratory exercise
- Y93.B Activities involving other muscle strengthening exercises
- Y93.C Activities involving computer technology and electronic devices
- Y93.D Activities involving arts and handcrafts
- Y93.E Activities involving personal hygiene and interior property and clothing maintenance
- Y93.F Activities involving caregiving
- Y93.G Activities involving food preparation, cooking and grilling
- Y93.H Activities involving exterior property and land maintenance, building and construction
- Y93.I Activities involving roller coasters and other types of external motion
- Y93.J Activities involving playing musical instrument
- Y93.K Activities involving animal care
- Y93.8 Activities, other specified
- Y93.9 Activity, unspecified

● **Y93.0 Activities involving walking and running**

Excludes1 Activity, walking an animal (Y93.K1)
Activity, walking or running on a treadmill (Y93.A1)

Y93.01 Activity, walking, marching and hiking
Activity, walking, marching and hiking on level or elevated terrain

Excludes1 activity, mountain climbing (Y93.31)

Y93.02 Activity, running

● **Y93.1 Activities involving water and water craft**

Excludes1 activities involving ice (Y93.2-)

Y93.11 Activity, swimming

Y93.12 Activity, springboard and platform diving

Y93.13 Activity, water polo

Y93.14 Activity, water aerobics and water exercise

Y93.15 Activity, underwater diving and snorkeling
Activity, SCUBA diving

Y93.16 Activity, rowing, canoeing, kayaking, rafting and tubing
Activity, canoeing, kayaking, rafting and tubing in calm and turbulent water

Y93.17 Activity, water skiing and wake boarding

Y93.18 Activity, surfing, windsurfing and boogie boarding
Activity, water sliding

Y93.19 Activity, other involving water and watercraft
Activity involving water NOS
Activity, parasailing
Activity, water survival training and testing

● **Y93.2 Activities involving ice and snow**

Excludes1 activity, shoveling ice and snow (Y93.H1)

Y93.21 Activity, ice skating
Activity, figure skating (singles) (pairs)
Activity, ice dancing

Excludes1 activity, ice hockey (Y93.22)

Y93.22 Activity, ice hockey

Y93.23 Activity, snow (alpine) (downhill) skiing, snow boarding, sledding, tobogganing and snow tubing

Excludes1 activity, cross country skiing (Y93.24)

Y93.24 Activity, cross country skiing
Activity, nordic skiing

Y93.29 Activity, other activity involving ice and snow
Activity, activity involving ice and snow NOS

● **Y93.3 Activities involving climbing, rappelling and jumping off**

Excludes1 activity, hiking on level or elevated terrain (Y93.01)
activity, jumping rope (Y93.56)
activity, trampoline jumping (Y93.44)

Y93.31 Activity, mountain climbing, rock climbing and wall climbing

Y93.32 Activity, rappelling

Y93.33 Activity, BASE jumping
Activity, building, Antenna, Span, Earth jumping

Y93.34 Activity, bungee jumping

Y93.35 Activity, hang gliding

Y93.39 Activity, other activity involving climbing, rappelling and jumping off

● **Y93.4 Activities involving dancing and other rhythmic movement**

Excludes1 activity, martial arts (Y93.75)

Y93.41 Activity, dancing
Coding Clinic: 2012, Q4, P108

Y93.42 Activity, yoga

Y93.43 Activity, gymnastics
Activity, rhythmic gymnastics

Excludes1 activity, trampolining (Y93.44)

Y93.44 Activity, trampolining

Y93.45 Activity, cheerleading

Y93.49 Activity, other involving dancing and other rhythmic movements

● **Y93.5 Activities involving other sports and athletics played individually**

Excludes1 activity, dancing (Y93.41)
activity, gymnastic (Y93.43)
activity, trampolining (Y93.44)
activity, yoga (Y93.42)

Y93.51 Activity, roller skating (inline) and skateboarding

Y93.52 Activity, horseback riding

Y93.53 Activity, golf

Y93.54 Activity, bowling

Y93.55 Activity, bike riding

Y93.56 Activity, jumping rope

Y93.57 Activity, non-running track and field events

Excludes1 activity, running (any form) (Y93.02)

Y93.59 Activity, other involving other sports and athletics played individually

Excludes1 activities involving climbing, rappelling, and jumping (Y93.3-)
activities involving ice and snow (Y93.2-)
activities involving walking and running (Y93.0-)
activities involving water and watercraft (Y93.1-)

● **Y93.6 Activities involving other sports and athletics played as a team or group**

Excludes1 activity, ice hockey (Y93.22)
activity, water polo (Y93.13)

Y93.61 Activity, American tackle football
Activity, football NOS

Y93.62 Activity, American flag or touch football

Y93.63 Activity, rugby

Y93.64 Activity, baseball
Activity, softball

Y93.65 Activity, lacrosse and field hockey
Coding Clinic: 2015, Q1, P9

Y93.66 Activity, soccer

Y93.67 Activity, basketball

Y93.68 Activity, volleyball (beach) (court)

Y93.6A Activity, physical games generally associated with school recess, summer camp and children
Activity, capture the flag
Activity, dodge ball
Activity, four square
Activity, kickball

Y93.69 Activity, other involving other sports and athletics played as a team or group
Cricket

● **Y93.7 Activities involving other specified sports and athletics**

Y93.71 Activity, boxing

Y93.72 Activity, wrestling

Y93.73 Activity, racquet and hand sports
Activity, handball
Activity, racquetball
Activity, squash
Activity, tennis

Y93.74 Activity, frisbee
Activity, ultimate frisbee

Y93.75 Activity, martial arts
Activity, combatives

Y93.79 Activity, other specified sports and athletics

Excludes1 sports and athletics activities specified in categories Y93.0-Y93.6

● **Y93.A Activities involving other cardiorespiratory exercise**
Activities involving physical training

Y93.A1 Activity, exercise machines primarily for cardiorespiratory conditioning
Activity, elliptical and stepper machines
Activity, stationary bike
Activity, treadmill

Y93.A2 Activity, calisthenics
Activity, jumping jacks
Activity, warm up and cool down

Y93.A3 Activity, aerobic and step exercise

Y93.A4 Activity, circuit training

Y93.A5 Activity, obstacle course
Activity, challenge course
Activity, confidence course

Y93.A6 Activity, grass drills
Activity, guerilla drills

Y93.A9 Activity, other involving other cardiorespiratory exercise

Excludes1 activities involving cardiorespiratory exercise specified in categories Y93.0-Y93.7

● **Y93.B Activity involving other muscle strengthening exercises**

Y93.B1 Activity, exercise machines primarily for muscle strengthening

Y93.B2 Activity, push-ups, pull-ups, sit-ups

Y93.B3 Activity, free weights
Activity, barbells
Activity, dumbbells

Y93.B4 Activity, pilates

Y93.B9 Activity, other involving other muscle strengthening exercises

Excludes1 activities involving muscle strengthening specified in categories Y93.0-Y93.A

● **Y93.C Activities involving computer technology and electronic devices**

Excludes1 activity, electronic musical keyboard or instruments (Y93.J-)

Y93.C1 Activity, computer keyboarding
Activity, electronic game playing using keyboard or other stationary device

Y93.C2 Activity, hand held interactive electronic device
Activity, cellular telephone and communication device
Activity, electronic game playing using interactive device

Excludes1 activity, electronic game playing using keyboard or other stationary device (Y93.C1)

Y93.C9 Activity, other involving computer technology and electronic devices

● **Y93.D Activities involving arts and handcrafts**

Excludes1 activities involving playing musical instrument (Y93.J-)

Y93.D1 Knitting and crocheting

Y93.D2 Sewing

Y93.D3 Furniture building and finishing
Furniture repair

Y93.D9 Activity, other involving arts and handcrafts

● **Y93.E Activities involving personal hygiene and interior property and clothing maintenance**

Excludes1 activities involving cooking and grilling (Y93.G-)
activities involving exterior property and land maintenance, building and construction (Y93.H-)
activity involving caregiving (Y93.F-)
activity, dishwashing (Y93.G1)
activity, food preparation (Y93.G1)
activity, gardening (Y93.H2)

Y93.E1 Activity, personal bathing and showering
Y93.E2 Activity, laundry
Y93.E3 Activity, vacuuming
Y93.E4 Activity, ironing
Y93.E5 Activity, floor mopping and cleaning
Y93.E6 Activity, residential relocation
Activity, packing up and unpacking involved in moving to a new residence
Y93.E8 Activity, other personal hygiene activity
Y93.E9 Activity, other household maintenance

● **Y93.F Activities involving person providing caregiving**
Activity involving the provider of caregiving
Y93.F1 Activity, caregiving involving bathing
Y93.F2 Activity, caregiving involving lifting
Y93.F9 Activity, other caregiving

● **Y93.G Activities involving food preparation, cooking and grilling**
Y93.G1 Activity, food preparation and clean up
Activity, dishwashing
Y93.G2 Activity, grilling and smoking food
Y93.G3 Activity, cooking and baking
Activity, use of stove, oven and microwave oven
Y93.G9 Activity, other activity involving cooking and grilling

● **Y93.H Activities involving property and land maintenance, building and construction**
Y93.H1 Activity, digging, shoveling and raking
Activity, dirt digging
Activity, raking leaves
Activity, snow shoveling
Y93.H2 Activity, gardening and landscaping
Activity, pruning, trimming shrubs, weeding
Y93.H3 Activity, building and construction
Y93.H9 Activity, other activity involving property and land maintenance, building and construction

● **Y93.I Activities involving roller coasters and other types of external motion**
Y93.I1 Activity, rollercoaster riding
Y93.I9 Activity, other involving external motion

● **Y93.J Activities involving playing musical instrument**
Activity involving playing electric musical instrument
Y93.J1 Activity, piano playing
Activity, musical keyboard (electronic) playing
Y93.J2 Activity, drum and other percussion instrument playing
Y93.J3 Activity, string instrument playing
Y93.J4 Activity, winds and brass instrument playing

● **Y93.K Activities involving animal care**

Excludes1 activity, horseback riding (Y93.52)

Y93.K1 Activity, walking an animal
Y93.K2 Activity, milking an animal
Y93.K3 Activity, grooming and shearing an animal
Y93.K9 Activity, other activity involving animal care

● **Y93.8 Other activity**
Y93.81 Activity, refereeing a sports activity
Y93.82 Activity, spectator at an event
Y93.83 Activity, rough housing and horseplay
Coding Clinic: 2015, Q1, P8
Y93.84 Activity, sleeping
Y93.85 Activity, choking game ◀
Activity, blackout game ◀
Activity, fainting game ◀
Activity, pass out game ◀
Y93.89 Activity, other specified

OGCR See Section I.C.20.c.

Do not assign Y93.9, Unspecified activity, if the activity is not stated.

● **Y93.9 Activity, unspecified**

Y95 Nosocomial condition

● **Y99 External cause status**

Note: A single code from category Y99 should be used in conjunction with the external cause code(s) assigned to a record to indicate the status of the person at the time the event occurred.

Y99.0 Civilian activity done for income or pay
Civilian activity done for financial or other compensation

Excludes1 military activity (Y99.1)
volunteer activity (Y99.2)

Y99.1 Military activity

Excludes1 activity of off duty military personnel (Y99.8)

Y99.2 Volunteer activity

Excludes1 activity of child or other family member assisting in compensated work of other family member (Y99.8)

Y99.8 Other external cause status
Activity NEC
Activity of child or other family member assisting in compensated work of other family member
Hobby not done for income
Leisure activity
Off-duty activity of military personnel
Recreation or sport not for income or while a student
Student activity

Excludes1 civilian activity done for income or compensation (Y99.0)
military activity (Y99.1)

Coding Clinic: 2012, Q4, P108

Y99.9 Unspecified external cause status

CHAPTER 21

FACTORS INFLUENCING HEALTH STATUS AND CONTACT WITH HEALTH SERVICES (Z00-Z99)

OGCR Chapter-Specific Coding Guidelines

21. Chapter 21: Factors influencing health status and contact with health services (Z00-Z99)

Note: The chapter specific guidelines provide additional information about the use of Z codes for specified encounters.

a. Use of Z codes in any healthcare setting

Z codes are for use in any healthcare setting. Z codes may be used as either a first-listed (principal diagnosis code in the inpatient setting) or secondary code, depending on the circumstances of the encounter. Certain Z codes may only be used as first-listed or principal diagnosis.

b. Z Codes indicate a reason for an encounter

Z codes are not procedure codes. A corresponding procedure code must accompany a Z code to describe any procedure performed.

c. Categories of Z Codes

1) Contact/Exposure

Category Z20 indicates contact with, and suspected exposure to, communicable diseases. These codes are for patients who do not show any sign or symptom of a disease but are suspected to have been exposed to it by close personal contact with an infected individual or are in an area where a disease is epidemic.

Category Z77, **Other contact with and (suspected) exposures hazardous to health,** indicates contact with and suspected exposures hazardous to health.

Contact/exposure codes may be used as a first-listed code to explain an encounter for testing, or, more commonly, as a secondary code to identify a potential risk.

2) Inoculations and vaccinations

Code Z23 is for encounters for inoculations and vaccinations. It indicates that a patient is being seen to receive a prophylactic inoculation against a disease. Procedure codes are required to identify the actual administration of the injection and the type(s) of immunizations given. Code Z23 may be used as a secondary code if the inoculation is given as a routine part of preventive health care, such as a well-baby visit.

3) Status

Status codes indicate that a patient is either a carrier of a disease or has the sequelae or residual of a past disease or condition. This includes such things as the presence of prosthetic or mechanical devices resulting from past treatment. A status code is informative, because the status may affect the course of treatment and its outcome. A status code is distinct from a history code. The history code indicates that the patient no longer has the condition.

A status code should not be used with a diagnosis code from one of the body system chapters, if the diagnosis code includes the information provided by the status code. For example, code Z94.1, Heart transplant status, should not be used with a code from subcategory T86.2, Complications of heart transplant. The status code does not provide additional information. The complication code indicates that the patient is a heart transplant patient.

For encounters for weaning from a mechanical ventilator, assign a code from subcategory J96.1, Chronic respiratory failure, followed by code Z99.11, Dependence on respirator [ventilator] status.

The status Z codes/categories are:

Z14 Genetic carrier
Genetic carrier status indicates that a person carries a gene, associated with a particular disease, which may be passed to offspring who may develop that disease. The person does not have the disease and is not at risk of developing the disease.

Z15 Genetic susceptibility to disease Genetic susceptibility indicates that a person has a gene that increases the risk of that person developing the disease.

Codes from category Z15 should not be used as principal or first-listed codes. If the patient has the condition to which he/she is susceptible, and that condition is the reason for the encounter, the code for the current condition should be sequenced first. If the patient is being seen for follow-up after completed treatment for this condition, and the condition no longer exists, a follow-up code should be sequenced first, followed by the appropriate personal history and genetic susceptibility codes. If the purpose of the encounter is genetic counseling associated with procreative management, code Z31.5, Encounter for genetic counseling, should be assigned as the first-listed code, followed by a code from category Z15. Additional codes should be assigned for any applicable family or personal history.

Z16 Resistance to antimicrobial drugs
This code indicates that a patient has a condition that is resistant to antimicrobial drug treatment. Sequence the infection code first.

Z17 Estrogen receptor status

Z18 Retained foreign body fragments

Z19 Hormone sensitivity malignancy status

Z21 Asymptomatic HIV infection status This code indicates that a patient has tested positive for HIV but has manifested no signs or symptoms of the disease.

Z22 Carrier of infectious disease Carrier status indicates that a person harbors the specific organisms of a disease without manifest symptoms and is capable of transmitting the infection.

Z28.3 Underimmunization status

Z33.1 Pregnant state, incidental This code is a secondary code only for use when the pregnancy is in no way complicating the reason for visit. Otherwise, a code from the obstetric chapter is required.

Z66 Do not resuscitate

This code may be used when it is documented by the provider that a patient is on do not resuscitate status at any time during the stay.

Z67 Blood type

Z68 Body mass index (BMI)
As with all other secondary diagnosis codes, the BMI codes should only be assigned when they meet the definition of a reportable diagnosis (see Section III, Reporting Additional Diagnoses).

Z74.01 Bed confinement status

Z76.82 Awaiting organ transplant status

Z78 Other specified health status

Code Z78.1, Physical restraint status, may be used when it is documented by the provider that a patient has been put in restraints during the current encounter. Please note that this code should not be reported when it is documented by the provider that a patient is temporarily restrained during a procedure.

Z79 Long-term (current) drug therapy

Codes from this category indicate a patient's continuous use of a prescribed drug (including such things as aspirin therapy) for the long-term treatment of a condition or for prophylactic use. It is not for use for patients who have addictions to drugs. This subcategory is not for use of medications for detoxification or maintenance programs to prevent withdrawal symptoms in patients with drug dependence (e.g., methadone maintenance for opiate dependence). Assign the appropriate code for the drug dependence instead.

Assign a code from Z79 if the patient is receiving a medication for an extended period as a prophylactic measure (such as for the prevention of deep vein thrombosis) or as treatment of a chronic condition (such as arthritis) or a disease requiring a lengthy course of treatment (such as cancer). Do not assign a code from category Z79 for medication being administered for a brief period of time to treat an acute illness or injury (such as a course of antibiotics to treat acute bronchitis).

Z88 Allergy status to drugs, medicaments and biological substances Except: Z88.9, Allergy status to unspecified drugs, medicaments and biological substances status

Z89 Acquired absence of limb

Z90 Acquired absence of organs, not elsewhere classified

Z91.0- Allergy status, other than to drugs and biological substances

Z92.82 Status post administration of tPA (rtPA) in a different facility within the last 24 hours prior to admission to a current facility Assign code Z92.82, Status post administration of tPA (rtPA) in a different facility within the last 24 hours prior to admission to current facility, as a secondary diagnosis when a patient is received by transfer into a facility and documentation indicates they were administered tissue plasminogen activator (tPA) within the last 24 hours prior to admission to the current facility. This guideline applies even if the patient is still receiving the tPA at the time they are received into the current facility. The appropriate code for the condition for which the tPA was administered (such as cerebrovascular disease or myocardial infarction) should be assigned first. Code Z92.82 is only applicable to the receiving facility record and not to the transferring facility record.

Z93 Artificial opening status
Z94 Transplanted organ and tissue status
Z95 Presence of cardiac and vascular implants and grafts
Z96 Presence of other functional implants
Z97 Presence of other devices
Z98 Other postprocedural states

Assign code Z98.85, Transplanted organ removal status, to indicate that a transplanted organ has been previously removed. This code should not be assigned for the encounter in which the transplanted organ is removed. The complication necessitating removal of the transplant organ should be assigned for that encounter.

See section I.C.19. for information on the coding of organ transplant complications.

Z99 Dependence on enabling machines and devices, not elsewhere classified

Note: Categories Z89-Z90 and Z93-Z99 are for use only if there are no complications or malfunctions of the organ or tissue replaced, the amputation site or the equipment on which the patient is dependent.

4) History (of)

There are two types of history Z codes, personal and family. Personal history codes explain a patient's past medical condition that no longer exists and is not receiving any treatment, but that has the potential for recurrence, and therefore may require continued monitoring.

Family history codes are for use when a patient has a family member(s) who has had a particular disease that causes the patient to be at higher risk of also contracting the disease.

Personal history codes may be used in conjunction with follow-up codes and family history codes may be used in conjunction with screening codes to explain the need for a test or procedure. History codes are also acceptable on any medical record regardless of the reason for visit. A history of an illness, even if no longer present, is important information that may alter the type of treatment ordered.

The history Z code categories are:

Z80 Family history of primary malignant neoplasm
Z81 Family history of mental and behavioral disorders
Z82 Family history of certain disabilities and chronic diseases (leading to disablement)
Z83 Family history of other specific disorders
Z84 Family history of other conditions
Z85 Personal history of malignant neoplasm
Z86 Personal history of certain other diseases
Z87 Personal history of other diseases and conditions
Z91.4- Personal history of psychological trauma, not elsewhere classified
Z91.5 Personal history of self-harm
Z91.8- Other specified personal risk factors, not elsewhere classified
Exception:
Z91.83, Wandering in diseases classified elsewhere
Z92 Personal history of medical treatment Except: Z92.0, Personal history of contraception Except: Z92.82, Status post administration of tPA (rtPA) in a different facility within the last 24 hours prior to admission to a current facility

5) Screening

Screening is the testing for disease or disease precursors in seemingly well individuals so that early detection and treatment can be provided for those who test positive for the disease (e.g., screening mammogram).

The testing of a person to rule out or confirm a suspected diagnosis because the patient has some sign or symptom is a diagnostic examination, not a screening. In these cases, the sign or symptom is used to explain the reason for the test.

A screening code may be a first-listed code if the reason for the visit is specifically the screening exam. It may also be used as an additional code if the screening is done during an office visit for other health problems. A screening code is not necessary if the screening is inherent to a routine examination, such as a pap smear done during a routine pelvic examination.

Should a condition be discovered during the screening then the code for the condition may be assigned as an additional diagnosis.

The Z code indicates that a screening exam is planned. A procedure code is required to confirm that the screening was performed.

The screening Z codes/categories:

Z11 Encounter for screening for infectious and parasitic diseases
Z12 Encounter for screening for malignant neoplasms
Z13 Encounter for screening for other diseases and disorders Except: Z13.9, Encounter for screening, unspecified
Z36 Encounter for antenatal screening for mother

6) Observation

There are **three** observation Z code categories. They are for use in very limited circumstances when a person is being observed for a suspected condition that is ruled out. The observation codes are not for use if an injury or illness or any signs or symptoms related to the suspected condition are present. In such cases the diagnosis/symptom code is used with the corresponding external cause code.

The observation codes are to be used as principal diagnosis only. **The only exception to this is when the principal diagnosis is required to be a code from category Z38, Liveborn infants according to place of birth and type of delivery. Then a code from category Z05, Encounter for observation and evaluation of newborn for suspected diseases and conditions ruled out, is sequenced after the Z38 code.** Additional codes may be used in addition to the observation code but only if they are unrelated to the suspected condition being observed.

Codes from subcategory Z03.7 Encounter for suspected maternal and fetal conditions ruled out, may either be used as a first-listed or as an additional code assignment depending on the case. They are for use in very limited circumstances on a maternal record when an encounter is for a suspected maternal or fetal condition that is ruled out during that encounter (for example, a maternal or fetal condition may be suspected due to an abnormal test result). These codes should not be used when the condition is confirmed. In those cases, the confirmed condition should be coded. In addition, these codes are not for use if an illness or any signs or symptoms related to the suspected condition or problem are present. In such cases the diagnosis/symptom code is used.

Additional codes may be used in addition to the code from subcategory Z03.7, but only if they are unrelated to the suspected condition being evaluated.

Codes from subcategory Z03.7 may not be used for encounters for antenatal screening of mother. *See Section I.C.21. Screening.*

For encounters for suspected fetal condition that are inconclusive following testing and evaluation, assign the appropriate code from category O35, O36, O40 or O41.

The observation Z code categories:

Z03 Encounter for medical observation for suspected diseases and conditions ruled out
Z04 Encounter for examination and observation for other reasons Except: Z04.9, Encounter for examination and observation for unspecified reason
Z05 Encounter for observation and evaluation of newborn for suspected diseases and conditions ruled out

7) Aftercare

Aftercare visit codes cover situations when the initial treatment of a disease has been performed and the patient requires continued care during the healing or recovery phase, or for the long-term consequences of the disease. The aftercare Z code should not be used if treatment is directed at a current, acute disease. The diagnosis code is to be used in these cases.

Exceptions to this rule are codes Z51.0, Encounter for antineoplastic radiation therapy, and codes from subcategory Z51.1, Encounter for antineoplastic chemotherapy and immunotherapy. These codes are to be first-listed, followed by the diagnosis code when a patient's encounter is solely to receive radiation therapy, chemotherapy, or immunotherapy for the treatment of a neoplasm. If the reason for the encounter is more than one type of antineoplastic therapy, code Z51.0 and a code from subcategory Z51.1 may be assigned together, in which case one of these codes would be reported as a secondary diagnosis.

The aftercare Z codes should also not be used for aftercare for injuries. For aftercare of an injury, assign the acute injury code with the appropriate 7th character (for subsequent encounter).

The aftercare codes are generally first-listed to explain the specific reason for the encounter. An aftercare code may be used as an additional code when some type of aftercare is provided in addition to the reason for admission and no diagnosis code is applicable. An example of this would be the closure of a colostomy during an encounter for treatment of another condition.

Aftercare codes should be used in conjunction with other aftercare codes or diagnosis codes to provide better detail on the specifics of an aftercare encounter visit, unless otherwise directed by the classification. Should a patient receive multiple types of antineoplastic therapy during the same encounter, code Z51.0, Encounter for antineoplastic radiation therapy, and codes from subcategory Z51.1, Encounter for antineoplastic chemotherapy and immunotherapy, may be used together on a record. The sequencing of multiple aftercare codes depends on the circumstances of the encounter.

Certain aftercare Z code categories need a secondary diagnosis code to describe the resolving condition or sequelae. For others, the condition is included in the code title.

Additional Z code aftercare category terms include fitting and adjustment, and attention to artificial openings.

Status Z codes may be used with aftercare Z codes to indicate the nature of the aftercare. For example code Z95.1, Presence of aortocoronary bypass graft, may be used with code Z48.812, Encounter for surgical aftercare following surgery on the circulatory system, to indicate the surgery for which the aftercare is being performed. A status code should not be used when the aftercare code indicates the type of status, such as using Z43.0, Encounter for attention to tracheostomy, with Z93.0, Tracheostomy status.

The aftercare Z category/codes:

Z42	Encounter for plastic and reconstructive surgery following medical procedure or healed injury
Z43	Encounter for attention to artificial openings
Z44	Encounter for fitting and adjustment of external prosthetic device
Z45	Encounter for adjustment and management of implanted device
Z46	Encounter for fitting and adjustment of other devices
Z47	Orthopedic aftercare
Z48	Encounter for other postprocedural aftercare
Z49	Encounter for care involving renal dialysis
Z51	Encounter for other aftercare **and medical care**

8) Follow-up

The follow-up codes are used to explain continuing surveillance following completed treatment of a disease, condition, or injury. They imply that the condition has been fully treated and no longer exists. They should not be confused with aftercare codes, or injury codes with a 7th character for subsequent encounter, that explain ongoing care of a healing condition or its sequelae. Follow-up codes may be used in conjunction with history codes to provide the full picture of the healed condition and its treatment. The follow-up code is sequenced first, followed by the history code.

A follow-up code may be used to explain multiple visits. Should a condition be found to have recurred on the follow-up visit, then the diagnosis code for the condition should be assigned in place of the follow-up code.

The follow-up Z code categories:

Z08	Encounter for follow-up examination after completed treatment for malignant neoplasm
Z09	Encounter for follow-up examination after completed treatment for conditions other than malignant neoplasm
Z39	Encounter for maternal postpartum care and examination

9) Donor

Codes in category Z52, Donors of organs and tissues, are used for living individuals who are donating blood or other body tissue. These codes are only for individuals donating for others, not for self-donations. They are not used to identify cadaveric donations.

10) Counseling

Counseling Z codes are used when a patient or family member receives assistance in the aftermath of an illness or injury, or when support is required in coping with family or social problems. They are not used in conjunction with a diagnosis code when the counseling component of care is considered integral to standard treatment.

The counseling Z codes/categories:

Z30.0-	Encounter for general counseling and advice on contraception
Z31.5	Encounter for genetic counseling
Z31.6-	Encounter for general counseling and advice on procreation
Z32.2	Encounter for childbirth instruction
Z32.3	Encounter for childcare instruction
Z69	Encounter for mental health services for victim and perpetrator of abuse
Z70	Counseling related to sexual attitude, behavior and orientation
Z71	Persons encountering health services for other counseling and medical advice, not elsewhere classified
Z76.81	Expectant mother prebirth pediatrician visit

11) Encounters for Obstetrical and Reproductive Services

See Section I.C.15. Pregnancy, Childbirth, and the Puerperium, for further instruction on the use of these codes.

Z codes for pregnancy are for use in those circumstances when none of the problems or complications included in the codes from the Obstetrics chapter exist (a routine prenatal visit or postpartum care). Codes in category Z34, Encounter for supervision of normal pregnancy, are always first listed and are not to be used with any other code from the OB chapter.

Codes in category Z3A, Weeks of gestation, may be assigned to provide additional information about the pregnancy. **Category Z3A codes should not be assigned for pregnancies with abortive outcomes (categories O00-O08), elective termination of pregnancy (code Z33.32), nor for postpartum conditions, as category Z3A is not applicable to these conditions.** The date of the admission should be used to determine weeks of gestation for inpatient admissions that encompass more than one gestational week.

The outcome of delivery, category Z37, should be included on all maternal delivery records. It is always a secondary code. Codes in category Z37 should not be used on the newborn record.

Z codes for family planning (contraceptive) or procreative management and counseling should be included on an obstetric record either during the pregnancy or the postpartum stage, if applicable.

Z codes/categories for obstetrical and reproductive services:

Z30	Encounter for contraceptive management
Z31	Encounter for procreative management
Z32.2	Encounter for childbirth instruction
Z32.3	Encounter for childcare instruction
Z33	Pregnant state
Z34	Encounter for supervision of normal pregnancy
Z36	Encounter for antenatal screening of mother
Z3A	Weeks of gestation
Z37	Outcome of delivery
Z39	Encounter for maternal postpartum care and examination
Z76.81	Expectant mother prebirth pediatrician visit

12) Newborns and Infants

See Section I.C.16. Newborn (Perinatal) Guidelines, for further instruction on the use of these codes.

Newborn Z codes/categories:

Z76.1	Encounter for health supervision and care of foundling
Z00.1-	Encounter for routine child health examination
Z38	Liveborn infants according to place of birth and type of delivery

13) Routine and administrative examinations

The Z codes allow for the description of encounters for routine examinations, such as, a general check-up, or, examinations for administrative purposes, such as, a pre-employment physical. The codes are not to be used if the examination is for diagnosis of a suspected condition or for treatment purposes. In such cases the diagnosis code is used. During a routine exam, should a diagnosis or condition be discovered, it should be coded as an additional code. Pre-existing and chronic conditions and history codes may also be included as additional codes as long as the examination is for administrative purposes and not focused on any particular condition.

Some of the codes for routine health examinations distinguish between "with" and "without" abnormal findings. Code assignment depends on the information that is known at the time the encounter is being coded. For example, if no abnormal findings were found during the examination, but the encounter is being coded before test results are back, it is acceptable to assign the code for "without abnormal findings." When assigning a code for "with abnormal findings," additional code(s) should be assigned to identify the specific abnormal finding(s).

Pre-operative examination and pre-procedural laboratory examination Z codes are for use only in those situations when a patient is being cleared for a procedure or surgery and no treatment is given.

The Z codes/categories for routine and administrative examinations:

Z00	Encounter for general examination without complaint, suspected or reported diagnosis
Z01	Encounter for other special examination without complaint, suspected or reported diagnosis
Z02	Encounter for administrative examination Except: Z02.9, Encounter for administrative examinations, unspecified
Z32.0-	Encounter for pregnancy test

14) Miscellaneous Z codes

The miscellaneous Z codes capture a number of other health care encounters that do not fall into one of the other categories. Certain of these codes identify the reason for the encounter; others are for use as additional codes that provide useful information on circumstances that may affect a patient's care and treatment.

Prophylactic Organ Removal

For encounters specifically for prophylactic removal of an organ (such as prophylactic removal of breasts due to a genetic susceptibility to cancer or a family history of cancer), the principal or first-listed code should be a code from category Z40, Encounter for prophylactic surgery, followed by the appropriate codes to identify the associated risk factor (such as genetic susceptibility or family history).

If the patient has a malignancy of one site and is having prophylactic removal at another site to prevent either a new primary malignancy or metastatic disease, a code for the malignancy should also be assigned in addition to a code from subcategory Z40.0, Encounter for prophylactic surgery for risk factors related to malignant neoplasms. A Z40.0 code should not be assigned if the patient is having organ removal for treatment of a malignancy, such as the removal of the testes for the treatment of prostate cancer.

Miscellaneous Z codes/categories:

Z28	Immunization not carried out Except: Z28.3, Underimmunization status
Z29	**Encounter for other prophylactic measures**
Z40	Encounter for prophylactic surgery
Z41	Encounter for procedures for purposes other than remedying health state Except: Z41.9, Encounter for procedure for purposes other than remedying health state, unspecified
Z53	Persons encountering health services for specific procedures and treatment, not carried out
Z55	Problems related to education and literacy
Z56	Problems related to employment and unemployment
Z57	Occupational exposure to risk factors
Z58	Problems related to physical environment
Z59	Problems related to housing and economic circumstances
Z60	Problems related to social environment
Z62	Problems related to upbringing
Z63	Other problems related to primary support group, including family circumstances
Z64	Problems related to certain psychosocial circumstances
Z65	Problems related to other psychosocial circumstances
Z72	Problems related to lifestyle **Note: These codes should be assigned only when the documentation specifies that the patient has an associated problem**
Z73	Problems related to life management difficulty
Z74	Problems related to care provider dependency Except: Z74.01, Bed confinement status
Z75	Problems related to medical facilities and other health care
Z76.0	Encounter for issue of repeat prescription
Z76.3	Healthy person accompanying sick person
Z76.4	Other boarder to healthcare facility
Z76.5	Malingerer [conscious simulation]
Z91.1-	Patient's noncompliance with medical treatment and regimen
Z91.83	Wandering in diseases classified elsewhere
Z91.89	Other specified personal risk factors, not elsewhere classified

15) Nonspecific Z codes

Certain Z codes are so non-specific, or potentially redundant with other codes in the classification, that there can be little justification for their use in the inpatient setting. Their use in the outpatient setting should be limited to those instances when there is no further documentation to permit more precise coding. Otherwise, any sign or symptom or any other reason for visit that is captured in another code should be used.

Nonspecific Z codes/categories:

Z02.9	Encounter for administrative examinations, unspecified
Z04.9	Encounter for examination and observation for unspecified reason
Z13.9	Encounter for screening, unspecified
Z41.9	Encounter for procedure for purposes other than remedying health state, unspecified
Z52.9	Donor of unspecified organ or tissue
Z86.59	Personal history of other mental and behavioral disorders
Z88.9	Allergy status to unspecified drugs, medicaments and biological substances status
Z92.0	Personal history of contraception

16) Z Codes That May Only be Principal/First-Listed Diagnosis

The following Z codes/categories may only be reported as the principal/first-listed diagnosis, except when there are multiple encounters on the same day and the medical records for the encounters are combined:

Z00	Encounter for general examination without complaint, suspected or reported diagnosis Except: Z00.6
Z01	Encounter for other special examination without complaint, suspected or reported diagnosis
Z02	Encounter for administrative examination
Z03	Encounter for medical observation for suspected diseases and conditions ruled out
Z04	Encounter for examination and observation for other reasons
Z33.2	Encounter for elective termination of pregnancy
Z31.81	Encounter for male factor infertility in female patient
Z31.83	Encounter for assisted reproductive fertility procedure cycle
Z31.84	Encounter for fertility preservation procedure
Z34	Encounter for supervision of normal pregnancy
Z39	Encounter for maternal postpartum care and examination
Z38	Liveborn infants according to place of birth and type of delivery
Z42	Encounter for plastic and reconstructive surgery following medical procedure or healed injury
Z51.0	Encounter for antineoplastic radiation therapy
Z51.1-	Encounter for antineoplastic chemotherapy and immunotherapy
Z52	Donors of organs and tissues Except: Z52.9, Donor of unspecified organ or tissue
Z76.1	Encounter for health supervision and care of foundling
Z76.2	Encounter for health supervision and care of other healthy infant and child
Z99.12	Encounter for respirator [ventilator] dependence during power failure

CHAPTER 21

FACTORS INFLUENCING HEALTH STATUS AND CONTACT WITH HEALTH SERVICES (Z00-Z99)

Note: Z codes represent reasons for encounters. A corresponding procedure code must accompany a Z code if a procedure is performed. Categories Z00-Z99 are provided for occasions when circumstances other than a disease, injury or external cause classifiable to categories A00-Y89 are recorded as 'diagnoses' or 'problems.' This can arise in two main ways:

(a) When a person who may or may not be sick encounters the health services for some specific purpose, such as to receive limited care or service for a current condition, to donate an organ or tissue, to receive prophylactic vaccination (immunization), or to discuss a problem which is in itself not a disease or injury.

(b) When some circumstance or problem is present which influences the person's health status but is not in itself a current illness or injury.

This chapter contains the following blocks:

Z00-Z13	Persons encountering health services for examination
Z14-Z15	Genetic carrier and genetic susceptibility to disease
Z16	Resistance to antimicrobial drugs
Z17	Estrogen receptor status
Z18	Retained foreign body fragments
Z19	Hormone sensitivity malignancy status ◀
Z20-Z29	Persons with potential health hazards related to communicable diseases ◀
Z30-Z39	Persons encountering health services in circumstances related to reproduction
Z40-Z53	Encounters for other specific health care
Z55-Z65	Persons with potential health hazards related to socioeconomic and psychosocial circumstances
Z66	Do not resuscitate status
Z67	Blood type
Z68	Body mass index (BMI)
Z69-Z76	Persons encountering health services in other circumstances
Z77-Z99	Persons with potential health hazards related to family and personal history and certain conditions influencing health status

PERSONS ENCOUNTERING HEALTH SERVICES FOR EXAMINATIONS (Z00-Z13)

Note: Nonspecific abnormal findings disclosed at the time of these examinations are classified to categories R70-R94.

Excludes1 examinations related to pregnancy and reproduction (Z30-Z36, Z39.-)

● **Z00 Encounter for general examination without complaint, suspected or reported diagnosis**

Excludes1 encounter for examination for administrative purposes (Z02.-)

Excludes2 encounter for pre-procedural examinations (Z01.81-)
special screening examinations (Z11-Z13)

● **Z00.0 Encounter for general adult medical examination**
Encounter for adult periodic examination (annual) (physical) and any associated laboratory and radiologic examinations

Excludes1 encounter for examination of sign or symptom - code to sign or symptom
general health check-up of infant or child (Z00.12.-)

● **Z00.00 Encounter for general adult medical examination without abnormal findings** A
Encounter for adult health check-up NOS
Coding Clinic: 2016, Q1, P37

● **Z00.01 Encounter for general adult medical examination with abnormal findings** A
Use additional code to identify abnormal findings
Coding Clinic: 2016, Q1, P36

● **Z00.1 Encounter for newborn, infant and child health examinations**

● **Z00.11 Newborn health examination**
Health check for child under 29 days old
Use additional code to identify any abnormal findings

Excludes1 health check for child over 28 days old (Z00.12-)

● **Z00.110 Health examination for newborn under 8 days old** N
Health check for newborn under 8 days old

● **Z00.111 Health examination for newborn 8 to 28 days old** N
Health check for newborn 8 to 28 days old
Newborn weight check

● **Z00.12 Encounter for routine child health examination**
Encounter for development testing of infant or child
Health check (routine) for child over 28 days old

Excludes1 health check for child under 29 days old (Z00.11-)
health supervision of foundling or other healthy infant or child (Z76.1-Z76.2)
newborn health examination (Z00.11-)

● **Z00.121 Encounter for routine child health examination with abnormal findings** P
Use additional code to identify abnormal findings
Coding Clinic: 2016, Q1, P34-35

● **Z00.129 Encounter for routine child health examination without abnormal findings** P
Encounter for routine child health examination NOS
Coding Clinic: 2016, Q1, P34

● **Z00.2 Encounter for examination for period of rapid growth in childhood** P

● **Z00.3 Encounter for examination for adolescent development state** P
Encounter for puberty development state

● **Z00.5 Encounter for examination of potential donor of organ and tissue**

Z00.6 Encounter for examination for normal comparison and control in clinical research program
Examination of participant or control in clinical research program

● **Z00.7 Encounter for examination for period of delayed growth in childhood**

● **Z00.70 Encounter for examination for period of delayed growth in childhood without abnormal findings** P

● **Z00.71 Encounter for examination for period of delayed growth in childhood with abnormal findings** P
Use additional code to identify abnormal findings

● **Z00.8 Encounter for other general examination**
Encounter for health examination in population surveys

Z01 Encounter for other special examination without complaint, suspected or reported diagnosis

Includes routine examination of specific system

Note: Codes from category Z01 represent the reason for the encounter. A separate procedure code is required to identify any examinations or procedures performed.

Excludes1 encounter for examination for administrative purposes (Z02.-)
encounter for examination for suspected conditions, proven not to exist (Z03.-)
encounter for laboratory and radiologic examinations as a component of general medical examinations (Z00.0-)
encounter for laboratory, radiologic and imaging examinations for sign(s) and symptom(s) - code to the sign(s) or symptom(s)

Excludes2 screening examinations (Z11-Z13)

Z01.0 Encounter for examination of eyes and vision

Excludes1 examination for driving license (Z02.4)

Z01.00 Encounter for examination of eyes and vision without abnormal findings
Encounter for examination of eyes and vision NOS

Z01.01 Encounter for examination of eyes and vision with abnormal findings
Use additional code to identify abnormal findings

Z01.1 Encounter for examination of ears and hearing

Z01.10 Encounter for examination of ears and hearing without abnormal findings
Encounter for examination of ears and hearing NOS

Z01.11 Encounter for examination of ears and hearing with abnormal findings

Z01.110 Encounter for hearing examination following failed hearing screening

Z01.118 Encounter for examination of ears and hearing with other abnormal findings
Use additional code to identify abnormal findings

Z01.12 Encounter for hearing conservation and treatment

Z01.2 Encounter for dental examination and cleaning

Z01.20 Encounter for dental examination and cleaning without abnormal findings
Encounter for dental examination and cleaning NOS

Z01.21 Encounter for dental examination and cleaning with abnormal findings
Use additional code to identify abnormal findings

Z01.3 Encounter for examination of blood pressure

Z01.30 Encounter for examination of blood pressure without abnormal findings
Encounter for examination of blood pressure NOS

Z01.31 Encounter for examination of blood pressure with abnormal findings
Use additional code to identify abnormal findings

Z01.4 Encounter for gynecological examination

Excludes2 pregnancy examination or test (Z32.0-)
routine examination for contraceptive maintenance (Z30.4-)

Z01.41 Encounter for routine gynecological examination
Encounter for general gynecological examination with or without cervical smear
Encounter for gynecological examination (general) (routine) NOS
Encounter for pelvic examination (annual) (periodic)
Use additional code:
for screening for human papillomavirus, if applicable (Z11.51)
for screening vaginal pap smear, if applicable (Z12.72)
to identify acquired absence of uterus, if applicable (Z90.71-)

Excludes1 gynecologic examination status-post hysterectomy for malignant condition (Z08)
screening cervical pap smear not a part of a routine gynecological examination (Z12.4)

Z01.411 Encounter for gynecological examination (general) (routine) with abnormal findings ♀
Use additional code to identify any abnormal findings ◀

Z01.419 Encounter for gynecological examination (general) (routine) without abnormal findings ♀

Z01.42 Encounter for cervical smear to confirm findings of recent normal smear following initial abnormal smear ♀

Z01.8 Encounter for other specified special examinations

Z01.81 Encounter for preprocedural examinations
Encounter for preoperative examinations
Encounter for radiological and imaging examinations as part of preprocedural examination

Z01.810 Encounter for preprocedural cardiovascular examination

Z01.811 Encounter for preprocedural respiratory examination

Z01.812 Encounter for preprocedural laboratory examination
Blood and urine tests prior to treatment or procedure

Z01.818 Encounter for other preprocedural examination
Encounter for preprocedural examination NOS
Encounter for examinations prior to antineoplastic chemotherapy

Z01.82 Encounter for allergy testing

Excludes1 encounter for antibody response examination (Z01.84)

Z01.83 Encounter for blood typing
Encounter for Rh typing

Z01.84 Encounter for antibody response examination
Encounter for immunity status testing

Excludes1 encounter for allergy testing (Z01.82)

Z01.89 Encounter for other specified special examinations

Z02 Encounter for administrative examination

Z02.0 Encounter for examination for admission to educational institution

Encounter for examination for admission to preschool (education)

Encounter for examination for re-admission to school following illness or medical treatment

Z02.1 Encounter for pre-employment examination

Z02.2 Encounter for examination for admission to residential institution

Excludes1 examination for admission to prison (Z02.89)

Z02.3 Encounter for examination for recruitment to armed forces

Z02.4 Encounter for examination for driving license

Z02.5 Encounter for examination for participation in sport

Excludes1 blood-alcohol and blood-drug test (Z02.83)

Z02.6 Encounter for examination for insurance purposes

Z02.7 Encounter for issue of medical certificate

Excludes1 encounter for general medical examination (Z00-Z01, Z02.0-Z02.6, Z02.8-Z02.9)

Z02.71 Encounter for disability determination

Encounter for issue of medical certificate of incapacity

Encounter for issue of medical certificate of invalidity

Z02.79 Encounter for issue of other medical certificate

Z02.8 Encounter for other administrative examinations

Z02.81 Encounter for paternity testing

Z02.82 Encounter for adoption services

Z02.83 Encounter for blood-alcohol and blood-drug test

Use additional code for findings of alcohol or drugs in blood (R78.-)

Z02.89 Encounter for other administrative examinations

Encounter for examination for admission to prison

Encounter for examination for admission to summer camp

Encounter for immigration examination

Encounter for naturalization examination

Encounter for premarital examination

Excludes1 health supervision of foundling or other healthy infant or child (Z76.1-Z76.2)

Z02.9 Encounter for administrative examinations, unspecified

OGCR Section II.C.21.c.6.

Observation

There are **three** observation Z code categories. They are for use in very limited circumstances when a person is being observed for a suspected condition that is ruled out. The observation codes are not for use if an injury or illnesses or any signs or symptoms related to the suspected condition are present. In such cases the diagnosis/symptom code is used with the corresponding external cause code.

The observation codes are to be used as principal diagnosis only. **The only exception to this is when the principal diagnosis is required to be a code from category Z38, Liveborn infants according to place of birth and type of delivery. Then a code from category Z05, Encounter for observation and evaluation of newborn for suspected diseases and conditions ruled out, is sequenced after the Z38 code.** Additional codes may be used in addition to the observation code but only if they are unrelated to the suspected condition being observed.

Codes from subcategory Z03.7 Encounter for suspected maternal and fetal conditions ruled out, may either be used as a first listed or as an additional code assignment depending on the case. They are for use in very limited circumstances on a maternal record when an encounter is for a suspected maternal or fetal condition that is ruled out during that encounter (for example, a maternal or fetal condition may be suspected due to an abnormal test result). These codes should not be used when the condition is confirmed. In those cases, the confirmed condition should be coded. In addition, these codes are not for use if an illness or any signs or symptoms related to the suspected condition or problem are present. In such cases the diagnosis/symptom code is used.

Additional codes may be used in addition to the code from subcategory Z03.7, but only if they are unrelated to the suspected condition being evaluated.

Codes from subcategory Z03.7 may not be used for encounters for antenatal screening of mother. *See Section I.C.21. Screening.*

For encounters for suspected fetal condition that are inconclusive following testing and evaluation, assign the appropriate code from category O35, O36, O40 or O41.

The observation Z code categories:

Z03 Encounter for medical observation for suspected diseases and conditions ruled out

Z04 Encounter for examination and observation for other reasons
Except: Z04.9, Encounter for examination and observation for unspecified reason

Z05 Encounter for observation and evaluation of newborn for suspected diseases and conditions ruled out

Z03 Encounter for medical observation for suspected diseases and conditions ruled out

This category is to be used when a person without a diagnosis is suspected of having an abnormal condition, without signs or symptoms, which requires study, but after examination and observation, is ruled out. This category is also for use for administrative and legal observation status.

Excludes1 contact with and (suspected) exposures hazardous to health (Z77.-)

newborn observation for suspected condition, ruled out (P00-P04)

person with feared complaint in whom no diagnosis is made (Z71.1)

signs or symptoms under study - code to signs or symptoms

Z03.6 Encounter for observation for suspected toxic effect from ingested substance ruled out

Encounter for observation for suspected adverse effect from drug

Encounter for observation for suspected poisoning

Z03.7 Encounter for suspected maternal and fetal conditions ruled out
Encounter for suspected maternal and fetal conditions not found
Excludes1 known or suspected fetal anomalies affecting management of mother, not ruled out (O26.-, O35.-, O36.-, O40.-, O41.-)

Z03.71 Encounter for suspected problem with amniotic cavity and membrane ruled out ♀ M
Encounter for suspected oligohydramnios ruled out
Encounter for suspected polyhydramnios ruled out

Z03.72 Encounter for suspected placental problem ruled out ♀ M

Z03.73 Encounter for suspected fetal anomaly ruled out ♀ M

Z03.74 Encounter for suspected problem with fetal growth ruled out ♀ M

Z03.75 Encounter for suspected cervical shortening ruled out ♀ M

Z03.79 Encounter for other suspected maternal and fetal conditions ruled out ♀ M

Z03.8 Encounter for observation for other suspected diseases and conditions ruled out

Z03.81 Encounter for observation for suspected exposure to biological agents ruled out

Z03.810 Encounter for observation for suspected exposure to anthrax ruled out

Z03.818 Encounter for observation for suspected exposure to other biological agents ruled out

Z03.89 Encounter for observation for other suspected diseases and conditions ruled out

Z04 Encounter for examination and observation for other reasons
Includes encounter for examination for medicolegal reasons
This category is to be used when a person without a diagnosis is suspected of having an abnormal condition, without signs or symptoms, which requires study, but after examination and observation, is ruled-out. This category is also for use for administrative and legal observation status.

Z04.1 Encounter for examination and observation following transport accident
Excludes1 encounter for examination and observation following work accident (Z04.2)

Z04.2 Encounter for examination and observation following work accident

Z04.3 Encounter for examination and observation following other accident

Z04.4 Encounter for examination and observation following alleged rape
Encounter for examination and observation of victim following alleged rape
Encounter for examination and observation of victim following alleged sexual abuse

Z04.41 Encounter for examination and observation following alleged adult rape A
Suspected adult rape, ruled out
Suspected adult sexual abuse, ruled out

Z04.42 Encounter for examination and observation following alleged child rape P
Suspected child rape, ruled out
Suspected child sexual abuse, ruled out

Z04.6 Encounter for general psychiatric examination, requested by authority

Z04.7 Encounter for examination and observation following alleged physical abuse

Z04.71 Encounter for examination and observation following alleged adult physical abuse A
Suspected adult physical abuse, ruled out
Excludes1 confirmed case of adult physical abuse (T74.-)
encounter for examination and observation following alleged adult sexual abuse (Z04.41)
suspected case of adult physical abuse, not ruled out (T76.-)

Z04.72 Encounter for examination and observation following alleged child physical abuse P
Suspected child physical abuse, ruled out
Excludes1 confirmed case of child physical abuse (T74.-)
encounter for examination and observation following alleged child sexual abuse (Z04.42)
suspected case of child physical abuse, not ruled out (T76.-)

Z04.8 Encounter for examination and observation for other specified reasons
Encounter for examination and observation for request for expert evidence

Z04.9 Encounter for examination and observation for unspecified reason
Encounter for observation NOS

Z05 Encounter for observation and evaluation of newborn for suspected diseases and conditions ruled out ◀
This category is to be used for newborns, within the neonatal period (the first 28 days of life), who are suspected of having an abnormal condition unrelated to exposure from the mother or the birth process, but without signs or symptoms, and which, after examination and observation, is ruled out. ◀
Excludes2 newborn observation for suspected condition, related to exposure from the mother or birth process (P00-P04) ◀

Z05.0 Observation and evaluation of newborn for suspected cardiac condition ruled out ◀

Z05.1 Observation and evaluation of newborn for suspected infectious condition ruled out ◀

Z05.2 Observation and evaluation of newborn for suspected neurological condition ruled out ◀

Z05.3 Observation and evaluation of newborn for suspected respiratory condition ruled out ◀

Z05.4 Observation and evaluation of newborn for suspected genetic, metabolic or immunologic condition ruled out ◀

Z05.41 Observation and evaluation of newborn for suspected genetic condition ruled out ◀

Z05.42 Observation and evaluation of newborn for suspected metabolic condition ruled out ◀

Z05.43 Observation and evaluation of newborn for suspected immunologic condition ruled out ◀

Z05.5 Observation and evaluation of newborn for suspected gastrointestinal condition ruled out ◀

Z05.6 Observation and evaluation of newborn for suspected genitourinary condition ruled out ◀

Z05.7 Observation and evaluation of newborn for suspected skin, subcutaneous, musculoskeletal and connective tissue condition ruled out ◀

Z05.71 Observation and evaluation of newborn for suspected skin and subcutaneous tissue condition ruled out ◀

Z05.72 Observation and evaluation of newborn for suspected musculoskeletal condition ruled out ◀

Z05.73 Observation and evaluation of newborn for suspected connective tissue condition ruled out ◀

● **Z05.8 Observation and evaluation of newborn for other specified suspected condition ruled out** ◀

● **Z05.9 Observation and evaluation of newborn for unspecified suspected condition ruled out** ◀

OGCR See Section II.C.21.c.8.

The follow-up codes are used to explain continuing surveillance following completed treatment of a disease, condition, or injury. They imply that the condition has been fully treated and no longer exists. They should not be confused with aftercare codes, or injury codes with 7th character "D," that explain ongoing care of a healing condition or its sequelae. Follow-up codes may be used in conjunction with history codes to provide the full picture of the healed condition and its treatment. The follow-up code is sequenced first, followed by the history code.

A follow-up code may be used to explain multiple visits. Should a condition be found to have recurred on the follow-up visit, then the diagnosis code for the condition should be assigned in place of the follow-up code.

The follow-up Z code categories:

Z08 Encounter for follow-up examination after completed treatment for malignant neoplasm

Z09 Encounter for follow-up examination after completed treatment for conditions other than malignant neoplasm

Z39 Encounter for maternal postpartum care and examination

● **Z08 Encounter for follow-up examination after completed treatment for malignant neoplasm**

Medical surveillance following completed treatment

Use additional code to identify any acquired absence of organs (Z90.-)

Use additional code to identify the personal history of malignant neoplasm (Z85.-)

Excludes1 aftercare following medical care (Z43-Z49, Z51)

● **Z09 Encounter for follow-up examination after completed treatment for conditions other than malignant neoplasm**

Medical surveillance following completed treatment

Use additional code to identify any applicable history of disease code (Z86.-. Z87.-)

Excludes1 aftercare following medical care (Z43-Z49, Z51)
surveillance of contraception (Z30.4-)
surveillance of prosthetic and other medical devices (Z44-Z46)

Coding Clinic: 2015, Q1, P8

OGCR Section II.C.21.c.5.

Screening

Screening is the testing for disease or disease precursors in seemingly well individuals so that early detection and treatment can be provided for those who test positive for the disease (e.g., screening mammogram).

The testing of a person to rule out or confirm a suspected diagnosis because the patient has some sign or symptom is a diagnostic examination, not a screening. In these cases, the sign or symptom is used to explain the reason for the test.

A screening code may be a first listed code if the reason for the visit is specifically the screening exam. It may also be used as an additional code if the screening is done during an office visit for other health problems. A screening code is not necessary if the screening is inherent to a routine examination, such as a pap smear done during a routine pelvic examination.

Should a condition be discovered during the screening then the code for the condition may be assigned as an additional diagnosis.

The Z code indicates that a screening exam is planned. A procedure code is required to confirm that the screening was performed.

The screening Z codes /categories:

Z11 Encounter for screening for infectious and parasitic diseases

Z12 Encounter for screening for malignant neoplasms

Z13 Encounter for screening for other diseases and disorders
Except: Z13.9, Encounter for screening, unspecified

Z36 Encounter for antenatal screening for mother

● **Z11 Encounter for screening for infectious and parasitic diseases**

Screening is the testing for disease or disease precursors in asymptomatic individuals so that early detection and treatment can be provided for those who test positive for the disease.

Excludes1 encounter for diagnostic examination - code to sign or symptom

● **Z11.0 Encounter for screening for intestinal infectious diseases**

● **Z11.1 Encounter for screening for respiratory tuberculosis**

● **Z11.2 Encounter for screening for other bacterial diseases**

● **Z11.3 Encounter for screening for infections with a predominantly sexual mode of transmission**

Excludes2 encounter for screening for human immunodeficiency virus [HIV] (Z11.4)
encounter for screening for human papillomavirus (Z11.51)

● **Z11.4 Encounter for screening for human immunodeficiency virus [HIV]**

● **Z11.5 Encounter for screening for other viral diseases**

Excludes2 encounter for screening for viral intestinal disease (Z11.0)

● **Z11.51 Encounter for screening for human papillomavirus (HPV)**

● **Z11.59 Encounter for screening for other viral diseases**

● **Z11.6 Encounter for screening for other protozoal diseases and helminthiases**

Diseases or infestations caused by parasitic worms

Excludes2 encounter for screening for protozoal intestinal disease (Z11.0)

● **Z11.8 Encounter for screening for other infectious and parasitic diseases**

Encounter for screening for chlamydia
Encounter for screening for rickettsial
Encounter for screening for spirochetal
Encounter for screening for mycoses

● **Z11.9 Encounter for screening for infectious and parasitic diseases, unspecified**

● **Z12 Encounter for screening for malignant neoplasms**

Screening is the testing for disease or disease precursors in asymptomatic individuals so that early detection and treatment can be provided for those who test positive for the disease.

Use additional code to identify any family history of malignant neoplasm (Z80.-)

Excludes1 encounter for diagnostic examination - code to sign or symptom

● **Z12.0 Encounter for screening for malignant neoplasm of stomach**

● **Z12.1 Encounter for screening for malignant neoplasm of intestinal tract**

● **Z12.10 Encounter for screening for malignant neoplasm of intestinal tract, unspecified**

● **Z12.11 Encounter for screening for malignant neoplasm of colon**

Encounter for screening colonoscopy NOS

● **Z12.12 Encounter for screening for malignant neoplasm of rectum**

● **Z12.13 Encounter for screening for malignant neoplasm of small intestine**

● **Z12.2 Encounter for screening for malignant neoplasm of respiratory organs**

● **Z12.3 Encounter for screening for malignant neoplasm of breast**

● **Z12.31 Encounter for screening mammogram for malignant neoplasm of breast**

Excludes1 inconclusive mammogram (R92.2)

Coding Clinic: 2015, Q1, P24

● **Z12.39 Encounter for other screening for malignant neoplasm of breast**

- **Z12.4 Encounter for screening for malignant neoplasm of cervix ♀**
  Encounter for screening pap smear for malignant neoplasm of cervix
  Excludes1 when screening is part of general gynecological examination (Z01.4-)
  Excludes2 encounter for screening for human papillomavirus (Z11.51) ◀
- **Z12.5 Encounter for screening for malignant neoplasm of prostate ♂**
- **Z12.6 Encounter for screening for malignant neoplasm of bladder**
- **Z12.7 Encounter for screening for malignant neoplasm of other genitourinary organs**
  - **Z12.71 Encounter for screening for malignant neoplasm of testis ♂**
  - **Z12.72 Encounter for screening for malignant neoplasm of vagina ♀**
    Vaginal pap smear status - post hysterectomy for non-malignant condition
    Use additional code to identify acquired absence of uterus (Z90.71-)
    Excludes1 vaginal pap smear status - post hysterectomy for malignant conditions (Z08)
  - **Z12.73 Encounter for screening for malignant neoplasm of ovary ♀**
  - **Z12.79 Encounter for screening for malignant neoplasm of other genitourinary organs**
- **Z12.8 Encounter for screening for malignant neoplasm of other sites**
  - **Z12.81 Encounter for screening for malignant neoplasm of oral cavity**
  - **Z12.82 Encounter for screening for malignant neoplasm of nervous system**
  - **Z12.83 Encounter for screening for malignant neoplasm of skin**
  - **Z12.89 Encounter for screening for malignant neoplasm of other sites**
- **Z12.9 Encounter for screening for malignant neoplasm, site unspecified**

- **Z13 Encounter for screening for other diseases and disorders**
  Screening is the testing for disease or disease precursors in asymptomatic individuals so that early detection and treatment can be provided for those who test positive for the disease.
  Excludes1 encounter for diagnostic examination - code to sign or symptom
  - **Z13.0 Encounter for screening for diseases of the blood and blood-forming organs and certain disorders involving the immune mechanism**
  - **Z13.1 Encounter for screening for diabetes mellitus**
  - **Z13.2 Encounter for screening for nutritional, metabolic and other endocrine disorders**
    - **Z13.21 Encounter for screening for nutritional disorder**
    - **Z13.22 Encounter for screening for metabolic disorder**
      - **Z13.220 Encounter for screening for lipoid disorders**
        Encounter for screening for cholesterol level
        Encounter for screening for hypercholesterolemia
        Encounter for screening for hyperlipidemia
      - **Z13.228 Encounter for screening for other metabolic disorders**
    - **Z13.29 Encounter for screening for other suspected endocrine disorder**
      Excludes1 encounter for screening for diabetes mellitus (Z13.1)
  - **Z13.4 Encounter for screening for certain developmental disorders in childhood** P
    Encounter for screening for developmental handicaps in early childhood
    Excludes1 routine development testing of infant or child (Z00.1-)
  - **Z13.5 Encounter for screening for eye and ear disorders**
    Excludes2 encounter for general hearing examination (Z01.1-)
    encounter for general vision examination (Z01.0-)
  - **Z13.6 Encounter for screening for cardiovascular disorders**
  - **Z13.7 Encounter for screening for genetic and chromosomal anomalies**
    Excludes1 genetic testing for procreative management (Z31.4-)
    - **Z13.71 Encounter for nonprocreative screening for genetic disease carrier status**
    - **Z13.79 Encounter for other screening for genetic and chromosomal anomalies**
  - **Z13.8 Encounter for screening for other specified diseases and disorders**
    Excludes2 screening for malignant neoplasms (Z12.-)
    - **Z13.81 Encounter for screening for digestive system disorders**
      - **Z13.810 Encounter for screening for upper gastrointestinal disorder**
      - **Z13.811 Encounter for screening for lower gastrointestinal disorder**
        Excludes1 encounter for screening for intestinal infectious disease (Z11.0)
      - **Z13.818 Encounter for screening for other digestive system disorders**
    - **Z13.82 Encounter for screening for musculoskeletal disorder**
      - **Z13.820 Encounter for screening for osteoporosis**
      - **Z13.828 Encounter for screening for other musculoskeletal disorder**
    - **Z13.83 Encounter for screening for respiratory disorder NEC**
      Excludes1 encounter for screening for respiratory tuberculosis (Z11.1)
    - **Z13.84 Encounter for screening for dental disorders**
    - **Z13.85 Encounter for screening for nervous system disorders**
      - **Z13.850 Encounter for screening for traumatic brain injury**
      - **Z13.858 Encounter for screening for other nervous system disorders**
    - **Z13.88 Encounter for screening for disorder due to exposure to contaminants**
      Excludes1 those exposed to contaminants without suspected disorders (Z57-Z77.-)
    - **Z13.89 Encounter for screening for other disorder**
      Encounter for screening for genitourinary disorders
  - **Z13.9 Encounter for screening, unspecified**

GENETIC CARRIER AND GENETIC SUSCEPTIBILITY TO DISEASE (Z14-Z15)

Z14 Genetic carrier
- **Z14.0 Hemophilia A carrier**
  - **Z14.01 Asymptomatic hemophilia A carrier**
  - **Z14.02 Symptomatic hemophilia A carrier**
- **Z14.1 Cystic fibrosis carrier**
- **Z14.8 Genetic carrier of other disease**

Z15 Genetic susceptibility to disease

Excludes1 chromosomal anomalies (Q90-Q99)

Includes confirmed abnormal gene

Use additional code, if applicable, for any associated family history of the disease (Z80-Z84)

- **Z15.0 Genetic susceptibility to malignant neoplasm**

  Code first if applicable, any current malignant neoplasm (C00-C75, C81-C96)

  Use additional code, if applicable, for any personal history of malignant neoplasm (Z85.-)
  - **Z15.01 Genetic susceptibility to malignant neoplasm of breast**
  - **Z15.02 Genetic susceptibility to malignant neoplasm of ovary ♀**
  - **Z15.03 Genetic susceptibility to malignant neoplasm of prostate ♂**
  - **Z15.04 Genetic susceptibility to malignant neoplasm of endometrium ♀**
  - **Z15.09 Genetic susceptibility to other malignant neoplasm**
- **Z15.8 Genetic susceptibility to other disease**
  - **Z15.81 Genetic susceptibility to multiple endocrine neoplasia [MEN]**

    Excludes1 multiple endocrine neoplasia [MEN] syndromes (E31.2-)
  - **Z15.89 Genetic susceptibility to other disease**

RESISTANCE TO ANTIMICROBIAL DRUGS (Z16)

Z16 Resistance to antimicrobial drugs

Note: The codes in this category are provided for use as additional codes to identify the resistance and non-responsiveness of a condition to antimicrobial drugs.

Code first the infection

Excludes1 Methicillin resistant Staphylococcus aureus infection (A49.02)
Methicillin resistant Staphylococcus aureus infection in diseases classified elsewhere (B95.62)
Methicillin resistant Staphylococcus aureus pneumonia (J15.212)
Sepsis due to Methicillin resistant Staphylococcus aureus (A41.02)

- **Z16.1 Resistance to beta lactam antibiotics**
  - **Z16.10 Resistance to unspecified beta lactam antibiotics**
  - **Z16.11 Resistance to penicillins**
    Resistance to amoxicillin
    Resistance to ampicillin
  - **Z16.12 Extended spectrum beta lactamase (ESBL) resistance**
  - **Z16.19 Resistance to other specified beta lactam antibiotics**
    Resistance to cephalosporins
- **Z16.2 Resistance to other antibiotics**
  - **Z16.20 Resistance to unspecified antibiotic**
    Resistance to antibiotics NOS
  - **Z16.21 Resistance to vancomycin**
  - **Z16.22 Resistance to vancomycin related antibiotics**
  - **Z16.23 Resistance to quinolones and fluoroquinolones**
  - **Z16.24 Resistance to multiple antibiotics**
  - **Z16.29 Resistance to other single specified antibiotic**
    Resistance to aminoglycosides
    Resistance to macrolides
    Resistance to sulfonamides
    Resistance to tetracyclines
- **Z16.3 Resistance to other antimicrobial drugs**

  Excludes1 resistance to antibiotics (Z16.1-, Z16.2-)
  - **Z16.30 Resistance to unspecified antimicrobial drugs**
    Drug resistance NOS
  - **Z16.31 Resistance to antiparasitic drug(s)**
    Resistance to quinine and related compounds
  - **Z16.32 Resistance to antifungal drug(s)**
  - **Z16.33 Resistance to antiviral drug(s)**
  - **Z16.34 Resistance to antimycobacterial drug(s)**
    Resistance to tuberculostatics
    - **Z16.341 Resistance to single antimycobacterial drug**
      Resistance to antimycobacterial drug NOS
    - **Z16.342 Resistance to multiple antimycobacterial drugs**
  - **Z16.35 Resistance to multiple antimicrobial drugs**

    Excludes1 Resistance to multiple antibiotics only (Z16.24)
  - **Z16.39 Resistance to other specified antimicrobial drug**

ESTROGEN RECEPTOR STATUS (Z17)

Z17 Estrogen receptor status

Code first malignant neoplasm of breast (C50.-)
- **Z17.0 Estrogen receptor positive status [ER+]**
- **Z17.1 Estrogen receptor negative status [ER-]**

RETAINED FOREIGN BODY FRAGMENTS (Z18)

Z18 Retained foreign body fragments

Includes embedded fragment (status)
embedded splinter (status)
retained foreign body status

Excludes1 artificial joint prosthesis status (Z96.6-)
foreign body accidentally left during a procedure (T81.5-)
foreign body entering through orifice (T15-T19)
in situ cardiac device (Z95.-)
organ or tissue replaced by means other than transplant (Z96.-, Z97.-)
organ or tissue replaced by transplant (Z94.-)
personal history of retained foreign body fully removed Z87.821
superficial foreign body (non-embedded splinter) - code to superficial foreign body, by site

- **Z18.0 Retained radioactive fragments**
  - **Z18.01 Retained depleted uranium fragments**
  - **Z18.09 Other retained radioactive fragments**
    Other retained depleted isotope fragments
    Retained nontherapeutic radioactive fragments
- **Z18.1 Retained metal fragments**

  Excludes1 retained radioactive metal fragments (Z18.01-Z18.09)
  - **Z18.10 Retained metal fragments, unspecified**
    Retained metal fragment NOS
  - **Z18.11 Retained magnetic metal fragments**
  - **Z18.12 Retained nonmagnetic metal fragments**
- **Z18.2 Retained plastic fragments**
  Acrylics fragments
  Diethylhexylphthalates fragments
  Isocyanate fragments
- **Z18.3 Retained organic fragments**
  - **Z18.31 Retained animal quills or spines**
  - **Z18.32 Retained tooth**
  - **Z18.33 Retained wood fragments**
  - **Z18.39 Other retained organic fragments**

◀ New ◀ Revised ~~deleted~~ Deleted Excludes 1 Excludes 2 Includes Use additional Code first Code also Unspecified
OGCR Official Guidelines ● Unacceptable Principal Diagnosis X Assign placeholder X ● Use Additional Character(s) ▶ Manifestation Code Coding Clinic

- **Z18.8 Other specified retained foreign body**
  - **Z18.81 Retained glass fragments**
  - **Z18.83 Retained stone or crystalline fragments**
    Retained concrete or cement fragments
  - **Z18.89 Other specified retained foreign body fragments**
- **Z18.9 Retained foreign body fragments, unspecified material**

HORMONE SENSITIVITY MALIGNANCY STATUS (Z19) ◀

- **Z19 Hormone sensitivity malignancy status** ◀
  Code first malignant neoplasm —*see* Table of Neoplasms, by site, malignant ◀
  Z19.1 Hormone sensitive malignancy status ◀
  Z19.2 Hormone resistant malignancy status ◀
  Castrate resistant prostate malignancy status ◀

PERSONS WITH POTENTIAL HEALTH HAZARDS RELATED TO COMMUNICABLE DISEASES (Z20-Z29)

- **Z20 Contact with and (suspected) exposure to communicable diseases**
  Excludes1 carrier of infectious disease (Z22.-)
  diagnosed current infectious or parasitic disease - see Alphabetic Index
  Excludes2 personal history of infectious and parasitic diseases (Z86.1-)
  - **Z20.0 Contact with and (suspected) exposure to intestinal infectious diseases**
    Z20.01 Contact with and (suspected) exposure to intestinal infectious diseases due to Escherichia coli (E. coli)
    - **Z20.09 Contact with and (suspected) exposure to other intestinal infectious diseases**
  - **Z20.1 Contact with and (suspected) exposure to tuberculosis**
  - **Z20.2 Contact with and (suspected) exposure to infections with a predominantly sexual mode of transmission**
  - **Z20.3 Contact with and (suspected) exposure to rabies**
  - **Z20.4 Contact with and (suspected) exposure to rubella**
  Z20.5 Contact with and (suspected) exposure to viral hepatitis
  Z20.6 Contact with and (suspected) exposure to human immunodeficiency virus [HIV]
  Excludes1 asymptomatic human immunodeficiency virus [HIV]
  HIV infection status (Z21)
  - **Z20.7 Contact with and (suspected) exposure to pediculosis, acariasis and other infestations**
  - **Z20.8 Contact with and (suspected) exposure to other communicable diseases**
    - **Z20.81 Contact with and (suspected) exposure to other bacterial communicable diseases**
      - **Z20.810 Contact with and (suspected) exposure to anthrax**
      Z20.811 Contact with and (suspected) exposure to meningococcus
      - **Z20.818 Contact with and (suspected) exposure to other bacterial communicable diseases**
    - **Z20.82 Contact with and (suspected) exposure to other viral communicable diseases**
      Z20.820 Contact with and (suspected) exposure to varicella
      Z20.828 Contact with and (suspected) exposure to other viral communicable diseases
    - **Z20.89 Contact with and (suspected) exposure to other communicable diseases**
  - **Z20.9 Contact with and (suspected) exposure to unspecified communicable disease**

Z21 Asymptomatic human immunodeficiency virus [HIV] infection status
HIV positive NOS
Code first Human immunodeficiency virus [HIV] disease complicating pregnancy, childbirth and the puerperium, if applicable (O98.7-)
Excludes1 acquired immunodeficiency syndrome (B20)
contact with human immunodeficiency virus [HIV] (Z20.6)
exposure to human immunodeficiency virus [HIV] (Z20.6)
human immunodeficiency virus [HIV] disease (B20)
inconclusive laboratory evidence of human immunodeficiency virus [HIV] (R75)
MCE: Questionable admission when principal dx

- **Z22 Carrier of infectious disease**
  Includes colonization status
  suspected carrier
  Excludes2 carrier of viral hepatitis (B18.-) ◀
  - **Z22.0 Carrier of typhoid**
  - **Z22.1 Carrier of other intestinal infectious diseases**
  - **Z22.2 Carrier of diphtheria**
  - **Z22.3 Carrier of other specified bacterial diseases**
    - **Z22.31 Carrier of bacterial disease due to meningococci**
    - **Z22.32 Carrier of bacterial disease due to staphylococci**
      - **Z22.321 Carrier or suspected carrier of Methicillin susceptible Staphylococcus aureus**
        MSSA colonization
      - **Z22.322 Carrier or suspected carrier of Methicillin resistant Staphylococcus aureus**
        MRSA colonization
    Z22.33 Carrier of bacterial disease due to streptococci
      - **Z22.330 Carrier of Group B streptococcus**
        Excludes1 Carrier of streptococcus group B (GBS) complicating pregnancy, childbirth and the puerperium (O99.82-) ◀
      - **Z22.338 Carrier of other streptococcus**
    - **Z22.39 Carrier of other specified bacterial diseases**
  - **Z22.4 Carrier of infections with a predominantly sexual mode of transmission**
  ~~Z22.5 Carrier of viral hepatitis~~
  ~~Z22.50 Carrier of unspecified viral hepatitis~~
  ~~Z22.51 Carrier of viral hepatitis B~~
  ~~Hepatitis B surface antigen [HBsAg] carrier~~
  ~~Z22.52 Carrier of viral hepatitis C~~
  ~~Z22.59 Carrier of other viral hepatitis~~
  - **Z22.6 Carrier of human T-lymphotropic virus type-1 [HTLV-1] infection**
  - **Z22.8 Carrier of other infectious diseases**
  - **Z22.9 Carrier of infectious disease, unspecified**

- **Z23 Encounter for immunization**
  Code first any routine childhood examination
  Note: Procedure codes are required to identify the types of immunizations given.

- **Z28 Immunization not carried out and underimmunization status**
  - **Includes** vaccination not carried out
  - **Z28.0 Immunization not carried out because of contraindication**
    - **Z28.01 Immunization not carried out because of acute illness of patient**
    - **Z28.02 Immunization not carried out because of chronic illness or condition of patient**
    - **Z28.03 Immunization not carried out because of immune compromised state of patient**
    - **Z28.04 Immunization not carried out because of patient allergy to vaccine or component**
    - **Z28.09 Immunization not carried out because of other contraindication**
  - **Z28.1 Immunization not carried out because of patient decision for reasons of belief or group pressure**
    - Immunization not carried out because of religious belief
  - **Z28.2 Immunization not carried out because of patient decision for other and unspecified reason**
    - **Z28.20 Immunization not carried out because of patient decision for unspecified reason**
    - **Z28.21 Immunization not carried out because of patient refusal**
    - **Z28.29 Immunization not carried out because of patient decision for other reason**
  - **Z28.3 Underimmunization status**
    - Delinquent immunization status
    - Lapsed immunization schedule status
  - **Z28.8 Immunization not carried out for other reason**
    - **Z28.81 Immunization not carried out due to patient having had the disease**
    - **Z28.82 Immunization not carried out because of caregiver refusal**
      - Immunization not carried out because of guardian refusal
      - Immunization not carried out because of parent refusal
      - **Excludes1** immunization not carried out because of caregiver refusal because of religious belief (Z28.1)
    - **Z28.89 Immunization not carried out for other reason**
  - **Z28.9 Immunization not carried out for unspecified reason**
- **Z29 Encounter for other prophylactic measures** ◀
  - **Excludes1** desensitization to allergens (Z51.6) ◀
    prophylactic surgery (Z40.-) ◀
  - **Z29.1 Encounter for prophylactic immunotherapy** ◀
    - Encounter for administration of immunoglobulin ◀
    - **Z29.11 Encounter for prophylactic immunotherapy for respiratory syncytial virus (RSV)** ◀
    - **Z29.12 Encounter for prophylactic antivenin** ◀
    - **Z29.13 Encounter for prophylactic Rho(D) immune globulin** ◀
    - **Z29.14 Encounter for prophylactic rabies immune globin** ◀
  - **Z29.3 Encounter for prophylactic fluoride administration** ◀
  - **Z29.8 Encounter for other specified prophylactic measures** ◀
  - **Z29.9 Encounter for prophylactic measures, unspecified** ◀

PERSONS ENCOUNTERING HEALTH SERVICES IN CIRCUMSTANCES RELATED TO REPRODUCTION (Z30-Z39)

- **Z30 Encounter for contraceptive management**
  - **Z30.0 Encounter for general counseling and advice on contraception**
    - **Z30.01 Encounter for initial prescription of contraceptives**
      - **Excludes1** encounter for surveillance of contraceptives (Z30.4-)
      - **Z30.011 Encounter for initial prescription of contraceptive pills** ♀
      - **Z30.012 Encounter for prescription of emergency contraception** ♀
        - Encounter for postcoital contraception
      - **Z30.013 Encounter for initial prescription of injectable contraceptive** ♀
      - **Z30.014 Encounter for initial prescription of intrauterine contraceptive device** ♀
        - **Excludes1** encounter for insertion of intrauterine contraceptive device (Z30.430, Z30.432)
      - **Z30.015 Encounter for initial prescription of vaginal ring hormonal contraceptive** ♀ ◀
      - **Z30.016 Encounter for initial prescription of transdermal patch hormonal contraceptive device** ◀
      - **Z30.017 Encounter for initial prescription of implantable subdermal contraceptive** ◀
      - **Z30.018 Encounter for initial prescription of other contraceptives** ♀
        - Encounter for initial prescription of barrier contraception ◀
        - Encounter for initial prescription of diaphragm ◀
      - **Z30.019 Encounter for initial prescription of contraceptives, unspecified** ♀
    - **Z30.02 Counseling and instruction in natural family planning to avoid pregnancy**
    - **Z30.09 Encounter for other general counseling and advice on contraception**
      - Encounter for family planning advice NOS
  - **Z30.2 Encounter for sterilization**
  - **Z30.4 Encounter for surveillance of contraceptives**
    - **Z30.40 Encounter for surveillance of contraceptives, unspecified**
    - **Z30.41 Encounter for surveillance of contraceptive pills** ♀
      - Encounter for repeat prescription for contraceptive pill
    - **Z30.42 Encounter for surveillance of injectable contraceptive** ♀
    - **Z30.43 Encounter for surveillance of intrauterine contraceptive device**
      - **Z30.430 Encounter for insertion of intrauterine contraceptive device** ♀
      - **Z30.431 Encounter for routine checking of intrauterine contraceptive device** ♀
      - **Z30.432 Encounter for removal of intrauterine contraceptive device** ♀
      - **Z30.433 Encounter for removal and reinsertion of intrauterine contraceptive device** ♀
        - Encounter for replacement of intrauterine contraceptive device

- **Z30.44 Encounter for surveillance of vaginal ring hormonal contraceptive device ♀ ◀**
- **Z30.45 Encounter for surveillance of transdermal patch hormonal contraceptive device ♀ ◀**
- **Z30.46 Encounter for surveillance of implantable subdermal contraceptive ♀ ◀**
  - Encounter for checking, reinsertion or removal of implantable subdermal contraceptive ◀
- **Z30.49 Encounter for surveillance of other contraceptives ♀**
  - Encounter for surveillance of barrier contraception ◀
  - Encounter for surveillance of diaphragm ◀
- **Z30.8 Encounter for other contraceptive management**
  - Encounter for postvasectomy sperm count
  - Encounter for routine examination for contraceptive maintenance
  - **Excludes1** sperm count following sterilization reversal (Z31.42)
    sperm count for fertility testing (Z31.41)
- **Z30.9 Encounter for contraceptive management, unspecified**

- **Z31 Encounter for procreative management**
  - **Excludes1** complications associated with artificial fertilization (N98.-)
    female infertility (N97.-)
    male infertility (N46.-)
  - **Z31.0 Encounter for reversal of previous sterilization**
  - **Z31.4 Encounter for procreative investigation and testing**
    - **Excludes1** postvasectomy sperm count (Z30.8)
    - **Z31.41 Encounter for fertility testing**
      - Encounter for fallopian tube patency testing
      - Encounter for sperm count for fertility testing
    - **Z31.42 Aftercare following sterilization reversal**
      - Sperm count following sterilization reversal
    - **Z31.43 Encounter for genetic testing of female for procreative management**
      - Use additional code for recurrent pregnancy loss, if applicable (N96, O26.2-)
      - **Excludes1** nonprocreative genetic testing (Z13.7-)
      - **Z31.430 Encounter of female for testing for genetic disease carrier status for procreative management ♀**
      - **Z31.438 Encounter for other genetic testing of female for procreative management ♀**
    - **Z31.44 Encounter for genetic testing of male for procreative management**
      - **Excludes1** nonprocreative genetic testing (Z13.7-)
      - **Z31.440 Encounter of male for testing for genetic disease carrier status for procreative management ♂**
      - **Z31.441 Encounter for testing of male partner of patient with recurrent pregnancy loss ♂** A
      - **Z31.448 Encounter for other genetic testing of male for procreative management ♂** A
    - **Z31.49 Encounter for other procreative investigation and testing**
  - **Z31.5 Encounter for genetic counseling**
  - **Z31.6 Encounter for general counseling and advice on procreation**
    - **Z31.61 Procreative counseling and advice using natural family planning**
    - **Z31.62 Encounter for fertility preservation counseling**
      - Encounter for fertility preservation counseling prior to cancer therapy
      - Encounter for fertility preservation counseling prior to surgical removal of gonads
    - **Z31.69 Encounter for other general counseling and advice on procreation**
  - **Z31.7 Encounter for procreative management and counseling for gestational carrier ◀**
    - **Excludes1** pregnant state, gestational carrier (Z33.3) ◀
  - **Z31.8 Encounter for other procreative management**
    - **Z31.81 Encounter for male factor infertility in female patient ♀**
    - **Z31.82 Encounter for Rh incompatibility status ♀**
      - **Coding Clinic: 2015, Q3, P40**
    - **Z31.83 Encounter for assisted reproductive fertility procedure cycle ♀**
      - Patient undergoing in vitro fertilization cycle
      - Use additional code to identify the type of infertility
      - **Excludes1** pre-cycle diagnosis and testing - code to reason for encounter
    - **Z31.84 Encounter for fertility preservation procedure**
      - Encounter for fertility preservation procedure prior to cancer therapy
      - Encounter for fertility preservation procedure prior to surgical removal of gonads
    - **Z31.89 Encounter for other procreative management**
  - **Z31.9 Encounter for procreative management, unspecified**

- **Z32 Encounter for pregnancy test and childbirth and childcare instruction**
  - **Z32.0 Encounter for pregnancy test**
    - **Z32.00 Encounter for pregnancy test, result unknown ♀**
      - Encounter for pregnancy test NOS
    - **Z32.01 Encounter for pregnancy test, result positive ♀** M
    - **Z32.02 Encounter for pregnancy test, result negative ♀**
  - **Z32.2 Encounter for childbirth instruction**
  - **Z32.3 Encounter for childcare instruction**
    - Encounter for prenatal or postpartum childcare instruction

- **Z33 Pregnant state**
  - **Z33.1 Pregnant state, incidental ♀** M
    - Pregnant state NOS
    - **Excludes1** complications of pregnancy (O00-O9A)
      pregnant state, gestational carrier (Z33.3) ◀
  - **Z33.2 Encounter for elective termination of pregnancy ♀** M
    - **Excludes1** early fetal death with retention of dead fetus (O02.1)
      late fetal death (O36.4)
      spontaneous abortion (O03)
  - **Z33.3 Pregnant state, gestational carrier ♀ ◀**
    - **Excludes1** encounter for procreative management and counseling for gestational carrier (Z31.7) ◀

- **Z34 Encounter for supervision of normal pregnancy**
  - **Excludes1** any complication of pregnancy (O00-O9A)
    encounter for pregnancy test (Z32.0-)
    encounter for supervision of high risk pregnancy (O09.-)
  - **Z34.0 Encounter for supervision of normal first pregnancy**
    - **Z34.00 Encounter for supervision of normal first pregnancy, unspecified trimester ♀** M
    - **Z34.01 Encounter for supervision of normal first pregnancy, first trimester ♀** M
    - **Z34.02 Encounter for supervision of normal first pregnancy, second trimester ♀** M
    - **Z34.03 Encounter for supervision of normal first pregnancy, third trimester ♀** M

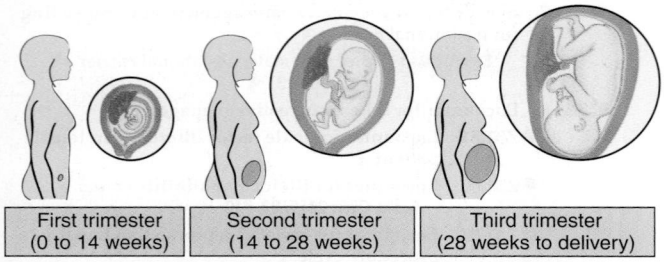

Figure 21-1 Trimesters. (From Shiland, Betsy J. Medical Terminology & Anatomy for ICD-10 Coding, ed 2, Mosby, 2015)

- **Z34.8 Encounter for supervision of other normal pregnancy**
  - **Z34.80 Encounter for supervision of other normal pregnancy, unspecified trimester ♀** M
  - **Z34.81 Encounter for supervision of other normal pregnancy, first trimester ♀** M
  - **Z34.82 Encounter for supervision of other normal pregnancy, second trimester ♀** M
  - **Z34.83 Encounter for supervision of other normal pregnancy, third trimester ♀** M
- **Z34.9 Encounter for supervision of normal pregnancy, unspecified**
  - **Z34.90 Encounter for supervision of normal pregnancy, unspecified, unspecified trimester ♀** M
  - **Z34.91 Encounter for supervision of normal pregnancy, unspecified, first trimester ♀** M
  - **Z34.92 Encounter for supervision of normal pregnancy, unspecified, second trimester ♀** M
  - **Z34.93 Encounter for supervision of normal pregnancy, unspecified, third trimester ♀** M

- **Z36 Encounter for antenatal screening of mother ♀** M

  Excludes1 abnormal findings on antenatal screening of mother (O28.-)
  diagnostic examination - code to sign or symptom
  encounter for suspected maternal and fetal conditions ruled out (Z03.7-)
  suspected fetal condition affecting management of pregnancy - code to condition in Chapter 15

  Excludes2 genetic counseling and testing (Z31.43-, Z31.5)
  routine prenatal care (Z34)

- **Z3A Weeks of gestation**

  Note: Codes from category Z3A are for use, only on the maternal record, to indicate the weeks of gestation of the pregnancy, if known. ◀

  Code first complications of pregnancy, childbirth and the puerperium (O00-O9A)

  Coding Clinic: 2013, Q2, P33

  - **Z3A.0 Weeks of gestation of pregnancy, unspecified or less than 10 weeks**
    - **Z3A.00 Weeks of gestation of pregnancy not specified ♀** M
    - **Z3A.01 Less than 8 weeks gestation of pregnancy ♀** M
    - **Z3A.08 8 weeks gestation of pregnancy ♀** M
    - **Z3A.09 9 weeks gestation of pregnancy ♀** M
  - **Z3A.1 Weeks of gestation of pregnancy, weeks 10-19**
    - **Z3A.10 10 weeks gestation of pregnancy ♀** M
    - **Z3A.11 11 weeks gestation of pregnancy ♀** M
    - **Z3A.12 12 weeks gestation of pregnancy ♀** M
    - **Z3A.13 13 weeks gestation of pregnancy ♀** M
    - **Z3A.14 14 weeks gestation of pregnancy ♀** M
    - **Z3A.15 15 weeks gestation of pregnancy ♀** M
    - **Z3A.16 16 weeks gestation of pregnancy ♀** M
    - **Z3A.17 17 weeks gestation of pregnancy ♀** M
    - **Z3A.18 18 weeks gestation of pregnancy ♀** M
    - **Z3A.19 19 weeks gestation of pregnancy ♀** M
  - **Z3A.2 Weeks of gestation of pregnancy, weeks 20-29**
    - **Z3A.20 20 weeks gestation of pregnancy ♀** M
    - **Z3A.21 21 weeks gestation of pregnancy ♀** M
    - **Z3A.22 22 weeks gestation of pregnancy ♀** M
    - **Z3A.23 23 weeks gestation of pregnancy ♀** M
    - **Z3A.24 24 weeks gestation of pregnancy ♀** M
    - **Z3A.25 25 weeks gestation of pregnancy ♀** M
    - **Z3A.26 26 weeks gestation of pregnancy ♀** M
    - **Z3A.27 27 weeks gestation of pregnancy ♀** M
    - **Z3A.28 28 weeks gestation of pregnancy ♀** M
    - **Z3A.29 29 weeks gestation of pregnancy ♀** M
  - **Z3A.3 Weeks of gestation of pregnancy, weeks 30-39**
    - **Z3A.30 30 weeks gestation of pregnancy ♀** M
    - **Z3A.31 31 weeks gestation of pregnancy ♀** M
    - **Z3A.32 32 weeks gestation of pregnancy ♀** M
    - **Z3A.33 33 weeks gestation of pregnancy ♀** M
    - **Z3A.34 34 weeks gestation of pregnancy ♀** M
    - **Z3A.35 35 weeks gestation of pregnancy ♀** M
    - **Z3A.36 36 weeks gestation of pregnancy ♀** M
    - **Z3A.37 37 weeks gestation of pregnancy ♀** M
    - **Z3A.38 38 weeks gestation of pregnancy ♀** M
      Coding Clinic: 2016, Q2, P34
    - **Z3A.39 39 weeks gestation of pregnancy ♀** M
  - **Z3A.4 Weeks of gestation of pregnancy, weeks 40 or greater**
    - **Z3A.40 40 weeks gestation of pregnancy ♀** M
    - **Z3A.41 41 weeks gestation of pregnancy ♀** M
    - **Z3A.42 42 weeks gestation of pregnancy ♀** M
    - **Z3A.49 Greater than 42 weeks gestation of pregnancy ♀** M

- **Z37 Outcome of delivery**

  This category is intended for use as an additional code to identify the outcome of delivery on the mother's record. It is not for use on the newborn record.

  Excludes1 stillbirth (P95)

  - **Z37.0 Single live birth ♀** M
    Coding Clinic: 2016, Q2, P34
  - **Z37.1 Single stillbirth ♀** M
  - **Z37.2 Twins, both liveborn ♀** M
  - **Z37.3 Twins, one liveborn and one stillborn ♀** M
  - **Z37.4 Twins, both stillborn ♀** M
  - **Z37.5 Other multiple births, all liveborn**
    - **Z37.50 Multiple births, unspecified, all liveborn ♀** M
    - **Z37.51 Triplets, all liveborn ♀** M
    - **Z37.52 Quadruplets, all liveborn ♀** M
    - **Z37.53 Quintuplets, all liveborn ♀** M
    - **Z37.54 Sextuplets, all liveborn ♀** M
    - **Z37.59 Other multiple births, all liveborn ♀** M

- **Z37.6 Other multiple births, some liveborn**
  - **Z37.60 Multiple births, unspecified, some liveborn ♀** M
  - **Z37.61 Triplets, some liveborn ♀** M
  - **Z37.62 Quadruplets, some liveborn ♀** M
  - **Z37.63 Quintuplets, some liveborn ♀** M
  - **Z37.64 Sextuplets, some liveborn ♀** M
  - **Z37.69 Other multiple births, some liveborn ♀** M
- **Z37.7 Other multiple births, all stillborn ♀** M
- **Z37.9 Outcome of delivery, unspecified ♀** M
  Multiple birth NOS
  Single birth NOS

- **Z38 Liveborn infants according to place of birth and type of delivery**
  This category is for use as the principal code on the initial record of a newborn baby. It is to be used for the initial birth record only. It is not to be used on the mother's record.
  Coding Clinic: 2015, Q2, P15
  - **Z38.0 Single liveborn infant, born in hospital**
    Single liveborn infant, born in birthing center or other health care facility
    - **Z38.00 Single liveborn infant, delivered vaginally** N
    - **Z38.01 Single liveborn infant, delivered by cesarean** N
  - **Z38.1 Single liveborn infant, born outside hospital** N
  - **Z38.2 Single liveborn infant, unspecified as to place of birth** N
    Single liveborn infant NOS
  - **Z38.3 Twin liveborn infant, born in hospital**
    - **Z38.30 Twin liveborn infant, delivered vaginally** N
    - **Z38.31 Twin liveborn infant, delivered by cesarean** N
  - **Z38.4 Twin liveborn infant, born outside hospital** N
  - **Z38.5 Twin liveborn infant, unspecified as to place of birth** N
  - **Z38.6 Other multiple liveborn infant, born in hospital**
    - **Z38.61 Triplet liveborn infant, delivered vaginally** N
    - **Z38.62 Triplet liveborn infant, delivered by cesarean** N
    - **Z38.63 Quadruplet liveborn infant, delivered vaginally** N
    - **Z38.64 Quadruplet liveborn infant, delivered by cesarean** N
    - **Z38.65 Quintuplet liveborn infant, delivered vaginally** N
    - **Z38.66 Quintuplet liveborn infant, delivered by cesarean** N
    - **Z38.68 Other multiple liveborn infant, delivered vaginally** N
    - **Z38.69 Other multiple liveborn infant, delivered by cesarean** N
  - **Z38.7 Other multiple liveborn infant, born outside hospital** N
  - **Z38.8 Other multiple liveborn infant, unspecified as to place of birth** N

- **Z39 Encounter for maternal postpartum care and examination**
  - **Z39.0 Encounter for care and examination of mother immediately after delivery ♀** M
    Care and observation in uncomplicated cases when the delivery occurs outside a healthcare facility
    Excludes1 care for postpartum complication - see Alphabetic index
  - **Z39.1 Encounter for care and examination of lactating mother ♀** M
    Encounter for supervision of lactation
    Excludes1 disorders of lactation (O92.-)
  - **Z39.2 Encounter for routine postpartum follow-up ♀** M

ENCOUNTERS FOR OTHER SPECIFIC HEALTH CARE (Z40-Z53)

Categories Z40-Z53 are intended for use to indicate a reason for care. They may be used for patients who have already been treated for a disease or injury, but who are receiving aftercare or prophylactic care, or care to consolidate the treatment, or to deal with a residual state

Excludes2 follow-up examination for medical surveillance after treatment (Z08-Z09)

- **Z40 Encounter for prophylactic surgery**
  Excludes1 organ donations (Z52.-)
  therapeutic organ removal - code to condition
  - **Z40.0 Encounter for prophylactic surgery for risk factors related to malignant neoplasms**
    Admission for prophylactic organ removal
    Use additional code to identify risk factor
    - **Z40.00 Encounter for prophylactic removal of unspecified organ**
    - **Z40.01 Encounter for prophylactic removal of breast**
    - **Z40.02 Encounter for prophylactic removal of ovary ♀**
    - **Z40.09 Encounter for prophylactic removal of other organ**
  - **Z40.8 Encounter for other prophylactic surgery**
  - **Z40.9 Encounter for prophylactic surgery, unspecified**

- **Z41 Encounter for procedures for purposes other than remedying health state**
  - **Z41.1 Encounter for cosmetic surgery**
    Encounter for cosmetic breast implant
    Encounter for cosmetic procedure
    Excludes1 encounter for plastic and reconstructive surgery following medical procedure or healed injury (Z42.-)
    encounter for post-mastectomy breast implantation (Z42.1)
  - **Z41.2 Encounter for routine and ritual male circumcision ♂**
  - **Z41.3 Encounter for ear piercing**
  - **Z41.8 Encounter for other procedures for purposes other than remedying health state**
  - **Z41.9 Encounter for procedure for purposes other than remedying health state, unspecified**

- **Z42 Encounter for plastic and reconstructive surgery following medical procedure or healed injury**
  Excludes1 encounter for cosmetic plastic surgery (Z41.1)
  encounter for plastic surgery for treatment of current injury - code to relevent injury
  - **Z42.1 Encounter for breast reconstruction following mastectomy** A
    Excludes1 deformity and disproportion of reconstructed breast (N65.1-)
  - **Z42.8 Encounter for other plastic and reconstructive surgery following medical procedure or healed injury**

Z43 Encounter for attention to artificial openings

Includes closure of artificial openings
passage of sounds or bougies through artificial openings
reforming artificial openings
removal of catheter from artificial openings
toilet or cleansing of artificial openings

Excludes1 artificial opening status only, without need for care (Z93.-)
complications of external stoma (J95.0-, K94.-, N99.5-)

Excludes2 fitting and adjustment of prosthetic and other devices (Z44-Z46)

Z43.0 Encounter for attention to tracheostomy

Z43.1 Encounter for attention to gastrostomy
Ex Z43.1

Z43.2 Encounter for attention to ileostomy

Z43.3 Encounter for attention to colostomy

Z43.4 Encounter for attention to other artificial openings of digestive tract

Z43.5 Encounter for attention to cystostomy

Z43.6 Encounter for attention to other artificial openings of urinary tract
Encounter for attention to nephrostomy
Encounter for attention to ureterostomy
Encounter for attention to urethrostomy

Z43.7 Encounter for attention to artificial vagina

Z43.8 Encounter for attention to other artificial openings

Z43.9 Encounter for attention to unspecified artificial opening

Z44 Encounter for fitting and adjustment of external prosthetic device

Includes removal or replacement of external prosthetic device

Excludes1 malfunction or other complications of device - see Alphabetical Index presence of prosthetic device (Z97.-)

Z44.0 Encounter for fitting and adjustment of artificial arm

Z44.00 Encounter for fitting and adjustment of unspecified artificial arm

Z44.001 Encounter for fitting and adjustment of unspecified right artificial arm

Z44.002 Encounter for fitting and adjustment of unspecified left artificial arm

Z44.009 Encounter for fitting and adjustment of unspecified artificial arm, unspecified arm

Z44.01 Encounter for fitting and adjustment of complete artificial arm

Z44.011 Encounter for fitting and adjustment of complete right artificial arm

Z44.012 Encounter for fitting and adjustment of complete left artificial arm

Z44.019 Encounter for fitting and adjustment of complete artificial arm, unspecified arm

Z44.02 Encounter for fitting and adjustment of partial artificial arm

Z44.021 Encounter for fitting and adjustment of partial artificial right arm

Z44.022 Encounter for fitting and adjustment of partial artificial left arm

Z44.029 Encounter for fitting and adjustment of partial artificial arm, unspecified arm

Z44.1 Encounter for fitting and adjustment of artificial leg

Z44.10 Encounter for fitting and adjustment of unspecified artificial leg

Z44.101 Encounter for fitting and adjustment of unspecified right artificial leg

Z44.102 Encounter for fitting and adjustment of unspecified left artificial leg

Z44.109 Encounter for fitting and adjustment of unspecified artificial leg, unspecified leg

Z44.11 Encounter for fitting and adjustment of complete artificial leg

Z44.111 Encounter for fitting and adjustment of complete right artificial leg

Z44.112 Encounter for fitting and adjustment of complete left artificial leg

Z44.119 Encounter for fitting and adjustment of complete artificial leg, unspecified leg

Z44.12 Encounter for fitting and adjustment of partial artificial leg

Z44.121 Encounter for fitting and adjustment of partial artificial right leg

Z44.122 Encounter for fitting and adjustment of partial artificial left leg

Z44.129 Encounter for fitting and adjustment of partial artificial leg, unspecified leg

Z44.2 Encounter for fitting and adjustment of artificial eye

Excludes1 mechanical complication of ocular prosthesis (T85.3)

Z44.20 Encounter for fitting and adjustment of artificial eye, unspecified

Z44.21 Encounter for fitting and adjustment of artificial right eye

Z44.22 Encounter for fitting and adjustment of artificial left eye

Z44.3 Encounter for fitting and adjustment of external breast prosthesis

Excludes1 complications of breast implant (T85.4-)
encounter for adjustment or removal of breast implant (Z45.81-)
encounter for initial breast implant insertion for cosmetic breast augmentation (Z41.1)
encounter for breast reconstruction following mastectomy (Z42.1)

Z44.30 Encounter for fitting and adjustment of external breast prosthesis, unspecified breast

Z44.31 Encounter for fitting and adjustment of external right breast prosthesis

Z44.32 Encounter for fitting and adjustment of external left breast prosthesis

Z44.8 Encounter for fitting and adjustment of other external prosthetic devices

Z44.9 Encounter for fitting and adjustment of unspecified external prosthetic device

Z45 Encounter for adjustment and management of implanted device

Includes removal or replacement of implanted device

Excludes1 malfunction or other complications of device - see Alphabetical Index
presence of prosthetic and other devices (Z95-Z97)

Excludes2 encounter for fitting and adjustment of non-implanted device (Z46.-)

Z45.0 Encounter for adjustment and management of cardiac device

Z45.01 Encounter for adjustment and management of cardiac pacemaker
Encounter for adjustment and management of cardiac resynchronization therapy pacemaker (CRT-P) ◀

Excludes1 encounter for adjustment and management of automatic implantable cardiac defibrillator with synchronous cardiac pacemaker (Z45.02)

Z45.010 Encounter for checking and testing of cardiac pacemaker pulse generator [battery]
Encounter for replacing cardiac pacemaker pulse generator [battery]
MCE: Questionable admission when principal dx

Z45.018 Encounter for adjustment and management of other part of cardiac pacemaker
MCE: Questionable admission when principal dx

Z45.02 Encounter for adjustment and management of automatic implantable cardiac defibrillator
Encounter for adjustment and management of automatic implantable cardiac defibrillator with synchronous cardiac pacemaker
Encounter for adjustment and management of cardiac resynchronization therapy defibrillator (CRT-D) ◀
MCE: Questionable admission when principal dx

Z45.09 Encounter for adjustment and management of other cardiac device
MCE: Questionable admission when principal dx

Z45.1 Encounter for adjustment and management of infusion pump

Z45.2 Encounter for adjustment and management of vascular access device
Encounter for adjustment and management of vascular catheters

Excludes1 encounter for adjustment and management of renal dialysis catheter (Z49.01)

Z45.3 Encounter for adjustment and management of implanted devices of the special senses

Z45.31 Encounter for adjustment and management of implanted visual substitution device

Z45.32 Encounter for adjustment and management of implanted hearing device

Excludes1 encounter for fitting and adjustment of hearing aide (Z46.1)

Z45.320 Encounter for adjustment and management of bone conduction device

Z45.321 Encounter for adjustment and management of cochlear device

Z45.328 Encounter for adjustment and management of other implanted hearing device

Z45.4 Encounter for adjustment and management of implanted nervous system device

Z45.41 Encounter for adjustment and management of cerebrospinal fluid drainage device
Encounter for adjustment and management of cerebral ventricular (communicating) shunt

Z45.42 Encounter for adjustment and management of neuropacemaker (brain) (peripheral nerve) (spinal cord)

Z45.49 Encounter for adjustment and management of other implanted nervous system device

Z45.8 Encounter for adjustment and management of other implanted devices

Z45.81 Encounter for adjustment or removal of breast implant
Encounter for elective implant exchange (different material) (different size)
Encounter removal of tissue expander without synchronous insertion of permanent implant

Excludes1 complications of breast implant (T85.4-)
encounter for initial breast implant insertion for cosmetic breast augmentation (Z41.1)
encounter for breast reconstruction following mastectomy (Z42.1)

Z45.811 Encounter for adjustment or removal of right breast implant

Z45.812 Encounter for adjustment or removal of left breast implant

Z45.819 Encounter for adjustment or removal of unspecified breast implant

Z45.82 Encounter for adjustment or removal of myringotomy device (stent) (tube)

Z45.89 Encounter for adjustment and management of other implanted devices

Z45.9 Encounter for adjustment and management of unspecified implanted device

Z46 Encounter for fitting and adjustment of other devices

Includes removal or replacement of other device

Excludes1 malfunction or other complications of device - see Alphabetical Index

Excludes2 encounter for fitting and management of implanted devices (Z45.-)
issue of repeat prescription only (Z76.0)
presence of prosthetic and other devices (Z95-Z97)

Z46.0 Encounter for fitting and adjustment of spectacles and contact lenses

Z46.1 Encounter for fitting and adjustment of hearing aid

Excludes1 encounter for adjustment and management of implanted hearing device (Z45.32-)

Z46.2 Encounter for fitting and adjustment of other devices related to nervous system and special senses

Excludes2 encounter for adjustment and management of implanted nervous system device (Z45.4-)
encounter for adjustment and management of implanted visual substitution device (Z45.31)

Z46.3 Encounter for fitting and adjustment of dental prosthetic device
Encounter for fitting and adjustment of dentures

Z46.4 Encounter for fitting and adjustment of orthodontic device

● **Z46.5 Encounter for fitting and adjustment of other gastrointestinal appliance and device**

Excludes1 encounter for attention to artificial openings of digestive tract (Z43.1-Z43.4)

● **Z46.51 Encounter for fitting and adjustment of gastric lap band**

● **Z46.59 Encounter for fitting and adjustment of other gastrointestinal appliance and device**

● **Z46.6 Encounter for fitting and adjustment of urinary device**

Excludes2 attention to artificial openings of urinary tract (Z43.5, Z43.6)

● **Z46.8 Encounter for fitting and adjustment of other specified devices**

● **Z46.81 Encounter for fitting and adjustment of insulin pump**

Encounter for insulin pump instruction and training

Encounter for insulin pump titration

Z46.82 Encounter for fitting and adjustment of non-vascular catheter

● **Z46.89 Encounter for fitting and adjustment of other specified devices**

Encounter for fitting and adjustment of wheelchair

● **Z46.9 Encounter for fitting and adjustment of unspecified device**

● **Z47 Orthopedic aftercare**

Excludes1 aftercare for healing fracture - code to fracture with 7th character D

Z47.1 Aftercare following joint replacement surgery

Use additional code to identify the joint (Z96.6-)

Z47.2 Encounter for removal of internal fixation device

Excludes1 encounter for adjustment of internal fixation device for fracture treatment - code to fracture with appropriate 7th character

encounter for removal of external fixation device - code to fracture with 7th character D

infection or inflammatory reaction to internal fixation device (T84.6-)

mechanical complication of internal fixation device (T84.1-)

● **Z47.3 Aftercare following explantation of joint prosthesis**

Aftercare following explantation of joint prosthesis, staged procedure

Encounter for joint prosthesis insertion following prior explantation of joint prosthesis

Coding Clinic: 2015, Q1, P17

Z47.31 Aftercare following explantation of shoulder joint prosthesis

Excludes1 acquired absence of shoulder joint following prior explantation of shoulder joint prosthesis (Z89.23-)

shoulder joint prosthesis explantation status (Z89.23-)

Z47.32 Aftercare following explantation of hip joint prosthesis

Excludes1 acquired absence of hip joint following prior explantation of hip joint prosthesis (Z89.62-)

hip joint prosthesis explantation status (Z89.62-)

Coding Clinic: 2015, Q1, P17

Z47.33 Aftercare following explantation of knee joint prosthesis

Excludes1 acquired absence of knee joint following prior explantation of knee prosthesis (Z89.52-)

knee joint prosthesis explantation status (Z89.52-)

● **Z47.8 Encounter for other orthopedic aftercare**

Z47.81 Encounter for orthopedic aftercare following surgical amputation

Use additional code to identify the limb amputated (Z89.-)

Z47.82 Encounter for orthopedic aftercare following scoliosis surgery

Z47.89 Encounter for other orthopedic aftercare

Coding Clinic: 2015, Q1, P8

● **Z48 Encounter for other postprocedural aftercare**

Excludes1 encounter for follow-up examination after completed treatment (Z08-Z09)

Excludes2 encounter for attention to artificial openings (Z43.-)

encounter for fitting and adjustment of prosthetic and other devices (Z44-Z46)

● **Z48.0 Encounter for attention to dressings, sutures and drains**

Excludes1 encounter for planned postprocedural wound closure (Z48.1)

● **Z48.00 Encounter for change or removal of nonsurgical wound dressing**

Encounter for change or removal of wound dressing NOS

● **Z48.01 Encounter for change or removal of surgical wound dressing**

Coding Clinic: 2015, Q4, P38

● **Z48.02 Encounter for removal of sutures**

Encounter for removal of staples

Coding Clinic: 2015, Q1, P6

Z48.03 Encounter for change or removal of drains

Z48.1 Encounter for planned postprocedural wound closure

Excludes1 encounter for attention to dressings and sutures (Z48.0-)

● **Z48.2 Encounter for aftercare following organ transplant**

Z48.21 Encounter for aftercare following heart transplant

CC when PDx is its own CC

Ex: D47.Z1, T86.20-T86.39, T86.850-T86.859, T86.90-T86.99, Z94.1, Z94.3, Z94.89-Z94.9

Z48.22 Encounter for aftercare following kidney transplant

CC when PDx is its own CC

Ex: D47.Z1, T86.10-T86.19, T86.850-T86.859, T86.90-T86.99, Z94.0, Z94.89-Z94.9

Z48.23 Encounter for aftercare following liver transplant

CC when PDx is its own CC

Ex: D47.Z1, T86.40-T86.49, T86.850-T86.859, T86.90-T86.99, Z94.4, Z94.89, Z94.9

Z48.24 Encounter for aftercare following lung transplant

CC when PDx is its own CC

Ex: D47.Z1, T86.810-T86.819, T86.850-T86.859, T86.90-T86.99, Z94.2, Z94.89-Z94.9

● **Z48.28 Encounter for aftercare following multiple organ transplant**

Z48.280 Encounter for aftercare following heart-lung transplant

CC when PDx is its own CC

Ex: See Z48.21

Z48.288 Encounter for aftercare following multiple organ transplant

● **Z48.29 Encounter for aftercare following other organ transplant**

Z48.290 Encounter for aftercare following bone marrow transplant

CC when PDx is its own CC

Ex: D47.Z1, D89.810-D89.813, T86.00-T86.09, T86.850-T86.859, T86.90-T86.99, Z94.9

Z48.298 Encounter for aftercare following other organ transplant

Z48.3 Aftercare following surgery for neoplasm
Use additional code to identify the neoplasm

Z48.8 Encounter for other specified postprocedural aftercare

Z48.81 Encounter for surgical aftercare following surgery on specified body systems
These codes identify the body system requiring aftercare. They are for use in conjunction with other aftercare codes to fully explain the aftercare encounter. The condition treated should also be coded if still present.
Excludes1 aftercare for injury - code the injury with 7th character D
aftercare following surgery for neoplasm (Z48.3)
Excludes2 aftercare following organ transplant (Z48.2-)
orthopedic aftercare (Z47.-)

Z48.810 Encounter for surgical aftercare following surgery on the sense organs

Z48.811 Encounter for surgical aftercare following surgery on the nervous system
Excludes2 encounter for surgical aftercare following surgery on the sense organs (Z48.810)

Z48.812 Encounter for surgical aftercare following surgery on the circulatory system
Coding Clinic: 2012, Q4, P96

Z48.813 Encounter for surgical aftercare following surgery on the respiratory system

Z48.814 Encounter for surgical aftercare following surgery on the teeth or oral cavity

Z48.815 Encounter for surgical aftercare following surgery on the digestive system
Coding Clinic: 2015, Q4, P38

Z48.816 Encounter for surgical aftercare following surgery on the genitourinary system
Excludes1 encounter for aftercare following sterilization reversal (Z31.42)

Z48.817 Encounter for surgical aftercare following surgery on the skin and subcutaneous tissue
Coding Clinic: 2015, Q1, P6

Z48.89 Encounter for other specified surgical aftercare

Z49 Encounter for care involving renal dialysis
Code also associated end stage renal disease (N18.6)

Z49.0 Preparatory care for renal dialysis
Encounter for dialysis instruction and training

Z49.01 Encounter for fitting and adjustment of extracorporeal dialysis catheter
Removal or replacement of renal dialysis catheter
Toilet or cleansing of renal dialysis catheter

Z49.02 Encounter for fitting and adjustment of peritoneal dialysis catheter

Z49.3 Encounter for adequacy testing for dialysis

Z49.31 Encounter for adequacy testing for hemodialysis

Z49.32 Encounter for adequacy testing for peritoneal dialysis
Encounter for peritoneal equilibration test

Z51 Encounter for other aftercare and medical care
Code also condition requiring care
Excludes1 follow-up examination after treatment (Z08-Z09)

Z51.0 Encounter for antineoplastic radiation therapy

Z51.1 Encounter for antineoplastic chemotherapy and immunotherapy
Excludes2 encounter for chemotherapy and immunotherapy for nonneoplastic condition-code to condition

Z51.11 Encounter for antineoplastic chemotherapy
Coding Clinic: 2015, Q3, P19

Z51.12 Encounter for antineoplastic immunotherapy

Z51.5 Encounter for palliative care

Z51.6 Encounter for desensitization to allergens

Z51.8 Encounter for other specified aftercare
Excludes1 holiday relief care (Z75.5)

Z51.81 Encounter for therapeutic drug level monitoring
Code also any long-term (current) drug therapy (Z79.-)
Excludes1 encounter for blood-drug test for administrative or medicolegal reasons (Z02.83)

Z51.89 Encounter for other specified aftercare
MCE: This code may be considered "acceptable" when a secondary diagnosis is also coded on the record.
Coding Clinic: 2012, Q4, P96-97

Z52 Donors of organs and tissues
Includes autologous and other living donors
Excludes1 cadaveric donor - omit code
examination of potential donor (Z00.5)
Coding Clinic: 2012, Q4, P100

Z52.0 Blood donor

Z52.00 Unspecified blood donor

Z52.000 Unspecified donor, whole blood

Z52.001 Unspecified donor, stem cells

Z52.008 Unspecified donor, other blood

Z52.01 Autologous blood donor

Z52.010 Autologous donor, whole blood

Z52.011 Autologous donor, stem cells

Z52.018 Autologous donor, other blood

Z52.09 Other blood donor
Volunteer donor

Z52.090 Other blood donor, whole blood

Z52.091 Other blood donor, stem cells

Z52.098 Other blood donor, other blood

Z52.1 Skin donor

Z52.10 Skin donor, unspecified

Z52.11 Skin donor, autologous

Z52.19 Skin donor, other

Z52.2 Bone donor

Z52.20 Bone donor, unspecified

Z52.21 Bone donor, autologous

Z52.29 Bone donor, other

Z52.3 Bone marrow donor

Z52.4 Kidney donor

Z52.5 Cornea donor

Z52.6 Liver donor
Coding Clinic: 2012, Q4, P100

- **Z52.8 Donor of other specified organs or tissues**
  - **Z52.81 Egg (Oocyte) donor**
    - **Z52.810 Egg (Oocyte) donor under age 35, anonymous recipient ♀**
      Egg donor under age 35 NOS
    - **Z52.811 Egg (Oocyte) donor under age 35, designated recipient ♀**
    - **Z52.812 Egg (Oocyte) donor age 35 and over, anonymous recipient ♀**
      Egg donor age 35 and over NOS
    - **Z52.813 Egg (Oocyte) donor age 35 and over, designated recipient ♀**
    - **Z52.819 Egg (Oocyte) donor, unspecified ♀**
  - **Z52.89 Donor of other specified organs or tissues**
  - **Z52.9 Donor of unspecified organ or tissue**
    Donor NOS

- **Z53 Persons encountering health services for specific procedures and treatment, not carried out**
  - **Z53.0 Procedure and treatment not carried out because of contraindication**
    - **Z53.01 Procedure and treatment not carried out due to patient smoking**
    - **Z53.09 Procedure and treatment not carried out because of other contraindication**
  - **Z53.1 Procedure and treatment not carried out because of patient's decision for reasons of belief and group pressure**
  - **Z53.2 Procedure and treatment not carried out because of patient's decision for other and unspecified reasons**
    - **Z53.20 Procedure and treatment not carried out because of patient's decision for unspecified reasons**
    - **Z53.21 Procedure and treatment not carried out due to patient leaving prior to being seen by health care provider**
    - **Z53.29 Procedure and treatment not carried out because of patient's decision for other reasons**
  - **Z53.3 Procedure converted to open procedure ◀**
    - **Z53.31 Laparoscopic surgical procedure converted to open procedure ◀**
    - **Z53.32 Thoracoscopic surgical procedure converted to open procedure ◀**
    - **Z53.33 Arthroscopic surgical procedure converted to open procedure ◀**
    - **Z53.39 Other specified procedure converted to open procedure ◀**
  - **Z53.8 Procedure and treatment not carried out for other reasons**
  - **Z53.9 Procedure and treatment not carried out, unspecified reason**

PERSONS WITH POTENTIAL HEALTH HAZARDS RELATED TO SOCIOECONOMIC AND PSYCHOSOCIAL CIRCUMSTANCES (Z55-Z65)

- **Z55 Problems related to education and literacy**
  Excludes1 disorders of psychological development (F80-F89)
  - **Z55.0 Illiteracy and low-literacy**
  - **Z55.1 Schooling unavailable and unattainable**
  - **Z55.2 Failed school examinations**
  - **Z55.3 Underachievement in school**
  - **Z55.4 Educational maladjustment and discord with teachers and classmates**
  - **Z55.8 Other problems related to education and literacy**
    Problems related to inadequate teaching
  - **Z55.9 Problems related to education and literacy, unspecified**
    Academic problems NOS

- **Z56 Problems related to employment and unemployment**
  Excludes2 occupational exposure to risk factors (Z57.-)
  problems related to housing and economic circumstances (Z59.-)
  - **Z56.0 Unemployment, unspecified**
  - **Z56.1 Change of job** A
  - **Z56.2 Threat of job loss**
  - **Z56.3 Stressful work schedule**
  - **Z56.4 Discord with boss and workmates**
  - **Z56.5 Uncongenial work environment**
    Difficult conditions at work
  - **Z56.6 Other physical and mental strain related to work**
  - **Z56.8 Other problems related to employment**
    - **Z56.81 Sexual harassment on the job**
    - **Z56.82 Military deployment status**
      Individual (civilian or military) currently deployed in theater or in support of military war, peacekeeping and humanitarian operations
    - **Z56.89 Other problems related to employment**
  - **Z56.9 Unspecified problems related to employment**
    Occupational problems NOS

- **Z57 Occupational exposure to risk factors**
  - **Z57.0 Occupational exposure to noise**
  - **Z57.1 Occupational exposure to radiation**
  - **Z57.2 Occupational exposure to dust**
  - **Z57.3 Occupational exposure to other air contaminants**
    - **Z57.31 Occupational exposure to environmental tobacco smoke**
      Excludes2 exposure to environmental tobacco smoke (Z77.22)
    - **Z57.39 Occupational exposure to other air contaminants**
  - **Z57.4 Occupational exposure to toxic agents in agriculture**
    Occupational exposure to solids, liquids, gases or vapors in agriculture
  - **Z57.5 Occupational exposure to toxic agents in other industries**
    Occupational exposure to solids, liquids, gases or vapors in other industries
  - **Z57.6 Occupational exposure to extreme temperature**
  - **Z57.7 Occupational exposure to vibration**
  - **Z57.8 Occupational exposure to other risk factors**
  - **Z57.9 Occupational exposure to unspecified risk factor**

- **Z59 Problems related to housing and economic circumstances**
  Excludes2 problems related to upbringing (Z62.-)
  - **Z59.0 Homelessness**
  - **Z59.1 Inadequate housing**
    Lack of heating
    Restriction of space
    Technical defects in home preventing adequate care
    Unsatisfactory surroundings
    Excludes1 problems related to the natural and physical environment (Z77.1-)
  - **Z59.2 Discord with neighbors, lodgers and landlord**
  - **Z59.3 Problems related to living in residential institution**
    Boarding-school resident
    Excludes1 institutional upbringing (Z62.2)
  - **Z59.4 Lack of adequate food and safe drinking water**
    Inadequate drinking water supply
    Excludes1 effects of hunger (T73.0)
    inappropriate diet or eating habits (Z72.4)
    malnutrition (E40-E46)
  - **Z59.5 Extreme poverty**
  - **Z59.6 Low income**
  - **Z59.7 Insufficient social insurance and welfare support**

- **Z59.8 Other problems related to housing and economic circumstances**
  - Foreclosure on loan
  - Isolated dwelling
  - Problems with creditors
- **Z59.9 Problem related to housing and economic circumstances, unspecified**

- **Z60 Problems related to social environment**
  - **Z60.0 Problems of adjustment to life-cycle transitions**
    - Empty nest syndrome
    - Phase of life problem
    - Problem with adjustment to retirement [pension]
  - **Z60.2 Problems related to living alone**
  - **Z60.3 Acculturation difficulty**
    - Problem with migration
    - Problem with social transplantation
  - **Z60.4 Social exclusion and rejection**
    - Exclusion and rejection on the basis of personal characteristics, such as unusual physical appearance, illness or behavior.
    - **Excludes1** target of adverse discrimination such as for racial or religious reasons (Z60.5)
  - **Z60.5 Target of (perceived) adverse discrimination and persecution**
    - **Excludes1** social exclusion and rejection (Z60.4)
  - **Z60.8 Other problems related to social environment**
  - **Z60.9 Problem related to social environment, unspecified**

- **Z62 Problems related to upbringing**
  - **Includes** current and past negative life events in childhood
    - current and past problems of a child related to upbringing
  - **Excludes2** maltreatment syndrome (T74.-)
    - problems related to housing and economic circumstances (Z59.-)
  - **Z62.0 Inadequate parental supervision and control**
  - **Z62.1 Parental overprotection**
  - **Z62.2 Upbringing away from parents**
    - **Excludes1** problems with boarding school (Z59.3)
    - **Z62.21 Child in welfare custody** P
      - Child in care of non-parental family member
      - Child in foster care
      - **Excludes2** problem for parent due to child in welfare custody (Z63.5)
    - **Z62.22 Institutional upbringing**
      - Child living in orphanage or group home
    - **Z62.29 Other upbringing away from parents**
  - **Z62.3 Hostility towards and scapegoating of child** P
  - **Z62.6 Inappropriate (excessive) parental pressure**
  - **Z62.8 Other specified problems related to upbringing**
    - **Z62.81 Personal history of abuse in childhood**
      - **Z62.810 Personal history of physical and sexual abuse in childhood**
        - **Excludes1** current child physical abuse (T74.12, T76.12)
        - current child sexual abuse (T74.22, T76.22)
      - **Z62.811 Personal history of psychological abuse in childhood**
        - **Excludes1** current child psychological abuse (T74.32, T76.32)
      - **Z62.812 Personal history of neglect in childhood**
        - **Excludes1** current child neglect (T74.02, T76.02)
      - **Z62.819 Personal history of unspecified abuse in childhood**
        - **Excludes1** current child abuse NOS (T74.92, T76.92)
    - **Z62.82 Parent-child conflict**
      - **Z62.820 Parent-biological child conflict**
        - Parent-child problem NOS
      - **Z62.821 Parent-adopted child conflict**
      - **Z62.822 Parent-foster child conflict**
    - **Z62.89 Other specified problems related to upbringing**
      - **Z62.890 Parent-child estrangement NEC**
      - **Z62.891 Sibling rivalry**
      - **Z62.898 Other specified problems related to upbringing**
  - **Z62.9 Problem related to upbringing, unspecified**

- **Z63 Other problems related to primary support group, including family circumstances**
  - **Excludes2** maltreatment syndrome (T74.-, T76)
    - parent-child problems (Z62.-)
    - problems related to negative life events in childhood (Z62.-)
    - problems related to upbringing (Z62.-)
  - **Z63.0 Problems in relationship with spouse or partner**
    - **Excludes1** counseling for spousal or partner abuse problems (Z69.1)
    - counseling related to sexual attitude, behavior, and orientation (Z70.-)
  - **Z63.1 Problems in relationship with in-laws**
  - **Z63.3 Absence of family member**
    - **Excludes1** absence of family member due to disappearance and death (Z63.4)
    - absence of family member due to separation and divorce (Z63.5)
    - **Z63.31 Absence of family member due to military deployment**
      - Individual or family affected by other family member being on military deployment
      - **Excludes1** family disruption due to return of family member from military deployment (Z63.71)
    - **Z63.32 Other absence of family member**
  - **Z63.4 Disappearance and death of family member**
    - Assumed death of family member
    - Bereavement
  - **Z63.5 Disruption of family by separation and divorce**
    - Marital estrangement
  - **Z63.6 Dependent relative needing care at home**
  - **Z63.7 Other stressful life events affecting family and household**
    - **Z63.71 Stress on family due to return of family member from military deployment**
      - Individual or family affected by family member having returned from military deployment (current or past conflict)
    - **Z63.72 Alcoholism and drug addiction in family**
    - **Z63.79 Other stressful life events affecting family and household**
      - Anxiety (normal) about sick person in family
      - Health problems within family
      - Ill or disturbed family member
      - Isolated family

- **Z63.8 Other specified problems related to primary support group**
  - Family discord NOS
  - Family estrangement NOS
  - High expressed emotional level within family
  - Inadequate family support NOS
  - Inadequate or distorted communication within family
- **Z63.9 Problem related to primary support group, unspecified**
  - Relationship disorder NOS

Z64 Problems related to certain psychosocial circumstances

- **Z64.0 Problems related to unwanted pregnancy ♀**
- **Z64.1 Problems related to multiparity ♀**
- **Z64.4 Discord with counselors**
  - Discord with probation officer
  - Discord with social worker

Z65 Problems related to other psychosocial circumstances

- **Z65.0 Conviction in civil and criminal proceedings without imprisonment**
- **Z65.1 Imprisonment and other incarceration**
- **Z65.2 Problems related to release from prison**
- **Z65.3 Problems related to other legal circumstances**
  - Arrest
  - Child custody or support proceedings
  - Litigation
  - Prosecution
- **Z65.4 Victim of crime and terrorism**
  - Victim of torture
- **Z65.5 Exposure to disaster, war and other hostilities**
  - **Excludes1** target of perceived discrimination or persecution (Z60.5)
- **Z65.8 Other specified problems related to psychosocial circumstances**
- **Z65.9 Problem related to unspecified psychosocial circumstances**

DO NOT RESUSCITATE STATUS (Z66)

Z66 Do not resuscitate
- DNR status

BLOOD TYPE (Z67)

Z67 Blood type
- Coding Clinic: 2015, Q3, P40

- **Z67.1 Type A blood**
  - **Z67.10 Type A blood, Rh positive**
  - **Z67.11 Type A blood, Rh negative**
- **Z67.2 Type B blood**
  - **Z67.20 Type B blood, Rh positive**
  - **Z67.21 Type B blood, Rh negative**
- **Z67.3 Type AB blood**
  - **Z67.30 Type AB blood, Rh positive**
  - **Z67.31 Type AB blood, Rh negative**
- **Z67.4 Type O blood**
  - **Z67.40 Type O blood, Rh positive**
  - **Z67.41 Type O blood, Rh negative**
- **Z67.9 Unspecified blood type**
  - **Z67.90 Unspecified blood type, Rh positive**
  - **Z67.91 Unspecified blood type, Rh negative**
    - Coding Clinic: 2015, Q3, P40

BODY MASS INDEX [BMI] (Z68)

OGCR Section I.B.14.

> General Coding Guidelines
>
> 14. Documentation for BMI, *Depth of* Non-pressure ulcers, Pressure Ulcer Stages, **Coma Scale,** *and NIH Stroke Scale*
>
> For the Body Mass Index (BMI), depth of non-pressure chronic ulcers, pressure ulcer stage, **coma scale, and NIH stroke scale (NIHSS) codes,** code assignment may be based on medical record documentation from clinicians who are not the patient's provider (i.e., physician or other qualified healthcare practitioner legally accountable for establishing the patient's diagnosis), since this information is typically documented by other clinicians involved in the care of the patient (e.g., a dietitian often documents the BMI, a nurse often documents the pressure ulcer stages, **and an emergency medical technician often documents the coma scale**). However, the associated diagnosis (such as overweight, obesity, **acute stroke,** or pressure ulcer) must be documented by the patient's provider. If there is conflicting medical record documentation, either from the same clinician or different clinicians, the patient's attending provider should be queried for clarification.
>
> The BMI, **coma scale, and NIHSS** codes should only be reported as secondary diagnoses.

Z68 Body mass index [BMI]
- Kilograms per meters squared

Note: BMI adult codes are for use for persons 21 years of age or older.

BMI pediatric codes are for use for persons 2-20 years of age. These percentiles are based on the growth charts published by the Centers for Disease Control and Prevention (CDC)

- **Z68.1 Body mass index (BMI) 19 or less, adult** A
  - Ex: E66.01-E66.1, E66.8-E66.9, Z68.1-Z68.54
- **Z68.2 Body mass index (BMI) 20-29, adult**
  - **Z68.20 Body mass index (BMI) 20.0-20.9, adult** A
  - **Z68.21 Body mass index (BMI) 21.0-21.9, adult** A
  - **Z68.22 Body mass index (BMI) 22.0-22.9, adult** A
  - **Z68.23 Body mass index (BMI) 23.0-23.9, adult** A
  - **Z68.24 Body mass index (BMI) 24.0-24.9, adult** A
  - **Z68.25 Body mass index (BMI) 25.0-25.9, adult** A
  - **Z68.26 Body mass index (BMI) 26.0-26.9, adult** A
  - **Z68.27 Body mass index (BMI) 27.0-27.9, adult** A
  - **Z68.28 Body mass index (BMI) 28.0-28.9, adult** A
  - **Z68.29 Body mass index (BMI) 29.0-29.9, adult** A
- **Z68.3 Body mass index (BMI) 30-39, adult**
  - **Z68.30 Body mass index (BMI) 30.0-30.9, adult** A
  - **Z68.31 Body mass index (BMI) 31.0-31.9, adult** A
  - **Z68.32 Body mass index (BMI) 32.0-32.9, adult** A
  - **Z68.33 Body mass index (BMI) 33.0-33.9, adult** A
  - **Z68.34 Body mass index (BMI) 34.0-34.9, adult** A
  - **Z68.35 Body mass index (BMI) 35.0-35.9, adult** A
  - **Z68.36 Body mass index (BMI) 36.0-36.9, adult** A
  - **Z68.37 Body mass index (BMI) 37.0-37.9, adult** A
  - **Z68.38 Body mass index (BMI) 38.0-38.9, adult** A
  - **Z68.39 Body mass index (BMI) 39.0-39.9, adult** A
- **Z68.4 Body mass index (BMI) 40 or greater, adult**
  - Ex: For category Z68.4 CC codes: E65-E66.1, E66.8-E66.9, Z68.1-Z68.54
  - **Z68.41 Body mass index (BMI) 40.0-44.9, adult** A
  - **Z68.42 Body mass index (BMI) 45.0-49.9, adult** A
  - **Z68.43 Body mass index (BMI) 50-59.9, adult** A
  - **Z68.44 Body mass index (BMI) 60.0-69.9, adult** A
  - **Z68.45 Body mass index (BMI) 70 or greater, adult** A

- **Z68.5 Body mass index (BMI) pediatric**
  - **Z68.51 Body mass index (BMI) pediatric, less than 5th percentile for age**
  - **Z68.52 Body mass index (BMI) pediatric, 5th percentile to less than 85th percentile for age**
  - **Z68.53 Body mass index (BMI) pediatric, 85th percentile to less than 95th percentile for age**
  - **Z68.54 Body mass index (BMI) pediatric, greater than or equal to 95th percentile for age**

PERSONS ENCOUNTERING HEALTH SERVICES IN OTHER CIRCUMSTANCES (Z69-Z76)

- **Z69 Encounter for mental health services for victim and perpetrator of abuse**

  Includes counseling for victims and perpetrators of abuse
  - **Z69.0 Encounter for mental health services for child abuse problems**
    - **Z69.01 Encounter for mental health services for parental child abuse**

      Z69.010 Encounter for mental health services for victim of parental child abuse P
    - **Z69.011 Encounter for mental health services for perpetrator of parental child abuse**

      Excludes1 encounter for mental health services for non-parental child abuse (Z69.02-)
    - **Z69.02 Encounter for mental health services for non-parental child abuse**

      Z69.020 Encounter for mental health services for victim of non-parental child abuse P
    - **Z69.021 Encounter for mental health services for perpetrator of non- parental child abuse**
  - **Z69.1 Encounter for mental health services for spousal or partner abuse problems**
    - **Z69.11 Encounter for mental health services for victim of spousal or partner abuse**
    - **Z69.12 Encounter for mental health services for perpetrator of spousal or partner abuse**
  - **Z69.8 Encounter for mental health services for victim or perpetrator of other abuse**
    - **Z69.81 Encounter for mental health services for victim of other abuse**

      Encounter for rape victim counseling
    - **Z69.82 Encounter for mental health services for perpetrator of other abuse**
- **Z70 Counseling related to sexual attitude, behavior and orientation**

  Includes encounter for mental health services for sexual attitude, behavior and orientation

  Excludes2 contraceptive or procreative counseling (Z30-Z31)
  - **Z70.0 Counseling related to sexual attitude**
  - **Z70.1 Counseling related to patient's sexual behavior and orientation**

    Patient concerned regarding impotence
    Patient concerned regarding non-responsiveness
    Patient concerned regarding promiscuity
    Patient concerned regarding sexual orientation
  - **Z70.2 Counseling related to sexual behavior and orientation of third party**

    Advice sought regarding sexual behavior and orientation of child
    Advice sought regarding sexual behavior and orientation of partner
    Advice sought regarding sexual behavior and orientation of spouse
  - **Z70.3 Counseling related to combined concerns regarding sexual attitude, behavior and orientation**
  - **Z70.8 Other sex counseling**

    Encounter for sex education
  - **Z70.9 Sex counseling, unspecified**
- **Z71 Persons encountering health services for other counseling and medical advice, not elsewhere classified**

  Excludes2 contraceptive or procreation counseling (Z30-Z31)
  sex counseling (Z70.-)
  - **Z71.0 Person encountering health services to consult on behalf of another person**

    Person encountering health services to seek advice or treatment for non-attending third party

    Excludes2 anxiety (normal) about sick person in family (Z63.7)
    expectant (adoptive) parent(s) pre-birth pediatrician visit (Z76.81)
  - **Z71.1 Person with feared health complaint in whom no diagnosis is made**

    Person encountering health services with feared condition which was not demonstrated
    Person encountering health services in which problem was normal state
    'Worried well'

    Excludes1 medical observation for suspected diseases and conditions proven not to exist (Z03.-)
  - **Z71.2 Person consulting for explanation of examination or test findings**
  - **Z71.3 Dietary counseling and surveillance**

    Use additional code for any associated underlying medical condition

    Use additional code to identify body mass index (BMI), if known (Z68.-)
  - **Z71.4 Alcohol abuse counseling and surveillance**

    Use additional code for alcohol abuse or dependence (F10.-)
    - **Z71.41 Alcohol abuse counseling and surveillance of alcoholic**
    - **Z71.42 Counseling for family member of alcoholic**

      Counseling for significant other, partner, or friend of alcoholic
  - **Z71.5 Drug abuse counseling and surveillance**

    Use additional code for drug abuse or dependence (F11-F16, F18-F19)
    - **Z71.51 Drug abuse counseling and surveillance of drug abuser**
    - **Z71.52 Counseling for family member of drug abuser**

      Counseling for significant other, partner, or friend of drug abuser
  - **Z71.6 Tobacco abuse counseling**

    Use additional code for nicotine dependence (F17.-)
  - **Z71.7 Human immunodeficiency virus [HIV] counseling**
  - **Z71.8 Other specified counseling**

    Excludes2 counseling for contraception (Z30.0-)
    counseling for genetics (Z31.5)
    counseling for procreative management (Z31.6-)
    - **Z71.81 Spiritual or religious counseling**
    - **Z71.89 Other specified counseling**
  - **Z71.9 Counseling, unspecified**

    Encounter for medical advice NOS

Z72 Problems related to lifestyle
Excludes2 problems related to life-management difficulty (Z73.-)
problems related to socioeconomic and psychosocial circumstances (Z55-Z65)

Z72.0 Tobacco use
Tobacco use NOS
Excludes1 history of tobacco dependence (Z87.891)
nicotine dependence (F17.2-)
tobacco dependence (F17.2-)
tobacco use during pregnancy (O99.33-)

Z72.3 Lack of physical exercise

Z72.4 Inappropriate diet and eating habits
Excludes1 behavioral eating disorders of infancy or childhood (F98.2.-F98.3)
eating disorders (F50.-)
lack of adequate food (Z59.4)
malnutrition and other nutritional deficiencies (E40-E64)

Z72.5 High risk sexual behavior
Promiscuity
Excludes1 paraphilias (F65)

Z72.51 High risk heterosexual behavior

Z72.52 High risk homosexual behavior

Z72.53 High risk bisexual behavior

Z72.6 Gambling and betting
Excludes1 compulsive or pathological gambling (F63.0)

Z72.8 Other problems related to lifestyle

Z72.81 Antisocial behavior
Excludes1 conduct disorders (F91.-)

Z72.810 Child and adolescent antisocial behavior P
Antisocial behavior (child) (adolescent) without manifest psychiatric disorder
Delinquency NOS
Group delinquency
Offenses in the context of gang membership
Stealing in company with others
Truancy from school

Z72.811 Adult antisocial behavior A
Adult antisocial behavior without manifest psychiatric disorder

Z72.82 Problems related to sleep

Z72.820 Sleep deprivation
Lack of adequate sleep
Excludes1 insomnia (G47.0-)

Z72.821 Inadequate sleep hygiene
Bad sleep habits
Irregular sleep habits
Unhealthy sleep wake schedule
Excludes1 insomnia (F51.0-, G47.0-)

Z72.89 Other problems related to lifestyle
Self-damaging behavior

Z72.9 Problem related to lifestyle, unspecified

Z73 Problems related to life management difficulty
Excludes2 problems related to socioeconomic and psychosocial circumstances (Z55-Z65)

Z73.0 Burn-out

Z73.1 Type A behavior pattern

Z73.2 Lack of relaxation and leisure

Z73.3 Stress, not elsewhere classified
Physical and mental strain NOS
Excludes1 stress related to employment or unemployment (Z56.-)

Z73.4 Inadequate social skills, not elsewhere classified

Z73.5 Social role conflict, not elsewhere classified

Z73.6 Limitation of activities due to disability
Excludes1 care-provider dependency (Z74.-)

Z73.8 Other problems related to life management difficulty

Z73.81 Behavioral insomnia of childhood

Z73.810 Behavioral insomnia of childhood, sleep-onset association type P

Z73.811 Behavioral insomnia of childhood, limit setting type P

Z73.812 Behavioral insomnia of childhood, combined type P

Z73.819 Behavioral insomnia of childhood, unspecified type P

Z73.82 Dual sensory impairment

Z73.89 Other problems related to life management difficulty

Z73.9 Problem related to life management difficulty, unspecified

Z74 Problems related to care provider dependency
Excludes2 dependence on enabling machines or devices NEC (Z99.-)

Z74.0 Reduced mobility

Z74.01 Bed confinement status
Bedridden

Z74.09 Other reduced mobility
Chairridden
Reduced mobility NOS
Excludes2 wheelchair dependence (Z99.3)

Z74.1 Need for assistance with personal care

Z74.2 Need for assistance at home and no other household member able to render care

Z74.3 Need for continuous supervision

Z74.8 Other problems related to care provider dependency

Z74.9 Problem related to care provider dependency, unspecified

Z75 Problems related to medical facilities and other health care

Z75.0 Medical services not available in home
Excludes1 no other household member able to render care (Z74.2)

Z75.1 Person awaiting admission to adequate facility elsewhere

Z75.2 Other waiting period for investigation and treatment

Z75.3 Unavailability and inaccessibility of health care facilities
Excludes1 bed unavailable (Z75.1)

Z75.4 Unavailability and inaccessibility of other helping agencies

Z75.5 Holiday relief care

Z75.8 Other problems related to medical facilities and other health care

Z75.9 Unspecified problem related to medical facilities and other health care

Z76 Persons encountering health services in other circumstances

Z76.0 Encounter for issue of repeat prescription
Encounter for issue of repeat prescription for appliance
Encounter for issue of repeat prescription for medicaments
Encounter for issue of repeat prescription for spectacles
Excludes2 issue of medical certificate (Z02.7)
repeat prescription for contraceptive (Z30.4-)

Z76.1 Encounter for health supervision and care of foundling

Z76.2 Encounter for health supervision and care of other healthy infant and child P
Encounter for medical or nursing care or supervision of healthy infant under circumstances such as adverse socioeconomic conditions at home
Encounter for medical or nursing care or supervision of healthy infant under circumstances such as awaiting foster or adoptive placement
Encounter for medical or nursing care or supervision of healthy infant under circumstances such as maternal illness
Encounter for medical or nursing care or supervision of healthy infant under circumstances such as number of children at home preventing or interfering with normal care

Z76.3 Healthy person accompanying sick person

Z76.4 Other boarder to healthcare facility
Excludes1 homelessness (Z59.0)

Z76.5 Malingerer [conscious simulation]
Person feigning illness (with obvious motivation)
Excludes1 factitious disorder (F68.1-)
peregrinating patient (F68.1-)

Z76.8 Persons encountering health services in other specified circumstances

Z76.81 Expectant parent(s) prebirth pediatrician visit
Pre-adoption pediatrician visit for adoptive parent(s)

Z76.82 Awaiting organ transplant status
Patient waiting for organ availability

Z76.89 Persons encountering health services in other specified circumstances
Persons encountering health services NOS

PERSONS WITH POTENTIAL HEALTH HAZARDS RELATED TO FAMILY AND PERSONAL HISTORY AND CERTAIN CONDITIONS INFLUENCING HEALTH STATUS (Z77-Z99)

Code also any follow-up examination (Z08-Z09)

Z77 Other contact with and (suspected) exposures hazardous to health
Includes contact with and (suspected) exposures to potential hazards to health
Excludes2 contact with and (suspected) exposure to communicable diseases (Z20.-)
exposure to (parental) (environmental) tobacco smoke in the perinatal period (P96.81)
newborn affected by noxious substances transmitted via placenta or breast milk (P04.-)
occupational exposure to risk factors (Z57.-)
retained foreign body (Z18.-)
retained foreign body fully removed (Z87.821)
toxic effects of substances chiefly nonmedicinal as to source (T51-T65)

Z77.0 Contact with and (suspected) exposure to hazardous, chiefly nonmedicinal, chemicals

Z77.01 Contact with and (suspected) exposure to hazardous metals

Z77.010 Contact with and (suspected) exposure to arsenic

Z77.011 Contact with and (suspected) exposure to lead

Z77.012 Contact with and (suspected) exposure to uranium
Excludes1 retained depleted uranium fragments (Z18.01)

Z77.018 Contact with and (suspected) exposure to other hazardous metals
Contact with and (suspected) exposure to chromium compounds
Contact with and (suspected) exposure to nickel dust

Z77.02 Contact with and (suspected) exposure to hazardous aromatic compounds

Z77.020 Contact with and (suspected) exposure to aromatic amines

Z77.021 Contact with and (suspected) exposure to benzene

Z77.028 Contact with and (suspected) exposure to other hazardous aromatic compounds
Aromatic dyes NOS
Polycyclic aromatic hydrocarbons

Z77.09 Contact with and (suspected) exposure to other hazardous, chiefly nonmedicinal, chemicals

Z77.090 Contact with and (suspected) exposure to asbestos

Z77.098 Contact with and (suspected) exposure to other hazardous, chiefly nonmedicinal, chemicals
Dyes NOS

Z77.1 Contact with and (suspected) exposure to environmental pollution and hazards in the physical environment

Z77.11 Contact with and (suspected) exposure to environmental pollution

Z77.110 Contact with and (suspected) exposure to air pollution

Z77.111 Contact with and (suspected) exposure to water pollution

Z77.112 Contact with and (suspected) exposure to soil pollution

Z77.118 Contact with and (suspected) exposure to other environmental pollution

Z77.12 Contact with and (suspected) exposure to hazards in the physical environment

Z77.120 Contact with and (suspected) exposure to mold (toxic)

Z77.121 Contact with and (suspected) exposure to harmful algae and algae toxins
Contact with and (suspected) exposure to (harmful) algae bloom NOS
Contact with and (suspected) exposure to blue-green algae bloom
Contact with and (suspected) exposure to brown tide
Contact with and (suspected) exposure to cyanobacteria bloom
Contact with and (suspected) exposure to Florida red tide
Contact with and (suspected) exposure to pfiesteria piscicida
Contact with and (suspected) exposure to red tide

Z77.122 Contact with and (suspected) exposure to noise

● Z77.123 **Contact with and (suspected) exposure to radon and other naturally occuring radiation**

Excludes2 radiation exposure as the cause of a confirmed condition (W88-W90, X39.0-)
radiation sickness NOS (T66)

● Z77.128 **Contact with and (suspected) exposure to other hazards in the physical environment**

● Z77.2 **Contact with and (suspected) exposure to other hazardous substances**

● Z77.21 **Contact with and (suspected) exposure to potentially hazardous body fluids**

● Z77.22 **Contact with and (suspected) exposure to environmental tobacco smoke (acute) (chronic)**
Exposure to second hand tobacco smoke (acute) (chronic)
Passive smoking (acute) (chronic)

Excludes1 nicotine dependence (F17.-)
tobacco use (Z72.0)

Excludes2 occupational exposure to environmental tobacco smoke (Z57.31)

● Z77.29 **Contact with and (suspected) exposure to other hazardous substances**
Coding Clinic: 2016, Q2, P34

● Z77.9 **Other contact with and (suspected) exposures hazardous to health**

● Z78 **Other specified health status**

Excludes2 asymptomatic human immunodeficiency virus [HIV] infection status (Z21)
postprocedural status (Z93-Z99)
sex reassignment status (Z87.890)

● Z78.0 **Asymptomatic menopausal state** ♀ A
Menopausal state NOS
Postmenopausal status NOS

Excludes2 symptomatic menopausal state (N95.1)

● Z78.1 **Physical restraint status**

Excludes1 physical restraint due to a procedure - omit code

● Z78.9 **Other specified health status**

● Z79 **Long term (current) drug therapy**

Includes long term (current) drug use for prophylactic purposes

Code also any therapeutic drug level monitoring (Z51.81)

Excludes2 drug abuse and dependence (F11-F19)
drug use complicating pregnancy, childbirth, and the puerperium (O99.32-)
long term (current) use of oral antidiabetic drugs (Z79.84) ◀
long term (current) use of oral hypoglycemic drugs (Z79.84) ◀

● Z79.0 **Long term (current) use of anticoagulants and antithrombotics/antiplatelets**

Excludes2 long term (current) use of aspirin (Z79.82)

Z79.01 **Long term (current) use of anticoagulants**

● Z79.02 **Long term (current) use of antithrombotics/ antiplatelets**

● Z79.1 **Long term (current) use of non-steroidal anti-inflammatories (NSAID)**

Excludes2 long term (current) use of aspirin (Z79.82)

● Z79.2 **Long term (current) use of antibiotics**

Z79.3 **Long term (current) use of hormonal contraceptives**
Long term (current) use of birth control pill or patch

Z79.4 **Long term (current) use of insulin**

● Z79.5 **Long term (current) use of steroids**

● Z79.51 **Long term (current) use of inhaled steroids**

● Z79.52 **Long term (current) use of systemic steroids**

● Z79.8 **Other long term (current) drug therapy**

● Z79.81 **Long term (current) use of agents affecting estrogen receptors and estrogen levels**

Code first, if applicable:
malignant neoplasm of breast (C50.-)
malignant neoplasm of prostate (C61)

Use additional code, if applicable, to identify:
estrogen receptor positive status (Z17.0)
family history of breast cancer (Z80.3)
genetic susceptibility to malignant neoplasm (cancer) (Z15.0-)
personal history of breast cancer (Z85.3)
personal history of prostate cancer (Z85.46)
postmenopausal status (Z78.0)

Excludes1 hormone replacement therapy (postmenopausal) (Z79.890)

● Z79.810 **Long term (current) use of selective estrogen receptor modulators (SERMs)**
Long term (current) use of raloxifene (Evista)
Long term (current) use of tamoxifen (Nolvadex)
Long term (current) use of toremifene (Fareston)

● Z79.811 **Long term (current) use of aromatase inhibitors**
Long term (current) use of anastrozole (Arimidex)
Long term (current) use of exemestane (Aromasin)
Long term (current) use of letrozole (Femara)

● Z79.818 **Long term (current) use of other agents affecting estrogen receptors and estrogen levels**
Long term (current) use of estrogen receptor downregulators
Long term (current) use of fulvestrant (Faslodex)
Long term (current) use of gonadotropin-releasing hormone (GnRH) agonist
Long term (current) use of goserelin acetate (Zoladex)
Long term (current) use of leuprolide acetate (leuprorelin) (Lupron)
Long term (current) use of megestrol acetate (Megace)

Z79.82 **Long term (current) use of aspirin**

● Z79.83 **Long term (current) use of bisphosphonates**

● Z79.84 **Long term (current) use of oral hypoglycemic drugs** ◀
Long term (current) use of oral antidiabetic drugs ◀

Excludes2 long term (current) use of insulin (Z79.4) ◀

● Z79.89 **Other long term (current) drug therapy**

● Z79.890 **Hormone replacement therapy (postmenopausal)**

Z79.891 **Long term (current) use of opiate analgesic**
Long term (current) use of methadone for pain management

Excludes1 methodone use NOS (F11.9-) ⇐
use of methodone for treatment of heroin addiction (F11.2-)

Z79.899 **Other long term (current) drug therapy**
Coding Clinic: 2015, Q4, P34, Q3, P21

- **Z80 Family history of primary malignant neoplasm**
  - **Z80.0 Family history of malignant neoplasm of digestive organs**
    Conditions classifiable to C15-C26
  - **Z80.1 Family history of malignant neoplasm of trachea, bronchus and lung**
    Conditions classifiable to C33-C34
  - **Z80.2 Family history of malignant neoplasm of other respiratory and intrathoracic organs**
    Conditions classifiable to C30-C32, C37-C39
  - **Z80.3 Family history of malignant neoplasm of breast**
    Conditions classifiable to C50.-
  - **Z80.4 Family history of malignant neoplasm of genital organs**
    Conditions classifiable to C51-C63
    - **Z80.41 Family history of malignant neoplasm of ovary**
    - **Z80.42 Family history of malignant neoplasm of prostate**
    - **Z80.43 Family history of malignant neoplasm of testis**
    - **Z80.49 Family history of malignant neoplasm of other genital organs**
  - **Z80.5 Family history of malignant neoplasm of urinary tract**
    Conditions classifiable to C64-C68
    - **Z80.51 Family history of malignant neoplasm of kidney**
    - **Z80.52 Family history of malignant neoplasm of bladder**
    - **Z80.59 Family history of malignant neoplasm of other urinary tract organ**
  - **Z80.6 Family history of leukemia**
    Conditions classifiable to C91-C95
  - **Z80.7 Family history of other malignant neoplasms of lymphoid, hematopoietic and related tissues**
    Conditions classifiable to C81-C90, C96.-
  - **Z80.8 Family history of malignant neoplasm of other organs or systems**
    Conditions classifiable to C00-C14, C40-C49, C69-C79
  - **Z80.9 Family history of malignant neoplasm, unspecified**
    Conditions classifiable to C80.1
- **Z81 Family history of mental and behavioral disorders**
  - **Z81.0 Family history of intellectual disabilities**
    Conditions classifiable to F70-F79
  - **Z81.1 Family history of alcohol abuse and dependence**
    Conditions classifiable to F10.-
  - **Z81.2 Family history of tobacco abuse and dependence**
    Conditions classifiable to F17.-
  - **Z81.3 Family history of other psychoactive substance abuse and dependence**
    Conditions classifiable to F11-F16, F18-F19
  - **Z81.4 Family history of other substance abuse and dependence**
    Conditions classifiable to F55
  - **Z81.8 Family history of other mental and behavioral disorders**
    Conditions classifiable elsewhere in F01-F99
- **Z82 Family history of certain disabilities and chronic diseases (leading to disablement)**
  - **Z82.0 Family history of epilepsy and other diseases of the nervous system**
    Conditions classifiable to G00-G99
  - **Z82.1 Family history of blindness and visual loss**
    Conditions classifiable to H54.-
  - **Z82.2 Family history of deafness and hearing loss**
    Conditions classifiable to H90-H91
  - **Z82.3 Family history of stroke**
    Conditions classifiable to I60-I64
  - **Z82.4 Family history of ischemic heart disease and other diseases of the circulatory system**
    Conditions classifiable to I00-I52, I65-I99
    - **Z82.41 Family history of sudden cardiac death**
    - **Z82.49 Family history of ischemic heart disease and other diseases of the circulatory system**
  - **Z82.5 Family history of asthma and other chronic lower respiratory diseases**
    Conditions classifiable to J40-J47
    Excludes2 family history of other diseases of the respiratory system (Z83.6)
  - **Z82.6 Family history of arthritis and other diseases of the musculoskeletal system and connective tissue**
    Conditions classifiable to M00-M99
    - **Z82.61 Family history of arthritis**
    - **Z82.62 Family history of osteoporosis**
    - **Z82.69 Family history of other diseases of the musculoskeletal system and connective tissue**
  - **Z82.7 Family history of congenital malformations, deformations and chromosomal abnormalities**
    Conditions classifiable to Q00-Q99
    - **Z82.71 Family history of polycystic kidney**
    - **Z82.79 Family history of other congenital malformations, deformations and chromosomal abnormalities**
  - **Z82.8 Family history of other disabilities and chronic diseases leading to disablement, not elsewhere classified**
- **Z83 Family history of other specific disorders**
  Excludes2 contact with and (suspected) exposure to communicable disease in the family (Z20.-)
  - **Z83.0 Family history of human immunodeficiency virus [HIV] disease**
    Conditions classifiable to B20
  - **Z83.1 Family history of other infectious and parasitic diseases**
    Conditions classifiable to A00-B19, B25-B94, B99
  - **Z83.2 Family history of diseases of the blood and blood-forming organs and certain disorders involving the immune mechanism**
    Conditions classifiable to D50-D89
  - **Z83.3 Family history of diabetes mellitus**
    Conditions classifiable to E08-E13
  - **Z83.4 Family history of other endocrine, nutritional and metabolic diseases**
    Conditions classifiable to E00-E07, E15-E88
    - **Z83.41 Family history of multiple endocrine neoplasia [MEN] syndrome**
    - **Z83.42 Family history of familial hypercholesterolemia** ◀
    - **Z83.49 Family history of other endocrine, nutritional and metabolic diseases**
  - **Z83.5 Family history of eye and ear disorders**
    - **Z83.51 Family history of eye disorders**
      Conditions classifiable to H00-H53, H55-H59
      Excludes2 family history of blindness and visual loss (Z82.1)
      - **Z83.511 Family history of glaucoma**
      - **Z83.518 Family history of other specified eye disorder**
    - **Z83.52 Family history of ear disorders**
      Conditions classifiable to H60-H83, H92-H95
      Excludes2 family history of deafness and hearing loss (Z82.2)
  - **Z83.6 Family history of other diseases of the respiratory system**
    Conditions classifiable to J00-J39, J60-J99
    Excludes2 family history of asthma and other chronic lower respiratory diseases (Z82.5)

- **Z83.7 Family history of diseases of the digestive system**
  Conditions classifiable to K00-K93
  - **Z83.71 Family history of colonic polyps**
    Excludes1 family history of malignant neoplasm of digestive organs (Z80.0)
  - **Z83.79 Family history of other diseases of the digestive system**

- **Z84 Family history of other conditions**
  - **Z84.0 Family history of diseases of the skin and subcutaneous tissue**
    Conditions classifiable to L00-L99
  - **Z84.1 Family history of disorders of kidney and ureter**
    Conditions classifiable to N00-N29
  - **Z84.2 Family history of other diseases of the genitourinary system**
    Conditions classifiable to N30-N99
  - **Z84.3 Family history of consanguinity**
  - **Z84.8 Family history of other specified conditions**
    - **Z84.81 Family history of carrier of genetic disease**
    - **Z84.82 Family history of sudden infant death syndrome** ◀
      Family history of SIDS ◀
    - **Z84.89 Family history of other specified conditions**

- **Z85 Personal history of malignant neoplasm**
  Code first any follow-up examination after treatment of malignant neoplasm (Z08)
  Use additional code to identify:
  alcohol use and dependence (F10.-)
  exposure to environmental tobacco smoke (Z77.22)
  history of tobacco dependence (Z87.891) ◀
  occupational exposure to environmental tobacco smoke (Z57.31)
  tobacco dependence (F17.-)
  tobacco use (Z72.0)
  Excludes2 personal history of benign neoplasm (Z86.01-)
  personal history of carcinoma-in-situ (Z86.00-)
  - **Z85.0 Personal history of malignant neoplasm of digestive organs**
    - **Z85.00 Personal history of malignant neoplasm of unspecified digestive organ**
    - **Z85.01 Personal history of malignant neoplasm of esophagus**
      Conditions classifiable to C15
    - **Z85.02 Personal history of malignant neoplasm of stomach**
      - **Z85.020 Personal history of malignant carcinoid tumor of stomach**
        Conditions classifiable to C7A.092
      - **Z85.028 Personal history of other malignant neoplasm of stomach**
        Conditions classifiable to C16
    - **Z85.03 Personal history of malignant neoplasm of large intestine**
      - **Z85.030 Personal history of malignant carcinoid tumor of large intestine**
        Conditions classifiable to C7A.022-C7A.025, C7A.029
      - **Z85.038 Personal history of other malignant neoplasm of large intestine**
        Conditions classifiable to C18
    - **Z85.04 Personal history of malignant neoplasm of rectum, rectosigmoid junction, and anus**
      - **Z85.040 Personal history of malignant carcinoid tumor of rectum**
        Conditions classifiable to C7A.026
      - **Z85.048 Personal history of other malignant neoplasm of rectum, rectosigmoid junction, and anus**
        Conditions classifiable to C19-C21
    - **Z85.05 Personal history of malignant neoplasm of liver**
      Conditions classifiable to C22
    - **Z85.06 Personal history of malignant neoplasm of small intestine**
      - **Z85.060 Personal history of malignant carcinoid tumor of small intestine**
        Conditions classifiable to C7A.01-
      - **Z85.068 Personal history of other malignant neoplasm of small intestine**
        Conditions classifiable to C17
    - **Z85.07 Personal history of malignant neoplasm of pancreas**
      Conditions classifiable to C25
    - **Z85.09 Personal history of malignant neoplasm of other digestive organs**
  - **Z85.1 Personal history of malignant neoplasm of trachea, bronchus and lung**
    - **Z85.11 Personal history of malignant neoplasm of bronchus and lung**
      - **Z85.110 Personal history of malignant carcinoid tumor of bronchus and lung**
        Conditions classifiable to C7A.090
      - **Z85.118 Personal history of other malignant neoplasm of bronchus and lung**
        Conditions classifiable to C34
    - **Z85.12 Personal history of malignant neoplasm of trachea**
      Conditions classifiable to C33
  - **Z85.2 Personal history of malignant neoplasm of other respiratory and intrathoracic organs**
    - **Z85.20 Personal history of malignant neoplasm of unspecified respiratory organ**
    - **Z85.21 Personal history of malignant neoplasm of larynx**
      Conditions classifiable to C32
    - **Z85.22 Personal history of malignant neoplasm of nasal cavities, middle ear, and accessory sinuses**
      Conditions classifiable to C30-C31
    - **Z85.23 Personal history of malignant neoplasm of thymus**
      - **Z85.230 Personal history of malignant carcinoid tumor of thymus**
        Conditions classifiable to C7A.091
      - **Z85.238 Personal history of other malignant neoplasm of thymus**
        Conditions classifiable to C37
    - **Z85.29 Personal history of malignant neoplasm of other respiratory and intrathoracic organs**
  - **Z85.3 Personal history of malignant neoplasm of breast**
    Conditions classifiable to C50.-
  - **Z85.4 Personal history of malignant neoplasm of genital organs**
    Conditions classifiable to C51-C63
    - **Z85.40 Personal history of malignant neoplasm of unspecified female genital organ ♀**
    - **Z85.41 Personal history of malignant neoplasm of cervix uteri ♀**
    - **Z85.42 Personal history of malignant neoplasm of other parts of uterus ♀**
    - **Z85.43 Personal history of malignant neoplasm of ovary ♀**
    - **Z85.44 Personal history of malignant neoplasm of other female genital organs ♀**
    - **Z85.45 Personal history of malignant neoplasm of unspecified male genital organ ♂**
    - **Z85.46 Personal history of malignant neoplasm of prostate ♂**
    - **Z85.47 Personal history of malignant neoplasm of testis ♂**

- **Z85.48 Personal history of malignant neoplasm of epididymis ♂**
- **Z85.49 Personal history of malignant neoplasm of other male genital organs ♂**

Z85.5 Personal history of malignant neoplasm of urinary tract
Conditions classifiable to C64-C68

- **Z85.50 Personal history of malignant neoplasm of unspecified urinary tract organ**
- **Z85.51 Personal history of malignant neoplasm of bladder**
- **Z85.52 Personal history of malignant neoplasm of kidney**

  Excludes1 personal history of malignant neoplasm of renal pelvis (Z85.53)

  - **Z85.520 Personal history of malignant carcinoid tumor of kidney**
    Conditions classifiable to C7A.093
  - **Z85.528 Personal history of other malignant neoplasm of kidney**
    Conditions classifiable to C64
- **Z85.53 Personal history of malignant neoplasm of renal pelvis**
- **Z85.54 Personal history of malignant neoplasm of ureter**
- **Z85.59 Personal history of malignant neoplasm of other urinary tract organ**

Z85.6 Personal history of leukemia
Conditions classifiable to C91-C95

Excludes1 leukemia in remission C91.0-C95.9 with 5th character 1

Z85.7 Personal history of other malignant neoplasms of lymphoid, hematopoietic and related tissues

- **Z85.71 Personal history of Hodgkin lymphoma**
  Conditions classifiable to C81
- **Z85.72 Personal history of non-Hodgkin lymphomas**
  Conditions classifiable to C82-C85
- **Z85.79 Personal history of other malignant neoplasms of lymphoid, hematopoietic and related tissues**
  Conditions classifiable to C88-C90, C96

  Excludes1 multiple myeloma in remission (C90.01)
  plasma cell leukemia in remission (C90.11)
  plasmacytoma in remission (C90.21)

Z85.8 Personal history of malignant neoplasms of other organs and systems
Conditions classifiable to C00-C14, C40-C49, C69-C75, C7A.098, C76-C79 ◀

- **Z85.81 Personal history of malignant neoplasm of lip, oral cavity, and pharynx**
  - **Z85.810 Personal history of malignant neoplasm of tongue**
  - **Z85.818 Personal history of malignant neoplasm of other sites of lip, oral cavity, and pharynx**
  - **Z85.819 Personal history of malignant neoplasm of unspecified site of lip, oral cavity, and pharynx**
- **Z85.82 Personal history of malignant neoplasm of skin**
  - **Z85.820 Personal history of malignant melanoma of skin**
    Conditions classifiable to C43
  - **Z85.821 Personal history of Merkel cell carcinoma**
    Conditions classifiable to C4A
  - **Z85.828 Personal history of other malignant neoplasm of skin**
    Conditions classifiable to C44
- **Z85.83 Personal history of malignant neoplasm of bone and soft tissue**
  - **Z85.830 Personal history of malignant neoplasm of bone**
  - **Z85.831 Personal history of malignant neoplasm of soft tissue**

    Excludes2 personal history of malignant neoplasm of skin (Z85.82-)
- **Z85.84 Personal history of malignant neoplasm of eye and nervous tissue**
  - **Z85.840 Personal history of malignant neoplasm of eye**
  - **Z85.841 Personal history of malignant neoplasm of brain**
  - **Z85.848 Personal history of malignant neoplasm of other parts of nervous tissue**
- **Z85.85 Personal history of malignant neoplasm of endocrine glands**
  - **Z85.850 Personal history of malignant neoplasm of thyroid**
  - **Z85.858 Personal history of malignant neoplasm of other endocrine glands**
- **Z85.89 Personal history of malignant neoplasm of other organs and systems**

Z85.9 Personal history of malignant neoplasm, unspecified
Conditions classifiable to C7A.00, C80.1

Z86 Personal history of certain other diseases
Code first any follow-up examination after treatment (Z09)

- **Z86.0 Personal history of in-situ and benign neoplasms and neoplasms of uncertain behavior**

  Excludes2 personal history of malignant neoplasms (Z85.-)

  - **Z86.00 Personal history of in-situ neoplasm**
    Conditions classifiable to D00-D09 ◀
    - **Z86.000 Personal history of in-situ neoplasm of breast**
    - **Z86.001 Personal history of in-situ neoplasm of cervix uteri ♀**
      Personal history of cervical intraepithelial neoplasia III [CIN III] ◀
    - **Z86.008 Personal history of in-situ neoplasm of other site**
      Personal history of vaginal intraepithelial neoplasia III [VAIN III] ◀
      Personal history of vulvar intraepithelial neoplasia III [VIN III] ◀
  - **Z86.01 Personal history of benign neoplasm**
    - **Z86.010 Personal history of colonic polyps**
    - **Z86.011 Personal history of benign neoplasm of the brain**
    - **Z86.012 Personal history of benign carcinoid tumor**
    - **Z86.018 Personal history of other benign neoplasm**
  - **Z86.03 Personal history of neoplasm of uncertain behavior**

- **Z86.1 Personal history of infectious and parasitic diseases**
  Conditions classifiable to A00-B89, B99
  Excludes1 personal history of infectious diseases specific to a body system sequelae of infectious and parasitic diseases (B90-B94)
  - **Z86.11 Personal history of tuberculosis**
  - **Z86.12 Personal history of poliomyelitis**
  - **Z86.13 Personal history of malaria**
  - **Z86.14 Personal history of Methicillin resistant Staphylococcus aureus infection**
    Personal history of MRSA infection
  - **Z86.19 Personal history of other infectious and parasitic diseases**
- **Z86.2 Personal history of diseases of the blood and blood-forming organs and certain disorders involving the immune mechanism**
  Conditions classifiable to D50-D89
- **Z86.3 Personal history of endocrine, nutritional and metabolic diseases**
  Conditions classifiable to E00-E88
  - **Z86.31 Personal history of diabetic foot ulcer**
    Excludes2 current diabetic foot ulcer (E08.621, E09.621, E10.621, E11.621, E13.621)
  - **Z86.32 Personal history of gestational diabetes ♀**
    Personal history of conditions classifiable to O24.4-
    Excludes1 gestational diabetes mellitus in current pregnancy (O24.4-)
  - **Z86.39 Personal history of other endocrine, nutritional and metabolic disease**
- **Z86.5 Personal history of mental and behavioral disorders**
  Conditions classifiable to F40-F59
  - **Z86.51 Personal history of combat and operational stress reaction** A
  - **Z86.59 Personal history of other mental and behavioral disorders**
- **Z86.6 Personal history of diseases of the nervous system and sense organs**
  Conditions classifiable to G00-G99, H00-H95
  - **Z86.61 Personal history of infections of the central nervous system**
    Personal history of encephalitis
    Personal history of meningitis
  - **Z86.69 Personal history of other diseases of the nervous system and sense organs**
- **Z86.7 Personal history of diseases of the circulatory system**
  Conditions classifiable to I00-I99
  Excludes2 old myocardial infarction (I25.2)
  personal history of anaphylactic shock (Z87.892)
  postmyocardial infarction syndrome (I24.1)
  - **Z86.71 Personal history of venous thrombosis and embolism**
    - **Z86.711 Personal history of pulmonary embolism**
    - **Z86.718 Personal history of other venous thrombosis and embolism**
  - **Z86.72 Personal history of thrombophlebitis**
  - **Z86.73 Personal history of transient ischemic attack (TIA), and cerebral infarction without residual deficits**
    Personal history of prolonged reversible ischemic neurological deficit (PRIND)
    Personal history of stroke NOS without residual deficits
    Excludes1 personal history of traumatic brain injury (Z87.820)
    sequelae of cerebrovascular disease (I69.-)
    Coding Clinic: 2012, Q4, P3
  - **Z86.74 Personal history of sudden cardiac arrest**
    Personal history of sudden cardiac death successfully resuscitated
  - **Z86.79 Personal history of other diseases of the circulatory system**

- **Z87 Personal history of other diseases and conditions**
  Code first any follow-up examination after treatment (Z09)
  - **Z87.0 Personal history of diseases of the respiratory system**
    Conditions classifiable to J00-J99
    - **Z87.01 Personal history of pneumonia (recurrent)**
    - **Z87.09 Personal history of other diseases of the respiratory system**
  - **Z87.1 Personal history of diseases of the digestive system**
    Conditions classifiable to K00-K93
    - **Z87.11 Personal history of peptic ulcer disease**
    - **Z87.19 Personal history of other diseases of the digestive system**
  - **Z87.2 Personal history of diseases of the skin and subcutaneous tissue**
    Conditions classifiable to L00-L99
    Excludes2 personal history of diabetic foot ulcer (Z86.31)
  - **Z87.3 Personal history of diseases of the musculoskeletal system and connective tissue**
    Conditions classifiable to M00-M99
    Excludes2 personal history of (healed) traumatic fracture (Z87.81)
    - **Z87.31 Personal history of (healed) nontraumatic fracture**
      - **Z87.310 Personal history of (healed) osteoporosis fracture**
        Personal history of (healed) fragility fracture
        Personal history of (healed) collapsed vertebra due to osteoporosis
      - **Z87.311 Personal history of (healed) other pathological fracture**
        Personal history of (healed) collapsed vertebra NOS
        Excludes2 personal history of osteoporosis fracture (Z87.310)
      - **Z87.312 Personal history of (healed) stress fracture**
        Personal history of (healed) fatigue fracture
    - **Z87.39 Personal history of other diseases of the musculoskeletal system and connective tissue**

- **Z87.4 Personal history of diseases of genitourinary system**
  Conditions classifiable to N00-N99
  - **Z87.41 Personal history of dysplasia of the female genital tract**
    Excludes1 personal history of intraepithelial neoplasia III of female genital tract (Z87.001, Z87.008) ◀
    personal history of malignant neoplasm of female genital tract (Z85.40-Z85.44)
    - **Z87.410 Personal history of cervical dysplasia ♀**
    - **Z87.411 Personal history of vaginal dysplasia ♀**
    - **Z87.412 Personal history of vulvar dysplasia ♀**
  - **Z87.42 Personal history of other diseases of the female genital tract ♀**
  - **Z87.43 Personal history of diseases of male genital organs**
    - **Z87.430 Personal history of prostatic dysplasia ♂**
      Excludes1 personal history of malignant neoplasm of prostate (Z85.46)
    - **Z87.438 Personal history of other diseases of male genital organs ♂**
  - **Z87.44 Personal history of diseases of urinary system**
    Excludes1 personal history of malignant neoplasm of cervix uteri (Z85.41)
    - **Z87.440 Personal history of urinary (tract) infections**
    - **Z87.441 Personal history of nephrotic syndrome**
    - **Z87.442 Personal history of urinary calculi**
      Personal history of kidney stones
    - **Z87.448 Personal history of other diseases of urinary system**
- **Z87.5 Personal history of complications of pregnancy, childbirth and the puerperium**
  Conditions classifiable to O00-O9A
  Excludes2 recurrent pregnancy loss (N96)
  - **Z87.51 Personal history of pre-term labor ♀**
    Excludes1 current pregnancy with history of pre-term labor (O09.21-)
  - **Z87.59 Personal history of other complications of pregnancy, childbirth and the puerperium ♀**
    Personal history of trophoblastic disease
- **Z87.7 Personal history of (corrected) congenital malformations**
  Conditions classifiable to Q00-Q89 that have been repaired or corrected
  Excludes1 congenital malformations that have been partially corrected or repair but which still require medical treatment - code to condition
  Excludes2 other postprocedural states (Z98.-)
  personal history of medical treatment (Z92.-)
  presence of cardiac and vascular implants and grafts (Z95.-)
  presence of other devices (Z97.-)
  presence of other functional implants (Z96.-)
  transplanted organ and tissue status (Z94.-)
  - **Z87.71 Personal history of (corrected) congenital malformations of genitourinary system**
    - **Z87.710 Personal history of (corrected) hypospadias ♂**
    - **Z87.718 Personal history of other specified (corrected) congenital malformations of genitourinary system**
  - **Z87.72 Personal history of (corrected) congenital malformations of nervous system and sense organs**
    - **Z87.720 Personal history of (corrected) congenital malformations of eye**
    - **Z87.721 Personal history of (corrected) congenital malformations of ear**
    - **Z87.728 Personal history of other specified (corrected) congenital malformations of nervous system and sense organs**
  - **Z87.73 Personal history of (corrected) congenital malformations of digestive system**
    - **Z87.730 Personal history of (corrected) cleft lip and palate**
    - **Z87.738 Personal history of other specified (corrected) congenital malformations of digestive system**
  - **Z87.74 Personal history of (corrected) congenital malformations of heart and circulatory system**
  - **Z87.75 Personal history of (corrected) congenital malformations of respiratory system**
  - **Z87.76 Personal history of (corrected) congenital malformations of integument, limbs and musculoskeletal system**
  - **Z87.79 Personal history of other (corrected) congenital malformations**
    - **Z87.790 Personal history of (corrected) congenital malformations of face and neck**
    - **Z87.798 Personal history of other (corrected) congenital malformations**
- **Z87.8 Personal history of other specified conditions**
  Excludes2 personal history of self harm (Z91.5)
  - **Z87.81 Personal history of (healed) traumatic fracture**
    Excludes2 personal history of (healed) nontraumatic fracture (Z87.31-)
  - **Z87.82 Personal history of other (healed) physical injury and trauma**
    Conditions classifiable to S00-T88, except traumatic fractures
    - **Z87.820 Personal history of traumatic brain injury**
      Excludes1 personal history of transient ischemic attack (TIA), and cerebral infarction without residual deficits (Z86.73)
    - **Z87.821 Personal history of retained foreign body fully removed**
    - **Z87.828 Personal history of other (healed) physical injury and trauma**
  - **Z87.89 Personal history of other specified conditions**
    Z87.890 Personal history of sex reassignment
    - **Z87.891 Personal history of nicotine dependence**
      Excludes1 current nicotine dependence (F17.2-)
    - **Z87.892 Personal history of anaphylaxis**
      Code also allergy status such as:
      allergy status to drugs, medicaments and biological substances (Z88.-)
      allergy status, other than to drugs and biological substances (Z91.0-)
    - **Z87.898 Personal history of other specified conditions**
      Coding Clinic: 2013, Q1, P21

- **Z88 Allergy status to drugs, medicaments and biological substances**
  - **Excludes2** allergy status, other than to drugs and biological substances (Z91.0-)
  - **Z88.0 Allergy status to penicillin**
  - **Z88.1 Allergy status to other antibiotic agents status**
  - **Z88.2 Allergy status to sulfonamides status**
    - **Coding Clinic: 2015, Q3, P23**
  - **Z88.3 Allergy status to other anti-infective agents status**
  - **Z88.4 Allergy status to anesthetic agent status**
  - **Z88.5 Allergy status to narcotic agent status**
  - **Z88.6 Allergy status to analgesic agent status**
  - **Z88.7 Allergy status to serum and vaccine status**
  - **Z88.8 Allergy status to other drugs, medicaments and biological substances status**
  - **Z88.9 Allergy status to unspecified drugs, medicaments and biological substances status**
- **Z89 Acquired absence of limb**
  - **Includes** amputation status
    postprocedural loss of limb
    post-traumatic loss of limb
  - **Excludes1** acquired deformities of limbs (M20-M21)
    congenital absence of limbs (Q71-Q73)
  - **Z89.0 Acquired absence of thumb and other finger(s)**
    - **Z89.01 Acquired absence of thumb**
      - **Z89.011 Acquired absence of right thumb**
      - **Z89.012 Acquired absence of left thumb**
      - **Z89.019 Acquired absence of unspecified thumb**
    - **Z89.02 Acquired absence of other finger(s)**
      - **Excludes2** acquired absence of thumb (Z89.01-)
      - **Z89.021 Acquired absence of right finger(s)**
      - **Z89.022 Acquired absence of left finger(s)**
      - **Z89.029 Acquired absence of unspecified finger(s)**
  - **Z89.1 Acquired absence of hand and wrist**
    - **Z89.11 Acquired absence of hand**
      - **Z89.111 Acquired absence of right hand**
      - **Z89.112 Acquired absence of left hand**
      - **Z89.119 Acquired absence of unspecified hand**
    - **Z89.12 Acquired absence of wrist**
      Disarticulation at wrist
      - **Z89.121 Acquired absence of right wrist**
      - **Z89.122 Acquired absence of left wrist**
      - **Z89.129 Acquired absence of unspecified wrist**
  - **Z89.2 Acquired absence of upper limb above wrist**
    - **Z89.20 Acquired absence of upper limb, unspecified level**
      - **Z89.201 Acquired absence of right upper limb, unspecified level**
      - **Z89.202 Acquired absence of left upper limb, unspecified level**
      - **Z89.209 Acquired absence of unspecified upper limb, unspecified level**
        Acquired absence of arm NOS
    - **Z89.21 Acquired absence of upper limb below elbow**
      - **Z89.211 Acquired absence of right upper limb below elbow**
      - **Z89.212 Acquired absence of left upper limb below elbow**
      - **Z89.219 Acquired absence of unspecified upper limb below elbow**
    - **Z89.22 Acquired absence of upper limb above elbow**
      Disarticulation at elbow
      - **Z89.221 Acquired absence of right upper limb above elbow**
      - **Z89.222 Acquired absence of left upper limb above elbow**
      - **Z89.229 Acquired absence of unspecified upper limb above elbow**
    - **Z89.23 Acquired absence of shoulder**
      Acquired absence of shoulder joint following explantation of shoulder joint prosthesis, with or without presence of antibiotic-impregnated cement spacer
      - **Z89.231 Acquired absence of right shoulder**
      - **Z89.232 Acquired absence of left shoulder**
      - **Z89.239 Acquired absence of unspecified shoulder**
  - **Z89.4 Acquired absence of toe(s), foot, and ankle**
    - **Z89.41 Acquired absence of great toe**
      - **Z89.411 Acquired absence of right great toe**
      - **Z89.412 Acquired absence of left great toe**
      - **Z89.419 Acquired absence of unspecified great toe**
    - **Z89.42 Acquired absence of other toe(s)**
      - **Excludes2** acquired absence of great toe (Z89.41-)
      - **Z89.421 Acquired absence of other right toe(s)**
      - **Z89.422 Acquired absence of other left toe(s)**
      - **Z89.429 Acquired absence of other toe(s), unspecified side**
    - **Z89.43 Acquired absence of foot**
      - **Z89.431 Acquired absence of right foot**
      - **Z89.432 Acquired absence of left foot**
      - **Z89.439 Acquired absence of unspecified foot**
    - **Z89.44 Acquired absence of ankle**
      Disarticulation of ankle
      - **Z89.441 Acquired absence of right ankle**
      - **Z89.442 Acquired absence of left ankle**
      - **Z89.449 Acquired absence of unspecified ankle**
  - **Z89.5 Acquired absence of leg below knee**
    - **Z89.51 Acquired absence of leg below knee**
      - **Z89.511 Acquired absence of right leg below knee**
      - **Z89.512 Acquired absence of left leg below knee**
      - **Z89.519 Acquired absence of unspecified leg below knee**
    - **Z89.52 Acquired absence of knee**
      Acquired absence of knee joint following explantation of knee joint prosthesis, with or without presence of antibiotic-impregnated cement spacer
      - **Z89.521 Acquired absence of right knee**
      - **Z89.522 Acquired absence of left knee**
      - **Z89.529 Acquired absence of unspecified knee**

◀ New ⇐ Revised ~~deleted~~ Deleted Excludes 1 Excludes 2 Includes Use additional Code first Code also Unspecified
OGCR Official Guidelines ● Unacceptable Principal Diagnosis X Assign placeholder X ● Use Additional Character(s) ▶ Manifestation Code Coding Clinic

- **Z89.6 Acquired absence of leg above knee**
  - **Z89.61 Acquired absence of leg above knee**
    Acquired absence of leg NOS
    Disarticulation at knee
    - **Z89.611 Acquired absence of right leg above knee**
    - **Z89.612 Acquired absence of left leg above knee**
    - **Z89.619 Acquired absence of unspecified leg above knee**
  - **Z89.62 Acquired absence of hip**
    Acquired absence of hip joint following explantation of hip joint prosthesis, with or without presence of antibiotic-impregnated cement spacer
    Disarticulation at hip
    - **Z89.621 Acquired absence of right hip joint**
    - **Z89.622 Acquired absence of left hip joint**
    - **Z89.629 Acquired absence of unspecified hip joint**
- **Z89.9 Acquired absence of limb, unspecified**

- **Z90 Acquired absence of organs, not elsewhere classified**
  Includes postprocedural or post-traumatic loss of body part NEC
  Excludes1 congenital absence - see Alphabetical Index
  Excludes2 postprocedural absence of endocrine glands (E89.-)
  - **Z90.0 Acquired absence of part of head and neck**
    - **Z90.01 Acquired absence of eye**
    - **Z90.02 Acquired absence of larynx**
    - **Z90.09 Acquired absence of other part of head and neck**
      Acquired absence of nose
      Excludes2 teeth (K08.1)
  - **Z90.1 Acquired absence of breast and nipple**
    - **Z90.10 Acquired absence of unspecified breast and nipple**
    - **Z90.11 Acquired absence of right breast and nipple**
    - **Z90.12 Acquired absence of left breast and nipple**
    - **Z90.13 Acquired absence of bilateral breasts and nipples**
  - **Z90.2 Acquired absence of lung [part of]**
  - **Z90.3 Acquired absence of stomach [part of]**
  - **Z90.4 Acquired absence of other specified parts of digestive tract**
    - **Z90.41 Acquired absence of pancreas**
      Code also exocrine pancreatic insufficiency (K86.81) ◀
      Use additional code to identify any associated:
      insulin use (Z79.4)
      diabetes mellitus, postpancreatectomy (E13.-)
      - **Z90.410 Acquired total absence of pancreas**
        Acquired absence of pancreas NOS
      - **Z90.411 Acquired partial absence of pancreas**
    - **Z90.49 Acquired absence of other specified parts of digestive tract**
  - **Z90.5 Acquired absence of kidney**
  - **Z90.6 Acquired absence of other parts of urinary tract**
    Acquired absence of bladder
  - **Z90.7 Acquired absence of genital organ(s)**
    Excludes1 personal history of sex reassignment (Z87.890)
    Excludes2 female genital mutilation status (N90.81-)
    - **Z90.71 Acquired absence of cervix and uterus**
      - **Z90.710 Acquired absence of both cervix and uterus ♀**
        Acquired absence of uterus NOS
        Status post total hysterectomy
      - **Z90.711 Acquired absence of uterus with remaining cervical stump ♀**
        Status post partial hysterectomy with remaining cervical stump
      - **Z90.712 Acquired absence of cervix with remaining uterus ♀**
    - **Z90.72 Acquired absence of ovaries**
      - **Z90.721 Acquired absence of ovaries, unilateral ♀**
      - **Z90.722 Acquired absence of ovaries, bilateral ♀**
    - **Z90.79 Acquired absence of other genital organ(s)**
  - **Z90.8 Acquired absence of other organs**
    - **Z90.81 Acquired absence of spleen**
    - **Z90.89 Acquired absence of other organs**

- **Z91 Personal risk factors, not elsewhere classified**
  Excludes2 contact with and (suspected) exposures hazardous to health (Z77.-)
  exposure to pollution and other problems related to physical environment (Z77.1-)
  occupational exposure to risk factors (Z57.-)
  personal history of physical injury and trauma (Z87.81, Z87.82-)
  - **Z91.0 Allergy status, other than to drugs and biological substances**
    Excludes2 allergy status to drugs, medicaments, and biological substances (Z88.-)
    - **Z91.01 Food allergy status**
      Excludes2 food additives allergy status (Z91.02)
      - **Z91.010 Allergy to peanuts**
      - **Z91.011 Allergy to milk products**
        Excludes1 lactose intolerance (E73.-)
      - **Z91.012 Allergy to eggs**
      - **Z91.013 Allergy to seafood**
        Allergy to shellfish
        Allergy to octopus or squid ink
      - **Z91.018 Allergy to other foods**
        Allergy to nuts other than peanuts
    - **Z91.02 Food additives allergy status**
    - **Z91.03 Insect allergy status**
      - **Z91.030 Bee allergy status**
      - **Z91.038 Other insect allergy status**
    - **Z91.04 Nonmedicinal substance allergy status**
      - **Z91.040 Latex allergy status**
        Latex sensitivity status
      - **Z91.041 Radiographic dye allergy status**
        Allergy status to contrast media used for diagnostic X-ray procedure
      - **Z91.048 Other nonmedicinal substance allergy status**
    - **Z91.09 Other allergy status, other than to drugs and biological substances**

- **Z91.1 Patient's noncompliance with medical treatment and regimen**
  - **Z91.11 Patient's noncompliance with dietary regimen**
  - **Z91.12 Patient's intentional underdosing of medication regimen**
    - *Code first underdosing of medication (T36-T50) with fifth or sixth character 6*
    - **Excludes1** adverse effect of prescribed drug taken as directed - code to adverse effect
      poisoning (overdose) - code to poisoning
    - **Z91.120 Patient's intentional underdosing of medication regimen due to financial hardship**
    - **Z91.128 Patient's intentional underdosing of medication regimen for other reason**
  - **Z91.13 Patient's unintentional underdosing of medication regimen**
    - *Code first underdosing of medication (T36-T50) with fifth or sixth character 6*
    - **Excludes1** adverse effect of prescribed drug taken as directed - code to adverse effect
      poisoning (overdose) - code to poisoning
    - **Z91.130 Patient's unintentional underdosing of medication regimen due to age-related debility**
    - **Z91.138 Patient's unintentional underdosing of medication regimen for other reason**
  - **Z91.14 Patient's other noncompliance with medication regimen**
    - Patient's underdosing of medication NOS
  - **Z91.15 Patient's noncompliance with renal dialysis**
  - **Z91.19 Patient's noncompliance with other medical treatment and regimen**
- **Z91.4 Personal history of psychological trauma, not elsewhere classified**
  - **Z91.41 Personal history of adult abuse**
    - **Excludes2** personal history of abuse in childhood (Z62.81-)
    - **Z91.410 Personal history of adult physical and sexual abuse** A
      - **Excludes1** current adult physical abuse (T74.11, T76.11)
        current adult sexual abuse (T74.21, T76.11)
    - **Z91.411 Personal history of adult psychological abuse** A
    - **Z91.412 Personal history of adult neglect** A
      - **Excludes1** current adult neglect (T74.01, T76.01)
    - **Z91.419 Personal history of unspecified adult abuse** A
  - **Z91.49 Other personal history of psychological trauma, not elsewhere classified**
- **Z91.5 Personal history of self-harm**
  - Personal history of parasuicide
  - Personal history of self-poisoning
  - Personal history of suicide attempt
- **Z91.8 Other specified personal risk factors, not elsewhere classified**
  - **Z91.81 History of falling**
    - At risk for falling
  - **Z91.82 Personal history of military deployment** A
    - Individual (civilian or military) with past history of military war, peacekeeping and humanitarian deployment (current or past conflict)
    - Returned from military deployment
  - ▶ ***Z91.83 Wandering in diseases classified elsewhere***
    - *Code first underlying disorder such as:*
      - Alzheimer's disease (G30.-)
      - autism or pervasive developmental disorder (F84.-)
      - intellectual disabilities (F70-F79)
      - unspecified dementia with behavioral disturbance (F03.9-)
  - **Z91.89 Other specified personal risk factors, not elsewhere classified**
- **Z92 Personal history of medical treatment**
  - **Excludes2** postprocedural states (Z98.-)
  - **Z92.0 Personal history of contraception**
    - **Excludes1** counseling or management of current contraceptive practices (Z30.-)
      long term (current) use of contraception (Z79.3)
      presence of (intrauterine) contraceptive device (Z97.5)
  - **Z92.2 Personal history of drug therapy**
    - **Excludes2** long term (current) drug therapy (Z79.-)
    - **Z92.21 Personal history of antineoplastic chemotherapy**
    - **Z92.22 Personal history of monoclonal drug therapy**
    - **Z92.23 Personal history of estrogen therapy**
    - **Z92.24 Personal history of steroid therapy**
      - **Z92.240 Personal history of inhaled steroid therapy**
      - **Z92.241 Personal history of systemic steroid therapy**
        - Personal history of steroid therapy NOS
    - **Z92.25 Personal history of immunosupression therapy**
      - **Excludes2** personal history of steroid therapy (Z92.24)
    - **Z92.29 Personal history of other drug therapy**
  - **Z92.3 Personal history of irradiation**
    - Personal history of exposure to therapeutic radiation
    - **Excludes1** exposure to radiation in the physical environment (Z77.12)
      occupational exposure to radiation (Z57.1)
  - **Z92.8 Personal history of other medical treatment**
    - **Z92.81 Personal history of extracorporeal membrane oxygenation (ECMO)**
    - **Z92.82 Status post administration of tPA (rtPA) in a different facility within the last 24 hours prior to admission to current facility**
      - *Code first condition requiring tPA administration, such as:*
        - acute cerebral infarction (I63.-)
        - acute myocardial infarction (I21.-, I22.-)
    - **Z92.83 Personal history of failed moderate sedation**
      - Personal history of failed conscious sedation
      - **Excludes2** failed moderate sedation during procedure (T88.52)

- **Z92.84 Personal history of unintended awareness under general anesthesia** ◀
  - **Excludes2** unintended awareness under general anesthesia during procedure (T88.53) ◀
- **Z92.89 Personal history of other medical treatment**

Z93 Artificial opening status
- **Excludes1** artificial openings requiring attention or management (Z43.-)
  complications of external stoma (J95.0-, K94.-, N99.5-)
- **Z93.0 Tracheostomy status**
- **Z93.1 Gastrostomy status**
- **Z93.2 Ileostomy status**
- **Z93.3 Colostomy status**
- **Z93.4 Other artificial openings of gastrointestinal tract status**
- **Z93.5 Cystostomy status**
  - **Z93.50 Unspecified cystostomy status**
  - **Z93.51 Cutaneous-vesicostomy status**
  - **Z93.52 Appendico-vesicostomy status**
  - **Z93.59 Other cystostomy status**
- **Z93.6 Other artificial openings of urinary tract status**
  Nephrostomy status
  Ureterostomy status
  Urethrostomy status
- **Z93.8 Other artificial opening status**
- **Z93.9 Artificial opening status, unspecified**

Z94 Transplanted organ and tissue status
- **Includes** organ or tissue replaced by heterogenous or homogenous transplant
- **Excludes1** complications of transplanted organ or tissue - see Alphabetical Index
- **Excludes2** presence of vascular grafts (Z95.-)
- **Z94.0 Kidney transplant status** CC
  Ex: D47.Z1, T86.10-T86.19, T86.850-T86.859, T86.90-T86.99, Z94.0, Z94.89-Z94.9
- **Z94.1 Heart transplant status** CC
  - **Excludes1** artificial heart status (Z95.812)
    heart-valve replacement status (Z95.2-Z95.4)
  Ex: D47.Z1, T86.20-T86.39, T86.850-T86.859, T86.90-T86.99, Z94.1, Z94.3, Z94.89-Z94.9
- **Z94.2 Lung transplant status** CC
  Ex: D47.Z1, T86.810-T86.819, T86.850-T86.859, T86.90-T86.99, Z94.2, Z94.89-Z94.9
- **Z94.3 Heart and lungs transplant status** CC
  CC when PDx is its own CC
  Ex: See Z94.1
- **Z94.4 Liver transplant status** CC
  Ex: D47.Z1, T86.40-T86.49, T86.850-T86.859, T86.90-T86.99, Z94.4, Z94.89, Z94.9
- **Z94.5 Skin transplant status**
  Autogenous skin transplant status
- **Z94.6 Bone transplant status**
- **Z94.7 Corneal transplant status**
- **Z94.8 Other transplanted organ and tissue status**
  - **Z94.81 Bone marrow transplant status** CC
    Ex: D47.Z1, D89.810-D89.813, T86.00-T86.09, T86.850-T86.859, T86.90-T86.99, Z94.9
  - **Z94.82 Intestine transplant status** CC
    Ex: D47.Z1, T86.830-T86.839, T86.90-T86.99, Z94.82, Z94.89-Z94.9
  - **Z94.83 Pancreas transplant status** CC
    Ex: D47.Z1, T86.850-T86.859, T86.890-T86.99, Z94.83, Z94.9
  - **Z94.84 Stem cells transplant status** CC
    Ex: D47.Z1, T86.850-T86.859, T86.90-T86.99, Z94.9
  - **Z94.89 Other transplanted organ and tissue status**
- **Z94.9 Transplanted organ and tissue status, unspecified**

Z95 Presence of cardiac and vascular implants and grafts
- **Excludes1** complications of cardiac and vascular devices, implants and grafts (T82.-)
- **Z95.0 Presence of cardiac pacemaker**
  Presence of cardiac resynchronization therapy (CRT-P) pacemaker ◀
  - **Excludes1** adjustment or management of cardiac device (Z45.0-) ◀
    adjustment or management of cardiac pacemaker (Z45.0)
    presence of automatic (implantable) cardiac defibrillator with synchronous cardiac pacemaker (Z95.810)
- **Z95.1 Presence of aortocoronary bypass graft**
  Presence of coronary artery bypass graft ◀
- **Z95.2 Presence of prosthetic heart valve**
  Presence of heart valve NOS
- **Z95.3 Presence of xenogenic heart valve**
- **Z95.4 Presence of other heart-valve replacement**
- **Z95.5 Presence of coronary angioplasty implant and graft**
  - **Excludes1** coronary angioplasty status without implant and graft (Z98.61)
- **Z95.8 Presence of other cardiac and vascular implants and grafts**
  - **Z95.81 Presence of other cardiac implants and grafts**
    Ex: For category Z95.81 CC codes: D47.Z1, T86.20-T86.39, T86.850-T86.99, Z94.1, Z94.3, Z95.811-Z95.812
    - **Z95.810 Presence of automatic (implantable) cardiac defibrillator**
      Presence of automatic (implantable) cardiac defibrillator with synchronous cardiac pacemaker
      Presence of cardiac resynchronization therapy defibrillator (CRT-D) ◀
      Presence of cardioverter-defribillator (ICD) ◀
    - **Z95.811 Presence of heart assist device** CC
    - **Z95.812 Presence of fully implantable artificial heart** CC
    - **Z95.818 Presence of other cardiac implants and grafts**
  - **Z95.82 Presence of other vascular implants and grafts**
    - **Z95.820 Peripheral vascular angioplasty status with implants and grafts**
      - **Excludes1** peripheral vascular angioplasty without implant and graft (Z98.62)
    - **Z95.828 Presence of other vascular implants and grafts**
      Presence of intravascular prosthesis NEC
- **Z95.9 Presence of cardiac and vascular implant and graft, unspecified**

- **Z96 Presence of other functional implants**
  - **Excludes2** complications of internal prosthetic devices, implants and grafts (T82-T85)
    fitting and adjustment of prosthetic and other devices (Z44-Z46)
  - **Z96.0 Presence of urogenital implants**
  - **Z96.1 Presence of intraocular lens**
    Presence of pseudophakia
  - **Z96.2 Presence of otological and audiological implants**
    - **Z96.20 Presence of otological and audiological implant, unspecified**
    - **Z96.21 Cochlear implant status**
    - **Z96.22 Myringotomy tube(s) status**
    - **Z96.29 Presence of other otological and audiological implants**
      Presence of bone-conduction hearing device
      Presence of eustachian tube stent
      Stapes replacement
  - **Z96.3 Presence of artificial larynx**
  - **Z96.4 Presence of endocrine implants**
    - **Z96.41 Presence of insulin pump (external) (internal)**
    - **Z96.49 Presence of other endocrine implants**
  - **Z96.5 Presence of tooth-root and mandibular implants**
  - **Z96.6 Presence of orthopedic joint implants**
    - **Z96.60 Presence of unspecified orthopedic joint implant**
    - **Z96.61 Presence of artificial shoulder joint**
      - **Z96.611 Presence of right artificial shoulder joint**
      - **Z96.612 Presence of left artificial shoulder joint**
      - **Z96.619 Presence of unspecified artificial shoulder joint**
    - **Z96.62 Presence of artificial elbow joint**
      - **Z96.621 Presence of right artificial elbow joint**
      - **Z96.622 Presence of left artificial elbow joint**
      - **Z96.629 Presence of unspecified artificial elbow joint**
    - **Z96.63 Presence of artificial wrist joint**
      - **Z96.631 Presence of right artificial wrist joint**
      - **Z96.632 Presence of left artificial wrist joint**
      - **Z96.639 Presence of unspecified artificial wrist joint**
    - **Z96.64 Presence of artificial hip joint**
      Hip-joint replacement (partial) (total)
      - **Z96.641 Presence of right artificial hip joint**
      - **Z96.642 Presence of left artificial hip joint**
        Coding Clinic: 2015, Q1, P16
      - **Z96.643 Presence of artificial hip joint, bilateral**
      - **Z96.649 Presence of unspecified artificial hip joint**
    - **Z96.65 Presence of artificial knee joint**
      - **Z96.651 Presence of right artificial knee joint**
      - **Z96.652 Presence of left artificial knee joint**
      - **Z96.653 Presence of artificial knee joint, bilateral**
      - **Z96.659 Presence of unspecified artificial knee joint**
    - **Z96.66 Presence of artificial ankle joint**
      - **Z96.661 Presence of right artificial ankle joint**
      - **Z96.662 Presence of left artificial ankle joint**
      - **Z96.669 Presence of unspecified artificial ankle joint**
    - **Z96.69 Presence of other orthopedic joint implants**
      - **Z96.691 Finger-joint replacement of right hand**
      - **Z96.692 Finger-joint replacement of left hand**
      - **Z96.693 Finger-joint replacement, bilateral**
      - **Z96.698 Presence of other orthopedic joint implants**
  - **Z96.7 Presence of other bone and tendon implants**
    Presence of skull plate
  - **Z96.8 Presence of other specified functional implants**
    - **Z96.81 Presence of artificial skin**
    - **Z96.89 Presence of other specified functional implants**
  - **Z96.9 Presence of functional implant, unspecified**

- **Z97 Presence of other devices**
  - **Excludes1** complications of internal prosthetic devices, implants and grafts (T82-T85)
    fitting and adjustment of prosthetic and other devices (Z44-Z46)
  - **Excludes2** presence of cerebrospinal fluid drainage device (Z98.2)
  - **Z97.0 Presence of artificial eye**
  - **Z97.1 Presence of artificial limb (complete) (partial)**
    - **Z97.10 Presence of artificial limb (complete) (partial), unspecified**
    - **Z97.11 Presence of artificial right arm (complete) (partial)**
    - **Z97.12 Presence of artificial left arm (complete) (partial)**
    - **Z97.13 Presence of artificial right leg (complete) (partial)**
    - **Z97.14 Presence of artificial left leg (complete) (partial)**
    - **Z97.15 Presence of artificial arms, bilateral (complete) (partial)**
    - **Z97.16 Presence of artificial legs, bilateral (complete) (partial)**
  - **Z97.2 Presence of dental prosthetic device (complete) (partial)**
    Presence of dentures (complete) (partial)
  - **Z97.3 Presence of spectacles and contact lenses**
  - **Z97.4 Presence of external hearing-aid**
  - **Z97.5 Presence of (intrauterine) contraceptive device ♀**
    - **Excludes1** checking, reinsertion or removal of implantable subdermal contraceptive (Z30.46) ◀
      checking, reinsertion or removal of intrauterine contraceptive device (Z30.43-) ◀
  - **Z97.8 Presence of other specified devices**

- **Z98 Other postprocedural states**
  - **Excludes2** aftercare (Z43-Z49, Z51)
    follow-up medical care (Z08-Z09)
    postprocedural complication - see Alphabetical Index
  - **Z98.0 Intestinal bypass and anastomosis status**
    - **Excludes2** bariatric surgery status (Z98.84)
      gastric bypass status (Z98.84)
      obesity surgery status (Z98.84)
  - **Z98.1 Arthrodesis status**
  - **Z98.2 Presence of cerebrospinal fluid drainage device**
    Presence of CSF shunt
  - **Z98.3 Post therapeutic collapse of lung status**
    Code first underlying disease
  - **Z98.4 Cataract extraction status**
    Use additional code to identify intraocular lens implant status (Z96.1)
    - **Excludes1** aphakia (H27.0)
    - **Z98.41 Cataract extraction status, right eye**
    - **Z98.42 Cataract extraction status, left eye**
    - **Z98.49 Cataract extraction status, unspecified eye**

- **Z98.5 Sterilization status**
  - **Excludes1** female infertility (N97.-)
    male infertility (N46.-)
  - **Z98.51 Tubal ligation status** ♀
  - **Z98.52 Vasectomy status** ♂ A
- **Z98.6 Angioplasty status**
  - **Z98.61 Coronary angioplasty status**
    - **Excludes1** coronary angioplasty status with implant and graft (Z95.5)
  - **Z98.62 Peripheral vascular angioplasty status**
    - **Excludes1** peripheral vascular angioplasty status with implant and graft (Z95.820)
- **Z98.8 Other specified postprocedural states**
  - **Z98.81 Dental procedure status**
    - **Z98.810 Dental sealant status**
    - **Z98.811 Dental restoration status**
      Dental crown status
      Dental fillings status
    - **Z98.818 Other dental procedure status**
  - **Z98.82 Breast implant status**
    - **Excludes1** breast implant removal status (Z98.86)
  - **Z98.83 Filtering (vitreous) bleb after glaucoma surgery status**
    - **Excludes1** inflammation (infection) of postprocedural bleb (H59.4-)
  - **Z98.84 Bariatric surgery status**
    Gastric banding status
    Gastric bypass status for obesity
    Obesity surgery status
    - **Excludes1** bariatric surgery status complicating pregnancy, childbirth, or the puerperium (O99.84)
    - **Excludes2** intestinal bypass and anastomosis status (Z98.0)
  - **Z98.85 Transplanted organ removal status**
    Transplanted organ previously removed due to complication, failure, rejection or infection
    - **Excludes1** encounter for removal of transplanted organ -code to complication of transplanted organ (T86.-)
  - **Z98.86 Personal history of breast implant removal**
  - **Z98.87 Personal history of in utero procedure**
    - **Z98.870 Personal history of in utero procedure during pregnancy** ♀
      - **Excludes2** complications from in utero procedure for current pregnancy (O35.7)
        supervision of current pregnancy with history of in utero procedure during previous pregnancy (O09.82-)
    - **Z98.871 Personal history of in utero procedure while a fetus**
  - **Z98.89 Other specified postprocedural states**
    - **Z98.890 Other specified postprocedural states** ◀
      Personal history of surgery, not elsewhere classified ◀
    - **Z98.891 History of uterine scar from previous surgery** ◀
      - **Excludes1** Maternal care due to uterine scar from previous surgery (O34.2-) ◀
- **Z99 Dependence on enabling machines and devices, not elsewhere classified**
  - **Excludes1** cardiac pacemaker status (Z95.0)
  - **Z99.0 Dependence on aspirator**
  - **Z99.1 Dependence on respirator**
    Dependence on ventilator
    Ex For category Z99.1 CC codes: J95.850, Z99.0-Z99.12, Z99.81-Z99.89
    - **Z99.11 Dependence on respirator [ventilator] status**
      Coding Clinic: 2015, Q1, P21
    - **Z99.12 Encounter for respirator [ventilator] dependence during power failure**
      - **Excludes1** mechanical complication of respirator [ventilator] (J95.850)
  - **Z99.2 Dependence on renal dialysis**
    Hemodialysis status
    Peritoneal dialysis status
    Presence of arteriovenous shunt for dialysis
    Renal dialysis status NOS
    - **Excludes1** encounter for fitting and adjustment of dialysis catheter (Z49.0-)
    - **Excludes2** noncompliance with renal dialysis (Z91.15) ◀
    Coding Clinic: 2016, Q1, P13
  - **Z99.3 Dependence on wheelchair**
    Wheelchair confinement status
    Code first cause of dependence, such as:
    muscular dystrophy (G71.0)
    obesity (E66.-)
  - **Z99.8 Dependence on other enabling machines and devices**
    - **Z99.81 Dependence on supplemental oxygen**
      Dependence on long-term oxygen
    - **Z99.89 Dependence on other enabling machines and devices**
      Dependence on machine or device NOS

Trust Elsevier
to provide your complete curriculum solution!

Content

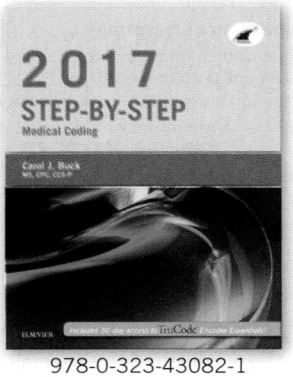

978-0-323-43082-1

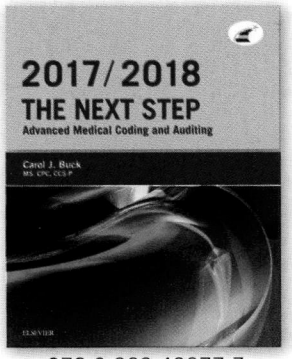

978-0-323-43077-7

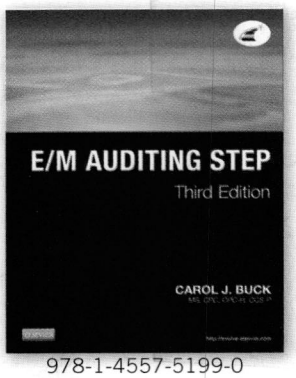

978-1-4557-5199-0

Study Tools

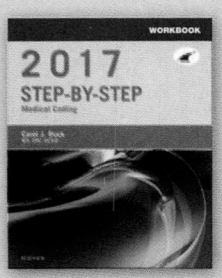

978-0-323-43080-7

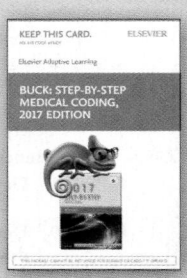

978-0-323-51071-4

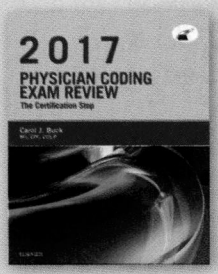

978-0-323-43122-4

evolve

More study tools available

Simulations

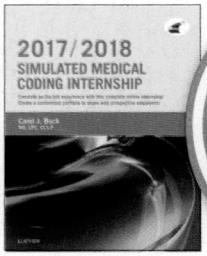

978-0-323-49772-5

Create a customized portfolio to show employers

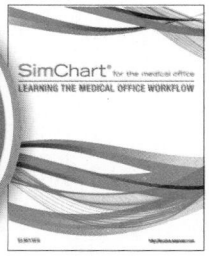

978-0-323-24195-3

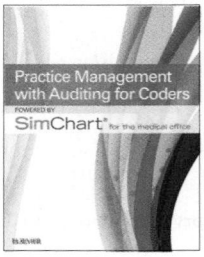

978-0-323-43011-1

Courses

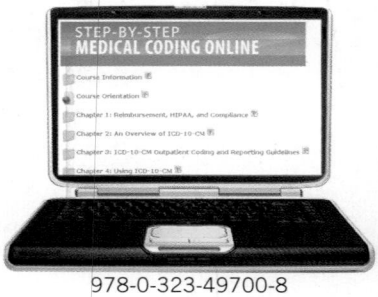

978-0-323-49700-8

Learn more at evolve.elsevier.com/education/medical-insurance-coding